Ballenger's
OTORHINOLARYNGOLOGY **17**
HEAD AND NECK SURGERY

DISEASES

OF THE

NOSE, THROAT AND EAR

MEDICAL AND SURGICAL

BY

WILLIAM LINCOLN BALLENGER, M.D.

PROFESSOR OF OTOLOGY, RHINOLOGY AND LARYNGOLOGY, COLLEGE OF PHYSICIANS AND SURGEONS,
DEPARTMENT OF MEDICINE, UNIVERSITY OF ILLINOIS; FELLOW OF THE AMERICAN
LARYNGOLOGICAL ASSOCIATION; FELLOW OF THE AMERICAN LARYNGOLOGICAL,
RHINOLOGICAL AND OTOLOGICAL ASSOCIATION; FELLOW OF AMERICAN
ACADEMY OF OPHTHALMOLOGY AND OTOLARYNGOLOGY, ETC.

ILLUSTRATED WITH 471 ENGRAVINGS AND 16 PLATES

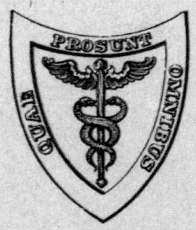

LEA & FEBIGER

PHILADELPHIA AND NEW YORK

1908

Ballenger's
OTORHINOLARYNGOLOGY **17**
HEAD AND NECK SURGERY

JAMES B. SNOW JR., MD, FACS
Professor Emeritus
Department of Otorhinolaryngology Head and Neck Surgery
University of Pennsylvania
Philadelphia, Pennsylvania
Former Director, National Institute on Deafness and
Other Communication Disorders
National Institutes of Health

P. ASHLEY WACKYM, MD, FACS, FAAP
John C. Koss Professor and Chairman
Department of Otolaryngology and
Communication Sciences
Medical College of Wisconsin
Milwaukee, Wisconsin

2009
BC Decker Inc

PEOPLE'S MEDICAL PUBLISHING HOUSE
SHELTON, CONNECTICUT

People's Medical Publishing House
2 Enterprise Drive, Suite 509
Shelton, CT 06484
Tel: 203-402-0646
Fax: 203-402-0854
E-mail: info@pmph-usa.com

PEOPLE'S MEDICAL PUBLISHING HOUSE

PMPH

BC Decker

© 2009 BC Decker Inc

08 09 10 11 12 / AOP / 9 8 7 6 5 4 3 2 1

ISBN 978-1-55009-337-7
Printed in India by Ajanta Offset and Packagings Limited
Managing Editor: Patricia Bindner; Cover Design: Elizabeth Hayden

Sales and Distribution

United States
BC Decker Inc
P.O. Box 785
Lewiston, NY 14092-0785
Tel: 905-522-7017; 800-568-7281
Fax: 905-522-7839; 888-311-4987
E-mail: info@bcdecker.com
www.bcdecker.com

Canada
McGraw-Hill Ryerson Education
Customer Care
300 Water St.
Whitby, Ontario L1N 9B6
Tel: 1-800-565-5758
Fax: 1-800-463-5885

Foreign Rights
John Scott & Company
International Publishers' Agency
P.O. Box 878
Kimberton, PA 19442
Tel: 610-827-1640
Fax: 610-827-1671
E-mail: jsco@voicenet.com

Japan
United Publishers Services Limited
1-32-5 Higashi-Shinagawa
Shinagawa-Ku, Tokyo 140-0002
Tel: 03 5479 7251
Fax: 03 5479 7307

UK, Europe, Middle East
McGraw-Hill Education
Shoppenhangers Road
Maidenhead
Berkshire, England SL6 2QL
Tel: 44-0-1628-502500
Fax: 44-0-1628-635895
www.mcgraw-hill.co.uk

*Singapore, Malaysia,Thailand, Philippines, Indonesia,
Vietnam, Pacific Rim, Korea*
McGraw-Hill Education
60 Tuas Basin Link
Singapore 638775
Tel: 65-6863-1580
Fax: 65-6862-3354

Australia, New Zealand
McGraw-Hill Australia
Pty Ltd Level 2, 82 Waterloo Road North Ryde,
NSW, 2113 Australia
Customer Service Australia
Phone: +61 (2) 9900 1800
Fax: +61 (2) 9900 1980
Email: cservice_sydney@mcgraw-hill.com

Customer Service New Zealand
Phone (Free Phone): +64 (0) 800 449 312
Fax (Free Phone): +64 (0) 800 449 318
Email: cservice@mcgraw-hill.co.nz

Brazil
Tecmedd Importadora E Distribuidora De Livros Ltda.
Avenida Maurílio Biagi, 2850
City Ribeirão, Ribeirão Preto – SP – Brasil
CEP: 14021-000
Tel: 0800 992236
Fax: (16) 3993-9000
E-mail: tecmedd@tecmedd.com.br

India, Bangladesh, Pakistan, Sri Lanka
CBS Publishers & Distributors
4596/1A-11, Darya Ganj
New Delhi-2, India
Tel: 23271632
Fax: 23276712
E-mail: cbspubs@vsnl.com

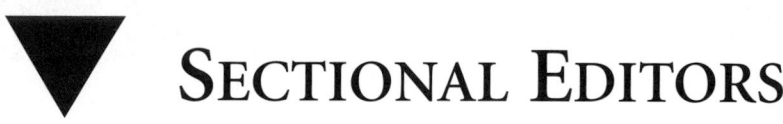

SECTIONAL EDITORS

OTOLOGY AND NEUROTOLOGY
P. Ashley Wackym, MD, FACS, FAAP
John C. Koss Professor and Chairman
Department of Otolaryngology and Communication Sciences
Medical College of Wisconsin
Milwaukee, Wisconsin

RHINOLOGY
Andrew P. Lane, MD
Associate Professor and Chief
Division of Rhinology and Sinus Surgery
Department of Otolaryngology–Head and Neck Surgery
Johns Hopkins University School of Medicine
Baltimore, Maryland

FACIAL PLASTIC AND RECONSTRUCTIVE SURGERY
John S. Rhee, MD, MPH
Associate Professor and Chief
Division of Facial Plastic and Reconstructive Surgery
Department of Otolaryngology and Communication Sciences
Medical College of Wisconsin
Milwaukee, Wisconsin

PEDIATRIC OTORHINOLARYNGOLOGY
J. Christopher Post, MD, PhD, FACS
Professor of Otolaryngology,
Microbiology and Immunology
Drexel University College of Medicine
President and Scientific Director
Center for Genomic Sciences
Allegheny-Singer Research Institute
Pittsburgh, Pennsylvania

LARYNGOLOGY AND BRONCHOESOPHAGOLOGY
Gayle E. Woodson, MD
Professor and Chief
Division of Otolaryngology–Head and Neck Surgery
Department of Surgery
Southern Illinois University
Springfield, Illinois

HEAD AND NECK SURGERY
Scott E. Strome, MD, FACS
Professor and Chair
Department of Otolaryngology–Head and Neck Surgery
University of Maryland Medical Center
Baltimore, Maryland

▼ PREFACE

It has been a great pleasure to be associated with John Jacob Ballenger in the production of several recent editions of this book and to work with Phillip Ashley Wackym in the development and execution of this centennial edition of Ballenger's Otorhinolaryngology Head and Neck Surgery. The central focus of the 17th Edition is the important role molecular medicine is playing in understanding the pathogenesis of disease and patient diagnosis and therapy in the first decade of the 21st century. The selection of the sectional editors and the senior authors for each chapter was based on their contribution of new knowledge to the subject matter of their sections and chapters through highly regarded research and their intellectual leadership of the specialty, thereby assuring that their contributions to this book are truly authoritative. The editorial aim was to encompass the important information in all of the specialties relating to disorders of hearing, balance, smell, taste, voice, speech and language that are the principal responsibilities of the 21st century otorhinolaryngologist head and neck surgeon and to organize and edit it into a comprehensive compendium with an absolute minimum of redundancy. In the last ten years, there has been a great deal of international cooperation in understanding and categorization of major disease entities and developing consensus on patient management based on these concepts; the fruits of these labors are to be found in the various sections of the book. The book is designed to satisfy the informational needs of developing specialists and specialists wanting to maintain their competence with a reader friendly source of contemporary knowledge. The extraordinary currency of this work is largely due to the short time between composition and printing which is a tribute to the publisher, Brian C. Decker, and his gifted staff. My gratitude goes foremost to Ashley Wackym for his leadership, creativity, brilliant intellect and just plain hard work but in full measure to the sectional editors, authors and illustrators who have made this centennial edition one that will give the reader information, pleasure and inspiration.

James B. Snow, Jr., M.D.
July 2008

▼ FOREWORD

One hundred years ago William Lincoln Ballenger at the University of Illinois College of Physicians and Surgeons wrote the great American classic, Diseases of the Nose, Throat and Ear. The 17th Edition embraces a tradition, which embodies clear and concise writing with complementary full color illustrative material. As the original author expressed in his Preface for the First Edition, the current editors have endeavored to include material that one would find in a "textbook and an atlas."

The editors have expanded this edition into 101 chapters, which offer a comprehensive compilation of the specialty of otorhinolaryngology head and neck surgery. The editors chose authors who are experts in their respective fields who have offered reliable and authoritative treatises of their subjects. Care was taken to present the scientific underpinnings of each discipline, which provide the basis for diagnosis and treatment. The authors have endeavored to include the evidence that underlies management of the disorders.

The addition of color plates throughout the chapters has added an important new dimension to this book distinguishing it in the field. The use of color not only conveys additional information rarely seen in a text of this magnitude but also enhances the appearance of the book. The illustration of surgical concepts and procedures in color carries on Ballenger's original idea of adding an "atlas" to the text.

The six sections of this book cover the field of Otorhinolaryngology Head and Neck Surgery with thoroughness that includes not only the breadth of the specialty but the depth of knowledge in each of the disciplines. As it has for the last 100 years, this book provides a valuable foundation for the library of all otorhinolaryngologists head and neck surgeons.

Richard A. Chole, M.D., Ph.D.
July 2008

INTRODUCTION

One hundred years. An interval that is longer than the vast majority of us will live. After I was asked to serve as an editor of the seventeenth edition of *Ballenger's Otorhinolaryngolgy Head and Neck Surgery*, with Dr. James B. Snow, Jr., I searched for and acquired a copy of the first edition of William Lincoln Ballenger's *Diseases of the Nose, Throat and Ear Medical and Surgical*, which was published in 1908. I read portions of the original book and spent much time thinking about our field, our progress and our future opportunities. It was an opportune time to do so. I was mid-career, approaching my fiftieth birthday and preparing to enter my second decade as a department chairman. My mentors and role models helped shape the person I am today; but, when Jim Snow asked me to work with him to develop the current edition, I was in the right time in my life and career to be able to try to synthesize what was needed for current and future students, young otorhinolaryngologists-head and surgeons and experienced surgeons who wanted to update their base of knowledge. Jim was the perfect person to lead me through this phase of my development. He is amazingly bright, organized, thoughtful and willing to be introspective. He has served as a brutally honest critic, enthusiastic supporter and father figure for me. Jim has taken my critical and analytical skills honed by Paul Ward, Brian McCabe, Bruce Gantz and Vicente Honrubia to another level, for which I will forever be grateful. We established a comfortable relationship in which each person could say exactly what was on his mind and then be confident that we would each incorporate the other's view point in improving the book—that goal was always foremost in our minds. Jim was generous in seeking my vision, perspective and judgment. He treated me as an equal, thereby facilitating our work, and I now understand how this contributed to making this book exceptional. During the course of the development of this book, it was also a traumatic and difficult personal journey for Jim. His wife of 53 years, Sallie Lee Ricker Snow, valiantly fought and gracefully succumbed to cancer. Sallie was exceptionally kind and thoughtful and engaged in our community. She completed Jim as a person, and her loss saddened all of us who knew her.

Looking at the first edition was amazing. What were our predecessors thinking? What clinical challenges were the greatest for them and how could they advance and develop the field? What was the world like a century ago?

The 1908 Nobel Prize in Physiology or Medicine was given to Ilya Ilyich Mechnikov of Russia and Paul Ehrlich of Germany in recognition of their work on immunity. Other notable events that year include: the first time the ball signifying the New Year was dropped in Times Square, New York; General Baden-Powell founded the Boy Scouts; Denmark, Germany, England, France, the Netherlands and Sweden signed the North Sea Accord; Mother's Day was celebrated for the first time; the Lusitania crossed the Atlantic in a record four days and 15 hours; Robert E. Peary sailed from New York on his expedition to the North Pole; Bulgaria declared independence from the Ottoman Empire; Henry Ford introduced the Model T automobile; Albert Einstein presented his quantum theory of light; and, at age three, Hsuan-T'ung (Henry Pu-Yi) became the last Emperor of China. Clearly much has changed in our world. It is also true that much has changed between the first and seventeenth editions of this book.

Although a tremendous amount of work was completed during the two years that I spent with Jim in designing and editing this book, I am proud to have played a role in this centennial edition of *Ballenger's Otorhinolaryngology Head and Neck Surgery*. I hope that all those using the printed book and its online version will benefit from its organization and content; and, more importantly, I hope that a multitude of patients will benefit from the information contained in this edition.

P. Ashley Wackym, M.D.
July 2008

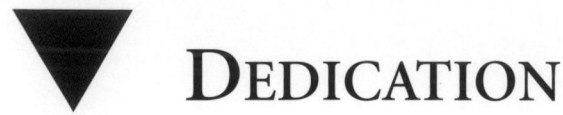 DEDICATION

This centennial edition is dedicated to Sallie Lee Ricker Snow, wife, mother, artist, friend and colleague, whose keen intellect and faithful companionship served as the inspiration for this and several recent editions.

James B. Snow, Jr., M.D.

This work is dedicated to my wife Jeremy and my son Ashton from whom I have stolen innumerable hours in pursuit of the highest standard of academic otorhinolaryngology-head and neck surgery, and Paul Ward—the teacher who has influenced me the most.

P. Ashley Wackym, M.D.

▼ Contents

▼ OTOLOGY AND NEUROTOLOGY
P. Ashley Wackym, MD: Sectional Editor

▼ HEAD AND NECK SURGERY
Scott E. Strome, MD: Sectional Editor

▼ CONTRIBUTORS

Arman Abdalkhani, MD
Resident
Department of Otolaryngology–Head and Neck Surgery
Stanford University School of Medicine
Stanford, California
*Embryology, Anatomy and Physiology of
the Nose and Paranasal Sinuses*

Sumit K. Agrawal, MD
Fellow (Otology/Neurotology)
Stanford University School of Medicine
Stanford, California
*Vestibular Schwannomas and Other
Skull Base Neoplasms*

Ian J. Alexander, MD
Fellow
Cosmetics Program
Facial Plastic Surgery and Otolaryngology
Geisinger Medical Center
Danville, Pennsylvania
Wound Healing and Flap Physiology

George Alexiades, MD
Associate Adjunct Professor
Department of Otolaryngology–Head and Neck Surgery
New York Eye and Ear Infirmary
New York, New York
*Microtia, Canal Atresia and Middle
Ear Anomalies*

John W. Alldredge, MD
Resident
Department of Otolaryngology–Head and Neck Surgery
University of North Carolina at Chapel Hill
Chapel Hill, North Carolina
*Endoscopic Surgery of the Skull Base, Orbits
and Benign Sinonasal Neoplasms*

Kenneth W. Altman, MD, PhD
Associate Professor
Department of Otolaryngology
Mount Sinai School of Medicine
New York, NY
*Laryngopharyngeal Reflux and Laryngeal Infections
and Manifestations of Systemic Diseases*

Bryan T. Ambro, MD, MS
Assistant Professor
Division of Facial Plastic and Reconstructive Surgery
Department of Otolaryngology–Head and Neck Surgery
University of Maryland Medical Center
Baltimore, Maryland
Rejuvenation of the Lower Face and Neck

Manali Amin, MD
Associate in Otolaryngology
Department of Otolaryngology
Children's Hospital of Boston
Boston, Massachusetts
Anatomy and Physiology of the Oral Cavity

Raghu S. Athré, MD
Resident
Department of Otolaryngology–Head and Neck Surgery
University of Texas Southwestern Medical Center at Dallas
Dallas, Texas
Cellular Biology of the Immune System

Nafi Aygun, MD
Assistant Professor
Division of Neuroradiology
Department of Radiology
Johns Hopkins University School of Medicine
Baltimore, Maryland
*Imaging of the Nasal Cavities, Paranasal Sinuses,
Nasopharynx, Orbits, Infratemporal Fossa,
Pterygomaxilliary Fissure and Base of Skull*

Shan R. Baker, MD
Professor and Chief
Division of Facial Plastic and Reconstructive Surgery
Department of Otolaryngology–Head and Neck Surgery
University of Michigan
Ann Arbor, Michigan
Nasal Reconstruction

Steven A. Bielamowicz, MD
Professor and Chief
Division of Otolaryngology
Director of Voice Treatment Center
Department of Surgery
The George Washington University
Washington, District of Columbia
Neurogenic Disorders of the Larynx

Nikolas H. Blevins, MD
Associate Professor
Division of Otology and Neurotology
Department of Otolaryngology–Head and Neck Surgery
Stanford University School of Medicine
Stanford, California
*Vestibular Schwannomas and Other
Skull Base Neoplasms*

Kofi O. Boahene, MD
Assistant Professor
Division of Facial Plastic and Reconstructive Surgery
Department of Otolaryngology–Head and Neck Surgery
Johns Hopkins University School of Medicine
Baltimore, Maryland
Local Flaps in Facial Reconstruction

William E. Brownell, PhD
Jake and Nina Kamin Chair and Professor
Bobby R. Alford Department of Otolaryngology–Head
and Neck Surgery
Baylor College of Medicine
Houston, Texas
Cochlear Biophysics

Brian B. Burkey, MD
Associate Professor
Vice Chairman for Clinical Affairs and Education
Department of Otolaryngology and Communication Sciences
Vanderbilt University Medical Center
Nashville, Tennessee
*Airway Control and Laryngotracheal
Stenosis in Adults*

Joseph A. Califano, III, MD
Associate Professor
Department of Otolaryngology–Head and Neck Surgery
Johns Hopkins University School of Medicine
Baltimore, Maryland
*Molecular Diagnostic Approaches to
Head and Neck Cancer*

Ricardo L. Carrau, MD
Associate Professor
Departments of Otolaryngology
and Neurological Surgery
Eye and Ear Institute
University of Pittsburgh School of Medicine
Pittsburgh, Pennsylvania
Trauma to the Larynx

Kenny H. Chan, MD
Professor and Chief
Division of Pediatric Otolaryngology
Department of Otolaryngology
University of Colorado Health Sciences Center
Aurora, Colorado
*Diseases of the Oral Cavity,
Oropharynx and Nasopharynx*

Andrei I. Chapoval, PhD
Assistant Professor
Department of Otorhinolaryngology–Head and Neck Surgery
University of Maryland Medical Center
Baltimore, Maryland
Immunotherapy for Head and Neck Cancer

Changhu Chen, MD
Assistant Professor
Division of Oncology
Department of Radiation Oncology
University of Colorado Health Sciences Center
Aurora, Colorado
Chemoradiation for Head and Neck Cancer

Douglas B. Chepeha, MD, MPH
Associate Professor
Department of Otolaryngology–Head and Neck Surgery
University of Michigan School of Medicine
Ann Arbor, Michigan
Neoplasms of the Oropharynx and Hypopharynx

Richard A. Chole, MD, PhD
Lindburg Professor and Head
Department of Otolaryngology
Washington University School of Medicine
St. Louis, Missouri
Chronic Otitis Media and Cholesteatoma
Headache and Facial Pain

Daniel I. Choo, MD
Associate Professor and Director
Division of Otology/Neurotology
Department of Otolaryngology–Head and Neck Surgery
University of Cincinnati
College of Medicine
Cincinnati, Ohio
Development of the Ear

Jacquelynne P. Cory, MD
Associate Professor
Director, ENT Allergy Program
Section of Otolaryngology Head and Neck Surgery
Department of Surgery
University of Chicago
Chicago, Illinois
Assessment of Nasal Function

Robin T. Cotton, MD
Director, Otolaryngology–Head and Neck Surgery
Director, Aerodigestive Sleep Center
Department of Pediatric Otolaryngology
Cincinatti Children's Hospital Medical Center
Cincinatti, Ohio
Airway Management in the Infant and Child

Mark S. Courey, MD
Professor, Director, Division of Laryngology
Department of Otolaryngology–Head and Neck Surgery
Director, UCSF Voice Center
University of California at San Francisco
San Francisco, California
Laryngoscopy

Ricardo Cristobal, MD, PhD
Clinical Fellow
Bobby R. Alford Department of Otolaryngology–Head and
    Neck Surgery
Baylor College of Medicine
Houston, Texas
Hair Cell Regeneration

Richard E. Davis, MD
Professor and Chief
Division of Facial Plastic Surgery
Department of Otolaryngology
University of Miami Leonard M. Miller School of Medicine
Miami, Florida
Rhinoplasty and Septoplasty

Laurence J. DiNardo, MD
Professor and Vice Chairman
Department of Otolaryngology–Head and Neck Surgery
Virginia Commonwealth University Medical Center
Richmond, Virginia
Nutrition and the Patient with Head
    and Neck Cancer

Robert A. Dobie, MD, FACS
Clinical Professor
Department of Otolaryngology–Head and Neck Surgery
University of California Davis
Sacramento, California
Idiopathic Sudden Sensorinerual Hearing Loss

Paul J. Donald, MD
Professor and Vice Chairman
Director, Center for Skull Base Surgery
Department of Otolaryngology–Head and Neck Surgery
University of California-Davis Health System
Sacramento, California
Facial Fractures

Joni K. Doherty, MD, PhD
Assistant Professor
Division of Otolaryngology–Head and Neck Surgery
Department of Surgery
University of California at san Diego
School of Medicine
San Diego, California
Molecular Biology of Hearing and Balance

Richard L. Doty, PhD
Professor
Department of Otolaryngology–Head and Neck Surgery
University of Pennsylvania School of Medicine
Philadelphia, Pennsylvania
Olfaction and Gustation

Karen Jo Doyle, MD, PhD
Professor in Residence
Department of Otolaryngology–Head and Neck Surgery
University of California Davis
Sacramento, California
Idiopathic Sudden Sensorineural Hearing Loss

Ward R. Drennan, PhD
Postdoctoral Fellow
Auditory Prosthesis Perception and
    Psychophysics Laboratories
Kresge Hearing Research Institute
University of Michigan School of Medicine
Ann Arbor, Michigan
*Cochlear Implant Coding Strategies
    and Device Programming*

Marc G. Dubin, MD, FACS
Assistant Professor
Department of Otolaryngology–Head and Neck Surgery
Johns Hopkins University School of Medicine
Baltimore, Maryland
*Revision Paranasal Sinus Surgery and
    Surgery of the Frontal Sinus*

Garth D. Ehrlich, PhD
Professor of Microbiology,
Immunology and Otolaryngology
Professor and Vice Chairman, Human Genetics
Drexel University College of Medicine
Executive Director
Center for Genomic Sciences
Allegheny-Singer Research Institute
Pittsburgh, Pennsylvania
Biofilms and Their Role in Ear and Respiratory Infection

Marc D. Eisen, MD, PhD
Assistant Clinical Professor
Division of Otolaryngology
Department of Surgery
University of Connecticut School of Medicine
Farmington, Connecticut
*Central Auditory Processing and
    Functional Neuroimaging*

Mark R. Elstad, MD
Professor
Department of Internal Medicine
University of Utah School of Medicine
Salt Lake City, Utah
Bronchology

Jose N. Fayad, MD
Associate
House Clinic
House Ear Institute
Los Angeles, California
*Microtia, Canal Atresia and
    Middle Ear Anomalies*

Adam E. Flanders, MD
Consultant/Neuroradiology
Professor of Rehabilitation Medicine
Division of Neuroradiology/ENT
Department of Radiology
Thomas Jefferson University Medical College
Philadelphia, Pennsylvania
*Imaging of the Oral Cavity, Pharynx,
    Salivary Glands and Neck*

David R. Friedland, MD, PhD
Associate Professor and Chief
Division of Otology and Neuro-Otologic Skull Base Surgery
Department of Otolaryngology and
    Communication Sciences
Medical College of Wisconsin
Milwaukee, Wisconsin
*Cranial and Intracranial Complications
    of Acute and Chronic Otitis Media*
*Menière Disease, Vestibular Neuritis,
    Benign Paroxyysmal Positional Vertigo,
    Superior Semicircular Canal Dehiscence
    and Vestibular Migraine*
Perilymphatic Fistulae

Rick A. Friedman, MD, PhD
Neurotologist, House Ear Clinic
Chief, Section on Hereditary Disorders of the Ear
House Ear Institute
Los Angeles, California
Hereditary Hearing Impairment
Molecular Biology of Hearing and Balance

John L. Frodel Jr, MD
Director, Cosmetics Program
Facial Plastic Surgery and Otolaryngology
Geisinger Medical Center
Danville, Pennsylvania
Wound Healing and Flap Physiology

Joseph M. Furman, MD, PhD
Professor of Otolaryngology and Neurology
Department of Otolaryngology
University of Pittsburgh
School of Medicine
Pittsburgh, Pennsylvania
Vestibular and Balance Rehabilitation

Richard R. Gacek, MD
Professor
Department of Otolaryngology–Head and Neck Surgery
University of Massachusetts Medical Center
Worcester, Massachusetts
Anatomy of the Auditory and Vestibular Systems

Brian R. Gastman, MD
Assistant Professor
Division of Facial Plastic Surgery
Department of Otorhinolaryngology–Head and Neck Surgery
University of Maryland Medical Center
Baltimore, Maryland
*Mechanisms of Immune Evasion of
    Head and Neck Cancer*

Joel A. Goebel, MD, FACS
Professor and Vice Chairman
Department of Otolaryngology–Head and Neck Surgery
Washington University School of Medicine
St. Louis, Missouri
Evaluation of the Vestibular System

Nira A. Goldstein, MD
Associate Professor
Division of Pediatric Otolaryngology
Department of Otolaryngology
State University of New York
Downstate Medical Center
Brooklyn, New York
Sleep Apnea in Children

Quinton S. Gopen, MD
Associate Surgeon
Brigham and Women's Hospital
Division of Otolaryngology
Children's Hospital of Boston
Boston, Massachusetts
*Autoimmune Inner Ear Disease and
    Other Autoimmune Diseases with
    Inner Ear Involvement*
Eustachian Tube Dysfunction

Steven L. Goudy, MD
Assistant Professor of Otolaryngology
Bill Wilkerson Center
Department of Otolaryngology and Communication Sciences
Vanderbilt University Medical Center
Nashville, Tennessee
*Airway Control and Laryngotracheal
    Stenosis in Adults*

Jennifer R. Grandis, MD, PhD, FACS
Professor and Vice Chair for Research
Department of Otolaryngology
University of Pittsburgh School of Medicine
Pittsburgh, Pennsylvania
*Targeted Therapeutic Approaches to
    Head and Neck Cancer*

Linda Grossheim, MD
Assistant Professor
Department of Radiation Oncology
Medical College of Wisconsin
Milwaukee, Wisconsin
Stereotactic Radiosurgery and Radiotherapy

James W. Hall III, PhD
Clinical Professor and Associate Chair
Department of Communicative Disorders
University of Florida
Gainesville, Florida
*Diagnostic Audiology, Hearing
    Instruments and Aural Habilitation*

Maureen T. Hannley, PhD
Associate Professor and Chief
Division of Research
Department of Otolaryngology and Communication Sciences
Medical College of Wisconsin
Milwaukee, Wisconsin
*Outcomes Research, Clinical Trials and
    Clinical Research*
*Physiology of the Auditory and
    Vestibular Systems*

Matthew B. Hanson, MD
Assistant Professor
Department of Otolaryngology
State University of New York
Downstate Medical Center
Brooklyn, New York
Diseases of the External Ear

Jeffrey P. Harris, MD, PhD, FACS
Professor and Chief
Division of Otolaryngology–Head and Neck Surgery
Department of Surgery
University of California at San Diego
San Diego, California
*Autoimmune Inner Ear Disease and Other
     Autoimmune Diseases with Inner Ear Involvement*

James M. Hartman, MD
Town and Country Head and Neck
Saint Louis, Missouri
Headache and Facial Pain

Bridget C. Hathaway, MD
Assistant Professor
Department of Otolaryngology
University of Pittsburgh
Pittsburgh, Pennsylvania
Trauma to the Larynx

Katherine D. Heidenreich, MD
Private Practice
Cleveland, Ohio
Evaluation of the Vestibular System

Peter A. Hilger, MD
Head/Neck Surgery Lions 5M
International Hearing Center
Department of Otolaryngology
University of Minnesota
Minneapolis, Minnesota
Local Flaps in Facial Reconstruction

Peter H. Hwang, MD
Associate Professor
Director, Stanford Sinus Center
Department of Otolaryngology–Head and Neck Surgery
Stanford University School of Medicine
Stanford, California
*Embryology, Anatomy and Physiology
     of the Nose and Paranasal Sinuses*

Robert K. Jackler, MD
Sewall Professor and Chair
Department of Otolaryngology–Head and Neck Surgery
Stanford University
Stanford, California
*Vestibular Schwannomas and Other
     Skull Base Neoplasms*

Alexis H. Jackman, MD
Assistant Professor
Department of Otolaryngology–Head and Neck Surgery
Albert Einstein College of Medicine
Montefiore Medical Center
Bronx, New York
Olfaction and Gustation

Margaret M. Jastreboff, PhD
Visiting Research Professor
Department of Audiology, Speech-Language
Pathology and Deaf Studies
Towson University
Towson, Maryland
Tinnitus and Decreased Sound Tolerance

Pawel J. Jastreboff, PhD, ScD, MBA
Professor
Department of Otolaryngology
Emory University
Atlanta, Georgia
Tinnitus and Decreased Sound Tolerance

Herman A. Jenkins, MD
Professor and Chairman
Department of Otolaryngology–Head and Neck Surgery
University of Colorado Health Science Center
Denver, Colorado
Otosclerosis

Michael M. Johns, MD
Assistant Professor
Director, Emory Voice Center
Department of Otolaryngology
Emory University School of Medicine
Atlanta, Georgia
Benign Laryngeal Lesions

Kristin N. Johnston, AuD
Instructor
Department of Communicative Disorders
University of Florida
Gainesville, Florida
*Diagnostic Audiology, Hearing
     Instruments and Aural Habilitation*

Jan L. Kasperbauer, MD
Professor
Department of Otolaryngology
Mayo Clinic
Rochester, Minnesota
*Management of Diseases of the Thyroid and
    Parathyroid Glands*

Elizabeth M. Keithley, PhD
Professor
Division of Otolaryngology–Head and Neck Surgery
Department of Surgery
University of California at San Diego
San Diego, California
*Autoimmune Inner Ear Disease and Other
    Autoimmune Diseases with Inner Ear Involvement*

Robert M. Kellman, MD
Professor and Chair
Department of Otolaryngology and
    Communication Sciences
SUNY Upstate Medical Center
Syracuse, New York
Neoplasms of the Anterior Skull Base

Margaret A. Kenna, MD, MPH
Associate Professor of Otology
    and Laryngology
Department of Otolaryngology
Harvard Medical School
Children's Hospital, Boston
Boston, Massachusetts
Anatomy and Physiology of the Oral Cavity

Raymond D. Kent, PhD
Professor, Communicative Disorders
Waisman Center
University of Wisconsin, Madison
Madison, Wisconsin
Disorders of Speech and Language

Joseph E. Kerschner, MD
Professor and Chief
Division of Pediatric Otolaryngology
Academic Vice Chairman
Department of Otolaryngology and
    Communication Sciences
Medical College of Wisconsin
Milwaukee, Wisconsin
Otitis Media and Middle Ear Effusions

Young-Ho Kim, MD, PhD
Associate Professor
Department of Otolaryngology–Head and Neck Surgery
Ajou University School of Medicine
Suwon, Korea
*Development, Anatomy and Physiology
    of the Larynx*

Charles P. Kimmelman, MD
Director
New York City Ear, Nose & Throat Center
993 Park Avenue
New York, New York
*Microtia, Canal Atresia and Middle Ear
    Anomalies*

Amit Kochhar, BS
Fellow
Department of Otolaryngology–Head and Neck Surgery
University of Iowa Carver College of Medicine
Iowa City, Iowa
Hereditary Hearing Impairment

Theda C. Kontis, MD
Facial Plastic Surgicenter, Ltd.
1838 Greene Tea Road
Baltimore, Maryland
*Rejuvenation of the Upper Face
    and Midface*
Scar Revision and Skin Resurfacing

Jamie A. Koufman, MD
The Voice Institute of New York
New York, New York
*Laryngopharyngeal Reflux and Laryngeal Infections
    and Manifestations of Systemic Diseases*

Dennis H. Kraus, MD
Director, Speech Hearing Center
Memorial Sloan-Kettering Cancer Center
New York, New York
Neoplasms of the Oral Cavity

Sharon G. Kujawa, PhD
Associate Professor
Department of Otology and Laryngology
Harvard Medical School
Boston, Massachusetts
Noise-Induced Hearing Loss

John F. Kveton, MD
46 Prince Street
New Haven, Connecticut
*Cranial and Intracranial Complications
    of Acute and Chronic Otitis Media*

Stephen Y. Lai, MD, PhD
Assistant Professor
Division of Head and Neck Surgery
Department of Otolaryngology
University of Pittsburgh School of Medicine
Pittsburgh, Pennsylvania
*Targeted Therapeutic Approaches to
    Head and Neck Cancer*

Anil K. Lalwani, MD
Mendik Foundation Professor and Chairman
Department of Otolaryngology
New York University Medical Center
New York, New York
Inner Ear Drug Delivery and Gene Therapy

Paul R. Lambert, MD
Professor and Chair
Department of Otolaryngology–Head and Neck Surgery
Medical University of South Carolina
Charleston, South Carolina
Presbyacusis and Presbyastasis

Andrew P. Lane, MD
Associate Professor and Chief
Director of Rhinology and Sinus Surgery
Department of Otolaryngology–Head and Neck Surgery
Johns Hopkins University School of Medicine
Baltimore, Maryland
*Revision Paranasal Sinus Surgery and
    Surgery of the Frontal Sinus*

Adam J. LeVay, MD
Resident
Section of Otolaryngology
Department of Surgery
Yale University School of Medicine
New Haven, Connecticut
Development, Anatomy and Physiology of the Larynx

Amy Anne Donatelli Lassig, MD
Assistant Professor
Department of Otolaryngology–Head and Neck Surgery
University of Minnesota Medical School
Minneapolis, Minnesota
Neoplasms of the Oropharynx and Hypopharynx

Charles J. Limb, MD
Assistant Professor
Department of Otolaryngology–Head and Neck Surgery
Johns Hopkins University School of Medicine
Baltimore, Maryland
*Central Auditory Processing and
    Functional Neuroimaging*

Todd A. Loehrl, MD
Professor and Chief
Division of Rhinology and Sinus Surgery
Department of Otolaryngology and
    Communication Sciences
Medical College of Wisconsin
Milwaukee, Wisconsin
Acute Rhinosinusitis and its Complications
*Robotic Surgery, Navigational Systems
    and Surgical Simulators*

Brenda L. Lonsbury-Martin, PhD
Professor
Department of Otolaryngology–Head and Neck Surgery
Loma Linda University
Loma Linda, California
Physiology of the Auditory and Vestibular Systems

Frank E. Lucente, MD
Professor and Chairman
Department of Otolaryngology
State University of New York
Downstate Medical Center
Brooklyn, New York
Diseases of the External Ear

Christy L. Ludlow, PhD
Senior Investigator
Laryngeal and Speech Section
Clinical Neuroscience Program
National Institute of Neurological Disorders and Stroke
Bethesda, Maryland
Neurogenic Disorders of the Larynx

Valerie J. Lund, MS, FRCS, FRCS(Ed)
Professor of Rhinology
Ear Institute
University College London
London, England
Acute and Chronic Nasal Disorders

Rodney P. Lusk, MD
Director
Boys Town Ear, Nose and Throat Institute
Boys Town National Research Hospital
Director of the Cochlear Implant Center
Omaha, Nebraska
Congenital Anomalies of the Larynx

Mahmood F. Mafee, MD
Professor
Department of Radiology
University of California, San Diego School of Medicine
San Diego, California
Imaging of the Temporal Bone

Lawrence J. Marentette, MD
Professor
Departments of Neurosurgery and Otolaryngology
University of Michigan Health System
Ann Arbor, Michigan
Neoplasms of the Anterior Skull Base

Bradley F. Marple, MD
Professor and Vice Chairman
Department of Otolaryngology–Head and Neck Surgery
University of Texas Southwestern Medical School
Dallas, Texas
Cellular Biology of the Immune System

Glen K. Martin, PhD
Professor
Department of Otolaryngology–Head and Neck Surgery
Loma Linda University
Loma Linda, California
Physiology of the Auditory and Vestibular Systems

Becky L. Massey, MD
Assistant Professor
Division of Head and Neck Oncology
Department of Otolaryngology and
    Communication Sciences
Medical College of Wisconsin
Milwaukee, Wisconsin
Neoplasms of the Anterior Skull Base

Rob McCammon, MD
Resident Physician
Division of Oncology
Department of Radiation Oncology
University of Colorado Health Sciences Center
Aurora, Colorado
Chemoradiation for Head and Neck Cancer

Bryan McIver, MB, PhD
Fellow in Endocrinology
The Mayo Clinic
Rochester, Minnesota
*Management of Diseases of the Thyroid and
    Parathyroid Glands*

Michael J. McKenna, MD
Professor
Department of Otolaryngology
Massachusetts Eye and Ear Infirmary
Harvard Medical School
Boston, Massachusetts
Otosclerosis

Cliff A. Megerian, MD
Professor and Vice-Chairman
Department of Otolaryngology–Head and Neck Surgery
Case Western Reserve School of Medicine
Cleveland, Ohio
Presbyacusis and Presbyastasis

Albert L. Merati, MD
Associate Professor
Chief of the Division of Laryngology
Department of Otolaryngology–Head and Neck Surgery
University of Washington
School of Medicine
Seattle, Washington
*Imaging of the Larynx, Trachea
    and Esophagus*

Saumil N. Merchant, MD
Gudren Larsen Eliasen and Nels Kristian Eliasen
Professor of Otology and Laryngology
Department of Otology and Laryngology
Harvard Medical School
Boston, Massachusetts
Reconstruction of the Middle Ear

James A. Merrell, MD
Resident
Department of Otolaryngology–Head and Neck Surgery
University of Cincinnati College of Medicine
Cincinnati, Ohio
Epistaxis

Elizabeth G. Miller, RD
Dietetics
Medical College of Virginia
Richmond, Virginia
*Nutrition of the Patient with
    Head and Neck Cancer*

John H. Mills, PhD
Professor
Department of Otolaryngology–Head and Neck Surgery
Medical University of South Carolina
Charleston, South Carolina
Presbyacusis and Presbyastasis

Lloyd B. Minor, MD
Andelot Professor and Director
Department of Otolaryngology–Head and Neck Surgery
Johns Hopkins University School of Medicine
Baltimore, Maryland
*Menière Disease, Vestibular Neuritis, Benign
    Paroxysmal Positional Vertigo, Superior
    Semicircular Canal Dehiscence and
    Vestibular Migraine*

Robert E. Morales, MD
Assistant Professor
Division of Neuroradiology
Department of Radiology
University of Maryland
Baltimore, Maryland
*Imaging of the Oral Cavity, Pharynx,
    Salivary Glands and Neck*

Murray D. Morrison, MD, FRCSC
Professor
Division of Otolaryngology
Department of Surgery
University of British Columbia
Vancouver, British Columbia
Muscle Misuse Disorders of the Larynx

Craig S. Murakami, MD
Clinical Associate Professor
Division of Facial Plastic and Reconstructive Surgery
Department of Otolaryngology–Head and Neck Surgery
University of Washington
Seattle, Washington
Rejuvenation of the Lower Face and Neck

Robert M. Naclerio, MD
Professor and Section Chief
Otolaryngology Head and Neck Surgery
Department of Surgery
University of Chicago Medical Center
Chicago, Illinois
Allergic Rhinitis

Shri Nadig, MD
Lecturer
Department of Otolaryngology–Head and Neck Surgery
Oregon Health & Science University
Portland, Oregon
Regional Flaps and Free Tissue Transfer

Joseph B. Nadol, Jr, MD
Walter Augustus Lecompte Professor and Chairman
Department of Otology and Laryngology
Chief of Otolaryngology
Massachusetts Eye and Ear Infirmary
Harvard Medical School
Boston, Massachusetts
Pathologic Correlates in Otology and Neurotology

Robert Nason, MD
Resident
Department of Otolaryngology
Washington University School of Medicine
St. Louis, Missouri
Chronic Otitis Media and Cholesteatoma

Hamish Nichol, MBChir
Professor Emeritus
Department of Psychiatry
University of British Columbia
Vancouver, British Columbia
Muscle Misuse Disorders of the Pharynx

Kaibao Nie, PhD
Acting Instructor
Department of Otolaryngology–Head and Neck Surgery
University of Washington
Seattle, Washington
*Cochlear Implant Coding Strategies
    and Device Programming*

John S. Oghalai, MD
Associate Professor
Bobby R. Alford Department of Otolaryngology–Head and
    Neck Surgery
Baylor College of Medicine
Houston, Texas
Cochlear Biophysics

Bert W. O'Malley Jr, MD
Gabriel Tucker Professor and Chair
Department of Otolaryngology–Head and Neck Surgery
University of Pennsylvania Health System
Philadelphia, Pennsylvania
*Robotic Surgery, Navigational Systems
    and Surgical Simulators*

Mark D. Packer, MD
Neurotology Fellow
Division of Neurotology
Department of Otolaryngology–Head and Neck Surgery
Ohio State University
Columbus, Ohio
Trauma to the Middle Ear, Inner, Ear and Temporal Bone

Shatul Parikh, MD
Resident
Department of Otolaryngology–Head and Neck Surgery
Emory University School of Medicine
Atlanta, Georgia
Benign Laryngeal Lesions

Simon C. Parisier, MD
Co-Director
Otolaryngology, Head and Neck Surgery
New York Eye and Ear Infirmary
New York, New York
*Microtia, Canal Atresia and Middle Ear
    Anomalies*

Nirmal P. Patel, MD
Garnett Passe Research Fellow
Department of Otolaryngology
New York University School of Medicine
New York, New York
Inner Ear Drug Delivery and Gene Therapy

Karen S. Pawlowski, PhD
Assistant Professor
Department of Otolaryngology–Head and Neck Surgery
University of Texas
Southwestern Medical Center at Dallas
Dallas, Texas
Ototoxicity

Myles L. Pensak, MD
H.B. Brody Professor and Chairman
Department of Otolaryngology–Head and Neck Surgery
University of Cincinnati College of Medicine
Cincinnati, Ohio
*Cranial and Intracranial Complications of
    Acute and Chronic Otitis Media*

Fred A. Pereira, PhD
Assistant Professor
Bobby R. Alford Department of Otolaryngology–Head and
    Neck Surgery
Huffington Center on Aging
Baylor College of Medicine
Houston, Texas
Hair Cell Regeneration

Randall L. Plant, MD
Department of Otolaryngology
Alaska Native Medical Center
Anchorage, Alaska
Neoplasms of the Nasopharynx

Dennis S. Poe, MD
Associate Professor of Otology and
    Laryngology
Harvard Medical School
Boston, Massachusetts
Eustachian Tube Dysfunction

David M. Poetker, MD, MA
Assistant Professor
Division of Rhinology and Sinus Surgery
Department of Otolaryngology and Communication Sciences
Medical College of Wisconsin
Milwaukee, Wisconsin
*Etiology of Infectious Diseases of the Upper
    Respiratory Tract*

Paul Popper, PhD
Associate Professor
Division of Research
Department of Otolaryngology and
    Communication Sciences
Medical College of Wisconsin
Milwaukee, Wisconsin
Hair Cell Regeneration

J. Christopher Post, MD, PhD, FACS
Professor of Otolaryngology,
Microbiology and Immunology
Drexel University College of Medicine
President and Scientific Director
Center for Genomic Sciences
Allegheny-Singer Research Institute
Pittsburgh, Pennsylvania
Biofilms and Their Role in Ear and Respiratory Infections
Otitis Media and Middle Ear Effusions

Gregory N. Postma, MD
Professor and Director
Center for Voice and Swallowing Disorders
Department of Otolaryngology
Medical College of Georgia
Augusta, Georgia
Esophagology

Ching-Lon Pui, MD
Professor
Department of Pediatrics
University of Tennessee
Health Sciences Center
Memphis, Tennessee
*Endoscopic Surgery of the Skull Base, Orbits,
    and Benign Sinonasal Neoplasms*

Vito C. Quatela, MD
Quatela Center for Plastic Surgery
Rochester, New York

David Raben, MD
Professor
Division of Oncology
Department of Radiation Oncology
University of Colorado
Health Sciences Center
Aurora, Colorado
Chemoradiation for Head and Neck Cancer

Vijay R. Ramakrishnan, MD
Staff Physician
Department of Otolaryngology–Head and Neck Surgery
University of Colorado Health Sciences Center
Aurora, Colorado
*Diseases of the Oral Cavity, Oropharynx
    and Nasopharynx*

Linda Rammage, PhD
Research Associate
Division of Otolaryngology
Department of Surgery
University of British Columbia
Vancouver, British Columbia
Muscle Misuse Disorders of the Larynx

John S. Rhee, MD, MPH
Associate Professor and Chief
Division of Facial Plastic and Reconstructive Surgery
Department of Otolaryngology and Communication Sciences
Medical College of Wisconsin
Milwaukee, Wisconsin
Facial Paralysis
Ostoplasty of the Prominent Ear
Rejuvenation of the Upper Face and Midface

Catherine J. Rees, MD
Assistant Professor and Medical Director
Center for Voice and Swallowing Disorders
Wake Forest University Baptist Medical Center
Winston-Salem, North Carolina
Esophagology

Gresham T. Richter, MD
Assistant Professor
Department of Otolaryngology–Head and Neck Surgery
University of Arkansas for Medical Sciences
Little Rock, Arkansas
Development of the Ear

Frederick C. Roediger, MD
Resident
Department of Otolaryngology–Head and Neck Surgery
University of California at San Francisco
San Francisco, California
Laryngoscopy

Sarah L. Rohde, MD
Resident
Department of Otolaryngology and Communication Sciences
Vanderbilt University Medical Center
Nashville, Tennessee
*Airway Control and Laryngotracheal
  Stenosis in Adults*

Peter S. Roland, MD
Professor and Chairman
Department of Otolaryngology–Head and Neck Surgery
University of Texas
Southwestern Medical Center at Dallas
Dallas, Texas
Ototoxicity

John J. Rosowski, PhD
Professor
Department of Otology and Laryngology
Harvard Medical School
Boston, Massachusetts
Reconstruction of the Middle Ear

Lee D. Rowe, MD
Associate Clinical Professor
Department of Otolaryngology–Head and Neck Surgery
Thomas Jefferson University Medical College
Philadelphia, Pennsylvania
Congenital Anomalies of the Head and Neck

Jay Rubinstein, MD, PhD
Professor and Director
Virginia Merrill Bloedel Hearing Research Center
Department of Otolaryngology–Head and Neck Surgery
University of Washington
Seattle, Washington
*Cochlear Implant Coding Strategies
  and Device Programming*

Christina L. Runge-Samuelson, PhD
Associate Professor and Co-Director
Koss Cochlear Implant Program
Department of Otolaryngology and
  Communication Sciences
Medical College of Wisconsin
Milwaukee, Wisconsin
Cochlear and Auditory Brainstem Implantation
Stereotactic Radiosurgery and Radiotherapy

Michael J. Rutter, MBChB
Associate Professor
Department of Otolaryngology–Head and Neck Surgery
University of Cincinnati College of Medicine
Director of Clinical Research
Children's Hospital of Cincinnati
Cincinnati, Ohio
Airway Management in the Infant and Child

Asli Sahin-Yilmaz, MD
Fellow
Section of Otolaryngology
Department of Surgery
University of Chicago
Chicago, Illinois
Allergic Rhinitis
Assessment of Nasal Function

Christine M. Sapienza, PhD
Professor and Chair
Department of Communication Sciences and Disorders
University of Florida
Gainesville, Florida
Assessment of Vocal Function

Clarence T. Sasaki, MD
Charles W. Ohse Professor and Chief
Section of Otolaryngology
Department of Surgery
Yale University School of Medicine
New Haven, Connecticut
*Development, Anatomy and Physiology
of the Larynx*

Rodney J. Schlosser, MD
Assistant Professor and Director,
Division of Rhinology and Sinus Surgery
Department of Otolaryngology
Medical University of South Carolina
Charleston, South Carolina
Chronic Rhinosinusitis and Polyposis

Dan H. Schulze, PhD
Associate Professor
Department of Microbiology and Immunology
University of Marlyand School of Medicine
Baltimore, Maryland
Immunotherapy for Head and Neck Cancer

Joseph M. Scianna, MD
Assistant Professor
Division of Head and Neck Surgery
Department of Otolaryngology
Loyola University
Maywood, Illinois
Primary Paranasal Sinus Surgery

Anthony P. Sclafani, MD
Professor and Director of Facial Plastic Surgery
The New York Eye and Ear Infirmary
New York, New York
*Microtia, Canal Atresia and
Middle Ear Atresia*

Brent A. Senior, MD, FACS, FARS
Associate Professor
Division of Rhinology, Allergy and Sinus Surgery
Department of Otolaryngology–Head and Neck Surgery
University of North Carolina at Chapel Hill
Chapel Hill, North Carolina
*Endoscopic Surgery of the Skull Base,
Orbits and Benign Sinonasal Neoplasms*

Melanie W. Seybt, MD
Resident
Department of Otolaryngology–Head and Neck Surgery
Medical College of Georgia
Augusta, Georgia
Esophagology

Clough Shelton, MD
Professor and Chief
Division of Otolaryngology–Head and Neck Surgery
Department of Surgery
University of Utah
Salt Lake City, Utah
Reconstruction of the Middle Ear

Mark G. Shrime, MD
Fellow
Department of Otolaryngology–Head and Neck Surgery
University of Toronto
Toronto, Ontario, Canada
Neoplasms of the Oral Cavity

Ian M. Smith, MD
Resident
Department of Otolaryngology–Head and Neck Surgery
Johns Hopkins University School of Medicine
Baltimore, Maryland
Molecular Diagnostic Approaches to Head and Neck Cancer

Marshall E. Smith, MD
Associate Professor
Division of Otolaryngology–Head and Neck Surgery
Department of Surgery
University of Utah
Salt Lake City, Utah
Bronchology

Richard J. H. Smith, MD
Professor and Vice Chairman
Department of Otolaryngology–Head and Neck Surgery
University of Iowa Health Care
Iowa City, Iowa
Hereditary Hearing Impairment

Timothy L. Smith, MD, MPH
Professor and Chief
Division of Rhinology
Department of Otolaryngology
Oregon Health & Science University
Portland, Oregon
Etiology of Infectious Diseases of the Upper Respiratory Tract

C. Arturo Solares, MD
Assistant Professor
Department of Otolaryngology
Medical College of Georgia
Augusta, Georgia
Neoplasms of the Larynx

James A. Stankiewicz, MD
Professor and Chairman
Department of Otolaryngology–Head and Neck Surgery
Loyola Medical Center
Maywood, Illinois
Primary Paranasal Sinus Surgery

Marshall Strome, MD, MS
Director Center for Head and Neck Oncology
Co-Director Head and Neck Transplantation Program,
    Center for Facial Reconstruction
St. Luke's–Roosevelt Hospital Centers
New York, New York
Neoplasms of the Larynx

Scott E. Strome, MD, FACS
Professor and Chair
Department of Otolaryngology–Head and Neck Surgery
University of Maryland Medical Center
Baltimore, Maryland
Immunotherapy for Head and Neck Cancer

Grant W. Su, MD
Instructor
Department of Ophthalmology
Medical College of Wisconsin
Milwaukee, Wisconsin
Acute Rhinosinusitis and Its Complications

Lucian Sulica, MD
Associate Professor
Department of Otorhinolaryngology
Weill Cornell Medical College
New York, New York
Laryngeal Paralysis

Aaron Sulman, MD
Assistant Professor
Department of Urology
Medical College of Wisconsin
Milwaukee, Wisconsin
Robotic Surgery, Navigational Systems and Surgical Simulators

Mohan Suntha, MD
Professor
Division of Oncology
Department of Radiation Oncology
University of Maryland School of Medicine
Baltimore, Maryland
Chemoradiation for Head and Neck Cancer

Thomas A. Tami, MD
Professor
Department of Otolaryngology
University of Cincinnati College of Medicine
Cincinnati, Ohio
Epistaxis

Rodney J. Taylor, MD
Assistant Professor
Division of General Otolaryngology
Department of Otolaryngology–Head and Neck Surgery
University of Maryland School of Medicine
Baltimore, Maryland
Diseases of the Salivary Glands

Theodoros N. Teknos, MD
Associate Professor
Department of Otolaryngology–Head and Neck Surgery
University of Michigan, Medical School
Ann Arbor, Michigan
Neoplasms of the Oropharynx and Hypopharynx

Jeffrey Tseng, MD
Resident
Department of Otolaryngology and Communication Sciences
Medical College of Wisconsin
Milwaukee, Wisconsin
Ostoplasty of the Prominent Ear

Galdino E. Valvassori, MD
Professor
Department of Radiology
University of Illinois, Chicago
Chicago, Illinois
Imaging of the Temporal Bone

P. Ashley Wackym, MD, FACS, FAAP
John C. Koss Professor and Chairman
Department of Otolaryngology and
    Communication Sciences
Medical College of Wisconsin
Milwaukee, Wisconsin
Cochlear and Auditory Brainstem Implantation
Facial Paralysis
Stereotactic Radiosurgery and Radiotherapy

Carter Van Waes, MD, PhD
Chief, Head and Neck Surgery Branch
Clinical Director
National Institute on Deafness and Other
    Communication Disorders
National Institutes of Health
Bethesda, Maryland
Molecular Biology of Squamous Cell Carcinoma

Lacey Washington, MD
Associate Clinical Professor
Department of Radiology/Cardiac
    and Thoracic Imaging
Duke University
Durham, North Carolina
Imaging of the Larynx, Trachea
    and Esophagus

Mark K. Wax, MD
Professor
Department of Otolaryngology–Head and Neck Surgery
Oregon Health & Science University
Portland, Oregon
Regional Flaps and Free Tissue Transfer

Gregory S. Weinstein, MD
Professor and Vice-Chairman
Director, Division of Head and Neck Surgery
Department of Otorhinolaryngology–Head and Neck Surgery
University of Pennsylvania
Philadelphia, Pennsylvania
Robotic Surgery, Navigational Systems
    and Surgical Simulators

D. Bradley Welling, MD, PhD
Professor and Chair
Department of Otolaryngology–Head and Neck Surgery
Ohio State University
Columbus, Ohio
Trauma to the Middle Ear, Inner Ear and Temporal Bone

Timothy S. Wells, MD
Assistant Professor
Department of Ophthalmology
Medical College of Wisconsin
Milwaukee, Wisconsin
Acute Rhinosinusitis and Its Complications

Judith A. White, MD, PhD
Section Head, Vestibular and Balance Disorders
Head and Neck Institute
Cleveland Clinic
Cleveland, Ohio
Evaluation of the Vestibular System

Susan L. Whitney, PhD, PT, NCS, FAPTA
Associate Professor
Departments of Physical Therapy
    and Otolaryngology
University of Pittsburgh School of Medicine
Pittsburgh, Pennsylvania
Vestibular and Balance Rehabilitation

David L. Witsell, MD, MHS
Associate Professor
Division of Otolaryngology–Head and Neck Surgery
Department of Surgery
Duke University Medical Center
Durham, North Carolina
Outcomes Research, Clinical Trials
    and Clinical Research

Jeffrey S. Wolf, MD, FACS
Assistant Professor
Department of Otolaryngology–Head and Neck Surgery
University of Maryland School of Medicine
Baltimore, Maryland
Diseases of the Salivary Glands

Aaron H. D. Wood, MD
Department of Otolaryngology–Head and Neck Surgery
University of Maryland School of Medicine
Baltimore, Maryland
Mechanisms of Immune Evasion of Head
    and Neck Cancer

Gayle E. Woodson, MD
Professor and Chief
Division of Otolaryngology–Head and Neck Surgery
Department of Surgery
Southern Illinois University
Springfield, Illinois
Assessment of Vocal Function

B. Tucker Woodson, MD, DABSM
Professor and Chief
Division of Sleep Medicine
Department of Otolaryngology and
    Communication Sciences
Medical College of Wisconsin
Milwaukee, Wisconsin
Sleep Medicine and Surgery

Bradford A. Woodworth, MD
Instructor
Department of Otorhinolaryngology–Head and Neck Surgery
University of Pennsylvania
Philadelphia, Pennsylvania
Chronic Rhinosinusitis and Polyposis

Robert F. Yellon, MD
Associate Professor, Co-Director and Co-Chief
Division of Pediatric Otolaryngology
Children's Hospital of Pittsburgh
Department of Otolaryngology
University of Pittsburgh School of Medicine
Pittsburgh, Pennsylvania
Deep Head and Neck Space Infections

David M. Yousem, MD, MBA
Professor of Radiology
Director of Neuroradiology
Division of Neuroradiology
Department of Radiology
Johns Hopkins University School of Medicine
Baltimore, Maryland
*Imaging of the Nasal Cavities, Paranasal Sinuses,
    Nasopharynx, Orbits, Infratemporal Fossa,
    Pterygomaxillary Fissure and Base of Skull*

Jeffrey W. Yu, MD
Research Fellow
Department of Otolaryngology
Washington University School of Medicine
St. Louis, Missouri
Headache and Facial Pain

OTOLOGY AND NEUROTOLOGY

1

Anatomy of the Auditory and Vestibular Systems

Richard R. Gacek, MD

The temporal bone (TB) is a complex portion of the skull base that contains the labyrinth with its nerve supply (cranial nerve VIII) and also other cranial nerves such as the facial, trigeminal, vagus, glossopharyngeal, spinal accessory, and hypoglossal nerves. A thorough knowledge of the gross and microscopic anatomy[1,2] of the TB and the physiology of the labyrinthine sense organs is essential for the specialist who strives for accuracy in diagnosis and precision in surgery of the TB. This knowledge is gained first from dissection of cadaveric whole TB specimens but is greatly enhanced by study of prepared histologic sections from normal and pathologic TB.

OSTEOLOGY

Four major components of the TB contribute to the skull base: the squamous, tympanic, mastoid, and petrous.

The *squamous* portion of the TB provides attachment for the temporalis muscle, which is bounded inferiorly by the temporal line (Figure 1). The temporal line provides an external landmark for the floor of the middle cranial fossa. The zygomatic process projects forward from the lower portion of this bone, and together they form the anterior border of the mandibular fossa, which receives the condyle of the mandible.

The *tympanic* portion of the TB is an incomplete cylindrical portion of the TB that, together with the squamosal portion, forms the medial part of the external auditory canal. This portion of the external auditory canal is 2 cm in length by 1 cm in diameter. Its anterior boundary is the posterior limit of the mandibular fossa; medially, its border is the tympanic membrane. The posterior part fuses with the mastoid component of the TB at the tympanomastoid suture. Failure in development of this part of the TB is responsible for congenital aural atresia, a form of conductive hearing loss correctable by surgery.

The major portion of the TB formed by the *mastoid* portion attributes its large size to extensive pneumatization. The mastoid process projects posteriorly and inferiorly behind the external auditory meatus and serves as the attachment for the sternocleidomastoid muscle. A deep groove in its inferior aspect houses the posterior belly of the digastric muscle, which is innervated by the facial nerve. The superior surface of the mastoid compartment is formed by a thin plate of bone known as the tegmen mastoidea. Posteriorly, it forms the anterior plate of the posterior cranial fossa and is indented by a groove for the sigmoid sinus. The superior and inferior petrosal sinuses travel medially along the superior and inferior aspects of this part of the TB.

The *petrous* portion of the TB forms its medial part inferior to the middle cranial fossa; posteriorly, it forms the anterior surface of the posterior cranial fossa (Figure 2). The superior surface of the petrous bone is highlighted by the prominence of the superior semicircular canal, a landmark in surgery within the middle cranial fossa. Anterior to this portion of the petrous bone is the hiatus for the greater superficial petrosal nerve, which joins with the geniculate ganglion of the facial nerve. In some temporal bones, this hiatus is enlarged, and the geniculate ganglion may be exposed in the middle cranial fossa. Anterior and medial to this region is a concave area for the semilunar ganglion of the trigeminal nerve. On the posterior surface of the petrous bone are several important landmarks. The most obvious aperture is the

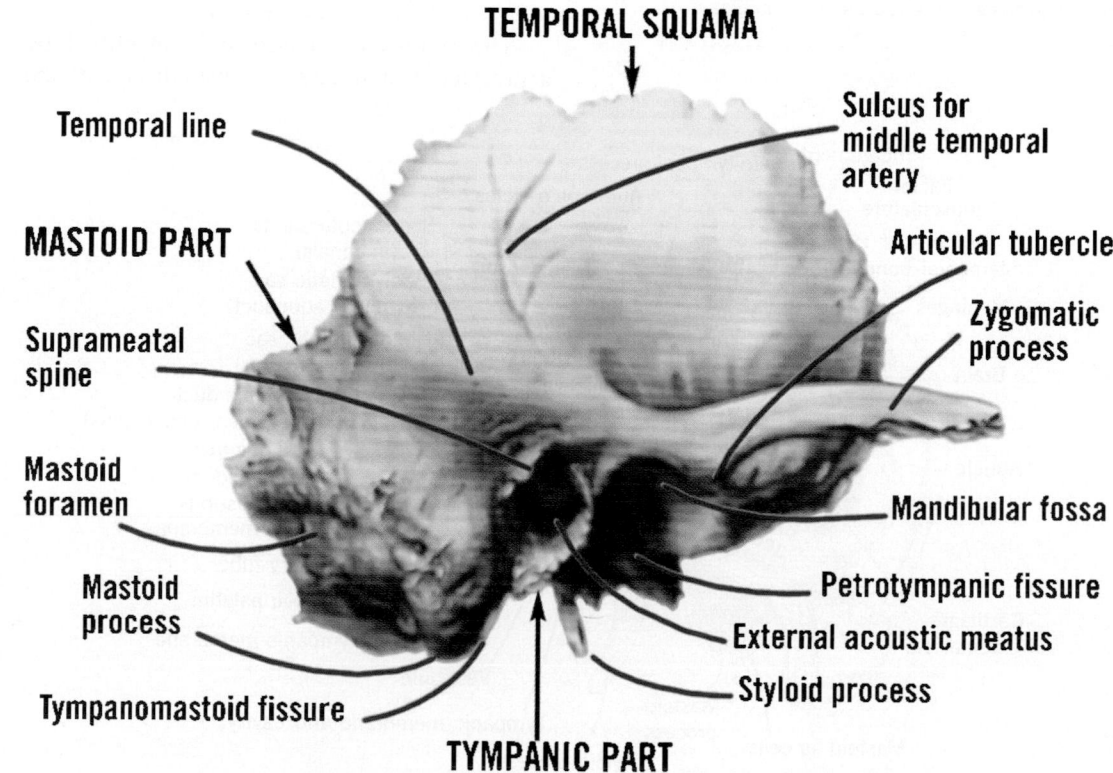

TEMPORAL SQUAMA

Temporal line

Sulcus for middle temporal artery

MASTOID PART

Articular tubercle

Zygomatic process

Suprameatal spine

Mastoid foramen

Mandibular fossa

Mastoid process

Petrotympanic fissure

External acoustic meatus

Styloid process

Tympanomastoid fissure

TYMPANIC PART

Figure 1 Right temporal bone, lateral view. (Reproduced with permission from reference 2.)

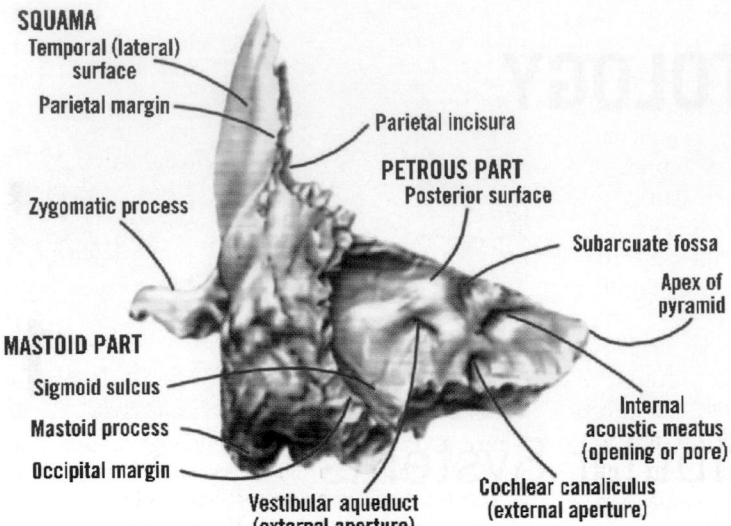

SQUAMA
Temporal (lateral) surface
Parietal margin
Parietal incisura
PETROUS PART
Posterior surface
Zygomatic process
Subarcuate fossa
Apex of pyramid
MASTOID PART
Sigmoid sulcus
Mastoid process
Occipital margin
Internal acoustic meatus (opening or pore)
Vestibular aqueduct (external aperture)
Cochlear canaliculus (external aperture)

Figure 2 Left temporal bone, posterolateral view. (Reproduced with permission from reference 2.)

internal auditory meatus (canal) that transmits the seventh and eighth cranial nerves as well as the labyrinthine artery or loop of the anterior inferior cerebellar artery (Figure 3). The lateral end (fundus) of the internal auditory canal (IAC) is divided horizontally by the falciform crest.[1,2] The superior compartment contains the facial nerve anteriorly and the superior division of the vestibular nerve posteriorly (Figure 4). The inferior compartment transmits the cochlear nerve anteriorly and the inferior division of the vestibular nerve posteriorly. The endolymphatic sac may be found in a depression covered by a bony shelf (operculum) anterior to the sigmoid groove. It narrows down into the vestibular aqueduct as the intraosseous endolymphatic sac. The depression for the semilunar ganglion and the fifth cranial nerve on the anterior surface of the petrous bone also carries the sixth cranial nerve through a dural canal referred to as Dorello's canal. These two nerves may be involved in inflammatory or neoplastic processes that occupy the petrous apex (PA) and are responsible for the clinical syndrome known as Gradenigo syndrome (fifth cranial nerve pain, diplopia from lateral rectus muscle palsy, and otorrhea).

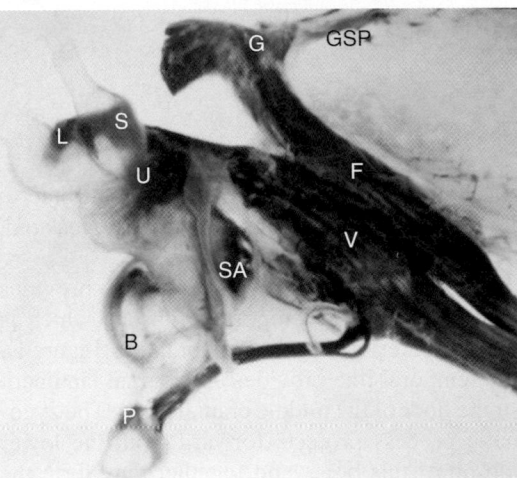

Figure 4 Human inner ear dissection with nerve supply demonstrates the relationship of the facial (F) and superior vestibular nerve (V) in the superior compartment of the internal canal. B = basal turn of cochlea; GSP = greater superficial petrosal nerve; G = geniculate ganglion; L = lateral canal crista; P = posterior canal crista; S = superior canal crista; SA = saccule; U = utricle.

AUDITORY SYSTEM

External Ear

The external or outer ear is that portion of the ear that is lateral to the tympanic membrane (Figure 5).[3] It consists of the external auditory canal as well as the auricle and cartilaginous portion of the ear.

The auricle is a semicircular plate of elastic cartilage characterized by a number of ridges or grooves. The major ridges of the auricle are the helix and antihelix, the tragus and antitragus, which surround the concha, which is the scaphoid depression posterior to the external auditory meatus. The cartilage of the external auditory meatus is continuous with that of the outer portion of the ear canal and auricle.

The external auditory canal is made up of a cartilaginous extension of the auricle in its outer half and the mastoid and tympanic portion of the TB in its medial half. It is bounded medially by the tympanic membrane and is lined with skin that is thin with little subcutaneous tissue medially but laterally contains numerous hair follicles and ceruminous and sebaceous glands. The bony external auditory canal averages 3.5 cm in length, with a diameter of 1 cm. The tympanic membrane is composed of three layers: the outer squamous cell epithelial layer, the medial mucosal layer facing the middle ear, and the fibrous layer or tunica propria, forming the substance of the tympanic membrane.[4] The fibrous layer gives the tympanic membrane its shape and consistency. Radial fibers of the tunica propria insert into the manubrium, circumferential fibers providing strength without interfering with vibration, whereas tangential fibers reinforce the architecture of the tympanic membrane. These physical characteristics are important for the vibratory characteristics necessary for sound transmission.

The tympanic membrane is identified by a prominent landmark, the manubrium of the

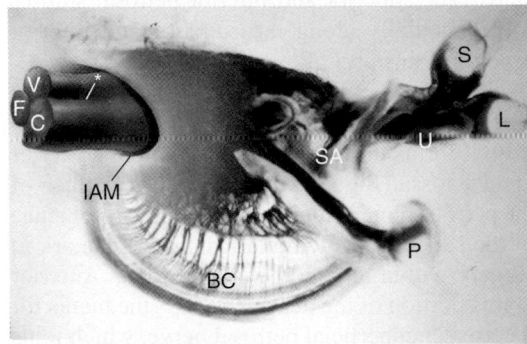

Figure 3 This orientation of the human inner ear dissection shows the anatomical relationship of the nerves and sense organs when viewed from the posterior surface of the temporal bone. IAM = internal auditory meatus; V = vestibular nerve trunk; C = cochlear nerve trunk; F = facial nerve; BC = basal turn of cochlea; SA = saccule; U = utricular nerve; S, L, P = superior, lateral, and posterior semicircular canal ampullae; * = cleavage plane between vestibular and cochlear nerve trunks.

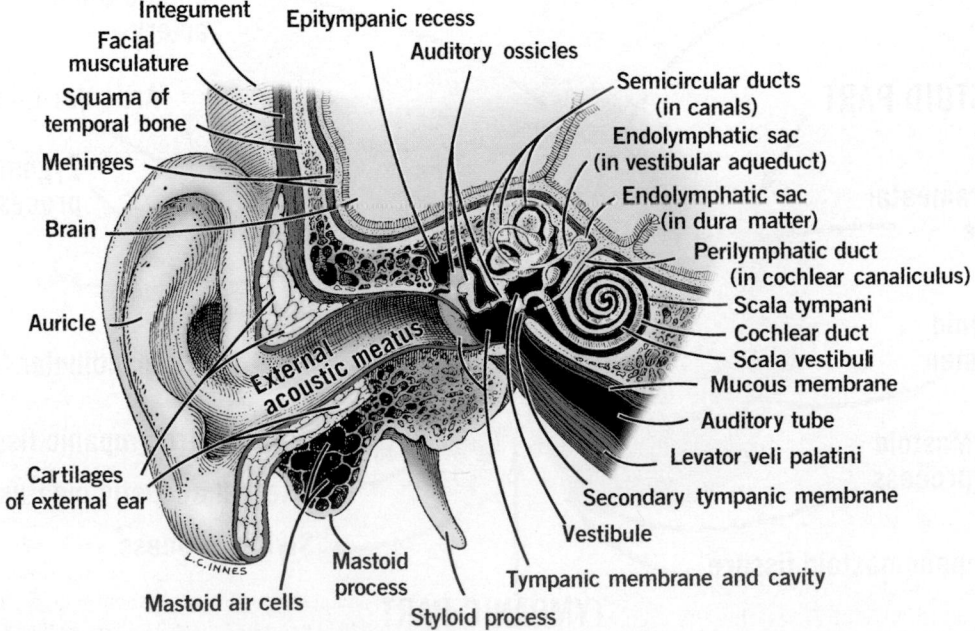

Integument
Facial musculature
Epitympanic recess
Auditory ossicles
Squama of temporal bone
Semicircular ducts (in canals)
Endolymphatic sac (in vestibular aqueduct)
Meninges
Endolymphatic sac (in dura matter)
Perilymphatic duct (in cochlear canaliculus)
Brain
Scala tympani
Cochlear duct
Scala vestibuli
Mucous membrane
Auricle
External acoustic meatus
Auditory tube
Levator veli palatini
Secondary tympanic membrane
Cartilages of external ear
Vestibule
Tympanic membrane and cavity
L.C.INNES
Mastoid process
Styloid process
Mastoid air cells

Figure 5 General relationship of parts of the ear (semidiagrammatic). (Reproduced with permission from reference 3.)

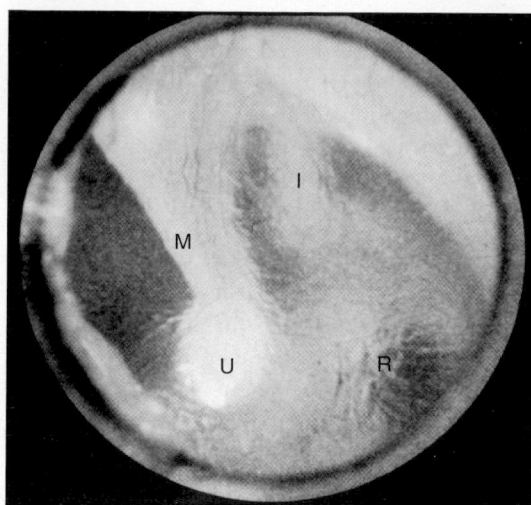

Figure 6 Photograph of a normal left tympanic membrane. I = long process of incus; M = malleus; R = round window niche; U = umbo.

malleus, which is limited superiorly by its lateral or short process and inferiorly by a rounded end referred to as the umbo (Figure 6). The umbo forms the deep apex of the conical shape formed by the tympanic membrane. The tympanic membrane is incomplete superiorly, where it lacks a fibrous layer in the portion superior to the short process of the manubrium.[5] Since it lacks a fibrous layer, this portion is called the pars flaccida (Shrapnell's membrane). The major or inferior portion of the tympanic membrane is referred to as the pars tensa.

Middle Ear

The space between the tympanic membrane and the bony capsule of the labyrinth in the petrous portion of the TB contains the ossicular chain with its associated muscles, the aperture of the eustachian tube, and the vascular system. The tympanic cavity is divided into the epitympanic, mesotympanic, and hypotympanic regions. The *hypotympanic* portion is that portion of the middle ear that lies inferior to the aperture of the eustachian tube and the round window niche (RWN). This portion of the middle ear contains various bony trabeculae and the bony covering of the jugular bulb. This bony surface may be dehiscent, exposing the jugular bulb in the hypotympanic region. Inferiorly, a small channel (the inferior tympanic canaliculus) transmits Jacobson nerve (a branch of cranial nerve IX).

The *mesotympanic* portion of the middle ear is limited superiorly by the horizontal portion of the facial canal and inferiorly by the RWN. This region contains the oval and round windows, the stapes bone, the stapedius muscle posteriorly, and the canal for the tensor tympani muscle anteriorly. The oval window is kidney bean shaped with a convex superior rim and a concave inferior rim. In the oval window, the footplate of the stapes bone is held in place by the annular ligament. The RWN forms a deep recess often covered with various mucous membrane configurations that obscure the round window membrane (RWM). The RWM is a fibrous

membrane covered with a layer of mucosa that is roughly kidney bean shaped, with a major component anterior and inferior and a minor component located posteriorly and horizontally in the RWN. Posteriorly, in the mesotympanum there are two bony recesses of clinical importance. The recess lateral to the vertical segment of the facial canal is called the facial recess. The space medial to the facial canal is called the sinus tympani (Figure 7). These two recesses are important clinically as they frequently harbor chronic middle ear infection and must be controlled in surgery. The facial recess also provides access to the middle ear space and RWN in those procedures in which the ear canal wall is preserved (ie, intact canal wall mastoidectomy, cochlear implantation). A bony projection from the facial canal (pyramidal eminence) contains the tendon of the stapedius muscle before its insertion into the neck of the stapes bone. The most anterior portion of the middle ear space is called the *protympanum* and is bordered superiorly by the orifice of the eustachian tube and anteriorly by the canal for the internal carotid artery (see Figure 7).

The *epitympanum* is the portion of the middle ear that is limited superiorly by the bony roof of the middle ear called the tegmen tympani. This bony landmark is continuous posteriorly as the tegmen mastoidea. The medial wall of the epitympanum is formed by the bony prominence of the lateral and superior semicircular canal ampullae as well as the epitympanic portion of the facial (fallopian) canal. The head and neck of the malleus and its articulation with the body and short process and a portion of the long process of the incus occupy most of the space in the epitympanum. These two ossicular masses are held in place by ligaments anteriorly and posteriorly to provide an axis of rotation for the ossicular chain (Figure 8). The epitympanic space communicates posteriorly through a narrow opening called the aditus ad antrum to the central mastoid tract of the mastoid cavity.

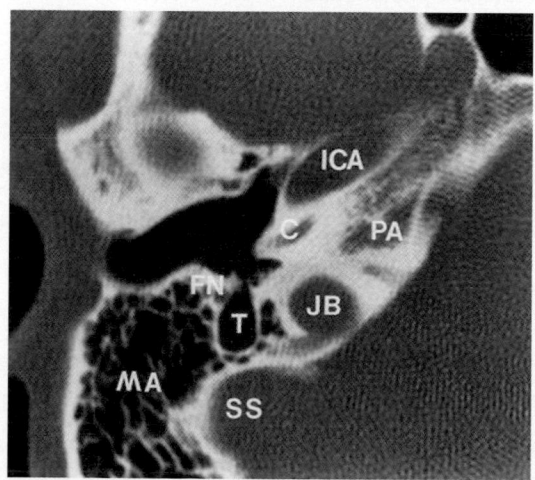

Figure 7 This axial computed tomographic scan of the temporal bone illustrates a normal mastoid cell system (MA), the horizontal segment of the internal carotid artery (ICA), the jugular bulb (JB), the sigmoid sinus (SS), and a nonpneumatized petrous apex (PA). C = basal turn of the cochlea; FN = facial nerve; T = sinus tympani.

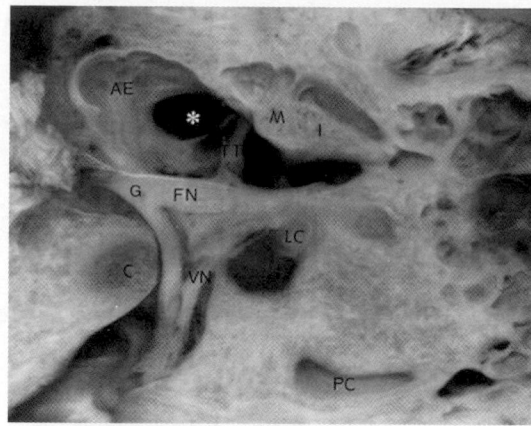

Figure 8 This horizontal cut through a celloidin-embedded temporal bone illustrates the relationship of the facial nerve (FN) to the superior division of the vestibular nerve (VN) in the internal auditory canal. The axis of rotation of the head of the malleus (M) and body of the incus (I) with their ligamentous attachments in the epitympanum is shown. AE = anterior epitympanic space ventilated into the protympanum (*); LC = lateral semicircular canal crista and ampulla; PC = posterior semicircular canal; C = endosteum of the cochlea (basal turn); TT = tensor tympani tendon; G = geniculate ganglion.

Anteriorly, the epitympanum is separated at the cochleariform process from an anterior epitympanic cell of variable size by a bony and mucous membrane barrier, which may completely or incompletely separate the two compartments. This anterior epitympanic space is formed by pneumatization from the protympanum (see Figure 8). The anterior epitympanic space is also important surgically as it may contain inflammatory tissue (ie, cholesteatoma) that has extended from the protympanum.

Auditory Ossicles. Sound pressure energy is transmitted from the tympanic membrane across the middle ear space by the ossicular chain composed of the malleus, incus, and stapes (Figure 9).[6] The head of the malleus and body of the incus function as a unit suspended by ligaments in the epitympanum. The tip of the long process of the incus articulates at a right angle with the head of the stapes so that the sound energy transmission initiated by medial displacement of the tympanic membrane is carried by the parallel displacement of the elongate processes of the malleus and incus to the head, crura, and footplate of the stapes (see Figure 9). Since the surface area of the tympanic membrane is larger than that of the stapes footplate by a ratio of 25 to 1, the sound pressure density in the oval window and the inner ear fluids is similarly increased. Maintaining this ratio by various reconstructive methods constitutes an important principle in middle ear surgery. The stapes therefore acts in a piston-like fashion in the oval window. The stapes bone is shaped like a stirrup with a head, neck, and footplate or base. The crura are bowed, the posterior one more so than the anterior, and fused with the footplate, which is formed from both otic capsule and periosteal bone. These auditory ossicles are controlled to some degree by two middle ear muscles, the tensor tympani and the stapedius. The tensor tympani muscle is housed in a bony semicanal in the anterior mesotympanum

LIGAMENTS AND MUSCLES

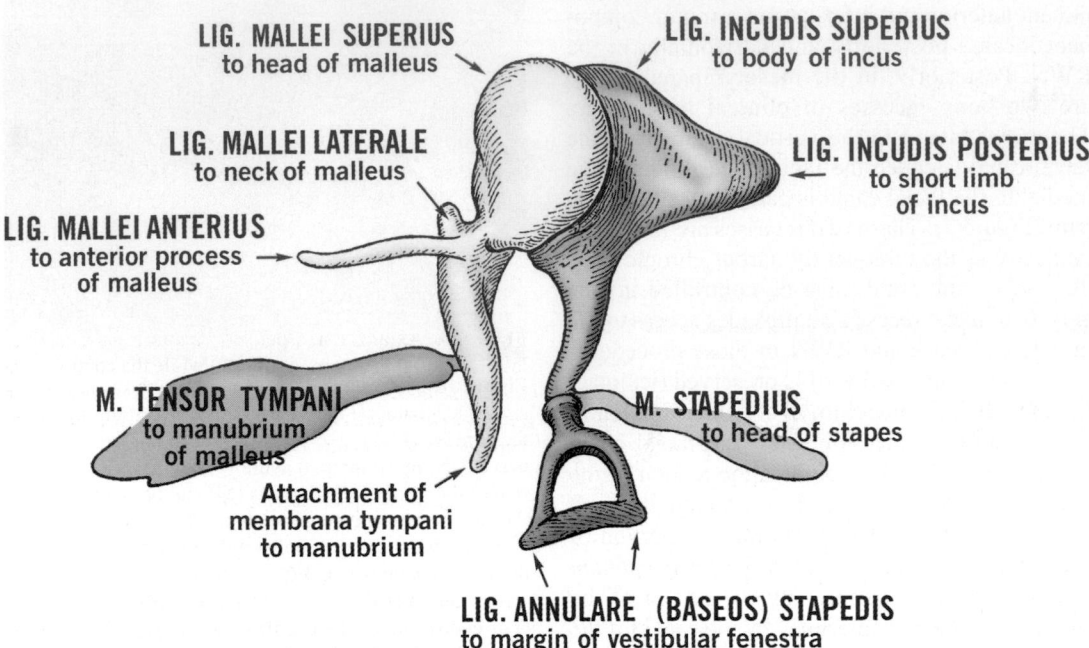

Figure 9 Auditory ossicles: their adult form and muscles and ligaments. (Reproduced with permission from reference 6.)

just superior to the orifice of the eustachian tube (Figure 10). The muscle converges posteriorly into a tendinous segment that is anchored at the cochleariform process and turns abruptly laterally to insert on the neck of the malleus. The tensor tympani is innervated by a branch of the fifth cranial nerve. Its motoneurons are located centrally in the parvocellular division of the trigeminal motor nucleus, and its action causes the drumhead to be pulled medially, thus raising the resonant frequency of the sound conduction system.

The stapedius muscle arises within either its own or the fallopian canal and is accompanied by

the motor portion of the facial nerve. It converges superiorly and anteriorly to form the stapedius tendon, which emerges through the pyramidal eminence to insert at the neck of the stapes. The stapedius muscle is innervated by a branch of the seventh nerve, and its motoneurons are located in the brainstem in the interface between the facial nucleus and the lateral superior olivary nucleus. Contraction of the stapedius muscle displaces the stapes posteriorly and attenuates sound transmitted by the ossicular chain. Since reflex contraction of the stapedius muscle is activated by sound, it is regarded as a protective mechanism for the cochlea.

Eustachian Tube. The eustachian tube is an essential communication between the nasopharynx and the middle ear (Figure 11). It is responsible for pneumatization of the middle ear and the mastoid and for maintaining normal pressure between the middle ear and the atmosphere. It represents the pharyngeal extension of the first

branchial arch and extends from the lateral wall of the nasopharynx.

The skeleton of the medial three-fourths of the eustachian tube is cartilage that is surrounded by soft tissue, adipose tissue, and respiratory epithelium. The cartilage of the eustachian tube, which is hook shaped on cross-section, is stabilized and displaced by contraction of the tensor veli palatini and levator veli palatini muscles on swallowing or yawning. The eustachian tube is thereby opened, allowing for pressure equalization. The lining epithelium of the cartilaginous portion is similar to that of the pharynx with pseudostratified columnar cell epithelium and many mucous glands. Posterior to the union of the cartilaginous and osseous portion of the eustachian tube where the isthmus is located, the mucosa undergoes transition to cuboidal or low columnar cell epithelium similar to the tympanic cavity epithelium. Neoplastic compression of the eustachian tube lumen near its pharyngeal orifice (Rosenmüller fossa) will cause fluid to fill the middle ear space (serous otitis media), usually in an adult patient (see Figure 11). Investigation of this occult region by endoscopy, radiologic imaging, and biopsy is necessary in such instances.

In some patients fullness in the ear, autophony without hearing loss and a normal eardrum may be produced by an overly patent eustachian tube. Such patency of the eustachian tube may be caused by a decrease in the fat cells surrounding its cartilaginous segment associated with weight loss.

Nerve Supply of the External and Middle Ear. The auricle and the external auditory canal receive the sensory nerve branches from the fifth nerve via the auriculotemporal nerve and the greater and lesser auricular nerves. Branches from the glossopharyngeal and vagus nerves also contribute to this innervation. The branch of the vagus nerve is referred to as Arnold nerve, which travels in the posterior part of the ear canal in the posterior part of the tympanomastoid suture. When this nerve is stimulated, it produces a cough reflex as when the external auditory canal is being cleaned with an instrument. It may also participate in heralding a neoplastic or infectious process in distant regions of the aerodigestive tract also innervated by the vagus nerve (ie, larynx, hypopharynx) when pain is referred to the ear.

The main innervation to the middle ear space is through the tympanic plexus and Jacobson nerve, which receives a major contribution from the glossopharyngeal nerve through the inferior tympanic canaliculus. This nerve travels in a bony sulcus or canal over the promontory along with the inferior tympanic artery anterior to the oval window and finally anteriorly to become the lesser superficial petrosal nerve. This nerve ultimately carries the fibers of the preganglionic neurons of the ninth nerve to the otic ganglion, where they synapse with postganglionic neurons and are carried over the auriculotemporal nerve to the parotid gland. The glossopharyngeal nerve provides sensory innervation to the

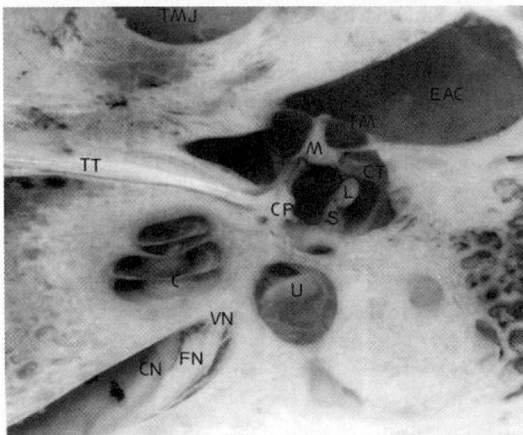

Figure 10 A more inferior cut through the same temporal bone as in Figure 8 demonstrates the cochlea (C), the utricular macula and its nerve (U), the cochlear nerve (CN), the facial nerve (FN), and vestibular nerves (VN) in the internal auditory canal. The muscle and tendon of the tensor tympani muscle (TT) overlie the cochlea as it turns laterally in the cochleariform process (CP) to attach near the neck of the malleus (M). The articulation of the long process (L) of the incus with the stapes head (S) can be seen in the mesotympanum. The chorda tympani nerve (CT) passes between the malleus and incus. TM = tympanic membrane; EAC = external auditory canal; TMJ = temporomandibular joint space.

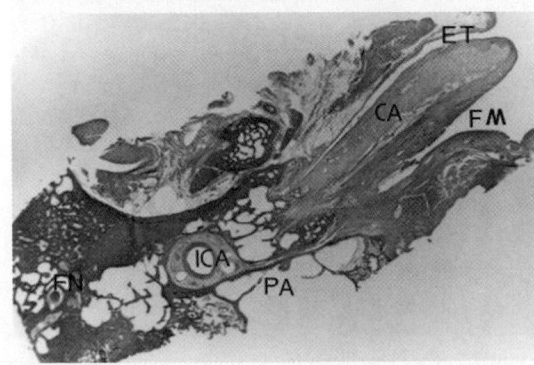

Figure 11 Low-power horizontal section through the eustachian tube (ET) as it passes into the protympanum. CA = cartilage of the ET; FM = fossa of Rosenmüller; ICA = internal carotid artery; FN = facial nerve; PA = petrous apex air cells.

pharyngeal tonsillar fossa and may be responsible for referred otalgia from neoplasms in this organ. Such referred ear pain is commonly encountered after tonsillectomy. Sympathetic fibers from the carotid plexus also contribute to the tympanic plexus. The chorda tympani nerve, which is a sensory branch of the facial nerve, will be discussed in the section "Facial Nerve."

Mastoid Compartment. The air cell system of the mastoid bone represents an extension of the air compartment in the middle ear from the first pharyngeal pouch. This process occurs in development of the TB and may result in a variable degree of pneumatization in the mastoid compartment (see Figure 7). Recurrent infection in the middle ear and mastoid has been identified as a factor that may limit the extent of pneumatization of the mastoid air cell system, whereas absence of such infection may favor full development of the air cell system. The air cells in the mastoid compartment extend from the aditus ad antrum in the epitympanum to the central mastoid tract (antrum) from which further extension in several directions may occur.[7] The *posterior superior* cell tract extends medially at the level of the superior semicircular canal toward the PA, and the *posterior medial* cell tract extends toward the PA at the level of the posterior semicircular canal. The *supralabyrinthine* cell system extends medially superior to the labyrinth, whereas the *retrofacial* cell system extends posteriorly and inferiorly along the bony ear canal to pneumatize the mastoid tip. These cell tracts may vary considerably and are important for the surgeon to know as a guide in tracing infection into deep recesses of the mastoid compartment and particularly the PA.

Normal structures may be aberrantly located near pneumatized portions of the TB where they may become important in adult life. Such are the arachnoid villi whose function is the circulation of cerebrospinal fluid (CSF) into the dural venous sinuses. Aberrant arachnoid villi in the middle or posterior cranial fossa may be located adjacent to the bone of pneumatized areas of the skull base where they may enlarge with time into arachnoid granulations which erode into the mastoid compartment in adult life (Figure 12). Their clinical presentation as spontaneous CSF otorrhea or rhinorrhea[8] offers timely diagnosis and treatment for the astute clinician (Figure 13). The prevention of intracranial morbidity (meningitis, brain abscess) from acute infection in these bony cavities is the goal of early recognition.

Cell tracts arising from the middle ear space are also important for the surgeon. These cell tracts, particularly those that may lead to air cell development in the PA, are those that course inferior to the labyrinth or those that extend around the canal of the internal carotid artery (see Figure 14). Extensive pneumatization in the development of the PA may create air cells that can become isolated when the cell tract is obliterated by bone or fibrous tissue leading to the formation of cholesterol cysts over a period of many years. Over time, these cysts erode the

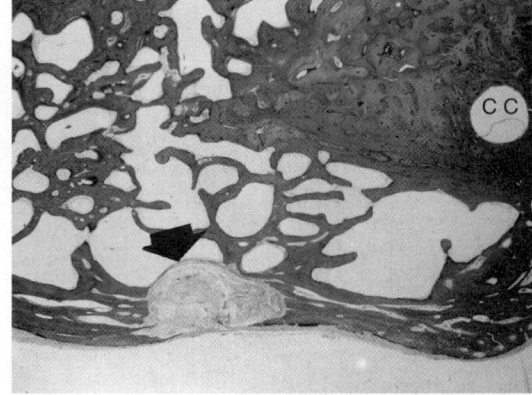

(A)

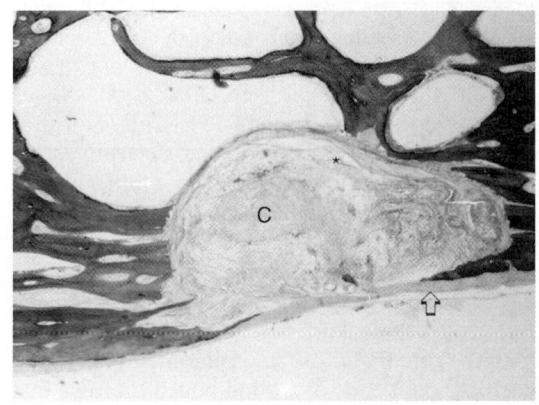

(B)

Figure 12 (A) Medium power view of an arachnoid granulation (*arrow*) located on the posterior surface of the temporal bone. CC = Crus Commune. (B) Higher power photo shows the arachnoid core (C) surrounded by the subarachnoid space (*) which contains spinal fluid. Arrow indicates the dura mater. Communication with the mastoid air cells is eminent.

surrounding bone and may reach considerable size in early or late adulthood. Compression of the trigeminal nerve and the sixth nerve near the PA may present a clinical picture similar to Gradenigo syndrome, which is the clinical manifestation of petrous apicitis.

The PA is of special interest because of a variety of lesions that may involve this region. The clinical manifestation may be subtle and requires a high index of suspicion to pursue the diagnosis.[9] Imaging (both computed tomography and

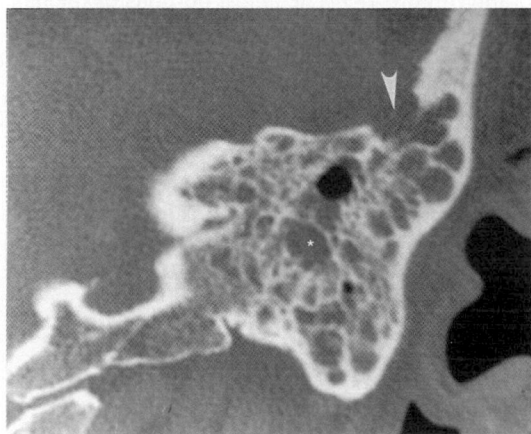

Figure 13 This coronal CT demonstrates filling of a mastoid compartment (*) with CSF from a middle fossa arachnoid granulation (*arrow*).

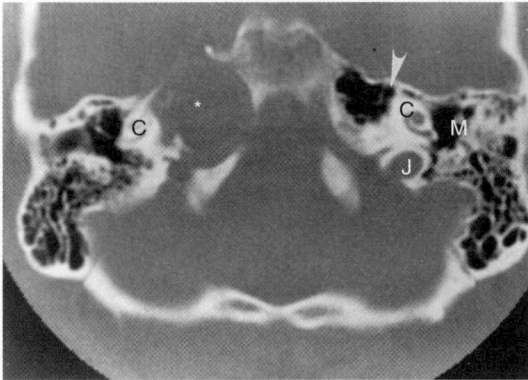

Figure 14 Axial CT in a patient with an expanding cholesterol cyst in the petrous apex (*) while the contralateral temporal bone illustrates pneumatization of the apex region (*arrow*) which leads to cyst formation. C = cochlea; M = mastoid compartment; J = jugular foramen.

magnetic resonance imaging) is especially sensitive to the identification of pathology in the PA. Since the composition of the PA can include air cells (see Figure 14), bone marrow (Figure 7), the internal carotid artery (Figure 7), and the cartilage of the foramen lacerum, the list of lesions that occur here is lengthy. Cholesterol cysts and congenital cholesteatomas are the most common; however, infection, bone marrow neoplasms, cartilage tumors, metastatic malignancies, neurogenic tumors, and aneurysms of the internal carotid artery have been reported. Clinical signs of a progressive lesion in the PA relate to nearby structures: eustachian tube obstruction, facial pain or anesthesia, and lateral rectus muscle palsy.

Inner Ear

The petrous portion of the TB houses the labyrinth with its attendant sensory structures responsible for auditory and balance function. Within the bony labyrinth is contained the membranous labyrinth, which represents a continuous series of epithelial-lined tubes and spaces of the inner ear containing endolymph and the sense organs of hearing and balance. The membranous labyrinth can be divided into three regions that are interconnected: the pars superior or the vestibular labyrinth with the exception of the saccule, the pars inferior (cochlea and the saccule), and the endolymphatic duct and sac. All the sense organs of the labyrinth have in common that they contain hair cells with rigid cilia and are innervated by afferent and efferent neurons.[10,11] Displacement of the cilia of the hair cells is responsible for opening potassium and calcium channels that initiate the electrical potential within the hair cell that is then leaked into the afferent neuron and carried to the brainstem.

Cochlea. The cochlear duct, the auditory portion of the labyrinth, extends approximately 35 mm.[12] The cochlear duct and associated sensory and supportive structures assume the form of a spiral similar to a snail shell of 2.5 to 2.75 turns (Figure 15).[13] This allows the long cochlear duct to be contained in a small space. A cross-section of a cochlear turn (Figure 16) demonstrates the essential structures in this sense organ. The scala

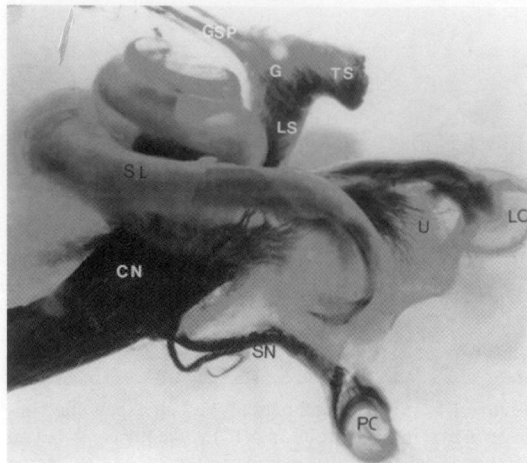

Figure 15 Photograph of a dissection of the human labyrinth and its nerve supply that demonstrates the 2 1/2 turns of the cochlear duct and the spiral ligament (SL). U = utricular nerve and macula; LC = lateral duct ampulla; PC = posterior duct ampulla; SN = singular nerve. Facial nerve: labyrinthine segment (LS) and tympanic segment (TS). G = geniculate ganglion; GSP = greater superficial petrosal nerve; CN = cochlear nerve. (Reproduced with permission from reference 13.)

media or cochlear duct containing endolymph is triangular in shape in cross-section. The basilar membrane forms the horizontal limb of the triangle, Reissner membrane, the superior limb, and the stria vascularis with spiral ligament on the vertical side. The cochlear duct is filled with a fluid referred to as endolymph, whereas the fluid in the scala vestibuli and scala tympani is perilymph. Perilymph of the two scalae communicates through the helicotrema at the apex of the cochlea (Figure 17). All the structures of the cochlear duct and, particularly, the basilar membrane have a morphologic gradient whereby the width of the basilar membrane is narrowest at the basal end and widest at the apex. The spiral ligament and epithelial elements in the organ of Corti also have a morphologic gradient from

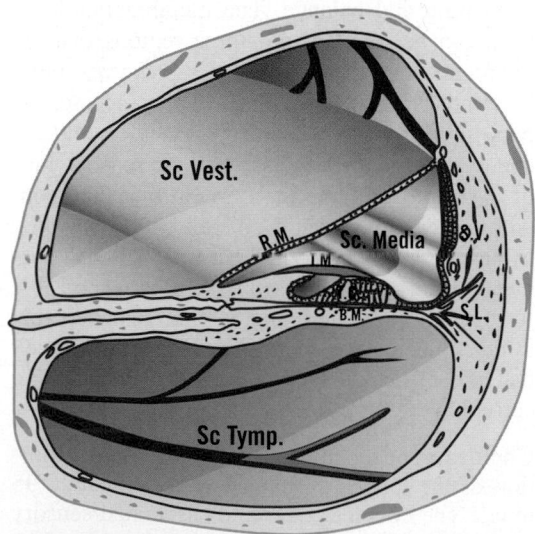

Figure 16 Section (diagrammatic) through the cochlea. Sc Vest = scala vestibuli; RM = Reissner membrane; Sc Media = scala media; TM = tectorial membrane; OC = organ of Corti; BM = basilar membrane; SV = stria vascularis; SL = spiral ligament; OSL = osseous spiral lamina; Sc Tymp = scala tympani.

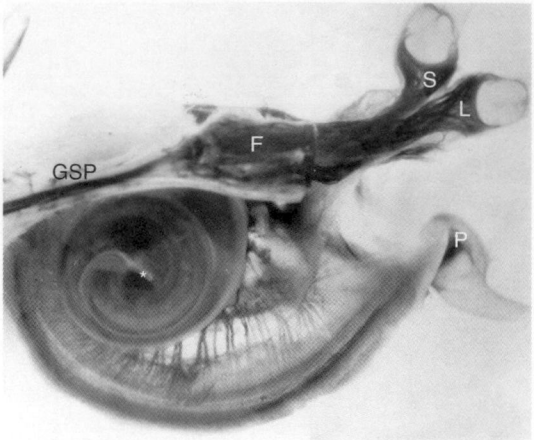

Figure 17 Human inner ear specimen viewed from the middle ear demonstrates communication of the vestibular and tympanic scalae at the helicotrema (*).

base to apex (see Figure 15). This morphologic gradient, to a large degree, determines the location of maximal stimulation of the basilar membrane and inner hair cells by a given tone or frequency that is introduced to the inner ear. In this way, high frequencies are located at the base and low frequencies at the apex, with the frequency scale laid out in an orderly fashion over the remainder of the basilar membrane. The cochlear duct ends in a blind pouch (cecum) that is located near the RWM.

Perilymph of the scala vestibuli fills the vestibule under the stapes footplate. This perilymphatic compartment extends up the scala vestibuli of the cochlea and communicates with the perilymph in the scala tympani, which extends down the cochlea to terminate at the RWM. The perilymphatic compartment also communicates with the subarachnoid space through the periotic duct by way of the cochlear aqueduct that is filled with a trabecular meshwork of connective tissue capable of allowing some exchange of CSF and perilymph. However, perilymph is primarily formed by filtration from the vascular network in the spiral ligament.

The organ of Corti is a complex sense organ that contains inner and outer hair cells and supporting cells resting on the basilar membrane, with the ciliated ends of the hair cells protruding into or near a covering structure, the tectorial membrane (Figure 18). The apical portions of the hair cells are anchored in the cuticular plate,[10] with the stereocilia (usually 100 to 150 per cell) protruding

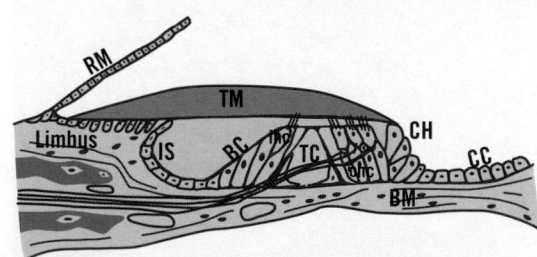

Figure 18 Detail of organ of Corti. RM = Reissner membrane; TM = tectorial membrane; IS = inner sulcus; BC = border cells; ihc = inner hair cells; TC = tunnel of Corti; ohc = outer hair cells; phc = phalangeal cells; CH = cells of Hensen; CC = cells of Claudius; BM = basilar membrane.

through the cuticular plate.[10–12] The stereocilia of the outer hair cells make contact with the tectorial membrane, whereas the stereocilia of the inner hair cells lie free in the endolymphatic space inferior to the tectorial membrane. There are a single row of inner hair cells and three to five rows of outer hair cells. These cells differ morphologically in that the inner hair cells are more flask shaped and tightly surrounded by supporting cells and have stereocilia that are arranged in a linear fashion, whereas the outer hair cells are columnar and incompletely surrounded by phalangeal or supporting cells lying free in the perilymph of the organ of Corti.[14] The stereocilia of the outer hair cells form an inverted "W," and a basal body representing a rudimentary kinocilium is located on the spiral ligament side of the ciliary tuft. The inner hair cells are supported by interphalangeal cells, whereas the outer hair cells are supported by Deiters cells inferiorly and laterally by Hensen cells. The tectorial membrane is anchored medially at the limbus and attached to the Hensen cells laterally by a fibrous net. The basilar membrane and tectorial membrane are displaced vertically by the traveling wave created by sound energy delivered to the oval window. Since the fulcrum of these two structures is separate, they will slide horizontally when stimulated, resulting in a shearing action between the tectorial membrane and the cuticular plate. The resultant displacement of stereocilia initiates an electrical event in the hair cell. The organ of Corti contains approximately 15,500 hair cells, with about 3,500 of them being inner hair cells and 12,000 being outer hair cells. These hair cells are innervated by afferent and efferent neurons in a complex but orderly manner.[15] The afferent neurons to the auditory sense organ are bipolar neurons referred to as spiral ganglion cells that are located in Rosenthal canal of the bony modiolus. Approximately 30,000 spiral ganglion cells innervate the human organ of Corti. The spiral ganglion takes the form of clusters of ganglion cells throughout the extent of the length of the cochlea. Ninety to 95% of the spiral ganglion neurons are type I neurons, which are large and myelinated and project a single dendrite directly to an inner hair cell.[14] Approximately 10 to 20 type I spiral ganglion cells innervate one inner hair cell (Figure 19). These form the major

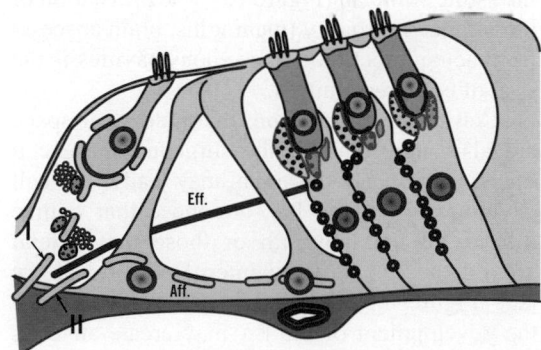

Figure 19 Schematic of the organ of Corti summarizing the efferent (*dark*) and afferent clear innervation termination. I = type I spiral ganglion cell afferents; II = type II spiral ganglia cell afferents.

afferent input from stimulation of the organ of Corti. Type I ganglion cells degenerate readily following injury to the dendrite. The remaining 5% of afferent neurons in the spiral ganglion are type II ganglion cells, which are smaller and unmyelinated and have very thin distal processes. The dendrites of these type II neurons cross the tunnel space along its floor enveloped by pillar cell processes and form spiral bundles between Deiters cells. These dendrites then course apically between Deiters cells to innervate several to many outer hair cells per type II dendrite. A type II ganglion survives following injury to its dendrite.

The axons of the spiral ganglion cells project to the cochlear nucleus complex, which has anteroventral and posteroventral divisions of the ventral cochlear nucleus and the dorsal cochlear nucleus. Each type I afferent neuron bifurcates and also sends a trifurcating branch to the dorsal cochlear nucleus in an orderly fashion according to frequency.[12] Apical turn neurons terminate in the most medial portion of the nuclear complex, whereas the basal turn neurons terminate laterally. Remaining frequency projections are ordered between these two regions of the cochlear nucleus. The central termination of the type II ganglion cells is not known largely because the small caliber axons are difficult to trace for long distances.

This frequency organization of the auditory pathway characterizes the remainder of the afferent pathway from end organ to cortex. Another feature of the afferent auditory pathway is that the numbers of neurons involved at the various nuclear way stations undergo a progressive increase from cochlear nucleus to the cortex.[16] Although there are 30,000 spiral ganglion cells in the monkey auditory nerve, 88,000 neurons are found in one cochlear nucleus in the primate. One superior olivary complex contains 34,000 neurons, whereas the nucleus of the lateral lemniscus has 38,000 neurons, and at the inferior colliculus level there are almost 400,000 neurons on each side and at the medial geniculate body 500,000 neurons. The auditory cortex has approximately 10 million neurons.

A brief description of the afferent auditory pathway follows (Figure 20).[17] The cells of the dorsal cochlear nucleus project axons to the dorsal acoustic stria, which crosses the midline and ascends in the contralateral lateral lemniscus to terminate in the dorsal nucleus of the lateral lemniscus and the inferior colliculus, particularly its inferior half. The cell bodies of the ventral cochlear nucleus project axons to the ipsilateral accessory and main superior olivary nuclei and to the medial dendrites of the contralateral accessory olive. The neurons of the accessory olive have bipolar dendrites arranged horizontally. This arrangement is favorable to receive input from projections of both cochlear nuclei. As such, it is an important nuclear "way-station" for determining sound localization. Some fibers of the intermediate and ventral cochlear striae travel beyond the superior olivary complex and enter the contralateral lateral lemniscus to terminate in the inferior colliculus. The superior olive

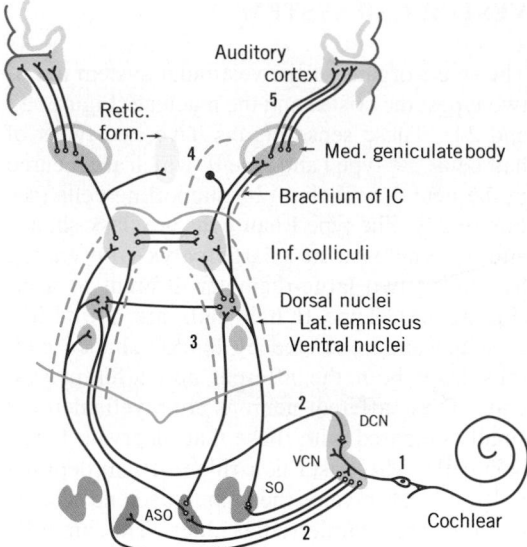

Figure 20 Diagram of the neuronal linkage that serves the afferent auditory pathway from one cochlea. Numerals indicate order of neuron units in the pathway. VCN = ventral cochlear nucleus; DCN = dorsal cochlear nucleus; SO = lateral superior olivary nucleus; ASO = accessory superior olivary nucleus; IC = inferior colliculus; Retic. form. = reticular formation. (Reproduced with permission from reference 17.)

is thought to function as both a relay station for the auditory pathway and as a reflex center. The best known reflex mediated through the superior olive is the stapedius reflex. Stapedius muscle motoneurons are located in the interface between the superior olivary and the facial nerve nuclei. The accessory superior olive projects bilaterally in the lateral lemnisci to terminate in the dorsal nuclei of the lateral lemnisci and the inferior colliculi. The lateral superior olive projects homolaterally in the lateral lemniscus to terminate in the dorsal nucleus of the lateral lemniscus and also in the inferior colliculus. No neurons from the superior olivary nuclei project beyond the inferior colliculus.

Projections from the inferior colliculus are primarily to the medial geniculate body. However, some projections to the medial geniculate body are received from the nuclei of the lateral lemniscus. All ascending neurons terminate in the medial geniculate body so that the final projection pathway to the auditory cortex, which is a major one, is from the medial geniculate body. Furthermore, the only commissural or interconnections between the two sides of the auditory pathway are at the superior olivary level, the level of the nuclei of the lateral lemniscus, and the inferior colliculus. No commissural projections are present superior to the inferior colliculus.

The ascending auditory pathway, although composed of four to five neurons in the linkage from end organ to auditory cortex and having an increasing volume of neural units active at each level, nevertheless is precisely organized according to the frequency scale and project bilaterally but predominantly in a contralateral pathway to the auditory cortex.

Efferent Auditory Pathways. Paralleling the afferent auditory pathway is a descending

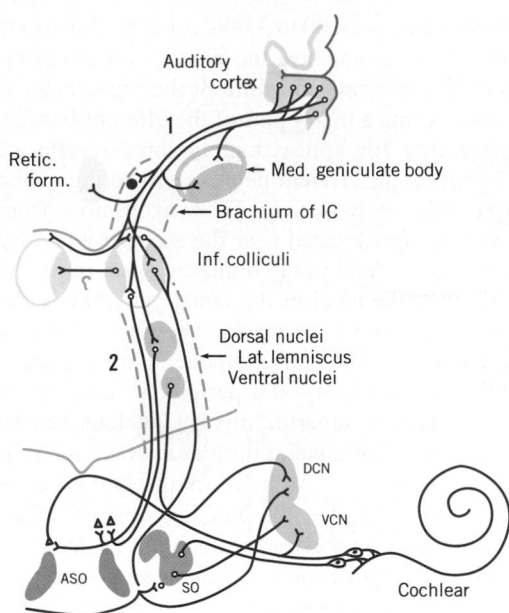

Figure 21 Diagram of the descending (efferent) auditory pathway. IC = inferior colliculus; DCN = dorsal cochlear nucleus; VCN = ventral cochlear nucleus; ASO = accessory superior olivary nucleus; SO = lateral superior olivary nucleus. (Reproduced with permission from reference 17.)

pathway originating in the auditory cortex and terminating in the end organ (Figure 21).[17] This pathway does not involve as many neurons as the ascending or afferent pathway but has the feature of extensive ramification and formation of many terminals, which contact a large number of neurons. Nevertheless, the efferent pathway does not make as many neural contacts in the auditory nuclei as the ascending pathway. The descending auditory pathway originates in the auditory cortex and initially projects to the inferior colliculus and the dorsal nucleus of the lateral lemniscus, with some termination in the medial geniculate body and the reticular formation.

The next neuron in the descending chain is located in peripheral regions of the inferior colliculus and the nuclei of the lateral lemniscus. These projections terminate in brainstem neurons that give rise to efferent neurons projecting to divisions of the cochlear nucleus and to neurons that give rise to the third and final neuron in the descending auditory pathway, the olivocochlear bundle, which innervates the organ of Corti.[18,19]

The olivocochlear bundle has both an ipsilateral and a contralateral limb or component (Figure 22). The neurons, which number

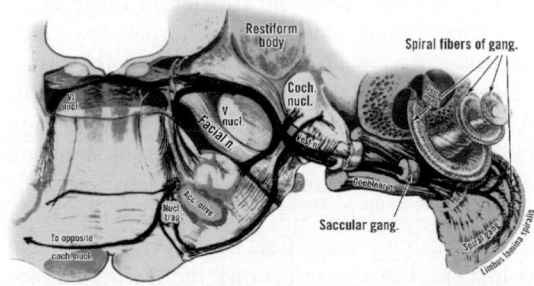

Figure 22 Drawing of the olivocochlear efferent pathway. See text for a description. (From reference 19.)

approximately 1,000 to 3,000, arise from neurons located within and near the superior olivary complex. The contralateral limb of the olivocochlear bundle forms a major part of the efferent bundle, accounting for approximately three-fourths of the number of efferent neurons projecting to the organ of Corti in one ear. These axons arise from small neurons located near the accessory olivary nucleus,[20] ascend in the brainstem, and cross the midline at the level of the facial genu below the floor of the fourth ventricle. They are joined by the smaller ipsilateral component, which arises from similar olivary and periolivary neurons of the ipsilateral superior olivary nucleus before joining the contralateral limb as it enters the vestibular nerve root. As it leaves the brainstem in the vestibular nerve, the bundle gives off collateral branches to the ventral cochlear nucleus and exits the vestibular nerve within the IAC just distal to the saccular ganglion. It then enters Rosenthal canal, where it travels perpendicular to the spiral ganglion cells and their dendrites, forming the intraganglionic or juxtaganglionic spiral bundle. The fibers from the efferent bundle are given off regularly as they ascend the cochlea. These fibers penetrate the habenulae perforatae in the osseous spiral lamina along with afferent dendrites to enter the organ of Corti. The differential termination of the efferent neurons from the ipsilateral and the contralateral limbs is as follows: the fibers from the ipsilateral efferent component terminate on type I afferent dendrites and their terminals below the inner hair cell. The contralateral limb of the efferent pathway crosses the tunnel space and ramifies extensively to terminate on several outer hair cells in the first and second rows in a wider area than the inner hair cells at that region (see Figure 19). The efferent innervation to outer hair cells is most extensive in the basal turn and decreases as the apex is reached.[21] This decrease is most noticeable in the outermost rows of outer hair cells of the organ of Corti. Whereas the inner hair cell type I neuron innervation provides the major afferent input to the cochlear nucleus, the efferent innervation of the outer hair cells is thought to alter mechanically the resistance at the outer hair cell level by contractile changes in the length of the outer hair cells. In this way, the sensitivity to sound stimulation of type I–innervated hair cells is modified. The predominant effect on auditory nerve transmission by stimulation of the efferent pathway has been to suppress the action potential in the auditory nerve.[22] It is thought that the outer hair cells with their type II afferent innervation and the efferent innervation sharpen the characteristic frequency discrimination of the organ of Corti. It is also probable that the hair cells, with their spontaneous and induced transition in length, may be responsible for otoacoustic emissions, which are small electrical potentials recorded from the ear.[23] In some patients in whom the inhibitory effect of the efferent system is lost (ie, surgery, infection), the facilitated otoacoustic emissions may be perceived as ringing in the ear (tinnitus).

VESTIBULAR SYSTEM

The sense organs of the vestibular system are of two types, the cristae and the maculae (Figures 23 and 24). These sense organs have two types of hair cells,[11,24] type I and type II, which are secured in the neural epithelium by supporting cells (see Figure 24). The type I hair cells are flask shaped and are enclosed in a large calyx-type ending by one or two large-diameter afferent neurons (Figure 25). Type II hair cells are cylindrical in shape and contacted by bouton-shaped endings from both the afferent and efferent systems. These afferent neurons are myelinated but small compared with those that innervate type I hair cells. The crista is a ridge of neuroepithelial cells that traverse the ampullated end of each membranous semicircular duct. The ampulla contains the sense organ for the detection of angular acceleration and deceleration[25] (see Figure 23). The hair cells in the crista ampullaris are arranged with the type I hair cells near the crest of the crista and type II hair cells near the slopes.[10,24] It is noteworthy that the hair cells in cristae of the semicircular ducts are oriented in

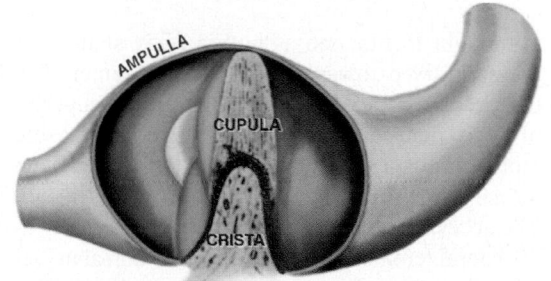

Figure 23 Section (diagrammatic) through the ampulla of a semicircular duct.

a single direction based on the alignment of their ciliary bundle.[10,24] The ciliary bundle of each vestibular hair cell consists of 100 to 150 stereocilia and a single kinocilium, which is located to one side of the stereocilia (see Figure 25). In the case of the horizontal semicircular duct, the kinocilium of each hair cell is located on the utricular side of the crista. In the vertical cristae (of the superior and posterior semicircular ducts), the kinocilia are located toward the nonampullated ends or away from the utricle (Figure 26). Sitting on top of the crista and reaching to the roof of the ampullary wall, even attached to it, is a gelatinous partition called the cupula, composed of mucopolysaccharides possessing an equal density to the endolymph, which surrounds it (see Figure 23). It is the displacement of the cupula that initiates through the hair cells an action potential in the neurons contacting the hair cells.[25,26] When the deflection of the cupula is toward the kinocilium, there is a depolarization of the hair cell neuron unit with an increase in the resting vestibular nerve action potential, whereas a deflection away from the kinocilium produces hyperpolarization or a decrease in the resting discharge of the vestibular neuron.[10] The semicircular ducts in each labyrinth are oriented to each of three planes in space, with the lateral semicircular duct cristae recording angular acceleration in a horizontal plane, whereas the posterior and superior (vertical) semicircular duct cristae record movement in the two vertical planes of space. In man, when the head is in the upright erect position, the anterior aspect of the lateral semicircular canal angles 30° upward from the horizontal plane. To induce complementary input to the vestibular nuclei, the canals of each bony labyrinth are coplanar; in other words, the

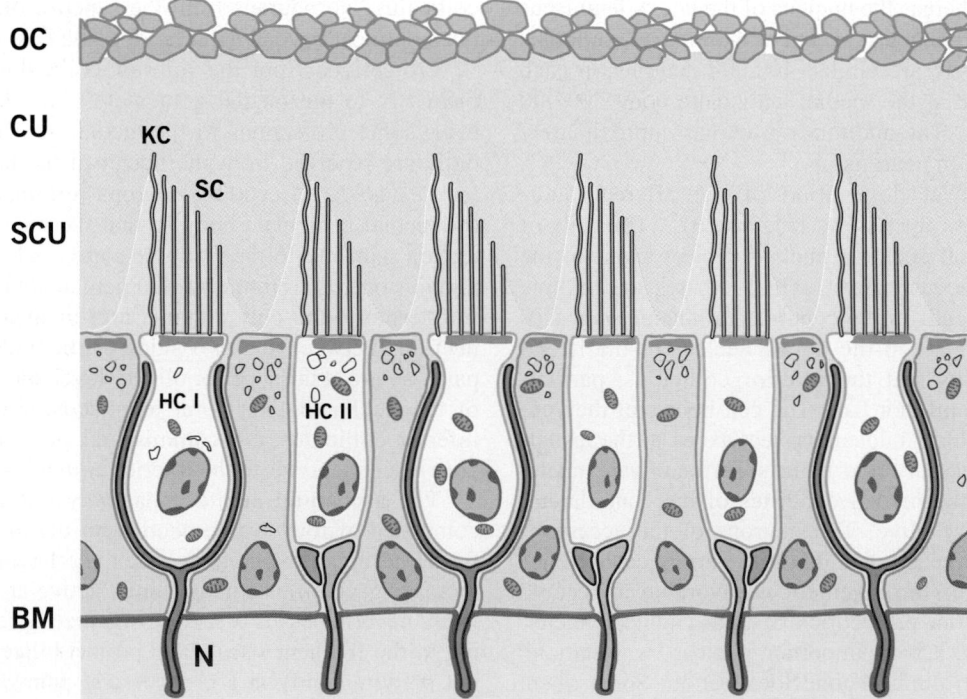

Figure 24 Schematic drawing of a cross-section of a macula. The gelatinous substance is divided into cupular (CU) and subcupular (SCU) layers. There are two types of hairs: kinocilia, labeled KC (one per hair cell), and stereocilia, labeled SC (many per hair cell). OC = otoconia; HC I = type I hair cell; HC II = type II hair cell; N = nerve fiber; BM = basement membrane; S = supporting cell.

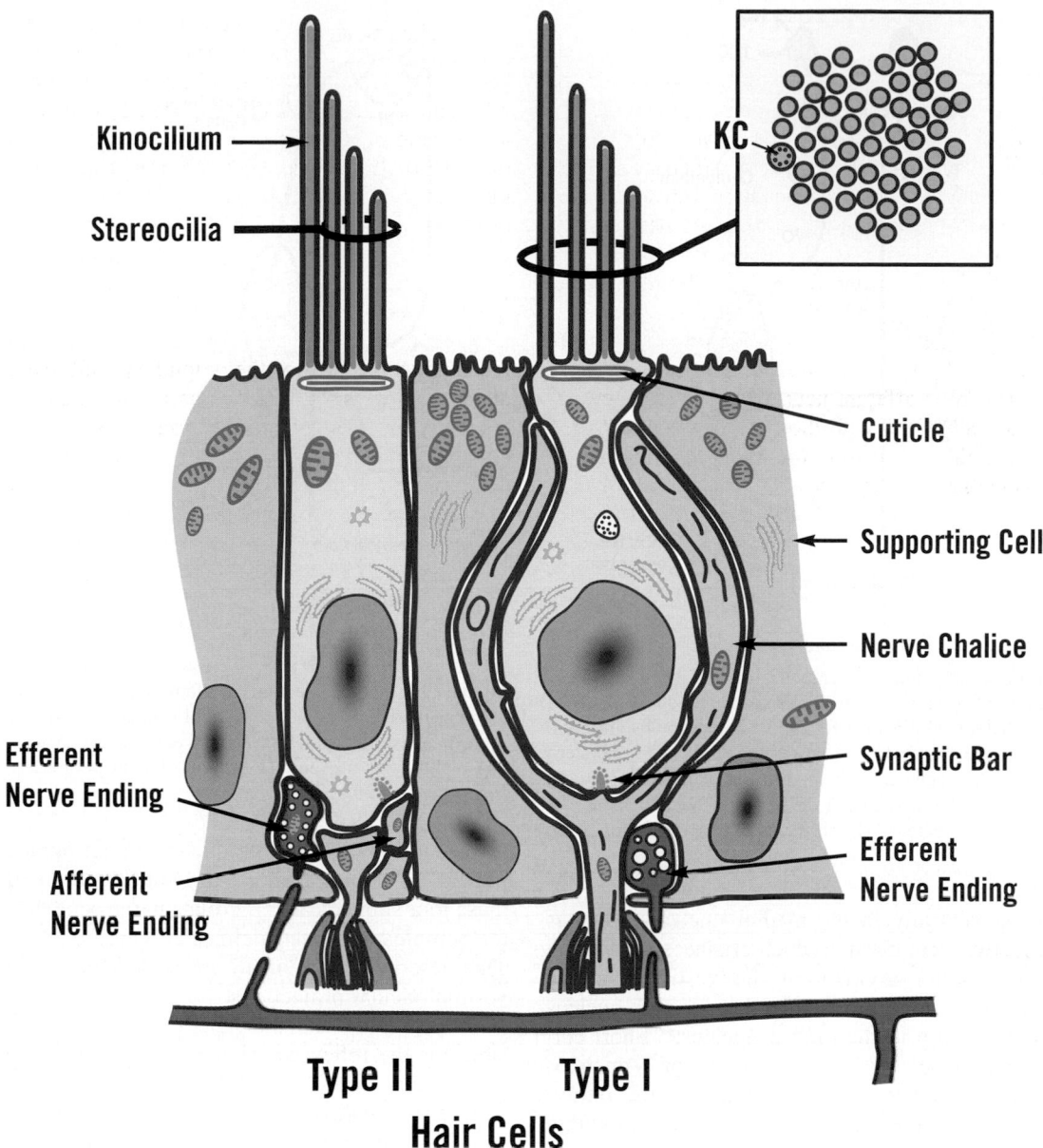

Figure 25 Diagram of the innervation pattern to the type I and type II vestibular hair cells.

The innervation of hair cells in the vestibular sense organs is by both afferent and efferent neurons (see Figure 25). The afferent neurons can be divided into three types, the large afferent neurons belonging to the large bipolar ganglion cells in Scarpa ganglia, which innervate type I hair cells with large calyx-like endings,[11,24] the smaller afferent bipolar neurons in Scarpa ganglia, which innervate type II hair cells with bouton-type terminals, and the dimorphic bipolar ganglion cells which innervate both type I and type II hair cells. Vestibular neurons have a high spontaneous activity with a higher range (90 to 100 spikes per second [sps]) in canal afferents than in macular afferents (60 to 70 sps). The large vestibular afferents characteristically show an irregular discharge pattern, whereas the smaller afferents have a regular pattern of discharge.[27] The pathological behavior of the large and small vestibular afferent neurons parallels that of the type I and type II spiral ganglion cells to the organ of Corti. Following injury to their dendrites (ie, labyrinthectomy), the large vestibular afferents undergo irreversible retrograde degeneration while the small afferents remain intact.[28] It seems probable that these two afferent neuronal populations to the auditory and vestibular sense organs have similar dependencies to peripheral trophic factors (ie, neurotrophins). The significance of such different afferent units is not known but implies a functional difference. The efferent neurons are also small in diameter and consist of unmyelinated axons. They penetrate the basement membrane of the neuroepithelium and ramify extensively to form bouton-like terminals filled with many synaptic vesicles on both type II hair cells and the calyces of type I hair cells.

The afferent neurons to the vestibular sense organs are bipolar neurons of Scarpa ganglia. There are approximately 18,000 to 19,000 ganglion cells in the human vestibular ganglia. The organization of the afferent neurons in the vestibular nerve has been elucidated.[29] The vestibular nerve has superior and inferior divisions, with the superior division innervating the cristae of the lateral and superior semicircular ducts and the utricle as well as a small portion of the saccule (Figure 27). The inferior division innervates the macula of the saccule and the posterior semicircular duct crista. The bipolar neurons innervating the lateral and the superior semicircular duct cristae travel in the most rostral (toward the facial nerve) portion of the vestibular ganglion. As they course centrally, they are joined by axons of the bipolar neurons innervating the posterior semicircular duct cristae to form the rostral portion of the vestibular nerve containing all semicircular duct afferents. The afferent neurons innervating the utricle bend caudally to join those of the saccule and form the caudal portion of the vestibular nerve as it reaches the brainstem. Between these two groups of neurons is located the parent efferent bundle for both the cochlear and vestibular efferent axons. Consistent with the innervation pattern in the cristae ampullaris, the large

posterior semicircular canal of one labyrinth is coplanar with the superior semicircular canal of the contralateral labyrinth. Because of the opposite polarization of hair cells in coplanar semicircular ducts (see Figure 26) following rotation in a given plane, one coplanar duct will be facilitated and its contralateral partner will be inhibited.[27]

Polarization of Cilia

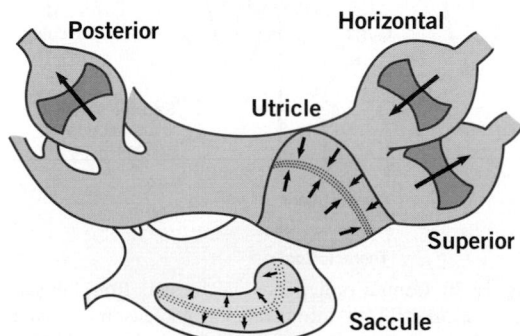

Figure 26 Diagram summarizing the orientation of hair cells in the vestibular sense organs based on the location of the kinocilium in the ciliary bundle.

The maculae are flat sense organs that are divided approximately in half by a line called the striola. The striola divides the macula into two halves, in which the hair cell ciliary polarization is in opposite directions (see Figure 26). In the macula of the utricle, the hair cells are oriented toward the striola, whereas in the saccule, hair cells are oriented away from the striola. Since the maculae project centrally to the vestibulospinal pathways primarily, but to a lesser extent to the vestibuloocular pathways, it is possible that the opposite polarization of regions in the maculae allows excitation and inhibition to antagonistic muscle groups. Type I hair cells seem to predominate near the striola, with type II hair cells furthermost from the striola. The cilia of the hair cells in the macular sense organs are covered by an otolithic membrane, gelatinous in makeup with otoconia composed of calcium carbonate crystals with a specific gravity of 2.71 embedded in the gelatinous blanket. The movement of the otoconial membrane by gravitational forces or inertial forces displaces the hairs of the hair cells, thus bringing about activity in their afferent nerve input.

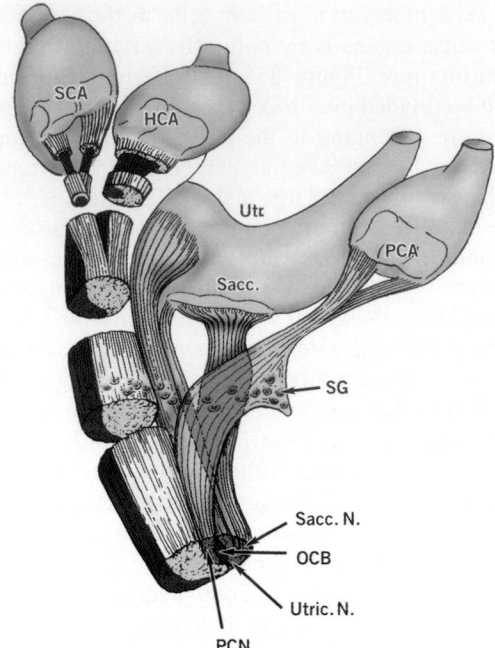

Figure 27 Drawing of the organization of bipolar neurons of the vestibular nerve. Ganglion cells in Scarpa ganglia (SG) that innervate the cristae converge into the rostral two-thirds of the nerve trunk as it approaches the brainstem. The ganglion cells that supply the utricular and saccular maculae occupy the caudal third of the vestibular nerve trunk. The cochlear and vestibular efferent axons are located at the interface of these two divisions. The dark portion of the vestibular nerve signifies the location of large neurons that supply type I hair cells in the superior and lateral duct cristae. SCA = superior canal ampulla; HCA = horizontal canal ampulla; PCA = posterior canal ampulla; Utr. = utricle; Sacc. = saccule; Sacc N. = saccular nerve; Utric N. = utricular nerve; PCN = posterior canal nerve; OCB = efferent bundle (cochlear and vestibular). (Reproduced with permission from reference 29.)

afferents travel up the center of the ampullary nerve to innervate type I hair cells at the crests of the cristae,[24,29] whereas the smaller fibers innervate the slopes and therefore surround the larger fibers in each ampullary nerve (see Figure 27). On the other hand, the distribution of the large and small afferents in the saccular and the utricular nerves is more dispersed since the division between the location of type I and type II hair cells in the maculae is not so clearly demarcated as in the cristae.

Central Vestibular Pathways

The division of duct afferents in the rostral one half to two-thirds in the vestibular nerve and utricular afferents in the caudal portion of the vestibular nerve is related to their termination in the major vestibular nuclei in the brainstem.[29] The semicircular duct afferents after bifurcating send an ascending branch to the superior vestibular nucleus and a descending branch with many collaterals to the rostral portion of the medial vestibular nucleus, with some collaterals to the ventral division of the lateral vestibular nucleus (Figure 28).[30] This projection is organized in the duct innervated by the inferior division terminates most medially in the superior nucleus and

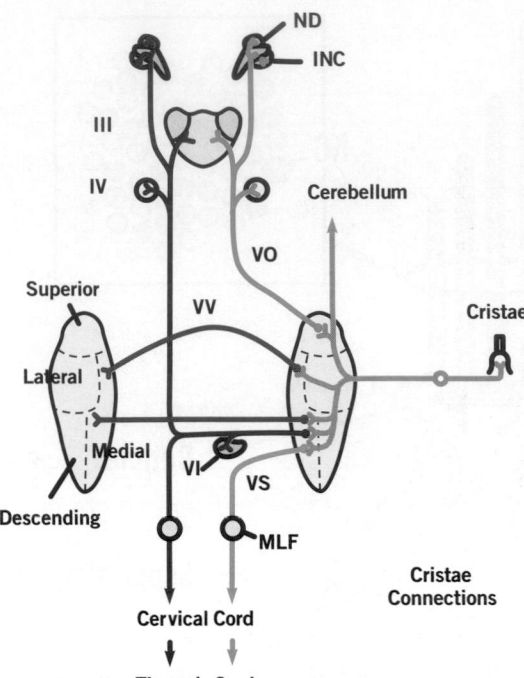

Figure 28 Diagram summarizing the central projections of afferents from the semicircular ducts. MLF = medial longitudinal fasciculus; VS = vestibulospinal; VV = commissural; VO = vestibuloocular; ND = nucleus of Darkeschewitch; INC = interstitial nucleus of Cajal III = oculomotor nucleus; VI = abducens nucleus; IV trochlear nucleus. (Reproduced with permission from reference 30.)

most ventrally in the medial nucleus, whereas the two semicircular duct cristae supplied by the superior division of the vestibular nerve terminate dorsolaterally in the superior nucleus and dorsally in the medial nucleus.[29] Short collaterals from the incoming axons of semicircular duct afferents also terminate on the intravestibular nerve nucleus, a small nucleus within the vestibular nerve root. The afferents from the utricular and saccular maculae also bifurcate, with their ascending ramus terminating in the lateral and medial nuclei and the descending branch to the descending and group Y vestibular nuclei (Figures 29 and 30).[30] The projection to the lateral nucleus is on neurons in the ventral division of the lateral vestibular nucleus and on large neurons in the rostral extension of the medial vestibular nucleus. The large neurons in the medial nucleus represent afferents to the abducens nucleus and to the subnucleus in the oculomotor nucleus, which innervates the medial rectus muscle. The latter projection pathway travels over the ascending tract of Deiters.[31] The saccular afferents also send terminations to the group Y nucleus, a minor nucleus that is located between the restiform body and the dorsal acoustic stria and the lateral vestibular nucleus. The group Y nucleus' major projection is to the contralateral group Y and superior nuclei.[32]

The oculomotor nucleus is the most complex nucleus serving extraoculomotor function. The organization of the four subnuclear groups of motor neurons had evaded precise description by traditional neuroanatomical methods employing the retrograde neuronal reaction following axon

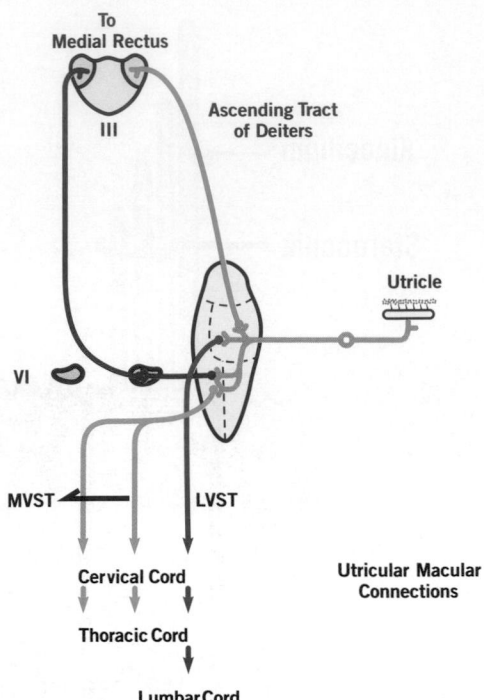

Figure 29 Central projections of afferents from the utricular macula. LVST = lateral vestibulospinal tract; MVST = medial vestibulospinal tract; III = oculomotor nucleus; VI = abducens nucleus. (Reproduced with permission from reference 30.)

transection. With the introduction of retrograde tracers of axon transport, the configuration of these four subnuclear cell groups in the oculomotor complex has been delineated (Figure 31).[33] This description has aided our understanding of vestibuloocular projections.

The projections of the major nuclei are responsible for the reflex connections of the duct and the macular afferents.[31,34–36] Second-order pathways are activated by duct afferents that project from the superior and medial vestibular nuclei and course in a parallel fashion to terminate in

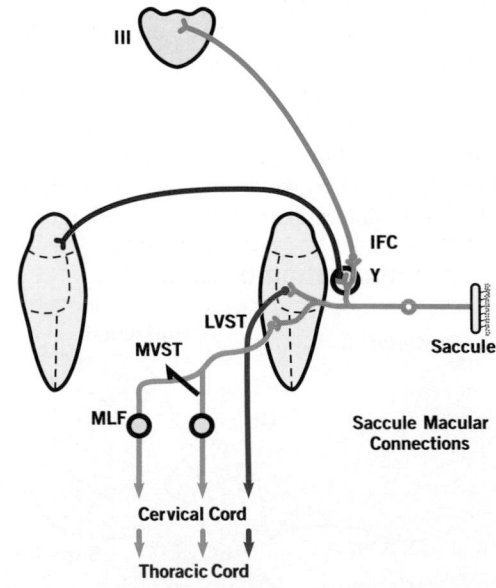

Figure 30 Central projections of afferents from the saccular macula. IFC = infracerebellar nucleus; Y = group Y nucleus; LVST = lateral vestibulospinal tract; MVST = medial vestibulospinal tract; MLF = medial longitudinal fasciculus; III = oculomotor nucleus. (Reproduced with permission from reference 30.)

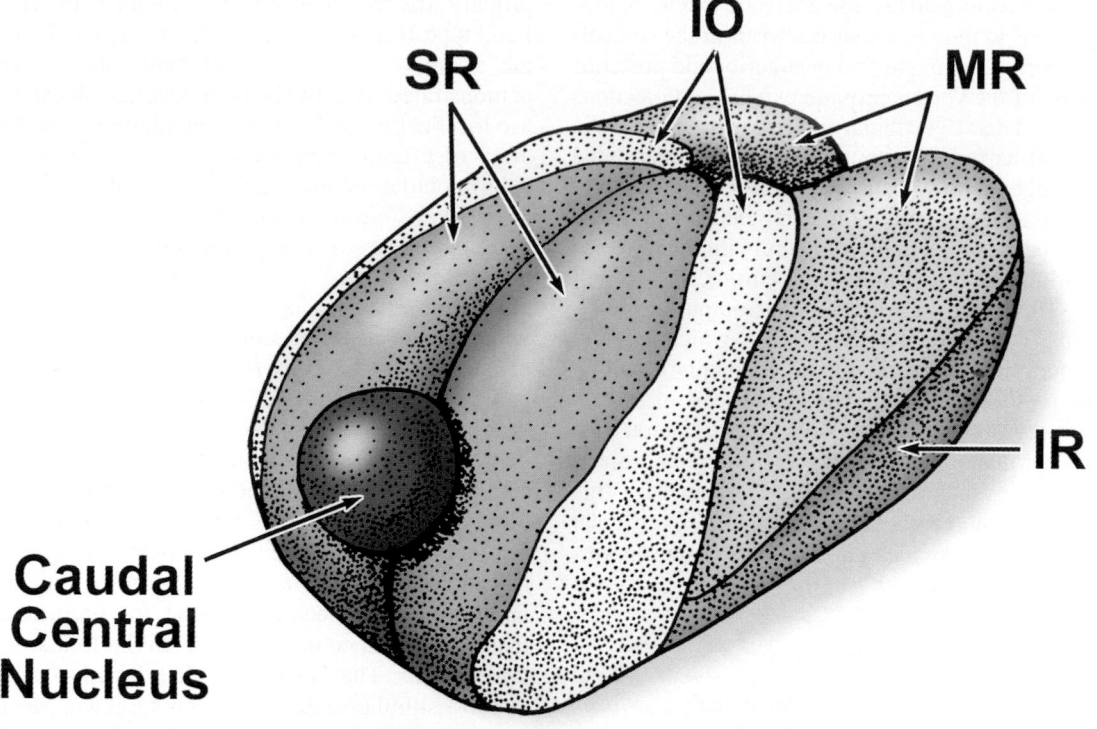

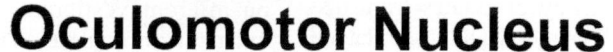

Oculomotor Nucleus

Figure 31 Drawing of a model of the oculomotor nucleus which demonstrates the organization of the subnuclei serving the superior rectus (SR), the inferior rectus (IR), the medial rectus (MR), and the inferior oblique (IO) muscles.

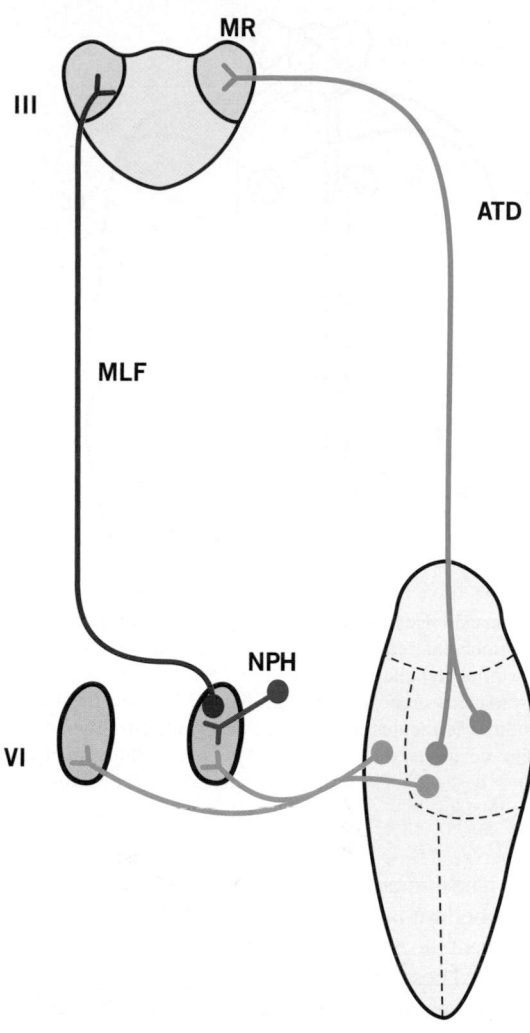

Figure 32 Central pathways for the horizontal vestibuloocular reflex. MR = medial rectus subnucleus; ATD = ascending tract of Deiters; MLF = medial longitudinal fasciculus; NPH = nucleus prepositus hypoglossi; III = oculomotor nucleus; VI = abducens nucleus.

the trochlear and oculomotor nuclei with rostral terminations in the nucleus of Darkeschewitch and the interstitial nucleus of Cajal (see Figure 28). These pathways travel in the medial longitudinal fasciculus (MLF), with the ipsilateral pathway from the superior nucleus being inhibitory and the contralaterally projecting pathway from the medial nucleus being excitatory.[34] They are responsible for the conjugate eye displacement manifesting as nystagmus from canal stimulation or destruction. Neurons from the medial vestibular nucleus project bilaterally to the abducens nuclei.[37] The ascending tract of Deiters projects from neurons in the ventral portion of the lateral vestibular nucleus to the subnucleus of the oculomotor nucleus, which supplies the medial rectus muscle. The vestibuloocular reflex pathway for horizontal eye movement is completed with an interneuron located in the abducens nucleus, which carries an excitatory charge to neurons serving the contralateral medial rectus muscle (Figure 32). The oculomotor pathways for horizontal[37] and vertical rotatory eye[38] movements are separate, with the latter located in more lateral portions of the brainstem (Figure 33), whereas the pathways involved in the horizontal eye movement are located beneath the floor of the fourth ventricle (see Figure 32). It is this organization of pathways for horizontal and vertical rotatory eye movements that explains the perversion of nystagmus when the lateral canal is stimulated (calorically) in patients with midline cerebellar or brainstem lesions. That is, instead of seeing a horizontal nystagmus, a vertical nystagmus is seen because the afferent pathways to the abducens nuclei are interrupted, whereas

those supplying the remaining extraocular muscles are intact.

The projections from the caudal vestibular nuclei, that is, the medial, descending, and entire lateral vestibular nuclei (both ventral and dorsal divisions), travel down the spinal cord to muscles of the trunk and limbs.[35,36] These projections join the vestibulospinal tract (VST) and make up the major output reflex pathway from the maculae, particularly the utricular macula (see Figures 29 and 30).

The major pathway is the lateral vestibulospinal tract (LVST), which arises from the large multipolar neurons in the lateral vestibular nucleus and to a lesser extent from the descending nucleus. This pathway is somatotopically organized so that the vestibulospinal projections to the cervical and upper thoracic regions arise from neurons in the anteroventral portion of the lateral vestibular nucleus, whereas the most caudal and sacral portions of the spinal cord are innervated by the multipolar neurons in the most dorsal and caudal portions of the lateral vestibular nucleus. Truncal and limb musculature of the intervening segments are organized in an orderly fashion between these extremes. This pathway provides excitatory tone to extensor muscles of the limbs. The medial vestibulospinal tracts (MVSTs) travel down the MLF and are largely inhibitory, although some facilitatory connections are made from the descending vestibular nucleus.[27] The projections through the MLF arise from the caudal portions of the medial and descending vestibular nuclei. Since they are largely inhibitory, they act synergistically with the innervation of neck and upper truncal mus-

cles excited by the LVST. The MVSTs extend down to the upper cord levels but do not reach the thoracic, lumbar, and sacral region levels reached by the LVST.

Other pathways exist in the vestibular nuclei that are of importance. One such pathway is the commissural pathway that interconnects the vestibular nuclei (see Figure 28). The major intervestibular or commissural projections are between the superior, medial, and descending vestibular nuclei.[32] A minor projection may exist between the lateral vestibular nuclei. As mentioned earlier, the group Y nucleus also forms a significant commissural projection to the contralateral group Y nucleus as well as the superior nucleus. The commissural pathways are largely inhibitory on second-order neurons activated by canal input. It is possible that they serve to potentiate the differential response arising from stimulation of coplanar canals. The commissural projections are important in the recovery of balance following ablation of one set of vestibular sense organs (labyrinthectomy). It has been demonstrated that the commissural pathways are largely responsible for providing the reactivation of input to the denervated side of the brainstem to approximate that in the intact half.[39]

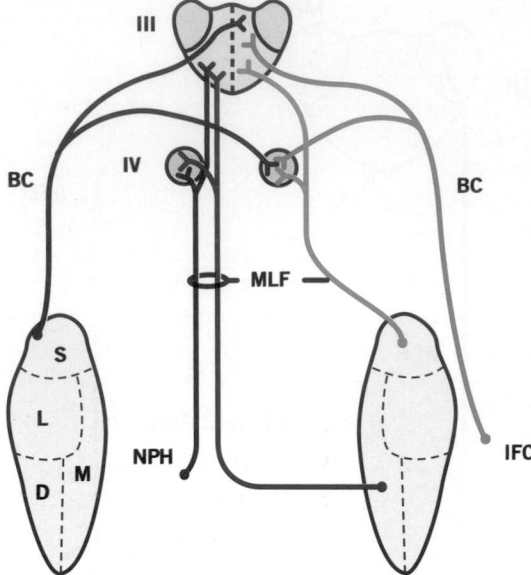

Figure 33 Central pathways for the vertical rotatory vestibuloocular reflex. BC = brachium conjunctivum; IFC = infracerebellar nucleus; IV = trochlear nucleus; NPH = nucleus prepositus hypoglossi; MLF = medial longitudinal fasciculus; III = oculomotor nucleus; S = superior vestibular nucleus; L = lateral vestibular nucleus; D = descending vestibular nucleus; M = medial vestibular nucleus.

The interaction of vestibular pathways with the cerebellum is emphasized by reference to certain areas of the cerebellum as the *vestibulocerebellum* (VC). These are the nodulus, uvula, flocculus, and ventral paraflocculus (see Figure 28). Other areas of the anterior and posterior lobes of the vermis are also included to a lesser extent. This association is based on the projection of the first- and second-order vestibular afferents to the cerebellar cortex by way of mossy fibers.[27] All canal afferents continue through the superior nucleus after termination there, to converge and terminate on neurons in the VC. Second-order neurons in the superior, medial, lateral, and descending nuclei relay input from the utricular and saccular maculae to the same areas. There is also some relay of canal input to the vestibular nuclei onto the cerebellum. The importance of such direct as well as relayed labyrinthine input to the cerebellum is not known but may have some bearing on different information coming in for modification of cerebellar output. For example, the relayed canal input may be modified by commissural inhibition before entering the cerebellum. Furthermore, other afferent input (spinal) may alter the labyrinthine (macular) input before relay to the cerebellum.

Input from the labyrinth and spinal cord, although important, is not the only source of inputting information to this important part of the vestibular system.[27] The visual system also has significant input to the flocculus and nodulus, where overlap with labyrinth input occurs. Therefore, interaction between vestibular and visual signals in the VC has firm anatomic and physiologic support. These various inputs to the VC probably determine the pattern of output from these regions, which will impact on neurons in the vestibular nuclei.

In a reciprocal fashion, there are extensive projections to the vestibular nuclei from the cerebellar cortex and nuclei.[35] The anterior and posterior parts of the vermis provide extensive projections to the lateral vestibular nucleus, particularly the dorsal half. The output of the VC is distributed throughout the vestibular nuclei, especially to those areas related to the cerebellar input. These cerebellar projections are entirely inhibitory since Purkinje cells are inhibitory neurons.

However, not all cerebellar output is inhibitory. The fastigial nucleus (FN), which receives labyrinthine input, exerts an excitatory effect on the vestibular nuclei. The caudal part of the FN projects to parts of all of the contralateral vestibular nuclei, whereas the rostral region projects to the ipsilateral nuclei. The FN can be a link between the cerebellar cortex and the vestibular nuclei that provides an excitatory input on vestibular neurons.

Efferent Vestibular Pathway

An efferent vestibular pathway has also been demonstrated in lower and higher mammalian forms.[20,40,41] This pathway originates from discrete populations of ipsilateral and contralateral neurons located lateral to the abducens nucleus near the medial vestibular nucleus[42] and projects to each vestibular labyrinth (Figure 34). The unmyelinated axons converge with the olivocochlear bundle as the vestibular root is reached in the brainstem. They travel with the olivocochlear bundle efferents through the vestibular nerve to the point where the vestibular ganglia are reached. At this point, the vestibular efferents diverge from the parent efferent bundle to break up into fascicles and individual axons that then disperse throughout the ampullary and macular nerve branches. They branch and ramify richly along their course within the nerve trunks and after penetration of the basement membrane in the neuroepithelium of the vestibular sense organs. Here they represent fine fibers that form many bouton-like vesiculated endings in termination on type II hair cells and the calyces encapsulating type I hair cells (see Figure 25), as well as on the primary afferent dendrites innervating both type I and type II hair cells. These fibers are cholinergic, as are the olivocochlear efferents, and can be demonstrated selectively with acetylcholinesterase localization techniques.[21] In addition, a wide array of efferent neuropeptides, which serve as neuromodulators, are expressed. Similarly there are a diverse group of muscarinic, nicotinic, and neuropeptide receptors expressed by hair cells and primary afferent neurons which receive the vestibular efferent input, thereby producing a wide array of neurophysiologic effects. The number of efferent neurons is relatively small compared with the number of afferent neurons in the vestibular nerve. In the cat, for the 8,000 afferent neurons, there are 200 to 300 efferent neurons that supply through their branching an almost equal number of efferent terminals to the number of afferent terminals in the sense organs. Although the number of vestibular efferents in the human labyrinth has not been determined, it is presumed that the imbalance in number is similar to that in lower forms. The function of the efferent system to the vestibular sense organs is not known. Most experimental studies indicate an inhibitory effect on afferent vestibular activity.[43] However, an excitatory effect has also been demonstrated in primates.[41] It is possible that the efferent effect is to raise or lower the resting activity level in vestibular afferents, thereby modifying their operating range. Unlike the efferent auditory pathway, the vestibular efferent pathway is represented by small neurons located near the medial vestibular nucleus, where they can be contacted by first-order afferents. Thus, a two-neuron reflex arc exists to type I hair cell afferent terminals and type II hair cell soma.

FLUIDS OF THE INNER EAR

As mentioned earlier, there are two fluid compartments of the inner ear, the endolymph and the perilymph. Endolymph is a fluid that has a similar ionic composition to intracellular fluid and fills the membranous auditory and vestibular labyrinth. Endolymph is formed by secretory cells in the stria vascularis and by dark cells near

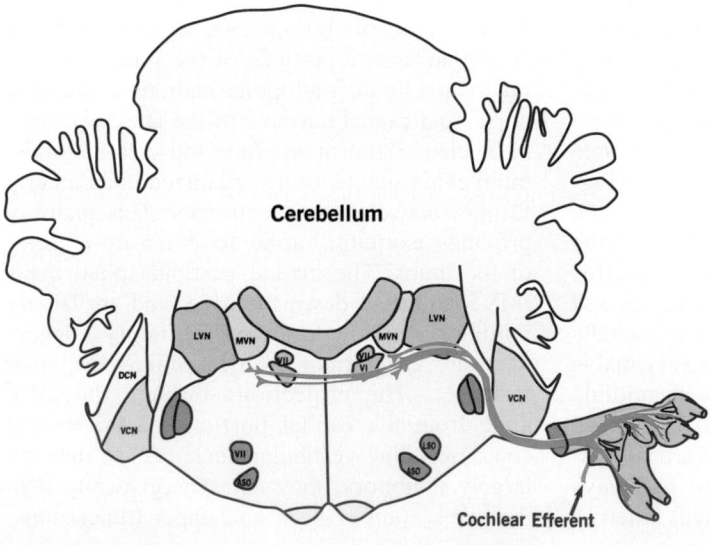

Figure 34 Diagram of the efferent vestibular pathway (*solid lines*) and efferent cochlear pathway (*stippled area*). LVN = lateral vestibular nucleus; MVN = medial vestibular nucleus; DCN, VCN = dorsal and ventral divisions of the cochlear nucleus; VII = genu of facial nerve; VI = abducens nucleus; ASO = accessory superior olivary nucleus; LSO = lateral superior olivary nucleus. (Reproduced with permission from reference 42.)

the ampullary ends of the semicircular ducts and the walls of the utricle. The endolymph is thought to be absorbed in the endolymphatic sac. Endolymph composition is characterized by a high potassium level and a low sodium level.[44] The membranous labyrinth is suspended within the bony labyrinth by a fine trabecular network in a space that is filled with perilymph. Perilymph, in contradistinction to endolymph, has an ionic composition similar to extracellular fluid, with low potassium and high sodium levels.[44] A comparison of the composition of the two fluids with that of serum and CSF is found in Table 1. This differential chemical makeup in the two fluid compartments is important to the establishment of a standing voltage surrounding the sense organs, which permits the generation of nerve impulse in the hair cell afferent neuron unit. Perilymph is secreted largely as the result of diffusion from the capillary network in the spiral ligament adjacent to the scala tympani with a smaller portion derived from CSF by way of the cochlear aqueduct.

BLOOD VESSELS OF THE EAR

Two major vessels have little or nothing to do with the vascular supply of the ear itself but are important in disorders and surgery of the TB. These are the sigmoid sinus and the internal carotid artery. The sigmoid sinus is a continuation of the lateral (transverse) sinus, which is formed by the superior sagittal sinus. It makes an indentation into the posterior fossa plate of the mastoid portion of the TB before taking an abrupt redundant turn on itself (jugular bulb) to exit through the jugular foramen accompanied by cranial nerves IX, X, and XI (see Figure 7). This structure is important as it may represent a lethal complication of bacterial mastoiditis (thrombophlebitis) when erosion of its bony covering occurs. The anatomy of the jugular bulb is particularly crucial to the diagnosis and surgical management of neoplasms, which originate in the bulb such as glomus jugulare tumors or schwannomas.

The internal carotid artery enters the TB just anterior to the jugular foramen and travels in a bony canal anterior to the middle ear space, first in a vertical direction and then in a horizontal anteromedial direction medial to the eustachian tube (see Figure 7). Its main clinical significance is as an important landmark in surgery of the PA and skull base. Rarely, an anomalous internal carotid artery may appear clinically to be a vascular neoplasm in the middle ear.

The circulatory networks of the external and middle ears and the inner ear are completely separate, with the one being supplied by the carotid system, whereas that of the labyrinth is derived from the vertebrobasilar system.[12] The external ear is supplied by the auriculotemporal branch of the superficial temporal artery and posterior auricular branches of the external carotid artery. The middle ear and mastoid are supplied by a different set of arterial branches from the external carotid system. The arterial branches to the middle ear space are the anterior tympanic branch from the internal maxillary artery, which enters through the petrotympanic fissure and travels along the eustachian tube and the semicanal for the tensor tympani. The middle meningeal artery gives off the superior tympanic branch that enters the middle ear through the petrosquamous fissure. The middle meningeal artery also gives off the superficial petrosal artery that travels with the greater superficial petrosal nerve and enters the facial canal at the hiatus. This vessel anastomoses with a branch of the posterior auricular artery, the stylomastoid artery, which enters the facial canal inferiorly through the stylomastoid foramen. A branch of the stylomastoid artery leaves the fallopian canal to travel through the canaliculus with the chorda tympani nerve to enter the middle ear. Finally, the inferior tympanic artery, a branch of the ascending pharyngeal artery, enters the middle ear through the tympanic canaliculus in the hypotympanum with the tympanic branch of the ninth nerve.

The vascular supply to the ossicles is derived from the anterior tympanic artery, the posterior tympanic artery, and branches from the plexus of vessels on the promontory. The most tenuous link in the ossicular chain as regards blood supply is the tip of the long process of the incus, which commonly undergoes necrosis secondary to conditions that compromise its blood supply.[45]

BLOOD SUPPLY TO THE INNER EAR

The blood supply to the inner ear is derived from the labyrinthine branch of the anterior inferior cerebellar artery off the basilar artery.[12] Occasionally, the internal auditory artery has a direct origin from the basilar artery. This vessel represents an end artery as it receives no known anastomosing arterial vessels. The internal auditory artery as it enters the IAC divides into three branches. The first branch, the anterior vestibular artery, supplies the semicircular ducts, utricle, and saccule. The second branch, the vestibulocochlear artery, supplies the saccule, utricle, posterior duct, and basal turn of the cochlea. Its third and terminal branch is the cochlear artery, which enters the modiolus, where it gives off the spiral vessels that form external and internal radiating arterioles. The internal radiating arterioles descend to supply the limbus as well as the basilar membrane and organ of Corti. The external radiating arteriole courses through the interscalar septum to supply the vascular arcades and capillaries of the stria vascularis. This arteriole anastomoses with the venous supply near the spiral prominence, with the venous return being along the floor of the scala tympani, where the veins merge with the collecting venules from the spiral vein to form the posterior spiral vein. This posterior spiral vein, or inferior cochlear vein, then travels along the scala tympani to exit at the cochlear aqueduct through a separate channel and enters the inferior petrosal sinus. The remainder of the labyrinth is drained by a venous system, which parallels to some degree the arterial system. Therefore, an anterior vestibular vein and the posterior vestibular vein drain the posterior duct ampulla as well as the saccule and a portion of the utricle and superior duct ampulla. These merge to join the vein at the cochlear aqueduct. The venous return from the semicircular ducts and the body of the utricle converge to form the vein at the vestibular aqueduct, which travels as the vein of the paravestibular aqueduct. This vein travels along with the intraosseous endolymphatic sac toward the extraosseous endolymphatic sac. This venous system drains into the sigmoid sinus.

FACIAL NERVE

The anatomy of the facial nerve and its branches are important in clinical practice not only because of the cosmetic effects of facial paralysis, whether it be by disease or surgical injury, but because the various components of facial nerve are important for the diagnosis and localization of lesions in the TB. The facial nerve has sensory function and autonomic afferent and efferent function, together with the motor function for the facial musculature. The neuronal pathway from the motor cortex to the facial nucleus is either two or three neurons in a mono- or disynaptic pathway. The motor control of the facial muscles is located at the inferior end of the presylvian gyrus. The area for facial musculature

Table 1 Chemical Composition of Inner Ear Fluids

Mean Value	Perilymph	Endolymph	Cap. Serum	CSF
Na^+ (meq/L)	143	12–16	141	141
K^+ (meq/L)	5.5–6.25	143.3 (140–160)	5.9	2.9
Protein (mg %)	200 (89–326)	150	7,170	30
Glucose (mg %)	104		104	67
Free cholesterol (mg %)	1.5			0.035
Total cholesterol (mg %)	12		28	
MDH (IU)	95.6–136		63.5	18.3
LDH (IU)	127–155		151	1.9
PO_3^- (mM/L)	0.72		0.95	0.36
Ca^{2+} (mM/L)	1.16	1.07	2.44	1.12
Lactate (mM/L)	6.78		4.63	3.94

Adapted from reference 44.

CSF = cerebrospinal fluid; LDH = lactate dehydrogenase; MDH = malate dehydrogenase.

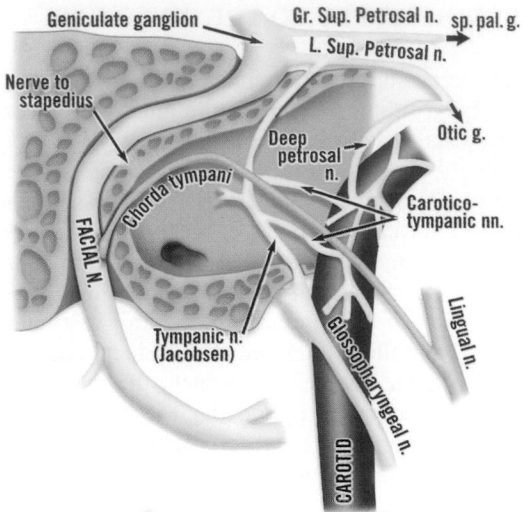

Figure 35 The facial nerve and its relationships (diagrammatic). Sp.pal.g. = sphenopalatine ganglion.

innervation is located near the area of innervation of laryngeal muscles. Although a modest corticonuclear projection exists, it is not the only higher pathway inputting the facial nucleus. Various extrapyramidal neurons located in the red nucleus as well as the periaqueductal gray nucleus also project to the facial nucleus. The projection to the facial nucleus is largely contralateral as are most corticobulbar projections, but there is bilateral innervation to the facial neurons supplying the frontalis muscle. The facial nerve consists of four major components: the motor component to the facial musculature, a sensory component to receptors in facial muscles as well as to the face, autonomic secretomotor and special sensory pathways. The motor component of the facial nerve is the largest component and arises from the facial nerve nucleus, which is located just caudal to the lateral superior olivary nucleus of the auditory system.[46] Immediately caudal to the facial nerve nucleus is the rostral limit of the nucleus ambiguus, which provides the motor innervation to the laryngeal musculature. It has been demonstrated in the cat with retrograde neuronal tracers that the regional facial muscle groups are supplied by groups of neurons within the facial nerve nucleus in a

medial and lateral arrangement.[46] The number of facial motoneurons has been estimated at approximately 10,000 to 20,000. As axons leave the facial nucleus, they travel in a dorsal direction to loop around the abducens nucleus under the floor of the fourth ventricle and then curve in a ventrolateral direction passing between the lateral superior olivary nucleus and the descending trigeminal root to emerge from the brainstem ventral to the eighth nerve. The nerve is joined by the nervus intermedius and travels in the IAC in its anterior and superior compartment. In this portion of the IAC, it has an intimate anatomic relationship with the superior division of the vestibular nerve, and indeed the nervus intermedius may travel within the vestibular nerve for a part of its intracanalicular course. At the distal end of the IAC, the facial nerve diverges in an anterolateral direction to enter the labyrinthine segment of the fallopian canal (see Figures 4 and 8). At the geniculate ganglion, it makes an acute bend near the floor of the middle cranial fossa to continue within the bony canal in its tympanic segment. The course within the labyrinthine segment of the fallopian canal is associated with an extension of the subarachnoid space. This extension of the subarachnoid space is usually limited by the location of the geniculate ganglion but in a small portion of TBs may extend into the tympanic portion of the fallopian canal. The greater superficial petrosal nerve emerges from the geniculate ganglion at the facial hiatus (see Figure 4) and courses along the floor of the middle cranial fossa between layers of dura to reach the foramen lacerum, where it joins with the carotid sympathetic nerves to form the vidian nerve in the vidian canal. The tympanic portion of the facial nerve travels superior to the oval window in a posterolateral direction to the level of the horizontal or lateral semicircular canal, where it makes a 90° turn in a ventral direction to continue as the mastoid portion of the facial nerve (Figure 35). After traveling the length of the vertical canal, the facial nerve emerges from the stylomastoid foramen to enter the parotid gland anterior to the mastoid tip. Before emerging from the stylomastoid foramen, the chorda

tympani nerve is given off through a bony canal in a retrograde direction toward the middle ear, where it passes between the long process of the incus and the neck of the malleus to enter the epitympanum and leave the middle ear space before joining the lingual nerve. The facial nerve provides innervation to the posterior belly of the digastric muscle just external to the stylomastoid foramen and then emerges into the parotid gland, where it gives rise to four to five branches providing innervation to the facial musculature. Although the motoneurons in the facial nerve are spatially organized within the nucleus, the fibers to the peripheral facial muscle groups are interspersed throughout the course of the facial nerve but gather together again on exiting the TB to provide the four to five distal branches supplying the regional facial musculature.[46]

General Sensory Component

An unknown number of sensory afferent neurons are intermixed with the motor axons in the facial nerve trunk. In an animal model (cat), approximately 15 to 20% of the nerve fibers in the medium to large fiber size persist even after total facial nerve transection in the cerebellopontine angle. It is not clear what peripheral receptors these afferents innervate. The possibilities are either spindles within the facial musculature or some sensory receptors in the skin, particularly the dermis.

Autonomic Secretomotor Neurons

Secretomotor or motor preganglionic neurons of the facial nerve are located in the superior salivary nucleus in the brainstem (Figure 36A). They travel in the nervus intermedius, with some traveling within the vestibular nerve trunk. Those traveling within the vestibular nerve leave in the vestibulofacial anastomosis in the distal part of the IAC to join the nervous intermedius as it travels with the facial nerve trunk in the meatal canal.[12] Some efferent preganglionic neurons pass through the geniculate ganglion to the foramen lacerum and the vidian canal. After leaving the vidian canal, they synapse with postganglionic neurons in the sphenopalatine ganglion that innervate the

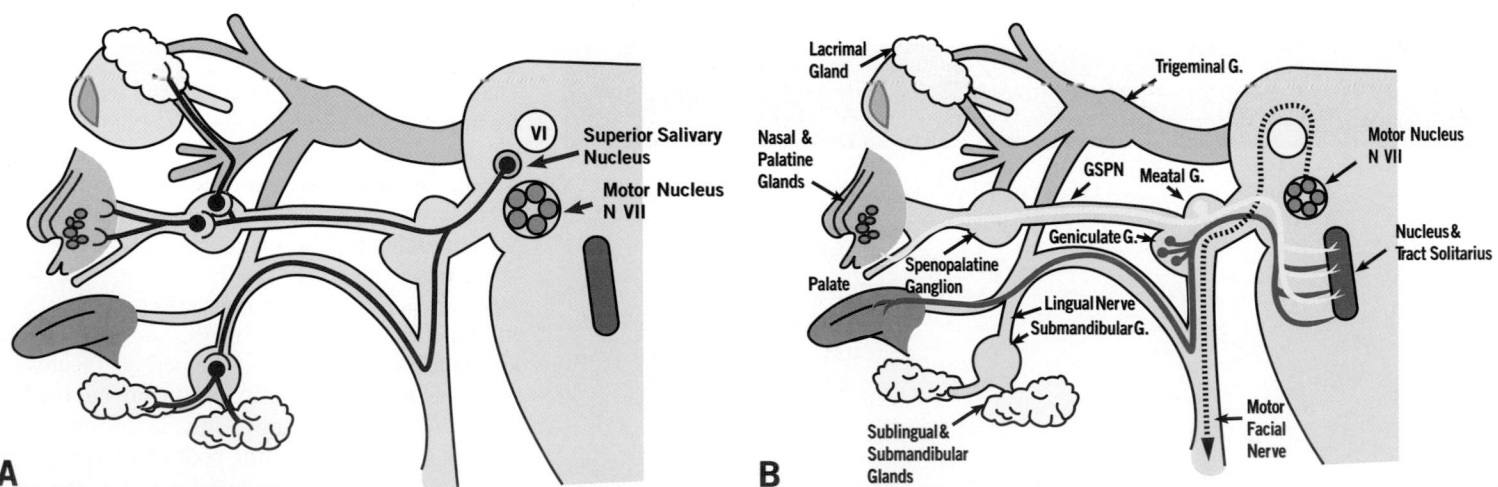

Figure 36 (A) Diagram of the autonomic secretomotor pathways associated with the facial nerve. (B) Diagram of the special sensory pathways in the facial nerve.

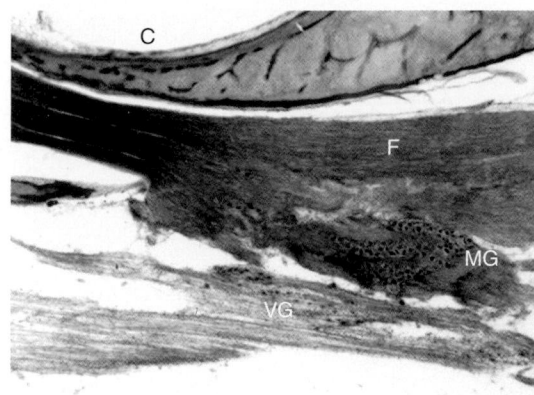

Figure 37 This horizontal section through the internal auditory canal illustrates the position of the meatal ganglion (MG) to the vestibular nerve ganglion (VG). C = cochlea.

lacrimal gland and secretory glands of the nose. Other preganglionic neurons travel within the sensory bundle of the facial nerve and leave with the chorda tympani nerve to join the lingual nerve, which carries them to the submandibular ganglion, where they synapse with postganglionic neurons, providing secretomotor function to the submandibular gland. The sensory bundle is located lateral to the motor component throughout the intratemporal course of the facial nerve.[12]

Special Sensory Function

Special sensory function for taste receptors in the anterior two-thirds of the tongue as well as the soft palate and nasopharyngeal mucosa are carried by unipolar ganglion cell masses in the facial nerve (Figure 36B). Taste receptors in the anterior two-thirds of the tongue are innervated by dendrites of the geniculate ganglion and travel by way of the lingual and the facial nerve trunk, where they are contained in the sensory bundle of the facial nerve to ganglion cells in the geniculate ganglion.[47] Axons of these ganglion cells pass into the brainstem in the nervus intermedius to reach the tractus and nucleus solitarius, where they terminate. Taste receptors in the oral cavity, primarily the soft palate and the nasopharynx, are supplied by afferent dendrites, which travel in the vidian nerve and the greater superficial petrosal nerve. They pass through the facial hiatus to join the nervus intermedius, which brings them to their ganglion cells in the meatal ganglion of the facial nerve within the IAC (Figure 37).[47,48] Axons of these neurons also enter the brainstem in the nervus intermedius to terminate in the tractus and nucleus solitarius. The meatal ganglion located within the IAC has special signifi-

cance in harboring neurotropic viruses (herpes virinae), which gain entry through nerve endings in the oral cavity.[49] After long latent periods, the viruses can be reactivated later in life to manifest as viral neuropathies (eg, Bell palsy, recurrent vertigo).

REFERENCES

1. Bast TH, Anson BJ. The Temporal Bone and the Ear. Springfield, IL: Charles C. Thomas; 1949.
2. Anson BJ, Donaldson JA. Surgical Anatomy of the Temporal Bone and Ear. Philadelphia, PA: WB Saunders; 1981.
3. Anson BJ, McVay CB. Surgical Anatomy, 5th edition. Philadelphia, PA: WB Saunders; 1981.
4. Lim DJ. Tympanic membrane. Electronmicroscopic observations. Part I. Pars tensa. Acta Otolaryngol (Stockh) 1968;66:181–98.
5. Lim DJ. Tympanic membrane. Part II: Pars flaccida. Acta Otolaryngol (Stockh) 1968;66:515–32.
6. Anson BJ. Morris' Human Anatomy, 12th edition. New York: McGraw-Hill; 1966.
7. Allam AF. Pneumatization of the temporal bone. Ann Otol Rhinol Laryngol 1969;78:49–64.
8. Gacek RR, Gacek MR, Tart R. Adult spontaneous cerebrospinal fluid otorrhea: Diagnosis and management. Am J Otol 1999;20:770–6.
9. Gacek RR. Diagnosis and management of primary tumors of the petrous apex. Ann Otol Rhinol Laryngol 975;84:1–20.
10. Wersall J, Flock A, Lundquist RG. Structural basis for directional sensitivity in cochlear and vestibular sensory receptors. Cold Spring Harbor Symp Quant Biol 1965;30:115–32.
11. Wersall J. Studies on the structure and innervation of the sensory epithelium of the cristae ampullares in the guinea pig. A light and electronmicroscope investigation. Acta Otolaryngol (Stockh) 1956;126:1–85.
12. Schuknecht HF. Pathology of the Ear, 2nd edition. Philadelphia, PA: Lea and Febiger; 1993.
13. Gacek RR. Membranous inner ear. Ann Otol Rhinol Laryngol 1961;70:974–5.
14. Spoendlin H, Schrott A. The spiral ganglion and the innervation of the human organ of Corti. Acta Otolaryngol (Stockh) 1990;105:403–10.
15. Spoendlin HH, Gacek RR. Electronmicroscopic study of the efferent and afferent innervation of the organ of Corti in the cat. Ann Otol Rhinol Laryngol 1963;72:660–87.
16. Chow KL. Numerical estimates of the auditory central nervous system of the rhesus monkey. J Comp Neurol 1951;95:159–75.
17. Gacek RR. Neuroanatomy of the auditory system. In: Tobias JV, editor. Foundations of Modern Auditory Theory, Volume 2. New York: Academic Press; 1972. p. 239–63.
18. Rasmussen GL. The olivary peduncle and other fiber projections of the superior olivary complex. J Comp Neurol 1946;84:141–220.
19. Rasmussen GL. Further observations of the efferent cochlear bundle. J Comp Neurol 1953;99:61–74.
20. Warr B, Guinan J, White JS. Organization of the efferent fibers: The lateral and medial olivocochlear systems. In: Altschuler RA, Hoffman GW, Bobbin RP, editors. Neurobiology of Hearing: the Cochlea. New York: Raven Press; 1986. p. 333–48.
21. Ishii D, Balogh K. Distribution of efferent nerve endings in the organ of Corti: Their graphic reconstruction in cochleae by localization of acetylcholinesterase activity. Acta Otolaryngol (Stockh) 1968;66:282–8.
22. Fex J. Efferent inhibition of the cochlea related to hair cell DC activity: Study of post-synaptic activity of the crossed olivocochlear fibers in the cat. J Acoust Soc Am 1967;41:666–75.
23. Kemp DT. Stimulated acoustic emissions from the human auditory system. J Acoust Soc Am 1978;64:1386–91.
24. Spoendlin H. Ultrastructural studies of the labyrinth in squirrel monkeys. In: Graybiel A, editor. Symposium on the Role of the Vestibular Organs in the Exploration of Space. Washington, DC: National Aeronautics and Space Administration; 1965. p. 7–22 (NASA SP-77).
25. Dohlman G. On the mechanism of transformation into nystagmus on stimulation of the semicircular canals. Acta Otolaryngol (Stockh) 1938;26:425–42.
26. Dohlman G. The shape and function of the cupula. J Laryngol Otol 1969;83:43–53.
27. Wilson VJ, Melville Jones G. Mammalian Vestibular Physiology. New York: Plenum Press; 1979.
28. Gacek RR, Schoonmaker J. Morphologic changes in the vestibular nerves and nuclei following labyrinthectomy in the cat: A case for the neurotrophin hypothesis in vestibular compensation. Acta Otolaryngol (Stockh) 1997;117:244–9.
29. Gacek RR. The course and central termination of first order neurons supplying vestibular end organs in the cat. Acta Otolaryngol (Stockh) 1969;254:1–66.
30. Gacek RR. Neuroanatomical correlates of vestibular function. Ann Otol Rhinol Laryngol 1980;89:1–5.
31. Gacek RR. Anatomical demonstration of the vestibuloocular projections in the cat. Laryngoscope 1971;81:1559–95.
32. Gacek RR. Location of commissural neurons in the vestibular nuclei of the cat. Exp Neurol 1978;59:479–91.
33. Gacek RR. Localization of neurons supplying the extraocular muscles in the kitten using horseradish peroxidase. Exp Neurol 1974;44:381–403.
34. Highstein SM. The organization of the vestibulo-oculomotor and trochlear reflex pathways in the rabbit. Exp Brain Res 1973;17:285–300.
35. Brodal A, Pompieano O, Walberg F. The Vestibular Nuclei and Their Connections, Anatomy and Functional Correlations. The Henderson Trust Lectures. Edinburgh, UK: Oliver and Boyd; 1962.
36. Pompieano O, Brodal A. The origin of vestibulospinal fibers in the cat. An experimental-anatomical study with comments on the descending medial longitudinal fasciculus. Arch Ital Biol 1957;95:166–95.
37. Gacek RR. Location of abducens afferent neurons in the cat. Exp Neurol 1979;64:342–53.
38. Gacek RR. Location of trochlear vestibule-ocular neurons in the cat. Exp Neurol 1979;66:692–706.
39. Precht W, Shimazu H, Markham CH. A mechanism of central compensation of vestibular function following hemilabyrinthectomy. J Neurophysiol 1966;29:996–1010.
40. Gacek RR. Efferent component of the vestibular nerve. In: Rasmussen GL, Windle WF, editors. Neural Mechanisms of the Auditory and Vestibular Systems. Springfield, IL: Charles C. Thomas; 1960. p. 276–84.
41. Goldberg JM, Fernandez C. Efferent vestibular system in the squirrel monkey, abstract. Neurosci Abstr 1977;3:543.
42. Gacek RR, Lyon M. The localization of vestibular efferent neurons in the kitten with horseradish per oxidase. Acta Otolaryngol (Stockh) 1974;77:92–101.
43. Klinke R, Schmidt CL. Efferent influence on the vestibular organ during active movements of the body. Pflugers Arch 1970;318:352–3.
44. Smith CA, Lowry OH, Wu ML. The electrolytes of the labyrinthine fluids. Laryngoscope 1954;64:141–53.
45. Alberti PW. The blood supply to the incudostapedial joint and the lenticular process. Laryngoscope 1963;73:605–15.
46. Gacek RR, Radpour S. Fiber orientation of the facial nerve: An experimental study in the cat. Laryngoscope 1982;92:547–56.
47. Gacek RR. On the duality of the facial nerve ganglion. Laryngoscope 1998;108:1077–86.
48. Gacek RR. Pathology of facial and vestibular neuronitis. Am J Otolaryngol 1999;20:202–10.
49. Gacek RR, Gacek MR. Meatal ganglionitis: Clinical pathologic correlation in idiopathic facial paralysis. Otorhinolaryngol Nova 1999;9:229–38.

2

Development of the Ear

Daniel I. Choo, MD
Gresham T. Richter, MD

The development of the ear has been an object of intense investigation for the past century. Housed within the temporal bone, the human ear is composed of 3 discreet but interdependent units: the external, middle, and inner ear. The function of these components is to conduct and translate sound efficiently into signals that can be interpreted by the brain. This process is highly dependent on the synergistic and complete development of each part. The external ear, composed of the pinna and external auditory canal (EAC), gathers and introduces sound to the eardrum, a thin elastic membrane connecting the external to the middle ear. The middle ear mechanically conducts and amplifies the sound to the inner ear through a lever system of 3 interconnected ossicles from lateral to medial: the malleus, incus, and stapes. An intimate connection between the malleus and tympanic membrane (TM) as well as the stapes and the oval window of the inner ear allows energy to be transmitted into a liquid medium. Waves within the inner ear, generated by movement of the stapes on the oval window, stimulate mechanoreceptors within the cochlea that are transduced into neural impulses.

The inner ear is derived from the otic vesicle, an invagination of ectoderm adjacent to the primitive hindbrain. The external and middle ear arise almost entirely from the first and second branchial (ie, pharyngeal) arches around the interposed first pharyngeal cleft and pouch. From these embryologic origins, development begins around 4 weeks of gestation and progresses via a continually adaptive array of molecular signals governed by specific genetic foci. Both animal and human studies have contributed to our understanding of the interplay of mechanical, molecular, and genetic forces involved in normal and abnormal ear growth. The complexity of this process, and the timing of each successive event, is not completely understood but leads to 1 of the most intricate organs of the human body.

EXTERNAL EAR

The basic structure of the external ear is a cup and funnel whose fundamental evolutionary role is to direct sound to the middle and inner ear at optimal resonant frequency. The architecture allows sound waves generated in an aerial environment to be focused onto an elastic membrane (TM) that ultimately assists in the coupling of sound into a liquid medium. The auricle (or pinna) is the cup whose components include the concha, helix, tragus, antitragus, antihelix, and lobule (Figure 1). The funnel, with its opening at the center of the auricle along the side of the head, is the elongated external auditory canal that connects the external environment to the TM. Despite a rather simple design, isolated defects in the development of these structures can lead to mild to moderate deficits in hearing. When not accompanied with middle or inner ear anomalies, surgical correction is often possible. However, basic understanding of external ear development is necessary before appropriate repair can be designed.

Mammalian head and neck structures develop as a result of graduated differentiation of embryologic soft tissues within the "pharyngeal apparatus." Sequential levels (1 to 5) of the pharyngeal apparatus are subdivided into 3 components known as the branchial (pharyngeal) arches, pouches, and clefts. The arches are the fundamental constituent from which structures arise from embryonic mesoderm: the building blocks of muscle and vascular elements, and the neural crest cells, which are the source of skeletal and neural elements. Embryologic disruption of a branchial arch can lead to congenital head and neck anomalies, for example, branchial clefts, cysts, sinuses, or fistulae. The first and second branchial arches are referred to as the mandibular and hyoid arches, respectively. As their names imply, they also contribute significantly to bony and soft tissue skull base and maxillofacial growth. Thus, malformations of the auricle often accompany craniofacial anomalies. The most common examples include Treacher Collins syndrome, Goldenhar syndrome, Nager syndrome (acrofacial dysostosis), and Kabuki syndrome.

Auricular Development

During the fifth to sixth week of development, the early auricle arises from a series of paired mesenchymal condensations around the first pharyngeal cleft referred to as the 6 hillocks of His (auricular hillocks). Debate has ensued regarding the origin of each hillock as they soon lose their identity in early development. However, it is now generally accepted that the first three hillocks arise from the first branchial arch and lead to the development of the tragus, helical root, and helical crus, respectively. The last 3 hillocks are thought to be second branchial arch derivatives that ultimately become the antihelix, antitragus, and lower helix and lobule. Figure 1 provides a schematic of the proposed auricular components from each hillock. Complex rearrangements and fusion of the hillocks camouflage the details of their individual contributions to the ear. Nonetheless, they become the cartilage and soft tissue of the external ear that is nearly fully developed by birth. Continued cartilage deposition and matrix formation occurs after birth to create a stronger and larger auricle. By 5 to 6 years

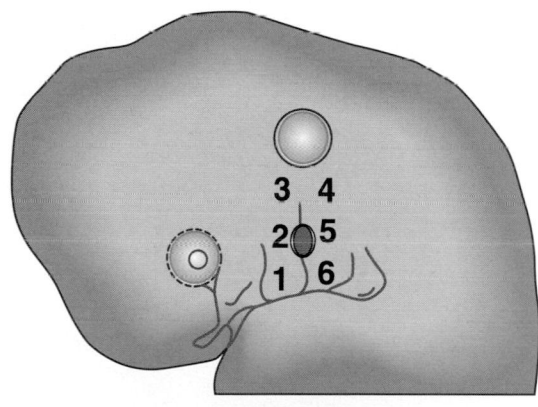

(A)

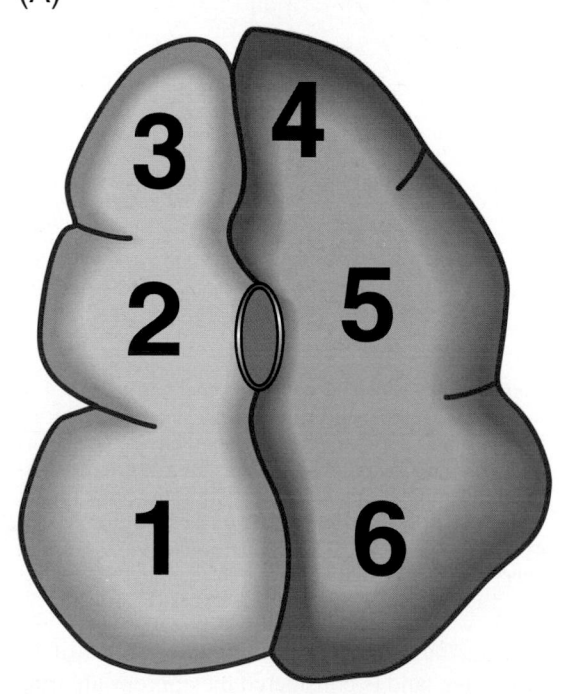

(B)

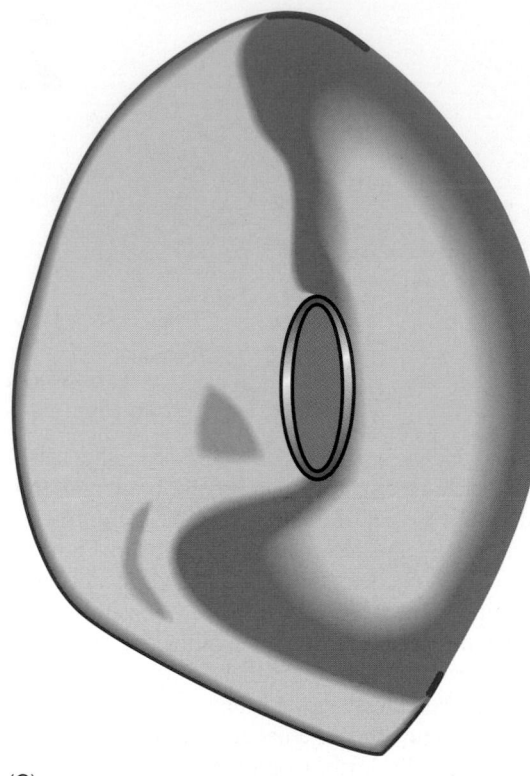

(C)

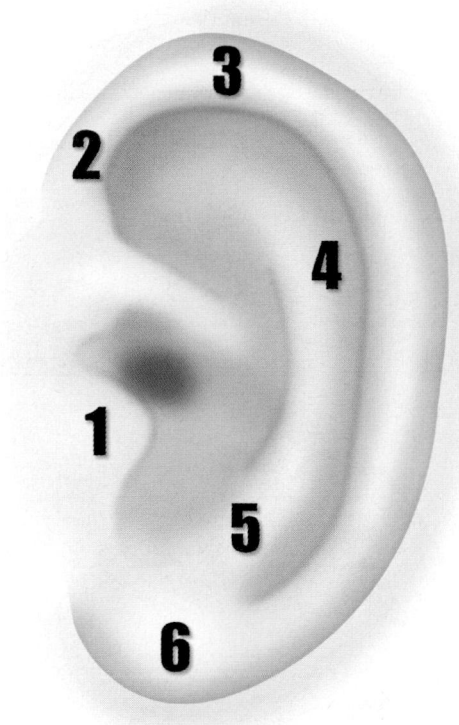

(D)

Figure 1 Development of the external ear. (A) At 4 to 6 weeks gestation, the external ear develops from six (three paired) mesenchymal condensations known as the auricular hillocks. (B) At approximately 8 to 9 weeks gestation, the hillocks rapidly fuse to form the primordia of the auricle. (C) The foundation of the future auricle is evident by 13 weeks. (D) The proposed parts of the auricle generated by the individual auricular hillocks are illustrated and are clearly seen in the 28 weeks embryo.

of age, the auricle is approximately 80% of its adult size, and is considered the appropriate time for surgical management of deformities without risk to future growth. Adult size is achieved by early adolescence.

Simultaneous development of mesenchymal precursors gives rise to the extrinsic (anterior, superior, and posterior) and intrinsic auricular muscles and blood supply. Sensory and motor branches of the fifth (arch I) and seventh (arch II) cranial nerves supply the external ear. While the muscles are controlled by the seventh cranial nerve (CNVII), the auriculotemporal nerve (CNV) and great auricular nerve (C2, C3) provide the majority of sensation to the tragus and the pinna. Sensory branches of the facial nerve (CNVII) and vagus (CNX) also provide sensation to the central and cranial portions of the external auditory canal, respectively.

The early embryonic pinna begins caudal to the growing mandible near the base of the neck. However, as synchronous first arch derivatives develop (mandible), the auricle is displaced more cephalad and posterior. By the end of the second trimester, the pinna will reach its adult location at the side of the head. It follows then that in syndromes with proposed arrested development of first and second branchial arch derivatives (eg, Treacher Collins syndrome, hemifacial microsomia, Nager syndrome, and Klippel-Feil syndrome), the auricle is retroverted, malformed, and set in a lower and more anterior position than the normal adult configuration. These deformities are frequently accompanied with middle ear malformations as its components also arise from the first and second pharyngeal arches. The relationship between ear and facial development is thereby evident in innumerable syndromes and teratogenic anomalies. Disturbances in external ear growth can also hallmark associated corporal defects. Thus, clinically a newborn with low set or dysmorphic ears should be explored for potential malformations or syndromes involving the face, limb, eye, heart, spine, or kidneys (eg, CHARGE, VATER, VACTERL, Townes-Brocks, Wildervanck, and branchio-oto-renal syndromes). Consultation with a genetics specialist is warranted as genetic numerators are frequently discovered in children with auricular malformations.

Failure of differentiation or fusion of the hillocks is thought to result in developmental malformations of the auricle including microtia, anotia, fistula, sinuses, and preauricular tags. Microtia occurs in approximately 0.03% of newborns and can be accompanied by canal stenosis, atresia, and ossicular abnormalities. Isolated cases are thought to arise sporadically, although autosomal recessive and autosomal dominant transmission patterns have been reported. Microtia is divided into 4 grades from a mild auricular deformity, with a small but recognizable pinna (grade I), to complete agenesis (anotia, grade IV). Grades II and III represent gradual reductions in pinna formation, from a rudimentary pinna found in grade II to complete loss of the pinna with only a malformed lobule (grade III) (Figure 2). Higher grade microtia are often associated with canal abnormalities. Eighty-five percent of microtia

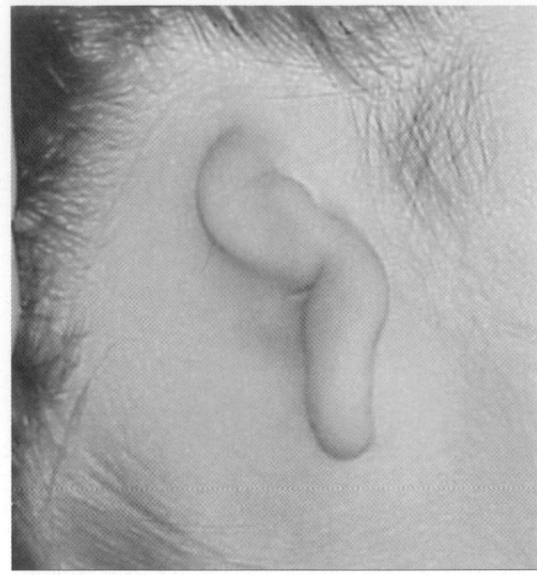

Figure 2 Grade III microtia showing a discrete earlobe with a cartilaginous and soft tissue rudiment. Grade III anomalies are likely to result from dysplastic or aplastic development of the auricular hillocks of the first two branchial arches at 5 to 6 weeks of gestation.

cases are unilateral, whereas bilaterality is more common in syndromic patients.

First branchial cleft anomalies are the result of early disruption of hillock fusion. They result in a duplicated EAC (type I) or persistent embryologic tract often communicating with the EAC (type II). These can present as periauricular swellings, tags, cysts, sinuses, or fistulae and consist of only ectodermal (as in type I anomalies) or ectodermal and mesodermal (type II) origin. Preauricular tags, the most common and benign ear deformity, are the result of supernumerary auricular hillock formation and can point to more serious anomalies of other parts of the body. Variations in the complex structure of the auricle can lead to minor malformations of the pinna or conchal bowl. The classic "lop" (prominent) and "cup" ear deformities are the result of exorbitant or disrupted cartilage formation of the helix and concha, respectively. Fetal alcohol syndrome, fetal positioning, teratogenic exposure (eg, thalidomide or isotretinoin), and maternal endocrinopathies have caused deformities of the external ear. Patients with Down syndrome frequently have hypoplastic and round ears. Regardless of cause, many auricular malformations and first cleft anomalies are surgically correctable problems.

External Auditory Canal and Tympanic Membrane

As the hillocks of His condense at around 6 weeks gestation, the first branchial cleft (groove), an ectoderm derivative nestled between the first two branchial arches, deepens to form the external auditory meatus (EAM). Simultaneously, the concha arises, in concert with the cartilaginous portion of the EAC, to create the cup and funnel form of the ear introitus.

Invagination of the first branchial cleft is coordinated with development of the tympanic ring, a mesenchymal first arch derivative that develops as a discrete unit in approximately the ninth week of gestation. This ring forms the peripheral framework of the future TM and bony EAC but is incomplete with a defect superiorly corresponding to the future notch of Rivinus.[1,2] Initially the tympanic ring develops along the superficial and lateral aspect of the temporal bone. The medial aspect of the first branchial cleft at this point becomes intimately attached to the ring's circumference. During the ninth to sixteenth week of gestation, as the ring dives deeper anteriorly and medially within the temporal bone, so does the adherent first branchial cleft. A meatal plug, a solid core of epithelial cells, follows as the cleft extends inward from the introitus toward the developing tympanic cavity. Proliferation of the ectodermal cells contributes to the meatal plug and assists in the medial expansion of the EAC. Furrowing ceases as a sheet of ectoderm (epithelium) comes in close contact with the endoderm of the lateral end of the first pharyngeal pouch that is simultaneously creating the future tympanic cavity (ie, tubotympanic recess). A mesenchymal contribution from the first arch remains between these 2 layers (Figure 3)[2a]. Ultimately, this component thins and differentiates to form the fibrous layer of the TM to include both outer radial and inner circular fibers. As the tympanic ring develops, it widens to consummate the future dimension and orientation of the bony EAC and TM.[1,2] The intimate layers of the first branchial cleft and pouch with the intervening mesenchyme of the first branchial arch ultimately become the final squamous, fibrous, and mucosal components of the TM at birth, the only ear structure that retains all 3 germ cell layers.

Formation of the EAC, however, is not complete until resorption of the epidermal plug. This process begins at approximately 21 weeks of gestation with proposed apoptosis and gradual hollowing of the EAC until only the most medial cells remain to form the outer (lateral) layer of the future TM. The process is thought to end by 28 weeks of gestation with the new EAC between the mastoid and the condylar fossa of the mandible. After birth, the tympanic ring continues to grow with ossification and lateral expansion to become the bony EAC. Although smaller in the infant, final dimensions of the EAC should approximate 8 mm in diameter and 2.5 cm in length to create a total volume of approximately 2 cm³. Failure of resorption during the end of the second and beginning of the third trimesters can lead to a continuum of pathology from partial stenosis, membranous atresia, to complete bony atresia of the EAC.

Congenital aural atresia occurs in 1:10,000 to 1:20,000 live births and occurs more frequently as unilateral cases (3:1), on the right side, and in males. A medial bony meatal plate remains in aural atresia and is juxtaposed to the developing tympanic cavity and replaces the TM. This contributes to a maximal conductive hearing loss found in these patients. The development of the manubrium malleus has also been shown to be intimately coordinated with the formation of

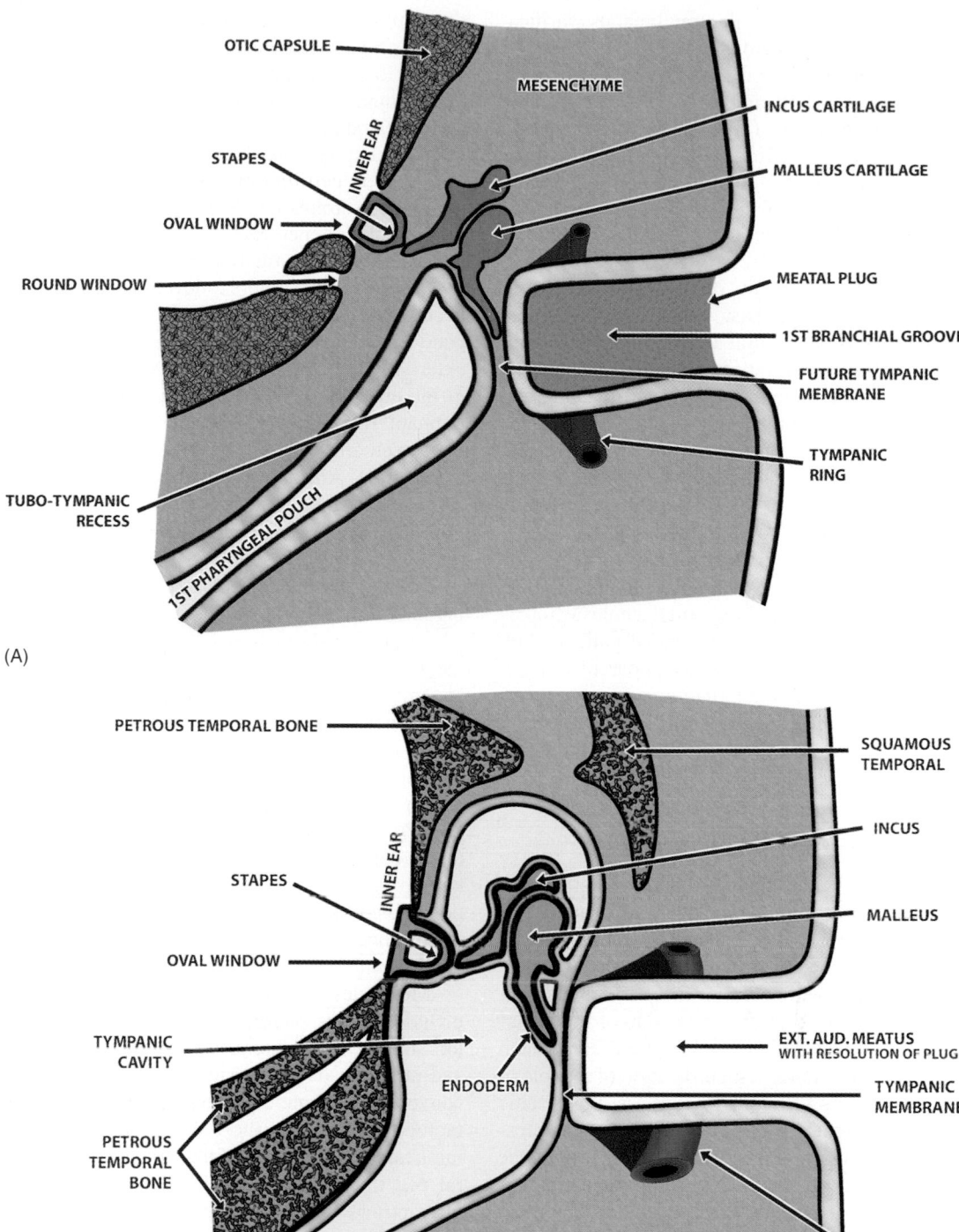

(A)

(B)

Figure 3 Drawing showing the development of the external auditory canal (EAC) and middle ear. Development of the external meatus, EAC, and middle ear space involves a complex process of ectodermal proliferation, cellular resorption, and coordinated maturation with the tubotympanic recess forming the tympanic membrane (TM) and middle ear cleft. The ectodermal cells at the dorsal end of the first branchial groove proliferate and expand medially. This solid core of ectodermal cells is referred to as the meatal plug (A). By the twenty-first week this meatal plug begins to hollow out, leaving the EAC lumen. Formation of the EAC is typically complete by the twenty-eighth week of gestation (B). Note that the medial-most ectoderm and endoderm of the tubotympanic recess interface in such a way that these two layers combine to form the TM (B). (Reference 2a.)

the medial EAC; and, despite the degree of canal deformity, defects in canal resorption are accompanied by lateral malleal anomalies.[3] Additional middle ear malformations also occur with complete aural atresia.

By birth, the TM is near adult size (9 mm in diameter); however, its position remains horizontal relative to the vertical axis of the adult TM. Distinction between the 2 components of the TM (pars flaccida and pars tensa) is also difficult in the newborn. Continued expansion and ossification of the tympanic ring during the first year postnatally leads to reorientation of the TM, formation of the lateral bony EAC, and closure of the notch of Rivinus with simultaneous clarification of the pars flaccida. In addition, expansion of the tympanic ring assists in closure of ventral embryologic tracts of the EAC and middle ear to the meninges (Hyrtl fissure) and parotid gland (foramen of Huschke). Retention of these structures has been blamed for some intracranial (meningitis, epidural abscess) and extracranial (parotitis) complications of otitis media due to infectious spread.

EAC development occurs subsequent to auricular morphogenesis. Accordingly, it is possible to see isolated aural atresia or stenosis without concomitant auricular deformities. This result suggests incomplete dissolution of the epidermal plug near the twenty-first to twenty-eighth week of gestation. In contrast, it is quite unusual to find severe auricular malformations without associated middle ear or EAC abnormalities, since this suggests disrupted development early in gestation. In a child with microtia, temporal bone imaging is appropriate to identify potential middle ear or canal defects. Congenital cholesteatomas may be found in the middle ear of patients with aural atresia without clinically apparent disease. Early discovery through imaging can prompt earlier surgical intervention and prevent potential adverse effects (see Chapter 62, "Microtia, Canal Atresia, and Middle Ear Anomalies").

Genetic and Molecular Determinants

Multiple genetic and molecular factors are involved in external ear development. Many appear to be equally distributed within middle and inner ear anlages and are involved in the coordinated development of these structures with the external ear. Significant overlap of molecular events in inner, middle, and external ear growth has made isolation and identification of the role of various factors difficult. Regardless, the genetic analysis of external ear malformations has blossomed from gene-targeting techniques and the identification of human syndromes affecting ear formation. The most notable is branchio-otorenal (BOR) syndrome that consists, as the name implies, of simultaneous ear, craniofacial, and renal defects. Ear anomalies including supernumerary tags, periauricular fistulae, microtia, and atresia, as well as dysplastic middle ear development have been associated with these patients. Haploinsufficiency of the *Eya1* gene causes BOR syndrome, and there are similar external ear anomalies identified in mice homozygous for *Eya1* null mutation.[4] Nonetheless, the role of *Eya1* remains unclear. Its presence in early cartilaginous condensations suggests that this is a fundamental element is ear cartilage formation. Malformations of the ossicular chain found in *Eya1* negative embryos also validate claims that ear cartilage growth (the embryonic source of early ossicular development) is dependent on this gene.[5]

Similarly, the *bmp5* gene, a member of the bone morphogenetic protein family, appears to be involved in late stages of pinna cartilage development. Specifically, positional cloning of the *bmp5* gene has been performed; it has been shown to be mutated in a strain of mice with small pinna (*short ear*, *se*). Condensations of ear cartilage and the perichondrium of differentiating cartilage express *bmp5*.[6] Mesenchymal condensation of ear cartilage during late development is defective in strains with *bmp5* mutant genes leading to foreshortened ears.

Extensive investigation into the *HOXa* family of genes in external ear development has also been performed. In particular, mutants in *Hoxa2* gene are associated with various anomalies of the external ear.[7] The normal pinna does not form in the absence of *Hoxa2* resulting in a microtic remnant. In addition, dose-dependent phenotypes have been created with differing levels of *Hoxa2* expression. Although considered important in early developmental stages of the pinna, the direct impact of *Hoxa2* on expression on external ear development remains unclear.[8] Nonetheless, some studies suggest that its fundamental role is defining the future identity of the second arch hillocks.

As previously mentioned, the development of the EAC is regulated in part by the formation and migration of the tympanic ring. This process appears independent of the formation of the pinna. Embryos with mutations of genetic determinants of the EAC have no associated external ear deformities. Specifically, *Goosecoid* (*Gsc*) and *Prx1* mutant embryos display absent EAC in the context of normal pinna. These genes are known regulators of tympanic ring condensation and endochondral ossification conferring the importance of tympanic ring elements in EAC formation.[2]

Molecules important in the formation of EAC include various secreted factors and their receptors that are simultaneously implicated in middle and inner ear development. *Endothelin-1* and its converting enzyme along with fibroblast growth factor 8 (*Fgf8*) are the most notable products implicated in formation of the tympanic ring, neural cell migration, and epithelial–mesenchymal interactions involved in external ear development.[2] Future identification and investigation of specific gene products found in auricular and EAC malformations will improve our understanding of the complex and coordinated development of the ear from its branchial arches and cleft.

MIDDLE EAR

Acoustic waves are transmitted as vibrations of the TM at the medial aspect of the EAC. These vibrations are amplified through a lever system of the middle ear ossicles. In total, sound is amplified 22 times from the air to the inner ear as a result of the size differential of the TM to the oval window (17:1), and the shape of the ossicular chain (malleus handle is 1.3 times longer than the long arm of the incus); hence the overall mechanical advantage is $1.3 \times 17 = 22$. Disruption of middle ear mechanics can thereby cause major conductive hearing losses. Discontinuity of the chain alone can maximize conductive deficits to 50 to 60 dB and this emphasizes the importance of normal middle ear and ossicular development.

The middle ear is located medial to the EAC and is composed of the air-filled tympanic cavity, the 3 ossicles and their ligamentous attachments, the eustachian tube orifice, the oval and round windows, the facial nerve and its chorda tympani branch, and 2 muscles that help dampen the mobility of the ossicular chain (tensor tympani muscle and stapedius muscle). The compartment is lined with mucosa and contained by the temporal bone that includes the squamous (superior), petrous (medial), tympanic (lateral), and mastoid (posterior) segments. The roof of the tympanic cavity is called the tegmen tympani and is composed of squamous bone that separates the middle ear from the middle cranial fossa. The lateral aspect of the tympanic cavity consists of the TM and its surrounding tympanic ring. All temporal bone segments, except the mastoid, develop prenatally and synchronous with the middle ear. As the middle ear expands postnatally so does the mastoid which maintains connection to the middle ear by a posterior air-filled, mucosal-lined space known as the aditus ad antrum. Bony growth of the mastoid is nearly complete by 3 years of age, but pneumatization and expansion continue into early adult life. Ossification of the temporal bone also proceeds well after birth and includes the lateral tympanic ring (medial EAC), that is initially cartilaginous and flexible until approximately 1 year of age.

Middle ear formation begins as a lateral and superior expansion of the first pharyngeal pouch between the first and second pharyngeal arches. Initially, this creates an endoderm-lined space known as the tubotympanic recess (see Figure 3). At 4 weeks gestation, progressive superior and lateral advancement of the recess eventually engulfs surrounding and loosely organized mesenchyme. By 7 weeks, a fluid-filled tympanic cavity or nascent middle ear has been shaped. The distal end of the tubotympanic recess remains connected to the developing nasopharynx and becomes the eustachian tube anteriorly as the second pharyngeal arch mesenchyme constricts and delineates it from the expanding tympanic cavity. Simultaneous ingrowth of the first pharyngeal cleft (early EAM), lateral to the tubotympanic recess, allows early interface of the medial recess endoderm with the ectoderm of the EAC to mark the boundaries of the future TM.

Pre- and postnatal orientation of the eustachian tube is shown to be horizontal. Eustachian tube dysfunction and concomitant otitis media commonly affecting infants and young children have been attributed to the horizontal position of the early eustachian tube. This theoretically prevents appropriate drainage and ventilation of the middle ear. Fortunately, gradual growth of the skull base and midface accommodates lengthening (17 mm in the child to 35 mm in the adult) and displacement of the tube vertically (45° in adulthood). This is accompanied with a reduced incidence of otitis media in childhood.

Although the ossicular chain is absent within the early tympanic cavity, it is already in construction from neural crest cells within the mesenchyme of the first and second pharyngeal arches above and lateral to the growing recess (Figure 4).[9] Specifically, around 5 to 6 weeks of gestation, the malleus head and neck along with the body and short process of the incus arise as a common ossicular mass from the first branchial (mandibular) arch. These first arch contributions are otherwise known as Meckel cartilage. At the same time, the stapes suprastructure, malleal manubrium, and long process of the incus stem from Reichert cartilage, elements derived from the second branchial (hyoid) arch. In contrast, the stapedial footplate and annular ligament of the stapes at the oval window of the inner ear develop from the otic capsule and anlage of the inner ear. By the sixteenth week of gestation, the ossicles reach adult size.

The tensor tympani and stapedius muscles also develop from the mesenchyme from the first and second branchial arches. Accordingly, their innervation corresponds to the nerve of each respective arch. The mandibular branch of the trigeminal nerve (CNV) supplies the tensor tympani, a muscle that extends from its bony canal near the eustachian tube to the malleal manubrium and attenuates mobility of the chain when stimulated by loud sounds. Similarly, the facial nerve (CNVII) provides motor branches to the stapedius muscle, which is activated at high sound intensity and limits the amplitude of the stapes.

Stapes development involves an additional process of complex morphogenesis as it begins as a blastema near 4.5 weeks of gestation. The facial nerve divides the blastema into the stapes, interhyale, and laterohyale. The interhyale becomes the stapedial muscle and tendon, whereas the laterohyale becomes the posterior wall of the middle ear and a portion of the fallopian (facial nerve) canal. The stapes suprastructure begins as a ring around the stapedial artery, a second arch derivative that ultimately regresses. Although rare, a persistent stapedial artery can result in significant

and unexplained conductive hearing losses. By the tenth week of gestation, the stapes assumes its more typical stirrup-like shape as the footplate develops in conjunction with the otic capsule.

Each ossicle begins as a cartilaginous condensation of neural crest derivatives of their respective arches and, within 4 weeks of their onset, become models for the future chain. Ossification of the entire chain starts around the sixteenth week of gestation as it quickly reaches adult size. Stapes ossification is delayed until 19 weeks of gestation. Ossicular remodeling is an adaptive process and continues throughout gestation and shortly after birth for the malleus and incus. Stapes growth and ossification is thought to be complete by the third trimester and does not appear to undergo remodeling postnatally.

As the ossicular chain develops, expansion of the mesenchyme- and mucoid-filled tympanic cavity continues laterally and superiorly. In the process, the pharyngeal endoderm divides into 4 sacs known as the saccus anticus, saccus posticus, saccus superior, and saccus medius. These sacs envelop the developing ossicular chain, pneumatize the middle ear, and become future spaces within the tympanic cavity. In the process, the middle ear ossicles, muscles, and ligaments and mastoid antrum become lined with endoderm (future cuboidal epithelium) derived from the first pharyngeal pouch. Simultaneously, blood supply is transmitted through numerous mucosal folds created at the junction of 2 sacs. Expansion of the tympanic cavity is nearly finished by approximately 30 weeks of gestation. Several mesenchymal elements differentiate into mucosal folds and permanent ligaments that suspend the ossicular chain. During the final (ninth) month of gestation, fine tuning of the tympanic cavity and its lining is complete. However, embryonic mesenchymal remnants and fluid can remain for several months after birth as they are slowly absorbed from the middle ear space. This can affect early chain mobility and be mistaken for otitis in the neonate. Theoretically, sufficient absorption shall have occurred by 2 months of age to allow for proper ossicular mobility.

Residual rests of epithelial cells within the tympanic cavity can give rise to an unusual but notable cause of hearing loss in the infant known as a congenital cholesteatoma. Retained amniotic epithelia, squamous differentiation of middle ear mucosal epithelium, or epithelial cells derived from the developing TM have been blamed for their occurrence. Despite the origin and in contrast to the acquired type, congenital cholesteatoma grow deep to the TM and most frequently in the anterior–superior quadrant. If untreated, these otherwise benign tumors can cause serious otic complications as a result of ossicular, labyrinthine, or fallopian canal bone destruction.

Further pneumatization of the epitympanum, middle ear, antrum, and petrous bone occurs during the latter part of the third trimester and early postnatal life as these cavities enlarge without deposition of additional bony matrix. Epithelium simultaneously covers the growing spaces. Pneumatization of the middle ear is nearly complete by the first year of life. The middle ear and antrum are of adult size in the infant. However, continued postnatal pneumatization of the mastoid leads to further lateral and posterior expansion of this bone. The styloid process, lateral to its respective foramen, also develops postnatally. Together, the growth of these structures assists in the protection of the facial nerve as it exits the stylomastoid foramen. In a neonate and infant, the facial nerve is subject to injury as it projects more superficially and laterally from the temporal bone. Facial weakness from the use of obstetric forceps and mastoid surgery has been reported and should incite extreme care in this region when operating on an infant less than 1 year of age.

The facial nerve is an integral component of the developing middle ear. Arising from the facial nucleus, the nerve enters the internal auditory meatus, travels via the fallopian canal to the geniculate ganglion, and takes a sharp turn posteriorly to enter the tympanic cavity. It traverses the middle ear as the tympanic (ie, horizontal) segment and travels above the oval window (and stapes) to abruptly take a posterior vertical course through the mastoid cortex. Along this second genu (turn), it becomes intimately associated with the stapes and its footplate. From the mastoid segment, the chorda tympani nerve projects through the posterior iter into the middle ear cleft to traverse between the incus and malleus and exit the anterior petrous bone through the Huguier canal. The chorda tympani nerve provides taste sensation to the anterior two-thirds of the tongue. In approximately 50% of cases, the bony canal of the tympanic segment of the facial nerve is congenitally dehiscent, a fact that has been attributed to facial nerve complications during middle ear surgery. An aberrant course of the facial nerve can also contribute to ossicular deformities and conductive hearing loss. For example, the facial nerve may override the oval window and lead to stapes malformations or discontinuity of the ossicular chain.

Although an overriding facial nerve is rare and can occur independent of other auricular

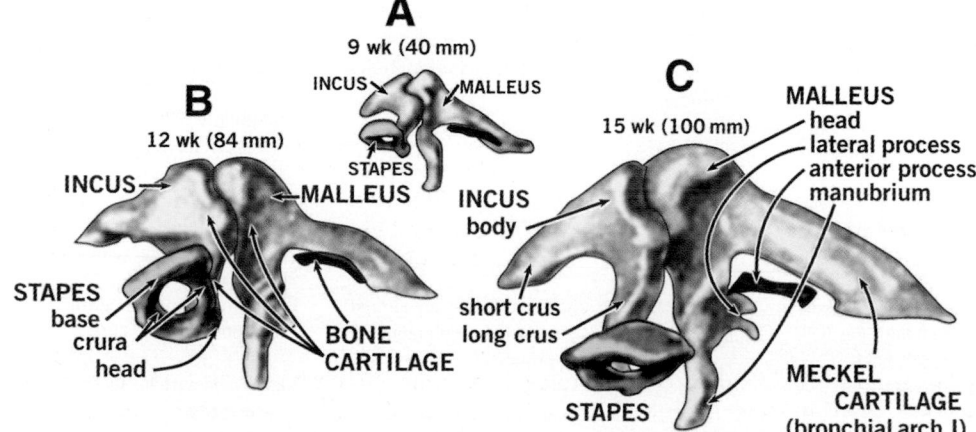

Figure 4 Ossicular development. (A) By the ninth week of gestation, the incus and malleus are still fused but begin to differentiate into individual structures. The stapes at this stage has developed beyond the stapes ring stage and more closely resembles the mature stirrup configuration. (B and C) By 12 to 15 weeks, the ossicles are more clearly differentiated and approximate adult size. Shortly following this stage, ossification begins at discrete centers of ossification. (Reproduced with permission from reference 9.)

anomalies, it is not an uncommon finding during the repair of aural atresia. Due to the disrupted development of the EAC, the mastoid segment of the temporal bone is juxtaposed to the glenoid fossa of the mandibular condyle in these patients. Disrupted ossicular development accompanies the external ear deformity. As a result, the facial nerve, unimpeded by the normal growth of the ossicular chain and EAC, dives sooner and more anterior within the middle ear to emerge from the stylomastoid foramen. Here, it can override the stapes or simply prevent risk-free reconstruction of the ossicular chain. Jahrsdoerfer and others have thereby created radiographic criteria to determine which candidates for aural reconstruction will have the best possible hearing outcome.[10] Those with an absent stapes, poorly aerated tympanic cavity or a significantly anomalous facial nerve at surgical risk within the space of the middle ear are considered poor candidates.

Anomalies of the middle ear often accompany those of the external ear. Naturally, syndromes affecting development of the first and second branchial arches have not only auricular and EAC deformities but impact the ossicular chain as they also arise from the same embryonic anlages. The middle ear cleft is commonly hypoplastic in the BOR syndrome, as can be the middle ear ossicles.[11] Crouzon disease is characterized by craniofacial abnormalities and hearing loss. The hearing loss is usually conductive owing to anomalies of the middle ear and atresia of the EAC. Other craniofacial disorders with hearing loss include Treacher Collins syndrome, Goldenhar syndrome and hemifacial microsomia, Nager syndrome, and Klippel-Feil syndrome. Early tests for conductive hearing losses are essential in these patients. Deformity of the malleus and incus, with coalescence into a common ossicular mass and adherence to an atretic bony meatal plate, is frequently found in these patients. Conductive hearing losses may be surgically correctable around 5 years of age when development of the mastoid and middle ear space is nearly complete. However, hearing losses should be addressed within 6 months of age using bone-conductive hearing devices to allow for appropriate auditory and speech development.

Intrinsic bone diseases can also influence development of the ossicular chain. Osteogenesis imperfecta is an autosomal dominant disorder with abnormal osteoblastic activity that can be accompanied by pathologic or iatrogenic fractures of the ossicles due to "weak" bones. Brittle bones also accompany osteopetrosis (Albers-Schoenberg disease) due to failed resorption of calcified cartilage leading to ossicular fractures with mixed hearing losses. Patients with syndromes restricting skeletal growth, such as achondroplasia, an autosomal dominant syndrome, can also have absent, fused, or foreshortened ossicular chains. Symphalangism syndrome, another autosomal dominant disorder, has aberrant bone fusion at interphalangeal joints and is associated with conductive hearing loss. The ear anomaly is attributable to the fixation of the

stapes to the petrous part of the temporal bone. Congenital otosclerosis occurs as a result of disrupted mesenchyme development at the junction of the otic capsule with the middle ear leading to fixation of the stapes to the oval window and a 20 to 40 dB conductive hearing loss. Another conductive disorder with fixation of the stapes is due to mutations of the X-linked DFN3, M genes, POU3F4/BRN4.[12] These disorders of middle ear morphogenesis along with their recently discovered aberrations in genetic and molecular factors are listed in Table 1.

Genetic and Molecular Determinants

The middle ear develops from condensations of neural crest cells within the mesenchyme of the first and second branchial arches. Mesenchymal–epithelial interactions are thought to coordinate the complex structure of the ossicular chain. Significant overlap exists with growth of the external ear as the temporal ring, tympanic membrane, and manubrium of the malleus involve a common wall. This is evident when examining genes responsible for development of the branchial arches. Early molecular and genetic studies on the middle ear involved extrapolation from avian models to mammals since these were easily manipulated during embryogenesis. However, precise mutations in the murine model have recently and dramatically expanded our knowledge of genetic and molecular determinants of middle ear growth.[2,13]

Molecular signals involved in branchial arch development have been confirmed to play a role in middle ear growth. Specifically, endothelin-1, Fgf8, and retinoic acid (RA) are required for appropriate maturation of the ossicular chain.[14] Targeted mutations in endothelin-1 and Fgf8 lead to profound underdevelopment to absence of first arch derivatives, namely, the malleus and incus. The stapes is also affected during endothelin-1 mutations but does not seem to be impacted significantly by defects in Fgf8 production. On the other hand, RA appears to have an affinity for stapes development, a structure arising predominantly from the second branchial arch, while conferring minimal if no deficits on malleus and incus formation when mutated.[14,15]

Homeobox transcription factors also appear to function as regulators of middle ear development but with less direct impact on specific branchial arches. Predominant and extensively studied factors include Prx1, Goosecoid (Gsc), Dlx1, and Dlx2. Prx1 appears to help establish location, size, and fate of neural crest condensations of future skeletal elements of the ossicular chain. Mutations in the Prx1 gene lead to egregious cartilaginous attachments from surrounding skeletal bone to the maldeveloped structures consistent with incus and stapes. Malleal growth is also affected by Prx1 mutations but may be the result of a disturbance in the coordinated development and insertion of the manubrium into the tympanic ring during TM and EAC development since these structures are also affected by mutations in this gene. Gsc is thought to regulate expression of molecules important in recruiting mesenchymal cells into skeletal condensations within the middle ear.[2,13] In contrast Dlx1 and

Table 1	Genes Involved in the Development of the Human Ear		
Syndrome/Disease	Gene	Type of Product	Structures Affected
Branchio-oto-(BO), branchio-oto-renal (BOR)	EYA1	Transcription coactivator	Atresia and stenosis of external auditory canal (EAC), malformed auricle
			Hypoplasia or absence of three ossicles
			Absent or abnormal semicircular canals and cochlea
Crouzon disease	FGFR2 FGFR3	Growth factor receptor	Atresia of EAC Malformation of ossicles
Craniosynostosis	FGFR3	Growth factor receptor	Sensorineural deafness
DFN3/ Gusher	POU3F4/ BRN4	Pou-domain transcription factor	Conductive hearing loss
			Abnormally wide connection between internal acoustic canal and the inner ear
			Stapes fixation
Pendred DFNB4	PENDRIN	Anion transporter	Sensorineural deafness Widened vestibular aqueduct Shortened cochlea
Proximal symphalangism (SYM1), multiple synostoses (SYNS1)	NOGGIN	Secreted factor, antagonist of bone morphogenetic proteins	Fixation of stapes to petrous part of temporal bone
Townes-Brocks	SALL1	C2H2 Zinc-fingered transcription factor	Malformed auricle, sensorineural hearing loss
Treacher Collins (mandibulofacial dysostosis)	TCOF1	Nucleolar trafficking protein	Atresia of EAC, malformed auricle
			Middle and inner ear anomalies

BO = branchio-oto; BOR = branchio-oto-renal; EAC = external auditory canal.

Dlx2 confer direct effects on skeletal morphogenesis of the incus and stapes with almost exclusive stapes deformities in *Dlx1* deficient mice.[16]

As previously mentioned, during external ear development, *Hoxa2* is critical for development of second branchial arch derivatives. Mutations in *Hoxa2* lead to duplication of first arch elements, the malleus and incus, within the middle ear. Theoretically, *Hoxa2* seems to be regulating the impact of molecular signals from surrounding structures on the fate of skeletal elements in the second branchial arch. Specifically, *Hoxa2* is thought to perform this function by acting as an inhibitor of mesenchymal determinants and thereby assisting in formation of the second arch derivatives in the middle ear.[13]

Investigation into genetic determinants of human disorders with conductive deficits has also led to discoveries of genes and their factors involved in middle ear growth (see Table 1). For example, Treacher Collins syndrome is an autosomal dominant disorder of craniofacial development associated with bilateral conductive hearing loss, and occasionally malformations of the inner ear have also been reported.[3] This syndrome is caused by mutations in the *TCOF1* gene that encodes for the nucleolar protein treacle.[17] *TCOF1* is widely expressed in fetal and adult tissues and is thought to function as a trafficking protein between the nucleolus and cytoplasm. Mutations in both *fibroblast growth factor receptor (FGFR) 2* and *3* have been shown to cause Crouzon disease.[18–20] A unique mutation in *FGFR3* has also been shown to cause craniosynostosis that is associated with deafness and abnormalities on radiographs of hands and feet.[21] The abnormal bone fusion at interphalangeal joints and the stapes associated with symphalangism in humans is most likely caused by an alteration of bone morphogenic protein (BMP) levels in those regions during development. This disorder is caused by mutations in *NOGGIN*, which encodes a secreted polypeptide that inactivates members of the transforming growth factor R family, in particular bone morphogenetic proteins (BMP-2 and -4).[22–24]

INNER EAR

The inner ear structures consist of a membranous fluid-filled labyrinth, which is derived from ectoderm, and a surrounding bony labyrinth (or otic capsule), which is derived from the mesoderm and neural crest surrounding the membranous labyrinth.

The membranous portion of the inner ear originates from a thickening of the ectoderm adjacent to the hindbrain known as the otic placode (Figure 5).[25] In humans, the otic placode is evident at the third week of embryonic development. The otic placode soon invaginates from the surface ectoderm to form an otic cup. By the end of the fourth week, the edges of the otic cup come together and fuse to form the otic vesicle/otocyst. At this developmental point, the inner ear is unique in generating a neural ganglion that is derived from its own primordial otocyst by allowing cells to delaminate from the anteroventromedial otocyst which coalesce to form the statoacoustic ganglion. These neurons then develop dendrites and axons that connect the sensory epithelia in the ear to the second-order auditory neurons.

Concomitant with this neural differentiation, the otocyst proper undergoes a complex morphogenesis, such that the gross anatomy of the membranous labyrinth is nearly mature by the end of the eighth week of gestation (Figure 6).[25] The first morphologic change in the otocyst is the outgrowth of the future endolymphatic duct and sac. This structure begins as a dorsal diverticulum that elongates and migrates medially. The remaining otocyst enlarges circumferentially and also elongates on a dorsal–ventral axis. From this time point onward, the inner ear can be divided morphologically, developmentally and, in terms of clinical relevance, into a superior and inferior region (ie, pars superior and pars inferior). The superior portion of the otocyst gives rise to the 3 semicircular ducts, their associated ampullae and the utricle. The inferior portion gives rise to the saccule and cochlea. The clinical significance of such delineation is that congenital malformation of the inner ear is often observed as defects of the pars inferior, that is, abnormalities of the cochlea and saccule.

The 3 semicircular ducts develop sequentially during the fifth week of gestation, starting with the superior duct and followed by the posterior and then lateral duct. The superior and posterior ducts differentiate from a vertical canal plate while the lateral duct differentiates from a lateral (horizontal) canal plate outgrowth. These plate-like outgrowths generate the mature semicircular ducts by fusing the central portions of each plate which then resorb, leaving behind a duct-like structure (see Figure 6). One end of the lateral and the common crus of the superior and posterior ducts open into the utricle while the other ends form a dilated structures (the ampullae) that house the actual sensory hair cell organs (the cristae ampullares) for each semicircular duct and open into the utricle. The 2 ampullae for the superior and lateral ducts form anteriorly near the junction of the ducts with the utricle, while the ampulla for the posterior duct is located at the posterior end of the duct (see Figure 6E).

The cochlea begins as an evagination from the ventral portion of the otocyst starting at around the fifth week of gestation. After extending ventrally, the cochlear duct begins coiling such that it has formed $1\frac{1}{2}$ turns by the eighth week, 2 turns by the tenth week, and has completed the normal $2\frac{1}{2}$ turns by 25 weeks of gestation.

The utricle and saccule start to form during the sixth week. As the cochlear duct extends, the opening between the saccule and cochlea becomes constricted and forms the narrow cochleosaccular duct. In the mature inner ear, two additional ducts are evident medially: the utricular and saccular ducts that connect to the endolymphatic duct (Figure 7).[26]

Development of the Sensory Organs

Six major sensory organs are present in the human inner ear. The organ of Corti is responsible for auditory function, while the remaining 5 other sensory organs are dedicated to vestibular function (the 3 cristae and the utricular and saccular maculae). The developmental origin of these sensory organs is unclear. Based on early studies of the chicken inner ear, it has been proposed that all sensory cells in the inner ear derive from a ventromedial region of the otic cup. Subsequent studies utilizing gene expression patterns as molecular markers for the developing sensory organs in the chicken and mouse have since revealed that expression of *bmp4* (bone morphogenetic protein 4), *Msx-1* (muscle segment homeobox 1), and *Lfng* (lunatic fringe) can mark several specific cell patches (as opposed to one) that ultimately differentiate into hair cell patches.[27,28] Similarly, in Xenopus experiments, time-lapsed, fluorescent labeling of various regions of the primitive otocyst show that all quadrants of the otocyst can contribute to sensory hair cells.[29]

Once the position and type of a sensory organ has been specified, morphologic differentiation follows, and the sensory epithelium can be identified by an increase in the thickness of the otic epithelium into a pseudostratified layer that later differentiates into sensory hair cells and

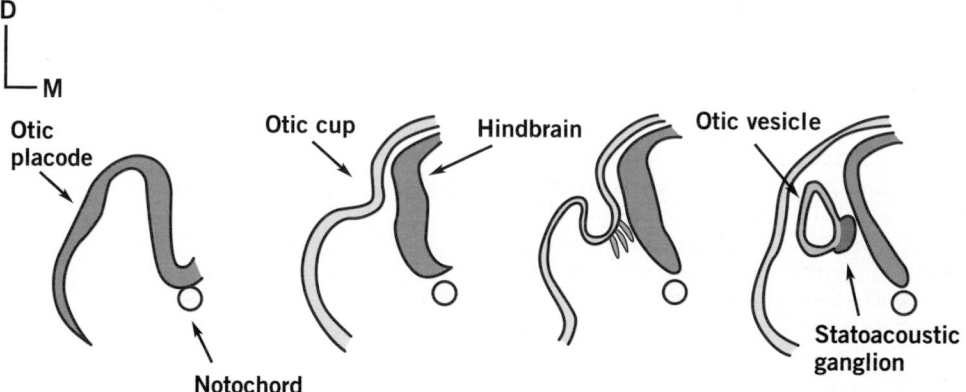

Figure 5 Diagram of coronal sections illustrating the development of the otocyst. Orientations: D = dorsal; M = medial. (Reproduced with permission from reference 25.)

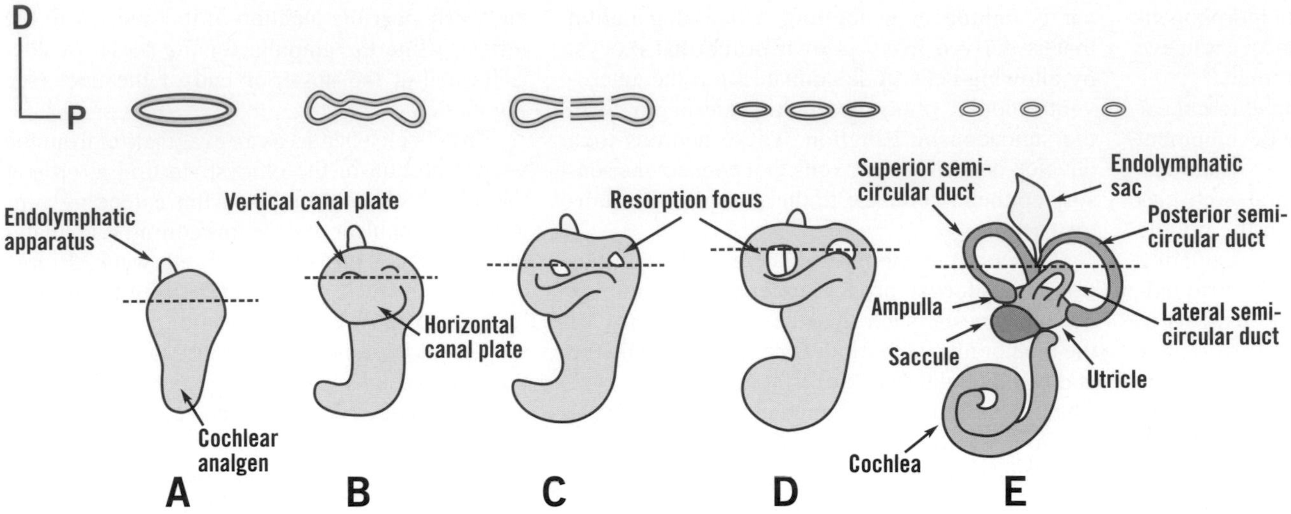

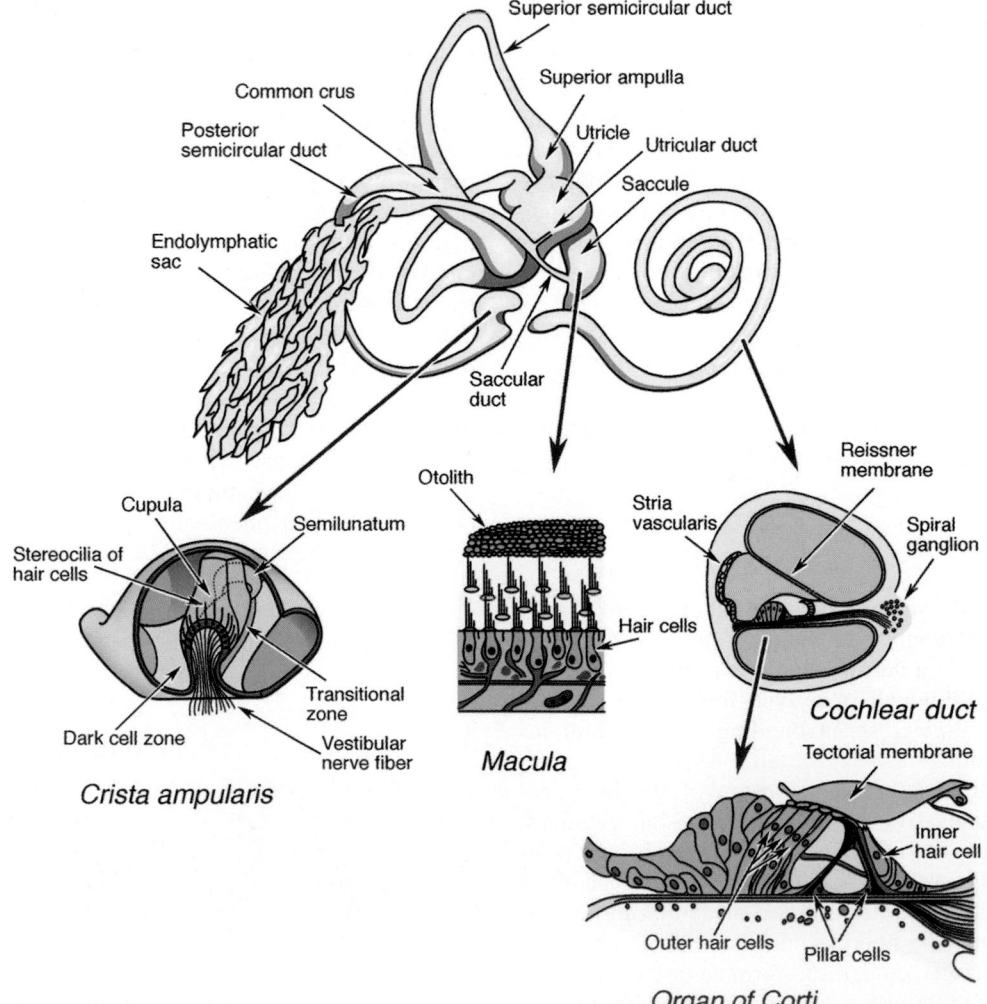

D
P

Endolymphatic apparatus

Vertical canal plate

Resorption focus

Horizontal canal plate

Cochlear analgen

A B C D E

Superior semi-circular duct

Endolymphatic sac

Posterior semi-circular duct

Ampulla

Saccule

Lateral semi-circular duct

Utricle

Cochlea

Figure 6 Diagram showing the development of the membranous labyrinth of the internal ear. (A–E) Lateral views of the left inner ear from the fifth to eighth weeks. The dotted lines represent the level of section for the diagrams shown in the upper panel, illustrating the development of the superior and posterior semicircular ducts. Orientations: D = dorsal; P = posterior. (Reproduced with permission from reference 25.)

supporting cells. The notch signaling pathway is used in a variety of tissues for generating cell type diversity and regulating differentiation during development. Genes in the notch signaling pathway have also been implicated in the determination of hair cells and supporting cells in the inner ear.[30,31] Mutation or deletion of the genes in this pathway have also been implicated in the determination of hair cells and supporting cells in the cochlea. Mutation or deletion of genes in this pathway resulted in the absence or aberrant number of sensory hair cells in zebrafish and mice.[31–34]

Cristae Ampullares. The sensory epithelium for the crista ampullaris elevates into a ridge-like fold where hair cells and supporting cells develop. Cells surrounding the sensory epithelium are secretory in function and are thought to generate the gelatinous cupula in which the stereocilia of the sensory hair cells are embedded. The mound-like elevation of the crista is evident by the eighth week of gestation, and the sensory structure is mature by the twenty-third week of gestation (see Figure 7).

Maculae. The maculae develop in a similar fashion as the cristae except the sensory epithelium is flat, and it is covered by an otolithic membrane that contains superficial calcareous deposits, the otoconia. The maculae appear to be fully differentiated between 14 and 16 weeks of gestation (see Figure 7).

Organ of Corti. The organ of Corti develops from the posterior wall of the cochlear duct. As the cochlear duct increases in length, the cross-sectional shape of the duct changes from round to oval to triangular (Figures 8).[25] The posterior wall develops into the sensory tissue, the organ of Corti; the anterior wall forms part of Reissner membrane; and the lateral wall forms the stria vascularis. The organ of Corti starts to differentiate at the basal region of the cochlear duct around the seventh week of gestation, whereas the epithelium in the apical turn is undifferentiated and pseudostratified at this age. By the twenty-fifth week of gestation, the organ of Corti is fully differentiated.

Development of the Statoacoustic Ganglion. Based on animal studies, neurons of the statoacoustic ganglion are thought to originate from the otic epithelium, whereas glial cells in the ganglion are derived from the neural crest.[35] Morphologic studies suggest that cells in the anteroventral lateral region of the otic cup/otocyst delaminate from the epithelium, migrate away from the otocyst, and undergo proliferation before aggregating to form the ganglion.[36] In parallel with the growth of the otocyst, the statoacoustic ganglion forms a pars superior and a pars inferior at about the time when the membranous labyrinth is divided into a dorsal vestibular and a ventral cochlear region. The pars superior of the ganglion provides the peripheral neural connections to the superior and lateral cristae and the macula of the utricle. The pars inferior gives rise to a distinct vestibular portion that innervates the macula of the saccule and posterior crista and the spiral ganglion that innervates the organ of Corti.

Helix loop helix transcription factors, such as *Neurogenin 1*, have been implicated in the

Figure 7 Diagram illustrating the anatomy of a mature membranous labyrinth and its sensory organs. (Reproduced with permission from reference 26.)

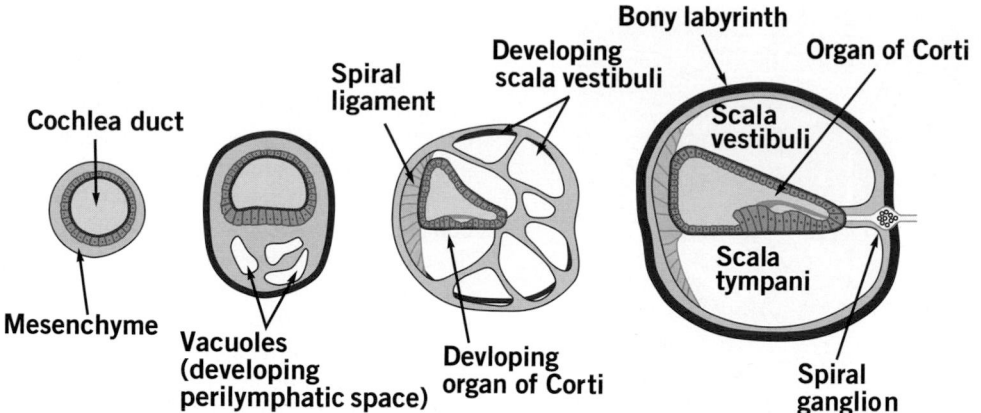

Figure 8 Diagram showing development of the bony labyrinth. Cross-sections through the cochlea showing the development of the organ of Corti, bony labyrinth, and perilymphatic spaces from the eighth to twelfth weeks of gestation. (Reproduced with permission from reference 25.)

formation of the statoacoustic ganglion. In mice with a deletion of *Neurogenin 1*, the statoacoustic ganglion fails to form.[37] Growth factors such as fibroblast growth factor 3 are also important for the formation of the vestibular ganglion in the mouse.[38] Once the neurons of the ganglion reach their final position and finish proliferation, they express high-affinity neurotrophin receptors and become dependent on neurotrophins secreted by the presumptive sensory organs in the membranous labyrinth. Mice with targeted deletion (knockout) of genes encoding brain-derived nerve growth factor or *Neurotrophin 3* or their respective receptors had a loss of ganglionic neurons and innervations to the sensory organs.[39] However, this trophic dependency of ganglionic neurons on their target tissues is not reciprocal. In the absence of afferent innervation, the differentiation of sensory hair cells appears unaffected, at least until birth.[40,41]

Bony Labyrinth Development. Concurrent with the development of the otocyst, the mesenchymal cells surrounding the otic vesicle differentiate into a cartilaginous otic capsule by the eighth week of gestation. As the membranous labyrinth enlarges, vacuoles appear in areas surrounding the otic epithelium as a result of programmed cell death. These vacuoles soon coalesce to form the perilymphatic space that is filled with perilymph. In the cochlea, the perilymphatic space develops in 2 divisions; the scala tympani forms before the scala vestibuli (see Figure 8).

Ossification of the cartilaginous capsule to form the bony labyrinth does not occur until the membranous labyrinth has acquired its adult size. Bone formation starts around the fifteenth week of gestation and ends by the twenty-first week with a total of 14 ossification centers. The first ossification center appears at the base of the cochlea where ossification occurs more rapidly than in the semicircular canals. In the vestibular portions of the inner ear, the membranous labyrinth continues to grow until approximately the twenty-first week of gestation. But by the twenty-third week of gestation, all the ossification centers have fused thus limiting any further growth in the membranous or bony labyrinth.

HUMAN EAR MALFORMATIONS AND MODELS OF MOLECULAR DEVELOPMENT

Many genes causing human deafness have been identified recently. In some cases, the functional deficit is the result of gross malformations of the external, middle, or inner ear or a combination of more than one of these components (Table 1). Examples of some of these syndromes are described in the molecular sections of the external and middle ears listed above and in the following paragraphs. Steel and Bussoli have reviewed syndromes that are associated with the lack of proper differentiation and functioning of sensory hair cells[42] (see Chapter 26, "Hereditary Hearing Impairment").

Branchio-Oto-Renal and Branchio-Oto Syndromes

The branchio-oto-renal (BOR) syndrome is an autosomal dominant disorder characterized by branchial arch anomalies (branchial cleft cysts and sinuses), ear malformations affecting the external, middle, and inner ear regions, and various renal anomalies ranging from undetectable (in the branchio-oto (BO) syndrome) to bilateral aplasia.[4] Hearing loss is the most common presenting symptom and occurs in 88% of patients with BOR syndrome.[11,43]

The most common external ear anomalies are preauricular pits and skin tags, but microtia and aural atresia are also noted in patients with BOR syndrome. The middle ear cleft is commonly hypoplastic in patients with BOR syndrome, as can be the middle ear ossicles. In the inner ear, aplasia or hypoplasia of the cochlea has been reported as a BOR phenotype (Figure 9). The vestibular portions of the inner ear similarly show absent or malformed semicircular canals. Depending on the ear phenotype, hearing loss can be sensorineural, conductive, or mixed, as seen in approximately one-half of the patients with BOR syndrome.[4]

The gene responsible for causing BOR and BO syndromes has been identified to be the human homolog of the Drosophila *eyes absent* (eya) gene.[11,42] The spectrum of malformations seen in BOR syndrome suggests a defect in the *EYA1* molecular pathway occurring sometime between the fourth and the tenth week of gestation. The types of DNA mutations identified in patients with BOR syndrome suggest that the developmental malformations result from reduced gene dosage.[11]

Mice with *eya1* also displayed similar severe external, middle, and inner ear defects suggesting that the functions of this protein in ear development are evolutionarily conserved.[5] In mice, *eya1* is specifically expressed in the early otocyst along the ventromedial wall and the adjacent statoacoustic ganglion.[44] At later embryonic time points, *EYA1* is expressed along the neuroepithelium that eventually gives rise to key cochlear structures, such as the inner and outer hair cells. In addition, *EYA1* is also expressed in the external and middle ear primordia. These results suggest that the encoded protein of *EYA1* plays a direct role in the formation of all three components of the ear in mice as well as in humans. Studies in Drosophila eye imaginal disks show that the *Eya* gene product is a transcriptional coactivator that acts as part of a complex with other transcription coactivators during eye morphogenenesis.[24]

Pendred Syndrome

Pendred syndrome is an autosomal recessive disorder classically characterized by deafness and goiter. The presence of goiter is usually variable in severity; however, most patients have a positive perchlorate discharge test indicative of a defective organification of iodine in the thyroid gland. The onset of deafness in the classically described syndrome is congenital, profound, and sensorineural in nature. Cochlear hypoplasia with poorly partitioned mid and apical turns, sometimes referred to as Mondini malformations, and enlarged vestibular aqueducts (EVAs) are often described in these patients.

The gene responsible for causing Pendred syndrome was identified using a positional cloning approach and was named *PENDRIN*.[45,46] Functional studies in Xenopus oocytes show that the encoded protein functions as a chloride/iodide transporter.[47] The clinical significance of this gene broadened when mutations in *PENDRIN* were also shown to cause autosomal recessive deafness that mapped to the locus of DFNB4, a recessive nonsyndromic form of deafness.[48] Expression and gene-targeting studies in mice have provided insights into the etiology of this disorder. In mice, *Pds* is activated during embryonic development of the inner ear. Its expression is restricted to nonsensory regions of the inner ear including the endolymphatic duct and sac, nonsensory regions of the utricle and saccule, and the external sulcus region in the cochlea.[45] *Pendrin* knockout mice are deaf and display variable defects of the vestibular structures.[49] However, the cause of inner ear dysfunction in these mice most likely is not attributable to structural malformations as implied by the human disorder. The membranous

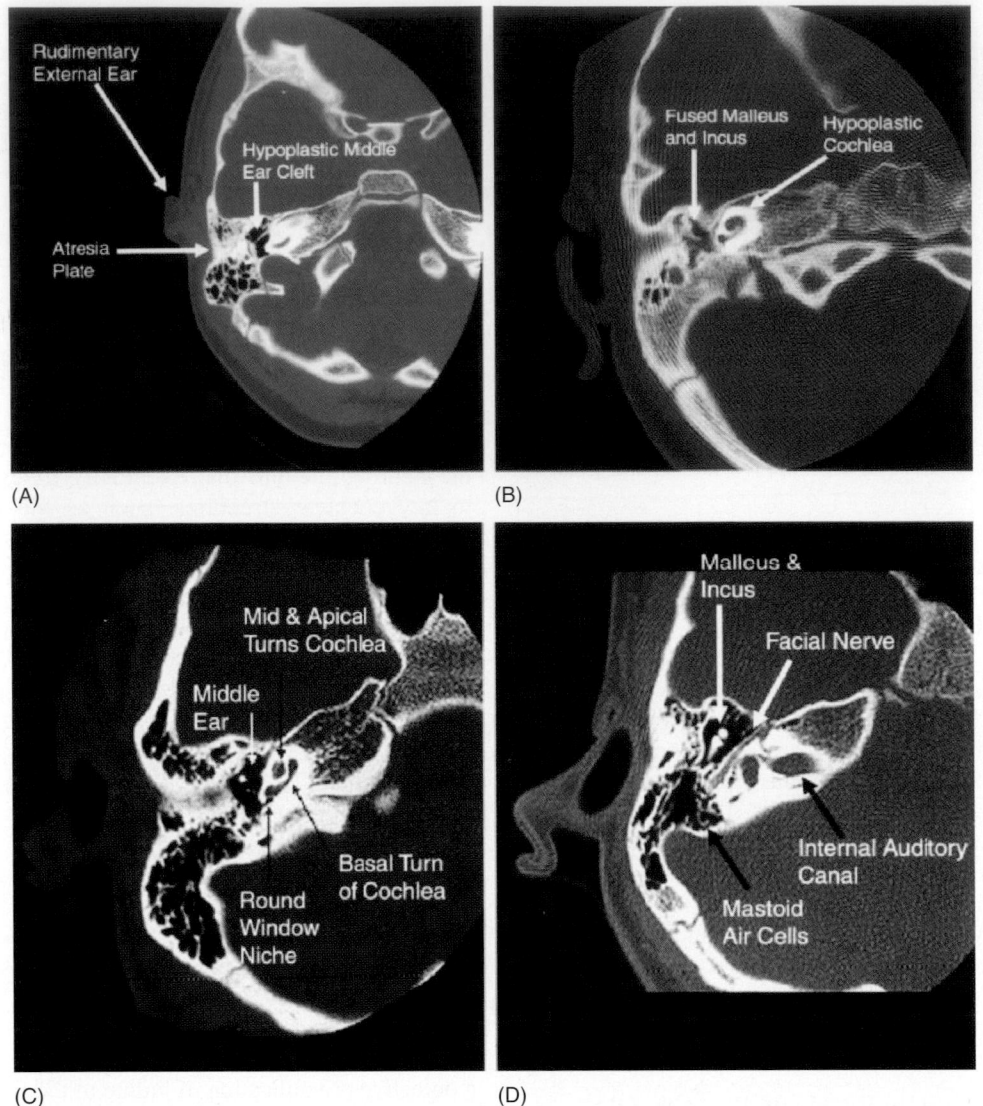

(A)   (B)

(C)   (D)

Figure 9 The external, middle, and inner ears are all potentially affected in branchio-oto-renal (BOR) syndrome. At the external ear level, auricular malformations vary from mild hypoplasia to complete aplasia. (A) A rudimentary ear lobe is apparent even on this axial computed tomographic (CT) scan of the temporal bones in a child with BOR syndrome. Note also the failure of development of an external auditory canal (aural atresia) and the associated small middle ear cavity. (B) Another patient with BOR syndrome demonstrates hypoplastic development of the cochlea with a discrete basal turn but poorly differentiated middle and apical turns appearing as a bulbous mass on high-resolution CT imaging. (C and D) Demonstrate normative CT imaging data with middle and inner ear structures labeled as shown.

labyrinth of the *Pds* knockout mice dilates during embryogenesis that is likely due to the disruption of normal endolymph homeostasis resulting from loss of the ion transport function of *Pds*. The sensory hair cells develop and appear normal at birth but degenerate later in life. This is thought to be due (again) to the loss of a normal inner ear fluid environment. It is likely that the etiology of human Pendred syndrome is similar to that of the *Pds* mutant mouse model, where the deficit lies in ionic imbalance of the endolymph rather than the structural malformation during development. The EVA associated with Pendred syndrome supports this hypothesis. Clinically, our knowledge base and understanding of the function of *PENDRIN* in the inner ear, the sequelae of loss of normal *PENDRIN* function, the mechanisms explaining associations of EVA and cochlear hypoplasia with *PENDRIN* mutations are steadily advancing. Mutant mice carrying mutations similar to those found in patients with Pendred syndrome will help to clarify this issue.

X-Linked Deafness Locus 3

X-linked DFN3 is caused by mutations in a member of the POU domain transcription factors, POU3F4/BRN4.[12] In mice, Pou3f4 is important for the development of the ear. Transcription of this gene is activated in mice at the otocyst stage in the mesenchymal cells surrounding the otocyst.[50] Pou3f4 knockout mice show a variety of deficits, including abnormal fibrocytes surrounding the cochlea, misshapen stapes, and shortened cochlea.[50,51] The deficits caused by mutations of this gene in humans are usually conductive in nature and can be corrected by surgery.

SUMMARY

A tremendous number of advances have been made over the past several years in identifying developmental ear anomalies (hearing loss, malformations, etc) and the molecular defects underlying those abnormalities. An in-depth

review of the various genetic causes of hearing loss overlaps with this discussion and is presented in Chapter 26, "Hereditary Hearing Impairment." However, it is worthwhile to point out that since many genetic causes of hearing loss present as congenital deafness, it is reasonable to speculate that the genetic mutations causing congenital hearing loss likely perturb the normal development of the inner ear in utero and are thus relevant to both abnormal and normal ear development. Through continued investigations into human manifestations (such as syndromic and nonsyndromic hearing loss), as well as continued research using animal models of human ear anomalies (eg, transgenic mouse models), marked advances in our understanding of human inner ear development will continue to emerge.

REFERENCES

1. Mallo M, Gridley T. Development of the mammalian ear: Coordinate regulation of formation of the tympanic ring and the external acoustic meatus. Development 1996;122:173–9.
2. Mallo M. Formation of the outer and middle ear, molecular mechanisms. Curr Top Dev Biol 2003;57:85–113.
2a. Goeringer GC. Development of the Ear. In: Lalwani AK, Grundfast KM, editors. Pediatric Otology and Neurotology. Philladelphia, PA: Lippincott-Ravin Publishers;1998.
3. Mallo M, Schrewe H, Martin JF, et al. Assembling a functional tympanic membrane: Signals from the external acoustic meatus coordinate development of the malleal manubrium. Development 2000;127:4127–36.
4. Vincent C, Kalatzis V, Abdelhak S, et al. BOR and BO syndromes are allelic defects of EYA1. Eur J Hum Genet 1997;5:242–6.
5. Xu PX, Adams J, Peters H, et al. Eya1-deficient mice lack ears and kidneys and show abnormal apoptosis of organ primordia. Nat Genet 1999;23:113–7.
6. King JA, Marker PC, Seung KJ, Kingsley DM. BMP5 and the molecular, skeletal, and soft-tissue alterations in short ear mice. Dev Biol 1994;166:112–22.
7. Chisaka O, Musci R, Capecchi M. Developmental defects of the ear, cranial nerves and hindbrain resulting from targeted disruption of the mouse homeobox gene Hox-1.6. Nature 1992;355:516–20.
8. Ohnemus S, Bobola N, Kanzler B, Mallo M. Different levels of Hoxa2 are required for particular developmental processes. Mech Dev 2001;108:135–47.
9. Anson BJ, Davies J, Duckert LG. Embryology of the ear. In: Paparella MM, Shumrick DA, editors. Otolaryngology, 3rd edition. Philadelphia, PA: WB Saunders; 1991.
10. Jahrsdoerfer RA, Yeakley JW, Aguilar EA, et al. Grading system for the selection of patients with congenital aural atresia. Am J Otol 1992;13:6–12.
11. Millman B, Gibson WS, Foster WP. Branchio-oto-renal syndrome. Arch Otolaryngol Head Neck Surg 1995;121:922–5.
12. de Kok YJ, van der Maarel SM, Bitner-Glindzicz M, et al. Association between X-linked mixed deafness and mutations in the POU domain gene POU3F4. Science 1995;267:685–8.
13. Mallo M. Formation of the middle ear: Recent progress on the developmental and molecular mechanisms. Dev Biol 2001;231:410–9.
14. Lohnes D, Mark M, Mendelsohn C, et al. Function of the retinoic acid receptors (RARs) during development (I). Craniofacial and skeletal abnormalities in RAR double mutants. Development 1994;120:2723–48.
15. Morriss-Kay GM, Ward SJ. Retinoids and mammalian development. Int Rev Cytol 1999;188:73–131.
16. Qiu M, Bulfone A, Ghattas I, et al. Role of the Dlx homeobox genes in proximodistal patterning of the branchial arches: Mutations of Dlx-1, Dlx-2, and -2 alter morphogenesis of proximal skeletal and soft tissue structures derived from the first and second arches. Dev Biol 1997;185:165–84.
17. Isaac C, Marsh KL, Paznekas WA, et al. Characterization of the nucleolar gene product, treacle, in Treacher Collins syndrome. Mol Biol Cell 2000;11:3061–71.
18. Meyers GA, Orlow SJ, Munro IR, et al. Fibroblast growth factor receptor 3 (FGFR3) transmembrane mutation in

Crouzon syndrome with acanthosis nigricans. Nat Genet 1995;11:462–4.

19. Reardon W, Wilkes D, Rutland P, et al. Craniosynostosis associated with FGFR3 pro250arg mutation results in a range of clinical presentations including unisutural sporadic craniosynostosis. J Med Genet 1997;34:632–6.

20. Wilkes D, Rutland P, Pulleyn LJ, et al. A recurrent mutation, ala391glu, in the transmembrane region of FGFR3 causes Crouzon syndrome and acanthosis nigricans. J Med Genet 1996;33:744–8.

21. Muenke M, Gripp KW, McDonald-McGinn DM, et al. A unique point mutation in the fibroblast growth factor receptor 3 gene (FGFR3) defines a new craniosynostosis syndrome. Am J Hum Genet 1997;60:555–64.

22. Gong Y, Krakow D, Marcelino J, et al. Heterozygous mutations in the gene encoding noggin affect human joint morphogenesis. Nat Genet 1999;21:302–4.

23. Holley SA, Neul JL, Attisano L, et al. The Xenopus dorsalizing factor noggin ventralizes Drosophila embryos by preventing DPP from activating its receptor. Cell 1996;86:607–17.

24. Pignoni F, Hu B, Zavitz KH, et al. The eye-specification proteins So and Eya form a complex and regulate multiple steps in Drosophila eye development. Cell 1997;91:881–91.

25. Moore KL. The Developing Human. Philadelphia, PA: WB Saunders; 1977. p. 45–80.

26. Schuknecht HF. Developmental Defects. An Pathology of the Ear, 2nd edition. Philadelphia, PA: Lea & Febiger; 1993. p. 115–89.

27. Wu D, Oh S. Sensory organ generation in the chick inner ear. J Neurosci 1995;16:6463–75.

28. Morsli H, Choo D, Ryan A, et al. Development of the mouse inner ear and its sensory organs. J Neurosci 1998;18:3327–35.

29. Kil SH, Collazo A. Origins of inner ear sensory organs revealed by fate map and time-lapse analyses. Dev Biol 2001;233:365–79.

30. Artavonis-Tsakonis S, Matsuno K, Fortini M. Notch signaling. Science 1995;268:225–32.

31. Bray S. Notch signalling in drosophila: Three ways to use a pathway. Semin Cell Dev Biol 1998;9:591–7.

32. Haddon C, Jiang Y, Smithers L, Lewis J. Delta-Notch signalling and the patterning of sensory cell differentiation in the zebra fish ear: Evidence from the mind bomb mutant. Development 1998;125:4637–44.

33. Lanford PJ, Lan Y, Jiang R, et al. Notch signalling pathway mediates hair cell development in mammalian cochlea. Nat Genet 1999;21:289–92.

34. Bermingham NA, Hassan BA, Price SD, et al. Math1: An essential gene for the generation of inner ear hair cells. Science 1999;284:1837–41.

35. D'Amico-Martel A, Noden DM. Contributions of placodal and neural crest cells to avian cranial peripheral ganglia. Am J Anat 1983;166:445–68.

36. Carney PR, Couve E. Cell polarity changes and migration during early development of the avian peripheral auditory system. Anat Rec 1989;225:156–64.

37. Ma Q, Anderson DJ, Fritzsch B. Neurogenin 1 null mutant ears develop fewer, morphologically normal hair cells in smaller sensory epithelia devoid of innervation. J Assoc Res Otolaryngol 2000;1:129–43.

38. Mansour S, Goddard J, Capecchi M. Mice homozygous for a targeted disruption of the proto-oncogene int-2 have developmental defects in the tail and inner ear. Development 1993;117:13–28.

39. Fritzsch B, Pirvola U, Ylikoski J. Making and breaking the innervation of the ear: Neurotrophic support during ear development and its clinical implications. Cell Tissue Res 1999;295:369–82.

40. Fritzsch B, Farinas I, Reichardt LF. Lack of neurotrophin 3 causes losses of both classes of spiral ganglion neurons in the cochlea in a region-specific fashion. J Neurosci 1997;17:6213–25.

41. Silos-Santiago I, Fagan AM, Garber M, et al. Severe sensory deficits but normal CNS development in newborn mice lacking TrkB and TrkC tyrosine protein kinase receptors. Eur J Neurosci 1997;9:2045–56.

42. Steel K, Bussoli T. Deafness genes: Expression of surprise. Trends Genet 1999;15:207–11.

43. Fraser FC, Sproule JR, Halal F. Frequency of the branchio-oto-renal (BOR) syndrome in children with profound hearing loss. Am J Med Genet 1980;7:341–9.

44. Kalatzis V, Sahly I, El-Amraoui A, Petit C. Eya1 expression in the developing ear and kidney: Towards the understanding of the pathogenesis of branchio-oto-renal (BOR) syndrome. Dev Dyn 1998;213:486–99.

45. Everett LA, Morsli H, Wu DK, Green ED. Expression pattern of the mouse ortholog of the Pendred's syndrome gene (Pds) suggests a key role for pendrin in the inner ear. Proc Natl Acad Sci U S A 1999;96:9727–32.

46. Kopp P. Pendred's syndrome: Identification of the genetic defect a century after its recognition. Thyroid 1999;9:65–9.

47. Scott DA, Wang R, Kreman TM, et al. The Pendred syndrome gene encodes a chloride-iodide transport protein. Nat Genet 1999;21:440–3.

48. Li XC, Everett LA, Lalwani AK, et al. A mutation in PDS causes non-syndromic recessive deafness. Nat Genet 1998;18:215–7.

49. Everett LA, Belyantseva IA, Noben-Trauth K, et al. Targeted disruption of mouse Pds provides insight about the inner-ear defects encountered in Pendred syndrome. Hum Mol Genet 2001;10:153–61.

50. Phippard D, Lu L, Lee D, et al. Targeted mutagenesis of the POU-domain gene Brn4/Pou3f4 causes developmental defects in the inner ear. J Neurosci 1999;19:5980–9.

51. Minowa O, Ikeda K, Sugitani Y, et al. Altered cochlear fibrocytes in a mouse model of DFN3 nonsyndromic deafness. Science 1999;285:1408–11.

3

Molecular Biology of Hearing and Balance

Joni K. Doherty, MD, PhD
Rick A. Friedman, MD, PhD

Our working knowledge of the inner ear at the molecular level has been attained through analyses of mutations that result in hearing and balance dysfunction. Investigation of a particular mutation to determine its genomic location and gene product can provide vast information in terms of inner ear molecular mechanisms. Genetic mutations affecting the inner ear are being intensely studied in both humans and animal models, resulting in an exponential increase in our understanding of the molecular biology of the middle and inner ear.

MOLECULAR METHODOLOGY

Molecular biology has been used to address many basic science questions in otology. In many cases, the potential exists for such studies to influence clinical care, currently and in the future. An exhaustive discussion of molecular techniques is beyond the scope of this chapter, but a brief discussion follows. During the 1980s, advances in molecular genetic technology led to a rapidly progressive increase in the number of molecular markers that facilitate linkage analysis. These markers are polymorphisms, which are variations in the genetic code between individuals. They can be silent, in terms of encoding the protein sequence, depending on their location, that is, at the third position of a codon, or can result in amino acid substitution, which is sometimes inconsequential to protein function. Because differences in sequence can alter restriction enzyme cleavage sites, they can define genetic locations and have enabled scientists to identify the approximate location of inherited mutations.

The first requirement for linkage analysis is a large family with an inherited defect, such as hearing loss. The second requirement is to identify useful deoxyribonucleic acid (DNA) markers that differ in individuals with versus without the disease phenotype, in order to establish linkage. The Human Genome Project has facilitated identification of useful DNA markers that can be used in screening. Once the location is identified, DNA within that chromosomal location is cloned and functionally analyzed, termed positional cloning. Positional cloning refers to identifying a gene by its location first, and then determining its function by expression analyses.

Advancements in gene cloning techniques, such as use of the polymerase chain reaction (PCR) to amplify, that is, produce many copies, a gene of interest and incorporate DNA cleavage sites that facilitate cloning, have facilitated expression and functional analyses. The PCR can be combined with a reverse transcription reaction (RT-PCR) to target and amplify sequences that are expressed in a single cell, such as an inner hair cell. These single cells can be laser-microdissected and subjected to RT-PCR using an oligo-dT primer that amplifies messenger ribonucleic acid (mRNA) selectively, since it targets the poly-A tail.[1]

Typically, cloning via PCR initially involves isolation of mRNA from a tissue of interest and construction of complementary DNA (cDNA) from this mRNA using a reverse transcriptase enzyme adapted from viruses (Figure 1) in a thermal cycling reaction, including a series of repeating denaturing steps, annealing steps, and elongation steps in sequence. An expression library can then be created by incorporating cleavage sequences at both ends of the cDNA via PCR. Screening of such expression libraries from isolated inner ear tissues has been a powerful tool to facilitate identification of genes that are important in those tissues. Genes can then be expressed in biologic systems, from bacteria to mammals, to determine their expression pattern, subcellular location, structure, and function (see http://www.genexpression.info). Indeed, much of the developmental and functional information we have obtained thus far has been from animal studies. Herein, we will review the biology of middle ear and inner ear at the molecular level, as it pertains to human diseases and disorders. We will begin by reviewing what is known about middle ear pathology and otitis media, and a discussion of the knowledge of the inner ear molecular mechanisms subserving specific functions will follow.

MOLECULAR PATHOGENESIS OF OTITIS MEDIA

Otitis media (OM) is a common cause of hearing loss worldwide. OM with effusion causes conductive hearing loss and can contribute to delayed speech development in children. Chronic OM can lead to conductive hearing loss and even sensorineural hearing loss, particularly if cholesteatoma erodes the labyrinth. Advances in diagnosis, research, and potential treatments for middle ear (ME) disease involve molecular biology as well. OM susceptibility has been shown to be genetically mediated.[2] The PCR has been instrumental in identifying microbes involved in OM, and quantitative PCR is utilized to measure middle ear responses to OM via cytokine production.[3,4] Immunoregulation has also been investigated using in situ hybridization and implantation of genetically modified microbes.[5,6]

Cloning bacterial genes has facilitated production of genetically engineered bacteria, including gene alterations or deletions, to investigate host interactions, virulence factors, and immunogenicity. These genetically altered bacteria can also be used to create vaccines. Host defense mechanisms are being studied via transgenic and knockout animal models.

Bacterial Adherence Factors in Otitis Media

The exact mechanisms by which bacteria attach to the mucosal surface of the ME are incompletely understood but likely involve receptor ligand-mediated interactions. The host receptor for *Streptococcus pneumoniae* is known to be Glc Nac1-3Gal,[2] yet the receptor for nontypable *Haemophilus influenza* (NTHi) is uncharacterized. While the receptor is yet to be identified, ligands include pilin (both 22 kD and 27.5 LKP1 kD, depending on serotype), a subunit of the surface appendage pilus that mediates hemagglutination,[7,8] and fimbrin (36.4 kD), a subunit of the surface appendage fimbria that is thinner than pilus and nonhemagglutinating.[8–10] Expression of the gene that encodes 27.5 kD LKP1 pilin in *Escherichia coli* mediates bacterial binding to the buccal mucosal surface and hemagglutination.[8] However, less than 5% of middle ear isolates expressed pili; therefore, their role in the pathogenesis of OM is unclear.[11] Conversely, 100% of NTHi isolates from chronic ME effusion were fimbriated.[12] Other potential ligands include high-molecular-weight outer membrane proteins (OMPs) (120 kD HMW-1 and HMW-2),[13] which may facilitate binding of bacteria to the epithelial cell surface. OMPs show significant sequence homology with fimbrin. Disruption of the fimbrin gene resulted in decreased virulence and lack of adherence to the epithelial cell surface in vitro.[10]

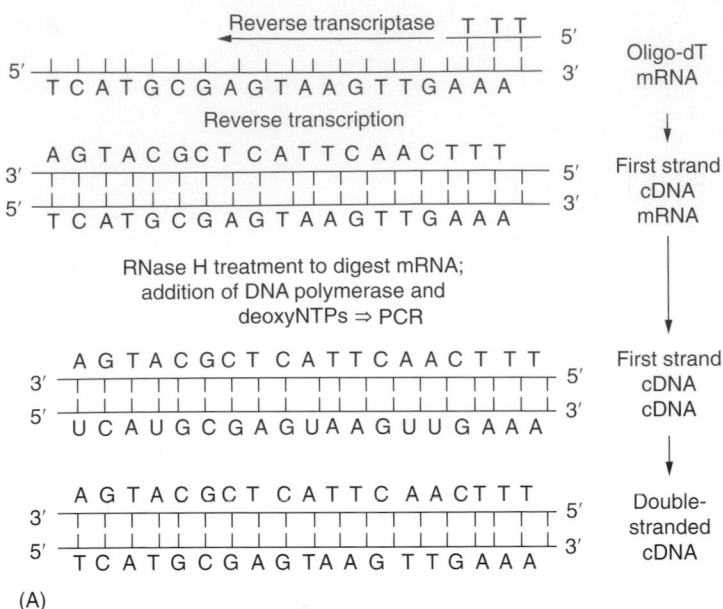

(A)

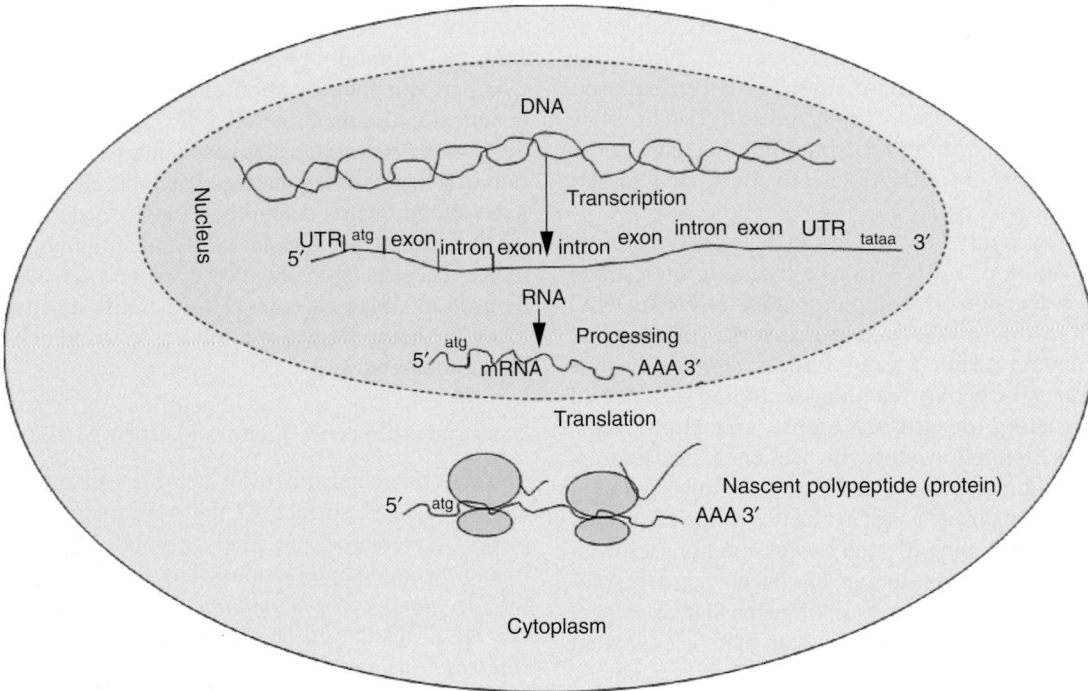

(B)

Figure 1 (A) Schematic illustration of gene expression in a cell. Nuclear DNA is transcribed into RNA, which is processed into mRNA via removal of intervening (intron) sequences and polyadenylation of the 3′ end. This mRNA is then transported out of the nucleus into the endoplasmic reticulum, where ribosomes are abundant (not shown). Multiple ribosomes translate a single mRNA strand into multiple proteins. Several factors regulate the amount of gene expression in terms of mRNA transcript and protein produced, including DNA promoter sequences, enhancer and modifier sites, mRNA transcript stability, and the affinity for ribosome binding to the 5′ untranslated (UTR) sequence upstream of the start codon (ATG). Additionally, RNA molecules form secondary structures, which can affect their processing and subsequent translation rate. (B) Schematic illustration of complementary deoxyribonucleic acid (cDNA) synthesis via reverse transcription-polymerase chain reaction (RT-PCR) method. Messenger ribonucleic acid (mRNA) isolated from a tissue or cell type of interest represents the expression array of genes for the particular tissue or cell type, for example, auditory hair cell. A virally derived reverse transcriptase enzyme "copies" this mRNA molecule into a complementary cDNA, and RNase H then digests the RNA and a DNA polymerase can replicate the cDNA molecules.

Virulence Factors in Otitis Media

Endotoxin is an important mediator in OM,[14] and type b *Haemophilus influenzae* displays phase variation of the endotoxin lipo-oligosaccharide (LOS), which allows it to switch expression from one of the two stable genotypes.[15] Phase variation of endotoxin expression is, in itself, a virulence factor and involves three *lic* genes, that enable a number of different LOS structures to be produced from a limited set of genes.[15,16] Loss of phase variation by gene inactivation affected the ability of *H. influenzae* to invade the bloodstream from respiratory epithelium.

Pneumolysin and autolysin are two pneumococcal proteins that contribute to the virulence of *S. pneumoniae*.[17] Insertional mutagenesis of the gene in *S. pneumoniae* resulted in decreased survival time intraperitoneally. Mouse studies with pneumococcal challenge have demonstrated that the role of autolysin appears to be in mediating release of pneumolysin from pneumococcal cytoplasm.[18]

Middle Ear Mucosal Response to Otitis Media

The ME mucosa has the unique capacity for hyperplasia in response to inflammation, as opposed to other mucosal surfaces within the aerodigestive tract. Normally, a simple cuboidal mucosa lines the ME. However, this can differentiate into a respiratory-type pseudocolumnar ciliated epithelium with goblet cells. Additionally, these cells undergo proliferation. What regulates these pathophysiologic processes is the topic of intense research aimed at improving treatment for acute and chronic OM.

Growth Factor and Cytokine Signaling

Extracellular growth factors bind and activate transmembrane receptors at the cell surface that induce intracellular signal transduction, initiating physiologic and pathophysiologic processes. RT-PCR has been utilized to investigate the expression of vascular endothelial growth factors (VEGFs) and their receptors, which are essential signaling molecules for angiogenesis. Oehl and Ryan found upregulation of several forms in rat ME mucosa following bacterial inoculation.[19] Angiogenic growth factors and their receptors were also identified in cholesteatoma.[20] Immunocytochemistry techniques have demonstrated expression of epidermal growth factor (EGF), fibroblast growth factor (FGF), platelet-derived growth factor, and keratinocyte growth factor.[21,22] Downstream intracellular signaling molecules involved in the process appear to include ras, *c*-jun, and p53.[21,23] Evidence for integrin signaling is suggested by the finding of increased tenascin in cholesteatoma keratinocytes,[24] and this molecule is involved with growth factor receptor cross talk signaling as well. Known downstream signaling effectors, including mitogen-activated protein (MAP) kinases have been investigated with respect to OM. Mucin upregulation induced by *H. influenzae* inoculation involves activation of a Rac-dependent MEKK-SEK-p38 MAP kinase pathway.[25] Additionally, radical oxygen species (ROS) may be involved in the inflammatory response via activation of p38 MAP kinase, leading to mucin transcription.[26] Mucin is a high-molecular-weight glycoprotein that is the major component of mucus. Overproduction of mucus in OM with effusion contributes to defective mucociliary clearance and recurrent infection and causes conductive hearing loss. Human ME epithelial cells express mucin from the *MUC1*, *MUC2*, *MUC5AC*, *MUC5B*, *MUC7*, and *MUC8* mucin genes.[27–29] The proinflammatory cytokine, tumor necrosis factor-alpha (TNF-α), induces upregulation of mucin in rat ME mucosa.[27]

Proinflammatory transcriptional regulation is also evident in upregulation of cytokines via nuclear factor kappa B (NF-κB). Proinflammatory cytokines, such as interleukins, are upregulated in response to ME inoculation. Their expression is induced rapidly, peaking at 6 hours, and declines by 24 hours following inoculation.[30] Interleukin-1 (IL-1) leads to downregulation of surfactant expression in the ME,[31] possibly contributing to contraction of the ME space with negative ME pressure, as is observed in early acute and in chronic OM. Conversely, anti-inflammatory and immunoregulatory cytokines are induced over a longer time course, lasting up to weeks after inoculation.[32,33] Nitric oxide (NO) synthesis is also increased, particularly in ME effusion.[34]

Host Defenses Against Otitis Media

Innate immunity defends tissues of the aerodigestive tract against microbial invasion. Epithelial cells lining the ME, eustachian tube, and nasopharyngeal tract express antimicrobial peptides, including lytic enzymes, defensins, lysozyme, lactoferrin, and collectins.[35] Defensins have broad-spectrum antimicrobial activity against bacteria, fungi, and even some enveloped viruses.[36] Human β-defensins 1 and 2 (HBD-1, HBD-2) are expressed in ME epithelium following contact with microorganisms or cytokine stimulation, and HBD-1 and 2 exhibit potent activity against gram-negative bacteria and candida but less activity against gram positives, such as *Staphylococcus aureus*.[37,38]

Lysozyme is another important molecule involved in innate immunity. It is produced in secretory cells of the mucosal epithelium and is increased in ME effusions. Polymorphonuclear leukocytes and macrophages also express lysozyme as an antimicrobial enzyme, and lysozyme is a component of human breast milk that exhibits anti-NTHi activity.[35]

Lactoferrin, an iron-binding glycoprotein detected in ME effusions, is also found in breast milk, secreted by exocrine glands, and released from neutrophilic granules during inflammation.[39] Lactoferrin secretion has been localized to the serous cells of eustachian tube glands,[40] and in the cuboidal and transitional cells of ME mucosal epithelium.[41]

Collectins are structurally and functionally related to complement protein C1q, the first component of the classic complement pathway. Collectins are thought to enable innate immunity via opsonization and complement activation.[42] Surfactant proteins A and D, classified as collectins, are expressed in the ME and eustachian tube, where they are likely involved in protection against OM pathogens, particularly in the tubotympanum.[35]

Otitis Media Pathogens: Antibiotic Resistance

Bacterial resistance is primarily enzymatic. The mechanism of ampicillin resistance is β-lactamase production, encoded within a large gene segment called transposon A,[43] mediated by alterations in bacterial penicillin-binding proteins (PBPs).[44,45]

The basis for *H. influenzae* type b resistance to chloramphenicol is largely due to acetyltransferase expression from a gene that is also located within a transposon.[46] Trimethoprin resistance results from overproduction of dihydrofolate reductase via chromosomal rearrangement.[47]

Vaccine Development in Otitis Media

Knowledge of the factors that mediate virulence and adhesion has enabled scientists to develop vaccines against these bacteria. The nucleotide sequence information and expression of several OMPs have facilitated the identification of domains that are conserved across strains. Together with mapping of epitope molecules, this has provided structural and functional information, which is critical in selecting antigens for vaccine development. Monoclonal antibody production against the OMP P26 is an example of utilizing this information for vaccine development, since scientists were able to identify the sequence of the region of P26 that conferred bactericidal antibody production by inoculation in a polyclonal model.[48] Pilin and fimbrin are also good candidates since antibodies directed at these proteins can prevent adhesion and reduce colonization and infection.[10,11]

Viral upper respiratory infections often precede OM, and PCR data confirmed that a significant number of ME effusions contained upper respiratory viruses.[49] In a chinchilla model, vaccination with attenuated influenza virus prevented pneumococcal OM after inoculation, indicating that the viral vaccine protected the animal from bacterial infection.[50] Clinical trials to that effect in children have been performed in Finland with promising results. However, viral vaccines are prone to being ineffective since they utilize surface antigens and viruses' surface proteins evolve rapidly and evade the host immune system. Use of interior viral proteins or viral DNA as vaccines may prove to be a more promising long-term solution.

Future Directions: Middle Ear Mucosa Gene Transfer

FGF-1 secreting ME mucosal cells have been successfully engineered via stable transfection and implanted into the subepithelial compartment.[6] Adenoviral vector transduction is another method of inducing expression of a transgene that has been successful in the rat neonatal and guinea pig ME.[51,52]

TECHNIQUES FOR THE IDENTIFICATION OF GENES INVOLVED IN HEARING AND BALANCE

The recent development of thousands of molecular tags for specific locations in the genome has dramatically enhanced the ability to link inherited disorders to their specific chromosomal location via recombination frequency analysis. When combined with information from prior localization studies of candidate genes or related animal mutations in the same chromosomal region, such linkage analysis has enabled the characterization of an increasing number of mutations that cause disorders of hearing. Well over 100 deafness loci have been identified to date. Our knowledge of the identity and function of these genes has grown almost exponentially over the last decade. Today, more than 10 genetic mutations leading to congenital hearing loss can be identified with genetic testing (http://www.genetests.com). This increased diagnostic capability has improved our ability to provide genetic counseling and, in the future, may lead to gene therapy for aural diseases. Gene identification also allows for investigation of function via animal studies utilizing homologous gene mutations, which can be genetically engineered.

The study of mouse genetics has been indispensable in terms of advancing knowledge about human development and disorders. Creating homologous mutations in experimental mouse models enables us to determine the function of genes mutated in human disorders. Techniques for developing animal models include creating transgenic animals, insertional mutagenesis, and site-directed mutagenesis.

Transgenic Animals

Insertion of a synthesized gene into the genome of a normal mouse embryo can result in the production of a transgenic mouse. The artificial gene is composed of a tissue-specific promoter sequence linked to the sequence coding for the protein of interest. This construct is then inserted into the fertilized mouse embryo through various means, including physical injection or retroviral transfection. If the transgene inserts into the genomic DNA and if the embryo survives, the adult mouse will pass the gene on to future generations (Figure 2). In any transgenic animal, if there are cells that express a transcription factor that interacts with the promoter, the gene product will be expressed in these cells and may affect their function.

Insertional Mutagenesis

In a small percentage of the offspring of transgenic animals, the transgene will be randomly inserted into another gene in the genome, resulting in a mutation and a phenotype change in the animal. This process is termed as insertional mutagenesis. The position of the mutated gene is now marked by the transgene, which can facilitate its localization and identification.

Site-Directed Mutagenesis

Site-directed mutagenesis or gene targeting relies on the process of insertional mutagenesis. Basically, a mutant gene that confers antibiotic resistance and disrupts expression of a normal protein is flanked by sequences of a gene to be disrupted, and then it is inserted into an embryonic stem cell (Figure 3). The cultured cell then divides, and through homologous recombination,

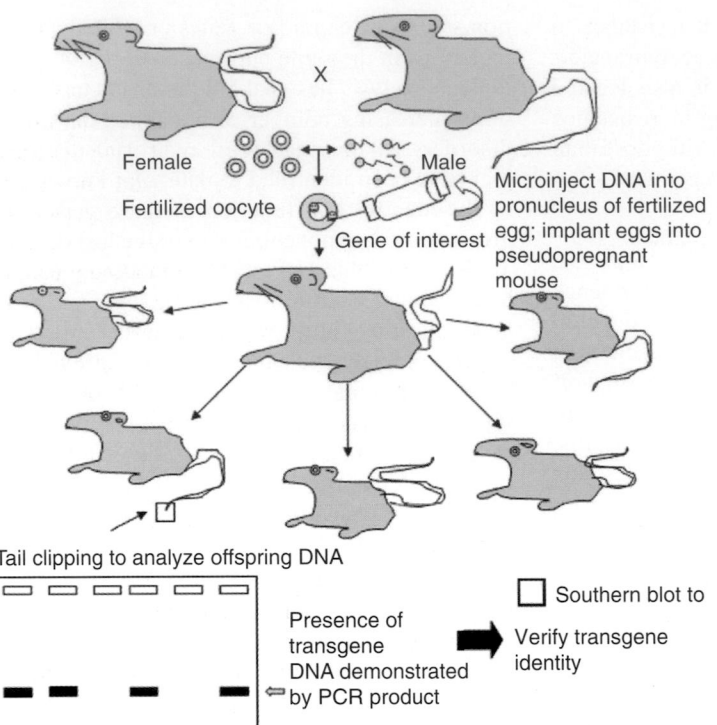

Female
Fertilized oocyte
Male

Microinject DNA into pronucleus of fertilized egg; implant eggs into pseudopregnant mouse

Gene of interest

Tail clipping to analyze offspring DNA

Presence of transgene DNA demonstrated by PCR product

☐ Southern blot to

Verify transgene identity

Figure 2 Schematic illustration transgenic mice production using the microinjection technique. Utilizing a promoter that normally directs routine gene expression in the tissue of interest, a transgene is constructed with the gene sequence to be studied and a termination sequence. Fertilized eggs are collected from the mated female, and the transgene is injected into one of the pronuclei. The injected eggs are implanted in a surrogate mother, in a pseudopregnant hormonal state. Offspring are assessed for transgene expression by PCR analysis of a tail clipping. The PCR products represent fragments of DNA incorporating the transgene or not, and the identity is verified via Southern blotting.

targeted insertional mutagenesis occurs and simultaneously results in both gene deletion and antibiotic resistance in some of the progeny cells (Figure 3C). The progeny cells are then selected for antibiotic resistance and inserted into a blastocyst, which is then implanted into the uterus of a mouse (Figure 3D). The resulting offspring mice are chimeric, and subsequent breeding of the mice in which the germline is affected will eventually generate some homozygous mutants if the mutation is not lethal. This method was used by Mansour and colleagues to generate mice with a mutation in the *int-2* gene, which encodes fibroblast growth factor 3 (FGF-3).[53] Prior to production of this mutant mouse, Represa and colleagues had shown that disruption of *int-2* expression in vitro prevented inner ear development.[54] The mutant mice created by Mansour and colleagues, however, had normal induction of the inner ear despite having decreased FGF-3 production, suggesting the existence of a redundant pathway for induction. Interestingly, these mice did have hearing and vestibular defects that correlated with multiple inner ear abnormalities, indicating that such an alternative pathway is inadequate for compensation of the defect and still results in aberrant development.

An alternative method for studying gene expression and function is the analysis of mutant mice with hearing and balance defects. This has also facilitated our current understanding of inner ear development. The process of inner ear development is governed by complex gene interactions, which regulate a series of ontogenetic events. Generally, mutations in genes that play a role early in otocyst induction and patterning result in gross malformations, while mutations in genes expressed later tend to result in subtle inner ear structural abnormalities, often limited to discreet elements of the sensory neuroepithelium

or dysregulation of inner ear homeostasis. Thus, phenotypic abnormalities can be used to predict the stage of development at which a particular gene is expressed. Some genes, however, display overlap in their developmental roles, such as those encoding *Delta* and *Jagged*—the Notch receptor ligands, as discussed below.[55]

Additionally, subtractive hybridization technique, using chicken embryos, has led to the rapid identification of several inner ear genes that are expressed during development as unique inner ear proteins. Among them are otoancorin, ß-tectorin, calbindin, type II collagen, and connexins.[56] Such genes are potential candidates for deafness genes based on their temporal expression, and several have subsequently been identified in humans in association with hereditary deafness.

Microarray Technology

Thousands of genes and their protein products are essential to the finely coordinated process of mammalian inner ear development and function. The study of the genetics of mammalian development and disease has relied upon the single gene methodological approach. This is a low throughput analysis that provides a finite look at the complex cascade of genetic events. Scientists have thus far been limited in their ability to see the genetic "big picture." A new technology has emerged, DNA microarray, and it is providing scientists with a means to scan the entire genome, on a single chip. This is opening the door to the discovery of the combinatorial genetic interactions that lead to the generation of an organ as complex as the inner ear.

A microarray is an ordered arrangement of DNA samples that, based upon complementary base pairing, provides a platform for matching defined and, as yet, undefined DNA samples. Microarrays consist of thousands of sample spots

(200 µm or less in diameter) linked to a particular medium (glass or nylon membranes). The use and analysis of microarrays requires highly specialized robotics and imaging systems. Each of these spots can be simultaneously probed by a known sequence, and through complementary base–pair interactions, these arrays provide an extremely high-throughput gene identification and or expression studies.

In general, microarrays can be found in two different varieties. In one, small fragments of cDNA are immobilized onto a solid surface (glass) and are exposed to a specific target allowing massive gene expression studies to occur in parallel. For example, variations in gene expression in a tissue of interest after delivery of a new drug can be studied using this technology. Similarly, the analysis of gene expression in a particular mutant mouse strain can be compared to the normal for a given tissue, giving insights into the developmental role played by the mutant gene in a particular process.

The other type of array involves the placement of oligonucleotide or peptide nucleic acid probes. These arrays are hybridized by a labeled DNA sample, and the abundance of complementary sequences is ascertained. This technology has become very useful for genetic testing. A "gene chip" can be created such that oligonucleotides associated with a particular mutation can be identified rapidly in at risk individuals. The state-of-the-art chips have opened a new era in human genetics. With the ability to scan the entire genome for single nucleotide polymorphisms (SNPs) across experimental and control cohorts, high-resolution genetic association studies are now possible (http://www.gene-chips.com/).

RNA Interference

RNA interference (also called "RNA-mediated interference," abbreviated RNAi) is a mechanism for RNA-guided regulation of gene expression in which double-stranded ribonucleic acid (dsRNA) inhibits the expression of genes with complementary nucleotide sequences. Conserved in most eukaryotic organisms, the RNAi pathway is thought to have developed as a form of innate immunity against viruses and also plays a major role in regulating development and genome maintenance.

The RNAi pathway is initiated by the enzyme dicer, which cleaves dsRNA to short double-stranded fragments of 20 to 25 base pairs. One of the two strands of each fragment, known as the *guide strand*, is then incorporated into the RNA-induced silencing complex (RISC) and base pairs with complementary sequences. The most well-studied outcome of this recognition event is a form of posttranscriptional gene silencing. This occurs when the guide strand base pairs with a mRNA molecule and induces degradation of the mRNA by argonaute, the catalytic component of the RISC complex. The short RNA fragments are known as small interfering RNA (siRNA) when they derive from exogenous

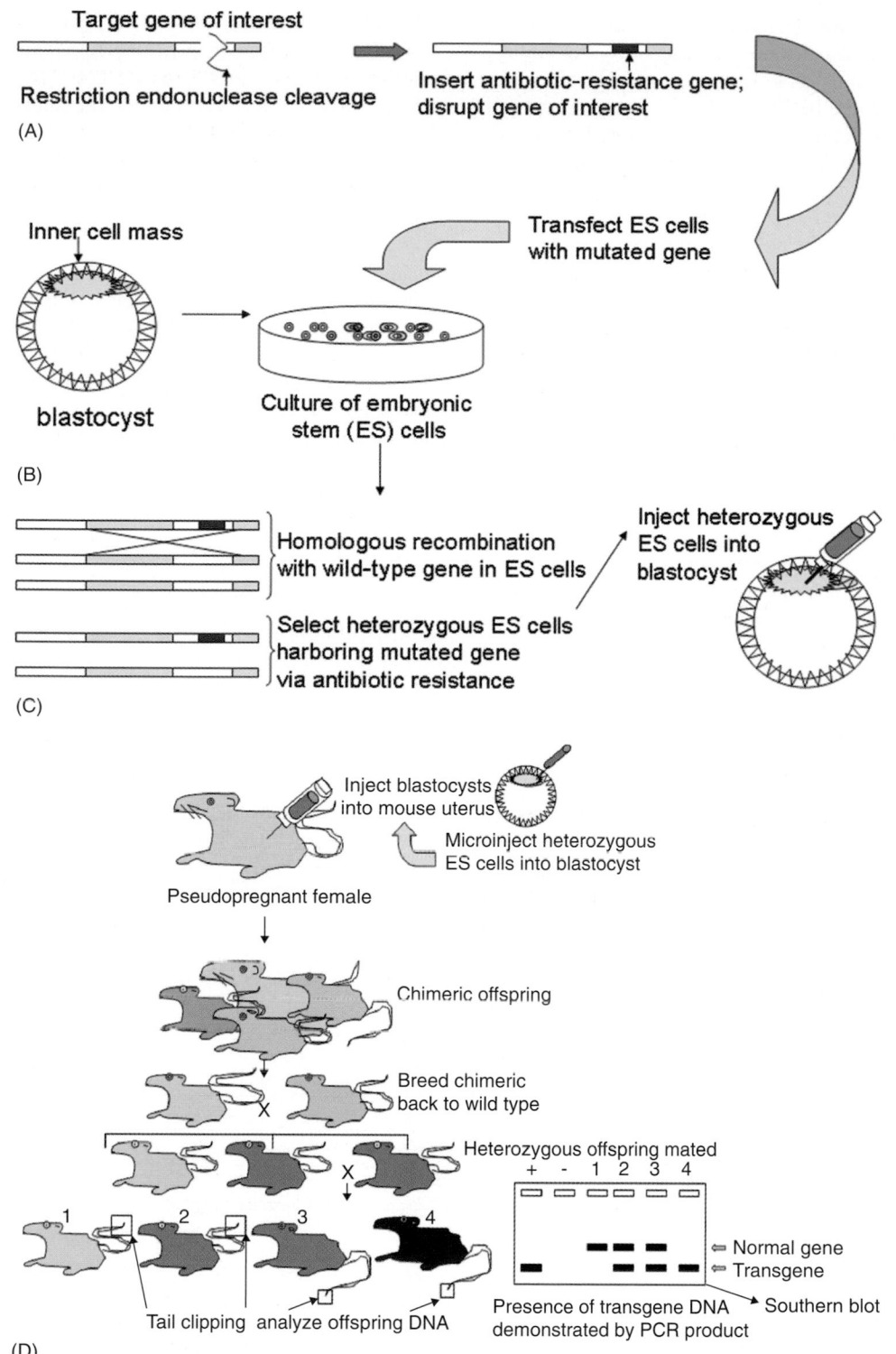

and will no doubt be applied to diseases affecting the head and neck region.

Two nucleotides overhang at each 3′ end with a 5′-phosphate moiety and a 3′-hydroxyl group characterize these small double-stranded RNAs. siRNAs can be constructed and transfected into mammalian cells allowing precise genetic interference or gene knock-down experiments. A limitation of siRNAs is their transient effects. Advances in recombinant technology now allow placement of a siRNA construct into an expression plasmid leading to longer half-lives.

As with any biological tool, siRNA studies present some challenges. These small RNA species may interact with a number of other cellular pathways leading to undesired or uncontrollable effects. Additionally, off-targeting, the process by which other, incompletely homologous sequences can be targeted, may lead to erroneous outcomes. Furthermore, in mammalian cells, siRNAs can induce an innate immune response if mistakenly recognized as a by-product of a double-stranded RNA virus.

Despite these challenges, RNAi and gene knock-down experiments are being successfully used in large-scale screens to define genetic pathways of disease and in therapeutic trials (http://www.nature.com/nature/journal/v431/n7006/full/nature02870.html).

INNER EAR DEVELOPMENT

The inner ear is a highly complex yet ordered structure in which induction and differentiation initiate the process of development, and maturation completes it. Studying gene expression during development in animal models has enabled identification of essential factors in each stage of inner ear development. Additionally, some of these observations have potential clinical implications.

Transcription Factors

The otic placode, which develops as an ectodermal thickening of either side of the neural plate in the hindbrain of mice at embryonic day 8.8 (E8.5), gives rise to all of the inner ear structures and cell types, except melanocytes and Schwann cells.[57] Transcription factor gene expression is thought to specify the patterning of inner ear development at this crucial stage.[58] Essential genes at this early stage that have been described include *Pax2*, *Hmx3*, *Hoxa1*, retinoic acid receptor (*RAR*), and *NeuroD1*.

***Otx1* and *Prx1/Prx2* Genes.** The horizontal semicircular canal is absent in *Otx1* mutants and in double mutants of *Prx1* and *Prx2*.[59] Targeted deletion of *Otx1* results in normal development of the cochlea and all other vestibular structures, while in double mutants of *Prx1/2*, the other semicircular canals are delayed in development.

***Pax* Gene.** Disruption of the *Pax* gene in mice results in cochlear agenesis with absence of the spiral ganglion, while the vestibular apparatus is unaffected.[60,61] *Pax3*, or paired box DNA-binding

Figure 3 Schematic illustration of (gene) targeting for construction of knockouts. (A) Embryonic stem (ES) cells are isolated from a blastocyst and cultured. (B) A gene-targeting molecule (plasmid) is constructed utilizing endogenous restriction endonuclease sequences/sites within the gene of interest to insert a sequence containing an antibiotic resistance gene, and this is transfected into ES cells. (C) ES cells undergo homologous recombination with the synthetic DNA, thus disrupting one copy of the gene of interest and conferring antibiotic resistance. Antibiotic-resistant cells are then selected and injected into a blastocyst, which is injected into a pseudo-pregnant mouse. (D) Chimeric offspring result and are back breeded to wild-type mouse to result in some heterozygotes (with respect to the knockout gene). Heterozygous mice are breeded to obtain a homozygous knockout mouse, which may be lethal.

sources and microRNA (miRNA) when they are produced from RNA-coding genes in the cell's own genome. The RNAi pathway has been particularly well studied in certain model organisms such as the nematode worm *Caenorhabditis elegans*, the fruit fly *Drosophila melanogaster*, and the flowering plant *Arabidopsis thaliana*.

The selective and robust effect of RNAi on gene expression makes it a valuable research tool, both in cell culture and in living organisms; synthetic dsRNA introduced into cells can induce suppression of specific genes of interest. RNAi may also be used for large-scale screens that systematically shut down each gene in the cell, which can help identify the components necessary for a particular cellular process or an event such as cell division. Exploitation of the pathway is also a promising tool in biotechnology and medicine, protein 3, encodes a transcription factor essential for proper migration of melanocytes and organization of the stria vascularis, and, thus, appears to play an essential role in endolymph production. *PAX3*, the human homologue, is mutated in Waardenburg syndrome type I (WS-I).

***Hmx3* Gene.** *Hmx3* is expressed in the inner ear as well as in the second branchial arch. Targeted deletion of *Hmx3* results in vestibular dysgenesis.[58] *Hmx3* appears to play a role in separation of the utricular and saccular maculae and development of the semicircular canals. The sensory organ within the horizontal semicircular canal is absent in *Hmx3* mutants.

***RAR* Genes.** Three genes encode RAR subtypes α, β, and γ that are expressed in the mouse embryonic inner ear and are important in otocyst development.[62,63] These RARs bind all trans retinoic acid, the major biologically active metabolite of vitamin A, as ligand and are activated to then bind retinoic acid response elements of target genes.

One such gene, which encodes bone morphogenic protein 4 (BMP4), plays a role in patterning of the semicircular canals (SCC). BMP4 downregulation by retinoic acid, mediated by RAR action at a promoter site of the second intron of the *BMP4* gene, affects SCC formation.[64]

Other genes involved in the retinoic acid signaling pathways are also essential, such as the mouse gene *Hoxa1*, a homeobox gene that is a putative downstream target of RAR.[65] Mutations in RAR-α and RAR-γ, together, result in severe vestibular and cochlear malformations which are similar to *Hoxa1*-deficient mice. *Hoxa1* mutants display inner ear dysmorphogenesis with variable defects in the vestibular and cochlear components. Although RARs are widely expressed in the mouse inner ear, phenotypic defects are not displayed unless two or more receptors are absent, as in compound null mutants.[66] This fact underscores the redundancy of such receptor isoforms.

Furthermore, RNA-encoding RAR-β has been found in the inner ear of embryonic mice.[67] In addition, when exposed to retinoic acid in vitro, embryonic supporting cells show premature differentiation into hair cells.[54] Retinoic acid or similar growth factors could thus eventually play a role in hair cell regeneration.

***BETA2/NeuroD1* Gene.** A basic helix-loop-helix transcription factor (bHLH TF) that is expressed in many cell types during development of the mammalian central nervous system is *BETA2/NeuroD1*. Its role in the inner ear is essential in that knockouts are deaf and have balance disorders, displayed by head tilting and circling.[68] Null mutations result in severely reduced numbers of cochlear and vestibular ganglion (CVG) cells in mice due to apoptosis after differentiation therefore, the role of *BETA2/NeuroD1* appears to be in CVG cell survival. Additionally, mutants have defects in cochlear duct differentiation and patterning, sensory epithelium, and dorsal cochlear nucleus cells.

***Math1* Gene.** Determination of auditory and vestibular hair cell fate is an early event in embryogenesis and has not been completely elucidated. In mice, the bHLH TF *Math1*, is expressed early in hair cell (HC) differentiation and *Math1* knockouts fail to develop HCs.[69] However, the fact that *Math1* is expressed in several cell lineages suggests that its role is contributory and essential but that it does not act alone in determining HC fate. It is likely that combinatorial coding in TF regulation of gene expression occurs as a unique process in specifying cell type and initiating differentiation.[70]

***POU-Domain* Genes.** At least two of the three members of the *Brn-3* subfamily of POU-domain regulatory *RF* genes also play a key role in auditory and vestibular sensory neuron development. The Brn-3.0 (or Brn-3a) and Brn-3.2 (or Brn-3b) proteins are expressed in some spiral ganglion and Scarpa ganglion cells. The Brn-3.1 (or Brn-3c) protein is essential for auditory and vestibular HC development and appears to function downstream of *Math1*. Brn-3.1 knockout mice are deaf and have impaired balance function due to absence of sensory HCs.[71,72] Localization studies in mice embryos have shown that *Brn-3.1* is expressed early in HC lineage after fate is determined but before HC morphology is distinguishable, and high-level expression continues throughout HC life. *Brn-3.1* knockouts display normal migration of HC precursors, but HCs degenerate and undergo apoptosis by embryonic day 18 in mice.[73] The human homologues are *POU4F3* and *POU3F4*, mutations of which lead to late-onset progressive nonsyndromic sensorineural hearing loss (SNHL). The *POU4F3* transcription factor may play a dual role. While the mouse homologue *Pou4f3* determines late hair cell differentiation, and mutations lead to hair cell death prior to complete differentiation, the human *POU4F3* is a dominant deafness gene (DFNA15), inducing adult-onset hearing loss. Thus, *POU4F3* may play a role in long-term HC survival in the human, but its role is clearly distinct from that in mice.[74]

SENSORY CELL DIFFERENTIATION AND DEVELOPMENT

Differentiation and development of the organ of Corti in mice arises from the "zone of nonproliferating cells" (ZNPC), induced by a synchronous exit from the cell cycle promoted by the cyclin-dependent kinase inhibitor p27 kip1.[75] Cell-cycle exit also seems to depend upon expression of *Notch1* and its ligand, *Jagged1*, which may define boundaries and patterning of sensory cell development in the cochlea,[75] since *Jagged1* and *Notch* mutants display abnormal patterning of the cochlea.[55,76]

Sensory cell fate determination is orchestrated by Notch-Delta signaling via lateral inhibition, which results in precise patterning of sensory neuroepithelia of the cochlea and vestibular apparatus. The website, http://www.ihr.mrc. ac.uk, provides a table of genes expressed in mice and humans during inner ear development.

Myosins in Inner Ear Development

The mouse mutant Shaker-2 carries a *Myosin XV* mutation, for which the homologous human deafness gene is *DFNB3*, which results in shortened stereocilia.[77] Myosin XVa localizes to the tips of stereocilia of the cochlear and vestibular hair cells, overlaps with the barbed ends of actin filaments, and extends into the apical plasma membrane. Myosin XVa is essential for the graded elongation of stereocilia in formation of the characteristic staircase pattern of the hair bundle[78] (Figure 4).

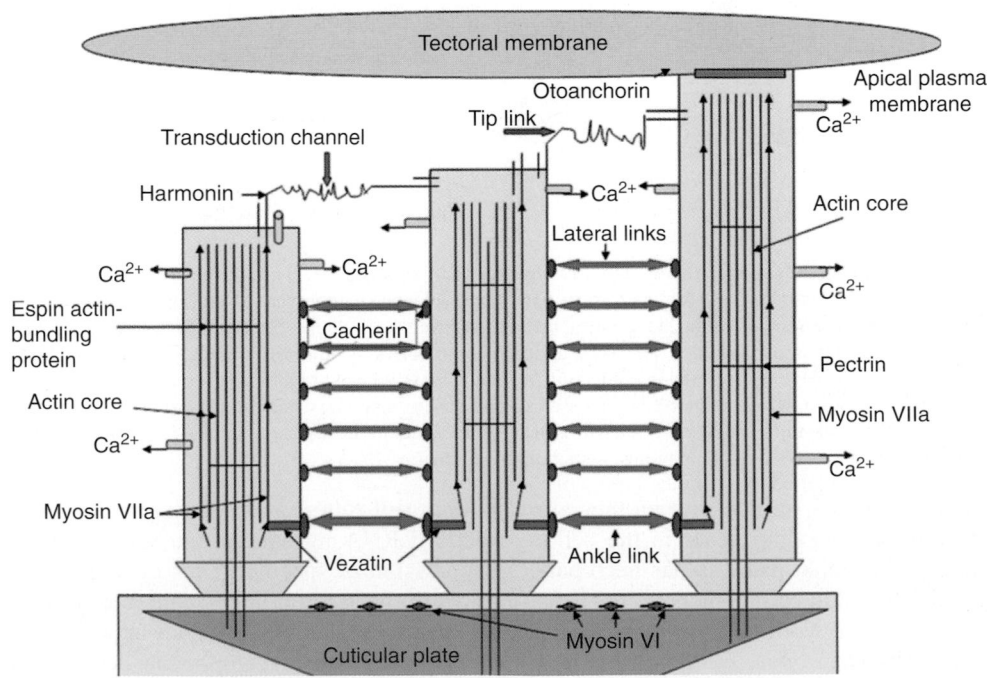

Figure 4 Schematic illustration of the top of an auditory hair cell with cilia attached to the cuticular plate and embedded in the tectorial membrane. This view illustrates some of the tip link molecules involved in regulating hair cell response to shearing forces, thus transducing mechanical energy into electroacoustical energy.

A *Myosin VI* null mutation causes the mouse mutant Snell waltzer, which displays fusion of the stereocilia at birth and subsequent hair cell degeneration. These findings, combined with immunofluorescence and electron microscopy studies, revealed the function of myosin VI as an anchor between the cuticular plate of stereocilia and the apical membrane of hair cells[79] (Figure 4).

Growth Factors in Inner Ear Development

Growth factors have been implicated in the development and survival of inner ear neurons. Nerve growth factor (NGF), brain-derived growth factor (BDGF), neurotrophin-3 (NT-3), basic fibroblast growth factor (bFGF), and transforming growth factor-β (TGF-β) have all been shown to be important in early and late cochlear and vestibular neuronal development.[80–83]

Both vestibular and cochlear HVs produce mRNA-encoding neurotrophic factors, especially BDNF and NT-3. Cochlear and vestibular neurite extension in vitro is inhibited with antisense oligonucleotides to BDNF and NT-3, but it is enhanced when NGF, BDNF, or NT-3 is added to the media.[84,85] In addition, mice have been bred with gene knockouts of the *BDNF* gene, the *NT-3* gene, and both genes.[85,86] BDNF knockout mice lose most vestibular as well as type II cochlear ganglion cells and outer HC afferents. *NT-3* knockouts lose type I cochlear ganglion cells in addition to inner HC afferent neurons. The mice without both genes lack vestibular and cochlear ganglion cells.[86] The importance of these neurotrophic factors for the survival of inner ear neurons suggests that they have the potential to protect these cells from degenerating. Therefore, they might have a role in preserving spiral ganglion neurons for stimulation by the cochlear implant.

Other growth factors which have been identified as key players in inner ear development via animal models are discussed below.

***Jagged/Delta* Gene.** Exit from the cell cycle is crucial for induction of differentiation and maturation. Cell-cycle exit in the cochlea seems to depend upon expression of *Notch1* and its ligands, *Jagged1/2* and *Delta*, which may define boundaries and patterning of sensory cell development.[75] Mutants in *Jagged1* and *Notch* display abnormal patterning of the cochlea.[55,76] Notch-Delta signaling plays a crucial role in primary cell fate determination through lateral inhibition. Early in development of the organ of Corti in chicks, Delta and Jagged expression by developing inner hair cells appears to result in lateral inhibition of hair cell differentiation, committing adjacent progenitor cells to the fate of supporting cells and possibly induces outer HC development as well. Later in development, expression of Delta and Jagged appears to inhibit both inner and outer HC differentiation.[87,88]

***Fgf3* Gene.** Although the fibroblast growth factor 3 (Fgf3) is expressed widely in both brain and ear tissues, the role it appears to play in inner ear morphogenesis involves the endolymphatic duct (ELD) and sac. *Fgf3* knockout mice display malformation of both the ELD and sac, among other abnormalities.[53,89]

***Neurogenin1* Gene.** Auditory and vestibular ganglion neurons fail to develop in mice with targeted deletion of *neurogenin1*.[90]

***Shh* Gene.** Mesenchymal–epithelial interactions appear to play an essential role in inner ear development, based on observations in mice. The protein product of sonic hedgehog (*Shh*) is secreted by notochord in early development and is essential for ventral otic derivatives, such as the cochlear duct and cochleovestibular ganglion.[91] *Shh* interacts with both *Pax2* and BMPs during otocyst development, where it may induce mesenchymal condensation to form the bony otic capsule. *Shh* knockouts display a poorly mineralized otic capsule that occasionally lacks semicircular canals.[91]

INNER EAR HOMEOSTASIS

Numerous studies have investigated genes involved in cochlear homeostasis and, in particular, the molecular basis of production and maintenance of ion gradients between cochlear fluids and cells. Such studies have particular relevance for disorders of fluid balance in the inner ear, including Meniere disease. Genes encoding isoforms of the ion channels, such as the sodium-potassium ATPase or the plasma membrane calcium ATPase (PMCA), are differentially expressed by cochlear cells within the spiral ligament and stria vascularis and the organ of Corti.[92] This is likely related to the uniquely high electrochemical gradient against which the stria vascularis must transport ions to maintain the endocochlear potential. Furuta and colleagues found that, in particular, inner hair cells express high levels of PMCA1 mRNA, while outer hair cells express high levels of PMCA2, suggesting that the calcium regulation requirements of the two cell types are distinct, owing to their different functions and sensitivities.[92]

Furthermore, the pendrin protein is involved in endolymph homeostasis through its role as an anion transporter in the inner ear. Targeted disruption of the *Pds* gene in mice leads to severe vestibular defects, endolymphatic hydrops with dilation of associated inner ear structures, reduced macular otoconia, and cochlear HC degeneration.[93] The finding of excess endolymph in such mice has led to the assumption that pendrin plays an essential role in endolymph resorption.

In contrast, two other ion transporters of the inner ear have been identified in mice as having an essential role in endolymph production: the Na-K-Cl cotransporter encoded by *Slc12a2*, which is expressed at the basolateral membrane of stria vascularis in marginal cells, and the potassium ion channel KCNE1 or Isk, which is expressed at the apical surface of strial marginal cells (Figure 5). In mice with targeted disruption of either gene, there is failure of endolymph production, resulting in endolymph compartment collapse, smaller than normal semicircular canals, and severe vestibular defects similar to those of *Pds* mutants.[94,95] Characterization of human homologues will likely expand our knowledge of related human audiovestibular disorders.

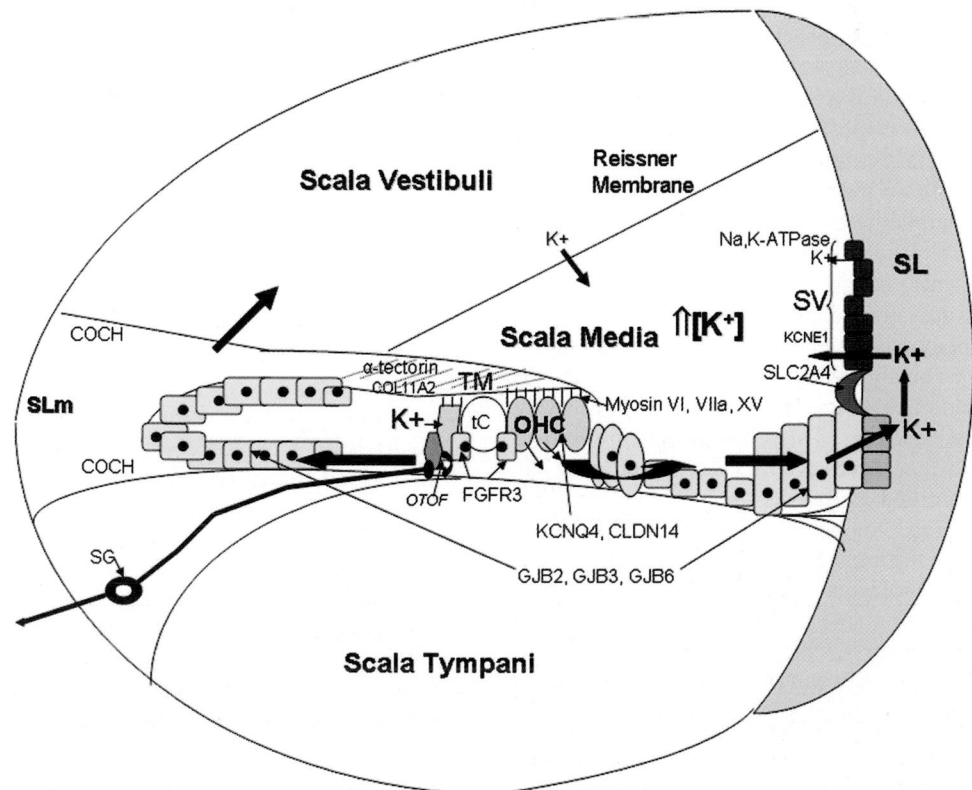

Figure 5 Schematic illustration of a cross-section through the cochlea displaying the endolymphatic compartment (scala media), perilymphatic compartments (scala vestibuli and scala tympani), and basilar membrane with the organ of Corti, containing the outer and inner hair cells and overlying tectorial membrane.

Connexins also play a crucial role in ion homeostasis in the inner ear via recycling of potassium ions to the endolymphatic compartment, as will be discussed in the nonsyndromic deafness section. For an overview of current connexin-related research, visit the URL: http://www.crg.es/deafness/.

Also of importance in inner ear homeostasis is the aquaporin (AQP) family of water channels. AQPs are transmembrane channel proteins that are expressed in many isoforms in the inner ear, including AQP2, AQP5, and AQP6. Their function in water transport and location in the inner ear suggest a role in maintaining endolymphatic fluid balance, and they may play a role in Meniere disease.[96,97] AQP activity may be regulated by antidiuretic hormone (ADH) or vasopressin, which is elevated in some patients with Meniere disease.[98]

MECHANOELECTRIC TRANSDUCTION

The hearing and balance sensory systems require mechanoelectrical transduction of sound and head movements. In the hearing process, a sound wave, a vibrational mechanical force, is transformed into an electrochemical signal that is transmitted as a nerve impulse to the brain. Investigation continues into the process of mechanoelectrical transduction, which is thought to occur as follows. When an acoustic stimulus is received, the stereociliary bundle on the apical surface of hair cells is deflected. The stereocilia are connected by filamentous structures at their tips, called tip links. These are at least partially composed of Cadherin 23 (CDH23) and Myosin-1c (MYO1C), as well as a calcium channel.[77,99–101] If the stereocilia are deflected toward the kinocilium, tension on these tip links activates a mechanically sensitive channel, and a transduction current is induced.[102,103] If the deflection is away from the kinocilium, the channel will close, and no current is produced. Evidence places the transduction channel, which is responsible for inducing the transduction current, on the stereocilia close to the tip links[103–105] (see Figure 4). If the stereocilia deflection is sustained, as frequently occurs in vestibular hair cells, then the cells appear to adapt actively, by readjusting the attachment site of the tip links.[106] This adaptation maintains an appropriate level of tension at the tip links and enables the HC to maintain sensitivity over a wide range of stereociliary positions. The molecule that serves as a transduction channel has been identified as transient receptor potential no mechanoreceptor potential C (TRPN1) in zebra fish,[107] but the human homologue has not yet been identified. Molecular studies have identified prestin[108] as a candidate molecule for regulating the tensioning process, which appears to be controlled by 120 kD myosin motors that attach to the tip links and slide along the actin filaments that form the core of stereocilia.[104,109–112]

Neurotransmission

By understanding the patterns of neurotransmission within the inner ear, a pharmacologic approach to some forms of tinnitus might be developed. The afferent neurotransmitter from the hair cell to the spiral ganglion neurons has not yet been identified. However, spiral ganglion and vestibular ganglion neurons strongly express genes encoding glutamate receptors of the α-amino-3-hydroxy-5-methyl-4-isoxazolepropionate (AMPA), N-methyl-D-aspartate (NMDA), and kainate families,[112–117] implicating a glutamate-like neurotransmitter. The olivocochlear efferent neurotransmitter that operates from the brainstem to the inner ear is primarily acetylcholine,[118] acting at nicotinic acetylcholine receptors[119] that are strongly expressed in hair cells.[120] Other receptors found in the cochlea include muscarinic acetylcholine, γ-aminobutyric acid (GABA), and adenosine triphosphate (ATP) receptors,[121–123] while olivocochlear efferent neurons express enkephalin mRNA.[115]

Fine-Tuning of the Auditory System: Outer Hair Cell Electromotility

The discovery of otoacoustic emissions has led to their use as a tool in infant hearing impairment screening, and audiologists use them widely as part of their battery of diagnostic testing.[124] The basis for otoacoustic emissions is the electromotile activity of outer hair cells, first discovered in 1985, and thought to be responsible for both sharp tuning of the basilar membrane frequency response and for increased auditory sensitivity. Deflection of the hair cell stereocilia leads to a change in membrane voltage. For the outer hair cells, unlike inner hair cells, this voltage response induces changes in cell length that affect the motion of the basilar membrane. Several candidates for the outer hair cell motor are under investigation, including AP-1-like proteins[125] and molecules containing a motif related to the S4 segment of voltage-gated ion channels,[126] both of which change shape in response to changes in membrane voltage. A more thorough discussion of these issues can be found in Chapter 7, "Cochlear Biophysics."

HUMAN EVIDENCE OF A MOLECULAR BASIS FOR HEARING AND BALANCE DYSFUNCTION

Hearing loss is the most common sensory impairment. At least 1 out of every 750 babies born in the United States has sensorineural hearing loss (SNHL). Demographic studies estimate that approximately 50% of all congenital deafness can be traced to inheritable factors, most due to single gene mutations, and at least 90% are inherited as autosomal recessive (AR) traits. Of these, approximately 30% are syndromic and 70% are nonsyndromic. Considerable progress has been made in identifying and characterizing these deafness genes.

During the 1980s, advances in molecular genetic technology led to a rapidly progressive increase in the number of molecular markers that facilitate linkage analysis. These markers, or polymorphisms, define genetic locations and have enabled scientists to identify the approximate location of inherited mutations. Thus, gene mapping began to be applied to familial deafness in the late 1980s, resulting in the first definitive information regarding the physical site and nature of the mutations affecting the inner ear. The recent development of thousands of molecular tags for specific locations in the genome has dramatically enhanced the ability to link inherited disorders to their specific chromosomal location via recombination frequency analysis. When combined with information from prior localization studies of candidate genes or related animal mutations in the same chromosomal region, such linkage analysis has enabled the characterization of an increasing number of mutations that cause disorders of hearing. More than 100 deafness loci have been identified. Our knowledge of the identity and function of these genes has grown almost exponentially over the last decade. Today, more than 10 genetic mutations leading to congenital hearing loss can be identified with genetic testing (see http://www.genetests.com for testing laboratory information). This has improved our ability to provide genetic counseling and, in the future, may lead to gene therapy for aural diseases. Gene identification also allows determination of function through animal studies of homologous gene mutations which can be genetically engineered.

Syndromic Hearing Impairment

Genetic mutations causing hearing impairment in association with other morphological or clinical features are referred to as syndromic hearing impairment genes. Syndromic deafness accounts for 30% of inherited congenital hearing loss.[127] Linkage analysis has been facilitated by the fact that affected individuals are more easily distinguishable from unaffected members within a given population or family with respect to a specific syndrome. The specific mutations causing Alport syndrome, Waardenburg syndrome, Usher syndrome, branchio-oto-renal (BOR) syndrome, Pendred syndrome, X-linked deafness with perilymph gusher, neurofibromatosis type 2 (NF2), and many other forms of syndromic deafness, as well as nonsyndromic deafness, have been determined, and many have been characterized, in terms of the molecular defect. The mitochondrial DNA mutation leading to inherited susceptibility to aminoglycoside-induced hearing loss has also been identified.[128] Although the molecular genetics of inherited deafness is discussed in detail in Chapter 26, "Hereditary Hearing Impairment," there are several disorders that merit further discussion in the context of molecular methodology.

Alport Syndrome. The first human mutation affecting the inner ear to be identified was that causing Alport syndrome, an X-linked disease associated with renal abnormalities and progressive hearing loss. The mutated gene was initially linked to Xq22–26 and was subsequently identified as that encoding the $\alpha 5$ chain of type IV collagen, which plays a critical role in the formation of basement membranes.[129] Six subtypes of Alport syndrome have since been identified: types II, III, and IV are X-linked while types I, V, and VI are inherited in an autosomal dominant (AD) fashion.[127]

Waardenburg Syndrome. WS can be inherited as an AD, AR, or sporadic mutation. WS-I is characterized by hearing loss and pigmentary abnormalities such as white forelock and heterochromia irides. WS type II (WS-II) is distinguished from WS-I by the presence of dystopia canthorum, which presents as lateral displacement of the medial canthi. The autosomal dominant WS-I defect was initially localized to the long arm of chromosome 2 (2q35–37) because of a de novo chromosomal malformation,[130] and then further linked to a gene near 2q37.[131] This locus is homologous to the *Pax3* gene in *Splotch* mice, which had been proposed as a murine equivalent of WS-I. Mutations in the *PAX3* gene of WS-I patients were subsequently shown to be responsible for WS-I and WS type III (WS-III).[132] *PAX3* encodes a transcription factor that regulates expression of other genes. The PAX3 protein product plays a regulatory role in melanocyte differentiation during embryogenesis when melanocytes migrate from the neural crest to various tissues, including the intermediate cells of the stria vascularis in the cochlea and the melanocytes apposing the dark cells of the vestibular labyrinth, where they are necessary for production of endolymph and the endolymphatic potential. In *VGA-9* mice, harboring a transgenic mutation of *Pax3* similar to that in *Splotch* mice (the murine equivalent of WS-I), the stria vascularis shows a lack of intermediate cells and disorganization of the basal layer. WS-II has not shown linkage to the region of chromosome 2 that includes *PAX3*, and WS-II appears to be caused by mutation of either the microphthalmia-associated transcription factor, *MITF* gene, which maps to 3p12.3–14.1, or *SNA12*, which is located at 8q11 and encodes the SLUG transcription factor.[127] Type IV Waardenburg (WS-IV) maps to still other sites: (1) 20q13.2–3, where the *EDN3* gene is located, encoding endothelin-3[133]; (2) 13q22, where *ENDRB* encodes the endothelin receptor, type B; and (3) 22q13, encoding the transcription factor SOX10. Endothelin signaling is involved in neuronal survival, and patients with WS-IV develop Hirschsprung disease (lack of autonomic innervation to the distal large colon) in addition to signs and symptoms of WS-II.[134]

Usher Syndrome. Usher syndrome (US) is inherited in an autosomal recessive fashion and is characterized by deafness and retinitis pigmentosa. Usher syndrome type I (US-I) is characterized by severe hearing loss and impaired vestibular function, while Usher syndrome type II (US-II) has less severe involvement of both. Additional subtypes based on severity and character of progression have been proposed: US-III and US-IV. Both US-I and US-II are genetically heterogeneous, with some US-I families linking to chromosome 14q32 and others linking to chromosome 11, and the *Shaker-1* mouse mutation, which maps to a region homologous to human 14q32, was shown to involve a gene-encoding myosin VII.[127] Based on this observation, *myosin VIIA* was subsequently identified as the gene responsible for US IB.[135] Although incompletely understood, the role of myosin VIIA in the inner ear appears to involve inner hair cell integrity.[136] Myosin VIIA localizes to the cross-links between adjacent stereocilia and at the cuticular plate of inner hair cells (see Figure 4). It has been postulated to play a role in adaptation, which is the process of maintenance of lateral tip link tension and restoration of hair cell sensitivity after depolarization.[77,99] Myosin VIIA can move upward on the actin core within stereocilia, and may connect with cadherin-catenin complexes via the primary decidual zone (PDZ) (uterine PDZ found in many cell junction–associated proteins) domain-containing protein, harmonin in an adaptation motor to maintain stereocilia tension as well as lateral link tension within hair cells (see Figure 4). Mutations in *harmonin* gene cause US IC.[137] US-IIa links to chromosome 1q41, where the gene product, named usherin, is encoded. Usherin contains laminin-EGF and fibronectin domains and, thus, likely functions in extracellular matrix interactions.[138–141] Overall, at least nine distinct chromosomal locations have been linked to the various forms of US.[127]

Pendred Syndrome. An autosomal recessive disorder characterized by deafness and euthyroid goiter results from mutation of the *PDS* gene, also called solute carrier 26A gene family (*SLC26A4*), which encodes the pendrin protein. Pendrin is a putative ion transport molecule that appears to function as an iodide (in the thyroid), chloride, bicarbonate, formate, and nitrate transporter.[142] Pendrin is discretely expressed in the endolymphatic duct and sac and utricle and saccule and on the apical surface of certain cells within the stria vascularis of the embryonic mouse. Pendrin appears to play a vital role in endolymph fluid homeostasis in the inner ear.[143] The spectrum of inner ear abnormalities associated with *PDS* mutations ranges from isolated enlarged vestibular aqueduct (EVA) to classic Mondini malformation, or incomplete partition type II with cystic apical and middle turns of the cochlea, lacking the interscalar septum, a mildly dilated vestibule, and EVA. Hearing is similarly variable, ranging from normal in early childhood to mild low frequency conductive loss to profound sensorineural hearing loss. Stepwise progression of hearing loss is the typical pattern, and there have been no reported cases with normal hearing beyond early childhood. In association with Pendred syndrome, euthyroid goiter, and a positive perchlorate discharge test are present.

Neurofibromatosis Type 2. Affecting 1 in 40,000 individuals, neurofibromatosis type 2 (NF2) is caused by a mutation at 22q12.2.[144] Individuals affected with NF2 characteristically develop bilateral vestibular schwannomas, inevitably leading to hearing loss and balance dysfunction. The NF2 mutation is also associated with schwannomas of other cranial nerves, meningiomas, and spinal tumors. NF2 is inherted in an autosomal dominant fashion, but approximately 50% of cases are sporadic. Mosaicism of *NF2* gene mutation also occurs in up to 25% of cases. The *NF2* gene encodes merlin, or schwannomin, an intracellular tumor suppressor protein expressed in Schwann cells. Merlin shares extensive homology with the erzin/radixin/moesin family, is negatively regulated by phosphorylation, likely mediated by p21-activated kinase 1 (PAK1), and translocates to the cytoplasmic cell membrane in a paxillin-dependent manner, where it binds to ErbB2.[145] ErbB2 is a growth factor receptor tyrosine kinase that couples with ErbB3 when stimulated by neuregulin binding and activates intracellular signaling cascades, such as MAP kinase and pAkt/PI3-K, thus mediating Schwann cell proliferation and survival. Merlin also has been shown to translocate to the nucleus where it may affect gene expression in Schwann cells.[145] However, the role of merlin as a tumor suppressor gene is still poorly understood.

Other Deafness Syndromes. Apert syndrome is AD or, more commonly, sporadic and results from mutation of the fibroblast growth factor receptor 2 (*FGFR2*) gene at 10q26. Congenital stapedial footplate fixation results in conductive hearing loss, and craniofacial deformities, as well as developmental delay, are secondary to craniosynostosis in Apert syndrome.[127]

Branchio-oto-renal syndrome is autosomal dominant in inheritance and is characterized by several branchial arch deformities, deafness, and renal anomalies. The mutation has been localized to a gene at 8q13.3, termed *EYA1* for the "eyes absent" phenotype associated with the orthological mutation in *Drosophila*.[146,147]

X-linked deafness with a perilymph gusher is an X-linked progressive mixed deafness associated with a perilymph gusher during stapes surgery, as the name implies. It was linked to Xq21.1 by examination of the cytogenetically visible deletion.[148–150] The gene causing X-linked mixed deafness with stapes fixation has recently been identified to encode a transcription factor, Brn-4, which is a member of the POU-domain family and extensively expressed during cochlear development.[151]

Other AD syndromic forms of hearing loss include Crouzon, DiGeorge, Goldenhar (oculoauricular vertebral dysplasia), osteogenesis imperfecta, Paget, Noonan, Pfeiffer, Stickler, Townes-Brocks, Treacher Collins, and velo-cardio-facial syndromes. Other AR syndromic hearing loss syndromes include Cockayne, Fanconi anemia A, Friedrich ataxia, Hurler, Jervell and Lange-Nielsen, osteopetrosis (Albers-Schonberg),

Refsum, Tay-Sachs, and xeroderma pigmentosum. X-linked syndromic deafness disorders include Charcot-Marie-Tooth, Hunter, Norrie, otofacial digital, and otopalatodigital syndromes. For a more complete and current review of syndromic deafness genes, please refer to the Online Mendelian Inheritance in Man website http://www.ncbi.nlm.nih.gov/omim/.

Nonsyndromic Hearing Impairment

While 30% of prelingual hearing impairment is syndromic, 70% is nonsyndromic hearing impairment (NHI).[152] NHI is a diagnosis that applies to patients who suffer genetic HI without associated phenotypic abnormalities, and it results from mutations in an estimated 100 genes. Linkage analysis is difficult in this group of patients due to the genetic heterogeneity. However, using relatively isolated populations and large families, linkage analysis has facilitated the identification of over 70 loci and cloning of more than 21 genes responsible for NHI. Identification of genetic mutations associated with HI enables genetic testing, precise diagnosis, and genetic counseling. Human temporal bone studies have revealed morphologic defects resulting from such mutations, providing speculative information on gene function. Animal studies utilizing homologous-targeted mutations facilitate experimental studies of gene function and have been the major tool in expanding our knowledge of inner ear protein functions. Since the number of DNA polymorphic markers for genetic NHI is increasing exponentially, up-to-date information can be found on the Hereditary Hearing Loss Homepage (http://dnalab-www.uia.ac.be/ dnalab/hhh).

Molecules Involved in Ion Homeostasis. Maintaining the endolymphatic potential within the cochlear duct is essential for normal HC function, and it is postulated that the potassium content in endolymph is highly regulated via a bimodal recycling pathway. According to the predominant theory, potassium is recycled both medially and laterally within the cochlea. The medial pathway involves the spiral limbus interdental cells medial to the organ of Corti, which recycle potassium ions (K^+) back into the scala media after auditory hair cell depolarization (see Figure 5; please refer to Chapter 1, "Anatomy of the Auditory and Vestibular Systems" for a description of cellular subtypes). The lateral pathway involves the supporting cells adjacent to hair cells within the organ of Corti, that recycle K^+ through the spiral ligament and stria vascularis back into the scala media (see Figure 5). Potassium recycling requires a network of ion channels and transporters, including gap junctions assembled by connexins, the anion transporter pendrin, and potassium channels KCNQ and KCNE.[152]

Connexins. Currently, *GJB2*, which encodes connexin 26, is recognized as the most frequent gene mutation associated with congenital HI. DFNA3, the dominantly inherited form, and DFNB1, the autosomal recessive mutation, account for up to 50% of cases of congenital HI. Although relatively small, with the entire coding sequence contained in one exon, over 50 mutations within the *GJB2* gene account for hearing loss. The most common is the 35delG mutation in European countries and the United States.[153] In contrast, the 235delC mutation accounts for 73% of *GJB2* mutations in the Japanese population.[154] The small coding region has facilitated genetic screening methods for *GJB2* mutations, which can now be done more rapidly and easily using microarray.[155] The role of connexin 26 in the inner ear is related to its function as a subunit of connexon gap junctions. Connexons are composed of hexameric connexin molecules forming a hemipore. The connexon hemipore of two adjacent cells will join to form a complete gap junction and allow intercellular diffusion of potassium ions. Other connexin proteins associated with NHI include connexin 30 (encoded by *GJB6*, associated with *DFNA3* and *DFNB1* loci), 31 (*DFNA2* locus, *GJB3* gene), and 43 (*GJA1*). Connexins form mostly homomeric connexons, but the heteromeric connexons of connexin 26 and connexin 32 are also expressed in the inner ear. Connexons appear to be essential for generation and maintenance of the endocochlear potential due to their role in K^+ recycling[156] (see Figure 5). There are two independent networks of intercellular connexons that seem to play an important role in recycling of K^+ ions: (1) the epithelial network within the basilar membrane adjacent to the organ of Corti both medially and laterally, and (2) the fibrocyte network which is present within the spiral limbus (medially) and spiral ligament (laterally) and includes the basal, intermediate and endothelial cells of the stria vascularis. The major pathway for K^+ recycling appears to involve the stria vascularis (see Figure 5), and connexons have been implicated as part of the structure required for this process, via transcellular circulation of K^+ through the spiral ligament and basal cells of the stria vascularis.[156]

Other Ion Transport Molecules. Another junctional protein important for fluid homeostasis in the inner ear is Claudin 14, a *CLDN14* gene product. Claudin 14 forms tight junctions within sensory epithelia of the cochlea and vestibular organs, and NHI results from mutation at the *DFNB29* locus[157] (see Figure 5).

PDS gene mutations that lead to EVA in isolation (ie, in absence of goiter or a positive perchlorate discharge test) are a form of NHI and are thought to be part of a continuum of diseases caused by the same gene, in which Pendred syndrome in association with Mondini malformation (as discussed above under section "Syndromic Hearing Impairment") is at the opposite end of the spectrum.[158] Expression studies in *Xenopus* oocytes as well as mammalian cells, including knockout studies in mice, indicate that pendrin function can support chloride/formate, chloride/hydroxide, chloride/bicarbonate, chloride/nitrate, and chloride/iodide ion exchange.[142]

Potassium channels in the inner ear are encoded by the *KCNQ1-4* and *KCNE1-4* genes. Splice variants from these genes are expressed as subunits of the various isoforms of potassium channels present throughout the mammalian inner ear.[159] Together, the KCNE and KCNQ subunits form a functional potassium channel. The KCNE1 (minK) subunit IsK regulates the pore-forming KvLQT1 α-subunit encoded by KCNQ1, which is expressed at the apical surface of marginal cells in the stria vascularis (see Figure 5). Mutation in any of these genes can result in deafness, presumably secondary to lack of endocochlear potential generation. These potassium channels are expressed in cardiac tissue as well; Jervell and Lange-Nielsen syndrome results from mutations in either KCNE1 or KCNQ1.[159,160] KCNQ4 is expressed by cochlear outer hair cells (OHCs) and vestibular type I hair cells. Several lines of evidence suggest that KCNQ4 channels are responsible for the resting K^+ current described in OHCs and type I hair cells, which likely influence their electrical properties. Furthermore, KCNQ4 is expressed in central auditory pathway nuclei, suggesting that defects in *KCNQ4*, which lead to DFNA2, contribute to both peripheral and central deafness.[161]

Transcription Factors: Developmental Regulation and Beyond. The POU-domain family of transcription factors contains the genes *POU4F3* and *POU3F4*, both of which have been identified in association with late-onset progressive NHI. These transcription factors are expressed in the late stages of inner ear development and are important for neuronal differentiation and survival. *POU3F4* is expressed in the otic capsule in mesenchyme of the cochlear and the vestibular primordial.[162] Mutations in *POU3F4* are associated with X-linked progressive mixed hearing loss (HL) due to stapes fixation with a progressive senosrineural hearing impairment (SNHI), termed *DFN3*.[148] It is associated with increased perilymphatic pressure and a "gusher" at stapedectomy. Conversely, *POU4F3* is expressed in developing cochlear and vestibular hair cells.[163] A family with a dominantly inherited mutation in the *POU4F3* gene encoding a truncated Brn-3.1 resulting in late-onset nonsyndromic sensorineural deafness has been identified, and the deafness gene termed *DFNA15*.[164]

Proteins with Unknown Function. A common form of AD low frequency nonsyndromic SNHI is caused by mutation of the *WFS1* gene designated DFNA6/14. *WFS1* encodes wolframin, a protein that localizes to the endoplasmic reticulum and is thought to play a role in protein sorting and trafficking, although the function is unknown.[165]

Cytoskeletal Proteins. Structural components of the cochlea and vestibular organs are highly organized, and their maintenance is essential for the function of hearing and balance, especially with respect to sensory hair cells. Mutation in many of the genes that encode cytoskeletal proteins within hair cells leads to NHI. These include (1) a conventional myosin, *MYH9*; (2) four unconventional myosins, *MYO3A*, *MYO6*, *MYO7A*, and *MYO15*; (3) stereocilin, a novel stereocilia-associated protein; (4) harmonin, a PDZ-domain protein; (5) a putative actin-polymerization protein, human homologue of the *Drosophila* diaphonus gene (*HDIA1*); and (6) a cadherin, *CDH23*.[152]

Stereocilia are the main structures responsible for mechanosensory transduction in auditory and vestibular hair cells. Stereocilia are cellular organelles that are organized into rows of increasing height and create the characteristic staircase pattern seen by electron microscopy. Unlike vestibular hair cells, auditory hair cells do not contain a "kinocilium." Stereocilia are exquisitely sensitive to mechanical vibration and can easily be damaged by overstimulation but undergo continuous renewal from tip to base to continue to function an entire lifetime.[166] Each stereocilium is composed of a rigid central structure containing several hundred parallel, polarized, and cross-linked actin filaments. Different members of the myosin family are present with these actin filaments in specific locations within stereocilia: myosin XVa (*MYO15A* gene product) is located at the tips, while myosin VIIa (encoded by *MYO7A*) is located alongside actin at cross-links of adjacent stereocilia, and myosin VI (gene product of *MYO6*) is present at the cuticular plate (see Figure 4). Myosins bind actin, forming the molecular motor units that generate movement via ATP hydrolysis. The *MYO7A* gene, also the causative gene mutation associated with US-IB, is associated with two forms of nonsyndromic deafness, DFNB2, an autosomal recessive disorder, and DFNA11, an autosomal dominant disorder.[135,167]

Harmonin, encoded by *USH1C* at 11p14-15.2, is associated with NHI via mutations linking to the *DFNB18* locus. Harmonin contains a PDZ domain, which suggests that it may function as an assembling protein. PDZ proteins organize protein complexes into their specific subcellular location, anchor transmembrane proteins, and recruit cytosolic signaling molecules, and may bind directly to the actin cytoskeleton.[137]

A putative actin-polymerizing protein is expressed as the gene product of *HDIA1*.[168] *HDIA1* is a formin gene family member, of which most are involved in cytokinesis and establishing cell polarity.

A novel cadherin-like protein is encoded by *CDH23*, which is also linked to Usher type 1D, and mutation at the *DFNB12* locus results in NHI. Cadherins form adherins junctions which are critically important during embryogenesis and organogenesis. Stereocilia organization is disrupted early during hair cell differentiation in mouse mutants.[169]

Synaptic Vesicle Trafficking. *OTOF* mutation, associated with *DFNB9*, is reported to be a frequent cause of recessive prelingual NHI in Spanish patients, and accounts for 4.4% of recessive prelingual NHI not due to *GJB2* (connexin 26) mutations.[170] *OTOF* encodes otoferlin, which has been identified as a calcium-triggered synaptic vesicle trafficking protein that interacts with syntaxin1 and synapsome-associated protein of 25 kD (SNAP25) of the synapsome-associated receptor (SNARE) complex for Ca^{2+}-dependent presynaptic vesicle exocytosis within inner hair cells. Otoferlin, therefore, appears to be important for afferent neural signaling, and mutations have also been found to be associated with auditory neuropathy.[171]

Extracellular Matrix Components. Overlying the auditory HCs within the organ of Corti is the tectorial membrane, which generates the shearing force that bends the stereocilia, opening transduction channels, and initiating depolarization. This comprises the mechanosensory transduction process that is necessary for hearing. Additionally, the tectorial membrane matrix acts as a second resonator and ensures that the outer hair cell bundles are displacement coupled to the sound stimulus. Thus, it facilitates optimal electromechanical feedback to the basilar membrane from outer hair cells.[172] The tectorial membrane consists of collagen fibers and a noncollagenous matrix containing mostly α- and β-tectorin.[152] Otoancorin mediates the attachment of the tectorial membrane to the apical surface of the hair cells (see Figure 4). *TECTA* encodes α-tectorin, *OTOA* encodes otoancorin, and *COL11A2* encodes the type XI collagen subunit 2. Mutation in any of these three genes results in SNHI, which can be dominant, recessive, NHI, or syndromic HI.[152]

COCH encodes cochlin, an extracellular matrix protein that is abundantly expressed throughout the inner ear, except in sensory hair cells.[173] Mutations in *COCH* at the DFNA9 locus lead to late-onset, progressive nonsyndromic HL (NHI), which is characterized by acidophilic mucopolysaccharide deposits in the cochlea and vestibular organs,[174] SNHI, and vestibular symptoms similar to Meniere disease.[52] Interestingly, only missense mutations of the *COCH* gene have been identified in association with DFNA9 NHL.[175]

Mitochondrial Deafness. Mitochondrial mutations have recently been identified in association with some maternally inherited hearing losses. These can result from heteroplasmic or homoplasmic states with respect to the mitochondrial DNA pool. Heteroplasmy refers to a mixture (usually two, but "multiplasmy" has been reported) of mitochondrial genotypes, while homoplasmy refers to a single mitochondrial genotype present in all of the cells of the body.[176] Mitochondrial mutations are associated with some forms of syndromic as well as NHI.

The systemic neuromuscular syndromes MELAS (mitochondrial encephalopathy, lactic acidosis, and stroke-like episodes), MERRF (mitochondrial encephalomyopathy with ragged red fibers), and Kearns-Sayre syndrome frequently present with hearing loss, among other symptom.[177] They are caused by heteroplasmic mitochondrial DNA mutations that manifest in nerves and muscle tissue where energy requirements are highest and, therefore, mitochondria are more abundant and active. Hearing loss results from generalized neuronal dysfunction.[178]

A form of inherited SNHI associated with diabetes mellitus results from several distinct heteroplasmic mutations in the mitochondrial transfer RNA (tRNA) genes. In these patients, hearing loss develops after diabetes but is of early onset with a severe phenotype. Interestingly, these include the A3243G mutation within the mitochondrial gene encoding $tRNA_{leu}$ (UUR), which is the same mutation that results in MELAS syndrome.[178]

A mitochondrial genome 1555A→G mutation within the gene encoding 12S ribosomal RNA is associated with aminoglycoside susceptibility to hearing loss. Additionally, a progressive high-frequency SNHL and permanent tinnitus, even in the absence of exposure to aminoglycosides, may occur in individuals harboring this mutation, which is, thus, a form of NHI.[179] Hearing loss presumably results from increased susceptibility to cochlear injury in response to various environmental factors.

Presbyacusis is thought to be inherited as a mitochondrial mutation, but the specific mutation(s) have yet to be identified. It is thought to involve at least one of the genes for the oxidative phosphorylation pathway, and the mitochondrial cytochrome oxidase II gene is a likely candidate.[176,180]

Besides the particular mutation in a single gene, other factors may modify the observed clinical phenotype. Such factors may include the genetic background, modifying genes, and environmental factors, such as noise exposure and ototoxicity. Modifying genes can influence the phenotype resulting from a given mutation at another locus. An extreme example is *DFNM1*, which acts as a dominant suppressor of DFNB26.[181] Modifier genes may explain why the level of HI can range from mild to profound with identical NH mutations, as well as the phenotypic variance of identical syndromic and mitochondrial mutations.[176]

Semicircular Canal Dysplasias

Another class of disorders resulting in SNHI, conductive HL, or mixed HL is semicircular canal dysplasia.[182] Although traditional hypotheses have held that semicircular canal dysplasias result from arrest in development during the sixth week of gestation, several cases of semicircular canals dysplasia or aplasia have been reported with normal cochlear development.[183,184] The majority are nonsyndromic, although 12.5% were associated with known syndromes in a series of 16 cases.[184] The genetic mutations leading to isolated semicircular canal abnormalities have yet to be identified. Additionally, there is a paucity of genetic disorders leading to isolated balance dysfunction, likely owing to compensation by the other sensory organs involved in the balance system: vision, proprioception, and central nervous system integration.

FUTURE CONSIDERATIONS

In the last decade, the dramatic increase in our knowledge of molecular biology of the inner ear has translated into a remarkable increase in diagnostic and treatment capabilities for inner ear disorders. One such possibility is the detection of gene mutations involved in hereditary deafness, and additional genes are being identified at an almost exponential pace. Of great interest is the potential for development of gene therapy and of the delivery systems that will enable clinicians to bypass the blood-perilymph barrier and directly administer various pharmacologic therapies to the inner ear. Gene therapy has been applied experimentally in the *shiverer* mouse, which shows deficits in the amplitude and latency of auditory evoked potential (AEP) responses secondary to a mutation in the myelin basic protein gene. Yoo and colleagues demonstrated improved AEP responses in a *shiverer* mouse in which a transgene coding for normal myelin basic protein was integrated into its genome.[185] Gene therapy of this nature might one day be applied to humans with genetic hearing impairment, with the use of in vitro fertilization.

Research efforts at gene therapy are concentrating on the delivery of gene products or genes to the adult system. The development of such delivery systems for the inner ear is being approached in several ways, and this topic is discussed in greater detail in Chapter 5, "Inner Ear Drug Delivery and Gene Therapy." The first approach is to infuse drugs directly into the inner ear with a microcatheter placed through the tympanic membrane, either against or through the round window membrane to gain entry into the scala tympani. This method has been used successfully in delivering neurotrophins to the scala tympani of guinea pigs to improve survival of

neurons after ototoxin-induced damage.[186] An alternative approach is to embed the drug of choice into a polymer that, once placed in the inner ear, would protect the drug from degradation and help to sustain its release at a specific rate.[187] This approach, however, requires a second operation to terminate the therapy. A third technique is to utilize carrier proteins that would link the drug of choice to endothelial cells lining the inner ear capillaries. These carrier proteins could facilitate the transportation of the drug across the endothelial cell barrier and release the drug into the endolymph or perilymph where the targeted cell population awaits. Early success with this technique has been achieved in brain when nerve growth factor was delivered across the blood-brain barrier utilizing an anti-transferrin antibody as the carrier protein.[188]

Other approaches of gene therapy utilize the techniques of molecular biology (Figure 6). Viral vectors that carry and express genes that encode therapeutic proteins or factors can be used to infect cochlear cells. The advantage of this approach is that the delivery of the inactivated viral vector requires only one procedure, and once transfection has occurred within the target site, the therapeutic factor can be continually produced. These viruses can be driven by specifically designed promoters but do not retain the ability to replicate. The viruses being investigated for this purpose include retroviruses, herpes viruses, adenoviruses, and adeno-associated viruses with each virus having different cell type specificity. An in vivo report in 1992 documented that a *Herpes simplex* viral vector, carrying a nerve growth factor gene, protected neurons of the dorsal root ganglion from the consequences of a traumatic injury.[191] Several laboratories are using herpes viruses and adenoviruses to induce gene expression in inner ear cells.[190–192]

Another approach is transplantation of cells that have been genetically modified to produce therapeutic factors. This method involves injecting genetically engineered cells into the inner ear where they can release the therapeutic factors in large quantities. These cells, however, must be incapable of reproducing, as uncontrolled proliferation and neoplastic processes might potentially be induced otherwise. Two studies have shown that genetically engineered fibroblasts could be used to deliver growth factors to the cochlear duct.[186,193] The tools of molecular biology will enable us to develop these and other delivery systems further. Please visit http://www.nlm.nih.gov/medlineplus/genesandgenetherapy.html for an up-to-date overview of progress in this area.

An emerging area is nanotechnology for drug delivery to the inner ear, among other tissues. Nanoparticles in the range of 1 to 100 nm in diameter can be coated with pharmacotherapeutics, in the form of DNA molecules, siRNAs, small molecules, or possibly even small peptides, for entry through the round window membrane into cells through the cell membrane or into tissues. The core may be composed of magnetic nanoparticles which are subject to manipulation when an external magnetic field is applied,[194] for instance, to facilitate uptake.[195]

Additionally, magnetic nanoparticles can be utilized to induce biomechanical force, as in the case of a middle ear implant that drives ossicular motion.[194] This model simulates the completely implantable middle ear amplifiers but is potentially more durable owing to its smaller size as it would require less power to operate.

Another example of nanotechnology applications for the inner ear is the ongoing development of a vestibular implant.[196] This resembles a gyroscope that senses angular motion, mimicking the semicircular canal sensation, and generates electrical pulses (mimicking those of the ipsilateral vestibular nerve activity during a similar angular motion) that stimulate the vestibular nerve.

An additional development is the micromechanical resonator array that is being designed as a completely implantable multiresonant transducer.[197] It would ideally perform the function of a "bionic" cochlea.

With advancing technologies from the both diagnostic and therapeutic fronts, we are approaching an era in which we may have the capability to alter genetic disease, with respect to hearing and balance dysfunction.

REFERENCES

1. Cristobal R, Wackym PA, Cioffi JA, et al. Assessment of differential gene expression in vestibular epithelial cell types using microarray analysis. Mol Brain Res 2005;133:19–36.
2. Anderson B, Svanborg-Eden C. Attachment of *Streptococcus pneumoniae* to human pharyngeal epithelial cells. Respiration 1989;55:49–52.
3. Post JC, Erlich GD. The impact of the polymerase chain reaction in clinical medicine. JAMA 2000;283:1544–6.
4. Melhus A, Ryan AF. Expression of cytokine genes during pneumococcal and nontypeable *Haemophilus influenza* acute otitis media in the rat. Infect Immun 2000;68:4024–31.
5. Ryan AF, Luo L. Expression of nitric oxide synthase in the mouse middle ear mucosa during immune-mediated

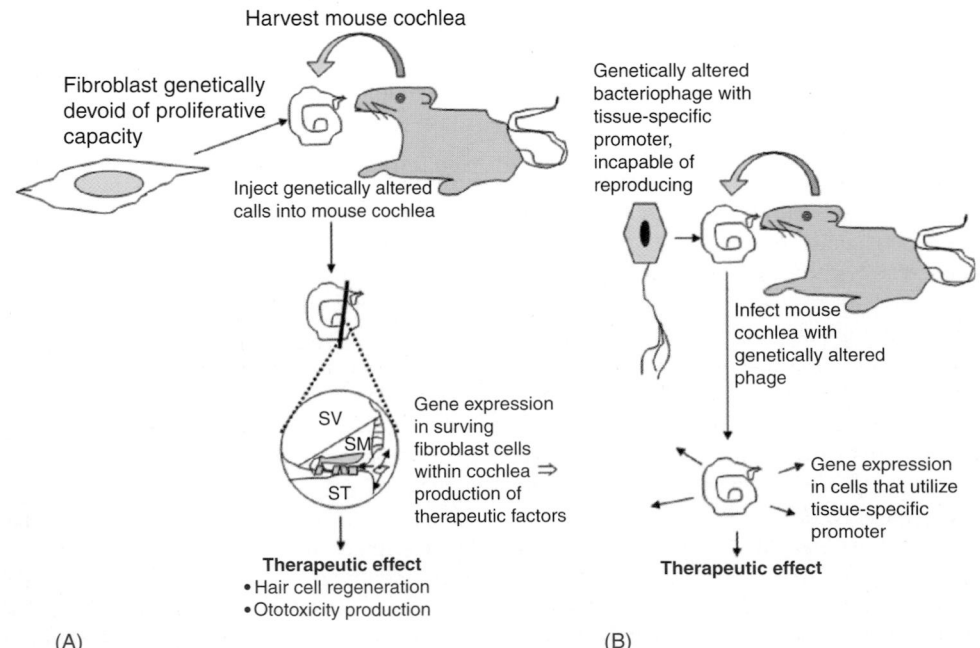

Harvest mouse cochlea

Fibroblast genetically devoid of proliferative capacity

Inject genetically altered calls into mouse cochlea

Genetically altered bacteriophage with tissue-specific promoter, incapable of reproducing

SV
SM
ST

Gene expression in surving fibroblast cells within cochlea ⇒ production of therapeutic factors

Infect mouse cochlea with genetically altered phage

Gene expression in cells that utilize tissue-specific promoter

Therapeutic effect
• Hair cell regeneration
• Ototoxicity production

Therapeutic effect

(A)

(B)

Figure 6 Schematic illustration of proposed gene delivery systems utilizing genetically engineered fibroblasts (A) and viruses constructed with tissue-specific promoters (B). Ideally, these methods will result in targeted molecular therapeutic delivery.

chronic otitis media. In: Tos M, Thomsen J, Balle V, editors. Recent Advances in Otitis Media. Amsterdam: Kugler; 2000. p. 112–6.
6. Ryan AF, Luo L, Baird A. Implantation of cells transfected with the FGF-1 gene induces middle ear mucosal proliferation. In: Lim DL, editor. Recent Advances in Otitis Media with Effusion. Amsterdam: Kugler; 1997. p. 248–50.
7. Coleman T, Grass S, Munson R. Molecular cloning, expression, and sequence of the pilin gene from nontypeable *Haemophilus influenzae* M37. Infect Immun 1991;59:1716–22.
8. Kar S, To SC, Brinton CC. Cloning and expression in *Escherichia coli* of LKP pilus genes from a nontypeable *Haemophilus influenzae* strain. Infect Immun 1990;58:903–8.
9. Bakaletz LO, Ahmed MA, Kolattukudy PE, et al. Cloning and sequence analysis of a pilin-like gene from an otitis media isolate of nontypeable *Haemophilus influenzae*. J Infect Dis 1992;165:S201–3.
10. Sirakova T, Kolattukudy PE, Murwin D, et al. Role of fimbriae expressed by nontypeable *Haemophilus influenzae* (NTHi) in the pathogenesis of and protection against otitis media and relatedness of the fimbrin subunit to outer membrane protein A. Infect Immun 1994;62:2002–20.
11. Brinton CC, Carter M, Derber DB, et al. Design and development of pilus vaccines for *Haemophilus influenzae* diseases. Pediatr Infect Dis J 1989;8:54–61.
12. Bakaletz LO, Tallan BM, Hoepf TM, et al. Frequency of fimbriation of nontypeable *Haemophilus influenzae* and its ability to adhere to chinchilla and human respiratory epithelium. Infect Immun 1988;56:331–5.
13. St. Geme JW, Falkow S, Barenkamp SJ. High-molecular-weight proteins of nontypeable *Haemophilus influenzae* mediate attachment to human epithelial cells. Proc Natl Acad Sci U S A 1993;90:75–9.
14. DeMaria TF, Yamaguchi T, Lim DJ. Quantitative cytologic and histologic changes in the middle ear after the injection of nontypeable *Haemophilus influenzae* endotoxin. Am J Otolaryngol 1989;10:261–6.
15. Weiser JN, Lindberg AA, Manning EJ, et al. Identification of chromosomal locus for expression of lipopolysaccharide epitopes in *Haemophilus influenzae*. Infect Immun 1989;57:3045–52.
16. Weiser JN, Williams A, Moxon ER. Phase-variable lipopolysaccharide structures enhance the invasive capacity of *Haemophilus influenzae*. Infect Immun 90;58:3455–7.
17. Berry AM, Paton JC, Hansman D. Effect of insertional inactivation of the genes encoding pneumolysin and autolysin on the virulence of *Streptococcus pneumoniae* type 3. Microb Pathog 1992;12:87–93.
18. Lock RA, Hansman D, Paton JC. Comparative efficacy of autolysin and pneumolysin as immunogens protecting mice against infection by *Streptococcus pneumoniae*. Microb Pathog 1992;12:137–43.
19. Oehl H, Ryan A. Expression of genes encoding growth factor receptors in middle ear mucosa [abstract]. In: Lim DJ, editor. Abstracts of the 7th International Symposium on Recent Advances in Otitis Media. FL: Ft. Lauderdale; 1999. p. 70.
20. Sudhoff H, Dazert S, Gonzales AM, et al. Angiogenesis and angiogenic growth factors in middle ear cholesteatoma. Am J Otol 2000;21:793–8.
21. Huang CC, Chen CT, Huang TS, Shinoda H. Mediation of signal transduction in keratinocytes of human middle ear cholesteatoma by ras protein. Eur Arch Otorhinolaryngol 1996;253:385–9.
22. Ishibashi T, Shinogami M, Kaga K, Fukaya T. Keratinocyte growth factor and receptor mRNA expression in cholesteatoma of the middle ear. Acta Otolaryngol 1997;117:714–8.
23. Shinoda H, Huang CC. Expression of c-jun and p53 proteins in human middle ear cholesteatoma: Relationship to keratinocyte proliferation, differentiation, and programmed cell death. Laryngoscope 1995;105:1232–7.
24. Schilling V, Lang S, Rasp G, et al. Overexpression of tenascin in cholesteatoma and external auditory meatal skin compared to retroauricular epidermis. Acta Otolaryngol (Stockh) 1996;116:741–6.
25. Li JD, Xu H, Wang B, et al. Signal transduction mechanisms involved in bacteria-induced mucin overproduction. In: Lim DJ, editor. Abstracts of the 7th International Symposium on Recent Advances in Otitis Media. FL: Ft. Lauderdale; 1999. p. 77.
26. Xu H, Wang B, Kim JH, et al. Oxygen radicals as second messengers for bacteria-induced up-regulation of mucin gene transcription. In: Lim DJ, editor. Abstracts of the 7th International Symposium on Recent Advances in Otitis Media. FL: Ft. Lauderdale; 1999. p. 255.
27. Lin J, Kawano H, Tsuboi Y, et al. Alterations of mucin gene expression in the transition of acute to mucoid otitis media. In: Lim DJ, editor. Abstracts of the 7th International Symposium on Recent Advances in Otitis Media. FL: Ft. Lauderdale; 1999. p. 72.
28. Hutton DA, Fogg FJ, Kubba H, et al. Heterogeneity in the protein cores of mucins isolated from middle ear effusions: Evidence for expression of different mucin gene products. Glycoconjugate J 1998;15:283–91.
29. Severn TL, Hutton DA, Birchall JP, Pearson JP. Mucin gene expression in human middle ear. In: Lim DJ, editor. Abstracts of the 7th International Symposium on Recent Advances in Otitis Media. FL: Ft. Lauderdale; 1999. p. 253.
30. Hebda PA, Alper CM, Doyle WJ, et al. Upregulation of messenger RNA for inflammatory cytokines in middle ear mucosa in a rat model of acute otitis media. Ann Otol Rhinol Laryngol 1998;107:501–8.
31. Chun YM, Li JD, Lim DJ. MEK1/2-MAPK pathway is involved in IL-1-induced down-regulation of surfactant B. In: Lim DJ, editor. Abstracts of the 7th International Symposium on Recent Advances in Otitis Media. FL: Ft. Lauderdale; 1999. p. 256.
32. Melhus A, Forseni M, Ryan AF. Molecular markers for bone formation during bacterial otitis media in the rat. In: Lim DJ, Bluestone CD, Casselbrant M, et al, editors. Recent Advances in Otitis Media with Effusion. Amsterdam: Kugler; 2000.
33. Bikhazi P, Luo L, Ryan AF. Expression of immunoregulatory cytokines during acute and chronic middle ear immune response. Laryngoscope 1995;105:629–34.
34. John EO, Nam TTK. Concentration of nitric oxide in middle ear effusion. In: Lim DJ, editor. Abstracts of the 7th International Symposium on Recent Advances in Otitis Media. FL: Ft. Lauderdale; 1999. p. 83.
35. Lim DJ, Chun YM, Lee HY, et al. Cell biology of tubotympanum in relation to pathogenesis of otitis media—a review. Vaccine 2000;19:S17–25.
36. Lehrer RI, Ganz T. Antimicrobial peptides in mammalian and insect host defense. Curr Opin Immunol 1999;11:23–7.
37. Takemura H, Kaku M, Kohno S, et al. Evaluation of susceptibility of gram-positive and gram-negative bacteria to human defensins by using radial diffusion assay. Antimicrob Agents Chemother 1996;40:2280–4.
38. Schroder JM, Harder J. Human beta-defensin-2. Int J Biochem Cell Biol 1999;31:645–51.
39. Vorland LH, Ulvatne H, Andersen J, et al. Lacoferricin of bovine origin is more active than lactoferricins of human, murine and caprine origin. Scand J Infect Dis 1998;30:513–7.
40. Hanamure Y, Lim DJ. Normal distribution of lysozyme- and lactoferrin-secreting cells in the chinchilla tubotympanum. Am J Otolaryngol 1986;7:410–25.
41. Park K, Lim DJ. Development of secretory elements in murine tubotympanum: Lysozyme and lactoferrin immunohistochemistry. Ann Otol Rhinol Laryngol 1993;102:385–95.
42. Lu J. Collections: Collectors of microorganisms for the innate immune system. Bioessays 1997;19:509–18.
43. Needham CA. *Haemophilus influenzae*: Antibiotic susceptibility. Clin Microbiol Rev 1988;1:218–27.
44. Clairoux N, Picard M, Brochu A, et al. Molecular basis of the non-beta-lactamase-mediated resistance to beta-lactam antibiotics in strains of *Haemophilus influenzae* isolated in Canada. Anti-microb Agents Chemother 1992;36:1504–13.
45. Malouin F, Bryan LE. DNA probe technology for detection of *Haemophilus influenzae*. Mol Cell Probes 1987;1:221–32.
46. Roberts MC, Swenson CD, Owens LM, Smith AL. Characterization of chloramphenicol-resistant *Haemophilus influenzae*. Antimicrob Agents Chemother 1980;18:610–5.
47. de Groot R, Campos J, Moseley SL, Smith AL. Molecular cloning and mechanisms of trimethoprim resistance to *Haemophilus influenzae*. Antimicrob Agents Chemother 1988;32:477–84.
48. Murphy TF, Kirkham C. Amino acid sequence of a surface-exposed epitope of the P6 outer membrane protein of nontypable *Haemophilus influenzae*. In: Lim DJ, editor. Abstracts of the Fifth International Symposium on Recent Advances in Otitis Media. FL: Ft. Lauderdale; 1993. p. 120–1.
49. Okamoto Y, Kudo K, Ishikawa K, et al. Presence of respiratory syncytial virus genomic sequences in middle ear fluid and its relationship to expression of cytokines and cell adhesion molecules. J Infect Dis 1993;168:1277–81.
50. Giebink GS. Studies of *Streptococcus pneumoniae* and influenzae virus vaccines in the chinchilla otitis media model. Pedriatr Infect Dis J 1989;8:S42–4.
51. Dazert S, Aletsee C, Brors D, et al. In vivo adenoviral transduction of the neonatal rat cochlea and middle ear. Hear Res 2001;151:30–40.
52. Mondain M, Restituito S, Vincenti V, et al. Adenovirus-mediated in vivo gene transfer in guinea pig middle ear mucosa. Hum Gene Ther 1998;9:1217–21.
53. Mansour SL, Goddard JM, Capecchi MR. Mice homozygous for a targeted disruption of the proto-oncogene INT-2 have developmental defects in the tail and ear. Development 1993;117:13–28.
54. Represa J, Leon Y, Miner C, Giraldez F. The Int-2 proto-oncogene is responsible for induction of the inner ear. Nature 1991;353:561–3.
55. Kiernan AE, Ahituv N, Fuchs H, et al. The Notch ligand Jagggedl is required for inner ear sensory development. Proc Natl Acad Sci U S A 2001;98:3873–8.
56. Heller S, Sheane CA, Javed Z, Hudspeth AJ. Molecular markers for cell types of the inner ear and candidate genes for hearing disorders. Proc Natl Acad Sci U S A 1998;95:11400–5.
57. Carney PR, Silver J. Studies on cell migration and axon guidance in the developing distal auditory system of the mouse. J Comp Neurol 1983;215:359–69.
58. Fekete DM, Wu DK. Revisiting cell fate specification in the inner ear. Curr Opin Neurobiol 2002;12:35–42.
59. Acampora D, Mazan S, Avantaggiato V, et al. Epilepsy and brain abnormalities in mice lacking the Otx1 gene. Nature Genet 1996;14:218–22.
60. Favor J, Sandulache R, Neuhauser-Klaus A, et al. The mouse Pax2(1Neu) mutation is identical to a human PAX2 mutation in a family with renal-coloboma syndrome and results in developmental defects of the brain, ear, eye, and kidney. Proc Natl Acad Sci U S A 1996;93:13870–5.
61. Torres M, Gomez-Pardo E, Gruss P. Pax2 contributes to inner ear patterning and optic nerve trajectory. Development 1996;122:3381–91.
62. Glass CK, Direnzo J, Kurokawa R, Han Z. Regulation of gene expression by retinoic acid receptors. DNA Cell Biol 1991;10:623–38.
63. Romand R, Sapin V, Dolle P. Spatial distributions of retinoic acid receptor gene transcripts in the prenatal mouse inner ear. J Comp Neurol 1998;393:298–308.
64. Thompson DL, Gerlach-Bank LM, Barald KF, Koenig RJ. Retinoic acid repression of bone morphogenetic protein 4 in inner ear development. Mol Cell Biol 2003;23:2277–86.
65. Romand R, Hashino E, Dolle P, et al. The retinoic acid receptors RARalpha and RARgamma are required for inner ear development. Mech Dev 2002;119:213–23.
66. Lohnes D, Mark M, Mendelsohn C, et al. Function of the retinoic acid receptors (RARs) during development (I). Craniofacial and skeletal abnormalities in RAR double mutants. Development 1994;120:2723–48.
67. Kelly M, Xu X-M, Wagner MA, et al. The developing organ of Corti contains retinoic acid and forms supernumary hair cells in response to exogenous retinoic acid in culture. Development 1993;119:1041–55.
68. Liu M, Pereira FA, Price SD, et al. Essential role of BETA2/NeuroD1 in development of the vestibular and auditory systems. Genes Dev 2000;14:2839–54.
69. Bermingham N, Hassan B, Price S, et al. Math1: An essential gene for the generation of inner ear hair cells. Science 1999;284:1837–41.
70. Ryan AF. Molecular studies of hair cell development and survival. Audiol Neurootol 2002;7:138–40.
71. Erkman L, McEvilly RJ, Luo L, et al. Role of transcription factors Brn-3.1 and 3.2 in auditory and visual system development. Nature 1996;381:603–6.
72. Xiang M, Gan L, Li D, et al. Essential role of POU-domain factor Brn-3c in auditory and vestibular hair cell development. Proc Natl Acad Sci U S A 1997;94:9445–50.
73. Xiang M, Gao WQ, Hasson T, Shin JJ. Requirement for Brn-3c in maturation and survival, but not in fate determination of inner ear hair cells. Development 1998;125:3935–46.
74. Fekete DM. Development of the vertebrate ear: Insights from knockouts and mutants. Trends Neurosci 1999;22:263–9.
75. Chen P, Johnson JE, Zoghbi HY, Segil N. The role of Math1 in inner ear development: Uncoupling the establishment of the sensory primordium from hair cell fate determination. Development 2002;129:2495–505.
76. Tsai H, Hardisty RE, Rhodes C, et al. The mouse slalom mutant demonstrates a role for Jagged1 in neuroepithelial patterning in the Organ of Corti. Hum Mol Genet 2001;10:507–12.
77. Friedman TB, Sellers JR, Avraham KB. Unconventional myosins and the genetics of hearing loss. Am J Med Genet 1999;89:147–57.
78. Belyantseva IA, Boger ET, Friedman TB. Myosin XVa localizes to the tips of inner ear sensory cell stereocilia and is essential for staircase formation of the hair bundle. Proc Natl Acad Sci U S A 2003;100:13958–63.
79. Avraham KB, Hasson T, Steel KP, et al. The mouse Snell's waltzer deafness gene encodes an unconventional myosin required for structural integrity of inner ear hair cells. Nature Genet 1995;11:369–75.

80. Lefebvre P, Staecker H, Weber T, et al. TGFB1 modulates bFGF receptor message expression in cultured adult auditory neurons. Neuro Report 1991;2:305–8.
81. Lefebvre P, Van De Water TR, Represa J, et al. Temporal pattern of nerve growth factor (NGF) binding in vivo and the in vitro effects of NGF on cultures of developing auditory and vestibular neurons. Acta Otolaryngol 1991; 111:304–11.
82. Lefebvre P, Van De Water TR, Weber T, et al. Growth factor interactions in cultures of dissociated adult acoustic ganglia: Neuronotrophic effects. Brain Res 1991; 567:306–12.
83. Lefebvre P, Van De Water TR, Staecker H, et al. Nerve growth factor stimulates neurite regeneration but not survival of adult auditory nerves in vitro. Acta Otolaryngol 1992;112:288–93.
84. Staecker H, Lefebvre P, Liu W, et al. Brain-derived neurotrophic factor and its influence on the otocyst. Abstr Assoc Res Otolaryngol 1993;16:26.
85. Ernfors P, Lee KF, Jaenisch R. Mice lacking brain-derived neurotrophic factor develop with sensory deficits. Nature 1994;368:147–50.
86. Ernfors P, Loriong J, Jaenisch R, Van De Water TR. Function of the neurotrophins in the auditory and vestibular systems: Analysis of BDNF and NT-3 gene knockout mice. Abstr Assoc Res Otolaryngol 1995;18:190.
87. Daudet N, Lewis J. Two contrasting roles for Notch activity in chick inner ear development: Specification of prosensory patches and lateral inhibition of hair-cell differentiation. Development 2005;132:541–51.
88. Eddison M, Le Roux I, Lewis J. Notch signaling in the development of the inner ear: Lessons from *Drosophila*. Proc Natl Acad Sci U S A 2000;97:11692–9.
89. McKay IJ, Lewis J, Lumsden A. The role of FGF-3 in early inner ear development: An analysis in normal and Kreisler mutant mice. Dev Biol 1996;174:370–8.
90. Ma Q, Chen Z, del Barco Barrantes I, et al. Neurogenin 1 is essential for the determination of neuronal precursors for proximal cranial sensory ganglia. Neuron 1998;20:469–82.
91. Liu W, Li G, Chien JS, et al. Sonic hedgehog regulates otic capsule chondrogenesis and inner ear development in the mouse embryo. Dev Biol 2002;248:240–50.
92. Furuta H, Luo L, Helper K, Ryan AF. Evidence for differential regulation of calcium by outer versus inner hair cells: Plasma membrane Ca-ATPase gene expression. Hear Res 1998;123:10–26.
93. Everett LA, Belyantseva IA, Noben-Trauth K, et al. Targeted disruption of mouse Pds provides insight about the inner-ear defects encountered in Pendred syndrome. Hum Mol Genet 2001;10:153–61.
94. Delpire E, Lu J, England R, et al. Deafness and imbalance associated with inactivation of the secretory Na-K-Cl co-transporter. Nature Genet 1999;22:192–5.
95. Letts VA, Valenzuela A, Dunbar C, et al. A new spontaneous mouse mutation in the Kcne1 gene. Mamm Genome 2000;11:831–5.
96. Couloigner V, Berrebi D, Teixeira M, et al. Aquaporin-2 in the human endolymphatic sac. Acta Otolaryngol 2004;124:449–53.
97. Fukushima M, Kitahara T, Fuse Y, et al. Changes in aquaporin expression in the inner ear of the rat after i.p. injection of steroids. Acta Otolaryngol Suppl 2004;553:13–8.
98. Ferrary E, Sterkers O, Couloigne V. Hormonal regulation of endolymph homeostasis. Abst Meniere's Symp 2005;2:39.
99. Hasson T, Gillespie PG, Garcia JA, et al. Unconventional myosins in inner-ear sensory epithelia. J Cell Biol 1997;137:1287–307.
100. Holt JR, Gillespie SK, Provance DW, et al. A chemical-genetic strategy implicates myosin-1c in adaptation by hair cells. Cell 2002;108:371–81.
101. Siemens J, Lillo C, Dumont RA, et al. Cadherin 23 is a component of the tip link in hair-cell stereocilia. Nature 2004;428:950–5.
102. Pickles J, Comis SD, Osborne MP. Cross-links between stereocilia in the guinea pig organ of Corti and their possible relation to sensory transduction. Hear Res 1984;15:103–12.
103. Assad J, Shepherd GMG, Corey DP. Tip-link integrity and mechanical transduction in vertebrate hair cells. Neuron 1991;7:985–94.
104. Gillespie P, Wagner MC, Huspeth AJ. Identification of a 120 kD hair-bundle myosin located near stereociliary tips. Neuron 1993;11:581–94.
105. Hackney C, Furness DN, Benos DJ, et al. Putative immunolocalization of the mechanoelectric transduction channels in mammalian cochlear hair cells. Proc Roy Soc B 1992;248:215–21.
106. Howard J, Hudspeth AJ. Mechanical relation of the hair bundle mediated adaptation in mechanoelectrical transduction by the bullfrog's saccular hair cells. Proc Natl Acad Sci U S A 1987;84:3064–8.
107. Sidi S, Friedrich R, Nicolson T. NomC TRP channel required for vertebrate sensory hair cell mechanotransduction. Science 2003;301:96–9.
108. Zheng J, Shen W, He DZ, et al. Prestin is the motor protein of cochlear outer hair cells. Nature 2000;405:149–55.
109. Hudspeth AJ, Gillespie PG. Pulling springs to tune transduction: Adaptation by hair cells. Neuron 1994;12:1–9.
110. Metcalf A, Chelliah Y, Hudspeth AJ. Molecular cloning of a myosin 1 beta isozyme that may mediate adaptation by hair cells of the bullfrog's internal ear. Proc Natl Acad Sci U S A 1994;91:11821–5.
111. Soc C, Derfler BH, Buyks GM, Corey DP. Molecular cloning of myosins from the bullfrog saccular macula: A candidate for the hair cell adaptation motor. Auditory Neurol 1994;1:63–75.
112. Kuriyama H, Albin RL, Altschuler RA. Expression of NMDA-receptor mRNA in the rat cochlea. Hear Res 1993;69:215–20.
113. Hunter C, Petralia RS, Vu T, Wenthold RJ. Expression of AMPA-selective glutamate receptor in morphologically-defined neurons of the mammalian cochlear nucleus. J Neurosci 1993;13:1932–46.
114. Niedzielski A, Wenthold RJ. Expression of AMPA, kainite and NMDA receptor subunits in cochlear and vestibular ganglia. J Neurosci 1995;15:2338–53.
115. Ryan A, Brumm D, Kraft M. Occurrence and distribution of non-NMDA glutamate receptor mRNAs in the cochlea. Neurol-Rep 1991;2:543–646.
116. Wenthold R, Martin MR. Neurotransmitters of the auditory nerve and central auditory system. In: Berlin C, editor. Hearing Science: Recent Advances. San Diego, CA: College-Hill Press; 1984. p. 342–69.
117. Li HS, Niedzielski AS, Beisel KW, et al. Identification of a glutamate/aspartate transporter in the rat cochlea. Hear Res 1994;78:235–42.
118. Housley GAJ. Direct measurement of the action of acetylcholine on isolated outer hair cells of the guinea pig cochlea. Proc R Soc Lond 1991;244:161–7.
119. Wackym PA, Popper P, Lopez I, et al. Expression of alpha 4 and beta 2 nicotinic acetylcholine receptor subunit mRNA and localization of alpha-bungarotoxin binding proteins in the rat vestibular periphery. Cell Biol Int 1995;19:291–300.
120. Luo L, Bennett T, Jung HH, Ryan AF. Developmental expression of alpha 9 acetylcholine receptor mRNA in the rat cochlea and vestibular inner ear. J Comp Neurol 1998;393:320–31.
121. Mockett BG, Housley GD, Thorne PR. Fluorescence imaging of extracellular purinergic receptor sites and putative ecto-ATPase sites on isolated cochlear hair cells. J Neurosci 1994;14:6992–7007.
122. Drescher D, Upadhyay S, Wilcox, Fex J. Analysis of muscarinic receptor subtypes in the mouse cochlea by means of PCR. J Neurochem 1992;59:765–7.
123. Drescher D, Green GE, Khan KM, et al. Analysis of GABA-A receptor subunits in the mouse cochlea by means of PCR. J Neurochem 1993;61:1167–70.
124. Kemp D. Stimulated acoustic emissions from within the human auditory system. J Acoust Soc Am 1978;64:1386–91.
125. Kalinec R, Kachar B. Inhibition of outer hair cell electromotility by sulfhydryl specific agents. Neurosci Lett 1993;157:231–4.
126. Ryan A, Housley GD. Molecular cloning of sequences containing S4-like regions from the rat organ of Corti. Abstr Mol Biol Hear Deafness 1992;74.
127. Friedman TB, Schultz JM, Ben-Yosef T, et al. Recent advances in the understanding of syndromic forms of hearing loss. Ear Hear 2003;24:289 302.
128. Hu D, Qui WQ, Wu BT, et al. Genetic aspects of antibiotic induced deafness: Mitochondrial inheritance. J Med Genet 1991;28:79–83.
129. Barker D, Hostikka SL, Zhou J, et al. Identification of mutations in the COL4A5 collagen gene in Alport syndrome. Science 1990;248:1224–7.
130. Ishikiriyama S, Tonoki H, Shibuya Y, et al. Waardenburg syndrome type I in a child with de novo inversion (2q35-q37.3). Am J Med Genet 1989;33:505–7.
131. Foy C, Newton V, Wellesley D, et al. Assignment of the locus for Waardenburg syndrome type I to human chromosome 2q37 and possible homology to Splotch mouse. Am J Hum Genet 1990;46:1017–23.
132. Hoth C, Milunsky A, Lipsky N, et al. Mutations in the paired domain of the human PAX3 gene caused Klein-Waardenburg syndrome (WSIII) as well as Waardenburg syndrome type I (WS-I). Am J Hum Genet 1993;52:455–562.
133. Edery P, Attie T, Amiel J, et al. Mutation in the endothelin-3 gene in the Waardenburg-Hirshsprung disease (Shah-Waardenburg syndrome). Nature Genet 1996; 12:442–4.
134. Hofstra RM, Osinga J, Tan-Sindhunata G, et al. A homozygous mutation in the endothelin-3 gene associated with a combined Waardenburg type 2 and Hirshsprung phenotype (Shah-Waardenburg syndrome). Nature Genet 1996;12:445–7.
135. Weil D, Blanchard S, Kaplan J, et al. Defective myosin VIIA gene responsible for Usher syndrome type 1B. Nature 1995;374:60–1.
136. Steel KP, Kros CJ. A genetic approach to understanding auditory function. Nature Genet 2001;27:143–9.
137. Verpy E, Leibovici M, Zwaenepoel I, et al. A defect in harmonin, a PDZ domain-containing protein expressed in the inner ear sensory hair cells, underlies Usher syndrome type 1C. Nature Genet 2000;26:51–5.
138. Kimberling W, Weston MD, Moller C, et al. Localization of Usher syndrome type II to chromosome 1q. Genomics 1990;7:245–9.
139. Lewis R, Otterud B, Stauffer D, et al. Mapping recessive ophthalmic diseases: Linkage of the locus for Usher syndrome type II to a DNA marker on chromosome 1q. Genomics 1990;7:250–6.
140. Kaplan J, Gerber S, Bonneau D, et al. A gene for Usher syndrome type I (USH1A) maps to chromosome 14q. Genomics 1992;14:979–87.
141. Kimberling W, Moller CG, Davenport S, et al. Linkage of Usher syndrome type gene (USH1B) to the long arm of chromosome 11. Genomics 1992;14:988–94.
142. Scott DA, Karniski LP. Human pendrin expressed in *Xenopus laevis* oocytes mediates chloride/formate exchange. Am J Physiol Cell Physiol 2000;278:C207–11.
143. Everett LA, Morsli H, Wu DK, Green ED. Expression pattern of the mouse ortholog of the Pendred syndrome gene (Pds) suggests a key role for pendrin in the inner ear. Proc Natl Acad Sci U S A 1999;96:9727–32.
144. Trofatter J, MacCollin MM, Rutter JL, et al. A novel moesin-radixin-like gene is a candidate for the neurofibromatosis 2 tumor suppressor. Cell 1993;72:791–800.
145. Fernandez-Valle C, Tang Y, Richard J, et al. Paxillin binds schwannomin and regulates its density-dependent localization and effect on cell morphology. Nature Genet 2002;31:354–62.
146. Abdelhak S, Kalatzis V, Heilig R, et al. A human homolog of the *Drosophila* eyes absent gene underlies branchio-oto-renal (BOR) syndrome and identifies a novel gene family. Nature Genet 1997;15:157–64.
147. Smith R, Coppage KB, Ankerstjerne JKB, et al. Localization of the gene for Branciootorenal syndrome to chromosome 8q. Genomics 1992;14:841–4.
148. Merry D, Lesko JG, Sosnoski DM, et al. Choroidermia and deafness with stapes fixation: A contiguous gene deletion syndrome in Xq21. Am J Hum Genet 1989;45:530–40.
149. Cremers F, Van De Pol TJR, Diergaarde PJ, et al. Physical fine mapping of the choroidema locus using Xq21 deletions associated with complex syndromes. Genomics 1989;4:41–6.
150. Bach I, Brunner HG, Beighton P, et al. Microdeletions in patients with gusher-associated, X-linked mixed deafness (DFN3). Am J Hum Genet 1992;50:38–44.
151. de Kok Y, Vander Maarel SM, Bitner-Glindzicz M, et al. Association between X-linked mixed deafness and mutations in the POU domain gene POU3F4. Science 1995;7:685–8.
152. Laer LV, Cryns K, Smith RJH, Van Camp G. Nonsyndromic hearing loss. Ear Hear 2003;24:275–88.
153. Kelsell DP, Di WI, Houseman MJ. Connexin mutations in skin disease and hearing loss. Am J Hum Genet 2001;68:559–68.
154. Abe S, Usami S, Shinkawa H, et al. Prevalent connexin 26 gene (GJB2) mutations in Japanese. J Med Genet 2000;37:41–3.
155. Usami S, Koda E, Tsukamoto K, et al. Molecular diagnosis of deafness: Impact of gene identification. Audiol Neurootol 2002;7:185–90.
156. Chang EH, Van Camp G, Smith RJH. The role of connexins in human disease. Ear Hear 2003;24:314–23.
157. Wilcox ER, Burton QL, Naz S, et al. Mutations in the gene encoding tight junction claudin-14 cause autosomal recessive deafness DFNB29. Cell 2001;104:165–72.
158. Usami S, Abe S, Weston MD, et al. Non-syndromic hearing loss associated with enlarged vestibular aqueducts is caused by PDS mutations. Hum Genet 1999;104:188–92.
159. Schmitt N, Schwarz M, Peretz A, et al. A recessive C-terminal Jervell and Lange-Nielsen mutation of the KCNQ1 channel impairs subunit assembly. EMBO J 2000;19:332–40.
160. Schultze-Barr E, Wang Q, Wedekind H, et al. KCNE1 mutations cause Jervell and Lange-Nielsen syndrome. Nature Genet 1997;17:267–8.

161. Kharkovets T, Hardelin J-P, Safieddine S, et al. KCNQ4, a K+-channel mutated in a form of dominant deafness, is expressed in the inner ear and the central auditory pathway. Proc Natl Acad Sci U S A 2000;97:4333–8.
162. Phippard D, Heydemann A, Lechner M, et al. Changes in the subcellular location of the Brn4 gene product precede mesenchymal remodeling of the otic capsule. Hear Res 1998;120:77–85.
163. Erkman L, McEvilly RJ, Luo L, et al. Role of transcription factors Brn-3.1 and Brn-3.2 in auditory and visual system development. Nature 1996;381:603–6.
164. Vahava O, Morell R, Lynch E, et al. Mutation in transcription factor POU4F3 associated with inherited progressive hearing loss in humans. Science 1998;279:1950–4.
165. Bespalova IN, Van Camp G, Bom S, et al. Mutations in the Wolfram syndrome 1 gene (WFS1) are a common cause of low frequency sensorineural hearing loss. Hum Molec Genet 2001;10:2501–8.
166. Schneider ME, Belyantseva IA, Azededo RB, Kachara B. Rapid renewal of auditory hair bundles. Nature 2002;418:837–8.
167. Lui XZ, Walsh J, Tamagawa Y, et al. Autosomal dominant non-syndromic deafness caused by a mutation in the myosin VIIA gene. Nature Genet 1997;17:268–9.
168. Lynch ED, Lee MK, Morrow JE, et al. Nonsyndromic deafness DFNA1 associated with mutation of a human homolog of the *Drosophila* gene diaphanous. Science 1997;278:1315–8.
169. Di Palma F, Holme RH, Bryda EC, et al. Mutations in Cdh23, encoding a new type of cadherin, cause stereocilia disorganization in waltzer, the mouse model for Usher syndrome type 1D. Nature Genet 2001;27:103–7.
170. Migliosi V, Modamio-Hoybjor S, Moreno-Pelayo MA, et al. Q829X, a novel mutation in the gene encoding otoferlin (OTOF), is frequently found in Spanish patients with prelingual nonsyndromic hearing loss. J Med Genet 2002;39:502–6.
171. Varga R, Kelley PM, Keats BJ, et al. Non-syndromic recessive auditory neuropathy is the result of mutations in the otoferlin (OTOF) gene. J Med Genet 2003;40:45–50.
172. Richardson RT, Wise A, O'Leary S, et al. Tracing neurotrophin-3 diffusion and uptake in the guinea pig cochlea. Hear Res 2004;198:25–35.
173. Ikezono T, Omori A, Ichinose S, et al. Identification of the protein product of the Coch gene (hereditary deafness gene) as the major component of bovine inner ear protein. Biochimica et Biophysica Acta 2001;1535:258–65.
174. Robertson NG, Lu L, Heller S, et al. Mutations in a novel cochlear gene cause DFNA9, a human nonsyndromic deafness with vestibular dysfunction. Nature Genet 1998;20:299–303.
175. Franzen E, Verstreken M, Verhagen WIM, et al. High prevalence of symptoms of Meniere's disease in three families with a mutation in the COCH gene. Hum Molec Genet 1999;8:1425–9.
176. Fischel-Ghodsian N. Mitochondrial deafness. Ear Hear 2003;24:303–13.
177. Sue CM, Lipsett LJ, Crimmins DS, et al. Cochlear origin of hearing loss in MELAS syndrome. Ann Neurol 1998;43:350–9.
178. Reardon W, Ross RJM, Sweeney MG, et al. Diabetes mellitus associated with a pathogenic point mutation in mitochondrial DNA. Lancet 1992;340:1376–9.
179. Usami S, Abe S, Kasai M, et al. Genetic and clinical features of sensorineural hearing loss associated with the 1555 mitochondrial mutation. Laryngoscope 1997;107:483–90.
180. Fischel-Ghodsian N, Bykhovskaya Y, Taylor K, et al. Temporal bone analysis of patients with presbycusis reveals high frequency of mitochondrial mutations. Hear Res 1997;110:147–54.
181. Riazuddin S, Castelein CM, Ahmed ZM, et al. Dominant modifier DFNM1 suppresses recessive deafness FNB26. Nature Genet 2000;26:431–4.
182. Llalwani AK. Evaluation of childhood sensorineural hearing loss in the post-genome world. Arch Otolaryngol Head Neck Surg 2002;128:88–9.
183. Parnes LS, Chernoff WG. Bilateral semicircular canal aplasia with near-normal cochlear development. Ann Otol Rhinol Laryngol 1990;99:957–9.
184. Yu KK, Mukherji S, Carrasco V, et al. Molecular genetic advances in semicircular canal abnormalities and sensorineural hearing loss: A report of 16 cases. Otolaryngol Head Neck Surg 2003;129:637–46.
185. Yoo T, Fujiyoshi T, Readhead C, Hood L. Restoration of auditory evoked potential by myelin basic protein (MBP) gene therapy in shiverer mice. Abstr Assoc Res Otolaryngol 1993;16:147.
186. Staecker H, Galinovic-Schwartz V, Liu W, et al. The role of the neurotrophins in maturation and maintenance of postnatal auditory innervation. Am J Otol 1996;17:486–92.
187. Leong K, D'Amore P, Marletta M, Langer R. Biodegradable polyanhydrides as drug-carrier matrices II. Biocompatibility and chemical reactivity. J Biomed Mater Res 1986;20:51–64.
188. Pardridge W. Receptor mediated peptide transport through the blood brain barrier. Endocr Rev 1986;7:314–30.
189. Federoff H, Geschwind MD, Geller AI, Kessler JA. Expression of NGF in vivo from a defective HSV-I vector prevents effects of axotomy on sympathetic ganglia. Proc Natl Acad Sci U S A 1992;89:1636–40.
190. Qun LX, Pirvola U, Saarma M, Ylikoski J. Neurotrophic factors in the auditory periphery. Ann N Y Acad Sci 1999;884:292–304.
191. Weiss MA, Frisancho JC, Roessler BJ, Raphael Y. Viral-mediated gene transfer in the cochlea. Int J Dev Neurosci 1997;15:577–83.
192. Dazert S, Battaglia A, Ryan AF. Transfection of neonatal rat cochlear cells in vitro with an adenovirus vector. Int J Dev Neurosci 1997;15:595–600.
193. Ryan A, Luo L. Delivery of a recombinant growth factor into the mouse inner ear by implantation of a transfected cell line. Abstr Assoc Res Otolaryngol 1995;18:47.
194. Kopke RD, Wassel RA, Mondalek, et al. Magnetic nanoparticles: Inner ear targeted molecule delivery and middle ear implant. Audiol Neurotol 2006;11:123–33.
195. Dormer K, Mamedova N, Kopke R, et al. Feasibility of superparamagnetic nanoparticles for drug delivery to the inner ear. Nanotech 2005;1:132–5.
196. Shkel AM, Zeng F-G. An electronic prosthesis mimicking the dynamic vestibular function. Audiol Neurotol 2006;11:113–22.
197. Bachman M, Zeng F-G, Xu T, Li G-P. Micromechanical resonator array for an implantable bionic ear. Audiol Neurotol 2006;11:95–103.

4

Physiology of the Auditory and Vestibular Systems

Brenda L. Lonsbury-Martin, PhD
Glen K. Martin, PhD
Maureen T. Hannley, PhD

AUDITORY SYSTEM

General Principles

Over the past three decades, major advances have occurred in our knowledge about how the ear achieves its high sensitivity, sharp frequency tuning, vast dynamic range, and precise temporal resolution. This accumulated wisdom has led to a new understanding about the unique functions of the inner hair cells (IHCs) and outer hair cells (OHCs) of the cochlea. Traditionally, the transfer of information about sounds from the environment to the higher centers of analysis in the central auditory nervous system was considered to be entirely a passive process. According to conventional thinking, the salient features of sound, including frequency, magnitude, and timing attributes, were principally encoded by peripheral processes and then simply passed relatively unaltered along the ascending system, from 1 structure to another, in a forward-moving manner. With the discoveries that the healthy ear can generate sounds in the form of otoacoustic emissions (OAEs) and that OHCs mechanically vibrate in response to depolarizing stimuli, the role of the cochlea in analyzing acoustic signals is now considered to represent an active process. Given the current view that the vibromechanical activity of the OHC along with certain aspects of its transduction properties underlie the generation of OAEs and the knowledge that a major portion of the cochlear efferent system innervates this particular class of hearing receptor, it is likely that central auditory centers also modify peripherally generated responses in an active manner. Thus, rather than conceptualizing the role of the auditory system as a passive analyzer of environmental sounds, the modern view is to consider it as an active participant in controlling acoustic information so that the most meaningful features are registered.

Auditory Apparatus

A traditional approach toward understanding the primary sensitivity, frequency tuning, and timing functions of the peripheral auditory system is to divide the periphery into 3 discrete parts. In this manner, the unique contributions that the external, middle, and inner ear, that is, cochlea, make to the overall analysis of sound can best be appreciated.

External Ear. The external ear or pinna of the mammal is regarded as a simple funnel that collects and crudely filters sound. Given the immobility of the human external ear, it is assumed that this frequency tuning function is performed passively. However, evidence from experimental studies suggests that the human pinna serves 2 functions: (1) it aids in sound localization, especially front-to-back and high-to-low distinctions, where interaural time differences provide no clues, and (2) along with the external ear canal, it increases acoustic pressure at the tympanic membrane in the 1.5 to 5 kHz range, which is the frequency range most important for speech perception. Evidence for the sound-localizing function of the human external ear includes the demonstration of accurate sound localization in patients with monaural hearing and the loss of this localization ability when the pinna of the hearing ear is strapped to the head. In addition, abnormally poor sound localization around an "imperfectly" remodeled pinna has been reported.[1]

In summarizing available data on the role that the external ear plays in boosting sound pressure at the tympanic membrane, Shaw described the contributions of the distinct parts of the head and neck and external ear by successively adding their different components in a model.[2] According to this classic analysis, shown in Figure 1, most of the individual components of the external ear provide complementary gains, resulting in a significant increase in sound pressure from approximately 2 to 7 kHz. When the overall additive effect is appreciated ("T" in Figure 1), it can be seen that at certain frequencies this gain is substantial, resulting in sound pressure increases on the order of 20 dB.

Studies of models of the human external ear suggest that the pinna extracts information about sound location by altering the transmission properties of different frequencies according to the location of the sound source relative to the pinna. For example, when the sound source is behind the ear, interference of directly transmitted sound with sound waves scattered off the pinna flange or helix alters the response in the 3 to 6 kHz range. Thus, the external ear modifies the spectrum of the incoming sound, allowing an individual to make judgments about the location of unknown sound sources. This localization ability suggests that the central part of the auditory system can use very subtle spectral cues in the analysis of environmental sounds.[3]

Middle Ear. Figure 2 outlines the anatomy of the middle and inner ears. The middle ear ossicles form a transmission pathway that conducts sound energy from the tympanic membrane, at the interface of the external and middle ear, to the oval window of the cochlea. The discussion of middle ear function is separated into two categories: (1) "impedance matching" between the air of the external environment and the fluids (perilymph and endolymph) of the cochlea and (2) the acoustic reflex of the middle ear muscle system. A third set of functions is served by the eustachian tube (pharyngotympanic tube), a narrow,

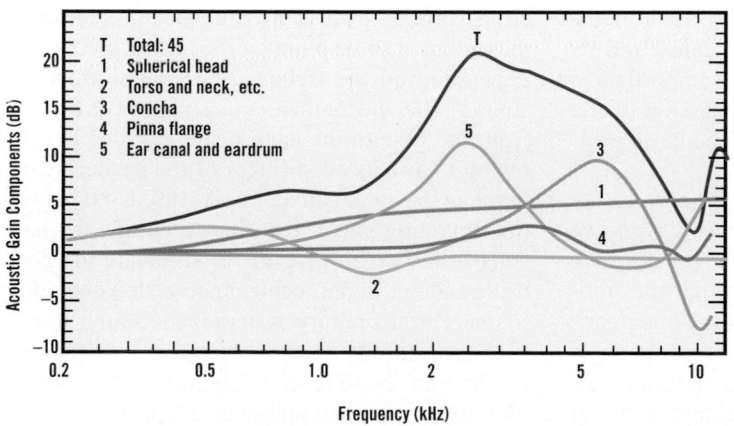

Figure 1 Pressure gain contributed by the individual components of the outer ear in humans. The total (T) curve plots the overall gain based on the addition of the various components in the order listed with the sound source positioned 45° from straight ahead. (Reprinted with permission from reference 2.)

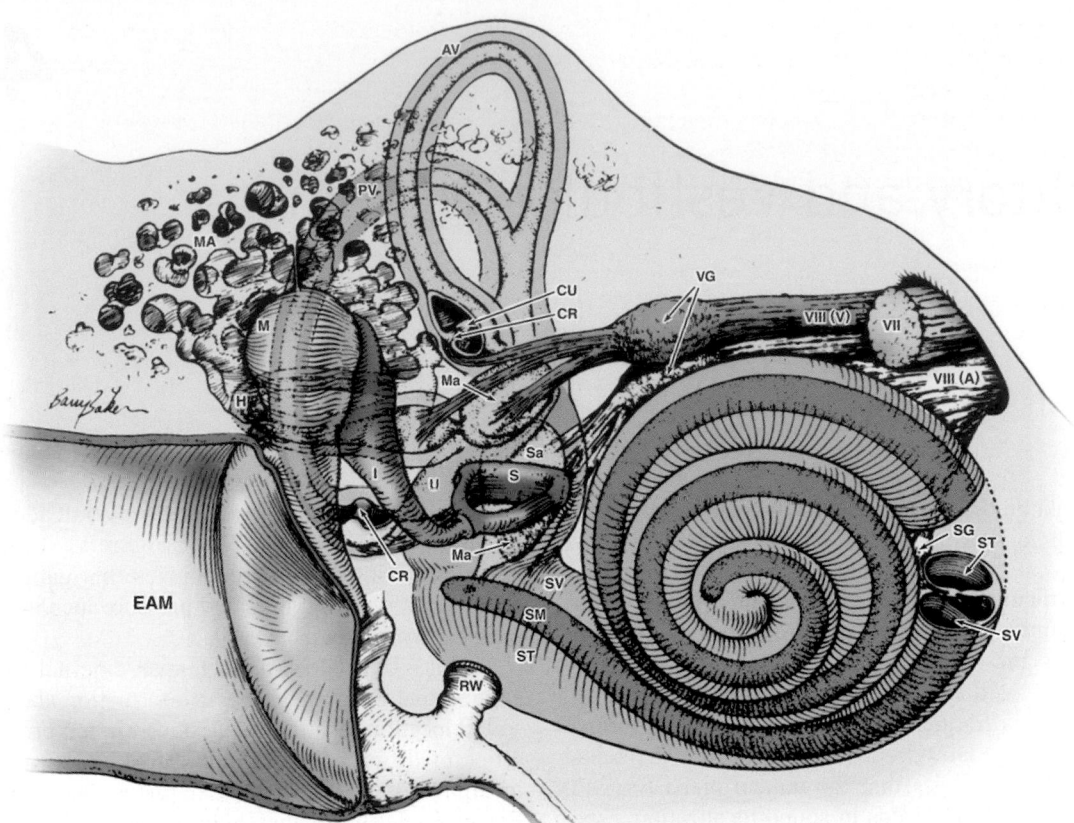

Figure 2 Schematic drawing of the inner ear (labyrinth), which consists of a series of tunnels within the petrous portion of the temporal bone. The osseous labyrinth (outer tunnel) is clear, and the membranous labyrinth (inner tunnel) is stippled. SV = scala vestibuli; ST = scala tympani; SM = scala media; SG = spiral ganglion, containing the cell bodies of the auditory nerve; VG = vestibular ganglia, containing the cell bodies of the vestibular nerve; VIII (A) = auditory part of the eighth cranial nerve; VIII (V) = vestibular part of the eighth cranial nerve; VII = facial nerve; Ma = macula; CU = cupula; CR = crista; Sa = sacculus; U = utriculus. Semicircular canals are labeled AV (anterior vertical), PV (posterior vertical), and H (horizontal). EAM = external auditory meatus; RW = round window; M = malleus; I = incus; S = stapes; MA = mastoid air cells in temporal bone.

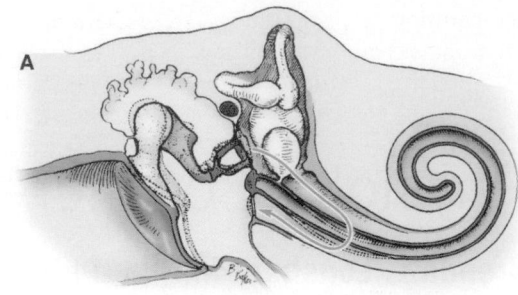

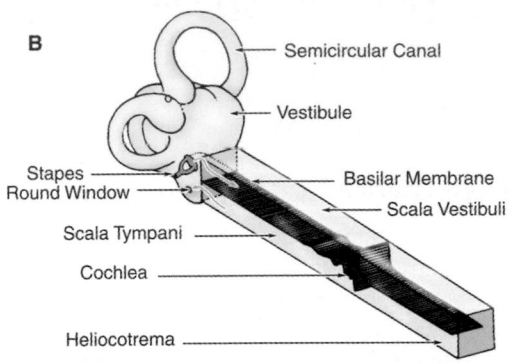

Figure 3 (A) Transmission of tympanic membrane movement to the cochlea via the ossicles. The system at rest is unstippled. The stippled ossicles and dashed cochlear partition illustrate the system when the tympanic membrane is pushed inward by a sound wave. (B) Inward pressure (*arrows*) initiates a traveling wave that migrates toward the apex of the cochlea (toward the helicotrema). This propagation depends largely on fluid coupling and the fact that the basilar membrane changes in stiffness, with the traveling wave moving from a region of highest stiffness (base) to a point of lower stiffness (apex). (Reproduced with permission from reference 4.)

osseocartilaginous channel connecting the middle ear space with the nasopharynx. These include ventilating the middle ear; equilibrating the air pressure in the middle ear with that of atmospheric pressure, thus permitting the tympanic membrane to stay in its most efficient neutral position; draining mucous secretions from the middle ear; and protecting the middle ear from reflux of nasopharyngeal and laryngopharyngeal secretions and from the disturbing awareness of one's own voice, breathing and other internal sounds (autophony). A discussion of eustachian tube anatomy, physiology, dysfunction, and treatment appears in Chapter 15, "Eustachian Tube Dysfunction."

The widespread use of surgical modification of middle ear structures to improve hearing and the usefulness of immittance audiometry make the concept of acoustic impedance and its relationship to middle ear function important to the clinician. Accordingly, the discussion of the middle ear begins by reviewing some basic principles of acoustic impedance.

Transmission of Acoustic Energy through the Middle Ear. Figure 3A diagrams the route for the transmission of sound energy through the middle ear into the cochlear portion of the inner ear.[4] The ossicular chain (see Figure 2), consisting of the malleus, incus, and stapes, can be thought of as a lever system. The tympanic membrane moves

the manubrium or handle of the malleus. In turn, the long process of the incus and manubrium moves together because the malleoincudal joint is essentially fixed. In contrast, the joint between the incus and the stapes is flexible. Therefore, because the stapes is fixed at its posteroinferior border, movement of the tympanic membrane causes it to rock in and out of the oval window. The changes in acoustic pressure caused by the stapes moving in and out of the oval window are transmitted instantaneously by the perilymph through the cochlear partition and then to the round window. This pressure transmission through the cochlear partition causes it to move either upward or downward, depending on the direction of the pressure change. The pressure change initiates a mechanical traveling wave, shown in Figure 3B, that reaches a maximum at some point on the basilar membrane depending on the frequency of the stimulating sound. The mechanical traveling wave moves from the base to the apex of the cochlea largely owing to a reduced stiffness of the basilar membrane in the apical direction. As discussed below, this traveling wave disturbance causes the hair cells in the organ of Corti to stimulate the dendritic endings of the cochlear nerve, thus signaling to the central auditory system that a sound stimulus has occurred.

At high sound levels of approximately 100 to 110 dB SPL (sound pressure level), the mode of

vibration of the ossicular chain changes. Thus, instead of rotating about its short axis, as shown in Figure 3A, the stapes footplate turns about its long axis.[5] Because this change results in less efficient sound transmission through the middle ear, it likely serves a protective function. Interestingly, the change in vibration mode occurs at the threshold of feeling, thus suggesting that the somatic sensation caused by excessive sounds may result from the detection of the altered ossicular vibration by middle ear bone and tendon receptors.

Impedance Matching by the Middle Ear. Hearing by terrestrial animals requires transmission of sound from an air to a fluid environment. A useful way to appreciate the problem in conducting sound effectively between two distinct media is to recall how difficult it is to listen to sounds produced even a few inches above the surface while swimming underwater. Thus, direct transmission of sound across an air/water boundary is extremely inefficient because the specific acoustic impedances of air and water differ greatly. Moreover, whenever energy is transmitted between media with different specific impedances, much of the energy is reflected back from the boundary between the two media. To help solve this problem, the middle ear matches reasonably well the impedances of the air with those of the cochlea and thereby greatly increases the efficiency of transmitting acoustic energy from the ambient environment into the cochlea.

The term impedance describes the opposition of a system to movement. Thus, the more force required to move a mechanical system at a given speed, the greater its impedance. Figure 4 illustrates the principles of mechanical impedance. The impedance of a mechanical system involves a complex relationship between the three physical parameters illustrated in Figure 4. Together, mass, stiffness, and resistance, that is, friction, determine the mechanical impedance of the middle ear system. Friction, the resistive component of impedance, consumes energy and is independent of the driving frequency. Stiffness and mass store energy; thus, they comprise the reactive component of impedance. For example, once the "fluid"-filled cylinder in Figure 4 is set in motion, it tends to continue because of inertia; and, if the spring representing stiffness is compressed, it tends to push backward.

Acoustic impedance represents a special type of mechanical impedance in which force is replaced by pressure, that is, force per unit area, and the system is driven by sound. Thus, Figure 4 could be converted into a diagram of an acoustic system by interposing a piston, or membrane, between the force and the mass.

When air conducts sound, the stiffness component of its acoustic impedance is determined by the elastic coupling between air molecules, the mass component is determined by the mass of the air molecules, and the frictional component is determined by frictional resistance between the molecules. Because water is much denser and less compressible than air, it might seem at first that mass and stiffness create the principal difference between the acoustic impedance of the cochlea and that of air. However, Figure 4 demonstrates that transmission of energy into the cochlea does not involve compression of the cochlear fluid itself. In addition, the elastic restorative forces of the cochlear partition and round window tend to cancel out the effect of the fluid's mass. Thus, the effective acoustic impedance of the cochlea is primarily resistive.[6]

As noted earlier, a primary function of the middle ear is to provide a means of "matching" the low impedance of air with the high cochlear impedance resulting from fluid flow and the distensibility of the cochlear membranes that separate the endolymph from the perilymph. Impedance matching by the middle ear is achieved by 3 factors: (1) the area of the tympanic membrane relative to the oval window, (2) the lever action of the middle ear ossicles, and (3) the shape of the tympanic membrane. The principles behind these factors are depicted in the 3 diagrams of Figure 5. By focusing the incident sound pressure from the large area of the tympanic membrane onto the small area of the oval window (Figure 5A), the effectiveness of energy transfer between the air of the external ear canal and the fluids of the cochlea is increased greatly. In the human, the area ratio of the tympanic membrane to the oval window is about 20 to 1. However, the tympanic membrane does not vibrate as a whole.[7] Thus, the effective area ratio is only about 14 to 1. The ossicular chain also contributes to the transformer role of the middle ear by a levering action that increases the vibration amplitude (Figure 5B). The ossicular chain lever ratio is around 1.3 to 1. A final factor influencing the efficiency of energy transfer depends on the conical shape of the tympanic membrane that allows a buckling action to occur (Figure 5C). The buckling motion of the tympanic membrane results in an increased force and decreased velocity to produce approximately a fourfold increase in the effectiveness of energy transfer.[8] Together, these actions of the middle ear system result in an estimated overall transformer ratio of 73 to 1.

Middle Ear Muscles. Mammals have 2 small skeletal muscles, the tensor tympani and the stapedius, which are attached to the ossicular chain. In primates, the stapedius muscle, which attaches to the stapes and is innervated by the stapedial branch of the facial nerve, contracts reflexively in response to intense sound stimuli. However, the tensor tympani muscle, which attaches to the malleus and is innervated by the trigeminal nerve, probably does not.[9] In laboratory animals such as the cat, rabbit, and guinea pig, both muscles contract in response to loud sound. However, the threshold of the tensor tympani is often higher than that of the stapedius muscle. A four-neuron reflex arc consisting of the afferent fibers of the auditory nerve, neurons of the ventral cochlear nucleus, neurons of the medial superior olive, and facial motoneurons comprises the stapedius reflex pathway illustrated in Figure 6 for the rabbit.[10] The reflex arc for the tensor tympani muscle is slightly different in that neurons of the ventral nucleus of the lateral lemniscus are also involved.[11] From the neural pathway depicted in Figure 6, it is clear that clinical abnormalities of

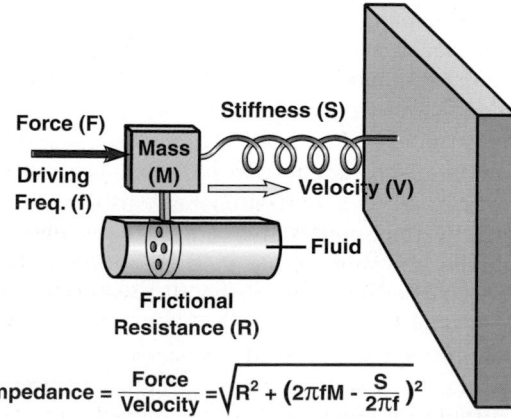

Figure 4 Principles of mechanical impedance. Frictional resistance is represented by a "dashpot"—a perforated piston operating inside a fluid-filled cylinder. The diagram could be converted to a representation of acoustic impedance by interposing a cylinder, or diaphragm, between the driving force (F) and the driven mass (M) and expressing the displacing input as pressure, that is, force per unit area.

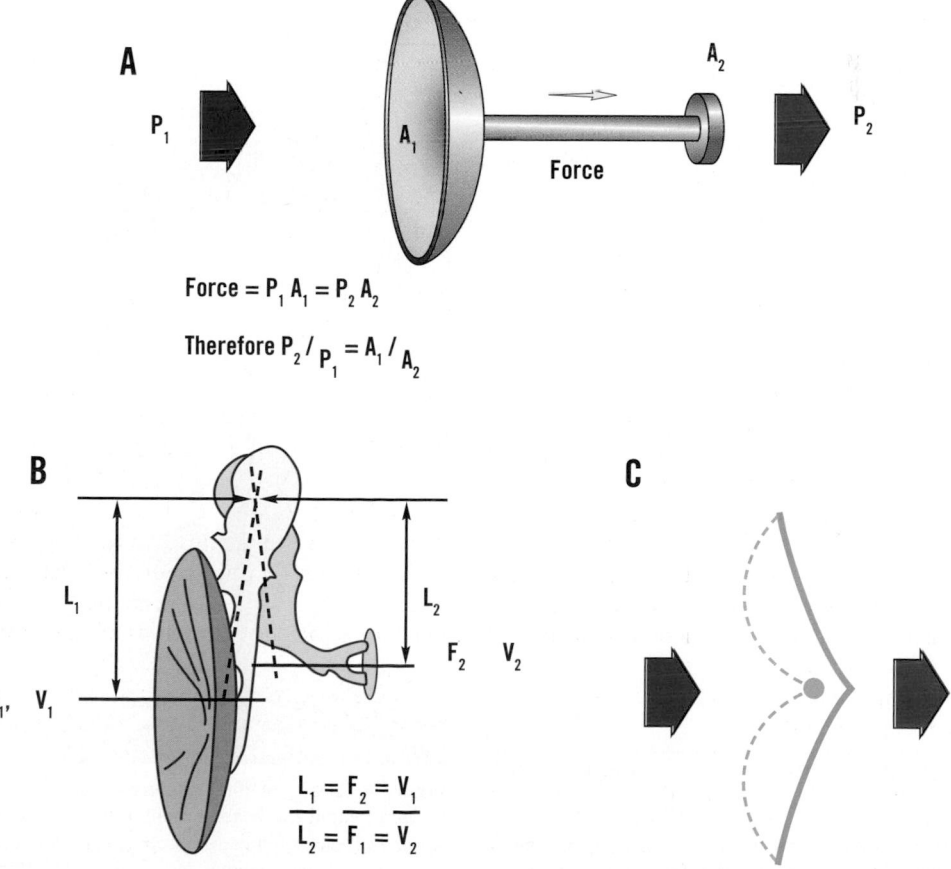

Figure 5 Illustration of the 3 principles of impedance matching performed by the middle ear. (A) The primary factor is the ratio of the area of the tympanic membrane to that of the oval window. (B) The lever action increases the force and decreases the velocity. (C) Buckling motion of the tympanic membrane also increases the force while reducing the velocity. (Reproduced with permission from reference 3.)

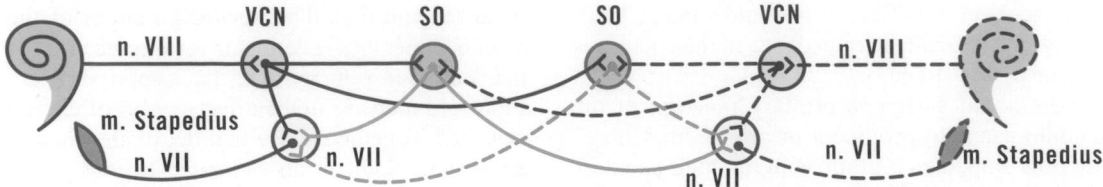

Figure 6 Neural pathway for the acoustic middle ear reflex in the rabbit. Reflex is mainly a chain of four neurons with a small ipsilateral three-neuron link. N. VIII = auditory nerve; N. VII = facial nerve; VCN = ventral cochlear nucleus; SO = superior olive; n. VII = facial nerve motoneuron. (Reproduced with permission from reference 10.)

the acoustic reflex primarily implicate pathology at the level of the lower brainstem.

In Figure 7, the sensitivity of the stapedius reflex in humans is plotted as a function of sound frequency. The reflex threshold curve evoked by pure tones parallels the audibility threshold curve but is about 80 dB above it.[12] Not surprisingly, because of their greater overall energy levels, broadband stimuli, for example, white noise, elicit the reflex more effectively than do pure tones.[13] Experimental evidence indicates that the stapedius reflex threshold decreases with increasing stimulus duration, with a time constant of about 200 ms.[14] This value approximates the time constant of temporal summation for the percepts of loudness and sensitivity. These findings, along with the clinical observation that the stapedius reflex exhibits "recruitment" in patients with cochlear hearing loss,[15] suggest that the acoustic reflex threshold correlates more with subjective loudness than with absolute stimulus intensity.

Contraction of the middle ear muscles can also be caused by nonauditory factors, including (1) spontaneous contractions, (2) body movements,[9] (3) vocalizations in which contractions begin prior to vocalization,[9] that is, prevocalization contractions, (4) movements of facial muscles involving only the tensor tympani,[9] (5) stimulation of the external ear canal,[16] and (6) voluntary contractions.[17]

As diagrammed in Figure 8, the stapedius muscle moves the stapes footplate medially into the oval window, whereas the tensor tympani muscle pulls the manubrium inward. The effects of these contractions on the transmission of pure tones through the middle ear[17,18] are illustrated in Figure 9. In summary, the transmission of low-frequency sounds is attenuated by contraction of either muscle,[13] but the stapedius is probably a somewhat better attenuator than the tensor tympani.

The function of the human acoustic reflex has been studied by recording (1) gross muscle potentials via the electromyogram,[9] (2) pressure changes in the external auditory canal,[19] and (3) acoustic immittance changes.[13,15] The clinical application of acoustic impedance measurements is known as immittance audiometry, with the terms "impedance" and "immittance" being interchangeable. In Figure 10, the time course is shown for the human stapedius reflex as recorded by the immittance change method. The latency or time to the first detectable change generally varies from

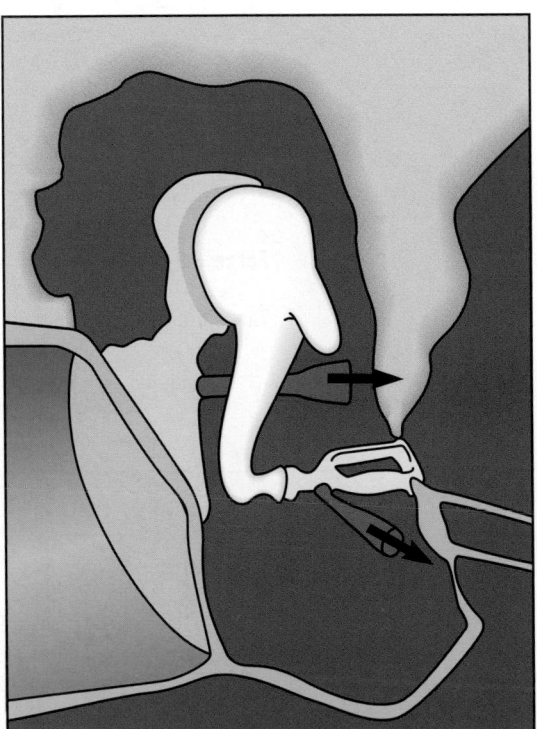

Figure 8 Action of the middle ear muscles. The view is from behind the head. The muscles are not drawn to scale. The tensor tympani muscle (*top arrow*) attaches to the handle of the malleus and pulls it medially, tensing the tympanic membrane. The stapedius muscle (*bottom arrow*) attaches to the neck of the stapes and pulls the posteroinferior border of the stapes footplate medially into the oval window.

10 to 30 ms, whereas the reflex decays over about 500 ms after the onset of the stimulus. The initial reduction in impedance is frequency dependent.

To date, acoustics-based clinical evaluations of middle ear function using immittance audiometry are an important part of the audiologic diagnostic test battery. However, they are not specific enough to represent independent diagnostic tests mainly because of limitations in the frequency range over which impedance is easily measured at the tympanic membrane and the wide variations in their normal values. Currently, several new techniques, ear canal reflectance[20] and tympanic membrane velocity measurements,[21] are being investigated to determine if they can act as more specific indicators of middle ear dysfunction. In particular, wideband energy reflectance measures of middle ear function are gaining in popularity in terms of their ability to describe better the contribution of an abnormal middle ear system to hearing problems.[22]

One major function of the middle ear muscles is to support and stiffen the ossicular chain.[13] In addition, because loud sounds are attenuated by the actions of the acoustic reflex, it is likely that another function of the reflex is to protect the inner ear against the damage that can be caused by overexposure to excessive sounds. This notion is supported by the results of a study investigating the amount of temporary threshold shift in patients suffering from acute Bell palsy, which represents a disease in which the stapedius muscle can be completely paralyzed.[23] These patients showed a greater threshold shift in the affected ear after exposures to low-frequency noise than in the opposite ear with a normal stapedius reflex. However, whether this protective effect is a "true" function of the stapedius reflex has been criticized on the basis that the continuous loud sounds against which the reflex is supposed to protect do not exist in nature.[24]

An alternative middle ear muscle function could be to attenuate low-frequency masking sounds that might otherwise interfere with auditory function. Contractions during chewing and other facial and body movements would attenuate the resultant internal body sounds, which are largely low frequency, while preserving sensitivity to high-frequency external sounds. The low-frequency attenuation produced by contractions prior to vocalization may also be functionally important. Observations that support a middle ear muscle role in vocalization and in speech discrimination are as follows: (1) patients with otosclerosis show significant deficits when administered the delayed feedback test for malingering,[25] (2) stutterers have a deficit in prevocalization middle ear muscle contraction,[26] and (3) absence of the stapedius reflex results in decreased speech discrimination when the level of speech is raised above 90 dB SPL in patients with seventh and eighth nerve disorders[26–28] and even in normal individuals.[29]

Cochlea. The cochlea performs two basic functions as (1) a transducer that translates sound

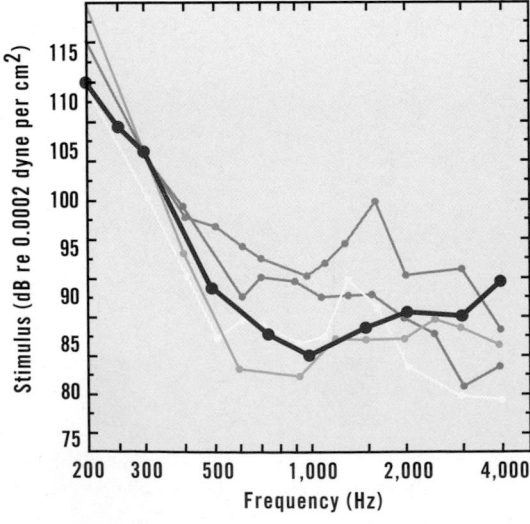

Figure 7 Sensitivity of the human acoustic reflex. Dashed lines from four subjects plot stimulus levels required to elicit an acoustic reflex with 10% of the maximum obtainable amplitude (measured with an immittance technique). The bold red line is the threshold of audibility raised 80 dB. (Reprinted with permission from reference 12.)

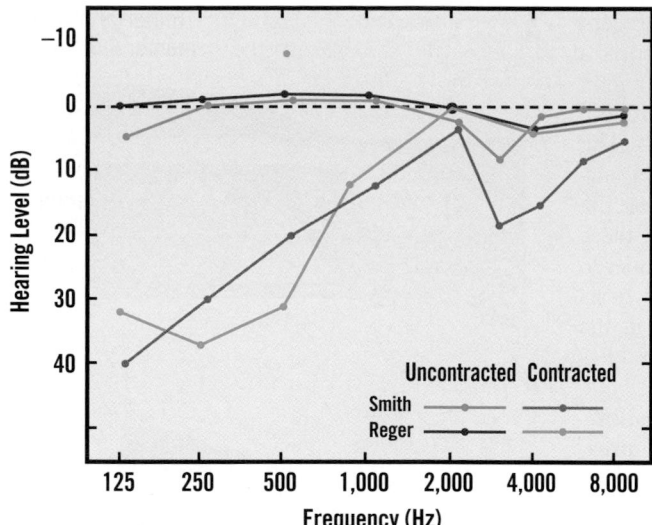

Figure 9 Effect of middle ear muscle contractions on pure-tone thresholds. The curves were obtained from normal subjects with the ability to voluntarily contract their middle ear muscles.[17,18] Although the effect of voluntary contraction may differ from the effect of normal involuntary contraction, the general observation that middle ear muscle contractions preferentially attenuate low frequencies is probably valid.

energy into a form suitable for stimulating the dendritic endings of the auditory nerve and (2) an encoder that programs the features of an acoustic stimulus so that the brain can process the information contained in the stimulating sound. Each of these functions is considered below.

Transducer Function. Anatomy. As shown in Figure 11A, the cochlea is divided into three tubes or scalae. The middle tube or scala media is the cochlear extension of the membranous labyrinth and is filled with a potassium (K^+)-rich, sodium (Na^+)-poor electrolyte fluid called endolymph.[30] The outer two tubes, the scala vestibuli and the scala tympani, fill the rest of the osseous labyrinth. They are separated by the scala media and filled with perilymph, a Na^+-rich, K^+-poor electrolyte fluid. When the cochlea is activated by sound, the scala media and its contents, bounded superiorly by Reissner membrane and inferiorly by the basilar

membrane, tend to move as a unit. This space is referred to as the "cochlear partition."[5]

The contents of scala media are illustrated in Figure 11B.[31] The auditory nerve fibers synapse at the bases of the hair cells of the organ of Corti. The dendrites of the auditory nerve enter the scala media through the habenulae perforatae, where they lose their myelin sheaths. The reticular lamina and the tectorial membrane are two membranes in the organ of Corti that are particularly critical in stimulus transduction. The reticular lamina, supported by the rods of Corti, resembles a stiff net with its webbing enmeshing

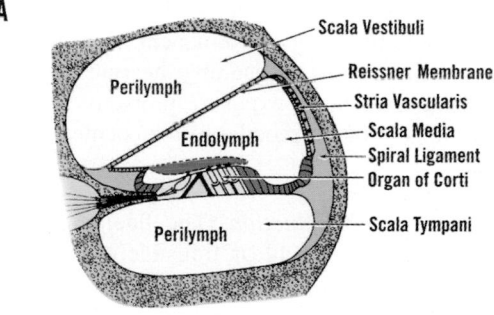

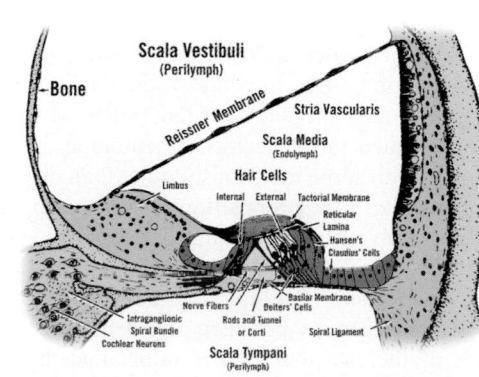

Figure 11 (A) Simplified drawing depicting a cross-section through one turn of the cochlea showing the three compartments (scalae). The middle compartment (scala media) is filled with K^+-rich endolymph. The other two compartments (scala tympani and scala vestibuli) are enclosed in the osseous labyrinth. These compartments are filled with Na^+-rich perilymph. (B) Semidiagrammatic representation of a cross-section of the guinea pig cochlear duct. (A reproduced with permission from reference 30; B reproduced with permission from reference 31.)

the apical surfaces of the hair cells. Together, the rods of Corti and the reticular lamina provide the skeletal support of the organ of Corti.

The boundary separating the high-K^+ and high-Na^+ electrolytes is formed by the reticular lamina. As diagrammed in Figure 12, tight junctions, which are generally thought to present a barrier against ionic diffusion, are observed by scanning electron microscopy (SEM) between all cells that face the endolymphatic space. Figure 12 also indicates that the junctions between non-sensory epithelium (eg, the cells of Hensen and Claudius, the cells lining the spaces of Nuel, and the cells of Reissner membrane) are not as "tight" (dotted line) as the junctions between the sensory cells and the basal cells (solid line) of the stria vascularis.[32] The fluid within the organ of Corti (ie, between the basilar membrane and the reticular lamina) has been termed cortilymph.[33] However, the fluid in this space is in free communication with the perilymph of scala tympani via relatively large channels through the basilar membrane.[34] Thus, cortilymph is probably identical to perilymph with respect to its electrolyte content. The tectorial membrane resembles a rather stiff, oval, gelatinous tube. It is attached to the limbus by a flexible membranous band that allows it to move up and down like the cover of a book.[35]

Mammals have 3 rows of OHCs. A fourth row of OHCs is seen in an occasional cross-section, especially in primates, but there is no well-defined fourth row.[36] There is only 1 row of IHCs. The fine fingerlike projections present on the apical surface of the hair cells are called stereocilia. The detailed arrangements of the stereocilia on the hair cell apices are unique to each class of receptor and are illustrated in the SEM of Figure 13.[37] The IHC stereocilia form a longitudinally oriented, relatively shallow curve, whereas the OHC cilia make a radially oriented

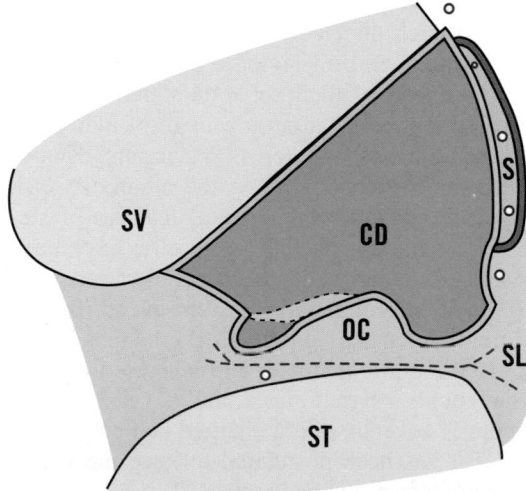

Figure 12 The perilymph/endolymph barriers around the scala media and stria vascularis. The dotted line represents "intermediate-to-tight" tight junctions, whereas the solid line represents "very tight" junctions. The circles represent blood vessels, all of which have tight junctions that separate them from the intracochlear spaces. SV = scala vestibuli; ST = scala tympani; CD = cochlear duct; OC = organ of Corti; S = stria vascularis; SL = spiral ligament. (Reproduced with permission from reference 32.)

Figure 10 Time course of human stapedius contractions in response to white noise (WN) and 2 kHz pure-tone stimuli. Bottom trace shows stimulus time course. The stimuli were 90 dB above normal threshold and were delivered to the right ear. The muscle contractions were recorded from the left ear by the acoustic immittance change method. (Records courtesy of Dr James Jerger.)

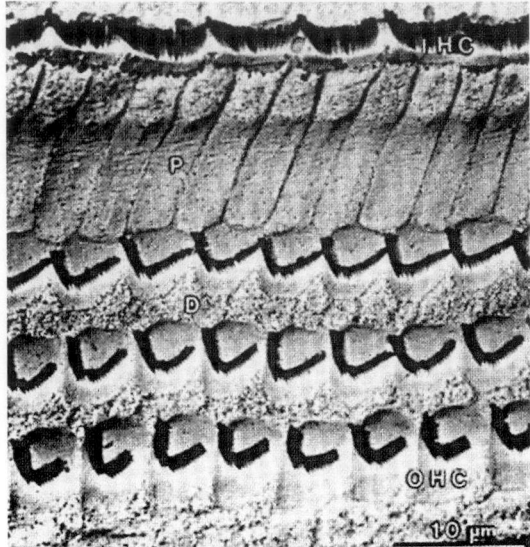

Figure 13 Scanning electron micrograph of the surface of the organ of Corti after removal of the tectorial membrane. A single row of inner hair cells (IHCs) has cilia arranged in a linear (or shallow "U") pattern, whereas the 3 rows of outer hair cells (OHCs) have stereocilia arranged in a "V" pattern. D = Deiters cells; P = pillar cells. (Reproduced with permission from reference 37.)

"V," with a notch at the apex marking the site of the missing kinocilium that degenerates embryonically during development of cochlear hair cells. The OHC stereocilia vary systematically in length in that they are longest at the apex of the V and shorten progressively from the apex to the distal limbs. Whereas the longest OHC stereocilia attach to the undersurface of the tectorial membrane, it is probable that the shorter cilia do not.[38] However, an interconnecting network of fine fibrils links the entire bundle of stereocilia, both laterally and from tip to tip, so that it moves as a unit.[39]

Until recently, little was known about stereocilia bundles. However, their importance in the transduction process has stimulated considerable research directed toward understanding the morphologic and physiologic properties of hair cell bundles and their separate stereocilia. The detailed structure and arrangement of individual hair cell bundles vary across species and even as a function of position along the organ of Corti. However, a number of general features of stereocilia bundles and individual cilia have been described, including (1) each bundle consists of 30 to 150 stereocilia arranged in several rows of decreasing length, (2) individual cilia range from 0.8 to 0.2 μm in diameter and increase in length from cochlear base to apex, and (3) each stereocilium is covered with a charged cell coat material that has been postulated to keep individual stereocilia from fusing together.[40]

Using various techniques, Flock and coworkers demonstrated that stereocilia contained the proteins actin and fimbrin.[41,42] Indeed, one theory was that stereocilia and their associated ion channels participate in an amplificatory process that sensitizes and sharpens hearing.[43] Although the unidirectional orientation of the actin filaments[44] initially suggested that these proteins served a

structural rather than a contractile role, recent evidence using immunofluorescence supports a rapid turnover of proteins of the stereocilia actin core[45] as well as the major membrane protein, that is, plasma membrane Ca^{2+}-ATPase-2. The latter plasma membrane component has a surprisingly brief half-life residency in stereocilia of approximately 5 to 7 hours.[46] Together, these observations demonstrate that stereocilia undergo continuous renewal, which may form the basis for developing a "replacement" therapy in the future for either salvaging damaged hair bundles or regrowing missing ones.

Other studies from the laboratories of Dallos[47] and Liberman[48] have demonstrated the presence of a third protein, prestin, in the plasma membrane of the OHC's lateral wall. In contrast to enzyme activity-based motors, prestin is a voltage-to-force converter that, by regulating changes in hair cell length in response to electric membrane potential variation, thus functions as the motor for OHC motility, enabling mechanical amplification of approximately 100-fold, or about a 40 dB gain in hearing sensitivity.

Functional studies of the mechanical properties of stereocilia showed that the cilia are stiff and pivot at their bases.[49] When too much force is applied, the stereocilia break as if they were brittle. Noise exposure studies have also demonstrated the vulnerability of stereocilia to damage.[40] That is, the tallest stereocilia are affected first by becoming floppy owing to alterations in their membrane and cytoskeleton. With continued noise exposure, the stereocilia fuse and then degenerate, resulting in permanent hearing loss. In fact, the earliest measurable hearing changes resulting from noise exposure probably involve alterations in the stereocilia of the cochlea's hair cells.[40]

Mechanical Transduction. The final mechanical event in the cochlear transduction process is the bending of the stereocilia, as illustrated in Figure 14. Basilar membrane deformation causes a shearing action between the reticular and tectorial membranes. Because the long OHC cilia are attached to both membranes, they are bent (Figure 14B). In contrast, the IHC cilia, and possibly also the shorter OHC cilia, which are not attached to the tectorial membrane, bend in response to some mechanism other than displacement shear. One proposition is that this process may involve fluid streaming between the sliding parallel plates formed by the reticular and tectorial membranes.[50] Fluid streaming would result from differences between the relative velocities of the two membranes rather than by their relative displacements. Thus, the IHCs may be velocity sensors and the OHCs displacement sensors.[51,52] However, other notions about the unique functions of OHCs versus IHCs have also been proposed.[53] For example, von Békésy noted that the shearing action between the 2 membranes could reduce the displacement amplitude of the stimulating energy while increasing its force.[5,54] Thus, the shearing action may serve to match

A

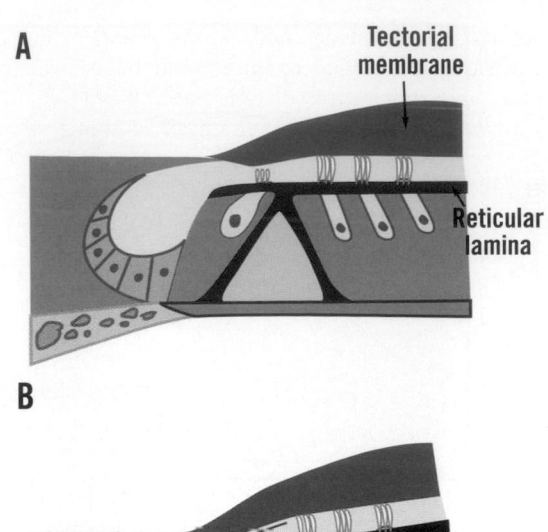

B

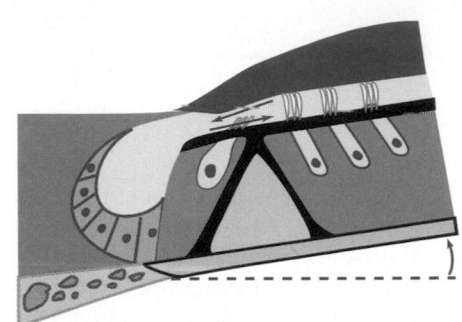

Figure 14 (A) Translation of basilar membrane displacement (as shown in Figure 3) into bending of the hair cell cilia. (B) Basilar membrane displacement (*arrow*) indicates the shearing action between the tectorial membrane and the reticular lamina bends the OHC cilia, which are attached to both structures. Streaming movement, imparted to the fluid between the reticular lamina and the tectorial membrane, may bend the inner hair cell cilia, which are not attached to the tectorial membrane. Inner hair cell cilia deflection may be longitudinal, that is, perpendicular to the page, rather than radial, as depicted.

the impedances of fluid and solid transmission media, just as the middle ear matches air and fluid impedances.

Electrical Potentials of the Cochlea. Using gross microelectrode methods, 3 cochlear bioelectric events have been studied extensively: (1) the endocochlear potential (EP), (2) the cochlear microphonic (CM), and (3) the summating potential (SP). Whereas the EP is present at rest, the CM and SP appear only when sound stimulates the ear.

Endocochlear Potential. The EP is a constant direct current (DC), +80 mV potential that can be recorded with an electrode in the scala media.[55] The majority of evidence indicates that the stria vascularis generates the EP.[56] Because it is extremely sensitive to anoxia and chemical agents interfering with oxidative metabolism,[56–58] its existence likely depends on the active metabolic ion pumping processes of the stria vascularis.[59] The anatomic distribution of the EP closely approximates the limits of the endolymphatic compartment formed by the tight junction boundaries shown in Figure 12. The augmentation of the voltage drop cross the apical ends of the hair cells that the EP provides is thought to be critically important in cochlear transduction.[60]

Cochlear Microphonics and Summating Potentials. When the appropriate stimulus is applied, most sensory end-organs generate bio-electric events called receptor potentials. These potentials differ from action potentials in that (1) they are graded rather than all or none, (2) they have no latency, (3) they are not propagated, and (4) they have no apparent postresponse refractoriness.[61] The SP and CM form the receptor potentials of the cochlea and can be recorded indirectly from gross electrodes on the round window or directly from the fluid spaces within the organ of Corti.

The CM reproduces the alternating current (AC) waveform of the stimulating sound (hence the name "microphonic"[62]). The SP, illustrated in the lowest inset at the top left of Figure 15,[63] represents the DC shift that follows the "envelope" of the stimulating sound.[64] As depicted in Figure 15, both the CM and SP are generated across the hair-bearing end of the hair cells.[55,65] Based on experimental findings, it is assumed that the generator site for the receptor potentials is at the apical tips of the stereocilia.[66]

The results of intracellular recordings from IHCs and OHCs suggest that IHCs generate the SP and the OHCs generate the CM.[53] Generation of the SP requires some form of rectification of the acoustic waveform, that is, alteration from a waveform that oscillates above and below the baseline to a waveform that is entirely above or below the baseline. It is reasonably straightforward to model the mechanical coupling of the free-floating IHC cilia in such a way as to produce the mechanical rectification. Thus, the concept

that the IHCs generate the SP fits well with what is known about the morphology of this class of hair cell. Other evidence, however, derived from recording in the fluid spaces of the cochlea with OHCs selectively damaged by kanamycin,[67] suggests that the both IHCs and OHCs contribute to the volume-recorded SP and CM. Indeed, this latter notion represents the current consensus of the field.[68]

Generation of the CM can be understood by examination of the resistance battery model of Davis[69] depicted in Figure 16. In this conceptualization, the EP serves as the "battery" that provides the driving force to move current through the high resistance of the reticular lamina in which the apical ends of the hair cells are embedded. The traveling wave displaces the basilar membrane, resulting in the deflection of the stereocilia and changes in hair cell resistance. Thus, hair cells acting as variable resistors modulate current flow across the reticular lamina to produce a time-varying potential, the CM, which follows the waveform of the input stimulus.[3]

Role of the Cochlear Potentials in Stimulus Transduction. Wever and Bray's discovery of the CM[70] led to the hypothesis that auditory nerve fiber endings are stimulated electrically.[71] However, studies with the transmission electron microscope (TEM) revealed that the morphology of the interfaces between the afferent nerve endings and the hair cell bases was unmistakably that of a chemical synapse. The chemical synapse-like

structures found there include (1) a synaptic cleft, that is, a uniform space between the hair cell and nerve fiber membranes, (2) synaptic vesicles, and (3) a synaptic bar in the form of an electron-dense disk surrounded by vesicles that resembles the synaptic ribbon of the retina.[72]

The presence of subcellular organelles consistent with a chemical synapse at the hair cell/auditory nerve junction supports the current view that a chemical transmitter released by the hair cell stimulates the auditory nerve endings.[73] Thus, cochlear receptor potentials are probably either directly involved in the cause-and-effect chain leading to chemical stimulation of the auditory nerve or are intimately related to a process that is directly involved but does not stimulate the auditory nerve fibers electrically.[69]

Current thinking about cochlear transduction, which originates primarily from the studies of Hudspeth,[73] is illustrated in Figure 17. In this formulation, displacement of the hair cell bundle opens the transduction channels located at the tips of the stereocilia to allow K^+ to flow into the cell. This influx of K^+ depolarizes the cell, causing calcium (Ca^{2+}) channels at the base of the hair cell to open, thus admitting Ca^{2+} into the cell. The Ca^{2+} ions, in turn, stimulate the transmitter vesicles to fuse with the hair cell membrane and release transmitter into the synaptic cleft. Transmitter substance then diffuses across the synaptic space to initiate action potentials in the adjacent auditory nerve fibers.

Cochlear Transmitters. One area of intense research interest in the study of cochlear transduction leading to intercellular communication has been the identification of the afferent transmitter substance that is released onto the primary afferent neurons at the bases of the IHCs and OHCs. In combination with these studies, other efforts have attempted to characterize the efferent neurotransmitter released on the hair cells and on afferent endings terminating on hair cells by efferent neurons originating in the brainstem. Recent evidence indicates that the afferent neurotransmitter is probably a single excitatory amino acid, or a structurally related compound, which is responsible for initiating auditory nerve action potentials. Besides this chemical transmitter substance, other chemicals, called neuromodulators,[74] that influence the action of the transmitter are also believed to be released into the synaptic cleft.[75]

In the search for neurotransmitters, several criteria have been established that are requisite for the identification of transmitter substances.[76] These criteria require that (1) the transmitter must produce the same response when applied to the synapse as the natural stimulation of presynaptic elements, (2) extraneous substances that alter natural synaptic transmission such as blocking agents should produce the same effect on the transmitter candidate, (3) stimulation of presynaptic elements should release the transmitter substance, (4) the transmitter substance must be shown to exist presynaptically, (5) enzymes responsible for the

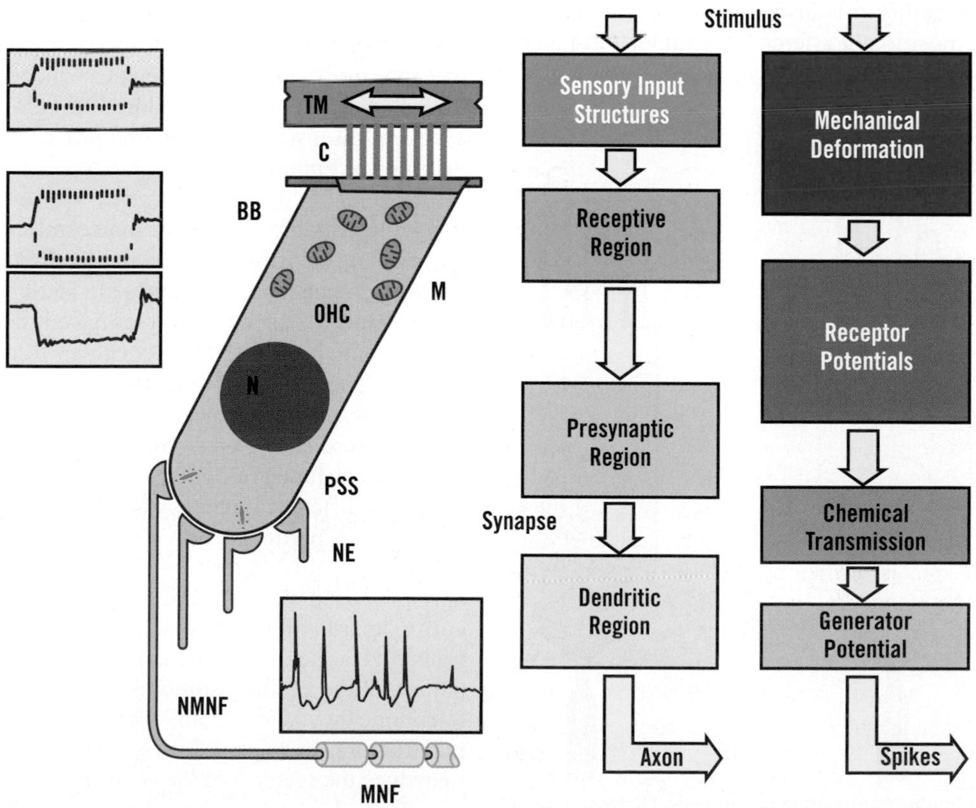

Figure 15 Generator sites of cochlear potentials (*upper left from top to bottom*: sound stimulus, cochlear microphonic, and summating potential) and functional diagram of the cochlear transducer mechanism (*right*). TM = tectorial membrane; C = cilia; OHC = outer hair cell body; N = cell nucleus; M = mitochondria; PSS = presynaptic structures; NE = afferent nerve endings; NMNF = nonmyelinated segment of nerve fiber; MNF = myelinated segment of nerve fiber; BB = basal body. (Reproduced with permission from reference 63.)

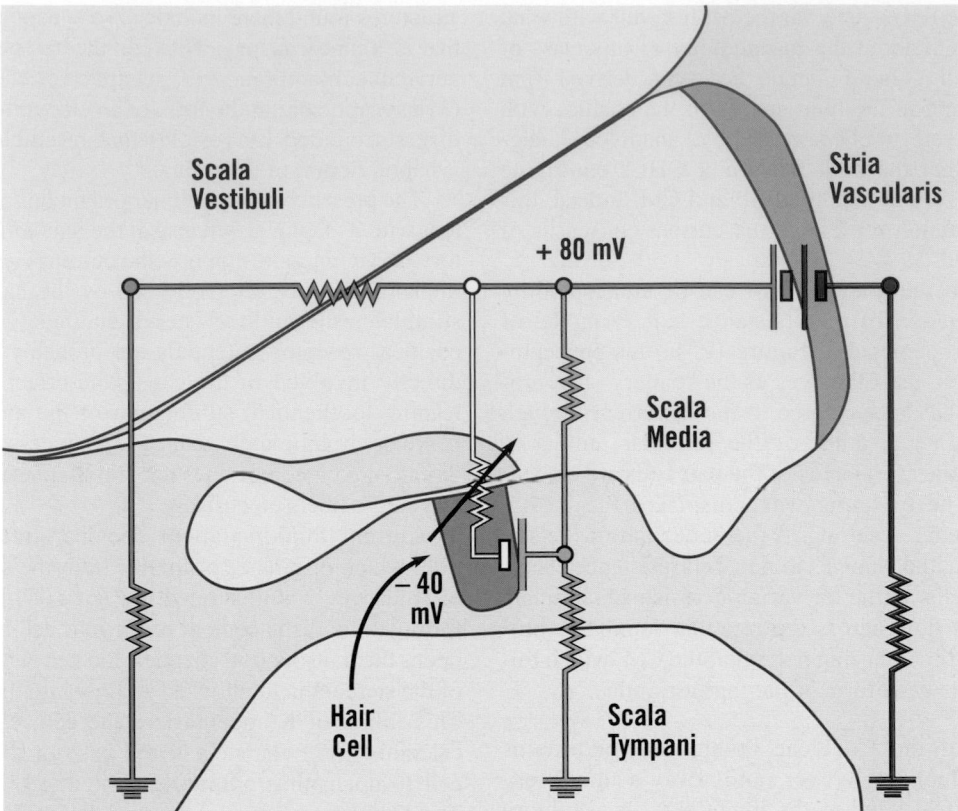

Figure 16 Diagram of Davis' battery model of transduction in which the positive endocochlear potential and negative intracellular potential provide the force to drive current through the variable resistances at the top of the hair cells. (Reprinted with permission from reference 3.)

synthesis of the transmitter candidate must be present, and (6) a mechanism must be demonstrated that can deactivate the transmitter once it has been released into the synaptic cleft. To date, concrete evidence for the auditory transmitter in the mammalian cochlea is scanty when compared

with the findings of other studies of the central nervous system. That is to say, all of the criteria have yet to be met for any candidate afferent transmitter substance. However, based on our present ability to satisfy the above criteria, one of the most likely afferent transmitter substances

is believed to be the excitatory amino acid glutamate,[77] and aspartate, too, represents a more recently documented potential candidate.[78]

Documentation regarding the efferent transmitter in the mammalian cochlea is considerably stronger with the most persuasive evidence favoring acetylcholine (ACh). The strongest support for ACh comes from a set of experiments demonstrating that anticholinergic compounds block the effects of efferent stimulation but do not influence afferent cochlear activity.[79] From other histochemical and immunostaining studies of the mammalian cochlea, there is considerable evidence for a GABAergic, that is, γ-aminobutyric acid, efferent innervation of the OHCs, as well as the IHC afferents, including (1) measurements of the uptake of tritiated GABA,[80] (2) immunostaining for glutamic acid decarboxylase,[81] and (3) immunostaining for GABA.[81] Interestingly, evidence that isolated OHCs stain for GABA[82] and that GABA application to isolated OHCs induces membrane hyperpolarization and membrane elongation[83] infers that the functional consequences of this candidate transmitter substance is inhibition of the electromechanical transduction process. For a more in-depth treatment of studies of cochlear transmitters, readers are encouraged to consult an excellent review.[84]

Coding in the Cochlea. The cochlea must encode acoustic features into properties of neural activity. The principal acoustic parameters to be encoded are frequency, intensity, and temporal pattern, whereas the basic biologic variables available for neural encoding are place, that is, the location of the activated cell, amount of neural firing, and temporal pattern of firing. Because they are the percepts most studied, the cochlear encoding of frequency and intensity is addressed below. For excellent discussions of temporal processing, see Frisina[85] or Eggermont.[86]

Frequency Coding. In the late nineteenth century, 2 opposing theories of frequency coding in the auditory periphery were proposed. These classic "place" and "frequency" theories have influenced subsequent thinking about cochlear frequency coding.[3] The place theory of Helmholtz held that the basilar membrane acts as if it were a series of tuned resonators, analogous to a set of piano strings. Each tuned resonator vibrates sympathetically to a different frequency and thus selectively stimulates a particular nerve fiber. Rutherford's frequency theory, later termed "telephone" theory, proposed that all frequencies activate the entire length of the basilar membrane, which transmits, essentially unchanged, the temporal pattern of the auditory stimulus. According to the telephone theory, it remains for more central neural structures to "decode" these temporal patterns to deduce the features of the acoustic stimulus.

Evidence for Place Coding: Mechanical and Neural Tuning Curves. Von Békésy used optical methods to make the first direct observations of the mechanical place analysis of

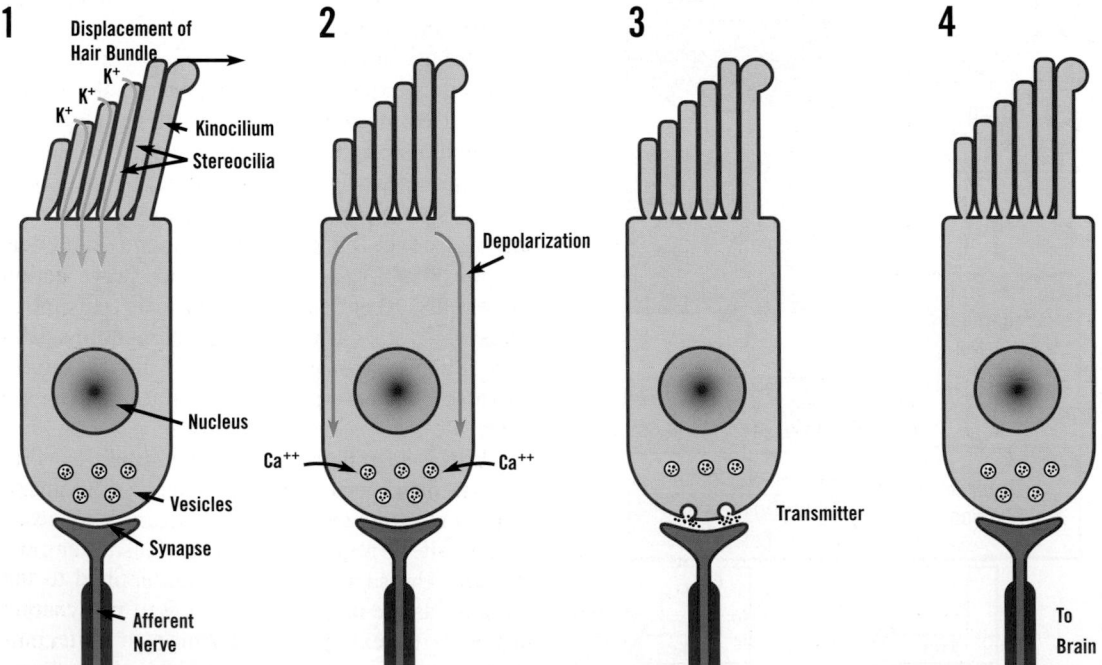

Figure 17 Schematic representation of the major steps involved in stimulus transduction in hair cells. Deflection of the hair bundle (1) opens the transduction channels to allow K$^+$ to flow into the hair cell. This results in a reduction of potential difference or depolarization. Depolarization spreads instantly to the lower part of the cell (2), causing Ca^{2+} channels to open. Ca^{2+} ions (3) cause transmitter vesicles to fuse with the basal part of the cell membrane. Fusing vesicles release transmitter substance into the synaptic cleft. (4) Transmitter diffuses across the synaptic cleft to initiate an action potential in the adjacent auditory nerve fiber. (Reproduced with permission from reference 73.)

stimulus frequency in the cochlea.[5] Subsequent observations using more sensitive techniques (eg, Mössbauer radioactive source, capacitive probe, laser interferometry) confirmed the general nature of von Békésy's results but, as discussed below, modified his conclusions with respect to several important details.[87]

The principal features of the mechanical responses that von Békésy observed are illustrated in Figure 18. Each pure-tone cycle elicits a traveling wave that moves along the cochlear partition from base to apex.[5] As it travels, the wave's amplitude increases slowly, passes through a maximum, and then declines rapidly (Figure 18A).[88] As the frequency of the stimulating tone is increased, the maximum of the traveling wave moves basally toward the oval window.

The inset at the bottom of Figure 18B illustrates the tuned behavior of the vibration of a specific locus on the cochlear partition that results from the traveling wave patterns generated by stimuli of different frequencies (4 plots above). The bottom plot of Figure 18B, called a cochlear mechanical tuning curve, was obtained by plotting the vibration amplitude of a single cochlear partition point against the exciting

frequency. The frequency that generates the maximum vibration of a specific place on the cochlear partition is that point's characteristic frequency (CF). Thus, the plot at the bottom of Figure 18B illustrates the mechanical tuning curve for a place on the cochlear partition with a CF of 150 Hz. Mechanical tuning curves at all cochlear partition locations have the same general shape, that is, a rapid falloff for frequencies above the CF (>150 Hz) and a gradual drop-off for frequencies below the CF (<150 Hz).

Microelectrode recordings from single hair cells and auditory nerve fibers yield an analog of the cochlear mechanical tuning curve. Figures 19 and 20, respectively, show examples of neural tuning curves obtained from primary auditory nerve fibers with traditional glass micropipets[89] and mechanical tuning curves for the 9 kHz point on the basilar membrane made by a laser-Doppler vibrometer for a number of vibration criteria.[90] Essentially, neural tuning curves are plots of response threshold against frequency (see Figure 19), and similar tuning curves can be recorded from single neurons throughout the auditory neural pathway. Note the relatively similar tuning capabilities of the nerve fiber with the

9 kHz CF (middle panel at the right of Figure 19), the most sensitive membrane velocity response (thick solid line of Figure 20) with respect to frequency selectivity (ie, the Q_{10dB} "tuning," at 10 dB above threshold, of ~2), and the tip-to-tail distance of about 80 dB.

The tuning curves of primary auditory nerve fibers have the same basic shape (ie, steep high-frequency slope, shallow low-frequency slope) as the mechanical tuning curves. Thus, the mechanical place code of the cochlea is clearly imprinted on the auditory nerve's neural response pattern.

Cochlear Tuning. Two characteristics of cochlear tuning are critical to the determination of its location and mechanism. First, the process by which filtering takes place is too rapid to permit a neural delay; thus, there is no possibility that tuning is sharpened by some sort of neural "lateral inhibition" analogous to that occurring at higher levels in the auditory pathway (see below).[91] The second important characteristic of cochlear filtering is that it is physiologically vulnerable. Almost all damaging agents, including hypoxia,[92] ototoxic drugs,[93] local mechanical damage,[94] and acoustic trauma[95] detune the neural tuning curves so that they closely approximate the broader mechanical tuning curves. As Figure 21 shows, the detuning by damaging agents occurs not only for neural tuning curves but also for mechanical tuning curves, SP tuning curves measured with electrodes placed intracellularly in IHCs, and psychophysical tuning curves from humans with cochlear deficits.[96,97] Until recently, the vulnerability of mechanical tuning curves was a controversial point. The first published "modern" mechanical tuning curves measured using Mössbauer and capacitive probe techniques were tuned about as poorly as von Bekesy's.[98] However, even at this early stage, the sharpness obtained by different laboratories differed.[99]

It has now become clear that the sharpness of cochlear mechanical tuning is extremely vulnerable and that, even when great care is taken, the surgical and other manipulations necessary to obtain mechanical tuning curves in experimental preparations unavoidably cause broadening of the mechanical frequency response.[87] Cochlear mechanical tuning curves obtained under conditions in which extreme precautions were taken to minimize cochlear damage have demonstrated tuning that is as sharp as that of neural tuning curves.[90] In addition, the existence of nonlinear behavior in the normal cochlear mechanical response has been confirmed. Thus, the sharpness of tuning observed at the primary neuron level is already accomplished at the level of the mechanical traveling wave.

The question remains, however, of how the physiologic vulnerable sharpening of mechanical tuning is accomplished. One critical consideration in answering this question is the calculation by Kim and coworkers that mechanically tuning a location on the basilar membrane requires the local addition of mechanical energy.[100] The discovery that OAEs are produced by the

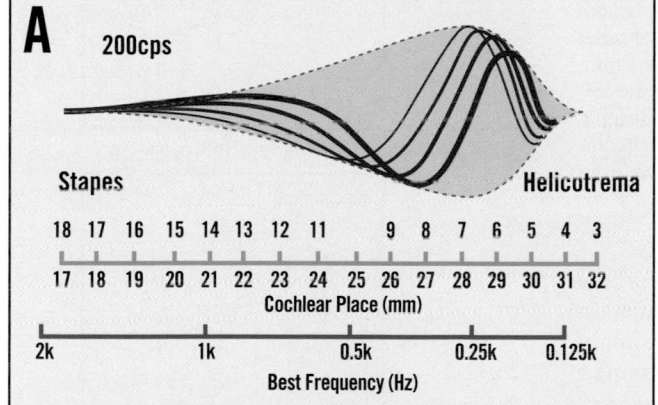

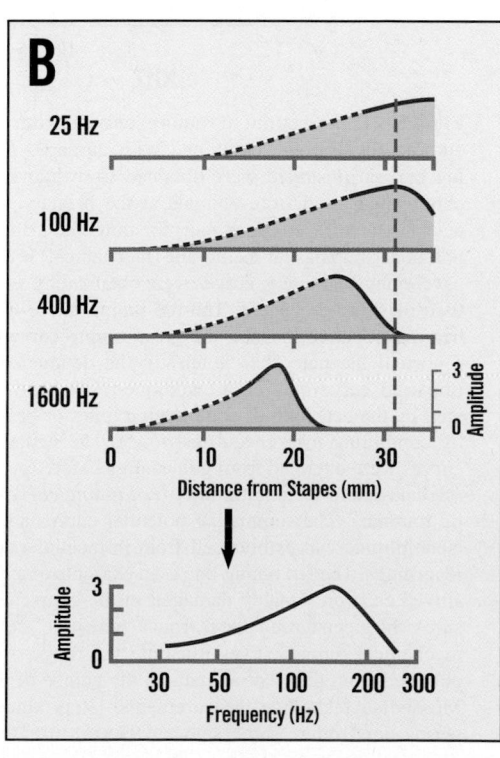

Figure 18 Mechanical place coding in the cochlea. (A) The cochlear partition is "uncoiled," showing the traveling wave response to a pure-tone stimulus. Vertical distance represents the amount of cochlear partition displacement. The 4 progressively darker lines show cochlear partition positions at 3 successive instants during 1 cycle of a 200 Hz stimulation tone. Darker lines represent later points in time. The fine dashed line shows the "envelope" of cochlear partition displacement. Scales at the bottom show linear distance along the cochlear partition measured from helicotrema (*upper scale*), from stapes (*middle scale*), and also in terms of 1 commonly used cochlear partition "frequency map" (*bottom scale*). Note the expected peak in displacement pattern envelope at about the 0.2 kHz point on the frequency map. (B) The top 4 curves are envelopes of traveling wave responses to pure-tone stimuli of varying frequencies. Each envelope depicts a point on the partition approximately 30 mm from the stapes (*vertical dashed line*). Only the upper half of the envelope traced in A is shown. At bottom, the response of a single cochlear point is plotted against frequency. This is the mechanical tuning curve of this point. (Reproduced with permission from references 5 and 88.)

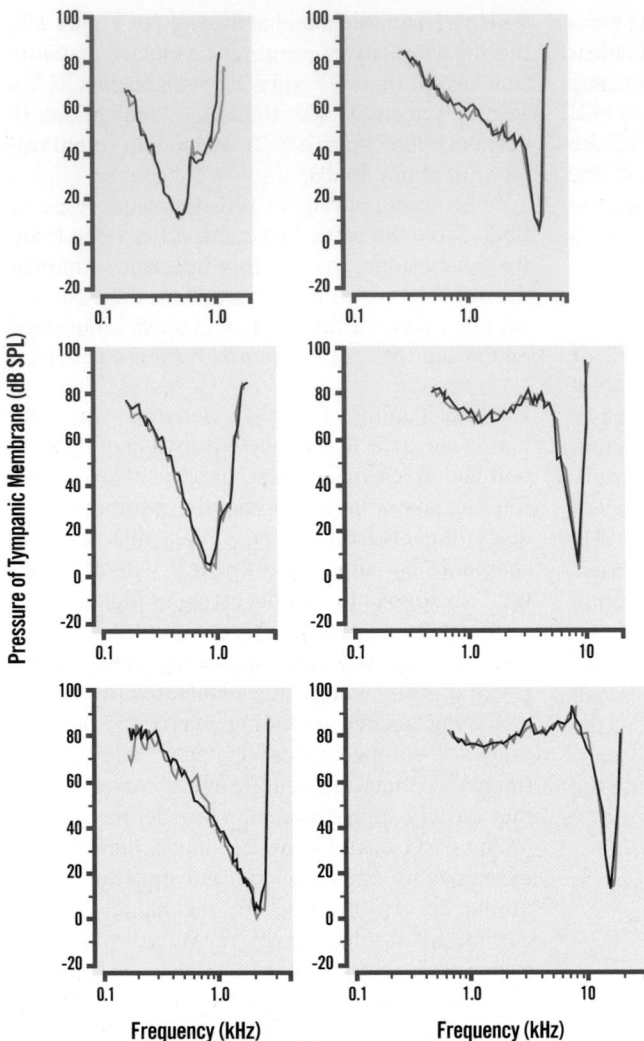

Pressure of Tympanic Membrane (dB SPL)

Frequency (kHz) Frequency (kHz)

Figure 19 Representative tuning curves (frequency threshold curves) of cat single auditory nerve fibers are shown for 6 distinct frequency regions. In each panel, 2 fibers from the same animal, of similar characteristic frequency and threshold, are shown, indicating the constancy of tuning under such circumstances. (Reproduced with permission from reference 89.)

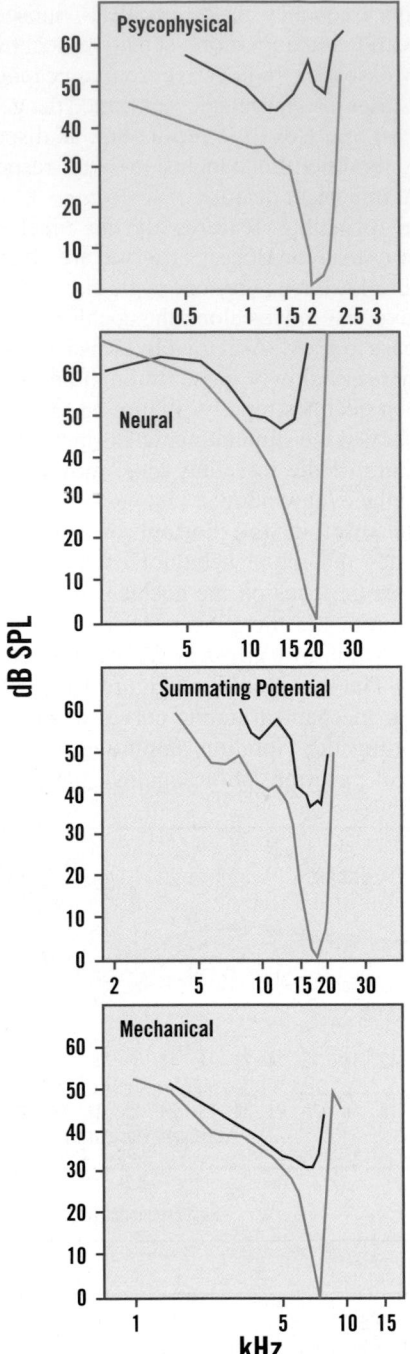

dB SPL

kHz

Figure 21 Collection of tuning curves from several authors illustrating "detuning" with damage. The tuning curves illustrated were obtained from humans (psychophysical) and from animals at the primary auditory neuron (neural), cochlear receptor potential (summating potential), and basilar membrane (mechanical) levels. The psychophysical tuning curves were obtained by a tone-on-tone masking procedure. The red tuning curve is from a hearing-impaired listener; the green tuning curve is from a normal listener. The "notch" in the detuned hearing-impaired curve may be a technique-related artifact created by the detection of combination tones or beats made by combining masker and test tones. The neural tuning curves were obtained from guinea pigs before (*green tuning curve*) and 20 minutes after (*red tuning curve*) acoustic trauma.[95] The summating potential curves are 10 μV isoamplitude curves obtained from intracellular hair cell recordings. The red tuning line is an example of an "insensitive" cell (presumably damaged in the course of exposure); the green tuning line is from a "sensitive" cell.[53] The mechanical tuning curves illustrate the range of results obtained from different animals in the course of Rhode's Mössbauer technique measurements. (Reproduced with permission from references 96 and 97.)

healthy cochlea[101] and can be recorded simply from human and animal ear canals provided indirect evidence for the presence of such a mechanical energy generator within the cochlea. The results of further studies on OAEs in vertebrates and more recent investigations of the biophysical properties of isolated OHCs have implicated micromechanical processes at the level of the OHCs as being responsible for the normal frequency selectivity of the cochlea.

The OAEs are traditionally classified into 2 general categories: those that are elicited with deliberate acoustic stimuli (evoked OAEs) and those that occur in the absence of stimulation (spontaneous OAEs). All OAEs can be simply recorded using conventional averaging techniques by a sensitive subminiature microphone assembly inserted snugly into the external auditory canal. Over the past several decades, 4 types of emissions, illustrated in Figures 22 and 23, have been studied extensively. These include the spontaneous OAE (SOAE), which is measured in the absence of acoustic stimulation (see Figure 22A); the stimulus frequency OAE (SFOAE), which is

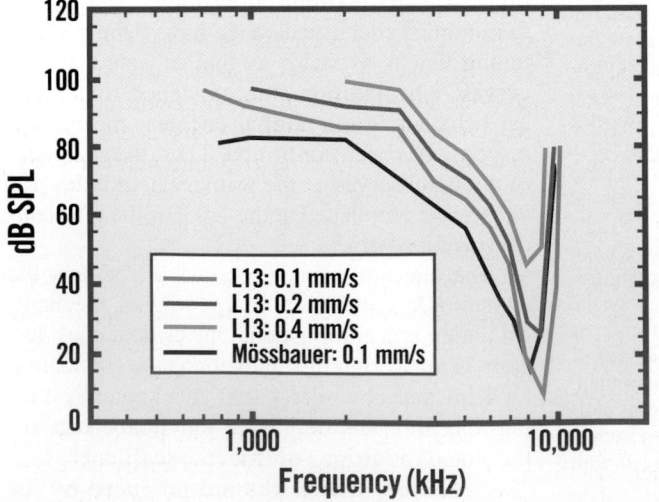

dB SPL

L13: 0.1 mm/s
L13: 0.2 mm/s
L13: 0.4 mm/s
Mössbauer: 0.1 mm/s

Frequency (kHz)

Figure 20 Isoresponse contours (*tuning curves*) for basilar membrane velocity responses to tone pips recorded from the chinchilla with the laser vibrometer (*blue, green and purple lines*). The ordinate indicates the sound pressure level required at any particular frequency to elicit a given velocity amplitude (0.1, 0.2, or 0.4 mm/s, indicated as the parameter). For the laser vibrometry responses, sound pressure levels were interpolated logarithmically using a series of isointensity contours for basilar membrane responses to tone pips. For comparison, a 0.1 mm/s tuning curve is shown, which is representative of results obtained using the Mössbauer technique (*red line*) at an approximately equivalent basilar membrane site in normal chinchilla. (Reproduced with permission from reference 90.)

evoked by a low-level, continuous pure tone (see Figure 22B); the transient evoked OAE (TEOAE), which is elicited by clicks or tone pips (see Figure 22C) and distortion-product OAE (DPOAE), which is elicited by 2 simultaneously applied pure tones (see Figure 23)[102] known as the lower- (f_1) and higher-frequency (f_2) primary tones.

The following facts support the notion that OAEs come from the cochlea and are related to the active frequency filtering process: (1) The frequency of the TEOAE varies considerably from subject to subject, and across subjects there is a systematic relationship between the emission's delay (ie, latency) and its frequency.[103] This suggests that the origin of OAEs is the cochlear bandpass filtering mechanism. (2) Stimulation of the crossed olivocochlear bundle (OCB), which preferentially provides efferent innervation to the OHCs, modulates the magnitude of OAEs.[104,105] (3) The emission is extremely sensitive to the detrimental effects of cochlear pathology, acoustic trauma, and ototoxic drugs.[105,106] The most parsimonious interpretation of the existence of the various OAE types, their duration, bandwidth, and delayed-onset characteristics and their relationship to the activity of the cochlear efferent system is that they originate in the OHCs, which possess a mechanical energy that generates the frequency-selective output of the cochlea.

Brownell and Zenner and their colleagues were the first to show that in in vitro preparations of mammalian hair cells OHCs display electromotility.[107,108] Using mechanical trituration to dissociate single OHCs from other organ of Corti tissues and video-enhanced imaging to visualize the isolated OHC directly, these investigators used both intracellular and transcellular electrical stimulation[107] or pharmacologic (K^+, cholinergic chemicals) agents[108] to elongate and shorten OHCs from their resting lengths. Because it has been demonstrated that hair cells possess both actin and myosin,[109] it was originally presumed that some aspect of the active motile mechanism is mediated, as in muscle, by interactions between these molecules. However, as more details developed about OHC electromotility, including the knowledge that they mechanically vibrate at frequencies up to at least 30 kHz, it became clear that a fast-acting motor molecule,[110] or some instantaneous physical phenomenon induced by an electrokinetic process,[111] formed the basis of the ability of the OHC to vibrate in response to changes in the receptor potential. Most recently, Zheng and colleagues tentatively identified a protein they called prestin as the motor protein of the OHC.[47] The detailed follow-up studies of these investigators further support the proposition that this membrane protein is the motor molecule responsible for the electromotility of OHCs.[112] Hair cell biophysics is discussed in Chapter 7, "Hair Cell Biophysics and Otoacoustic Emissions."

Inner Versus Outer Hair Cell Function. Figure 24 illustrates the salient characteristics of IHC and OHC anatomy,[113] and Figures 25 and 26 illustrate their afferent and efferent innervation, respectively. There are many differences between IHCs and OHCs in terms of their morphology, biochemistry, physiology, and afferent and efferent innervation patterns. Phylogenetically, OHCs are much younger than IHCs, being present only in the mammalian cochlea. In keeping with their relative phylogenetic youth, OHCs develop later embryologically,[114] are more easily compromised by various damaging agents, and have many unique characteristics that distinguish them from hair cells in other mechanoreceptor systems.

It seems clear that the OHCs and IHCs are functionally different, but our concept of the nature of this difference is changing. The classic view that the relatively insensitive IHC system carries the frequency place code, whereas the OHCs comprise a sensitive low-level detector system that has poor place-coding ability, has been abandoned in favor of more recent notions based on the active biomechanical functioning of the organ of Corti. That the OHCs possess effector abilities supports the proposal of Kim that these receptors are bidirectional transducers capable of converting acoustic energy into neural energy, that is, mechanoelectrical transduction, and electrical into mechanical energy, that is, electromechanical transduction.[115] Kim elaborated on this notion by postulating the existence of 2 distinct but parallel cochlear subsystems that use OHCs as the modulators and IHCs as the carriers of auditory information.[115] Table 1 presents a summary of a comparison of the 2 subsystems.

There is good evidence that the vulnerable filter sharpening described previously involves some kind of interaction between the IHCs and

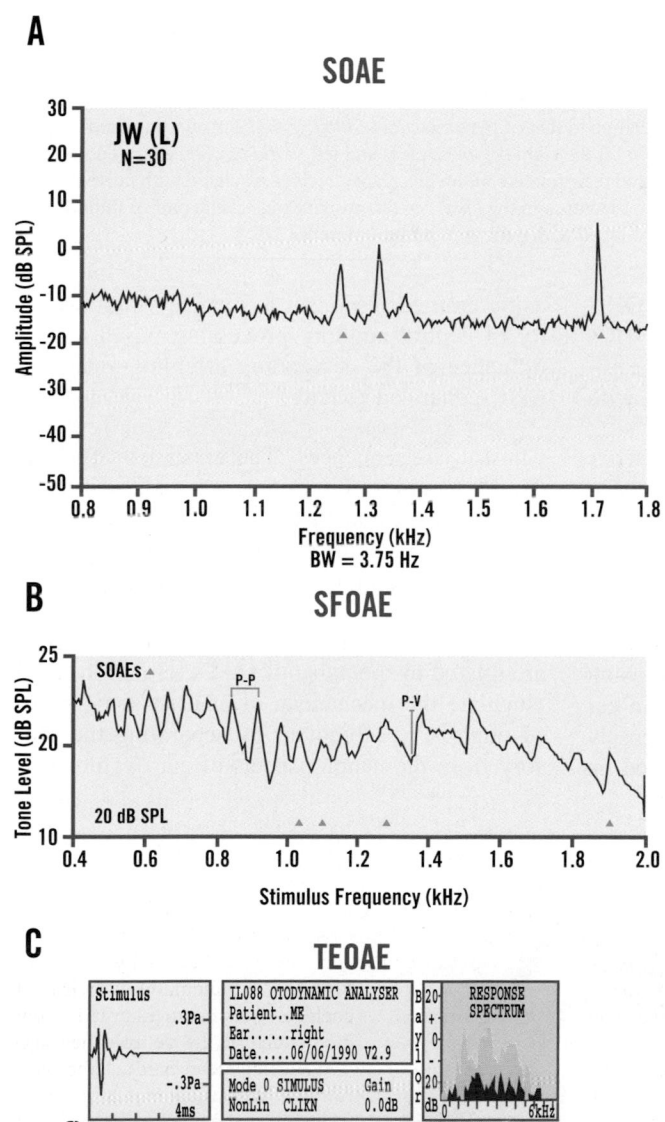

A

SOAE

JW (L)
N=30

B

SFOAE

SOAEs ▲

P-P

P-V

20 dB SPL

C

TEOAE

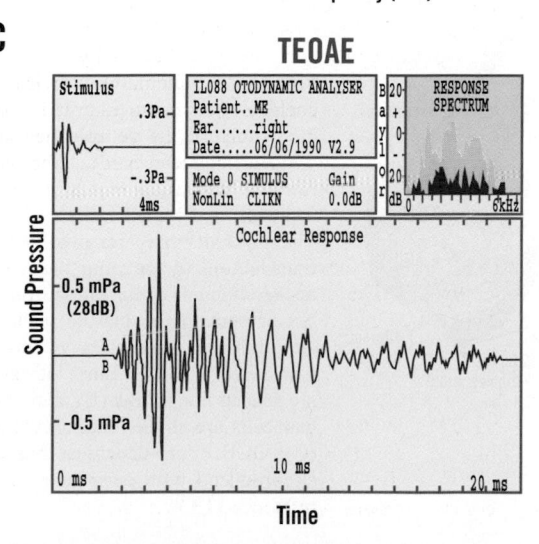

Figure 22 Examples of 3 types of otoacoustic emissions (OAEs). (A) Spectrum of the sound pressure level in the ear canal of a 26-year-old woman showing 4 spontaneous OAEs (SOAEs) within the 0.8 to 1.8 kHz frequency range. Spectral average was based on 30 samples. Arrowheads = frequencies of SOAEs. (B) Ear canal record for a 23-year-old man evoked by a continuous 20 dB SPL pure tone swept slowly (150 s) from 0.4 to 2 kHz. Peaks (P) and valleys (V) in the trace indicate regions of stimulus frequency OAE (SFOAE) activity in which the elicited returning emitted response moves in and out of phase with the sweeping tone. Arrowheads = frequencies of coexisting SOAEs. (C) An example of the ILO88 Otodynamic Analyser record displayed on screen and in hard copy form, which includes visual representations of the temporal course of 2 averages of the poststimulus response acquired by separate buffers (*below*), the form of the eliciting stimulus (*above left*), in this case a click based on an 80 μs rectangular pulse with a peak level of about 82 dB SPL, and a spectrum (*above right*) of the response showing both the emission (*orange*) and background noise (*red*) components. Basic information concerning the patient and stimulus mode is noted (*above center*). (Reproduced with permission from reference 219.)

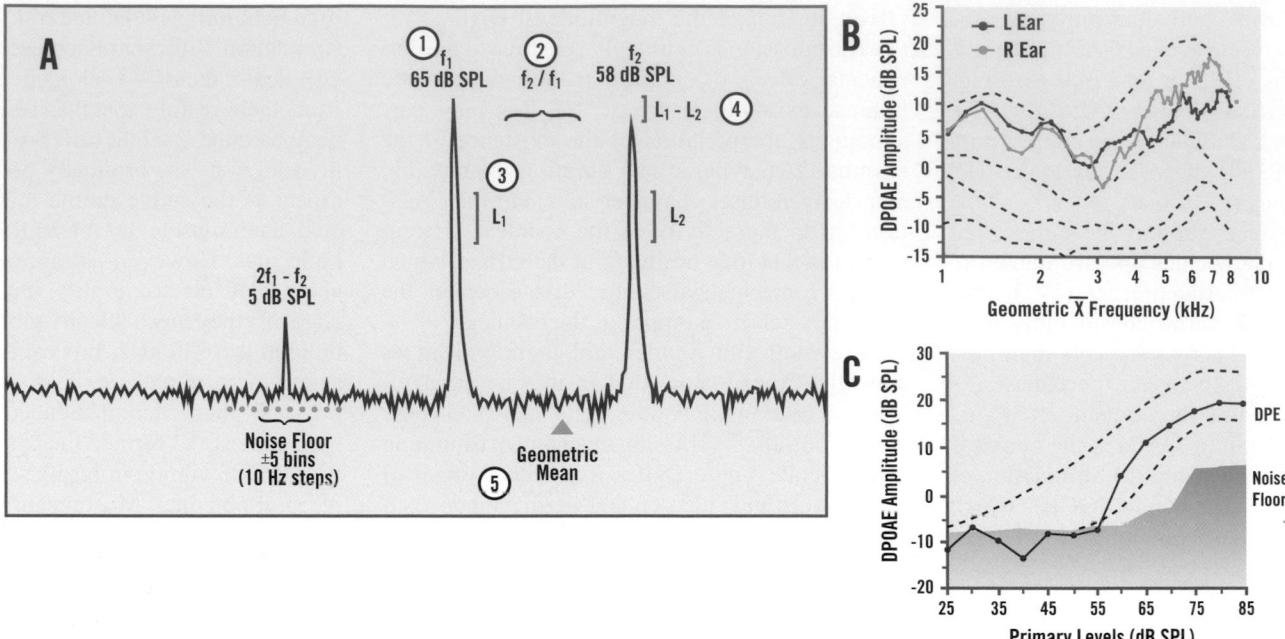

Figure 23 Distortion-product otoacoustic emissions (DPOAEs). (A) DPOAE at $2f_1-f_2$ is shown in the spectrum of the ear canal sound. Note the position of the geometric mean frequency (5) with respect to the primary tones (f_1, f_2) and the frequency range over which the noise floor (NF) is measured relative to that of the emission (*dotted region* surrounding the DPOAE frequency). (B) A typical DPOAE frequency/level function or "DP-gram" elicited by 75 dB SPL primaries is shown for the right (*open circles*) and left (*solid circles*) ears of a normal-hearing individual. The pairs of long (*above*) and short (*below*) dotted lines represent the ranges of average activity and their related NF levels, respectively, associated with normal function. (C) A typical response/growth or input/output curve depicts the growth of the DPOAE (DPE) with progressive increases in the levels of the primary tones. The pair of dotted lines above depicts the normal range of emission levels, whereas the striped lines below represent the average NF. (Reproduced with permission from reference 102.)

OHCs including the following: (1) selective damage to OHCs causes detuning of neural tuning curves (Figure 27),[116] which presumably are from IHC fibers; (2) crossed OCB stimulation, which presumably affects only OHCs (see below), strongly depresses the auditory nerve's click-evoked, whole-nerve, or compound action potential (CAP), which apparently originates entirely from IHC fibers; (3) crossed OCB stimulation also reduces the amplitude of the receptor potential recorded intracellularly from IHCs[117]; (4) crossed OCB stimulation as well reduces the firing rate and synchronization index[118] and shifts the dynamic range of auditory nerve fibers[119]; and (5) a trapezoid acoustic stimulus elicits from an auditory nerve fiber a spike train with a complex

time course, suggesting combined IHC and OHC influences, whereas selective damage to OHCs by kanamycin treatment simplifies the trapezoidal response pattern in a way compatible with isolated IHC influence.[51]

The precise mechanism by which OHCs influence the response of IHCs is unknown at this time. However, because the physiologically vulnerable cochlear filter-sharpening process appears to involve basilar membrane vibrations, the mechanism requires that the OHCs directly influence the mechanical vibration of the basilar membrane. A corollary to this conclusion is that the OAEs recorded from the human ear canal reflect OHC function. Indeed, 1 intensely studied subfield of OAE research is focused on

using emitted responses to evaluate the normality of central auditory processing based on the influence of the descending efferent system on OHC-generated activity.[120,121]

Clinical Consequences. The existence of a vulnerable cochlear filtering process and a related cochlear emission that can be recorded noninvasively have some important implications for our understanding of pathophysiologic processes in the cochlea. First, although it is unlikely that the majority of cases exhibiting severe tinnitus are related to spontaneous OAEs, emissions may elucidate the mechanism of at least some kinds of tinnitus.[122] Moreover, by separating the sensory from the neural aspects of ear dysfunction,

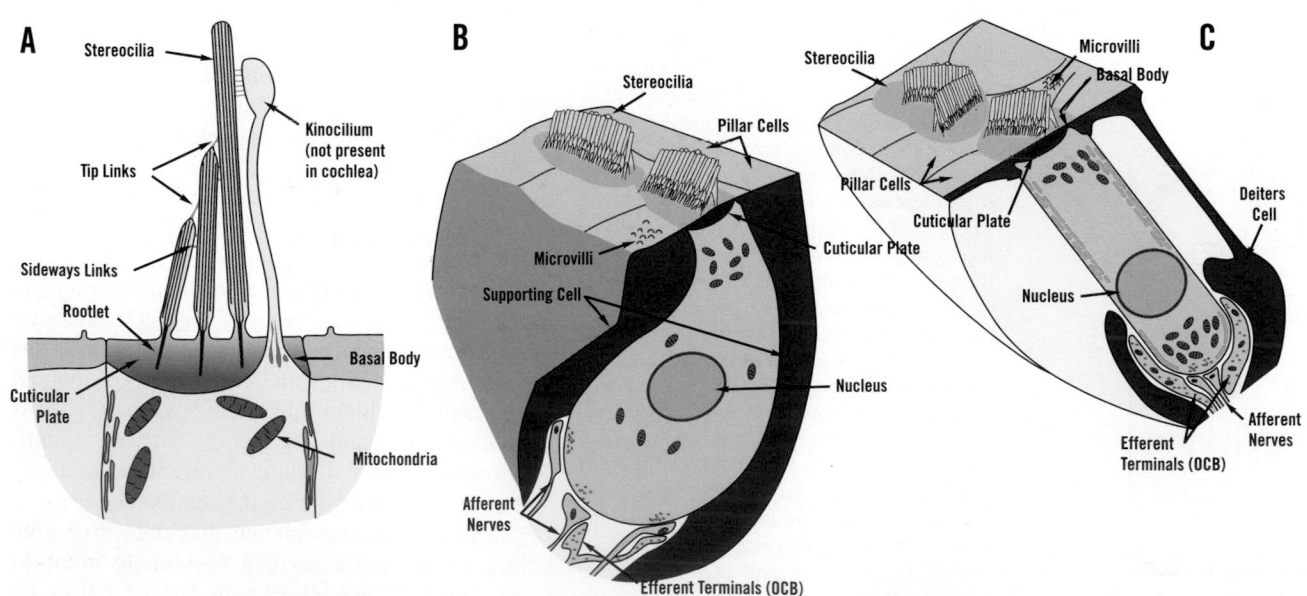

Figure 24 Schematic drawing of cochlear hair cells. (A) The common structures on the apical portion of acousticolateral hair cells include rows of stereocilia that are graded in height and joined by cross-links. The tip links may be involved in transduction by opening the transducer channels. The kinocilium is not present in the mature cochlea, although it is present in vestibular hair cells. (B and C) Inner hair cells are shaped like a flask (B), and outer hair cells are shaped like a cylinder (C). OCB = olivocochlear bundle. (Reproduced with permission from reference 113.)

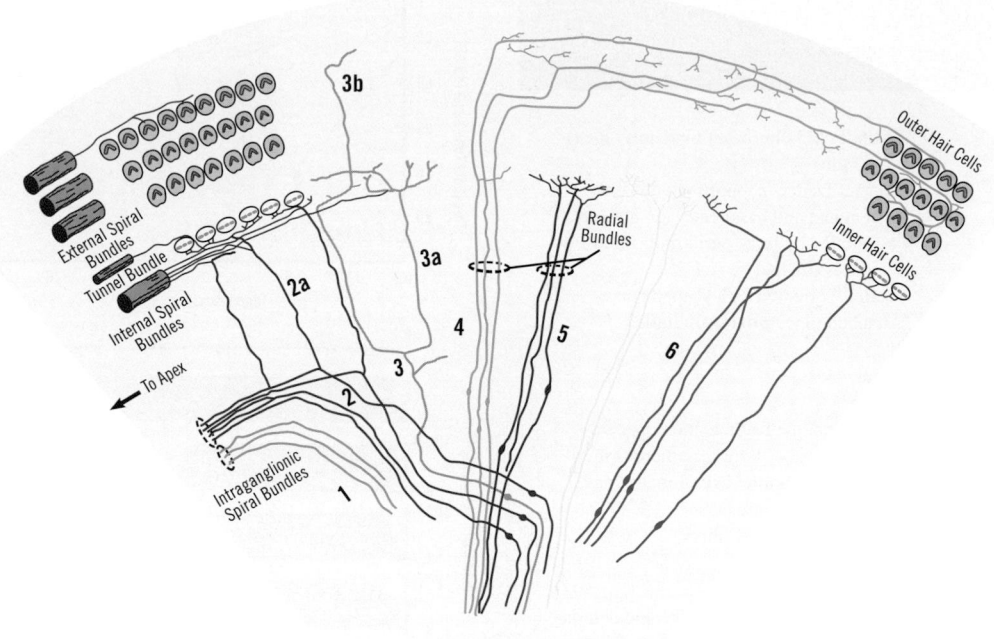

Figure 25 Diagram of the cochlea's afferent innervation pattern. The view is through Reissner membrane, looking down on the organ of Corti. Principal fiber bundles are 1 and 2, intraganglionic spiral bundles (fibers labeled "1" are efferent olivocochlear fibers); 2a and 3a = internal spiral fibers; 4 = external spiral fibers, traveling in radial bundle to innervate outer hair cells (OHCs); 5 and 6 = radial fibers, innervating inner hair cells (IHCs). The "V" shape of cilia pattern on the OHCs and the shallower "U" pattern on the IHCs are shown in the upper corners of the diagram. (Reproduced with permission from reference 131.)

OAEs may reveal the critical underlying causes of some common but puzzling otologic diseases such as Meniere disease[123] and sudden idiopathic sensorineural hearing loss.[124] Second, as shown in Figure 28, detuning of the neural response in cochlear pathologic conditions may also explain recruitment.[125] As previously described, detuning caused by cochlear pathology eliminates the low-threshold, sharply tuned tip region of the tuning curve but preserves the high-threshold tail region. Elimination of the tip region raises threshold, but preservation of the tail region preserves neural responsiveness at high intensities. Thus, the loudness function (bottom right plot) is made abnormally steep because threshold is elevated. However, at high intensities, loudness is normal because a normal number of neurons are responding.

Evidence for Telephone Coding. The aforementioned evidence for place coding has not invalidated Rutherford's telephone theory because there is also considerable evidence for a telephone code at low frequencies. For example, cochlear tuning becomes progressively poorer as frequency is lowered, and below about 100 Hz, there are no cochlear partition amplitude maxima and no tuned auditory units.[126] Thus, the physiologically observed frequency place code becomes progressively worse as frequency is lowered.

A neural telephone code has been demonstrated that, in contrast to the place code, becomes progressively better as frequency is lowered. Analyzing the spike discharges of single auditory nerve fibers to low-frequency stimulation demonstrated "phase-locking" to the individual cycles of the eliciting tone that preserves the temporal firing pattern.[127] Compiling large

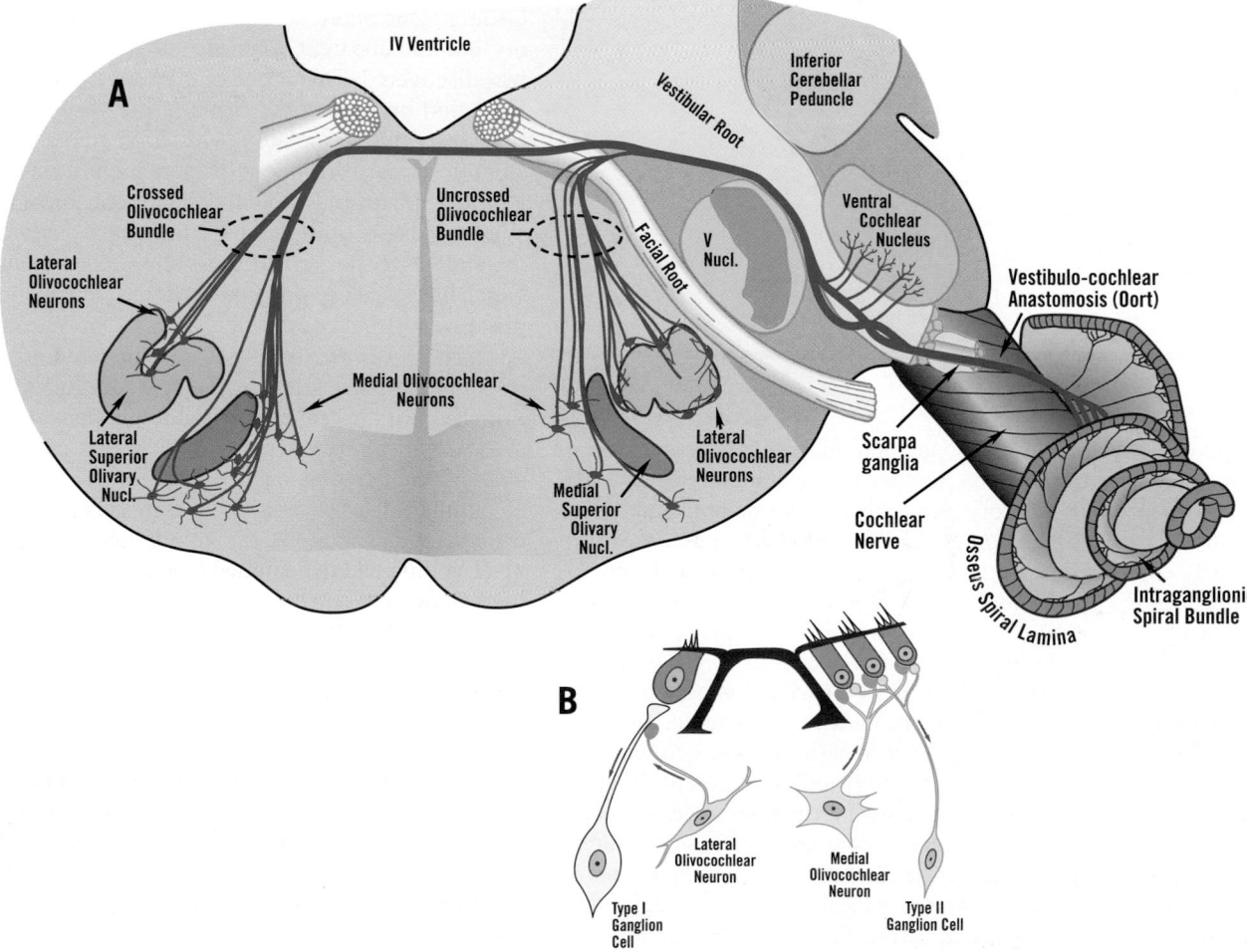

Figure 26 The descending auditory system. (A) Origination in the brainstem, distribution, and termination within the cochlea of the olivocochlear bundle efferent fibers of the cat. (B) Organization of the lateral and medial olivocochlear (OC) systems. Lateral OC neurons project to the region beneath the inner hair cells, where they form axodendritic contacts on the dendrites of type I spiral ganglion cells. Medial OC neurons project to the region beneath the outer hair cells and synapse directly with them. (A reproduced with permission from reference 143; B reproduced with permission from reference 167.)

Table 1 Differences between Inner and Outer Hair Cells

	Inner Hair Cells	Outer Hair Cells
Anatomy (see Figure 24)		
Cell shape	Flask (35 μm × 10 μm)	Cylinder [25 μm (base) to 45 μm (apex) × 7 μm]
Relation to supporting cells	Closely approximated to inner phalangeal cell processes	Contact Deiters supporting cells only at apical and basal ends and are surrounded by large perilymph-filled spaces of Nuel
Cilia	Longitudinally oriented shallow curve Not obviously attached to tectorial membrane	Radially oriented "V"-shaped curve Attached to tectorial membrane
Location of cell nucleus	Central	Basal
Organelles	Resemble hair cells in other systems	Several unique features including submembrane cisternae, numerous mitochondria parallel to cell membrane, Hensen bodies
Afferent innervation (see Figure 25)	Convergent via radial fibers 95% of fibers in auditory nerve come from IHCs	Divergent via spiral fibers
	All published nerve fiber studies are probably from IHCs	No convincing neurophysiologic demonstration of population of nerve fibers from OHCs
	Nerve endings plentiful and show typical chemical synapse morphology	Nerve endings relatively sparse; morphology differs from chemical synapse
Efferent innervation (see Figure 26)	Small neurons near LSO	Large neurons near MSO
	Primarily ipsilateral via uncrossed olivocochlear bundle	Primarily contralateral via crossed olivocochlear bundle
	Small endings primarily on afferent nerve terminals	Large endings on OHCs
	Acetylcholinesterase activity poorly visualized	Acetylcholinesterase activity easily visualized
	Enkephalin-like immunoreactivity	Aspartate aminotransferase immunoreactivity
	Distributed evenly along cochlear length	Distributed preferentially in middle and basal cochlea
Physiology		
Resting membrane potential	−35 to 45 mV	−70 mV
Basal cells		
AC receptor potential	0.6 mV	3 mV
DC receptor potential	12 mV	Immeasurable
Apical cells		
AC receptor potential	10 mV	5 mV
DC receptor potential	5 mV	3 mV
Biochemistry		
Intracellular glycogen	Scarce	Plentiful

IHCs = inner hair cells; OHCs = outer hair cells; LSO = lateral superior olive; MSO = medial superior olive.

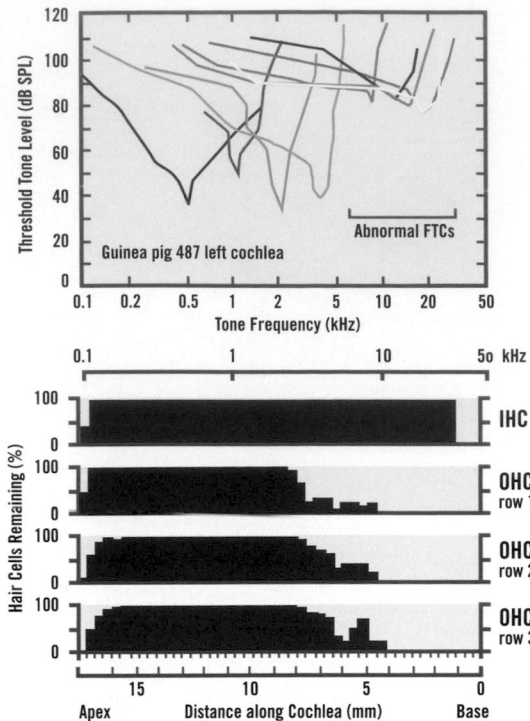

Figure 27 Correlation between detuning of neural tuning curves and outer hair cell (OHC) damage. The results are shown from a kanamycin-treated guinea pig in which the inner hair cells (IHCs) were intact throughout the cochlea. In the high-frequency region, however, OHCs were damaged, and frequency tuning curves (FTCs), presumably from fibers coming from this region, were detuned. This result suggests that the OHCs participate in the process by which cochlear tuning curves are sharpened. (Reproduced with permission from reference 116.)

numbers of single-unit spikes into spike discharge histograms showed an impressive ability of single auditory unit discharges to reproduce the waveform of the stimulating sound. The upper limit of this phenomenon is generally estimated at about 4 kHz, but critical inspection of quantitative single-unit data suggests that phase locking becomes poor at around 2.5 kHz.[128]

Another line of evidence supporting the importance of the encoding of phase or timing information comes from the outcome of studies of the responses of auditory nerve fibers to speech sounds. The work of Kiang addressed the limitations of fiber discharge rate place encoding in neurally representing the frequency components in speech signals, especially those of moderate to high intensities.[129] More recently, the single-unit population studies of Sachs and Young on the representation of speech sounds in hundreds of auditory nerve fibers have demonstrated that the temporal pattern of fiber discharges in the form of phase locking provides considerable information about the frequency content of the stimulus at all levels of stimulation.[130] These population measures of temporal synchrony were based on Fourier transforms of period histograms from fibers with CFs near each frequency component of the sound. Such measures were combined to provide discharge rate profiles for groups of active nerve fibers. Because information concerning rate, timing, and place is represented in these measures, these spectra provide details concerning temporal fine structure from a localized cochlear region and thus represent a type of temporal place code.

"Telephone Place" Theory of Frequency Coding. One shortcoming of the telephone theory became apparent when neural refractoriness was discovered. This process imposed a physical limitation on nerve fiber firing at the very short time intervals associated with high-frequency stimuli. Thus, to reconcile in part the effects of neural refractoriness on the telephone theory, Wever published an auditory frequency coding theory, which he termed the volley theory, but which has since become known as the "telephone place" or "frequency place" theory.[131] Wever advanced an interesting evolutionary argument in support of the telephone place code theory. Primitive ears (as found in fish, amphibians, and lower reptiles) are telephone coders that cannot analyze high frequencies because of the inherent limitation of the rate at which nerve fibers can respond. Therefore, as evolution progressed, place coding had to be added to allow analysis of high frequencies, which are important in sound localization and directionality.

Our use of sounds in communication is greatly aided by our keen sensitivity to the frequency region between 1 to 4 kHz, and although our sensitivity falls off beyond 4 kHz, we still depend on the higher frequencies for many of our discriminations of consonants and sharp transients. The appearance and elaboration of the place principle for frequency representation, therefore, was a major event in the evolution of the ear.[131]

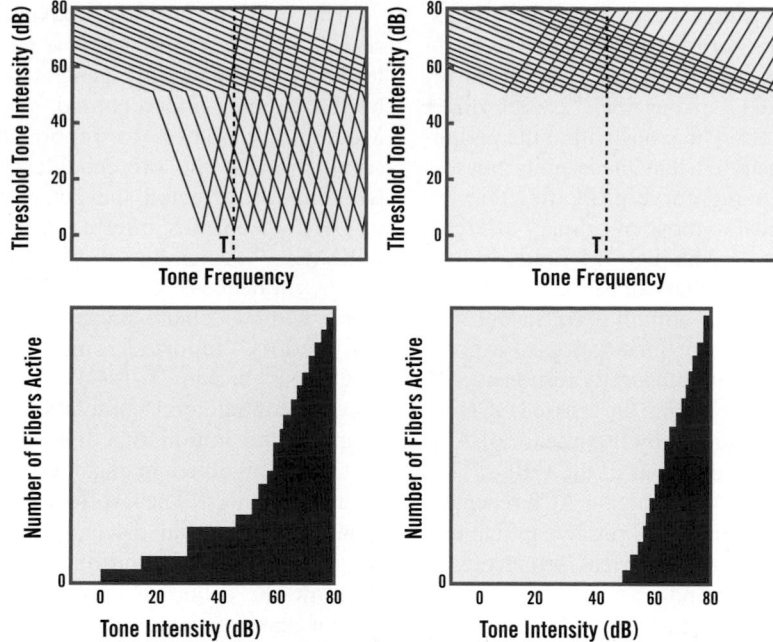

Figure 28 Possible explanation of recruitment (elevated threshold and abnormal growth of loudness) based on detuning with pathology. Solid diagrams at bottom depict increase in number of active auditory nerve fibers as tone level is increased in normal (*left*) and abnormal (*right*) ears. The tone's frequency (T) is indicated by the dashed line in the upper diagram. Because the effect of disease is to remove the sharply tuned "tips" but leave the broadly tuned "tails" relatively unaffected, the threshold of the pathologic cochlea is increased. However, as tone level is increased into the normal tail regions, the number of active fibers responding becomes normal; hence, loudness grows abnormally rapidly from the elevated threshold. (Reproduced with permission from reference 126.)

Intensity Coding. Loudness is the approximate subjective correlate of the physical dimension of sound intensity. It is generally assumed that the neural correlate of loudness is the amount of nervous activity, with the amount factor meaning the total number of action potentials delivered by a population of nerve fibers over a given time period. Thus, loudness is encoded as a combination of the number of fibers firing and the rate at which they are firing.

Figure 29 compares plots of stimulus level versus single auditory nerve fiber firing rates (left) and stimulus level versus subjective loudness (right).[132] The agreement in the general shapes of the curves supports the view that the amount of auditory nerve firing encodes loudness. On closer scrutiny, however, it is apparent that firing rate changes only over a 20 dB sound intensity range, whereas loudness varies over a 100 dB range. This limited dynamic range is a general property of all primary auditory neurons.[133]

The obvious way to solve this loudness-encoding problem is to assume that additional nerve fibers are "recruited" as stimulus level is increased. This process would increase the total number of discharges per unit time by increasing the number of fibers firing rather than the firing rate for an individual fiber. However, most studies of auditory nerve single units agree that the thresholds of the nerve fiber population fall within a relatively restricted stimulus range, that is, within 20 to 30 dB of behavioral threshold.[134] Thus, there is no possibility of recruiting additional fibers as sound level is increased more than 60 dB above threshold. The fiber recruitment hypothesis also creates problems for frequency place coding because adding new respond-

ing fibers as stimulus level is increased would quickly require the spread of activity to fibers of adjacent CFs. This tradeoff between the ability to recruit new fibers and the ability to place code is especially bothersome for explaining the perception of complex sounds for which multiple

frequencies must be distinguished simultaneously. Thus, the dynamic range problem becomes apparent.[135] The dynamic range of auditory nerve fibers, that is, the range over which the spike rate changes as stimulus level is altered, is too narrow to account for (at least in simple terms) the extent over which the human ear discriminates sound levels.

Several subsequent observations shed light on the dynamic range problem. Evans and Palmer discovered that approximately two-thirds of the cells in the dorsal cochlear nucleus (DCN) had dynamic ranges that extend to well over 100 dB and thus could easily "code" loudness over the necessary sound intensity range.[136] However, the problem of the input pathway to these DCN cells remains to be resolved. In addition, some auditory nerve units have been found that do, after all, have wide dynamic ranges, but these are only a minority of the total auditory nerve fiber population.[137] Other studies have also demonstrated that relative degrees of phase locking[138] of different frequency components in complex sounds could code the relative intensity levels of the frequency components. However, because phase locking does not occur above 3 to 4 kHz, this mechanism could not account for the loudness coding of high frequencies.

Another approach to the dynamic range problem is the concept of an automatic gain control operating at the input of the auditory system.[135] Such a control mechanism would feed back a decreased gain command signal to the input to maintain the cochlear output within an acceptable operating range. Possibilities for such a control

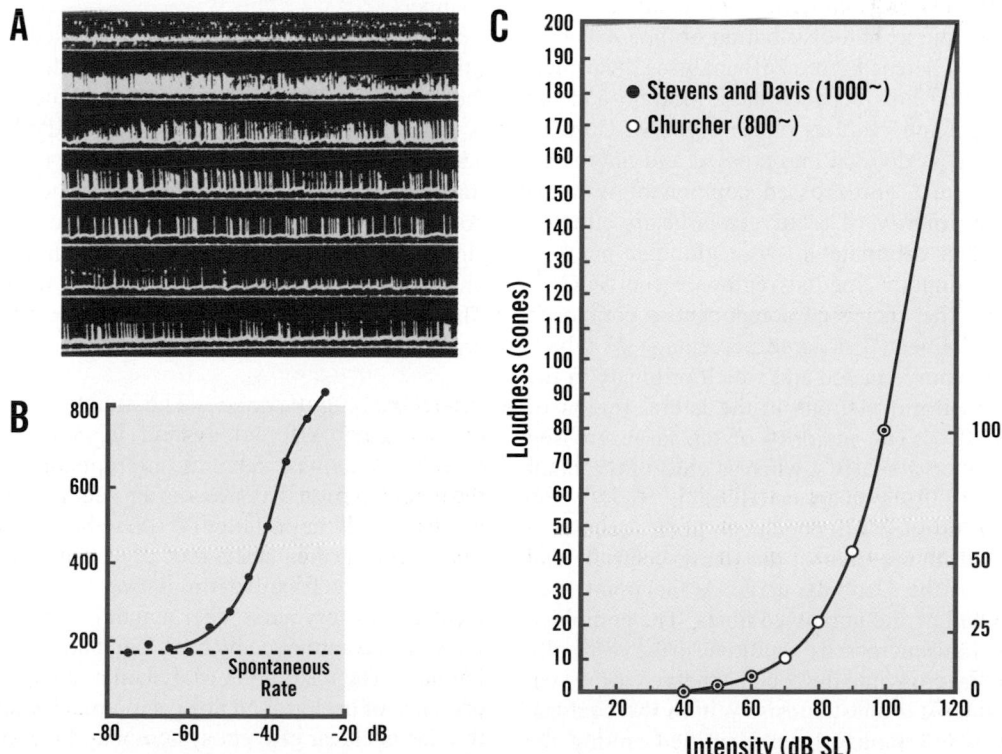

Figure 29 Effects of sound intensity on subjective loudness (*right*) and auditory nerve fiber firing rate (*left*). The shapes of the curves are similar, but the dynamic range of the single auditory nerve fiber is much narrower than that of the auditory system as a whole. Above the auditory nerve firing rate curve (B) are single-fiber responses to sounds of progressively increasing levels (A). Subjective loudness curve from Gulick (1971) noted in the legend for Figure 21. (Auditory nerve curve reprinted with permission from reference 132.)

system include the middle ear reflex and the olivocochlear efferent system.

Finally, Liberman classified auditory nerve fibers into 3 functional subclasses according to spontaneous discharge rate as low-, medium-, and high-firing units.[139] Whereas high spontaneous rate (SR) fibers exhibited low thresholds and restricted dynamic ranges of about 20 dB, the medium and low SR units displayed higher thresholds and dynamic ranges as great as 60 dB. Thus, it is possible that although fewer in number than the high SR fibers, the low and medium SR fibers are available to encode the higher intensity sounds.[140]

Viemeister concluded from his review of the psychophysical and physiologic literature relevant to intensity encoding in auditory nerve fibers that a localized rate code "seems theoretically possible and, at present, appears to be the best candidate for a general intensity code."[141] The conclusion that rate information from a frequency-specific population of active nerve fibers provides the neural basis for a code of stimulus intensity is consistent with the findings discussed above concerning the encoding of high-level speech sounds by a population of auditory nerve fibers that possibly exhibit low to intermediate spontaneous firing rates.

Efferent Auditory System. *Anatomy.* Rasmussen established the existence of a chain of descending auditory neurons that links auditory cortex to hair cells and that parallels the classic afferent projection pathway (discussed below).[142] The OCB, the final link in the descending chain, originates in the superior olivary complex (SOC).

Figure 26A summarizes schematically the origins, course, and distribution of the OCB to 1 cochlea, whereas Figure 26B analyzes the principal relationships between the 2 afferent and the 2 efferent innervations of the organ of Corti.[143] The OCB is divided into crossed and uncrossed components. The crossed component is composed primarily of relatively large myelinated fibers that originate in large globular neurons surrounding the medial region of the SOC.[144] Most of the uncrossed component is composed of small fibers,[145] a large percentage of which may be unmyelinated and which originate in the small fusiform neurons in the lateral region of the SOC.[144] The majority of the large crossed fibers innervate OHCs, whereas most of the small uncrossed fibers innervate IHCs.[144]

The crossed olivocochlear fibers decussate just beneath the floor of the fourth ventricle and then enter the vestibular nerve. At this point, they are joined by the uncrossed fibers. The combined crossed and uncrossed fibers travel in the vestibular nerve and cross into the cochlear nerve via the vestibulocochlear anastomosis. Within the cochlea, efferent fibers have been identified among the external spiral fibers (3b in Figure 25), the tunnel spiral fibers, and the internal spiral fibers.[146]

Physiology. In cases in which olivocochlear axons have been labeled histochemically and traced following single nerve fiber recordings, the labeled fibers terminate beneath OHCs in cochlear regions with best frequencies corresponding to the CFs of the fiber.[147] Such direct recordings from efferent axons within the periphery have demonstrated that these units possess thresholds and tuning curve properties that are essentially identical to those of primary afferents with similar CFs.[147] Although the proportion of olivocochlear neurons that can be excited by ipsilateral and contralateral stimuli is consistent with the predominant efferent innervation to a given cochlea, many units are binaurally responsive.[148]

The effects of stimulating the crossed OCB are almost certainly mediated by the release of ACh as the major neurotransmitter at the OHCs,[149] as noted above. In turn, ACh acts on ACh receptors (AChRs) located on the OHC postsynaptic membrane to modulate the electrical properties of the OHCs. Elgoyhen and associates established that ACh acts on nicotinic AChRs (nAChRs) containing the alpha9 (α9) subunit, which mediates synaptic transmission between the cholinergic olivocochlear fibers and the OHCs.[150] It has long been known that stimulating the crossed OCB in the floor of the fourth ventricle causes depression of the auditory nerve's response to sound stimulation, that is, the CAP, and a simultaneous increase in the amplitude of the CM.[151] It is likely that the α9 nAChR subunit mediates such efferent inhibition because an α9 knockout mouse model showed no suppression of either CAPs or DPOAEs by electrically stimulating the OCB at the floor of the fourth ventricle.[152] It was further shown that the α9 nAChR protein opens its ion channel via associated Ca^{2+}-activated K^+ channels.[153]

Much less is known about the uncrossed OCB. Stimulation of the uncrossed bundle decreases the click-evoked CAP amplitude, but the effect is much less than for the crossed bundle.[118] In addition, unlike the crossed bundle, the terminations of the uncrossed bundle do not show high concentrations of acetylcholinesterase,[154] and curare does not block the effect of stimulating the uncrossed bundle (although strychnine does).[149] Thus, the uncrossed system may not be cholinergic.

Functional Significance. The function of the olivocochlear efferent system is, at present, largely unknown. Several attempts to demonstrate functional deficits after sectioning the crossed OCB have failed.[155] A series of more recent studies has systematically examined the effects of electrically stimulating the crossed OCB on auditory nerve fiber dynamic ranges that have been compressed by broadband noise stimulation.[119] The restoration of dynamic range in the presence of background noise supports the notion that the cochlear efferent system may function to improve the ability to discriminate complex signals, that is, the signal-to-noise ratio. However, the hypothesis that the olivocochlear system primarily provides some sort of input gating mechanism may not be completely correct.

The most recent and unexpected effect of stimulating the crossed OCB is a decrease in the levels of OAEs that are generated mechanically by the cochlea and recorded in the ear canal. Mountain was first to report that electrical stimulation of the olivocochlear efferent system directly affected the active nonlinearities in OHC mechanics inferred from decreases in DPOAEs.[104] A number of other studies evaluating the influence of contralateral acoustic stimulation with wideband noise on OAEs recorded ipsilaterally reported small reductions in TEOAEs[120] and in $2f_1$-f_2 DPOAEs.[156] The influence of contralateral stimulation on OAEs also supports the notion that the cochlear efferent system is involved in the modulation of OHC micromechanics. These effects, along with the reductions in neural discharge rate and tuning, suggest that the function of the crossed OCB is to allow the central auditory system to govern the mechanical properties of the basilar membrane by controlling the vulnerable cochlear tuning mechanism previously discussed. Because detuning a frequency bandpass system increases damping, the detuning effect of the crossed OCB could be useful as a method of improving auditory temporal resolution, for example, to improve speech perception. The consensus view at present is that the active transduction process[157] is regulated in some way through efferent innervation of the OHCs.[111] Also, as noted above, the olivocochlear efferent system may also contribute toward extending the dynamic range of the auditory system.[158]

In addition, other experimental results suggest that the olivocochlear system may help protect against acoustic trauma.[158] In this work, it was discovered that the amount of threshold shift induced by overstimulation of 1 ear could be reduced by the presentation of a simultaneous tone to the contralateral ear, thus inferring that activating the efferent system reduced the effects of overexposure. 1 intriguing line of current research on the traumatic effects of noise exposure is the notion of "training" the cochlea to become less susceptible to damaging sounds.[159–161] One common protocol to induce the training (or conditioning or toughening) effect is to apply daily, moderate-level sound exposures to reduce injury from a subsequent high-level noise exposure.[162] Although the underlying mechanism(s) responsible for the trained protective effect is, at present, unknown, the most likely site is the crossed cochlear efferent system.[163,164] Indeed, LePage demonstrated that loud sound induces a mechanical baseline shift in the position of the cochlear partition.[165] It is highly probable that such a gain control system is effected by cochlear efferents.

Central Auditory Pathway

Each of the 5 primary senses sends information into the brain via 2 separate pathways: a direct or specific pathway and a nonspecific pathway. The nonspecific pathway involves structures in the core of the neuraxis, collectively known as the reticular system. In the reticular system, all sensory modalities share the same gross neural structures (hence the name nonspecific). Ascent via the nonspecific structures is multisynaptic and hence is characterized by long delay times.

The direct pathways for each sensory modality are separate and involve long axonal processes, with a minimal number of synapses; consequently, compared with the indirect pathway, transmission along the direct pathways involves minimal delay times. The synapses of the direct pathways tend to congregate in well-defined neural structures called nuclei. Clinically, lesions of the central auditory system are localized according to their level in the direct projection pathway. Therefore, the following discussion emphasizes this pathway.

Anatomy. Figure 30 diagrams the direct auditory projection pathway. The numbers in each nucleus indicate neuronal order (determined by the number of synapses). The auditory projection pathway is more complex than the pathways of other sensory systems, possibly because it developed relatively late on the phylogenetic scale and had to incorporate pieces of other already developed neuronal systems. Although the basic wiring diagram depicted in Figure 30 has remained relatively unchanged for many years, it should be emphasized that within the last half century, a number of advances have been made in the development of methods for describing neuronal connectivity.[166] These breakthroughs have relied on the discovery that, when certain amino acids, conjugated enzymes (eg, horseradish peroxidase-conjugated lectin from soy bean), sugars, or immunocytochemicals (eg, polyclonal or monoclonal antibodies) are injected into a neu-

ronal or fluid (eg, cochlear duct) region of interest, they will be taken up by the cells or nerve fiber endings in this region and transported by the normal cellular process of axonal transport in both retrograde and anterograde directions. Other techniques make use of such labels as lipophilic dyes (eg, dilinoleyl-tetramethylindocarbocyanine or DiI), which can be retrogradely transported in fixed tissue by diffusion.

Visualization of the location of cellular projections or the cellular/subcellular location of labeled substances at the light and electron microscope levels is achieved either by autoradiography, in the case of radioactive compounds, or by catalyzation of histochemical reactions, which are typically viewed under epifluorescence or dark-field optics. With recent refinement of these tract tracing and cell component-labeling techniques using immunohistochemical markers, virtually all projection pathways and cell types of the auditory system have been described. Lagging far behind our description of the connections of the neural pathway for hearing is our understanding of how this network of interconnections interacts to produce our complex auditory sensations. Presented below is a brief description of the major projections of the auditory pathway sufficient for the clinician to understand the transfer of information within the auditory system, without consideration of the many lesser connections revealed by modern immunocytochemical staining techniques. The reader is referred to several comprehensive reviews that provide more details of the intricate interconnections of the central auditory system.[167,168]

Cochlear Nucleus. Central processing of the information carried in the auditory nerve begins in the cochlear nucleus (CN), the first obligatory synapse for all nerve fibers. On entering the CN, the auditory portion of the eighth nerve bifurcates into two branches, one that sends fibers to synapse in the anteroventral cochlear nucleus (AVCN) and one that synapses in the posteroventral cochlear nucleus (PVCN) and dorsal cochlear nucleus (DCN). The distribution of fibers within the CN is not random but follows an orderly pattern of tonotopic projection throughout the nucleus, with low-frequency fibers projecting ventrally and high-frequency fibers distributed

dorsally. Thus, both neurophysiologic and anatomic observations show that cochlear place is represented in an orderly manner throughout the projection pathways of the central auditory system.[169] The security of tonotopic organization is also apparent in the multiple representation of the stimulus frequency domain. For example, typically, along any 1 penetration of a microelectrode trajectory within a principal nucleus, there are 2 or more breaks in the orderly progression of best frequencies. Thus, as in the direct projection pathways of all sensory systems, multiple representation of the receptor surface occurs. It is likely that nerve fiber branching in the various nuclei, as described for the CN, is the anatomic basis of this multiple frequency representation.[170]

All auditory nerve fibers display relatively uniform response characteristics to pure-tone stimuli compared to the activity of CN cells when categorized by the use of a poststimulus time histogram (PSTH).[134] The PSTH plots the number of nerve discharges that occur in small time bins within the period that begins slightly before and extends throughout the duration of the stimulus. PSTHs are shown for an auditory nerve fiber and various CN cells in Figure 31.[171] The CN consists of at least 9 different cell types described for their anatomic characteristics revealed by various staining techniques.[172] It can be seen from the unit activity patterns of Figure 31 that the uniform response characteristics of auditory nerve fibers are soon elaborated by the various cells of the CN to produce a variety of response types named after the patterns seen in the PSTH.[173] When examined in the frequency intensity domain, some CN cells exhibit complex response patterns that describe regions of excitation and inhibition produced by a pure-tone stimulus. An example of such complex response patterns by cells in the CN is shown in Figure 32.[174]

Three fiber pathways project information from the CN to higher brainstem centers. These fiber tracts include the ventral (trapezoid body), intermediate, and dorsal acoustic striae. The ventral acoustic stria, originating from AVCN and PVCN regions, projects ventrally and medially to send fibers ipsilaterally to the lateral superior olive (LSO) and the medial superior olive (MSO) and then to the medial nucleus of the trapezoid body (MTB). The fibers then cross the

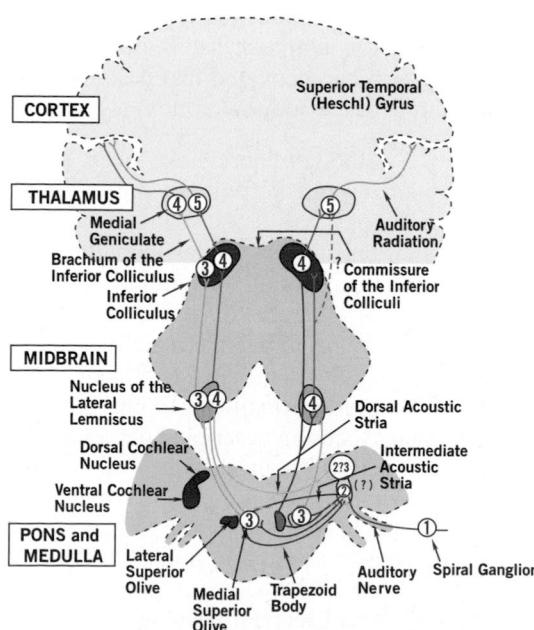

Figure 30 Diagram of the direct auditory projection pathway. Numbers indicate the approximate neuron order as determined by the number of synapses traversed. Dashed lines labeled with question marks indicate 2 areas of uncertainty: (1) whether the dorsal cochlear nucleus primarily contains second- or third-order neurons and (2) whether any nerve fibers bypass the inferior colliculus.

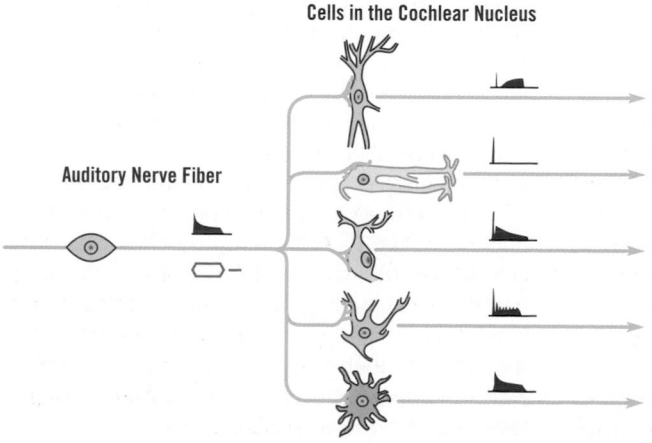

Figure 31 Diagram showing the diverse single-unit response types obtained from cells in the cochlear nucleus compared to the uniform response pattern found for fibers of the auditory nerve. The poststimulus time histograms were obtained by presenting short 25 to 50 ms tone bursts at the unit's characteristic frequency. Response types from top to bottom are pauser, on₁, primary like with notch, chopper, and primary like. Cell types presumably associated with these response patterns from top to bottom are pyramidal, octopus, globular, multipolar, and spherical. (Reproduced with permission from reference 171.)

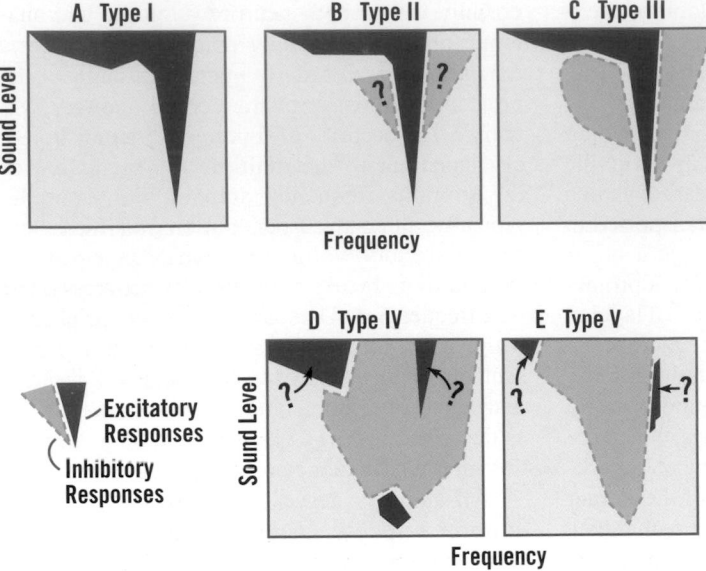

Figure 32 Tuning curves of excitation and inhibition in the cat cochlear nucleus are shown in order of increasing amounts of inhibition (A–E). Purely excitatory responses as in A are predominant in the anteroventral cochlear nucleus. Greater amounts of inhibition are found toward the dorsal cochlear nucleus (D and E). Question marks show variable or uncertain features. (Reproduced with permission from reference 174.)

midline to terminate on the contralateral MSO and MTB but do not innervate the LSO on the opposite side. Thus, for any 1 ear, connections are bilateral only to the MSO and MTB.[175] The intermediate acoustic stria, the primary output of the PVCN, sends some fibers ipsilaterally to a group of cells around the superior olivary complex (SOC) called the periolivary nucleus (PON), whereas other fibers ascend in the lateral lemniscus (LL). This pathway also crosses the midline to innervate the same structures on the contralateral side. Fibers of the intermediate acoustic stria, which enter the LL, synapse within the nucleus.

The dorsal acoustic stria, the principal output of the DCN, bypasses the SOC to synapse in the contralateral dorsal nucleus of the LL and the inferior colliculus (IC).[174]

Superior Olivary Complex. The SOC is composed of the LSO, MSO, MTB, and PON. The SOC receives fibers from both CNs and consequently receives information from both ears. This feature allows this group of nuclei to monitor the arrival time and level of sounds to both ears and provides the cues for the localization of sound in space based on the stimulus arrival time and intensity to both ears.[174] In fact, localization of sound in the horizontal plane provides the most straightforward relationships that have been observed between central auditory single-unit behavior and psychophysical function. As sound to 1 ear is made progressively louder or earlier than sound to the opposite ear, some SOC units change abruptly from inhibitory to facilitatory response patterns. By assuming a facilitatory contralateral input and an inhibitory ipsilateral input (or vice versa), the neurophysiologic behavior of these units can be explained. Thus, slight binaural differences in level and/or arrival time provide the auditory cues for localization of sound in the horizontal plane (sound lateralization). The acoustic image is located on the side of the louder or earlier sound. As a whole, the SOC represents the lowest level in the auditory system at which binaural processing takes place.[175] However, at all levels in the

auditory projection pathway above the trapezoid body, there are units that are sensitive to binaural time and level differences.[176,177]

Lateral Lemniscus. The LL is the major ascending projection from the CN and SOC to the IC and contains both contralateral and ipsilateral fibers from lower auditory brainstem structures. Although there are 3 distinct nuclei within the LL, historical emphasis has been simply on its function as a connection between the SOC and IC. Recently, these nuclei have received more attention in attempts to define their role in auditory processing.[178]

Inferior Colliculus. The IC receives synapses from the majority, if not all, of the fibers projecting from the lower auditory nuclei. The 3 neuronal areas that make up the IC are the central, external, and pericentral nuclei. The predominant termination zone for the ascending auditory projections is in the ventrolateral region of the central nucleus. This region receives inputs from the SOC and a heavy contralateral input from the DCN. Other major projections come ipsilaterally from the MSO and bilaterally from the LSO. The function of the IC is far from completely understood, with many neurons exhibiting complex excitatory–inhibitory interactions. A simple view is that the IC integrates the frequency analysis features of the DCN with the localization abilities of the SOC.[174]

Medial Geniculate. The medial geniculate (MG) is the thalamic relay nucleus for auditory information. All auditory projections from the IC to the auditory cortex pass through the MG. This nucleus is also composed of 3 divisions, the ventral, dorsal, and medial nuclei.[179] The ventral nucleus receives heavy ipsilateral projections from the ventrolateral portion of the central nucleus of the IC. This portion of the MG projects to the AI, AII, and EP regions of the auditory cortex (see below). Again, a wide variety of single-unit response types have been recorded in the MG. In attempting to understand the MG's role in auditory processing, special efforts have been made to examine MG single-unit responses

to complex sounds. Thus, David and associates[180] and Keidel[181] demonstrated that MG neurons in the unanesthetized cat were responsive only to specific parameters of complex speech sounds. In general, it has been extremely difficult to attribute specific feature extraction capabilities to neurons in the higher auditory nuclei that cannot be explained by complex responses already present at the level of the CN.

Auditory Cortex. The auditory cortex has been most extensively studied in the cat and can be divided into 3 areas based on similarity of Nissl stained cytoarchitectural details.[182] These include a primary area AI, a secondary area AII, and a remote projection region EP. In human and nonhuman primates, the primary auditory projection area is located in the temporal lobe but hidden by the sylvian fissure. The ventral division of the MG projects almost entirely to AI,[183] which can be considered the primary auditory cortex. Surrounding auditory areas receive projections from all divisions of the MG. Like the auditory relay nuclei, the auditory cortex is also tonotopically organized. As might be expected by the many intricate interconnections of the auditory system prior to input arriving at the cortex, the understanding of cortical processing has been a complex and difficult task. One approach to solving the problem of cortical function has been the use of ablation studies in which the auditory cortex is removed after training an animal to perform a specific auditory task. These studies have demonstrated that cortical ablation does not result in a complete loss of function as do similar lesions in the visual system. In fact, for many simple tasks, no long-term deficits can be detected.[181] Based on these results, it is reasonable to assume that the auditory cortex is involved in numerous details of more complex auditory processing. Consequently, it is unlikely that 1 simple unifying concept will be uncovered that describes the functional role of the auditory cortex.

Summary. Although there have been many studies of single-unit activity in the auditory nuclei over the past half century, they have thus far yielded few unifying principles about the data-processing mechanisms of the auditory nervous system. However, a number of recent studies suggest that, in many instances, the brain makes use of patterns of activity distributed over many cells to extract relevant information.[170] Consequently, if future studies focus on describing the responses of individual cells without viewing their participation, as a whole, in some functional unit, they may be doomed to result in failure as a means of understanding central auditory processing.

Auditory-Evoked Electrophysiologic Responses

Modern averaging techniques have made it possible to record from humans, with surface electrodes, electrical responses reflecting the entire auditory pathway, from cochlea to cortex.[184,185] Clinical applications of this technique have expanded rapidly and are routine in most otolaryngology clinics today. In this section, some basic physiologic principles are discussed on which the clinical applications of auditory-evoked potentials are based.

Two major classes of human auditory-evoked potentials generated by acoustic transients (clicks) are used clinically. One class is recorded with an electrode located as close to the cochlea as possible, that is, either extratympanic (eg, located on the external ear canal skin) or transtympanic (eg, penetrating the eardrum to rest on the medial wall of the middle ear).[186] Tests based on this class of auditory-evoked potentials have been termed electrocochleography (ECochG). The second class of auditory-evoked potentials is recorded between one electrode located on the vertex and another near the external ear, for example, either on the mastoid or earlobe. This latter class of evoked potentials has been subdivided conventionally according to their onset latency range into early, middle, and late responses.

Electrocochleographic Responses: Whole-Nerve Compound Action Potential, Cochlear Microphonic, Summating Potential. *Description of the Responses.*

Figure 33 shows a typical example of cochlear and auditory nerve click-evoked potentials recorded from the ear canal. Evoked responses to clicks of opposite polarity are shown in Figure 33A. The whole-nerve CAP has 2 or more ear canal negative peaks designated N_1, N_2, N_3 (N_2 and N_3 not labeled here), and so forth. Each peak lasts about 1 ms and, in normal ears, N_1 is always the larger peak. In Figure 33B, the CM appears as a series of sinusoidal oscillations, typically about 3 kHz, on the leading edge of the N_1 peak. The SP in Figure 33C appears as an ear canal negative hump on the leading edge

of the N_1 peak, with the CM oscillations superimposed.

The auditory nerve CAP (see Figure 33A) is the sum of the synchronous firing of single-fiber auditory nerve fibers as seen by the distant recording electrode as illustrated in Figure 34.[187] The single-unit spikes are triggered by the passage of the cochlear traveling wave. Thus, spikes from basal (high-frequency) fibers appear at the recording electrode earlier than spikes from apical (low-frequency) fibers. Because the degree to which single neural unit responses contribute to the evoked potential is determined largely by their synchrony, high-frequency (basal) fibers contribute more effectively to the whole-nerve CAP and also to the evoked auditory brainstem response (ABR) than do low-frequency fibers.

This principle leads to several important conclusions for clinical applications: (1) Broadband-click–evoked CAPs preferentially reflect high-frequency fiber activity, and, as a corollary, high-frequency clicks are more effective generators of auditory-evoked potentials than low-frequency clicks.[188] (2) High-frequency hearing loss caused by selective removal of basal units tends to bias the broadband-click–evoked CAP and ABR toward more apical units. Therefore, high-frequency cochlear deficits prolong N_1 peak latencies.[188] (3) A low-frequency deficit does not cause a corresponding basalward shift because of the already existing heavy bias toward basal units in the normal response. Therefore, low-frequency cochlear deficits have no apparent effect on CAP and ABR latencies. Because the CM response follows the waveform of basilar membrane vibration, it reverses polarity when click polarity is reversed, whereas the envelope-following SP does not. The neural response also maintains the same polarity. Thus, adding together responses

to opposite polarity clicks cancels out the polarity-reversing CM and allows a better view of the SP (see Figure 33C). In contrast, subtracting the condensation and rarefaction responses preserves the CM, while canceling the SP and most of the CAP (see Figure 33B).

The cochlear receptor potentials (CM, SP) can also be separated from the CAP because receptor potentials are nonrefractory and do not adapt, whereas neural responses do. Thus, masking and increasing click rate are often used in clinical testing to depress selectively the neural response while preserving the CM and SP.

Reliable methods for separation of the SP from the other cochlear potentials have made this response useful in the diagnosis of Meniere disease.[189] A number of studies have demonstrated that the SP is enlarged in a certain percentage of patients with Meniere disease.[190] Evidence supporting the notion that SP enlargement is specifically related to endolymphatic hydrops is provided by observations that manipulations expected to reduce fluid accumulation within the endolymphatic space, for example, administration of hyperosmotic agents such as glycerol, often shrink abnormally enlarged SPs.[191]

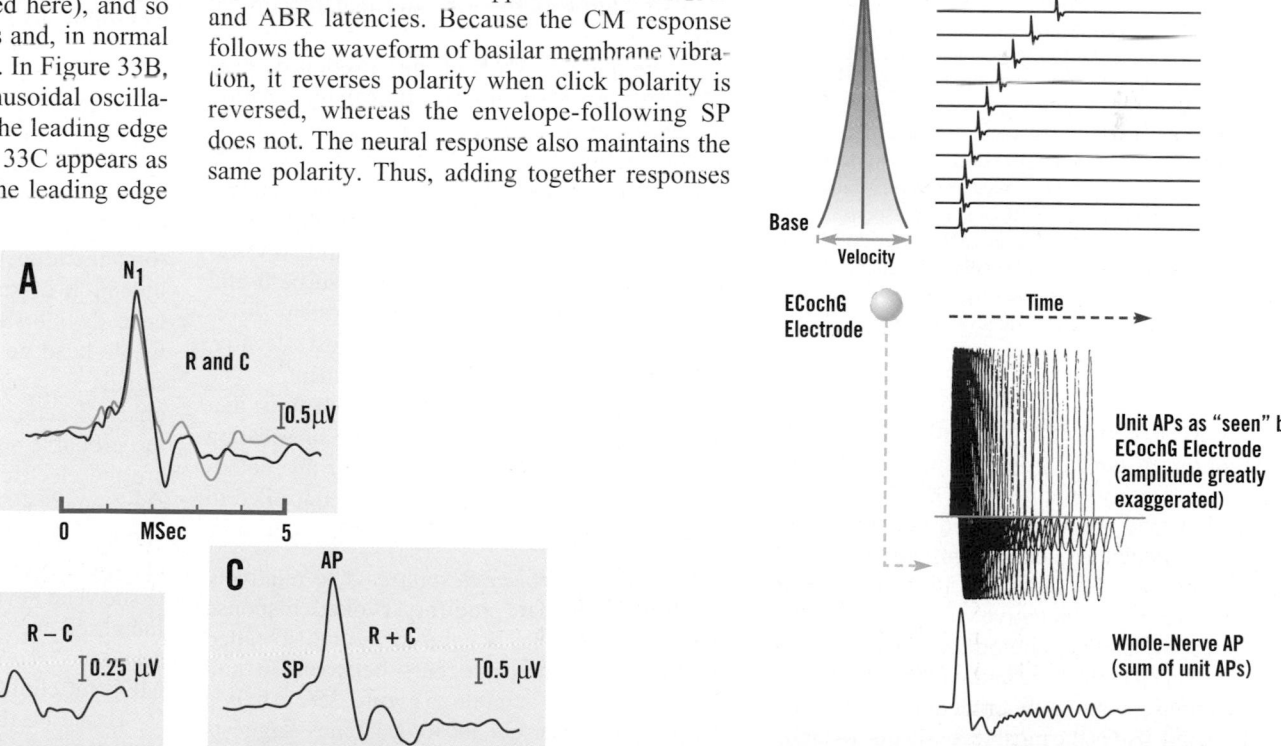

Figure 34 Summation of the single-unit spikes (amplitude exaggerated) picked up by a distant electrocochleographic (ECochG) electrode to form the whole-nerve compound action potential (CAP). Note that the highly synchronized spikes from the basal end of the cochlea sum more effectively than the poorly synchronized spikes from the apical end of the cochlea. The records of unit action potentials (APs) and the whole-nerve CAP at the bottom are from a simplified computer experiment. (Reproduced with permission from reference 187.)

Figure 33 Examples of cochlear and auditory nerve electrical responses to clicks recorded from the human outer ear canal. The cochlear potentials are the cochlear microphonic (CM) and summating potential (SP). (A) The whole-nerve compound action potential typically has a large negative peak (N_1). R and C are shown as separate condensation (*dashed line*) and rarefaction (*solid line*) rectangular-pulse click responses recorded from the outer ear canal with a nasion "reference" electrode. (B) R – C is the waveform produced by subtracting C from R responses. (C) R + C is the waveform produced by adding C and R responses. Upward deflections represent negativity at the ear canal, and time scale zeroes are set at the leading edge of the rectangular pulse driving the ear speaker. Click rate was 8/s; click level was 115 dB peak equivalent SPL. Each C and R response was the average of 1,000 single sweeps.

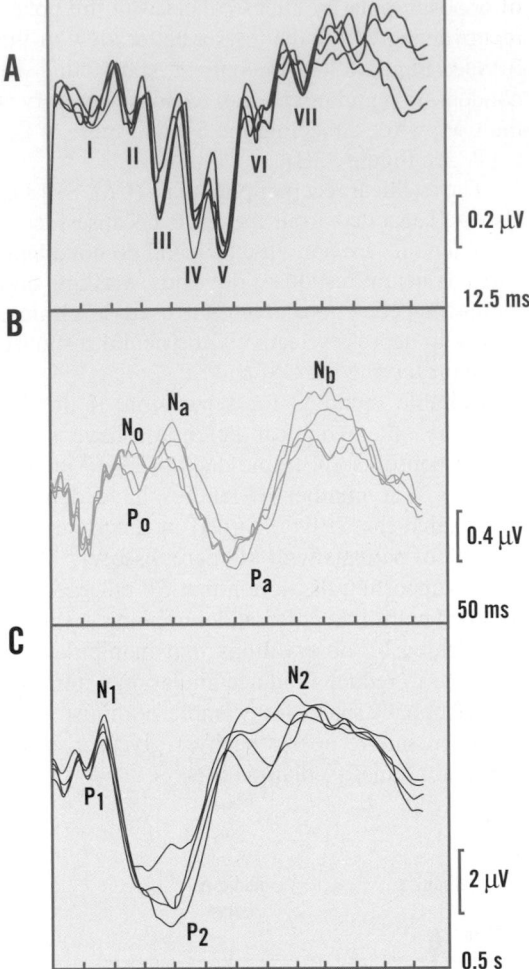

Figure 35 Averaged human click-evoked potentials, recorded with vertex-mastoid electrodes. Upward deflection represents negativity at the vertex. From top to bottom, the time base is slowed to demonstrate progressively later responses. (A) Auditory brainstem response (with the polarity opposite to the response recorded with a nasopharyngeal electrode). (B) Middle latency response. (C) Late "vertex" auditory-evoked response. Each tracing represents the average of 1,024 single responses. Several tracings are superimposed in each record to give an idea of variability. Roman numerals and letters identify individual peaks of the various responses according to accepted convention. (Reproduced with permission from reference 185.)

Vertex-Recorded Auditory-Evoked Potentials.
Description of the Responses. Figure 35 shows examples of early (A), middle (B), and late (C) vertex-recorded auditory-evoked potentials generated by broadband clicks. Commonly used peak designations are also shown. In all traces, upward deflection represents negative voltage at the vertex ("referred" to an electrode on the mastoid). Note the differences in the time and voltage scales. The early response, commonly termed the ABR, is the smallest and also is the most recently discovered.

Auditory Brainstem Response. An example of an ABR is shown in Figure 35A, in which the peaks of this response are labeled with Roman numerals I to VII. It can be seen that the ABR occurs approximately between 1 and 8 ms after stimulus onset. Wave V is typically the largest and most robust of the potentials, and waves beyond V are seldom used clinically. Studies in humans[192] and animals[193] suggest that wave V is generated at the LL. Thus, the ABR is probably not useful in detecting abnormalities at or above the level of the IC.[194] However, for the lower brainstem, the ABR is one of the best audiologic tests for detecting dysfunction.

The ABR is 1 of the most frequently used auditory-evoked potential procedures because the variables that affect this response have been well described, and it provides a good measure of cochlear sensitivity and retrocochlear status. Clinically, the response can be interpreted by quantitative measures of peak latencies, interpeak intervals, and interpeak latency differences. In addition, the presence or absence of the various waves is noted as well as waveform morphology.[195]

Middle Latency Response. The middle latency response (MLR), labeled N_0, P_0, N_a, P_a, and so forth (Figure 35B), occurs between 8 and 40 ms after the auditory stimulus.[196] In animals, wave P_a appears to be generated in the primary auditory cortex by cortical elements on the side contralateral to stimulation.[197] However, in humans, P_a seems to be generated in both hemispheres, even with monaural stimulation. Human cortical mapping localizes this potential to the region of the sylvian fissure,[198] whereas studies based on clinical correlations indicate involvement of thalamocortical projections to the primary auditory area located along Heschl gyrus in the genesis of this response. Site-of-lesion studies suggest that wave N_a originates in the midbrain, including such structures as the MG and thalamocortical projections.[198]

Although the MLR is not used nearly as frequently as ABR, useful clinical information can be obtained from this response, particularly in conjunction with ABR testing. The MLR is robust at all frequencies including low frequencies below 1,000 Hz and, consequently, offers a complementary index of high- and low-frequency hearing.[199] The MLR can also be useful in assessment of central auditory system disorders, neurologic evaluation, and, most recently, as a tool for cochlear implant assessment.[200] The most significant disadvantage of MLR is that subject variables such as sleep state or sedation can severely reduce the amplitude of this potential. Thus, behavioral state must be controlled to obtain meaningful results.

Late Auditory-Evoked Response. The relatively high-amplitude late auditory-evoked response (LAER), labeled P_1, N_1, and so forth (also called the vertex potential), occurs between 50 and 250 ms after the stimulus (Figure 35C). It is a cortical response, but its long latency suggests that the LAER is not generated within the primary auditory cortex but rather that it originates in the associative cortex.[185] These potentials are often dependent on the subject's state of alertness and consequently have received little use in clinical situations.

Auditory Brain Mapping. One technique that is receiving considerable attention as a new and potentially powerful diagnostic tool is the use of auditory brain mapping. Methods for this procedure are highly similar to those used to obtain the traditional evoked responses already described. The primary difference is that brain mapping simultaneously records the electrical activity from an array of scalp electrodes. Although this mass of data could be viewed as many evoked potentials, the human observer cannot readily interpret such a massive amount of data. Therefore, brain mapping was developed using computer-processing techniques to provide a visual display of the potential fields among all of the electrodes simultaneously. This method reduces the data into a multicolored or shaded plot in which intense activity is usually given the most brilliant color or the darkest shading. An example of the typical electrode placements and the derivation of a simple brain map are shown in Figure 36. With this type of visual output, patterns of activity in normal patients can be established and abnormalities easily visualized in pathologic cases. Computer techniques also allow the clinician to view the patterns of activity throughout the duration of the stimulus to produce a motion picture of the evoked electrical activity that occurred over time. This method allows for the visualization of the spatiotemporal patterns of brain activity. Because the data are stored in the computer, a number of advanced mathematical processing methods, which permit further refinement of the data, can be applied to aid in the detection of subtle abnormalities. For more information on this topic, the reader is referred to these comprehensive reviews.[201,202]

Magnetoencephalography. Magnetoencephalography (MEG) involves the completely noninvasive recording of weak cerebral magnetic fields, which represent about 1 part in 109 of the earth's geomagnetic field, outside the head.[203] The neuromagnetic technique was made possible by the invention of superconducting quantum interference device (SQUID) magnetometers. Using a whole-head neuromagnetometer, magnetic brain signals are averaged by time locking them to the onset of acoustic stimulation. It is assumed that the probable sources of cerebral magnetic fields are the electric currents in the synapses of synchronously activated cortical pyramidal neurons, and the sinks or volume currents, to complete the electrical circuit, are generated in the surrounding tissue. The development of multichannel systems increased the speed and convenience of neuromagnetic recording and made it feasible to apply MEG for clinical purposes.

Based on the accurate spatiotemporal resolution of whole-head MEG, Hari and Lounasmaa have been instrumental in applying MEG to investigate the activity of the auditory projection areas, particularly with respect to language-related sites.[203] A schematic illustration of a typical experimental setup for auditory measurements is illustrated in Figure 37 and shows the relationship of the SQUID to the patient's head. The inset above indicates the isocontours across the scalp for the

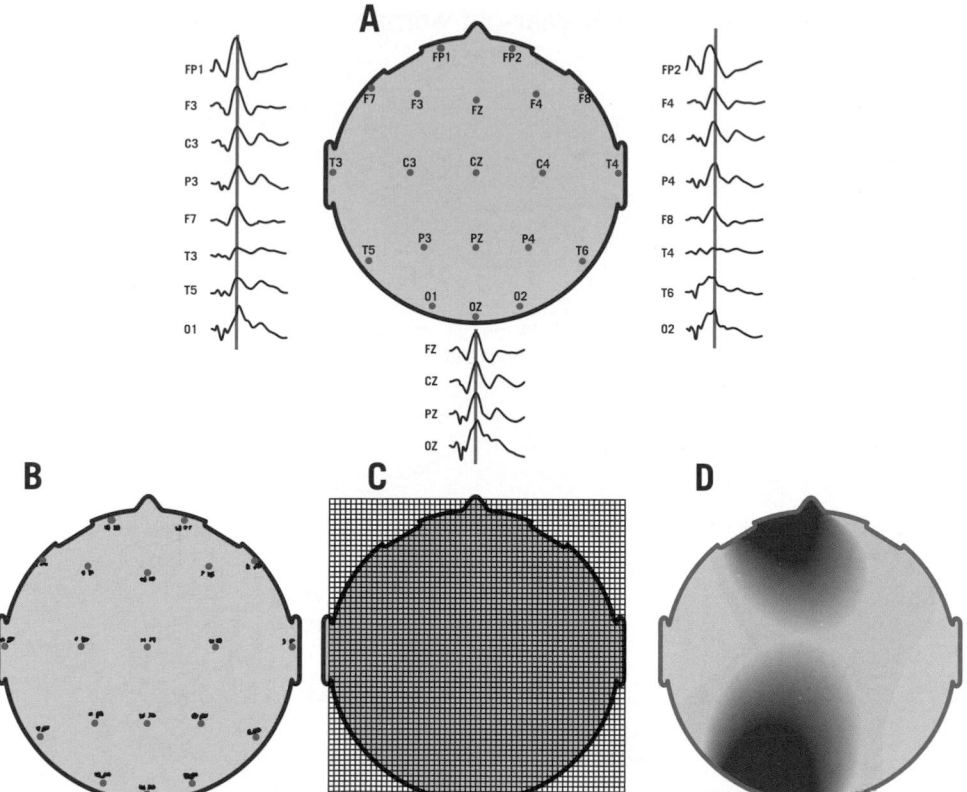

Figure 36 Example of the construction of topographic images from evoked potential data. (A) Individual-evoked potentials are shown at the electrode locations indicated in the diagram. (B) Mean voltages are shown for the time interval 192 ms after the stimulus. (C) Head region is divided into a 64 × 64 matrix to produce 4,096 spatial domains. Each spatial domain is assigned a voltage derived by linear interpolation from the 3 nearest recording locations. (D) A visual image constructed by fitting a discrete-level, equal-interval intensity scale to the points of C. Although a visual-evoked potential was used to create this topographic map, the same procedure is used for mapping auditory data. (Reprinted with permission from reference 201.)

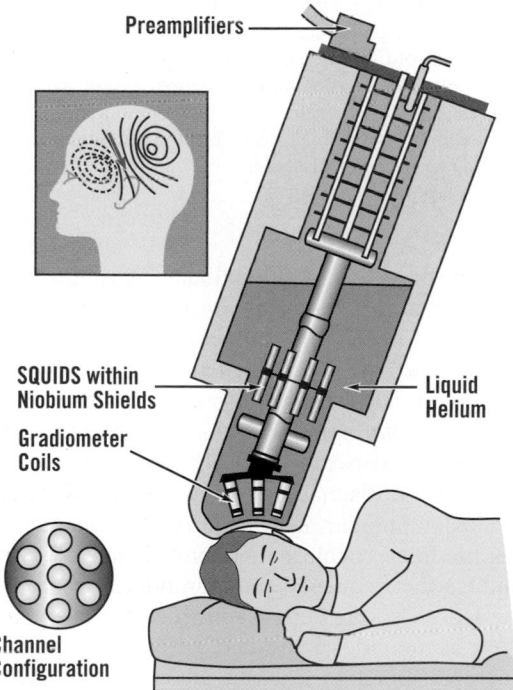

Figure 37 Schematic illustration of a typical experimental setup for auditory measurements using magnetoencephalography. The most important parts of the seven-channel DC SQUID instrument are shown, with the midpoints of the different channels separated by 36.5 mm. The insert above depicts isocontours across the scalp for the radial component of the magnetic field, generated by an active area in the auditory cortex. The arrow illustrates the location of the equivalent current dipole. (Reproduced with permission from reference 203.)

component of the magnetic field, which is generated by the active region of the auditory cortex. An example of the averaged magnetic responses from measurement sites anterior (above) and posterior (below) to the sylvian fissure of the right hemisphere, that is, along the superior surface of the temporal lobe, are shown for 1 subject for a spoken word (solid line) and noise bursts (dashed lines) on the left side of Figure 38. The right side of Figure 38 illustrates the effects of increasing the duration of the onset of the word in another subject. It is clear that sound evokes a complex magnetic waveform, which lasts several hundred milliseconds after stimulus onset. Interesting and clinically useful data have been obtained about the perception of speech of deaf patients with cochlear prostheses by examining the activity of their auditory cortices with MEG.[204] Information

of this real-time sort implies that neuromagnetic recording may be used to assess functional disorders in more detail than what is possible by other clinical evidence; thus, it is likely to become an important diagnostic tool of the future.

Neuroimaging. The beginning of in vivo imaging in awake and behaving subjects has revolutionized the ability to relate structure to function, particularly in the human brain. For example, 3-dimensional magnetic resonance imaging (MRI) provides detailed static images of the in vivo brain, with spatial resolution on the order of cubic millimeters. Other functionally related techniques in neuroimaging such as positron emission tomography and functional MRI provide excellent spatial and temporal resolutions for recording changes in regional blood flow and cellular metabolism during auditory stimulation. These techniques have been used to study a number of central auditory processes, including speech perception,[205,206] revealing tinnitus-related abnormalities in brain function.[207,208] Although these individual functional imaging approaches still have some limitations, the results are converging to improve our understanding of the neural processes underlying both normal and pathologic auditory function. Central auditory processing and functional neuroimaging are discussed in Chapter 8, "Central Auditory Processing and Functional Neuroimaging."

Evoked Otoacoustic Emissions. One of the principal benefits of OAEs with respect to clinical testing is that they provide an objective and noninvasive measure of cochlear activity, which is completely independent of retrocochlear activity. In particular, OAEs measure the functional responses of OHCs that are uniquely sensitive to agents that damage hearing. Kemp,[101] the pioneer investigator into the basic features of OAEs, has also been instrumental in establishing 1 class of evoked emissions, the click-based TEOAE (see Figure 22C), as a potentially useful diagnostic indicator of various ear diseases including Meniere disease[123] and acoustic neurinoma.[209] In addition, Kemp and Ryan have also established the use of the click-evoked OAE as a method of screening for hearing dysfunction in newborns.[210]

Because of the frequency specificity of the eliciting pure tones, DPOAEs (see Figure 23)

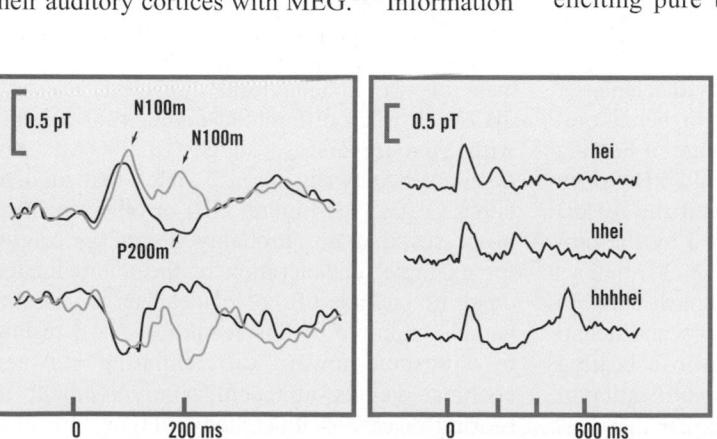

Figure 38 Averaged magnetic responses from the auditory cortex. (A) Averaged magnetic response (*n* = 120) to "hei" words (*red lines*) and noise bursts (*green lines*) from the right hemisphere in one subject; the upper curves are from an anterior and the lower ones from a posterior measurement location near the ends of the sylvian fissure. The passband was 0.05 to 70 Hz. (B) Effect of increasing the duration of "h" in another subject. (Reproduced with permission from reference 204.)

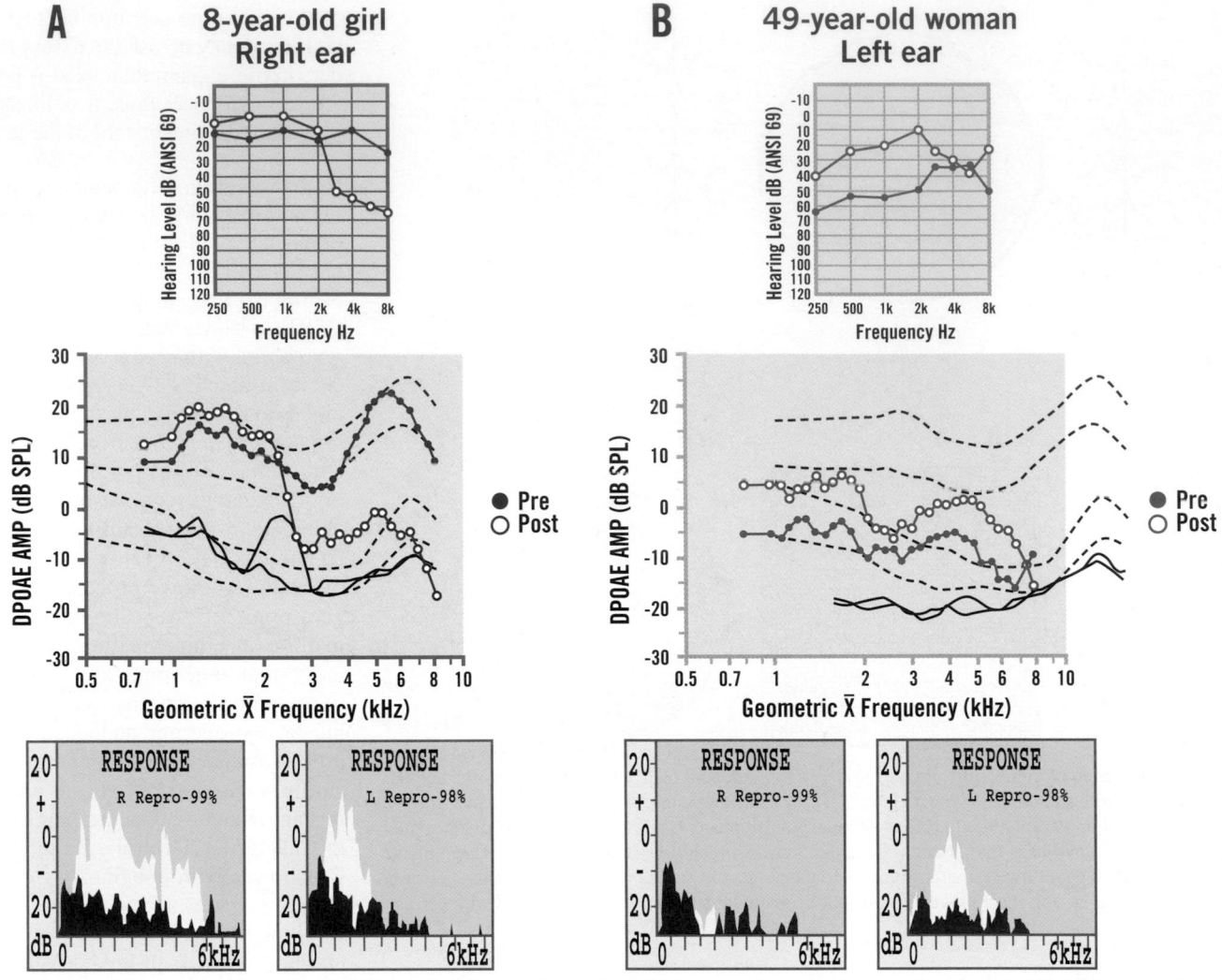

Figure 39 Conventional audiograms (*top*), distortion-product otoacoustic emission (DPOAE) frequency/level or DP-gram functions (*middle*) relating emission magnitude to stimulus frequency, in 0.1 octave steps from 0.8 to 8 kHz, for primary tone levels of 75 dB SPL, and click-evoked transient evoked otoacoustic emissions (OAEs) (*bottom*) elicited by the "default" mode of the ILO88 Otodynamic Analyser. (A) Behavioral hearing and evoked OAE findings for the right ear of an 8-year-old girl comparing pre- (*solid circles*) versus posttreatment (*open circles*) responses following a course of antineoplasm therapy with cisplatin. Immittance and speech testing results were normal for the baseline session and were not tested during the posttreatment examination. (B) Audiometric and OAE results for the left ear of a 49-year-old woman for 2 test sessions separated by about 2 weeks. The patient complained of a fluctuating hearing loss, tinnitus, aural fullness, and episodic dizziness of several months duration. Immittance findings were normal, whereas the speech discrimination score and speech reception threshold improved from 72 to 96% and 55 to 25 dB HL, respectively, at the last evaluation period (*open circles*). (Reproduced with permission from reference 211.)

also have a beneficial clinical applicability. This stimulus-related frequency specificity permits DPOAEs to be measured after averaging the responses to only a few stimuli. Thus, under computer control, the fine resolution of DPOAEs in both the stimulus frequency and level domains permits the precise determination of the boundary between normal and abnormal OHC function. Data from our laboratory illustrate this feature of DPOAEs in the plots of Figure 39A,[211] which show the development of ototoxicity during a course of antineoplasm therapy with cisplatin. Comparing the OAE findings with behavioral hearing (top), note the abrupt change in hearing and emission activity between 2 and 3 kHz (open circles), which accurately followed the 40 dB loss in hearing sensitivity produced by the ototoxic agent.

Based on their ability to distinguish between the relative contribution that sensory and neural components of the cochlea make to a hearing loss, OAEs promise to facilitate identification of the anatomic substrate of complex ear diseases.

For example, the records shown in Figure 39B represent a typical pattern of audiometric loss in early Meniere disease, which is accompanied by thresholds that are >40 dB HL and, not unexpectedly, no TEOAEs (bottom left) and abnormally low-level DPOAEs (solid circles). Together, these results imply that the OHC system is involved in this patient's disease. However, other patients with Meniere disease, who show a similar hearing loss, can demonstrate rather robust DPOAEs, even for test frequencies for which behavioral thresholds are >50 dB HL.[212] Such differential findings for patients with Meniere disease suggest that OAEs can distinguish between disease states that involve either OHCs (see Figure 39B) or other cochlear processes that are probably neural in origin, for example, degeneration of the unmyelinated dendritic endings of the cochlear nerve. A comparable example of this feature of OAE testing to contribute toward differentiating between cochlear versus noncochlear involvement in hearing disease is illustrated in Figure 40 for 2

patients diagnosed with vestibular schwannomas. The patient in Figure 40A displays the expected outcome for OAE testing in the presence of a retrocochlear disease. That is, in the presence of a moderate hearing loss on the tumor side (solid circles), both TEOAEs and DPOAEs are measurable. However, it is clear for the patient in Figure 40B, diagnosed with a right-sided (open circles) vestibular schwannoma, that the tumor has modified cochlear function in a manner that mimics the frequency configuration of the hearing loss. Thus, in certain retrocochlear disorders such as tumors of the cerebellopontine angle, cochlear function can be adversely affected, probably owing to compromise of the vascular supply to the inner ear. One benefit of OAE testing illustrated in Figure 39B is its sensitivity to changes in hearing status, which are mediated by the OHC system. In this instance, at the time the patient returned for follow-up testing (open circles), her hearing had improved, particularly over the low-frequency test range. The 20 to 30 dB improvement in low-frequency hearing was

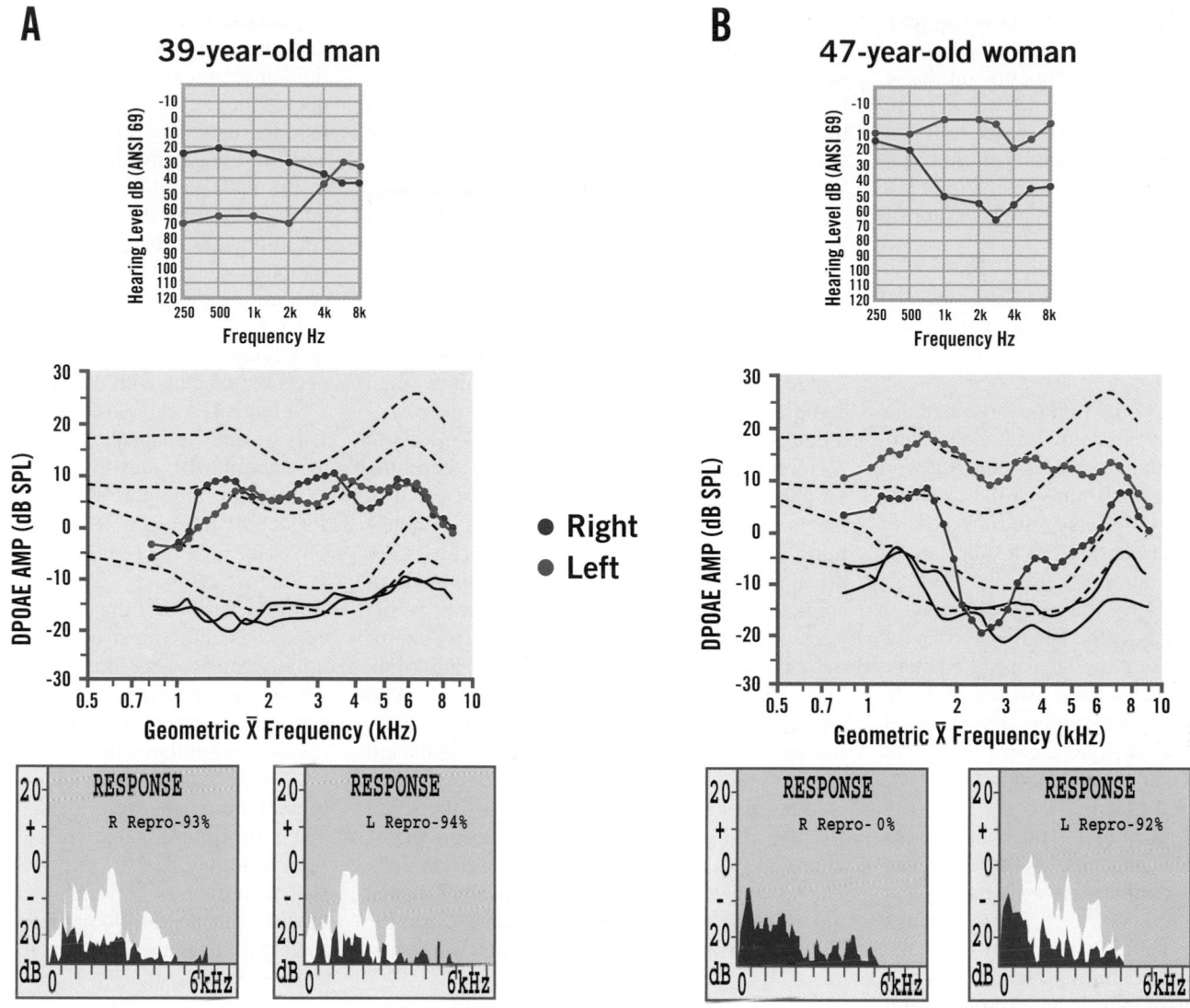

Figure 40 Audiometric and otoacoustic emission findings for 2 patients with vestibular schwannomas confirmed by magnetic resonance imaging. (A) A 39-year-old man with a vestibular schwannoma on the left side who had normal tympanograms but absent reflexes bilaterally. Although speech testing was normal for the right ear (*open circles*), the speech discrimination score and speech reception threshold were 0% and 70 dB HL, respectively, for the involved left ear (*solid circles*). (B) A 47-year-old woman with a right-sided vestibular schwannoma. Whereas her tympanograms were normal, the only measurable acoustic reflex threshold was for ipsilateral stimuli at 1 kHz. Speech testing was normal for the left ear, whereas the right ear was associated with a speech discrimination score of 60% and a speech reception threshold of 35 dB HL. (Reproduced with permission from reference 211.)

mirrored by a similar increase in DPOAEs and by the ability to now measure TEOAEs.

In addition to the clinical applications noted above for OAEs, a number of studies have also demonstrated the utility of using emitted responses to understand the fundamental basis of common cochlear lesions, including the effects of noise-induced hearing loss,[213] hereditary hearing impairment,[214] congenital hearing disorders,[212] ototoxicity,[215] bacterial meningitis,[216] and presbyacusis[217] on both TEOAEs and DPOAEs. The interested reader is encouraged to refer to these comprehensive reviews concerning the strengths and limitations of the clinical application of OAEs.[218,219]

Exactly how OAEs in general arise and how they are propagated in the cochlea is still a matter of debate. Recent experimental and theoretical findings suggest that there may be 2 mechanisms of OAE generation.[220–223] SOAEs, TEOAEs, and SFOAEs probably arise predominantly as reflection OAEs via coherent linear reflection from impedance discontinuities (ie, out of place OHCs, disarranged stereocilia) distributed along the cochlear partition. DPOAEs

likely result mainly from distortion processes due to the nonlinear interaction between the f_1 and f_2 primary tones at their "overlap" region on the basilar membrane. Knight and Kemp[221,222] established the terms "wave-fixed" and "placed-fixed" OAEs to describe the corresponding emission sources that are physically associated with either fixed structures (ie, reflection emissions) or the traveling-wave peak (ie, distortion emissions) within the cochlea, respectively. Moreover, it is probable that the electromotility of the OHCs has a closer association with the generation of SOAEs, TEOAEs, and SFOAEs than DPOAEs. Rather, DPOAEs appear to be generated principally in the nonlinear aspects of the OHC transduction process, probably involving the opening and closing of transduction channels at the tips of the OHC stereocilia. This analysis may explain why following the administration of furosemide in experimental preparations, DPOAEs evoked by high-level primaries typically persist.[224] Thus, with ototoxicity, the fundamental processes underlying OHC nonlinearity in the form of somatic electromotility are probably only minimally damaged. However, the

"cochlear amplifier" gain[71] associated with basilar membrane vibration is severely reduced or absent due to a decrease in the driving voltage across the cell membrane, which was prevented from developing normally by insufficient stimulation of the nonlinearity located in the OHC stereocilia. For high-level primary tones, then, the low or absent gain is overcome and DPOAEs can again be observed. Such an explanation is supported by the findings of Liberman and colleagues,[48] using mutant mice lacking the molecular motility motor protein, prestin. Specifically, with prestin deletion, OHC microvibrations were not necessary for the production of high-level DPOAEs.

However, although there is general agreement with respect to the existence of two OAE generators, a growing debate concerns the role of reverse propagation of OAEs within the cochlea. That is, it is commonly believed that the cochlea emits sounds through backward traveling waves. However, based mainly on the relationship between OAE latencies and the specificity of origin location,[225–227] the possibility of compressive waves propagating through cochlear fluids is being actively investigated. In any case, the lively discussions noted above are leading to focused experiments on these issues. Most certainly, by developing a more complete understanding of OAE generation and propagation processes, the resulting more exact interpretation of emissions will vastly improve the clinical utility of this intriguing measure of cochlear function.

VESTIBULAR SYSTEM

General Principles

The nonauditory part of the inner ear (termed the vestibular apparatus) consists of 2 functional subdivisions: (1) the semicircular ducts consisting of 2 vertical and 1 horizontal and (2) the otolithic organs consisting of the saccule and the utricle. The semicircular ducts respond to head rotation, that is, angular acceleration, whereas the otolithic organs are stimulated by the effects of gravity and linear acceleration of the head. The primary function of the utricle is to signal head position relative to gravity. Ablation of the saccule produces a less significant deficit than ablation of the utricle; hence, the function of the saccule is less well defined than that of the utricle. In fact, it has been proposed that the saccule is a low-frequency auditory receptor.[228] However, a series of systematic studies using single-unit recordings have revealed that saccular nerve fibers respond only to linear acceleration.[229–231] These findings suggest that the saccular system provides the high-level vertical acceleration signals required to elicit the motor response necessary to land optimally from a fall.[232]

Conventionally, the vestibular system is regarded as one of 3 sensory systems that function to maintain body balance and equilibrium. The other 2 are the somatosensory (chiefly proprioceptive) and visual systems. Loss of proprioception, for example, as in tabes dorsalis, or vision causes more significant balance and equilibrium difficulty than does loss of vestibular function. With bilateral vestibular function loss, difficulties occur only when 1 of the other systems is disrupted, for example, when walking in the dark or on a soft surface, or when balance must be maintained under particularly difficult conditions, for example, walking on a narrow beam.[233] Thus, in humans, under physiologic conditions, the vestibular system is probably the least important of the 3 balance and equilibrium sensory systems. The most significant functional deficits occur when the vestibular system suffers acute, asymmetric damage and generates "false" head position or head rotation signals.

Vestibular Apparatus

The top portion of Figure 2 illustrates the general anatomic plan of the vestibular apparatus. There are many similarities with cochlear anatomy. For example, both end-organs are located in a tunnel that is hollowed out of the petrous portion of the temporal bone (embryologically, both organs come from the same tunnel). The tunnel is divided into an outer perilymph-filled bony labyrinth and an inner endolymph-filled membranous labyrinth. In addition, as in the cochlea, the receptor cells of the vestibular apparatus are ciliated, and these cilia extend into a gelatinous matrix.

The 3 semicircular canals are oriented orthogonally or at right angles to each other. They can be thought of as lying in a bottom corner of a box. The horizontal (or lateral or external) canal is in the plane of the bottom of the box, and the anterior-vertical (or superior) and posterior-vertical (or posterior) canals are in the planes of the 2 sides of the box. In humans, the entire canal complex is tilted upward about 30°. In the physiologic position, the head is bent forward about 30° from the earth's horizontal plane; therefore, the 30° upward tilt puts the horizontal canal in the horizontal position under everyday conditions.[234] The superior and posterior canals are oriented in vertical planes that form an angle of approximately 45° with the sagittal head plane. Each semicircular canal lies parallel to one of the canals in the opposite vestibular labyrinth. Thus, the right horizontal canal is coplanar with the left horizontal canal, whereas the right superior and posterior canals are coplanar with the left posterior and superior canals, respectively.

The sensory epithelia or cristae of the semicircular ducts are located in enlarged areas, referred to as ampullae, at one end of each duct. The nonampullated ends of the vertically oriented superior and posterior ducts connect to form the common crus. The bony vestibular aqueduct originates in the vestibule, that is, the entrance to the inner ear, and connects to the cerebrospinal fluid space medially. Within the vestibular aqueduct is the fibrous endolymphatic duct that establishes a route between the membranous vestibule and the cranial meninges, where the duct ends in the endolymphatic sac. The utriculosaccular duct, connecting the utricle and saccule, permits communication between the saccule and endolymphatic duct. Although there is no agreement concerning the site of endolymph absorption, it is likely that the K^+-rich fluid is absorbed in the endolymphatic sac.[235] The ductus reuniens connects the saccule with the cochlear duct.

Figure 41A shows the anatomy of the crista.[236] It is a saddle-shaped mound of tissue, attached to the ampullar wall at right angles to the long axis of the ampulla. The hair cells are on the surface of the crista. The ampullar nerve fibers travel through the center of the crista to synapse at the hair cell bases. The hair cell cilia protrude from the surface of the crista into the fan-shaped cupula, a gelatinous structure consisting of mucopolysaccharides within a keratin framework.[237] The cupula partitions the semicircular duct by covering the top of the crista and extending to the opposite ampullar wall.

The sacculus and utriculus are 2 sacs in the membranous labyrinth, located in the vestibule. Their receptor organs, called maculae, can be seen in Figure 41B,[238] as patches of epithelia on the membranous labyrinth walls. The utricular macula lies on the floor of the utricle approximately in the plane of the horizontal semicircular

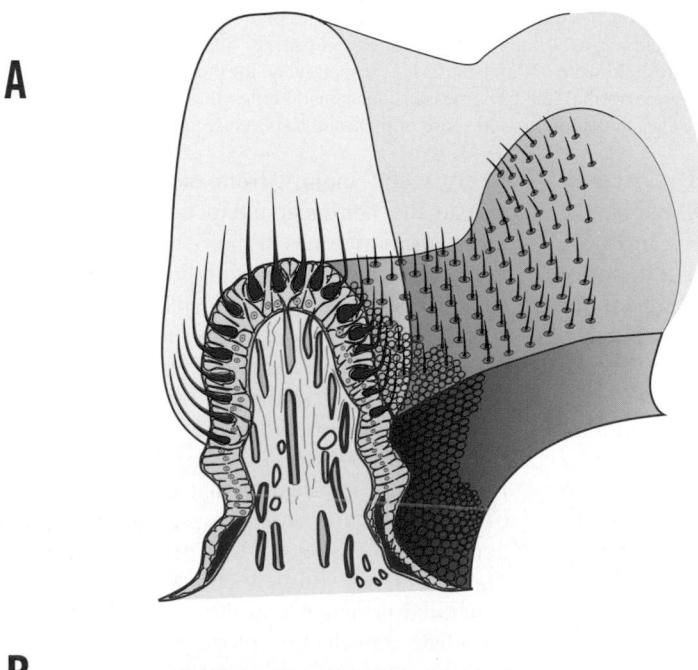

A

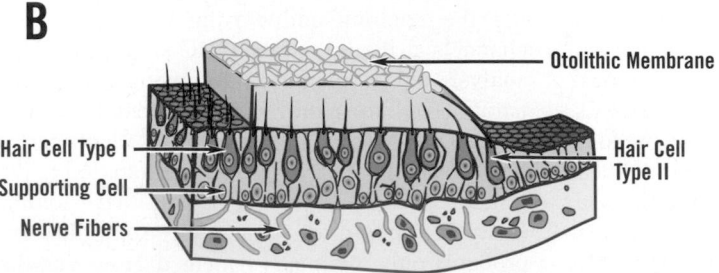

B

Otolithic Membrane

Hair Cell Type I

Supporting Cell

Hair Cell Type II

Nerve Fibers

Figure 41 Sensory receptors of the vestibular system. (A) Schematic drawing of the crista ampullaris illustrating the sensory cells, their hair bundles (cilia) that protrude into the cupula, and their innervating nerve fibers. (B) Schematic drawing of a macula, showing how the cilia of the hair cells are embedded in a gelatinous membrane to which are attached calcium carbonate crystals, that is, otoconia. (A reproduced with permission from reference 236; B reproduced with permission from reference 238.)

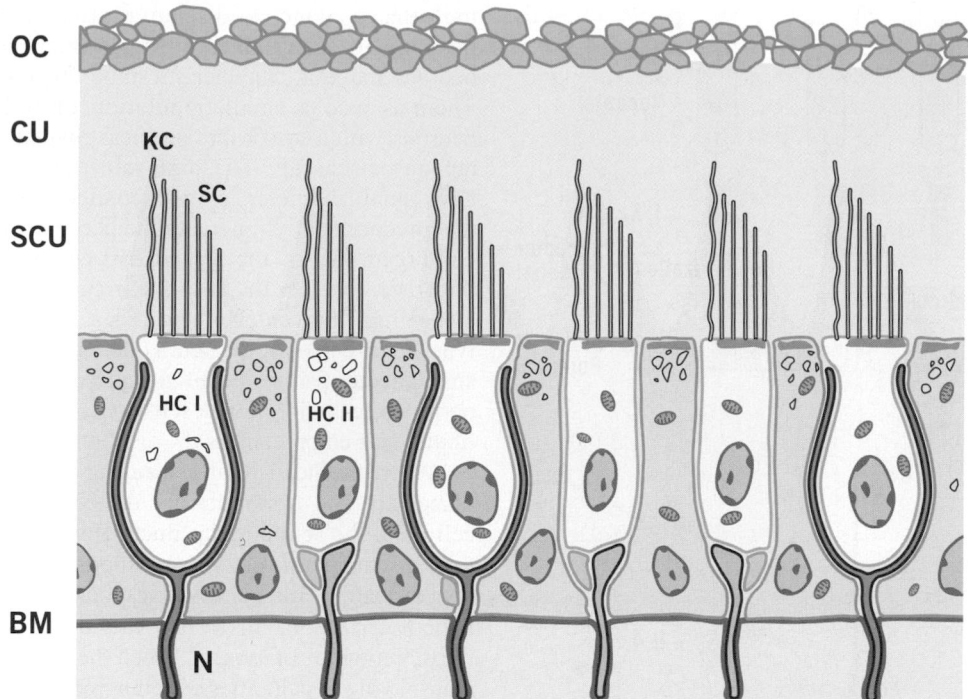

OC
CU
SCU
KC
SC
HC I
HC II
BM
N

Figure 42 Schematic drawing of a cross-section of a macula. The gelatinous substance is divided into cupular (CU) and subcupular (SCU) layers. There are two types of cilia: kinocilia, labeled KC (one per hair cell), and stereocilia, labeled SC (many per hair cell). OC = otoconia; HC I = type I hair cell; HC II = type II hair cell; N = nerve fiber; BM = basement membrane; S = supporting cell.

also demonstrated 2 types of cilia: stereocilia and kinocilia[244–246] (Figure 43B). Each hair cell has only 1 motile kinocilium and a bundle of 60 to 100 stereocilia.

Stereocilia are relatively rigid, club-like rods, varying systematically in length in a "pipe organ" fashion that extend at the apical end of the hair cell, from a dense cuticular plate that consists of actin and myosin.[59] They are not homogeneous, as was originally thought. Rather, they contain longitudinally oriented microfilaments[247] composed of actin.[41] The membrane enveloping the stereocilia is a thickened continuation of the hair cell cuticular membrane.[247] The stereocilia are constricted at their base and, when deflected, move like stiff rods pivoting around the basal constricted area.[49] Interconnections between stereocilia via fibrils or tip links have been demonstrated.[248]

Kinocilia end in basal bodies, located just beneath the hair cell membrane. Within each kinocilium, there are 9 peripherally arranged double-tubular filaments, positioned regularly around two centrally located tubular filaments. This 9-plus-2 tubule pattern is found in many motile cilia, for example, respiration epithelia, oviduct epithelium, unicellular flagellates.[249] Stereocilia are coupled to the kinocilium and to each other so that during deflection, all cilia are stimulated as 1 bundle.[66]

On each hair cell, the single kinocilium is located to 1 side of the bundle of stereocilia. In both maculae and cristae, hair cells in the same area tend to have kinocilia on the same side of the stereocilia bundle. Thus, the vestibular sensory epithelium has a morphologic directional polarization[244] that is determined by the direction of the cilia alignment. Figure 43C illustrates the directional polarization of the utricular macula. The kinocilia all tend to point toward a line of demarcation called the striola, or linea alba, running across the approximate center of the macula. In the saccule, the kinocilia point away from the striola. In the horizontal duct crista, kinocilia point toward the utricle, whereas in the pair of vertical cristae, they point away from the utricle. Thus, vertical and horizontal cristae are morphologically polarized in opposite directions.[241]

Transduction and Coding

Mechanical Events. As in the cochlea, the final mechanical event in vestibular transduction is the bending of the hair cell cilia. Figure 44 illustrates transduction by the macula. When the macular surface is tilted, the heavy otoliths tend to slide downward, carrying the gelatinous membrane and attached cilia with them.

The 6 semicircular ducts consist of a circular, narrow-bore tube in the temporal bone filled with fluid called endolymph. The tube originates from and returns to a reservoir (the utricle), but each duct may be thought of, for practical purposes, as a fluid ring. When the head undergoes an angular acceleration, the fluid is left behind because of its inertia. This causes the endolymph to flow relative to the duct and to push on the

canal. The saccular macula lies on the anteromedial wall of the saccule and is oriented principally in the vertical plane.

Figure 42 shows the structure of the macula. It consists of hair cells that are surrounded by supporting cells. The hair cell cilia are attached to a gelatinous otolithic membrane. On the top of the gelatinous membrane is a layer of calcium carbonate crystals called statoconia or otoliths. The otoliths are denser than the surrounding endolymph,[239] hence their ability to respond to gravity and inertial forces.

Figure 43 summarizes in a schematic form some TEM observations of vestibular hair cell morphology. First, as shown by Figure 43A, there are 2 types of hair cells in both the macula and the crista.[240] Type I hair cells are flask-shaped and have "chalice"-type afferent nerve endings that surround all but the hair-bearing end.

Efferent nerve terminals synapse with the afferent calyx near its base. Type II hair cells have a cylindrical or test tube shape and have several small bouton-type nerve endings that represent both afferent and efferent innervation only at the cell's base. Type I hair cells are concentrated in the central apex of the crista and the central part of the macula; type II hair cells are more numerous toward the peripheral region of the end-organ.[241] Although significant amounts of filamentous actin occur at the apical surfaces of both the sensory cells and the supporting cells in the hair cell-containing regions of the vestibular organs,[242] motile properties such as the fast rates of lengthening and shortening, which have been observed for cochlear OHCs, have not been shown for vestibular hair cells. However, there is some evidence that slow motility is exhibited by type II hair cells.[243] The electron microscope has

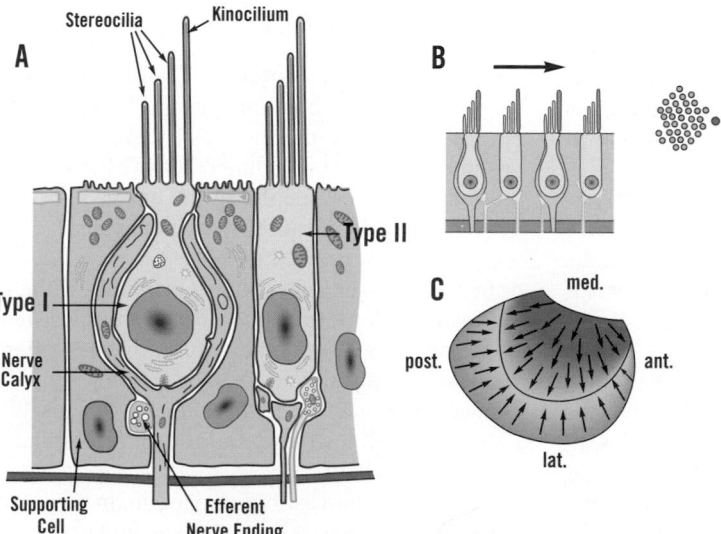

A Stereocilia Kinocilium
Type II
Type I
Nerve Calyx
Supporting Cell
Efferent Nerve Ending

B

C med. post. ant. lat.

Figure 43 Microanatomy of the vestibular hair cells. (A) Schematic drawing of the 2 vestibular hair cell types. (B) Diagram showing morphologic polarization of the hair cells. Arrow shows the direction of cilia bending that produces excitation. At right is a cross-section through the hair-bearing end of the hair cell showing many stereocilia (*open circles*) and 1 kinocilium (*filled circle*). (C) A diagrammatic surface view of the human utricular macula. Arrows indicate direction of polarization. Dashed line is the linea alba. (A reproduced with permission from reference 260; B and C reproduced with permission from references 240 and 246.)

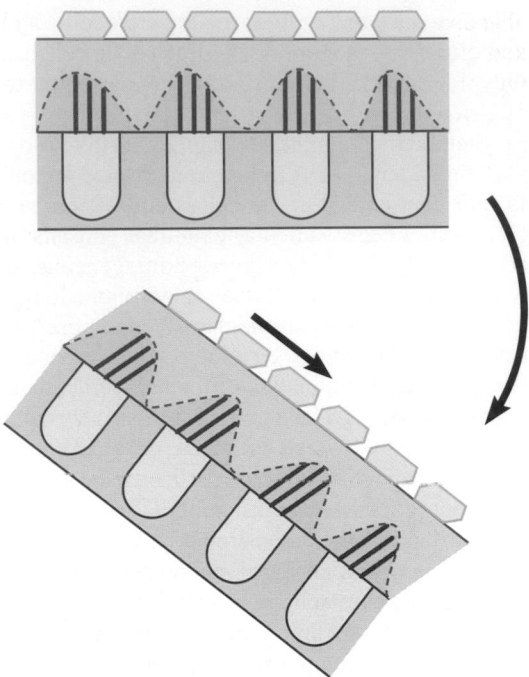

Figure 44 Diagrammatic representation of the bending of the hair cell cilia by the otoconia in tilting the head.

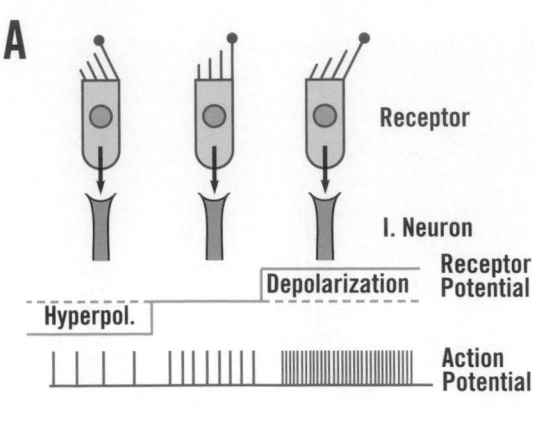

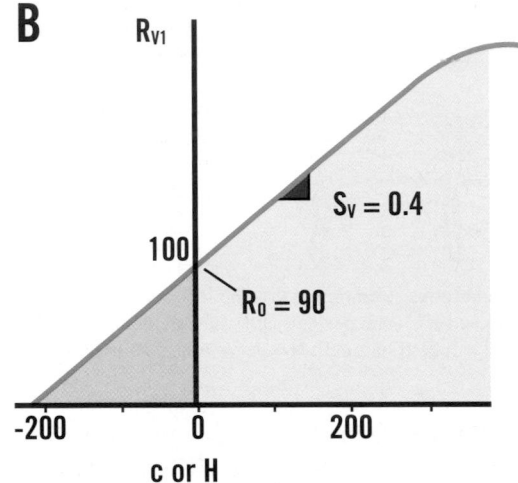

Figure 45 Motion transduction by vestibular hair cells. (A) At rest there is a resting rate of action potential discharge in the primary vestibular afferents (*center*). Shearing forces on the hair cells cause either depolarization (*right*) or hyperpolarization (*left*), depending on whether the stereocilia are deflected toward or away from the kinocilium (indicated by longest cilium, with beaded end), respectively. This modulates the discharge rate in the vestibular nerve as shown below (action potential). (B) Vestibular nerve discharge rate (R_{v1}) is 90 spikes/s at rest (R_o) in the squirrel monkey and changes approximately linearly with cupula deflection (c). When the latter is expressed in equivalent head velocity (H), the slope of the line Sv is about 0.4 (spikes/s)/(deg/s) for the average vestibular afferent fiber. (Part A reproduced with permission from reference 255; Part B reproduced with permission from reference 256.)

cupula, which lies across the duct blocking it. The cupula is attached to the ampulla wall around its entire periphery and billows, like a sail, under endolymph pressure.[250,251] Normal deflections are tiny, in the range of 0.01 to 0.3 mm.[252] The subsequent strain on the hair cells by the bending of their cilia embedded in the cupula creates a generator potential that modulates the discharge rate of primary vestibular afferent fibers.

The overall behavior of the cupula and duct was first described by Steinhausen.[253] If c is some measure of cupular (and thus endolymph) displacement, the force balance equation for the duct is:

$$m[c(d^2c/dt^2)] + r[c(dc/dt)] + kc = m[H(d^2H/dt^2)]$$

where m represents the net, equivalent moment of inertia of the endolymph, r is the lumped effect of viscous drag on fluid flow (c), k represents the stiffness of the gelatinous cupula, and H is the head velocity. The term $m[H(d^2H/dt^2)]$ is the driving force on the endolymph owing to head acceleration. During most natural head movements, the inertial reactance, $m[c(d^2c/dt^2)]$, and the cupular restoring force, kc, are small compared to the viscous term, $r[c(dc/dt)]$, because the narrowness of the tube creates a high resistance to flow. Consequently, the above equation can be reduced to:

$$r[c(dc/dt)] = m[H(d^2H/dt^2)]$$

or, integrating both sides:

$$c = m/r \, [H(dH/dt)].$$

Thus, the discharge rate, which is proportional to cupular deflection, carries a signal into the central nervous system proportional to head velocity, not acceleration. In other words, a constant head acceleration applies a constant force on the endolymph, causing it to flow at a constant velocity.

Consequently, cupula position, the integral of flow, must be proportional to head velocity, that is, the integral of head acceleration.

In the squirrel monkey, the typical resting discharge rate is 90 spikes/s.[254] The discharge rate increases for deflection of the cupula in 1 direction and decreases in the other. On the abscissa of Figure 45B, $B(dH/dt)$ may be substituted for c, in which case the slope of the line, Sv, for the average fiber is 0.4 (spikes/s)/(deg/s).[255,256] Thus, the signal sent from the duct to the brainstem on the average fiber for most normal head movements is $90 + 0.4 \, [H(dH/dt)]$.

Response of Primary Vestibular Neurons. Microelectrode studies in higher mammals have demonstrated the following characteristics of primary vestibular neuron activity. For example, most of the primary vestibular neurons called regular units exhibit a high (~100/s) and remarkably uniform spontaneous discharge rates.[257] When listening to such spikes on a loudspeaker, the neurons make a characteristic motorboat sound. There is also a small population of irregular neurons with a lower rate and less regular spontaneous discharge. The high-rate regular units have small diameter, slowly conducting axons that predominantly innervate the periphery of the end-organ, that is, the type II hair cell region of the crista, whereas the low-rate irregular neurons come from the center of the crista, where most type I hair cells are located.[229] The high, regular spontaneous firing rate of the primary neurons permits the bidirectional sensitivity of the vestibular hair cell receptors.

When the head rotates, causing cupular displacement and a stimulatory deflection of hair cell cilia, the semicircular duct afferents change their discharge rate above, in response to hair cell depolarization, and below, in response to hair cell hyperpolarization, the resting rate depending on the direction of rotation.[258] When the head rotates sinusoidally at velocities encountered during normal function, the ampullar nerve discharge rate varies sinusoidally, as shown in Figure 46. The phase relationship between head position and head velocity, which displays a phase lag of about 90°, is such that the maximum discharge rate occurs at the head's 0 crossing, that is, at the head's maximum velocity. Thus, the ampullar afferent discharge rate codes head angular velocity. The adequate stimulus is actually angular acceleration, but the hydrodynamics of the semicircular duct system are such that the head's acceleration is integrated to give a velocity output.[259]

Similarly, with the macular afferents, accurate coding by discharge rate of the head's position relative to gravitational vertical can be demonstrated in all species. The more complex orientation of the macular hair cells makes directional correlates more difficult to establish than for semicircular duct afferents. However, Fernandez and Goldberg[229] studied large populations of saccular and utricular neurons and were able to demonstrate neural "sensitivity vectors" among the neuronal populations that corresponded to the relative orientations of the saccular and utricular maculae.

Central Vestibular Pathway

Anatomy. *Primary Afferent Connections.* The vestibular system functions primarily as an afferent reflex input to the motor system. In general, vestibular pathway–mediated reflexes involve 3 muscular systems, including the extrinsic oculomotor, cervical, and antigravity pathways.

As might be expected, the semicircular ducts, or the rotation sensors, connect primarily with the extrinsic oculomotor and cervical muscles, that is, the muscles that compensate for head rotation, whereas the otolithic organs, or position sensors, connect primarily with the antigravity muscles. Figure 47 outlines these major central vestibular connections.[260]

Scarpa, or the vestibular, ganglia, in the internal auditory canal, within the vestibular portion

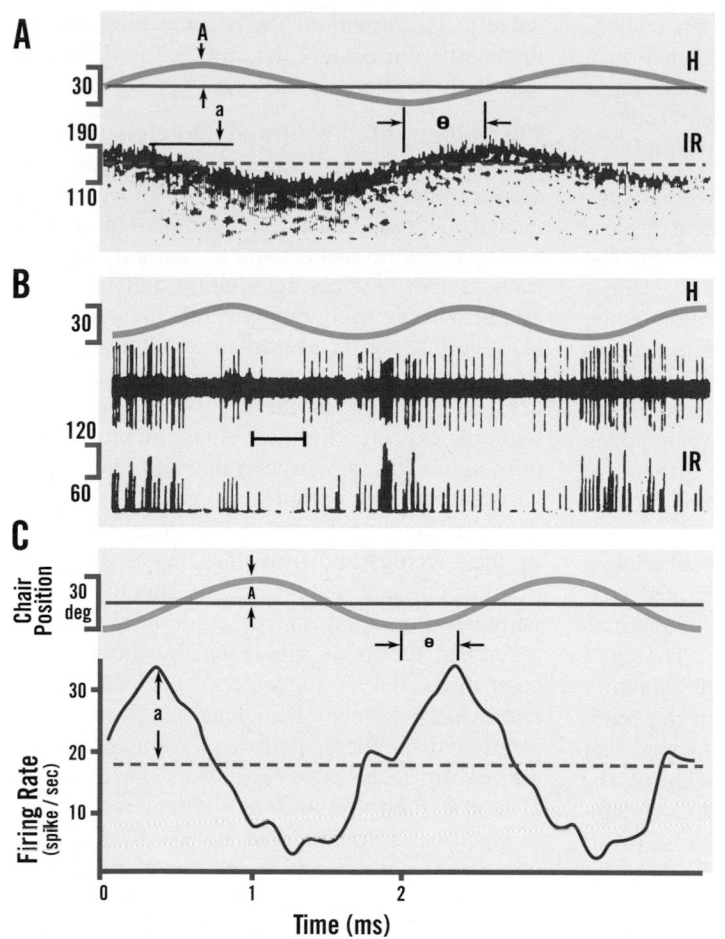

Figure 46 Peripheral vestibular neuron responses to sinusoidal rotation stimulation in the alert monkey. (A) A regular (high-rate) neuron. (B) An irregular (IR) neuron. Sinusoidal curve (H) plots head position. The records immediately below the sinusoidal traces show intervals between neuronal spikes. The height of vertical bars on these records is proportional to the interval between spikes. Because 1 of these bars occurs for every spike, their frequency reflects the frequency of the recorded spikes. (C) Response of unit in B averaged over 10 cycles; 0 is the phase lag of firing rate (ie, the shortest interval between spikes), which occurs at about the 0 crossing of the head-position signal. Thus, firing rate at the output of the semicircular duct is related most closely to head velocity.

able area beneath the floor of the fourth ventricle and lies across the pontomedullary boundary. On entering the brainstem, the vestibular axons bifurcate into the ascending rostral and descending caudal divisions.

The vestibular nuclear complex, as shown in Figure 47, consists of 4 distinct subnuclei: (1) the superior (Bechterew or angular), (2) lateral (Deiters), (3) medial (Schwalbe or principal or triangular), and (4) inferior (spinal or descending) nuclei.[261] There is recent anatomic evidence that the nucleus prepositus hypoglossi, which is classically thought to relate to taste sensation, has strong efferent and afferent vestibulo-oculomotor connections, through the medial longitudinal fasciculus (MLF), and cerebellar projections. In addition, microelectrode recordings from awake monkeys have demonstrated that prepositus neurons fire in relation to both vestibularly and visually induced eye movements.[262] Studies on the activity of ocular motoneurons in alert monkeys have shown that the neural commands for all conjugate eye movements (vestibular, optokinetic, saccadic, and pursuit) have both velocity and position commands.[263]

The vestibular input to prepositus is disynaptic and reciprocally organized, that is, ipsilateral input is excitatory, whereas contralateral input is inhibitory. In addition, if cells in the monkey's nucleus prepositus hypoglossi are lesioned with kainic acid, the monkey's eye movements only reflect the velocity command.[264] A great amount of neurophysiologic evidence indicates that the position command is obtained from the velocity command by the mathematical process of integration. That is, a neural network located in the nucleus prepositus hypoglossi integrates, in the mathematical sense, velocity-coded signals; thus, the prepositus is included in the diagram of the vestibular nuclear complex in Figure 47.

As indicated in Figure 47, each subnucleus has a unique set of connections with the periphery and with specific regions of the central nervous system including the spinal cord, cerebellum, and brainstem oculomotor nuclei (III, IV, VI). Most of the semicircular duct afferents terminate in the superior nucleus and rostral portion of the medial vestibular nucleus. Both of these nuclei, in turn, project to the oculomotor nuclei of the extraocular muscles via the ascending MLF. The superior nucleus projects only to the ipsilateral MLF, whereas the medial nucleus projects bilaterally. The medial nucleus, via the medial vestibulospinal tracts in the descending MLF, also sends bilateral descending projections to spinal anterior horn cells that control the cervical musculature.[265] Thus, the input and output of the superior and medial vestibular nuclei provide a possible anatomic basis for the nystagmus and head-turning-reflex responses to semicircular duct stimulation (see below).

The otolith organs, particularly the utricles, project primarily to the inferior nucleus and caudal part of the lateral nucleus. Outputs from these nuclei, in turn, project downward to the ventral horn region throughout the length of the spinal

of the eighth nerve, contain the bipolar ganglion cell bodies of the first-order vestibular neurons. The vestibular nerve can be divided into superior and inferior divisions that innervate the sensory epithelia of the ducts and otolithic end-organs. The superior portion innervates the cristae of the superior and horizontal semicircular

ducts, the utricular macula, and a small region of the saccular macula. The inferior division of the vestibular nerve innervates the crista of the posterior semicircular duct and the remaining part of the saccular macula. Centrally, all first-order vestibular neurons synapse in the vestibular nuclear complex, which occupies a consider-

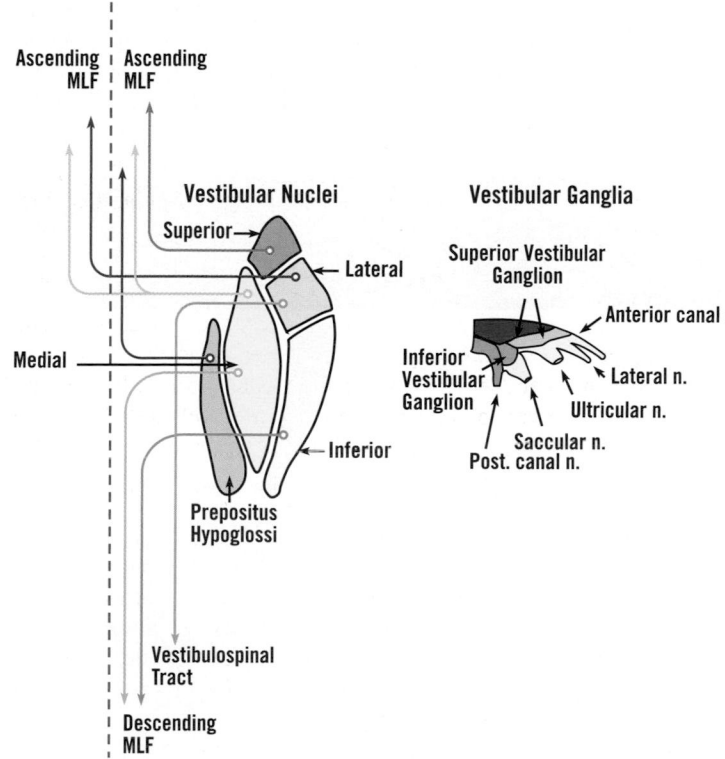

Figure 47 Diagram of major connections between primary vestibular neurons in the vestibular ganglia and the vestibular nuclei. Also shown are major outflows from the vestibular nuclei. Vestibulocerebellar connections are excluded. MLF = medial longitudinal fasciculus. (The primary afferent connections are modified from reference 261.)

cord via the lateral vestibulospinal tract. Thus, the afferent and efferent connections of the lateral vestibular nucleus provide a possible anatomic basis for antigravity muscle responses in the limbs (extensors of the legs and flexors of the arms) to postural change. The otolith organs have relatively sparse connections to the extraocular muscles. These may be the connections that produce the ocular counter-rolling response to head tilt.[266]

Efferent Innervation of the Vestibular System. The vestibular organs in all vertebrates receive efferent innervation originating in brainstem nuclei. Although there are relatively few parent efferent neurons, their axons branch to innervate more than 1 end-organ and also ramify extensively in the neuroepithelium of the individual organs. By means of this divergent innervation pattern, efferent fibers provide a major source of synaptic input to type II hair cells, afferent calyces, and other unmyelinated afferent processes. In nonvestibular organs, efferent activation typically reduces afferent activity by hyperpolarizing the hair cell receptor. In contrast, efferent responses in vestibular organs are more heterogeneous. For example, in fish and mammals, there is an excitation of afferents, whereas in frogs and turtles, both excitation and inhibition are observed. In addition, there are variations in the efferent responses of vestibular afferents innervating different parts of the neuroepithelium, which differ in their responses to natural stimulation. Moreover, efferent neurons receive convergent inputs from several vestibular and nonvestibular receptors and also respond in association with active head movements. On the basis of the discharge properties of efferent neurons, one of their proposed functions is that they switch the vestibular organs from a postural to a volitional mode. For a more detailed review of the vestibular efferent system, see a recent summary by Goldberg.[267]

Vestibulocerebellar Connections. *Primary Vestibular Fibers.* Primary vestibular neurons project not only to the vestibular nuclei but also to the cerebellum. Most of these fibers are distributed to the ipsilateral flocculus and nodulus and the medially located uvula.[268] Because of this innervation by primary vestibular fibers, these 3 cerebellar areas have been termed collectively the vestibulocerebellum. As discussed below, the primary vestibular input to the vestibulocerebellum appears to be important in controlling the vestibulo-oculomotor reflex (VOR). Moreover, the primary vestibular input to the vestibulocerebellum and the climbing fiber input from the inferior olive appear to be important in controlling the VOR.

Secondary Vestibular Fibers. The vestibulocerebellum receives secondary fibers primarily from the medial and inferior vestibular nuclei but also from the other divisions. In addition, the fastigial nucleus and the cortex of the vermis receive a strong, somatotopically organized projection from

the lateral vestibular nucleus. Since this nucleus is the primary origin of the vestibulospinal tract, connections to it from the cerebellum are probably important in regulating antigravity reflexes that help to maintain an upright body posture.[269]

Projections to Cerebral Cortex. Whether the vestibular system has a direct cortical projection has long been a controversial question. The functional corollary to this question is whether we can consciously appreciate a sensation owing to vestibular stimulation. This question also has generated debate because most of the subjective sensations produced by vestibular stimulation, for example, vertigo, are secondary to motor reflex or to autonomic responses, and it is difficult or impossible to separate a primary vestibular sensation from the secondary sensations.[232]

Experiments employing electrical stimulation of the vestibular nerve have demonstrated relatively short-latency localized cortical responses in both the cat and the monkey.[270] The cat's vestibular area is adjacent to both the auditory and the somatosensory fields, but in the monkey, and possibly in the human, it is located near the face area of the somatosensory field on the postcentral gyrus. Deecke and colleagues[271] demonstrated that the ventroposteroinferior (VPI) nucleus is the thalamic relay for the vestibulocortical projection. The VPI nucleus lies adjacent to the thalamosomatosensory representation of the face. Prior to this study, the function of the VPI nucleus was unknown.

Vestibular Influence on Postural Control. The main unit for the control of tone in the trunk and extremity muscles is the myotactic reflex. These reflexes of the antigravity muscles are under the combined excitatory and inhibitory influence of multiple supraspinal centers. Two of these supraspinal centers are facilitatory, that is, the lateral vestibular nucleus and rostral reticular formation, and 4 are inhibitory centers including the pericruciate cortex, basal ganglia, cerebellum, and cau-

dal reticular formation. The balance of input from these different centers determines the degree of tone in the antigravity muscles.

Physiology of Vestibular Nuclei. *General Characteristics of Neuronal Responses.* Microelectrode studies of responses of vestibular nucleus neurons to electrical stimulation of individual ampullary nerves and to "natural" stimuli, such as those involving rotation and tilt, have established the following general characteristics: (1) Neurons can be classified as tilt responders (otolith units) or rotation responders (duct units). (2) The locations of these 2 types correspond with that expected from the anatomic projections of otolithic and semicircular duct afferents to the vestibular nuclear complex. Thus, the tilt responders are found primarily in the areas innervated by the sacculus and utriculus, that is, the inferior nucleus and caudal part of lateral nucleus, whereas the rotation responders are found mainly in the areas innervated by the semicircular ducts, that is, the superior nucleus and the rostral part of medial nucleus. (3) Among the rotation responders, pathways from individual ducts seem to be preserved. Thus, for example, a neuron that responds to vertical rotation or to electrical stimulation of a vertical ampullary nerve does not respond to horizontal rotation or to stimulation of a horizontal ampullary nerve and vice versa.

Classification of Neuronal Response Types. Both duct and otolithic vestibular nucleus units preserve the basic properties of the primary afferent input, but some respond in the same direction, for example, ipsilateral horizontal rotation increases firing rate; others respond in the opposite direction. A few of the vestibular nucleus neurons respond with either inhibition or facilitation in both directions. Table 2 outlines the characteristics of the duct units. The type I units, exhibiting a primary response pattern, are innervated by the ipsilateral labyrinth, whereas the type II units,

Table 2 Characteristics of Duct Responding Units in Vestibular Nuclei

	Input Side	Response Directionality	Response Time Course	Latency	Gain	Spontaneous Activity
Type I (67%)	Ipsilabyrinth	Same as primary afferent	—	—	—	—
Kinetic (56%)	Ipsilabyrinth	Same as primary afferent	Fast decay	Long (multisynaptic)	High	None
Tonic (11%)	Ipsilabyrinth	Same as primary afferent	Slow decay	Short (monosynaptic)	Low	High level
Type II (29%)	Contralabyrinth	Opposite of primary afferent				
Type III (3%)	?	Facilitated both directions				
Type IV (<1%)	?	Inhibited both directions				

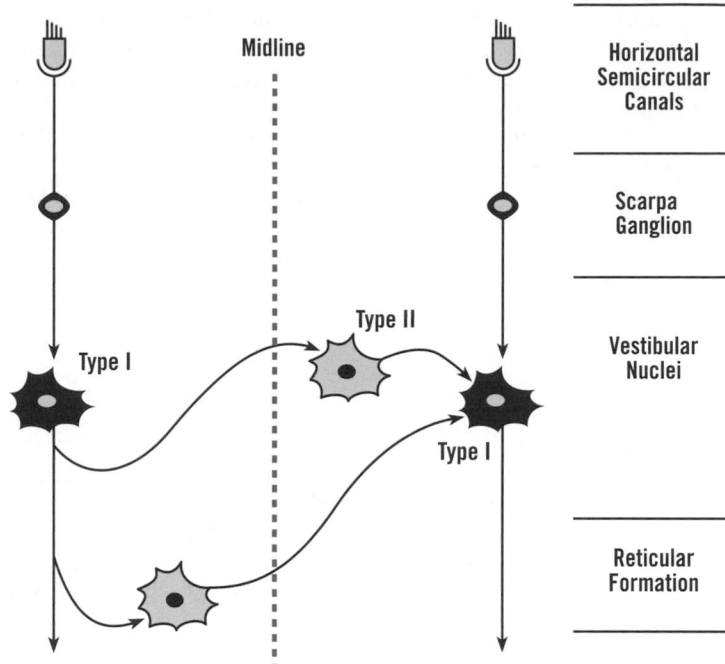

Figure 48 Interrelation of type I and type II secondary vestibular neurons. Dark neurons are excitatory, and light neurons are inhibitory. (Reproduced with permission from reference 255.)

showing response patterns that are opposite to those of the primary units, are innervated by the contralateral labyrinth.

The analogous classification for otolith responders subdivides all types into (1) "a" units, which increase firing on ipsilateral tilt; (2) "b" units, which decrease firing on ipsilateral tilt; (3) "y" units, which increase firing in response to tilt in both directions; and (4) "o" units, which decrease firing by tilt in both directions. Analogous to the duct units, the relative populations of these units are a > b > y > o.[272]

Commissural Inhibition and Vestibular Compensation. Many of the contralateral (type II) semicircular duct responses listed in Table 2 are abolished when a midline dorsal brainstem incision is made that interrupts the vestibular crossing fibers. Thus, the "opposite-primary" type II responses are likely elicited by inhibitory input from type I neurons of the opposite labyrinth. Figure 48 summarizes the simplest of the probable neuronal interconnections responsible for this contralateral inhibition.[255]

The commissural inhibitory system is also important in the mechanism of compensation following labyrinthectomy. Thus, immediately after labyrinthectomy, the type I units on the labyrinthectomized side show no spontaneous activity and do not respond to rotation. However, within a few days, the deafferented type I units regain their spontaneous activity and, via inhibition from the contralateral pathway, also regain their normal response to rotation. The mechanisms by which this recovery process occur are unknown, but a contributing factor is the lowered threshold of the deafferented type I neuron for contralateral input.[273] In animal studies, the course of compensation is affected by exercise,[274] visual experience,[275] and drugs.[276] Thus, as a rule, stimulants accelerate and sedatives slow compensation.[275] Fetter and Zee showed further that visual experience was not necessary for the acquisition or for the maintenance of this recovery process.[275]

If a second labyrinthectomy is performed after compensation for the first labyrinthectomy, the animal again develops signs of acute unilateral vestibular loss with nystagmus directed toward the previously operated ear, that is, a condition referred to as Bechterew compensatory nystagmus.[277] That is, the overall effect is as if the first labyrinthectomy had not occurred. Compensation after the second labyrinthectomy is slightly faster than the first but still requires several days. For a recent review on the molecular mechanisms underlying vestibular compensation, see the summary by Darlington and Smith.[278]

Vestibulo-Oculomotor Reflex. Although there are neural connections between the maculae and the extraocular muscles, they are less important in humans, both functionally and clinically, than are the semicircular duct connections. This discussion of the VOR will therefore focus on the reflex connection between the semicircular ducts and the extraocular muscles.

An important function of the semicircular ducts is to provide afferent input to the VOR that generates eye movements that compensate for head movements by maintaining a stabilized visual image on the retina during rotation. Such eye adjustments are called compensatory eye

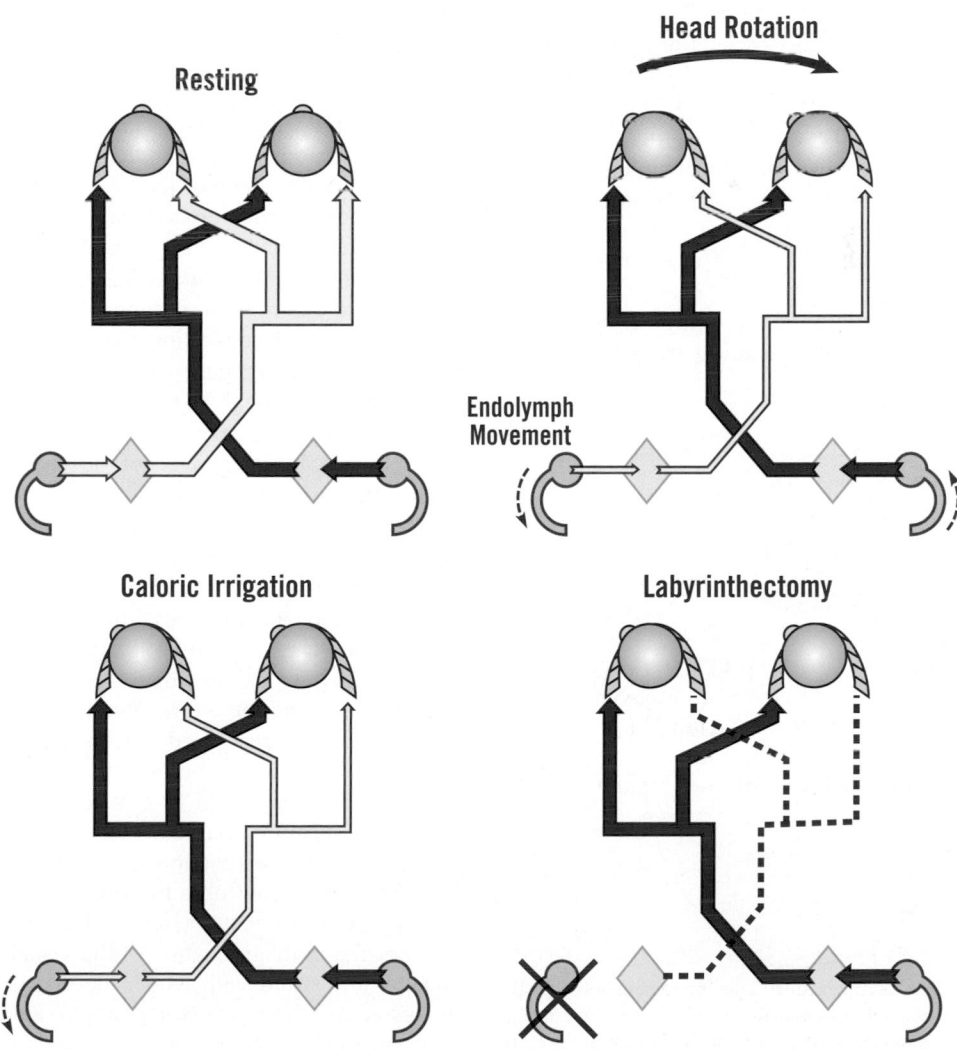

Figure 49 Generation of the vestibular (slow) phase of different kinds of nystagmus. The thickness of the lines connecting the semicircular duct to the extraocular muscles is proportional to the intensity of neural discharge along the nerve pathways.

movements. Figure 49 diagrams the neural connections that stabilize gaze during head movement.

Anatomic Connections. The VOR is subserved by a three-neuron pathway. That is, motions detected by the end-organ are transduced into neural impulses that are sent via the vestibular nerve to the vestibular nuclei and rostrally through the ascending MLF to the oculomotor nuclei of the extraocular muscles. Secondary vestibulo-ocular connections via the reticular formation have been described, but functionally these are less important than the "direct" three-neuron MLF vestibulo-ocular pathway.

Inhibitory crossed connections at the levels of both vestibular and oculomotor nuclei, which were described above, probably also participate in the VOR. The crossed inhibitory oculomotor connections subserve antagonistic extraocular muscles.[279] These inhibitory interconnections are important in the formation of conjugate eye movements.

Functional Connections. A number of investigations have uncovered many details of the facilitatory and inhibitory interactions between neurons of the vestibular nuclear complex and motoneurons of the extraocular eye muscles. For a review, the reader is referred to Wilson and Melvill-Jones.[272] However, in older experiments, the effect of mass stimulation of individual ampullary nerves on eye movements provided the clinician with the most useful integrative concepts of the functional organization of the VOR. The results of all of these ampullary nerve-stimulating experiments agree on the principle, illustrated by Figure 49, that stimulation of an ampullary nerve generates conjugate eye movements away from the side stimulated and in the plane of the duct stimulated.

This principle allows a straightforward description of the events leading from endolymph

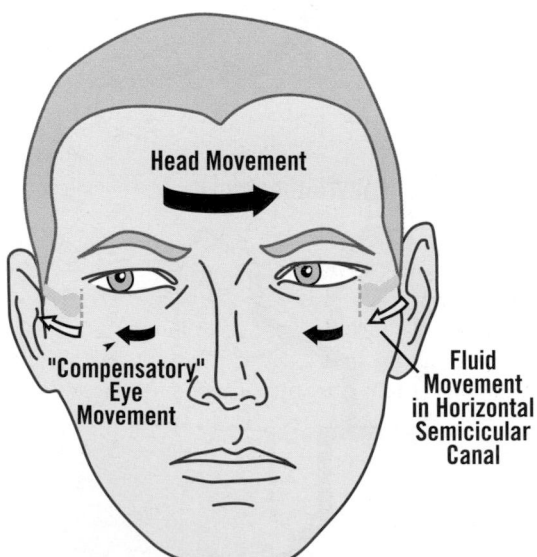

Figure 50 A compensatory eye movement initiated by the horizontal semicircular ducts. The eyes move in the direction of endolymph movement. If rotation of the head is continued at an ever-increasing speed, the compensatory eye movement becomes the slow phase of a rotational nystagmus.

movement in the horizontal duct to the compensatory eye movement depicted in Figure 50: (1) Head movement to the left generates endolymph movement to the right in the left duct. This is toward the ampulla and therefore increases the ampullary nerve discharge rate. (2) The increased ampullary nerve output, according to the aforementioned rule, causes conjugate eye deviation away from the side stimulated, that is, to the right, which is opposite to the direction of head movement. (3) Similarly, head movement to the left generates ampullofugal movement in the right duct, which decreases neural output. (4) Decreased neural output inhibits the extraocular muscles, thus causing the eyes to deviate conjugately to the left, which provides a neural output that is synergistic to the conjugate right-eye deviation, generated by the output of the opposite duct. Figure 49 (upper right) depicts this sequence of events.

Functionally, the VOR provides more than a simple one-to-one transfer of information from the semicircular duct to the extraocular muscles. It should be recalled that the response of the ampullary nerves reflects head velocity, yet the ocular rotation, at the vestibular reflex output, reflects head position. Therefore, at some point in the transfer from vestibular input to ocular output, some form of neural integration must occur that converts the velocity signal at the input into the displacement signal at the output. The location of this integrator, as noted above, is the nucleus prepositus hypoglossi.[264]

Control of the Gain of the Vestibulo-Oculomotor Reflex. In studies of the VOR, the concept of gain is important. Gain of the VOR is simply the amplitude of eye rotation divided by amplitude of the head rotation. Generally, amplitudes of eye and head rotation are expressed as angles.

Because eye rotation is supposed to be equal and opposite to head rotation, that is, to compensate fully and leave gaze steady, it might seem at first that the ideal VOR gain would be –1. However, there are many real-life situations for which the ideal VOR gain is not –1. Functionally, such situations can be divided into long-term (ie, slow) and short-term (ie, fast) adjustments. The short-term or fast VOR gain adjustments occur in the course of visual tracking tasks, in which both the head and the eyes follow the fixation target at varying relative velocities. For example, in a tracking task in which the head and eyes must move in the same direction, the VOR must be completely suppressed. In the clinical test situation, this visual suppression of the VOR is observed as suppression of caloric or rotational nystagmus during visual fixation.

An example of functionally beneficial long-term VOR gain control is the situation in which a prescription for new glasses has been received. The change in magnification of the visual image changes the speed with which the visual image moves across the retina (for example, increasing magnification would increase the speed of movement of retinal images). Therefore, to maintain a stable retinal image after new glasses have been

obtained, the VOR gain must be adjusted for the new magnification levels. Such adjustments have been demonstrated experimentally in humans by testing the VOR rotational response in the dark after long-term periods of wearing highly corrective lenses.[280]

An extreme example of the plasticity of the VOR gain is provided by adjusting to reversing prisms. Reversing prism glasses cause a normal visual image to be reversed right to left; hence, movement of the visual image, when the head or eyes are rotated horizontally, is exactly opposite of normal. Even in this extreme example, humans and other animals have been shown to function normally after a few days of wearing the prisms,[281,282] even in situations requiring visually controlled movements during head movements, for example, mountain climbing.[283] Testing the VOR in humans after a few days of wearing reversing prisms has demonstrated actual reversal, that is, conversion of a negative to a positive gain, of the VOR.[284]

There is strong evidence that the vestibulocerebellum plays an important role in both short-[285] and long-term[286] control of the VOR gain. The strong primary vestibular afferent projection to the vestibulocerebellum and equally strong projection from the vestibulocerebellum to the oculomotor portion of the vestibular nuclear complex have already been described. There is also a strong input to the vestibulocerebellum from the retina by way of the inferior olivary climbing fibers. Most of these visual units detected in the vestibulocerebellum are "movement detectors."[287] They are thus ideally suited to provide information on "retinal slip" of the visual image, which is needed to modify VOR gain control. The visual and vestibular inputs to the cerebellum converge on the Purkinje cells of the flocculus cortex. Furthermore, experiments on alert monkeys, in which rotation of the animal's visual environment and its head were controlled independently, showed that visual and vestibular inputs modulate Purkinje cell outputs in ways exactly appropriate for the functionally useful control of the VOR gain.

Ablation experiments further support the role of the flocculonodular lobes in control of VOR gain. It has been demonstrated, for example, that removal of the vestibulocerebellum eliminates suppression of caloric nystagmus by visual fixation.[288] An analogous failure of fixation suppression (FFS) of nystagmus is also observed in humans with cerebellar lesions.[289] However, clinical data suggest that FFS can be produced by lesions in the brainstem and, less frequently, cerebral hemispheres, as well as the cerebellum.[290]

Robinson reported the results of a notable ablation experiment that demonstrates the role of the flocculus in causing long-term or plastic changes in VOR gain.[282,286] Specifically, cats wore reversing prisms for several days, and VOR gain was measured each day by rotating the cats in the dark. After several days, as expected, VOR gain dropped from 0.9 to 0.1. When the vestibulocerebellum was removed, the VOR gain promptly increased to about 1.2. Furthermore, it proved impossible to reinstate the VOR gain decrease by continued wearing of prisms after removal of the vestibulocerebellum. In addition, Miles and colleagues uncovered results in the monkey that implicated synaptic changes at other sites, especially in the brainstem.[290] More recently, Lisberger provided further evidence that the modifiable synapses were located between vestibular primary afferents and those second-order and/or possibly third-order vestibular neurons that also received synapses from Purkinje cells.[291] Finally, Luebke and Robinson reversibly silenced the flocculus of alert cats adapted to either high- or low-gain VOR.[292] This reversible floccular shutdown did not alter the adapted VOR gain, yet the animals were subsequently unable to modify their VOR gain, while the flocculus was silenced.

Clinical Considerations of Vestibular Reflexes

General Pattern. It has been stated that the vestibular system functions primarily as an afferent input for motor reflexes and that, at rest, most primary vestibular neurons have high and remarkably regular spontaneous discharge rates. For the purposes of the following clinically oriented discussion, the spontaneous vestibular neuronal activity will be referred to as the resting discharge.

Normally, with the head at rest in the neutral position, the resting discharges in the 2 vestibular nerves are equal. Vestibulomotor reflexes are elicited when inputs from the 2 vestibular end-organs or their central projections are made unequal, that is, they are unbalanced. Such unbalancing can occur by an abnormality involving one side to a greater degree than the other. In this case, we term the resultant vestibular reflex spontaneous. Vestibular input from the 2 sides can also be unbalanced by stimulating 1 or both of the vestibular end-organs. In this case, the resultant vestibular reflex is termed "induced."

When a vestibular input imbalance is unusually large or prolonged, a constellation of stereotyped responses occurs.[293] These responses are head turning, falling (or swaying), past pointing, vertigo representing a sensation of rotation, and nystagmus involving a rhythmic back-and-forth eye movement, with alternate slow phases in one direction and fast phases in the opposite direction. These slow and fast eye movements are termed the slow and fast phases of vestibular nystagmus. The head turning, falling, past pointing, and nystagmus slow phase are all in the same direction, that is, away from the ear with the greater output. In this discussion, the reference is to the nystagmus slow or vestibular phase. The clinical convention is to designate nystagmus direction by the fast of central phase, presumably because these movements can be easily observed. Thus, the indicated reflex directions may be the opposite of those to which the reader is accustomed. Fast-phase nystagmus is in the direction of the angular acceleration VOR. The rotation sensation, or vertigo, may be referred either to the subject's body, that is, subjective vertigo, or to the environment, that is, objective vertigo. If the body rotates, it is in the same direction as the nystagmus slow phase; if the environment rotates, it is in the opposite direction.

Methods of Eliciting. Vestibular responses can be generated by rotational, caloric, or galvanic stimulation of the vestibular periphery. The caloric and rotational responses are discussed in the following section. The galvanic vestibular response occurs when electrical current is applied to the head in the vicinity of the ear.[289] Electrical current applied in this manner elicits the entire constellation of vestibular responses except vertigo. Interestingly, however, some subjects may report a slight sense of disorientation. If the current is positive, the nystagmus slow-phase, past-pointing, and body-sway responses are toward the stimulated ear; in contrast, if the current is negative, these responses are away from the stimulated ear.

Because the galvanic stimulus probably acts at a retrolabyrinthine location, that is, either vestibular nerve, Scarpa ganglia, or a more central location, it has been suggested as a means of differentiating vestibular end-organ from vestibular nerve lesions. However, this procedure has not found widespread clinical acceptance, possibly because of uncertainty over the exact locus of action. For example, patients with their vestibular nerves sectioned intracranially still have a recognizable body-sway galvanic response,[294] suggesting that at least part of the action of the galvanic stimulus is central to the vestibular nerve, that is, at the level of the brainstem or possibly cerebellum.

Vestibular Nystagmus. Vestibular nystagmus occurs when the semicircular duct system is overstimulated. For example, if the head is continuously rotated in one direction at an ever-increasing speed, the semicircular duct–initiated compensatory eye movement becomes repeatedly interrupted by rapid, snap-back movements and hence becomes a rotational nystagmus. Because the relatively slow compensatory eye movement phase of the nystagmus comes from the semicircular duct system, it is called the vestibular or slow phase of the nystagmus. Conversely, because the fast, snap-back eye movement comes from the brain, it is called the central or fast phase of the nystagmus. Caloric nystagmus is produced by a temperature change in the region of the vestibular apparatus.

In the clinical laboratory, this temperature change is usually produced by running cool or warm water into the external auditory canal. The temperature change is conducted through bone to the semicircular canals. Since the horizontal semicircular canal is closest to the irrigating water, it is the most affected; hence, caloric nystagmus is almost entirely in the horizontal plane.

Figure 51 illustrates the generation of caloric nystagmus. The subject is in the supine position, with his head elevated 30° to bring the horizontal canal into the vertical position. The cold caloric irrigation cools the endolymph in part of the horizontal duct. This cooled endolymph becomes slightly denser than the surrounding endolymph and thus falls, causing the eyes to rotate toward the irrigated ear. This vestibular eye movement is repeatedly interrupted by a compensatory rapid central eye movement in the opposite direction. A cold caloric nystagmus is thus created, with its slow phase toward and its fast phase away from the irrigated ear.

Although the slow phase is the vestibular phase of vestibular nystagmus, it is the clinical convention to designate the direction of the vestibular nystagmus by the direction of the fast phase. This convention, as noted above, originated because the fast phase is easier to observe than the slow phase.

Neural Mechanisms of Nystagmus. Figure 49 diagrams the neural mechanisms of different kinds of vestibular nystagmus.[295] This Figure shows the physiologic rather than the anatomic form of the horizontal VOR system. It is drawn to reflect the fact that increased neural activity from a horizontal semicircular duct rotates the eyes horizontally away from the duct.[295]

At rest, both ducts generate equal neural activity, which represents the resting discharge described above. Unbalancing the vestibular inputs from the 2 ears generates vestibular nystagmus if the imbalance is prolonged. Caloric and rotational stimuli unbalance the vestibular input via the normal transducer action of the semicircular ducts. Lesioning 1 labyrinth by surgery or disease causes a pathologic imbalance by eliminating or reducing the resting discharge on the involved side.

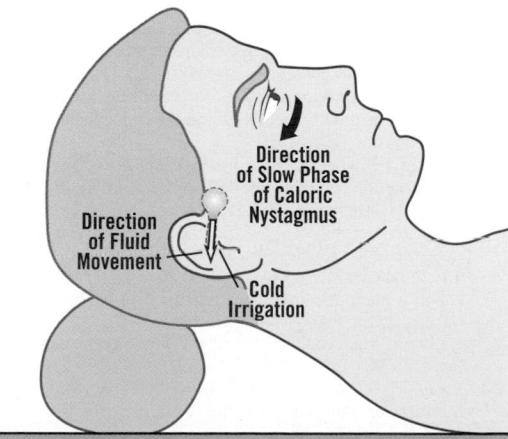

Direction of Slow Phase of Caloric Nystagmus

Direction of Fluid Movement

Cold Irrigation

Figure 51 The mechanism of cold caloric nystagmus. The density of the cooled portion of the endolymph is increased, causing it to fall, thereby producing endolymph movement. The slow phase of the caloric nystagmus is in the direction of endolymph movement.

REFERENCES

1. Shaw EA, Teranishi R. Sound pressure generated in an external-ear replica and real human ears by a nearby point source. J Acoust Soc Am 1968;44:240–9.
2. Shaw EAG. The external ear. In: Keidel WD, Neff WD, editors. Handbook of Sensory Physiology, Volume V/1. Auditory System, Anatomy Physiology (Ear). New York: Springer-Verlag; 1974. p. 455–90.

3. Pickles JO. An Introduction to the Physiology of Hearing. New York: Academic Press; 1982.

4. Zweig G, Lipes R, Pierce JR. The cochlear compromise. J Acoust Soc Am 1976;59:975–82.

5. von Békésy G. Experiments in Hearing. Translated and edited by EG Wever. New York: McGraw-Hill; 1960.

6. Moller AR. An experimental study of the acoustic impedance of the middle ear and its transmisssion properties. Acta Otolaryngol (Stockh) 1965;60:129–49.

7. Tonndorf J, Khanna SM. The role of the tympanic membrane in middle ear transmission. Ann Otol Rhinol Laryngol 1970;79:743–53.

8. Khanna SM, Tonndorf J. Tympanic membrane vibration in cats studied by time-averaged holography. J Acoust Soc Am 1972;51:1904–20.

9. Salomon G, Starr A. Electromyography of middle ear muscles in man during motor activities. Acta Neurol Scand 1963;39:161–8.

10. Moller AR. Auditory Physiology. New York: Academic Press; 1983. p. 154–8.

11. Borg E. On the neuronal organization of the acoustic middle ear reflex. A physiological and anatomical study. Brain Res 1973;49:101–23.

12. Moller AR. The sensitivity of contraction of the tympanic muscles in man. Ann Otol Rhinol Laryngol 1962;71:86–95.

13. Moller A. Acoustic reflex in man. J Acoust Soc Am 1962;34:1524–34.

14. Djupesland G, Zwislocki JJ. Effect of temporal summation on the human stapedius reflex. Acta Otolaryngol (Stockh) 1971;71:262–5.

15. Jerger J. Clinical experience with impedance audiometry. Arch Otolaryngol 1970;92:311–24.

16. Klockhoff IH. Middle ear muscle reflexes in man. Acta Otolaryngol Suppl (Stockh) 1961;164:1.

17. Reger SN. Effect of middle ear muscle action on certain psychophysical measurements. Ann Otol Rhinol Laryngol 1960;69:1179–98.

18. Smith HD. Audiometric effects of voluntary contraction of the tensor tympani muscles. Arch Otolaryngol 1943;38:369–72.

19. Holst HE, Ingelstedt S, Örtegren V. Ear drum movements following stimulation of the middle ear muscles. Acta Otolaryngol Suppl (Stockh) 1963;182:73–84.

20. Keefe DH, Bulen JC, Arehart KH, Burns EM. Ear-canal impedance and reflection coefficient in human infants and adults. J Acoust Soc Am 1993;94:2617–38.

21. Goode RL, Ball G, Nishihara S, Nakamura K. Laser Doppler vibrometer (LDV)—a new clinical tool for the otologist. Am J Otol 1996;17:813–22.

22. Feeney MP, Sanford CA. Age effects in the human middle ear: Wideband acoustical measures. J Acoust Soc Am 2004;116:3546–58.

23. Zakrisson JE, Borg E, Diamant H, Miller AR. Auditory fatigue in patients with stapedius muscle paralysis. Acta Otolaryngol (Stockh) 1975;79:228–32.

24. Simmons FB. Perceptual theories of middle ear muscle function. Ann Otol Rhinol Laryngol 1964;73:724–40.

25. Harford ER, Jerger JF. Effect of loudness recruitment on delayed speech feedback. J Speech Hear Res 1959;2:361–8.

26. Borg E, Zakrisson JE. The activity of the stapedius muscle in man during vocalization. Acta Otolaryngol (Stockh) 1973;79:325–33.

27. McCandless G, Schumacher MH. Auditory dysfunction with facial paralysis. Arch Otolaryngol 1979;105:271–4.

28. Hannley M, Jerger J. PB rollover and the acoustic reflex. Audiology 1981;20:251–8.

29. Dorman M, Hannley M, Lindholm J. Vowel identification in the absence of the acoustic reflex: Performance-intensity characteristics. J Acoust Soc Am 1987;81:562–4.

30. Salt AN, Konishi T. The cochlear fluids: Perilymph and endolymph. In: Altschuler RA, Hoffman DW, Bobbin RP, editors. Neurobiology of Hearing: The Cochlea. New York: Raven Press; 1986. p. 109–22.

31. Davis H. Advances in the neurophysiology and neuroanatomy of the cochlea. J Acoust Soc Am 1962;34:1377–85.

32. Jahnke K. The fine structure of freeze-fractured intercellular junctions in the guinea pig inner ear. Acta Otolaryngol Suppl (Stockh) 1975;336:1–40.

33. Engstrom H. The cortilymph, the third lymph of the inner ear. Acta Morphol Neer Scand 1960;3:195–204.

34. Nadol JB. Intercellular fluid pathways in the organ of Corti of cat and man. Ann Otol Rhinol Laryngol 1979;88:2–11.

35. Steele KP. Tectorial membrane. In: Altschuler RA, Hoffman DW, Bobbin RP, editors. Neurobiology of Hearing: The Cochlea. New York: Raven Press; 1986. p. 123–37.

36. Smith CA. Structure of the cochlear duct. In: Naunton RF, Fernandez C, editors. Evoked Electrical Activity in the Auditory Nervous System. New York: Academic Press; 1978. p. 3–19.

37. Harrison RV, Hunter-Duvar IM. An anatomical tour of the cochlea. In: Jahn AF, Santos-Sacchi J, editors. Physiology of the Ear. New York: Raven Press; 1988. P. 159–199.

38. Lim DJ. Fine morphology of the tectorial membrane: Its relationship to the organ. Corti Arch Otolaryngol 1972;96:199–215.

39. Flock A. Physiological properties of sensory hairs in the ear. In: Evans EF, Wilson JP, editors. Psychophysics and Physiology of Hearing. New York: Academic Press; 1977. p. 15–25.

40. Nielsen DW, Slepecky N. Stereocilia. In: Altschuler RA, Hoffman DW, Bobbin RP, editors. Neurobiology of Hearing: The Cochlea. New York: Raven Press; 1986. p. 23–46.

41. Flock A, Cheung HC. Actin filaments in sensory hairs of inner ear receptor cells. J Cell Biol 1977;75:339–43.

42. Flock A, Bretscher A, Weber K. Immunohistochemical localization of several cytoskeletal proteins in inner ear sensory and supporting cells. Hear Res 1982;7:75–89.

43. Hudspeth AJ, Choe Y, Mehta AD, Martin P. Putting ion channels to work: Mechanoelectrical transduction, adaptation, and amplification by hair cells. Proc Natl Acad Sci U S A 2000;97:11765–72.

44. Slepecky N, Chamberlain SC. Distribution and polarity of actin in the sensory hair cells of the chinchilla cochlea. Cell Tissue Res 1982;224:15–24.

45. Rzadzinska AK, Schneider ME, Davies C, et al. An actin molecular treadmill and myosins maintain stereocilia functional architecture and self-renewal. J Cell Biol 2004;164:887–97.

46. Grati M, Schneider ME, Lipkow K, et al. Rapid turnover of stereocilia membrane proteins: Evidence from the trafficking and mobility of plasma membrane Ca^{2+}-ATPase 2. J Neurosci 2006;6386–95.

47. Zheng J, Shen W, He DZ, et al. Prestin is the motor protein of cochlear outer hair cells. Nature 2000;405:149–55.

48. Liberman MC, Gao J, He DZ, et al. Prestin is required for electromotility of the outer hair cell and for electromotility. Nature 2002;419:300–4.

49. Flock A, Flock B, Murray E. Studies on the sensory hairs of receptor cells in the inner ear. Acta Otolaryngol (Stockh) 1977;83:85–91.

50. Steele CR. A possibility for sub-tectorial membrane fluid motion. In: Moller AR, editor. Basic Mechanisms in Hearing. New York: Academic Press; 1973. P. 69–90.

51. Dallos P, Billone MC, Durrant JD, et al. Cochlear inner and outer hair cells: Functional differences. Science 1972;177:356–8.

52. Jia S, Dallos P, He DZ. Mechanoelectric transduction of adult inner hair cells. J Neurosci 2007;27:1006–14.

53. Russell IJ, Sellick PM. The responses of hair cells to low frequency tones and their relationship to the extracellular receptor potentials and sound pressure level in the guinea pig cochlea. In: Syka J, Aitkin L, editors. Neuronal Mechanisms of Hearing. New York: Plenum Press; 1981. P. 3–15.

54. von Bekesy G. Shearing microphonics produced by vibrations near the inner and outer hair cells. J Acoust Soc Am 1953;25:786–90.

55. Tasaki I, Davis H, Eldredge DH. Exploration of cochlear potentials in guinea pig with a microelectrode. J Acoust Soc Am 1954;26:765–73.

56. Tasaki I, Spyropoulos CS. Stria vascularis as source of endocochlear potential. J Neurophysiol 1959;22:149–55.

57. Konishi T, Kelsey E. Effect of cyanide on cochlear potentials. Acta Otolaryngol (Stockh) 1968;65:381–90.

58. Tawackoli W, Chen GD, Fechter LD. Disruption of cochlear potentials by chemical asphyxiants, cyanide, and carbon monoxide. Neurotoxicol Teratol 2001;23:157–65.

59. Wangemann P. Supporting sensory transduction: Supporting cochlear fluid homeostasis and the endocochlear potential. J Physiol 2006;576:11–21.

60. Tasaki I, Fernandez C. Modification of cochlear microphonics and action potentials by KCl solution and by direct currents. J Neurophysiol 1952;15:497–512.

61. Davis H, Derbyshire AJ, Lurie JH, Saul LJ. The electric response of the cochlea. Am J Physiol 1934;107:311–32.

62. Tasaki I, Davis H, Legouix JP. The space-time pattern of the cochlear microphonic (guinea pig) as recorded by differential electrodes. J Acoust Soc Am 1952;24:502–19.

63. Dallos P. The Auditory Periphery. New York: Academic Press; 1973.

64. Davis H, Deatheridge BH, Eldredge DH, Smith CA. Summating potentials of the cochlea. Am J Physiol 1958;195:251–61.

65. Konishi T, Yasuno T. Summating potential of the cochlea in the guinea pig. J Acoust Soc Am 1963;35:1448–52.

66. Hudspeth AJ. Extracellular current flow and the site of transduction by vertebrate hair cells. J Neurosci 1982;2:1–10.

67. Dallos P, Cheatham MA. Production of cochlear potentials by inner and outer hair cells. J Acoust Soc Am 1976;60:510–2.

68. Durrant JD, Wang J, Ding DL, Salvi RJ. Are inner or outer hair cells the source of summating potentials recorded from the round window? J Acoust Soc Am 1998;104:370–7.

69. Davis H. A model for transducer action in the cochlea. Cold Spring Harb Symp Quant Biol 1965;30:181–90.

70. Wever EG, Bray CW. Action currents in the auditory nerve in response to acoustical stimulation. Proc Natl Acad Sci U S A 1930;16:344–500.

71. Davis H, Tasaki I, Goldstein R. The peripheral origin of activity with reference to the ear. Cold Spring Harb Symp Quant Biol 1952;17:143–54.

72. Brownell WE. Cochlear transduction: An integrative model and review. Hear Res 1982;6:335–60.

73. Hudspeth AJ. The hair cells of the inner ear. Sci Am 1983;248:54–64.

74. LeBlanc CS, Fallon M, Parker MS, et al. Phosphorothioate oligodeoxynucleotides can selectively alter neuronal activity in the cochlea. Hear Res 1999;135:105–12.

75. Puel J-L. Chemical synaptic transmission in the cochlea. Prog Neurobiol 1995;47:449–76.

76. Werman R. Criteria for identification of a central nervous system transmitter. Comp Biochem Physiol 1966;18:745–66.

77. Kuriyama H, Jenkins O, Altschuler RA. Immunocytochemical localization of AMPA selective glutamate receptor subunits in the rat cochlea. Hear Res 1994;80:233–40.

78. Jager W, Goiny M, Herrera-Marschitz M, et al. Sound-evoked efflux of excitatory amino acids in the guinea-pig cochlear in vitro. Exp Brain Res 1998;121:425–32.

79. Bobbin RP, Bledsoe SC, Jenison GL. Neurotransmitters of the cochlea and lateral line organ. In: Berlin CI, editor. Hearing Science: Recent Advances. San Diego: College-Hill Press; 1984. p. 159–80.

80. Schwartz IR, Ryan AF. Uptake of amino acids in the gerbil cochlea. In: Altschuler RA, Hoffman DW, Bob-bin RP, editors. Neurobiology of Hearing: The Cochlea. New York: Raven Press; 1986. p. 173–90.

81. Fex J, Altschuler RA. Neurotransmitter-related immunocytochemistry of the organ of Corti. Hear Res 1986;22:249–63.

82. Plinkert PK, Mohler H, Zenner HP. A subpopulation of outer hair cells possessing GABA receptors with tonotopic organization. Arch Otorhinolaryngol 1989;246:417–22.

83. Gitter AH, Zenner HP. Gamma-aminobutyric acid receptor activation of outer hair cells in the guinea pig cochlea. Eur Arch Otorhinolaryngol 1992;249:62–5.

84. Eybalin M. Neurotransmitters and neuromodulators of the mammalian cochlea. Physiol Rev 1993;73:309–73.

85. Frisina RD. Subcortical neural coding mechanisms for auditory temporal processing. Hear Res 2001;158:1–27.

86. Eggermont JJ. Between sound and perception: Reviewing the search for a neural code. Hear Res 2001;157:1–42.

87. LePage EL, Johnstone BM. Nonlinear mechanical behaviour of the basilar membrane in the basal turn of the guinea pig cochlea. Hear Res 1980;2:183–9.

88. Greenwood DD. Critical bandwidth and the frequency coordinates of the basilar membrane. J Acoust Soc Am 1961;33:1344–56.

89. Liberman MC, Kiang NYS. Acoustic trauma in cats. Cochlear pathology and auditory-nerve activity. Acta Otolaryngol Suppl (Stockh) 1978;358:1–63.

90. Ruggero MA, Rich NC. Application of a commercially manufactured Doppler-shift laser velocimeter to the measurement of basilar-membrane vibration. Hear Res 1991;51:215–30.

91. Moller AR. Studies of the damped oscillatory response of the auditory frequency analyzer. Acta Physiol Scand 1970;78:299–314.

92. Evans EF. Auditory frequency selectivity and the cochlear nerve. In: Zwicker E, Terbardt E, editors. Facts and Models in Hearing. New York: Springer-Verlag; 1974. p. 118–29.

93. Kiang NYS, Moxon EC, Levine RA. Auditory nerve activity in cats with normal and abnormal cochleas. In: Wolstenhome GEW, Knight J, editors. Ciba Symposium on Sensorineural Hearing Loss. London: Churchill Press; 1970. p. 241–68.

94. Robertson D. Cochlear neurons: Frequency selectivity altered by perilymph removal. Science 1974;186:153–5.

95. Cody AR, Johnstone BM. Single auditory neuron response during acute acoustic trauma. Hear Res 1980;3:3–16.

96. Gulick WL. Hearing, Physiology and Psychophysics. New York: Oxford University Press; 1971

97. Rhode WS. Cochlear partition vibration—recent views. J Acoust Soc Am 1980;67:1696–1703.

98. Johnstone BM, Boyle AJ. Basilar membrane vibration examined with the Mossbauer technique. Science 1967;158:389–90.

99. Rhode WS. Measurement of vibration of the basilar membrane in the squirrel monkey. Ann Otol Rhinol Laryngol 1974;83:619–25.

100. Kim DO, Neely ST, Molnar CE, Matthews JW. An active cochlear model with negative damping in the partition: Comparison with Rhode's ante- and post-mortem observations. In: van den Brink G, Bilsen FA, editors. Psychophysical, Physiological, and Behavioral Studies in Hearing. Delft, The Netherlands: Delft University Press; 1980. p. 7–14.
101. Kemp DT. Stimulated acoustic emissions from within the human auditory system. J Acoust Soc Am 1978;64:1386–91.
102. Lonsbury-Martin BL, Whitehead ML, Martin GK. Clinical applications of otoacoustic emissions. J Speech Hear Res 1991;34:964–81.
103. Wit HP, Ritsma RJ. Evoked acoustical responses from the human ear: Some experimental results. Hear Res 1980;2:253–61.
104. Mountain DC. Changes in endolymphatic potential and crossed olivocochlear bundle stimulation alter cochlear mechanics. Science 1980;210:71–2.
105. Engdahl B, Kemp DT. The effect of noise exposure on the details of the distortion-product otoacoustic emissions in humans. J Acoust Soc Am 1996;99:1573–87.
106. Allen GC, Tiu C, Koike K, et al. Transient-evoked otoacoustic emissions in children after cisplatin chemotherapy. Otolaryngol Head Neck Surg 1998;118:584–8.
107. Brownell WE, Bader CR, Bertrand D, de Ribaupierre Y. Evoked mechanical responses of isolated cochlear outer hair cells. Science 1985;227:194–6.
108. Zenner HP, Zimmermann U, Schmitt U. Reversible contraction of isolated mammalian cochlear hair cells. Hear Res 1985;18:127–33.
109. Flock A. Hair cells, receptors with a motor capacity? In: Klinke R, Hartman R, editors. Hearing, Physiological Bases and Psychophysics. New York: Springer-Verlag; 1983. p. 2–7.
110. Dallos P, Evans BN, Hallworth R. Nature of the motor element in electrokinetic shape changes of cochlear outer hair cells. Nature 1991;350:155–7.
111. Brownell WE. Outer hair cell electromotility and otoacoustic emissions. Ear Hear 1990;11:82–92.
112. Oliver D, He DZ, Klocker N, et al. Intracellular anions as the voltage sensor of prestin, the outer hair cell motor protein. Science 2001;292:2340–3.
113. Pickles JO. An Introduction to the Physiology of Hearing, 2nd edition. New York: Academic Press; 1988.
114. Rubel EW. Ontogeny of structures and function in the vertebrate auditory system. In: Jacobson M, editor. Handbook of Sensory Physiology, Volume IX. Development of Sensory Systems. New York: Springer-Verlag; 1978. p. 135–237.
115. Kim DO. Functional roles of the inner- and outerhair-cell subsystems in the cochlea and brainstem. In: Berlin CI, editor. Hearing Science: Recent Advances. San Diego: College-Hill Press; 1984. p. 241–62.
116. Evans EF, Harrison RV. Correlation between cochlear outer hair cell damage and deterioration of cochlear nerve tuning properties in the guinea pig. J Physiol 1976;256:43–4.
117. Brown MC, Nuttal AL, Masta RI. Intracellular recordings from cochlear inner hair cells: Effects of stimulation of the crossed olivocochlear efferents. Science 1983;222:69–72.
118. Gifford ML, Guinan JJ. Effects of crossed-olivocochlear-bundle stimulation on cat auditory nerve fiber responses to tones. J Acoust Soc Am 1983;74:115–23.
119. Winslow RL, Sachs MB. Effect of electrical stimulation of the crossed olivocochlear bundle on auditory nerve response to tones in noise. J Neurophysiol 1987;57:1002–21.
120. Collet L. Use of otoacoustic emissions to explore the medial olivocochlear system in humans. Br J Audiol 1993;27:155–9.
121. Berlin CI, Hood LJ, Hurley A, Wen H. Contralateral suppression of otoacoustic emissions: An index of the function of the medial olivocochlear system. Otolaryngol Head Neck Surg 1994;110:3–21.
122. Penner MJ. An estimate of the prevalence of tinnitus caused by spontaneous otoacoustic emissions. Arch Otolaryngol Head Neck Surg 1990;116:418–23.
123. Fetterman BL. Distortion-product otoacoustic emissions and cochlear microphonics: Relationships in patients with and without endolymphatic hydrops. Laryngoscope 2001;111:946–54.
124. Schweinfurth JM, Cacace AT, Parnes SM. Clinical applications of otoacoustic emissions in sudden hearing loss. Laryngoscope 1997;107:1457–63.
125. Evans EF. The sharpening of cochlear frequency selectivity in the normal and abnormal cochlea. Audiology 1975;14:419–42.
126. Evans EF. The frequency response and other properties of single fibers in the guinea-pig cochlear nerve. J Physiol 1972;226:263–87.
127. Brugge JF, Anderson DJ, Hind JE, Rose JE. Time structure of discharges in single auditory nerve fibers of the squirrel monkey in response to complex periodic sounds. J Neurophysiol 1969;32:386–401.
128. Rose JE, Brugge JF, Anderson DJ, Hind JE. Phase-locked response to low-frequency tones in single auditory nerve fibers of the squirrel monkey. J Neurophysiol 1967;30:769–93.
129. Kiang NY. Processing of speech by the auditory nervous system. J Acoust Soc Am 1980;68:830–5.
130. Sachs MB, Young ED. Encoding of steady state vowels in the auditory nerve: Representation in terms of discharge rate. J Acoust Soc Am 1979;66:470–9.
131. Wever EG. Theory of Hearing. New York: John Wiley & Sons Press; 1949. p. 484.
132. Katsuki Y, Sumi T, Uchiyama H, Watanabe T. Electric responses of auditory neurons in cat to sound stimulation. J Neurophysiol 1958;21:569–88.
133. Kiang NYS, Watanabe T, Thomas EC, Clark LF. Discharge Patterns of Single Fibers in the Cat's Auditory Nerve. Cambridge, MA: Massachusetts Institute of Technology Press; 1965. MIT research monograph no. 35.
134. Kiang NYS. A survey of recent developments in the study of auditory physiology. Ann Otol Rhinol Laryngol 1968;77:656–75.
135. Evans EF. The dynamic range problem: Place and time coding at the level of the cochlear nerve and nucleus. In: Syka J, Aitkin L, editors. Neuronal Mechanisms of Hearing. New York: Plenum Press; 1981. p. 69–85.
136. Evans EF, Palmer AR. Responses of units in the cochlear nerve and nucleus of the cat to signals in the presence of bandstop noise. J Physiol 1975;252:60P–2P.
137. Palmer AR, Evans EF. On the peripheral coding of the level of individual frequency components of complex sound levels. Exp Brain Res 1979;2:19–20.
138. Young ED, Sachs MB. Representation of steady-state vowels in the temporal aspects of the discharge patterns of populations of auditory-nerve fibers. J Acoust Soc Am 1979;66:1381–403.
139. Liberman MC. Auditory-nerve response from cats raised in low-noise chamber. J Acoust Soc Am 1978;63:442–55.
140. Kawase T, Liberman MC. Spatial organization of the auditory nerve according to spontaneous discharge rate. J Comp Neurol 1992;319:312–8.
141. Viemeister NF. Intensity coding and the dynamic range problem. Hear Res 1988;34:267–74.
142. Rasmussen GL. Anatomic relationships of the ascending and descending auditory systems. In: Fields WS, Alford BR, editors. Neurological Aspects of Auditory and Vestibular Disorders. Springfield, MA: Charles C. Thomas Press; 1964. p. 1–19.
143. Warr WB, Guinan JJ, White JS. Organization of the efferent fibers: The lateral and medial olivocochlear systems. In: Altschuler RA, Hoffman DW, Bobbin RP, editors. Neurobiology of Hearing: The Cochlea. New York: Raven Press; 1986. p. 333–48.
144. Warr WB. The olivocochlear bundle: Its origins and terminations in the cat. In: Naunton RF, Fernandez C, editors. Evoked Electrical Activity in the Auditory Nervous System. New York: Academic Press; 1978. p. 43–63.
145. Iurato S, Smith CA, Eldredge DH, et al. Distribution of the crossed olivocochlear bundle in the chinchilla's cochlea. J Comp Neurol 1978;182:57–76.
146. Spoendlin HH, Gacek RR. Electronmicroscopic study of the efferent and afferent innervation of the organ of Corti in the cat. Ann Otol Rhinol Laryngol 1963;72:660–86.
147. Liberman MC, Brown MC. Physiology and anatomy of single olivocochlear neurons in the cat. Hear Res 1986;24:17–36.
148. Liberman MC. Response properties of cochlear efferent neurons: Monaural vs. binaural stimulation and the effects of noise. J Neurophysiol 1988;60:1779–98.
149. Le Prell CG, Bledsoe SC, Bobbin RP, Puel J-L. Neurotransmission in the inner ear: Functional and molecular analyses. In: Jahn AF, Santos-Sacchi J, editors. Physiology of the Ear, 2nd edition. San Diego: Singular/Thompson Learning Press; 2001. p. 575–611.
150. Elgoyhen AB, Johson DS, Boulter J, et al. Alpha 9: An acetylcholine receptor with novel pharmacological properties expressed in rat cochlear hair cells. Cell 1994;79: 705–15.
151. Desmedt JE. Physiological studies of the efferent recurrent auditory system. In: Keidel WD, Neff WD, editors. Handbook of Sensory Physiology, Volume V/2. Physiological (CNS), Behavioral Studies, Psychoacoustics. New York: Springer-Verlag; 1974. p. 219–46.
152. Vetter DE, Liberman MC, Mann J, et al. Role of alpha 9 nicotinic ACh receptor subunits in the development and function of cochlear efferent innervation. Neuron 1999;23:93–103.
153. Fuchs PA. Synaptic transmission at vertebrate hair cells. Curr Opin Neurobiol 1996;6:514–9.
154. Ishii D, Balogh K. Distribution of efferent nerve endings in the organ of Corti. Their graphic reconstruction in cochleae by localization of acetyl-cholinesterase activity. Acta Otolaryngol (Stockh) 1968;66:282–8.
155. Igarashi M, Cranford JL, Nakai Y, Alford BR. Behavioral auditory function after transection of crossed olivo-cochlear bundle in the cat. IV. Study of pure-tone frequency discrimination. Acta Otolaryngol (Stockh) 1979;87:79–83.
156. Moulin A, Collet L, Duclaux R. Contralateral auditory stimulation alters acoustic distortion products in humans. Hear Res 1993;65:193–210.
157. Davis H. An active process in cochlear mechanics. Hear Res 1983;9:79–90.
158. Geisler CD. Hypothesis on the function of the crossed olivocochlear bundle. J Acoust Soc Am 1974;56:1908–9.
159. Cody AR, Johnstone BM. Temporary threshold shift modified by binaural acoustic stimulation. Hear Res 1982;6: 199–205.
160. Canlon B. The effect of acoustic trauma on the tectorial membrane, stereocilia, and hearing sensitivity: Possible mechanisms underlying damage, recovery, and protection. Scand Audiol Suppl 1988;27:1–45.
161. Franklin DJ, Lonsbury-Martin BL, Stagner BB, Martin GK. Altered susceptibility of $2f_1$-f_2 acoustic-distortion products to the effects of repeated noise exposure in rabbits. Hear Res 1991;53:185–208.
162. Dagli S, Canlon B. The effect of repeated daily noise exposure on sound-conditioned and unconditioned guinea pigs. Hear Res 1997;104:39–46.
163. Brown MC, Kujawa SG, Liberman MC. Single olivocochlear neurons in the guinea pig. II. Response plasticity due to noise conditioning. J Neurophysiol 1998;79:3088–97.
164. Canlon B, Fransson A, Viberg A. Medial olivocochlear efferent terminals are protected by sound conditioning. Brain Res 1999;850:253–60.
165. LePage EL. Frequency-dependent self-induced bias of the basilar membrane and its potential for controlling sensitivity and tuning in the mammalian cochlea. J Acoust Soc Am 1987;82:139–54.
166. Heimer L, Robards MJ. Neuroanatomical Tract-Tracing Methods. New York: Plenum Press; 1981. p. 171–205.
167. Spangler KM, Warr WB. The descending auditory system. In: Altschuler RA, Bobbin RP, Clopton BM, Hoffman DW, editors. Neurobiology of Hearing: The Central Auditory System. New York: Raven Press; 1991. p. 27–45.
168. Helfert RH, Snead CR, Alschuler RA. The ascending auditory pathways. In: Altschuler RA, Bobbin RP, Clopton BM, Hoffman DW, editors. Neurobiology of Hearing: The Central Auditory System. New York: Raven Press; 1991. p. 1–25.
169. Moore JK. Cochlear nuclei: Relationship to the auditory nerve. In: Altschuler RA, Hoffman DW, Bobbin RP, editors. Neurobiology of Hearing: The Cochlea. New York: Raven Press; 1986. p. 283–301.
170. Phillips DP. Introduction to the central auditory nervous system. In: Jahn AF, Santos-Sacchi J, editors. Physiology of the Ear, 2nd edition. San Diego: Singular/Thompson Learning Press; 2001. p. 613–38.
171. Kiang NYS. Stimulus representation in the discharge patterns of auditory neurons. In: Tower DB, editor. The Nervous System, Volume 3. Human Communication and Its Disorders. New York: Raven Press; 1975. p. 81–96.
172. Lorenté de No R. Anatomy of the eighth nerve: I. The central projection of the nerve endings of the internal ear. Laryngoscope 1933;43:1–38.
173. Brawer JR, Morest DK, Kane EC. The neuronal architecture of the cochlear nucleus of the cat. J Comp Neurol 1974;155:251–300.
174. Young ED. Response characteristics of neurons of the cochlear nucleus of the cat. In: Berlin CI, editor. Hearing Science: Recent Advances. San Diego: College-Hill Press; 1984. p. 423–60.
175. Goldberg JM, Brown PB. Response of binaural neurons of dog superior olivary complex to dichotic tonal stimuli: Some physiological mechanisms of sound localization. J Neurophysiol 1969;32:613–36.
176. Thompson GC. Structure and function of the central auditory system. Semin Hear 1983;4:81.
177. Brugge JF, Anderson DJ, Aitkin LM. Responses of neurons in the dorsal nucleus of the lateral lemniscus of cat to binaural tonal stimulation. J Neurophysiol 1970;33:441–58.
178. Schofield BR, Cant NB. Ventral nucleus of the lateral lemniscus in guinea pigs: Cytoarchitecture and inputs from the cochlear nucleus. J Comp Neurol 1997;379:363–85.
179. Morest DK. The neuronal architecture of the medial geniculate body of the cat. J Anat 1964;98:611–30.
180. David E, Keidel WD, Katlert S, et al. Decoding processes in the auditory system and human speech analysis. In: Evans EF, Wilson JP, editors. Psychophysics and Physiology of Hearing. New York: Academic Press; 1977. p. 509–16.
181. Keidel WD. Information processing in the higher parts of the auditory pathway. In: Zwicker E, Terhardt E, editors.

Facts and Models in Hearing. New York: Springer-Verlag; 1974. p. 216–26.
182. Rose JE. The cellular structure of the auditory region of the cat. J Comp Neurol 1949;91:409–39.
183. Winer JA, Diamond IT, Raczkowski D. Subdivisions of the auditory cortex of the cat: The retrograde transport of horseradish peroxidase to the medial geniculate body and posterior thalamic nuclei. J Comp Neurol 1977;176: 387–417.
184. Coats AC. On electrocochleographic electrode design. J Acoust Soc Am 1974;56:708–11.
185. Picton TW, Hillyard SA, Krausz HI, Galabos R. Human auditory evoked potentials. I. Evaluation of components. Electroencephalogr Clin Neurophysiol 1974;36:179–90.
186. Haapaniemi J, Laurikainen E, Johansson R, Karjalainen S. Transtympanic versus tympanic membrane electrocochleography in examining cochleovestibular disorders. Acta Otolaryngol Suppl (Stockh) 2000;543:127–9.
187. Elberling C. Simulation of cochlear action potentials recorded from the ear canal in man. In: Ruben RJ, Elberling C, Salomon G, editors. Electrocochleography. Baltimore: University Park Press; 1976.
188. Coats AC. Electrocochleography: Recording techniques and clinical applications. Semin Hear 1986;7:24766.
189. Ferraro JA, Tibbils RP. SP/AP area ratio in the diagnosis of Meniere's disease. Am J Audiol 1999;8:21–8.
190. Wuyts FL, Van de Heyning PH, Van Spaendonck M, et al. Rate influences on tone burst summating potential amplitude in electrocochleography: Clinical (a) and experimental (b) data. Hear Res 2001;152:1–9.
191. Moffat DA, Gibson WP, Ramsden RT, et al. Transtympanic electrocochleography during glycerol dehydration. Acta Otolaryngol (Stockh) 1978;85:158–66.
192. Moller AR. Physiology of the ascending auditory pathway with special reference to the auditory brainstem response (ABR). In: Pinheiro ML, Musiek FE, editors. Assessment of Central Auditory Dysfunction: Foundations and Clinical Correlates. Baltimore: Williams and Wilkins; 1985.
193. Wada S, Starr A. Generation of auditory brainstem responses. III. Effects of lesions of the superior olive, lateral lemniscus, and inferior colliculus on the ABR in guinea pig. Electroencephalogr Clin Neurophysiol 1983;56:352–66.
194. Musiek FE, Gollegly KM, Kibbe KS, Verkest SB. Current concepts on the use of ABR and auditory psychophysical tests in the evaluation of brain stem lesions. Am J Otol 1988;9:25–35.
195. Hosford-Dunn H. Auditory function tests. In: Cummings CW, Fredrickson JM, Harker LA, et al, editors. Otolaryngology— Head and Neck Surgery. St. Louis: CV Mosby; 1986.
196. Kaga K, Hink RF, Shimada Y, Suzuki J. Evidence for a primary cortical origin of a middle latency auditory evoked potential in cats. Electroencephalogr Clin Neurophysiol 1980;50:254–66.
197. McGee TJ, Ozdamar O, Kraus N. Auditory middle latency responses in the guinea pig. Am J Otolaryngol 1983;4:116–22.
198. Scherg M, Von Cramer D. Topographical analysis of auditory evoked potentials: Derivation of components. In: Nodar R, Barber C, editors. Evoked Potentials. Stoneham, MA: Butterworth Press; 1984.
199. Fifer RC, Sierra-Irizzary B. Clinical applications of the auditory middle latency response. Am J Otol 1988;9:47–56.
200. Kileny PR, Kemink JL. Electrically evoked middle-latency auditory potentials in cochlear implant candidates. Arch Otolaryngol Head Neck Surg 1987;113:1072–7.
201. Duffy FH. Auditory brain mapping. In: Jahn AF, Santos-Sacchi J, editors. Physiology of the Ear. New York: Raven Press; 1988. P. 507–518.
202. Baran JA, Long RR, Musiek FE, Ommaya A. Topographic mapping of brain electrical activity in the assessment of central auditory nervous system pathology. Am J Otol 1988;9:72–6.
203. Hari R, Lounasmaa OV. Recording and interpretation of cerebral magnetic fields. Science 1989;244:432–6.
204. Hari R, Pelizzone M, Makela JP, et al. Neuromagnetic responses from a deaf subject to stimuli presented through a multi-channel cochlear prosthesis. Ear Hear 1988;9: 148–52.
205. Zatorre RJ, Belin P. Spectral and temporal processing in human auditory cortex. Cereb Cortex 2001;11:946–53.
206. Shaywitz BA, Shaywitz SE, Pugh KR, et al. Sex differences in the functional organization of the brain for language. Nature 1995;373:607–9.
207. Melcher JR, Sigalovsky IS, Guinan JJ, Levine RA. Lateralized tinnitus studied with functional magnetic resonance imaging: Abnormal inferior colliculus activation. J Neurophysiol 2000;83:1058–72.
208. Cacace AT, Tasciyan T, Cousins JP. Principles of functional magnetic resonance imaging: Application to auditory neuroscience. J Am Acad Audiol 2000;11:239–72.
209. Filipo R, Delfini R, Fabiani M, et al. Role of transient-evoked otoacoustic emissions for hearing preservation in acoustic neuroma surgery. Am J Audiol 1997;18:746–9.
210. Kemp DT, Ryan S. The use of transient evoked otoacoustic emissions in neonatal hearing screening programs. Semin Hear 1993;14:30–45.
211. Balkany TJ, Telischi FF, Lonsbury-Martin BL, Martin GK. Otoacoustic emissions in clinical practice. Am J Otol 1994;15:29–38.
212. Martin GK, Ohlms LA, Franklin DJ, et al. Distortion-product otoacoustic emissions in humans: III. Influence of sensorineural hearing loss. Ann Otol Rhinol Laryngol 1990;147:30–42.
213. Hotz MA, Probst R, Harris FP, Hauser R. Monitoring the effects of noise exposure using transiently evoked otoacoustic emissions. Acta Otolaryngol (Stockh) 1993;113:478–82.
214. Fiore C, Cagini C, Menduno P, et al. Evoked otoacoustic emissions behaviour in retinitis pigmentosa. Doc Ophthalmol 1994;87:167–76.
215. Zorowka PG, Schmitt HJ, Gutjahr P. Evoked otoacoustic emissions and pure tone threshold audiometry in patients receiving cisplatinum therapy Int J Pediatr Otorhinolaryngol 1993;25:73–80.
216. Fortnum H, Farnsworth A, Davis A. The feasibility of evoked otoacoustic emissions as an in-patient hearing check after meningitis. Br J Audiol 1993;27:227–31.
217. Stover L, Norton SJ. The effects of aging on otoacoustic emissions. J Acoust Soc Am 1993;94:2670–81.
218. Hall JW, Baer JE, Chase PA, Schwaber MK. Clinical application of otoacoustic emissions: What do we know about factors influencing measurement and analysis? Otolaryngol Head Neck Surg 1994;110:22–38.
219. Lonsbury-Martin BL, Martin GK, Balkany T. Clinical applications of otoacoustic emissions. In: Lucente FE, editor. Highlights of the Instructional Courses. Alexandria, VA: American Academy of Otolaryngology—Head and Neck Surgery; 1994. p. 343–55.
220. Shera CA, Guinan JJ, Jr. Evoked otoacoustic emissions arise by two fundamentally different mechanisms: A taxonomy for mammalian OAEs. J Acoust Soc Am 1999;105:782–98.
221. Knight RD, Kemp DT. Indications of different distortion product otoacoustic emission mechanisms from a detailed f_1,f_2 area study. J Acoust Soc Am 2000;107:457–73.
222. Knight RD, Kemp DT. Wave and place fixed DPOAE maps of the human ear. J Acoust Soc Am 2001;109:1513–25.
223. Shera CA (2004). Mechanisms of mammalian otoacoustic emission and their implications for the clinical utility of otoacoustic emissions. Ear Hear 2004;25:86–97.
224. Whitehead ML, Lonsbury-Martin BL, Martin GK. Evidence for two discrete sources of $2f_1$-f_2 distortion-product otoacoustic emission in rabbit: II. Differential physiological vulnerability. J Acoust Soc Am 1992;92:2662–82.
225. Ren T. Reverse propagation of sound in the gerbil cochlea. Nat Neurosci 2004;7:333–4.
226. Ruggero MA. Comparison of group delays of $2f_1$-f_2 distortion product otoacoustic emissions and cochlear travel times. Acoust Res Let Online 2004;5:143–7.
227. Siegel JH, Cerka AJ, Recio-Spinoso A, et al. Delays of stimulus-frequency otoacoustic emissions and cochlear vibrations contradict the theory of coherent reflection filtering. J Acoust Soc Am 2005;18:2434–43.
228. Igarashi M, Miyata L, Alford BR. Utricular ablation and dysequilibrium in squirrel monkeys. Acta Otolaryngol (Stockh) 1972;74:66–72.
229. Fernandez C, Goldberg JM. Physiology of peripheral neurons innervating otolith organs of the squirrel monkey. I. Response to static tilts and to long-duration centrifugal force. J Neurophysiol 1976;39:970–84.
230. Fernandez C, Goldberg JM. Physiology of peripheral neurons innervating otolith organs of the squirrel monkey. II. Directional selectivity and force-response relations. J Neurophysiol 1976;39:985–95.
231. Fernandez C, Goldberg JM. Physiology of peripheral neurons innervating otolith organs of the squirrel monkey. III. Response dynamics. J Neurophysiol 1976;39: 996–1008.
232. Wendt GR. Vestibular functions. In: Stevens SS, editor. Handbook of Experimental Psychology. New York: John Wiley & Sons; 1951. p. 1191–223
233. Cogan DG. Some objective and subjective observations on the vestibulo-ocular system. Am J Ophthalmol 1958;45: 74–8.
234. de Beer GR. Presidential address: How animals hold their heads. Proc Linn Soc Lond 1947;159:125–39.
235. Juhn SK. Biochemistry of the Labyrinth: A Manual. Rochester, MN: American Academy of Ophthalmology and Otolaryngology; 1973.
236. Wersäll J. Studies on the structure and innervation of the sensory epithelium of the cristae ampullaris in the guinea pig. Acta Otolaryngol Suppl (Stockh) 1956;126:1–185.
237. Dohlman GF. Critical review of the concept of cupula function. Acta Otolaryngol Suppl (Stockh) 1980;376:1–30.
238. Iurato S. Submicroscopic Structure of the Inner Ear. Oxford (England): Pergamon Press; 1967. p. 219–25.
239. Carlstrom D, Engstrom H, Hjorth S. Electron microscopic and x-ray diffraction studies of statoconia. Laryngoscope 1953;63:1052–7.
240. Wersäll J, et al. Ultrastructure of the vestibular end organs. In: De Reuck AVS, Knight J, editors. Myotatic, Kinesthetic and Vestibular Mechanisms. Boston, MA: Little, Brown Press; 1968. p. 105–16.
241. Spoendlin H. Ultrastructure of the vestibular sense organ. In: Wolfson RJ, editor. The Vestibular System and Its Diseases. Philadelphia, PA: University of Pennsylvania Press; 1966.
242. Anniko M, Thornell LE, Virtanen I. Cytoskeletal organization of the human inner ear. IV. Expression of actin in vestibular organs. Acta Otolaryngol Suppl (Stockh) 1987;437:5–76.
243. Zenner HP, Zimmermann U. Motile responses of vestibular hair cells following caloric, electrical or chemical stimuli. Acta Otolaryngol (Stockh) 1991,111:291–7.
244. Wersäll J, Flock A, Lundquist PG. Structural basis for directional sensitivity in cochlear and vestibular sensory receptors. Cold Spring Harb Symp Quant Biol 1965;30: 115–32.
245. Engstrom H, Bergstrom B, Ades HW. Macula utriculi and macula saculi in the squirrel monkey. Acta Otolaryngol Suppl (Stockh) 1972;301:75–126.
246. Lindeman HH, Ades HW, Bredberg G, Engstrom H. The sensory hairs and the tectorial membrane in the development of the cat's organ of Corti. Acta Otolaryngol (Stockh) 1971;72:229–42.
247. Tilney LG, DeRosier DJ, Mulroy MJ. The organization of actin filaments in the stereocilia of cochlear hair cells. J Cell Biol 1980;86:244–59.
248. Assad JA, Shepherd GM, Corey DP. Tip link integrity and mechanical transduction in vertebrate hair cells. Neuron 1991;7:985–94.
249. Spoendlin H. Receptor ultrastructure. In: De Reuck AVS, Knight J, editors. Symposium on Hearing Mechanisms in Vertebrates. Boston, MA: Little, Brown Press; 1968. p. 89–119.
250. Hillman DE, McLaren JW. Displacement configuration of semiciruclar canal cupulae. Neuroscience 1979;4:1989–2000.
251. McLaren JW, Hillman DE. Displacement of semicircular canal cupula during sinusoidal rotation. Neuroscience 1979;4:2001–8.
252. Oman CM, Young LR. Physiological range of pressure difference and cupula deflections in the human semicircular canal: Theoretical considerations. Prog Brain Res 1972;37:529–39.
253. Steinhausen W. The cupula. Z Hals Nas Ohrenh 1931;29:211–6.
254. Goldberg JM, Ferenadez C. Physiology of peripheral neurons innervating semicircular canal of the squirrel monkey. I. Resting discharge and response to constant angular accelerations. J Neurophysiol 1971;34:635–60.
255. Baloh R, Honrubia V. Clinical Neurophysiology of the Vestibular System, 2nd edition. Philadelphia: FA Davis; 1990. p. 63–70.
256. Zee DS, Leigh RJ. The Neurology of Eye Movements, 2nd edition. Philadelphia: FA Davis; 1991.
257. Goldberg JM, Fernandez C. Vestibular mechanisms. Ann Rev Physiol 1975;37:129–62.
258. Keller EL. Behavior of horizontal semicircular canal afferents in alert monkey during vestibular and optokinetic stimulation. Exp Brain Res 1976;24:459–71.
259. Fernandez C, Goldberg JM. Physiology of peripheral neurons in innervating semicircular canals of the squirrel monkey. II. Response to sinusoidal stimulation and dynamics of peripheral vestibular system. J Neurophysiol 1971;34:661–75.
260. Brodal A. Neurological Anatomy in Relation to Clinical Medicine. New York: Oxford University Press; 1969.
261. Carpenter MG. Human Neuroanatomy, 7th edition. Baltimore: Williams and Wilkins; 1976. p. 463–4.
262. Baker R. The nucleus prepositus hypoglossi. In: Brooks BA, Bajandas FJ, editors. Eye Movements. New York: Plenum Press; 1977.
263. Keller EL. The behavior of eye movement motoneurons in the alert monkey. Bibl Ophthalmol 1972;82:7–16.
264. Cannon SC, Robinson DA. Loss of the neural integrator of the oculomotor system from brainstem lesions in monkey. J Neurophysiol 1987;57:1383–409.

265. Wilson VJ, Wylie RM, Marco LA. Organization of the medial vestibular nucleus. J Neurophysiol 1968;31:166–75.

266. Miller EF, Graybiel A. A comparison of ocular counter rolling movements between normal persons and deaf subjects with bilateral labyrinthine defects. Ann Otol Rhinol Laryngol 1963;72:885–93.

267. Goldberg JM. Afferent diversity and the organization of central vestibular pathways. Exp Brain Res 2000;130:277–97.

268. Kotchabhakdi N, Walberg F. Primary vestibular afferent projections to the cerebellum as demonstrated by retrograde axonal transport of horseradish peroxidase. Brain Res 1978;142:142–6.

269. Kotchabhakdi N, Walberg F. Cerebellar afferent projections from the vestibular nuclei in the cat: An experimental study with the method of retrograde axonal transport of horseradish peroxidase. Exp Brain Res 1978;31:591–604.

270. Fredrickson JM, Frigge U, Scheid P, Kornhuber HH. Vestibular nerve projection to the cerebral cortex of the rhesus monkey. Exp Brain Res 1966;2:318–27.

271. Deecke L, Schwartz DW, Fredrickson JM. The vestibular thalamus in the rhesus monkey. Adv Otorhinolaryngol 1973;19:210–9.

272. Wilson VJ, Melvill-Jones G. Mammalian Vestibular Physiology. New York: Plenum Press; 1979.

273. Precht W, Shimazu H, Markham CH. A mechanism of central compensation of vestibular function following hemilabyrinthectomy. J Neurophysiol 1966;29:996–1010.

274. Igarashi M, Levy JK, O-Uchi T, Reschke MF. Further study of physical exercise and locomotor balance compensation after unilateral labyrinthectomy in squirrel monkeys. Acta Otolaryngol (Stockh) 1981;92:101–5.

275. Fetter M, Zee DS. Recovery from unilateral labyrinthectomy in rhesus monkey. J Neurophysiol 1988;59:370–93.

276. Brandt T. Management of vestibular disorders. J Neurol 2000;247:491–9.

277. Bechterew W. Ergebnisse der Durchschneidung des N. acusticus, nebst Eroerterung der Bedeutung der semicirculaeren Canaele fuer das Koerpergleichgewicht. Pfluegers Arch Ges Physiol 1883;30:312–47.

278. Darlington CL, Smith PF. Molecular mechanisms of recovery from vestibular damage in mammals: Recent advances. Prog Neurobiol 2000;62:313–25.

279. Highstein SM. Abducens to medical rectus pathway in the MLF: A possible cellular basis for the syndrome of internuclear ophthalmoplegia. In: Brooks BA, Bajandas FJ, editors. Eye Movements. New York: Plenum Press; 1977.

280. Gauthier GM, Robinson DA. Adaptation of the human vestibulo-ocular reflex to magnifying lenses. Brain Res 1975;92:331–5.

281. Miles FA, Fuller JH. Adaptive plasticity in the vestibulo-ocular responses of the rhesus monkey. Brain Res 1974;80:512–6.

282. Robinson DA. Adaptive gain control of the vestibulo-ocular reflex by the cerebellum. J Neurophysiol 1976;39:954–69.

283. Kohler I. Experiments with goggles. Sci Am 1962;206:62–84.

284. Melvill-Jones G, Davies PRT, Gonshor A. Long-term effects of maintained vision reversal: Is vestibulo-ocular adaptation either necessary or sufficient? In: Baker R, Berthoz A, editors. Control of Gaze by Brainstem Neurons, Volume 1. Developments in Neuroscience. Amsterdam: Elsevier/North-Holland Biomedical; 1977.

285. Miles FA. The primate flocculus and eye-head coordination. In: Brooks BA, Bajandas FJ, editors. Eye Movements. New York: Plenum Press; 1977. p. 75–92.

286. Robinson DA. Is the cerebellum too old to learn? In: Brooks BA, Bajandas FJ, editors. Eye Movements. New York: Plenum Press; 1976. p. 65–73.

287. Simpson J, Alley KE. Visual climbing fiber input to rabbit vestibulo-cerebellum: A source of direction-specific information. Brain Res 1974;82:301–8.

288. Honrubia V, Koehn WW, Jenkins HA, Fenton WH. Effect of bilateral ablation of the vestibular cerebellum on visual-vestibular interaction. Exp Neurol 1982;75:616–26.

289. Sato Y, Kato I, Kawasaki T, et al. Failure of fixation suppression of caloric nystagmus and ocular motor abnormalities. Arch Neurol 1980;37:35–8.

290. Miles FA, Braitman DJ, Dow BM. Long-term adaptive changes in primate vestibuloocular reflex. IV. Electrophysiological observations in flocculus of adapted monkeys. J Neurophysiol 1980;43:1477–93.

291. Lisberger SG. The neural basis for learning of simple motor skills. Science 1988;242:728–35.

292. Luebke AE, Robinson DA. Gain changes of the cat's vestibulo-ocular reflex after flocculus deactivation. Exp Brain Res 1994;98:379–90.

293. McNally WJ, Stuart WA. Physiology of the Labyrinth. Chicago: American Academy of Ophthalmology and Otolaryngology; 1967.

294. Benson AJ, Jobson PH. Body sway induced by a low frequency alternating current. Int J Equilib Res 1973;3: 55–61.

295. Cohen B. Vestibulo-ocular relations. In: Bach-y-Rita P, Collins CC, Hyde JE, editors. The Control of Eye Movements. New York: Academic Press; 1971. p. 105–48.

5

Inner Ear Drug Delivery and Gene Therapy

Anil K. Lalwani, MD
Nirmal P. Patel, MD

Over the past quarter century, there has been an expanding interest in directed therapy to address inner ear disorders as indirect, systemic therapy has shown limited success and significant morbidity. Intratympanic (IT) therapy has several potential advantages over conventional systemic therapy including increased therapeutic concentrations in the inner ear, reduced side-effect profiles, cost effectiveness by avoiding surgery, use when systemic therapy is contraindicated, and lastly as a salvage for failure of systemic therapy. Experimentally, as reviewed below, investigators have shown that intratympanic and intracochlear therapy is feasible and efficacious. In this chapter, the core of knowledge regarding delivery of material into the inner ear and its therapeutic consequences will be reviewed.

ROUND WINDOW MEMBRANE

The anatomy and physiology of the round window membrane (RWM) are covered in Chapter 1, "Anatomy of the Auditory and Vestibular Systems," and Chapter 4, "Physiology of the Auditory and Vestibular Systems"; however, the aspects of the RWM that are relevant to intratympanic therapy are reviewed here.

Anatomy of the Round Window Membrane

The RWM is a three-layered structure that protects the inner ear from middle ear pathology and facilitates active transport. There is an outer epithelial layer that faces the middle ear, a central connective tissue layer, and an inner epithelial layer interfacing with the scala tympani. The outer epithelial layer is continuous with the promontory. Mucoperiosteal folds from the neighboring epithelium can sometimes obstruct the round window niche, forming a "false" RWM. Other reactive changes, such as scarring from middle ear infections or surgery, may also lead to adhesions that obstruct the RWM. In a study of 202 cadaveric ears to determine the amount and nature of RWM obstruction, Alzamil and Linthicum identified RWM obstruction in one-third of ears.[1] In their series, 21% had false RWMs, 10% had fibrous plugs, and 1.5% had fatty plugs. These obstructions may explain why a proportion of patients treated with intratympanic therapy have no beneficial effect or require multiple pharmacotherapeutic courses to achieve treatment goals.

Permeability

A large range of substances are able to cross the RWM, including various antimicrobials, corticosteroids, anesthetics, water, ions, and macromolecules, including bacterial toxins. Several factors contribute to the RWM permeability, including size, charge, the morphology of the compound, and the thickness of the RWM. Size has proven to be a factor in permeability, as 1 μm spheres cross the RWM, but 3 μm spheres do not. Furthermore, substances with a molecular weight of less than 1,000 kD diffuse across the RWM fairly rapidly, whereas substances over 1,000 kD are transported by pinocytosis. Charge of the ion can also impact its ability to traverse the RWM; for example, it has been noted that cationic ferritin crosses the RWM, but anionic ferritin does not. Finally, increased thickness of the RWM will decrease permeability of substances. Whereas the average thickness of the human RWM is between 10 and 30 μm, its thickness can double in inflammatory conditions.

Kinetics

Delivery of therapeutic agents across the RWM displays a nonuniform distribution in the perilymph. Concentrations of the delivered agent are usually high in the basal turn in close proximity to the RWM and low in the apical turn. The permeability of the substance across the RWM and the rate of its clearance from the perilymph are the two major factors that determine the dispersion of substances in perilymph. Perilymph clearance includes a combination of clearance to blood, clearance to other scalae, uptake or binding by cells, or metabolism by cochlear tissues. Therefore, knowing the RWM permeability and clearance rates of a given agent will permit simulation of its perilymphatic distribution with reasonable accuracy.

Using these observations, Salt and Ma described the development of a computer-simulated model of drug distribution in the perilymphatic space (http://otowustl.edu/cochlea/). An example of the power of this program is demonstrated in a study by Plontke and colleagues, in which a model of gentamicin kinetics in the perilymph closely approximated published in vivo kinetics data by adjusting parameters defining RWM permeability, perilymphatic clearance, and interscala drug exchange.[2] They were able to establish

that intratympanically administered gentamicin spreads from the RWM to the vestibule by diffusion through the scala rather than the helicotrema. The study also suggested that drug concentrations and distribution in the perilymph were substantially influenced by the delivery method and the duration of exposure of the drug to the RWM.

Importantly, distribution kinetics alone may not account for the widely observed phenomenon of disproportionate basal turn damage in aminoglycoside toxicity; inherent susceptibility of the basal hair cells to ototoxicity may contribute. Sha and colleagues investigated the base-to-apex sensitivity of hair cells to aminoglycoside toxicity by dissecting cells from different turns of the organ of Corti and subjecting them to the same degree of aminoglycoside exposure.[3] After 5 hours of exposure, 70% of the basal cells were no longer viable, whereas only 10% of the apex cells were damaged. Therefore, the greater inherent susceptibility of the basal hair cells to aminoglycoside damage in part determines the pattern of base-to-apex toxicity.

Delivery Methods

For a typical intratympanic injection, the patient lies flat with the affected ear facing the ceiling. Local anesthetic, such as 88% phenol, is then applied to the tympanic membrane. A myringotomy is necessary, as there should be a vent for air to escape the middle ear space as it is filled with fluid. The injection should be administered slowly and directed into the posterior half of the middle ear toward the round window, so that the solution pools around the round window niche. The patient should remain with the injected ear toward the ceiling for around 15 to 30 minutes. Some protocols call for multiple injections over a short period of time. Under these circumstances, it is useful to place a tympanostomy tube after the initial myringotomy.

Advances in microendoscopes may significantly increase the ease and accuracy of intratympanic drug delivery. Plontke and colleagues described the development of a 1.2 mm endoscope that incorporates a thin fiber optic, a working/laser channel (0.3 mm), and a suction/irrigation channel (0.27 mm).[4] This new device allows several manipulations to occur at once, including direct observation of the RWM, lysis of adhesions (if present), and application of medications directly to the RWM.

Intratympanic injection is inherently inaccurate as the injected medication can leak down the eustachian tube, escape out of the external auditory canal, or be sequestered in the middle ear. Therefore, the amount of medication delivered potentially changes with each patient and each dose. In an attempt to address this problem, several static sustained release vehicles have been developed. For instance, a dry 2 × 3 mm Gelfoam (Upjohn, Kalamazoo, MI) pledget can be placed directly in the round window niche (Figure 1). The treatment compound can be injected directly onto the Gelfoam pad. Because of the slow dissipation of Gelfoam, this can be repeated several times. A Gelfoam slurry can also be used to suspend the medicine. A two-component fibrin glue system may also be used (Red Cross-Holland Laboratory, College Park, MD). The first component of the glue is deposited in the round window niche. The other component is mixed with the medicine. The two are mixed in situ and subsequently solidified, allowing the medicine to be slowly released from the glue onto the RWM. A final alternative as an inner ear delivery suspension is hyaluronic acid (Healon, Advanced Medical Optics Inc., Santa Ana, CA) which has been demonstrated to cause less ototoxic damage compared to fibrin or Gelfoam.[5]

The ultimate degree of pharmacokinetic control can be achieved with the use of mechanical sustained release devices. These devices allow researchers to manipulate inner ear kinetic curves reliably by changing the rate and amount of dose delivered to the RWM. There are two devices that are currently approved for use in humans and have been studied in clinical trials: the Silverstein MicroWick (Micromedics, Eaton, MN) and the IntraEar Microcatheter (Durect, Cupertino, CA). The Silverstein MicroWick is made of polyvinyl acetate and measures 1 × 9 mm long, small enough to fit through a tympanostomy tube (Figure 2). The wick absorbs medication which can be instilled into the external auditory canal by the patient at home and delivers it to the RWM. This device has been used to deliver corticosteroids and gentamicin in human clinical trials. The IntraEar Microcatheter consists of an electronic pump (Disetronics, Minneapolis, MN) connected to a catheter tip that is placed directly on the RWM. Implantation of the Microcatheter is more invasive and requires the elevation of a tympanomeatal flap. This device has also been extensively tested in human subjects for both corticosteroid and gentamicin therapy to the inner ear.

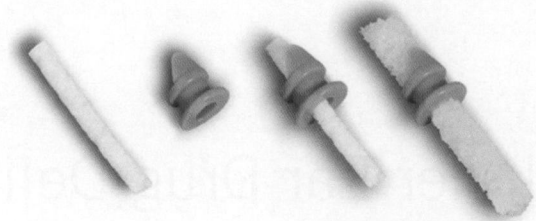

Figure 2 Silverstein otowick. The wick is used in combination with a ventilation tube to deliver agents to the round window membrane.

Several new therapeutic agents, such as neurotrophins, require chronic or continuous application. This presents a serious challenge from a delivery point of view. In an attempt to address the need for a long-term delivery device, Praetorius and colleagues developed a fully implantable micropump system.[6] The device is made from pure titanium, polyethylene, and silicone and is designed for life-long implantation in humans. To place the device, a cavity is drilled in the mastoid bone to house the pump and reservoir system, a procedure that is similar to the one used to place cochlear implants or implantable hearing devices.

Intratympanic Corticosteroids

The two principal indications for intratympanic (IT) corticosteroids are sudden sensorineural hearing loss (SSNHL) and Ménière's disease. The pathogenesis, pathophysiology, and diagnostic criteria for these indications are subject to controversy; furthermore, the mechanisms of action of corticosteroids in the inner ear are incompletely understood. Therefore, a comprehensive evaluation of the use of IT corticosteroids as a treatment for these conditions is exceedingly difficult. Table 1 summarizes the relative anti-inflammatory and sodium retention properties, relative to hydrocortisone duration and equivalent dose of various corticosteroids.

Mechanism of Action. Corticosteroids help mitigate the destructive processes caused by the immune response. Corticosteroids decrease the number of circulating blood leukocytes and inhibit the formation and liberation of inflammatory mediators, therefore, decreasing the damage from an inflammatory response, whether the response is secondary to mechanical, hypoxic, ischemic, infectious, or autoimmune causes. In addition to modulation of the immune response, corticosteroids are linked to several other biological effects in the inner ear, including ion homeostasis, functioning as apoptosis inhibitors, antioxidants, signal transducers in the neuroepithelial regions of the inner ear, and vasoactive agents that increase cochlear blood flow. To understand their various roles and potential target tissues, the presence and distribution of glucocorticoid receptors in the inner ear have been extensively studied. The distribution of corticosteroid receptors is not uniform, and this differential expression in the inner ear may explain, in part, their spectrum of functions.

Pharmacokinetics. IT administration yields much higher concentrations of corticosteroids

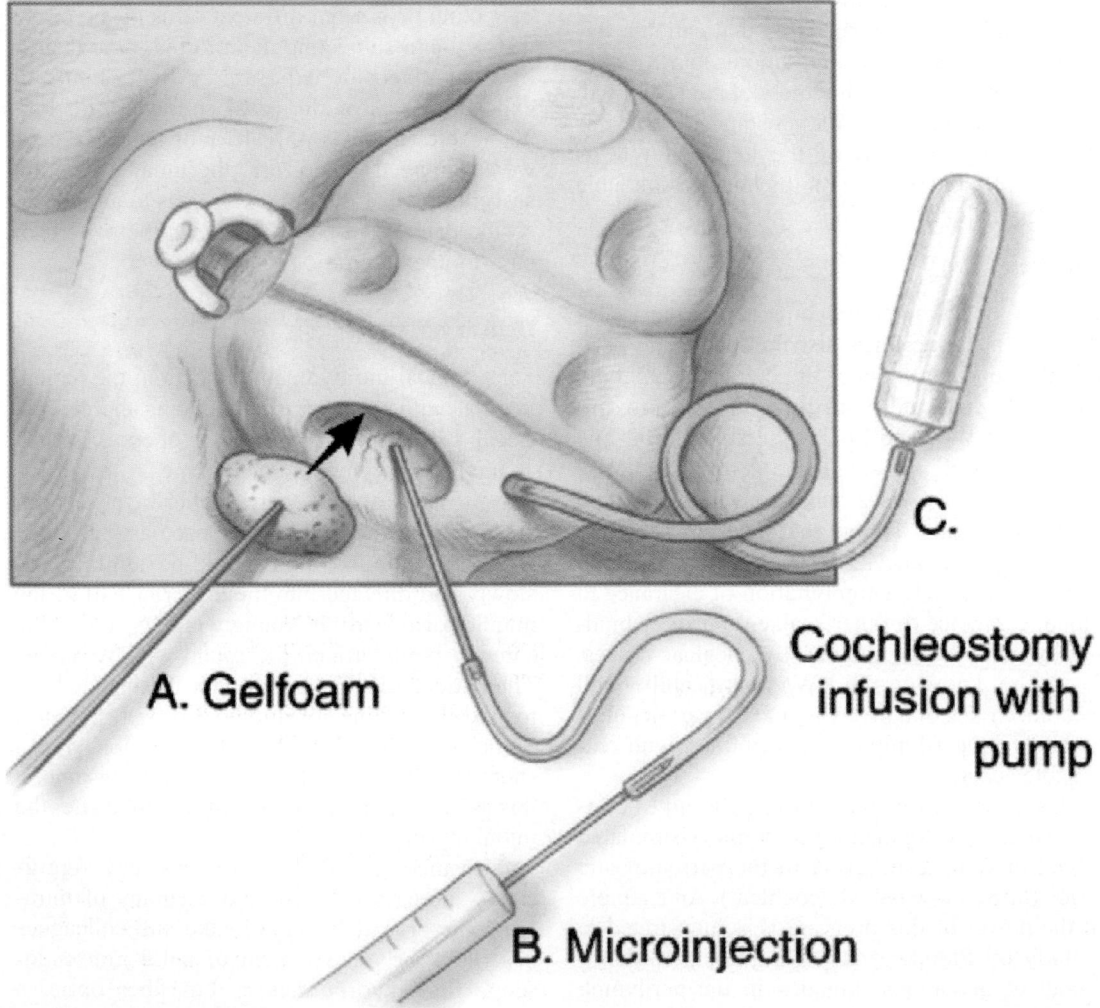

A. Gelfoam

B. Microinjection

C. Cochleostomy infusion with pump

Figure 1 Routes of delivery for inner ear therapy. A variety of routes are available to introduce a drug or gene therapy vector to the cochlea. These include direct instillation of the agent through an intact round window membrane with a gelatin sponge (A), direct injection through the round window membrane (B), and infusion with osmotic mini-pump through cochleostomy (C). (Published with permission, copyright © 2007 Anil K. Lalwani, MD.)

Table 1 Anti-inflammatory and Sodium Retention Properties of Various Corticosteroids Relative to Hydrocortisone

Corticosteroid	Anti-inflammatory Properties	Sodium Retention Properties	Duration Equivalent Dose (mg)
Betamethasone	0.6		
Cortisone	0.8	0.8	S 25
Hydrocortisone	1.0	1.0	S 20
Prednisone	4.0	0.8	I 5
Prednisolone	4.0	0.8	I 5
Methylprednisolone	5.0	0.5	I 4
Triamcinolone	5.0		I 4
9α-Fluorocortisol	10.0	125.0	S
Dexamethasone	25.0		L 0.75

Short (S) = 8 to 12 h t° 1/2; intermediate (I) = 12 to 36 h t° 1/2; long (L) = 36 to 72 h.

in the inner ear than either intravenous (IV) or oral administration. Parnes and colleagues compared IV and IT administration of hydrocortisone, methylprednisolone, and dexamethasone (short-, intermediate-, and long-acting corticosteroids, respectively).[7] While all the three corticosteroids successfully penetrated the blood-labyrinthine barrier, there was a much higher concentration of corticosteroids in inner ear tissues with IT administration. Methylprednisolone had the highest concentration and longest duration in perilymph and endolymph of the three compounds.

Systemic Corticosteroids

Currently, systemic corticosteroids are the treatment of choice for sudden sensorineural hearing loss and acute vestibular vertigo. IT corticosteroid delivery without controlled study may be premature as there may be certain biological effects that can only be achieved with systemic corticosteroids. For example, it is well established that corticosteroids decrease peripheral blood leukocytes. These cells enter the inner ear through the endolymphatic sac, the immunocompetent organ of the inner ear. Local administration may be incapable of stopping this system-wide process. Yang and colleagues developed a model of labyrinthitis induced by delayed hypersensitivity to keyhole limpet hemocyanin (KLH) that mimics a full scale, cell-mediated immune response.[8] They found that IT dexamethasone was ineffective in reducing inflammatory infiltrate after KLH challenge. This situation represents the risk of using IT corticosteroids alone for inner ear disease, rather than in combination with oral or IV corticosteroids.

Sudden Sensorineural Hearing Loss

Systemic and IT corticosteroid therapy have been used for treatment of sudden sensorineural hearing loss (SSNHL). The major prognostic factors predicting response to treatment for SSNHL are initial severity of hearing loss and time between onset and treatment. There is a high spontaneous recovery rate of 30 to 60%, therefore treatment efficacy of any intervention has to be greater than the spontaneous recovery rate. Oral corticosteroid therapy within the first 2 weeks has shown recovery rates approaching 80% and decreasing with

a greater interval between onset and treatment. Due to the high initial response to oral corticosteroids, few practitioners have attempted to use IT corticosteroids, and most IT corticosteroid trials enroll patients who have failed oral treatment.

Dallan and colleagues reported results of a trial of IT corticosteroids for patients with SSNHL who had failed to improve after high-dose systemic corticosteroids.[9] The protocol consisted of transtympanic injection of 62.5 mg/mL methyl-prednisolone for eight patients with no controls. The results showed a pure tone average improvement of 10 dB or greater in 75% of patients. The authors argue that while this improvement seems modest, this is in a cohort of patients who would otherwise be considered refractory to corticosteroid treatment.

Chandrasekhar and colleagues published results from a 10-patient series treated with IT dexamethasone.[10] The dexamethasone concentration and number of IT injections varied among patients, and several patients were taking oral medications in addition to IT-administered corticosteroids, making outcomes difficult to assess. However, of the 10 patients treated, 6 experienced hearing improvements greater than 10 dB. Parnes and colleagues reported results from a similar series of 13 patients with sudden hearing loss treated with IT corticosteroids.[7] Of the 13 patients treated, 6 showed hearing improvements of 10 dB or more.

Meniere Disease

Meniere disease in some cases may be due to immune dysfunction, therefore corticosteroids are occasionally used in Meniere disease treatment protocols. Itoh and Sakata reported the first IT corticosteroid protocol in 1987, in which 4 to 5 weekly injections of 2 mg of dexamethasone were administered to 61 patients with unilateral Meniere disease.[11] This protocol resulted in vertigo relief in 80% of patients and tinnitus reduction in 74% of patients. Subsequently, additional studies have used IT corticosteroids to treat Meniere disease, some with results more promising than others.

Sennaroglu and colleagues placed tympanostomy tubes in 24 patients with Meniere disease with intractable vertigo and applied five drops of 1 mg/mL dexamethasone solution into the middle

ear space every other day for 3 months, which was administered at home by the patient.[12] This protocol resulted in a vertigo control rate of 72%, improved hearing in 17%, decreased tinnitus in 75%, and reduced aural fullness in 75%. To their credit, the authors acknowledge that their results may be confounded by a placebo effect secondary to the tympanostomy tubes.

Arriaga and Goldman presented short-term hearing results of Meniere disease patients who underwent an IT corticosteroid protocol with placement of Gelfoam and injection of an 8 mg dose of dexamethasone mixed with hyaluron.[13] The only parameter recorded was a 1-month postoperative audiogram. Results showed 33% improvement in hearing and 20% deterioration in hearing. The largest drop in hearing was a 20 dB loss with the speech discrimination score dropping from 88 to 24%. This patient also had severe Meniere disease symptoms during testing, including nausea, vomiting, and vertigo.

In a rare controlled trial, Silverstein and colleagues conducted a prospective, randomized, double-blind, crossover trial of IT dexamethasone and placebo in 17 patients with Meniere disease.[14] All patients had stage IV Meniere disease by the Shea classification (they no longer had vertigo and had poor hearing and significant fullness and tinnitus). They received IT injection of either placebo or 0.2 to 0.3 mL of a 1:1 mixture of 16 mg/mL dexamethasone and sodium hyaluronate. This protocol was performed for 3 consecutive days. Three weeks after the initial treatment, the groups received their crossover treatment. The parameters recorded were audiometric data, ENG recordings, and tinnitus evaluations. The IT corticosteroids provided no significant benefit over placebo in any of the parameters recorded. However, a selection bias in this severely diseased patient population may not be present in other studies, leaving open the possibility that IT corticosteroids may be useful in less severe cases. Regardless, evidence is needed to support a role for IT corticosteroids in Meniere disease.

Dosing for Administration of Intratympanic Corticosteroids

The most widely used corticosteroid for IT protocols is dexamethasone, followed by methyl-prednisolone. IT dexamethasone preparations vary from as little as 1 mg/mL to as high as 25 mg/mL. Most IT methylprednisolone studies use a 62.5 mg/mL solution. The amount of solution injected (0.3 to 0.5 mL) is designed to fill the middle ear space.

Side Effects of Treatment

The side effects of long-term systemic corticosteroid use are well known and include compromise of the immune system leading to infections, osteoporosis, peptic ulcers, hypertension, myopathy, cataract formation, impaired healing, psychological effects, sleep impairment, and avascular necrosis. In contrast, IT corticosteroids are characterized by minor local morbidities.

Several preclinical studies have documented that IT corticosteroids cause no morphological or functional compromise in animal models.[15] Human clinical trials have reported relatively benign side-effect profiles. There are several reports of decreased hearing in human clinical trials of Meniere disease patients, but it is unclear whether this is a side effect of treatment or part of the natural course of the disease. There have also been reports of tympanic membrane perforations and otitis media secondary to the perfusion process.[16]

Conclusions on the Use of Intratympanic Corticosteroids

There is currently no consensus on the mechanism of action of corticosteroids in the inner ear. Furthermore, there is insufficient experience with IT corticosteroids to advocate its routine use in autoimmune hearing loss, SSNHL, or Meniere disease. IT corticosteroids may prove to have a role in SSNHL unresponsive to oral corticosteroids or as an adjuvant to oral corticosteroids in acute settings.

Intratympanic Gentamicin

In 1957, Schuknecht published his work on IT administration of streptomycin for Meniere disease.[17] Although loss of hearing was almost as common as the resolution of vertigo, his work sets the stage for the development of modern IT chemical ablation protocols. It was not until the mid-1970s that Beck and Schmidt described a low-dose strategy that departed from the goal of total vestibular ablation.[18] They compared a high-dose ablative protocol with a low-dose, low injection frequency protocol, and found that while vertigo control was essentially the same, the hearing loss rate decreased from 58 to 15%. This improvement rekindled interest in IT gentamicin therapy.

Mechanism of Action. Despite the widespread belief that gentamicin is selectively toxic to vestibular hair cells, the literature does not fully support this assertion. Several researchers have shown that gentamicin and streptomycin cause parallel and dose-dependent damage to both vestibular and cochlear hair cells.[19–20] The clinical finding of significant correlation between loss of caloric response and hearing loss following gentamicin exposure further betrays the notion of selective vestibular toxicity.

If there is no selective vestibular toxicity, how is it that clinicians have achieved good vertigo control with minimal hearing loss? In part, the answer may lie in pharmacokinetics. Hoffer and colleagues compared the kinetic profiles of IT injection versus microcatheter delivery of gentamicin and correlated these data to the functional changes.[21] Despite the fact that the total dose in both methods was roughly equal, the resulting morphological changes were quite different. Intratympanic injection led to erratic changes, sometimes causing obliteration of auditory

functioning within 4 hours, and in other cases showing significantly delayed ototoxic effects. In contrast, controlled perfusion by microcatheter caused predictable and uniform damage. Hoffer and colleagues explain that this may be due to two different patterns of hair cell loss which included a necrotic pattern associated with rapid and high-dose perfusion and an apoptotic pattern associated with slower or chronic perfusion.[22] Therefore, in addition to the amount of gentamicin that accumulates in the perilymph over time, the nature of the distribution curve, timing of the peak, and total dose determine morphological and functional consequences of aminoglycoside exposure.

The alternative explanation for gentamicin's selective vestibular effect is the proposal that gentamicin primarily affects secretory, rather than sensory cells: the "dark cell theory." Vestibular dark cells are important in creating and maintaining ionic homeostasis in the inner ear since they transport potassium from extracellular environments to the endolymph. Several studies have documented that aminoglycosides induce structural and functional alteration of these dark cells.[23] This damage is thought to alter the ionic homeostasis of the inner ear in such a way that it restores the ionic dysregulation of endolymphatic hydrops. Hilton and colleagues examined secretory and sensory cells in response to aminoglycoside challenge and found no significant changes in dark cells, despite extensive damage in both cochlear and vestibular hair cells.[19] If dark cells are responsible for the selective effect of gentamicin, this has yet to be established in any preclinical models.

There is overwhelming clinical evidence that vestibular ablation is not required for vertigo control.[24] These observations have caused a shift in strategy from vestibular ablation to "chemical alteration." This term describes the clinical goal of balancing vertigo control and hearing loss.

Pharmacokinetics. Intratympanic gentamicin kinetics in the perilymph follows a one-compartment model. Gentamicin rapidly diffuses across the RWM; therefore, the kinetics of gentamicin in perilymph are largely determined by the method of delivery. IT injection has a faster absorption phase, demonstrates higher peak concentrations, and exhibits significantly more variability in all measurements than sustained release delivery methods. In pharmacokinetic studies, large value ranges and standard deviations are characteristic of IT injection delivery.

The pharmacokinetic data generated in animal models appear to fit what occurs in humans. Becvarovski and colleagues devised an in vivo human pharmacokinetic study by recruiting patients who were undergoing either translabyrinthine surgery or labyrinthectomy and exposed them to gentamicin intraoperatively through the facial recess.[25] In these patients, there was rapid diffusion of gentamicin into the perilymph that peaked after 30 minutes. After this peak, concentrations were in a stable range until the limit of their experiment at 110 minutes. While there was no evidence of gentamicin in the cerebrospinal

fluid (CSF), gentamicin was detected in serum shortly after administration, for example, 1 to 2 hours. In summary, this study confirms that rapid diffusion of gentamicin across the round window occurs in humans. Furthermore, this study indicates that the elimination of gentamicin involves crossing the blood-labyrinthine barrier, since gentamicin was detected in the serum shortly after administration.

Clinical Protocols. There are three basic strategies used in IT gentamicin therapy: fixed, titrated, and sustained release protocols. Fixed protocols use a specific dose and number of injections in all patients. Titration protocols adjust the total dose delivered to a predetermined end point, such as paralytic nystagmus, decreased tandem gait, subjective disequilibrium, or more simply relief from vertigo. The supposed advantage of fixed protocols is that each patient receives the same treatment, making outcomes easier to interpret across individuals. The flexible structure of titrated protocols supposedly allows for more control of the ototoxic effects of gentamicin, thereby decreasing the risk of hearing loss.

Much of the controversy in IT gentamicin therapy in the 1990s concerned a form of fixed protocol known as a "shotgun" protocol. The "shotgun" protocol was popularized by Nedzelski and colleagues in 1992.[26] The protocol called for three daily injections for 4 consecutive days of 26.7 mg/mL gentamicin and resulted in a vertigo control rate of 94% and hearing loss rate of 26%. The main argument against the "shotgun" protocols is that they lead to higher rates of hearing loss that is often profound. Atlas and Parnes have pointed out that in "shotgun" protocols, the proportion of patients who experience hearing loss greater than 30 dB (10 to 24%) is much higher than the proportion seen in titration protocols (0 to 4%).[27]

Recently, "hybrid" protocols have been introduced. Quaranta and colleagues used a fixed schedule of two 0.5 mL IT injections of 20 mg/mL gentamicin solution spaced 1 week apart.[28] Patients who did not achieve vertigo control after the first two doses were offered additional doses, up to a total of four doses. This was a prospective study with a control group who refused treatment. At the 2-year follow-up point, the vertigo control rate was 93% versus 47% for the nontreated group. Hearing loss was 7% for the treated group versus 47% for the nontreated group.

Microcatheter delivery method has been advocated to provide sustained gentamicin levels in the perilymph. Schoendorf and colleagues used a pump and microcatheter to deliver 40 mg/d of gentamicin to the RWM.[29] The treatment was continued at this fixed rate until vestibular symptoms appeared (in essence, a titration protocol). While vertigo control was achieved in most patients, 8 of 11 patients treated became deaf.

In a study that epitomizes the microdose, slow perfusion rate strategy, Hoffer and colleagues reported the 2-year results of 27 patients who underwent microcatheter gentamicin therapy.[21]

The study used a solution of 10 mg/mL, at 1 μL/h for 10 days resulting in total dose of 2.4 mg. This strategy achieved vertigo control in 93% of patients, hearing loss in only 4%, tinnitus relief in 63%, and elimination of aural pressure in 74%. Surprisingly, 96% of patients had no decrease in vestibular function.

Practical Considerations. *Delivery.* The argument for using IT injections is that it is the simplest, most cost-effective, and least invasive method of delivery, and from published studies, it provides comparable vertigo control and hearing preservation rates to sustained release protocols. The argument for using sustained release mechanisms is that they may produce lower rates of hearing loss, allow for standardization across individuals, leading to more predictable and uniform results.

Dose. There is no minimum safe dose for IT gentamicin; the lowest documented IT gentamicin dose to produce hearing loss is 0.24 mg. Low-dose protocols use the pediatric formulation of gentamicin, a 10 mg/mL preparation. The adult preparation of 40 mg/mL is often diluted to 30 mg/mL. Comparing outcomes between 30 and 40 mg/mL IT gentamicin preparations has found that both cohorts had similar vertigo control and hearing loss rates, but the 40 mg/mL cohort required fewer injections to achieve these results.

Interval. The injection interval depends on the end point chosen for the study. There is increasing support for spacing the injections over a period of at least a week, primarily because of the delayed onset of gentamicin toxicity. The typical deafferentation syndrome only occurs 3 to 5 days after injection.

Complications. The complication of IT gentamicin treatment is hearing loss. Risk factors for hearing loss have been inconsistently identified across studies, partially due to the substantial differences in protocols. As noted above, Atlas and Parnes argue that "shotgun" protocols result in substantial rates of hearing loss greater than 30 dB (10 to 24%) whereas titration methods report low rates of substantial hearing loss (0 to 3.5%).[27]

Hearing loss reporting in gentamicin trials does not distinguish whether the deficit is due to drug-induced toxicity or the natural consequence of Meniere disease. The long-term hearing outcome for untreated Meniere disease has been reported to be around 30% with medical therapy. This figure is close to the hearing loss rates reported by most IT gentamicin trials. The interesting implication is that any IT gentamicin trial that significantly beats this 30% hearing loss rate of untreated patients may represent an actual prevention of hearing loss.

Acute vestibular deafferentation syndrome should be an anticipated outcome of treatment, and in this sense is not strictly a complication. Acute vestibular deafferentation syndrome, also known as acute chemical labyrinthine upset, is the consequence of unilaterally injuring the vestibular apparatus. This phenomenon usually occurs 3 to 5 days after the injection, with symptoms including vertigo, nausea, oscillopsia, and disequilibrium. Patients can readily distinguish these symptoms from their typical Meniere disease–related symptoms. Gradual resolution occurs in 2 to 4 weeks in most patients.

Indications and Contraindications. The indication for IT gentamicin treatment is the cohort of patients with Meniere disease that have failed conservative therapy and have recurrent vertigo. Conservative therapy consists of a diuretic and diet restrictions (salt, caffeine) and is effective in 70% of cases. Most practitioners only begin to consider IT gentamicin therapy after conservative therapy has failed for at least 1 year. After this time, low-pressure pulse therapy, IT corticosteroids, IT gentamicin, and endolymphatic sac surgery are considered. Sennaroglu and colleagues argued that it is reasonable to try using IT corticosteroids before using IT gentamicin.[12] In a prospective study that compared IT dexamethasone ($n = 24$) versus gentamicin ($n = 16$), they found that vertigo control rates were 72 and 75%, respectively. However, IT gentamicin was considerably more cochleotoxic than IT corticosteroids. Labyrinthectomy and vestibular nerve section are reserved for only the most severe and refractory cases.

Some practitioners recommend that elderly patients be treated with caution, as central compensation for peripheral vestibular loss is less effective in this cohort. Bilateral Meniere disease (incidence of 15 to 30%) is considered by some to be a contraindication for unilateral IT gentamicin treatment, because if hearing loss results from treatment, the remaining ear may be vulnerable to hearing loss as a natural course of the disease. Patients with no serviceable hearing in the problematic ear are generally considered candidates for labyrinthectomy, but it seems reasonable that the low-morbidity, low-cost IT gentamicin protocol be attempted in these patients before surgery is considered.

There is some debate as to whether otologic surgery is a contraindication to IT gentamicin treatment. Initial studies demonstrated poor vertigo control after endolymphatic surgery. However, more recent work has achieved the opposite effect with complete vertigo control and no effect on hearing outcomes in a cohort of five patients following endolymphatic surgery.[30] The importance of this debate is that several practitioners advocate endolymphatic shunt procedures before resorting to IT gentamicin when treating intractable vertigo in Meniere disease patients.

Conclusions on the Use of Intratympanic Gentamicin. In a meta-analysis by Cohen-Kerem and colleagues of studies that used IT gentamicin as the only method of treatment and reported results according to American Academy of Otolaryngology-Head and Neck Surgery Foundation guidelines for Meniere disease, they found that, from an inclusion group of 15 studies, complete class A control was achieved in 74.7% of patients and complete or substantial class B control was achieved in 92.7% of patients.[31] Furthermore, the success rate of vertigo control was not affected by treatment regimen (fixed vs titrated), and hearing level and word recognition scores did not seem to be adversely affected by either treatment regimen when compared to control groups. Similar analyses have found comparable vertigo control rates with increased deafness.[32] Using these data, IT gentamicin using low dose with long inter-therapy intervals could justifiably become the treatment of choice for medically recalcitrant Meniere disease, especially when hearing is poor in the affected ear.

GENE THERAPY OF THE INNER EAR

The simple and powerful objective of gene transfer technology is to introduce a "therapeutic gene," for example, a normal version of the defective gene, into appropriate target cells of the affected individual. Expression of the exogenous "therapeutic gene" would alter the target cell and the clinical phenotype.

Both viral and nonviral vectors have been used to transfer and express genes in the inner ear of animal models. Individual virions represent a highly efficient means of introducing the viral genome into the nuclei of target cells followed by the use of the cellular machinery to express the viral genes. These viral agents have been adapted for the purpose of gene transfer by altering their genome so that they can no longer replicate within the transduced cell and lead to cellular lysis. These replication defective viruses are engineered to function solely to introduce the desired gene into the nuclei of target cells. Viral vectors have been developed from both DNA (eg, adenovirus, adeno-associated virus and herpes simplex virus) and RNA (eg, retrovirus and influenza viruses).

Viral Vectors in Intracochlear Gene Therapy

Feasibility of gene therapy for inner ear pathology was initially demonstrated through intracochlear transgene expression using the guinea pig as an animal model.[33] A viral vector derived from the adeno-associated virus (AAV) was used to deliver a marker transgene to the cochlea via steady state infusion using an osmotic mini-pump. Based upon expression of the marker transgene encoding a bacterial enzyme β-galactosidase, the AAV vector was found to transduce the spiral limbus, spiral ligament, spiral ganglion, and the organ of Corti. Subsequent studies investigating intracochlear gene transfer have characterized a variety of different vectors for their efficacy and safety as well as their mode of introduction into the cochlea.

The adenoviral (Ad) vector represents one of the well-characterized viral vectors used for intracochlear gene transfer. The attributes of the adenoviral vector for gene transfer include its capacity to carry large transgenes (8 kB), generating them at high titer in both dividing and nondividing cells. The major disadvantage associated with the use of first generation Ad vector was the strong immune response that it elicited. Subsequent development of adenoviral vectors has generated attenuated viruses with complete deletion of viral protein sequences, leaving a vector with all the advantages and diminishing, if not eliminating, its immunogenicity.[34]

A lentiviral vector, based on the human immunodeficiency virus (HIV), can integrate into the chromosome of both dividing and nondividing or mitotically quiescent cells leading to a potentially stable, long-term expression of a transgene spliced into the viral vector. Thus, the postmitotic cochlea neuroepithelia and the spiral ganglion neurons (SGNs) represent suitable targets for a stable long-term transgene expression via lentivirus-mediated gene transfer. Restricted transduction of cell types confined to the periphery of the perilymphatic space by the lentivirus is ideal for stable production of gene products secreted into the perilymph (Figure 3).

Nonviral Vectors for Intracochlear Gene Transfer

In addition to viral vectors, cationic lipid vesicles or liposomes have also been used for intracochlear gene transfer. The liposome, coupled to the transgene integrated within a plasmid vector, binds to the plasma membrane of the target cells, releasing the DNA into the cytoplasm where it is eventually incorporated into the host genome. Liposome vectors are nonimmunogenic and are easy to produce. Furthermore, the DNA introduced into the host cell is incorporated by recombination, so there is little risk of insertional mutagenesis. The drawback of liposome vectors is a low transfection rate compared with other vectors. The feasibility of inner ear gene transfer with liposome vectors has been demonstrated. The attributes of the vectors that have been used in intracochlear gene transfer are summarized in Table 2.

Suitable Animal Models for Gene Therapy of the Inner Ear

Preliminary studies in intracochlear gene therapy used the guinea pig as the animal model due to the relatively large size of its cochlea compared to mice and rats and the ease of surgical manipulation in this species. Subsequent studies are shifting their focus toward the mouse as the preferred model. The mouse genome is the most extensively characterized of all mammalian model organisms.

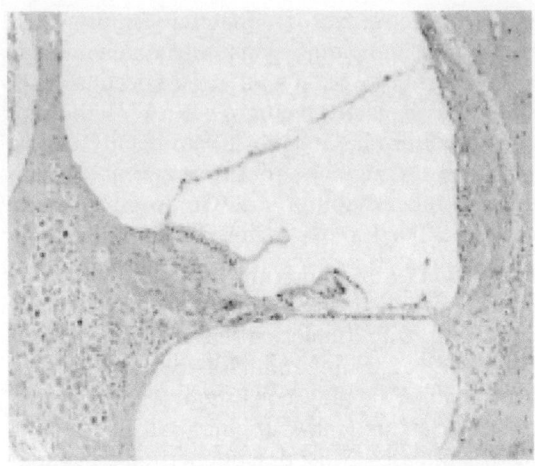

(A)

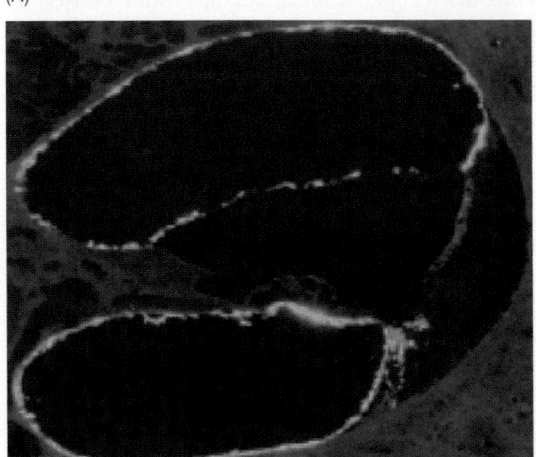

(B)

Figure 3 Intracochlear transgene expression in the guinea pig. Expression of the transgene is dependent on a variety of factors including the choice of vector. The expression of the transgene using a liposome vector (A) and a lentivirus vector (B) is shown, respectively. With the use of liposomes, ß-galactosidase (β-gal) transgene expression is seen in the stria vascularis, spiral ligament, Reissner membrane, spiral ganglion cells, and the organ of Corti (A). In contrast, with the use of a lentivirus, green fluorescent protein (GFP) transgene expression is limited to spiral ligament, Reissner membrane, and the lining of the scala vestibuli and scala tympani (B). (Published with permission, copyright © 2007 Anil K. Lalwani, MD.)

The intrinsic value of the mouse as a model in hearing research is seen in the availability of a number of mutant mice with inherited hearing loss. These mutant mice have been well characterized, and the genetic basis of their hearing loss is identified. Furthermore, established in vitro and in vivo rodent models for ototoxic sensorineural damage to the inner ear exist.

Delivery Modalities for Gene Therapy of the Inner Ear

Local biological transfer to the inner ear is feasible because of its relatively closed anatomy. However, developing a delivery method for genetic vectors/cells to the inner ear without causing local destruction and concomitant hearing loss is a significant obstacle. The general strategy behind these delivery modalities is to introduce the transgene-carrying vector into the inner ear fluid, enabling its diffusion to the surrounding tissues. Most of the delivery methods introduce the gene into the perilymphatic fluid. These methods include microinjection via the round window membrane, microinjection or mini-osmotic pump infusion following cochleostomy, and diffusion across the round window membrane after local Gelfoam placement (Figure 1). Gene transfer vectors have also been introduced into the endolymphatic fluid through injection into the endolymphatic sac or into the scala media following cochleostomy.

Histologically, introduction of viral vectors with a mini-osmotic pump was characterized by an inflammatory response and connective tissue deposition at the basal turn adjacent to the cochleostomy site, with associated increase of auditory brainstem response (ABR) thresholds at higher frequencies.[35] Systemic dexamethasone-induced immunosuppression has also been shown to largely protect the inoculated ear from threshold shift and appears to improve Ad vector–based gene expression.[36]

A much less traumatic alternative to cochleostomy is microinjection through the round window membrane. Histologically, cochleae microinjected through the round window demonstrate after 2 weeks intact cochlear cytoarchitecture and an absence of inflammatory response with no hearing dysfunction.

To avoid potential hearing loss associated with the direct manipulation of the cochlea, gene transfer vectors and stem cells have also been delivered through the vestibular apparatus via semicircular canal fenestration to the perilymph and through the endolymphatic sac to the endolymph.

As a treatment for spiral ganglion neuronal damage, the direct delivery of vectors to the auditory nerve is feasible. Access to the auditory nerve is routinely achieved in the human patient for neoplasm removal and treatment of incapacitating vertigo. The modiolus and the auditory nerve have been successfully accessed in animal models.

Table 2 Characteristics of Gene Transfer Vectors Used in the Inner Ear								
Vector	Genome	Insert Size	Site	Efficiency	Cell Division	Expression	Advantages	Disadvantages
Adeno-associated virus	SsDNA	4.5 kB	Genome	Variable	Not required	Permanent	No human disease	Difficult to produce
Retrovirus	RNA	6–7 kB	Genome	Low	Required	Permanent	Suited for neoplastic cells	Insertional mutagenesis
Adenovirus	DsDNA	7.5 kB	Episome	Moderate	Not required	Transient	Ease of production	Inflammatory response
Herpes simplex virus	DsDNA	10–100 kB	Episome	Moderate	Not required	Transient	Neural tropism	Human disease
Plasmid	RNA/DNA	Unlimited	Episome	Very low	Not required	Transient	Safe, easy production	Low transfection
Liposome	RNA/DNA	Unlimited	Episome	Very low	Not required	Transient	Safe, easy production	Low transfection

The potential for surgical trauma, inflammation, and hearing loss associated with infusion or microinjection techniques has led to the investigation of a less invasive delivery method to the cochlea. The potential to deliver a variety of vectors across an intact round window membrane by loading vectors onto a Gelfoam patch has been explored. Adenovirus and liposome vectors but not the AAV vector have successfully transfected cochlear tissues.

Preclinical Applications of Gene Therapy

The preclinical applications of gene transfer in the inner ear have focused upon four broad areas. The first application was to demonstrate the protective effects of various neurotrophins and growth factors in certain ototoxic circumstances. Secondly, gene therapy technology has been used to introduce antioxidant gene overexpression as a technique of ameliorating aminoglycoside-induced oxidative stress. Finally, gene transfer technology has been used to induce the differentiation of nonsensory organ of Corti cells toward hair cell fates, a preliminary step toward hair cell regeneration.

Certain neurotrophins and growth factors, including brain-derived neurotrophic factor (BDNF), neurotrophin-3 (NT-3), and glial cell line–derived neurotrophic factor (GDNF), have been expressed within the cochlea as transgenic products. These agents have served to protect sensory hair cells and the primary auditory neurons against atrophy and degeneration. Staecker and colleagues, in 1998, used a herpes simplex virus-1 (HSV-1) vector to deliver BDNF to the inner ear and assessed its protective effect against neomycin.[37] This gene therapy group demonstrated a 94.7% salvage rate for SGNs, in contrast to a 64.3% loss of SGNs in control animals.

Both in vitro and in vivo models have been used to test the protective effect of AAV-mediated BDNF expression.[38] A significant survival of SGNs in cochlear explants transduced with AAV-BDNF and challenged with aminoglycoside relative to controls was observed. In the in vivo experiment, animals infused with AAV-BDNF with an osmotic mini-pump displayed enhanced SGN survival. The protection from AAV-BDNF therapy was region-specific; there was protection at the basal turn of the cochlea but not in the middle or apical turn. The authors proposed that this regional selectivity is a pharmacokinetic phenomenon.

NT-3-mediated protection against cisplatin-induced ototoxicity has been documented using an HSV-1-derived viral vector. The efficacy of the vector was established in an in vitro study, in which HSV-1-mediated transfer of NT-3 (demonstrated by production of NT-3 mRNA proteins and by reporter gene expression) conferred increased survival to cochlear explants after cisplatin exposure.[39] These HSV-1 effects were confirmed in an in vivo model, in which HSV-1-mediated transfer of NT-3 to SGNs suppressed cisplatin-induced apoptosis and necrosis.

The efficacy of an Ad vector carrying the GDNF gene (Ad.GDNF) to protect against a variety of ototoxic insults has been established. When administered prior to aminoglycoside challenge, Ad.GDNF significantly protects cochlear and vestibular hair cells from death. Pretreatment with Ad.GDNF also provides significant protection against noise-induced trauma and transient cochlear ischemia.[40–41] Finally, Ad.GDNF enhances SGN survival when administered 4 to 7 days after ototoxic deafening with aminoglycosides.

Antioxidants represent a potential therapeutic tool to counter the destructive effects of reactive oxygen species that are considered to be triggered by aminoglycoside-induced ototoxicity.[42–43] Recently, inner ear gene therapy has been used to corroborate the protective effects of antioxidants against aminoglycoside-mediated ototoxicity.[44] Catalase and superoxide dismutase (SOD2) were introduced into the cochleae of guinea pigs, which were subsequently challenged with kanamycin and ethacrynic acid. The catalase and SOD2-expressing animals preserved their auditory brainstem thresholds and had significantly less hair cell loss when compared to control animals.

Inner ear gene therapy has also been used to verify the molecular "switch" responsible for turning on the genetic program for supporting cell differentiation toward a hair cell fate. Math 1 is a basic helix loop helix transcription factor that is a master regulator gene in hair cell differentiation during cochlear development. To convert supporting, nonsensory cells phenotypically to hair cells *Math 1* gene overexpression was used.[45] Following Ad vector introduction, *Math 1* transgene expression occurred mostly in supporting cells. Furthermore, 30 to 60 days following the transfer, rudimentary hair cells were identified with electron microscopy, and myosin VIIa was immunohistochemically verified in ectopic locations near the organ of Corti. These "new" immature hair cells appeared to act as target sites for axon fibers that extended over a 50 µm range toward the newly formed ectopic hair cells. These results have been extended by introducing *Math 1* into supporting cells of deafened guinea pigs through adenovirus transfection.[46] Transfected animals showed phenotypically normal inner hair cells and a recovery of ABR levels to normal. These findings demonstrate the potential of gene therapy to coax a damaged mammalian ear toward regeneration via phenotypic transdifferentiation of nonsensory cells in the organ of Corti.

Risks and Limitations of Inner Ear Gene Therapy

Major risk factors associated with the introduction of either genes or cells into the inner ear are twofold: damage to the cochlear structure and function as a consequence of the delivery modality and the relative safety of the biological material transferred. Delivery modalities that prevent damage to the cochlear structure and function have been described above. The safety of the gene transfer agent is determined by assessing its immunogenicity, toxicity, and unwanted dissemination of the therapeutic agent outside of the target region.

Utilizing AAV as the gene therapy vector, transgene expression within the contralateral cochlea of the AAV perfused animal has been observed, albeit much weaker than within the directly perfused cochlea.[33] Expression of the transgene away from the intended target site, that is, within the contralateral cochlea, raises concern about the risks associated with dissemination of the virus from the target tissue. The appearance of the virus, distant from the site of infection, may be due to its hematogenous dissemination to near and distant tissues. However, this is unlikely due to the absence of the viral vector in near and distant tissues. Other possible explanations include migration of AAV via the bone marrow space of the temporal bone or via the CSF space to the contralateral ear.[47] The perilymphatic space into which the virus was perfused is directly connected to the CSF via the cochlea aqueduct; transgene expression within the contralateral cochlea aqueduct has been demonstrated following introduction of the viral vector in the ipsilateral cochlea. Collectively, these results suggest that potential routes for AAV dissemination from the infused cochlea are via the cochlea aqueduct or by extension through the temporal bone marrow spaces.

Conclusions on Gene Therapy in the Inner Ear

A critical step forward toward the eventual application of gene therapy for hearing disorders has been accomplished: viral and nonviral vectors have been shown to be able to introduce and express exogenous genes into the peripheral part of the auditory system. Future refinements will include the development of newer hybrid vectors that assimilate the infectivity and stability of the viral vectors and the safety of liposomes. The hybrid vectors will largely replace the current generation of vectors. The preferred mode of introduction of gene therapy vectors will be those that minimize tissue damage and hearing loss, such as microinjection or application of the vector at the RWM. Safety concerns, specially regional and distant dissemination of the therapeutic agent, will have to be monitored and minimized.

REFERENCES

1. Alzamil KS, Linthicum FH, Jr. Extraneous round window membranes and plugs: Possible effect on intratympanic therapy. Ann Otol Rhinol Laryngol 2000;109:30–2.
2. Plontke SK, Wood AW, Salt AN. Analysis of gentamicin kinetics in fluids of the inner ear with round window administration. Otol Neurotol 2002;23:967–74.
3. Sha SH, Taylor R, Forge A, Schacht J. Differential vulnerability of basal and apical hair cells is based on intrinsic susceptibility to free radicals. Hear Res 2001;155:1–8.
4. Plontke SK, Plinkert PK, Plinkert B, et al. Transtympanic endoscopy for drug delivery to the inner ear using a new microendoscope. Adv Otorhinolaryngol 2002;59:149–55.
5. Sheppard WM, Wanamaker HH, Pack A, et al. Direct round window application of gentamicin with varying delivery vehicles: A comparison of ototoxicity. Otolaryngol Head Neck Surg 2004;131:890–6.

6. Praetorius M, Limberger A, Muller M, et al. A novel microperfusion system for the long-term local supply of drugs to the inner ear: Implantation and function in the rat model. Audiol Neurootol 2001;6:250–8.

7. Parnes LS, Sun AH, Freeman DJ. Corticosteroid pharmacokinetics in the inner ear fluids: An animal study followed by clinical application. Laryngoscope 1999;109:1–17.

8. Yang GS, Song HT, Keithley EM, Harris JP. Intratympanic immunosuppressives for prevention of immune-mediated sensorineural hearing loss. Am J Otol 2000;21:499–504.

9. Dallan I, Bruschini L, Nacci A, et al. Transtympanic steroids as a salvage therapy in sudden hearing loss: Preliminary results. ORL J Otorhinolaryngol Relat Spec 2006;68:247–52.

10. Chandrasekhar SS, Rubinstein RY, Kwartler JA, et al. Dexamethasone pharmacokinetics in the inner ear: Comparison of route of administration and use of facilitating agents. Otolaryngol Head Neck Surg 2000;122:521–8.

11. Itoh A, Sakata E. Treatment of vestibular disorders. Acta Otolaryngol Suppl 1991;481:617–23.

12. Sennaroglu L, Sennaroglu G, Gursel B, Dini FM. Intratympanic dexamethasone, intratympanic gentamicin, and endolymphatic sac surgery for intractable vertigo in Meniere's disease. Otolaryngol Head Neck Surg 2001;125:537–43.

13. Arriaga MA, Goldman S. Hearing results of intratympanic steroid treatment of endolymphatic hydrops. Laryngoscope 1998;108:1682–5.

14. Silverstein H, Isaacson JE, Olds MJ, et al. Dexamethasone inner ear perfusion for the treatment of Meniere's disease: A prospective, randomized, double-blind, crossover trial. Am J Otol 1998;19:196–201.

15. Himeno C, Komeda M, Izumikawa M, et al. Intracochlear administration of dexamethasone attenuates aminoglycoside ototoxicity in the guinea pig. Hear Res 2002;167:61–70.

16. Gianoli GJ, Li JC. Transtympanic steroids for treatment of sudden hearing loss. Otolaryngol Head Neck Surg 2001;125:142–6.

17. Schuknecht HF. Ablation therapy in the management of Meniere's disease. Acta Otolaryngol Suppl 1957;132:1–42.

18. Beck C, Schmidt CL. 10 years of experience with intratympanally applied streptomycin (gentamycin) in the therapy of Morbus Meniere. Arch Otorhinolaryngol 1978;221:149–52.

19. Hilton M, Chen J, Kakigi A, et al. Middle ear instillation of gentamicin and streptomycin in chinchillas: Electrophysiological appraisal of selective ototoxicity. Clin Otorhinolaryngol Allied Sci 2002;27:529–35.

20. Wanamaker HH, Slepecky NB, Cefaratti LK, Ogata Y. Comparison of vestibular and cochlear ototoxicity from transtympanic streptomycin administration. Am J Otol 1999;20:457–64.

21. Hoffer ME, Kopke RD, Weisskopf P, et al. Use of the round window microcatheter in the treatment of Meniere's disease. Laryngoscope 2001;111:2046–9.

22. Lang H, Liu C. Apoptosis and hair cell degeneration in the vestibular sensory epithelia of the guinea pig following a gentamicin insult. Hear Res 1997;111:177–84.

23. Ge X, Shea JJ, Jr. Scanning electron microscopic observation of dark cells after streptomycin perfusion of the vestibule in guinea pigs. Scanning Microsc 1995;9:283–8.

24. Diamond C, O'Connell DA, Hornig JD, Liu R. Systematic review of intratympanic gentamicin in Meniere's disease. J Otolaryngol 2003;32:351–61.

25. Becvarovski Z, Bojrab DI, Michaelides EM, et al. Round window gentamicin absorption: An in vivo human model. Laryngoscope 2002;112:1610–3.

26. Nedzelski JM, Schessel DA, Bryce GE, Pfleiderer AG. Chemical labyrinthectomy: Local application of gentamicin for the treatment of unilateral Meniere's disease. Am J Otol 1992;13:18–22.

27. Atlas J, Parnes LS. Intratympanic gentamicin for intractable Meniere's disease: 5-year follow-up. J Otolaryngol 2003;32:288–93.

28. Quaranta A, Aloisi A, De Benedittis G, Scaringi A. Intratympanic therapy for Meniere's disease. High-concentration gentamicin with round-window protection. Ann N Y Acad Sci 1999;884:410–24.

29. Schoendorf J, Neugebauer P, Michel O. Continuous intratympanic infusion of gentamicin via a microcatheter in Meniere's disease. Otolaryngol Head Neck Surg 2001;124:203–7.

30. Gouveris H, Lange G, Mann WJ. Intratympanic gentamicin treatment after endolymphatic sac surgery. Acta Otolaryngol 2005;125:1180–3.

31. Cohen-Kerem R, Kisilevsky V, Einarson TR, et al. Intratympanic gentamicin for Meniere's disease: A meta-analysis. Laryngoscope 2004;114:2085–91.

32. Chia SH, Gamst AC, Anderson JP, Harris JP. Intratympanic gentamicin therapy for Meniere's disease: A meta-analysis. Otol Neurotol 2004;25:544–52.

33. Lalwani AK, Walsh BJ, Reilly PG, et al. Development of in vivo gene therapy for hearing disorders: Introduction of adeno-associated virus into the cochlea of the guinea pig. Gene Ther 1996;3:588–92.

34. Amalfitano A, Parks RJ. Separating fact from fiction: Assessing the potential of modified adenovirus vectors for use in human gene therapy. Curr Gene Ther 2002;2:111–33.

35. Carvalho GJ, Lalwani AK. The effect of cochleostomy and intracochlear infusion on auditory brain stem response threshold in the guinea pig. Am J Otol 1999;20:87–90.

36. Ishimoto S, Kawamoto K, Stover T, et al. A glucocorticoid reduces adverse effects of adenovirus vectors in the cochlea. Audiol Neurootol 2003;8:70–9.

37. Staecker H, Gabaizadeh R, Federoff H, Van De Water TR. Brain-derived neurotrophic factor gene therapy prevents spiral ganglion degeneration after hair cell loss. Otolaryngol Head Neck Surg 1998;119:7–13.

38. Lalwani AK, Han JJ, Castelein CM, et al. In vitro and in vivo assessment of the ability of adeno-associated virus-brain-derived neurotrophic factor to enhance spiral ganglion cell survival following ototoxic insult. Laryngoscope 2002;112:1325–34.

39. Chen X, Frisina RD, Bowers WJ, et al. HSV ampliconmediated neurotrophin-3 expression protects murine spiral ganglion neurons from cisplatin-induced damage. Mol Ther 2001;3:958–63.

40. Hakuba N, Watabe K, Hyodo J, et al. Adenovirus-mediated overexpression of a gene prevents hearing loss and progressive inner hair cell loss after transient cochlear ischemia in gerbils. Gene Ther 2003;10:426–33.

41. Yamasoba T, Schacht J, Shoji F, Miller JM. Attenuation of cochlear damage from noise trauma by an iron chelator, a free radical scavenger and glial cell line-derived neurotrophic factor in vivo. Brain Res 1999;815:317–25.

42. McFadden SL, Ding D, Salvemini D, Salvi RJ. M40403, a superoxide dismutase mimetic, protects cochlear hair cells from gentamicin, but not cisplatin toxicity. Toxicol Appl Pharmacol 2003;186:46–54.

43. Takumida M, Popa R, Anniko M. Free radicals in the guinea pig inner ear following gentamicin exposure. ORL J Otorhinolaryngol Relat Spec 1999;61:63–70.

44. Kawamoto K, Sha SH, Minoda R, et al. Antioxidant gene therapy can protect hearing and hair cells from ototoxicity. Mol Ther 2004;9:173–81.

45. Kawamoto K, Ishimoto S, Minoda R, et al. Math1 gene transfer generates new cochlear hair cells in mature guinea pigs in vivo. J Neurosci 2003;23:4395–400.

46. Izumikawa M, Minoda R, Kawamoto K, et al. Auditory hair cell replacement and hearing improvement by Atoh1 gene therapy in deaf mammals. Nat Med 2005;11:271–6.

47. Kho ST, Pettis RM, Mhatre AN, Lalwani AK. Safety of adeno-associated virus as cochlear gene transfer vector: Analysis of distant spread beyond injected cochleae. Mol Ther 2000;2:368–73.

6

Hair Cell Regeneration

Ricardo Cristobal, MD, PhD
Paul Popper, PhD
Fred A. Pereira, PhD

Hearing loss is a disability that affects approximately 1.7% of children under age 18. The incidence increases with age: approximately 31% of people over the age of 65 and 40 to 50% of people 75 years and older have hearing loss.[1] According to World Health Organization estimates from 2005, approximately 278 million people worldwide have moderate to profound hearing loss in both ears. In a large majority of cases, hearing loss is the result of degeneration and death of hair cells and their associated spiral ganglion cells. This can result from accumulated or acute exposure to excessive noise, including loud work environments, increased use of portable electronic devices, and other loud noises, such as gunfire or explosions. Other common causes include infections and the use of ototoxic drugs. Hearing loss can impose a heavy social and economic burden on individuals, families, communities, and countries.

Children with hearing impairment often experience delayed development of speech, language, and cognitive skills, which may result in slow learning and difficulty progressing in school. In adults, hearing impairment and deafness often make it difficult to obtain, perform, and keep employment. As a result of hearing impairment, both children and adults may suffer from social stigmatization and isolation. The cost of special education and lost employment due to hearing impairment can also impose a substantial economic burden. Furthermore, loss of hair cells in the vestibular end organs of the inner ear can lead to balance disorders with significant associated morbidity and change in quality of life, particularly in the elderly.

Ultimately, the treatment of sensorineural deafness will require maintenance, repair, or regeneration of the structures involved. In a simplified model, restoration of inner ear function requires anatomical restoration of the hair cells of the sensory epithelia and associated structures and the formation of new, functional, and meaningful connections between hair cells and afferent and efferent neural elements. For some time it was thought that the vertebrate inner ear sensory epithelium lacked the ability to regenerate. However, over the past 25 years this concept gradually changed as studies in several different vertebrate species demonstrated various degrees of hair cell regeneration following acute loss of preexisting hair cells. In general, the term regeneration is used to describe mitotic division of progenitor cells within the tissue and their differentiation into mature specialized cells capable of restoring normal function. Yet in certain tissues such as peripheral nerves, the term regeneration refers to regrowth of neuronal axons without an intervening cell division. In the inner ear, sensory epithelia hair cell regeneration refers to restoration of the hair cell population and is thought to result from various mechanisms, individually or in combination: (1) proliferation of hair cell progenitors through mitotic division; (2) transdifferentiation of surrounding supporting cells; (3) repair of partially damaged hair cells; and (4) migration and differentiation of nonsensory epithelial cells.

Multiple experimental protocols have been designed to investigate the biological processes of hair cell origin, proliferation, and differentiation following the destruction of preexisting hair cells. In in vivo models, hair cells have been damaged with laser beams (fish lateral line organ hair cells), ototoxic drugs (vestibular and auditory hair cells), or with sound trauma (auditory hair cells). These experiments provided information about the existence and degree of hair cell regeneration in the normal adult vertebrate under physiologic conditions. In in vitro organ culture experiments, hair cells have been damaged with laser beams or with ototoxic drugs, and the process of regeneration has been evaluated directly, with time-lapse video microscopy, or indirectly, in histological preparations of organs fixed at different times after treatment. One characteristic of organ culture conditions is that the relative contributions to new hair cell formation of systemic factors such as inflammation cells and mediators are eliminated. But, in a third group of experimental protocols, the sensory epithelia of adult and developing ears were dissociated and dispersed cells were cultured, minimizing the effects of the normal physical and chemical interactions that occur between contiguous cells in the putative tissue. In all 3 experimental paradigms, mitotic tracers have allowed quantification of the process of cell division and subsequent differentiation. Newer lines of hair cell regeneration research have focused on the identification of genes that trigger the cellular program of hair cell development. Research on inner ear development has produced considerable information regarding extracellular soluble molecules that regulate the process of cell differentiation, cell–cell contact proteins that regulate patterning of the sensory epithelia, and intracellular signaling pathways and transcription factors that control the cell cycle. This information has proved invaluable in understanding hair cell regeneration in the adult animal. Progress also has been made in understanding the mechanisms that govern hair cell survival and repair. Attenuation of hair cell death has been achieved with the application of neurotrophic factors, antioxidants and antiapoptotic agents. The immune system has also been shown to play an important role in this process.[2]

Studies in the last few years have demonstrated that the inner ear sensory epithelia of adult mammals contain stem cells capable of dividing indefinitely and of generating multiple cell types. This has raised hopes for restoring damaged inner ears by stimulating these cells in the putative epithelium or by transplanting these cells into the damaged ear to replace lost hair cells. This exciting and promising discovery also affords new avenues for investigating the molecular mechanisms that govern hair cell formation. This chapter reviews the field of hair cell regeneration as it has evolved over the past quarter century. A large body of literature has been produced during this time period.

VERTEBRATE INNER EAR ANATOMICAL ORGANIZATION

The inner ear of vertebrates contains vestibular organs capable of sensing gravitational pull, vibrations of the ground, linear and angular acceleration of the head and auditory organs that detect sound pressure waves. Both the auditory and the vestibular end organs have specialized patches of neurosensory epithelia that transduce mechanical stimuli into chemical signals, which are ultimately conveyed to the brain through the afferent innervation. The general organization of the vestibular sensory epithelia is common to all vertebrate organs and consists of sensory hair cells, supporting cells, afferent and efferent nerve terminals, and a membrane overlying the apical surface of the cells (Figure 1). The hair cells are the mechanotransducers: they have specialized stereocilia in the apical portion of the cell that are deflected during appropriate mechanical stimulation. This leads to depolarization or hyperpolarization of the cell's membrane and results in change in neurotransmitter release and consequent modulation of the afferent neuron activity. The basal firing rate of afferent neurons increases or decreases with hair cell depolarization or hyperpolarization, respectively.

In the vestibular epithelia of higher vertebrates, 2 types of hair cells with different morphological characteristics and electrophysiological properties have been identified: type I hair cells, which are surrounded by cup-shaped, chaliceal afferent nerve endings and which are thought to be more highly differentiated; and, type II hair cells, which receive only bouton-type afferent nerve endings. The hair cells occupy the portion of the epithelium closest to the lumen and rest on their surrounding supporting cells. Unlike hair cells, the supporting cell bodies in the vestibular sensory epithelia are tightly packed together and rest on the basal membrane, with their nuclei aligned adjacent to it. Their cytoplasms span the entire thickness of the epithelium, from the basal lamina to the lumen of the end organ and are interspersed between hair cells so that two hair cells never touch each other.

The avian vestibular system is structurally, developmentally, and functionally similar to the mammalian vestibular system.[3] Discovery of hair cell regeneration in the avian vestibular epithelia led to speculation and demonstration that hair cell regeneration takes place in the mammalian vestibular system as well.[4] The auditory epithelium on the other hand has evolved separately in birds and mammals and has different structural organization[5] (Figure 2). In humans, the auditory epithelia contain 3 rows of outer hair cells and 1 row of inner hair cells. The supporting cells surround the hair cells and fluid filled spaces in a more intricate arrangement. Structural and possibly molecular differences among classes may account for the capability of spontaneous regeneration of the avian but not the mammalian auditory epithelia. While the hair cells and afferent neurons have been the subject of intense investigation for many years, the supporting cells have been assumed to play mostly a structural role and have received little attention. Recent studies on hair cell regeneration have suggested that supporting cells contribute to the generation of new hair cells in the adult vertebrate ear, and this has raised the level of interest in this cell type.

HAIR CELL REGENERATION

Fish and Amphibians

For many years, it was believed that vertebrates were born with the full complement of inner ear hair cells, and that those lost throughout the life of the animal were never replaced. However, quantitative studies performed in 1981 demonstrated that 80% of the inner ear hair cells in adult sharks are produced in the postnatal period.[6] The majority of the new hair cells are produced in a germinal zone at the edges of the epithelia. This original study sparked a great deal of interest in the production of hair cells beyond the embryonic period. Cell division and postnatal production of new hair cells in the peripheral growth zone of the inner ear sensory epithelia was documented next in amphibians by demonstrating the incorporation of mitotic tracers into dividing epithelial cells and the subsequent localization of the tracer in newly formed hair cells.[7] The natural next step was to investigate the possibility of hair cell regeneration following loss of preexisting ones.

Fish and amphibians have a specialized organ along the sides of their bodies termed the lateral line, which is stimulated by water currents and micromovements around their body (Figure 3). Immediately beneath the skin are hair cells that are similar to their inner ear counterparts. This organ provides an optimal model for direct visualization of hair cell formation in live animals. Time-lapse videomicroscopy of the lateral line was carried out following selective ablation of hair cells with a laser microbeam.[8] This provided the first direct evidence of an increased rate of supporting cell division and subsequent differentiation of the progeny into supporting cells and new hair cells. Other in vivo studies delivered gentamicin to the bullfrog perilymphatic space and established a dose that induces complete hair

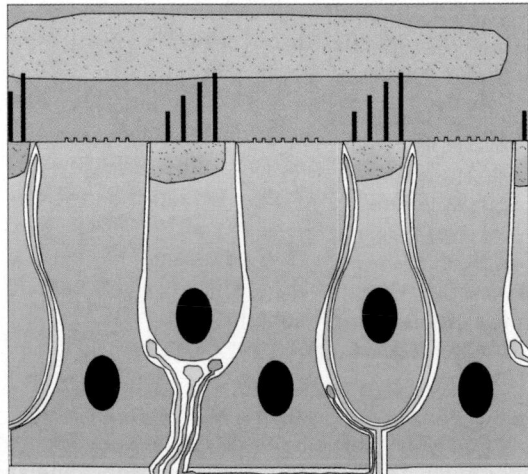

Figure 1 Graphic representation of the general organization of the vertebrate vestibular sensory epithelia. Supporting cells rest on the basal membrane with their nuclei basally oriented and aligned. Their cytoplasm spans the full thickness of the epithelium. Hair cells rest on the supporting cells. Type I hair cells are flask shaped and are surrounded by chaliceal afferent nerve endings. Type II hair cells are cylindrical and receive bouton-type afferent nerve endings. Efferent nerve endings are bouton-type endings that contact both chaliceal endings and type I hair cells. Gel matrix rests over the kinocilia.

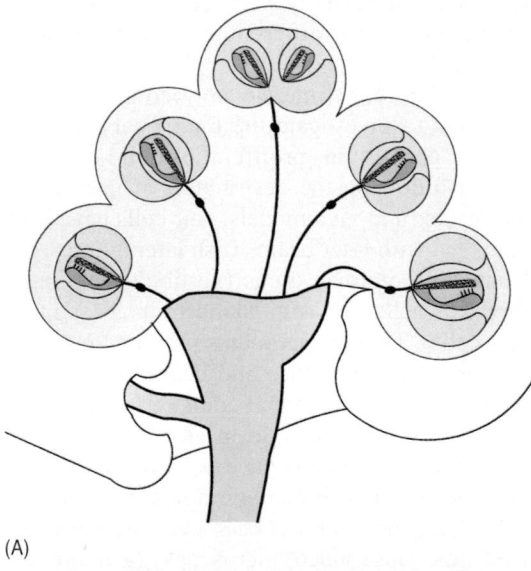

(A)

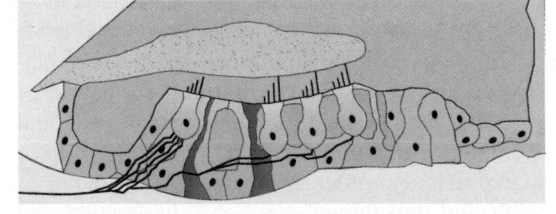

(B)

Figure 2 Depiction of the mammalian auditory organ. (A) The cochlear sensory epithelium is coiled around an axis, the modiolus, which contains the neuronal cell bodies. (B) The cochlear hair cells form 1 row of inner hair cells that receive the majority of the afferent innervation and 3 rows of outer hair cells. The inner and outer hair cells are separated by supporting cells and fluid-filled tunnels.

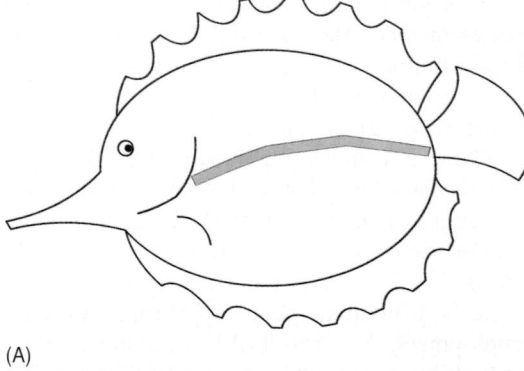

(A)

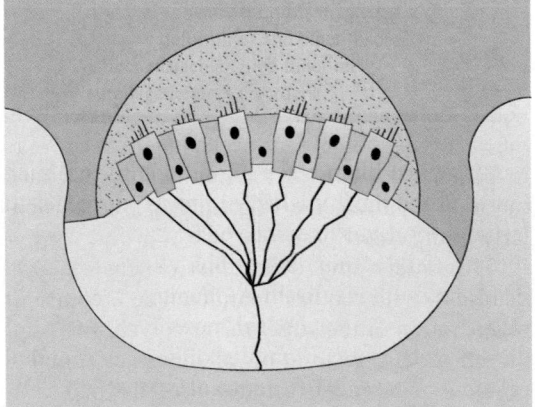

(B)

Figure 3 Representation of the lateral line of fishes. (A) The lateral line spans the length of the animal body (*dark line*). (B) Magnified cross section of 1 canal, illustrating the structure of the sensory organ, composed mainly of hair cells, supporting cells, afferent nerves, and a gelatinous cupula overlying the epithelium. This organ is sensitive to sound pressure waves and to movement of the surrounding fluid.

cell destruction with minimal disruption of other components of the sensory epithelium.[9] After a time there was recovery of the hair cell number and restoration of vestibular afferent response to stimuli, suggesting that new functional connections do indeed form between afferent neurons and the regenerated sensory hair cells.[10]

In parallel studies, vestibular sensory epithelia of bullfrogs were microdissected, and cells dissociated and placed in culture. The in vitro preparation allowed direct microscopic documentation of supporting cell division and asymmetrical differentiation of the progeny into hair cells and round cells. This demonstrated that vestibular sensory epithelia of adult animals contain precursor cells capable of generating new hair cells and that mitotic division is a mechanism for new hair cell formation in vitro.[11]

Birds

Avian Vestibular System. The avian vestibular system is an easy model to work with and has remarkable similarities in structure and function to its mammalian counterpart. Unlike fish and amphibians, the vestibular sensory epithelia of adult birds lack a peripheral area of growth. Early regeneration studies in the avian vestibular epithelium demonstrated in vivo continuous production of new hair cells at a low rate in all regions of the intact sensory epithelia.[12,13] Similarly, formation of both supporting cells and hair cells was demonstrated in organ cultures of normal postnatal chicken utricles.[14] In another study, the degree of cell proliferation was shown to increase in damaged sensory epithelia. Young chickens treated with streptomycin injections to induce hair cell damage underwent a significant increase in the rate of supporting cell proliferation, which was followed by complete anatomical restoration of the epithelium.[15] In a subsequent study, sheets of sensory epithelia were isolated from the utricles of chicks and cultured in serum-free media and in media that contained serum. The proliferation of epithelial supporting cells was assayed using the mitotic tracer bromodeoxyuridine. Similar levels of supporting cell proliferation were observed in epithelia maintained in serum-free and serum-containing media, suggesting that the vestibular epithelia of birds contain all the mitogens necessary for the continued proliferation of epithelial supporting cells.[16]

Recovery of function was investigated in vivo in 4- to 8-day-old chicks treated with intramuscular streptomycin for 5 days. Within 1 week, the vestibular hair cell density decreased to 40% of normal, and there was no measurable vestibulo-ocular reflex (VOR) gain. In the subsequent 2 weeks, the average hair cell density increased along with the average VOR gain and phase. By 8 to 9 weeks after the ototoxic insult, the hair cell density and the VOR parameters had returned to normal values. The VOR recovery correlated better with the rise in type I than type II hair cell density. Furthermore, when comparing hair cell density within the control and treated organs, this study found that epithelia with similar hair cell density had a range of VOR gains. The study

suggested that several factors, such as degree of repair of stereocilia, efficacy of hair cell synapses on afferent fibers, and the extent of compensation by central vestibular pathways also contribute to the recovery of VOR gain.[17]

Avian Auditory System. The auditory peripheral organ of birds, the basilar papilla, evolved independently from its mammalian counterpart and is structurally different.[18] In chickens, this organ contains a long spatula-shaped strip of epithelium bearing supporting cells and hair cells. Its sensory cells have been classified into tall hair cells, which have elongated morphology and are arranged along the superior neural side of the epithelium, and short hair cells, which are wide and short and are located along the inferior abneural side of the epithelium (Figure 4). As in the mammalian inner ear, there appears to be a division of labor between these 2 cell types, with the tall hair cells receiving predominantly afferent innervation and the short hair cells receiving efferent innervations. The characteristics and the innervation patterns of these 2 cell types suggest that they are analogous to the inner and outer hair cells, respectively, of the mammalian cochlea.[19] The supporting cells rest on the basilar lamina and have narrow, elongated cytoplasm in between the hair cells. Unlike the mammalian cochlea, there are no tunnels or spaces within the avian auditory sensory epithelia.

In vivo auditory hair cell regeneration studies in birds have focused on the restoration of the inner ear sensory epithelia following acoustic trauma or ototoxic drug administration. Excessive pure-tone stimulation results in hair cell damage that follows a tonotopical or frequency-specific distribution.[20] In general, the short hair

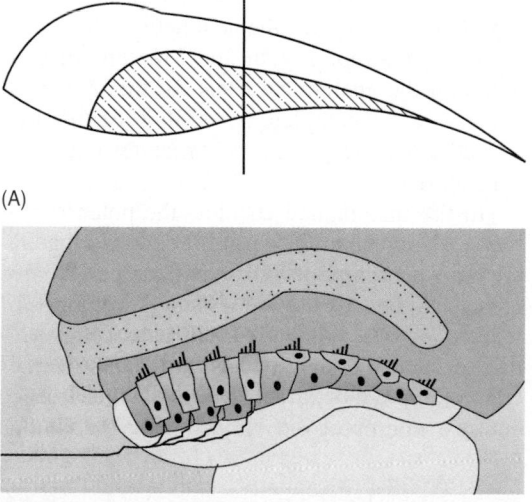

(A)

(B)

Figure 4 Schematic of the structure of the avian auditory organ. (A) The organ has a long spatulated shape. The short hair cells are localized in the inferior shaded area, and the tall hair cells are in the remaining superior region. Straight line represents level of cross section in panel B. (B) Drawing of a cross section of the avian basilar papilla demonstrating the tall hair cells in the superior aspect of the epithelium. These cells receive the afferent innervation. The short hair cells are in the inferior aspect of the epithelium and do not receive afferent innervation. The tectorial membrane lies over both cell types.

cells in the inferior or abneural portion of the epithelium of the respective frequency-sensitive area were preferentially damaged.[19] As the duration of the noise exposure increased, the position of damage shifted to the neural portion of the epithelium containing the tall hair cells. In animals treated with a mitotic tracer, new hair cells bearing the mitotic marker were observed at later time periods, demonstrating that mitotic division of precursor cells contributed significantly to the process of regeneration.[20,21]

Hair cell regeneration in the avian cochlea has also been studied following ototoxic damage.[22] With lower doses of ototoxic agents, the hair cells in the proximal or basal region of the epithelium, representing high frequency pitch location, were most affected. Larger doses of the drug or longer administration periods affected progressively lower frequency hair cells. The anatomical and/or physiological causes for this differential sensitivity remain unclear. Administration of a mitotic tracer allowed demonstration that only the cells in the damaged region of the epithelium entered the S phase of the cell cycle and underwent division.[23] A reliable organ culture preparation of the chick basilar papilla has been developed,[24] and this allowed confirmation of these findings under direct microscopic observation.[25]

It is encouraging that following noise-induced trauma or ototoxic auditory epithelia damage, there is recovery of auditory thresholds in association with restoration of the normal organ structure. Pure-tone–induced trauma results in threshold shifts of 50 to 70 dB in the frequencies around the stimulus.[26,27] Ultrastructural studies revealed that the localized lesion induced by pure-tone exposures resulted in damage to the tectorial membrane, changes in surface organization of the papilla, and loss of short hair cells. In chickens, the threshold shift recovered to 9.4 dB hearing loss on average by only 3 days after exposure.[26,28] While many new hair cells reappear within these 3 days, their immature stereocilia are still not coupled to the restored tectorial membrane. Thus, the initial recovery has been attributed to restoration of the tectorial membrane overlying the unaffected tall hair cells, allowing it to couple to and stimulate the cells.[29] This is not surprising since nearly all the afferent innervation of the basilar papilla is associated with the tall hair cells. A low degree of recovery continued over the subsequent 10 days, up to a final permanent threshold shift of about 5 dB. Further measurements of threshold sensitivity and frequency selectivity in the nucleus magnocellularis correlated recovery of function with structural recovery of the basilar papilla, suggesting that the source of the threshold shift was restricted to the cochlea.[30] Behavioral studies, which reflect a response to an acoustic signal and which are considered a more sensitive measurement of recovery, agreed with the findings and the time course of recovery of earlier-evoked potential studies.[31,32]

Ototoxicity studies allowed evaluation of recovery of auditory function without the confounding factors of damage to the tectorial membrane and selective hair cell subtype sensitivity inherent in acoustic trauma studies. Following aminoglycoside administration, both tall and short hair cells from the basilar papilla are affected, with a predilection for the basal aspect of the papilla, as described earlier. One study measured the cochlear nucleus evoked potential thresholds in neonatal chickens after gentamicin treatments. There was immediate isolated high frequency threshold shift with progression over the ensuing 5 weeks to involve the entire frequency range tested (0.25 to 5 kHz). Hearing loss correlated well with the time course of hair cell damage. Early loss of hair cells in the basal or high frequency aspect of the cochlea also progressed in the apical direction over the following weeks in a pattern that matched the threshold shift across frequencies. Sixteen to 20 weeks after treatment, robust recovery of thresholds was found for low and mid-frequencies, with a significant residual high frequency hearing loss.[33] The pattern of functional recovery matches the structural recovery of hair cells in the basilar papilla of hatchling chickens[34] and was slightly faster in Bengalese finches.[35] The hair cell density was found to be normal in the long term. The residual high frequency shift was associated with disorganization in the basal cochlea, residual regenerated hair cell functional immaturity, and shortcomings in the synaptic reconnections of nerve fibers with the regenerated hair cells.[36]

In summary, the avian inner ear has the capability to regenerate hair cells following acoustic trauma or ototoxic damage. Furthermore, there is recovery of function of the auditory organs. The slower recovery of auditory function after gentamicin exposure when compared to acoustic trauma is thought to be related to the fact that hair cell loss is prolonged and the newly regenerated tall hair cells need to be reconnected with the afferent nerve fibers.

Mammals

In mammals, the vestibular epithelia are morphologically similar to those of the lower vertebrates, leading to speculation that hair cell regeneration could take place in the mammalian vestibular end organs as well. In a seminal in vivo study from 1993, mature guinea pigs were treated with gentamicin.[4] Scanning electron micrographs and thin section histological preparations demonstrated loss of utricular hair cells. Four weeks after completion of the treatment, a large number of cells with immature hair bundles in multiple stages of development were identified in the epithelia. The lost type I hair cells were replaced by cells with the morphological appearance of type II hair cells. This study demonstrated an unexpected capacity for hair cell regeneration in vivo in the mature mammalian inner ear. In parallel studies, explants of the utricular maculae of guinea pigs and of humans (this was the first regeneration study in human inner ear sensory epithelia) were placed in culture and treated with aminoglycoside antibiotics at doses that killed the hair cells.

Supporting cell proliferation was documented under these conditions. After 4 weeks in culture, the epithelia contained new cells with some phenotypical characteristics of immature hair cells.[37]

Multiple studies investigating hair cell formation in the mammalian vestibular end organs followed. In the normal untreated adult guinea pig, utricle cells carrying immature-appearing stereocilia were identified, representing 0.7% of the utricular hair cell population.[38] This study suggested that some degree of hair cell replacement may be an active process in the vestibule of adult mammals. In the chinchilla, administration of gentamicin to the perilymphatic space resulted in direct damage to the hair cells.[39] This was followed by postmitotic formation of new hair cells and complete restoration of the hair cell density 8 weeks after treatment. In another study gentamicin was injected transtympanically in guinea pigs, and the epithelia were evaluated with scanning electron microscopy up to 10 months after treatment.[40] A significant degree of hair cell loss, predominantly type I, was found in the first 4 weeks after treatment. Only limited long-term recovery of mature hair bundles was found, and it did not result in complete restoration of the epithelium. Type I hair cells were found to be more susceptible to ototoxic damage than type II hair cells. In summary, studies agree that the vestibular sensory epithelia of mammals have some regenerative capability, albeit low.[41-43]

Recovery of vestibular function in mammals following damage to the hair cells was documented in two additional studies. In one study, guinea pigs were treated with streptomycin until postrotatory nystagmus response was eliminated. The response was completely reestablished within 22 days along with recovery of the expression of a hair cell marker.[44] Another study in humans reported return of vestibular function after treatment with streptomycin for Ménière disease although the anatomical basis for this remained unclear, and incomplete penetration of the drug as well as recovery of neural structures may have contributed.[45]

In the mammalian cochlea, the potential for hair cell regeneration in embryonic and neonatal mouse organs of Corti maintained in vitro has also been examined.[46] Small numbers of hair cells were killed by laser microbeam irradiation, and the subsequent recovery processes were monitored by direct differential interference contrast microscopy combined with continuous

time-lapse video recordings. Replacement hair cells were observed to develop in lesion sites in embryonic cochleae and, on rare occasions, in neonatal cochleae. In embryonic cochleae, replacement hair cells developed from preexisting cells that changed from their normal developmental fates without any intervening mitosis. In neonatal cochleae, epithelial lesions were created with a laser beam resulting in an average of at least 3 damaged hair cells per lesion. Of 245 lesions analyzed, only 11 apparently regenerated hair cells and a single hair cell labeled by a mitotic tracer were observed. The results indicated that the organ of Corti can replace lost hair cells during embryonic development. The ability to generate new hair cells in the neonate was only anecdotal.

In vivo, hair cell regeneration in the mammalian cochlea was investigated in 9-day-old rat pups.[47] The animals received amikacin injections for 7 consecutive days and were sacrificed at intervals up to 90 days postinjection. At 21 and 35 days after treatment, atypical cells bearing tufts of microvilli and resembling immature hair cells were observed in the outer hair cell region. The cells in the inner hair cell area lacked stereocilia but had afferent and efferent innervations. The study suggested that the cochlea only regenerates incompletely and does not reach the mature morphology.

In summary, in mammals there is evidence for only partial recovery of hair cells in the vestibular system. Only 2 reports of associated recovery of function are available. The evidence for spontaneous hair cell recovery in the cochlea is, thus far, unclear. Recent studies, though, have been successful at stimulating new cochlear hair cell formation through modification of the expression of the Math 1 transcription factor genes, as will be reviewed later in the chapter.[48-49] The ability to regenerate the inner ear of different vertebrate species is summarized in Table 1.

MECHANISMS FOR HAIR CELL RECOVERY

The origin of the recovered hair cells is still debated, and multiple mechanisms for hair cell regeneration have been proposed. Several experimental protocols have been designed and demonstrated partial or complete recovery of hair cell density through precursor cell proliferation, supporting cell transdifferentiation, hair

Table 1 Hair Cell Regeneration in Vertebrate Species

Species and Organ	Continuous Hair Cell Formation	Proliferation after Damage	Spontaneous Hair Cell Regeneration	Recovery of Function
Fish and amphibian inner ear and lateral line	+	+	+	+
Bird vestibular organs	+	+	+	+
Bird auditory organs	−	+	+	++++
Mammalian vestibular organs	−	+	+/−	+++
Mammalian auditory organs	−	−	−	+/−

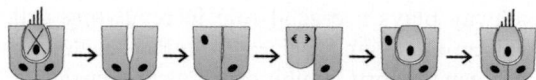

Figure 5 Schematic of hair cell regeneration through supporting cell proliferation. Following death and extrusion of a hair cell, the adjacent supporting cells expand to seal the luminal surface of the epithelium. Next one supporting cell divides and gives rise to a new hair cell that replaces the lost one.

cell repair, cell migration, and a combination of the above.

Supporting Cell Proliferation

This mechanism consists of proliferation of supporting cells and differentiation of the progeny into hair cells and supporting cells (Figure 5). Avian inner ear regeneration studies have demonstrated upregulation of supporting cell proliferation around the region of hair cell loss under multiple conditions: in vivo in the chick utricle following ototoxic damage,[50] in organ cultures of the basilar papilla after laser ablation,[25] and in the basilar papilla in vitro,[51] and in vivo after ototoxic damage.[52] In mammals, cultures of guinea pig and human utricles treated with neomycin in the presence of the mitotic tracer tritiated thymidine led to the appearance of labeled nuclei in the basal aspect of the epithelia 2 to 6 days after treatment.[37] By 4 weeks some labeled cells had migrated to the apical aspect of the epithelium. A number of these apical labeled cells went on to develop immature hair bundles, demonstrating postmitotic hair cell formation. Upregulation of supporting cell proliferation has also been demonstrated in the chinchilla following ototoxic damage.[35]

Supporting Cell Transdifferentiation

Another proposed mechanism for new hair cell formation is the conversion of the phenotype of supporting cells to hair cells without intervening mitosis (Figure 6). Abundant evidence supporting this mechanism is available. In vivo studies investigating morphological changes in the chick basilar papilla suggest that ototoxicity leads to an initial wave of hair cell formation through transdifferentiation, followed by a second, slower wave of mitotic new hair cell formation.[53] In other in vivo studies, chicks were treated with an ototoxic drug followed by the mitotic blocker Ara-C. This was followed by formation of immature new hair cells, suggesting a direct change of the supporting cell phenotype.[54] In mammalian studies, guinea pigs received a transtympanic injection of gentamicin and a mitotic tracer.

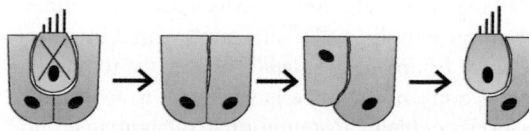

Figure 6 Schematic of hair cell regeneration through supporting cell transdifferentiation. Following loss and extrusion of a hair cell, the surrounding supporting cells expand to fill the gap and seal the epithelial surface. Next one of the adjacent supporting cells changes its phenotype and transforms into a mature hair cell.

Soon after treatment, light and scanning electron microscopy techniques allowed demonstration of a variable degree of hair cell loss, while the supporting cell density remained constant. Subsequently, a small number of cells in the supporting cell region incorporating the mitotic tracer were identified, indicating a low degree of cell proliferation. Also, new immature hair cells without the tracer were noted to emerge, suggesting that new hair cell formation during this time period was due to supporting cell transdifferentiation rather than proliferation.[41]

Hair Cell Repair

The hair cell repair theory proposes that hair cells are only partially damaged following an insult. The damaged hair cells become sequestered below the reticular lamina and are internalized among the supporting cells. These cells may then remain dedifferentiated or regrow an apical process that regains contact with the surface of the organ (Figure 7). Direct videomicroscopic documentation for this mechanism was obtained in cultures of bullfrog saccule following ablation of hair cells with a laser pulse.[55]

In cultures of neonatal rat utricles, destruction of hair cells by ototoxic agents was followed by recovery of the hair cell number. While the supporting cell number remained constant, the degree of cell proliferation was limited and far below the number of recovered hair cells, suggesting that other mechanisms besides proliferation led to hair cell regeneration.[43] Furthermore, this study presented ultrastructural evidence for hair cell repair and regrowth of the stereociliary tuft. Other morphological studies have demonstrated hair cell repair in the mammalian cochlea.[56,57] In organ cultures of the newborn mouse organ of Corti, hair cells damaged mechanically or with a laser pulse: (1) lost their stereocilia but survived at the surface of the organ; (2) retained contact with the reticular lamina but were overgrown by the processes of the supporting cells; or, (3) became internalized among the supporting cells and either remained dedifferentiated or resurfaced with newly formed apical processes.

Cell Migration

In the basilar papilla of chickens, localized destruction of both hair cells and supporting cells with severe acoustic trauma was followed initially by replacement of the lost cells by a layer of flattened epithelial cells.[58] These cells are thought

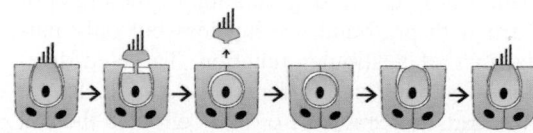

Figure 7 Drawing representing the process of hair cell regeneration through cell repair. Following damage to a hair cell, the stereocilia are extruded and the hair cell becomes sequestered from the reticular lamina. The supporting cells reclose the gap. The hair cell may survive internalized by the supporting cells, or it may regain contact with the reticular lamina and regrow an apical process.

to derive from the hyaline cells or cuboidal cells normally located along the inferior abneural edge of the basilar papilla.[59] Thus, hyaline cell migration may be involved in maintenance or repair of the severely damaged cochlea (Figure 8).

REGULATION OF HAIR CELL FORMATION: MOLECULAR ASPECTS

During mammalian embryogenesis, cochlear hair cells and supporting cells have common cellular precursors.[60–63] The formation of a cellular mosaic of sensory hair cells and nonsensory cells is a highly regulated developmental event involving cell fate decisions, coordinated cell division, pattern formation, and differentiation.[63] Much of the research in regeneration revolves around the identification of master, regulatory genes that control the processes of patterning and hair cell formation, as have been shown in other systems. Controlled manipulation of these genes may lead to hair cell recovery.

Extracellular Signals

Research has focused on signaling mechanisms that regulate the decision to commit to mitotic division or to remain quiescent.

Soluble Factors. Multiple growth factors and hormones that might promote hair cell formation have been investigated. When intact basilar papillae are co-cultured with aminoglycoside-damaged papillae, the intact papillae experience increased rates of incorporation of the mitotic tracer, tritiated thymidine, suggesting that a diffusible factor is released by the injured papillae that stimulates cell proliferation.[64] In dissociated cell culture preparations of the bullfrog, supporting cells express receptors for brain-derived neurotrophic factor (BDNF), and basic fibroblast growth factor (bFGF).[65] In the same preparation, bFGF induces cell proliferation early after dissociation, while BDNF exerted its effect only at a later time and contributed to promoting hair cell differentiation and survival. In the chick vestibular epithelium, insulin-like growth factor 1 stimulates DNA synthesis in a dose-dependent manner.[66] Retinoic acid and bFGF have also been implicated in the control of the cell cycle in the avian sensory epithelia.[65] In mammals, transforming growth factor alpha (TGFα) and epidermal growth factor (EGF), in the presence of insulin,

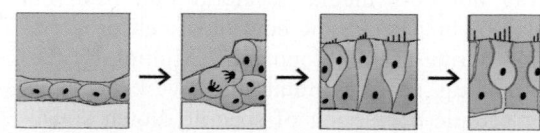

Figure 8 Representation of the process of hair cell regeneration in avians through cell migration. Following noise exposure and loss of hair cells and supporting cells, the hyaline or cuboidal cells on the inferior abneural area of the organ migrate to cover the exposed basilar membrane. Next hyaline or cuboidal cells proliferate. Proliferating cells begin differentiation into hair cells and supporting cell lineages. The new cells express the mature hair or supporting cell phenotype.

stimulate cell proliferation in adult mouse vestibular epithelial cultures.[67,68] Receptors for heregulin, a member of the EGF family, are widely expressed in vestibular and auditory sensory epithelia in neonatal and adult mouse inner ears. Heregulin-α, however, stimulates cell proliferation in organotypic cultures of neonatal, but not adult, mouse utricular sensory epithelia.[69] Thus, this factor may play a role in growing/developing but not in differentiated/quiescent epithelia. Studies evaluating the role of BDNF in the utricle of the chinchilla ear after ototoxic damage suggested that it may be involved in the maintenance of the vestibular ganglia and contribute to neurite outgrowth to new and repaired hair cells.[70] A variety of other trophic factors regulating the cell cycle in the developing and mature inner ear have been described.[71]

Cell–Cell Contact. Cell–cell contact interactions are crucial for cell cycle regulation in the sensory epithelia. In cultures of small pieces of chicken utricular epithelia, the degree of cell proliferation was inversely related to local cell density.[72]

N-cadherin is a protein belonging to a family of transmembrane molecules that mediate calcium-dependent intercellular adhesion. Cadherins are involved in controlling morphogenetic movements of cells during development and regulating cell surface adhesion. In cultures of chicken inner ear sensory epithelia, binding of microbeads coated with a function-blocking antibody to N-cadherin inhibited ongoing cell proliferation.[72] The growth of epithelial cells was also affected by the density of extracellular matrix molecules.

Notch and its ligands, Delta, Serrate, and Jagged, are cytoplasmic membrane proteins that mediate cell–cell contact interactions. The Notch pathway mediates 3 types of developmental processes: (1) lateral inhibition between neighboring cells; (2) lineage decisions (determination of cell fate between two daughter cells); and (3) boundary formation (such as between sensory and nonsensory epithelia).[73] Transient administration of Notch ligands to the adult rat brain resulted in expansion of the stem cell population.[74] In mice, genes encoding the receptor protein Notch1 and its ligand, Jagged-2, are expressed in alternating cell types in the developing sensory epithelium.[75] Genetic deletion of Jag2 results in a significant increase in sensory hair cells, presumably as a result of a decrease in Notch activation. More recent studies suggested that the Notch pathway not only mediates lateral inhibition but also participates in the control of cell proliferation during ear development.[76] Multiple studies involving genetic mutations, overexpression, or ectopic expression of specific Notch signaling cascade protein genes in the inner ear sensory epithelia demonstrated formation of supernumerary hair cells and/or supporting cells. In these models, new cells arose from expansion of the precursor cell pool, secondary division of the precursor cells, proliferation and transdifferentiation into hair cells, or the recruitment and differentiation of adjacent nonsensory cells.[77] In summary, cell density, cell–cell contact signaling and the composition of the extracellular matrix are essential factors in the regulation of hair cell formation.

Intracellular Signaling Pathway

Downstream from the processes above, the intracellular signaling pathways regulate cell proliferation and differentiation in the sensory epithelium.

Cell Cycle Regulation. Cell cycle regulation requires the appropriately coordinated activities of various cyclins and cyclin-dependent kinases, which are tightly regulated by multiple effector proteins. One family of regulator proteins is the Cip/Kip family of molecules (cyclin-dependent kinase inhibitory protein/kinase inhibitory protein). This family includes the protein p27kip1, which was recently discovered in supporting cells of the organ of Corti.[78] P27Kip1 plays a critical role in cell cycle arrest and in maintaining the differentiated phenotype of sensory epithelial cells during development and is the first known marker for the patch of epithelial cells destined to become sensory epithelium.[78] Interestingly, developing hair cells downregulate p27kip1 while supporting cells continue to express it. Mice that lack p27kip1 continue to develop hair cells and supporting cells beyond the normal period.[78,79] Moreover, supporting cells in mice lacking p27kip1 can generate new cochlear hair cells after acoustic trauma-induced hair cell loss. Thus, release of the inhibition of the cell cycle induced by these molecules in a controlled fashion may allow the regeneration of hair cells in the adult auditory sensory epithelia. In a recent study, supporting cells from the adult mouse cochlea were purified and cultured in vitro under conditions that support growth and differentiation of embryonic cochlear sensory progenitors.[80] Some supporting cells downregulated the cell cycle inhibitor p27kip1 and transdifferentiated into hair cells, suggesting that this gene may be important for repressing regeneration in the adult mammalian cochlea.

Another gene involved in cell cycle control, the retinoblastoma (*Rb*) gene, is required for cell-cycle exit and to prevent reentry into cell cycle of embryonic mammalian hair cells.[81,82] However, the role of the *Rb* gene in postnatal hair cells is unknown. In mice with deletion of the *Rb* gene, hair cells continue to divide and can transduce mechanical stimuli in the early postnatal period.[83] However, in adult life these mice exhibit progressive degeneration of the organ of Corti with profound hearing loss but only partial loss of vestibular function. Targeted deletion of another cyclin-dependent kinase, Ink4d, also leads to reentrance of hair cells into the cell cycle and hair cell death, with subsequent hearing loss.[83] The mitogen-activated protein kinase (MAPK) intracellular signaling pathways transduce a large variety of external signals, leading to a wide range of cellular responses, including growth, differentiation, inflammation, and apoptosis. Studies in birds demonstrated that MAPK pathway plays a crucial role in regulating cell cycle in the avian inner ear.[84] In the developing rat organ of Corti, inhibition of cyclin-dependent kinases resulted in differentiation of precursor cells without an intervening mitosis, suggesting their participation in normal development of the organ of Corti.[85]

Hair Cell Differentiation. Math 1 is a transcription factor that is expressed in the developing sensory epithelia of the inner ear at early embryonic stages. In a recent study, Math 1–null mutant mice were generated and had complete lack of hair cells and supporting cells.[62] This study suggested that *Math 1* serves to initiate inductive signals that regulate the overall formation of both hair and supporting cells from the sensory epithelia at the very early stages of development, and that it is necessary for hair cell formation.[86] In another study, neonatal rat cochlear organ cultures were transfected with the *Math 1* gene; overexpression of this factor in nonsensory cells adjacent to the sensory epithelia led to their differentiation into hair cells.[87] Similar findings were obtained in vivo in the normal adult guinea pig cochlea following *Math 1* gene transfer,[48] demonstrating that *Math 1* expression is sufficient for hair cell differentiation. Newly formed hair cells resulted in improved hearing thresholds.[88] However, the morphology of these regenerated or transdifferentiated hair cells was at a poor level, suggesting that better control of *Math 1* expression (timing and level) during delivery may be critical.[89] Moreover, other pathways may be involved and require simultaneous regulation. Another transcription factor, Hes1, has been shown to negatively regulate hair cell differentiation by antagonizing *Math 1*.[90] Taken together these studies demonstrate that forced expression of Math1 in the mammalian adult inner ear may lead to differentiation of supporting cells into hair cells. Effective regeneration of the cochlea, however, is likely to require the generation of new supporting cells as well as hair cells. Co-transfection experiments in postnatal rat explant cultures show that overexpression of Hes1 prevents hair cell differentiation induced by *Math 1*, further supporting the role of *Math 1* in hair cell formation.

Other factors important for hair cell formation have also been discovered and may represent important targets for hair cell regeneration genetic therapies. The transcription factor *Brn-3.1* is expressed in the inner ear hair cells throughout life and is necessary for their development. Mice with mutation of both copies of the *Brn-3.1* gene had complete deafness due to no identifiable cochlear hair cells and greatly reduced numbers of spiral ganglia cells.[91] In mice with a mutation of only 1 copy of the *Brn-3.1* gene, the remaining intact copy of the gene is sufficient to maintain a normal cochlea.[92] A mutation in the human homologue of this gene has been shown to be related to adult-onset sensorineural hearing loss.[93]

In summary, studies to date have unveiled multiple signaling pathways involved in hair cell formation. They highlight the importance of coordinated expression of all genes involved in the cell cycle control, including those that regulate patterning of the epithelium and those that inhibit cell proliferation, as well as those that enhance it.

NEW LINES OF RESEARCH: STEM CELLS

As stated earlier, only anecdotal evidence of hair cell regeneration in the mammalian cochlea has been produced to date. This has led to the search for new ways to restore the hair cell population in damaged auditory organs. In 1998 human embryonic stem cell lines were isolated and expanded for the first time.[94,95] This generated a tremendous amount of interest in embryonic and adult stem cells and their potential for treating diseases involving the loss of specific cell types, including hair cell loss in the inner ear sensory epithelia. The use of this technology has resulted in great progress in our understanding of the process of hair cell formation in the developing and regenerating ear.

Definition and Properties of Stem Cells

Stem cells are primitive, undifferentiated cells that are defined according to functional criteria: they must have the ability to self-renew and the ability to differentiate into more than 1 cell type. During stem cell division, at least 1 of the daughter cells must remain a stem cell to maintain the lineage, while the other daughter cell may differentiate or remain as a stem cell.

Stem cells can be found in embryonic and adult tissues. During development, as the divisions progress from the fertilized oocyte, the cells become progressively restricted in the cell types that they can produce and in their ability to proliferate.[96] Initial totipotent cells formed from the first postfertilization cleavages are able to develop into complete new animals. In mammals, this capacity is lost as the early morula matures to form the late morula and blastula. The latter has an outer layer of cells, the trophoectoderm, and an inner layer of cells, the inner cell mass. Pluripotent embryonic stem cells (ESCs) can be established from the inner cell mass and are used extensively in stem cell research (Figure 9). The cells from the inner cell mass are capable of generating cells from all 3 layers of the embryo: the endoderm or inner layer, the mesoderm or middle layer, and the ectoderm or outermost layer. The latter gives rise to multiple tissues including skin and adnexa, neural tissue and the inner ear epithelia and associated nerve

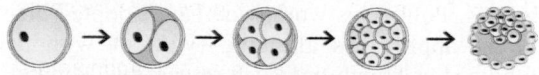

Figure 9 Representation of the formation of the inner cell mass as the fertilized oocyte divides multiple times to form the morula. Next the blastula is formed. This hollow sphere contains the inner cell mass (*shaded cells*). Human cells from this region are used for embryonic stem cell research.

supply. Inner cell mass cells placed in culture and exposed to the proper biochemical signals are able to divide indefinitely and to generate the different cell types in the body, which makes them great candidates for developmental and regeneration research. Other fetal tissues including umbilical cord and placenta have been used to obtain fetal stem cells that develop into various organs. Stem cells are also found in adult tissues. As development proceeds, cells go through a series of restrictions in potency until they become committed to different cellular fates. As they do, rare cells are set aside in specific tissues that maintain a high proliferational and developmental potential, the so called somatic stem cells (SSCs) that are found in embryonic and adult tissues and organs. The number of adult stem cells in tissues may be extremely small. In addition, adult stem cells proliferate at fairly low rates compared to ESCs, making expansion of these cells more challenging. Progenitor cells (PCs) are cell types intermediate between the stem cells and mature cells. They are in transit and amplifying stages that have multilineage differentiation capacity but lack the ability for unlimited self-renewal. The highest burden of cell division is placed on the PCs.

Cell differentiation has traditionally been regarded as a one-way avenue, and SSCs and PCs were thought to be restricted in the cell types they can produce.[96] However, several recent reports have concluded that committed progenitor cells can actually transform to generate cell types of further stem cell systems. Cultured murine neuronal stem cells from embryonic and adult brains have been shown to repopulate the hematopoietic system of irradiated mice and produce a variety of blood cell types[97] and, when injected into blastocysts, to generate multiple other tissue cells.[98] However, unexpected spontaneous fusion of embryonic stem cells with hematopoietic or neural stem cells has also been observed, making it possible that the observed cell products are, in fact, the result of fusion.[99,100] Multiple other examples supporting the hypothesis of stem cell plasticity have recently been published.

Stem Cell Research

Mouse ESCs have been used for research for nearly one-quarter century and have enabled greater understanding of basic principles of stem cell biology. They have also led to the now common technique of "knockout mice," which are mice genetically engineered to eliminate the expression of a particular gene.

In the inner ear, ESCs provide a unique opportunity to study in vitro the genetic and molecular nature of cell fate and the environmental cues that induce specific cell fate commitment and differentiation. Understanding these processes may allow us to manipulate hair cell regeneration in vivo by means of the application of soluble factors or by activating specific gene expression programs through gene therapy. Furthermore, stem cells could be transplanted into the inner ear, where damaged sensory epithelia may provide the proper signals to trigger incorporation of stem cells into the epithelia and new hair cell formation.

Certain caveats must be kept in mind in designing and interpreting stem cell research. In general, in vitro exposure of cells to factors that mimic in vivo conditions has been thought to exert similar effects[101] and allow identification of signals that trigger progression through the cell cycle and differentiation. However, in reality, the putative conditions and endogenous signals converging in the damaged epithelia in vivo are much more complex and may themselves lead to changes in transplanted stem cells. These transformed stem cells may respond differently to the exogenous or endogenous signals and undergo uncontrolled division and tumorigenesis. Also, the efficacy of new stem cell–derived treatments may depend on the degree of damage and amount of tissue scarring, which may be a function of the length of time elapsed between the time of injury and the treatment.

Stem Cell Research in the Vertebrate Inner Ear

Many important issues regarding stem cell research and inner ear hair cell regeneration remain incompletely understood, including: (1) the existence of stem cells in the inner ear; (2) our ability to direct stem cells from the inner ear or from a different source to differentiate into the hair cell lineage in vitro; and (3) the presence in the damaged inner ear of cues capable of inducing stem cell differentiation (either with stem cells from the inner ear or from another source).

To date, these questions have been addressed in multiple studies. In a recent study, utricular sensory epithelia of adult mice were dissociated and cells were cultured in vitro at low density. Within a few days, spheres of cells containing stem cells were identified in the preparation.[102] Although stem cells were not identified directly in the inner ear of adult mammals in this study, it demonstrated that some cells within the vestibular end organs have the ability to behave as stem cells following dissociation and culture. Furthermore, these stem cells were induced to express multiple hair cell markers in vitro under the appropriate conditions.[102] While these results are encouraging, the degree to which these new hair cells are able to fully mature phenotypically and functionally remains unclear. In another study utricular organ cultures of rats were treated with gentamicin and rat otocyst stem cells were added to the media.[103] These cells integrated into the utricular epithelia and expressed the hair cell marker calretinin, suggesting that the damaged utricle may contain or release the cues required for inducing the incorporation of stem cells and their differentiation into hair cells. In in vivo studies, cultured spheres of neural cells containing stem cells were transplanted into intact neonatal rat cochleas. This resulted in significant cell migration along the cochlea; expression of differentiation markers of neurons, astrocytes and oligodendrocytes; and incorporation of a few cells into the sensory epithelia with acquisition of differentiating hair cell phenotype.[104] Such results were unexpected since no damage was induced to the epithelia prior to transplantation and differentiation cues might be absent. Furthermore, neurospheres may be a poor model for predicting stem cell attributes since they consist of heterogeneous populations of cells, and only a small proportion of these are truly "stem-like."[105] On the other hand, the fact that efficiency of hair cell formation was poor in a neonatal ear argues against the efficiency of transplanting stem cells from a different lineage and led the authors to propose that it may be more reasonable to use stem cells originating from the cochlea, rather than from the hippocampus, to replace hair cells in the inner ear.

The early otic placode possesses extensive autonomy and does not require additional external signals to form all major inner ear cell types.[106,107] In a recent study, Li and colleagues proposed that ESCs could be induced to differentiate into hair cell progenitors at a stage equivalent to the otic placodes.[108] ESCs were cultured in the presence of EGF, insulin-like growth factor and bFGF. New cells expressing otic placode and otic vesicle markers were generated. Next, the growth factors were withdrawn from the culture media, and the cells were further induced to differentiate into hair cell-like cells expressing a variety of markers including Math 1, Brn-3.1 and myosin VIIA, and supporting cell-like cells expressing the marker p27kip1.

The aforementioned studies suggest the presence of stem cells in the adult mammalian vestibular organs. In the cochlea, on the other hand, the existence of such cells was demonstrated in small numbers.[80,109,110] The exact origin has been attributed to the the lesser epithelial ridge of the postnatal rat cochlea[111] and to the pillar and Hensen cells of the adult mouse.[80]

Challenges of Stem Cell Therapy

Currently, severe to profound hearing loss as a result of hair cell loss is treated with cochlear implantation. When considering stem cell transplant, the advantages and disadvantages over cochlear implantation must be carefully weighed.

Cochlear Implantation Considerations. Cochlear implantation has the advantage of providing the ability to stimulate the auditory neurons directly in a tonotopic fashion. The device can be reprogrammed over time should auditory sensitivity or function change. A great wealth of information is available on the outcomes of the surgical procedure and the auditory performance of implanted patients, with more than 59,000 people worldwide having received cochlear implants.[1] On the other hand as Raz points out, this treatment is far from ideal.[112] Cochlear implantation is discussed in Chapter 32, "Cochlear and Brainstem Implantation," and Chapter 33, "Cochlear Implant Coding Strategies and Device Programming."

Stem Cell Technology Considerations. The ability to restore the natural tissue by transplanting stem cells would eliminate many of the concerns related to cochlear implantation, including risks, costs, and performance. Multiple challenges must still be overcome.

Tumorigenesis. The fact that tumors may often originate from stem cells[113] has led to concerns regarding uncontrolled proliferation of transplanted stem cells incorporated into the damaged epithelium, as well as those that get incorporated into other nondamaged areas of the inner ear. Tumorigenesis can occur early after transplantation or, conceivably, several years later. Due to their shorter lifespan, this possibility cannot be evaluated in animal models. Furthermore, as pointed out in studies demonstrating fusion of stem cells with other cell types following transplantation,[114] the cell products of fusion may have altered cell cycle control and undergo uncontrolled proliferation. A possible strategy to overcome uncontrolled proliferation is to predifferentiate stem cells along the hair cell or neuronal pathway prior to transplantation, thus decreasing their proliferative capability and ensuring that transplanted cells acquire the desired phenotype. Predifferentiated cells, however, have lesser ability to migrate and integrate into tissues and may not be as effective in replenishing lost hair cells. Cell proliferation in stem cells could possibly be regulated by inserting suicide genes into the stem cells under the control of a promoter that can be turned on with pharmacotherapy. Another concern is that transplanted cells could migrate out of the inner ear into adjacent structures, such as the brain, and fail to differentiate, disrupting the local tissues.

Graft-versus-Host Disease. The use of nonautologous human ESCs also raises the question of HLA incompatibility and graft-versus-host disease. This would require lifetime immune suppression therapy, which also carries significant risks of infection and tumor formation. An alternative would be to use autologous stem cells from cord-banked blood or autologous adult stem cells if, and when, these become available. Other alternatives include the use of nuclear transfer techniques, in which the nucleus of a somatic cell is transferred into a blastocyst cell to create embryonic stem cells with the genetic information of the host. Finally, another option is the creation of stem cell banks with human leukocyte antigen-typed cells.

Biological Contamination. Mouse ESCs have been routinely grown on a layer of mouse embryonic fibroblasts, which inhibited cell differentiation. However, recently the use of the cytokine leukemia inhibitory factor (LIF) has eliminated the need for the feeder layers. In human ESC cultures, it remains unclear whether LIF can replace the feeder layers. This raises serious concern regarding cross-contaminating human cells with mouse pathogens by growing the human cells on mouse feeder layers or with culture media conditioned by mouse cells.

Genetic Mutations. The transplanted ESCs must be carefully genetically screened, and the presence of mutations in genes pertaining to deafness or any other disorder must be ruled out before any type of transplantation can take place. A standard of test protocol must be in place before cell transplantation can be routinely performed.

Transplantation Issues. Different approaches have been proposed for the delivery of cells to the damaged inner ear. The endolymphatic space can be accessed through a transmastoid approach to the endolymphatic sac or the semicircular canals. The cells delivered through these approaches would have to travel a fair distance to reach the target, the damaged cochlear epithelia. The endolymphatic space could theoretically also be accessed through the basilar membrane, either through a transmastoid transfacial recess approach to the cochlea, similar to cochlear implantation surgery, or through the external auditory canal, tympanic membrane and round or oval window. This route would require the development of appropriately designed precision tools. So far, the incorporation of the cells into the damaged regions of the sensory epithelium in experimental models, has had poor efficiency.[104] The endolymph is so rich in potassium ions that it is toxic to the nerve endings on the basolateral membrane of the hair cells. When a hair cell dies in response to trauma, 2 of the 4 surrounding supporting cells undergo rapid expansion of the apical cytoplasmic domain while sealing the reticular lamina against a leak of fluids.[115,116] This prevents mixing of perilymph and endolymph and is essential for maintaining the endocochlear potential. In these conditions, survival of transplanted cells in this environment and migration through the apical surface of the epithelium may be diminished. Finally, neural stem cells delivered intravenously have been used successfully in animal models to target tumors with little accumulation in normal tissues,[117] demonstrating that stem cells can migrate following gradients of cytokines or other soluble molecules. However, to date, our understanding of the molecules that bring about this process in the ear is poor.

Ethical Issues. Human ESCs are derived at a point when the fertilized zygote has developed into a hollow sphere of cells, the blastocyst. The process of deriving the stem cells thus destroys a developing embryo. While the potential for medical benefits deriving from stem cell technology is theoretically tremendous, no clinical benefit has derived to date. This research has generated strong opinions for, or against, this technology, based on differing cultural, moral, and religious beliefs. Politicians worldwide have adopted different approaches allowing (with or without funding) or prohibiting such research.[118] Parallel research currently focuses on the development of stem cell lines from adult tissues, bypassing ethical concerns dealing with experimentation on embryonic tissue. In a recent study, functional neural stem cells were derived from adult bone marrow, indicating the great potential for this technology as well.[119]

OTHER LINES OF RESEARCH: MOLECULAR GENETICS

A great deal of research effort has recently been focused on elucidating the genes for cell cycle regulation molecules, cell surface receptors, and transcription factors that participate in hair cell formation and patterning of the inner ear sensory epithelia. These studies have taken advantage of global gene expression profiling techniques, the development of immortalized cell lines of inner ear epithelia at different stages of differentiation, and gene therapy techniques.

Global Gene Expression Profiling Technology[48,49,120]

The Human Genome Project has been the most significant undertaking in recent molecular biology. This project focused on enumerating the basic components of human biology (such as genes, genomes, and proteomes) and describing rudimentary aspects of behavior in an attempt to deconstruct the biological processes into their molecular components. Such essential information will provide the basis for mapping gene activity into biological and physiological processes, thereby shifting the focus from lists of genes to pathways, networks, molecular machines, organelles and eventually, the cell itself as a unit of work. The development of microarray and other high throughput technologies has made it possible to measure the relative abundance of mRNA from thousands of genes per experiment. These technologies have allowed comparison of gene expression differences in regenerating versus nonregenerating avian papillae[121–125] and the identification of multiple genes that may be targets for pharmacological upregulation of the process in vivo. In a recent study, laser capture microdissection of individual hair cells and supporting cells allowed elucidation of the gene expression profiles of these individual cell populations in the inner ear sensory epithelia.[126] Furthermore, cells can be labeled with immunocytochemistry for specific markers and individually captured for analysis of gene expression patterns within subpopulations of cells with similar morphological characteristics, but different functional phenotypes.

Cell Lines

One of the impediments for studying global gene expression in the regenerating inner ear sensory epithelia is the paucity of cells at the different stages of differentiation in this tissue. The Immortomouse is a transgenic animal in which any cell can be induced to proliferate continuously or to differentiate in vitro. Taking advantage of this property, different cell lines have been derived by cloning individual cells from the Immortomouse (Charles River Laboratories, Wilmington, MA) (transgenic H2Kb-tsA58 mouse) embryonic inner ear at different stages of development and

from the adult inner ear sensory epithelia.[127–130] This has allowed analysis of gene expression in cultured cells from the inner ear at different stages of differentiation[131] or at different times after aminoglycoside ototoxicity.[132] The protocols for turning these cells into hair cells have been published recently.[133] Furthermore, techniques have been developed that allow labeling of dissociated hair and supporting cell precursors from the embryonic cochlea and purification with flow cytometry.[134] These new technologies should enable substantial progress to be made in understanding the process of hair cell formation.

Gene Therapy

In a recent study, adult guinea pigs were deafened with systemic administration of ototoxic drugs, leading to complete loss of hair cells in the high- and mid-frequency regions of the cochlea. The gene for Math 1, a transcription factor that regulates hair cell formation, was delivered using adenoviral vectors infused into the cochlea. This resulted in new hair cell formation with substantial restoration of hearing thresholds, demonstrating that delivery of crucial genes for hair cell formation may induce restoration of auditory organ structure and function.[88] For further information on gene therapy, see Chapter 5, "Inner Ear Drug Delivery and Gene Therapy."

CONCLUSIONS

Studies over the past quarter century have produced extensive evidence of hair cell regeneration in nonmammalian vertebrate vestibular and auditory organs and generated a wealth of knowledge on the mechanisms that regulate the process. Although regeneration occurs to a modest degree in the mammalian vestibular sensory epithelia, no evidence, to date, of spontaneous hair cell regeneration has been produced in the mammalian cochlea sensory epithelia. However, recent stem cell and gene transfer research has resulted in hair cell formation and auditory threshold recovery in the damaged auditory epithelia. Although multiple essential questions remain unanswered, the large advances in this field over this short period of time may well lead to successful strategies for anatomical and functional restoration of the organ of Corti. Clinical applications of this technology will surely follow. Other lines of research are currently needed, such as the development of therapies to increase resistance of hair cells to damage and to enhance the repair of injured hair cells in the organ of Corti.

REFERENCES

1. NIDCD. Statistics about Hearing Disorders, Ear Infections, and Deafness [Web page]. Available at: http://www.nidcd.nih.gov/health/statistics/hearing.asp. Accessed October 1, 2006.
2. Raphael Y. Cochlear pathology, sensory cell death and regeneration. Br Med Bull 2002;63:25–38.
3. Walshe P, Walsh M, McConn Walsh R. Hair cell regeneration in the inner ear: A review. Clin Otolaryngol Allied Sci 2003;28:5–13.
4. Forge A, Li L, Corwin JT, Nevill G. Ultrastructural evidence for hair cell regeneration in the mammalian inner ear. Science 1993;259:1616–19.
5. Manley GA, Koppl C. Phylogenetic development of the cochlea and its innervation. Curr Opin Neurobiol 1998;8:468–74.
6. Corwin JT. Postembryonic production and aging in inner ear hair cells in sharks. J Comp Neurol 1981;201:541–53.
7. Corwin JT. Perpetual production of hair cells and maturational changes in hair cell ultrastructure accompany postembryonic growth in an amphibian ear. Proc·Natl Acad Sci USA 1985;82:3911–15.
8. Balak KJ, Corwin JT, Jones JE. Regenerated hair cells can originate from supporting cell progeny: Evidence from phototoxicity and laser ablation experiments in the lateral line system. J Neurosci 1990;10:2502–12.
9. Carranza A, Lopez I, Castellano P, et al. Intraotic administration of gentamicin: A new method to study ototoxicity in the crista ampullaris of the bullfrog. Laryngoscope 1997;107:137–43.
10. Hernandes JD, Hoffman LF, Lopez I. Recovery of vestibular afferent responses associated with hair cell regeneration following gentamicin ototoxicity in the bullfrog. Abstr Assoc Res Otolaryngol 1996;19:30.
11. Cristobal R, Lopez I, Chiang S, et al. Hair cell formation in cultures of dissociated cells from the vestibular sensory epithelium of the bullfrog. Am J Otol 1998;19:660–8.
12. Jørgensen JM, Mathiesen C. The avian inner ear. Continuous production of hair cells in vestibular sensory organs, but not in the auditory papilla. Naturwissenschaften 1988;75:319–20.
13. Roberson DF, Weisleder P, Bohrer PS, Rubel EW. Ongoing production of sensory cells in the vestibular epithelium of the chick. Hear Res 1992;57:166–74
14. Oesterle EC, Tsue TT, Reh TA, Rubel EW. Hair-cell regeneration in organ cultures of the postnatal chicken inner ear. Hear Res 1993;70:85–108.
15. Weisleder P, Rubel EW. Hair cell regeneration after streptomycin toxicity in the avian vestibular epithelium. J Comp Neurol 1993;331:97–110.
16. Warchol ME. Supporting cells in isolated sensory epithelia of avian utricles proliferate in serum-free culture. Neuroreport 1995;6:981–4.
17. Carey JP, Fuchs AF, Rubel EW. Hair cell regeneration and recovery of the vestibuloocular reflex in the avian vestibular system. J Neurophysiol 1996;76:3301–12.
18. Gleich O, Dooling RJ, Manley GA. Inner-ear abnormalities and their functional consequences in Belgian Waterslager canaries (Serinus canarius). Hear Res 1994;79:123–36.
19. Cotanche DA, Lee KH, Stone JS, Picard DA. Hair cell regeneration in the bird cochlea following noise damage or ototoxic drug damage. Anat Embryol 1994;189:1–18.
20. Corwin JT, Cotanche DA. Regeneration of sensory hair cells after acoustic trauma. Science 1988;240:1772–4.
21. Ryals BM, Rubel EW. Hair cell regeneration after acoustic trauma in adult Coturnix quail. Science 1988;240:1774–6.
22. Cruz RM, Lambert PR, Rubel EW. Light microscopic evidence of hair cell regeneration after gentamicin toxicity in chick cochlea. Arch Otolaryngol Head Neck Surg 1987;113:1058–62.
23. Bhave SA, Stone JS, Rubel EW, Coltrera MD. Cell cycle progression in gentamicin-damaged avian cochleas. J Neurosci 1995;15:4618–28.
24. Frenz DA, Yoo H, Liu W. Basilar papilla explants: A model to study hair cell regeneration-repair and protection. Acta Otolaryngol 1998;118:651–9.
25. Warchol ME, Corwin JT. Regenerative proliferation in organ cultures of the avian cochlea: Identification of the initial progenitors and determination of the latency of the proliferative response. J Neurosci 1996;16:5466–77.
26. McFadden EA, Saunders JC. Recovery of auditory function following intense sound exposure in the neonatal chick. Hear Res 1989;41:205–15.
27. Adler HJ, Kenealy JF, Dedio RM, Saunders JC. Threshold shift, hair cell loss, and hair bundle stiffness following exposure to 120 and 125 dB pure tones in the neonatal chick. Acta Otolaryngol 1992;112:444–54.
28. Saunders JC, Adler HJ, Pugliano FA. The structural and functional aspects of hair cell regeneration in the chick as a result of exposure to intense sound. Exp Neurol 1992;115:13–7.
29. Cotanche DA. Regeneration of the tectorial membrane in the chick cochlea following severe acoustic trauma. Hear Res 1987;30:197–206.
30. Cohen YE, Saunders JC. The effects of sound overexposure on the spectral response patterns of nucleus magnocellularis in the neonatal chick. Exp Brain Res 1993;95:202–12.
31. Niemiec AJ, Raphael Y, Moody DB. Return of auditory function following structural regeneration after

acoustic trauma: Behavioral measures from quail. Hear Res 1994;79:1–16.
32. Marean GC, Burt JM, Beecher MD, Rubel EW. Hair cell regeneration in the European starling (*Sturnus vulgaris*): Recovery of pure-tone detection thresholds. Hear Res 1993;71:125–36.
33. Tucci DL, Rubel EW. Physiologic status of regenerated hair cells in the avian inner ear following aminoglycoside ototoxicity. Otolaryngol Head Neck Surg 1990;103:443–50.
34. Girod DA, Tucci DL, Rubel EW. Anatomical correlates of functional recovery in the avian inner ear following aminoglycoside ototoxicity. Laryngoscope 1991;101:1139–49.
35. Woolley SM, Wissman AM, Rubel EW. Hair cell regeneration and recovery of auditory thresholds following aminoglycoside ototoxicity in Bengalese finches. Hear Res 2001;153:181–95.
36. Smolders JW. Functional recovery in the avian ear after hair cell regeneration. Audiol Neurootol 1999;4:286–302.
37. Warchol ME, Lambert PR, Goldstein BJ, et al. Regenerative proliferation in inner ear sensory epithelia from adult guinea pigs and humans. Science 1993;259:1619–22.
38. Lambert PR, Gu R, Corwin JT. Analysis of small hair bundles in the utricles of mature guinea pigs. Am J Otol 1997;18:637–43.
39. Tanyeri H, Lopez I, Honrubia V. Histological evidence for hair cell regeneration after ototoxic cell destruction with local application of gentamicin in the chinchilla crista ampullaris. Hear Res 1995;89:194–202.
40. Walsh RM, Hackney CM, Furness DN. Regeneration of the mammalian vestibular sensory epithelium following gentamicin-induced damage. J Otolaryngol 2000;29: 351–60.
41. Rubel EW, Dew LA, Roberson DW. Mammalian vestibular hair cell regeneration. Science 1995;267:701–7.
42. Warchol ME, Lambert PR, Goldstein BJ, et al. Response to: Mammalian vestibular hair cell regeneration. Science 1995;267:704–6.
43. Zheng JL, Keller G, Gao WQ. Immunocytochemical and morphological evidence for intracellular self-repair as an important contributor to mammalian hair cell recovery. J Neurosci 1999;19:2161–70.
44. Meza G, Solano-Flores LP, Poblano A. Recovery of vestibular function in young guinea pigs after streptomycin treatment. Glutamate decarboxylase activity and nystagmus response assessment. Int J Dev Neurosci 1992;10:407–11.
45. Glasscock ME, III, Johnson GD, Poe DS. Streptomycin in Meniere's disease: A case requiring multiple treatments. Otolaryngol Head Neck Surg 1989;100:237–41.
46. Kelley MW, Talreja DR, Corwin JT. Replacement of hair cells after laser microbeam irradiation in cultured organs of corti from embryonic and neonatal mice. J Neurosci 1995;15:3013–26.
47. Lenoir M, Vago P. Does the organ of Corti attempt to differentiate new hair cells after antibiotic intoxication in rat pups? Int J Dev Neurosci 1997;15:487–95.
48. Kawamoto K, Ishimoto S, Minoda R, et al. Math1 gene transfer generates new cochlear hair cells in mature guinea pigs in vivo. J Neurosci 2003;23:4395–4400.
49. Shou J, Zheng JL, Gao WQ. Robust generation of new hair cells in the mature mammalian inner ear by adenoviral expression of Hath1. Mol Cell Neurosci 2003;23:169–79.
50. Tsue TT, Watling DL, Weisleder P, et al. Identification of hair cell progenitors and intermitotic migration of their nuclei in the normal and regenerating avian inner ear. J Neurosci 1994;14:140–52.
51. Stone JS, Leaño SG, Baker LP, Rubel EW. Hair cell differentiation in chick cochlear epithelium after aminoglycoside toxicity: In vivo and in vitro observations. J Neurosci 1996;16:6157–74.
52. Stone JS, Rubel EW. Temporal, spatial, and morphologic features of hair cell regeneration in the avian basilar papilla. J Comp Neurol 2000;417:1–16.
53. Roberson DW, Alosi JA, Cotanche DA. Direct transdifferentiation gives rise to the earliest new hair cells in regenerating avian auditory epithelium. J Neurosci Res 2004;78:461–71.
54. Adler HJ, Raphael Y. New hair cells arise from supporting cell conversion in the acoustically damaged chick inner ear [published erratum appears in Neurosci Lett 1996;210:73]. Neurosc Lett 1996;205:17–20.
55. Gale JE, Meyers JR, Periasamy A, Corwin JT. Survival of bundleless hair cells and subsequent bundle replacement in the bullfrog's saccule. J Neurobiol 2002;50:81–92.
56. Sobkowicz HM, August BK, Slapnick SM. Post-traumatic survival and recovery of the auditory sensory cells in culture. Acta Otolaryngol 1996;116:257–62.
57. Sobkowicz HM, August BK, Slapnick SM. Cellular interactions as a response to injury in the organ of Corti in culture. Int J Dev Neurosci 1997;15:463–85.
58. Cotanche DA, Messana EP, Ofsie MS. Migration of hyaline cells into the chick basilar papilla during severe noise damage. Hear Res 1995;91:148–59.
59. Girod DA, Rubel EW. Hair cell regeneration in the avian cochlea: If it works in birds, why not in man? Ear Nose Throat J 1991;70:343–50.
60. Fekete DM. Cell fate specification in the inner ear. Curr Opin Neurobiol 1996;6:533–41.
61. Fekete DM. Making sense of making hair cells. Trends Neurosci 2000;23:386.
62. Bermingham NA, Hassan BA, Price SD, et al. Math1: An essential gene for the generation of inner ear hair cells. Science 1999;284:1837–41.
63. Fekete DM, Muthukumar S, Karagogeos D. Hair cells and supporting cells share a common progenitor in the avian inner ear. J Neurosci 1998;18:7811–21.
64. Tsue TT, Oesterle EC, Rubel EW. Diffusible factors regulate hair cell regeneration in the avian inner ear. Proc Natl Acad Sci U S A 1994;91:1584–88.
65. Cristobal R, Popper P, Lopez I, et al. In vivo and in vitro localization of brain-derived neurotrophic factor, fibroblast growth factor-2 and their receptors in the bullfrog vestibular end organs. Brain Res Mol Brain Res 2002;102:83–9.
66. Oesterle EC, Tsue TT, Rubel EW. Induction of cell proliferation in avian inner ear sensory epithelia by insulin-like growth factor-I and insulin. J Comp Neurol 1997;380:262–74.
67. Lambert PR. Inner ear hair cell regeneration in a mammal: Identification of a triggering factor. Laryngoscope 1994;104:701–18.
68. Yamashita H, Oesterle EC. Induction of cell proliferation in mammalian inner-ear sensory epithelia by transforming growth factor alpha and epidermal growth factor. Proc Natl Acad Sci U S A 1995;92:3152–5.
69. Hume CR, Kirkegaard M, Oesterle EC. ErbB expression: The mouse inner ear and maturation of the mitogenic response to heregulin. J Assoc Res Otolaryngol 2003;4:422–43.
70. Popper P, Lopez I, Beizai P, et al. Expression of BDNF and TrkB mRNAs in the crista neurosensory epithelium and vestibular ganglia following ototoxic damage. Brain Res 1999;846:40–51.
71. Oesterle EC, Hume CR. Growth factor regulation of the cell cycle in developing and mature inner ear sensory epithelia. J Neurocytol 1999;28:877–87.
72. Warchol ME. Cell density and N-cadherin interactions regulate cell proliferation in the sensory epithelia of the inner ear. J Neurosci 2002;22:2607–16.
73. Weir J, Rivolta MN, Holley MC. Notch signaling and the emergence of auditory hair cells. Arch Otolaryngol Head Neck Surg 2000;126:1244–8.
74. Androutsellis-Theotokis A, Leker RR, Soldner F, et al. Notch signalling regulates stem cell numbers in vitro and in vivo. Nature 2006;442:823–6.
75. Lanford PJ, Lan Y, Jiang R, et al. Notch signalling pathway mediates hair cell development in mammalian cochlea. Nat Genet 1999;21:289–92.
76. Kiernan AE, Cordes R, Kopan R, et al. The Notch ligands DLL1 and JAG2 act synergistically to regulate hair cell development in the mammalian inner ear. Development 2005;132:4353–62.
77. Tang LS, Alger HM, Pereira FA. COUP-TFI controls Notch regulation of hair cell and support cell differentiation. Development 2006;133:3683–93.
78. Chen P, Segil N. p27(Kip1) links cell proliferation to morphogenesis in the developing organ of Corti. Development 1999;126:1581–90.
79. Lowenheim H, Furness DN, Kil J, et al. Gene disruption of p27(Kip1) allows cell proliferation in the postnatal and adult organ of corti. Proc Natl Acad Sci U S A 1999;96:4084–8.
80. White PM, Doetzlhofer A, Lee YS, et al. Mammalian cochlear supporting cells can divide and trans-differentiate into hair cells. Nature 2006;441:984–7.
81. Frolov MV, Dyson NJ. Molecular mechanisms of E2F-dependent activation and pRB-mediated repression. J Cell Sci 2004;117:2173–81.
82. Taylor R, Forge A. Developmental biology. Life after deaf for hair cells? Science 2005;307:1056–8.
83. Sage C, Huang M, Vollrath MA, et al. Essential role of retinoblastoma protein in mammalian hair cell development and hearing. Proc Natl Acad Sci U S A 2006;103:7345–50.
84. Witte MC, Montcouquiol M, Corwin JT. Regeneration in avian hair cell epithelia: Identification of intracellular signals required for S-phase entry. Eur J Neurosci 2001;14:829–38.
85. Malgrange B, Knockaert M, Belachew S, et al. The inhibition of cyclin-dependent kinases induces differentiation of supernumerary hair cells and Deiters' cells in the developing organ of Corti. FASEB J 2003;17:2136–8.
86. Woods C, Montcouquiol M, Kelley MW. Math1 regulates development of the sensory epithelium in the mammalian cochlea. Nature Neurosci 2004;7:1310–8.
87. Zheng JL, Gao WQ. Overexpression of Math1 induces robust production of extra hair cells in postnatal rat inner ears. Nature Neurosci 2000;3:580–6.
88. Izumikawa M, Minoda R, Kawamoto K, et al. Auditory hair cell replacement and hearing improvement by Atoh1 gene therapy in deaf mammals. Nature Med 2005;11: 271–6.
89. Tang LS, Montemayor C, Pereira FA. Sensorineural hearing loss: Potential therapies and gene targets for drug development. Life 2006;58:1–6.
90. Zheng JL, Shou J, Guillemot F, et al. Hes1 is a negative regulator of inner ear hair cell differentiation. Development 2000;127:4551–60.
91. Erkman L, McEvilly RJ, Luo L, et al. Role of transcription factors Brn-3.1 and Brn-3.2 in auditory and visual system development. Nature 1996;381:603–6.
92. Keithley EM, Erkman L, Bennett T, et al. Effects of a hair cell transcription factor, Brn-3.1, gene deletion on homozygous and heterozygous mouse cochleas in adulthood and aging. Hear Res 1999;134:71–6.
93. Vahava O, Morell R, Lynch ED, et al. Mutation in transcription factor POU4F3 associated with inherited progressive hearing loss in humans. Science 1998;279:1950–4.
94. Thomson JA, Itskovitz-Eldor J, Shapiro SS, et al. Embryonic stem cell lines derived from human blastocysts [erratum appears in Science 1998;282:1827]. Science 1998;282:1145–7.
95. Shamblott MJ, Axelman J, Wang S, et al. Derivation of pluripotent stem cells from cultured human primordial germ cells [erratum appears in Proc Natl Acad Sci U S A 1999;96:1162]. Proc Natl Acad Sci U S A 1998;95: 13726–31.
96. Dazert S, Aletsee C, Brors D, et al. Regeneration of inner ear cells from stem cell precursors—a future concept of hearing rehabilitation? DNA Cell Biol 2003;22:565–70.
97. Bjornson CR, Rietze RL, Reynolds BA, et al. Turning brain into blood: A hematopoietic fate adopted by adult neural stem cells in vivo. Science 1999;283:534–7.
98. Clarke DL, Johansson CB, Wilbertz J, et al. Generalized potential of adult neural stem cells. Science 2000;288:1660–3.
99. Terada N, Hamazaki T, Oka M, et al. Bone marrow cells adopt the phenotype of other cells by spontaneous cell fusion. Nature 2002;416:542–5.
100. Ying QL, Nichols J, Evans EP, Smith AG. Changing potency by spontaneous fusion. Nature 2002;416: 545–8.
101. Loebel DA, Watson CM, De Young RA, Tam PP. Lineage choice and differentiation in mouse embryos and embryonic stem cells. Dev Biol 2003;264:1–14.
102. Li H, Liu H, Heller S. Pluripotent stem cells from the adult mouse inner ear. Nat Med 2003;9:1293–9.
103. Kim TS, Kojima K, Nishida AT, et al. Expression of calretinin by fetal otocyst cells after transplantation into damaged rat utricle explants. Acta Otolaryngol Suppl 2004;551:34–8.
104. Ito J, Kojima K, Kawaguchi S. Survival of neural stem cells in the cochlea. Acta Otolaryngol 2001;121:140–2.
105. Parker MA, Anderson JK, Corliss DA, et al. Expression profile of an operationally-defined neural stem cell clone. Exp Neurol 2005;194:320–32.
106. Swanson GJ, Howard M, Lewis J. Epithelial autonomy in the development of the inner ear of a bird embryo. Dev Biol 1990;137:243–57.
107. Corwin JT, Cotanche DA. Development of location-specific hair cell stereocilia in denervated embryonic ears. J Comp Neurol 1989;288:529–37.
108. Li H, Roblin G, Liu H, Heller S. Generation of hair cells by stepwise differentiation of embryonic stem cells. Proc Natl Acad Sci U S A 2003;100:13495–500.
109. Malgrange B, Belachew S, Thiry M, et al. Proliferative generation of mammalian auditory hair cells in culture. Mech Dev 2002;112:79–88.
110. Doetzlhofer A, White PM, Johnson JE, et al. In vitro growth and differentiation of mammalian sensory hair cell progenitors: A requirement for EGF and periotic mesenchyme. Dev Biol 2004;272:432–47.
111. Zhai S, Shi L, Wang BE, et al. Isolation and culture of hair cell progenitors from postnatal rat cochleae. J Neurobiol 2005;65:282–93.
112. Raz Y. Clinical applications for embryonic stem cells: Ideas from an otolaryngologist. Daytona Beach, FL: Association for Research in Otolaryngology Midwinter Conference; 2004. p. 28–36.
113. Reya T, Morrison SJ, Clarke MF, Weissman IL. Stem cells, cancer, and cancer stem cells. Nature 2001;414:105–11.
114. Alvarez-Dolado M, Pardal R, Garcia-Verdugo JM, et al. Fusion of bone-marrow-derived cells with Purkinje neurons, cardiomyocytes and hepatocytes. Nature 2003;425: 968–73.

115. Raphael Y, Altschuler RA. Reorganization of cytoskeletal and junctional proteins during cochlear hair cell degeneration. Cell Motil Cytoskeleton 1991;18:215–27.

116. Lenoir M, Daudet N, Humbert G, et al. Morphological and molecular changes in the inner hair cell region of the rat cochlea after amikacin treatment. J Neurocytol 1999;28:925–37.

117. Brown AB, Yang W, Schmidt NO, et al. Intravascular delivery of neural stem cell lines to target intracranial and extracranial tumors of neural and non-neural origin. Hum Gene Ther 2003;14:1777–85.

118. Walters L. Human embryonic stem cell research: An intercultural perspective. Kennedy Inst Ethics J 2004;14:3–38.

119. Bonilla S, Silva A, Valdes L, et al. Functional neural stem cells derived from adult bone marrow. Neurosci 2005;133:85–95.

120. Holley MC. Hair cell re-growth. Int J Pediatr Otorhinolaryngol 2003;67:S1–5.

121. Hawkins RD, Bashiardes S, Helms CA, et al. Gene expression differences in quiescent versus regenerating hair cells of avian sensory epithelia: Implications for human hearing and balance disorders. Hum Mol Genet 2003;12:1261–72.

122. Gong TW, Hegeman AD, Shin JJ, et al. Identification of genes expressed after noise exposure in the chick basilar papilla. Hear Res 1996;96:20–32.

123. Gong TW, Hegeman AD, Shin JJ, et al. Novel genes expressed in the chick otocyst during development: Identification using differential display of RNA. Int J Dev Neurosci 1997;15:585–94.

124. Kanzaki S, Kawamoto K, Oh SH, et al. From gene identification to gene therapy. Audiol Neurootol 2002;7:161–4.

125. Lomax MI, Huang L, Cho Y, et al. Differential display and gene arrays to examine auditory plasticity. Hear Res 2000;147:293–302.

126. Cristobal R, Wackym PA, Cioffi JA, et al. Assessment of differential gene expression in vestibular epithelial cell types using microarray analysis. Brain Res Mol Brain Res 2005;133:19–36.

127. Barald KF, Lindberg KH, Hardiman K, et al. Immortalized cell lines from embryonic avian and murine otocysts: Tools for molecular studies of the developing inner ear. Int J Dev Neurosci 1997;15:523–40.

128. Lawlor P, Marcotti W, Rivolta MN, et al. Differentiation of mammalian vestibular hair cells from conditionally immortal, postnatal supporting cells. J Neurosci 1999;19:9445–58.

129. Rivolta MN, Holley MC. Cell lines in inner ear research. J Neurobiol 2002;53:306–18.

130. Rivolta MN, Grix N, Lawlor P, et al. Auditory hair cell precursors immortalized from the mammalian inner ear. Proc R Soc Lond B Biol Sci 1998;265:1595–603.

131. Rivolta MN, Halsall A, Johnson CM, et al. Transcript profiling of functionally related groups of genes during conditional differentiation of a mammalian cochlear hair cell line. Genome Res 2002;12:1091–9.

132. Kalinec GM, Webster P, Lim DJ, Kalinec F. A cochlear cell line as an in vitro system for drug ototoxicity screening. Audiol Neurootol 2003;8:177–89.

133. Rivolta MN, Li H, Heller S. Generation of inner ear cell types from embryonic stem cells. Methods Mol Biol 2006;330:71–92.

134. Doetzlhofer A, White P, Lee YS, et al. Prospective identification and purification of hair cell and supporting cell progenitors from the embryonic cochlea. Brain Res 2006;1091:282–8.

7

Cochlear Biophysics

William E. Brownell, PhD

John S. Oghalai, MD

OVERVIEW: BIOPHYSICS AND THE INNER EAR

Physics deals with matter and energy and the interaction between the two. This chapter describes the biophysics underlying energy transduction by cochlear hair cells. Transduction is the conversion of one type of energy to another. The cochlea converts sound-evoked vibrations into neural information that is transmitted to the brain via the auditory nerve. The cochlea can detect mechanical movements at the eardrum that are less than the size of a hydrogen atom, and encodes the temporal features of those movements with a precision that allows us to discriminate which ear receives the sound first to within 20 microseconds. The conversion of acoustic energy to neural (electrochemical) energy occurs in the hair cells. The mechanical vibration of hair cell stereocilia results in a change of hair cell transmembrane electrical potential and ultimately leads to the secretion of an excitatory neurotransmitter that activates an eighth nerve fiber. Outer hair cells (OHCs) have both sensory and motor functions. Sensory receptor potentials are produced by the bending of the stereociliary bundle. The receptor potentials are converted directly into mechanical force by the membranes of the outer hair cell lateral wall. This electromechanical force counteracts viscous-damping forces within the fluid-filled environment of the inner ear, and it provides the basis of the cochlear amplifier that enhances sensitivity and frequency selectivity. One side effect that can be measured clinically is otoacoustic emissions.

High-Frequency Force Production in the Ear

Sound waves arriving at the external ear pass through the ear canal and displace the tympanic membrane. The sound vibrations are transmitted through the bones of the middle ear and create pressure differences in the cochlea. The pressure differences between cochlear compartments produce a traveling wave along the elastic basilar membrane (Figure 1). Auditory nerve fibers at a given location in vertebrate hearing organs respond most vigorously to sounds at a specific frequency. Systematic differences in geometry, elastic properties, and mass of the basilar membrane and cochlear partition result in a frequency

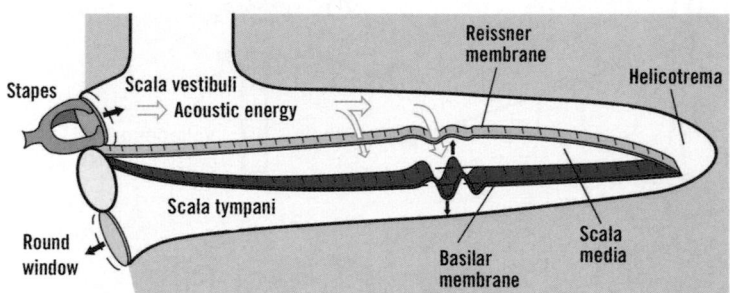

Figure 1 Diagram of uncoiled cochlea showing the traveling wave. (Adapted from reference 1.)

mapping along the length of the cochlea. The topographic mapping of best frequencies is called "tonotopic" and is retained in the central nervous system (CNS) auditory structures. Factors that impose limits on the frequency at which inner ear structures can vibrate set the frequency limits of hearing.

Vertebrate hearing organs are fluid filled, and fluids impose a damping force on vibrations. Fluid or viscous damping is directly proportional to the velocity of the vibrating structures so that the damping force resisting differential movements (such as the bending of stereocilia) increases proportionally with frequency. It becomes more difficult for animals to hear as frequency increases unless there is a mechanism to counteract viscous damping. Diverse strategies to mechanically counteract fluid damping and increase the upper frequency limit of hearing are found in animal ears and involve the production of a "negative damping" force. It is likely that force production by the stereociliary bundle was the negative-damping strategy used for the relatively low-frequency hearing of early vertebrates. When mammals appeared over 220 million years ago, they adopted a different mechanism associated with the lateral wall of their cylindrically shaped OHCs. The ability of the OHC to counteract viscous damping is referred to as the cochlear amplifier. The amplification is a function of the magnitude of the vibration, operating with the greatest gain for low-intensity sounds. The result is a compressive nonlinearity that improves the sensitivity and frequency selectivity of hearing.

HAIR CELLS

Hair cells are polarized epithelial cells that get their name from the stereociliary bundle on their apical surface (Figure 2). The stereocilia are giant microvilli arranged in three rows that increase in length toward the side of the cell located away from the central axis (the modiolus) of the cochlear spiral (Figure 3). Stereocilia have a dense inner core of tightly packed actin filaments that send a bundle of rootlets into a matrix of cytoskeletal proteins known as the cuticular plate located at the base of the stereociliary bundle (Figure 4). Just lateral to the center of the tallest row and located in the cytoplasm adjacent to the cuticular plate is a basal body which is all that remains of a single kinocilium that was present during early development but is resorbed as the organ of Corti matures (see Figure 2). During development, the kinocilium is thought to establish the morphologic polarization of the stereociliary bundle. The morphologic polarization then determines the physiologic polarization.

Mechanoelectrical transduction (MET) channels located in the wall of the stereocilia are hypothesized to be tethered to adjacent stereocilia by "tip links" (see Figure 2). The deflection of the stereocilia toward the tallest row causes the tip links to pull on the MET channels and open them. Deflection in the other direction releases the tension of the tip links, causing the transduction channels to close. Thus bending the bundle in the direction of the tallest row leads to entry of K^+ and Ca^{+2} ions from the endolymph into the hair cell. This causes depolarization of the hair cell. Bending the bundle in the opposite direction closes the channels and the hair cell hyperpolarizes. The stereociliary bundle has an axis of symmetry that runs through the basal body perpendicular to the rows (see Figure 4). Bending the bundle parallel to the axis modulates the flow of ions into the hair cell. Bundle deflection perpendicular to the axis of symmetry results in no change in membrane potential. The magnitude of the voltage change produced by a stereociliary

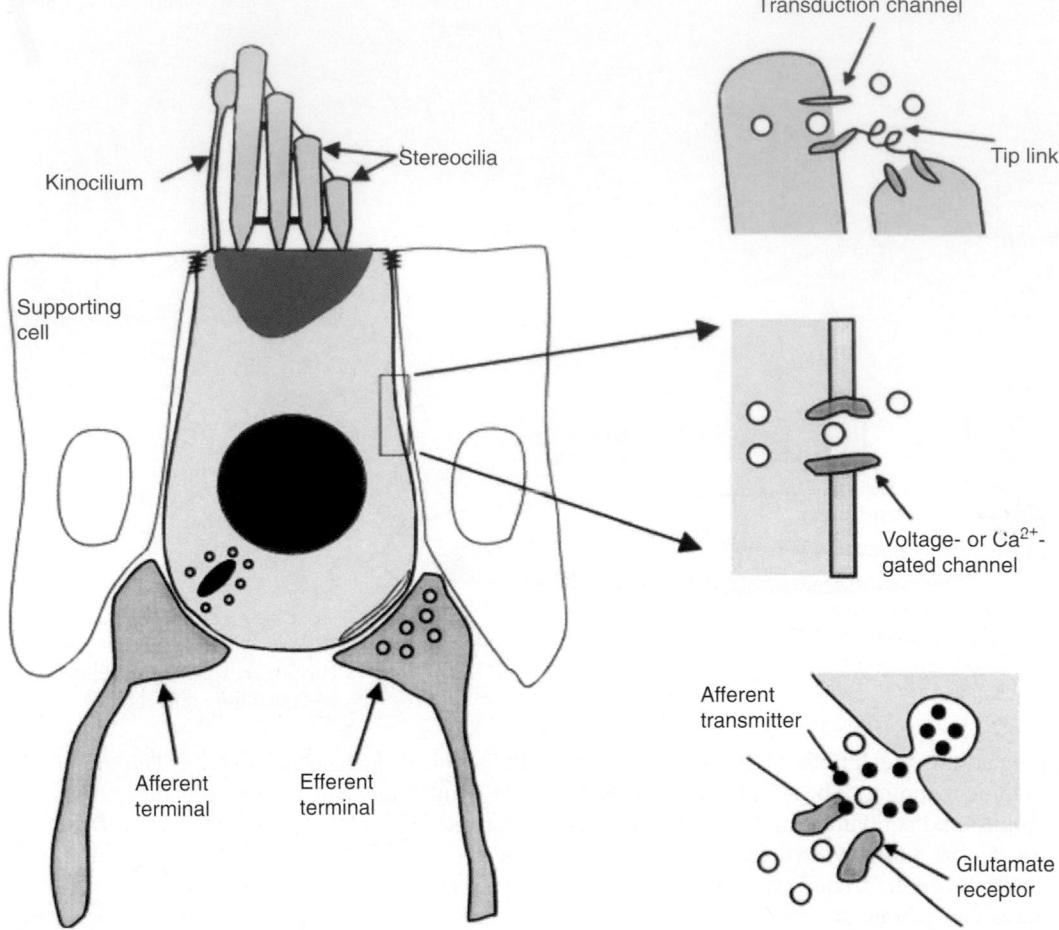

Figure 2 An immature cochlear hair cell. (Published with permission, copyright © 2007, W.E. Brownell, PhD, and J.S. Oghalai, MD.)

deflection toward the modiolus (which closes MET channels) is less than that of an equivalent deflection away from the modiolus (which opens MET channels). This nonlinearity results from the various voltage- and calcium-dependent ion channels in the hair cell's basolateral plasma membrane that shape the relation between current and voltage.

ORGAN OF CORTI

The sensory epithelium of the cochlea is called the organ of Corti. It consists of hair cells supported by an elegant matrix of cellular and acellular structures (see Figure 3). There are 3 rows of OHCs and a single row of inner hair cells (IHCs). The IHCs are located nearer the central axis of the cochlear spiral while the OHCs are further away. Both inner and outer hair cells are mechanoreceptors, but only IHC receptor potentials trigger afferent nerve activity sending signals to the brain. The fact that more than 10 afferent nerve fibers receive information from a single inner hair cell tells us that there is ample redundancy and added security for information transfer to the CNS. OHCs have the specialized role of enhancing the micromechanical tuning of the basilar membrane. They do this by generating a mechanical force in response to the receptor potential changes produced by bending the stereociliary bundle. The force alters the vibrations

of the organ of Corti and refines the stimulation of the IHCs, thereby enhancing the perception and discrimination of the high-frequency sounds. There are about 12,000 hair cells (3,000 IHCs and 9,000 OHCs) in a normal human cochlea. This is a small number of cells when compared to the hundreds of millions of sensory cells found in the sensory epithelia of the retina, nose, or skin. Physics helps to understand the reason for the much smaller number of hair cells. The auditory system must detect small mechanical vibrations. Newtonian mechanics tells us that detecting a small force requires that the detection mass must be as small as possible. Similar considerations suggest that the benefits of small mass for the detection of rapid, low energy

mechanical events may scale to the molecular level where assemblies of smaller molecules would be favored.

TECTORIAL MEMBRANE

The stereociliary bundles of the OHCs are embedded in the tectorial membrane (see Figure 3). The tectorial membrane is an extracellular matrix, which contains at least 3 types of collagen and the noncollagenous glycoproteins: α-tectorin, β-tectorin, and otogelin. The organization of these proteins within the tectorial membrane is anisotropic in that they project radially away from the central axis of the cochlea. Within the body of the tectorial membrane, a laminated striated sheet matrix is formed from 7 to 9 nm diameter filaments. The lower fibrous layer near the hair cells (Kimura membrane) consists of collagen organized in bundles of straight 20 nm diameter filaments. The marginal band at the lateral edge of the tectorial membrane and the cover net bundles on the top of the tectorial membrane contain anastomosing networks of thick collagen fibrils. Alpha- and beta-tectorin are thought to play a role in crosslinking collagen fibers. The role of otogelin is unclear at this time.

The development of the tectorial membrane occurs in concert with the development of the organ of Corti and differentiation of hair cells during embryogenesis. The greater epithelial ridge begins to give rise to inner hair cells and the lesser epithelial ridge begins to give rise to outer hair cells. The tectorial membrane matrix is secreted by supporting cells within the greater and lesser epithelial ridge. Eventually, the inner sulcus cells under the medial aspect of the tectorial membrane resorb, leaving it attached medially only to the spiral limbus and stretching across the surface of the organ of Corti. Once the cochlea has fully developed, the tectorial membrane is thought to remain inert with little protein turnover.

Hair cell stereocilia deflection is coordinated by the tectorial membrane. The tips of OHC stereociliary bundles are embedded in the tectorial membrane. When sound is transmitted to the inner ear, the organ of Corti vibrates up and

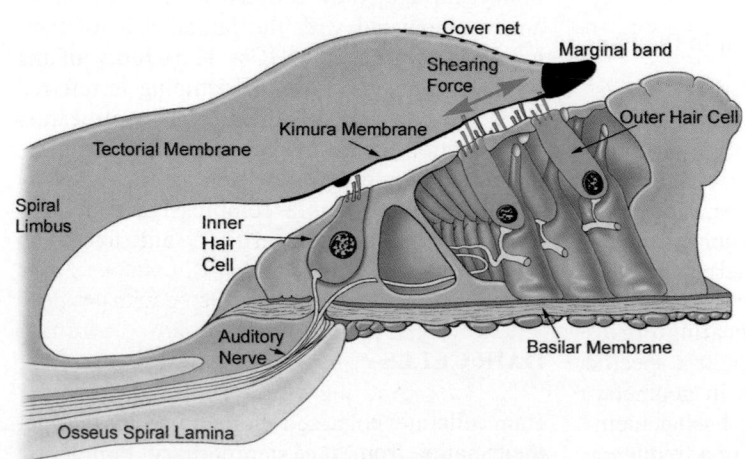

Figure 3 The organ of Corti. The central axis or modiolus of the spiraling cochlea is to the left of the drawing. (Adapted from reference 2.)

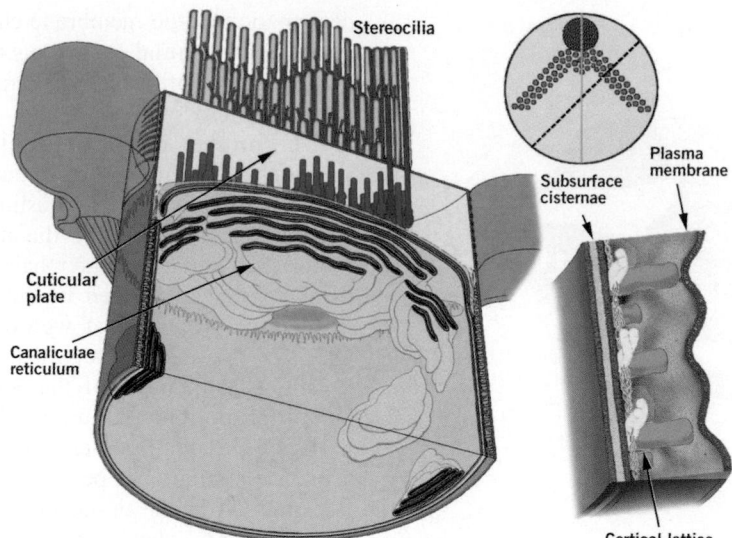

Stereocilia

Plasma
membrane

Subsurface
cisternae

Cuticular
plate

Canaliculae
reticulum

Cortical lattice

Figure 4 Three-layer organization in the apical pole and the lateral wall of the cochlear outer hair cell. The plasma membrane is the outermost layer in both locations. The innermost layer is composed of a membrane-bound organelle called the canaliculae reticulum in the apex and the subsurface cisterna in the lateral wall. In between the membranes is a cytoskeletal structure called the cuticular plate in the apex and the cortical lattice in the lateral wall. Insert on the lower right portrays a high power rendering of the outer hair cell lateral wall. Insert at upper right is a view looking down on the apical end; the green line shows the axis of symmetry which defines the anatomical and functional polarization of the stereociliary bundle; the dashed line shows the plane at which the outer hair cell has been opened. (Adapted from reference 3.)

However, the extent to which this causes clinically relevant hearing loss is unknown.

OUTER HAIR CELLS

OHCs have a cylindrical shape (see Figures 3–5). They vary in length from approximately 12 µm at the basal or high-frequency end of the cochlea to >90 µm at the low-frequency end. Their diameter at all locations is approximately 9 µm, which is slightly larger than the diameter of a red blood cell. Their apical end is capped with a rigid cuticular plate which anchors the stereocilia. Their synaptic end is a hemisphere containing the nucleus along with synaptic structures. Each of these 3 regions (the apical stereociliary bundle, middle cylinder, and hemispheric base) has a specific function. The top and the bottom of the OHC perform functions that are common to all hair cells. The stereociliary bundle at the top of the cell is responsible for converting the mechanical energy of sound into electrical energy. Afferent and efferent synaptic structures are found at the base of the OHC. While the function of the OHC afferent synapse is unknown, the efferent synapse modulates the cochlear amplifier. The elongated cylindrical portion of the outer hair cell is where electrical energy is converted into mechanical energy.[4] This function is unique to the OHC. No other hair cell (nor any other kind of cell) is able to change its length at acoustic frequencies in response to electrical stimulation. This electromotility can be greater than 1% of the cell's original length if the electrical stimulation is large.

The Outer Hair Cell Is Pressurized

In contrast to the other cells in the body which have a cytoskeleton to maintain their shape the OHC is a hydrostat. A hydrostat is a mechanical structure in which an elastic shell is inflated by a pressurized fluid core. The OHC cytoplasm is slightly hyperosmotic relative to the cochlear fluids, and the resulting osmotic pressure inflates the cell. A rigid internal skeleton such as that found in other cells would impede electromotility, so it is not surprising that no long-chain polymerized proteins exist within the axial core of the OHC. The turgidity of the OHC renders it mechanically strong enough to transmit force to the rest of the organ of Corti. Pressurized cells are common in the plant kingdom but are rarely found in cells of the animal kingdom. Plant cells, such as those found at the base of a tree, are highly pressurized. This allows the cells to hold the weight of the tree and still be flexible enough to bend and not shatter in a wind. Most of the cells in our body will not tolerate internal pressure because the membrane that encloses them would rupture. The OHC membrane is reinforced with a highly organized actin-spectrin cytoskeleton just underneath the plasma membrane (see Figures 4 and 5). This cortical lattice determines the cylindrical shape of the OHC when it is inflated by the hyperosmotic fluid core. The nature of the osmolytes is unknown at this time.

down (see Figure 1). Since the basilar membrane is attached both medially and laterally, the area of maximal vibration is near the third row of OHCs. In contrast the tectorial membrane is fixed only at the spiral limbus. Movement of the basilar membrane up and down, induced by sound waves within the cochlear fluids, causes a shearing force to deflect the hair cell stereocilia (see Figure 3). Displacement of the cochlear partition upward deflects stereocilia away from the central cochlear axis and opens MET channels. Movement in a downward direction deflects the stereocilia toward the central cochlear axis and closes MET channels. The OHCs feed back mechanical forces, enhancing the vibrations of the cochlear partition. A normal tectorial membrane is necessary for normal cochlear amplifier function.

While OHC stereociliary movements can be directly linked to movements of the cochlear partition, the movements of the IHC stereocilia are not as straightforward. IHC stereociliary bundles are not directly connected to the tectorial membrane, but they are in close proximity to it. As a consequence of this anatomy, the fluid space around the stereociliary bundles (the subtectorial space) is constrained, and the fluid movement makes a major contribution to IHC stereociliary deflection. Current models include the fact that OHC electromotility may act to "pump" fluid back and forth within the subtectorial space.

Mutations that affect the tectorial membrane cause hearing loss. Most tectorial membrane mutations have been found within the gene for alpha-tectorin (*Tecta*). Alpha-tectorin is a large modular protein composed of an N-terminal entactin G1-like domain, a central region containing 3 full and 2 partial von Willebrand factor (vWF) type D repeats, and a C-terminal

zona pellucida (ZP) domain. To date, 9 different mutations in *Tecta* that cause hearing loss have been identified. All are point mutations and cause nonsyndromic sensorineural hearing loss; some are autosomal dominant, and some are autosomal recessive. Mutations in the ZP domain are associated with moderate hearing loss in the middle frequencies that tends to remain stable over time, that is, a cookie-bite audiogram. On the other hand, mutations in the vWF domains tend to cause progressive, high-frequency hearing loss.

Hearing loss due to tectorial membrane protein mutations is due to alterations in cochlear biophysics. Changing the proteins that constitute the tectorial membrane changes its shape and mechanical properties, and this produces cochlear dysfunction. For example, if the mutant tectorial membrane does not interface with the OHC stereocilia, loss of the cochlear amplifier will occur. This will lead to elevated auditory brainstem response (ABR) thresholds, widened tuning curves, and reduced distortion product otoacoustic emissions (DPOAE). On the other hand, if the tectorial membrane interfaces with the OHCs, but is farther away from the IHC stereocilia than normal, there will be elevated ABR thresholds but normal DPOAE responses and normal tuning curve sharpness.

Little is known about age-related or other degenerative processes affecting the tectorial membrane. Ultrastructural studies in aged rats have shown a reduced number of collagen fibers in the tectorial membrane associated with progressive hearing loss. Another study has shown that aged rats have a distorted tectorial membrane that is detached from the organ of Corti. Therefore, it appears as though age-related degeneration of the tectorial membrane can occur in mammals.

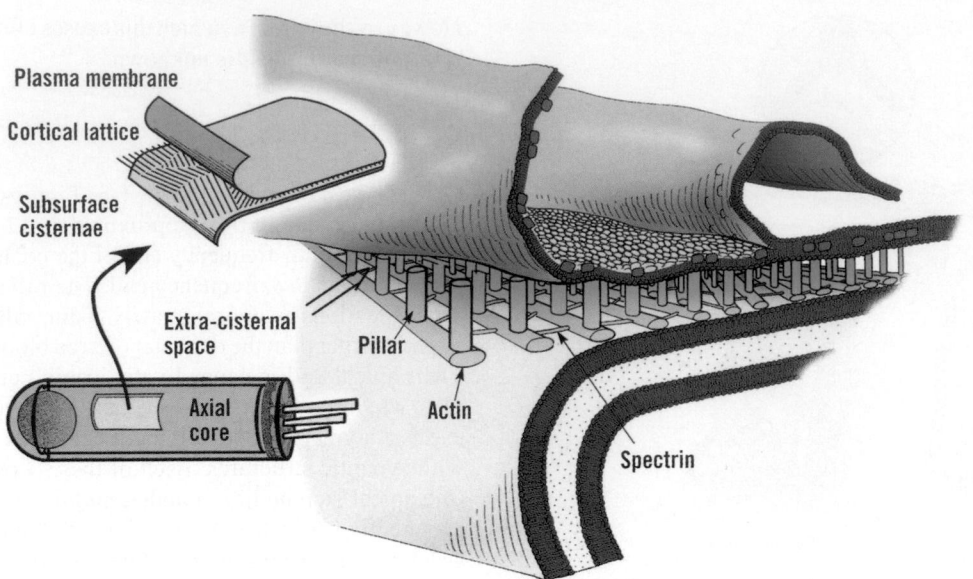

Figure 5 Diagram of the outer hair cell showing organization of lateral wall components. (Adapted from reference 5.)

The Lateral Wall

The lateral wall of the OHC is about 100 nm thick and contains the plasma membrane, the cortical lattice, and an intracellular organelle called the subsurface cisterna (SSC). Electron microscopy reveals the presence of hexagonally packed particles within the lateral wall plasma membrane. The composition and function of the particles has not been identified. Cortical lattice actin filaments are oriented circumferentially around the cell and are cross-linked by spectrin molecules. Actin is less compliant than spectrin. This is why OHC length changes are greater than diameter changes. Pillars tether the actin-spectrin network to the plasma membrane, but their molecular composition has not yet been identified. The plasma membrane may be rippled between adjacent pillar molecules (Figure 6).[6]

The SSC structurally resembles endoplasmic reticulum, but it can be stained with both endoplasmic reticulum and Golgi body markers. It does not belong to the plasma membrane–endoplasmic reticulum–Golgi membrane pool but instead appears to be a part of a membrane pool that includes the canaliculae reticulum (see Figure 4), a structure that occurs in ion-transporting epithelia. The membranes of the canaliculae reticulum are contiguous with those of the SSC as well as the outer membrane of mitochondria. The molecular composition of the SSC (its phospholipid composition and complement of integral membrane proteins) and the content of the narrow approximately 20 nm lumen lying between the inner and outer SSC membranes have not been identified. The SSC partitions the cytoplasm into two domains, the axial core and the extracisternal space. The axial core is the larger of the compartments, and it contains only a few structures, such as most of the cell's complement of mitochondria, which are located adjacent to the lateral wall. This partitioning may help to maintain the OHC's cytoskeletal organization.

The Outer Hair Cell Membrane Motor Involves Prestin and Intracellular Chloride

OHC electromotility involves a membrane-based motor mechanism in the plasma membrane of the lateral wall. The mechanical force generated by the plasma membrane is communicated to the ends of the cell both hydraulically and via the cortical lattice. The motor mechanism is piezoelectric-like in that mechanical

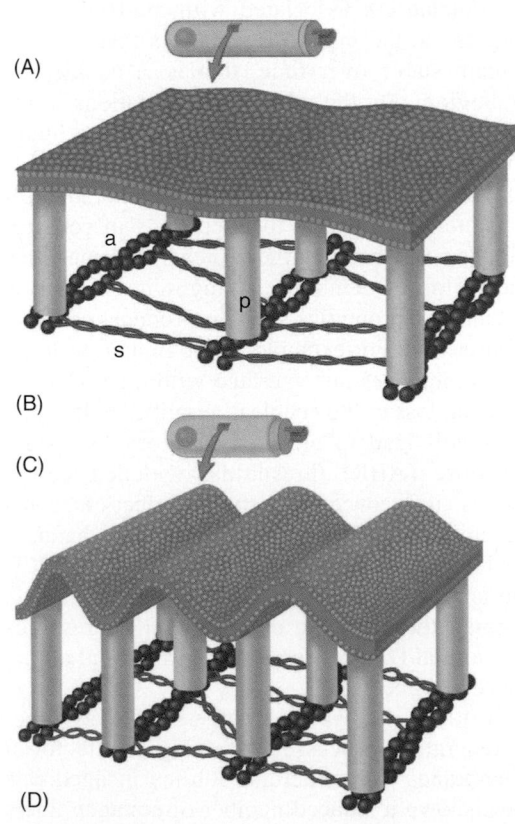

Figure 6 Postulated nanoscale membrane rippling within the lateral wall of the outer hair cell (OHC). Pillars (p) actin filaments (a) spectrin (s). (A and C) The OHC when hyperpolarized and depolarized respectively. (B and D) Alterations in membrane curvature are associated with electromotile length changes. (From reference 6.)

deformation of the membrane changes the transmembrane potential (direct piezoelectric effect) while electromotility is comparable to converse piezoelectricity.[7]

The protein prestin and intracellular chloride ions are required for optimal performance of the membrane motor. Prestin (Slc26A5) is a necessary component of the membrane-based motor that underlies outer hair cell electromotility. It was discovered by subtractive cloning to identify proteins that were expressed in the OHCs but not the IHCs (which are nonmotile).[8] Prestin is a member of the Slc26A family of anion transporters with up to 12 transmembrane helices. The family member with the closest sequence similarity is pendrin Slc26A4. Pendrin is expressed in the tissue forming the membranous labyrinth where it may be involved in the maintenance of the unique endolymphatic fluids (Figure 7). When prestin is in a membrane, a displacement charge movement into and out of, as opposed to through, the membrane can be measured. The prestin-associated charge movement is the accepted electrical signature of electromotility. Intracellular anions such as chloride and bicarbonate appear to be the charge carrier. The involvement of anions is consistent with prestin's membership in the SLC26A family of anion transporters. Computational (informatic) analysis of the amino acid sequence of prestin and close family members indicate those regions of the proteins that are highly conserved in the prestins from different mammals. These include 2 sets of residues at the extracellular ends of transmembrane helices 1 and 2. Membrane electromotility and prestin-associated charge movement are blocked by single point mutations in these residues.

The dependence of electromotility and the prestin-associated charge movement on the material properties of the membrane has long been known. Changes in membrane tension shift the voltage dependence of both electromotility and the charge movement. The membranous nature of the motor mechanism is highlighted by altering the lipid profiles of cell membranes. The voltage charge movement function can be shifted over a 100 mV range by adding or depleting cholesterol in the membrane while the total amount of charge moved is not affected. Reduction of membrane cholesterol in the living cochlea eliminates DPOAEs while cholesterol enrichment results in a small (~3 dB) increase followed by the elimination of DPOAEs. The nature of these lipid–protein interactions requires further exploration and may be related to gender differences in hearing sensitivity and cochlear amplification.

STRIA VASCULARIS

The energy required for OHC mechanoelectrical and electromechanical transduction is provided by the stria vascularis (see Figure 7). This structure forms the outer wall of the scala media and is located within the spiral ligament. It is

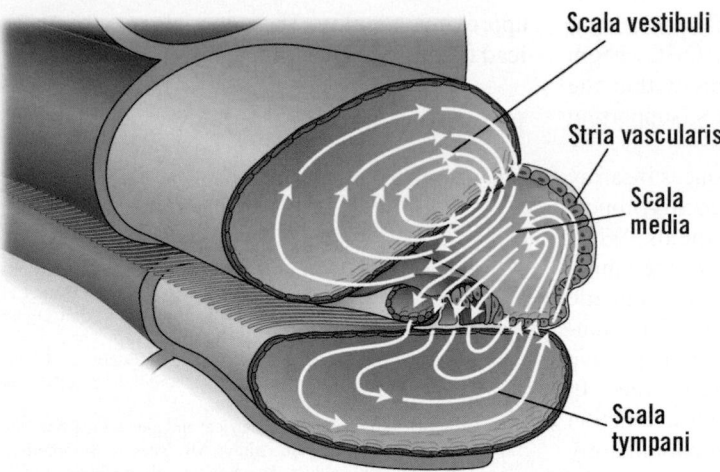

Scala vestibuli

Stria vascularis

Scala media

Scala tympani

Figure 7 Cross-section of the cochlea. There are 3 fluid-filled chambers: the scala vestibuli and scala tympani are connected at the apex of the cochlea and contain perilymph, and the scala media contains endolymph. The stria vascularis maintains the endolymphatic potential and drives the silent current (*arrows*). (Adapted from reference 9.)

highly vascular and metabolically active; it maintains the high potassium concentration within the scala media. The stria vascularis acts as a battery whose electrical current powers hearing. It is the energy source for both the production of receptor potentials and OHC electromotility. In addition to elevated potassium concentrations in the scala media, it creates a positive potential within the endolymph relative to the perilymph and increases the electrochemical gradient that drives a constant flow of K^+ ions from the endolymph into the hair cells. The resulting "silent current" is modulated as hair cell stereocilia are deflected. Depolarizing OHC receptor potentials are dominated by an increase in potassium ion movement into the cell which differs from most other cells where depolarization is based primarily on the entry of extracellular sodium ions. Because OHCs do not experience an intracellular sodium ion increase, they do not require energetically expensive ion pumps. Further independence from adenosine triphosphate (ATP) is obtained because the OHC membrane–based motor is piezoelectric-like. It converts the energy in the transmembrane electric field into mechanical energy and does not use cellular stores of ATP. Reducing ATP requirements for both the sensory and the motor functions of the OHC decreases the need for oxidative phosphorylation consistent with the relatively poor vascularization of the organ of Corti. The sensitivity of the human ear would allow it to hear blood flowing in the organ of Corti. By having the energy-generating apparatus for hearing in the stria vascularis, the ear can detect lower energy sounds without interference from the blood supply. After passively exiting the OHCs, potassium ions are recycled back to the stria vascularis by diffusion through the perilymph and through supporting cells via gap junctions. The gap junction proteins are called connexins, and mutations of their genes result in sensorineural hearing loss. Connexin mutations are the most common mechanism of genetic hearing loss.

OUTER HAIR CELL SYNAPTIC STRUCTURE AND FUNCTION

The importance of the OHC's motor role is reflected in the afferent and efferent synapses found at the cell's basal pole. The few afferent synapses found at the base of an OHC do not appear to excite the auditory nerve fibers that they contact while the efferent synapses are capable of modulating OHC force generation.

Afferent Synapses

Presynaptic dense bodies (synaptic ribbons) touch presynaptic thickenings of afferent synapses and are surrounded by synaptic vesicles (see Figure 2). There are fewer synaptic ribbons in OHCs than in IHCs; and, in some species, they are missing in adult OHCs. There is no evidence that the OHC afferent synapses activate the eighth nerve fibers they contact. There is only one study in which an eighth nerve fiber was reconstructed after intracellular recording and found to terminate on an OHC. The fiber did not fire action potentials in response to acoustic stimuli. The absence of acoustically evoked activity in nerve fibers coming from the OHC is consistent with the absence of evidence for vesicle membrane recycling at the OHC afferent synapse. Those afferent eighth nerve fibers that innervate OHCs may communicate information to the CNS but it is unlikely to be encoded in spike train activity.

Efferent Synapses

The OHC synaptic pole is dominated by efferent synapses. Postsynaptic cisternae are found in the cytoplasm adjacent to the postsynaptic thickening of efferent synapses. Most of the efferent endings originate from neurons located in the contralateral medial olivary complex. The end result of stimulating the efferent fibers is to decrease the sensitivity of afferent nerve fibers from the IHCs. Since these efferent fibers innervate the OHCs and not the IHCs, they perform their function indirectly through an effect on OHC force production. The synapse is cholinergic and cell shortening was observed when acetylcholine (ACh) was iontophoretically applied to isolated OHCs. It was later found that ACh modulates the magnitude of the OHC's electrically evoked movments.

The novel heteromeric nicotinic receptors at the efferent synapse contain both α9- and α10-subunits, which may activate cell-signaling

pathways that alter mechanical properties of cytoskeletal proteins in the OHC lateral wall. A family of small guanosine triphosphatases (GTPases) regulates the polymerization and depolymerization of cytoskeletal proteins, and studies that have biochemically dissected the action of several of these GTPases, specifically Rac, Rho, and Cdc42, suggest that signaling triggered by the nicotinic receptor at the efferent synapse may regulate the mechanical properties of the OHC lateral wall.

ACTIVE PROCESSES IN HEARING

Enhanced Frequency Selectivity

OHC electromotility is important in overcoming viscous damping and allowing the ear to hear high frequencies. It also enhances frequency selectivity. The mechanical tuning of the cochlea based only on passive mechanical properties such as mass and stiffness cannot explain the exquisite frequency selectivity of human hearing or the frequency selectivity that can be measured from individual auditory nerve fibers. OHC electromotility allows the human ear to discriminate between sounds that are very close in frequency. The reason for this can be understood by considering a simple mechanically tuned system, the playground swing. The frequency at which a swing vibrates is determined by the length of the rope. Its tuning may be appreciated when attempting to push it at a frequency other than the natural frequency of the swing. When pushed at a different frequency, the system requires considerably more energy to affect movement at that frequency.

A child sitting passively on a swing is an example of a passive, in contrast to an active, system. To understand what is meant by an active system, one need only recall one's own early experiences on a swing. After a short time, one learned how to make the swing go higher and higher by pumping energy into the system through a combination of kicking your legs and tilting your upper body. Not only could one make the swing go high, but one probably experimented with kicking at a frequency other than the natural (passive) best frequency. When one did, one found that the magnitude of the swing was rapidly attenuated. The "active" system with one pumping had become effectively more narrowly tuned than the original system in which one just sat on the swing. Narrow tuning is also a feature of the inner ear where the active pumping of the OHCs greatly improves the mechanical tuning of the inner ear vibrations. Not only is the amplitude of the vibrations enhanced at the best frequency, but they are suppressed for frequencies near best frequency.

Otoacoustic Emissions

One consequence of having an active, nonlinear system is that oscillations can occur even when no energy is coming into the system from the outside. This happens in the cochlea, and the resulting sound vibrations can be measured in the ear canal. These are called spontaneous otoacoustic emissions and are only observed in living ears. Other types of otoacoustic emissions can be measured as well, including distortion product otoacoustic emissions and transient-evoked otoacoustic emissions. These can be triggered as needed by playing certain types of sound stimuli into the ear and are, therefore, more useful clinically than the measurement of spontaneous otoacoustic emissions. Measuring otoacoustic emissions has become an important diagnostic tool for determining if OHCs are working, particularly in newborn hearing screening.

Sensorineural hearing loss is a common clinical problem and has many different causes, including noise exposure, ototoxicity, and age-related hearing loss (presbyacusis). The common site of pathology for all of these conditions within the inner ear is the OHC. The attachments of OHC stereocilia to the tectorial membrane can be broken, even with mild noise exposure. This reduces the ability of OHC electromotility to provide positive feedback, leading to a temporary hearing loss. With further damage, the actin core of the OHC stereocilia can fracture. With enough trauma, hair cell death occurs and a permanent

hearing loss results because mammalian cochlear hair cells do not regenerate. After OHCs begin to degenerate, additional structures within the cochlea die as well, including IHCs, supporting cells, and auditory nerve cells.

A low level of trauma that produces disarray of both inner and outer hair cell stereocilia proportionally elevates tuning curve thresholds. When OHCs are lost, only the sharp peak of the tuning curve is lost. Loss of IHCs produces a dramatic elevation in tuning curve thresholds. OHC damage blocks the cochlear amplifier, but the passive tuning properties of the cochlea are retained. In contrast, IHC damage reduces cochlear function overall. In summary, OHCs are predominantly responsible for the cochlear amplifier while the IHCs are responsible for signal detection to provide afferent input.

CONCLUSIONS

Throughout this chapter simple physical principles have been used to explain the biophysics of the cochlea at the microscopic and molecular level. More sophisticated application of the same concepts leads to mathematical models that better

approximate reality. These models may someday lead to improved hearing health.

REFERENCES

1. Geisler CD. From Sound to Synapse: Physiology of the Mammalian Ear. New York: Oxford University Press; 1988. p. 56.
2. Brownell WE. How the ear works—nature's solutions for listening. Volta Review 1999;99:9–28.
3. Brownell WE. On the origins of outer hair cell electromotility. In: Berlin CI, Hood LJ, Ricci AJ, editors. Hair Cell Micromechanics and Otoacoustic Emissions. San Diego: Delmar Learning; 2002. p. 25–46.
4. Brownell WE, Spector AA, Raphael RM, Popel AS. Micro- and nanomechanics of the cochlear outer hair cell. Annu Rev Biomed Eng 2001;3:169–94.
5. Brownell WE, Popel AS. Electrical and mechanical anatomy of the outer hair cell. In: Palmer AR, Rees A, Summerfield AQ, Meddis R, editors. Psychophysical and Physiological Advances in Hearing. London: Whurr; 1998. p. 89–96.
6. Oghalai JS, Zhao HB, Kutz JW, Brownell WE. Voltage- and tension-dependent lipid mobility in the outer hair cell plasma membrane. Science 2000;287:658–61.
7. Brownell WE. The piezoelectric outer hair cell. In: Eatock RA, Popper AN, Fay RR, editors. Vertebrate Hair Cells, Springer Handbook of Auditory Research. New York: Springer; 2006. p. 313–47.
8. Dallos P, Fakler B. Prestin, a new type of motor protein. Nat Rev Mol Cell Biol 2002;3:104–11.
9. Oghalai JS, Brownell WE. Anatomy and physiology of the Ear. In: Lalwani AK, editor. Current Diagnosis and Treatment in Otolaryngology—Head and Neck Surgery. New York: McGraw-Hill; 2004. p. 611–30.

Central Auditory Processing and Functional Neuroimaging

Charles J. Limb, MD
Marc D. Eisen, MD, PhD

INTRODUCTION

Whereas the structures that comprise the auditory periphery, including the external auditory apparatus and cochlea, provide us with the ability to hear, it is the auditory cortex that enables us to understand what we hear, providing us with auditory cognition. In the hierarchy of neural processing centers for sound perception, it is the cerebral cortex that ultimately permits auditory cognition—the conscious awareness of the acoustic environment. The emergence of new functional neuroimaging techniques, especially functional magnetic resonance imaging (fMRI), has provided unprecedented access to the study of the brain, allowing researchers to delineate both neuroanatomical substrates and functional roles of auditory processing centers. This chapter reviews the key components of the network of central neural structures for sound processing and highlights critical data obtained through an array of novel methods.

METHODS OF INVESTIGATION

Anatomical Methods

Traditional methods of elucidating anatomical–functional correlates in the human central nervous system were based primarily on lesion studies of individuals with behavioral or cognitive deficits, typically after central nervous system damage (whether due to stroke, tumor, or trauma), with postmortem anatomical analysis. Part of the difficulty in elucidating the mechanisms of human auditory processing deals with the inherent interspecies variability, which makes comparisons between humans and animal models challenging. Compared to most other mammals, humans are sensitive to a relatively lower frequency spectrum and lack the specialized auditory abilities (eg, echolocation) found in certain species. Hence, while animal research in auditory processing has flourished, the applicability of results from animal work to our understanding of human sound perception has been variable.

The development of anatomical imaging methods, including X-ray, computed tomography, and magnetic resonance, ushered in dramatic increases in the ability of physicians and scientists to study the human brain. Yet, these methods were anatomical rather than functional in nature—they provided static images of the brain at rest and required inferences and assumptions for one to make any functional correlations. The recent introduction of functional imaging modalities has truly revolutionized our ability to draw functional–anatomic correlations. By measuring neural activity, functional imaging has provided unprecedented access into the inner workings of the human brain.

Functional Methods: Positron Emission Tomography

Positron emission tomography, or PET scanning, was developed shortly after computed tomography scanning. In PET, radionuclides are coupled to a tracer agent introduced intravenously into a patient's bloodstream concurrent with the acquisition of data. These radionuclides have a spontaneous emission of positrons, which annihilate with electrons present in the study subject, in a manner proportional to the pharmacodynamics of the molecule to which the radionuclide is attached, thereby allowing measurements of local blood flow or metabolic activity. The annihilation of positrons and electrons causes a release of energy in opposite directions, which is subsequently detected by scintillator/photomultiplier tubes arranged concentrically around the brain. Based on differences in timing of coincidence detection, it is possible to calculate the exact location from where the energy was emitted, thus localizing the putative neural event. It should be emphasized here that neural blood flow and neural activity are not necessarily the same. Herein lies one of the crucial limitations of both PET scanning and functional MRI methods which both rely on local increases in blood flow as a marker of increased neural activity. While the correlation between blood flow and neural activity is widely accepted,[1] it is an acknowledged limitation of the methods that the measurement of neuronal activity is indirect rather than direct, and that the anatomic variance in vasculature can cause artificial differences between subjects as well as provide an absolute physical limit (ie, the distance between the vessel and neuron) to the accuracy of activity measurement, since these methods typically detect metabolic activity within the nearest blood vessel rather than the nearest neuron. Furthermore, both neuronal inhibition and excitation require increases in local metabolism and blood flow, and therefore the two cannot be discerned with this modality.

There are several types of available radionuclide-tracer combinations, the most commonly used being 18-fluorodeoxyglucose (^{18}FDG) and $H_2^{15}O$, that have widely varying pharmacokinetics and thus provide widely differing types of data. ^{18}FDG has primarily been employed as a marker of increased glucose consumption and, by extension, metabolic activity and is therefore useful for detecting regions of abnormally high uptake, such as the case of many cancers, including tumors of the head and neck.[2] For auditory experiments, the most useful agent has been $H_2^{15}O$, which involves the administration of a modified water molecule with a relatively short (123 seconds) half-life. During the roughly 2-minute time period of radionuclide stability, subjects typically undergo an imaging scan during which an experimentally controlled task or stimulus is introduced.[3] The neural activity over the entire interval is accumulated during each acquisition period. Therefore, in $H_2^{15}O$ PET, the acquired functional images represent a *condensation* of neural activity over the preceding 2-minute interval. By inference, this half-life represents the limit in temporal resolution that can be achieved using this method. For auditory stimuli, which frequently vary from millisecond to millisecond, the temporal limitations of PET must be considered in both experimental design as well as data interpretation.

Functional Methods: Functional Magnetic Resonance Imaging

Functional MRI (fMRI) is based upon a modification of traditional MRI methods, which measure intrinsic differences in magnetic properties between adjacent tissues, thereby providing a high level of anatomical detail that has been extremely useful for all medical disciplines. In MRI, subjects are placed within a high-strength magnetic field (typically 0.5 to 1.5 T), inducing magnetic alignment of protons within the body, and then an orthogonal magnetic field is applied, causing the magnetic dipoles to "flip" sideways. As the second magnetic field is extinguished, the flipped dipoles decay to their original aligned orientation with a decay constant that is tissue-specific and measurable, ultimately producing a high-quality MR image. Unlike traditional MRI methods, functional MRI does not produce a high-quality anatomical image. Rather, it employs technology that allows extremely fast (~2 to 5 seconds) imaging throughout the entire brain. This speed is achieved through a method known as echo planar imaging (EPI),[4] which is a process that quickly applies and diminishes the magnetic cross-field, measuring extremely small differences in decay. Using EPI, multiple series of brain images can be acquired in a relatively brief time period, allowing comparison of different neural responses to experimentally controlled stimuli.

In fMRI, no intravenous agent is typically administered. Rather, the method relies on an endogenous contrast agent. fMRI relies on the fact that deoxyhemoglobin is a ferromagnetic molecule, unlike oxyhemoglobin. Active neurons require greater amounts of oxygen and produce subsequently higher amounts of deoxyhemoglobin. However, it has been found that the relative increase in blood flow outweighs the relative increase in deoxyhemoglobin. Therefore, there is a net decrease in the local amount of deoxyhemoglobin in areas of heightened neural activity.[5,6] By utilizing the magnetic properties of deoxyhemoglobin, it was determined that differences in deoxyhemoglobin related to changes in neural activity could be detected using MRI. This method, known as blood-oxygen-level-dependent (BOLD) contrast imaging, has been the cornerstone of functional MRI methods.[7] Because no ionizing radiation is administered (therefore removing the constraints of radiation exposure to subjects), no intravenous agent is required, the acquisition speed is extraordinarily fast (thereby improving temporal resolution), and the spatial resolution is very good (typically around 3 mm^3 on average), fMRI has largely supplanted PET scanning as the dominant method of functional neural imaging.

Once functional imaging data are obtained, several processing steps are required prior to analysis of the data. While a detailed discussion of data processing methods in functional imaging is beyond the scope of this chapter, the reader should be familiar with the need to correct for head movement artifact, to normalize differences both within and between subjects (usually to a template brain), and to apply smoothing algorithms that improve our ability to identify clusters of neural activity. This process thus allows comparisons to be made between brains of different sizes and shapes and employs a standardized stereotaxic coordinate system to allow for accurate localization of regions of activity.[8]

To construct useful functional neuroimaging maps, the method of subtractive analysis (typically referred to as *contrast analysis*) is employed, usually through the process of general linear modeling analysis.[9] In the simplest type of contrast analysis, a baseline level of activity is measured with the subject at rest (or performing some other control condition) for an extended period of time, referred to as a *block*. During the same scanning session, images are also acquired with the subject exposed to an experimental condition (eg, listening to an auditory stimulus). The images from the baseline condition are subtracted out from the images obtained during the experimental condition, presumably allowing identification of those regions of neural activity specific to the experimental task. Using variations on this methodology, researchers have been able to employ fMRI to both substantiate existing claims as well as derive new insights into the way the brain processes sound.

Limitations of Functional Imaging Methods

Both PET scanning and fMRI have inherent practical and theoretical limitations. In PET scanning, a radionuclide must first be available for administration. Given the short half-life of $H_2^{15}O$, this requires that the agent is produced on site, with the use of a cyclotron. The cost associated with this modality is therefore quite expensive. Because ionizing radiation is administered, PET scanning is less useful in children and for experiments in which repeated acquisition of data from a subject is required. Because the half-life is also fairly long (2 minutes), the spatiotemporal resolution of PET is relatively poor. fMRI is widely available, since it requires only a modification of existing MRI technology. However, fMRI is also an exceptionally noisy technology, with background scanner noise levels approaching 130 dB SPL. For auditory experiments, this noise level is a clear limitation and requires several assumptions to be made in the evaluation of auditory stimuli processing or the use of specialized data acquisition paradigms which can reduce the number (but improve the quality) of data sets acquired in a session. Also, the powerful magnetic fields employed by fMRI limit the use of indwelling devices, such as cochlear implants, thereby excluding this important patient population from participation in fMRI experiments.

CENTRAL AUDITORY PROCESSING

It should be stated at the outset that our understanding of how sound is actually perceived in all of its complexity is quite limited. Although we have a good deal of information regarding the various processing stages that occur along the auditory pathways, it still remains a mystery how these signals ultimately produce an accurate percept that enables cognition. Functional imaging methods, however, hold the most promise in terms of identifying those areas of the brain that are actively engaged during these tasks and will hopefully continue to shed new light on this fascinating process.

Once sound enters the cochlea, the process of acoustic-to-neural conversion begins. That is, sound, which is composed of waves of vibrational energy, induces neural stimulation within the cochlea, leading to hair cell initiation of neurotransmission. From this point onward, the process of auditory perception ceases to be an acoustic phenomenon and is entirely neural. The central auditory system is responsible for analyzing these incoming neural impulses and then filtering, encoding, recoding, and distributing them to the appropriate neural centers (Figure 1).[10] While much of auditory cognition per se takes place in the auditory cortex, many baseline processes required for complex perception take place in the brainstem, such as the encoding of multiple frequency channels and binaurally driven calculations needed for sound localization.

Cochlear Nucleus

The peripheral auditory mechanism collects, filters, and disperses sound in a frequency-specific pattern known as *tonotopy*. This tonotopic arrangement that begins in the cochlea is maintained throughout the auditory system as it ascends through subcortical and cortical processing stages. The auditory brainstem is the first synaptic relay station of the central auditory pathway. The auditory nerve enters the brainstem at the pontomedullary junction, where its axons synapse within the *cochlear nucleus*. The cochlear nucleus is subdivided anatomically into two principal components, the dorsal cochlear nucleus (DCN) and the ventral cochlear nucleus (VCN). Each individual auditory nerve fiber branches within the cochlear nucleus and travels to the DCN and VCN in an orderly arrangement that preserves the tonotopic gradient established in the cochlea. The processing that occurs in the cochlear nucleus (and throughout the auditory brainstem) is dependent largely upon the cell type upon which each neuron synapses as well as upon the nature of the physical and physiological coupling between

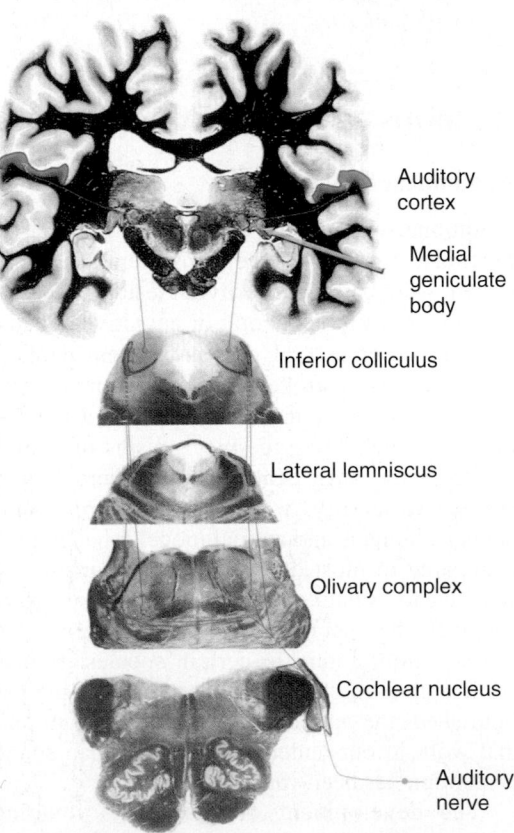

Auditory cortex

Medial geniculate body

Inferior colliculus

Lateral lemniscus

Olivary complex

Cochlear nucleus

Auditory nerve

Figure 1 The ascending central pathways of the auditory system. Although most basic aspects of sound processing occur in the brainstem, it is the auditory cortex that enables sound perception. (Modified from reference 10.)

presynaptic and postsynaptic neurons; different classes of recipient cells have intrinsically different neuronal response properties and therefore relay incoming auditory signals in varying fashion to upstream processing sites. The VCN contains large synapses that are tightly coupled with the postsynaptic recipient (the spherical bushy cells), thereby constituting a form of fail-safe synaptic transmission that is believed to be important in sound localization. The DCN receives fewer inputs directly from the auditory nerve than the VCN but is thought to be important in spectral tuning and is characterized by strong inhibitory influences among DCN neurons.

The effects of auditory deprivation on the cochlear nucleus are significant. It has been shown that primary synapses of the auditory nerve within the cochlear nucleus, especially the endbulb of Held, undergo an atrophy of their complex 3-dimensional structure that appears to limit the neural connectivity between the afferent auditory nerve input and the recipient cochlear nucleus (Figure 2).[11–13] Furthermore, the few synapses that do exist appear to have undergone hypertrophy of their size upon examination via electron microscopy, perhaps to compensate for the limited neural connectivity that exists between these malformed neurons. In a landmark study attesting to the importance of cochlear implantation, Ryugo and colleagues showed that early cochlear implantation in the deaf white cat led to synaptic rescue, with a restoration of normal synaptic morphology following a period of sustained

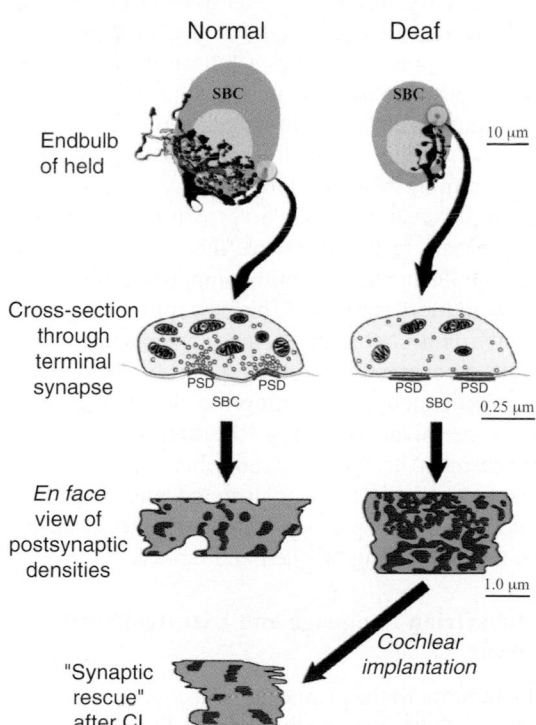

Figure 2 "Synaptic rescue" in deaf white cats following cochlear implantation. This figure shows light microscopic and ultrastructural changes seen within the anteroventral cochlear nucleus of deaf animals and indicates how these changes affect the total area of synaptic transmission. Serial reconstructions of synaptic transmission areas show normalization of synaptic transmission regions (postsynaptic densities) following cochlear implantation at an early age. (Adapted from references 11 and 13.)

implant use.[14] It has been also shown that synaptic development in the auditory brainstem takes place during early life and likely corresponds to a so-called critical period during which auditory synaptic connections may form and after which neuroplastic changes (including those responsible for proper sound transmission) are limited.

Superior Olivary Complex

One of the computational demands on the auditory brainstem is that of spatial sound source localization. This challenge is hampered by the fact that (unlike the visual system) there is no physical representation of 3-dimensional sound space within the auditory periphery. The superior olivary complex (SOC) is thought to be the first location in the ascending auditory pathway in which bilateral peripheral inputs converge, and this feature supports the notion that the SOC processes differences between binaural input, which are necessary for proper sound localization to occur. In simplified terms, the ability to localize sound is based on differences in both amplitude (or level) and timing between right and left ears. A sound that is closer to the right side, for example, will stimulate the right ear both earlier and with greater intensity than it will stimulate the left ear, due to the head shadow effect and greater physical distance required for the sound wave to travel. Using these differences, the auditory brainstem can subserve localization of sound with great accuracy, particularly in certain animal species like the barn owl that can hunt for prey using auditory cues alone. Within the SOC, neurons are ideally suited to perform the function of binaural comparison, allowing computations based on interaural timing differences (intensity level differences are likely calculated in the inferior colliculus). Certain neurons in the medial nucleus of the SOC have been found to serve as "coincidence detectors," in which simultaneous binaural input is required to stimulate a neural response in the postsynaptic cell.[15]

Lateral Lemniscus

The lateral lemniscal nuclei receive input from the lower nuclei and transmit them (mostly contralateral) to the inferior colliculus via the lateral lemniscus pathways. The inferior aspect of the lemniscus is less prominent in humans compared to that in animals equipped with echolocation. The superior (dorsal) lemniscal nucleus is more prominent and is involved in spatial localization. This pathway incorporates postsynaptic neurons traveling from the cochlear nuclei and SOC and processes them for presentation to the inferior colliculus, where they can be integrated.

Inferior Colliculus

The inferior colliculus (IC) plays an important, albeit less well-understood, role in the integration of auditory input and receives direct inputs from all of the nuclei in the auditory brainstem via the lateral lemniscus. The largest processing nucleus within the IC is called the central nucleus. The IC

subsequently provides input to the auditory thalamus. Although the inferior colliculus has a relatively limited number of cell types, the neuronal response properties within the IC have been found to be quite diverse, including both excitatory and inhibitory interactions that modulate both ascending and descending activity, as well as activity to the contralateral IC.[16] There is significant evidence to suggest that the IC plays a crucial role in spectral processing of sound, in addition to the calculation of interaural intensity differences.[17] In a technically challenging functional neuroimaging experiment, Melcher and colleagues studied the auditory brainstem activity within the IC of patients suffering from unilateral versus bilateral tinnitus (Figure 3).[18] In this study, it was determined that patients with unilateral tinnitus had increased activity within the IC compared to patients without tinnitus, thereby suggesting a link between aberrant brainstem activity within the IC (triggered by peripheral deafferentation through hair cell loss or damage) and the development of tinnitus.[18] This finding also sheds light as to why transection of the auditory nerve ordinarily does not relieve patients of their tinnitus.

Medial Geniculate Nucleus

The medial geniculate nucleus (or body) is the portion of the thalamus that receives all incoming auditory input that has been integrated by the

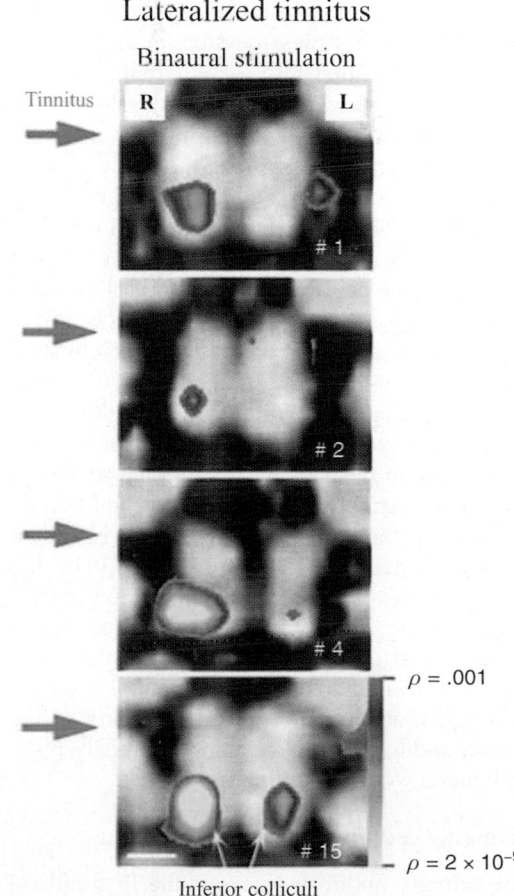

Figure 3 Functional MRI data showing abnormal activation in the inferior colliculus of patients suffering from unilateral tinnitus. (Reprinted with permission from reference 18.)

inferior colliculus and subsequently presents it to primary auditory cortex. Neurons within the medial geniculate nucleus demonstrate sharp tuning curves, consistent with the fact that the cortical processing of sound retains the tonotopic organization established in the cochlea. The medial geniculate nucleus is divided into 3 principal portions anatomically, with ventral, dorsal, and medial components. Inputs to the "core" areas of the primary auditory cortex primarily come from the ventral component of the medial geniculate nucleus. Further, studies in primates have shown that the posterodorsal division of the medial geniculate nucleus is the primary input to the rostromedial area of the "belt" area of primary auditory cortex, whereas the anterodorsal division is the primary input to the caudomedial "belt" area.[19] The primary auditory cortex also communicates in descending reciprocal fashion with the medial geniculate nucleus (ventral subdivision). The functional implication of these pathways is poorly understood.

THE AUDITORY CORTEX

Numerous organizational schemes have been used to describe the components of the human cerebral cortex. The organization scheme of Brodmann[20] has been widely used to depict the parcellation of the brain into smaller functional units although functional imaging experiments have begun to reveal the oversimplified nature of these schemes, with an increasing trend away from relying upon Brodmann's classification. Anatomically, the brain is divided into lobes (frontal, temporal, occipital, parietal), and it is also likely that discrete neural systems (eg, limbic system) exist to serve specific functions. Of the cortical lobes, the temporal, occipital, and parietal lobes are all thought to subserve somatosensory functions, while the frontal lobe is thought to have an executive role in the coordination and control of activity within the somatosensory lobes. Indeed, it is the prefrontal cortex, more than any neural area, which demonstrates the greatest degree of expansion during hominid evolution. The auditory cortex is housed within the temporal lobe, much of it hidden within the Sylvian fissure (and seen only after lateral retraction of the temporal lobe). More specifically, the human auditory cortex is located along the superior temporal gyrus. As will be discussed, however, cortical areas outside the temporal lobe (eg, inferior parietal lobule) are known to be critical in the cognition of complex auditory stimuli. Perhaps most importantly, it should be noted that our current understanding of the human auditory cortex remains essentially poor, with much work remaining to be done.

Primary Auditory Cortex

The primary auditory cortex is the first cortical stage of auditory processing, found in all mammals (often referred to as A1). The primary auditory cortex receives inputs primarily from the medial geniculata nucleus of the thalamus (MGv),

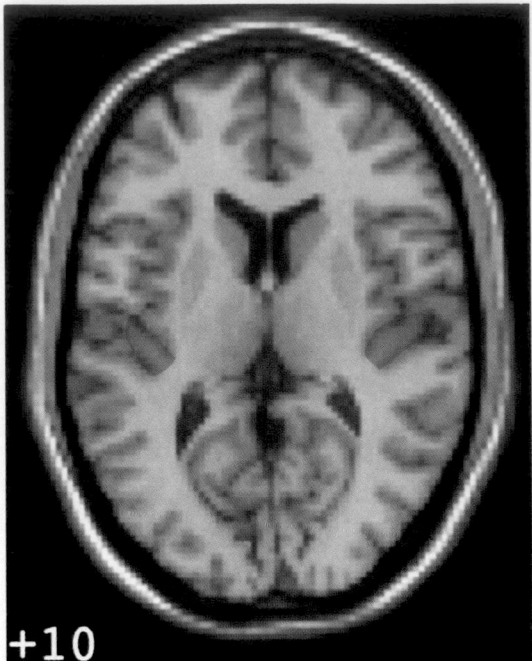

Figure 4 Axial view of anatomical T1-weighted MRI image at level $z = +10$ (Montreal Neurologic Institute coordinate system). The image shows the transverse temporal gyrus, or Heschl gyrus, highlighted in red bilaterally. This area contains the primary auditory cortex.

and it is thought to be located on the superior temporal plane, along the transverse temporal gyrus, also known as Heschl gyrus and Brodmann area 41 (Figure 4).

From seminal work by Kaas and Hackett (primarily in the macaque monkey model), it has been determined that an area known as the *core* (which consists of 3 main areas: A1, rostral, and rostrotemporal) receives primary input from the thalamus and has connections with a surrounding region of secondary auditory processing areas (known as the *belt*, which is itself bordered laterally by *parabelt* regions). The core is known to have a tonotopic arrangement.[21] There are several lines of evidence to support that this organization is consistent in other primates and humans. In humans, cytoarchitectonic, myeloarchitectonic, and histochemical data support the fact that the core is likely to be primary in nature, as this combination of characteristics is found only in 2 other areas of the brain, namely the primary visual areas and primary somatosensory areas.[22] In contrast, the belt and parabelt regions are nonprimary in nature but instead receive most of their projections directly from the primary core regions immediately adjacent to them.

All auditory processing (whether the sound is linguistic, environmental, or musical in nature) relies on the integrity of this primary processing phase. Even at this early stage of cortical processing, differences can be seen both anatomically and functionally in the primary auditory cortex of individuals with high levels of auditory training. More specifically, Heschl gyrus was found to have a significantly greater degree of activity (determined by magnetoencephalography) as well as significantly greater volumetric measurements in musicians as compared to nonmusicians.[23] In

this study, psychometric analysis also revealed a correlation between the size of Heschl gyrus and musical aptitude, implying the interesting notion that the size of Heschl gyrus may serve as a marker of musical ability.

Auditory Association Cortex

Once primary input to the auditory brain is processed and received by the core/belt/parabelt regions, it undergoes a secondary stage of auditory processing in areas known as auditory association cortex (also referred to as secondary auditory cortex) (Figure 5). The identification of functional roles of auditory association cortex has been controversial and challenging. However, it is generally accepted that this portion of auditory cortex lies along the superior temporal plane, posterior to Heschl gyrus, in an area known as the planum temporale (PT). The PT is thought to be involved in the processing of complex auditory stimuli, such as speech and music. These stimuli typically have both spectral and temporal components of complex, evolving patterns that change constantly. The PT is thought to provide the neural substrate through which the challenging calculations of spectrotemporal pattern identification and segregation (eg, separation and tracking of competing sounds presented from multiple sources) are performed.[24] In anatomical studies of the planum temporale in musicians with absolute pitch, which is the ability to identify a musical pitch without the use of a reference note, this region was found to demonstrate leftward asymmetry, ultimately determined to be the product of decreased PT size in those with absolute pitch.[25] Studies such as these encouraged scientists away from the notion that the PT was an area dedicated to language processing and broadened the notion to include complex auditory stimuli of which language was one specific example. Although the diverse functions of the PT remain to be described, there may be a role for the PT in the temporal comparison of successive auditory patterns. The perception of sound, which is a continuum of energy presented over time, necessarily involves a certain amount of working memory to integrate the significance of successive events (eg, the first syllable of a word must be remembered when heard for the second syllable to be interpreted meaningfully), and the PT may provide the computational means of accomplishing this demanding task.[24]

Perisylvian Language and Extratemporal Areas

In addition to the primary and secondary auditory areas of the cortex, there are additional extratemporal regions that also play critical roles in auditory processing (Figure 6). The most well-described of these areas is a focal portion of the left frontal operculum that was identified by Carl Broca in 1861, often referred to as Broca area, or Brodmann area 42 and classically considered to be necessary for speech production. Closely related to this region is a portion of the inferior

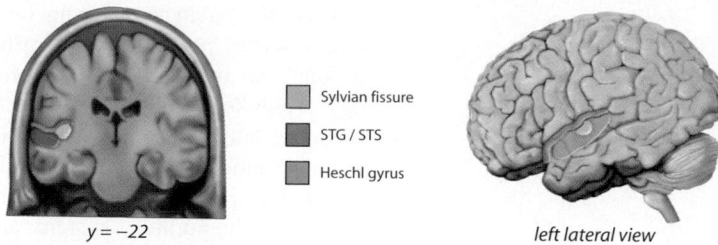

Figure 5 Primary and secondary auditory cortical regions. The left image shows an MRI film ($y = -22$) with colored regions depicting the locations of the Sylvian fissure (*green*), superior temporal gyrus (STG) and sulcus (STS) (*blue*), and Heschl gyrus (*orange*). Heschl gyrus (transverse temporal gyrus) contains the primary auditory core and it is located medially; it can be seen by reflecting the temporal lobe laterally at the Sylvian fissure. The secondary auditory cortical regions are located within the belt and parabelt regions, along the STG. The right image shows a three-dimensional view of the brain with surface renderings of the primary and secondary auditory regions and Sylvian fissure. (Reprinted from reference 28.)

parietal lobule described by Wernicke in 1876 as a language receptive region. The classical perisylvian language areas are those regions that are clustered around the Sylvian fissure that are thought to be crucial for language processing; and although these regions may not be wholly responsible, they are certainly critical for language perception.

Recent functional neuroimaging studies have revealed that the simple division of language processing into these subdivisions is overly simplistic, and that there are numerous areas of the brain involved in language production.[26] In terms of cortical demands, it is likely that the primary and secondary auditory areas process the incoming auditory stimuli into identifiable temporal and pitch patterns that are relayed to extratemporal portions of the brain where the cognitive assessment of awareness and significance takes place. In addition, there are numerous connections between auditory and "nonauditory" portions of the brain, including the visual, motor, limbic, somatosensory systems, and prefrontal cortex. Although these regions are considered nonauditory in nature, it is highly likely that they play

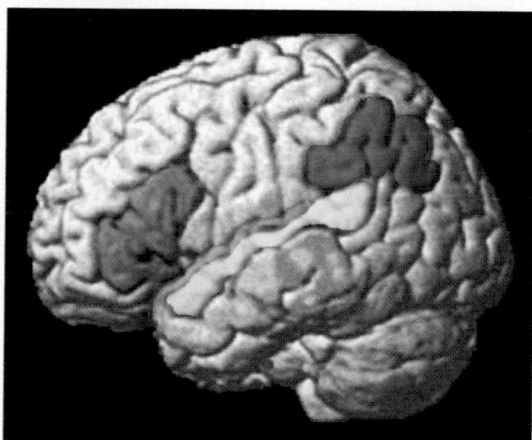

Figure 6 Left lateral view of the human brain with perisylvian language areas highlighted. The blue area of the frontal operculum corresponds to the area traditionally known as Broca area, whereas the red area of the inferior parietal lobule corresponds to the traditional Wernicke area. The yellow region shows the superior temporal gyrus, and the green line depicts the line of the Sylvian fissure as well as the superior temporal plane along which the main auditory processing areas are located.

critically important roles in cognitive awareness of sound, particularly those of a complex nature, such as speech and music.

Hemispheric Lateralization

As suggested by the left hemispheric specialization for language processing, the neural processing of sound is not necessarily a symmetric process, even though the similar neural substrates are present in both hemispheres. In right-handed individuals, language processing clearly occurs in a left hemispheric dominant fashion, leading individuals to suggest the notion of a right-ear advantage for speech in right-handed individuals, given the contralateral routing of neural signals in the ascending pathway. It has also been shown that this asymmetry is even present within the primary auditory cortex. In a functional neuroimaging study of passive sound perception, individuals listened to auditory stimuli that varied in either spectral or temporal domains. The results of this study showed that primary auditory cortices were activated in both sides, but that there was relatively greater activity within the left primary auditory cortex for temporal variation and relatively greater activity within the right primary auditory cortex for spectral variation (Figure 7).[27] This study has been supported by other investigations using music as a complex auditory stimulus, which have shown that in right-handed individuals, processing for rhythmic (temporal) patterns is left-hemisphere dominant, whereas processing for melody (spectral) patterns is right-hemisphere dominant.[28]

CENTRAL AUDITORY PROCESSING DISORDERS

Patients who demonstrate impairment of sound discrimination, localization, or comprehension in the face of normal cochlear and auditory nerve function are considered to have a central auditory processing disorder. The implication of such disorders is that the auditory nerve faithfully conveys all of the timing, spectral, and intensity information about the sound stimulus but that upstream deficits in the brainstem or cortex preclude adequate processing of the sound. Adequate processing is

required for language acquisition and comprehension. In addition, however, impairment in central auditory processing has been implicated in more global behavioral disorders.

Assessing Central Auditory Processing

Central auditory processing can be assessed with a complement of behavioral and electrophysiological testing. Behavioral tests can assess complex and subtle processing abilities but require intelligent, compliant patients for reliable testing. Behavioral tests of central auditory processing can be grouped 3 into types. One involves tests of binaural fusion, where stimuli to both ears need to be compiled. These include tests of sound localization, detection of sound level thresholds in one ear with concurrent masking noise presented to the other ear, and comprehension of speech stimuli alternating rapidly between the two ears. These tasks rely on brainstem auditory centers, and impairment implies brainstem lesions. Another type involves presenting distorted speech. Recorded speech is sped up (accelerated), slowed down (decelerated), or low-pass filtered and then presented to the subject. Deficits on these comprehension tasks are associated with temporal lobe lesions.[29] A third type involves presenting different, conflicting (typically speech-like) acoustic stimuli simultaneously to the two ears, termed "dichotic" listening tasks. With conflicting sounds presented to the two ears, the sound contralateral to the dominant hemisphere is typically suppressed. With hemispheric cortical lesions, however, the contralateral ear is typically suppressed regardless of dominance.[30] These central auditory processing behavioral tests can be complicated, however, by peripheral auditory impairment and, in the case of conductive or sensorineural hearing loss, need to be interpreted cautiously.[31]

Auditory Evoked Potentials and Central Processing

Electrophysiological tests of central auditory processing have the substantial advantage of being free from the bias and criterion inherent in behavioral testing. Their limitation, however, is that interpretation of the tests tends to be difficult and relies to some degree on the test reader's judgment. Potentials recorded from scalp surface electrodes evoked by auditory stimuli are typically grouped by their latencies as being either early, middle, or late.

Early potentials occur within 10 ms of the auditory stimulus and represent the auditory brainstem response (ABR). Waves I, III, and V are the most robust and are thought to reflect synchronous activity in the auditory nerve (I), the projection from the ventral cochlear nucleus to the superior olivary complex (III), and the contralateral lateral lemniscus or inferior colliculus (V).[32]

Middle latency responses occur typically between 10 and 50 ms following the auditory stimulus. These responses are generated by both

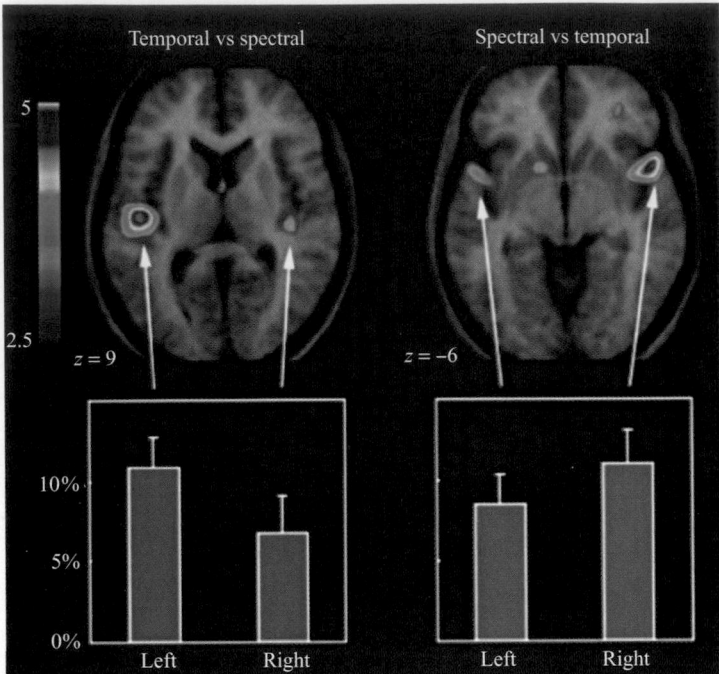

Figure 7 PET scan data showing relatively left lateralization of activity within primary auditory cortex for temporally varying stimuli, compared to spectrally varying stimuli, which show right lateralization of primary auditory cortex activity. Note that these images show right and left sides in anatomic (rather than radiologic) convention. (Reprinted from reference 27.)

subcortical and primary auditory areas within the temporal lobe. Long latency responses occur between 50 and 500 ms after the auditory stimulus and are generated by the auditory cortex. Because the auditory cortex receives bilateral projections, only bilateral deafness abolishes these potentials. Changes in these potentials are thus diagnostic of central auditory pathology. One long latency response that is used is the P-300 (ie, latency of 300 ms). Its amplitude and latency correlate with attention to auditory stimuli and auditory cognitive processing.[33]

Recognizing differences in sound stimuli, that is, discrimination, is another component of central auditory processing. An electrophysiological measure of sound discrimination is the mismatch negativity response (MMN). When a simple stimulus is presented repeatedly in a series, the MMN is recorded when the frequency of the stimulus is changed.[34–35] The MMN is elicited even when the subject is not attending to the stimuli.[36] The MMN is therefore a useful tool for studying cortical auditory discrimination, even in patients who have difficulty undergoing behavioral testing.[37]

Specific Central Auditory Processing Disorders

Several fairly common neurologic and psychiatric disorders have been associated with deficits in central auditory processing.

Schizophrenia. Sensory gating refers to the suppression of central auditory processing to subsequent external sounds while previously presented sounds are being processed. Deficits of auditory sensory gating result in "sensory overload" and disruption of higher-order processing. An electrophysiological measure of auditory sensory gating is the P50 event-related potential. P50 is a middle-latency potential found in the auditory evoked response to a click stimulus. Suppression

of the P50 amplitude occurs in normal subjects to clicks presented closely in time.[38] Impaired suppression of P50 has been demonstrated in schizophrenic patients and their relatives,[39] suggesting that a deficit in auditory sensory gating underlies schizophrenia.

Autism. Autism spectrum disorder (ASD), is a phenotypically heterogeneous diagnostic category characterized by variable impairment in social interaction, communication, and the presence of restrictive or stereotyped patterns of behavior.[40] Autistic subjects have shown superior pitch memory, discrimination, labeling, and tone from chord disembedding,[41] but a failure to attend to the sounds, like speech, to which normal children favor. An interpretation of these studies is that autism is associated with abnormal sound discrimination and orienting function.

Stroke. Hearing complaints in stroke victims are typically overshadowed by more prominent complaints involving other neurological systems. Furthermore, the auditory deficits in hemispheric strokes are likely to be subtle. Nonetheless, stroke can certainly result in central auditory processing deficits, especially in elderly patients.[42] Insular stroke is associated with temporal resolution and sequencing deficits in auditory processing.[43]

Alzheimer's Disease. Patients with Alzheimer's disease can demonstrate central auditory processing deficits that appear to be independent of cognitive decline and may even precede the onset of dementia diagnosis by many years.[44]

CONCLUSIONS

Central auditory processing is responsible for interpreting and integrating the "raw" data of sound stimuli from two ears into meaningful sensations of the sounds around us. Delineating human central auditory pathways and structures

has its origins in correlating behavioral abnormalities with postmortem identification of brain lesions—an inherently low-resolution methodology. With technological advancements in PET scanning and fMRI, however, we can "see" the brain in action in live human subjects and with much finer resolution. Such methods have been applied to the auditory system, and details about how we process sounds have begun to be decoded. As we begin to understand how and where complex sounds are processed in the normal listener, we can begin to pinpoint abnormalities in the pathway that may be associated with auditory processing disorders. As such, we have seen that several common neuropsychiatric disorders may have central auditory processing abnormalities as their root cause. As functional imaging technology advances, researchers will undoubtedly gain tremendous new insights into the mysterious phenomenon of auditory cognition.

REFERENCES

1. Raichle ME. Circulatory and Metabolic Correlates of Brain Function in Normal Humans. Bethesda, MD: American Physiological Society; 1987. p. 643–74.
2. Reivich M, Kuhl D, Wolf A, et al. The [18F] fluorodeoxyglucose method for the measurement of local cerebral glucose utilization in man. Circ Res 1979;44:127–37.
3. Raichle ME, Martin WR, Herscovitch P, et al. Brain blood flow measured with intravenous H2(15)O. II. Implementation and validation. J Nucl Med 1983;24:790–8.
4. Bandettini PA, Wong EC, Hinks RS, et al. Time course EPI of human brain function during task activation. Magn Reson Med 1992;25:390–7.
5. Fox PT, Raichle ME, Mintun MA, Dence C. Nonoxidative glucose consumption during focal physiologic neural activity. Science 1988;241:462–4.
6. Fox PT, Raichle ME. Focal physiological uncoupling of cerebral blood flow and oxidative metabolism during somatosensory stimulation in human subjects. Proc Natl Acad Sci U S A 1986;83:1140–4.
7. Ogawa S, Lee TM, Kay AR, Tank DW. Brain magnetic resonance imaging with contrast dependent on blood oxygenation. Proc Natl Acad Sci U S A 1990;87:9868–72.
8. Talairach J, Tournoux J. Co-planar Stereotaxic Atlas of the Human Brain: An Approach to Medical Cerebral Imaging. New York: Thieme; 1988.
9. Friston KJ, Holmes AP, Worsley KJ, et al. Statistical parametric maps in functional imaging: A general linear approach. Hum Brain Map 1995;2:189–210.
10. De Armond SJ, Fusco MM, Dewey MM. Structure of the Human Brain: A Photographic Atlas. New York: Oxford University Press; 1989.
11. Redd EE, Pongstaporn T, Ryugo DK. The effects of congenital deafness on auditory nerve synapses and globular bushy cells in cats. Hear Res 2000;147:160–74.
12. Ryugo DK, Pongstaporn T, Huchton DM, Niparko JK. Ultrastructural analysis of primary endings in deaf white cats: Morphologic alterations in endbulbs of Held. J Comp Neurol 1997;385:230–44.
13. Shepherd RK, Meltzer NE, Fallon JB, Ryugo DK. Consequences of deafness and electrical stimulation on the peripheral and central auditory system. In: Waltzman SB, Roland JT, Jr, editors. Cochlear Implants. New York: Thieme;2006. p. 25–39.
14. Ryugo DK, Kretzmer EA, Niparko JK. Restoration of auditory nerve synapses in cats by cochlear implants. Science 2005;310:1490–2.
15. Yin TC, Chan JC. Interaural time sensitivity in medial superior olive of cat. J Neurophysiol 1990;64:465–88.
16. Davis KA. Spectral processing in the inferior colliculus. Int Rev Neurobiol 2005;70:169–205.
17. Delgutte B, Joris PX, Litovsky RY, Yin TC. Receptive fields and binaural interactions for virtual-space stimuli in the cat inferior colliculus. J Neurophysiol 1999;81:2833–51.
18. Melcher JR, Sigalovsky IS, Guinan JJ, Jr, Levine RA. Lateralized tinnitus studied with functional magnetic resonance imaging: Abnormal inferior colliculus activation. J Neurophysiol 2000;83:1058–72.

19. de la Mothe LA, Blumell S, Kajikawa Y, Hackett TA. Thalamic connections of the auditory cortex in marmoset monkeys: Core and medial belt regions. J Comp Neurol 2006;496:72–96.

20. Brodmann K. Vergleichende Lokalisationslehre der Grosshirnrinde in ihren prinzipien Dargestellt auf Grund des Zellaufbaus. Leipzig Germany, Barth; 1909.

21. Kaas JH, Hackett TA, Tramo MJ. Auditory processing in primate cerebral cortex. Curr Opin Neurobiol 1999;9: 164–70.

22. Morosan P, Rademacher J, Schleicher A, et al. Human primary auditory cortex: Cytoarchitectonic subdivisions and mapping into a spatial reference system. Neuroimage 2001;13:684–701.

23. Schneider P, Scherg M, Dosch HG, et al. Morphology of Heschl's gyrus reflects enhanced activation in the auditory cortex of musicians. Nat Neurosci 2002;5:688–94.

24. Griffiths TD, Warren JD. The planum temporale as a computational hub. Trends Neurosci 2002;25:348–53.

25. Keenan JP, Thangaraj V, Halpern AR, Schlaug G. Absolute pitch and planum temporale. Neuroimage 2001;14: 1402–8.

26. Braun AR, Guillemin A, Hosey L, Varga M. The neural organization of discourse: An H2 15O-PET study of narrative production in English and American sign language. Brain 2001;124:2028–44.

27. Zatorre RJ, Belin P. Spectral and temporal processing in human auditory cortex. Cereb Cortex 2001;11:946–53.

28. Limb CJ. Structural and functional neural correlates of music perception. Anat Rec A Discov Mol Cell Evol Biol 2006;288:435–46.

29. Hausler R, Levine RA. Auditory dysfunction in stroke. Acta Otolaryngol (Stockh) 2000;120:689–703.

30. Eustache F, Lechevalier B, Viader F, Lambert J. Identification and discrimination disorders in auditory perception: A report on two cases. Neuropsychologia 1990;28:257–70.

31. Neijenhuis K, Tschur H, Snik A. The effect of mild hearing impairment on auditory processing tests. J Am Acad Audiol 2004;15:6–16.

32. Melcher JR, Kiang NY. Generators of the brainstem auditory evoked potential in cat. III: Identified cell populations. Hear Res 1996;93:52–71.

33. Salamat MT, McPherson DL. Interactions among variables in the P300 response to a continuous performance task. J Am Acad Audiol 1999;10:379–87.

34. Sams M, Paavilainen P, Alho K, Naatanen R. Auditory frequency discrimination and event-related potentials. Electroencephalogr Clin Neurophysiol 1985;62: 437–48.

35. Winkler I, Reinikainen K, Naatanen R. Event-related brain potentials reflect traces of echoic memory in humans. Percept Psychophys 1993;53:443–9.

36. Naatanen R, Simpson M, Loveless NE. Stimulus deviance and evoked potentials. Biol Psychol 1982;14:53–98.

37. Seri S, Cerquiglini A, Pisani F, Curatolo P. Autism in tuberous sclerosis: Evoked potential evidence for a deficit in auditory sensory processing. Clin Neurophysiol 1999;110:1825–30.

38. Adler LE, Pachtman E, Franks RD, et al. Neurophysiological evidence for a defect in neuronal mechanisms involved in sensory gating in schizophrenia. Biol Psychiatry 1982;17:639–54.

39. Nagamoto HT, Adler LE, Waldo MC, et al. Gating of auditory response in schizophrenics and normal controls. Effects of recording site and stimulation interval on the P50 wave. Schizophr Res 1991;4:31–40.

40. American Psychiatric Association. Diagnostic and Statistical Manual of Mental Disorders, 4th edition. Washington, DC: American Psychiatric Press; 1994. p. 1163–6.

41. Heaton P. Pitch memory, labelling and disembedding in autism. J Child Psychol Psychiatry 2003;44:543–51.

42. Hariri MA, Lakshmi MV, Larner S, Connolly MJ. Auditory problems in elderly patients with stroke. Age Ageing 1994;23:312–6.

43. Bamiou DE, Musiek FE, Stow I, et al. Auditory temporal processing deficits in patients with insular stroke. Neurology 2006;67:614–9.

44. Gates GA, Beiser A, Rees TS, et al. Central auditory dysfunction may precede the onset of clinical dementia in people with probable Alzheimer's disease. J Am Geriatr Soc 2002;50:482–8.

9

Diagnostic Audiology, Hearing Instruments and Aural Habilitation

James W. Hall III, PhD
Kristin N. Johnston, AuD

Within the past quarter century, dramatic advances in technology and techniques have contributed to more powerful audiologic test batteries and more effective management options for pediatric and adult populations. With auditory brainstem response (ABR) and otoacoustic emissions (OAEs), newborn infants can be screened for hearing impairment within days after birth and managed audiologically within the next critical 6 months. New techniques and strategies for the assessment of auditory function in adults have also been introduced in recent years. Pure-tone audiometry, immittance measurements (tympanometry and acoustic reflexes), and calculation of word recognition scores continue to be important for hearing assessment, and the traditional audiogram remains useful in summarizing the results of basic audiologic assessment. Clinical audiology, however, now also includes other behavioral and electrophysiological test procedures. For example, electrocochleography (ECochG) can contribute to the diagnosis of Menière disease. ABR offers a readily accessible, and relatively inexpensive, means for identification of retrocochlear auditory dysfunction. A variety of speech and nonspeech behavioral measures and several cortical auditory evoked responses are available for clinical assessment of central auditory nervous system dysfunction and associated auditory processing disorders. Finally, OAEs, because of their unique sensitivity and specificity to cochlear dysfunction, have become the latest addition to the clinical audiologic test battery.

The otolaryngologist is in a pivotal position to identify children and adults at risk for hearing loss, work closely with audiologists in diagnostic hearing assessment, and contribute to timely and appropriate medical or surgical intervention. In this chapter, we summarize current techniques and strategies for hearing assessment of adults, with an emphasis on the application of a test battery approach that maximizes diagnostic accuracy and efficiency, while minimizing test time and costs. The chapter includes a review of current hearing instrument technology for management of hearing impairment when other medical interventions do not or cannot rectify the hearing impairment and is a summary of pediatric audiologic habilitation approaches. At the end of the chapter, we define in a glossary common audiologic terms and abbreviations.

THE BASIC AUDIOLOGIC TEST BATTERY

Pure-Tone Audiometry

Pure-tone audiometry, the most common hearing test, is a measure of hearing sensitivity utilizing sinusoid stimuli at octave frequencies from 250 up to 8,000 Hz, and usually two inter-octave frequencies (3,000 and 6,000 Hz). The normal hearing, young (under 20 years) ear responds to frequencies from 20 to 20,000 Hz. Test results are graphed on an audiogram. Two common audiogram versions are illustrated in Figure 1. All audiograms include, minimally, a graph for plotting hearing threshold levels (HTLs) as a function of the frequency of pure-tone signals, although the exact format and symbols may vary.

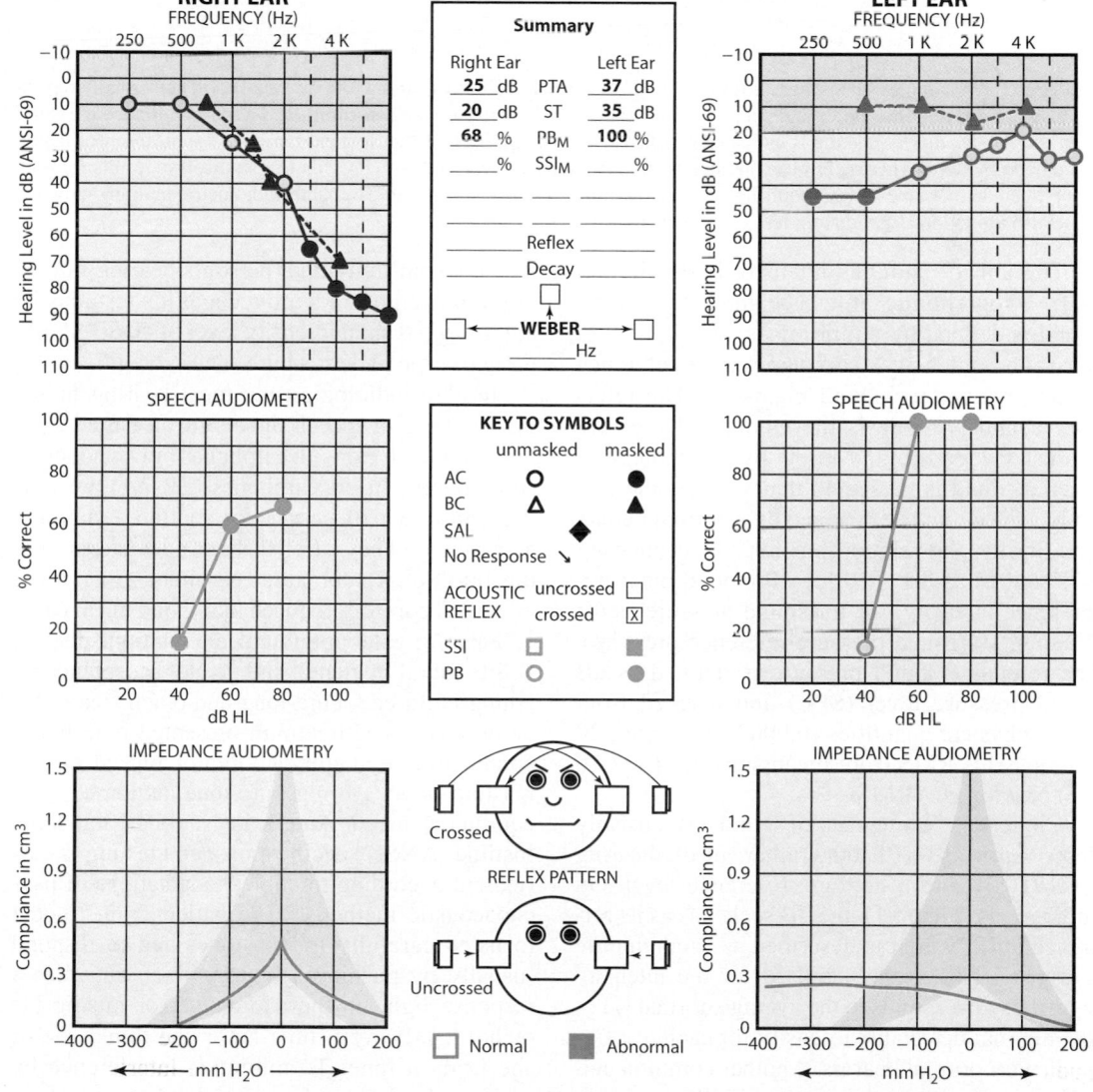

(A)

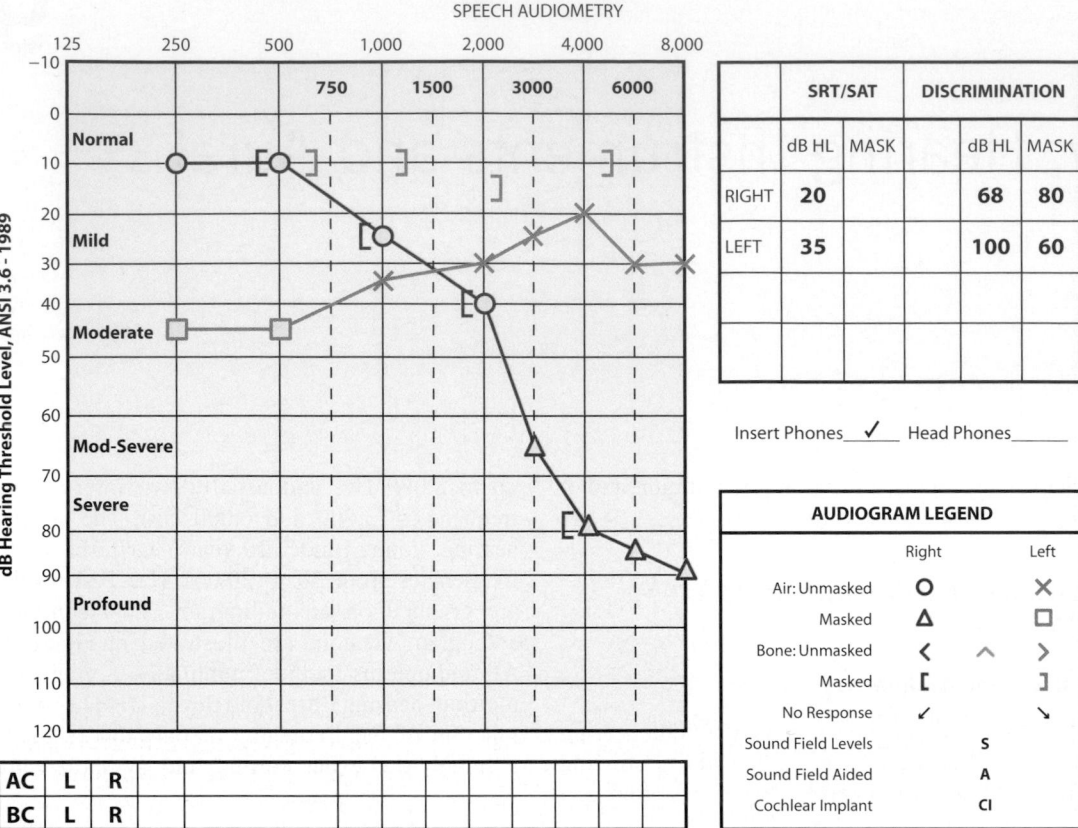

Figure 1 Two examples of audiogram formats. (A) This format includes sections for graphically and numerically reporting results for pure-tone audiometry (*top portion*), speech audiometry (*middle portion*), and aural immittance measurement (*bottom portion*). Masking is indicated by filled symbols. Findings for the right ear represent a typical sensorineural audiometric pattern, whereas left ear findings typify a conductive hearing loss. (B) This format displays results for both ears plotted on the same graph, requiring a separate symbol system for each ear. The same audiometric findings shown in A are also plotted in B, producing less clear analysis.

The unit of stimulus intensity is the decibel (dB), a logarithmic unit. The intensity of any sound is defined by a ratio of its sound pressure (or sound intensity) compared to a reference sound pressure (or sound intensity). The reference sound pressure is the amount of pressure against the eardrum, caused by air molecules when a sound is presented that vibrates the eardrum and can just be detected by a normal human ear. Briefly, the relationship for sound intensity is described as dB = 10 log 10 (sound intensity/reference intensity), or for sound pressure as dB = 20 log 10 (sound pressure/reference pressure). The reference sound pressure is defined as dB sound pressure level (SPL) and derived from 1 to 2 physical quantities (0.0002 dynes/cm^2, 20 micropascals RMS (root mean square) or 2 × 10 (−5) Newtons/m^2 RMS.

Clinically, the intensity of sound is not usually described in dB SPL but, rather, in dB hearing level (HL), with a biologic reference level. On audiograms (Figure 1), the dB scale has as its reference 0 dB, which is described as "audiometric 0 (zero)." This is the standard for the intensity level that corresponds to the average normal HTL, the minimal detectable intensity for each test frequency for normal hearers. Another common unit for expressing sound intensity is dB sensation level (SL) which is intensity of the stimulus in dB above an individual person's hearing threshold. For example, a word recognition test may be administered at an intensity level of 40 dB SL (40 dB above the patient's pure-tone average).

In adult audiologic assessment, hearing thresholds for tonal or speech signals are measured separately for each ear with earphones (air-conduction stimulation). Insert earphones (ER-3A) are now the transducer of choice for routine audiologic assessment. They offer distinct advantages over the traditional supraaural earphones, including increased comfort, reduced likelihood of ear canal collapse, greater interaural attenuation, disposability (aural hygiene), and greater acceptance by young children.[1] Pure-tone audiometry can also be performed with stimuli presented by a bone-conduction oscillator or vibrator placed on the mastoid bone. During pure-tone audiometry, all equipment meets American National Standards Institue (ANSI) specifications, and testing is carried out according to clinical adaptations of psychoacoustic methods.[2] The patient is instructed to listen carefully for the tones and to respond (usually by pushing a button which activates a response light on the audiometer or raising his or her hand) every time he or she thinks, he or she hears a tone. To minimize interference by ambient background acoustic noise, pure-tone audiometry should always be carried out with the patient in a double-walled, sound-treated room meeting ANSI specifications.[1,3]

For adults, the clinically normal region on the audiogram is from 0 to 20 dB HL. The normal region for children is more limited because even mild hearing loss can interfere with speech and language acquisition. Pediatric hearing threshold levels exceeding 15 dB may be considered abnormal. Thresholds in the 20 to 40 dB HL region constitute a mild hearing loss, 40 to 60 dB HL thresholds define a moderate loss, and threshold levels greater than 60 dB HL are considered a severe hearing loss.[1] As a reference, the intensity level of whispered speech close to the ear is less than 25 dB HL, conversational speech is in the 40 to 50 dB HL region, and a shouted voice within a foot of the ear is at a level of about 80 dB HL. The essential frequencies for understanding speech are in the 500 through 4,000 Hz region although higher frequencies also contribute to discrimination between certain speech sounds. Hearing sensitivity within the "speech frequency" region is traditionally summarized by calculating the pure-tone average, or PTA (hearing thresholds for 500, 1,000, and 2,000 Hz divided by 3 and reported in dB).

The validity of audiometric results depends on whether the patient's responses result from stimulation of the test ear. If a sound of greater than 40 dB HL is presented to 1 ear via standard earphones with supraaural (resting on the outer ear) cushions, it is possible that the acoustic energy will cross over from 1 side of the head to the other and stimulate the nontest ear. The mechanism for the crossover is presumably bone-conduction stimulation caused by vibration of the earphone cushion against the skull at high stimulus intensity levels. The amount of sound intensity needed before the crossover occurs is a reflection of interaural attenuation, that is, the sound insulation between the 2 ears provided by the head. Interaural attenuation is usually about 50 dB for lower test frequencies and 60 dB for higher test frequencies (such as those contributing to the ABR). Interaural attenuation is considerably higher for insert earphones.[1] With bone-conduction stimulation, interaural attenuation is very limited (at most 10 dB). Clinically, one must assume that interaural attenuation for bone-conducted signals is 0 dB. That is, any sound presented to the mastoid bone of 1 ear by a bone-conduction vibrator may be transmitted through the skull to either or both inner ears. Actual perception of this bone-conducted signal will, of course, depend on the patient's sensorineural hearing sensitivity in each ear.

Masking is the audiometric technique used to eliminate participation of the nontest ear whenever air- and bone-conduction stimulation exceeds interaural attenuation. An appropriate noise (narrow band noise for pure-tone signals and speech noise for speech signals) is presented to the nontest ear when the stimulus is presented to the test ear. With adequate masking, any signal crossing over to the nontest ear is masked by the noise. Selection of appropriate masking is sometimes difficult, especially when there is bilateral hearing impairment. The otolaryngologist should always attempt to verify that appropriate masking was used in interpreting audiologic results.

Comparison of the hearing thresholds for air versus bone-conduction signals is useful in classifying type of hearing loss, that is, whether a hearing loss is sensorineural (no air-bone gap), conductive (normal bone conduction and a loss by air conduction), or mixed (loss by bone conduction with a superimposed air- vs bone-conduction gap). *Configuration* refers to hearing loss as a function of the test frequency. With the sloping configuration, hearing is better for low frequencies and poorer for higher frequencies. High-frequency deficit hearing loss is the most common pattern associated with a sensorineural hearing impairment. A rising configuration is typified by relatively poor hearing for lower frequency stimuli and better hearing for the high frequencies. The rising configuration can result from varied types of middle ear pathology. One exception to the typical association of conductive hearing loss with rising configuration is Menière disease, which is discussed in Chapter 28, "Menière Disease, Vestibular Neuritis, Benign Paroxysmal Positional Vertigo, Superior Semicircular Canal Dehiscence, and Vestibular Migraine." Menière disease includes cochlear pathology that produces a rising configuration. A flat audiometric configuration is often recorded from patients with mixed hearing loss, that is, when both sensorineural and conductive components are present.

Speech Audiometry

Speech audiometry measures how well a person hears and understands speech signals. Speech audiometry procedures are used routinely to measure hearing sensitivity (thresholds in dB) for words or to estimate word recognition, for example, speech discrimination, ability. Spondee reception threshold (SRT), also referred to as the speech reception threshold (SRT) or speech threshold (ST), is the softest intensity level at which a patient can correctly repeat words approximately 50% of the time. Spondee words, 2-syllable words with equal stress on each syllable, for example, airplane, baseball, cowboy, are presented to the patient monaurally via earphones. The technique is equivalent to the method for determining pure-tone thresholds described previously.

Because the PTA indicates hearing threshold levels in the speech frequency region and ST or SRT is measured with a speech signal, close agreement between the PTA and the ST is expected. If the difference between PTA and ST exceeds ±7 dB, there is reason to suspect that 1 or both of the measures are invalid. An unusually good ST relative to PTA, for example, ST of 5 dB and PTA of 45 dB should immediately alert the tester to the possibility of a nonorganic hearing loss, as in malingering. With cooperative adult patients, particularly if pure-tone hearing thresholds are within the normal region from 500

to 4,000 Hz, there is probably little or no clinical benefit in measuring speech thresholds. Test time can be saved, with no loss of diagnostic information, by excluding speech threshold measurement from the test battery for such patients.

The common clinical approach for estimating a person's ability to hear and understand speech is speech recognition for phonetically balanced (PB) words.[1] Usually, a list of 25 or 50 single-syllable words is presented to the patient via earphones at 1 or more fixed intensity levels, and the percentage of words correctly repeated by the patient is calculated by the tester. One ear is tested at a time. Within the list of words, specific speech sounds (phonemes) occur approximately as often as they would in everyday conversation, that is, they are "phonetically balanced." Traditionally, these words were spoken into a microphone by the tester, while the level was monitored with a VU (volume unit) meter. Then, the words were routed to the patient through the audiometer after selection of the test ear and desired intensity level. This is, however, an outdated and poor clinical practice since it lacks standardization and consistency and increases the variability of test outcome. With adult patients, it is almost always possible and always preferable to use professionally produced (and commercially available) speech materials presented via compact disk player and an audiometer.[1] Diagnostic speech audiometry utilizing more sophisticated materials, for example, spectrally degraded or temporally distorted speech, or speech in noise materials, is feasible for assessment of the central auditory system.[1,4]

Immittance Measurement

Introduction. *Aural immittance (impedance) measures* are an important part of the basic audiometry test battery. Immittance is a term derived from the terms for 2 related techniques for assessing middle ear function (impedance and admittance), techniques which have been applied clinically since 1970.[5] A detailed discussion of the principles of immittance measurement is not within the scope of this chapter; however, this

has been reviewed by Hall and Mueller.[1] Briefly, the external ear canal is sealed with a soft rubber probe tip. Connected to the probe tip is a device producing a tone which is delivered toward tympanic membrane. Middle ear impedance or admittance is calculated from the intensity and other physical properties, for example, phase, of the tone in the ear canal. A middle ear (tympanic membrane and ossicular system) with low impedance (higher admittance) more readily accepts the acoustic energy of the probe tone, whereas a middle ear with abnormally high impedance (lower admittance) due, for example, to fluid within the middle ear space tends to reject energy flow. Thus, impedance (admittance) characteristics of the middle ear system can be inferred objectively with this quick and noninvasive technique, and then related to well-known patterns of findings for various types of middle ear pathologies.

Tympanometry. Tympanometry is the continuous recording of middle ear impedance as air pressure in the ear canal is systematically increased or decreased. The technique is a sensitive measure of tympanic membrane integrity and middle ear function (Figure 2). Compliance (the reciprocal of stiffness) of the middle ear, the dominant component of immittance, is the vertical dimension of a tympanogram. Tympanometry is popular clinically because it requires minimal technical skill and less than a minute to perform. Because aural immittance measurement is an electrophysiologic (vs behavioral) method, it does not depend on cooperation of the patient. Importantly, it is a sensitive measure of middle ear function. Tympanometry patterns, in combination with audiogram patterns, permit differentiation among and classification of middle ear disorders.

James Jerger in 1970 described what has become the most clinically widespread approach for describing tympanograms.[5] There are 3 general tympanogram types: A, B, and C. The normal, or type A, tympanogram has a distinct peak in compliance within 0 to −100 mm of water pressure (decapascals or daPa) in the ear canal (shown in Figure 2). To be classified as normal,

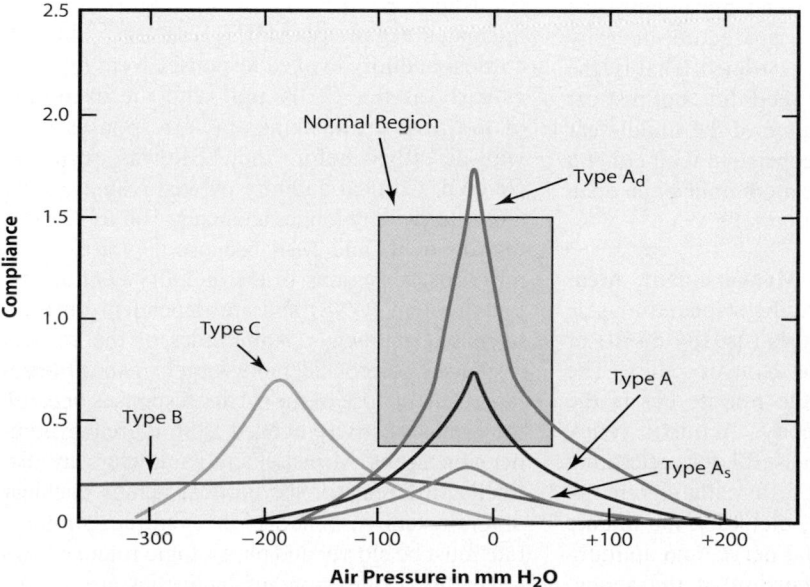

Figure 2 Classification system for tympanograms. (Adapted from reference 5.)

the location of the compliance peak on the pressure dimension, and the height of the peak, must be within the normal range, indicated in Figure 2 by the stippled area. With a type B tympanogram, there is no peak in compliance but, rather, a flat pattern with little or even no apparent change in compliance as a function of pressure in the ear canal. This pattern is most often associated with fluid within the middle ear space, for example, otitis media, although other middle ear pathologies may give rise to a type B tympanogram as well. Type C tympanograms also have a distinct peak in compliance (as with the type A), but the peak is within the negative pressure region beyond –150 mm H_2O decapascal (daPa). This pattern is usually found in patients with eustachian tube dysfunction and inadequate ventilation of the middle ear space, and often precedes the type B tympanogram in the development of otitis media.

The type A_s (Figure 2) is a variation of the type A tympanogram. The "s" stands for shallow. Peak compliance is below the lower normal limits of compliance. That is, middle ear impedance is abnormally high. The type A_s pattern is typically recorded from patients with fixation of the ossicular chain, including those with the diagnosis of otosclerosis. In contrast, with an unusually steep and high-compliance tympanogram (type A_d for deep), the peak may actually exceed the upper compliance limits of the equipment. The A_d tympanogram type is recorded from patients with disruption of the ossicular chain, which leaves the middle ear extremely mobile and hypercompliant, that is, very little impedance. In the absence of serious hearing loss, however, this tympanogram pattern is usually associated with minor tympanic membrane abnormality, such as scarring. During the initial portion of the tympanometry procedure, high positive or negative pressure is introduced into the ear canal. This essentially decouples the middle ear system from the measurement. If the aural immittance device records an abnormally large equivalent volume of air, for example, 2 cm or more in an adult or twice the volume that was recorded for the other ear, between the probe tip and presumably the eardrum at this stage in the procedure, integrity of the eardrum should be questioned. That is, the aural immittance device is recording not just ear canal volume but also volume of the middle ear space. This test finding is consistent with either a perforation of the tympanic membrane or an open (patent) middle ear ventilation tube.

Acoustic Stapedial Reflex Measurement. Measurement of contractions of the stapedial muscle to high sound intensity levels (usually 80 dB or greater) is the basis of the acoustic reflex. The stapedial muscle within the middle ear is the smallest muscle in the body. Acoustic reflex measurement is clinically useful for estimating hearing sensitivity and for differentiating among sites of auditory disorders, including the middle ear, inner ear, eighth cranial nerve, and auditory brainstem. The afferent portion of the acoustic reflex arc is the eighth cranial nerve. There are complex brainstem pathways leading from the cochlear nucleus on the stimulated side to the region of the motor nucleus of the seventh (facial) nerve on both sides (ipsilateral and contralateral to the stimulus) of the brainstem. The efferent portion of the arc is the seventh nerve innervating the stapedial muscle. When the stapedial muscle contracts, the result is increased stiffness (decreased compliance) of the middle ear system. This small change in compliance following stapedius muscle contraction (within 10 ms) is detected by the probe and aural immittance device.

Measurement of the acoustic reflex is useful clinically because it can quickly provide objective information on the status of the auditory system from the middle ear to the brainstem. Distinctive acoustic reflex patterns for ipsilateral and contralateral stimulation and measurement conditions characterize middle ear, cochlear, eighth nerve, brainstem, and even facial nerve dysfunction (see "faces" in lower portion of Figure 1A). Comparison of acoustic reflex threshold levels—the lowest stimulus intensity level that activates the reflex—for tonal versus noise signals permits estimation of the degree of cochlear hearing impairment.[1] This technique is especially valuable in children and difficult-to-test patients.

AUDITORY EVOKED RESPONSES

Introduction

Auditory evoked responses are electrophysiological recordings of responses to sounds.[6] With proper test protocols, the responses can be recorded clinically from activation of all levels of the auditory system, from the cochlea to the cortex. More than a dozen subtypes of auditory evoked responses can be recorded beyond the brainstem, from auditory regions of the thalamus, hippocampus, internal capsule, and cortex. Prominent among the cortical evoked responses measured for clinical purposes are the auditory middle latency response (AMLR), the auditory late response (ALR), the P300 response, and the mismatch negativity (MMN) response.[1,6] In fact, cortical auditory evoked responses were reported as early as the 1930s and, with the exception of the MMN, all of the above responses were well-described before the ABR was even discovered. Cortical auditory evoked responses are characterized by longer latencies (100 to 300 ms) than ECochG and ABR because they arise from more rostral regions of the auditory central nervous system (CNS) and are dependent on multisynaptic pathways. Amplitudes of the cortical responses are considerably larger (2 to 20 times larger) than those of the earlier responses because they reflect activity evoked from a greater number of neurons. Measurement parameters are distinctly different for the cortical versus cochlear or brainstem responses. For example, stimulus rate must be slower and physiologic filter settings lower. As a rule, stimulus intensities are moderate, rather than high. Cortical evoked responses are best elicited with longer duration, and therefore frequency-specific, tonal stimuli, rather than the click stimuli that are optimal for evoking ECochG and ABR. The analysis time must, of course, extend beyond the expected latency of the response (>300 ms) for the cortical responses. Recording electrode sites also are different for the cortical responses, with more emphasis on scalp sites over each cerebral hemisphere and less concern about electrode sites near the ears.

Auditory Brainstem Response

Among the many auditory evoked responses, the ABR (often referred to by neurologists as the brainstem auditory evoked response or BAER) and ECochG are applied most often clinically.[6] An ABR recording is shown schematically in Figure 3. The ABR is generated with transient acoustic stimuli (clicks or tone bursts) and detected with surface electrodes (discs) placed on the forehead and near the ears (earlobe or within external ear canal). Using a computer-based device, it is possible to present rapidly, for example, at rates of 20 to 30 per second, thousands of sound stimuli and to average reliable ABR waveforms in a matter of minutes. Automated devices are now available for special clinical applications, for example, newborn hearing screening. The anatomic generators of the ABR components have been studied extensively.[6] Waves I through V arise from the eighth cranial nerve and auditory regions in the caudal and rostral brainstem (Figure 4). Wave I clearly represents the synchronously stimulated compound action potentials from the distal part of the eighth cranial nerve. Wave II may also arise from the eighth nerve, but at the proximal end near the brainstem. Waves I and II are generated by structures ipsilateral to the ear stimulated. All later ABR waves have multiple generators within the auditory brainstem. Wave III, which is usually prominent, is generated within the caudal pons, with likely contributions from the cochlear nuclei, the trapezoid body, and the superior olivary complex. The largest and most rostral component of the ABR (wave V) is generated in the region of the lateral lemniscus as it approaches the inferior colliculus, presumably mostly on the side contralateral to the ear stimulated.

The first objective in ABR waveform analysis is to assure that the response is reliably recorded. Minimally, 2 replicated waveforms should be averaged. If the response is not highly replicable, modifications in the test protocol should be made, and then potential technical problems must be considered and systematically ruled out. When a replicable response is confirmed, absolute latencies for each replicable wave component and relative (interwave) latencies between components are calculated in milliseconds (ms). These latency data for each ear are assessed for symmetry and also compared to appropriate normative data. With regard to symmetry, ABR wave V should be within 0.4 ms between ears, that is, an interaural latency difference of >0.4 ms for wave V is a

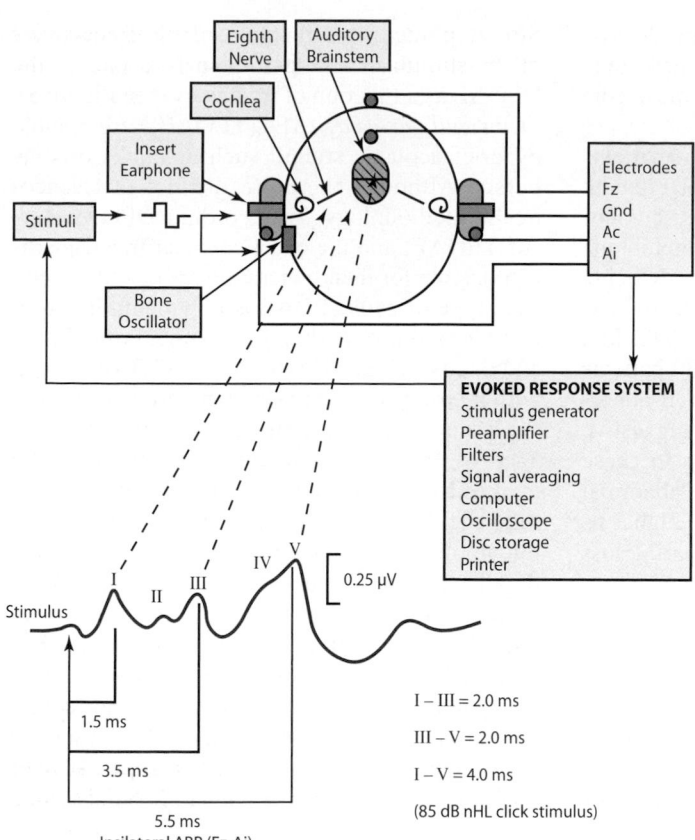

Figure 3 Schematic of the instrumentation used for recording the auditory brainstem response (ABR) and major relations between auditory anatomy and waveform components. A simple strategy for analysis of ABR waveform in neurodiagnosis is also shown.

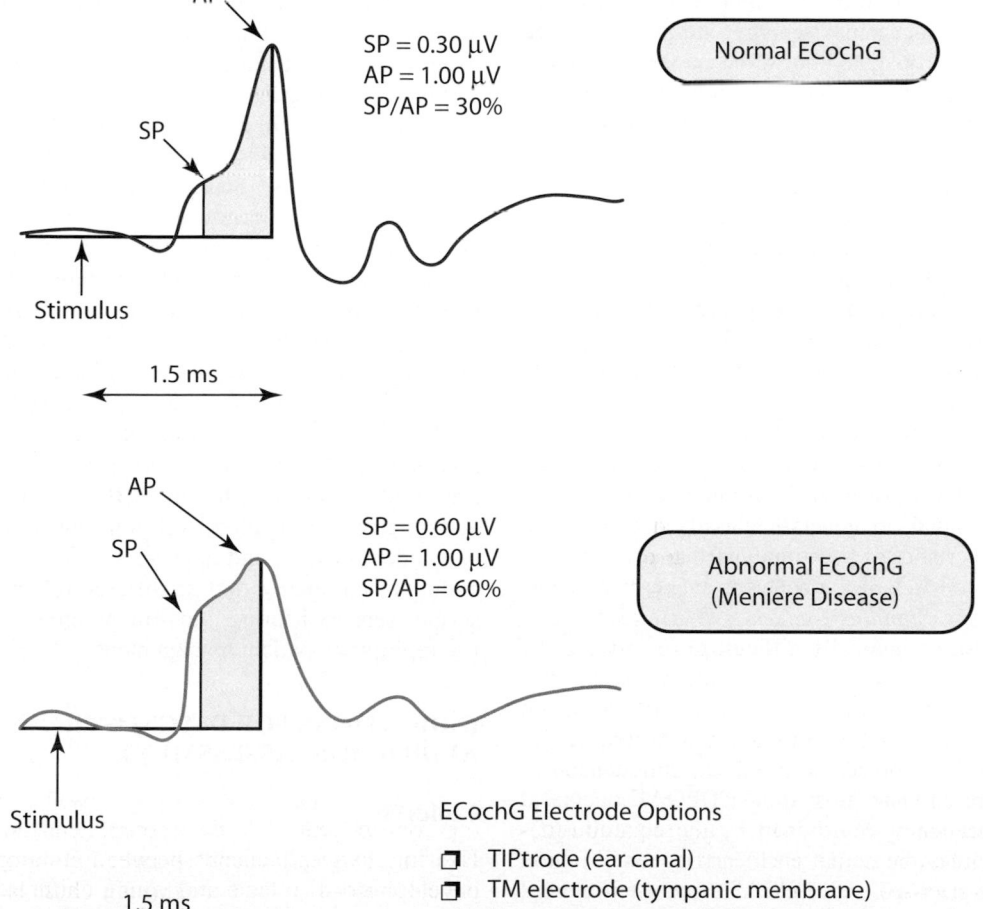

Figure 4 Electrocochleography (ECochG) waveforms illustrating normal relation of summating potential (SP) and action potential (AP) and abnormally enlarged SP/AP relation in a patient with Menière disease. Absolute and relative amplitude values for the SP and AP components, and the criteria for definition of a normal response, vary significantly for different electrode sites (ear canal vs tympanic membrane vs promontory).

sign of retrocochlear auditory dysfunction on the side with longer latency values. Common ABR waveform patterns are illustrated in Figure 3. A well-formed and clear wave I at a delayed latency value for the maximum stimulus intensity level is characteristic of a conductive or mixed hearing loss. When wave I is small and poorly formed, but interwave latency values are within normal limits (the wave I–V latency value is less than 4.60 ms), a high-frequency sensory (cochlear) hearing loss is suspected. Delayed interwave latency values are the signature of retrocochlear auditory dysfunction. Abnormal delays between the early wave components, for example, I–III, are consistent with posterior fossa lesions involving the eighth nerve and/or lower brainstem, whereas a prolonged III–V latency suggests intra-axial auditory brainstem dysfunction.

A primary goal in any diagnostic ABR is to record a clear and reliable wave I component. Wave I serves as the benchmark for peripheral auditory function. Subsequent interwave latencies offer indices of retrocochlear (eighth nerve and brainstem) function that are relatively unaffected by conductive or sensory hearing loss. The likelihood that a wave I will be recorded is enhanced by the use of either ear canal (TIPtrode) or tympanic membrane electrode designs, along with alterations of the test protocol, such as a slower stimulus rate, rarefaction stimulus polarity, and maximum stimulus intensity level. Reports on ABR dating back to the late 1970s confirmed that waveforms evoked by high intensity yielded neurodiagnostic information on cochlear and retrocochlear auditory function and could be applied in the identification of retrocochlear disorders, for example, vestibular schwannomas, with a hit rate exceeding 95%. With the development of sophisticated neuroradiological techniques, such as computed tomography (CT) or magnetic resonance imaging (MRI) with enhancement, reports of normal ABR findings among patients with very small posterior fossa tumors have appeared in the literature. These are clearly false-negative ABR outcomes in patients at risk for retrocochlear auditory dysfunction due, usually, to very small intracanicular vestibular schwannomas. On the other hand, false-positive outcomes for CT and MRI have also been reported for patients with normal ABRs and no surgical evidence of tumor.[1,6] ABR continues to be a readily available, relatively inexpensive, and reasonably sensitive procedure for initial diagnostic assessment of eighth nerve and auditory brainstem status in patients with retrocochlear signs and symptoms. ABR is also valuable in electrophysiological monitoring of the eighth nerve and auditory brainstem function during certain neurotologic operations, for example, vestibular neurectomy, auditory brainstem implant placement, or posterior fossa tumor removal.

Auditory Steady State Response

The auditory steady state response (ASSR) is an electrophysiological technique that is useful for estimation of auditory thresholds in infants and young children.[6] The ASSR is elicited with pure-tone (steady state) signals that are rapidly modulated or changed in amplitude and, usually, frequency. Fast stimulus modulation rates, for example, >80 Hz, are utilized when the ASSR is recorded from children who are sedated or lightly anesthetized. As with ABR measurement, sedation or anesthesia is necessary in recording the ASSR from children to eliminate the deleterious effects on response detection of muscle or movement-related measurement artifact. ASSR measurement is now possible with commercially available evoked response systems used also for ABR assessment. The ASSR offers 3 potential advantages over the ABR for auditory assessment of young children. First, because the response is elicited with pure-tone (steady state), rather than transient (very brief) stimuli, it is possible to present stimuli with intensity levels up to 120 to 125 dB HL. Second, depending on the extent of the modulation, especially the frequency modulation, the stimuli used to elicit the ASSR can be rather frequency specific and valuable for electrophysiological estimation of the audiogram. Finally, the analysis of either the phase and/or the frequency content of brain activity elicited by the modulated pure-tone signals is fully automated and independent of the skills and experience of the tester. Clinical experience confirms that the ASSR complements the ABR in the electrophysiological assessment of auditory function of infants. Each technique has its advantages and disadvantages, but together the ABR and ASSR offer a powerful diagnostic duo for early assessment of hearing in children in the era of universal newborn hearing screening.

Electrocochleography

For over 30 years, ECochG has been applied in the assessment of peripheral auditory function.[6] Currently, ECochG is performed most often for intraoperative monitoring of cochlear and eighth nerve status and in the diagnosis of Ménière disease. Optimal ECochG waveforms are recorded from a small needle electrode placed through the tympanic membrane on to the promontory although tympanic membrane and, to a lesser extent, ear canal electrode locations are also clinically useful. Stimulus and acquisition parameters for recording ECochG have been well-defined for decades.[6] The 3 major components of the ECochG are the cochlear microphonic (CM), the summating potential (SP), and the action potential (AP). The CM and SP reflect cochlear bioelectric activity, whereas the AP is generated by synchronous firing of distal afferent eighth nerve fibers and is equivalent to ABR wave I (Figure 4). The typical ECochG analysis technique in neurotology requires determination of the amplitude of the SP and the AP from a common baseline. Then, the ratio of the SP/AP is calculated and reported in percent. Normal SP/AP ratio ranges and cutoffs in percentage have been reported for each electrode type. Abnormal SP/AP ratio values are defined as >50% for the ear canal electrode type (the TIPtrode), >40% for the tympanic membrane electrode, and >30% for the transtympanic needle electrode type.[1,6]

The characteristic ECochG finding for patients with Ménière disease is an abnormal enlargement of the relation between the SP and AP component amplitudes. With the tympanic membrane electrode technique, sensitivity of ECochG in the diagnosis of endolymphatic hydrops is reported as 57%, whereas specificity is 94% in a series of 100 patients.[7] Only 3 out of 30 patients yielded false-positive findings. Thus, an abnormally enlarged SP/AP ratio is highly suggestive of endolymphatic hydrops according to these data. In this study, the likelihood of an abnormal ECochG SP/AP ratio was statistically higher as hearing loss increased and when the hearing loss fluctuated.

OTOACOUSTIC EMISSIONS

OAEs are low intensity sounds produced by the cochlea in response to an acoustic stimulus.[8] A moderate intensity click stimulus, or an appropriate combination of two tones, can evoke outer hair cell movement or motility. Outer hair cell motility affects basilar membrane biomechanics, resulting in a form of intracochlear energy amplification, as well as cochlear tuning for more precise frequency resolution. The outer hair cell motility generates mechanical energy within the cochlea which is propagated outward, via the middle ear system and the tympanic membrane, to the ear canal. Vibration of the tympanic membrane then produces an acoustic signal, that is, the OAE, which can be measured by a sensitive microphone. There are two broad classes of otoacoustic emissions: spontaneous and evoked. *Spontaneous* OAEs (SOAEs), present in only about 70% of persons with normal hearing, are measured in the external ear canal when there is no external sound stimulation. A significant gender effect for SOAE has been confirmed with females demonstrating SOAE at twice the rate of males.

Evoked OAEs, elicited by moderate levels (50 to 80 dB SPL) of acoustic stimulation in the external ear canal, are generally classified according to characteristics of the stimuli used to elicit them or characteristics of the cochlear events that generate them. *Stimulus-frequency* OAEs (SFOAEs), which are technically difficult to record, are the least studied of the evoked otoacoustic emissions. *Distortion-product* OAEs (DPOAEs) are produced when 2 pure-tone stimuli at frequencies f_1 and f_2 are presented to the ear simultaneously (Figure 5). The most robust DPOAE occurs at the frequency determined by the equation $2f_1-f_2$ whereas the actual cochlear frequency region that is assessed with DPOAE is between these 2 frequencies and probably close to the f_2 stimulus for recommended test protocols. With all of the 5 FDA-approved instruments that are commercially available for recording DPOAE, amplitude as detected in the ear canal and described in dB SPL is plotted as a function of the frequencies of the stimuli in a DPgram, that is, a plot of the DPOAE as a function of frequency (see Figure 5). *Transiently evoked* OAEs (TEOAEs) are elicited by brief acoustic stimuli such as clicks or tone bursts. Although there are distinct differences in the methodology for recording DPOAE versus TEOAE, and the exact cochlear mechanisms responsible for their generation are also different, each type of evoked OAE is now being incorporated into routine auditory assessment of children and adults.[8] Clinical applications of OAEs, along with their rationale, are summarized in Table 1.

When outer hair cells are structurally damaged or at least nonfunctional, OAE cannot be evoked by acoustic stimuli. Among patients with mild cochlear dysfunction, OAE may be recorded but amplitudes are below normal limits for some or all stimulus frequencies. Importantly, some patients with abnormal OAE, consistent with cochlear dysfunction, will have normal pure-tone audiograms. An example is a patient with the symptom of tinnitus, yet a normal audiogram. Abnormal OAEs are expected in the frequency region represented by the tinnitus. Up to 30% of a population of outer hair cells may be damaged without substantially affecting the simple audiogram. In such cases, however, abnormal OAE findings are invariably recorded. The noninvasive nature of OAE recording, coupled with their accuracy and objectivity in assessing cochlear, in particular outer hair cell, function suggests diverse potential clinical applications, ranging from auditory screening to the diagnosis of sensorineural hearing loss.

Among the more important clinical contribution of OAEs in children is the identification and diagnosis of auditory neuropathy. First described regularly in the literature in the mid-1990s as clinical equipment for OAE measurement became widely available auditory neuropathy is hearing impairment secondary to eighth cranial nerve pathology that is not related to a tumor or other neoplasm.[6,8] Since OAEs originate from the outer hair cells and are, therefore, "preneural," OAEs are typically normal in patients with auditory neuropathy, even with evidence of severe to profound hearing loss by the ABR or pure-tone audiometry. As detailed by Rapin and Gravel,[9] early identification and appropriate diagnosis of auditory neuropathy, and its differentiation from serious sensory hearing impairment, are essential for appropriate patient management.

INDICATIONS FOR DIAGNOSTIC AUDIOLOGIC ASSESSMENT

Children

Hearing loss influences speech and language development of infants and young children, and these effects begin within the first 6 months of life.[10] Even mild peripheral hearing deficits among preschool- and school-age children interfere with educational development. Therefore, early identification of hearing loss, coupled

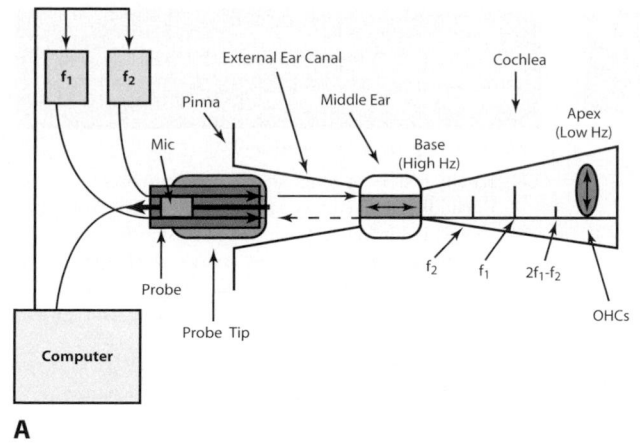

A

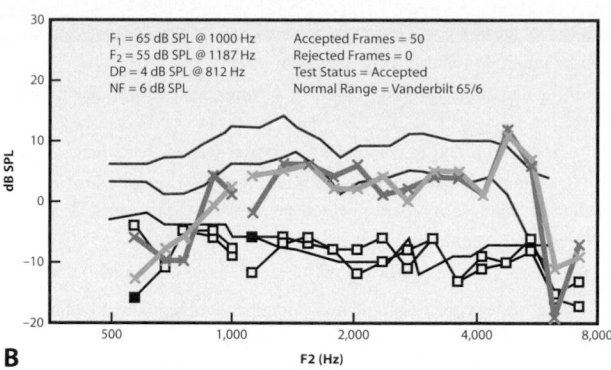

B

Figure 5 (A) Schematic illustration of the generation of distortion product otoacoustic emissions (DPOAEs) from outer hair cells within the cochlea. (B) DPgram recorded for patient with normal hearing in the lower frequencies, and a mild sensory hearing impairment (25 to 35 dB HL) secondary to noise exposure in the 3,000 to 6,000 Hz region. Replicated plots of DPOAE amplitude in dB SPL are shown as a function of the frequency of the stimuli (the geometric mean of the f_1 and f_2) in a "DPgram." Noise levels as a function of frequency are indicated in the lower portion of the DPgram. NF = noise floor.

with timely and appropriate intervention and management, is necessary for a child to reach his or her full communicative and educational potential.[11] A number of factors put children at risk for hearing impairment. Table 2 summarizes risk factors for hearing impairment identified by the 2000 Joint Committee on Infant Hearing.[12] Otolaryngologists and audiologists must coordinate efforts in properly and promptly assessing and managing pediatric hearing impairment. Currently, the most effective strategy for infant hearing screening, that is, with the highest degree of sensitivity and specificity, is the application of a combination of automated OAEs and automated ABR technologies.[13]

In addition to peripheral hearing impairment secondary to common causes, such as conductive hearing loss with otitis media or sensorineural hearing loss in ototoxicity, the otolaryngologist must also consider the possibility of auditory processing disorders (APDs) in children. According to a recent Consensus Conference report,[4] APDs are defined as "deficits in the processing of information that is specific to the auditory modality." Often APDs are related to central auditory nervous system dysfunction. Common risk factors for APDs in school-age children include:

- teacher concern about hearing despite a normal audiogram,
- academic underachievement,
- recurrent middle ear disease,
- suggestion of APD on language evaluation,
- poor response to language treatment,
- attention deficit disorder (ADD) with or without hyperactivity,
- reading delay or disorder,
- learning disabilities, and
- history of neurological insult, for example, head injury and neonatal asphyxia.

There are now a variety of behavioral and electrophysiological measures for diagnosis of APD.[1,14,15] Electrophysiological procedures were outlined above. Among them, cortical evoked responses are especially appropriate for evaluation of APD.[6] The behavioral procedures include measures of detection, for example, auditory integration tasks, and suprathreshold discrimination,

for example, temporal ordering tasks and identification, for example, recognition of speech signals from phonemes to sentences, presented monotically, diotically, and dichotically.[4] Speech and nonspeech materials for assessment of APDs are available in CD format from multiple commercial sources.[1,14,15]

Adults

In adults, risk factors for central auditory nervous system dysfunction include, but are not limited to, advanced age; history or clinical evidence of stroke, head injury, and brain neoplasms; Alzheimer disease; and other disorders affecting the central nervous system. In general, it is a good clinical policy always to consider the possibility of central auditory dysfunction when a patient's hearing complaints exceed expectations based on the audiogram.

HEARING AIDS

Introduction

A *hearing aid* is an assistive device that delivers an amplified acoustic signal into the ear canal.[3] Some form of amplification has for centuries been used to overcome the deleterious effects of a hearing impairment on communication. The most simplistic "hearing aid" is easily made by cupping ones' hand behind the ear. This technique is effective because it helps channel the acoustic signal into the ear canal. Another simple means for improving the reception of an acoustic signal is to move closer to the sound source. When the distance between the listener and the sound source is doubled, the acoustic intensity is reduced by 6 dB at the listener. Similarly, a reduction in the distance by one-half increases the intensity by 6 dB. When the acoustic signal is an electronic device, such as a television or radio, reception can be easily enhanced by adjusting the volume control to make a more intense signal. All of these methods enhance the reception of a particular acoustic signal and demonstrate that amplification is often an effective means of improving one's ability to hear. Amplification can be used to improve hearing in many forms of hearing impairment. Cochlear and auditory

brainstem implants are discussed in Chapter 32, "Cochlear and Brainstem Implantation."

Electronic hearing aids enhance the signal strength by amplifying the acoustic signals that reach its microphone. Hearing aid design has evolved rapidly with advances in electronics becoming smaller, reliable, and more efficient. Some of today's hearing aids are small enough to fit completely within the ear canal, and some have advanced technological features, such as digital signal processing, that can significantly improve listening in noise. One noteworthy aspect of hearing aid design is that only a single disposable button-type battery of less than 1.5 V powers most units.[3] Average battery life ranges between 10 and 14 sixteen-hour days.

Electronic hearing aids consist of 3 basic components: a microphone, an amplifier, and a receiver, with each component housed in a casing designed to fit behind or in the ear. The microphone is located externally and is activated by miniscule fluctuations in air pressure caused by the sound source. These vibrations are converted into an electrical impulse and delivered to the amplifier. At this stage, the signal is amplified and filtered. The altered signal is delivered to the receiver, which converts the electronic impulse into an acoustic signal. The amplified acoustic signal is delivered to the ear canal for reception of the signal by the wearer.

Types of Hearing Aids

Hearing aids are classified in 2 general ways. The first is by the style of the hearing aid, which usually refers to the size and location of the hearing aid and the hearing aid receiver relative to the ear. The second is by the technological features of the device.

Hearing Aid Styles. The most commonly used hearing aid styles (although other types do exist) are the behind-the-ear (BTE), open-fit in-the-ear (ITE), in-the-canal (ITC), and completely-in-the-canal (CIC) hearing instruments. Figure 6 shows a hearing aid representing each of these major styles.

Behind-the-ear hearing aids are aptly named because the body of the hearing aid lies on the posterosuperior aspect of the auricle. The receiver

Table 1 Clinical Applications of Otoacoustic Emissions (OAEs) and Their Rationale

Application	Rationale
Newborn hearing screening	OAEs can be recorded reliably from newborn infants
	OAE recording can be performed in nursery setting (test performance may be affected by noise)
	Normal OAEs are recorded in persons with normal sensory (cochlear) function
	OAEs are abnormal in persons with even mild degrees of sensory hearing loss; the main objective of screening is to detect sensory hearing impairment
	OAE recording may require a relatively brief test time
	OAE measurement may be performed by nonaudiologic personnel (ie, at reduced cost)
Pediatric audiometry	OAE recording is electrophysiologic and not dependent on patient behavioral response
	OAEs assess cochlear function specifically (behavioral audiometry and ABR are dependent also on the status of the central auditory nervous system)
	OAEs can be recorded from sleeping or sedated children
	OAE recording requires a relatively short test time
	OAEs provide ear-specific audiologic information
	OAEs provide frequency-specific audiologic information
	OAEs are a valuable contribution to the "crosscheck principle"*
Diagnosis of central auditory processing disorders	OAE recording is electrophysiologic and not dependent on patient behavioral response
	OAEs are a sensitive means of ruling out cochlear (outer hair cell) dysfunction
Assessment in suspected functional hearing loss	OAE recording is electrophysiologic and not dependent on patient behavioral response
	Normal OAEs invariably imply normal sensory function
	OAEs provide frequency-specific audiologic information
Differentiation of cochlear versus retrocochlear auditory dysfunction	OAEs are site specific for cochlear (sensory) auditory dysfunction
	In combination with ABR, OAEs can clearly distinguish sensory versus neural auditory disorders
Monitoring ototoxicity	OAEs are site specific for cochlear (sensory) auditory dysfunction
	Ototoxic drugs exert their effect on outer hair cell function; OAEs are dependent on outer hair cell integrity
	OAE recording is electrophysiologic and not dependent on patient behavioral response; can be recorded from patients who, owing to their medical condition, are unable to perform behavioral audiometry tasks or from infants and young children
	OAEs can detect cochlear dysfunction before it is evident by pure-tone audiometry
	OAEs provide frequency-specific audiologic information
Tinnitus	OAEs are site specific for cochlear (sensory) auditory dysfunction
	OAEs can provide objective confirmation of cochlear dysfunction in patients with tinnitus and normal audiograms
	OAEs provide frequency-specific audiologic information that may be associated with the frequency region of tinnitus
Noise/music exposure	OAEs are site specific for cochlear (sensory) auditory dysfunction
	Excessive noise/music intensity levels affect outer hair cell function; OAEs are dependent on outer hair cell integrity
	OAEs can provide objective confirmation of cochlear dysfunction in patients with normal audiograms
	OAE findings are associated with cochlear frequency specificity, ie, "tuning"; musician complaints of auditory dysfunction can be confirmed by OAE findings, even with a normal audiogram
	OAEs can provide an early and reliable "warning sign" of cochlear dysfunction owing to noise/music exposure before any problem is evident in the audiogram

Adapted from reference 8. ABR = auditory brainstem response.

* The crosscheck principle in pediatric audiology is that the results of any single audiologic test should not be relied on without independent corroboration or crosscheck from another audiologic test.

Table 2 Joint Committee on Infant Hearing Screening 2000 Indicators Associated with Sensorineural Hearing Loss

Birth through age 28 d (neonate)

Family history of congenital or delayed-onset childhood hereditary sensorineural hearing loss

Congenital infection, such as toxoplasmosis, syphilis, rubella, cytomegalovirus, and herpes

Craniofacial anomalies including abnormalities of the pinna and ear canal, absent philtrum, and low hairline.

Birth weight less than 1,500 g (3.3 lb); hyperbilirubinemia at level requiring exchange transfusion

Ototoxic medications including but not limited to the aminoglycosides (eg, gentamicin, tobramycin, kanamycin, streptomycin) used in multiple courses or in combination with loop diuretics

Bacterial meningitis

Apgar scores of 0 to 4 at 1 min or 0 to 6 at 5 min

Mechanical ventilation lasting 5 d or longer

Stigmata or other findings associated with a syndrome known to include sensorineural and/or conductive hearing loss (eg, Waardenburg's or Usher's syndrome).

Age 29 d through 2 yr (infant)

Parent caregiver concern regarding hearing, speech, language, and/or developmental delay

Bacterial meningitis and other infections associated with sensorineural hearing loss

Ototoxic medications including but not limited to chemotherapeutic agents or aminoglycosides used in multiple courses or in combination with loop diuretics

Recurrent or persistent otitis media with effusion for at least 3 mo

For use with infants (age 29 d through 3 yr) requiring monitoring of hearing

Indicators associated with delayed-onset sensorineural hearing loss

Family history of hereditary childhood hearing loss

In utero infections (eg, cytomegalovirus, rubella, syphilis, herpes, or toxoplasmosis)

Neurofibromatosis 2 and neurodegenerative disorders

Indicators associated with conductive hearing loss

Recurrent or persistent otitis media with effusion

Anatomic deformities and other disorders that affect eustachian tube function

Neurodegenerative disorders

is coupled to the ear canal by a piece of acoustic tubing attached to a custom-made ear mold, as illustrated in Figure 6A. A recently introduced BTE style is the open-fit mold described below. BTE hearing aids are extremely flexible because of their design. Due to the amount of available space within the body of the BTE hearing aid for electronic components, any degree of hearing loss, ranging from mild to profound, and con-figuration of hearing loss can be managed with a BTE device. A defective unit can be replaced by removing the tubing and ear mold assembly and by attaching it to a new or repaired unit. Changes in the size of the auricle in individual patients are inexpensively accommodated by making a new ear mold. In other words, it is not necessary to modify the body of the hearing aid. For these reasons, the BTE style is a popular choice for children. In addition, the ear mold can be made of material varying in density from hard (lucite) to soft (silicone). The choice of ear mold material can significantly add to the comfort and flexibility of the instrument. A disadvantage of the BTE instrument, however, is the location of the microphone. The ideal location of a microphone would be deep in the ear canal using the natural resonance of the auricle and ear canal. However, the microphones of BTE instruments are generally located above the auricle and oriented anteriorly. The loss of natural cues must be compensated by the hearing aid. One advantage of this microphone placement is the availability of a directional microphone, a technology further discussed in a later section of this chapter. Because of the acoustic, and perhaps cosmetic, advantages

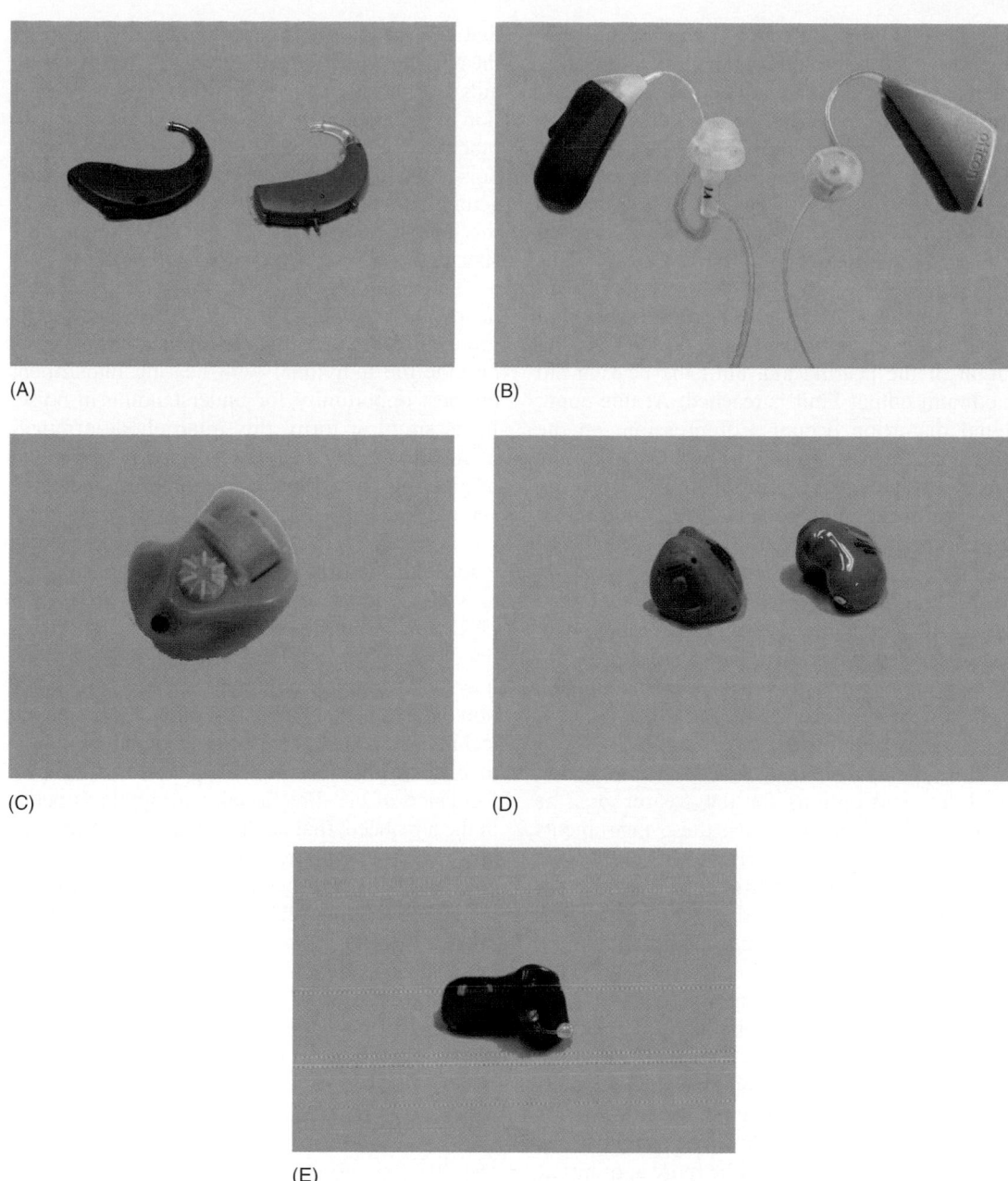

Figure 6 Examples of major hearing instrument styles. The five types of hearing instruments are: (A) behind-the-ear (BTE); (B) open-fit; (C) in-the-ear (ITE); (D) in-the-canal (ITC); and (E) completely-in-the-canal (CIC).

of open-fit BTE hearing aids, and further advantages associated with the open-fit design, market share of the BTE style in annual hearing aid sales is increasing.

Open-fit hearing aids use a BTE design for housing the electronics. Open-fit hearing aids were designed to benefit individuals with high-frequency hearing loss and essentially normal hearing in the lower frequency range, a common configuration for hearing loss, especially in older adults. Traditional BTE and other custom-made hearing aids can be problematic for people with this type of hearing loss for a couple of reasons. One reason is the occlusion effect, an acoustic phenomenon that results in increased gain for low-frequency sounds when the ear is occluded with a fitted ear mold or custom-made hearing aid. The occlusion effect most often interferes with the hearing aid wearer's perception of his or her own voice, a common complaint among hearing aid wearers with traditionally fit BTE

and custom-made hearing aids. Open-fit hearing instruments do not utilize the custom ear mold assembly typical of traditional BTE hearing instruments. A cone- or dome-shaped piece rests in the ear canal just before the second bend of the ear canal (Figure 6B). This earpiece has an open design and deep insertion allowing some sounds to enter the ear naturally while maximizing the natural resonance of the concha and auricle. The earpiece connects to a slim tube and ear hook assembly connected to the BTE device. Some benefits of the open-fit design include more pleasant perception of one's voice because it can be heard more naturally through the open design earpiece, and gain is not inappropriately applied to the low frequencies. Open-fit hearing aids tend to be cosmetically appealing because the BTE case is often much smaller than the traditional BTE case, and the tube and earpiece used are small and deeply inserted making them much less conspicuous (Figure 6B). One drawback of this

style of hearing aid is a fitting range that is limited to high-frequency hearing loss.

In-the-ear hearing aids are housed completely within a custom-made ear mold designed to fit in the auricle and ear canal (Figure 6C). The body of the hearing aid, completely filling the concha, contains most of the electronic components, including the battery and a volume control. The anterosuperior portion of the ITE hearing aid fits into the helix of the auricle inferior to the triangular fossa and functions primarily to keep the instrument in place. The microphone is frequently located within this portion of the instrument. The medial portion fits partially in the ear canal and contains the receiver. ITE hearing aids are completely self-contained, with no tubing or ear mold assembly. The hearing aid is essentially built into the ear mold. Properly fit ITE hearing aids are appropriate for mild to severe losses of hearing. The location of the microphone close to the level of the ear canal is an advantage of the ITE style. Additionally, an ITE hearing aid can include directional microphones. Despite these advantages and its cosmetic appeal, the ITE hearing aid style does have at least 3 disadvantages. First, the size of the instrument within the auricle minimizes the use of the natural acoustic resonance of the external ear. Second, when the instrument must be repaired or replaced at an off-site facility, that is, the manufacturer, the patient must get by without the hearing aid for a number of days. A BTE loaner may be provided when coupled with a temporary ear mold, but this is usually not an acceptable alternative. Finally, ITE hearing aids may be difficult for some patients to insert and remove, especially for individuals with decreased manual dexterity skills.

In-the-canal hearing aids fit primarily into the ear canal (Figure 6D). Only the faceplate of the hearing aid is visible in the concha of the ear. A properly fitted ITC hearing aid may accommodate up to a moderately severe hearing loss. The location of the microphone is at the opening of the ear canal taking advantage of the acoustic properties of most of the auricle. Also, these devices are inserted deeper within the external ear canal than ITE hearing aids, producing an increase in gain of about 5 dB. Some ITC hearing aids can include directional microphones. However, the availability of this desirable feature depends on the size of the faceplate of the hearing aid. Although the size of the ITC instrument is an acoustic advantage, there are a couple of disadvantages. Since the hearing aid casing making contact with the ear serves to hold the hearing aid in place, the smaller ITC device more easily becomes dislodged and lost. The small size of ITC hearing aids makes them more difficult to insert and remove, hindering use by those with manual dexterity limitations.

Completely-in-the-canal (CIC) hearing aids are the smallest of the hearing aid styles and, therefore, often the most cosmetically appealing (Figure 6E). CIC hearing aids are inserted deeply into the ear canal by the patient and are essentially invisible to the casual observer. With the CIC hearing instrument design, the receiver is located past the second bend of the ear canal, and the medial end of the hearing aid is within 5 mm of the tympanic membrane. A CIC hearing aid has a nylon fish line-type cord attached to its lateral surface to aid in retrieval of the instruments from the ear canal. Because of its size and microphone location, these devices have a number of advantages. These advantages include a reduction in the occlusion effect, ease of use on the telephone, no problems with wind noise on the microphone, an increase in gain by as much as 15 dB, and enhancement of the acoustic effects of the auricle and ear canal. Unfortunately, CIC devices are not without disadvantages. Practical drawbacks include problems obtaining and maintaining a good seal with the external ear canal and associated acoustic feedback, increased repair problems related to blockage with cerumen, difficulty inserting and removing the device from the ear canal, increased expense, reduction in the number of advanced technological features, and an inability to provide adequate amplification for persons with severe hearing losses. Another disadvantage of this hearing aid style is that its small size prevents the use of directional microphones as the microphone ports require a certain amount of space between them to achieve directionality. There is simply not enough space for multiple microphones on the faceplate of a CIC hearing aid.

Hearing Aid Technology. Within the past decade, hearing aid technology has advanced tremendously.[3] Hearing aids today have many advanced components and features. We will now review briefly some of the more important developments in hearing aid technology. In addition, there are many published and internet sources of current hearing aid technology.

Disposable and instant fit hearing aids are a relatively recent development to emerge on the hearing aid market. These devices have attracted increased attention because they can be fit immediately while the patient is in the office, without the need to ship ear mold impressions to a laboratory or the manufacturer. The products are available in a wide range of sizes, from BTE to CIC instruments. An advantage of these devices is their significantly reduced price in comparison to custom-made products. The disposable hearing aids have an added benefit in that there is never a need to replace the battery, since the entire hearing aid is replaced after 40 days. However, these devices may only be appropriate for milder degrees of hearing impairment, rendering those individuals with severe and profound hearing losses ineligible for this technology.

Conventional or analog hearing aids are the least technologically sophisticated of the custom-made hearing aids. An analog hearing aid receives the acoustic signal from the microphone, converts it into an electrical signal, amplifies and filters it according to the individual's hearing loss, and reconverts it into an acoustic signal that is delivered to the ear canal. With this type of technol-ogy, the audiologist selects a matrix for the hearing aid, which determines its overall gain, slope, and maximum output. Relatively few adjustments can be made directly by the physician, hearing aid dispenser, or audiologist. These minor adjustments may be made by screwdriver controls known as "trim pots." Typically, these devices provide linear amplification, although some do provide some form of compression. Linear amplification in hearing aids produces the same amount of gain regardless of the input signal. As the input signal increases in intensity, so does the resulting output of the hearing aid, until the hearing aid maximum output limit is reached. At this point, signal distortion occurs. Compression, on the other hand, helps eliminate the problem of distortion created by linear hearing aids. With a hearing aid containing compression circuitry, the amount of gain provided by the hearing aid depends on the intensity of the incoming signal. Signals at greater intensity level are amplified less than those with lower intensities. This reduction in gain decreased distortion as the signal approaches the maximum output provided by the hearing aid. Typically, these instruments have a volume control that may be adjusted by the user.

Programmable hearing aids provide increased flexibility and options for the wearer. Just as in conventional hearing aids, these instruments have analog amplifiers. However, unlike the conventional hearing instruments, programmable devices can be modified in the audiologist's office via a computer or hand-held programmer. The programming allows for increased flexibility in shaping the frequency response, output limitations, compression characteristics, and enhanced features provided by the hearing aid. Additionally, many of the programmable devices offer multiple memories or programs. The utilization of these multiple programs allows the patient access to different settings that may be more appropriate for various listening environments, for example, quiet versus noisy. The multiple programs may be accessed via a remote control or a switch on the hearing instrument.

Digital hearing aids are the most popular hearing aid technology available today, and the market share continues to increase. A digital hearing aid processes the acoustic signal differently than an analog instrument. In digital processing, the acoustic signal is converted into a digital or binary code, minimizing the possibility for distortion of the signal. The signal is then amplified and converted back to an acoustic signal that is delivered to the ear canal through the receiver. Digital devices offer a number of advantages, including increased flexibility of shaping the frequency response of the instrument, feedback suppression capabilities, improved sound quality, decreased battery drain, and less internal circuit noise. Like programmable hearing instruments, digital devices may have multiple memories and can be adjusted via a computer or hand-held programmer. The memories may be also be accessed via a remote control or a switch on the hearing instrument. Most manufacturers currently market advanced hearing aids that change the program automatically based on the noise levels in the environment. These hearing aids also usually have some form of noise reduction to reduce sounds such as wind noise that may otherwise be unnecessarily amplified. The goal of noise reduction technology is to reduce unwanted sounds and increase the speech signal. To achieve this goal, the device must acoustically sort out the speech signal from a background of noise.

The major complaint of persons with sensorineural hearing loss is the inability to hear in background noise. Currently, *directional microphones* provide the individual with hearing impairment the best opportunity for understanding in noise. In its simplest form, this microphone arrangement allows the wearer to differentiate sound originating from the front, which is where the sound source is usually located, from sound coming from the rear, which is usually where noise is located. Multiple microphones may result in 5 to 8 dB of improvement in signal-to-noise ratio (SNR) in comparison to standard, omnidirectional microphones.[16] The improvement in SNR may result in improvement in speech recognition by as much as 60%. Directional microphone technology is available in conventional, programmable, and digital hearing aids. However, the performance of the directional hearing aid is better in the advanced, that is, digital devices. Additionally, directional microphone technology is available in BTE instruments through half-shell ITE instruments. However, the improvement in noise is greater in the larger styles. In some advanced hearing aids, adaptive directionality is available, allowing the hearing aid to analyze the direction of speech versus noise signal sources with automatic appropriate adjustment of the hearing aid.

Indications for Amplification

Hearing aids are indicated whenever it can be demonstrated that the patient's ability to communicate will be significantly improved through the use of amplification. A hearing aid is not recommended under the following conditions:

- Effective medical treatment can be implemented to restore normal hearing
- Hearing aid use would exacerbate pathology or interfere with treatment for it
- A hearing aid fails to improve the ability of the patient to communicate

A common myth is that amplification is of no benefit in the case of sensorineural hearing loss. While there is no evidence correlating the use of a hearing aid with restoration or treatment of the impaired auditory system, hearing aids are routinely used to offset the negative effects of sensory hearing impairment. Sensory hearing loss accounts for 90% of all types of hearing loss. More than 95% of all hearing aids are purchased by patients with sensorineural hearing loss. Amplification is an effective means of improving the communicative abilities of individuals with sensory hearing impairment, as attested by hundreds of research articles published in the last 50 years.

Amplification is an extremely effective means of improving the hearing of patients with conductive hearing loss. A hearing aid is clearly not an acceptable alternative to effective medical treatment of a pathological condition, but it may be utilized after the course of treatment to offset residual hearing impairment. Residual conductive hearing loss is commonly present following placement of an ossicular prosthesis, for example. In this case, a hearing aid is often an effective means for further improving hearing sensitivity. In contrast, a hearing aid is rarely of benefit for patients with retrocochlear (neural or central) auditory disorders. In some cases, amplification may actually exacerbate the effects of the disorder. The use of amplification must also be carefully evaluated in all cases of central impairment. However, there are alternatives for these patients. Perhaps the most common approach is the recommendation of an assistive listening device, like an FM system, for improvement of speech understanding by significantly enhancing the speech signal in relation to background noise. FM technology can be effective in the management of persons with hearing impairment and also as a treatment option for children with auditory processing disorders. Representative types of FM technology are shown in Figure 7. With any type of FM device, the primary objective is to increase the SNR for the listener. That is, the speaker's voice is enhanced in comparison to background sounds. A personal FM device (see Figure 7A and B) is most effective for an individual person, for example, a single child with APD in the classroom. However, classroom FM systems (Figure 7D) provide benefit to many children at minimal cost. Even modest improvements in the signal-to-noise ratio, for example, 5 dB, are associated with large improvements in speech perception and communication.

Benefits of Amplification

It is readily apparent that the utilization of amplification can significantly improve the communicative ability of an individual with hearing impairment. However, recent research has revealed additional benefits in psychosocial and functional health measures.[17] These studies have shown that individuals utilizing amplification reported less depressive feelings, richer social relationships, and less anxiety and paranoia. Additionally, and perhaps as a result of improved communicative psychosocial functioning, these individuals noted improvements in their physical health status. Hence, the utilization of amplification has the potential to improve significantly the quality of life of an individual with hearing impairment.

Monaural versus Binaural Amplification

A great deal of research has been devoted to the following question: if hearing loss is bilateral, are 2 hearing aids better than 1? The intuitive answer is, of course, that 2 hearing aids would best offset the effects of a hearing loss in both ears. The question persists, however, because some patients choose monaural fittings, although this is becoming more uncommon. This decision is usually based on cosmetic or financial reasons, although some patients claim to hear just as well with 1 hearing aid as with 2, and others appear to hear better with a single instrument.

The benefits of binaural amplification have been well documented in the aural literature.[3] The most commonly cited benefits are as follows:

- improved word identification, particularly in adverse listening conditions,
- improved localization of the sound source,
- a sense of "balanced hearing,"

- the need for less gain,
- elimination of the head shadow effect, and
- increased perception of high-frequency consonants.

In addition to these advantages, recent studies document the effects of auditory deprivation in unaided ears. The research indicates that, with a monaural hearing aid fitting, word identification scores in the unaided ear decrease over time relative to the scores in the aided ear. In contrast, decrements are not observed in either ear in a binaural fitting. Further, limited recovery in word identification is observed following the provision of amplification to the deprived ear.

With regard to this evidence, binaural amplification should be recommended unless specifically contraindicated. Valid contraindications to binaural amplification are as follows:

- unilateral hearing loss,
- medical complication in 1 ear,
- 1 ear cannot be effectively aided due to insufficient residual hearing, and
- binaural amplification results in diminished word identification performance.

Rehabilitation of Unilateral Hearing Loss

Contralateral routing of signal (CROS) is a hearing aid technology for people with unilateral hearing, that is, the other ear is unaidable. There are 2 implementations of this strategy: CROS and BiCROS (bilateral contralateral routing of signal).

Using this technology, a receiver resembling a hearing instrument worn on the unaidable side, and the microphone within the device picks up sound from that side and sends it to another instrument at the better ear. The sound is delivered to the better ear via a wire around the posterior part of the neck or wirelessly via FM radio transmission.

The CROS implementation is for an individual who has relatively normal hearing in the better side and has hearing that is too poor to be aided on the worse side. The receiving BTE device on the worse side transmits the sound to a device on the better side. The user hears the amplified sound from the unaidable side in their best ear. The user hears the sound delivered to the better ear naturally, without amplification, via an open hearing aid mold.

The BiCROS implementation is for a patient with unaidable hearing on 1 side and with some hearing loss in their better ear. It is similar to the CROS system, except that the device on the better side is a hearing aid fitted to rehabilitate the hearing loss in the better ear, and it is also capable of receiving the sound transmitted from the CROS aid on the other side. There are 2 advantages of CROS and BiCROS technologies: (1) elimination of the head shadow effect results in an improved ability to hear sounds arriving to the worse ear, and (2) the user can have improved cues for sound localization.

Another alternative to the CROS system is what used to be referred to as a bone-anchored

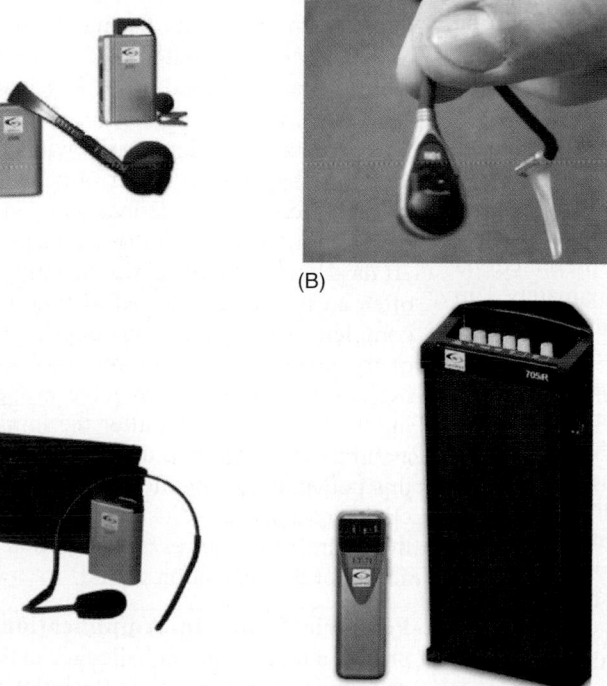

(A)

(B)

(C)

(D)

Figure 7 Examples of FM systems (assistive listening devices). (A) Conventional personal FM device. (B) Phonak EduLink personal device. (C) Desktop FM device. (D) Classroom FM device.

hearing aid (BAHA). The Baha sound processor (Entific Medical Systems, Cochlear Americas, Englewood, CO; http://www.entific.com) is based on the principle of direct bone conduction (DBC). The Baha system uses a combination of sound processor attached to a percutaneous abutment and osseointegrated fixture. The vibrating Baha transducer is directly connected to the skull via the abutment and fixture and via DBC stimulates the better hearing cochlea. Currently, the United States Food and Drug Administration (FDA) has approved the use of this system with single-sided deafness, as well as to rehabilitate individuals with unilateral conductive hearing loss due to congenital aural atresia and in the setting of chronic ear disease when chronic infection prevents the use of a traditional air-conduction hearing aid.

Hearing Aid Selection

The selection of an appropriate hearing aid requires a combination of factors. First, it is essential that the practitioner thoroughly assess the patient's motivation, concerns, communicative goals, and listening needs before selecting a hearing instrument. Issues like cosmetics, dexterity, and financial constraints may significantly limit the style and technological options. Additionally, one's communicative goals or typical listening environment may dictate the need for a directional microphone or other advanced features. To aid in this endeavor, the use of self-assessment inventories, which will be discussed in the following section, may be of benefit.

To aid in the selection of a hearing aid, multiple researchers have developed *prescriptive formulae* that are based on audiometric thresholds or suprathreshold information.[3] The goal of these formulae is to provide the listener with the optimum-aided speech intelligibility possible. However, formulae are not expected to be a panacea but, rather, are intended to provide the dispenser with a valid approximation, a logical starting point. From here, minimal modifications should be required. Currently, there are a number of prescriptive formulae available, but no standard has been adopted.

Assessment of Hearing Aid Outcomes

Whenever treatment is rendered, some measure of efficacy of the service should be performed. In the age of managed care, it is exceedingly important to document the success (or failure) of rehabilitation services, that is, treatment outcome. Currently, there are a number of means to assess of the efficacy of amplification, which include electroacoustic analysis, functional gain measures, real-ear measures, and self-assessment inventories. Each of these procedures will be discussed briefly in the following sections.

Electroacoustic Analysis. When hearing instruments are received from the manufacturer, and before they are dispensed to the patient, it is essential that the devices be evaluated to determine if they are functioning appropriately.[3] According to the American Speech Language Hearing Association (ASHA), hearing devices should be assessed via an *electroacoustic analysis* according to the ANSI S3.22 standard as well as a listening check.[18] With the first test, the hearing aid is attached to a 2 cm^3 coupler and placed in a test box that analyzes the sound pressure present within this cavity that is produced by the hearing aid receiver. The electroacoustic analysis provides information regarding the gain characteristics of the hearing aid at each frequency, the frequency response, the maximum output, battery drain, and distortion of the hearing aid. The results can then be compared to the specifications of the hearing instrument provided by the manufacturer. If discrepancies occur, the hearing instrument should be returned to the manufacturer for repair or replacement.

Additionally, a listening check of the instruments should be performed. This check will provide information regarding the sound quality, circuit noise, and any intermittent function of the devices. Once again, if problems are noted, the devices should be returned to the manufacturer.

Functional Gain Measures. *Functional gain measures* are designed to assess the realistic benefit the patient derives from his hearing instruments, by determining behaviorally the amount the hearing aid improves the patient's thresholds of audibility.[3] Utilizing a speech signal and/or warble tones, the procedure is conducted in the sound field (ie, in a sound booth with the signals presented via loud speakers) to determine the difference in the patient's aided and unaided hearing thresholds. Although functional gain measures are designed to assess the patient's "real world" benefit, the procedure is plagued by serious limitations, including poor test-retest reliability, limited frequency response information, lack of maximum output information, and a dependence on the patient's behavioral responses.

Real-Ear Measures. *Real-ear measures* are currently the most accepted means of verifying hearing aid performance.[3,19] Real-ear measurement systems use a specially designed probe microphone to measure the sound pressure in the ear canal at the eardrum. The probe microphone is inserted along the side of the patient's ear canal into a position located within 6 to 8 mm of the tympanic membrane. A broadband noise, speech composite noise, or tonal series is presented via a loudspeaker that is located approximately 1 m away from the patient. Measurements are made and graphically displayed with and without the hearing aid in place. Aided test results are usually compared to unaided results, and the hearing aid is then adjusted to match the prescribed target. At a minimum, real-ear measurement should be conducted at an input level of 60 to 70 dB SPL, which is typical of average conversational speech. Additionally, the saturation level of the hearing aid should be determined to ensure that the maximum output of the hearing aid is set below the patient's threshold of uncomfortable loudness. For nonlinear hearing aids, testing at a high input level (80 to 85 dB SPL) and a low input level (50 dB SPL) should also be included. At each of these input levels, the patient's feedback regarding the volume of the input signal should be solicited.

Self-Assessment Inventories. Perhaps the most compelling evidence of the success of a hearing aid fitting comes directly from the patient. After a brief period of hearing aid use, most adult patients are quite capable of determining whether the prescribed amplification has improved their ability to hear. This is understandable, considering that the vast majority of individuals who purchase hearing aids cope with the hearing impairment for many years before deciding to pursue amplification. After little experience wearing the new hearing aids, most patients are able to describe precisely the listening situations in which their hearing aids are effective or ineffective. To quantify the valuable patient report, a number of self-assessment inventories have been developed for use by audiologists and hearing aid dispensers.[3] These inventories are widely used to evaluate the initial fitting and the effectiveness of subsequent modifications.

Patient Accommodation to Amplification. An individual with hearing impairment requires a period of adjustment to become accustomed to wearing hearing aids. The average patient has developed a hearing loss over a period of years before deciding to pursue amplification. During this time period, considerable adaptation has occurred in the central auditory system.[20] The sudden introduction to amplified sound initiates compensatory neurophysiologic changes that may take 5 to 6 weeks to develop fully. Within this time period, adjustments to the hearing instruments are often needed to assist the patient in the process of accommodation. Many hearing aid programs encourage patients to utilize a wearing schedule that gradually extends the length of time that the hearing aids are worn each day. Some programs also restrict hearing aid use to quiet listening environments during the initial period of accommodation with systematic exposure to more demanding conditions as accommodation progresses.

A common problem arises when a patient is initially unhappy with the performance of the hearing aid. According to federal law, an individual may return a hearing aid to the dispenser within 30 days for a refund. Unfortunately, 30 days is often an insufficient period of time to allow for complete accommodation and/or modification of the instruments. Therefore, prospective hearing aid patients should receive proper counseling before, during, and after the initial fitting to avoid making a premature decision. To address this potential hearing aid fitting challenge, some clinicians allow an adjustment period longer than the federal law requires in recognition of the variability of the adaptation period.

Pediatric Issues in Amplification. Children present a unique set of challenges in the selection and fitting of amplification. Potential problems to be addressed include the small size of children's ears in comparison to adult ears, noncompliance of some children, the increased demands in their communication needs, the important impact of the accuracy of the hearing aid fitting on the successful acquisition of speech and language, and often a lack of complete audiometric data required to make these decisions. To address these challenges, audiologists have developed a special set of standards for selecting and fitting hearing aids for young children. As noted earlier in the chapter, BTE instruments are the most popular hearing aid style for children as they permit maximum flexibility. First, the BTE design allows for an inexpensive means for accommodating changes in the size of the auricle and ear canal as the child grows. As these adjustments are made over time, the child can continue to use the hearing instrument. Second, BTE devices are more resistant to feedback problems due to the increased distance between the microphone and the receiver. Furthermore, utilizing an ear mold with thick tubing may also decrease the likelihood of feedback. Third, the BTE style offers options that contribute to the retention of the hearing aid within the ear canal, like wire retention attachments, kiddie tone hooks, and Huggie-Aids. Finally, a BTE hearing instrument offers many additional technological features that may not be available on smaller styles.

In addition to the style of hearing aid, a number of other hearing aid options and features should be considered. Every hearing aid dispensed to a child should have several options, including direct audio input, the telecoil feature, and microphone/telecoil options. These features offer the advantage of maximum adaptability with assistive listening devices, such as FM systems. Additionally, tamper-resistant volume controls and battery doors should be considered. For maximum flexibility, digital hearing aids with feedback suppression, programmable features, and multiple memories that offer both omnidirectional and directional microphone technology are added assets. Finally, due to the likelihood of the hearing instruments becoming lost or damaged in young hands, a loss and damage insurance policy is highly encouraged.

Noting the difficulties in fitting and the communication needs of young children, Richard Seewald developed a prescriptive formula called the desired sensation level (DSL).[21] This hearing aid fitting approach calculates a prescriptive target for average conversational speech and maximum output of the hearing instrument from a variety of sources, using either pure-tone thresholds obtained via behavioral audiometry under headphones or frequency-specific electrophysiological, for example, ABR or ASSR, estimations of auditory thresholds. Additionally, if hearing aid verification and adjustments cannot be made utilizing real-ear measures in the child's ear canals, the adjustments may be made using a 2 cm^3 coupler in the hearing aid test box by using real-ear-to-coupler differences (RECDs). RECD is the decibel difference between the level of sound in the ear canal versus the level that is measured in the 2 cm^3 coupler. RECD is determined by taking an unaided measurement in the child's ear canal. If this measurement cannot be obtained, the formula provides average RECDs for children of various ages. Hence, with this prescriptive formula, appropriate amplification can be provided with little dependence on the cooperation of the child.

ADVISING THE PARENTS OF YOUNG CHILDREN WITH HEARING IMPAIRMENT

General Guidelines

It is important to maintain an understanding and an appreciation for the various educational options and communication modalities available to the families of children with hearing impairments.[22] Since otolaryngologists are 1 of the professionals responsible for the identification and the professionals responsible for the diagnosis of hearing impairments, they are often the first, if not only, resource that the parent has for information regarding these difficult choices. The debate over the best communication mode and training approach has raged since the fourteenth century. Unfortunately, no single communication modality is right for all children.[23] Rather, decisions must be made on an individual basis taking into account issues like the characteristics of the child, that is, age of diagnosis and accompanying learning disabilities, available community resources, and the commitment of the family to the child and the chosen communication modality. A basic review of the various communication options are presented, and the major methods are summarized in Table 3. There are, of course, a number of variations in these methodologies.

Oral Approaches. Two major forms of oral English instruction in practice today are the *auditory-verbal approach* and the *auditory-oral approach*. These 2 approaches are based on the idea that all children with hearing impairment can realistically attain receptive and expressive language competence regardless of the degree of hearing loss. The auditory-verbal philosophy places an emphasis on the child's residual hearing through the use of amplification with the goal of developing listening skills through natural communication. With this approach, the child is placed in mainstream education beginning in preschool years. The auditory-oral approach, on the other hand, emphasizes the development of amplified residual hearing and spoken language, utilizing speech-reading cues as a supplement to the auditory signal. With this approach, the child is usually enrolled in an oral education program until he/she can be appropriately mainstreamed.

Both these approaches have their pros and cons. The biggest benefit of each program is the possibility that the child will develop effective access to the hearing world. Geers and Moog revealed that children who attended oral education programs attained better speech production, speech perception, and overall spoken language skills than those students who attended total communication programs.[23] Additionally, evidence suggests that students educated with oral approaches attain literacy scores twice the national average for children with hearing impairments. Unfortunately, the success of these programs is heavily dependent on early identification of the hearing loss and early intervention with amplification, as

Table 3 Summary of Strengths and Limitations of Various Approaches for Auditory Habilitation of Children with Hearing Impairment and Deafness

Educational Option	Benefits	Limitations
Auditory-verbal	Greatest access to hearing world	Dependent on early identification and intervention
	Better speech production, speech perception, and spoken language	Isolation from the deaf community
	Higher literacy rates	
	Early mainstream education	
Auditory-oral	Greatest access to hearing world	Dependent on early identification and intervention
	Better speech production, speech perception, and spoken language	Isolation from the deaf community
	Higher literacy rates	
Cued speech	Reading and writing skills on par with hearing peers	Few educational programs available
		Few transliterators
	Access to hearing world	Isolation from the deaf community
Total communication	Allows the child access to all means of communication	Few programs put this into practice
		May overstimulate the child
Bilingual-bicultural	Designed to teach language and culture of the deaf and hearing communities	Little information available regarding its success
	Promotes increased literacy and academic skills	
Signing exact English	Uses English syntax and grammatical features	Denial of deaf culture
American sign language	Natural mode of communication for the deaf child	Syntax not conducive to the development of English language
	Allows membership in the deaf community and may improve self-confidence	

well as consistent, quality aural habilitation training. A major drawback to these approaches is isolation from the deaf community due to a lack of training in sign language. For a readable review of oral education for hearing impaired children, the reader is referred to a book entitled *Practical Guide to Quality Interaction with Children Who Have Hearing Loss* authored by Morag Clark, a woman who has successfully implemented such programs in developed and developing countries around the world.[24] Because of the rapid implementation of universal infant screening programs and the resulting early identification of profound hearing loss, most deaf children undergo cochlear implantation before 18 months of age, with many children undergoing cochlear implantation before 12 months of age. Consequently, most children with cochlear implants are entering mainstream educational environments by the first grade. Cochlear implantation is addressed in Chapter 32, "Cochlear and Brainstem Implantation" and Chapter 33, "Cochlear Implant Coding Strategies and Device Programming."

Manual Approaches. In stark contrast to the aforementioned oral educational strategies are the *manual approaches.* American Sign Language (ASL) is the common language of the deaf community. It is a vast lexicon of hand shapes and motions, or signs, with its own syntax and grammar. Additionally, ASL places a heavy emphasis on the facial expressions and body language of the signer. It is a unique language, having no simple translation to the oral English language. Proponents of ASL believe that it is an easier, more natural mode of communication for the child with hearing loss. Additionally, ASL facilitates membership into and acceptance by the deaf community, with the resultant capability for improving the child's self-esteem and confidence. A major limitation of ASL, however, is syntax that is not conducive to development of the English language, a feature that may hinder spoken language and literacy skill acquisition.

In an attempt to alleviate the difficulties in learning English language through manual communication, educators developed English-based sign systems. The most popular form of the English-based sign systems is Signing Exact English (SEE or SEE2). SEE2 utilizes much of the same vocabulary as ASL but adds grammatical features and follows English syntax. This system is primarily geared toward preschool and lower elementary school children to provide them access to English instruction during the language learning years. Opponents of this system believe that it is a denial of deaf culture, by inflicting the standards of the hearing world on the deaf child.

Bilingual–Bicultural Approach. Momentum has been growing for the development of *bilingual–bicultural education* for children who are deaf. This approach is designed to educate the child in the mores, customs, and practices, as well as the language, of the hearing world and the deaf culture. In these programs, the child is taught ASL as his or her first language, providing a base for which English is later taught. Early access to language is designed to promote increased literacy and academic skills. However, since these programs are relatively new, little information is available regarding their long-term success in developing effective communication in children with hearing impairment.

Combination Approaches. A combination of the oral and manual approaches is referred to as a combination approach. The most popular combination approach is *total communication.* Total communication involves the use of 1 or more modes of communication at any given time in the child's educational program, whether it be manual, oral, auditory only, or written. The design of this approach is to utilize whatever communication modality is most appropriate for the child at that stage of development or for that given situation, allowing the child access to all means of communication. Despite its promise, the total communication approach has serious limitations. Few programs actually put this philosophy into practice due to biases of the instructor and the difficulty of combining all of these methods at the same time. Additionally, the utilization of all of these modalities may overstimulate the child and, therefore, actually interfere with the development of communication.

A less popular combination approach is *cued speech.* Cued speech is a visual communication system that employs 8 hand shapes placed at 4 different locations near the mouth. These hand shapes are designed to supplement spoken language and speech reading cues, since many sounds may not be visible or distinguishable by watching the lips. The purpose of the cued speech approach is to allow the child to see and hear the English language as it is spoken. Limitations of the cued speech approach are that few programs provide this type of education and few "transliterators" (individuals that cue what an instructor says) are available. Additionally, persons who learn cued speech are unable to communicate with the deaf community, unless they also learn ASL.

A variety of educational methods are, therefore, available to the individual with hearing impairment. For the vast majority of families, the important decision about the educational approach to be used for their child is made during a period of emotional turmoil. Parents naturally view the identification of a hearing impairment as a loss of their dream of a normal child and may grieve accordingly. Unfortunately, a lack of understanding of the hearing loss, its implications, and remedial interventions can only exacerbate this emotional reaction. Although most parents want to receive this information, few professionals offer the supportive counseling and information needed for parents to make appropriate and timely decisions regarding educational strategies.[25]

The concept of critical period of development during which the CNS exhibits maximal plasticity is central to any discussion about the education of the individual with hearing impairment. It is reasonable to ask the question: should one attempt to maximize language development or focus on the use of residual hearing within a given time period? With the recent implementation of universal newborn hearing screening, it is logical to ask if early identification and management results in a significant improvement in the acquisition of communication skills. Yoshinaga-Itano and colleagues provided compelling evidence that children with hearing loss who are identified prior to 6 months of age and who receive immediate intervention have greater language development, better receptive and expressive vocabulary, and higher social–emotional aspects of communication development than infants who are identified later, regardless of the degree of hearing loss or mode of communication.[10,26] Additionally, no significant differences in language development were noted in terms of time of identification for those children identified after 6 months. This finding suggests that auditory and language stimulation within the first 6 months of life is critical for CNS development.

In summary, each of the currently available educational methods has proponents and opponents. Whenever appropriate, and with the support of the parents and other caregivers, otolaryngologists should encourage and facilitate maximal use of residual hearing and language development in an attempt to help hearing-impaired children reach their full communicative potential. It is essential that the otolaryngologist provide the parent with supportive, unbiased information regarding the benefits and limitations of the aforementioned modalities. No matter what the family's educational decision, early intervention services should be highly encouraged. Indeed, with early identification and intervention for hearing loss, that is, before the child is 6 months old, the development of effective communication is greatly enhanced independent of the educational approach.

GLOSSARY

ABLB Alternate binaural loudness balance. A traditional diagnostic auditory procedure for detecting "loudness recruitment" used in differentiating cochlear versus retrocochlear auditory dysfunction in unilateral hearing loss. The task is to balance the sensation of loudness for the better versus poorer hearing ear. Loudness recruitment is a cochlear auditory sign.

ABR (BAER) Auditory brainstem response. Electrical activity, evoked (stimulated) by brief-duration sounds that arises from the eighth cranial nerve and auditory portions of the brainstem. The ABR is usually recorded from the surface of the scalp and external ear with disc-type electrodes and processes with a fast signal averaging computer. ABR wave components are labeled with Roman numerals (eg, I, III, V) and described by the latency after the stimulus (in msec) and the amplitude from one peak to the following trough (in microvolts).

AC Air conduction. Audiometric signals presented via earphones to the ear canal.

Air-bone gap The difference in pure-tone thresholds for air- versus bone-conducted signals. With calibrated audiometers, the normal ear and the sensorineurally impaired ear show no air-bone gap, whereas conductive hearing losses are characterized by an air-bone gap.

ASL American Sign Language. A manual mode of communication that is commonly used by the deaf community.

Audiologist A hearing care professional who is educated and trained clinically to measure auditory system function and to provide nonmedical management to persons with auditory and communicative impairments. Minimal educational requirements for audiologists are a master's degree and certification and/or state licensure.

BC Bone conduction. Audiometric signals presented via an oscillator to the skull (eg, mastoid bone or forehead).

BCL Bekesy Comfortable Level. A Bekesy audiometry procedure conducted at a comfortable loudness level versus threshold level.

Bekesy audiometry An audiometric procedure performed with a Bekesy audiometer for differentiating cochlear versus retrocochlear auditory dysfunction. Bekesy audiometry is based on the comparison of responses to pulsed versus continuous tones varied across a wide frequency range. Four patterns of Bekesy responses were classified by Jerger.

BOA Behavioral observation audiometry. A pediatric behavioral audiometry procedure in which motor responses to sounds, for example, eye opening, head turning, are detected by a trained observer.

BTE Behind-the-ear hearing aid design.

CIC Completely-in-the-canal hearing aid design.

Configuration Term used to describe the shape or pattern of an audiogram, that is, how hearing loss varies as a function of the audiometric test frequency. There are 3 main configurations: rising (low-frequency loss), sloping (high-frequency loss), and flat.

CROS Contralateral routing of signals. A hearing aid configuration in which a microphone is located on the poorer ear and the sounds are transduced and delivered electrically to the normal or mildly impaired ear.

Crossover Sound stimulus presented to 1 ear (the test ear) travels around the head (by air conduction) or across the head (by bone conduction) to stimulate the other (nontest) ear. See interaural attenuation.

dB HL A decibel scale referenced to accepted standards for normal hearing (0 dB is average normal hearing for each audiometric test frequency).

dB nHL A decibel scale used in auditory brainstem response measurement referenced to average behavioral threshold for the click stimulus of a small group of normal hearing subjects.

dB SL Sound intensity is described in reference to an individual patient's behavioral threshold for an audiometric frequency or some other measure of hearing threshold, for example, the speech reception threshold.

dB SPL A decibel scale referenced to a physical standard for intensity (eg, 0.0002 dynes/cm^2).

Dichotic Simultaneous presentation of a different sound to each ear.

DPOAE Distortion product otoacoustic emission.

DPgram (DPOAEgram) A graph of distortion product otoacoustic emission amplitude in the ear canal (in dB SPL) as a function of the frequencies of the stimulus tones (in Hz).

ECochG Electrocochleography. Evoked responses originating from the cochlea (the summating potential, or SP, and the cochlear microphonic, or CM) and the eighth cranial nerve (the action potential or AP).

ENG Electronystagmography. A test of vestibular function in which nystagmus is recorded with electrodes placed near the eyes during stimulation of the vestibular system.

ENoG Electroneuronography. Myogenic activity recorded from the facial muscles, usually in the nasolabial fold, in response to electrical stimulation of the facial nerve as it exits the stylomastoid foramen.

FM system A device in which the acoustic information received by a remote microphone is transmitted via FM radio waves to a receiver utilized by the listener.

ITC In-the-canal hearing aid design.

ITE In-the-ear hearing aid design.

Interaural attenuation Insulation to the crossover of sound (acoustic or mechanical energy) from 1 ear to the other provided by the head. Interaural attenuation varies depending on whether the signal is presented by air conduction (interaural attenuation >40 dB) or bone conduction (interaural attenuation <10 dB). Insert earphones offer maximum interaural attenuation.

Malingering Feigning or exaggerating a hearing impairment. Also referred to as functional or nonorganic hearing loss.

Masking (masker) A controlled background noise presented usually to the nontest ear in an audiometric procedure to prevent a response from the nontest ear (due to crossover when interaural attenuation is exceeded).

Masking dilemma A problem encountered in audiometric assessment of patients with severe conductive hearing loss. The level of masking noise necessary to overcome the conductive component and adequately mask the nontest ear exceeds interaural attenuation levels. The masking noise may then cross over to the test ear, and mask the signal (eg, pure tone or speech). In the masking dilemma, enough masking is too much masking. The masking dilemma can be reduced by the use of insert earphones. The SAL test is also helpful for measuring ear-specific bone-conduction hearing thresholds in patients presenting the masking dilemma.

MCL Most comfortable level. The intensity level of a sound that is perceived as comfortable.

MLD Masking level difference. An audiometric procedure which compares a threshold response with masking noise presented in-phase versus out-of-phase with a pure-tone or speech signal. Release from masking is a normal phenomenon reflecting auditory brainstem integrity.

OAE Otoacoustic emissions. Sounds generated by energy produced by the outer hair cells in the cochlea and detected with a microphone placed within the external ear canal.

PB Phonetically balanced. Word lists developed in the late 1940s which contains all the phonetic elements of general American English speech that occurs with the approximate frequency of their occurrence in conversational speech.

PI Performance-intensity. A measure of speech recognition or understanding as a function of the intensity level of the speech signal. See rollover.

PTA Pure-tone average. The arithmetic average of hearing threshold levels for 500, 1,000, and 2,000 Hz, or the speech frequency region of the audiogram. The PTA should agree within ±7 dB of the speech reception threshold (SRT).

RECD Real-ear to coupler difference. This is the decibel difference between the level of sound in the ear canal versus the level that is measured in the 2 cm^3 coupler.

Rollover A decrease in speech recognition performance (in percent correct) at high signal intensity levels versus lower levels. Rollover is an audiometric sign of retrocochlear auditory dysfunction.

SAL Sensory acuity level. An audiometric procedure developed by James Jerger (1970) for assessing bone-conduction hearing in patients with serious conductive hearing loss. Air-conduction thresholds are determined without masking and then with masking presented by bone conduction to the forehead. The size of the masked shift in hearing thresholds corresponds to the degree of conductive hearing loss component.

SAT (SDT) Speech awareness threshold (speech detection threshold). The lowest intensity level at which a person can detect the presence of a speech signal. The SAT approximates the best hearing level in the 250 to 8,000 Hz audiometric frequency region.

SEE2 Signing Exact English. A manual form of communication that utilizes most of the same vocabulary as ASL but adds grammatical features and follows English syntax.

SSI Synthetic sentence identification. A measure of central auditory function which involves identification of syntactically incomplete sentences (a closed set of 10 sentences) presented simultaneously with a competing message (an ongoing story about Davy Crockett).

SSW Staggered spondaic word test. A measure of central auditory function developed by Katz that utilizes spondee words presented dichotically.

SISI Short increment sensitivity index. A clinical procedure developed by Jerger for assessing the ability to detect a 1 dB increase in intensity. High SISI score is consistent with cochlear auditory dysfunction.

S/N Signal-to-noise. The signal-to-noise ratio is the difference between the intensity level of a sound or electrical event and background acoustic or electrophysiologic energy.

SRT   Speech reception threshold. The lowest intensity level at which a person can accurately identify a speech signal (eg, two syllable spondee words). See PTA.

SSPL   Saturation sound pressure level. A measure of the maximum power output (MPO) of the hearing aid.

Telecoil   An option on a hearing aid that enables it to receive the electromagnetic signals directly from the telephone. This option may be utilized to reduce the presence of feedback while the wearer is using the telephone.

TEOAEs   Transient evoked otoacoustic emissions. OAE elicited by brief (click or tone burst) stimuli.

Tone decay test   A clinical measure of auditory adaption in which a tone is presented continuously to a hearing-impaired ear until it becomes inaudible. There are numerous versions of tone decay tests. Excessive tone decay is a sign of retrocochlear auditory dysfunction.

TROCA   Tangible reinforcement operant conditioning audiometry. A pediatric behavioral audiometry technique that reinforces a response to auditory signals with food. TROCA is used mainly with mentally retarded or developmentally delayed children.

UCL/LDL   Uncomfortable level or loudness discomfort level. The intensity level of a sound that is perceived as too loud.

VRA   Visual reinforcement audiometry. A pediatric behavioral audiometry procedure that reinforces localization responses to acoustic signals with a visual event (eg, an animal playing).

REFERENCES

1. Hall JW, III, Mueller HG, III. Audiologists' Desk Reference, Volume I: Diagnostic Audiology Principles, Procedures & Protocols. San Diego, CA: Singular Publishing Group; 1997. p. 113–68.
2. Carhart R, Jerger JF. Preferred method for clinical determination of pure-tone thresholds. J Speech Hear Dis 1959;24:330–45.
3. Mueller HG, III, Hall JW, III. Audiologists' Desk Reference Volume II. Amplifiication, Management, and Rehabilitation. San Diego, CA: Singular Publishing Group; 1998.
4. Jerger J, Musiek F. Report of the consensus conference on the diagnosis of auditory processing disorders in school-aged children. J Am Acad Audiol 2000;11:467–74.
5. Jerger JF. Clinical experience with impedance audiometry. Arch Otorhinol 1970;92:11–24.
6. Hall JW, III. New Handbook of Auditory Evoked Responses. Boston, MA: Allyn & Bacon; 2007.
7. Pou AM, Hirsch BE, Durrant JD, et al. The efficacy of tympanic electrocochleography in the diagnosis of endolymphatic hydrops. Am J Otol 1996;17:607–11.
8. Hall JW, III. Handbook of Otoacoustic Emissions. San Diego, CA: Singular Publishing Group; 2000.
9. Rapin I, Gravel J. "Auditory neuropathy": Physiological and pathologic evidence calls for more diagnostic specificity. Int J Ped Otorhinol 2003;67:707–28.
10. Yoshinaga-Itano C, Sedley AL, Coulter DK, Mehl AL. Language of early- and later-identified children with hearing loss. Pediatrics 1998;102:1161–71.
11. Hall JW, III. Screening for and assessment of infant hearing impairment. J Perinatol 2000;20:S113–21.
12. Joint Committee on Infant Hearing. Year 2000 position statement: Principles and guidelines for early hearing detection and intervention. Am J Audiol 2000;9:9–29.
13. Hall JW, III, Smith SD, Popelka GR. Newborn hearing screening with combined otoacoustic emissions and auditory brainstem responses. J Am Acad Audiol 2004;15:414–25.
14. Hall JW, III. Central auditory processing disorder (CAPD) in Y2K. Hear J 1999;52:35–42.
15. Report of the Task Force on (Central) Auditory Processing Disorders (APD). American Speech Language and Hearing Association. (www.asha.org), April 2005.
16. Valente M, Fabry DA, Potts LG. Recognition of speech in noise with hearing aids using dual microphones. J Am Acad Audiol 1995;6:440–9.
17. Crandell CC. Hearing aids: Their effects on functional health status. Hear J 1998;51:2–6.
18. ASHA ad hoc committee on hearing aid selection and fitting. Guidelines for hearing aid fitting for adults. ASHA 1997;40:123–30.
19. Mueller G, Hawkins D, Northern J. Probe Microphone Measurements: Hearing Aid Selection and Assessment. San Diego, CA: Singular Publishing Group; 1992. p. 251–68.
20. Hurley R. Onset of auditory deprivation. J Am Acad Audiol 1999;10:529–34.
21. Seewald R. The desired sensation level (DSL) method for hearing aid fitting in infants and children. Phonak Focus 1995;20:3–19.
22. Reamy CE, Brackett D. Communication methodologies: options for families. Otolaryngol Clin N Am 1999;32:1103–16.
23. Geers A, Moog J. Speech perception and production skills of students with impaired hearing from oral and total communication education settings. J Speech Hear Res 1992;35:1384–93.
24. Clark M. A practical guide to quality interaction with children who have hearing loss. San Diego: Plural Publishing; 2007, in press.
25. Kricos P. The counseling process: Children and parents. In: Alpiner J, McCarthy P, editors. Rehabilitative Audiology: Children and Adults. Baltimore: Williams and Wilkins; 1993. p. 211–33.
26. Yoshinaga-Itano C. Benefits of early intervention for children with hearing loss. Otolaryngol Clin N Am 1999;32:1089–102.

10

Evaluation of the Vestibular System

Joel A. Goebel, MD
Judith A. White, MD, PhD
Katherine D. Heidenreich, MD

The human vestibular system is responsible for sensing angular head acceleration and maintaining objects in visual focus during rapid impulsive head motion and detecting gravity and impulsive linear acceleration for accurate control of balance. It can be subdivided into peripheral and central components.[1] The peripheral component consists of the vestibular end organs (semicircular canals, utricle, and saccule) and the superior and inferior divisions of the vestibular nerve. The central component refers to the vestibular nuclei, their ascending and descending pathways, and higher centers in the brainstem and cerebellum which integrate signals that ultimately impart our sense of spatial orientation.

Derangements in the vestibular system can manifest unusual sensations that can be difficult to describe clearly, and, therefore, diagnose accurately. As a result, the catchall phrase "dizziness" has been used to describe symptomatology in patients who have true disorders of the vestibular system but may also include those whose underlying pathology is of an entirely different organ system. Understanding how to evaluate the integrity of the vestibular system and its relationship to visual and proprioceptive inputs is important because dizziness is the ninth most common complaint patients report to their primary care physicians, representing an enormous investment in healthcare dollars and medical personnel time.[2] A systematic approach to the patient with dizziness will be presented which includes the history, physical examination, and laboratory testing that point to an underlying disorder of the peripheral component of the vestibular system will be reviewed in this chapter.

OBTAINING THE HISTORY

A comprehensive history is the single most valuable part of the evaluation of the patient with dizziness. This is best achieved by a written questionnaire filled out well in advance of the patient visit and a careful oral follow-up to their responses during the examination. Initially, patients are asked to describe their symptom without using the word "dizzy" and then the questioning rapidly focuses in on key symptoms of vestibular dysfunction. Vague complaints like "dizziness" warrant further clarification to determine if the patient really means vertigo, lightheadedness, specific visual disturbances, imbalance, feelings of dissociation, or poor concentration. Investing the time to distinguish between these symptoms often helps to narrow the differential diagnosis considerably.

Vertigo is a term often used to describe dizziness, but there is a lack of consensus—even among otologists—regarding its precise meaning.[3] In general, vertigo should be reserved to describe the false illusion of rotational motion of the environment. Therefore, ask the patient specifically, "Do things spin in front of your eyes when you are dizzy?" Although vertigo strongly points to vestibular dysfunction, it is by no means pathognomonic and has been reported to occur in the setting of migraine, postural orthostatic hypotension, and stroke.[4-6]

Some patients with chronic or uncompensated vestibular disease do not experience the spinning characteristic of vertigo but instead describe a sensation of visual blurring of their environment with rapid head movements or during ambulation. This symptom is consistent with oscillopsia and should raise concern for bilateral peripheral vestibular hypofunction or poorly compensated unilateral injury.

Eliciting a history of fainting, "blacking out," or syncope suggests an underlying cardiac cause and practically excludes vestibular disorders which never manifest loss of consciousness. Reports of imbalance, difficulty ambulating, stumbling, or frank ataxia should raise concern for neurological disorders, particularly degenerative conditions of the cerebellum. Feelings of dissociation, inattention, lightheadedness, or a generalized sense of ill-being are nonspecific and neither implicate nor exclude an underlying vestibular component.

Once the clinician has elicited as specific a description of the dizziness as possible, attention should be directed toward determining the true duration and frequency of the symptom. Is the symptom constant or episodic? If the latter is the case, how long is each episode? In general, patients tend to overestimate the duration of vertigo and may initially report vertigo that lasted for hours but, when pressed, really mean seconds followed by hours of nausea or mild disequilibrium. Being able to discern the true length of the symptom has significant diagnostic implications. For example, the vertigo of benign paroxysmal positional vertigo (BPPV) lasts seconds, compared to minutes to 2 hours in Menière disease, and >12 hours in vestibular neuritis. For additional information regarding these disorders see Chapter 28, "Menière Disease, Vestibular Neuritis, Benign Paroxysmal Positional Vertigo, Superior Semicircular Canal Dehiscence, and Vestibular Migraine."

An understanding of the events surrounding the onset of symptoms can be valuable by helping to identify activities that are known risk factors or triggers for the development of certain vestibular disorders. First, determine what the patient was doing immediately prior to the onset of symptoms by asking, "What exactly were you doing when the first episode occurred?" for example, rolling over in bed versus sitting quietly in a chair. Next, inquire about unusual antecedent events that may have occurred in hours to days leading up to onset of symptoms. Head trauma would predispose a patient to develop BPPV or postconcussive vestibulopathy. Travel by airplane with complaints of "ear popping" raise concern for perilymphatic fistula from inner ear barotrauma. An uneventful boat cruise followed by persistent rocking sensation on land suggests mal de debarquement syndrome. Recent recreational diving activity can lead to alternobaric vertigo, perilymphatic fistula, or inner ear decompression sickness.

Associated symptoms should be noted next. It is important to document any auditory symptoms such as hearing change or loss, tinnitus, or aural fullness. Focal neurologic symptoms such as visual loss, headache, numbness, and weakness should be inquired about specifically. Provoking factors such as position change, pressure changes, for example, sneezing or lifting, or loud noises should be addressed as well. It is safe to say that documented prolonged loss of consciousness is never attributable to vestibular dysfunction although a brief vasovagal episode is possible. A summary of symptoms associated with peripheral vestibular disease is included in Table 1.

A thorough review of the patient's past medical and surgical history is important because it establishes risk factors and impacts on the likelihood of some diagnoses. The acute onset of prolonged, debilitating vertigo in a patient with

Table 1 Historical Aspects of Dizziness

	Peripheral Vestibular Disease	Central Nervous System Disease	Orthostasis	Psychogenic
Sensation	Vertigo—unilateral disease Oscillopsia—bilateral disease Trouble walking in dark—bilateral disease	Vertigo Imbalance Incoordination	Lightheadedness	Lightheadedness Vertigo "in my head"
Time course	Seconds—benign paroxysmal positional vertigo Minutes—Ménière disease Hours—vestibular neuritis	Minutes—vertebrobasilar insufficiency Variable—migraine Constant—tumor, multiple sclerosis	Seconds	Constant
Position related	Yes—benign paroxysmal positional vertigo	Variable	Yes—arising	No
Motion related	Yes	Variable	No	Yes
Nausea/vomiting	Yes	Variable	No	Variable
Hearing loss/tinnitus	Yes—Ménière disease	Rare	No	No
Sound sensitive	Yes—Ménière disease, superior semicircular canal dehisence	Yes—migraine	No	No
Light sensitive	No	Yes—Migraine	No	No
Alteration of consciousness	No	Possible	Possible	No

a history of cardiac arrhythmias, diabetes, poorly controlled hypertension, or known coagulopathy should heighten concern for acute cerebrovascular pathology, like cerebellar infarction, a true vestibular emergency. An otologic source of the dizziness is more likely in a patient with a history of chronic otitis media, prior ear surgery, or exposure to vestibulotoxic medications like aminoglycosides. A history of oncologic disease treated with chemotherapy may lead to imbalance from peripheral neuropathy or to bilateral peripheral hypofunction from exposure to otovestibulotoxic agents like cisplatinum.

Inquiry for history of migraine should be made in any patient presenting for evaluation of recurrent dizziness as it is increasingly recognized as a cause of episodic vestibular symptoms. One study found unexplained episodic dizziness in approximately 25% of patients meeting defined criteria for migraine.[7] Because the term "migraine" is often used indiscriminately to refer to any severe headache, familiarity with migraine classification criteria is helpful in making the diagnosis of migraine-associated dizziness (MAD); and these criteria are outlined in Table 2. Vestibular symptoms in MAD may precede headache, occur variably (most commonly), or be totally unrelated to headache.[8] The duration of vestibular symptoms ranges broadly from minutes to days, and any nystagmus observed can have peripheral, central, or mixed features. Photophobia during the attack is highly suggestive of MAD with or without cephalgia. Additional criteria for MAD have been proposed by Neuhauser and colleagues and are listed in Table 3.[9]

OFFICE EXAMINATION OF THE PATIENT WITH DIZZINESS

Physical examination of the patient with dizziness begins with a general assessment of overall health, followed by careful review of vital signs obtained by the nurse. Blood pressure and pulse should be taken with the patient in a sitting, lying, and then standing position to elicit postural cardiovascular instability. Orthostatic hypotension is defined as either a drop in systolic blood pressure of

20 mm Hg or a decline in diastolic blood pressure of 10 mm Hg.[10] However, failure to elicit postural orthostatic changes does not rule out a neurocardiogenic cause of dizziness, as this screening test is not always reproducible and can miss delayed forms of orthostatic intolerance picked up by more sensitive methods like tilt table testing.[11,12]

Table 2 International Classification of Headache Disorders II (ICHD-II): Criteria for Migraine without Aura (1.1) 2004[13]

At least 5 attacks fulfilling criteria B–D
A. Headache attacks lasting 4 to 72 h (untreated or unsuccessfully treated)
B. Headache has at least 2 of the following characteristics:
  1. Unilateral location
  2. Pulsating quality
  3. Moderate or intense intensity
  4. Aggravation by or causing avoidance of routine physical activity (eg, walking or climbing stairs)
C. During headache at least 1 of the following:
  1. Nausea and/or vomiting
  2. Photophobia and phonophobia
D. Not attributed to another disorder

ICHD-II (2004) criteria for basilar-type migraine (1.2.6)
A. At least 2 attacks fulfilling criteria B–D
B. Aura consisting of at least 2 of the following fully reversible symptoms, but no motor weakness:
  1. Dysarthria (slurred speech)
  2. Vertigo (dizziness)
  3. Tinnitus (illusory noise)
  4. Hypacusia (reduced hearing)
  5. Diplopia (double vision)
  6. Simultaneous bilateral visual aura in both temporal and nasal fields
  7. Ataxia (imbalance)
  8. Decreased level of consciousness
  9. Simultaneous bilateral paresthesias
C. At least 1 of the following:
  1. At least 1 aura symptom develops gradually over 5 or more min and/or different aura symptoms occur in succession for 5 or more min
  2. Each aura symptom lasts for at least 5 min but not greater than 60 min
D. Headache fulfilling criteria for ICHD-II migraine without aura begins during the aura or follows aura within 60 min
E. Not attributed to another disorder

A careful otologic examination should be performed next. Tuning fork testing at 512 Hz is a rapid and simple assessment of the conductive and sensorineural components of hearing utilizing the Weber and Rinne tests. Careful visualization of the tympanic membrane with pneumatic otoscopy is undertaken to exclude active infections, chronic effusion, cholesteatoma, or structural disease. A positive fistula test occurs when nystagmus and/or vertigo are induced by applying positive and negative pressure to the external auditory canal and can be seen in otosyphilis, perilymphatic fistula, or superior semicircular canal dehiscence.

Cranial nerves II–XII are evaluated with attention to gross visual acuity, ocular motion in the 9 cardinal directions of gaze (neutral, up, down, left, right, up and left, down and left, up and right, down and right), ocular alignment, facial sensation to light touch, facial movement, palate elevation, shoulder shrug and head turn, and tongue motion. At this point, the physician performs a specialized oculomotor and vestibulo-ocular examination and evaluation of posture and gait. It is important that this examination be systematic and progress in a logical fashion from the seated to lying to standing position as each aspect of eye movement, coordination, and gait is assessed (Table 4).

Spontaneous Nystagmus

To begin the examination, spontaneous nystagmus is examined in the seated patient in neutral

Table 3 Neuhauser Criteria for Migrainous Vertigo

1. Recurrent episodic vestibular symptoms (attacks)
2. Migraine headache meeting International Headache Society (HIS) 1988 criteria
3. At least 1 of the following migrainous symptoms during at least 2 of these attacks:
  • Migraine-type headache
  • Visual or other auras
  • Photophobia
  • Phonophobia
4. Other causes ruled out by appropriate investigations

Table 4 The Comprehensive Examination of the Patient with Dizziness

	Peripheral Vestibular Disease	Central Nervous System/Peripheral Nervous System Disease	Orthostasis	Psychogenic
Spontaneous nystagmus	Horizontal/rotary Direction fixed Suppressed with fixation	Horizontal or vertical Direction changing Enhanced with fixation	None	None
Gaze nystagmus	Horizontal/rotary Direction fixed Enhanced in direction of fast phase	Horizontal or vertical Direction changing	None	None
Smooth pursuit	Normal for age	Saccadic pursuit	Normal for age	Normal for age
Saccades	Normal for age Inaccurate Slow Delayed	Disconjugate—multiple sclerosis Cerebellar Brainstem Variable	Normal for age	Normal for age
Fixation suppression of per-rotary nystagmus	Normal	Poor—flocculus	Normal	Normal
Head impulse test	Refixation saccade to side of lesion	Normal	Normal	Normal
Postheadshake nystagmus	Horizontal/rotary Toward intact side-common Toward lesioned side—occasional	Vertical with horizontal headshake	Normal	Normal
Dynamic visual acuity	>3-line reduction from static acuity with headshake	Variable	<3-line reduction	<3-line reduction
Hyperventilation	Nystagmus—rare	Lightheaded	Lightheaded	Very lightheaded
Pneumatic otoscopy/sound	Elevation/intorsion ipsilateral eye— superior semicircular canal dehiscence	None	None	None
Positional testing Positioning testing	Horizontal nystagmus—common Geotropic torsional upbeat nystagmus—posterior canal Benign paroxysmal positional nystagmus Horizontal nystagmus—lateral canal BPPN	Horizontal or vertical nystagmus None	None None	None None
Limb coordination	Normal for age	Incoordination	Normal for age	Normal for age
Limb vibrotactile/proprioceptive sensation	Normal for age	Reduced	Normal for age	Normal for age
Romberg-firm surface	Normal—eyes open Normal or mildly reduced—eyes closed	Markedly reduced Eyes closed > eyes open	Normal for age	Normal for age
Tandem Romberg	Reduced	Markedly reduced	Variable	Variable
3″ in foam eyes closed	Reduced	Reduced	Normal	Normal
Gait observation	Normal or slight deviation	Marked ataxia Poor initiation	Normal for age	Inconsistent

gaze both with and without visual fixation. Fixation can be removed with use of Frenzel lenses in either the optical or infrared versions. In most cases, there are no spontaneous eye movements, and gaze is stable. In a small percentage of individuals, congenital nystagmus is present, horizontal in direction, pendular or jerk in waveform, and diminishes with vergence or without fixation. Nystagmus due to a peripheral vestibular abnormality is horizontal rotary, direction-fixed, and decreases with visual fixation, a phenomenon known as fixation suppression. In most instances, the nystagmus beats with the fast phase toward the stronger on nonpathologic ear and increases in intensity with gaze in the direction of the fast phase (Alexander's law). On the other hand, spontaneous nystagmus of central origin is purely horizontal or vertical, enhances with fixation and, in cases of periodic alternating nystagmus, changes direction without change in gaze. Failure of fixation suppression occurs when nystagmus does not decrease or becomes worse with fixation and is a strong predictor of central pathology within the flocculus of the cerebellum. This can be confirmed by rotating the patient in an examination chair while he or she views his or her outstretched thumb and observing for any nystagmus not suppressed by a head-fixed target.

Gaze Testing

After evaluation for spontaneous nystagmus is performed, the patient is asked to fixate on the examiner's finger held in an eccentric gaze position. In normal subjects, there is no gaze-evoked eye movement. Nystagmus that is provoked on eccentric gaze at 20° from center should be noted for its intensity, direction, and persistence. Unidirectional nystagmus that increases while gazing in the direction of the fast phase (Alexander's law) implies a peripheral cause. In contrast, gaze-evoked nystagmus which beats in the direction of gaze is indicative of floccular lesions or central effects of sedative and anticonvulsive medications.

Smooth Pursuit Testing

Ocular motility can be influenced by preexisting strabismus, which should be noted prior to onset of this portion of the examination. The value of the oculomotor examination lies in its ability to detect central oculomotor abnormalities, which will then affect the sensitivity and specificity of the vestibular examination that will follow. The ability to follow accurately a slowly moving target requires foveal vision and intact occipital cortices and oculomotor brainstem nuclei.

To assess smooth pursuit, the examiner slowly moves a finger or pen 20 to 40°/s in both the lateral and vertical planes at a comfortable distance in front of the patient using best corrected vision, for example, glasses or contact lenses. Finger movement that is too rapid will elicit rapid catch-up saccades and is the most frequent error in performing this examination. Restrict testing to the central 30° of vision (15° to the left and 15° to the right or up and down) to avoid provoking end-gaze physiologic nystagmus. Normal pursuit eye movements are smooth and accurately track the target. Saccadic breakup of pursuit is significant and can suggest visual problems, especially in the elderly, attentional problems or central pathology of the pursuit pathways in the brainstem, occipital cortex, or cerebellum.

Saccade Testing

The capability to fixate conjugately on a new visual target is generated by the saccadic system in the frontal motor cortex and brainstem. Saccades are tested in both vertical and horizontal planes and are characterized by their accuracy, velocity, and latency. The patient is instructed to look rapidly back and forth between two fingers presented 15 to 20° lateral or vertical to neutral eye position. Several repetitions are optimal in each direction (right, left, up, and down). Accurate saccades will demonstrate conjugate movements of the eyes without target overshoot or undershoot. Cerebellar disease may cause saccadic overshoots or undershoots. If the adducting eye moves slowly while the abducting eye overshoots or exhibits nystagmus, an internuclear ophthalmoplegia (INO) is present, and further evaluation for multiple sclerosis or other central brainstem pathology should be undertaken.

Vestibulo-Ocular Reflex Testing

Office testing of the vestibulo-ocular reflex (VOR) is performed using the head thrust, headshake, and dynamic visual acuity tests. The VOR is a 3-neuron arc that stabilizes vision during high velocity impulsive head movements. Office assessment of VOR by rotating the examination chair while having the patient wear Frenzel lenses to eliminate fixation can provide a rough estimate of vestibular function but lacks a standardized stimulus. The most widely used bedside test of the VOR is the head thrust test, which was developed by Halmagyi and Curthoys to enable evaluation of the high-frequency VOR for each ear individually.[14] The patient is placed facing the examiner with the head tilted down about 30° to place the lateral semicircular canals in earth horizontal position. The examiner grasps the patient's head in both hands and asks the patient to keep their gaze on the examiner's nose. The head is slowly rotated back and forth laterally until an unexpected high velocity, low amplitude thrust is made to bring the head from lateral to midline. The normal patient keeps the eyes on the examiner's nose without difficulty. The patient with a significantly weak peripheral vestibular system cannot stabilize vision in this situation, and the eyes slide past the target and are redirected to the examiners nose with a compensatory saccade immediately after the thrust. This abnormality is seen when the thrust is in the direction of the weak ear in unilateral lesions and in both directions with bilateral deficits (Figure 1).

Headshake testing is performed by rotating the patient's head at 2 Hz in the horizontal or vertical plane for 20 to 30 seconds using Frenzel lenses and examining the eyes for postheadshake nystagmus. If present, postheadshake nystagmus beats in the plane of head rotation toward the stronger ear. However, in Ménière's disease and other acute vestibular losses, the nystagmus may beat toward the affected or unaffected ear depending on the state of compensation. Vertical nystagmus after horizontal headshaking is indicative of central brainstem pathology.

Dynamic visual acuity (DVA) is assessed by comparing the change in visual acuity induced with a high velocity, low amplitude headshake. Under normal circumstances, the VOR stabilizes the image on the fovea well enough to preserve acuity to within 3 lines of static acuity as measured on a standard Snellen eye chart with best-corrected vision. In cases of bilateral vestibular loss, retinal slip occurs and dynamic acuity

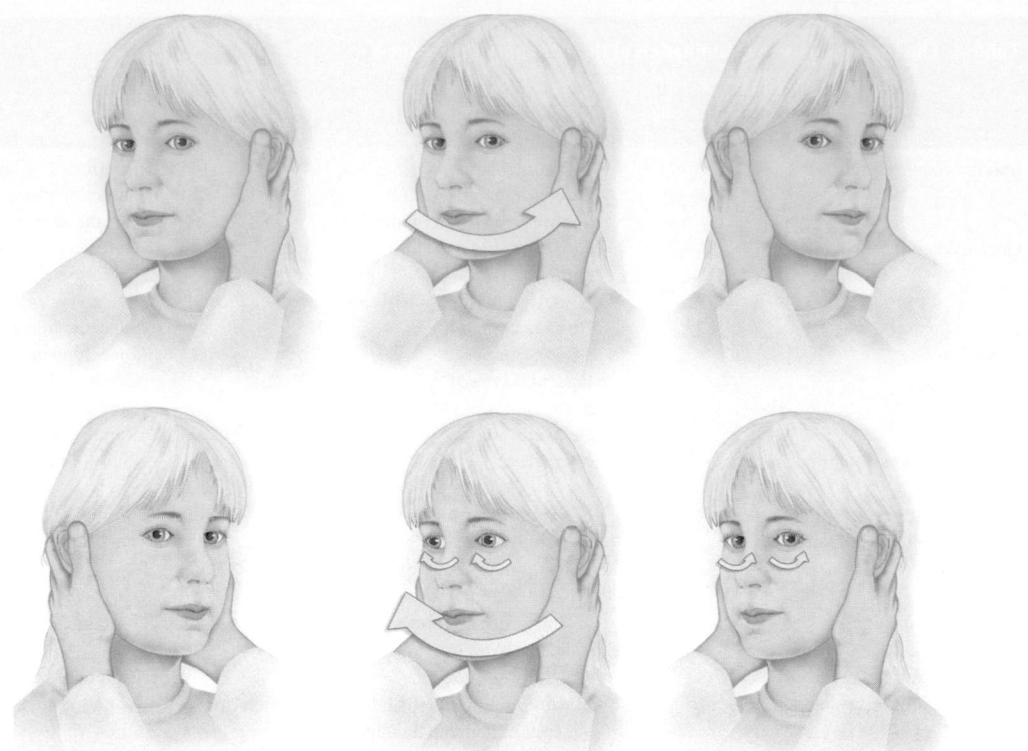

Figure 1 Halmagyi-Curthoys head thrust test. Note normal gaze stability with head thrust left and impaired gaze stability with head thrust right, requiring a compensatory refixation saccade to bring gaze back to center after head thrust. (Reprinted with permission. Copyright © 2004. The Cleveland Clinic Foundation. All rights reserved.)

is severely impaired. However, poor DVA scores may also be seen in cases of unilateral loss with poor central compensation.

Positional and Positioning (Dix-Hallpike) Testing

After the examiner has finished the oculomotor and VOR tests, the patient is placed in a variety of recumbent positions and any resultant nystagmus is noted. The most common positioning test is the Dix-Hallpike test which is used to identify posterior canal benign paroxysmal positional nystagmus (BPPN). During this maneuver, the patient's head is turned 45° to one side while he or she is seated. The patient is then moved quickly to a supine position with the neck slightly extended and the head remaining turned. When the undermost ear is affected, a geotropic upbeat nystagmus is seen after a variable latency period. The patient is then brought back up to a sitting position, and the nystagmus is often noted to reverse direction. The maneuver is then performed on the other side. The characteristic nystagmus occurs after a delay of several seconds, declines after 10 to 30 seconds, and diminishes with repeated positional testing in the same sitting (Figure 2).

For static positional testing, the patient is initially placed in a supine position with eyes open and Frenzel lenses in place, and any nystagmus is noted for direction and intensity. The head is rotated to the right lateral position for 10 seconds, brought back to midline for 10 seconds, and rotated to the left lateral position for 10 seconds before being returned to midline. The patient then returns to sitting. Although positional nystagmus had previously been considered nonlocalizing, this maneuver detects horizontal nystagmus that

may be related to lateral canal benign paroxysmal positional vertigo. Lateral canal BPPV affects about 15% of patients with BPPV and may not be detected in Dix-Hallpike positioning.[15] The paroxysmal positional nystagmus in lateral canal BPPV usually has less latency and a longer duration than that typically seen in posterior canal BPPV. It changes direction depending on the portion of the canal involved and the direction of the head. Geotropic (beating toward the ground, ie, leftward in left ear down and rightward in right ear down positions) nystagmus suggests canalithiasis in the distal lateral canal, with the strongest nystagmus in the affected ear down position (Figure 3). Apogeotropic nystagmus beats toward the uppermost ear in lateral supine position and suggests material proximal to or adherent to the cupula (Figure 4).

Posture and Gait Testing

The neurotologic office examination is completed with assessment of postural stability, gait, and cerebellar function. Finger-to-nose and heel-to-shin testing and rapid alternating movements are examined as indicated. In appropriate patients (older patients, diabetics, and those complaining of leg numbness or clumsiness), vibration sense is tested at the ankle and compared to the wrist. A Rydel-Seiffer graduated or other 128 Hz tuning fork may be used. Decreased lower extremity vibration sense suggests neurologic processes, such as peripheral neuropathy. Proprioception is assessed with toes up or toes down positioning. A survey of reflexes and motor strength may be included as needed if deficits are suspected.

Postural control is assessed by observing static stance and dynamic gait. The Romberg

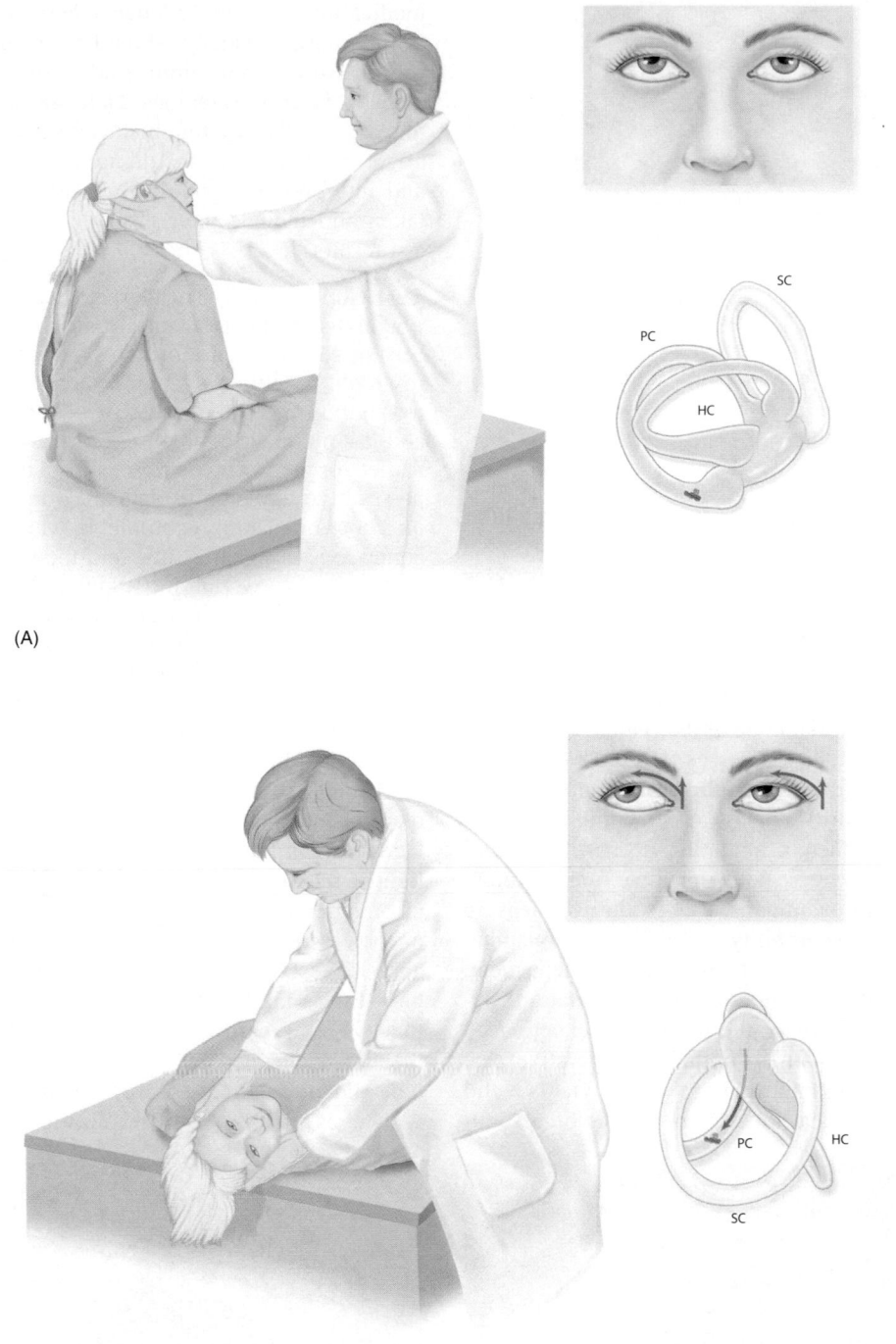

(A)

(B)

Figure 2 (A) Initial position for a right Dix-Hallpike maneuver. The head is turned 45° to the right prior to moving the patient to the lying position. No nystagmus is seen (see insert). (B) Final right Dix-Hallpike position. If posterior canalithiasis is present, an upward geotropic nystagmus is noted. (Reprinted with permission. Copyright © 2004. The Cleveland Clinic Foundation. All rights reserved.)

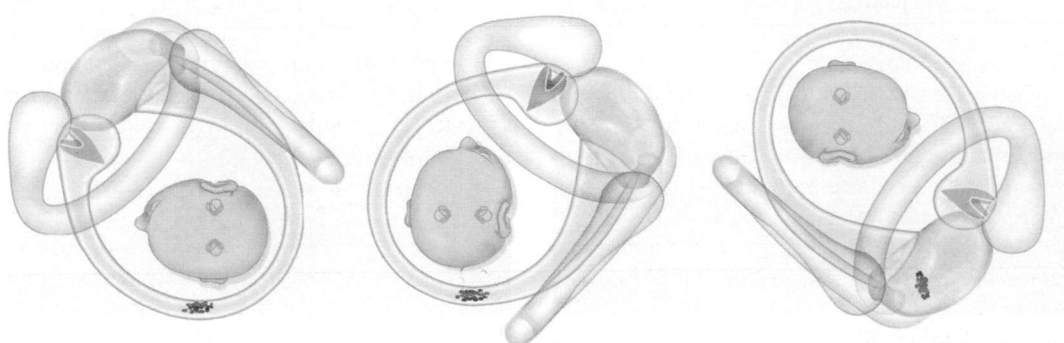

Figure 3 Geotropic lateral semicircular canal benign paroxysmal positional vertigo. (Reprinted with permission. Copyright © 2004. The Cleveland Clinic Foundation. All rights reserved.)

test is performed with the patient standing feet together and eyes open and closed and primarily assesses proprioceptive input. However, a tandem Romberg stance or Romberg stance on a 4" compliant foam pad distorts somatosensation and with eyes closed places emphasis on vestibulospinal inputs for balance (Figure 5). Patients with poorly compensated vestibular loss show increased sway on foam eyes closed whereas bilateral loss patients freely fall into the examiner's outstretched arms. Finally, observation of gait is done to observe any signs of ataxia, extrapyramidal signs, musculoskeletal dysfunction, or exaggeration. Since there is no true "vestibular" gait, the purpose of this part of the examination is to look for confounding factors other than vestibular loss. In some instances, however, patients may deviate toward the side of a vestibular lesion during a marching stance test known as the Fukuta or Unterberger test.

DIAGNOSTIC TESTING

Comprehensive Audiometry

An audiogram remains one of the most helpful tests in the clinical evaluation of the patient with dizziness. It is important that a comprehensive test is performed which includes air and bone conduction thresholds with adequate masking, word recognition testing at appropriate presentation levels, tympanometry, and acoustic reflex testing including reflex decay. Asymmetric sensorineural hearing loss (>10 dB at two or more frequencies or >15 dB at any one frequency), word recognition scores (>10% difference between ears), absent reflexes with normal tympanometry and adequate air and bone thresholds and reflex decay are indications to consider a retrocochlear evaluation. Low-frequency sensorineural hearing loss is suspicious for endolymphatic hydrops whereas a low-frequency conductive loss with normal tympanogram and reflexes is seen in cases of superior semicircular canal dehiscence syndrome. Although a normal audiogram does not eliminate a labyrinthine or cochleovestibular nerve source of vertigo, an abnormal test frequently supports it.

Other tests of audiometric function involve evoked response protocols which include auditory brainstem response (ABR), otoacoustic emissions (OAE), and electrocochleography (ECochG). Auditory brainstem testing in patients with dizziness is primarily used to measure the integrity of eighth nerve function in suspected cases of neoplasm, vascular compression, or degenerative diseases. Otoacoustic emissions are used to document cochlear outer hair cell function. Finally, ECochG using either external auditory canal or transtympanic electrodes measures the summating potential (SP) to action potential (AP) ratio or absolute SP amplitude to either click or tone stimuli and is supportive but not solely diagnostic of endolymphatic hydrops.[16] Details of these audiometric tests can be found in Chapter 9, "Diagnostic Audiology, Hearing Instruments, and Aural Habilitation."

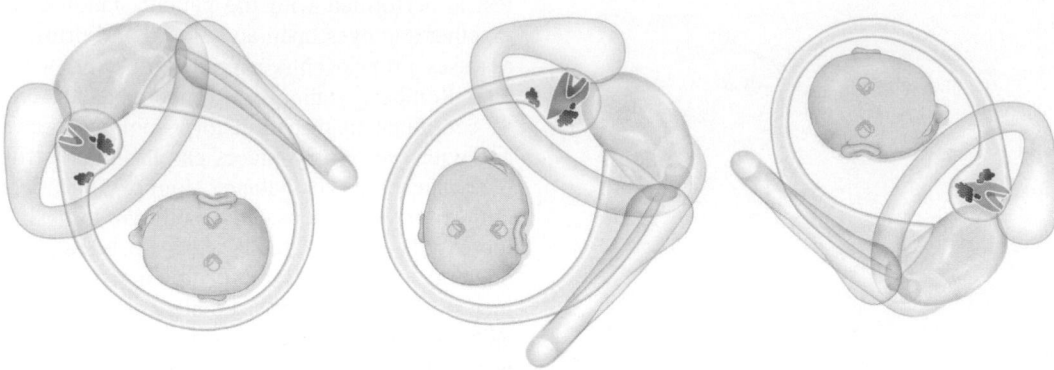

Figure 4 Apogeotropic lateral semicircular canal benign paroxysmal positional vertigo. (Reprinted with permission. Copyright © 2004. The Cleveland Clinic Foundation. All rights reserved.)

Vestibular Function Testing

Formal vestibular testing in the laboratory may not be needed in every patient seen for a vestibular evaluation. Diagnoses that can be readily established based on history and examination findings alone in the office obviate the need for further testing. The classic example of this is benign paroxysmal positional vertigo, which can be diagnosed during positioning testing and treated without further studies.

Quantitative vestibular function testing should be chosen by the informed physician based on the quantitative information each test can provide, as well as by the inherent limitations and sensitivity of each test. As a general rule, the history and physical examination provide the physician with a qualitative diagnosis; and, therefore, the primary role of laboratory tests is to document and quantify the suspected deficits. Vestibular function tests can also serve to assess the degree of compensation following vestibular injury, to follow compensation over time, and to quantify function prior to vestibular ablative procedures.

The traditional vestibular test battery assesses the oculomotor system, positional and positioning testing, low-frequency VOR caloric responsiveness, multi-frequency VOR gain, phase and symmetry, vestibular–visual interaction and postural control. Note that none of the standard vestibular laboratory studies assesses vertical canal function (aside from Dix-Hallpike testing for posterior canal BPPV) or otolith function. There are also other inherent limitations to vestibular testing. These tests are not a substitute for a thorough history and examination. They do not measure the degree of disability in a patient complaining of dizziness. They are human operator-dependent, and, therefore, computerized interpretation systems cannot replace the role of the experienced operator in obtaining optimal, cooperative performance from the patient which yields valid and reliable data. Finally, the results of vestibu-

lar testing can be influenced by factors such as medications, making adequate patient preparation essential. Patients should be instructed to refrain from antihistamines, alcohol, sedatives, and PRN benzodiazepines 24 to 48 hours prior to testing. Other routine medications which may affect test sensitivity should not be discontinued, and interpretation should note all medications taken and include their possible effects on the test results.

Test Conventions. To interpret accurately vestibular test data, it is important to understand certain test conventions. Nystagmus refers to rhythmic repetitive eye movements. Vestibular nystagmus is characterized by a distinct slow and fast phase. The direction of the nystagmus is named for the fast phase as seen from the patient's perspective. Nystagmus data are often presented on a horizontal strip recording, in which the horizontal axis designates time and the vertical axis represents eye deviation. Rightward nystagmus (fast component to the right, slow component to the left) appears on a strip recording as a sharp upward deflection followed by a gradual deflection downward. Strength of nystagmus is calculated by measuring the degrees that the eye moves in 1 second during the slow phase.

There are several methods employed to record nystagmus with advantages and disadvantages to each method. Visual inspection in room light is the simplest, least expensive method but affords the least sensitivity as patients can fixate on objects in the room, which can diminish or abolish vestibular nystagmus. Electrooculography (EOG) uses surface skin electrodes around the eye to record changes in the strength of the field generated by the corneoretinal potential, and nystagmus is recorded in the dark or with eyes closed. EOG resolution is 1°/s and

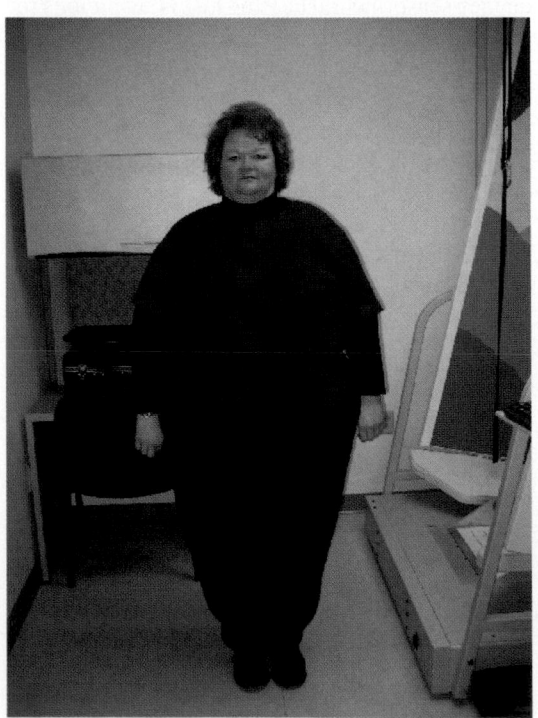

(A)

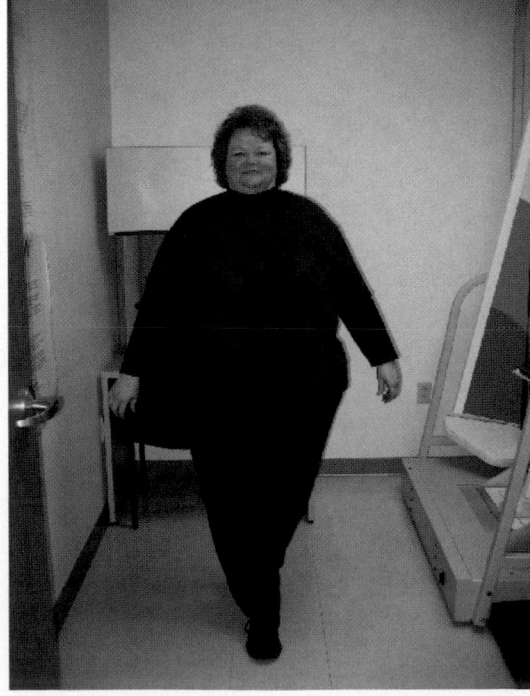

(B)

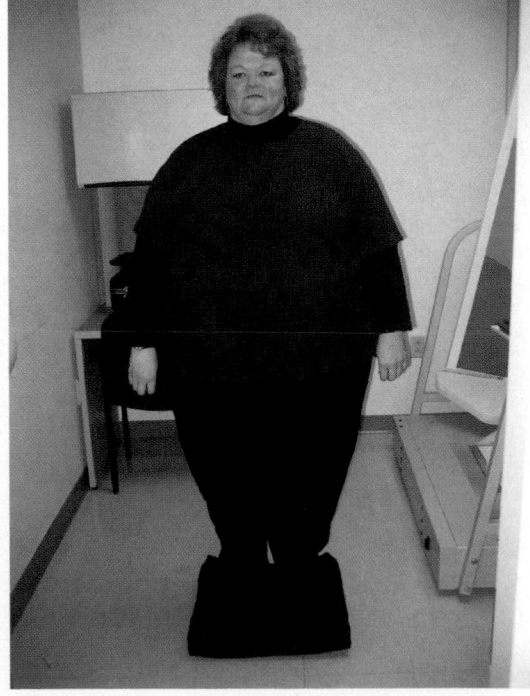

(C)

Figure 5 (A) Standard Romberg test on firm surface. (B) Tandem Romberg test on firm surface. (C) Foam Romberg test on compliant surface. As proprioceptive cues are altered in (B) and (C), vestibular input to balance becomes more important.

recording bandwidth is narrow (35 Hz), but electrical and muscle interference from blinking decreases sensitivity. Infrared video oculography (IR-VOG) uses infrared recording cameras placed in goggles in front of the eyes, which must be kept open for the examination. Resolution is high (0.1°), but bandwidth is limited by present recording speed technology which currently exceeds 100 Hz. This limitation does not usually affect the accuracy of clinical vestibular testing, but more advance infrared systems are available at a considerably the higher cost for research applications of high velocity eye movements. The most complex technique utilizes magnetic search coils placed on the sclera, and offers high resolution (0.02°), high recording speed, and the ability to record torsional nystagmus. However, search coils are expensive, run the risk of corneal abrasion, and recording time is limited to 60 minutes following application of topical anesthetic eye drops.

Oculomotor Testing. Bedside oculomotor testing was discussed briefly in the previous section on physical examination. Laboratory oculomotor testing is similar; but, in addition to assessment of pursuit, saccade, spontaneous, and gaze-evoked nystagmus, optokinetic nystagmus may also be evaluated. The oculomotor tests should be performed first in the vestibular test battery in order to identify abnormalities and to ensure that nystagmus can be recorded accurately during later vestibular stimulation.

Calibration is performed first and is important for computerized interpretation systems to ensure accurate measurement of the amplitude and direction of nystagmus throughout testing. It is done by having the patient look at fixed points 1 m away, including center, left (27 cm), and right (27 cm). These lateral points correspond to approximately 15° of eccentric gaze. Calibration errors are the most common reason caloric responses appear "reversed."

Spontaneous nystagmus is recorded with the patient sitting comfortably and is recorded with and without visual fixation. A small light located inside the infrared goggle or projected on the wall is illuminated for fixation testing. Vestibular nystagmus is characterized by a persistent horizontal unidirectional nystagmus that diminishes at least 50% with fixation. As already noted, vestibular nystagmus may appear stronger when the patient directs their gaze in the direction of the fast phase (Alexander's law). It is usually seen in the acute period following a unilateral vestibular loss, and the fast phase beats away from the affected ear.

Spontaneous nystagmus that does not have these important characteristics (unidirectional, horizontal, diminishes with fixation and worsens with gaze in the direction of the fast phase) should be considered potentially central. This includes vertical nystagmus (upbeat or downbeat), direction changing nystagmus (Figure 6), irregular or disconjugate nystagmus, or nystagmus that worsens with fixation (Figure 7). Alcohol and certain medications such as sedatives

Spontaneous Gaze Test

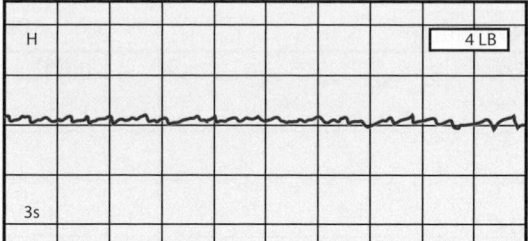

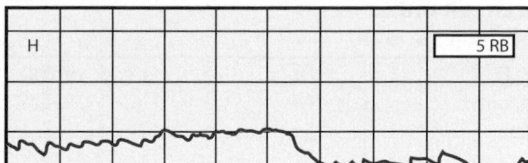

Scale = 10 degrees x 1 second

Figure 6 Direction changing spontaneous nystagmus of central origin. The nystagmus beats leftward with fixation then rightward without fixation.

and anticonvulsants may cause atypical spontaneous nystagmus.

A search for gaze-evoked nystagmus is undertaken next. Rightward, leftward, upward, and downward gaze are assessed by having the patient look 15 to 30° of eccentric gaze. Having the patient look any further than 15 to 30° may provoke normal end-gaze physiologic nystagmus. In general, gaze-evoked nystagmus is indicative of central pathology but may occur in the setting of patients who have recently consumed alcohol or are on anticonvulsants. Figure 8 demonstrates a central gaze-evoked nystagmus. In extreme cases, gaze-evoked nystagmus can interfere with the patient's ability to follow visually a moving object, as seen in Figure 9.

Next, saccades which are extremely high acceleration eye movements which volitionally redirect sight, or reflexively gaze toward a startling stimulus are tested. When assessing saccades, 4 parameters are of particular interest: latency, accuracy, peak velocity, and conjugacy. Latency refers to the delay between the presentation of the stimulus and beginning of the saccade and is usually 200 ms in normal subjects. Prolonged latency can be secondary to inattention, advanced age, or central pathology. Saccadic inaccuracy can be described as overshoot (hypermetria) or undershoot (hypometria). Hypometria must be severe and reproducible to be considered abnormal. Hypermetric responses are more significant even if slightly abnormal and suggest midline cerebellar injury. Any disconjugate saccade abnormality is considered significant. For example, internuclear ophthalmoplegia (INO) is a central disorder which causes slowing in the adducting eye and overshooting or gaze-evoked nystagmus in the abducting eye during attempted saccades. Bilateral INO is most commonly associated with lesions of the median longitudinal fasciculus in conditions like

multiple sclerosis whereas unilateral INO can be seen in brainstem lesions or infarction.

Pursuit eye movements enable clear viewing of slowly moving objects in the visual environment by allowing the eye to focus the image on the fovea. Gain refers to the match of peak eye speed to target speed. Pursuit performance is highly affected by age, alertness, attention, and cooperation. Asymmetric pursuit or gain that is significantly reduced may reflect an underlying central or visual disorder. In some instances, gain can be so abnormal that saccadic interruption of smooth pursuit is observed, giving a "stair step" appearance on the eye movement tracing termed saccadic pursuit (Figure 10).

Optokinetic nystagmus is a combination of pursuit (foveal vision) and optokinetic (extrafoveal) systems. It is best seen when the moving stimulus surrounds the patient in an environment without fixed visual reference points. In the vestibular laboratory, such visual stimuli are best presented in the rotary chair booth surrounding the seated patient, and the ability of the eye movements to follow the visual stimuli is recorded as gain. Typically, optokinetic nystagmus abnormalities will be associated with other oculomotor system abnormalities; and, as in all oculomotor test abnormalities, asymmetric responses are more likely to represent localized central pathology such as acute unilateral parieto-occipital lesions.

In summary, oculomotor tests can be particularly valuable for detecting central pathology but are affected by age, vision, medication, alertness, and cooperation. Thus, interpret oculomotor abnormalities cautiously and recognize that central pathologic patterns are usually evident on several of the tests. Bilateral findings are less often central in origin than are unilateral asymmetric findings. The demonstration of an intact oculomotor system during oculomotor

Spontaneous Nystagmus

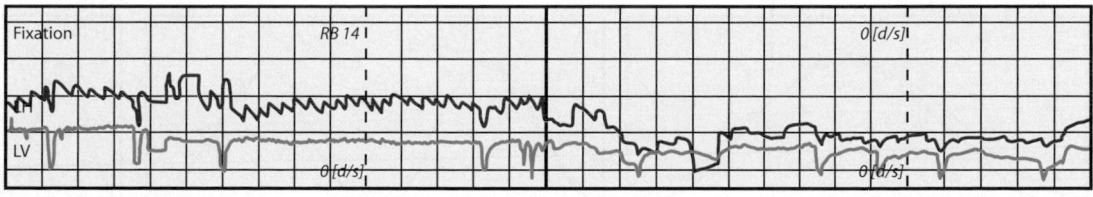

Scale = 10 degrees x 1 second

Figure 7 Spontaneous rightward beating central nystagmus. The nystagmus is recorded only during fixation and disappears without fixation.

Spontaneous Gaze Test

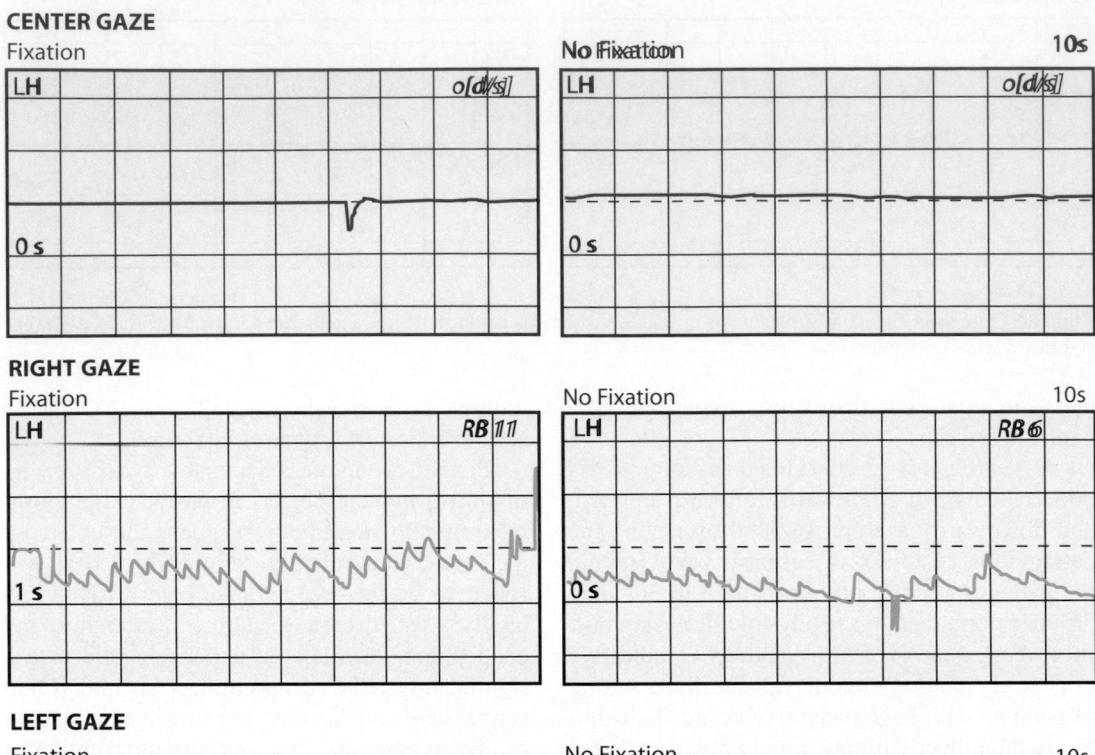

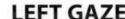

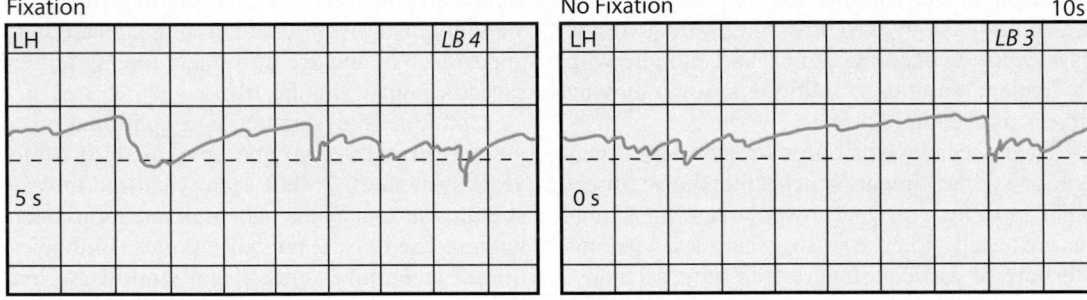

Scale=10 degrees x 1 second

Figure 8 Gaze-evoked nystagmus of central origin. No nystagmus is observed on central gaze, whereas a right beating nystagmus is seen on rightward gaze and a left beating nystagmus is observed with left gaze.

testing allows valid interpretation of the vestibular responses obtained during the next steps vestibulo-ocular testing and caloric testing. A sample normal oculomotor computer-generated report is seen in (Figure 11).

Positional and Positioning Testing. Positional and positioning testing was addressed earlier in the bedside/office physical examination section. Formal testing in a laboratory is essentially identical, and therefore is not discussed in detail. As laboratory testing is typically performed in the absence of the interpreting clinician, it is useful to record the nystagmus seen during posi-

tional and positioning testing and to replay it during interpretation by the physician. This permits greater sensitivity in identifying torsional eye movements, which are not accurately analyzed by commonly used computerized systems which record only horizontal and vertical eye movements.

Caloric Testing. Caloric testing of the VOR compares responses of the left with the right lateral semicircular canal; and, therefore, it is notable for being the only vestibular test that provides lateralizing information. It should also be noted that caloric testing evaluates only the

lowest frequency response of the VOR (about 0.003 Hz); and, therefore, any interpretation of abnormal function should not be extrapolated to higher frequencies or vertical canal or otolith function.

Testing is conducted with the patient placed supine in the darkness with the head of bed elevated 30°. This effectively brings the lateral semicircular canal into a vertical orientation. Standardized warm (44°C) and cool (30°C) stimuli are applied to the external auditory canal, in an alternating bithermic manner, that is, left warm (LW), right warm (RW), left cold (LC), right cold (RC). Water is the most dependable stimulus and can be directly irrigated into the external auditory canal (open loop), or used in a "closed loop" balloon system when prior surgery, infection, or tympanic membrane perforation precludes direct instillation of water. An air caloric stimulation is easier to use but may provide a less reliable and even paradoxical stimulus using warm air with a moist canal or tympanic membrane perforation due to evaporation.

A warm caloric test transmits heat to the lateral semicircular canal, causing endolymph to rise and flow toward the cupula (ampullopetal flow). This is stimulatory to the lateral canal, and nystagmus is generated with the fast phase beating toward the tested ear. The cool caloric stimulus effectively cools endolymph, making it more dense and causing it to fall away from the cupula (ampullofugal flow), which is inhibitory. This generates nystagmus away from the tested ear. The mnemonic devices, COWS (cold-opposite, warm-same), is a simple way to remember the association. Jonkees' formula is used to calculate differences in caloric responses between the ears, where % caloric paresis = $100 \times [(LC + LW) - (RC + RW)/(LC + LW + RC + RW)]$. An 18 to 30% difference is considered significant and varies between laboratories and type of stimulation (open water, closed-loop water, or air). The strength of leftward nystagmus to rightward nystagmus can also be calculated:

% directional preponderance (DP) = $100 \times [(LC + RW) - (RC + LW)/(LC + LW + RC + RW)]$

Greater than 30% directional preponderance of nystagmus is considered abnormal, although this is a rather nonspecific finding in isolation. An example of graphic caloric results is shown in (Figure 12).

Fixation is tested following peak caloric nystagmus measurement. The patient is instructed to stare at a strong fixed light, which should cause nystagmus to decrease by at least 50% after 2 seconds. After 10 seconds of fixation, the patient is returned to darkness and nystagmus should rebound. Failure of fixation suppression is a strong central sign and would be expected to be seen consistently throughout caloric (and VOR) testing when there is true central pathology. Isolated failure of fixation is generally disregarded.

If caloric responses are low or absent, ice water irrigation should be tested. Ice water is

PURSUIT HORIZONTAL

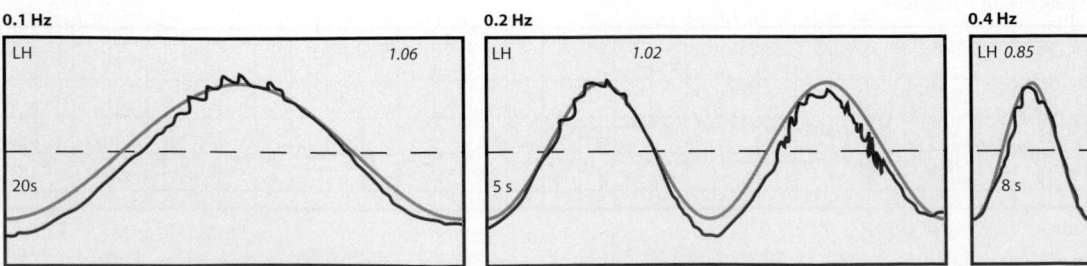

Figure 9 Right gaze-evoked nystagmus interfering with smooth pursuit tracking.

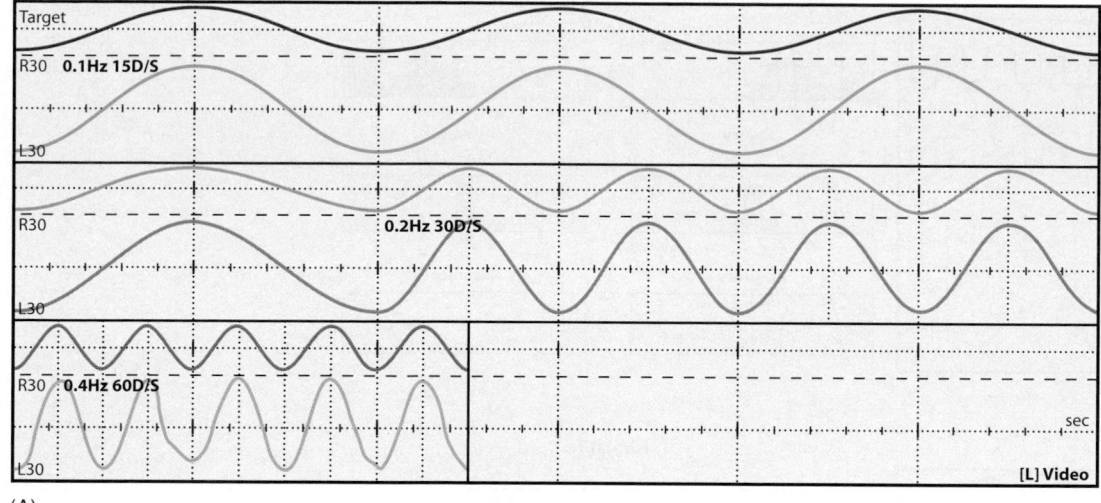

(A)

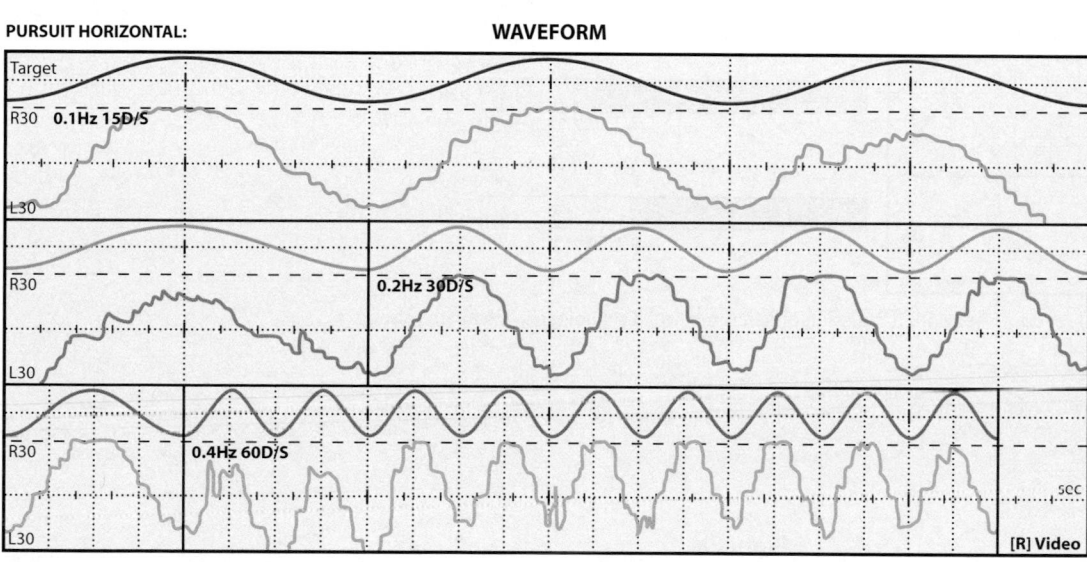

(B)

Figure 10 (A) Normal smooth pursuit.(B) Saccadic pursuit. Note stair-step pattern. (Used with permission of Micromedical Technologies, Chatham, illinois.)

a stronger stimulus than either cold or warm water and may be used with the patient supine or prone. In the supine position, it causes ampulofugal flow of endolymph, an inhibitory stimulus that leads to nystagmus away from the tested ear. If the patient is placed prone, the vertical orientation of the lateral canal has effectively been inverted, and ice water would cause ampulopetal flow of endolymph, generating nystagmus toward the tested ear. This alteration in ice water–generated nystagmus direction may be a helpful sign when an overlying spontaneous nystagmus makes interpretation of low-amplitude ice water–induced nystagmus problematic; the patient can be tested in both prone and supine positions to determine if there is a measurable vestibular response.

Despite its ability to provide lateralizing information, calorics represent a rather imprecise test in the vestibular armamentarium. As mentioned, caloric testing assesses only low-frequency responses (0.003 Hz), far below physiologic frequencies encountered during active head or body movement. Moreover, caloric responses are subject to anatomic variability and conductivity of

the external auditory canal, medication effects (sedatives, benzodiazepines, antihistamines, alcohol, and anticonvulsants), and patient arousal and compliance. For this reason, caloric testing results must be interpreted with caution. Isolated caloric asymmetry in the face of normal VOR testing without positional or positioning nystagmus may suggest either a problem with the test itself or a compensated peripheral weakness and is unlikely to explain any recent symptoms the patient is experiencing. Reduced bilateral caloric responses (total eye speeds for all 4 caloric irrigations less than 20°/s) may raise concern for bilateral peripheral hypofunction but may also represent unilateral dysfunction with central inhibition of the intact side, poor mental tasking, or technical issues with temperature transfer. In such instances, multifrequency VOR testing in the rotary chair helps to distinguish between these possibilities.[16]

Rotary Chair Testing of the Vestibulo-Ocular Reflex. The VOR stabilizes vision during high velocity head movements. When the head is rotated to the left, the eyes turn to the right to

allow vision to remain centered on the target. Conversely, right head rotation results in a leftward movement of the eyes to remain centered on the target.

VOR testing via rotary chair is the only standardized physiologic method that assesses the vestibulo-ocular system at multiple frequencies (0.01 to 1.0 Hz). At these frequencies, the VOR is generated by both the right and left vestibular systems working in tandem; and, therefore, its results can be used to assess for both compensation following unilateral loss and extent of bilateral loss. During rotary chair testing, the body is passively rotated en bloc with the patient's head immobilized in a headholder. Frequencies between 0.01 and 1.0 Hz are generated by a computer and presented as sinusoidal chair movement. On a time strip, the movement of the chair appears as a sinusoid moving left and right. The slow phase of the eye movements can be recorded on the same strip, but the eyes will appear as a mirror image of the chair, moving rightward with left rotation of the chair and leftward with right chair rotation (Figure 13). Standard computerized VOR summary analysis is shown in Figure 14.

Three VOR parameters of interest are measured during sinusoidal rotary chair testing: gain, phase, and symmetry. Gain is a measure of how closely the eye movements match the head (chair) movement, with a perfect match resulting in a gain of 1. Phase measures the timing of eye versus chair movement and is best calculated as a difference in degrees at the 0 crossing during low-frequency testing. Symmetry compares the gain of eye movements during rightward versus leftward head rotation. In normal individuals, gain increases toward 1, phase decreases toward 0, and symmetry is preserved with increasing frequency. In patients with acute unilateral loss, gain is moderately decreased, phase is abnormally increased, and asymmetry may be seen, especially in cases with spontaneous nystagmus. With compensation, gain variably recovers, phase usually remains increased, and symmetry abates. With bilateral loss, gain is so low that phase and asymmetry are incalculable.

An alternate approach for rotational testing is to spin the patient in one direction as a constant speed (100 to 300°/s) and observe the resultant nystagmus slow phase velocity both during rotation (per-rotary) and after an abrupt stop (post-rotary). During the initial acceleration of the step velocity test, the VOR generates nystagmus in the direction of rotation which decays at a certain rate dependent on cupular deflection and central velocity storage of the cupular signal. After an abrupt stop, nystagmus is generated in similar fashion in the opposite direction. A measure called "time constant" refers to the time in seconds it takes for the initial nystagmus to decline to 37% of its initial value. In normal individuals, this time constant is of the order of 12 to 15 seconds and reflects intact central velocity storage of the peripheral cupular signal. In cases of vestibular disease, central velocity

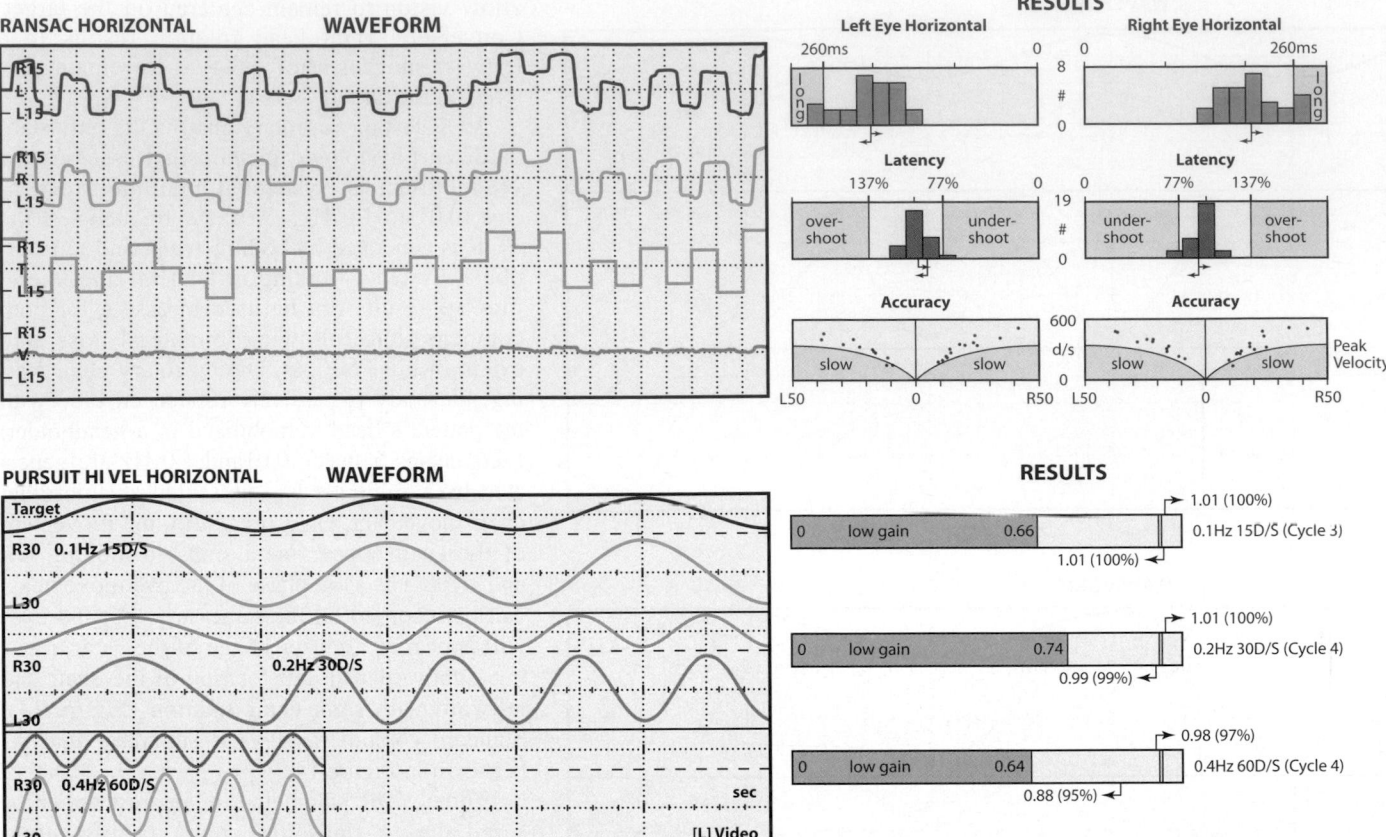

Figure 11 Normal oculomotor test battery computer-generated report. (Used with permission of Micromedical Technologies, Chatham, illinois.)

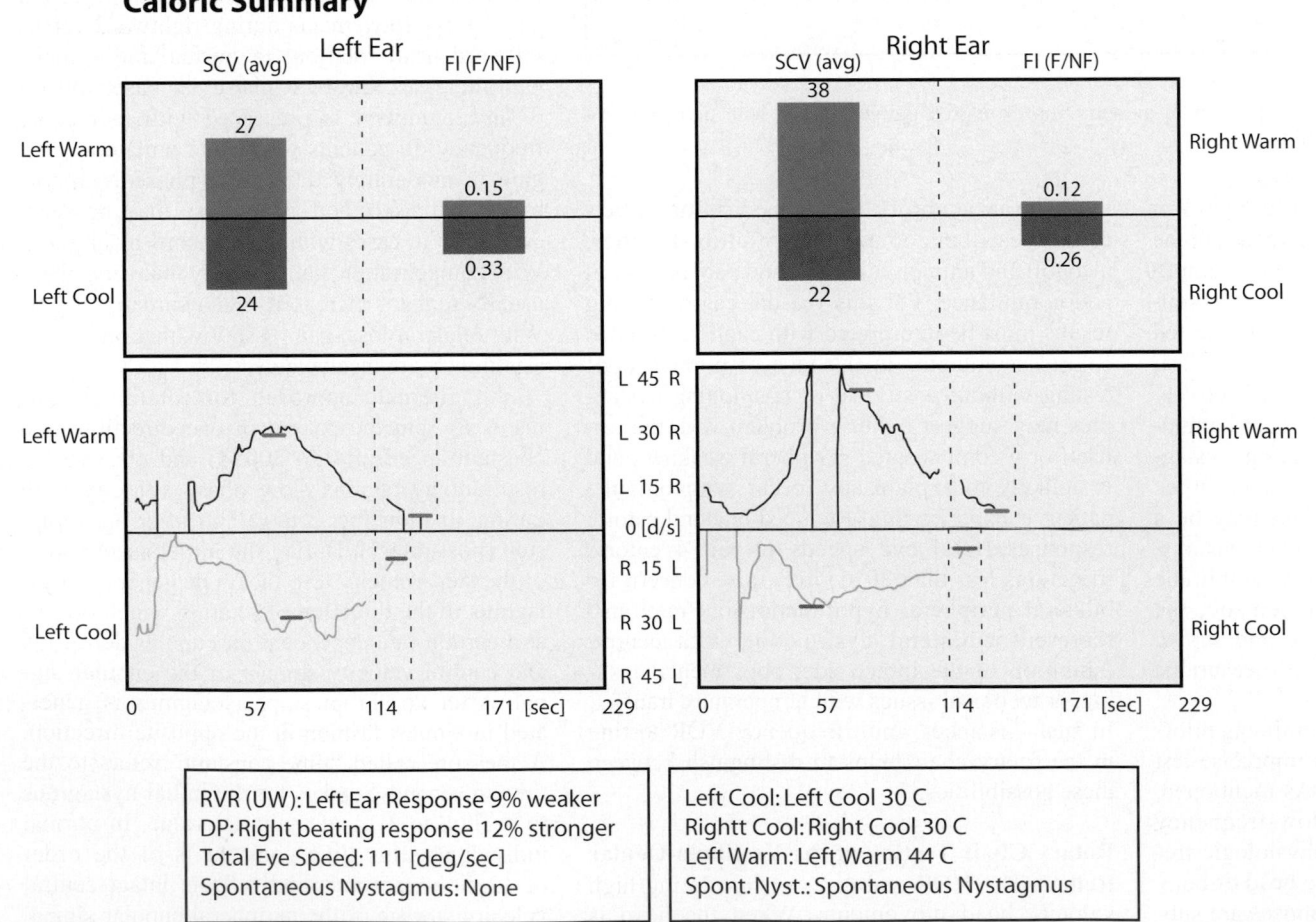

Figure 12 Normal graphic caloric results. (Used with permission of Micromedical Technologies, Chatham, illinois.)

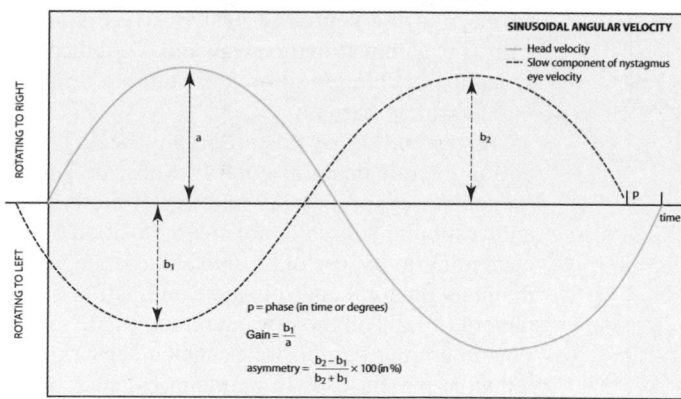

Figure 13 Vestibulo-ocular reflex (VOR) sinusoidal gain, phase a and b asymmetry measures.

Rotational Chair Summary

VOR Summary

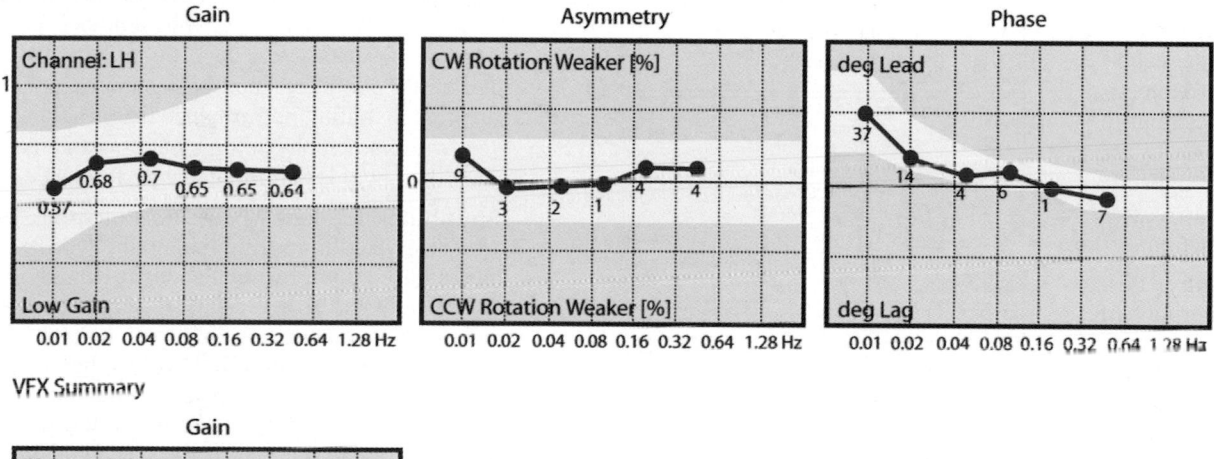

VFX Summary

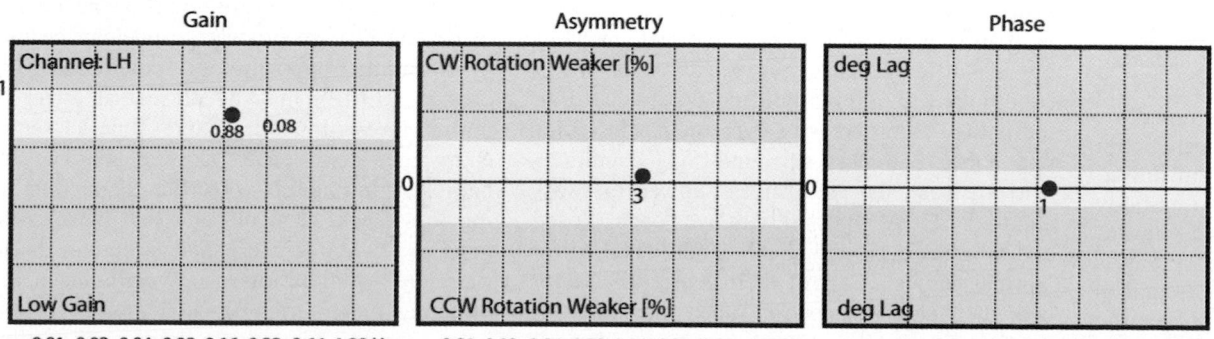

Asymmetry and Phase results are not calculated for Gains less than 0.2

Figure 14 Standard computerized rotational chair vestibulo-ocular reflex (VOR) summary analysis. (Graphic results display used with permission of Micromedical Technologies, Chatham, illinois.)

storage is disabled, and the time constant reverts to the cupular value of <6 seconds. Both time constant and phase are sensitive markers of vestibular dysfunction.

Rotary chair testing of the VOR is performed in the dark to eliminate visual fixation. Visual stimuli are included in two additional portions of the test, fixation and visual–vestibular interaction testing. During vestibulo-ocular fixation (VFIX), a steady light rotating with the subject is used to test for the expected (>50%) decrease in vestibulo-ocular gain during visual fixation. During visual–vestibular (VVOR) interaction, earth-fixed visual stimuli are used to increase the perceived motion of the subject by stimulating both the VOR and the optokinetic systems. Since the VOR works best at higher frequencies and the optokinetic system at lower frequencies, the union of these 2 systems during VVOR testing in normal subjects yields unity gain, 0 phase, and no asymmetry across all frequencies. \ pathology or poor vision can affect the integration of visual and vestibular inputs, resulting in abnormal fixation suppression during VFIX testing and/or VOR enhancement during VVOR testing.

Limitations of rotary chair testing include cost of the systems, limitation to earth-vertical stimulation of only the lateral semicircular canals and limitations of peak velocity and frequency due to problems with head and body restraint in the chair. Enhancements to standard protocols are being investigated, including eccentric dynamic testing and off-vertical-axis-rotation to assess otolith function and canal–otolith interaction.

Computerized Dynamic Posturography. Postural control involves a complex interplay of visual, proprioceptive, and vestibular input. Computerized dynamic posturography (CDP) tests static postural control in a series of conditions designed to emphasize or minimize each of these inputs. The somatosensory system detects contact force and motion between the feet and contact surface and utilizes tactile, deep pressure, joint receptor, and muscle proprioceptive input to influence static posture in a "bottom-up fashion" via the ankle joint. Under normal conditions, the somatosensory system dominates balance control. Firm, fixed surfaces favor the somatosensory system, and classic Romberg testing utilizes these features by testing postural control on a stable surface with eyes closed. The visual system relies on visual cues from the environment to assist in maintaining upright posture. It may be affected by decreased vision, or inappropriate dependence on visual stimuli, for example, standing next to a moving bus and perceiving sway. The vestibular system usually functions to allow head and eye movements that are independent in most situations and functions as a "top down" system for gaze stabilization and head-on-body coordination. In situations of decreased proprioceptive and visual input, the vestibular system is crucial for maintaining upright postural control. Patients with bilateral vestibular hypofunction have great difficulty maintaining postural control on compliant surfaces in the dark, such as deep carpeting or uneven landscape.

Conditions

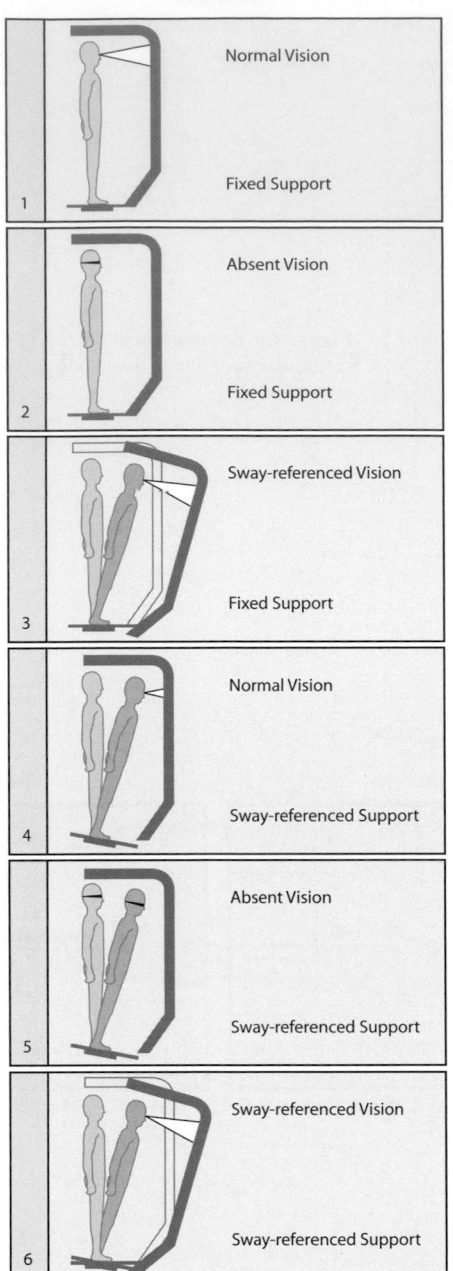

Figure 15 Computerized dynamic posturography sensory organization test (SOT) conditions. SOT conditions 1 to 3 performed with stable support surface and SOT conditions 4 to 6 performed with sway-referenced support surface. (Courtesy of NeuroCom International Inc, Clackamas, OR.)

CDP presents 6 differing conditions to maximize or minimize input from the somatosensory, visual, and vestibular systems (Figure 15). Postural sway is assessed using force plate technology in 6 different sensory organization test (SOT) conditions 1 to 6. Initially using a fixed platform, the patient is tested with eyes open, closed, or with a swaying visual surround (SOT conditions 1 to 3). Next, the platform is allowed to sway, and the tests are repeated with eyes open, closed and swaying surround (SOT conditions 4 to 6). Normal subjects control their center of gravity over their base of support. When movement of the feet is not allowed, subjects generally will fall if swaying is greater than about 12.5° in the anterior–posterior direction (termed the limits of

stability). Patients are compared to age-matched norms, and the degree of peak sway is reported with 100% indicating no sway and 0% indicating sway approaching the limits of stability or a fall into the safety harness.

Interpretation of posturography begins with noting overall postural control. Subscale scores on somatosensory, visual and visual preference, and vestibular subscales are noted. Position of the center of gravity, use of hip and ankle strategies to maintain postural control, and examination of the pattern of falls on the raw data tracings are made. Posturography demonstrates which sensory systems the patient uses to maintain balance, but it does not directly assess deficits in those systems. Thus, a low score on the vestibular subscale (SOT conditions 5 and 6) suggests either that the patient is not using vestibular input when appropriate to maintain posture (late falls on the raw data) or that vestibular input may be deficient (early falls on the raw data) (Figure 16). Hence, CDP uniquely assesses the functional use of the vestibular system to achieve postural control and is best included in a comprehensive vestibular test battery for patients with complaints of postural instability. An additional use of posturography is to identify patients with "aphysiologic" performance on various test conditions. Patients who fail easier conditions and pass harder conditions are demonstrating performance that is not consistent with known physiologic patterns and may be identified by this pattern of test performance.[17]

Vestibular-Evoked Myogenic Potential. Vestibular-evoked myogenic potential (VEMP) testing is based upon residual acoustic sensitivity of the saccule and serves as a screening test of saccular otolith function. VEMPs can be elicited by air conduction stimuli (click or tone burst), bone conduction stimuli, or galvanic stimulation. Most commonly, click stimuli are used, and changes in the static contraction of the ipsilateral sternocleidomastoid muscle are measured via electromyography.

A normal VEMP response consists of a biphasic wave, with a positive peak (P1) and a negative peak (N1). It is of short latency, with P1 normally occurring within 13 to 15 milliseconds of the stimulus, while N1 occurs within 21 to 24 milliseconds. Normal click-evoked VEMP thresholds fall within 85 to 90 dB SPL and are present in normal individuals younger than 60 years of age.[18–19]

Abnormal VEMP responses may be indicative of certain disease processes and may be useful in differentiating pathologic conditions. Click-evoked VEMPS may be present at lower than normal thresholds in ipsilateral superior semicircular canal dehiscence[20] (Figure 17). They may be absent in patients with true conductive hearing loss (such as in otosclerosis) with air-bone gaps as low as 8.75 dB, and in certain diseases like late Menière disease, vestibular neuritis affecting the inferior division of the vestibular nerve, acoustic neuroma, or peripheral vestibular hypofunction (including iatrogenic hypofunction due to intratympanic gentamicin).[21–23] It should

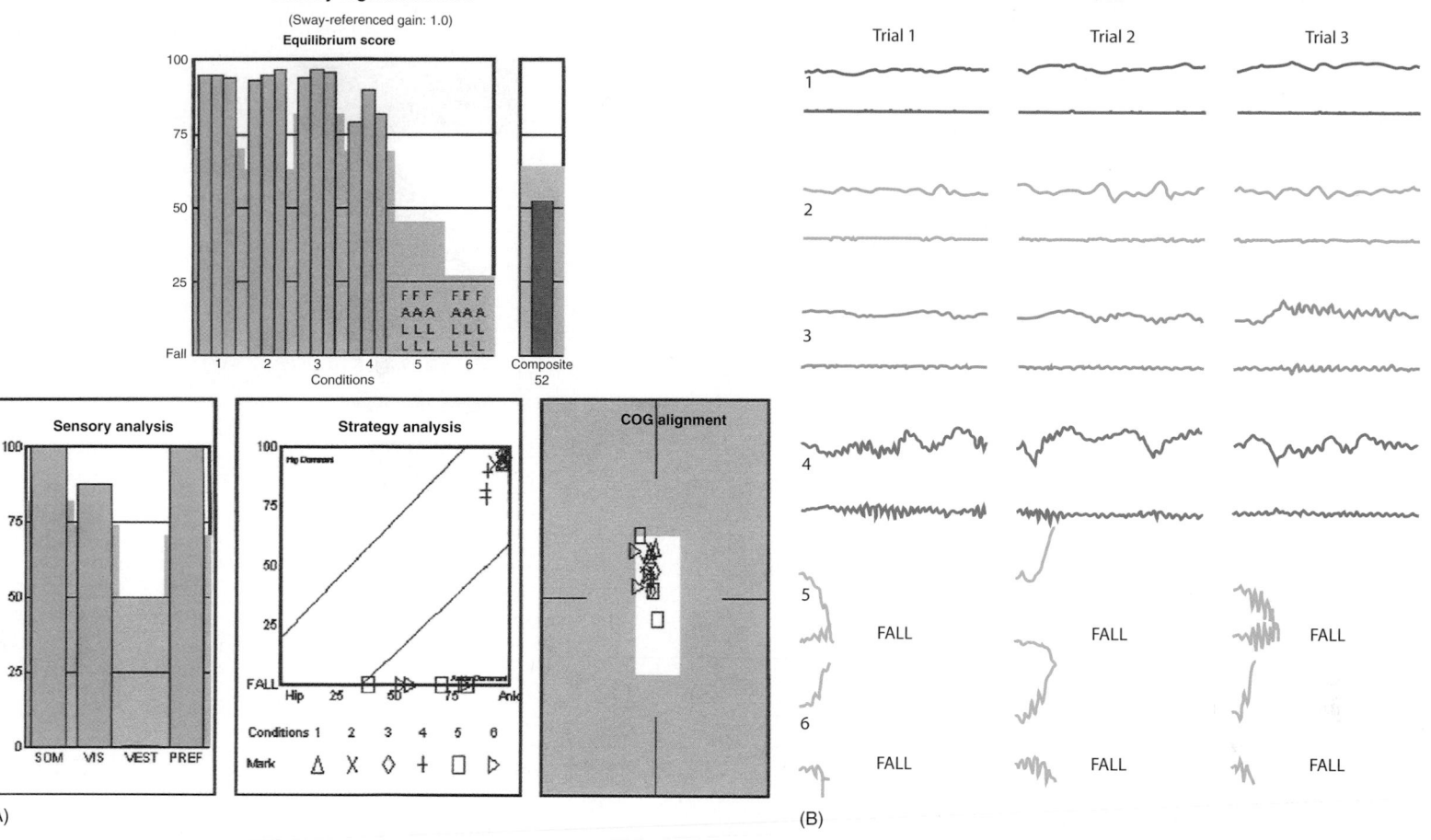

Figure 16 (A) Graphic display of computerized dynamic posturography sensory organization test (SOT) results in a patient with a vestibular loss pattern. (B) Raw sway data for the same patient showing early falls under SOT conditions 5 and 6 consistent with loss of vestibular cues. (Courtesy of NeuroCom International Inc, Clackamas, OR.)

be noted that normal subjects older than 60 years may have absent click VEMPs; and, thus, their absence in these patients, being evaluated for dizziness, must be interpreted carefully and should not be used solely to guide diagnosis and treatment.[19]

Eccentric Dynamic Subjective Visual Vertical. The otolith organs (utricle and saccule) detect linear acceleration, in contrast to the semicircular canals which detect angular acceleration. Linear vectors of force can be applied to each utricle by rotating a subject around a vertical axis while the subject is eccentrically displaced 4 cm. This centers 1 utricle on the axis of rotation and subjects the other side to a linear force vector. While rotating, the patient feels as if they are being pushed outward toward the side of displacement (similar to standing on the edge of a merry-go round). The response of each utricle can be contrasted when the subject is rotated with the right ear displaced laterally versus the left ear displaced laterally.

One response mediated by the utricles is the assessment of visual vertical. In the dark, a subject is asked to move a light bar until it appears vertical. The accuracy of the subject's placement is recorded. This technique can be affixed to the rotary chair to provide subjective visual vertical assessment during eccentric rotation. This protocol allows for comparison of right and left utricular function.[24]

Off Vertical Axis Rotation. Research applications use off vertical axis rotation (OVAR) to tilt the entire rotary chair unit and allow for analysis of gravitational forces on utricular function in rotating subjects.[25] This method can be visualized as a spinning holiday tree tilting from side to side in its base. OVAR testing requires complex chair construction and interpretation and is mainly utilized by research laboratories.

Vestibular Test Battery Interpretation. Interpretation begins with a review of oculomotor testing performance. Central oculomotor abnormalities are usually obvious and recurrent (see the discussion included in the section "Oculomotor Testing" of this chapter). Demonstration of normal oculomotor function allows assessment to progress to the next level.

Next, check for spontaneous nystagmus. Spontaneous nystagmus may affect results on oculomotor, caloric, VOR symmetry, and directional preponderance. Note any spontaneous nystagmus, and consider its effect on the aforementioned tests. Caloric asymmetry is assessed next. Caloric asymmetry in our laboratory is defined by a greater than 28% difference between ears as calculated with Jonkees' formula. The next task of the interpreter, once a caloric asymmetry is noted, is to determine if this is an acute uncompensated unilateral loss, a partially compensated loss, or a compensated loss. The following pattern suggests acute uncompensated peripheral vestibular loss:

1. Spontaneous horizontal nystagmus away from the affected ear that decreases at least 50% with fixation.
2. Positional or positioning nystagmus away from the affected ear, especially if seen in several positions.
3. Gaze-evoked unidirectional horizontal nystagmus worse in the direction of gaze away from the affected ear.
4. Asymmetric vestibulo-ocular reflex (VOR) gain decreased with rotation toward the affected side.
5. Low-frequency VOR phase elevation may be present (variable).
6. VOR gain may be normal or reduced.
7. Posturography may show a vestibular pattern of deficit.

In contrast, a unilateral caloric loss which is fully compensated is associated with

1. no spontaneous nystagmus;
2. no gaze-evoked nystagmus;
3. minimal positional and positioning nystagmus (less than 6°/s and not present in several positions);
4. symmetric VOR gain;
5. low-frequency VOR phase elevation may be present (variable);
6. normal VOR gain;
7. normal posturography;
8. asymmetric caloric responses.

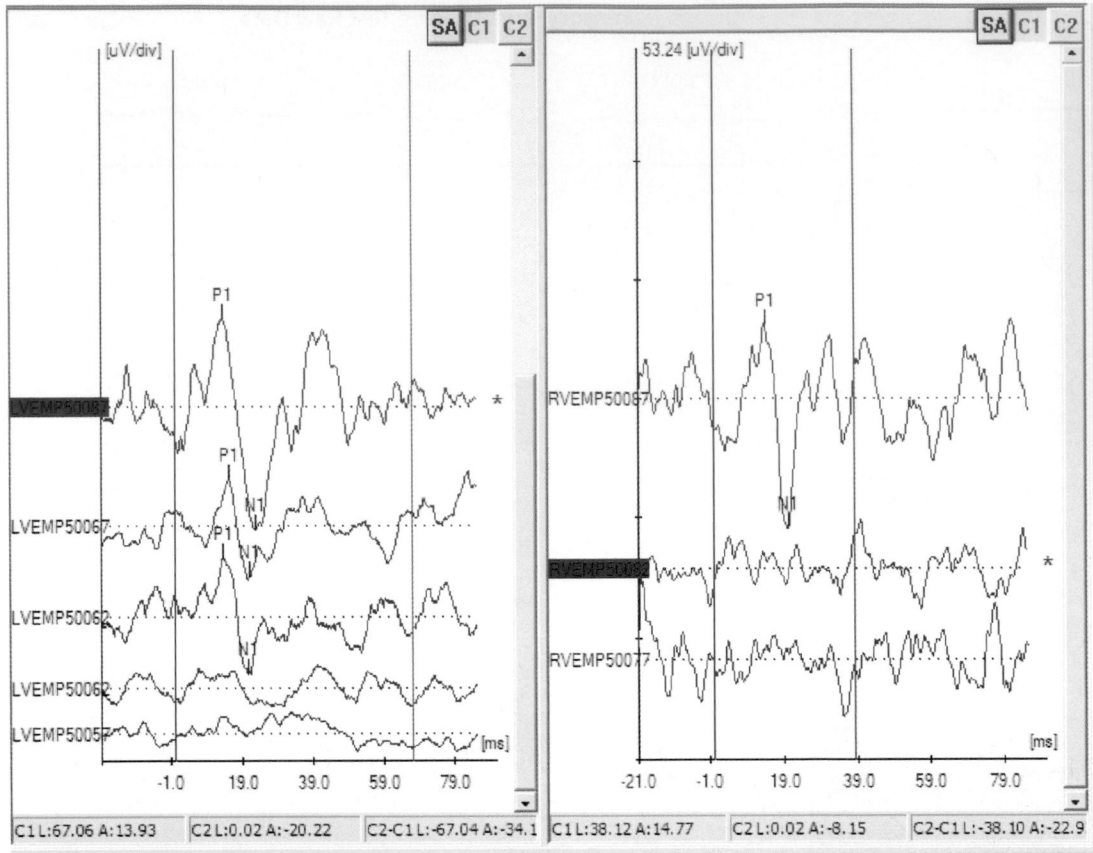

Figure 17 Vestibular-evoked myogenic potential (VEMP) at 500 Hz in a patient with left superior semicircular canal dehiscence. Note the normal response to the loudest clicks (top tracing) in both ears and the abnormal response to lower intensities in the left ear.

Patterns that are a mixture or acute uncompensated and compensated features are described as partially compensated.

Bilateral vestibular hypofunction is suggested by caloric responses less than 22°/s total eye speed and confirmed by rotary chair VOR that is 2 or more standard deviations below normal.[26] The time constant on impulse testing is less than 5 seconds, and sinusoidal VOR testing results indicate reduced VOR gain (at 0.05 Hz <0.20; at 0.2 Hz <0.21; at 1.0 Hz <0.62). Medication effects must be excluded.

REFERENCES

1. Baloh RW, Honrubia V. Clinical Neurophysiology of the Vestibular System, 2nd edition. Philadelphia: FA Davis and Company; 1990. p. 130–73.
2. Kroenke K, Arrington ME, Mangelsdorff AD. The prevalence of symptoms in medical outpatients and the adequacy of therapy. Arch Intern Med 1990;150:1685–9.
3. Blakley BW, Goebel J. The meaning of the word "vertigo." Otolaryngol Head Neck Surg 2001;125:147–50.
4. Neuhauser H, Leopold M, von Brevern M, et al. The interrelations of migraine, vertigo, and migrainous vertigo. Neurology 2001;56:436–41.
5. Newman-Toker DE, Camargo CA, Jr. "Cardiogenic vertigo"—true vertigo as the presenting manifestation of primary cardiac disease. Nat Clin Pract Neurol 2006;2:167–72.
6. Low PA, Opfer-Gehrking TL, McPhee BR, et al. Prospective evaluation of clinical characteristics of orthostatic hypotension. Mayo Clin Proc 1995;70:617–22.
7. Baloh RW. Neurotology of migraine. Headache 1997;37:615–21.
8. von Brevern M, Zeise D, Neuhauser H, et al. Acute migrainous vertigo: Clinical and oculographic findings. Brain 2005;128:365–74.
9. Neuhauser H, Leopold M, von Brevern M, et al. The interrelations of migraine, vertigo and migrainous vertigo. Neurology 2001;56:436–41.
10. Freeman R. Assessment of cardiovascular autonomic function. Clin Neurophysiol 2006;117:716–30.
11. Ward C, Kenny RA. Reproducibility of orthostatic hypotension in symptomatic elderly. Am J Med 1996;100:418–22.
12. Gibbons CH, Freeman R. Delayed orthostatic hypotension: a frequent cause of orthostatic intolerance. Neurology 2006;67:8–9.
13. Headache Classification Committee. The international classification of headache disorders. Cephalalgia 2004;24:1–160.
14. Halmagyi GM, Curthoys IS. A clinical sign of canal paresis. Arch Neurol 1988;45:737–9.
15. White J, Coale K, Catalano P, Oas J. Diagnosis and management of lateral semicircular canal benign positional vertigo. Otolaryngol Head Neck Surg 2005;133:278–84.
16. Fife TD, Tusa RJ, Furman JM, et al. Assessment: Vestibular testing in adults and children. Report of the Therapeutic and Technology Assessment Subcommittee of the American Academy of Neurology. Neurology 2000;55:1431–41.
17. Goebel JA, Sataloff RT, Hanson JM, et al. Posturographic evidence of non-organic sway patterns in normal subject patients and suspected malingerers. Otolaryngol Head Neck Surg 1997;117:293–302.
18. Rauch SD. Vestibular evoked myogenic potentials. In: Jackler RK, Brackmann DE, editors. Neurotology, 2nd edition. Philadelphia: Elsevier Mosby; 2005. p. 270–2.
19. Welgampola MS, Colebatch JG. Characteristics and clinical applications of vestibular-evoked myogenic potentials. Neurology 2005;64:1682–8.
20. Streubel SO, Cremer PD, Carey JP, et al. Vestibular-evoked myogenic potentials in the diagnosis of superior canal dehiscence. Acta Otolaryngol 2001;545:41–9.
21. Bath AP, Harris N, McEwan J. Effect of conductive hearing loss on the vestibulocollic reflex. Clin Otolaryngol 1999;24:181–3.
22. De Waele C, Tran Ba Huy P, Diard JP, et al. Saccular dysfunction in Meniere's patients. A vestibular-evoked myogenic potential study. Ann N Y Acad Sci 1999;871:392–7.
23. Murofushi T, Matsuzaki M, Mizuno M. Vestibular evoked myogenic potentials in patients with acoustic neuromas. Arch Otolaryngol Head Neck Surg 1998;124:509–12.
24. Kingma H. Function tests of the otolith or statolith system. Curr Opin Neurol 2006;19:21–5.
25. Furman JM, Schlor RH, Schumann TL. Off-vertical axis rotation: a test of the otolith-ocular reflex. Am Otol Rhinol Laryngol 1992;101:643–50.
26. Baloh RW, Halmagyi GM. Disorders of the Vestibular System. New York: Oxford University Press; 1996.

11

Imaging of the Temporal Bone

Mahmood F. Mafee, MD, FACR
Galdino E. Valvassori, MD, FACR

The temporal bone is unique in the human body because it contains, in the small volume of a cubic inch (petrous bone), a concentration of vital osseous and membranous structures surrounded by a more or less extensive system of petromastoid pneumatic cells. Because of the different densities of its bony components and of the air and fluid-filled spaces around and within it, the temporal bone lends itself to accurate visualization and assessment by various imaging modalities.[1–10]

Conventional radiography, computed tomography (CT), magnetic resonance imaging (MRI), and arteriography are the techniques currently used to study the temporal bone and auditory-vestibular pathways.[2–30] Familiarity with clinical applications of these varied modalities is essential for requesting the proper imaging study.

CONVENTIONAL RADIOGRAPHY

Today, the use of conventional radiography is limited to evaluation of the mastoid pneumatization and assessment of the position and integrity of cochlear implant electrodes and gross evaluation of the temporomandibular joint (TMJ). Only 3 projections are of practical interest: the lateral or Schüller projection, the frontal or transorbital, and the oblique or Stenvers projection. The other special projections have historic significance but no useful clinical application.

Schuller or Rungstrom Projection

The Schüller projection is a lateral view of the mastoid obtained with a cephalocaudad angulation of the X-ray beam of 25° to 30°. The patient's head is turned so that the sagittal plane of the skull becomes parallel to the tabletop and the side under examination is closer to the film. Proper centering is obtained by placing the external auditory meatus of the side to be examined 1 cm above the center of the film or of the tabletop.

The extent of the pneumatization of the mastoid, distribution of the air cells, and degree of aeration and status of the trabecular pattern are the main features of this projection (Figure 1). The anterior plate of the vertical portion of the sigmoid sinus groove (corresponding to the most lateral part of the posterior aspect of the petrous pyramid) casts an almost vertical line, slightly concave posteriorly in its upper portion, superimposed on the air cells. At its upper

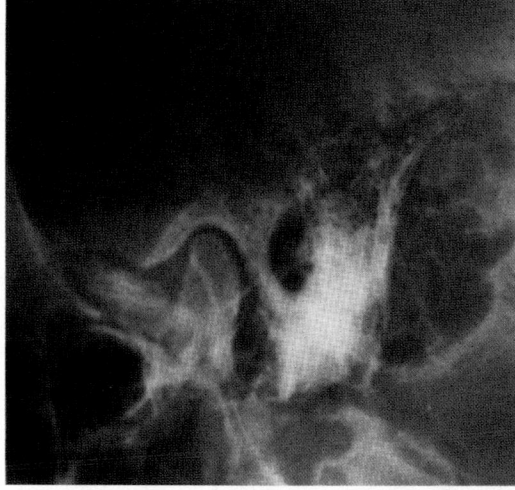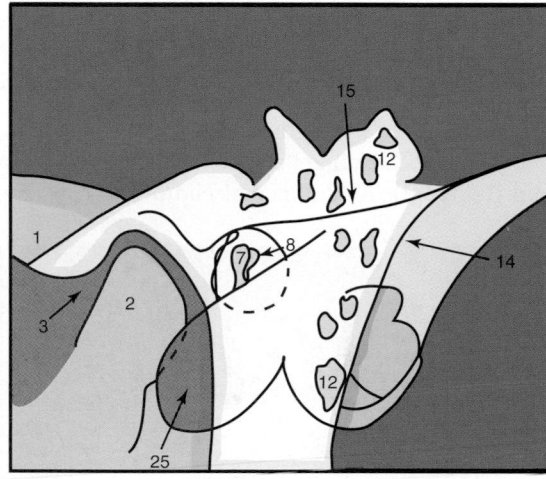

Figure 1 Schüller projection. (1) Root of the zygomatic process, (2) condyle of the mandible, (3) temporomandibular joint, (7) malleus, (8) incus, (12) air cells, (14) anterior plate of the sigmoid sinus, (15) dural plate, and (25) petrous apex.

extremity, this line joins another line that slopes gently forward and downward to form the sinodural angle of Citelli. The latter line is produced by the superior aspect of the lateral portion of the petrous pyramid. The more medial portion of the superior petrous ridge, from the arcuate eminence to the apex, has been displaced downward by the angulation of the X-ray beam and casts a line that extends forward and downward, crossing the epitympanic area, and more anteriorly, the neck of the mandibular condyle. Above this line, the upper portion of the attic with the head of the malleus is usually visible. Finally, the TMJ joint is outlined.

Transorbital Projection

The transorbital projection can be obtained with the patient's face either toward or away from the film. The patient's head is flexed on the chin until the orbitomeatal line is perpendicular to the tabletop. For better details, each side should be obtained separately, and the central X-ray beam should be directed at the center of the orbit of the side under examination and perpendicular to the film.

The petrous apex is outlined clearly but foreshortened because of its obliquity to the plane of the film. The internal auditory canal (IAC) is

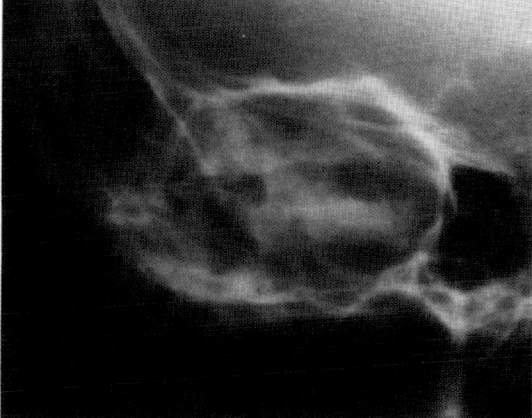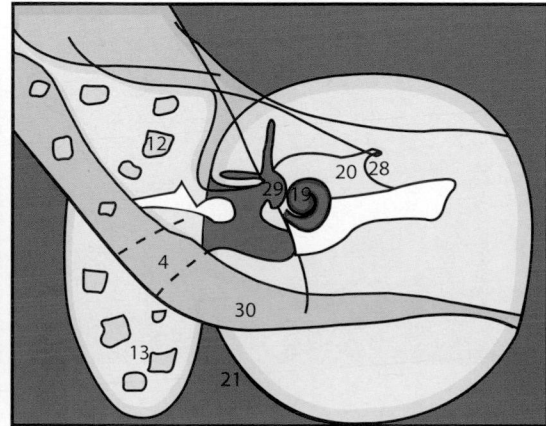

Figure 2 Transorbital projection. (4) External auditory canal, (12) air cells, (13) mastoid process, (19) cochlea, (20) internal auditory canal, (21) orbital rim, (28) medial lip of the posterior wall of the internal auditory canal, (29) vestibule, and (30) base of the skull.

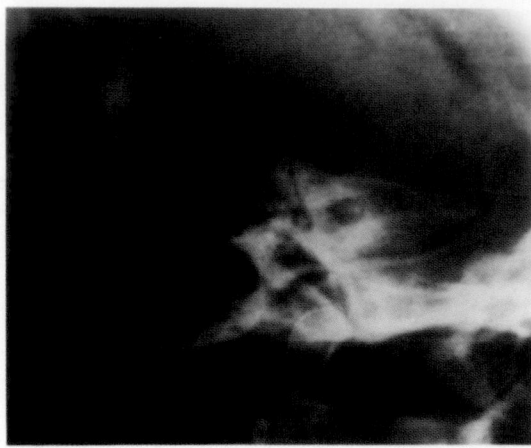
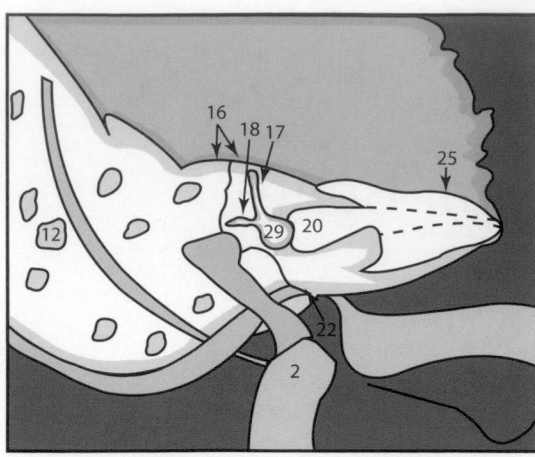

Figure 3 Stenvers projection. (2) Condyle of the mandible, (12) air cells, (16) arcuate eminence, (17) superior semicircular canal, (18) horizontal semicircular canal, (20) internal auditory canal, (22) basilar turn of the cochlea, (25) petrous apex, and (29) vestibule.

visualized in its full length as a horizontal band of radiolucency extending through the petrous pyramid (Figure 2). At the medial end of the canal, the free margin of the posterior wall casts a well-defined and smooth margin, concave medially. Often, the radiolucent band of the IAC seems to extend medially to the lip of the posterior wall into the petrous apex. This band is not caused by the IAC but is produced by the medial extension of the upper and lower lips of the porus (opening) of the canal and by the interposed groove. Lateral to the IAC, the outline (radiolucency) of the vestibule and of the superior and horizontal semicircular canals are usually detectable. The apical and middle coils of the cochlea are superimposed on the lateral portion of the IAC, whereas the basilar turn is visible underneath it and the vestibule.

Stenvers Projection

The patient is positioned facing the film, with the head slightly flexed and rotated 45° toward the side opposite the 1 under examination. The lateral rim of the orbit of the side under investigation should lie in close contact with the tabletop. The X-ray beam is angulated 14° caudad.

The entire petrous apex is visualized in its full-length lateral to the orbital rim (Figure 3). The porus of the IAC seen on face appears as an oval-shaped radiolucency open medially and limited laterally by the free margin of the posterior canal wall. Lateral to the porus, the IAC appears foreshortened. The vestibule and semicircular canals, especially the superior, which lies in this projection in a plane parallel to the film, are usually recognizable. On the outside, the entire mastoid is outlined, with the mastoid process free from superimpositions.

COMPUTED TOMOGRAPHY (CT)

CT is the imaging study of choice for the assessment of intratemporal pathology.[3–14] CT is also very good for the evaluation of retrolabyrinthine pathology; however, MRI in this respect is superior to CT scanning.[16,17,24–28] CT is a radiographic technique that allows measurement of small differentials of absorption coefficients of X-ray not recognizable to such extent by previously available recording or displaying systems.

The scan is initiated at a chosen level, and the X-ray tube, collimated to a thin or pencil beam, rotates around the patient. The transmitted X-rays are picked up by detectors arrayed along the circumference of the tube trajectory and converted into electronic current that is amplified and transmitted to the computer for storing and processing. The computer analyzes these data and develops an image on a matrix of picture element (pixel) where the brightness of each point is proportional to its attenuation coefficient.

Spatial resolution of CT is measured by the volume of tissue represented by the displayed pixel. In the later generation of multidetector CT scanners, spatial resolution has been reduced to 0.1 cu mm by a special software reconstruction technique of the area of interest. Narrowing the collimator of the X-ray beam and the aperture of each detector has reduced the slice thickness to 0.625 mm or less.

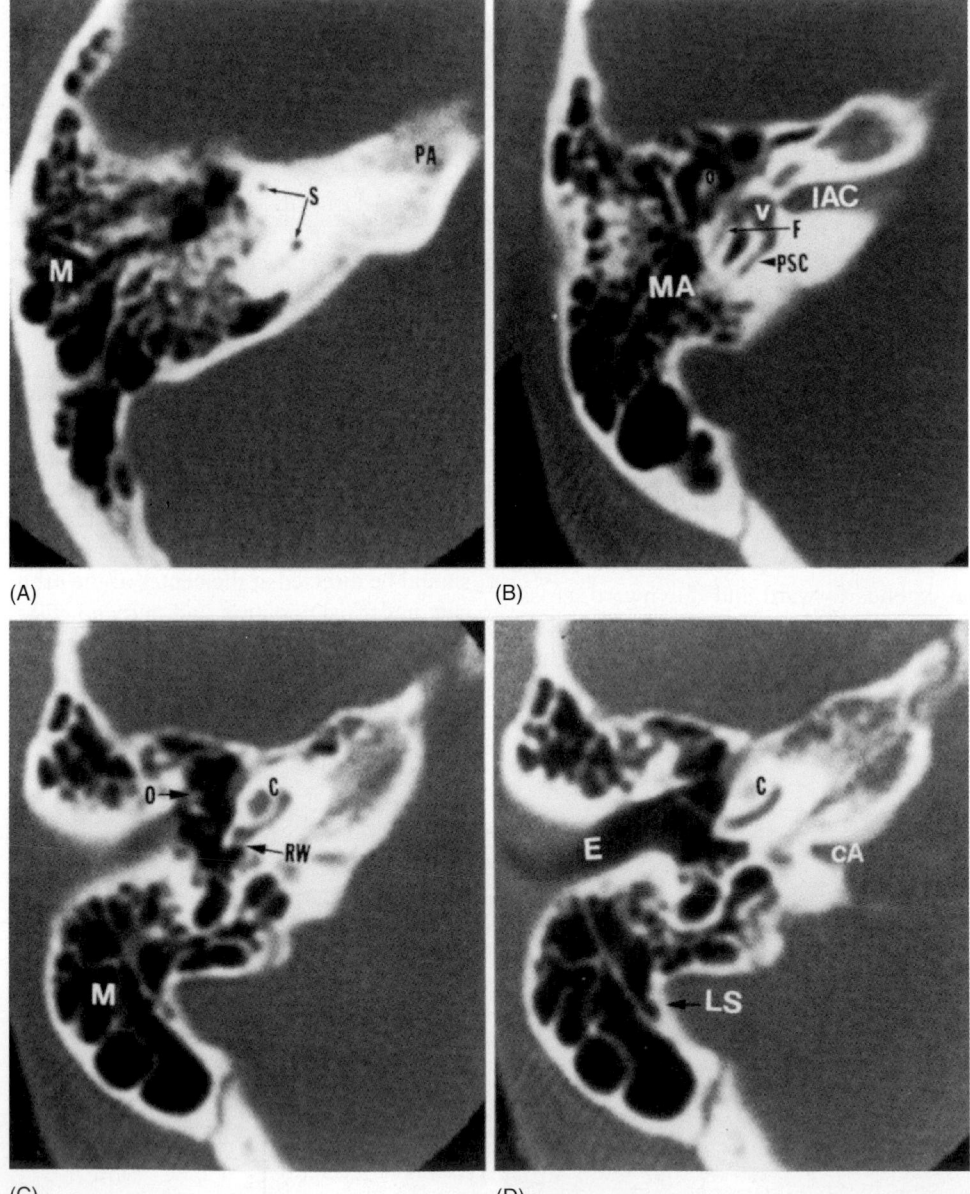

Figure 4 Horizontal computed tomographic sections of a normal right temporal bone, in sequence from top to bottom. (A) M = mastoid; PA = petrous apex; S = superior semicircular canal. (B) F = facial nerve canal; IAC = internal auditory canal; MA = mastoid antrum; O = ossicles; PSC = posterior semicircular canal; V = vestibule. (C) C = cochlea; RW = round window. (D) CA = cochlear aqueduct; E = external auditory canal; LS = lateral sinus plate.

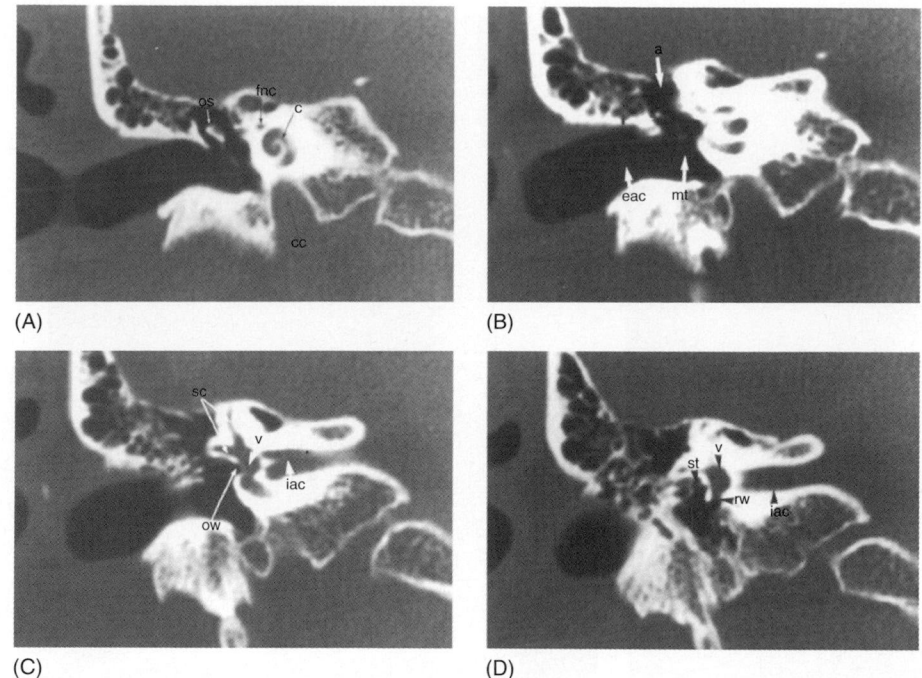

Figure 5 Coronal computed tomographic sections of a normal right temporal bone in sequence from front to back. (A) C = cochlea; CC = carotid canal; fnc = facial nerve canal; OS = ossicles. (B) a = attic; eac = external auditory canal; i = incus; mt = mesotympanum. (C) iac = internal auditory canal; OW = oval window; SC = semicircular canals; V = vestibule. (D) rw = round window; st = sinus tympani.

Enhancement of the lesion after intravenous administration of iodine-based contrast material allows the recognition of vascularity of lesions, such as a glomus tumor, and vascular structures, such as the jugular bulb and the internal carotid artery. Further differentiation of the type of lesions can be obtained by CT angiography (CTA) or by CT dynamic scanning, in which 6 or more consecutive scans of a single preselected section demonstrating the mass are obtained in a few seconds. The exposure starts simultaneously with the bolus injection of 30 to 45 mL of iodine-based contrast material. A curve, characteristic of the type of lesion, is obtained by plotting the amount of enhancement expressed in CT numbers versus time. A glomus tumor shows a high peak and rapid wash-in and wash-out phases. A schwannoma or meningioma often shows a delayed wash-out phase. Following the development of CTA, CT dynamic study is infrequently used.

CT Projections of the Temporal Bone

Horizontal or Axial Projection. This is the basic projection of the CT study. It is comfortable for the patient who lies supine on the table, and is easy to obtain and reproduce. It allows a good

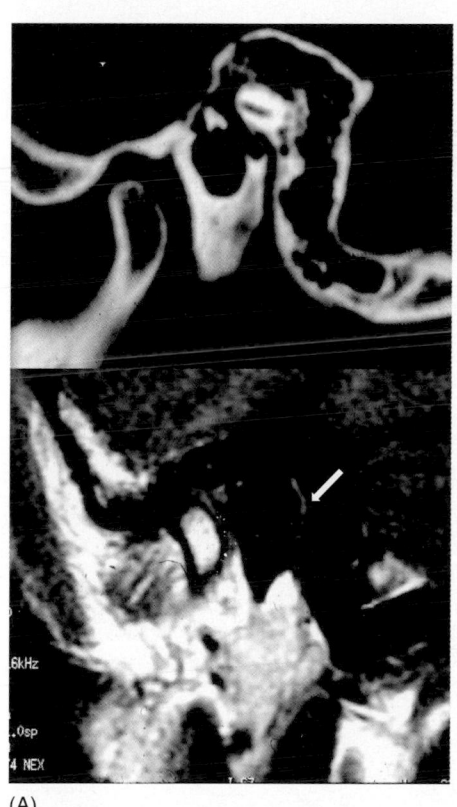

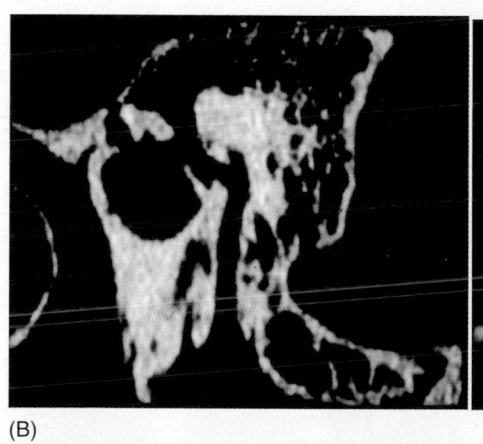

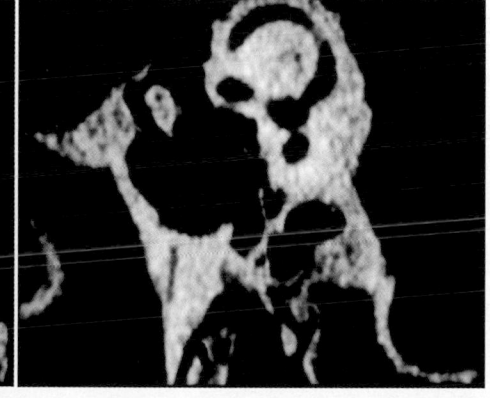

(B)

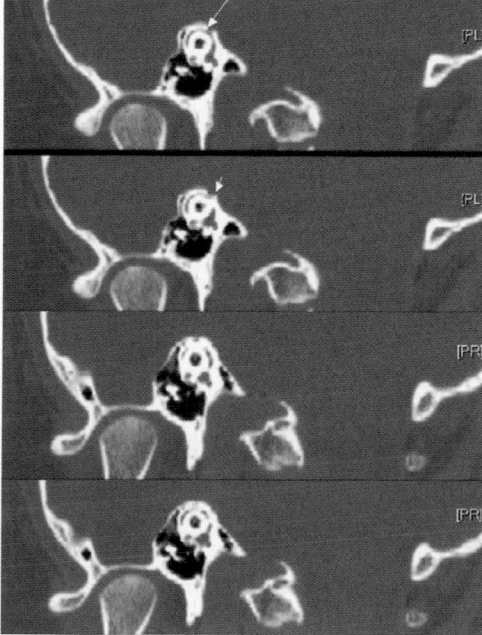

Figure 11-6. *A*, Direct sagittal CT scan (*top*), showing the TMJ, malleus, incus, lateral semicircular canal and facial canal. T$_1$-weighted sagittal MR scan (*bottom*) showing facial nerve (*long arrow*) and stapedius muscle (*short arrow*). *B*, Sagittal reformatted CT scans, showing malleus, incus, facial canal, and intact cortex of superior semicircular canal. *C*, Sagittal reformatted CT scans, showing a focal bony dehiscence of the superior semicircular canal (arrows). *D*, Sagittal reformatted CT scans showing dehiscence of superior semicircular canal (arrow). Note normal contralateral side (*bottom*).

(A)

(C)

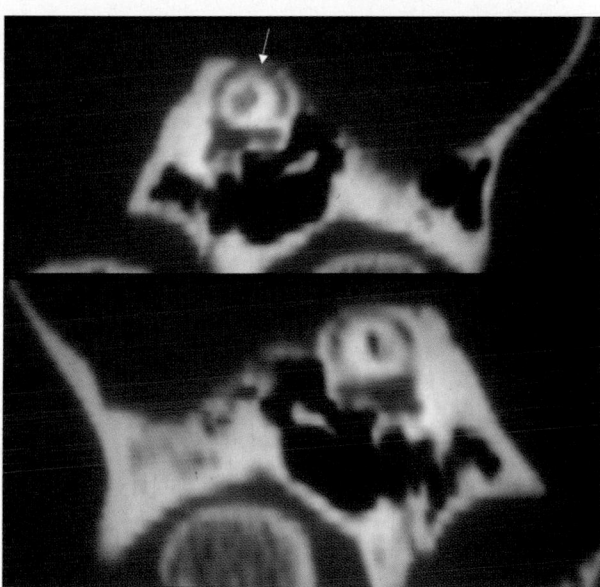

(D)

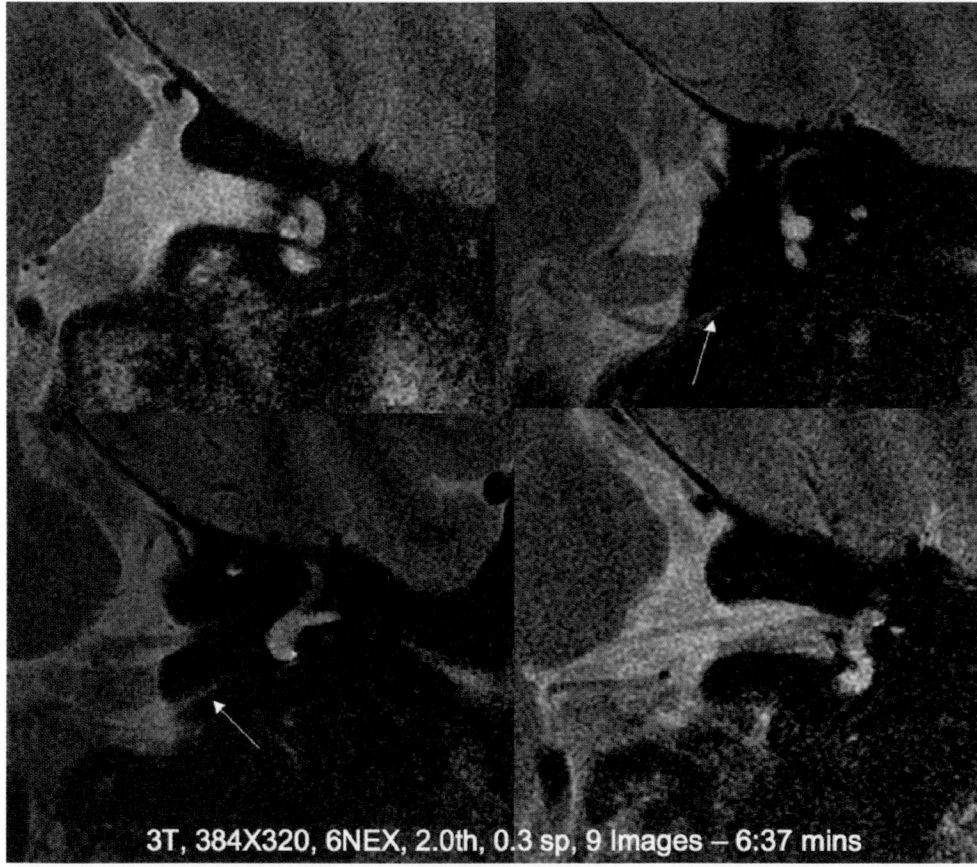

(A)

(B)

3T, 384X320, 6NEX, 2.0th, 0.3 sp, 9 Images – 6:37 mins

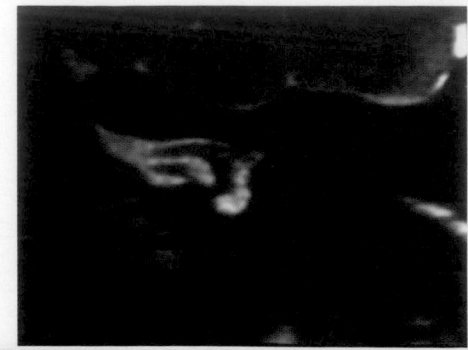

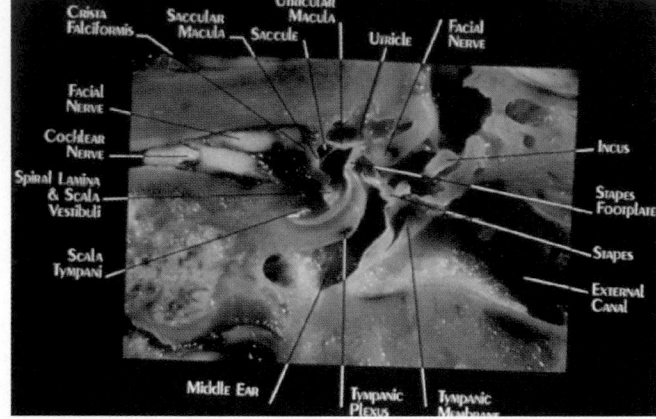

Crista Falciformis · Saccular Macula · Saccule · Utricular Macula · Utricle · Facial Nerve · Facial Nerve · Cochlear Nerve · Spiral Lamina & Scala Vestibuli · Scala Tympani · Incus · Stapes Footplate · Stapes · External Canal · Middle Ear · Tympanic Plexus · Tympanic Membrane

(C)

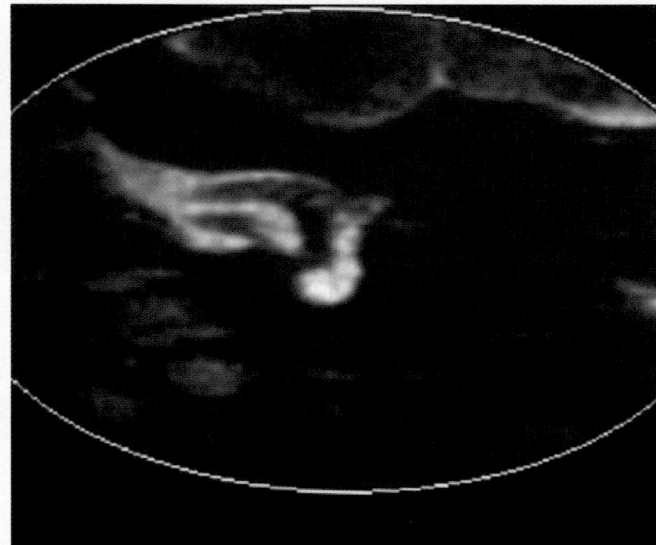

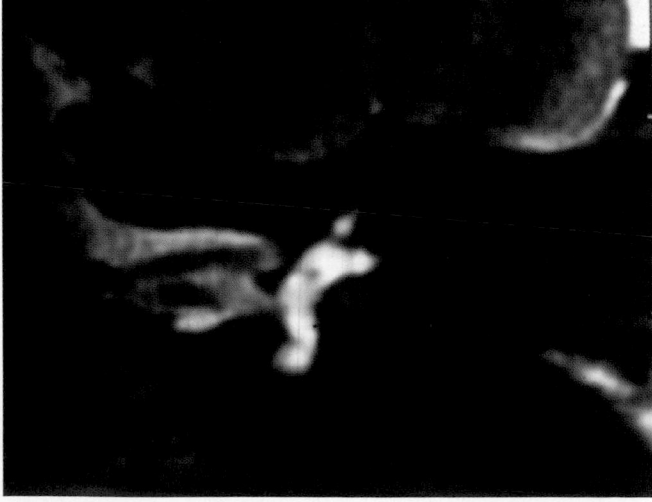

(D)

Figure 7 (A) Axial T$_2$-weighted MR scan, obtained with a 3T MR unit, showing high definition of otic labyrinth. Note scala tympani, scala vestibuli, cochlear and vestibular nerves, facial nerve, vestibule, posterior and lateral semicircular canals, common crus, and endolymphatic duct (*arrow*). (B) Coronal T$_2$-weighted MRI scans, obtained with 3T MR unit, showing otic labyrinth, cochlear, vestibular and facial nerves, and cochlear aqueduct (*arrow*). (C) Coronal T$_2$-weighted MRI scan (*top*) and coronal macrosection of temporal bone (*bottom*). Note cochlear and facial nerve on MR scan (*top*). (D) Coronal T$_2$-weighted scans showing cochlear and facial nerves (*top*) and inferior and superior vestibular nerves (*bottom*).

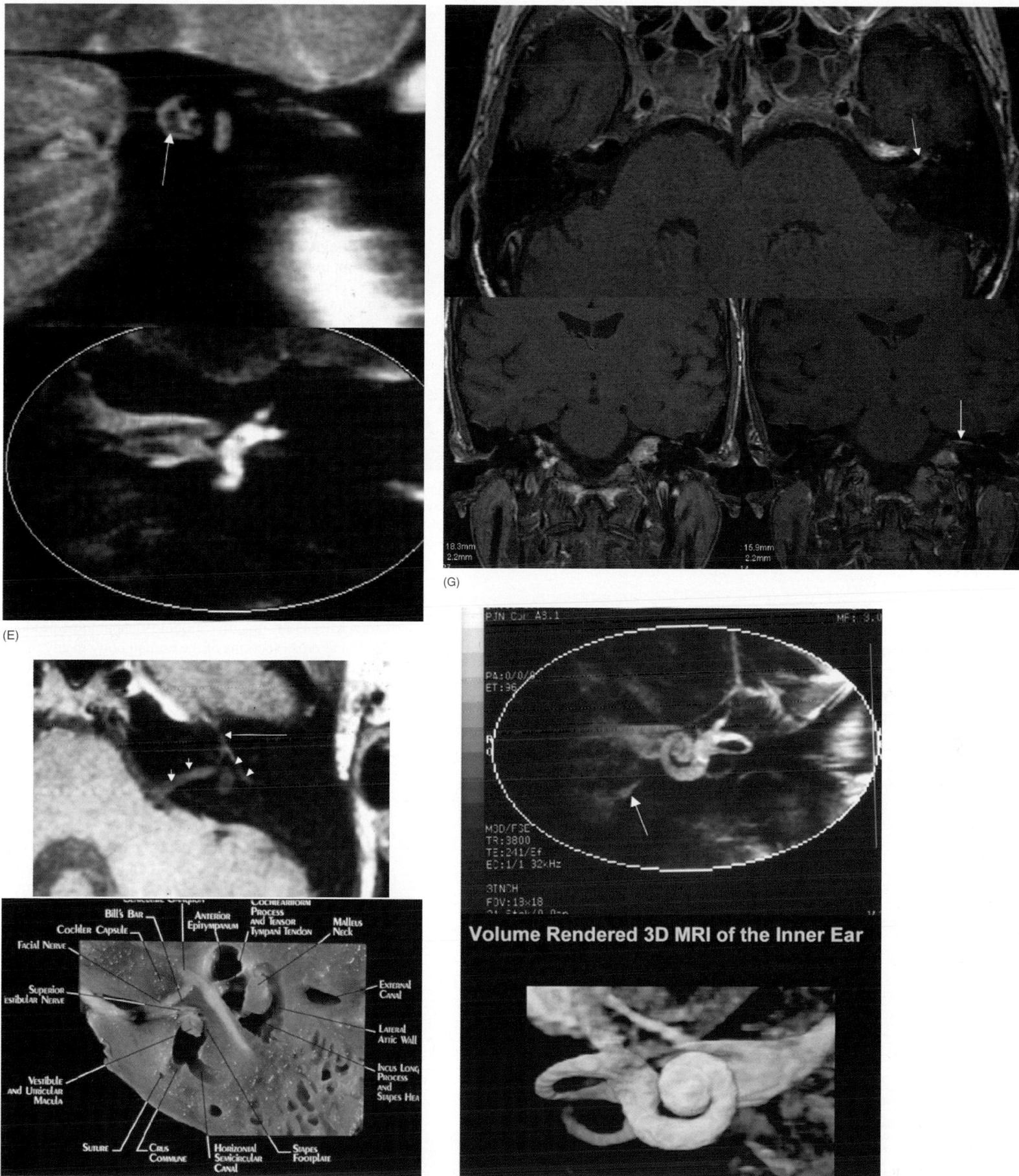

(E) Sagittal T₂-weighted MR scan of IAC (*top*) showing inferior vestibular nerve (*arrow*), superior vestibular nerve above it, cochlear nerve in anterior inferior compartment of IAC, and facial nerve above the cochlear nerve. Coronal T₂-weighted MR scan showing vestibule, ampulla of superior semicircular canal, and vestibular nerves within the IAC. (F) Axial T₁-weighted MR scan (*top*) showing facial nerve (*short arrows*), greater superficial petrosal nerve (*long arrow*), and superior vestibular nerve behind the facial nerve within the IAC. Horizontal macrosection of temporal bone, showing structures of the inner and middle ears. (G) Axial (*top*) and coronal (*bottom*) enhanced T1-weighted MR scans showing facial nerves. Note abnormal enhancement on the left (*arrows*) in this patient with viral neuronitis of facial nerve. (H) Maximum intensity projection (MIP) 3D MRI of normal inner ear (*top*) and volume rendered 3D MRI of the normal inner ear. Note cochlear aqueduct (*arrow*).

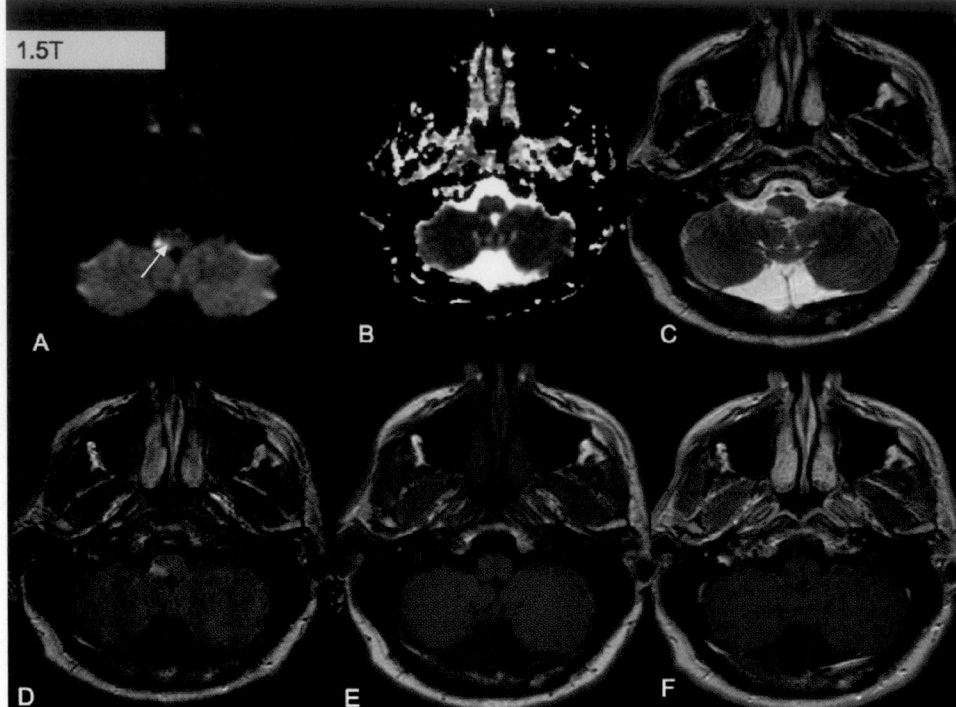

Figure 8 Acute infarct involving cochlear nuclei axial DWI (A), ADC map (B), T_2-weighted (C), flair (D), unenhanced T_1-weighted (E), and enhanced T_1-weighted (F) showing an acute infarct involving the right inferior cerebellar peduncle (*arrow*), where the ventral and dorsal nuclei of cochlear nerve are located. This few days-old infarct is best depicted on DW1 (*arrow*).

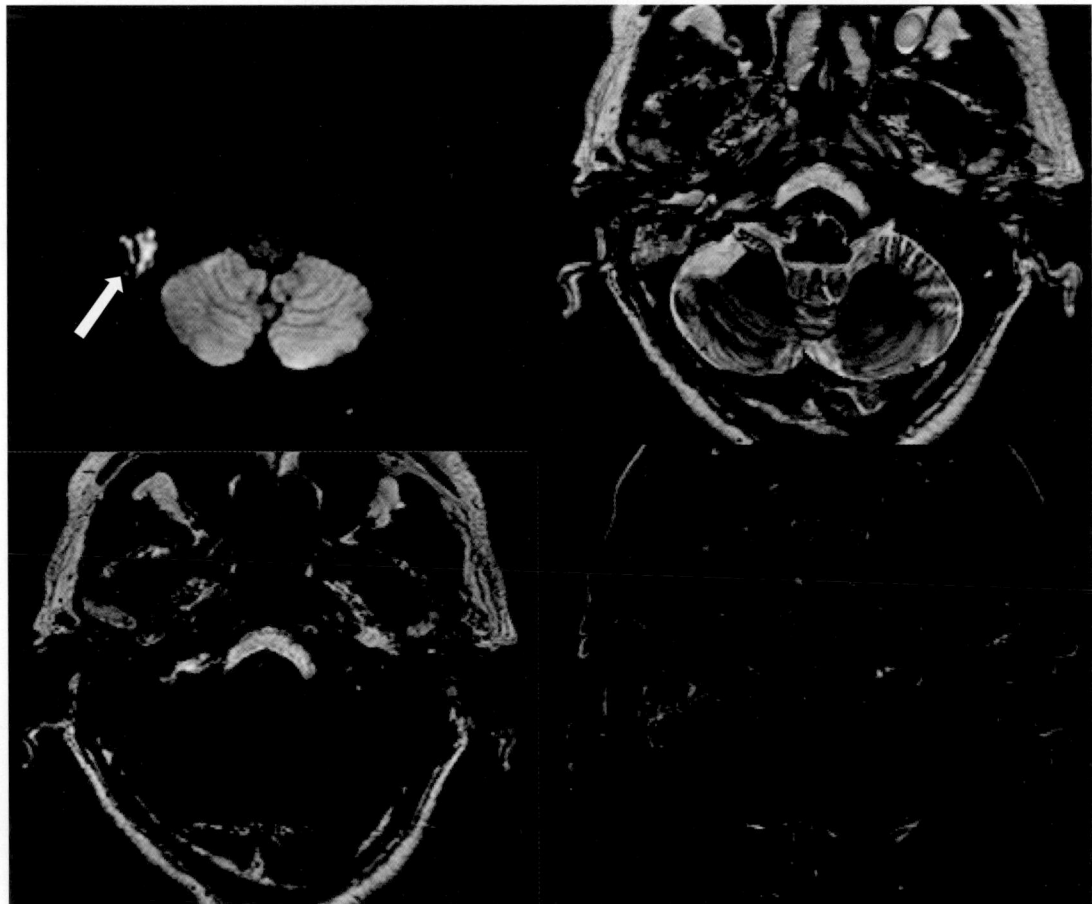

Figure 9 Acute otomastoiditis with antral abscess. Axial DWI (*top left*), T_2-weighted (*top right*), unenhanced T_1-weighted (*bottom left*), and enhanced T_1-weighted (*bottom right*) MR scans showing an antral abscess (*arrow*) in this patient with coalescent mastoiditis. The abscess is hyperintense on DWI (*arrow*) and shows no enhancement on enhanced T_1-weighted MR scan. Note enhancement of granulation tissue around abscess cavity.

demonstration of the external, middle, and inner ear (Figure 4), except for the structures parallel to the plane of section, such as the tegmen.

Coronal or Frontal Projection. The patient lies on the table, either prone or supine, with the head extended. The gantry of the scanner is often tilted to compensate for an incomplete extension of the head. This projection is indispensable to complement the axial sections (Figure 5) but often difficult to obtain, particularly in young children and older patients.

Sagittal or Lateral Projection. It is impossible or extremely difficult to obtain direct sagittal sections.[8] However, computer-reconstructed sagittal images can be obtained from the raw data collected for the horizontal sections. This is particularly true if fast or spiral CT is used, and thin sections at 1 to 0.625 mm increments are obtained. Although these images are not as satisfactory as the direct sections, they are always sufficient for the demonstration of the mastoid segment of the facial canal, the vestibular aqueduct, cortical outline of superior semicircular canal (Figure 6), other parts of otic labyrinth, carotid canal, jugular fossa, external auditory canal (EAC), and TMJ.

MAGNETIC RESONANCE IMAGING (MRI)

MRI is an imaging modality capable of producing cross sections of the human body in any plane without exposing the patient to ionizing radiation. MR images are obtained by the interaction of hydrogen nuclei (protons) of the human body with a high static magnetic field and radio frequency pulses. The strength of the MR signal to be converted into imaging data depends on the concentration of the free hydrogen nuclei or protons and on 2 magnetic relaxation times, T1 and T2, which are tissue specific. One of the characteristics of MR is the possibility of changing appearance and therefore information of the images by changing the contribution of the T1 and T2 relaxation times. This is accomplished by varying the time between successive pulses (TR or repetition time) and the time that the emitted signal or echo is measured after the pulse (TE or echo time).

Examination is performed with the patient supine and the plane extending from the tragus to the inferior orbital rim perpendicular to the tabletop. Different projections (views) are obtained by changing the orientation of the magnetic field gradients without moving the patient's head. Axial, coronal, and sagittal projections are usually obtained.

T1-weighted (T1W) images obtained by a short TR (400 to 1,000 ms) and TE (20 to 30 ms) offer the best anatomical delineation. T2-weighted (T2W) images obtained with long TR (1,500 to 4,000 ms) and TE (80 to 120 ms) better differentiate normal from pathologic tissues. Proton-weighted (PD) or spin-density-weighted MR images are obtained with long TR (1,500 to 4,000 ms) and short TE (20 to 30 ms). PD images are a kind of balanced

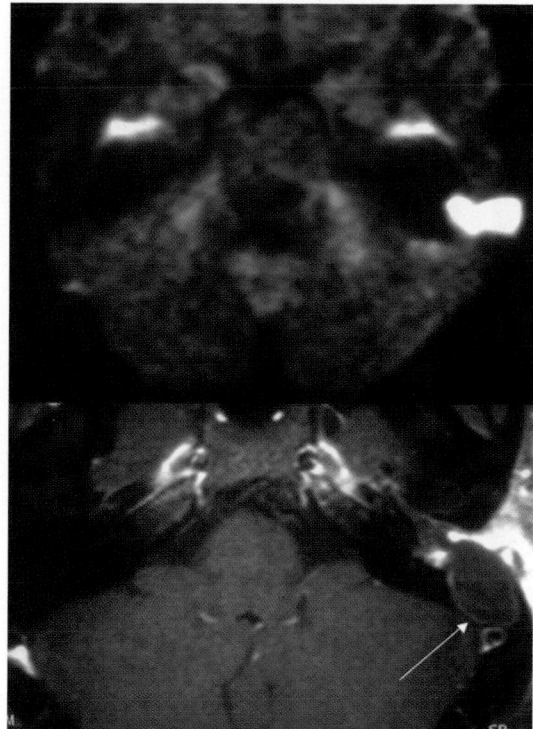

Figure 10 Cholesteatoma. Axial DW1 (*top*) and enhanced axial T₁-weighted (*bottom*) MR scans showing a large cholesteatoma (*arrow*). Note that cholesteatoma appears hyperintense on DWI.

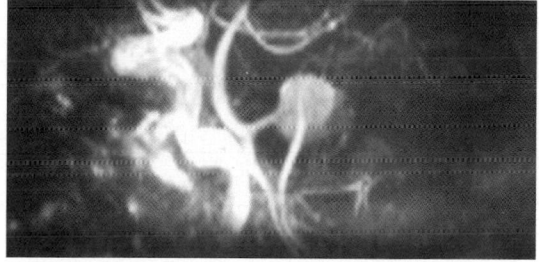

Figure 11 Magnetic resonance angiography demonstrating an aneurysm (A) of the left vertebral artery. The aneurysm may compress the acoustic nerve and mimics acoustic neurinoma.

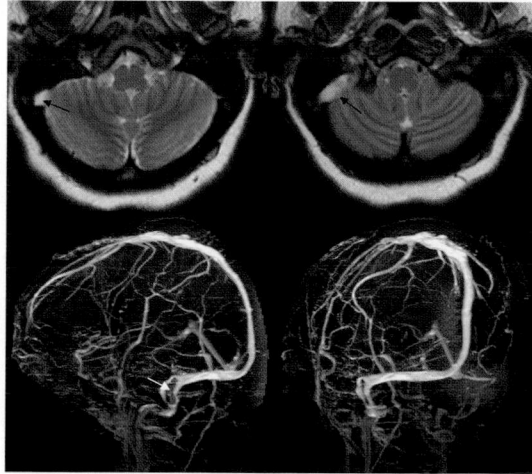

Figure 12 Thrombosis of sigmoid sinus. Axial T₂-weighted MR scans (*top*) showing hyperintensity of the sigmoid sinus (*arrow*) due to thrombosis. Sagittal MRV scans (*bottom*) showing the thrombus (*arrow*).

images between T1W and T2W MR images, not frequently used in routine MR studies.

Air, cortical bone, and calcifications contain few free protons and therefore appear in the images as dark areas of no signal. Fat and body fluid are rich in free protons and produce signals to be detected. Tissues with short T1 relaxation time such as fat appear hyperintense (bright) on T1W and hypointense (dark) on T2W spin-echo (SE) MR images. Water and tissues with long T1 and T2 relaxation times, such as cerebrospinal fluid and vitreous, appear hypointense on TIW and hyperintense on T2W SE pulse sequences.

Fast-moving blood in arterial vessels usually appear as areas of signal void (dark) because the stimulated protons of the circulating blood have moved out of the selected section before their emitted signals can be detected. Because cortical or nondiploic bone and air emit no signal, the normal mastoid, EAC, and middle ear appear in the MR images as dark areas without pattern or structures within them. At times malleus and incus can be recognized because of their bone marrow. The petrous pyramid is equally dark except for a gray or white cast of the inner ear structures and IAC, produced by the fluid within their lumens (Figure 7). The marrow of petrous apex appears hyperintense on T1W MR images.

Pathologic processes are demonstrated by MRI whenever the hydrogen density and relaxation times of the pathological tissues are different from the normal. The T1 and in particular T2 relaxation times of pathologic tissue will be longer than those of normal tissue. The intravenous injection of paramagnetic contrast agents (gadolinium DPTA (diethylenetriaminepentaacetic acid) and gadolinium chelate) has improved the recognition and differentiation of pathological processes. Because the contrast material does not penetrate the intact blood–brain barrier, normal brain does not enhance except for structures such as the stalk of pituitary gland and choroid plexus that lack a complete blood–brain barrier. Enhancement of brain lesions occurs whenever the blood–brain barrier is disrupted, provided there is sufficient blood flow to the lesions. Extra-axial lesions such as meningiomas, neurofibromas, and schwannomas as well as most intra-axial lesions cause disturbance of the blood–brain barrier and therefore undergo a moderate to marked enhancement.

Diffusion-Weighted Imaging (DWI)

Diffusion is a process in which molecules are mixing together via the action of random collisions (the so-called Brownian motion) among themselves and with other molecules or structures such as cell membrane. When the diffusion process is the same in all directions, it is called isotropic diffusion. When the diffusion process is not appearing the same in all directions (*x*, *y*, and *z*), it is referred to as anisotropic diffusion. The apparent diffusion coefficient (ADC) is a diffusion coefficient that is determined by displacement of diffusion along a particular direction.

DWI is a new powerful pulse sequence which is obtained using an SE pulse sequence that has been modified by using diffusion sensitizing gradients. DWI is able to detect an ischemic region of the brain within seconds/minutes following the onset of a stroke. A superacute infarct appears hyperintense on DWI and hypointense on ADC, reflecting marked diffusion restriction of water molecules in infracted brain (Figure 8). DWI has been found to be very useful in the MRI diagnosis of other lesions besides brain ischemia. Intracranial and extracranial abscesses (Figure 9), cholesteatomas (epidermoids), lymphoma, medulloblastoma, esthesioblastoma, and some other lesions may demonstrate restriction on DWI, appearing hyperintense on DWI scans and hypointense on ADC scans (Figure 10).

Fluid, blood, and soft tissue masses within the temporal bone are identified readily with MRI as areas of abnormal intensity. The exact location, extent, and involvement of bony structures such as the ossicles, scutum, and labyrinthine capsule cannot be detected, however. For this reason, CT remains the study of choice for the assessment of middle ear, otic capsule, and intratemporal bony pathology.

The images shown in this chapter were obtained with a superconducting magnet and a magnetic field of 15,000 gauss or 1.5 tesla (T). Some of the MR images have been obtained with a 3T MR unit. The higher the magnetic field, the higher the signal-to-noise ratio, and therefore, the thinner the sections can be obtained. A further improvement in details has been accomplished for structures close to the surface of the body by the use of surface receiver coils.

Magnetic Resonance Angiography (MRA)

Gradient-echo (GE) techniques and flow-encoding gradients have enabled the development of MRA. Time-of-flight (TOF) angiography is a GE technique in which the stationary tissues within the imaging plane are saturated with the radiofrequency pulses so that they will not produce a signal.[24] Blood flowing within the same plane is unsaturated and will be the only tissue to produce a signal. Three-dimensional (3D) TOF MRA is used for intracranial angiography, and 2-dimensional (2D) TOF MRA is used for cervical angiography. 2D-TOF is used for intracranial MR venography.

Phase-contrast (PC) angiography is acquired differently. Instead of saturating the stationary tissues with radiofrequency pulses, a bipolar gradient of magnetization is applied to the entire slice, first with a positive value and then with a negative value. In the stationary tissues, the 2 opposite gradients cancel each other out. In the flowing blood, however, the 2 opposite gradients cannot cancel out each other because the blood will have moved to a different plane in the region before the inverse gradient is applied.

The obtained slices are reconstructed into projection images, which can be rotated in different planes to separate vessels and eliminate superimposition. MRA of the intracranial

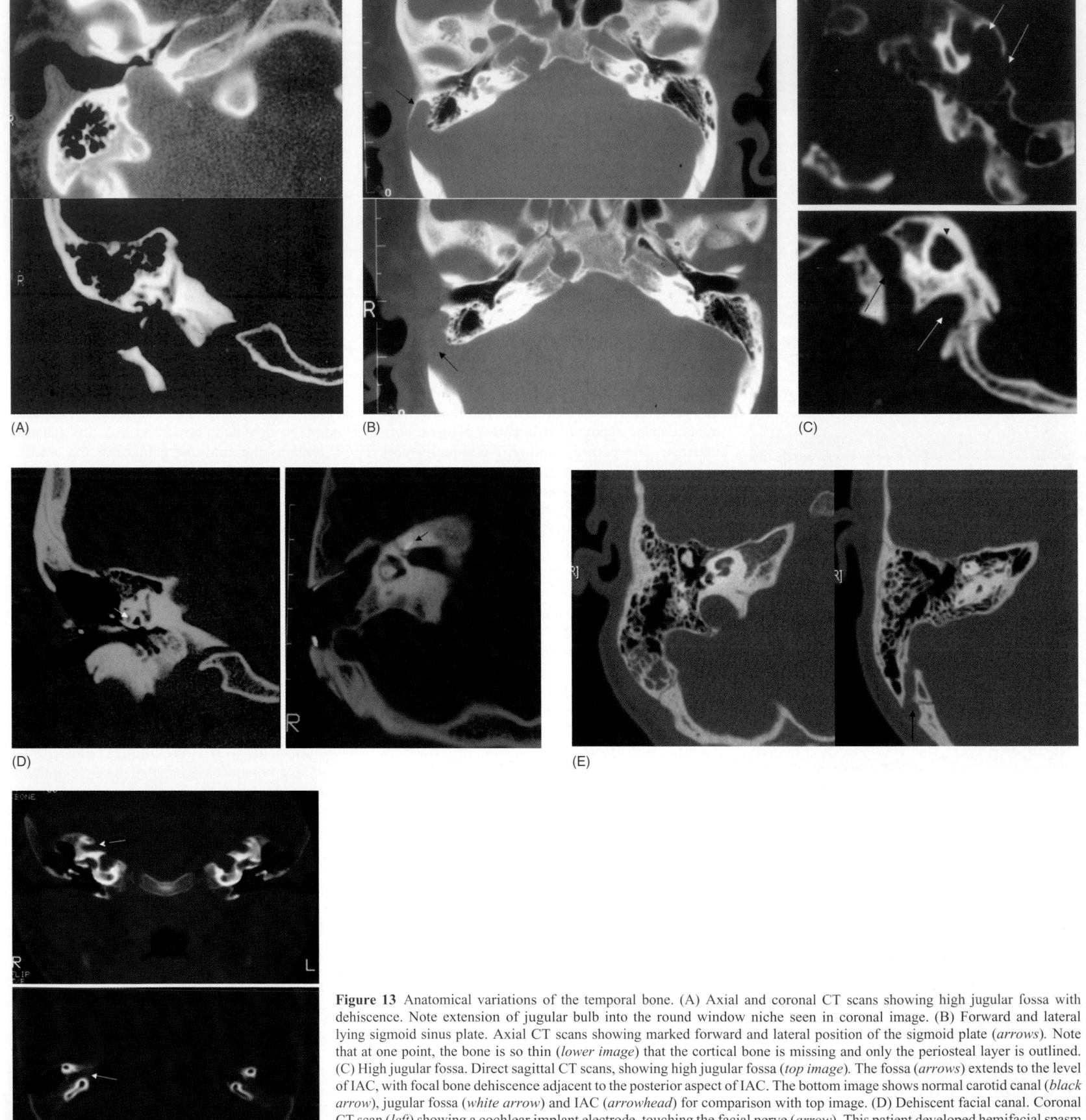

(A)

(B)

(C)

(D)

(E)

(F)

Figure 13 Anatomical variations of the temporal bone. (A) Axial and coronal CT scans showing high jugular fossa with dehiscence. Note extension of jugular bulb into the round window niche seen in coronal image. (B) Forward and lateral lying sigmoid sinus plate. Axial CT scans showing marked forward and lateral position of the sigmoid plate (*arrows*). Note that at one point, the bone is so thin (*lower image*) that the cortical bone is missing and only the periosteal layer is outlined. (C) High jugular fossa. Direct sagittal CT scans, showing high jugular fossa (*top image*). The fossa (*arrows*) extends to the level of IAC, with focal bone dehiscence adjacent to the posterior aspect of IAC. The bottom image shows normal carotid canal (*black arrow*), jugular fossa (*white arrow*) and IAC (*arrowhead*) for comparison with top image. (D) Dehiscent facial canal. Coronal CT scan (*left*) showing a cochlear implant electrode, touching the facial nerve (*arrow*). This patient developed hemifacial spasm following activation of the implant. Axial CT scan (*right*) showing a cochlear implant (*arrow*) adjacent to the labyrinthine segment of the facial canal. This patient also developed facial dysfunction following activation of the electrode. (E) Large emissary mastoid canal. Axial CT scans showing congenital deformity of the malleus and incus and a prominent mastoid emissary canal (*arrow*). (F) Large petromastoid (subarcuate) canal. Coronal (*top*) and axial (*bottom*) CT scans of an infant, showing a large petromastoid canal (*arrows*). The enlarged canal gives the appearance of pseudodouble IAC.

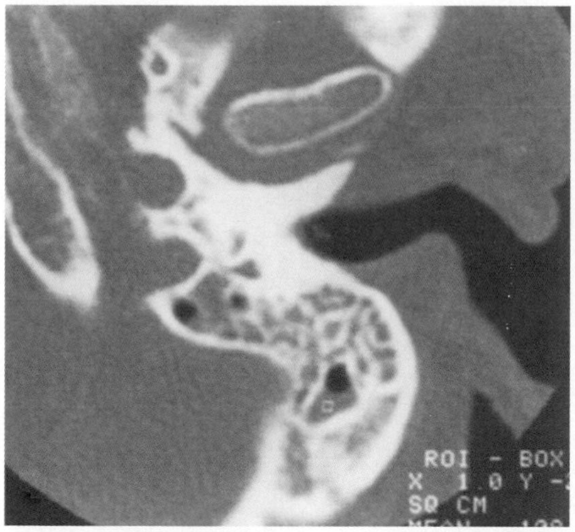

(A)

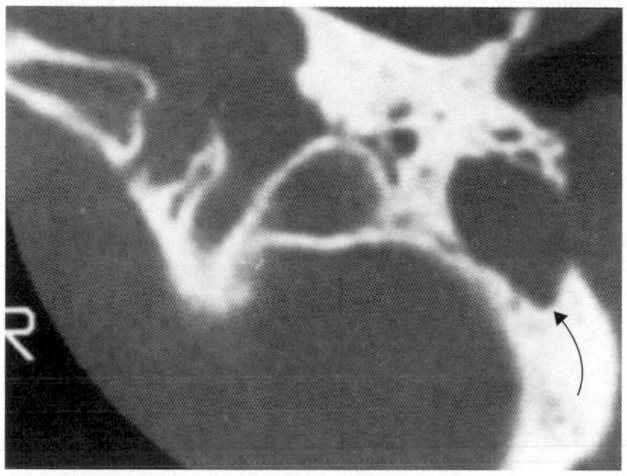

(B)

Figure 14 (A) Acute mastoiditis. This axial computed tomographic (CT) section of the left mastoid shows clouding and air-fluid levels within the air cells. The trabecular pattern is intact. (B) Coalescent mastoiditis, axial CT section of the left mastoid. A large coalescent cavity is noticed in the mastoid (arrows) with erosion of the outer cortex and formation of a subperiosteal abscess.

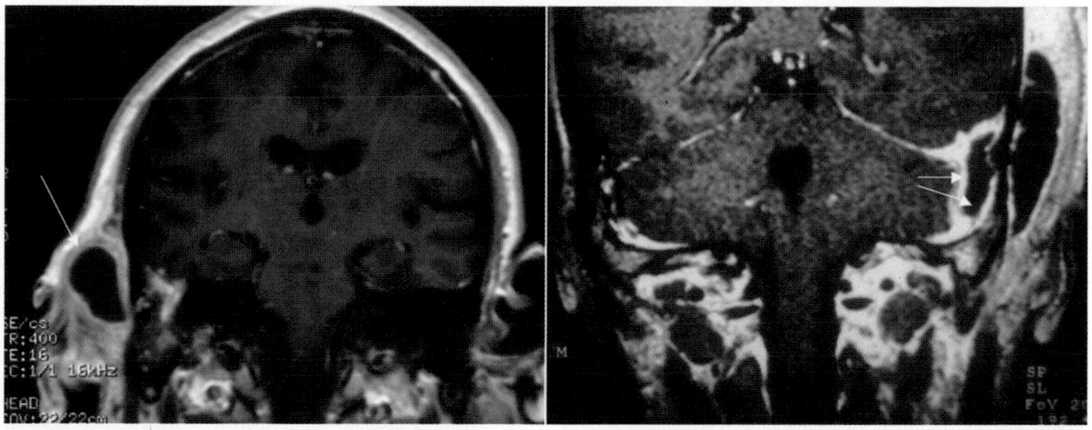

(A)

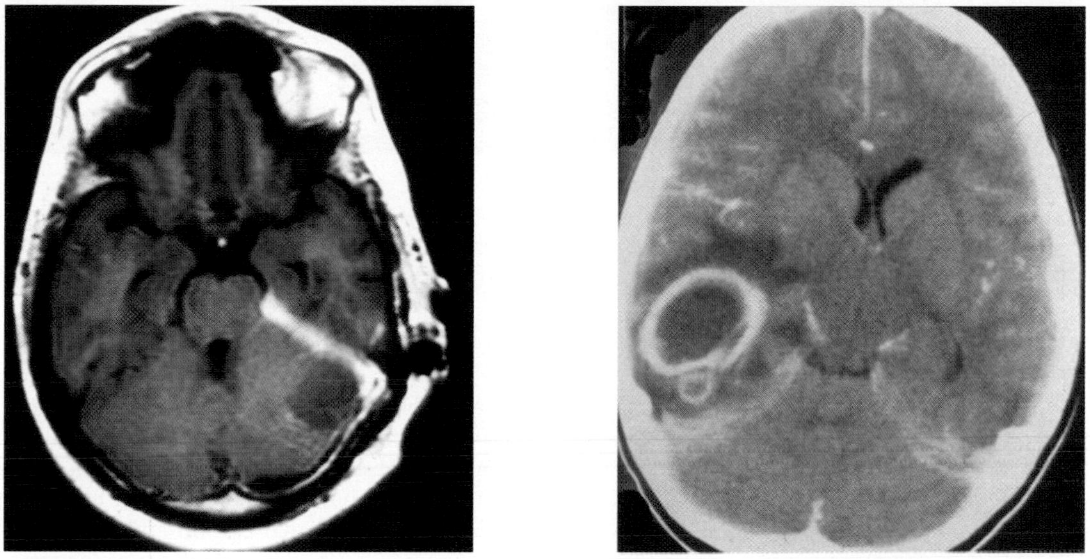

(B)

Figure 15 (A) Otogenic perisinus (sigmoid) abscess. Enhanced coronal T_1-weighted MR scans showing a large mastoid abscess (*single arrow*) and a large perisinus abscess (*double arrows*) in another patient. Note also a mastoid subperiosteal abscess in the patient with perisinus abscess. (B) Otogenic cerebellar and temporal lobe abscesses are enhanced. Enhanced T1W MR (left) CT scan (right) showing cerebellar and temporal lobe abscesses in two different patients.

vasculature has been particularly useful in the demonstration of intracranial vascular anatomy and pathology such as vascular stenosis, aneurysms in the region of the circle of Willis (Figure 11), and arteriovenous malformation (AVM), for example, dural AVM that may not be visible on routine SE images. Magnetic resonance venography (MRV) is essential to show dural sinus thrombosis (Figure 12). MRA of the extracranial circulation provides excellent information about the patency of the carotid and vertebral arteries. These vessels may be compressed or displaced by neck masses and their lumens stenosed or obstructed by thrombosis, dissection, or atheromatous plaques.

Conventional angiography is seldom required for the diagnosis of vascular tumors or anomalies within or adjacent to the temporal bone. Arteriography is, however, mandatory for identifying the feeding vessels of lesions, usually glomus tumors, whenever embolization or surgical ligation is contemplated. Subtraction is necessary to delineate the vascular mass and feeding vessels, which are otherwise obscured by the density of the surrounding temporal bone. The

injection should be performed in the common carotid artery to visualize both internal and external carotid circulation. Selective external carotid and vertebral injections are often performed to evaluate the tumor's feeding vessels and the anatomy of collateral circulation if embolization is planned.

Retrograde jugular venography is no longer used for the diagnosis of a high jugular bulb or its occlusion by a mass. 2-D TOF MRV and contrast-enhanced SPGR (spoiled gradient-recalled) imaging and pulse sequence venography are excellent to evaluate dural sinus and jugular bulb (Figure 12).

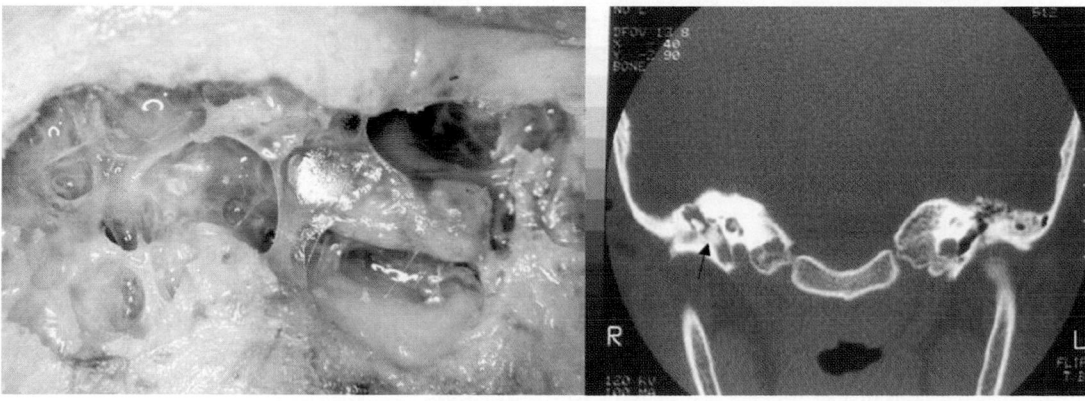

Figure 16 Chronic adhesive otomastoiditis. Macroscopic tissue section and coronal CT scan of a different patient with chronic otomastoiditis. Note contracted middle ear due to scarring, sclerotic malleus, and a large calcification (*arrow*) in the mesotympanum due to tympanosclerosis.

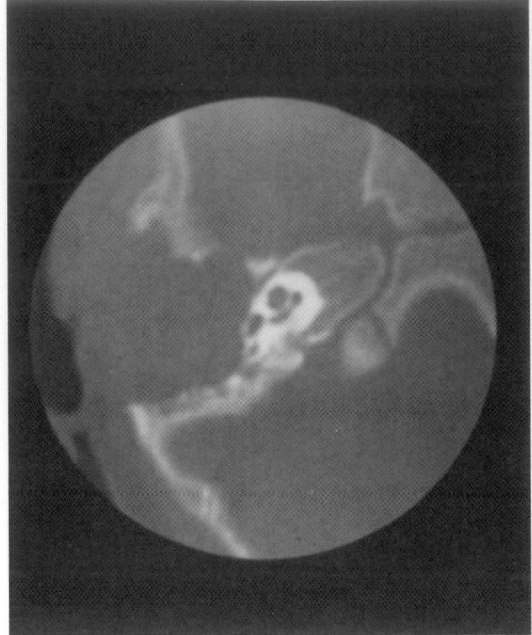

(A)

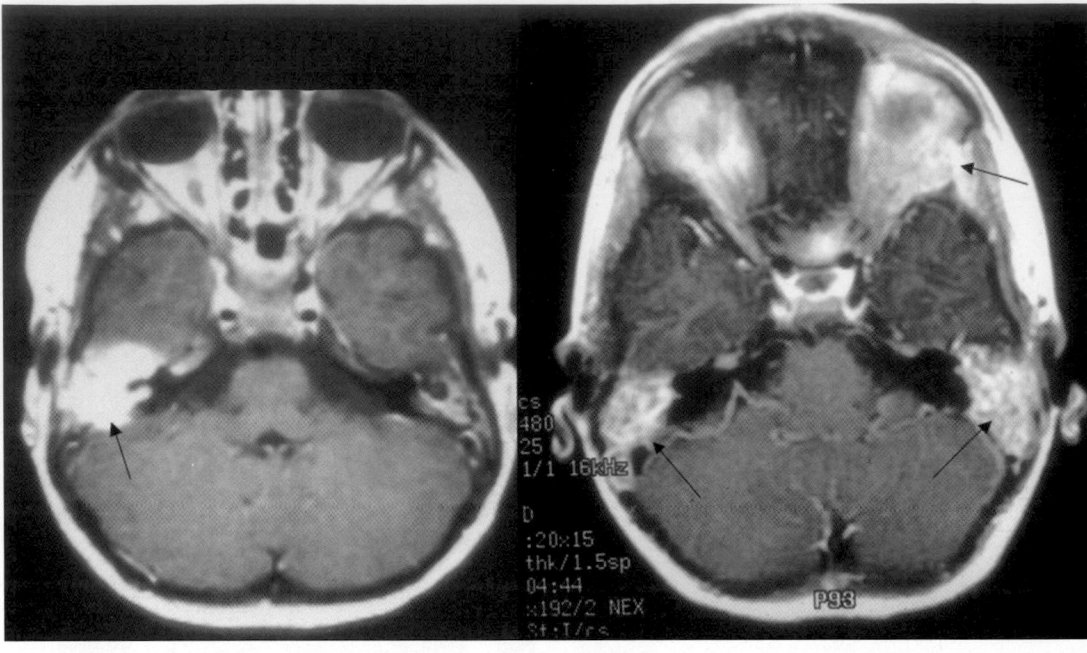

(B)

Figure 17 (A) Eosinophilic granuloma, axial computed tomographic section of the right ear. A large lytic lesion involves the right mastoid, external auditory canal, and middle ear. A soft tissue mass fills the cavity. (B) Langerhans cell histiocytosis and rhabdomyosarcoma. Enhanced axial T_1-weighted MR scans showing an enhancing rhabdomyosarcoma of right temporal bone (*arrow*) and bilateral enhancing Langerhans cell histiocytosis (*arrow*) in another patient. Note also involvement of lateral orbit (*upper arrow*) in patient with histiocytosis.

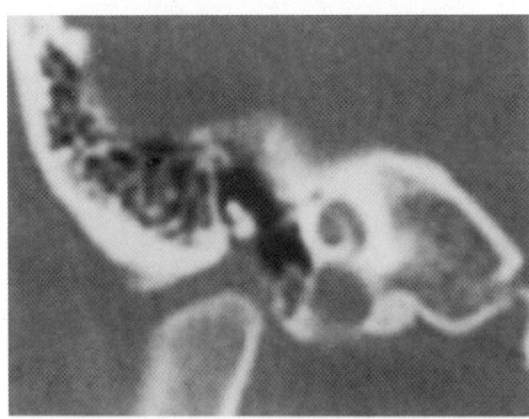

(A)

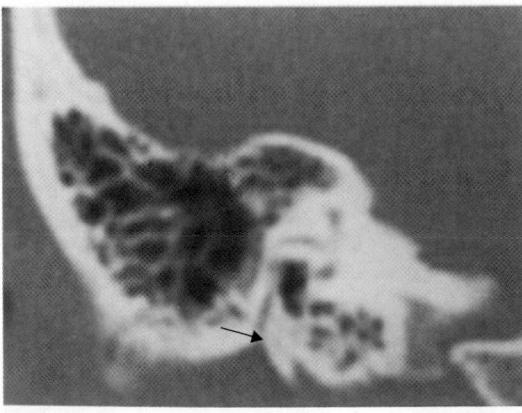

(B)

Figure 18 Agenesis of the right external auditory canal, coronal computed tomographic sections. (A) The external auditory canal is absent and the mandibular condyle is displaced posteriorly and lies lateral to the atretic plate. The middle ear cavity is aerated and near normal in size, but the head of the malleusz and body of the incus appear malformed and fused. (B) The mastoid is well pneumatized and clear. The vertical segment of the facial canal is rotated slightly outward (arrow).

ANATOMICAL VARIATIONS

Recognition of anatomical variation of the temporal bone is important. These include the forward-lying sigmoid sinus plate, dehiscent jugular dome with the jugular bulb protruding into the hypotympanum, ectopic internal carotid artery coursing into the middle ear, aberrant course of the internal carotid artery, dehiscent facial canal, enlarged subarcuate (petromastoid) canal, prominent Hyrtl fissure, prominent groove for superior petrosal vein, dehiscence of the tegmen tympani and antri, and widened geniculate fossa (Figure 13A–F). In aberrant course of the internal carotid artery, the absence of vertical segment of the internal carotid artery results in the lateral coursing of the artery. The vertical petrous portion is represented by the enlarged inferior tympanic artery. A persistent stapedial artery may be found in patients with an aberrant internal carotid artery. The persistent stapedial artery on its way to become the middle meningeal artery results in enlargement of the proximal portion of the tympanic segment of the facial canal. In these patients, the foramen spinosum through which the middle meningeal artery passes may be absent.

PATHOLOGIC CONDITIONS

The pathologic conditions of the ear and temporal bone will be reviewed by anatomic location. Seven sites of involvement are considered: mastoid, EAC, middle ear, inner ear, petrous pyramid, facial nerve canal, and cerebellopontine angle region.

Mastoid

Conventional views, and CT, and MRI are used for the study of this region.

Acute Mastoiditis. The early findings of acute mastoiditis are diffuse and homogeneous clouding of the middle ear cavity and mastoid air cells, and often air-fluid levels within the air cells (Figure 14A). With the progression of the process, the mastoid trabeculae become first demineralized and then destroyed, with formation of coalescent areas of suppuration and subperiosteal abscess over the outer cortex of mastoid (Figure 14B). Involvement of the posterior sinus plate often leads to thrombophlebitis of the sigmoid or lateral sinus and to perisinus as well as posterior fossa abscesses (Figure 15), whereas erosion of the tegmen may lead to extension of the infection into the middle cranial fossa.

Chronic Mastoiditis. The mastoid is often poorly pneumatized, and the mastoid antrum and mastoid air cells appear nonhomogeneously cloudy. Reactive mucosal thickening and new bony formation produces thickening of the trabeculae (Figure 16), which may lead to complete obliteration of the air cells (sclerotic mastoiditis).[6]

Eosinophilic Granuloma (Langerhans Cell Histiocytosis). Lytic lesions of variable size are observed in the mastoid, petrous, external ear, and temporal squama in eosinophilic granuloma. In the involved areas, the trabecular pattern is partially or completely erased and the mastoid cortex may be thinned out, destroyed, or expanded (Figure 17).[2]

External Auditory Canal (EAC)

CT is the study of choice for the evaluation of EAC, but MRI may add useful information whenever the lesion extends outside the confines of the canal into the adjacent structures (Figures 18–22).

Congenital Malformations. Microtia and atresia of varying degrees are often associated with

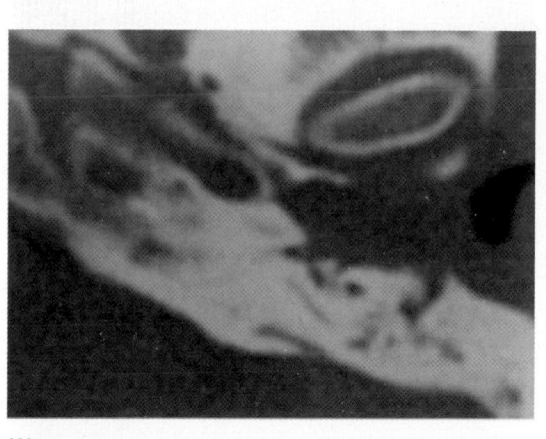

(A)

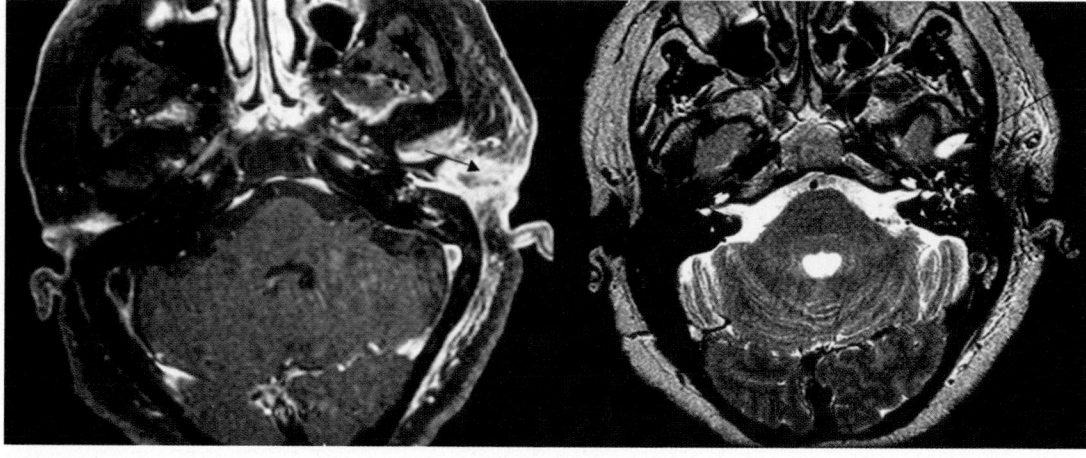

(B)

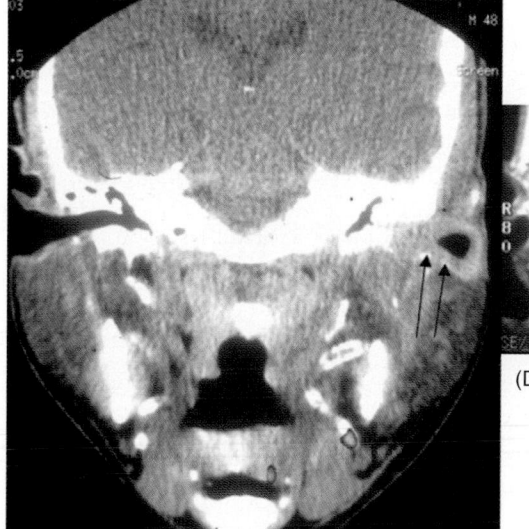

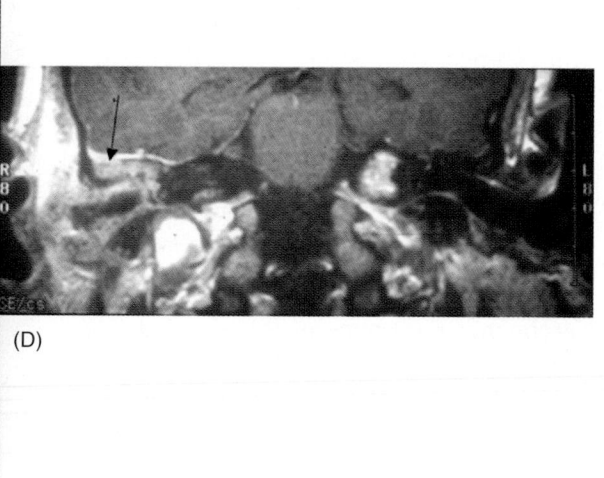

(D)

(C)

Figure 19 (A) Necrotizing external otitis. Axial computed tomographic section of the left ear. There is erosion of the anterior wall of the external auditory canal with stenosis of the lumen of the canal caused by soft tissue swelling. The infection has spread into the middle ear. (B) Necrotizing external otitis. Axial enhanced T_1-weighted (*left*) and T_2-weighted (*right*) scans showing marked enhancement of tissue around left external auditory canal (*arrow*). Note fluid in the TM joint, depicted on T_2-weighted image (*arrow*). (C) Necrotizing external otitis and carcinoma of left EAC. Coronal enhanced CT scan showing increased thickening and enhancement (*double arrows*) in this patient with necrotizing external otitis. Note extension of disease along the adjacent fascial planes and base of skull. (D) Coronal enhanced T_1-weighted MR scan in another patient with carcinoma of right EAC. Note increased soft tissue thickening and enhancement similar to necrotizing external otitis. Note extension of carcinoma along dura (*arrow*).

dysplasia of the EAC. The degree of malformation of the EAC varies from complete agenesis of the tympanic bone (Figure 18) and EAC to stenosis of its lumen and atresia (atretic bony plate) of an otherwise well-developed EAC. The malleus

may be fused to the atretic plate. The small tissue tag and pit frequently observed in patients with atresia of the EAC often have no topographic relationship to the underlying mastoid and middle ear.

Trauma. Fractures of the EAC are the result of a longitudinal fracture of the temporal bone, direct trauma to the anterior wall after a blow to the mandible, or projectile missiles such as bullets or metallic fragments from industrial accidents. Longitudinal fractures usually pass from the temporal squama into the superior canal wall.[2,15] The fracture often extends to the anterior canal wall and TMJ.

Necrotizing External Otitis. This condition, also known as malignant external otitis, is an acute osteomyelitis of the temporal bone that occurs in debilitated, diabetic, and immunosuppressed patients, and is usually caused by the *Pseudomonas* bacterium. The infection starts in the EAC and spreads rapidly to the other portions of the temporal bone and adjacent areas. CT reveals initially increased soft-tissue thickening and later on erosion of the bony external canal, particularly of its floor, and stenosis of the lumen of the canal caused by soft-tissue swelling. The infection may then spread inferiorly along the undersurface of the temporal bone to involve the facial nerve at the stylomastoid foramen, anteriorly to the temporomandibular fossa, and parotid space, posteriorly to the mastoid, and medially into the middle ear, and petrous pyramid and base of the skull (Figure 19).[2]

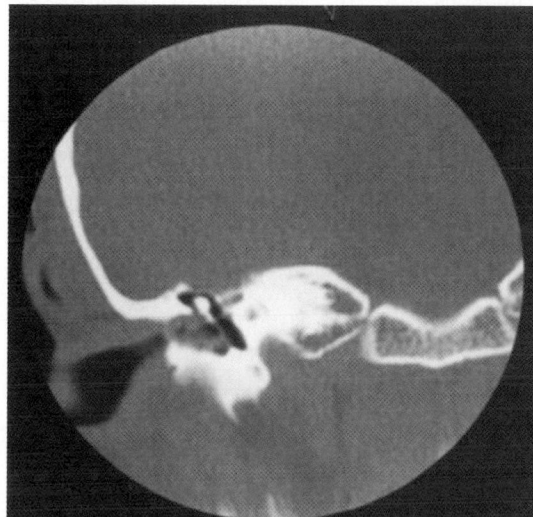

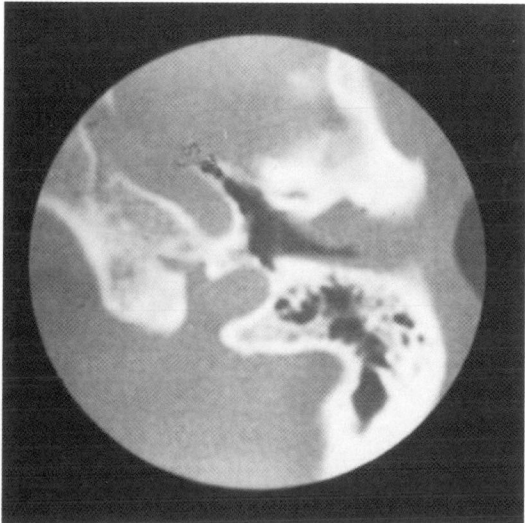

Figure 20 External auditory canal cholesteatoma, coronal section of the right ear. The cholesteatoma fills and obstructs the bony external auditory canal. The cholesteatoma erodes the inferior margin of the lateral wall of the attic and extends into the attic lateral to the ossicles.

Figure 21 Carcinoma of the left external auditory canal, axial computed tomographic section. The anterior wall of the external auditory canal is eroded by an adjacent soft tissue mass. The lesion does not extend into the middle ear cavity.

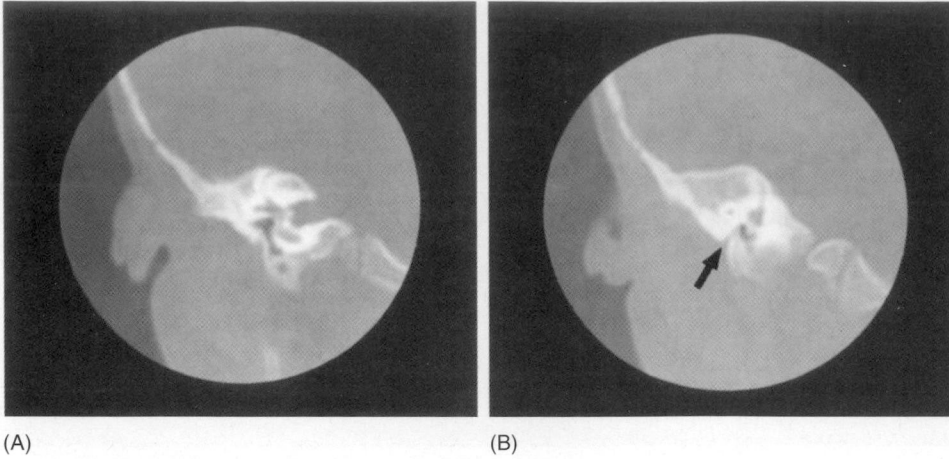

(A)   (B)

Figure 22 Congenital malformation of the right external and middle ears, coronal computed tomographic sections. (A) Agenesis of the external auditory canal with hypoplasia of the middle ear. (B) Notice the lack of development of the mastoid pneumatization and the outward rotation of the vertical segment of the facial canal (*arrow*).

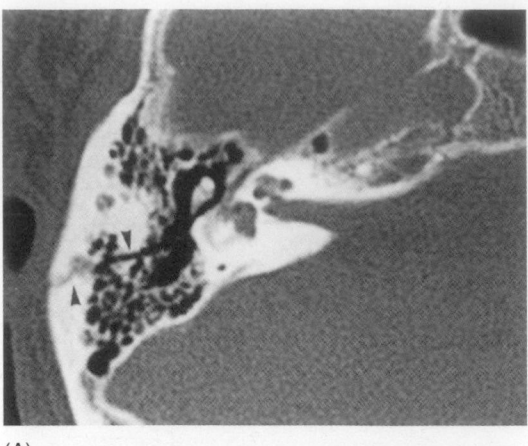

(A)

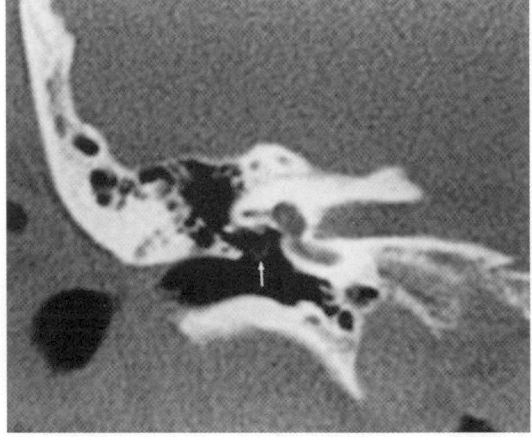

(B)

Figure 25 Longitudinal fracture of the right temporal bone. (A) Axial and; (B) coronal computed tomographic sections. A fracture extends from the mastoid cortex to the region of the aditus (*black arrows*). The head of the malleus and the body of the incus are in normal relationship, but the incudostapedial joint is disrupted (*white arrows*).

EAC Cholesteatoma. Cholesteatoma of the EAC is caused either by blockage of the EAC, with consequent accumulation of epithelial debris (keratosis obliterans), or by dyskeratosis with localized accumulation of debris on the floor of the canal (invasive keratitis). In the first type, a soft tissue mass fills and expands the canal medial to the site of stenosis or obstruction (Figure 20). In the second type, the lumen of the canal is patent, but areas of bony erosion and scalloping are demonstrated in the involved portion of the canal. When the cholesteatoma is large and erodes the annulus, it may extend into the middle ear cavity and mastoid.[2]

Carcinoma. Carcinoma of the temporal bone usually arises in the EAC epithelium. The CT findings vary with the extent of the lesion. In an early lesion, portions of the bony wall of the EAC are eroded (Figure 21). When further destruction occurs, the neoplasm may spread anteriorly into the temporomandibular fossa; posteriorly into the mastoid, where it often reaches the facial canal; and medially into the middle ear, jugular fossa, petrous pyramid, and labyrinth. Extension into the mastoid and petrous pyramid causes a typical moth-eaten appearance because of infiltration of the bone.

Middle Ear and Ossicular Chain

CT is the study of choice for pathologic processes that arise in the middle ear and involve the ossicular chain. Because granulation tissue enhances after the injection of paramagnetic agents, MRI with contrast is useful in some cases to differentiate granulation tissue from fluid and cholesteatoma, which have a similar density in CT images.

Congenital Malformations. Malformations of the middle ear space vary from minor hypoplasia to complete agenesis. In the majority of cases with an atretic EAC, the middle ear cavity is near normal in size and aerated. The head of the malleus and the body of the incus are often fused (Figure 13A) and fixed to the atretic plate at the level of the malleus neck. If the middle ear cavity is grossly hypoplastic, the malleus and incus form a rudimentary amalgam that is often in an ectopic position (Figure 22). A congenital anomaly may be confined to the ossicular chain, which may be malformed or fixed. Malformations of the stapes superstructures and fixation of the stapes footplate are not uncommon isolated defects. The jugular bulb sometimes projects into the hypotympanum or mesotympanum. The bulb

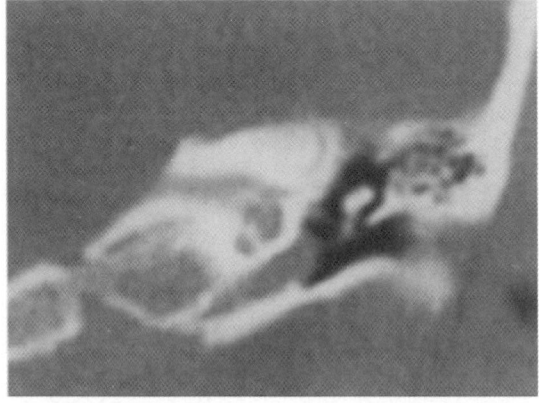

(A)

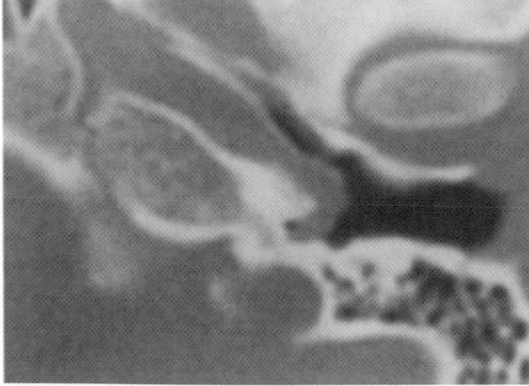

(B)

Figure 23 Ectopic left internal carotid artery. Coronal (A) and axial (B) computed tomographic sections. The ectopic carotid artery courses throughout the entire length of the middle ear cavity. Notice the absence of the vertical portion of the carotid canal normally seen underneath the cochlea and of the bony wall dividing the anterior part of the mesotympanum from the horizontal segment of the carotid canal.

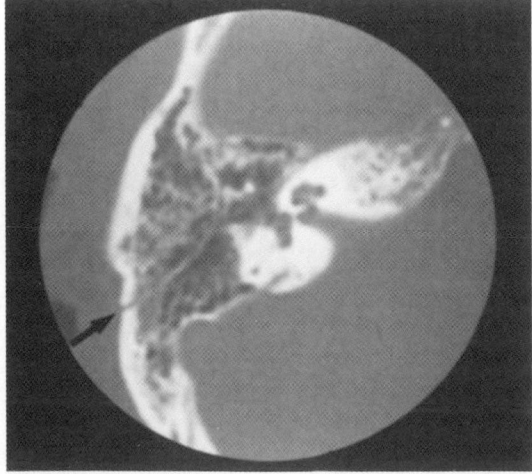

Figure 24 Longitudinal fracture of the right temporal bone, axial computed tomographic section. The longitudinal fracture extends from the cortex of the posterior portion of the mastoid to the posterosuperior canal wall (*arrow*). The fracture reaches the attic and disrupts the ossicular chain. The body of the incus is displaced laterally and posteriorly.

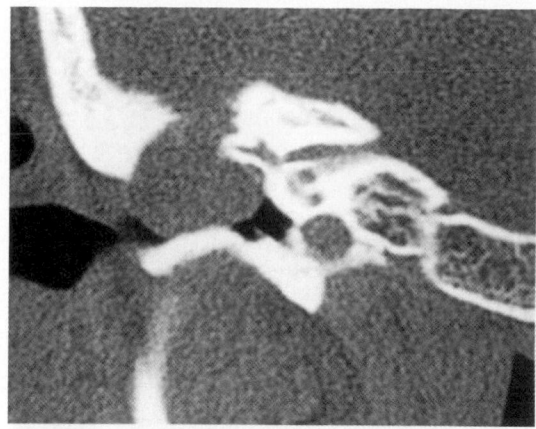

(A)

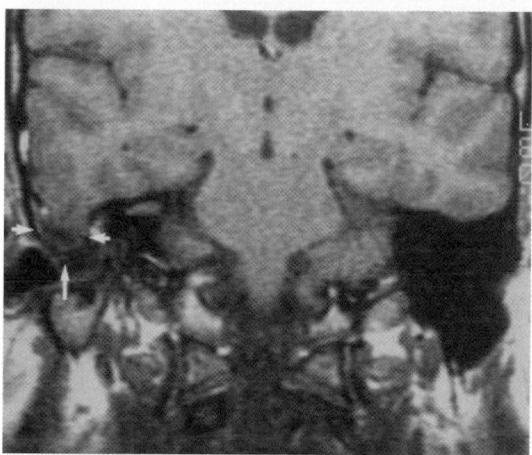

(B)

Figure 26 Meningoencephalocele, after modified radical mastoidectomy. (A) Coronal computed tomographic section showing a large defect in the tegmen of the cavity with a soft tissue mass underneath it. (B) T1W coronal magnetic resonance image clearly identifying the soft tissue mass (*arrow*) as a brain herniation.

may be covered by a thin bony shell or may be exposed in the middle ear, often in contact with the medial surface of the tympanic membrane, and thus mimicking a glomus tumor. Whenever

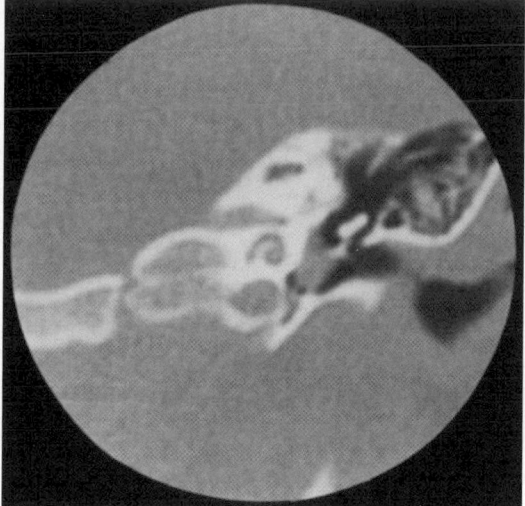

Figure 28 Left congenital cholesteatoma, coronal computed tomographic section. A well-defined soft tissue mass lies in the mesotympanum and extends from the intact tympanic membrane to the promontory. The remainder of the middle ear cavity and the mastoid are well aerated.

the diagnosis is in doubt, we perform MRV and enhanced SPGR pulse sequence. The intratemporal segment of the carotid artery may take an ectopic or an aberrant course through the middle ear. In these cases, the CT examination shows a soft tissue mass extending throughout the entire length of the middle ear cavity to regain its normal position in the petrous apex (Figure 23). The vertical portion of the carotid artery, rather than being located underneath the cochlea, enters temporal bone through an enlarged inferior tympanic artery canal in the floor of the posterior part of the hypotympanum. MRA may be used to confirm the anomalous course of the artery.

Trauma. The middle ear cavity is usually involved in longitudinal fractures of the temporal bone.[7] CT permits precise evaluation of the course of the fracture and status of the ossicular chain (Figure 24, 25). A fracture line may disappear at

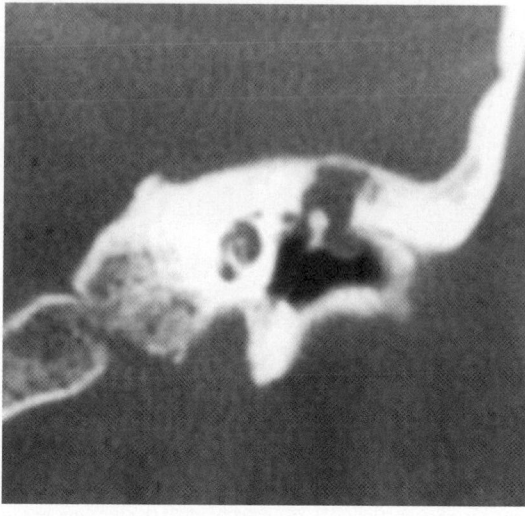

Figure 29 Left attic cholesteatoma, coronal computed tomographic section. The lateral wall of the attic is eroded by a soft tissue mass extending into the attic lateral to the ossicles. A polyp protrudes into the external auditory canal through a perforation of the pars flaccida of the tympanic membrane.

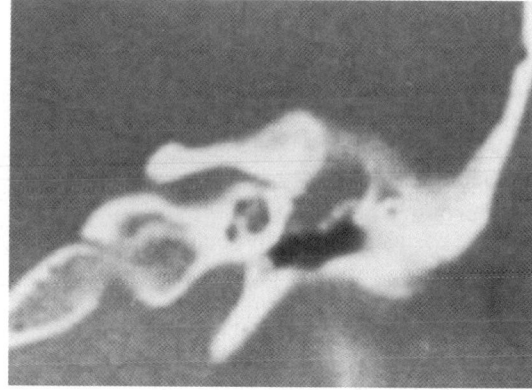

Figure 30 Left cholesteatoma, pars tensa perforation type, coronal computed tomographic section. The cholesteatoma extends into the attic medial to the ossicles and displaces the ossicles laterally.

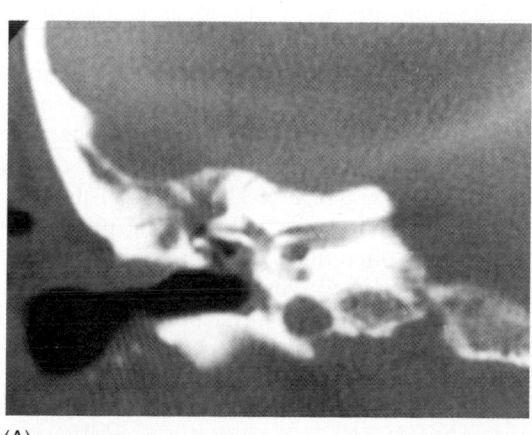

(A)

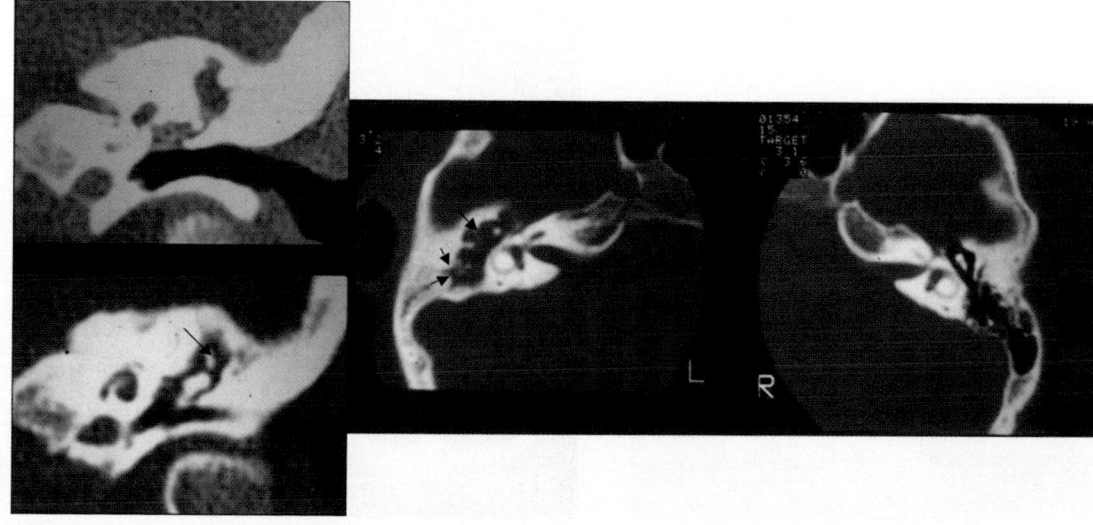

(B)

Figure 27 (A) Right chronic otitis media, coronal computed tomographic section. The tympanic membrane is thickened and retracted. The mesotympanum is markedly contracted, and the mastoid air cells appear cloudy. The lateral wall of the attic and incudostapedial junction is intact. (B) Tympanosclerosis. Coronal CT scan (*left*) showing sclerotic mastoid, contracted middle ear, sclerotic ossicles, and calcification (*arrow*) due to tympanosclerosis. Axial CT scans (*right*) showing an atticoantral cholesteatoma (*arrows*) of the right ear. Note left ear for comparison. Note that only a piece of the matter is present on the right ear.

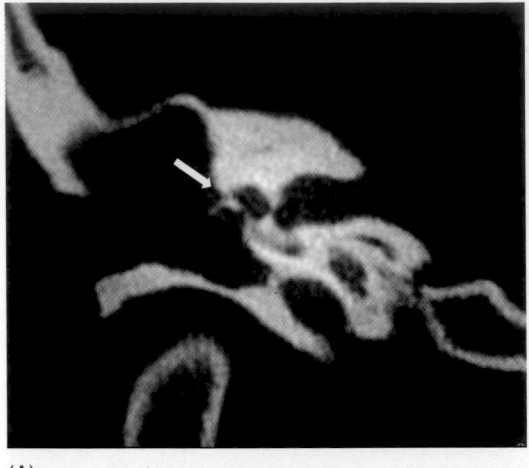

(A)

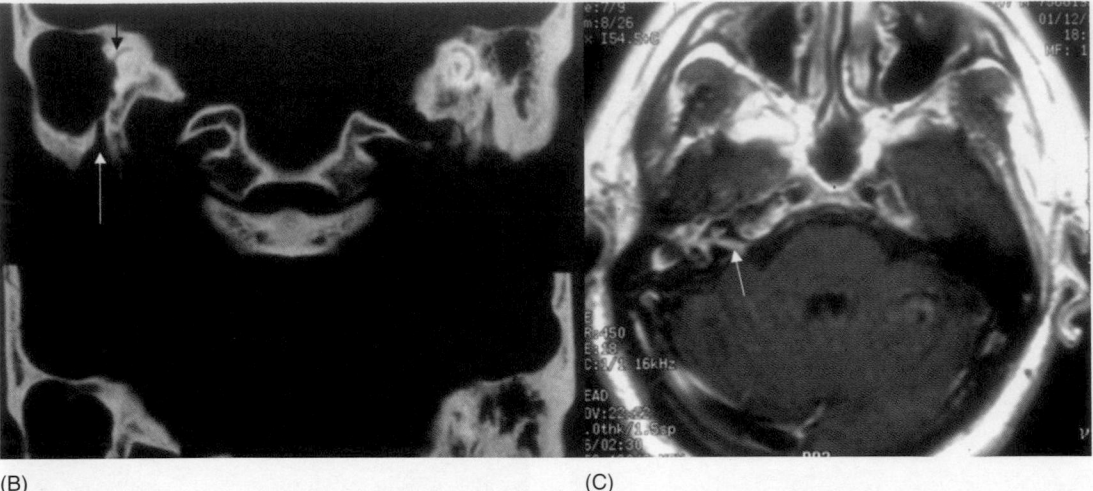

(B)   (C)

Figure 31 (A) Right cholesteatoma with labyrinthine fistula. Coronal computed tomographic section: a soft tissue mass fills the attic, eroding the ossicles and the lateral aspect of the horizontal semicircular canal (*arrow*). (B) Cholesteatoma eroding facial canal and posterior semicircular canal. Coronal CT scans (*left*) showing a large acquired cholesteatoma. Note erosion of posterior semicircular canal (*black arrow*) and erosion of mastoid segment of facial canal (*white arrow*). (C) Enhanced axial T_1-weighted MR scan showing an infected cholesteatoma extending into the IAC (*arrow*). The abnormal enhancement of IAC and labyrinth is due to infection.

a certain level only to reappear a few millimeters distant. This apparent gap is not caused by interruption of the fracture line but rather by a change in its course so that the fracture becomes invisible in some of the sections. The tegmen is usually involved, and cerebrospinal fluid (CSF) otorrhea or rhinorrhea occurs whenever the dura is torn. Anterior extension of the fracture may reach the eustachian tube, which becomes obstructed. Conductive hearing loss is usually secondary to disruption of the ossicular chain (Figure 24, 25). The body of the incus is usually rotated and displaced superiorly, posteriorly, and laterally. Interruption at the incudostapedial area results from a fracture of the lenticular process of the incus or the stapes superstructure and from a dislocation of the incudostapedial joint.

Meningocele and Meningoencephalocele. A soft tissue mass contiguous to a defect in the

tegmen of the mastoid suggests the possibility of a meningocele or meningoencephalocele. If the brain and meninges herniate into the small space of the antrum or epitympanum, the constant pulsation of the CSF is transmitted through the walls of the meningocele to cause a gradual resorption of the surrounding bony walls. CT demonstrates the bony defect in the tegmen and a soft tissue mass filling the mastoid cavity (Figure 26). This soft tissue lesion cannot be reliably differentiated from a recurrent cholesteatoma since the absorption coefficients of both lesions are similar. A more definite diagnosis of meningoencephalocele is reached by injecting, by means of lumbar puncture, a small amount of myelographic contrast that will diffuse in the subarachnoid space and produce an enhancement of the herniated CSF mass. The differentiation between a meningocele and a cholesteatoma may also be made with MR. On MR, cholesteatoma appears as a

lesion of low to intermediate signal in the T1W and high signal intensity in T2W images.[10] A meningocele will have the same characteristics as CSF: low signal intensity in T1W and high intensity in the T2W images. On DWI, cholesteatoma appears hyperintense while meningocele remains hypointense. On MR, meningoencephaloceles have the same characteristics of the adjacent brain, which are quite different from a cholesteatoma (Figure 26).

Acute Otitis Media. In acute otitis media, the CT images demonstrate a nonspecific and diffuse clouding of the middle ear cavity. Occasionally, on CT scans, air bubbles may be seen within the middle ear. The tympanic membrane is often swollen and bulges externally.

Chronic Otitis Media. There are 2 types of chronic otitis media which can be differentiated with imaging studies. In chronic suppurative otitis media, a partial, nonhomogeneous clouding of the middle ear cavity is caused by granulation tissue, polyps, and fluid or pus. Because the tympanic membrane is perforated, some aeration of the middle ear space may be present. Erosion of the long process of the incus is a common finding, whereas erosion of the body of the incus and the head of the malleus is rare unless a cholesteatoma is present. In chronic adhesive otitis media, the middle ear space is contracted because of retraction of the tympanic membrane on the promontory (Figure 27). The handle of the malleus is foreshortened, and the long process of the incus is often thinned out or eroded. In these cases, the retracted tympanic membrane may be attached to the head of the stapes with formation of a natural myringostapediopexy.

Tympanosclerotic deposits are recognizable by CT whenever they are sufficiently large and calcified. The deposits appear as punctate or linear densities within the tympanic membrane or the mucosa covering the promontory. Large deposits of tympanosclerosis in the attic may surround and fix the ossicles.

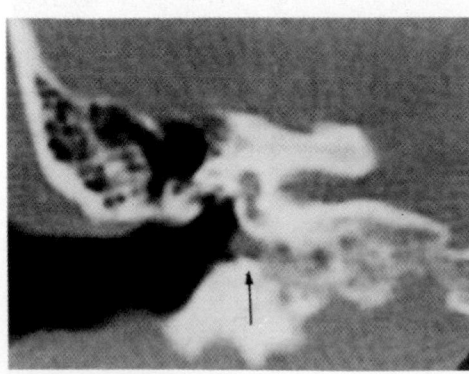

(A)

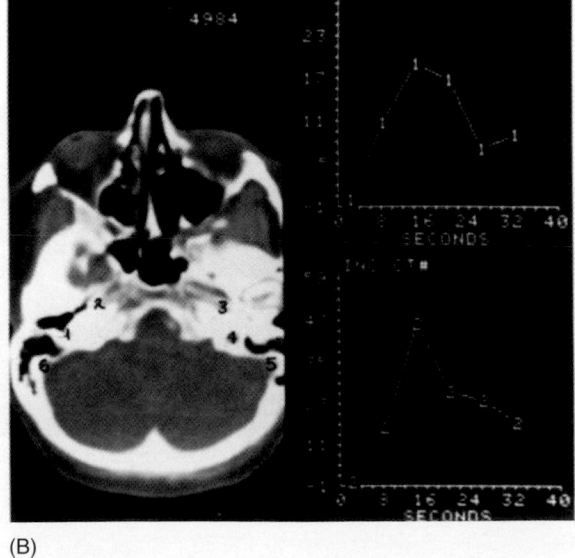

(B)

Figure 32 Right glomus tympanicum. (A) Coronal computed tomographic (CT) section showing a small soft tissue mass in the lower portion of the middle ear cavity (*arrow*). (B) Dynamic CT study of the preselected section at the level of the mass. Graphic display of the circulation in the tumor (1) and internal carotid artery (2). Notice the high peak of the tumor at arterial time.

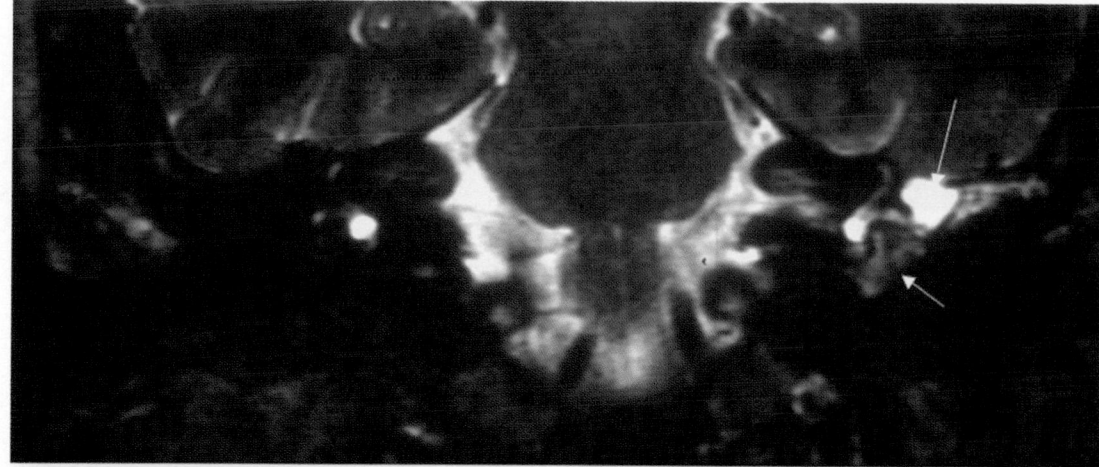

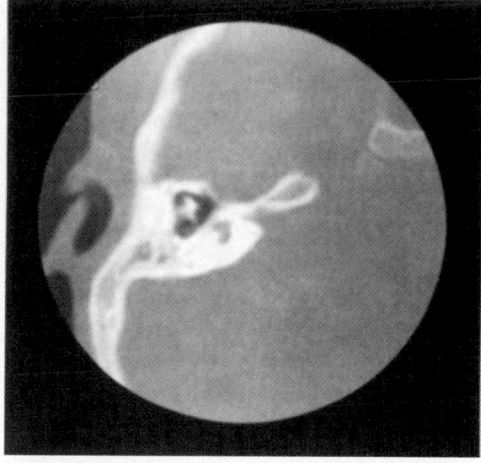

(A)

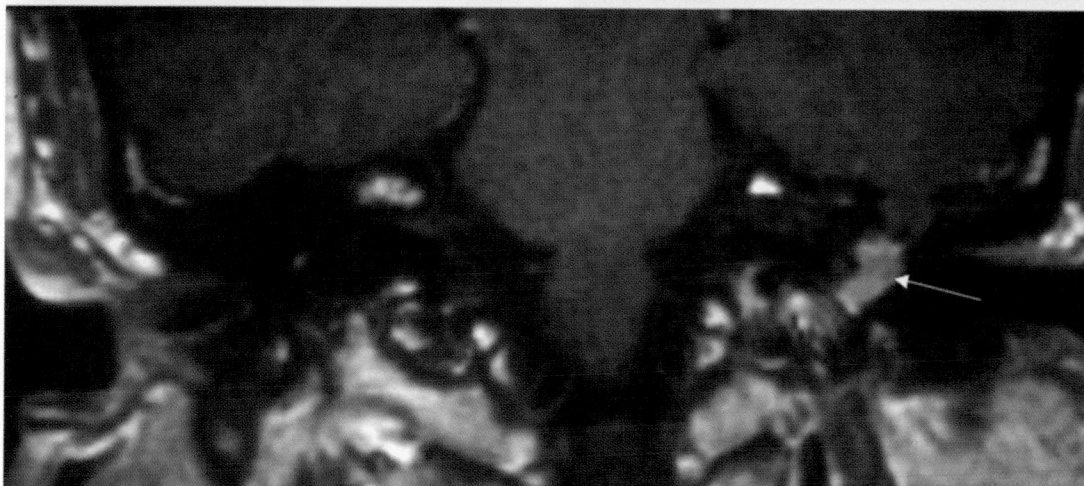

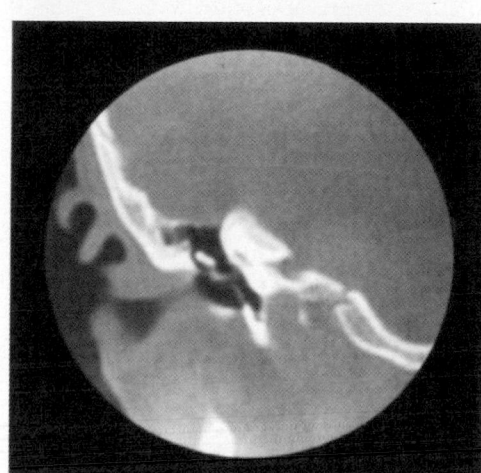

(B)

Figure 33 Glomus tympanicum. Coronal T$_2$-weighted (*top*) MRI scan showing fluid in the attic (*long arrow*) and a mass in the mesotympanum (*short arrow*). Coronal enhanced T$_1$-weighted MR scan (*bottom*) showing enhancing glomus tympanicum (*arrow*).

Figure 36 Michel malformation of the right inner ear structures. Axial (A) and coronal (B) computed tomographic sections. The middle ear cavity is normal, but the petrous pyramid is hypoplastic. The cochlea is absent or markedly hypoplastic. Notice the cavity in the region of the vestibule with rudimentary semicircular canals.

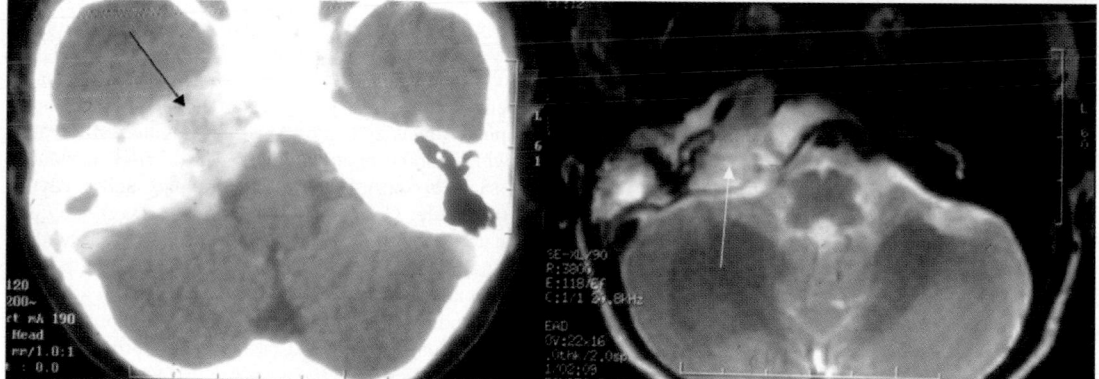

Figure 34 Rhabdomyosarcoma. Enhanced axial CT scan and axial T$_2$-weighted MR scan showing a rhabdomyosarcoma involving the petrous apex (*arrows*).

around the facial nerve canal and in the mastoid (least common).

Acquired cholesteatomas produce a soft tissue mass mainly in the attic or in the middle ear, resulting in typical erosion of the lateral attic wall, posterosuperior canal wall, and ossicles.[3,7,9] If the middle ear cavity is aerated, the soft tissue mass is well-outlined (Figures 29–30). When fluid or inflammatory tissue surrounds the cholesteatoma, the margin of the mass is obscured because the X-ray densities of cholesteatoma, inflammatory tissue, and fluid are similar. MRI with contrast may be useful in these cases to differentiate the enhancing granulation tissue from fluid and cholesteatoma. On DWI, cholesteatoma appears hyperintense while fluid and granulation tissues appear hypointense. Different patterns of X-ray findings are observed. Cholesteatomas that arise from retraction of the pars flaccida of the tympanic membrane produce erosion of the anterior portion of the lateral wall of the attic and of the anterior tympanic spine (Figure 29). The lesion extends into the attic lateral to the ossicles, which may become medially displaced.

Cholesteatomas arising from retraction of the pars tensa, usually from the posterosuperior

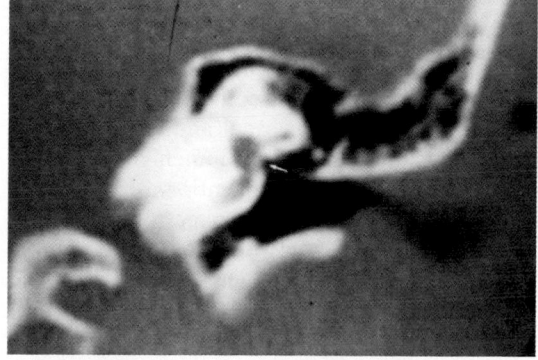

Figure 35 Stapedial otosclerosis, 20° coronal oblique section of the left ear. The footplate of this stapes appears thickened (*arrow*).

Cholesteatoma. Congenital cholesteatomas appear as well-defined soft tissue masses often adjacent to the tensor tympani tendon, handle of the malleus, or long process of the incus, and produce an outward bulge of the intact tympanic membrane (Figure 28).[10] The middle ear and mastoid air cells appear otherwise well-aerated. If there is an accompanying serous otitis media related to obstruction of the eustachian tube, the fluid may obscure the mass as the entire tympanic cavity becomes cloudy. If the lesion extends into the attic, the medial or the lateral wall of the attic may be eroded. Other sites of congenital cholesteatomas (epidermoid) are in the petrous apex,

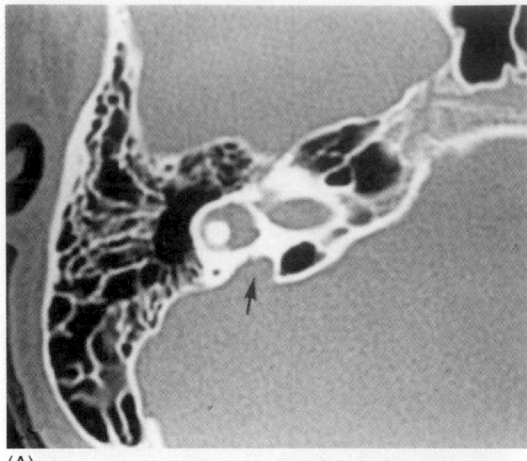

(A)

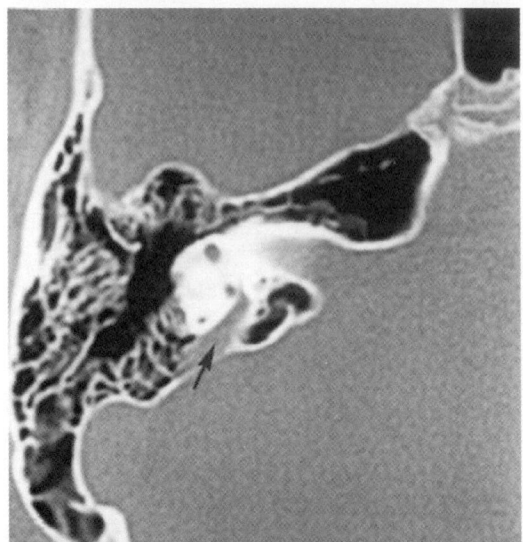

(B)

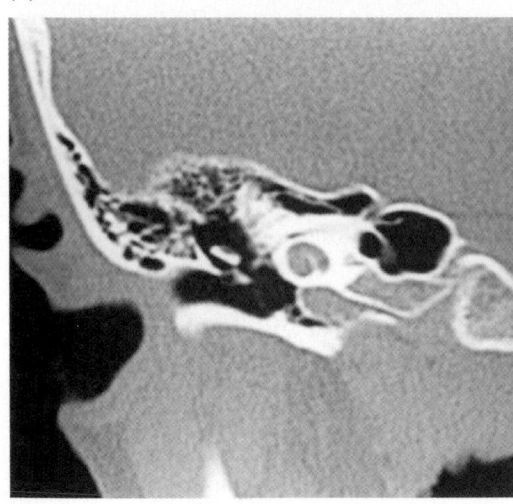

(C)

Figure 37 Mondini malformation of the right inner ear structures. (A) and (B) Axial sections showing a short but wide vestibular aqueduct (*arrows*) and a moderate dilation of the vestibule. (C) Coronal computed tomographic section. The cochlea appears normal in size, but the bony partitions between the cochlear coils are hypoplastic, causing the appearance of an empty cochlea.

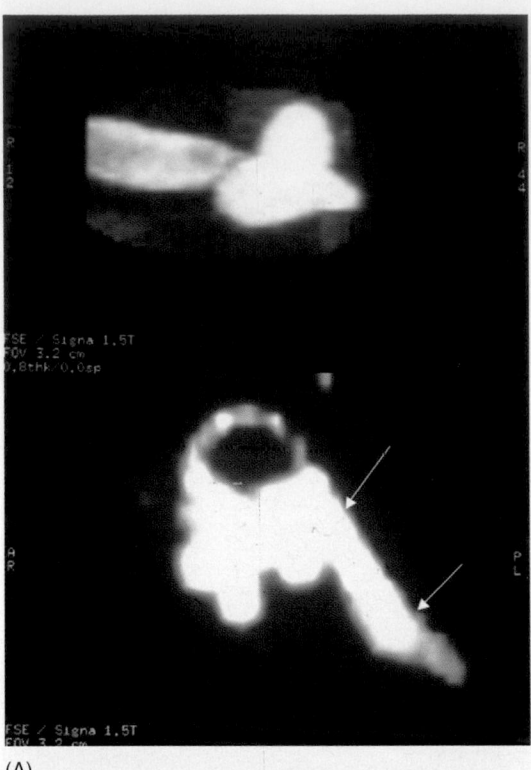

(A)

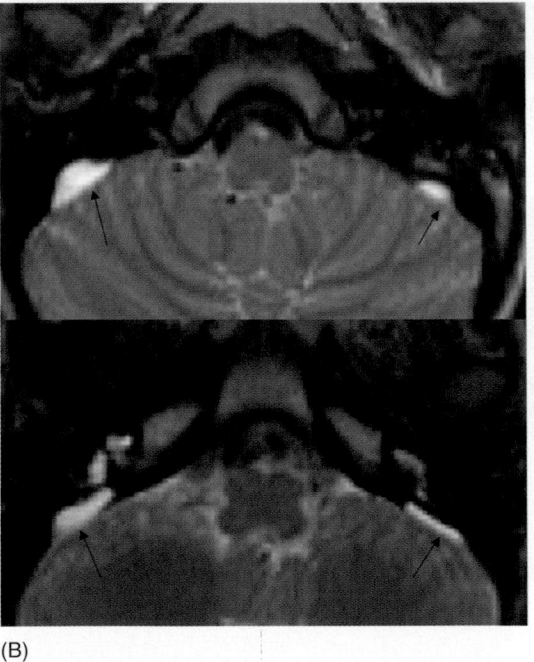

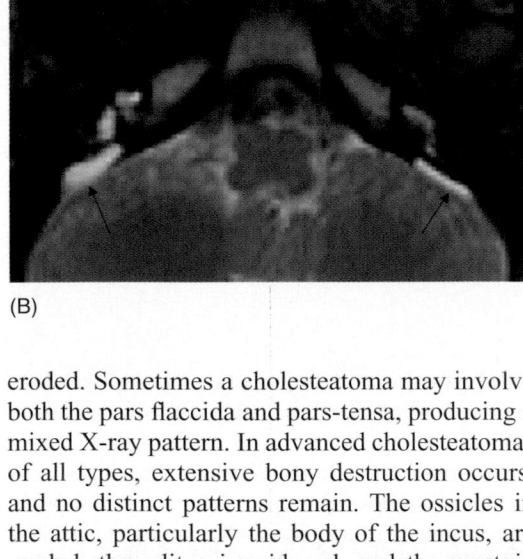

(B)

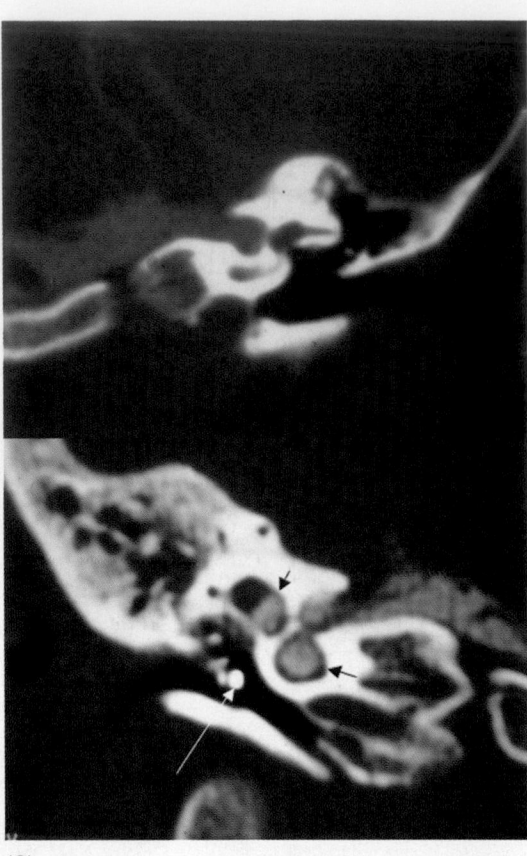

(C)

Figure 38 (A) Volume rendered 3D MRI showing a Mondini anomaly (*top*) and a Mondini anomaly with large endolymphatic duct and sac (*bottom*). The endolymphatic system (*arrows*) is very large. (B) Enlarged bilateral endolymphatic ducts and sacs. Axial T$_2$-weighted MR scans, showing marked bilateral enlarged endolymphatic ducts and sacs (*arrows*). (C) Mondini anomaly and perilymphatic fistula. Coronal CT cisternogram (*top*) showing iodinated contrast in the CPA cistern as well as within the IAC. There is no contrast in the vestibule, because this is a normal ear. Coronal CT cisternogram in a patient with Mondini anomaly (*bottom*), showing the presence of iodinated contrast in the IAC, as well as abnormal contrast in the cystic vestibule (*upper black arrow*), in the cystic cochlear (*lower black arrow*) and within the middle ear. Note ventilating tube (*white arrow*) in this patient with clinical diagnosis of serous fluid in the middle ear.

margin of the membrane, appear as a soft tissue mass in the middle ear eroding the long process of the incus and extending into the attic medial to the ossicles which may be displaced laterally (Figure 24). The lateral wall of the attic is usually intact, but the posterosuperior canal wall is often eroded. Sometimes a cholesteatoma may involve both the pars flaccida and pars-tensa, producing a mixed X-ray pattern. In advanced cholesteatomas of all types, extensive bony destruction occurs, and no distinct patterns remain. The ossicles in the attic, particularly the body of the incus, are eroded; the aditus is widened; and the mastoid antrum becomes enlarged, cloudy, and smooth in outline because of erosion of the air cells lining the walls of the antrum. Further extension into the mastoid causes destruction of the trabeculae with formation of large cavities. Erosion of the tegmen may lead to meningeal and intracranial complications. Labyrinthine fistulas occur most commonly in the lateral portion of the horizontal semicircular canal. The CT sections show flattening of the normal convex contour of the horizontal semicircular canal and erosion of the bony capsule covering the lumen of the canal (Figure 31). Further complications of cholesteatoma are extension into the petrous pyramid, which usually occurs in well-pneumatized bones, and erosion of the facial canal, which may lead to facial paralysis (Figure 31B, C).

Neoplasms. Osteomas are frequent in the EAC, but also rarely occur in the middle ear, where they may cause conductive hearing loss by impinging

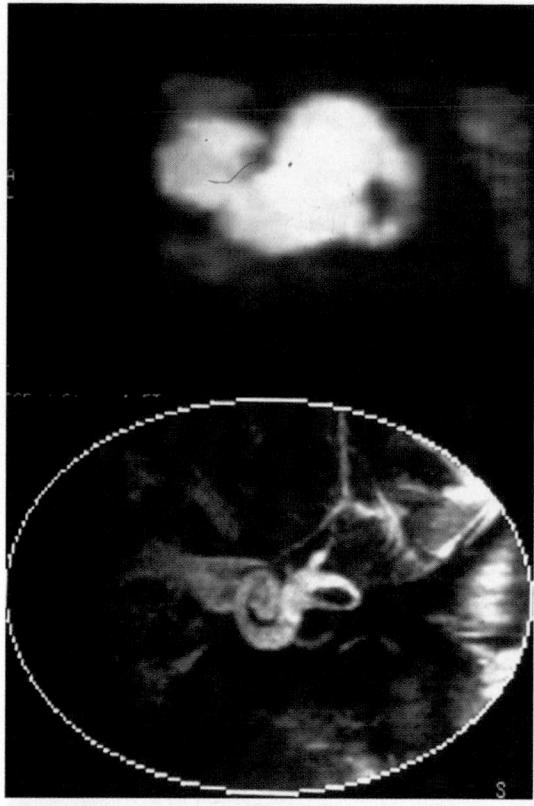

Figure 39 Mondini anomaly. Volume rendered 3D MRI showing Mondini anomaly (*top*) and a normal labyrinth (*bottom*).

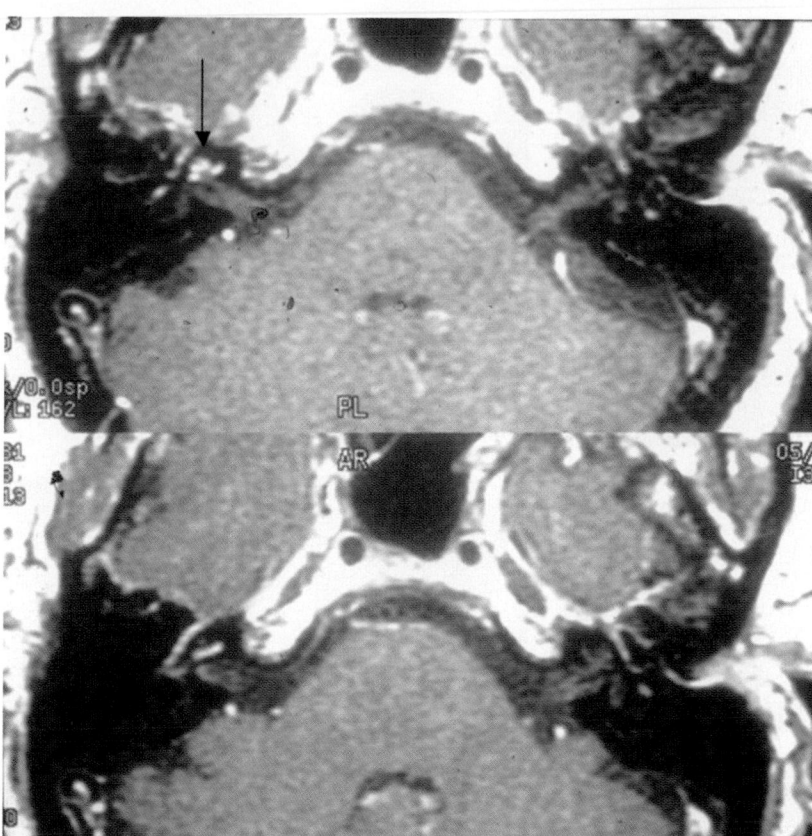

Figure 42 Labyrinthitis. Enhanced axial T_1-weighted MR scan showing enhancement of right cochlea (*arrow*) related to viral labyrinthitis.

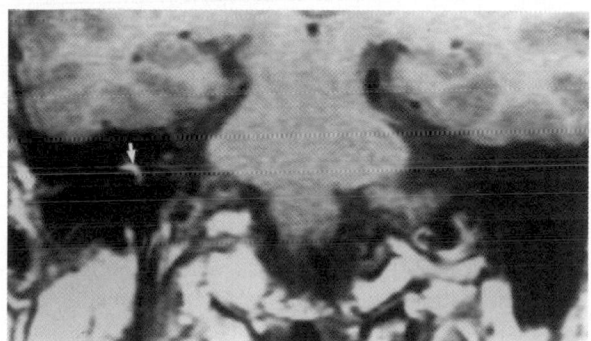

Figure 40 Labyrinthine concussion with bleeding. This T_1 coronal MR section shows an area of high signal intensity within the right vestibule (*arrow*) and adjacent portion of the semicircular canals.

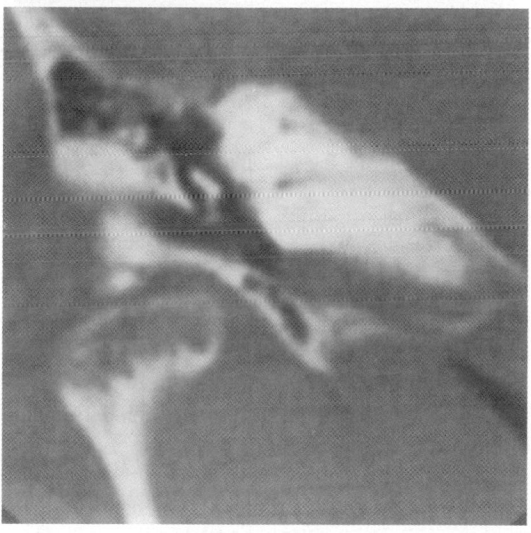

Figure 43 Obliterative labyrinthitis, coronal computed tomographic section of the right ear. Notice the complete bony obliteration of the cochlear lumen.

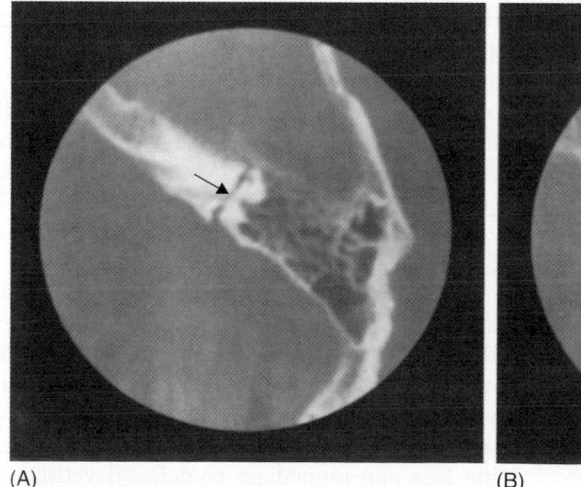

(A)   (B)

Figure 41 Transverse fracture of the left petrous pyramid. (A) and (B) Axial computed tomographic sections. The fracture (arrows) extends from the superior part of the petrous ridge to the undersurface of the temporal bone crossing the superior semicircular canal, vestibule, and promontory of the cochlea.

on the ossicular chain. Glomus tumors, also called chemodectomas or nonchromaffin paragangliomas, arise in the middle ear or jugular fossa from minute glomus bodies. Glomus tympanicum tumors arise from glomus bodies along Jacobson nerve on the promontory. The CT sections reveal a soft tissue mass of variable size, usually in the lower portion of the middle ear cavity (Figure 32A). As the lesion enlarges, it may cause a lateral bulge of the tympanic membrane, smooth erosion of the promontory, and involvement of the mastoid and hypotympanic air cells. If the lesion erodes into the jugular fossa, it becomes indistinguishable from a glomus jugulare. A dynamic CT study of a preselected section showing the tumor mass generates a curve with a high arterial peak (Figure 32B)

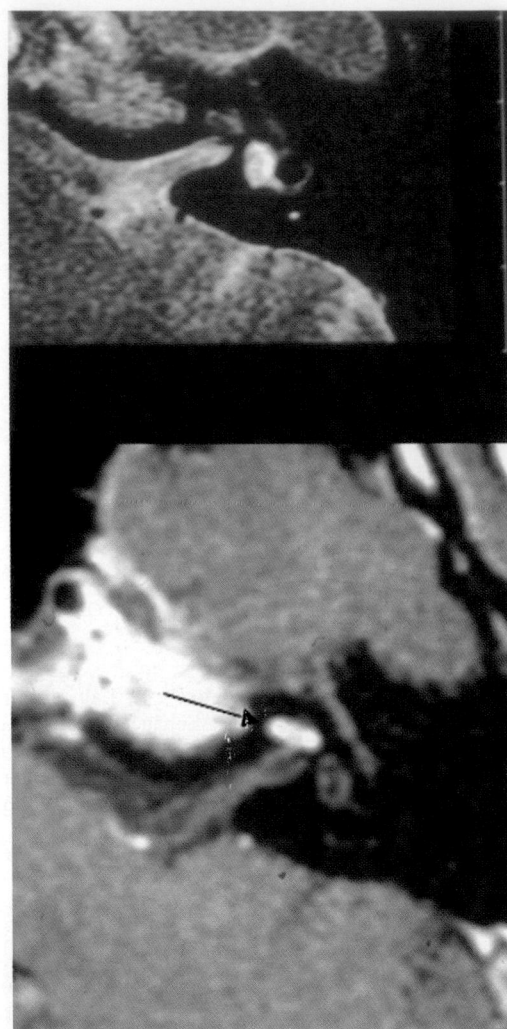

Figure 44 Labyrinthine schwannoma. Axial T$_2$-weighted (*top*) and enhanced axial T$_1$-weighted (*bottom*) MR scan showing an enhancing mass (*arrow*) within the cochlea. This was presumed to be a cochlear schwannoma.

rather than the high but delayed venous peak of a high jugular bulb.[18,23] On T2W and unenhanced T1W MRI, glomus tympanicum may not be differentiated from fluid or cholesteatoma. However, on contrast-enhanced T1W; MRI, glomus tumors show marked enhancement hence they can be readily recognized (Figure 33). On sensitive MR sequences such as GE and MRA, glomus tumors appear hyperintense, reflecting their nature of increased vascularity. Selective arteriography with subtraction is indicated to identify feeding vessels before embolization. Squamous cell carcinomas extend into the middle ear from the EAC. Adenocarcinoma and adenomas are rare and produce nonspecific soft tissue masses. Erosion of the walls of the middle ear is a feature in keeping with adenocarcinoma.

Rhabdomyosarcoma is the most common malignant mesenchymal tumor of childhood. Common primary sites include the head and the neck (45%), trunk (40%), and extremities (15%).[14] In the temporal bone, the neoplasm may arise within the middle ear, EAC, mastoid, petrous region, or adjacent to eustachian tube. On CT and MRI, the tumor appears as a soft tissue mass, often associated with bone erosion. There will be marked contrast enhancement on enhanced CT and MRI

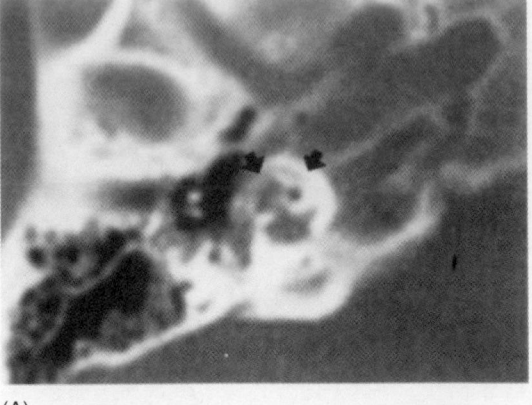

(A)

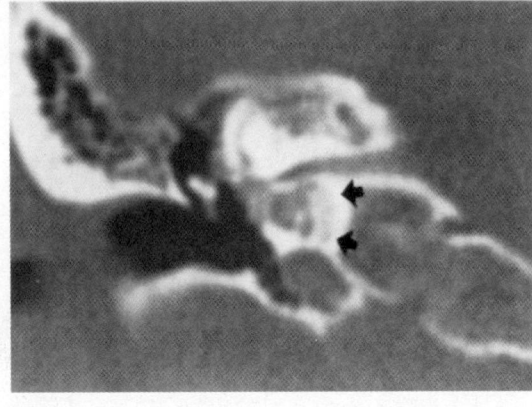

(B)

Figure 45 Cochlear otosclerosis. Axial (A) and coronal (B) computed tomographic sections. Multiple spongiotic foci are noted in the cochlear capsule with formation of a double ring (*arrows*).

scans. At times, aggressive fibromatosis as well as modular fasciitis may mimic rhabdomosarcoma of the mastoid and EAC. Langerhans cell histiocytosis of the mastoid, middle ear, and petrous apex may simulate rhabdomyosarcoma (Figure 34).

Otospongiosis and Otosclerosis. The middle layer of the otic capsule is composed of com-

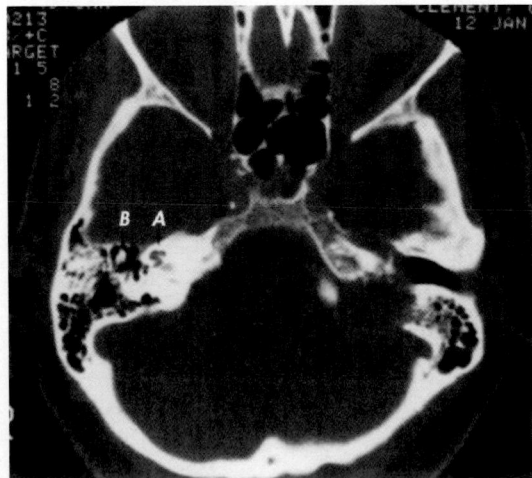

Figure 46 Left glomus jugulare tumor, axial computed tomographic section. The posterior aspect of the left temporal bone in the region of the jugular fossa is eroded. A soft tissue mass extends into the middle ear cavity through a large defect in its posterior wall. (A) = cochlea; (B) = ossicles, on the right side.

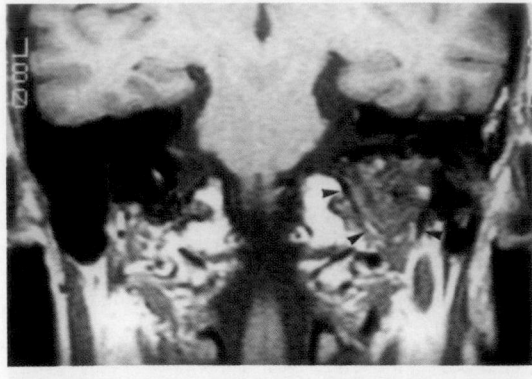

(A)

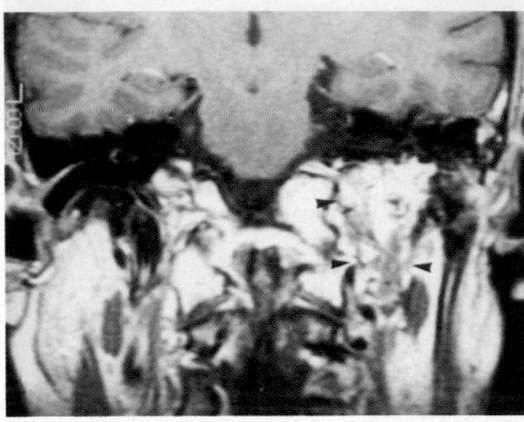

(B)

Figure 47 Glomus jugulare tumor. Coronal T$_1$-weighted magnetic resonance image (A) prior to and (B) after injection of contrast. A large and enhancing soft tissue mass (*arrowheads*) is present in the region of the left jugular fossa. The tumor extends into the lower portion of the middle ear cavity and erodes the undersurface of the petrous pyramid. Multiple areas of signal void, produced by high flow blood vessels, are seen within the tumor mass, producing the so-called "salt and pepper" appearance.

bined intrachondral and endochondral bone. The intrachondral bone is composed of irregular areas of calcified hyaline cartilage that contain true bone within the original cartilage lacunae.[13] The histogenesis of the middle layer of otic capsule is noteworthy because it has no counterpart in the human skeleton. It is in the avascular, ivory-hard, endochondral bone that the pathologic process of otospongiosis arises. Otosclerosis that involves the oval window causes fixation of the stapes and consequent conductive hearing loss.[2,13] In active otosclerosis or otospongiosis, the margin of the oval window becomes decalcified so that the window seems larger than normal. In mature otosclerosis, the oval window becomes narrowed (Figure 35) or closed, and in severe cases the entire oval window niche is obliterated by calcified otosclerotic foci. The CT assessment may be useful before surgery in some cases to confirm the clinical diagnosis, and in some bilateral cases for selection of the ear on which to operate. More important is the study of the expected anatmical variations, and post-stapedectomy ear for determining the cause of recurrent or persistent hearing loss and immediate or delayed vertigo. CT can demonstrate protrusion of the prosthesis into the vestibule, reobliteration of the oval window with fixation of the prosthesis, dislocation of the

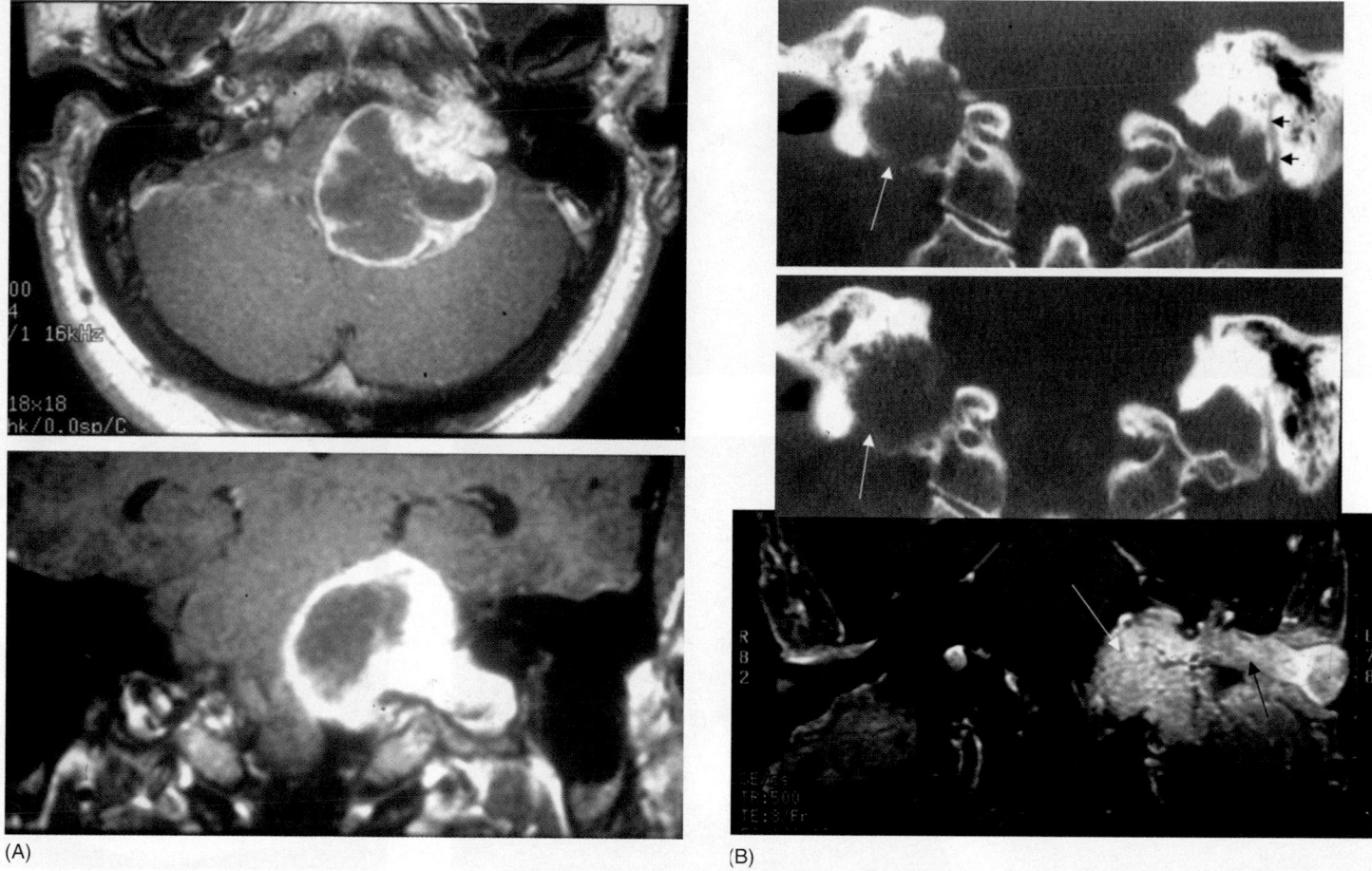

Figure 48 (A) Jugular fossa schwannoma. Enhanced axial (*top*) and coronal (*bottom*) T$_1$-weighted MR scans showing a large jugular schwannoma, extending into the posterior fossa. (B) Jugular fossa paraganglioma. Coronal CT scans (*top*) showing a large right glomus jugulare (*arrows*), resulting in destruction of the mastoid segment of facial canal. Note normal left facial canal (*black arrows*). Enhanced T$_1$-weighted coronal MR scan in another patient, showing a large glomus jugulare (*white arrow*). Note extension into middle ear (*black arrow*) and into EAC.

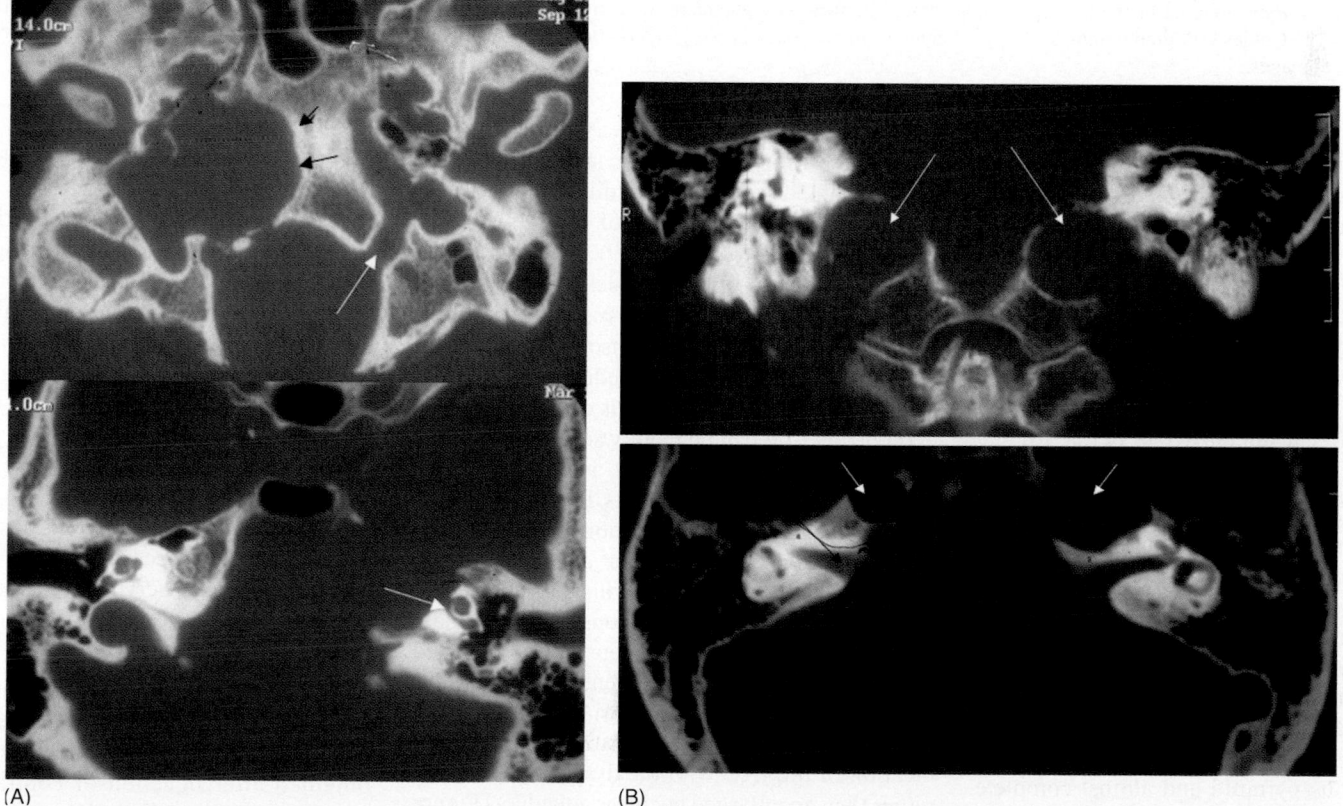

Figure 49 (A) Petrous apex cholesteatoma and cholesterol granuloma. Axial CT scan (*top*) showing a large expansile mass involving right petrous bone. Note erosion of clivus (*black arrows*) and right hypoglossal canal. Note normal left hypoglossal canal (*white arrow*). This was due to a cholesterol granuloma. Axial CT scan (*bottom*) showing a similar destructive and expansile lesion, involving left petrous bone in another patient. This was due to a primary petrous apex cholesteatoma. Note erosion of cochlea (*arrow*). (B) Coronal (*top*) and axial (*bottom*) CT scans in another patient showing bilateral cholesterol granulomas (*arrows*) of the petrous apices.

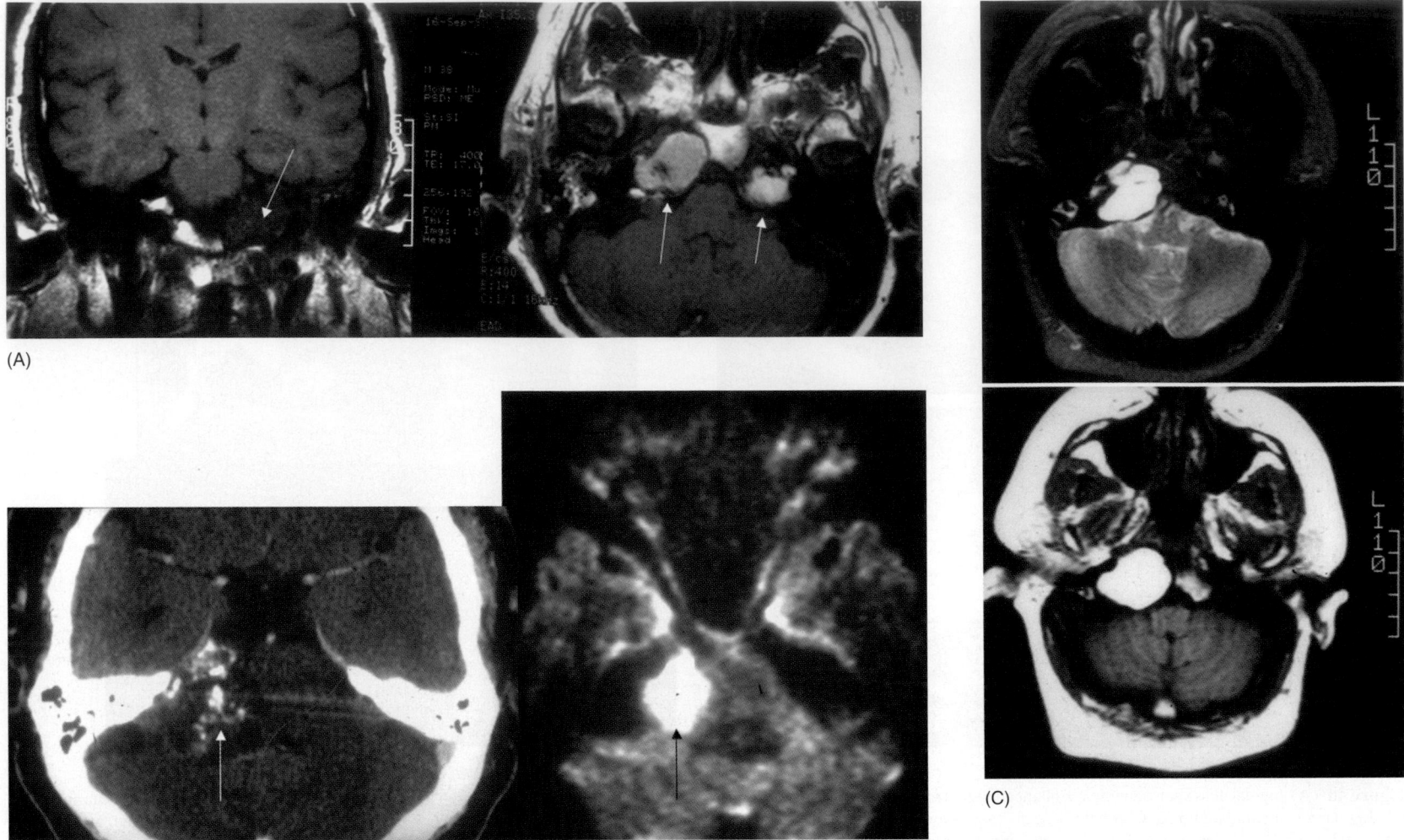

Figure 50 (A) Cholesteatoma and cholesterol granuloma. Coronal T_1-weighted (*left*) showing a petrous cholesteatoma (*arrow*) axial T_1-weighted (*right*) showing bilateral cholesterol granulomas (*arrows*). Cholesteatoma appears hypointense while cholesterol granulomas appear hyperintense. (B) Primary cholesteatoma (epidermoid cyst). Axial CT scan (*left*) showing a large CPA mass (*arrow*) compatible with an epidermoid. Note calcifications, which are not common in epidermoid cysts. Axial DWI (*right*) showing characteristic hyperintensity of epidermoid cyst. (C) Cholesterol granuloma. Axial T_2-weighted (*top*) and axial T_1-weighted (*bottom*) MR scans showing characteristic hyperintensity of cholesterol granuloma on T_1- and T_2-weighted images.

medial end of the prosthesis from the oval window, air within the vestibule, and separation of the lateral end of the prosthesis from the incus or necrosis of the long process of the incus.

Inner Ear

Both CT and MRI are used for the study of the inner ear structures. CT is better for the study of the labyrinthine capsule; MRI is better for the assessment of the membranous labyrinth and neurovascular structures of the IAC.

Congenital Anomalies. Most cases of congenital sensorineural hearing loss have abnormalities limited to the membranous labyrinth and therefore not demonstrable with present imaging studies.[11] Defects in the otic capsule are visible by CT. Anomalies may involve a single structure or the entire capsule. The most severe anomaly is the Michel type, which is characterized by hypoplasia of the petrous pyramid and almost complete lack of development of the inner ear structures (Figure 36). A less severe but more common malformation is the Mondini defect, which is characterized by hypoplasia or absence of the bony

partitions within the cochlear turns, a short but wide vestibular aqueduct and dilation of the vestibule, and ampullated ends of the semicircular canals[2,11,12] (Figure 37, 38, 39). Enlargement of the vestibular aqueduct, hypoplasia of the cochlea and IAC, and deformity of the vestibule and semicircular canals may occur as isolated anomalies. Dilation of the cochlear aqueduct is extremely rare. If the cochlear aqueduct is enlarged, the lateral portion of it can be readily seen on CT scans. The medial end of it is quite wide and can be several millimeters in size. Its lateral portion is considered enlarged if it is more than 1 mm in diameter. An enlarged cochlear aqueduct may be responsible for CSF gush, which rarely occurs during a stapedectomy for congenital footplate fixation or otosclerosis. CSF gushing or repeated episodes of meningitis in patients with the Mondini deformity or Mondini variants of inner ear dysplasia is often related to abnormal communication of the IAC with the dysplastic inner ear rather than an enlarged cochlear aqueduct (Figure 38C).

Trauma. Bleeding within the lumen of the inner ear structures may occur after trauma. If bleeding

occurs due to concussion without actual fracture, MR may be indicated to confirm the diagnosis. Methemoglobin appears as a bright signal in both T1 and T2 MR images (Figure 40). The inner ear structures are seldom crossed by longitudinal fractures of the temporal bone but are usually involved in transverse fractures. These fractures typically cross the petrous pyramid at a right angle to the longitudinal axis of the pyramid and extend from the dome of the jugular fossa to the superior petrous ridge (Figure 41). Laterally located transverse fractures involve the promontory, vestibule, horizontal and posterior semicircular canals, and occasionally the tympanic segment of the facial nerve canal. Medially situated fractures involve the vestibule, cochlea, fundus of the IAC, and common crus.

Labyrinthitis. Enhancement within the lumen of the bony labyrinth (perilymphatic and membranous labyrinth) is often observed in MRI obtained after injection of contrast material in patients with acute bacterial and viral labyrinthitis and sometimes in patient with sudden deafness (Figure 42). Chronic labyrinthitis varies from a localized reaction caused by a fistula of the bony

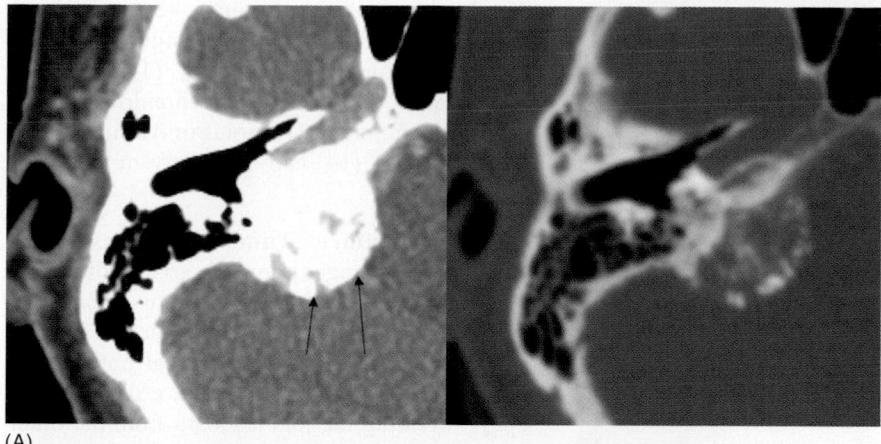

(A)

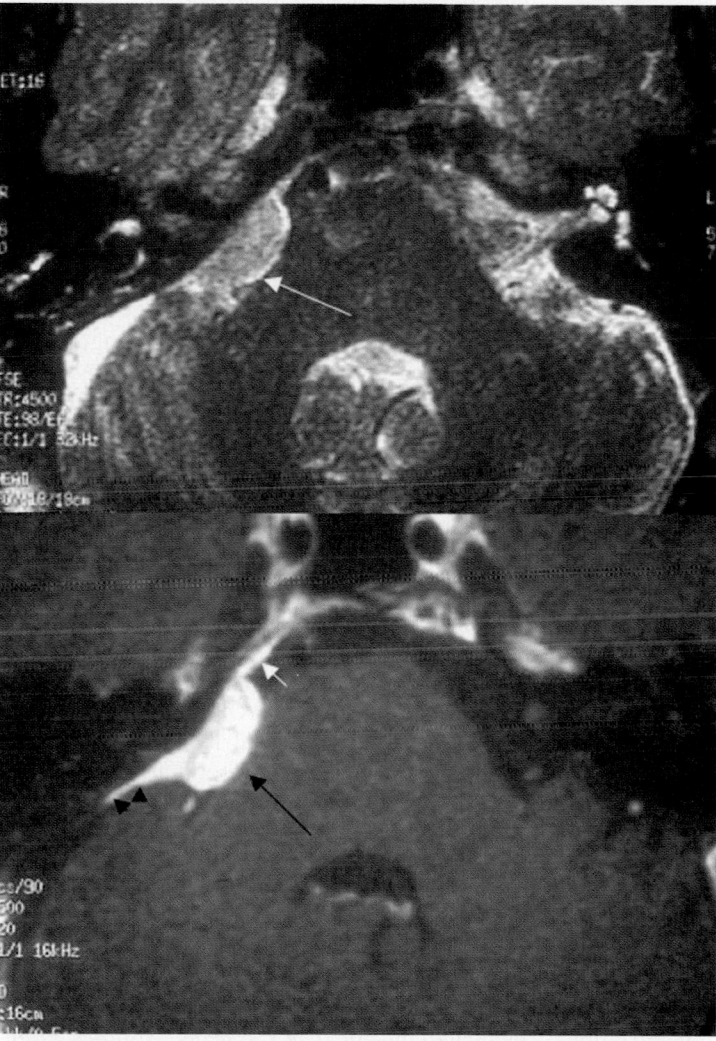

(B)

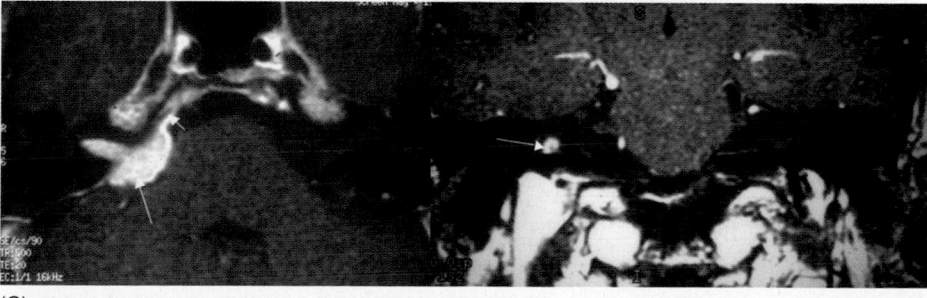

(C)

Figure 51 (A) CPA meningioma. Axial CT scans showing a markedly calcified CPA meningioma (*arrows*). (B) CPA meningioma. Axial T$_2$-weighted (*top*) and enhanced axial T$_1$-weighted (*bottom*) MR scans showing a CPA meningioma (*arrows*). Note dural tail (*small arrows*). (C) Axial enhanced T$_1$-weighted and coronal enhanced T$_1$-weighted MR scans showing a CPA meningioma extending into IAC and a small meningioma arising within IAC (*arrows*).

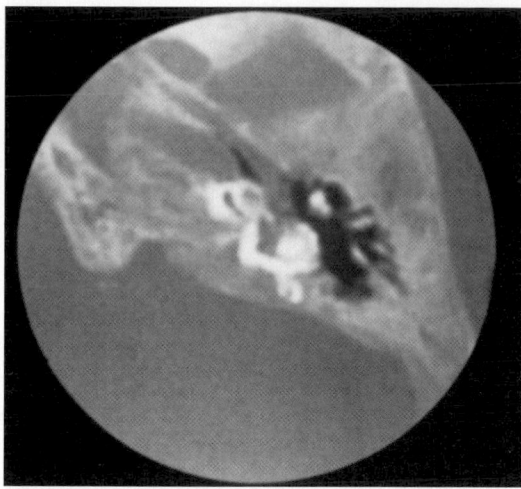

Figure 52 Paget disease, axial section of the left temporal bone. Notice the severe demineralization of the petrous pyramid and mastoid with thinning of the otic capsule, particularly of the cochlea.

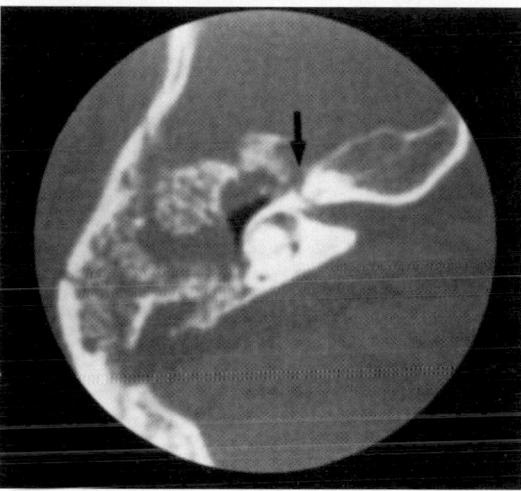

Figure 53 Longitudinal fracture of the right temporal bone, axial computed tomographic section. The fracture passes from the mastoid through the attic into the petrous pyramid anterior to the labyrinth. The fracture reaches and involves the facial canal at its anterior genu (*arrow*).

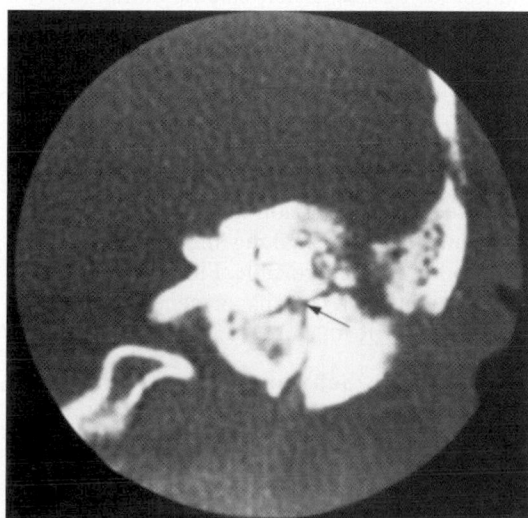

Figure 54 Comminuted fracture of the left mastoid, coronal computed tomographic section. Multiple fractures are noticed in the mastoid. One of the fractures passes underneath the posterior semicircular canal and transects the vertical segment of the facial canal (*arrow*).

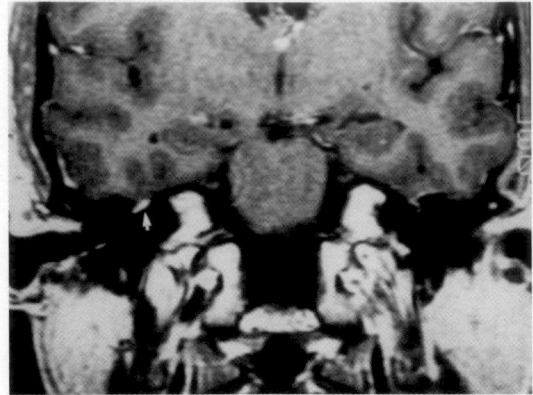

(A)

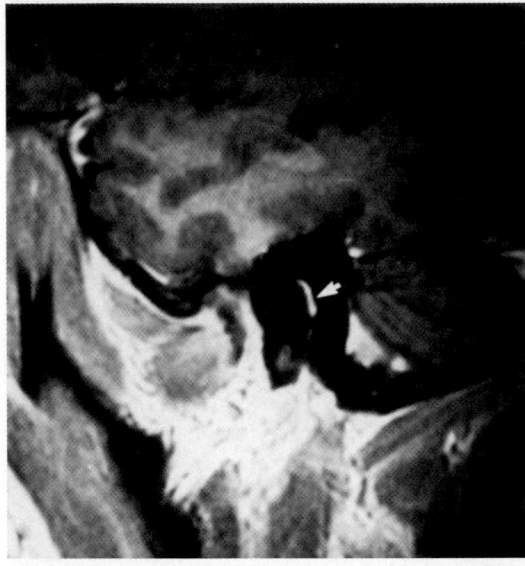

(B)

Figure 55 Facial neuritis. Coronal (A) and sagittal (B) T₁-weighted magnetic resonance images after injection of contrast material. There is enhancement of the right facial nerve in the regions of the anterior genu and proximal portion of the mastoid segment (*arrows*).

labyrinth to a diffuse process. The lumen of inner ear is partially or totally filled with granulation and fibrous tissues. Later, calcific obliteration of the bony labyrinth may occur, which may lead to a partial or complete bony obliteration (labyrinthitis ossificans) of its lumen (Figure 43). Whereas the bony obliteration of the inner ear is readily identified by CT, fibrous obliteration is recognizable only by MRI. In the T2W images, the high signal seen within the normal inner ear structures is absent, therefore making the involved structures no longer recognizable. Fibrous obliteration will appear as area of enhancement on postgadolinium T1W MR images.

Labyrinthine Schwannomas. In the past, small schwannomas have been found within the vestibule and cochlea during postmortem dissections of the temporal bones or during labyrinthectomies. These lesions are usually not recognizable by CT but are well demonstrated as small enhanced masses in MR examinations particularly if performed after injection of contrast material[22,27] (Figure 44). The CT and MRI characteristics of labyrinthine pathol-

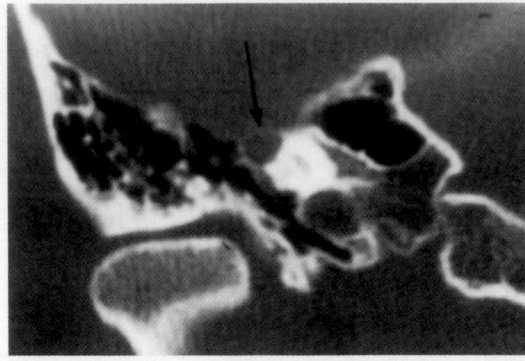

(A)

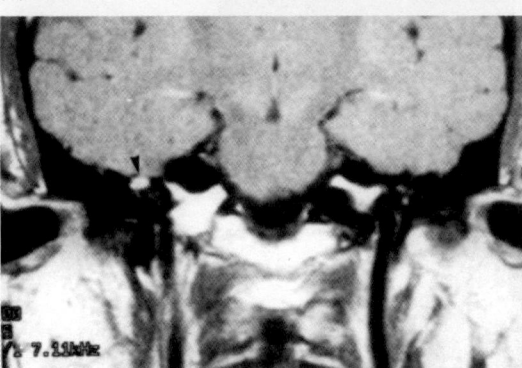

(B)

Figure 56 Facial neurinoma. (A) Coronal computed tomographic section revealing expansion of the right facial canal at the anterior genu (*arrow*). (B) The coronal T₁-weighted magnetic resonance image section obtained after injection of gadolinium diethylenetriamine pentaacetic acid shows the actual enhancing tumor mass (*arrowhead*).

ogy were first reported in 1990 by Mafee and colleagues.[27]

Otospongiosis and Otosclerosis. Osteosclerosis involving the cochlear capsule is often responsible for sensorineural hearing loss by an unknown mechanism. Cochlear otosclerosis is caused by progressive enlargement of the perifenestral foci or by single or multiple foci in other locations in the cochlear capsule. The CT findings vary with the stage of maturation of the process. In the active or spongiotic phase, small areas of demineralization are first observed in the normally sharp contour of the capsule.[13] These foci may enlarge and become confluent, producing large areas of demineralization and finally complete dissolution of the capsule. In the mature or sclerotic stage, localized or diffuse areas of thickening of the capsule are present.[2,13] A typical sign of active cochlear otosclerosis is the "double ring" caused by confluent spongiotic foci within the thickness of the capsule (Figures 45A and B).

Petrous Pyramid

Primary tumors of the petrous bone involve a number of solid and cystic lesions, the more common of which are (1) primary cholesteatoma (epidermoid), (2) cholesterol granuloma, (3) meningocele, (4) mucocele (least common), (5) meningioma, (6) glomus tumor,

(7) schwannoma/neurofibroma, (8) lymphoma (multiple myeloma), (9) Langerhans cell chondroblastoma histiocytosis, (10) rhabdomyosarcoma (children), (11) chondrosarcoma, chondroblastoma (12) chondromyxoid tumor, (13) chordoma, (14) carotid aneurysm, and (15) metastases.[2,20]

Glomus Jugulare Tumors. Glomus jugulare tumors (paragangliomas) arise from minute glomus bodies (chemoreceptors) found in the jugular fossa.[2,4,18,23,25] The typical CT findings include erosion of the cortical outline and enlargement of the jugular fossa, erosion of the septum dividing the jugular fossa from the outer opening of the carotid canal, and erosion of the hypotympanic floor with extension of the tumor in the middle ear cavity (Figure 46). As the lesion enlarges, the posterioinferior aspect of the entire petrous pyramid becomes eroded, as well as the adjacent aspect of the occipital bone including the hypoglossal canal. Large tumors protrude extradurally in the posterior cranial fossa and inferiorly below the base of the skull along the jugular vein. These extensions are better demonstrated by MRI in which the tumor appears in both T1W and T2W images as a mass of medium signal intensity containing several small areas of signal void produced by blood vessels[19,23,25] (Figure 47). After the injection of contrast material, the tumor undergoes a moderate to marked enhancement. The signal intensity of the glomus tumor is differentiated easily from the surrounding intra- and extracranial structures. In addition, MRI allows determination of displacement, encroachment, narrowing, or obstruction of the jugular vein and internal carotid artery because these large vessels are well-visualized with no need for invasive vascular procedures. Jugular venography and carotid arteriography are replaced by MRA and MRV and seldom needed, and carotid arteriography is limited to pre-embolization studies.

Jugular Fossa Schwannoma. Jugular fossa schwannoma and neurofibroma are the second most common jugular fossa masses. These lesions can be readily detected by CT including OTA and MRI scanning (Figure 48). MRI is preferred as the outline of the mass and its extent is better evaluated on MR than CT scans. At times extension of a posterior cranial fossa meningioma or metastasis to the jugular fossa may simulate a jugular fossa neuroma or glomus jugulare tumor.

Congenital Cholesteatomas and Cholesterol Granulomas. Congenital cholesteatomas (epidermoids) may arise in the petrous pyramid. In the CT images, the involved area of the pyramid appears expanded by a cyst-like low-density lesion[9,10,21,26] (Figure 49), which often reaches and erodes the IAC and labyrinth. A CT study with infusion shows no enhancement of the mass except for its thin capsule. With CT, a congenital cholesteatoma of the petrous apex is difficult to differentiate from a cholesterol granuloma cyst that occurs in extensively pneumatized petrous

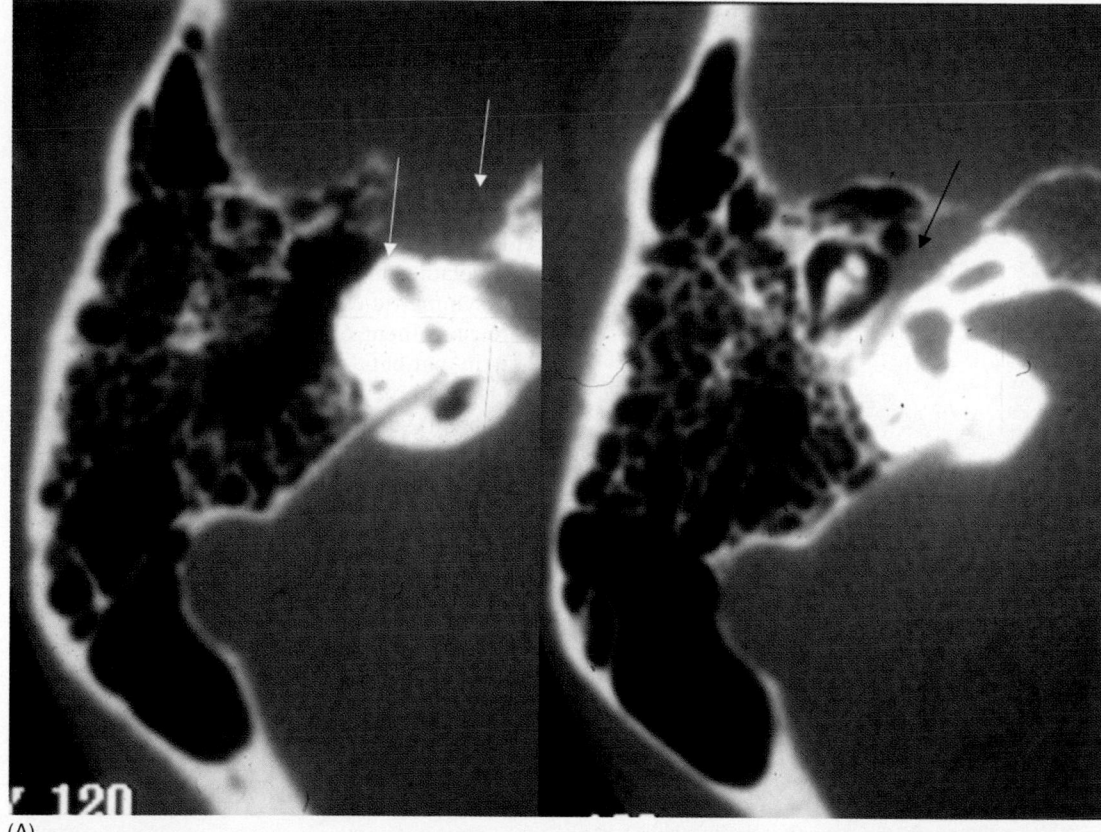

(A)

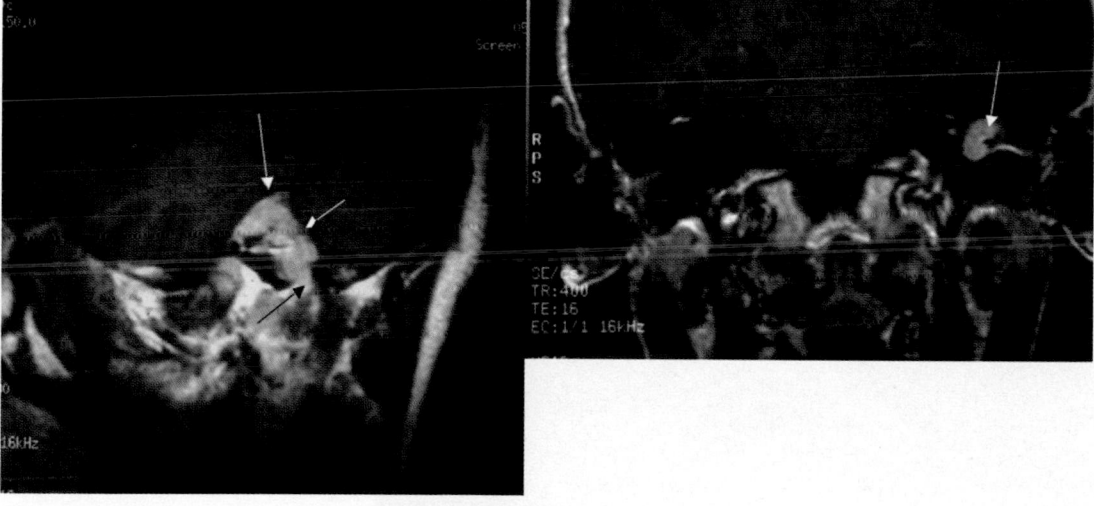

(B)

Figure 57 (A) Facial neuroma. Axial CT scans showing enlargement of facial canal (*arrows*) due to a facial neuroma. (B) Coronal enhanced T₁-weighted MR scans showing an enhancing facial neuroma (*arrows*).

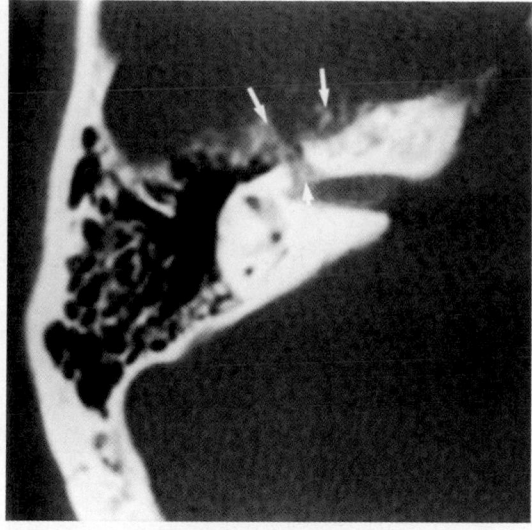

(A)

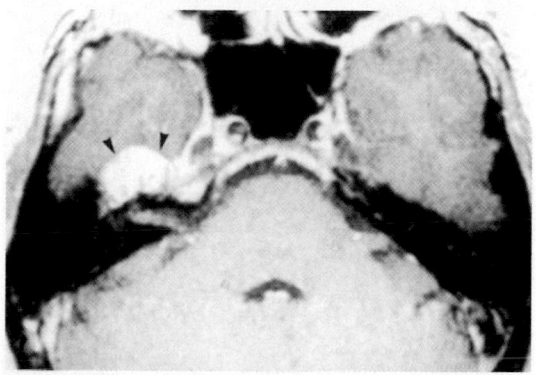

(B)

Figure 58 Hemangioma, right petrous pyramid. (A) Axial computed tomographic section. (B) Axial T₁-weighted magnetic resonance image after contrast. The anterior aspect of the right petrous pyramid is eroded by an enhancing soft tissue mass (*arrowheads*) extending into the attic, labyrinthine segment of the facial nerve canal, and fundus of the internal auditory canal. Note the characteristic bony spiculation within the tumor mass (*arrows*).

pyramids. The 2 lesions can be differentiated with MR because congenital cholesteatomas produce a signal of medium intensity in the T1W images and high intensity in T2W, whereas cholesterol granulomas have a similar high signal in both T1W and T2W sequences (Figure 50). In addition, areas of hypointensity are observed in cholesterol granulomas produced by deposits of hemosiderin or blood of varied ages. Epidermoid cysts may be intradural and adjacent to the cerebellopontine angle. Petrous epidermoids as well as intradural epidermoid cysts demonstrate diffusion restriction on DWI, being hyperintense on DWI and hypointense on ADC mapping sequence. Epidermoid cysts also appear hyperintense on fluid attenuated inversion recovery

(FLAIR) MR pulse sequence. Both DWI and FLAIR pulse sequences differentiate epidermoid cysts from arachnoid cysts and meningoceles.

Meningiomas. Meningiomas arise from the arachnoid cap cells of the meningeal covering around the temporal bone and from the meningeal extension into the IAC (Figure 51). The latter mimics, both clinically and in imaging, the appearance of a vestibular schwannoma. Meningiomas that arise from the petrous ridge are usually recognizable in the CT images as highly enhancing masses producing hyperostotic or lytic changes in the adjacent petrous pyramid. Unlike neurogenic tumors, calcifications are frequently seen in meningiomas (Figure 51A). With en

plaque meningiomas, only the bony changes may be recognizable. MRI obtained after injection of paramagnetic contrast demonstrates a strong and usually homogeneous enhancement of the tumor. En plaque meningiomas are recognizable as areas of enhancing meningeal thickening.

Paget Disease. Paget disease often affects the calvarium and the base of the skull including the petrous pyramids. The disease usually spreads from the petrous apex laterally and produces a typical washed-out appearance of the involved pyramid caused by extensive demineralization (Figure 52). The IAC is usually involved first, followed by the otic capsule, which becomes first thinned out and then completely erased. In the late stage of the disease, deposition of irregularly mineralized bone occurs and results in thickening of the petrosa, narrowing of the IAC, and fixation of the footplate of the stapes.

Facial Nerve

CT is the study of choice for imaging the facial canal. The examination should be performed in

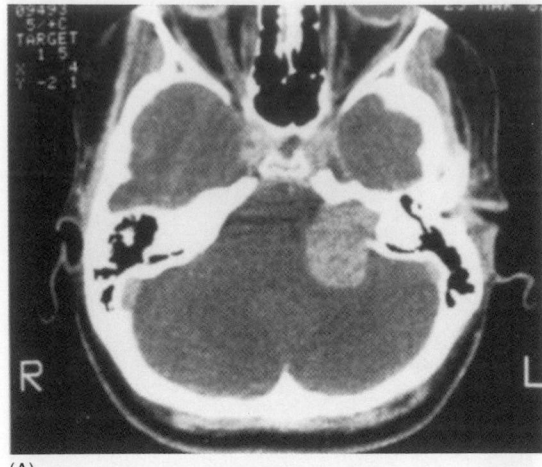

(A)

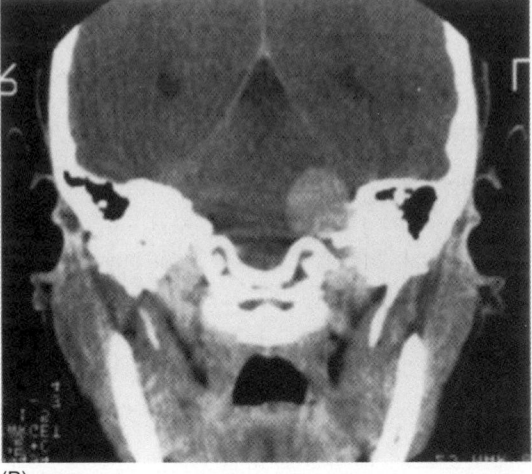

(B)

Figure 59 Left vestibular schwannoma, postinfusion study. (A) Horizontal enhanced CT section. (B) Coronal CT section. The left internal auditory canal appears grossly expanded and eroded. A large enhancing tumor mass fills the canal and the cerebellopontine cistern. Notice the displacement to the right of the brainstem and fourth ventricle.

2 or 3 planes to visualize the various segments of the canal. MRI makes the facial nerve itself genieculate ganglion visible, particularly when the nerve is pathologic. Additional imaging examples of facial nerve disorders are found in Chapter 34, "Facial Paralysis."

Congenital Anomalies. Congenital anomalies involve the size and course of the facial canal. The canal may be partially or completely absent, hypoplastic, or unusually narrow. Minor variations of the course of the facial nerve are common and of no clinical significance. More severe anomalies should be identified to avoid serious damage of the nerve during surgery. The horizontal segment may be displaced inferiorly to cover the oval window or lie exposed adjacent to the promontory. In congenital atresia of the EAC, the mastoid segment of the facial canal is rotated laterally and anteriorly. The rotation varies from minimal obliquity to a true horizontal course (Figures 13B and 18B).

Trauma. Traumatic lesions of the intratemporal portion of the facial nerve occur in approxi-

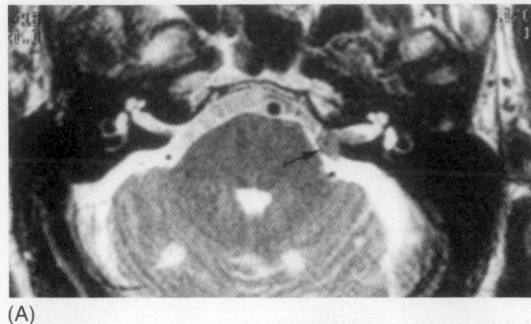

(A)

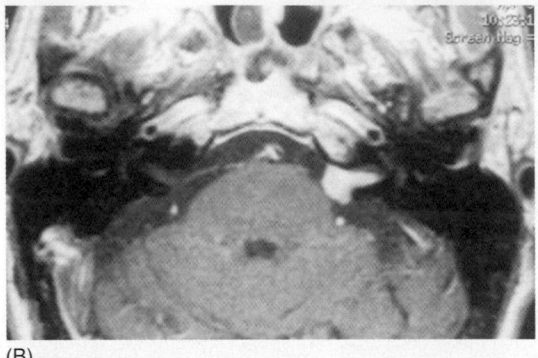

(B)

Figure 60 Left vestibular schwannoma. Axial magnetic resonance images. (A) T2W fast spin echo. Note that the tumor is well seen in the fast spin echo image (A) as a filling defect within the bright signal of the cerebrospinal fluid (*arrow*). (B) T1W postcontrast. An enhancing soft tissue mass fills the left internal auditory canal and protrudes into the cerebellopontine cistern.

mately 20% of longitudinal fractures of the temporal bone and 50% of transverse fractures. The most common site of involvement in longitudinal fractures is the anterior genu (Figures 53 and

54), and in transverse fractures the labyrinthine or intracanalicular segments. The facial nerve may be transected by the fracture, compressed, sheared by a depressed fragment of the canal wall, or simply contused by the violent shock.

Facial Neuritis. Moderate bilateral enhancement of the normal facial nerve, particularly in the region of its anterior genu, is often observed in MRI obtained after injection of contrast material.

Asymmetric enhancement of the facial nerve more prominent on the paralyzed side is common in patients with Bell palsy and Ramsay Hunt syndrome. In Bell palsy, the involvement is segmental and usually confined to the anterior genu and adjacent labyrinthine and tympanic segments. In Ramsay Hunt syndrome, the involvement by the herpes zoster virus is more uniform and often extends to the part of the nerve within the IAC (Figure 55), associated with abnormal enhancement of Scarpa ganglion and vestibular nerves.

In viral neuritis, the nerve is usually not thickened. In sarcoidosis, the involvement is similar to Bell palsy, but the nerve is moderately thickened. In sarcoidosis and Lyme disease, facial nerve involvement may be bilateral.

Neoplasms. Although primary neoplasms of the facial nerve are rare, facial neuromas are the most common (Figure 56). Even rarer, facial neuromas may be congenital. Facial neuromas can cause thickening of the nerve and expansion of the canal (Figure 46A). Further enlargement of the lesion can result in erosion of the bony canal, extension into the middle ear space, and involvement of the mastoid and petrous pyramid (Figure 57A). MRI is the study of choice to depict a facial neuroma

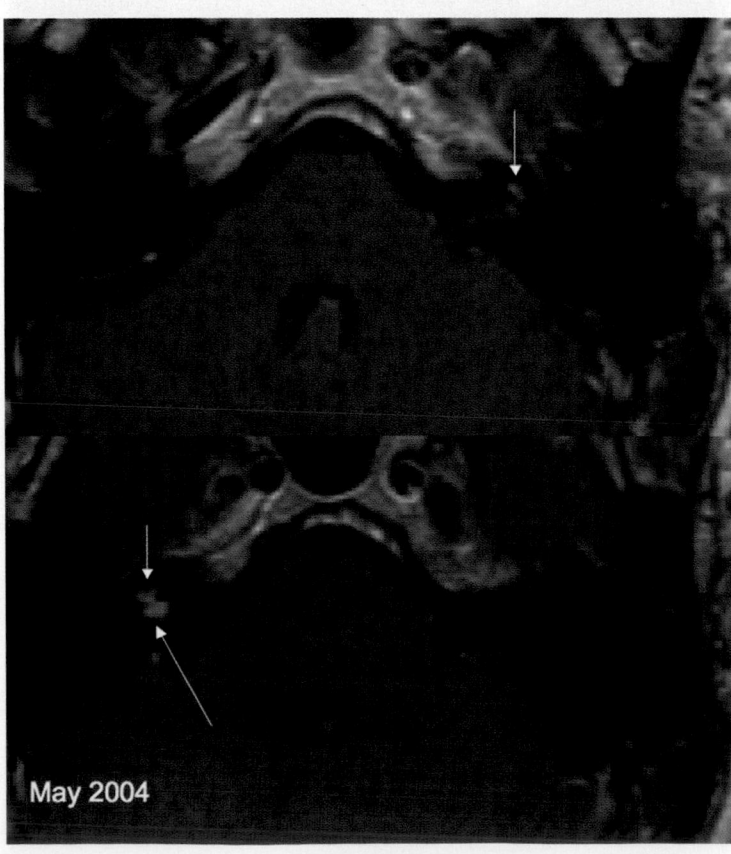

Figure 61 Small vestibular schwannoma. Enhanced axial T$_1$-weighted MR scans showing small right vestibular schwannoma (*large arrow*) and bilateral cochlear schwannomas (*small arrows*).

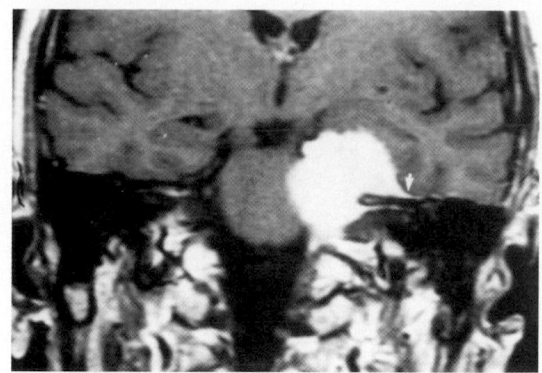

Figure 62 Meningioma coronal T$_1$-weighted magnetic resonance image section after injection of contrast material. A large enhancing mass extends above and below the left side of the tentorial notch. The tumor spares the internal auditory canal. Notice the lateral en plaque extension of the lesion (*arrow*).

and to differentiate facial nerve neuromas from other lesions. The mass has a nonspecific low signal in T1W and high signal in T2W images and shows marked enhancement in T1W MR images obtained after injection of gadolinium DPTA (Figure 57B). Facial neuromas arising from the geniculate region of facial nerve and those arising from greater superficial petrosal nerve and facial nerve hemangioma (Figure 58) may present as a small or large extra-axial mass in the middle cranial fossa. The facial nerve, particularly its vertical segment, may be involved by carcinoma arising in the parotid gland and extending into the temporal bone. This is found particularly with adenoid cystic carcinomas which have a tendency for perineural and perivascular spread.

Cerebellopontine Angle

Vestibular Schwannomas. Vestibular schwannomas account for 80 to 90% of the tumors of the cerebellopontine angle.[2] These neoplasms usually arise within the IAC, which becomes enlarged. Expansion of the IAC, shortening of its posterior wall, and erosion of the crista falciformis are well visualized in high-definition CT images targeted for bone. Both sides should always be examined to compare differences. Vestibular schwannomas are often missed on plain CT scans because the neoplasm is isodense to the surrounding brain and usually is not surrounded by edema. After infusion of iodinated contrast material, the mass enhances and may become visible (Figure 59). Intracanalicular lesions and cisternal masses smaller than 0.5 cm usually are not visualized with CT scanning. Before the development of the MRI technique, small vestibular schwannomas were diagnosed with CT pneumocisternography.[2,28–30]

MRI is the study of choice for diagnosis of vestibular schwannomas without exposing the patient to ionizing radiation and without the necessity for spinal puncture. The neoplasm appears in the T1W images brighter than CSF and isointense to gray matter. In the T2W MR images, the neoplasms are brighter than brain. Large masses are easily identified in both sequences, but small lesions can be detected only in the T1W images because in the T2W they may be obscured by the hyperintense CSF. A final diagnosis of small neoplasms is achieved by injecting intravenously paramagnetic contrast agents. Gadolinium DPTA concentrates in the tumor produces a shortening of the T1 relaxation time with consequent marked increase of the MR signal in the T1W images (Figures 60 to 61). Vestibular schwannomas as small as 2 mm can be diagnosed by this technique.[2,28]

Meningioma. Meningiomas account for approximately 3 to 7% of the cerebellopontine angle tumors. The lesion has signal intensity less than the brain in the T1W MRI sequences. In the T2W MR images, the lesion has variable signal characteristics, ranging from slight to moderate hyperintensity. After intravenous injection of paramagnetic contrast material, meningiomas show in the T1W MR images a marked increase in signal intensity similar to that seen in vestibular schwannomas. Unlike the latter neoplasm, which is centered at the IAC, meningiomas usually are centered in the cerebellopontine angle anterior to the IAC and spare the ICA. Meningiomas show increased thickening and enhancement of the adjacent dura (so-called dural tail), which is an important imaging finding favoring the diagnosis of meningiomas (Figure 62). Unlike schwannomas, which are often round and globular in shape, meningiomas have a broad base with the dura. At times cerebellopontine angle meningiomas may enter the IAC, or they may arise within the IAC, mimicking an intracanalicular schwannoma (Figure 51C), Metastasis may mimic primary tumors of TAC (Figure 63).

Endolymphatic Sac Neoplasms and Fibro-Osseous Lesions of the Temporal Bone and TMJ

Endolymphatic Sac Neoplasms. Primary adenomatous lesions of the temporal bone are rare neoplasms.[31–35] In 1989, Heffner described 20 cases of a type of papillary cystic adenocarcinoma in which the neoplasm destroyed a large portion of the posterior petromastoid part of the

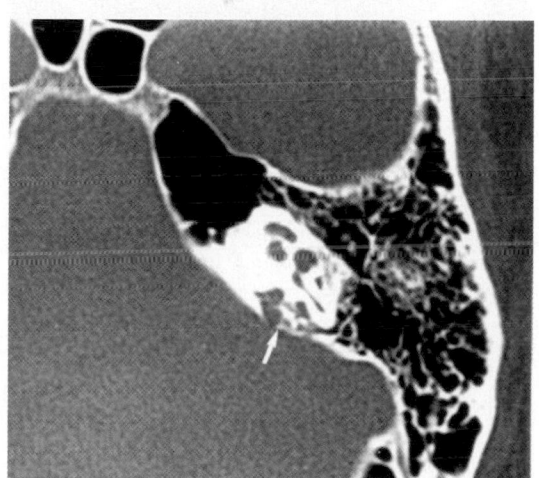

(A)

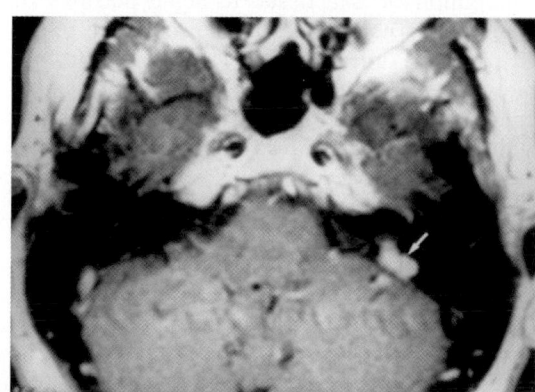

(B)

Figure 64 Endolymphatic sac tumor. (A) Axial CT section of the left petrous pyramid. There is erosion of the posterior aspect of the petrous pyramid in the region of the endolymphatic sac with the formation of an irregular cavity (*arrow*). (B) T$_1$ axial magnetic resonance image. The tumor mass enhances after injection of contrast (*arrow*).

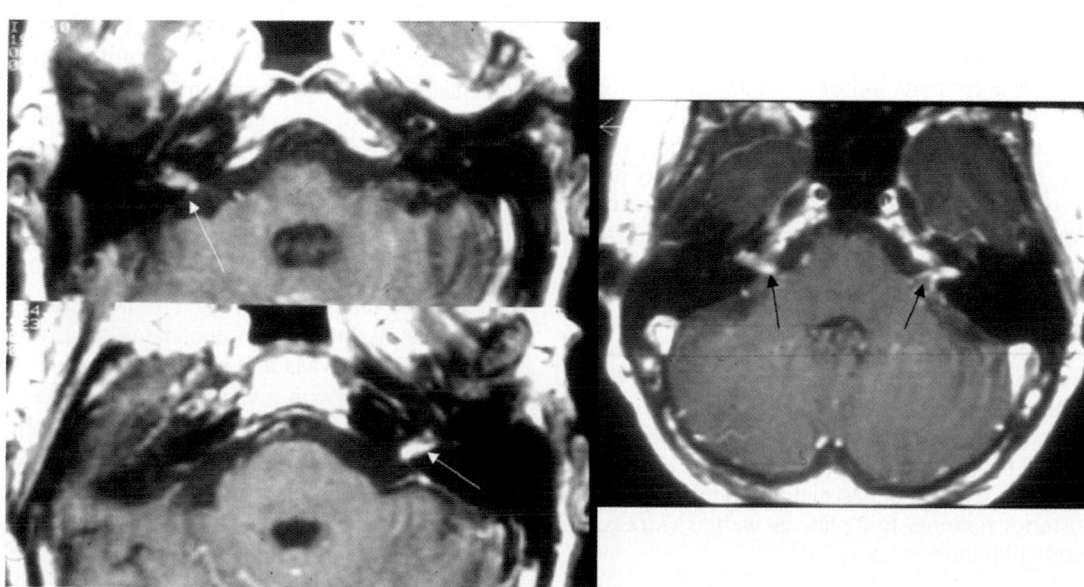

Figure 63 Metastasis into IAC. Axial enhanced T$_1$-weighted MR scans (*left*) showing metastasis (*arrows*) into bilateral IACS from primary lung cancer. Axial enhanced T$_1$-weighted MR scan showing metastasis into IACS from primary shoulder malignant melanoma (*arrows*).

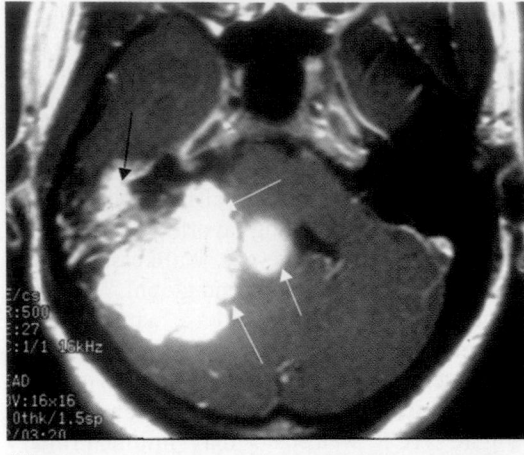

(A)

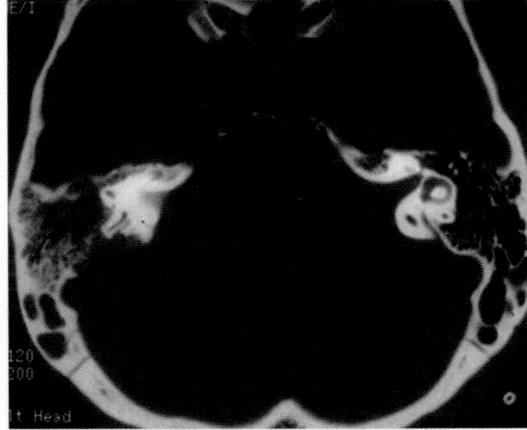

(B)

Figure 65 Endolymphatic sac tumor. (A) Axial enhanced T₁-weighted MR scan showing a round enhancing mass (*arrows*). Note tumor extension into the right middle ear (*black arrow*). (B) Axial CT scan. Same patient showing marked destruction of right petromastoid plate and vestibular aqueduct. Note normal left vestibular aqueduct (*arrow*).

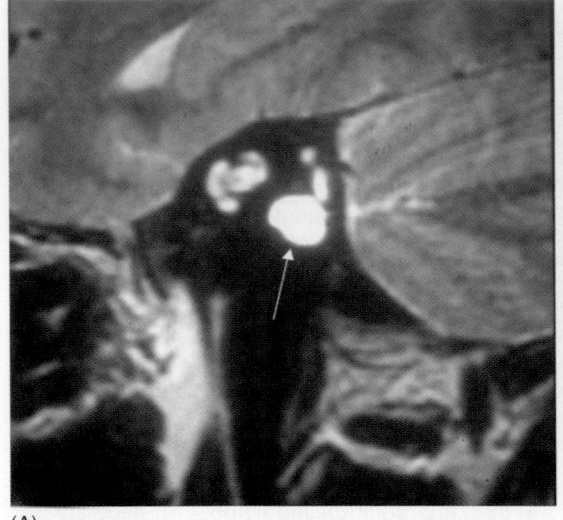
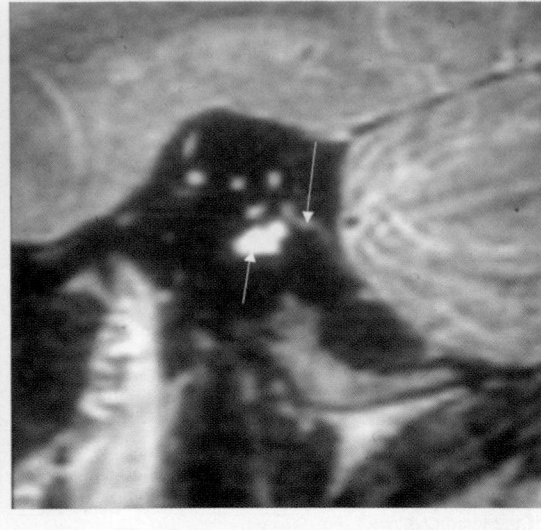

(A)

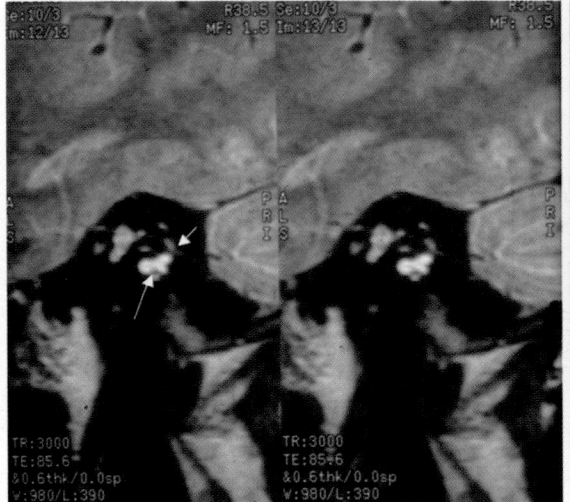
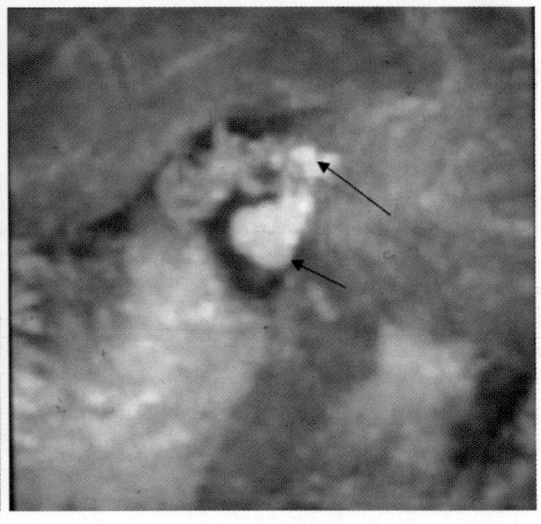

(B)

Figure 66 (A) Papillary adenocarcinoma of temporal bone. Sagittal T₂-weighted MR scans showing a mass (*arrows*) arising in the sublabyrinthine region. Note normal endolymphatic duct and sac (*upper arrow*). (B) Sagittal T₂-weighted MR scans (*left*) and volume-rendered 3D MR image showing the tumor (*arrows*) and normal endolymphatic duct (*short white arrow*).

temporal bone and included a prominent extension into the posterior cranial fossa.[31] Patient histories indicated a slow growth rate of the lesions. There were resemblances of the normal distal endolymphatic sac tissue to some portions of many of the neoplasms. Tissue submitted to the US Armed Forces Institute of Pathology from a rare case of papillary adenomatous neoplasm of endolymphatic sac origin, reported by Hassard and colleagues had a strong similarity to the larger, destructive neoplasms reviewed by Heffner. In his final analysis, Heffner concluded that the neoplasms in his series grew slowly, but the neoplasms manifested a destructive, infiltrating growth into the temporal bone. Heffner preferred to diagnose them as low-grade papillary adenocarcinoma. Because the neoplasms were epithelial and manifested a distinctive destructive growth along the posterior-medial petromastoid portion of the temporal bone, Heffner inferred that the endolymphatic sac seems an ideal location to give rise to these neoplasms with their combined intrabony and posterior fossa components. These neoplasms characteristically cause destruction of the vestibular aqueduct and at times marked erosion of the petromastoid plate.

There may be extension of the neoplasm into the jugular fossa and middle ear cavity. There may be fine or coarse calcifications present within these neoplasms. The neoplasm may be solid or a combination of solid and cystic components. There will be moderate to marked contrast enhancement on CT and MRI scans (Figures 64 to 66). Some of the neoplasms may arise from sublabyrinthine mastoid air cells mucosal glands with intact endolymphatic sac and vestibular aqueduct. Bilateral neoplasms have been reported in patients with Von Hippel-Lindau disease. Other rare neoplasms found in the temporal bone, such as mucoepidermoid and adenoid cystic carcinoma, may have similar CT and MRI findings to low-grade papillary adenocarcinoma of endolymphatic sac origin. These neoplasms should be included in the differential diagnosis of destructive or nondestructive tumors about the posterior petromastoid plate as well as extraaxial cerebellopontine tumors.

Fibro-Osseous Lesions of the Temporal Bone and TMJ. The temporal bone and TMJ can be affected by a variety of benign and

malignant conditions, including fibrous dysplasia, osteoma, osteochondroma, osteoblastoma, chondroblastoma, chondrosarcoma (Figure 67), osteogenic sarcoma, chondromyxoid tumor, osteoclastoma (true giant cell tumor), aggressive fibromatosis, and synovial chondromatosis.[36,37] Fibrous dysplasia, osteoma, osteochondroma, and osteoblastoma have characteristic CT and MRI findings limited to the involved bone without involvement of the surrounding soft tissue. Chondroblastoma and chondrosarcoma are rare neoplasms of the temporal bone and TMJ, resulting in bone destruction and an enhancing heterogeneous mass in the TMJ and squamous portion of the temporal bone with invasion into the adjacent soft tissues. Fine or coarse calcification may be present. Osteogenic sarcoma typically involves the mastoid process and is associated with periosteal reaction and bone formation in the involved surrounding soft tissue. Osteoclastomas typically result in marked expansion of involved bone and most often occur in the squamous portion of the temporal bone and its articular fossa. On MRI and CT, osteoclastomas contain multiple hemorrhagic

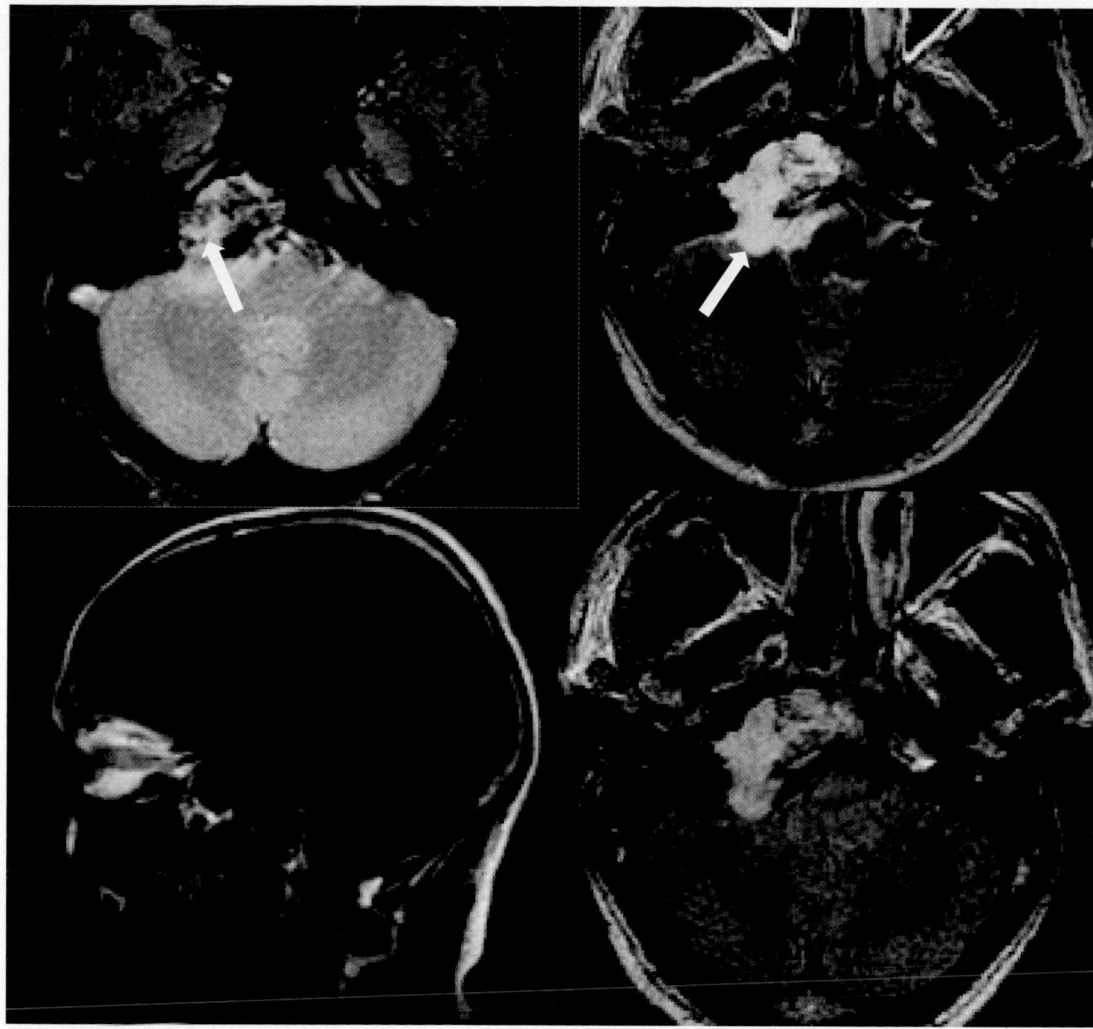

Figure 67 Chondrosarcoma. Axial enhanced T_1-weighted and coronal enhanced T_1-weighted MR scans showing a large CPA chondrosarcoma (*arrows*).

cystic components, simulating the appearance of an "aneurysmal bone cyst."

REFERENCES

1. Valvassori, GE, Buckingham RA. Tomography and Cross Sections of the Ear. Philadelphia: WB Saunders Co.; Stuttgart: Georg Thieme Verlag; 1975.
2. Valvassori GE. Imaging of the temporal bone. In: Mafee MF, Valvassori GE, Becker M, editors. Imaging of the Head and Neck, 2nd edition. Stuttgart: Georg Thieme Verlag; 2005. p. 3–133.
3. Mafee MF, Kumar A, Yannias DA, et al. Computed tomography of the middle ear in the evaluation of cholesteatoma and other soft tissue masses: Comparison with pluridirectional tomography. Radiology 1983;148:465–72.
4. Mafee MF, Valvassori GE, Dobben GD. The role of radiology in surgery of the ear and skull base. Otolaryngol Clin North Am 1982;15:723–53.
5. Mafee MF, Singleton EL, Valvassori GE, et al. Acute otomastoiditis and its complications: Role of CT. Radiology 1985;54:391–7.
6. Mafee MF, Almi K, Kahen HL, et al. Chronic otomastoiditis: A conceptual understanding of CT findings. Radiology 1986;160:193–200.
7. Mafee MF, Levin BC, Applebaum EL. Cholesteatoma of the middle ear and mastoid: A comparison of CT scan and operative findings: Otolaryngol Clin North Am 1988; 21:265–93.
8. Cundiff JG, Djalilian HR, Mafee MF. Bilateral Sequential petrous apicitis secondary to an anaerobic bacterium. Otolaryngology-Head and Neck Surgery 2006;135:969–971.
9. Mafee MF. MRI and CT in the evaluation of acquired and congenital cholesteatomas of the temporal bone. J Otolaryngol 1993;22:239–48.
10. Mafee MF, Kumar A, Heffner D. Epidermoid cyst (cholesteatoma) and cholesterol granuloma of the temporal bone and epidermoid cysts affecting the brain. Neuroimaging Clin North Am 1994;4:561–78.
11. Curtin HD. Congenital malformation of the ear. Otolaryngol Clin North Am 1988;21:317–36.
12. Mafee MF, Charletta D, Kumar A, Belmont H. Large vestibular aqueduct and congenital sensorineural hearing loss. AJR Am J Neuroradiol 1992;13:805–19.
13. Mafee MF, Valvassori GE, Deitch RL, et al. Use of CT in the evaluation of cochlear otosclerosis. Radiology 1985;156:703–8.
14. Conneely MF, Mafee MF. Orbital rhabdomyosarcoma and simulating lesions. Neuroimaging Clin N Am 2005; 15: 121–36.
15. Phelps PD, Lloyd GAS, editors. Traumatic lesions of the temporal bone. In: Radiology of the Ear. Oxford: Blackwell Scientific Publications; 1983. p. 68–75.
16. Harnsberger HR, Dahlen RT, Shelton C, et al. Advanced techniques in magnetic resonance imaging in the evaluation of the large endolymphatic duct and sac syndrome. Laryngoscope 1995;105:1037–42.
17. Casselman JW, Kuhweide R, Ampe W, et al. Pathology of the membranous labyrinth: Comparison of T1- and T2-weighted and gadolinium-enhanced spin-echo and 3DFT-CISS imaging. AJR Am J Neuroradiol 1993;14:59–69.
18. Mafee MF, Valvassori GE, Kumar A, et al. Tumors and tumor-like conditions of the middle ear and mastoid: Role of CT and MRI. Otolaryngol Clin North Am 1988; 21:349–75.
19. Rodgers GK, Applegate L, De la Cruz A, et al. Magnetic resonance angiography: Analysis of vascular lesions of the temporal bone and skull base. Am J Otolaryngol 1993;14:56–62.
20. Mafee MF. Base of the skull. In: Mafee MF, Valvassori GE, Becker M, editors. Imaging of the Head and Neck, 2nd edition. New York: Thieme; 2005. p. 295–349.
21. Mafee MF, Aimi K, Valvassori GE. CT in the diagnosis of primary tumors of the petrous bone. Laryngoscope 1984;94:1423–30.
22. Mafee MF. MR imaging of intralabyrinthine schwannoma, labyrinthitis, and other labyrinthine pathology. Otolaryngol Clin North Am 1995;28:407–30.
23. Mafee MF, Valvassori GE, Shugar MA, et al. High resolution and dynamic sequential computed tomography. Use in the evaluation of glomus, complex tumors. Arch Otolaryngol 1983;109:691–5.
24. Pisaneschi MJ, Mafee MF, Samii M. Applications of MR angiography in head and neck pathology. Otolaryngol Clin North Am 1995;28:543–61.
25. Mafee MF, Raofi B, Kumar A, et al. Glomus faciale, glomus jugulare, glomus tympanicum, glomus vagale, carotid body tumors, and simulating lesions. Radiol Clin North Am 2000;83:1059–76.
26. Pisaneschi MJ, Langer B. Congenital cholesteatoma and cholesterol granuloma of the temporal bone: Role of magnetic resonance imaging. Top Magn Reson Imaging 2000; 11:87–97.
27. Mafee MF, Lachenaure CS, Kumar A, et al. CT and MRI of intralabyrinthine schwannoma: Report of two cases and review of the literature. Radiology 1990; 174: 395–400.
28. Mafee MF. Acoustic neuroma and other acoustic nerve disorders. Role of MRI and CT: An analysis of 238 cases. Semin Ultrasound CT MR 1987;8:256–83.
29. Mafee MF, Meyer DH, Hill JH. Neuroradiologic evaluation of patients with central auditory lesions. Otolaryngol Clin North Am 1985;18:223–63.
30. Mafee MF, Kumar A, Valvassori GE, et al. Diagnostic potential of CT in neurotological disorders. Laryngoscope 1985;95:505–14
31. Heffner DK. Low-grade papillary adenocarcinoma of endolymphatic sac. Cancer 1989;64:2292–302.
32. Hassard AD, Boudreau SF, Cron CE. Adenoma of the endolymphatic sac. J Otolaryngol 1984;13:213–6.
33. Mafee MF, Weer L, Mafee RF. Imaging of vestibular aqueduct, endolymphatic duct and sac and adenocarcinoma of probable endolymphatic sac origin. Riv Neuroradiol 1995;8:951–61.
34. Mafee MF, Shah H. Endolymphatic sac tumors and papillary adenocarcinoma of the temporal bone: Role of MRI and CT. Iran J Radiol 2005;1:53–60.
35. Mukherji SK, Albernaz VS, Low W, et al. Papillary endolymphatic sac tumors: CT, MR imaging and angiographic findings in 20 patients. Radiology 1997;202:801–8.
36. Mafee MF. Temporomandibular joint. In: Mafee MF, Valvassori GE, Becker M, editors. Imaging of the Head and Neck, 2nd edition. New York: Thieme; 2005. p. 477–507.
37. Rao V, Bacelar MT. MR imaging of temporomandibular joint. Neuroimag Clin N Am 2004;14:761–75.

12

Pathologic Correlates in Otology and Neurotology

Joseph B. Nadol, Jr, MD

INTRODUCTION

Otopathology is important not only for the understanding of the pathogenesis and pathophysiology of otologic disease but also as a critical method for evaluating the results of medical and surgical interventions for such disorders.

SURGERY FOR OTOSCLEROSIS

Residual and Recurrent Conductive Hearing Loss

Primary stapedectomy can be expected to close the preoperative air-bone gap to within 10 dB in approximately 90% of cases.[1] However, over time the mean air-bone gap tends to increase, causing at least some degree of recurrent conductive hearing loss.[2,3] Furthermore, the success rate as measured by closure of the air-bone gap to within 10 dB in revision stapedectomy is considerably lower than in primary stapes surgery with a mean of approximately 50%.[4] The causes for both residual and recurrent conductive hearing loss can be validated by temporal bone histopathology in patients who had undergone stapes surgery during life.

Residual Conductive Hearing Loss. The most common causes for failure to close the air-bone gap to within 10 dB at the time of primary stapedectomy include unrecognized or untreated fixation of the malleus, unrecognized obliteration of the round window by otosclerosis, malposition of the stapes prosthesis resulting in inadequate transmission of sound from the tympanic membrane to the oval window, and adhesions in the middle ear as a consequence of surgical intervention.

Fixation of the Malleus. Fixation of the malleus occurs in the epitympanum (Figure 1) and can be the result of developmental disorders, chronic otitis media, and trauma, including previous surgery. Fisch and his colleagues suggested that at least partial fixation of the malleus at the anterior mallear ligament may occur in up to 38% of stapes procedures which undergo revision.[5] In an otopathologic study, Oktay and colleagues identified a much lower incidence, that is, in 4 out of 52 specimens with otosclerotic fixation of the stapes footplate.[6] In a study of 279 consecutive stapes operations, both primary and revision, Lesinski identified an incidence of malleus fixation of 4%.[7]

In a series of clinical and histopathologic cases, Harris and colleagues identified an air-bone gap ranging from less than 10 to 28 dB as caused by fixation of the malleus.[8] In a histologic study of 1,108 temporal bones, which otherwise demonstrated a normal middle ear, bony fixation of the malleus was found in 14 cases and almost always unilaterally.[9] Fixation was most common at the lateral epitympanic wall and did not include the ligaments of the malleus. Otosclerosis did not seem to be a predisposing factor. The use of preoperative laser doppler vibrometry may be an adjunct to pneumo-otoscopy for preoperative diagnosis of fixation of the malleus.[10]

Obliteration of the Round Window. Although it is known that the round window is a site of predilection for otosclerosis (Figure 2),[11,12] this finding is not commonly reported as a cause of residual conductive hearing loss following primary stapedectomy.[4] Clinically, otosclerosis in the area of the round window may be obvious at the time of surgery. However, confirmation of complete closure of the round window, necessary for production of residual conductive hearing loss, is difficult to determine by otomicroscopy. Therefore, most authors would suggest completion of a stapedectomy in suspected round window obliteration, but not if it had been identified as present at a previous operation.

Malpositioning of Stapes Prosthesis and Formation of Cicatrix in the Middle Ear. Residual conductive hearing loss may also be caused by inadequate size of the fenestration of the footplate, the angle of the incus attachment prosthesis with the footplate resulting in friction of the prosthesis against the margin of fenestration, or by a prosthesis that is too short.

Superior Semicircular Canal Dehiscence. Although the usual presenting symptom of dehiscence of the superior semicircular canal (Figure 3)[13] is vestibular disturbance, conductive hearing loss has also been reported.[14–17]

Recurrent Conductive Hearing Loss. Most authors agree that after stapedectomy, the postoperative mean air-bone gap increases over time, producing some degree of conductive hearing loss in many patients.[2,3] In a series of 279 consecutive cases of revision stapes surgery, Lesinski identified displacement of the prosthesis out of the oval window and/or fixation of the prosthesis against the otic capsule or residual footplate (81%) as the most common causes of recurrent conductive hearing loss.[7] The most common cause of displacement of the prosthesis was erosion of the incus.

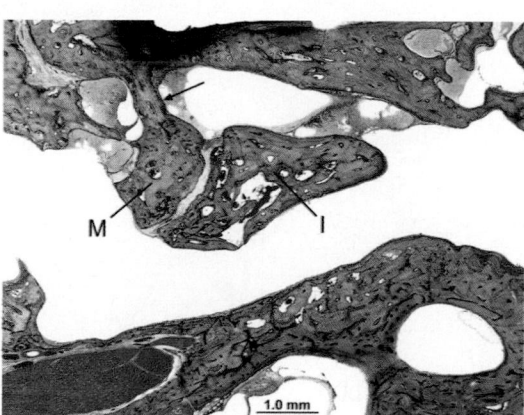

Figure 1 Residual conductive hearing loss after stapedectomy. This 81-year-old woman with bilateral otosclerosis underwent a right stapedectomy 11 years prior to death. A conductive hearing loss persisted after surgery. The cause of the residual conductive hearing loss could be attributed to fixation of the head of the malleus (M) to the anterolateral wall of the epitympanum (*arrow*) by lamellar bone. Otosclerosis was found at the oval window niche, and the stapes prosthesis was in good position. I = incus

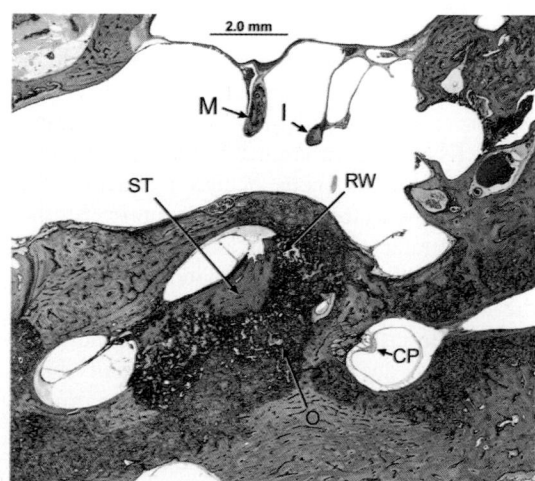

Figure 2 Residual conductive hearing loss after stapedectomy. This 65-year-old woman suffered a bilateral progressive hearing loss caused by otosclerosis. She underwent a right stapedectomy at age 42. Although there was a 20 dB improvement in hearing following stapedectomy, a large residual air-bone gap persisted. The stapes prosthesis was in good position. There was a large otosclerotic focus (O) involving the cochlear labyrinth extending to the endosteum and with total obliteration of the round window niche (RW) with extension to the adjacent scala tympani (ST) of the basal turn. CP = crista of the posterior semicircular canal; I = incus; M = malleus.

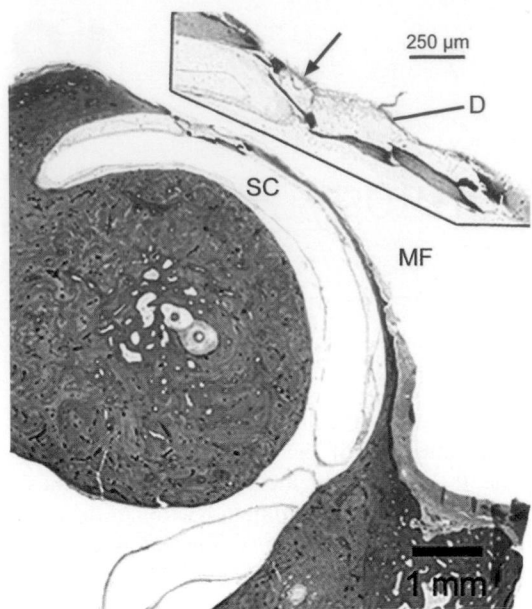

Figure 3 Bony dehiscence of the superior semicircular canal. This vertically sectioned temporal bone demonstrates a very thin bony layer between the arch of the superior semicircular canal (SC) and the middle fossa (MF). As seen in the inset, the dura (D) seemed to be intact. Although there is some artifactual fracture of the thin bone, in one area (*arrowhead*) only periosteum of the superior semicircular canal separates the canal from the middle fossa. (Adapted from reference 13.)

In a meta-analysis, Han and colleagues[4] identified erosion of the incus as a common surgical finding (43% of cases) in revision stapes surgery for recurrent conductive loss. Other causes of recurrent conductive hearing loss include new bone growth at the oval window or displacement of the prosthesis over time to the margin of the oval window niche.

Other studies have reported histopathologic findings after stapedectomy.[18–23]

Resorption of Incus. The pathogenesis of resorption of the incus is unknown. The histopathology (Figures 4 and 5) suggests the presence of a resorptive osteitis with small amounts of granulation tissue and inflammatory cells. Although resorption of the incus occurs frequently following stapedectomy, it may occur from other causes. In fact, Lannigan and colleagues suggested that there is an age-related resorption of the normal incus.[24] Similarly, Imauchi and colleagues described in a patient with conductive hearing loss due to ossicular discontinuity bilateral spontaneous resorption of the long process of the incus.[25] Experimental studies suggest that osteoclastic bone resorption in the temporal bone, including the incus, is enhanced in osteoprotegerin deficient mice.[26]

New Bone Growth at Oval Window. In two histopathologic studies,[27,28] a total of five cases were described with new bone formation at the oval window following stapedectomy and resulting in refixation of the stapes prosthesis. In all five cases the primary stapedectomy had required drill out of obliterative otosclerosis in the oval window niche. Furthermore, the histopathology of the new bone formation following primary stapedectomy

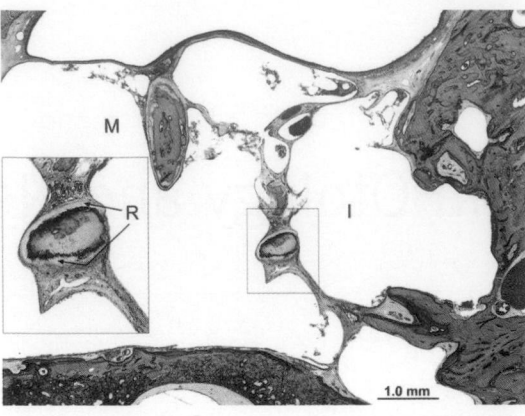

Figure 4 Incus resorption following stapedectomy. This 65-year-old woman had a progressive bilateral mixed hearing loss starting early in life. She underwent a right stapedectomy at age 42 using a Teflon wire piston. Although there was initial improvement in hearing, over the years a conductive hearing loss recurred. Although the prosthesis remained in appropriate position, there was evidence of resorption (R) of the incus (I) at the site of the wire crimp. M = malleus.

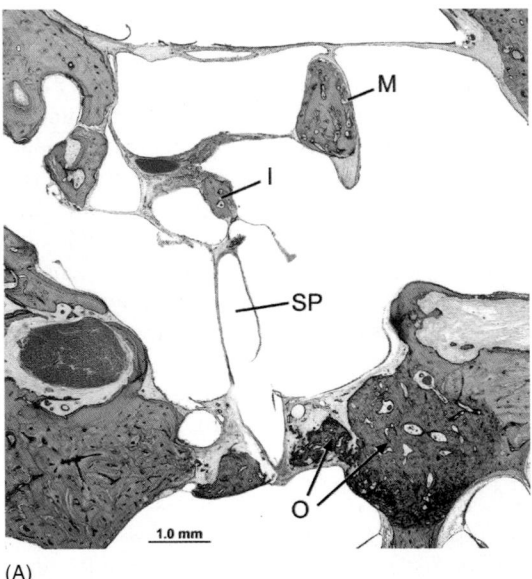

(A)

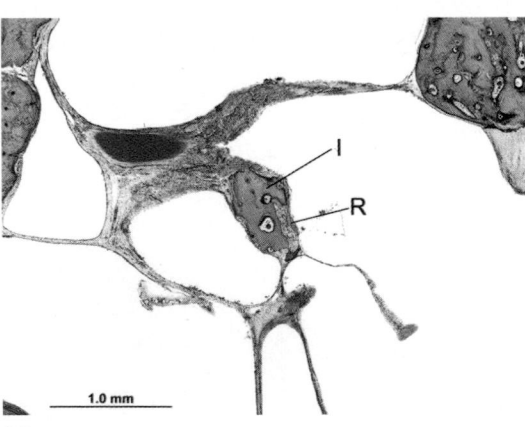

(B)

Figure 5 Incus resorption following stapedectomy. This 80-year-old man with bilateral otosclerosis underwent a left stapedectomy at age 66 using a Teflon wire incus to oval window prosthesis. (A) The outline of the stapes prosthesis (SP), malleus (M), and incus (I) are seen. Otosclerosis (O) is visible within the footplate and anterior to the stapediovestibular joint. (B) Resorptive osteitis (R) of the incus (I) is seen near the wire crimp.

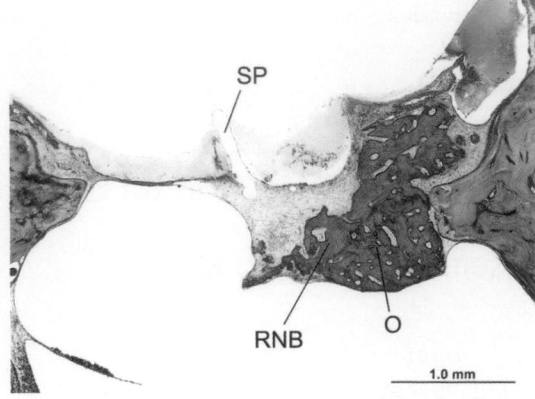

Figure 6 New bone formation after "drill out" of footplate and oval window niche. This 70-year-old man suffered bilateral otosclerosis. At age 56, he underwent a right stapedectomy. Obliterative otosclerosis of the oval window was identified, and the footplate and oval window were saucerized using a microdrill. A gel wire prosthesis was then inserted. Initial closure of the air-bone gap occurred. However, at age 66 there was a recurrent 20 dB conductive hearing loss on the right. The outline of the gel wire stapes prosthesis (SP) is seen. At the oval window, in proximity to the stapes prosthesis, there is not only otosclerosis (O) but also reparative new bone formation (RNB).

appeared to be lamellar new bone rather than progression of otosclerosis (Figure 6). This would suggest that extensive drilling in the oval window may induce reparative new bone formation following stapedectomy. Therefore, a somewhat larger than normal fenestra should be made to accommodate for postoperative new bone formation when confronted by obliterative otosclerosis.

Displacement of the Prosthesis. A stapes prosthesis may migrate with the passage of time following primary stapedectomy resulting in inefficient sound transmission and the development of recurrent conductive hearing loss. This may be the result of resorption of the incus, but it has also been seen in cases of total stapedectomy in which an otherwise well positioned prosthesis migrated to the margin of the oval window (Figure 7).

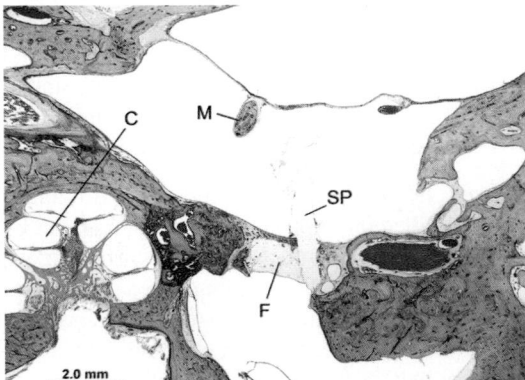

Figure 7 Displacement of stapes prosthesis following stapedectomy. This 57-year-old woman with known bilateral otosclerosis underwent a right stapedectomy at age 45 using a fat-stainless steel wire prosthesis. A total removal of the stapes footplate was performed. Postoperative audiometry demonstrated closure of the air-bone gap. The outline of the stapes prosthesis (SP) and the fatty tissue graft (F) in the oval window are seen. The stapes prosthesis has become marginalized to the posterior aspect of the oval window niche. C = cochlea; M = malleus.

Complications of Stapes Surgery

Although the success rate for primary stapedectomy in closing the air-bone gap to within 10% has been reported as 90% or better, complications other than residual or recurrent conductive hearing loss may occur following stapedectomy. Such complications include perilymphatic gusher, trauma to the inner ear including delayed endolymphatic hydrops, and suppurative labyrinthitis.

Perilymphatic Gusher. Although the most common association of perilymphatic gusher is with x-linked mixed deafness with congenital fixation of the stapes footplate and perilymphatic gusher[29,30] which has been recently associated with the *POU3F4* gene (DFN-3),[31] it is certainly not exclusive to this diagnosis. A congenital defect in the modiolus has been demonstrated as the etiology of a perilymphatic gusher (Figure 8).[32] Thus, perilymphatic gushers have been identified at cochlear implantation in a variety of congenital malformations of the inner ear, including common cavity deformities (widely patent communication between the cochlea and vestibule), and Mondini malformations.[33] Although CT scanning of the temporal bone may identify a defect in the modiolus, which predisposes to a perilymphatic gusher,[34] this abnormality is not always identified.[35]

Surgical Trauma to the Inner Ear. Surgical trauma to the inner ear may occur during stapedectomy in the process of fenestration of

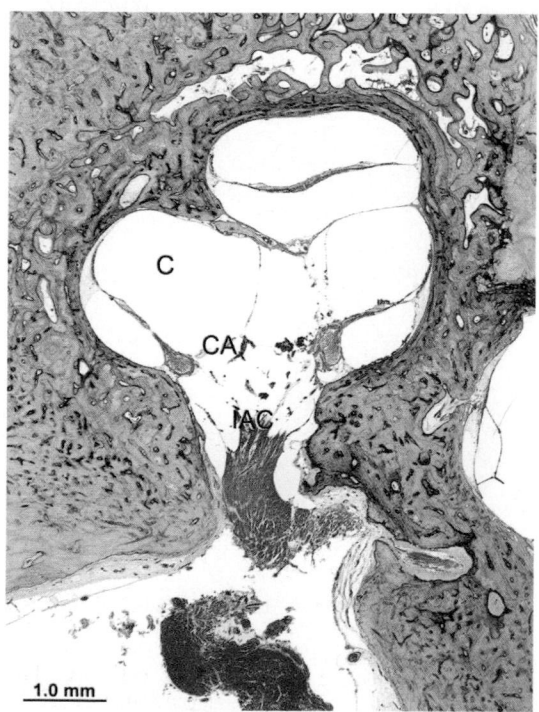

Figure 8 Anatomic potential for perilymphatic gusher. This 2.5-year-old boy with otopalatodigital syndrome had multiple temporal bone anomalies including an incompletely formed cribrose area (CA) between the cochlea (C) and the internal auditory canal (IAC) providing a large communication between the perilymphatic and cerebrospinal fluid spaces.

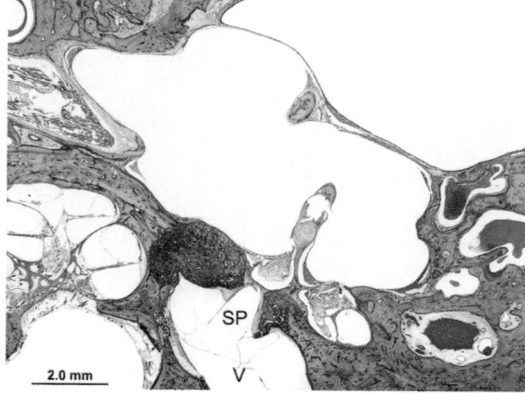

(A)

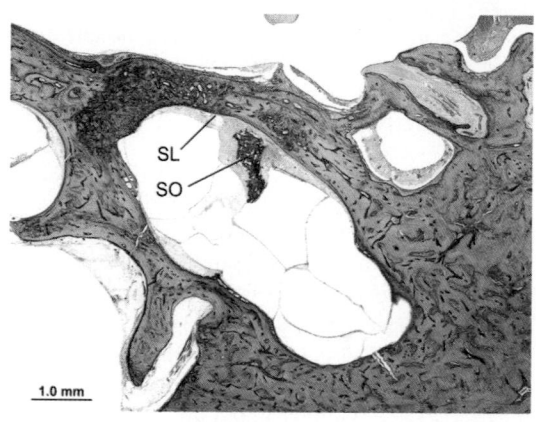

(B)

Figure 9 Surgical trauma to the inner ear secondary to stapedectomy. This 55-year-old woman with otosclerosis underwent a right stapedectomy at age 41. Obliterative otosclerosis was identified, and a "drill out" of the oval window was done using a microdrill. A stapes prosthesis was inserted. Postoperatively there was no significant change in her hearing. However, 8 months following surgery a sudden sensorineural loss occurred without vertigo. At age 49, the speech discrimination in the right ear began to decrease and she had occasional episodes of vertigo. (A) The silhouette of the stapes prosthesis (SP) is seen deep within the vestibule (V). (B) In the hook region of the basal turn, between the round and oval windows a spicule of otosclerotic bone (SO) was found impaling the spiral ligament (SL). There was marked endolymphatic hydrops and severe neurosensory degeneration presumably secondary to surgical trauma.

the footplate or the insertion of a prosthesis. A common mechanism appears to be subluxation of part of, or the entire, stapes footplate into the vestibule and direct damage to the saccular wall. An excessively long stapes prosthesis or plunging of the prosthesis during insertion may cause similar injury to the saccular wall (Figure 9). Trauma to the inner ear may result in severe vertigo and either immediate or delayed sensorineural hearing loss. Delayed endolymphatic hydrops is a well-known complication of surgical trauma to the inner ear.[36–38]

Suppurative Labyrinthitis. Suppurative labyrinthitis and/or meningitis has been reported in the interval 20 days to 5 years after stapes surgery.[39–43] Histologic evidence would suggest that an open communication between the middle ear and the perilymphatic space is responsible for most cases (Figure 10).

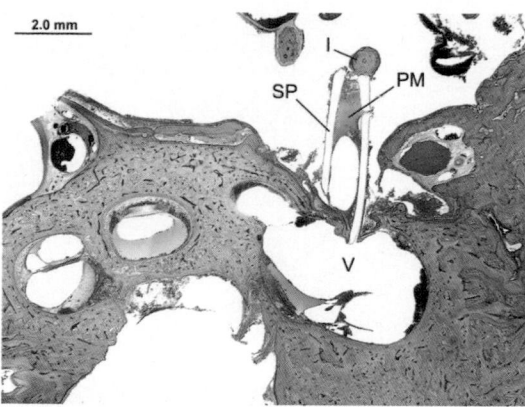

Figure 10 Suppurative labyrinthitis following stapedectomy. This 39-year-old man had a slowly progressive bilateral hearing loss. A left stapedectomy was performed at age 37, and a polyethylene tube was used between the lenticular process of the incus and residual fragments of the footplate. At 20 months after stapedectomy while on a trip at high elevations, he experienced several brief attacks of vertigo; and 2 years following the stapes procedure during an upper respiratory infection, he developed an acute suppurative otitis media complicated by fever, headache, ataxia, and meningitis and died 2 days later. The outline of the polyethylene tube stapes prosthesis (SP) can be seen between the incus (I) and the vestibule (V). There is an open communication between the vestibule and the middle ear within the lumen of the polyethylene tube which contained purulent material (PM) secondary to the acute otitis media. Inflammatory cells were also seen within the vestibule.

SURGERY FOR CHRONIC OTITIS MEDIA

Causes of Failure

The goals of mastoid surgery for chronic otitis media are the: (1) elimination of disease to produce a safe, dry ear; (2) alteration of the anatomy of the mastoid and middle ear to prevent recurrent disease; and (3) reconstruction in the form of ossiculoplasty and tympanoplasty to restore serviceable hearing if possible.[44,45] Failure of the first two goals will result in either recurrent cholesteatoma and/or recurrent suppuration. Failure rates of primary mastoidectomy range from 3 to 26%.[45] The reasons for failure of primary surgery as judged by surgical findings at revision mastoidectomy are multiple, including residual recurrent cholesteatoma,[46] or recurrent granulation and suppuration.[47] The following are examples of various factors resulting in failure of primary mastoidectomy.

Aditus Block. As in other organ systems, sequestration of disease behind an obstruction may lead to residual or recurrent chronic otitis media. In canal wall up mastoidectomy in which the aditus ad antrum is preserved and expanded through the use of a posterior tympanotomy, obstruction of this communication may result in a recurrent inflammatory reaction (Figure 11).

The Symptomatic (Draining) Mastoid Bowl. The creation of a canal wall down mastoid bowl may result in recurrent drainage, even in the absence of cholesteatoma. There is no better clinical evidence for the fact that surgical technique alone may result in recurrent

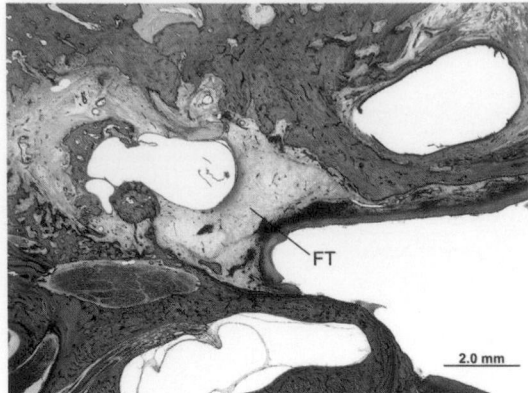

Figure 11 Aditus block following canal wall up tympanomastoidectomy. This 62-year-old man underwent a canal wall-up tympanomastoidectomy at age 50. Despite the presence of a posterior tympanotomy and placement of a silastic implant between the middle ear and antrum at the time of surgery, dense fibrous tissue (FT) was found in the aditus ad antrum causing obstruction and inflammatory cells within the mastoid.

suppuration of the mastoid bowl than the experience of some patients with the fenestration procedure. In this procedure, the creation of a canal down mastoid bowl to create a fenestration of the lateral semicircular canal in many cases resulted in chronic suppuration in ears in which there was none preoperatively.[48] The causes of recurrent drainage are multiple and include sequestration of inflammation within residual air cells, poorly exenterated mastoid air cells (Figure 12), and the presence of a high facial ridge. Cells that are most commonly instrumental in recurrent infection include cells located in the tegmen and in the sinodural angle, mastoid tip, facial recess, and hypotympanum.[49] In addition, skin against bone is inherently unstable and may result in ulceration and granulation within the mastoid bowl (Figure 13).

Residual disease in infralabyrinthine or hypotympanic cells (Figure 14) may in and of itself result in otitis media.[49]

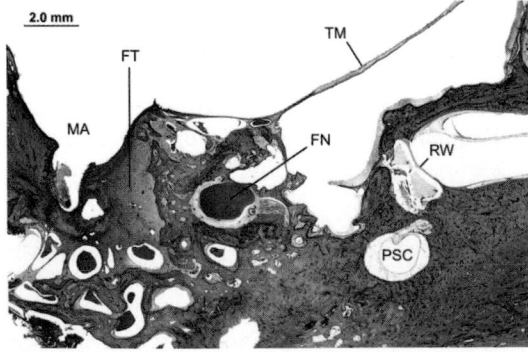

Figure 12 Incompletely exenterated mastoidectomy and high facial ridge. This 79-year-old man had a history of mastoidectomy for acute mastoiditis in childhood on the left side. At age 77, recurrent pain and swelling occurred over the left mastoid, and revision mastoidectomy was done. Many air cells remained within the mastoid (MA), and dense fibrous tissue (FT) containing cystic space was found within the exenterated portion of the mastoid. The bone lateral to the descending segment of the facial nerve (FN) was not lowered to the level of the facial nerve. PSC = posterior semicircular canal; RW = round window; TM = tympanic membrane.

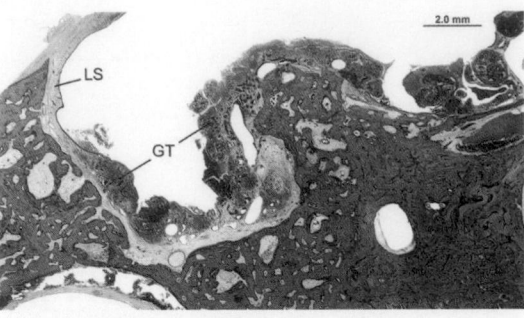

Figure 13 The symptomatic mastoid bowl. This 67-year-old woman underwent a modified radical mastoidectomy on the right side at age 59. Operative findings included granulation and thickened mucosa but not cholesteatoma. Following surgery, the right ear continued to discharge despite medical management. In much of the mastoid bowl, the lining skin (LS) has become ulcerated and replaced by granulation tissue (GT).

Reconstructive Materials

In the course of either canal wall up or canal wall down mastoidectomy, a variety of materials and techniques are used to accomplish the goals of mastoid surgery previously described. These include the use of obliteration pedicles, autologus bone grafts or cartilage grafts, and a variety of total ossicular replacement prostheses (TORPs) and partial ossicular replacement prostheses (PORPs) constructed of biocompatible materials.

Obliteration Pedicles. A variety of obliteration pedicles have been used to minimize the size of a canal wall down mastoid cavity and also to provide a stable soft tissue barrier between the skin and the underlying bone. Some surgeons have advocated the use of musculoperiosteal flaps, either superiorly or inferiorly based. However, these flaps have a distinct tendency to atrophy over time (Figure 15), decreasing their efficacy. As a result, others have recommended fibroperiosteal flaps[50] and the use of bone pate.[51] The use of fibromuscular flaps based on named vessels such as the wing flap[52] or the temporoparietal fascial flap[53] may result in better preservation of the obliterative bulk and a more stable mastoid bowl.

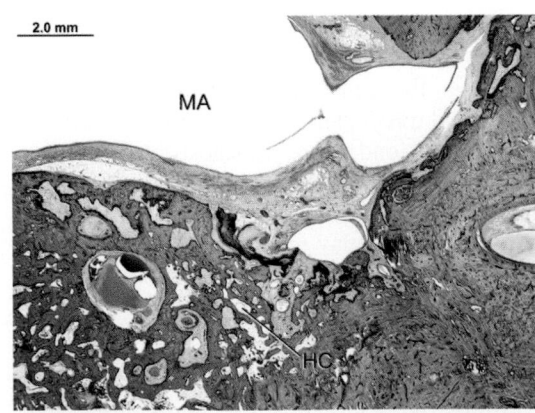

Figure 14 Sequestration and infection of hypotympanic cells. This 67-year-old woman underwent a left modified radical mastoidectomy at age 59 for an attic perforation and cholesteatoma. Underlying an intact epithelialized mastoid bowl (MA) unexenterate cells of the hypotympanum (HC) had become sequestered and in part filled with fibrous tissue.

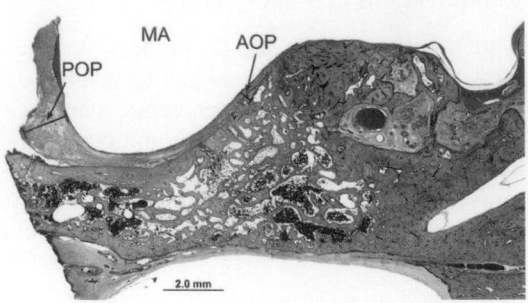

Figure 15 Obliterative musculofascial pedicle. This 76-year-old woman underwent a canal wall down tympanomastoidectomy at age 61 for chronic otitis media with granulation but without cholesteatoma. An inferiorly based musculofascial flap was used to obliterate the mastoid. There is a large canal wall down mastoidectomy bowl (MA). The posterior aspect of the obliteration pedicle (POP) is thicker than the more anterior portion (AOP) presumably due to postoperative atrophy over time.

Ossicular Replacement Prostheses. In an effort to reconstruct the ossicular chain, a variety of materials have been used as replacement materials over the years, including autologous bone or cartilage grafts and synthetic materials, including Plastipore, ceramic, and hydroxyapatite prostheses. Histologic study of ossicular implants in human subjects demonstrate that bone grafts derived from ossicles of cortical bone maintain their morphologic structure for many years and are slowly replaced by new bone growth (Figure 16). Although cartilage grafts persist without significant inflammatory response, they tend to lose tensile strength and to be resorbed

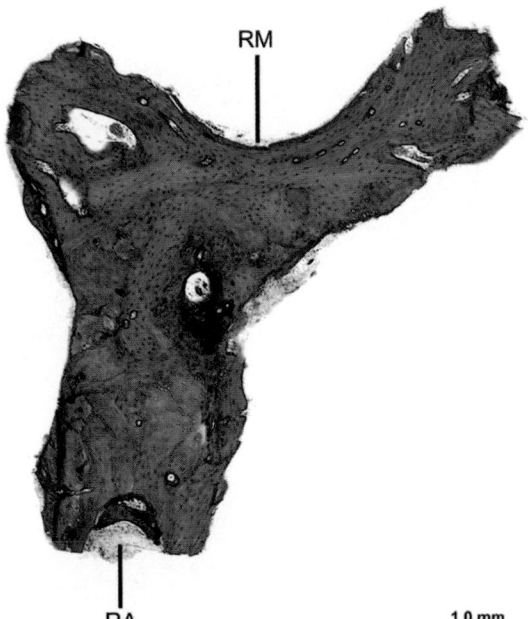

Figure 16 Incus autograft. This 46-year-old man underwent an autologous incus interposition between the capitulum of the stapes and the manubrium of the malleus. Because a large air-bone gap persisted postoperatively, the procedure was revised to 2 years later. The incus graft had become ankylosed to the promontory and also embedded in fibrous tissue. The incus strut has retained its shape including the recess to receive the manubrium (RM) and the recess to articulate with the capitulum (RA). The bone graft had become revascularized with new blood vessels, and over 75% of the bone had been remodeled as evidence by the presence of living osteocytes.

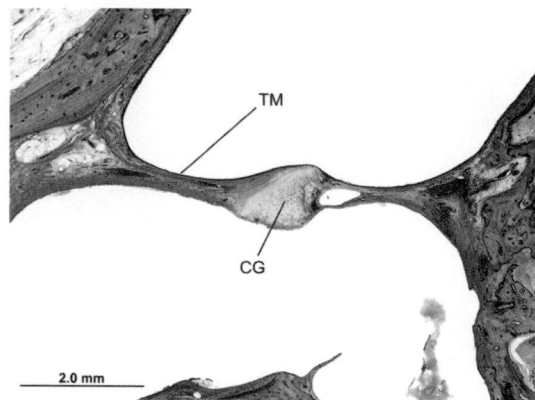

Figure 17 Autologous cartilage graft. This 62-year-old man underwent a right canal wall up tympanomastoidectomy at age 50. According to the operative notes, a cartilage graft was placed between the footplate and the grafted tympanic membrane. At the time of death, there was a 40 dB conductive hearing loss on the right side. The tympanic membrane (TM) consisted of a thick fascial graft. Embedded within it was a cartilage graft (CG). No living chondrocytes were found within the graft, and the extension from the tympanic membrane to the footplate was no longer present presumably because of postoperative resorption.

over time (Figure 17). Cartilage therefore can be effectively used to prevent retraction of the tympanic membrane or as an interposition between a synthetic ossicular reconstruction prosthesis and tympanic membrane; however, it is not ideal as a primary ossicular replacement graft.

Plastipore prostheses elicit a very vigorous foreign-body giant-cell reaction (Figure 18) which results in resorption with time and perhaps predisposes to extrusion. Prostheses made of hydroxyapatite seem to invoke less foreign-body giant-cell reaction and tend to be encapsulated over time, with little evidence of bony ingrowth.[54,55]

Lessons Learned From Histopathology on Limitations on Hearing Reconstruction in Chronic Otitis Media

Although the major limitation to successful ossicular reconstruction and hearing restoration in surgery for chronic otitis media appears to be persistent dysfunction of the eustachian tube resulting in a poorly aerated or nonaerated middle ear, the biologic response to chronic otitis media

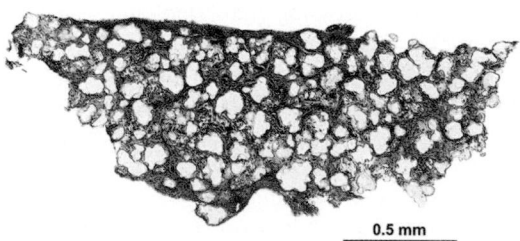

Figure 18 Plastipore total ossicular replacement prosthesis (TORP). This 53-year-old man underwent a type III tympanoplasty using a plastipore TORP as a major columella between footplate and tympanic membrane at age 32. A revision type III major columella was performed 21 years later, and the previously placed prosthesis was submitted for histologic study. It was found to be somewhat short and displaced anterior to the footplate. There was cellular and fibrous tissue ingrowth into the interstices of the prosthesis and the presence of multiple multi-nucleated giant cells.

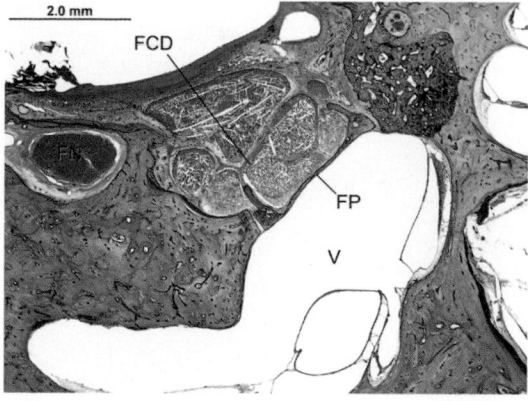

Figure 19 Fibrocystic degeneration of oval window niche. This 76-year-old woman underwent a left tympanomastoidectomy at age 59 for chronic otitis media with granulation. The malleus and incus were removed. Postoperatively a severe conductive loss was identified at least partially attributable to fibrocystic degeneration (FCD) filling the oval window niche. FN = facial nerve; FP = stapes footplate; V = vestibule.

and related surgery may also result in interference with hearing restoration. The principal processes appear to be fibrocystic sclerosis and fibro-osseous sclerosis. Thus, as a result of chronic inflammatory change associated with chronic otitis media, fibrous tissue may be deposited in a submucosal plane causing sequestration and obstruction of previously pneumatized spaces. This is particularly critical in the area of the oval window (Figure 19) and round window (Figure 20).

Osteitic Complications of Chronic Otitis Media

The resorptive osteitis that may occur in chronic otitis media with or without cholesteatoma may result in fistulization of the vestibular labyrinth (Figure 21) or the cochlea (Figure 22) either at the otic capsule or due to osteolysis of the footplate (Figure 23).

Complications of Surgical Intervention in Chronic Otitis Media

In addition to failure to control chronic otitis media, surgical intervention may result in iatrogenic damage or trauma to the facial nerve (Figure 24), accidental fenestration of the

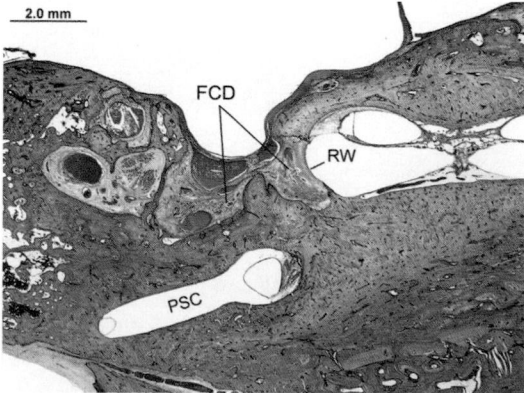

Figure 20 Fibrocystic degeneration of round window. In the same patient as described in Figure 19, there was also fibrocystic degeneration (FCD) within the niche of the round window (RW). PSC = posterior semicircular canal.

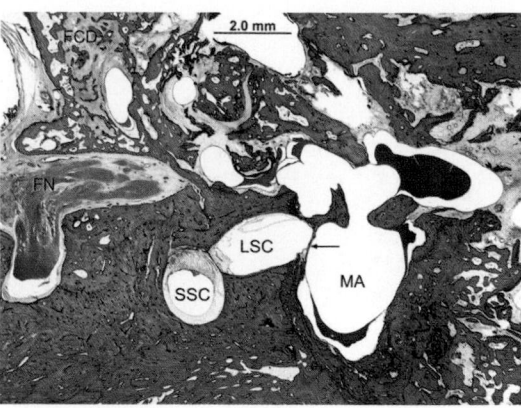

Figure 21 Dehiscence of the lateral semicircular canal in chronic otitis media. This 76-year-old woman had a long history of chronic suppurative otitis media of the right ear. Histologically there was an attic retraction lined by squamous epithelium, fibrocystic obliteration (FCD) of the epitympanum, and mastoid and erosion of the posterior part of the bony labyrinth (arrow) extending to the endosteum of the lateral semicircular canal (LSC). FN = facial nerve; MA = mastoid ; SSC = superior semicircular canal.

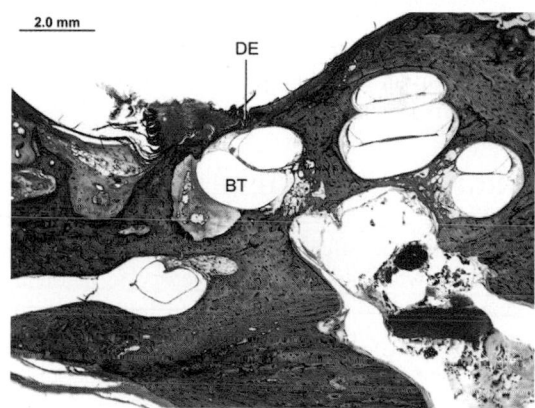

Figure 22 Pathologic dehiscence of cochlea. This 71-year-old man with longstanding bilateral chronic suppurative otitis media underwent a canal wall down mastoidectomy of the left ear at age 55. A large cholesteatoma was found with exposure of the middle fossa dura and thinning of the otic capsule over the promontory. Within the large mastoid bowl, there was dehiscence (DE) of the basal turn of the cochlea (BT). The adjacent spiral ligament contained an inflammatory infiltrate, and the adjacent organ of Corti was atrophied.

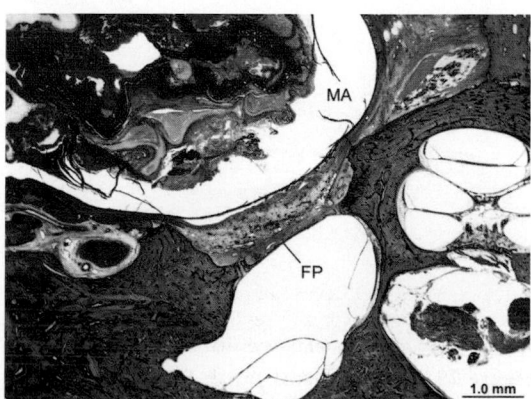

Figure 23 Erosion of stapes footplate. In the left ear of a patient described in Figure 22, there was marked pathologic thinning of the stapes footplate (FP) underlying fibrous tissue separating it from the mastoid bowl (MA).

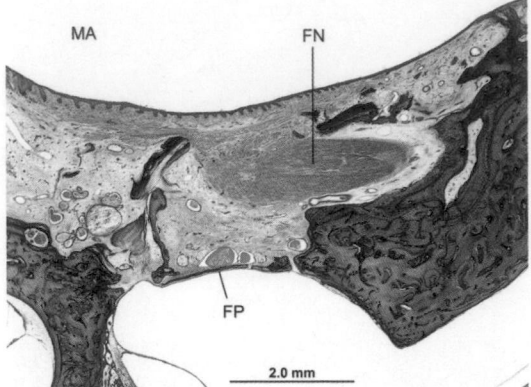

Figure 24 Surgical trauma to the horizontal segment of the facial nerve. This 60-year-old man suffered from chronic otitis media. At the age of 48, a right canal wall down tympanomastoidectomy was performed. Immediately following surgery, a right facial palsy was noted. Decompression of the facial nerve was performed 5 days later. The facial nerve was found to be intact but edematous. There was some recovery of facial movement, although there was permanent paresis. In the region of the stapes footplate (FP), some fibers of the facial nerve (FN) seemed to course in an irregular fashion into the fibrous tissue between the footplate and the mastoid bowl (MA) representing aberrant regeneration.

lateral semicircular canal (Figures 25 and 26), fenestration of the cochlea or fracture or luxation of the stapes (Figures 27 and 28).

SURGERY FOR MENIERE SYNDROME

Surgery may be offered to patients with Meniere syndrome which has been refractory to medical management and which can be attributed to one ear. Surgical techniques can be categorized by their ability to preserve cochlear function in the operated ear and those which are destructive of both cochlear and vestibular function. Examples include decompression of the endolymphatic sac as a function-sparing procedure and labyrinthectomy as a destructive procedure.

Decompression of the Endolymphatic Sac

The goal of decompression or shunting of the endolymphatic sac has been to decrease the

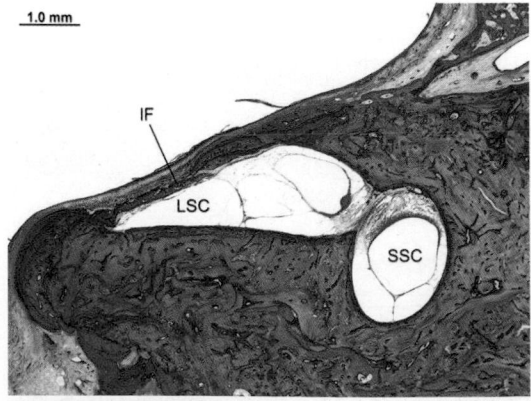

Figure 25 Surgical trauma to the lateral semicircular canal. In the same patient described in Figure 22, there is an iatrogenic infracture (IF) of the wall of the lateral semicircular canal (LSC) with fragments of bone depressed into the canal lumen and with surrounding fibrosis. SSC = superior semicircular canal.

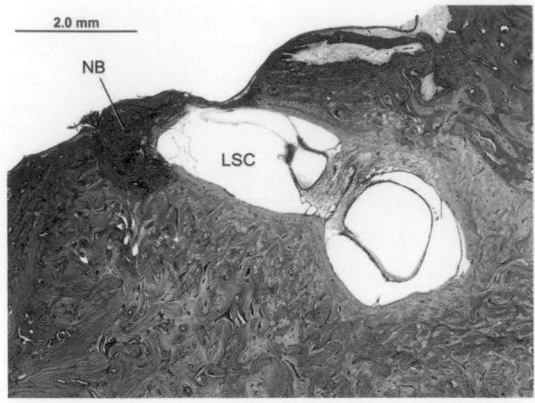

(A)

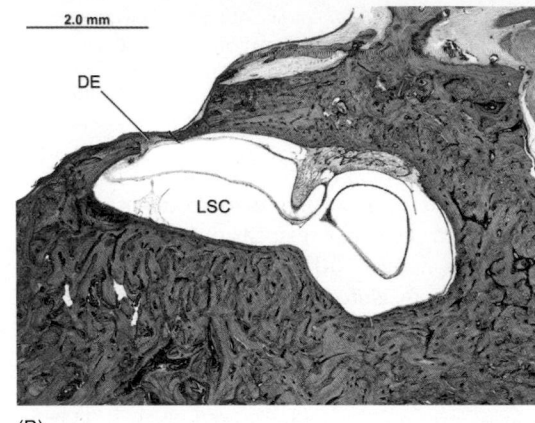

(B)

Figure 26 Iatrogenic dehiscence of lateral semicircular canal. This 55-year-old man with chronic suppurative otitis media of the left ear underwent a canal wall down tympanomastoidectomy at age 42 for cholesteatoma. Postoperatively he was vertiginous and was found to have nystagmus which subsided over several days. (A) Surgical trauma to the lateral semicircular canal (LSC) was seen with evidence of new bone growth (NB). (B) Persistent dehiscence (DE) of the lateral semicircular canal (LSC) was found.

volume of endolymph within the inner ear due to the hydropic state in Meniere syndrome. Surgery of the endolymphatic sac was introduced to otologic surgery by Georges Portmann[56] and a number of variations have been proposed in subsequent years, including establishment of shunts between the lumen of the sac and the subarachnoid space or the mastoid air cell system.

Although many authors continue to report a high incidence of relief of vestibular symptoms

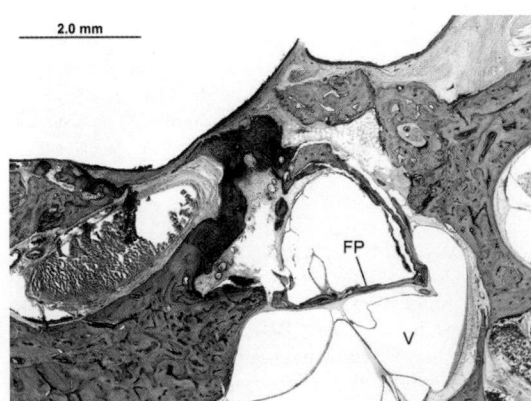

Figure 27 Iatrogenic subluxation of the stapes footplate. As a result of the surgery described in Figure 26, iatrogenic subluxation of the stapes, including the footplate (FP), into the vestibule (V) was also found.

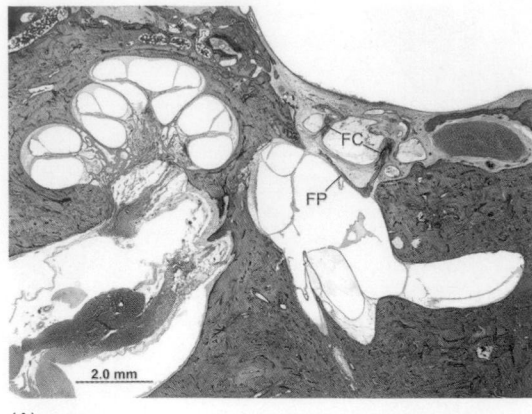

(A)

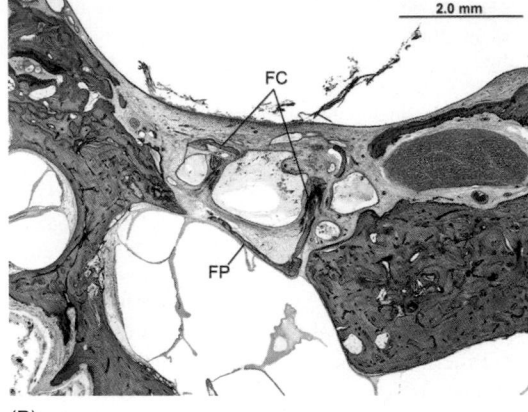

(B)

Figure 28 Iatrogenic fracture of stapes footplate and endolymphatic hydrops. This 76-year-old woman underwent a canal wall down tympanomastoidectomy at age 50 with postoperative vertigo and sensorineural hearing loss. (A) The anterior third of the stapes footplate (FP) is missing and replaced with fibrous tissue. Frag ments of the stapes crura (FC) are embedded in connective tissue in the oval window niche. There is endolymphatic hydrops in of the cochlea and saccule. (B) The oval window area is shown at higher magnification demonstrating missing anterior third of the footplate (FP) and presumably surgically fractured fragments of the superstructure (FC) embedded in fibrous tissue in the oval window.

using endolymphatic sac procedures,[57,58] others could find no difference between excision of the endolymphatic sac and a shunting procedure between the sac and mastoid.[59] Furthermore, a series of papers by Thompson and colleagues has suggested on the basis of a double-blind study that patients undergoing endolymphatic sac shunt surgery benefited significantly from a placebo effect.[60–62] These authors could show no significant difference between shunt and sham surgery.

Only a few cases of endolymphatic sac surgery have been studied histopathologically. In one, the histologic findings in three patients who had undergone endolymphatic/subarachnoid shunt for Meniere syndrome were reported.[63] A fibrous tissue response, presumably the result of the surgery in the area of the shunt, was observed. The feasibility of achieving permanent shunting between the subarachnoid space or the mastoid air cell system and the endolymphatic sac was questioned by Schuknecht resulting in the speculation that the effectiveness of the surgical procedure was more related to labyrinthine insult than true shunting of endolymph (Figure 29).[64]

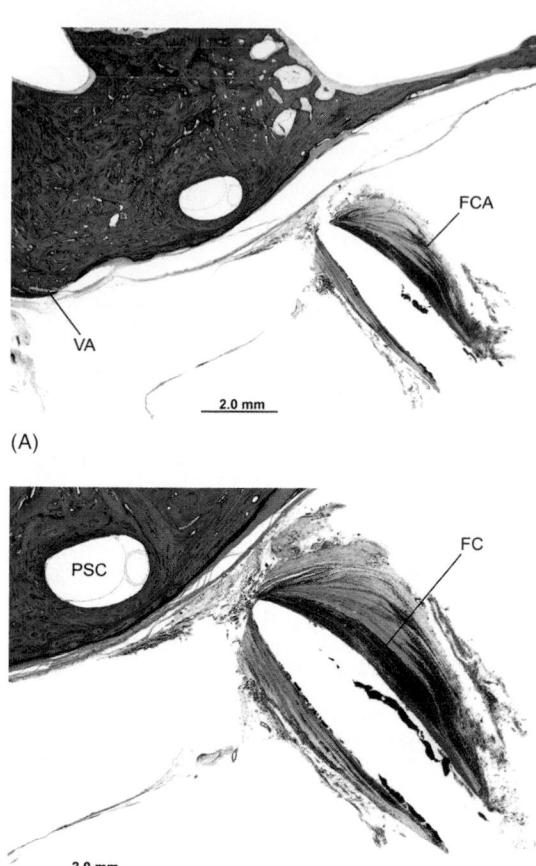

(A)

(B)

Figure 29 Endolymphatic decompression and drainage of the endolymphatic sac. This 91-year-old man had a clinical history of bilateral Meniere syndrome and underwent bilateral endolymphatic subarachnoid shunts. Following this surgery the patient had less in the way of attacks of vertigo but continued to have a progressive sensorineural hearing loss. Severe endolymphatic hydrops was confirmed histologically in both of cochleae and vestibular systems. (A) There was a dense fibrous capsule (FCA) around a foreign body, presumably silastic near the vestibular aqueduct (VA). (B) The fibrous capsule (FCA) around the foreign body and an intense mononuclear cell reaction are seen. PSC = posterior semicircular canal.

Labyrinthectomy

Labyrinthectomy is a method of ablating vestibular function in unilateral Meniere syndrome in which there is no useful residual cochlear function and in which there has been a failure of medical management. Unilateral vestibular ablation can be achieved by sectioning of the vestibular nerve or by transmastoid or transcanal labyrinthectomy. The surgical goal is total ablation of unilateral vestibular function.[65] A transcanal route was introduced by Lempert in 1948 and modified by Schuknecht.[66] A transmastoid approach for labyrinthectomy provides a wider field and therefore more assurance that the neuroepithelium of the vestibular system has been completely ablated.[67] Linthicum and colleagues presented histologic evidence that in some cases of transcanal labyrinthectomy a postoperative traumatic neuroma of the vestibular nerve may develop, potentially delaying or preventing vestibular compensation following labyrinthectomy.[68] These authors therefore suggested that vestibular neurectomy in conjunction

with labyrinthectomy will likely provide a more complete ablation. Indeed Schuknecht reported that incomplete ablation of the vestibular end organs occurred in 10 of 24 cases studied following transcanal labyrinthectomy (Figure 30).[69] In labyrinthectomy by any route, creating a soft tissue barrier between the subarachnoid space and perilymphatic spaces and the middle ear is essential (Figure 31).

COCHLEAR IMPLANTATION

Cochlear implantation has become the standard of care for rehabilitation of individuals with severe to profound sensorineural hearing loss in both ears. Histopathology of temporal bones from patients who in life had undergone cochlear implantation has shed light both on immediate and delayed changes in the inner ear as a consequence of the implant device and provided some insight into the histopathologic correlates

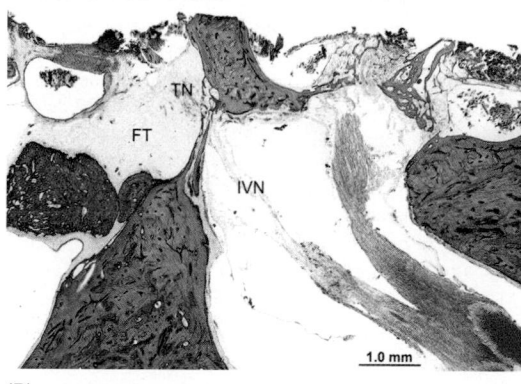

(A)

(B)

Figure 30 Labyrinthectomy. This 87-year-old woman with Meniere syndrome of the left ear underwent a postauricular transmastoid labyrinthectomy at age 69. Because postoperatively ice water caloric testing induced nystagmus in the left ear, the patient underwent a transcanal revision labyrinthectomy and singular neurectomy. The saccule and utricle were visualized and removed. The cristae were totally degenerated and the utricle missing. (A) The superior aspect of the vestibule was occupied by fibrous tissue and bone. The superior division of the vestibular nerve (SVN) was partially atrophied. However, there was a traumatic neuroma (TN) on the vestibular side of the cribrose area. (B) At the saccular level, the saccular macula and part of the vestibule were replaced by fibrous tissue (FT). The inferior vestibular nerve (IVN) was partially atrophied. However, there was a traumatic neuroma (TN) embedded in the fibrous tissue on the vestibular side of the cribrose area.

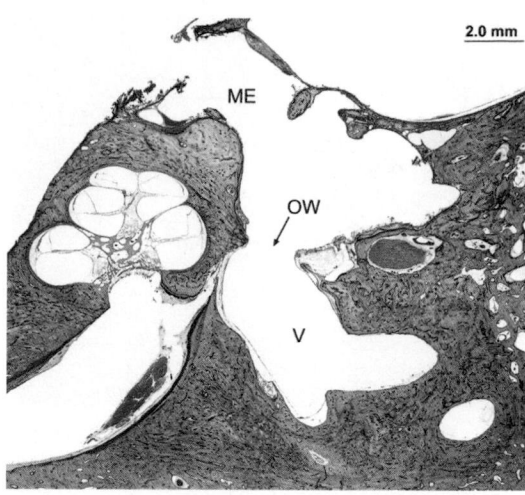

Figure 31 Labyrinthectomy. This 71-year-old woman suffered Meniere syndrome of the right ear beginning at age 50. A right transcanal labyrinthectomy was performed at age 57 which resulted in complete resolution of her vertiginous episodes. At the oval window (OW) the vestibule (V) is widely open and is in continuity with the middle ear (ME).

of success of cochlear implantation as measured by speech recognition scores.

Immediate and Delayed Changes

Histopathologic study of the temporal bones from patients who in life had undergone implantation has demonstrated a variety of immediate and delayed changes in the inner ear. Immediate changes may include fracture-dislocation of the osseous spiral lamina (Figure 32) and dissection of the lateral cochlear wall (Figure 33).[70] Delayed changes include new bone and fibrous tissue (Figures 34 and 35) in the cochlea and around the implanted electrode.

Bacterial meningitis has been reported as an infrequent complication of cochlear implantation.

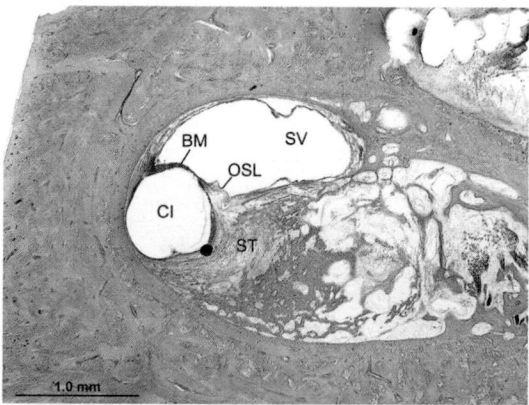

Figure 32 Fracture-dislocation of osseous spiral lamina following cochlear implantation. This 72-year-old man was profoundly deaf secondary to meningitic labyrinthitis at the age of 20 years. Preoperative computed tomography scan at age 64 demonstrated no evidence of new bone within the inner ear. At age 65, he underwent a cochlear implantation using a Symbion device (Richards Medical Company, Bartlett, TN) in the right ear. The electrode array was inserted with no resistance reported by the operating surgeon. In the basal turn of the cochlea the outline of the cochlear implant (CI) is seen in the scala tympani. The basilar membrane (BM) and part of the osseous spiral lamina (OSL) were displaced toward the scala vestibuli (SV). The rest of the scala tympani (ST) was filled with new bone and fibrous tissue.

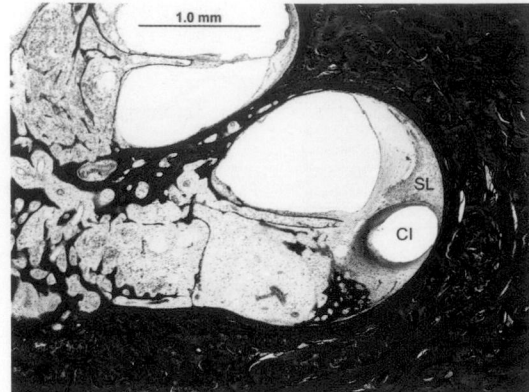

Figure 33 Dissection of lateral cochlear wall secondary to cochlear implantation. This 91-year-old man underwent a left cochlear implantation at age 80 because of profound sensorineural hearing loss secondary to bilateral Meniere syndrome. A Nucleus 22 channel device (Cochlear Corporation, Englewood, CO) was placed in the scala tympani. A full insertion was accomplished. His NU-6 (Northwestern University 6) scores were 15%. He used the device until the time of his death. The outline of the cochlear implant (CI) can be seen in the basal turn. It was embedded in a fibrous capsule within the spiral ligament (SL) of the lateral cochlear wall.

To date, the pathogenesis of meningitis is unclear. Histologic study of the tissue seal and biologic response around the cochlear implant has demonstrated a very robust fibrous and osseous reaction to several types of implants and no obvious communication between the middle and inner ear (Figures 34 and 35).[71] In addition, a significant inflammatory cellular response, including mononuclear leukocytes, histiocytes, and foreign body giant cells were present in over 50% of the implanted specimens (Figure 36). This may result in a local immune compromise.[72]

Correlates of Success with the Implant

Khan and colleagues demonstrated that despite significant trauma to the cochlea, the mean spiral ganglion cell count for implanted and impaired nonimplanted ears were not significantly different,

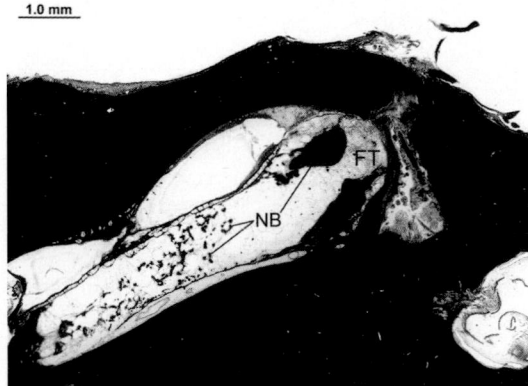

Figure 34 New bone and fibrous tissue following cochlear implant. This 74-year-old woman underwent a right cochlear implantation at age 59 for bilateral profound sensorineural hearing loss secondary to ototoxicity. A Nucleus 22 channel device (Cochlear Corporation, Englewood, CO) was inserted. For the remainder of her life, she used the cochlear implant with a stable NU-6 (Northwestern University 6) word score of approximately 25%. In the basal turn there was new bone (NB) and fibrous tissue (FT) near the cochleostomy site.

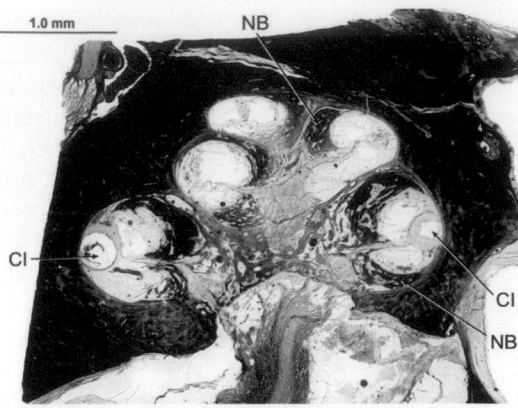

Figure 35 New bone formation around a cochlear implant. This 67-year-old man suffered a bilateral profound sensorineural loss at age 65 secondary to transverse temporal bone fractures. At age 65, he underwent a right cochlear implantation using a Nucleus 22 channel device (Cochlear Corporation, Englewood, CO). Full insertion was achieved. At 2 years after cochlear implantation his open-set monosyllabic word score was 30% using the implant. The cochlear implant electrode array (CI) can be seen in the basal turn. There is new bone (NB) in the perilymphatic scalae of all turns.

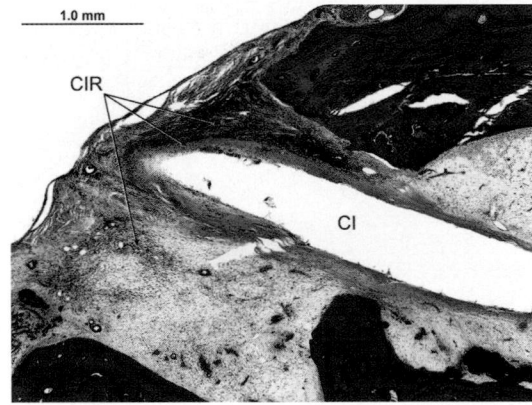

Figure 36 Cellular immune response to presence of cochlear implant. This 91-year-old man, profoundly deaf bilaterally secondary to Meniere syndrome, underwent a left cochlear implant at age 80 using a Nucleus 22 device (Cochlear Corporation, Englewood, CO). His NU-6 (Northwestern University 6) word scores were approximately 15%. He used his device until the time of his death. There was an intense cellular immune response (CIR), consisting of mononuclear and multinucleated giant cells, found along the implant track (CI).

particularly in the basal turn of the cochlea.[72] In addition, the segmental and total spiral ganglion cell counts of the implanted ears were not significantly correlated with word recognition scores[73] although some correlation of numbers of surviving spiral ganglion cells and psychophysical measures has been identified.[74]

In summary, continued histologic study of human temporal bones will provide insight into the pathogenesis of otologic disease and, in addition, as illustrated in this chapter, will provide important data concerning the consequences of medical and surgical intervention.

REFERENCES

1. Shea JJ, Jr. Forty years of stapes surgery. Am J Otol 1998;19:52–5.
2. Portmann D, Arramon-Tucoo JF. Stapedectomy and microstapedotomy in the treatment of otospongiosis: A comparative study. Rev Laryngol Otol Rhinol (Bord) 1989;110:317–22.
3. Langman AW, Jackler RK, Sooy FA. Stapedectomy: Long-term hearing results. Laryngoscope 1991;101:810–4.
4. Han WW, Incesulu A, McKenna MJ, et al. Revision stapedectomy: Intraoperative findings, results, and review of the literature. Laryngoscope 1997;107:1185–92.
5. Huber A, Koike T, Wada H, et al. Fixation of the anterior mallear ligament: Diagnosis and consequences for hearing results in stapes surgery. Ann Otol Rhinol Laryngol 2003;12:348–55.
6. Oktay MF, Cureoglu S, Schachern PA, et al. Histologic changes in the anterior mallear ligament and the head of the malleus in otosclerosis. Otolaryngol Head Neck Surg 2006;134:232–5.
7. Lesinski SG. Causes of conductive hearing loss after stapedectomy or stapedotomy: A prospective study of 279 consecutive surgical revisions. Otol Neurotol 2002;23:281–8.
8. Harris JP, Mehta RP, Nadol JB, Jr. Malleus fixation: Clinical and histopathologic findings. Ann Otol Rhinol Laryngol 2002;111:246–54.
9. Subotic R, Mladina R, Risavi R. Congenital bony fixation of the malleus. Acta Otolaryngol (Stockh) 1998;118:833–6.
10. Rosowski JJ, Mehta RP, Merchant SN. Diagnostic utility of laser-Doppler vibrometry in conductive hearing loss with normal tympanic membrane. Otol Neurotol 2003;24:165–75.
11. Stewart TJ, Belal A. Surgical anatomy and pathology of the round window. Clin Otolaryngol Allied Sci 1981;6:45–62.
12. Schuknecht HF, Barber W. Histologic variants in otosclerosis. Laryngoscope 1985;95:1307–17.
13. Carey JP, Minor LB, Nager GT. Dehiscence of thinning of bone overlying the superior semicircular canal in a temporal bone survey. Arch Otolaryngol Head Neck Surg 2000;126:137–47.
14. Mikulec AA, Poe DS, McKenna MJ. Operative management of superior semicircular canal dehiscence. Laryngoscope 2005;115:501–7.
15. Rosowski JJ, Songer JE, Nakajima HH, et al. Clinical, experimental, and theoretical investigations of the effect of superior semicircular canal dehiscence on hearing mechanisms. Otol Neurotol 2004;25:323–32.
16. Mikulec AA, McKenna MJ, Ramsey MJ, et al. Superior semicircular canal dehiscence presenting as conductive hearing loss without vertigo. Otol Neurotol 2004;25:121–9.
17. Minor LB, Carey JP, Cremer PD, et al. Dehiscence of bone overlying the superior canal as a cause of apparent conductive hearing loss. Otol Neurotol 2003;24:270–8.
18. Himi T., Igarashi M., Kataura A. Temporal bone histopathology over 15 years post-stapedectomy. Acta Otolaryngol (Stockh) Suppl 1988;447:126–34.
19. Schuknecht HF, Jones DD. Stapedectomy. Postmortem findings. Ann Otol Rhinol Laryngol 1979;88:1–43.
20. Schuknecht HF, McGee TM, Igarashi M, et al. Stapedectomy. Postmortem studies. Arch Otolaryngol 1964;79:437–46.
21. Subotic R, Kaufman RS. Human temporal bone findings post stapedectomy: A review of ten cases. Acta Otolaryngol (Stockh) 1971;71:385–91.
22. Gibbin KP. The histopathology of the incus after stapedectomy. Clin Otolaryngol 1979;4:343–54.
23. Nadol JB, Jr. Histopathology of residual and recurrent conductive hearing loss after stapedectomy. Otol Neurotol 2001;22:162–9.
24. Lannigan FJ, O'Higgins P, Oxnard CE, McPhie P. Age related bone resorption in the normal incus: A case of maladaptive remodelling? J Anat 1995;186:651–5.
25. Imauchi Y, Karino S. Yamasoba T. Acquired atrophy of the long process of the incus. Otolaryngol Head Neck Surg 2005;132:156–8.
26. Kanzaki S, Ito M, Takada Y, et al. Resorption of auditory ossicles and hearing loss in mice lacking osteoprotegerin. Bone 2006;39:414–9.
27. Lindsay JR. Histologic findings following stapedectomy and polyethylene tube inserts in the human. Ann Otol Rhinol Laryngol 1961;70:785–807.
28. Nadol, JB, Jr. Histopathology of residual and recurrent conductive hearing loss after stapedectomy. Otol Neurotol 2001;22:162–9.
29. Nance WE, Setleff R. McLeod A, et al. X-linked mixed deafness with congenital fixation of the stapedial footplate and perilymphatic gusher. Birth Defects Orig Artic Ser 1971;07:64–9.
30. Phelps PD, Reardon W, Pembrey M, et al. X-linked deafness, stapes gushers and a distinctive defect of the inner ear. Neuroradiol 199;33:326–30.
31. Friedman RA, Bykhoyskaya Y, Tu G, et al. Molecular analysis of the POU3F4 gene in patients with clinical and radiographic evidence of X-linked mixed deafness with perilymphatic gusher. Ann Otol Rhinol Laryngol 1997;106:320–5.

32. Schuknecht HF, Reisser C. The morphologic basis for perilymphatic gushers and oozers. Adv Otorhinolaryngol 1988;39:1–12.

33. Graham JM, Phelps PD, Michaels L. Congenital malformations of the ear and cochlear implantation in children: Review and temporal bone report of common cavity. J Laryngol Otol Suppl 2000;25:1–14.

34. McFadden MD, Wilmoth JG, Mancuso AA, Antonelli PJ. Preoperative computed tomography may fail to detect patients at risk for perilymph gusher. ENT J 2005;84:770,772–4.

35. Michel O, Breunsbach J, Matthias R. Congenital cerebrospinal fluid pressure labyrinth. HNO 1991;39:486–90.

36. Shea JJ, Jr, Ge X, Orchik DJ. Traumatic endolymphatic hydrops. Am J Otol 1995;16:235–40.

37. Schuknecht HF. Delayed endolymphatic hydrops. Ann Otol Rhinol Laryngol 1978;87:743–8.

38. Nadol JB, Jr, Weiss AD, Parker SW. Vertigo of delayed onset after sudden deafness. Ann Otol Rhinol Laryngol 1975;84:841–6.

39. Rutledge LJ, Lewis ML, Sanabria F. Fatal meningitis related to stapes operation. Report of a case with temporal bone study. Arch Otolaryngol 1963;78:637–41.

40. Wolff D. Untoward sequelae eleven months following stapedectomy. Ann Otol Rhinol Laryngol 1964;73:297–304.

41. Matz GJ, Lockhart HB, Lindsay JR. Meningitis following stapedectomy. Laryngoscope 1968;78:56–63.

42. Palva T, Palva A, Karja AJ. Fatal meningitis in a case of otosclerosis operated upon bilaterally. Arch Otolaryngol 1972;96:130–7.

43. Benitez JT. Stapedectomy and fatal meningitis. A human temporal bone study. ORL Otorhinolaryngol Relat Spec 1977;39:94–100.

44. Nadol JB, Jr. Causes of failure of mastoidectomy for chronic otitis media. Laryngoscope 1985;95:410–3.

45. Nadol JB, Jr. Revision mastoidectomy. Otolaryngol Clin North Am 2006;39:723–40.

46. Syms MJ, Luxford WM. Management of cholesteatoma: Status of the canal wall. Laryngoscope 2003;113:443–8.

47. Merchant SN, Wang P, Jang CH, et al. Efficacy of tympanomastoid surgery for control of infection in active chronic otitis media. Laryngoscope 1997;107:872–7.

48. Rambo JH. Mastoid surgery: Effect of retained mucosa on healing. Ann Otol Rhinol Laryngol 1979;88:701–7.

49. Nadol JB, Jr, Krouse JH. The hypotympanum and infralabyrinthine cells in chronic otitis media. Laryngoscope 1991;101:137–41.

50. Ramsey MJ, Merchant SN, McKenna MJ. Postauricular periosteal-pericranial flap for mastoid obliteration and canal wall down tympanomastoidectomy. Otol Neurotol 2004;25:873–8.

51. Sheehy JL. Bone pate collecting device. Otolaryngol Head Neck Surg 1980;88:472.

52. Black B. Mastoidectomy elimination: Obliterate, reconstruct or ablate? Am J Otol 1998;19:551–7.

53. Cheney ML, Megerian CA, Brown MT, et al. The use of the temporoparietal fascial flap in temporal bone reconstruction. Am J Otol 1996;17:137–42.

54. Bahmad F, Merchant SN. Histopathology of ossicular grafts and implants in chronic otitis media. Ann Otol Rhinol Laryngol 2007;116(3):181–91.

55. Merchant SN, Nadol JB, Jr. Histopathology of ossicular implants. Otolaryngol Clin North Am 1994;27:813–33.

56. Portmann G. Vertigo. Surgical treatment by opening the saccus endolymphaticus. Arch Otolaryngol 1927;6:309–15.

57. Pensak ML, Friedman RA. The role of endolymphatic mastoid shunt surgery in the managed care era. Am J Otol 1998;19:337–40.

58. Durland WF, Jr, Pyle GM, Connor NP. Endolymphatic sac decompression as a treatment for Meniere's disease. Laryngoscope 2005;115:1454–7.

59. Welling DB, Pasha R, Roth LJ, Barin K. The effect of endolymphatic sac excision in Meniere disease. Am J Otol 1996;17:278–82.

60. Thomsen J, Bretlau P, Tos M, Johnsen NJ. Placebo effect in surgery for Meniere's disease. A double-blind, placebo-controlled study on endolymphatic sac shunt surgery. Arch Otolaryngol 1981;107:271–7.

61. Thomsen J, Bretlau P, Tos M, Johnsen NJ. Placebo effect in surgery for Meniere's disease: Three-year follow-up. Otolaryngol Head Neck Surg 1983;91:183–6.

62. Bretlau P, Thomsen J, Tos M, Johnsen NJ. Placebo effect in surgery for Meniere's disease: A three-year follow-up study of patients in a double blind placebo controlled study on endolymphatic sac shunt surgery. Am J Otol 1984;5:558–61.

63. Belal A, Jr, House WF. Histopathology of endolymphatic subarachnoid shunt surgery for Meniere's disease. Am J Otol 1979;1:37–44.

64. Schuknecht HF. Pathology of Meniere's disease as it relates to the sac and tack procedures. Ann Otol Rhinol Laryngol 1977;86:677–82.

65. Pulec JL. Labyrinthectomy; indications, technique and results. Laryngoscope 1974;84:1552–73.

66. Schuknecht HF. Ablation therapy for the relief of Meniere's disease. Laryngoscope 1956;66:859–70.

67. Graham MD, Colton JJ. Transmastoid labyrinthectomy indications. Technique and early postoperative results. Laryngoscope 1980;90:1253–62.

68. Linthicum FJ, Jr, Alonso A, Denia A. Traumatic neuroma. A complication of transcanal labyrinthectomy. Arch Otolaryngol 1979;105:654–5.

69. Schuknecht HF. Behavior of the vestibular nerve following labyrinthectomy. Ann Otol Rhinol Laryngol 1982;9:16–32.

70. Nadol JB, Jr, Shiao JY, Burgess BJ, et al. Histopathology of cochlear implants in humans. Ann Otol Rhinol Laryngol 2001;110:883–91.

71. Nadol JB, Jr, Eddington DK. Histologic evaluation of the tissue seal and biologic response around cochlear implant electrodes in the human. Otol Neurotol 2004;25:257–62.

72. Khan AM, Handzel O, Damian D, et al. Effect of cochlear implantation on residual spiral ganglion cell count as determined by comparison with the contralateral nonimplanted inner ear in humans. Ann Otol Rhinol Laryngol 2005;114:381–5.

73. Khan AM, Handzel O, Burgess BJ, et al. Is word recognition correlated with the number of surviving spiral ganglion cells and electrode insertion depth in human subjects with cochlear implants? Laryngoscope 2005;115:672–7.

74. Khan AM, Whiten DM, Nadol JB, Jr, Eddington DK. Histopathology of human cochlear implants: Correlation of psychophysical and anatomical measures. Hear Res 2005;205:83–93.

13

Outcomes Research, Clinical Trials, and Clinical Research

Maureen Hannley, PhD
David L. Witsell, MD, MHS

Sir Francis Bacon, Renaissance author, courtier, and father of inductive reasoning, observed that the true essence of progress is in the application of scientific knowledge for enhancing the human condition.[1] Today we express that same expectation by calling for studies that bridge the bench-to-bedside gap. In the past half-century new challenges to the healthcare system have been presented by deadly new viruses, antibiotic-resistant strains of bacteria, and broad societal and environmental changes that have altered disease epidemiology, raising medical, social, legal, and economic issues. These challenges have been paralleled by rapid advances in biomedical and information technology, vaccines to protect against many infectious diseases, the Human Genome Project, an explosion in the volume of medical literature, and increasing demands for evidence of the effectiveness, quality and outcome of the care provided to patients.

Rather than solving patient care decisions or creating consensus on disease management, however, these achievements in biomedical science and technology have paradoxically *increased* uncertainty and practice variation among healthcare providers by offering a constantly expanding menu of choices. Patient-oriented research, once limited largely to randomized clinical trials conducted in large academic medical centers by highly trained physician-scientists, is now being done in greater numbers by community-based practitioners who are motivated to find answers to the problems they encounter in daily clinical practice, make a contribution to their specialty, and take an active role in generating evidence about the effectiveness of otolaryngology interventions for providers, patients, and their colleagues in other specialties.

In this chapter we will use clinical vignettes to illustrate how questions that arise in an otolaryngology practice can be used to guide the selection of an appropriate study design, the strengths and weaknesses of each, and some representative studies using that design. Finally, we will briefly discuss the trend in evidence-based medicine and how it will affect the practice of otolaryngology–head and neck surgery.

THE RESEARCH QUESTION: THE CORE OF THE PROCESS

A well-constructed, *focused research question* is paramount in the clinical research process. The nature and structure of the research question will determine the research design and the types of statistics needed to analyze the data collected. Do you want to know about associations, correlations, risk factors related to a group of patients or to a treatment, the sensitivity or specificity of a diagnostic test, or how commonly a clinical event occurs? These questions can be formed into a focused research question using the *PICO format*.[2] Using this paradigm, the well-constructed research question has four parts.

Patient or Problem of Interest

How would you describe a group of patients similar to yours? What are the most important characteristics in addition to the primary diagnosis? You may want to specify an age range, ethnicity, or gender if that is important to the condition.

Intervention, Prognostic Factor, or Exposure

What treatment, intervention, or diagnostic test is being considered? What risk factor is at issue that may influence the prognosis?

Comparison

Is there an alternative treatment or test you would like to compare? Comparisons are not always strictly necessary, depending on the nature of the question.

Outcome

What are you hoping to accomplish, measure, or improve? Be specific as to what your goal is; a quantifiable goal is preferable.

Closely related to the specification of the focused research question is the decision about whether to take a passive role in observing the events and their effects on the study subjects by designing an *observational study* or to take a more active role and design a prospective *experimental study* and examine the effects of an intervention in a clinical trial.[3] We will examine the characteristics, advantages and disadvantages, with some examples of each of these options in the following sections.

OBSERVATIONAL RESEARCH

As its name implies, observational research is one in which the investigator takes an essentially passive role in the research process, simply *observing* events taking place in study subjects under various conditions and configurations, thus determining how exposure to certain risk factors influences the probability of developing a disease or disorder of interest. The risk factors may be endogenous, such as genetic or familial history, or exogenous, related to environmental, lifestyle, or other medical intervention factors. This is in contrast to experimental studies, such as clinical trials, where the investigator applies an intervention and studies its effects under controlled circumstances. Observational studies may be prospective or retrospective; the three most common types are cross-sectional studies, cohort studies, and case-control studies.

Cross-Sectional Studies

At the tenth reunion of their medical school class, two good friends and colleagues who trained in otolaryngology strike up a conversation about their practices. Dr Cold, who now lives in Wisconsin, has been extremely busy caring for children with ear infections and has inserted over 60 pairs of tympanostomy tubes in the last month of January. His friend, Dr Warm, who lives in Florida, comments that while he has seen an increase in children with ear infections (which he usually does in January), he does not think that it is nearly as great as Dr Cold's. Their discussion prompts the following research question:

Is the prevalence of young children with otitis media in a multispecialty practice in Wisconsin who receive tympanostomy tubes different than the prevalence of children with otitis media in a multispecialty practice in Florida who receive tympanostomy tubes during the same time period?

Each physician decides to return to his multispecialty group and review the charts of all children between the ages of 6 months and 3 years seen by the group in January. They decide to record the primary diagnosis noted in the chart, allergies, age of first ear infection (if they had one), and whether they were breastfed. No patient identifiers are recorded. These are their results:

	Florida Group	Wisconsin Group
Children seen	1,000	2,000
Ear infections	150	500
Allergies	300	400
Average age of first infection	12 mo	10.5 mo
Breastfed	200	400

Our clinicians have a convenient sample that lends itself to a simple retrospective *cross-sectional study*, sometimes called a *prevalence study*. Prevalence is the number of persons with a given disease at any specified point in time and is arrived at by a simple calculation:

Prevalence = number of people with the disease/number of people at risk

Our two classmates can readily compare the prevalence of wintertime otitis media in their respective practices. In the Florida practice, the prevalence is *150/1,000* or *0.15* (15 cases per 100). In the Wisconsin practice, the prevalence is *500/2,000* or *0.25* (25 cases per 100). Dr Cold's impression that his caseload of otitis media is higher in Wisconsin is justified—at least for the month that was examined. A variation of this kind of study would be to examine *period prevalence*, by calculating the prevalence over a longer period of time, usually 1 year. Here, the period prevalence is calculated as follows[4]:

Period prevalence = number of people with disease during the time period/number of people at risk during the time period

Gathering these data would also allow the investigators to calculate quarterly prevalences and to examine the question of whether there are seasonal fluctuations in the disease that correspond to certain predictors of interest.

A cross-sectional design can help provide information about the association of variables of interest [such as number of children who have otitis media with effusion (OME) at a particular time] with other factors (such as season of the year) that may be predictors, although it cannot establish causality. However, seasonal trends in disease recurrence or exacerbation in established cases could be readily examined by a cross-sectional chart review, with the understanding that this is not a random sample and that *existing* disease may not be representative of *all cases* of the same disease. A cross-sectional study would answer the question "What is happening?" with relative ease and low cost.

Cross-sectional studies have several advantages: they are relatively inexpensive; they are fast (no waiting for the outcome to occur); and there is no loss to follow-up. The results of a cross-sectional study can sometimes serve as the baseline study for a prospective cohort study (see next section) by revealing *associations* (*not* correlations or evidence of causality) of interest. For example, if there were peaks in OME prevalence in the spring or fall that corresponded with peaks of environmental ragweed or other pollens, it would be natural to study allergy as a risk factor for OME. However, they have limitations as well: they provide only a snapshot in time of the condition of interest and thus may be misleading if one is interested in the natural history of a disease or in the disease process in general. It is difficult to choose appropriate, nonbiased control groups for cross-sectional studies, and, as previously noted, the affected group may not be representative of the entire population.

Cohort Studies

> Dr Cold enlists his colleague in pediatrics, Dr Snow, to explore further the natural history of ear infections and to try to identify possible risk factors that may predispose patients to the development of ear infections which may begin to explain why they have a higher incidence of otitis media than children in Dr Warm's practice. Since children in Milwaukee spend more time indoors and are closely grouped at daycare in the winter compared to Florida children who continue to play outside, they believe that daycare may be a risk factor for ear problems.
>
> Drs Cold and Snow decide to examine this idea in their practice and follow two groups of patients for 1 year. At the first well-child visit, Dr Snow will ask the parent if their child will be going to daycare or not. This determination will divide the children into two groups. The two groups of children are checked every 3 months, or more often if an ear infection occurs. Dr Cold confirms the presence or absence of an ear infection in children every month.
>
> Drs Cold and Snow determine that children in daycare have more ear problems than children cared for at home.

In a cohort study patients who have a particular disease are recruited into a study based on whether they have had exposure to a particular risk factor. A cohort study is also called an *incidence study*. Incidence is the number of *new cases* in a fixed time period and is calculated as:

Incidence = number of new cases in fixed time period/number of people at risk

The risk factor may be environmental, genetic, behavioral, traumatic, or even a treatment. These individuals are then followed over time for the *occurrence of an outcome of interest*. A different focused research question would be developed for this type of study:

> What is the incidence of recurrent acute otitis media in young children who are in daycare compared with those cared for at home in a specified time interval after treatment?

For this question, the outcome of interest is the number of documented episodes of acute otitis media in a specified time interval after the treatment. Here, we would select a group of children with histories of recurrent acute otitis media and group them according to their daycare environment. The cohort of "exposed" children (E) are in group daycare; the cohort of "unexposed" children (N) are cared for at home. These numbers are then easily analyzed to determine the relative risk for the "E" and "N" groups.

If "e" designates the children in the group care cohort who develop future infections and "n" designates the children in the home care cohort who develop future infections, the relative risk is calculated as:

$$(e/E)/(n/N)$$

It is important to consider the possible contribution of *confounding factors* in collecting and analyzing the data from any clinical research study. A confounding factor is one that could be related both to the outcome and to the risk factor and thus could be considered responsible for some or all of the observed effect. In this example, the investigator would want to examine other factors, such as exposure to second-hand smoke and predisposing conditions such as craniofacial anomalies to determine whether these factors were disproportionately represented in one cohort. Statistical procedures are necessary to help analyze the impact of confounding factors in analysis of the data.

The cohort study is one of the best designs for studying the course of a disease or risk factors. When biases and confounding factors are minimized, it is a powerful design to provide strong evidence for the time sequence between outcomes and risk factors. However, it can be expensive and time-consuming when serial data collection is involved, and it is not especially useful for rare diseases because of the difficulty in gathering an adequate sample size. Finally, because this is an observational study, *causation* cannot be proved since other factors invariably will affect the outcome; the best the investigator can do is to be meticulously aware of those factors and to control for them to the greatest extent possible.

Case-Control Studies

> Meanwhile, Dr Warm and his colleague Dr Sun embark upon their own study to examine whether children of large families have more ear problems than single-child families. They review the charts of the previous year's patients who had tympanostomy tube insertion and children who only had a visit for vaccinations. They match each patient who had tympanostomy tubes inserted with one from the vaccination group on age, ethnicity, daycare setting, and a few other factors. They contact each patient's family and determine how many siblings the child has in the house. They divide the whole group of patients by "only-child families" and "multisibling families."
>
> They find that 50% of the children with tympanostomy tubes insertion had larger families, while 45% of the vaccination children had larger families.
>
> | 100 patients with ear tubes | 100 vaccination patients |
> | --- | --- |
> | 50 had large families | 45 had large families |
>
> Odds ratio of having tympanostomy tubes if you have a large family is:
>
> 50/45 or 1.1

Most case-control studies tend to be *retrospective*: they identify a group of individuals with the condition of interest and another without the same condition (ideally matched on critical variables such as age, gender, ethnicity, etc), and look backward in time to determine differences in predictor variables that might explain why one group developed the disease and the other did not. This is a standard epidemiological approach for risk factors determination.

Another excellent example of a simple case-control study appears in the following abstract. The focused research question might be constructed in the following way:

> Do children who swim regularly develop otitis media more frequently than children matched for age, sex, and race who do not swim?

To determine the influence of swimming on the incidence of otitis media in children, the authors designed a case-control survey involving 32 children, aged 1 to 4 years, who were participating in swimming classes. Thirty control subjects were matched for age, race, and sex. The participants were pooled from the general pediatrics clinic and toddler swimming classes in Nassau County, NY. Parents completed a questionnaire gathering data over a 12-week study period during the winter months. Information was gathered regarding demographics, number of ear infections, history and frequency of swimming during the study period, presence of head submersion, daycare center attendance, allergies, chronic medical conditions, otolaryngology consultations, ear surgery, and air travel. Forty-three percent of nonswimmers compared with 19% of swimmers had one or more ear infections during the study period ($p < .02$). The remaining factors surveyed did not differ significantly between groups. A review of the literature yielded two studies suggesting that swimming may have a beneficial effect on eustachian tube function and may indirectly decrease the occurrence of otitis media. Based on these findings, the authors conclude that there appears to be no basis to the commonly held belief that swimming may induce or exacerbate otitis media. In fact, the converse may be true.[5]

In this example, the cases were the children who developed otitis media and the controls were those who did not. The investigators were testing the validity of a theory that swimming is a risk factor for the development of otitis media. The major feature of a case-control study is that the groups are identified on the basis of an outcome of interest (in this case, otitis media) and the search for exposure to a putative cause (in this case, swimming) is retrospective. Stated differently, the case-control study looks backward in time to detect possible causes or risk factors that occur in the history of the cases but not in the history of the controls to answer the question "What happened to cause this outcome?"

The case-control study is the quickest and least expensive of the observational study designs and is also the most useful for investigating a preliminary hypothesis about risk factors that may be associated with an outcome or condition of interest, although it does not establish the sequence of events. For rare diseases or conditions that develop over a long time, the case-control study is by far the best choice. It is not without its limitations, however: because it is retrospective, it is difficult to exercise appropriate controls, and it is subject to the largest number of biases, including sampling bias, measurement bias, and observer bias. It also depends on recall or on existing records, both of which may be imperfect and lead to error. Case-control studies do not provide indications of prevalence, incidence, or excess risk, although they are useful in estimating the odds ratio, a good approximation of relative risk.[4]

The relative merits of these three designs of observational research are summarized in Table 1.

Table 1 Advantages and Disadvantages of the Major Observational Study Designs

Design	Advantages	Disadvantages
Cross-sectional	• May study several outcomes • No one exposed to causal agent or denied therapy • Relatively short duration • Inexpensive • A good first step for a cohort study • Yields prevalence and relative prevalence data	• Does not establish sequence of events • Does not establish causality • Not feasible for rare predictors or rare outcomes • Potential confounders may not be equally distributed • Does not yield incidence or relative risk • Groups may have different sample sizes, resulting in loss of statistical efficiency
Cohort All	• Establishes sequence of events • Can study several outcomes • Number of outcome events grows over time • Yields incidence, relative risk, excess risk	• Often requires large sample sizes • Less feasible for rare outcomes
Prospective	• More control over subject selection • More control over measurement • Avoids bias in measuring predictors	• More expensive • Longer duration
Retrospective	• Less expensive • Shorter duration	• Less control over subject selection • Less control over measurements
Multiple cohort	• Useful when distinct cohorts have different or rare exposures	• Potential for bias and confounding from sampling several populations
Case-control	• Useful for studying rare conditions • Short duration • Relatively inexpensive • Relatively small • Yields odds ratio (usually a good approximation of relative risk unless the outcome is common) • Usually requires fewer subjects than for cross-sectional studies	• Potential for bias and confounding from sampling two populations • Relies on recall or records to establish exposure • Does not establish sequence of events • Potential survivor bias • Limited to one outcome variable • Does not yield prevalence, incidence, or excess risk

Adapted from references 3 and 4.

EXPERIMENTAL RESEARCH

Following these three observational studies, Drs Cold, Snow, Warm, and Sun win the funding for a large grant to explore further the relationship of ear infections and number of children in their daytime play environment. Stated in the PICO format, they want to know:

In newborn babies who have two working parents, will home care compared to daycare decrease the number of ear infections during the first year of life?

They conduct an experimental study in which first newborn children of young double-income families are randomized to home care or daycare. If they are home-cared, the grant pays for a qualified babysitter to care for the child in the child's home. If they are randomized to daycare, the grant pays for the child to be in a qualified daycare with at least eight children. The study follows each child for 1 year, and each child visits their pediatrician and has an ear exam every 2 weeks. Ear infections are documented and treated according to standard of care.

The number of ear infections is counted and compared for each group.

Clinical trials are the most widely recognized form of experimental clinical research. They may be controlled or uncontrolled, randomized or nonrandomized, blinded or nonblinded, but all have in common the feature that an experimental drug or procedure is introduced to the patient and its effect on the patient's condition is observed prospectively; thus, they provide the most compelling evidence of a *causal relationship* between a treatment and an effect. One of the earliest randomized controlled clinical trials was conducted by Scottish physician James Lind in the mid-eighteenth century, who daily gave citrus fruits to a pair of British sailors suffering from scurvy aboard the *HMS Salisbury*; five other similarly affected pairs of sailors received different treatments. Only the group treated with citrus fruits recovered from their disease, establishing the evidence for a causal link between vitamin C deficiency and scurvy and leading to a simple treatment and prevention of this debilitating disease. Lind's study was published and recognized, but the translation of research into practice was even slower 250 years ago: it was not until some 40 years after publication of *A Treatise on Scurvy* that the British Navy issued an order for a daily ration of lime juice to sailors on long sea voyages, almost immediately wiping out scurvy from the British Fleet and Naval hospitals.[4]

Not every clinical question, of course, lends itself to investigation by means of a clinical trial, and questions involving surgical management are notoriously difficult to investigate using this methodology. Sackett has gone so far as to say that because they are so expensive and cumbersome, clinical trials should be undertaken only when six criteria are fulfilled: (1) the trial needs to be done; (2) the question posed is both appropriate and unambiguous; (3) the trial architecture is valid; (4) the subject inclusion/exclusion criteria strike a balance between efficiency and generalizability; (5) the trial protocol is feasible; and (6) the trial administration is effective.[6]

But how does one know when a clinical trial "needs to be done"? The US Food and Drug Administration (FDA) requires evidence of the safety and efficacy of new drugs, devices, and other medical products that will be approved for use in medical and dental settings for specific indications before they can be placed on the market. *Efficacy* refers to the impact of an intervention in a clinical trial, indicating that the intervention has the desired ability to produce an expected effect, for example, a new antibiotic kills bacteria. Efficacy differs from *effectiveness*, which relates to the impact of the intervention in "real world" situations when it is used with a broader range of patients than those who participated in the clinical trial, and who may have comorbid conditions that require the use of other medications. Stated differently, efficacy studies are focused on determining whether the *compound/intervention works* in the expected way; effectiveness studies focus on whether the *patient is clinically and functionally better* to a worthwhile degree as a result of the intervention, on some range of systematic objective, subjective, and outcomes measures.[7]

Drugs may be used for indications other than those for which they were approved ("off-label" use). Clinical trials are needed when the efficacy of the off-label treatment is unclear; the treatment is moderately different from the standard treatment; or when the frequency or severity of adverse effects associated with the new treatment is unclear. A clinical trial is *not* needed when the new treatment is unequivocally superior to the standard treatment. Nonetheless, because randomized clinical trials have achieved a reputation as the gold standard for the methodical assessment of treatment efficacy and adverse effects, they have become the lynchpin on which evidence-based medicine rests, as we shall see in a later section.

Basic Requirements of a Clinical Trial

Under most ordinary circumstances, a clinical trial has the following characteristics: (1) it is prospective; (2) it involves human subjects; (3) it has both intervention and control groups; (4) subjects are randomized into the intervention and control groups; and (5) the subjects, and sometimes the investigators (as well as other participants in the trial), are masked (or blinded) as to the group assignment of the subjects.[8] The latter is not always possible in surgical, behavioral, and some device trials but is frequently possible with drug trials.

The central legal, moral, and ethical requirement of clinical trials—and all other clinical research involving human subjects—is *informed consent*. Patients must be fully aware that they are participating in a research study and must

know what the potential risks and benefits are, what the procedure is, what is expected of them, what they can expect as a result of participating in the study; and they must *freely consent* to participate once they know all of the above. There are well-defined elements that must appear in every informed consent. These are presented in Table 2.

Informed consent documents should be written in such a way as to translate complex scientific and medical terms into easily understood language and be written in the patient's native or preferred language. Care should be taken to avoid making any concrete or implied assurances of benefit or effectiveness of the interventions on the trial. It is important that the informed consent be signed, dated, and witnessed to demonstrate that consent was obtained before treatment began.

The Ethics of Clinical Trials

When the topic of ethics in clinical trials is raised, the most polarizing issue is that of *randomization*, particularly if the comparison treatment is a placebo or nonactive drug. Random assignment to intervention groups gives all subjects the same chance of receiving each possible treatment, and it serves several important purposes. It constitutes a means of assigning patients to treatments in a way that is free of personal bias, and it forms the basis for the statistical tests that will be used to test the underlying hypotheses. Most importantly, randomization distributes the variables, both measured and unobserved (and possibly unknown) among the groups in a chance, and therefore in an impartial manner. It is another way of ensuring lack of bias and permitting unambiguous statistical analysis and interpretation of group data.[9]

Unfortunately, many clinicians and even more patients are uncomfortable with the concept of random assignment to treatment arms; only 3% of all cancer patients in the United States participate in clinical trials![10] Both physician and patient want the best possible treatment to be administered, whether it is new or the standard of care, and the prospect of receiving an "inferior" treatment by chance assignment is troubling. This has given rise to the principle of *clinical equipoise*: patients should be entered into a randomized controlled

clinical trial only if there is substantial uncertainty within the expert medical community about which intervention is superior and both interventions appear to offer the same probability of benefit for treatment of the disease under study.[11]

Not every clinical trial is placebo-controlled, nor should it be.[12] Many authorities agree that placebos should be used as a control only under the following circumstances:

- There is no standard treatment available for the disease being studied;
- The standard treatment is ineffective or unproven to be effective;
- The standard treatment is inappropriate for this particular clinical trial;
- Placebo has been reported to be relatively effective in treating the disease/condition of interest;
- The disease process is characterized by frequent exacerbations and remissions;
- Allowing concomitant treatment shown to be effective on an as-needed basis;
- In a population of patients who are refractory to standard treatment and for whom no standard second-line treatment exists; or
- When testing an add-on treatment to standard therapy when all subjects receive all treatments that would be prescribed; and
- "Escape clauses" or points are designed into the protocol.[13]

The ethical principles governing the conduct of clinical trials are discussed in detail in *The Belmont Report*,[14] a document based on the work of the National Commission for the Protection of Human Subjects of Biomedical and Behavioral Research. It identifies three fundamental ethical principles for all human subject research—*respect for persons*, *beneficence*, and *justice*. Those principles remain the basis for the US Department of Health and Human Services, human subject protection regulations and are an essential reference for institutional review boards. Among the topics covered in this report are the use of vulnerable populations who may not be able to give fully informed consent (eg, mentally retarded, demented, or psychotic patients) or who are subject to coercion and thus may not

Table 2 Elements of Informed Consent

- Statement that the study involves research, explanation of purpose of research, expected duration of subject's participation, description of procedures, identification of procedures that are experimental
- Description of reasonably foreseeable risks or discomfort to patient
- Description of potential benefits to patient or others that can be reasonably expected
- Disclosure of appropriate alternative treatments that could be advantageous
- Description of extent to which confidentiality of records identifying patient will be maintained
- Explanation of any compensation; whether medical treatments available in case of injury; where to get further information
- Statement that participation is voluntary
- Anticipated circumstances under which subject's participation may be terminated
- Any additional costs to the patient that may result from participation in the research
- Consequences of subject's decision to withdraw from research
- Statement that significant new findings will be revealed to subject
- Number of anticipated subjects in study

Source: http://www.fda.gov/oc/ohrt/irbs/informedconsent.html#general.

be autonomous (eg, impoverished, addicted, or imprisoned patients); and the important principle that in all cases the benefits of the trial should be maximized and the potential risks minimized.

The Surgical Clinical Trial

There is little question that randomized controlled clinical trials are the most effective ways to evaluate new pharmacologic interventions, but controversy still attends their role in nonpharmacologic interventions, such as surgery. A surgical trial is unique in that the expertise of the surgeon becomes an integral part of the intervention, unlike drug and device trials, where the physician is the case manager, but the treatment efficacy depends on the pharmacologic compound or on device technology rather than on the physician's skill. In a traditional surgical trial, the patient is randomized to Procedure A or Procedure B; randomizing patients to one of the procedure arms requires the assumption that the surgeon has equal expertise in the interventions under evaluation and that all participating surgeons have comparable expertise.

An alternative to the traditional randomized trial is the *expertise-based trial*, in which patients are randomized to clinicians with expertise in Procedure A or to clinicians with expertise in Procedure B, and the clinicians perform only the procedure in which they are expert. Devereaux and colleagues in 2005 presented a cogent argument and multiple clinical illustrations of the ways in which the expertise-based design will enhance the validity, applicability, feasibility, and ethical integrity of randomized controlled trials in surgery.[15]

The potential for bias in favor of one surgical approach over another is significant in surgical trials: surgical expertise takes training and experience to develop and surgeons tend to primarily use a single surgical approach to treat specific problems. If, as Devereaux and colleagues demonstrate, surgeons with expertise in, for example, an endoscopic approach treat 70% of the patients in both groups A and B and surgeons with expertise in, for example, an open approach treat 30% of those in both groups A and B, the trial results will be biased in favor of the endoscopic approach. Devereaux refers to this type of bias as *differential expertise bias* and suggests that its potential is high in surgical trials for three reasons. First, measures are rarely instituted to ensure that the number of participating surgeons with expertise in each procedure is equal. Second, there is usually no assurance that participating surgeons have reached the asymptote of their learning curves for the procedures under evaluation, and outcomes usually continue to improve with extensive experience. This is especially true if new devices or procedures are being compared to an existing standard of care. Third, even if these two problems are overcome, one of the procedures may be more technically challenging; thus, surgeons who have to acquire expertise in the more challenging procedure will remain less proficient than those who are learning the less technically challenging

procedure or who are already proficient in one procedure. In this situation the trial will be biased toward the latter.

One important advantage of the expertise-based design for randomized surgical clinical trials is that the consent process can inform patients that, regardless of the procedure to which they are assigned, a surgeon with specific expertise will perform the surgery. This may not always be the case in traditional randomized surgical trials, and it is a significant ethical consideration.

Clinical Trial Phases

Clinical trials are generally described in terms of their *phase*, a descriptor that designates the overall purpose of the trial. *Phase I* trials are small trials of 20 to 80 patients designed to study the toxic and pharmacologic effects of a new treatment that has been studied in an animal model but which now needs to be tested in humans. Phase I trials are either done in healthy volunteers or in patients with severe or terminal illnesses who have failed accepted treatments. *Phase II* trials generally involve 100 to 200 patients to expand study of the treatment effect on a disease; dose-response parameters are obtained, as well as safety data. *Phase III* trials are large-scale, randomized, tightly controlled trials designed to study the efficacy of the experimental treatment in a rigidly defined sample of patients. Usually conducted as a multicentered trial, the treatment is compared to a standard of care treatment to determine which is more effective. Phase III trials may also be planned to test the efficacy of an established drug for a new (non-FDA-approved) indication. If a standard treatment is not available, a placebo may be used as a comparison. Considerable controversy has surrounded some surgical trials, where sham procedures have been conducted on patients randomized into the control group.[16–18] The *Phase IV* trial involves postmarketing surveillance of the drug in the general population and may be structured more as an effectiveness study, including use of the drug in combination with other drugs or in patients with comorbidities. Phase IV trials (and other forms of clinical research) may also be conducted using patient outcomes and quality-of-life instruments to assess a more global impact of the intervention on the patient's life.

OUTCOMES RESEARCH

Outcomes research goes beyond the traditional epidemiological assessment of objective biological signs or measurements that have been accepted as valid surrogates for patient well-being and focuses on the systematic evaluation of all the disease- and intervention-related outcomes that are relevant to patients: mortality, morbidity, complications, symptom reduction, functional status improvement, and health-related quality of life.[19] Outcomes assessment has also come to encompass the patient experience with the healthcare system, processes, and providers. Outcomes are

generally classified using the simple mnemonic of *six D's*: *D*eath, *D*isease, *D*isability, *D*iscomfort, *D*issatisfaction, and *D*ollars. This concept captures four distinct paradigms for studying the outcome of healthcare, reflecting the interests of the various groups of stakeholders in the healthcare cycle (healthcare providers, patients, employers and insurance carriers, and policymakers)[2]:

- The medical/epidemiological perspective (*death and disease*)
- The social psychological perspective, concerned with functional status and health-related quality of life (*disability and discomfort*)
- The consumer or customer service perspective (*dissatisfaction*)
- The economic perspective (*dollars*)

These perspectives are not independent but often are closely interrelated: For example, morbidity resulting from surgical complications and requiring hospital readmission will have an impact on quality of life, disability or loss of employment productivity, and cost of care, and will likely result in some level of dissatisfaction. The types of parameters studied under each of these attributes are shown in Figure 1.

Measurement of Outcomes

There are several different ways to categorize outcome measures. The broadest scheme describes outcome measures as being either *generic (or general)* or *disease-specific*. As their name implies, the generic measures are generalizable across health conditions, practice settings, and types of treatments. They may be applied to most patient populations and are widely used to measure health-related quality of life (HRQOL), activities of daily life (ADL), mental health, role disability, pain, and feelings of well-being. Some well-known generic instruments are the Quality of Well-Being Index[20] and the 36-item short-form health survey (SF-36).[21] While these measures are sensitive to the impact produced by serious diseases such as cancer, however, they are relatively insensitive to the effects of less serious conditions such as rhinosinusitis, mild to moderate hearing impairment, or laryngeal disorders. Disease-specific outcomes capture more detailed information about function directly related to the condition of interest and make it more straightforward to attribute change to treatment response. There are a number of well-known disease-specific outcome measures in otolaryngology—head and neck surgery, including those examples shown in Table 3, which is not meant to be comprehensive.

Some measures are linked temporally to the disease or intervention process and thus enjoy a high degree of specificity with respect to health outcomes; recovery from a surgical procedure, for example, or changes that occur early in the natural history of the disease. Other measures occur later in the process and are more subject to the influence of external factors; life satisfaction, for example, will certainly be affected by health status but will also be influenced by unrelated social, economic, and psychological factors.[22] HRQOL,

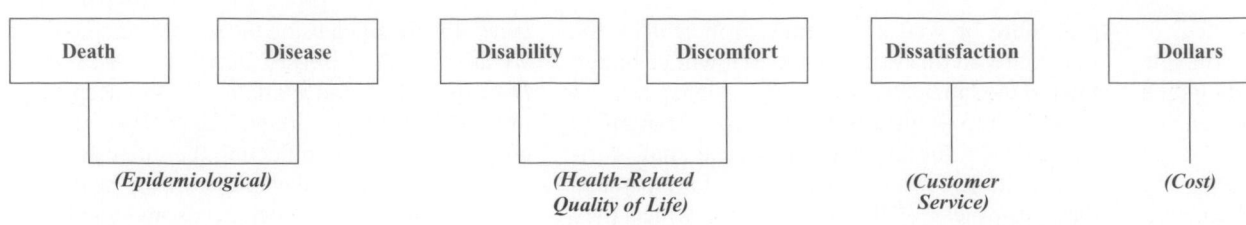

Figure 1 Six D's of outcomes. (Adapted from reference 2.)

the patient's perception of how a disease affects their physical, social, and emotional function,[23] is inescapably individual and subjective and may vary widely among patients with the same disease stage, severity, and symptoms. This being the case, the *difference* or *change* in disease-related quality of life following intervention is the more meaningful parameter to track.

Selecting an Outcome Measure

When selecting an outcome measure for use in a study, investigators should be aware of three major characteristics of the instrument. First, an outcome measure should have evidence of its *validity* or the ability to measure what it is supposed to measure. Second, there should be evidence of its *responsiveness* or the ability to detect clinically and socially important differences when change has indeed occurred. Third, there should be evidence of its *reliability* or the ability to provide consistent values between and within subjects. Further, the outcome measure should have these characteristics defined within the population of interest. For example, the OM-6[24] is valid, responsive, and reliable for otitis media, but not for acute otitis externa or other ear diseases such as mastoiditis.

Two additional attributes are important to evaluate when selecting an outcome measure. The late Dr Alvan Feinstein described the *sensibility* of an outcomes instrument as "enlightened common sense," characterized by a clear purpose and framework, an easily understood and interpreted output scale, and content validity.[25] The final attribute to consider is the *burden* imposed by its use. Burden, of course, is defined by the experience of the user. Lengthy health outcome surveys create a time burden; placing that burden on the patient rather than on a busy, distracted office staff relieves the staff of the time and effort necessary to retrieve medical data or compound their paperwork and may enhance their willingness to participate in clinical research studies. These five attributes are summarized in Table 4.

Medical Outcomes and Patient Outcomes

The emergence of health services and outcomes research has brought about recognition that medical outcomes and patient outcomes are not always directly correlated: a very positive medical outcome in terms of controlling disease may carry very unwelcome patient outcomes in terms of quality of life, social, or mental function. For example, tracheostomy is quite effective in controlling severe obstructive sleep apnea and some dangerous associated conditions such as cardiac dysrhythmias, hypertension, and blood oxygen desaturation. Patients, however, now have to deal with care and protection of the stoma, effect on communication, and body image factors, and those issues will impact their perceived quality of life. Patients' satisfaction with their medical care has been shown to be directly associated with how effectively that care reduces the symptoms they view as most important or troublesome, even if those symptoms are not the most medically significant.[26]

Application of Outcomes and Effectiveness Research

Driven by geographic variations in practice patterns and utilization, rising healthcare costs, the proliferation of information technology that has motivated patients to take more active roles in the decision process about their healthcare, and the demand by payers for evidence to support the effectiveness and quality of medical and surgical interventions, medical and patient outcomes, and effectiveness research has assumed an increasingly important role in the American healthcare system. Because outcomes and effectiveness research has evolved to reflect the interests of

---

Table 3 Selected Disease-Specific Outcome Measures in Otolaryngology—Head and Neck Surgery

Rhinosinusitis
Sino-nasal outcomes test (SNOT-20)
Chronic sinusitis survey (CSS)
Sino-nasal assessment questionnaire (SNAQ-11)
Rhinosinusitis disability index (RDI)
Rhinosinusitis QOL survey

Sleep-disordered breathing
Obstructive sleep disorders-6 (OSD-6)
Obstructive sleep apnea-18 (OSA-18)
Epworth sleepiness scale (ESS)
Empirical sleepiness scale
Functional outcomes of sleep questionnaire (FOSQ)
Sleep disorders questionnaire (SDQ)
Sleep apnea quality of life index (SAQLI)
Snore outcome survey

Head and neck cancer
Univ of Washington quality of life instrument (rev.) (UW-QOL-R)
Quality of life radiation therapy instrument (QOL-RTI)
Neck dissection impairment index
EORTC quality of life – HN-35
Functional assessment of cancer therapy (FACT – HN)
MD Anderson dysphagia inventory (MDADI)
Head and neck quality of life scale

GERD/EERD
Reflux symptom index (RSI)
Reflux questionnaire (ReQuest)
Supraesophageal reflux questionnaire
GERD symptom frequency questionnaire (GSFQ)

Otitis media
Otitis media – 6 (OM-6)
Chronic ear survey (CES)
TAP-QOL
OM-CSI, OM-FSQ, OMD

Meniere disease
Meniere disease outcomes questionnaire (MDOQ)
Meniere disease patient-oriented symptom-severity index (MD-POSI)

Hearing loss
Hearing satisfaction scale (HSS)
Effectiveness of auditory rehabilitation scale (EAR)
Hearing handicap inventory for the elderly (HHI-E)
Hearing disability handicap scale (HDHS)

Tinnitus
Tinnitus handicap inventory (THI)
Tinnitus severity questionnaire (TSQ)

Vertigo/dizziness
Dizziness handicap inventory (DHI)
Vertigo symptom scale (VSS)
Vestibular activities of daily living (VADL)
UCLA dizziness questionnaire (UCLA-DQ)

Facial paralysis
Facial clinimetric evaluation scale (FACE)
Facial disability index (FDI)

Voice disorders
Voice handicap index (VHI)
Voice outcome survey (VOS)

Adenotonsillitis
Tonsil and adenoid health symptom index (TAHSI)

Nasal obstruction
Nasal obstruction symptom evaluation scale (NOSE)

Allergic rhinitis
Rhinoconjunctivitis quality of life questionnaire (RQLQ)
Rhinitis symptom utility index (RSUI)
Pediatric allergic disease quality of life questionnaire (PADQLQ)

Table 4   Selecting an Outcomes Instrument

Characteristic	Discrimination	Prediction	Evaluation
Sensibility			
Purpose and framework	Taps clinically and socially significant dimensions of health	Taps the dimension of health associated with predicted outcome	Taps the dimension of health related to change in health
Comprehensible output	Low level of scale that can be interpreted in a uniform manner	Scale output that correlates with predicted outcome	High level of scale output that provides a number of health outcome gradations
Content validity	Content has universal application	Content validated by statistical methods	Content has clinical significance
Reliability	Measure provides consistent values between subjects	Measure provides consistent values between and within subjects	Measurement provides consistent values within subjects
Validity	Emphasis on construct validity at one point in time	Emphasis on accuracy of the measure in predicting an outcome	Emphasis on the association with other external criteria
Responsiveness	Not relevant	Not relevant	Power to detect clinically and socially important differences
Burden			
Data collection	Burden in collecting data generally low	Intermediate in terms of data collection burden	Highest data collection burden because of follow-up
Scoring	Simple scoring systems	More difficult scoring systems	Most complex scoring systems
Resources	Requires the fewest resources	Intermediate in terms of resource demand	Requires the most resources

Adapted from reference 2.

major stakeholders in the healthcare process, it offers distinct advantages to each:

- It helps *healthcare providers* understand the importance and therapeutic value of the practitioner–patient relationship, design and evaluate more efficient ways to deliver healthcare, and improve informed consent procedures.
- It helps *patients* develop realistic expectations about disease and treatment, participate in treatment decisions that will have an impact on their quality of life, and provide feedback to their physicians and nurses on their satisfaction with the quality of care they have received.
- It helps *healthcare delivery systems* develop guidelines based on relative probabilities of explicit outcomes and patient preferences; analyze the cost-effectiveness of primary care versus specialty care based on long-term outcomes; determine the most significant factors in patient satisfaction for quality improvement programs; and establish evidence-based indications for care to develop appropriate utilization rates.
- *Insurance companies* use the results of clinical research to standardize and validate healthcare evaluation parameters, develop objective methodologies to define "appropriate" versus "unnecessary" levels of care, and increasingly, determine reimbursement policies.
- *Health regulatory agencies* apply the results of outcomes and effectiveness research to develop a balanced view of quality, cost, and access for national healthcare, project societal and workplace impact of disease prevention and treatment, and increase their awareness of demographic variables and their impact on patterns of health care.

Far from being isolated from the realities of clinical practice, clinical research of all kinds is now inextricably linked to progress in medical diagnosis, prognosis, and management; health policy and regulation, licensing and certification;

and reimbursement. Research can answer the nagging clinical questions that arise in a practice; the answers form the evidence base to document the quality and effectiveness of interventions in otolaryngology—head and neck surgery.

EVIDENCE-BASED MEDICINE

Evidence-based medicine is the integration of clinical expertise, patient values, and the *best evidence available* into the decision-making process for patient care. Clinical expertise refers to the clinician's cumulated experience, education, and clinical skills. The patient brings to the encounter his or her own personal and unique concerns, expectations, and values. The best evidence is usually found in clinically relevant research that has been conducted using sound methodology.[6] The evidence, of itself, is never a deciding factor, but it can be a powerful tool in supporting the patient care process and in other aspects of organized medicine.

Medical decision making based on the triad of these three factors represents a fundamental paradigm shift in medicine, requiring new skills of the physician, including efficient literature searching and the application of formal rules of evidence evaluating the clinical literature. Clinical research of all kinds is far more common today than it was 50 years ago: In 1960 randomized clinical trials were sporadic and outcomes research as a discipline did not exist.[27] Clinical decisions were made on the basis of clinical experience and understanding of related biology and pathophysiology; patients were not expected to have a role in the decision process. An essential premise underlying this new paradigm is the acknowledgment of the uncertainties of clinical medicine, which continue to grow with the exponential growth of medical literature, new technologies, the linking of reimbursement to outcome and effectiveness, and an increasingly litigious society.

As the volume of literature has grown, presenting evidence for and against the effectiveness of interventions and the assessment of diagnostic tests and prognosis, a new field has emerged, focused on systematically evaluating the validity of the clinical evidence and summarizing the evidence. At the center of this new field is a hierarchy of research designs, arranged in descending order of quality and increasing probability of bias. Randomized controlled clinical trials appear near the top of the hierarchy (high quality, low bias); individual case reports and retrospective case series toward the bottom (lower quality, higher probability of bias). The steps in this hierarchy have come to be referred to as "levels of evidence,"[28] and are widely used for a variety of applications, ranging from publications to development of practice guidelines to reimbursement criteria.

Evidence-based medicine is a skilled, multistep process that exceeds the scope of this chapter. Given the empowerment of healthcare consumers through access to a greater body of information about disease treatment and prevention on the World Wide Web and a continuously expanding literature, readers are encouraged to pursue this subject and put it into use in their practices. Some excellent resources are:

- Straus SE, Richardson WS, Glasziou P, Haynes RB. Evidence-Based Medicine: How To Practice and Teach EBM, 3rd edition. New York: Elsevier/Churchill Livingstone; 2005.
- Glasziou P, Del Mar C, Salisbury J. Evidence-Based Medicine Workbook. Finding and Applying the Best Evidence to Improve Patient Care. London: BMJ Books; 2003.
- Guyatt G, Rennie D, editors. Users' Guides to the Medical Literature. A Manual for Evidence-Based Clinical Practice. Chicago: AMA Press; 2002.

Clinical research is an extension of the medical care process, based on formulating a question and making structured, systematic observations to answer the question. The rewards lie in advancing knowledge, broadening your understanding of the impact of disease on patients, introducing variety to clinical practice, and contributing to your specialty.

REFERENCES

1. Gelijns AC, Thier SO. Medical technology development: An introduction to the innovation–evaluation nexus. In: Gelijns, AC, editor. Modern Methods of Clinical Investigation. Washington, DC: National Academy Press; 1990. p. 1–15.
2. Radosevich DM, Kalambokidis-Werni TL. A Practical Guidebook for Implementing, Analyzing, and Reporting Outcomes Measurements. Bloomington, MN: Stratis Health; 1997.
3. Hulley SB, Cummings SR, Browner WS, et al. Designing Clinical Research, 2nd edition. Baltimore: Lippincott Williams & Wilkins; 2001.
4. Streiner DL, Norman GR. PDQ Epidemiology. Hamilton, Ontario: BC Decker Inc.; 1998.
5. Robertson, LM, Marino RV, Namjoshi S. Docs swimming increase the incidence of otitis media? J Am Osteopath Assoc 1997;97: 150–2.
6. Sackett DL. On some prerequisites for a successful clinical trial. In: Shapiro SH, Louis TA, editors. Clinical Trials. New York: Marcel Dekker; 1983. p. 65.
7. Rosenfeld RM. Outcomes Research. DRF Clinical Research Workshop. Bethesda, MD, March, 2006.
8. McKneally MF, McPeek B, Mosteller F, Neugebauer EAM. Clinical trials. In: Troidl H, McKneally MF, Mulder DS, et al., editors. Surgical Research: Basic Principles and Clinical Practice, 3rd edition. New York: Springer-Verlag; 1998. p. 197–209.
9. http://www.worldscibooks.com/lifesci/etextbook/p131/p131_chap1_4.pdf, accessed 2 October 2006.
10. http://www.cancer.gov/clinicaltrials/resources/basicworkbook/page6, accessed 4 October 2006.
11. Freedman B. Equipoise and the ethics of clinical research. N Engl J Med 1987;317:141–5.
12. Smith GC, Pell JP. Parachute use to prevent death and major trauma related to gravitational challenge: Systematic review of randomized controlled trials. BMJ 2003; 327:1459–61.
13. Spilker B. Guide to Clinical Trials. New York: Raven Press; 1991. p. 62.
14. http://ohsr.od.nih.gov/guidelines/belmont.html, accessed 5 October 2006.
15. Devereaux PJ, Bhandari M, Clarke M, et al. Need for expertise based randomized controlled trials. BMJ 2005; 330:88 98.
16. Kim SY, Frank S, Holloway R, et al. Science and ethics of sham surgery: A survey of Parkinson disease researchers. Arch Neurol 2005;62:1357–60.
17. Miller FG. Sham surgery: An ethical analysis. Sci Eng Ethics 2004;10:157–66.
18. London AJ, Kadane JB. Placebos that harm: Sham surgery controls in clinical trials. Stat Methods Clin Res 2002;11:413–27.
19. Wennberg JE. What is outcomes research? In: Gelijns AC, editor. Modern Methods of Clinical Investigation. Washington, DC: National Academy Press; 1990. p. 33–46.
20. Kaplan RM, Bush JW. Health-related quality of life measurement for evaluation research and policy analysis. Health Psychol 1982;1:61–80.
21. Ware JE, Sherbourne CD. The MOS 36-item short-form health survey (SF-36). Med Care 1992;30:473–483.
22. Brenner MH, Curbow B, Legro MW. The proximal-distal continuum of multiple health outcome measures: The case of cataract surgery. Med Care 1995:33:AS236–44.
23. Guyatt GH, Feeny DH, Patrick DL. Measuring health-related quality of life. Ann Int Med 1993;118:622–9.
24. Rosenfeld RM, Goldsmith AJ, Tetlus L, Balzano A. Quality of life for children with otitis media. Arch Otolaryngol Head Neck Surg 1997;123:1049–54.
25. Feinstein AR. Clinimetrics. New Haven, CT: Yale University Press; 1987.
26. Stewart MG, Sicard MW, Piccirillo JF, Diaz-Marchan PJ. Severity staging in chronic sinusitis: Are CT scan findings related to patient symptoms? Am J Rhinol 1999;13:161–7.
27. Evidence-Based Medicine Working Group. Evidence-based medicine. A new approach to teaching the practice of medicine. JAMA 1992;268:2420–5.
28. Centre for Evidence-Based Medicine. Levels of evidence and grades of recommendations. http://cebm.jr2.ox.ac.uk/docs/, accessed 18 November 1999.

14

Diseases of the External Ear

Frank E. Lucente, MD
Matthew Hanson, MD

The external ear is composed of the auricle and the external auditory canal and is a frequent source of patient complaints in otolaryngology. External ear problems can range from the deceptively simple, such as earwax impactions and foreign bodies to severe and life-threatening problems such as malignancy or invasive infection. Often the presenting symptoms of the 2 extremes may be indistinguishable; and the otolaryngologist must rely on a thorough evaluation, appropriate testing, and a high index of suspicion to ensure the appropriate treatment of the patient. This chapter presents an overview of diseases of the external ear, primarily infectious and inflammatory disorders.

ANATOMY AND PHYSIOLOGY

The fundamental function of the external ear is the conduction of sound. The shape of the auricle, or pinna, and the canal provide a small degree of amplification which is greatest at normal speech frequencies. The auricle also provides a degree of selective directionality to hearing, favoring sounds coming from in front of the listener. The entire external ear complex provides approximately 5 dB of gain (depending on the frequency) and the greatest gain is for sounds coming from a 45° angle from the front of the individual and at frequencies of 500 to 6,000 Hz.[1] In addition to its acoustic function, the external ear is protective, allowing the delicate structures of the middle and internal ear to lie deeply embedded in the skull and safe from trauma and environmental insults. The auricle also has important bearing on the aesthetic aspects of facial appearance, but this is discussed in greater detail in Chapter 52, "Otoplasty for the Prominent Ear."

The canal itself can be further divided into a lateral, cartilaginous portion and a medial, bony portion (Figure 1). The epithelium of the canal is stratified squamous epithelium, ie, skin. Over the medial bony portion, the skin is thin and applied directly to the periosteum of the bone. In this portion, there are no skin appendages, glands or hairs; and the close approximation of the periosteum makes this area very sensitive. The lateral cartilaginous portion has considerably thicker skin with a generous adventitia and numerous appendages, including hairs, sebaceous glands, and modified apocrine ceruminous glands.

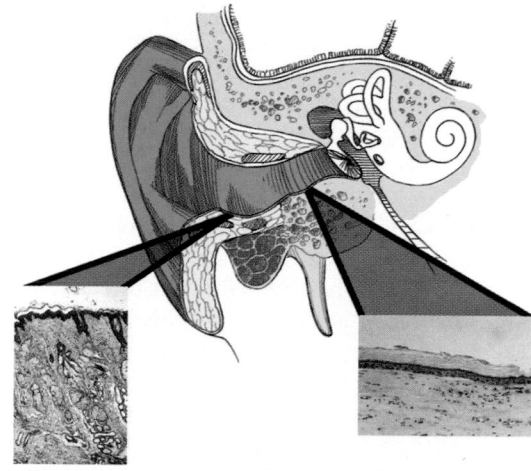

Figure 1 Coronal section of the ear canal with magnification of the skin of the cartilaginous and osseous canals. (Published with permission, copyright © 2008, P.A. Wackym, MD.)

As a skin-lined, blind-ended cul-de-sac, the external canal would seem to be at risk for accumulation of the desquamated keratin debris normally created by skin. In fact, however, the ear canal skin has a migratory property that gives it a self-cleaning mechanism. The first studies of the migratory nature of desquamated canal skin were published by Blake in 1882.[2] Alberti in 1964 further characterized this mechanism and measured the rate of migration at 0.07 mm/d.[3] As the stratum corneum approaches the cartilaginous portion of the canal, it is lifted up by the action of the hairs and the secretions of the sebaceous and ceruminous glands. This mass of desquamated skin cells and secretions blankets the outer portions of the ear canal and slowly migrates out of the ear canal as what is commonly known as earwax.

Earwax has many properties that make it protective of the ear canal. It is hydrophobic, providing a barrier to the penetration of water (and water-borne organisms) to the deeper areas of the ear canal. It is sticky, trapping dust, dirt, and pollen and pushing these out of the ear. It is acidic, having a pH of around 6.5. This not only suppresses the growth of many bacteria and fungi but also makes the human ear an unwelcoming place to vermin such as insects and mites that can be so troublesome in other species. Lastly, the ceruminous secretions contain lysozyme and immunoglobulin G, providing the substance with a true antibiotic character. Indeed,

most infectious and inflammatory problems with the external canal have a common origin in the excessive cleaning of the ear and the removal of this vital protective substance.

It has long been noticed that earwax has significant variation across races. Asians tend to have a dry, flaky wax, while a wet, sticky wax predominates in Africans and Caucasians. Studies of the Mendelian inheritance of wax type has shown the wet variety to be the dominant trait. The ceruminous glands are closely related to the lactiferous glands of the breast, and studies have also shown that the incidence of breast cancer is considerably lower in persons with the dry wax type. Genetic linkage studies mapped the locus for the gene to the pericentromeric region of chromosome 16.[4] A single nucleotide polymorphism in a gene known as *ABCC11* has been found to be the determinant of wet/dry wax type. This gene, located at 16q12.1, codes for a transmembrane protein in the ATP-binding cassette protein class, a class of proteins involved in transmembrane transport. Disorders of genes in this class are implicated in a host of chronic diseases. A single switch at base pair 538 from a guanine moiety to an arginine changes wet wax into dry. Homozygotes for the arginine substitution have dry wax, while those with a guanine will have wet.[5] The clinical relevance of this may bear on understanding the role of apocrine secretions and their relation to breast cancer.

Earwax Removal

Earwax is a beneficial substance and does not routinely need to be cleaned or removed. In some persons, however, the earwax does not extrude but becomes impacted in the canal preventing the normal transmission of sound. Overzealous use of cotton-tipped swabs is the usual underlying cause, but some patients do demonstrate excessive production of wax, produce an abnormally hard or tenacious wax or have impaired migration and extrusion. And, even though a small amount of wax is not pathologic, the otolaryngologist may need to remove it to perform a complete examination of the eardrum. As such, removal of earwax is one of the most frequently performed procedures.

Many different strategies have been tried over the years for earwax removal, but they basically fall into 1 of 3 categories: manual removal, irrigation, and chemical dissolution. Many patients will require a combination of all 3 stratagems. Manual removal using suction (#5 or #7 Frazier tips) and microinstruments (ring curette, right angle hook) under microscopic visualization is the preferred method of the authors. This affords the least traumatic removal and does not risk the worsening of underlying pathology, such as cholesteatoma or tympanic membrane perforations that may lie beneath the wax. Irrigation is used frequently in both primary care and specialty settings. Lukewarm water (to prevent caloric stimulation) is instilled using a large syringe (Figure 2). The auricle is pulled back to straighten the canal and the water is directed to the roof of the ear canal, not directly at the eardrum. A basin is held below the ear to catch the irrigant and wax. Although irrigation is a mostly effective and a time-honored technique, it does put the patient at risk for injury. The irrigation is done, of necessity, blindly, and too much force may damage the canal skin or tympanic membrane. If underlying pathology is present, such as a cholesteatoma or perforation, the introduction of water may worsen the situation and hasten severe infection. Overall, the use of irrigation for cleaning out earwax should be discouraged.

Chemical dissolution does not so much remove the wax as much as soften it. This facilitates its removal by manual disimpaction, irrigation, or the natural extrusion over time. The simplest chemical in use is over-the-counter 4% hydrogen peroxide. Cheap and readily available, hydrogen peroxide will effectively soften wax over a brief period of time. Because of its aqueous nature it may not penetrate deeply into the wax, and its use may cause a keratinolytic epidermal reaction that may lead to infection. Carbamine peroxide is a mineral oil-based peroxide solution and is widely available over the counter under a number of brand names (Debrox being the best known). The mineral oil-base allows much greater penetration of the substance into the wax, and there is generally no epidermal reaction. Ceruminex, (triethanolamine polypeptide oleate-condensate), prescription medication, is a useful softening agent in office situations. This medication is a keratinolytic that will effectively soften earwax in about 45 minutes. It is usually recommended that it be instilled in the office and

suctioned out completely with the softened wax. This medication is not meant for patient use and should never be given for home-instillation. The keratinolytic action causes a severe inflammatory reaction with repeated use and frequently predisposes the patient to acute infection. Roland and colleagues compared the efficacy of carbamine peroxide and Ceruminex in a randomized, controlled trial against a placebo control and found no significant benefit of either over saline.[6] Other substances have also been used for earwax dissolution, including liquid ducosate (Colace), mineral oil, and others. Most are probably safe, but there are no studies of the long-term safety and efficacy of these treatments. A Cochrane Database Sytematic Review in 2003 found the data to be insufficient to make any recommendations regarding the role of cerumenolytics.[7]

One treatment touted for earwax removal by herbalists and other advocates of alternative medicine is "ear candling." In this practice, a wax cone is inserted into the ear and lit on fire and allowed to burn down. It is to be extinguished when the candle has burned down to less than three inches. It is claimed that the earwax is melted and drawn up into the candle by the flame, allowing it to be removed with the extinguished candle. The efficacy of this treatment is doubtful, especially for deeply impacted wax, and it is obviously unsafe. There are reports of significant burns resulting from this practice, and it is to be strongly discouraged.[8]

Symptoms of External Ear Disease

Disease of the external ear can present with a limited number of symptoms: pain, pruritus, aural fullness, and hearing loss. Diplacusis and autophonia can also be noted, but are rarely the presenting complaints. Otorrhea, either purulent or bloody, will often be the symptom associated with more advanced disease.

It is important to have a systematic way of evaluating the patient presenting with ear pain. Otalgia, essentially, has 3 possible sources: the ear, something else that is close to the ear, or something distant that is causing referred pain in the ear. All parts of the ear, external, middle, and inner, can be potential sources of otalgia (inner least of all). Clinical assessment of these areas by careful history and examination will usually reveal or rule out an aural source. The temporomandibular joint (TMJ), lying just anterior to the ear canal, is a frequent source of otalgia. Referred otalgia may result from a number of sources ranging from dental irritation to esophageal malignancies. As such, a complete history and otorhinolaryngologic examination is absolutely necessary in evaluating the patient with otalgia.

Much the same can be said regarding the sensation of pruritus and aural fullness, in terms of their possible sources. Both can result from aural, adjacent, and referred sources. TMJ disease will frequently result in a "full" sensation in the ear, and itchy ears can be a referred sensation due to nasal allergies. Hearing loss, on the other hand,

is obviously aural in nature and has its own diagnostic paradigm. As with otalgia, any of these symptoms would require a complete history and otorhinolaryngologic physical examination to evaluate for distant, referred sources.

Foreign Bodies and Insects

One of the most common presenting complaints involving the external canal is the presence of a foreign body. Adults will typically know the nature of the object in the ear, whereas in children it may be incidentally found by a pediatrician. Pain is occasionally present, but more often the patient complains of hearing loss or a full feeling in the ear. In most adults, the object can be easily removed in the office under microscopic visualization using a combination of suction, alligator forceps or a right-angle hook. Deeply impacted objects in adults or foreign bodies in an uncooperative child may best be removed in the operating room. Hard, round objects, such as beads, present a particular challenge, as they may not present an easily grasped aspect. Often a right-angle hook can be passed deep to the object or a large suction can be used to engage the object and draw it out.

One particularly disturbing foreign body is a live insect, such as a cockroach (Figure 3). More of a problem in urban areas, these patients will note severe pain in the ear. Most insects do not have the ability to crawl backward and cannot turn around in the canal. Meanwhile, the acidic wax layer may irritate them. This will usually cause them to crawl incessantly against the eardrum causing the severe pain. A great deal of relief is often obtained by just killing the insect. This can usually be done by instilling alcohol or lidocaine solution. Mineral oil can also be used but often makes the carcass brittle and difficult to remove in 1 piece. Once the insect is dead, it can be removed in the office similarly to removal of any foreign body.

Injury and Thermal Trauma

The exposed position of the pinna makes it a frequent site of trauma. Injuries fall into 4 broad categories: sharp trauma or lacerations, avulsions, blunt trauma, and thermal trauma. In dealing with any injury, one must remember the "ABCs" and

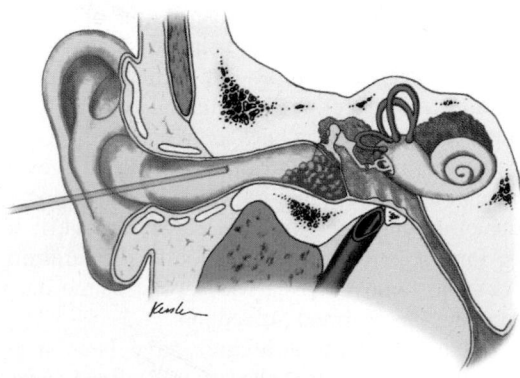

Figure 2 Irrigation of earwax.

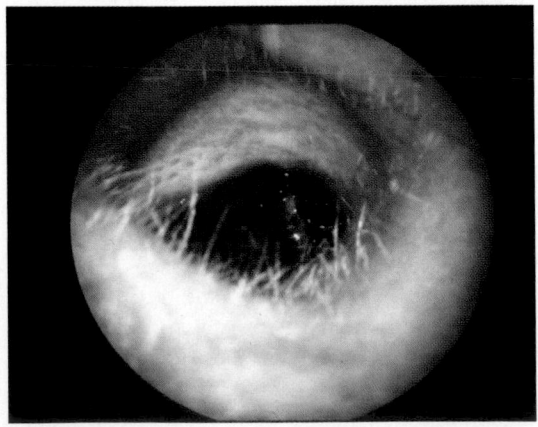

Figure 3 Insect in the external canal.

consider the risks of deeper injury. An apparently simple laceration of the tragus may in fact involve laceration of the facial nerve. An auricular hematoma from a baseball bat injury may also show "Battle sign" indicating a deeper skullbase fracture.

Lacerations and Avulsions. Lacerations of the pinna can often be challenging to repair. It is an established surgical principle that wound edges should be cleaned and debrided back to healthy, clean tissue. In lacerations of the auricle, however, too excessive debridement may result in loss of too much tissue, possibly resulting in greater tension of the closure and risk of a poor cosmetic result. Nonetheless, wound edges must be aggressively cleaned to remove any bacteria, dirt, or debris.

Closure of full-thickness lacerations of the auricle must be planned to provide a cosmetic, durable repair. The cartilage should be reapproximated with a very fine permanent monofilament suture placed through the perichondrium and cartilage. Care should be taken to approximate all layers of tissue closely, including the inner and outer layers of skin. Even apparently clean wounds of the pinna should receive antibiotic coverage to prevent perichondritis. If the laceration is the result of a human or animal bite, this, too, should affect the choice of antibiotic coverage.

Lacerations become even more problematic if portions of the pinna have become completely avulsed. If available, the avulsed portion should be reattached, essentially making it a full-thickness composite graft. Platelet inhibitors, anticoagulants, hyperbaric oxygen, and surgical leeches have all been used to enhance the survival of these reattached pieces. If the entire pinna is avulsed, microvascular re-anastomosis may be required. If the avulsed portion is not available for reimplantation, the wound may be closed primarily or allowed to close by secondary intent, with formal reconstruction performed when the wound is stable.

Auricular Hematoma. Blunt injury to the auricle may result in the formation of an auricular hematoma. This is a not-uncommon injury in sports, particularly in wrestlers and boxers, and is the primary reason for use of headgear in these sports. Injury to a perichondrial blood vessel results in blood accumulation in the subperichondrial space, elevating the perichondrium off of the cartilage. If not drained, this separation of the cartilage from its blood supply may result in cartilage necrosis. The trapped blood and injured perichondrium will eventually organize into a fibrocartilagenous mass, creating the deformity known as "cauliflower ear." Once a cauliflower ear is formed, there is little that can be done to return the ear to its prior, normal state. Therefore, auricular hematomas must be evaluated and addressed as soon as possible following the injury, preferably within 72 hours.

The long-recommended treatment involves evacuation of the hematoma and application of a pressure dressing to prevent reaccumulation of the blood[9] (Figure 4). Wide incision with a scalpel is the preferred means of drainage. Incisions should be placed parallel to the helix in the scapha. After drainage and removal of clot and fibroneocartilage, bolster dressings should be applied. This is usually done with dental rolls applied to both sides of the auricle and secured with through and through permanent sutures. These bolsters are usually left in place for 7 to 10 days.

Some feel that incision and bolstering is unnecessary and an auricular hematoma can be managed by needle aspiration. Indeed, many published series have advocated needle aspiration, only using incision and bolstering for recurrent cases. A Cochrane Database Systematic Review of the literature was unable to find adequate data to suggest a clearly defined best treatment, so further study is needed.[10]

Burns. Burns represent a major source of trauma to the external ear. Thermal burns are traditionally classified as first, second, and third degree. First-degree burns are essentially scald injuries and result in little necrosis, but a great deal of inflammation and considerable pain. Treatment of first-degree burn is usually minor; nonsteroidal medications for pain and emollient creams. The burn usually heals with no scar. Second-degree burns are partial thickness burns that will lead to epidermolysis and blistering. These, too, are often treated expectantly with nonsteroidal antiinflammatory medications. Gentle cleansing and application of antibiotic ointments are recommended. Third-degree burns are full thickness and are generally anesthetic. These are treated the same way as second-degree burns but are much more likely to result in significant tissue loss and require reconstructive intervention. In all types

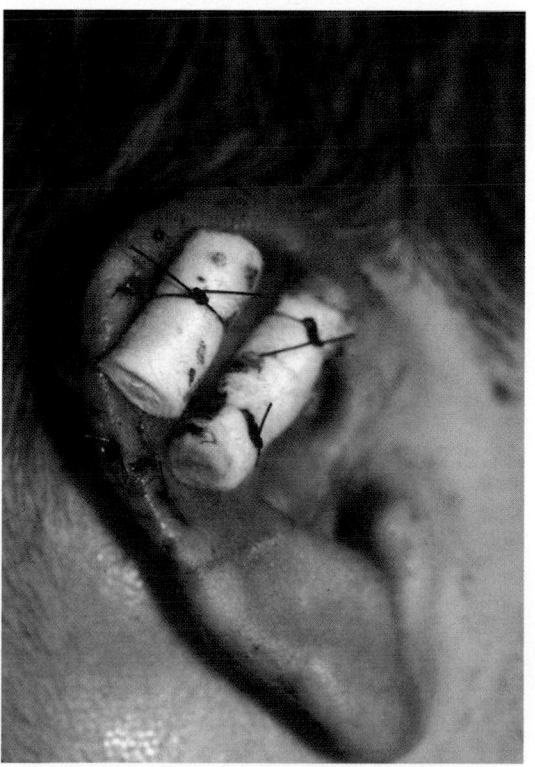

Figure 4 Bolstering of auricular hematoma.

of burns to the auricle, pressure on the auricle should be avoided, and the patient may need to wear a protective cup or bolster. Adequate analgesics should be administered to all patients with burns.

One common risk of auricular burn is the risk of perichondritis. This disorder was thought to occur in up to 25% of all second- and third-degree burns of the ear and may result in significant loss of cartilage if not recognized and immediately addressed. With the greater awareness of this issue and the use of topical antibiotic ointments, the risk of this disorder has fallen to around 3%. It is usually caused by Pseudomonas and often develops 2 to 4 weeks following the initial injury. In the initial phase there is redness, pain, and swelling, and this represents a perichondritis. Intravenous antibiotics are often successful in this stage. The later stage is characterized by abscess formation and will generally result in significant cartilage loss if not addressed. Because of the avascular nature of this stage, intravenous antibiotics alone are ineffective and surgical drainage is needed. Multiple incisions are made and aggressive local care is needed for full control.

Frostbite. The exposed position of the auricle also puts it at risk for frostbite. Prolonged exposure to temperatures less than 0°C results in anesthesia, pallor, and ice crystal formation within the tissue. With thawing, endothelial damage results in severe edema and sludging of blood, increasing the risk of necrosis. Still later, erythema develops around the demarcated tissue. The demarcated tissue may eventually slough and reconstruction may be needed. Nonsteroidal antiinflammatory medications, corticosteroids, aloe vera, and heparinization have all been recommended in the early stages to prevent necrosis, but no controlled studies have proven their roles.

In the acute setting, it is recommended that the area be gently thawed by application of moist cotton pledgets slightly warmer than body temperature. Radiant heat is not recommended. Just as with burns, compressive dressings should be avoided and antibiotic creams should be applied.

A rare late result of auricular frostbite is auricular ossification. The results from replacement of the elastic cartilage of the auricle with bone. This results in a rigid, ossified auricle that is uncomfortable to the patient and may prevent examination of the eardrum with a speculum. Aside from this, the condition is benign and there is no treatment. Repeated exposures may be a factor in this disorder.

Inflammatory and Infectious Disorders

The vast majority of patient complaints involving the external ear are going to involve inflammatory or infectious disorders. The close proximity of the canal skin to the exquisitely sensitive periosteum can often make this a painful disorder. Failure to diagnose and treat such a disorder adequately can result in prolonged discomfort and potentially life-threatening spread of infection.

Acute Otitis Externa (AOE). AOE or acute external otitis is an acute, usually bacterial, infection of the skin of the external auditory canal (Figure 5). In its later stages it presents with severe pain in the affected ear and will frequently be associated with drainage and decreased hearing, but early infection may cause only itching and fullness. The clinician will usually note pain on manipulation of the pinna with erythema and swelling of the ear canal skin. Often, the skin of the bony external canal will be spared. Often the swelling of the canal skin prevents full evaluation of the drumhead, making it uncertain whether the eardrum is intact and the middle ear is not involved with the infection as well. The infection may also cause excessive skin desquamation, resulting in the accumulation of a large amount of keratin debris in the canal.

The initial therapy should include a thorough cleaning of the canal. Not only can the debris prevent an adequate examination, but the debris in the canal will harbor microorganisms and prevent adequate penetration of drops. The importance of this often-overlooked step cannot be overstated as it is a frequent cause of therapy failures. After cleaning, the treatment usually involves the use of topical treatments in drop form. In situations in which the canal swelling prevents adequate penetration of the drops, a sponge wick can be used. Placed dry and compressed in the canal, the wick will swell in response to the instilled drops. A wick provides 2 important actions: first, it draws the antibiotic down into the canal to the site of infection; second, it puts pressure on the walls of the canal to decrease the swelling. A wick, like any other packing, can turn into a nidus for infection so should be removed or changed after a few days.

Otic Antibiotic Preparations. The general treatment of AOE is with the use of antibiotic otic drops. Over the years, many preparations have been on the market (Table 1). In ancient times, ear infections were treated by the instillation of vinegar into the ear. The acetic acid lowers the pH of the ear canal and suppresses the growth of the usual AOE pathogens of pseudomonas and staphylococcus. It will also suppress the growth of most fungal microorganisms as well. A number of commercially available otic preparations are acids

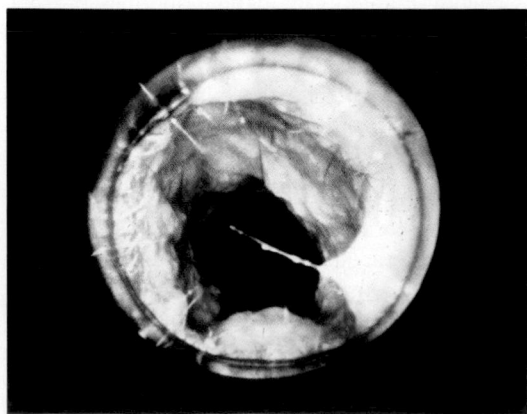

Figure 5 Acute otits externa.

Table 1 Common Otic Antibiotic Preparations		
Product Names	Active Agents	Cost of Trade (Generic)
Acetasol, Vosol, Domeboro	Acetic acid, Boric acid	US$31 ($22)
Acetasol-HC, Vosol-HC	Acetic acid and hydrocortisone	US$110 (US$24)
Cortisporin Otic Sol'n/Susp	Neomycin, polymyxin-B, hydrocortisone	US$89 (US$46)
Floxin Otic	Ofloxacin	US$71 (NA)
Cipro-HC Otic	Ciprofloxacin and hydrocortisone	US$125 (NA)
Ciprodex Otic	Ciprofloxacin and dexamethasone	US$125 (NA)

Adapted from reference 11.

and are meant to work in this way, eg, Domeboro (boric acid) and Acetasol (acetic acid).

For many years, the preferred otic drop preparation was a combination drop containing neomycin, polymyxin-B, and hydrocortisone. Sold under a number of brand names, most notably "Cortisporin," this otic drop was usual sold in 2 forms: a mineral oil-based liquid and an aqueous suspension. The mineral oil-based drop had excellent penetration in small canals and those filled with debris but could be quite painful if the drop entered the middle ear through an unknown perforation or tube. The aqueous suspension was better tolerated in open ears but had a strong tendency to leave a white, filmy debris, the suspended solid crystals of hydrocortisone, which is insoluble in water. This filmy debris would often be mistaken for a fungal overgrowth, and the patient would be placed on an additional antibiotic.

These 2 antibiotics and a corticosteroid preparation have enjoyed a long history of success in the treatment of AOE. The neomycin, an aminoglycoside, had high activity against staphylococcus species and moderate activity against pseudomonas. The polymyxin B had strong activity against pseudomonas as well as staphylococcus. The hydrocortisone would lessen the inflammation, opening the ear and relieving the pain. The neomycin and polymyxin-B, however, both have a long-known toxicity to the inner ear when used systemically. This raised some concern about their extensive use in ears, often in situations in which there is perforation or a ventilating tube. No cases of certain eardrop-related ototoxicity have ever been documented, and chronic infection itself is a risk to hearing, so it is difficult to make a case that these preparations are dangerous, especially considering their decades of popular use.

Otic drops containing quinolone solutions were brought to the market in the 1990s. These contained either ofloxacin (Floxin Otic) or ciprofloxacin (Cipro-HC Otic or CiproDex, both also contain a corticosteroid). These drops offered an antibiotic with known effectiveness against the common microorganisms encountered in AOE with no known risk of ototoxicity. Heavily marketed, these drops soon became the most frequent treatment used in AOE. Unfortunately, a steady increase in quinolone resistance has been seen in both staphylococcus and pseudomonas microorganisms. In some areas, less than half of all cultures of pseudomonas aeruginosa will be

sensitive to quinolones. In addition, these drops often lack other characteristics, such as a lower pH, that suppresses the growth of other microorganism, such as fungus.

To address the issue of the appropriate treatment of AOE, a committee from the American Academy of Otolaryngology Head and Neck Surgery developed evidence-based treatment guidelines for this disorder.[11] Although antibiotic drops were shown to give significantly higher symptomatic and bacteriologic cure rates, no difference could be demonstrated between the various preparations.

When to Use Systemic Antibiotics. Most AOE can adequately be treated with debridement and otic antibiotic preparations. In some situations, systemic antibiotics should be added. If the patient is diabetic or otherwise immune-suppressed, systemic treatment will be another barrier to deeper and more life-threatening spread of the infection. In a patient in whom the swelling of the canal has become so profound that a wick has had to be placed, systemic antibiotics will ensure adequate penetration of coverage.

"Malignant" Necrotizing Otitis Externa. Malignant otitis externa represents an invasive bone infection involving the external canal (Figure 6). The nomenclature of this disorder is confusing to patients. The traditional name, coined initially by Chandler in 1968,[12] is "malignant" otitis externa, reflecting its life-threatening nature. The term "malignant" is usually applied to neoplasia, so there is confusion about its use in this nonneoplastic disorder. Since bone necrosis is a feature of this disorder, the term "necrotizing" otitis externa is often preferred.

Whatever name is used, it is a serious and life-threatening infection. Mortality for necrotizing otitis externa has been measured as high as 20%. With increased awareness of the disease and aggressive treatment (including the availability of effective oral antibiotics), the mortality now is less than 1%. This disease occurs when the infectious agent of AOE penetrates to deeper tissue to involve bone and deeper fascial planes. Although it is usually initially limited to the temporal bone and its adjacent structures, it can spread medially to become a full-fledged osteomyelitis of the base of the skull. As it advances, it will cause dysfunction of the cranial nerves as their foramina are involved. Infection can also spread to the subarachnoid space resulting in meningitis. Mortality is often due to intracranial

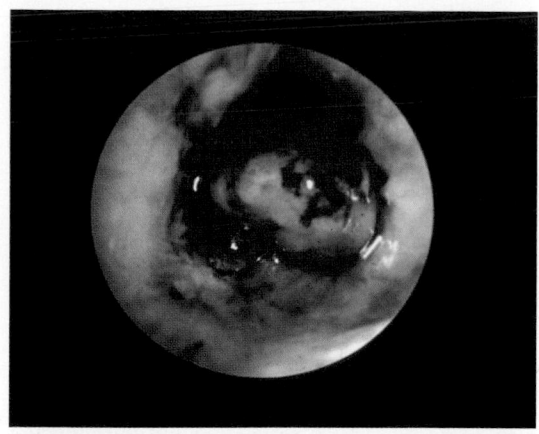

(A)

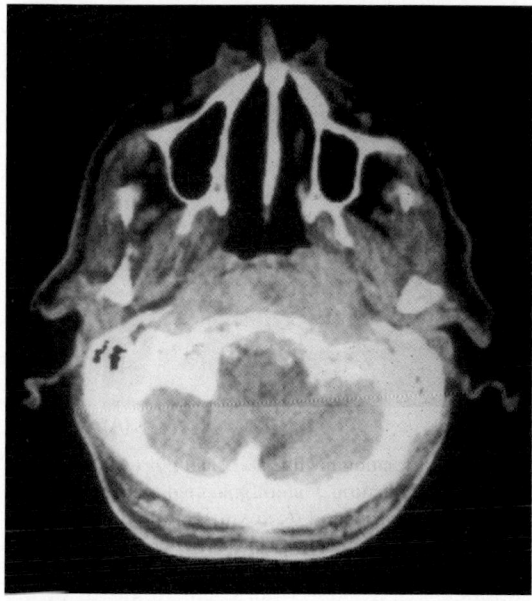

(B)

Figure 6 (A) Necrotizing otitis externa, granulation tissue in canal. (B) CT scan showing opacification of mastoid and nasopharyngeal mass.

infection or aspiration secondary to lower cranial nerve dysfunction.

Patients with necrotizing otitis externa are typically older and diabetic. They may also be otherwise immune-suppressed. They present with severe, boring pain in the ear with associated drainage. There is usually a prolonged course, and often they will have been treated with one or several courses of topical antibiotics. They may rarely present with a facial paralysis or other lower cranial nerve involvement. In diabetics, they may note an elevation in their blood sugar and increased difficulty in controlling their diabetes. On examination, granulation tissue is often seen in the canal, usually on the floor and adjacent to the bony-cartilagenous junction. Biopsy of this tissue should be taken to ensure the absence of malignancy, which can present in a similar fashion.

Further workup should begin with a culture of the drainage in an attempt to identify the offending microorganism, usually pseudomonas. Fungal culture should be obtained as well. A high-definition computed tomography (CT) scan of the temporal bones may show areas of

bone erosion but is normal in many early cases. MRI has also been recommended, usually showing fatty streaking in the precondylar space but is fairly nonspecific and does not show bone detail like the CT.

In general, diagnosis is confirmed using radionucleotide scanning. A technecium-99 bone scan will show increased uptake in the involved area, confirming that bone in the area is rapidly being metabolized. This may be the most sensitive test for necrotizing otitis externa, but this uptake will remain present for months to years following the resolution of the infection, making it a poor examination to monitor treatment. A Gallium-67 scan, showing areas of active infection, will have increased uptake early in the disease and will clear as the infection is controlled. Both the bone scan and the Gallium scan are ordered initially; the bone scan confirming the diagnosis by demonstrating bone involvement; and the Gallium scan to confirm the infectious process. The Gallium scan is then used to monitor the effectiveness of the treatment. The erythrocyte sedimentation rate can also be monitored to assess the resolution of infection.

The treatment, in addition to debridement of the granulation tissue and rigorous control of blood sugar, is to use topical and systemic antibiotics directed against pseudomonas. Before the availability of the quinolones, this usually meant an aminoglycoside (such as gentamicin) in combination with an antipseudomonal penicillin (such as piperacillin) or a third-generation cephalosporin. These treatments could only be given intravenously, and a 6-week course was usually required. This usually meant a prolonged hospital stay and some degree of vestibular impairment due to the aminoglycoside. The quinolones, such as ciprofloxacin, provided excellent pseudomonal coverage in an oral form, allowing most necrotizing otitis externa to now be treated on an outpatient basis.[13] In most cases, the patient will be started on an oral quinolone for a 6-week course. This antibiotic regimen may be altered based on the results of the culture and the effectiveness of the therapy, as determined by a Gallium scan 6 weeks after starting therapy.

Surgery is required in only rare cases of necrotizing otitis externa. In earlier years, aggressive surgery had been attempted to remove necrotic bone. Results of this intervention were often disappointing as it often facilitated the spread of the disease. Nowadays, surgical intervention is avoided as it may hasten the spread of infection and is only used after failure of a more prolonged, conservative approach.

Otomycosis. Fungal infections are frequently involved in inflammatory processes of the ear canal (Figure 7). Unlike bacterial infections, pain seems to be an uncommon complaint in these disorders, where the usual complaint is pruritus. Often they are asymptomatic. A variety of fungal microorganisms are involved.

Much of the time, fungus found in the ear canal is saprophytic, meaning it feeds off of

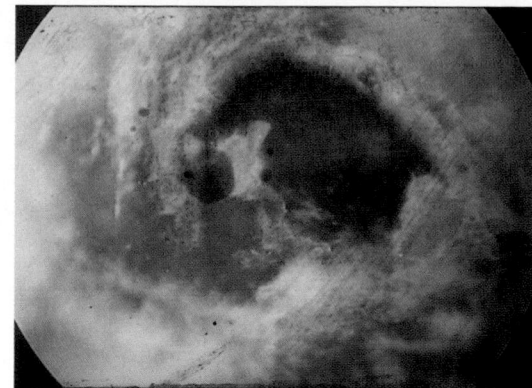

Figure 7 Otomycosis.

other material. This most often occurs in cases of chronic suppurative otitis media where the pus serves as a food source for the fungus. In such cases, the fungus involved, usually aspergilllus, is not a true infective pathogen. The drainage and infection are due to the middle ear pathology, and the fungus a mere saprophyte. Debridement of granulation and necrotic tissue and treatment of the underlying suppuration will usually resolve the fungal overgrowth. Saprophytes, however, can become invasive infectious microorganisms when there is significant immune suppression or impaired circulation. Invasive fungal infections can be rapidly fatal and require aggressive treatment. Often their presentation is identical to that of necrotizing otitis externa. The fungal hyphae often spread in the endothelial layer of the blood vessels, causing hypoperfusion and necrosis (as seen in mucormycosis). Aggressive surgical debridement, correction of immune suppression, and high-dose amphotericin B are the only available options and a severe trial for these already frail patients.

Another common fungal infection found in the external ear is due to *Candida* species. Patients may complain of pruritus, a smelly discharge from the ear and a hearing loss due to the accumulated debris. Pain is uncommon and usually points to another abnormality. Candidal infections are also more saporphytic in nature. They are characterized by a large amount of cheesy, white debris in the canal. The underlying canal skin may be slightly edematous and erythematous, but it is rarely as severe as that seen in AOE. Very often, these candidal overgrowths are the result of overuse of newer antibiotic otic drops. Otic quinolone preparations will suppress bacteria and allow overgrowth of the resident *Candida* species. Complete debridement, acidifying drops, and, occasionally, instillation of antifungal creams or ointments, eg, nystatin, will frequently be curative.

Some external ear complaints will be due to dermatophyte infection. These microorganisms, notorious as a cause of athlete's foot and ringworm, will cause severe ear itching and scaling of the canal skin. Dermatophytes are usually treated with acidifying drops with corticosteroid and on occasion may need more directed antifungal treatment.

One interesting aspect of dermatophyte infection is the risk of the allergic dermatophytid or "id" reaction. This phenomenon, not uncommon with dermatophytes, is a local inflammatory skin reaction caused by an infection some distance away.[14] This sometimes occurs in the external ear. A patient will present with chronic itching and scaling of the canal that does not respond to any local therapy. Canal scrapings viewed with a potassium hydroxide (KOH) preparation fail to show any microorganisms. Often, additional questioning will reveal the presence of a troublesome dermatophyte infection such as an athlete's foot. Successful treatment of the primary dermatophyte infection will often result in clearing of the id reaction as well.

Viral External Otitis. The external ear can also be inflamed due to herpetic viral outbreaks. These generally present as a painful vesicular eruption following a dermatomal pattern. Herpes zoster and simplex are the most common microorganisms. When such a herpetic outbreak is associated with a facial paralysis, it is termed Ramsay Hunt syndrome (see Chapter 34, "Facial Paralysis"). Tzanck preparations will often confirm the herpetic nature of the outbreak, but this is rarely needed in obvious outbreaks. Treatment is usually with an antiviral medication, such as Valtrex (valciclovir), with analgesics being given for the pain. Outbreaks may be followed by prolonged periods of neuralgia, the care of which is largely supportive.

Noninfectious Ear Canal Inflammation. Not all otitis externa is due to infectious microorganisms. Often, canal inflammation is the result of an allergic or cutaneous condition. This will frequently present identically to, and be treated as, a bacterial or fungal otitis externa. Its true nature may not be determined until after multiple treatment failures or recurrences. Further complicating the distinction is the fact that these conditions may respond nicely to the corticosteroid component of antibiotic ear drops. Additionally, such cutaneous conditions lead to recurrent infection, further blurring this distinction. Seasonal or environmental variation and the associated atopic picture will often support this diagnosis.

Unlike otitis externa, however, pain is less common than itching. Typically one will see thickening of the skin of the lateral aspect of the canal skin with hyperkeratosis and scaling. It may appear identical to a dermatophyte infection and a KOH preparation should be considered to differentiate the disorders. Such patients may have a history of psoriasis involving other areas of the body. Alternatively such cutaneous inflammation may be seborrheic or eczematous, with crusted, weepy skin. Such chronic inflammation may result in the gradual narrowing of the external meatus and stenosis of the ear canal.

For most of these cutaneous disorders, conservative therapy involves the use of corticosteroid-containing drops or creams. Since it is the lateral part of the canal and conchal bowl that are most frequently involved, a small amount of corticosteroid cream dabbed on the fingertip can be easily applied to the affected areas. If conservative therapy fails to provide significant relief, biopsy should be considered. Referral to a dermatologist should be considered for conservative treatment failures and when there are concomitant systemic lesions.

Granular myringitis. Granular myringitis is a poorly defined disorder characterized by chronic inflammation and weeping on the surface of the tympanic membrane.[15] Although cultures may frequently demonstrate a dominant microorganism, it tends to recur despite appropriate antibiotic therapy. The chronic inflammation results in the gradual deposition of scar tissue, resulting in marked thickening of the tympanic membrane and gradual stenosis of the external canal (Figure 8). The disease course usually spans over many years, with frequent bouts of itching and drainage, and progressive conductive hearing loss due to the thickening drumhead. The problem often ceases when the scar tissue deposition reaches the cartilaginous canal.

Treatment of this disorder should be fairly aggressive. Granulation tissue on the drumhead should be cauterized with silver nitrate or trichloroacetic acid, and the infection treated with acetic acid/corticosteroid drops. Antifungal, antibiotic, and antiseptic drops should be considered. Cultures should be taken to direct therapy.

In situations in which the stenosis has progressed to a significant conductive hearing loss, surgical treatment may be needed. This procedure involves dissecting the deposited scar off of the canal wall and the fibrous layer of the tympanic membrane, which can usually be found intact. Denuded areas are then grafted with split-thickness skin grafts harvested from behind the ear or from the undersurface of the upper part of the arm. Packing of some sort is used to stent the canal open and maintain the skin grafts in place. When healed, this procedure often returns the eardrum to a normal appearance. Nonetheless, the patient may frequently again develop granular myringitis and start the process all over again.

Disorders of Keratin Migration

As mentioned earlier, the keratin layer of the ear canal skin has a migratory characteristic. As the outer layers mature, they move laterally and are

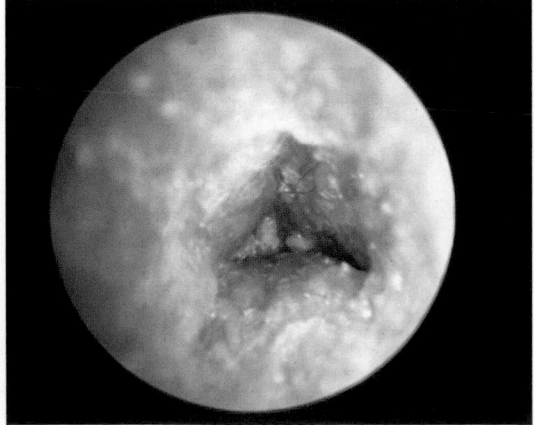

Figure 8 Medial canal stenosis due to granular myringitis.

finally desquamated out of the meatus by the action of the ceruminous and sebaceous glands. Occasionally this process is disrupted resulting in a neoplastic-like accumulation of keratin debris in the canal. Like cholesteatoma of the middle ear, this keratin accumulation can cause resorption of bone with resultant anatomic changes of the ear canal.

Keratosis Obturans. Keratosis obturans occurs when this migratory pattern of keratin maturation ceases or is in some way blocked.[16] Patients with keratosis obturans usually complain only of a hearing loss, but pain, pruritus, or drainage may also be noted. The keratin plug initially appears like a "run-of-the-mill" wax impaction, but as it is removed the true keratinous nature of the lesion can be seen. In the deeper part of the canal, large accumulations of white, cheesy keratin are removed. Frequently, bone absorption will result in a dramatic widening of the medial canal, which can result in dehiscence of the fallopian canal in the external ear. As such, caution should be used as the keratin is dissected from the underlying, viable tissue.

Keratosis obturans can occur in 2 forms, a primary form and a secondary form. The patients with the secondary form are typically older and are more often male. In this form, a long-standing plug of hard, dense wax results in effective blockage of the keratin migration. Patients with the primary form typically develop the problem when younger than 40 years, and it represents a primary dysfunction in epithelial migration. There is an equal sex predilection, and it is more common in African-Americans. Removal of the keratin plug is often curative, but the patient may need to be seen on a regular basis to remove accumulated keratin before it becomes impacted.

Canal Cholesteatoma. Keratoma obturans must be distinguished from the much rarer entity of canal cholesteatoma.[17] Canal cholesteatomas have a histologic similarity with those found in the middle ear but are not associated with middle ear disease. A canal cholesteatoma typically forms on the floor of the external canal. There is often a localized sequestration of necrotic bone with keratin accumulation often surrounding this sequestrum. There may be a cystic keratin "pearl" on the floor of the ear canal. These lesions may sometimes be small, and office debridement (often requiring local anesthesia) is curative. At other times, the lesion may be extensive and require operative canaloplasty and, occasionally, mastoidectomy.

The exact pathophysiology that leads to this type of cholesteatoma is unknown. One theory suggests that the process is initiated by some insult (infectious or traumatic) that results in a localized area of necrosis within the bony tympanic ring. The body walls off this necrotic area, and skin grows underneath it, resulting in the cholesteatoma. Another theory is that trauma, such as self-instrumentation of the ear for relief of pruritus, causes skin laceration and inversion of the epithelial lining. The buried keratin layer no longer migrates as in healthy canal skin and gradually develops the keratin accumulation characteristic of cholesteatoma. Some other canal cholesteatomas may be caused by retraction pockets into dehiscent mastoid air cells. These cholesteatomas typically occur on the posterior wall and are associated with well-pneumatized mastoids.

Congenital Sinuses, Cysts, and Skin Tags

Sinuses, cysts, and skin tags are congenital lesions associated with the embryologic development of the external ear (Figure 9). The more common of these lesions are the preauricular sinuses and pits. These lesions are due to a failure of the union of the hillocks from the first and second branchial arches. Typically, a small pit is found in the skin just anterior to the tragus, and there may be an underlying cyst. These cysts may occasionally become infected or have a foul-smelling drainage, in which case surgical excision should be considered. Excision is performed with an elliptical preauricular incision with primary closure. There is usually a sinus tract found on the deep aspect of the cyst that can usually be traced to the helical cartilage. Care must be taken to dissect out the entire cyst and sinus tract to prevent recurrence.

Related to these lesions are the first branchial cleft anomalies, ie, cysts and sinuses. These lesions are usually lined by squamous epithelium and may have sinus tracts connecting to the middle ear. These lesions were classified by Work[18] as either type I or type II. Type I lesions usually present as a cyst located behind the meatus, sometimes within the conchal bowl. Surgical excision is usually curative but is usually reserved only for those cysts that become repeatedly infected. Again, careful dissection of the associated sinus

tract is necessary to prevent recurrence. Type II lesions typically occur in the preauricular area and may involve the facial nerve and the parotid gland. Surgical excision of these lesions requires great care.

Accessory auricular skin tags usually present at birth as a prominence just anterior to the tragus. It is usually sporadic but may be familial. The sole issue with these lesions is cosmetic, and surgical removal is curative.

Any congenital ear malformation, from a preauricular skin tag to complete microtia, can be a finding in branchio-oto-renal (BOR) syndrome.[19] This autosomal dominant disorder is characterized by congenital ear abnormalities (external, middle, or inner), branchial cleft anomalies (sinuses, cysts, or pits) and renal abnormalities (ranging from mild hypoplasia to complete absence).[20] This disorder has been linked to a mutation in the *EYA1* gene, on the q arm of chromosome 8 (8q13.8). This gene is the human analog of the drosophila "eyes absent" gene and codes for a protein that is involved in the regulation of differentiation. Genetic testing is available for this gene and should be considered in patients with auricular and branchial anomalies, especially if they are familial or associated with sensorineural hearing loss (see Chapter 26, "Hereditary Hearing Impairment)" for additional information.

Benign Neoplasms and Tumor-Like Soft Tissue Lesions of the External Ear

The external ear, which is fundamentally a skin appendage, is prone to a number of neoplasms that may occur anywhere on the skin. Other lesions are unique to the ear. Identification by characteristic presentation and appearance is the rule, but biopsy should always be considered when the exact nature of the lesion is uncertain.

Keloids. A keloid is a very firm, round, painless mass that typically occurs at a site of trauma, most typically the site of ear piercing. It occurs as a result of such trauma in susceptible individuals, who are most often of African descent. These "hypertrophic scars" are totally benign, and the main problem that they present is cosmetic disfigurement. Small lesions can typically be treated with vigorous massage and pressure, with intralesional triamcinolone (Kenalog) injections for refractory cases. Large lesions require surgical excision, usually with primary closure. Massage and intralesional corticosteroid should be used after postoperative healing to prevent recurrence of the lesion.

Chondrodermatitis Nodularis Chronica Helicus. Chondrodermatitis nodularis chronica helicus presents as an exquisitely painful, discrete nodule usually involving the rim of the helix. The lesion is tender, and patients will most often complain that they cannot sleep on that side or use a telephone on that ear due to the pain induced by such activity. Similar lesions may be found in the meatus or conchal bowls of hearing-aid users and may prevent the patient from using the aid. On

initial presentation, the lesion may not be easily differentiated from a basal cell or squamous cell carcinoma, but it tends not to grow larger than a few millimeters. Histologically there will be surface ulceration with pseudoepitheliomatous hyperplasia in very close contact to the sensitive perichondrium. The underlying cartilage is usually nonvital, and it is thought that the skin and perichondrial reaction is secondary to this cartilage necrosis. It is believed that perichondrial irritation due to trauma or chronic pressure is the initiating factor. Surgical excision, including the involved perichondrium and nonvital cartilage (which has a distinctly whiter appearance than normal cartilage) is usually curative.

Gouty Tophi. Gouty tophi may accompany systemic gout and may affect any part of the auricle. This is usually a painful, discrete nodule covered with a thin, vascular, orange skin that may discharge a white, creamy material. This is a manifestation of the systemic disease, and treatment is, therefore, medical and involves the use of urate-lowering medications.

Inflammatory Polyps. In most cases, inflammatory polyps do not come from the external canal but usually originate in the middle ear and extend

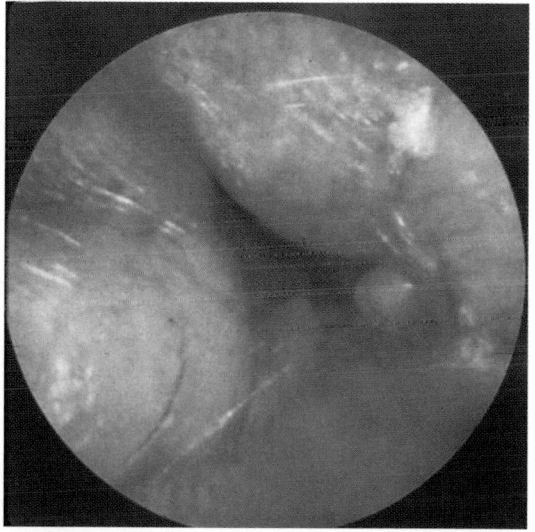

(A)

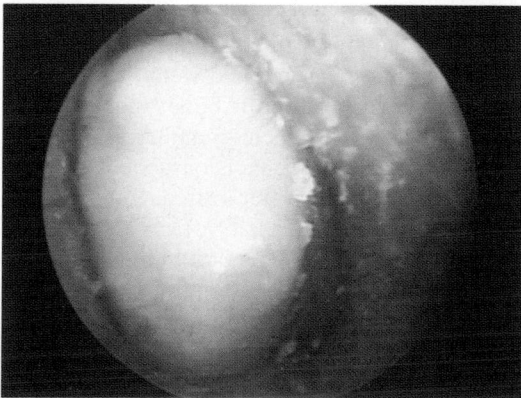

(B)

Figure 10 Exostosis versus osteoma. (A) Exostosis. These lesions are found medially, are usually multiple and bilateral, and sessile. (B) Osteoma. Osteomas are unilateral, singular, found more laterally in the canal, and have a pedunculated appearance.

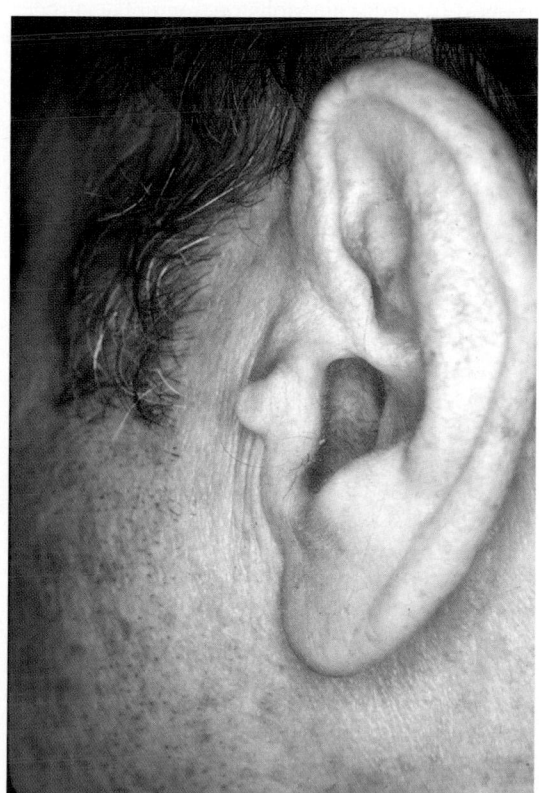

Figure 9 Preauricular skin tag.

into the external canal through a perforation. Exuberant, friable inflammatory proliferation with purulent discharge is the typical appearance. Histologically there is a dense infiltration of plasma cells. Although classically associated with chronic inflammatory disease of the middle ear, these lesions can be associated with more aggressive neoplasia. Imaging, usually with CT, is usually indicated and biopsy should be considered based on the results of such imaging. For purely inflammatory polyps, topical antibiotic drops, preferably containing a corticosteroid should cause their involution, but systemic antibiotics should be considered as well.

Cystic Lesions. Several varieties of skin cysts may present in the external ear. This includes sebaceous cysts, epidermal cysts, and dermoid cysts. They are typically nontender and largely asymptomatic unless they are infected or enlarge to the point that they affect hearing. Surgical excision is curative.

Osteoma and Exostosis. The most common bony tumors found in the external ear are exostoses and osteomas[21] (Figure 10). These lesions can be distinguished clinically by the following characteristics: exostoses are typically found deep in the canal, often adjacent to the tympanic membrane, whereas osteomas typically occur more laterally, near the bony-cartilagenous junction; there are usually multiple exostoses, often on both sides, whereas osteomas are typically single and almost never bilateral; exostoses typically have a broad base whereas osteomas often have a single, pedunculated stalk; and exostoses are typically located more superiorly in the canal whereas osteomas typically are attached posteriorly. Histologically, they are vastly different in appearance. Exostoses have a hard, laminated appearance with multiple parallel layers of subperiosteal bone with no medullary cancellous portion. Osteomas have a more neoplastic appearance, with areas of dense, skin-covered laminar bone with a central portion of cancellous bone, bone marrow, and fibrous tissue.

Exostoses are strongly associated with participation in water sports and are sometimes called "swimmer's nodules" or "surfer's ear." It is believed they result from irritation of the deep periosteum of the ear by cold water, resulting in the increased deposition of bone by the periosteum. The lesions are benign and typically need no treatment. Surgical excision should be considered if the lesions result in frequent infections or impactions, if their size affects the hearing (primarily due to wax retention), or if their presence prevents the proper fitting of a hearing aid. Caution should be taken in this surgery in regard to the facial nerve, as it may be shallow in the posterior-medial ear canal, and there are reports of iatrogenic facial nerve injury in these cases.

Osteomas, on the other hand, will almost always require removal. Their location more lateral makes them more obstructing and problematic. If they have a small stalk, as is almost always the case, they can often be easily removed

in the office. The base is infiltrated with 1% lidocaine with 1:100,000 epinephrine and a small, firm tool such as a Freer elevator is used to "snap" the osteoma off at its base. Hemostasis can be obtained with a small cotton pledget or oxidized cellulose (Surgicel), and the base allowed to granulate in. Larger, more sessile osteomas will require surgical removal in an operative setting.

Other Benign Neoplasms. In addition to the above mentioned lesions, there may be many other types of benign neoplasms that arise from the external ear. Any benign neoplasm arising from skin or its appendages particularly glands, bone or cartilage can be found on occasion in the external canal. As would be expected, most benign neoplasms will be well-circumscribed, painless masses. Excisional biopsy is usually curative.

Malignant Neoplasms of the External Ear

Maligant neoplasms of the external ear are a particular challenge to the otolaryngologist–head and neck surgeon. The vast majority of these neoplasms are skin-derived, and sun exposure and fair skin are the obvious risk factors. Basal cell and squamous cell carcinomas arising from auricular skin make up about 44% of all neoplasms of the external ear.[22] Skin cancer involving the ear makes up 6% of all skin cancers. Squamous cell carcinoma is the most common type of such malignancy, making around 60% of all external ear malignancies.[23] This is in contrast to elsewhere on the body, where basal cell predominates and makes up 90% of skin malignancies. On the sun-exposed skin of the auricle, basal cell carcinoma is indeed more common than squamous cell. In the ear canal, basal cell carcinoma is rare. Squamous cell carcinoma of

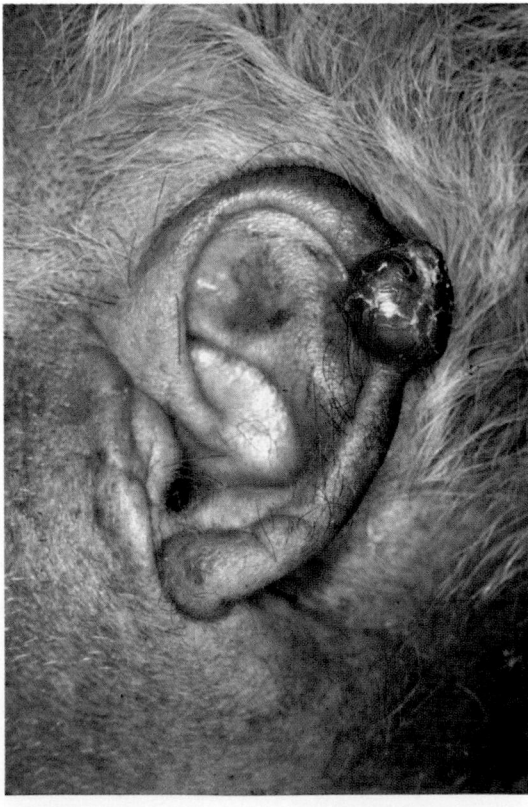

Figure 11 Basal cell carcinoma of the auricle.

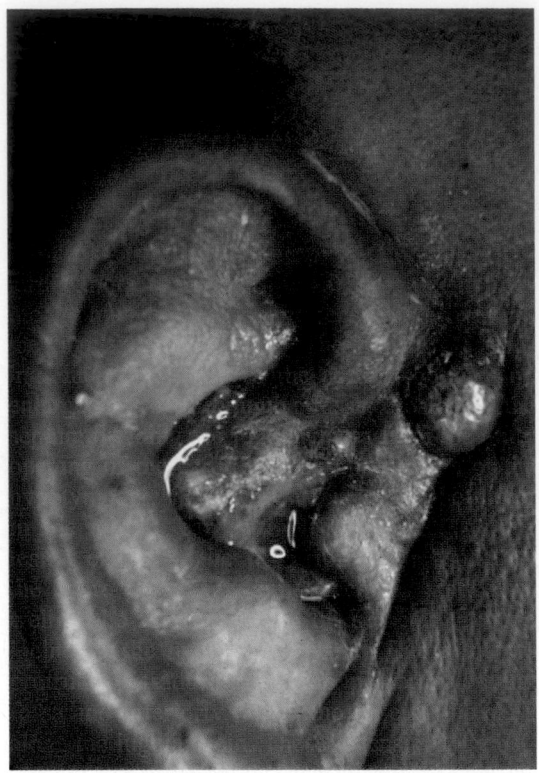

Figure 12 Squamous cell carcinoma of the auricle.

the canal may not only be a result of sun exposure but also of chronic infections, trauma, radiation, and chronic dermatitis.

Basal cell carcinoma (Figure 11) has the typical appearance of a pearly nodule, possibly with central ulceration and surrounding telangectasia. These painless lesions rarely metastasize but may spread to deeper tissues via embryonic tissue planes. Diagnosis is made by biopsy, which is often curative if the entire lesion can be easily excised. Larger lesions and biopsies with positive margins are best treated with Mohs micrographic surgery (MMS). This technique relies on intraoperative pathologic evaluations and re-resection in positive areas until margins are free of disease. This has the advantages of complete neoplasm removal and maximal sparing of normal tissue. Reconstruction of such defects is described in Chapter 57, "Scar Revision and Skin Resurfacing."

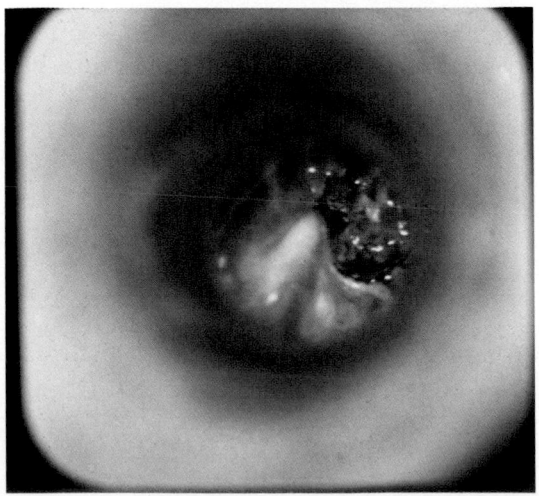

Figure 13 Squamous cell carcinoma of the external auditory canal.

Squamous cell carcinoma of the auricle usually appears similar to its appearance in other areas of the body: an indurated, scaly, maculopapular area with possible ulceration (Figure 12). Wide excision or Mohs surgery is recommended, but the metastatic potential is markedly higher with squamous cell carcinoma, so selective neck dissection or sentinel node biopsy may be indicated.

Unlike squamous cell carcinoma of the auricle, squamous cell carcinoma of the canal tends to be a much more problematic disease (Figure 13). Patients with this problem in this location tend to be younger, averaging 52 to 55 years, as opposed to 65 to 70 years in squamous cell carcinoma of the auricle, are predominantly male, and have fewer skin cancer risk factors. Chronic ear complaints such as pain, drainage (bloody and/or purulent), and pruritus are not uncommon. Often, diagnosis is delayed due to prolonged attempts to treat what appears to be an infectious condition, and biopsy is recommended when putative ear canal inflammation fails to respond to appropriate treatment. The carcinoma tends to be infiltrative and poorly defined and histologically less differentiated than those found on the auricle. Facial paralysis may be a presenting symptom. These tumors are classified with the TMN system recommended by Arriaga and colleagues, commonly referred to as the Pittsburgh system[24] (Table 2). Surgery is the preferred treatment modality and is usually extensive and disfiguring. Radiotherapy is a useful adjunct in more advanced disease.[25] This is discussed in Chapter 92, "Chemoradiation for Head and Neck Cancer."

In addition to basal cell and squamous cell carcinomas, a variety of malignant neoplasms may affect the external ear. Malignant melanoma, sarcomas of the bony or cartilaginous framework

Table 2 TNM Tumor Staging System for Carcinoma of the External Auditory Canal*

T1	Tumor limited to ear canal with no bone erosion
T2	Tumor with slight bone erosion, but not full thickness
T3	Full thickness bone erosion or extension to middle ear, mastoid, or glenoid fossa or with facial paralysis
T4	Tumor with involvement of cochlea, petrous apex, or dura

*Nodal stage (N) and metastases (M) are classified as elsewhere in the head and neck

and adenocarcinoma of the cerumen glands can be considered primary malignancies of the external ear. Salivary neoplasms of the parotid gland or the middle ear may involve the external ear by direct extension. The external ear may even be the site of metastases from distant primary neoplasms. For this reason, a high index of suspicion should be maintained, and biopsy should be considered for any lesion or in a situation in which a seemingly infectious process does not respond to appropriate therapy.

REFERENCES

1. Weiner FM, Ross DA. The pressure distribution in the auditory canal in a progressive sound field. J Acoust Soc Am 1946;18:401–8.
2. Blake CJ. Progressive growth of the dermoid coat of the tympanic membrane. Am J Otol 1882;4:266–8.
3. Alberti PWR. Epithelial migration of the tympanic membrane. J Laryngol Otol 1964;78:808–30.
4. Tomita H, Yamada K, Ghadami M, et al. Mapping of wet/dry earwax locus to the pericentromeric region of chromosome 16. Lancet 2002;359:2000 2.
5. Yoshiura K, Kinoshita A, Ishida T, et al. A SNP in the ABCC11 gene is the determinant of human earwax type. Nat Genet 2006;38:324–30.
6. Roland PS, Eaton DA, Gross RD, et al. Randomized, controlled trial of Ceruminex and Murine earwax removal products. Arch Otolaryngol Head Neck Surg 2004;130:1175–7.
7. Burton MJ, Doree CJ. Eardrops for the removal of earwax. Cochrane Database Syst Rev 2003;3:CD0004400.
8. Seely DR, Quigley SM, Langman AW. Ear candles-efficacy and safety. Laryngoscope 1996;106:1226–9.
9. Gernon WH. The care and management of acute hematoma of the external ear. Laryngoscope 1980;90:881–5.
10. Jones SE, Mahendran S. Interventions in auricular haematoma Cochrane Database Syst Rev 2004;2:CD004166.
11. Rosenfeld RM, Brown L, Cannon CR, et al. Clinical practice guideline: Acute otitis externa. Otolaryngol Head Neck Surg 2006;134:S4–23.
12. Chandler JR. Malignant external otitis. Laryngoscope 1968;78:1257–94.
13. Levenson MJ, Parisier SC, Dolitsky J, et al. Ciprofloxacin: The drug of choice for malignant otitis externa. Laryngoscope 1991;101:821–4.
14. Derebery J, Berliner KI. Foot and ear disease: A dermatophytid reaction in otology. Laryngoscope 1996;106:181–6.
15. Stoney P, Kwok P, Hawke M. Granular myringitis: A review. J Otolaryngol 1992;21:129–35.
16. Corbridge RJ, Michaels L, Wright T. Epithelial migration in keratosis obturans. Am J Otolaryngol 1996;17:411–4.
17. Sismanis A, Huang CE, Abedi E, Williams GH. External canal cholesteatoma. Am J Otol 1986;7:126–9.
18. Work WP. New concepts in first branchial cleft defects. Laryngoscope 1972;82:1581–93.
19. Fraser FC, Sproule JR, Halal F. Frequency of branchio-oto-renal (BOR) syndrome in children with profound hearing loss. Am J Med Genet 1980;7:341–9.
20. Chang CH, Menezes M, Meyer NC, et al. Branchio-oto-renal syndrome: The mutation spectrum in EYA1 and its phenotypic consequences. Hum Mutat 2004;23:582–9.
21. Fenton JE, Turner J, Fagan PA. A histopathologic review of temporal bone exostoses and osteomata. Laryngoscope 1996;105:624–8.
22. Thawley SE, Panje WR. Comprehensive Management of Head and Neck Tumors. Philadelphia: WB Saunders; 1986.
23. Shockley WW, Stucker FJ. Squamous cell carcinoma of the external ear: A review of 75 cases. Otolaryngol Head Neck Surg 1987;97:308–12.
24. Arriaga M, Curtin H, Takahashi H, et al. Staging proposal for external auditory meatus carcinoma based on pre-operative clinical examination and computed tomography findings. Ann Otol Rhinol Laryngol 1990;90:714–21.
25. Moody SA, Hirsch BE, Myers EN. Squamous cell carcinoma of the external auditory canal: An evaluation of a staging system. Am J Otol 2000;21:582–8.

15

Eustachian Tube Dysfunction

Dennis S. Poe, MD
Quinton Gopen, MD

The eustachian tube performs the critical roles of aeration and drainage for the middle ear cavity. It also protects the middle ear from reflux of sound and material from the nasopharynx. Proper function of this tubular organ is required for optimal conduction of sound through the middle ear cavity. Since its initial description by Eustachius in the mid-1500s, much has been learned of its anatomy, physiology, and pathology.[1] This chapter provides a comprehensive review of the eustachian tube anatomy, physiology, and pathology, including both eustachian tube dysfunction and patulous eustachian tube.

HISTORY

Although the eustachian tube was first mentioned by Alcmaeon of Sparta in 400 BC,[1] Bartolomeus Eustachius is credited with its discovery in 1562 when he published a detailed description of its structure and function.[2] Valsalva went on to characterize the eustachian tube into cartilaginous and osseous parts and was the first to describe the importance of the tensor veli palatini muscle in opening the eustachian tube.[3] He also described the Valsalva maneuver, a technique which remains clinically relevant to this day. Toynbee furthered our understanding of the eustachian tube through an extensive investigation of the peritubal muscles,[4] and Politzer played a pivotal role in delineating the eustachian tube and its role in middle ear pathology.[1]

ANATOMY

The eustachian tube courses from the middle ear cavity proximally to the nasopharynx distally. The distal portion is comprised of a cartilaginous skeleton whereas the proximal skeleton is osseous. The osseous portion constitutes approximately one-third of the entire length of the eustachian tube. The osseous portion is funnel shaped with the wide end of the funnel extending from the anterior aspect of the middle ear cavity. The narrow end of the funnel, also termed the isthmus, is the narrowest point of the eustachian tube and is located just proximal to the junction of the bony and cartilaginous segments of the eustachian tube. The osseous portion is normally patent and does not open and close dynamically as does the cartilaginous portion.[5] The cartilaginous distal two-thirds

of the eustachian tube courses from the isthmus into the nasopharynx. It comprises a single segment of cartilage attached along its superior edge to the basisphenoid bone. Although the cartilaginous portion closer to the osseous eustachian tube segment remains fixed in its position, the more distal end of the cartilage as it enters the nasopharynx has dynamic movement. The distal end of this cartilage protrudes into the nasopharynx and is termed the medial cartilaginous lamina. The medial cartilaginous lamina is mobile and allows the orifice of the eustachian tube to open as it medially rotates during tubal dilation. The medial cartilaginous lamina provides the framework for the torus tubarius, a mobile structure also known as the posterior cushion or posterior medial wall which comprises part of the eustachian tube orifice (Figure 1). The eustachian tube orifice is mainly comprised of the lateral cartilaginous lamina, an immobile structure also known as the hook or "J" portion of the eustachian tube orifice. The remainder of the eustachian tube orifice is completed by a fibrous membrane. It is firmly attached to the basisphenoid bone. The eustachian tube orifice lies between the medial cartilaginous lamina and the lateral cartilaginous lamina (Figure 1). Just posterior to the medial cartilaginous lamina is the fossa of Rosenmuller, an important space containing lymphoid tissue and is medial to the internal carotid artery. The adenoid pad lies just medial to the fossa of Rosenmuller and occupies the midline of the nasopharynx (Figure 1).[6]

The pediatric eustachian tube has many critical differences from the mature adult eustachian tube. Several studies have demonstrated that the

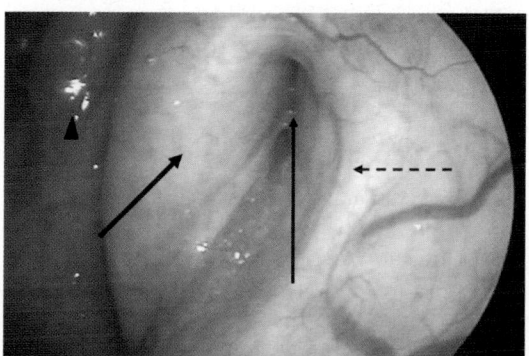

Figure 1 Normal left eustachian tube, closed position. Adenoid (*arrowhead*), posterior cushion (*thick arrow*), orifice, valve closed (*thin arrow*), lateral cartilaginous lamina (*dashed arrow*).

pediatric eustachian tube is anatomically smaller than the adult eustachian tube. For example, the cross-sectional area including the width and the length of the cartilaginous eustachian tube lumen was significantly smaller in children than in adults.[7] The length of the eustachian tube was nearly half as long in infants when compared to adults (21 mm at 3 months vs. 37 mm in adult).[8] The eustachian tube reaches adult length of 31 to 38 mm typically at 7 years of age.[9] Another important difference in eustachian tube development is the angle at which the tube courses from the middle ear space to the nasopharynx. In children, the tube courses horizontally, whereas in adults the tube is much more dependent and has an angle closer to 45° from the horizontal.[10] Other differences include cartilage volume, Ostmann fat pad, mucosal folds, luminal glands, and middle ear volume in children compared to adults (Table 1).[11]

PHYSIOLOGY

Although the osseous portion of the eustachian tube remains patent and is not dynamic, the cartilaginous portion of the eustachian tube remains closed in its resting state and only opens for brief periods of time. This blocks gastric reflux from entering into the middle ear as well as prevents autophony, an abnormally loud perception of one's own voice, breathing, and other internal sounds. Autophony of voice can be disturbingly loud when sound energy during vocalizations passes internally into the middle ear space. The tensor veli palatini muscle has significant bulk which when the muscle is relaxed serves to obliterate the eustachian tube orifice. Additionally, the mucosa and submucosa lining the eustachian tube are quite elastic and serve to decrease the eustachian tube lumen. The anterolateral wall of the eustachian tube contains a collection of fat, termed Ostmann fat pad, which also aids in closure of the eustachian tube orifice along with the rigid lateral cartilaginous lamina. The combination of mucosa, submucosa, Ostmann fat pad, and tensor veli palatine muscle, in effect, comprise a "valve" within the cartilaginous tubal lumen with the mucosal surfaces in apposition during closure.

Importantly, brief intermittent periods of eustachian tube dilation must occur in normal individuals for ventilation. These brief periods of tubal dilation and patency result from contractions of

Table 1 Developmental Differences between the Anatomy of the Eustachian Tube and Middle Ear in Infants Compared with Adults

Anatomic Feature of the Eustachian Tube and Middle Ear	Infant Anatomic Feature Compared to the Adult
Length of tube	Shorter
Angle of tube to horizontal plane	10° vs 45°
Angle/length of tensor veli palatini to cartilage	Variable vs stable angle, shorter attachment
Lumen	Smaller area and volume
Cartilage volume	Less
Cartilage cell density	Greater
Elastin at hinge portion of cartilage	Less
Ostmann fat pad	Relatively wider
Mucosal folds	Greater
Lumen glands	Variable type
Connective tissue lateral to tube	Different
Middle ear volume	Smaller

Adapted from reference 1.

the peritubular musculature (Figure 2). There are four peritubal muscles: tensor veli palatini, levator veli palatini, salpingopharyngeus, and the tensor tympani. The most important muscle for opening the eustachian tube is the tensor veli palatini muscle.[12,13] This muscle predominantly originates from the basisphenoid bone and to a smaller degree from the lateral cartilaginous lamina. It courses inferiorly and anteriorly, passing mostly deep around the pterygoid hamulus, and then inserting into the soft palate. It runs longitudinally along the cartilaginous portion of the eustachian tube. When this muscle contracts, the eustachian tube is pulled open by a laterally directed force onto the membranous eustachian tube wall. An extension of the tensor veli palatini muscle, termed the dilator tubae muscle, originates along the anterolateral membranous wall of the eustachian tube and aids in opening the lumen of the tube.

The levator veli palatini muscle is also important in opening the eustachian tube. This muscle has its origin in the base of the temporal bone and inserts into the soft palate. It forms a sling and courses under the inferior aspect of the medial cartilaginous lamina and floor of the membranous eustachian tube. When this muscle contracts, it results in elevation of the soft palate as well as medial rotation of the medial cartilaginous lamina, both important steps toward opening the eustachian tube orifice.

A slow-motion video evaluation of eustachian tube opening was performed and has identified four distinct phases involved in eustachian tube opening.[14] The first phase involves elevation of the soft palate along with medial rotation of the medial cartilaginous lamina and the posteromedial wall. This occurs by contraction of the levator veli palatini muscle and results in the initial dilation of the nasopharyngeal orifice. The levator veli palatini then remains contracted throughout all four phases of eustachian tube opening and may serve as a scaffold that aids the tensor veli palatini action to dilate the valve to the open position. The second phase occurs as the superior pharyngeal constrictor muscle contracts which results in a medial displacement of the lateral pharyngeal wall. This results in a transient narrowing of the eustachian tube orifice. The third phase involves contraction of the tensor veli palatini muscle which dilates the eustachian tube orifice from a laterally directed traction on the membranous eustachian tube wall. The fourth and final phase is when the tensor veli palatini maximally contracts resulting in an effacement of the anterolateral eustachian tube orifice with maximal opening. The eustachian tube orifice has a rounded appearance during maximal dilation. The entire four-phase process of eustachian tube opening lasts for roughly 400 ms.[6]

Tubal dilation propagates from the nasopharyngeal orifice proximally into the "valve" toward the bony isthmus. Tubal closure reverses the process beginning proximally and progressing distally, resulting in a pumping action that clears the middle ear space and eustachian tube of secretions.[13] Tubal closure occurs by sequential relaxation of the tensor veli palatini and the levator veli palatini musculature, and the eustachian tube orifice once again returns to its resting configuration with a convex bulge along its anterolateral wall.[15]

The eustachian tube dilates during deglutition or yawning. Investigators have suggested that the autonomic nervous system provides the control for intermittent, involuntary dilations of the eustachian tube through baroreceptors and chemoreceptors found within the middle ear cavity.[16,17]

When the eustachian tube is closed, an ongoing exchange of gas occurs between the middle ear cavity and the mucosa. Venous blood contains a lesser amount of dissolved nitrogen and also has a slightly lower pressure compared to atmospheric pressure. This results in a large gradient between the overall pressure and the partial pressure of nitrogen. Consequently, nitrogen slowly diffuses into the venous blood from the middle ear. This leads to a steady absorption of gas from the middle ear resulting in an increased negative pressure within the middle ear space relative to the ambient atmosphere. Each gas within the middle ear space has a different solubility constant for diffusion into the mucosa. Carbon dioxide diffuses most readily, approximately 40 times greater than nitrogen. Oxygen is roughly twice as soluble as nitrogen. Accordingly, carbon dioxide and oxygen may play a greater role in short-term pressure effects (more soluble) when compared to nitrogen which is theorized to have a more important role in long-term effects.[18] This negative pressure formed by gases diffusing out of the middle ear and mastoid spaces and into the mucosal lining and capillaries continues to build until the eustachian tube periodically opens (Figure 3).

Surfactants have been identified in the eustachian tube and the middle ear cavity where they facilitate the exchange of gases across mucosal barriers and allow for easier opening of the eustachian tube orifice.[19] Surfactants are defined as any substance which results in a decreased surface tension. Surfactants found within the body are phospholipids which serve to facilitate air-fluid exchange, most importantly in the lungs but also within the middle ear and mastoid spaces.

Aeration of the middle ear space occurs when the eustachian tube opens and nasopharyngeal air, generally at atmospheric pressure, is exchanged with the middle ear gases allowing for an equalization of pressure on both sides of the tympanic membrane. The eustachian tube opens approximately 1.4 times each minute for a duration of 0.4 to 0.5 seconds, usually with a swallow or yawn. The tube does not dilate open with every swallow or yawn. Between openings, there is a net absorption of middle ear gases that results in a progressively negative pressure in the middle ear space that ranges between 0 and –50 cm H_2O in healthy awake adults.[20]

In addition to middle ear aeration, the eustachian tube also serves as a drainage pathway for fluid buildup within the middle ear. Middle ear secretions or infection are removed by two primary mechanisms. The first mechanism involves mucociliary clearance, much akin to the pulmonary system. The inferior or dependent portion of the eustachian tube is lined by columnar ciliated epithelium, in contrast to the osseous and superior portions of the eustachian tube which are lined by cuboidal respiratory epithelium.[13,21] These ciliated epithelial cells provide a mucociliary elevator to push debris and secretions down the eustachian tube and into the nasopharynx. The second mechanism of clearance involves muscular pumping. Muscular pumping of the eustachian tube occurs as the tubal valve progressively closes from the isthmus toward the nasopharyngeal orifice when the tensor veli palatini muscle relaxes.[13] This works synergistically

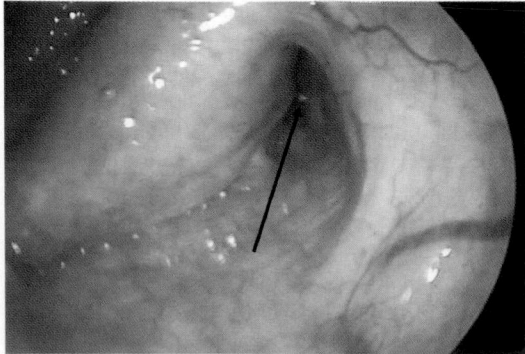

Figure 2 Normal left eustachian tube, open position. Valve dilated open (*arrow*).

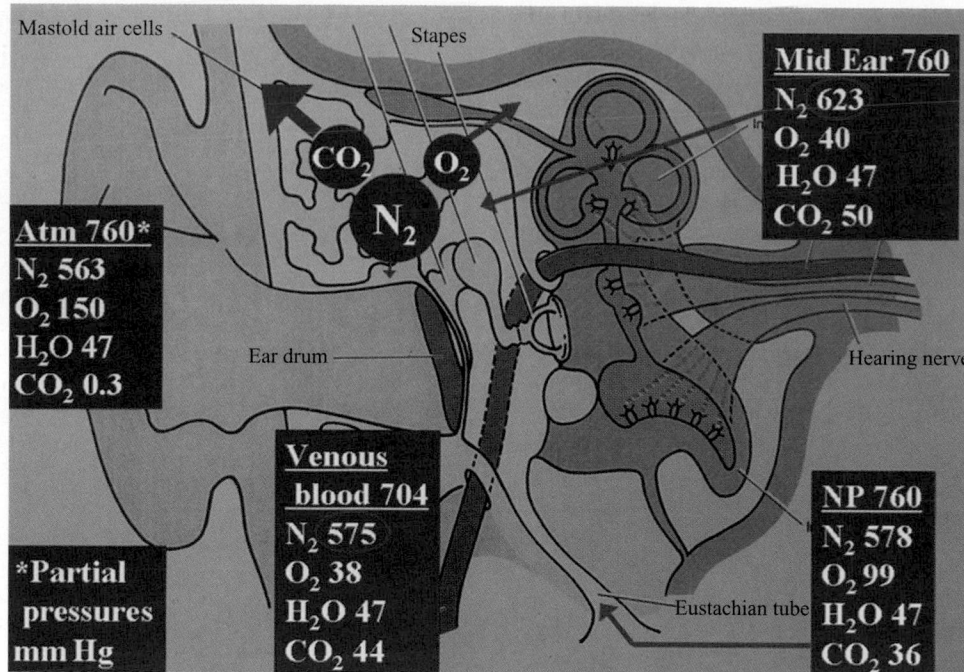

Figure 3 Middle ear gas exchange. (Artwork reproduced with permission from Medtronic Xomed, Inc., Jacksonville, FL.)

along with mucociliary clearance to propel fluids and debris down the eustachian tube and out the orifice within the nasopharynx where they can be swallowed or expectorated.

The third role of the eustachian tube is to prevent gastroesophageal reflux from penetrating into the middle ear cavity and to block the passage of sound from entering the middle ear cavity during speech. As the eustachian tube remains closed for all but brief intermittent periods of time, the primary mechanism for prevention of reflux of fluid and sound is mechanical blockage due to a closed lumen. During the brief periods of time when the tube is open, reflux of sound and fluid is limited by a back pressure of air within the middle ear space, the so-called gas cushion effect.[12]

EVALUATION

Evaluation of patients with suspected eustachian tube dysfunction begins with a comprehensive history and physical examination. History should focus on any disorders which could lead to edema or inflammation of the eustachian tube, such as laryngopharyngeal reflux, allergies, Samter triad (asthma, nasal polyposis, and aspirin sensitivity) or sinusitis. Disorders affecting ciliary motility such as cystic fibrosis and Kartagener syndrome should be diagnosed. Prior operations, particularly a history of adenoidectomy, should be elicited. In children, otitis media is associated with cigarette smoke exposure, wood burning stoves, and participation in group daycare facilities.[22] Inquiry should be made about excessive respiratory tract infections, immune deficiency, food or environmental allergies, or a family history of eustachian tube problems. Social history should include questions about smoking and secondhand exposures to smoke which have a

detrimental effect on mucosal ciliary clearance. A detailed list of medications is important and should focus on any nasal preparations including topical corticosteroids and oxymetazoline (Afrin), allergy medications, and hormonal replacement therapies.

Examination is comprehensive and includes a thorough head and neck evaluation with particular focus on otoscopy as well as nasopharyngoscopy. Otoscopy is best performed using the binocular microscope and the tympanic membrane should be inspected for any retraction, retraction pockets, cholesteatoma, perforations, atelectasis, tympanosclerosis, or effusions. Pneumatic otoscopy is particularly important, looking for evidence of tympanic membrane retractions and the degree of retraction and negative middle ear pressure. Insufflation of a retraction helps to determine if there is active negative middle ear pressure that may indicate compromise of eustachian tube function. If the retraction has become adherent but the surrounding tympanic membrane moves equally well with positive or negative insufflation, the adhesion may be a remnant of past tubal dysfunction, a factor that could be important in deciding whether surgical intervention is indicated for the retraction. Audiologic assessment is indicated and begins with pure-tone audiometry to assess for conductive or sensorineural hearing loss. Tympanograms are also obtained to ascertain the resting middle ear pressure.

Endoscopic examination of the eustachian tube is important to determine the nature of tubal dysfunction. It is best performed with an endoscope positioned close to the nasopharyngeal orifice of the eustachian tube with the view directed down its longitudinal axis, approximately 45° superiorly to the floor of the nasal cavity. Examination during swallows and yawns reveals the mucosal folds within the valve of the cartilaginous portion

of the eustachian tube unfolding in full view during the dilation and closing processes.

Endoscopic examination should include both nasopharyngoscopy and laryngoscopy. Nasopharyngoscopy can be accomplished with either rigid or flexible scopes passed through the nasal passages. Although rigid scopes allow for the best images and clarity, flexible scopes are often better tolerated by patients. Optimal patient position is sitting upright in a chair. The patient is anesthetized with topical spray consisting of lidocaine 4% mixed with an equal contribution of phenylephrine 4%. The initial examination is most commonly performed with a flexible endoscope to survey all of the nasal cavity, nasopharynx, pharynx, hypopharynx, and larynx. Nasal mucosa is also inspected for any signs of allergies, inflammation, granulomatous disease, or other pathology. The larynx is examined for evidence of laryngopharyngeal reflux such as inflammation of the arytenoid and interarytenoid web, false or true vocal folds, and especially the subglottic space. When using a flexible scope, the eustachian tube lumen is best seen through the contralateral naris by curving it posteriorly around the posterior edge of the vomer. The endoscope is positioned as close to the eustachian tube orifice as possible and directed along the long axis of the tubal lumen. Rigid endoscopy is then done for more directed detailed inspection. A 4 mm rigid 30° or 45° endoscope is quite useful in evaluation of the eustachian tube orifice. In the relaxed, closed state, the valve mucosa takes on an S-shaped curve within the lumen. During dilation, the valve becomes rounded. Patients with a patulous eustachian tube are seen to have a concave or scaphoid defect where the normal anterolateral wall bulge exists.

Dynamic endoscopic inspection of the eustachian tube orifice is important in differentiating whether the cause of dysfunction may be a mucosal or obstructive problem versus a muscular dilatory failure. Tubal dysfunction is classified as either an obstructive or dynamic disorder. Patients are initially asked to repeat the consonant "k" several times under direct visualization to assess the quality of palatal elevation and to assess the levator veli palatini muscle's ability to rotate the posterior cushion medially. The valve does not dilate during this maneuver. To evaluate normal dilation, the patient is instructed to do a series of swallows. To evaluate maximal dilatory effort, the patient is instructed to do a series of yawns. The tube should be seen going from the closed S position into a rounded open lumen and relax back to its resting closed state.

Slow-motion video endoscopy is also used to evaluate eustachian tube opening, particularly for patients with chronic tubal dysfunction. Images captured on video are reviewed in slow motion to evaluate the eustachian tube dynamics in detail. Each of the four phases of eustachian tube opening along with the dynamic function of both the tensor veli palatini and levator veli palatini can be isolated and evaluated using this technique.

Eustachian Tube Function Tests

A number of tests have been employed using either positive or negative pressure through the external auditory canal or nasopharynx to assess eustachian tube function. None of these tests have gained widespread use as they all lack clinical significance. The forced response test measures the pressure needed to open the eustachian tube, and a patent ventilation tube or tympanic membrane perforation is required. The external auditory canal is sealed using a tympanometry probe, and the pressure is increased until the eustachian tube opens resulting in a sudden decompression. The inflation–deflation test uses a tympanometry probe to record and vary pressure as the patient swallows in an attempt to open the eustachian tube. Both the forced response test and the inflation–deflation test were used to evaluate pediatric patients prior to tympanoplasty in one study.[23] Although good eustachian tube function did correlate with a favorable outcome for tympanoplasty, poor eustachian tube function did not correlate with poor outcomes for tympanoplasty.[23]

Another test of eustachian tube function, sonotubometry, takes measurements of the eustachian tube opening using a speaker which produces a tone inside the nose and mouth. A microphone is placed within the external auditory canal such that opening of the eustachian tube can be detected as an increase in the sound reception from the nasopharynx. Unfortunately, difficulties with signal-to-noise ratio have limited its clinical use.

Tubomanometry records impedance tympanometry of the external auditory canal during swallowing while the mouth is closed and the nose is sealed with a probe that increases the nasopharyngeal pressure. Investigators have correlated higher tubal opening pressures with middle ear pathology, but its clinical utility remains limited.[24]

PATHOLOGY AND TREATMENT

In general, impairment of tubal function can be divided into two main categories: the tube cannot open properly or the tube remains inappropriately patent. Eustachian tube dysfunction commonly, and as used throughout this chapter, refers to tubal dysfunction when the eustachian tube cannot open properly. Patulous eustachian tube describes the condition when the tubal orifice remains inappropriately patent. Both entities are reviewed below.

Eustachian Tube Dysfunction

Eustachian tube dysfunction can result from anatomical obstructions or physiologic causes. Tubal dysfunction appears to be due to: (1) hereditary factors as seen in strong family histories of ear disease, (2) mucosal inflammation and edema with obstruction or failure of dilation, and (3) muscular problems causing dilatory dynamic dysfunction.

Anatomical obstructions must be ruled out, particularly in patients presenting with unilateral symptoms. Malignant masses resulting in obstruction include nasopharyngeal carcinoma, lymphoma, and chondrosarcoma. Serous otitis media is the second most common presentation of nasopharyngeal carcinoma after a neck mass. Benign causes of mechanical obstruction include adenoid hypertrophy, mucus retention cysts, Tornwaldt cysts, or synechiae from adenoidectomy and other surgical procedures.

Physiologic blockage of the eustachian tube is more common than anatomical obstruction. Physiologic dysfunction most often results from mucosal inflammation, possibly due to allergies or laryngopharyngeal reflux.[9] The allergic response of the mucosa lining the eustachian tube results in edema, narrowing of the lumen, and consequent dysfunction (Figures 4 and 5). This can occur at the eustachian tube orifice or along the entire length of the eustachian tube. Laryngopharyngeal reflux into the eustachian tube orifice and lumen similarly results in mucosal edema, inflammation, narrowing, and dysfunction. Tobacco use results in a loss of the normal ciliary clearance of the eustachian tube and frequently causes eustachian tube dysfunction. Hormonal influences on the eustachian tube can be observed in pregnancy, particularly in the third trimester when progesterone levels are peaking. Progesterone has a direct effect on the mucosa with ensuing edema and occasional dysfunction.

Once eustachian tube dysfunction begins and the eustachian tube can no longer open properly, negative pressure builds within the middle ear

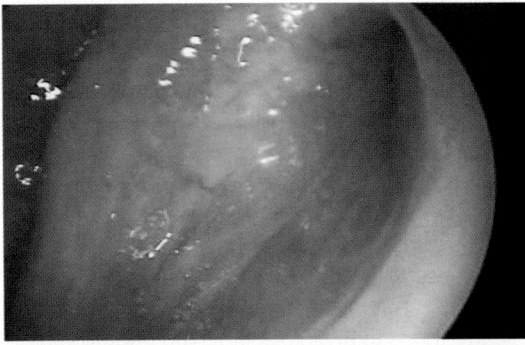

(A)

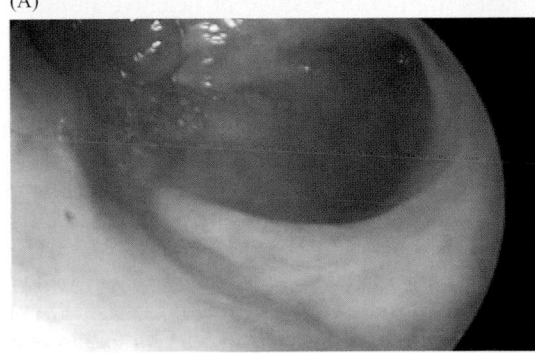

(B)

Figure 4 Eustachian tube dysfunction. (A) This endoscopic image demonstrates mild inflammation of the left eustachian tube orifice in the resting position. (B) This endoscopic image demonstrates mild inflammation of the left eustachian tube orifice in the dilated position.

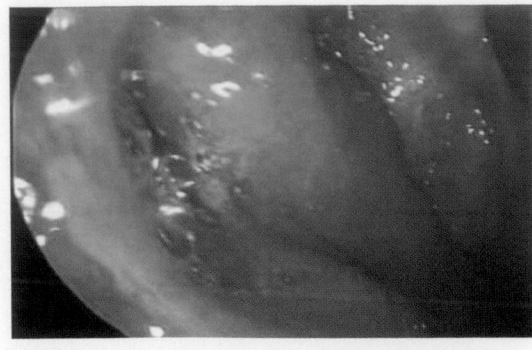

(A)

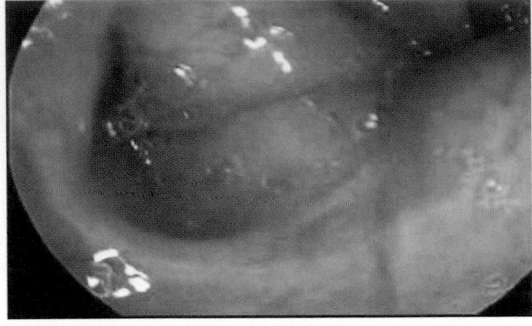

(B)

Figure 5 Eustachian tube dysfunction. (A) This endoscopic image demonstrates moderate inflammation of the right eustachian tube orifice in the resting position. (B) This endoscopic image demonstrates moderate inflammation of the right eustachian tube orifice in the dilated position.

space. This results in the symptom of aural fullness along with varying degrees of conductive hearing loss. The negative middle ear pressure may lead to other sequelae, including retraction pocket formation, tympanic membrane perforation, atelectasis, cholesteatoma, serous otitis media, and chronic otitis media.

Chronic feeling of fullness in the ear associated with a normal-appearing mobile tympanic membrane, absence of any retraction or effusion, and a normal tympanogram should not be interpreted as eustachian tube dysfunction. Instead, a search for other causes of fullness, blockage, or otalgia is indicated and should include evaluation of the temporomandibular joint as the most common cause followed by superior semicircular canal dehiscence syndrome and endolymphatic hydrops.

Evidence is mounting that eustachian tube dysfunction results from dysfunction along the cartilaginous portion of the eustachian tube. Using slow-motion video analysis, 40 adult patients were evaluated with the identification of significant pathology and compromise of tubal dilation within the cartilaginous portion. Eighty-three percent had mucosal edema and 74% had reduced anterolateral wall movement. Muscular dysfunction was demonstrated and typically involved the tensor veli palatini muscle. Weakness of the tensor veli palatini muscle may also cause a decrease in anterolateral wall dilatory movement. However, several cases of levator veli palatini muscle dysfunction were also identified.[15]

Slow-motion video endoscopy has revealed examples of hyper- or hypofunction of the tensor veli palatini or levator veli palatini muscles resulting in dynamic dysfunction of tubal dilation. Weak efforts by either muscle result in incomplete dilation of the valve. Excessive contraction may create a bulky mass effect that can paradoxically block the valve dilation just at the moment it should be opening. In some cases, there is a lack of coordination between the muscle contractions. For example, the levator veli palatini may relax prematurely leaving the valve partially closed by the time the tensor veli palatini begins its contraction (Figure 6). A hypertrophic adenoid pad does not need to cover the tubal orifice at rest to cause a significant functional obstruction. During the swallowing process, contraction of the pharyngeal constrictors can compress an otherwise nonobstructive adenoid into the posterior cushion of the eustachian tube and force it anteriorly to close the tubal orifice at the time it should be dilating open.[15] Nguyen and colleagues demonstrated that adenoidectomy for relief of otitis media with effusion was most effective when adenoid tissue was in contact with the posterior cushions of the eustachian tube orifices.[25] These findings would be consistent with the dynamic observations of pharyngeal constriction acting to push the adenoid into the posterior cushions as a mechanism causing tubal dysfunction.

The treatment of eustachian tube dysfunction depends upon identification of the underlying causality. Laryngopharyngeal reflux should be treated with dietary modifications such as

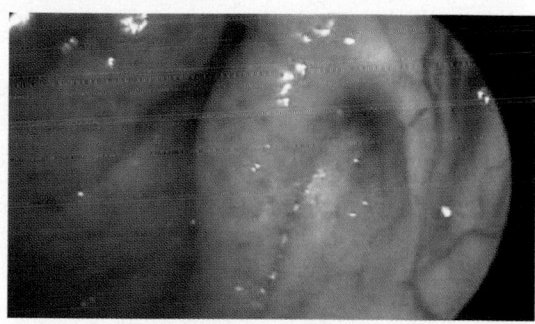

(A)

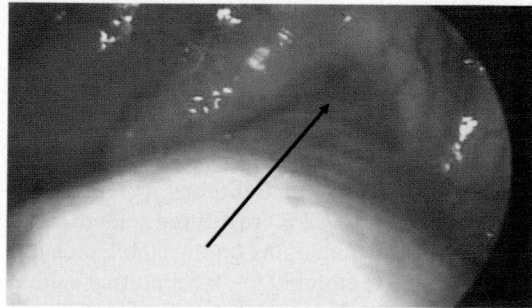

(B)

Figure 6 Eustachian tube dysfunction. (A) This endoscopic image demonstrates the left eustachian tube orifice in the resting position. (B) This endoscopic image demonstrates the same left eustachian tube orifice as seen in A, being paradoxically closed during tubal dilation due to the levator veli palatini muscle blocking the valve orifice (*arrow*).

avoiding foods that relax the lower esophageal sphincter and that promote acid production. Consideration should be given to acid-reducing agents such as proton pump inhibitors taken daily or twice daily and H_2 blockers at bedtime. Refractory cases may be managed by sleeping on an inclined bed, and ultimately, fundoplication may be considered.

Any history or findings of allergies should be investigated. Avoidance of the offending allergen can be effective but may not always be possible. Oral second-generation antihistamines, nasal corticosteroid sprays, or combination therapy may be effective in reducing allergic manifestations. Refractory cases may require immunotherapy.

Management of anatomical obstructions is tailored to the causality. Nasopharyngeal carcinoma is often treated with radiation therapy, and benign masses such as hypertrophic adenoid tissue can be excised. Infections are treated with the appropriate antibiotics. Recurrent infections should prompt a search for underlying nasal or sinus disease, immunosuppression or immunodeficiency, or primary mucosal disorders (eg, Samter triad, Wegener granulomatosis). Granulomatous disease is typically treated with immunosuppressants.

Surgical Management of Eustachian Tube Dysfunction. In the event that thorough investigation of underlying medical conditions and maximal medical therapy fail to resolve otitis media or atelectasis, surgical intervention is indicated. Tympanostomy tubes are effective in the treatment of serous otitis media and may prevent retraction of the tympanic membrane, atelectasis, and other sequelae of eustachian tube dysfunction. If the effusion or inflammation continues despite a tube in place, it raises the suspicion of a primary mucosal disorder rather than just a eustachian tube problem. Thick proteinaceous "glue-like" effusions that repeatedly occlude the lumen of the ventilating tube often will respond to oral or topical corticosteroids and may represent a primary mucosal problem. In cases of long-term persistent eustachian tube dysfunction, repeated placement of ventilating tubes may become necessary. In such cases, larger flanged tubes such as "T" tubes or subannular semipermanent tubes may be indicated. Longer duration tubes raise the risk of permanent perforation of the tympanic membrane.

For adult cases of medically refractory eustachian tube dysfunction and need for repeated tympanostomy tubes, eustachian tuboplasty is currently being studied. It appears to be most effective when the underlying medical conditions have been brought under control but there is irreversible mucosal disease causing functional obstructive dysfunction of dilation. Laser tuboplasty with removal of redundant edematous tissue along the posteromedial eustachian tube orifice has been shown to be an effective alternative for patients with chronic otitis media with effusion who have received numerous prior tympanostomy tubes with or without significant

atelectasis.[26,27] The operation involves laser debulking of posterior cushion luminal mucosa and submucosa down to the medial cartilaginous lamina from the free margin at the nasopharyngeal opening and extending proximally up to the valve (Figures 7 and 8). The extent of valve mucosa treated depends on preoperative evaluation with slow-motion video endoscopy to reveal the dynamics of the obstruction. Even after successful surgery, patients must remain vigilant about continuing medical therapy for their underlying condition. If they stop allergy or reflux therapy, the effusion may recur. In general, the operation has been well tolerated and without significant complications; however, long-term results and controlled studies need to be completed to determine the ultimate role of the procedure in the treatment of refractory otitis media due to chronic eustachian tube dysfunction. Further research must be done on the physiology and pathophysiology of tubal function in children before tuboplasty surgery would be recommended for pediatric cases.

Patulous Eustachian Tube

The condition known as patulous eustachian tube occurs when the eustachian tube remains patent for variable periods of time outside of the normal brief interval of opening which occurs during deglutition or yawning. When the eustachian tube is inappropriately open, patients typically present complaining of loud and disturbing autophony of their voice and nasal breathing sounds as well as aural fullness. Most patients describe the symptoms as if they are speaking within a barrel and complain of severe echoing with speech. Physicians can simulate the symptoms for themselves by listening through their stethoscopes while they speak and breathe with their mouth directly over the diaphragm. Unfortunately, many patients will simply state that they have a "blocked ear," prompting their physicians to treat them inappropriately for obstructive eustachian tube dysfunction for prolonged periods of time. The condition may arise spontaneously or occur with exercise, probably from dehydration or decongestion from exercise related hormones. When patients lie down or compress their ipsilateral internal jugular vein, the symptoms usually abate due to venous engorgement and closure of the patulous tube. Symptoms are often intermittent and can last from minutes to hours, or in extreme cases, persist continuously throughout daytime hours. Patients may note that symptoms are worse with nasal decongestants and improved with upper respiratory tract infections. Often, symptoms follow a dramatic and substantial weight loss such as with postpregnancy, cachectic diseases, dietary weight loss, and bariatric surgery. In the senior author's experience, one-third of cases of patulous eustachian tube have a substantial history of weight loss, one-third have an associated systemic rheumatologic disorder, and the remaining third are idiopathic.

Patulous eustachian tube must be confirmed by physical examination. Unfortunately, symptoms

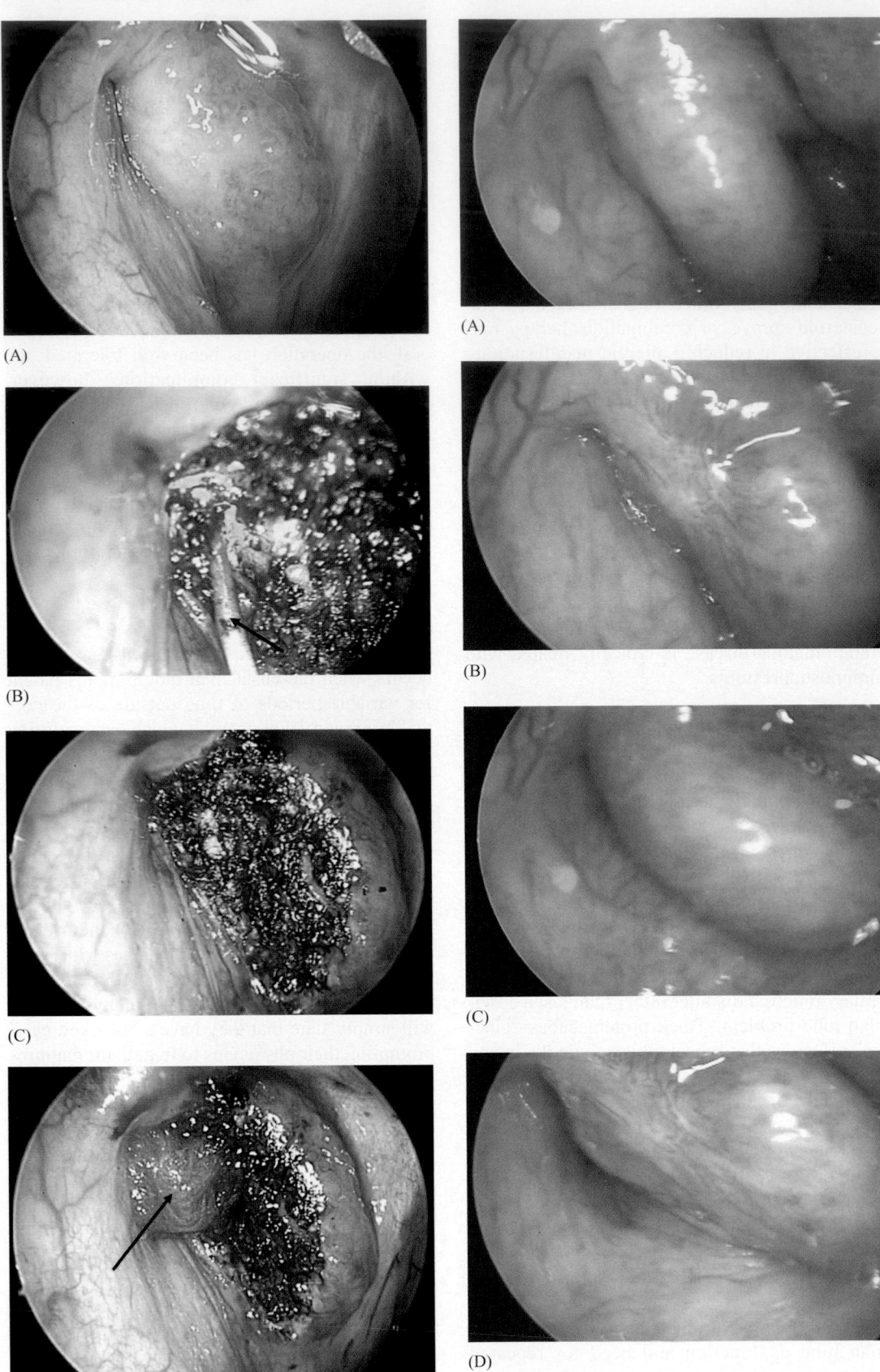

(A)

(B)

(C)

(D)

Figure 7 Right laser eustachian tuboplasty. (A) This endoscopic image demonstrates a eustachian tube orifice with eustachian tube dysfunction. (B) This endoscopic image demonstrates use of the KTP laser (*arrow*) in removal of the redundant edematous tissue along the posteromedial eustachian tube orifice. (C) This endoscopic image demonstrates complete excision of the redundant edematous tissue along the posteromedial eustachian tube orifice. (D) This endoscopic image demonstrates placement of a Merogel™ sponge (*arrow*) soaked in sulfa 10% and prednisolone 0.2% into the valve orifice.

Figure 8 Right laser eustachian tuboplasty. (A) Preoperative, resting position. (B) Six months postoperative, resting position. (C) Preoperative, dilated position. (D) Six months postoperative, dilated position.

are often intermittent, and if the patient is not having active autophony during the evaluation, the condition can be missed. If the patient is suspected of having patulous eustachian tube and is not having autophony on arrival for clinical evaluation, the patient should exercise (eg, walking up and down stairs) for several minutes in an

attempt to elicit the symptoms. The patient can be instructed to breathe deeply in and out through the ipsilateral nasal cavity, occluding the contralateral nares during the otoscopic examination. While the autophony is present, examination will demonstrate excursions of the tympanic membrane that move synchronously with ventilations, a condition that is pathognomonic for the patulous eustachian tube. The condition often resolves due to venous congestion in the supine position, such that the evaluation should be performed while the patient is sitting upright.

Endoscopic evaluation of the eustachian tube may aid in the diagnosis. Patients with patulous eustachian tube typically have tissue loss longitudinally through the valve that can be seen as a concave or scaphoid defect along the superior aspect of the anterolateral wall. The senior author's surgical experience has revealed that the loss of tissue volume can involve mucosa, submucosa, Ostmann fat, tensor veli palatini muscle, lateral cartilaginous lamina, or any combination of these. Endoscopy will show a concave defect in the anterolateral wall at the nasopharyngeal orifice during resting examination. However, this can be misleading as many patients, particularly thin individuals, will have similar mucosal gaps on examination. The tube must be examined for the defect which continues longitudinally throughout the full length of the valve as revealed during sustained yawn efforts. Most of the time, the full length of the valve is not easily examined up to the bony-cartilaginous junction so that endoscopic examination alone is not usually reliable.

Treatment of patulous eustachian tube is centered on thickening the mucus or restoring the bulk of the eustachian tube valve. If the patient is on any decongestants or topical nasal corticosteroid sprays, these should be discontinued. Weight gain is only recommended if the patient is malnourished. Good hydration can be effective and may be supplemented with nasal saline drops or irrigations. Drops can be instilled during the day anytime symptoms occur. Patients should be instructed to direct their nose vertically, place the drops, then tilt the head 45° laterally to maximize the contact with the tubal orifice. Placing the head in a dependant position for a few minutes is usually effective, at least temporarily. Autophony may often occur during prolonged speaking and unobtrusive neck compression of the ipsilateral internal jugular vein may relieve symptoms for some time. Although not FDA approved, "off-label use" of estrogen nasal drops -[Premarin 25 mg injectable SECULE (registered trademark to designate a vial containing an injectable preparation in dry form) diluted in 30 ml normal saline] or estradiol nasal drops (Depo-Estradiol 5 mg injectable ampule diluted in 30 ml normal saline), three drops TID for a 6-week trial period can lead to localized hypertrophy around the eustachian tube orifice that may improve or resolve symptoms. Topical irritants, such as aspirin or boric acid powder insufflated onto the nasopharyngeal orifice can cause a localized inflammatory edema around the orifice and are usually effective. Unfortunately, the benefits are generally short-lived. Ongoing daily topical irritant therapy such as chlorine-based nasal drops may prolong the efficacy if the patients tolerate the treatment. Potassium iodine [ie, saturated solution of potassium iodide (SSKI)] has been used with some efficacy to thicken mucous secretions. Ventilation tube placement may provide some relief but in only half of patients.[28] Ventilating tubes are generally effective in relieving the sensation of patulous excursions of the tympanic membrane during breathing but rarely control the more disturbing symptom of autophony.

Early attempts at surgical correction of the patulous eustachian tube involved peritubal injections of tetrafluoroetheylene (Teflon) paste which typically gave transient relief. Injections were directed into the posterior cushion or floor of the tubal lumen. The practice was largely discontinued after several deaths occurred after inadvertent intracarotid injections. Intranasal placement of a needle into the inferior tubal orifice brought the needle into a direct line with the internal carotid artery. Since the patulous defect has more recently been identified in the anterolateral wall, new attempts at injection have been made. However, since the tissue planes around the anterolateral wall, especially around the tensor veli palatini muscle, are very loosely applied, they do not hold the material in place resulting in spread of material from the basisphenoid to the parapharyngeal space.[29]

Complete occlusion of the eustachian tube is very effective in relieving patulous symptoms, but an effusion occurs that generally must be managed with long-term ventilation with tympanostomy tubes. Occlusion can be accomplished by transnasal or middle ear approaches.

More recently, endoscopic approaches are being developed for reconstruction of the patulous defect while preserving eustachian tube function. The authors have found that a combined endoscopic transnasal and transoral approach can provide reliable long-term resolution of symptoms. The technique implants conchal cartilage grafts into the concave anterolateral defect to create a normal convex shape that will restore the competency of the valve (Figure 9). The mucosal incision is sutured closed to maintain the graft position and special instrumentation is recommended for the technique (see Figure 9). Although long-term data are not yet available, patients followed for 5 years demonstrate that the procedure is efficacious and does not lead to recurrence of symptoms or the development of eustachian tube dysfunction. In the senior author's series, 14 patients, most of whom were treated with cadaveric dermal implants (Alloderm), had 93% efficacy in reducing symptoms resulting in 43% of patients completely satisfied. For the 57% of patients not completely satisfied, an additional procedure to bulk up the anterolateral wall further was offered to the patients.[29] Alloderm is known to lose a significant amount of volume over time, and much improved results are now being seen

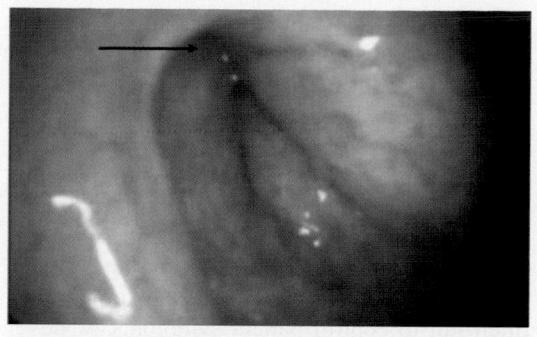

(A)

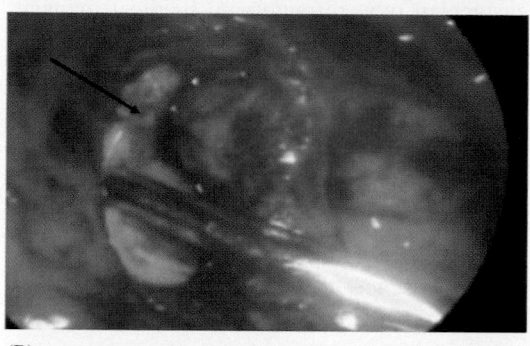

(B)

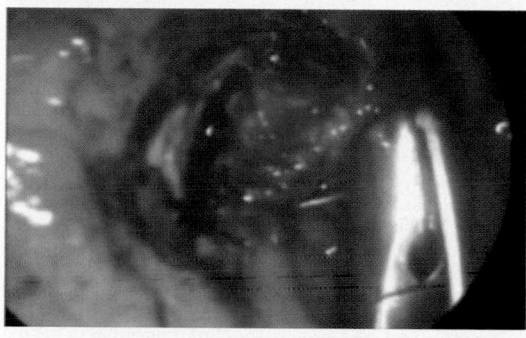

(C)

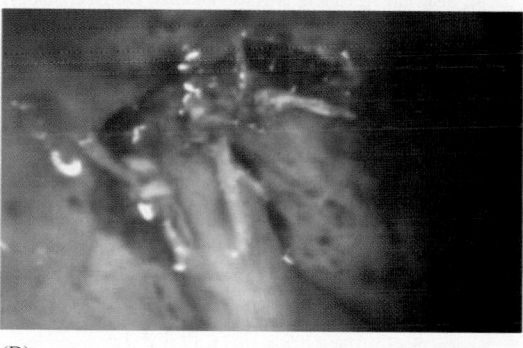

(D)

Figure 9 Right patulous eustachian tube reconstruction. (A) This endoscopic image demonstrates the valve with the characteristic concave anterolateral wall (*arrow*) seen in patients with patulous eustachian tubes. (B) This endoscopic image demonstrates a conchal cartilage graft (*arrow*) inserted into the anterolateral wall within a submucosal pocket. (C) This endoscopic image demonstrates suturing of the incision. (D) This endoscopic image demonstrates the incision after suture closure.

using cartilage grafts. This patulous eustachian tube reconstruction provides an efficacious low-risk alternative for patients suffering from patulous eustachian tube which prove refractory to medical management (Figure 10).

Finally, it is important to recognize that another common cause of autophony is superior

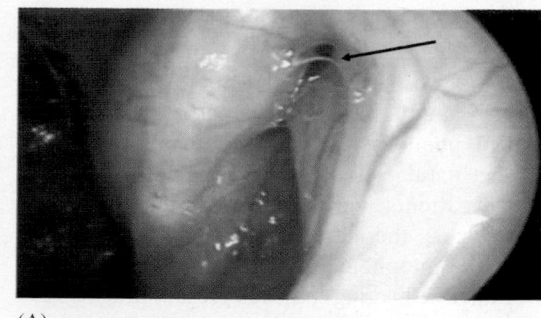

(A)

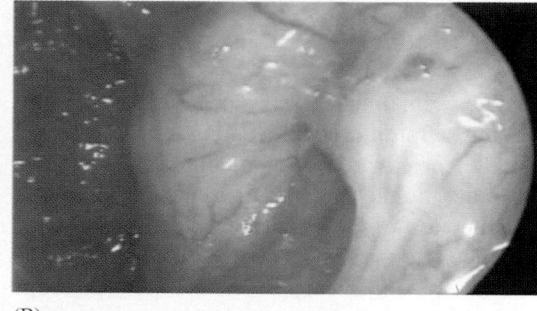

(B)

Figure 10 Right patulous eustachian tube reconstruction. (A) Preoperative view. This endoscopic image demonstrates the characteristic concave defect (*arrow*) seen within the anterolateral wall of the valve. (B) Postoperative view. This endoscopic image demonstrates repair of the concave defect within the anterolateral wall.

semicircular canal dehiscence syndrome (third window syndrome). Patients describe a "blockage" or fullness of the ear and autophony in terms indistinguishable from patulous eustachian tube symptoms. The perception of bone conducted sounds are abnormally enhanced in superior semicircular canal dehiscence syndrome creating autophony which can also include sounds from chewing, footsteps, and even eye movements. An important point of differentiation is that nasal breathing is not typically amplified in superior semicircular canal dehiscence syndrome but is amplified and equally bothersome to patients with patulous eustachian tube. Furthermore, autophony in superior semicircular canal dehiscence syndrome is often sudden in onset followed by a persistence of the symptoms except at night. Patulous eustachian tube patients usually have more intermittent or fluctuating symptoms with some periods of relief.

Another confusing similarity between the two disorders is that in both the autophony can be relieved by supine or head-down positioning. The most critical distinction between superior semicircular canal dehiscence syndrome and patulous eustachian tube is made on the physical examination of the tympanic membrane while the patient reports ongoing active autophony. Excursions of the tympanic membrane will be pathognomonic for patulous eustachian tube while the absence of the excursions during autophony effectively rules out that condition. Other causes for autophony must be sought and superior semicircular canal dehiscence syndrome would be a prime suspect with endolymphatic hydrops a distant alternative. Superior semicircular canal dehiscence syndrome may also be associated with low-frequency conductive hearing loss, a supranormal bone conducting threshold above 0 dB in low frequencies, intact stapedius reflex, vertigo, hearing distortion, Tullio phenomenon, and torsional nystagmus with a fistula test. In the senior author's series of 18 patients with superior semicircular canal dehiscence, the most common presenting symptom was autophony occurring in 94% of patients. Conductive hearing loss was present in only 72% of patients.[29]

CONCLUSIONS

The eustachian tube plays a central role in maintaining aeration and preventing reflux into the middle ear cavity as well as draining secretions from the middle ear cavity into the nasopharynx. Dysfunction of the eustachian tube occurs when the tube cannot open properly or when the tube remains patent at inappropriate times (patulous eustachian tube). In a search for an underlying cause, larygopharyngeal reflux, allergies, primary mucosal disease such as Samter triad or granulomatous disease, and mechanical obstructions such as hypertrophic tissue, benign tumors, and malignant neoplasms should be considered. When the eustachian tube cannot open properly, negative pressure builds within the middle ear resulting in aural fullness and a conductive hearing loss. This can lead to other sequelae such as retraction pockets, tympanic membrane perforation, atelectasis, serous otitis media, and cholesteatoma. Treatment should be directed toward the underlying medical condition and will successfully relieve the dysfunction in the majority of cases. Medically refractory dysfunction is managed with tympanostomy tubes. If eustachian tube dysfunction persists in spite of multiple tube placements over time or adequate medical management, irreversible mucosal disease is probably responsible; and eustachian tuboplasty surgery may be indicated for adults.

Patulous eustachian tube can cause disturbing but physiologically harmless autophony and aural fullness. A concave defect in the anterolateral wall of the tubal valve and patulous excursion of the tympanic membrane will be seen during autophony symptoms. Medical therapies for patulous eustachian tube include weight gain if appropriate, hydration, saline- or estrogen-based nasal drops, chlorine-based nasal drops, and mucus thickening medications. Tympanostomy tubes often fail to control patient symptoms. A novel surgical technique for the treatment of patulous eustachian tube refractory to medical management has been developed and involves augmenting the anteromedial eustachian tube orifice with cartilage or alloplastic materials.

Semicircular canal dehiscence syndrome can also present with autophony, aural fullness, and commonly conductive hearing loss. Patients with superior semicircular canal dehiscence syndrome will not have autophony to respirations. There will be absence of excursions of the tympanic membrane with nasal breathing during autophony.

REFERENCES

1. Bluestone CD. Introduction. In: Bluestone CD, editor. Eustachian Tube Structure, Function, Role in Otitis Media. London, Ontario: BC Decker Inc; 2005. p. 1–9.
2. Eustachius B, editor. Epistola de auditus organis. In: Opuscula Anatomica. Venice: Luchinus; 1564. p. 153.
3. Canalis R. Valsalva's contribution to otology. Am J Otolaryngol 1990;11:420–7.
4. Toynbee J. On the muscles that open the eustachian tube. Proc R Soc Med 1853;6:286–91.
5. Hopf J, Linnarz M, Gundlach P, et al. Microendocopy of the eustachian tube and the middle ear. Indications and clinical application. Laryngorhinootologie 1991;70:391–4.
6. Poe DS. Eustachian tube function and dysfunction. In: Hamid M, Sismanis A, editors. Medical Otology and Neurotology: A Clinical Guide to Auditory and Vestibular Disorders. New York: Thieme; 2006. p. 110–22.
7. Suzuki C, Balaban CD, Sando I, et al. Postnatal development of eustachian tube: A computer-aided 3-D reconstruction and measurement study. Acta Otolaryngol (Stockh) 1998; 118:837–43.
8. Ishijima K, Sando I, Balaban CD, et al. Length of the eustachian tube and its postnatal development: Computer-aided three-dimentional reconstruction and measurement study. Ann Otol Rhinol Laryngol 2000;109:542–8.
9. Proctor B. Anatomy of the eustachian tube. Arch Otolaryngol 1973;97:2–8.
10. Proctor B. Embryology and anatomy of the eustachian tube. Arch Otolaryngol 1967;86:503–14.
11. Bluestone CD. Anatomy. In: Bluestone CD, editor. Eustachian Tube Structure, Function, Role in Otitis Media. London, Ontario: BC Decker Inc; 2005. p. 25–50.
12. Bluestone CD. Physiology. In: Bluestone CD, editor. Eustachian Tube Structure, Function, Role in Otitis Media. London, Ontario: BC Decker Inc; 2005. p. 51–65.
13. Honjo I, Hayashi M, Ito S, Takahashi H., Pumping and clearance function of the eustachian tube. Am J Otolaryngol 1985;6:241–4.
14. Poe DS, Pyykko I, Valtonen H, Silvola J. Analysis of eustachian tube function by video endoscopy. Am J Otol 2000;21:602–7.
15. Poe DS, Abou-Halawa A, Abdel-Razek O. Analysis of the dysfunctional eustachian tube by video endoscopy. Otol Neurotol 2001;22:590–5.
16. Eden AR, Gannon PJ. Neural control of middle ear aeration. Arch Otolaryngol Head Neck Surg 1987;113:133–7.
17. Rockley TJ, Hawke WM. The middle ear as a baroreceptor. Acta Otolaryngol (Stockh) 1992;112:816–23.
18. Tideholm B. Middle ear cleft pressure. In: Ars B, editor. Fibrocartilaginous Eustachian Tube Middle Ear Cleft. The Hague, Netherlands: Kugler Publications; 2003. p. 49–56.
19. Grace A, Kwok P, Hawke M. Surfactant in middle ear effusions. Otolaryngol Head Neck Surg 1987;96:336–40.
20. Mondain M, Vidal D, Bouhanna S, Uziel A. Monitoring Eustachian tube opening: Preliminary results in normal subjects. Laryngoscope 1997;107:1414–.
21. Sando I, Takahashi H, Matsune S, Aoki H. Localization of function in the eustachian tube: A hypothesis. Ann Otol Rhinol Laryngol 1994;103:311–4.
22. Bluestone CD. Epidemiology. In: Bluestone CD, editor. Eustachian Tube Structure, Function, Role in Otitis Media. London, Ontario: BC Decker Inc; 2005. p. 11–24.
23. Manning SC, Cantekin EI, Kenna MA, Bluestone CD. Prognostic value of eustachian tube function in pediatric tympanoplasty. Laryngoscope 1987;97:1012–6.
24. Martin C, Chelikh L, Prades J, et al. Functional study of the auditory tube (eustachian tube) in otitic pathology by tubomanometry. In: Tos M, Thomsen J, Balle V, editors. Otitis Media Today. Proceedings of the Third Extraordinary Symposium on Recent Advances in Otitis Media. The Hague, Netherlands: Kugler Publications; 1999. p. 281–6.
25. Nguyen LH, Manoukian JJ, Yoskovitch A, Al-Sebeih KH. Adenoidectomy: Selection criteria for surgical cases of otitis media. Laryngoscope 2004;114:863–6.
26. Poe DS, Metson RB, Kujawski O. Laser eustachian tuboplasty: A preliminary report. Laryngoscope 2003;113:583–91.
27. Poe DS, Grimmer JF, Metson R. Laser eustachian tuboplasty: Two-year results. Laryngoscope 2007;117:23–37.
28. Luxford WM, Sheehy JL. Myringotomy and ventilation tubes: A report of 1568 ears. Laryngoscope 1982;92:1293–7.
29. Poe DS. Diagnosis and management of the patulous eustachian tube. Otol Neurotol 2007;28:668–770.

16

Otitis Media and Middle-Ear Effusions

J. Christopher Post, MD, PhD

Joseph E. Kerschner, MD

THE PROBLEM OF OTITIS MEDIA

The late Sylvan Stool, MD, aptly summarized the area of otitis with the term "Otitis media (OM) with confusion." While intensive clinical and basic studies have begun to clarify this common disease, many areas of controversy remain. These areas include the following: Do patients with acute otitis media (AOM) require antibiotic therapy? Does chronic OM adversely impact development of speech and language? and When should surgical intervention be considered? The treatment of otorrhea is controversial, and the relationship between allergy and OM is completely muddled. There is even a fundamental disagreement as to whether chronic OM is primarily an inflammatory or an infectious process. The terminology is not standardized, and the accuracy of diagnosis in the hands of primary care providers is around 50%. This chapter will highlight these areas of controversy, while attempting to provide the practitioner with practical guidelines regarding the management of patients OM and middle-ear (ME) effusions.

OM is a worldwide pediatric healthcare problem. OM is the most common reason that an ill child visits a physician in the United States. Children from age 6 months to 2 years are most commonly affected, and almost all children will have an episode of OM by age 3 years, with over half having three or more episodes. The incidence of OM increased 250% from 1975 to 1990, an increase attributable to improved diagnostic efficacy, the increased number of children in daycare and, perhaps, the increased prevalence of allergic children. The American Academy of Pediatrics states that over 5 million AOM cases occur annually in US children, with about 30 million annual visits to healthcare providers.

OM is the most common indication for prescribing antibiotics, which results in more than 10 million annual antibiotic prescriptions representing 25% of all antibiotic prescriptions. Fifty percent of antibiotics for preschoolers in the United States are prescribed for ear infections. The overprescription of antibiotics is considered a major driver of the development of antibiotic resistance and there is a great concern regarding the overprescribing of antibiotics. The combination of multiple independent antibiotic selective pressures, together with the high rates of transmission within the daycare population generates an environment which is conducive to the development of multiple drug-resistant bacteria.

Surgical management of OM is the most common reason to administer a general anesthetic to a child. Treatment of OM costs over 5 billion dollars a year in the United States.[1] While the majority of cases of OM are self-limited, OM can result in hearing loss, language delay, or serious extracranial or intracranial complications. Thus, there exist important public health reasons to develop alternate antiinfective strategies, that is, vaccines, which can be used to combat ME pathogens.

There is little consensus concerning risk–benefit ratios of available medical and surgical treatments. Legitimate concerns regarding the overprescription of antibiotics have led to a bias for beneficial societal outcomes, that is, reduction of antimicrobial-resistant microorganisms, at the expense of the individual patient and family. Studies that evaluate treatment strategies use limited outcome measures and often fail to include important considerations, including the pain and suffering of the sick child, the role OM plays in limiting women's participation in the workforce, loss of wages as the result of caring for a sick child, parental distress and familial disruption, the disproportional adverse impact on lower socioeconomic and minority populations, the likelihood of long-term consequences of OM, and even the potential for decreased lifetime earning potential of a child with cognitive delays associated with prolonged, inadequately treated OM.

OM is the most common cause of acquired hearing loss in the pediatric population. The role of OM, and the associated hearing loss, in adversely impacting speech and language development, school performance, psychosocial development, and cognitive ability has been the focus of intense study, resulting in over 100 publications. While the results of these studies have been mixed, it is clear that the adverse impact is disproportionately large for children with developmental delay, special populations, or children with existing hearing loss not due to OM. There is a school of thought that the risk of cognitive and functional damage is not as great as previously believed. Unfortunately, these beliefs have translated into a more nihilistic approach to the treatment of OM, without much thought being given to the impact on the child's overall well-being. Fortunately, a growing number of researchers are evaluating the impact of OM on the overall health and well-being of the child, rather than taking a more proscribed course. These studies indicate that children with chronic OM have significantly decreased quality of life (QOL) scores when compared with unaffected controls.[2]

The epidemiology, pathophysiology, treatment, and impact of OM have been widely studied, but several fundamental issues challenge almost every effort in each of these areas (Table 1).

HISTORY OF OM

OM has long been recognized as a common disease and until the late nineteenth century, it was associated with a high complication rate, major morbidity, and frequent mortality. Ancient temporal bone osteopathology studies have provided evidence regarding the prevalence of ear disease in various ancient populations.[3] Skulls obtained from throughout the world show evidence of acute and chronic OM in the Aleutians, Peru,

Table 1 Challenges Associated with Otitis Media Research	
High rate of spontaneous resolution, necessitating large sample sizes	Overly narrow focus on one outcome measure
Poor ascertainment of disease	Failure to consider cost-effectiveness, ie, one therapy may cost more than another but is still better if it is more efficacious
Insufficient intensity of disease surveillance	
Reliance upon culture data, and failing to understand that "no growth by culture" does not equate with "absence of microorganism"	Determination of otitis media burden by chart review or parental report, rather than by prospective serial examinations by validated otoscopists
Differences in study design, methodology, and scope	Extrapolation from narrow study groups to the overall population
	Investigator bias

Chile, Iran, Egypt, and Central Europe, with some of the skulls over 8,000 years old. Hippocrates described the disease in 450 BC.

Treatments for OM have been known since Byzantine times, and included herbs, animal and mineral substances applied as eardrops or poultices. Ventilating the ME space has long been recognized as beneficial in the treatment of OM. Valsalva described the eponymous maneuver in 1704, and Toynbee's realization that eustachian tube (ET) dysfunction was associated with negative ME pressure and hearing loss led to efforts to aerate the ME actively via the ET, generally with catheterization of the ET. Politzer's method of insufflation of the ME through the ET with the Politzer bag without the use of a catheter was a great advance.

Tympanocentesis as a treatment for OM came about when Jean Riolan the Younger inadvertently punctured a patient's tympanic membrane (TM) while attempting to clean the canal, which fortunately resulted in the patient's hearing improving. Given the recognition of the spontaneous healing tendencies of the TM, many techniques were devised to obtain a more permanent opening. A wide variety of materials, including catgut, whalebone rods, and gold foil were placed into the TM in efforts to maintain patency. Unfortunately, TM perforation was performed indiscriminately by unprincipled and inexpert practitioners and fell into disfavor for decades. Tympanocentesis was reintroduced by Schwartze, the director of the 25-bed Königliche Universitäts-Ohtrenklinik (the Royal University Ear Clinic) in Halle, and Armstrong popularized the use of ear tubes in the twentieth century.

Nasopharyngeal radium irradiation has been used to reduce hypertrophied lymphoid tissue, with the goal of treating ET dysfunction or OM in groups as disparate as military aviators, submariners, and children. After World War II, nasopharyngeal radium irradiation became a popular treatment for pediatric hearing loss and chronic ear infections. Estimates of the number of children treated range from 500,000 to 2.5 million. This treatment modality is no longer used given the potential for the development of malignancies.

DEFINITIONS, ETIOLOGY, AND PATHOGENESIS OF OM

Confusion regarding terminology continues, and care must be taken to strike a balance between differentiating among clinically significant diagnoses and splintering the diagnoses into numerous varieties with insignificant differences. OM is best thought of as representing a continuum of disease states, all characterized by the accumulation of fluid in the ME space. OM can be broadly divided into three major types: (1) AOM, a purulent effusion with constitutional symptoms such as fever or pain; (2) OM with effusion (OME), the presence of fluid in the ME in the absence of constitutional symptoms other than hearing loss or balance problems; and (3) chronic suppurative

OM (CSOM), drainage (otorrhea) through a perforated TM or tympanostomy tube (TT). AOM and OME are interrelated, in that most episodes of OME are preceded by an episode of AOM. In both AOM and OME, ME effusion is present, which may be serous, a thin, watery liquid, mucoid, a thick, viscous, mucus-like liquid, or purulent.

The most likely cause of OM is a sequence of events: acute OM is initiated by a viral infection which damages the ciliated mucosa of the upper respiratory tract and permits pathogenic bacteria to invade the ME space through retrograde movement from the nasopharynx through the ET. These bacteria elicit potent inflammatory responses from the ME mucosa as well as infiltrating leukocytes. Compromise of the ET is a major component of OM. The ET ventilates the ME by equilibrating the pressure between the ME space and the nasopharynx, drains the ME of secretions, and protects the ME from excessive sound pressure and reflux of secretions. ME effusions can result from nasopharyngeal secretions entering the ME space and can also result from inadequate ventilation of the ME. ME underpressures can lead to the development of effusions, that is, the *hydrops ex vacuo* theory. The relatively horizontal positioning of the ET in the young child's skull base is thought to increase the child's susceptibility to reflux of secretions from the nasopharynx into the ME cleft.

OM generally takes place in young children with a relatively immature immune system. This lack of development in this patient population, coupled with anatomic disadvantages in the developing ET explains the susceptibility of young children to OM. In older children selective IgG2 and IgG4 subclass deficiencies can predispose to repeated episodes of OM, and patients with persistent OM should be evaluated for deficits in immunoregulatory function.

A variety of viruses can be isolated from ME effusions, including rhinovirus, respiratory syncytial virus, influenza virus, adenovirus, parainfluenza virus, and enterovirus. The major role of viruses in OM appears to be setting the stage for a subsequent bacterial infection. Viruses can invade the ME space, generating an inflammatory response, which results in effusion. Viruses also compromise the ET's ability to protect the ME by impairing mucociliary clearance and, in addition, enhance bacterial adherence and provoke the production of inflammatory mediators. It is not clear that viruses alone can cause AOM, and studies that rely solely on viral culture techniques have presented an incomplete picture. Not surprisingly, it is clear that the use of nucleic amplification techniques greatly enhances the yield of bacterial identification in ME effusions. Using culture, antigen detection and nucleic acid amplification, a co-infection with bacteria and viruses can be found in almost all cases of OM.[4] Increased exposure to viral and bacterial pathogens is felt to be the reason that daycare attendance increases a child's risk of developing OM.

AOM elicits potent inflammatory responses from the cells of the ME mucosa as well as from infiltrating leukocytes. These mediators have a

wealth of inter-related biological effects and play an active role in ME inflammation. Inflammatory mediators can impair mucociliary clearance, produce fever, increase bacterial adherence, activate leukocytes, and regulate antibody formation. A large number of inflammatory mediators have been studied in association with AOM, including prostaglandins, and cytokines such as interleukin (IL)-1beta, IL-6, and IL-8, IL-10, and tumor necrosis factor alpha (TNF-alpha). Local inflammatory mediators such as inflammatory cells, lysozymes, and oxidative metabolic products, also play a role. Chapter 3, "Molecular Biology of Hearing and Balance," contains a broader discussion of the molecular biology of OM.

While allergic events, may lead to congestion, there is no convincing evidence that upper respiratory allergies are a primary etiologic event in the development of OM. Allergies can lead to nasal congestion and obstruction and ET edema and dysfunction, with resulting negative pressure in the ME and compromised ventilation of the ME space. Inflammatory mediators can be released by mucosal mast cells following the interaction of antigen and specific IgE antibody, resulting in ET obstruction and subsequent transudation of fluid into the ME space.

Microbiology of AOM

Streptococcus pneumoniae, Haemophilus influenzae, and *Moraxella catarrhalis* are the predominant bacterial species isolated from the effusions of AOM. Other pathogens that are isolated from AOM effusions include group A *Streptococcus* and *Staphylococcus aureus. Alloiococcus otitidis* is a bacterium that is being isolated from effusions of AOM and OME with increasing frequency. *Alloiococcus otitidis* is most readily identified by the polymerase chain reaction, as it grows poorly in culture. While the role of this bacterium in otitis is unclear, a recent report that specific ME immune responses are induced suggests that the microorganism may be a true pathogen.[5] Young infants can have gram-negative enteric microorganisms such as *Escherichia coli, Klebsiella*, and *Enterobacter* species, and *Pseudomonas aeruginosa*. Microorganisms that are rarely involved in OM include *Mycoplasma pneumoniae, Chlamydia trachomatis, Corynebacterium diphtheriae, Mycobacterium tuberculosis*, nontuberculous *Mycobacteria*, and *Clostridium tetani*.

Microbiology of Chronic OME

OME has historically been considered to be an inflammatory process, as only 30% of effusions were positive for bacteria by culture using standard techniques. Over the past decade, there has been a growing body of evidence that "no growth" by culture does not equate with "absence of microorganism." Using nucleic acid amplification strategies, it has been shown that the majority of "sterile" ME effusions actually contain DNA and messenger RNA from the three major pathogens of OM, as well as *A. otitidis*. These findings led to the advancement of the mucosal biofilm paradigm, which postulates that chronic OME is due to the persistence of a bacteria biofilm on the ME mucosa. A recent report has demonstrated the presence of mucosal biofilms with confocal laser scanning microscopy in the vast majority of OME and recurrent OM ME mucosa biopsy specimens, while no biofilms were found in control specimens.[6]

Epidemiology

Understanding the epidemiology of OM serves as a foundation to help the clinician in making good management decisions, particularly surgical decisions, for the individual child. Consequently, the epidemiology of OM has been the focus of much investigatory effort. Despite the difficulties in OM research mentioned previously, considerable progress has been made, providing information that allows clinicians to help families identify mutable risk factors and assist with changing or ameliorating these risk behaviors. Clearly, the clinician would be more apt to intervene surgically in a child who had the first episode of OM at age 3 months, spends 40 hours a week in daycare, and has significant hearing loss with language delay (Table 2).

DIAGNOSIS OF OM

As a group, otolaryngologists–head and neck surgeons are more accurate in the diagnosis when compared to pediatricians and general practitioners. Using video-recorded otoscopic examinations, including pneumatic otoscopy of the TM, to ascertain the ability to differentiate among AOM, OME, and normal, pediatricians and general practitioners made the correct diagnosis only half the time.[7] Pediatric residents perform even more poorly. Given the recent trend toward withholding antibiotics, it is imperative that better diagnostic acumen be developed.[8] A cloudy, bulging or clearly immobile TM are some of the most useful signs for diagnosing acute OM, and a distinctly red TM increases the likelihood of OM significantly.[9] Tympanometry, acoustic reflectometry, and selective use of tympanocentesis can be helpful in establishing the diagnosis and guiding therapy in refractory cases.

History

The diagnosis of OM is frequently not as straightforward as might be thought. The history is generally obtained, not from the patient, but from the caregiver, the symptoms of fever and irritability are neither sensitive nor specific, the physical examination can be hampered by cerumen occluding the external auditory canal, and the patient is often uncooperative. An upper respiratory infection may precede the onset of OM. Signs and symptoms include fever, ear pain, irritability, inconsolable crying, changes in eating or sleeping habits, malaise, vomiting and diarrhea, and occasionally tugging at the ear. A recent meta-analysis demonstrated that ear pain is the most useful symptom, while fever, upper respiratory tract symptoms, and irritability were less specific. The older child may note fullness in the ear as well as decreased hearing in the affected ear. Children with OME are generally asymptomatic except for hearing loss or problems with balance.

Physical Examination

It is time well spent to gain the trust of the child before proceeding with the examination. Ensure that you have washed your hands; not only is this good infectious disease practice, but warm hands will elicit less of a response from an apprehensive child. Rest assured that the caregiver takes note if you do not wash your hands. Correct

Table 2 Factors That Have Been Consistently Observed to Increase a Child's Risk of Developing Otitis Media, with Suggested Explanations for the Observation, and Potential Intervention Strategies for Amelioration*

Factors That Increase a Child's Risk of Otitis Media	Suggested Explanations for the Observation	Potential Intervention Strategies for Amelioration
Viral upper respiratory infections	Compromised mucociliary clearance	Develop vaccinations against the most common viruses; good hand-washing
Craniofacial abnormalities, including cleft palate, and Down syndrome	A deficiency in the functioning of the eustachian tube	Early surgical intervention in patients demonstrating difficulties with otitis media
Repeated exposure to other children	Increased exposure to resistant microorganisms	The total number of children in the daycare is an important variable, particularly for the child less than 1 yr
Strong family history of otitis media	Various human leukocyte antigen subtypes predispose to otitis media	
Early age of onset of otitis media	Genetic susceptibility, or early exposure to robust pathogens	Consider colonizing the infant with beneficent bacteria
Lack of breastfeeding	The infant's immature immune system is bolstered by IgA antibodies in the breast milk. Breast milk also contains a variety of nonspecific defense factors contributing to its antimicrobial effect. Breastfeeding protects against nasopharyngeal colonization of bacteria associated with otitis media	Prenatal education emphasizing the benefits of breastfeeding
Tobacco exposure	A meta-analysis of 36 studies demonstrated a consistent relationship between parental smoking and the development otitis media	Advise families of the dangers of passive smoking and provide specific strategies to help quit
Gastroesophageal reflux	Chronic irritation of nasopharyngeal or middle-ear mucosa, with decreased ciliary efficiency	Treatment of gastroesophageal reflux disease may reduce the incidence and severity of otitis media
Lower socioeconomic status	Increased exposure to pathogens, delayed access to healthcare	Societal changes to improve access to health care
Season of the year, with highest rates observed during winter months	Increased infectious rates of viral agents	Development of viral vaccinations
Age less than 2 yr	Less well-developed immunologic defenses and immature eustachian tubal factors, including anatomical alignment, structure, and function.	
Native American, Inuit, and Indigenous Australian children	Eustachian tube dysfunction	
Immune deficiency disorders, such as HIV	Increased susceptibility to infectious agents	Immunoglobulin transfusion
Failure to receive pneumococcal vaccine	Immunization with a multivalent, conjugated pneumococcal vaccine	
Presence of oral or nasally placed tubes	Reduced ciliary clearance of pathogens	Remove tubes as soon as medically feasible

*Note that understanding these aspects of the OM epidemiology suggest strategies to reduce or prevent OM: breastfeeding, avoidance of upper respiratory infections, avoidance of tobacco smoke, and vaccination with a pneumococcal vaccine. The most important sociodemographic risk factors for otitis media appear to be low socioeconomic status and repeated exposure to large numbers of other children. Other epidemiological aspects, including gender, race, pacifier use, and feeding practices, are less clear.

positioning of the child is essential. Most children can be easily examined if they are held in the caregiver's lap, with the child's back against the caregiver's front. Instruct the caregiver to hold the child's arms and body with one arm, and the turned head with the other. Holding the child's feet between the caregiver's knees provides an extra margin of safety for the examiner. Conversely, infants can be placed in the prone position on the examining table. Have an assistant hold the infant's arms extended on each side of the head, parallel to the long axis of the body, this way one person can hold both the infant's head and arms simultaneously. If the child is small, the examiner can hold the child's body secure by gently leaning on the child's torso and hips. Occasionally, a third restrainer is necessary. The use of a papoose or other restraining device becomes less frequent with experience. Cerumen can be cleaned from the external canal by use of a curette, or by lavage, if you are certain that the TM is intact. Most cerumen impactions are the result of misguided parental efforts to clean the external auditory canal with cotton swabs, displacing the wax medially.

Examination of the TM. The most common method for diagnosing OM is examination of the TM with an otoscope. Otoscopes are of two basic types, surgical or operating and diagnostic. Surgical otoscopes have a moveable lens that allows access to the external auditory canal. This type of otoscope allows for cerumen removal using a curette, and for tympanocentesis. The diagnostic otoscope has a lens and light source enclosed in a larger head and has an attached tubing and rubber bulb for the performance of pneumatic otoscopy. This type of otoscope provides for an airtight seal when the speculum is placed into the external auditory canal. Care must be taken not to place the speculum too deeply into the canal, to avoid causing the child pain. If a satisfactory seal cannot be obtained, the use of a rubber-tipped speculum or sheathing the tip of the speculum with a sleeve of rubber tubing can help.

A normal TM is translucent, with the observer able to distinguish the short and long processes of the malleus and occasionally the incus. The TM is concave medially, pearly gray in color, and will readily move with insufflation. To diagnose OM, the observer should look for abnormalities of color, translucency, contour, and mobility. Thus, the TM may appear erythematous, whitish, or yellow. The drumhead may be opaque or bulging. Purulent otorrhea is indicative of a TM that ruptured as the result of AOM. In OME, the observer may note either air-fluid levels or air bubbles deep to the TM. The TM may be retracted, and the TM will be dull gray or amber, and nonerythematous, unless the child is crying.

Common sources of error in diagnosis include mistaking an erythematous TM due to the child's crying for an infection, failure to perform insufflation, failure to perform insufflation correctly, pumping the bulb of the pneumatic otoscope as though the observer were trying to inflate a truck

tire is contraindicated, and failure to restrain the uncooperative patient adequately.

An assessment of the TM mobility by pneumatic otoscopy will greatly enhance the accuracy of diagnosis.[10] To perform pneumatic otoscopy, hold the otoscope in one hand with the bulb under your thumb and rest your hand against the child's head, so that if the child moves, the tip of the speculum does not lacerate the ear canal. Using the other hand to steady the child's head, ensure that a seal is achieved between the tip of the speculum and the external auditory canal. Gently squeeze the bulb with your thumb. As the bulb is alternately squeezed gently and released, the response of the TM to both positive and negative pressure can be assessed. A normal TM will readily move medially in response to positive pressure, and laterally in response to negative pressure. If an effusion is present, the TM movement will be dampened.

While complete immobility almost guarantees the diagnosis of otitis, in the absence of a TM perforation, decreased mobility is a more common finding. Unfortunately the technique is operator-dependent and is often not used by pediatricians or general practitioners.[11] Diagnostic accuracy is improved with a structured approach to teaching otoscopy and by validating clinicians either with myringotomy or videotaped otoendoscopic examinations.

Tympanometry is an objective measurement of the compliance of the TM and is analogous to TM mobility during pneumatic otoscopy. Tympanometry can be a useful adjunct in the diagnosis of otitis but cannot distinguish between AOM and OME. Tympanometry is a simple, rapid, noninvasive test that provides information about TM compliance in electroacoustic terms, using a tympanometer. A known sound pressure is applied in a sealed volume between the external auditory canal and the TM, and the air pressure in the ear canal is varied above and below atmospheric pressure. The TM reflects the sound pressure, and the tympanometer measures the energy of the reflected sound signal at these different pressures. The mobility of the TM is maximal when air pressures are equal medially and laterally. In the normal condition, the air pressure on each side of the TM is already equalized via the ET, and the TM mobility (compliance) will be at its maximum when the tympanometer provides no change in pressure to the external auditory canal (0 decapascal pressure). If the ME has an effusion, the TM mobility is dampened, and the compliance will be decreased. If the ME has negative pressure, the compliance will be greatest when the tympanometer creates a negative pressure in the external auditory canal equal to the negative pressure in the ME space. TM mobility will also be decreased if the mobility of the ossicular chain is stiffened as in otosclerosis or if the TM itself is stiffened as in tympanosclerosis. The tympanometer produces a curve known as a tympanogram, which graphically displays compliance on the y-axis and pressure (from negative to atmospheric to positive) on the x-axis in decapascals (daPa).

Tympanograms are generally classified into one of three categories: Type A, a normal curve characterized by a steep gradient, with a sharp peak. Type B, a flat tracing that indicates decreased TM compliance across a broad range of air pressures. The most common reason for a Type B tracing with a "normal" volume is ME effusion. A Type B tracing with a "large" volume indicates a TM perforation or patent ear tube. Normal volume for a child is around 1 mL. Type C, indicates significant negative pressure in the ME space, which correlates with a retracted TM. A type C tympanogram is suggestive of impaired ventilatory function of the ET and may indicate a transition between a normal ear and an ear with a ME effusion. Overall, a Type C tympanogram is relatively nonspecific.

Tympanometry is not as accurate in infants (6 months of age and younger), as the skin and cartilage in the external auditory canal are quite lax and will move in response to changing air pressure (producing a Type A tympanogram), even though the ME may have an ME effusion.

Future Diagnostic Modalities. A variety of new technologies are being investigated to determine their role in the diagnosis of otitis. A-mode ultrasonography has been used to detect ME effusion. In one preliminary study, ultrasound identified the presence or absence of effusion in 96% of cases and could distinguish between serous and mucoid effusions with 100% accuracy. However, it could not distinguish between mucoid and purulent effusion.[12]

MEDICAL MANAGEMENT OF OM

The treatment of OM continues to undergo transformation. From the days of unbridled antibiotic use for acute disease and month after month of "treatment" for OME, there is an increasing emphasis on a more nuanced approach, with a decreased reliance on antibiotic use in uncomplicated OM and an increased emphasis on the clinical setting rather than a "one-drug-fits-all" approach. The decreased emphasis on antibiotics is directly related to the increasing rates of bacterial antimicrobial resistance, particularly in young children attending daycare.

Guidelines have been developed by the American Academy of Pediatrics and the American Academy of Family Physicians to help the clinician choose the appropriate course of action. The Institute of Medicine defines guidelines as "systematically developed statements to assist practitioner and patient decisions about appropriate healthcare for specific clinical circumstances." The goals of the OM guidelines are to promote the judicious use of antibiotics in an effort to protect their therapeutic advantage. It is also thought that several million antibiotic prescriptions can be avoided annually by the use of guidelines. While these guidelines are helpful, they tend to be narrowly drawn and couched with disclaimers and leave great latitude in the practice pattern of the individual physician (Table 3).

Table 3 Guidelines on the Management of Acute Otitis Media from the American Academy of Pediatrics and the American Academy of Family Physicians*

- To reliably diagnose acute otitis media, the physician should confirm a history of abrupt onset (<48 h) of middle-ear effusion and inflammation.
- The management of acute otitis media should include assessment of pain. If pain is present, the clinician should provide treatment to reduce it, eg, acetaminophen or ibuprofen.
- Observation without antibiotics is an appropriate option for selected children with uncomplicated acute otitis media based on diagnostic certainty, age, severity of illness, and certainty of follow-up.
- If the decision is made to treat with an antibiotic, amoxicillin remains the initial antibiotic of choice for most children.
- Lack of response within 48–72 h requires reassessment to confirm acute otitis media. If confirmed in a child initially managed with observation, an antibiotic should be prescribed. If initial management was with an antibiotic, an alternative antibiotic should be prescribed.
- Physicians should encourage acute otitis media prevention through reduction of risk factors.

*The guidelines are limited to otherwise healthy children from 2 months to 12 years of age, who have not had a recurrence of acute otitis media (AOM) within 30 days or AOM with underlying chronic otitis media with effusion. The diagnosis of AOM should include recent onset of illness, presence of middle-ear effusion, and signs or symptoms of middle-ear inflammation. Antibiotics should be used for children age six months or younger, or for older children with severe symptoms, generally defined as temperature greater than 39° with severe otalgia. Note that the key to success of these guidelines is accuracy in diagnosis, particularly the use of pneumatic otoscopy and close follow-up of the child.

Several considerations argue against the with-holding of antibiotics from children with AOM: (1) children will resolve their symptoms more quickly with antimicrobial treatment; (2) antimicrobial treatment reduces the number of suppurative complications and withholding antibiotics can lead to an increase in suppurative complications (Table 4); (3) primary care physicians lack diagnostic precision and follow-up may be variable; (4) multiple follow-up visits are not possible for many families; (5) leaving the final decision to administer antibiotics in the hands of lay people is an abdication of the responsibilities of the physician; and (6) in today's medicolegal climate, the onus of responsibility for a child developing a devastating complication as the result of an easily

Table 4 The Use of Antibiotics for the Treatment of Acute Otitis Media Markedly Reduced the Incidence of Suppurative Complications

- Historically, acute otitis media has had a high complication rate, major morbidity, and frequent mortality.
- The Hospital for Sick Children in Toronto ended its first century with a logo depicting a child with a mastoid dressing.
- In 1927, one patient died on average every 2 wk at the Charite Hospital in Berlin from complications of otitis, including labyrinthitis, meningitis, sinus thrombosis, and brain abscess.[28]
- The introduction of antibiotic therapy in the 1930s ushered in an era of marked reduction in complications from acute otitis media and chronic suppurative otitis media with the mortality rate from mastoiditis falling from 2/100,000 to less than 1/10,000,000.
- Otitis media and complications accounted for 27% of all pediatric admissions to Bellevue Hospital in New York City in 1932.[29]
- Before the use of antibiotics, the rate of mastoiditis following acute otitis media was between 5 and 10%.[30]
- Antibiotic treatment has reduced the incidence of facial palsy as a complication of otitis media from 0.5 to 0.005%.[31]

treatable disease may fall directly on the individual physician.

Bacterial Resistance

Bacteria have evolved multiple mechanisms to develop resistance to antimicrobial agents, including reducing antibiotic penetration through the bacterial membrane, metabolic bypass, active efflux pumps to eliminate antibiotics from the bacteria, inactivation of antibiotics by specific enzymes, for example, beta-lactamase, and alteration of the antibacterial target site. Bacteria can develop antibiotic resistance via nucleic acid mutation, bacterial generations are measured in minutes, or horizontal transfer of genetic material occurs via plasmids or transposons. Bacterial biofilms also provide phenotypic resistance to antibiotics, and enhance nucleic acid transfer among bacteria.

In the United States, approximately 40% of strains of nontypable *H. influenzae* and almost all strains of *M. catarrhalis* are resistant to amoxicillin because of the production of beta-lactamase, or less commonly, alterations in penicillin-binding proteins.[13] This resistance can be overcome by the use of a beta-lactamase inhibitor, such as clavulanate, or by using a beta-lactamase-stable antibiotic. Approximately half of the strains of *S. pneumoniae* are penicillin-nonsusceptible, mediated by alternations in penicillin-binding proteins. This mechanism of resistance can be overcome by increased concentration of antibiotic.[13]

Selection of Antimicrobials for AOM

Studies have shown that antibiotic treatment of AOM shows a modest but significant impact on the disease, with earlier resolution and a reduction in the frequency of persistent disease and suppurative complications. Having said that, antibiotic use varies from 31% of patients in the Netherlands to 98% in the United States, although there are some indications that this percentage of patients receiving antibiotics for AOM in the United States is dropping. Given that tympanocentesis is generally not used in the management of uncomplicated

AOM, the infectious agent in the individual case can only be surmised. Thus, the treatment of the vast majority of AOM episodes is empiric, based upon a historic knowledge of the major pathogens in AOM, that is, *S. pneumoniae*, *H. influenzae*, and *M. catarrhalis*, and their antimicrobial resistance patterns (Table 5). Other considerations include the clinical setting, tolerability, concentrations achieved in the ME, and cost. Compliance with antibiotic regimens is enhanced by selecting agents that require less frequent dosing, such as one or two times a day, and by prescribing shorter, 5 days or less, treatment courses, although shorter courses of antibiotics are still controversial.

Amoxicillin remains the drug of choice for the treatment of uncomplicated OM. Limitations of amoxicillin include inactivation by the beta-lactamases, eg, nontypable *H. influenzae* and most strains of *M. catarrhalis*, and penicillin-resistant strains of *S. pneumoniae*. Indications for second-line medications include a failure, or history of failure, to respond to amoxicillin, penicillin allergy or culture results indicating the presence of a resistant microorganism. A Therapeutic Working Group convened by the United States Centers for Disease Control and Prevention recommended that children who fail initial therapy with amoxicillin be treated with amoxicillin-clavulanate, cefuroxime axetil or intramuscular ceftriaxone, although there was criticism of the group's methodology and conclusions. Tympanocentesis and culture can help guide effective therapy in recalcitrant cases. The follow-up interval for AOM should be individualized. Young patients and patients with continued pain should be seen within a few days, while 2 to 4 weeks may be adequate for older children. Parents should be educated that the presence of fluid in an asymptomatic child at the initial follow-up visit is not an indication for additional antibiotic treatment.

A number of other antibiotics that have been used in the past for the treatment of AOM. These include trimethoprim sulfa, clarithromycin, cephalexin, cefaclor, erythromycin ethylsuccinate and sulfisoxazole acetyl, and azithromycin, all of which have fallen out of favor due to high rates of antimicrobial resistance in common OM pathogens. The use of macrolides should be avoided in the treatment of OM. A variety of other treatments have been tried in the past, including decongestants, antihistamines, prostaglandin inhibitors, corticosteroids, and various methods of ME insufflation, however good evidence for efficacy is lacking. Although there is likely some small advantage, antibiotic treatment is no longer recommended in resolving OME.

Amoxicillin prophylaxis (20 mg/kg/d) has been shown to be effective for the prevention of OM in the past, however, this practice leads to the development of resistant microorganisms, particularly pneumococci, is less likely to be effective in the current environment of resistant microorganisms and is not currently recommended as a routine approach for recurrent AOM. Prophylaxis should only be used in those children who are not surgical candidates or are immunocompromised.

Table 5 Antibiotic Choices from the National Guideline Clearinghouse*

First-Line Medication

Category	Drug	Usual Pediatric Dosage
Penicillin derivative	Amoxicillin	Low risk: 40 mg/kg/d High risk: 80 to 90 mg/kg/d divided b.i.d. if not low risk or treatment failure of lower dose (effective against resistant *S. pneumoniae*)

Second-Line Medication

Category	Drug	Usual Pediatric Dosage
Penicillin derivative	Amoxicillin/clavulanate potassium	>3 mo of age: 45 mg/kg/d in divided doses q 12 h; amoxicillin/ clavulanate (90/6.4 mg/kg/d in two divided doses for 10 d)
Cephalosporin, second generation	Cefuroxime axetil	250 mg b.i.d. × 10 d or 30 mg/kg/d in divided doses b.i.d. × 10 d
	Cefprozil	15 mg/kg/d q 12 h
	Ceftriaxone sodium	50 mg/kg intramuscular injection (not to exceed 1 g) prescribe one dose for new onset otitis media and a 3-d course for a truly resistant pattern of otitis media or if oral treatment cannot be given
	Loracarbef	30 mg/kg/d in divided doses q 12 h
Cephalosporin, third generation	Cefdinir	7 or 14 mg/kg q 12 h
	Cefixime	8 mg/kg/d as a single dose or 4 mg/kg
	Cefpodoxime proxetil	5 mg/kg q 12 h (max 400 mg/d) × 5 d

*Low risk is defined as children over two year of age, with no history of chronic or recurrent otitis media (OM) and no antibiotics for the past three months. The use of multiple courses of empiric, broad-spectrum antibiotics should be avoided. Five days of therapy should be considered in cases of uncomplicated OM, and 10 days in resistant cases.

Table 6 Guidelines on the Management of Otitis Media with Effusion from the American Academy of Family Physicians; American Academy of Otolaryngology–Head and Neck Surgery; American Academy of Pediatrics Subcommittee on Otitis Media with Effusion*

- Document the laterality, duration of effusion, and presence and severity of associated symptoms at each assessment
- Distinguish and more promptly evaluate the child at risk for speech, language, or learning problems
- Manage an uncomplicated case with watchful waiting for 3 mo from the date of effusion onset or diagnosis
- Test the child's hearing when otitis media with effusion persists for 3 mo or longer, or when language delay, learning problems, or a significant hearing loss are suspected
- Not-at-risk children with persistent otitis media with effusion should be reexamined at 3- to 6-mo intervals until the effusion resolves, or significant hearing loss is identified
- Tympanostomy tubes are the preferred initial procedure

*The guidelines are limited to children aged 2 months through 12 years with or without developmental disabilities or underlying conditions. As in the case of acute otitis media, the guidelines strongly recommend that pneumatic otoscopy be employed. Adenoidectomy should not be performed with the initial set of tubes unless nasal obstruction or chronic adenoiditis is present; repeat surgeries should consist of adenoidectomy and myringotomy, with or without tube insertion. The guidelines recommend against tonsillectomy alone or myringotomy alone, antihistamines and decongestants, or the routine use of antimicrobials or corticosteroids. No recommendations were made for complementary or alternative medicine, or for allergy management, based on a lack of evidence of efficacy.

This group includes patients with human immunodeficiency virus (HIV), cyclic neutropenia, Wegener granulomatosis, and Shwachman–Diamond syndrome (severe neutropenia and frequent suppurative infections).

Modification of OM risk factors should be an important part of the management. Practitioners should ensure that children with a history of recurrent OM have an annual influenza vaccination and have received the pneumococcal conjugate vaccine. Families should be encouraged to discontinue smoking and to consider alternative childcare strategies than group daycare, which may not be feasible for many families. In families with a strong history of OM, the benefits of breastfeeding in limiting OM should be discussed. Comorbid conditions, such as rhinitis or allergy, should be managed, using environmental control measures, pharmacologic therapy, and allergen immunotherapy. The current guidelines for the management of OME are presented in Table 6.

Selection of Antibiotics for Otorrhea

Otorrhea is generally well treated with ototopical antibiotic drops alone. In refractory cases, culture should be considered to rule out associated fungal infection, and occassionally systemic antibiotics may be beneficial. Postoperative otorrhea is not uncommon after the placement of TT in patients that have ME fluid at the time of their tube placement.[14] This postoperative otorrhea can be reduced with intraoperative ME irrigation and the use of topical otic drops. Pathogens associated with acute otorrhea are those associated with AOM, particularly in younger children, while *Pseudomonas* spp. are more common in older children. Chronic otorrhea is more commonly associated with *Pseudomonas* spp. and *Staphlococcus aureus*. Medical treatment, including topical medications, systemic antibiotics, and aural toilet is generally adequate, however mastoidectomy should be considered in refractory cases or if a cholesteatoma is present. Repair of chronic perforations should be performed once the infectious process has been resolved.

Complementary and Alternative Medicine Treatments of OM

Our society is increasingly interested in complementary and alternative medicine (CAM) treatments for medical conditions, and OM is no exception. Given the propensity of otitis to spontaneously resolve, these treatments may appear to be successful, however, well-designed studies demonstrating efficacy are few in number, and the results are inconclusive. Homeopathy, chiropractic manipulation, acupuncture, Qigong, that is, an ancient Chinese breathing exercise with meditation, and a large number of herbs have been recommended for AOM, including garlic and Sai-rei-to, that is, a herb used in Kampo, or Japanese herbal medicine. Herbal eardrops include calendula (marigold flowers), St John's wort, mullein flower, and garlic, while Echinacea is widely believed to alleviate upper respiratory symptoms, despite several studies to the contrary. Dietary manipulations include adding foods rich in antioxidants and omega-3 fatty acids. Probiotics such as lactobacillus and xylitol, a sugar alcohol, that may interfere with bacterial adherence have been advocated, and may actually be of value in reducing bacterial adherence to mucosa.

Vaccine Strategies

Otolaryngology has a history of diseases vanquished by vaccination, including diphtheria and epiglottis, as two examples. It is hoped that OM will one day be added to this list. Administration of the pneumococcal conjugate vaccine results in a fairly substantial reduction in OM secondary to the included serotypes, and a more modest reduction in total episodes of OM. Use of the pneumococcal vaccination has now made *H. influenzae* the most frequently isolated bacteria in AOM.[15] It is likely that the frequency of nonvaccine serotypes being isolated from children with OM will increase.[16] Development of effective vaccinations against nontypable *H. influenzae* and *M. catarrhalis* have proven more challenging. Viral vaccinations may prove useful in the prevention of OM, particularly against respiratory syncytial virus (RSV), influenza virus, and parainfluenza virus.[17]

SURGICAL MANAGEMENT OF OM

Patient Selection

The surgical treatment of OM can be extremely efficacious in patients refractory to medical management. Using a validated instrument, children with OME or recurrent OM had improvement in their QOL after placement of TT.[18] Surgery offers a treatment pathway for the child that does not contribute to the emergence of antibiotic-resistant bacteria.[19] Parents overwhelmingly perceive that their child's health has improved after the placement of tubes and are satisfied with the results of the operation.[20] To the extent possible, clinicians should explain to the child what is involved in the procedure, and there are a variety of children's books available that can help with this task. A tour of the operating facility conducted preoperatively can be helpful in allaying parental and patient anxiety.

Myringotomy and Tympanocentesis

Myringotomy can be useful in a variety of clinical settings, including the relief of severe otalgia or hyperpyrexia. Myringotomy is indicated in cases of OM complicated by facial paralysis, mastoiditis, or labyrinthitis and can be helpful in obtaining effusion for culture in cases of persistent disease. Otolaryngologists should have a low threshold for performing myringotomy in immunologically compromised children or as a part of a septic workup in infants. Myringotomy alone as a treatment for OM is not effective, as the myringotomy site will rapidly close.

Myringotomy with TT Placement

Myringotomy with TT placement is the most common operation performed on children requiring general anesthesia in the United States. In one study, almost 7% of US children had tubes inserted by age 3 years.[21] Indications for tubes include chronic OME, recurrent AOM, ET dysfunction, and persistent TM retraction pockets. Tubes are also used to ensure adequate drainage in the treatment of suppurative complications of OM. With careful patient selection, the placement of tubes can be expected to resolve conductive hearing loss due to fluid, treat the balance disorders associated with OM, reduce the frequency, severity and duration of OM episodes, and reduce the incidence of long-term sequelae of chronic ear disease. The greatest risk to the child revolves around the risk of general anesthesia. Other factors to weigh include the cost and chronic TM changes, including persistent perforations, the percentage of which is low.

The timing to placement of TT for patients with chronic OME and recurrent OM will be affected by a number of factors. These include risk factors for OM, family history, tolerance or allergies to antibiotic therapy, craniofacial structure, underlying hearing loss, and associated developmental status. In OME, some patients may have relatively asymptomatic disease and can be monitored for a period of time with close follow-up to assess for development concerning anatomic abnormalities, that is, retraction pocket, TM adhesion, cholesteatoma, or hearing loss. In patients with OME, hearing loss frequently develops, and even small levels of persistent bilateral hearing loss has the potential to impact negatively patient development, especially those with underlying developmental concerns or speech delay. Interestingly, most studies which have demonstrated a smaller impact of OME on development have specifically excluded patients with underlying developmental or anatomic considerations or socioeconomic disadvantages and have focused on patient populations with less severe disease such as unilateral OME.[22] Patients who tend to be referred to otolaryngologists–head and neck surgeons for consideration of TT placement often have more severe disease as well as considerations related to development and language.

There has been a great deal of interest in performing the myringotomy with various lasers, including the carbon dioxide and ND-Yag lasers. A laser myringotomy can provide relatively short-term ventilation of ME space. Proponents tout the advantage of performing the laser myringotomy with a local anesthetic in the office setting without general anesthesia, thus reducing the risk and cost of the procedure. Variable success of disease resolution and family satisfaction seem to have limited the appeal of this procedure. There is no evident clinical benefit to using the laser to perform a myringotomy and then placing a tube. Additional indication for laser myringotomy include elimination of ME fluid before auditory testing, barotraumas, ET construction, or tympanocentesis to obtain a culture of ME fluid.[23]

Adenoidectomy

There is good evidence that adenoidectomy is an effective treatment for recurrent or persistent OM. Adenoidectomy should not be chosen as the initial surgical treatment for OM, unless there are clear indications, such as persistent nasal obstruction or chronic adenoiditis. Most otolaryngologists–head and neck surgeons will recommend an adenoidectomy if a second set of TT is needed. Adenoidectomy is thought to be effective either by improving ET function or by removing a reservoir for bacteria. Recent work demonstrating the presence of bacterial biofilms in the adenoid lends credence to the latter.[24]

COMPLICATIONS OF OM

Impact of OM on Language Development

A child's language development is a wonderfully complex interweave of genetic and environmental factors. The impact of OM, or more precisely the hearing loss associated with OM, on a child's development has been the subject of intense investigation and passionate debate for years. While it is clear that language development can be hindered by moderate or profound hearing loss, or by lesser degrees of loss that are permanent, the exact impact of mild or fluctuating hearing loss on language development remains unclear. The average hearing loss associated with OM is 15 to 50 dB between 500 and 4,000 Hz, which are the most important frequencies for speech reception.

There are many challenges to research in this area, including accuracy of diagnosis, determination of outcome measurements of language and cognition, influence of gender, and short-term duration of follow-up. Controlling for other influencers of language development, including a nonnurturing environment and cognitive deficits, is difficult. The effects of intermittent hearing loss associated with OM may be subtle and long term. Deleterious effects on phonological representations and working memory have been noted, along with degradation of communicative skills, particularly in a noisy background. A long-term study of over 1,000 children from the United Kingdom demonstrated that the developmental sequelae of OM remained significant for a decade.[25]

Other complications of OME include dizziness, clumsiness, and balance problems which generally improve with the insertion of tubes.[26] Children with bilateral OM did poorly compared to controls on the Peabody Developmental Motor Scales, which tests balance and locomotion skills. There is also an association between OM and learning disabilities.

Children with cleft palate, mental retardation, educational difficulties, or underlying sensorineural hearing loss are particularly at risk for the adverse effects of OM on language and social development. Children with Down syndrome and cleft palate benefit from aggressive management of their ear disease, but families should be counseled that they will have more episodes of otorrhea with tubes.

Central auditory processing disorder (CAPD) is an auditory-specific perceptual deficit located in the higher auditory pathways that underlies many learning problems in school-age children. CAPD cannot be identified by standard audiometric evaluations, and diagnosis requires specific tests employing temporal and frequency distortion and dichotic challenges. The conductive loss associated with OME may play a role in the development of CAPD.

Given our current inability to identify the child with the potential for long-term problems, the prudent clinician will ensure that a child with a prolonged history of OM is evaluated for hearing acuity and will have a high degree of suspicion regarding language delay. Speech and language intervention should be considered once the hearing loss has been corrected. Conversely, children with language or speech problems should be evaluated for OM and aggressively managed. Children from lower socioeconomic backgrounds or with mothers with marginal communication skills are at particular risk.

Additional complications of OM are considered in Chapter 17, "Chronic Otitis Media and

Cholesteatoma," and Chapter 18, "Cranial and Intracranial Complications of Acute and Chronic Otitis Media."

RESEARCH DIRECTIONS IN OM

As outlined in this chapter, there are many aspects of OM that are incompletely understood. Challenges abound in diagnosis, treatment, and management. Controversies exist in the timing of intervention or even the need for intervention at all. The basic pathophysiology is beginning to be understood, but there is a great deal of work to be done.

Animal Models of OM

A variety of animal models have been developed to investigate various aspects of OM, including the chinchilla, rat, guinea pig, gerbil, cat, ferret, and cynomolgus (*Macaca fascicularis*), and rhesus monkeys. While there is no one perfect animal model of OM, these models allow for focused investigations and sequential observations. The chinchilla's suitability to OM research has made it perhaps the most widely used animal model for this disease although its widely patulous ET makes it a poor choice for ET studies. The gerbil is an important model for the study of cholesteatoma. The rat is a useful model for secretory OM in studies investigating the role of allergy in OM, and in vaccines trials while its high incidence of naturally occurring OM mandates that results be interpreted with caution. The guinea pig is useful in studying immune-mediated OM, while the cat is used to study ET function and ME changes secondary to OM. Monkeys are excellent models for studying ET function, with rhesus monkeys useful in studying gas absorption process in the ME cavity and the cynomolgus monkey used to study chronic suppurative OM. The ferret's susceptibility to influenza A virus and the close similarity of its ET function to that of the human make a good model to study the relationship of upper respiratory infections and ET dysfunction.

Genetics of OM

The fact that almost every child will have an episode of OM was taken by most observers to indicate that there was not a genetic predisposition to the development of the disease. However, the broad recognition that susceptibility to infectious disease can be genetically determined along with OM-specific evidence from twin studies, particularly the landmark Casselbrant and colleagues studies,[26,27] as well as epidemiological, immunological, and animal studies, have led to the recognition that susceptibility to OM is, at least in part, determined by the genetics of the host. The identification of susceptibility genes will help identify children at increased risk, will provide a clearer understanding of the pathophysiology, and inform new treatment modalities.

Some of the challenges of identifying the OM genes include: (1) It is most likely that numerous genes influence the development of OM, that is, there is not one "OM gene;" (2) multi-generational families with clear diagnoses of OM are not common; and (3) there is likely a high degree of heterogeneity in phenotypes, particularly among various population groups. Despite these challenges, several factors work in the investigators' favor: (1) no *a priori* knowledge of specific susceptibility genes or inheritance patterns is necessary; (2) the human genome sequence is known; (3) genetic markers such as single nucleotide polymorphisms are available; and (4) multiple small families, rather than a few large families, can be used for mapping.

Relationship Between the Host and Bacteria

The relationship between infectious agents and the host is a complex one. The nasopharynx of children is colonized by bacteria that can interact in both an antagonistic and synergistic fashion by a variety of mechanisms, including the production of bacteriocins (a protein toxin produced and released by bacteria that inhibits the growth of similar bacteria). These interactions help maintain balance in the normal endogenous flora. Many children tolerate colonization of the nasopharyx with *S. pneumonia, H. influenzae*, or *M. catarrhalis* without developing OM. How these bacteria change from colonizers to pathogens is poorly understood, but the changes appear to be triggered by viral infections. Preferential colonization of the nasopharynx with microorganisms that have interfering capability, such as alpha-haemolytic streptococci, *Peptostreptococcus anaerobius*, and *Prevotella melaninogenica*, may help prevent the establishment of pathogenic bacteria in the nasopharynx.

In all, these current directions in OM research and an approach based on molecular and cellular techniques will not only provide a broader understanding of the pathogenesis of OM but also novel intervention strategies.

REFERENCES

1. Klein JO. The burden of otitis media. Vaccine 2000;19:S2–8.
2. Nadol JB, Jr, Staecker H, Gliklich RE. Outcomes assessment for chronic otitis media: The Chronic Ear Survey. Laryngoscope 2000;110:32–5.
3. Loveland CJ, Pierce LC, Gregg JB. Ancient temporal bone osteopathology. Ann Otol Rhinol Laryngol 1990;99:146–54.
4. Ruohola A, Meurman O, Nikkari S, et al. Microbiology of acute otitis media in children with tympanostomy tubes: Prevalences of bacteria and viruses. Clin Infect Dis 2006;43:1417–22.
5. Harimaya A, Takada R, Himi T, et al. Evidence of local antibody response against Alloiococcus otitidis in the middle ear cavity of children with otitis media. FEMS Immunol Med Microbiol 2007;49:41–5.
6. Hall-Stoodley L, Hu FZ, Gieseke A, et al. Direct detection of bacterial biofilms on the middle-ear mucosa of children with chronic otitis media. JAMA 2006;296:202–11.
7. Pichichero ME, Poole MD. Comparison of performance by otolaryngologists, pediatricians, and general practioners on an otoendoscopic diagnostic video examination. Int J Pediatr Otorhinolaryngol 2005;69:361–6.
8. Klein JO. Management of otitis media: 2000 and beyond. Pediatr Infect Dis J 2000;19:383–7.
9. Rothman R, Owens T, Simel DL. Does this child have acute otitis media? JAMA 2003;290:1633–40.
10. Kaleida PH, Fireman P. Diagnostic assessment of otitis media. Clin Allergy Immunol 2000;15:247–62.
11. Preston K. Pneumatic otoscopy: A review of the literature. Issues Compr Pediatr Nurs 1998;21:117–28.
12. Discolo CM, Byrd MC, Bates T, et al. Ultrasonic detection of middle ear effusion: A preliminary study. Arch Otolaryngol Head Neck Surg 2004;130.1407–10.
13. Guidelines for the management of otitis media with effusion. Pediatrics 2004;113:1412–29.
14. Poetker DM, Lindstrom DR, Patel NJ, et al. Ofloxacin otic drops vs. neomycin-polymyxin B otic drops as prophylaxis against early postoperative tympanostomy tube otorrhea. Arch Otolaryngol Head Neck Surg 2006;132:1294–8.
15. Pichichero ME. Pathogen shifts and changing cure rates for otitis media and tonsillopharyngits. Clin Pediatr 2006;45:493–502.
16. Pelton SI. Acute otitis media in the era of effective pneumococcal conjugate vaccine: Will new pathogens emerge? Vaccine 2000;19:S96–9.
17. Greenberg DP, Hoberman A. Vaccine prevention of acute otitis media. Curr Allergy Asthma Rep 2001;1:358–63.
18. Rosenfeld RM, Goldsmith AJ, Tetlus L, Balzano A. Quality of life for children with otitis media. Arch Otolaryngol Head Neck Surg 1997;123:1049–54.
19. Bluestone CD. Role of surgery for otitis media in the era of resistant bacteria. Pediatr Infect Dis J 1998;17:1090–8.
20. Urben SL, Nichols RD. Tympanostomies with tubes: The parent perspective. Laryngoscope 1996;106:1269–73.
21. Kogan MD, Overpeck MD, Hoffman HJ, Casselbrant ML. Factors associated with tympanostomy tube insertion among preschool-aged children in the United States. Am J Public Health 2000;90:245–50.
22. Paradise JL, Campbell TF, Dollaghan CA, et al. Developmental outcomes after early or delayed insertion of tympanostomy tubes. N Engl J Med 2005;353:576–86.
23. Cook SP, Deutsch ES, Reilly JS. Alternative indications for laser-assisted tympanic membrane fenestration. Lasers Surg Med 2001;28:320–3.
24. Zuliani G, Carron M, Gurrola J, et al. Identification of adenoid biofilms in chronic rhinosinusitis. Int J Pediatr Otorhinolaryngol 2006;70:1613–7.
25. Bennett KE, Haggard MP, Silva PA, Stewart IA. Behaviour and developmental effects of otitis media with effusion into the teens. Arch Dis Child 2001;85:91–5.
26. Casselbrant ML, Furman JM, Mandel EM, et al. Past history of otitis media and balance in four-year-old children. Laryngoscope 2000;110:773–8.
27. Casselbrant ML, Mandel EM, Fall PA, et al. The heritability of otitis media: A twin and triplet study. JAMA 1999;282:2125–30.
28. Bergmann K. Fatal complications of otitis 60 years ago. HNO 1995;43:478–81.
29. Bakwin H, Jacobinzer H. Prevention of purulent otitis media in infants. J Pediatr 1939;14:730–6.
30. Giebink GS, Le CT. Risk of mastoiditis in typical otitis media not managed by antibiotics. Lancet 1982;1:111.
31. Ellefsen B, Bonding P. Facial palsy in acute otitis media. Clin Otolaryngol Allied Sci 1996;21:393–5.

17

Chronic Otitis Media and Cholesteatoma

Richard A. Chole, MD, PhD
Robert Nason, MD

Otitis media (OM) is broadly defined as inflammation from any cause of the middle ear. This process may involve any of the contiguous pneumatized portions of the temporal bone such as the mastoid or petrous apex. In the United States, it is the most common reason for visits to the pediatrician and is the disease most commonly treated with antibiotics. Overall, healthcare costs related to OM account for approximately $4 billion annually.[1]

In light of this broad definition, OM is classified along a temporal continuum. Acute otitis media (AOM) refers to the rapid onset of middle ear inflammation with its attendant signs and symptoms; this process is termed recurrent AOM (RAOM) when four or more acute episodes occur in a one year period. If fluid accumulates behind an intact tympanic membrane (TM), this process is referred to as otitis media with effusion (OME), secretory otitis media, or "glue ear." The etiology of OME is unclear, but evidence points to eustachian tube dysfunction (primary or secondary), viral infection, or inflammatory sequelae of AOM as probable causes. OME is defined as chronic should the effusion persist for more than 3 months. Chronic OME should be distinguished from "chronic otitis media" (COM). The latter term refers to intractable pathology of greater than 3 months duration within the middle-ear system in the setting of a permanent TM defect. If persistent otorrhea is present, the term chronic suppurative otitis media (CSOM) is applied. TM defects include retraction pockets, atelectasis, and perforations secondary to infection, trauma, or surgery, for example, tympanostomy tubes.

COM can be further subclassified into those cases with or without aural cholesteatoma. Cholesteatomas, the majority of which are complications of COM, are epidermal inclusion cysts within the pneumatized portions of the temporal bone. Cholesteatoma can be classified as either congenital or acquired with the latter variant being further divided into primary or secondary forms to be defined later in the chapter.

EPIDEMIOLOGY AND RISK FACTORS OF COM

OM is most common in the winter and least common in the summer months.[1] Some studies have demonstrated male predominance while incidence rates of OM among white and black American children have shown no differences.[2] Native American and Eskimo populations, however, do experience higher rates of OM. The highest incidence of AOM occurs in the 6- to 11-month age group with ~75% of all infants experiencing an episode by 12 months of age. Furthermore, those children who have their first episode of AOM before 12 months of age are significantly more likely to experience RAOM compared to those who do not. Despite prevalence rates of OME that approach 90% in some populations, studies have demonstrated that the vast majority of cases of AOM and OME resolve spontaneously and without sequelae.[3]

Epidemiological data on COM is elusive due to varying definitions by authors. In regard to CSOM, the highest prevalence rates are found in children of Alaskan Inuits, Native Americans, and Australian Aborigines (7 to 46%). Industrialized countries such as the United States and the United Kingdom boast rates of less than 1%.[4] Sade and others demonstrated that only half of the 200 patients that they studied could remember an acutely painful ear associated with otorrhea; rather, 40% of patients noticed only a slow, gradual onset of otorrhea and possible hearing loss.[5] This explained an average elapsed time of 10 years before disease onset and consultation with an otolaryngologist. Interestingly, one-third of these patients were found to have disease in the contralateral ear. In following 493 patients an average of 6.5 years after surgery for COM, Vartainen and others determined that only 37% of patients had structurally normal contralateral ears whereas only 64% of contralateral ears exhibited normal hearing.[6] Tympanosclerosis and atrophy of the pars tensa were the most common physical findings in the contralateral ear. These findings underscore the morbidity and insidious nature of COM.

Risk factors for OM include mechanical obstruction of the eustachian tube (eg, sinusitis, adenoid hypertrophy, nasopharyngeal carcinoma), immunodeficiency (primary or acquired), ciliary dysfunction, congenital midfacial anomalies (eg, cleft palate, Down syndrome), and gastroesophageal reflux.[7] Environmental factors such as number of hours spent in child daycare, passive exposure to smoke, lack of breastfeeding in infancy, and low socioeconomic status have all been implicated in higher OM rates.[1] Significant risk factors for CSOM include history of RAOM, parents with histories of COM, and crowded daycare settings.[8] No studies have established links between CSOM and breastfeeding, gender, or smoke exposure. Allergy has been implicated as a risk factor since some studies have demonstrated allergens to cause eustachian tube and nasal obstruction; however, middle-ear effusions were never seen to develop. Furthermore, studies involving antihistamines, directed at an allergic cause for OM, have failed to show any benefit in alleviating OME.[2]

Recent studies now highlight genetic predisposition to OM. Casselbrant and colleagues, in a prospective study of 168 sets of twins and 7 sets of triplets, have demonstrated a significantly higher correlation for proportion of time with middle-ear effusion in monozygotic twins compared to dizygotic twins.[9] Furthermore, in patients suffering from RAOM due to *Streptococcus pneumoniae*, polymorphisms have recently been found in antibody receptors to certain IgG subclass molecules which inhibit leukocyte phagocytosis of antibody-coated bacteria.[10] Failure to kill invading bacteria would permit both disease establishment and progression. Other studies point to polymorphisms in cytokine production as predisposing to OM. Respiratory syncytial virus (RSV) is commonly found in OME and AOM isolates and is regarded as a copathogenic factor in OM from the standpoint of specific eustachian tube dysfunction and generalized upper airway edema. In one study of 77 infants with RSV, Gentile and others demonstrated an association between low interferon-gamma (IFN-γ) production and OM.[11] Thus, patients with this polymorphism would possess increased risk of developing OM and its sequelae.

MICROBIOLOGY OF COM

Bacteria reach the middle ear via the external auditory canal in the presence of a TM defect or retrograde through the nasopharnyx. It is well established that *Streptococcus pneumoniae* is the most common microorganism isolated from AOM samples, followed by *Haemophilus influenzae*, *Moraxella catarrhalis*, and group A streptococci. These same microorganisms have been isolated from chronic OME samples with polymerase chain reaction (PCR) techniques, demonstrating at the very least the presence of bacterial genomic DNA in effusion samples.[12]

The bacteria isolated in COM and infected cholesteatomas differ markedly from those found in AOM or chronic OME. In CSOM isolates, aerobic and anaerobic bacteria are involved, coexisting in half of cases. The most common aerobic bacteria isolated are *Pseudomonas aeruginosa*, *Staphylococcus aureus*, and other gram-negative bacilli, for example, *Escherichia coli*, *Proteus* species, and *Klebsiella* species. *Pseudomonas aeruginosa* is known to reside in the moist environment of the external auditory canal, whereas *S. aureus* is universally harbored within human nares. The proximity of these bacteria reflects the likelihood of their eventual presence within the middle ear, either as contaminants or bonafide pathogens. *Bacteroides* spp. and *Fusobacterium* spp. are the most common anaerobic bacteria isolated. Furthermore, fungi are frequently found within CSOM samples, specifically *Aspergillus* spp. and *Candida* spp. There is some speculation that fungi may result as overgrowth after initial treatment with antibiotic drops.

PATHOGENESIS OF COM

COM is characterized by pathological findings consistent with irreversible inflammatory changes within the middle ear and mastoid. The sequence of events which result in these changes are unclear mostly due to the silent nature of this disease and, hence, the amount of time that elapses before attention is sought. In a temporal bone study of chronically infected ears with either intact or perforated TMs, da Costa and colleagues demonstrated almost universal presence of both granulation tissue and ossicular bony changes in either group.[13] This highlights the fact that significant disease may exist despite the presence of an intact TM.

Undoubtedly, dysfunction of the eustachian tube plays a prominent role in both AOM and COM. The eustachian tube opens to the contraction of the tensor veli palatini muscle during swallowing and, under physiologic conditions, is responsible for clearance of middle ear secretions into the nasopharynx, prevention of nasopharyngeal secretions from refluxing into the middle ear, and pressure equalization between the middle ear and the external environment. Obstruction of the eustachian tube functionally (eg, cleft palate, paradoxical constriction) or mechanically (eg, mucoid secretions, edema, neoplasm, nasogastric tube, adenoid hypertrophy) results in lowering of the normally negative middle ear pressure due to increased nitrogen absorption into middle ear subepithelial mixed venous blood. This results in transudation of serous fluid into the middle ear cleft. Also, nasopharyngeal bacteria are more readily introduced into the middle ear upon tubal opening as they are in the settings of a shorter tube (eg, infant) or a perforated TM. Other factors thought to promote tubal dysfunction are gastroesophageal reflux or virally induced ciliary transport deficiencies of middle ear secretions by middle ear epithelium.

Once bacteria enter the middle ear via the nasopharynx or a TM defect, bacterial replication ensues within a serous effusion. Concomitantly, an immune response is triggered within an intact host, releasing immune and inflammatory mediators into the middle ear space. The hyperemia and polymorphonuclear leukocyte-dominated acute inflammatory phase gives way to a chronic phase, characterized by a shift toward mononuclear cellular mediators (eg, macrophages, plasma cells, lymphocytes), persistent edema, and granulation tissue. Furthermore, metaplasia of the middle ear epithelium may occur, converting cuboidal epithelium to a pseudostratified columnar epithelium capable of increased mucoid secretion.[14] Granulation tissue becomes increasingly fibrotic, eventually forming adhesions to important structures within the middle ear. This can disturb aeration of the antrum and mastoid by decreasing space between the ossicles and mucosa which separate the middle ear from the antrum. Chronic obstruction leads to irreversible changes within both bone and mucosa of these structures.

Whether COM results as a continuation of AOM is a matter of debate. On 1 hand, AOM is much more prevalent than COM and most perforations secondary to AOM resolve spontaneously and without consequences. On the other hand, studies have shown degeneration of the fibrous layers of the TM lamina propria in the setting of OME or RAOM, thereby weakening this structure.[5] In a study by Yoon and colleagues of temporal bones with or without OM, retraction of the TM was not found at all in those samples without OM.[15] In the OM group, however, retraction was present in the OME group (2.1%) and to a significantly greater degree in those samples with COM (19.5%). Exposure of a progressively weakening TM to increased negative middle ear pressure in the setting of eustachian tube dysfunction would drive the TM medially, causing retraction pockets (see Figure 1). Further TM weakening or destruction may result in middle-ear atelectasis, adhesive otitis, perforation, and acquired cholesteatoma.

MIDDLE EAR ATELECTASIS AND ADHESIVE OM

Middle ear atelectasis is a variant of COM and refers to TM retraction onto the promontory and ossicles of the middle ear (see Figure 2). The most likely reason for this phenomenon is increased negative middle ear pressure from eustachian tube dysfunction.

To accommodate for an increase in negative middle ear pressure, the drumhead moves medially to decrease middle ear volume. This action is in accordance with Boyle's law which states that pressure multiplied by volume must be constant.

Further medial displacement is possible if TM atrophy occurs with loss of the fibrous layer; this is usually secondary to repeated infection or persistent middle ear effusion.[5] Obliteration of the middle ear space may be complete or partial but, importantly, is potentially reversible and does not involve changes to the lining middle ear mucosa. Should a medially retracted TM completely obliterate the middle ear space and irreversibly replace the normal mucosa by adhering to the bony promontory, the term adhesive OM is applied. Several authors have included atelectasis and adhesive OM in a staging system of TM retraction with each stage representing progressive loss of the TM fibrous layer: stage I, retracted TM; stage II, retraction with contact of the incus; stage III, middle ear atelectasis; stage IV, adhesive OM.[5,16] Ossicular contact from such retraction may cause bony erosion, particularly of the long process of the incus and the stapes.

Another important factor in the development of atelectasis and COM is mastoid pneumatization. The mastoid is a pneumatized space connected to the middle ear which is invariably hypopneumatized in the setting of COM. Like the middle ear, it also behaves as a pressure buffer to counteract pressure changes within the middle ear (ie, Boyle's law). In this closed system, Sadé and others have demonstrated that smaller mastoids

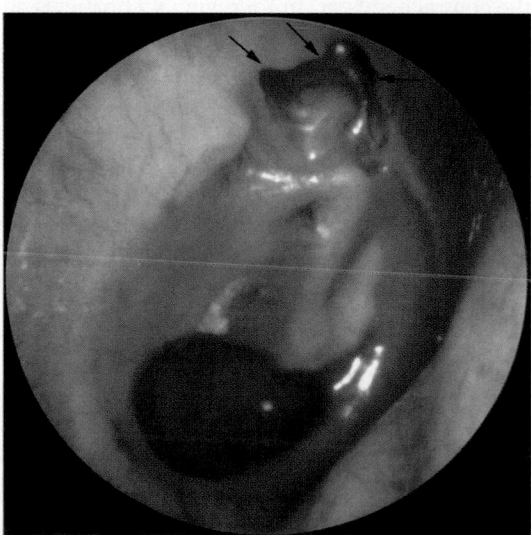

Figure 1 Severe chronic otitis media with effusion with extreme pars flaccida retraction and an attic retraction pocket (*arrows*). In this photo there is also retraction of the inferior portion of the pars tensa.

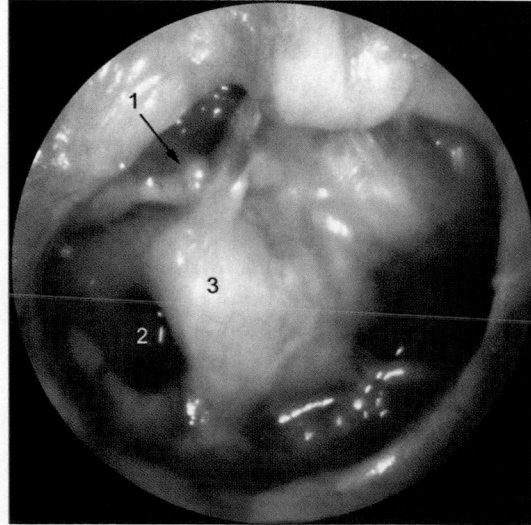

Figure 2 Severe middle ear atelectasis due to chronic eustachian tube dysfunction. In this case, the thinned tympanic membrane is adherent to the stapes (1), the round window niche (2) and the promontory (3). (Adapted from reference 17.)

are the weakest pressure buffers, thereby increasing the sensitivity of the TM to increased negative middle ear pressures.[18] Thus, the TM is more prone to displacement in COM which may help explain why atelectatic drums can also balloon out in the same patient.[19]

Unequivocally, patients with chronic middle ear disease have poorly aerated mastoids. Controversy exists as to whether chronic infection leads to mastoid maldevelopment or whether smaller, maldeveloped mastoids predispose to COM. In support of the former theory, a recent 5-year follow-up study of infants with RAOM or chronic OME treated with tympanostomy tubes demonstrated that those requiring increased numbers of ventilation tubes, increased frequency of tubes, and with pars tensa retraction had significantly decreased mastoid air cell system sizes.[20]

COM with Tympanostomy Tubes

Tympanostomy tubes have been used as a means of mitigating middle ear effusions, retractions, and atelectasis in the hope of achieving return of the TM to its normal physiologic position. As defined earlier, COM can occur from a spontaneous TM perforation or as a result of tympanostomy tube placement. As many as 80% of patients experience at least 1 episode of otorrhea after tube placement and approximately 5% of patients experience chronic tympanostomy tube otorrhea.[21] Antibiotic topical solutions administered at the time of tube placement decreases the incidence of postoperative otorrhea.[22] Furthermore, silver oxide-impregnated tympanostomy tubes have been shown to decrease subsequent otorrhea by 50%.[23] In cases of CSOM, the same microorganisms as found in COM populations are isolated. Unfortunately, it remains unclear whether ventilation tubes propagate chronic infections. In support of this possibility, a small percentage of TM perforations persist after tympanostomy tube removal. Also, the recent identification of biofilms within tympanostomy tubes would invariably lead to chronicity and difficulty in eradicating any established infection.[24,25]

CHOLESTEATOMA

The term cholesteatoma was first coined by Johannes Müller in 1838 to describe what we now understand to be epidermal inclusion cysts of the pneumatized portions of the temporal bone.[26] As such, keratinizing stratified squamous epithelium is found ectopically within the middle ear, an area typified by low cuboidal epithelium. The squamous epithelium comprises the "matrix" of the cholesteatoma which rests above the "perimatrix" that contains inflamed fibrous tissue. In contrast to the name, cholesteatomas do not contain fat or cholesterol within their matrices. Their appearance, described as "pearly tumors" by Cruveilhier in 1829, relates rather to the desquamated keratin debris produced by the squamous epithelium which lines these cysts.[27] Other than the congenital variant, cholesteatomas are usually

the result of COM and, therefore, possess its attendant inflammatory changes such as granulation tissue. In studies by da Costa and Sadé, approximately 10% of COM ears were complicated by cholesteatoma.[5,13] The significance of cholesteatoma is based upon its propensity to erode the bony structures of the temporal bone.

Epidemiology of Cholesteatoma

The exact prevalence of cholesteatoma is not known. Acquired cholesteatoma complicates approximately 10% of COM cases and is more likely to arise from COM ears with TM perforations than those without perforations.[13] The annual incidence of cholesteatoma is low, ranging from 3 to 12 cases per 100,000 population. It is slightly more common in males and Caucasians and rarely seen in Asian populations. Although the Alaskan Inuit population has a large predilection for COM, they, interestingly, have low prevalence rates for cholesteatoma. Reasons for this are unclear. Children typically present approximately at 5 years of age with congenital variants and at 10 years with acquired cholesteatomas.[28]

Pathogenesis of Cholesteatoma

Cholesteatoma can be classified as either congenital or acquired. Acquired cholesteatomas are further divided into primary or secondary forms. Cholesteatomas can also be classified according to their sites of origin. Attic cholesteatomas begin from pars flaccida retraction and usually spread to the aditus or mastoid. Sinus cholesteatoma refers to those arising from posterosuperior retraction or perforation of the pars tensa. Tensa cholesteatoma refers to cholesteatoma arising from retraction of the entire pars tensa.

Congenital Cholesteatoma. When cholesteatoma arises behind an intact TM without history of otorrhea, the term congenital cholesteatoma is used (see Figure 3). Congenital cholesteatomas arise from keratinizing epithelium within the middle ear cleft. Unfortunately, the origin of this epithelium is the source of much speculation; furthermore, proof of causation has not

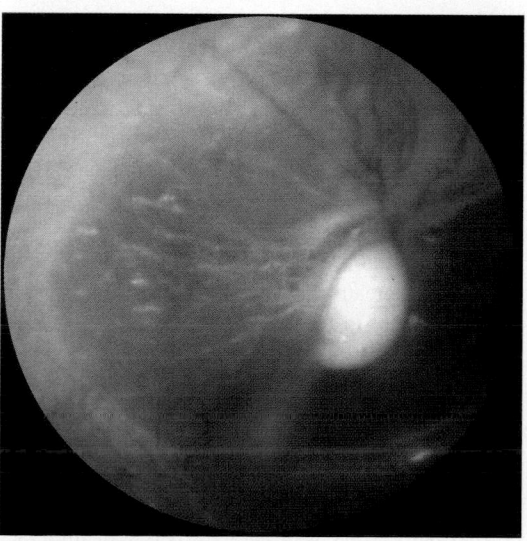

Figure 3 Congenital cholesteatoma.

been established from any of the proposed theories. It is possible that middle ear mucosa may undergo squamous metaplasia or that external canal squamous epithelium may migrate through TM microperforations. Another possibility is that of middle ear space deposition of desquamated epithelial cells from amniotic fluid during fetal development. Yet another theory proposes that squamous epithelial cells may implant onto the malleus or incus from early TM retraction. The most widely accepted theory is that of failure of involution of keratinizing epithelium. It has been established that small tufts of squamous epithelium are normally found within the anterosuperior portion of the middle ear cleft; furthermore, these tufts undergo normal transition into normal middle ear mucosa. In support of this theory, Michaels discovered squamous tufts that he termed "epidermoid formations" in the anterosuperior portion of the middle ear in 37 of 68 temporal bones from fetuses between 10 and 33 weeks of gestation.[29] These epidermoid formations have also now been found in infants and children. Failure of the epidermoid formation to involute could possibly account for the anterosuperior location of most congenital cholesteatomas.

Congenital cholesteatomas typically develop in the anterosuperior quadrant of the middle ear; thereafter, they spread to the posterosuperior quadrant and gain access to the antrum and mastoid. A useful classification system developed by Potsic and others exists in which stage advancement correlates directly with risk of residual disease: stage I, cholesteatoma limited to one quadrant; stage II, involving multiple quadrants without ossicular involvement; stage III, ossicular involvement without mastoid extension; stage IV, mastoid involvement.[30]

Acquired Cholesteatoma. Primary acquired cholesteatoma refers to cholesteatoma that arises from simple retraction of the pars flaccida (see Figure 4). Secondary acquired cholesteatoma refers to cholesteatoma that arises in the setting of TM perforation, usually in the posterosuperior quadrant of the middle ear (see Figure 5). There are 4 main theories proposed to account for acquired cholesteatoma etiopathogenesis: (1) TM invagination; (2) migration of epithelium through a TM perforation; (3) basal cell hyperplasia; and (4) squamous metaplasia (see Figure 6). A fifth mechanism, implantation, is also established and requires little explanation. In the case of implantation, squamous epithelial cells are displaced into the middle ear space either iatrogenically (eg, tympanoplasty, tympanostomy tube placement) or traumatically. This is an uncommon mechanism; for example, the prevalence of cholesteatoma following ventilation tube placement is less than 1%.

Invagination Theory. This theory is widely accepted as the most likely mechanism for primary acquired or attic cholesteatomas. In this setting, the TM becomes retracted further medially into the middle ear secondary to increased negative middle ear pressure. The reasons for

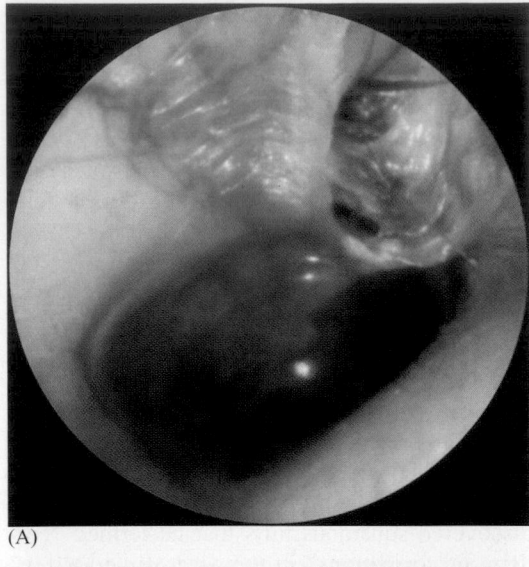

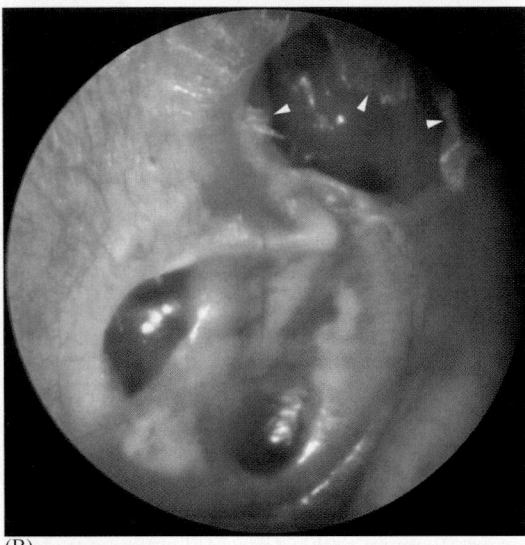

Figure 4 Primary acquired cholesteatoma. Arrowheads denote attic retration.

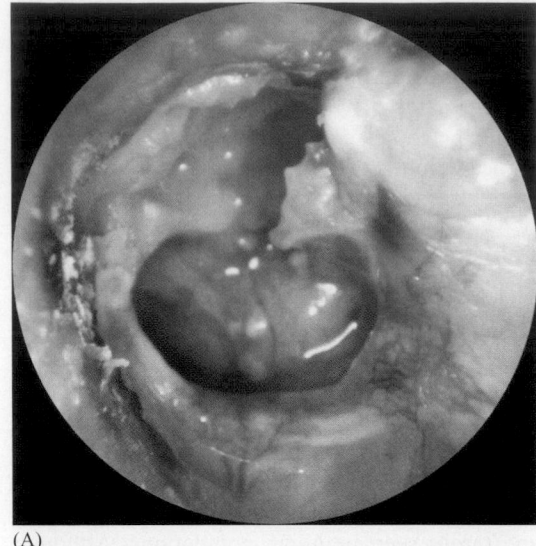

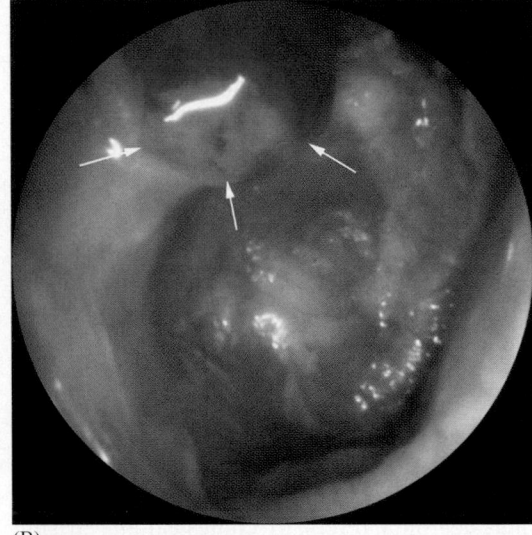

Figure 5 Secondary acquired cholesteatoma. Granulation tissue is very common (*arrows*).

medial displacement are the same as those that have been established for COM in general: eustachian tube dysfunction, inflammation, TM atrophy, and poor mastoid pneumatization. Wolfman and Chole, for example, demonstrated cholesteatoma development in 75% of gerbils 16 weeks after experimental bilateral eustachian tube obstruction.[31] Although this process typically occurs in the pars flaccida due to its inherent weakness from lack of a fibrous layer, any portion of the TM can be involved. As the retraction pocket progressively deepens, the squamous epithelial cells lining the retraction pocket continually release keratin debris into its center. This is compounded by alteration of normal epithelial cell migration that results in a functionally closed cyst that can no longer drain its desquamated keratin debris. Instead, the growing cyst expands into the middle-ear system and gives the prototypical appearance of a posterosuperior TM defect. Although the TM is intact in the case of a retraction pocket, it may give the appearance of a marginal perforation. Retraction pockets, especially of the attic, must be considered precursors to cholesteatoma and demand close observation.

Epithelial Invasion. Squamous epithelium of the external auditory canal and the outer margin of the TM has the ability to migrate into the middle ear across TM perforations. It has also been established that epithelium will advance until confronted by another epithelial surface, a term called contact inhibition. If middle ear mucosa either along the medial portion of the TM or further into the middle ear space were to be disrupted by inflammation, infection, or trauma in the setting of a TM defect, the mucocutaneous junction could theoretically shift into the middle ear space. In support of this theory, van Blitterswijk and others determined that cytokeratin (CK) 10, an intermediate filament protein and marker of squamous epithelium, could be found in external meatal epidermis and cholesteatoma matrix but not in middle ear mucosa.[32] Marginal perforations are understood to be more likely to lead to epidermal ingrowth than central perforations, most likely because perforation at this site exposes the middle ear mucosa and bony canal wall structures to the external ear canal. Central TM perforations, however, should not be disregarded as safe ears. In a recent analysis of central TM perforations from COM patients,

38% of perforations were found to have significant epidermal ingrowth with the mucocutaneous junction located beyond the inner surface of the perforation.[33] This rate is comparable to studies involving both marginal and central perforations.

Basal Cell Hyperplasia. In 1925, Lange observed that keratinizing epithelial cells of the pars flaccida could invade the normally inaccessible subepithelial space to form attic cholesteatomas.[34] Furthermore, Huang and colleagues have shown that TM injury via propylene glycol application results in middle ear epithelial ingrowth in a chinchilla model.[35] For keratinzing epithelial cells to reach the lamina propria of the TM and form epithelial cones, they must travel through disruptions of the basal lamina.[36] Once within the subepithelial connective tissue, entrapped epithelial cones are equivalent to microcholesteatomas, essentially keratin-producing cysts with the potential to expand and form larger cholesteatomas. Upon secondary perforation of the TM, a typical attic cholesteatoma would be seen.

Squamous Metaplasia. Chronically infected or inflamed tissues are known to undergo metaplastic transformation (eg, esophagus, bronchus). Similarly, the cuboidal epithelium of the middle ear may undergo transformation into keratinizing epithelium. Keratinizing squamous epithelium has been found in middle ear biopsies of pediatric patients with OM as well as in middle ears of rats deprived of vitamin A.[37] However, progression to cholesteatoma has yet to be established.

Inflammation and Hyperproliferation. The epithelium of cholesteatoma, while not neoplastic, is hyperproliferative. Involucrin, the precursor to cornified envelope formation at the uppermost layers of the epidermis, is found only in high suprabasal layers of normal skin. In cholesteatoma, however, involucrin is found in all suprabasal layers, resulting in much higher accumulation of keratin within a larger portion of the epidermis. Studies have also demonstrated increased expression of proliferative markers in basal and suprabasal layers of the epidermis: CK 4, CK 5/6, CK 10, CK 13/16, epidermal growth factor receptor (EGFR), keratinocyte growth factor (KGF), and Ki-67.[28] Abnormal distribution of p53, c-jun, and, c-myc expression are also implicated in the hyperproliferative process. Recently, studies using cDNA array technology have identified many more genes with possible roles in cholesteatoma development.[38] These include calgranulin A/B, thymosin, and extracellular matrix protein-1.

Another important factor in the hyperproliferative process is the invariable presence of chronic inflammation. The stroma of the cholesteatoma possesses fibroblasts, Langerhans cells, mast cells, activated lymphocytes, macrophages, and keratinocytes. Furthermore, keratinocytes produce large amounts of keratin. Inflammation with or without infection recruits these cell types to create a milieu with increased concentrations of proinflammatory cytokines. Such an environment is known to stimulate basal keratinocytes

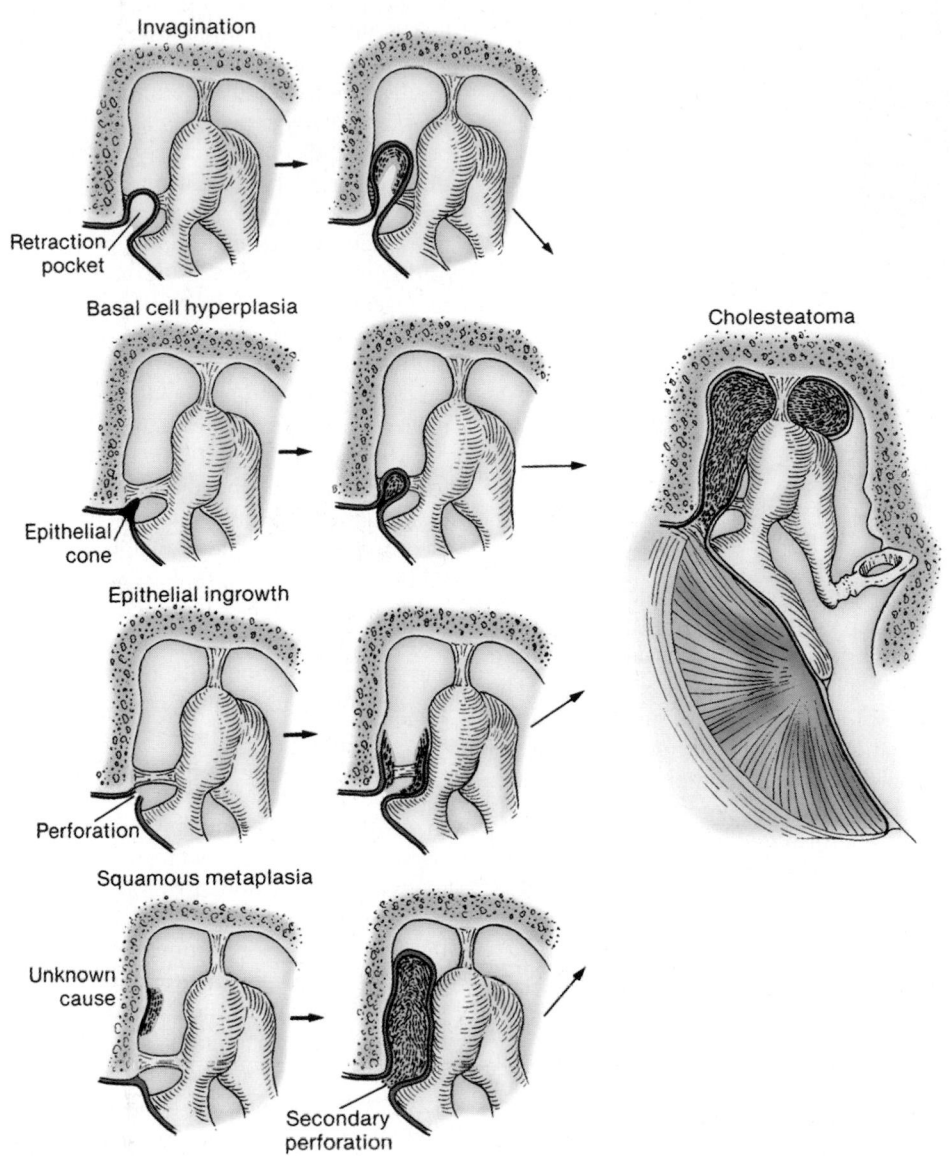

Figure 6 Acquired cholesteatoma pathogenesis.

a dynamic organ constantly being remodeled to achieve both calcium homeostasis and structural integrity. Matrix synthesis is carried out by osteoblasts while osteoclasts dictate resorption. Osteoclasts are multinucleated specialized cells of the macrophage/monocyte family which arise from the fusion of mononuclear precursors that have attached to bone. More importantly, they are the cell capable of bone resorption in the human body.[42] Pathologic conditions which favor inappropriate osteoclast activation overturn this balance and result in excess erosion of bony structures. In established cases of COM with or without cholesteatoma, bone erosion is almost invariably present and represents the major source of morbidity. As opposed to pressure necrosis or proteolytic factor secretion by components of the cholesteatoma matrix, it is now clear that resorption occurs, as in other inflammatory conditions, via the action of osteoclasts.

Recently, osteoclast formation from precursor cells has been discovered to be under the control of 2 essential cytokines: receptor activator of nuclear factor-κB ligand (RANKL) and macrophage colony-stimulating factor (M-CSF). Normally, osteoblasts produce M-CSF and RANKL to initiate osteoclast formation by engaging the c-Fms and RANK receptors on osteoclast precursors, respectively (see Figure 7).

In pathologic conditions, other cell types participate in the production of these cytokines. An important inhibitor of this process is osteoprotegrin (OPG), a soluble decoy receptor of the tumor necrosis factor (TNF) superfamily that competes with RANK for RANKL (see Figure 7). Jeong and others have recently demonstrated nonspecific overall higher counts of RANKL-producing cells in cholesteatoma compared to normal postauricular skin; conversely, normal skin had a significantly higher rate of cells expressing OPG.[43] These results reveal that cholesteatoma tissue possesses an increased RANKL/OPG ratio due to inflammation and very likely potentiates osteoclastogenesis.

A hallmark feature of COM with or without cholesteatoma is chronically inflamed tissue near bony structures. As such, inflammatory cytokines (eg, interleukin-1 (IL-1), IL-6, tumor necrosis factor-alpha (TNF-α)) and prostaglandins are elaborated in a microenvironment composed of keratinocytes, macrophages, lymphocytes, fibroblasts, osteoblasts, and other cell types. These cytokines are upregulated in cholesteatoma tissue and are also known to promote osteoclastogenesis by either direct or indirect effects on osteoclasts. IL-1 and TNF-α, for example, promote osteoclast formation, increase osteoclast survival, and increase bone resorption by mature osteoclasts. In addition to osteoblasts, lymphocytes (eg, B and T cells) contribute largely to inflammatory osteolysis by generating RANKL themselves (both soluble and membrane-bound) in the inflammatory microenvironment.[44]

Infected cholesteatomas are known to act aggressively and erode bone more quickly. Elevated levels of bacterial virulence factors likely

into active proliferation and lead to cholesteatoma growth.

Biofilms. In addition to being found within tympanostomy tubes, biofilms have also recently been demonstrated within human cholesteatoma and COM middle ear epithelium.[39,40] Biofilms are bacterial aggregates in which planktonic, free-floating bacteria join other bacteria to form sessile, stationary communities. In the environment, most bacteria exist as biofilms. Via quorum sensing genes, bacteria communicate with one another to express genes and products that afford protection to the community as a whole. This translates into lower total energy requirements, increased ability to survive in otherwise inhospitable niches, and encasement in matrices composed mostly of polysaccharides and extracellular DNA. This community is in constant flux, with microorganisms detaching and rejoining when opportunities or energy needs arise. The extracellular matrix dramatically decreases antibiotic penetration, thereby minimizing bacterial exposure to these drugs. Furthermore, bacteria in biofilms are

capable of altering their individual phenotypes, switching to those possessing increased antibiotic resistance. In turn, the presence of a biofilm within an infection leads to extreme difficulty in cure and invariable chronicity, as antibiotics usually prove ineffective in the long run.

In the setting of a biofilm infection, antigenic bacterial components such as lipopolysaccharide (LPS) or peptidoglycan would be intermittently reintroduced into the middle ear system by re-entrant bacteria, establishing chronicity of infection and inflammation. This scenario, for example, could explain why, after antibiotic administration, purulent otorrhea typically recurs in infected cholesteatomas or colonized tympanostomy tubes. This inflammatory microenvironment would exert its effects on downstream middle ear and cholesteatoma components, further propagating the well-known consequences of COM and cholesteatoma.

Bone Resorption

It is estimated that 10% of the total bone content is replaced per year in adult humans.[41] Bone is

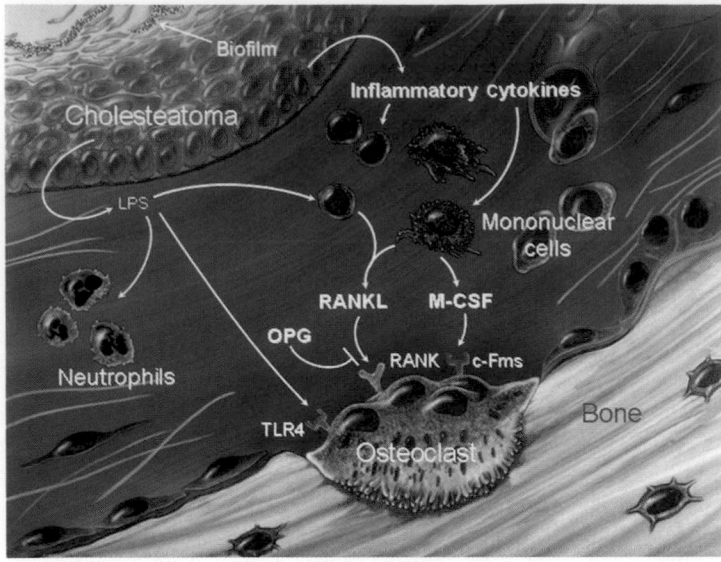

Figure 7 Signaling mechanisms involved in inflammatory osteolysis.

play key roles in this phenomenon. Biofilms also contribute to increased concentrations of virulence factors since they represent a safe niche from which bacteria or their antigenic components can re-emerge (see Figure 7). In support of this Peek and others have recently demonstrated higher concentrations of LPS in samples from patients with otorrhea and bone resorption secondary to cholesteatoma.[45] LPS is the main antigenic component of gram-negative bacterial cell walls (eg, *Pseudomonas aeruginosa*) and is a well-characterized virulence factor known to powerfully stimulate the immune system.

Eukaryotic microorganisms use a family of receptors called toll-like receptors (TLRs) to sense diverse populations of microbial pathogens. TLRs recognize common bacterial structures, allowing quick tailor-made responses to pathogens. Studies have recently demonstrated that TLR4 is the TLR responsible for detecting LPS from gram-negative bacteria. Via TLR4, LPS is known to promote the release of inflammatory cytokines from monocytes, osteoblasts, and lymphocytes (see Figure 7). LPS is also known to induce RANKL release by certain cell types and to promote osteoclast formation. The mechanisms by which this occurs is currently under investigation.

COMPLICATIONS OF COM AND CHOLESTEATOMA

The most common complication of COM is conductive hearing loss, typically ranging from 20 to 60 dB. This may be caused by one of many noninfectious sequelae of COM, namely TM perforation, middle-ear atelectasis, tympanosclerosis, ossicular disruption, and cholesteatoma. Although conductive hearing loss predominates, infectious and inflammatory components may also be transmitted to the inner ear via the round window resulting in cochlear damage and hearing loss. Other important noninfectious sequelae include facial paralysis and cholesterol granuloma. Infectious complications include subperiosteal abscess, mastoiditis, CSOM,

labyrinthitis, petrositis, and intracranial infection, eg, encephalitis, meningitis, brain parenchymal abscess, subdural empyema, sigmoid sinus thrombophlebitis, extradural abscess. The significance of hearing loss and subsequent auditory deprivation, especially in children, remains a major topic of interest. Although poorer attention, speech perception, and expression skills have been demonstrated in children, the final impact on their language and cognitive development remains unclear.

The main complications accounting for the morbidity of cholesteatoma arise from destruction of nearby bony structures. These include the ossicles, the otic capsule, facial nerve canal, tegmen tympani, and tegmen mastoideum. Infections of cholesteatomas are also a common complication and tend to be recurrent. This results in purulent otorrhea and inflammatory damage to structures that infected cholesteatoma tissue may abut. Conductive hearing loss typically results from erosion of the incus. Erosion of the otic capsule, most commonly involving the lateral semicircular canal, can result in labyrinthine fistula, vertigo, or infectious sequelae such as suppurative labyrinthitis. Fistula, labyrinthitis or cochlear erosion may result in sensorineural hearing loss. Facial nerve paralysis may result from nerve invasion after erosion through the facial nerve canal or from infectious involvement of cholesteatoma tissue that abuts the facial nerve. Cerebrospinal fluid leakage and brain herniations can result from erosion of either tegmen.

Diagnosis of COM

The diagnosis of COM with or without cholesteatoma is usually made based on the history and physical examination. Evaluation should elicit prior history of middle ear disease and surgical interventions. Although COM and cholesteatoma may be diagnosed incidentally in asymptomatic patients, symptoms including hearing loss, otorrhea, otalgia, nasal obstruction, tinnitus, and vertigo may prompt the patient to seek medical attention. Of these presenting symptoms, hearing loss and otorrhea are by far the most common.

CSOM presents with a profuse, viscous otorrhea that is intermittent in nature. On the other hand, patients with infected cholesteatoma present with small amounts of foul-smelling, purulent otorrhea. Otalgia usually represents a secondary external otitis and will conceal underlying pathology of the middle ear. For this reason, follow-up evaluation with thorough canal debridement is imperative after an acute flare-up to properly visualize middle-ear pathology. Alternatively, pain may represent an intracranial sequela of cholesteatoma. Other symptoms of possible sequelae include bloody otorrhea in advanced disease, vertigo from a labyrinthine fistula, facial nerve paralysis, or neurologic symptoms from intracranial spread.

The diagnosis of COM and aural cholesteatoma can usually be made on otomicroscopic examination given that the ear is properly cleansed of debris and drainage. It is also important to evaluate the nasopharynx in these patients, as eustachian tube dysfunction is a common cause of COM in many cases. In regard to the ear, the microscope will allow visualization of the drumhead to identify perforations, retraction pockets, cholesteatoma, and granulation tissue. If a TM perforation is present and large enough, middle ear mucosa may be assessed for evidence of inflammation and infection; furthermore, some or all of the ossicles may be visible and assessed for erosion, fixation, or disruption. A primary acquired cholesteatoma will be seen in the posterosuperior portion of the TM as a pearl-white defect containing keratin debris, whereas a secondary acquired cholesteatoma will be found next to a TM perforation (see Figures 4 and 5). Alternatively, a congenital cholesteatoma may be seen as a white mass behind the anterosuperior quadrant of an intact TM if discovered before secondary TM perforation (see Figure 3).

Granulation tissue is the most common finding associated with COM and is a consequence of inflammation (see Figure 5). Sometimes polyps herald the presence of cholesteatoma; they represent granulation tissue at the junction between the cholesteatoma and eroding bone and may be seen extending as far as the external meatus in advanced cases.

Most commonly, patients complain of progressive unilateral worsening of their hearing status. Audiometric evaluation including air and bone thresholds as well as speech discrimination testing is imperative. Test results can additionally be correlated with Weber and Rinne tests performed with a 512 Hz tuning fork. The reduction in hearing is determined by the extent of middle ear disease as related to the status of the TM, ossicles, and the middle-ear mucosa. A perforation of the TM will result in a conductive hearing loss of about 15 dB, whereas a loss of 50 dB is possible if a TM perforation is accompanied by disruption of the ossicular chain. Perforations of the posterior TM that expose the round window membrane will also result in more severe conductive hearing loss because the TM no longer shields the round window from sound, the so-called "baffle effect." Conductive hearing loss will also result from changes to the ossicles. Erosion of ossicles with subsequent discontinuity may result from atelectasis, adhesive OM, inflammation, or cholesteatoma growth. Alternatively, ossicular fixation may be the root cause. Fixation of the stapes footplate is well known to occur in cases of middle ear tympanosclerosis that has reached the oval window. Additionally, fixation of the incudostapedial joint arises commonly as a postinflammatory consequence. If granulation tissue within the middle ear space inhibits ossicular mobility, conductive hearing loss can also be expected. Of note, granulation tissue or cholesteatoma that has eroded much of the ossicular chain may only cause minimal hearing loss if sound is able to be transmitted through these lesions to reach the inner ear via the stapes or footplate.

In any patient with findings suggestive of COM or cholesteatoma, and especially those presenting with vestibular symptoms, pneumatic otoscopy is imperative. A positive fistula test characterized by vertigo and nystagmus suggests inner ear involvement and need for urgent intervention.

Imaging. Although imaging is usually unnecessary for uncomplicated cases of COM or cholesteatoma due to eventual surgical exposure, high-resolution computed tomography (CT) and magnetic resonance imaging (MRI) of the temporal bones may provide supplementary information. In addition to complementing the clinical examination, imaging characterizes the extent of disease and may also identify cholesteatoma in asymptomatic patients. Although CT is considered the "gold standard" for imaging cholesteatoma, it lacks specificity due to difficulty in distinguishing cholesteatoma from granulation tissue or edema, especially when bony erosion is absent. On CT, cholesteatoma will appear as a lesion with smooth, sharp margins that does not enhance upon intravenous contrast administration (see Figure 8). When bone erosion is concurrently identified, CT can identify a nondependent mass as cholesteatoma with 80% specificity. CT is also useful in highlighting surrounding anatomical features such as temporal bone pneumatization or the presence of a low-lying tegmen mastoideum. Furthermore, it is extremely useful in revision cases in delineating altered anatomy and recurrent disease.

On MRI, cholesteatoma will appear with low signal intensity on T1-weighted images and high signal intensity on T2-weighted images (see Figure 9).

In addition to being nonspecific in diagnosing cholesteatoma like CT, air and bone are indistinguishable on MRI making delineation of bony details difficult. However, if intracranial complication is suspected, eg, lateral sinus thrombosis, MRI with gadolinium is extremely valuable due to its superiority in visualizing soft tissue densities. It is also effective in diagnosing disease extension into the petrous apex.

Tympanosclerosis

Tympanosclerosis refers to the deposition of acellular hyalin within the TM or middle ear

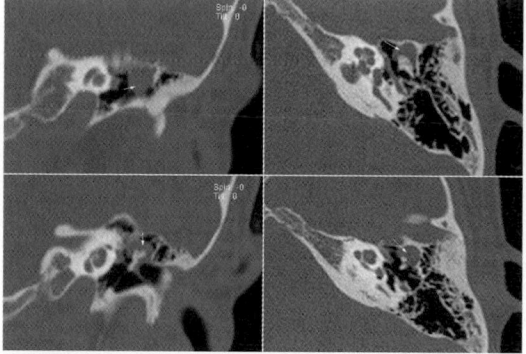

Figure 8 High resolution computed tomographic imaging of a left-sided primary acquired cholesteatoma. Note the cholesteatoma, seen as a soft tissue density mass (white arrow), enveloping the middle ear ossicles on both axial (right) and coronal (left) images.

submucosa as a result of OM or trauma. Sometimes, tympanosclerotic lesions are also calcified. If the process is isolated to the TM, the term myringosclerosis is used. On otoscopic examination, white crescent- or horseshoe-shaped plaques are seen in the TM (see Figure 9). Most cases are incidentally identified and asymptomatic. If tympanosclerosis extends into the middle ear cleft, however, the ossicles are at risk and conductive hearing loss may occur (see Figure 10).

Pathogenesis. Tympanosclerosis results as a consequence of RAOM, COM, or tympanostomy tube placement. In one study by Jaisinghani and others, 52 (35%) of 150 temporal bones from COM patients demonstrated myringosclerosis.[46] In a study of 146 children with bilateral OME who were treated with adenoidectomy, right-sided tympanostomy tube placement, and left-sided myringotomy, Tos and Stangerup demonstrated that 59% of right ears that underwent tube placement had tympanosclerosis while only 13% of left-sided ears had the same finding.[47]

The exact pathogenesis of tympanosclerosis remains unclear. Microscopically, tympanosclerosis is characterized by acellular hyaline degeneration of the lamina propria of the TM, middle ear, and mastoid mucosa. This may progress to

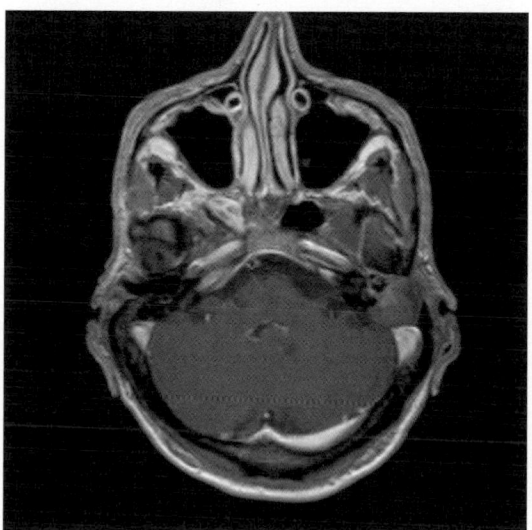

Figure 9 Magnetic resonance imaging of cholesteatoma involving the left temporal bone.

calcium deposition. Furthermore, both cartilage and bone formation may occur within these lesions. It is generally accepted that infectious or inflammatory injury to the TM or mucosa is the inciting event in the pathogenesis of tympanosclerosis. One possible mechanism is degeneration of fibroblasts which are known to progressively accumulate in these plaques. Fibroblasts accumulate cytosolic matrix vesicles rich in calcium, phosphate, and alkaline phosphatase. These vesicles eventually merge with the cell membrane and are released extracellularly upon fibroblast cell death. Continued accumulation leads to calcification of the collagen matrix.

Hypercalcemia in itself may be a contributing factor since de Carvalho Leal and others recently demonstrated that rats given a calcium-rich diet developed tympanosclerosis more frequently after *S. pneumoniae* middle ear infection than rats maintained on normal calcium content diets.[48] Another possible mechanism is dystrophic calcification of degenerated collagen fibers after an infectious or inflammatory insult (eg, AOM, OME). In contrast to the belief that tympanosclerosis arises from infectious or inflammatory insult, Wielinga and colleagues showed that sterile middle ear effusions secondary to eustachian tube obstruction was enough to incite tympanosclerotic plaque formation.[49] In their study, infected effusions caused almost complete replacement of the lamina propria with a dense connective tissue of normal cellularity; hence, no plaque formation was seen. Another possibility is autoimmune injury. Schiff and colleagues induced tympanosclerotic plaque formation after iatrogenic TM trauma in guinea pigs that were passively immunized with antisera to lamina propria.[50]

Treatment. Tos and Stangerup demonstrated that tympanosclerosis secondary to tympanostomy tube placement resulted in an inconsequential conductive hearing loss of less than 0.5 dB.[47] Should tympanosclerosis involve the middle ear cleft, however, involvement of the ossicles and middle ear mucosa is likely to occur. New bone growth usually involves the attic where fixation of the malleus and incus may occur. Tympanosclerosis involving the oval window leads to stapes fixation and conductive hearing loss.

Tympanoplasty and ossicular reconstruction may be performed to treat tympanosclerosis. Vincent and others reported recently that stapedotomy with reconstruction resulted in reduction of the air-bone gap to less than 20 dB in 70% of patients and 10 dB in 39% of patients.[51] In a review of 135 cases of tympanosclerosis with an average preoperative air-bone gap of 30.9 dB treated mainly by-stage operations, Teufert and De La Cruz reported that the air-bone gap was reduced to less than 20 dB in 65% with ossicular fixation even after 10 years of follow-up.[52] There were no dead ears in this group of patients, and only patient experienced partial sensorineural hearing loss. Gormley, however, showed that

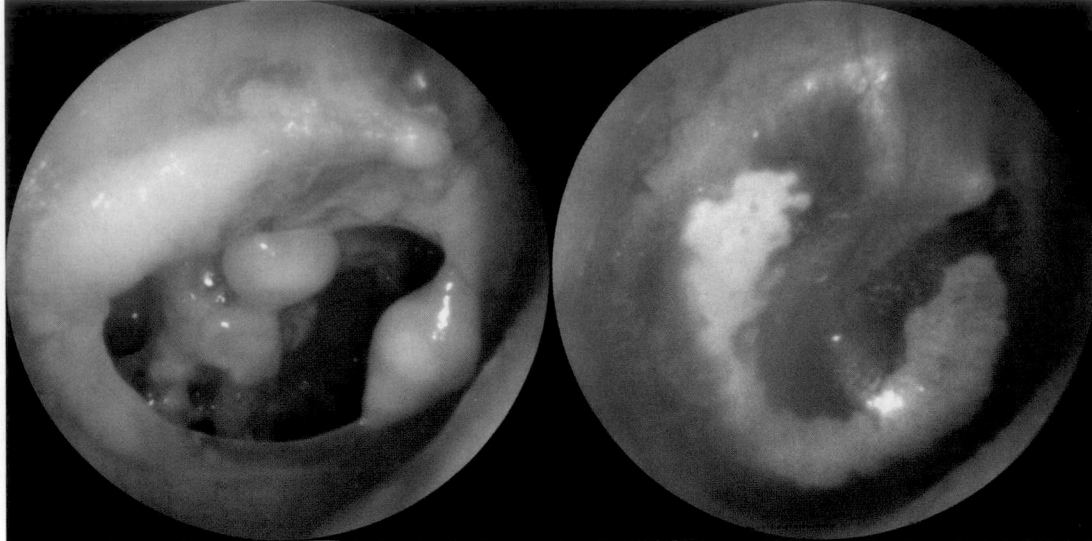

Figure 10 Tympanosclerosis (*left*) and myringoslcerosis (*right*).

dead ears resulted from stapedectomy and only 7% of patients had an air-bone gap of less than 21dB on long-term follow-up, citing recurrence of disease as problematic.[53] Significant risk of sensorineural hearing loss may result from either cochlear erosion of the disease process or from surgery due to the extensive dissection required in affected ears.

Cholesterol Granuloma

Cholesterol granuloma of the temporal bone is a brownish-yellow and mucoid lesion first described by Manasse in 1894.[54] Also called cholesterol cyst, blue drum membrane, blue dome cyst, cholestrin pseudocyst, or black cholesteatoma by some experts, cholesterol granuloma of the temporal bone arises as a consequence of COM in as many as 20% of temporal bones. In a study of 144 temporal bones from patients with COM, 21% of the 28 samples with TM perforations and 12% of the 116 samples without TM perforations revealed tympanosclerosis.[13] Although it may occur in any pneumatized portion of the temporal bone, it is most commonly found in the petrous apex and represents the most common primary lesion of this site. It is essentially a sterile foreign-body reaction to cholesterol crystals and, therefore, may arise in any part of the body. Although most common in the temporal bone, it has also been demonstrated in sites such as the paranasal sinuses, jaw, lungs, pleura, mediastinum, orbit, testes, and kidney.

Pathogenesis. Although the etiology is unclear, cholesterol granuloma arises from the same factors which lead to COM. It commonly coexists with both mucoid middle ear effusion and TM retraction, likely the result of increased negative middle ear pressure from disrupted aeration and drainage. Negative pressure and inflammation lead to hemorrhage into the area. Breakdown of erythrocyte membranes releases cholesterol, initiating crystal formation and a sterile inflammatory reaction. Microscopically, multinucleated foreign-body giant cells are seen

engulfing and surrounding cholesterol crystals. Inflammation leads to eventual granulation tissue formation, and repeated hemorrhage results in a lesion which grows in size.

Diagnosis. Cholesterol granuloma may be completely asymptomatic. Conversely, it may present by mass effect with symptoms such as hearing loss, tinnitus, vertigo, or facial twitching. Otoscopic examination may reveal a brownish-yellow, viscous lesion in the middle ear. If the lesion is not visible within the middle ear and likely involving the petrous apex, radiographic imaging greatly aids in diagnosis and preoperative planning. On CT, cholesterol granuloma has smooth borders, is isodense to brain parenchyma and does not enhance with intravenous contrast due to it avascularity. MRI is most helpful and usually establishes the diagnosis. The lesion is characterized by hyperintensity on both T1- and T2-weighted images and does not enhance after gadolinium administration. The unique hyperintensity on T1-weighted images is thought to be related to crystal presence, protein content, and hemorrhage. Should cholesterol granuloma coexist with cholesteatoma, it might be differentiated by the fact that cholesteatoma shows high signal intensity only on T2-weighted images.

Treatment. The form of treatment for cholesterol granuloma is based upon its location within the temporal bone as well as the patient's hearing status. Recurrence of surgically excised cholesterol granuloma is not uncommon, and, therefore, conservative treatment is generally warranted for uncomplicated cholesterol granuloma of the middle ear cleft or mastoid. If aeration of the middle ear system is unaffected, observation may be employed. Should cholesterol granuloma exist in the setting of poor middle ear ventilation and drainage, ventilation tubes are warranted. Small, asymptomatic lesions of the petrous apex may be followed with serial CT or MRI. Surgical approaches for symptomatic lesions of the petrous apex include middle cranial fossa, infratemporal fossa type B, infralabyrinthine, transcanal

infracochlear, transsphenoidal, and retrosigmoid approaches. Goals of surgery are to achieve drainage and aeration.

Management of COM

Medical. Most infected perforations can be managed conservatively with topical antibiotics and regular aural toilet. A clean external meatus is needed to ensure proper drug penetration into the middle ear mucosa. The antibiotics chosen should have efficacy in eradicating *Pseudomonas aeruginosa* and *Staphylococcus aureus*, the most common pathogens in COM cases. Importantly, studies have recently shown that approximately 20% of *Pseudomonas* isolates in European and American hospitals now demonstrate ciprofloxacin resistance.[55] In a recent review, Macfadyen and others determined that topical quinolone antibiotics were superior to systemic antibiotics in the management of otorrhea in patients with uncomplicated CSOM.[56] Also, topical quinolones have been shown to be superior to topical nonquinolones in several reviews; a recent evidence-based review by Manolidis demonstrated at least equal efficacy to topical aminoglycoside antibiotics.[57]

Topical antibiotics offer the advantage of minimizing possibility of bacterial resistance because their concentration at the site of infection exceeds the pathogen's minimal inhibitory concentration to such a degree that eradication is faster and more complete. Furthermore, topical antibiotics bypass the systemic circulation and result in significantly fewer adverse systemic effects. Topical antibiotics combined with corticosteroids in suspension form are also frequently employed. However, this combination has never been formally compared to antibiotic treatment alone. It is believed that corticosteroids alleviate edema, thereby allowing increased penetration of the antibiotic. Topical antiseptics such as boric acid, aluminum acetate, and povidine-iodine have also been used with good results. Antiseptics such as borate and antibiotics including chloramphenicol, sulfamethoxazole, and amphotericin may also be applied via insufflation in powder form; this technique is particularly useful in the setting of epitheliitis and moist mastoid cavities.

In those with recurrent or chronic infections, cultures should be obtained to direct antimicrobial therapy; if possible, cultures should be obtained from the middle ear to avoid possible contaminating flora, particularly *P. aeruginosa* from the external auditory canal. Systemic antibiotics may be administered according to culture and sensitivity results. Another useful option in patients with recalcitrant otorrhea is irrigation of the affected ear with half-strength acetic acid solution (eg, distilled vinegar diluted 1:1 with water) prior to otic antibiotic drop application.

The status of the round window and the risk associated with potentially ototoxic agents must be appreciated in the clinical decision-making process. The round window membrane serves as the major route by which toxins reach the inner ear, likely due to its accessibility to fluids pooling in the hypotympanum. In the setting of COM, the round window membrane thickens and is characterized by decreased permeability, affording some level of protection from ototoxic drugs. This is in contradistinction to the initial stages of active inflammation in which the membrane increases in permeability. Systemic aminoglycosides are well known for their ototoxic effects; whether topical administration of aminoglycosides cause similar toxicity has not been established and only isolated cases of vestibular and cochlear damage have been reported. The ototoxic potential of aminoglycosides should make them second-line agents unless quinolones are contraindicated or sensitivities call for them as first-line agents. Whereas studies have established the safety of topical quinolones, systemic administration is not approved in children less than 12 years of age due to reports of arthrotoxicity in young animals. This causation may be tenuous as comprehensive review of 31 previous reports showed no quinolone-associated arthropathy in over 7,000 children and adolescents who received ciprofloxacin, ofloxacin, or nalidixic acid.[58] Other agents shown to have ototoxic effects after topical administration include propylene glycol, chloramphenicol, polymyxin B, chlorhexidine, ethanol, and povidine-iodine.

Surgical Considerations. When conservative medical management has failed to control COM an individual often becomes a candidate for a surgical procedure. Surgical judgement as to whether a procedure should be performed is multifactorial. The surgeon must keep in mind the benefits and risks in a particular patient given their general medical condition. Surgical risks in elderly, diabetic or immunocompromised patients may trump an otherwise indicated procedure for COM.

Surgical procedures on the only hearing ear can be considered when COM is progressive and unrelenting and the purpose of the procedure is to halt progression (eg, progressively enlarging cholesteatoma or progressively destructive COM without cholesteatoma). Surgery on the only hearing ear is also indicated when there are central complications or threatening central complications. However, surgical procedures for correction of conductive hearing loss as a result of COM are not indicated.[59,60]

If a surgical procedure is required, the choice of the surgical procedure depends on the nature and extent of disease. In COM without cholesteatoma, the procedure should be designed to provide aeration of the middle ear, attic, antrum, and mastoid air cell spaces, as well as closure of the TM. These procedures may require a mastoidectomy with or without facial recess approach for the purposes of removing pathological mucosa, removing granulation tissue, and providing aeration of the mastoid. Atticotomy is rarely indicated for COM without cholesteatoma. Tympanoplasty is often accompanied by conservative mastoid procedures.

When a surgical procedure is chosen for COM with cholesteatoma, the nature and extent of the cholesteatoma must also be kept in consideration. Cholesteatoma limited to the attic area, especially those that are completely lateral to the head of the malleus and body of the incus, may be dealt with through an atticotomy approach with planned reconstruction of the scutal defect.

Cholesteatomas extending into the antrum and mastoid and those extending medially past the ossicular heads are most appropriately handled with a complete mastoidectomy and facial recess approach so that the cholesteatoma can be removed in its entirety. This approach, as described below, can allow excellent visualization of the entire cholesteatoma and its involvement of the attic, antrum, and mastoid.

Reconstruction of the hearing mechanism in intact canal wall procedures leads to a more physiologically normal middle ear. This procedure has the drawback of potentially leaving keratinizing epithelium in a closed mastoid which is not amenable to physical examination. The judgment as to whether or not to leave a canal wall intact depends on the surgeon's estimate of the adequacy of removal of the cholesteatoma matrix as well as patient reliability factors.

When extensive cholesteatomas involve the antrum and mastoid and an intact canal wall procedure cannot be performed safely, the posterior ear canal may be removed and the surgical procedure converted into canal wall down procedure with an open mastoid cavity. Recurrences of cholesteatomas when the canal wall is down are visible to the examining surgeon and are more easily detected and treated than in the intact canal wall procedure. Indications for the canal wall down procedure include destruction of the posterior canal wall by cholesteatoma, an extremely small sclerotic mastoid, recalcitrant recurrent cholesteatoma and "cholesteatosis" (widespread patches of keratinizing epithelium in which the cholesteatoma matrix has interdigitated into so many areas in the mastoid that physical removal is impossible).

Tympanoplasty. Tympanoplasty for TM perforation and ossicular reconstruction is usually performed when chronic inflammation is controlled or sometimes in conjunction with a procedure to remove pathological mucosa and granulation tissue from the mastoid. The techniques of TM repair and ossicular reconstruction do not differ from those used in cases of traumatic or postoperative injury to the tympanum and are presented in Chapter 19, "Reconstruction of the Middle Ear."

Compete Mastoidectomy. Complete mastoidectomy is performed on patients with suspected mastoid cholesteatoma or in COM without cholesteatoma in the presence of blockage (ie, attic, aditus ad antrum), chronic unremitting inflammation, cholesterol granuloma or when chronic granulation tissue is present.

A cortical mastoidectomy is performed with exposure of the antrum and incus (see Figure 11).[61]

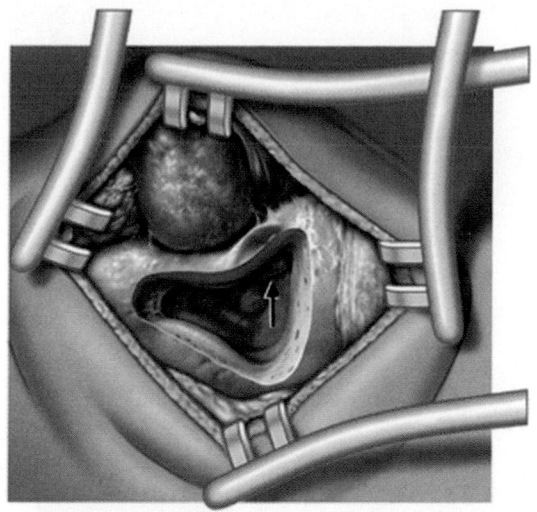

Figure 11 A complete mastoidectomy is performed by removing the cortex of the mastoid bone and exposing the antrum. Adequate exposure requires visualization of the incus (*arrow*). (Adapted from reference 61.)

Atticotomy for Cholesteatoma. Cholesteatomas that are limited to the attic region may be removed through either an atticotomy approach with reconstruction of the attic defect or by an intact canal wall mastoidectomy. If an atticotomy procedure is used, the entire cholesteatoma sac must be exposed and removed meticulously (see Figure 12). The defect must be reconstructed with a tragal or conchal cartilage graft.

Intact Canal Wall Mastoidectomy. An intact canal wall mastoidectomy has the advantage of preserving the normal anatomy of the entire posterior ear canal without need for scutum removal and recontruction (see Figure 13). This procedure is most often performed in cases of primary acquired cholesteatoma when the cholesteatoma involves the attic and antrum. Complete cortical mastoidectomy is performed, and the mastoid antrum is entered. Care is taken to preserve the cholesteatoma matrix as dissection is continued around the periphery of the matrix. Ideally, a primary acquired cholesteatoma can be removed

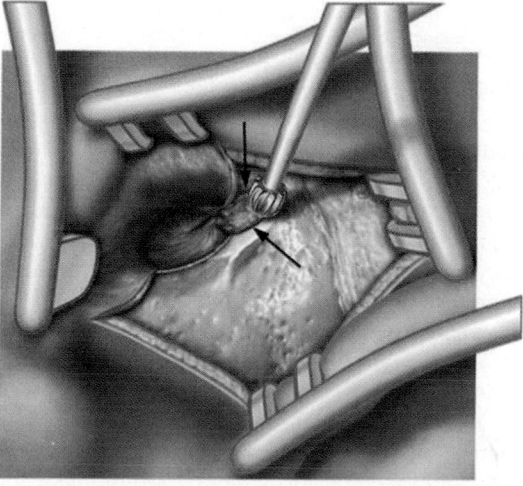

Figure 12 In cases in which a primary cholesteatoma is limited to the attic, lateral to the incus, without attic obstruction, an atticotomy may be performed transcanal (*arrows*). After the cholesteatoma is removed, the defect must be reconstructed; tragal cartilage is usually the best option. (Adapted from reference 61.)

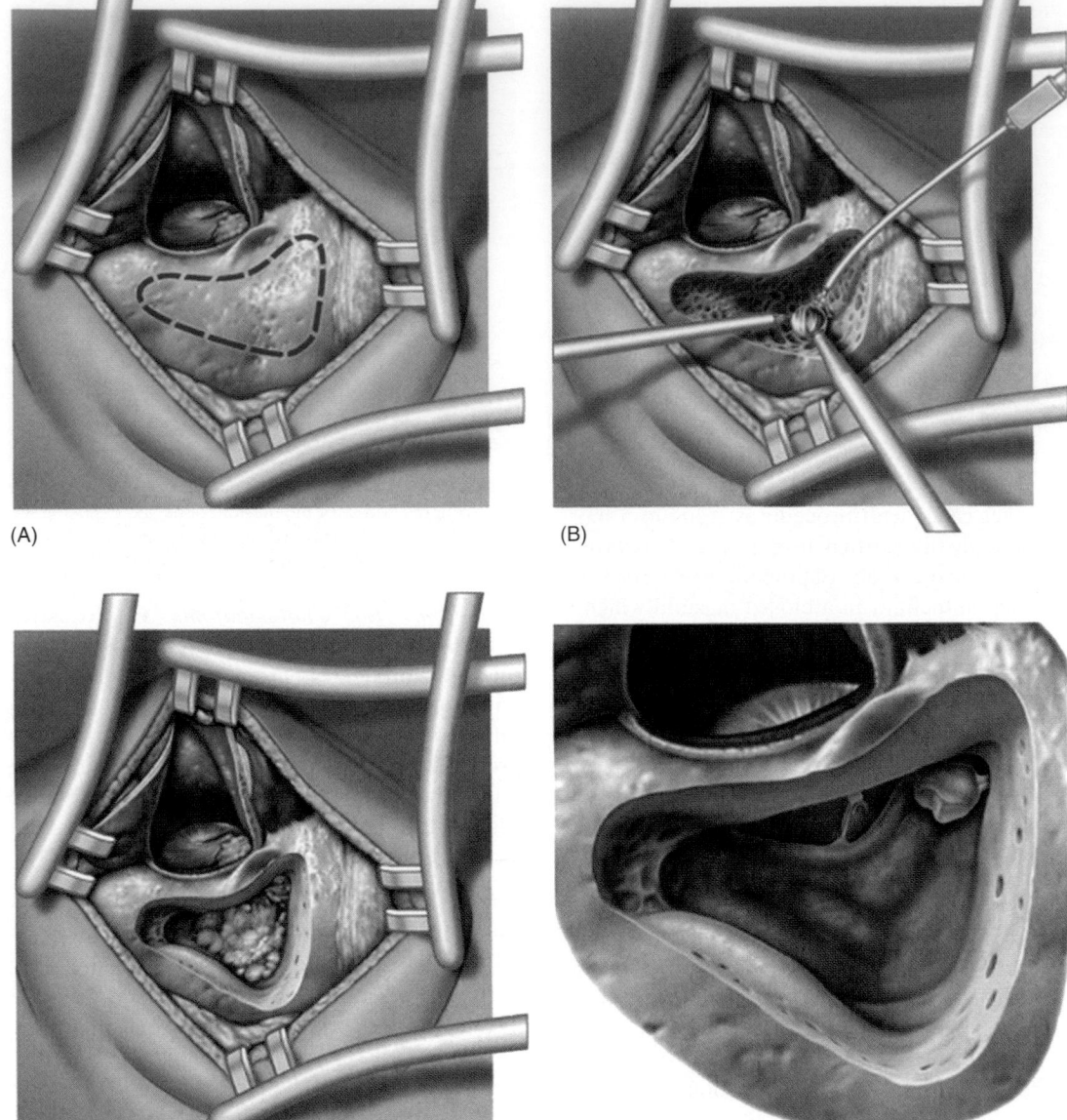

(A)   (B)

(C)   (D)

Figure 13 (A) and (B). An intact canal wall procedure is done by first performing a complete mastoidectomy. (C) The extent of the cholesteatoma must be visualized by removing as much of the overlying bone as possible. In most cases the cholesteatoma involves the facial recess and the recess must be opened posteriorly. In this case, the incus was involved and removed. (D) The facial nerve is identified in its course through the mastoid by thinning the overlying bone sufficiently. (Adapted from reference 61.)

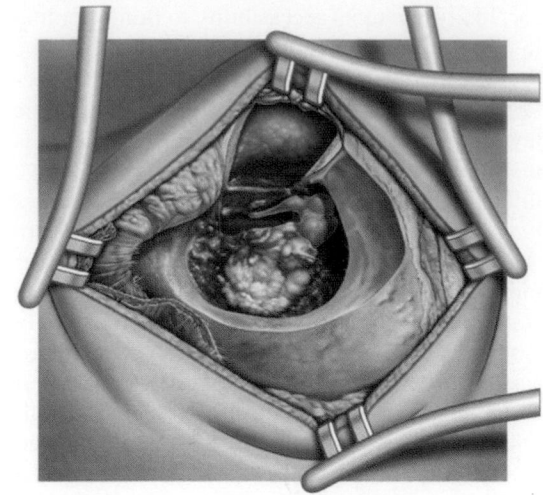

Figure 14 Extensive cholesteatomas that cannot be removed entirely with an intact canal wall procedure require the removal of the posterior ear canal down to the level of the fallopian canal. (Adapted from reference 61.)

any air cells which may lie lateral to the sigmoid sinus. In most cases of canal wall down mastoidectomy, the mastoid air cells of the mastoid tip are exenterated completely and the tip removed. Removal of the mastoid tip in a canal wall down mastoidectomy minimizes the possibility of forming a deep troublesome mastoid cavity inferiorly.

The mastoid cavity can be further minimized with closure techniques utilizing bone chips ("bone pâté"). Bone can be used to obliterate deeper portions of the mastoid cavity, especially behind the labyrinth. These bone chips must be covered by viable tissue. The surgeon may also choose to employ a Palva flap (postauricular subcutaneous tissue), rotated over the bone chips, to provide a smooth lining for the mastoid cavity (see Figure 16). Meatoplasty is always performed with a canal wall down mastoidectomy and is often appropriate for intact canal wall procedures.

The ultimate goal of a canal wall down mastoidectomy is to create an ear in which the meatus

without interrupting the matrix until final removal is appropriate. This minimizes the chance of leaving small fragments of keratinizing epithelium which may lead to recurrence. When the cholesteatoma is extremely extensive, the matrix is attenuated and there is difficulty in removing the matrix from underlying bony tissues. The surgeon may often elect to perform a "second look operation" for recurrences 6 to 12 months later. Alternatively, a canal wall down procedure may be selected when complete removal of the matrix is not possible.

When performing an intact canal wall procedure, there is no necessity for removing all air cells and mucosa, nor is there a requirement for smoothing the margins of the cavity (saucerization). The surgical approach for the intact canal wall procedure, therefore, is quite different from the canal wall down procedure in that the former preserves normal mucosa and trabecular anatomy

that aid in healing and re-pneumatization of the mastoid. This is in contrast to the canal wall down procedure in which all air cells should be exenterated and the mastoid cavity widely saucerized to minimize compartmentalization of the cavity (see Figure 14).

Canal Wall Down Mastoidectomy. When a canal wall down mastoidectomy is chosen, it is critical to exenterate all possible air cells since mucosa originating from air cells can harbor and trap disease. Furthermore, this mucosa can become secretory and form a moist and troublesome mastoid cavity. The bone lateral to the fallopian canal should be removed (the so-called facial ridge) to minimize the possibility that debris and inflammatory material can be harbored within the cavity posterior to the facial nerve (see Figure 15).

Additionally, the mastoid cortex lateral to the sigmoid sinus should be thinned to obliterate

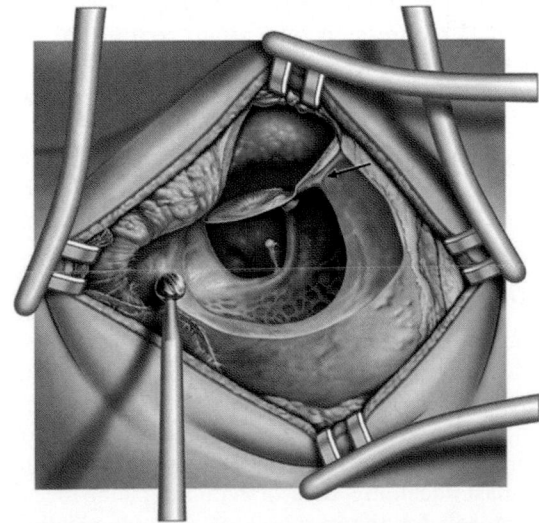

Figure 15 Canal wall down mastoidectomy with lowering of the facial ridge. In canal wall down procedures, the bone lateral to the facial nerve should be thinned (*arrow*). The margins of the mastoidectomy defect should be rounded and saucerized and the tip removed. (Adapted from reference 61.)

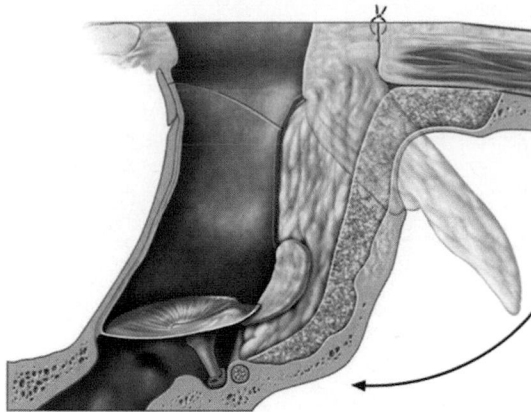

Figure 16 Mastoid obliteration using a bone chips ("bone pâté") and a Palva flap. (Adapted from reference 61.)

is large enough for easy examination and provides appropriate ventilation of the external canal and mastoid cavity. Furthermore, the resultant mastoid cavity should be small and lined with healthy keratinizing epithelium. A canal wall down mastoidectomy is often accompanied by reconstruction of the middle ear and a tympanoplasty. One alternative reconstructive approach to leaving the canal wall down is to remove it en bloc after an intact canal wall procedure and to replace it for reconstructive purposes.[62]

REFERENCES

1. Daly KA, Hunter LL, Giebink GS. Chronic otitis media with effusion. Pediatr Rev 1999;20:85–93; quiz 94.
2. Bluestone CD. Studies in otitis media: Children's Hospital of Pittsburgh-University of Pittsburgh progress report–2004. Laryngoscope 2004;114:1–26.
3. Bluestone CD, Klein JO. Otitis Media and Eustachian Tube Dysfunction. Philadelphia: Saunders; 2003. p. 474–685.
4. Verhoeff M, van der Veen EL, Rovers MM, et al. Chronic suppurative otitis media: A review. Int J Pediatr Otorhinolaryngol 2006;70:1–12.
5. Sade J, Berco E. Atelectasis and secretory otitis media. Ann Otol Rhinol Laryngol 1976;85:66–72.
6. Vartiainen E, Kansanen M, Vartiainen J. The contralateral ear in patients with chronic otitis media. Am J Otol 1996; 17:190–2.
7. Lieu JE, Muthappan PG, Uppaluri R. Association of reflux with otitis media in children. Otolaryngol Head Neck Surg 2005;133:357–61.
8. Fliss DM, Shoham I, Leiberman A, Dagan R. Chronic suppurative otitis media without cholesteatoma in children in southern Israel: Incidence and risk factors. Pediatr Infect Dis J 1991;10:895–9.
9. Casselbrant ML, Mandel EM. Genetic susceptibility to otitis media. Curr Opin Allergy Clin Immunol 2005;5:1–4.
10. Straetemans M, Wiertsema SP, Sanders EA, et al. Immunological status in the aetiology of recurrent otitis media with effusion: Serum immunoglobulin levels, functional mannose-binding lectin and Fc receptor polymorphisms for IgG. J Clin Immunol 2005;25:78–86.
11. Gentile DA, Doyle WJ, Zeevi A, et al. Cytokine gene polymorphisms moderate illness severity in infants with respiratory syncytial virus infection. Hum Immunol 2003;64: 338–44.
12. Post JC, Preston RA, Aul JJ, et al. Molecular analysis of bacterial pathogens in otitis media with effusion. JAMA 1995;273:1598–1604.
13. da Costa SS, Paparella MM, Schachern PA, et al. Temporal bone histopathology in chronically infected ears with intact and perforated tympanic membranes. Laryngoscope 1992;102:1229–36.
14. Kerschner JE, Meyer TK, Burrows A. Chinchilla middle ear epithelial mucin gene expression in response to inflammatory cytokines. Arch Otolaryngol Head Neck Surg 2004;130:1163–7.
15. Yoon TH, Schachern PA, Paparella MM, Aeppli DM. Pathology and pathogenesis of tympanic membrane retraction. Am J Otolaryngol 1990;11:10–7.
16. Tos M, Poulsen G. Attic retractions following secretory otitis. Acta Otolaryngol 1980;89:479–86.
17. Chole RA, Forsen JW. Color Atlas of Ear Disease, 2nd edition. Hamilton, Ontario: B.C. Decker; 2002.
18. Sade J. The buffering effect of middle ear negative pressure by retraction of the pars tensa. Am J Otol 2000;21:20–3.
19. Sade J. Hyperectasis: The hyperinflated tympanic membrane: The middle ear as an actively controlled system. Otol Neurotol 2001;22:133–9.
20. Valtonen HJ, Dietz A, Qvarnberg YH, Nuutinen J. Development of mastoid air cell system in children treated with ventilation tubes for early-onset otitis media: A prospective radiographic 5-year follow-up study. Laryngoscope 2005;115:268–73.
21. Oberman JP, Derkay CS. Posttympanostomy tube otorrhea. Am J Otolaryngol 2004;25:110–7.
22. Baker RS, Chole RA. A randomized clinical trial of topical gentamicin after tympanostomy tube placement. Arch Otolaryngol Head Neck Surg 1988;114:755–7.
23. Chole RA, Hubbell RN. Antimicrobial activity of silastic tympanostomy tubes impregnated with silver oxide. A double-blind randomized multicenter trial. Arch Otolaryngol Head Neck Surg 1995;121:562–5.
24. Post JC. Direct evidence of bacterial biofilms in otitis media. Laryngoscope 2001;111:2083–94.
25. Bothwell MR, Smith AL, Phillips T. Recalcitrant otorrhea due to Pseudomonas biofilm. Otolaryngol Head Neck Surg 2003;129:599–601.
26. Müller J. Über den Feineren Bau und die Formen der Krankhaften Geschwülste. Berlin: Reimer G; 1838.
27. Cruveilhier LJB. Anatomie Pathologique du Corpus Humani. Paris: JB Balliere; 1829.
28. Olszewska E, Wagner M, Bernal-Sprekelsen M, et al. Etiopathogenesis of cholesteatoma. Eur Arch Otorhinolaryngol 2004;261:6–24.
29. Michaels L. An epidermoid formation in the developing middle ear: Possible source of cholesteatoma. J Otolaryngol 1986;15:169–74.
30. Potsic WP, Samadi DS, Marsh RR, Wetmore RF. A staging system for congenital cholesteatoma. Arch Otolaryngol Head Neck Surg 2002;128:1009–12.
31. Wolfman DE, Chole RA. Experimental retraction pocket cholesteatoma. Ann Otol Rhinol Laryngol 1986;95:639–44.
32. van Blitterswijk CA, Grote JJ. Cytokeratin expression in cholesteatoma matrix, meatal epidermis and middle ear epithelium. A preliminary report. Acta Otolaryngol 1988; 105:529–32.
33. Oktay MF, Cureoglu S, Schachern PA, et al. Tympanic membrane changes in central tympanic membrane perforations. Am J Otolaryngol 2005;26:393–7.
34. Lange WL. Über bei Enstehung der Mittlohrcholesteatome. Z Hals Nas Ohrenheilk 1925;11:250.
35. Huang CC, Shi GS, Yi ZX. Experimental induction of middle ear cholesteatoma in rats. Am J Otolaryngol 1988; 9:165–72.
36. Chole RA, Tinling SP. Basal lamina breaks in the histogenesis of cholesteatoma. Laryngoscope 1985;95:270–5.
37. Chole RA, Frush DP. Quantitative Studies of Eustachian Tube Epithelium during Experimental Vitamin A Deprivation and Reversal. Amsterdam: Kugler Publishing; 1982.
38. Kwon KH, Kim SJ, Kim HJ, Jung HH. Analysis of gene expression profiles in cholesteatoma using oligonucleotide microarray. Acta Otolaryngol 2006;126:691–7.
39. Chole RA, Faddis BT. Evidence for microbial biofilms in cholesteatomas. Arch Otolaryngol Head Neck Surg 2002;128:1129–33.
40. Hall-Stoodley L, Hu FZ, Gieseke A, et al. Direct detection of bacterial biofilms on the middle-ear mucosa of children with chronic otitis media. JAMA 2006;296:202–11.
41. Alliston T, Derynck R. Medicine: Interfering with bone remodelling. Nature 2002;416:686–7.
42. Teitelbaum SL. Osteoclasts: What do they do and how do they do it? Am J Pathol 2007;170:427–35.
43. Jeong JH, Park CW, Tae K, et al. Expression of RANKL and OPG in middle ear cholesteatoma tissue. Laryngoscope 2006;116:1180–.
44. Kawai T, Matsuyama T, Hosokawa Y, et al. B and T lymphocytes are the primary sources of RANKL in the bone resorptive lesion of periodontal disease. Am J Pathol 2006;169:987–98.
45. Peek FA, Huisman MA, Berckmans RJ, et al. Lipopolysaccharide concentration and bone resorption in cholesteatoma. Otol Neurotol 2003;24:709–13.
46. Jaisinghani VJ, Paparella MM, Schachern PA, Le CT. Tympanic membrane/middle ear pathologic correlates in chronic otitis media. Laryngoscope 1999;109:712–6.
47. Tos M, Stangerup SE. Hearing loss in tympanosclerosis caused by grommets. Arch Otolaryngol Head Neck Surg 1989;115:931–5.
48. de Carvalho Leal M, Ferreira Bento R, da Silva Caldas Neto S, et al. Influence of hypercalcemia in the formation of tympanosclerosis in rats. Otol Neurotol 2006;27:27–32.
49. Wielinga EW, Peters TA, Tonnaer EL, et al. Middle ear effusions and structure of the tympanic membrane. Laryngoscope 2001;111:90–5.
50. Schiff M, Poliquin JF, Catanzaro A, Ryan AF. Tympanosclerosis. A theory of pathogenesis. Ann Otol Rhinol Laryngol Suppl 1980;89:1–16.
51. Vincent R, Oates J, Sperling NM. Stapedotomy for tympanosclerotic stapes fixation: Is it safe and efficient? A review of 68 cases. Otol Neurotol 2002;23:866–72.
52. Teufert KB, De La Cruz A. Tympanosclerosis: Long-term hearing results after ossicular reconstruction. Otolaryngol Head Neck Surg 2002;126:264–72.
53. Gormley PK. Stapedectomy in tympanosclerosis. A report of 67 cases. Am J Otol 1987;8:123–30.
54. Manasse P. Über Granulationsgeschwülste mit Fremdkörperriesenzellen. Virchows Arch 1894;136:245.
55. Leibovitz E. The use of fluoroquinolones in children. Curr Opin Pediatr 2006;18:64–70.
56. Macfadyen CA, Acuin JM, Gamble C. Systemic antibiotics versus topical treatments for chronically discharging ears with underlying eardrum perforations. Cochrane Database Syst Rev 2006:CD005608.
57. Manolidis S, Friedman R, Hannley M, et al. Comparative efficacy of aminoglycoside versus fluoroquinolone topical antibiotic drops. Otolaryngol Head Neck Surg 2004;130:S83–8.
58. Burkhardt JE, Walterspiel JN, Schaad UB. Quinolone arthropathy in animals versus children. Clin Infect Dis 1997;25:1196–1204.
59. Schuknecht HF, Gacek RR. Surgery on only-hearing ears. Trans Am Acad Ophthalmol Otolaryngol 1973;77:ORL 257–66.
60. Chandler JR, Freeman J. Otologic surgery in patients with one hearing ear only. Laryngoscope 1972;82:848–63.
61. Hildmann H, Sudhoff H. Middle Ear Surgery. Cambridge: Springer; 2006.
62. Gantz BJ, Wilkinson EP, Hansen MR. Canal wall reconstruction tympanomastoidectomy with mastoid obliteration. Laryngoscope 2005;115:1734–40.

Cranial and Intracranial Complications of Acute and Chronic Otitis Media

David R. Friedland, MD, PhD

Myles L. Pensak, MD

John F. Kveton, MD

Inflammation and pains of the ear lead sometimes to insanity and death.—Celsus, 25 AD

The European and American otologic literature of the nineteenth and preantibiotic twentieth centuries well document the fear and anxiety provoked by intracranial complications associated with aural infection of either acute or chronic nature. Reading before the California State Medical Society in April of 1916 and subsequently published in the California State Journal of Medicine, the prominent otologist Edward Sewall presented a detailed assessment of otitic meningitis.[1] Included in this seminal text is a detailed review of the regional anatomy, confounding factors, and ultimately the need for prompt assessment and management. "The purulent process in the temporal bone that causes brain disease begins in the tympanum, labyrinth, or adjacent pneumatic cavities. Prompt evacuation of pus that has accumulated here is the safeguard that the surgeon must bear in mind while using his best judgment for the advantage of the patient." Although the advent of antibiotics has greatly reduced the incidence of such disease, it is precisely because they are rare and potentially fatal that the clinician must be familiar with complications of acute and chronic otitis media (Table 1).

ANATOMY

Temporal bone anatomy is discussed in detail in Chapter 1, "Anatomy of the Auditory and Vestibular Systems;" however, we emphasize that the irregular and complex osteology of the bony skull base produces a number of preformed pathways that enable the extension of disease into the intracranial compartment. The multiple neural and vascular structures that traverse the temporal bone and petrous ridge provide avenues for infectious extension which we will discuss briefly in this section.

Osteology

Infection of the ear canal or middle ear may expand beyond the confines of the local environs through preformed pathways. The fissures of Santorini allow for external auditory canal infections to extend anteriorly into the parotid gland. From there passage may provide for extension into the infratemporal fossa, parapharyngeal space, masticator space, and neck along with the lymphatic drainage from the parotid system.

Medially, infections within the mesotympanic space may pass into the adjacent tympanic recesses and cavities, including the hypotympanum where the jugular bulb and jugular fossa may be seeded. Anteriorly, these infections may extend into the protympanum and track along the internal carotid artery and eustachian tube. Should the roof of the eustachian tube become violated, spread into Glasscock triangle (bounded by the greater superficial petrosal nerve, the mandibular division of the trigeminal nerve and a line between the foramen spinosum and the arcuate eminence) along the middle fossa floor may occur. Continued anterior extension may track along the route of the greater superficial petrosal nerve while posterior extension may involve the geniculate ganglion (Figure 1).

If a significant air cell tract is present in Kawase triangle (actually a quadrangular area bounded anteriorly by the mandibular division of the trigeminal nerve posteriorly by the arcuate eminence, laterally by the greater superficial petrosal nerve, and medially by the superior petrosal sinus), anterior extension may involve the trigeminal nerve while involvement of the apex and Dorello canal may precipitate a classic Gradenigo syndrome resulting in abducens nerve paralysis. Medial extension within Kawase triangle may result in invasion of the superior petrosal sinus. Propagation of infection anteriorly may seed the cavernous sinus while posterior extension will result in sigmoid sinus involvement. Finally, with aggressive destructive processes, violation of the internal auditory canal and otic capsule may result in suppurative labyrinthitis and anacusis.

Mesotympanic pathology extending posteriorly may involve the sinus tympani within the roof of which lays the fallopian canal and facial nerve. Cephalic extension into the epitympanum may seed the aditus ad antrum, the central mastoid air cell tract and, thus, the air cell system of the petrous ridge. Infection leading from the central mastoid air cell system will track along well-defined pathways including the pre- and postsigmoid tracts, the sinodural, retrolabyrinthine, infralabyrinthine, supralabyrinthine, retrofacial, subarculate, and apical cells. Extra temporal involvement may ultimately invade accessory air cells including the zygomatic root, styloid process, and occipital bone.

Vasculature

Knowledge of the venous anatomy of the peripetrous architecture is of vital importance (Figure 2). The sigmoid sinus and jugular bulb

Table 1 Cranial and Intracranial Complications of Otitis Media[2,3,23,39,60,67]	
Cranial Complications	**Intracranial Complications**
Mastoiditis	Meningitis
Facial nerve paralysis	Venous thrombosis
Subperiosteal abscess	Intracranial abscess
Petrous apicitis	Epidural abscess
Labyrinthitis	Subdural empyema
Labyrinthine fistulae	Brain abscess
Cerebrospinial fluid leak/ encephalocele	Otitic hydrocephalus

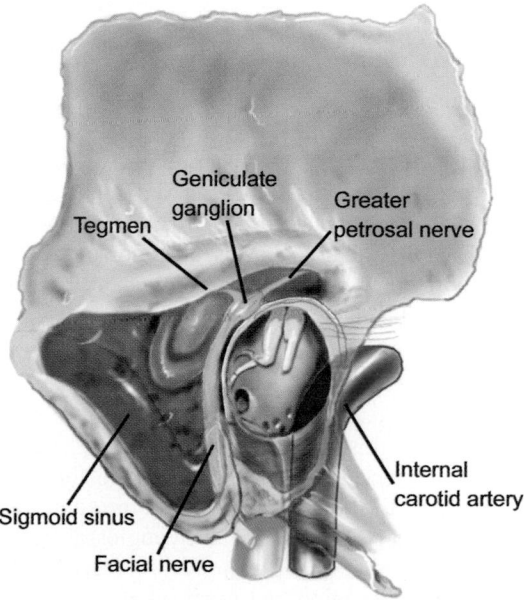

Figure 1 Relationship of the temporal bone to local neural and vascular structures. Infections within the middle ear and mastoid can propagate along these pathways and lead to cranial and intracranial complications. (Published with permission, copyright © 2007 D.R. Friedland, MD, PhD.)

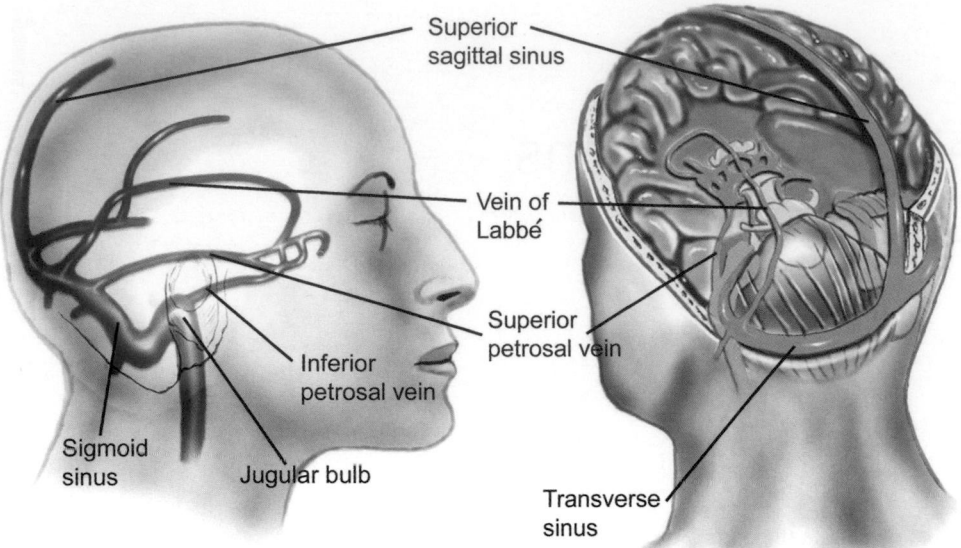

Figure 2 Venous anatomy around the temporal bone and posterior fossa. Complications of acute and chronic otitis media include thrombophlebitis of the sigmoid sinus which can extend proximally and distally to contiguous and anastamosing veins. (Published with permission, copyright © 2007 D.R. Friedland, MD, PhD.)

occupy central positions within the temporal bone and thus involvement of these structures may result in a thrombophlebitis. Antegrade extension of infection propagates inferiorly into the jugular vein itself. Mastoid involvement may extend to the sigmoid sinus and it is not uncommon to find granulations over an exposed sigmoid sinus in coalescent mastoiditis. Such a finding may be an early process in the progression to sigmoid sinus thrombophlebitis. Continued retrograde involvement may impact the transverse sinus, torcula, and the vein of Labbé (inferior anastomotic vein). Emissary veins along the posterior petrous ridge may be sources of spread of infection to the posterior fossa dura. Furthermore, temporal venous channels may result in temporal lobe seeding by either retrograde propagation of infected clot or emboli.

The carotid sheath is relatively resistant to infection but may serve as a conduit for skull base osteomyelitis. The carotid canal represents a preformed pathway as the artery enters the skull base anterior to the jugular bulb, rises superiorly ventral to the cochlea, turns along the floor of the eustachian tube and the temporal fossa before entering the intradural intracranial compartments at the level of foramen lacerum. Natural dehiscences along the artery's osseous course provide areas for entry of infection leading to abscess, osteomyelitis, and extradural seeding.

Neural Structures

Infection spreading along neural pathways may follow the glossopharyngeal, vagus, or spinal accessory nerves as they pass through the pars nervosa of the jugular foramen before entering the upper cervical neck. The hypoglossal nerve and hypoglossal canal are rarely involved with intracranial infection and paralysis of this nerve portends an ominous course in cases of skull base osteomyelitis. In general, the facial and vestibulocochlear nerves remain fairly protected through their course within the internal auditory canal.

However, the facial nerve is at risk in the tympanic segment because of frequent dehiscences in the bone of the fallopian canal. There is also potential involvement of the vertical facial nerve due to either mastoid disease or involvement of the sinus tympani.

MICROBIOLOGY

The microorganisms involved in cranial and intracranial complications of otitis media generally reflect the bacteriology of the primary infection (Table 2). Bacteria commonly associated with acute otitis media are well documented and include *Streptococcus pneumoniae*, *Haemophilus influenzae*, and *Moraxella catarrhalis*.[2] Other microorganisms causing acute otitis media include *Staphylococcus aureus*, *S. pyogenes* and, in infants under 6 months of age, *Escherichia coli*. Complications of acute otitis media are more likely to remain intratemporal, and treatment of such disorders should focus on these microorganisms. Mastoiditis, the most common complication of acute otitis media, has similar causative microorganisms, but the clinician must also direct treatment toward *Pseudomonas aeruginosa*, coagulase negative staphylococci, *Proteus* species, and anaerobes.[3,4] Meningitis, the most common intracranial complication of acute otitis media is most commonly caused by *S. pneumoniae*.[5,6] The advent of multivalent pneu-

mococcal vaccines may shift this microbiological spectrum as nontypeable *H. influenzae* becomes a more prevalent cause of acute otitis media.[7]

Chronic otitis media has a different microbial profile than acute ear infections (Table 2). *S. aureus* and *P. aeruginosa* are the typical infective agents.[8,9] Coagulase negative staphylococci and *Proteus* species are also frequently seen. *Klebsiella* species and mixed gram-negative microorganisms and anaerobes may also be found. A significant percentage of cultures of acute and chronic otitis media and their associated complications are sterile.[4,6,10,11] Biofilms in chronic otitis media may also affect culture results and require polymerase chain reaction techniques to identify the pathogens. Many patients with complications of aural infections have been on antibiotics prior to presentation with a cranial or intracranial process and this may affect culture results. The choice of antibiotic should take into account the susceptibility of the microorganism and the ability of the antibiotic to cross the blood–brain barrier (Table 3).

DIAGNOSIS

Physical Examination

The history and physical examination remain the cornerstones of an early diagnosis of cranial and intracranial complications associated with otitic infections.[12] A history of a change in alertness or behavior may indicate extratemporal extension of disease or infection. Diminished cognitive responses such as alterations in arousal, somnolence, wakefulness, reduced response to verbal or physical stimulation, or impaired consciousness require emergent assessment. New onset seizures or emesis should also be addressed with haste.

The patient may give a history of an ear infection that has been treated with antibiotics and even myringotomy and tube placement. A history of chronic perforation may be present but does not ensure that the mastoid is aerated. Masked mastoiditis can occur if the antrum is blocked by inflammatory tissue, yet the middle ear may appear relatively free from disease.[13] New onset otorrhea, headache, vertigo, and hearing loss despite treatment are symptoms and signs of severe otitis and impending or early complication.[2] Facial weakness, spiking fevers, vomiting, and changes in alertness suggest extension of disease beyond the tympanum and require urgent evaluation.

The physical examination must include a general head and neck examination and a thorough

Table 2 Common Pathogens	
Acute Otitis Media[2]	Chronic Otitis Media and Mastoiditis[4,8]
Streptococcus pneumoniae	*Staphylococcus aureus*
Haemophilus influenzae	Coagulase negative staphylococci
Moraxella catarrhalis	*Pseudomonas aeruginosa*
Streptococcus pyogenes (group A)	*Staphylococcus epidermidis*
Staphylococcus aureus	*Proteus* species
Escherichia coli (infants)	*Klebsiella* species
	Mixed infection with anaerobes and aerobes

Table 3 Diffusion of Antimicrobials into the Cerebrospinal Fluid[83]		
Excellent	**Good with Meningeal Inflammation**	**Poor or Unpredictable**
Chloramphenicol	Ampicillin	Amikacin
Cefotaxime	Ceftriaxone	Benzathine penicillin
Metronidazole	Ceftazidime	Erythromycin/azithromycin
Rifampin	Cefuroxime	Gentamicin
Sulfonamides	Ciprofloxin	Moxifloxacin
Trimethoprim–sulfa	Fluconazole	Tetracycline
	Imipenem (seizure risk)	Tobramycin
	Nafcillin	Vancomycin
	Penicillin G	
	Piperacillin	
	Timentin	

neurologic evaluation. Visual acuity changes and oculomotor deficits may indicate intracranial complications such as otitic hydrocephalus or petrous apicitis. Facial paresthesia suggests extension to the cavernous sinus and possible thrombophlebitis. Facial paralysis may occur with involvement of the nerve anywhere along its path through the temporal bone. Hearing loss beyond the conductive loss of middle ear involvement may herald a labyrinthitis or labyrinthine fistula. Vertigo may suggest a similar complication. Lower cranial deficits such as dysphagia, voice changes, shoulder weakness, or tongue deviation may indicate jugular bulb involvement, thrombophlebitis, or skull base osteomyelitis.

The external ear and neck needs careful examination. A protuberant auricle may suggest mastoid edema from an underlying mastoiditis or presence of a subperiosteal abscess. Upper neck swelling and tenderness may represent a Bezold abscess, reactive lymphadenopathy, or jugular vein thrombosis. Signs of distal septic emboli from the latter, characteristic of Lemierre syndrome (postangial sepsis), should be noted.[14] External otitis may represent extension of disease beyond the middle ear, and granulation tissue, typically in the floor of the canal, may indicate malignant otitis externa, ie, skull base osteomyelitis.

The tympanic membrane should be inspected. It may be bulging, opaque or perforated. Approximately 50% of patients with intracranial complications will have had prior otorrhea.[6] Cultures of purulent discharge should be taken and sent for gram stain, aerobic and anaerobic culture and sensitivities, and examination for fungus and acid-fast bacilli. Granulation tissue at the tympanic membrane may suggest underlying cholesteatoma. Mastoid palpation can reveal tenderness and fluctuance may be present in patients with abscess or cortical erosion. Tuning fork testing may distinguish a sensorineural from a conductive loss. Romberg and tandem gait may reveal ataxia which suggests intracranial involvement. Cerebellar signs should also be checked with rapid alternating hand movements and finger-to-nose testing. Nystagmus or a positive head-thrust refixation saccade may indicate labyrinthine involvement.

Radiographic Imaging

The mainstay of evaluation of cranial and intracranial complications of otitic infection is the computed tomography (CT) scan.[15,16] The CT scan should be performed with contrast to delineate areas of abscess and inflammation as well as reveal flow voids in thrombosed vessels. Aeration of the mastoid should be noted. A sclerotic mastoid suggests an acute exacerbation of chronic ear disease which should increase suspicion for underlying cholesteatoma and focus attention on direct or disseminated intracranial extension. A well-developed mastoid may be found in acute otitis media with associated mastoiditis, and local cranial complications are more likely. Meningitis is more common with acute otomastoiditis. Meningitis is not readily apparent on CT scan, and magnetic resonance imaging (MRI) should be performed before lumbar puncture (LP).

CT bone windows will delineate the osteology of the temporal bone and demonstrate coalescence in the mastoid, dehiscence of the tegmen tympani or tegmen mastoidea, erosion into the sigmoid sinus, and extension of disease through the lateral or medial cortex of the mastoid cavity. The clinician should not focus solely on the temporal bone disease and must also evaluate the entire scan. The brain and intracranial cavity should be examined for intraparenchymal brain abscess, abscess around the dural layers, ventricular dilatation suggestive of hydrocephalus, and abscesses or flow voids within the transverse, sigmoid and jugular veins. The neck should be evaluated for lymphadenopathy, necrotic or abscessed lymph nodes, deep neck space infections, or Bezold abscess. Localized edema and inflammation of tissue around the temporal bone may suggest a skull base osteomyelitis.

MRI is useful in evaluating for the intracranial complications of acute or chronic otitis media.[17] Dural enhancement and thickening suggests meningitis and is usually along the side of ear involvement. Brain abscesses may be difficult to see in the early stages but localized cerebral edema may suggest an impending abscess. In later stages, brain abscesses are easily seen on MRI. Intracranial and venous abscesses are also quite apparent. A magnetic resonance venogram (MRV) can also be included in the MR evaluation and helps to identify venous thrombosis and the extent of involvement. Localized tissue edema and cellulitis from skull-base osteomyelitis can be more impressive on MRI as compared to findings on CT.

Lumbar Puncture

Suspicion of infection within the spinal fluid compartment requires a LP. Prior to the LP the patient should undergo neuroradiographic evaluation to assess for hydrocephalus or brain compression from intracranial abscess or pneumocephaly. On physical examination, the presence of papilledema is an ominous finding and necessitates caution and neurologic consultation before the LP is done. LP performed in the face of elevated cerebrospinal fluid (CSF) pressure may lead to brain herniation and death. An opening pressure should be obtained to assess for increased intracranial pressure. In meningitis, normal CSF flow and reabsorption is inhibited, and intracranial pressure increases. The CSF in meningitis typically shows a low glucose level but elevated white blood cell count and protein levels. Culture should be performed for bacterial and fungal growth. Polymerase chain reaction techniques can be used for detection and identification of the microorganism causing the infection including viruses, prions, and tuberculosis.[18]

Radionucleotide Bone Scans

In cases of malignant otitis externa, skull base osteomyelitis, or osteoradionecrosis of the temporal bone with attendant infection, both gallium-67 and technetium-99 scans have been used. These scans provide evidence of an acute inflammatory process and the ability to monitor response to treatment. Gallium will provide a short-term assessment for the response to acute-phase antibiotics and/or surgical drainage, while the technetium scans will provide a longer-term evidence of the resolution of infection. Bone scans are not commonly used in current management as CT and MRI provide high-resolution images of bone involvement and tissue inflammation.

CRANIAL COMPLICATIONS

Mastoiditis

Mastoiditis denotes inflammation with the mastoid air cell system. Almost all cases of acute otitis media will have radiographic evidence of mastoid fluid or mucosal thickening which represent inflammation.[19] In uncomplicated middle-ear infection, concurrent mastoid involvement should not be considered a complication of acute otitis media and is not a surgical disease. If inflammatory tissue obstructs the aditus ad antrum self-sustaining acute mastoiditis may be followed by chronic mastoiditis. The incidence of acute mastoiditis may be increasing due to resistant bacterial strains.[20]

Acute mastoiditis can cause systemic signs of infection such as fever and malaise. Mastoid tenderness and localized reactive lymphadenopathy is commonly present. In the child with a thin mastoid cortex there may be erythema and/or edema of the overlying mastoid soft tissue. This leads to the unilateral protuberant ear characteristic of this disease. In the adult with a thicker cortex, local pain may occur, and tenderness may be the only external sign. Typically, in the early stages of mastoiditis, there are concurrent signs of acute infection in the middle ear, and antibiotic therapy alone may be all that is necessary. Aggressive intravenous antibiotic use, especially in children, should be considered. Myringotomy will release pus from the middle ear, remove the nidus of inflammation and should be strongly considered on initial presentation. A complete head and neck examination is critical to identifying impending other cranial and intracranial complications and establishing a baseline upon which to gauge response to therapy.

If the aditus block and mastoid inflammation persist, fluid within the mastoid air cells will become increasingly purulent and lead to worsening mucosal edema and venous stasis. The subsequent acidosis and osteoclast activity causes decalcification of bony septae and coalescence of air cells into a confluent cavity (Figure 3). This coalescent mastoiditis may develop despite antibiotic treatment and myringotomy. The middle-ear infection may appear to have resolved by this time, but the blocked antrum walls off the mastoid from drainage. Antibiotic therapy may be less effective under these circumstances, and the clinician must be attuned to signs and symptoms of such a masked mastoiditis.[13] In the patient with chronic otitis media, antral block may lead to acute or coalescent mastoiditis despite the presence of a perforation or resolution of otorrhea. Cholesteatoma in chronic otitis media may cause mastoid outlet obstruction and serve as the potential nidus of infection.

There is no definitive algorithm for the treatment of acute or coalescent mastoiditis. The efficacy of modern antimicrobials and the relative efficiency in which disease progression can be radiographically monitored make initial medical therapy of uncomplicated acute and coalescent mastoiditis the preferred option. The early performance of a myringotomy may prevent the development of complications of acute mastoiditis

and need for further surgery.[4] Failure to improve despite aggressive medical management (including myringotomy with or without tympanoplasty tube placement), the development of other cranial or intracranial complications, or the presence of complications on admission is an indication for mastoid surgery.[4] For uncomplicated mastoiditis, the need for mastoidectomy despite admission and intravenous antibiotic therapy is about 10%.[21,22] In patients with intracranial complications, the mastoidectomy rate is much higher and can be up to 70%.[4,21]

The mastoidectomy for complicated acute or coalescent mastoiditis is a difficult operation. There is typically friable granulation tissue throughout the mastoid, antrum, and middle ear. The granulations may be so thick as to prevent the insertion of a ventilation tube. The abundant tissue distorts the anatomy, makes visualization difficult and can cause local bone erosion. Dehiscence of the sigmoid sinus, facial nerve, or labyrinthine fistulae is not uncommon. Cholesteatoma is commonly encountered in chronic otitis media and may cause similar bone destruction and involvement of vital structures.[23] Drainage of the mastoid, removal of granulation tissue, and restoration of normal ventilatory pathways should be the goal of the operation. Continuation of antibiotic therapy postoperatively for weeks can eradicate residual disease.

Facial Paralysis

Facial nerve paralysis secondary to acute or chronic otitis media represents only about 3 to 5% of all occurrences of acquired facial weakness.[24,25] Paralysis from Bell palsy, trauma, herpes zoster oticus, ie, Ramsay Hunt syndrome or *Borrelia burgdorferi*, ie, Lyme disease, is more prevalent.[24] Nevertheless, it is imperative that the physician carefully inspects the ear for the presence of middle-ear infection or masked mastoiditis.[26] The facial nerve paralysis in acute otitis media has usually been present for less than a week whereas

facial paralysis in chronic otitis media may have been present a much longer period.[24] The severity of the facial palsy in acute and chronic otitis media varies with almost all patients having at least House-Brackmann grade III and 30 to 50% having total facial paralysis.[24,27]

The cause of facial paralysis with acute otitis media is not clear. Historically, direct pressure on an exposed nerve has been considered a principal cause. However, formal explorations do not consistently reveal fallopian canal dehiscences.[27] A neurotoxic effect of the infection, entering the fallopian canal through natural dehiscences or vessel channels, is considered a more likely cause.[28] Alternatively, there may be recrudescence of latent herpes virus in previously exposed individuals. In chronic otitis media with facial paralysis, there is a high incidence of cholesteatoma.[23,25,29] Direct exposure and pressure on the facial nerve by cholesteatoma are commonly seen. The rate of development of facial paralysis may be rapid if there has been an acute infection but may be slow in onset if secondary to gradual expansion of cholesteatoma.[23]

In acute otitis media, treatment should consist of systemic antibiotics and myringotomy with or without tympanostomy tube insertion. There does not appear to be a need for mastoidectomy and facial nerve decompression in acute otitis media.[24] In chronic otitis media, however, surgical exploration is indicated as the vast majority harbor cholesteatoma.[23,29,30] Decompression of the facial nerve is performed in most series, however, finding at mastoidectomy an entirely intact fallopian canal may result in a similar outcomes.[23–25,27] Removal of cholesteatoma and granulation tissue along the course of the tympanic and mastoid segments of the facial nerve early in the infectious process may improve recovery.[24,25]

The outcome in patients with acute otitis media is generally excellent with the vast majority returning to a House-Brackmann grade I with appropriate treatment. In chronic otitis media, the outcomes are more variable.[24,29] Factors that may determine final facial function include the duration of facial paralysis before presentation and the presence of cholesteatoma at exploration. Facial palsies of greater than 1 year may not show any appreciable improvement after surgical intervention, and the presence of cholesteatoma increases the incidence of residual weakness.[24] Involvement at the geniculate ganglion has a worse prognosis than isolated tympanic or mastoid infection.[31] Facial paralysis and its management are discussed in Chapter 34, "Facial Paralysis."

Subperiosteal Abscess

Infection within the mastoid can extend through the cortex and form a subperiosteal abscess in the upper neck.[32] The absence of full mastoid development in young children may make this age group more resistant to the development of this complication.[33] However, hematogenous spread through venous perforators may provide

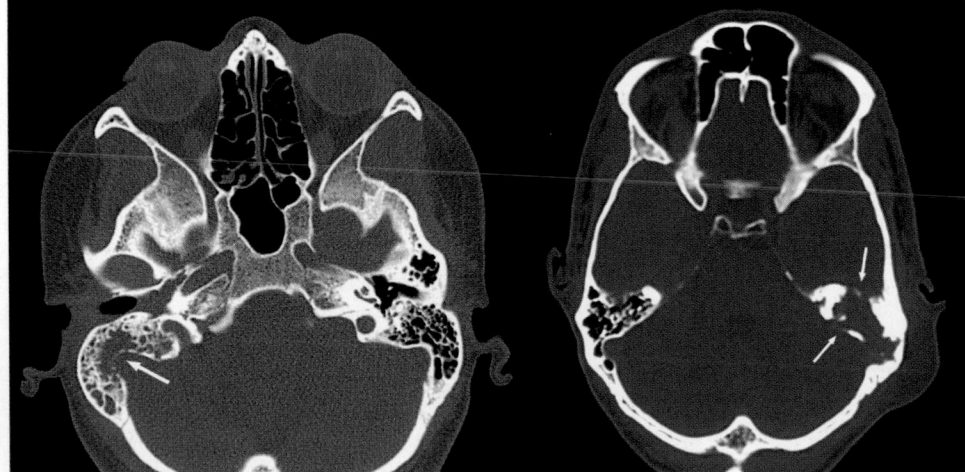

Figure 3 Computed tomography scan of the temporal bones in acute coalescent mastoiditis. On the left, the trabecular structure of the mastoid is progressively being eroded and posterior extension to the sigmoid sinus is imminent (*arrows*). On the right, progression of mastoiditis has led to complete coalescence of the mastoid and erosion into the posterior and middle fossae (*arrows*). (Published with permission, copyright © 2007 D.R. Friedland, MD, PhD.)

an alternate route for infection to access the subperiosteal space. There are three principal classes of subperiosteal abscess defined by their site of formation.

The lateral mastoid subperiosteal abscess is often referred to as simply a "subperiosteal abscess" as it is most common and typically forms over the superficial cortex of the mastoid (Figure 4). In this location the subperiosteal abscess often, but not consistently, presents with a protuberant auricle, postauricular fluctuance and tenderness, and occasionally spontaneous drainage.[32] In contrast, formation of an abscess on the medial side of the mastoid at the digastric ridge has more subtle clinical signs. These patients may complain of, or show signs of, pain along the sternocleidomastoid muscle and have a palpable mass in the infra-auricular region. This is the Bezold abscess and may progress to involve deeper neck spaces if not recognized promptly. The least common abscess is the zygomatic root subperiosteal abscess. This may cause preauricular swelling and malocclusion due to involvement of the glenoid fossa.

Treatment of subperiosteal abscess includes intravenous antibiotics, incision and drainage of the abscess, and mastoidectomy. Separate incisions may be needed for each approach. A myringotomy can also be performed to improve ear drainage from the middle ear, and cultures should be taken of pus in the subperiosteal abscess. Purulent fluid from a neck abscess should also be sent for acid-fast bacillus (AFB) smear and culture. There have been rare reports of successful treatment with intravenous antibiotics without mastoidectomy, but this is not recommended by the authors. A review of patients with Bezold abscesses found that many of them also have other cranial and intracranial complications, and a prompt mastoidectomy may also help prevent further complications.[33]

Petrous Apicitis

The progressive inflammatory processes that lead to acute mastoiditis can also affect the petrous pyramid (Figure 5). When the pneumatized and marrow containing spaces of the petrous apex become infected, potential routes of drainage can become obstructed and lead to persistent infection. Even if the middle ear and mastoid have been cleared of infection, the petrous apex may still harbor walled-off infection. The lower incidence of acute petrous apicitis as compared to mastoidectomy is attributable to the lower incidence of petrous apex pneumatization in the normal condition thus restricting one route of potential extension of infection.[17] Venous channels to the petrous apex may provide additional pathways for dissemination of infection.[34]

Petrous apicitis should be suspected if an ipsilateral retrobulbar or deep aural pain persists despite clearance of disease from the middle ear and mastoid.[35] The pain of petrous apicitis may be from local dural involvement or proximity to Meckel cave and the trigeminal sensory ganglion. The classic triad of Gradenigo syndrome consisting of retrobulbar pain, abducens palsy, and suppurative otorrhea is rarely fully present.[35,36] Horner syndrome may also be present due to involvement of sympathetic nerves around the petrous portion of the internal carotid artery. One or more of these symptoms in association with cochleo-vestibular findings, facial weakness or signs of systemic infection should prompt careful evaluation. A CT scan can demonstrate petrous opacification, coalescence, or disruption of local architecture.[37] The postcontrast T1 MRI can demonstrate granulation tissue in the petrous apex and around the carotid artery or involving Meckel cave.[17]

The treatment for petrous apicitis is expeditious removal of the source of infection. Myringotomy with or without tube placement, mastoidectomy, and intravenous antibiotics are recommended.[36,38] Corticosteroid use may be beneficial if cranial neuropathies are present although this had not been definitively studied. If

drainage of the petrous apex becomes necessary, several routes have been defined. These include transnasal/transsphenoidal drainage if the anatomy is favorable, although a transtympanic subcochlear drainage is the least invasive route via the petrous ridge. Because numerous cell tracts will allow passage to the petrous apex, CT scanning of the temporal bone will provide preoperative visualization for potential routes of access.

Labyrinthitis

Inflammation within the labyrinth associated with acute and chronic otitis media produces hearing loss and vertigo. The two principal forms of labyrinthitis that may develop are serous labyrinthitis and suppurative labyrinthitis. Serous labyrinthitis is thought to involve the translocation of bacterial toxins or inflammatory mediators to the inner ear without invasion of the labyrinth by the bacterial pathogen. In contrast, suppurative labyrinthitis is a fulminant bacterial infection within the inner ear. Labyrinthitis is more commonly associated with acute otitis media.[39]

Serous labyrinthitis typically presents with sudden onset vertigo in the setting of acute otitis media. It is less commonly found with chronic otitis media but can also be secondary to meningitis. Infectious or inflammatory elements in meningitis can follow the cochlear aqueduct to enter the inner ear and lead to labyrinthitis ossificans.[40] The most common microorganism in meningitis-induced hearing loss is *S. pneumoniae*.[41] The diagnosis of labyrinthitis is typically clinical, but inflammation in the labyrinth can be visualized with postcontrast T1-weighed MR scans.[17] The treatment of acute serous labyrinthitis secondary to acute otitis media is myringotomy and antibiotics. Mastoidectomy may be necessary if disease persists or progresses to suppurative labyrinthitis. Hearing loss with serous labyrinthitis is rarely profound and can improve following the resolution of infection. Vertigo and imbalance, as in vestibular neuritis, may persist for several months but is rarely permanent.

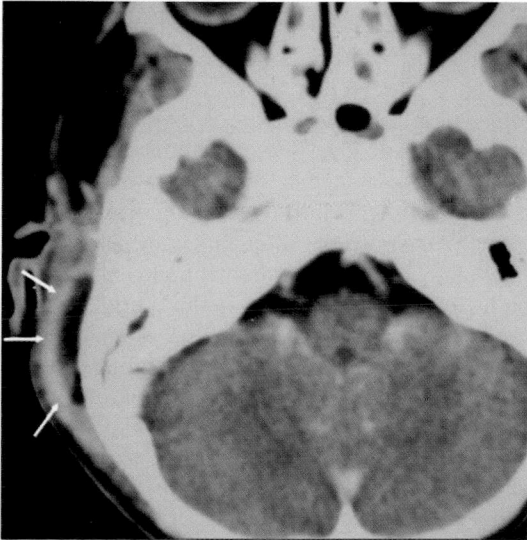

Figure 4 Computed tomography scan with contrast of the temporal bone demonstrating a rim-enhancing abscess over the mastoid. Notice there is no coalescence of the ipsilateral mastoid as most extratemporal complications spread via venous thromboemboli. (Published with permission, copyright © 2007 M.A. Michel, MD.)

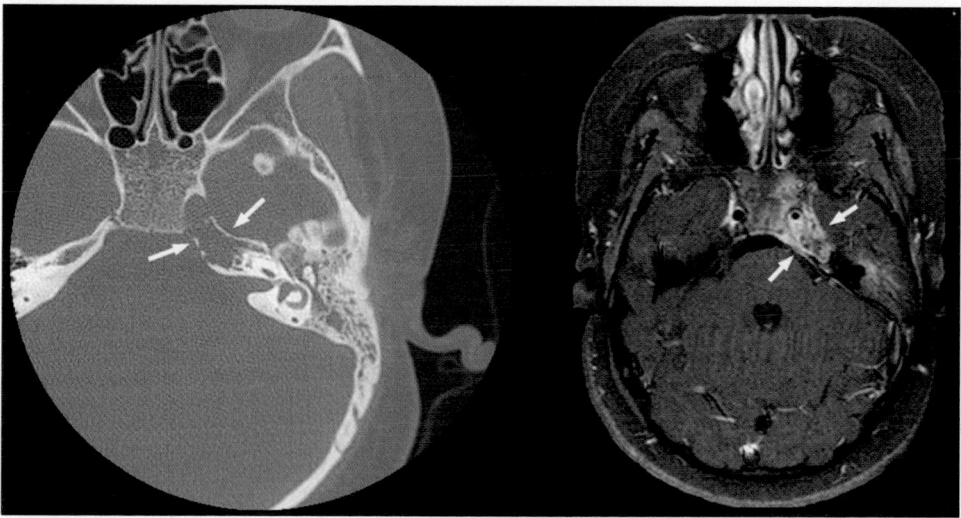

Figure 5 Computed tomography scan, left, of the temporal bones demonstrates coalescence and opacification in the left petrous apex (*arrows*). Magnetic resonance imaging, right, shows local inflammation around the cavernous sinus which can cause abducens palsy or trigeminal paresthesias.

Suppurative labyrinthitis represents invasion of the inner ear by the bacterial organisms. It is thought that entry to the inner ear is via the round window membrane although other potential routes include otic capsule fistulae and venous channels.[42] Suppurative labyrinthitis can progress to meningitis and intracranial abscess.[43] The hearing loss with suppurative labyrinthitis is usually severe to profound and has a poor prognosis for recovery. Treatment for this condition includes myringotomy and intravenous antibiotics with a low threshold for mastoidectomy based upon clinical examination. In rare occasions the labyrinth may require surgical drainage to control intracranial disease.[44] Corticosteroids are a consideration in labyrinthitis to reduce inflammation, improve hearing outcomes, and prevent labyrinthitis ossificans (Figure 6). Their use depends on the entire clinical picture.

Labyrinthine Fistula

Labyrinthine fistula is almost exclusively reported in association with chronic otitis media and cholesteatoma,[45–47] although otic capsule defects have been seen in noncholesteatomatous ear disease.[48,49] The incidence of labyrinthine fistula in chronic otitis media is approximately 10%.[45,46,49] The most commonly affected canal is the lateral (or horizontal) semicircular canal, but involvement of the posterior and superior canals as well as other regions of the labyrinth and cochlea have been reported.[45,47,49] The existence of a labyrinthine fistula is highly correlated with concurrent involvement of the facial nerve, with tegmen defects, and with ossicular erosion.[49,50]

The clinical history is typical for chronic otitis media and cholesteatoma with only subtle differences between patients with or without labyrinthine fistulae. While a labyrinthine fistula may cause dizziness, most patients with labyrinthine fistulae do not have imbalance. Rather, patients may present with intermittent vertigo or with the Tullio phenomenon in which they report vertigo and oscillopsia with loud noises or aural pressure changes. Signs of a fistula may be evoked clinically by the application of pressure to the ear with pneumatic otoscopy, ie, Hennebert sign. The direction of eye movements during the fistula test may help identify which semicircular canal is involved, but a high-resolution CT scan will provide better definition of the extent of the cholesteatoma and otic capsule defects.

Management of a labyrinthine fistula due to chronic otitis media and cholesteatoma is surgical and typically requires a canal wall down mastoidectomy. The region of suspected fistula should be approached carefully, and the cholesteatoma matrix left over the area until the rest of the operation is completed. This protects the inner ear from inadvertent suctioning and from the debris created by the drill. Once the remainder of the cholesteatoma and infection has been removed, the fistula is addressed. Typically, the cholesteatoma can be gently elevated off the membranous labyrinth, and constant irrigation will prevent excess perilymph leakage.[51] The defect can be sealed with combinations of fascia, perichondrium and bone dust.[49,51] Alternative management is to leave the cholesteatoma matrix over the fistula and externalize the matrix of the cholesteatoma by radical mastoidectomy. This approach is not preferred as the Tullio phenomenon may persist if the dehiscence is not addressed, and the remaining matrix may have continued toxic effects on the inner ear. Hearing loss and vestibulopathy are potential outcomes of the operation, but complete removal of the cholesteatoma does not appear to entail a significant additional risk to the inner ear.[49,51]

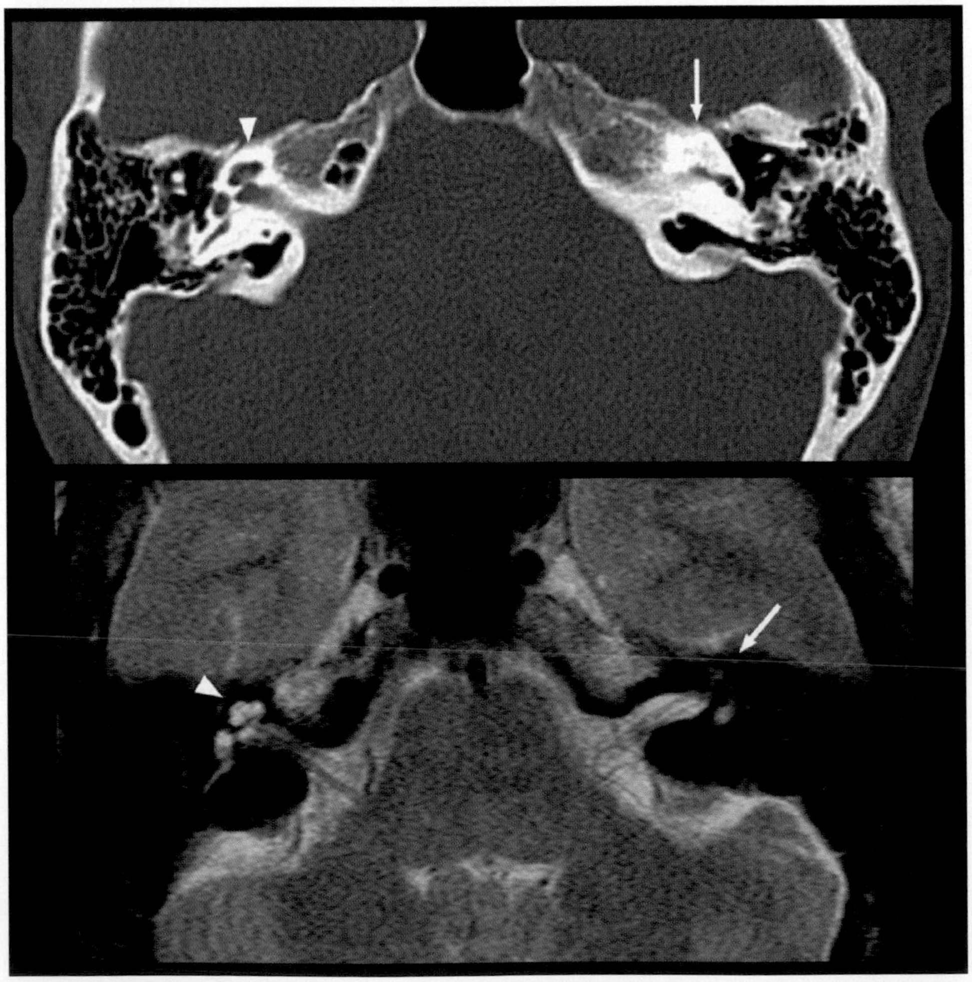

CSF Leak and Encephalocele

A tegmen dehiscence sufficient to cause a CSF leak or encephalocele is a rare complication of acute otitis media. More commonly, a spontaneous CSF leak is mistaken for acute otitis media and identified after myringotomy and tube placement.[52,53] In chronic otitis media, however, the recurrent episodes of inflammation may lead to thinning of the tegmen and ultimately tearing of the middle or posterior fossa dura. A tegmen dehiscence is more common in the presence of cholesteatoma and may allow for encephalocele formation.[23,54] Following appropriate antibiotic coverage, the leak should be sealed via a transtemporal or intracranial approach.[55,56] For leaks managed via the intracranial route, either extradural or intradural repairs may be performed.

INTRACRANIAL COMPLICATIONS

Meningitis

Meningitis is the most common intracranial complication of acute otitis media in children and adults.[57,58] In recent years, *S. pneumoniae* has replaced *H. influenzae* type B as the most common organism identified in childhood meningitis.[5,57,59] This change in microbial profile is likely secondary to the introduction of the HiB vaccine.[59] Access to the intracranial space and CSF may be by any of the aforementioned anatomical pathways. In acute otitis media, entry into the CSF via the labyrinth and cochlear aqueduct is more likely in congenital abnormalities of the inner ear such as Mondini malformation. Infection may also spread hematogenously through venous channels or directly through bony dehiscences in the middle and posterior fossa plates. Dehiscences predisposing to bacterial meningitis may arise from chronic otitis media, cholesteatoma, encephalocele, or trauma.

The mortality from bacterial meningitis ranges from 5%, to as high as 30%, in some series.[59–62] Factors associated with an unfavorable outcome are advanced age, a positive blood

Figure 6 Computed tomography scan, top, and magnetic resonance imaging, bottom, of the temporal bones in a patient with left labyrinthitis ossificans postmeningitis. The cochlea on the right (*arrowheads*) is clearly visible in both images, but the left cochlea is ossified and lacks a fluid filled lumen (*arrows*).

culture, tachycardia, a low CSF leukocyte count, and severe mental status changes on admission. The occurrence of meningitis from complications of otitis media or sinusitis portends a worse outcome. Meningitis from *S. pneumoniae* carries a worse prognosis for survival than meningococcal meningitis.[62]

Patients with meningitis typically complain of severe headache but this is not a particularly specific symptom. More specific for meningitis are complaints of fever, neck stiffness, and altered mental status which comprise the classic triad of meningitis. This triad is not usually present in its entirety on initial presentation,[63,64] however, at least two of four symptoms, ie, headache plus the triad, can be found in over 95% of patients with bacterial meningitis.[62] In addition to assessing temperature and general mental status, examination for meningitis typically focuses on identifying meningeal irritation and its effect on neck mobility.

Nuchal rigidity can be assessed by asking the patient to touch the chin to the chest or to move the chin alternately from shoulder to shoulder. Kernig sign is the presence of back or leg pain when the patient is in the supine position and one leg is passively flexed at the hip and then extended at the knee. Brudzinski sign is also performed in the supine position and involves passively flexing the neck. A positive sign is the observation of reflexic bilateral hip and knee flexion to lift the legs. These tests are commonly used but appear to have poor sensitivity for detecting meningitis.[63] Therefore, the absence of these findings should not influence the decision to perform further evaluation in the patient suspected of having meningitis.

Meningitis signs in association with acute or chronic otitis media may also reflect other intracranial complications such as brain abscess or venous thrombophlebitis. Obtaining a CT scan with contrast is critical for evaluating a patient for these conditions and also serves to determine whether the performance of a LP is contraindicated. MRI scans can also rule out other intracranial pathology and demonstrate dural enhancement and thickening suggestive of meningitis.

The LP is the mainstay of diagnosing meningitis. CSF should be sent for cytology, chemistry, and smear and culture. The CSF may be turbid. Opening pressures may be elevated due to alterations in CSF circulation with meningeal inflammation. Cytology shows elevated white cells (generally >100 cells/μL) and increased neutrophils in bacterial meningitis. Microorganisms may be tentatively identified on Gram stain and the chemistry may demonstrate a low glucose and high protein in bacterial infections as opposed to viral meningitis. The cultures can demonstrate and identify the microorganism but may show no growth if antibiotics have been previously administered.

Treatment consists of early administration of intravenous antibiotics. A delay in antibiotic administration may be associated with an increased long-term mortality.[63] The antibiotic should be broad spectrum and cover potentially resistant microorganisms. The usual initial regimen consists of ceftriaxone or cefotaxime which have good CSF penetration in the presence of inflammation. Vancomycin is recommended to cover resistant microorganisms but may be discontinued if culture and sensitivity so indicate. In older patients without penicillin allergy, ampicillin is recommended to cover for *Listeria monocytogenes,* but this is more likely in community-acquired meningitis rather than otitic meningitis.

Corticosteroids are strongly recommended early in the course of meningitis to reduce the incidence of subsequent hearing loss and overall mortality in children and adults, respectively.[63,65,66] Dexamethasone dosing varies in reports but is between 0.4 and 1.5 mg/kg/d in children and about 10 mg every 6 hours in the adult over the first 4 days of treatment.[65] Timing appears critical, and the first dose should be administered just before, or with, the initial dose of antibiotics. Corticosteroids may alter the blood–brain barrier and affect antibiotic levels in the CSF. The cephalosporins do not appear to be affected, but vancomycin levels may be reduced. Few adverse side effects have been noted from corticosteroid use in meningitis.

In acute otitis media, antibiotic therapy alone can control the meningitis and clear the middle ear of infection.[21] Myringotomy should be performed immediately in the patient with a sudden change in mental status. Surgical management of the mastoid should be undertaken to remove the nidus of infection in cases of chronic otitis media or additional cranial and intracranial complications. Continued assessment clinically and radiographically during the course of treatment is necessary to identify further complications and ensure that surgical intervention is undertaken expeditiously.

Venous Thrombosis

Septic thrombophlebitis may obstruct the venous drainage system adjacent to the petrous pyramid. Sigmoid sinus thrombophlebitis is the second most common intracranial complication of otitis media and has a mortality rate of about 10%.[60,67,68] The process generally starts with an acute or chronic otitis media that progresses to involve the sigmoid sinus directly. Erosion of bone over the sigmoid sinus and deposition of granulation tissue along the vein are commonly seen. In some cases there is no violation of the bone around the sigmoid sinus suggesting that thrombosis of emissary veins may provide a route for disease extension. Proximal propagation of inflammation and clot may involve the transverse sinus and torcula. Distal propagation can cause obstruction of the jugular bulb and jugular vein. The thrombus commonly progresses to involve one or more of these sites by the time of diagnosis.[68] In the rare occasion when obstruction crosses the midline, an acute intracranial event may lead to severe and rapid central venous obstruction, hydrocephalus, intracranial edema, and death.

Presenting symptoms and signs are variable, and the classic picket fence spiking fevers may not be present. Headache and otalgia are usually present with rare exception.[68–71] Other symptoms include otorrhea, mental status changes, nausea or emesis, and photophobia. The examination may reveal an intact or perforated tympanic membrane, purulent drainage, edema of the skin of the ear canal, and soft tissue changes over the mastoid. Griesinger sign is erythema, edema, and tenderness over the posterior part of the mastoid process due to septic thrombosis of mastoid emissary veins indicating thrombophlebitis of the sigmoid sinus.[68–71] Involvement of the jugular foramen may cause paresis of the glossopharyngeal, vagus, and spinal accessory nerves. Rarely, abducens palsy has been observed.

Neuroradiographic evaluation with contrast-enhanced CT or MRI will show a reduction in flow, ie, flow void, at the site of occlusion (Figure 7). A CT venogram or MRV can be used for definitive diagnosis and to assess progression of the thrombosis or recanalization over time.[37,71] CT and MRI should also be used to evaluate the patient for other cranial and intracranial complications as these are commonly found in conjunction with sigmoid sinus thrombosis.[69] LP should be performed to assess intracranial pressure and to evaluate for concurrent meningitis. Digital pressure over the nonoccluded internal jugular vein may cause a rise in CSF pressure whereas compression of the occluded side will have no effect, ie, Toby–Ayer–Queckenstedt test. Elevated intracranial pressure with sigmoid sinus thrombosis is characteristic of otitic hydrocephalus.

Treatment consists of broad-spectrum intravenous antibiotics and an urgent complete mastoidectomy. In addition to covering the usual aural pathogens such as *Streptococcus* species and *Staphylococcus* species, therapy should include coverage for mixed flora such as *Bacteroides* species and *Proteus* species.[69,70] During mastoidectomy, granulations and inflammation overlying the sigmoid sinus should be removed. Surgical intervention directed at the thrombosed vessels is controversial. Some authors have recommended thrombectomy, ligation, or resection of the sigmoid sinus.[68,70] Others have noted that conservative management of the sinus is equally effective.[69,72] Additionally, the employment of anticoagulation remains controversial.[71] In patients in whom there appears to be a seeding of the distal venous architecture and the potential for embolic phenomenon impacting the cardiovascular system, utilization of anticoagulant medication is warranted. Additionally, septic emboli that continue to shower distal sites may necessitate the extirpation or ligation of the involved venous structures in the neck.

Intracranial Abscess

Bacteria can spread from the temporal bone to the intracranial compartment and establish distinct loci of infection. Abscesses can form in the epidural space, between the dura and arachnoid

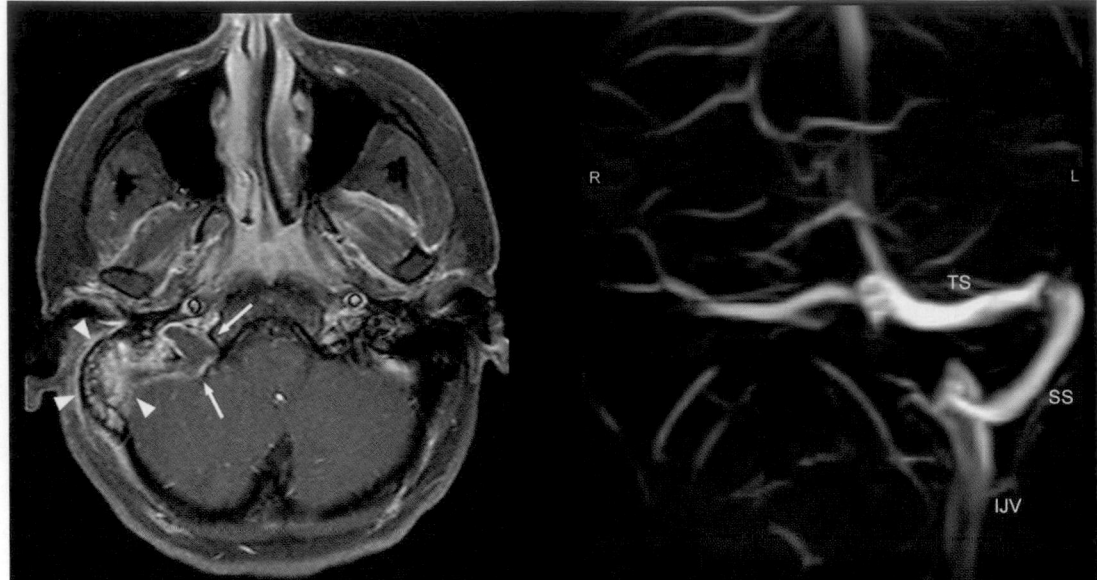

Figure 7 Magnetic resonance imaging (*left*) of the temporal bone demonstrating mastoiditis (*arrowheads*) and thrombophlebitis of the right sigmoid sinus and jugular bulb (*arrows*). Note the enhancement around the jugular bulb due to local granulation tissue. A magnetic resonance venogram (*right*) shows diminished flow in the right transverse sinus (TS) and lack of flow in the sigmoid sinus (SS) and internal jugular vein (IJV). These vessels are clearly defined on the left side. (Published with permission, copyright © 2007 D.R. Friedland, MD, PhD.)

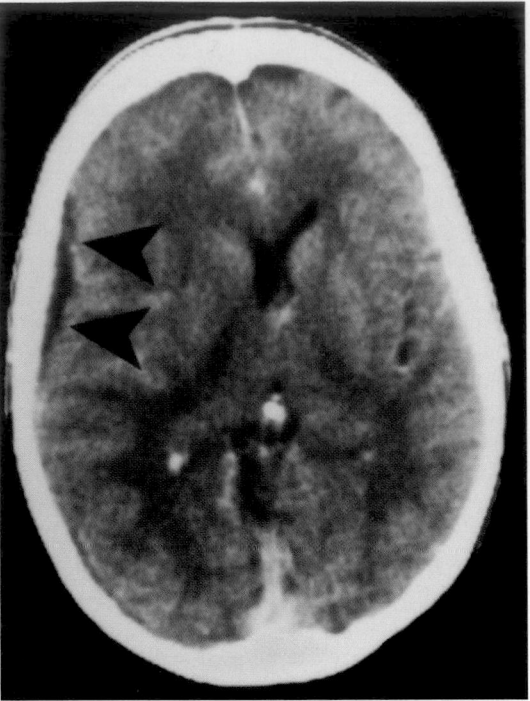

Figure 9 Computed tomography scan of the brain with contrast demonstrating a collection of hypointense pus in the subdural space overlying the right cerebral cortex (*arrowheads*). These infections are called subdural empyemas because they develop in potential spaces rather than form distinct abscesses capsules. Subdural empyemas typically form along the tentorium cerebelli and interhemispheric fissure. (Published with permission, copyright © 2007 P.A. Wackym, MD.)

(subdural space), or within the substance of the cerebrum or cerebellum. Even though these intracranial abscesses are all serious, they have different prognoses requiring specific and expeditious therapies.

Epidural Abscess. Direct extension of middle ear or mastoid infection tissue through the bony confines of the temporal bone into the middle or posterior fossae leads to an epidural abscess (Figure 8). Bone erosion can be caused by coalescence, cholesteatoma, or granulation tissue. Localized granulation tissue and purulent material may remain fairly quiescent for a protracted period of time before manifesting as an epidural

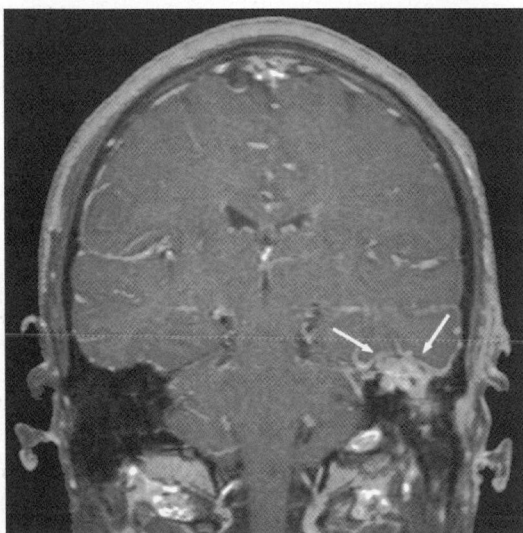

Figure 8 Coronal computed tomography scan of the temporal bones and brain demonstrating direct extension of infection in the left mastoid to the epidural space of the middle fossa (*arrows*). Epidural abscesses typically form by direct extension and may also occur in the posterior fossa around the sigmoid sinus, ie, perisinus abscess. (Published with permission, copyright © 2007 D.R. Friedland, MD, PhD.)

abscess. Silent epidural abscesses, found only at exploration, have been reported.[73,74] The abscess may form along either the posterior fossa dura or adjacent to the superior petrosal vein and the middle fossa dura. Epidural abscess formation around the sigmoid sinus is referred to as a perisinus abscess.

Symptoms are variable and can be quite mild. Chronic low-grade fevers and a dull headache often are the only clinical symptoms. Resolution of acute otitis media may occur inspite of persistent mastoid infection and provide a false sense of improvement. Granulation tissue in the tympanum should raise the suspicion of an impending complication.[75] Exacerbations of infection may lead to invasion of venous structures around the epidural abscess. On the left side, inflammation around the vein of Labbé may occur with the patient presenting with speech difficulties and aphasia. CT scan with contrast can demonstrate bone erosion along the posterior or middle fossae and rim enhancement of the epidural abscess. Gadolinium enhanced MRI can be used to identify intracranial abscess and thrombosis of surrounding vessels. Treatment is surgical and entails mastoidectomy with direct drainage of the abscess. Cultures should be taken to direct antibiotic therapy.

Subdural Empyema. Infection in the potential space between the dural and pia-arachnoid layers can produce a localized collection of pus more accurately referred to as subdural empyema rather than an abscess (Figure 9). Subdural empyema is the least common complication of otitis media and is seen more commonly with sinusitis and trauma.[76] It was found in only 1 of 70 patients with complications of chronic otitis media and 1 of 68 patients with complications of acute otitis media.[4,60] Although rare, it is one of the most

serious of the otitic intracranial complications. Mortality rates are as high as 15% in recent years, and permanent morbidity in the form of seizures and neurological deficits can occur in over 30% of survivors.[77]

The clinical presentation is usually rapidly progressive and severe. Meningitic signs of fever, headache, altered mental status, and emesis are typically present and can progress within 48 hours to seizures, focal neurological deficits, and coma.[77] Contrast-enhanced CT scan can demonstrate a widened subdural space and resultant flattening of surrounding cerebral sulci.[37] Subdural empyema of otitic origin will generally form along the tentorium cerebelli and the interhemispheric fissure.[37] MRI may demonstrate changes in the surrounding cerebral cortex which can become edematous or necrotic and cause a mass effect.[78] Diffusion weighted images can distinguish subdural empyema by its high signal from the mixed signal appearance of epidural abscesses.[79]

Surgical drainage of the abscess and decompression of the brain should be undertaken by a neurosurgeon emergently. Concurrent mastoidectomy and myringotomy are performed to address the source of infection. Parenteral antibiotics should provide broad coverage and, based upon findings in subdural empyema from sinusitis, be directed at microorganisms more common in chronic rather than acute ear disease.[77] Cultures obtained during drainage of the subdural empyema should direct further antimicrobial treatment.

Brain Abscess. Spread of otitic infection beyond the meninges can lead to the formation of cellulitis (cerebritis) and abscess within the brain parenchyma (Figure 10). Generally resultant from retrograde thrombophebitis, brain abscesses consist of a focal mass and localized signs reflective of the site of invasion. Cerebellar, as well as, temporal lobe abscesses have historically been reported as resulting from uncontrolled and untreated mastoiditis.[80] Brain abscesses due to otitis media form almost exclusively ipsilateral to the ear infection. Otitic sources account for 10 to 20% of all brain abscesses.[10,81,82] Age of presentation appears to be bimodal with brain abscesses of all causes occurring most commonly in children younger than 10 years and in adults between 30 and 50 years.[81,82] Mortality from brain abscesses is about 10% in the modern era of CT and antibiotics.[80,83,84]

Symptoms and signs of brain abscess are dependent on the stage of development of the abscess. There is a period of early and late stage cerebritis which occurs over the first week to 10 days following entry of bacteria to the brain.[80,85] During the early period, an inflammatory response develops around the thrombophlebitic vessels and, as the infection progresses, the late stage heralds the body's attempt to restrict the infection to one region of the brain. The cerebritis stage may present with headache, fluctuating temperatures, depressed mental status, and generalized malaise. The late stage cerebritis, when the infection is being isolated by the body, can be mistaken for recovery as symptoms may seem to improve or abate. In the second week following infection the localized inflammation becomes purulent and is encapsulated forming a discrete abscess. The encapsulation stage is heralded by signs of suddenly increased intracranial pressure due to the mass effect of the abscess.[79,80]

The complete classic triad of headache, fever, and focal neurological deficits is rarely seen, and other findings are vomiting, seizures, change in mental status, papilledema, and meningism. As with other intracranial complications, immuno-compromised patients, including diabetics, those being treated for active HIV infection, and those individuals on chemotherapeutic regimens may have a paucity of symptoms.

Typically, otitis media has been identified and treated by the late cerebritis stage and may appear to improve along with the clinical symptoms. A sudden worsening of symptoms should prompt radiographic evaluation with contrast-enhanced CT scan. Areas of low attenuation may be all that is seen in the cerebritis stage. Rim-enhancing abscess will be apparent as disease progresses to the encapsulation stage. CT will also demonstrate mass effect, hydrocephalus, and other intracranial complications of otitis media. MR imaging can demonstrate surrounding areas of edema, dural changes suggestive of meningitis, flow in the venous system, and CSF flow in the ventricular system. Diffusion weighted MRI scans can distinguish abscesses from other lesions of the central nervous system (CNS) due to restricted diffusion in pyogenic lesions.[79] LP is not useful in evaluating for brain abscess and rarely provides a microorganism for identification.[82]

Treatment of brain abscess of otitic origin requires mastoidectomy to address the source of infection. Myringotomy or tube placement can be performed concurrently. Otologic surgery should be performed after the patient is neurologically and medically stabilized. Broad-spectrum antibiotics should be started as aerobic and anaerobic microorganisms are commonly seen.[81,82,84] Neurosurgical consultation should be sought urgently regarding management of the abscess. Medical therapy in the early stage may abort encapsulation

and abscess formation. Small abscesses, high risk patients, multiple abscesses, or those with a good response to initial therapy may be managed without neurosurgical intervention.[80–82] Serial CT or MRI scans should be performed to monitor for abscess growth. Aspiration of the abscess is the most common surgical intervention and can be performed stereotactically, through a burr hole, or open craniotomy[10,81,86] Aspiration is primarily to decompress the abscess and provide a sample for microorganism identification. Surgical excision of the abscess is rarely necessary but cerebellar abscesses should be aggressively managed as they portend a worse outcome due to potential CSF obstruction.[80]

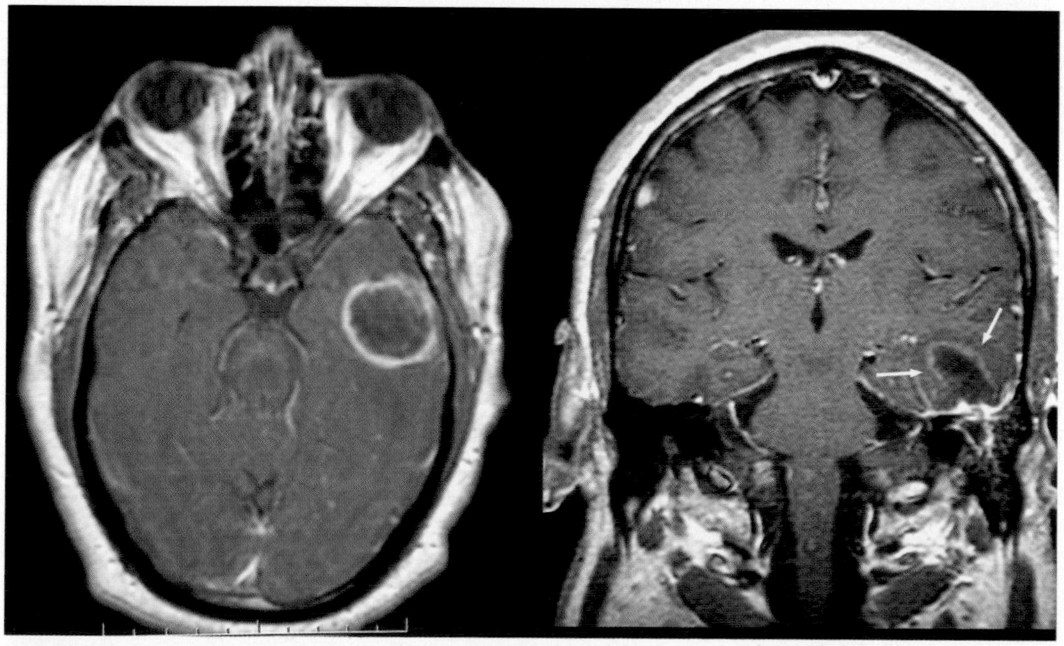

Otitic Hydrocephalus. Otitic hydrocephalus is an increase in CSF pressure in the presence of acute or chronic otitis media. By definition, otitic hydrocephalus is not secondary to brain abscess or meningitis. It is, however, almost exclusively associated with sigmoid sinus thrombosis although not all cases of venous thrombosis show increases in intracranial pressure. Thrombosis of the central venous sinuses can impede absorption of CSF and raise intracranial pressures.[87] Ventricular dilation does not occur as the pathways for CSF circulation remain patent.

Patients typically present with headache, visual changes, and emesis. They may also exhibit changes in mental status, changes in wakefulness, and dizziness or imbalance. On physical examination, there is evidence of acute or chronic otitis media and commonly an abducens nerve palsy.[88] Fundoscopic examination reveals papilledema, but the presence of papilledema does not always imply an increased CSF pressure. An MRI should be performed to assess other intracranial complications, and the MRI or MRV will clearly demonstrate a sigmoid sinus thrombosis.[89] LP should be performed in suspicious cases and an opening pressure of greater than 240 mm H_2O with normal CSF chemistry and cytology is diagnostic.[88]

Treatment should be directed at the underlying otitis media and sigmoid sinus thrombosis. There may be potential benefit to reestablishing flow in a fully thrombosed sigmoid sinus by thrombectomy, but this is controversial. Regulation of intracranial pressure and protection of the optic nerve with corticosteroids, diuretics, or serial LPs should be considered. Ophthalmologic consultation and monitoring of visual acuity and visual fields are recommended.

Figure 10 Magnetic resonance imaging showing a well-encapsulated brain abscess of otitic origin in the left temporal lobe. The coronal image shows an abscess in the early encapsulation phase (*arrows*) forming over an inflamed mastoid. Brain abscesses of otitic origin typically form in the ipsilateral temporal lobe or cerebellum. (Published with permission, copyright © 2007 D.R. Friedland, MD, PhD.)

REFERENCES

1. Sewall E. Otitic meningitis. Calif State J Med 1917; 15:206–12.
2. Agrawal S, Husein M, MacRae D. Complications of otitis media: An evolving state. J Otolaryngol 2005;34:S33–9.
3. Go C, Bernstein JM, de Jong AL, et al. Intracranial complications of acute mastoiditis. Int J Pediatr Otorhinolaryngol 2000;52:143–8.
4. Luntz M, Brodsky A, Nusem S, et al. Acute mastoiditis—the antibiotic era: A multicenter study. Int J Pediatr Otorhinolaryngol 2001;57:1–9.
5. Barry B, Delattre J, Vie F, et al. Otogenic intracranial infections in adults. Laryngoscope 1999;109:483–7.

6. Migirov L, Kronenberg J. Mastoidectomy for acute otomastoiditis: Our experience. Ear Nose Throat J 2005;84:219–22.
7. Block SL, Doern GV, Pfaller MA. Oral beta-lactams in the treatment of acute otitis media. Diagn Microbiol Infect Dis 2007;57:S19–30.
8. Suzuki K, Nishimura T, Baba S. Current status of bacterial resistance in the otolaryngology field: Results from the Second Nationwide Survey in Japan. J Infect Chemother 2003;9:46–52.
9. Aslam MA, Ahmed Z, Azim R. Microbiology and drug sensitivity patterns of chronic suppurative otitis media. J Coll Physicians Surg Pak 2004;14:459–61.
10. Roche M, Humphreys H, Smyth E, et al. A twelve-year review of central nervous system bacterial abscesses; presentation and aetiology. Clin Microbiol Infect 2003;9:803–9.
11. Migirov L, Kronenberg J. Bacteriology of mastoid subperiosteal abscess in children. Acta Otolaryngol 2004;124:23–5.
12. Nissen AJ, Bui H. Complications of chronic otitis media. Ear Nose Throat J 1996;75:284–92.
13. Holt GR, Gates GA. Masked mastoiditis. Laryngoscope 1983;93:1034–7.
14. Masterson T, El-Hakim H, Magnus K, et al. A case of the otogenic variant of Lemierre's syndrome with atypical sequelae and a review of pediatric literature. Int J Pediatr Otorhinolaryngol 2005;69:117–22.
15. Shanley DJ, Murphy TF. Intracranial and extracranial complications of acute mastoiditis: Evaluation with computed tomography. J Am Osteopath Assoc 1992;92:131–4.
16. Antonelli PJ, Garside JA, Mancuso AA, et al. Computed tomography and the diagnosis of coalescent mastoiditis. Otolaryngol Head Neck Surg 1999;120:350–4.
17. Dobben GD, Raofi B, Mafee MF, et al. Otogenic intracranial inflammations: Role of magnetic resonance imaging. Top Magn Reson Imaging 2000;11:76–86.
18. Thomson RB, Jr, Bertram H. Laboratory diagnosis of central nervous system infections. Infect Dis Clin North Am 2001;15:1047–71.
19. Schachern P, Paparella MM, Sano S, et al. A histopathological study of the relationship between otitis media and mastoiditis. Laryngoscope 1991;101:1050–5.
20. Antonelli PJ, Dhanani N, Giannoni CM, et al. Impact of resistant pneumococcus on rates of acute mastoiditis. Otolaryngol Head Neck Surg 1999;121:190–4.
21. Zanetti D, Nassif N. Indications for surgery in acute mastoiditis and their complications in children. Int J Pediatr Otorhinolaryngol 2006;70:1175–82.
22. Taylor MF, Berkowitz RG. Indications for mastoidectomy in acute mastoiditis in children. Ann Otol Rhinol Laryngol 2004;113:69–72.
23. Greenberg JS, Manolidis S. High incidence of complications encountered in chronic otitis media surgery in a U.S. metropolitan public hospital. Otolaryngol Head Neck Surg 2001;125:623–7.
24. Makeham TP, Croxson GR, Coulson S. Infective causes of facial nerve paralysis. Otol Neurotol 2007;28:100–3.
25. Savic DL, Djeric DR. Facial paralysis in chronic suppurative otitis media. Clin Otolaryngol Allied Sci 1989;14:515–7.
26. Fukuda T, Sugie H, Ito M, et al. Bilateral facial palsy caused by bilateral masked mastoiditis. Pediatr Neurol 1998;18:351–3.
27. Hyden D, Akerlind B, Peebo M. Inner ear and facial nerve complications of acute otitis media with focus on bacteriology and virology. Acta Otolaryngol 2006;126:460–6.
28. Joseph EM, Sperling NM. Facial nerve paralysis in acute otitis media: Cause and management revisited. Otolaryngol Head Neck Surg 1998;118:694–6.
29. Yetiser S, Tosun F, Kazkayasi M. Facial nerve paralysis due to chronic otitis media. Otol Neurotol 2002;23:580–8.
30. Kangsanarak J, Fooanant S, Ruckphaopunt K, et al. Extracranial and intracranial complications of suppurative otitis media. Report of 102 cases. J Laryngol Otol 1993;107:999–1004.
31. Chu FW, Jackler RK. Anterior epitympanic cholesteatoma with facial paralysis: A characteristic growth pattern. Laryngoscope 1988;98:274–9.
32. Spiegel JH, Lustig LR, Lee KC, et al. Contemporary presentation and management of a spectrum of mastoid abscesses. Laryngoscope 1998;108:822–8.

33. Marioni G, de Filippis C, Tregnaghi A, et al. Bezold's abscess in children: Case report and review of the literature. Int J Pediatr Otorhinolaryngol 2001;61:173–7.
34. Gadre AK, Brodie HA, Fayad JN, et al. Venous channels of the petrous apex: Their presence and clinical importance. Otolaryngol Head Neck Surg 1997;116:168–74.
35. Chole RA, Donald PJ. Petrous apicitis. Clinical considerations. Ann Otol Rhinol Laryngol 1983;92:544–51.
36. Lutter SA, Kerschner JE, Chusid MJ. Gradenigo syndrome: A rare but serious complication of otitis media. Pediatr Emerg Care 2005;21:384–6.
37. Vazquez E, Castellote A, Piqueras J, et al. Imaging of complications of acute mastoiditis in children. Radiographics 2003;23:359–72.
38. Goldstein NA, Casselbrant ML, Bluestone CD, et al. Intratemporal complications of acute otitis media in infants and children. Otolaryngol Head Neck Surg 1998;119:444–54.
39. Leskinen K, Jero J. Acute complications of otitis media in adults. Clin Otolaryngol 2005;30:511–6.
40. Tinling SP, Colton J, Brodie HA. Location and timing of initial osteoid deposition in postmeningitic labyrinthitis ossificans determined by multiple fluorescent labels. Laryngoscope 2004;114:675–80.
41. Dodge PR, Davis H, Feigin RD, et al. Prospective evaluation of hearing impairment as a sequela of acute bacterial meningitis. N Engl J Med 1984;311:869–74.
42. Trinidad A, Ramirez-Camacho R, Garcia-Berrocal JR, et al. Labyrinthitis secondary to experimental otitis media. Am J Otolaryngol 2005;26:226–9.
43. Durisin M, Stover T, Leinung M, et al. Otogenic cerebellar abscess due to purulent labyrinthitis and defect of the superior semicircular canal and its propagation through the endolymphatic sac. Eur Arch Otorhinolaryngol 2007.
44. Wetmore RF. Complications of otitis media. Pediatr Ann 2000;29:637–46.
45. Magliulo G, Terranova G, Varacalli S, et al. Labyrinthine fistula as a complication of cholesteatoma. Am J Otol 1997;18:697–701.
46. Jang CH, Merchant SN. Histopathology of labyrinthine fistulae in chronic otitis media with clinical implications. Am J Otol 1997;18:15–25.
47. Gersdorff MC, Nouwen J, Decat M, et al. Labyrinthine fistula after cholesteatomatous chronic otitis media. Am J Otol 2000;21:32–5.
48. de Zinis LO, Campovecchi C, Gadola E. Fistula of the cochlear labyrinth in noncholesteatomatous chronic otitis media. Otol Neurotol 2005;26:830–3.
49. Grewal DS, Hathiram BT, Dwivedi A, et al. Labyrinthine fistula: A complication of chronic suppurative otitis media. J Laryngol Otol 2003;117:353–7.
50. Manolidis S. Complications associated with labyrinthine fistula in surgery for chronic otitis media. Otolaryngol Head Neck Surg 2000;123:733–7.
51. Herzog JA, Smith PG, Kletzker GR, et al. Management of labyrinthine fistulae secondary to cholesteatoma. Am J Otol 1996;17:410–5.
52. Brown NE, Grundfast KM, Jabre A, et al. Diagnosis and management of spontaneous cerebrospinal fluid-middle ear effusion and otorrhea. Laryngoscope 2004;114:800–5.
53. Patel RB, Kwartler JA, Hodosh RM, et al. Spontaneous cerebrospinal fluid leakage and middle ear encephalocele in seven patients. Ear Nose Throat J 2000;79:372-3, 76–8.
54. Lundy LB, Graham MD, Kartush JM, et al. Temporal bone encephalocele and cerebrospinal fluid leaks. Am J Otol 1996;17:461–9.
55. Wootten CT, Kaylie DM, Warren FM, et al. Management of brain herniation and cerebrospinal fluid leak in revision chronic ear surgery. Laryngoscope 2005;115:1256–61.
56. Abramson M, McMurtry JG, Kadis G. Combined otoneurosurgical approach to patients with chronic ear disease and cerebrospinal otorrhea. Laryngoscope 1979;89:918–21.
57. Migirov L, Duvdevani S, Kronenberg J. Otogenic intracranial complications: A review of 28 cases. Acta Otolaryngol 2005;125:819–22.
58. Kangsanarak J, Navacharoen N, Fooanant S, et al. Intracranial complications of suppurative otitis media: 13 years' experience. Am J Otol 1995;16:104–9.
59. Husain E, Chawla R, Dobson S, et al. Epidemiology and outcome of bacterial meningitis in Canadian children: 1998-1999. Clin Invest Med 2006;29:131–5.

60. Dubey SP, Larawin V. Complications of chronic suppurative otitis media and their management. Laryngoscope 2007;117:264–7.
61. Osma U, Cureoglu S, Hosoglu S. The complications of chronic otitis media: Report of 93 cases. J Laryngol Otol 2000;114:97–100.
62. van de Beek D, de Gans J, Spanjaard L, et al. Clinical features and prognostic factors in adults with bacterial meningitis. N Engl J Med 2004;351:1849–59.
63. Fitch MT, van de Beek D. Emergency diagnosis and treatment of adult meningitis. Lancet Infect Dis 2007;7:191–200.
64. Durand ML, Calderwood SB, Weber DJ, et al. Acute bacterial meningitis in adults. A review of 493 episodes. N Engl J Med 1993;328:21–8.
65. van de Beek D, de Gans J, McIntyre P, et al. Corticosteroids for acute bacterial meningitis. Cochrane Database Syst Rev 2007:CD004405.
66. Manolidis S, Johnson R. Do corticosteroids prevent hearing loss in pediatric bacterial meningitis? An analysis of the evidence. Ear Nose Throat J 2006;85:586–92.
67. Hafidh MA, Keogh I, Walsh RM, et al. Otogenic intracranial complications. A 7-year retrospective review. Am J Otolaryngol 2006;27:390–5.
68. Manolidis S, Kutz JW, Jr. Diagnosis and management of lateral sinus thrombosis. Otol Neurotol 2005;26:1045–51.
69. Syms MJ, Tsai PD, Holtel MR. Management of lateral sinus thrombosis. Laryngoscope 1999;109:1616–20.
70. Iseri M, Aydin O, Ustundag E, et al. Management of lateral sinus thrombosis in chronic otitis media. Otol Neurotol 2006;27:1098–103.
71. Bradley DT, Hashisaki GT, Mason JC. Otogenic sigmoid sinus thrombosis: What is the role of anticoagulation? Laryngoscope 2002;112:1726–9.
72. Singh B. The management of lateral sinus thrombosis. J Laryngol Otol 1993;107:803–8.
73. Rosen A, Ophir D, Marshak G. Acute mastoiditis: A review of 69 cases. Ann Otol Rhinol Laryngol 1986;95:222–4.
74. Bizakis JG, Velegrakis GA, Papadakis CE, et al. The silent epidural abscess as a complication of acute otitis media in children. Int J Pediatr Otorhinolaryngol 1998;45:163–6.
75. Park H, Jang H, Shim D, et al. Surgical management of acute mastoiditis with epidural abscess. Acta Otolaryngol 2006;126:782–4.
76. Wackym PA, Canalis RF, Feuerman T. Subdural empyema of otorhinological origin. J Laryngol Otol 1990;104:118–22.
77. Osborn MK, Steinberg JP. Subdural empyema and other suppurative complications of paranasal sinusitis. Lancet Infect Dis 2007;7:62–7.
78. Weisberg L. Subdural empyema. Clinical and computed tomographic correlations. Arch Neurol 1986;43:497–500.
79. Ferreira NP, Otta GM, do Amaral LL, et al. Imaging aspects of pyogenic infections of the central nervous system. Top Magn Reson Imaging 2005;16:145–54.
80. Sharma BS, Gupta SK, Khosla VK. Current concepts in the management of pyogenic brain abscess. Neurol India 2000;48:105–11.
81. Yen PT, Chan ST, Huang TS. Brain abscess: With special reference to otolaryngologic sources of infection. Otolaryngol Head Neck Surg 1995;113:15–22.
82. Kao PT, Tseng HK, Liu CP, et al. Brain abscess: Clinical analysis of 53 cases. J Microbiol Immunol Infect 2003;36:129–36.
83. Yogev R, Bar-Meir M. Management of brain abscesses in children. Pediatr Infect Dis J 2004;23:157–9.
84. Carpenter J, Stapleton S, Holliman R. Retrospective analysis of 49 cases of brain abscess and review of the literature. Eur J Clin Microbiol Infect Dis 2007;26:1–11.
85. Brand B, Caparosa RJ, Lubic LG. Otorhinological brain abscess therapy–past and present. Laryngoscope 1984;94:483–7.
86. Barlas O, Sencer A, Erkan K, et al. Stereotactic surgery in the management of brain abscess. Surg Neurol 1999;52:404–10; discussion 11.
87. Stam J. Thrombosis of the cerebral veins and sinuses. N Engl J Med 2005;352:1791–8.
88. Kuczkowski J, Dubaniewicz-Wybieralska M, Przewozny T, et al. Otitic hydrocephalus associated with lateral sinus thrombosis and acute mastoiditis in children. Int J Pediatr Otorhinolaryngol 2006;70:1817–23.
89. Omer Unal F, Sennaroglu L, Saatci I. Otitic hydrocephalus: Role of radiology for diagnosis. Int J Pediatr Otorhinolaryngol 2005;69:897–901.

Reconstruction of the Middle Ear

Saumil N. Merchant, MD
John J. Rosowski, PhD
Clough Shelton, MD

INTRODUCTION

Tympanoplasty is a surgical procedure designed to reconstruct the sound transmission mechanism of the middle ear. The modern era of tympanoplasty was ushered in during the 1950s with the pioneering work of Wullstein[1] and Zollner.[2] Subsequently, many other otologic surgeons contributed to the development and refinement of techniques of tympanoplasty. The most common indication for tympanoplasty is to repair a defect of the middle ear caused by chronic otitis media (COM). Tympanoplasty is also indicated for the repair of middle ear defects resulting from other causes such as trauma and neoplasms. Tympanoplasty may be combined with mastoidectomy performed for control of infection in COM. Techniques to repair traumatic lesions of the middle ear are described in Chapter 21, "Trauma to the Middle Ear, Inner Ear, and Temporal Bone" and mastoidectomy procedures are described in Chapter 17, "Chronic Otitis Media and Cholesteatoma." This chapter focuses on tympanoplasty in COM.

PHYSIOLOGIC PRINCIPLES OF TYMPANOPLASTY

It is helpful to review the functions of the normal middle ear to understand the physiologic basis of successful tympanoplasty. The tympanic membrane(TM)-ossicular system of the normal ear amplifies the sound pressure at the oval window compared to the sound pressure in the ear canal; this amplification is termed "the middle ear gain." The gain provided by the average normal ear is only about 20 dB (a factor of 10).[3] Most of the gain is a result of the TM to stapes footplate area ratio: the TM gathers force over its surface and the ossicles couple the gathered force to the smaller footplate of the stapes. Only about 2 dB of gain is provided by the ossicular lever that results from the difference in length of the rotating malleus and incus lever arms, (manubrium vs. incus long process). Some of the amplification provided by the area and lever ratios is used to overcome the stiffness, mass and damping within the TM and ossicular system, so the resultant gain is smaller than expected from calculations based on anatomy and also varies with frequency.[3]

The middle ear cavity (the air space behind the TM) enables motion of the TM and ossicles by providing a compressible air cushion. When sound in the ear canal strikes the TM, most of the gathered force is used to move the TM, ossicles and the cochlear fluids, but about one-third to one-tenth of the gathered force acts to compress and rarify the air in the enclosed cavity. The result is a sound pressure within the cavity that is 10 to 20 dB lower than the ear canal sound pressure[4] and a trans-tympanic difference in sound pressure that is proportional to the drive on the TM and the ossicles.

The increase in sound pressure relative to the ear canal delivered by the stapes in combination with the relative decrease in middle ear cavity sound pressure are important, since the cochlea responds to a difference in the sound pressure between the oval and round windows.[5] Since sound can vary in both its magnitude and relative phase, it is important to understand that the sound-pressure difference at the cochlear windows is affected by differences in the magnitudes and phases of the individual sounds at the windows. One simplification is that differences in magnitude can overwhelm differences in phase. In the normal ear, the difference in magnitude between the sounds acting on the two windows is at least 30 dB. The middle ear gain increases the pressures at the oval window by 20 dB, and sound pressure acting on the round window is the middle ear cavity pressure, which is at least 10 dB smaller than the ear canal sound stimulus. In the normal ear and after successful tympanoplasty, the magnitude of sound pressure at the oval window is significantly greater than that at the round window, and under these circumstances, differences in phase have little effect on determining the window pressure difference.[6]

It follows from this discussion that the goal of a tympanoplasty should be to restore the difference in sound pressure at the cochlear windows, by (1) reconstructing a TM-ossicular system to amplify the sound pressure at the oval window, and (2) reducing the sound pressure at the round window by placing a reconstructed TM, and an air-filled middle ear space between the ear canal and the round window. In reconstructing the TM-ossicular system, the surgeon should concentrate on restoring the TM-to-stapes area ratio rather than the less important ossicular lever. It is noteworthy that other considerations require that the reconstructed stapes footplate should have an area similar to that of the normal stapes,[7] so that minimizing footplate area to maintain a "normal" area ratio is not a viable reconstructive philosophy. It should also be clear that establishing an aerated middle ear cavity that allows motion of the reconstructed TM and reduces the sound pressure acting on the round window is a prerequisite for the success of any tympanoplasty.

PREOPERATIVE CONSIDERATIONS

Tympanoplasty can be considered when there is a conductive hearing loss of 30 dB or greater in an ear with COM that has good cochlear function. It can also be considered for repair of a TM perforation to eliminate the need for water precautions. Tympanoplasty carries a small risk of inducing a sensorineural hearing loss. Therefore, an only hearing ear or much better hearing ear is a contraindication for tympanoplasty.

Surgical decision-making in a patient with COM must be individualized. Several factors should be considered including the hearing levels in the diseased and contralateral ear, the pathology and activity of COM, and the age, general health and medical condition of the patient. These factors must be modified by the experience and talent of the otologic surgeon.

At the outset, it is critical to make an accurate diagnostic assessment of the type and nature of COM in each patient when contemplating tympanoplasty. First, one should distinguish between COM with and without cholesteatoma. Patients with cholesteatoma generally need a mastoidectomy or atticotomy to eradicate the cholesteatoma in addition to tympanoplasty to restore hearing. In such cases, tympanoplasty could be combined with mastoidectomy or be performed at a second stage (see later under staging). Patients who have COM without cholesteatoma may be conveniently divided into three categories: *active* COM, characterized by a perforated TM with otorrhea, *inactive* COM, characterized by a dry perforation, and *inactive COM with frequent reactivation*, characterized by ears that drain intermittently.[8] Active COM without cholesteatoma should be treated medically to control infection and eliminate otorrhea, thus converting the process to inactive COM. Expectant observation for 4 to 6 months is recommended, and if the ear remains dry, then elective tympanoplasty may be performed. Failure of medical management in active COM without cholesteatoma generally indicates the presence of irreversible disease in the middle ear and mastoid (typically granulation tissue) and is best treated by combining mastoidectomy with tympanoplasty. Inactive COM with frequent reactivation needs attention to inciting events such as water exposure. If there are no obvious predisposing events, then mastoidectomy is generally recommended in conjunction with tympanoplasty to eliminate infection and granulation in the mastoid tracts, antrum, and epitympanum. Failure to recognize and treat cholesteatoma or potential infection in the middle ear and mastoid is a common cause of failed tympanoplasty.

Children under 5 years of age are not good candidates for tympanoplasty because of risk of subsequent failure from otitis media and poor eustachian tube function. For the elderly and for adults with serious medical problems, one has to determine whether the benefits of surgery outweigh the risks of anesthesia.

Patients with a history of multiple failed tympanoplasty procedures are likely to have insurmountable hurdles, including nonfunctioning eustachian tubes, middle ear fibrosis, and tendency for failure of TM grafts and extrusion of prostheses. In such patients, the goal of chronic ear surgery should be to make the ear safe and dry, and hearing improvement should be achieved by amplification or a bone-anchored hearing aid, rather than additional tympanoplasty surgery.

PREOPERATIVE EVALUATION

The preoperative evaluation should include a complete otologic and medical history, otologic and head and neck examination, and audiometric evaluation. Evaluation using an otomicroscope can provide a wealth of useful information to the trained eye. The size and shape of a perforation should be noted, which in conjunction with the extent of anterior canal wall convexity will help to determine the appropriate surgical approach. A retraction pocket of the pars tensa or pars flaccida with retention of keratin debris signifies a cholesteatoma. Signs of infection may be obvious, such as pooling of pus in the middle ear, or subtle, such as minute granulations at the margins of a perforation. As previously noted, the presence of a cholesteatoma or infection may signify the need to consider an atticotomy or mastoidectomy in addition to the tympanoplasty to eradicate the infection.

Otomicroscopic examination can also help one to assess the integrity of the ossicular chain. Malleus mobility can be evaluated by pneumatic otoscopy if the TM is intact. A perforation may allow for inspection of the continuity of the incus and stapes. Chalky white plaques of tympanosclerosis around the oval window may signify fixation of the footplate, in which case a second-stage stapedectomy may be necessary.

A functioning eustachian tube is critical to the success of tympanoplasty. However, tests of tubal function that can be used preoperatively as a reliable predictor of surgical success do not exist.[9,10] Indirect indicators for poor eustachian tube function include bilateral disease, chronic serous otitis media in the contralateral ear, fibrocystic obliteration of the middle ear and mastoid air spaces, uncontrolled rhinosinusitis, cleft palate, and other skull base abnormalities.

Preoperative audiologic evaluation should include a pure tone audiogram with adequate masking and speech discrimination testing. Assessment of the audiometric profile can help the clinician anticipate middle ear pathology which in turn can help in preoperative planning and counseling. Perforations of the TM result in a predominantly low frequency conductive hearing loss that is roughly proportionate to the size of the perforation.[11] An air-bone gap that is disproportionately large for a given perforation may indicate ossicular discontinuity or fixation. A piece of cigarette paper or gelfilm coated with ointment may be placed over the perforation with assessment of hearing before and after application of the patch. Lack of hearing improvement after placing the patch indicates ossicular problems such as fixation or discontinuity.

Ossicular discontinuity in the presence of an intact TM results in a relatively flat, 60-dB air-bone gap on audiometry. Ossicular discontinuity in the presence of a perforation gives a somewhat smaller air-bone gap of about 40 to 50 dB. Resorption of the incudostapedial joint and its replacement by a fibrous band may result in an air-bone gap that is greater at the higher frequencies than at the lower frequencies and may be manifest as fluctuating hearing loss with better hearing thresholds when the ear is autoinflated. Lateral displacement of the TM and incus by autoinflation causes the fibrous band to become taut, improving sound transmission.

An air-bone gap in a patient with an intact, healthy TM and an aerated middle ear usually indicates ossicular fixation. Stapes fixation due to tympanosclerosis or otosclerosis can result in an air-bone gap of up to 50 to 60 dB. In contrast, isolated fixation of the malleus head usually results in an air-bone gap of no more than 20 to 30 dB. Less commonly, lesions of the inner ear (such as superior semicircular canal dehiscence or an enlarged vestibular aqueduct) can present with an air-bone gap mimicking ossicular fixation.[12] Distinguishing features of air-bone gaps caused by such inner ear lesions are: (1) bone conduction thresholds below 2,000 Hz may be better than 0 dB (-5 to -15 dB); hence it is important for the audiologist to determine true bone conduction thresholds in ears with an air-bone gap rather than terminate testing when a threshold of 0 dB is attained; (2) the stapedial (acoustic) reflex is present, as opposed to ears with ossicular lesions where the reflex is abolished; and (3) thresholds for the vestibular evoked myogenic potential (VEMP) test are lower than normal. High-resolution computed tomography (CT) will help confirm a suspected diagnosis of an inner ear lesion such as superior semicircular canal dehiscence or enlarged vestibular aqueduct.

CLASSIFICATION AND SURGICAL TECHNIQUES

We present a modified version of Wullstein's original classification. Tympanoplasties are classified as types I–V, wherein type I involves reconstruction of only the TM, while types II–V involve reconstruction of the ossicular chain with or without repair of the TM. Table 1 lists the various types of tympanoplasty, which are discussed in more detail below.

Tympanoplasty may be performed under local or general anesthesia, and via a transcanal, endaural, or postauricular incision. The choice of incision depends on several factors including the nature of the anticipated pathology and reconstruction, the desired degree of exposure of the tympanic cavity, the state of the patient's ear canal and external auditory meatus, whether additional mastoid or atticotomy procedures are contemplated, and preference of the otologic surgeon. Informed consent should also be obtained. A large number of tympanoplasty methods and techniques have been described over the past five decades. This chapter provides an overview of basic techniques.

Type I Tympanoplasty

Type I tympanoplasty refers to repair of the TM without altering the ossicular system. The procedure includes exploration of the middle ear to inspect and ensure normality of the ossicles. *Myringoplasty* refers to repair of the TM alone, without inspection of the ossicular chain. A large variety of tissue grafts have been described for type I tympanoplasty including temporalis fascia, perichondrium, cartilage, periosteum, ear lobe adipose tissue, etc.[13] Furthermore, a large number of techniques have been described for repair of perforations, depending on the size and location of the perforation. Type I tympanoplasty is the most commonly performed tympanoplasty.

For small posterior perforations or small central perforations, a commonly used technique is the medial onlay grafting technique, also called the underlay technique (Figures 1A and 2). The edges of the perforation are freshened with a sharp pick, followed by elevation of a tympanomeatal flap. The medial surface of the TM remnant is inspected under high magnification to identify and remove squamous epithelium that may have migrated through the perforation onto the medial surface of the TM. The ossicles are inspected and their mobility is confirmed. It may be necessary to remove a small amount of bone of the ear canal near the annulus in the posterior-superior quadrant to obtain an adequate view of the incus and stapes. A tissue graft such as that made of temporalis fascia is trimmed to approximately double the area of the perforation and then placed medial to the TM. The middle ear is filled with pledgets of gelfoam to support the graft on its undersurface.

Table 1 Classification of Tympanoplasty

Type I	Repair of the tympanic membrane without altering the ossicular chain
Type II	Repair of the ossicular chain with restoration of the lever mechanism
Type III, minor columella	Repair of the ossicular chain by placing a graft from the stapes capitulum to the tympanic membrane or manubrium
Type III, major columella	Repair of the ossicular chain using a single graft interposed between a mobile footplate and the tympanic membrane or manubrium
Type III, stapes columella	Repair of the ossicular chain by placing a tympanic membrane graft directly onto the capitulum of the stapes
Type IV	A mobile stapes footplate remains directly exposed to incoming sound from the ear canal, while a tissue graft is placed to acoustically shield the round window membrane from sound
Type Va	Fenestration of the lateral semicircular canal so as to bypass an ankylosed stapes footplate
Type Vb	Identical to a type IV, except that the stapes footplate is removed and the oval window is sealed by a tissue graft

The perforation is approached via an endaural or postauricular incision. The skin of the bony ear canal is elevated and either preserved for replacement at the end, or resected if skin grafting is utilized. The bony ear canal is then enlarged (canalplasty) using liberal irrigation to avoid overheating the tympanic bone. Care is taken to avoid trauma to the capsule of the temporomandibular joint and its contents. In the lateral onlay technique (also called overlay tympanoplasty), all epithelium is removed from the surface of the TM remnant, while preserving its fibrous layer. A graft of temporalis fascia is then placed on the lateral surface of the TM remnant but with a slit made in the graft, so that the graft goes deep to the manubrium and can be wrapped around the neck of the malleus. In the total drum replacement technique, the entire remnant of the TM is

If the perforation is in the anterior half of the TM or if the perforation is of a subtotal or total nature, then the medial onlay technique described above may fail because the anterior edge of the graft falls away from and fails to adhere to the anterior remnant of the TM. In such cases of large or anteriorly situated perforations, two techniques that can be utilized are the lateral onlay technique or the technique of total drum replacement (Figure 1B). Both techniques are similar and are described below. While technically demanding, both methods are extremely reliable with graft-take rates in excess of 95%.

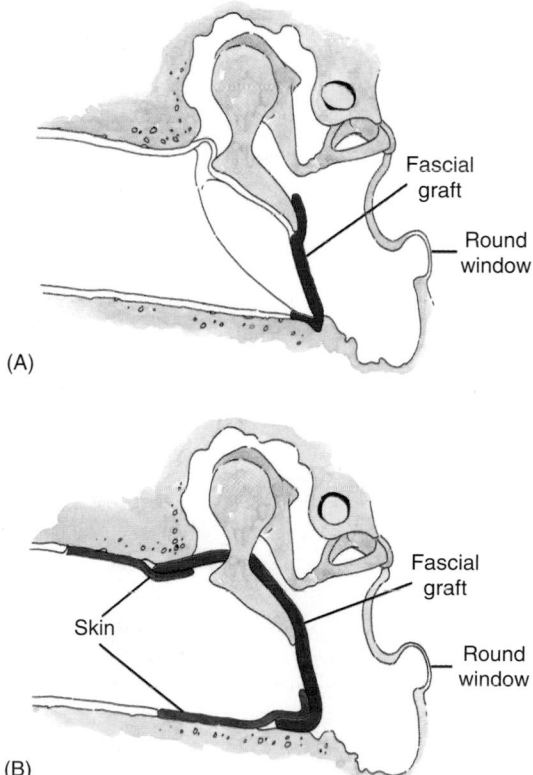

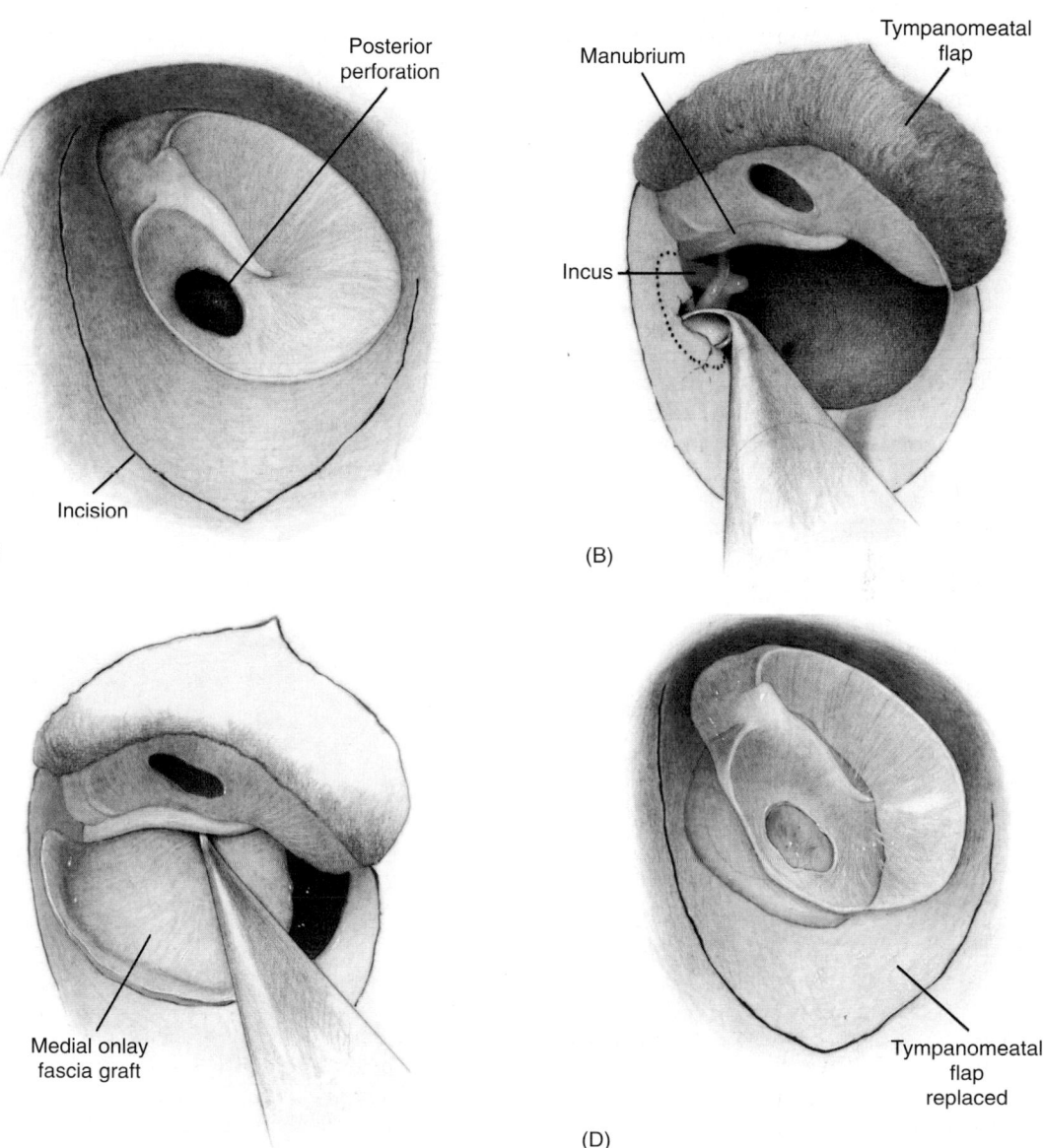

Figure 1 Type I tympanoplasty: repair of a tympanic membrane perforation with a tissue graft in the presence of an intact and mobile ossicular chain. (A) Schematic showing repair of a small perforation of the tympanic membrane with a medial onlay fascial graft (also called an underlay graft). (B) Schematic showing repair of the entire tympanic membrane with temporalis fascia (total drum replacement). (Published with permission, copyright © 2006 S.N. Merchant.)

Figure 2 Type I tympanoplasty by the medial onlay grafting (also called underlay) technique. Schematics depict surgical view of right tympanic membrane. (A) Showing incision made in skin of posterior canal wall. This is followed by elevation of a tympanomeatal flap which is reflected anteriorly. (B) The middle ear is inspected and the ossicles are palpated to confirm integrity of the ossicular chain. If necessary, the bony sulcus tympanicus is removed as depicted by the dotted line to improve visualization of the ossicular chain. (C) A graft of temporalis fascia is placed so that it will be on the medial aspect of the tympanomeatal flap. (D) The tympanomeatal flap is replaced. Gelfoam packing is usually used to fill the tympanic space between the graft and the medial wall of the middle ear, which helps to hold the graft in place against the under surface of the tympanic membrane. (Published with permission, copyright © 2006 S.N. Merchant.)

removed. A graft of temporalis fascia is trimmed to an appropriate size that will bridge the entire tympanic space and reflect approximately 3 mm onto the walls of the bony canal. A slit in the graft enables the graft to be placed medial to the manubrium and be wrapped around the neck of the malleus. The remainder of the procedure is similar in both techniques. The exposed bony canal is covered with canal skin that was saved initially, or with split-thickness skin grafts harvested from the upper arm. In this manner, all raw surfaces of the ear canal are covered with epithelium. This is followed by carefully packing the ear canal to hold the reconstruction in place. The success of the lateral onlay and total drum replacement techniques depends on recreating a sharp anterior tympanomeatal angle so as to prevent blunting, as well as placing the fascia graft medial to the manubrium to prevent lateralization of the graft. Blunting refers to proliferation of fibrous tissue in the anterior tympanomeatal angle, which interferes with mechanics of the TM and the manubrium, resulting in conductive hearing loss. As an alternative to fascia, thin AlloDerm (LifeCell Corporation Branchburg, NJ) can be used.

Type II Tympanoplasty

Type II tympanoplasty refers to repair of the TM and ossicular system with restoration of the lever mechanism, which is a normal function of the malleus and incus (Figure 3). The most common indication is osteitic resorption of the distal part of the long process of the incus. Often, the area of the resorption is replaced by a fibrous band. The fibrous band is resected with scissors or a laser. Continuity of the ossicular chain can be restored in one of several ways, including a bone strut, a synthetic prosthesis, or otologic cement. If there is any doubt about the stability or adequacy of the mechanical coupling of the reconstruction, the incus should be removed and continuity restored by a type III procedure (see below).

Type III Tympanoplasty

Type III tympanoplasty restores sound conduction to the oval window by one of the following three types of columellar reconstructions- minor columella, major columella, or stapes columella, each of which is considered separately:

Tympanoplasty type III, minor columella. A minor columella procedure consists of placing a graft or prosthesis from the stapes capitulum to the TM or manubrium (Figure 4). A synthetic columella of this type is termed a partial ossicular replacement prosthesis (PORP). A minor columella is suitable for reconstructing an ear with an intact posterior canal wall and a mobile stapes with its superstructure. A minor columella may be the only procedure, as in an elective tympanoplasty, or may be combined with a canal wall up or down mastoidectomy for COM.

A variety of autograft, homograft, and alloplastic prostheses are available for minor columellar reconstructions. A readily available reconstructive material is an autologous ossicle, either the body of the incus or the head of the malleus. The ossicular graft is sculpted to suitable dimensions using the operating microscope and small burs, along with liberal irrigation with

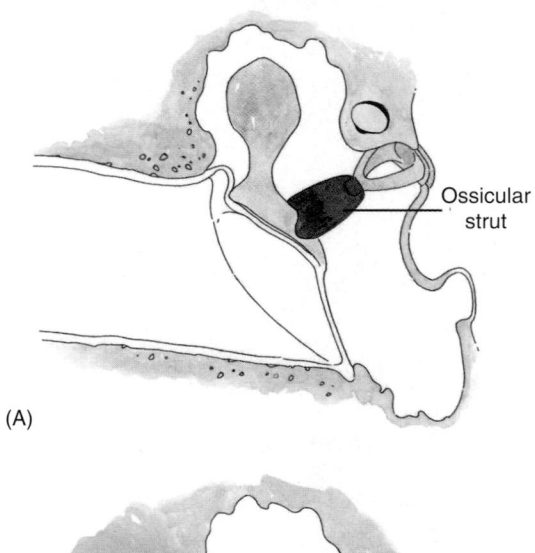

(A)

saline to avoid thermal injury. A facet is drilled to accommodate the stapes capitulum, and a groove is created on the opposite side to accept the manubrium (Figure 4A). If the manubrium is missing or too far anterior (when compared to the stapes) for a stable assembly, the strut is brought from the stapes capitulum to the TM. It is important to make the ossicle strut small enough so that it is not too close to the bony tympanic sulcus, promontory or facial canal to prevent ankylosis of the strut to these structures. If autologous ossicles are not available, a minor columella can be fashioned from autologous cortical bone. Studies have shown that autogenous ossicular and cortical bone grafts behave in a similar manner and retain their morphologic size, shape, and contour for extended periods of time, at least up to 30 years and probably much longer. They do not incite formation of exuberant new bone nor do they show excessive resorption of bone in the absence of infection.[14] They demonstrate varying amounts of replacement of nonviable bone by new bone through a slow process of creeping substitution.

A PORP can be used as an alternative to an autograft or homograft ossicle (Figure 4B). A large variety of PORPs have been described, which differ in the material used to make the PORP or in the shape and size of the PORP.[15] PORPs made of porous polyethylene, hydroxyapatite or titanium are popular in contemporary otologic practice. A buffer of thin cartilage (0.5 mm or less in thickness) is often interposed between a PORP and the TM to decrease the potential for extrusion.

Tympanoplasty type III, major columella. A major columella is a reconstruction interposed between the stapes footplate and TM or manubrium (Figure 5). It is performed in cases where the stapes crurae are missing and the footplate is intact and mobile. A major columella made of synthetic material is termed a total ossicular

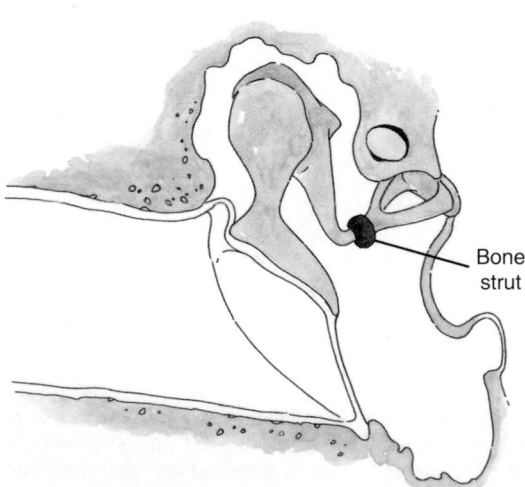

Figure 3 Type II tympanoplasty, which implies reestablishing the lever mechanism of the ossicular chain. Schematic shows a small bone strut interposed between the long process of the incus and stapes capitulum. (Published with permission, copyright © 2006 S.N. Merchant.)

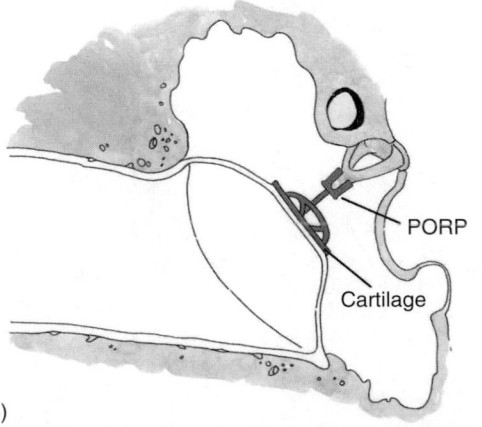

(B)

Figure 4 Type III tympanoplasty, minor columella. The reconstruction consists of interposing a sculptured bone strut (A) or a partial ossicular replacement prosthesis (PORP) (B) between the stapes head and manubrium or tympanic membrane. A thin slice of cartilage is generally placed between a PORP and tympanic membrane to act as a buffer and minimize extrusion of the PORP. (Published with permission, copyright © 2006 S.N. Merchant.)

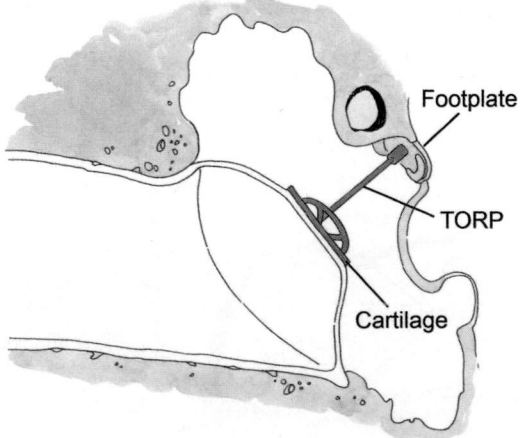

Figure 5 Type III tympanoplasty, major columella. A major columella is a single reconstructive strut that bridges the space from the footplate to the tympanic membrane or manubrium. Total ossicular replacement prostheses (TORPs) are generally preferable to bone struts which have a tendency to ankylose to the walls of the oval window niche. A thin slice of cartilage is usually placed between the TORP and tympanic membrane to act as a buffer and minimize extrusion of the TORP. (Published with permission, copyright © 2006 S.N. Merchant.)

replacement prosthesis (TORP). A major columellar reconstruction may be the only procedure performed, or it may be combined with a canal wall up or canal wall down mastoidectomy. An ossicular or cortical bone strut fashioned as a major columella has a risk of delayed ankylosis of the strut to the fallopian canal or to the promontory. It is also difficult to fashion such as a strut with precision. In general, better results are achieved with a TORP. As is the case with minor columellas, a variety of TORPs are available, and reconstructions can be performed from the footplate to the TM or to the manubrium, if the latter is present. A thin slice of cartilage (0.5 mm or less in thickness) is often placed between the TORP and the TM to decrease the chance for extrusion.

Tympanoplasty type III, stapes columella. A stapes columellar reconstruction involves placing the TM graft directly on the capitulum of the stapes (Figure 6). The procedure is usually done in association with a canal wall down mastoidectomy for active COM. The posterior bony canal wall is removed to the level of the facial nerve. The new tympanic cavity (cavum major) is limited superiorly by the tensor tympani semicanal and tympanic segment of the facial nerve and posteriorly by the mastoid segment of the facial nerve. The mastoid cavity and epitympanum are usually obliterated with pedicled or free muscle-fascial grafts, supplemented with bone pâté (Figures 6 to 8). The procedure is usually combined with enlargement of the ear canal (canalplasty) and the external auditory meatus (meatoplasty). It has been shown that placing a large, thin slice of cartilage (0.5 mm or less in thickness) between the fascial graft and the stapes capitulum improves the postoperative hearing results of this reconstruction, probably because of an improved area ratio.[16]

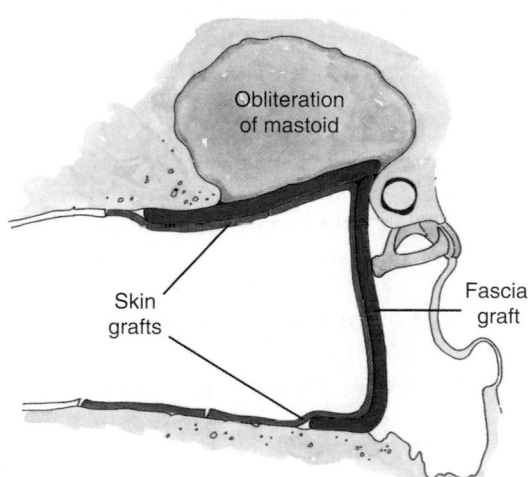

Figure 6 Type III tympanoplasty, stapes columella. A graft of temporalis fascia bridges across the tympanic cavity and is placed in direct contact with the stapes head. The procedure is usually done in conjunction with a canal wall down mastoidectomy. The mastoid cavity and epitympanum are usually obliterated with pedicled or free muscle-fascial grafts, supplemented with bone pâté. Unepithelialized surfaces are covered with skin grafts. (Published with permission, copyright © 2006 S.N. Merchant.)

Mastoidectomy

Mastoidectomy is often combined with tympanoplasty, as described above. A canal wall up mastoidectomy consists of removal of disease from the mastoid, while preserving the posterior wall of the bony external auditory canal. The cells of the mastoid are exenetrated by surgical drilling. The limits of surgery are the tegmental plate superiorly, the sinodural angle posterosuperiorly, the sigmoid sinus plate posteriorly, the bony canal wall anteriorly, and the bony semicircular canals medially. The epitympanum is opened by enlarging the aditus ad antrum. A posterior tympanotomy is often performed by opening the facial recess, which enables removal of disease. A canal-wall down mastoidectomy consists of removal of the posterior bony canal wall so that the external auditory canal, mastoid, and epitympanum become one common cavity. The bony canal wall is lowered to the level of the facial nerve. Thorough exenteration of cells of the mastoid is necessary for success of the procedure. This includes removal of cells of the mastoid tip, the sinodural angle, and the tegmental area. The size of the resulting mastoid bowl is often reduced by obliterating the mastoid cavity. A variety of options are available for obliteration including bone pâté and free or pedicled flaps of soft tissue.

Type IV Tympanoplasty

In type IV tympanoplasty, the stapes footplate is allowed to remain directly exposed to incoming sound from the ear canal, and a tissue graft is placed to acoustically shield the round window membrane from sound (Figure 7). The air space that is enclosed between the acoustic shield and the round window is called the cavum minor. The cavum minor is aerated via the eustachian tube. A type IV procedure is suitable when there is a canal wall down mastoidectomy and the TM, malleus, incus, and stapes superstructure are missing but the footplate is mobile. The footplate is usually covered by a thin split-thickness skin graft and the round window is acoustically shielded by a stiff graft, comprised of thick (1 mm) cartilage and temporalis fascia.[6] A stiff graft will help to maximize the sound-pressure difference between the oval and round windows.

Type V Tympanoplasty

The type V operation is used to bypass an ankylosed stapes footplate and is performed as a second-stage procedure after eradication of active COM. There are two subtypes: (1) The type Va procedure is the original Wullstein type V and consists of fenestration of the lateral semicircular canal to bypass the ankylosed stapes footplate; and (2) The type Vb is similar to a type IV, except the stapes footplate is removed and the oval window is sealed by a tissue graft, usually made of adipose tissue (Figure 8). Type Va procedures are rarely performed, having been largely supplanted by type Vb operations.

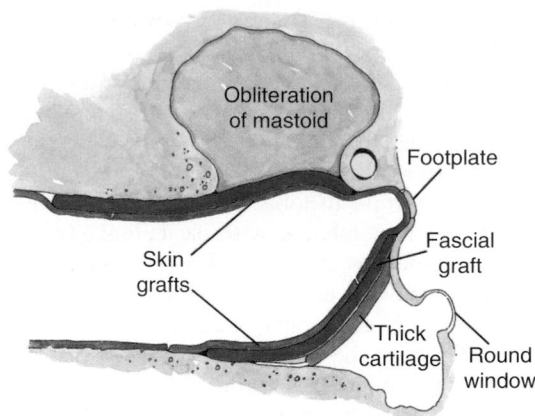

Figure 7 Type IV tympanoplasty. This procedure requires a canal wall down tympanomastoidectomy and may be performed when all ossicles are missing, but the footplate is mobile. A thin split-thickness skin graft lines the oval window niche. The hypotympanum and round window are acoustically protected by a stiff graft of fascia and thick cartilage. The air space lateral to the round window (cavum minor) is aerated via the eustachian tube. The mastoid cavity and epitympanum are usually obliterated with pedicled or free muscle-fascial grafts, supplemented with bone pâté. Unepithelialized surfaces are covered by skin grafts. (Published with permission, copyright © 2006 S.N. Merchant.)

SPECIAL CONSIDERATIONS: STAGING

Staging refers to performing the tympanoplasty reconstruction in two operations, usually 6 to 12 months apart. Staging can be considered for three different indications. (1) A two-stage procedure is almost always indicated when the stapes is fixed. The first stage consists of eradication of active disease from the middle ear and mastoid and repair of a TM perforation. The second stage consists of a stapedectomy and is performed provided the ear is dry, aerated, and free of disease. It is unwise to perform a stapedectomy at the first stage, because of the risk of iatrogenic labyrinthitis and meningitis, and subsequent

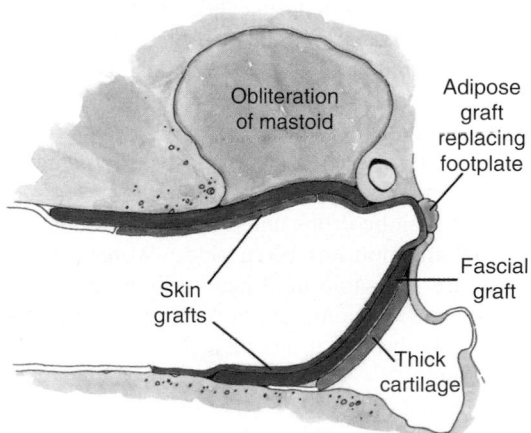

Figure 8 Type Vb tympanoplasty. This is similar to a type IV, except that the footplate which is fixed is removed, and replaced by a graft of adipose tissue. This procedure is done many months after the eradication of the active COM with a successful mastoidectomy. The mastoid cavity and epitympanum have usually been obliterated with pedicled or free muscle-fascial grafts, supplemented with bone pate. (Published with permission, copyright © 2006 S.N. Merchant.)

sensorineural hearing loss. (2) A two-stage procedure is also performed when there is a high risk of residual cholesteatoma at the time of the first procedure. The first stage consists of removal of the cholesteatoma and repair of the TM. The second stage consists of re-exploration of the middle ear and mastoid to look for residual cholesteatoma and is combined with ossiculoplasty. (3) A two-stage operation has also been advocated in patients with extensive mucous membrane destruction of the tympanic cavity due to COM. The first stage consists of elimination of disease, sealing the middle ear with a tissue graft and placing plastic sheeting over the denuded middle ear. The objective of the first stage is to obtain a well-healed ear with a mucosa lined, aerated middle ear cleft so that ossicular reconstruction may be performed later at a second stage under ideal circumstances. Considerable difference of opinion exists among experienced otologists in regard to this third indication for staging.[17] There are experienced otologists who perform the entire procedure in one stage. Every effort is made to eliminate disease and maximize hearing results at the first operation. Should the hearing results be unsatisfactory and the postoperative status regarding aeration of the middle ear and control of suppuration satisfactory, a revision operation for hearing can be done. In this rationale, revisions are not necessary in many cases; therefore, a second procedure is avoided.

POSTOPERATIVE CARE AND COMPLICATIONS

Surgical packing is placed within the ear canal at the end of the procedure to hold the TM and other grafts in place. A variety of packing materials are in contemporary use including gelfoam, antibiotic-corticosteroid ointments, and dressings made of strips of silk or rayon cloth filled with antibiotic-soaked cotton. Prophylactic antibiotic coverage is usually given during surgery and continued for 7 to 10 days postoperatively. The surgical packing is removed 1 to 2 weeks postoperatively. The patient is instructed to avoid nose-blowing and vigorous physical activity for 2 weeks after surgery. Further treatment consists of cleaning and removing debris as well as applying antiseptic or antibiotic drops until complete healing and epithelialization has taken place. Water precautions are advisable until healing is complete. A postoperative audiogram is performed when the ear is fully healed, usually 2 to 4 months after the operation.

The major intraoperative complications are injury to the cochlea, the vestibular system, and the facial nerve. The risk of partial or total sensorineural hearing loss after tympanoplasty ranges from 1 to 5%.[18,19] Etiologic factors for sensorineural hearing loss include avulsion or subluxation of the stapes footplate, laceration of the round window membrane, or acoustic trauma due to instrumentation of the ossicles. Injury to the facial nerve occurs most often at the level of

the oval window.[20] Abnormal dehiscence of the fallopian canal can be expected in up to 25% of cases with COM in this region. Therefore, avoidance of aggressive manipulations or dissection in the oval window niche area is important. Intraoperative facial nerve electromyography provides useful adjunctive information during the surgical dissection adjacent to a dehiscent facial nerve and therefore can be useful to the surgeon to minimize the risk of facial nerve injury.

Postoperative complications include hematoma formation, infection, graft failure with reperforation, stenosis of the external auditory canal or meatus, displacement or extrusion of an ossicular prosthesis, iatrogenic cholesteatoma due to implantation of squamous epithelium, and recurrent COM. Long-term follow-up is advisable to monitor the ear and for early detection of complications or recurrent disease.

RESULTS

Surgery of the middle ear and mastoid is very successful in controlling infection in COM, with success rates in excess of 80 to 90%. On the other hand, improvement in hearing after tympanoplasty is rather modest. Hearing results are determined by the extent of initial damage to the TM and ossicles, and whether or not the tympanic cavity becomes properly aerated after tympanoplasty.[21]

Restoration of aeration of the tympanic cavity after the operation is the single most important determinant of a successful tympanoplasty. Unfortunately, the otologic surgeon does not have control over whether an ear will become aerated postoperatively or not. Nonaerated ears due to middle ear fibrosis or eustachian tube dysfunction demonstrate large conductive hearing losses of 40 to 60 dB, regardless of the type of tympanoplasty that has been performed. Therefore, the confounding effect of nonaeration must be removed to accurately analyze and compare the results of various types of tympanoplasties.

Patients undergoing type I tympanoplasty have the best outcome, with a greater than 90% probability for successful take of the graft and 80 to 90% probability for a postoperative airbone gap of 20 dB or less. Hearing results are less satisfactory when the ossicular chain is diseased. When ossiculoplasty is performed, hearing results are better if there is an intact stapes superstructure. Long-term closure of the air-bone gap to less than 20 dB occurs in 40 to 70% of cases in which the stapes is intact, and in only 20 to 55% of cases in which the stapes superstructure is missing.[6]

One can also consider the effect of a canal wall down mastoidectomy on the hearing result. From an acoustical perspective, a canal wall down mastoidectomy results in a significant reduction of the size of the residual middle ear air space. Experimental studies have shown that this reduction should not create any significant hearing loss as long as the middle ear remains

aerated.[4] Indeed, clinical studies involving large numbers of patients have revealed no significant differences between canal wall up and canal wall down mastoidectomy for comparable ossicular pathology.[21–23]

CHALLENGES FOR FUTURE RESEARCH

Tympanoplasty is unique compared with surgery elsewhere in the body because of the constraints imposed by a combination of factors, including the pathology of COM, the unpredictable nature of wound healing, and the need for a functioning tympano-ossicular system. Otologists routinely place TM and ossicular grafts in a recipient middle ear that is hostile as a result of active or arrested inflammatory disease. TM grafts have to be in contact with air over a relatively large portion of their surface areas and must derive nourishment and blood supply from small parts of the graft in contact with the canal wall. Furthermore, ossicular grafts and prostheses must couple well at their ends to bone or soft tissue but must remain suspended in air elsewhere to transmit sound effectively. Therefore, it is not surprising that functional success after tympanoplasty is determined not only by a surgeon's technical skill and judgment, but also by other factors, such as the mechanics and acoustics of the reconstruction[6,24] and the biology and pathology of chronic ear disease.[25]

COM poses a particular challenge in that postoperative mucosal fibrosis, *neo*-osteogenesis, and development of negative static pressure in the middle ear with nonaeration of the middle ear can occur over the course of months or years.[25] These host responses have a detrimental effect on the hearing result, which is not apparent in the short term. It is instructive to note that the few studies in the literature that assess long-term hearing loss show a progressive and systematic decline in the initial hearing gain, as a function of time. For example, a study of 832 ossiculoplasty procedures found that 77% of ears had an air-bone gap of 20 dB or less at 6 months, but the same measure declined to 42% at 5 years.[23] An improved understanding of the biology and pathology of COM would provide fruitful avenues for research to improve upon today's results after tympanoplasty.

ACKNOWLEDGEMENTS

We are grateful for the support provided by Mr. Axel Eliasen, Mr. Lakshmi Mittal and the National Institutes of Health.

REFERENCES

1. Wullstein H. The restoration of the function of the middle ear in chronic otitis media. Ann Otol Rhinol Laryngol 1956;65:1020–41.
2. Zollner F. The principles of plastic surgery of the sound-conducting apparatus. J Laryngol Otol 1955;69:637–52.
3. Puria S, Peake WT, Rosowski JJ. Sound-pressure measurements in the cochlear vestibule of human-cadaver ears. J Acoust Soc Am 1997;101:2754–70.

4. Whittemore KR, Merchant SN, Rosowski JJ. Acoustic mechanisms: Canal wall-up versus canal wall-down mastoidectomy. Otolaryngol Head Neck Surg 1998;118:751–61.

5. Voss SE, Rosowski JJ, Peake WT. Is the pressure difference between the oval and round windows the effective acoustic stimulus for the cochlea? J Acoust Soc Am 1996;100:1602–16.

6. Merchant SN, Ravicz ME, Voss SE, et al. Toynbee Memorial Lecture 1997 - Middle-ear mechanics in normal, diseased and reconstructed ears. J Laryngol Otol 1998; 112:715-31.

7. Rosowski JJ, Merchant SN. A mechanical and acoustical analysis of middle-ear reconstruction. Am J Otol 1995;16:486–97.

8. Nadol JB, Jr. Chronic otitis media. In: Nadol JB, McKenna MJ, editors. Surgery of the Ear and Temporal Bone, 2nd edition. Philadelphia: Lippincott Williams and Wilkins; p. 199–218.

9. Bluestone CD, Cantekin EI. Panel on experiences with testing eustachian tube function. Ann Otol Rhinol Laryngol 1981;90:552–62.

10. Sheehy JL. Testing eustachian tube function. Ann Otol Rhinol Laryngol 1981;90:562–4.

11. Mehta RP, Rosowski JJ, Voss SE, et al. Determinants of hearing loss in perforations of the tympanic membrane. Otol Neurotol 2006;27:136–43.

12. Mikulec AA, McKenna MJ, Ramsey MJ, et al. Superior semicircular canal dehiscence presenting as conductive hearing loss without vertigo. Otol Neurotol 2004; 25:121–9.

13. Rizer F. Tympanoplasty: A historical review and a comparison of techniques. Laryngoscope 1997;107:1–36.

14. Merchant SN, Nadol JB, Jr. Histopathology of ossicular implants. Otolaryngol Clin North Am 1994;27:813–33.

15. Yung MW. Editorial Review: Literature review of alloplastic materials in ossiculoplasty. J Laryngol Otol 2003; 117:431–6.

16. Merchant SN, McKenna MJ, Mehta RP, et al. Middle-ear mechanics of type III tympanoplasty (stapes columella): II. Clinical studies. Otol Neurotol 2003;24:186–94.

17. Sheehy JL, Shelton C. Tympanoplasty: To stage or not to stage. Otolaryngol Head Neck Surg 1991;104:399–407.

18. Palva T, Karja J, Palva A. Immediate and short term complications of chronic ear surgery. Arch Otolaryngol 1976; 102:137–9.

19. Tos M, Lau T, Plate S. Sensorineural hearing loss following chronic ear surgery. Ann Otol Rhinol Laryngol 1984; 93:403–9.

20. Green JD, Shelton C, Brackmann DE. Iatrogenic facial nerve injury during otologic surgery. Laryngoscope 1994;104:922–6.

21. Merchant SN, Rosowski JJ, McKenna MJ. Tympanoplasty. Op Tech Otolaryngol Head Neck Surg 2003;14:224–36.

22. Brackmann DE, Sheehy JL, Luxford WM. TORPS and PORPS in tympanoplasty: Review of 1042 operations. Otolaryngol Head Neck Surg 1984;92:32–7.

23. Colletti V, Fiorino FG, Sittoni V. Minisculptured ossicle grafts versus implants: Long-term results. Am J Otol 1987;8:553–9.

24. Goode RL, Nishihara S. Experimental models of ossiculoplasty. Otolaryngol Clin N Am 1994;27:663–75.

25. Schuknecht HF. Pathology of the Ear, 2nd edition. Philadelphia: Lea and Febiger; 1993.

20

Otosclerosis

Herman A. Jenkins, MD
Michael J. McKenna, MD

The term otosclerosis is derived from the Greek words for "hardening of the ear." While first recognized as a pathological entity by Valsalva[1] early in the eighteenth century, it was not until the mid-nineteenth century with the observations of authors such as Magnus,[2] von Tröltsch,[3] Politzer,[4] and Toynbee[5] that the clinical presentation of the disease was clearly defined. During the twentieth century, its audiometric features were identified. Today, otosclerosis is recognized as an alteration in bony metabolism that is exclusive to the endochondral bone of the otic capsule.[6,7] The ongoing process of resorption and redeposition of bone results in fixation of the ossicular chain and a conductive hearing loss.

PREVALENCE

Otosclerosis occurs most commonly among Caucasians with an incidence of 1%, followed by Asians at 0.5%.[8,9] It is far less common in African-Americans. Guild, in postmortem examinations of temporal bones, found evidence of a higher prevalence rate histologically, with 8.3% of Caucasians and 1% of African-Americans manifesting the disease.[10] Although occurring in all age groups, the usual clinical presentation varies from second to fifth decade of life. There is a female predominance of 2:1, and bilateral disease occurs in 80% of patients. Approximately 20 to 30% develops a progressive sensorineural hearing loss with no reliable preventative measures available.

HISTOPATHOLOGY

Histologically, the otosclerotic process is divided into two phases. Bone resorption and increased vascularity characterize the early phase. As the mature collagen content diminishes, the bone acquires a spongy appearance (otospongiosis).[11] On hematoxylin-eosin staining it assumes a bluish coloration, referred to as the blue mantles of Manasse.[12] In the late phase, the reabsorbed bone is replaced with dense sclerotic bone, thus the name otosclerosis (Figure 1).

When involving the stapes, otosclerosis often starts from the fissula ante fenestrum, although focal lesions involving the posterior annular ligament are also seen. In general, the disease progresses from an anterior focal lesion to complete

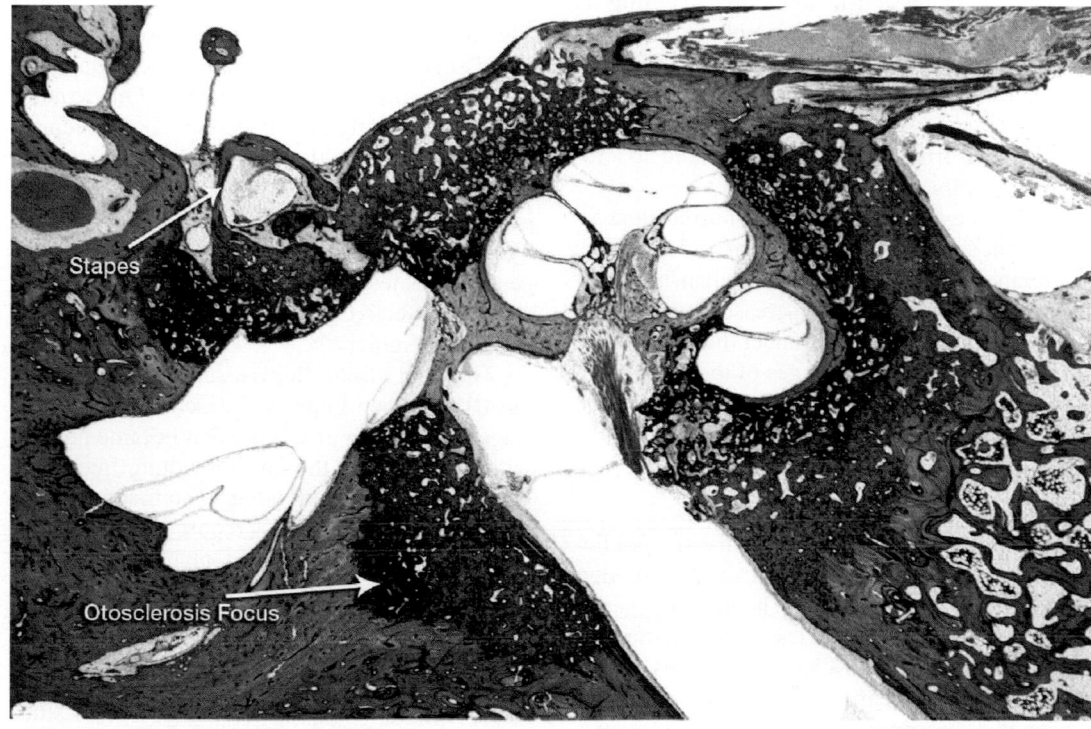

Figure 1 Histological picture of otosclerosis. The otosclerosis has immobilized and stapes and has involved nearly the entire otic capsule.

footplate involvement and, in more advanced cases, may fill the oval window niche entirely with new bone (obliterative otosclerosis). In contrast, the round window is less frequently involved, and complete obliteration a rare finding. Involvement of the cochlea can result in sensorineural hearing loss.

ETIOLOGY

Various causes of the disease and evidence for inflammatory or infective relationships have been reported. A genetic component has been long recognized and generally accepted as being dominant in transmission with incomplete penetrance.[13,14] Current understanding points to the marked heterogeneity of the genetic pattern. Six different loci have been identified as associated with otosclerosis (Table 1).[15–20] Identified sites are associated with genes involved in the regulation of collagen, cartilage and bone homeostasis, and growth suppression and intracellular communication.[21]

The expression of COL1A1, Type 1 collagen gene has been implicated strongly in osteogenesis imperfecta and osteoporosis, both sharing lesions in the otic capsule and many clinical presentations similar to otosclerosis.[22–27] While roles for autoimmunity have been suggested, data remains inconclusive.[28–30]

Recent investigations have evaluated the potential role of infective agents in otosclerosis. The measles virus has been implicated, with viral particles, antigens, and RNA found in active otosclerosis foci.[31–39] Elevated titers of IgG specific for measles virus antigens have been found in the perilymph of patients with otosclerosis.[40] While the evidence is compelling, the actual role of the measles virus in manifesting or inciting the disease remains to be established.

Table 1 Otosclerosis Associated Genetic Loci1[5–20]

OTSC1 on chromosome 15q25–q26
OTSC2 on chromosome 7q34–q36
OTSC3 on chromosome 6p21.3–p22.3
OTSC4 on chromosome 16q21–q23.2
OTSC5 on chromosome 3q22–q24
Monogenic nonsyndromic, not linked to the above, or
  to COL1A1 or 2

The contributions of the endocrine system to manifestation of otosclerosis is unclear. While clinically implicated anecdotally, the role of estrogen and parathyroid hormone (PTH) has not been proven but warrants further investigation.[41]

CLINICAL PRESENTATION

The clinical presentation of otosclerosis is that of a progressive conductive hearing loss in an adult, thought to occur in less than 20% of genetically affected individuals. Some note improved speech understanding in noisy environment, known as the paracusis of Willis. Tinnitus is the second most common complaint reported. Vestibular symptoms are uncommon. Sensorineural hearing loss may be associated with the conductive changes in the disease. However, an isolated sensorineural hearing loss due to otosclerosis is rare.

Physical examination shows a normal appearance of the external auditory canal and tympanic membrane. Schwartze sign, a reddish hue over the promontory caused by increased in vascularity of the bone immediately under the periosteum, may be seen in the early stages of the disease but is not present in all cases.

LABORATORY TESTING

Depending on the stage of the disease, audiometric studies show typically a mild to moderate conductive hearing loss. The air-bone gap is wider at the lower frequencies. The Carhart notch is characteristic of otosclerosis and this apparent sensorineural hearing loss at 2 kHz is spurious since bone conduction in the mid frequency range is not reliable. Stapes fixation interferes with the bone conduction of the acoustic signal, and the bone conduction thresholds are reduced 10 to 15 dB after stapes surgery. With progression of the conductive loss, the Rinne tuning fork test demonstrates bone conduction to be greater than air conduction, and the Weber test lateralizes to the affected side. The tympanogram is either depressed (As) or normal. The stapedial reflex may be normal in the early stages but cannot be elicited as stapes fixation proceeds. Speech reception threshold and speech discrimination are often normal, except in cases of cochlear involvement. Clinically, other diagnostic studies such as high-resolution computed tomography (CT) and magnetic resonance imaging (MRI) are of little use in evaluation of otosclerosis. With high-resolution CT, however, one may be able to identify the sclerotic lesion.

MEDICAL MANAGEMENT

Medical management of otosclerosis remains controversial and is primarily directed at maturing the involved bone and decreasing osteoclastic activity. Shambaugh and Scott[42] introduced use of sodium fluoride as treatment, based on its success in osteoporosis. However, this required high doses, and the efficacy has yet to be clearly established. Bisphosphonates that inhibit osteoclastic activity and cytokine antagonists that inhibit bone resorption may offer hope for the future. At present, no medical treatment is recommended on a consistent basis. Hearing aids, however, do offer an effective means of nonsurgical management of hearing loss in otosclerosis.

SURGICAL MANAGEMENT

History

The history of surgery for otosclerosis dates back to Kessel in 1877 with early attempts at mobilization and extraction of the stapes.[43] Other otologists subsequently attempted similar procedures, notably Miot in 1890, who described an extensive experience with successful operations and suggested various techniques.[44] However, the report by Siebenmann at the beginning of the twentieth century was less encouraging and condemned the surgery, effectively ending these early ventures into stapes surgery.[45]

The field of otosclerosis surgery lay dormant until 1938 when Lempert[46] described the single-stage fenestration procedure that became popular with otologists of the era, rekindling interest in surgery for stapedial fixation. The focus returned to the stapes with Rosen's report of stapes mobilization and the restoration of hearing.[47] Shea introduced the technique of stapes extraction with tissue coverage of the oval window and polyethylene strut reconstruction of the stapes in the 1950s, ushering in the modern approach to stapes surgery.[48] In the intervening years since the reintroduction of this procedure, techniques have changed slightly and new materials for reconstruction have been introduced; however, the principles remain basically the same.

The surgical goal in otosclerosis is restoration of the sound transmission mechanism from the tympanic membrane, going through the ossicular chain to the oval window membrane, bypassing the resistance of the fixed stapes footplate. Today, a variety of techniques are used to correct for stapes footplate fixation. Generally, the stapes arch is removed, and either a perforation or a partial to complete removal of the footplate is performed. A prosthetic implant is employed to connect the incus to the oval window.

Patient Selection

Surgical selection of patients is based on audiologic findings and physical examination. Preferred are patients with normal middle ear aeration, free of any infection or tympanic membrane perforation and with a Rinne test that demonstrates bone conduction to be greater than air conduction. When bilateral disease presents, the worse hearing ear is treated first, followed by the other ear, typically at least 6 months later. The performance of stapes surgery on an only hearing ear should be done with great trepidation.

Informed Consent

Preoperative consent is obtained, informing the patient of the risks of hearing loss, vertigo, injury to the facial nerve, loss or alteration of taste, tympanic membrane perforation, prosthesis extrusion or displacement, and residual conductive hearing loss. Singers and musicians are informed of possible change in quality of sound perception that may affect their professional performance. Individuals who are exposed or plan to be involved in activities associated with rapid and/or considerable change in pressure, such as SCUBA diving and piloting a nonpressurized airplane, are advised that their risk for postoperative hearing loss during these activities may be greater following stapedectomy.

Preoperative Treatment

Surgery may be performed under either general or local anesthesia. With improvements in anesthesia in recent decades, more otologists are now using general. Use of any anticoagulants during the 2 weeks prior to the surgery should be avoided, including antiinflammatory agents. Muscle relaxants in conjunction with anesthetic agents are not recommended, because of their effect on the facial nerve activity. Perioperative antibiotics are at the surgeon's discretion, but antiemetic agents are recommended should nausea and vomiting occur.

Whether a general or local anesthesia is employed, injections of local anesthetics should be administered in such a manner as to avoid unintentional involvement of the facial nerve medial to the mastoid tip. Sterility of the operative field is of paramount importance, since a direct connection to the labyrinth is established during parts of the operation. Routinely, surgical site preparation includes installation of preparation solution into the external auditory canal. Facial nerve activity is monitored by direct vision of the face through a transparent occlusive drape, or an electromyographic monitor, should stapedectomy be performed using general anesthesia.

Surgical Technique

Stapes surgery may be performed via an endaural or anterior incisural incision. The endaural incision requires use of a speculum held stationary, either manually or with a speculum holder assembly. In contrast, the anterior incisural incision is held open using one or two self-retaining retractors, eliminating the need to operate through a speculum. The cosmetic result is good as the incision is rarely noticeable. The latter also provides direct access to the tragal cartilage, should a perichondrial graft be desired.

Regardless of the approach, a tympanomeatal flap is raised, the annulus identified, and hemostasis established, prior to entering the middle-ear space. A 1% lidocaine with 1:100,000 epinephrine or a 1:1,000 epinephrine soaked piece of Gelfoam or small cotton ball is used in this step. The tympanomeatal flap is elevated anteriorly, and the chorda tympani nerve is dissected free toward the malleus. A portion of the scutum should be curetted to expose the incus and the incudostapedial joint. Fixation of the stapes is determined by palpation of the malleus, while viewing the suprastructure and footplate of the stapes.

Prior to any footplate work, the distance between the mid-shaft of the long process of the incus and the footplate is measured (Figure 2). The incudostapedial joint is separated, and the stapedial tendon is severed. The stapes suprastructure is fractured inferiorly and removed from the middle ear (see Figure 2).[49]

Establishing contact with the perilymphatic space may be done in several ways. The trend within the last two decades has moved to smaller fenestra to protect the inner ear as much as possible. Typically, either a small fenestra is created, or the footplate is partially removed. When the surgeon removes the entire footplate, a stapedectomy is performed. Depending on the training and preference of the otologist, the posterior half or the entire footplate is removed (Figure 3). In the partial stapedectomy technique demonstrated, the footplate is fractured in half, with the posterior portion being removed. A perichondrial graft from the tragus or a vein graft is placed over the defect, and the prosthesis is positioned over it and secured to the incus.

In the stapedotomy technique, a perforation in the footplate is made, just large enough to allow passage of the prosthesis (Figure 4). In the technique popularized by Fisch, a perforation is gradually enlarged with a hand-held drill to 0.6 mm in diameter. The stapes replacement prosthesis of choice is placed in the perforation and attached to the incus. The length of the prosthesis used is slightly longer (0.25 mm) than the measured length between the incus and footplate to ensure contact with the perilymph space and prevent displacement during the healing process. The addition of fresh clotted blood to the area also helps reduce the risk of a perilymphatic fistula.

Many otologists have advocated use of laser in performing a stapedotomy. The advantage of the laser is decreased mechanical manipulation of the suprastructure and the footplate. The thermal effect is negligible.[50] The disadvantage is the additional time, expense, and instrumentation needed. Perkins and Curto popularized a combination laser stapedotomy with tissue coverage of the perforation[51] (Figure 5). A vein graft is placed over a drilled hole in a Teflon block. A prosthesis is placed in the hole, and the vein graft allowed to dry and become adherent to the prosthesis. Rosettes of charred bone are created by the laser and gently removed with a pick. The prosthesis with adherent graft is positioned over the fenestra with the tip projecting into the vestibule and then positioned under the incus.

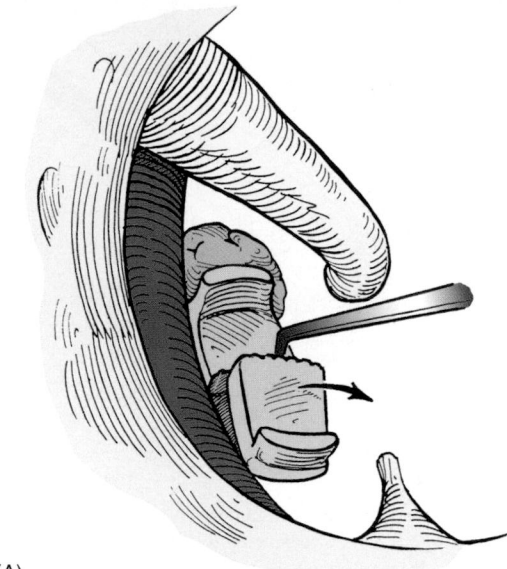

(A)

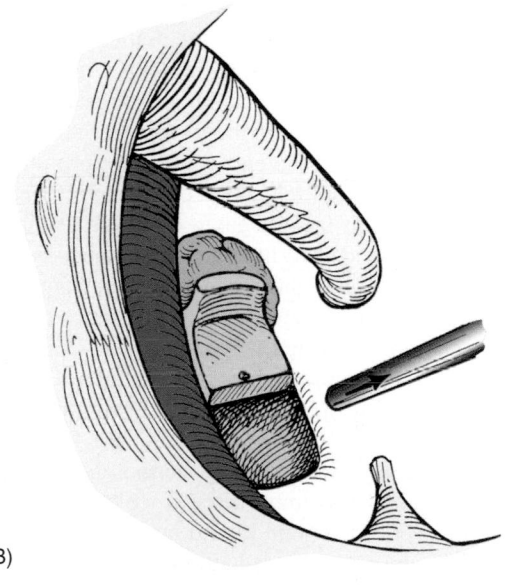

(B)

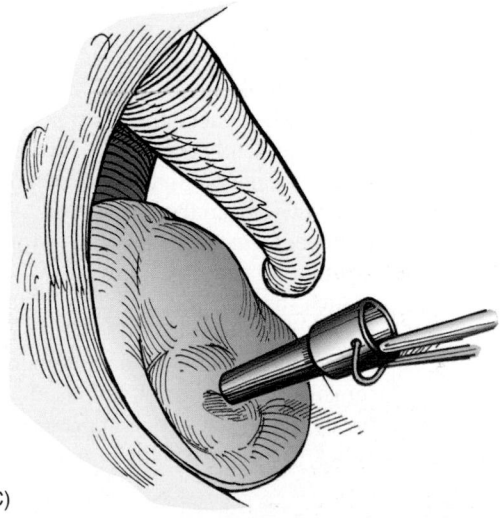

(A)

(B)

Figure 2 (A) Proper measuring technique for a stapes prosthesis. (B) Fracturing the superstructure of the stapes. (Adapted from reference 49.)

(C)

Figure 3 (A) Partial stapedectomy with extraction of the footplate. (B) Aspiration technique: place suction away from the fenestration. (C) Placement of a prosthesis over a perichondrial graft. (Adapted from reference 49.)

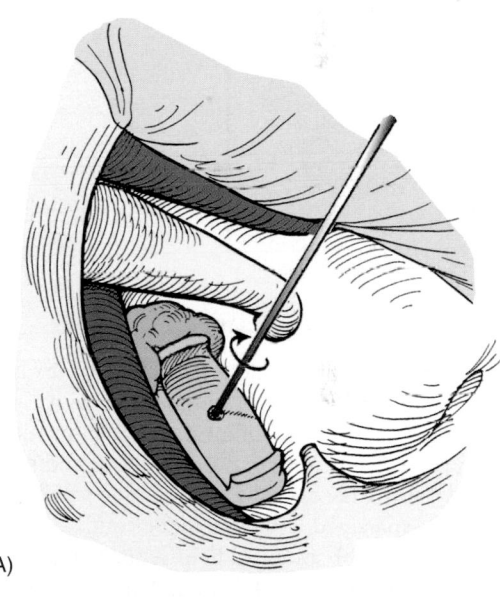

(A)

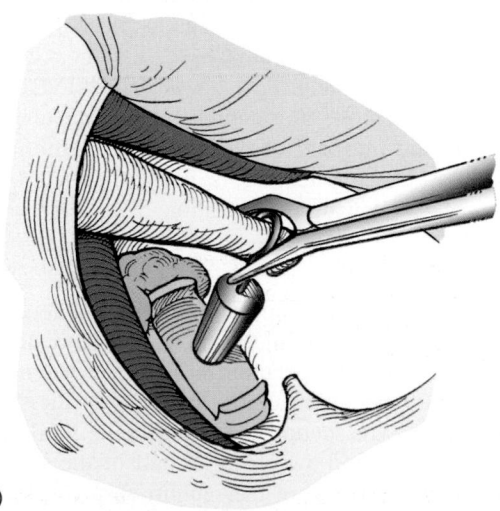

(B)

Figure 4 Stapedotomy technique. (A) Fenestration of footplate by a graduated series of perforators. (B) Placement of prosthesis in the fenestra with crimping to incus. (Adapted from reference 49.)

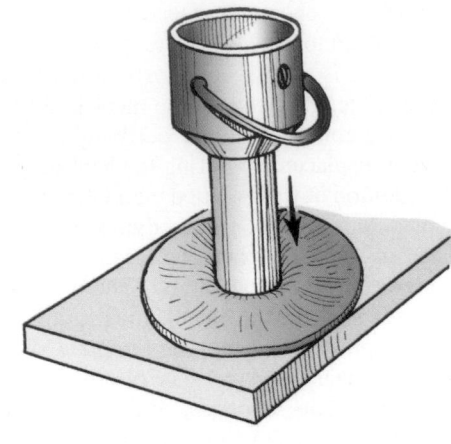

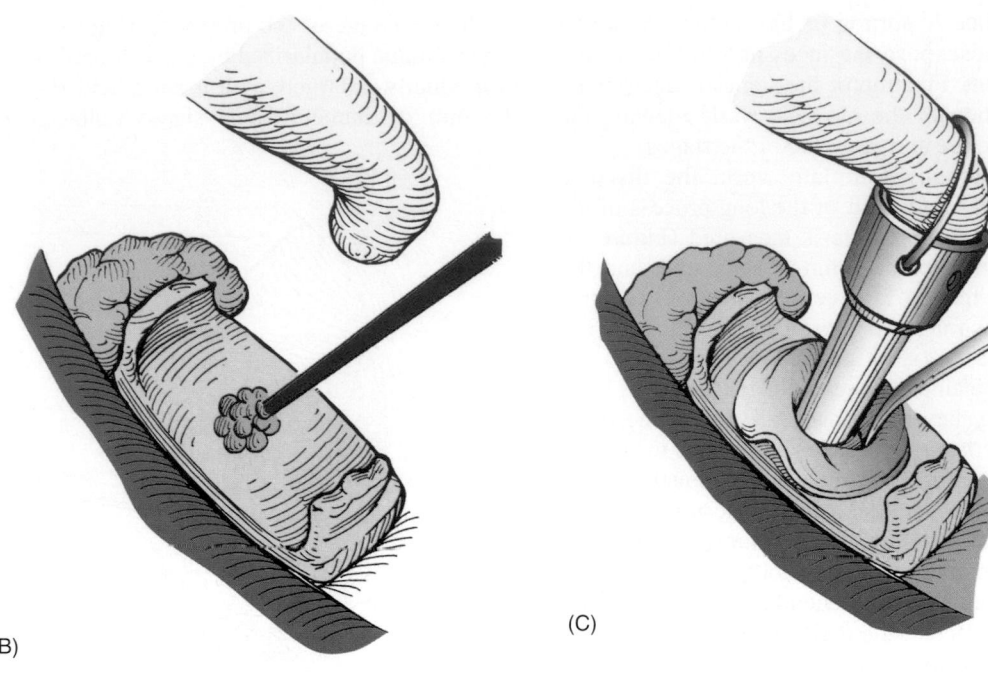

(B)

(C)

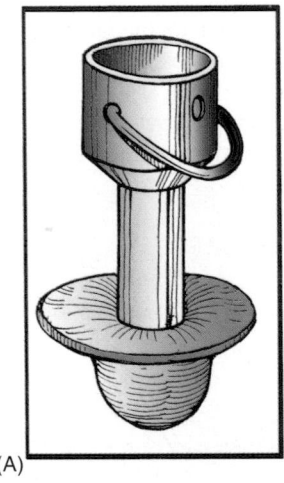

(A)

Figure 5 Stapedotomy technique with vein graft. (A) Graft adheres to the prosthesis by drying in a well (*top*), and the adherent graft can be seen (*bottom*). (B) Laser stapedotomy with rosette formation. (C) Prosthesis and graft in place. (Adapted from reference 49.)

Postoperative Management

Postoperatively, the patient is sent home to bed and requested to remain on light activity for several days to allow initial healing. Pain management requires mild oral medication, and antibiotics are not necessary. Postoperative vertigo or nausea is managed with antiemetics and sedation as needed. Stool softeners help reduce straining, decreasing the chance of forming a perilymph fistula. Patients are cautioned against nose blowing and sneezing with mouth closed.

Postoperative follow-up is scheduled at 1 week to remove any suture or packing and to assess the integrity of the tympanic membrane. Repeat hearing testing is performed at 4 to 8 weeks following the operation.

Pitfalls

Pitfalls of stapes surgery include inadequate exposure and anatomical variations. The endaural incision and speculum produces a narrower opening when compared to the anterior incisural approach. The scutum can cover the long process of the incus and the posterior half of the stapes. Adequate removal of the scutum ensures proper visualization of the footplate in the crucial stage of footplate perforation and prosthesis placement. Greater exposure is obtained if the superior limit of the tympanomeatal flap is carried forward to the

area of the short process of the malleus. Reflecting the tympanic membrane forward with visualization of the malleus handle adds greatly to the ease of performance of the procedure. An aberrant location of the facial nerve may prohibit a stapedectomy, and relocation of the nerve, which carries a risk of facial weakness and paralysis, is not recommended. With a dehiscent facial canal, the nerve has a higher chance of being injured. Surgical judgment dictates when a stapes operation should be aborted.

Advanced otosclerosis with obliteration of the oval window requires drilling of the footplate and significant experience with temporal bone anatomy. Sclerotic obstruction of the round window is of less importance since only a small opening over the round window is necessary to allow proper cochlear function. Drilling out the round window often results in a severe hearing loss and is avoided.

If the footplate should be displaced into the vestibule, attempts should be made to remove it. However, this should be done, only if one can easily grasp the edge and gently remove it. Never go "fishing" for a bony fragment that has descended into the vestibule away from the annular rim.

During the stapedectomy, the protective function of the stapedial muscle is destroyed. A new technique in which the stapedial muscle is left in place and the posterior crus of the down-fractured suprastructure is shaped and used as autologous stapes replacement graft has been proposed and used. The efficacy of this technique in preserving the acoustic reflex is controversial.

Results

Otosclerosis surgery has withstood the test of time since its reinstitution in the early 1950s. Shea in his review of 40 years of stapes surgery reported

closure to within 10 dB of the preoperative bone conduction level in over 95% of patients.[52] This changed little over the next several years. Glasscock and colleagues reported over 91% closure to within 5 dB.[53] Both groups reported significantly less success in revision surgery. Persson and colleagues contrasted stapedectomy and stapedotomy in the review of their series.[54] They demonstrated that partial and total stapedectomy had better results at all frequencies with the exception of 4 kHz. However, the hearing results in this group tended to deteriorate more quickly than the stapedotomy patients. Others have reported similar preservation of high frequencies with stapedotomy.[55] Results in the training situation demonstrate significantly less success.[56] A definite learning curve in stapes surgery occurs after training.[57] The overall accepted rate of anacusis following stapes surgery is in the range of 1 to 2%.[55]

Complications

Complications of stapedectomy surgery are both immediate and delayed in nature. Immediate complications are those occurring during the operation, for example, facial nerve injury, vertigo and/or hearing loss, or persistent postoperative perilymphatic leakage from the oval window. Bed rest and light activities are recommended for vertiginous patients, and most recover shortly after surgery. Changes in or loss of taste may result from excessive manipulation or injury to chorda tympani nerve. Labyrinthitis, though possible, occurs rarely under sterile conditions.

Delayed postoperative complications, including fistula formation,[58] granuloma,[59] and prosthesis dislocation have been reported. Immediate treatment with antibiotics and rest is recommended. Re-exploration should be entertained to correct the fistula, should vertigo persist. Granuloma formation can occur for unknown reasons and in the best of settings. Keeping all foreign material, such as glove powder and bone dust, away from the footplate area may decrease the chances of development of a granuloma. A dislocated prosthesis requires re-exploration and revision.

REFERENCES

1. Valsalva AM. Opera, Hoc est, Tractatus de Aure Humana. Venice: Pitteri; 1735.
2. Magnus A. Uber Verlauf und Sektionsbefund eines Falles von hochgradiger und eigenthumlicher Gehorstorung. Arch Ohrenheilk 1876;11:244–51.
3. von Tröltsch A. Treatise on the Disease of the Ear Including the Anatomy of the Organ. New York: Wiliam Wood; 1869.
4. Politzer A. Uber primare Erkrankung der knochernen Labyrinthkapsel. Z Ohrenheilk 1894;25:309–27.
5. Toynbee J. Diseases of the Ear. Philadelphia: Blanchard and Lea; 1860.
6. Chole RA, McKenna M. Pathophysiology of otosclerosis. Otol Neurotol 2001;22:249–57.
7. Wang PC, Merchant SN, McKenna MJ, et al. Does otosclerosis occur only in the temporal bone? Am J Otol 1999; 20:162–5.
8. Morrison AW. Genetic factors in otosclerosis. Ann R Coll Surg Engl 1967;41:202–37.
9. Altmann F, Glasgold A, Macduff JP. The incidence of otosclerosis as related to race and sex. Ann Otol Rhinol Laryngol 1967;76:377–92.
10. Guild SR. Histologic otosclerosis. Ann Otol Rhinol Laryngol 1944;53:246.
11. Siebenmann, F. Demonstration mikroscopischer und makroscpischer paraparate von otospongiosis progressiva. Papers Internat Otol Cong 1912;9:207.
12. Manasse, P. Neue Untersuchungen zur otosklerosenfrage. Ztschr Ohrenh 1992;82:76.
13. Larson A. Otosclerosis: A genetic and clinical study. Acta Otolaryngol 1960;154:1–86.
14. Causse JR, Causse JB. Otospongiosis as a genetic disease. Early detection, medical management, and prevention. Am J Otol 1984;5:211–23.
15. Tomek MS, Brown MR, Mani SR et al. Localization of a gene for otosclerosis to chromosome 15q25–q26, Hum Mol Genet, 1998;7:285–90.
16. Van Den Bogaert K, Govaerts PJ, Schatteman I, et al. A second gene for otosclerosis, OTSC2, maps to chromosome 7q34–36. Am J Hum Genet 2001;68:495–500.
17. Chen W, Campbell CA, Green GE, et al. Linkage of otosclerosis to a third locus (OTSC3) on human chromosome 6p21.3–22.3. J Med Genet 2002;39:473–7.
18. Brownstein Z, Goldfarb A, Levi H, et al. Chromosomal mapping and phenotypic characterization of hereditary otosclerosis linked to the OTSC4 locus. Arch Otolaryngol Head Neck Surg 2006;132:416–24.
19. Van Den Bogaert k, De Leenheer EMR, Chen W, et al. A fifth locus for otosclerosis, OTSC5, maps to chromosome 3q22–24. J Med Genet 2004;41:450–3.
20. Iliadou V, Van Den Bogaert K, Eleftheriades N, et al. Monogenic nonsyndromic otosclerosis; audiological and linkage analysis in a large Greek pedigree. Int J Pediatr Otorhinolaryngol 2006;70:631–7.
21. Stankovic KM, McKenna MJ. Current research in otosclerosis. Curr Opin Otolaryngol Head Neck Surg 2006,14:347–51.
22. McKenna MJ, Kristiansen AG, Tropitzsch AS. Similar COL1A1 expression in fibroblasts from some patients with clinical otosclerosis and those with type 1 osteogenesis imperfecta. Ann Otol Rhinol Laryngol 2002;111:184–9.
23. McKenna MJ, Kristiansen AG, Bartley ML, et al. Association of COL1A1 and otosclerosis: Evidence for a shared genetic etiology with mild osteogenesis imperfecta. Am J Otol 1998;19:604–10.
24. McKenna MJ, Nguyen-Huynh AT, Kristiansen AG. Association of otosclerosis with Sp1 binding site polymorphism in COL1A1 gene: Evidence for a shared genetic etiology with osteoporosis. Otol Neurotol 2004;25:447–50.
25. Clayton AE, Mikulec AA, Mikulec KH, et al. Association between osteoporosis and otosclerosis in women. J Laryngol Otol 2004;118:617–21.
26. Nager GT. Osteogenesis imperfecta of the temporal bone and its relation to otosclerosis. Ann Otol Rhinol Laryngol 1981;97:585–93.
27. Pedersen U, Melsen F, Elbrond O, Charles P. Histopathology of the stapes in osteogenesis imperfecta. J Laryngol Otol 1985;99:451–8.
28. Yoo TJ, Tomoda K, Stuart, et al. Type II collagen-induced autoimmune otospongiosis: A preliminary report. Ann Otol Rhinol Laryngol 1983;92:103–8.
29. Bujia J, Alsalameh S, Jerez R, et al. Antibodies to minor cartilage collagen type IX in otosclerosis. Am J Otol 1994;15:222–4.
30. Lolov, Sr, Edrev GE, Kyurkchiev SD, et al. Elevated autoantibodies in sera from otosclerotic patients are related to the disease duration. Acta Otolaryngol 1998;118:375–80.
31. Niedermeyer HP, Arnold W. Otosclerosis: A measles virus associated inflammatory disease Acta Otolaryngol 1995;115:300–3.
32. McKenna MJ, Mills BG, Galey FR, Linthicum FH, Jr. Filamentous structures morphologically similar to viral nucleocapsids in otosclerotic lesions in two patients. Am J Otol 1986;7:25–8.
33. McKenna MJ, Mills BG. Immunohistochemical evidence of measles virus antigens in active otosclerosis. Otolaryngol Head Neck Surg 1989;101:415–21.
34. McKenna MJ, Kristiansen AG, Haines J. Polymerase chain reaction amplification of a measles virus sequence from human temporal bone sections with active otosclerosis. Am J Otol 1996;17:827–30.
35. McKenna MJ, Mills BG. Ultrastructural and immunohistochemical evidence of measles virus in active otosclerosis. Acta Otolaryngol 1990;:130–139; discussion 139–140.
36. Niedermeyer HP, Arnold W. Otosclerosis: A measles virus associated inflammatory disease. Acta Otolaryngol 1995;115:300–3.
37. Arnold W, Sedlmeier R, Wiest I, et al. Progress in basic research of otosclerosis. Otolaryngol Pol 2000; 54:281–3.
38. Karosi T, Konya J, Szabo LZ, Sziklai I. Measles virus prevalence in otosclerotic stapes footplate samples. Otol Neurotol 2004;25:451–6.
39. Vrabec JT, Coker NJ. Stapes surgery in the United States. Otol Neurotol 2004;25:465–9.
40. Lolov, SR, Edrev GE, Kyurkchiev SD, Kehayov IR. Elevated autoantibodies in sera from otosclerotic patients are related to the disease duration. Acta Otolaryngol 1998; 118:375–80.
41. Hultcrantz M, Simonoska R, Stenberg AE. Estrogen and hearing: A summary of recent investigations. Acta Otolaryngol 2006;126:10–4.
42. Shambaugh GE, Jr, Scott A. Sodium fluoride for arrest of otosclerosis. Arch Otol 1964;80:263.
43. Kessel, J. Uber das ausschneiden des trommelfelles und mobilisierin des steigbugels. Arch F Ohrenh1877;12:237.
44. Miot C. De la mobilization de L'etrier. Rev de laryng 1880;7:225.
45. Siebenmann F. Sur le traitement chirurgical de la sclerose otique, Congr Int de Med Sect d'Otol 1900;13:170.
46. Lempert J. Improvement in hearing in cases of otosclerosis: A new, one stage surgical technic. Arch Otolaryngol 1938;28:42.
47. Rosen, S. Palpation of the stapes for fixation. Arch Otolaryngol 1952;56:610.
48. Shea JJ, Jr. Fenestration of the oval window. Ann Otol Rhinol Laryngol 1958;67:932.
49. Coker NJ, Jenkins HA. Atlas of Otologic Surgery. Philadelphia: WB Saunders; 2001.
50. Coker NJ, Ator GA, Jenkins HA, et al. Carbon dioxide laser stapedotomy, thermal effects in the vestibule. Arch Otolaryngol. 1985;111:605–11.
51. Perkins R, Curto FS, Jr. Laser stapedotomy: A comparative study of prosthesis and seals. Laryngoscope 1992; 102:1321–7.
52. Shea JJ, Jr. Forty years of stapes surgery. Am J Otol 1998; 19:52–5.
53. Glasscock ME III, Storper IS, Haynes DS, Bohrer PS. Twenty-five years of experience with stapedectomy. Laryngoscope 1995;105:899–904.
54. Persson P, Harder H, Magnuson B. Hearing results in otosclerosis surgery after partial stapedectomy, total stapedectomy and stapedotomy. Acta Otolaryngol 1997; 117:94–9.
55. Kursten R, Schneider B, Zrunek M. Long-term results after stapedectomy versus stapedotomy. Am J Otol 1994; 15:804–6.
56. Backous DD, Coker NJ, Jenkins HA. Prospective study of resident-performed stapedectomy. Am J Otol 1993; 14:451–4.
57. Hughes GB. The learning curve in stapes surgery. Laryngoscope 1991;101:1280–4.
58. Goodhill V. Variable oto-audiologic manifestations of perilymphatic fistulae. Rev Panam Otorhinolaringol Bronchoesofagol 1967;1:100–9.
59. Harris I, Weiss L. Granulomatous complications of oval window fat grafts. Laryngoscope 1962;72:870–85.

21

Trauma to the Middle Ear, Inner Ear and Temporal Bone

D. Bradley Welling, MD, PhD
Mark D. Packer, MD

Trauma to the ear is a natural consequence of the innate sense of protection of the eyes and face. We instinctively turn away from approaching insult exposing one ear or the other to projectiles, blows, blasts, etc. The pinna and temporal bone encase and deflect injury from deeper middle and inner ear structures and contribute to the scalp and skull that protect the central hearing and balance pathways. The fragile middle ear is readily damaged when affronted by foreign objects introduced through the outer ear, as well as by the larger forces that are required to disrupt the inner ear. In a world where technology produces exposure to new heights, depths, speeds, and pressures that increase the risk of damage to ear structures, new technology may also allow preventative measures to avert damage and novel treatment options when such has occurred. The objective of this chapter is to provide information that will aid in diagnosis and treatment, and will guide future endeavors that may be necessary when the technology of protection does not exceed the forces of destruction.

More than a space of anatomical structures, the outer and middle ear is a system that captures ambient sound pressure waves that are transduced into the inner ear. This normally efficient transfer of information is dependent on an intact, taut tympanic membrane (TM) and an intact, mobile ossicular chain that traverses an air-filled medium. Trauma disrupts this system in several different ways. The end result of trauma to the TM and middle ear structures is a compromise in the efficient handling of sound information and potential breach of the sealed inner ear structures.

The middle ear is secondarily affected by trauma to the nose, mid-face, and paranasal sinuses. Congestion, blood, edema, and fracture of those regions surrounding the nasopharynx can inhibit eustachian tube function that is responsible for maintaining middle ear pressure and aeration. Resultant negative pressure from a disrupted eustachian tube can induce secretion that manifests as a middle ear effusion and conductive hearing loss. Blunt force applied to the mandible can be transmitted through the glenoid fossa fracturing the tympanic bone and rupturing the TM or disrupting the ossicles.

Trauma to the middle ear, inner ear, and temporal bone, as well as the central pathways of hearing, balance, and facial function are dealt with systematically in a lateral to medial approach. Sources, instruments, and mechanisms of trauma vary, and the understanding of each is central to management decisions and determining prognostic outcome information. Whether a product of blunt trauma, penetrating trauma or barotrauma, the magnitude of force applied to the ear differs widely, as does the outcome.

Foreign bodies within the external auditory canal (EAC) can pose a threat to the middle ear as well. They obscure visualization and may penetrate the TM, disrupt the ossicular chain, and create fistulae of the oval or round window membranes. Small batteries deserve particular attention as liquifactive necrosis can cause burns that affect surrounding bone and can extend into the middle ear and mastoid. They damage tissue by pressure necrosis, low-voltage burns, and alkaline corrosion. Corticosteroid drops that enhance burns if applied prior to battery extraction, facilitate reepithelialization of ulcers once the battery is removed.[1]

MIDDLE EAR TRAUMA

Penetrating objects vary from the misguided cotton tip applicator, hairpin, key, or pencil, to the more directed injury from picks and knives. Injury is usually localized and often has a predictable path. Pain, conductive and/or sensory hearing loss, disequilibrium, tinnitus, and rarely dysgeusia or facial nerve paresis may occur. Delayed infection, otorrhea, and subsequent cholesteatoma formation may result.

Visualization of the extent of damage is necessary. Otomicroscopic removal of debris and blood gives an optimal assessment. If evidence of inner ear penetration, for example, vertigo, nystagmus, or sensorineural hearing loss (SNHL) is present, an examination under anesthesia may be necessary. Up to 88% of traumatic perforations of the TM heal spontaneously within 3 to 10 months.[2–4] The rate of spontaneous healing is inversely related to the size of the perforation. Sensorineural, mixed, or conductive hearing loss may complicate perforations. The latter may be due to the perforation alone or may be associated with ossicular chain disruption in 4 to 33% of cases. Ossicular chain disruption without perforation may result in losses up to 50 dB. In a prospective study of 62 perforations, Mehta and colleagues examined the effect of perforation on hearing.[2] They found that the location of perforation did not significantly affect hearing, while the size of the perforation was directly proportional to the amount of conductive loss. Their findings argue against the "phase cancellation effect" of a posterior perforation overlying the round window as location-specific differential losses were not apparent. Hearing loss was frequency specific with larger losses in the lower frequencies.

Evidence of inner ear injury includes vertigo, hearing loss, or ongoing tinnitus. Nystagmus and sensorineural loss may be associated with perilymphatic fistula (PLF), although fistula may be difficult to differentiate from labyrinthine concussion. Weber and Rinne testing following debridement and documentation of symptoms are important to help guide further audiometric testing and to determine the necessity or urgency of middle ear exploration.

In most conditions, early management of acute perforations is directed toward facilitating spontaneous closure. This may require debridement of the canal with unfurling of medialized squamous cell epithelium associated with flaps or tears. The placement of a paper patch on the TM provides a scaffold for healing and helps splint mobile flaps from falling medially. Ongoing research shows potential application of a multitude of techniques from laser welding to growth factor solutions to promote TM closure, for example, fibrin gel, cyanoacrylates, calcium alginate patches, transforming growth factor beta-1 (TGF ß-1), epidermal growth factor (EGF) releasing film, and keratinocyte/basic fibroblast/platelet-derived growth factors. Topical nonototoxic antibiotic drops may be used to treat associated infection and inflammation. Whether or not the addition of corticosteroids to the solution promotes or inhibits healing is not clearly defined.

Perforations that do not heal spontaneously within 3 to 10 months may require tympanoplasty to reduce the risk of chronic infection or cholesteatoma. Additionally, if conductive hearing loss persists, exploration may be warranted. In Kronenberg and colleagues' series of 147 perforations, the risk of postinjury cholesteatoma was limited to patients whose perforations did not heal within 10 months.[4] A postinjury audiogram is necessary to delineate and document associated SNHL prior to any recommended surgical repair. Tympanoplasty and ossicular chain reconstruction are discussed in Chapter 19, "Reconstruction of the Middle Ear."

INNER EAR TRAUMA

Traumatic penetration of the TM may be complicated by fistulae of the oval or round window. A PLF can result from direct blast or penetrating forces that may also dislocate or fracture the ossicles, or by barotrauma or blunt forces exerting their energy indirectly through the ossicular chain. Pressure exerted on an intact TM transmitted along an intact ossicular chain strain the round or oval window coverings as TM perforations have been shown to be protective against fistula formation in animal studies.

Barotrauma

Barotrauma occurs due to pressure differentials between the atmosphere and the middle ear. Pressure differentials develop when diving, during air travel, in hypo- and hyperbaric chambers, and to a lesser extent along mountain paths, and in fast moving elevators. The pressure volume relationship of a gas is defined by Boyle gas law. Pressure (P) times volume (V) is equal to a constant (k) which varies with the mass and temperature of a gas, $PV = k$. This applies to trapped gases as can occur in the middle ear due to a dysfunctional eustachian tube, or the EAC when completely occluded by cerumen or foreign bodies. As pressure increases, volume decreases maintaining the constant.

As ambient pressure drops in ascent, air trapped in the EAC by a foreign body expands causing pressure against the lateral surface of the TM. Air expansion in the middle ear space egresses via the eustachian tube. The middle ear pressure decreases in relation to the gas trapped by canal occlusion creating a pressure gradient across the TM. The TM bows medially which causes pain, and possible rupture relieves pressure if the differential becomes great enough. Alternatively, as ambient pressures increases with descent as occurs in diving obstructing objects are moved medially. Lateral forces push objects against the relative vacuum of trapped ear canal air potentially damaging the TM, middle, and inner ear.

The reverse situation occurs in an open canal when air is trapped in the middle ear by eustachian tube obstruction or dysfunction. The air volume trapped within the middle ear expands unopposed by the decreased ambient pressure in the ear canal at altitude. The TM bows outward, the round window membrane bows medially, and the stapes footplate lateralizes in suit. Pain from the displaced TM can be relieved by actively opening the eustachian tube with an insufflation maneuver, or by swallowing, or yawning to contract the tensor veli palatini muscle. Too forceful an opening of the eustachian tube exacerbates the situation and can outwardly tear the TM or oval window ligament or implode the round window membrane. Similar maneuvers if ineffective in overcoming eustachian tube closure can elevate intracranial pressure. This pressure transmitted through the internal auditory canal (IAC) or a patent cochlear aqueduct can raise perilymphatic pressures and theoretically outwardly rupture the oval or round window coverings (Figure 1). On descent, increasing air or water pressure lateral to the TM and negative pressure from contracted trapped air medial to the TM, move the ossicular chain against the footplate that shifts fluid toward the round window and the round window membrane bows outward into the niche. Otalgia, mucosal congestion, rupture of small blood vessels, and effusion can result from the negative pressure within the middle-ear space. Autoinsufflation replenishes the middle-ear air and equalizes pressures across the TM. If equalization of the differential forces does not occur, either the TM, the round window membrane, or the oval window ligament may rupture and relieve the pressure. Perforations of the TM offer immediate relief of pain and are generally small and inconsequential to hearing and balance function. Perforations of the oval or round windows on the other hand can be a source of immediate SNHL or vestibular symptoms.

Mirza and Richardson reviewed the effects of barotrauma on air travelers. Ear symptoms, mostly pressure, but also pain, dizziness, tinnitus, hemorrhage, and hearing loss in flight were found to be as high as 71% in subjective questionnaires.[5] Otoscopic evidence of barotrauma is much less prevalent than symptoms manifesting in 10% of adult travelers, and 22% of children. The prevalence of perforation of the TM in passengers of commercial airlines is rarely reported. A randomized placebo-controlled treatment of adults with pseudoephedrine 120 mg administered 30 minutes prior to descent decreased symptoms of pain and pressure by 52% whereas another study showed no significant change in symptoms using topical nasal oxymetazoline hydrochloride 0.05%. In a third study, pseudoephedrine did not significantly diminish symptoms in children.[5,6]

"Alternobaric vertigo" is the illusion of motion brought on by differential middle-inner ear pressure between ears. This condition occurs with unequal clearing of pressure in the middle ears during diving or flying and has been reported in sleep apnea patients treated with nasal continuous positive air pressure (CPAP). This is most often managed by equalizing middle ear pressure with autoinsufflation, ie, the Valsalva maneuver. Management of recurring symptoms is directed at ruling out unilateral nasopharyngeal pathology, treatment of related sinonasal pathology, and medical methods to improve eustachian tube function. Rarely pressure equalization tubes may be necessary to allow continued CPAP treatment.

When compared with middle ear pressure fluctuations that occur during CPAP treatment and commercial flight, barotrauma using self-contained underwater breathing apparatus (SCUBA), during unpressurized flight, or occurring with exposure to blast overpressures are due to greater sustained pressure differentials and larger peak intensity levels. The result is a much higher propensity to cause damage to ear structures. The symptoms are more severe, and the otoscopic examination more revealing. Perforations of the TM are managed expectantly as with penetrating perforations. Close observation over 6 to 12 months is warranted to monitor closure, rule out cholesteatoma formation, and to ensure hearing and balance function reverts to normal. Unresolved dizziness, vertigo, imbalance, nausea, and vomiting are suggestive of PLF.

Middle ear barotrauma associated with SCUBA diving generally occurs with exposure to increasing water pressure, upon descent. Most injuries occur in shallow water where the pressure differentials are greatest. Water volume does not compress and does not follow Boyle's gas law, but the air within the middle ear does. The increasing water pressure in the ear canal pushes the TM medially and is not equalized by the compressing volume of air behind the eardrum. Otalgia can develop in as little as 3 ft of water, and the eustachian tube can become entirely dysfunctional and locked at 4 ft. If the pressure differential is not relieved, TM rupture

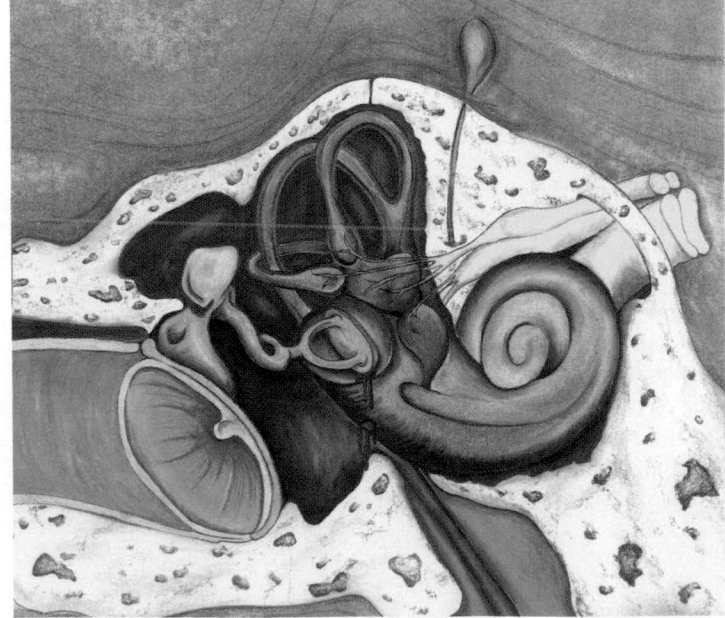

Figure 1 Schematic depiction perilymphatic fluid leak through the annular ligament, at the oval window, or through a ruptured round window membrane.

can occur within 5 ft of the surface. Cortes and colleagues reported a dive-related temporal lobe injury manifesting as acute otalgia and persistent headache.[7] CT findings of hemorrhage and pneumocephalus in the epidural space and adjacent temporal lobe where documented. Forceful auto-insufflation could theoretically rupture thin bone of the tegmen tympani. A reported rate of 52% dehiscence of the tegmen tympani in 100 temporal bones of 50 routine autopsies could explain the transmittal of air into the epidural spaces with Politzerization or baropressure and clarify the route of intracranial communication even without rupture of the tegmen.

Inner ear decompression sickness (DCS) is a separate entity that generally manifests during or within 24 hours of SCUBA or unpressurized aircraft ascent. This occurs as nitrogen gas, which is normally compressed into solution in serum at atmospheric pressure, bubbles out of solution with decreasing ambient pressures. Neurotologic symptoms of tinnitus, pain, hearing loss, and vertigo may occur related to occlusion of the labyrinthine microcirculation. Severe neurologic or respiratory symptoms of cerebral or pulmonary edema may complex the situation. The otoscopic examination is usually normal. Diagnosis is presumed based on temporal association with a recent ascent, and treatment for dive-related DCS is immediate recompression in a hyperbaric chamber to three times the depth at which symptoms occurred with a more gradual ascent. If prophylaxis for high-altitude DCS with a carbonic anhydrase inhibitor fails, patients are treated with 100% oxygen and immediate descent to sea level.

Perilymphatic Fistula

PLF must be considered when a documented pressure exposure, head trauma, or posterosuperior quadrant TM perforation is complicated by symptoms of SNHL, vertigo, tinnitus, and headache. PLF was first described to explain similar symptoms in patients after stapedectomy; however, trauma is the most common cause followed by iatrogenic exposure of the vestibule or membranous labyrinth. Additionally, events that raise intracranial pressure such as straining, nose blowing, coughing, or sneezing have been linked to PLF formation. Minor head trauma without loss of consciousness was seen in 36% of 350 patients with purported PLF, and whiplash injury alone was presumptively responsible for 33% of 102 cases of suggested fistulae.[8]

The constellation of the symptoms of PLF as well as association with trauma mimics other pathology such as labyrinthine concussion, traumatic Meniere disease, and cervical vertigo. Glasscock and colleagues and Seltzer and colleagues independently showed an extremely high incidence of SNHL and vestibular symptoms in surgically confirmed cases.[9,10] SNHL ranged from 83 to 90%, and vestibulopathy was manifest in 77 to 80%. A history of Tullio phenomenon, ie, vertigo brought on by loud noises is useful diagnostic information.

When the history and symptom complex leave the diagnosis in question the diagnosis may be suspected based on physical examination findings. Nystagmus brought on with pneumatic otoscopy is considered a positive fistula test. Audiometry may also confirm the side of pathology if hearing loss is present, although it is unable to distinguish a fistula from the more commonly seen labyrinthine concussion. It can be helpful distinguishing round window fistulae from superior semicircular canal dehiscence as the latter may result in a pattern of conductive hyperacusis. Videonystagmography (VNG) may show dysfunction even with a normal audiogram. Findings may be side specific, but not necessarily pathology specific. Electrocochleography has been reported to show an elevation of the summating potential to the action potential (SP/AP ratio) in an active PLF. This finding is quite nonspecific and would be anticipated in active or posttraumatic endolymphatic hydrops as well.

High-resolution (<1 mm cuts) computerized tomography (HRCT) may show fistulae. Veillon and colleagues studied 800 temporal bone fractures.[11] They were readily able to identify trauma to the oval and round windows and discuss findings suggestive of PLF. The more common oval window trauma may be diagnosed by following fracture lines, identifying stapedial fracture, and/or displacement of the footplate. Even subtle displacement is picked up when the plane of the footplate falls out of parallel with the tympanic segment of the facial nerve canal. A footplate within the vestibule, or air bubbles within the vestibule or cochlea are less subtle signs of PLF.

Round window fracture was only seen in 2.5% of all 600 fractures, but in 20% of the translabyrinthine fractures. The round window niche is normally an air space, and hence black on CT. When one-third or more of the recess is grayed by fluid, PLF was diagnosed and surgically confirmed in 14 of 16 patients with only one false-positive, and one false-negative result. One hundred temporal bone CT examinations from patients with chronic otitis media were reviewed to assess the prevalence of round window recess secretions. The round window niche rarely had fluid when the middle ear was normally aerated and other recesses were dry. Acute findings following blunt trauma might expect to be confounded by blood, inflammation, and effusion depending on the timing of the examination. Imaging of temporal bones associated with barotrauma overlying serous otitis media would be expected to be an unusual situation. Imaging the round window could be repeated after 3 months when effusions should be resolved if no fracture was seen at the outset and if symptoms of PLF persist. Other authors have a less encouraging opinion regarding the utility of CT in the diagnosis of PLF and view imaging evidence of PLF as unreliable and expensive.[12] Further evidence is necessary to validate or refute its utility.

Magnetic resonance imaging (MRI) is rarely of value or utility in acute trauma; but, for persistent symptoms, it may reveal contusion of the labyrinth as seen by diffusion of gadolinium within the labyrinth on T1 sequencing and a usual normal loss of signal on T2 sequencing. MRI does have other applications in defining dural defects, meningoencephaloceles, and examining the course of the facial nerve and other IAC and retrocochlear structures.

PLF management remains controversial possibly due to the historical difficulty in specifically identifying the pathology. Other diagnostic means, such as fluorescence endoscopy and beta-2 transferrin analysis of suspect fluid, among others are described in the otologic literature, but exploratory tympanotomy based on a high suspicion of fistula remains the current standard of both diagnosis and treatment. Identification of perilymph-specific proteins will likely be of great value in definitive diagnosis. Conservative initial management is advocated with bed rest, avoidance of provocative maneuvers, for example, cough, sneeze, strain, and observation for 24 to 72 hours. Exploratory tympanotomy with closure of the fistula site is warranted for severe persistent symptoms, positive findings on HRCT, or complications such as meningitis. Weber and colleagues reported the outcome of fistula exploration and repair in 137 children that had not shown improvement with conservative management.[13] Hearing was stabilized in 83%, improved in 10%, worsened in 3%, and 4% were lost to follow up. All vestibular complaints stopped within 24 hours of surgery.

Surgical treatment of PLF is accomplished by exploration of the round window membranes after elevation of a tympanomeatal flap. The ossicular chain is surveyed and palpated for integrity. Fractures, dislocations, and disarticulations are accounted but left undisturbed. Meticulous hemostasis, and topical adrenalin are helpful to ensure that any fluid welling up within the oval or round windows is not dripping in from above. The window regions should be observed for at least 5 minutes looking for accumulation of clear fluid consistent with perilymph. Fat, fascia, perichondrium, or vein may be used to close off both windows. Associated ossicular abnormalities may then be addressed using standard tympanoplasty methods as discussed in Chapter 19, "Reconstruction of the Middle Ear." Newer ionomeric and other cements and bone mimicking pastes (hydroxyapatite, Bone Bource, and Mimix) may prove useful in reconstructing fractured and dislocated ossicles (Figure 2). PLFs are discussed in Chapter 25, "Perilymphatic Fistulae."

TEMPORAL BONE TRAUMA

Trauma to the inner ear, other than that sustained by transmission through middle ear structures as with pressure and blast trauma, requires greater forces, and generally manifests both clinically and radiographically as identifiable temporal bone fractures. These high-energy impact injuries

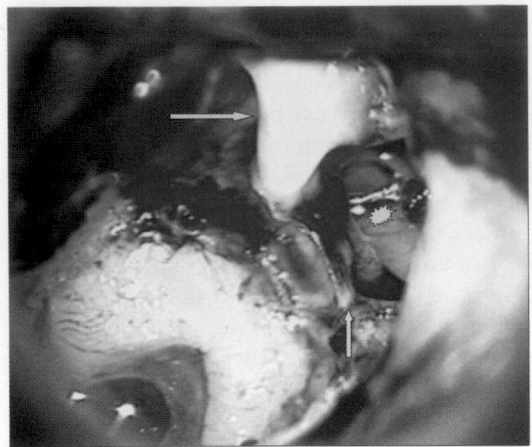

Figure 2 Intraoperative photograph showing repair of a foreshortened fractured incus to an intact stapes superstructure using Mimix hydroxyapatite cement. Horizontal arrow at Mimix repair; vertical arrow at the stapedial tendon; star within the arch of the stapes and over the footplate.

are generally seen associated with damage to other organs and systems and may be of secondary or tertiary importance as assessed by the triaging team. Forces sufficient to fracture the skull, temporal bone, and skull base can also result in injury to the central nervous system (CNS) and cervical spine, which must be evaluated and stabilized prior to temporal bone considerations. Inner ear trauma can be complicated by SNHL, vestibulopathy, facial nerve injury, cerebrospinal fluid (CSF) leak, and CNS insult that affect hearing and balance tracts, nuclei, and cortical centers within the brain.

Modeling of the complex three-dimensional (3-D) anatomy of the temporal bone is difficult, and the effect of blunt impact sustained, in light of the potential multifaceted mechanical insult from motor vehicle crashes, accidents, and assault, can be difficult to predict in the lab. Anatomical changes are reflected in injury patterns to the skull. Infants' head to total body proportional weight decreases from 15% to the adult head to body proportional weight of 3 to 6%. Newborn accidents yield more blows to the vertex. The newborn skull is composed of plates and has approximately 4% of the adult skull stiffness. At 6 to 8 years the stiffness is about 75%. Skull bones do not lose strength with age like long bones in the body. Brain material shrinks with age, but also becomes more fragile. Temporal squamosa is thinner than parietal, occipital, and frontal regions, but, according to the Society of Automotive Engineers, require similar forces to fracture; 5,000 to 6,000 newtons, or 850 g at 18 mph.[14]

Trauma registries and temporal bone CT data have been reviewed to assess the incidence of temporal bone fractures in patients treated for closed head injury or traumatic brain injury, relative to associated skull fracture, mechanism of injury, and other epidemiological information.[15–19] Temporal bone fracture was seen in 3 to 5% of traumatic brain injury. Skull fracture was seen in 23 to 66%. Basilar skull fracture was identified in 40 to 75%, and temporal bone fracture was associated with 18 to 40% of these. Temporal bone

fractures occurred predominantly in men (71 to 81%), as a result of blunt trauma (87 to 90%), and were unilateral (85 to 90%). The mechanism of injury in 45 to 47% was motor vehicle related (one-third of these were motorcycle crashes), followed by falls/accidents in 31 to 33%, and assault in 11 to 12%. Six to 10% were related to gun shot wounds. Fractures were also associated with intracranial injuries in 56% of one large study that lists a 16% neurosurgical procedure rate. Death from related injuries was as high as 18.7% in patients with temporal bone fractures.

Initial hospital-based evaluation and management of patients with temporal bone fractures generally happens in the emergency department by emergency physician, or a general/trauma surgeon or team. Trauma patients are assessed according to advanced trauma life support protocol. Along with cervical spine imaging, standard CT trauma protocols for head injury usually are carried out at 5 mm intervals. Consultation is requested for neurosurgical and other more urgent intracranial, vascular, thoracic, abdominal, and open orthopedic injuries. Treatment and stabilization of these injuries often happen prior to requesting evaluation by an otolaryngologist as temporal bone fracture itself is not often life threatening, and otologic symptoms may be masked or not expressed due to obtundation. The otolaryngologist is consulted based on the temporal location of the known or suspect fracture or for complications related to the injury, or to evaluate other areas of the head and neck. The initial assessment should include a thorough head and neck examination. Inspection of the EAC, TM, and middle ear may require debridement.

Temporal Bone Fracture

Temporal bone fractures occur along lines of limited resistance between foramina that weaken its mechanical strength. These fracture lines may disrupt the intervening structures causing edema, hematoma, bleeding, conductive or SNHL, dizziness, CSF leak, and facial paralysis. Access to previously closed spaces can result in infection including meningitis and CNS abscess. Disruption of the carotid artery can manifest as exsanguination by bleeding from the nose or ear or cerebrovascular compromise. Hemotympanum and or blood in the EAC was associated with temporal bone trauma in up to 90% of patients.[15] Twenty-six of 113 suspected fractures had a combination of audiometric SNHL, and vertigo or nystagmus. This combination was associated with fracture in 100% of cases. The initial head CT showed the fracture 67 to 79% of the time. Blood behind the TM or within the EAC had a positive predictive value (PPV) for fracture of 86%, and when combined with a positive head CT the PPV was 99%. HRCT confirmed suspected fractures in 79% and ruled out fracture in 11 to 21%.

Normal extrinsic sutures and intrinsic fissures and channels of the complicated temporal bone anatomy may be misinterpreted as fractures on trauma imaging[12] (Figure 3). "Pseudofractures"

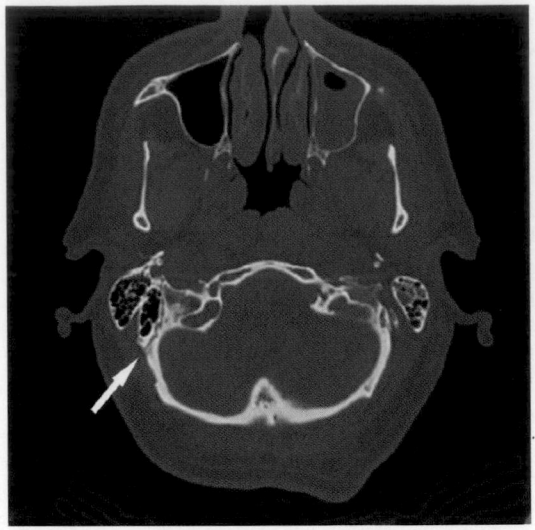

Figure 3 Temporal bone computed tomography (CT) image in the axial plane of the right occipito-mastoid suture line occasionally mistaken for temporal bone fracture.

extrinsically separate the temporal bone from adjacent bones at the parieto-occipital, the temporo-occipital, and the occipito-mastoid sutures. Intrinsic fissures along the tympanosquamous, tympanomastoid, and petrotympanic junctions may be similarly misleading. Several structures transit through channels of the temporal bone that may be misread as fracture including: the cochlear aqueduct, glossopharyngeal sulcus, vestibular aqueduct, petromastoid canal of the subarcuate artery, singular canal, mastoid canaliculus transmitting Arnold branch of the tenth cranial nerve from the jugular foramen, and the inferior tympanic canaliculus that houses Jacobsen nerve. Awareness of the course of these normal structures, and comparison to the contralateral temporal bone, provides for astute and accurate diagnoses.

Whether or not HRCT is necessary or useful is debated. In an interesting study, Ishman and Friedland showed the referral rate of patients with temporal bone fractures to the otolaryngology services was only 43%.[16] The audiology service was contacted in 58% of cases. When consulted, two-thirds of otolaryngologists surveyed always or almost always evaluated the temporal bone further with HRCT. One-third based imaging requests on clinical symptoms for surgical planning. Otolaryngologists and neuroradiologists alike consider HRCT of the temporal bone as the most appropriate radiology study in temporal bone trauma, and many feel that it is a necessary part of the evaluation of a patient with a temporal bone fracture, particularly for patient counseling or surgical planning.

Traditionally temporal bone fractures were categorized by their orientation with relation to the long axis of the petrous ridge based on postmortem examinations and animal studies.[15] This classification scheme, as based on developing imaging technology was leaving fracture distinction largely up to clinical judgment. With widespread access to HRCT, temporal bone fracture patterns are more fully appreciated. The following discussion revolves around the accuracy of the longitudinal and transverse typing of fractures.

Longitudinal fractures run parallel to the long axis of the petrous ridge. These were extensions of fractures from the temporal skull that were initiated by lateral or temporo-parietal blows and run through the foramen lacerum parallel to the eustachian tube and IAC (Figure 4). They comprised 70 to 90% of all temporal bone fractures and were seen with facial nerve injury 10 to 25% of the time.[16,17] Lacerations of the EAC extending into tears of the TM were seen, and hearing loss was generally due to perforation of the TM or ossicular discontinuity. Anterior fractures were associated with a low incidence of middle meningeal artery laceration causing epidural hematoma formation.[12]

Transverse fractures are thought to originate at the vestibular aqueduct and run perpendicular across the petrous pyramid (Figure 5). Traditionally these accounted for 10 to 30% of fractures and were caused by occipito-frontal blows.[16,17] They were associated with signs and symptoms of hemotympanum, SNHL, vertigo, nystagmus; and facial nerve paresis in 38 to 50% of the patients. Subtypes of medial and lateral helped explain SNHL.[12] Medial fractures traversed the fundus of the IAC and resulted in complete and permanent SNHL. Lateral subtypes fractured the cochlea or vestibule, and SNHL was incomplete and fluctuant related to PLF.

Retrospective temporal bone series have shown that fractures do not often fit into the classical scheme. Fractures that did not fit the generalized class have been referred to as mixed, and recent review place 35 to 75% of fractures in this category, while 38 to 64% could be described as longitudinal and 0 to 23% as transverse.[15,16,18,19] Several authors feel that fracture nomenclature should better reflect important inner ear anatomical structures and predict potential risk of complication by their involvement. To this end authors have attempted to classify fractures as otic capsule sparing versus otic capsule violating, petrous

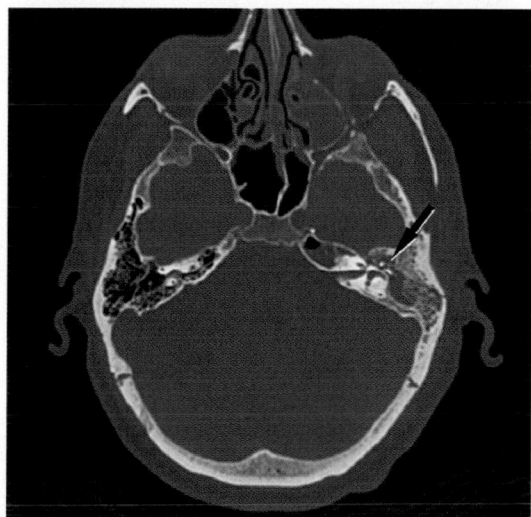

Figure 4 Axial computed tomography (CT) image with black arrow showing an incudo-malleolar separation resulting from an otic capsule sparing longitudinal temporal bone fracture.

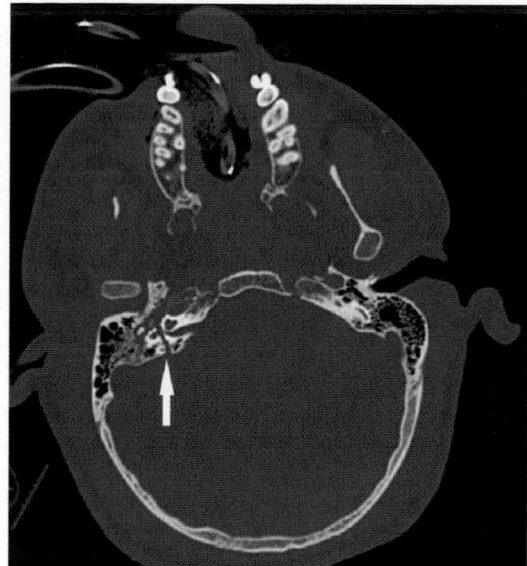

(A)

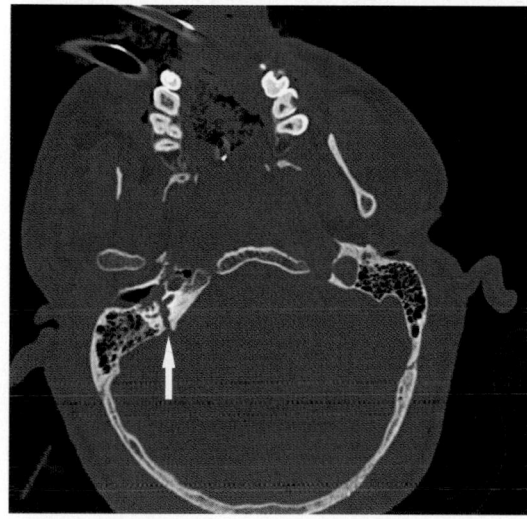

(B)

Figure 5 Axial computed tomography (CT) of an otic capsule violating transverse fracture in a patient with immediate facial nerve paralysis. (A) Arrow at fracture diastasis through the superior vestibule transecting the distal labyrinthine segment of the facial nerve. The incudo-malleolar joint is intact. (B) Fracture line originating near the endolymphatic sac, extending through the posterior semicircular canal and creating a prominent hemotympanum.

versus nonpetrous, or labyrinthine versus nonlabyrinthine. Fractures involving the otic capsule, ie, cochlea, vestibule, or semicircular canals, are reported in only 0.7 to 6.7% of patients.[15,16,18,19] When the otic capsule is violated, the risk of facial nerve paralysis is more than two times greater than when the otic capsule is spared, the risk of CSF leak is four times greater, and the risk of SNHL is seven times greater. Conductive hearing loss in otic capsule sparing fractures is as high as 56% whereas the rate in otic capsule violating fractures was 20% but dropped to 5% when reexamined after 7 weeks.

Fractures are best seen on axial imaging, which is often the only direct examination available in the trauma setting. With thin collimation axial imaging (0.5 to 0.75 mm), it is possible to reconstruct multiplanar and 3-D images that approximate direct coronal and sagittal examinations. These

provide excellent identification of fracture involvement of the labyrinth, IAC, facial nerve, and ossicles. Schuknecht and Graetz felt that 3-D imaging would make a useful contribution in up to 29% of fracture patients.[18] Symptom and outcome correlation, as well as the cost, benefit, and utility of HRCT diagnostics impacting management, are subjects of debate.[14–16,18] Fractures can be defined with great precision, but the question is whether that knowledge affects the patient's outcome or provides crucial management information. Retrospective review of trauma data bases comparing initial head CT with follow up HRCT further correlating these with complications and interventions has been used to evaluate the indications for HRCT.

Kahn and colleagues estimated that HRCT was clinically warranted in approximately 10% of cases of temporal bone fracture.[15] The clinical picture of blood in the EAC or behind the TM along with a positive head CT, was an excellent indicator of fracture. A definitive CT diagnosis of fracture did not alter the clinical management. HRCT did not play a role in the management of 30 out of 39 patients with facial nerve paresis in a series of 105 fractures. It did provide complimentary localizing information in those patients who were surgical candidates by timing and degree of weakness. Of 11 patients with carotid canal fractures on HRCT, 1 was symptomatic, 6 had angiography, and only the single symptomatic patient was shown to have carotid injury. Resnick and colleagues reviewed 230 skull base fractures, 55 of which involved the carotid canal.[20] Thirty-three underwent an angiogram, and only the 6 symptomatic patients were shown to have injury. HRCT for hearing loss was not helpful unless the loss persisted more than 7 to 8 weeks, was fluctuant, mixed or associated with otorrhea. Kahn and colleagues proposed that HRCT is a useful expenditure when the clinical examination is unreliable, for the unusual clinical course, or for surgical planning. If the clinical examination is reliable, initial head CT is helpful, and the patient follows an expected course, HRCT may not add practical information (Figure 6).

The majority of blunt temporal bone fractures are managed expectantly. Complications which may require surgery include facial nerve

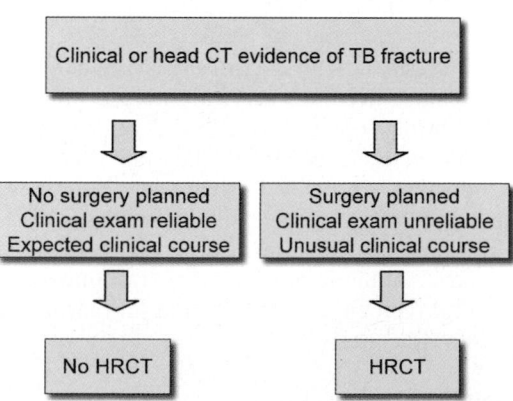

Figure 6 Decision algorithm for obtaining high-resolution computed tomography (HRCT) in patients with temporal bone (TB) fractures.

paralysis, hearing loss, vertigo, and CSF leak. Delayed complications consist of meningitis, abscess, pseudomeningocele, and posttraumatic cholesteatoma. Published rates for blunt injuries that require surgical intervention indicate facial nerve involvement in 7 to 40%, CSF leak in 11 to 45%, and hearing loss in 24 to 66%.[16,19] Surgical intervention is more commonly necessary with penetrating fractures of the temporal bone. Gunshot wounds show higher rates of complication and are associated with a higher incidence of intracranial damage and death.

Penetrating Trauma

A discussion of penetrating trauma to the temporal bone requires a certain understanding of ballistics keeping in mind a general dictum of emergency medical management to "treat the injury, not the weapon." The degree of tissue damage is determined by the velocity and design of the projectile, and the physical properties of the tissue that it disrupts. Weapons are considered low velocity if they project a missile at less than 1,000 feet per second (f/s), mid velocity between 1,000 and 2,000 f/s, and high velocity if they exceed 2,000 f/s. Handguns, and shotguns are generally low-velocity weapons unless fired at close range. Rifles usually project high-velocity missiles. Skin is penetrated by a projectile at about 163 f/s, while bone requires 213 f/s to fracture. Acceleration of fractured bone or fragmentation of the missile in contact with bone can produce numerous secondary missiles.

Tissue damage is caused by laceration, crush, cavitation, and shock waves. Low-velocity injuries cause damage by lacerating and/ or crushing tissues. Cavitation follows mid- to high-velocity missiles traveling at greater than 1,000 f/s. A permanent cavity is formed by the bullet path, and a temporary cavity is created by the acceleration of the tissue in the wake of the missile. Shock waves that can reach 200 atmospheres of pressure are formed by tissue compression before and to the sides of the projectile. Tissue damage is dependent on the density and elastic properties of the tissue. More damage occurs in tissues with greater specific gravities, and less damage in those with higher elasticity.

Acute management of ballistic injury is similar to management of other open wounds and fractures requiring initial basic life support assessment with control of airway and life-threatening bleeding, cervical spine evaluation and control, copious irrigation, debridement of devitalized tissue, and sterile dressing. Predictors of infection are delay in treatment, gross contamination of the wound, significant tissue devitalization, open fractures, and larger or multiple wounds. Antibiotic prophylaxis is recommended for high-velocity, shotgun, and intraarticular gunshot fractures.

Facial Nerve Paralysis

Trauma causes 3 to 5% of all facial weakness.[21] The incidence of facial palsy is 1,000 to 1,250 per 5 million per year, and 1 per 5 million per year for bilateral facial nerve paresis. Facial nerve injury is noted in 7 to 40% of patients with temporal bone fractures. Historically the injury occurs along the labyrinthine segment in 80% of medial transverse fractures, and in the perigeniculate region of laterally based transverse fractures.[22] The perigeniculate region is involved up to 94% of the time in longitudinal fractures.[23] Eighty-seven percent of gunshot fractures affect the nerve along the descending mastoid segment.[24] Intracranial injury coincides with 22% of temporal bone fractures, higher when bilateral or gunshot related.

Early evaluation of facial function is the most telling sign of the extent of nerve damage. Patients with complete paralysis, immediate or delayed, within 14 days have a poor prognosis for satisfactory recovery. The mechanism of immediate paralysis is thought to be due to crush, traction or bony fragment laceration or contusion of the nerve at the fracture site. Delayed paralysis is seen less often, but attributed to edema, arterial spasm, thrombosis, intraneural hematoma, or external compression. Delayed injuries manifest approximately 4 to 5 days after injury and recover adequately in 94%.[25,26]

As noted above, the otolaryngologist is not always involved in initial triage and treatment and often must rely on the examination of the trauma responders who may be focused on more pressing injuries. Referrals also lag the injury because evaluation of facial function in the first few days can be confounded by the patient's level of consciousness, facial edema and dressings that can give the illusion of retained facial function and residual muscle tone. Bilateral facial nerve injury may also be overlooked because of symmetry. Coexisting symptoms of hearing loss and vertigo are easily overlooked for similar reasons. The first neurotologic examination averages 3 to 5 days postinjury.

If facial weakness does not progress to paralysis [House–Brackmann (HB) grade II to V], prognosis is good; and care is supportive focused on ensuring adequate eye protection to avoid corneal abrasion and ulceration. The injury is neurapraxia, a conduction block with myelin damage that spares the axon, or axonotmesis where the axon is transected with retention of the perineurium and epineurium. Wallerian degeneration occurs in axonotmetic injuries in the distal nerve segment in 3 to 10 days (Figure 7). Regeneration of the distal nerve ensues at 1 to 2 mm/d, and return of full function is seen in up to 94%.[21,26–28] Immediate facial nerve paralysis is likely due to neurotmesis and surgical intervention is warranted. When facial function is observed to diminish completely within 6 days, prognosis is less sure and consideration of decompression is debated.

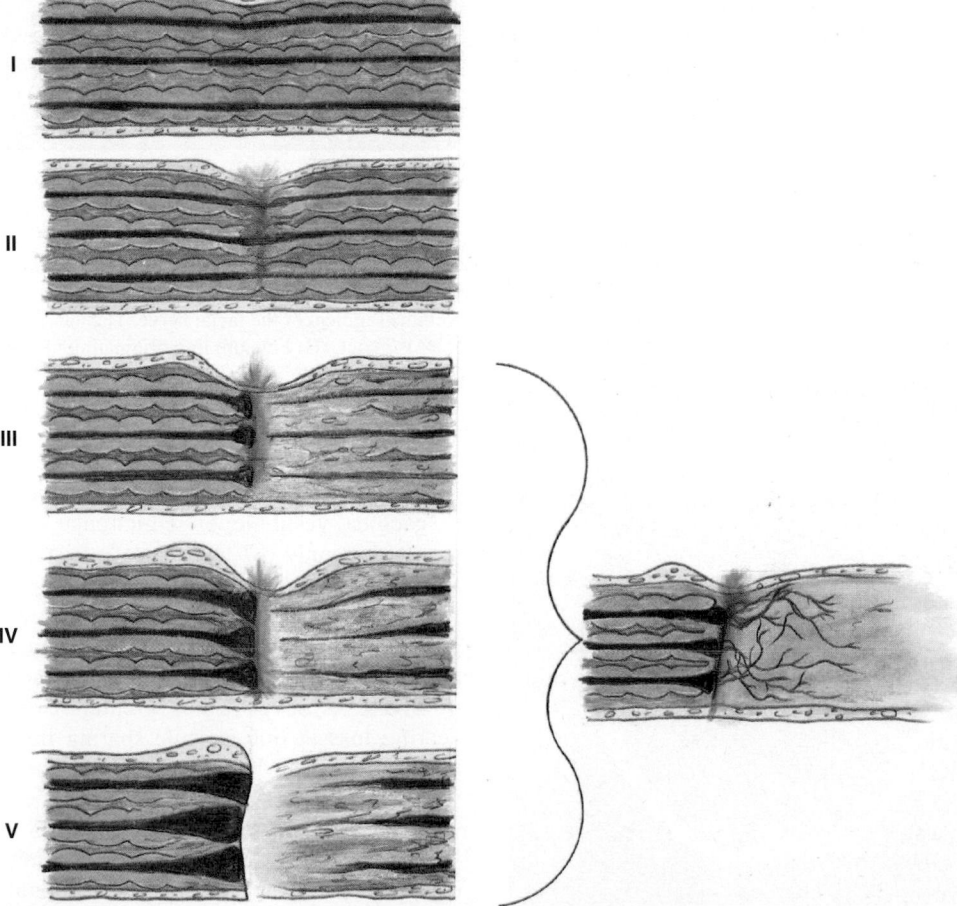

Figure 7 Examples of increasing severity of nerve injuries. (I) and (II) show neurapraxia, nerve compression without damage to the sheath or axon. (III) and (IV) show axonotmesis, disruption of the axon with ensuing Wallerian degeneration but without disruption of the perineurium or epineurium. (V) depicts neurotmesis which is disruption of the axon with its perineurium, epineurium, and its nerve sheath with complete transection.

Electrophysiological Testing. Further information about the extent and location of the injury can be obtained through electrophysiological and imaging studies. Neurofunction testing of the damaged distal segment of the nerve should be normal in neuropraxic injuries but may also give false-negative results if performed prior to Wallerian degeneration with more severe damage. Nerve excitability testing (NET) is a bedside test whereby nerve conduction is evaluated with a Hilger monitor, and the minimal stimulation intensity of the damaged side is compared to that of the normal side. Greater than 3.5 mA difference is considered clinically significant and leads to more objective testing. If tested within 3 to 21 days, electroneuronography (ENoG) is a reliable test.[27,28] This is also a comparison study that requires a functional contralateral nerve. The amplitude of nerve conduction velocity stimulated at the stylomastoid foramen and detected with surface electrodes at the nasolabial fold correlates with denervation, severe injury, and poor prognosis if >95% reduction in amplitude occurs on the affected side.

ENoG information is extrapolated from data pulled from Bell palsy research for which there is good untreated natural history record correlating timing of viral injury with electrophysiologic and functional results.[23,26–28] Some cases of blunt temporal bone trauma may be expected to follow a similar pathophysiologic course, but one would expect to see the possibility of more diverse and devastating injury patterns following traumatic facial nerve injury. As yet, there are no published reports showing the untreated functional results of facial nerve injury due to injuries in any substantial number of patients with >95% degeneration of the facial nerve by ENoG. Prognosis has been presumed to follow the observations of patients with Bell palsy, as ENoG is a measurement of functional conduction along the damaged distal nerve. The proportional difference in electrical output from side to side theoretically correlates with the percent of damaged neural motor units; but, until the natural history is studied prospectively, the correlation of ENoG findings with functional recovery will remain undetermined.

Spontaneous and volitional electromyography (EMG) provides useful information regarding nerve status. EMGs are of greatest prognostic value in patients with delayed paralysis and can be used for cases with bilateral paralysis.[23,26,28] They require more sophisticated equipment, technical support, and training to read. Voluntary potentials equate to neural integrity, ie, no transection, and an intact motor endplate. Reassuring polyphasic regeneration potentials may be seen on spontaneous EMG after 21 days from injury and can be seen 8 to 12 weeks prior to clinical movement. Positive waves and fibrillation potentials are more ominous. EMG can be used to rule out fibrosis of the nerve–muscle interface that precludes nerve repair benefit in long standing paralysis.

Continued slight motion, <95% ENoG degeneration, or voluntary potentials should prompt further observation as partial nerve damage

spontaneously healed offers better outcome than nerve grafting. When nerve recovery is in question, corticosteroid therapy offers theoretical benefit if not medically contraindicated. Corticosteroid treatment within 3 days of paresis for Bell palsy offered a higher and faster rate of recovery of facial function and increased the likelihood of complete facial recovery. High-dose methylprednisolone was shown to be detrimental to wound healing compared to the usual dosage.[21] EMG testing after 6 months allows sufficient time for distal nerve healing to manifest clinically or may show electrical signs of healing that will determine further planning.

Imaging. Imaging to localize injury for surgical planning is important. This information is extremely useful for patients with gunshot wounds and bilateral paralysis or unilateral fractures with immediate facial paralysis.[15,21,28] Paralysis in gunshot injuries may be seen without CT evidence of disruption due to ballistic heat or shock properties, or the bone may be comminuted to the point that the location of the injury cannot be found. HRCT with the contribution of EMG and clinical judgment has the greatest impact on decision-making in patients seen late in the course of their injuries.[23] Imaging in the axial and direct coronal planes should be obtained when possible. Dehiscence of the middle third of the tympanic segment of the fallopian canal occurs in 41 to 74% and leaves the nerve vulnerable to heat injury, fragments, or spicules.[22] The labyrinthine segment is the narrowest division averaging 1.2 mm in diameter and has been shown to be involved in up to 96% of some paralysis series.

Surgical indications, timing, and approach have been controversial subjects. CT imaging showing fracture, diastasis, or bony spicules along the course of the nerve with >95% degeneration within 14 days by ENoG together are indications for exploration with decompression or nerve repair.[19,26] We advocate for intervention as soon as the patient's status permits. Ongoing denervation of >95% by ENoG and fibrillation potentials instead of regeneration patterns on EMG portend a poor prognosis. Site of injury information correlated with audiometric findings will help plan the surgical approach.

MRI may be useful to follow the course of the facial nerve to identify injury in patients with late referral or who show no improvement primarily, and to exclude other unsuspected pathology such as a facial nerve schwannoma or tumor invasion. Some caution should be exercised however as enhancement in the geniculate and proximal tympanic segment of the facial nerve due to a rich perineural venous plexus has been documented in patients without facial nerve dysfunction.[22] Abnormal thickening of the nerve may be seen in conjunction with strong gadolinium enhancement on T1-weighted sequences at sites of injury. Posttraumatic labyrinthine enhancement is due to facial nerve prolapse. Facial nerve enhancement can be seen up to 2 years postinjury but does not directly correlate

with electrophysiologic findings. Most series concur that the perigeniculate region is the area most often injured.[19,22,26–29] Retrograde injury was seen by intrameatal enhancement on T1-weighted sequences in 92% of 22 traumatic palsies.[18] Fisch found perigeniculate involvement in 94% of longitudinal fractures that he decompressed through a middle cranial fossa (MCF) approach.[27] Dural enhancement along the anterior border of the pyramid without facial nerve enhancement may indicate trauma leading to facial nerve injury even without other imaging signs of nerve damage.[22]

Timing of Management. Review of management patterns shows a consensus that facial nerve repair is beneficial for immediate posttraumatic facial paralysis when surgically addressed within the first 2 weeks of injury, although other philosophies exist.[19,26,28,29] Fisch has advocated immediate exploration only for those with delayed paralysis that reach >90% degeneration within 6 days of injury.[23,27] He proposed that this pattern is due to the development of an intraneural hematoma that would benefit from decompression. The same argument might be made for neural edema. He delayed exploration of immediate palsies by 3 to 4 weeks, as they were often associated with other injury. Waiting allowed the patient to stabilize and tolerate a procedure better and cleared the anatomy improving surgical visibility. Most controversy has revolved around what to do with facial paralysis outside of the 14-day window. With patient access delayed for various reasons, patients that show evidence of nerve injury on HRCT by bony impingement or obvious fracture disruption and displacement of the nerve may still benefit from surgical repair.[26] Patients without apparent disruption or impingement and those without immediate paralysis or with unknown timing of progression to >95% degeneration fall into a gray zone.

Short of complete transaction, the type of nerve injury has no clear effect on facial outcome. Integrity of the partially injured nerve yields a better outcome than cable grafting, and interposition results are similar if performed prior to significant muscle atrophy and fibrosis of the motor endplates, which takes place within 12 to 18 months of the injury. Awaiting a functional recovery is an option. Prolonged delays can increase the risk of traumatic neuroma formation, ear infection, scarring, and fibrosis around the nerve that may affect the functional outcome. Late exploration and decompression of those with severe head trauma, or without recovery seen late for other reasons have been reportedly successful and may be managed based on HRCT and EMG findings.[26–29] As nerve regeneration rates average 1 to 2 mm/d, if no clinical evidence of recovery is supported by a lack of volitional EMG responses at 9 months with passive fibrillation rather than regeneration potentials, exploration with nerve repair is warranted. If the function of the motor endplate is uncertain, EMG stimulation is useful to demonstrate muscular contraction proving residual function at the distal nerve muscle interface prior to grafting.

Quaranta and colleagues retrospectively studied 13 patients who underwent surgical decompression 27 to 90 days post injury.[29] All fractures resulted in immediate paralysis from lateral impact motor vehicle accidents. All showed >90% denervation within 6 days and >95% at the time of surgery. The fracture location in all cases was the perigeniculate region from five transverse, three longitudinal, and five mixed fractures. Interpretation of audiometric testing revealed conductive hearing loss in 69%, SNHL in 8%, and mixed loss in 23%. All patients were decompressed through a transmastoid extralabyrinthine approach. Exploration showed additional labyrinthine injury in 15% and mastoid pathology in 23%. Pathology encountered was edema in 62%, hematoma in 23%, and a bony spicule in 38%. Facial function in the 9 patients followed over 1 year showed HB grades I or II in 7 of 9 patients, and III in the other 2.

Ulug and Ulubil prospectively looked at 10 patients with 11 facial nerve paralyses operated on 14 to 75 days after trauma.[23] Surgery on 9 patients was delayed more than 21 days. The timing of the first neurotologic examination was 5 to 50 days obviating utility of ENoG in all but 1 patient. Surgery was based on HRCT and EMG findings. Sixty-three percent of fractures were longitudinal and were decompressed through the MCF, 37% were mixed and underwent combined middle fossa and transmastoid decompression. No postoperative hearing deterioration ensued. Pathology encountered showed fibrosis in the region of the geniculate ganglion in five, bony spicule impingement at the geniculate ganglion in two, disruption and laceration at the greater superficial petrosal nerve in two, and edema around the geniculate ganglion in two. Facial outcome in 9 of 10 patients was HB grade I or II, and was HB III in 1.

Surgical Approach. Approaches to the traumatized facial nerve are individualized by surgeons, as no universal guidelines have been adopted. Most advocate surgical approach based on fracture location and hearing status, others on type of nerve injury or repair expected, others on fracture orientation, and some others attempt to decompress all nerve injuries through the same approach. Most agree that decompression or nerve repair on the side of profound hearing loss warrants a translabyrinthine approach. This allows exposure of the nerve along its entire length with access to reroute and graft as necessary. The caveat being that with expanding indications for cochlear implantation, the slightest amount of cochlear reserve justifies great care to preserve the eighth cranial nerve.

Controversy lies in the extent of decompression necessary and whether or not an "adequate" decompression can be accomplished via the chosen route. Findings show involvement of the perigeniculate region in the majority of cases. The geniculate ganglion is not bony covered 16

to 18% of the time, which is important in MCF exposure of the nerve.[22] For patients with serviceable hearing, a combined transmastoid and MCF operation can also expose the length of the nerve for decompression and allow access for cable grafting as necessary.

Some authors advocate a "less invasive" approach and feel that adequate exposure for decompression can be frequently accomplished through the transmastoid extra-labyrinthine operation.[19,28,29] This entails a complete canal wall up mastoidectomy with isolation of the facial nerve from the stylomastoid foramen to the labyrinthine segment. After opening of the aditus ad antrum and identifying the short process of the incus, the incus is disarticulated and removed. The head of the malleus is removed through a posterior tympanotomy. The epitympanum and cog are drilled, thinning the tegmen tympani, which offers exposure of the labyrinthine segment of the facial nerve and geniculate ganglion. Proponents of this approach feel that it offers sufficient decompression of the intratympanic segment of the facial nerve to the geniculate ganglion without a craniotomy and cite review series supporting adequate outcomes.

The disadvantages of this approach are that it is insufficient access for repair of a transected nerve proximal to the first genu of the facial nerve, and the surgeon may be unable to expose the fundus in up to 40% of cases, the labyrinthine segment of nerve is hidden behind and poses risk of injury to the tympanic segment, and the incus is necessarily dislocated for exposure potentially compounding facial nerve injury with hearing loss.[23,26–29] Fisch argues that the extent of decompression of a perigeniculate injury should be from the meatal foramen to the stylomastoid foramen. This is based on animal studies, imaging data, and surgical experience showing that intraneural edema and demyelination extend proximal from the site of injury. The retrograde effect is suspected to be due to a damming effect on axoplasmic flow at the level of the narrow lumen of the entrance of the fallopian canal. The facial nerve occupies greater than 80% of the cross-sectional area of the surrounding facial canal between the meatal foramen and geniculate fossa, and less than 75% of the facial canal lumen in the more distal segments of the canal. This offers a slight buffering effect that may reduce the risk of extensive axonal injury. The medial extent of decompression should include the meatal segment to help avoid progressive fibrosis of the traumatized nerve and ossification of the fallopian canal, and offers the best chance for good restoration of facial function.[23,26,27]

Twenty to 50% of gunshot wounds to the head involve the temporal bone and are associated with a higher rate of vascular and CNS injury than blunt trauma.[24] Penetrating trauma resultant in facial nerve paralysis is most often immediate, and exploration shows that most are total or near-total facial nerve transections. Damage is mostly seen in the descending mastoid segment. Wounds have a high incidence of infection. In a review

of 98 patients whose facial nerves were injured by gunshot wounds, Bento and de Brito showed that physiologic testing was only indicated in two patients.[24] Eighty-one required cable grafting, 14 underwent hypoglossal to facial reanimation, 2 were repaired with an end-to-end anastomosis, and 1 had decompression only. Sixty-five percent had HB grade III or IV, and 35% had V or VI function. Only 1 patient was conducive to decompression and had a grade I outcome (1%). The treatment of choice was an open mastoidectomy with meatoplasty in 63 of 98. MCF exposure was added in four to facilitate grafting. Thirty-five patients were treated with canal-wall down mastoidectomy, fat obliteration of the cavity, and closure of the EAC to protect the sural nerve graft if all foreign bodies were removed and the pinna was not damaged. Thirty-five percent of these were revised for infection. They found that an open mastoid with meatoplasty had a lower incidence of infection (10%) and subsequent cholesteatoma formation.

Opening of the nerve sheath is also controversial.[26,28] Recommendations have been made for a bony decompression without opening the nerve sheath based on a review that showed lower recovery in the sheath opening arm compared with a bony decompression arm and an observation arm. It was proposed that opening the nerve sheath might further damage axonal elements and compound injury. The study had low numbers and was retrospective and nonrandomized. Also, decompression stopped at the geniculate area in a transmastoid procedure; and, therefore the labyrinthine segment was not decompressed.

If less than 50% of the nerve is found to be disrupted, at the time of exploration, decompression of the nerve proximal and distal to the site of injury is warranted. If the extent of nerve injury is greater than 50%, repair with end-to-end anastomosis or cable grafting is advocated although any remaining axonal connections should not be disrupted to minimize synkinesis (Figure 8). Eighty-two percent result in HB grade III or IV function.[26] Rerouting the tympanic segment of the facial nerve can offer 1 cm of latitude to accomplish an end-to-end anastomosis. The easy access and good approximate size match of the greater auricular nerve makes it an ideal source for grafting. If unavailable, the sural nerve is an alternative donor cable graft. If no return of function is noted within 12 months of nerve grafting, consideration of a partial hypoglossal to facial nerve reinnervation may be considered. More detailed discussion of facial paralysis, facial nerve repair and rehabilitation of facial nerve dysfuction is found in Chapter 34, "Facial Paralysis."

Cerebrospinal Fluid Leak

The enchondral bone of the inner ear is mature at birth. The low metabolic activity of the otic capsule accounts for its lack of bony healing with trauma. Micro- and macro-fractures heal by fibrous repair rather than neo-osteogenesis with callus formation. Bony exchange in the perilymphatic

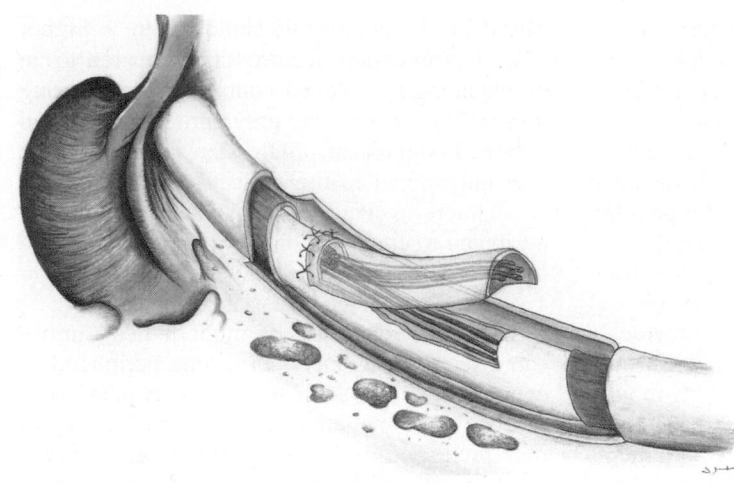

Figure 8 Partial transaction shown repaired by cable grafting of transected fibers, yet not disrupting the intact nerve fibers to minimize synkinesis.

regions gradually increases in a centrifugal pattern to the periphery of the labyrinth where bone turnover approximated normal healing patterns. Inhibition of bony healing is greater around the cochlea and vestibule than around the semicircular canals. This healing pattern may explain the 15 to 20% traumatic CSF leak rate found in otic capsule violating fractures. Poorly sealed microfractures may also explain cases of latent meningitis seen years after trauma.

CSF leaks in general are categorized as traumatic or nontraumatic. The majority are traumatic related to head injury and surgery.[30,31] In a retrospective series of 92 leaks, 32% were related to head injury, 58% were iatrogenic, 8% were spontaneous, and 2% related to osteolytic erosion from chronic otomastoiditis.[30] Otorhinorrhea was a presenting sign in 94%. Meningitis occurred in 16.3% with 11 of 15 related to iatrogenic trauma and only one to head trauma. Hearing loss was not an informative symptom because most of the patients developed the leak subsequent to vestibular schwannoma surgery, but profound hearing loss is seen in a high percentage of otic capsule violating fractures.

Clinically, CSF otorhinorrhea is reproduced with provocative maneuvers, ie, Valsalva maneuver or jugular venous compression. A steady flow of clear rhinorrhea brought on by leaning the patient forward is a positive reservoir sign. Reproducible clear otorhinorrhea in the postsurgical or head trauma patient on physical examination is suggestive of a CSF leak and obtainable in 78 to 87% of head injured patients with a CSF leak.[30] When the diagnosis is in doubt, the fluid can be tested for a halo sign, glucose content, or more specifically for beta-2 transferrin. Glucose multireagent strip testing can yield false-positive confirmation in 45 to 75%. Transferrin is converted to beta-2 transferrin by the enzyme neuraminidase which is only found in CSF, vitreous humor, and perilymph.

HRCT with and without gadolinium is the most helpful study for identifying the most likely site of leak. HRCT without contrast has been shown to detect the site of leak in 70% of traumatic CSF leaks.[30] Cisternography and radionuclide studies do not show anything that was not evident on CT imaging; however, intrathecal administration of radiopaque contrast material prior to HRCT can be useful. MR may be useful to delineate dural defects with soft tissue herniation and is indicated if CT does not explain cranial nerve injury to rule out hematoma. The common sites of leakage are along the tegmen, through or around the labyrinth, or along the posterior fossa plate. The site of CSF leakage depends on fracture orientation, the surgical route if iatrogenic, and presence of inner-ear malformations when spontaneous.

Most traumatic CSF leaks heal spontaneously. In a study by Savva and colleagues, 24 of 29 head injury patients with CSF leaks were managed successfully with observation and measures to prevent CSF pressure spikes such as bed rest with head of bed elevation, avoidance of cough and sneezing, diuretics, and stool softeners. Brodie and Thompson showed 78% of 122 traumatic leaks healed with conservative management.[19] Seven to 12% required a lumbar drain or serial lumbar taps to decrease intracranial pressure. CSF drained too rapidly can cause tension pneumocephalus. Intracranial inflammation from meningitis, trauma, blood, or surgery can impair CSF resorption elevating intracranial pressure. Surgical intervention should be considered for the 6 to 10% of traumatic CSF leaks that do not seal spontaneously within 7 to 10 days.

Prospective double-blind studies from the neurosurgical literature maintain that prophylactic antibiotic treatment of traumatic skull base CSF leak does not prevent the onset of meningitis. Brodie performed a meta-analysis of six retrospective reviews that individually found prophylactic antibiotic treatment of traumatic CSF fistula ineffective.[32] Collectively they showed that the combined numbers correlated a significant decrease in cases of meningitis with prophylactic treatment of traumatic CSF leaks. Meningitis ensued in untreated controls at a rate of 8 to 10%, and 2.5% in those receiving prophylaxis. The risk of meningitis increased in patients with leaks that did not seal within 7 days and in patients who had concurrent infections. In a more recent retrospective review of 122 traumatic leaks, Brodie and colleagues again showed an elevated risk of meningitis in patients whose leak persisted beyond 7 days and in those with concurrent infections. No cases of meningitis were seen in patients without a concurrent infection who were treated with an adequate antibiotic. The authors advocate prophylactic antibiotics for patients with fracture-related CSF leaks.

Iatrogenic CSF leaks more commonly necessitate surgical repair.[30] Only one spontaneous closure was seen in a series of 53 iatrogenic leaks. Surgical intervention was recommended if spontaneous closure did not occur within 3 to 4 days. Seventy-nine percent were controlled through a transmastoid re-exploration. Repair is again dictated by site of injury and hearing status.[30,31] Historically, many methods have been used to repair CSF fistulae. Adhesives, such as isobutyl-2-cyanoacrylate and fibrin glue with dural patching or transtympanic glue combined with lumbar drain for isolated leaks have been described. Muscle, fascia, perichondrium, and fat as well as several regional flaps have been utilized to prevent or stop leaks. Persistent leaks since Hitselberger described the use of fat strips have been rare. Multilayer closure supported with autologous grafts, for example, fat, fascia, muscle, showed an 81% 2-year success rate that was increased to 100% when artificial material, for example, bone wax, Oxycell cotton, gelfoam, was added to the closure in 16 of 16 repairs. Bone wax has been associated with osteomyelitis in other surgical fields, but its use in the temporal bone has not caused this complication. Bone wax mixed with Oxycell cotton provides a sturdy yet conforming sealant for open mastoid air cells and to plug the eustachian tube. Dural defects may be plugged with soft tissue and supported by fascia. If the dural opening is greater than 1 cm in diameter, support with cartilage or bone is suggested along with filling the mastoid with fat and covering the mastoid with fascia. For multiple tegmen defects, or those greater than 2 cm, MCF exposure should be considered.

When conservative measures fail, re-exploration and fat repacking and they have serviceable hearing, Glasscock and colleagues have recommended the middle fossa approach to expose and pack the eustachian tube.[31] Air cells that track below the IAC toward the hypotympanum and eustachian tube have been identified and are impossible to identify through a transmastoid approach.[33] For those with nonserviceable hearing, the transcochlear approach to obliterate these cell tracts is effective. Blind sac closure of the lateral EAC in conjunction with obliteration of the middle ear and eustachian tube may be necessary. This requires full eversion of the sac and complete removal of all squamous cell epithelium from the EAC and TM.

Hearing Loss

Hearing loss is documented in 24 to 66% of patients suffering temporal bone fracture and may occur by different mechanisms.[15,16,19,29] In a study of 820 temporal fracture patients, hearing loss was conductive in 21%, mixed in 22%, and sensorineural in 57%.[19] Only 3% had profound loss, and 1 patient had bilateral profound SNHL. Most conductive losses dissipated with time or were lost to follow-up, and 5 patients with conductive deficits underwent ossicular chain reconstruction for sustained loss. Hearing loss is likely under reported because it is a subjective symptom that may be masked by clouded sensorium, treatment conditions, or may be deferred to later assessment. Legal challenges regarding hearing loss have spurred review of the history of SNHL complicating head trauma.[34-36]

Conductive hearing loss as discussed is explained by damage to or obstruction of the outer- or middle ear structures. Many resolve over time. Patients who sustain conductive losses attributed to acquired canal stenosis, perforation of the TM, tympanosclerosis causing ossicular adhesions, ossicular fracture and dislocations, and posttraumatic cholesteatoma, may benefit from surgical repair or reconstruction (Figure 9).

Direct trauma to the auditory pathway causing SNHL may be obvious, such as fractures through the otic capsule or the eighth cranial nerve or central damage along cortical auditory pathways. Indirect damage may result from secondary hemorrhage/hematoma, edema, ischemia, hypoxia, and infection that damage hair cells. Direct damage may cause permanent injury while other injuries may show greater resiliency. Damage may be transient as with labyrinthine concussion, show fluctuating symptoms related to PLF and posttraumatic endolymphatic hydrops, or trend to progression with fibrosis related to healing.

Enlarged vestibular aqueduct (EVA) syndrome may predispose to transient, fluctuating or persistent SNHL with even minor trauma.[37] This syndrome is the most common congenital ear abnormality seen on CT affecting up to 14% of children with SNHL. There is an average gap of 22 months from the diagnosis of hearing loss to the specific identification of the anomaly with CT. This gap without the protective information for vigilant avoidance of minor trauma leaves children vulnerable to hearing loss from minor insult. Progressive hearing loss was seen in 22%, and fluctuating loss in 39% of 77 patients with EVA.[37] Progressive deficits in pure tone average were less than 20 dB in 92%. In this study group,

4% had vestibular symptoms, 4% gave a history of antecedent head trauma, and 4% were explored for PLF and all were found to be negative. The authors felt that the low incidence of trauma related hearing loss was due to counseling efforts and reflects a falsely low incidence of trauma-associated hearing loss, but also possibly the protective effect of avoidance of trauma.

Another theory for progressive loss is traumatic autoimmune damage through activation of preexisting conditions or exposure of previously naïve proteins to the immune system.[38] Corticosteroid responsive hearing loss mimicking rapidly progressive autoimmune losses have been anecdotally reported. These reports were in patients with Meniere disease undergoing endolymphatic sac procedures, which confounds the issue given Meniere disease may have possible autoimmune cause in some patients. Further elucidation of this theory is necessary to draw direct conclusions.

Posttraumatic SNHL may be due to the synergistic effects of acoustic trauma, physical trauma, systemic physiologic abnormalities, and ototoxic medicines. Some SNHL persists beyond the 6-month time frame expected for resolution of concussion. Segal and colleagues reviewed audiograms and medical records from 1,741 ears in patients with hearing loss.[34] They imposed a highly selective process that excluded patients with skull or temporal bone fracture, or those with closed head injury. Their strictly defined inclusion criteria minimized the influence of other diseases or age-related hearing loss. The investigators completed a 4-year posttrauma study of the group with a goal of identifying the time course and pattern of trauma induced hearing degeneration. Any change in the severity of the initial 655 mild losses, 701 moderate losses, and 385 severe losses took place in the first year after trauma. The minor changes that did occur showed an increase in the proportion of mild loss, and a decrease in the proportion of severe loss. No significant changes happened after the first year. Bergemalm followed a smaller group to look at long-term hearing outcomes.[35] The subjects included more severe trauma including fracture and CNS injury. They followed 43 patients for 2 to 13 years.

Significantly poorer thresholds with a higher risk of progression occurred as compared to an atraumatic age-matched control group. Hearing loss in 74% of the study group progressed. When stratified, significant progression in hearing loss was only noted in the patients diagnosed with skull fractures. Patients whose hearing loss was attributed to contusion did not progress. The progression with fracture victims was not limited to 1 year and was noted across all frequencies.

The violent nature of modern head injury can affect hearing anywhere along peripheral or central pathways. With anatomical evaluation by otoscopy and imaging one can explain how injury may predispose to hearing and balance dysfunction, and it may help prompt testing but cannot determine the severity of hearing loss. Evaluation of inner ear and central function is difficult at the bedside. Otoscopic examination along with whisper, Weber and Rinne tuning fork, and otoacoustic emissions testing may be correlated to offer simple gross determination of sensorineural injury, although acute testing is often confounded with mixed conductive loss and SNHL. Formal audiometric analysis as well as tuning fork testing requires a certain cognitive level of functioning and mobility. Often traumatic brain injury leaves patients unable to participate in traditional behavioral audiometric testing even past the acute phase of their injuries. Coexisting impairment may make it difficult for the patient or the caregiver to recognize the silent handicap of hearing loss. Auditory brainstem response (ABR) testing can be accomplished in these difficult patients and lead to hearing rehabilitation that will facilitate directed therapy and overall recovery.[36]

Sensory function can be evaluated by electrocochleography if the EAC and middle ear are free from obstruction. ABR electrophysiologically tests the neural hearing, displaying five waves that fall along the hearing pathway. Evoked stimuli travel between the eighth cranial nerve, cochlear nucleus, superior olivary complex, lateral lemniscus, and the inferior colliculus on their way to the auditory cortex. Potentials are recorded representing ipsilateral as well as contralateral synapses. Prolonged latencies or poor waveform morphology can identify neural injury. In a patient that cannot participate in behavioral audiometry, the entire hearing pathway can still be evaluated by otoscopy, tympanometry, otoacoustic emissions as long as the middle ear is aerated, ABR, and may be correlated with CT and MR imaging to combine anatomical and physiologic testing to determine hearing status.

Although there are patients who experience bilateral profound hearing loss after head trauma, it is rare.[19] When this occurs, however, successful rehabilitation through cochlear implantation can be achieved, provided that the cochlear nerve remains intact. The US Food and Drug Administration (FDA) warns of an increased risk of meningitis in cochlear implants placed in patients with temporal bone fracture, but the risk is reduced by preoperative administration of the pneumococcal vaccine, for example, Pneumovax 23. HRCT

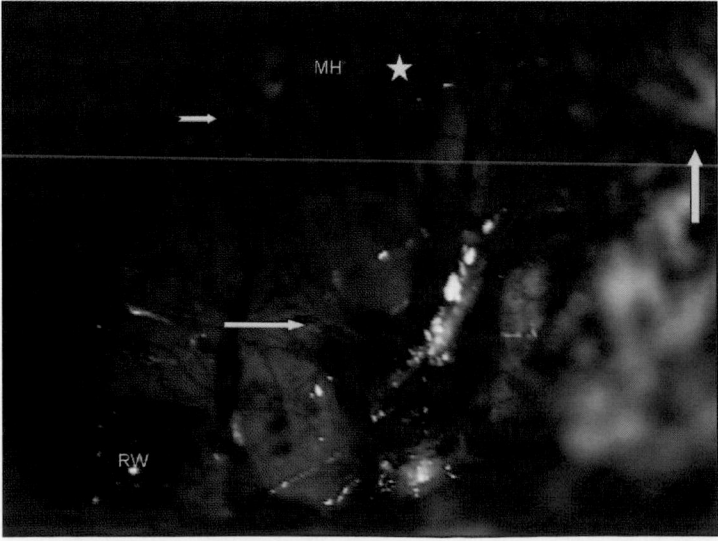

Figure 9 Intraoperative photo showing disarticulation of the incudomalleolar joint (*). The head of the malleus (MH) is retracted anteromedially. The body of the incus is retracted posteroinferiorly with an intact incudo-stapedial joint. Fracture of the stapes superstructure is seen with the anterior crus avulsed from the oval window niche (*horizontal arrow*) and the stapedial tendon (*black arrow*). A longitudinal fracture line is seen extending laterally from the scutum (*vertical arrow*). Notched arrow at manubrium. RW = round window.

imaging is important to rule out IAC fracture and labyrinthitis ossificans. High-resolution T2-weighted MRI may even be more sensitive to determine patency of the cochlea. Promontory stimulation helps determine cochlear nerve integrity, and if negative bilaterally, suspicion of disrupted cochlear nerves should prompt consideration of an auditory brainstem implant. Cochlear and brainstem implants are discussed in Chapter 32, "Cochlear and Brainstem Implantation." Facial nerve stimulation has been reported to be a greater problem in patients with cochlear implant with temporal bone fractures than in patients deaf from other causes, although otosclerosis may also predispose to facial nerve stimulation. Overt or even microfractures of the otic capsule allowing leak of current affecting the facial nerve may explain this occurrence.

POSTTRAUMATIC VESTIBULOPATHY

Traumatic disequilibrium is a common and usually self-limited entity following head injury. Postconcussive syndrome is reported in 40 to 60% of head injured patients.[39,40] Interestingly, it seems to be unrelated to the severity of the injury. Symptoms are often vague. Those related to the vestibulocochlear system include dizziness, vertigo, hearing loss, tinnitus, and noise sensitivity. Spontaneous resolution of symptoms occurs within 3 to 9 months in the majority of patients but may persist past 1 year in 8 to 15%. Elderly patients may especially show lingering symptoms of chronic disequilibrium due to either increased susceptibility to shearing axonal injury or to coexistent sensory deficit. When symptoms are suspect or motivated by secondary gain, dynamic posturography is useful in identifying cases of malingering. Vestibular rehabilitation is useful for those with profound or protracted symptoms.

Ernst and colleagues looked at posttraumatic vestibular symptoms.[39] They categorized primary and secondary disorders in a prospective study of posttraumatic vertigo in patients with mild head injury. Primary disorders stratified as labyrinthine concussion in 29%, PLF in 10%, and cervicogenic vertigo in 19% of patients. The secondary disorders included otolithic disturbances in 8%, delayed endolymphatic hydrops in 19%, and canalolithiasis in 14%. Most patients, 74%, were successfully treated by directed habituation training and or medical or surgical interventions for more discrete symptoms.

Hoffer and colleagues categorized patients with dizziness following mild head trauma into three groups: posttraumatic vestibular migraine, 41%, positional vertigo, 28%, and spatial disorientation, 19%.[40] 12% of the total group could not be categorized. They prospectively treated 58 patients with vertigo following mild traumatic brain injury with 6 to 8 weeks of vestibular rehabilitation. Those with symptoms of positional vertigo and vestibular migraine responded well to therapy and returned to work within 1 to 8 weeks, respectively. Abnormal static posture and dynamic posturography findings were signs of spatial disorientation that were not seen in the positional vertigo and migraine-associated dizziness groups. Those in the spatial disorientation category followed a more protracted course averaging 39 weeks to resolution of symptoms with 4% remaining symptomatic past 1 year.

Electronystagmographic testing is typically normal in postconcussive disequilibrium. Symptoms are self-limited but can be distressing. Supportive treatment with reassurance is generally adequate with vestibulosuppressant medications reserved for intractable nausea and vomiting, and then withdrawing these drugs as soon as possible to allow for central compensation for the balance disability. Vestibular rehabilitation stressing vestibulo-ocular and vestibulo-spinal exercises have also been shown to accelerate recovery. Associated audiometric threshold shifts are often temporary but must be monitored with follow-up testing.

Concussive injury to the membranous labyrinth or brain may exacerbate pre existing Meniere disease or vestibular migraine, or may produce syndromes that mimic these processes and cause vertigo. When vertigo more discretely falls into classical diagnostic schemes, medical and surgical treatment can be applied to those symptom complexes. Posttraumatic benign positional vertigo evoked by specific head positioning with observation of fatigueable geotropic nystagmus on the Dix–Hallpike maneuver is treated with canalith repositioning maneuvers. Fluctuating or persistent audiovestibular symptoms of posttraumatic endolymphatic hydrops may respond to dietary salt restriction and diuretic therapy. Posttraumatic migraine syndrome may benefit from an occipital nerve block for cervicogenic pain, or from medication used for prophylaxis of idiopathic migraine, propranolol, or amitriptyline. As previously discussed, surgical exploration should be considered for management when overt signs and symptoms of a PLF are present.

REFERENCES

1. Skinner DW, Chui P. The hazards of "button-sized" batteries as foreign bodies in the nose and ear. J Laryngol Otol 1986;100:1315–8.
2. Mehta RP, Rosowksi JJ, Voss SE, et al. Determinants of hearing loss in perforations of the tympanic membrane. Otol Neurotol 2006;27:136–43.
3. Kristensen S, Juul A, Gammelgaard NP, Rasmussen OR. Traumatic tympanic membrane perforations: Complications and management. ENT J 1989;68:503–16.
4. Kronenberg J, Ben-Shoshan J, Wolf M. Perforated tympanic membrane after blast injury. Am J Otol 1993;14:92–4.
5. Mirza S, Richardson H. Otic barotraumas from air travel. J Laryngol Otol 2005;119:366–70.
6. Stangerup SE, Tjernstrom O, Klokke M, et al. Point prevalence of barotitis in children and adults after flight, and the effect of autoinflation. Aviat Space Environ Med 1998;69:45–9.
7. Cortes MD, Longridge NS, Lepawsky M, Nugent RA. Barotrauma presenting as temporal lobe injury secondary to temporal bone rupture. AJNR Am J Neuroradiol 2005;26:1218–9.
8. Kim S, Kazahaya K, Handler S. Traumatic perilymphatic fistulas in children: Etiology, diagnosis and management. Int J Pediatr Otorhinolaryng 2001;60:147–53.
9. Glasscock M, Hart M, Rosdeutscher J. Traumatic perilymphatic fistula: How long can symptoms persist? Am J Otol 1992;13:333–8.
10. Seltzer S, McCabe B. Perilymph fistula: The Iowa experience. Laryngoscope 1986;96:37–49.
11. Veillon F, Riehm S, Emachescu B, et al. Imaging of the windows of the temporal bone. Semin Ultrasound CT MR 2001;22:271–80.
12. Swartz JD. Temporal bone trauma. Semin Ultrasound CT MR 2001;22:219–28.
13. Weber P, Bluestone C, Perez B. Surgical Outcome of Perilymphatic Fistula Surgery. Annual Meeting of the American Otological, Rhonological and Laryngological Society, Los Angeles, April, 1993.
14. Yoganandan N, Pintar F. Biomechanics of temporo-parietal skull fracture. Clin Biomech 2004;19:225–39.
15. Kahn JB, Stewart MG, Diaz-Marchan PJ. Acute temporal bone trauma: Utility of high-resolution computed tomography. Am J Otol 2000;21:743–52.
16. Ishman SL, Friedland DR. Temporal bone fractures: Traditional classification and clinical relevance. Laryngoscope 2004;114:1734–41.
17. Schuknecht B, Graetz K. Radiologic assessment of maxillofacial, mandibular, and skull base trauma. Eur Radiol 2005;15:560–8.
18. Dahiya R, Keller JD, Litofsky NS, et al. Temporal bone fractures: Otic capsule sparing versus otic capsule violating clinical and radiographic considerations. J Trauma 1999;47:1079–83.
19. Brodie HA, Thompson HC. Management of complications from 820 temporal bone fractures. Am J Otol 1997;18:188–97.
20. Resnick DK, Subach BR, Marion DW. The significance of carotid canal involvement in basilar cranial fracture. Neurosurgery 1997;40:1177–81.
21. Li J, Goldberg G, Munin M, et al. Post traumatic bilateral facial palsy: A case report and literature review. Brain Injury 2004;18:315–20.
22. Jager L, Reiser M. CT and MR imaging of the normal and pathologic conditions of the facial nerve. Eur J Radiol 2001;40:133–46.
23. Ulug T, Ulubil SA. Management of facial paralysis in temporal bone fractures: A prospective study analyzing 11 operated fractures. Otolaryngol Head and Neck Surg 2005;26:230–8.
24. Bento RF, de Brito RV. Gunshot wounds to the facial nerve. Otol Neurotol 2004;25:1009–13.
25. McKennan KX, Chole RA. Facial paralysis in temporal bone trauma. Am J Otol 1992;13:167–72.
26. Chang CYJ, Cass SP. Management of facial nerve injury due to temporal bone trauma. Am J Otol 1999;20:96–114.
27. Fisch U. Facial paralysis in fractures of the petrous bone. Laryngoscope 1974;84:2141–54.
28. Darrouzet V, Duclos JY, Liguoro D, et al. Management of facial paralysis resulting from temporal bone fractures: Our experience in 115 cases. Otolaryngol Head and Neck Surg 2001;125:77–84.
29. Quaranta A, Campobasso G, Piazza F, et al. Facial nerve paralysis in temporal bone fractures: Outcomes after late decompression surgery. Acta Otolaryngol 2001;121:652–5.
30. Savva A, Taylor MJ, Beatty CW. Management of cerebrospinal fluid leaks involving the temporal bone: Report on 92 patients. Laryngoscope 2003;113:50–6.
31. Giddings NA, Brackmann DE. Surgical treatment of difficult cerebrospinal fluid otorhinorrhea. Am J Otol 1994;15:781–4.
32. Brodie HA. Prophylactic antibiotics for posttraumatic cerebrospinal fluid fistulae. A meta-analysis. Arch Otolaryngol Head Neck Surg 1997;123:749–52.
33. Grant IL, Welling DB, Oehler MC, Baujun MA. Transcochlear repair of persistent cerebrospinal fluid leaks. Laryngoscope 1999;109:1392–6.
34. Segal S, Eviatar E, Berenholz L, et al. Dynamics of sensorineural hearing loss after head trauma. Otol Neurotol 2002;23:312–5.
35. Bergemalm PO. Progressive hearing loss after closed head injury: A predictable outcome? Acta Otolaryngol 2003;123:836–45.
36. Lew HL, Lee EH, Miyoshi Y, et al. Brainstem auditory-evoked potentials as an objective tool for evaluating hearing dysfunction in traumatic brain injury. Am J Phys Med Rehabil 2004;83:210–5.
37. Madden C, Halsted M, Benton C, et al. Enlarged vestibular aqueduct syndrome in pediatric population. Otol Neurotol 2003;24:625–32.
38. Ochoa VM, Weider DJ. Development of autoimmune sensorineural hearing loss after endolymphatic sac decompression: Two case reports. Otol Neurotol 2003;24:279–82.
39. Ernst A, Basta D, Seidl RO, et al. Management of posttraumatic vertigo. Otolaryngol Head and Neck Surg 2005;132:554–8.
40. Hoffer ME, Gottshall KR, Moore R, et al. Characterizing and treating dizziness after mild head trauma. Otol Neurotol 2004;25:135–8.

22

Noise-Induced Hearing Loss

Sharon G. Kujawa, PhD

Noise-induced hearing loss (NIHL) is common, its consequences currently not amenable to medical treatment, and its impact on communication and quality of life, significant. Theoretically, NIHL is entirely preventable; in practice, exposure to high-level sound is one of the most common causes of permanent, sensorineural hearing loss and inner ear damage. NIHL usually accumulates gradually with repeated exposure to high-level sound, although a single traumatic exposure can have immediate and permanent outcomes. NIHL is influenced by many factors, both related to the exposure itself and to characteristics of the individual that shape vulnerability to NIHL. In spite of numerous attempts to regulate exposure and to educate, there is mounting concern that NIHL prevalence is increasing, and reaching younger ears. Given the aging of our society, the co-existence of noise-induced and age-related hearing losses (AHLs) in the same ears will impact an increasingly larger proportion of the population and the societal burden will grow.

NIHL is thus of significant epidemiological concern. The National Institutes of Health, the Centers for Disease Control and Prevention, the World Health Organization (WHO), the European Commission, and many organizations with more focused missions all identify NIHL as a strategic target area for their efforts.

This chapter will review effects of high-level sound (for simplicity, noise) on the ear. In its description of structural and functional consequences of noise exposure, and of the variables that shape outcomes, it will rely heavily on animal models, as they provide the opportunity for strict experimental control and provide access to the underlying histopathology. The chapter will describe methods and outcomes of surveillance programs for NIHL in the human. Finally, it will address current management and treatments on the horizon that may prevent or reduce NIHL and inner ear damage.

PREVALENCE OF NIHL

Opportunities for noise exposure are commonplace in work and recreational activities. The WHO describes exposure to excessive noise as *"the major avoidable cause of permanent hearing impairment worldwide."*[1] In the United States, estimates cited by the National Institute on Deafness and Other Communication Disorders suggest that 10 million individuals already

have permanent NIHL and that 30 million more are exposed daily to potentially damaging sound.[2] Occupational sources of exposure are problematic worldwide.[3] In the United States, NIHL is among the most common reasons workers seek medical attention for workplace injury and among the most common reasons they seek compensation.[4] Auditory-related disabilities were the second most common type claimed by veterans of US military service who initiated compensation in 2003.[5] On an annualized basis, monthly compensation payments to veterans with hearing loss as their major disability were ~$660 million and payments for tinnitus were ~$190 million in 2004.

NOISE-INDUCED PATHOPHYSIOLOGY AND HISTOPATHOLOGY

It should not be surprising that a system optimized to respond to exquisitely small displacements would suffer compromise, for example, sensitivity loss and structural damage, when exposed to displacements orders of magnitude greater. Although NIHL is common in the human, characterization of physiologic and histologic outcomes is limited by incomplete and often retrospective assessment of cumulative noise dose, numerous confounding influences that cannot be readily controlled and may not be apparent, and of course, limited access to tissue. Thus, much of what we know about the effects of noise on the ear has been characterized in animal models, and most of this work has concentrated on noise-induced loss of threshold sensitivity and histopathologic correlates of that loss.

Pathophysiology: Temporary and Permanent Threshold Shifts

Noise exposure can produce temporary and permanent effects on function. Noise-induced sensitivity alterations that resolve on a timescale of hours to a few days after exposure are termed temporary threshold shifts (TTS). Such shifts tend to recover exponentially with postexposure time and reach a steady state, such that "final" permanent threshold shifts (PTS) are attained with a time course similar to that shown in Figure 1.[6,7] Details of the magnitude and frequency extent of the functional compromise and the recovery time course are related to the frequency composition, level, temporal characteristics, and duration of the exposure and are shaped by the vulnerabilities of the individual as discussed later in this chapter.

Typically, threshold shifts secondary to shorter, lower-level exposures (those producing threshold shifts of about 40 dB or less when assayed at short postexposure times), resolve in this timeframe. The long-term impact of such apparently reversible insult is currently unresolved. As exposure becomes more significant, initial shifts increase, time to recovery is prolonged and, of course, shifts may become permanent.

Sensitivity losses apparent at longer postexposure times are termed PTS. As an example, Figure 2 displays temporary and permanent ABR threshold shifts in the same ears of young CBA/CaJ mice 24 hours and 2 weeks following octave-band noise exposure. Here, lower levels of exposure (94, 97 dB) produced milder degrees of TTS which have largely recovered by 2 weeks, except for a small residual shift apparent at high frequencies after 97 dB exposure. Noise exposures at 100 and 103 dB SPL resulted in progressively larger TTSs that spread across an increasingly greater extent of the frequency range tested. In such ears, a significant, but more frequency restricted PTS remained 2 weeks after exposure. PTS grows rapidly with exposure level in most mammalian species. In the example provided here, this rapid growth is evident: a 3 dB increase in the level of a single, 2-hour exposure (97 to 100 dB), yielded a nominally 40 dB difference in measured PTS.

Noise-induced threshold shifts are often observed to be greatest not at the frequency of exposure but rather, approximately one-half octave above it, particularly for narrow band (including pure tone) and higher-level exposures. Such an upward shift of functional compromise is apparent in Figure 2. The "half-octave shift"

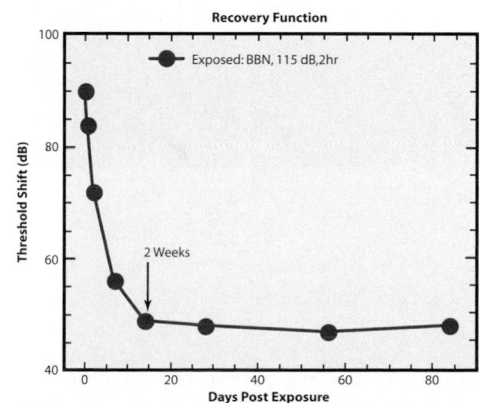

Figure 1 Postexposure threshold shift dynamics. (Adapted from reference 6.)

94
97
100
103
Threshold Shift (dB)
noise band
24 hr
2 wk
Frequency (kHz)
0
10
20
30
40
50
60
4
6
8
10
30
50

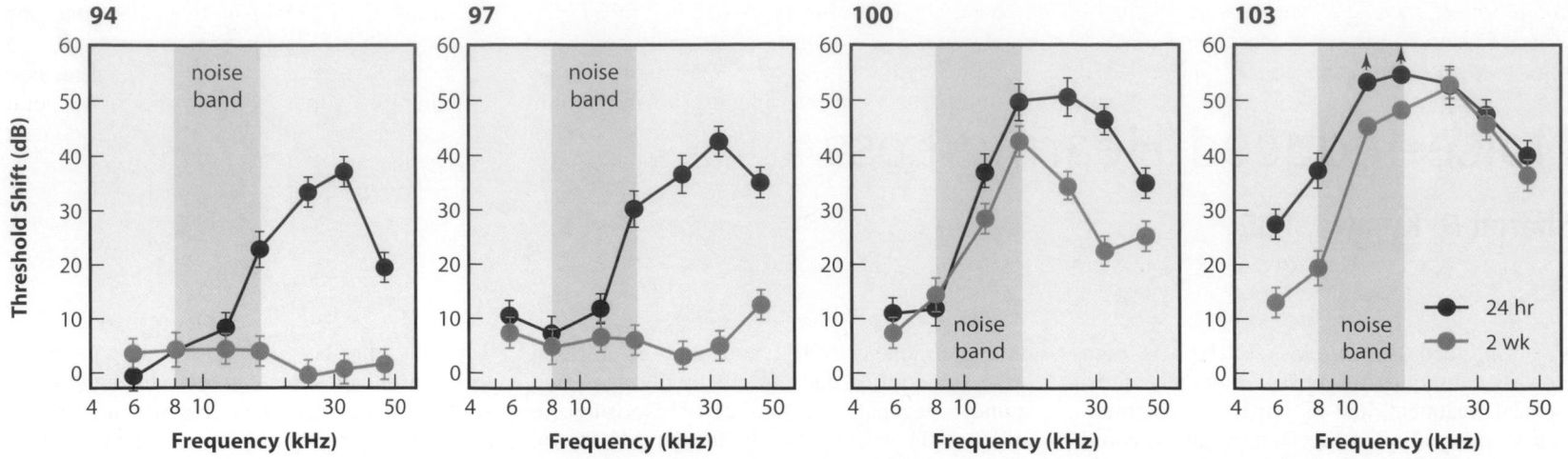

Figure 2 Noise-induced threshold shifts assayed by auditory brainstem response (ABR) 24-hour and 2-week postexposure (8 to 16 kHz octave noise band, 94 to 103 dB SPL, 2 hours) in CBA/CaJ mice (n = 8 to >100) exposed at 4 to 6 weeks of age. At highest exposure level, ABR metric saturates at some frequencies; points at which >50% of responses were absent are noted by up arrows. Data are expressed as mean shifts ± SE relative to strain- and age-matched, unexposed controls. (Kujawa, unpublished data.)

originates in the nonlinear mechanical response of the basilar membrane to high-level sound. Evidence of this upward shift of sensitivity loss can be seen in the basilar membrane response[8] and in electrophysiological[9,10] and behavioral[10,11] responses to sound, and histopathology can be documented in correspondingly shifted cochlear places.[12,13] In addition to this tonotopically "appropriate" injury, the literature provides clear examples of threshold shifts and cochlear lesions which are tonotopically "inappropriate" with respect to the frequency content of the exposure.[14] Most often, these lesions are observed in the extreme base or "hook" region of the cochlea, which demonstrates greater vulnerability to insult. As exposure bandwidth increases, maximum injury can be greatest in basal cochlear regions.

Although the threshold shifts shown in Figure 2 for a murine model reveal little variability among identically exposed, age- and strain-matched animals within groups, it is important to note that vulnerability to noise-induced TTS, PTS, and cochlear structural injury demonstrates dramatic variability among animals heterogeneous for genetic background, exposure age, gender, and certain other variables. It is reasonable to suspect that such factors contribute materially to apparent noise vulnerability differences observed in humans. Such individual differences will be addressed later in this chapter.

Histopathology: Temporary and Permanent Injury

Assessment of noise-induced histopathology reveals that many cell types in the cochlea can be

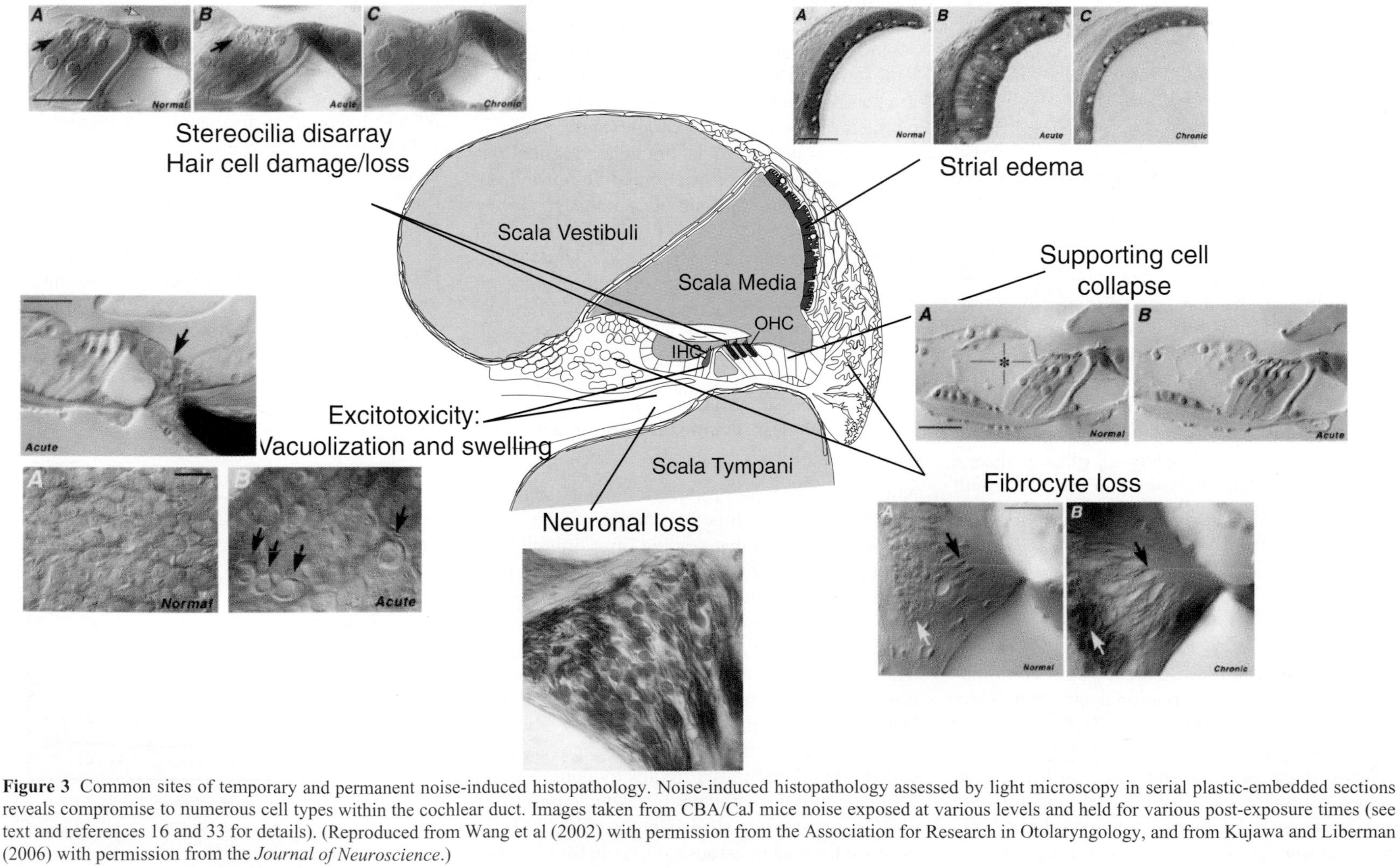

Stereocilia disarray
Hair cell damage/loss
Strial edema
Scala Vestibuli
Scala Media
Supporting cell collapse
OHC
IHC
Excitotoxicity:
Vacuolization and swelling
Scala Tympani
Fibrocyte loss
Neuronal loss
A
B
C
Normal
Acute
Chronic

Figure 3 Common sites of temporary and permanent noise-induced histopathology. Noise-induced histopathology assessed by light microscopy in serial plastic-embedded sections reveals compromise to numerous cell types within the cochlear duct. Images taken from CBA/CaJ mice noise exposed at various levels and held for various post-exposure times (see text and references 16 and 33 for details). (Reproduced from Wang et al (2002) with permission from the Association for Research in Otolaryngology, and from Kujawa and Liberman (2006) with permission from the *Journal of Neuroscience*.)

compromised by sound overexposure (Figure 3). Hair cell stereocilia damage, evidence of swelling and vacuolization in the inner hair cell (IHC) area, hair cell loss, collapse of supporting cells, strial compromise, fibrocyte loss, and neuronal loss all have been identified in noise-exposed ears.[15,16,33] Although there is overlap in the histologic underpinnings of TTS and PTS, the mechanisms underlying a large but reversible threshold shift, eg, 40 dB at 12 hours post exposure, and a comparable permanent threshold shift, eg, 40 dB at 2 weeks post exposure, are widely regarded to be fundamentally different, and attempts to predict the latter from the former have been largely disappointing.[17] In the sections that follow, the focus is on recurring themes of damage and loss, apparent in many species and for a range of exposures.

At short post-exposure times, histologic examination frequently reveals alterations to hair cell stereocilia.[18–20] Stereocilia deflection changes tip-link tension, opening mechanically gated transduction channels. High-level sound can cause disarray of the stereocilia bundle, fusion of its elements, and can break tip links as shown in Figure 4A. Stereocilia damage or loss has been correlated both in its distribution and degree with the frequency extent and degree of functional compromise, assayed by threshold shift metrics.[16,21]

The afferent synapse between IHCs and peripheral terminals of spiral ganglion cells (Figure 4B) is glutamatergic, and a type of glutamate excitotoxicity appears to be a ubiquitous aspect of the cochlea's acute response to noise. Sound overexposure resulting in massive transmitter release can tax postsynaptic receptors and glutamate clearance mechanisms leading to classic signs of glutamate excitotoxicity.[22] If an ear is fixed 0-12 h after an acoustic overexposure, there is often evidence of vacuole formation and swelling of afferent dendrites under the IHCs and swelling of spiral ganglion cells and/or their satellite cell sheaths in Rosenthal canal (Figure 3). Histologic evidence for excitotoxicity is visible whether the exposure produces a temporary threshold shift (TTS) only, or has both temporary and permanent components, and can be present even if no hair cell loss will eventually ensue.[16] Excitotoxic injury seen acutely may have long-term consequences. Puel and colleagues[23] have suggested that such changes may underlie the neuronal degeneration seen in a subset of human ears with presbycusis.

Swelling of the stria vascularis (Figure 3) is an acute consequence of noise exposure with as yet unclear functional consequences.[16,24] The stria vascularis, as the name implies, is a highly vascular tissue located at the cochlear lateral wall. It plays an important role in maintaining the ionic environment and the endocochlear potential (EP) which are, in turn, crucial for the normal transduction processes of the hair cells. Such fundamental

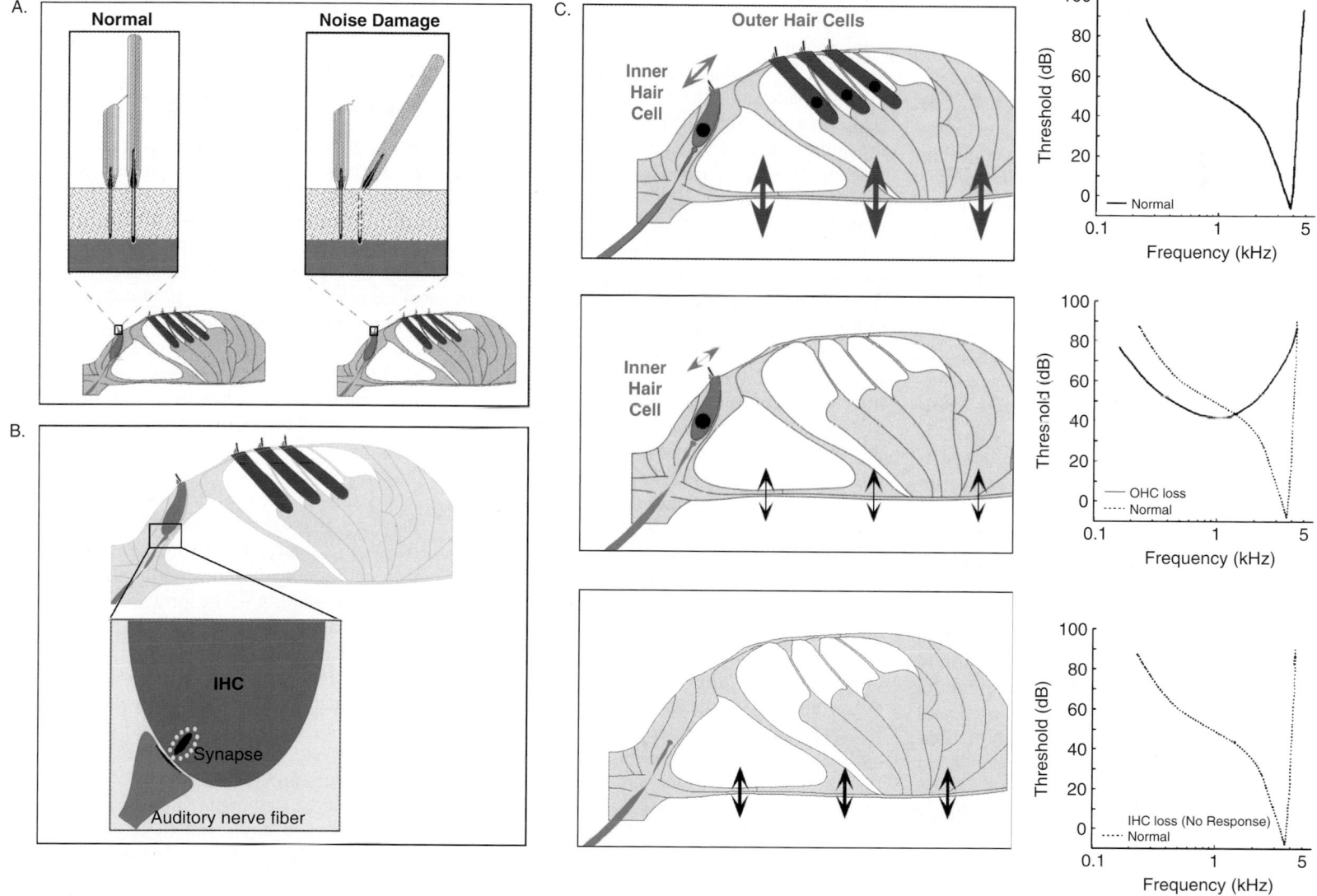

Figure 4 Acute and chronic consequences of noise-induced hair cell compromise. Panel A. Noise-induced damage to hair cell stereocilia can include disarray, fusion or loss of individual stereocilia comprising the bundle on the hair cell's apical surface, and breakage of the fine tip links that connect the individual stereocilia. Such changes can occur where no other obvious ultrastructural changes are visible and can contribute materially to noise-induced threshold shifts. Panel B. Synaptic transmission between IHCs and dendrites of type 1 SGCs takes place at ribbon synapses, where released glutamate activates AMPA receptors on the post-synaptic membrane. Mechanisms for glutamate clearance and receptor regulation maintain optimum responsiveness; however, with acoustic overstimulation, release of neurotransmitter may exceed such regulatory processes and induce dendritic damage, presumably through glutamate excitotoxicity. Panel C. Organ of Corti schematics and idealized threshold tuning curves are shown for 3 cochlear conditions: top panel—the normal condition, in which there is a full complement of outer and inner hair cells and a sensitive and sharply tuned response; middle panel with noise-induced OHC loss, and associated loss of the physiologically-assisted amplification of low-level sounds resulting in a less sensitive and more broadly tuned response; bottom panel now adding IHC loss which prevents communication with neural elements, resulting in no acoustic responses from this cochlear region. (Organ of Corti schematics courtesy of MC Liberman).

contributions to normal cochlear function suggest that noise-induced compromise to the stria should have functional consequences.[25,26] Although the EP recovers quickly from the effects of noise, degeneration of strial marginal and interdental cells may contribute to threshold shifts in the steady state.[27]

Supporting cell collapse can also be evident in the acute post-exposure period, and reversible components of such structural alteration have been associated with reversible effects on cochlear potentials in guinea pigs[28] and in chinchillas.[13] Reversible changes to supporting cell architecture (at least to highest levels of exposure) were also seen in ears with TTS in a recent survey of noise effects in mice (Figure 3).[16]

Histopathology evident weeks to months after exposure can be quite different from that seen in the acute post-exposure period. Cells damaged by noise can degenerate rather quickly. Hair cells damaged during exposure, for example, may degenerate, being replaced by nonsensory (supporting) cells which form a phalangeal "scar" on the surface of the cochlear sensory epithelium.[29]

There is wide agreement that the hair cells, especially the outer hair cells (OHCs), are particularly vulnerable to noise-induced injury and that their compromise is a primary contributor to post-exposure changes in function.[21,25,30,31] OHCs amplify motion patterns, enhancing the cochlear mechanical response to low-level signals. IHCs serve as traditional sensory receptors. Noise-induced OHC loss elevates thresholds and broadens tuning (Figure 4C). Noise-induced IHC loss eliminates cochlear communication with afferent neurons altogether, resulting in unresponsive regions, as Figure 4C.

Noise-induced histopathology often originates with focal OHC damage and loss, and for more significant exposures, IHC, and supporting cell compromise. Degeneration of myelinated afferent neurons and spiral ganglion cells can follow as a secondary consequence to IHC loss,[32] although it also can occur in ears without such loss (Figure 3).[33] It is nevertheless clear that frank hair cell loss is not obligatory, even in ears with PTS on the order of 40 to 50 dB. Threshold shifts of this magnitude can be explained entirely by stereocilia damage.[19] In mice, stereocilia damage seen in acute ears often persisted and was the most functionally important structural change underlying PTS.[16]

The functional significance of certain cellular changes and details of their postexposure appearance in different species remains under active investigation in many laboratories. Fibrocyte loss in the spiral ligament (Figure 3), for example, is seen commonly in noise-exposed ears of mice.[16,33] Loss of these cells has currently unknown effects on auditory sensitivity; ears with large fibrocyte losses may demonstrate minimal threshold shifts and vice versa. It has been suggested that fibrocytes of the lateral wall may be involved in an endolymph K^+ recycling pathway that is particularly crucial during acoustic overstimulation. In this role, K^+ ions entering and leaving the OHCs are subsequently shuttled through the fibrocytes and finally back to the stria vascularis.[34]

FACTORS INFLUENCING NIHL RISK

The appearance, nature, and degree of noise-induced functional and structural compromise depend on various characteristics of the exposure, the individual, and interactions between the 2. In the sections that follow, such variables will be briefly reviewed.

Variables Related to Noise Exposure

Efforts to establish risk of NIHL in individuals and in populations rely heavily on characterizations of the exposures themselves. Although straightforward in laboratory studies, obtaining reliable work and/or recreational exposure estimates for individuals and groups is a comparatively daunting task. In quantifying exposures to human ears in occupational settings, exposure assessments often focus on sound level and duration. Sound-level measurements, including those acquired by wearable noise "dosimeters" usually are made using the "A" frequency weighting scale, to approximate the frequency response of the human ear. The resulting sound level is designated in dBA. A metric of particular interest is the "noise dose," in which the overall level is integrated over the entire time of exposure. Because such information is most frequently captured in relation to work-related noise monitoring, noise dose is commonly specified relative to a full-shift (8 hour) time-weighted average (TWA).

Exposure variables related to frequency composition, level, temporal pattern, and duration of the exposure, however, all can influence the risk of NIHL and cochlear histopathology. In brief, the mechanical properties and tonotopic arrangement of the cochlear sensory epithelium and the frequency content of the exposure combine to determine the base-to-apex places of overstimulation and the frequency range of hearing loss produced by the exposure. As the level of the noise increases, risk of temporary and permanent hearing loss and inner ear damage also increase. As seen previously in Figure 2, exposure level also influences the frequency range of the noise-induced insult, as higher-level exposures (over)-stimulate a broader extent of the cochlear epithelium. Risk of noise-induced compromise increases with exposure duration. A time-for-intensity trading relationship exists for many exposures, such that the higher the level, the shorter the time before insult. Such generalities are influenced, however, by temporal characteristics of exposure, including whether exposures are intermittent or continuous.

For exposures equal in total energy, those delivered in interrupted fashion are associated with less PTS than continuous exposures. The periods of quiet appear to afford some protection against the noise-induced insult, as long as the noise off time is of sufficient duration. In contrast, impulsive noise is more hazardous to hearing than continuous noise of the same spectrum and intensity. An important variable appears to be the degree of amplitude kurtosis in the noise exposure stimulus.[35] Detailed treatments of exposure parameter influences on NIHL and cochlear histopathology can be found elsewhere.[5,36,37]

Acoustic Trauma

To this point, the focus has been on consequences of more or less continuous exposure. NIHL can result, however, from short duration, even single exposure to a particularly damaging sound, for example, explosion, gunshot or firecracker, commonly termed an acoustic trauma. Here, the mechanical insult may produce different patterns of structural damage, frequency patterns of functional involvement may shift, and recovery patterns may be altered from those seen after chronic exposure with longer duration, less intense sound. Structural compromise may include tympanic membrane rupture and injury to middle-ear structures as well as damage to the inner ear. Significant and permanent hearing loss is a common result.

Exposure History and NIHL

Bridging the transition between variables related to the exposure and those intrinsic to the individual is the observation that risk of NIHL may be shaped by an individual's history of particular kinds of exposure. Substantial reduction of threshold shifts (protection) has been seen for a variety of chronic noise-exposure protocols, collectively referred to as "conditioning" or "toughening" of the ear. These protective effects of sound-exposure history have been studied with a number of different paradigms; however, the protocols fall into 2 main classes. In 1 case, animals are conditioned by daily exposure to a moderately intense sound, which, by itself, causes little or no permanent damage. Then, after a variable rest period, they are given a traumatic exposure of shorter duration; usually, 1 with the same spectrum as the conditioning stimulus but applied at a higher sound pressure.[38,39] The protection observed is that animals sound conditioned before frank overexposure show less PTS (and/or cochlear damage) than those overexposed without conditioning pretreatment. In a second type of experiment, here is 1 type of exposure stimulus, usually a mildly traumatic one, which is delivered in daily doses (eg, 6 hours on, 18 hours off).[40] The "toughening" observed in this paradigm is that thresholds measured each day, immediately postexposure, improve as the number of daily doses increases. However, in most such studies, thresholds measured immediately *before* each exposure progressively deteriorate, and the animals demonstrate PTS (and/or permanent cochlear damage) weeks after the daily exposures are terminated.[41] Thus the toughening consists of an observed decrease in a compound threshold shift (CTS) consisting of a small, increasing PTS and a larger, decreasing TTS component.

Coexposures. Risk of developing an NIHL may be increased for noise-exposed individuals who receive certain therapeutic drugs like aminoglycosides and cisplatin, and for individuals working in certain industrial and military settings that likely expose them to certain chemical agents, eg, solvents, chemical asphyxiants, heavy metals. Such agents can interact with noise and add to or even potentiate NIHL. Some produce hearing loss on their own and, when delivered to a noise-exposed individual, contribute in an additive fashion to NIHL. Other agents potentiate the effects of the noise on hearing and histopathology, in some cases doing so with little or no effect on hearing of their own; Such co-exposure synergies are well described in the toxicology literature and perhaps easier to identify and quantify, as the effects of 2 chemicals with the same target organs or sharing the same metabolic pathway may be more easily predicted and prevented.[42]

Variables Related to the Individual

Hearing losses recorded in noise-exposed ears are highly variable in human populations. This variability may arise from differences in noise exposure as described above, as well as other intrinsic and environmental variables that produce hearing loss on their own or alter susceptibility to NIHL. Many variables have been considered over the years.[43] Aiding these efforts, low-variance murine models have been used to characterize genetic influences on NIHL susceptibility; and, with genetic variability minimized, effects of other individual variables on NIHL outcomes may be isolated as well, as discussed below. Such work promises to translate to the human, as genetic influences on NIHL and other susceptibilities are clarified.

Genetic Influences on Noise Susceptibility.

Many investigators have turned to animal models to characterize effects of noise on the ear without certain of the confounding variables inherent when studying NIHL in humans. Although the additional experimental control possible with such approaches can reduce variability, for example, by careful specification and control of exposure parameters, variability among identically exposed, outbred animals can remain high.[44] Noise-induced sensitivity loss and cochlear histopathology within inbred strains of mice, in contrast, show comparatively small variability, suggesting that genetic differences contribute to interindividual NIHL vulnerability differences.

Within-strain NIHL phenotype homogeneity has facilitated characterization of between-strain NIHL susceptibility differences. At some ages and with certain levels of noise exposure, mice from some inbred strains, for example, 129S6SvEvTac and MOLF/Ei, demonstrate remarkable resistance to NIHL,[7,45] whereas mice from other strains (B6, BALB/cJ) can show dramatic vulnerability.[46] Since animals of a given strain are genetically identical, these phenotype differences may provide important clues to mechanisms contributing to such vulnerability differences. Moreover, given the similarities between mouse and human auditory systems and mouse and human genomes, such findings may provide important clues to human NIHL susceptibility.[47]

Age-at-Exposure. There has long been general agreement that a period of heightened sensitivity to insult from noise or ototoxic drugs exists during and even beyond the period of obvious structural and functional maturation of the cochlea.[48] Elimination of genetic variation, however, uncovers dramatic effects of age-at-exposure on vulnerability to noise; effects that do not asymptote until young adulthood.[33,49] This vulnerability cannot be explained by differences in baseline sensitivity, nor can they be accounted for by differences in transfer through the middle ear.[50] Additional work will be required to identify mechanisms contributing to these NIHL vulnerability shifts with age.

Efferent Influences. The olivocochlear (OC) system of neurons comprises a descending system that originates in the brainstem superior olivary complex and projects to the cochlea where it directly or indirectly shapes responsiveness. Based on observations that OC activation can control the OHC-based cochlear amplifier to make the cochlea less sensitive, 1 proposed role for the efferents is that they may protect the inner ear from damage due to high-level sound.[51] In support, NIHL, whether assayed acutely or chronically, is greater in ears in which OC pathways have been sectioned, their actions blocked pharmacologically, or in mouse models in which the receptors mediating these OC effects have been genetically disabled. Such experimental manipulations continue to provide important clues regarding the relative contributions of medial OC versus lateral OC neurons to the protection and the mechanisms by which they exert their protective influence.[52]

Individual differences in the magnitude of this efferent-mediated protection may contribute to NIHL variability. Investigators have shown, using a DPOAE-based assay of efferent response strength, that reflex strength in noise-exposed guinea pigs was inversely correlated with the degree of hearing loss after subsequent noise exposure.[53] These data suggest that the well-known distinction between "tough' and "tender" ears may arise, at least in part, from differences in OC reflex strength. Since OC reflexes can be assayed noninvasively using otoacoustic emissions (OAEs), a screen for NIHL vulnerability may be possible for human application.

EVALUATION AND MANAGEMENT OF NIHL IN HUMANS

Behavioral thresholds for pure tones are the most commonly employed metric for assaying the effects of noise on hearing in clinical and occupational settings. Pure-tone threshold audiometry has served as the standard assay of hearing sensitivity in humans for many decades. Measurement protocols are standardized and validated. Such measurements form the basis of population sensitivity norms against which individual sensitivity can be assessed. Moreover, NIHL risk models, upon which every existing noise exposure standard is based, utilize audiometric data.

The Audiometric "Noise Notch"

Probably the most clearly recognizable audiometric pattern of permanent hearing loss is that commonly seen in human ears with a history of noise exposure. The pattern takes the form of a notched reduction in sensitivity which reaches a maximum between 3,000 and 6,000 Hz. Hearing may be quite normal at lower test frequencies and often demonstrates substantial recovery at 8 kHz[54] (Figure 5). There can be substantial variation in the specifics of this configuration; in a given ear, it is influenced by the many variables already discussed, as well as any other pathology that might be present.

Several explanations have been offered for the noise-notch hearing loss configuration. Noises to which human ears are often exposed are broadband signals. These signals are shaped (some frequencies amplified, others filtered out) by passage through the external and middle ears.[55] Vulnerabilities of cochlear regions stimulated by these signals, and even frequency-dependent attenuation of those noises that may activate the acoustic reflex, also have been cited as contributing to the observed hearing loss pattern in human ears. Reports of different frequency foci for noise-induced threshold shifts usually can be traced to differences in the frequency composition of the exposure or differences in the system through which the noise has passed.

No universally accepted metric for NIHL exists; however, the 3 to 6 kHz notch is so often seen in noise-exposed ears that it has been taken as a proxy measure for noise-exposure history.[56,57] Specifics of its use in this manner are controversial and are problematic for those tasked with assigning cause and determining compensation for individual cases of NIHL. The general observation, particularly if accompanied by a reported noise-exposure history in work and/or recreational activities, nevertheless has broad clinical utility in the differential diagnosis of NIHL from other causes, for example those with genetic, ototoxic, and age-related underpinnings. Several methods have been proposed to aid identification and quantification of these so-called noise notches.[56,58]

Are OAEs a More Sensitive Indicator?

To increase sensitivity to subtle changes in function, particularly those occurring early for a given individual exposed to noise, some investigators and clinicians have turned to OAEs. OAEs are sensitive and objective measures of cochlear function, and their sensitivity to noise-induced OHC compromise, in particular, makes them a

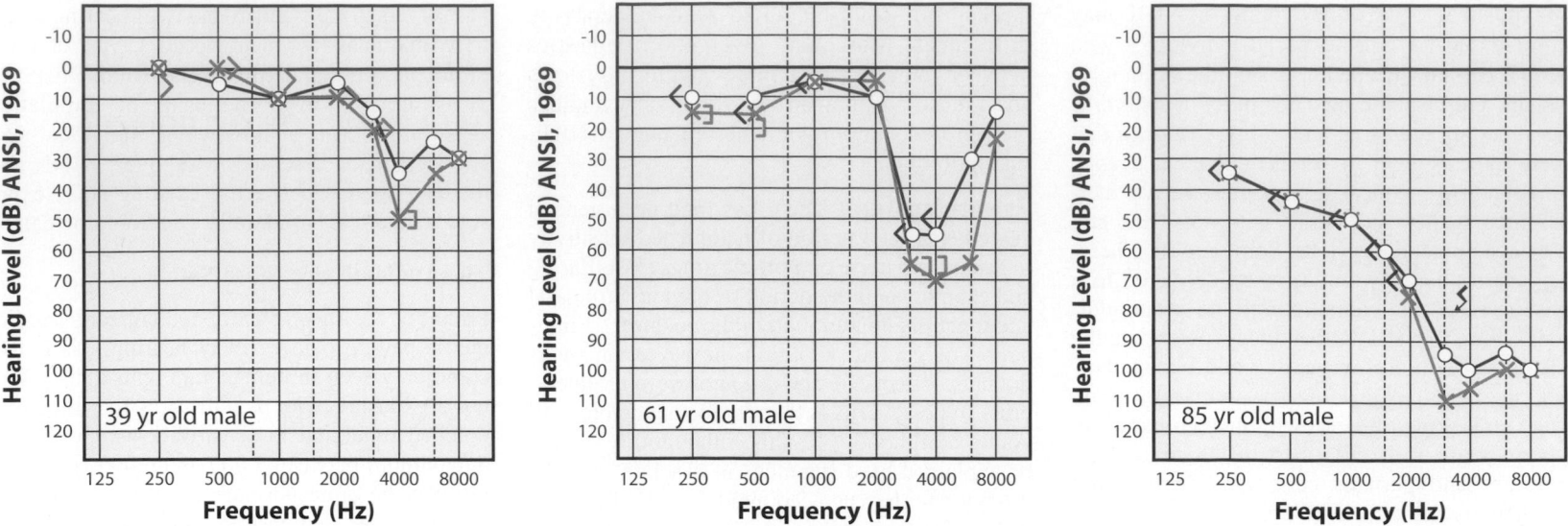

Figure 5 Audiometric pure tone thresholds recorded for three males with history of noise exposure. Shown in each panel is the commonly observed notched reduction in sensitivity, maximum in the region of 3 to 6 kHz. The panel on the right provides an example of the common coexistence of age-related and noise-induced loss in the same ear and the challenges presented by their separation.

potentially good candidate for monitoring early effects of noise exposure of OHCs. Indeed, several investigations have presented evidence that OAEs may demonstrate noise-induced shifts earlier than conventional pure tone thresholds.[59] The potential for OAEs to provide early warning of cochlear insult suggests that these noninvasively recorded responses may be of value in hearing conservation efforts.

Delayed Consequences of Noise Exposure

Once an ear has been compromised by noise, a question with significant clinical and public health importance is whether the insult influences future changes in hearing; for example, those that accrue with age. In the human, NIHL and AHL often coexist in the same ear, and current clinical and medical–legal evaluations often require allocation of noise-induced versus age-related components of such aggregate hearing losses.[60] Methods commonly used to aid such allocations treat these components as though they add independently (allowing some compression for large shifts) in their contribution to the aggregate hearing loss.[61–63] Work by Miller and colleagues appears to support this notion, showing asymptote of threshold shifts between several weeks and several months postexposure[6] (see Figure 1). If original noise-induced shifts remain stable, age-related changes would be expected to add to the preexisting hearing loss. Few animal studies, however, have followed the NIHL for extended postexposure times, that is, spanning time windows over which AHL sets in.

Two recent studies in aging humans challenge the view that NIHL and AHL are independent, suggesting, rather, that prior NIHL exacerbates subsequent AHL.[56,64] In the Gates study, males with audiometric configurations suggesting prior noise exposure (stereotypic 3 to 6 kHz noise notch) showed ongoing, 15-year threshold shifts with age that were smaller in the region of the original noise notch (presumably related to large

preexisting hearing loss and cochlear damage) but were greater in frequency regions below the notch than males without notches. This finding was confirmed in an analysis of the annual decline of pure-tone thresholds in aging men with, versus without, reported histories of occupational noise exposure. In contrast, a recent longitudinal study, threshold shifts over 3- to 11.5-year time spans were not significantly different for individuals with and without reported histories of noise exposure.[65] Thus, although there is general agreement that AHL often includes a component that can be attributed to noise exposure, characterizing NIHL–AHL relationships in humans has proven difficult.

Recent work in a low-variance mouse model[33] has tested the issue directly and provided support for the notion that there can be significant, delayed effects of noise exposure. In these studies, prior exposure set in motion a slow cascade of events leading to an exaggerated AHL and dramatic primary neuronal degeneration when followed to old age. Such findings may have significance in the consideration of noise risk assessment for human populations.

Beyond Sensitivity Loss

Depending on the magnitude of the hearing loss, its distribution in the frequency domain, and the degree and nature of the underlying histopathology, effects on auditory performance can range from subtle to profound. Audiometric threshold changes that have been the focus of discussion here clearly have downstream consequences that can impair performance on suprathreshold listening tasks like listening to speech. Pure-tone audiograms are imperfect reflections of these performance limits.[66] Comprehensive management of the individual with significant NIHL thus should include a more comprehensive assessment of the functional consequences of their sensitivity loss to provide appropriate treatment recommendations.

OCCUPATIONAL NOISE EXPOSURE

A major source of noise exposure for many individuals is in connection with work-related activities, and substantial effort has gone into development and implementation of regulations designed to protect workers from exposure to hazardous levels of noise.

Permissible Exposure Limits

Models relating exposure level and duration to risk of NIHL have been in place for many years,[67] and have been incorporated into existing models developed to predict NIHL.[68] The current 8-hour steady-state noise exposure standard used in many industrial settings uses a value of 90 dBA, measured at the location of the unprotected ear of the exposed individual.[69] Some agencies, however, have adopted a more stringent 85 dBA, 8-hour TWA.[70] How do such maximum allowable exposures relate to those of different durations or levels? Commonly, exchange rates [5 dB (OSHA), 3 dB (NIOSH)] are employed to describe trading relationships between exposure level and time predicted to yield equivalent noise dose and hazard. Thus, using OSHA's 5-dB exchange rate, a 90-dBA exposure is allowed for 8 hours; for 95 dBA, exposure time must be reduced to 4 hours, with continued halving of duration such that a 115-dBA exposure is allowed for only 15 minutes. A recent review of findings in humans[5] reports that safety data support the use of the more stringent 85 dBA 8-hour exposure limit and 3 dB exchange rate, concluding that chronic exposure (8 h/d, 40-hour work week, for years) to noises exceeding this 85 dBA TWA pose significant risk to human hearing, with risk of NIHL increasing as the TWA increases beyond this value.

Exposure Estimation

Noise exposures traditionally have been assessed using a full-shift TWA assigned to a particular job title or work group. This approach can reasonably be used in steady-state, continuous noise environments for stable groups of workers but is not particularly useful for intermittent and variable noise exposures and nonconstant work tasks and workers. Thus, task-based exposure assessment strategies have been employed in certain industries, for example, construction. Task-based methods have distinct advantages over full-shift methods in that they can target measurements on those tasks with the greatest exposure level or variability and allow for exposure level estimation for a whole range of task combinations and exposure durations. Error using such task-based estimates is largely due to high variability in noise levels between individuals doing the same task or between tasks conducted in different circumstances by the same individual.[71]

Exposure estimation can be particularly challenging among groups in which the use and attenuation of hearing protection devices (HPDs) is variable. Among 44 construction workers utilizing foam insert earplugs, the mean attenuation was 20 ± 10 dB, demonstrating a wide range of HPD effectiveness as applied by these individuals. Furthermore, among 557 construction work shifts assessed for noise exposure and simultaneous HPD use, the mean percent of time HPDs were used during exposures above 85 dBA was only 17.1% (range, 0 to 100%; SD of 34.9%), again demonstrating large variability in use time among construction workers. The variability in personal HPD attenuation and time of use contributes substantially to error in assigning individual exposures[72] and, of course, to protective benefit received from such devices, as will be discussed later.

Recreational Sources of Exposure

There is little disagreement that the potential exists for nonoccupational exposures to cause NIHL. Some have argued that a growing prevalence of such exposures may contribute to the apparent overall NIHL prevalence stability and even growth in the face of significant regulation of exposure on the job.[73] NIHL has been reported in a significant proportion of young children not receiving occupational exposures.[57] Such concerns have been heightened in recent years as personal stereo systems have become more or less permanently attached to the ears of their wearers. Putting such concerns in perspective, however, Rabinowitz and colleagues found no evidence for increased hearing loss prevalence in a large group of young adults over a two-decade period.[74]

Nevertheless, there are many potentially dangerous sources of exposure for individuals of all ages.[75] Other work has investigated whether such nonoccupational exposures add materially to risk of NIHL for occupationally noise-exposed workers.[76,77] In general, reports suggest that nonoccupational sources represent high noise levels for some individuals, but they often account for little total exposure time. Such findings were recently supported by studies of Neitzel and coworkers for noise-exposed workers in various construction trades.[73,78] They concluded that, for most workers, little additional risk is incurred from nonoccupational exposures, as these constitute a small proportion of the noise exposures they receive.

HEARING CONSERVATION AND EDUCATION

Prudent safety practices, bolstered by government regulations in some settings, have fostered the implementation of hearing conservation programs to protect the hearing of workers at risk for NIHL. Such programs include provisions for noise-level surveys, engineering and administrative controls to reduce high-level sound at its sources (equipment) and to limit exposure time of individuals to high-level sound, training and use of personal HPDs, and hearing monitoring through serial audiometry. Currently, OSHA regulations require the establishment of such hearing conservation programs in settings where noise levels exceed 85 dBA. In most settings, efforts have concentrated on regular audiometric screening and on use of HPDs.

Education on dangers and sources of hazardous noise should be an integral part of any hearing conservation program and should be widely available to the general public. Signs and symptoms of overexposure should be described, the usually gradually progressive and insidious nature of the accompanying hearing loss emphasized, and the permanent and significant consequences of noise damage made clear. Although use of HPDs would significantly reduce NIHL risk both on and off the job, it is clear that, in practice, there are many barriers that limit their effectiveness. Training in effective and consistent use of HPDs should be an integral part of any hearing conservation effort. Noise reduction ratings can be employed to help guide choices; ultimately, however, the most effective HPDs are those that will be consistently and correctly worn.

Efforts to make such messages widely available have been aided in recent years by electronic (web-based) information, sponsored by various governmental, professional, and concerned private entities. Such media also provide a means to assay the public's knowledge and behavior regarding NIHL. Unfortunately, recent work suggests that awareness of the hazard by some who may be at significant risk is low.[79] Responses to a web-based survey of attitudes and knowledge regarding NIHL from exposure to loud music revealed that, while a majority of those responding had experienced tinnitus and hearing loss following exposure to loud music, most expressed little concern. Most also indicated that education on the risks of NIHL from loud music could motivate them to protect their ears. Web-based educational tools may be an effective avenue for transmitting such information.

TREATMENTS ON THE HORIZON

Currently, hearing aids are the most common form of treatment used in the management of the permanent sensorineural hearing loss that arises secondary to noise exposure. Many individuals can realize significant benefit from such devices. There are others, however, for whom benefit from hearing aids is limited. Moreover, such treatment cannot address hearing loss prevention or minimize hearing loss progression. Even with optimal device fitting, they cannot increase a damaged ear's basic capacity.

Recent advances in the pharmacology and molecular biology of hearing are paving the way for new and powerful possibilities for preventing or minimizing hearing loss. In the future, drug treatments arising from these discoveries may be used to minimize damage to cellular constituents from postexposure processes that lead to their demise, or they may be used to promote the regrowth or replacement of cells lost to compromise from any number of inner ear insults, including noise exposure.

Work in animal models is progressing. Compounds have been identified that target several cellular processes associated with noise-induced damage, and certain of these compounds have demonstrated promise in protecting against the threshold shifts and cochlear damage that can result from exposure.

REFERENCES

1. WHO. Fact sheet: Deafness and hearing impairment, 2007. WHO Media Center. http://www.who.int/mediacentre/factsheets/fs300/en/index.html
2. NIDCD. National Institute on Deafness and other Communication Disorders: Fact sheet - noise- induced hearing loss. NIH Pub. No. 97–4233, April; 1999.
3. Nelson DI, Nelson RY, Concha-Barrientos M, Fingerhut M. The global burden of occupational noise-induced hearing loss. Am J Indus Med 2005;48:446–58.
4. Daniell WE, Fulton-Kehoe D, Cohen M, et al. Increased reporting of occupational hearing loss: Workers' compensation in Washington State. 1984–1998. Am J Indus Med 2002;42:502–10.
5. Humes LE. Noise and military service: Implications for hearing loss and tinnitus In: Humes LE, Joellenbeck LM, Durch JS, editors. Committee on Noise-Induced Hearing Loss and Tinnitus Associated with Military Service from World War II to the Present Medical Follow-up Agency. Washington, DC: The National Academies Press; 2006.
6. Miller JD, Watson CS, Covell WP. Deafening effects of noise on the cat. Acta Otolaryngol Suppl 1963;176:1–91.
7. Yoshida N, Hequembourg SJ, Atencio CA, et al. Acoustic injury in mice: 129/SvEv is exceptionally resistant to noise-induced hearing loss. Hear Res 2000;141:97–106.
8. Ruggero MA, Rich NC, Recio A. The effect of intense stimulation on basilar-membrane vibration. Aud Neurosci 1996;2:329–45.
9. Lonsbury-Martin BL, Meikle MB. Neural correlates of auditory fatigue. Frequency dependent changes in activity of single cochlear nerve fibers. J Neurophysiol 1978;41:987–1006.
10. Cody AR, Johnstone BM. Acoustic trauma: Single neuron basis for the "half-octave shift." J Acoust Soc Am 1981;70:707–11.
11. Davis H, Morgan, CT, Hawkins JE, et al. Temporary deafness following exposure to loud tones and noise. Acta Otolaryngol Suppl 1950;88:4–57.

12. Johnsson LG, Hawkins JE, Jr. Degeneration patterns in human ears exposed to noise. Ann Otol Rhinol Laryngol 1976;85:725–39.

13. Nordmann AS, Bohne BA, Harding GW. Histopathological differences between temporary and permanent threshold shift. Hear Res 2000;139:13–30.

14. Fried MP, Dudek SE, Bohne BA. Basal turn cochlear lesions following exposure to low-frequency noise. Trans Am Acad Opthalmol Otolaryngol 1976;82:285–98.

15. Saunders JC, Dear SP, Schneider ME. The anatomical consequences of acoustic injury: A review and tutorial. J Acoust Soc Am 1985;78:833–60.

16. Wang Y, Hirose K, Liberman MC. Dynamics of noise-induced cellular injury and repair in the mouse cochlea. J Assoc Res Otolaryngol 2002;3:248–68.

17. Melnick W. Human temporary threshold shift (TTS) and damage risk. J Acoust Soc Am 1991;90:147–54.

18. Mulroy MJ, Whaley EA. Structural changes in auditory hairs during temporary deafness. Scan Electron Micros 1984;11:831–40.

19. Liberman MC, Dodds LW. Acute ultrastructural changes in acoustic trauma: Serial-section reconstruction of stereocilia and cuticular plates. Hear Res 1987;26:45–64.

20. Pickles JO, Osborne MP, Comis SD. Vulnerability of tip links between stereocilia to acoustic trauma in the guinea pig. Hear Res 1987;25:173–83.

21. Liberman MC, Dodds LW. Single-neuron labeling and chronic cochlear pathology III. Stereocilia damage and alterations of threshold tuning curves. Hear Res 1984;16:55–74.

22. Pujol R, Puel JL. Excitotoxicity, synaptic repair and functional recovery in the mammalian cochlea: A review of recent findings. Ann N Y Acad Sci 1999;884:249–54.

23. Puel JL, d'Aldin C, Ruel J, et al. Synaptic repair mechanisms responsible for functional recovery in various cochlear pathologies. Acta Otolaryngol 1997;117:214–8.

24. Santi PA, Duvall AJ. Stria vascularis pathology and recovery following noise exposure. ORL J Otorhinolaryngol Relat Spec 1978;86:354–61.

25. Liberman MC, Kiang NY-S. Acoustic trauma in cats, cochlear pathology and auditory-nerve activity. Acta Otolaryngol 1978;358:5–63.

26. Schulte BA, Schmiedt RA. Lateral wall Na, K-ATPase and endocochlear potentials decline with age in quiet-reared gerbils. Hear Res 1992;61:35–46.

27. Hirose K, Liberman MC. Lateral wall histopathology and endocochlear potential in the noise-damaged mouse cochlea. J Assoc Res Otolaryngol 2003;4:339–52.

28. Flock A, Flock B, Fridberger A, et al. Supporting cells contribute to control of hearing sensitivity. J Neurosci 1999;19:4498–4507.

29. Raphael Y, Altschuler RA. Reorganization of cytoskeletal and junctional proteins during cochlear hair cell degeneration. Cell Motil Cytoskeleton 1991;18:215–27.

30. McGill TJ, Schuknecht HF. Human cochlear changes in noise induced hearing loss. Laryngoscope 1976;86:1293–1302.

31. Robertson D, Johnstone BM. Acoustic trauma in the guinea pig cochlea: Early changes in ultrastructure and neural threshold. Hear Res 1980;3:167–79.

32. Bohne BA, Harding GW. Degeneration in the cochlea after noise damage: Primary versus secondary events. Am J Otol 2000;21:505–9.

33. Kujawa SG, Liberman MC. Acceleration of age-related hearing loss by early noise exposure: Evidence of a misspent youth. J Neurosci 2006;26:2115–23.

34. Spicer SS, Schulte BA. The fine structure of spiral ligament cells relates to ion return to the stria and varies with place-frequency. Hear Res 1996;100:80–100.

35. Qiu W, Hamernik RP, Davis B. The kurtosis metric as an adjunct to energy in the prediction of trauma from continuous, nonGaussian noise exposures. J Acoust Soc Am 2006;120:3901–3906.

36. Borg E, Canlon B, Engstrom B. Noise-induced hearing loss. Literature review and experiments in rabbits. Morphological and electrophysiological features, exposure parameters and temporal factors, variability and interactions. Scand Audiol Suppl 1995;40:1–147.

37. Henderson D, Hamernik RP. Impulse noise: Critical review. J Acoust Soc Am 1986;80:569–84.

38. Canlon B. Protection against noise trauma by pre-exposure to a low level acoustic stimulus. Hear Res 1988;34:197–200.

39. Kujawa SG, Liberman MC. Conditioning-related protection from acoustic injury: Effects of chronic deefferentation and sham surgery. J Neurophysiol 1997;78:3095–3106.

40. Clark WW, Bohne BA, Boettcher FA. Effect of periodic rest on hearing loss and cochlear damage following exposure to noise. J Acoust Soc Am 1987;82:1253–64.

41. Boettcher FA, Spongr VP, Salvi RJ. Physiological and histological changes associated with the reduction in threshold shift during interrupted noise exposure. Hear Res 1992;62:217–36.

42. Fechter LD. Promotion of noise-induced hearing loss by chemical contaminants. J Toxicol Environ Health Part A 2004;67:727–40.

43. Henderson D, Subramaniam M, Boettcher FA. Individual susceptibility to noise-induced hearing loss: An old topic revisited. Ear Hear 1993;14:152–68.

44. Cody AR, Robertson D. Variability of noise-induced damage in the guinea pig cochlea: Electrophysiological and morphological correlates after strictly controlled exposures. Hear Res 1983;9:55–70.

45. Candreia C, Martin GK, Stagner BB, Lonsbury-Martin BL. Distortion product otoacoustic emissions show exceptional resistance to noise exposure in MOLF/Ei mice. Hear Res 2004;194:109–17.

46. Davis RR, Kozel P, Erway LC. Genetic influences in individual susceptibility to noise: A review. Noise Health 2003;5:19–28.

47. Van Laer L, Carlsson PI, Ottschytsch N, et al. The contribution of genes involved in potassium-recycling in the inner ear to noise-induced hearing loss. Hum Mutat 2006;27:786–95.

48. Bock GR, Saunders JC. A critical period for acoustic trauma in the hamster and its relation to cochlear development. Science 1977;197:396–8.

49. Henry KR. Lifelong susceptibility to acoustic trauma: Changing patterns of cochlear damage over the life span of the mouse. Audiology 1983;22:372–83.

50. Rosowski JJ, Brinsko KM, Tempel BL, Kujawa SG. The aging of the middle ear in 129S6/SvEvTac and CBA/CaJ mice: Measurements of umbo velocity, hearing function, and the incidence of pathology. J Assoc Res Otolaryngol 2003;4:371–83.

51. Reiter ER, Liberman MC. Efferent-mediated protection from acoustic overexposure: Relation to slow effects of olivocochlear stimulation. J Neurophysiol 1995;73:506–14.

52. Darrow KN, Maison SF, Liberman MC. Selective removal of lateral olivocochlear efferents increases vulnerability to acute acoustic injury. J Neurophysiol 2007;97:1775–85.

53. Maison SF, Liberman MC. Predicting vulnerability to acoustic injury with a noninvasive assay of olivocochlear reflex strength. J Neurosci 2000;20:4701–7.

54. Cooper JC, Owen JH. Audiologic profile of noise-induced hearing loss. Arch Otolaryngol 1976;102:148–50.

55. Rosowski JJ. The effects of external- and middle-ear filtering on auditory threshold and noise-induced hearing loss. J Acoust Soc Am 1991;90:124–35.

56. Gates GA, Schmid P, Kujawa SG, et al. Longitudinal threshold changes in older men with audiometric notches. Hear Res 2000;141:220–8.

57. Niskar AS, Kieszak SM, Holmes AE, et al. Estimated prevalence of noise-induced hearing threshold shifts among children 6 to 19 years of age: The third national health and nutrition examination survey, 1988–1994. Pediatrics 1991;108:40–3.

58. Rabinowitz PM, Galusha D, Slade MD, et al. Audiogram notches in noise-exposed workers. Ear Hear 2006;27:742–50.

59. Lapsley Miller JA, Marshall L, Heller LM, Hughes LM. Low-level otoacoustic emissions may predict susceptibility to noise-induced hearing loss. J Acoust Soc Am 2006;120:280–96.

60. Dobie RA. The relative contributions of occupational noise and aging in individual cases of hearing loss. Ear Hear 1992;13:19–27.

61. ISO. Acoustics-determination of occupational noise exposure and estimation of noise-induced hearing impairment. Geneva: International Organization for Standardization, ISO, 1990; 1999.

62. Mills JH, Boettcher FA, Dubno JR. Interaction of noise-induced permanent threshold shift and age-related threshold shift. J Acoust Soc Am 1997;101:1681–6.

63. ACOM. Occupational noise-induced hearing loss. J Occup Med 1989;31:996–1001.

64. Rosenhall U. The influence of ageing on noise-induced hearing loss. Noise Health 2003;5:47–53.

65. Lee FS, Matthews LJ, Dubno JR, Mills JH. Longitudinal study of pure-tone thresholds in older persons. Ear Hear 2005;26:1–11.

66. Halpin C. The tuning curve in clinical audiology. Am J Audiol 2002;11:56–64.

67. Passchier-Vermeer W. Hearing loss due to continuous exposure to steady-state broad-band noise. J Acoust Soc Am 1974;56:1585–93.

68. ANSI. Determination of occupational noise exposure and estimation of noise-induced hearing impairment. New York, NY: American National Standards Institute, Inc. 1996; Report No.: S3.44–1996.

69. OSHA. Occupational Noise Exposure: Hearing Conservation Amendment. Final Rule. 29 C.F.R. 1910.95. Federal Register 1983;48:9738–85.

70. NIOSH. Criteria for a recommended standard: Occupational noise exposure. NIOSH Publication No. 98–126; 1998.

71. Seixas NS, Sheppard L, Neitzel R. Comparison of task-based estimates with full-shift measurements of noise exposure. AIHA J 2003;64:823–9.

72. Neitzel R, Seixas N. The effectiveness of hearing protection among construction workers. J Occup Environ Hyg 2005;2:227–38.

73. Neitzel R, Seixas N, Goldman B, Daniel W. Contributions of non-occupational activities to total noise exposure of construction workers. Ann Occup Hyg 2004;48:463–73.

74. Rabinowitz PM, Slade MD, Galusha D, et al. Trends in the prevalence of hearing loss among young adults entering an industrial workforce 1985 to 2004. Ear Hear 2006;27:369–75.

75. Clark W. Noise exposure from leisure activities: A review. J Acoust Soc Am 1991;90:171–81.

76. Johnson DL, Farina ER. Description of the measurement of an individual's continuous sound exposure during a 31-day period J Acoust Soc Am 1977;62:1431–5.

77. Schori T, McGatha E. A real-world assessment of noise exposure Sound Vib. 1978;12:24–30.

78. Neitzel R, Seixas N, Olson, J, et al. Nonoccupational noise: Exposures associated with routine activities. J Acoust Soc Am 2004;115:237–45.

79. Chung JH, Des Roches CM, Meunier J, Eavey RD. Evaluation of noise-induced hearing loss in young people using a web-based survey technique. Pediatrics 2005;115:861–7.

23

Ototoxicity

Peter S. Roland, MD
Karen S. Pawlowski, PhD

Ototoxicity can be broadly defined as damage of the inner ear by a toxin. The damage can occur in the cochlea, vestibular apparatus, and/or auditory nerve, and the toxin can be any number of substances. The most commonly used ototoxic substances are drugs administered to treat potentially life-threatening conditions where other treatment options have failed or are unavailable. Some of these ototoxic substances do not become ototoxic unless other conditions are present at time of administration, which predisposes the patient to the ototoxicity. Risk factors associated with potentially ototoxic substances have been identified and will be discussed in this chapter, along with monitoring practices designed to minimize the ototoxic effect during drug administration and improve patient outcome once ototoxicity has been detected. This chapter will cover effects of systemically and topically applied drugs that have been shown to induce ototoxicity.

SYSTEMICALLY INDUCED OTOTOXICITY

Both auditory and vestibular symptoms can occur in ototoxicity. The symptoms of cochlear ototoxicity from systemic administration typically include bilateral hearing loss and tinnitus (the sensation of sound when none is present). Vestibular ototoxicity causes a loss of the sense of balance, dizziness, lightheadedness, faintness, unsteadiness, and/or nystagmus. The symptoms can be temporary, subsiding after the ototoxic substance has been cleared from the body, or they can be permanent.

When hearing loss from ototoxicity becomes permanent, the first detectable symptom is increased auditory thresholds for high frequency sounds. This change is often unnoticed by the patient until lower frequencies become involved. Although not always the case, the outer hair cells of the organ of Corti are commonly the first cells that exhibit signs of intoxication. Early outer hair cell loss can be demonstrated morphologically in both human tissue and animal models. Injury ranges from damaged stereocilia on the surface of the hair cell to complete loss of the hair cell with only supporting cells remaining (Figure 1). Severe damage includes inner hair cell loss with associated loss of spiral ganglion cells (Figures 2 and 3). In electrophysiological

studies, damage first manifests as a reduction in evoked otoacoustic emissions (OAEs), compound action potentials (CAPs), and/or auditory brainstem responses (ABR). The reduction is typically first seen in high frequency responses. Although not typical, in some cases of cochlear ototoxicity, such as that occurring after carboplatin

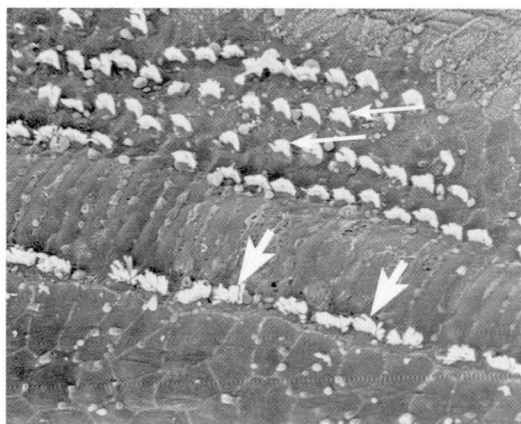

(A)

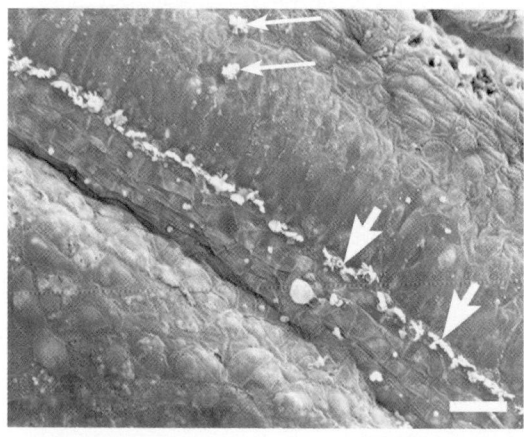

(B)

Figure 1 Scanning electron micrographs of the organ of Corti from an adult human after cisplatin administration. Comparatively normal organ of Corti is seen in the mid cochlear region (A) with three to four rows of outer hair cell stereocilia (*thin arrows*) and a fairly complete row of inner hair cell stereocilia (*thick arrows*). As with most cases of cochlear ototoxicity, damage is first seen in the basal region of the organ of Corti (B). Typically with mild or acute cochlear ototoxicity, damage is limited to the outer hair cell region. Only a few bundles of outer hair cell stereocilia (*thin arrows*) remain in this region. Yet, the row of inner hair cell stereocilia in this region remains fairly intact (*thick arrows*). Calibration bar = 10 μm. (Published with permission, copyright © 2007, C.G. Wright.)

administration, degeneration begins within the inner hair cells. Carboplatin adversely affects the central and peripheral nervous systems and may

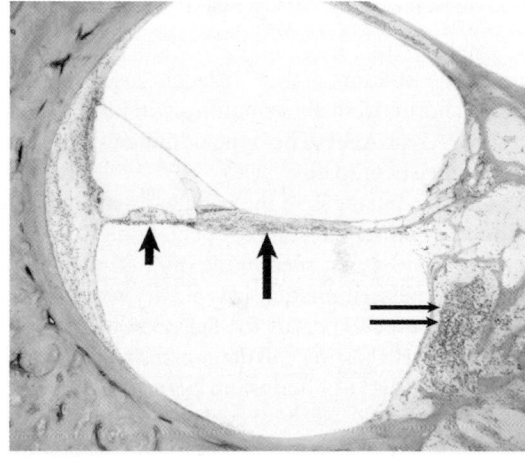

(A)

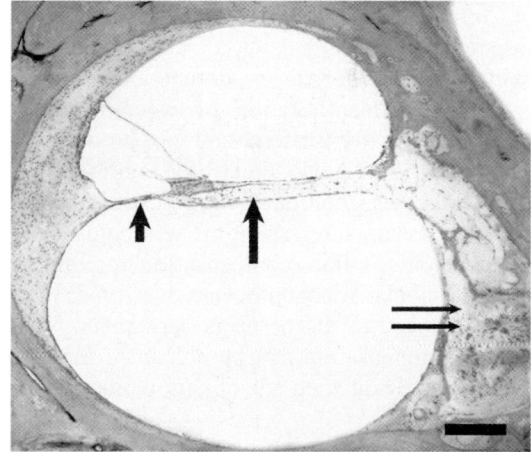

(B)

Figure 2 Temporal bone horizontal sections from the upper basal turn of the cochlear duct of two adult humans. (A) A cross section from a 60-year-old diabetic individual. The organ of Corti (*short thick arrow*), nerve fibers in the osseous spiral lamina (*long thick arrow*), and cell bodies of the spiral ganglion within Rosenthal canal (*double arrow*) appear intact. (B) A section demonstrating changes often seen after chronic or severe ototoxicity in a 67-year-old individual who suffered from chronic alcohol intoxication. The organ of Corti in this region of the cochlea has degenerated to a single row of cuboidal cells, no longer recognizable as organ of Corti tissue (*short thick arrow*). Few nerve fibers remain in the osseous spiral lamina (*long thick arrow*), and few spiral ganglion cell bodies remain within Rosenthal canal (*double arrow*). Calibration bar = 0.5 mm.

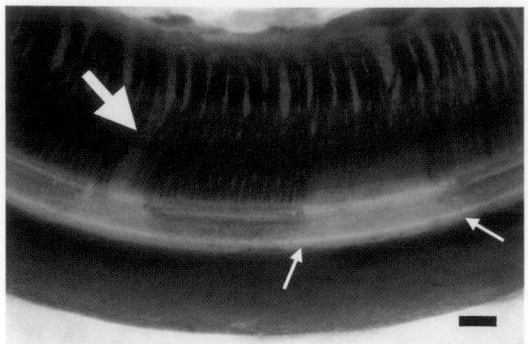

Figure 3 Light microscopic view of an osmium tetroxide stained surface preparation from an adult who had been administered cisplatin. The mid-basal portion of the organ of Corti and osseous spiral lamina is represented here. Ototoxicity can be seen as patchy losses of organ of Corti structures (*between small arrows*) and in some areas (*large arrow*) a corresponding loss of myelinated nerve fibers. Calibration bar = 40 μm. (Published with permission, copyright © 2007, C.G. Wright.)

injure the auditory nerve. In such cases, OAEs may be normal, but abnormalities will be detected in the CAP or ABR. This type of deficit is known as auditory neuropathy.

Ototoxic changes in the cochlear nerve or the auditory brainstem resemble cochlear ototoxicity, ie, hearing loss first seen in the high frequencies, but speech discrimination is typically worse than what would be expected for the level of hearing loss. The ABR testing can demonstrate damage to the auditory nerve or brainstem by increased latencies of later peaks, as these peaks are generated by the auditory nerve or brainstem nuclei. The body can only compensate for the mildest forms of hearing loss, in which only a small region of the organ of Corti is affected. More severe forms of hearing loss require hearing aids or cochlear implants to help compensate for the loss of function.

Vestibular manifestations of systemic ototoxicity are typically bilateral and can be detected with caloric testing, electronystagmography (ENG), or via rotational chair testing, all of which assess the integrity of the vestibulo-ocular reflex (VOR). Often, compensation for loss of some vestibular function occurs over time, even if the damage to the tissue is permanent. Vestibular compensation can be enhanced through professionally directed rehabilitation programs.

Temporary Ototoxicity

Many ototoxic drugs typically cause only temporary hearing loss, known as "temporary threshold shift" (TTS). Other temporary affects can include tinnitus or vertigo. These effects may occur as a direct consequence of the drug's effects on the sensory organ or on other components of the inner ear that are required for organ function. For instance, loop-inhibiting diuretics have been shown to cause temporary cochlear dysfunction.[1] In this type of ototoxicity either the "stiffness" of outer hair cells is affected, directly affecting the organ of Corti; or the stria vascularis is affected, resulting in strial edema, loss of endolymphatic potassium and a corresponding reduction in endocochlear potential. The reduc-

tion in endolymphatic potassium concentrations and the endocochlear potential leads to a loss of transduction in the organ of Corti. Whether the effect occurs at the outer hair cell or the stria vascularis, the result is an elevation of auditory thresholds. Under normal circumstances, once the loop-inhibiting diuretic clears the blood stream, normal thresholds are restored.

Substances that cause temporary ototoxicity are often used to treat serious disease. Therefore they are administered to fairly ill patients with multiple medical problems in whom an otherwise temporary ototoxic effect may become permanent. For example, loop-inhibiting diuretics are administered to patients with renal insufficiency.[2] This leads to an increase in the blood levels of the drug beyond the threshold for permanent ototoxicity.

Combining administration of multiple drugs, which when administered individually and at low concentrations are nontoxic, can also result in permanent ototoxicity. For example, when low doses of aminoglycoside antibiotics are administered to a patient who is also receiving loop-inhibiting diuretics, the ototoxic effects are synergistic. Patient age can also be a risk factor for increased ototoxicity.[3]

TOPICAL OTOTOXICITY

Severe inner ear damage encompassing large areas of sensory cell loss, obvious neural degeneration, and significantly reduced auditory function has been repeatedly demonstrated in animals following middle ear application of commercially available otic drops.[4] Therefore, ototoxicity should be considered a possible side effect of topical drug applications to the human ear. Since these affects are local, ototoxicity due to topical agents is limited to the side of application. The symptoms of cochlear topical ototoxicity (hearing loss) are similar to those seen in systemic cochlear ototoxicity but are limited to the treated ear. Unilateral hearing loss has less severe consequences than bilateral hearing loss because only one ear is needed for adequate function in most hearing conditions. Conversely, manifestations of vestibular ototoxicity may be more severe after unilateral topical application because the injury to the vestibular system is asymmetric. Normal vestibular function relies on symmetrical input from both ears. Acute asymmetric vestibular loss is associated with significant discomfort for several days following the insult. Severe rotatory vertigo, uncommon following systemic ototoxicity (which is usually a symmetrical loss), is not unusual after unilateral injury from topical aminoglycoside treatment of the middle ear.

MONITORING FOR OTOTOXICITY

Audiologic monitoring for ototoxicity can detect changes early during administration of potentially ototoxic drugs to allow for altered treatment plans and help prevent permanent losses. The standard test battery for audiologic monitoring

include a baseline pure tone audiogram, speech discrimination testing, and OAEs.[5] Follow-up can usually be limited to pure tone air-conduction thresholds, unless there is a change in hearing threshold. In which case, repeating the test battery is recommended.

Tests for OAEs measure an involuntary response created by outer hair cell activity in the cochlea. The tests are relatively inexpensive, quick and do not rely on patient response, making them especially useful in monitoring ototoxicity in patients that are unable to provide reliable behavioral responses.[6] Monitoring OAEs can detect alterations in outer hair cell activity before the lesion is sufficiently large for detection by a standard audiogram. There are several types of OAEs, but transient evoked otoacoustic emissions (TOAEs) and distortion product otoacoustic emissions (DPOAEs) are most commonly used to monitor ototoxicity. TOAEs are occasionally used when DPOAEs cannot be obtained. TOAES have broader spectra, less frequency-specific responses than DPOAEs and, therefore, are less sensitive to small lesions along the organ of Corti. DPOAEs can often be recorded in subjects with a higher degree of hearing loss and can detect lesions at higher frequencies.

In addition to monitoring for hearing loss, vestibular monitoring should also be performed when administering potentially ototoxic medications to detect vestibulotoxicity early and allow for intervention prior to the development of irreversible injury. There are no widely accepted protocols to test for vestibulotoxicity. However, there are a number of both qualitative and quantitative tests that are commonly used to assess vestibular function. The integrity of the VOR is commonly used to detect changes in the vestibular end-organ and some central nervous system pathways.[7] There are two neural pathways involved in the VOR, the pathway from the eighth nerve to position-vestibular-pause cells (PVP) to oculomotor nuclei and the pathway from the eighth nerve to floccular target neurons (FTN) to oculomotor nuclei, with additional input to the FTN from the cerebellum.

In practice, the VOR is elicited either by caloric testing or by use of a rotational chair. For caloric testing, warm and cool liquids or air are placed into the external ear canal to cause unequal heating/cooling of the inner ear, which results in bulk fluid movement within the vestibular system, triggering the VOR. Rotational chair testing uses a more "natural" stimulus with a range of quantifiable stimuli (rotational speed) that results in a quantifiable result. The VOR response can be elicited at several different physiological rotational frequencies. The response for each rotational frequency can be quantified.

The ENG is a widely used test battery that includes measurement of spontaneous nystagmus, caloric testing, testing for benign positional vertigo, the ability to suppress nystagmus by visual fixation, an optokinetic test, a gaze test, a sinusoidal tracking test, and the saccade test (which tests the ability for the eye to rapidly fix and refix its point of fixation). ENG can be used to test for vestibulotoxicity.[8]

ENG testing can also be combined with computerized dynamic posturography (CDP), also known as platform posturography. CDP measures the movement of the patient's center of gravity as visual and somatosensory cues are altered.[9]

Many of these vestibular tests require that the subject be brought to a specific testing facility. In cases where this is not practical, bedside assessments can be performed. Dynamic visual acuity (DVA) testing, or oscillopsia testing, assesses the function of the VOR.[10] To perform DVA, the head is passively oscillated at a frequency of about 1 to 2 Hz during which time the subject is asked to read the lowest line of a Snellen eye chart at 20 ft. A drop in visual acuity of more than two lines suggests a significant bilateral vestibular loss.

High frequency horizontal head thrust maneuver is done by quickly turning the subject's head while the subject is fixing on a midline target. In patients with unilateral vestibular dysfunction, this maneuver will elicit a corrective saccade toward the side with hypofunction.

Patients with unilateral vestibular lesions exhibit postheadshake nystagmus (post-HSN).[11] Post-HSN is observed immediately following vigorous horizontal headshake when visual fixation is eliminated with Frenzel glasses. Since post-HSN is an involuntary response, it is useful in discriminating between psychogenic dizziness and peripheral vestibular dysfunction.

Although clinical tests for semicircular canal function have been available for years, clinically useful tests for function of the otolith organs have been difficult to devise. The vestibular evoked myogenic potential (VEMP), is currently being developed to detect abnormal function in the saccule and/or the inferior vestibular nerve.[12] The VEMP can be evoked by loud click or tone burst. The response of the sternocleidomastoid muscle is recorded using an electrode on the skin surface covering the muscle. VEMP uses low-frequency sound to stimulate the saccule first; the response is transmitted through the vestibular nerve to the vestibular nuclei and on to the medial vestibulospinal tract and the sternocleidomastoid muscle. An absent or significantly reduced VEMP would indicate a lesion somewhere along the neural pathway between the saccule to the muscle, and other tests can be used to rule out muscle and spinal tract dysfunction.

Occasionally, toxicity affects the auditory neural components while the hair cells remain intact. This is called auditory neuropathy.[13] In these patients, a change may be noted in the basic audiologic assessment, while no change is seen in OAEs. The best test for monitoring auditory nerve ototoxic effects is the ABR. ABR measurement can be used to observe the activity of the auditory nerve and the auditory brainstem up to the inferior colliculus. Changes in ABR will also occur without changes in OAEs if the toxicity is within the inner hair cells.

OTOTOXIC DRUGS

A variety of drugs have been shown to be ototoxic (Table 1). Their mode of action and ototoxic effects differ. Below are classes of ototoxic drugs and the characteristics of specific drugs in their classification.

Salicylates

Acetylsalicylic acid (aspirin) can cause reversible ototoxicity, usually manifesting as a mild to moderate hearing loss and tinnitus.[14] Aspirin-associated hearing loss is due to reversible enzyme inhibition, and symptoms typically clear 24 to 72 hours after cessation of the drug. Permanent damage to the organ of Corti in humans is rare, but administration of 5 to 10 g/d can cause a permanent hearing loss and abolish spontaneous OAEs in animals.[15]

Nonsteroidal AntiInflammatory Agents (NSAIDS)

NSAIDs have ototoxic side effects that are similar to aspirin.[14] Examples of commonly used NSAIDs are ibuprofen, naproxen, and indomethacin.

Quinine

As is true of aspirin, hearing loss is generally temporary with quinine ototoxicity but cases of permanent hearing loss have been reported. In addition to producing hearing loss and tinnitus, quinine intoxication can result in temporary vertigo. Hearing loss from quinine administration is bilateral, initially affecting the higher frequencies, with a characteristic notch at 4 kHz. Permanent effects of quinine administration have been reported in patients receiving prolonged daily doses of 200 to 300 mg. Quinine administration is used as an initial treatment of severe *Plasmodium falciparum* malaria.[16]

Heavy Metals

Chronic lead and mercury toxicity cause little histopathologic change in the inner ear, but nonetheless produce subclinical changes in hearing, observed by slight, but significant lengthening of ABR peak latencies.[17–20] This indicates these substances have a more dramatic effect on neural processing than on the organ of Corti transduction process although some changes in hair cell function have been seen in vitro. The effects occur either within the auditory nerve (auditory neuropathy) or within the brainstem and midbrain (central auditory processing disorder).

Loop Diuretics

Ethacrynic acid, bumetanide, piretanide, azosemide, ozolinone, indacrinone, torasemide, and furosemide have all been implicated as systemic ototoxic agents.[21] These organic compounds have potent saliuretic effects on the loop of Henle in the kidney. They also exert effects on the Na^+/K^+-ATPase in the stria vascularis, reducing the endocochlear potential and the endolymphatic K^+

concentrations within the inner ear. This typically leads to a temporary auditory threshold shift that recovers as the drug is cleared from the body.[1] Under certain conditions, as in combination with even low doses of other potentially ototoxic drugs or in neonates, hearing loss from loop diuretics can be permanent. Deafness associated with ethacrynic acid therapy has been reported to occur in seven patients per 1,000 treated.[22]

Cancer Chemotherapeutic Agents: Cisplatin, Carboplatin, Iron Chelating Agents, and Vinca Alkaloids

Cisplatin ototoxicity, like the aminoglycoside antibiotics, typically causes high frequency sensorineural hearing loss in a dose-dependent manner.[23] However, unlike the aminoglycosides, cisplatin administration rarely causes vestibular dysfunction. The most susceptible cell type within the inner ear for most platinum compounds is the outer hair cell. The principal mode of action is an alteration of DNA transcription, leading to cell death through a combination of necrosis and apoptosis.

Although carboplatin is used in a manner similar to cisplatin, the most susceptible cell type within the inner ear differs.[24] Carboplatin administration can cause inner hair cell damage, leading to abnormal synaptic activity or complete inner hair cell loss, resulting in changes known as auditory neuropathy.

Vinca alkaloids are antineoplastic drugs that are often administered in combination with drugs like cisplatin. Vinca alkaloids include several drugs derived from the periwinkle plant, vincristine, vinblastine, and the semisynthetic vinorelbine. The chief mode of action for these drugs is interference with outer hair cell metabolism.[25]

Iron chelators, such as deferoxamine, are used to alleviate the affects of acute iron intoxication or chronic iron overload due to repeated transfusions. Iron chelators can cause mild to moderate high frequency sensorineural hearing loss, which is more commonly seen in younger patients and patients receiving higher dosages. In some instances, this loss has been shown to be reversible upon cessation of drug administration.

Aminoglycoside Antibiotics

Earlier studies suggest an incidence of ototoxicity from aminoglycosides of up to 41% of subjects treated, but more recent studies indicate an incidence of 5 to 7%.[26,27] This discrepancy may reflect a change in treatment protocols and a reduction in the use of the more ototoxic aminoglycosides, such as streptomycin.

There are a number of aminoglycoside antibiotics in clinical use; examples include streptomycin, dihydrostreptomycin, neomycin, tobramycin, kanamycin, gentamicin, netilmicin, and amikacin. All share common characteristics in their chemical structure and biological activity but differ in their ototoxic potential. Hair cells are the cellular target for aminoglycoside antibiotics in the ear.[28] Outer hair cells seem to be the most vulnerable to attack, but inner hair cells

Table 1   List of Common Ototoxic Substances, Type of Damage Produced, Mechanisms of Action, and Agents with Synergistic Effects

Toxin	Commonly Used Forms	Type of Damage	Mechanism of Action	Possible Synergistic Effects
Salicylates and nonsteroidal anti-inflammatory drugs	Aspirin, NSAIDs, Ibuprofen (Advil, Motrin), Naproxen (Aleve), magnesium salicylate (Doan's Pills), Celebrex	Temporary tinnitus and sensorineural hearing loss, permanent loss can occur with high doses	Increases spontaneous activity in the auditory nerve, decreases outer hair cell turgor and reduces capacitance, reduces cochlear blood flow	
Quinine	Jesuit bark	Similar to salicylates, plus vertigo	Similar to salicylates	
Heavy metals	Methyl mercury, lead	Permanent hearing loss with increased wave I-V interwave latency	Neural toxicity by inhibition of Na^+/K^+ ATPase activity	
Loop diuretics	Ethacrynic acid, furosemide, bumetinide	Temporary hearing loss across frequencies	Hair cell permeability changes and disruption of Na^+/K^+ ATPase	Aminoglycoside antibiotics, renal failure, neonates
Cancer agents	Cisplatin, carboplatin, iron chelating agents, vinc alkaloids	Permanent high frequency hearing loss, typically no vestibular symptoms	Alteration of DNA transcription in hair cells, interference with hair cell metabolism	
Aminoglycoside antibiotics	Streptomycin, dihydrostreptomycin, neomycin, tobramycin, kanamycin, gentamicin, netilmicin, amikacin	Permanent high frequency hearing loss, vestibular symptoms	Disruption of protein synthesis in hair cells	Loop diuretics, renal failure, acoustic insult, aging, vancomycin and associated drugs, inherited mitochondrial defects
Macrolide antibiotics	Erythomycin, azithromycin, clarithomycin	Temporary hearing loss, typically no tinnitus or vestibular symptoms	May have central or peripheral neural effects; shown to be toxic to hair cells and reduce endocochlear potential in animals	Age, HIV
Polymyxins, colymycin, and chloramphenicol	Polymyxin, colymycin or polymyxin E, chloramphenicol	Permanent sudden sensorineural hearing loss after systemic or topical application	Unknown for ears, but they affect bacteria by disrupting cell membrane integrity	
Vancomycin and vancomycin analogs	Vancomycin, teichoplanin, daptomycin, norvancomycin	Temporary hearing loss in most cases, permanent hearing loss occurs when administered with other potentially ototoxic drugs	Unknown	Aminoglycoside antibiotics
Antifungal medications	Azoles, clotrimazole, miconazole, nystatin, tolnaftate, gentian violet, cresylate, preparations containing propylene glycol	Permanent middle and inner ear toxicity after topical application	Unknown	
Disinfectants and antiseptics	Chlorohexidine, alcohols, iodine containing skin preparations, benzalkonium chloride	Permanent severe sensorineural hearing loss plus vestibular symptoms	Unknown	

can be affected with higher doses or with a longer period of drug treatment. Typically, these drugs affect the high frequencies first.[4,27,29,30] The drugs selectively concentrate in hair cells when present in the perilymphatic space. These drugs can be found within the inner ear minutes after systemic application, and they can remain in inner ear fluids for months after treatment.

Apoptosis appears to be the most likely pathway for cell death in aminoglycoside antibiotic ototoxicity. The antibacterial action of aminoglycoside antibiotics relies on their ability to disrupt protein synthesis within bacterial cells through binding to the cellular ribosomes (mRNA). The disruption of protein synthesis affects protein turnover and leads to cell death. In the mammalian hair cell, the most likely mode of cell death after aminoglycoside intoxication is via interference in cell metabolism, creating reactive oxygen species (ROS) free radicals that cause oxidative damage to the cell leading to apoptotic death.

Maternally Inherited Aminoglycoside-Induced Deafness. A high incidence of aminoglycoside antibiotic-induced hearing loss is especially likely in individuals with an inherited defect in their mitochondrial rRNA.[29] Unlike eukaryotic cell DNA, which is a product of both parent's DNA, mitochondrial DNA is passed directly from mother to child. Therefore, mitochondrial defects are maternally inherited. Mitochondrial rRNA closely resembles prokaryotic mRNA in structure, making them a more likely target for aminoglycoside binding than the RNA produced by the nucleus of hair cell. In patients carrying certain mitochondrial mutations (12S rRNA mutations), the structure of the mitochondrial rRNA resembles that of the bacterial ribosome even more. This closer resemblance increases the potential for aminoglycoside binding to the rRNA, which in turn, increases the potential for ototoxic effects to the hair cells after aminoglycoside exposure.

One mitochondrial mutation shown to increase aminoglycoside ototoxicity is the 1555 A→G (A1555G) mutation in the 12S rRNA gene.[30] This mutation has been most commonly reported in families of Asian descent; however it has also been detected in a large family of Arab–Israeli descent. This mutation has not been found in the American or Swiss populations.[29,30] In addition to an increased sensitivity to aminoglycoside antibiotic ototoxicity, individuals carrying the A1555G mutation are also more likely to develop hearing loss over time, without exposure to aminoglycoside antibiotics. This finding indicates the mutation compromises the hair cell to a greater extent than just rendering it more vulnerable to aminoglycoside antibiotic intoxication.

Macrolide Antibiotics

Administration of the macrolide antibiotic erythromycin has been reported to cause temporary hearing loss, which is not accompanied by tinnitus or vestibular symptoms.[31] There is some indication that erythromycin can have either central or peripheral neural effects on the auditory system. While there is clinical evidence of temporary ototoxic effects after systemic administration, the strongest evidence for an ototoxic effect to involve the inner ear comes from animal studies. Cochlear hair cell loss has been demonstrated after topical (middle ear) application, and a temporary reduction in endocochlear potentials in guinea pigs was seen after systemic delivery of the drug.[32] Patients with renal failure, hepatic impairment, and patients who have undergone renal transplantation are most susceptible to macrolide antibiotic ototoxicity. In transplant patients, there is a clear correlation between dosage and effect. The higher and/or longer dosage regimens have been shown to affect hearing.

Azithromycin and clarithromycin are newer-generation macrolide antibiotics that have shown some temporary ototoxic effects in patients compromised by HIV or age. Ototoxicity appears after prolonged administration of doses between 500 to 600 mg/d. Most often the hearing improved after reducing the dose to 300 mg/d.[33]

Polymyxins, Colymycin, and Chloramphenicol

These ototoxic agents are naturally occurring agents made from soil-dwelling microbes. Polymyxins are a group of closely related antibiotic substances produced by a soil dwelling, spore forming, rod, *Bacillus polymyxa*.[34] Colymycin is a similar agent to the polymyxins. It is also know as Polymyxin E. Colymycin is produced by another soil-dwelling microorganism, *B. colistinus*. Chloramphenicol is produced by the soil dwelling microorganism, *Streptomyces venezuelae*.

The polymyxins and colymycin produce an antibacterial effect by disrupting the integrity of the bacterial cell membrane. They are effective against gram-negative bacteria. Chloramphenicol affects many bacterial species: aerobic and anaerobic, gram-positive and gram-negative. The action of chloramphenicol is more bacteriostatic than bactericidal, as it inhibits protein synthesis within the bacterial cell.

The first reported case of ototoxicity from chloramphenicol was in 1959 after *systemic* administration of high doses of the drug. Sudden sensorineural hearing loss occurred shortly after drug administration. The first reported case of ototoxicity from *topical* application of chloramphenicol was in 1964. The drug was administered as a mixture of 1% ethylaminobenzoate and nearly 100% propylene glycol, given drop wise into the ear canal of a person with a perforated tympanic membrane due to chronic suppurative otitis media. In this case, it is not clear whether the ototoxicity was due to the chloramphenicol or the propylene glycol, which is also ototoxic when in contact with the middle ear.[4]

Like chloramphenicol, polymyxins are highly ototoxic when administered topically.[4] However, no ototoxicity has been reported with systemic administration of these drugs.

Vancomycin and Vancomycin Analogs

Vancomycin is a glycopeptide whose antibiotic actions were first used clinically in the late 1950s. Its potential ototoxicity limited its use until the 1980s when it was shown to be beneficial in the treatment of resistant S*taphylococcus aureus* infections.[35]

Reports of vancomycin ototoxicity are varied. Usually patients experiencing ototoxic effects during vancomycin treatment have resolution once the treatment is stopped. Permanent effects occur when the patients have other conditions that contribute to the ototoxic outcome, or when other potentially ototoxic drugs were given during treatment.

Animal studies of the effects of vancomycin administration on inner ear functions have shown little evidence of ototoxicity when the drug is administered alone. But, when combined with aminoglycosides or tobramycin, vancomycin administration can result in a significant ototoxic effect.

Several analogs of vancomycin have been developed: teichoplanin, daptomycin, and norvancomycin. To date, ototoxicity has not been demonstrated, but since these drugs resemble vancomycin chemically, they should be considered potentially ototoxic.[36]

Antifungal Medications

Otomycosis has been defined as a fungal infection of the external auditory canal, the middle ear, or open mastoid cavities.[37] Although this condition is not as common as bacteria-associated external otitis and otitis media, it is a significant problem in cultures where swimming in natural bodies of water is a common practice (swimmer's ear) or in areas with tropical and subtropical climates. Patients who have increased susceptibility to fungal infections, such as HIV or chemotherapy patients are at higher risk for otomycosis. The choice of antifungal medications used for treatment in the past has been varied and not based on scientific data. There is no US Food and Drug Administration approved otic preparation specifically for otomycosis, and only a few animal studies have assessed potential toxicity of antifungal agents applied topically to the external or middle ear.

Tom and colleagues reported no discernible evidence of ototoxicity in guinea pigs when he examined several antimycotic agents: the azoles, clotrimazole, miconazole; the polyene nystatin; or tolnaftate.[38] However, middle ear and inner ear toxicity has been demonstrated in guinea pig studies designed to assess toxic effects of several other types of medications used to treat otomycosis, ie, the antiseptics gentian violet and Cresylate™ and preparations containing the solvent propylene glycol.

Disinfectants and Antiseptics

Disinfectants and antiseptics used to help sterilize the skin preoperatively have been shown to be ototoxic if they enter the middle ear.[39] Preoperative use of chlorohexidine has been implicated in several cases of severe sensorineural hearing loss after otologic surgery. Since then, permanent ototoxic effects have b een shown after middle ear application of chlorohexidine in several different animals, using several different means to determine the effects including morphological changes and cochlear and vestibular electrophysiology. Alcohols and some iodine-containing skin preparations have also been shown to be ototoxic when applied to the middle ear in animals.

Benzalkonium chloride, a quaternary ammonium compound, is a substance shown to cause irritation to corneal and middle ear tissues at the typical concentrations used.[40] In addition, Aursnes demonstrated inner ear ototoxicity in middle ear applications of 0.1% concentrations of benzalkonium chloride with or without a 70% ethanol base.

REFERENCES

1. Ding D, McFadden SL, Woo JM, Salvi RJ. Ethacrynic acid rapidly and selectively abolishes blood flow in vessels supplying the lateral wall of the cochlea. Hear Res 2002;173:1–9.
2. Pillay VK, Schwartz FD, Aimi K, Kark RM. Transient and permanent deafness following treatment with ethacrynic acid in renal failure. Lancet 1969;1:77–9.
3. Grigor RR, Spitz PW, Furst DE. Salicylate toxicity in elderly patients with rheumatoid arthritis. J Rheumatol 1987;14:60–6.
4. Roland PS, Rybak L, Hannley M, et al. Animal ototoxicity of topical antibiotics and the relevance to clinical treatment of human subjects. Otolaryngol Head Neck Surg 2004;130: S57–78.
5. Campbell KCM, Kelly E, Targovnik N, et al. Audiologic monitoring for potential ototoxicity in a phase I clinical trail of a new glycopeptide antibiotic. J Am Acad Audiol 2003;14:157–69.
6. Tas A, Yagiz R, Tas M, et al. Evaluation of hearing in children with autism by using TEOAE and ABR. Autism 2007;11:73–9.
7. O'Leary DP, Davis LL, Li S. Predictive monitoring of high-frequency vestibulo-ocular reflex rehabilitation following gentamicin ototoxicity. Acta Otolaryngol 1995;520 Pt1:202–4.
8. Bath AP, Walsh RM, Bance ML, Rutka JA. Ototoxicity of topical gentamicin preparations. Laryngoscope 1999;109:1088–93.
9. Rama-Lopez J, Perez N, Martinez Vila E. Dynamic posture assessment in patients with peripheral vestibulopathy. Acta Otolaryngol 2004;124:700–5.
10. Schubert MC, Migliaccio AA, Della Santina CC. Dynamic visual acuity during passive head thrusts in canal planes. J Assoc Res Otolaryngol 2006;7:329–38.
11. Weiss AH, Phillips JO. Congenital and compensated vestibular dysfunction in childhood: An overlooked entity. J Child Neurol 2006;21:572–9.
12. Young YH. Vestibular evoked myogenic potentials: Optimal stimulation and clinical application. J Biomed Sci 2006;13:745–51.
13. Mills DM. Determining the cause of hearing loss: Differential diagnosis using a comparison of audiometric and otoacoustic emission responses. Ear Hear 2006;27:508–25.
14. Jung TT, Rhee CK, Lee CS, et al. Ototoxicity of salicylate, nonsteroidal antiinflammatory drugs, and quinine. Otolaryngol Clin North Am 1993;26:791–810.
15. Cazals Y. Auditory sensori-neural alterations induced by salicylate. Prog Neurobiol 2000;62:583–631.
16. Mishra SK, Mohanty S, Mohanty A, Das BS. Management of severe and complicated malaria. J Postgrad Med 2006;52:281–7.
17. Liang GH, Jarlebark L, Ulfendahl M, Moore EJ. Mercury (Hg2+) suppression of potassium currents of outer hair cells. Neurotoxicol Teratol 2003;25:349–59.

18. Liang GH, Jarlebark L, Ulfendahl M, et al. Lead (Pb2+) modulation of potassium currents of guinea pig outer hair cells. Neurotoxicol Teratol 2004;26:253–60.

19. Counter SA. Neurophysiological anomalies in brainstem responses of mercury-exposed children of Andean gold miners. J Occup Environ Med 2003;45:87–95.

20. Counter SA, Buchanan LH. Neuro-ototoxicity in Andean adults with chronic lead and noise exposure. J Occup Environ Med 2002;44:30–8.

21. Rybak LP. Ototoxicity of loop diuretics. Otolaryngol Clin North Am 1993;26:829–44.

22. Anonymous. Boston Collaborative Drug Surveillance Program: Drug induced deafness: A comparative study. JAMA 1973;224:515–16.

23. So HS, Park C, Kim HJ, et al. Protective effect of T-type calcium channel blocker flunarizine on cisplatin-induced death of auditory cells. Hear Res 2005;204:127–39.

24. Thomas JP, Lautermann J, Liedert B, et al. High accumulation of platinum-DNA adducts in strial marginal cells of the cochlea is an early event in cisplatin but not carboplatin ototoxicity. Mol Pharmacol 2006;70:23–9.

25. Scott AR, Prepageran N, Rutka JA. Iron chelating and other chemotherapeutic agents: The vinca alkaloids. In: Roland PS, Rutka JA, editors. Ototoxicity. Hamilton, Ontario: BC Decker Inc.; 2004. p. 78–81.

26. Sataloff J, Wagner S, Menduke H. Kanamycin ototoxicity in healthy men. Arch Otolaryngol 1964;80:413–7.

27. Gurtler N, Schmuziger N, Kim Y, et al. Audiologic testing and molecular analysis of 12S rRNA in patients receiving aminoglycosides. Laryngoscope 2005;115:640–4.

28. Jiang H, Sha SH, Schacht J. Kanamycin alters cytoplasmic and nuclear phosphoinositide signaling in the organ of Corti in vivo. J Neurochem 2006;99:269–76.

29. Prezant TR, Agapian JV, Bohlman MC, et al. Mitochondrial ribosomal RNA mutation associated with both antibiotic-induced and non-syndromic deafness. Nat Genet 1993;4:289–94.

30. Usami S, Abe S, Kasai M. Genetic and clinical features of sensorineural hearing loss associated with the 1555 mitochondrial mutation. Laryngoscope 1997;107:483–90.

31. Brumett RE. Ototoxic liability of erythomycin and analogues. Otolaryngol Clin North Am 1993;26:811–9.

32. Kobayashi T, Rong Y, Chiba T, et al. Ototoxic effect of erythromycin on cochlear potentials in the guinea pig. Ann Otol Rhinol Laryngol 1997;106:599–603.

33. Brown BA, Griffith DE, Girard W, et al. Relationship of adverse events to serum drug levels in patients receiving high-dose azithromycin for mycobacterial lung disease. Clin Infect Dis 1997;24:958–64.

34. Rybak LP, Krishna S. Chloramphenicol, colymycin, and polymyxin. In: Roland PS, Rutka JA, editors. Ototoxicity. Hamilton, Ontario: BC Decker Inc.; 2004. p. 128–33.

35. Brummett RE. Ototoxicity of vancomycin and analogues. Otolaryngol Clin North Am 1993;26:821–8.

36. Gao W, Zhang S, Liu H, et al. Ototoxicity of a new glycopeptide, norvancomycin with multiple intravenous administrations in guinea pigs. J Antibiot (Tokyo) 2004;57:45–51.

37. Paulose KO, Al Khalifa S, Shenoy P, Sharma RK. Mycotic infection of the ear (otomycosis): A prospective study. J Laryngol Otol 1989;103:30–35.

38. Tom LWC, Elden LM, Marsh RR. Topical antifungals. In: Roland PS, Rutka JA, editors. Ototoxicity. Hamilton, Ontario: BC Decker Inc.; 2004. p. 134–9.

39. Perez R, Freeman S, Sohmer H, Sichel JY. Vestibular and cochlear ototoxicity of topical antiseptics assessed by evoked potentials. Laryngoscope 2000;110:1522–7.

40. Aursnes J. Ototoxic effect of quaternary ammonium compounds. Acta Otolaryngol 1982;93:421–33.

24

Idiopathic Sudden Sensorineural Hearing Loss

Robert Dobie, MD
Karen Jo Doyle, MD, PhD

DEFINITION, CLINICAL PRESENTATION, AND PROGNOSIS

Idiopathic sudden sensorineural hearing loss (ISSNHL) is a term that requires little elaboration. Most patients describe waking up with hearing loss that was not present the night before, or they can identify the time of day when hearing loss began. Nevertheless, the literature reflects a consensus to consider onset over a period of less than 3 days as "sudden."

Hearing loss, whether sudden or more gradual in onset, can obviously range from barely detectable to profound, but, once again, a convention has evolved: ISSNHL is generally defined as demonstrating a threshold change for the worse of at least 30 dB in at least three contiguous audiometric frequencies. Occasionally, this change can be assessed by comparing current to prior audiograms. More often, the affected ear is compared with the unaffected ear, assuming that the two ears were equal before. Fortunately, ISSNHL is almost always unilateral.

According to Byl, ISSNHL affects about 1 person per 10,000 per year[1]; this would correspond to over 25,000 cases per year in the United States. In contrast, Hughes and colleagues estimate only 4,000 cases per year in the United States.[2] All ages and both sexes are affected; the peak ages are 30 to 60 years.[3]

Tinnitus is usually present (>90%), and vertigo is frequent, either spontaneous (as in acute vestibular neuronitis) or as isolated positional vertigo.[4,5] Sixty-five percent of patients recover completely with or without treatment, most within 2 weeks.[6] Low-frequency losses have a better prognosis than high-frequency losses; of course, this is true of all types of rapidly progressive or fluctuating sensorineural hearing loss (SNHL), not just ISSNHL.[7]

ETIOLOGY

Since ISSNHL is, by definition, idiopathic, the cause of any individual case is not known. Nevertheless, there has been considerable speculation about viral and vascular causes, with rather more evidence for the former than the latter.

Viral

Many otologists believe that viral infection (or reactivation of latent viruses) is the most important cause of ISSNHL. The circumstantial evidence for that belief can be summarized as follows: (1) Many viral diseases, for example, mumps, can cause congenital or sudden SNHL, (2) Cochlear histopathology after these diseases resembles that seen after ISSNHL, (3) Patients with ISSNHL often demonstrate immunologic evidence for viral infection, (4) Viruses such as herpes simplex may lie dormant in neural tissue for years and have been identified in human spiral ganglia.

Intrauterine viral infection may damage many organ systems. The rubella (German measles) virus caused thousands of cases of congenital deafness during a 1964 to 1965 epidemic[8]; most were associated with a syndrome that included eye, heart, and brain abnormalities. Since the introduction of the mumps–measles–rubella (MMR) vaccine, the congenital rubella syndrome has virtually disappeared in the United States.

At present, the most important viral cause of congenital deafness is cytomegalovirus (CMV), a member of the herpes virus family. CMV has been cultured from the inner ear[9] and causes cochlear lesions in experimentally infected animals.[10] Congenital CMV syndrome includes deafness and lesions of the eye, brain, liver, and spleen.[11] It is important to note, however, that most CMV-infected neonates do not demonstrate the full-blown CMV syndrome. Indeed, "asymptomatic" CMV infection causes more hearing loss than "symptomatic" (syndromic) CMV infection. Neonatal CMV screening has shown an infection rate (virus cultured from urine) of 1.3%[12]; 10% of these cases had either congenital or progressive hearing loss. Most of the babies who had (or developed) hearing loss were otherwise healthy and would have been missed by conventional high-risk criteria for congenital hearing loss. No vaccine is yet available to reduce or eliminate hearing loss from CMV.

Neonatal herpes simplex virus (HSV) infection is associated with hearing loss in about 10% of cases.[13]

Mumps (viral parotitis) is the prototypical example of sudden unilateral hearing loss in childhood. Rare since the widespread use of the MMR vaccine, mumps deafness occurred in about 5 of every 10,000 mumps cases[14] and was usually unilateral. Like CMV, the mumps virus has been cultured from the inner ear[15] and causes cochlear lesions in experimental animals.[16] Measles

(rubeola virus) accounted for 3 to 10% of bilateral deafness in children prior to the MMR vaccine.[17]

The varicella-zoster (or herpes zoster) virus causes chickenpox in children and shingles in adults. When the geniculate ganglion is involved, with facial paralysis plus auricular bullae, it is called herpes zoster oticus (HZO) or Ramsay Hunt syndrome. About 6% of HZO cases exhibit SNHL,[18] making HZO probably the most common type of hearing loss in adults in which a viral cause is reasonably certain. Herpes zoster viral deoxyribonucleic acid (DNA) has been identified in temporal bone tissue taken from a patient with HZO and sudden hearing loss.[19]

Human immunodeficiency virus (HIV) may cause hearing loss directly but more commonly makes the host more susceptible to other viruses, many of which (CMV, HSV, adenovirus) have been cultured from the HIV-infected inner ear,[20] as well as to other infectious agents.

Schuknecht and Donovan first showed that ears from patients who had suffered ISSNHL demonstrated atrophy of the organ of Corti and tectorial membrane and spiral ganglion losses; these findings were similar to those seen in cases (mumps, measles) known to be caused by viral infections and different from the cochlear pathology (fibrous and osseous proliferation) seen after ischemic disease.[21] However, more recent temporal bone histopathologic studies by Merchant and colleagues[22] from 15 ears with ISSNHL from the same laboratory showed similar findings, and the authors suggested that there was no direct evidence of viral cochleitis, such as viral particles by electron microscopy. They support a separate etiologic factor for ISSNHL, pathologic activation of cellular stress pathways involving nuclear factor-kappaB within the cochlea.

Given the possible otopathologic similarity between ISSNHL and hearing loss of known viral origin, investigators looked for immunologic evidence of viral infection in ISSNHL. Veltri and colleagues showed that patients with ISSNHL frequently had seroconversion (increasing antibody levels) for several viruses, including mumps, influenza (which may have been coincidental), measles, HSV, rubella, and CMV.[23] Wilson focused specifically on HSV, noting that 16% of ISSNHL patients showed seroconversion compared with only 4% of controls.[24] The identification of DNA from HSV in human spiral ganglion,[25] and the development of an animal model for HSV neurolabyrinthitis[26,27] that responds to antiviral drug treatment, have added to suspicion that this virus may be an important cause of ISSNHL. Pitkaranta and colleagues noted that there are many negative serologic studies, failing to implicate HSV or other viruses, but also noted that long-dormant neurotropic viruses can reactivate and cause localized disease without triggering changes in systemic immunoglobulin levels.[28] This is true for herpetic cold sores, for example, and may also be true for diseases such as ISSNHL, Bell palsy, and vestibular neuronitis. Unfortunately, the difficulty of inner ear culture or biopsy makes proving this hypothesis in individual cases impossible.

Vascular

Diseases of blood vessels affect many organ systems and constitute some of the most important causes of death and disability in developed countries. Risk factors for vascular disease include diabetes, hypertension, obesity, and hyperlipidemia; controlling these risk factors can reduce the incidence of heart attacks, strokes, blindness, kidney failure, and premature death. Equally important, but uncontrollable, risk factors include age, sex, and family history. Since no organ can survive without adequate blood supply and since vascular disease affects so many different organ systems, it is natural that investigators have looked for evidence that SNHL is linked to vascular disease or to its risk factors. Despite the intensity of their efforts, the evidence is extremely weak.

In other organ systems, vascular disease may cause either gradual or sudden/stepwise deterioration of function. Congestive heart failure may develop insidiously in some patients, whereas others have sudden-onset myocardial infarctions. Even when the disease process, for example, atherosclerotic narrowing of arterial lumen, is gradual, the symptoms and signs of dysfunction are often sudden, when a critical point is reached or a new event such as thrombosis or embolism totally shuts off blood flow. If vascular disease is important for a particular organ, for example, the cochlea, one should expect it to cause both sudden and gradual changes in function.

Unfortunately, otologists cannot yet measure cochlear blood flow in clinical practice, so whether a person (or an ear) has cochlear ischemia cannot be determined. Reliance must be placed on correlations between hearing loss and vascular disease risk factors (or established vascular disease elsewhere in the body) and to a lesser extent on histopathologic evidence.

Consideration can begin with age-related hearing loss (ARHL). Age is not really a cause of SNHL but rather an association; still, after excluding common causes of SNHL (noise, head injury, etc), the hearing loss of the vast majority of people with adult-onset SNHL cannot be labeled any more precisely than to call it age-related. If vascular disease was an important component of ARHL, it might be expected that patients, and longitudinal studies of ARHL, would describe stepwise progression with substantial asymmetry as one ear suffers ischemic events whereas the other escapes, at least for a while. The rarity of such reports in ARHL should already cast doubt on the vascular hypothesis, but those doubts can momentarily be put aside and one might ask whether vascular disease and its risk factors are correlated with ARHL. For example, do diabetics have more hearing loss than nondiabetics of the same age and sex? The extensive literature addressing this issue has been reviewed and can best be described as inconclusive.[29] If vascular disease is responsible for some proportion of ARHL, its contribution is small.

Focusing on patients presenting with ISSNHL, are some of these cases attributable to "vascular accidents" such as thrombosis, embolism, or hemorrhage affecting the cochlea? If vascular disease caused a substantial fraction of ISSNHL, the incidence of ISSNHL would be expected to be much higher in men than in women and to rise sharply with age; however, neither is true. Frequent recurrences and, over time, bilaterality would also be expected, yet most people who suffer ISSNHL have only one event, affecting only one ear. Studies of vascular disease and risk factors have shown only that diabetics with ISSNHL have a poorer prognosis,[30,31] not that any of these factors predict the likelihood of suffering ISSNHL.

None of this proves that vascular disease is totally irrelevant to ISSNHL. Inner ear hemorrhages with sudden deafness do occur rarely in patients with leukemia, sickle cell disease, and thalassemia,[32-34] although the temporal bone histopathologic findings after hemorrhage or ischemia are very different from those seen in patients who have suffered ISSNHL, as previously discussed. Sudden SNHL may[35] or may not[36] be an occasional complication of cardiopulmonary bypass surgery presumably owing to emboli. Patients with sudden hearing loss have significantly more blood MTHFR (methylenetetrahydrofolatereductase) gene polymorphisms and factor V Leiden mutations than in control patients, these deficiencies being risk factors for thrombovascular disease.[37,38] Until otologists are able to assess cochlear blood flow reliably and noninvasively in their patients, we will not know much about the role of vascular disease in ISSNHL (or SNHL in general); at this point in time, it appears to be somewhere between small and negligible.

Other

Simmons postulated that double inner ear membrane breaks could be responsible for some cases of ISSNHL,[39] and it is hard to prove that he was wrong, but there is little evidence that he was right either. The only temporal bone evidence of cochlear membrane ruptures has been associated with barotrauma.[40] Because Simmons hypothesized that one of these membrane breaks would involve the oval or round window, producing a perilymphatic fistula (PLF), there was a wave of enthusiasm in the 1980s for middle ear exploration, looking for PLF, in patients with ISSNHL. Today, most otologists believe that PLFs do occur, causing SNHL and dizziness, but almost exclusively in the context of identifiable barotraumas: after scuba diving, violent nose blowing, or extreme exertion during breath holding, for example, weight lifting with improper technique. In the absence of such a history, few otologists would diagnose membrane breaks and/or PLF in sudden SNHL or recommend therapy appropriate to such a diagnosis including bed rest and/or middle ear exploration.

DIFFERENTIAL DIAGNOSIS

As shown in Table 1, there are dozens of otologic and systemic disorders have been associated with sudden SNHL. Many of these disorders, for example, Meniere disease or autoimmune inner ear disease, typically cause rapidly progressive or fluctuating hearing loss rather than truly sudden loss. The more important identifiable causes of sudden SNHL (by definition, these are not "idiopathic") are clinically easy to diagnose, for example, meningitis, acoustic trauma, head injury. Others, such as multiple sclerosis, are usually missed when sudden SNHL is the first manifestation. In areas where Lyme disease is endemic, it is probably wise to ask patients with sudden SNHL about recent rash or arthralgia.

INVESTIGATIONS

Patients presenting with sudden unilateral hearing loss without obvious antecedent cause should

---

Table 1 Causes of Sudden Sensorineural Hearing Loss

Infectious
- Meningitis
- Labyrinthitis (bacterial, fungal, viral, parasitic, spirochetal)

Traumatic
- Head injury (with/without fracture)
- Barotrauma (without/without perilymph fistula)
- Acoustic trauma
- Iatrogenic injury

Neoplastic
- Vestibular schwannoma
- Metastases (to meninges or temporal bone)
- Hematologic malignancies (leukemia, myeloma)

Immunologic
- Autoimmune inner ear disease
- Systemic immune diseases (Cogan syndrome, Wegener granulomatosis, polyarteritis, temporal arteritis)

Ototoxic

Vascular (see text)

Neurologic
- Multiple sclerosis
- Focal pontine ischemia

Metabolic
- Disturbance of iron metabolism
- Renal failure/dialysis

Miscellaneous
- Meniere disease
- Functional hearing loss

Adapted from reference 2.

receive a careful otologic history and examination, as well as an audiologic assessment (including the Stenger test to detect functional hearing loss). Otoacoustic emissions (OAEs) are sometimes present (implying sparing of outer hair cells) in ISSNHL,[41] but it is unclear whether OAE testing is clinically useful, that is, whether the results can assist in selecting therapy.

Routine blood testing in ISSNHL is of dubious value. Children with ISSNHL, although rare, should receive a complete blood count as a screening test for leukemia. If there are clinical cues pointing toward Lyme disease, confirmatory testing is indicated. Patients with symptoms of systemic disease should probably be referred to an internist rather than receive blood tests selected by an otolaryngologist. If corticosteroid therapy is being considered in a patient who has not been tested for diabetes recently, a blood glucose test is probably in order.

About 1% of patients presenting with sudden SNHL have vestibular schwannomas,[42] and even complete recovery of hearing loss does not completely rule out this diagnosis. When hearing in the affected ear is poorer than the opposite ear, magnetic resonance imaging (MRI) with gadolinium contrast injection is the most appropriate study to detect or rule out a tumor. The poorer ear is commonly defined as having asymmetry in two or more pure-tone thresholds of 15 dB or more or asymmetry in speech discrimination scores of 15%.[43] For patients who cannot have an MRI, alternative strategies include serial audiometry, auditory brainstem response testing, or computed tomographic testing, which could detect larger tumors.

The increasingly frequent use of MRI in cases of sudden SNHL has shed additional light on the etiology. Precontrast films can document inner ear hemorrhage in the rare cases associated with hematologic disorders.[33] Soon after the onset of hearing loss, gadolinium enhancement of the cochlea is seen in typical cases of ISSNHL, probably owing to a transiently leaky blood-brain barrier.[44] Six months or more after onset, no fibrotic or osseous proliferation (such as would be expected after ischemic damage) could be identified.[45]

INTERVENTIONS

Corticosteroids

Wilson and colleagues showed, in a randomized clinical trial, that patients receiving oral corticosteroids achieved substantial recovery, defined as more than 50% recovery vis-à-vis the uninvolved ear, more frequently than patients receiving placebo.[46] This benefit was apparent only for "moderate" degrees of loss (Figure 1); 78% of patients in this category who received corticosteroids recovered at least half of their loss, compared with 38% of those who received placebo. Patients with mid-frequency losses did well with or without corticosteroids; those with profound losses did poorly regardless of treatment. This study

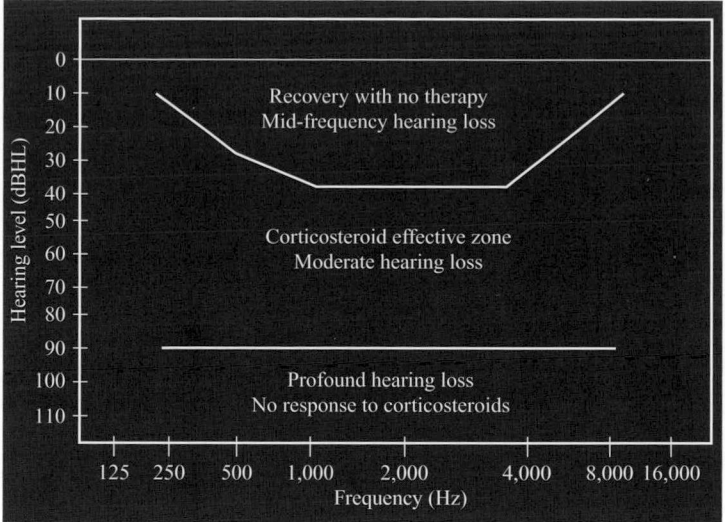

Figure 1 Audiometric categories predicting corticosteroid responsiveiness (after reference 46). Patients with mid-frequency losses, most of which are more severe than shown in this figure but always with better hearing in the low- and high frequencies than in the mid-frequencies, always recovered without treatment (*n* = 14). Patients with profound losses (>90 dB, all frequencies) did poorly with or without corticosteroids (*n* = 34). The remaining patients (*n* = 74) were in the "corticosteroid-effective" zone.

is the only randomized trial of corticosteroid treatment of ISSNHL; subsequent clinical trials use oral corticosteroids as the control group for comparison to alternative treatment.

Subsequent studies have validated the efficacy of oral corticosteroid treatment for ISSNHL. A nonrandomized study by Moskowitz and colleagues showed benefits similar to those seen in the Wilson and colleagues' study (89% recovery with corticosteroids, 44% recovery without treatment).[47] Most otologists offer oral corticosteroids to patients with ISSNHL who have no contraindications, for example, diabetes, active duodenal ulcer, tuberculosis. Higher-dose prednisone, 60 mg/d for 9 days, followed by a 5-day taper, and treatment within 2 weeks of the onset are associated with clinically significant hearing recovery as compared to lower doses and later treatment.[48]

Recently, corticosteroids injected into the middle ear space have been used as a salvage treatment for patients with ISSNHL failing oral corticosteroid treatment. Most of these studies have been uncontrolled[49] but hint that a minority of patients could benefit from this treatment.[50,51] Xenellis and colleagues published the only randomized clinical trial comparing intratympanic corticosteroid injections to no treatment in patients who were initially treated with 10 days of intravenous corticosteroid but did not benefit.[52] They found that patients treated with four intratympanic injections of methylprednisolone over 2 weeks had improvement in the pure-tone average (14.9 dB), which was statistically better than the control group, which did not improve. Clinical trials employing intratympanic corticosteroid injection as first-line treatment for ISSNHL are in progress.

Antiviral Drugs

Useful oral antiviral drugs have been available in recent years but have yet to be found helpful for patients with ISSNHL. Two prospective, randomized, double-blind clinical trials exist in which acyclovir combined with oral prednisolone[53] or valacyclovir combined with prednisone[54] was compared to placebo combined with corticosteroid. Neither study could demonstrate

that the addition of the antiviral agent improved outcome in hearing levels.

Other Treatments

The vascular hypothesis is extremely popular in Europe, where treatments such as oral pentoxifylline and intravenous dextran (intended to reduce blood viscosity),[55,56] apheresis (intended to remove low-density lipoprotein cholesterol from the blood),[57,58] carbogen (a mixture of 10% carbon dioxide and 90% oxygen),[59–61] and papaverine (intended to dilate blood vessels) are often used. None of these has been shown to be superior to placebo.

Other medications having antioxidant properties have been studied, such as magnesium, ginkgo biloba, and vitamin E.[62–64] These randomized trials typically combine antioxidant treatment/placebo with carbogen inhalation and corticosteroid and conclude that the addition of antioxidant improves hearing outcomes.

When a cause for sudden SNHL is found (see Table 1), the case is not idiopathic, and the treatment should depend on the diagnosis. The management of persistent tinnitus and hearing loss, when recovery is incomplete, is nonspecific. Some patients choose to try hearing aids, but, for most, sympathetic counseling is the best approach.

REFERENCES

1. Byl F. Sudden hearing loss: Eight years' experience and suggested prognostic table. Laryngoscope 1984;94:647–66.
2. Hughes GB, Freedman MA, Haberkamp TJ, Guay ME. Sudden sensorineural hearing loss. Otolaryngol Clin North Am 1996;29:393–405.
3. Megighian D, Bolzan M, Barion U, Nicolai P. Epidemiological considerations in sudden hearing loss: A study of 183 cases. Arch Otorhinolaryngol 1986;243:250–3.
4. Karlberg M, Halmagyi GM, Buttner U, Yavor RA. Sudden unilateral hearing loss with simultaneous ipsilateral posterior semicircular canal benign paroxysmal positional vertigo. Arch Otolaryngol Head Neck Surg 2000;126:1024–9.
5. Fetterman BL, Saunders JE, Luxford WM. Prognosis and treatment of sudden sensorineural hearing loss. Am J Otol 1996;17:529–36.
6. Mattox DE, Simmons FB. Natural history of sudden sensorineural hearing loss. Ann Otol Rhinol Laryngol 1977;86:463–80.
7. Dobie RA. Drug treatments for sensorineural hearing loss and tinnitus. In: Berlin CI, editor. Neurotransmissions and Hearing Loss: Basic Science, Diagnosis and Management. San Diego: Singular; 1997. p. 147–59.

8. Trybus RJ, Karchmer MA, Kerstetter PP, Hicks W. The demographics of deafness resulting from maternal rubella. Am Ann Deaf 1980;125:977–84.

9. Davis LE, James CG, Fiber F, McLaren LC. Cytomegalovirus isolation from a human inner ear. Ann Otol Rhinol Laryngol 1979;88:424–6.

10. Keithley EM, Woolf NK, Harris JP. Development of morphological and physiological changes in the cochlea induced by cytomegalovirus. Laryngoscope 1989;99:409–14.

11. Stagno S, Reynolds DW, Amos CS, et al. Auditory and visual defects resulting from symptomatic and subclinical congenital cytomegaloviral and toxoplasma infections. Pediatrics 1977;59:669–78.

12. Hicks T, Fowler K, Richardson M, et al. Congenital cytomegalovirus infection and neonatal auditory screening. J Pediatr 1993;123:779–82.

13. Dahle AJ, McCollister FP. Audiological findings in children with neonatal herpes. Ear Hear 1988;9:256–8.

14. Everberg G. Deafness following mumps. Acta Otolaryngol 1957;48:397–403.

15. Westmore GA, Pickard BH, Stern H. Isolation of mumps virus from the inner ear after sudden deafness. BMJ 1979;1:14–5.

16. Tanaka K, Fukuda S, Terayama Y, et al. Experimental mumps labyrinthitis in monkeys (*Macaca irus*) – immunohistochemical and ultrastructural studies. Auris Nasus Larynx 1988;15:89–96.

17. Tieri L, Masi R, Marsells P, PInelli V. Sudden deafness in children. Int J Pediatr Otorhinolaryngol 1984;7:257–64.

18. Harbert F, Young IM. Audiologic findings in Ramsay Hunt syndrome. Arch Otolaryngol 1967;85:632–9.

19. Wackym PA. Molecular temporal bone pathology: II. Ramsay Hunt syndrome (herpes zoster oticus). Laryngoscope 1997;107:1165–75.

20. Davis LE, Rarey KE, McLaren LC. Clinical viral infections and temporal bone histologic studies of patients with AIDS. Otolaryngol Head Neck Surg 1995;113:695–701.

21. Schuknecht HF, Donovan ED. The pathology of idiopathic sudden sensorineural hearing loss. Arch Otorhinolaryngol 1986;243:1–15.

22. Merchant SN, Adams JC, Nadol JB. Pathology and pathophysiology of idiopathic sudden sensorineural hearing loss. Otol Neurotol 2005;26:151–60.

23. Veltri RW, Wilson WR, Sprinkle PM, et al. The implication of viruses in idiopathic sudden hearing loss: Primary infection or reactivation of latent viruses? Otolaryngol Head Neck Surg 1981;89:137–41.

24. Wilson WR. The relationship of the herpes virus family to sudden hearing loss: A prospective clinical study and literature review. Laryngoscope 1986;96:870–7.

25. Schulz P, Arbusow V, Strupp M, et al. Highly variable distribution of HSV-1-specific DNA in human geniculate, vestibular and spiral ganglia. Neurosci Lett 1998;252:139–42.

26. Stokroos RJ, Albers FW, Schirm J. The etiology of idiopathic sudden sensorineural hearing loss. Experimental herpes simplex virus infection of the inner ear. Am J Otol 1998;19:447–52.

27. Stokroos RJ, Albers FW, Schirm J. Therapy of idiopathic sudden sensorineural hearing loss: Antiviral treatment of experimental herpes simplex virus infection of the inner ear. Ann Otol Rhinol Laryngol 1999;108:423–8.

28. Pitkaranta A, Vasama J-P, Julkunen I. Sudden deafness and viral infections. Otorhinolaryngol Nova 1999;9:190–7.

29. Dobie RA. Medical-legal evaluation of hearing loss, 2nd edition. San Diego: Singular; 2001.

30. Wilson WR, Laird N, Moo-Young G, et al. The relationship of idiopathic sudden hearing loss to diabetes mellitus. Laryngoscope 1982;92:155–60.

31. Weng S-F, Chen Y-S, Hsu C-J, et al. Clinical features of sudden sensorineural hearing loss in diabetic patients. Laryngoscope 2005;115:1676–80.

32. Schuknecht HF, Chasin WD. Inner ear hemorrhage in leukemia. A case report. Laryngoscope 1965;75:662–8.

33. Vakkalanka S, Ey E, Goldenberg RA. Inner ear hemorrhage and sudden sensorineural hearing loss. Am J Otol 2000;21:764–5.

34. Tavin ME, Rubin JS, Camacho FJ. Sudden sensorineural hearing loss in haemoglobin SC disease. J Laryngol Otol 1993;107:831–3.

35. Plasse HM, Mittleman M, Frost JO. Unilateral sudden hearing loss after open heart surgery: A detailed study of seven cases. Laryngoscope 1981;91:101–9.

36. Ness JA, Stakilsicz JA, Kaniff T, et al. Sensorineural hearing loss associated with aortocoronary bypass surgery: A prospective analysis. Laryngoscope 1993;103:589–93.

37. Capaccio P, Ottaviani F, Cuccarini V, et al. Sudden hearing loss and MTHFR 677C>T/1298A>C gene polymorphisms. Genet Med 2005;7:206–8.

38. Görür K, Buncer U, Eskandari G, et al. The role of factor V Leiden and prothrombin G20210a mutations in sudden sensorineural hearing loss. Otol Neurotol 2005; 26:599–601.

39. Simmons FB. The double-membrane break syndrome in sudden hearing loss. Laryngoscope 1979;89:59–66.

40. Gussen R. Sudden hearing loss associated with cochlear membrane rupture. Two human temporal bone reports. Arch Otolaryngol 1981;107:598–600.

41. Sakashita T, Minowa Y, Hachikawa K, et al. Evoked otoacoustic emissions from ears with idiopathic sudden deafness. Acta Otolaryngol 1991;:66–72.

42. Shaia FT, Sheehy JL. Sudden sensori-neural hearing impairment: A report of 1,220 cases. Laryngoscope 1976;86:389–98.

43. Ruckenstein MJ, Cueva RA, Morrison DH, Press G. A prospective study of ABR and MRI in the screening for vestibular schwannomas. Am J Otol 1996;17:66–72.

44. Mark AS, Seltzer S, Nelson-Drake J, et al. Labyrinthine enhancement on gadolinium-enhanced magnetic resonance imaging in sudden deafness and vertigo: Correlation with audiologic and electronystagmographic studies. Ann Otol Rhinol Laryngol 1992;101:459–64.

45. Albers FWJ, Demerynck KMNP, Casselman JW. Three-dimensional magnetic resonance imaging of the inner ear in idiopathic sudden sensorineural hearing loss. ORL J Otorhinolaryngol Relat Spec 1994;56:1–4.

46. Wilson WR, Byl FM, Laird N. The efficacy of steroids in the treatment of idiopathic sudden hearing loss. A double-blind clinical study. Arch Otolaryngol 1980;106:772–6.

47. Moskowitz D, Lee KJ, Smith HW. Steroid use in idiopathic sudden sensorineural hearing loss. Laryngoscope 1984; 94:664–6.

48. Slattery WH, Fisher LM, Iqbal Z, Liu N. Oral steroid regimens for idiopathic sudden sensorineural hearing loss. Otolaryngol Head Neck Surg 2005;132:5–10.

49. Doyle KJ, Bauch C, Battista R, et al. Intratympanic steroid treatment: A review. Otol Neurotol 2004;25:1034–9.

50. Banerjee A, Parnes LS. Intratympanic corticosteroids for sudden idiopathic sensorineural hearing loss. Otol Neurotol 2005;26:878–81.

51. Slattery WH, Fisher LM, Iqbal Z, et al. Intratympanic steroid injection for idiopathic sudden hearing loss. Otolaryngol Head Neck Surg 2005;133:251–9.

52. Xenellis J, Papadimitriou N, Nikolopoulos T, et al. Intratympanic steroid treatment in idiopathic sudden sensorineural hearing loss: A control study. Otolaryngol Head Neck Surg 2006;134:940–5.

53. Westerlaken BO, Stokroos RJ, Dhooge IJ, et al. Treatment of idiopathic sudden sensorineural hearing loss with antiviral therapy: A prospective, randomized, double-blind clinical trial. Ann Otol Rhinol Laryngol 2003;112:993–1000.

54. Tucci DL, Farmer JC, Kitch RD, Witsell DL. Treatment of sudden sensorineural hearing loss with systemic steroids and valacyclovir. Otol Neurotol 2002;23:301–8.

55. Kronenberg J, Almagor M, Bendet E, Kushnir D. Vasoactive therapy versus placebo in the treatment of sudden hearing loss: A double-blind clinical study. Laryngoscope 1992;102:65–8.

56. Probst R, Tschopp K, Ludin E, et al. A randomized, double-blind, placebo-controlled study of dextran/pentoxifylline medication in acute acoustic trauma and sudden hearing loss. Acta Otolaryngol 1992;112:435–43.

57. Suckfull M, Thiery J, Schorn K, et al. Clinical utility of LDL-apheresis in the treatment of sudden hearing loss: A prospective, randomized study. Acta Otolaryngol 1999;119:763–6.

58. Ramunni A, Quaranta N, Saliani MT, et al. Does a reduction of adhesion molecules by LDL-apheresis have a role in the treatment of sudden hearing loss? Ther Apher Dial 2006;10:282–6.

59. Fisch U. Management of sudden deafness. Otolaryngol Head Neck Surg 1983;91:3–8.

60. Kallinen J, Laurikainen E, Laippala, Grenman R. Sudden deafness: A comparison of anticoagulant therapy and carbogen inhalation therapy. Ann Otol Rhinol Laryngol 1997;106:22–6.

61. Edamatsu H, Hasegawa M, Oku T, et al. Treatment of sudden deafness: Carbon dioxide and oxygen inhalation and steroids. Clin Otolaryngol Allied Sci 1985;10:69–72.

62. Gordin A, Goldenberg D, Golz A, et al. Magnesium: A new therapy for idiopathic sudden sensorineural hearing loss. Otol Neurotol 2002;23:447–51.

63. Burschka MA, Hassan HA, Reineke T, et al. Effect of treatment with Ginkgo biloba extract EGb 761 (oral) on unilateral idiopathic sudden hearing loss in a prospective randomized double-blind study of 106 outpatients. Eur Arch Otorhinolaryngol 2001;258:213–9.

64. Joachims HZ, Segal J, Golz A, et al. Antioxidants in treatment of idiopathic sudden hearing loss. Otol Neurotol 2003;24:572–5.

25

Perilymphatic Fistulae

David R. Friedland, MD, PhD

Perilymphatic fistulae (PLFs) are abnormal connections between the middle ear space and perilymphatic compartment of the inner ear. Such connections may be congenital, traumatic, spontaneous, postsurgical, or the result of otologic disease such as cholesteatoma. Clinical presentation may include sudden or fluctuating hearing loss, disequilibrium, episodic vertigo, tinnitus, and aural fullness. This chapter will review the various forms of PLFs, their diagnosis and management, with particular attention being paid to the controversial entity of spontaneous PLF.

HISTORY AND BACKGROUND

The first widespread use of the term "perilymph fistula" began in the 1960s shortly after the introduction of stapedectomy surgery. Steffen and colleagues reported on delayed postoperative symptoms consisting of hearing loss, tinnitus, and vertigo.[1] In a significant number of these patients leakage of perilymph from the oval window was observed on middle ear exploration. Additional reports of poststapedectomy fistula associated with the constellation of symptoms of hearing loss and/or vertigo followed.[2] Shortly thereafter, perhaps due to the awareness of the signs and symptoms of fistulae postsurgically, reports of nonsurgically related PLFs appeared. Manuscripts detailed evidence of congenital PLFs with leakage at the stapes footplate.[3,4] In 1968, Fee reported on 3 patients with posttraumatic signs of fistulae who demonstrated perilymph leak from the oval window on exploration.[5] Two years later, Stroud and Calcaterra reported on 1 pediatric and 3 adult cases of spontaneous PLFs apparently caused by episodes of increased intracranial pressure.[6] The noise- and pressure-induced symptoms of some of their patients invoke consideration of superior semicircular canal dehiscence as a potential alternative explanation. Even at that time the difficulty in distinguishing PLF from other ear diseases such as Meniere disease was acknowledged.

Case reports of spontaneous PLFs continued until enough experience had been achieved to evaluate large series of explorations and treatments. Two classic studies by Shelton and Simmons and later Rizer and House found negative exploration rates for spontaneous PLFs of 50 to 60%.[7,8] All patients underwent patching around the oval window and improvement was noted in 64 to 68% of those with PLFs and in 29 to 44% of those with negative explorations. High negative exploration rates raised questions as to the validity and existence of spontaneous PLFs, and contentious manuscripts appeared decrying their existence.[9,10] Others began to look more critically at difficulties with diagnosis and the role of surgery in evaluation and treatment.[11]

Investigators of spontaneous PLFs performed anatomic studies of the temporal bone for natural conduits for the potential egress of perilymph. Kohut and colleagues described the histology of the fissula ante fenestrum, a region of the otic capsule just anterior to the oval window. They found this region to contain a loose fibrous matrix in 5 patients with PLFs and postulated it could allow for the passage of perilymph.[12] Kohut and colleagues later reported on a surgically confirmed and treated case of PLF whose temporal bone upon bequeathal demonstrated an unobstructed fissula ante fenestrum with an intact "patch" on the middle ear side.[13] In control temporal bones, in contrast, they reported that the fissula ante fenestrum is closed by bone or cartilage. A radiographically definable "cochlear cleft" has subsequently been reported in approximately 34% of temporal bones and was postulated to represent the fissula ante fenestrum.[14] Visualization of this region decreased with age suggesting a developmental reduction in the prominence of the fissula ante fenestrum. Correlation of this radiographic finding with the incidence of clinically suspected PLF has not been performed.

Other investigators revisited an early twentieth century concept of otic capsule microfissures as being potential conduits for perilymph leakage. Harada and colleagues in 1981 and later Sato and associates in 1993, found round window and oval window microfissures in a significant percentage of temporal bone specimens.[15,16] They found these fissures to increase in length and number with age and proposed that they could represent weak points in the bony labyrinth. El Shazly and Linthicum in 1991, in contrast, felt microfissures were common occurrences and had no clinical significance.[17] Correlation of microfissures with PLFs was indirectly addressed by Kamerer and colleagues, and this concept remains one potential route of communication between the middle and inner ears.[18]

An alternative anatomical argument for the development of PLFs has focused on the cochlear aqueduct as a potential conduit for transmitting cerebrospinal fluid (CSF) pressure to the inner ear. This would lead to the "explosive" form of PLF as postulated by Goodhill.[19] Kerth and Allen in 1963 and later Beentjes in 1972 showed in animal models that CSF pressure changes are transmitted through the cochlear aqueduct to the perilymphatic space.[20,21] In 1991 Weider and colleagues reported a patient with PLF noted to have an unusually large cochlear aqueduct both radiographically and on exploration.[22] Also in 1991, Jackler and Hwang contested the concept of an enlarged cochlear aqueduct and found the lateral component to be fairly consistent and small.[23]

At present there is little overall consensus regarding the anatomical basis for spontaneous PLFs. The fissula ante fenestrum is considered the most likely source of perilymph leakage, but many surgeons will patch the region of the round window as well. It is not clear whether explosive forces transmitted from the CSF or implosive forces through the middle ear exploit postulated otic capsule weakness.

PATIENT PRESENTATION

Individuals with PLFs may have a myriad of symptoms that often overlap the complaints of patients with other ear disorders. The most common presentation is the triad of hearing loss, vertigo, and tinnitus (Table 1). Given these symptoms, it is easy to see how a PLF can be confused with Meniere disease, labyrinthitis, and even vestibular migraine. A detailed history regarding the patient's aural symptoms is thus critical to determining the potential for a PLF and the need for further evaluation or exploration.

Hearing loss is one of the most common symptoms in reported series of PLF patients. Looking at confirmed leaks based on surgical exploration, Seltzer and McCabe found over

Table 1 Presenting Symptoms of Perilymphatic Fistula

Vestibular symptoms
- Chronic disequilibrium
- Episodic vertigo

Hearing loss
- Sudden hearing loss
- Fluctuating hearing
- Progressive hearing loss

Tinnitus

Aural Fullness

80% of individuals to have some form of hearing loss.[24] Their most common finding was fluctuations in speech discrimination. Shelton and Simmons found hearing loss in just over 50% of patients but no diagnostic pattern on the audiogram.[7] Rizer and House also found hearing loss in approximately 50% of patients with the majority of these occurring suddenly.[8] A large series reported by Fitzgerald and colleagues found hearing loss or fluctuation in 35% of patients.[25]

Vestibular complaints are the most common reason for seeking medical attention among PLF patients. Shelton and Simmons found approximately 75% of their patients with vestibular dysfunction, and 90% of Fitzgerald's patients also complained of vestibular problems.[7,25] Black and colleagues found vestibular symptoms to be the most common complaint with a sense of disequilibrium predominating.[26] Seltzer and McCabe noted vestibular symptoms consisting of chronic disequilibrium punctuated by attacks of vertigo.[24] In the House Ear Clinic series, dizziness was found in 46% of the patients, roughly the same incidence as those with hearing loss.[8] The duration of vestibular symptoms and the number of physicians seen for evaluation are typically higher in PLF patients than in other ear conditions. The mean duration of symptoms until diagnosis with PLF is about 3 to 4 years.

Tinnitus has been commonly reported as an associated symptom in PLF but is not considered to be associated with PLF if it occurs in isolation. In fact, any single ear symptom in the absence of other findings or complaints is uncommon in PLF. The vast majority of patients have all components of the triad, namely, hearing loss, vestibular symptoms, and tinnitus. An association of this triad with aural fullness is also commonly reported in PLF patients.[27] This makes it difficult to distinguish PLF from Meniere disease. In both disorders, symptoms appear suddenly, are often episodic, and with time, can be progressive or fluctuating. PLF, however, is more commonly associated with inciting events such as head trauma, sneezing, barotrauma from airplanes or SCUBA diving, and straining. Yet, in most series at least half of the patients do not recall or note a precipitating event. In clinical practice, the author focuses on establishing a diagnosis of Meniere disease (see Chapter 28, "Ménière Disease, Vestibular Neuritis, Benign Paroxysmal Positional Vertigo, Superior Semicircular Canal Dehiscence, and Vestibular Migraine"); and, if the patient does not fall into a category of definite or probable Meniere disease, consideration is given to a PLF as a possible alternative cause.

EVALUATION AND DIAGNOSTIC TESTING

The diagnosis of PLF is difficult due to the lack of unique symptoms or a definitive test. Diagnosis is largely based on the combination of a suspicious history, an array of ear symptoms, exclusion of other disorders and compatible findings on

Table 2 Diagnostic Methods Used for Evaluation of Perilymphatic Fistula

Audiometric assessment
- Document sensorineural hearing loss
- Assess for inner ear conductive hearing loss
- Consider performing with suspected ear up

Fistula test
- Subjective dizziness with pneumatic otoscopy
- Observed nystagmus with pneumatic otoscopy (Hennebert sign)
- Enhanced by use of Electronystagmography/ Videonystagmography (ENG/VNG) recording

Posturography
- Can enhance by performing fistula test during posturography

Electrocochleography
- Sensitive during active perilymph leak

Electronystagmography/Videonystagmography (ENG/VNG)
- Can identify a unilateral weakness
- Can combine with fistula test for greater sensitivity

Vestibular Evoked Myogenic Potentials (VEMPs)
- May have lower thresholds with PLF (rule out superior semicircular canal dehiscence)

Fluorescein
- Intrathecal injection may label perilymph (not FDA approved in the United States)
- Add to local anesthetic to distinguish from perilymph

Protein markers
- Compare overall protein concentration to serum and CSF (slow, expensive)
- Beta-2-transferrin (may indicate CSF rather than perilymph)
- Beta-trace protein (in early stages of investigation)

operative exploration with microscopy
- Large leak my indicate CSF (congenital, traumatic)
- May need to look for a long time; two surgeons observing may help
- Increase pressure: Valsalva, jugular compression, Trendelenburg position

Endoscopy
- Avoids potential contamination by local anesthetic
- Very low rate of positive exploration with endoscopy

diagnostic tests (Table 2). Symptoms such as hearing loss and dizziness are common to many ear lesions and care must be taken not to overlook more prevalent disorders for the allure of this surgically addressable entity. Although no one test is diagnostic, objective testing can raise one's suspicion of PLF and rule out alternative diagnoses.

Audiologic Assessment

Audiologic assessment should be carried out to document hearing loss at the time of presentation. This should be performed on all individuals in whom the diagnosis of PLF is entertained because hearing loss occurs in over 50% of those with a fistula but is the primary complaint in only one-fourth. Serial assessments can also serve to document hearing fluctuation and should include tests of word discrimination. No definitive audiometric pattern has been associated with PLF but low frequency sensorineural hearing loss may suggest Meniere disease as an alternative diagnosis. A low frequency conductive loss pattern

should raise the suspicion of superior semicircular canal dehiscence especially if it is a pseudo-conductive loss manifest by lower than normal bone conduction thresholds rather than increased air conduction thresholds. Conductive hearing losses have also been reported in PLF presumably due to air in the labyrinth. As such, a recommendation has been made for performing the hearing testing in the lateral decubitus position with the affected ear up to enhance detection of an inner ear conductive loss.[28] However, this has not been proven to be a diagnostically sensitive or specific test for PLF.

Fistula Test

Pressure sensitivity is a hallmark of PLF and many authors have reported on the use of the fistula test and the relevance of a positive Hennebert sign in diagnosis. Pressure is typically applied to one ear with pneumatic otoscopy, and the patient's eyes observed for induced nystagmus. The patient can also be questioned for the elicitation of a sense of disequilibrium in lieu of observed nystagmus. Modifications of this test have been proposed including the use of Frenzel lenses or with electronystagmography/videonystagmography (ENG/VNG) monitoring. Pressure can be applied with a tympanometer, and the response monitored objectively with VNG goggles. Others have performed the fistula test with the patient standing with eyes closed to increase subjective sensitivity or even with the patient on a posturography platform to enhance detection of altered vestibulospinal reflexes.

The utility of fistula testing is debatable as many studies have found it to lack in both sensitivity and specificity. Healy and colleagues along with Seltzer and McCabe showed a positive fistula test in only 25% of patients with confirmed fistulas on exploration.[24,29] Rizer and House found no difference in positive fistula test rates between those with a fistula and those without.[8] Vartiainen and coworkers demonstrated a positive fistula test in only 33% of patients with confirmed fistulae although there was only an 8% positive test rate in those without fistula.[30] Hain and Ostrowski found the fistula test to lack sensitivity for diagnosing PLF.[31] In particular, they concluded that a positive fistula test may raise one's suspicion of a PLF, but the lack of nystagmus or subjective dizziness on pneumatic otoscopy did not indicate the absence of a fistula.

Electrocochleography (EcoG)

ECoG has been studied as a potential test for diagnosing PLFs. A guinea pig model showed abnormal EcoG summating potential to action potential (SP/AP) ratio in the acute phase after creating a fistula that reverted to normal once the fistula healed.[32] Clinically, intraoperative ECoG was found to be abnormal in patients with fistulae only while suctioning around the round window.[33] Patching of the round window niche in these patients led to relief of symptoms. Arenberg and colleagues in 1988 using ECoG as a screening test found abnormalities in only about 50% of patients with surgically confirmed fistulae.[34] Further, ECoG was unable to distinguish between vestibular symptoms due to a fistula and those related to Meniere disease. Fitzgerald noted SP/AP ratios >0.40 on ECoG in approximately 66% of patients undergoing patching procedures.[35] There was a strong bias in his series toward patients with simultaneous cochlear hydrops which he felt was a result of a PLF as well as being associated with Meniere disease. ECoG, therefore, does not appear to be specific for PLF, but abnormal results during maneuvers causing the egress of perilymph can increase suspicion.

ENG and VNG Test Battery

ENG/VNG testing is the predominant method for objective vestibular evaluation. This test battery, and particularly the caloric testing, can identify a unilateral vestibular weakness, which may raise the suspicion of an inner ear insult and direct the clinician's attention toward one ear. As noted above, ENG/VNG ocular monitoring can also be used to enhance the sensitivity of the fistula test for determining the presence of pressure-induced nystagmus. ENG alone is not particularly specific for identifying the presence of a fistula or for distinguishing PLFs from other ear disorders.

Posturography

Due to the high prevalence of chronic disequilibrium in patients with fistulae, posturography has been frequently employed in patient evaluation. Whereas posturography can identify disorders of balance, it cannot distinguish a fistula from other lesions. Black and colleagues have pioneered the simultaneous application of pressure to the external ear canal, that is, the fistula test, during dynamic posturography.[36] Their results suggest a greater ability to detect pressure-related abnormalities than the fistula test alone. The majority of those studies were performed before the identification of the similarly pressure-sensitive entity of superior semicircular canal dehiscence which must be kept in mind. Low-frequency sound application has also been suggested as a useful provocative stimulus during posturography for identifying PLF. However, positive test results have also been seen in Meniere disease and non-PLF inner ear hypofunction.[37]

Vestibular Evoked Myogenic Potentials (VEMPs)

VEMPs have reemerged as an important test of vestibular function due to the significant threshold changes seen with superior semicircular canal dehiscence. Although not systematically tested, VEMPs may be useful in PLF as many symptoms of pressure sensitivity are found in common between these two clinical conditions. A recent report found lowered VEMP thresholds in a series of patients without radiographic evidence of superior semicircular canal dehiscence.[38] Consideration should be given to the possible presence of a PLF in such situations.

Detection of Perilymph

The absence of definitive clinical tests to diagnose PLFs has led some clinicians to look for other means of confirming the presence of perilymph in the middle ear. This has been achieved by direct means such as surgical or endoscopic exploration of the middle ear or by indirect means such as testing middle ear exudate for markers of perilymph. As with diagnostic tests, no single protocol to date has proven definitive, and controversy regarding some of these methods persists.

Fluorescein. Fluorescein is a commonly used labeling dye for detecting fistulas and leaks. It has most commonly been used in otorhinolaryngology head and neck surgery as an intraoperative marker to detect CSF leak during sinus surgery. It was shown in the 1940s and 1950s that fluorescein could enter the labyrinth by way of the cochlear aqueduct from the CSF. However, Gehrking and colleagues found that clinically apparent labeling of perilymph as seen through the round window membrane on microendoscopy was rare and occurred in less than 10% of patients.[39] Further, when directly inspecting perilymph at stapedectomy, they saw no fluorescence. Further damping the enthusiasm for use of intrathecal fluorescein has been the high rate of nervous system complications when administered quickly or in high concentrations. Currently, fluorescein is not Food and Drug Administration (FDA) approved for intrathecal use in the United States.

Alternative uses of fluorescein for identifying PLFs have been explored. It was initially thought that perilymph could be labeled by transudation of fluorescein across the cochlear vasculature after intravenous injection. This observation, however, was later contested and shown to be due to intravascular retention of fluorescein and transillumination of vascular mucosa.[40,41] Another use of fluorescein is as a label for injected local anesthetic. In this manner, fluid noted in the middle ear upon exploration could be distinguished from the injected local anesthetic. Arenberg and Wu found that labeled local anesthetic entered the middle ear in all their cases.[42] When they did not use local anesthetic but explored the ear with endoscopy, all ears were dry and no fluid of any form was found. Thus, many early reports of perilymph leak could represent local anesthetic contamination of the surgical field.

Protein Markers. Perilymph differs from serum and CSF in average protein concentration. Attempts at characterizing overall protein composition can be time consuming and dependent upon pure samples undiluted by anesthetic or mucosal transudate.[43,44] Identification of specific protein markers has largely focused on beta-2-transferrin, a protein considered to be present in perilymph and CSF but absent from serum. There is doubt, however, as to the natural occurrence of beta-2-transferrin in perilymph. Levenson and colleagues collected 13 samples of perilymph during cochlear implantation or stapedectomy and found only two to be positive for beta-2-transferrin.[45] All four of their control CSF samples were positive. Similar findings were reported by Buchman and coworkers who showed only a 29% sensitivity of beta-2-tranferrin testing for perilymph.[46] Thus, the beta-2-transferrin protein may not be useful for identifying PLF. Another protein under investigation as a marker of perilymph leak is beta-trace protein (prostaglandin D synthase) which is present in CSF but generally absent in serum.[47] Further investigation is needed to determine whether this can be used as a reliable marker or if it is fraught with the lack of specificity found with beta-2-transferrin.

Beta-2-transferrin may be useful in patients with congenital PLF in whom there may be CSF in the leak rather than pure perilymph. Concordance between positive observation of a PLF on exploration and positive beta-2-transferrin testing of middle ear fluid in congenital PLF is approximately 26%.[48] Approximately 10% of patients with no visible leak but a history suspicious for PLF may also have a positive beta-2-transferrin test. There is a higher incidence of positive beta-2-transferrin testing in children with congenital otic capsule or middle ear abnormalities. This suggests that CSF pressure transmitted to the inner ear may cause perilymph and CSF leakage at natural or acquired otic capsule weaknesses in children with congenital malformations.

Exploration. Direct surgical exploration for the presence of leaking perilymph has, since the earliest recognition of this entity, been the mainstay of diagnosing PLFs. A 1991 national survey of PLFs by House and colleagues found an overall positive exploration rate of approximately 50%.[11] This survey included a subset of surgeons who had never identified a leak and an equal subset who never failed to identify a leak. Similarly, a review of exploration outcomes in the 1980s and 1990s found an average positive exploration rate of 55%.[2] Thus, only half of patients clinically suspected as having a leak have such on exploration, and the reliability of directly seeing perilymph has been challenged.

The total volume of perilymph is less than a tenth of a milliliter and identifying such a small volume in a moist field is difficult. If larger volumes are identified they likely represent CSF that is consistent with congenital PLF which may be due to inner ear malformations. Indeed, positive exploration rates in children appear to be higher than those reported for adults.[49] To detect the small volumes associated with spontaneous fistulae, authors have suggested long periods of microscopic examination, looking for shifts in the light reflex, use of the Trendelenburg position, Valsalva maneuver, jugular vein compression, mineral oil to trap fluid at the oval and round windows, and the inspection of the ear by two surgeons.

As noted earlier, injected local anesthetic can enter the middle ear prior to raising a tympanomeatal flap and be mistaken for perilymph. Thus, labeling the anesthetic with fluorescein has been tried, but an alternative approach is not to use injected anesthetics. The use of topical anesthetics on the tympanic membrane and exploration by endoscopy to avoid canal injections has been reported. Interestingly, the rate of positive exploration by endoscopy is far lower than that by operative microscopy. In a report by Poe and Bottrill the positive exploration rate was 0% including notation that 48 consecutive endoscopies for PLF failed to find a leak.[50] Another report suggests limited utility of endoscopy in identifying PLFs.[51]

Currently, there are no definitive diagnostic tests for PLF or universally accepted tests for the detection of perilymph in the middle ear. Even surgical exploration with microscopic observation is considered unreliable for confirming the presence of a spontaneous leak. The observation of perilymph leak at an otic capsule fracture secondary to trauma or leakage around the oval window following stapedectomy is considered more reliable but may also suffer from the bias of expectation. A history suspicious for PLF and exclusion of other ear diseases remain the best diagnostic criteria for spontaneous PLFs.

MANAGEMENT

Medical and conservative therapies for the treatment of PLFs are similar to those used for CSF leaks. Namely, bed rest with head elevation and the avoidance of straining or other pressure increasing activities are prescribed. The use of lumbar drain to reduce CSF pressure further in PLF has not been reported. Interestingly, ventriculoperitoneal shunting (VPS) has been used, particularly for those patients whose PLF may be related to intracranial hypertension. Recent reports suggest that VPS may be useful for the control of chronic symptoms of dizziness in these situations.[52,53] The incidence of improvement following medical and conservative therapies for PLF is not known; and, similar to CSF leaks, failure to respond typically prompts surgical intervention.

Surgical treatment for PLF consists of patching the areas of fistula along the otic capsule. Given that the positive exploration rate for PLF is quite low, most surgeons will place tissue patches at the oval and round windows regardless of intraoperative findings.[54] Tissues that have been used as patches include fat, fascia, perichondrium, temporalis muscle, and areolar tissue.[2,49] Several reports suggest areolar tissue and perichondrium are superior to fat, and there have been reports of failure with fascia. Some surgeons have bolstered their patches with fibrin glue, fibrinogen, thrombin or Avitene (microfibrillar collagen hemostatic agent) and have even made use of the argon laser for sealing the graft in place. Postoperative instructions for patients undergoing patching

Table 3 Efficacy of Surgical Intervention

Vestibular Symptoms or Hearing Loss Outcomes	Percent of Patients Improving
Vestibular symptoms	
Healy and colleagues[29]	100%
Seltzer and McCabe[24]	94%
Black and colleagues[26]	84–89%
Fitzgerald and colleagues[25]	87%
House and colleagues[11]	72–78%
Weber and colleagues[49] (pediatric)	91%
Of those with positive PLF on exploration	71%
Hearing loss	
Rizer and House[8]	13–18%
Fitzgerald and colleagues[25]	40%
Healy and colleagues[29]	45%
Shelton and Simmons[7]	Rare
Hearing stabilized	50%
Seltzer and McCabe[24]	49%
Hearing stabilized	40%
Black and colleagues[26]	15%
Hearing stabilized	67%
Weber and colleagues[49] (pediatric)	8.7%
Hearing stabilized	83.5%

procedures should be similar to those for stapedectomy in which the inner ear is opened. Limitations on straining, nose blowing, bending, lifting, and immediate postoperative airplane travel should be advised.

Outcomes of surgical management are generally good and reported improvement in vestibular symptoms range from 71 to 100% (Table 3). Hearing improvement is less common and rarely exceeds 50% of patients in most series. Stabilization of hearing is seen in a similar percentage of patients, but further progression of hearing loss or loss at surgery can approach 25%. Objective testing, even in patients who improve, may not change postoperatively. Black and coworkers found no changes in ENG or rotational chair testing but did see improvement in performance on dynamic posturography in about 30% of patients.[26] Meyerhoff found return of ECoGs to normal SP/AP ratios in 21 of 24 patients following patching procedures.[55] Given the fairly low morbidity and risk associated with patching procedures, surgical management may be recommended in cases where PLF is a diagnostic consideration. Appropriate consent and discussion of controversies with the patient are essential.

SUMMARY

The goal of this chapter has been to present the salient features of PLFs that will aid in the diagnosis and management of these disorders particularly in patients with antecedent inciting events such as implosive or explosive trauma and prior stapedectomy. Also, congenital inner ear malformations predisposing to CSF/perilymph leakage are relevant to this discussion. Less clear

are patients with spontaneous PLF for whom there is little overall consensus regarding occurrence, pathophysiology, diagnosis, and treatment. It is imperative for the reader to assimilate the information presented and to use his or her own medical judgment in evaluating complaints of dizziness and hearing loss with regard to the differential diagnosis of PLF.

REFERENCES

1. Steffen TN, Sheehy JL, House HP. The slipped strut problem. Ann Otol Rhinol Laryngol 1963;72:191–205.
2. Friedland DR, Wackym PA. A critical appraisal of spontaneous perilymphatic fistulas of the inner ear. Am J Otol 1999;20:261–76; discussion 276–9.
3. Crook JP. Congenital fistula in the stapedial footplate. South Med J 1967;60:1168–70.
4. Rice WJ, Waggoner LG. Congenital cerebrospinal fluid otorrhea via a defect in the stapes footplate. Laryngoscope 1967;77:341–9.
5. Fee GA. Traumatic perilymphatic fistulas. Arch Otolaryngol 1968;88:477–80.
6. Stroud MH, Calcaterra TC. Spontaneous perilymph fistulas. Laryngoscope 1970;80:479–87.
7. Shelton C, Simmons FB. Perilymph fistula: The Stanford experience. Ann Otol Rhinol Laryngol 1988;97:105–8.
8. Rizer FM, House JW. Perilymph fistulas: The House Ear Clinic experience. Otolaryngol Head Neck Surg 1991;104:239–43.
9. Schuknecht HF. Myths in neurotology. Am J Otol 1992;13:124–6.
10. Shea JJ. The myth of spontaneous perilymph fistula. Otolaryngol Head Neck Surg 1992;107:613–6.
11. House JW, Morris MS, Kramer SJ, et al. Perilymphatic fistula: Surgical experience in the United States. Otolaryngol Head Neck Surg 1991;105:51–61.
12. Kohut RI, Hinojosa R, Ryu JH. The histologic characteristics of the core of the fissula ante fenestram. Acta Otolaryngol(Stockh) Suppl 1991;481:158–62.
13. Kohut RI, Hinojosa R, Thompson JN, et al. Idiopathic perilymphatic fistulas. A temporal bone histopathologic study with clinical, surgical, and histopathologic correlations. Arch Otolaryngol Head Neck Surg 1995;121:412–20.
14. Chadwell JB, Halsted MJ, Choo DI, et al. The cochlear cleft. Am J Neuroradiol 2004;25:21–4.
15. Harada T, Sando I, Myers EN. Microfissure in the oval window area. Ann Otol Rhinol Laryngol 1981;90:174–80.
16. Sato H, Takahashi H, Sando I. Bony dehiscence between singular canal and round window niche. Laryngoscope 1993;103:78–81.
17. El Shazly MA, Linthicum FH, Jr. Microfissures of the temporal bone: Do they have any clinical significance? Am J Otol 1991;12:169–71.
18. Kamerer DB, Sando I, Hirsch B, et al. Perilymph fistula resulting from microfissures. Am J Otol 1987;8:489–94.
19. Goodhill V. Sudden deafness and round window rupture. Laryngoscope 1971;81:1462–74.
20. Kerth JD, Allen GW. Comparison of the perilymphatic and cerebrospinal fluid pressures. Arch Otolaryngol (Stockh) 1963;77:581–85.
21. Beentjes BI. The cochlear aqueduct and the pressure of cerebrospinal and endolabyrinthine fluids. Acta Otolaryngol (Stockh) 1972;73:112–20.
22. Weider DJ, Saunders RL, Musiek FE. Repair of a cerebrospinal fluid perilymph fistula primarily through the middle ear and secondarily by occluding the cochlear aqueduct. Otolaryngol Head Neck Surg 1991;105:35–9.
23. Jackler RK, Hwang PH. Enlargement of the cochlear aqueduct: Fact or fiction? Otolaryngol Head Neck Surg 1993;109:14–25.
24. Seltzer S, McCabe BF. Perilymph fistula: The Iowa experience. Laryngoscope 1986;96:37–49.
25. Fitzgerald DC, Getson P, Brasseux CO. Perilymphatic fistula: A Washington, DC, experience. Ann Otol Rhinol Laryngol 1997;106:830–7.
26. Black FO, Pesznecker S, Norton T, et al. Surgical management of perilymphatic fistulas: A Portland experience. Am J Otol 1992;13:254–62.
27. Goto F, Ogawa K, Kunihiro T, et al. Perilymph fistula – 45 case analysis. Auris Nasus Larynx 2001;28:29–33.
28. Hazell JW, Fraser JG, Robinson PJ. Positional audiometry in the diagnosis of perilymphatic fistula. Am J Otol 1992;13:263–9.

29. Healy GB, Strong MS, Sampogna D. Ataxia, vertigo, and hearing loss. A result of rupture of inner ear window. Arch Otolaryngol 1974;100:130–5.

30. Vartiainen E, Nuutinen J, Karjalainen S, et al. Perilymph fistula – a diagnostic dilemma. J Laryngol Otol 1991;105:270–3.

31. Hain TC, Ostrowski VB. Limits of normal for pressure sensitivity in the fistula test. Audiol Neurootol 1997;2:384–90.

32. Campbell KC, Parnes L. Electrocochleographic recordings in chronic and healed perilymphatic fistula. J Otolaryngol 1992;21:213–7.

33. Aso S, Gibson WP. Perilymphatic fistula with no visible leak of fluid into the middle ear: A new method of intraoperative diagnosis using electrocochleography. Am J Otol 1994;15:96–100.

34. Arenberg IK, Ackley RS, Ferraro J, et al. ECoG results in perilymphatic fistula: Clinical and experimental studies. Otolaryngol Head Neck Surg 1988;99:435–43.

35. Fitzgerald DC. Perilymphatic fistula and Meniere's disease. Clinical series and literature review. Ann Otol Rhinol Laryngol 2001;110:430–6.

36. Black FO, Lilly DJ, Peterka RJ, et al. The dynamic posturographic pressure test for the presumptive diagnosis of perilymph fistulas. Neurol Clin 1990;8:361–74.

37. Selmani Z, Ishizaki H, Pyykko I. Can low frequency sound stimulation during posturography help diagnosing possible perilymphatic fistula in patients with sensorineural hearing loss and/or vertigo? Eur Arch Otorhinolaryngol 2004;261:129–32.

38. Modugno GC, Magnani G, Brandolini C, et al. Could vestibular evoked myogenic potentials (VEMPs) also be useful in the diagnosis of perilymphatic fistula? Eur Arch Otorhinolaryngol 2006;263:552–5.

39. Gehrking E, Wisst F, Remmert S, et al. Intraoperative assessment of perilymphatic fistulas with intrathecal administration of fluorescein. Laryngoscope 2002;112:1614–8.

40. Poe DS, Gadre AK, Rebeiz EE, et al. Intravenous fluorescein for detection of perilymphatic fistulas. Am J Otol 1993;14:51–5.

41. Bojrab DI, Bhansali SA. Fluorescein use in the detection of perilymphatic fistula: A study in cats. Otolaryngol Head Neck Surg 1993;108:348–55.

42. Arenberg IK, Wu CM. Fluorescein as an easy, low-cost, indirect, or reverse intraoperative marker to rule out perilymph versus local injection. Am J Otol 1996;17:259–62.

43. Woodson BT, Fujita S, Mawhinney TP, et al. Perilymphatic fistula: Analysis of free amino acids in middle ear microaspirates. Otolaryngol Head Neck Surg 1991;104:796–802.

44. Silverstein H. Rapid protein test for perilymph fistula. Otolaryngol Head Neck Surg 1991;105:422–6.

45. Levenson MJ, Desloge RB, Parisier SC. Beta-2 transferrin: Limitations of use as a clinical marker for perilymph. Laryngoscope 1996;106:159–61.

46. Buchman CA, Luxford WM, Hirsch BE, et al. Beta-2 transferrin assay in the identification of perilymph. Am J Otol 1999;20:174–8.

47. Michel O, Petereit H, Klemm E, et al. First clinical experience with beta-trace protein (prostaglandin D synthase) as a marker for perilymphatic fistula. J Laryngol Otol 2005;119:765–9.

48. Weber PC, Bluestone CD, Kenna MA, et al. Correlation of beta-2 transferrin and middle ear abnormalities in congenital perilymphatic fistula. Am J Otol 1995;16:277–82.

49. Weber PC, Bluestone CD, Perez B. Outcome of hearing and vertigo after surgery for congenital perilymphatic fistula in children. Am J Otolaryngol 2003;24:138–42.

50. Poe DS, Bottrill ID. Comparison of endoscopic and surgical explorations for perilymphatic fistulas. Am J Otol 1994;15:735–8.

51. Selmani Z, Pyykko I, Ishizaki H, Marttila TI. Role of transtympanic endoscopy of the middle ear in the diagnosis of perilymphatic fistula in patients with sensorineural hearing loss or vertigo. ORL J Otorhinolaryngol Relat Spec 2002;64:301–6.

52. Weider DJ, Roberts DW, Phillips J. Ventriculoperitoneal shunt as treatment for perilymphatic fistula: A report of six cases. Int Tinnitus J 2005;11:137–45.

53. Lollis SS, Weider DJ, Phillips JM, Roberts DW. Ventriculoperitoneal shunt insertion for the treatment of refractory perilymphatic fistula. J Neurosurg 2006;105:1–5.

54. Hughes GB, Sismanis A, House JW. Is there consensus in perilymph fistula management? Otolaryngol Head Neck Surg 1990;102:111–7.

55. Meyerhoff WL. Spontaneous perilymphatic fistula: Myth or fact. Am J Otol 1993;14:478–81.

26

Hereditary Hearing Impairment

Richard J.H. Smith, MD
Amit Kochhar, BS
Rick A. Friedman, MD, PhD

Hearing impairment may be classified etiologically as either inherited or acquired and temporally as either prelingual (congenital) or postlingual (late in onset). Although useful, these types of classification belie the complex interaction of genetics and environment that make the study of hearing impairment, particularly late-in-onset deafness, difficult. For example, although presbyacusis and noise-induced hearing loss might be dismissed as the end result of accumulated age and environmental trauma, animal studies have shown that genetic predisposition is an important determinant of final outcome. By focusing on congenital hereditary hearing loss, the confounding effects of environment are minimized, and our understanding of aural development and auditory function is simplified.

Approximately 50% of congenital deafness is inherited,[1,2] and among school-aged children, 1 child in 650 to 2,000 has some form of hereditary deafness.[3,4] As the incidence of deafness owing to infectious and iatrogenic causes diminishes, and as our ability to diagnose abnormalities improves, the relative importance of hereditary factors as causes of deafness increases.

PATTERNS OF INHERITANCE

Genetic information is passed from one generation to the next encoded in the human genome. The human genome comprises 46 chromosomes, 22 pairs of autosomes, and the sex chromosomes, XY in males and XX in females. The autosomes vary in size and can be arranged by karyotype from largest to smallest (Figure 1). Variances in shape are caused by the centromere, which divides a chromosome into two arms. A chromosome is described as metacentric if the centromere is in the center, submetacentric if it is off center or acrocentric if it is near the end. The shorter of the two arms is designated "p" (for petite), and the longer arm is designated "q." Chromosomes are further labeled by the banding pattern that is produced by staining (see Figure 1A and B). Band patterns are distinct for each chromosome and are individually numbered (7q31 refers to chromosome 7, long arm, band 3, 1).

Individuals inherit half of their autosomal chromosomes from their father and half from

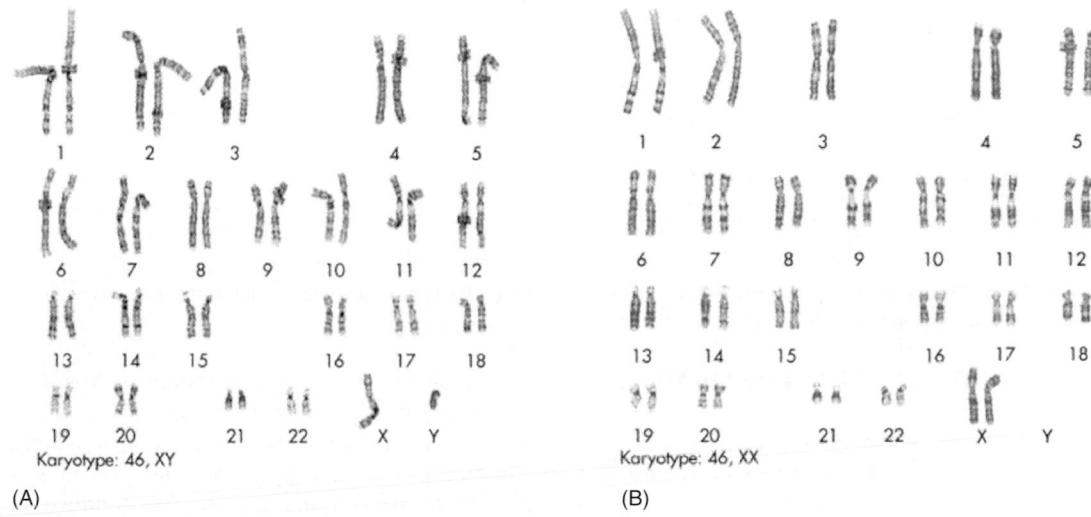

Figure 1 (A) Male karyotype, 23, XY. (B) Female karyotype, 23, XX.

their mother. Therefore, every gene exists as a pair, with 1 copy of paternal origin and the other copy of maternal origin. Each copy is referred to as an allele. The alleles of a gene pair may be identical, or subtle differences may be present. If the alleles are identical, and individual is said to be homozygous for that gene pair; alternatively, if the alleles are different, an individual is said to be heterozygous. For example, if a gene has two possible alleles, A and A′, and an AA′ by AA′ mating occurs, the progeny will have genotypes AA, AA′, or A′A′. If normal function of this gene is essential for normal hearing and A′ encodes an allele of the gene that is associated with hearing impairment, deafness may result. If progeny with genotypes AA′ or A′A′ are hearing impaired, one can assume that A′ is dominant over A. Alternatively, if all progeny have normal hearing except those with genotypes A′A′, one can assume that A′ is recessive with respect to A. In the first case, both parents will be hearing impaired, whereas in the second case, only A′A′ will be hearing impaired. These patterns of allele segregation are referred to as autosomal dominant and autosomal recessive inheritance, respectively (Figure 2A and B).

Deafness caused by genes on the X chromosome is usually inherited as an X-linked recessive trait (Figure 2C). The deafness is rarely penetrant in a carrier female, but half of all sons are affected, and half of all daughters are carriers.

If the affected gene is inherited through the father, there are no affected offspring, although all daughters are carriers. Mitochondrial deafness is inherited only through the mother,[5,6] and sons and daughter may be affected equally.

When hereditary deafness is classified by mode of inheritance, 60 to 70% of cases are autosomal recessive, 20 to 30% are autosomal dominant, and 2% are X-linked.[2,7] In nearly 33% of cases, other phenotypic characteristics cosegregate with the hearing loss. These types of hearing impairment are known as "syndromic" and make the unequivocal diagnosis of hereditary deafness much easier. Typically a wide range of phenotypes occurs, even in individuals carrying the same deafness-causing mutation, a phenomenon known as variable expressivity. An affected individual may exhibit a few, some, or all of the phenotypic manifestations typically associated with a particular genetic abnormality. On rare occasions, an individual may have no abnormal physical findings, and the genetic mutation is said to be nonpenetrant. In the absence of cosegregating physical findings, inherited deafness is said to be "nonsyndromic." Nonsyndromic deafness is subclassified by mode of inheritance as DFNA, DFNB, or DFN for dominant, recessive, or X-linked, respectively, (DFN for *deafness*). Loci are numbered in order of discovery. Mitochondrial deafness is designated by mutation type.

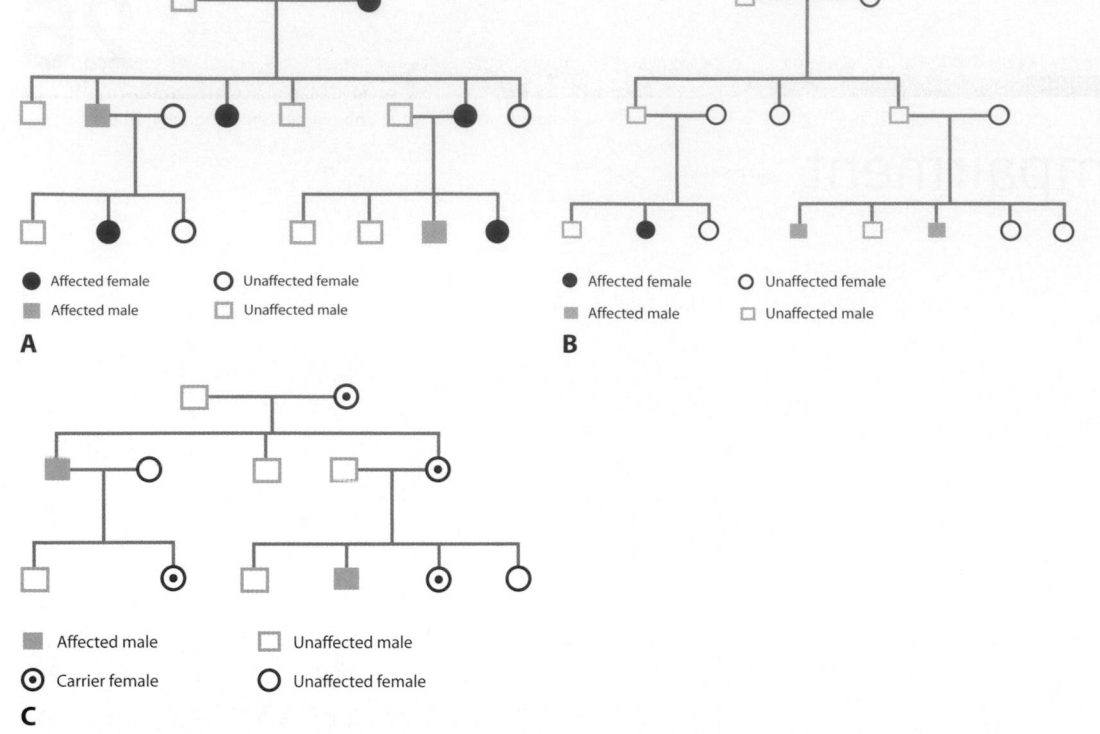

A

- ● Affected female
- ○ Unaffected female
- ■ Affected male
- □ Unaffected male

B

- ● Affected female
- ○ Unaffected female
- ■ Affected male
- □ Unaffected male

C

- ■ Affected male
- □ Unaffected male
- ⊙ Carrier female
- ○ Unaffected female

Figure 2 (A) Typical pedigree of autosomal dominant inheritance. (B) Typical pedigree of autosomal recessive inheritance. (C) Typical pedigree of X-linked recessive inheritance.

SYNDROMIC HEARING IMPAIRMENT

Over 400 forms of syndromic deafness have been described in which hearing loss is an intrinsic part. Though many classifications exist, one of the more useful is based on the involved organ system (Table 1). Some of the more common forms of syndromic hearing impairment are discussed in more detail with particular reference to recent advances in the understanding of their genetic basis (Table 2).

Autosomal Dominant Hearing Impairment

Branchio-Oto-Renal Syndrome (BOR). In 1864, Heusinger first recognized an association between hearing impairment, preauricular pits, and branchial fistulae. However, it was not until a century later that Melnick and Fraser comprehensively described the specific phenotypes. The BOR was defined to include hearing loss, auricular malformations, branchial arch remnants, and renal anomalies.[9,10] Table 3 outlines the most common features of BOR syndrome. These include cup-shaped pinnae, preauricular pits, branchial fistulae, and mild renal anomalies; however, preauricular tags, lacrimal duct stenosis, renal aplasia or agenesis, a constricted palate, a deep overbite and a long, narrow face may also be seen (Figure 3).

BOR syndrome is now recognized as one of the more common forms of autosomal dominant syndromic hearing impairment. It has an estimated incidence of 1:40,000 and has been reported in 2% of profoundly deaf children.[11] Penetrance is high, but incomplete and variable expressivity has been documented between and within families.[12–14] No anticipation or parent of origin effect has been implicated in the transmission of BOR

syndrome.[15,16] Hearing impairment is found in 70 to 93% of affected persons; however, age of onset may vary from early childhood to young adulthood. The severity of hearing loss ranges from mild to profound and may be conductive, sensorineural, or mixed.[2,3,7,17,18]

The first BOR gene was mapped to chromosome 8 in 1992[19,20] and the causative gene, *EYA1*, was cloned in 1997. This gene is the human

homolog of the *Drosophila* eyes absent gene (*eya*), and its expression pattern suggests a critical role in the development of all components of the inner ear. In the kidney, murine *Eya1* also plays a critical role in the development of the metanephric cells surrounding the "just divided" ureteric branches.[21]

Identification of a second locus associated with BOR syndrome was achieved in 1998 on chromosome 1q31. This confirmed previously hypothesized thoughts of genetic heterogeneity within BOR syndrome.[22] In 2003, yet another locus for BOR was isolated on chromosome 14q and this time a new causative gene was cloned, *SIX1*.[23,24] Like *EYA1*, *SIX1* is also involved the development of both the ear and kidney and is believed to be downstream of *EYA1*.

As of July 2006, 117 different mutations of *EYA1* had been associated with BOR syndrome. A full list of the mutations is available on the Pendred/BOR web page (www.medicine.uiowa. edu/pendredandbor/). However, only 30 to 40% of patients affected with BOR syndrome have known mutations in *EYA1*, and the number of patients with *SIX1* mutations is still unknown. Work is currently underway to identify new mutations that may be involved in the molecular pathology leading to the BOR phenotype.

Crouzon Syndrome (CS). In 1912, Crouzon defined an autosomal dominant syndrome characterized by cranial synostosis, hypertelorism, exophthalmos, parrot-beaked nose, short upper lip, hypoplastic maxilla, and a relative mandibular prognathism.[25,26] CS is the most distinctive and common autosomal dominant disorder of the craniofacial complex.[27] It represents

Table 1 Classification of Syndromic Hearing Impairment

System Involved	Examples	Phenotypic Features
Cardiac	Jervell and Lange-Nielsen syndrome	Prolonged QT interval, sudden death
Craniofacial/cervical	Apert syndrome	Craniosynostosis, syndactyly
	Goldenhar syndrome	Oculoauriculovertebral dysplasia
	Crouzon disease	Craniosynostosis
	Treacher Collins syndrmoe	Mandibulofacial dysostosis
	Pierre Robin syndrome	Micro-/retrognathia, cleft palate
Chromosomal abnormalities	Down syndrome (trisomy 21)	Flat facial profile, oblique palpebral fissures, mental retardation
	Turner syndrome	Short stature, amenorrhea, webbed neck
Endocrine	Pendred syndrome	Goiter
	Diabetes mellitus and deafness	Diabetes mellitus
Integumentary	Waardenburg syndrome	Dystopia canthorum, pigmentary anomalies of hair and skin
	Neurofibromatosis 1	Café-au-lait spots, neurofibromas
	Neurofibromatosis 2	Bilateral acoustic schwannomas
Metabolic	Hurler's syndrome	Dwarfism, hepatosplenomegaly, corneal clouding
	Hunter syndrome	Dwarfism, hepatosplenomegaly
Nervous	Charcot-Marie-Tooth disease	Progressive neuropathic (peroneal) muscular atrophy
Ocular	Usher syndrome	Retinitis pigmentosa
	Alström syndrome	Retinal degeneration, diabetes mellitus, infantile obesity
Renal	Alport syndrome	Hereditary nephritis
	Branchio-oto-renal syndrome	Branchial and renal anomalies
Skeletal abnormalities	Osteogenesis imperfecta	Blue sclera, fractures

Table 2. Selected Causes of Syndromic Hearing Impairment with Genetic Features

Syndrome/Disease	Locus	Gene	Function of Encoded Protein
Alport	Xq22	COL4A5	Specific components of glomerular basement membrane within the kidney; in the
	2q36-2q37	COL4A3	cochlea, they are found in basilar membrane, parts of spiral ligament, and
	2q36-2q37	COL4A4	the stria vascularis
Biotinidase deficiency	3p25	BTD	Enzyme allows the body to use and to recycle the B vitamin biotin
Branchio-oto-renal			
BOR1	8q13.3	EYA1	Human homologs of *Drosophila* eyes absent gene and sine oculis;
BOR2?	1q31	Unknown	Both play a role in the development of all components of the
BOS3	14q	SIX1	inner ear
Congenital fixation of the stapes with perilymphatic gusher (DFN3?)	Xq21.1	POU3F4	Transcription factor expressed in developing otic vesicle
Crouzon	10q25-26	FGFR2	Member of the tyrosine kinase receptor superfamily; has high affinity for peptides that signal the transduction pathway for mitogenesis, cellular differentiation, and embryogenesis
Jervell and Lange-Nielsen			
JLNS1	11p15.5	KCNQ1	Subunits of a voltage-gated potassium channel protein; important for endolymph
JLNS2	21q22.1-q22.2	KCNE1	homeostasis
Neurofibromatosis			
NF2	22q12	NF2	Merlin, a tumor suppressor
Norrie	Xp11.3	NDP	Norrin, suggested to regulate vascularization of the cochlea and retina
Pendred	7q21-34	PDS	Chloride-iodide transporter
Stickler			
STL1	12q13.11-13.2	COL2A1	Fibrillar collagens arrayed in a quarter staggered fashion; extracellular matrix
STL2	1p21	COL11A1	components
STL3	6p21.3	COL11A2	
	6q13	COL9A1	
Treacher Collins	5q32-q33.1	TCOF1	Highly phosphorylated nucleolar protein; a nuclear transcription factor
Usher			
USH1A	14q32	Unknown	Unconventional myosin—moves actin filaments using actin-activated adenosine
USHIB	11q13.5	MYO7A	triphosphatase; maintains stereocilia integrity
USH1C	11p15.1	USH1C	Harmonin, which may function as a rafting protein in gating complexes in the stereocilia
USH1D	10q22.1	CD.H23	Important for the formation of tight junctions.
USH1E	21q21	Unknown	Human homolog of the mouse protocadherin Pcdh15. Believed to be essential for
USH1F	10q21-22	PCDH15	normal cochlear and retinal function
USH1G	17q24-25	SANS	Suggested to be involved in the functional network formed by harmonin, cadherin 23 and myosin VIIa that is required for cohesion of the growing hair bundle.
USH2A	1q41	USH2A	Usherin, a protein with both laminin epidermal growth factor and fibronectin type III domains. Expressed in cochlea and cell of the outer nuclear layer of retina
USH2B	3p23-24.2	Unknown	Calcium-binding G protein-coupled receptor.
USH2C	5q14.3-q21.3	VLGR1	Expressed in the central nervous system
USH3	3q21-q25	USH3A	Clarin-1. 4 transmembrane domain protein. Expression detected in retina, skeletal muscle, testis, and olfactory epithelium. In mouse inner ear, expression was specific to the inner and outer hair cells of the organ of Corti and to the spiral ganglion cells
Waardenburg			A DNA binding protein that is believed to regulate the expression of other genes;
WS1	2q35	PAX3	mutation result in neural crest-derived melanocyte deficiency
			Homodimeric transcription factor
WS2	3p14.1-p12.3	MITF	Zinc finger protein transcription factor thought to play an essential role in the
		SNAI2	development of neural crest-derived human cell lineages
			As above
WS3	2q35	PAX3	A receptor involved in the formation of an endothelin signaling pathway
WS4	13q22	EDNRB	
			A transcription factor
WS4	20q13.2-q13.3	EDN3	Required for development of early neural crest-derived progenitor cells
WS4	22q13	SOX10	

Adapted from reference 8.

Table 3 Phenotypic Manifestations of Branchio-Oto-Renal Syndrome

Phenotypic Anomaly	Percentage Affected
Hearing loss	73–93
Conductive	23–33*
Sensorineural	17–29*
Mixed	35–52*
Preauricular pits	70–82
Branchial fistulae	49–84
Renal anomalies	9–75
Pinna anomalies	36–62
External auditory canal stenosis	2–29
Preauricular tags	8–13
Lacrimal duct aplasia	5–11
Retrognathia	4–16
Cleft palate	2–5

*Percentage affected in those with hearing loss.

approximately 4.8% of cases of craniosynostosis at birth and occurs with an estimated prevalence of 16.5 per million births.[28] One-third of affected persons have a conductive hearing loss secondary to external or middle ear abnormalities, and there is frequently an associated sensorineural component.[29]

Mutations in fibroblast growth factor receptor genes (*FGFR*) are implicated in a number of craniosynostosis syndromes including CS.[30] They are tyrosine kinases that span the cell membrane and are important in mitogenesis and cell migration, development, and differentiation. Molecular analysis identified mutations in *FGFR2* on chromosome 10q25-26[31] as being responsible for CS in approximately 50% of affected patients.[32,33] As for the unidentified mutations, genetic heterogeneity has been observed in other craniosynostosis

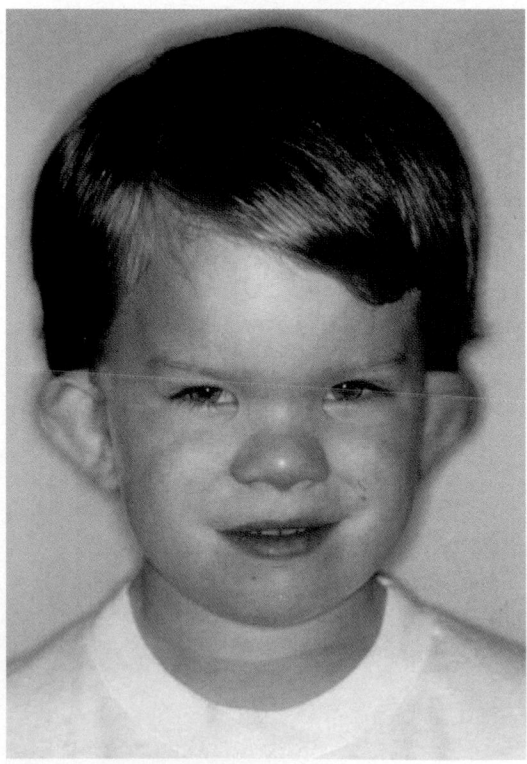

Figure 3 Child with branchio-oto-renal syndrome. Note failure of development of the antihelical folds resulting in prominent ears.

syndromes (Apert and Pfeiffer syndromes), and may play a role in CS as well.

Neurofibromatosis 2 (NF2). NF2 is a central form of neurofibromatosis characterized by bilateral vestibular schwannomas. Other features include meningiomas, spinal cord dorsal root schwannomas, and posterior subcapsular cataracts. Criteria for diagnosis include 1 of the following[34]: (1) bilateral internal auditory canal/cerebellopontine angle tumors; (2) a first-degree relative with NF2 and a unilateral eight nerve tumor; (3) a first-degree relative with NF2 and 2 of the following: neurofibroma, meningioma, glioma, schwannoma, or juvenile posterior subcapsular lenticular opacity. Vestibular schwannomas most commonly present with auditory sequelae. They are typically slow growing and cause gradual deterioration in hearing as well as impairment of vestibular and other cranial nerve function.[35]

The causative gene encodes a protein called merlin that shows similarity to a group of cell membrane–cytoskeleton protein linkers that regulate cell adhesion and morphogenesis. Studies indicate that it may act as a regulator of growth, motility, and cellular remodeling.[36] Inactivation of merlin in the mouse by targeted mutagenesis produces a variety of malignant tumors with a high rate of metastasis, suggesting that merlin also functions as a tumor suppressor.[37,38] It appears that there is some genotype/phenotype correlation as truncating or inactivating mutations lead to severe phenotypes with an earlier age of onset, whereas missense mutations are associated with milder disease and a later age of onset.[39,40]

Stickler Syndrome. STL, also known as hereditary arthro-ophthalmopathy, is an autosomal dominant disorder of collagen connective tissue characterized by marfanoid features, spondyloepiphyseal dysplasia, joint hypermobility, midface hypoplasia, severe myopia, and varying degrees of Robin sequence (cleft palate, micrognathia, and glossoptosis). Because of the substantial risk for retinal detachment, ophthalmologic assessment is mandatory. Approximately 15% of affected patients also have a mixed hearing loss.[41–43]

Gene linkage studies have demonstrated considerable genetic heterogeneity in STL, with known mutations in genes for type II collagen. *COL2A1, COL11A2,* and *COL11A1* are implicated in STL1, STL2, and STL3, respectively, and there is evidence for at least 1 additional STL locus.[44–47] Because *COL11A2* is not expressed in the eye, persons affected with STL2 do not have myopia. Approximately two-thirds of STL cases are associated with *COL2A1* gene mutations. However, there is considerable variability in expression, and knowing the mutation genotype has not been found to assist in prediction of phenotype severity for STL.[48,49]

Treacher Collins Syndrome (TCS). TCS is a disorder of craniofacial development affecting structures derived from the first branchial arch. It is characterized by midface hypoplasia,

micrognathia, macrostomia, colobomas of the lower eyelids, downward slanting palpebral fissures, cleft palate, and conductive hearing loss owing to external and middle ear abnormalities.[50] Inner ear abnormalities are rare although enlargement of the utricle and aplasia of the horizontal semicircular canal have been reported.[51] The incidence of TCS is about 1 in 50,000 live births[52] with wide intrafamilial variation yet small intersibling variation.[20]

The TCS locus has been mapped to chromosome 5q33.1.[53] The causative gene, *TCOF1*, encodes a protein called treacle that is structurally related to nucleolar phosphoproteins and may play a role in nuclear-cytoplasmic transport.[54] Up to 60% of affected persons have *TCOF1* mutations with the majority leading to the introduction of a premature termination codon that generates truncated proteins. These truncated proteins are then mislocalized within the cell during development of the affected structures.[24,55–57] The observation that these mutations are spread throughout the gene and lead to premature stop codons suggests that the developmental anomalies result from haploinsufficiency of *TCOF1*. The role of *TCOF1* in the inner ear is still unknown.

In 2004, *TCOF* mutations were identified in 28 of 36 patients with a clinically unequivocal diagnosis of TCS. Although there was inter- and intrafamilial variation ranging from mild to severe, there were no genotype/phenotype correlations. Four clinically unaffected parents were heterozygous for the *TCOF1* mutation leading to the conclusion that modifying factors are important for phenotypic expression.[58]

Waardenburg Syndrome (WS). The WS, first comprehensively described in 1951,[59] is a genetically heterogeneous condition with a wide clinical spectrum and a very high degree of phenotypic expressivity in each of its forms. WS is an autosomal dominant disorder with an incidence of 1 in 40,000 that manifests with sensorineural deafness and pigmentation defects of the hair, skin, and iris.[60] Common to the various WS types is a deficiency of melanocytes, which are neural crest derivatives. This deficiency is responsible for the pigmentation defects and also for the high incidence of deafness, secondary to the loss of melanocytes from the stria vascularis.[61]

WS is classified into 4 types, depending on the presence or absence of additional symptoms (see Table 2). The 2 most common forms, type 1 (WS1) and type 2 (WS2), are distinguished by the presence or absence of dystopia canthorum, respectively. The presence of limb abnormalities distinguishes the severe type 3 WS (WS3, Klein–Waardenburg syndrome) from WS2. Type 4 WS is referred to as Shah–Waardenburg or Waardenburg–Hirschsprung disease (WS4) and is characterized by the presence of aganglionic megacolon.

Formal clinical criteria have been adopted to diagnose WS1, and criteria have been suggested for WS2, although the clinical definition of WS2 covers any auditory–pigmentary syndrome that cannot be clearly classified (Table 4). As such,

Table 4 Diagnostic Criteria for Waardenburg Syndrome Type 1

Major Criteria*	Minor Criteria
Sensorineural hearing loss	Congenital leukoderma (areas of hypopigmented skin)
Pigmentary disturbance of the iris	Synophrys or medial eyebrow flare
Complete heterochromia	
Partial or segmental heterochromia	
Hypoplastic blue eyes	
Hair hypopigmentation (white forelock)	Broad, high nasal root
Dystopia canthorum (W > 1.95)	Alae nasi hypoplasia
Affected first-degree relative	Premature graying of hair (before 30 yr)

*An affected individual must have at least 2 major criteria or 1 major criterion and 2 minor criteria. Criteria for Waardenburg syndrome type 2 have been suggested that include premature graying as a major criterion instead of dystopia canthorum. W = Waardenburg index.

WS2 includes a mixed collection of melanocyte defects and is likely to exhibit considerable genetic heterogeneity. Aside from dystopia canthorum, all features of WS1 and WS2 show marked interfamilial and intrafamilial variability.[62,63]

Dystopia canthorum is the most common feature of WS1 and results from fusion of the eyelids medially leading to a reduction in the visible sclera medial to the iris (Figure 4). Hearing loss occurs in over 60% of cases of WS1 and in over 80% of WS2 cases. The loss is typically sensorineural, prelingual, and nonprogressive and varies from mild to profound with profound bilateral loss being most common.

Mutations in the *PAX3* gene, a member of the paired class of homeodomain family of transcription factors, are responsible for WS1 and WS3.[64–66] Some WS2 cases are associated with mutations in the microphthalmia-associated transcription factor (*MITF*) gene[67] or with the SLUG/snail-related zinc-finger transcription factor (*SNAI2*) gene.[68] The WS4 phenotype can result from mutations in the endothelin B receptor gene (*EDNRB*)[69,70] the gene for its ligand, endothelin-3 (*EDN3*)[71,72] or the Sry-box 10 (*SOX10*) gene, a co-transcription factor that functions during neural crest development.[73]

Several lines of evidence suggest that a functional relationship exists between these WS-related transcriptional factors. Numerous different allele variants in these genes have been reported as causing deafness.

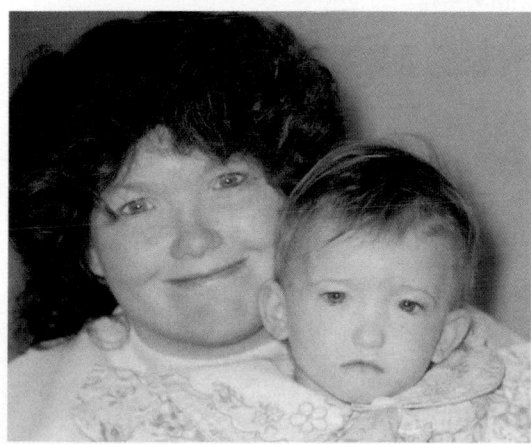

Figure 4 Mother and child with Waardenburg syndrome (WS). Note the characteristic dystopia canthorum of WS1. The child exhibits heterochromia iridis.

Autosomal Recessive Syndromic Hearing Impairment

Biotinidase Deficiency. Biotinidase deficiency is a preventable autosomal recessive form of hereditary hearing loss. A mutation in the biotinidase gene (*BTD*), located on chromosome 3p25, causes a deficiency in the enzyme required for the normal recycling of the vitamin biotin.[74] Thus infants with severe deficiency (<10% of normal serum enzyme activity) are dependent on dietary sources of biotin to meet their nutritional requirements. Without early recognition and prompt initiation of biotin therapy, affected infants will typically develop skin rashes, seizures, hair loss, hypotonia, vomiting, and acidosis within the first few months of life. This may leave the infant with varying degrees of neurological sequelae, including mental retardation, seizures, coma, and death.[75–77]

If untreated, 75% of affected infants develop hearing loss, which can be profound, and persists despite the subsequent initiation of treatment.[78] Since the symptoms of the disease, including the hearing loss, can be completely prevented by presymptomatic diagnosis and the administration of supplemental biotin, this disease has been included in many newborn screening programs throughout the world.[79–81] The incidence of affected homozygotes with severe enzyme deficiency is about 1 in 60,000.[82]

Jervell and Lange-Nielsen Syndrome (JNLS). In 1957, Anton Jervell and his associate Fred Lange-Nielsen published the first report on a familial disorder characterized by the presence of a markedly prolonged QT interval, congenital deafness, and a high incidence of sudden cardiac death in childhood.[83] Today, JLNS is characterized by profound prelingual sensorineural hearing loss, syncope, and sudden death secondary to a prolonged QT interval signifying a defect in cardiac repolarization. Diagnostic criteria include a QTc >440 ms in males and >460 ms in females. JLNS may account for 1 in 1,000 children with profound deafness, and in Norway, where it was first described, the estimated prevalence is 1 in 200,000.[84] Syncopal attacks are usually associated with exertion or emotion such as fear, and without prompt diagnosis and care by a cardiologist, may precipitate sudden cardiac death. Treatment with drugs such as beta-adrenergic blockers or devices that help to regulate heart rate may reduce the high mortality rate of JLNS.

JLNS is caused by a homozygous or compound heterozygous mutation in either 1 of 2 genes, *KCNQ1* and *KCNE1*. These genes encode subunits of voltage-gated potassium channel proteins.[85–87] However, there is likely to be considerable genetic heterogeneity as mutations have not been identified in a number of families with JLNS. Persons related to JLNS affected patients may be heterozygous for JLNS mutations and can have a prolonged QT interval in the absence of hearing loss. These individuals are prone to life-threatening arrhythmias, thus, genetic counseling should be offered to affected persons and their families to diminish potential morbidity and mortality.[84]

Pendred Syndrome (PS). Pendred syndrome, the most common syndromic form of deafness, is an autosomal recessive disorder associated with developmental abnormalities of the cochlea, congenital sensorineural hearing loss, and diffuse thyroid enlargement (goiter). It is believed to account for up to 10% of all hereditary hearing impairment. Prevalence estimates range from 1 to 7.5 per 100,000 newborns, suggesting that it may cause up to 7.5% of all childhood deafness.[88,89] Hearing loss in PS is prelingual, and in at least 80% of patients is associated with structural defects of the temporal bone and inner ear that include dilation of the vestibular aqueduct and the Mondini defect of the cochlea, respectively (Figure 5).[90,91] Hearing loss is usually profound but can be variable in onset, rapidly progressive, and even unilateral. Goiter may be apparent at birth but typically presents in mid-childhood. The thyroid defect involves organification of iodine and can be diagnosed by administering perchlorate, which releases unbound iodide from thyroid follicular cells. Despite this abnormality, affected individuals usually remain euthyroid.

PS is caused by mutations in *PDS*, the gene that encodes pendrin. Pendrin is a transmembrane protein of 780 amino acids, predicted to have either 11 or 12 membrane spanning domains.[92] It is a member of the solute carrier 26A gene family (*SLC26A*), a group of genes involved in sulfate anion transport. However, functional studies suggest pendrin is primarily involved in the transport of iodine and chloride ions and mediates the exchange of chloride and formate, properties that suggest tissue-specific function.[93]

PDS mRNA is expressed in the thyroid, kidney, and cochlea.[93] In the thyroid gland, pendrin has been immunolocalized to the apical membrane of the thyroid follicular cells,[94,95] where it may allow intracellular iodide to pass into the colloid space to be bound to thyroglobulin. In the kidney, pendrin seems to function as a chloride/formate exchanger in the proximal tubule[96] and, in the intercalated cells of the cortical collecting duct, has an essential role in bicarbonate secretion.[97] The role of pendrin in the inner ear is less clear. It has been hypothesized that the chloride transport function of pendrin is important in the homeostasis of the endolymph with ionic

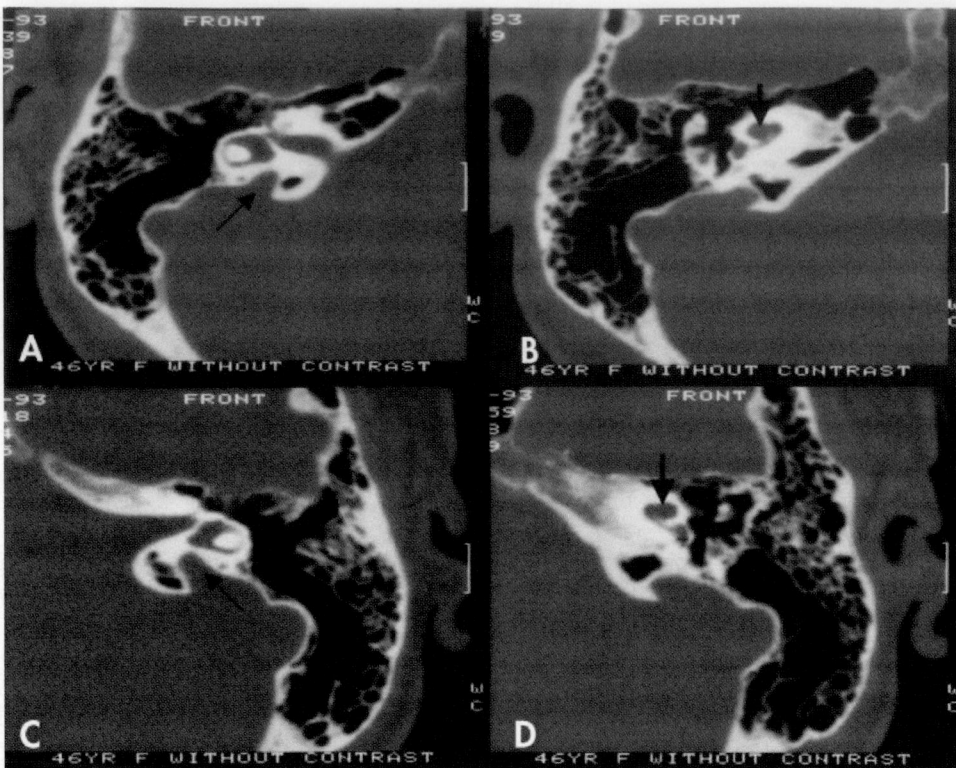

Figure 5 Axial computed tomograms of temporal bones in a patient with Pendred syndrome (A and B, left temporal bone; C and D, right temporal bone), illustrating dilated vestibular aqueducts (*small arrows*) and Mondini dysplasia (*large arrows*). The normal 2.5 turns of the cochlea are replaced by 1.5 turns in Mondini dysplasia.

imbalance potentially responsible for auditory developmental malformation.[98]

Over 50 different deafness-causing *PDS* mutations have been reported that are distributed throughout the coding sequence, having been identified in 18 of 21 exons. The majority of mutations are missense, with a smaller number of insertions, deletions, frameshift, and splice site mutations also having been reported.[68,69,99–104] The wide distribution of mutations and lack of clustering to any domain of the gene, together with the variable phenotype, serve to compound efforts to correlate phenotype with genotype. Mutations in *PDS* are also known to cause certain forms of nonsyndromic deafness.

Usher Syndrome (USH).   USH is one of the most common autosomal recessive syndromic forms of hearing impairment. Characterized by bilateral sensorineural hearing loss and visual loss secondary to retinitis pigmentosa (RP), it is responsible for 50% of all deaf-blindness in the United States and an estimated 3 to 10% of all congenital deafness.[105] The prevalence is estimated to range from 2 to 6.2 per 100,000.[106]

Three different clinical classifications exist for USH based on presentation (Table 5). USH1 and USH2 are most common, whereas USH3 is quite rare, accounting for only 5 to 15% of all USH.[107,108] In USH1, hearing loss is severe to profound across all frequencies, vestibular function is absent, and RP presents during childhood. Hearing aids are usually not helpful, but recently cochlear implantation has shown to be beneficial for some.[109] USH1 patients primarily integrate into the Deaf community. The degree

of hearing loss in patients with USH2 increases from moderate in the low frequencies to severe in the high frequencies and remains stable. USH2 patients have normal vestibular function, and the age of onset for RP is usually during the teenage years. Carefully fitted hearing aids work well in this population and persons affected with USH2 may communicate orally. USH3 is distinguished from USH1 and USH2 by the progressive nature of its hearing loss. The age of onset for RP and the degree of vestibular dysfunction in USH 3 are both variable.

A degeneration of cochlear hair cells and rod photoreceptor cells underlies the hearing loss and RP observed in USH. Hair cells of the ear and photoreceptor cells of the eye share similar structural features such as cilia and microvilli,[110] thus deciphering the molecular bases of USH may help to explain the biological processes involving these and other common structures.[111] Visual impairment usually begins as night blindness with constriction of the visual fields accompanying the loss in visual acuity. By the fifth decade, 40% of USH affected persons are blind; and, by the seventh decade 70% are blind.[112,113] Electroretinography (ERG) may uncover early RP and

should be considered in all cases of congenital deafness to identify early USH.[114]

Usher syndrome demonstrates considerable clinical and genetic heterogeneity. Eleven different loci have been mapped, and specific mutations in 7 genes have been associated with USH. For at least 3 of these genes, some mutations cause USH while others result in nonsyndromic hearing loss. Seven different USH1 loci (USH1A to USH1G), 3 USH2 loci (USH2A to USH2C), and only 1 USH3 locus have been identified.[115–120] Six of the relevant genes have been cloned: *MYO7A, USH1C, CDH23, PCDH1S, SANS,* and *USH2A* and their mutations cause USH1B, USH1C, USH1D, USH1F, USH1G, and USH2A, respectively.[121–126]

MYO7A is an unconventional myosin expressed mainly in inner and outer hair cells that causes 75% of USH1 in the form of USH1B. Extensive studies in *MYO7A* suggest that it has a role in transport and adhesion of membrane-associated proteins at apical surfaces of cells and, in the inner ear, it may be essential for adhesion between stereocilia. In the eye, it is localized to microvilli projections in retinal pigmentary epithelial cells and photoreceptor cells.[127,128] Mutations in this gene also cause DFNB2 and DFNA11. The *USH1C* gene encodes a PDZ domain-containing protein called harmonin, which may function as a rafting protein in gating complexes within stereocilia.[122] Several mutations have been found in USH1C patients, and *USH1C* has also been associated with DFNB18. USH1D is the second most common form of USH1, and its gene *CDH23* is a member of the cadherin gene family whose encoded protein is important for the formation of tight junctions. Mutations in this gene also cause DFNB12.

USH2A accounts for 70% of all Usher syndrome patients. The *USH2A* gene encodes a protein designated usherin, which has both laminin epidermal growth factor and fibronectin type III domains.[123,124] *USH2As* transcript is expressed primarily in the cochlea and the cells of the outer nuclear layer of the retina.[129] The 2299delG-allele variant is the most frequent mutation and is found in greater than 20% of USH2A patients in Europe and the United States as well as some persons with USH3.[130]

X-Linked Syndromic Hearing Impairment

Alport Syndrome (AS).   In 1927, Alport reported that deafness was a feature of a previously described familial nephropathy that caused uremia in males but spared females.[131]

Table 5 Clinical Characteristics of Usher Syndrome			
Type	Hearing Loss	Vestibular Response	Onset of Retinitis Pigmentosa
I	Profound HI from birth	Absent	First decade
II	Moderate HI from birth	Normal	First or second decade
III	Progressive HI	Variable	Variable

HI = hearing impairment.

Progressive glomerulonephritis, sensorineural hearing loss, and specific eye findings characterize AS, which can be inherited as an X-linked or autosomal disorder. To facilitate diagnosis, four clinical criteria were established in 1988.[132] In the presence of unexplained hematuria, a person can be considered affected if 3 of the following criteria are met: (1) a positive family history of hematuria or chronic renal failure; (2) electron microscopic renal biopsy evidence of AS; (3) characteristic eye signs of anterior lenticonus, white macular flecks, or both; and (4) high frequency sensorineural hearing loss.

Since light microscopy of renal biopsy specimens is usually normal in children and because findings are nonspecific in adults, electron microscopy is essential. This degree of resolution reveals splitting of segmental areas of the glomerular basement membrane, accompanied by thickening and electron-lucent areas that contain dense granulations. Serial biopsies will demonstrate progressive deterioration.[133] The eye findings characteristic of AS are rarely noted in childhood and may become apparent only with renal failure. These include anterior lenticonus (conical projection of the anterior surface of the lens), macular flecks, and peripheral coalescing flecks. The progressive myopia caused by anterior lenticonus is considered by some authors to be sufficient to diagnose AS.[134] Hearing loss is postlingual, progressive, and sensorineural.

The typical male with X-linked AS presents with hematuria at age 3 to 4 years, often following an upper respiratory tract infection. Toward the end of the first decade, hearing loss is detectable, and in the mid-teens, hypertension develops. By 25 years of age, over 90% of affected males have abnormal renal function.[133] The clinical course in female carriers is much more variable. Most are clinically asymptomatic through life. Although nearly all have evidence of microscopic hematuria, about one-third will have macroscopic hematuria. One-third will develop hypertension, whereas the risk of chronic renal failure may be as high as 15%.

X-linked AS is caused by mutations in COL4A5, a member of the type IV collagen gene family.[135] In a comprehensive review of the type IV collagen mutations, Lemmink and colleagues reported more than 160 different AS-causing mutations in COL4A5.[136] The mutation spectrum is broad. About 15% of affected males have large COL4A5 deletions; and, in 30%, a variety of missense and nonsense mutations are found. In many patients, however, no mutations are identified. Thus, development of a predictive genetic test is extremely difficult.

Congenital Fixation of the Stapes Footplate with Perilymphatic Gusher. X-linked mixed deafness type 3 (DFN3) is the X-recessive mixed deafness syndrome with congenital fixation of the stapes footplate with perilymphatic gusher.[137,138] The term perilymphatic gusher refers to a heavy flow of perilymph after the stapedial footplate has been surgically opened to replace a fixed stapes.[139] The gushing perilymph consists of

cerebrospinal fluid (CSF) which has access to the vestibule because of the lateral widening of the bony internal acoustic canal. Stapes gusher can be a major complication because it may lead to long-term dizziness/disequilibrium and cause a greater hearing loss.[140] Computerized tomography shows dilation of the internal auditory meatus with an abnormal communication between the subarachnoid space and the cochlear endolymph.

In 1995, the locus for DFN3 was successfully mapped to Xq21.1. Affected males were found to carry mutations involving a DNA binding regulatory gene, POU3F4,[141] and may have either a mixed hearing or sensorineural deafness. Carrier females may show a mild hearing loss and less severe abnormalities of the inner ear.

Norrie Disease. The diagnosis of Norrie disease can be difficult. Classic features include specific ocular symptoms (pseudotumor of the retina, retinal hyperplasia, hypoplasia and necrosis of the inner layer of the retina, cataracts, and phthisis bulbi), progressive sensorineural hearing loss, and mental disturbance, although less than one-half of patients are hearing impaired or mentally retarded. The Norrie gene encodes for a protein of 133 amino acids that has homologies at the C-terminus to a group of proteins including mucins. The high proportion of new mutations is an expected finding for an X-linked disorder with greatly reduced male reproductive fitness.[142] It is suggested that the norrin protein regulates vascularization of the cochlea and retina.[8,143]

Mitochondrial Syndromic Hearing Impairment

Hearing loss may be associated with numerous syndromic mitochondrial diseases. Most frequent are the acquired mitochondrial neuromuscular syndromes and maternally inherited diabetes mellitus associated with deafness.

Kearns–Sayre Syndrome (KSS). In 1958 Kearns and Sayre first described the triad of chronic progressive external ophthalmoplegia, retinitis pigmentosa, and atrioventricular block.[144] KSS is a rare multisystem disorder that usually begins in the first or second decade. Mixed hearing loss may be an additional feature. Patients with KSS typically show a 45 to 75% deletion of the total mitochondrial DNA (mtDNA).[145]

Maternally Inherited Diabetes and Deafness (MIDD). MIDD is caused by transition of A to G in the tRNA$^{LEU(RUU)}$ gene at position 3,243 of the mtDNA (also known to cause mitochondrial myopathy, encephalopathy, lactic acidosis, and stroke-like episodes (MELAS) syndrome).[146,147] MIDD is characterized by both diabetes mellitus and hearing impairment believed to result from impaired oxidative phosphorylation.[148] The auditory defect is a progressive, bilateral, sensorineural hearing loss that first affects high frequencies.[149] It is found in over 60% of these patients and usually develops after the onset of diabetes. MIDD may also be associated with macular dystrophy, cardiomyopathy, neuromuscular, and psychiatric manifestations as well as

renal deficiency. Both implantable hearing aids and cochlear implantation have been successful in rehabilitating these patients.[150]

Recent evidence supports the notion that patients with MIDD may present with 2 distinct phenotypes (MIDD1, MIDD2) that may be related to a variable severity of the disease.[151] Compared with patients with MIDD2, those with MIDD1 are younger at onset of diabetes by 9 years on average, and the age at onset was below 35 years twice more often.

Mitochondrial Myopathy, Encephalopathy, Lactic Acidosis, and Stroke-Like Episodes Syndrome (MELAS). The clinical characteristics of the MELAS syndrome are episodic vomiting, seizures, and recurrent cerebral insults resembling strokes and causing hemiparesis, hemianopsia, or cortical blindness.[152,153] Hearing loss occurs in approximately 30% of patients[143] and in the majority, a sudden, stepwise loss of hearing occurs usually in association with stroke-like episodes.[154,155] Patients with MELAS syndrome may also present with sensorineural hearing loss that usually affects the higher frequencies.[156,157] Bilateral hearing loss is a well-recognized feature in affected patients, and the common histopathological finding is atrophy of the stria vascularis.[158]

Myoclonic Epilepsy with Ragged Red Fiber Myopathy (MERRF). The phenotype of MERRF varies greatly with pedigree and is characterized by myoclonus, epilepsy, and ataxia. Dementia, optic atrophy, and deafness occur frequently with a variable degree of hearing loss.[8] A total of 80 to 90% of patients with MERRF have their disease as a result of an A to G mutation at nucleotide 8344.[159] Biochemically, the mutation produces multiple deficiencies in the enzyme complexes of the respiratory chain, most prominently involving reduced nicotinamide adenine dinucleotide-coenzyme Q (NADH-CoQ) reductase (complex I) in cytochrome c oxidase (COX) (complex IV), consistent with a defect in translation of all mtDNA genes.[160,161]

NONSYNDROMIC HEARING IMPAIRMENT

Over 80 different nonsyndromic hearing impairment loci have been mapped, and a number of the relevant genes have been cloned. The protein products of these genes include ion channels, membrane proteins, transcription factors, and structural protein.[8]

Autosomal Dominant Nonsyndromic Hearing Impairment

Autosomal dominant modes of inheritance account for 15% of all cases of nonsyndromic hearing impairment (ADNSHI) with 21 different genes identified to date.[8,162] The typical phenotype is 1 of postlingual hearing loss that starts in the second to third decades of life and progresses until it is moderate to severe in degree. However, frequencies that are initially affected may vary.

For example, DFNA1, DFNA6, DFN14, and DFN15 are characterized by a low frequency hearing loss that progresses to involve the remaining frequencies. With other loci, hearing loss starts in the mid-or high-frequencies before progressing. The DFNA3, DFNA12, and DFNA23 phenotypes are exceptional as they are congenital hearing losses on which age-related changes become superimposed. Many of the genes for ADNSHI have been cloned (Table 6); however, the complexity is underlined by the fact that several of the genes are involved in both dominant and recessive nonsyndromic deafness or in both nonsyndromic and syndromic deafness.[8,163]

Autosomal Recessive Nonsyndromic Hearing Impairment

Up to 85% of cases of nonsydromic hearing loss are inherited in a recessive Mendelian fashion (ARNSHI).[164] The typical phenotype is more severe than in ADNSHI, accounts for the majority of cases of congenital profound deafness, and is almost exclusively due to cochlear defects.[165] An exception is DFNB8 as it presents as a postlingual, progressive hearing loss. To date, 54 ARSNHI loci have been identified and 23 genes cloned (Table 7).[8] The first locus was published in 1994, 6 years after the first X-linked locus and 2 years after the first dominant locus were reported.[166] Three years later, the gene responsible for DFNB1, GJB2 (gap junction beta 2), was discovered.[167] This gene encodes connexin 26 (Cx26), one of a class of proteins involved in gap junction formation. A group of 6 connexins oligomerize to form a hexamer (connexon) in the plasma membrane. Two connexons dock to form a transmembrane channel that links neighboring cells and facilitates the exchange of molecules up to 1 kDa in size.[168] Connexons are important for the recycling of potassium ions into the cochlear endolymph through the network of gap junctions that extends from the epithelial supporting cells to the fibrocytes of the spiral ligament and to the epithelial marginal cells of the stria vascularis.[169,170] Ion homeostasis is essential for normal hearing, and mutations in several genes encoding connexins or ion channels lead to hereditary deafness.[171]

The most significant discovery in the field of genetic deafness to date has been the finding that mutations in Cx26 are responsible for over half of the moderate-to-profound congenital deafness in many world populations.[172,173] In certain regions of the Mediterranean, the prevalence may be as high as 79%, although studies in India and Pakistan reveal a much lower incidence.[174,175] Numerous different deafness-causing allele variants have been identified. In the United States and much of northern Europe, the most prevalent mutation is the deletion of a single guanine nucleotide from a sequence of six guanines at position 30 to 35. Referred to as the 35delG mutation, this shift in codon reading frame results in premature termination of translation.[172] In the midwestern United States, the carrier rate for this mutation is 2.5%, whereas the carrier rate for all

deafness-causing Cx26 mutations is 3%.[176] In the Mediterranean population, the carrier rate for the 35delG mutation is even higher and approaches 3.5 to 4.0%, implying that deafness due to homozygosity for this mutation could affect as many as 1 in 2,500 newborns in these populations.[177,178] Other "common" mutations are found in different populations, such as the 167delT mutation in

Table 6 Autosomal Dominant Nonsyndromic Hearing Impairment Genes Cloned

Locus	Location	Gene	Function of Encoded Protein
DFNA1	5q31	DIAPH1	Regulates polymerization of actin, a major component of the cytoskeleton of inner ear hair cells
DFNA2	1p34	GJB3	Connexin 31, gap junction protein important for intercellular communication
		KCNQ4	Form functional potassium channel; found only in outer hair cells
DFNA3	13q12	GJB2 GJB6	Gap junction proteins important for intercellular communication
DFNA4	19q13	MYH14	Nonmuscle myosin that interact with cytoskeletal actin and regulate cytokinesis, cell motility, and cell polarity
DFNA5	7p15	DFNA5	Function unknown
DFNA6	4p16.3	WFS1	May contribute to ion regulation in the inner ear; function unknown
DFNA8	11q22-24	TECTA	Interacts with β-tectorin to form noncollagenous matrix of tectorial membrane
DFNA9	14q12-q13	COCH	Extracellular matrix protein
DFNA10	6q22-q23	EYA4	Transcription co-activator; expressed during development of inner ear and important for maintenance of normal hearing; also expresses in heart
DFNA11	11q12.3-q21	MYO7A	Moves actin filaments using actin activated adenosine triphosphatase, maintains stereocilia integrity; present in inner and outer hair cells
DFNA12	11q22-q24	TECTA	As above
DFNA13	6p21	COL11A2	An α-chain polypeptide subunit of type XI collagen, a minor fibrillar collagen; important to structure and function of tectorial membrane; cochlear function unknown
DFNA14	4p16	WFS1	As above
DFNA15	5q31	POU4F3	Transcription factors; development regulators for determination of cellular phenotypes; expressed only in hair cells
DFNA17	22q	MYH9	Nonmuscle myosin in the organ of Corti, subcentral region of the spiral ligament, and Reissner membrane; function unknown
DFNA20	17q25	ACTG1	Actin protein proposed to help stabilize the cytoskeleton in hair cells
DFNA22	6q13	MYO6	Unconventional myosin that plays a role in moving molecules and small packages called vesicles within cells; helps to maintain stereocilia integrity
DFNA26	17q25	ACTG1	Actin protein proposed to help stabilize the cytoskeleton in hair cells
DFNA28	8q22	TFCP2L3	Transcription factor; expressed in many epithelial tissues, including cells lining the cochlear duct during development
DFNA36	9q13-q21	TMC1	Transmembrane channel located in the inner ear that may play a role in converting sound waves to nerve impulses; function unknown
DFNA39	4q21.3	DSPP	Active at low levels in the inner ear, and may play a role in normal hearing; function unknown
DFNA48	12q13-q14	MYO1A	Unconventional myosin that plays a role in moving molecules and small packages called vesicles within cells; function within the inner ear is unknown

Adapted from reference 8.

Ashkenazi Jews,[179] 235delC in Japanese,[180] and R143W in Africans,[181] suggesting founder events. Approximately 90 different GJB2 mutations have so far been reported to be associated with recessive, nonsyndromic hearing loss.[182,183]

These discoveries had an immediate application within clinical practice. In many populations, a definitive diagnosis can be made in 50% of cases of suspected hereditary hearing loss. The ability to establish causality affects recurrence

risk estimates and makes genetic counseling an essential part of the evaluation of hereditary deafness. However, it is important to note that the degree of hearing loss in 1 child with Cx26 related deafness cannot be used to predict the degree of deafness in another offspring. There can be enough intrafamilial variability to make 1 affected child a candidate for cochlear implantation, whereas a sibling effectively uses hearing aids (Figure 6).[184]

X-Linked Nonsyndromic Hearing Impairment

X-linked nonsyndromic hearing impairment is rare and makes up only 1 to 3% of nonsyndromic hearing loss (Table 8). It exhibits considerable phenotypic heterogeneity, but most affected males have a congenital hearing loss, which can vary from severe to profound. Hearing loss is mild to moderate in carrier females. The losses associated with DFN1 and DFN6 may be progressive.[164]

Mitochondrial Nonsyndromic Hearing Impairment

The first genetic defect causing nonsyndromic sensorineural hearing loss was isolated in 1993 and was a mitochondrial mutation.[185] Various other mitochondrial DNA (mtDNA) mutations have been identified that produce progressive, nonsyndromic, and symmetric bilateral hearing impairment. Nonsyndromic deafness mtDNA mutations are frequently homoplasmic or at high levels of heteroplasmy, suggesting a high threshold for pathogenicity.[186] Phenotyping expression of these mtDNA mutations requires the involvement of nuclear modifier genes, environmental factors, or mitochondrial haplotypes (polymorphisms).[78] Mitochondrial mutations may play a role in age-related hearing loss and have been implicated in a type of nonsyndromic deafness associated with increased susceptibility to aminoglycoside ototoxicity.[187]

Age-Related Hearing Loss.   Age-related hearing loss (presbyacusis) is a condition associated with acquired heteroplasmic mitochondrial mutations. Since mitochondrial DNA mutations, and the resulting loss of oxidative phosphorylation activity, seem to play an important role in the aging process,[188] it is likely that acquired mitochondrial mutations in the auditory system may also lead to age-related hearing loss.

Ueda and colleagues detected high rates of mitochondrial DNA deletions in lymphocytes of persons with idiopathic sensorineural hearing loss and noted that the number of deletions increased with increasing hearing loss.[189] They posited that at least some cases of sensorineural hearing loss should be categorized as a mitochondrial phosphorylation disease. Temporal bone studies have also shown that a proportion of people with age-related hearing loss have a significant load of mitochondrial DNA mutations in auditory tissue when compared to controls with great individual

Table 7 Autosomal Recessive Nonsyndromic Hearing Impairment Genes Cloned

Locus	Location	Gene	Function of Encoded Protein
DFNB1	13q12	GJB2 (Cx26)	Gap junction protein important for intercellular communication
DFNB2	11q13.5	MYO7A	Moves actin filaments using actin activated adenosine triphosphatase, maintains stereocilia integrity; present in inner and outer hair cells
DFNB3	17p11.2	MYO15A	Constitutes a class of myosins designated XV; necessary for actin organization in cell as well as development and maintenance of stereocilia
DFNB4	7q31	SLC26A4	Chloride iodide transport protein
DFNB6	14q12	TMIE	Function unknown
DFNB7	9q13-q21	TMC1	Transmembrane channel located in the inner ear that may play a role in converting sound waves to nerve impulses; function unknown
DFNB8	21q22	TMPRSS3	Function unknown
DFNB9	2p22-p23	OTOF	Involved in calcium ion-triggered synaptic vesicle plasma membrane fusion
DFNB10	21q22.3	TMPRSS3	As above
DFNB11	9q13-q21	TMC1	As above
DFNB12	10q21-q22	CDH23	Important for the formation of tight junctions.
DFNB16	15q21-q22	STRC	Thought to be important for the integrity of stereocilia; function unknown
DFNB18	11p14-15.1	USH1C	Harmonin, which may function as a rafting protein in gating complexes in the stereocilia
DFNB21	11q	TECTA	Interacts with β-tectorin to form noncollagenous matrix of tectorial membrane
DFNB22	16p12.2	OTOA	Specific to the inner ear, located at the interface between the apical surface of the sensory epithelia and their overlying acellular gels
DFNB23	10p11.2-q21	PCDH15	Human homolog of the mouse protocadherin Pcdh15. Believed to be essential for normal cochlear and retinal function
DFNB28	22q13	TRIOBP	Binding protein involved with neural tissue development and controlling actin cytoskeleton organization, cell motility and cell growth
DFNB29	21q22	CLDN14	Important for tight junction formation
DFNB30	10p12.1	MYO3A	Actin-dependent motor protein expressed specifically in retina and cochlea
DFNB31	9q32-q34	WHRN	Calmodulin dependent serine kinase; interaction with myosin 15A is believed to be a key event in hair bundle morphogenesis
DFNB36	1p36.3	ESPN	Binds to actin and helps to maintain stereocilia integrity
DFNB37	6q13	MYO6	Unconventional myosin that plays a role in moving molecules and small packages called vesicles within cells; helps to maintain stereocilia integrity
DFNB67	6p21.1-p22.3	TMHS	Tetraspan membrane protein of hair cell stereocilia

Adapted from reference 8.

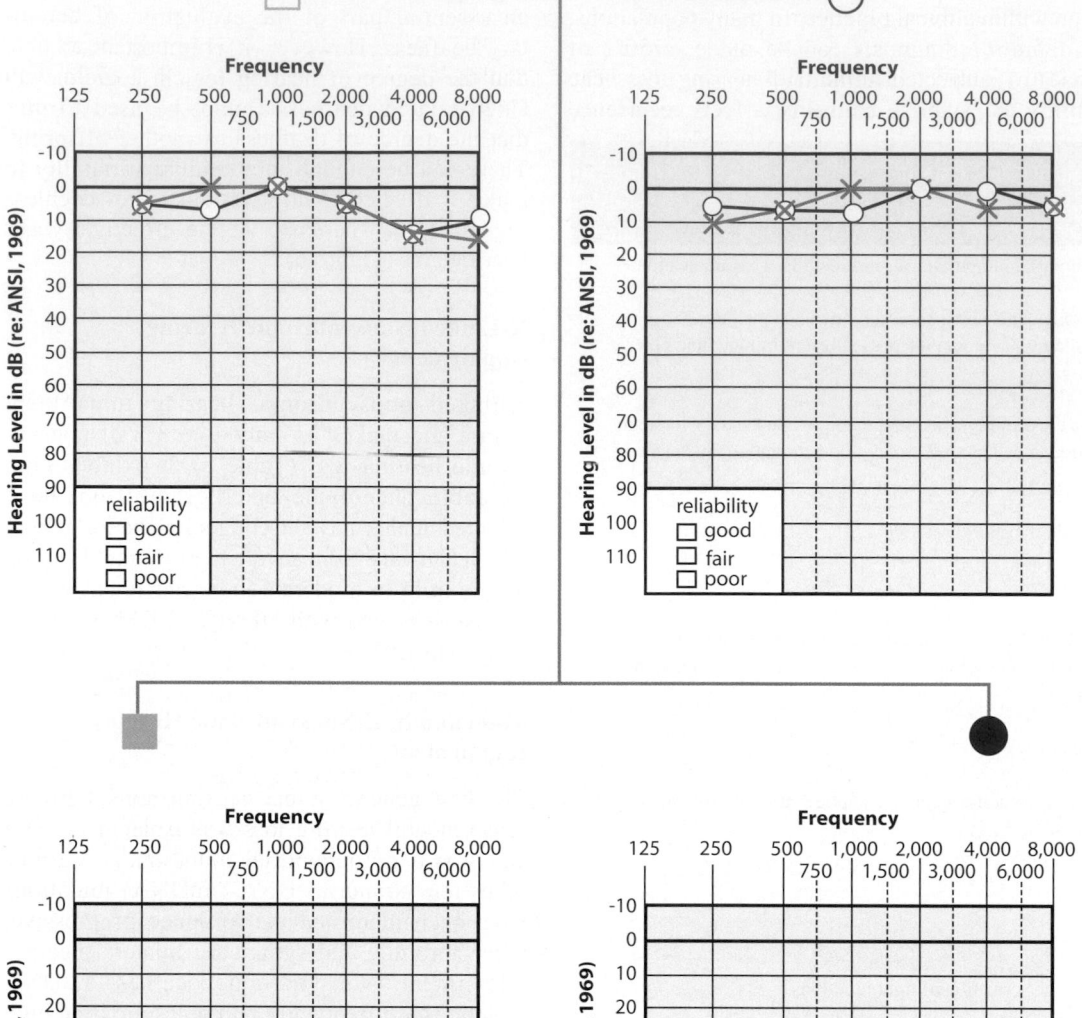

Figure 6 A pedigree of 2 siblings homozygous for the 35delG mutation in GJB2. Both parents have normal hearing. One sibling exhibits a profound sensorineural hearing loss and the other only a moderate hearing loss.

variability in both quantity and cellular location of these mutations.[190,191]

Familial Aminoglycoside Ototoxicity. Aminoglycoside antibiotics exert their antibacterial effects by binding to the 16S ribosomal RNA (rRNA) in the 30S subunit of the bacterial ribosome, thus leading to mistranslation or premature termination of protein synthesis.[192–194] However, use of these drugs can frequently lead to toxicity involving the renal, auditory, and vestibular systems[195,196] due to concentration in renal tubular cells and in the perilymph and endolymph of the inner ear.[197,198] Renal damage is usually reversible, however, the auditory and vestibular ototoxicity are often not.

In the United States alone, close to 4 million courses of aminoglycosides are administered each year.[199] It is estimated that at least 2 to 5%, and in some studies up to 25%, of patients treated with these antibiotics develop clinically significant hearing loss.[200–202] Numerous studies have documented that aminoglycoside hypersensitivity is often maternally transmitted[100] suggesting that mtDNA mutation(s) are involved in aminoglycoside ototoxicity.[203,204] Sequence analyses of the mitochondrial genome in patients with aminoglycoside ototoxicity have led to the identification of several ototoxic mtDNA mutations in the 12S rRNA gene: insertion or deletion at position 961, A1555G, and C1494T mutations.[205]

The 961 mutation localizes at the C-cluster of a region between loop 21 and 22 of 12S rRNA.[206] This region is not very evolutionarily conserved, nor is its function well defined specifically for possible interaction with aminoglycosides in bacterial homologs. Alteration of the tertiary or quaternary structure of this rRNA by the 961 mutation may indirectly affect the binding of aminoglycosides. Alternatively, this alteration may result in a mitochondrial translational defect.[207]

The A1555G mutation is one of the most common causes of aminoglycoside-induced deafness.[208–212] This mutation is homoplasmic in the affected or at-risk individual. The A1555G mutation is located at a highly conserved region of the 12S rRNA that is an essential part of the decoding site of the small ribosomal subunit[213–215] and is important for the action of aminoglycosides.[216–218] In particular, this mutation makes the 12S rRNA more similar to bacterial rRNA and thus a target for aminoglycoside binding.[208] This new G-C pair in 12S rRNA is also expected to create a binding site for aminoglycosides, which facilitates interaction with these drugs.[219] In the United States, over 15% of persons with aminoglycoside-induced hearing loss carry this mutation, a point of major clinical relevance for the prevention of aminoglycoside hearing loss.[220]

Recently, a homoplasmic C-to-T transition at position 1494 (C1494T) in the 12S rRNA gene was found in a large Chinese family with maternally transmitted aminoglycoside-induced and nonsyndromic deafness.[221] Maternal members of this family showed variable severity and age of onset for the hearing impairment. The C1494T mutation is expected to form a novel 1494U-A1555 base-pair, in the same position created by the deafness-linked A1555G mutation, at the highly conserved A-site of 12S rRNA. Since this site has been implicated as the main target of aminoglycoside toxicity, it is anticipated that this alteration in the tertiary structure of 12S rRNA may lead to sensitivity to aminoglycosides.

CLINICAL DIAGNOSIS OF HEARING IMPAIRMENT

History

An evaluation should be conducted as soon as hearing loss is suspected. Directed questions should focus on prenatal, perinatal, and postnatal history, specifically reviewing maternal illnesses, drug use, alcohol intake, and smoking. Recognized risk factors for hearing loss in the

Table 8 X-Linked Nonsyndromic Hearing Impairment Genes Cloned			
Locus	Location	Gene	Function of Encoded Protein
DFN1	Xq22	*TIMM8A*	A translocase involved in the import of metabolite transporters from the cytoplasm into the mitochondrial inner membrane

Adapted from reference 8.

perinatal period include low birth weight, prematurity, time spent in a neonatal intensive care unit, hyperbilirubinemia, sepsis, use of ototoxic medications, and birth hypoxia.[222–225] Risk factors in the postnatal period include viral illnesses such as mumps and measles as well as bacterial meningitis.[226] A record of speech and language milestones can establish whether the hearing loss is pre- or postlingual. However, even deaf infants coo and babble naturally up to the age of 6 months. A history of poor motor development may also indicate vestibular dysfunction.

An inquiry into hearing loss in first- and second-degree relatives is essential, especially if the loss started before the age of 30 years. Consanguinity or common origins from ethnically isolated areas should increase suspicion of hereditary deafness.[227,228] If there are a number of family members with hearing loss, constructing a pedigree may delineate the mode of inheritance.

Physical Examination

The majority of cases of hereditary hearing impairment are nonsyndromic, thus physical findings are often absent. However, even in cases of syndromic hearing impairment, physical findings may be subtle or hard to identify. Hence, the physical examination should include a general inspection and orderly evaluation of all systems. Careful notation should be made for hair color, the presence of a white forelock, facial symmetry, and skull shape. Fundoscopy and eye color and relative position should also be noted, taking specific biometric measurements in suspected cases of WS1. The ears should be examined for auricular pits or sinuses and skin tags. Note the shape and size of the pinnae, and check for abnormalities of the external ear canal and tympanic membrane. Observe the neck for branchial anomalies and thyroid enlargement as well as the oral cavity for possible clefts. Note the number, size, and shape of the digits and complete a thorough inspection of the skin for areas of pigmentation/hypopigmentation and café-au-lait spots. Do a complete neurologic examination, including tests of gait and balance to assess for vestibular function.

Audiology

In 2000, the Joint Committee on Infant Hearing endorsed universal newborn hearing screening (UNHS)[229] to provide hearing screening to all newborns before the age of 1 month, with confirmation of hearing loss in infants who do not pass the initial, or a subsequent screening, through an audiologic evaluation by the age of 3 months. Most children identified through this program have parents with normal hearing.

Hearing loss can be identified by several different complementary methods. Following the guidelines from the National Institutes of Health, all states in the United States have adopted UNHS, but testing algorithms and requirements vary. Another test of choice for infants and young children with suspected hearing impairment is the auditory brainstem response, which gives accurate hearing thresholds from 1 to 4 kHz.[230]

It is important to note that the UNHS may fail to identify children with progressive hearing loss, which accounts for approximately 15% of preschool children with SNHL.[231] The UNHS test is only the first step in a successful and cost-effective program. The main goal is early diagnosis and management, normal language development, and long-term success after intervention.

In older children or adults, a standard audiogram can be obtained. The presence or absence of hearing loss in other family members should be documented by formal audiometric testing.

Laboratory Testing

Laboratory testing should be individualized and directed toward the suspected diagnosis on the basis of history, physical examination, and age of the patient (Table 9). Such testing may include an IgM antibody assay in the first few years of life to assess the possibility of intrauterine infection, testing for hemoglobinopathies as these may be associated with SNHL, urinalysis and renal function tests in children with possible Alport syndrome, thyroid testing to rule out a deficiency, TSH and a perchlorate discharge test in suspected Pendred syndrome, and an evaluation of metabolic disorders such as lysosomal storage diseases.[231] An electrocardiogram to assess the QT interval should be performed if there is a history of syncopal episodes or a family history of sudden infant death syndrome (SIDS), as might be seen in JLNS.

Any evaluation of hearing loss requires a multidisciplinary approach, which should include counseling and support for parents. A recent survey revealed that identification of the cause of the hearing loss is the highest priority of parents who learn that their child is hearing impaired.[232]

Genetic Testing

In addition to UNHS and a general medical evaluation, genetic testing can provide direct benefits for patients and their families.[233] Defining the cause of a patient's hearing impairment through genetic testing will accomplish the following: (1) avoid unnecessary and costly testing; (2) allow accurate recurrence risk counseling; (3) dispel incorrect notions of what caused the hearing impairment; and (4) offer limited prognostic information and guide future medical management.

Samples used for testing can include peripheral blood and tissues, but also less invasive samples such as buccal cells obtained with a swab or part of the blood spots collected for newborn screening. Mutation scanning methods need to be fully optimized to create reproducible results. Depending on the technique, conditions, and level of expertise, some of these methods are general screening methods and can therefore miss certain mutations. Sequencing is the most all-inclusive method for it can detect almost all point mutations as well as small deletions and insertions.[234]

Table 9 Evaluation by Age of Onset

Type of Evaluation	Neonate/Infant	Child/Adolescent	Adult
To rule out acquired causes of HI	High-risk register Viral titers Viral cultures (urine, throat) Syphilis serology	Viral titers Syphilis serology	Viral titers Syphilis serology
Audiology and vestibular testing	Impedance testing ABR testing Otoacoustic emissions	Impedance testing Behavioral audiometry Conventional audiometry ABR Balancing testing	Impedance testing Conventional audiometry Cortical evoked response audiometry Electronystagmographic testing
Chromosomal karyotyping	Dysmorphic features History of miscarriage	Dysmorphic features Mental retardation	
Radiology	Temporal bone CT Renal ultrasonography	Temporal bone CT Renal ultrasonography	Temporal bone CT MRI of CP angle if hearing asymmetry
Ophthalmologic testing	Fundoscopy (CMV retinopathy)	Fundoscopy ERG	Fundoscopy ERG
Neurologic tests		Syndromes associated with mental retardation	Ataxia and neuropathies
Cardiac testing	ECG (Jervell and Lange-Nielsen syndrome)	ECG	
Dental evaluation		Osteogenesis imperfecta	
Renal evaluation	Ultrasonography (BOR)	Urine protein (Alport syndrome) Urine dermatan sulfate, heparin suppurate (mucopolysaccharidoses)	Urine protein Ultrasonography

HI = hearing impairment; ABR = auditory brainstem response; CT = computed tomography; MRI = magnetic resonance imaging; CP = cerebellopontine; CMV = cytomegalovirus; ERG = electroretinography; ECG = electrocardiography; BOR = branchio-oto-renal syndrome.

Radiology

Every patient with unexplained hearing loss should also have a renal ultrasound and neuroimaging of the temporal bone. Computed tomography is the best radiologic test for the evaluation of hearing impairment with the incidence of anatomic abnormalities, such as Mondini malformation or dilated vestibular aqueduct, ranging from 6.8 to 28.4%.[235,236] An MRI may be used to visualize the acoustic nerve, exclude aplasia, and rule out infectious inner ear destruction and is especially important before cochlear implant surgery.[225]

Other Consultations

An ophthalmologic opinion should be obtained in all children with severe-to-profound hearing impairment as half of children with severe to profound hearing loss have concomitant ocular abnormalities.[237] Although most of these abnormalities are refractive errors, the correction of which is essential, ERG may uncover signs of early RP. Referral to a clinical geneticist should be requested to ensure that parents and patients adequately understand the issues such as recurrence risk.

Management of Hearing Impairment

Hearing impairment is the only sensory defect that can be treated successfully even if the hearing loss is complete. Early identification of hearing impairment in infants and young children is essential for the development of age-appropriate speech and language skills. Children whose hearing losses are identified and in whom intervention is instituted before 6 months of age show that an almost age-appropriate level of language skills can be accomplished.[234,238] The level of habilitative intervention that is required depends on the degree of hearing impairment. Counseling of the family, proper hearing aid selection, hearing aid fitting, and continued audiologic assessment are important. While very few families now choose for their child to not receive a cochlear implant, the vast majory of children with prelingual or postlingual deafness now receive cochlear implants to rehabilitate syndromic and nonsyndromic hearing impairment, which has proven to be highly beneficial.[239] The criteria for cochlear and auditory brainstem implantation are reviewed in Chapter 32, "Cochlear Implantation." Schools that are focused on auditory oriented education are emerging as optimal for developing early speech and language acquisition and production, although total communication programs using combinations sign language and oral–aural remain as options. It is important for the physician to remain supportive of parental choice regarding the means for rehabilitation.

A variety of support systems exist, particularly on the World Wide Web. In the United States, the National Institute on Deafness and other Communication Disorders disseminates information on hearing impairment to professionals and families on their website, http://www.nidcd.nih.gov.

The site also contains information for individuals interested in supporting and participating in research projects and lists resources and links to other organizations.

FUTURE DEVELOPMENTS

Rapid advances in genetics and molecular biology have transformed the field of hearing loss and deafness. Genetic tests are now less expensive than ever before and available to the general population, thus making detection and treatment of hearing impairment possible for infants as young as 1 month. Furthermore, it has become easier to identify patients who are at risk for environmental damage to their hearing from noise, drugs and aging, and they too can be cared for accordingly. Molecular testing is beginning to become the first step in determination of the underlying etiology of hearing impairment and the use of these tests may impact management decisions by better defining therapeutic and habilitative options. As clinical management becomes more sophisticated, continued growth in science and technology will allow physicians to offer new, practical, and effective treatments for sensorineural hearing impairment.

REFERENCES

1. Morton NE. Genetic epidemiology of hearing impairment. Ann NY Acad Sci 1991;630:16–31.
2. Marazita ML, Ploughman LM, Rawlings B, et al. Genetic epidemiological studies of early-onset deafness in the U.S. school-age population. Am J Genet 1993;46:486–91.
3. Sank D, Kallman FJ. The role of heredity in early total deafness. Volta Rev 1963;65:461.
4. Brown KS. The genetics of childhood deafness. In: McConnell F, Ward PH, editors. Deafness in Childhood. Nashville, TN: Vanderbilt University Press; 1967. p. 177–202.
5. Anderson S, Bankier AT, Barrell BG, et al. Sequence and organization of the human mitochondrial genome. Nature 1981;290:457–65.
6. Jaber L, Shohat M, Bu X, et al. Sensorineural deafness inherited as a tissue specific mitochondrial disorder. J Med Genet 1992;29:86–90.
7. Grundfast KM. Hereditary hearing impairment in children. Adv Otolaryngol Head Neck Surg 1993;7:29–43.
8. Van Camp G, Smith RJH. Hereditary hearing loss home page. Available at http://webhost.ua.ac.be/hhh/. Accessed July 2006.
9. Melnick M, Bixler D, Silk K, et al. Autosomal dominant branchiootorenal dysplasia. Birth Defects Original Article Ser 1975;5:121–8.
10. Fraser FC, Ling D, Clogg D, Nogrady B. Genetic aspects of the BOR syndrome-branchial fistulas, ear pits, hearing loss, and renal anomalies. Am J Med Genet 1978;2:241–52.
11. Fraser FC, Sproule JR, Halal F. Frequency of the branchio-oto-renal (BOR) syndrome in children with profound hearing loss. Am J Med Genet 1980;7:341–9.
12. Heimler A, Lieber E. Branchio-oto-renal syndrome: Reduced penetrance and variable expressivity in four generations of a large kindred. Am J Med Genet 1986;25:15–27.
13. Konig R, Fuchs S, Dukiet C. Branchio-oto-renal (BOR) syndrome: Variable expressivity in a five-generation pedigree. Eur J Pediatr 1994;153:446–50.
14. Stratakis CA, Lin J-P, Rennert OM. Description of a large kindred with autosomal dominant inheritance of branchial arch anomalies, hearing loss and ear pits, and exclusion of the branchio-oto-renal (BOR) syndrome gene locus (chromosome 8q13.3). Am J Med Genet 1998;79:209–14.
15. Chen A, Francis M, Ni L, et al. Phenotypic manifestations of branchiootorenal syndrome. Am J Med Genet 1995;58:365–70.
16. Smith RJ, Schwartz C. Branchio-oto-renal syndrome. J Commun Disord 1998;31:411–20.
17. Cremers CWRJ, Fikkers-van Noord M. The earpits-deafness syndrome: Clinical and genetic aspects. Int J Pediatr Otorhinolaryngol 1980;2:309–22.
18. Gimsing S, Dyrmose J. Branchio-oto-renal dysplasia in three families. Ann Otol Rhinol Laryngol 1986;95:421–6.
19. Kumar S, Cremers CW, Kenyon JB, et al. Autosomal dominant branchio-oto-renal syndrome—localization of a disease gene to chromosome 8q by linkage in a Dutch family. Hum Mol Genet 1992;1:491–5.
20. Smith RJH, Ankerstjerne JKE, Capper DT, et al. Localization of the gene for branchio-oto-renal syndrome to chromosome 8q. Genomics 1992;14:843–4.
21. Kalatzis V, Sahly I, El Amraoui A, Petit C. Eya1 expression in the developing ear and kidney: Towards the understanding of the pathogenesis of branchio-oto-renal (BOR) syndrome. Dev Dyn 1998;213:486–99.
22. Kumar S, Deffenbacher K, Marres HA, et al. Genomewide search and genetic localization of a second gene associated with autosomal dominant branchio-oto-renal syndrome: Clinical and genetic implications. Am J Hum Genet 2000;5:1715–20.
23. Ruf RG, Berkman J, Wolf MT, et al. A gene locus for branchio-otic syndrome maps to chromosome 14q21.3-q24.3. J Med Genet 2003;40:515–9.
24. Ruf RG, Xu PX, Silvius D, et al. SIX1 mutations cause branchio-oto-renal syndrome by disruption of EYA1-SIX1-DNA complexes. Proc Natl Acad Sci USA 2004;101:8090–5.
25. Crouzon O. Dystose cranio-faciale hereditaire. Bull Mem Soc Med Hop Paris 1912;33:545–5.
26. Carinci F, Avantaggiato A, Curioni C. Crouzon syndrome: Cephalometric analysis and evaluation of pathogenesis. Cleft Palate Craniofac J 1994;31:201–9.
27. Cohen MM, editor. Craniosynostosis: Diagnosis, Evaluation and Management. New York: Raven Press;1986. p. 480.
28. Cohen MM, Krieborg S. Birth prevalence studies of the Crouzon syndrome: Comparison of direct and indirect methods. Clin Genet 1992;41:12–5.
29. Orvidas LJ, Fabry LB, Diavoca S, McDonald TJ. Hearing and otopathology in Crouzon syndrome. Laryngoscope 1999;109:1372–5.
30. Hollway GE, Suthers GK, Hann EA, et al. Mutation detection in FGFR2 craniosynostosis syndromes. Hum Genet 1997;99:251–5.
31. Reardon W, Winter RM, Rutland P, et al. Mutations in the fibroblast growth factor receptor 2 gene causes Crouzon syndrome. Nat Genet 1994;8:98–103.
32. Rutland P, Pulleyn LJ, Reardon W, et al. Identical mutations in the FGFR2 gene cause both Pfeiffer and Crouzon syndrome phenotypes. Nat Genet 1995;9:173–6.
33. AbBou-Sleiman PM, Apessos A, Harper JC, et al. Pregnancy following preimplantation genetic diagnosis for Crouzon syndrome. Mol Hum Reprod 2002;8:304–9.
34. NIH consensus Development Conference. Neurofibromatosis: Conference statement. Arch Neurol 1988;45:475–8.
35. Yohay K. Neurofibromatosis types 1 and 2. 1 Neurologist 2006;2:86–93.
36. Gijtenbeek JM, Gabreels-Festen AA, Lammens M, et al. Mononeuropathy multiplex as the initial manifestation of neurofibromatosis type 2. Neurology 2001;56:1766–8.
37. Trofatter JA, MacCollins MM, Rutter JL, et al. A novel moesin-, ezrin-, radixin-like gene is a candidate for the neurofibromatosis 2 tumor suppressor. Cell 1993;72:791–800.
38. Gusella JF, Ramesh V, MacCollin M, Jacoby LB. Merlin: The neurofibromatosis 2 tumor suppressor. Biochim Biophys Acta 1999;1423:M29–36.
39. Kluwe L, Mautner VF. A missense mutation in the NF2 gene results in moderate and mild clinical phenotypes of neurofibromatosis type 2. Hum Genet 1996;97:224–7.
40. Evans DG, Trueman L, Wallace A, et al. Genotype/phenotype correlations in type 2 neurofibromatosis (NF2): Evidence for more severe disease associated with truncating mutations. J Med Genet 1998;35:450–5.
41. Knowlton RG, Weaver EJ, Struyk AF, et al. Genetic linkage analysis of hereditary arthro-opthalmopathy (Stickler Syndrome) and the type II collagen procollagen gene. Am J Hum Genet 1989;45:681–8.
42. Ahmad NN, Ala-Kokko L, Knowlton RG, et al. Stop codon in the procollagen II gene (COL2A1) in a family with Stickler syndrome (arthro-opthalmology). Procl Natl Acad Sci U S A 1991;88:6624–7.
43. Winterpracht A, Hilbert M, Schwarze U, et al. Kniest and Stickler dysplasia phenotypes caused by collagen type II gene (COL2A1) defect. Nat Genet 1993;3:323–6.
44. Williams CJ, Ganguly A, Considine E, et al. A-2→G transition at the 3′ acceptor splice site of IVS17 characterizes the COL2A1 gene mutation in the original Stickler syndrome kindred. Am J Med Genet 1996;63:461–7.

45. Vikkula M, Mariman EC, Lui VC, et al. Autosomal dominant and recessive osteochondrodysplasias associated with the COL11A2 locus. Cell 1995;80:431–7.

46. Richards AJ, Yates JR, Williams R, et al. A family with Stickler syndrome type 2 has a mutation in the COL11A1 gene resulting in the substitution of glycine 97 by valine in alpha 1 (XI) collagen. Hum Mol Genet 1996;5:1339–43.

47. Wilkin DJ, Mortier GR, Johnson CL, et al. Correlation of linkage data with phenotype in eight families with Stickler syndrome. Am J Med Genet 1998;80:121–7.

48. Lisi V, Guala A, Lopez A, et al. Linkage analysis for prenatal diagnosis in a familial case of Stickler syndrome. Genet Couns 2002;13:163–70.

49. Liberfarb RM, Levy HP, Peter SR, et al. The Stickler syndrome: Genotype/phenotype correlation in 10 families with Stickler syndrome resulting from 7 mutations in the type II collagen gene locus COL2A1. Genet Med 2003;5:21–7.

50. Rovin S, Dachi SF, Borenstein DB, Cotter WB. Mandibulofacial dysostosis, a familial study of five generations. J Pediatr 1964;65:215–21.

51. Sando I, Hemenway WG, Morgan WR. Histopathology of the temporal bones in mandibulofacial dysostosis. Trans Am Acad Ophthalmol Otolaryngol 1968;72:913–24.

52. Jahrsdoerfer RA, Jacobson JT. Treacher Collins syndrome: Otologic and auditory management. J Am Acad Audiol 1995;6:93–102.

53. Jabs EW, Li X, Coss CA, et al. Mapping Treacher Collins syndrome locus to 5q31.3-q33.3. Genomics 1991;11:193–8.

54. Isaac C, Marsh KL, Paznekas WA, et al. Characterization of the nucleolar gene product, treacle, in Treacher Collins syndrome. Mol Biol Cell 2000;11:3061–71.

55. Edwards SJ, Gladwin AJ, Dixon MJ. The mutational spectrum in Treacher Collins syndrome reveals a predominance of mutations that create a premature-termination codon. Am J Hum Genet 1997;60:515–24.

56. Wise CA, Chiang LC, Paznekas WA, et al. TCOF1 gene encodes a putative nucleolar phosphoprotein that exhibits mutations in Treacher Collins syndrome throughout its coding region. Proc Nat Acad Sci U S A 1997;94:3110–5.

57. Marsh KL, Dixon J, Dixon MJ. Mutations in Treacher Collins syndrome gene lead to mislocalization of the nucleolar protein treacle. Hum Mol Genet 1998;1795–800.

58. Teber OA, Gillessen-Kaesbach G, Fischer S, et al. Genotyping in 46 patients with tentative diagnosis of Treacher Collins syndrome revealed unexpected phenotypic variation. Europ J Hum Genet 2004;12:879–90.

59. Waardenburg PJ. A new syndrome combining developmental anomalies of the eyelids, eyebrows, and nose root with pigmentary defects of the iris and head hair and with congenital deafness. Am J Hum Genet 1951;3:195–253.

60. Read AP, Newton VE. Waardenburg syndrome. J Med Genet 1997;34:656–65.

61. Steel KP, Barkway C. Another role for melanocytes: Their importance for normal stria vascularis development in the mammalian inner ear. Development 1989;107:453–63.

62. Farrer LA, Grundfast KM, Amos J, et al. Waardenburg syndrome (WS) type I is caused by defects at multiple loci, one of which is near ALPP on chromosome 2: First report of the WS consortium. Am J Hum Genet 1992;50:902–13.

63. Liu XZ, Newton VE. Hearing loss and Waardenburg's syndrome: Implications for genetic counselling. J Laryngol Otol 1990;104:97–103.

64. Baldwin CT, Hoth CF, Amos JA, et al. An exonic mutation in HuP2 paired domain gene causes Waardenburg's syndrome. Nature 1992;355:637–8.

65. Tassabehji M, Read AP, Newton VE, et al. Waardenburg's syndrome patients have mutations in the human homologue of Pax-3 paired box gene. Nature 1992;355:635–6.

66. Hoth CF, Milunsky A, Lipsky N, et al. Mutations in the paired domain of the human PAX3 gene cause Klein–Waardenburg syndrome (WS-III) as well as Waardenburg syndrome type I (WS-I). Am J Hum Genet 1993;52:455–62.

67. Tassabehji M, Newton VE, Read AP. Waardenburg syndrome type 2 caused by mutations in the human microphthalmia (MITF) gene. Nat Genet 1994;8:251–5.

68. Sánchez-Martín M, Rodríguez-García A, Pérez-Losada J, et al. SLUG (SNAI2) deletions in patients with Waardenburg disease. Hum Mol Genet 2002;11:3231–6.

69. Puffenberger EG, Hosoda K, Washington SS, et al. A missense mutation of the endothelin-B receptor gene in multigenic Hirschsprung's disease. Cell 1994;79:1257–66.

70. Syrris P, Carter ND, Patton MA. Novel nonsense mutation of the endothelin-B receptor gene in a family with Waardenburg–Hirschsprung disease. Am J Med Genet 1999;87:69–71.

71. Edery P, Attie T, Amiel J, et al. Mutation of the endothelin-3 gene in the Waardenburg–Hirschsprung phenotype (Shah–Waardenburg syndrome). Nat Genet 1996;12:442–4.

72. Hofstra RM, Osinga J, Tan-Sindhunata G, et al. A homozygous mutation in the endothelin-3 gene associated with a combined Waardenburg type 2 and Hirschsprung phenotype (Shah–Waardenburg syndrome). Nat Genet 1996;12:445–7.

73. Pingault V, Bondurand N, Kuhlbrodt K, et al. SOX10 mutations in patients with Waardenburg–Hirschsprung disease. Nat Genet 1998;18:171–3.

74. Pomponio RJ, Reynolds TR, Cole H, et al. Mutational hotspot in the human biotinidase gene causes profound biotinidase deficiency. Nat Genet 1995;11:96–8.

75. Wolf B, Grier RE, Allen RJ, et al. Biotinidase deficiency: The enzymatic defect in late-onset multiple carboxylase deficiency. Clin Chim Acta 1983;131:273–81.

76. Wolf B, Grier RE, Allen RJ, et al. Phenotypic variation in biotinidase deficiency. J Pediat 1983;103:233–7.

77. Wolf B, Heard GS, Weissbecker KA, et al. Biotinidase deficiency: Initial clinical features and rapid diagnosis. Ann Neurol 1985;18:614–7.

78. Wolf B, Spencer R, Gleason T. Hearing loss is a common feature of symptomatic children with profound biotinidase deficiency. J Pediatr 2002;140:242–6.

79. Wolf B. Disorders of biotin metabolism. In: Scriver CR, Beaudet AL, Sly WS, Valle D, editors. The Metabolic and Molecular Bases of Inherited Disease, volume II. New York: McGraw-Hill; 1995. p. 3151–80.

80. Heard GS, Annison EF. Gastrointestinal absorption of vitamin B-6 in the chicken (Gallus domesticus). J Nutr 1986;116:107–20.

81. Wolf B. Worldwide survey of neonatal screening for biotinidase deficiency. J Inherit Metab Dis 1991;14:923–7.

82. Nance W. The genetics of deafness. Men Ret Dev Disabil Res Rev 2003;9.109–19.

83. Jervell A, Lange-Nielsen F. Congenital deaf-mutism, functional heart disease with prolongation of the Q-T interval and sudden death. Am Heart J 1957;54:59–68.

84. Tranebjaerg L, Bathen J, Tyson J, Bitner-Glindzicz M. Jervell and Lange-Nielsen syndrome: A Norwegian perspective. Am J Med Genet 1999;89:137–46.

85. Neyroud N, Tesson F, Denjoy I, et al. A novel mutation in the potassium channel gene KVLTQ1 causes Jervell Lange-Nielsen cardioauditory syndrome. Nat Genet 1997;15:186–9.

86. Schulze-Bahr E, Wang Q, Wedekind H, et al. KCNE1 mutations cause Jervell and Lange-Nielsen syndrome. Nat Genet 1997;17:267–8.

87. Tyson J, Tranebjaerg L, Bellman S, et al. IsK and KvLQT1: Mutation in either of the two subunits of the slow component of the delayed rectifier potassium channel can cause Jervell and Lange-Nielsen syndrome. Hum Mol Genet 1997;6:2179–85.

88. Fraser GR. Association of congenital deafness with goiter (Pendred's syndrome): A study of 207 families. Ann Hum Genet 1965;28:201–49.

89. Marres HA. Congenital abnormalities of the inner ear. In: Ludman H, Wright T, editors. Diseases of the Ear. Bath (U K): Arnold & Oxford University Press; 1998. p. 288–96.

90. Phelps PD, Coffey RA, Trembath RC, et al. Radiological malformations of the ear in Pendred syndrome. Clin Radiol 1998;53:268–73.

91. Reardon W, O'Mahoney CF, Trembath R, et al. Enlarged vestibular aqueduct: A radiological marker of pendred syndrome, and mutation of the PDS gene. QJM 2000;93:99–104.

92. Everett LA, Glaser B, Beck JC, et al. Pendred syndrome is caused by mutations in a putative sulphate transporter gene (PDS). Nat Genet 1997;17:411–22.

93. Scott DA, Wang R, Kreman TM, et al. The Pendred syndrome gene encodes a chloride-iodide transport protein. Nat Genet 1999;21:440–3.

94. Royaux IE, Suzuki K, Mori A, et al. Pendrin, the protein encoded by the Pendred syndrome gene (PDS), is an apical porter of iodide in the thyroid and is regulated by thyroglobulin in FRTL-5 cells. Endocrinol 2000;141:839–45.

95. Bidart JM, Mian C, Lazar V, et al. Expression of pendrin and the Pendred syndrome (PDS) gene in human thyroid tissues. J Clin Endocrinol Metab 2000;85:2028–33.

96. Scott DA, Karniski LP. Human pendrin expressed in Xenopus laevis oocytes mediates chloride/formate exchange. Am J Physiol 2000;278:C207–11.

97. Royaux IE, Wall SM, Karniski LP, et al. Pendrin, encoded by the Pendred syndrome gene, resides in the apical region of renal intercalated cells and mediates bicarbonate secretion. Proc Natl Acad Sci U S A 2001;98:4221–6.

98. Everett LA, Belyantseva IA, Noben-Trauth K, et al. Targeted disruption of mouse Pds provides insight about the inner-ear defects encountered in Pendred syndrome. Hum Mol Genet 2001;10:153–61.

99. Campbell C, Cucci RA, Prasad S, et al. Pendred syndrome, DFNB4, and PDS/SLC26A4 identification of eight novel mutations and possible genotype–phenotype correlations. Hum Mutat 2001;17:403–11.

100. Coyle B, Reardon W, Herbrick JA, et al. Molecular analysis of the PDS gene in Pendred syndrome. Hum Mol Genet 1998;7:1105–12.

101. Usami S, Abe S, Weston MD, et al. Non-syndromic hearing loss associated with enlarged vestibular aqueduct is caused by PDS mutations. Hum Genet 1999;104:188–92.

102. Coucke PJ, Van Hauwe P, Everett LA, et al. Identification of two mutations in the PDS gene in an inbred family with Pendred syndrome. J Med Genet 1999;36:475–7.

103. Li XC, Everett LA, Lalwani AK, et al. A mutation in PDS causes non-syndromic recessive deafness. Nat Genet 1998;18:215–7.

104. Gonzales Trevino O, Karamanoglu Arseven O, Ceballos CJ, et al. Clinical and molecular analysis of three Mexican families with Pendred's syndrome. Eur J Endocrinol 2001;144:585–93.

105. Rosenberg T, Haim M, Hauch AM, Parving A. The prevalence of Usher syndrome and other retinal dystrophy-hearing impairment associations. Clin Genet 1997;51:314–21.

106. Keats B, Corey DP. The Usher syndromes. Am J Med Genet 1999;89:158–166.

107. Grondahl J, Mjoen S. Usher syndrome in four Norwegian counties. Clin Genet 1986;30:14–28.

108. Kimberling WJ, Moller CG, Davenport SL, et al. Usher syndrome: Clinical findings and gene localization studies. Laryngoscope 1989;99:66–72.

109. Loundon N, Marlin S, Busquet D, et al. Usher syndrome and cochlear implantation. Otol Neurotol 2003;24:216–21.

110. Petit C. Usher syndrome: From genetics to pathogenesis. Annu Rev Genom Hum Genet 2001;2:271–97.

111. Keats B, Savas S. Genetic heterogeneity in Usher syndrome. Am J Med Genet 2004;130A:13–6.

112. Fishman GA, Kumar A, Joseph ME, et al. Usher's syndrome. Ophthalmic and neuro-otologic findings suggesting genetic heterogeneity. Arch Ophthalmol 1983;101:1367–74.

113. Cherry PM. Usher's syndrome. Ann Ophthalmol 1973;5:743–52.

114. Young NM, Mets MB, Hain TC. Early diagnosis of Usher syndrome in infants and children. Am J Otol 1996;17:30–4.

115. Kaplan J, Gerber S, Bonneau D, et al. A gene for Usher syndrome type 1 (USH1) maps to chromosome 14q. Genomics 1992;14:979–88.

116. Smith RJ, Lee EC, Kimberling WJ, et al. Localization of two genes for Usher syndrome type I to chromosome 11. Genomics 1992;14:995–1002.

117. Sankila EM, Pakarinen L, Kaariainen H, et al. Assignment of an Usher syndrome type III (USH3) gene to chromosome 3q. Hum Mol Genet 1995;4:93–8.

118. Wayne S, Der Kaloustian VM, Schloss M, et al. Localization of the Usher syndrome type ID gene (USH1D) to chromosome 10. Hum Mol Genet 1996;5:1689–92.

119. Kimberling WJ, Weston MD, Moller C, et al. Localization of Usher syndrome type II to chromosome 1q. Genomics 1990;7:245–9.

120. Hmani M, Ghorbel A, Boulila-Elgaied A, et al. A novel locus for Usher syndrome type II, USH2B, maps to chromosome 3 at p23-24.2. Eur J Hum Genet 1999;7:363–7.

121. Weil D, Blanchard S, Kaplan J, et al. Defective myosin VIIA gene responsible for Usher syndrome type 1B. Nature 1995;374:60–1.

122. Verpy E, Leibovici M, Zwaenepoel I, et al. A defect in harmonin, a PDZ domain-containing protein expressed in the inner ear sensory hair cells, underlies Usher syndrome type 1C. Nat Genet 2000;26:51–5.

123. Eudy JD, Weston MD, Yao S, et al. Mutation of a gene encoding protein with extracellular matrix motifs in Usher syndrome type IIa. Science 1998;280:1753–7.

124. Weston MD, Eudy JD, Fujita S, et al. Genomic structure and identification of novel mutations in usherin, the gene responsible for Usher syndrome type IIa. Am J Hum Genet 2000;66:1199–210.

125. Kikkawa Y, Shitara H, Wakana S, et al. Mutations in a new scaffold protein Sans cause deafness in Jackson shaker mice. Hum Mol Genet 2003;12:453–61.

126. Weil D, El Amraoui A, Masmoudi S, et al. Usher syndrome type I G (USH1G) is caused by mutations in the gene encoding SANS, a protein that associates with the USH1C protein, harmonin. Hum Mol Genet 2003;12:463–71.

127. Boeda B, El-Amraoui A, Bahloul A, et al. Myosin VIIa, harmonin and cadherin 23, three Usher I gene products that cooperate to shape the sensory hair cell bundle. EMBO J 2002;21:6689–99.

128. Siemens J, Kazmierczak P, Reynolds A, et al. The Usher syndrome proteins cadherin 23 and harmonin form a complex by means of PDZ-domain interactions. Proc Natl Acad Sci U S A 2002;99:14946–51.

129. Huang D, Eudy JD, Uzvolgyi E, et al. Identification of the mouse and rat orthologs of the gene mutated in Usher syndrome type IIA and the cellular source of USH2A mRNA in retina, a target tissue of the disease. Genomics 2002;80:195–203.

130. Liu XZ, Hope C, Liang CY, et al. A mutation (2314delG) in Usher syndrome type IIA gene: High prevalence and phenotypic variation. Am J Hum Genet 1999;64:1221–5.

131. Alport AC. Hereditary familial congenital haemorrhagic nephritis. Br Med J 1927;1:504–6.

132. Flinter FA, Cameron JS, Chantler C, et al. Genetics of classic Alport's syndrome. Lancet 1988;2:1005–7.

133. Flinter F. Alport's syndrome. J Med Genet 1997;34:326–30.

134. Govan J. Ocular manifestations of Alport's syndrome: A hereditary disorder of basement membranes? Br J Ophthalmol 1983;67:493–503.

135. Barker DF, Hostikka SL, Zhou J, et al. Identification of mutations in the COL4A5 collagen gene in Alport syndrome. Science 1990;248:1224–7.

136. Lemmink HH, Schroder CH, Monnens LA, Smeets HJ. The clinical spectrum of type IV collagen mutations. Hum Mutat 1997;9:477–99.

137. Nance WE, Setleff R, McLeod A, et al. X-Linked mixed deafness with congenital fixation of the stapedial footplate and perilymphatic gusher. Birth Defects Orig Artic Ser 1971;7:64–9.

138. Cremers CW, Hombergen GC, Scaf JJ, et al. X-linked progressive mixed deafness with perilymphatic gusher during stapes surgery. Arch Otolaryngol 1985;111:249–54.

139. Glasscock ME. The stapes gusher. Arch Otolaryngol 1973;98:82–91.

140. Cremers CW, Snik AF, Huygen PL, et al. X-linked mixed deafness syndrome with congenital fixation of the stapedial footplate and perilymphatic gusher (DFN3). Adv Oto-rhino-laryngol 2002;61:161–7.

141. De Kok YJM, van der Maarel SM, Bitner-Glindzicz M, et al. Association between X-linked mixed deafness and mutations in the POU domain gene POU3F4. Science 1995;267:685–8.

142. Berger W, van de Pol D, Warburg M, et al. Mutations in the candidate gene for Norrie disease. Hum Mol Genet 1992;1:461–5.

143. Rehm HL, Zhang DS, Brown MC, et al. Vascular defects and sensorineural deafness in a mouse model of Norrie disease. J Neurosci 2002;22:4286–92.

144. Kearns TP, Sayre GP. Retinitis pigmentosa, external ophthalmoplegia and complete heart block. Arch Ophthalmol 1958;60:280–9.

145. Zeviani M, Moraes CT, DiMauro S, et al. Deletions of mitochondrial DNA in Kearns-Sayre syndrome. Neurology 1988;38:1339–46.

146. Kadowaki H, Tobe K, Mori Y, et al. Mitochondrial gene mutation and insulin-deficient type of diabetes mellitus. Lancet 1993; 341:893–4.

147. van den Ouweland J, Lemkes H, Ruitenbeek W, et al. Mutation in mitochondrial tRNA (Leu)((UUR)) gene in a large pedigree with maternally transmitted type II diabetes mellitus and deafness. Nat Genet 1992;1:368–71.

148. Guillausseau PJ, Massin P, Dubois-LaForgue D, et al. Maternally inherited diabetes and deafness: A multicenter study. Ann Intern Med 2001;134:721–8.

149. Tamagawa Y, Kitamura K, Hagiwara H, et al. Audiologic findings in patients with a point mutation at nucleotide 3,243 of mitochondrial DNA. Ann Otol Rhinol Laryngol 1997;106:338–42.

150. Raut V, Sinnathuray AR, Toner JG. Cochlear implantation in maternally inherited diabetes and deafness syndrome. J Laryngol Otol 2002;116:373–5.

151. Guillausseau PJ, Dubois-Laforgue D, Massin P, et al. Heterogeneity of diabetes phenotype in patients with 3243 bp mutation of mitochondrial DNA (maternally inherited diabetes and deafness or MIDD). Diabetes Metabol 2004;30:181–6.

152. Pavlakis SG, Phillips PC, DiMauro S, et al. Mitochondrial myopathy, encephalopathy, lactic acidosis, and stroke-like episodes: A distinctive clinical syndrome. Ann Neurol 1984;16:481–8.

153. Montagna P, Gallassi R, Medori R, et al. MELAS syndrome: Characteristic migrainous and epileptic features and maternal transmission. Neurology 1988;38:751–4.

154. Donovan TJ. Mitochondrial encephalomyopathy: A rare genetic cause of sensorineural hearing loss. Ann Otol Rhinol Laryngol 1995;104:786–92.

155. Chinnery PF, Elliott C, Green GR, et al. The spectrum of hearing loss due to mitochondrial DNA defects. Brain 2000;123:82–92.

156. Swift AC, Singh SD. Hearing impairment and the Kearns–Sayre syndrome. J Laryngol Otol 1998;102:626–7.

157. Vernham GA, Reid FM, Rundle PA, Jacobs HT. Bilateral sensorineural hearing loss in members of a maternal lineage with a mitochondrial point mutation. Clin Otolaryngol Allied Sci 1994;19:314–9.

158. Nadol J, Merchant SN. Histopathology and molecular genetics of hearing loss in the human. Int J Pediatr Otorhinolaryngol 2001;61:1–15.

159. Shoffner JM, Wallace DC. Mitochondrial genetics: Principles and practice (Editorial). Am J Hum Genet 1992;51:1179–86.

160. Wallace DC, Zheng X, Lott MT, et al. Familial mitochondrial encephalomyopathy (MERRF): Genetic, pathophysiological, and biochemical characterization of a mitochondrial DNA disease. Cell 1988;55:601–10.

161. Bindoff LA, Desnuelle C, Birch-Machin MA, et al. Multiple defects of the mitochondrial respiratory chain in a mitochondrial encephalopathy (MERRF): A clinical, biochemical and molecular study. J Neurol Sci 1991;102:17–24.

162. Van Laer L, McGuirt WT, Yang T, et al. Autosomal dominant nonsyndromic hearing impairment. Am J Med Genet 1999;89:167–74.

163. Petersen MB. Non-syndromic autosomal dominant deafness. Clin Genet 2002;62:1–13.

164. Lalwani AK, Castelein CM. Cracking the auditory genetic code: Nonsyndromic hereditary hearing impairment. Am J Otol 1999;20:115–32.

165. Petit C. Genes responsible for human hereditary deafness: Symphony of a thousand. Nat Genet 1996;14:385–91.

166. Guilford P, Ben Arab S, Blanchard S, et al. A non-syndromic form of neurosensory, recessive deafness maps to the pericentromeric region of chromosome 13q. Nat Genet 1994;6:24–8.

167. Kelsell DP, Dunlop J, Stevens HP, et al. Connexin 26 mutations in hereditary nonsyndromic sensorineural deafness. Nature 1997;387:80–3.

168. Kumar NM, Gilula NB. The gap junction communication channel. Cell 1996;84:381–8.

169. Holt JR, Corey DP. Ion channel defects in hereditary hearing loss. Neuron 1999;22:217–9.

170. Steel KP. The benefits of recycling. Science 1999;285:1363–4.

171. Rabionet R, Gasparini P, Estivill X. Molecular genetics of hearing impairment due to mutations in gap junction genes encoding beta connexins. Hum Mutat 2000;16:190–202.

172. Denoyelle F, Weil D, Maw MA, et al. Prelingual deafness: High prevalence of a 30delG mutation in the connexin 26 gene. Hum Mol Genet 1997;6:2173–7.

173. Maw MA, Allen-Powell DR, Goodey RJ, et al. The contribution of the DFNB1 locus to neurosensory deafness in a Caucasian population. Am J Hum Genet 1995;57:629–35.

174. Gasparini P, Estivill X, Volpini V, et al. Linkage of DFNB1 locus to neurosensory autosomal-recessive deafness in Mediterranean families. Eur J Hum Genet 1997;5:83–8.

175. Fukushima K, Ramesh A, Srisailapathy CR, et al. Consanguineous nuclear families used to identify a new locus for recessive non-syndromic hearing loss on 14q. Hum Mol Genet 1995;4:1643–8.

176. Green GE, Scott DA, McDonald JM, et al. Carrier rates in Midwestern United States for GJBS mutations causing inherited deafness. JAMA 1999;281:2211–6.

177. Estivill X, Fortina P, Surrey S, et al. Connexin-26 mutation in sporadic and inherited sensorineural deafness. Lancet 1998;351:394–8.

178. Antoniadi T, Rabionet R, Kroupis C, et al. High prevalence in the Greek population of the 35delG mutation in the connexin 26 gene causing prelingual deafness. Clin Genet 1999;55:381–2.

179. Morell RJ, Kim HJ, Hood LJ, et al. Mutations in the connexin 26 gene (GJB2) among Ashkenazi Jews with nonsyndromic recessive deafness. NEJM 1998;339:1500–5.

180. Fuse Y, Doi K, Hasegawa T, et al. Three novel connexin 26 gene mutations in autosomal recessive non-syndromic deafness. NeuroReport 1999;10:1853–7.

181. Brobby GW, Muller-Myshok B, Hortsmann RD. Connexin 26 R143W mutation associated with recessive nonsyndromic sensorineural deafness in Africa. NEJM 1998;338:548–50.

182. Ballana E, Ventayol M, Rabionet R, et al. Connexins and Deafness Homepage. Available at http://www.crg.es/deafness.

183. Petersen MB, Willems PJ. Non-syndromic, autosomal recessive deafness. Clin Genet 2006;69:371–92.

184. Lefebvre PP, Van de Water TR. Connexins, hearing and deafness: Clinical aspects of mutations in the connexin 26 gene. Brain Res Rev 2000;32:159–62.

185. Fischel-Ghodsian N. Mitochondrial deafness mutations reviewed. Hum Mutation 1999;13:261–70.

186. Guan MX. Molecular pathogenetic mechanism of maternally inherited deafness. Ann NY Acad Sci 2004;1011:259–71.

187. Fischel-Ghodsian N. Mitochondrial mutations and hearing loss: Paradigm for mitochondrial genetics. Am J Hum Genet 1998;62:15–9.

188. Nagley P, Zhang C, Martinus RD, et al. Mitochondrial DNA mutations and human aging: Molecular biology, bioenergetics, and redox therapy. In: DiMauro S, Wallace DC, editors. Mitochondrial DNA in Human Pathology. New York: Raven Press; 1993.

189. Ueda N, Oshima T, Ikeda K, et al. Mitochondrial DNA deletion is a predisposing cause for sensorineural hearing loss. Laryngoscope 1998;108:580–4.

190. Fischel-Ghodsian N, Bykhovskaya Y, Taylor K, et al. Temporal bone analysis of patients with presbycusis reveals high frequency of mitochondrial mutations. Hear Res 1997;110:147–54.

191. Bai U, Seidman MD, Hinojosa R, Quirk WS. Mitochondrial DNA deletions associated with aging and possibly presbycusis: A human archival temporal bone study. Am J Otol 1997;18:449–53.

192. Chambers HF, Sande MA. The aminoglycosides. In: Hardman JG, Limbird LE, Molinoff PB, et al., editors. The Pharmacological Basis of Therapeutics. New York: McGraw-Hill; 1996. p. 1103–221.

193. Davies J, Davis BD. Misreading of ribonucleic acid code words induced by aminoglycoside antibiotics. J Biol Chem 1968;243:3312–6.

194. Noller HF. Ribosomal RNA and translation. Annu Rev Biochem 1991;60:191–227.

195. Lortholary O, Tod M, Cohen Y, Petitjean O. Aminoglycosides. Med Clin North Am 1995;79:761–87.

196. Sande MA, Mandell GL. Antimicrobial agents. In: Gilman AG, Rall TW, Nies AS, Taylor P, editors. Goodman and Gilman's the Pharmacological Basis of Therapeutics. 8th edition. Elmsford, NY: Pergamon Press; 1990. p. 1098–116.

197. Henley CM, Schacht J. Pharmacokinetics of aminoglycoside antibiotics in blood, inner ear fluids and their relationship to ototoxicity. Audiology 1988;27:137–46.

198. Vrabec DP, Cody DT, Ulrich JA. A study of the relative concentrations of antibiotics in the blood, spinal fluid and perilmphy in animals. Ann Otol Rhino Laryngol 1965;74:689–705.

199. Price KE. Aminoglycoside research 1975–1985: Prospects for development of improved agents. Antimicrob Agents Chemother 1986;29:543–48.

200. Moore RD, Smith CR, Lietman PS. Risk factors for the development of auditory toxicity in patients receiving aminoglycosides. J Infect Dis 1984;149:23–30.

201. Prazic M, Salaj B. Ototoxicity with children caused by streptomycin. Audiology 1975;14:173–6.

202. Rybak LP. Drug ototoxicity. Annu Rev Pharmacol Toxicol 1986;26:79–99.

203. Hu DN, Qui WQ, Wu BT, et al. Genetic aspects of antibiotic induced deafness: Mitochondrial inheritance. J Med Genet 1991;28:79–83.

204. Higashi K. Unique inheritance of streptomycin-induced deafness. Clin Genet 1989;35:433–6.

205. Guan MX. Molecular pathogenetic mechanism of maternally inherited deafness. Ann NY Acad Sci 2004;1011:259–71.

206. Neefs JM, Van de Peer Y, De Rijik P, et al. Compilation of small ribosomal subunit RNA sequences. Nucleic Acids Res 1991;19:1987–2015.

207. Li R, Xing G, Yan M, et al. Cosegregation of C-insertion at position 961 with A1555G mutation of mitochondrial 12S rRNA gene in a large Chinese family with maternally inherited hearing loss. Am J Med Genet 2004;124A:113–7.

208. Prezant TR, Agapian JV, Bohlman MC, et al. Mitochondrial ribosomal RNA mutation associated with both antibiotic-induced and nonsyndromic deafness. Nat Genet 1993;4:289–94.

209. Fischel-Ghodsian N, Prezant TR, Bu X, et al. Mitochondrial ribosomal RNA gene mutation in a patient with sporadic aminoglycoside ototoxicity. Am J Otolaryngol 1993;4:399–403.

210. Hutchin T, Haworth I, Higashi K, et al. A molecular basis for human hypersensitivity to aminoglycoside antibiotics. Nucleic Acids Res 1993;21:4174–9.

211. Estivill X, Govea N, Barcelo E, et al. Familial progressive sensorineural deafness is mainly due to the mtDNA A1555G mutation and is enhanced by treatment with aminoglycosides. Am J Hum Genet 1998;62:27–35.

212. Fischel-Ghodsian N. Genetic factors in aminoglycoside toxicity. Ann NY Acad Sci 1999;884:99–109.

213. Zimmermann RA, Thomas CL, Wower J. Structure and function of rRNA in the decoding domain and at

the peptidyltransferase center. In: Hill WE, Moore PB, Dahlberg A, et al, editors. The Ribosome: Structure, Function and Evolution. Washington, DC: American Society of Microbiology; 1990. p. 331–47.

214. Gregory ST, Dahlberg AE. Nonsense suppressor and anti-suppressor mutations at the 1409–1491 base pair in the decoding region of Escherichia coli 16S rRNA. Nucleic Acid Res 1995;23:4234–8.

215. Chernoff YO, Vincent A, Liebman SW. Mutations in eukaryotic 18S ribosomal RNA affect translational fidelity and resistance to aminoglycoside antibiotics. EMBO J 1994;13:906–13.

216. Moazed D, Noller HF. Transfer RNA shields specific nucleotides in 16S ribosomal RNA from attack by chemical probes. Cell 1986;47:985–94.

217. Recht MI, Fourmy D, Blanchard SC, et al. RNA sequence determinants for aminoglycoside binding to an A-site rRNA model oligonucleotide. J Mol Biol 1996;262:421–36.

218. Fourmy D, Recht MI, Blanchard SC, et al. Structure of the A-site of *Escherichia coli* 16S ribosomal RNA complexed with an aminoglycoside antibiotic. Science 1996;274:1367–71.

219. Hamasaki K, Rando RR. Specific binding of aminoglycosides to a human rRNA construct based on a DNA polymorphism which causes aminoglycoside-induced deafness. Biochemistry 1997;36:12323–8.

220. Fischel-Ghodsian N, Prezant TR, Chaltraw WE, et al. Mitochondrial gene mutation is a significant predisposing factor in aminoglycoside ototoxicity. Am J Otolaryngol 1997;18:173–8.

221. Zhao H, Li R, Wang W, et al. Maternally inherited aminoglycoside-induced and nonsyndromic deafness is associated with the novel C1494T mutation in the mitochondrial 12S rRNA gene in a large Chinese family. Am J Hum Genet 2004;74:139–52.

222. Gerber S. Review of a high-risk register for congenital or early onset deafness. Br J Audiol 1990;24:347–56.

223. Sutton GJ, Rowe S. Risk factors for childhood sensorineural hearing loss in the Oxford region. Br J Audiol 1997;31:39–54.

224. Bamiou DE, Macardle B, Bitner-Glindzicz M, Sirimanna T. Aetiological investigations of hearing loss in childhood: A review. Clin Otolaryngol 2000;25:98–106.

225. Davis A, Wood S. The epidemiology of hearing impairment: Factors relevant to planning of services. Br J Audiol 1992;26:77–90.

226. Linthicum FH. Viral causes of sensorineural hearing loss. Otolaryngol Clin North Am 1978;11:29–33.

227. Basil A. Childhood sensorineural hearing loss in consanguineous marriages. J Audio Med 1994;3:151–9.

228. Naeem Z, Newton V. Prevalence of sensorineural hearing loss in Asian children. Br J Audiol 1996;30:332–9.

229. Guilford P, Ben Arab S, Blanchard S, et al. Joint Committee on Infant Hearing; American Academy of Audiology; American Academy of Pediatrics; American Speech-Language-Hearing Association; Directors of Speech and Hearing Programs in State Health and Welfare Agencies. Year 2000 position statement: Principles and guidelines for early hearing detection and intervention programs. Pediatrics 2000;106:798–817.

230. Tomaski SM, Grundfast KM. A stepwise approach to the diagnosis and treatment of hereditary hearing loss. Pediatr Clin North Am 1999;46:35–48.

231. Hone SW, Smith RJ. Medical evaluation of pediatric hearing loss: Laboratory, radiographic, and genetic testing. Otolaryngol Clin North Am 2002;35:751–64.

232. Baroch KA. Universal newborn hearing screening: Fine-tuning the process. Curr Opin Otolaryngol Head Neck Surg 2003;11:424–7.

233. ACMG. Genetics evaluation guidelines for the etiologic diagnosis of congenital hearing loss. Genetic Evaluation of Congenital Hearing Loss Expert Panel. ACMG statement. Genet Med 2002;4:162–71.

234. Schrijver I. Hereditary non-syndromic sensorineural hearing loss: Transforming silence to sound. J Mol Diagn 2004;6:275–84.

235. Zalzal GH, Shott SR, Towbin R, Cotton RT. Value of CT scan in the diagnosis of temporal bone diseases in children. Laryngoscope 1986;96:27–32.

236. Bamiou D, Phelps P, Sirimanna T. Temporal bone computed tomography findings in bilateral sensorineural hearing loss. Int J Pediatr Otorhinolaryngol 1999;51:91–9.

237. Green GE, Smith RJ, Bent JP, Cohn ES. Genetic testing to identify deaf newborns. JAMA 2000;284:1245.

238. Downs MP, Yoshinaga-Itano C. The efficacy of early identification and intervention for children with hearing impairment. Pediatr Clin North Am 1999;46:79–87.

239. Nikolopoulos TP, O'Donoghue GM. Cochlear implantation in adults and children. Hosp Med 1998;59:46–9.

27

Autoimmune Inner Ear Disease and Other Autoimmune Diseases with Inner Ear Involvement

Jeffrey P. Harris, MD, PhD
Quinton Gopen, MD
Elizabeth Keithley, PhD

AUTOIMMUNE INNER EAR DISEASE (AIED)

Scientific Basis

The idea that immunity might participate in the causation of inner ear disease has only recently become accepted. Using the brain as a model, the inner ear was initially viewed as an immunologically "privileged" site, separated from cellular and humoral immunity by a blood–labyrinthine barrier. Apart from inner ear inflammation associated with viral or bacterial labyrinthitis, it seemed inconceivable that the immune system could operate within the bony labyrinth. However, experiments beginning in the 1980s demonstrated that antigen introduced into the inner ear of naïve or systemically primed animals resulted in a brisk systemic immune response as well as a local one.[1–4] Moreover, antigen introduced into the inner ear of a systemically immunized animal resulted in hearing loss and even profound deafness owing to a vigorous secondary immune response (Figure 1).[2,5,6] The endolymphatic sac also becomes inflamed (Figure 2) and has been implicated as a site of local immune cell processing within the inner ear.[7–9] The magnitude of these responses was dependent on an intact endolymphatic sac since ablation of the sac or even

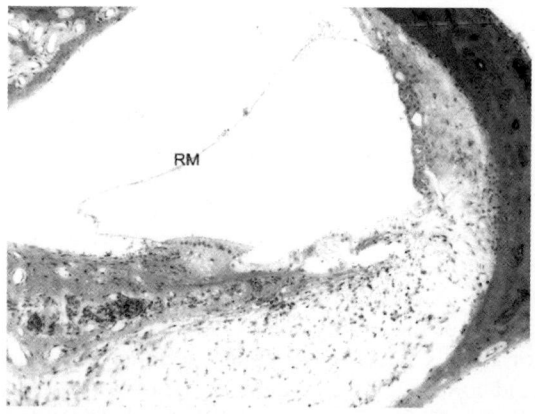

Figure 1 Photomicrograph of the middle turn of an inflamed guinea pig cochlea (20× original magnification). The scala tympani contains inflammatory cells and fibrotic tissue, and the position of Reissner membrane (RM) suggests endolymphatic hydrops. Toluidine blue staining.

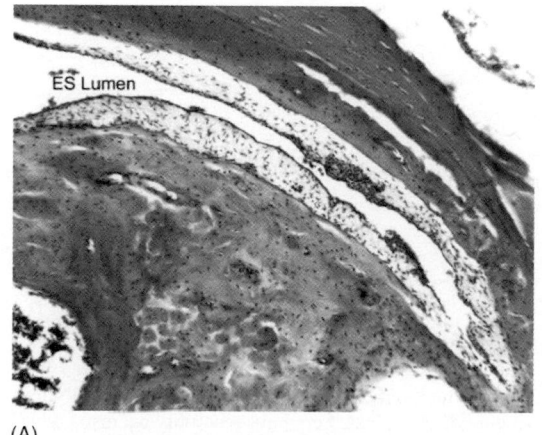

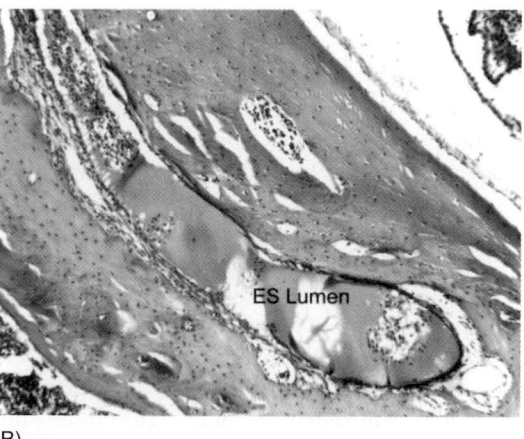

Figure 2 (A) Photomicrograph of a normal endolymphatic sac (ES) in the guinea pig inner ear. Hematoxylin and eosin-stained paraffin section (20× original magnification). (B) Photomicrograph of an ES from a guinea pig with cochlear inflammation following cochlear challenge with a foreign protein to which the animal was sensitized (20× original magnification).

blockage of the endolymphatic duct reduced inner ear immune responses.[8,9] Experiments then demonstrated that the inner ear, although protected by systemic immunity, was damaged by bystander injury when cell-mediated immunity became involved. For example, systemic immunity can protect the inner ear from viral infection through circulating antiviral antibodies.[10,11] If, however, there is a cellular response to viral inoculation of a naïve animal, there is hearing loss and cochlear damage. This damage can be reduced by systemic immunosuppression.[12] The route of entry of the inflammatory cells into the inner ear following antigen or viral challenge of the inner ear appears predominantly to be via the spiral modiolar vein (SMV) (Figure 3). During the inflammatory response, this vein takes on characteristics of an activated venule and expresses intercellular adhesion molecule-1 (ICAM-1) on the endothelial cell surface that facilitates the passage of circulating immunocompetent cells into the scala tympani.[13–16] Once within the inner ear, these cells divide,[16] release inflammatory mediators, and set in motion events that lead to cellular proliferation and eventually osteoneogenesis (Figure 4).[6] Shortly after entering the cochlea, hearing loss occurs.[17] Endolymphatic hydrops often accompanies these end-stage reactions (see Figure 4). Of

note, after the single inoculation of antigen, cells may continue to be stimulated, undergoing cell division for up to 6 weeks.[18]

Clinical Studies

In 1979, McCabe first brought attention to a possible discrete clinical entity when he presented a series of patients with bilateral, progressive hearing loss showing improvement following

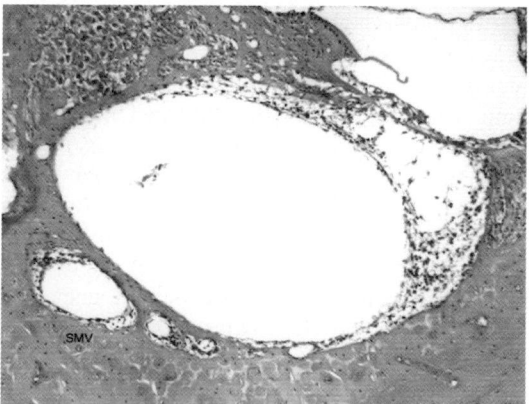

Figure 3 Photomicrograph of the middle turn of an inflamed guinea pig cochlea. Extravasated immunocompetent cells can be seen within the bony channel surrounding the SMV and its tributary on their way to the scala tympani.

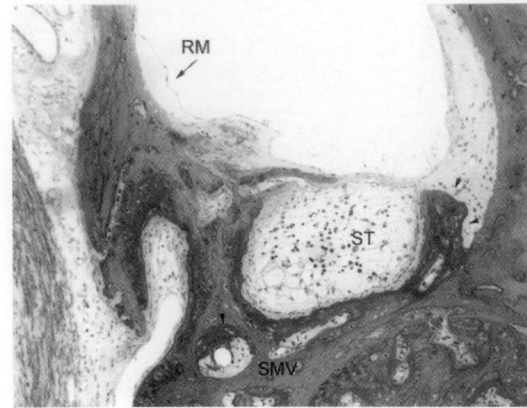

Figure 4 Photomicrograph of the middle turn of an inflamed guinea pig cochlea 4 weeks following challenge with a foreign protein to which the animal was sensitized. The scala tympani still contains infiltrated inflammatory cells, but the fibrotic matrix has begun to ossify both within the scala tympani (ST) and around the SMV (*arrowheads*). The location of Reissner membrane (RM) indicates severe hydrops.

treatment with corticosteroids.[19] Although others had over the years described patients with ear-related illnesses associated with systemic immune disorders,[20–22] none had collected such a large series or speculated that these patients might have an organ-specific illness. Since that time, autoimmunity has been proposed as a cause for other inner ear disorders, including Ménière disease,[23] sudden sensorineural hearing loss (SNHL),[24] and acute vertigo.[25] A relationship between inner ear disorders and systemic autoimmune disease has also been documented. A number of systemic autoimmune disorders, such as polyarteritis nodosa, systemic lupus erythematosus (SLE), relapsing polychondritis, ulcerative colitis, and Wegener granulomatosis include auditory and vestibular symptoms.[26] Moreover, some patients with suspected AIED have either presented with or later developed systemic autoimmune diseases.[27,28]

Unlike other organs and tissues, the inner ear is not amenable to biopsy for the expressed intent of investigating the underlying immunopathogenesis of purported autoimmune disorders affecting it. What little histopathology has been published from patients with suspected AIED shows fibrosis and/or bone deposition in the labyrinth, consistent with the late sequelae of inflammation.[29–32] Specific immune reactivity against inner ear antigens is often detected in patients with suspected AIED, but the results vary. Lymphocyte migration assays using inner ear tissue as a target have been disappointing, providing, at best, low stimulation indexes.[33] More promising results have been obtained with Western blotting. Significantly, more patients with suspected AIED show reactivity against a 68 kD antigen (Figure 5) than do match normal-hearing or rheumatic controls.[28,34] AIED has also been associated with reactivity against antigens of different molecular weights, especially 45 to 50, 30, and 20 kD.[35] Although reactivity of patient sera against tissue sections of the inner ear has produced reproducible inner ear labeling,[36] it

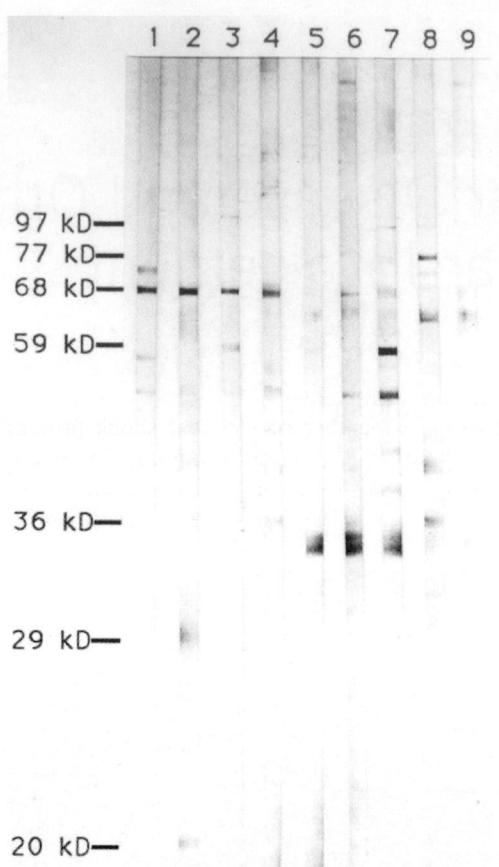

Figure 5 Western blot indicating reactivity of patient sera against antigens extracted from bovine inner ear tissue. Lanes 1 to 3 and 5 to 8 are sera from patients with sensorineural hearing loss. Sera have reactivity against a 68 kD protein or 33 to 35 kD proteins. There is also reactivity with 77, 52, and 58 kD antigens. Lane 4 is serum from a patient with giant cell arteritis and lane 9 is from a normal-hearing individual. (Reproduced with permission from reference 34.)

does not appear to be as practical or as useful as immunoblotting. A number of animal studies have supported an autoimmune cause for some types of SNHL. Immunization of animals with crude extracts of inner ear tissues results in hearing loss in approximately one-third of subjects.[37] Circulating monoclonal antibodies against inner ear tissues also produce hearing loss.[38] Animal models of systemic autoimmune disease, such as the MRL-Faslpr mouse model of SLE, display hearing loss.[39]

EPIDEMIOLOGY

AIED is a rare disorder, but the true incidence remains unknown. Although patients of all ages have been described with the disorder, the disease most commonly affects middle-aged adults. Men and women are affected at equal rates. No racial predilection has been identified, although the majority of reports are in Caucasian individuals.

Etiology

Because of the relative rarity of this condition and its recent recognition, as noted above, very few temporal bones with a diagnosis of AIED have been evaluated. More studies have assessed

the inner ears of patients with systemic autoimmune disorders. Sone and colleagues assessed 14 temporal bones from seven individuals with SLE.[40] The duration of disease and ages varied widely. The most consistent findings were hair cell and spiral ganglion cell loss. However, unusual accretions were observed in the stria vascularis of 6 of 14 temporal bones. Animal models have been valuable adjuncts in the study of AIED since the antigen and immunization history can be rigorously controlled, and histopathology is routinely available. Initial studies using immunization of guinea pigs with bovine inner ear extracts resulted in the development of hearing loss and mild inflammatory changes in the inner ears of a subset of animals.[37] More recent work has confirmed these findings and indicated that the hearing losses induced by this procedure tend to be modest. Bouman and colleagues found that immunization of animals with swine inner ear extracts produced modest declines in compound action potentials recorded from the guinea pigs 2 and 6 weeks after immunization but no changes in the cochlear microphonic.[35] This suggests that the events responsible for hearing loss occurred at the level of the inner hair cell and/or spiral ganglion neuron rather than at the level of the outer hair cell. Hearing losses were associated with increased Western blot reactivity to 68 kD and other antigens.[35]

Immunization with specific proteins has also resulted in hearing loss. Based on the observation that myelin protein P0 was associated with immunoreactivity against a 30 kD inner ear protein in patients with AIED,[41] Matsuoka and colleagues immunized mice with purified bovine P0.[42] They observed an approximately 10 dB hearing loss and a monocellular infiltrate in the eighth nerve within the cochlear modiolus. Experimental autoimmune encephalomyelitis can be induced by immunization with the neuronal S-100β calcium-binding protein and by passive transfer of T cells sensitized to this antigen. Based on this earlier finding, Gloddek and colleagues found that passive transfer of S-100β-reactive T cells produced a 10 dB hearing loss in rats as well as a cellular infiltrate into the perilymph.[43,44]

A monoclonal antibody raised against cochlear tissues of approximately 68 kD that specifically reacts with supporting cells in the organ of Corti has been shown to produce high frequency hearing loss in mice carrying the hybridoma.[38] More recently, Nair and colleagues infused this antibody into the cochlear perilymph using an osmotic minipump.[45] After 13 days, an approximately 20 dB hearing loss developed, associated with minor losses of hair cells.

To explore the origin of lymphocytes in the region of the endolymphatic sac and the reaction of T cells to self-antigens in the inner ear, Iwai and colleagues used a model of graft-versus-host disease.[46] T cells from C57BL/6 mice injected into the systemic circulation of BALB/c mice infiltrated and proliferated in the perisaccular region surrounding the endolymphatic sac, but not into other regions of the inner ear. These findings confirm the role of the endolymphatic sac region in mediating immunity in the inner ear, as well as the communication of the normal sac with circulating lymphocytes. This provides an additional foundation for autoimmunity as an etiology in disorders involving the sac, such as Ménière disease.

Animal models have also been used to study the relationship between systemic autoimmune disease and the inner ear. The MRL-Faslpr mouse is used as a model of SLE owing to the accumulation of autoreactive T cells normally eliminated by Fas-mediated apoptosis. This model also displays progressive hearing loss. Ruckenstein and colleagues found that the most striking inner ear pathology in this model was observed in the stria vascularis,[39] with progressive, hydropic degeneration of intermediate cells, consistent with the strial pathology observed in human SLE temporal bones as described above.[40] In addition, Ruckenstein and Hu observed the deposition of both complement-fixing and noncomplement-fixing antibodies in the stria vascularis and, to a lesser extent, in other structures.[47] All antibodies were bound to the capillary walls and were not associated with signs of inflammation. The same group found that systemic treatment with dexamethasone suppressed antibody deposition within the stria and other structures of the inner ear.[39] However, the treatment failed to suppress strial degeneration and hearing loss, suggesting that perhaps the hearing loss seen in these animals had a genetic basis. In contrast to this result, Wobig and colleagues found that systemic prednisolone treatment protected hearing in MRL-Faslpr mice.[48] The Palmerston-North mouse is also employed as a model of SLE with hearing loss. These animals develop abnormal mineralization of connective tissue in the region of the eighth nerve root within the modiolus. However, there is no deposition of antibody in or cellular infiltration of the cochlea in this strain.[49] As better imaging becomes available, the localization of inflammatory processes to specific regions of the inner ear should become possible. Having this information will certainly improve our diagnostic capability as well as our knowledge of the basic pathogenesis of this disorder.

Diagnosis

Diagnosis of AIED is still problematic. There is no universally accepted set of diagnostic criteria or diagnostic test for a condition that appears to have several independent causes. In general, in all cases of idiopathic, rapidly progressive, bilateral hearing loss, AIED should be suspected. However, there is no doubt that involvement of the second ear may occur months or even years after presentation of symptoms in the first ear. Hearing loss may be manifested as either diminished hearing acuity, decreased discrimination, or both, and may fluctuate over time. In bilateral Ménière disease, with its triad of vestibular dysfunction, low-tone, fluctuant hearing loss, and tinnitus, AIED should also be suspected, especially when

the second ear becomes affected within a short period of time. Aside from an empiric trial with high-dose corticosteroids showing improved inner ear function, Western blot assays are currently the most widely used category of diagnostic test for AIED. The initial assays used for this purpose were based on proteins extracted from bovine inner ear tissue, and inner ear extracts are still used. Reactivity to an approximately 68 kD antigen was detected in a significant proportion of patients with AIED and Ménière disease.[28,34,50–52] This, or an antigen with shared epitopes, was later shown to be present in kidney and to be a member of the heat shock protein (HSP) family.[53,54] Reactivity against inner ear antigens of other molecular weights, especially in the 45, 30, and 20 kD ranges, has frequently been reported.[35,41] Few of these other antigens have been characterized or found to be present in statistically significant proportions of hearing loss versus control populations. For example, studies examining the antigenic profile of inner ear tissues consistently demonstrate a multitude of antigens against which human sera reacts; however, these bands seen on Western blot failed to reach significance when carefully matched against controls.[34,50,55] Immunoreactivity to a 30 kD antigen has been associated with myelin protein P0.[42] The 68 kD antigen has been associated with HSP 70, and immunoreactivity against the bovine HSP 70 (bHSP 70) has been found to be correlated with AIED.[53] However, preabsorption with bHSP 70 does not remove all reactivity to the 68 kD inner ear antigen,[53] and immunization of animals with HSP 70 does not appear to produce hearing loss.[56] Antibodies against other antigens have also been implicated. Several investigators have reported that immunoreactivity to inner ear proteins with molecular weights in the 42 to 45 kD range is also positively correlated with AIED, although with a lower level of specificity than the 68 kD protein or HSP 70. For example, Atlas and colleagues found that positive Western blots against 68 and/or 42 to 45 kD inner ear proteins were present in significantly more patients with Ménière disease than in normal controls, whereas reactivity against 35 to 36 and 20 kD proteins was not different in the two groups.[52] Moreover, reactivity appeared to be related to disease state in that patients with active disease (at least one episode of vertigo within 1 month) were significantly more likely to be positive than those with inactive disease. Other specific antigenic targets have also been studied. Modugno and colleagues observed antithyroid antibodies in 27% of patients with benign paroxysmal positional vertigo, significantly more than were observed in a group of normal controls.[57] Using immunoblotting and enzyme-linked immunosorbent assay, Yamawaki and colleagues observed antibodies against the sulfoglucuronosyl glycolipid SGLPG, but not SGPG, in 37 of 74 patients with AIED, as compared with only 3 of 56 pathologic and 2 of 28 healthy controls.[58] In a negative result, Lopez-Gonzalez and colleagues found that anti-type II collagen antibodies and stimulation indexes

were unrelated to idiopathic or SNHL or Ménière disease.[59]

In one of the few prospective studies attempting to correlate the significance of Western blotting for the 68 kD antigen with response to treatment, Moscicki and colleagues found that a positive result for 68 kD was associated with a 75% rate of hearing improvement with corticosteroids, compared with 18% of patients who were Western blot negative.[51] In this study, disease activity was an important predictor of a positive antibody response and response to treatment. Eighty-nine percent of patients with active bilateral progressive hearing loss had a positive 68 kD antibody, whereas patients with inactive disease were uniformly negative.

A number of other studies have focused on the diagnostic utility of antibodies against HSP 70. In a retrospective case series, Hirose and colleagues evaluated a variety of assays for systemic autoimmune disease, as well as a Western blot assay against bHSP 70, for their utility in predicting the responsiveness of rapidly progressive SNHL to corticosteroids.[60] Again in this study, positivity in the HSP 70 blot assay was the best predictor of corticosteroid responsiveness in AIED. Although the sensitivity was low (42%), the specificity was 90% and the positive predictive value was 91%. Bloch and colleagues tested the serum of 52 patients with bilateral, progressive, idiopathic hearing loss or Ménière disease in Western blot assays to recombinant bHSP 70 and recombinant human HSP 70.[61] Reactivity against recombinant bHSP 70 was observed in 40 of 52 patients. Only 12 also reacted to recombinant human HSP 70. They also tested the positive sera against a panel of recombinant peptide fragments of bHSP 70. Reactivity was observed to widely separate epitopes. However, most positive patients reacted preferentially or only to an amino acid segment from the carboxy terminus of rbHSP (recombinant bovine), aa 427–461. Within this dominant epitope, the bovine peptide differs from the corresponding human peptide by only one amino acid. Western blotting has also been used to explore the possibility that a subset of patients has Ménière disease with an immunologic basis. Gottschlich and colleagues demonstrated that 32% of patients with Ménière disease were anti-68 kD positive.[34] Rauch and colleagues reported that anti-HSP 70 antibodies were found in 47% of patients with Ménière disease and that level increased to 58% when the disease was bilateral.[62] Recently, however, Rauch and colleagues had a similar level of sensitivity in 134 patients with Ménière disease but a much lower level of specificity owing to a relatively high level of reactivity in blood donor control sera.[63] This high rate of positivity in the control serum was unexplained and contradicts the previously low level of positives in control sera as well as those high rates of positivity reported by others.[28,54,62] Serial serum samples revealed no correlation between antibody level and the clinical course of the disease. These observations led them to question the clinical utility of the HSP 70 assay in Ménière disease. The answer to whether a subset of patients with classic Ménière disease is immune mediated is currently unclear.

A number of investigators have reacted patient sera against tissue sections to detect immunoreactivity against inner ear antigens. This technique has been used on a research basis since the 1980s, when Arnold and colleagues reported a high degree of labeling within the cochlea with patient serum.[64] Bachor and colleagues detected immunoreactivity to rat cochlear sections in 14 of 15 patients showing progressive or sudden hearing loss in the cochlea opposite an ear deafened by trauma or inflammation.[65] Using rat cryosections of the inner ear, Arbusow and colleagues detected antibodies against vestibular sensory epithelia in 8 of 12 patients with idiopathic bilateral vestibular pathology as compared with 1 of 22 healthy controls and 0 of 6 patients with systemic autoimmune disease.[66] Ottaviani and colleagues detected immunoreactivity against endothelial cells using sections of rat kidney tissue in 8 of 15 patients with sudden hearing loss, as compared with 2 of 14 normal controls.[67] Helmchen and colleagues observed positive, but low, levels of immunoreactivity against inner ear sections using serum from patients with Cogan syndrome.[68] However, unlike anticorneal antibodies, the anticochlear immunoreactivity levels were not correlated with disease stage.

Classification of Autoimmune Inner Ear Disease

During the quarter century since McCabe's article on AIED was published,[19] many patients have been diagnosed and treated for rapidly progressive SNHL and many have had their hearing maintained or even improved with treatment. As a result of the growing experience with patients with corticosteroid sensitive hearing loss, a pattern has begun to emerge that warrants a classification scheme to better sort out patients as they present with inner ear dysfunction. Although the following classification scheme is intended specifically for that purpose, it is likely that over the next few years it will be further refined:

Type 1: Organ (Ear) specific

- Rapidly progressive bilateral SNHL
- All age ranges, although middle age is most common
- No other clinical evidence of systemic autoimmune disease
- Positive Otoblot (Western blot 68 kD or HSP 70)
- Negative serologic studies (antinuclear antibody (ANA), erythrocyte sedimentation rate, rheumatoid factor (RF), C1q binding assay, etc)
- Greater than 50% response rate to high-dose corticosteroids

Type 2: Rapidly progressive bilateral sensorineural hearing loss with systemic autoimmune disease

- Rapidly progressive bilateral SNHL
- Hearing loss often greatest with flare of autoimmune condition

- Other autoimmune condition is present (eg, SLE, ulcerative colitis, polyarteritis nodosa, vasculitis, rheumatoid arthritis, or Sjögren syndrome)
- Otoblot may be positive or negative
- Serologic studies will be positive in accordance with the illness (eg, ANA-high titers, RF positive, and circulating immune complexes)
- Corticosteroid responsive and may be managed with targeted therapies for underlying illness

Type 3: Immune-mediated Ménière disease

- Bilateral, fluctuating SNHL with vestibular symptoms that may predominate
- Subset of patients with delayed contralateral endolymphatic hydrops or recent instability of better-hearing ear in a patient with burned out Ménière disease
- Otoblot positive 37 to 58%; may show presence of circulating immune complexes
- Corticosteroid responsive; may require long-term immunosuppression owing to relapses

Type 4: Rapidly progressive bilateral sensorineural hearing loss with associated inflammatory disease (chronic otitis media, Lyme disease, otosyphilis, serum sickness)

- Evidence of profound drop in hearing with long-standing chronic otitis media
- May show inflammation of the tympanic membrane, with perforations
- Hearing loss progresses despite treatment of the infectious agent (treponemal or rickettsial)
- Otoblot negative; serologic tests for the underlying disease may be positive; patient should be evaluated for granulomatous disease and vasculitis by biopsy if tissue is available
- Corticosteroid responsive and may require long-term immunosuppression
- Serum sickness has been reported after vaccinations, although anecdotal

Type 5: Cogan syndrome

- Sudden onset of interstitial keratitis and severe vestibuloauditory dysfunction
- Otoblot negative for 68 kD but positive for 55 kD antigen
- Responds to high-dose corticosteroids, although becomes resistant over long term

Type 6: Autoimmune inner ear disease-like

- Young patients with idiopathic, rapidly progressive, bilateral SNHL leading to deafness
- Severe ear pain, pressure, and tinnitus
- Otoblot and all serology negative
- May have an unrelated, nonspecific inflammatory event that initiates ear disease
- Not responsive to immunosuppressive drugs, although they are tried

Treatment

Once a diagnosis of AIED is established or considered highly presumptive, high-dose prednisone is the mainstay of treatment for this condition. Early institution of 60 mg of prednisone daily

for a month is now widely used, as short-term or lower-dose long-term therapy has either been ineffective or fraught with the risk of relapse. Prednisone is then tapered slowly if a positive response to therapy is obtained. If, during the taper, hearing suddenly falls, reinstitution of high-dose prednisone is indicated. One sensitive predictor of imminent relapse can be the appearance of loud tinnitus in one or both ears. If patients show corticosteroid responsiveness but attempts at taper result in relapse, the addition of a cytotoxic drug should be considered. Methotrexate held promise initially; but, in an exhaustive multiinstitutional study, it failed to be effective in maintaining hearing improvement achieved with prednisone therapy.[69] Cyclophosphamide (Cytoxan) remains an effective agent, but its side effects are prohibitive. For patients with severe hearing losses, positive 68 kD Western blots, and nonresponsiveness to prednisone therapy, consideration should be given to a trial of cyclophosphamide.[27] At oral doses of 1 to 2 mg per day taken each morning with liberal amounts of fluid, the risk of hemorrhagic cystitis or drug effects on the bladder can be minimized. The patient should be monitored closely for toxicity with complete blood counts, platelets, blood urea nitrogen, creatinine, liver function tests, and urinalysis. Cyclophosphamide should not be administered to children, and the risk of permanent sterility should be outlined. If, on the other hand, no response to high-dose prednisone is achieved, and the patient is 68 kD Western blot negative, it may be futile to continue potentially toxic drugs, with little evidence for AIED as the cause. As this field continues to evolve, there are, however, no hard and fast rules, and a practitioner may be justified in trying cytotoxic drugs on an empiric basis because unrelenting progressive deafness is a serious handicap for a previously normal hearing person. Luetje recommended plasmapheresis for difficult to manage patients,[70] and this can be a useful adjunct to the above-mentioned immunosuppressive drugs. Based on animal studies, tumor necrosis factor (TNF) blocking agents are being investigated for efficacy in treating AIED. Etanercept (Enbrel) was evaluated in a placebo controlled study but found to be no better than placebo for the treatment of AIED.[71] Other TNF blocking agents such as infliximab (Remicade) and adalimumab (Humira) may prove efficacious but await clinical evaluation. Rituximab (Rituxan), an antibody against selected B cells, is currently undergoing a clinical trial at the University of California, San Diego for its efficacy in treating patients with AIED.

Parnes and colleagues noted that local corticosteroids appear to be more effective in the treatment of other autoimmune disorders, such as corneal inflammation owing to Cogan syndrome.[72] They, therefore, investigated the pharmacokinetics of hydrocortisone, methylprednisone, and dexamethasone in perilymph and endolymph after oral, intravenous, or intratympanic administration. Dexamethasone was found to be largely excluded from the cochlea by the blood–labyrinthine barrier. Both methylprednisone and hydrocortisone reached inner ear fluid after systemic administration, attenuated presumably by the blood–labyrinthine barrier. Much higher levels of all three drugs were observed in cochlear fluid after intratympanic administration, with rapid declines over a 6- to 24-hour period. Similar results were noted by Chandrasekhar and colleagues.[73] Parnes and colleagues also reported that repeated intratympanic administration of corticosteroids in a small series of patients with hearing loss of diverse origins was followed by improvement in some patients, but no control group was included.[72] In contrast, Yang and colleagues found that local immunosuppression had no effect on experimental immune-mediated SNHL in an animal model.[74] It should be noted that local effects are not, of course, the only basis for the therapeutic efficacy of immunosuppressants. By decreasing peripheral blood leukocytes, these agents reduce the population of cells that can be recruited to the inner ear to participate in immune and inflammatory damage. An experiment designed to prevent entry of cells into the cochlea using antibodies to ICAM-1 did show a reduced number of infiltrated inflammatory cells in the cochlea following antigen challenge.[75] Although the inflammation was not entirely prevented, such a strategy may be worth pursuing. An analogous situation exists for ocular immune disorders such as uveitis. Despite the greater accessibility of the eye to topical drugs than the inner ear, ophthalmologists would never consider local therapy in lieu of high-dose corticosteroids for these disorders. Perhaps a lesson taken from their experience might lessen the enthusiasm that currently exists for treatment solely by local middle ear corticosteroid instillation.

OTHER AUTOIMMUNE DISEASES WITH INNER EAR INVOLVEMENT

A number of systemic autoimmune conditions have been associated with inner ear damage (Table 1). Although the majority of these conditions have vasculitis in their pathogenesis, other conditions involving connective tissue, bowel, and exocrine glands have been associated with AIED.

Table 1 Systemic Autoimmune Diseases with Inner Ear Involvement

Disease
Cogan syndrome*
Susac syndrome*
Wegener granulomatosis
Temporal arteritis
Behçet disease
Systemic lupus erythematosus
Relapsing polychondritis
Rheumatoid arthritis
Scleroderma
Sjögren syndrome
Inflammatory bowel disease

*Requires inner ear involvement for diagnosis.

Cogan Syndrome

The first reports what is now known as Cogan syndrome came from Morgan and Baumgartner, who described a patient with nonsyphilitic interstitial keratitis and audiovestibular dysfunction.[76] However, Cogan went on to describe four patients with the same presentation.[77] This disease is now commonly referred to as Cogan syndrome. Cogan syndrome is a rare autoimmune disease of young adults with a peak incidence in the third decade of life. It affects males and females equally with a strong predilection for Caucasians.[78]

Cogan syndrome presents with aural, ocular, and systemic features. Patients often have constitutional symptoms as the first sign of the disease, which include headache, malaise, and myalgias. Other systemic features variably present include gastrointestinal involvement (bleeding), cardiac involvement (aortic insufficiency), renal involvement (proteinuria, hematuria), respiratory involvement (pleural effusion, cough, dyspnea), and skin involvement (nodules, rash).[79] Patients frequently report a preceding upper respiratory tract infection. In the majority of patients, aural symptoms precede ocular symptoms. Tinnitus comes first, followed by progressive fluctuating SNHL in one or both ears. If the disease initially presents with unilateral involvement, the condition quickly progresses within days to involve both ears. Ocular symptoms include photophobia, tearing, redness and eye pain, all of which are usually bilateral. The classic finding in Cogan syndrome is interstitial keratitis. A critical criterion is that the patient does not have syphilis, an infection which can lead to an identical presentation to that of Cogan syndrome.

Diagnosis is accomplished with the clinical picture as delineated above and a negative test for syphilis. An audiologic assessment will document the characteristic SNHL. An ophthalmologic examination including a slit lamp examination is required to identify interstitial keratitis. Laboratory testing may reveal an elevated erythrocyte sedimentation rate, leukocytosis, or anemia.

Treatment is with high-dose corticosteroids. Without treatment, the hearing loss will progress over several months, leaving the majority of patients deaf. However, the prognosis for hearing recovery is quite good if aggressive corticosteroid therapy is initiated early in the disease.[78,80] Vestibular symptoms are more difficult to manage and are often refractory to treatment with corticosteroids.[81] Ophthalmic symptoms often respond to corticosteroid drops. If the patient does not respond to corticosteroid treatment, consideration to second line agents, such as cyclophosphamide or methotrexate, should be given.

Susac Syndrome

Susac syndrome was first described by John Susac in 1979.[82] It has also been termed SICRET (small infarctions of cochlear, retinal, and encephalic tissue) and RED-M (retinopathy, encephalopathy, deafness, and associated microangiopathy).

It is an autoimmune microangiopathy of unknown cause that typically affects the small blood vessels of the retina, cochlea, and brain and results in a triad of encephalopathy, branch retinal artery occlusions, and hearing loss. Susac syndrome affects women three times as often as men, with an age range of 8 to 59 years. No racial predilection has been identified.[83] It is considered a rare disorder, with fewer than 100 case reports in the world literature.

The clinical course is characterized by episodic exacerbations of hearing loss, encephalopathy, and/or visual loss. Symptoms persist for several years, but this is highly variable. Headaches often precede any organic brain impairment, which can include confusion, memory loss, psychiatric disturbances, or seizures. Hearing loss is typically acute, bilateral, and asymmetric. The hearing loss is sensorineural and usually involves the lower frequencies, although high-frequency losses have been documented.[83] The hearing loss fluctuates, and some recover without residual deficits while others are left with profound hearing loss.[84] Tinnitus often precedes or accompanies the hearing loss. Vestibular symptoms are also often present and include vertigo, ataxia, and gait impairment. Visual loss is usually mild and transient in nature.[85]

Diagnosis is based on the clinical picture, ophthalmologic evaluation, laboratory testing, and magnetic resonance imaging. Patients require a fundoscopic examination to evaluate for branch retinal artery occlusions. The retinopathy can be extensive or occult, confounding diagnosis.[83] Retinal fluorescein angiography is extremely useful in demonstrating branch retinal artery occlusions. Magnetic resonance imaging in Susac syndrome always reveals corpus callosum involvement. White matter lesions are typically small and multifocal and frequently enhance in the acute stage. Deep gray matter involvement can also be seen and is reported in 70% of cases.[85] Lesions are typically multiple, small, hyperintense foci on T2 images that enhance with contrast in both the white and gray matter. There is no correlation between the lesions evident on magnetic resonance imaging and the extent of the clinical encephalopathy. Cerebral arteriography findings are almost always normal, as the involved precapillary arterioles are beyond the resolution of the arteriogram.[83]

Biopsies of lesions have shown small artery sclerosis with a mononuclear perivascular infiltrate and microinfarctions, but without necrotizing vasculitis.[86] Other laboratory testing is nonspecific. The cerebrospinal fluid may show an elevated protein level with mild pleocytosis. No coagulopathy has been identified.[85]

Therapy usually begins with antiplatelet agents such as aspirin, as well as calcium channel blockers such as nimodipine. If the symptoms progress, high-dose methylprednisolone is employed. Failure of corticosteroids usually leads to initiation of treatment with cyclophosphamide. Anticoagulation has no role in treatment for the disorder.[85] Some investigators have advocated treatment with immunoglobulins as well as plasmapheresis.[87] The prognosis is variable, but to date no deaths directly attributable to Susac syndrome have been documented.[88] One case has had recurrence after remission.[86]

Although both Cogan syndrome and Susac syndrome require inner ear manifestations as one of the diagnostic criteria, the remaining systemic autoimmune conditions have only occasional inner ear involvement. Many of these conditions share vasculitis as their underlying pathology.

Wegener Granulomatosis

Wegener granulomatosis is a vasculitis of small blood vessels, which leads to pulmonary, renal, and aural manifestations. Patients often present with cough and hemoptysis. The kidney involvement is glomerulonephritis, which leads to hematuria and proteinuria. Middle ear effusions are common from granulomatous involvement of the eustachian tubes or the middle ear space. Granulomatous involvement of the middle ear space can also result in chronic otorrhea with tympanic membrane perforation, conductive hearing loss due to ossicular chain involvement, and rarely facial paralysis.[89] AIED is also occasionally seen in the disorder, with SNHL found in 8% of patients in one large study.[90] Although the disease is fatal if untreated, the prognosis is good with appropriate therapy. Cyclophosphamide along with prednisone are standard therapy, with the corticosteroid discontinued after adequate control of the disease, whereas the cyclophosphamide is continued for 1 year. Patients with SNHL also benefit from this therapy, with many demonstrating an improvement in hearing levels.[90]

Temporal Arteritis

Temporal arteritis, also known as giant cell or cranial arteritis, is another vasculitis which may produce inner ear dysfunction. Temporal arteritis is a vasculitis of large vessels with a predilection for the superficial temporal artery. Typical presentation is in an elderly patient with headaches and pain in the jaw when chewing. Untreated patients have a substantial risk of developing blindness. AIED occurs in 12% of patients diagnosed with temporal arteritis[91] and is readily treatable with an oral corticosteroid.

Behçet Disease

Behçet disease is a vasculitis which results in recurrent aphthous ulcers, genital lesions, ocular injury, and skin eruptions. It often occurs in young adults. Inner ear manifestations are common. Two recent studies demonstrated a high proportion of SNHL (32 to 55%) as well as vestibulopathy (30%).[92,93] Corticosteroids are useful in the treatment of AIED associated with Behçet disease. Remicade (infliximab) has had excellent results in maintaining remission in Behçet disease, but has not been evaluated for its efficacy for the treatment of AIED in the disorder.[94]

Systemic Lupus Erythematosus

SLE is an autoimmune condition, which results in both direct cytotoxic cell damage and vasculitis from immune complex depositions. Although the disease is diverse in its manifestations, the most common presentation includes fever, anorexia, arthralgias, alopecia, malar rash, and visceral organ involvement, most often of the kidney. It most commonly involves young women, with a racial predilection for African Americans, Hispanics, and Asians. Patients with SLE have an increased incidence of AIED,[95] and those with antiphospholipid antibodies have an even higher risk to have SNHL, presumably from vascular occlusion.[96] Treatment for AIED related to the disorder is with corticosteroids, but patients with antiphospholipid antibodies may also benefit from anticoagulation.[97]

Relapsing Polychondritis

Relapsing polychondritis is an autoimmune disorder directed against cartilage. Typically, the auricle, nose, and trachea are involved, although joints can also be affected. Ocular involvement is not uncommon. A key feature of the disorder is that the lobule of the auricle is spared from the inflammatory process, as it possesses no cartilage. AIED is frequently present and can be manifested by either sudden SNHL or a slow gradual decline in hearing. The hearing loss may be unilateral or bilateral and varies in severity.[98] Vestibular dysfunction, such as vertigo, ataxia, or disequilibrium, is commonly present. The treatment for AIED related to this disorder is a corticosteroid.

Rheumatoid Arthritis

Rheumatoid arthritis is an autoimmune disorder directed at the synovial tissues and most commonly seen in young women. Presentation is with joint pain along with anorexia, fever, and malaise. Although the ossicular joints can be involved in the disorder, leading to a conductive hearing loss, a high incidence of SNHL has been identified in patients with rheumatoid arthritis. The majority of these patients have a slowly progressive bilateral SNHL.[99,100] Corticosteroid treatment is reserved for patients with sudden or fluctuating SNHL.

Scleroderma

Scleroderma is an autoimmune disorder directed against connective tissue, as well as capillaries. It most commonly involves women in their fifth decade of life. As the skin sustains injury by the autoimmune process, it becomes thickened and fibrosed. Raynaud phenomenon is quite common. SNHL has been identified in 20% of patients with scleroderma in a large, prospective study.[101] Corticosteroids are not considered effective in the disorder and have not been evaluated in their efficacy for treating AIED related with the disease. Only cyclophosphamide has been evaluated for the treatment of SNHL in this disorder, with highly variable results.[102]

Sjögren Syndrome

Sjögren syndrome is an autoimmune disorder directed against the exocrine glands. The salivary and lacrimal glands are primarily involved, and patients consequently present with dry mouth (xerostomia) and dry eyes (xerophthalmia). The lack of saliva can lead to dysphagia and dental caries, whereas the lack of tears can lead to corneal abrasions and loss of visual acuity. A 20% incidence of SNHL has been found in this disorder in two large studies.[103,104] Currently, corticosteroids and other immunosuppressants have not been proven efficacious in treating AIED related to Sjögren syndrome.

Inflammatory Bowel Disease

Inflammatory bowel disease encompasses ulcerative colitis as well as Crohn disease. Both conditions involve an autoimmune injury to the bowel mucosa, which leads to bloody diarrhea, abdominal pain, and anorexia. Presentation is usually in young adults and there is a slight female predominance. Sudden and slowly progressive SNHL vestibulopathy, as well as, have been identified in patients with inflammatory bowel disease.[105] High-dose corticosteroids are the treatment of choice for AIED related to inflammatory bowel disease. Infliximab (Remicade) is a new anti–TNF-α agent which holds promise in the treatment of inflammatory bowel disease as well as its associated AIED.

SUMMARY

Debate continues as to whether AIED exists as a separate entity. Some authors prefer to refer to this condition as immune-mediated inner ear disease. Clearly, the evidence for specific autoimmunity is indirect. Hearing and vestibular problems that are diagnosed as autoimmune in origin are often responsive to corticosteroids. Although this suggests that the condition involves inflammation, one cannot infer the involvement of specific immunity. The fact that inner ear disease is often present in systemic autoimmune disorders provides strong evidence that autoimmune processes can damage the labyrinth, but does not speak to the issue of organ-specific disease. Animal models of hearing loss and/or vestibular dysfunction secondary to immunization with inner ear antigens provide stronger evidence of specific autoimmunity.

AIED is difficult to diagnose. Although it is generally agreed that the condition should be bilateral and rapidly progressive, the involvement of the second ear may take months or even years to occur. Although rapidly progressing conditions are more readily held to be autoimmune, AIED is increasingly considered as a potential cause of Ménière disease and as a less likely cause of sudden hearing loss. Improved diagnostic tests are clearly required. No one test appears to be positive in more than 30 to 40% of patients who otherwise fit the criteria for autoimmune disease. One possible explanation for this is that rapidly progressive SNHL has a number of different causes, including autoimmune, viral, genetic, developmental, vascular, and perhaps metabolic. Many of these cannot be separated by their presentation; therefore, it would not be unusual or unexpected for many of these patients to have negative antibody testing, and some who were not autoimmune, for example, those with a viral origin, might even improve with corticosteroids. Another possibility is that autoimmunity exists to a variety of inner ear antigens. Given the variety of autoimmune disorders that can affect the inner ear, the variety of antigens with which sera from patients with AIED will react, and the fact that immunization with a variety of proteins can lead to hearing loss in animal models, this would appear to be a strong possibility.

The usefulness of Western blotting for antibodies directed against the 68 kD or HSP 70 antigen as diagnostic assay seems clear, although there is little evidence to support an etiologic role for HSP 70. It is possible that HSP 70 shares one or more epitopes with an inner ear antigen, although reactivity to widely variable epitopes of HSP 70 argues against this. Alternatively, HSP 70 immunoreactivity may all be a well-correlated epiphenomenon, perhaps produced by immunization of self-proteins during inflammatory responses arising from other causes. Lastly, initial studies with serum tested by Western blotting were accomplished with the use of 68 kD inner ear tissue as the target antigen. After the recognition that HSP 70 showed results similar to 68 kD by several investigators, a number of groups have adopted HSP 70 as the target for immunologic testing. In fact, this may be the wrong approach if HSP 70 merely shares epitopes with but is not the actual antigen in 68 kD inner ear immunoreactivity. Future studies will certainly improve our knowledge of the actual antigenic target(s) involved in AIED. Despite uncertainty over etiology and difficulties in diagnosis, this condition is frequently responsive to treatment with immunosuppressive drugs. Since there are few forms of SNHL that can be treated other than symptomatically, AIED represents a unique opportunity to reverse SNHL and vestibular disorders. For this reason alone, the diagnosis should be considered when symptoms are appropriate, and both clinical and basic research on this condition is warranted.

REFERENCES

1. Harris JP. Immunology of the inner ear: Response of the inner ear to antigen challenge. Otolaryngol Head Neck Surg 1983;91:18–32.
2. Harris JP. Immunology of the inner ear: Evidence of local antibody production. Ann Otol Rhinol Laryngol 1984;93:157–62.
3. Harris JP, Ryan AF. Immunobiology of the inner ear. Am J Otolaryngol 1984;5:418–25.
4. Harris JP, Woolf NK, Ryan AF. Elaboration of systemic immunity following inner ear immunization. Am J Otolaryngol 1985;6:148–52.
5. Woolf NK, Harris JP. Cochlear pathophysiology associated with inner ear immune responses. Acta Otolaryngol 1986;102:353–64.
6. Ma C, Billings P, Harris JP, Keithley EM. Characterization of an experimentally induced inner ear immune response. Laryngoscope 2000;110:451–6.
7. Wackym PA, Friberg U, Linthicum FH, Jr, et al. Human endolymphatic sac: Morphologic evidence of immunologic function. Ann Otol Rhinol Laryngol 1987;96:276–81.
8. Tomiyama S, Harris JP. The endolymphatic sac: Its importance in inner ear immune responses. Laryngoscope 1986;96:685–91.
9. Tomiyama S, Harris JP. The role of the endolymphatic sac in inner ear immunity. Acta Otolaryngol 1987;103:182–8.
10. Harris JP, Woolf NK, Ryan AF, et al. Immunologic and electrophysiological response to cytomegaloviral inner ear infection in the guinea pig. J Infect Dis 1984;150:523–30.
11. Woolf NK, Harris JP, Ryan AF, et al. Hearing loss in experimental cytomegalovirus infection of the guinea pig inner ear: Prevention by systemic immunity. Ann Otol Rhinol Laryngol 1985;94:350–6.
12. Darmstadt GL, Keithley EM, Harris JP. Effects of cyclophosphamide on the pathogenesis of cytomegalovirus-induced labyrinthitis. Ann Otol Rhinol Laryngol 1990;99:960–8.
13. Harris JP, Fukuda S, Keithley EM. Spiral modiolar vein: Its importance in inner ear inflammation. Acta Otolaryngol 1990;110:357–65.
14. Stearns GS, Keithley EM, Harris JP. Development of high endothelial venule-like characteristics in the spiral modiolar vein induced by viral labyrinthitis. Laryngoscope 1993;103:890–8.
15. Takahashi M, Harris JP. Analysis of immunocompetent cells following inner ear immunostimulation. Laryngoscope 1988;98.1133–8.
16. Suzuki M, Harris JP. Expression of intercellular adhesion molecule-1 during inner ear inflammation. Ann Otol Rhinol Laryngol 1995;104:69–75.
17. Keithley EM, Woolf NK, Harris JP. Development of morphological and physiological changes in the cochlea induced by cytomegalovirus. Laryngoscope 1989;99:409–14.
18. Chen MC, Harris JP, Keithley EM. Immunohistochemical analysis of proliferating cells in a sterile labyrinthitis animal model. Laryngoscope 1998;108:651–6.
19. McCabe BF. Autoimmune sensorineural hearing loss. Ann Otol Rhinol Laryngol 1979;88:585–9.
20. Schiff M, Brown M. Hormones and sudden deafness. Laryngoscope 1974;84:1959–81.
21. Clemis JD, Mastricola PG, Schuler-Vogler M. Sudden hearing loss in the contralateral ear in postoperative acoustic tumor: Three case reports. Laryngoscope 1982;92:76–9.
22. Teryama Y, Saski Y. Studies on experimental allergic (isoimmune) labyrinthitis in guinea pigs. Acta Otolaryngol 1963;58:49–61.
23. Hughes GB, Barna BP, Kinney SE, et al. Autoimmune endolymphatic hydrops: Five-year review. Otolaryngol Head Neck Surg 1988;98:221–5.
24. Moskowitz D, Lee KJ, Smith HW. Steroid use in idiopathic sudden sensorineural hearing loss. Laryngoscope 1984;94:664–6.
25. Ariyasu L, Byl FM, Sprague MS, Adour KK. The beneficial effect of methylprednisone in acute vestibular vertigo. Arch Otolaryngol Head Neck Surg 1990;166:700–3.
26. Harris JP, Ryan AF. Fundamental immune mechanisms of the brain and inner ear. Otolaryngol Head Neck Surg 1995;112:639–53.
27. McCabe BF. Autoimmune inner ear disease. In: Bernstein J, Ogra P, editors. Immunology of the Ear. New York: Raven Press; 1987. p. 427–35.
28. Harris JP, Sharp PA. Inner ear autoantibodies in patients with rapidly progressive sensorineural hearing loss. Laryngoscope 1990;100:516–24.
29. Schuknecht HF. Ear pathology in autoimmune disease. Adv Otorhinolaryngol 1991;46:50–70.
30. Hoistad DL, Schachern PA, Paparella MM. Autoimmune sensorineural hearing loss: A human temporal bone study. Am J Otolaryngol 1998;19:33–9.
31. Jenkins HA, Pollak AM, Fisch U. Polyarteritis nodosa as a cause of sudden deafness: A human temporal bone study. Am J Otolaryngol 1981;2:99–107.
32. Keithley EM, Chen MC, Linthicum FH. Clinical diagnoses associated with histologic findings of fibrotic tissue and new bone in the inner ear. Laryngoscope 1998;108:87–91.
33. Hughes GB, Barna BP, Kinney SE, et al. Predictive value of laboratory tests in "autoimmune" inner ear disease: Preliminary report. Laryngoscope 1986;96:502–5.
34. Gottschlich S, Billings PB, Keithley EM, et al. Assessment of serum antibodies in patients with rapidly progressive sensorineural hearing loss and Ménière disease. Laryngoscope 1995;105:1347–52.
35. Bouman H, Klis SF, Meeuwsen F, et al. Experimental autoimmune inner ear disease: An electrocochleographic and histophysiologic study. Ann Otol Rhinol Laryngol 2000;109:457–66.
36. Soliman AM, Zanetti F. Improvements of a method for testing autoantibodies in sensorineural hearing loss. Adv Otorhinolaryngol 1988;39:13–7.
37. Harris JP. Experimental autoimmune sensorineural hearing loss. Laryngoscope 1987;97:63–76.
38. Nair TS, Raphael Y, Dolan DF, et al. Monoclonal antibody induced hearing loss. Hear Res 1995;83:101–13.
39. Ruckenstein MJ, Sarwar A, Hu L, et al. Effects of immunosuppression on the development of cochlear disease in the MRL-Fas(lpr) mouse. Laryngoscope 1999;109:626–30.
40. Sone M, Schachern PA, Paparella MM, Morizono N. Study of systemic lupus erythematosus in temporal bones. Ann Otol Rhinol Laryngol 1999;108:338–44.
41. Cao MY, Gersdorff M, Deggouj N, et al. Detection of inner ear disease autoantibodies by immunoblotting. Mol Cell Biochem 1995;146:157–63.
42. Matsuoka H, Cheng KC, Krug MS, et al. Murine model of autoimmune hearing loss induced by myelin protein P0. Ann Otol Rhinol Laryngol 1999;108:255–64.
43. Gloddek B, Lassmann S, Gloddek J, Arnold W. Role of S-100beta as potential autoantigen in an autoimmune disease of the inner ear. J Neuroimmunol 1999;101:39–46.
44. Gloddek B, Gloddek J, Arnold W. A rat T-cell line that mediates autoimmune disease of the inner ear in the Lewis rat. ORL J Otorhinolaryngol Relat Spec 1999;61:181–7.
45. Nair TS, Prieskorn DM, Miller JM, et al. KHRI-3 monoclonal antibody-induced damage to the inner ear: Antibody staining of nascent scars. Hear Res 1999;129:50–60.
46. Iwai H, Tomoda K, Sugiura K, et al. T cells infiltrating from the systemic circulation proliferate in the endolymphatic sac. Ann Otol Rhinol Laryngol 1999;108:1146–50.
47. Ruckenstein MJ, Hu L. Antibody deposition in the stria vascularis of the MRL-Fas(lpr) mouse. Hear Res 1999;127:137–42.
48. Wobig RJ, Kempton JB, Trune DR. Steroid-responsive cochlear dysfunction in the MRL/lpr autoimmune mouse. Otolaryngol Head Neck Surg 1999;121:344–7.
49. Khan DC, DeGagne JM, Trune DR. Abnormal cochlear connective tissue mineralization in the Palmerston North autoimmune mouse. Hear Res 2000;142:12–22.
50. Shin SO, Billings PB, Keithley EM, Harris JP. Comparison of anti-heat shock protein 70 (anti-hsp70) and anti-68-kD inner ear protein in the sera of patients with Ménière's disease. Laryngoscope 1997;107:222–7.
51. Moscicki RA, San Martin JE, Quintero CH, et al. Serum antibody to inner ear proteins in patients with progressive hearing loss. JAMA 1994;272:611–6.
52. Atlas MD, Chai F, Boscato L. Ménière's disease: Evidence of an immune process. Am J Otol 1998;19:628–31.
53. Billings PB, Keithley EM, Harris JP. Evidence linking the 68 kilodalton antigen identified in progressive sensorineural hearing loss patient sera with heat shock protein 70. Ann Otol Rhinol Laryngol 1995;104:181–8.
54. Bloch DB, San Martin JE, Rauch SD, et al. Serum antibodies to heat shock protein 70 in sensorineural hearing loss. Arch Otolaryngol Head Neck Surg 1995;121:1167–71.
55. Yamanobe S, Harris JP. Inner ear specific autoantibodies. Laryngoscope 1993;103:319–25.
56. Trune DR, Kempton JB, Mitchel CR, Heferneider SH. Failure of elevated heat shock protein 70 antibodies to alter cochlear function in mice. Hear Res 1998;116:65–70.
57. Modugno GC, Pirodda A, Ferri GG, et al. A relationship between autoimmune thyroiditis and benign paroxysmal positional vertigo? Med Hypoth 2000;54:614–5.
58. Yamawaki M, Ariga T, Gao Y, et al. Sulfoglucuronosyl glycolipids as putative antigens for autoimmune inner ear disease. J Neuroimmunol 1998;84:111–6.
59. Lopez-Gonzalez MA, Lucas M, Sanchez B, et al. Autoimmune deafness is not related to hyperreactivity to type II collagen. Acta Otolaryngol (Stockh) 1999;119:690–4.
60. Hirose K, Wener MH, Duckert LG. Utility of laboratory testing in autoimmune inner ear disease. Laryngoscope 1999;109:1749–54.
61. Bloch DB, Gutierrez JA, Jr, Guerriero V, et al. Recognition of a dominant epitope in bovine heat-shock protein 70 in inner ear disease. Laryngoscope 1999;109:621–5.
62. Rauch SD, San Martin JE, Moscicki RA, Bloch KJ. Serum antibodies against heat shock protein 70 in Ménière's disease. Am J Otol 1995;16:648–52.
63. Rauch SD, Zurakowski D, Bloch DB, Bloch KJ. Anti-heat shock protein 70 antibodies in Ménière's's disease. Laryngoscope 2000;110:1516–21.
64. Arnold W, Pfaltz R, Altermatt HJ. Evidence of serum antibodies against inner ear tissues in the blood of patients with certain sensorineural hearing disorders. Acta Otolaryngol 1985;99:437–44.
65. Bachor E, ten Cate WJ, Gloddek B, Ehsani N. Immunohistochemical detection of humoral autoantibodies in patients

with hearing loss in the last hearing ear. Laryngorhinootologie 2000;79:131–4.

66. Arbusow V, Strupp M, Dieterich M, et al. Serum antibodies against membranous labyrinth in patients with "idiopathic" bilateral vestibulopathy. J Neurol 1998;245:132–6.

67. Ottaviani F, Cadoni G, Marinelli L, et al. Anti-endothelial autoantibodies in patients with sudden hearing loss. Laryngoscope 1999;109:1084–7.

68. Helmchen C, Arbusow V, Jager L, et al. Cogan's syndrome: Clinical significance of antibodies against the inner ear and cornea. Acta Otolaryngol 1999;119:528–36.

69. Harris JP, Weisman MH, Derebery JM, et al. Treatment of corticosteroid-responsive autoimmune inner ear disease with methotrexate: A randomized controlled trial. JAMA 2003;290:1875–83.

70. Luetje CM. Theoretical and practical implications for plasmapheresis in autoimmune inner ear disease. Laryngoscope 1989;99:1137–46.

71. Cohen S, Shoup A, Weisman M, Harris J. Etanercept treatment for autoimmune inner ear disease: Results of a pilot placebo-controlled study. Otol Neurotol 2005;26:903–7.

72. Parnes LS, Sun AH, Freeman DJ. Corticosteroid pharmacokinetics in the inner ear fluids: An animal study followed by clinical application. Laryngoscope 1999;109:1–17.

73. Chandrasekhar SS, Rubinstein RY, Kwartler JA, et al. Dexamethasone pharmacokinetics in the inner ear: Comparison of route of administration and use of facilitating agents. Otolaryngol Head Neck Surg 2000;122:521–8.

74. Yang GS, Song HT, Keithley EM, Harris JP. Intra-tympanic immunosuppressives for prevention of immune-mediated sensorineural hearing loss. Am J Otol 2000;21:499–504.

75. Takasu T, Harris JP. Reduction of inner ear inflammation by treatment with anti-ICAM-1 antibody. Ann Otol Rhinol Laryngol 1997;106:1070–5.

76. Morgan RF, Baumgartner CF. Ménière's's disease complicated by recurrent interstitial keratitis. Excellent result following cervical ganglionectomy. West J Surg 1934;42:628.

77. Cogan DG. Syndrome of nonsyphilitic interstitial keratitis and vestibuloauditory symptoms. Arch Ophthalmol 1945;33:144–9.

78. Morgan GJ, Hochman R, Weider DJ. Cogan's Syndrome: Acute vestibular and auditory dysfunction with interstitial keratitis. Am J Otolaryngol 1984;5:258–61.

79. McDonald TJ, Vollertsen RS, Younge BR. Cogan's syndrome: Audiovestibular involvement and prognosis in 18 patients. Laryngoscope 1985;95:650–4.

80. Peeters GJ, Cremers CW, Pinckers AJ, Hoefnagels WH. Atypical Cogan's syndrome: An autoimmune disease? Ann Otol Rhinol Laryngol 1986;95:173–5.

81. Ndiaye IC, Rassi SJ, Wiener-Vacher SR, Cochleovestibular impairment in pediatric Cogan's syndrome. Pediatrics 2002;109:38.

82. Susac JO, Hardman JM, Selhorst JB. Microangiopathy of the brain and retina. Neurol 1979;29:313–6.

83. Gross M, Eliashar R. Update on Susac's syndrome. Curr Opin Neurol 2005;18:311–4.

84. Bateman ND, Johnson IJ, Gibbin KP. Susac's syndrome: A rare cause of fluctuating sensorineural hearing loss. J. Laryngol Otol 1997;111:1072–4.

85. Susac JO. Susac's syndrome. Am J Neurorad 2004;25:351–2.

86. Petty GW, Engel AG, Younge BR, et al. Retinocochleocerebral vasculopathy. Medicine 1998;77:12–40.

87. Lammouchi TM, Bouker SM, Grira MT, Benammou SA. Susacs syndrome. Saudi Med J 2004;25:222–4.

88. Plummer C, Rattray K, Donnan GA, Basilli S. An unusual disease presenting at an unusual age: Susac's syndrome. J Clin Neurosci 2005;12:99–100.

89. Macias JD, Wackym PA, McCabe BF. Early diagnosis of otologic Wegener's granulomatosis using the serologic marker C-ANCA. Ann Otol Rhinol Laryngol 1993;102:337–41.

90. McCaffrey TV, McDonald TJ, Facer GW, DeRemee RA. Otologic manifestations of Wegener's granulomatosis. Otolaryngol Head Neck Surg 1980;88:586–93.

91. Malmvall BE, Bengtsson BA. Giant cell arteritis. Clinical features and involvement of different organs. Scand J Rheumatol 1978;7:154–8.

92. Erdinc AK, Harputluoglu U, Oghan F, Baykal B. Behcet's disease and hearing loss. Auris Nasus Larynx 2004;31:29–33.

93. Kulahli I, Balci K, Koseoglu E, et al. Audio-vestibular disturbances in Behcet's patients: Report of 62 cases. Hear Res 2005;203:28–31.

94. Yates PA, Michelson JB. Behcet disease. Int Ophthalmol Clin 2006;46:209–33.

95. Paira SO. Sudden senorineural hearing loss in patients with systemic lupus erythematosus or lupus like syndrome and antiphospholipid antibodies. J Rheumatol 1998;25:2476–7.

96. Agarwal K, Thomas N, Taneja V, et al. Plasma exchange in a child with systemic lupus erythematosus antiphospholipid antibodies and profound deafness. Ann Trop Paediatr 2002;22:109–10.

97. Mora R, Mora F, Passali FM, et al. Restoration of immune-mediated sensorineural hearing loss with sodium enoxaparin: A case report. Acta Otolaryngol Suppl 2004;552:25–8.

98. Kumakiri K, Sakamoto T, Karahashi T, et al. A case of relapsing polychondritis preceded by inner ear involvement. Auris Nasus Larynx 2005;32:71–6.

99. Ozturk A, Yalcin S, Kaygusuz I, et al. High frequency hearing loss and middle ear involvement in rheumatoid arthritis. Am J Otolaryngol 2004;25:411–7.

100. Takatsu M, Higaki M, Kinoshita H, et al. Ear involvement in patients with rheumatoid arthritis. Otol Neurotol 2005;26:755–61.

101. Kastanioudakis I, Ziavra N, Voulgari PV, et al. Ear involvement in systemic lupus erythematosus patients: A comparative study. J Laryngol Otol 2002;116:103–7.

102. Sule SD, Wigley FM. Update on management of scleroderma. Bul Rheum Dis 2000;49:1–4.

103. Boki KA, Ioannidis JP, Segas JV, et al. How significant is sensorineural hearing loss in primary Sjogren's syndrome? An individually matched case–control study. J Rheumatol 2001;28:798–801.

104. Ziavra N, Politi EN, Kastanioudakis I, et al. Hearing loss in Sjogren's syndrome patients. A comparative study. Clin Exp Rheumatol 2000;18:725–8.

105. Kumar BN, Smith MS, Walsh RM, Green JR. Sensorineural hearing loss in ulcerative colitis. Clin Otolaryngol Allied Sci 2000;25:143–5.

28

Menière Disease, Vestibular Neuritis, Benign Paroxysmal Positional Vertigo, Superior Semicircular Canal Dehiscence, and Vestibular Migraine

David R. Friedland, MD, PhD
Lloyd B. Minor, MD

INTRODUCTION

Dizziness is one of the most frequent symptoms prompting referral to an otolaryngologist–head and neck surgeon. Dizziness, however, takes many forms, and it is up to the otolaryngologist–head and neck surgeon to decipher the nature of the dizziness and whether it represents an otologic pathology or the patient requires evaluation by other specialties, such as neurology, cardiology, or even psychiatry. If the dizziness is otologic in nature, it is the role of the otolaryngologist to determine the cause of the disorder and the appropriate treatment. One of the most important components in the evaluation of dizziness is the patient's history.

It is critical in the history taking process to understand what the patient means by the term "dizzy." Patients will use the term "dizzy" to describe lightheadedness, wooziness, fatigue, disconnectedness, disequilibrium, imbalance, as well as vertigo. Vertigo is the sensation of inappropriate motion, most commonly rotational or spinning in nature, but also applicable to sensations of being pulled or pushed in one direction. According to the Committee on Hearing and Equilibrium of the American Academy of Otolaryngology–Head and Neck Surgery, vertigo is the sensation of motion when no motion is occurring relative to Earth's gravity.[1] Vertigo may be perceived by the patient as "the world moving around me" or as "spinning inside my head." Some patients may not relate a sensation of spinning when recounting episodes of vertigo, but a history of intensity such that walking was not feasible should be considered significant. Vertigo is the most common sensation referable to otologic forms of dizziness, and it is thus important to distinguish vertigo from the other common uses of the word dizzy.

It is also important in the history taking process to determine the temporal pattern of a patient's dizziness. That is, does the dizziness last for seconds, minutes, hours, or days; does it occur daily, weekly or at longer intervals; was it a single episode or multiple similar attacks? Also, the clinician must piece apart an episode of dizziness and determine whether there was a few seconds of vertigo with a subsequent hour of malaise or a full hour of vertigo. The most useful information from the patient's history that will assist in determining the cause of dizziness will frequently come from answers to the following 5 questions: (1) Does the patient have vertigo? (2) Are the patient's symptoms episodic or continuous? (3) If the symptoms are episodic, what is their duration? (4) Are the symptoms positional in character? and (5) Are there associated auditory symptoms? By carefully questioning and requestioning the patient an accurate picture of the symptoms can be developed which will help to distinguish attacks of Menière disease from those of vestibular neuritis, benign paroxysmal positional vertigo (BPPV), vestibular migraine or superior semicircular canal dehiscence. This chapter will focus on these disorders and describe the typical presentations, characteristic features, and pitfalls in diagnosis and management.

VESTIBULAR PHYSIOLOGY

It is not the purpose of this chapter to review vestibular physiology (see Chapter 4, "Physiology of the Auditory and Vestibular Systems"), but it is important to understand the basic premise of peripheral vestibular input to the central nervous system to understand the disorders discussed. Each vestibular end organ maintains a bascline of spontaneous activity which is transmitted centrally via the vestibular division of the eighth cranial nerve to the vestibular nuclei. The brainstem and cerebellum integrate and compare the input from both sides to determine aspects of head motion including direction, distance, and velocity. Motion in the direction and plane of a semicircular canal causes an increase in activity in that canal along with a decrease of activity in its paired canal on the opposite side. For example, a head rotation to the left, in the horizontal or yaw plane, causes an increase in the discharge rate of vestibular-nerve afferents innervating the left horizontal canal and a decrease in the discharge rate of afferents innervating the right horizontal canal. The difference in activity between the ears is centrally computed, and the eyes move to the right the appropriate distance. The purpose of the vestibulo-ocular reflex (VOR) which is controlled by this neural information arising in the labyrinth is to maintain the stability of images on the retina during head movements. In so doing, the VOR enables us to maintain steady fixation on objects even during head movements.

Sudden changes in unilateral vestibular activity will likewise provoke eye movements according to the canal and side affected. If the change in activity is nonphysiologic, such as loss of unilateral function due to vestibular neuritis, the brain receives mismatched input. That is, there is abnormal input from the affected canal suggesting head motion, but the input from the rest of the body is inconsistent with actual motion. This asymmetry in activity from the 2 labyrinths results in nystagmus: a rapid, to-and-fro motion of the eyes with slow and fast components. The slow component (sometimes referred to as slow phase) represents the eye movement elicited by the VOR. The fast component (the direction of nystagmus) represents a correction for this erroneous movement of the eye. For example, loss of neural activity in the right labyrinth is interpreted as a head movement to the left because of the asymmetry in resting rate between the two sides with activity in the left horizontal canal being much higher than that in the right horizontal canal. The VOR that results from such a pattern of activation consists of an eye movement reflective of the asymmetry in resting rate and in this case causes a slow phase to the right. The fast component of nystagmus to the left occurs because of the limit of the oculomotor range such that a resetting movement is required to bring the eye back toward the center. The direction of the nystagmus is named with respect to the fast component. This nystagmus is visible to the observer and is experienced by the patient as repetitive movements of the visual field. The nystagmus due to asymmetries in neural activity between the two labyrinths typically displays three cardinal features: (1) it is a horizontal–torsional nystagmus with fast components that beat toward the side of increased activity, (2) the nystagmus can be reduced when the patient fixates on an object in the external environment, and (3) the nystagmus increases in amplitude when the patient looks in the direction of the fast component and is decreased when the patient looks in the direction of the slow component.

MENIÈRE DISEASE

The link between symptoms of vertigo and imbalance and the inner ear was first established in 1861 by Prosper Menière although the patients that he described may not have had the syndrome that is currently known by his name.[2] Menière syndrome can occur following injuries to the labyrinth as can occur following measles or rubella infections. When the symptom complex occurs without any known underlying cause, it is frequently referred to as Menière disease. Hallpike and Cairns, in 1938, clarified the pathophysiology of this disorder and demonstrated "endolymphatic hydrops" as an associated feature of Menière disease.[3] Often overlooked is work by Portmann a decade earlier who proposed the endolymphatic sac as a cause of Menière disease and even performed the first endolymphatic sac decompression in humans.[4] Currently, Menière disease is recognized as a primary otologic disorder characterized by fluctuating hearing loss, episodic vertigo, tinnitus and aural fullness. Unfortunately, the nuances that differentiate Menière disease from other otologic disorders are often overlooked and Menière disease is frequently misdiagnosed, almost always being overdiagnosed rather than missed.

The American Academy of Otolaryngology–Head and Neck Surgery Committee on Equilibrium and Balance has issued guidelines for the proper diagnosis and classification of Menière disease.[1] This report defines key properties of the symptoms of Menière disease and establishes diagnostic categories to be used for reporting on Menière disease and to guide treatment decisions. The report stresses the triad of vertigo, hearing loss, and tinnitus in defining the syndrome and recognizes idiopathic endolymphatic hydrops as the physiologic cause.

Vertigo is a mandatory symptom in the accurate diagnosis of Menière disease. The vertigo should be rotational, recurrent (ie, 2 or more distinct episodes), last from 20 minutes to 24 hours and occur spontaneously. The latter indicates that there should be no provoking stimulus such as head position or specific activity as occurs with BPPV or superior semicircular canal dehiscence. The vertigo should also occur in the absence of other neurologic symptoms such as parasthesias or visual scotomas, which would be more consistent with vestibular migraine. The vertigo is of such intensity that complaints of associated nausea and/or vomiting are common.

The hearing loss of Menière disease must be sensorineural and typically involves the low frequencies. The hearing loss should fluctuate and

a stronger case for Menière disease can be made if fluctuations are documented with audiometric testing on at least 1 occasion. The hearing loss is typically unilateral and usually increases in severity with time. Profound hearing loss in affected ear(s) occurs in only 1 to 2% of severely affected patients.[5] Those patients with bilateral profound sensorineural hearing loss as a consequence of Menière disease are benefited from cochlear implantation.[6] Lermoyez, in 1919, described improvement in hearing thresholds in some patients associated with an attack of vertigo.[7]

A common associated feature of hearing loss is a sense of pressure in the ear. Aural fullness is frequently noted in Menière disease and often gets worse leading up to or concurrent with attacks. There may also be baseline aural fullness on the affected side.

The tinnitus of Menière disease is generally low pitched and is often described as a rumble, machine sound, ocean/seashell sound, hum, or low buzzing. It should be distinguished from the common high pitched steady tone tinnitus usually seen with hearing loss due to presbyacusis. The tinnitus should localize to one side and be consistent with the suspected side of involvement based upon audiometric and vestibular testing. Commonly the tinnitus increases in volume during, or leading up to, attacks of vertigo. Care should be taken to distinguish this form of tinnitus from the bilateral or "head-buzzing" tinnitus common in migraine sufferers or those with panic attack.

The diagnosis of Menière disease includes possible, probable, definite, and certain categories (Table 1). Possible Menière disease has the vertigo of Menière disease without documented hearing loss or has hearing loss characteristic of the disorder without true episodic vertigo. This category is akin to the outdated terms of cochlear

Menière disease or vestibular Menière disease, and other disorders should be excluded. Possible Menière disease is just that, possible, and it should be explained as such to the patient and the initiation of therapy or observation carefully weighed. Often patients with a single episode of vertigo or an unexplained hearing loss will be erroneously labeled with Menière disease and detrimentally carry that diagnosis with them in all future physician contacts. It is the authors' opinion that "possible Menière disease" is a diagnosis in evolution and follow-up examinations and tests should be used to rule-in or rule-out Menière disease before initiating therapy.

Probable Menière disease is a category in which both cochlear and vestibular signs and symptoms are present. There should be at least 1 episode of vertigo and at least 1 occasion of hearing loss that has been documented with audiometric testing. The vertigo should be a discrete episode of rotation but does not necessarily need to fulfill the strict criterion of duration. The duration of the vertigo should, however, factor into the differential diagnosis to distinguish BPPV, vestibular migraine, vestibular neuritis, or superior semicircular canal dehiscence. Tinnitus or aural pressure in the suspected ear is a diagnostic criterion for probable Menière disease. Other causes for the patient's symptoms should be excluded.

Definite Menière disease has all the symptomatic features as described above, but the vertigo should be recurrent with discrete, spontaneous episodes lasting greater than 20 minutes. Hearing loss on at least 1 occasion should be documented with audiometric testing. Tinnitus or aural pressure is present in the affected ear and commonly fluctuates in intensity with attacks. Other causes for the symptoms should be excluded. If a patient with this history expires and histopathologic confirmation of endolymphatic hydrops is present then this represents a case of certain Menière disease.

Presentation

The patient with Menière disease will most commonly seek treatment for attacks of vertigo. Less often is the patient seeking evaluation for unilateral hearing loss, and uncommon is the patient with Menière disease seeking evaluation for isolated tinnitus. This pattern is principally due to the severity associated with the presentation of each of these aural symptoms. The vertigo of Menière disease is quite intense and typically lasts hours. That it recurs, often without warning, is particularly troublesome to the patient and prompts immediate evaluation. The hearing loss of Menière disease is typically low frequency, moderate, and fluctuating with initial attacks showing recovery to or near baseline. This hearing loss may initially be considered by some physicians to be due to eustachian tube dysfunction or serous otitis media. It is not until such attacks recur or fail to return to baseline that referral and specialty evaluation is initiated. The tinnitus of

---

Table 1 Classification of Menière Disease[1]

Possible Menière disease
  Episodic vertigo of the Menière type without documented hearing loss, or
  Sensorineural hearing loss, fluctuating or fixed, with disequilibrium but without definitive episodes
  Other causes excluded

Probable Menière disease
  One definitive episode of vertigo
  Audiometrically documented hearing loss on at least one occasion
  Tinnitus or aural fullness in the treated ear
  Other causes excluded

Definite Menière disease
  Two or more definitive spontaneous episodes of vertigo 20 min or longer
  Audiometrically documented hearing loss on at least 1 occasion
  Tinnitus or aural fullness in the treated ear
  Other causes excluded

Certain Menière disease
  Definite Menière disease, plus histopathologic confirmation

Menière disease is usually low frequency and less intrusive than that seen with noise exposure and presbyacusis. It is also unusual to develop Menière disease-type tinnitus without hearing loss or vertigo; and, thus, it is rare that tinnitus is the principal presenting complaint.

The patient with Menière disease is typically between the ages of 40 and 60 years.[8] A slight female to male preponderance (1.3:1) in the prevalence of Menière disease has been reported. Menière disease most commonly presents as a disorder affecting 1 ear.[9] Subsequent involvement of the contralateral ear has been reported to vary between 2 and 78%.[10] Lack of consensus about diagnostic criteria and varying lengths of time over which patients were followed are likely to be responsible for this wide range of values. A typical finding from longitudinal studies is that involvement of both ears occurs in about 20 to 30% of patients. A recent retrospective review of a large series of patients with Menière disease revealed that 11% of patients had bilateral disease at the time of diagnosis with an additional 12% developing Menière disease in the contralateral ear after initial diagnosis in one ear. The average time interval for conversion from unilateral to bilateral Menière disease was 7.6 years.[8]

Evaluation and Diagnostic Testing

There is no single test or group of tests that can be used to make the diagnosis of Menière disease. The patient's history as well as the findings on audiometric testing offer the most useful information.

A significant reduction of the caloric response in the affected ear has been observed in 48 to 74% of patients with Menière disease, and the caloric response is absent in the affected ear in 6 to 11% of patients.[11,12] When rapid, rotatory accelerations in the planes excitatory for each of the 6 semicircular canals were used to test the function in each canal, it was found that responses were most often normal in all canals (including the horizontal canal) even when the caloric response was diminished.[13] This preservation of function when evaluated with the head thrust in comparison to diminished function when evaluated with the caloric test may have one or more of the following explanations. Menière disease may have more adverse effects on the mechanisms controlling low frequency responses (tested by the caloric stimulus) in comparison to responses to stimuli that have high frequency, velocity, and acceleration (tested by the head thrust test). In this case, the low velocity and acceleration of endolymph movement resulting from a caloric stimulus would be insufficient to generate a normal response. However, the high velocity and acceleration of endolymph flow resulting from a head thrust would be adequate to generate a compensatory eye response. A second possibility is that the response to head velocity by vestibular nerve afferents in Menière disease is diminished for stimuli of both high and low frequency amplitudes, but the central gain for inputs of high frequency and amplitude is greater.

Electrocochleography has also been used in the diagnosis of Menière disease although interpretation of the findings remains a topic of controversy. The cochlea responds to repeated presentations of sound with a summating potential (SP) and an action potential (AP). The SP has been reported to be larger and more negative in patients with Menière disease.[14] This is thought to reflect the distention of the basilar membrane into the scala tympani causing an increase in the normal asymmetry of its vibration.[15] The utility of electrocochleography in the identification of Menière disease has been questioned.[16]

Treatment

There is no proven cure for Menière disease, and current therapy is directed at reduction of associated symptoms. The optimal treatment should stop vertigo, abolish tinnitus, and reverse hearing loss. Unfortunately, long-term hearing impairment does not seem amenable to treatment.[17] Most previous studies of the effects of therapy have analyzed the treatment of the most distressing aspect of Menière disease: vertigo.

Medical regimens aimed at prevention of vertigo are directed at decreasing the production and/or accumulation of endolymph. Salt restriction and diuresis are believed by many to be the best medical therapy for Menière disease.[18] These treatment measures have been reported to control vertigo in 58% of patients and to stabilize hearing in 69%.[19] Other studies, conducted using double-blind methodology, have shown no effect of diuretics.[20] Corticosteroids, administered orally and/or through intratympanic injection, have also been used in the management of the auditory and vestibular consequences of Menière disease.[21-23]

Vertigo persists despite optimal medical therapy in approximately 10% of patients with Menière disease.[24,25] Other forms of treatment are indicated in such situations. Surgical procedures performed on the endolymphatic sac are designed to decompress the sac and/or to drain endolymph from it. These procedures typically lead to complete resolution of vertigo in 50 to 75% of patients.[26-28] Recurrence of vertigo is common in patients followed up to 10 years. The efficacy of endolymphatic sac procedures has been questioned based upon comparisons involving sham surgery.[29,30]

In individuals failing medical therapy and/or sac surgery, definitive treatment for vertigo consists of one of several modalities of vestibular deafferentation with or without hearing preservation. Selective vestibular neurectomy, performed via a middle cranial fossa or posterior cranial fossa approach, has also been used to achieve control of vertigo in >90% of patients in whom this symptom was intractable.[31] The potential complications of these procedures, although uncommon, include hearing loss, facial nerve paralysis, cerebrospinal fluid (CSF) leak, and headache. Excellent control of vertigo is also achieved with surgical labyrinthectomy although remaining hearing in the operated ear is sacrificed.

Intratympanic aminoglycosides have long been used in the treatment of Menière disease. Schuknecht, in 1957, using streptomycin, and Lange, in 1976, using gentamicin, gave multiple intratympanic injections of these antibiotics each day until patients developed disequilibrium or until caloric responses were abolished.[32,33] Vertigo was controlled in most of these patients (100% in Schuknecht's series; 88% in Lange's series), but the rates of sensorineural hearing loss attributed to the aminoglycosides were unacceptably high (62 and 48%, respectively). Subsequent reductions in the number and frequency of doses have resulted in control of vertigo in 70 to 90% of patients and a reduction in the incidence of sensorineural hearing loss attributable to gentamicin.[34] Most recently, it has been shown that a single intratympanic injection of gentamicin is effective in the control of vertigo in most patients.[35] The long-term hearing outcome with these low dose gentamicin protocols is comparable to the hearing outcome in patients with Menière disease whose symptoms are medically managed.[35,36]

Recent studies have identified changes in vestibular function after intratympanic gentamicin; and, in so doing, these investigations are providing new insights into the mechanism through which gentamicin leads to control of vertigo. Carey and colleagues, in 2002, studied vestibular function as measured by caloric tests and by the 3-dimensional angular VOR (AVOR) elicited by rapid rotary head thrusts in the planes of the semicircular canals before and after low doses of intratympanic gentamicin.[13] Analyses of the AVOR were based upon the head thrust test.[37]

Subjects with complete surgical unilateral vestibular destruction (SUVD) on one side fail to maintain visual fixation on a target when the head undergoes a rapid rotation toward the lesioned side. The test relies on Ewald's second law which specifies that there is a greater effect from *excitation* of a semicircular canal than from *inhibition* of a canal.[38] When the head is horizontally rotated toward the intact side in the head thrust test, the horizontal canal on the intact side is excited. The usual—but small—contribution of inhibition from the canal on the lesioned side is missing, but the response (eye velocity) generated by the excited canal is sufficient to yield an AVOR that is compensatory and only minimally changed. However, when the head is horizontally rotated toward the lesioned side, the horizontal canal on the intact side is inhibited. Without the large excitatory contribution from the horizontal canal on the lesioned side, the asymmetry between excitation and inhibition becomes manifest, and the AVOR is noncompensatory. On clinical examination this noncompensatory AVOR is manifested as a delay in the eye-movement response followed by a rapid, corrective eye movement that brings the eye back to the target.

The head thrust test has been quantitatively validated using magnetic search coil recordings of eye and head movements. AVOR gain values (the ratio of eye to head velocity) near 1.0 have been demonstrated in normal subjects.[39] Subjects with SUVD have markedly diminished gains for head thrusts that would excite the canals on the lesioned side.[40] Head thrusts in the planes of the vertical semicircular canals likewise demonstrate hypofunction and can even isolate hypofunction affecting only 1 canal.[41]

Quantitative evaluation of the three-dimensional AVOR in response to head thrusts has shown that patients with intractable vertigo due to unilateral Menière disease typically have symmetric gains of the horizontal VOR prior to intratympanic gentamicin. In contrast, a reduction of the caloric responses from the affected ear is seen in approximately 75% of these same patients. When tested after treatment with intratympanic gentamicin, a reduced horizontal canal gain for rapid head movements that were excitatory for the horizontal canal on the treated side was noted in each subject. Figure 1 shows the representative head (dashed gray) and eye (solid gray) velocity traces for a 38-year-old woman with a 3-year history of episodic vertigo as well as right fluctuating sensorineural hearing loss and tinnitus. Her caloric tests showed a 23% right unilateral vestibular weakness. Each panel of Figure 1 shows the traces of the subject's eye and head velocities for head thrusts that excited the indicated canal. For example, the panels in the column labeled "Ipsi" show the AVOR for head thrusts that excited the canals on the side affected with Menière disease. For ease of comparison, the signs of the eye and head velocity traces have been given as positive values in all panels. Figure 2 shows data from the same subject tested 49 days after a single injection of gentamicin into the right middle ear. She did not experience any further episodes of vertigo after the single dose. Following gentamicin treatment, her caloric tests showed a 92% unilateral vestibular weakness on the right side. Her AVOR data also showed marked decrements in the gains for head thrusts that excited any of the treated canals. Her AVOR gains for excitation of the contralateral canals also changed, but much less. This slight reduction in gain attributed to excitation of the contralateral canals is due to a reduction in the inhibitory contribution to the response from semicircular canals on the treated side.

AVOR gains for head thrusts that excite canals on the gentamicin-treated side exceeded those seen for the same stimuli in subjects with SUVD and gain asymmetries were smaller after gentamicin than after SUVD. This finding indicates that gentamicin is not producing a complete loss of vestibular function on the treated side. Electrophysiological studies in chinchillas have shown that gentamicin administered intratympanically in a manner similar to that used in humans produces a marked reduction in the sensitivity of afferents to motion. Resting discharge rate, although somewhat reduced after gentamicin treatment, is preserved as are the groups of afferents that can be distinguished based upon discharge regularity.[42]

Reduction in the gain of the AVOR for head thrusts that are excitatory for semicircular canals on the treated side have been shown to be correlated with control of vertigo following a single intratympanic injection of gentamicin.[43] Patients treated with intratympanic gentamicin may develop recurrent episodes of vertigo 6 to 18 months after treatment. These recurrences are treated successful with an additional intratympanic injection of gentamicin.

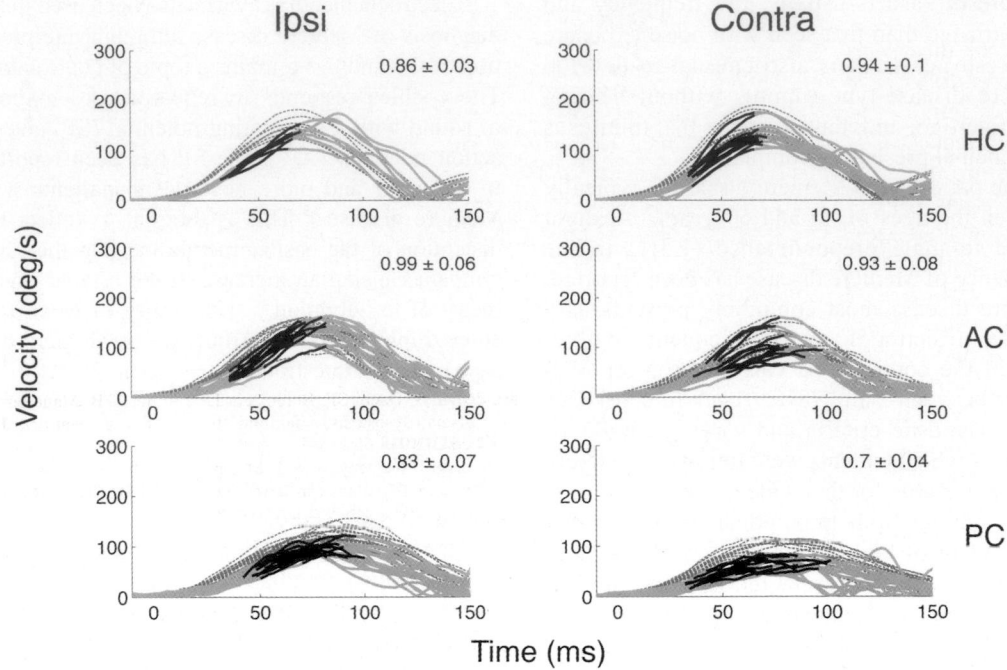

Figure 1 Responses to head thrusts in a patient tested immediately before intratympanic gentamicin treatment. Each panel shows head velocity (*light gray dashed*) and eye velocity (*dark gray and black*) for rotations in the excitatory direction for each semicircular canal (AC = anterior canal, HC = horizontal canal, PC = posterior canal). Data from 8 to 12 stimulus repetitions are shown for each canal. Head velocity has been inverted to permit a direct comparison of the stimulus and the response. The interval over which gain was analyzed (30 ms prior to peak head velocity) is shown in black for each trace. The eye velocity before and after this analysis interval is shown in dark gray. A gain value was calculated as eye/head velocity for every point in time during the analysis interval. The response gain for each stimulus repetition was defined as the maximum gain value during the interval of analysis. The response gain (mean ± SD for all stimulus repetitions) is given in each panel's upper right corner. (Published with permission from reference 13.)

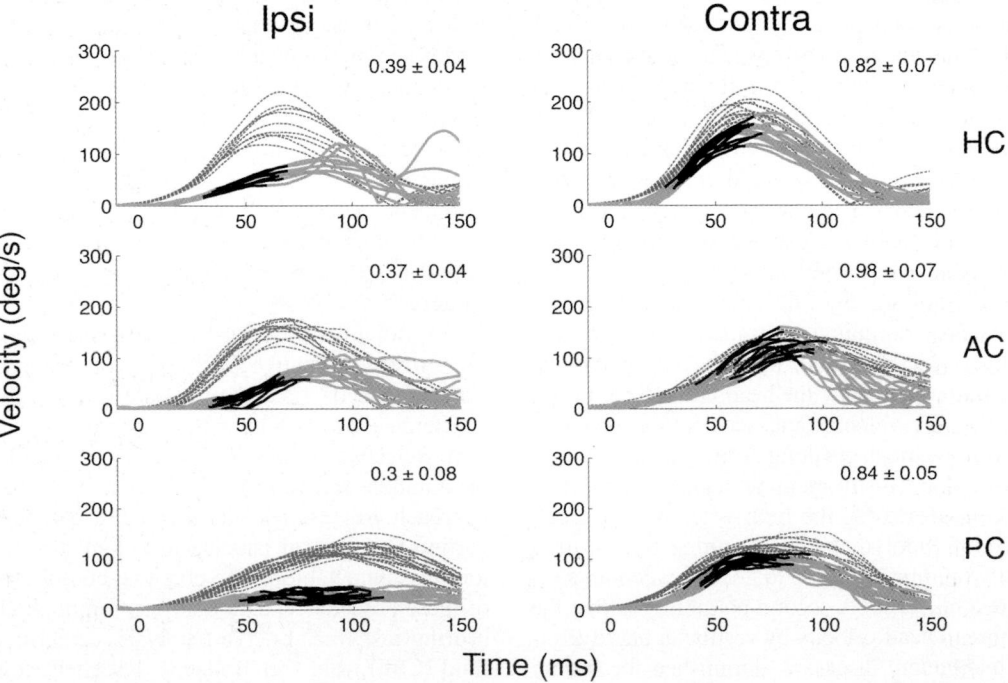

Figure 2 Responses to head thrusts that excited each of the six semicircular canals in the same patient as in Figure 1 measured 49 days after a single intratympanic injection of gentamicin. Panels, traces, and gain values are as described for Figure 1. (Published with permission from reference 13.)

Summary

Menière disease remains a highly debilitating disorder for many patients. Theories of pathogenesis remain incomplete. Treatment is based upon effects of the symptoms on patients' quality of life. Progress in the treatment of Menière disease has led to the development of effective treatment protocols involving intratympanic injection of gentamicin (low dose) in patients for whom vertigo has not been controlled by medical measures. Ongoing research is providing a greater understanding of the effects of gentamicin on vestibular function and of the mechanisms through which gentamicin leads to control of vertigo. Future directions for research related to Menière disease include genetic studies to define specific genotypes that may be associated with the development of the inner ear abnormalities. Investigations of mechanisms of inner ear injury and of autoimmune disorders that affect the ear should also help to understand the underlying cellular pathophysiology.

VESTIBULAR NEURITIS

One of the most common causes of dizziness for which an individual seeks emergency attention is vestibular neuritis. Overall, vestibular neuritis is the second most common cause of vertigo arising from a disorder of the labyrinth with an incidence of about 3.5 per 100,000 population per year.[44] The presenting symptoms and signs include sudden onset of sustained rotatory vertigo (lasting days to weeks), spontaneous nystagmus (with fast phase components beating toward the unaffected ear), and postural imbalance.

Various theories have been proposed to account for the cause of vestibular neuritis including inflammation of the vestibular nerve and ischemia of the labyrinth. Many of the histological features of vestibular neuritis when evaluated in postmortem studies are similar to those observed in other sensory epithelia in known viral disorders. Herpes simplex virus type 1 (HSV-1) DNA has been detected on autopsy with the use of polymerase chain reaction in about two of three human vestibular ganglia.[45] Reactivation of a latent infection with HSV-1 is an often-cited mechanism to account for the occurrence of vestibular neuritis.

Vestibular neuritis appears to affect the superior division of the vestibular nerve more commonly than the inferior division. Anatomic differences between the bony channels of the superior and inferior vestibular nerves may make the superior division more susceptible to injury.[46] The superior division has a longer course through bone than does the inferior division. The superior division could, therefore, be more susceptible to ischemic injury and entrapment.

Because of the putative association of the disorder with reactivation of HSV-1, the condition is sometimes referred to as vestibular neuronitis. The caloric test in vestibular neuritis most commonly reveals a reduced response on the affected side. In contrast, a vestibular evoked myogenic potential (VEMP) can be elicited from the affected ear in 61 to 88% of people affected with vestibular neuritis.[47] The VEMP response appears to arise from the sacculus so preservation of this response provides evidence that function of the inferior vestibular nerve and its end organs are intact. Also, quantitative assessment of the three-dimensional properties of the spontaneous nystagmus and of the vestibuloocular reflex evoked by rotations in the planes of different semicircular canals indicate that function in the posterior canal on the affected side is typically preserved whereas that in the horizontal and superior canals is diminished.[48]

Presentation

Due to the intensity of the vertigo, many patients are initially seen in the emergency room, treated supportively and discharged with instructions to follow-up with an otolaryngologist. These patients will complain of severe dizziness and vertigo, will have difficulty walking, will have nausea and commonly emesis and will try to remain still with their eyes closed so not to exacerbate their symptoms. Nystagmus will be present and in most cases beats toward the nonaffected ear as the insult results in loss of vestibular function on the affected side. In irritative cases of vestibular neuritis, the nystagmus may beat toward the affected ear, but this is rare.[49] The patient should be made to walk, however difficult it may be, as severe gait ataxia strongly raises the suspicion of a central cerebrovascular event such as cerebellar infarction. In a recent review of a large number of patients with isolated cerebellar infarction, 10% of patients (25/240) were noted to have a clinical picture that closely resembled vestibular neuritis.[50] The territory of the posterior inferior cerebellar artery (PICA) was most commonly involved in these patients. All these patients with infarction in the PICA territory had a normal head thrust test and normal caloric test in the affected ear. In practice, the possibility of brainstem or cerebellar infarct must be considered in any patient presenting with the acute onset of vertigo. Cranial magnetic resonance imaging (MRI) with diffusion weighted images should be performed when indicated based upon clinical suspicion of an infarct.

Hearing should be intact in cases of vestibular neuritis. The presence of hearing loss in the affected ear may indicate labyrinthitis, an acute Menière disease attack or infarct of the brainstem or cerebellum (often in the territory of the anterior inferior cerebellar artery).

The intense vertigo of acute vestibular neuritis can last from hours to days and rarely weeks. The patient is commonly first seen by an otolaryngologist in the subacute phase that lasts weeks, or occasionally months, following the initial attack. This phase is characterized by imbalance and disequilibrium that noticeably improves over this time. Patients will have sensitivity to motion and may avoid head turns and rapid movements. They may develop brief attacks of vertigo that are not as intense as the initial attack. Vestibular rehabilitation during this phase may speed recovery.[51]

At the end of the subacute phase the patient will be near their baseline balance function but may notice small disturbances of equilibrium with rapid motions or in challenging environments. If evaluated for dizziness at this late stage, a diagnosis of vestibular neuritis is based largely on a suspicious history of severe vertigo within the prior months to year. Additional testing, as described below, may also demonstrate a unilateral weakness confirming an insult to the inner ear. Commonly in this stage anxiety plays a major role in the patients' perception of their debility.[52] A significant portion of patients with acute vertigo will develop anxiety regarding their balance and potential for having recurring vertigo.[53–55] They will often limit activities such as driving, withdraw socially and become intensely fixated on any abnormal sensation of equilibrium. A multidisciplinary approach to treating these patients is necessary, and consideration should be given for early psychological intervention in any vestibular neuritis patient with a dependent or insecure personality type.[53,54]

It is rare for vestibular neuritis to recur. A recent retrospective review of 103 patients in whom vestibular neuritis was diagnosed identified a second occurrence 29 to 39 months after the first episode in only 2 patients.[56] The contralateral ear was affected in both of these patients, and vertigo was less distressing than the initial episode in both patients.

Although vestibular neuritis typically affects only the superior vestibular nerve, isolated involvement of the inferior division with diminished function in the posterior canal and sacculus but preserved function in the lateral and superior canals has been identified in some patients.[57] BPPV can occur following vestibular neuritis in cases where function in the inferior vestibular nerve is preserved.[58]

Evaluation and Diagnostic Testing

Physical Examination. Findings on physical examination will generally depend upon the stage of vestibular neuritis. In the acute phase, the examiner will note spontaneous nystagmus with a directional component that depends upon the affected semicircular canals. In the case of vestibular neuritis affecting the superior vestibular nerve, the fast phases will consist of horizontal and torsional components beating toward the unaffected ear. There may also be an up beating component reflecting preservation of function in the posterior canal on the affected side. The directional components of the nystagmus are reflective of Ewald's first law, which states that the eyes move in the plane of the affected semicircular canal(s).

Alexander's law is obeyed, and the nystagmus will increase in amplitude with gaze toward the horizontal fast phase component, which is usually toward the nonaffected ear. The nystagmus should suppress with visual fixation but may be of such intensity as to be reduced in amplitude but remain noticeable. Direction changing nystagmus and lack of visual suppression should raise the suspicion of a central event and prompt imaging for stroke evaluation. The presence of ataxia is also suggestive of central vestibular dysfunction or, rarely, a drug reaction.

Hearing should be checked during the acute phase, but this may only be feasible with tuning forks due to the severe nausea and emesis experienced by these patients. The Weber test will help to determine a unilateral loss of hearing, and the Rinne test will suggest whether that loss is sensorineural or conductive. A hearing loss is inconsistent with vestibular neuritis, and the practitioner should consider labyrinthitis, Menière disease, perilymphatic fistula, or acute otitis media among otologic causes of acute cochleovestibular symptoms.

The spontaneous nystagmus has usually resolved in the subacute phase although nystagmus may be observed with gaze toward the unaffected ear (Alexander's law). Evidence for a recent unilateral vestibular insult can be identified with the Halmagyi maneuver or head-thrust test.[59] In this test, the patient is asked to fixate on a point, for example, the examiner's nose, and the head is rapidly turned approximately 15% to 1 side in the horizontal plane. If there is a weakness, the patient will exhibit a refixation or "catch-up" saccade as the eyes jump back to the fixation point. In the normal condition, the eyes will remain fixed on the target due to the rapidity of the vestibular-ocular reflex. The horizontal canal is most commonly tested although head thrusts in the oblique planes can be performed to test the superior and posterior semicircular canals. Beyond the subacute phase, the head thrust examination may be positive in uncompensated cases. However, this most commonly returns to near normal due to peripheral vestibular recovery and central compensation.[60] A residual unilateral vestibular paresis may be detected clinically with the head shake test.[61,62] With Frenzel lenses on, the head is rotated left and right along the horizontal plane at about 1 to 2 Hz for 10 to 15 seconds. This takes advantage of Ewald's second law, which states that the range of encoding of motion is greater for activation than for inhibition of a semicircular canal. This repetitive maneuver thus loads each horizontal canal with compounding excitatory activity. At the end of the head shake, this activity discharges and will control eye movements. If both sides have equivalent function, the eyes will remain stable. If one side has vestibular paresis, the discharge from the good side will predominate and horizontal nystagmus toward the good ear will be observed.

Electronystagmography/Videonystagmography (ENG/VNG). Objective testing can be used to identify the unilateral vestibular hypofunction characteristic of vestibular neuritis. Caloric testing showing an asymmetry is consistent with a history of unilateral vestibular insult. This test is more sensitive than either head thrust or head shake for identifying such an asymmetry.[62] The ENG/VNG battery of tests can also be used to assess for the presence of BPPV which occurs often after vestibular neuritis. In the acute and subacute phases, ENG/VNG can identify and document spontaneous and gaze evoked nystagmus as well as determine their direction thus helping to identify the affected side.

Imaging. The acute phase of vestibular neuritis is of such severity and duration that clinical examination alone may not be sufficient to rule-out central vascular events. Thus, computed tomography (CT) scan is the initial imaging test of choice to look for an acute hemorrhage involving the brainstem or cerebellum. MRI of the internal auditory canals during an acute phase of vestibular neuritis may show subtle enhancement of the superior vestibular nerve at the region of Scarpa ganglion.[63] Beyond the acute phase, MRI with gadolinium enhancement is most useful for evaluating for other intracranial lesions that could account for an attack of vertigo or prolonged vestibular dysfunction. T1-weighted images with contrast can demonstrate the presence of vestibular schwannoma. Sudden vertigo is the initial presenting sign for vestibular schwannoma in approximately 15% of cases although its prevalence in vestibular schwannoma is about 40%.[64] It is rare in isolation and usually accompanies hearing loss. The presence of Chiari I malformation, cerebellar tumor, cerebellopontine angle arachnoid cyst, old brainstem infarct, or vascular loop can also be identified with MRI.

Management. Supportive treatment should also be given during the acute phase of vestibular neuritis. Patients should be hydrated if they are having significant emesis and provided antiemetics. Several medications can be used for nausea including the phenothiazines: prochlorperazine (Compazine), and promethazine (Phenergan); the antidopaminergic metoclopramide (Reglan); and the 5-HT receptor antagonist odansetron (Zofran). The authors prefer phenergan as it can be administered by intramuscular injection acutely and can be provided as a suppository if emesis continues as an outpatient. Vestibular suppressants can also be prescribed to attenuate the severity of the attack. Commonly emergency room and primary care physicians will use meclizine (Antivert) which commonly has side effects of urinary retention and sedation. Its efficacy has not been established for either acute phase vertigo or chronic disequilibrium although it can be effective for motion sensitivity.[65] Low dose valium is an effective vestibular suppressant, and minimally sedating dosages of 2 mg every 6 hours as needed can be provided. Attempts should be made to wean the patient off of vestibular suppressants as soon as possible to allow central compensation of the unilateral hypofunction.

The use of corticosteroids and antiviral medications in the treatment of vestibular neuritis has been investigated in a prospective randomized double-blind study. Placebo was compared with methylprednisolone, valcyclovir, and combination therapy of methylprednisolone and valcyclovir.[66] Methylprednisolone dosage was 100 mg daily for the first 3 days tapered by approximately 20 mg every 3 days for a total treatment time of 22 days. Valcyclovir was administered as 1,000 mg three times per day for 1 week. This study showed a significant benefit of corticosteroids but no added benefit of antiviral therapy nor any benefit of antiviral therapy alone. Some authors, however, have advocated antiviral therapy for recurrent vestibular neuritis and recommended intratympanic application of the antiviral medication if oral therapy fails to control symptoms.[67]

Once the patient has entered the subacute phase of their attack, vestibular rehabilitation exercises should be recommended. VOR exercises can speed central compensation for the unilateral weakness, and the interaction with a therapist through this stage can be reassuring to many patients. Those patients who are more distant from their acute attack but have evidence of continued failure to achieve compensation can also benefit from vestibular rehabilitation.[68] Patients experiencing chronic daily disequilibrium should be evaluated for psychogenic dizziness triggered by the initial neurotologic disorder. Additionally, an attack of vestibular neuritis may exacerbate underlying psychiatric or anxiety disorders.[55]

VESTIBULAR MIGRAINE

Vestibular migraine (migraine-associated dizziness) is an extremely common disorder afflicting approximately 17% of women and 6% of men in the United States. Although typically considered by many physicians and lay public alike to be a disorder of headache, migraine commonly manifests numerous additional neurological symptoms. Among these are disturbances of vision, parasthesias, fatigue, disordered thought, and disturbances of balance. Vestibular migraine is often misdiagnosed, specifically it is underdiagnosed, and should be considered in any patient presenting with dizziness, vertigo, or disequilibrium.

Migraine is classified into several subtypes by the International Headache Society (IHS).[69] Of importance to the otolaryngologist are migraine without aura and migraine with aura which has subcategories of basilar migraine, typical aura with migraine headache, and typical aura with nonmigraine headache and without headache (Table 2). To diagnose migraine without aura, the patient must have a headache lasting 4 hours to 3 days with at least 2 of the following 4 symptomatic characteristics: unilateral site, pulsating quality, moderate to severe in intensity or aggravation by physical activity. In addition, the headache phase must also be associated with nausea and/or vomiting, or photophobia or phonophobia. Migraine with aura has at least 3 of the following 4 features: at least 1 fully reversible neurological symptom suggesting brainstem or cortical dysfunction; at least 1 symptom developing

Table 2 Migraine Classification International Classification of Headache Disorders, Edition 2 (ICHD-II)[69]

ICHD-II Code	Diagnosis/Classification
1.	Migraine
1.1	Migraine without aura
1.2	Migraine with aura
1.2.1	Typical aura with migraine headache
1.2.2	Typical aura with nonmigraine headache
1.2.3	Typical aura without headache
1.2.6	Basilar-type migraine
1.3	Childhood periodic syndromes (migraine precursors)
1.3.3	Benign paroxysmal vertigo of childhood
1.5	Complications of Migraine
1.5.3	Persistent aura without infarction
1.6	Probable migraine (with or without aura)

gradually over >4 minutes or 2 symptoms in succession, for example, visual changes followed by nausea; neurological symptoms lasting <1 hour; or headache following the neurological symptoms within 1 hour.

The association between migraine and vestibular symptoms has been well established.[70,71] In practice, however, it is common to find patients and even some consulting neurologists resistant to the idea that dizziness may be related to migraine, particularly in headache free periods. While vestibular symptoms are present in over 50% of migraineurs, attacks of vertigo do not always occur with headache.[72] In fact, vestibular attacks occurred consistently in association with headache, that is, true aura, in only 24% of patients studied by Neuhauser and colleagues.[73] Thus, the majority of vestibular attacks occur in headache-free intervals. Indeed, vestibular symptoms may be the only sign of recurrent migraine in a patient with a distant history of severe headaches. It is not uncommon to be presented with a middle-aged woman with new onset dizziness in the absence of headache but with a history of headache or migraine as a teenager. This patient will also commonly have a family history of migraine or headache in first-degree relatives.

Presentation

The patient with vestibular migraine may present in several ways. The individual with migraine with aura will typically report discrete attacks of vertigo, usually lasting minutes to hours, associated with nausea that can occur before, concurrent or following the onset of dizziness. They will also note fatigue and commonly photophobia. Phonophobia, osmophobia, tinnitus, and a sense of hearing impairment are also not unusual. The hearing loss and tinnitus may suggest Menière disease but during migraine are typically bilateral. Further, the hearing loss is less of a threshold shift than a sense of not processing auditory information. Additionally, the tinnitus is often high

pitched or a roaring within the head rather than the classic Menière disease low pitched sound localized to one ear. Following or toward the end of these symptoms, the patient will develop headache or a sense of pressure in their head. They will typically sleep several hours and note that they awaken symptom-free and at baseline.

The episodic and intense form of vestibular migraine, that is , migraine with aura, is often difficult to distinguish from Menière disease but due to the recurrent nature, duration of symptoms and associated neurological complaints can usually be distinguished from BPPV, vestibular neuritis, or even panic attacks.[71,74] Complicating the differential diagnosis can be the lack of severe headache with these episodes. Specific questioning of the patient, however, can often reveal forms of attenuated headache such as head pressure, scalp parasthesias or neck pain and stiffness, that is, migraine classification 1.2.2: typical aura with nonmigraine headache.

The more common, but more difficult to diagnose, presentation of vestibular migraine is that which occurs without headache or with less distinct episodes of vertigo. Approximately 50% of vertigo attacks related to migraine occur in headache free intervals.[75] Additionally, migraine dizziness is often nonepisodic with complaints of chronic disequilibrium and waves of increasing severity that may crescendo to vertigo or severe imbalance. Other descriptions of dizzy attacks include lightheadedness, a swimming or drunk feeling, floating, or a sensation of disconnectedness from the environment. There may be postural complaints, but they often differ from BPPV on testing. Migraine postural sensitivities do not generally have a latency of onset and persist without fatigue during maneuvering. Nystagmus may or may not be present during postural changes, and the direction of nystagmus should be correlated with the vestibular labyrinth orientation to identify peripheral origin.

Patients with vestibular migraine will commonly note attacks provoked by visual stimuli and motion.[73] They will often have difficulties in stores with long and wide aisles and fluorescent lighting. Visually challenging situations such as watching a train pass, watching scrolling movie credits or a news ticker, or watching video games may provoke dizziness. Crowds may similarly pose problems. Repetitive activities such as computer work, particularly transcribing papers, and gardening may precipitate attacks or worsening of baseline dizziness. Approximately 50% of migraineurs will note histories of childhood car sickness, avoidance of amusement park rides, or sea-sickness. Oftentimes such sensitivity will have abated in adulthood, but recurred at the time of presentation.

The occurrences of attacks or exacerbations are often timed to the menstrual cycle or reflect irregularities in menstruation. Clusters of attacks may occur around menarche, pregnancy, and the perimenopausal period. Hormone replacement therapies or changes in an established regimen should be noted. Other strong stimulants for

vestibular migraine include stress, foods, weather changes, and travel.[76] Attacks tend to cluster around holidays, and they represent good temporal references in acquiring a history. These likely are due to stress of holiday activities, travel and dietary changes, most notably chocolate, red wine, and smoked meats such as ham. Commonly patients will note the onset of attacks after a period of intense stress such as the hospitalization of a family member or moving. The attack may represent a "decompression" of built up stress and anxiety. Travel by car, especially as a passenger, is very stimulating and is more troublesome than airplane travel. Boat trips and cruises can precipitate attacks and may lead to chronic migrainous-like disequilibrium after disembarking, the aptly named "mal de debarquement" syndrome.[77]

Many of these patients will show signs of depressed mood or heightened anxiety. It is not clear whether the migrainous dizziness is a symptom of their psychological disorder, an antecedent and triggering factor for the development of mood disturbance, or a separate but associated psychopathology.[55] Commonly, patients with chronic dizziness will have seen a psychiatrist, psychologist, or therapist and will readily admit to having an "anxious" personality. A history of panic disorder is also not unusual. In these anxious patients, it is important to get a detailed vestibular history. One can often find that the first attack was the most severe and of greater intensity and duration than those following. Careful questioning may reveal this primary attack to be consistent with vestibular neuritis and a prolonged compensation period. Postvestibular neuritis BPPV may have also been present and caused exacerbation of anxieties related to vestibular function. At the time of presentation, the patient has had months of various forms of dizziness and developed significant fear of having attacks in public.[53,54] Once the VOR has recovered and the BPPV has been treated or spontaneously resolved, the patient is left with a severe mood disorder and anxiety which serves as the predominant trigger for their dizziness. They appear to have attacks of vestibular migraine with chronic disequilibrium and of anxiety filling the interval periods. Indeed, in the susceptible patient, a peripheral vestibular insult such as vestibular neuritis may be a sufficient stressor to provoke the onset of vestibular migraine.

Diagnostic criteria based upon clinical presentation have been proposed for vestibular migraine.[78] This proposal is similar to the Menière disease classification and notes 2 categories of vestibular migraine, definite, and probable (Table 3). The patient with "definite" vertigo due to migraine should have moderate or severe episodic vestibular symptoms, a current or previous history of migraine according to IHS criteria, symptoms of headache, photophobia, phonophobia, visual or other auras on at least two occasions of vertigo, and other potential causes ruled out. The patient with "probable" vertigo due to migraine is similar, but the requirement for

Table 3 Classification of Vestibular Migraine[78]

Definite migrainous vertigo
  Recurrent episodic vestibular symptoms of at least
    moderate severity*
  Current or previous history of migraine according to
    the criteria of the International Headache Society
  One of the following migrainous symptoms during
    at least 2 vertiginous attacks:
    Migrainous headache
    Photophobia
    Phonophobia
    Visual or other auras
  Other causes ruled out by appropriate investigations

Probable migrainous vertigo
  Recurrent episodic vestibular symptoms of at least
    moderate severity*
  One of the following:
    Current or previous history of migraine according
      to the criteria of the International Headache
      Society
    Migrainous symptoms during ≥2 attacks of
      vertigo
    Migraine-precipitants before vertigo in more than
      50% of attacks: food triggers, sleep
      irregularities, hormonal changes
    Response to migraine medications in more than
      50% of attacks
  Other causes ruled out by appropriate investigations

*Rotational vertigo or subjective sense of motion that may be
spontaneous or positional, or may be provoked or aggravated
by head motion. Moderate vestibular symptoms = interfere
with but do not prohibit daily activities; severe vestibular
symptoms = cannot continue daily activities.

specific aura-like symptoms is relaxed. Rather, a probable diagnosis requires episodic vertigo with any of these four characteristics: a history of migraine by IHS criteria, migrainous neurologic symptoms with vertigo, vertigo precipitated by classic migraine triggers at least 50% of the time, or a 50% response to migraine medications.

Evaluation and Diagnostic Testing

The diagnosis of vestibular migraine is based upon a compatible history and the exclusion of primary aural disease. Specifically, vestibular migraine should be distinguished from Menière disease.[74,79] Such distinction can be difficult and even Prosper Menière recognized the similarity in his original treatise when writing "persons who are subject to migraine often present symptoms analogous to those which we have described."[80] There may be a pathophysiological relationship between migraine and Menière disease creating a continuum of symptoms in which some patients fall into a gray zone. There may also be an increased incidence of Menière disease in patients with a history of migraine; and, thus, both disorders may coexist.[79] Diagnostic testing is thus often directed at distinguishing Menière disease and other aural disorders from migraine.

Audiometric Testing. There is no characteristic audiometric pattern associated with migraine. The phonophobia commonly complained of during migrainous vertigo attacks should prompt audiometric evaluation to assess for threshold changes that could account for hearing loss or hyperacusis complaints. The principal utility of audiometric evaluation is to look for asymmetries of hearing that may suggest retrocochlear pathology, a history of labyrinthitis, ototoxicity, or Menière disease. The presence of a low frequency sensorineural hearing loss or documentation of fluctuating sensorineural loss is strongly suggestive of Menière disease and will aid in distinguishing these entities.

Electronystagmography/Videonystagmography. A complete ENG evaluation may be useful in the diagnosis of vestibular migraine. Unilateral weakness on caloric testing may be present in up to 60% of vertiginous migraine patients.[71] This may reflect insult to the labyrinth by the underlying pathophysiological process of migraine or may indicate a prior attack of vestibular neuritis that may have precipitated the current symptoms (see above discussion). Migraine may also result in ischemic injury to the inner ear.[81] Ocular motor testing in the ENG battery often shows abnormalities on tracking tests, and nystagmus with postural changes may also be present.[82] Dix-Hallpike testing will help to distinguish BPPV, and persistence of nystagmus without fatigue, or subjective symptoms without nystagmus, is more consistent with migraine. Optokinetic testing may induce more severe dizziness, nausea, and headache in migraineurs.[83] Rotary chair testing may show an elevated gain on visually enhanced VOR (VVOR) in migraineurs as compared to normal controls.[84]

Imaging. MRI scans are useful for ruling out other central lesions that may cause disequilibrium and vertigo. These include vestibular schwannoma, posterior fossa arachnoid cysts, Chari I malformation, atrophy and microvascular changes associated with aging, and cerebellar degeneration. Newer generation MRI scanners with increased magnet strength have been used to show gray matter changes in patients with migraine as compared to controls.[85] Functional MRI scanning has also shown differences between normals and migraine sufferers.[86] Thus, it may one day be possible to use imaging to make a diagnosis of migraine directly rather than to have the diagnosis be one of exclusion.

Management

Treatment for vestibular migraine should be tailored to whether the attacks are episodic or whether symptoms are more chronic in nature. Further, the frequency of episodic attacks will determine the form of intervention or whether any treatment may be necessary. That is, an individual with a single episode every few months may be reassured that no other disorder exists and may be willing to have the periodic attack and avoid medications. However, someone with weekly attacks will typically desire some form of intervention as do individuals with more chronic symptoms.

Diet Modification. Treatment for all individuals with vestibular and classic migraine should include dietary modifications. Many individuals prone to migraine are sensitive to specific foods and drinks and these should be avoided during migraine-prone periods (Table 4). Cured and preserved meats that use sodium nitrates are particularly strong stimulants as are red wines, peanuts, aged cheeses, and chocolate. Tyramine containing foods have traditionally been considered migraine sensitizers and include those mentioned above and also ripe bananas, beans and legumes, pickled fish, liver, and yeast. Caffeine and caffeine withdrawal may be migraine sensitizing as are fatty fried foods, citrus fruits, and additives such as monosodium glutamate (MSG), nitrites, sulfites, and aspartame. Patients should be counseled that the migraine response to these foods does not represent allergy, and they may not be sensitive to the migraine provoking activities of these substances at all times. Concomitant migraine stimulants, such as stress or travel may bring out the sensitization to these foods. Adherence to a migraine diet is sufficient in some patients to relieve their symptoms completely.

Stress reduction/Biofeedback/Psychotherapy. Patients with chronic dizziness and punctuated exacerbations characteristic of vestibular migraine often have associated psychological problems of anxiety and depression.[55,87] Regardless of which disorder was antecedent, both conditions need to be addressed. In addition to medications that may work on the pathogenesis of both migraine and anxiety/depression, the help of a therapist may be beneficial. Some patients need formal behavioral psychotherapy to address depression or significant anxiety. Others may benefit from learning biofeedback and stress reduction methods to cope with exacerbations of their dizziness or situations which seem to bring on further attacks. Many patients with longstanding vestibular disorders will benefit from counseling due to the disruption

Table 4 Food Triggers for Migraine

Alcoholic drinks: red wines, beer, champagne,
  vermouth
Anchovies
Aspartame, nitrites, sulfites, food dyes, additives
Avocados
Broad, lima, and other beans
Caffeine containing products
Caffeine withdrawal
Cheeses which have been aged, ie, cheddar
Chicken livers
Chocolate
Citrus fruits, bananas
Cured or dried meats (hot dogs, bacon, ham, and
  salami)
Dairy products, ice cream
Fatty or fried foods
Meat and vegetable extracts
Monosodium glutamate (MSG)
Nuts, peanuts, and peanut butter
Pickled herrings
Sauerkraut
Yeast, sourdough breads
Yogurt, sour cream

in normal social interactions and family dynamics that such a chronic condition incurs.

Vestibular Rehabilitation. Vestibular rehabilitation is an effective treatment for most causes of peripheral vestibulopathy, and patients with idiopathic and posttraumatic vestibular migraine have likewise shown subjective and objective improvement.[88] Migraine sufferers, however, may not subjectively improve as much as patients with other vestibular disorders.[89] Specifically, migraine sufferers appear to perceive their handicap as worse than matched controls despite similarities in overall function. This is consistent with the increased prevalence of anxiety and depression among these patients and a distorted perception of self and their interaction with their environment. Vestibular rehabilitation should be used in this population but may require more frequent visits and higher levels of support and encouragement from the therapist. Additionally, many of these patients will benefit from additional psychological supportive measures.

Pharmacotherapy. Migraine is treated with 2 broad categories of medications: abortive and prophylactic. Abortive medications are taken at the first sign of an attack to stop the physiological process, shorten the time of disability and reduce the severity of the episode. Most abortive medications fall into the category of triptans (migraine drugs that have triptan in their names) which are labeled as contraindicated in the treatment of basilar-like migraine. The 2004 IHS migraine classification considers vertigo only as a symptom of basilar-like migraine and does not recognize vertigo separately as an aura symptom for migraine with or without headache.[69] Recognition of vestibular migraine as a separate entity is increasing, and reclassification of this syndrome will allow the performance of studies to investigate the safety and efficacy of abortive medications in this condition.[78,90] Such reclassification and studies would also remove the potential medicolegal ramifications of using triptans to abort attacks of vestibular migraine. Limited reports of trials of triptans in migraineurs with vertigo are mixed.[71]

Vertigo is often the first sign of a migrainous attack, and abortive medications may stop the ensuing headache but will not necessarily attenuate the more troublesome vertigo. Antivertiginous medications or antiemetics may be of benefit during an attack. Medications used for vestibular neuritis such as the phenothiazines: prochlorperazine (Compazine), and promethazine (Phenergan), the antidopaminergic metoclopramide (Reglan), or diazepam (Valium) can reduce symptoms. However, for most patients with vestibular migraine the use of prophylactic medications to prevent attacks is preferred. For those patients with elements of chronic dizziness, a prophylactic medication will also ensure daily dosing. Currently there are several FDA-approved medications for migraine prophylaxis and nearly 100 off-label medications commonly employed.[91]

Propranolol and timolol (beta blockers) are FDA-approved for use in migraine prophylaxis.

Other beta-blockers such as nadolol, atenolol, and metoprolol have also been used, but are not explicitly approved for migraine. Twice daily dosing or extended release tablets are recommended to ensure consistently therapeutic drug levels. Dosing can be tapered upward over several weeks and titrated to efficacy and Side effects. Beta-blockers are contraindicated in patients with active asthma, moderate to severe chronic obstructive pulmonary disease, bradycardia, secondary and tertiary AV (atriventricular) block, severe peripheral vascular disease, and brittle diabetes. Side effects of beta-blockers include orthostatic hypotension and dizziness, and patients should be counseled to this regard. A good response would be reduction of attacks by 50%, and the medication can be tapered off over several weeks if there is complete remission for 6 months.

Among the calcium channel blockers, verapamil is FDA-approved for the treatment of migraine, and it has shown reasonable efficacy with few side effects. Flunarizine has effectiveness equivalent to that of propranolol.[92] Other calcium channel blockers, such as nimodipine, nifedipine, and diltiazem have been tried with little data to support their use over established treatments. Dosing is typically tapered upward, and therapeutic efficacy is at least 240 mg daily. Side effects include constipation and cardiac arrhythmias, and these medications should not be used in patients with bradycardia and heart block. Conflicting reports link calcium channel blockers to increased risk of cancer, and this should be considered particularly in pediatric patients.

Tricyclic amine antidepressants have a good track record of efficacy in migraine treatment. This class of drug includes amitriptyline, nortriptyline, imipramine, trimipramine, doxepin, dothiepin, clomipramine, and protriptyline. Amitriptyline (Elavil) has well-documented efficacy for migraine, as does nortriptyline (Pamelor). These drugs are sedating and thus useful in patients with sleep disturbance in addition to migraine since they are typically taken before bedtime. Tricyclic antidepressants are also useful in patients with depression as either a coexistent or resultant phenomenon of their dizziness. Dosing of amitriptyline usually starts at 10 mg nightly and can be increased weekly up to a dose of 50 mg daily. These medications can cause blurred vision, dry mouth, constipation, urinary retention, gastroesophageal reflux disease, and weight gain. The selective serotonin reuptake inhibitor (SSRI) class of antidepressants has been considered for migraine prophylaxis, but clinical trials are disappointing.[93] Paroxetine may be effective in patients with anxiety disorder as a component of their symptoms.

Other medications that have been used for migraine include benzodiazepines, in particular the longer acting clonazepam (Klonopin). This medication may be useful in patients with anxiety and panic disorder as part of their symptom complex. Acetazolamide (Diamox) has been proposed and may be effective in those with

Menière-like attacks as well as those with familial migraine syndromes. Anticonvulsants represent a more recent option for migraine prophylaxis and divalproex sodium (Depakote) and topiramate (Topamax) are FDA-approved for migraine prevention. Depakote can be started at low doses (250 mg to 500 mg daily) and, if effective, only limited liver enzyme surveillance may be necessary. Side effects include weight gain, nausea, sedation and tremor. Topamax is usually started at 25 mg daily and tapered upward to 100 mg/d with clinical response seen within one month. Unlike Depakote, Topamax can cause weight loss but must be used with caution in patients with a history of renal calculi. Gabapentin (Neurontin) has also been frequently used in migraine prophylaxis and has a good safety profile. Minimal dosage should be 600 mg/d and dosages at 2,400 mg/d have been well tolerated and shown good effectiveness for migraine.[94]

Summary

Vestibular migraine is a common disorder manifested by recurrent spontaneous attacks of dizziness. Its presentation may be similar to Menière disease but typically lacks the full constellation of ear-specific signs and symptoms. Diagnosis is made by history, a high index of suspicion, and subsequent exclusion of primary aural pathology. Multiple treatment options are available, but effective therapy also requires attention to associated psychological conditions. Increasing experience and diagnostic criteria regarding migrainous vertigo will aid in better defining this disorder and appropriate interventions.

BENIGN PAROXYSMAL POSITIONAL VERTIGO

BPPV is the most common aural cause of vertigo. Due to its propensity for spontaneous remission, it probably occurs in far more people than present to an otolaryngologist for evaluation. The diagnosis of BPPV can be strongly suspected based upon the characteristic history. The specific finding of nystagmus triggered by changes in head position and having the classic directional and time-dependent features establishes the diagnosis of BPPV with certainty. Treatments are very effective, and both patient and physician satisfaction with management and treatment outcomes are high.

Unlike many other causes of dizziness which arise from abnormalities in cellular physiology, BPPV is essentially an anatomical condition with physiological findings precisely related to the anatomical and structural events. Otoconia (calcium carbonate crystals that are normally a part of the otoconial membrane) from the utricle and saccule become dislodged and migrate into the semicircular ducts. The posterior semicircular duct is most commonly affected because of its dependent location in the labyrinth. Otolith crystals that freely float within the semicircular duct produce the condition referred to as canalithiasis and represent the vast majority of all cases of BPPV. Motion of these crystals, by gravitational forces with changes in head position, accounts for the characteristic short-lived, but intense vertiginous episodes of BPPV. Crystals that become adherent to the cupula or reside against the cupula opposite the duct lumen, produce the condition of cupulolithiasis. Cupulolithiasis can present with discrete vertigo but also with position or head motion induced dizziness. Cupulolithiasis may occur more commonly in the lateral (horizontal) semicircular duct whereas canalithiasis is by far more common in the posterior semicircular duct. Diagnosis of BPPV typically involves reproduction of symptoms by causing otolith crystal motion within the affected semicircular duct and treatment is directed at relocating those crystals back into the vestibule. Although the lesion is in the membranous labyrinth, in clinical parlance, reference is made to the semicircular canal rather than the semicircular duct.

The predominant canal affected by BPPV is the posterior semicircular canal, which accounts for 80 to 90% of all cases. The next most commonly affected canal is the horizontal semicircular canal which accounts for about 10% of cases and the least affected is the anterior canal only involved in 2% of cases.[58] As discussed above, the incidence of canal involvement in BPPV is likely related to the anatomical orientation of the semicircular canals: it is easiest for otolith crystals to "fall" into the posterior semicircular canal and most difficult for them to displace superiorly into the anterior semicircular canal. BPPV can affect more than 1 semicircular canal simultaneously and can also present bilaterally. Classic BPPV is that which involves the posterior semicircular canal, and the presentation, diagnosis, and treatment are presented below. This section will also address the less common variants of BPPV and their distinctive characteristics aiding in diagnosis.

Presentation

The majority of patients with classic BPPV will present with descriptions of discrete episodes of vertigo induced by specific head motions. Typical head motions include turning over in bed or looking up. Other motions involve bending to look under something with the affected ear down. Common activities that precipitate vertigo are reaching to retrieve an object from a high shelf (ie, top shelf sign), changing a light bulb, rinsing one's hair in a shower or getting into and out of bed. Occupationally, nurses report vertigo with changing intravenous solution bags, plumbers with looking under a sink, and mechanics with looking under a car.

Cupulolithiasis similarly presents with complaints of dizziness and disequilibrium with rapid head turns or with orientation of the dependent ear and canal relative to gravity. Common activities provoking symptoms include checking the blind spot for traffic or looking under objects with the affected ear down. Positional complaints of dizziness should be distinguished from orthostatic symptoms such as dizziness and lightheadedness that occur when returning to an upright position. Cupulolithiasis appears to most commonly affect the lateral canal which tends to provoke a strong vestibular response; and, thus, symptoms can be quite severe.

A distinguishing feature between BPPV and other vestibular disorders such as Menière disease or vestibular migraine is the lack of spontaneous occurrence. BPPV is an anatomic disorder and, thus, must be provoked by motion, in most cases specific movements. The movement that provokes an attack of BPPV should also be consistent. That is, the patient should note symptoms with a specific change in head position on more than one instance and ideally on multiple occasions. While patients with Menière disease or vestibular migraine may be motion sensitive, it is not usually a specific motion that elicits their symptoms but rather repetitive activity. Additionally, patients with Menière disease or migraine are often sensitive to visual stimuli from environmental movement whereas patients with BPPV must have a change in head position to provoke symptoms.

The duration of vertigo attacks with BPPV should be less than 1 minute and are often less than 30 seconds. Many patients have continued malaise after the attack of vertigo and it is important to separate the temporal pattern of these symptoms on history. The natural reaction to sudden dizziness with head position changes is to move the head back into a neutral position. Such a motion can reverse the direction of otolith crystal movement and also provoke vertigo which may add to the duration of symptoms. Often patients have difficulty estimating time while they are experiencing vertigo, and histories of BPPV attacks lasting 5 to 10 minutes are not uncommon.

Patients may also report a period of time during which symptoms are active and interval periods of no dizziness. BPPV commonly has periods of spontaneous remission and recurrence. In the patient reporting dizziness for 1 year, for example, it is important to obtain a history of the following: when attacks were prevalent, if there were periods when attacks abated, when the attacks recurred, and when the last attack occurred. In the patient with a strong history for BPPV but whose last attack occurred weeks ago the physical examination and testing may be nondiagnostic. Recurrent clusters of attacks, seasonally related attacks or attacks around the menstrual cycle are consistent with other vestibular disorders such as Menière disease or vestibular migraine.

The onset of recurrent attacks of BPPV can commonly be temporally related to an episode of head trauma.[58] Posttraumatic BPPV can occur immediately or may be delayed by weeks or months. The head trauma does not necessarily need to be severe to elicit BPPV, but BPPV is quite common after skull base fracture. BPPV is usually in the traumatized ear but not exclusively, and evaluation of both ears is important. Patients may recall striking their head or falling hard but not requiring medical attention shortly before the onset of symptoms. Postconcussive syndrome also has a strong component of postural dizziness and sensitivity to motion. The physical examination and vestibular testing are important in distinguishing these entities (see below).

BPPV is also common after attacks of vestibular neuritis and generally strikes within a year of the initial insult. Postneuritis BPPV is almost always in the same ear. The pathophysiology leading to BPPV may involve injury to the otolith organs caused by the neuritis or by an underlying vascular event with subsequent release. A common history is of a severe attack of vertigo lasting hours to days and necessitating an emergency room visit. This is followed by weeks of disequilibrium, gradual improvement, and then a period of full recovery before the sudden onset of short-lived episodic vertigo when lying down. As noted in other sections of this chapter, this can be quite disturbing and lead to, or exacerbate, anxiety and psychogenic-related dizziness. It is useful when counseling a patient with an attack of vestibular neuritis to warn about future attacks of vertigo, that is, BPPV. Stressing the benign nature of BPPV and the efficacy of treatments can assuage fears that vestibular neuritis has recurred.

BPPV also appears to commonly affect older individuals particularly those with histories of hypertension and hyperlipidemia.[95] It may occur after upper respiratory infections, but it is not known whether BPPV is related to viral insult or impulse head motion with sneezing. BPPV also occurs without any obvious risk factor or antecedent event. It can occur at any age but should not be confused with benign paroxysmal vertigo of childhood (BPVC). The latter is not felt to be related to displaced otolith crystals but rather appears to be a pediatric migraine-associated vertigo syndrome.

Evaluation and Diagnostic Testing

Characteristic findings on the physical examination are used to establish the diagnosis of BPPV. The examination should exclude acute middle ear disease or the presence of cholesteatoma. Acute otitis media can cause dizziness but more commonly causes disequilibrium, which may be confused with BPPV. Labyrinthine fistula due to cholesteatoma may cause position-related symptoms due to gravitationally induced movement of the keratoma. Tuning fork testing can identify a sensorineural loss, which may be suggestive of Menière disease. An apparent conductive loss can be found on tuning fork testing in superior semicircular canal dehiscence. A unilateral hearing loss may indicate a prior attack of labyrinthitis and, thus, unilateral vestibular hypofunction.

Dix-Hallpike Maneuver. The mainstay of the physical examination for diagnosing BPPV is the Dix-Hallpike test.[96] This test is typically performed with the patient wearing Frenzel lenses but the intensity of nystagmus commonly seen in BPPV does not usually require suppression of visual fixation. The patient sits upright at the edge of an examination table, and the head is turned 45° to the tested ear. The patient is then rapidly reclined with the head hanging over the edge of the examination table (Figure 3). This places the posterior semicircular canal in the tested ear in the vertical plane, which causes maximal stimulation in most cases of canalithiasis. The patient's eyes are examined for geotropic up beating nystagmus. That is, the fast phase of the nystagmus should beat vertically toward the vertex of the head. A torsional component of the nystagmus is also observed with torsional fast phases beating toward the test ear (ie, the ear nearer the ground). This nystagmus is due to the ampullofugal motion of the particles in the posterior canal, which is excitatory for the posterior canal. Each side is tested independently and the affected ear is the one toward the ground at the time of positive response.

The nystagmus of BPPV should also follow rules consistent with the anatomic pathology of the disorder. There should be a period of latency prior to the onset of nystagmus or subjective dizziness. This is typically a few seconds but it may take as long as 20 to 30 seconds for gravity to accelerate otolith particles sufficiently to cause vestibular stimulation. The vertigo and nystagmus should crescendo (corresponding to motion of the cupula of the posterior canal), and decrescendo as the particles settle in the dependent portion of the canal. Once the particles stop moving, the stimulus is removed, deflection of the cupula ends, and the patient should no longer experience vertigo nor should the examiner observe nystagmus. If either persists, an alternative diagnosis, particularly central pathology, should be entertained. BPPV should also fatigue. That is, repeated applications of the Dix-Hallpike test should lead to diminishing subjective and objective response. The fatigue of the nystagmus may be due to dispersion of the crystals within the canal.

BPPV may occasionally affect semicircular canals other than the posterior canal. The incidence of horizontal canal BPPV is between 10 and 15% while the anterior canal is affected in less than 5% of cases. In these cases, the Dix-Hallpike test may not be positive or will give results divergent from those expected with posterior canal BPPV. If the anterior canal is affected, the Dix-Hallpike maneuver will cause excitatory ampullofugal particle motion when the affected ear is up (Figure 3). This will generate nystagmus opposite of that seen in classic BPPV, but with similar latency and fatigability. Specifically, the examiner will see down-beating nystagmus with torsional components directed toward the opposite side. If the torsional component is not strong, purely vertical, down-beating nystagmus may be observed.[97,98]

If the horizontal semicircular canal is affected, Dix-Hallpike positioning may not provoke otolith crystal motion at all due to the orientation of the canal and cupula relative to the ground during this maneuver (Figure 3). Symptoms can be elicited by having the patient lie supine with the head elevated at 30° and quickly rotating the head 90° to the side. This maneuver orients the horizontal canal orthogonal to the ground and maximizes the movement of otolith particles in the lumen (Figure 4). It also maximizes the gravitational pull on otolith crystals relative to the cupula in cases of cupulolithiasis. Cupulolithiasis is commonly associated with horizontal semicircular canal BPPV.

Horizontal semicircular canal BPPV may cause symptoms with the head turned in either direction.[99] The nystagmus elicited may beat toward (geotropic) or away from (apogeotropic) the downward ear depending on the presence of canalithiasis or cupulolithiasis. In canalithiasis, head rotation toward the affected ear will cause ampullopetal particle movement in the lateral canal leading to horizontal nystagmus beating toward the dependent ear (ie, geotropic). Head rotation away from the affected ear will cause ampullofugal particle motion, which results in inhibition of the horizontal canal and nystagmus beating away from the affected ear. Since

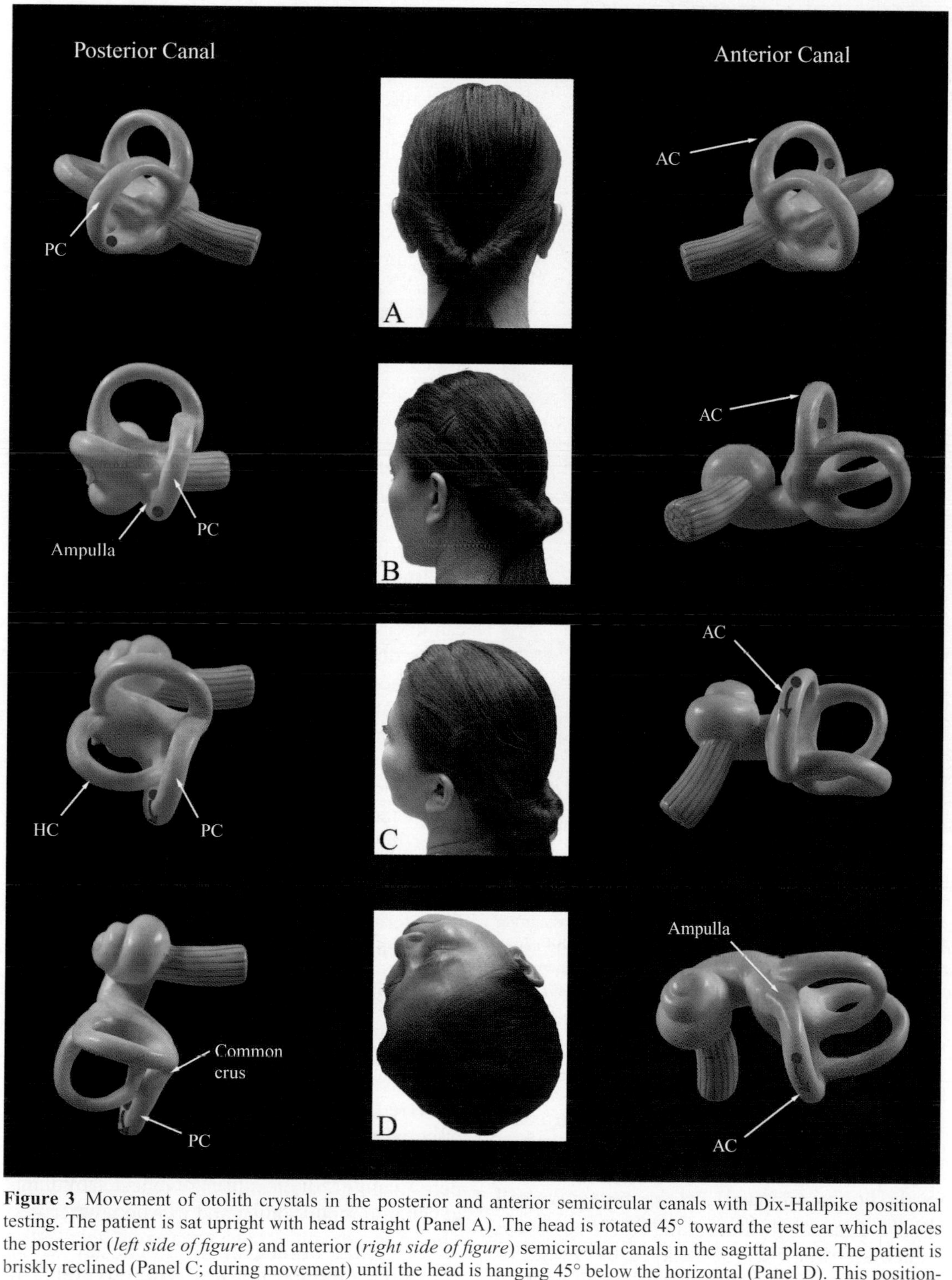

Figure 3 Movement of otolith crystals in the posterior and anterior semicircular canals with Dix-Hallpike positional testing. The patient is sat upright with head straight (Panel A). The head is rotated 45° toward the test ear which places the posterior (*left side of figure*) and anterior (*right side of figure*) semicircular canals in the sagittal plane. The patient is briskly reclined (Panel C; during movement) until the head is hanging 45° below the horizontal (Panel D). This positioning induces ampullofugal motion of otolith crystals (*red dot*) in the posterior canal (PC) which causes canal excitation and classic geotropic (ie, toward the ground) and up beating nystagmus (ie, toward the vertex of the head). In BPPV of the anterior canal (AC), Dix-Hallpike positioning also causes excitation, which leads to apogeotropic nystagmus with a down-beating component. The horizontal canal (HC) is not favorably positioned in this maneuver to cause significant activation. (Published with permission, copyright © 2007 D.R. Friedland, MD, PhD.)

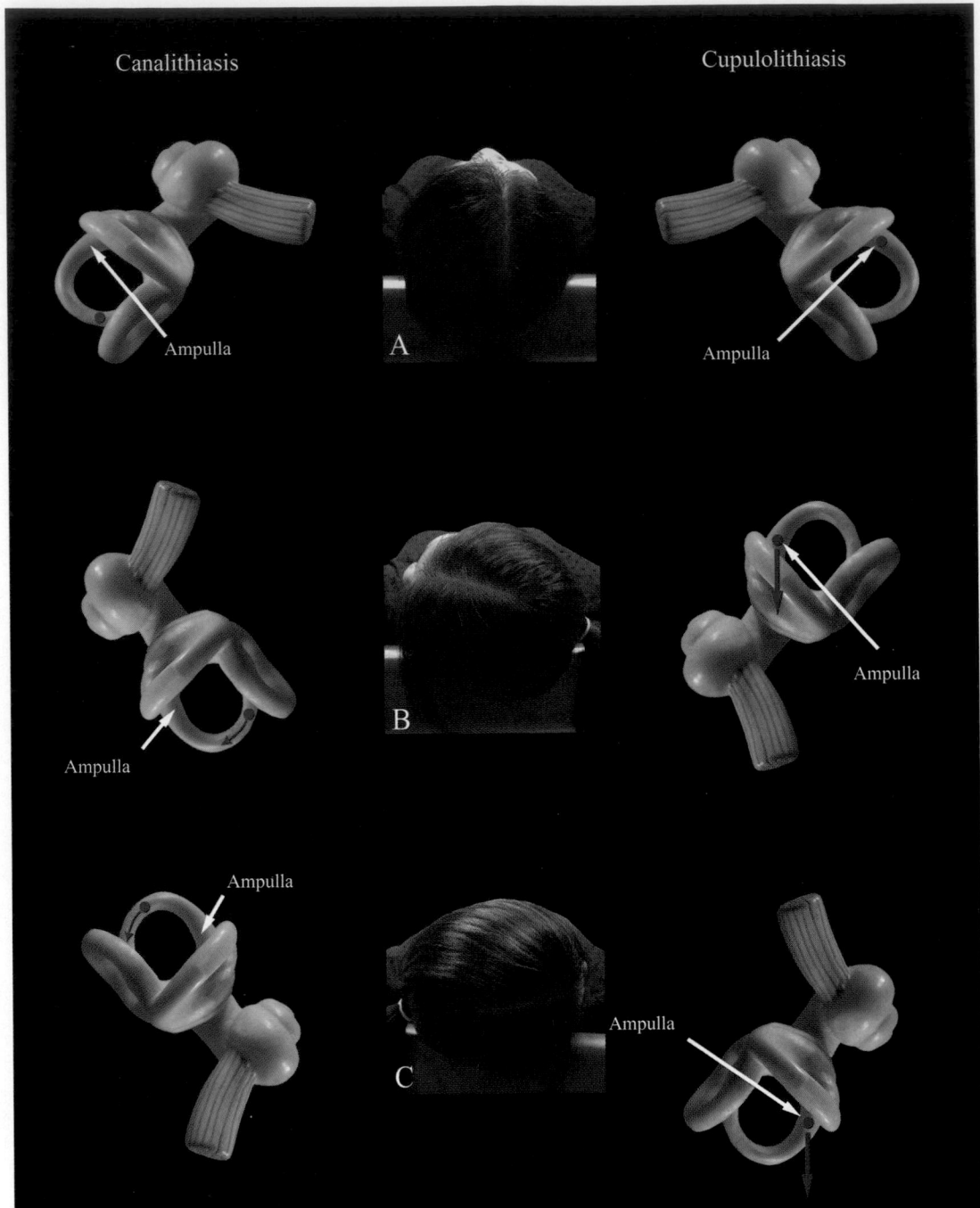

Canalithiasis

Cupulolithiasis

Ampulla

Ampulla

A

Ampulla

Ampulla

B

Ampulla

Ampulla

Ampulla

C

Ampulla

Figure 4 Movement of otolith crystals and deflection of the cupula in horizontal canal BPPV. In canalithiasis, head rotation toward the affected canal leads to excitation of the canal and geotropic nystagmus (ie, toward the ground). Head rotation away from the affected ear causes inhibition of activity and nystagmus away from the affected ear, which will also appear as geotropic. The ear that is dependent during the maneuver causing more intense symptoms or nystagmus is considered the affected ear. In cupulolithiasis, the displaced otolith crystals are adherent to the end organ and cause gravity dependent deflection. Opposite of canalithiasis, the direction of nystagmus with the affected ear up or down will appear as apogeotropic. (Published with permission, copyright © 2007 D.R. Friedland, MD, PhD.)

the affected ear is up, this will also appear to be geotropic. Thus, it is not possible to determine the affected ear simply by direction of nystagmus. The affected ear is typically the ear that is toward the ground in the position that elicits the most pronounced nystagmus or worse vertigo.[99]

In cupulolithiasis of the horizontal canal, the observed nystagmus is opposite that of canalithiasis. With the affected ear down, gravitational pull on the particles adherent to the cupula causes ampullofugal deflection of the stereocilia, which is inhibitory in the horizontal canal (Figure 4). The resultant nystagmus is thus away from the

dependent affected ear, and the examiner observes horizontal nystagmus beating away from the ground (ie, apogeotropic). When the affected ear is up, the pull on the particles will cause ampullopetal deflection of the cupula (excitatory for the horizontal canal) and the nystagmus will also be apogeotropic (ie, toward the affected ear). As in canalithiasis, the intensity of the nystagmus or subjective sensation of dizziness can be used to determine the affected ear.

The nystagmus in horizontal canal BPPV often begins with a shorter latency, increases in magnitude while maintaining the test position,

and is less susceptible to fatigue with repetitive testing than the vertical–torsional nystagmus in posterior canal BPPV. The increased amplitude and duration of the horizontal nystagmus may reflect action of the central velocity storage mechanisms, which perseverate signals from the vestibular periphery, especially those arising from the horizontal canal.

Electronystagmography/Videonystagmography. Although the physical examination is often quite sensitive and specific for classic posterior canal BPPV, the full battery of ENG/VNG testing is important in evaluating the patient with a history consistent with BPPV. Positional testing may elicit nystagmus in lateral or supine positions but not in Dix-Hallpike positioning and would alert the clinician to potential horizontal canal BPPV. The ENG/VNG test can also characterize and document the fatigability and duration of nystagmus during positioning. If ENG/VNGs are performed prior to the patient seeing the physician, Dix-Hallpike testing with the physician may be negative. Documented nystagmus on the prior ENG/VNG in conjunction with a consistent history can prompt appropriate therapy. The degree of nystagmus on ENG/VNG with positional testing can be used to determine the affected ear in horizontal canal BPPV.

The absence of recordable nystagmus in the presence of subjective dizziness on positional ENG/VNG can reassure the examiner of negative objective findings and lead to evaluation for central abnormality such as Chiari I malformation, orthostatic hypotension, postconcussive syndrome or migraine. The oculomotor and nystagmus tests may find abnormalities of gaze that can interfere with the interpretation of eye movements during Dix-Hallpike testing. The caloric component of ENG/VNG testing can identify a unilateral vestibular hypofunction, which may suggest an antecedent vestibular neuritis as the inciting event leading to the development of BPPV. Recall that vestibular neuritis typically affects the superior vestibular nerve, which innervates the anterior and horizontal semicircular canals. BPPV most commonly afflicts the posterior semicircular canal, which is innervated by the inferior vestibular nerve and will retain function after vestibular neuritis.

Management

The main treatment option for BPPV is to reposition the otolith particles out of the semicircular ducts or cupula. Canalith repositioning is the preferred first step in therapy and is often very effective. Additional medical, pharmacological, and surgical options are reserved for the small percentage of patients that fail repeated attempts at canalith repositioning and in whom other vestibular abnormalities have been excluded.

Canalith Repositioning Maneuvers. The mainstay of treatment for classic posterior canal canalithiasis is the Epley maneuver.[100] In this maneuver, the free floating otolith crystals are sequentially advanced through the posterior canal until they are released into the utricle at the common crus (Figure 5).[102] Initially the patient is reclined with the head turned 45° toward the affected side and extended back just as in the Dix-Hallpike test. The patient is maintained in this position until nystagmus and subjective sensations of vertigo have fully passed. The minimum time that the patient should be in this position is 30 seconds. The patient's head is then rapidly rotated 90° toward the opposite side so that the unaffected ear is down. This would be the same position as if performing a Dix-Hallpike test on the contralateral ear. The patient may experience vertigo as the otolith crystals move further along the posterior canal. After complete cessation of nystagmus and/or vertigo the patient is rotated another 90° away from the affected ear so that the eyes are looking directly at the ground. This aligns the common crus vertically with respect to gravity allowing the crystals to fall into the utricle and out of the posterior duct. After approximately 30 seconds, the patient is seated upright.

Some clinicians use a vibration device placed on the mastoid during the maneuver to facilitate otolith crystal migration. Also, some physicians will repeat the Dix-Hallpike test immediately after performance of the Epley maneuver to confirm satisfactory treatment. The overall success of the canalith repositioning maneuver is greater than 75% and over 90% of patients will respond well to repeated maneuvers.[103–105] The patient should be instructed to refrain from lying flat for at least 24 to 48 hours. Sleeping with the head elevated at 45° during this time is recommended. Although these postural restrictions are commonly employed, recent studies suggest no difference in recurrence rates between patients with imposed restrictions and those without.[106,107]

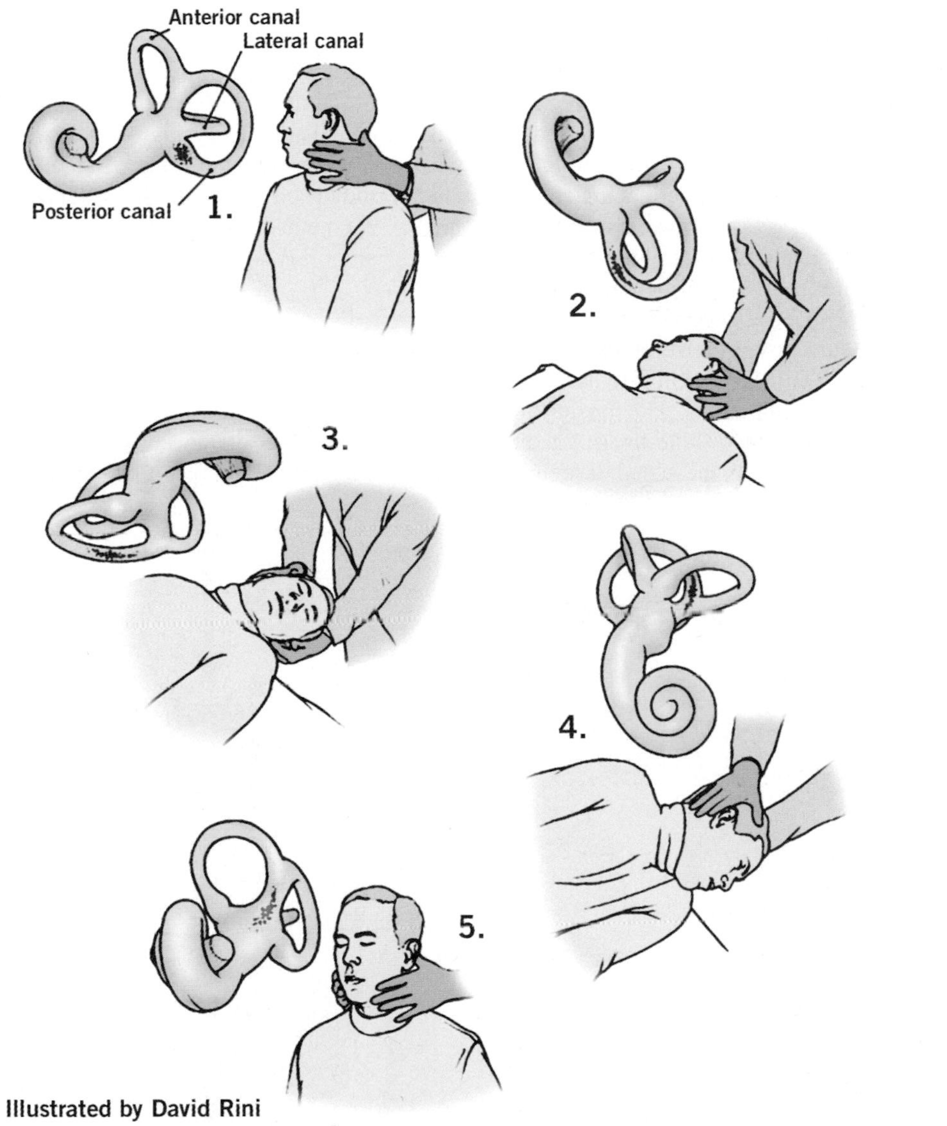

Anterior semicircular canal BPPV is a rare entity, but also responds well to canalith repositioning.[105] The maneuver is the same as for posterior semicircular canal BPPV but should be performed starting with the affected ear up.[108] For example, treatment of right anterior semicircular canal BPPV would entail the performance of an Epley maneuver starting with the left ear down and rotating toward the patient's right. Occasionally, treatment of BPPV can release otolith crystals into a different semicircular canal and thus repeat therapies should be preceded by confirmatory Dix-Hallpike testing to re-identify the affected ear and semicircular canal. Treatment of bilateral BPPV is best performed in stages, and the authors will treat the subjectively worse ear or canal first and address the second site 1 to 2 weeks later after confirming resolution of initial symptoms.

Other repositioning maneuvers for the treatment of canalithiasis include the Semont liberatory maneuver.[109] The patient is rapidly moved laterally from a sitting position to a position with the affected ear down on the treatment table. After 4 minutes the patient is rapidly swung over to the opposite side so that the affected ear is pointing upward. This maneuver is more time consuming and difficult to perform than the Epley maneuver, but has similar success rates with over 90% of patients responding after four sessions.[110] The Semont maneuver may be beneficial in patients not responding to the Epley maneuver and, due to the sudden impulse with position changes, may be effective in dislodging material in cupulolithiasis.

An alternative to repositioning maneuvers are the Brandt-Daroff exercises which the patient performs at home.[111] The patient is instructed to sit on the edge of the bed and lie laterally to the affected side with the head slightly rotated upward similar to the positioning in the Semont maneuver. The patient remains in this position for 30 seconds before sitting up for 30 seconds and repeating the maneuver to the opposite side for another 30 seconds. The patient performs five sets of these maneuvers three times daily for 7 to 10 days. Excellent response has been noted to these exercises, and cure rates are not statistically different from those achieved with canalith repositioning.[112] This exercise may cause central habituation to the position induced vertigo rather than relocation of the otolith crystals from the semicircular canals. Brandt–Daroff exercises may also be useful in preventing the recurrence of BPPV.

Illustrated by David Rini

Figure 5 Canalith repositioning maneuver for treatment of BPPV affecting the posterior semicircular canal. Panel 1 shows a patient with right posterior canal BPPV. The patient's head is turned to the right at the beginning of the canalith repositioning maneuver. The *inset* shows the location of the debris near the ampulla of the posterior canal. The diagram of the head in each inset shows the orientation from which the labyrinth is viewed. In Panel 2, the patient is brought into the supine position with the head extended below the level of the table. The debris falls toward the common crus as the head is moved backward. In Panel 3, the head is moved approximately 180° to the left while keeping the neck extended with the head below the level of the table. Debris enters the common crus as the head is turned toward the contralateral side. In Panel 4, the patient's head is further rotated to the left by rolling onto the left side until the patient's head faces down. Debris begins to enter the utricle. In Panel 5, the patient is brought back to the upright position. Debris collects in the utricle. Illustration by David Rini. (Published with permission from reference 101.)

Horizontal Canal Benign Paroxysmal Positional Vertigo.

Canalith repositioning for horizontal canal BPPV deserves separate mention as this canal is oriented orthogonal to the posterior and superior semicircular canals and thus not affected by the Epley maneuver. The recommended canalith repositioning maneuver for horizontal canal canalithiasis is the Lempert 360° roll.[113] The patient starts supine, and the head is rotated 90° to the unaffected side every 30 to 60 seconds. The first turn is 90° to the side so that the unaffected ear is down. With the head stable the patient turns his/her body prone in preparation for the next steps. Subsequently the patient's head is rotated another 90° so the face is directly toward the ground and then another 90° so that the affected ear is down, and then the patient returns to the upright position. The Lempert maneuver has demonstrated success for geotropic horizontal BPPV, but has not proven as effective in apogeotropic BPPV.[99] Geotropic horizontal canal BPPV may also have a high rate of spontaneous remission.[114] Additional therapies for apogeotropic BPPV can include Brandt–Daroff exercises and other liberatory or habituation maneuvers.[99] Overall, however the success rate in treating apogeotropic horizontal canal BPPV is approximately 50%. Recurrences and long-term failures should be examined for potential conversion to classic posterior canal BPPV after performance of repositioning maneuvers.

Pharmacologic Therapy. Pharmacologic management of BPPV is directed principally at suppressing the vestibular response and alleviating nausea associated with vertigo. Pharmacologic therapy does not treat the underlying cause of BPPV. The symptoms of BPPV can be treated similar to those of vestibular neuritis with low dose valium and antiemetics such as the phenothiazines (eg, Phenergan or Compazine). Symptoms of cupulolithiasis, which may include chronic disequilibrium due to inertial changes in the cupula,

can be addressed with longer acting vestibular suppressants such as clonazepam (ie, Klonopin) or with medications for motion sensitivity such as meclizine (Antivert). Pharmacologic therapy should not be used in management of symptoms in BPPV. Instead, repositioning maneuvers as described above should be used to address the underlying cause. Diazepam (Valium) can be used prior to canalith repositioning maneuvers in the extremely sensitive or anxious patient.

Surgical Management. Failure of repositioning maneuvers to alleviate symptoms in BPPV are rare. In such cases consideration should be given to surgical interventions to ablate responses from the offending semicircular canal. One approach is to transect the posterior ampullary (singular) nerve, which provides innervation to the posterior semicircular canal. In this method, a tympanomeatal flap is elevated to expose the round window niche and the bony overhang is removed. Subsequently, bone of the otic capsule just inferior to the round window membrane is drilled away to expose the singular nerve where it is transected. Singular neurectomy, as developed and performed by Gacek, has been effective and safe in treating BPPV with over 96% of patients experiencing complete relief of symptoms.[115,116] However, in other surgeons' hands, singular neurectomy has had an unacceptably high rate of sensorineural hearing loss and has largely been abandoned.[117]

The currently preferred method of surgically addressing BPPV is semicircular canal occlusion or plugging.[118,119] The posterior canal is exposed and thinned (blue-lined) via a transmastoid approach, and the canal is gently entered

to avoid disruption of the endolymphatic membrane. The canal is plugged with bone chips, fascia, or fibrous tissue which can be further bolstered with bone wax or fibrin glue. Postoperative hearing loss is generally temporary and persistent sensorineural hearing loss is rare.[119–121] This technique can be theoretically applied to any affected semicircular canal and has been utilized to treat therapy resistant geotropic horizontal canal BPPV.[122] Canal plugging has also been applied to the superior semicircular canal for superior semicircular canal dehiscence as described later in this chapter.

Summary

BPPV is an anatomical disturbance within the vestibular labyrinth caused by displacement of otoconia to the semicircular ducts. The posterior semicircular canal is most commonly affected followed by the horizontal and anterior semicircular canals. Specific changes in head position will lead to gravity-induced motion of displaced otoconia relative to the ampulla and cause canal-specific nystagmus and vertigo. Treatment involves repositioning of the otolith crystals into the utricle and is highly effective. Surgical management of BPPV is reserved for canalith repositioning failures and is rarely needed.

SUPERIOR SEMICIRCULAR CANAL DEHISCENCE SYNDROME

Dehiscence of bone overlying the superior semicircular canal can result in a syndrome of vestibular

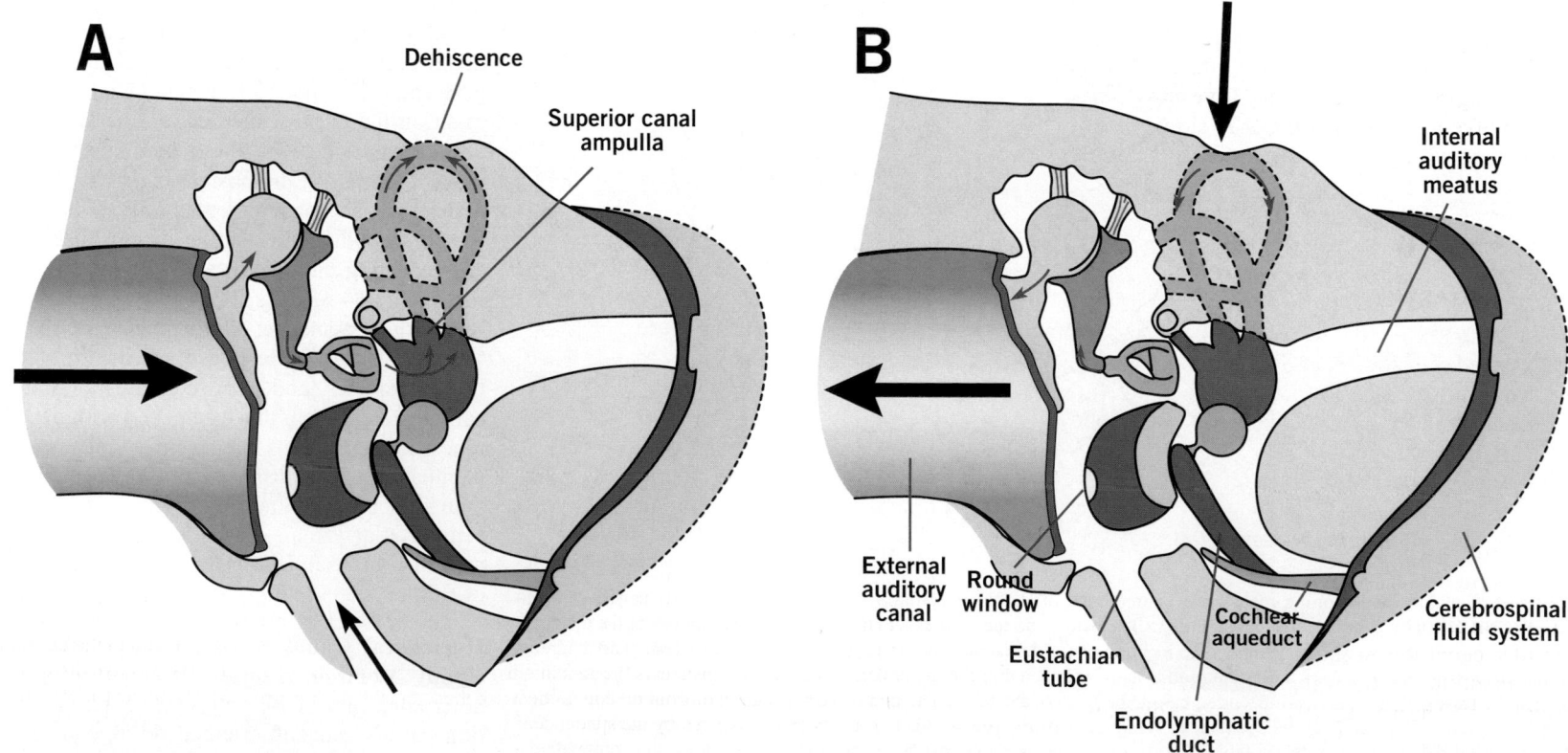

Figure 6 Pressure changes inducing nystagmus in superior semicircular canal dehiscence syndrome. (A) Positive pressure in the external auditory canal causes bulging of the membranous canal into the cranial cavity and ampullofugal flow. (B) Negative pressure in the external auditory canal causes bulging of the cranial contents into the superior canal and ampullopetal flow. (Published with permission from reference 123.)

and auditory abnormalities.[123–125] The vestibular abnormalities include vertigo and oscillopsia induced by loud sounds or by stimuli that change middle ear or intracranial pressure. These patients may exhibit a Tullio phenomenon (eye movements induced by loud sounds) or Hennebert sign (eye movements induced by pressure in the external auditory canal). They may also experience chronic disequilibrium. The auditory abnormalities include an apparent conductive hearing loss (manifested as an air-bone gap on audiometry that is not due to middle ear pathology), autophony, and pulsatile tinnitus. A recent report described the clinical manifestations of superior semicircular canal dehiscence in 65 patients.[126] Vestibular manifestations were present in 60 and exclusively auditory manifestations without vestibular symptoms or signs were noted in five patients. The auditory symptoms and signs may be subtle and may not prompt a patient to seek medical evaluation. The overall incidence of auditory compromise in the absence of vestibular symptoms and signs may, therefore, be higher than that suggested by the findings in this study.

The pathophysiology of superior semicircular canal dehiscence can be understood in terms of the effects of the dehiscence in creation of a "third mobile window" into the inner ear (Figure 6). Under normal circumstances, sound pressure enters the inner ear through the stapes footplate in the oval window and, after passing around the cochlea, exits through the round window. The presence of a dehiscence in the superior semicircular canal allows this canal to respond to sound and pressure stimuli. The direction of the evoked eye movements support this mechanism. Loud sounds, positive pressure in the external auditory canal, and Valsalva maneuver against pinched nares cause ampullofugal deflection of the superior semicircular canal, which results in excitation of afferents innervating this canal. The evoked eye movements can involve a nystagmus that has slow components directed upward with torsional motion of the superior pole of the eye away from the affected ear. Conversely, negative pressure in the external auditory canal, Valsalva against a closed glottis, and jugular venous compression cause ampullopetal deflection of the superior canal which results in inhibition of afferents innervating this canal. The evoked eye movements in these situations are typically in the plane of the superior semicircular canal but in the opposite direction (downward with torsional motion of the superior pole of the eye toward the affected ear).

Vestibular Manifestations of Superior Semicircular Canal Dehiscence

In a recent report of 65 patients with superior semicircular canal dehiscence, vestibular symptoms were identified in 60 patients (41 males and 19 females).[126] The age range at the time of diagnosis was 13 to 70 (median = 41; mean = 43) years. The right ear alone was affected in 27 patients and the left ear alone in 23 patients. There were 10 patients with vestibular symptoms and signs and

CT findings indicative of bilateral superior semicircular canal dehiscence. Vestibular symptoms induced by loud sounds were noted in 54 (90%) patients and pressure-induced symptoms (coughing, sneezing, and straining) were present in 44 (73%). There were 40 (67%) patients who had both sound- and pressure-induced symptoms.

In these 60 patients with vestibular symptoms associated with superior semicircular canal dehiscence, vestibular signs associated with superior semicircular canal dehiscence were present in 57 (90%). The vestibular signs in these 57 patients could be grouped into 4 categories. Sound-evoked eye movements were noted in 46 (82%) patients. A sound-induced tilt of the head in the plane of the superior canal was noted in 11 (20%) patients. There were 42 (75%) patients with eye

movements induced by Valsalva maneuvers. Eye movements evoked by pressure in the external auditory canal were noted in 26 (45%) patients. A sign in only one of these 4 categories was noted in 17 (27%) patients. Signs in two categories were noted in 16 (29%) patients. Signs in 3 categories were noted in 20 (36%) patients. Signs in all 4 categories were noted in four (7%) patients.

The eye movements induced by sound and pressure stimuli can have an important role in making the diagnosis.[123,127] These stimuli often lead to a nystagmus. The direction of the slow phase components of this nystagmus can be understood based upon the action of these sound and pressure stimuli on the affected superior canal. These eye movement findings have been

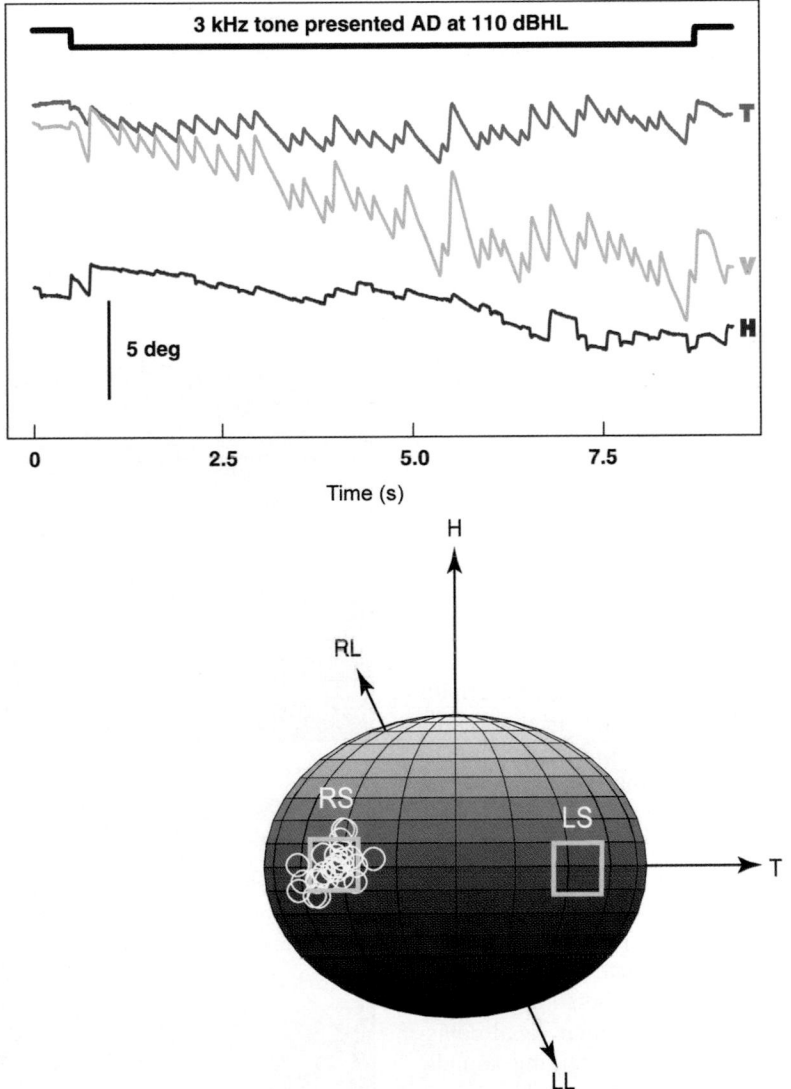

Figure 7 Nystagmus induced by 3 kHz tone at an intensity of 110 dB in the right ear (AD) of a 33-year-old woman with right superior semicircular canal dehiscence syndrome. *Upper panel*: Torsional (T), vertical (V), and horizontal (H) eye position recorded with the scleral search coil technique from the right eye. The time during which the tone was presented is indicated by the stimulus marker at the top. Positive directions for the horizontal, vertical, and torsional axes are defined as left, down, and clockwise (rotation of the superior pole of the patient's eye toward her right side). In response to the tone in her right ear, the patient developed a nystagmus with upward, counterclockwise slow phases consistent with excitation of the right superior canal. *Lower panel*: The axis of slow phase eye velocity corresponding to the data plotted in the upper panel. The sphere represents the patient's head, as viewed from the right side. The positive direction of the horizontal axis (H) travels upward from the top of the head, the torsional axis straight ahead from the patient's nose, and the vertical axis (which is obscured by the sphere) from the patient's left ear. The axis of the slow phase eye movement expected for excitation of each of the right superior (RS), left superior (LS), right lateral (RL), and left lateral (LL) semicircular canals is shown based upon the orientation of the canals. The box around the axis of each superior canal indicates the region (±2 SD) from the mean orientation of that axis. Each light circle represents the mean observed eye velocity axis for one slow phase of nystagmus. (Published with permission from reference 128.)

documented with three-dimensional search coil techniques and can be observed on clinical examination (Figure 7). Frenzel lenses (×20 magnifying lenses that blur images and preclude visual fixation in patients wearing the lenses) should be used for this examination because visual fixation can lead to suppression of the evoked eye movements. An enlarged, low threshold click-evoked VOR has also been noted in superior semicircular canal dehiscence.[129]

Auditory Manifestations of Superior Semicircular Canal Dehiscence

Auditory symptoms and signs in patients with superior semicircular canal dehiscence have also been described.[125,130] Symptoms indicative of hyperacusis for bone-conducted sounds were found in 31 of 60 patients with vestibular manifestations of superior canal dehiscence.[126] These symptoms included hearing heartbeat or eye movements in the affected ear and hearing the impact of the feet during walking or running. There were 30 of these patients with autophony in the affected ear. The Weber tuning fork test (512 Hz) typically lateralizes to the affected ear when auditory symptoms are present in cases of superior semicircular canal dehiscence.

Autophony may be a prominent complaint in patients with superior semicircular canal dehiscence. Patients can hear their voice loudly in the affected ear and may avoid singing or speaking above a soft conversational level of voice because of the discomfort in the affected ear that is brought on by these activities.[124,131] An increased sensitivity to bone-conducted sounds appears to be the mechanism responsible for the auditory symptoms in these patients. Autophony can also be caused by a patulous eustachian tube.[132] A loss of tissue within the cartilaginous portion of the eustachian tube is thought to cause abnormal patency of the tube that results in abnormally loud perception of a person's own voice. The autophony resulting from superior semicircular canal dehiscence tends to be unremitting from the time of onset whereas autophony due to patulous eustachian tube may be more intermittent. A further difference in the characteristics of autophony in the two conditions is that patulous eustachian tube results in autophony that is equally loud for the spoken voice and for breathing sounds. Autophony in superior semicircular canal dehiscence is typically absent for breathing sounds. Finally, otoscopy in patients with patulous eustachian tube who are experiencing autophony will demonstrate patulous excursions of the tympanic membrane with nasal breathing, especially if the contralateral naris is closed. An more thorough discussion of the differences between the two disorders can be found in Chapter 15, "Eustachian Tube Dysfunction."

It is likely that the same mechanism responsible for the vestibular abnormalities also underlies the auditory manifestations.[133] The third mobile window allows acoustic energy to be dissipated through the dehiscence. Direct experimental

evidence in support of this mechanism has been provided from studies performed in a chinchilla model of superior semicircular canal dehiscence. The sound-induced velocity measured within the perilymph or endolymph of a superior semicircular canal dehiscence demonstrated sound flow through the dehiscence. Measurements of the cochlear potential showed that superior semicircular canal dehiscence causes an increase in the bone-conducted sound.

Bone conduction thresholds on audiometry in patients with superior semicircular canal dehiscence can be less than 0 dB normal hearing level (NHL) because these individuals have better hearing via bone. An air-bone gap can, therefore, exist in these individuals even though their air conduction thresholds are in the normal range.[125,130] Distinguishing an air-bone gap on audiometry due to superior semicircular canal dehiscence from an air-bone gap due to middle ear pathology is important in determining the appropriate treatment options.

Several reports have discussed the air-bone gaps in patients initially thought to have otosclerosis but who were subsequently found to have superior semicircular canal dehiscence.[124,130,134] Air conduction thresholds did not improve in these patients following stapes replacement surgery. Earlier studies have described "inner ear conductive hearing loss" in patients with a conductive hearing impairment on audiometry but no evidence of tympanic membrane or ossicular abnormality found on exploratory middle ear surgery.[135] Superior semicircular canal dehiscence now appears to be one cause of such inner ear conductive hearing loss. The acoustic reflex test provides a useful screening test in the identification of patients in whom the conductive hearing loss on audiometry may be due to superior semicircular canal dehiscence rather than to a middle ear problem such as otosclerosis. The acoustic reflex is the contraction of the stapedial muscle in response to a sudden loud sound. Even mild limitation of the motion of the ossicles abolishes this reflex. Thus, patients with intact acoustic reflex responses and an air-bone gap on audiometry should undergo further investigation for superior semicircular canal dehiscence, such as a high resolution CT scan of the temporal bones.

The air-bone gap that is frequently noted on the audiogram of patients with superior semicircular canal dehiscence is typically greatest at the lower frequencies (250 to 1,000 Hz). Laser-Doppler vibrometer measurements of sound-induced umbo velocity in patients with superior semicircular canal dehiscence have revealed hypermobility of

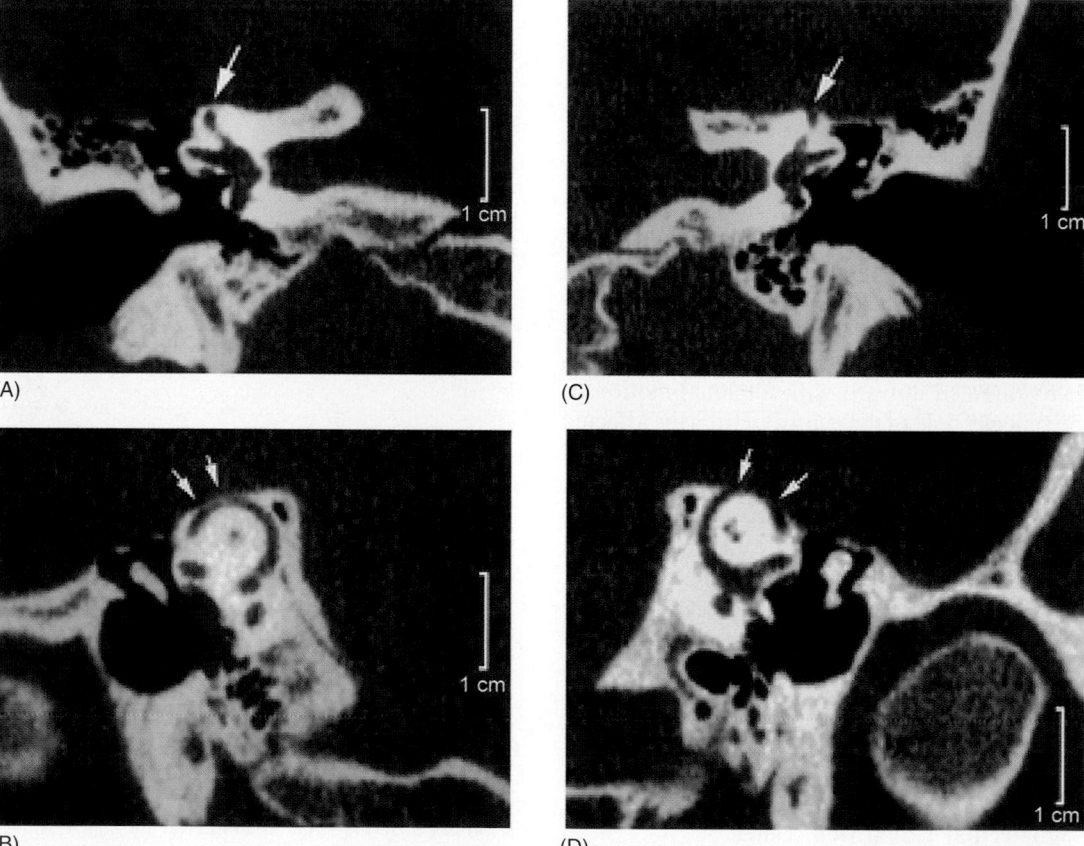

(A) (C)

(B) (D)

Figure 8 Computed tomographic images of the temporal bones in a 37-year-old man with left superior semicircular canal dehiscence syndrome. He developed vertigo, oscillopsia, and eye movements in the plane of the left superior semicircular canal in response to tones of 500 to 1,000 Hz at 110 dB HL in the left ear. Dehiscence of the bone over the left superior semicircular canal was confirmed at surgery. (A) Coronal 0.5 mm-collimated CT scan through right temporal bone demonstrates an intact layer of bone (*arrow*) over the superior canal. (B) Multiplanar reformation in an oblique sagittal orientation confirms the presence of an intact but thin layer of bone (*arrows*) over the right superior canal. (C) Coronal 0.5 mm collimated CT scan through the left temporal bone demonstrates dehiscence of bone (*arrow*) over the left superior canal. (D) Multiplanar reformation in an oblique sagittal orientation through the left temporal bone demonstrates an area of dehiscence (*arrows*) over the left superior canal. (Published with permission from reference 138.)

the tympanic membrane. The pattern of changes in velocity and angle on laser-Doppler vibrometry in these patients is similar to that noted in ears with ossicular interruption.[133]

Further studies will be required to determine why some patients with superior semicircular canal dehiscence have exclusively vestibular abnormalities, some exclusively auditory effects, and others both vestibular and auditory manifestations. Factors that may contribute to differences in the auditory and/or vestibular manifestations of superior semicircular canal dehiscence include whether or not the cochlear aqueduct is patent and the relative compliance of the round window membrane. One patient in a recent clinical series was noted to have exclusively auditory manifestations at the time superior semicircular canal dehiscence was identified but later developed vestibular symptoms and signs.[126]

Vestibular Evoked Myogenic Potentials Responses

Patients with superior semicircular canal dehiscence syndrome have a lowered threshold for eliciting a VEMP response in the ear(s) affected by the disorder.[131,136,137] The VEMP response can also have a larger than normal amplitude in superior semicircular canal dehiscence. The mechanism responsible for these abnormalities in the VEMP response in patients with superior canal dehiscence is most likely related to the "third mobile window" created by the dehiscence. The dehiscence creates a low impedance pathway that increases the sensitivity of vestibular receptors to sound and pressure stimuli.

Temporal Bone Computed Tomography Scans in the Diagnosis of Superior Semicircular Canal Dehiscence

High resolution temporal bone CT scans have been used to identify dehiscence of bone overlying the superior canal (Figure 8). The parameters used for these CT scans are important for maximizing the specificity of the scans. Conventional noncontrast enhanced temporal bone CT scans are performed with 1.0 mm collimation, and images are displayed in the axial and coronal planes. These scans have a relatively low specificity (high number of false positives) in the identification of superior semicircular canal dehiscence because of the effects of partial volume averaging. The specificity and positive predictive value of these scans are improved when 0.5 mm collimated helical CT scans are performed with reformation of the images in the plane of the superior canal.[138] Even with these improved CT methods, imaging alone should never be used to make the diagnosis of superior semicircular canal dehiscence. Instead, the diagnosis should be based upon the findings on CT imaging in conjunction with the physiological tests, characteristic symptoms, and findings on clinical examination.

CT studies have shown that the thickness of bone overlying the intact superior semicircular canal in a patient with unilateral dehiscence is significantly less than that found in individuals without superior semicircular canal dehiscence.[139] This finding and observations from a review of 1,000 histologically processed temporal bones sectioned in a plane perpendicular to the petrous ridge suggest an underlying developmental or congenital abnormality that leads to the dehiscence.[140] The onset of symptoms and signs associated with this syndrome has typically occurred during adulthood. Patients in whom the normal thickness of bone fails to develop may then manifest the syndrome when the abnormally thin layer of bone is disrupted by trauma or is eroded over time as a consequence of the pressure from the overlying temporal lobe.

Surgical Repair of Superior Semicircular Canal Dehiscence

Many patients with superior semicircular canal dehiscence are not debilitated by the disorder and are able to avoid the stimuli that elicit the symptoms and signs. These patients may not need any specific treatment for the disorder. In other patients, symptoms such as sound- or pressure-induced vertigo, pulsatile oscillopsia, and chronic disequilibrium may be disabling. Surgical repair of superior semicircular canal dehiscence was initially described by Minor and colleagues.[123] The success of surgical procedures to correct the dehiscence has been confirmed by others.[141] The surgery is typically performed through the middle cranial fossa approach (Figure 9). The surgical procedure has involved either canal plugging with obliteration of the canal lumen with fascia and bone or canal resurfacing that involves covering the dehiscence with fascia and a bone graft but without plugging of the canal lumen. Recent comparisons of surgical outcomes in patients who underwent either canal plugging or resurfacing (without plugging of the canal lumen) revealed

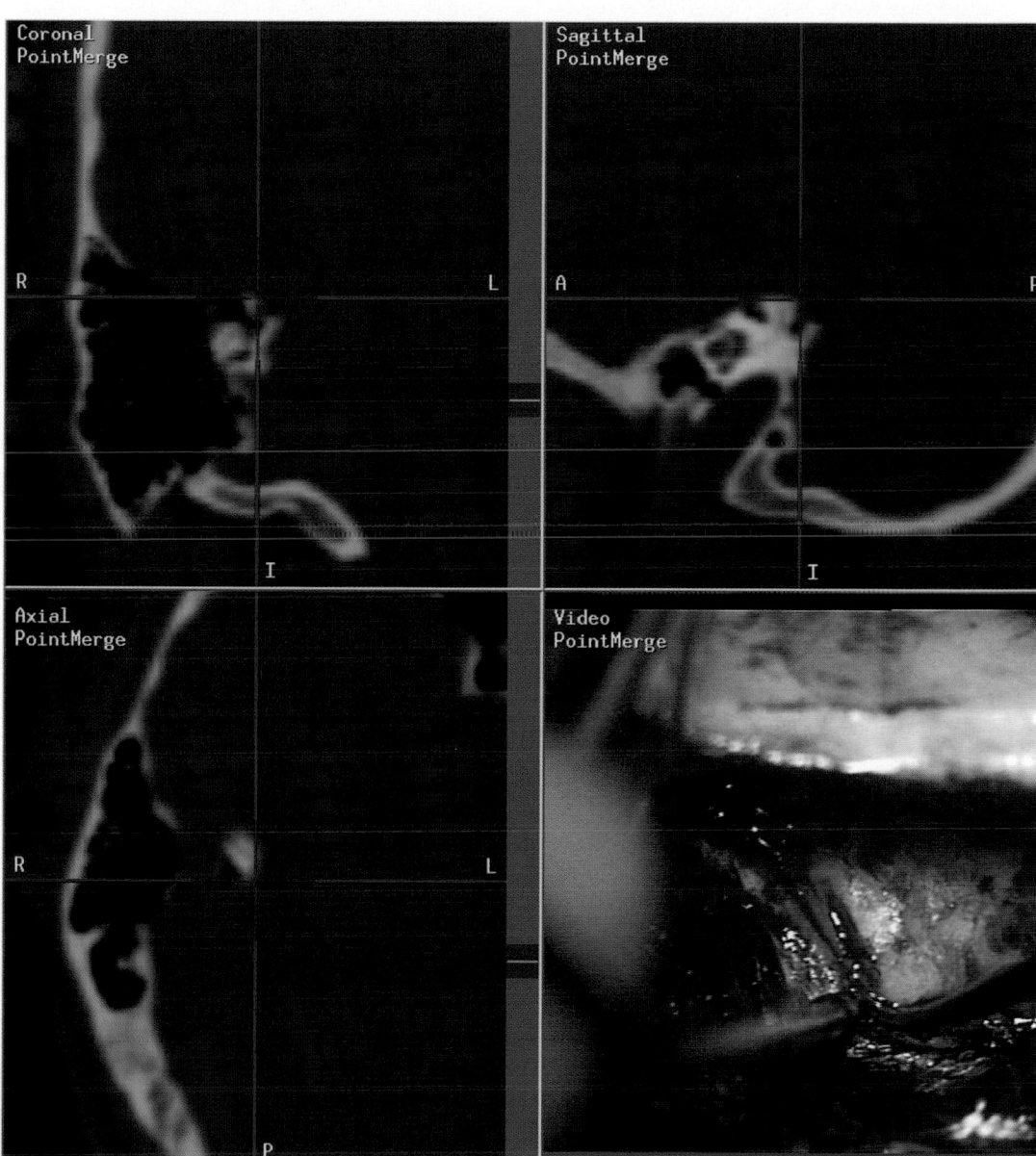

Figure 9 Intraoperative images from a right middle cranial fossa approach used to plug the superior semicircular canal for repair of superior semicircular canal dehiscence in a 41-year-old man with superior semicircular canal dehiscence syndrome on the right side. This image shows identification of the superior semicircular canal. The CT images in 3 planes (coronal, sagittal, and axial) are shown. The lower right panel shows the simultaneous image through the operative microscope. Note that the probe being detected by the navigation system is located immediately posterior to the superior semicircular canal as shown on both the axial CT image and the axial image through the operative microscope.

that complete resolution of vestibular symptoms and signs is more commonly obtained with canal plugging than with resurfacing alone.[126,142]

Primary middle fossa repair of superior semicircular canal dehiscence is associated with a low incidence of sensorineural hearing loss and, in some cases, can lead to normalization of conductive hearing loss.[143] Revision middle fossa repair or previous stapes surgery may be associated with postoperative sensorineural hearing loss. A recent study of the function of individual semicircular canals before and after surgical correction of superior semicircular canal dehiscence has shown reduction in the function of the operated superior canal but the function of other ipsilateral semicircular canals is typically preserved.[144]

REFERENCES

1. Committee on Hearing and Equilibrium guidelines for the diagnosis and evaluation of therapy in Meniere's disease. Otolaryngol Head Neck Surg 1995;113:181–5.
2. Baloh RW. Prosper Meniere and his disease. Arch Neurol 2001;58:1151–6.
3. Hallpike CS, Cairns H. Observations on the pathology of Meniere's syndrome. J Laryngol Otol 1938; 53: 625–55.
4. Lustig LR, Lalwani AK. The history of Meniere's disease. Otolaryngol Clin North Am 1997;30:917–45.
5. Stahle J. Advanced Meniere's disease. A study of 356 severely disabled patients. Acta Otolaryngol 1976;81:113–9.
6. Lustig LR, Yeagle J, Niparko JK, et al. Cochlear implantation in patients with bilateral Meniere's syndrome. Otol Neurotol 2003;24:397–403.
7. Lermoyez M. Le vertige qui fait entendre (angiospasme labyrinthique). Presse Medicale 1919;27:1–3.
8. House JW, Doherty JK, Fisher LM, et al. Meniere's disease: Prevalence of contralateral ear involvement. Otol Neurotol 2006;27:355–61.
9. Kitahara M. Bilateral aspects of Meniere's disease. Meniere's disease with bilateral fluctuant hearing loss. Acta Otolaryngol 1991;485:74–7.
10. Balkany TJ, Sires B, Arenberg IK. Bilateral aspects of Meniere's disease: An underestimated clinical entity. Otolaryngol Clin North Am 1980;13:603–9.
11. Black FO, Kitch R. A review of vestibular test results in Meniere's disease. Otolaryngol Clin North Am 1980;13:631–42.
12. Stahle J, Klockhoff I. Diagnostic procedures, differential diagnosis and general conclusions. In: Pfaltz CR, editor. Controversial aspects of Meniere's disease, New York: George Thieme; 1986. p. 71–86.
13. Carey JP, Minor LB, Peng GC, et al. Changes in the three-dimensional angular vestibulo-ocular reflex following intratympanic gentamicin for Meniere's disease. J Assoc Res Otolaryngol 2002;3:430–43.
14. Orchik DJ, Shea JJ, Jr, Ge X. Transtympanic electrocochleography in Meniere's disease using clicks and tonebursts. Am J Otol 1993;14:290–4.
15. Ferraro J, Best L, Arenberg IK. The use of electrocochleography in the diagnosis, assessment, and monitoring of endolymphatic hydrops. Otolaryngol Clin North Am 1983;16:69–82.
16. Campbell KC, Harker LA, Abbas PJ. Interpretation of electrocochleography in Meniere's disease and normal subjects. Ann Otol Rhinol Laryngol 1992;101:496–500.
17. Kinney SE, Sandridge SA, Newman CW. Long-term effects of Meniere's disease on hearing and quality of life. Am J Otol 1997;18:67–73.
18. Jackson CG, Glasscock ME, III, Davis WE, et al. Medical management of Meniere's disease. Ann Otol Rhinol Laryngol 1981;90:142–7.
19. Klockhoff I, Lindblom U. Meniere's disease and hydrochlorothiazide (Dichlotride)—A critical analysis of symptoms and therapeutic effects. Acta Otolaryngol 1967;63:347–65.
20. van Deelen GW, Huizing EH. Use of a diuretic (Dyazide) in the treatment of Meniere's disease. A double-blind crossover placebo-controlled study. ORL J Otorhinolaryngol Relat Spec 1986;48:287–92.
21. Parnes LS, Sun AH, Freeman DJ. Corticosteroid pharmacokinetics in the inner ear fluids: An animal study followed by clinical application. Laryngoscope 1999;109:1–17.

22. Shea JJ, Jr, Ge X. Dexamethasone perfusion of the labyrinth plus intravenous dexamethasone for Meniere's disease. Otolaryngol Clin North Am 1996;29:353–8.
23. Barrs DM, Keyser JS, Stallworth C, et al. Intratympanic steroid injections for intractable Meniere's disease. Laryngoscope 2001;111:2100–4.
24. Glasscock ME, III, Gulya AJ, Pensak ML, et al. Medical and surgical management of Meniere's disease. Am J Otol 1984;5:536–42.
25. Brown JS. A ten year statistical follow-up of 245 consecutive cases of endolymphatic shunt and decompression with 328 consecutive cases of labyrinthectomy. Laryngoscope 1983;93:1419–24.
26. Brackmann DE, Nissen RL. Meniere's disease: Results of treatment with the endolymphatic subarachnoid shunt compared with the endolymphatic mastoid shunt. Am J Otol 1987;8:275–82.
27. Monsell EM, Wiet RJ. Endolymphatic sac surgery: Methods of study and results. Am J Otol 1988;9:396–402.
28. Moffat DA. Endolymphatic sac surgery: Analysis of 100 operations. Clin Otolaryngol Allied Sci 1994;19:261–6.
29. Thomsen J, Bretlau P, Tos M, et al. Placebo effect in surgery for Meniere's disease. A double-blind, placebo-controlled study on endolymphatic sac shunt surgery. Arch Otolaryngol 1981;107:271–7.
30. Thomsen J, Bretlau P, Tos M, et al. Endolymphatic sac-mastoid shunt surgery. A nonspecific treatment modality? Ann Otol Rhinol Laryngol 1986;95:32–5.
31. Glasscock ME, III, Thedinger BA, Cueva RA, et al. An analysis of the retrolabyrinthine vs. the retrosigmoid vestibular nerve section. Otolaryngol Head Neck Surg 1991;104:88–95.
32. Schuknecht HF. Ablation therapy in the management of Meniere's disease. Acta Otolaryngol 1957;132:1–4.
33. Lange G. Ototoxische antibiotika in der behandlung des morbus Meniere. Ther Woche Wochensch Prakt Med 1976;26:1–6.
34. Blakley BW. Update on intratympanic gentamicin for Meniere's disease. Laryngoscope 2000;110:236–40.
35. Harner SG, Driscoll CL, Facer GW, et al. Long-term follow-up of transtympanic gentamicin for Meniere's syndrome. Otol Neurotol 2001;22:210–4.
36. Wu IC, Minor LB. Long-term hearing outcome in patients receiving intratympanic gentamicin for Meniere's disease. Laryngoscope 2003;113:815–20.
37. Halmagyi GM, Curthoys IS. A clinical sign of canal paresis. Arch Neurol 1988;45:737–9.
38. Ewald J. Physiologische Untersuchungen uber das Endorgan des Nervus Octavus. Wiesbaden, Germany: Bergmann; 1892. p. 325.
39. Aw ST, Haslwanter T, Halmagyi GM, et al. Three-dimensional vector analysis of the human vestibuloocular reflex in response to high-acceleration head rotations. I. Responses in normal subjects. J Neurophysiol 1996;76:4009–20.
40. Aw ST, Halmagyi GM, Haslwanter T, et al. Three-dimensional vector analysis of the human vestibuloocular reflex in response to high-acceleration head rotations. II. responses in subjects with unilateral vestibular loss and selective semicircular canal occlusion. J Neurophysiol 1996;76:4021–30.
41. Aw ST, Halmagyi GM, Pohl DV, et al. Compensation of the human vertical vestibulo-ocular reflex following occlusion of one vertical semicircular canal is incomplete. Exp Brain Res 1995;103:471–5.
42. Hirvonen TP, Minor LB, Hullar TE, et al. Effects of intratympanic gentamicin on vestibular afferents and hair cells in the chinchilla. J Neurophysiol 2005;93:643–55.
43. Lin FR, Migliaccio AA, Haslwanter T, et al. Angular vestibulo-ocular reflex gains correlate with vertigo control after intratympanic gentamicin treatment for Meniere's disease. Ann Otol Rhinol Laryngol 2005;114:777–85.
44. Sekitani T, Imate Y, Noguchi T, et al. Vestibular neuronitis: Epidemiological survey by questionnaire in Japan. Acta Otolaryngol 1993;503:9–12.
45. Arbusow V, Schulz P, Strupp M, et al. Distribution of herpes simplex virus type 1 in human geniculate and vestibular ganglia: Implications for vestibular neuritis. Ann Neurol 1999;46:416–9.
46. Gianoli G, Goebel J, Mowry S, et al. Anatomic differences in the lateral vestibular nerve channels and their implications in vestibular neuritis. Otol Neurotol 2005;26:489–94.
47. Welgampola MS, Colebatch JG. Characteristics and clinical applications of vestibular-evoked myogenic potentials. Neurology 2005;64:1682–8.
48. Fetter M, Dichgans J. Vestibular neuritis spares the inferior division of the vestibular nerve. Brain 1996;119:755–63.
49. Matsuzaki M, Kamei T. Stage-assessment of the progress of continuous vertigo of peripheral origin by means of

spontaneous and head-shaking nystagmus findings. Acta Otolaryngol 1995;519:188–90.
50. Lee H, Sohn SI, Cho YW, et al. Cerebellar infarction presenting isolated vertigo: Frequency and vascular topographical patterns. Neurology 2006;67:1178–83.
51. Strupp M, Arbusow V, Maag KP, et al. Vestibular exercises improve central vestibulospinal compensation after vestibular neuritis. Neurology 1998;51:838–44.
52. Godemann F, Schabowska A, Naetebusch B, et al. The impact of cognitions on the development of panic and somatoform disorders: A prospective study in patients with vestibular neuritis. Psychol Med 2006;36:99–108.
53. Godemann F, Koffroth C, Neu P, et al. Why does vertigo become chronic after neuropathia vestibularis? Psychosom Med 2004;66:783–7.
54. Godemann F, Linden M, Neu P, et al., A prospective study on the course of anxiety after vestibular neuronitis. J Psychosom Res 2004;56:351–4.
55. Staab JP, Ruckenstein MJ. Which comes first? Psychogenic dizziness versus otogenic anxiety. Laryngoscope 2003;113:1714–8.
56. Huppert D, Strupp M, Theil D, et al. Low recurrence rate of vestibular neuritis: A long-term follow-up. Neurology 2006;67:1870–1.
57. Halmagyi GM, Aw ST, Karlberg M, et al. Inferior vestibular neuritis. Ann N Y Acad Sci 2002;956:306–13.
58. Prokopakis EP, Chimona T, Tsagournisakis M, et al. Benign paroxysmal positional vertigo: 10-year experience in treating 592 patients with canalith repositioning procedure. Laryngoscope 2005;115:1667–71.
59. Halmagyi GM, Aw ST, Cremer PD, et al. Impulsive testing of individual semicircular canal function. Ann N Y Acad Sci 2001;942:192–200.
60. Palla A, Straumann D. Recovery of the high-acceleration vestibulo-ocular reflex after vestibular neuritis. J Assoc Res Otolaryngol 2004;5:427–35.
61. Tseng HZ, Chao WY. Head-shaking nystagmus: A sensitive indicator of vestibular dysfunction. Clin Otolaryngol Allied Sci 1997;22:549–52.
62. Guidetti G, Monzani D, Civiero N. Head shaking nystagmus in the follow-up of patients with vestibular diseases. Clin Otolaryngol Allied Sci 2002;27:124–8.
63. Karlberg M, Annertz M, Magnusson M. Acute vestibular neuritis visualized by 3-T magnetic resonance imaging with high-dose gadolinium. Arch Otolaryngol Head Neck Surg 2004;130:229–32.
64. Myrseth E, Moller P, Wentzel-Larsen T, et al. Untreated vestibular schwannomas: Vertigo is a powerful predictor for health-related quality of life. Neurosurgery 2006;59:67–76; discussion 67–76.
65. McGee SR. Dizzy patients. Diagnosis and treatment. West J Med 1995;162:37–42.
66. Strupp M, Zingler VC, Arbusow V, et al. Methylprednisolone, valacyclovir, or the combination for vestibular neuritis. N Engl J Med 2004;351:354–61.
67. Gacek RR, Gacek MR. Antiviral therapy of vestibular ganglionitis. Adv Otorhinolaryngol 2002;60:124–36.
68. Topuz O, Topuz B, Ardic FN, et al. Efficacy of vestibular rehabilitation on chronic unilateral vestibular dysfunction. Clin Rehabil 2004;18:76–83.
69. ICHD-II, Headache Classification Subcommittee of the International Headache Society: The International Classification of Headache Disorders, 2nd edition. Cephalalgia 2004;24:1–160.
70. Baloh RW. Neurotology of migraine. Headache 1997;37:615–21.
71. Eggers SD. Migraine-related vertigo: Diagnosis and treatment. Curr Neurol Neurosci Rep 2006;6:106–15.
72. Kayan A, Hood JD. Neuro-otological manifestations of migraine. Brain 1984;107:1123–42.
73. Neuhauser HK, Radtke A, von Brevern M, et al. Migrainous vertigo: Prevalence and impact on quality of life. Neurology 2006;67:1028–33.
74. Shepard NT. Differentiation of Meniere's disease and migraine-associated dizziness: A review. J Am Acad Audiol 2006;17:69–80.
75. Brantberg K, Trees N, Baloh RW. Migraine-associated vertigo. Acta Otolaryngol 2005;125:276–9.
76. Zivadinov R, Willheim K, Sepic-Grahovac D, et al. Migraine and tension-type headache in Croatia: A population-based survey of precipitating factors. Cephalalgia 2003;23:336–43.
77. Hain TC, Hanna PA, Rheinberger MA. Mal de debarquement. Arch Otolaryngol Head Neck Surg 1999;125:615–20.
78. Lempert T, Neuhauser H. Migrainous vertigo. Neurol Clin 2005;23:715–30.
79. Radtke A, Lempert T, Gresty MA, et al. Migraine and Meniere's disease: Is there a link? Neurology 2002;59:1700–4.

80. Atkinson M, Meniere's original papers [Reprinted with an English translation together with commentaries and biographical sketch.]. Acta Otolaryngol Suppl 1961;162:3–77.

81. Lee H, Lopez I, Ishiyama A, et al. Can migraine damage the inner ear? Arch Neurol 2000;57:1631–4.

82. Dieterich M, Brandt T. Episodic vertigo related to migraine (90 cases): Vestibular migraine? J Neurol 1999;246:883–92.

83. Drummond PD. Triggers of motion sickness in migraine sufferers. Headache 2005;45:653–6.

84. Arriaga MA, Chen DA, Hillman TA, et al. Visually enhanced vestibulo-ocular reflex: A diagnostic tool for migraine vestibulopathy. Laryngoscope 2006;116:1577–9.

85. Rocca MA, Ceccarelli A, Falini A, et al. Diffusion tensor magnetic resonance imaging at 3.0 Tesla shows subtle cerebral grey matter abnormalities in patients with migraine. J Neurol Neurosurg Psychiatry 2006;77:686–9.

86. Rocca MA, Colombo B, Pagani E, et al. Evidence for cortical functional changes in patients with migraine and white matter abnormalities on conventional and diffusion tensor magnetic resonance imaging. Stroke 2003;34:665–70.

87. Staab JP. Chronic dizziness: The interface between psychiatry and neuro-otology. Curr Opin Neurol 2006;19:41–8.

88. Gottshall KR, Moore RJ, Hoffer ME. Vestibular rehabilitation for migraine-associated dizziness. Int Tinnitus J 2005;11:81–4.

89. Wrisley DM, Whitney SL, Furman JM. Vestibular rehabilitation outcomes in patients with a history of migraine. Otol Neurotol 2002;23:483–7.

90. Crevits L, Bosman T. Migraine-related vertigo: Towards a distinctive entity. Clin Neurol Neurosurg 2005;107:82–7.

91. Loj J, Solomon GD. Migraine prophylaxis: Who, why, and how. Cleve Clin J Med 2006;73:793–4, 797, 800–1 passim.

92. Diener HC, Matias-Guiu J, Hartung E, et al. Efficacy and tolerability in migraine prophylaxis of flunarizine in reduced doses: A comparison with propranolol 160 mg daily. Cephalalgia 2002;22:209–21.

93. Landy S, McGinnis J, Curlin D, et al. Selective serotonin reuptake inhibitors for migraine prophylaxis. Headache 1999;39:28–32.

94. Mathew NT. Antiepileptic drugs in migraine prevention. Headache 2001;41:S18–24.

95. von Brevern M, Radtke A, Lezius F, et al. Epidemiology of benign paroxysmal positional vertigo. A population-based study. J Neurol Neurosurg Psychiatry 2006; Epub ahead of print.

96. Dix MR, Hallpike CS. The pathology, symptomatology and diagnosis of certain common disorders of the vestibular system. Ann Otol Rhinol Laryngol 1952;61:987–1016.

97. Lopez-Escamez JA, Molina MI, Gamiz MJ. Anterior semicircular canal benign paroxysmal positional vertigo and positional downbeating nystagmus. Am J Otolaryngol 2006;27:173–8.

98. Bertholon P, Bronstein AM, Davies RA, et al. Positional down beating nystagmus in 50 patients: Cerebellar disorders and possible anterior semicircular canalithiasis. J Neurol Neurosurg Psychiatry 2002;72:366–72.

99. White JA, Coale KD, Catalano PJ, et al. Diagnosis and management of lateral semicircular canal benign paroxysmal positional vertigo. Otolaryngol Head Neck Surg 2005;133:278–84.

100. Epley JM. The canalith repositioning procedure: For treatment of benign paroxysmal positional vertigo. Otolaryngol Head Neck Surg 1992;107:399–404.

101. Hullar TE, Minor LB: Vestibular physiology and disorders of the labyrinth. In: Glasscock ME, Gulya AJ, editors.

102. Surgery of the Ear, 5th edition. Hamilton: BC Decker, 2002. p. 83–103.

102. Furman JM, Cass SP. Benign paroxysmal positional vertigo. N Engl J Med 1999;341:1590–6.

103. von Brevern M, Seelig T, Radtke A, et al. Short-term efficacy of Epley's manoeuvre: A double-blind randomised trial. J Neurol Neurosurg Psychiatry 2006;77:980–2.

104. Woodworth BA, Gillespie MB, Lambert PR. The canalith repositioning procedure for benign positional vertigo: A meta-analysis. Laryngoscope 2004;114:1143–6.

105. Korres S, Balatsouras DG, Ferekidis E. Prognosis of patients with benign paroxysmal positional vertigo treated with repositioning manoeuvres. J Laryngol Otol 2006;120:528–33.

106. Moon SJ, Bae SH, Kim HD, et al. The effect of postural restrictions in the treatment of benign paroxysmal positional vertigo. Eur Arch Otorhinolaryngol 2005;262:408–11.

107. Marciano E, Marcelli V. Postural restrictions in labyrintholithiasis. Eur Arch Otorhinolaryngol 2002;259:262–5.

108. Viirre E, Purcell I, Baloh RW. The Dix-Hallpike test and the canalith repositioning maneuver. Laryngoscope 2005;115:184–7.

109. Semont A, Freyss G, Vitte E. Curing the BPPV with a liberatory maneuver. Adv Otorhinolaryngol 1988;42:290–3.

110. Levrat E, van Melle G, Monnier P, et al. Efficacy of the Semont maneuver in benign paroxysmal positional vertigo. Arch Otolaryngol Head Neck Surg 2003;129:629–33.

111. Brandt T, Daroff RB. Physical therapy for benign paroxysmal positional vertigo. Arch Otolaryngol 1980;106:484–5.

112. Cohen HS, Kimball KT. Effectiveness of treatments for benign paroxysmal positional vertigo of the posterior canal. Otol Neurotol 2005;26:1034–40.

113. Lempert T, Tiel-Wilck K. A positional maneuver for treatment of horizontal-canal benign positional vertigo. Laryngoscope 1996;106:476–8.

114. Sekine K, Imai T, Sato G, et al. Natural history of benign paroxysmal positional vertigo and efficacy of Epley and Lempert maneuvers. Otolaryngol Head Neck Surg 2006;135:529–33.

115. Gacek RR. Transection of the posterior ampullary nerve for the relief of benign paroxysmal positional vertigo. Ann Otol Rhinol Laryngol 1974;83:596–605.

116. Gacek RR, Gacek MR. Results of singular neurectomy in the posterior ampullary recess. ORL J Otorhinolaryngol Relat Spec 2002;64:397–402.

117. Kos MI, Feigl G, Anderhuber F, et al. Transcanal approach to the singular nerve. Otol Neurotol 2006;27:542–6.

118. Parnes LS, McClure JA. Posterior semicircular canal occlusion for intractable benign paroxysmal positional vertigo. Ann Otol Rhinol Laryngol 1990;99:330–4.

119. Agrawal SK, Parnes LS. Human experience with canal plugging. Ann N Y Acad Sci 2001;942:300–5.

120. Parnes LS, McClure JA. Posterior semicircular canal occlusion in the normal hearing ear. Otolaryngol Head Neck Surg 1991;104:52–7.

121. Pulec JL. Ablation of posterior semicircular canal for benign paroxysmal positional vertigo. Ear Nose Throat J 1997;76:17–22, 24.

122. Horii A, Imai T, Mishiro Y, et al. Horizontal canal type BPPV: Bilaterally affected case treated with canal plugging and Lempert's maneuver. ORL J Otorhinolaryngol Relat Spec 2003;65:366–9.

123. Minor LB, Solomon D, Zinreich JS, et al. Sound- and/or pressure-induced vertigo due to bone dehiscence of the superior semicircular canal. Arch Otolaryngol Head Neck Surg 1998;124:249–58.

124. Minor LB, Superior canal dehiscence syndrome. Am J Otol 2000;21:9–19.

125. Minor LB, Carey JP, Cremer PD, et al. Dehiscence of bone overlying the superior canal as a cause of apparent conductive hearing loss. Otol Neurotol 2003;24:270–8.

126. Minor LB. Clinical manifestations of superior semicircular canal dehiscence. Laryngoscope 2005;115:1717–27.

127. Cremer PD, Minor LB, Carey JP, et al. Eye movements in patients with superior canal dehiscence syndrome align with the abnormal canal. Neurology 2000;55:1833–41.

128. Minor LB, Cremer PD, Carey JP, et al. Symptoms and signs in superior canal dehiscence syndrome. Ann NY Acad Sci 2001;942:259–73.

129. Aw ST, Todd MJ, Aw GE, et al. Click-evoked vestibulo-ocular reflex: Stimulus-response properties in superior canal dehiscence. Neurology 2006;66:1079–87.

130. Mikulec AA, McKenna MJ, Ramsey MJ, et al. Superior semicircular canal dehiscence presenting as conductive hearing loss without vertigo. Otol Neurotol 2004;25:121–9.

131. Watson SR, Halmagyi GM, Colebatch JG. Vestibular hypersensitivity to sound (Tullio phenomenon): Structural and functional assessment. Neurology 2000;54:722–8.

132. Poe DS. Diagnosis and management of the patulous eustachian tube. Otol Neurotol. 2007;28:668–77.

133. Rosowski JJ, Songer JE, Nakajima HH, et al. Clinical, experimental, and theoretical investigations of the effect of superior semicircular canal dehiscence on hearing mechanisms. Otol Neurotol 2004;25:323–32.

134. Halmagyi GM, Aw ST, McGarvie LA, et al. Superior semicircular canal dehiscence simulating otosclerosis. J Laryngol Otol 2003;117:553–7.

135. House JW, Sheehy JL, Antunez JC. Stapedectomy in children. Laryngoscope 1980;90:1804–9.

136. Brantberg K, Bergenius J, Tribukait A. Vestibular-evoked myogenic potentials in patients with dehiscence of the superior semicircular canal. Acta Otolaryngol 1999;119:633–40.

137. Streubel SO, Cremer PD, Carey JP, et al. Vestibular-evoked myogenic potentials in the diagnosis of superior canal dehiscence syndrome. Acta Otolaryngol 2001;545:41–9.

138. Belden CJ, Weg N, Minor LB, et al. CT evaluation of bone dehiscence of the superior semicircular canal as a cause of sound- and/or pressure-induced vertigo. Radiology 2003;226:337–43.

139. Hirvonen TP, Weg N, Zinreich SJ, et al. High-resolution CT findings suggest a developmental abnormality underlying superior canal dehiscence syndrome. Acta Otolaryngol 2003;123:477–81.

140. Carey JP, Minor LB, Nager GT. Dehiscence or thinning of bone overlying the superior semicircular canal in a temporal bone survey. Arch Otolaryngol Head Neck Surg 2000;126:137–47.

141. Mikulec AA, Poe DS, McKenna MJ. Operative management of superior semicircular canal dehiscence. Laryngoscope 2005;115:501–7.

142. Friedland DR, Michel MA. Cranial thickness in superior canal dehiscence syndrome: Implications for canal resurfacing surgery. Otol Neurotol 2006;27:346–54.

143. Limb CJ, Carey JP, Srireddy S, et al. Auditory function in patients with surgically treated superior semicircular canal dehiscence. Otol Neurotol 2006;27:969–80.

144. Carey JP, Migliaccio AA, Minor LB. Semicircular canal function before and after surgery for superior canal dehiscence. Otol Neurotol 2006; Epub ahead of print.

29

Presbyacusis and Presbyastasis

John H. Mills, PhD
Cliff A. Megerian, MD
Paul R. Lambert, MD

Presbyacusis, defined generally as age-related hearing loss, and presbyastasis, defined generally as age-related balance disorders, are high prevalence problems today and will be even more prevalent in the immediate future. According to the National Center for Health Statistics in the quarter century between 1976 and 2000, the number of persons below age 75 increased by 23%, the number between age 75 and 84 increased by 57%, and the number over age 84 increased by 91%. Indeed, by the year 2030, the elderly will comprise 32% of the population, an increase of 250%. A total of 60 to 80% of these older persons will have clinically significant hearing and balance problems. Because of the increasing number of older Americans, high prevalence problems such as age-related hearing and balance problems and other chronic disabling conditions (vision, arthritis) will place extensive, novel, and expensive demands on the health care system.[1]

TERMINOLOGY OF PRESBYACUSIS

There are several definitions of the term presbyacusis. Indeed, even the spelling is an issue, that is, presbyacusis versus presbycusis. Here we use "presbyacusis." It is used loosely to describe a seemingly endless list of genetic, environmental, and disease states that can cause hearing loss in an older person. Often presbyacusis is used to refer to hearing loss purely caused by the natural process of aging. More often, hearing loss is called presbyacusis if the person is beyond the fifth decade, without consideration of disease, genetics, or other factors. In many studies, older persons are considered homogeneous and are grouped regardless of hearing levels or are grouped if their hearing loss exceeds an arbitrary criterion.

Some of the confusion associated with the use of the term can be eliminated or reduced by the appropriate use of the terms presbyacusis, socioacusis, and nosoacusis.[2] A generic definition of presbyacusis is age-related hearing loss that is the effect of aging in combination with life-long exposures to nonoccupational noise, ototoxic agents, diet, drugs, exercise, and other miscellaneous factors. It is conceptually useful to view presbyacusis as a mixture of acquired auditory stresses, trauma, and otological diseases superimposed upon an intrinsic, genetically controlled, aging process. A more restrictive, precise definition of presbyacusis is hearing loss that increases as a function of chronologic age and is attributable to "aging" per se. This "purely aging" hearing loss probably has a genetic basis. It may be correlated with age-related deterioration or declines in other senses, especially balance, vision, and touch.

Socioacusis is defined as the hearing loss produced by exposure to nonoccupational noise in combination with lifestyle factors such as diet and exercise. Nosoacusis is the hearing loss attributable to diseases with ototoxic effects.[2] Thus, the hearing loss assessed in a person into the fifth decade and beyond is the combined effects of aging, nosoacusis, socioacusis, and possibly, for many persons, exposure to occupational noise. Oftentimes it is important for medical and legal reasons to differentiate presbyacusis from socioacusis, nosoacusis, and occupational hearing loss.

Some laboratory (with animals) and field studies suggest that hearing losses caused by exposure to noise are additive (in decibels) with the hearing loss attributed to presbyacusis (in the strict sense of the word). A small sensorineural hearing loss (SNHL) of 25 dB at age 25, for example, seemingly has little social or medical relevance; however, by age 70, a hearing loss of 25 dB caused almost entirely by the aging process is added to the existing SNHL. The result is a moderate-to-severe SNHL of 50 dB. In other words, a seemingly minor hearing loss at a young age becomes a severe loss when the effects of presbyacusis become evident.

Rules for combining hearing losses attributable to presbyacusis, nosoacusis, and socioacusis are not always straightforward. In the medicolegal assessment of hearing loss, it is assumed that presbyacusis effects (aging plus socioacusis plus nosoacusis) add in decibels to the hearing loss produced by noise. As stated above, this approach is supported by some laboratory and field data for groups of subjects under a limited set of conditions; however, for individual subjects and for complicated noise exposures, there are few data available. As a consequence, the procedures for the allocation of hearing loss into different components, as required by many medicolegal questions, are controversial.[3]

TERMINOLOGY OF PRESBYASTASIS

The vestibular system, like the auditory system, undergoes a progressive decline over the lifetime of an individual. However, there exists a number of important distinctions between these 2 age-related disorders that renders the description, characterization and measurement of age-related vestibular disorders much more difficult than age-related hearing loss. The term presbyacusis is a well-accepted term used daily among members of the medical community, unlike the analogous term "presbyastasis" which is used to characterize disequilibrium of aging. This is likely due in part to the difficulty in accurately measuring the latter condition. Hearing loss of age or any etiology can be accurately measured with audiometric testing not only in magnitude, but also qualitatively along frequency ranges. For example, one can be reasonably sure that a complaint of hearing loss with audiometric evidence of a high frequency hearing loss harbors a deficiency at the level of the basilar turn of the cochlea and the magnitude of this loss can be measured in decibels. Conversely, the complaint of "dizziness" or "vertigo" can be the result of a myriad of abnormalities that may or may not even involve the vestibular system. Even after a detailed history has been taken and the patient's complaints point to a vestibular issue, it is often difficult to arrive at the conclusion that 1 particular portion of the vestibular system gives rise to the symptomatology. This is not necessarily the case in well-demarcated conditions such as benign paroxysmal positional vertigo (BPPV) or vestibular neuritis in a young healthy patient, but more so in the elderly patient presenting to the clinician with complaints of chronic imbalance or "constant vertigo." This is due to the fact that for the most part, normal hearing requires the proper function of the cochlear end-organ whereas proper balance and stable gait necessitate a choreographed interplay between not only the vestibular end organs, and also the visual, proprioceptive, musculoskeletal, and central nervous systems (CNSs). Thus most complaints of imbalance associated with aging are in reality a "multisystem decay" involving the systems previously mentioned, but can even include the cardiac and endocrine systems when issues related to orthostatic hypotension confound the clinical picture.

Terminology is also an issue that remains a challenge to accurate diagnosis and treatment. Many patients and referring physicians will report "dizziness" regardless of whether the patient harbors true rotatory vertigo or postural hypotension (lightheadedness). Also contributing to the paucity of information that accurately describes patterns of age-related vestibular loss with clinical correlation are the challenges associated with quantifying functional deficits. Electronystagmography can indirectly measure the activity of only 1 (lateral semicircular canal ampulla) of 5 vestibular neuroepithelial organs, whereas audiometry measures dynamic range of all useful auditory function. A number of newer tests have emerged which allow physicians to begin collecting and quantifying additional vestibular functional parameters including dynamic platform posturography, rotatory chair testing, videonystagmography (VNG), and vestibular evoked myogenic potentials (VEMP). In time these testing modalities will likely lead to a better understanding of the types and patterns of vestibular decline in the aging population and its relationship to presbyastasis overall. These will only yield clinical dividends, however, when a more thorough understanding emerges regarding the delicate interplay between the vestibular system and the rest of the body. The majority of this chapter will focus on the evidence that directly pertains to specific, measurable vestibular pathology that plays an integral role in presbyastasis.

EPIDEMIOLOGY OF PRESBYACUSIS

Over the past quarter century, there has been a significant epidemiologic effort to describe hearing levels as a function of chronologic age. Two sets of data have survived extensive scrutiny and are now part of an international standard, International Standards Organization (ISO) 1999, "Acoustics: Determination of Occupational Noise Exposure and Estimation of Noise-Induced Hearing Impairment." Figure 1A shows age-related permanent threshold shifts at audiometric frequencies for males and females. These data are referred to as Database A in the ISO 1999 standard and are considered to represent highly screened subjects. That is, the data in Figure 1A represent "pure aging" effects as well as socioacusis. Most of the hearing loss attributable to occupational hearing loss has been eliminated, although a small nosoacusic effect may be present. Figure 1B gives epidemiologic data, referred to as Database B in the ISO 1999 standard, which are considered to reflect "pure aging" effects, socioacusis, some nosoacusis, and some effects attributable to occupational hearing loss. As shown in Figure 1, hearing loss in the higher frequencies is measurable by age 30; it increases systematically to age 60 (and beyond), is largest at 4 and 6 kHz, and is much larger in males than in females. There are also significant differences between Figure 1A (Database A), and Figure 1B (Database B), presumably owing to differences in

subject selection. Small effects caused by occupational noise and nosoacusis were eliminated in Database A. Significant debate exists currently about the appropriateness and validity of Database A and B, particularly in a medicolegal context involving the assessment of occupational noise-induced hearing loss.

Data from Figure 1A and B, have been replotted in Figure 2 to show the average hearing loss at 0.5, 1, 2, and 3 kHz as a function of chronologic age. The mean hearing loss at these particular audiometric test frequencies is especially meaningful because this combination of test frequencies comprises those used in the computation of hearing handicap as recommended by the American Academy of Otolaryngology—Head and Neck Surgery (AAO-HNS). As Figure 2 shows, hearing loss increases systematically from age 20 through age 75. There are at least 2 remarkable features to Figure 2. One is that the largest difference between the worst case (males, Database B) and best case (females, Database A) is about 5 dB. One could suggest, perhaps strongly, that much of the ongoing debate about Database A and B is "much ado about nothing," that is, 5 dB. This line of thinking is supported by the fact that, even at age 75, the hearing loss is only about 20 dB. According to the AAO 1979 definitions of hearing handicap, the average hearing loss at 0.5, 1, 2, and 3 kHz must exceed 25 dB to be considered a hearing handicap. In other words, according

to the data of Figure 2 and the AAO-HNS 1979 definition of hearing handicap, substantially less than 50% of the population, male or female, have a hearing handicap even at age 75.

Other less selective epidemiologic data suggest that the prevalence of hearing handicap among older persons is substantially higher than that indicated by the epidemiologic data used in the ISO 1999 standard. Using 1,662 subjects from the famous Framingham study of cardiovascular

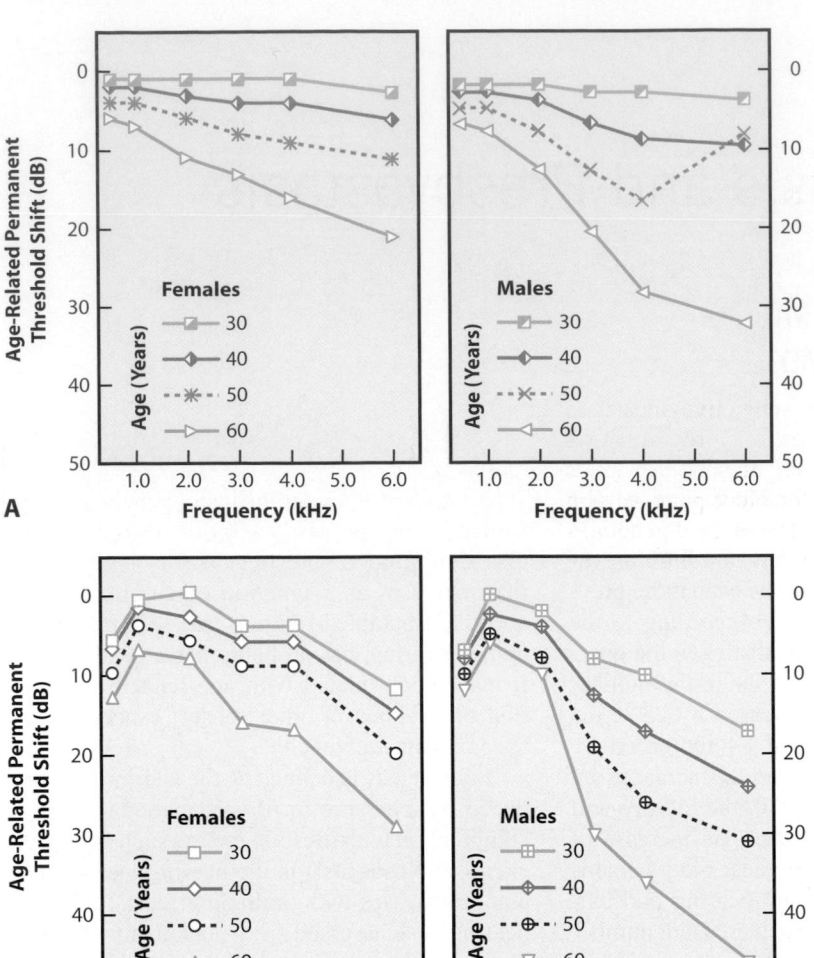

A

B

Figure 1 Epidemiologic data showing hearing levels and chronologic age from an international standard, ISO 1999. The top panel (A) is referred to as Database A and represents a sample that was highly screened to eliminate the potential influence of the effects of noise. The bottom panel (B) is also from ISO 1999 and is referred to as Database B. This sample is less well screened than A and may contain data from persons with a history of exposure to noise.

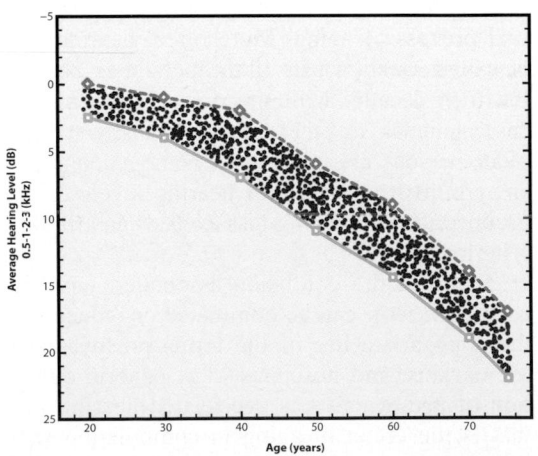

Figure 2 Data from Figure 1 have been replotted to show the average hearing level at 0.5, 1, 2, and 3 kHz as a function of age. The shaded area represents the difference between the best case, that is, the women of Database A, and the worst case, that is, the men of Database B.

disease, Gates and colleagues[4] reported that 55% met or exceeded the AAO 1979 medicolegal definition of hearing handicap. The difference between the results of Gates and colleagues and those of ISO 1999 reflect sampling differences and the inclusion of subjects older than age 75 in the Gates and colleagues sample.

In addition to an audiologic assessment, hearing handicap can be assessed more subjectively using questionnaires such as the Hearing Handicap Inventory for the Elderly.[5] The correspondence between objective, audiologic measures of hearing handicap and subjective measures from self-reports and questionnaires suggests that the AAO-HNS measure of handicap tends to overestimate handicap for older persons with mild-to-moderate hearing losses and to underestimate handicap for older persons with severe hearing losses. Of course, there are many reasons for discrepancies between subjective and audiologic estimates of hearing handicap. One general rule emerges from questionnaires and epidemiologic studies of hearing handicap in older persons, namely, that the pure-tone average (PTA) of 0.5, 1, 2, and 3 kHz must exceed about 30 dB before most older persons consider themselves to have a hearing problem. Thus, there are indeed millions of older hearing-handicapped persons in the United States.

Although much of the discussion has centered on the audiometric frequencies from 0.5 to 3 kHz, 1 of the more dramatic features of age-related hearing loss is the decline of auditory sensitivity at higher frequencies.[6,7] Figure 3A shows increasing hearing loss from age 20 to 29 to age 50 to 59 for test frequencies at and above 8 kHz. By age 50 to 59, the hearing loss at 16 kHz is greater than 60 dB. Figure 3B shows longitudinal threshold changes (the same group of observers) over the age range of 70 to 81 years, including thresholds for test frequencies up to 8 kHz. Hearing levels at 4 and 8 kHz exceed 50 dB by age 70 and at 8 kHz exceed 70 dB by age 79. Hearing loss at frequencies above 8 kHz is even more pronounced and is not predictable by hearing levels in the 1 to 4 kHz range.[8] Clearly, there is a dramatic age-related decline in auditory sensitivity at high frequencies. It appears that hearing loss starts in the second decade (or earlier) in the frequency range between 16 and 20 kHz, proceeds systematically in magnitude in the 16 kHz region, and spreads systematically downward in the frequency domain. By the eighth decade, the hearing loss is moderate to severe, even at 1 and 2 kHz.

The interpretation of epidemiologic data that show a loss of high frequency sensitivity at 16 to 20 kHz, when 10- and 19-year-olds are compared with 20- to 29-year-olds, is not straightforward. One point of view is that these age-related changes in hearing thresholds, as well as systematic declines in the number of outer hair cells starting at birth and continuing throughout the lifetime of the individual,[9] are genetically determined, age-dependent events. That is, these age-related events are totally endogenous in origin. They are independent of exogenous

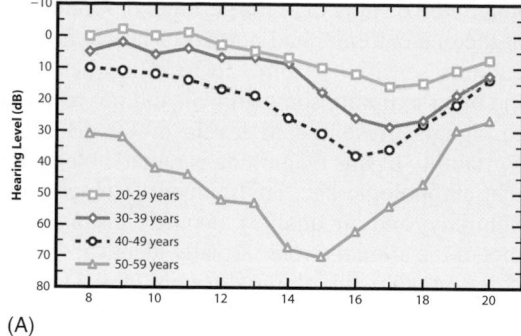

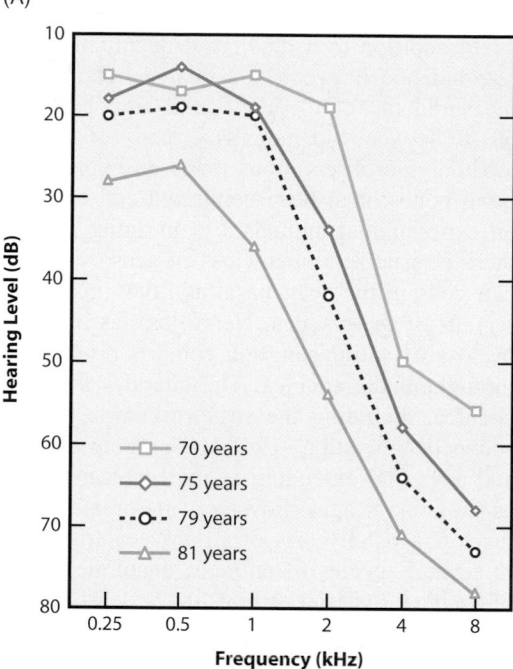

(B)

Figure 3 Hearing loss at high frequencies. (A) Hearing levels above 8 kHz over the age range 20 to 59 years. (B) Hearing levels from 0.25 to 8 kHz covering the age range 70 to 81 years, measured longitudinally. (Adapted from references 6 and 7.)

factors such as diet, exposure to environmental noise (socioacusis), and disease (nosoacusis).

As part of the Framingham heart study, Gates and colleagues have estimated the role of genetics in age-related hearing loss.[10] Their heritability estimates suggest that as much as 55% of the variance associated with age-related hearing loss is attributable to the effect of genes. A twin study reported heritability coefficients as high as 61%.[11] These heritability estimates of age-related hearing loss are similar in magnitude to those reported for hypertension and hyperlipidemia, are much stronger in women than in men, and can be used to support the point of view that age-related changes in the ear and hearing reflect the combined effect of genetics, socioacusis, and nosoacusis. In some views of presbyacusis, socioacusis is given a major role, almost surely because of the famous Mabaan study.[12]

A hearing survey of Mabaans, a tribe located in a remote and undeveloped part of Africa, showed exceptionally good auditory sensitivity for males and females in their sixth to ninth decades. In addition to the lack of exposure to occupational noise, no exposure to firearms, and exposure only to low levels of environmen-

tal noise, the Mabaans were reported to lead a low-stress lifestyle, have a low-fat diet, and have a low prevalence of cardiovascular disease. This study was quoted widely in lay and professional publications and became the scientific basis for the thesis that persons in Western industrialized societies were at risk of significant hearing loss because of socioacusis. Subsequent data from the Easter Islands were consistent with the Mabaan data thus confirming the importance of low stress, low noise levels, low-fat diet, and low prevalence of cardiovascular disease.[13]

EPIDEMIOLOGY OF PRESBYASTASIS

In contrast to age-related hearing loss, there are no international standards which quantitatively describe age-related vestibular disorders. The relevant data come mostly from clinical studies. In 1953, Droller and Pemberton noted that approximately 50% of otherwise self-sufficient English subjects in their middle to late 60s experience a balance problem.[14] Similarly, another study showed that 50% of patients in a geriatric clinic admitted to dizziness, however on closer questioning, more than 90% noted that their symptoms were "postural" and were most problematic with changes in head or body position and were devoid of the sensation of rotation. True rotatory vertigo was present in only one-third of the group.[15] As patients age further, balance-related problems become more pervasive. In a study conducted among patients in an outpatient medical clinic, "dizziness" was the most common presenting complaint in patients 75 years of age or older and is a central issue related to the occurrence of falls and hip fractures.[16] Although sometimes, specific causes of dizziness are found (such as BPPV) most patients are found to have multifactorial issues otherwise known as presbyastasis (disequilibrium of aging) or multisystem balance decline. Belal and Glorig reviewed the clinical findings of 740 patients at the House Ear Institute presenting with a complaint of dizziness and noted that nearly 80% did not have a specific vestibular diagnosis and hence classified them as having presbyastasis.[17] The fact that multifactorial balance deficits are clearly known to affect the aging population coupled with the fact that the aging population is expanding are central reasons why falls are a major factor in fatal and nonfatal injuries for persons 65 years of age and older.[18,19]

LABORATORY STUDIES: PRESBYACUSIS IN HUMANS AND ANIMALS

In the discussion which follows, the focus will largely be on the auditory periphery with only minor consideration given to the auditory CNS. Of the many investigations of presbyacusis, perhaps the most quoted and most extensive source of histopathologic data are the temporal bone studies of Schuknecht and colleagues.[20] From a number of studies of human temporal bones, they have identified 4 types or categories of presbyacusis: (1) sensory, characterized by atrophy and degeneration of the sensory and supporting cells; (2) neural, typified by loss of neurons in the cochlea and CNS; (3) metabolic, characterized by atrophy of the lateral wall of the cochlea, especially the stria vascularis; and (4) mechanical, where the inner ear changes its properties with a resulting inner ear conductive hearing loss. Each of these categories was hypothesized to have a characteristic audiometric configuration, that is, sloping, flat, and therefore to be audiometrically identifiable. In subsequent studies, considerable difficulty was encountered in correlating the audiometric configuration with histopathologic observations and in differentiating 1 type of presbyacusis from another on the basis of the audiometric configuration.[21] The problem is that the audiometric configurations of older persons do not form clearly defined categories, and histopathologic changes at the level of light and electron microscopy are almost always observed at multiple sites in a given aging ear.

In 1993, Schuknecht and Gacek revised the traditional categories of presbyacusis described above.[22] The revision was based on hundreds of observations of human temporal bones and is summarized: (1) Sensory cell losses are the least important type of loss in the aged; (2) neuronal losses are constant and predictable expressions of aging; (3) atrophy of the stria vascularis is the predominant lesion of the aging ear; (4) no anatomical correlation for a gradual descending hearing loss reflect a cochlear conductive loss; and (5) 25% cannot be classified using light microscopy.

This conclusion by Schuknecht and Gacek is important for at least 2 reasons. One is that the significance of sensory cell losses is deemphasized in presbyacusis. The second is that the dominance of strial degeneration is emphasized. These 2 points bring a consensus to human temporal bone results and those obtained from experiments with animals. In many species of animals, auditory thresholds estimated from electrophysiologic potentials arising from the auditory nerve and brainstem increase as a function of chronologic age.[23] The age-related decline in auditory function occurs in animals who are born and reared in acoustically controlled environments where sound levels rarely exceed 40 dBA. In addition to control of the acoustic environment, none of the animals received antibiotics or other drugs. Conductive hearing loss was eliminated as a potential source of the measured hearing loss. Clearly, environmental noise, drugs, disease, and trauma did not have a causative role in the hearing losses observed in the aging animals. Thus, the notion that presbyacusis is not an aging effect per se but the combined effect of socioacusis and nosoacusis is not supported by laboratory experiments with several species of animals.

Perhaps the most dramatic feature of age-related hearing loss in laboratory animals is the variability between animals. For example, in a longitudinal study of aging gerbils, some animals, at the one extreme, had normal or nearly normal auditory sensitivity from 1 to 16 kHz, whereas at the other extreme, some animals did not respond to signals presented at levels of 80 dB SPL. Variability of this magnitude is remarkable given that chronologic age, environment (temperature, humidity, and air quality), acoustic history, and diet of the animals were virtually identical. These data and others involving different inbred strains of mice are consistent with human data showing a strong genetic role in age-related hearing loss.

In addition to a qualitative/quantitative correspondence between age-related hearing loss measured in aging rodents and audiograms of 60- to 70-year-old humans,[23] many of the histopathologic observations made on human temporal bones have been confirmed and extended on experimental animals.[24–26] In aging rodents, there is usually a small loss of sensory (outer) hair cells in the most basal and the most apical regions of the cochlea. Nerve loss, as indicated by loss of spiral ganglion cells, is pronounced throughout the cochlea. The lateral wall of the cochlea, including the stria vascularis, usually shows degeneration originating in both the base and apex and extending to midcochlear regions as the animal ages; however, in some animals, there is a patchy loss of stria vascularis. Thus, in several species of animals, anatomic studies of cochlear material demonstrate at least 3 of the histopathologic conditions described in humans by Schuknecht and colleagues, namely, sensory, neural, and metabolic presbyacusis.[20] In animals, all 3 types are usually present in each animal.

As with humans, the most prominent (dominant) type of presbyacusis in laboratory animals (with the exception of mice, C57) is the metabolic category.[25–30] In addition to age-related, systematic degeneration of the stria vascularis starting in both the apex and base of the cochlea and proceeding to the midcochlear region, is a loss of the protein Na, K-adenosine triphosphatase (Na, K-ATPase). The stria vascularis and underlying spiral ligament have a prominent role in generating electrochemical gradients and regulating fluid and ion homeostasis in the cochlea. In accordance with its name, the stria is heavily vascularized and has an extremely high metabolic rate. Conceivably, alterations in strial microvasculature could compromise cochlear blood flow and ultimately lead to strial degeneration. Histopathologic studies on aging gerbil have provided strong evidence for vascular involvement in age-related hearing loss. Morphometric analyses of lateral wall preparations stained to contrast blood vessels (Figure 4) have revealed losses of strial capillary area in aged animals.[26,27] The vascular pathology first presented as small focal lesions mainly in the apical and lower basal turns and progressed with age to encompass large regions at both ends of the cochlea. Remaining strial areas were highly correlated with normal microvasculature and with the endocochlear potential (EP, described below).[27] Not surprisingly, areas of complete capillary loss invariably correlated with regions of

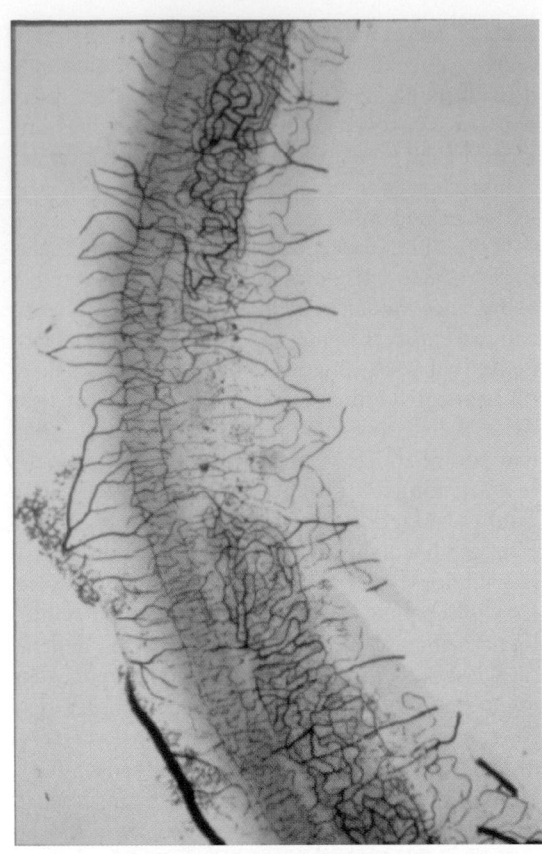

Figure 4 Surface preparation of stria vascularis/lateral wall dissection from an old gerbil stained with diaminobenzidine for endogeneus peroxidase to contrast with blood vessels (×100 original magnification). The strial capillary bed overlies vessels of the spiral ligament. The slide shows substantial atrophy of the capillary bed. (Adapted from reference 27.)

strial atrophy. Subsequent ultrastructural analysis has revealed a significant thickening of the basement membrane,[28] which is accompanied by an increase in the deposition of laminin and an abnormal accumulation of immunoglobulin, as shown histochemically.[29,30] Thus, considerable support exists for the major involvement of strial microvasculature in age-related degeneration of the stria vascularis; however, the question of what constitutes the initial injury remains unanswered. Although it is tempting to speculate that atrophy of the stria vascularis occurs secondarily to vascular insufficiency resulting from capillary necrosis, the reverse could very well be true. While the sequence of events is not clear, substantial data indicate that age-related alterations in the lateral wall of the cochlea (stria vascularis and spiral ligament) affect the mechanoelectric transduction process, which is dependent upon the development and maintenance of transcellular potassium gradients[25] and the 80 to 100 mV EP of scala media.

The 2 most prominent changes in the physiologic properties of the aging ear are reductions/losses of the EP and losses of auditory nerve function as indicated by increased thresholds of the compound action potential (CAP) of the auditory nerve.[31] Slopes of input–output functions of the CAP in aging animals are decreased even when the loss of auditory thresholds is only 5 to 10 dB. In other words, as the signal intensity is increased, the amplitude of the CAP increases by a fraction of that observed in young animals with normal hearing or young animals with noise-induced or drug-induced hearing losses. These shallow input–output functions of the CAP are also reflected in shallow input–output functions of auditory brain-stem responses (ABRs). Thus, what appears to be abnormal function of the auditory brainstem in older animals possibly reflects only the abnormal output of the auditory nerve. The reduced amplitudes of action potentials observed in aging ears are probably reflective of asynchronous or poorly synchronized neural activity in the auditory nerve. The pathologic basis of asynchronized activity in the auditory nerve is unknown but probably involves the nature of the synapse between individual auditory nerve fibers and the attachment to the inner hair cell, primary degeneration of spiral ganglion cells, and reductions in the EP, which are described below.

The EP, that is, the 80 to 100 mV DC resting potential in the scala media of the cochlea, is often reduced significantly and proportionally to losses/degeneration of the stria vascularis.[25] Reductions in EP produce elevations in auditory thresholds, about 1 dB reduction in threshold for every 1 mV reduction in EP in the base of the cochlea. In the apex thresholds declined only about 20 dB even for large reductions in EP.[32]

Most importantly, the audiometric configuration of threshold shifts produced by reductions of EP is strikingly similar to the audiometric configurations observed in aging animals and aging non-noise exposed humans (Figure 1). Thus, the correspondence between EP shifted thresholds in aged animals and in aged, nonnoise exposed humans suggests a common mechanism, namely a reduction in the EP. It is hypothesized that the EP produces the voltage or power to the cochlear amplifier which has a gain of 20 dB or so apically increasing to as much as 60 to 70 dB in the base of the cochlea. Thus, age-related hearing loss as shown by the audiogram can be explained almost entirely by age-related degeneration of the lateral wall with a resultant disruption in potassium recycling and a reduction in EP. Moreover, in aging experimental animals, hearing losses can be reduced/eliminated by introducing a DC voltage into scala media and raising a low EP, that is, 15 mV, to a value approaching 60 to 70 mV. Thresholds of the CAP can be improved by as much as 40 dB in aging animals and 60 dB in animals where the EP has been reduced by the application of furosemide.[32] Efforts to develop a hearing aid based on current injection into scala media are in progress.[33]

A significant difference between the physiology of the aging ear and the ear with noise-induced or drug-induced injury of the cochlea involves the nonlinear phenomenon of two-tone rate suppression, that is, activity of the auditory nerve elicited by 1 tone is suppressed or eliminated by the addition of a second tone of different frequency.[31] In ears of quiet-reared aging animals, the mechanism of two-tone rate suppression

appears to remain intact even for threshold shifts of 30 dB. In contrast, noise-and drug-exposed animals with minimal injury of the cochlea, and minimal threshold shifts, reduction or complete loss of two-tone rate suppression may be the first indicator of injury of the cochlea, usually outer hair cells. These data are an excellent indicator that the pathologic basis of age-related hearing loss is fundamentally different from the pathologic basis of most forms of noise-induced or drug-induced hearing loss.

Otoacoustic emissions, both transient evoked and distortion product, are nonlinear phenomena that are assumed to reflect the integrity of sensory cells, especially outer hair cells. Given this assumption, one would expect to find very high correlations between loss of outer hair cells and changes in otoacoustic emissions; however, inconsistent relations among distortion products, threshold measures, and sensory cell pathology have been reported from widely different types of experiments. Indeed, there are reports of normal emissions in the presence of missing outer hair cells as well as reduced emissions in the presence of a complete complement of outer hair cells.[34] In the aging ear of experimental animals with a minimal, if any, loss of outer hair cells, distortion-product emissions are reduced somewhat in amplitude but are clearly present and robust.[35] In aging human ears, transient emissions are present in about 80% of persons with a PTA hearing level better than 10 dB, present in about 50% with PTA of 11 to 26 dB, and absent in about 80% with a PTA greater than 26 dB. Thus, the presence of a transient otoacoustic emission suggests excellent hearing levels for most persons, whereas its absence reveals very little. Indeed, the major application of otoacoustic emissions may be in hearing screening of infants.

A recent development is the association of mitochondrial deoxyribonucleic acid (mtDNA) deletions with aging in general and with SNHL and age-related hearing loss.[36,37] Ueda and colleagues, using DNA specimens extracted from peripheral blood leukocytes, found a higher rate of mtDNA deletions in patients with SNHL than in controls.[38] Seidman, in a rat study, tied mtDNA deletions to presbyacusis and mtDNA deletions to reactive oxygen metabolites (ROMs).[39] These are highly toxic molecules that can damage mitochondrial DNA, resulting in the production of specific mtDNA deletions. Thus, compounds that block or scavenge ROMs should attenuate age-related hearing loss. Rats were assigned to treatment groups including controls, caloric restriction, and treatment with several antioxidants, including vitamins E and C, and were allowed to age in a controlled environment. The calorie-restricted groups maintained the best hearing, the lowest quantity of mtDNA deletions in brain and ear tissues, and the least amount of outer hair cell loss. The antioxidant-treated subjects had better hearing than the controls and a slight trend for fewer mtDNA deletions. The controls had the poorest hearing, the most mtDNA deletions, and the most outer hair cell loss. These data suggest

that nutritional and pharmacologic strategies may prove to be an effective treatment that would limit age-related increases in ROM production, reduce mtDNA deletions, and thus reduce age-related hearing loss. ROMs (or reactive oxygen species) and oxidative stress have also been implicated in noise-induced hearing loss, ototoxic hearing loss, and cumulative injury that presents as age-related hearing loss. It is speculated that there is a genetic impairment of antioxidant protections that leads to the production of both age-related and noise-induced hearing loss by placing the cochlea in a state of vulnerability.[40,41] Although an age-related hearing loss gene has been identified, the murine Ahl mutation,[42,43] the discovery of the molecular/genetic basis of presbyacusis and SNHL in general are just beginning.[44]

In summary, animal experiments conducted under strict conditions show age-related declines in auditory function that indicate a "pure" aging hearing loss. Most of the pathologic anatomy associated with this "pure aging" hearing loss is in the cochlea, where the dominant pathology is degeneration of the stria vascularis. In experimental animals, most of the hearing loss can be accounted for by anatomic, physiologic, and biochemical changes in the auditory periphery. Indeed, there is no need to include the auditory CNS in an explanation of age-related hearing loss, even when the criterion measure of age-related hearing loss is derived from potentials arising from the auditory brainstem.

Explanations of age-related changes in auditory brainstem potentials in terms of alterations in the auditory periphery run counter to the current dogma that there is a significant, perhaps dominant, component of presbyacusis that involves degeneration of the auditory CNS. Indeed, there are significant, age-related changes in the auditory CNS involving subtle to gross changes in anatomy and neurochemistry. One prominent change is a reduction in γ-aminobutyric acid (GABA) affecting neural inhibition. Another is increases in the release of aspartate in the cochlear nucleus following cochlear injury and leads to increased excitatory neurotransmission. The role of the CNS in age-related hearing loss is almost surely substantial; however, the focus here is on the auditory periphery. Nearly all changes observed in auditory brainstem potentials can be explained by alterations in the auditory periphery.

PERCEPTION OF AUDITORY SIGNALS AND SPEECH

In addition to age-related declines in auditory sensitivity, there are age-related declines in differential sensitivity for intensity, frequency, and time. Until recently, these age-related declines in the basic properties of the ear and hearing were almost always measured in older persons with significant hearing losses. Thus, it was nearly impossible to separate the effects of a hearing loss from the effects of aging. Recently, however, both discrimination in intensity and discrimination in frequency have been shown to decline with age only at low frequencies and independently of any hearing loss.[45] These results are important because they are negative effects measured in the presence of normal hearing and may very well represent age-related declines in information processing capability. It remains unclear whether these age-related declines represent age-related effects of the auditory periphery or CNS.

The term "phonemic regression" was coined to describe a disproportionate difficulty in speech perception relative to the magnitude of hearing loss of older persons. Later, many studies of speech discrimination and other complex listening tasks showed results with older subjects that were difficult to explain solely on the basis of the audiogram alone. With the ready availability of many published articles showing degenerative changes in the auditory brainstem and cortex of older persons, there evolved a viewpoint that a significant component of age-related hearing loss is attributable to the decline of the auditory CNS. Of course, the auditory CNS is involved in age-related hearing loss; however, the extent of the involvement of the CNS in presbyacusis is currently receiving much debate.

Perhaps the largest qualitative/quantitative description of speech discrimination as a function of age and hearing loss is provided by Jerger from the clinical records of 2,162 patients.[46] Figure 5 shows percent correct on phonetically balanced (PB) words as a function of chronologic age. The parameter on the figure is the PTA of 0.5, 1, and 2 kHz. Figure 5 shows that speech discrimination declines systematically as a function of chronologic age; however, the decline with age is dramatically dependent on hearing loss. That is, for subjects with very little hearing loss (less than 30 dB), the decline with age is measurable but small through age 70. On the other hand, for subjects with moderate-to-severe hearing losses, the decline with age is noteworthy, particularly for persons between the ages of 45 and 85 with hearing losses of 40 to 49 dB, 50 to 59 dB, and 60 to 69 dB. In other words, when hearing loss as indicated by the PTA is held constant, speech discrimination scores decreased between the ages of 50 and 80 for moderate (greater than 40 dB) to severe (60 dB) hearing losses. In contrast, age had very little effect as long as the PTA is less than about 30 to 39

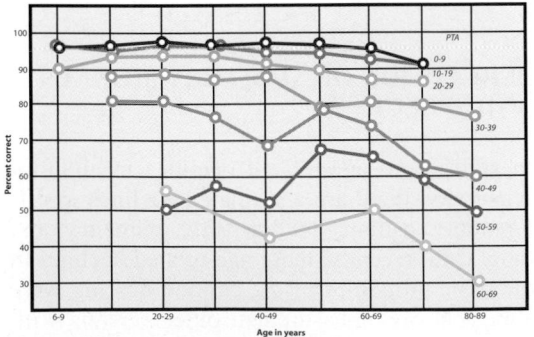

Figure 5 Speech discrimination (PB words) as a function of age with average hearing loss at 0.5, 1, and 2 kHz as parameter. PB = phonetically balanced; PTA = pure-tone average. (Adapted from reference 46.)

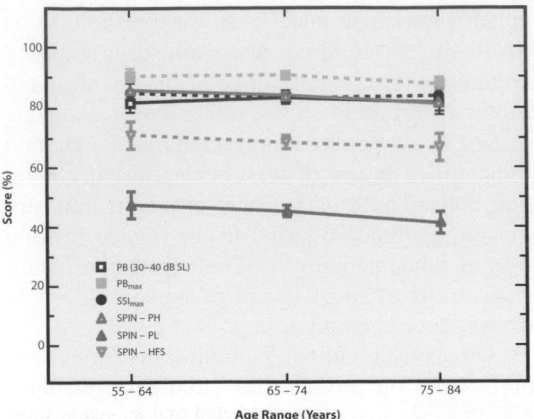

Figure 6 Speech discrimination as a function of age for different speech material. Hearing level is the same for each age group. HFS = hearing for speech; PB = phonetically balanced; PH = high probability; PL = low probability; SPIN = speech perception in noise; SSI = synthetic sentence identification. (Adapted from reference 47.)

dB. A remarkable and perhaps the most noteworthy feature of Figure 5 is that persons over the age range of 50 to 80 perform as well as 25 year olds as long as their average hearing loss at 0.5, 1, and 2 kHz is less than 35 dB or so.

Performance on tests of speech discrimination by older persons is shown (Figure 6) for PB words, 3 versions of the Speech Perception in Noise (SPIN) test, and synthetic sentence identification (SSI).[47] Subjects in whom hearing levels were nearly identical (±3 dB) were placed into 3 age groups over the range from 55 to 84 years. Statistical analysis of the speech discrimination data showed that performance on all tests was not affected by age. That is, when hearing levels were equated, there were no age-related declines in performance on tests of speech discrimination in persons over the age range of 55 to 84 years. Additional analyses using partial correlations, showed significant gender effects, that is, significant declines with age for males in word recognition, SSI, and SPIN in high-context sentences. Age-related declines were not observed for females.

There are many additional studies of speech discrimination using background noises, degraded speech signals, reverberation, and other variations that resulted in more difficult listening tasks than the usual speech discrimination test, which is done in quiet listening conditions.[48] Many of these studies show age-related effects; however, the interpretation of many of these data showing age-related declines in auditory behavior is not straightforward because the subjects usually have significant hearing loss, as indicated by the audiogram. Accordingly, some persons believe that there is a large CNS component to presbyacusis, whereas others believe and have shown that speech discrimination by older persons is predictable given the audiometric hearing loss and the audibility of the speech material. Indeed, as much as 95% of the variance in speech discrimination results can be accounted for on the basis of the audiogram.[49]

Whereas speech recognition in a monaural task can usually be predicted accurately from audiometric data in persons regardless of age, recent longitudinal suggests there are significant age-related declines in word recognition that are not predictable.[50] In a 15-to 20-year longitudinal study of age-related hearing loss, word recognition in 256 persons across the age range of 68 to 84 years was predicted from audiometric measures and compared to actual performance (Figure 7). Word recognition performance was underestimated by 3 to 4% from 68 years to about 70 to 72 years whereas at about age 75 years, performance was overestimated. In other words, word recognition in adults 75 years and older decreased significantly and nonpredictably from audiometric measures. Moreover, the decline in word recognition occurred at a constant, linear rate of 0.8% per year. It is important to note that these data are from well-trained older persons who have been participating in auditory listening experiments for up to 20 years. It is also the case that a significant history of noise exposure was not a factor as the results from noise exposed and nonnoise exposed were virtually identical.

In addition to the results observed for 75 year and older subjects described above, there are many age-related declines in auditory behavior that are not strongly associated with auditory thresholds. This is most evident using binaural (dichotic) listening tasks and right ear versus left ear performance under poor signal-to-noise conditions. In many of these binaural experiments using older subjects, age-related declines are observed that are clearly independent of peripheral hearing loss, and individual differences between subjects are sometimes dramatic.[51]

AUDITORY EVOKED POTENTIALS

With the development of straightforward techniques to measure evoked potentials arising from the auditory nerve, brainstem, and auditory cortex, there has been significant progress in evaluating the aging auditory nervous system of human subjects. In regard to the ABRs, most studies show age-related declines in the amplitude of wave V, which should be interpreted to reflect peripheral hearing loss rather than changes in the brainstem. Even in older persons with excellent hearing levels, ABR waveforms are of "poor quality" and reduced amplitude, probably reflecting pathology of the cochlea and auditory nerve as well as a reduction in synchronized neural activity. For young subjects with normal and abnormal hearing, auditory thresholds measured behaviorally are about 10 dB better than auditory thresholds estimated from the ABR. For aging subjects, this behavioral/ABR disparity is 20 dB, reflecting the poor quality/low amplitude of the ABR. Other evoked potentials show inconsistent results. The P300 arising from the auditory cortex shows age-related declines, whereas the amplitude-modulated following response may remain unaffected by aging. In contrast, the frequency-modulated following response may be enhanced in older subjects, perhaps reflecting the

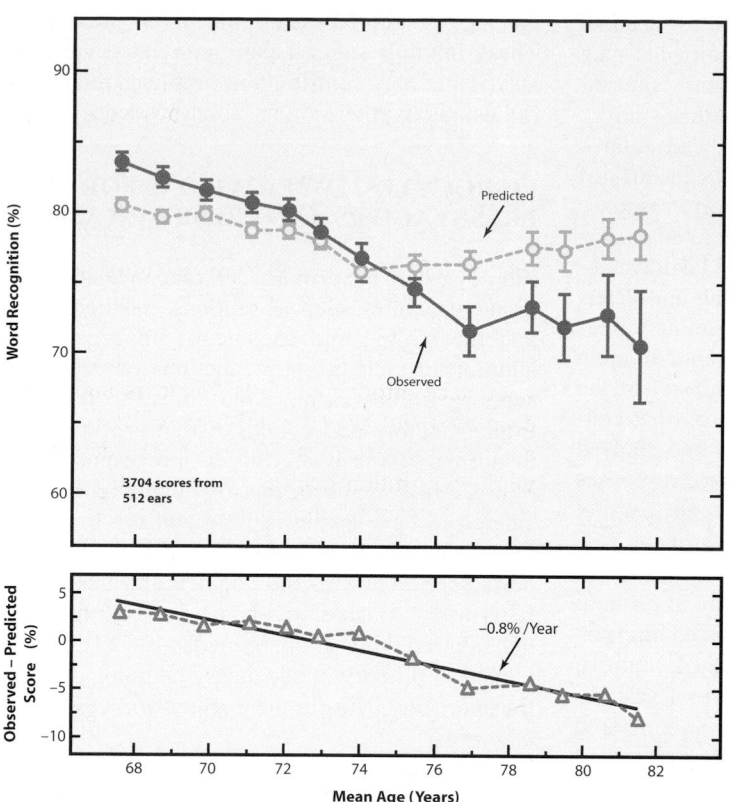

Figure 7 (A) Mean observed word-recognition scores (*filled*) and mean predicted scores (*open*) obtained during 13 consecutive laboratory visits plotted against mean subject age during those visits. Observed scores appear to be declining with age. Scores predicted by an audibility-based model, the articulation index, are also declining, as predicted from changes in speech audibility over time, independent of age. (B) Mean differences between observed and predicted scores. Scores at younger ages are better than predicted and scores at older ages, for example, >75 years, are worse than predicted. The observed-predicted difference function (*solid line*) has a negative slope, so that as subjects age, their observed scores deviate increasingly from predicted scores at a rate of 0.8% per year. The linear fit of these data suggests that this decline does not accelerate with age. Thus, word recognition in quiet declines significantly with age more than would be predicted by declines in pure-tone thresholds. (Adapted from reference 50.)

cristae lost type I cells with advancing age at a significantly greater rate than the maculae.

Otoconia

Otoconia are normally cylindrical calcite rods with a tripartite flat endplate at each pole and vary regularly in size. Ross and colleagues showed that aging is associated with a decrease in the number of otoconia, especially in the saccule.[58] They were shown to degenerate in a posteroanterior direction across the macula and take on a fibrous, hollowed-out appearance. During the sixth decade of life, the furrows become deepened with a loss of the original surface and pits of degeneration appear toward the middle of the rod. As normal crystalline substance is reabsorbed, some rods are cleaved in half.[58] A recent animal study in aged rats revealed similar findings with pitted, fissured ,and broken otoconia with preservation of terminal facets.[59] The clinical relevance of these observations may be reflected in data that shows BPPV increases in incidence exponentially as a function of age.[60] There does not appear to be any evidence, however, that standard repositioning maneuvers have any less efficacy in this age group.[61]

Vestibular Ganglia

An integral part of the vestibular system are the bipolar neurons that relay information from the sensory neuroepithelium to the vestibular nerve and the central vestibular nuclei and evidence exists that this anatomical component of the system, like all others, appears to undergo deterioration which contributes to the overall problem of disequilibrium. Park and colleagues utilized assumption free stereology techniques in the study of 20 serially sectioned archival human temporal bones specimens with no history of vestibular pathology from donors aged 2 to 88 years.[62] They were able to show that in youth, the human has a roughly constant number of cells at about 28,952. However, from ages 30 to 60 a decline begins such that patients older than 60 level off at approximately 23,349 cells which remains stable and demonstrates another anatomical basis for age-related imbalance.[62] A similar study confirmed that total ganglion cell count declines as a function of age at an average rate of 57 cells per year with a decline that appears to be significantly greater in the superior division compared to the inferior division.[63]

Primary Afferent Axons and Dendrites

Bergstrom studied freshly dissected human vestibular nerves from humans of varying ages and noted a reduction in fiber density beginning at age 40. Myelinated thick fibers from the cristae demonstrated the greatest loss.[64] This correlated well with the 40% hair cell loss noted in the cristae by Engstrom and colleagues[53] and another study by Richter which noted a dramatic reduction in the number of neuronal cell bodies in Scarpa ganglia noted to occur after age 50.[65] Amyloid

well-documented age-related decline in GABA. Although much of this research is in progress, it appears that evoked potentials produced by short-duration signals (onset responses such as ABR and CAP) are decreased in amplitude in older subjects, whereas those evoked potentials produced at higher levels in the CNS by long-duration signals may be unaffected or even increased in amplitude. Age-related increases could reflect a number of factors, including efforts by the CNS to compensate for peripheral deficits or age-related changes in the excitatory/inhibitory balance of the auditory CNS.

LABORATORY STUDIES: PRESBYASTASIS IN HUMANS AND ANIMALS

As in other parts of the nervous system, cells in the vestibular system do not undergo regeneration after they are lost to trauma or expected cellular loss associated with aging. Although there exists plasticity of the CNS which allows for modification and compensation of gait and balance control as the vestibular end organs undergoes decline, the resulting histological hallmarks of aging become visible and are similar to the cochlea in presbyacusis. These are generally characterized by a loss of sensory neuroepithelium, loss of primary afferent fibers and cells bodies within the sensory ganglion.[52] Details of research data pertaining to particular portions of the vestibular system have been studied and are presented below.

Sensory Neuroepithelium

An important study by Engstrom and colleagues in elderly monkeys and humans sheds a great deal of light on the neuroepithelial consequences

of aging.[53] Hair cell loss was found to be reduced by as much as 40% in the epithelium of the cristae and 20% on the maculae using transmission electron microscopy. Type I hair cells were more susceptible than Type II hair cells and as the former is more abundant at the top of cristae, it gives the light-microscopic appearance of neuroepithelial thinning. Concurrent with the death of hair cells are those of supporting cells which develop fibrillotubular and vesicular structures before death. Even surviving sensory and supporting cells appear to have irregularities which appear as abnormal intracellular laminated structures at the level of the basement membrane. Other signs of damage to sensory cells identified by this study include intracellular vesicles and irregular patchy changes in the synaptic membranes of type I cells and their afferent calyces.[53] Degenerative changes within the hair cell system show the tendency for accumulation of lipofuscin inclusions in sensory cells and supporting cells, but also disarrangement of cilia, increased fragility of cilia, and the formation of giant cilia are noted consequences of aging.[54] Similarly, intraneuroepithelial cysts have been shown in the maculae and cristae of elderly subjects which appear either as pale blue inclusions in near-normal sized cells or larger eccentrically placed structures.[52,55,56] Quantitative studies have been recently more feasible using differential interference contrast microscopy and have allowed for unambiguous identification of hair cells in the vestibular system. Merchant and colleagues performed serial section counting of hair cells in normal temporal bones that ranged in age from birth to 100 years of age.[57] At birth the ratio of type I to type II hair cells in the cristae was 2.4:1 and in the maculae it was 1:3.1. They found a highly significant age-related decline in all sense organs; however, they showed that the deposits, associated with degeneration of nerve cells are insoluble deposits that stain with amyloid and are associated with nerve degeneration. Fuji and colleagues sectioned the vestibulocochlear nerve at various points and found that in the aging human, amyloid bodies are concentrated to the limiting glial portion of the nerve and become increasingly larger in the sixth, seventh, and eighth decades of life.[66]

Central Nervous System

In an attempt to correlate central neurologic pathology with presbyastasis, Lopez and colleagues utilized computer-based microscopy to determine neuronal counts, nuclear volume, and neuronal density in postmortem specimens of the human vestibular nuclear complex (VNC) as a function of age.[67] Using 15 subjects aged 40 to 93 years of age the 4 vestibular nuclei were studied and a linear model revealed approximately a 3% neuronal loss per decade. Interestingly, neuronal loss as a percentage of the total number of neurons was greatest in the superior vestibular nucleus and least in the medial vestibular nucleus. There was a corresponding increase in giant neurons, which were felt to be due an accumulation of lipofuscin deposits in the cell somata. This was an important finding as studies of other brainstem nuclei had failed to show an age-related neuronal loss.[67] Whitman and colleagues compared postmortem brain specimens from 6 patients with disequilibrium of aging and 4 control subjects. In comparison with controls, the study group had prominent frontal atrophy and ventriculomegaly, but lacked any difference in other gross pathology such as infarcts or areas of necrosis.[68] Histologically the frontal lobes had markedly reactive astrocytes and increased arteriolar wall thickness (sclerosis index) in those with presbyastasis. This study furthers interest into the concept that atherosclerosis is a predisposing risk factor for multifactorial balance decline associated with aging.[68]

INFLUENCE OF AGE ON VESTIBULAR FUNCTION TESTING

The accumulation of anatomical deficits, which clearly characterize degeneration of the peripheral and central vestibular system and the associated CNS have a myriad of effects on balance and function. Some of these are measurable with objective testing, while other aspects of this decline are not. Electronystagmography (ENG) and videonystagmography (VNG) are the most commonly used tests of vestibular function and visual tracking. Some reports indicate age-related changes beginning after age 50 in saccade, pursuit, and optokinetic studies to the point at which saccade latency and velocity thresholds deviate by 10 to 20 ms and 10° to 20° per second, respectively, for each decade over 50.[69–71] The vestibulo-ocular response (VOR) was carefully measured in a larger study comparing aging effects on auditory and vestibular responses. The study revealed a significant amplitude-dependent decrease in gain and increase in phase lead of the VOR and a significant decrease in the gain of vestibular responses at low frequency sinusoidal stimulation over a 5-year longitudinal study.[72] Another study of the VOR using head autorotation testing revealed abnormalities in 86% of elderly volunteers.[73] However, caloric response as a function of age has been harder to characterize. In a study of caloric tests in 102 healthy subjects between ages 11 and 70, Mulch and Petermann showed that although the absolute values of nystagmus parameters are dependent upon age, there is no decrease in the intensity of the reaction with age.[74] A more recent study has confirmed and extended these findings and showed that the slow phase velocity of caloric responses does not decline with age and does not parallel the age-related physiological decline of the vestibular system as a whole.[75] However, asymmetric vestibular decline may play a role in postural control. In a study of elderly fall-related hip fracture patients compared to age-matched controls, postheadshake nystagmus (indicative of vestibular asymmetry) measured by VNG was compared between the two groups.[76] Those predisposed to falls had a significantly higher frequency of postheadshake nystagmus and a corresponding significant increase in postural sway and hence problems with balance and stability.[76] This may be due to earlier research that shows that unilateral vestibular hypofunction has deleterious consequences to postural sway due to dysregulation of the vestibulospinal reflex (VSR).[77] The authors postulate that vestibular asymmetry, while easily compensated for by central mechanisms in the young and healthy are more disturbing to balance and gait in those with decreased ability for central compensation such as age-related disorders of the proprioceptive and visual systems. Indeed this was confirmed in a recent study of "multisensorial decay" in 40 elderly patients with imbalance in which 85% were found to have marked impairment of the somatosensory system and 40% had visual problems.[78] The vestibulocollic reflex (VCR) has also shown deterioration in aged patients. Welgampola and Colebatch measured the VCR in 70 healthy adults aged 25 to 85 using 100 dB clicks, forehead taps, and galvanic stimulation. Beginning at age 60, average click evoked response amplitudes decrease with age at 25 to 30% per decade with the most marked effects noted using click and galvanic stimulation, a likely correlate of known hair cell decline associated with the aging maculae.[79] The otolithic organs not only stabilize the head and surrounding musculature during postural changes, they also appear to increase muscle sympathetic nerve activity (MSNA), which plays a role in regulating blood pressure during orthostatic stress. MSNA, arterial blood pressure, and heart rate responses were measured in older and younger subjects who were subjected to head-down rotation testing (which engages the otolithic organs) and results revealed that stimulation of the otolithic organs increased sympathetic tone in all age groups, but aged patients could not regulate MSNA in the face of altered orthostatic blood pressure.[80] These findings suggest that age-related vestibular decline may contribute to problems related to orthostatic hypotension or "light-headedness."

FIBROCYTES: IMPLICATIONS FOR PRESBYACUSIS AND PRESBYASTASIS

Fibrocytes are the primary cell type in connective tissue structures such as tendons and ligaments and the stroma and capsule of all organs. In addition to their primary functions of structural support, fibrocytes have the ability to produce trophic factors and cytokines that are involved in normal tissue homeostasis and responses to injury. Although fibrocytes are not normally considered to have a role in fluid and ion transport mechanisms, a large body of evidence now supports such a role in the cochlea and vestibular labyrinth.[81] Indeed, evidence is accumulating that altered potassium homeostasis is directly related to primary or secondary pathology of ion transport fibrocytes in the cochlea and vestibular labyrinth.[82]

Fibrocytes in the spiral ligament and spiral limbus of the cochlea, and presumably in the vestibular system as well, undergo continuous replacement and have the capacity to increase their proliferation in response to injury.[83] This suggests the presence of a population of adult stem/progenitor cells capable of self-renewal, although such cells have not been identified as yet. Fibrocytes and other connective tissue elements in the ear, including cartilage and bone, develop from periotic mesenchyme of mesodermal origin.[84] Engraftment of cells derived from clonal hematopoietic stem cells has been demonstrated in regions corresponding to the location of fibrocytes and mesenchymal cells in the irradiated cochlea.[85] This finding suggests the alternative possibility that bone marrow stem/precursor cells are continuously seeded to the inner ear throughout life and can serve as a source of fibrocyte progenitors. These results raise the intriguing possibility of reversing disorders associated with cochlear and vestibular fibrocytes and aging via the manipulation of endogenous stems cells or the introduction of exogenous stem cells or both.

PRESBYACUSIS: ALLEVIATION/ TREATMENT

Assuming that any problems with the external and middle ear are diagnosed and treated, that other medical issues are under control, and a diagnosis of presbyacusis in the general sense, the best treatment currently available is a hearing aid. The successful use of hearing aids by older persons and the hearing impaired in general is mixed. There is a literature of substantial magnitude that reports on the successful or unsuccessful use of hearing aids by the elderly. Many older persons who would clearly benefit from an aid do not use one. The reasons for not using an aid or being a dissatisfied user include cost, stigma of a hearing handicap and of being old, difficulty in manipulating controls, and too little benefit, particularly in the presence of background noise.

In a large group of older persons ($N = 516$) who are participants in a longitudinal study of age-related hearing loss, 53% ($n = 272$) are candidates for a hearing aid. Candidacy by very conservative audiologic criteria is a speech reception threshold greater than 30 dB in the better ear or hearing level greater than 40 dB at 3 and 4 kHz in the better ear. Using these criteria, nearly half ($n = 131$ of 272) of those who are considered to be excellent candidates have never tried a hearing aid, and only 38% ($n = 104$ of 272) of candidates were successful hearing aid users. Thirty-seven persons (~10%), for one or several reasons, were dissatisfied hearing aid users. Of those who did not meet the conservative criteria for a hearing aid ($n = 244$), our clinical judgment suggested that at least 40 to 50% of these persons would benefit from an aid. Clearly, the older persons in our longitudinal study were uninformed about hearing aids, poorly served, or underserved. Our experience is confirmed.[86] Indeed, it is our opinion that as a result of excellent advances in hearing aid technology in combination with improved fitting techniques, nearly every older hearing-impaired person should be considered a potential candidate for a hearing aid.

In the case of bilateral severe hearing loss not helped significantly by hearing aids, cochlear implants are indicated regardless of age. Current criteria are hearing no better than 50% or fewer key words in test sentences in the best aided condition in the worst ear and 60% in the best ear.[86] With current cochlear implant technology, the majority of patients experience excellent speech understanding in quiet. Speech discrimination in a noisy background as well as the appreciation of music remains problematic. An area of active interest to address these current limitations involves electroacoustic stimulation, that is, the combination of a shorter electrode (20 mm or less) with a hearing aid in the same ear. This paradigm is considered for individuals with residual low frequency hearing (rehabilitated with acoustical speech processing) and severe high frequency SNHL (rehabilitated with the electrical speech processing). The ability to preserve low frequency hearing after short electrode insertion and enhanced speech recognition in noise have been demonstrated in a small group of patients.[87]

PRESBYASTASIS: ALLEVIATION/ TREATMENT

The first objective when faced with a elderly patient who describes disequilibrium issues with or without vertigo is to assess the immediate risk of danger to the patient by virtue of a fall. Simple neurotologic, Romberg, and gait testing can give a reliable picture as to whether immediate referral to rehabilitation is needed for assistive gait strategies such as the use of a cane, walker, or wheelchair. Once this has been determined, a detailed historic

review is needed to evaluate the presence of neurological or other medical problems that may be affecting coordination, muscle strength, and balance. Cardiovascular issues are reviewed including blood pressure stability during orthostatic challenge. The potential for advanced cerebrovascular disease causing vertebrobasilar disease or transient ischemic attacks (TIAs) is investigated by review of imaging and carotid duplex studies. Vision status should then be reviewed along with a close review of medications, which the patient may be taking. An effort to remove unnecessary vestibular suppressants will often yield immediate benefits to the patient. Orthopedic issues, such as knee, hip, or spine arthritis should be accounted for as these contribute to a decline in proprioceptive function and muscle strength. Specific questions directed at determining the presence of vertigo should ensue in an effort to rule out more acutely treatable issues such as BPPV, Meniere disease, and perilymphatic fistula. This is coupled with an otoneurologic examination that includes positional testing and an audiometric evaluation. Once this is complete, specific vestibular testing can be obtained including VNG and posturography. Typically at this time, in the absence of a particular system issue that warrants immediate intervention, the presbyastasis patient is best served by vestibular rehabilitation therapy. Referral to a physical therapy group that has experience with specific protocols for balance retraining in the elderly patient will likely reduce the risk of falls and improve mobility, confidence, and quality of life.[88]

ACKNOWLEDGMENTS

Preparation of this chapter was supported by NIH (P01 DC00422) and CO6 RR014516 from the Extramural Research Facilities Program of the National Center for Research Resources.

REFERENCES

1. Kashima ML, Goodwin WJ, Jr, Balkany T, Casiano RR. Special Considerations in managing geriatric patients. In: Cummings CW, Flint PW, Harker LA, et al., editors. Otolaryngology Head & Neck Surgery, 4th edition. Philadelphia: Elsevier Mosby; 2005. p. 355–66.
2. Ward WD. Effects of noise exposure on auditory sensitivity. In: Neff DW, editor. Handbook of Physiology. Section 9: Reactions to Environmental Agents. Bethesda, MD: American Physiology Society; 1977. p. 1–15.
3. Dobie RA. Medical-Legal Evaluation of Hearing Loss. Albany, NY: Singular Thomson Learning; 2001.
4. Gates GA, Cooper JC, Kannel WB, Miller NJ. Hearing in the elderly: The Framingham cohort, 1983–85. Ear Hear 1990;11:247–56.
5. Matthews LJ, Lee FS, Mills JH, Schum DJ. Audiometric and subjective assessment of hearing handicap. Arch Otolaryngol Head Neck Surg 1990;116:1325–30.
6. Stelmachowicz PG, Beauchaine KA, Kalberer A, Jesteadt W. Normative thresholds in the 8- to 20-kHz range as a function of age. J Acoust Soc Am 1989;86:1384–91.
7. Moller MB. Hearing in 70 and 75 year old people: Results from a cross-sectional and longitudinal population study. Am J Otolaryngol 1981;2:22–9.
8. Matthews LJ, Lee FS, Mills JH, Dubno JR. Extended high-frequency thresholds in older adults. J Speech Lang Hear Res 1997;40:208–14.
9. Bredberg G. Cellular pattern and nerve supply of the human organ of Corti. Acta Otolaryngol Suppl 1968;236:1–135.
10. Gates GA, Couroupmitree NN, Myers RH. Genetic associations in age-related hearing thresholds. Arch Otolaryngol Head Neck Surg 1999;125:654–9.
11. Garringer HJ, Pankratz ND, Nichols WC, Reed T. Hearing impairment susceptibility in elderly men and the DFNA18 locus. Arch Otolaryngol Head Neck Surg 2006;132:506–10.
12. Rosen S, Bergman M, Plester D, et al. Presbycusis study of a relatively noise-free population in the Sudan. Ann Otol Rhinol Laryngol 1962;71:727–37.
13. Goycoolea MV, Goycoolea HG, Farfan CR, et al. Effect of life in industrialized societies on hearing in natives of Easter Island. Laryngoscope 1986;96:1391–6.
14. Droller H, Pemberton J. Vertigo in a random sample of elderly people living in their homes. J Laryngol Otol 1953;67:689–94.
15. Babin RW. Effects of aging on the auditory and vestibular systems. In: Cummings CW, Fredrickson JM, Harker LA, et al., editors. Otolaryngology Head and Neck Surgery, 2nd edition. St. Louis: CV Mosby Co; 1993. p. 3017–30.
16. Keil CH, Smith MC. Office Based Ambulatory Care for Patients 75 Years and Over: National Ambulatory Medical Care Survey, 1980, Vital Health Statistics; 1985. U.S. Department of Health and Human Services publication PHS 85.
17. Belal A, Jr, Glorig A. Dysequilibrium of ageing (presbyastasis). J Laryngol Otol 1986;100:1037–41.
18. American Academy of Orthopaedic Surgeons. Don't Let a Fall Be Your Last Trip. Rosemont, IL: AAOS; 1997.
19. Fatalities and injuries from falls among older adults—United States, 1993–2003 and 2001–2005. MMWR Weekly 2006;55:1221–4.
20. Schuknecht HF. Pathology of the Ear. Cambridge, MA: Harvard University Press; 1974.
21. Suga F, Lindsay JR. Histopathological observations of presbyacusis. Ann Otol Rhinol Laryngol 1976;85:169–76.
22. Schuknecht HF, Gacek MR. Cochlear pathology in presbycusis. Ann Otol Rhinol Laryngol 1993;102:1–16.
23. Mills JH, Schmiedt RA, Kulish LF. Age-related changes in auditory potentials of mongolian gerbil. Hear Res 1990;46:301–10.
24. Willcott JF. Aging and the Auditory System: Anatomy, Physiology, and Psychophysics. San Diego: Singular Publishing Group; 1991.
25. Schulte BA, Schmiedt RA. Lateral wall Na, K-ATPase and endocochlear potentials decline with age in quiet-reared gerbils. Hear Res 1992;61:35–46.
26. Gratton MA, Schulte BA. Alterations in microvasculature are associated with atrophy of the stria vascularis in quiet-aged gerbils. Hear Res 1995;82:44–52.
27. Gratton MA, Schmiedt RA, Schulte BA. Age-related decreases in endocochlear potential are associated with vascular abnormalities in the stria vascularis. Hear Res 1996;102:181–90.
28. Thomopoulos GN, Spicer SS, Gratton MA, Schulte BA. Age-related thickening of basement membrane in stria vascularis capillaries. Hear Res 1997;111:31–41.
29. Sakaguchi N, Spicer SS, Thomopoulos GN, Schulte BA. Increased laminin deposition in capillaries of the stria vascularis of quiet-aged gerbils. Hear Res 1997;105:44–56.
30. Sakaguchi N, Spicer SS, Thomopoulos GN, Schulte BA. Immunoglobulin deposition in thickened basement membranes of aging strial capillaries. Hear Res 1997;108:83–91.
31. Schmiedt RA, Mills JH, Adams JC. Tuning and suppresion in auditory nerve fibers of aged gerbils raised in quiet or noise. Hear Res 1990;45:221–36.
32. Schmiedt RA, Lang H, Okamura HO, Schulte BA. Effects of furosemide applied chronically to the round window: A model of metabolic presbyacusis. J Neurosci 2002;22:9643–50.
33. Johnson T, Carson M, Spelman F, et al. Electrodes and stimulators for strial presbycusis. Presented at The Neural Interfaces Workshop, NIDCD/NINDS; November 2004, Washington, DC.
34. Hamernick R, Qiu W. Correlations among evoked potential thresholds, distortion product otoacoustic emissions and hair cell loss following various noise exposures in the chinchilla. Hear Res 2000;150:245–57.
35. Boettcher FA, Gratton MA, Schmiedt RA. Effects of age and noise on hearing. Occup Med 1995;10:577–91.
36. Kujoth GC, Hiona A, Pugh TD, et al. Mitochondrial DNA mutations, oxidative stress, and apoptosis in mammalian aging. Science 2005;309:481–4.
37. Pickles JO. Mitochondria, cell death, and deafness: Will it be possible to prevent presbyacusis? Acoust Austr 2006;34:31–6.
38. Ueda N, Oshima T, Ikeda K, et al. Mitochondrial DNA deletion is a predisposing cause for sensorineural hearing loss. Laryngoscope 1998;108:580–4.
39. Seidman MD. Effects of dietary restriction and antioxidants on presbyacusis. Laryngoscope 2000;110:727–38.

40. Ohlemiller KK, McFadden SL, Ding D-L, et al. Targeted mutation of the gene for cellular glutathione peroxidase (Gpx1) increases noise-induced hearing loss in mice. J Assoc Res Otolaryngol 2000;1:243–54.

41. McFadden SL, Ding D, Burkard RF, et al. Cu/Zn SOD deficiency potentiates hearing loss and cochlear pathology in aged 129, CD-1 mice. J Comp Neurol 1999;413:101–12.

42. Li HS. Genetic influences on susceptibility of the auditory system to aging and environmental factors. Scand Audiol 1992;:1–39.

43. Erway LC, Willott JF. Genetic susceptibility to noise-induced hearing loss. In: Axelsson A, editor. A Scientific Basis of Noise-Induced Hearing Loss. New York: Thieme; 1996. p. 56–64.

44. Keithley EM, Canto C, Zheng QY, et al. Age-related hearing loss and the ahl locus in mice. Hear Res 2004;188:21–8.

45. He NJ, Dubno JR, Mills JH. Frequency and intensity discrimination measured in a maximum-likelihood procedure from young and aged normal-hearing subjects. J Acoust Soc Am 1998;103:553–65.

46. Jerger J. Audiological findings in aging. Adv Otorhinolaryngol 1973;20:115–24.

47. Dubno JR, Lee FS, Matthews LJ, Mills JH. Age-related and gender-related changes in monaural speech recognition. J Speech Lang Hear Res 1997;40:444–52.

48. Dubno JR, Dirks DD, Morgan DE. Effects of age and mild hearing loss on speech recognition in noise. J Acoust Soc Am 1984;76:87–96.

49. Humes LE, Christopherson L, Cokely C. Central auditory processing disorders in the elderly: Fact or fiction? In: Katz J, Stecker N, Henderson D, editors. Central Auditory Processing. St. Louis: Mosby Year Book; 1992. p. 141–9.

50. Dubno JR, Lee F, Matthews LJ, et al. Longitudinal changes in speech recognition in older persons. J Speech Hear Res, in press.

51. Jerger J. Behavioral studies of auditory aging. In: Vaughan N, Fausti S, editors. Seminars in Hearing. New York: Thieme; 2006. p. 243–63.

52. Babin RW, Harker LA. The vestibular system in the elderly. Otolaryngol Clin North Am 1982;15:387–93.

53. Engstrom H, Ades HW, Engstrom B, et al. Structural changes in the vestibular epithelia in elderly monkeys and humans. Adv Otorhinolaryngol 1977;22:93–110.

54. Rosenhall U, Rubin W. Degenerative changes in the human vestibular sensory epithelia. Acta Otolaryngol 1975;79:67–80.

55. Richter E. Quantitative study of Scarpa's ganglion and vestibular sense organs in endolymphatic hydrops. Ann Otol Rhinol Laryngol 1981;90:121–5.

56. Rosenthal U. Epithelial cysts in the human vestibular apparatus. J Laryngol Otol 1974;88:105–12.

57. Merchant SN, Velaquez-Villasenor L, Tsuji K, et al. Temporal bone studies of the human peripheral vestibular system. Normative vestibular hair cell data. Ann Otol Rhinol Laryngol Suppl 2000;181:3–13.

58. Ross MD, Peacor D, Johnsson LG, Allard LF. Observations on normal and degenerating human otoconia. Ann Otol Rhinol Laryngol 1976;85:310–26.

59. Jang YS, Hwang CH, Shin JY, et al. Age-related changes on the morphology of the otoconia. Laryngoscope 2006;116:996–1001.

60. Herdman SJ, Tusa RJ. Assessment and treatment of patients with benign paroxysmal positional vertigo. In: Herdman SJ, editor. Vestibular Rehabilitation, 2nd edition. Philadelphia: FA Davis Co; 1994.

61. Girardi M, Konrad HR. Imbalance and falls in the elderly. In: Cummings CW, Flint PW, Harker LA, et al., editors. Otolaryngology Head & Neck Surgery, 4th edition. Philadelphia: Elsevier Mosby; 2005. p. 3199–206.

62. Park JJ, Tang Y, Lopez I, Ishiyama A. Age-related change in the number of neurons in the human vestibular ganglion. J Comp Neurol 2001;431:437–43.

63. Velazquez-Villasenor L, Merchant SN, Tsuji K, et al. Temporal bone studies of the human peripheral vestibular system. Normative Scarpa's ganglion cell data. Ann Otol Rhinol Laryngol Suppl 2000;181:14–9.

64. Bergstrom B. Morphology of the vestibular nerve. II. The number of myelinated vestibular nerve fibers in man at various ages. Acta Otolaryngol 1973;76:173–9.

65. Richter E. Counts of neurons in Scarpa's ganglion from human temporal bones. Abstr Assoc Res Otolaryngol 1979;2:28.

66. Fujii M, Goto N, Okada A, et al. Distribution of amyloid bodies in the aged human vestibulocochlear nerve. Acta Otolaryngol 1996;116:566–71.

67. Lopez I, Honrubia V, Baloh RW. Aging and the human vestibular nucleus. J Vestib Res 1997;1:77–85.

68. Whitman GT, DiPatre PL, Lopez IA, et al. Neuropathology in older people with disequilibrium of unknown cause. Neurology 1999;53:375–80.

69. McPherson DL, Whitacker SL. Disequilibrium of aging. In: Goebel JA, editor. Practical Management of the Dizzy Patient. Philadelphia: Lippincott Williams & Wilkins; 2001. p. 269–98.

70. Shepard NT, Telian SA. Practical Management of the Balance Disorder Patient. San Diego: Singular Publishing Group, Inc; 1996.

71. Konrad HR, Girardi M, Helfert R. Balance and aging. Laryngoscope 1999;109:1454–60.

72. Enrietto JA, Jacobsen KM, Baloh RW. Aging effects on auditory and vestibular responses: A longitudinal study. Am J Otolaryngol 1999;20:371–8.

73. Hirvonen TP, Aalto H, Pyykko I, et al. Changes in vestibular-ocular reflex of elderly people. Acta Otolaryngol Suppl 1997;529:108–10.

74. Mulch G, Petermann W. Influence of age on results of vestibular function tests: Review of literature and presentation of caloric test results. Ann Otol Rhinol Laryngol Suppl 1979;88:1–17.

75. Mallinson AI, Longridge NS. Caloric response does not decline with age. J Vestib Res 2004;14:393–6.

76. Kristinsdottir EK, Jarnio GB, Magnusson M. Asymmetric vestibular function in the elderly might be a significant contributor to hip fractures. Scandin J Rehab Med 2000;32:56–60.

77. Norre ME, Forrez G, Beckers A. Vestibular dysfunction causing instability in aged patients. Acta Otolaryngol 1987;104:50–5.

78. Barozzi S, Giuliano DA, Giordano GP, Cesarani A. Dynamic stabilometric findings in equilibrium disorders of the elderly. Acta Otorhinolaryngol Ital 2005;25:220–3.

79. Welgampola MS, Colebatch JG. Vestibulocollic reflexes: Normal values and the effect of age. Clin Neurophysiol 2001;112:1971–9.

80. Monahan KD, Ray CA. Vestibulosympathetic reflex during orthostatic challenge in aging humans. Am J Physiol Regul Integr Comp Physiol 2002;283:R1027–32.

81. Spicer SS, Schulte BA, Adams JC. Immunolocalization of NA+, K+-ATPase and carbonic anhydrase in the gerbil's vestibular system. Hear Res 1990;43:205–18.

82. Spicer SS, Schulte BA. Differentiation of inner ear fibrocytes according to their ion transport related activity. Hear Res 1991;56:53–64.

83. Lang H, Schulte BA, Schmeidt RA. Effects of chronic furosemide treatment and age on cell division in the adult gerbil inner. J Assoc Res Otolaryngol 2003;4:164–74.

84. Lang H, Fekete DM. Lineage analysis in the chicken inner ear shows differences in clonal dispersion for epithelial, neurons and mesenchymal cells. Devel Biol 2001;234:120–37.

85. Lang H, Yasuhira E, Schmeidt R, et al. Contribution of bone marrow hematopoietic stem cells to adult mouse inner ear: Mesenchymal cells and fibrocytes. J Comp Neurol 2006;497:187–201.

86. Gates GA, Mills JH. Presbycusis. Lancet 2005;366:1111–20.

87. Gantz BJ, Turner C, Gfeller KE, Lowder MW. Preservation of hearing in cochlear implant surgery: Advantages of combined electrical and acoustical speech processing. Laryngoscope 2005;115:798–802.

88. Shepard NT, Telian SA, Smith-Wheelock M, Raj A. Vestibular and balance rehabilitation therapy. Ann Otol Rhinol Laryngol 1993;102:198–205.

30

Vestibular and Balance Rehabilitation

Susan L. Whitney, PhD, PT
Joseph M. Furman, MD, PhD

The concept of vestibular rehabilitation, that is, providing exercises for patients with dizziness and balance disorders, was first documented in the literature in the 1940s when Cooksey and Cawthorne worked together to develop an exercise program that was useful for patients with dizziness.[1,2] They suggested that the exercises were very effective in ameliorating dizziness symptoms and employed physical and mental exercise plus occupational therapy.[1,2] Their exercises included many different forms of eye–head coordination movements while incorporating balance activities. Approximately 40 years later, Norre and DeWeerdt suggested that exercise, in the form of repeating the dizziness provoking movements (habituation training) could decrease symptoms.[3] Shepard and Telian[4] and Horak[5] in the early 1990s provided evidence that vestibular rehabilitation was effective in patients with vestibular disorders. More recently, evidence suggests that various diagnostic groups may have different outcomes.[6–9]

Vestibular rehabilitation is a generic term that is used by physical therapists and occupational therapists to describe exercises that are provided to enhance balance function and reduce dizziness. Physical therapists focus on exercises to enhance balance, increase strength and range of motion, and improve coordination and walking. Occupational therapists focus on activities of daily living, instrumental activities of daily living, and driving skills.

Most of the therapists who treat patients with balance and vestibular disorders have prior experience working with patients with nonvestibular neurologic disorders. An interest in learning and a desire to treat people with vestibular dysfunction is a necessity. The practitioners who perform vestibular rehabilitation should have an understanding of the underlying anatomy and physiology of the inner ear and brain. Patients with vestibular disorders require more time than typical patients seen in therapy because of their comorbid conditions. They are also more likely to fall than those in the general community, so heightened vigilance is required while they perform their exercise programs, often requiring close supervision for safety.

Generally, it is thought that patients adapt, habituate or use sensory substitution to recover from a vestibular insult. Fatigue, bed rest, fear, and anxiety have all been implicated in slow recovery after a vestibular insult, most likely related to decreased activity of the patient. Movement appears to be a key factor in recovery in both primates and humans. Vestibulo-ocular reflex (VOR) adaptation has been hypothesized to be potentiated by either retinal slip or a visual position error stimulus.[10] Thus, many of the exercises employed by therapists (Table 1) attempt to stimulate retinal slip, to promote adaptation of the VOR. Since VOR efficiency decreases with unilateral hypofunction, a goal of vestibular rehabilitation is to increase the VOR gain, that is, the ratio of eye velocity to head velocity, to near unity. With the VOR gain closer to 1, vision improves and usually patients will report less dizziness. Figure 1A through C illustrates diagrammatically the process of recovering symmetric vestibulo-ocular signals following a unilateral peripheral vestibular injury.

Although there is no convincing evidence in the literature that habituation, through the use of repeated movements decreases dizziness, its use continues today because it seems to provide relief. For habituation to be successful, it appears to be very important to have patients focus on visual targets as they perform the exercises. Also patients should be exposed to more difficult visual conditions as they improve.

Sensory substitution is used for patients who either have minimal or no remaining vestibular function. The goal of sensory substitution is for the patient to use remaining senses, that is, somatosensory and visual signals, to help orient the body in space. These strategies are particularly helpful in patients with bilateral vestibular hypofunction and in those who have multisensory disequilibrium.

VESTIBULAR DISORDERS

Peripheral Vestibular Disorders

UNILATERAL VESTIBULAR LOSS. Patients with peripheral vestibular dysfunction, with the exclusion of those with bilateral vestibular loss, generally have better outcomes than those who have central vestibular dysfunction. Patients with benign paroxysmal positional vertigo (BPPV) have the best prognosis.

Unilateral peripheral loss is amenable to treatment with vestibular rehabilitation. Patients with unilateral loss who have minimal symptoms are usually considered to have compensated "well." However, there is evidence that the compensation is not complete.[11] Bowman reported that all patients with unilateral vestibular loss continue to have remaining complaints.[11] Even those with minimal symptoms are not symptom free and continue to have permanent deficits in balance function.[12]

Table 1 Common Exercises Provided to Patients in a Vestibular Rehabilitation Program

Balance exercises
Single leg stance
Romberg standing (eyes open → eyes closed → eyes open with head movement → eyes closed with head movement) progressing to a semitandem stance eventually to standing in tandem Romberg
Standing on a folded towel → to standing on a thin pad → standing on a foam pad → standing on the pad marching standing on the pad with head movements with eyes open; repeating the progression with eyes closed

Eye/head exercises
Focusing on a target and moving the head to the right and left
Focusing on a target and moving the head up and down

- Progressing the speed (slow to fast)
- Varying the distance (both close and far)
- Varying the patient position (seated, standing, marching, Romberg, semitandem Romberg, tandem Romberg, and walking)
- Varying the background (simple, plain, complex, eg, with stripes, a moving visual scene)

Sensory substitution exercises
Saccadic exercises
Imaginary target exercise (focus on a target, close eyes and try to remember where the target is located, move head, and then open and try to maintain the eyes on the original target). Vary the amount of head movement and try the exercise in different directions.
Exercises to increase strength in the distal musculature, especially the feet, eg, towel curls (with the toes, grab the towel and attempt to move it under the arch of the foot).

Gait exercises
Walking at different speeds
Walking while moving the head up/down or right/left
Walking and pivoting
Walking while focused on a target in the distance
Walking on a compliant surface

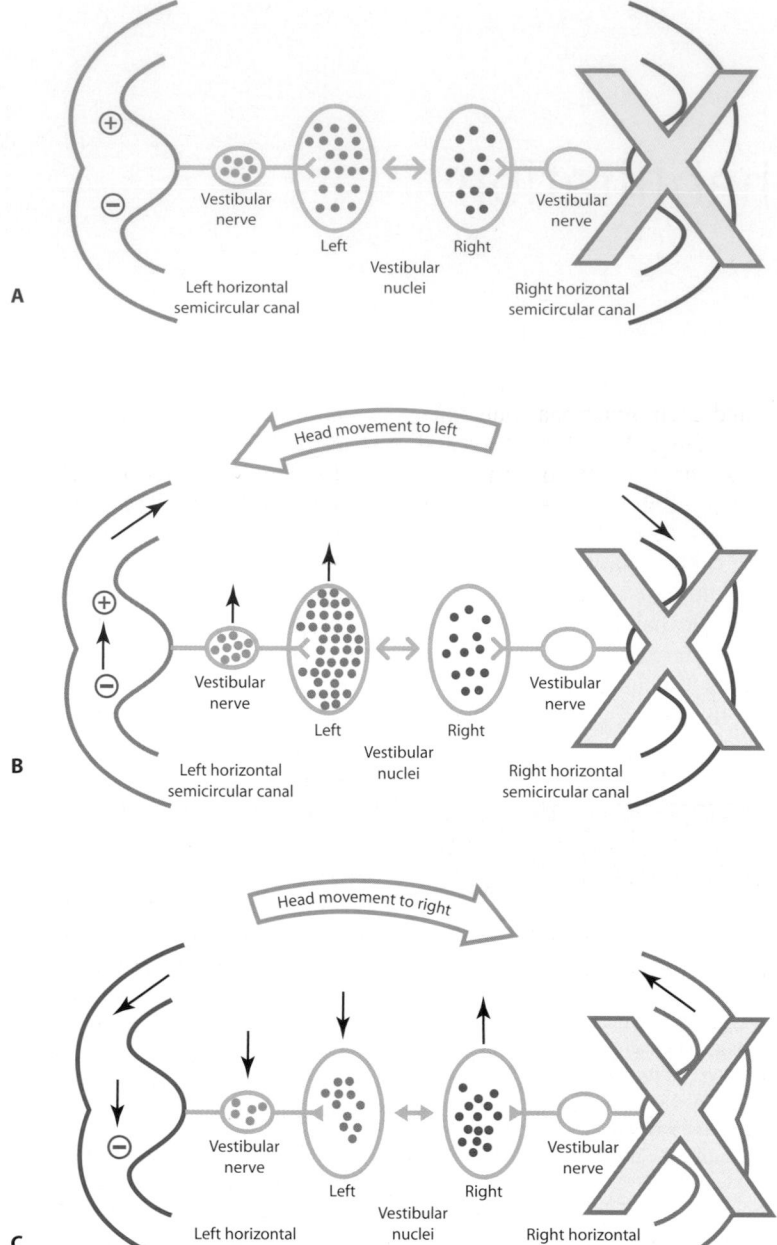

Figure 1 When a peripheral vestibular injury is chronic, in this case on the right, the CNS is able, through vestibular compensation, to restore partially the lost resting activity within the deafferented vestibular nucleus, and thus reduce the asymmetry of neural activity between the vestibular nuclei at rest (A) and partially restore the function of the vestibulo-ocular reflex (VOR). (B) Movement toward the intact ear. (C) Movement toward the lesioned ear. (Republished with permission of reference 13.)

Patients with unilateral vestibular loss who remain symptomatic note particular difficulty with strenuous activities, bright lights, noise, confined spaces, open spaces, and busy environments.[11] Also, such patients are often concerned that they might be injured as the result of a fall. Patients with obsessive–compulsive tendencies also poorly compensate from vestibular insults.[11]

Even though it has been previously suggested that patients with peripheral vestibular disorders make a full recovery, there is emerging evidence that this is not true. Vestibular neuritis, labyrinthitis, and vestibular ablative procedures all appear to result in some functional deficits, even after vestibular rehabilitation.[14] Patients should be advised that they may continue to have some

functional limitations even after "successful" vestibular rehabilitation.

Bilateral Vestibular Loss. Patients with bilateral vestibular loss exhibit significant functional impairments as a result of their disorder. Unlike many people with unilateral vestibular loss, patients with bilateral loss may be unable to stand or ambulate on uneven surfaces, often require an assistive device for ambulation and usually cannot walk in dimly lit or darkened environments without being very unstable or falling. The amount of improvement that can be expected from vestibular rehabilitation is dependent upon the amount of residual vestibular function. Those people with greater remaining vestibular function have the best prognosis. Patients with little

to no vestibular function fall frequently and have significant complaints of oscillopsia, gait ataxia, and often require an assistive device during ambulation.

Recent avenues of research in vestibular rehabilitation for patients with bilateral vestibular loss include the vibrotactile vest,[15] the vestibular implant (similar to the cochlear implant which is being developed in primates),[16] and the Brainport device.[17] These devices are designed to provide a postural control signal that the brain can utilize in lieu of the damaged labyrinth(s).

Exercise programs for patients with bilateral vestibular loss typically focus on substituting for the loss of vestibular function by increasing reliance on either the visual or the somatosensory systems. If there is any indication that there is remaining VOR function, VOR exercises are initiated (Figure 2). Also, head–eye coordination exercises are prescribed to activate the

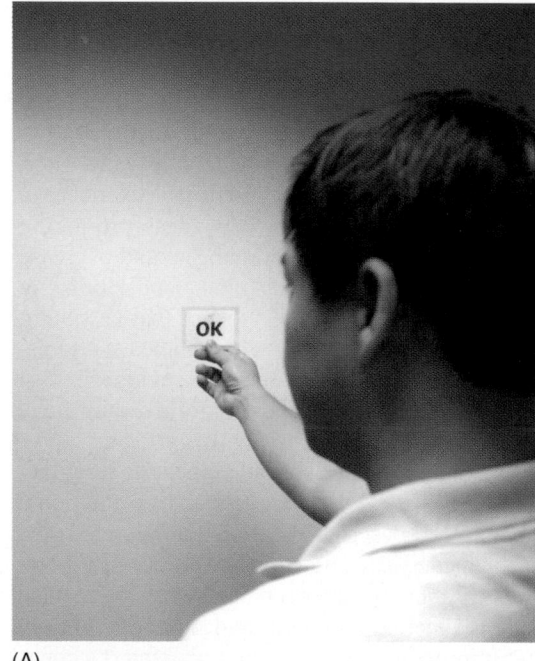

(A)

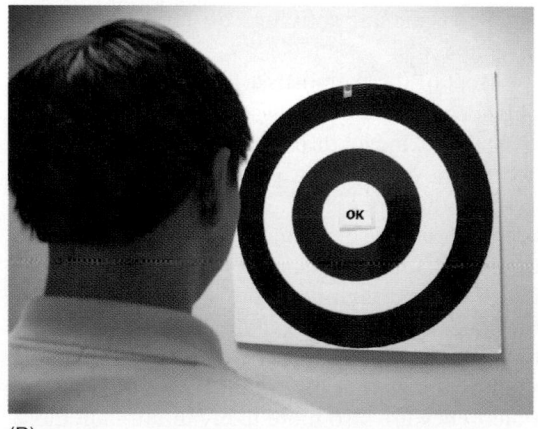

(B)

Figure 2 The patient is focusing on a target and moving his head to the right and left while keeping the object in focus. (A) Note the plain background to initiate the exercise. (B) Note that the background has high contrast. Patients are progressed from performing the exercise from a blank background (A) to a high contrast background (B) as their symptoms improve.

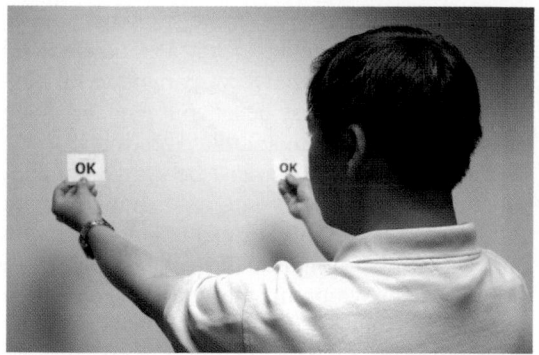

Figure 3 The patient is asked to focus on a target. Then the patient is asked to move the eyes to the target in the left hand, followed by head movement so that the patient is directly looking directly at the target. The patient is then asked to repeat the same eye movement to the object held in the right hand followed by the head movement back to the right target.

cervico-ocular reflex to optimize any remaining sensory systems that can compensate for the loss of vestibular sensory inputs (Figure 3).

When patients have multisensory disequilibrium, their ability to overcome the loss of vestibular dysfunction is lessened, affecting overall prognosis. Visual impairments resulting from glaucoma, macular degeneration, and diabetes are relatively common disorders seen in older adults that will adversely affect outcome after vestibular loss. Even the use of bifocals or trifocals can affect prognosis, as older adults with bifocals have been reported to fall more frequently than those seniors who do not wear glasses.[18] The use of bifocals and trifocals also makes eye–head coordination exercises more difficult, as it is not possible to keep the target in focus throughout the exercise. Because multisensory disequilibrium can be so much more debilitating than bilateral vestibular loss alone, vestibular ablative procedures such as intratympanic gentamycin injections should be considered more likely to produce chronic disequilibrium in patients with comorbid sensory disorders.

Central Vestibular Disorders

It is not evident what the frequency of central vestibular disorders is in the literature. From our tertiary vestibular clinic, the percentage of patients with central vestibular dysfunction that present to our vestibular physical therapy clinic is approximately 40%. Reports of people with central vestibular dysfunction in tertiary balance and vestibular clinics is between 7 and 45%,[4,19,20] yet little is known about the effect of physical rehabilitation on their outcomes. There are no randomized controlled trials to support the use of vestibular rehabilitation for patients with central vestibular dysfunction. However, recent evidence suggests that changes occur with gait, dizziness, and balance after rehabilitation.[4,6,19,21]

Central vestibular disorders include damage to the vestibular nuclei, vestibulocerebellum, perihypoglossal nuclei, or to the vestibulospinal, vestibulocollic, vestibulo-autonomic, and vestibule–cerebral pathways.[22] The vestibular nuclei are major sensory processing centers that receive input not only from the peripheral vestibular system, but also from the visual and somatosensory systems. If there is damage to the vestibular nuclear complex, postural control, eye movement, and orientation of the body in space may be compromised.

Damage to the cerebellum, especially the flocculonodular lobe, will impede the ability of the brain to adapt/compensate for either a central or a peripheral vestibular insult. If there is damage to the vestibular-cerebellar loop, recovery is impaired even in patients with peripheral vestibular damage[23] and their functional outcomes will be adversely affected. Patients with central vestibular diagnoses that have improved following vestibular rehabilitation include those with migraine dizziness, head trauma, cervical vertigo, anxiety-related dizziness, and cerebellar stroke.

The most common central vestibular disorder is migraine dizziness, which is also known as migraine-associated dizziness, or vestibular migraine. Migraine dizziness occurs with a prevalence of approximately 6.5%[24] and sometimes presents as migraine without headache. Migraine dizziness is a diagnosis of exclusion. Specific criteria have been developed to help guide the clinician in making the diagnosis of migraine dizziness.[25] A sensation of vertigo, head pressure, and situational dizziness are all common characteristics of patients with migraine dizziness with or without headache. Duration of symptoms in patients with migraine dizziness is variable.[26] Rehabilitation for patients with migraine dizziness must be done with great care, as these patients best optimize their progress with a combination of medication and exercise.[27] If patients with migraine are pushed to perform eye–head exercises without the benefit of medication, they often experience a worsening of symptoms and therapy may fail.

People with migraine dizziness have poorer emotional outcome scores on the Dizziness Handicap Inventory (DHI) than age-matched subjects with vestibular disorders, but no migraine.[9] Patients with migraine dizziness continue to experience emotional complaints from their migrainous disorder, even as their physical function improves. Even having a remote history of migraine appears to affect adversely vestibular rehabilitation outcome,[9] suggesting that it is important to determine if a patient has had migraines in the past when evaluating a patient.

Patients with migraine dizziness often complain of having an increase in symptoms in wide, open spaces, in large grocery stores with many products, and around crowds of people. Exposure to complex visual environments is often part of the therapy program, yet often patients cannot tolerate these complex environments without medication to help to control their symptoms. Gradual exposure to complex visual environments is a key principle leading to recovery. A physician/therapist team helps to optimize recovery.

Approximately 30% of patients with head trauma experience dizziness.[28] The dizziness complaints may be of short or long duration (seconds to years), depending on the cause. Symptoms may be perceived as dizziness, lightheadedness, or a sensation of spinning and even complaints of intense head pressure. After head trauma, people may experience dizziness from cervical injuries, damage to the peripheral labyrinth (unilateral dysfunction, BPPV, perilymphatic fistula, and posttraumatic endolymphatic hydrops), damage to the central vestibular structures (vestibular nuclei, cerebellum, and other structures), or damage to both peripheral and central structures. Preexisting central or peripheral dysfunction impedes functional recovery after vestibular insults from head injury.

Patients who have experienced head trauma are often difficult to rehabilitate because of their comorbid impairments. The International Classification of Diseases of the World Health Organization—10 or the ICD-10 diagnostic criteria for postconcussion syndrome describe a history of head trauma *with* loss of consciousness preceding symptom onset by a maximum of 4 weeks. Patients must have 3 of the following: headache, dizziness, malaise, fatigue, noise intolerance, irritability, depression, anxiety, or emotional libility. In addition, they must also have a minimum of 3 symptoms from these categories: (1) subjective concentration, memory, or intellectual difficulties without neuropsychological evidence of marked impairment; (2) insomnia, reduced alcohol tolerance, or preoccupation with above symptoms; and (3) fear of brain damage with hypochondriacal concern and adoption of a sick role. Patients with postconcussion disorder are more challenging rehabilitation candidates because of the above.

Patients with posttraumatic dizziness often have difficulty remembering the exercises provided, making compliance difficult. Any of the above symptoms have the potential to slow recovery that could occur with a vestibular rehabilitation program. A supportive family is needed for optimal functional recovery, as the patient often does not remember nor are they motivated to perform exercises that might make them dizzy because of their head injury.

Cervical vertigo has been discussed in the literature for over 100 years, yet the diagnostic criteria for cervical vertigo are not well-established. Whiplash injuries may result in cervical vertigo, with or without associated head injury. Furman and Cass[29] have defined cervical vertigo as "A nonspecific sensation of altered orientation in space and disequilibrium originating from abnormal afferent activity from the neck."

The cervical receptors provide inputs to the vestibulospinal track that travel to the vestibular nuclei, resulting in an accurate representation of the neck in space. The cervico-ocular reflex is not always used in humans,[30] but it has been suggested that it is helpful in the rehabilitation of patients with unilateral and bilateral vestibular loss with its ability to provide information of neck positioning. Disruption of cervical afferents has resulted in changes in postural stability, mild ataxia, visual disturbance, and dizziness that can last minutes to hours usually associated with a change of head position. It has been reported that decreasing neck pain and increasing neck range of motion decreases dizziness in patients experiencing cervical dizziness or vertigo.[31]

There is no definitive test to make the diagnosis of cervical vertigo, and the diagnosis of cervical vertigo is controversial. There are 2 tests suggested as helping to make the diagnosis of cervical vertigo: the head-fixed-body-turned maneuver and the smooth pursuit neck torsion test. The head-fixed-body-turned maneuver stimulates the neck without stimulating the labyrinths and may result in nystagmus and dizziness.[32] The smooth pursuit neck torsion test has recently been used to assess patients with whiplash injury.[3] The patient is placed in the neutral neck starting position and then is turned 45° to the right and left. Pursuit gain is calculated and compared between neutral and 45° of rotation with a sensitivity of 90% and a specificity of 91% in patients with dizziness.[33]

Vertigo can sometimes be elicited by extension and rotation of the cervical spine. However, without a history of trauma, it is not likely to be cervical vertigo. Endo and colleagues suggest that hyperextension combined with rotation of the cervical spine may result in a cerebellar infarction or vertebrobasilar insufficiency.[34] Although rare, vertigo, or dizziness associated with extension and rotation of the neck and accompanied by neurologic signs and symptoms should be carefully examined. Therapists must report neurologic signs and symptoms to the referring physician immediately and discontinue treatment until the cause of the symptoms has been investigated.

Patients with central vestibular disorders often improve with vestibular rehabilitation, but there is less improvement than in patients with peripheral vestibular disorders.[35] Patients with a central disorder diagnosis demonstrate better outcomes than patients with both central and peripheral vestibular disorders.[35] The length of treatment time is generally longer in patients with central vestibular disorders compared to those with peripheral disorders.[36]

Medication that decreases dizziness or pain may be necessary for patients with severe complaints to comply with an exercise program. Space and motion symptoms experienced with migraine or a vestibular disorder may need to be controlled pharmacologically for rehabilitation to progress. Communication among the patient, physician, and physical therapist appears to provide optimal recovery of function in this complex group of patients.

Central and Peripheral Vestibular Disorders

Many studies have combined results from people with peripheral vestibular disorders with results from people with central vestibular disorders, making it difficult to determine outcomes in either group.[4,14,19,37] Meli and colleagues recently reported on a group of people with either peripheral or central vestibular disorders and suggested that patients improved an average of 15 points on the DHI after rehabilitation and improved to a mean score of 22 (another decrease in score of 3 points) 6 months postrehabilitation.[14] Jacobson and Newman reported that a clinically significant change score on the DHI was 18 points, suggesting that 6 months postrehabilitation the average DHI score change was 18 points.[38] Seventy percent of the patients in Meli and colleagues study[14] had a DHI score between 0 and 30 at the conclusion of their rehabilitation program, which Whitney and colleagues have reported as being "mildly" impaired. Scores between 0 and 10 would be considered normal, so even 6 months postrehabilitation, patients had not returned to baseline "normal."

Space and Motion Symptoms

One can almost always improve a patient's balance, which is less true for their dizziness. Patients with dizziness who have "space and motion" complaints or visual vertigo are more difficult to treat. Patients with space and motion symptoms often complain of having difficulty walking in "busy" visual environments and may even start to avoid life situations that provoke their dizziness symptoms, such as refusing to go to a shopping mall or to ride a bus or train.

Space and motion symptoms are often associated with patients with panic/anxiety disorders and those with migraine, but the same complaints can also occur with unilateral hypofunction. There are patients who have space and motion symptoms who are incapacitated by the symptoms, yet they have no history of either panic/anxiety or migraine.

Many patients with uncompensated peripheral vestibular dysfunction have space and motion discomfort,[39] leaving them to feel disabled. They may become symptomatic during typical daily activities such as going to the grocery store, to visit family, or to a shopping mall. Even if their balance improves, these patients continue to feel limited because they are not comfortable in large groups or in situations where there is a lot of background motion. Empirically, it appears that those who complain of space and motion discomfort have a poorer recovery, yet Pavlou and colleagues[40] reported that there were improvements in space and motion discomfort after simulator-based therapy, which provides the patient with desensitization exposure through visual motion during exercises, in a group of people with chronic unilateral hypofunction.

REHABILITATION CONCEPTS

The sooner rehabilitative movement is begun following a vestibular insult, the quicker the functional recovery.[41] Patients with vestibular disorders have a tendency not to move, as moving increases their symptoms. Logically, one would stop or decrease head and body movements to decrease symptoms. The strategy of decreasing movement to feel better is not a good one and may actually delay recovery. Patients with vestibular disorders must be encouraged to move early and move a lot to stimulate recovery.

Care and experience must be utilized in constructing an exercise program for patients with vestibular dysfunction. For example, people with central vestibular impairments often complain of more constant symptoms that may or may not be related to changes of head position. They may have constant, intense symptoms of vertigo, nausea, and/or dizziness and may complain of difficulty with their vision. Head pain and head pressure are common complaints. The use of medication in conjunction with physical therapy is effective.[38] Decreasing the severe symptoms is often necessary to begin the rehabilitation program, as movement increases some patients' complaints of dizziness and vertigo.

Once some of the symptoms are managed medically, the patient is able to begin and make use of the rehabilitative exercise program. Exercises must begin slowly, and later the speed of the exercise is increased. In patients with central vestibular dysfunction, the progression is often slower than in patients with peripheral vestibular disorders. Bright lights, visually complex stimuli, and noise often bother people with vestibular dysfunction, so methods to decrease external stimuli while performing the exercises are employed as part of the exercise prescription.

Referral Patterns

People with various vestibular disorders appear to improve with rehabilitation (Table 2). Patients with vestibular disorders should be referred to a physical or occupational therapist who is knowledgeable about the management and care of patients with balance and vestibular disorders.[14] Experience with patients with balance and vestibular disorders most likely changes the rehabilitation outcome, as the entire person must be treated for optimal results. Both physical and psychological well-being are important variables in the outcome of patients with balance and vestibular dysfunction.[42]

Finding a therapist who is interested in treating patients with balance and vestibular dysfunction can sometimes be a daunting task. We typically quiz therapists about their knowledge and interest in treating our patients prior to referral. Other methods sometimes employed include checking web sites that list therapists who are interested in the treatment of patients with balance and vestibular disorders. The web site method does not insure that the person is an expert but is more effective than sending the patient to the local therapy office without any assurance of quality.

Most therapists who have expertise in the treatment of people with balance and vestibular dysfunction have some long-term rehabilitation experience. In addition, some of the physical therapists may be board certified neurologic clinical

Table 2 Patients with Disorders that Might Benefit from Vestibular Physical Therapy

Vestibular schwannoma (acoustic neuroma)
Benign paroxysmal positional vertigo
Bilateral vestibular loss
Cerebellar degeneration
Cerebellar stroke
Cerebellar tumors
Cervical vertigo
Head injury
Labyrinthitis
Meniere disease
Migraine-related dizziness
Multisensory disequilibrium
Orthostatic tremor
Ototoxcity
Panic disorder and dizziness
Perilymphatic fistula
Spinocerebellar atrophy
Vestibular neuritis

specialists (NCS). Similar to physician board certification, those who have an NCS as part of their credential have demonstrated that they have above entry-level expertise in the treatment of patients with neurologic dysfunction. Part of the NCS examination includes content area in vestibular rehabilitation.

Poor Candidates for Vestibular Rehabilitation

There are several key indicators that one can use to predict patient outcomes after a vestibular event. Patients with certain comorbid conditions often have a poorer recovery after a vestibular insult (Table 3). Even with comorbid conditions, vestibular rehabilitation can help aid in recovery or compensation for the vestibular event. Those patients who have conditions included in Table 3 will improve but lesser than those patients who have fewer key comorbidities. It is very important to explain to all patients that when one or both vestibular labyrinths are impaired, that they may continue to have some nagging problems, such as walking in grocery stores, bending over, driving on a freeway, and moving their head quickly.[11]

Age alone does not appear to be a major factor in recovery, but fear of falling, which is common in older persons, may affect the willingness of patients to challenge their balance and to experience additional dizziness episodes. Those who are afraid of falling may require more visits to a physical therapy clinic because they may be afraid to perform exercises at home that challenge their balance.

In patients with central vestibular dysfunction, Brown and colleagues reported that the central diagnostic group who improved the least were those with cerebellar dysfunction, probably because the cerebellum plays a key role in VOR adaptation.[6] Any preexisting visual or somatosensory deficit will impede recovery. Persons with diabetes may experience both visual and somatosensory deficits, which will impede recovery. When all three balance receptors (visual, somato-

sensory, and vestibular) are impaired, recovery is compromised. A history of a childhood strabismus or ocular misalignment is often overlooked until the person experiences a vestibular insult. The visual impairments, often forgotten from childhood, appear to make compensation from a vestibular injury more difficult.

There is insufficient evidence to state that patients with certain diagnoses should not have a trial of physical or occupational therapy. Improvements are noted in patients who demonstrate poor prognostic signs, yet their improvement is often lesser than what is usually expected. Being reasonable when explaining potential outcomes is important so that the patient does not feel like a treatment failure. Compliance with all exercises and instructions, with any of the conditions listed in Table 3, may still result in a rehabilitation disappointment for the patient and the family.

Presenting Complaints

Some patients complain of a balance problem or dizziness, and others will have both dizziness and balance complaints. Patients who are only dizzy are usually provided with exercises that promote VOR adaptation in various situations, both in static and more dynamic positions. Those who complain of having balance problems alone are often asked to perform exercises in more difficult positions and postures, but are usually not routinely asked to perform VOR exercises.

Patients who have both vestibular and balance complaints will be treated with both eye–head adaptation exercises and balance exercises in increasingly more difficult situations. One must use care with patients with both dizziness and a balance problem, as they may be at a higher risk for falling.

Table 3 Factors that Suggest Poor Compensation after a Vestibular Insult

Age may have an indirect effect on outcome (older adults may be more fearful, weaker)
Comorbid CNS and labyrinthine dysfunction
Cerebellar dysfunction
CNS depressant drugs
Comorbid neurological dysfunction, eg, Parkinson disease, stroke, diabetes
Distal lower extremity somatosensory disturbance
Fatigue
Fear of falling or fear of moving
Migraine or past history of migraine
Musculoskeletal dysfunction
Preexisting visual dysfunction (either congenital or acquired)
Psychiatric comorbidity (eg, panic disorder, agoraphobia, anxiety, obsessive–compulsive disorder, and perfectionistic personality)
Severity of the vestibular insult (bilateral disease is more debilitating than unilateral loss)
Surgery that reduces mobility
Visual difficulty such as cataracts, visual loss, bifocals, trifocals, macular degeneration, glaucoma, and ocular misalignment
White matter disease

Exercise Progression

Typically, the progression of positions and mobility during exercises is as follows: supine (if the patient is grossly unstable or fearful), sitting, standing, to more difficult standing positions (Romberg, semitandem, and then tandem Romberg), and lastly during gait. Exercises are performed with eyes open and sometimes with eyes closed, depending on the capabilities of the patient. Walking programs and specific actions during walking (turning, stepping over and around objects, bending over while walking, or even looking up or down) are incorporated into the exercise program as the patient improves. Head movements progress from slow to fast, and the distance of targets while performing exercises is varied from close to far.

It appears optimal to begin the exercise program at the highest level of difficulty that the patient can tolerate, rather than go through a specific exercise progression from supine to walking. Typically, the physical therapist will customize the exercise program to target the specific patient deficits identified in the physical therapy examination. Shepard and Telian reported more effective results with a customized versus a generic exercise program.[4] Horak and colleagues have also reported that customized balance exercises were more effective than a generic exercise program or medication in patients with peripheral vestibular dysfunction.[5]

Whether they have 1 or more presenting problems (balance, dizziness, or both), patients will still receive some benefit from performing the prescribed exercises. A patient who refuses to perform any exercise will not improve with rehabilitation. Primates who moved little after surgery did not improve until they were permitted to move about their cages. Movement is critical to a positive rehabilitation outcome.

VESTIBULAR REHABILITATION ASSESSMENT AND TREATMENT

People referred to physical therapy for vestibular disorders are usually seen one-on-one by physical therapists. The physical therapy assessment generally requires 1 hour or more during which subjective and objective testing is necessary to evaluate a patient with balance and/or vestibular dysfunction adequately.

The subjective history is very important to a physical therapist, as the patient's story will often dictate treatment and will also provide direction as to which clinical tests are necessary. Key questions are asked during the subjective history related to movements or situations that increase or decrease dizziness symptoms. Physical therapists develop a physical therapy diagnosis by the end of the assessment. Often the medical diagnosis and the physical therapy diagnosis will match, but not always. Physical therapists are concerned about functional limitations and how well patients are able to participate in their community and within their home environment.

Typically, the questions asked during the subjective history are similar or identical to what the physician might ask to make the medical diagnosis, but the information is placed in a slightly different context. Physical therapists are concerned with how to help patients overcome their disability. However, the medical diagnosis is important and will shape the rehabilitation program. Different exercises and treatment interventions will be employed depending on the presenting diagnosis. Communication of physician findings to the therapist will only enhance the care of the patient and allow the therapist to develop a more effective customized exercise program.

Key aspects of the subjective history include determining the intensity and duration of the symptoms and whether the symptoms are episodic or constant. Associated symptoms (nausea, vomiting) with their dizziness or vertigo are also determined. Questions such as does your dizziness increase with rolling over, moving from supine to sitting, moving from sitting to standing, walking in a grocery store, reading, and walking while moving the head are typically asked to determine what increases symptoms and to develop a treatment plan.

Duration, frequency, latency, and fatigability are all factors that are considered during the collection of the subjective history. Often patients are asked to rate their dizziness symptoms at rest and indicate what is the "best" and "worst" dizziness rating within the last 24 hours on a perceived dizziness scale (0 to 10 or 0 to 100). The dizziness rating provides an indication as to whether the patient has constant symptoms or if they are episodic and also provides information related to the magnitude of the perceived dizziness. Very high scores are often associated with severe dysfunction, possibly of central origin or of comorbid psychiatric dysfunction.

Information about vision, ear status (tinnitus, aural fullness, and pain), past and present medical history, past fall incidents, motions that provoke symptoms, and medication use all help guide the physical therapy intervention. The use of bifocals or trifocals makes a person at higher risk for falling, due to impaired depth perception. Similarly, a unilateral cataract or poor unilateral outcome following extraction and lens implantation can contribute to impaired depth perception. Preexisting visual disorders can impede recovery after a vestibular disorder, making rehabilitation more difficult.

Ear complaints such as tinnitus or aural fullness are important signs and need to be documented. If either are new symptoms, the symptoms need to be reported to the referring physician. One must also ask the patient about whether their dizziness symptoms are associated with nausea and/or vomiting and whether there is any family history of ear disease or similar presenting symptoms.

Obtaining a history of any falls can help guide intervention. Patients who have fallen more than 2 times in the past 6 months are at risk for a future fall event. Care should be given to guard the patient closely during any standing or walking tests, as they are at risk for falling during the examination especially when asked to perform advanced balance tasks.

Postural assessment, vital signs, and visual inspection of the eyes at rest are helpful to determine a baseline for intervention. Standing balance is assessed by having patients stand in the Romberg, tandem Romberg, and in single leg stance. Patients should be assessed while standing on a complaint surface with their eyes open and closed. The durations that the patient can maintain positions are documented. Stepping in place on foam is sometimes attempted, but is considered an advanced skill.

In addition, gait testing is performed to determine what deficits require remediation during ambulation. Patients are often asked to walk at different speeds and to move their heads while ambulating to determine what their functional deficits are during dynamic gait activities. Subjects are asked to perform the four-item Dynamic Gait Index (DGI),[43] as it has been shown to be a valid but shorter version of the DGI developed by Shumway-Cook and Woollacott.[44]

Typically, patients with vestibular dysfunction walk with little trunk rotation. Some patients with vestibular dysfunction, especially those with bilateral vestibular loss, may have a wide-based gait. Many patients are unable to turn their head while ambulating without a loss of balance. Also, pivoting during walking is often difficult. Some patients will develop musculoskeletal dysfunction such as neck stiffness because of dizziness provoked by head movement. Patients will generally move their heads less, which can result in a loss of range of motion.

Specific vestibular related tests, such as the head thrust test, head shake test, vibration-induced nystagmus, checking for phorias and tropias, observing extraocular movements, the Dix-Hallpike maneuver, computerized dynamic posturogrpahy, and dynamic visual acuity are typically performed during the physical therapy assessment (see Chapter 10, "Evaluation of the Vestibular System"). Sensory testing is very important during the assessment as disorders of sensation will affect outcome and complicate the rehabilitation process. Proprioception, light touch, and vibration are typically tested in all subjects.

Coordination testing is sometimes warranted, especially for those patients who present with ataxia or with central nervous system signs (CNS) or symptoms. Range of motion, especially in the neck and lower extremities, may affect outcome. Stiffness and lack of motion in the trunk, legs, and neck may make it more difficult to rehabilitate a patient. Exercises may be more difficult for the patient to perform if they have reduced range of motion. Decreased range of motion in the lower extremity may predispose patients to falls.

The timed "up & go" test is performed on all patients to determine fall risk.[45] Scores of greater than 11.1 seconds in patients with balance and vestibular disorders have been related to reports of falls.[46] The 5 times sit to stand test is easily performed and is helpful in determining lower extremity strength and balance.[47] Those subjects who cannot rise from a chair independently are at high risk for a future fall.[47]

Gait speed is especially helpful in older adults with vestibular dysfunction and is recorded for future comparison. Walking slowly has been related to increased fall risk. One of the typical goals of physical therapy intervention is to increase gait speed over the course of rehabilitation.

Vestibular Rehabilitation Therapy Outcome Measures

Several common outcome measures are available to assess the benefit of rehabilitation. The DHI has been used extensively to help quantify changes in perceived disability from dizziness.[39] Patients answer 25 questions that require them to decide whether they are always, sometimes, or never bothered by dizziness during the 25 activities or circumstances included as part of the questionnaire.

The DHI scale (scores range from 0 to 100) is easy to interpret, with lower scores indicating less dysfunction. Scores between 0 and 30 denote mild disability, 31 to 60 moderate, and >60 severe handicap.[48] The DHI is a helpful tool to determine if the patient's perceived disability has changed over the course of treatment. In addition to a total score, the DHI provides 3 subscores: emotional, functional, and physical. As the DHI decreases over time, the expectation would be that the patient's function is also improving. Very high DHI scores (>80) may be indicative of the need for a psychologic or psychiatric consultation. Scores >80 indicate that almost everything bothers the patient, suggesting that motion-provoked dizziness is only one of their problems.

The Activities-specific Balance Confidence (ABC) scale was initially developed to grade subjectively grade fear of falling.[49] The ABC scale consists of 16 questions that the patient rates on a 0 to 100% scale in increments of 10. Higher scores indicate greater confidence. Scores of <67 have been related to high fall risks and scores <50 have been related to older adults who are homebound or significantly functionally impaired.[50,51] The total score is calculated by adding up all of the percentage scores and dividing by 1,600. Changes in the ABC score have been noted after vestibular rehabilitation, suggesting that patients feel more confident with their balance. A positive change of 10 or more has been suggested to be clinically significant in patients with vestibular disorders.[9]

Gait speed and the Timed "Up & Go" test are both powerful measures of gait performance that help gauge recovery. In older adults, changes of 0.1 m/s in gait speed are considered to be clinically significant.[52] Both measures are easy to collect and provide quantifiable evidence of change over time from the physical therapy intervention.

The four-item DGI is helpful in identifying impaired gait during dynamic activities.[43]

Exercise Program

The frequency of physical therapy intervention visits ranges from 2 to 3 times a week to weekly and in some institutions the visits occur once every 2 weeks. Optimal frequency of visits is unknown. It has been suggested that patients who are older and/or fearful are less likely to follow though with the home exercise program and, therefore, should be seen more frequently face-to-face. Repeat visits are required to ensure that the patients are performing the exercises correctly. Patients can be performing the exercises incorrectly, as they do not always remember what they were instructed to do, even when they were provided with a written exercise prescription. Many of the eye–head exercises are complex and may require repetition for the patient to perform them correctly.

The exercises are done both in the physical therapy clinic and at home. The home exercises are essential for recovery, as the frequency of visits to the clinic is probably not adequate to cause changes in function. Figure 4 demonstrates a typical exercise that a patient might be asked to perform at home. Safety is always emphasized with the exercise prescription. Customized exercises have been shown to be better than a list of generic exercises.[4] Most therapists suggest that patients perform the exercises 2 to 3 times per day.

If the patient is continuing to work, 3 exercise sessions a day is usually unreasonable. Often the dose of the exercise must be adapted based on the patient's tolerance. The patient may need to spread out the exercise session over several hours to be able to tolerate the exercise without too much residual dizziness. Generally, most patients are told to use an analog scale (with some maximum score negotiated between the therapist and the patient). The patient is instructed to modify how they are doing the exercises if their symptoms remain 20 to 30 minutes after completion. If they become significantly symptomatic, the patient should be encouraged to contact the therapist, and the exercise program will most likely be modified over the telephone or they will be told to stop the exercise until the next session if they are particularly symptomatic.

Most patients with peripheral vestibular disorders are treated over a 2- to 3-month period or less. However, patients with central vestibular disorders or with bilateral hypofunction should be treated for longer periods of time. It is important that the patient continues to make positive functional changes through the treatment period, otherwise therapy is not considered helpful. Occasionally, if the patient becomes too symptomatic while performing the exercises, the therapist will contact the physician to see if a CNS or vestibular suppressant is necessary to assure exercise compliance, with the goal of decreasing or eliminating the use of the medication over time.[53]

Improvements Noted after Vestibular Physical Therapy

Patients undergoing vestibular physical therapy often demonstrate improvements in postural control, as measured via computerized dynamic posturography, gait tasks, gait speed, a negative Dix-Hallpike test, dizziness rating, quality of life, or even timed standing tasks. The DHI is used to determine if there are positive changes in the patients perceived handicap after the rehabilitation process. The ABC is used to determine if the patient's confidence related to fall risk has improved over the course of rehabilitation. Baseline dizziness at discharge is also compared to baseline dizziness symptoms to determine if the patient has improved.

Not all patients return to "normal" on the above tasks, but generally there are documentable improvements in performance on balance tasks. Changes in time to perform a task or enhanced stability during standing and walking tasks are most commonly recorded as outcome measures. Changes in postural control have been documented in patients with peripheral and/or central vestibular disorders.[4,5,6,21,38]

The DHI has been used to quantify change in dizziness over time. Not all patients improve by a clinically significant amount of 18 or more points on the DHI. Few patients get worse with rehabilitation, yet there are some who do not change even after having diligently performing their exercises. At this time, it is impossible to predict who will improve and who will not after a course of rehabilitation.

CONCLUSIONS

The ultimate goal of vestibular rehabilitation is to help patients with balance disorders return to work or to return to being a productive member of their community. Careful progression of exercises and monitoring are important to provide feedback to the patient and to keep them motivated. It is difficult to persuade patients that sometimes making themselves dizzy is advantageous. The therapist's experience in dealing with patients with dizziness probably improves patient compliance and eventual outcome.

REFERENCES

1. Cawthorne T. The physiological basis for head exercises. J Chart Soc Physiother 1944;3:106–7.
2. Cooksey FS. Rehabilitation in (provoked) vestibular injuries. Proc R Soc Med 1946;39.
3. Norre ME, De Weerdt W. Positional vertigo treated by postural training vestibular habituation training. Agressologie 1981;22:37–44.
4. Shepard NT, Telian SA. Programmatic vestibular rehabilitation. Otolaryngol Head Neck Surg 1995;112:173–82.
5. Horak FB, Jones-Rycewicz C, Black FO, et al. Effects of vestibular rehabilitation on dizziness and imbalance. Otolaryngol Head Neck Surg 1992;106:175–80.
6. Brown KE, Whitney SL, Marchetti GF, et al. Physical therapy for central vestibular dysfunction. Arch Phys Med Rehabil 2006;87:76–81.
7. Cohen HS, Kimball KT. Decreased ataxia and improved balance after vestibular rehabilitation. Otolaryngol Head Neck Surg 2004;130:418–25.
8. Herdman SJ, Blatt P, Schubert MC, et al. Falls in patients with vestibular deficits. Amer J Otol 2000;21:847–51.
9. Wrisley DM, Whitney SL, Furman JM. Vestibular rehabilitation outcomes in patients with a history of migraine. Laryngoscope 2002;23:483–7.
10. Eggers SD, De Pennington N, Walker MF, et al. Short-term adaptation of the VOR: Non-retinal-slip error signals and saccade substitution. Ann N Y Acad Sci 2003;1004:94–110.
11. Bowman A. Psychological and visual-perceptual explanations of poor compensation following unilateral vestibular loss. School of Psychology Doctoral Dissertation. The University of Sydney, Sydney; 2004. p. 130–41.
12. Redfern MS, Jennings JR, Martin C, et al. Attention influences sensory integration for postural control in older adults. Gait Posture 2001;14:211–6.
13. Furman JM, Cass SP. Vestibular Disorders: A Case Study Approach, 2nd edition. New York: Oxford University Press; 2002.
14. Meli A, Zimatore G, Badaracco C, et al. Vestibular rehabilitation and 6-month follow-up using objective and subjective measures. Acta Otolaryngol 2006;126:259–66.
15. Peterka RJ, Wall C, III, Kentala E. Determining the effectiveness of a vibrotactile balance prosthesis. J Vestib Res 2006;16:45–56.
16. Merfeld DM, Gong W, Morrissey J, et al. Acclimation to chronic constant-rate peripheral stimulation provided by a vestibular prosthesis. IEEE Trans Biomed Eng 2006;53:2362–72.
17. Danilov Y, Tyler M. Brainport: An alternative input to the brain. J Integr Neurosci 2005;4:537–50.
18. Lord SR, Dayhew J, Howland A. Multifocal glasses impair edge-contrast sensitivity and depth perception and increase the risk of falls in older people. J Am Geriatr Soc 2002;50:1760–6.
19. Badke MB, Shea TA, Miedaner JA, et al. Outcomes after rehabilitation for adults with balance dysfunction. Arch Phys Med Rehab 2004;85:227–33.
20. Whitney SL, Wrisley D, Furman JM. Concurrent validity of the Berg Balance Scale and the Dynamic Gait Index in people with vestibular dysfunction. Physiother Res Int 2003;8:178–86.
21. Suarez H, Arocena M, Suarez A, et al. Changes in postural control parameters after vestibular rehabilitation in patients with central vestibular disorders. Acta Otolaryngol (Stockh) 2003;123:143–7.
22. Furman JM, Whitney SL. Central causes of dizziness. Phys Ther 2000;80:179–87.
23. Furman JM, Balaban CD, Pollack IF. Vestibular compensation in a patient with a cerebellar infarction. Neurology 1997;48:916–20.

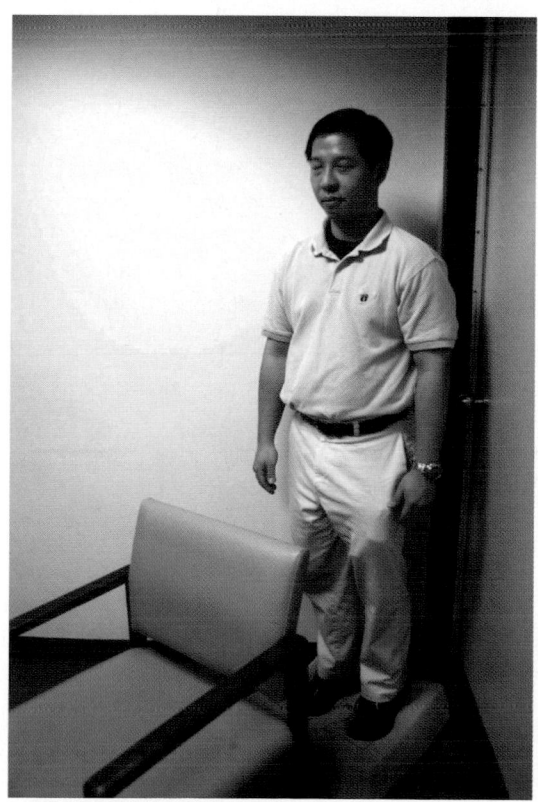

Figure 4 The patient is asked to stand on a couch cushion in a corner with a chair in front of them with their eyes open or closed. This exercise is often given to patients who have difficulty walking on uneven surfaces.

24. Stewart W, Breslau N, Keek PE. Comorbidity of migraine and panic disorder. Neurology 1994;44:23–7.

25. Neuhauser H, Leopold M, von Brevern M, et al. The interrelations of migraine, vertigo, and migrainous vertigo. Neurology 2001;56:436–41.

26. Cass SP, Furman JM, Ankerstjerne JKP, et al. Migraine-related vestibulopathy. Ann Otol Rhinol Laryngol 1997;106:182–9.

27. Johnson GD. Medical management of migraine-related dizziness and vertigo. Laryngoscope 1998;108:1–28.

28. Ingebrigtsen T, Waterloo K, Marup-Jensen S, et al. Quantification of post-concussion symptoms 3 months after minor head injury in 100 consecutive patients. J Neurol 1998;245:609–12.

29. Furman JM, Cass SP. Vestibular Disorders: a Case Study Approach. New York: Oxford University Press; 2003. p. 360.

30. Schubert MC, Das V, Tusa RJ, et al. Cervico-ocular reflex in normal subjects and patients with unilateral vestibular hypofunction. Otol Neurotol 2004;25:65–71.

31. Karlberg M, Magnusson M, Malmstrom EM, et al. Postural and symptomatic improvement after physiotherapy in patients with dizziness of suspected cervical origin. Arch Phys Med Rehab 1996;77:874–82.

32. Fitz-Ritson D, Assessment of cervicogenic vertigo. J Manipul Physiol Ther 1991;14:193–8.

33. Tjell C, Rosenhall U. Smooth pursuit neck torsion test: A specific test for cervical dizziness. Amer J Otol 1998;19:76–81.

34. Endo K, Ichimaru K, Shimura H, et al. Cervical vertigo after hair shampoo treatment at a hairdressing salon: A case report. Spine 2000;25:632–4.

35. Shepard NT, Telian SA, Smith-Wheelock M, et al. Vestibular and balance rehabilitation therapy. Ann Otol Rhinol Laryngol 1993;102:198–205.

36. Konrad HR, Tomlinson D, Stockwell CW, et al. Rehabilitation therapy for patients with disequilibrium and balance disorders. Otolaryngol Head Neck Surg 1992;107:105–8.

37. Cowand JL, Wrisley DM, Walker M, et al. Efficacy of vestibular rehabilitation. Otolaryngol Head Neck Surg 1998;118:49–54.

38. Jacobson GP, Newman CW. The development of the Dizziness Handicap Inventory. Acta Otolaryngol (Stockh) 1990;116:424–7.

39. Jacob R, Woody SR, Clark DB, et al. Discomfort with space and motion: A possible marker of vestibular dysfunction assessed by the Situational Characteristics Questionnaire. J Psychopathol Behav Assess 1993;15:299–32.

40. Pavlou M, Lingeswaran A, Davies RA, et al. Simulator based rehabilitation in refractory dizziness. J Neurol 2004;251:983–95.

41. Bamiou DE, Davies RA, McKee M, et al. Symptoms, disability and handicap in unilateral peripheral vestibular disorders. Effects of early presentation and initiation of balance exercises. Scand Audiol 2000;29:238–44.

42. Johansson M, Akerlund D, Larsen HC, et al. Randomized controlled trial of vestibular rehabilitation combined with cognitive-behavioral therapy for dizziness in older people. Otolaryngol Head Neck Surg 2001;125:151–6.

43. Marchetti GF, Whitney SL. Construction and validation of the 4-item dynamic gait index. Phys Ther 2006;86:1651–60.

44. Shumway-Cook A, Woollacott M. Motor Control: Theory and Practical Applications. Baltimore: Williams and Wilkins; 1995. p. 220–1.

45. Podsiadlo D, Richardson S. The timed "Up & Go": A test of basic functional mobility for frail elderly persons. J Am Geriatr Soc 1991;67:387–9.

46. Whitney SL, Marchetti GF, Schade A, et al. The sensitivity and specificity of the Timed "Up & Go" and the Dynamic Gait Index for self-reported falls in persons with vestibular disorders. J Vestib Res 2004;14:397–409.

47. Lord S, Murray S, Chapman K, et al. Sit-to-Stand performance depends on sensation, speed, balance, and psychological status in addition to strength in older people. J Gerontol 2002;57A:M539–43.

48. Whitney SL, Wrisley DM, Brown KE, et al. Is perception of handicap related to functional performance in persons with vestibular dysfunction? Otol Neurotol 2004;25:139–43.

49. Powell LE, Myers AM. The Activities-specific Balance Confidence (ABC) Scale. J Gerontol A Biol Sci Med Sci 1995;50A:M28–34.

50. Lajoie Y, Girard A, Guay M. Comparison of the reaction time, the Berg Scale and the ABC in non-fallers and fallers. Arch Gerontol Geriatr 2002;35:215–25.

51. Myers AM, Fletcher PC, Myers AH, et al. Discriminative and evaluative properties of the activities-specific balance confidence (ABC) scale. J Gerontol Ser A Biol Sci Med Sci 1998;53:M287–94.

52. Perera S, Mody SH, Woodman RC, et al. Meaningful change and responsiveness in common physical performance measures in older adults. J Am Geriatr Soc 2006;54:743–9.

53. Hain TC, Uddin M. Pharmacological treatment of vertigo. CNS Drugs 2003;17:85–100.

31

Tinnitus and Decreased Sound Tolerance

Pawel J. Jastreboff, PhD, ScD, MBA
Margaret M. Jastreboff, PhD

TINNITUS

Tinnitus is commonly described as a perception of sound that is not related to an external acoustic source or electrical stimulation.[1] National Center for Health Statistics categorizes tinnitus as chronic if it lasts at least 3 months.[2] It is an extremely common condition, but only a fraction of those who experience tinnitus are significantly disturbed by it.[3–5] Moreover, it has been shown that perception of tinnitus can be evoked in 94% of young, healthy subjects by putting them in a sufficiently low level of sound.[6] A recent experiment has confirmed this effect.[7] Although there is a lack of objective measures of tinnitus, no clear agreement as to the efficient way to help those suffering with tinnitus and many unanswered questions, significant progress has been made over the past quarter century in the tinnitus field. Still, most patients are given the unfortunate advice: "Learn to live with it."

Tinnitus is not a disease. It is a symptom that, similar to pain, headache, or fever, can vary in severity and can affect patients' lives to varying degrees. Sounds described by patients have different spectra and loudness, can change in loudness and type of sound, and can persist or be transient.[1,3] Tinnitus can be annoying to those who experience it and lead to a vicious circle whereby the tinnitus becomes the center of attention in patients' lives. Additionally, tinnitus can exist independently or as part of a complex medical condition.[8] The cause is unclear and no specific site or molecular or cellular mechanism has been proven to be responsible for the initiation and continuation of tinnitus. Tinnitus affects people of all ages.[2]

Frequently, tinnitus is accompanied by decreased sound tolerance and hearing loss.[2,3,5,8–10] Decreased sound tolerance includes hyperacusis and/or misophonia. There is no consensus regarding the testing of loudness discomfort levels (LDLs) to evaluate the problem, and there are only limited normative data.[11,12] The prevalence and epidemiology of hyperacusis are not well documented, and its etiology and mechanisms are poorly understood. Hyperacusis can occur alone or as an adjunct to complex medical conditions. Gradual desensitization can lead to the successful treatment of the problem.[13]

Definitions

Writings about tinnitus can be found in ancient documentation of Babylonian, Egyptian, Greek, Indian, and Assyrian medicine. Throughout the world, a variety of terms have been used to describe a ringing, tinkling (Latin, tinnire), buzzing, whistling, or unpleasant sound (French, acouphnes) in the ears or in the head, leaving us with the two most commonly used terms, tinnitus (in English) and acufenos (in Spanish). The historical review of tinnitus may be found in a number of publications, particularly those by Stephens.[14–16]

There is no precise, short, and distinctive definition of tinnitus. Today, commonly used definitions of tinnitus focus on different characteristics. Definitions that are based on patients' experiences describe tinnitus as: ringing, buzzing, the sound of escaping steam, hissing, humming, cricket-like, or noise in the ears.[1,5] Tinnitus as "a phantom auditory perception" represents a physiologic definition of tinnitus pointing out a lack of a physical acoustic stimulus related to tinnitus.[17,18] There is also the definition proposed by the Committee on Hearing, Bioacoustics and Biomechanics of the US National Research Council: "a conscious experience of sound that originates in the head" of its owner.[1]

Etiology, Prevalence, and Epidemiology

The results of studies conducted in numerous places around the world have shown a significant variability in the estimation of tinnitus prevalence in the general population.[3–5,19–23] Recent epidemiological data confirmed previous findings, pointing to even higher prevalence of bothersome tinnitus in the United States of about 8% compared with the 4% previously reported.[2] A total of 6 to 17% of the general population experience tinnitus lasting for a period of at least 5 minutes. About 3 to 7% of the general population seek help for their tinnitus, and 0.5 to 2.5% report that tinnitus has severe effect upon their life.[1,3–5,23] The prevalence of tinnitus in adults with hearing problems is high (59 to 86%), and it is estimated that tinnitus is present in 50% of patients with sudden hearing loss, 70% with presbyacusis, and 50 to 90% with noise-induced hearing loss.[2,24]

The prevalence of tinnitus increases significantly with aging, except in the highest age group when it declines,[2] but people of all ages experience tinnitus.[3,5,10,25] Although frequently not reported, children are also affected by tinnitus, and the estimated prevalence is similar to that reported in adults. Nodar, in a sample of 2,000 children, reported the average prevalence of 15%, with 13.3% for children with normal hearing and 58.6% with hearing loss.[26] Similar data were reported by others with a general prevalence in the range of 15 to 29% in healthy children and approximately 50% in children with otologic problems or hearing loss.[27,28] A significant proportion of children reported having problems with tinnitus including: sleep disturbance (42%), problems with concentration (47%), and sensitivity to sound (33%).[29] In younger healthy children (age 5 to 16 years), 29% have tinnitus and 9.6% reported their tinnitus as troublesome.[27] Recent data from a survey performed in Turkey on school children revealed that 15.1% of children had tinnitus, which was typically high pitched, of soft loudness, and described as ringing.[30] A study performed in Italy showed that out of 1,100 children, 34% of them had tinnitus and 6.5% complained about it,[31] and a study from Sweden showed 8.7% self-reported tinnitus and 17.1% self-reported decreased sound tolerance.[32]

Extensive studies have been performed in an attempt to link various factors with tinnitus prevalence.[1–3,10,19] Hearing loss, specifically the extent of high frequency impairment in the worse ear, is one of the main predicting factors for tinnitus.[3] Conductive hearing loss seems to be a separate factor,[33] and noise exposure has been correlated with tinnitus as well.[19] Tinnitus is also experienced by those with normal hearing; 18% of tinnitus patients were reported to have normal hearing.[33]

Other factors do not appear to be correlated with tinnitus. Pregnancy has been shown to increase significantly the probability of tinnitus.[34] Neither smoking, coffee, nor alcohol has been shown to increase tinnitus prevalence directly.[35,37] Severity of tinnitus is associated with severity of anxiety and depression,[38] and tinnitus seems to affect patients' cognitive abilities.[39,40] The main risk factors associated with the presence of tinnitus are age, male sex, lower level of education, lower annual income, being a military service veteran, poor general health status, being obese, significant hearing loss, exposure at work for more than 15 hours per week to loud sound, exposure to impulse noise, and daily smoking cigarettes.[2] Interestingly, being in the managerial or administrative or technical sales occupational group as well as moderate alcohol consumption were associated with reduced risk for tinnitus.[2]

Mechanisms and Models

Our knowledge of the mechanisms of tinnitus is still limited and based more on theoretical speculations than on strong research data or stringent clinical studies. Past models were focused on peripheral mechanisms in the auditory system,[41–50] whereas recent models tend to involve or even focus on processing information within the central auditory pathways and central nervous system.[17,41,51,52] Although the molecular and genetic basis for tinnitus is not known, brain-derived neurotrophic factor (BDNF) and the activity-dependent cytoskeletal protein (Arg3.1/arc) have been found to be potentially related with acoustic trauma induced tinnitus at both peripheral and central levels.[53] The neurophysiologic model of tinnitus combines all levels and differentiates between the perception of tinnitus versus tinnitus-induced activation of nonauditory structures in the brain.[9,17,42,43,54] The discordant damage/dysfunction theory of the generation of the tinnitus signal postulates that the tinnitus signal is generated at the level of dorsal cochlear nucleus as a result of imbalanced activation coming from outer and inner hair cells.[13,17] Specifically, when outer hair cells are dysfunctional at a certain region of the basilar membrane and inner hair cells in the same region are still working, this yields disinhibition in the dorsal cochlear nucleus and thereby generation of the tinnitus signal.[42] This theory explains many tinnitus conundrums[17,42] and is accumulating support from experimental data.[55–60] Table 1 summarizes the approaches to the mechanisms of tinnitus.

Tinnitus as a Symptom of Medically Treatable Diseases

Tinnitus may also be a part of more complex medical conditions, and some of these are identified in Table 2.

DECREASED SOUND TOLERANCE

Tinnitus is frequently accompanied by decreased sound tolerance, that is, oversensitivity to sound,[4,8,17,22,80–84] which, in many cases, is a sum of hyperacusis and misophonia.[80,85]

Definitions

There is no generally accepted definition for decreased sound tolerance to suprathreshold sounds although a variety of terms have been proposed, with hyperacusis used most frequently. According to Stedman's Medical Dictionary,[86] hyperacusis is defined as "Abnormal acuteness of hearing due to increased irritability of the sensory neural mechanism. Syn: auditory hyperesthesia,"

Table 1 Main Concepts Related to Proposed Mechanisms of Tinnitus

Structures involved
  Auditory system
    Periphery (cochlea, auditory nerve)
    Central auditory pathways
  Auditory and central nervous system
Manifestation of tinnitus-related neuronal activity
  Increase in spontaneous activity
  Modification in temporal patterns of discharges, including bursting activity
  Synchronization of the activity between neurons
Proposed mechanisms responsible for the emergence of tinnitus-related neuronal activity
  Abnormal coupling between neurons
  Local decrease of spontaneous activity enhanced by lateral inhibition
  Discordant damage/dysfunction of outer and inner hair cells
  Unbalanced activation of Type I and II auditory nerve fibers
  Abnormal neurotransmitter release from inner hair cells
  Decreased activity of the efferent system
  Mechanical displacement within the organ of Corti
  Abnormalities in transduction processes
  Various aspects of calcium function
  Physical/biochemical stress on the auditory nerve
  Enhanced sensitivity of the auditory pathways after decreased auditory input
  Hypoxia and ischemia in the cochlea
  Neuronal plasticity and cortical reorganization
  Cortical reorganization of tonotopic maps and hypersynchrony
  Somatosensory-auditory interaction
Level of interest
  Molecular-ion channels, synapses, cellular membranes
  Single neuron-processing information within one cell
  Neuronal assemblies-interaction within group of cells
  System-interaction between various systems in the brain
Somatosounds
  Included as "objective tinnitus"
  Separated with name tinnitus reserved to auditory phantom perception

Adapted from references 24, 42–45, and 61–76.

Table 2 Medical Conditions That May Be Associated with Tinnitus

Conductive hearing losses
  Otitis media, cerumen impaction
  Ossicular stiffness/discontinuity
  Otosclerosis
Sensorineural hearing losses
  Meniere disease
  Presbyacusis
  Cochlear otosclerosis
  Vestibular schwannoma
  Sudden hearing loss
Hormonal changes
  Pregnancy, menopause
  Thyroid dysfunction
Some medications or withdrawal from them
Somatosounds
  Produced by structures adjacent to the ear
    Pulsatile
      Neoplasm
      Arterial
      Venous
      Beginning of intracranial hypertension
      Great vessel bruits
    Nonpulsatile
      Tensor tympani myoclonus
      Tensor veli palatini myoclonus
      Patulous eustachian tube
  Produced by structures in the ear
    Spontaneous otoacoustic emissions
  Produced by joint abnormalities
    Temporomandibular joint disorders

Adapted from references 42 and 77–79.

with hyperesthesia defined as "Abnormal acuteness of sensitivity to touch, pain, or other sensory stimuli" or, according to American Heritage Dictionary, as "An abnormal or pathological increase in sensitivity to sensory stimuli, as of the skin to touch or the ear to sound."[87] It has been recognized that decreased sound tolerance might reflect physical discomfort or be related to a fear of sound.[8]

We proposed the approach to decreased sound tolerance based on neurophysiology, recognizing the systems that can be involved: the auditory system, both peripheral and central parts, and the limbic and autonomic nervous systems and consequently propose the following definitions. Hyperacusis is defined as abnormally strong reactions to sound occurring within the auditory pathways. At the behavioral level, it is manifested by a subject experiencing physical discomfort as a result of exposure to moderate/weak sound

that would not evoke such reaction in the average population. The strength of a reaction is linked to the physical characterization of a sound, for example, its spectrum and intensity. Misophonia is defined as abnormally strong reactions of the autonomic and limbic systems without abnormally high activation of the auditory system, resulting from enhanced connections between the auditory and limbic systems. At the behavioral level, patients have a generally negative attitude to sound (misophonia, from Greek: miso meaning strong dislike, hate) or could specifically be afraid of sound (phonophobia; phobia, fear). In this classification, phonophobia is a specific case of misophonia. The strength of a reaction will be only partially determined by the physical characterization of a sound and will depend on the patient's previous evaluation of a sound, for example, potential threat, beliefs that it can be harmful, the patient's psychological profile, and the context in which the sound is presented.

Note that neither hyperacusis nor misophonia have any relation to the threshold of hearing, which can be normal or can reflect hearing loss.

Most frequently, decreased sound tolerance results from a combination of hyperacusis and misophonia. It is important to assess the presence and the extent of both phenomena in a patient as each needs to be treated using different methods. Terms used in the literature do not differentiate these problems; and, since the reported decreased sound tolerance is typically dominated by hyperacusis, we will use the term hyperacusis in describing reports in the literature.

Additionally, note that the term recruitment is not related to a decreased sound tolerance or hyperacusis. Recruitment refers to unusually rapid growth of loudness as the level of a tone is increased, occurs in association with hearing loss, and is purely a cochlear phenomenon. It might coexist with hyperacusis, but there is no functional link between these two phenomena.

Prevalence and Epidemiology of Decreased Sound Tolerance

There are limited data available on the prevalence of hyperacusis. Questionnaires provide an assessment of hyperacusis prevalence in the general population. Recent data gathered from 10,349 randomly selected subjects showed that 15.3% reported hyperacusis.[22] Patients being evaluated for other otologic problems frequently undergo audiologic evaluation, which involves assessment of speech discomfort level and puretone LDLs. There are no good normative data. Several studies indicated that in the normal population, LDLs are in the range of 90 to 110 dB SPL, with varied results depending on the specific method used, for example, stimuli: pure tone, warble tone, noise; presentation: free field, insert earphones, headphones; and instructions given to patients.[11,88–90] Moreover, these measurements are not part of a routine audiological evaluation. The results tend to cluster within 95 to 110 dB sound pressure level (SPL) for frequencies from 500 to 8,000 Hz, which correspond to approximately 90 to 100 dB hearing level (HL).[11,88,91]

Hyperacusis and tinnitus frequently coexist, and it has been postulated that in some patients, hyperacusis might actually be a pretinnitus state.[17] Approximately 60% of tinnitus patients exhibit decreased sound tolerance, with about 30% requiring specific treatment for hyperacusis.[80,92–94] Conversely, study of 100 patients with hypersensitivity to sound showed that 86% of them suffered from tinnitus.[95] Considering the clinical observation that approximately 30% of tinnitus patients required treatment for hyperacusis and 86% of hyperacusis patients reported tinnitus and accepting that about 4 to 5% of the general population have clinically significant tinnitus, it is possible to estimate that significant hyperacusis exists in approximately 1 to 1.5% of the general population. An even larger proportion has some hyperacusis that, although detectable in questionnaires, is not sufficiently strong to initiate intervention.

EVALUATION OF TINNITUS

We do not have any objective method to detect and measure tinnitus. Therefore, interview and psychoacoustic characterization are typical approaches in clinical practice, sometimes expanding into the direction of physiologic testing. New advances in research offer the possibility to detect tinnitus in an objective manner using imaging techniques[96–99] or magnetoencephalography.[18] These techniques are promising but

Table 3 Methods Used for Evaluation of Tinnitus

Interview/questionnaires
Psychoacoustic
　Perceptual location
　Pitch
　Loudness
　Maskability
　Postmasking effects
Physiologic
　Otoacoustic emissions
　Efferent-mediated suppression of otoacoustic emissions
　Spontaneous auditory nerve activity
　Auditory brainstem responses
　Late cortical potentials
　Positron emission tomography/single photon emission tomography
　Functional magnetic resonance imaging
　Magnetoencephalography

Adapted from references 80 and 100–107.

cannot yet be implemented into clinical practice owing to their complexity and cost. Table 3 lists the methods used for evaluation of tinnitus.

Problems Evoked by Tinnitus

As tinnitus can present as part of a complex medical condition, a complete medical evaluation is needed to exclude all medically treatable problems that can be linked to tinnitus. Even though tinnitus is classified as a symptom and not a disease, it does require treatment as it can cause significant emotional and somatic distress and can significantly influence patients' quality of life, particularly if allowed to become a chronic problem. The list of reported associated complaints is long and includes emotional problems, such as irritation, annoyance, anxiety, stress and depression; hearing problems such as difficulty with speech comprehension; and somatic problems such as headache, neck pain, and jaw pain.[1,8,108,109] Tinnitus can be intrusive and may cause difficulty with sleep and concentration and a decreased ability to participate in everyday activities and social events; it may also create problems in relationships. A detailed interview, aimed at characterizing the specifics and degree of tinnitus impact on the patient's life, coupled with an otolaryngologic evaluation, provides the most thorough assessment and allows the practitioner to address all of the issues that need to be considered, including potential intervention of a psychologist or psychiatrist to accompany the commencement of a specific tinnitus oriented treatment.

Hyperacusis and Misophonia as a Problem

Decreased sound tolerance can have an extremely strong effect on patients' lives and can be even more debilitating than tinnitus. Whereas tinnitus may affect attention, sleep, work, and life enjoyment and make social contact less rewarding, hyperacusis can prevent people from exposing themselves to louder environments and therefore prevent them from working and interacting

socially; it can also control a patient's life. In extreme cases, patients do not leave their homes, and their lives and the lives of their families are controlled by the issue of avoidance of sound. Misophonia can have similar effects; and, since it is inevitable in all cases with significant hyperacusis, misophonia further enhances the effects of hyperacusis.

Decreased Sound Tolerance as a Symptom of Medical Conditions

Hyperacusis has been linked to a number of medical conditions (Table 4).

Etiology and Potential Mechanisms of Decreased Sound Tolerance

In the majority of cases, the cause of hyperacusis is unknown. Hyperacusis has been linked to sound exposure (particularly short, impulse noise), head injury, stress, medications, and some medical conditions. The lack of strong epidemiologic data and animal models of hyperacusis prevents proving the validity of any potential mechanism responsible for hyperacusis.

At the peripheral level, it is possible to speculate that the abnormal enhancement of vibratory signals within the cochlea by the outer hair cells might result in overstimulation of the inner hair cells and subsequently results in hyperacusis.[17] Indeed, in some cases, it is possible to observe high amplitude distortion product otoacoustic emissions and distortion products evoked by low level primaries.[124] The presence of asymmetric hyperacusis[80] might indicate a peripheral mechanism since central mechanisms would more likely act similarly on both sides.

Laboratory research has shown that damage to the cochlea or a decrease in the auditory input results in a decrease of the threshold of response in a significant proportion of neurons in the ventral cochlear nucleus and inferior colliculus.[125] Studies with evoked potentials indicated abnormal increase of the gain in the auditory pathways after such manipulations.[126] Some of the medical conditions listed in Table 4 can be linked to the central processing of signals and modification of the level of neuromodulators as possible

Table 4 Medical Conditions Linked to Hyperacusis

Tinnitus
Williams syndrome
Bell palsy
Lyme disease
Ramsay Hunt syndrome
Stapedectomy
Perilymphatic fistula
Head injury
Migraine
Depression
Withdrawal from benzodiazepines
Cerebrospinal fluid hypertension
Addison disease
Translabyrinthine excision of a vestibular schwannoma

Adapted from references 80 and 110–123.

factors inducing or enhancing hyperacusis. Moreover, serotonin has been implicated in hyperacusis,[127] and a case report indicated that serotonin reuptake inhibitors might be helpful for hyperacusis.[119]

Mechanisms of misophonia could involve enhancement of the functional links between the auditory and limbic systems, both at the cognitive and subconscious levels.[17] Alternatively, a tonic high level of activation of the limbic and autonomic nervous systems may result in strong behavioral reactions to moderate sounds.[54,128]

Methods of Evaluation of Decreased Sound Tolerance

Whereas there is no one clearly accepted method for the evaluation of decreased sound tolerance, hyperacusis, and misophonia, there is a general agreement that LDLs provide a good estimation of the problem. There are several variants of the protocols of LDL evaluation with various features, for example, continuous, pulsed, or beeps of sound; pure tone; narrow-band noise.[89,129,130] The approach we are pursuing incorporates modifications of the standard procedure[88] aimed at obtaining results dominated by hyperacusis by decreasing the effects of the misophonic component to a minimum. To achieve this, a situation is created during testing in which patients have the feeling of full control over the maximal sound level to which they will be exposed.[80] A detailed interview is needed with each patient to determine the relative contribution of hyperacusis and misophonia to decreased sound tolerance, reflected in decreased values of LDLs. As normative data are not uniform and there is substantial individual variability (even while using one method) in measuring LDL,[90] it is advisable to pay attention to the potential presence of hyperacusis when average across the frequencies LDL values are lower than 95 to 100 dB HL.

REVIEW OF TREATMENTS

The list of approaches and techniques attempted to help with patients tinnitus is long. Table 5 lists the most commonly used of these treatments.

Antireassurance

Over the years, the most common advice given to tinnitus patients has been, "Nothing can be done—go home and learn to live with it."[9,82] This is actually a powerful form of negative counseling, sufficient on many occasions to convert a person who just experiences tinnitus to a patient who suffers from it.[17,81,85]

Pharmacotherapy

Many pharmacologic agents have been considered for tinnitus treatment[8,133–135] (Table 6) but no single, effective, specific, secure, and reliable drug has yet to be identified.[67,136–142] In this respect, strong consideration must be given to the side effects of pharmacologic treatments, such as tolerance, dependence, and withdrawal effects. Recent reviews of randomized clinical trials of drugs for tinnitus have shown that all studied drugs have failed to prove their efficacy, as compared with a placebo.[133,143] Future double-blind randomized studies, with proper outcome measurements and adequate sample size, might identify some promising pharmacologic agents.[144–147]

Surgery

Surgery can offer help to some patients with somatosound, conductive hearing loss, and Meniere disease.[8] However, there is no specific surgical procedure shown to be consistently effective for tinnitus that does not have a clear surgically treatable cause. Neither transection nor microvascular decompression of the auditory nerve, promoted in the past,[148,149] has proven to be effective.[77,150,151]

Sound Therapies

A wide variety of therapies focused on sound is used, for example, music therapies, auditory discrimination therapy, pink noise therapy, desensitization, dynamic tinnitus mitigation system, phase shift tinnitus reduction, auditory integration training, masking relief therapy, neuromonics, and tinnitus retraining therapy (TRT).[13,152–155] They are based on various presumed mechanisms of sound action on tinnitus and implement different sounds and counseling. Sound modifications may involve varying intensity within a short

time, different intensities for specific stages of treatment, phase modifications, or complex processing of the sound. It is not clear which type of sound processing and protocol of sound use are optimal. For the majority of methods, results were not published in peer-reviewed journals and there are not sufficiently strong data from systematic studies to determine which of these methods might be effective in alleviating tinnitus.

Specific sound therapy is used as an integral part of TRT to achieve consistent and prolonged weakening of tinnitus signal and desensitization of the auditory system, with type and protocol of the sound used based on the neurophysiologic model of tinnitus.[13] According to the neurophysiologic model of tinnitus, any sound is better than silence, as long as it does not annoy, create discomfort, or damage hearing. Counseling appropriate to a given implementation of sound therapy is important as well.

Electrical Suppression

Electrical suppression of tinnitus was first reported in 1855.[156] Over the years, many different approaches have been attempted, and methods based on electrical stimulation are still of interest (Table 7).[156,157] Three new variants of electrical stimulation for tinnitus have been introduced over the last several years. The first involves deep brain stimulation, sometimes performed for movement disorder and chronic pain.[158] Anecdotal reports of patients receiving deep brain stimulation initiated an investigation that demonstrated that, indeed, some patients experienced a decrease in their tinnitus with deep brain stimulation.[159] A second approach involves high frequency electrical stimulation of the cochlea performed by placing an electrode on the promontory or via a cochlear implant.[160] A third approach involves direct electrical stimulation of the auditory cortex via electrodes placed on the auditory cortex.[161]

All these approaches are at an early stage of investigation. Only intracochlear or promontory stimulation has shown consistent and positive results in approximately 50% of patients.[157,162,163] Other approaches were less effective.[156] Although

---

Table 5 Review of Treatments for Tinnitus

Antireassurance
Pharmacology
Surgery
Electrical stimulation
Sound therapies
Psychological approaches
Tinnitus retraining therapy
Other approaches
  Biofeedback
  Temporomandibular joint treatment
  Acupuncture
  Hyperbaric oxygen therapy
  Homeopathy
  Magnets

Adapted from references 77, 131, and 132.

Table 6 Drugs Frequently Prescribed for Treatment for Tinnitus

Local anesthetics (lidocaine, procaine, tocainide, flecainide)
Sedatives (diazepam, flurazepam, oxazepam, alprazolam)
Antidepressants (nortriptyline, trimipramine)
Anticonvulsants (carbamazepine, clonazepam, aminooxyacetic acid, lamotrigine, baclofen)
Vasodilators (niacin)
Calcium channel blockers (nimodipine, nifedipine)
Others (misoprostol, zinc, betahistine, cinnarizine, caroverine, melatonin, furosemide, ginkgo biloba)

Adapted from references 8 and 134.

Table 7 Conditions Used in Electrical Stimulation for Suppression of Tinnitus

Sites of stimulation
  Behind the ear lobe/around the ear
  Mastoid
  Near cheeks
  External auditory canal
  Promontory
  Tympanic membrane
  Round window
  Intracochlear
Type of stimulus
  Direct current/positive pulses
  Alternating current
  Amplitude-modulated high-frequency carrier
Electrodes
  Acute/chronic

Adapted from references 156 and 157.

positive direct/pulsed current can provide tinnitus suppression,[164] it has no clinical application as it would damage the cochlea if used for a prolonged period of time.

Transcranial Magnetic Stimulation (TMS)

TMS uses short pulses of a powerful magnetic field to stimulate the brain cortex. The method, primarily used for psychiatric disorders (but not approved by the United States Food and Drug Administration [FDA]), has recently been investigated for tinnitus.[165,166] The magnetic field easily crosses the skull and induces a strong electrical field, perpendicular to the magnetic field, which in turn activates neurons in the cortex. As such, the final effect is electrical stimulation of the cortex. The relative position of the axons and dendrites of neurons to the evoked electrical field is crucial and depending on this relationship one group of neurons can be activated while another in the same area will not be activated. Consequently, changing the angle of the magnetic coil will modify which neurons are going to be stimulated within the active area, which is about 1 inch. in diameter. Moreover, as the cortex is highly convoluted, only some parts will be activated. All these factors, combined with the fact that the auditory cortex is in deeper part of a sulcus, create a challenge to achieve repetitive, stable results while using this method for tinnitus.

In addition to immediate effects longer lasting consequences are of clinical interest. There are two types of TMS differentiated by the frequency of stimulation. When higher frequency is used, TMS has an inhibitory effect on cortical activity reflected in immediate attenuation of tinnitus perception, which lasts only for a limited period of time.[167] When low frequency (1 Hz) stimulation is used over a period of days, this presumably evokes plastic changes in the cortical areas and their connections with subcortical centers. The initial effect might be absence of tinnitus or the tinnitus might even increase; but, over a period of time, the tinnitus is attenuated and its effects may last for some time.

The strong positive aspect of TMS is that it does not require opening the skull and can be done on conscious subjects easily, which have encouraged its use and a number of studies of its effect on tinnitus.[165,168,169] The results showed a statistically significant attenuation of tinnitus and a decrease in the negative impact of tinnitus. It is still not clear, however, to what extent this improvement has practical clinical value and how long it can be sustained.[166,170–172] There is concern as well regarding permanent changes induced in the brain by TMS and, therefore, the safety of the method.

Masking

The use of an external sound to cover tinnitus and, thus, bring immediate relief to patients, known as masking, was first used in 1825 by Itard.[14] At the end of the 1970s, Vernon and Schleuning revisited this idea and introduced the first commercial masker.[173,174] Initial reports proclaimed high success of maskers,[175,176] but the approach did not withstand the test of time.[133,134] One of the problems was the criterion used in evaluating the effectiveness of masking; for example, if the masker was still in use after 6 months, it was counted as a success.[175,176] Obviously, patients may continue using maskers even while not getting relief from their tinnitus. Presently, this method of alleviation of tinnitus is rarely used.

Recently, the term masking has been redefined, as Henry and colleagues have proposed, to use the term masking for therapy utilizing any sound which brings immediate relief, disregarding if perception of tinnitus is covered or not.[155] They described no specific counseling, only instruction about sound setting following the above definition. This therapy, which should be more appropriately labeled as a "relief therapy" utilizes sound levels close to those used in a variety of sound-based therapies, including TRT. While not as effective as TRT, it can be helpful for some patients, particularly those with a low level of tinnitus severity.[155]

Psychology

Psychological management of chronic tinnitus can be helpful for some patients.[177] As tinnitus affects patients' well-being, the application of cognitive behavioral therapies may have a positive impact on the quality of life by improving their ability to cope with tinnitus. Cognitive therapies, behavioral modifications, coping strategies, cognitive distraction, and minimizing distress are examples of the psychological approach.[178–180] Of particular interest seems to be methods of cognitive behavioral therapy (CBT).[181] Recent meta-analysis of all controlled, randomized clinical trials listed in the Cochrane ENT Group Trials Register, the Cochrane Central Register of Controlled Trials, MEDLINE and EMBASE identified six trials involving 285 patients and showed that while there were no effect of CBT on the subjective loudness of tinnitus or on depression, but cognitive behavioral therapy improved significantly quality of life.[182] Prospective study of 434 patients treated with integrative behavioral medicine treatment show significant improvement as well.[179]

NEUROPHYSIOLOGIC MODEL OF TINNITUS AND TINNITUS RETRAINING THERAPY

More than a decade and half has passed since the introduction of the neurophysiologic model of tinnitus and, based on it, treatment, which is known as TRT.[9,183–185] Several observations led to the neurophysiological model of tinnitus and hyperacusis. It is known that tinnitus induces distress in only about 20% of those who perceive it.[2,3,5,10] There is no correlation among the psychoacoustic characterization of tinnitus, tinnitus-induced distress, and the treatment outcome.[186] The experiment by Heller and Bergman showed that the perception of tinnitus cannot be pathologic since essentially everyone experiences it when put in a sufficiently quiet environment as evidenced by the emergence of tinnitus in 94% of people without prior tinnitus when isolated for several minutes in an anechoic chamber.[6] This phenomenon has been recently confirmed.[7] These observations strongly argue that the auditory system plays a secondary role, and other systems in the brain are dominant in clinically relevant tinnitus, that is, tinnitus that creates discomfort and annoyance and requires intervention.

Analysis of the problems reported by tinnitus patients, who exhibit a strong emotional reaction to its presence, a high level of anxiety, and psychosomatic problems, indicated that the limbic and autonomic nervous systems are crucial in individuals with clinically relevant tinnitus. It was postulated that the sustained activation of the limbic and autonomic nervous systems is essential in creating distress and, therefore, clinically relevant tinnitus.[17]

Tinnitus-related neuronal activity is processed by the parts of the central nervous system involved in memory and attention. It is possible to distinguish several feedback loops, with two major categories: loops involving the conscious perception of tinnitus and those that act at a subconscious level (Figure 1), with the subconscious loop dominant in most patients.[9,54] It is further suggested that the activation of the limbic and autonomic nervous systems by tinnitus-related neuronal activity follows the principles of conditioned reflexes.[54,85]

The processing of tinnitus-related neuronal activity occurs in a dynamic balance scenario, with continuous modification of the weight of synaptic connections. Both learning and memory have a physiologic basis in the modification of the strength of synaptic connections.[187] A continuous presence of tinnitus, combined with attention given to it, results in plastic modifications of synaptic connections, yielding the modification of receptive fields corresponding to the tinnitus signal and its subsequent enhancement.[42,54,188] This postulate has been proven using magnetoencephalography.[18]

Whereas the initial signal provided by the auditory system is needed to start the cascade of events, its strength is irrelevant, as the extent of activation of the limbic and autonomic nervous systems depends on the strength of negative associations linked to tinnitus and the susceptibility of the feed-back loops to modification.[189] It appears that tinnitus-related neuronal activity may result from compensatory processes that occur within the cochlea and the auditory pathways to minor dysfunction at the periphery.[17,42]

Notably, once plasticity-related modifications of neuronal connections occur, the peripheral signal itself may become of little importance, as is similarly observed in chronic pain.[43] Indeed, there are clear similarities between tinnitus and chronic pain, including the phenomenon of prolonged exacerbation of tinnitus as a result of exposure to sound, which is observed in some patients.[85,92]

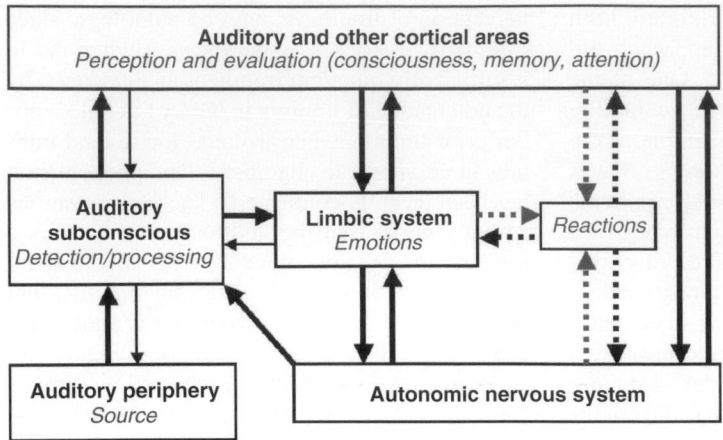

Figure 1 The neurophysiologic model of tinnitus.

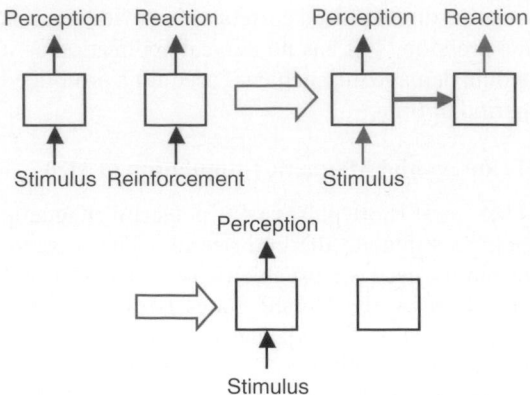

Figure 2 Principles of establishing conditioned reflexes and their passive extinction.

The neurophysiologic model includes several systems of the brain involved in analysis of clinically relevant tinnitus. All levels of the auditory pathways, starting from the cochlea through the subcortical centers and ending at the auditory cortex, are essential in creating the perception of tinnitus.[17] When subjects are not bothered or annoyed by tinnitus, auditory pathways are the only pathways involved, and tinnitus-related neuronal activity is constrained within the auditory system. Therefore, although subjects are perceiving tinnitus, they are not disturbed by it.[3,54,189]

In approximately 20% of those with tinnitus, strong negative emotions are induced, which, in turn, evoke a variety of physiological defense mechanisms of the brain. The limbic and autonomic nervous systems play a crucial role, and improper activation of these systems by tinnitus-related neuronal activity results at the behavioral level in the problems described by patients. The connections between the auditory, limbic, and autonomic systems with various cortical areas, as proposed in the neurophysiological model of tinnitus,[8,9,17,42,54,93] are outlined in Figure 1.

The model points out that the sustained activation of the limbic and autonomic nervous systems is responsible for the distress induced by clinically relevant tinnitus. Activation of both systems can be achieved through two routes branching at the level of thalamus (medial geniculate body). The first includes stimulation of the autonomic and limbic systems from higher level cortical areas, which are involved in our awareness, verbalization, and beliefs, called high, conscious or cortical in the neurophysiologic model of tinnitus.[9] The signal is passed from the medial geniculate body to the auditory cortices and then down to the amygdala. The second arises from the subconscious level, is called low subconscious or subcortical in the model, and provides stimulation from the lower level auditory centers, specifically linking directly the medial geniculate body with the amygdala and involves the extra-lemniscal auditory pathways.[69] These two paths are called the "high road" and the "low road."[190]

At the early stage of tinnitus, the high loop is dominant, and activation of the limbic and autonomic nervous systems are due to cognitive processing of the information and thinking about tinnitus. Later this loop and corticothalamic and corticolimbic interaction might still play a role in activation of the limbic and autonomic nervous systems. This postulate is supported by an analysis of spontaneous magnetoencephalography activity in tinnitus and control subjects which revealed enhancement of gamma band activity in tinnitus subjects and allows prediction of the laterality of tinnitus perception[72] as well by other studies assessing function of the limbic system in patients with tinnitus[191,192] and an animal model.[193]

Once negative associations with tinnitus are initiated, the low loop is automatically created and becomes dominant. The low loop does not involve cognition and is controlled by principles governing conditioned reflexes. Consequently, it is fast and activates the limbic and autonomic nervous systems before the higher loop may potentially modify reactions. Furthermore, conditioned reflexes cannot be modified by conscious thinking. Therefore, even though the patient may be totally convinced that tinnitus is benign, the negative reactions to the tinnitus signal will still occur.

The activation going through these two routes changes the strength of synaptic connections, enhancing the stimulation of the limbic and autonomic nervous systems by the tinnitus-related neuronal activity during the process of the development of tinnitus as a clinical problem. The question of how the neutral signal of tinnitus can evoke persistent strong distress can be answered by the principles of conditioned reflexes.[194] Basically, to create a conditional reflex, the temporal coincidence of sensory stimuli with negative (or positive) reinforcement is sufficient[183,189,194,195] (Figure 2). This initial association can be coincidental, without any real dependence. These types of associations of sensory stimuli are constantly created in normal life.

As long as the sensory stimulus is limited in time and there is no functional link between stimulus and reinforcement, this conditioned reflex will gradually disappear (habituate) owing to passive extinction of the reflex (the sensory stimulus is present but is not accompanied by a reinforcement) (see Figure 2). Since the 1930s, habituation has been defined as "The extinction of a conditioned reflex by repetition of the conditioned stimulus … the method by which the nervous system reduces or inhibits responsiveness during repeated stimulation."[194] Habituation of perception of this stimulus will follow in the same manner as for all unimportant stimuli.[13]

Notably, there are two different types of habituation. The first, habituation of reaction, is defined as "disappearance of a reaction to a neutral stimulus due to its repetitive appearance without reinforcement."[196] The second, habituation of perception, occurs when awareness of this particular stimulus disappears (Figure 3).[9] Habituations of reaction and perception are natural processes. Habituation is a crucial characteristic of brain function necessitated by the brain's inability to perform two tasks requiring complete attention simultaneously.

When forced to carry out two tasks concurrently that require full consciousness, the brain uses its function of task switching by actually devoting consciousness to only one task at a time. The brain areas involved in task switching have been indicated by a functional magnetic resonance imaging study.[197] If forced to monitor all of the incoming sensory stimuli, our brain would not be able to perform any tasks, except that of switching perception from one sensory stimulus to the other, ultimately paralyzing us in our actions.

To solve this problem, the central nervous system screens and categorizes all stimuli at the subconscious level. If the stimulus is new and unknown, it is passed to a higher cortical level where it is perceived and evaluated. However, in the case of a stimulus to which we have previously been exposed, the stimulus is compared with patterns stored in memory. If the stimulus was classified as unimportant and does not require action, it is blocked at the subconscious level of the auditory pathways and does not produce any reactions or reach the level of awareness. The reaction to this stimulus and its perception is habituated. In everyday life, habituation occurs to the majority of sensory stimuli surrounding us.

However, if a specific stimulus was once classified as important and, on the basis of comparison with the patterns stored in memory, was linked to something unpleasant or dangerous, this stimulus is perceived and attracts attention. Furthermore, the sympathetic part of the autonomic

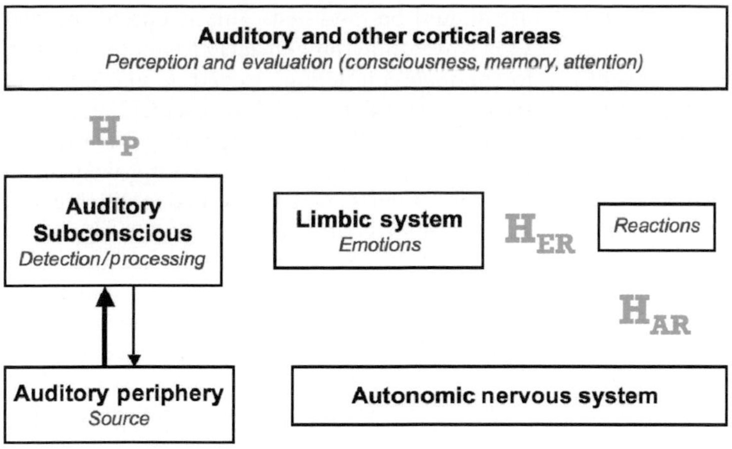

Auditory and other cortical areas
Perception and evaluation (consciousness, memory, attention)

H_P

Auditory Subconscious
Detection/processing

Limbic system
Emotions

H_{ER}

Reactions

H_{AR}

Auditory periphery
Source

Autonomic nervous system

Figure 3 Habituation of autonomic (H_{AR}) and emotional reactions (H_{ER}), and habituation of perception (H_P).

nervous system is activated, inducing reaction to this stimulus (frequently of the "fight or flight" category), which further reinforces memory patterns associated with this stimulus. Consequently, if the previous assessment of the importance of a stimulus has been confirmed, this specific stimulus becomes even more important; and its next appearance will result in faster identification, even in the presence of other competing stimuli, preventing the habituation of this stimulus. In the case of auditory stimuli, our auditory system becomes tuned to recognizing specific patterns of sound that have negative links. Under such conditions, the natural habituation of the tinnitus signal becomes impossible. In everyday life, this results in people having problems with their work, concentration, and sleep.

A simplistic description of the above process can be outlined to a patient as increased concern for tinnitus results in an increase of its significance, which ultimately increases the amount of time a person pays attention to it. This is a classic feedback loop or the "vicious circle" scenario, which increases patients' level of distress up to the limit of mental and physical endurance. At this stage, the patient will move from acute tinnitus, which can be easily relieved by proper counseling, into a chronic stage, which is much more difficult to deal with.

In the case of tinnitus, it is impossible to remove the reactions induced by the excitation of the sympathetic autonomic nervous system or even change them in a substantial manner. The solution to achieve the passive extinction of the conditioned reflex, in which both stimulus (tinnitus) and negative reinforcement are continuously present, is to decrease the magnitude of this negative reinforcement over a period of time. This will result in partial weakening of the reflex, but has to be applied consistently to yield positive effects. Moreover, it is fundamental that patients understand these principles so that the enhancement of this reflex by inducing too much verbal thinking and beliefs can be minimized.

Once activation of the autonomic nervous system is lowered, this decreases negative reinforcement to a signal that is continuously present and gradually decreases the strength of the conditioned reflex. This causes further decreases in the reaction. Once tinnitus has achieved a neutral status, its habituation is inevitable as the brain is continuously habituating to all types of stimuli, providing that they are not significant.

Consequently, retraining counseling (the first component of TRT) is oriented toward reclassification of tinnitus into a category of neutral stimuli and removal of the patient's negative associations with tinnitus. This is accomplished by educating the patients that their tinnitus results from a normal compensatory mechanism, which occurs in the auditory system, to typically minor changes in the cochlea. As part of counseling, it is also important to demystify the mechanisms through which tinnitus may affect a patient's life. Counseling in TRT is a teaching session aimed at providing patients with a new frame of reference by explaining potential mechanisms of tinnitus generation, neurophysiologic mechanisms through which tinnitus is influencing various aspects of their lives, and that by activating a naturally occurring mechanism of brain function (habituation and the plasticity underlying it), it is possible to achieve primarily habituation of the tinnitus-induced reaction of the brain and the body and secondarily habituation of the tinnitus perception. The clear goal of achieving an active and selective block of tinnitus-induced reactions is set for the patients.

The second component of TRT is sound therapy aimed at deceasing the strength of tinnitus signal in a systematic manner over the period of time of the treatment.[128,183] It is based on the following feature of brain function. All our senses are working on the principle of differences of the stimuli from the background, and the perceived strength of a signal is not linked directly to the physical strength of a stimulus. Presently, we cannot easily suppress tinnitus-related neuronal activity, but by increasing background neuronal activity, we are effectively decreasing the strength of this signal, which activates the limbic and autonomic nervous systems and which is being processed in all of the centers involved. There is no simple proportional relationship between the differences in tinnitus and background neuronal activity and the reactions induced by it. Nonetheless, we can achieve a decrease of reactions induced by the tinnitus and, through this, facilitate extinction of the conditioned reflex.

It is important to analyze the theoretical relationships existing between the physical intensity of sound and its effectiveness on tinnitus habituation (Figure 4). Five principles influence this relationship[128,183,184,198]: (1) stochastic resonance (enhancement of the signal by adding low level noise); (2) dependence of the signal's strength on its contrast with the background; (3) total suppression of the signal, preventing any retraining and consequently habituation; (4) partial suppression ("partial masking"), which does not prevent retraining but does make it more difficult as the training is performed on a different stimulus than the original; and (5) activation of limbic and autonomic nervous systems by too loud or unpleasant sounds, yielding an increase in tinnitus and contracting habituation.

It is intuitive that if the sound level is significantly below the threshold level of detection, there is no basis to believe that it asserts any effect on the auditory system and tinnitus. On the other hand, when external sound becomes strong enough to suppress detection of tinnitus-related neuronal activity, by definition, any kind of retraining (including habituation) is prevented because the brain cannot change reactions to a stimulus it cannot detect.

When the sound level is still below but close to the threshold of detection, the phenomenon of stochastic resonance, that is, addition of a low level of noise can decrease the threshold of detection of the stimulus and enhance it when the stimulus is weak and close to the threshold of detection, comes into play.[199] The presence of stochastic resonance has been shown at the level of hair cells and the auditory nerve, and preliminary data indicate its effect on the loudness of tinnitus.[198,200,201] The effective sound level inducing stochastic resonance covers a range of about 15 dB, beginning from about –9 dB below the threshold of detection of the additional noise. Thus, owing to stochastic resonance, by adding low level external noise, for example, by using sound generators set at the threshold of hearing,

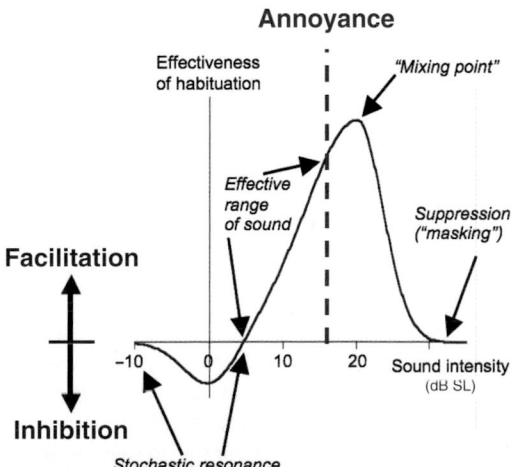

Figure 4 Functional dependence of habituation effectiveness on physical intensity of a sound. Notice the need to avoid sound levels close to the threshold of hearing, those inducing partial or total suppression and those evoking annoyance.

paradoxical enhancement of the tinnitus signal may occur. This will, in turn, make habituation more difficult. The results of a study in which a comparison was performed among groups with counseling only (including advice on using environmental sounds), counseling combined with sound generators set at the threshold of hearing, and counseling combined with sound generators set close to the "mixing" point fully support the prediction of the importance of stochastic resonance. The group that performed the worst was the one with the sound level set close to the threshold of hearing, whereas the group that performed the best was the one with the sound level set at the "mixing point," with the counseling-only group in the middle.[202]

When sound level is increased further, the mechanism involving the decreased difference between the tinnitus signals and background neuronal activity becomes the dominant factor. As with all perception, the difference between signal and background plays a dominant role. By decreasing the difference between the tinnitus-related neuronal activity and the background ongoing neuronal activity, the effective strength of the tinnitus signal decreases, and this weaker signal is passed to the higher level cortical areas and, most importantly, to the limbic and autonomic nervous systems. This helps in initiating and sustaining the process of passive extinction of conditioned reflexes that link tinnitus to negative reactions.[54,183] As the background activity is the sum of spontaneous and evoked activities, a decrease in the difference between the tinnitus signal and the background neuronal activity can be achieved by exposing patients to additional external sound.

This principle, if working alone, would imply that we should use a sound that is as intense as possible. Two other factors (3 and 4), however, become dominant. First, once the tinnitus signal is suppressed, by definition habituation will not occur owing to the lack of a signal to habituate (principle 3). Second, when the sound level surpasses the threshold of partial tinnitus suppression ("partial masking"), it will modify not only the intensity but also the quality (spectrum) of the tinnitus signal. Then retraining of neuronal networks will occur to the modified tinnitus signal and not to the original one. Owing to the generalization principle, that is, reaction can be induced to stimuli similar to the original, with the strength depending on the difference between the original and the modified signals, some habituation may still occur. The higher the external sound is above the threshold of partial masking, the smaller its contribution to habituation. Finally, once a level of total suppression is reached, the effectiveness of habituation is decreased to zero as the brain is unable to retrain to an undetectable signal.

The optimal setting of the sound level is different when hyperacusis is the dominant or the only problem. In this situation, the effect of stochastic resonance is of secondary importance to the primary need not to stimulate the auditory system sufficiently. Patients start with a sound level closer to their threshold but as high as their sound sensitivity allows, with the aim to be above the range of stochastic resonance. Once a partial reversal of hyperacusis is achieved, the sound level can be increased rapidly to address tinnitus directly. At this point, the rules previously outlined for patients with tinnitus should be followed.

Beneficial effects of the use of sound have been recently supported by results of experiments in which animals were exposed to a damaging sound level, which caused hearing loss and presumably tinnitus. Three groups of animals were studied: control, which were exposed to standard low level laboratory sound background, and two groups, which were subsequently exposed for several weeks to continuous broad-band, low, or high frequency sound. Control animals and animals exposed to low frequency continuous sound exhibited modification of the spontaneous activity recorded from the auditory cortex linked to tinnitus.[203] Neuronal activity recorded from animals exposed to continuous high frequency sound was, however, similar to activity recorded from animals which were not exposed to damaging sound and which did not have tinnitus.[66,74] These data support a postulate that continuous broad band sound may reverse tinnitus-related changes in the neuronal activity of the auditory cortex.

The need to preserve stimulation in the low frequency range yields a strong recommendation for people who have relatively normal low frequency hearing to be provided with devices or hearing aids with fittings as open as possible. It is not sufficiently appreciated that in the normal acoustic environment there is a high proportion of low frequency sounds, below 200 Hz, which provide constant stimulation of the auditory pathways. Since the majority of patients have relatively normal hearing in this frequency range, they benefit from this stimulation. Consequently, blocking the ear canal with closed ear molds decreases the auditory input, and many patients experience enhancement of tinnitus when their ears are blocked.

Note that even the best hearing aids act as earplugs in low frequencies when they are the in-the-canal type or are fitted with a closed mold as they are unable to reproduce frequencies below 200 to 250 Hz owing to restriction based on the physics of sound generation by a loudspeaker. Note that hearing aids for patients with tinnitus are used primarily as a part of sound therapy to provide extra amplification of background sounds and only secondarily for communicative purposes. Other tools may also be used to enrich the auditory background, such as nature sounds, neutral music, or tabletop sound generators.

Both counseling and sound use are dependent on patient categorization, and issues related to sound are summarized in Table 8. This categorization provides general guidance for treatment with TRT.[92,184] During the process of treatment, patients may move from one category to another, for example, hyperacusis can be totally eliminated and consequently the patient may move from category 3 to 1, and recommendations regarding sound use should be modified. This is one of the reasons why follow-up contacts are important; first, to continue counseling, second, to check patient status; and third, to modify protocol, if necessary.

Typically, the first effects of TRT are seen in about 3 months, with clear improvement in about 6 months, and many patients achieve a high level of control of their tinnitus by about 12 months.[81,85,92,206,207] Patients are advised to follow the TRT protocol for at least 9 months to prevent a relapse. Improvement in hyperacusis is typically faster than for tinnitus, however the time course of improvement in misophonia is similar to that observed for tinnitus and reflects similarity of mechanisms and centers involved for both phenomena.[13] The results from other centers and ours using TRT show satisfactory results in over 80% of patients.[202,206,208–213]

TREATMENTS FOR HYPERACUSIS

Treatments for hyperacusis go into two contrary directions. First, the most common approach is to advise patients to avoid sound and use ear protection. This is based on reasoning that because patients became sensitive to sound, this may indicate that they are more susceptible to sound exposure and consequently they need extra protection. Patients easily embrace this philosophy and start to protect their ears, even to the extent of using earplugs in quiet environments. Unfortunately, this approach actually makes the auditory system even more sensitive and further exacerbates hyperacusis.[214]

The second approach involves the desensitization of patients by exposure to a variety of sounds. The desensitization approach has been promoted for some time with a variety of protocols and types of sounds used, such as the recommendation of using sound with certain frequencies removed, short exposures to moderately loud sound, or prolonged exposures to low level sounds.[84,85,215] According to principles of the neurophysiologic model of tinnitus, the latter approach is recommended and is used as part of TRT. Note, that the misophonic component cannot be removed by desensitization, and a separate approach needs to be implemented.

Tinnitus Retraining Therapy for Decreased Sound Tolerance

TRT can help patients with both tinnitus and hyperacusis, and the presence of hyperacusis is one of the crucial factors in categorization of the patients (Table 8) and determining the optimal protocol for their treatment. It is recommended that if hyperacusis is present, it has to be treated first. Although TRT offers only a treatment for tinnitus rather than a cure, it can, in some patients with decreased sound tolerance, totally remove hyperacusis and misophonia, thus providing a cure for these conditions.[92,93,184]

In some patients, tinnitus and hyperacusis are two manifestations of the same internal mechanisms of increased gain within the auditory

Table 8 Categories of Patients with Tinnitus and Hyperacusis

Category	Impact on Life	Tinnitus	Significant Hearing Loss	Hyperacusis	Prolonged Sound-Induced Exacerbation	Counseling	Instrumentation
0	Low	Present				Abbreviated, with special care to avoid presentation that tinnitus can be worse than in specific case.	No wearable devices necessary
1	High	Present				Extensive, focused on mechanisms involved in tinnitus generation and in inducing reactions.	SG set, if possible, at a mixing point
2	High	Present	Present			Extensive, focused on mechanisms linking tinnitus and hearing loss.	Combi or HA with stress on enrichment of the auditory background
3	High	Not relevant	Not relevant	Present		Extensive, focused on mechanisms of decreased sound tolerance. When hearing loss is present as well, mechanisms linking it with decreased sound tolerance and tinnitus are discussed.	SG only in cases of normal hearing. Combi (or HA) when significant hearing loss present.
4	High	Not relevant	Not relevant	Present	Present	Extensive, highly individualized with discussion of potential medical problems.	SG set at the threshold; slow increase of sound level.

Abbreviations: Impact on life—the extent tinnitus and/or hyperacusis influence patient's life; Prolonged sound-induced exacerbation of tinnitus/hyperacusis—when the effects persists to the following day or longer; Significant hearing loss—having a significant impact on patient's life; SG = sound generators; Combi = combination instruments; HA = hearing aids. Common treatment for each category involves counseling and the use of enriched auditory background. Sound used in sound therapy is always set below annoyance level. Note that the presence of misophonia, which is treated concurrently, does not affect categorization. Adapted from reference 204. Details of Tinnitus Retraining Therapy implementation are presented elsewhere.[13,205]

pathways, and the improvement in hyperacusis results in the improvement in tinnitus as well. Moreover, the removal of hyperacusis yields a decrease in general anxiety and stress, which, in combination with proper counseling, significantly facilitates tinnitus habituation.

A few parameters of the TRT protocol are of specific importance in treating patients with hyperacusis: avoidance of silence and continued exposure to sound are even more important than for patients with tinnitus only. The level of sound should be better controlled during the treatment, which necessitates the use of wearable sound generators. The sound used should never induce discomfort or annoyance.

The setting of sound generators for hyperacusis is more complex than for tinnitus treatment. There might be a need for a low setting of initial sound level, which might bring patients to the range of effects of stochastic resonance. The use of real-ear measurements, as a guide in setting and checking sound level for all patients with instrumentation during initial and follow-up visits, is crucial in the case of patients with hyperacusis.

The method of desensitization works on the auditory system and consequently will not affect misophonia, which needs to be addressed using active extinction of conditioned reflexes between the auditory and limbic systems. This is achieved in practice by instructing patients to engage systematically in activities involving sound as a fundamental component and that are pleasant, for example, such as actively listening to music following a specific protocol.[94]

CONCLUSIONS

Tinnitus and hyperacusis are still challenging topics to study and symptoms to treat. Many questions remain unanswered. Mechanisms of tinnitus and hyperacusis are speculative and not yet proven. We do not yet have objective methods for detection and evaluation of tinnitus. We believe that the neurophysiologic model of tinnitus and TRT provide a promising approach that may ultimately result in a better understanding of tinnitus and in providing greater help to patients with tinnitus and hyperacusis.

REFERENCES

1. McFadden D. Tinnitus: Facts, Theories, and Treatments. Washington, DC: National Academy Press; 1982.
2. Hoffman HJ, Reed GW. Epidemiology of tinnitus. In: Snow JB, editor. Tinnitus: Theory and Management. Hamilton, London: BC Decker; 2004. p. 16–41.
3. Coles RRA. Epidemiology, aetiology and classification. In: Vernon JA, Reich G, editors. Proceedings of the Fifth International Tinnitus Seminar. Portland, OR: American Tinnitus Association; 1996. p. 25–30.
4. Pilgramm M, Rychlick R, Lebisch H, et al. Tinnitus in the Federal Republic of Germany: A representative epidemiological study. In: Hazell JWP, editor. Proceedings of the Sixth International Tinnitus Seminar. London: Ed Hazell Publishing THC; 1999. p. 64–67.
5. Davis A, El Refaie A. Epidemiology of tinnitus. In: Tyler RS, editor. Tinnitus Handbook. San Diego: Singular Publishing; 2000. p. 1–23.
6. Heller MF, Bergman M. Tinnitus in normally hearing persons. Ann Otol 1953;62:73–93.
7. Tucker DA, Phillips SL, Ruth RA, et al. The effect of silence on tinnitus perception. Otolaryngol Head Neck Surg 2005;132:20–4.
8. Jastreboff PJ, Gray WC, Mattox DE. Tinnitus and hyperacusis. In: Cummings CW, Fredrickson JM, Harker LA, et al, editors. Otolaryngology Head & Neck Surgery. St. Louis: Mosby; 1998. p. 3198–222.
9. Jastreboff PJ. Tinnitus habituation therapy (THT) and tinnitus retraining therapy (TRT). In: Tyler R, editor. Tinnitus Handbook. San Diego: Singular Publishing; 2000. p. 357–76.
10. Davis A. The aetiology of tinnitus: Risk factors for tinnitus in the UK population—A possible role for conductive pathologies? In: Vernon JA, Reich G, editors. Proceedings of the Fifth International Tinnitus Seminar. Portland, OR: American Tinnitus Association; 1996. p. 38–45.
11. Sherlock LP, Formby C. Estimates of loudness, loudness discomfort, and the auditory dynamic range: Normative estimates, comparison of procedures, and test–retest reliability. J Am Acad Audiol 2005;16:85–100.
12. Knobel KA, Sanchez TG. Loudness discomfort level in normal hearing individuals. Pro Fono 2006;18:31–40.
13. Jastreboff PJ, Hazell JWP. Tinnitus Retraining Therapy: Implementing the Neurophysiological Model. Cambridge: Cambridge University Press; 2004.
14. Stephens D. A history of tinnitus. In: Tyler RS, editor. Tinnitus Handbook. San Diego: Singular Publishing; 2000. p. 437–48.
15. Feldmann H. History of tinnitus research. In: Shulman A, editor. Tinnitus Diagnosis/Treatment. Philadelphia: Lea & Febiger; 1991. p. 3–37.
16. Feldmann H. Pathophysiology of tinnitus. In: Kitahara M, editor. Tinnitus: Pathophysiology and Management. Tokyo: Igaku-Shoin; 1988. p. 7–35.
17. Jastreboff PJ. Phantom auditory perception (tinnitus): Mechanisms of generation and perception. Neurosci Res 1990;8:221–54.
18. Muhlnickel W, Elbert T, Taub E, Flor H. Reorganization of auditory cortex in tinnitus. Proc Natl Acad Sci U S A 1998;95:10340–3.
19. Axelsson A, Ringdahl A. Tinnitus—A study of its prevalence and characteristics. Brit J Audiol 1989;23:53–62.
20. Leske MC. Prevalence estimates of communicative disorders in the U.S.A.: Language, learning and vestibular disorders. ASHA 1981;23:229–37.
21. George RN, Kemp S. A survey of New Zealanders with tinnitus. Br J Audiol 1991;25:331–6.
22. Fabijanska A, Rogowski M, Bartnik G, Skarzynski H. Epidemiology of tinnitus and hyperacusis in Poland. In: Hazell JWP, editor. Proceedings of the Sixth International Tinnitus Seminar. London: Ed Hazell Publishing THC; 1999. p. 569–71.
23. Siwiec H. Epidemiology of tinnitus in Lublin district. In: Hazell JWP, editor. Proceedings of the Sixth International Tinnitus Seminar. London: Ed Hazell Publishing THC; 1999. p. 572–3.
24. Spoendlin H. Inner ear pathology and tinnitus. In: Feldmann H, editor. Proceedings III International Tinnitus Seminar. Karlsruhe: Harsch Verlag; 1987. p. 42–51.
25. Holgers KM, Juul J. The suffering of tinnitus in childhood and adolescence. Int J Audiol 2006;45:267–72.
26. Nodar RH. Tinnitus aurium in school age children: A survey. J Audiol Res 1972;12:133–5.
27. Mills RP, Albert DM, Brain CE. Tinnitus in childhood. Clin Otolaryngol 1986;11:431–4.
28. Mills RP, Cherry JR. Subjective tinnitus in children with otological disorders. Int J Pediatr Otorhinolaryngol 1984;7:21–7.
29. Gabriels P. Children with tinnitus. In: Vernon JA, Reich G, editors. Proceedings of the Fifth International Tinnitus Seminar. Portland, OR: American Tinnitus Association; 1996. p. 270–5.
30. Aksoy S, Akdogan O, Gedikli Y, Belgin E. The extent and levels of tinnitus in children of central

Ankara. Int J Pediatr Otorhinolaryngol 2007;71: 263–8.

31. Savastano M. Characteristics of tinnitus in childhood. Eur J Pediatr 2006 Nov 16 [Epub ahead of print].

32. Widen SE, Erlandsson SI. Self-reported tinnitus and noise sensitivity among adolescents in Sweden. Noise Health 2004;7:29–40.

33. Stouffer JL, Tyler RS. Characterization of tinnitus by tinnitus patients. J Speech Hear Disord 1990;55:439–53.

34. Gurr P, Owen G, Reid A, Canter R. Tinnitus in pregnancy. J Clin Otolaryngol 1993;18:294–7.

35. Kemp S, George RN. Diaries of tinnitus sufferers. Brit J Audiol 1992;26:381–6.

36. Zelman S. Correlation of smoking history with hearing loss. JAMA 1973;223:920.

37. Ronis ML. Alcohol and dietary influences on tinnitus. J Laryngol Otol 1984;98:242–6.

38. Zoger S, Svedlund J, Holgers KM. Relationship between tinnitus severity and psychiatric disorders. Psychosomatics 2006;47:282–8.

39. Rossiter S, Stevens C, Walker G. Tinnitus and its effect on working memory and attention. J Speech Lang Hear Res 2006;49:150–60.

40. Hallam RS, McKenna L, Shurlock L. Tinnitus impairs cognitive efficiency. Int J Audiol 2004;43:218–26.

41. Langner G, Wallhdusser-Franke E. Computer simulation of a tinnitus model based on labelling of tinnitus activity in the auditory cortex. In: Hazell JWP, editor. Proceedings of the Sixth International Tinnitus Seminar. London: Ed Hazell Publishing THC; 1999. p. 20–5.

42. Jastreboff PJ. Tinnitus as a phantom perception: Theories and clinical implications. In: Vernon J, Moller AR, editors. Mechanisms of Tinnitus. Boston: Allyn & Bacon; 1995. p. 73–94.

43. Moller AR. Pathophysiology of severe tinnitus and chronic pain. In: Hazell JWP, editor. Proceedings of the Sixth International Tinnitus Seminar. London: Ed Hazell Publishing THC; 1999. p. 26–31.

44. Tonndorf J. The analogy between tinnitus and pain: A suggestion for a physiological basis of chronic tinnitus. Hearing Res 1987;28:271–5.

45. Tonndorf J. Stereociliary dysfunction, a case of sensory hearing loss, recruitment, poor speech discrimination and tinnitus. Acta Otolaryngol 1981;91:469–79.

46. Kiang NYS, Moxon EC, Levine RA. Auditory-nerve activity in cats with normal and abnormal cochleas. In: Wolstenholme GEW, Knight J, editors. Ciba Foundation Symposium on Sensorineural Hearing Loss. London: Churchill; 1970. p. 241–73.

47. Salvi RJ, Ahroon WA. Tinnitus and neural activity. J Speech Hear Res 1983;26:629–32.

48. Penner MJ. Two-tone forward masking patterns and tinnitus. J Speech Hear Res 1980;23:779–86.

49. Moller AR. Pathophysiology of tinnitus. Ann Otol Rhinol Laryngol 1984;93:39–44.

50. Eggermont JJ. On the pathophysiology of tinnitus; A review and a peripheral model. Hear Res 1990;48:111–23.

51. Zenner HP, Pfister M, Birbaumer N. Tinnitus sensitization: Sensory and psychophysiological aspects of a new pathway of acquired centralization of chronic tinnitus. Otol Neurotol 2006;27:1054–63.

52. Ma WL, Hidaka H, May BJ. Spontaneous activity in the inferior colliculus of CBA/J mice after manipulations that induce tinnitus. Hear Res 2006;212:9–21.

53. Tan J, Ruttiger L, Panford-Walsh R, et al. Tinnitus behavior and hearing function correlate with the reciprocal expression patterns of BDNF and Arg3.1/arc in auditory neurons following acoustic trauma. Neuroscience 2007;145:715–26.

54. Jastreboff PJ. The neurophysiological model of tinnitus and hyperacusis. In: Hazell JWP, editor. Proceedings of the Sixth International Tinnitus Seminar. London: Ed Hazell Publishing THC; 1999; p. 32–8.

55. Kaltenbach JA, Rachel JD, Mathog TA, et al. Cisplatin-induced hyperactivity in the dorsal cochlear nucleus and its relation to outer hair cell loss: Relevance to tinnitus. J Neurophysiol 2002;88:699–714.

56. Job A, Raynal M, Kossowski M. Susceptibility to tinnitus revealed at 2 kHz range by bilateral lower DPOAEs in normal hearing subjects with noise exposure. Audiol Neurootol 2007;12:137–44.

57. Kaltenbach JA. Summary of evidence pointing to a role of the dorsal cochlear nucleus in the etiology of tinnitus. Acta Otolaryngol Suppl 2006;556:20–6.

58. Kaltenbach JA. The dorsal cochlear nucleus as a participant in the auditory, attentional and emotional components of tinnitus. Hear Res 2006;216–217:224–34.

59. Ozimek E, Wicher A, Szyfter W, Szymiec E. Distortion product otoacoustic emission (DPOAE) in tinnitus patients. J Acoust Soc Am 2006;119:527–38.

60. Kaltenbach JA, Zhang J, Finlayson P. Tinnitus as a plastic phenomenon and its possible neural underpinnings in the dorsal cochlear nucleus. Hear Res 2005;206:200–26.

61. Pujol R. Neuropharmacology of the cochlea and tinnitus. In: Aran J-M, Dauman R, editors. Tinnitus 1991. Proceedings IV International Tinnitus Seminar. Amsterdam: Kugler Publications; 1992. p. 103–7.

62. Zenner H-P, Ernst A. Cochlear-motor, transduction and signal-transfer tinnitus. Europ Arch Otolaryngol 1993;249:447–54.

63. LePage EL. A model for cochlear origin of subjective tinnitus: Excitatory drift in the operating point of inner hair cells. In: Vernon J, Moller AR, editors. Mechanisms of tinnitus. Boston: Allyn & Bacon; 1995. p. 115–47.

64. Jastreboff PJ. Processing of the tinnitus signal within the brain. In: Vernon JA, Reich G, editors. Proceedings of the Fifth International Tinnitus Seminar. Portland, OR: American Tinnitus Association; 1996. p. 58–67.

65. Eggermont JJ. Correlated neural activity as the driving force for functional changes in auditory cortex. Hear Res 2007 Jan 16 [Epub ahead of print].

66. Eggermont JJ. Cortical tonotopic map reorganization and its implications for treatment of tinnitus. Acta Otolaryngol Suppl 2006;556:9–12.

67. Eggermont JJ. Tinnitus: Neurobiological substrates. Drug Discov Today 2005;10:1283–90.

68. Mazurek B, Haupt H, Georgiewa P, et al. A model of peripherally developing hearing loss and tinnitus based on the role of hypoxia and ischemia. Med Hypoth 2006;67:892–9.

69. Moller AR. Neural plasticity in tinnitus. Prog Brain Res 2006;157:365–72.

70. Moller AR. Pathophysiology of tinnitus. Otolaryngol Clin North Am 2003;36:249–56.

71. Moller AR, Rollins PR. The non-classical auditory pathways are involved in hearing in children but not in adults. Neurosci Lett 2002;319:41–4.

72. Weisz N, Muller S, Schlee W, et al. The neural code of auditory phantom perception. J Neurosci 2007;27:1479–84.

73. Weisz N, Wienbruch C, Dohrmann K, Elbert T. Neuromagnetic indicators of auditory cortical reorganization of tinnitus. Brain 2005;128:2722–31.

74. Norena AJ, Eggermont JJ. Enriched acoustic environment after noise trauma abolishes neural signs of tinnitus. NeuroReport 2006;17:559–63.

75. Sanchez TG, da Silva LA, Brandao AL, et al. Somatic modulation of tinnitus: test reliability and results after repetitive muscle contraction training. Ann Otol Rhinol Laryngol 2007;116:30–5.

76. Heinz MG, Issa JB, Young ED. Auditory-nerve rate responses are inconsistent with common hypotheses for the neural correlates of loudness recruitment. J Assoc Res Otolaryngol 2005;6:91–105.

77. Perry BP, Gantz BJ. Medical and surgical evaluation and management of tinnitus. In: Tyler R, editor. Tinnitus Handbook. San Diego: Singular Publishing; 2000. p. 221–41.

78. Baguley DM, Humphriss RL, Axon PR, Moffat DA. The clinical characteristics of tinnitus in patients with vestibular schwannoma. Skull Base 2006;16:49–58.

79. Mackenzie I, Young C, Fraser WD. Tinnitus and Paget's disease of bone. J Laryngol Otol 2006;120:899–902.

80. Jastreboff PJ, Jastreboff MM, Sheldrake JB. Audiometrical characterization of hyperacusis patients before and during TRT. In: Hazell JWP, editor. Proceedings of the Sixth International Tinnitus Seminar. London: Ed Hazell Publishing THC; 1999. p. 495–8.

81. Jastreboff PJ, Gray WC, Gold SL. Neurophysiological approach to tinnitus patients. Am J Otol 1996;17:236–40.

82. Jastreboff PJ, Hazell JWP. A neurophysiological approach to tinnitus; Clinical implications. Brit J Audiol 1993;27:1–11.

83. Wolk C, Seefeld B. The effects of managing hyperacusis with maskers (noise generators). In: Hazell JWP, editor. Proceedings of the Sixth International Tinnitus Seminar. London : Ed Hazell Publishing THC; 1999. p. 512–4.

84. Hazell JWP, Sheldrake JB. Hyperacusis and tinnitus. In: Aran J-M, Dauman R, editors. Tinnitus 1991. Proceedings IV International Tinnitus Seminar. Amsterdam: Kugler Publications; 1992. p. 245–8.

85. Jastreboff PJ, Jastreboff MM. Tinnitus retraining therapy (TRT) as a method for treatment of tinnitus and hyperacusis patients. J Am Acad Audiol 2000;11:156–61.

86. Stedman's Concise Medical Dictionary, 27th edition. Hagerstown, MD: Lippincott Williams & Wilkins; 2004.

87. The American Heritage Dictionary, 3rd edition. Cambridge, MA: The Learning Co; 1994.

88. Hood JD, Poole JP. Tolerable limit to loudness: It's clinical and physiological significance. J Acoust Soc Am 1966;40:47–53.

89. Cox RM, Alexander GC, Taylor IM, Gray GA. The countour test of loudness perception. Ear Hear 1997;18:388–400.

90. Byrne D, Dirks D. Effects of acclimatization and deprivation on non-speech auditory abilities. Ear Hear 1996;17:29S–37.

91. Stephens SD, Anderson C. Experimental studies on the uncomfortable loudness level. J Sp Hear Res 1971;14:262–70.

92. Jastreboff PJ. Categories of the patients and the treatment outcome. In: Hazell JWP, editor. Proceedings of the Sixth International Tinnitus Seminar. London: Ed Hazell Publishing THC; 1999. p. 394–8.

93. Jastreboff PJ. Tinnitus. The method of Pawel J. Jastreboff. In: Gates GA, editor. Current Therapy in Otolaryngology Head and Neck Surgery. St. Louis: Mosby; 1998. p. 90–5.

94. Jastreboff MM, Jastreboff PJ. Decreased sound tolerance and tinnitus retraining therapy (TRT). Austr NZ J Audiol 2002;21:74–81.

95. Anari M, Axelsson A, Elies W, Magnusson L. Hypersensitivity to sound—Questionnaire data, audiometry and classification. Scand Audiol 1999;28:219–30.

96. Lockwood AH, Salvi RJ, Coad ML, et al. The functional neuroanatomy of tinnitus: Evidence for limbic system links and neural plasticity. Neurology 1998;50:114–20.

97. Melcher JR, Sigalovski I, Levine RA. Tinnitus-related fMRI activation patterns in human auditory nuclei. In: Hazell JWP, editor. Proceedings of the Sixth International Tinnitus Seminar. London: Ed Hazell Publishing THC; 1999. p. 166–70.

98. Lockwood AH, Wack DS, Burkard RF, et al. The functional anatomy of gaze-evoked tinnitus and sustained lateral gaze. Neurology 2001;56:472–80.

99. Andersson G, Lyttkens L, Hirvela C, et al. Regional cerebral blood flow during tinnitus: a PET case study with lidocaine and auditory stimulation. Acta Otolaryngol 2000;120:967–72.

100. Jastreboff PJ, Ikner CL, Hassen A. An approach to objective evaluation of tinnitus in humans. In: Aran J-M, Dauman R, editors. Tinnitus 1991. Proceedings IV International Tinnitus Seminar. Amsterdam: Kugler Publications; 1992. p. 331–40.

101. Penner MJ. Linking spontaneous otoacoustic emissions and tinnitus. Br J Audiol 1992;26:115–23.

102. Lind O. Transient-evoked otoacoustic emissions and contralateral suppression in patients with unilateral tinnitus. Scand Audiol 1996;25:167–72.

103. McKee GJ, Stephens SD. An investigation of normally hearing subjects with tinnitus. Audiology 1992;31:313–7.

104. Jacobson GP, Calder JA, Newman CW, et al. Electrophysiological indices of selective auditory attention in subjects with and without tinnitus. Hear Res 1996;97:66–74.

105. Jacobson GP, Ahmad BK, Morgan J, et al. Auditory evoked cortical magnetic field (M100–M200) measurements in tinnitus and normal groups. Hearing Res 1991;56:44–52.

106. Martin WH, Schwegler JW, Shi J, et al. Developing an objective measurement tool for evaluating tinnitus: Spectral averaging. In: Vernon JA, Reich G, editors. Proceedings of the Fifth International Tinnitus Seminar. Portland, OR: American Tinnitus Association; 1996. p. 127–34.

107. Henry JA, Zaugg TL, Schechter MA. Clinical guide for audiologic tinnitus management I: Assessment. Am J Audiol 2005;14:21–48.

108. Hallberg LR-M, Erlandsson SI. Tinnitus characteristics in tinnitus complainers and noncomplainers. British J Aud 1993;27:19–27.

109. Hebert S, Lupien SJ. The sound of stress: Blunted cortisol reactivity to psychosocial stress in tinnitus sufferers. Neurosci Lett 2007;411:138–42.

110. Adour KK, Wingerd J. Idiopathic facial paralysis (Bell's palsy): Factors affecting severity and outcome in 446 patients. Neurology 1974;24:1112–6.

111. Fallon BA, Nields JA, Burrascano JJ, et al. The neuropsychiatric manifestation of Lyme borreliosis. Psychiatr Quart 1992;63:95–117.

112. Nields JA, Fallon BA, Jastreboff PJ. Carbamazepine in the treatment of Lyme disease-induced hyperacusis. J Neuropsychiatry Clin Neurosci 1999;11:97–99.

113. Klein AJ, Armstrong BL, Greer MK, Brown FR. Hyperacusis and otitis media in individuals with Williams syndrome. J Speech Hear Disord 1990;55:339–44.

114. Wayman DM, Pham HN, Byl FM, Adour KK. Audiological manifestations of Ramsay Hunt syndrome. J Laryngol Otol 1990;104:104–8.

115. McCandless GA, Goering DM. Changes in loudness after stapedectomy. Arch Otolaryng 1974;100:344–50.

116. Fukaya T, Nomura Y. Audiological aspects of idiopathic perilymphatic fistula. Acta Otolaryngol Suppl 1988;456:68–73.

117. Waddell PA, Gronwall DMA. Sensitivity to light and sound following minor head injury. Acta Neurologica Scand 1984;69:270–6.

118. Vingen JV, Pareja JA, Storen O, et al. Phonophobia in migraine. Cephalgia 1998;18:243–9.
119. Gopal KV, Daly DM, Daniloff RG, Pennartz L. Effects of selective serotonin reuptake inhibitors on auditory processing: Case study. J Am Acad Audiol 2000;11:454–63.
120. Lader M. Anxiolytic drugs: Dependence, addiction and abuse. Eur Neuropsychopharmacol 1994;4:85–91.
121. Oen JM, Begeer JH, Staal-Schreinemachers A, Tijmstra T. Hyperacusis in children with spina bifida; A pilot-study. Eur J Pediatr Surg 1997;46:479–80.
122. Henkin RI, Daly RL. Auditory detection and perception in normal man and in patients with adrenal cortical insufficiency:effect of adrenal cortical steroids. J Clin Invest 1968;47:1269–80.
123. Blomberg S, Rosander M, Andersson G. Fears, hyperacusis and musicality in Williams syndrome. Res Dev Disabil 2006;27:668–80.
124. Jastreboff PJ, Mattox DE. Treatment of hyperacusis by aspirin. Assoc Res Otolaryngol Abs 1998;21:207.
125. Boettcher FA, Salvi RJ. Functional changes in the ventral cochlear nucleus following acute acoustic overstimulation. J Acoust Soc Am 1993;94:2123–34.
126. Gerken GM. Alteration of central auditory processing of brief stimuli: A review and a neural model. J Acoust Soc Am 1993;93:2038–49.
127. Marriage J, Barnes NM. Is central hyperacusis a symptom of 5-hydroxytryptamine (5-HT) dysfunction? J Laryngol Otol 1995;109:915–21.
128. Jastreboff PJ. Optimal sound use in TRT—Theory and practice. In: Hazell JWP, editor. Proceedings of the Sixth International Tinnitus Seminar. London : Ed Hazell Publishing THC; 1999. p. 491–4.
129. Ricketts TA, Bentler RA. The effect of test signal type and bandwidth on the categorical scaling of loudness. J Acoust Soc Am 1996;99:2281–7.
130. Hawkins DB, Walden BE, Montgomery A, Prosek RA. Description and validation of an LDL procedure designed to select SSPL90. Ear Hear 1987;8:162–9.
131. Bennett M, Kertesz T, Yeung P. Hyperbaric oxygen for idiopathic sudden sensorineural hearing loss and tinnitus. Cochrane Database Syst Rev 2007;1:CD004739.
132. Bennett M, Kertesz T, Yeung P. Hyperbaric oxygen therapy for idiopathic sudden sensorineural hearing loss and tinnitus: A systematic review of randomized controlled trials. J Laryngol Otol 2005;119:791–8.
133. Dobie RA. Clinical trials and drug therapy for tinnitus. In: Snow JB, editor. Tinnitus: Theory and Management. Hamilton, London: BC Decker; 2004. p. 266–77.
134. Dobie RA. A review of randomized clinical trials in tinnitus. Laryngoscope 1999;109:1202–11.
135. Berninger E, Nordmark J, Alvan G, et al. The effect of intravenously administered mexiletine on tinnitus—A pilot study. Int J Audiol 2006;45:689–96.
136. Salembier L, De Ridder D, Van de Heyning PH. The use of flupirtine in treatment of tinnitus. Acta Otolaryngol Suppl 2006;556:93–5.
137. Baldo P, Doree C, Lazzarini R, et al. Antidepressants for patients with tinnitus. Cochrane Database Syst Rev 2006;4: CD003853.
138. Robinson SK, Viirre ES, Stein MB. Antidepressant therapy in tinnitus. Hear Res 2006 Sep 12 [Epub ahead of print].
139. Robinson SK, Viirre ES, Bailey KA, et al. Randomized placebo-controlled trial of a selective serotonin reuptake inhibitor in the treatment of nondepressed tinnitus subjects. Psychosom Med 2005;67:981–8.
140. Bauer CA, Brozoski TJ. Effect of gabapentin on the sensation and impact of tinnitus. Laryngoscope 2006;116:675–81.
141. Smith PF, Zheng Y, Darlington CL. Ginkgo biloba extracts for tinnitus: More hype than hope? J Ethnopharmacol 2005;100:95–9.
142. Smith PF, Darlington CL. Drug treatments for subjective tinnitus: Serendipitous discovery versus rational drug design. Curr Opin Investig Drugs 2005;6:712–6.
143. Witsell DL, Hannley MT, Stinnet S, Tucci DL. Treatment of tinnitus with gabapentin: A pilot study. Otol Neurotol 2007;28:11–5.
144. Khan M, Gross J, Haupt H, et al. A pilot clinical trial of the effects of coenzyme Q10 on chronic tinnitus aurium. Otolaryngol Head Neck Surg 2007;136:72–7.
145. Zoger S, Svedlund J, Holgers KM. The effects of sertraline on severe tinnitus suffering—A randomized, double-blind, placebo-controlled study. J Clin Psychopharmacol 2006;26:32–9.
146. Azevedo AA, Figueiredo RR. Tinnitus treatment with acamprosate: Double-blind study. Rev Bras Otorrinolaringol (Engl Ed) 2005;71:618–23.
147. Guitton MJ, Wang J, Puel JL. New pharmacological strategies to restore hearing and treat tinnitus. Acta Otolaryngol 2004;124:411–5.
148. Pulec JL. Tinnitus: Surgical therapy. Am J Otol 1984;5:479–80.
149. Moller MB, Moller AR, Jannetta PJ, Jho HD. Vascular decompression surgery for severe tinnitus: Selection criteria and results. Laryngoscope 1993;103:421–7.
150. Berliner KI, Shelton C, Hitselberger WE, Luxford WM. Acoustic tumors: Effect of surgical removal on tinnitus. Am J Otol 1992;13:13–7.
151. Baguley DM, Humphriss RL, Axon PR, Moffat DA. Change in tinnitus handicap after translabyrinthine vestibular schwannoma excision. Otol Neurotol 2005;26: 1061–3.
152. Argstatter H, Plinkert P, Bolay HV. Music therapy for tinnitus patients: An interdisciplinary pilot study of the Heidelberg Model. HNO 2006 Nov 3 [Epub ahead of print] German.
153. Nickel AK, Hillecke T, Argstatter H, Bolay HV. Outcome research in music therapy: A step on the long road to an evidence-based treatment. Ann N Y Acad Sci 2005;1060:283–93.
154. Herraiz C, Diges I, Cobo P, et al. Auditory discrimination therapy (ADT) for tinnitus managment: Preliminary results. Acta Otolaryngol Suppl 2006;556:80–3.
155. Henry JA, Schechter MA, Zaugg TL, et al. Outcomes of clinical trial: Tinnitus masking vs. tinnitus retraining therapy. JAAA 2006;17:104–32.
156. Dauman R. Electrical stimulation for tinnitus supression. In: Tyler R, editor. Tinnitus Handbook. San Diego: Singular Publishing; 2000. p. 377–98.
157. Hazell JWP, Jastreboff PJ, Meerton LE, Conway MJ. Electrical tinnitus suppression: Frequency dependence of effects. Audiol ogy 1993;32:68–77.
158. Olanow CW, Brin MF, Obeso JA. The role of deep brain stimulation as a surgical treatment for Parkinson's disease. Neurology 2000;55:60–66.
159. Martin WH, Shi Y-B, Burchiel KJ, Anderson VC. Deep brain stimulation efects on hearing function and tinnitus. In: Hazell JWP, editor. Proceedings of the Sixth International Tinnitus Seminar. London : The Tinnitus and Hyperacusis Centre; 1999. p. 68–72.
160. Rubinstein JT, Tyler RS, Johnson A, Brown CJ. Electrical suppression of tinnitus with high-rate pulse trains. Otol Neurotol 2003;24:478–85.
161. De Ridder D, De Mulder G, Verstraeten E, et al. Primary and secondary auditory cortex stimulation for intractable tinnitus. ORL J Otorhinolaryngol Relat Spec 2006;68:48–54.
162. Tyler RS. Tinnitus in the profoundly hearing-impaired and the effects of cochlear implants. Ann Otol Rhinol Laryngol Suppl 1995;165:25–30.
163. Tyler RS, Kelsay D. Advantages and disadvantages reported by some of the better cochlear-implant patients. Am J Otol 1990;11:282–9.
164. Portmann M, Cazals Y, Negrevergne M, Aran JM. Temporary tinnitus suppression in man through electrical stimulation of the cochlea. Acta Otolaryngol 1979;87:294–9.
165. Langguth B, Hajak G, Kleinjung T, et al. Repetitive transcranial magnetic stimulation and chronic tinnitus. Acta Otolaryngol Suppl 2006;556:102–4.
166. Pridmore S, Kleinjung T, Langguth B, Eichhammer P. Transcranial magnetic stimulation: potential treatment for tinnitus? Psychiatry Clin Neurosci 2006;60:133–8.
167. Fregni F, Marcondes R, Boggio PS, et al. Transient tinnitus suppression induced by repetitive transcranial magnetic stimulation and transcranial direct current stimulation. Eur J Neurol 2006;13:996–1001.
168. Londero A, Langguth B, De Ridder D, et al. Repetitive transcranial magnetic stimulation (rTMS): A new therapeutic approach in subjective tinnitus? Neurophysiol Clin 2006;36:145–55.
169. Langguth B, Eichhammer P, Kreutzer A, et al. The impact of auditory cortex activity on characterizing and treating patients with chronic tinnitus—First results from a PET study. Acta Otolaryngol Suppl 2006;556:84–8.
170. Rossi S, De CA, Ulivelli M, et al. Effects of repetitive transcranial magnetic stimulation on chronic tinnitus. A randomised, cross over, double blind, placebo-controlled study. J Neurol Neurosurg Psychiatry 2007 Feb 21 [Epub ahead of print].
171. Plewnia C, Bartels M, Gerloff C. Transient suppression of tinnitus by transcranial magnetic stimulation. Ann Neurol 2003;53:263–6.
172. De Ridder D, Verstraeten E, Van der KK, et al. Transcranial magnetic stimulation for tinnitus: Influence of tinnitus duration on stimulation parameter choice and maximal tinnitus suppression. Otol Neurotol 2005;26:616–9.
173. Vernon J. Attemps to relieve tinnitus. J Am Audiol Soc 1977;2:124–31.
174. Vernon J, Schleuning A. Tinnitus: A new management. Laryngoscope 1978;88:413–9.
175. Schleuning AJ, Johnson RM, Vernon JA. Evaluation of a tinnitus masking program: A follow-up study of 598 patients. Ear Hear 1980;1:71–4.
176. Johnson RM. The masking of tinnitus. In: Vernon JA, editor. Tinnitus Treatment and Relief. Boston: Allyn and Bacon; 1998. p. 164–86.
177. Wilson PH, Henry JL. Psychological management of tinnitus. In: Tyler R, editor. Tinnitus Handbook. San Diego: Singular Publishing; 2000. p. 263–79.
178. Caffier PP, Haupt H, Scherer H, Mazurek B. Outcomes of long-term outpatient tinnitus-coping therapy: Psychometric changes and value of tinnitus-control instruments. Ear Hear 2006;27:619–27.
179. Goebel G, Kahl M, Arnold W, Fichter M. 15-year prospective follow-up study of behavioral therapy in a large sample of inpatients with chronic tinnitus. Acta Otolaryngol Suppl 2006;556:70–9.
180. Andersson G, Juris L, Classon E, et al. Consequences of suppressing thoughts about tinnitus and the effects of cognitive distraction on brain activity in tinnitus patients. Audiol Neurootol 2006;11:301–9.
181. Wilson PH. Classical conditioning as the basis for the effective treatment of tinnitus-related distress. ORL J Otorhinolaryngol Relat Spec 2006;68:6–11.
182. Martinez DP, Waddell A, Perera R, Theodoulou M. Cognitive behavioural therapy for tinnitus. Cochrane Database Syst Rev 2007;1:CD005233.
183. Jastreboff PJ. How TRT derives from the neurophysiological model. In: Hazell JWP, editor. Proceedings of the Sixth International Tinnitus Seminar. London: Ed Hazell Publishing THC; 1999. p. 87–91.
184. Jastreboff PJ, Jastreboff MM. Tinnitus retraining therapy. In: Baguley D, editor. Perspectives in Tinnitus Management. New York: Thieme; 2001. p. 51–63.
185. Jastreboff PJ, Jastreboff MM. Tinnitus retraining therapy: A different view on tinnitus. ORL J Otorhinolaryngol Relat Spec 2006;68:23–29.
186. Jastreboff PJ, Hazell JWP, Graham RL. Neurophysiological model of tinnitus: Dependence of the minimal masking level on treatment outcome. Hearing Res 1994;80: 216–32.
187. Albus JS. A theory of cerebellar function. Math Biosci 1971;10:25–61.
188. Bartels H, Staal MJ, Albers FW. Tinnitus and neural plasticity of the brain. Otol Neurotol 2007;28:178–84.
189. Jastreboff PJ, Jastreboff MM. The neurophysiological model of tinnitus and its practical implementation: Current status. In: Myers EN, Bluestone CD, Brackman DE, et al, editors. Advances in Otolaryngology—Head and Neck Surgery, Volume 15. St. Louis: Mosby; 2001. p. 135–47.
190. LeDoux JE. Emotion circuits in the brain. Annu Rev Neurosci 2000;23:155–84.
191. De Ridder D, Fransen H, Francois O, et al. Amygdalohippocampal involvement in tinnitus and auditory memory. Acta Otolaryngol Suppl 2006;556:50–3.
192. Muhlau M, Rauschecker JP, Oestreicher E, et al. Structural brain changes in tinnitus. Cereb Cortex 2006;16:1283–8.
193. Mahlke C, Wallhausser-Franke E. Evidence for tinnitus-related plasticity in the auditory and limbic system, demonstrated by arg3.1 and c-fos immunocytochemistry. Hear Res 2004;195:17–34.
194. Konorski J. Conditioned Reflexes and Neuronal Organization. Cambridge: Cambridge University Press; 1948.
195. Konorski J. Integrative Activity of the Brain. Chicago, IL: University of Chicago Press; 1967.
196. Thompson RF, Donegan NH. Learning and memory. In: Adelman G, editor. Encyclopedia of Neuroscience. Boston: Birkhauser; 1987. p. 571–4.
197. Koechlin E, Basso G, Pietrini P, et al. The role of the anterior prefrontal cortex in human cognition. Nature 1999;399:148–51.
198. Jastreboff PJ, Jastreboff MM. Potential impact of stochastic resonance on tinnitus and its treatment. Assoc Res Otolaryngol Abs 2000;23:5542.
199. Ehrenberger K, Felix D, Svozil K. Stochastic resonance in cochlear signal transduction. Acta Otolaryngol 1999;119:166–70.
200. Jaramillo F, Wiesenfeld K. Mechanoelectrical transduction assisted by Brownian motion: A role for noise in the auditory system. Nat Neurosci 1998;1:384–8.
201. Morse RP, Evans EF. Enhancement of vowel coding for cochlear implants by addition of noise. Nat Med 1996;2:928–32.
202. McKinney CJ, Hazell JWP, Graham RL. An evaluation of the TRT method. In: Hazell JWP, editor. Proceedings of the Sixth International Tinnitus Seminar. London: Ed Hazell Publishing THC; 1999. p. 99–105.
203. Komiya H, Eggermont JJ. Spontaneous firing activity of cortical neurons in adult cats with reorganized tonotopic

map following pure-tone trauma. Acta Otolaryngol 2000;120:750–6.

204. Jastreboff PJ, Jastreboff MM. Tinnitus and decreased sound tolerance: Theory and treatment. In: Hughes G, Pensak M, editors. Clinical Otology. New York: Thieme Medical Publishers, in press.

205. Jastreboff PJ. Tinnitus retraining therapy. In: Snow JB, editor. Tinnitus: Theory and Management. Hamilton, London: BC Decker; 2004. p. 295–309.

206. Bartnik G, Fabijanska A, Rogowski M. Our experience in treatment of patients with tinnitus and/or hyperacusis using the habituation method. In: Hazell JWP, editor. Proceedings of the Sixth International Tinnitus Seminar. London: Ed Hazell Publishing THC; 1999: 415–7.

207. Jastreboff MM, Payne L, Jastreboff PJ. Effectiveness of tinnitus retraining therapy in clinical practice. In: Abstr 8th International Tinnitus Seminar; 2005.

208. Sheldrake JB, Hazell JWP, Graham RL. Results of tinnitus retraining therapy. In: Hazell JWP, editor. Proceedings of the Sixth International Tinnitus Seminar. London: Ed Hazell Publishing THC; 1999:292–6.

209. Heitzmann T, Rubio L, Cardenas MR, Zofio E. The importance of continuity in TRT patients: Results at 18 months. In: Hazell JWP, editor. Proceedings of the Sixth International Tinnitus Seminar. London: Ed Hazell Publishing THC; 1999. p. 509–11.

210. Herraiz C, Hernandez FJ, Plaza G, de los Santos G. Long-term clinical trial of tinnitus retraining therapy. Otolaryngol Head Neck Surg 2005;133:774–9.

211. Jastreboff PJ, Jastreboff MM, Mattox DE. Statistical analysis of the progress of tinnitus treatment during tinnitus retraining therapy (TRT). Association for Research in Otolaryngology. 2001;24: 21630.

212. Mazurek B, Fischer F, Haupt H, et al. A modified version of tinnitus retraining therapy: Observing long-term outcome and predictors. Audiol Neurootol 2006;11: 276–86.

213. Suchova L. Tinnitus retraining therapy—The experiences in Slovakia. Bratisl Lek Listy 2005;106:79–82.

214. Formby C, Sherlock LP, Gold SL. Adaptive plasticity of loudness induced by chronic attenuation and enhancement of the acoustic background. J Acoust Soc Am 2003;114:55–8.

215. Vernon J, Press L. Treatment for hyperacusis. In: Vernon JA, editor. Tinnitus Treatment and Relief. Boston: Allyn and Bacon; 1998. p. 223–7.

32

Cochlear and Auditory Brainstem Implantation

P. Ashley Wackym, MD
Christina L. Runge-Samuelson, PhD

The development and improvement of cochlear auditory prostheses have radically improved the management of children and adults with profound hearing loss. Rapid evolution in the candidacy criteria and the technology itself has resulted in large numbers of individuals who have benefited from implantation. Likewise, the introduction of three device manufacturers into the United States marketplace has accelerated the research and development of these auditory prostheses. In this chapter, the evaluation and expectations for both children and adults will be presented, as will the similarities and differences between all three available devices in the United States. The Advanced Bionics Corporation's (Sylmar, CA) HiResolution Bionic Ear (HiRes 90K) device, Cochlear Corporation's (Englewood, CO) Nucleus Freedom device with the Contour electrode (CI24RE (CA)), and the Med-El Corporation's (Durham, NC) Pulsar$_{CI}$^{100} and Sonata$_{TI}$^{100} devices, as well as various electrode options and external hardware, will be discussed. Surgical techniques and frontiers of applications with auditory prostheses, such as combined electro-acoustic stimulation, rehabilitation of asymmetric hearing loss, bilateral cochlear implantation, and auditory brainstem implantation will be analyzed.

GENERAL BACKGROUND

Cochlear implants are auditory prostheses designed to link an internal device interfaced with the auditory nerve to an external device that uses a specific speech coding strategy to translate acoustic information into electrical stimulation. For the majority of causes of deafness, the auditory hair cells are lost or dysfunctional. The bipolar spiral ganglion neurons and their primary afferent dendrites remain intact, to varying degrees based on etiology, and are available for direct electrical stimulation by the cochlear implant. The tonotopic organization of the cochlea is emulated by orienting the electrode contacts toward the modiolus within the scala tympani and assigning frequencies to specific electrodes along the length of the electrode array such that electrical stimulation corresponding to the highest pitches are delivered within the basal region of the cochlea while electrical stimulation corresponding to the lowest pitches are

delivered within the apical region of the cochlea. The electrical impulses directly depolarize the primary afferent neurons, effectively bypassing the dysfunctional hair cells. All 3 device manufacturers use an external processor that encodes speech based on the features that are critical for word understanding in normal listeners, and these features are discussed in Chapter 33, "Cochlear Implant Coding Strategies and Device Programming." There have been over 70,000 individuals who have received cochlear implants and these devices are now reliably enabling speech comprehension in the vast majority of appropriate cochlear implant recipients.

Prelingually deafened children acquire speech and language through central plasticity resulting from stimulation by auditory prostheses. Some prelingually deafened adults are appropriate cochlear implant recipients, but have more limited central plasticity that is required for auditory pathway development and processing. Postlingually deafened children and adults, as well as those with severe to profound hearing loss, who derive marginal benefit from hearing aids, are appropriate cochlear implant candidates. Detailed review of the current candidacy criteria for children and adults will follow.

PATIENT EVALUATION

There are several issues that can be generalized to both children and adults, and others that are specific to each of these groups. In this section we will address the common issues, followed by the specific adult and pediatric issues.

Otologic/Medical Evaluation and Imaging

The medical evaluation begins with a detailed collection of the patient's history, followed by physical examination. The otologic history includes age of onset, progression, bilaterality of the hearing loss; risk factors for hearing loss (eg, noise exposure, ototoxicity, trauma), and ear infection and surgery. History of possible vestibular dysfunction includes delayed walking, difficulty in riding a bicycle, or difficulty maintaining balance while walking with eyes closed or in the dark. A thorough family history is important, including the age of onset, severity and rate of progression of any hearing loss.

Genetic Hearing Loss. The etiology of the hearing loss is an important consideration. Profound hearing loss and deafness, while clear symptoms, have a heterogeneous group of causes. Of the genetic causes, over 400 forms of syndromic hearing loss have been described, and the list of nonsyndromic loci now exceeds 80,[1] many of which are discussed in Chapter 26, "Hereditary Hearing Impairment."

Congenital deafness occurs in approximately one in every 1,000 children, and at least 60% of these children have hereditary causes of the deafness.[2] It is estimated that 70% of all hereditary hearing losses are nonsyndromic; nearly 80% of which are inherited in an autosomal recessive fashion.[3] To date, 54 autosomal recessive, 24 autosomal dominant, and 8 X-linked loci have been characterized for nonsyndromic sensorineural hearing loss (NSHL).[1] Several mitochondrial DNA variants have also been implicated.[1] Studies indicate that up to 50% of all NSHL cases are due to a mutation in a single gene encoding connexin 26 (Cx26).[4] The gene coding for Cx26 (gap junction protein beta 2 or *GJB2*) is located at locus DFNB1 on human chromosome 13q12. The coding sequence of the protein is contained in a single exon that can be easily analyzed using sequencing methods.[5]

Gap junctions facilitate communication between adjacent cells by providing a channel for diffusion of ions, second messengers, and metabolites.[6,7] Gap junctions are composed of an integral membrane protein called connexin, which can oligomerize to form single-membrane channels called connexons. Each connexon is composed of 6 connexin subunits arranged radially around a central opening, and in some cases can be composed of multiple types of connexins (heteromeric).[8,9] Cx26 and connexin 30 (Cx30) are examples of different connexins that are capable of forming functional heteromeric connexon channels.[10,11] Connexins are members of a multigene family composed of 20 different connexins with distinct tissue-specific distributions. Cx26 and Cx30 are coexpressed in many tissues including the cochlea where they are thought to provide a means of returning K$^+$ ions to the endolymph after hair cell stimulation. A single genetic mutation, the deletion of a guanine within a stretch of six guanines at nucleic acid position 35 (35delG) resulting in premature chain termination, represents the majority of mutated Cx26 alleles among Caucasians worldwide.[12,13] Carrier rates for this allele have been well described and are estimated to be 2.5% in the general population with a total carrier rate for all Cx26 mutations at 3.01%.[14]

Cx26 mutations that are associated with other specific ethnic groups have also been described. Examples include 167delT which has a carrier rate as high as 7.5% in the Ashkenazi Jewish population,[15] and 235delC with a 0.5 to 1% carrier rate in Korean and Japanese populations.[16–19] The 235delC mutation has also been seen in individuals of Chinese decent.[20] Recent studies implicated connexin 30 (gap junction beta 6 or *GJB6*) in connexin-related hearing loss, and it is expressed in the same inner ear tissues as Cx26 and is also located on human chromosome 13q12.[11] A large deletion of 342 kb that involves most of the Cx30 gene plus ~340 kb of upstream sequence is the second most common connexin mutation (after 35delG) in some NSHL populations.[11] Cx26 mutations are not associated with other comorbidity. Children with Cx26 mutations, if implanted early, are typically excellent performers with their devices.[21]

Genetic syndromal deafness represents a small proportion of all profound hearing impairment; however, there are typically other considerations to be made when these individuals are being considered for cochlear implantation. While there are over 400 genetic syndromes that include hearing loss, most syndromic deafness is confined to a limited number of syndromes.[22] There are only 2 common autosomal recessive forms of syndromic deafness: Pendred syndrome (deafness, wide vestibular aqueduct, and thyroid dysfunction) and Usher syndrome (deafness, blindness due to retinitis pigmentosa, with or without vestibular dysfunction). Jervell and Lange-Nielsen syndrome (deafness and sudden death syndrome due to prolonged QT interval) occurs in families with strong histories or in population isolates. It is, however, important to consider when preparing to bring a child to the operating room when there is a family history of deafness and cardiac death. Unfortunately, the electrocardiogram (ECG) is not entirely sensitive or specific for this syndrome[23]; however, referral to a cardiologist for evaluation and treatment is essential for any deaf child with prolongation of the QT interval on an ECG, history of syncopal episodes, or a family history of prolonged QT interval. Neurofibromatosis type 2 (NF2) is usually diagnosed between the ages of 10 and 30 years, and these individuals can express the phenotype of bilateral acoustic neuromas, which is an important issue to consider when developing a management algorithm. If 1 of the tumors is removed while small and if the cochlear nerve is preserved, despite losing functional hearing, cochlear implantation is appropriate if a several year interval has been observed indicating that a recidivistic tumor will not compromise the cochlear nerve. Otherwise auditory brainstem implantation is an appropriate alternative and will be discussed later.

The previous 4 syndromic disorders are not readily diagnosed at birth by history and physical examination. The most common dominant syndromes resulting in deafness are Stickler syndrome, branchio-oto-renal syndrome, and Waardenburg syndrome. When physical examination or history suggests a syndromic hearing loss, online resources have been developed to help the physician during the evaluation process.[24]

Auditory Neuropathy/Auditory Dys-synchrony. Over several years evidence has gradually emerged regarding the existence of a hearing disorder that does not fit into the standard conductive, mixed, or sensorineural hearing loss categories. Relatively recently, the diagnosis of auditory neuropathy/auditory dys-synchrony (AN/AD) has been specified as a hearing disorder in which outer hair cell function is normal in conjunction with absent or abnormal auditory neural responses, which is indicative of poor neural synchrony.[25] Reports on the incidence of AN/AD symptoms range from 0.5[26] to 1.3%[27] of the population suspect for hearing loss and 15% of those with absent auditory brainstem responses,[27] who are otherwise consistent with those with severe-to-profound sensorineural hearing losses. Behavioral audiometric thresholds may or may not be within normal limits and can fluctuate over time, and speech perception in patients with AN/AD is often much poorer than the behavioral thresholds would predict. There are many possible reasons for poor auditory neural synchrony, including, but not limited to, dysfunction of inner hair cells, of the inner hair cell-spiral ganglion nerve synapse, or of the auditory nerve itself.

The variety of etiologies in AN/AD results in a heterogeneous population. Starr and colleagues reported the diagnoses from 70 patients with AN/AD as fitting into the following categories: 40% hereditary, often associated with Charcot-Marie-Tooth disease; 20% with a mix of causes including toxic-metabolic (ie, anoxia, hyperbilirubinemia), immune, and infectious; and 40% idiopathic.[28]

Recent investigations have examined the genetic aspects of nonsyndromic AN/AD. Nonsyndromic AN/AD heritability has been documented as X-linked,[29] autosomal dominant,[30,31] and autosomal recessive.[29,32,33] Mitochondrial mutations with AN/AD have also been reported.[34] In a large family of European descent, a gene responsible for late-onset, progressive, autosomal dominant AN/AD (Locus AUNA1) has been mapped to chromosome 13q 14–21.[30] Starr and colleagues reported on extensive audiologic and psychoacoustic tests performed on members of this family and indicated that the auditory processing abnormalities in the members with AN/AD were different than for those who have cochlear-sensory deficit and those who have auditory nerve degeneration.[31] Three affected family members had received cochlear implants, and all received considerable benefit with their devices compared to their preimplant performance. Although multiple individuals with AN/AD were present within this family, typical individuals with AN/AD seen clinically are either

isolated, that is, a child in a family or may be two siblings in a family. Therefore, based on these studies, AN/AD is more likely to be recessively than dominantly inherited.

In studies of consanguineous Lebanese families with prelingual severe-to-profound NSHL, a gene was identified on chromosome 2p22–23,[35] the locus of which was named DFNB9.[35–37] DFNB9 has been identified as an autosomal recessive locus associated with sensorineural hearing loss[35–39] and more recently with AN/AD.[32,33,40] Yasunaga and colleagues identified the causative gene for DFNB9 which they termed otoferlin (*OTOF*) due to the sequence and structural homology *OTOF* shared with the spermatogenesis factor *Fer-1* in *C. elegans*.[36] In the 4 unrelated Lebanese families with DFNB9, a nonsense mutation in *OTOF* was found which was homozygous in all affected individuals and heterozygous in their parents, consistent with a recessive inheritance pattern. Such a mutation was not found in 106 unrelated, unaffected Lebanese individuals. Recent investigations of families of Spanish,[33,41] European,[32,40,42] and Turkish[43] origin have determined that mutations in the *OTOF* gene are associated with clinical findings of AN/AD.

The *OTOF* gene has 48 exons, or coding regions, and has both short and long isoforms in humans.[44] There are 6 and three C2 domains on the long and short *OTOF* isoforms, respectively, and it is hypothesized that these C2 domains are instrumental in binding calcium and subsequent synaptic vesicle docking.[36,44] Strong otoferlin expression in mouse tissue samples has been found in cochlear inner hair cells, vestibular type I sensory cells, and brain tissue, while no or little otoferlin expression has been observed in the outer hair cells, supporting cells, and spiral ganglion cells.[36] Due to the potential for synaptic involvement and the inner hair cell expression findings, *OTOF* is considered an excellent candidate for underlying some cases of recessive AN/AD. To date, there have been 23 coding variants (affecting 16 exons) identified in *OTOF* which are considered to be pathologic.[40]

Audiologic findings for patients identified with DFNB9 commonly present with prelingual onset, severe-to-profound hearing loss[32,33,35,37,38,40–43]; however, there are instances of *OTOF* mutations associated with moderate-to-severe hearing loss and even with temperature-sensitive AN/AD that leads to exacerbation of hearing loss when febrile.[40,45]

While the spectrum of *OTOF* mutations and associated phenotypes are emerging, there have been reports of intervention outcomes for individuals with *OTOF* mutations. In the few cases available, hearing aid use has not demonstrated benefit whereas cochlear implantation has been considered successful.[33,42,46]

In general, fitting AN/AD patients with hearing aids may not provide sufficient benefit for communication, as amplification provides increased sound intensity but does not have the capability to contribute to improved neural synchrony. After careful evaluation and when recommended, electrical stimulation with cochlear implants holds promise as a treatment option for individuals who are severely hearing impaired from AN/AD,[47,48] and has been successful in our clinical experience. However, cochlear implantation may be contraindicated in individuals in whom neural function is compromised.

Acquired Deafness. In young children, many acquired forms of deafness cannot be easily differentiated from genetic deafness. Prenatal infection with TORCH microorganisms (toxoplasmosis, syphilis, rubella, cytomegalovirus (CMV), and herpes) is commonly associated with deafness. This spectrum of infections can result in reduced ganglion cell counts, cognitive dysfunction and abnormal position of the facial nerve, all issues limiting the effectiveness of cochlear implants or increasing the risk of cochlear implant surgery. Prematurity and low birth weight, low Apgar scores, and hyperbilirubinemia can all be associated with deafness and, because of the central auditory processing abnormalities associated with these conditions, expectations for performance outcome following cochlear implantation should be tempered. Similarly, there can be rehabilitation needs and problems with these multiply disabled children.

Autoimmune inner ear disease, first described by McCabe in 1979, is typically rapidly progressive in nature and is often associated with some of the best possible outcomes in postlingual patients receiving cochlear implants, largely due to the well-preserved primary afferent neuron population and the short duration of deafness. While it is unusual that patients with bilateral Meniere disease lose enough hearing to require cochlear implantation, these patients typically perform at excellent levels with an implant, likely due to the relatively high level of residual hearing.

There are many inherited or acquired diseases affecting the temporal bone that can produce severe to profound hearing loss requiring cochlear implantation. Examples of these disease processes include: otosclerosis, Paget disease, Camurati–Engelmann disease,[49] and meningitis with secondary labyrinthitis ossificans. Aside from the potential difficulty in electrode insertion, the reduction in bone density often leads to unwanted sequelae such as facial nerve stimulation due to current spread outside of the cochlea. These challenges impact the postoperative programming of the device.

Although rare, bilateral temporal bone fractures resulting in deafness can be rehabilitated with cochlear implants. Early implantation should be performed to avoid cochlear fibrosis. If imaging studies suggest trauma to the auditory nerve, it is important to determine if the auditory nerve is functional using promontory electrical stimulation while recording electrically evoked auditory brainstem responses (ABR). The use of auditory brainstem implantation in this clinical setting has been reported in Europe[50]; however, the first such application of this technology in the United States occurred recently as will be discussed later.

Physical Examination. All adults or children with profound hearing loss should have a complete physical examination. This should include features commonly associated with syndromic deafness. Important features include branchial cleft pits, cysts or fistulae, preauricular pits, telecanthus, heterochromia, white forelock, pigmentary anomalies, profound myopia, pigmentary retinopathy, goiter, and craniofacial abnormalities. It is also important to keep in mind that each of these genetic features can have variable expressivity, thereby limiting the specific phenotype.

Chronic Suppurative Otitis Media. Cochlear implantation was initially viewed as contraindicated in young children with chronic suppurative otitis media (CSOM) because of the potential risk of infection.[51] However, selective retrospective studies have shown that the prevalence and severity of OM does not increase following implantation,[52,53] leading surgeons to advocate cochlear implantation if the ear is dry at the time of implantation.

At present, there is no general consensus regarding the management of patients with CSOM with severe to profound hearing loss requiring cochlear implantation. Some surgeons advocate a two-stage operative approach; the first operation involves a radical mastoidectomy (if not already performed), eustachian tube obliteration, and mastoid cavity obliteration with oversewing of the ear canal. Cochlear implantation is performed at a later time, usually 2 to 6 months postobliteration.[54] The major risk of mastoid obliteration is the formation of cholesteatoma, which must be carefully monitored on a long-term basis. Other authors advocate an individualized management strategy: (1) patients with a dry tympanic membrane perforation receive a first-stage myringoplasty followed by implantation in 3 months; (2) patients with cholesteatoma or an unstable mastoid cavity receive a radical mastoidectomy and obliteration followed months later by a second-stage cochlear implantation; (3) patients with a stable cavity receive one-stage cavity obliteration and electrode implantation.[55] Finally, some practitioners advocate treating radical mastoid cavities with a one-stage operative approach that includes oversewing the external auditory canal and cochlear implantation without obliteration or reduction of the cavity.[56,57] Luntz and colleagues have described a treatment algorithm with multiple steps aimed at resolving the draining ear.[58] Using this strategy, cochlear implantation is performed at the completion of any step if the ear is dry. The existence of multiple protocols for managing cochlear implant candidates with CSOM reflects the problematic nature of this disease process. Regardless of the management protocol, all patients currently receive selected antimicrobial prophylaxis immediately prior to implantation.

Microbial biofilms are a common if not normal phenomena in nature, however in the clinical arena biofilm formation is associated with increased morbidity and mortality.[59,60] Biofilms are characterized by a complex 3-dimensional architecture with a network of adherent cells connected by water channels and encapsulated within an extracellular matrix.[61] Biofilms are recalcitrant to antibiotics, antiseptics, and industrial biocides. Possible mechanisms include (1) restricted penetration of drugs through the matrix; (2) phenotypic changes resulting from a decreased growth rate or nutrient limitation; and (3) surface-induced expression of resistance genes. While there is an extensive literature on bacterial biofilms, little attention has been paid to medically relevant fungal biofilms, despite the fact that yeasts are the third leading cause of catheter-related infections, with the second highest colonization to infection rate and the highest crude mortality. Transplantation procedures, immunosuppression, use of chronic indwelling catheters, and prolonged intensive care unit stays are salient risk factors for fungal disease.[62] Biomedical devices including: stents, shunts, and prostheses (voice, heart valve, knee, etc); implants (breast, lens, dentures, etc); endotracheal tubes; pacemakers; and various types of catheters have been shown to support colonization and biofilm formation by *Candida*.[63] Antifungal therapy alone has been shown to be insufficient for cure, requiring removal of the biomedical device.[64]

Since the advent of antibiotics in the 1940s, many authors have reported fungal overgrowth following antibacterial therapy.[65] Although bacteria usually cause CSOM, fungal infection or overgrowth is surprisingly common. One prospective study in CSOM patients reported growth of *Candida* species in 10% of ears with purulent otorrhea and in 35% of ears treated for purulence with topical ciprofloxacin for 3 weeks.[66] Furthermore, another study in which cultures were obtained from ears with ventilation tubes and otorrhea before and after a 10-day course of topical ofloxacin ear drops (Floxin) or oral amoxicillin/clavulanate demonstrated a 5% incidence of *Candida* superinfections in the amoxicillin/clavulanate group but negligible incidence in the ofloxacin group.[67,68] These results confirm the findings of an earlier study in which the incidence of *Candida* was significantly greater for patients treated with amoxicillin/clavulanate compared to a group treated with topical ofloxacin. We have had 1 case of fungal colonization of a cochlear implant with *Candida albicans*.[69] No guidelines have been proposed for dealing with episodes of otitis media in the early postoperative period. During this time interval, the physical barrier created by the fibrous sealing of the cochleostomy is in the process of being laid down; and, thus, the electrode array provides direct access to the inner ear. An infection of the middle ear during this period may easily extend along the electrode array, induce damage to the auditory nerve, and possibly lead to biofilm formation, requiring immediate removal of the implant. In addition, this puts the patient at higher risk for further spread of infection into the intracranial space and subsequent meningitis.[70] The high prevalence of bacterial biofilms in chronic otitis media have been recently demonstrated,[71] and bacterial biofilms have also been demonstrated in cases of infected cochlear implants that required explantation.[72] Biofilms are discussed in Chapter 71, "Biofilms."

Imaging. Preoperative high-resolution temporal bone computed tomography (CT) scans, without contrast, should be performed on all cochlear implant candidates. Determination of intact internal auditory canals (IACs), normalcy of the cochlea, primary or secondary bone diseases affecting the cochlea, and presence of a wide vestibular aqueduct represents an important data set to complete. Many children with congenital deafness will be found to have an associated cochlear malformation, typically dilated vestibule, wide vestibular aqueduct, cochlear hypoplasia or a common cavity.[73] When congenital or acquired narrow IACs are identified on preoperative CT scanning, primary afferent innervation may be lacking and cochlear implantation is therefore contraindicated (Figures 1 and 2).[49,74] Another important finding to identify is a wide vestibular aqueduct which when present is an indication to perform preoperative magnetic resonance imaging (MRI) (Figure 3). This is an important preoperative consideration since this abnormality is associated with an abnormal communication between the cerebrospinal fluid (CSF) space and the cochlea. Clinically, this is often associated with a "perilymph gusher," and sealing of the cochleostomy with pericranium or fascia is particularly important to avoid meningitis following acute suppurative otitis media. Hypoplastic cochleas are associated with shorter length and range in character from a common cavity to an incomplete partition at the apical region of the cochlea (Figure 4). In children with auditory neuropathy/auditory dys-synchrony, MRI should be performed since up to 18% of these children can have small or absent cochlear nerves despite normal IAC size as demonstrated with CT.[75] Other anomalies such as the abnormal course or position of the facial nerve and round window niche occur. With the exception of an absent auditory nerve or IAC, most malformed cochleas can be implanted with a sufficient number of electrodes to provide open-set (unlimited word or sentence possibilities) speech perception.

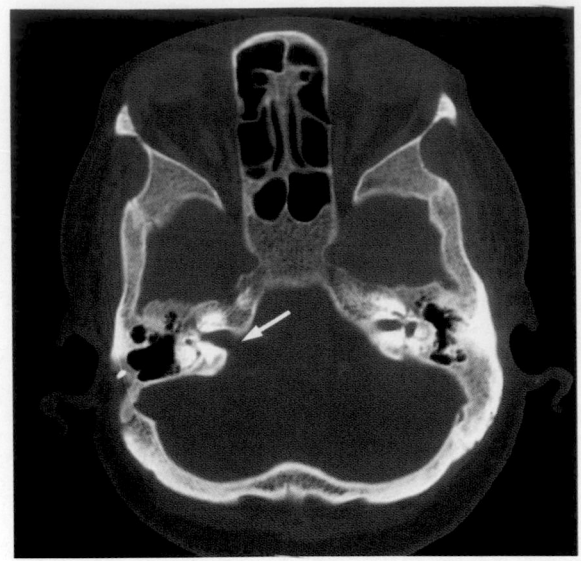
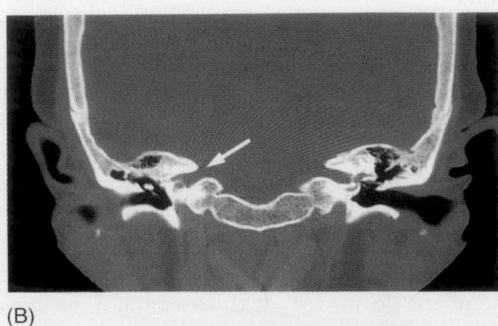
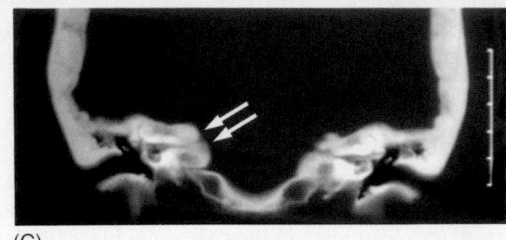

Figure 2 CT scans of skull and temporal bones in two patients with Camurati–Engelmann disease. (A) Patient 1, axial view demonstrating patent IAC (*arrow*). Note in this view, and in the coronal view, thickened bones of the cranium and skull base. This patient underwent cochlear implantation. (B) Patient 1, coronal view demonstrating patent IAC (*arrow*). (C) Patient 2, coronal view. Arrows indicate markedly narrowed IAC. Note thickened bones of the cranium. (Published with permission, copyright © 2000 Annals Publishing Company, reference 49.)

Labyrinthitis ossificans can occur after meningitis, particularly when *Streptococcus pneumoniae* is the infecting mocroorganism.[76] Whereas temporal bone CT can show complete ossification well (Figure 5), MRI can provide complementary information when partial ossification has occurred (Figure 6). T2-weighted MRI sequences are particularly useful in determining whether a scala tympani with partial ossification or fibrosis contains perilymph (Figure 6).

High-resolution temporal bone CT scanning can also be helpful in sorting out issues related to device dysfunction or when unexpectedly poor outcome occurs. Figure 7 shows the temporal bone containing a Med-El C40+ device in a patient who has otosclerosis and the new onset of facial nerve stimulation. The reduced bone density and lucency seen around the otic capsule resulting from her advanced cochlear otosclerosis allowed current to spread from the cochlea to the facial nerve. Figure 8 shows the temporal bone of a young child whose performance was unexpectedly low and who was also noted to have facial nerve stimulation with cochlear implant use. After his referral to our center for evaluation, a

high-resolution temporal bone CT was obtained. The CT scan showed a malformed cochlea with an incomplete partition at the apex and the electrode tip leaving the cochlea and extending into the IAC. This type of cochlear malformations is typically associated with a thin partition between the modiolus and the IAC.

EVALUATION OF ADULT COCHLEAR IMPLANT CANDIDATES

The benefits of cochlear implantation have increased substantially over the last quarter century due to changes in technology and expanded candidate criteria. Consideration for cochlear implantation in adults still requires careful assessment to (1) determine preimplant hearing aid fitting and performance, (2) compare a candidate's preimplant performance with that of current implant recipients, (3) provide a recommendation for or against cochlear implantation, (4) select an ear for implantation, and (5) determine appropriate expectations that will guide the counseling of prospective patients, which is critical for user satisfaction.

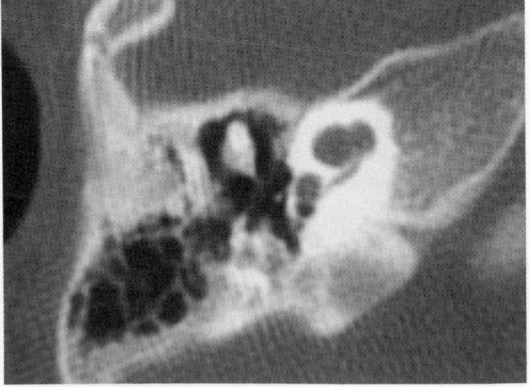

Figure 1 High-resolution temporal bone axial CT scan using a bone window algorithm shows a right ear with an absent IAC and grossly malformed cochlea. (Published with permission, copyright © 2007 P.A. Wackym, MD.)

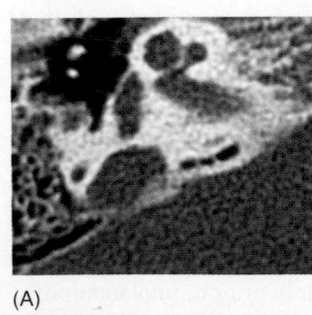
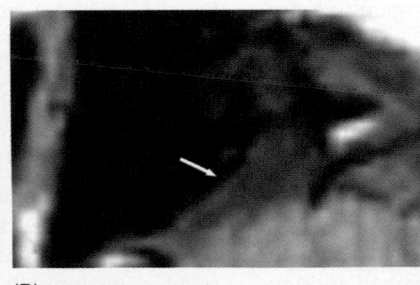
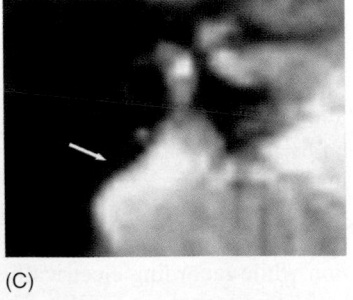

Figure 3 Wide vestibular aqueduct syndrome. (A) High-resolution temporal bone axial CT scan using a bone window algorithm shows a right ear with a grossly widened vestibular aqueduct containing the endolymphatic sac (*center left*). (B) Axial T1-weighted MRI shows that the contents of the wide vestibular aqueduct are isodense with CSF (*arrow*). (C) Axial T2-weighted MRI shows bright signal consistent with CSF (*arrow*). (Published with permission, copyright © 2007 P.A. Wackym, MD.)

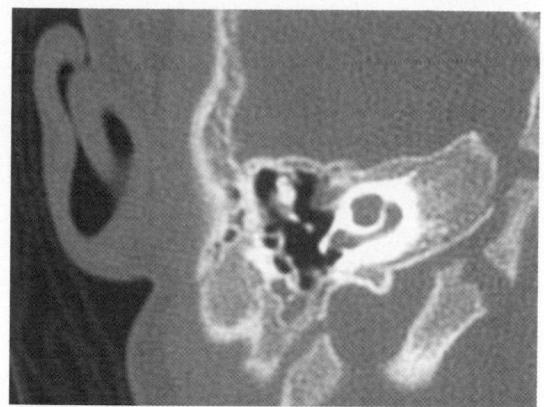

Figure 4 High-resolution temporal bone axial CT scan using a bone window algorithm shows a right ear with a malformed cochlea. Basal turn of the cochlea is normal; however, there is an incomplete partition and bulbous apical portion of the cochlea. Round window and its niche are normal. (Published with permission, copyright © 2007 P.A. Wackym, MD.)

Current Adult Selection Criteria

Food and Drug Administration (FDA) approved guidelines for cochlear implantation vary slightly with different clinical trials depending on the manufacturer's submission and labeling aims. Guidelines also change over time, in part, due to findings that cochlear implant recipients' average scores are higher than individuals with better hearing or word recognition. Current adult selection criteria in the most recent clinical trials include (1) severe or profound hearing loss with a pure-tone average (PTA) of 70 dB HL, (2) use of appropriately-fit hearing aids or a trial with amplification, (3) aided scores on open-set sentence tests of <50%, (4) no evidence of central auditory lesions or lack of an auditory nerve, and (5) no evidence of contraindications for surgery in general or cochlear implant surgery in particular. Additionally, cochlear implant centers generally recommend at least 1 to 3 months of hearing aid use, realistic expectations by the patient and family members, and willingness to comply with follow-up procedures as defined by the center.

The goal of the evaluation process is to determine whether an individual would perform as well with appropriately-fit hearing aids as with a cochlear implant. In addition to comparing the candidate's performance with average cochlear implant users, it is important to compare the candidate with cochlear implant users who are matched for such factors as length of profound hearing loss or useable residual hearing, which are known factors that contribute to the variance in patient performance. In other words, if a candidate has had recent onset of profound hearing loss, it is more appropriate to compare him or her to the top 25% of cochlear implant users. Likewise, if a candidate has had no hearing aid use for 20 years and long-term deafness, it is more appropriate to compare that individual to the lower 25% of implant recipients' performance. However, even with the most educated guess of cochlear implant outcome for a given individual and the knowledge that detection levels can be improved, specific postimplant results cannot be guaranteed, and this principle must be effectively communicated to potential candidates.

Adult Audiologic Protocol. For adults, sound detection and speech perception abilities are assessed to determine candidacy. Preoperatively, patients are evaluated with a battery of measures while using hearing aids, and the results are compared to the most recent average and range of cochlear implant performance. Preoperative measures are also repeated postimplant for longitudinal monitoring of patient performance. Single-subject research designs are often implemented in clinical trials in which each patient serves as his or her control, primarily due to the large variability within the population of cochlear implant candidates and users. The selection of preoperative test measures, therefore, should also take into consideration comparative postimplant measures.

Preimplant audiologic tests include unaided and aided detection thresholds for pure-tone and warble-tone stimuli, respectively. Unaided thresholds are obtained in each ear individually, and aided detection thresholds may be obtained monaurally as well as binaurally. Although there are no aided detection level criteria, it is helpful to determine aided levels as one aspect of appropriate hearing aid fitting and for comparison

to expected postimplant sound-field detection thresholds. For some patients, aided testing can also reveal recruitment, that is, unusual sensitivity to loud sounds, that may limit benefit from amplification due to the inability to incorporate needed hearing aid gain.

Aided speech perception abilities are often assessed in both monaural and binaural conditions, depending on the use of amplification in each ear. Speech perception measures are conducted in the sound field, typically at a presentation level of 60 dB SPL and include open-set recorded

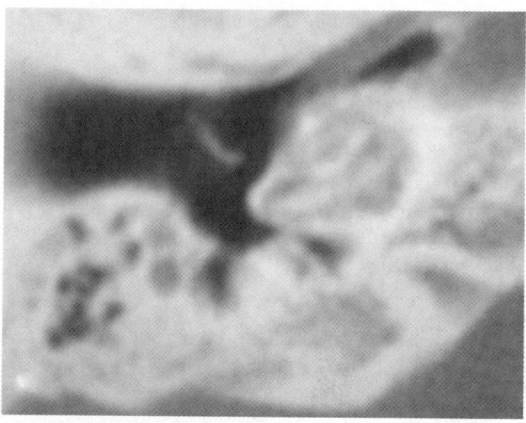

(A)

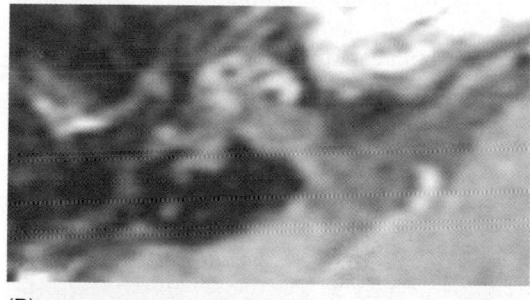

(B)

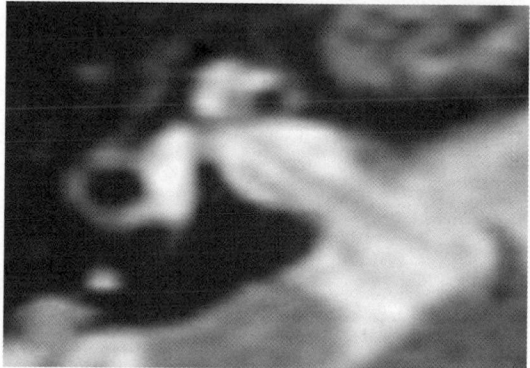

(C)

Figure 6 Incomplete labyrinthitis ossificans after meningitis, with partial obliteration of the right cochlea. The left cochlea was also partially ossified (not shown). This patient was subsequently implanted with bilateral HiRes 90K devices with full electrode insertions. (A) High-resolution temporal bone axial CT scan using a bone window algorithm shows the right ear with an incompletely ossified cochlea. However, determination of cochlear patency requires MRI demonstration of fluid within the scala tympani. (B) Axial T1-weighted MRI scan shows partial fibrosis of the right cochlea. (C) Axial T2-weighted MRI scan shows fluid within the right cochlea; however, the basal turn of the cochlea was completely ossified (absence of fluid). (Published with permission, copyright © 2007 P.A. Wackym, MD.)

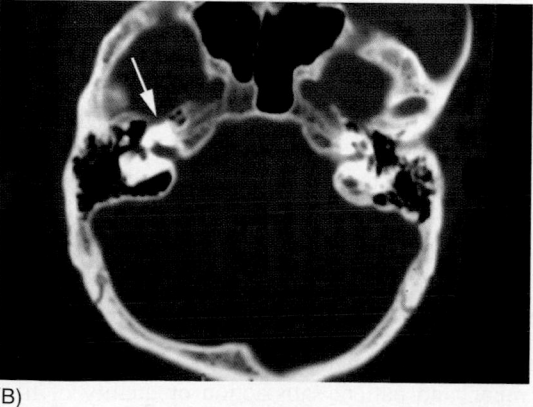

(A)   (B)

Figure 5 Labyrinthitis ossificans after meningitis, with complete obliteration of the right cochlea. (A) Axial T2-weighted MRI scan shows complete absence of fluid within the right cochlea (*arrow*). Compare to left cochlea, which remains patent. (B) High-resolution temporal bone axial CT using a bone window algorithm shows the right ear with the completely ossified cochlea (*arrow*). (Published with permission, copyright © 2007 P.A. Wackym, MD.)

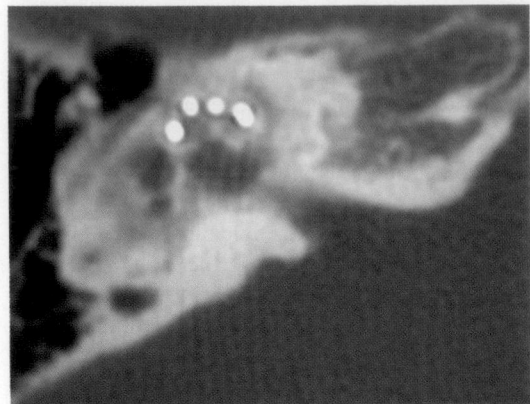

Figure 7 High-resolution temporal bone axial CT scan using a bone window algorithm shows a right ear with a well-positioned electrode array (Med-El C40+) within a cochlea affected by otosclerosis. Note the reduced density of the otic capsule bone and the lucency surrounding the otic capsule (*center, top right*). This patient was experiencing facial nerve stimulation with cochlear implant use due to current spread through the otic capsule to the facial nerve. (Published with permission, copyright © 2007 P.A. Wackym, MD.)

presentations of words and sentences in quiet, and if appropriate, in noise. In the best-aided condition, the assessment of individual ears provides critical information for determining which ear to implant for unilateral implantation. In addition, the best-aided condition, whether it be either ear alone or both ears together, provides information about the candidate's maximum performance for comparison with cochlear implant performance.

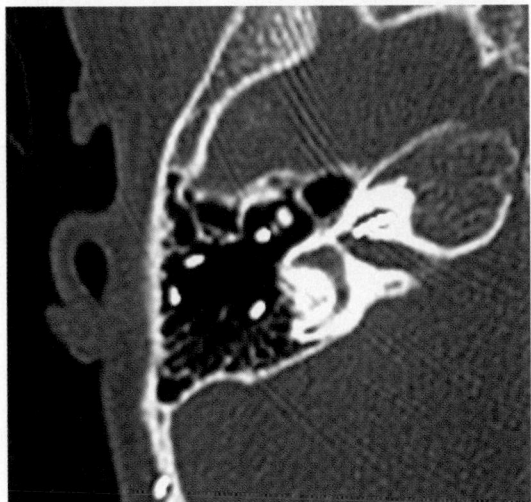

Figure 8 High-resolution temporal bone axial CT using a bone window algorithm shows a right ear with a cochlear implant electrode array that has broken through the cochlea/modiolar wall to enter the internal auditory canal (CII Bionic Ear with HiFocus 1j electrode). The implanting surgeon, at another institution, did not recognize that the child had an incomplete partition at the apex of the cochlea. This malformation can be associated with a thin bony wall between the cochlea and the modiolus. This child was performing at a level lower than expected with his cochlear implant and had facial nerve activation with implant use, which led to the CT scan to evaluate the electrode position. The child's second side was implanted with a HiRes 90K device, and the initial device was removed and replaced with a HiRes 90K device, resolving his facial nerve stimulation problem. (Published with permission, copyright © 2007 P.A. Wackym, MD.)

Word and sentence recognition tests included in the Minimum Speech Test Battery (MSTB) for Adult Cochlear Implant Users are used at many cochlear implant centers to assess performance. The MSTB is a set of compact disc recordings designed to provide word and sentence tests for the pre- and postimplant evaluation of speech recognition, regardless of implant device. The Consonant-Nucleus-Consonant (CNC) Monosyllable Word Test[77] assesses single-syllable word recognition. One CNC list contains 50 monosyllabic words presented in an open-set format. The CNC Words were among the original set of words from which the Northwestern University Auditory Test 6 (NU6) Monosyllabic Word Test[78] were taken.

The presentation of auditory-only sentence lists from the Hearing in Noise Test (HINT)[79] evaluates each patient's ability to understand sentence material in quiet or in the presence of background noise. Each HINT list is phonemically balanced and contains 10 sentences recorded by a male speaker that are equivalent in the features of length, intelligibility, and naturalness. When the sentences are presented in noise, the signal-to-noise (S/N) ratio typically used is +10 dB, although this ratio can be adjusted to make the test condition more or less difficult. For patients with some open-set speech recognition for words and/or sentences preoperatively, the Bamford–Koval–Bench (BKB) Sentences[80] may be administered in an adaptive procedure (ie, BKB SIN; sentences-in-noise). In this condition, the sentences are presented at a fixed presentation level, for example, 65 dB SPL, and the noise is varied for S/N ratios between +20 and −5. Clinical observations suggest that, when testing adults, scores on open-set word and sentence measures, particularly in the presence of noise when appropriate, are more reflective of patient satisfaction with hearing aids and more useful for determining cochlear implant candidacy than unaided and/or aided detection thresholds.

As performance with cochlear implants continues to improve due to advances in technology and broadening candidacy criteria, it is recommended that speech perception performance be assessed with measures that approximate everyday listening. Study findings by Skinner and colleagues[81] and our cochlear implant team[82] suggest that speech recognition tests be presented at 60 rather than 70 dB SPL to determine implant candidacy. These findings have resulted in the use of 60 dB SPL in United States clinical trials and general clinical practice across centers. Additional steps toward the use of measures that approximate everyday listening include the presence of background noise, variation in speaker gender and rate, and variation in the location of the speaker.

Following the evaluation of sound detection and speech perception, other areas of assessment may include vestibular testing, tinnitus assessment, and patient satisfaction or quality of life questionnaires.

Outcome Expectations for Adults. Almost all patients demonstrate improved sound detection

with their cochlear implants compared to their preoperative performance with hearing aids, and this is especially evident in the high-frequency range. Average postoperative sound-field detection thresholds for warble-tone stimuli are approximately 25 to 30 dB HL for frequencies 250 through 4,000 Hz.[82]

When determining patients' expectations for cochlear implant performance and when counseling patients preimplant, it is important to stay abreast of both the average speech perception performance of cochlear implant recipients as well as the range of performance. In a recent study of 78 of adult cochlear implant users, 26 each with the Clarion, Nucleus, and Med-El device, the average CNC word scores at 70, 60, and 50 dB SPL were 42, 39, and 24%, respectively.[82] In this same group of subjects, the mean HINT scores at 70, 60, and 50 dB SPL were 72, 73, and 57%, respectively. When the HINT was presented at 60 dB SPL in the presence of speech spectrum noise at a S/N ratio of +10, the average score for this subject sample was 48%. These results represent average performance; however, there was a great deal of variation in scores for individuals, ranging from 0 to 100% for most measures. In general, patients perform less well on single-syllable word tests compared to sentence tests, and less well in the presence of noise than in quiet. There are many cochlear implant users who are able to understand sentences without lipreading cues and, therefore, can converse on the telephone. Although the primary objective of speech coding strategies is the perception of speech, some patients also enjoy music.

The majority of postlingually deafened adults demonstrate significant pre- to postoperative improvements on open-set speech perception measures, often as early as 1 month postimplant. Compared to postlingual affected adults, some prelingually affected adults, defined as having onset of profound or severe-to-profound hearing loss at less than 3 to 6 years of age (depending on the respective study), demonstrate open-set speech recognition, although the percentage is smaller and often the length of device use needed to achieve this is longer. Although the average postoperative scores for individuals with prelingual hearing loss are generally lower compared to those with postlingual hearing loss, there have been significant pre- to postoperative improvements in speech perception reported for this group.[83] Therefore, adults with prelingual onset of severe-to-profound hearing loss may be appropriate candidates for cochlear implantation.

Providing that older patients are enjoying relatively good health, there presently is no upper age limit for cochlear implantation. Audiologic results for cochlear implant users ages 65 to 80 years indicate significant improvements for both pre- to postoperative comparisons[84,85] and for varied speech stimulus presentation levels.[82] Although increased age is not a contraindication for cochlear implant candidacy, it will be important to study the effects of aging on implant performance and determine whether additional preimplant central auditory assessment is warranted to ensure positive outcomes.

Current Trends that Affect Adult Cochlear Implant Candidacy

Combined Electrical and Acoustic Stimulation. For patients with more residual hearing preimplant than the average cochlear implant candidate, performance is expected to be better. In addition, some patients have considerable residual hearing in the lower frequencies (ie, 250 and 500 Hz), but little measurable hearing for frequencies at 1,000 Hz and above. In these patients, it is difficult to obtain good aided benefit in the high frequencies with a hearing aid while maintaining appropriate gain in the lower frequencies where little, if any, amplification is needed. The ability to understand speech is consequently compromised by the inability to detect and/or discriminate important high-frequency sounds. Also, low-frequency sounds may be masked or distorted by the power needed in the high frequencies. These findings have led to the investigation of combined electrical and acoustic stimulation (EAS), such that the basal end of the cochlea receives electrical signals that are complemented by acoustic signals received at the apical portion of the cochlea. To use EAS, the low-frequency residual hearing must be preserved when the electrode array is inserted in the cochlea (Figure 9). This is obtained by using shortened electrode arrays (20 mm for the Med-El device, and 10 mm for the Nucleus Hybrid device) inserted into the scala tympani and specific surgical techniques designed to make the electrode insertion as atraumatic as possible. These modifications include: controlled opening and no direct suctioning of perilymph from the scala tympani; avoidance of perilymph contamination by blood and debris; use of nonototoxic topical antibiotics, corticosteroids, and lubricant (hyaluronic acid) during insertion; and immediate sealing of the cochleostomy after insertion using fascia. Speech perception findings reported thus far suggest improved performance in the combined EAS condition compared to either stimulation condition alone and compared to preimplant performance.[86] Additionally, recent data suggest that speech perception performance while listening in the presence of noise, including multitalker babble, is superior in the combined EAS condition compared to that of traditional cochlear implant users under the same adverse listening conditions.[87,88] It is likely that future candidacy may include patients with more low-frequency hearing which is therefore a consideration during patient evaluation. Both Cochlear Corporation's and Med-El Corporation's devices designed to combine acoustic and electrical hearing are presently in clinical trials.

Rehabilitation of Asymmetric Hearing Loss. There are a large number of patients who have lost hearing in 1 ear and are not traditional cochlear implant candidates. These patients vary in the amount of hearing in their functional ear, ranging from normal hearing to severe hearing loss associated with marginal hearing aid benefit. As more experience has been gained with implantation of patients with more residual hearing and patients who benefit from hearing aid use in the nonimplanted ear[86] the concept of cochlear implantation to rehabilitate asymmetric hearing loss is being considered. A small-scale multicenter clinical trial is presently underway, and the results will no doubt stimulate additional interest in this new application.

Binaural Cochlear Implants. Traditionally, individuals have received cochlear implants in 1 ear only. With the implementation of clinical trials with bilateral implantation and the benefits of binaural implantation being realized, current candidacy decisions now include whether to receive 2 implants rather than 1. Outcomes data regarding the benefits of binaural implantation continue to emerge, and clear benefits in sound localization and listening in noise have been published.[47] Specifically, studies have shown that binaural implants provide a "head shadow" effect for listening to speech in the presence of other noise or competing speakers. This occurs because 1 ear is "shadowed" from the noise source when speech and noise come from different directions, allowing the ear with the better S/N ratio to do the listening. Other binaural advantages occur when information from both ears is combined to improve listening. Binaural summation effects have been reported whereby performance is improved in the binaural condition compared to either monaural condition when speech and noise are in the front.[89] Binaural squelch effects have been reported less frequently to date, but in some cases, improvement in performance has been shown by adding the ear nearer the noise source.[90] Both binaural summation and binaural squelch effects rely on successful bilateral interaction of the brainstem and central auditory system nuclei, whereas the head shadow effect is simply a physical phenomenon created by the listener's head. We have found that presentation of more difficult auditory stimuli helps to demonstrate the improved benefit obtained by patients tested in the binaural condition compared to that with their better performing cochlear implant.[91]

Binaural implantation in adults recently completed clinical trials at a number of centers and with each of the cochlear implant manufacturers in the United States. It has now become the norm for patients to inquire about the possibility of binaural implantation and receive bilateral cochlear implants if they so desire. Because results have been generally positive and the majority of bilateral recipients indicate a strong preference for bilateral over unilateral implant use, it is now the case that binaural implantation has become a part of the candidacy decision.

Factors that Affect Adult Cochlear Implant Performance

The most common preimplant factors that affect performance for adults include hearing experience (eg, amount of residual hearing, length of profound hearing loss, and hearing history for each ear), age at onset of profound hearing loss (particularly if prior to age 3 years), age at implant (particularly if 75 years and older), cognitive/central abilities, and motivation to hear. Postimplant factors that contribute to performance levels may include length of cochlear implant use, stability of threshold and comfort levels used for device programming, and lifestyle. The need for auditory skills and social interaction in the environment can be a greater issue for those who are not in the work force or who live alone (often the elderly) since they have less practice listening.

Ear Selection in Adult Unilateral Cochlear Implant Candidates

Cochlear implant teams have different philosophies about the selection of the ear for implantation. Some believe that the poorer ear should be chosen for implantation while others consistently choose the better ear. Generally speaking, with a normally developed cochlea, we expect the ear with the shortest length of deafness, better acoustic detection thresholds, acoustic hearing at more frequencies, and better word recognition, to be the better ear for cochlear implantation. At our center, 74% of adults have a cause that includes progressive hearing loss compared to 18% with

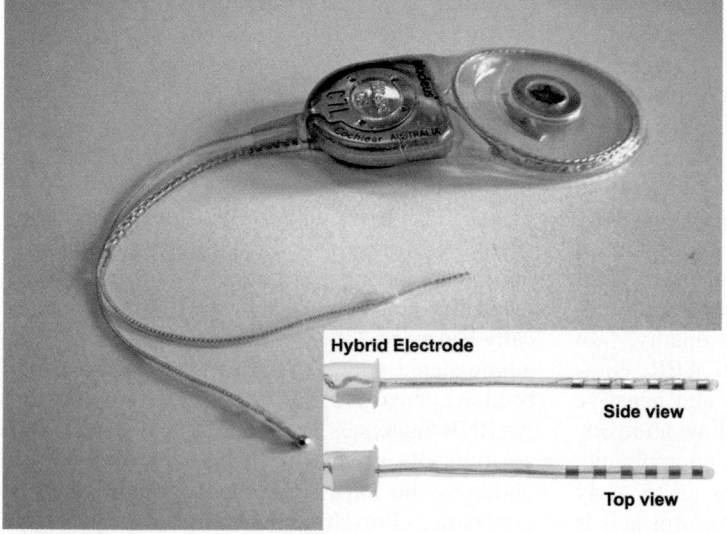

Figure 9 General appearance of the Nucleus Hybrid device for electroacoustic stimulation. Note the receiver/stimulator, removable magnet, loop antenna, separate ground electrode, and 10 mm electrode array. Inset shows the side and top view of the array that is designed to minimize electrode insertion trauma and preserve residual hearing. (Published with permission, copyright © 2007 Cochlear Americas.)

sudden bilateral hearing loss and 8% with congenital bilateral hearing loss. Although at times there is no ear difference, given the complexities in hearing history and ear asymmetry that can exist with progressive hearing loss, it can be difficult to know which ear is the better to select for unilateral implantation. If there has never been a response to acoustic stimulation in one ear, we select the other ear for implantation. Given that there is no medical reason to do otherwise, if either ear is a reasonable choice for implantation, we typically determine whether a hearing aid on the contralateral ear would be beneficial in conjunction with the cochlear implant. If so, we recommend implantation of the poorer ear with hearing aid use on the other side. If neither ear can continue to use a hearing aid, then we generally implant the better ear. If either ear can continue to use a hearing aid equally well, we choose the ear to implant based on handedness, patient preference, or other nonotologic reasons.

Recommendations for Referral for Adult Cochlear Implant Evaluation

At our center, we suggest the following referral criteria for cochlear implant evaluation for adults. Referral to a cochlear implant center does not mean that the individual is necessarily going to receive a cochlear implant, but that an evaluation is recommended to determine whether a cochlear implant would be beneficial. If the individual meets the following criteria, an evaluation is suggested. The criteria are (1) unaided thresholds of 70 dB HL or poorer at 1,000 Hz and above in the better ear, even if hearing levels at 250 and 500 Hz are better; (2) unaided word discrimination <70%; and (3) frustration on the part of the patient due to communication difficulties, even with appropriate hearing aid use.

EVALUATION OF PEDIATRIC COCHLEAR IMPLANT CANDIDATES

Cochlear implants have been available for children ages 2 to 17 years since 1990. Originally, children who were candidates for cochlear implantation typically had profound bilateral sensorineural hearing loss with PTA thresholds of 100 dB HL or greater, often with corner audiograms. These children also displayed aided sound-field thresholds well below the range of average conversational speech and typical speech detection thresholds at and above 60 dB HL. During early clinical trials, pediatric candidates were not able to understand words when using their hearing alone, even with high-gain hearing aids and well-fitted earmolds. Since then, candidacy criteria have changed and technology has improved, both of which have influenced benefit. As with adults, consideration for cochlear implantation still requires careful assessment to (1) determine preimplant fitting of hearing aids and baseline performance, (2) compare a candidate's preimplant performance with that of current implant users, (3) provide a recommendation

for or against cochlear implantation, (4) select an ear for implantation, and (5) determine appropriate expectations that will guide the counseling of prospective families.

Current Pediatric Selection Criteria

The selection criteria for children vary slightly depending on the respective FDA approved clinical trial and/or criteria recommended by the cochlear implant center. Generally speaking, the subject selection criteria include the following: (1) 12 months through 17 years of age; (2) profound sensorineural hearing loss (unaided PTA thresholds of 90 dB HL or greater); (3) minimal benefit from hearing aids, defined as <20 to 30% on single-syllable word tests, or for younger children, lack of developmentally appropriate auditory milestones measured using parent report scales; (4) no evidence of central auditory lesions or lack of an auditory nerve; and (5) no evidence of contraindications for surgery in general or cochlear implant surgery in particular. Additionally, cochlear implant centers generally recommend at least 3 to 6 months of hearing aid use, unless cochlear ossification is noted or anticipated; realistic expectations by family members; enrollment in a postoperative rehabilitation program that supports the use of cochlear implants and the development of auditory skills; and willingness on the part of the family to comply with follow-up procedures as defined by the center.

Pediatric Audiologic Protocol. As with adults, children are assessed preoperatively with a battery of sound detection and speech perception measures while using hearing aids, and this baseline is compared to the most recent average and range of cochlear implant performance. For children, speech perception measures assess a wide range of auditory skills from sound detection to recognition of words and sentences. Measures are selected that are developmentally appropriate for the child's age, language level, and auditory ability. Although the audiologic assessment will play a key role in candidacy, with children other factors may influence the candidacy decision and/or postimplant outcome, and therefore a multidisciplinary team approach is advised.

Prior to cochlear implant evaluation, most children will have an ABR test as an objective measure of the status of the peripheral and brainstem auditory system. With an ABR, acoustic click stimuli are presented to assess auditory sensitivity to each ear. Children who are implant candidates typically have no response to acoustic stimuli at the limits of the testing equipment, suggesting with reasonable accuracy hearing loss in the profound range. Another group of children that can display absent or abnormal ABR findings are those with auditory neuropathy.[25] In these cases of absent or abnormal ABR, comparison of positive (condensation) and negative (rarefaction) polarity stimuli will show an inversion of the peaks of the cochlear microphonic. The cochlear microphonic appears as an early latency response on the ABR waveform and is

indicative of outer hair cell function. Otoacoustic emission testing can also be used as a measure of outer hair cell function. Due to the prevalence of children diagnosed with AN/AD,[92] and the number of these children who have received cochlear implants,[93] our current protocols for electrophysiologic assessment include otoacoustic emission and ABR testing, since these measures are sensitive to cochlear and auditory nerve function, respectively. The diagnosis of auditory neuropathy does not necessarily preclude a child from cochlear implant candidacy.

Unaided detection thresholds for pure-tone stimuli are obtained in individual ears using standard clinical procedures. Aided thresholds are obtained in the binaural condition, and if possible, the monaural conditions. For young children who are unable to participate in speech perception tasks, both unaided threshold testing and electrophysiologic measures become important criteria for cochlear implantation. Since we know the limitations of hearing aids, if we are confident in the reliability of the unaided threshold levels, we can predict with some certainty the eventual aided benefit. Using hearing aids, the measurement of sound detection levels, and when possible, speech perception abilities, can provide confirmation of the unaided thresholds. Although 1 criterion for pediatric candidacy is profound hearing loss, published reports and clinical experience both indicate that adults with severe hearing losses perform well with cochlear implants, therefore we might expect the same outcome for children with similar severe hearing losses. With respect to children with AN/AD, unaided detection levels vary considerably and may not be predictive of aided levels or speech perception abilities.

Tests of speech perception assess a range of skills depending on the child's auditory abilities and language level. Closed-set measures include a small number of choices that are provided to the child either as objects or pictures (eg, Early Speech Perception Test or ESP).[94] Monosyllable, spondee and/or trochee words are spoken with audition alone (no visual cues), and the child is asked to select the object or picture that represents the stimulus. With open-set measures of word and sentence recognition, no choices are provided. The child repeats the words or sentences presented in quiet or in the presence of background noise. For example, using the Lexical Neighborhood Test (LNT),[95] 50 monosyllabic words are presented that are either "easy," occurring with high frequency in the English language and having few lexical neighbors, or "hard," occurring less frequently and with many lexical neighbors. For children with vocabulary levels that approximate a 5-year old, the Phonetically Balanced Kindergarten (PBK) Test[96] can be administered which includes 50 words, and has been in clinical use for many years. Recordings of the BKB Sentences[80] and the HINT-C Sentences[79] are typically used in the evaluation process for children who have some language and auditory experience. For children who are too young to participate in speech perception measures, parent interview scales are administered. The Meaningful Auditory Integration Scale (MAIS)[48] asks questions of parents or family members related to the child's spontaneous awareness of sound and use of audition in a meaningful way at home, school, or other natural environments.

Other Evaluations for Pediatric Cochlear Implant Candidates. For children, the results of speech production assessments are good indicators of hearing history and whether the child has learned to use his or her residual hearing. Language evaluations are also important since the ultimate goal of cochlear implantation is effective communication. Neither of these areas of assessment dictates candidacy, but they contribute to the confirmation of hearing levels and expected preimplant communication coincident with auditory experience. Results also are used to monitor either pre- or postimplant performance over time and to develop rehabilitation goals for educators, clinicians and parents.

A psychological evaluation is obtained to assess the child's verbal and nonverbal intelligence, attention and memory skills, and visual-motor integration. When considering a child for a cochlear implant, counseling the family preimplant, and planning for possible rehabilitative needs postimplant, it is important to know the cognitive abilities of the child. If the child is gifted, for example, then expecting average cochlear implant performance may be an underestimation. Likewise, if the child has a developmental delay, this will affect rate and eventual level of performance with the implant; and counseling may be directed toward more conservative expectations. Differentiating the influence of deafness and cochlear implantation from other disabilities or diagnoses, such as developmental delay, autism, attention deficit disorder, or learning disabilities can be difficult. These issues are addressed in the psychological evaluation preimplant and influence the recommendation for or against cochlear implantation, provide guidance for counseling families, and assist in rehabilitative planning.

Success with a cochlear implant can be influenced by the collaboration of individuals working with the child (parents, educators, and therapists). A team effort is best initiated during the preimplant process and sets the stage for later communication between the individuals on the implant team and the child's educators and family. Early cultivation of communication is important for a variety of reasons, including confirmation of the child's test results and use of residual hearing, discussion of areas of concern, sharing effective test-taking and rehabilitative strategies, setting expectations, and identification of postimplant rehabilitation resources and goals.

Outcome Expectations for Children. Auditory detection levels with a cochlear implant are expected to be similar to those for adults, which are approximately 25 dB HL for frequencies 250 through 4,000 Hz. These detection levels allow access to information that is important for the development of auditory skills and communication. As with adults, when determining expectations, it is important to stay informed of the average and range of pediatric cochlear implant performance.

In a publication by Geers and colleagues,[97] the results of 181 prelingual deaf children, implanted prior to age 5 years who had used their cochlear implants for an average of 5 years, were reported for the outcome areas of speech perception, speech production, spoken language, total language, and reading. The average scores reported for several measures are as follows: ESP-spondee 85%, ESP-monosyllable 79%, LNT-easy 48%, LNT-hard 44%, and BKB sentences 57%. Children who were good speech perceivers were also the children who exhibited superior performance for measures of speech intelligibility, language, and reading. Half of the children were enrolled in oral communication programs and the other half were enrolled in programs using total communication. Those children enrolled in educational environments that emphasized auditory and spoken language development had the highest scores on speech perception, speech production, and language measures. In this study, subjects were implanted between 1992 and 1994, mostly using the Nucleus 22 and SPEAK coding strategy; therefore, the most recent cochlear implant technology and candidacy criteria were not represented.

Studies conducted with children indicate that earlier implantation is associated with higher performance for a given time period postimplant,[98] that preimplant unaided residual hearing influences performance and the development of speech perception skills postimplant,[99] and that there is a steady increase in performance over time that does not plateau during the first 3 to 5 years of implant use.[100]

Based on research studies and clinical experience, we describe below general expectations for children with onset of deafness of less than 1 year based on their age at implantation. Expectations for children *implanted at age 2 years and before* include the potential for communication skill development at rates similar to normal-hearing peers, potential for speech to be easily understood by strangers, reduced or possible elimination of language delay, attendance at a neighborhood school with minimal support services by kindergarten or first grade, and increased likelihood of becoming an auditory/oral communicator. Expectations for children *implanted before the age of 4 years* include substantial improvement in speech perception, increased vocalizations/verbalizations at early stages postimplant, auditory behaviors evident before they can be formally measured, speech production skills reflective of auditory abilities, and language delays that are reduced. For children *implanted between 4 and 5 years*, expectations include improvement in speech perception with excellent closed-set performance and varied open-set abilities, improvements in speech production, use of hearing to support improvements in language, and reduced dependence on visual cues for communication.

For children *implanted at or after age 6 years*, we expect improved auditory detection abilities, improvements in speech perception that entail good closed-set abilities but limited open-set skills, possible improvements in speech production, and continued dependence on visual cues for communication. Generally, children implanted at an older age require more time to reach their potential with the device than those implanted at younger ages.

In addition, for children with progressive or sudden onset of hearing loss, we expect excellent progress with cochlear implantation and achievement of these skills with a shorter duration of cochlear implant use. Likewise, for children with some residual hearing preimplant, we also expect higher levels of performance in relatively shorter periods of time. As discussed regarding adults, it is important to match expectations with reasonable appropriate outcomes for children based on their hearing history, age at implantation, and nonaudiologic factors.

Current Trends that Affect Pediatric Cochlear Implant Candidacy

Binaural Cochlear Implants. Far beyond what has been experienced with adult patients, the majority of major cochlear implant centers are now performing bilateral cochlear implantation of children in the majority of children. Reports in children have followed similar trends as those for adults, with improvements in the ability to recognize speech in noise and to localize a sound source. The ability to follow large spatial changes in speaker location is a critical skill for academic learning in the classroom setting, as is the ability to follow rapid changes between speakers in a smaller space, such as in a small group setting at school or during a conversation with multiple speakers at home. Bilateral implantation is desirable for young children during the critical period for the development of spoken communication. To study the observed clinical benefits reported by parents and teachers and observed by clinicians caring for these children, there are several multicenter investigations of bilateral cochlear implantation in children currently underway in North America and Europe. Due to the longer periods required for speech language development in young children, these trials are designed to extend a minimum of 5 years. Based on the findings in these trials, the circumstances for which we would recommend bilateral implants for children will be evident.

Factors that Affect Pediatric Cochlear Implant Performance

The most common preimplant factors that affect performance for children include age at implantation, hearing experience (age at onset of profound hearing loss, amount of residual hearing, progressive nature of the hearing loss, aided levels, and consistency of hearing aid use), training with amplification (in the case of some residual hearing), presence of other disabilities, and parent and family support. Postimplant factors that contribute to performance levels include length of cochlear implant use, rehabilitative training, and family support. Communication mode is also a documented variable that affects postimplant outcome, where children in programs and homes that focus on the development of spoken language perform higher than children in programs without this emphasis.[97] Children using total communication at school and home can achieve substantial levels of performance; however, this achievement will be less likely if an emphasis on auditory skill development and spoken communication is not included with the use of sign language.

Ear Selection in Pediatric Cochlear Implant Candidates

For children whose parents elect for their child to receive a single cochlear implant, the selection of the ear for unilateral implantation follows the same logic as discussed earlier for adults. At our center, the pediatric population differs from the adults in that fewer children have an etiology of progressive hearing loss (22%), compared to those with congenital bilateral hearing loss (65%), or sudden onset of bilateral hearing loss (13%). In general, this results in fewer children having ear asymmetries or patterns of change in hearing over time; therefore, there are fewer children with ear differences. Since we encourage the use of a contralateral hearing aid postimplant if at all possible, we select the ear for implantation that is least likely to benefit from amplification. All things being equal, we select the right ear to capture the possible advantage of contralateral, left hemisphere specialization for speech recognition.[101]

Recommendations for Referral for Pediatric Cochlear Implant Evaluation

At our center, we suggest the following referral criteria for cochlear implant evaluation for children. As mentioned previously with adults, referral to a cochlear implant center does not mean that a child is necessarily going to receive a cochlear implant, but that an evaluation is recommended to determine whether a cochlear implant would be beneficial. If the child meets 1 or more of the following criteria, an evaluation is suggested. The criteria are (1) unaided thresholds of 90 dB HL or poorer at 2,000 Hz and above in the better ear, even if hearing levels at 250 and 500 Hz are better; (2) aided levels in the better ear poorer than 35 dB HL, especially at 4,000 Hz; (3) no response for ABR testing in both ears or no response for 1 ear and responses at elevated levels in the other ear; (4) parents are frustrated with their child's development of auditory and/or communication skills; (5) progressive hearing loss with detection levels at or near the profound range at 2,000 Hz and above; or (6) evidence of severely impairing auditory neuropathy/dys-synchrony. There is no lower age limit for evaluation; age at implantation is a critical factor that influences postimplant performance, and children who may be too young for the operation are not too young for evaluation.

DEVICE SELECTION

All cochlear implant systems include external and internal hardware. The external equipment includes a microphone, a speech processor, and a transmission system. The internal device includes a receiver/stimulator and electrode array.

In general, an external microphone picks up sound and speech in the environment and sends the information to a speech processor, either the body-worn (BW) or ear-level type. The speech processor converts the sounds into electrical signals, which are sent across the skin via radio frequency transmission to the internal receiver/stimulator. The transmission of the signal occurs when there is successful alignment of the external magnet housed in the transmitter with the internal magnet housed in the receiver/stimulator. The receiver/stimulator decodes the signals and delivers them to the electrodes positioned within the cochlea. The electrodes stimulate the auditory nerve, and the signal is sent along the auditory pathway to the auditory cortex. A description of the most recent available equipment for each cochlear implant manufacturer used by patients in the United States is provided below.

Internal Receiver Stimulators and Electrode Designs

Nucleus Freedom with Contour Advance Electrode. The Nucleus Freedom device with Contour Advance electrode [CI24RE(CA)] consists of an internal receiver/stimulator that uses a flexible silicone housing surrounding a titanium case. The overall dimensions are 58.2 × 33.0 mm, and is 6.2 mm at the thickest point where the electronics are encased in titanium; however, the portion designed to remain on the surface of the skull ranges from 4.7 to 3.6 mm thick. The Nucleus Freedom device with the Contour Advance electrode is shown in Figures 10 and 11. The magnet is removable/replaceable and allows for MRI studies with magnets up to 1.5 T, after removal of the magnet. The electrode design is a perimodiolar electrode and is preformed to conform to the modiolus. There is a stylet that is positioned within this electrode array and maintains the electrode in a straight configuration, until its removal during the operation. The electrode array is curved, consisting of 22 half-banded platinum electrodes, variably spaced

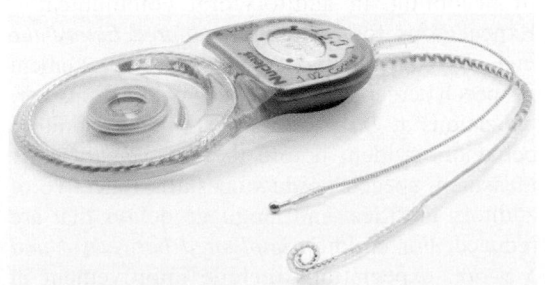

Figure 10 General appearance of the Nucleus Freedom device with the Contour Advance electrode. Note the receiver/stimulator, removable magnet, loop antenna, separate ground electrode, and electrode array. (Published with permission, copyright © 2007 Cochlear Americas.)

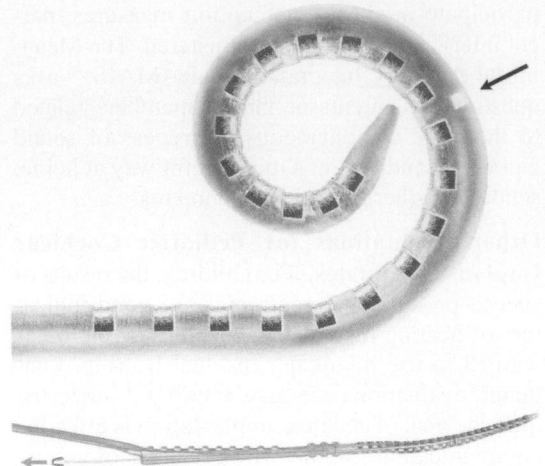

Figure 11 Nucleus Contour Advance electrode after (*top*) and before (*bottom*) stylet removal. The electrode array has a more linear configuration before stylet removal. The electrode is advanced until the white marker (*long arrow*) is located at the level of the cocheostomy. The electrode is then advanced off of the stylet by holding the stylet with a forceps and inserting the electrode. Removal of the stylet (*short arrow*) allows the electrode to return to the precurved configuration of the array, which places the electrode contacts in a perimodiolar position. (Published with permission, copyright © 2007 Cochlear Americas.)

over 15 mm. The diameter of the intracochlear portion ranges from 0.5 to 0.8 mm. Overall, the length of the electrode array distal to the first of 3 silicon marker rings is 24 mm; however, the electrode is designed to be inserted 22 mm, and a platinum band is present at this position to use as a guide for depth of insertion. The half-banded electrodes face the modiolus with a width of 0.3 mm, and a geometric area ranging from 0.28 to 0.31 mm². In addition to the electrodes, there are 10 support bands that together with the stylet stiffen the electrode array. Of all available electrodes on the market, this is the stiffest electrode and consequently, is relatively easy to insert. The greatest disadvantage of this current electrode design is that once the stylet has been removed, it cannot be replaced. This is problematic should the electrode insertion be difficult because of anatomic variations, in which case the back-up device would be required. Manual positioning of the electrode tip within the opening of the cochleostomy is performed and guiding the tip into this position is facilitated by the use of a claw-shaped instrument held in the dominant hand. Once the electrode tip is retained within the opening of the cochleostomy, bimanual advancement of the electrode array using 2 claw-shaped instruments held opposing each other, as close to the cochleostomy as possible, facilitates advancement of the electrode array within the scala tympani. There is a white marker incorporated along the electrode that is used to determine when the electrode array should be advanced off of the stylet until complete insertion has been achieved. The Nucleus Contour electrode array has 3 silastic bands outside of the electrode array that represent the proximal limit and these should remain outside of the cochleostomy. Once this level is reached, the remainder of the stylet is withdrawn and discarded. The electrode is then maintained in a perimodiolar position.[102]

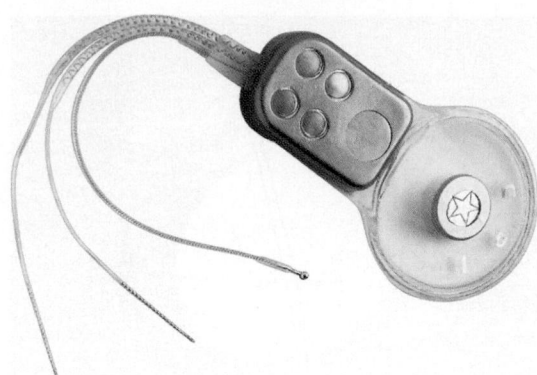

Figure 12 General appearance of the Nucleus device with double electrodes for use in patients with cochlear ossification. Note the receiver/stimulator, removable magnet, loop antenna, separate ground electrode, and the dual electrode arrays, each with 11 contacts over a length of 8.5 mm. (Published with permission, copyright © 2007 Cochlear Americas.)

The Nucleus device also has a second electrode design, a double electrode array to be used for implantation of severely ossified cochleas (Figure 12). The configuration for this includes two electrode arrays, each with 11 contacts within a length of 8.5 mm. A depth gauge is used to determine whether the standard or double array is appropriate.

HiRes 90K. The Advanced Bionics Corporation system includes the HiRes 90K receiver/stimulator (Figure 13) and a choice of 2 electrodes; the HiFocus 1j array or the Helix array. The receiver/stimulator uses a flexible silicone housing surrounding a titanium case, the overall dimensions are 28 × 56 mm, and the thickest point is 5.5 mm where the electronics are encased in titanium; however, the portion designed to remain on the surface of the skull is only 2.5 mm thick. The HiRes 90K system has a removable magnet that has been approved by the FDA to allow for an MRI with a field strength of up to 1.5 T, providing

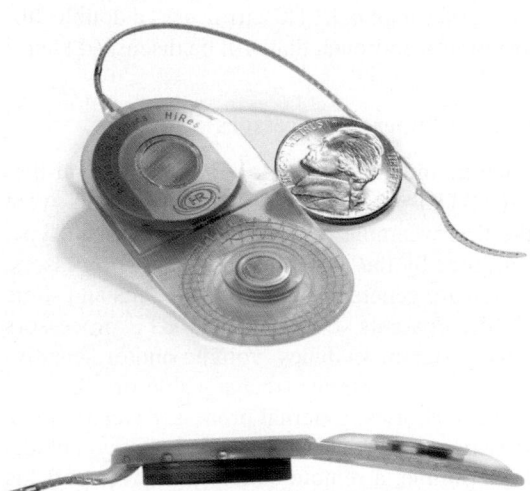

Figure 13 General appearance of the HiRes 90K Bionic Ear device with the 1j electrode. Note the receiver/stimulator with tapered edge at the front of the implant, removable magnet, loop antenna, and electrode array (*top*). The side view shows the low profile of the portion of the device that is located on the surface of the skull (*bottom*). (Published with permission, copyright © 2007 Advanced Bionics Corporation.)

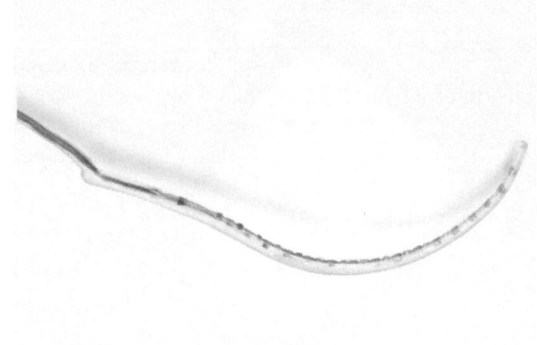

(A)

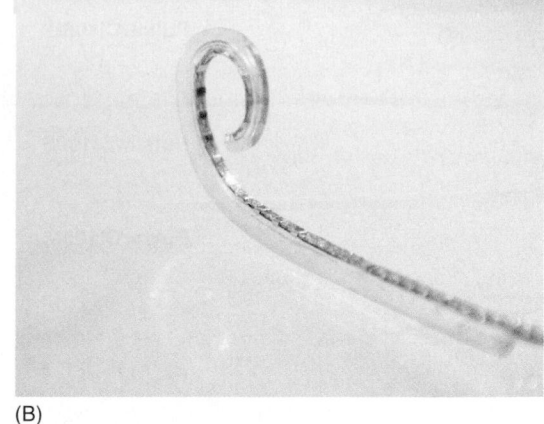

(B)

Figure 14 Photographs of the HiFocus 1j and Helix electrodes. (A) The 1j electrode is banana-shaped and has flat contacts oriented toward the modiolus. The raised partitions shown in the inset, between electrode contacts, are designed to reduce electrode interactions. (B) The Helix electrode uses the same flat contact configuration with the raised partitions but is precurved to place the electrode array in a perimodiolar position after insertion. (Published with permission, copyright © 2007 Advanced Bionics Corporation.)

that the magnet has been removed. The HiFocus 1j electrode system is shown in Figure 14. This electrode is "banana-shaped" and curved toward the modiolus, consisting of 16 contacts, spaced every 1.1 mm over 17 mm. The diameter of the intracochlear portion ranges from 0.6 to 0.8 mm. The length of the electrode array inserted into the cochlea is 23 mm. The electrodes face the modiolus with a width of 0.4 mm and length of 0.5 mm. The HiFocus 1j electrode system utilizes an insertion tube through which the insertion tool allows advancement of the electrode array. Both a metal (outer diameter of 1.5 mm) insertion tube and a Teflon (outer diameter of 2 mm) insertion tube are included, and selection is based on surgeon preference; however, the metal tube provides greater stability. Gentle pressure along a thumb-driven advancement mechanism is required to insert the electrode. Should errors occur during electrode insertion, the electrode is easily reloaded into the insertion tube, and additional electrode insertion attempts can be completed until the electrode insertion has been achieved.

The HiFocus Helix electrode system is shown in Figure 14. This electrode is designed to be perimodiolar in location after insertion. The array consisting of 16 contacts spaced every 0.85 mm over 13 mm. The diameter of the intracochlear portion ranges from 0.6 to 1.1 mm. The length of the electrode array inserted into the cochlea is 24.5 mm. The electrodes face the modiolus with a width of 0.4 and length of 0.5 mm. The HiFocus Helix electrode system utilizes a preloaded stylet assembly by which the electrode array is advanced. Should errors occur during electrode insertion, the electrode is easily reloaded into the insertion stylet assembly, and additional electrode insertion attempts can be completed until the electrode insertion has been achieved. This is in contrast to the Nucleus Contour Advance perimodiolar electrode that cannot be reloaded after removal of the stylet.

Med-El Pulsar$_{CI}$^{100} and Sonata$_{TI}$^{100}. The Med-El Pulsar$_{CI}$^{100} system uses a receiver/stimulator that is housed in a ceramic case that is 26.5 mm at

the base, 23.7 mm at the end, and 4 mm thick (Figure 15). The Pulsar$_{CI}$^{100} system has FDA approval for use with MRI at 0.2 T causing no additional risk to the patient or significant impact on the device or image quality, except for the magnet-induced artifact surrounding the internal magnet. In Europe, many patients with Med-El implants have safely undergone MRI studies with 1.0 and 1.5 T scanners.[103] The Med-El system has 6 separate electrode designs (Figures 16 and 17). The standard electrode is the longest electrode available in the marketplace and is tapered in design. Twelve pairs of electrode bands are distributed over the 31.5 mm electrode array length. The contacts are spaced over 26.4 mm with 2.4 mm between each contact. There is also a FLEXeas array (20.9 mm) available for applications such as EAS; for cochleas that are partially ossified, a compressed electrode is available; and

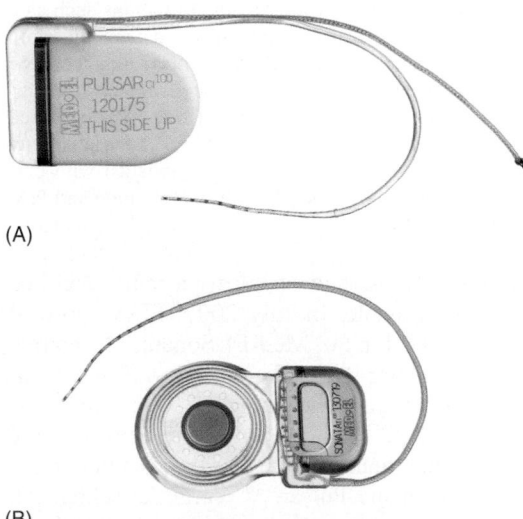

(A)

(B)

Figure 15 (A) General appearance of the Med-El Pulsar$_{CI}$^{100} device. The internal device is housed in a ceramic case containing the receiver/stimulator, internal magnet, and loop antenna. (B) General appearance of the Med-El Sonata$_{TI}$^{100} device. The internal device is housed in silastic and has a similar configuration for the receiver/stimulator, internal magnet, and loop antenna as does the Nucleus Freedom and HiRes 90K devices. (Published with permission, copyright © 2007 Med-El Corporation.)

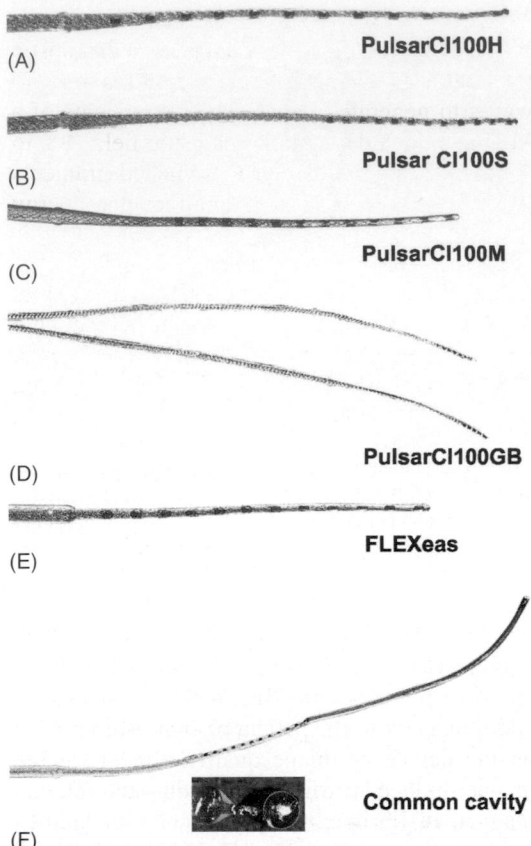

(A) PulsarCl100H

(B) Pulsar Cl100S

(C) PulsarCl100M

(D) PulsarCl100GB

(E) FLEXeas

(F) Common cavity

Figure 16 Six electrode designs available for the Med-El Pulsar$_{CI}^{100}$ and Sonata$_{TI}^{100}$ cochlear implants. (A) Standard 31.5 mm electrode with the electrode contacts distributed over 26.4 mm. When ossification is encountered during creation of the cochleostomy, use of the ITD allows determination of whether to open the standard electrode array or 1 of the 2 shorter arrays or the split electrode array. (B) The compressed array distributes the electrode contacts over 13 mm. (C) The medium array distributes the electrode contacts over 21 mm. (D) The split array has 1 with 5 pairs of electrode contacts, while the other has 7 pairs of electrode contacts. (E) For hearing preservation and application of electroacoustic stimulation the FLEXeas electrode is designed to be thin and 20.9 mm in length. (F) For severe cochlear malformations such as a common cavity, the custom-manufactured common cavity electrode can be used. This electrode array uses the basic compressed electrode with a nonfunctional silastic extension terminating in a platinum ball (inset) which is used to place the electrode array via a double labyrinthotomy technique as shown in Figure 17. (Published with permission, copyright © 2007 Med-El Corporation and P.A. Wackym, MD.)

for severely ossified cochleas, a split electrode array is available. In July 2007, FDA approval was granted for the Med-El Sonata$_{TI}^{100}$ internal device (Figure 15). The Sonata$_{TI}^{100}$ Cochlear Implant contains the same I^{100} electronics as the Pulsar$_{CI}^{100}$ device, but the electronics are encased in a titanium housing that is smaller and thinner than the Pulsar$_{CI}^{100}$ ceramic casing. All Med-El electrode arrays are compatible with the Sonata$_{TI}^{100}$. The receiver coil and internal magnet are positioned outside of the electronics package in flexible silicone, although the magnet is not removable for MRI. The Sonata$_{TI}^{100}$ is also MRI-compatible in the United States at 0.2 T without magnet removal.

If ossification of the cochlea is encountered during the opening of the cochleostomy, the use

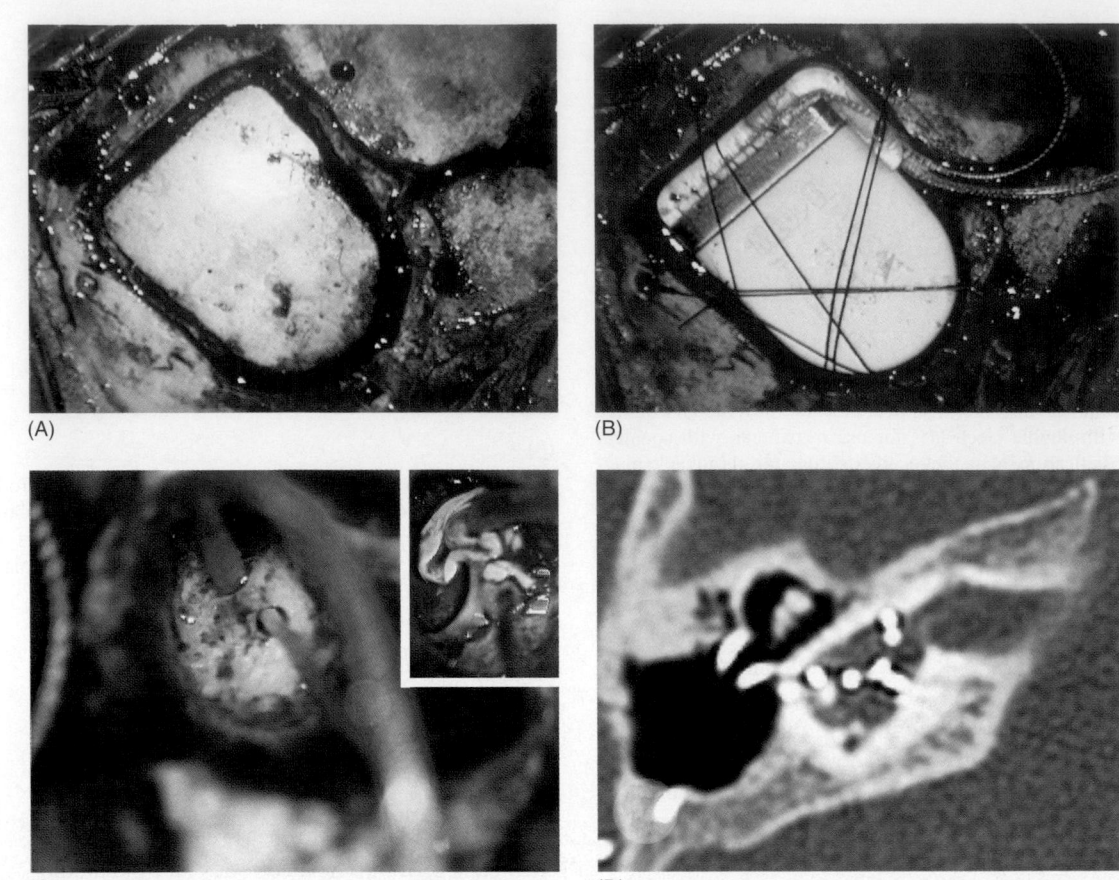

(A) (B) (C) (D)

Figure 17 Cochlear implantation in a common cavity malformation. (A) Craniotomy with the bone island technique. (B) The Med-El internal receiver/stimulator secured with three 3-0 nylon sutures. (C) The common cavity electrode was inserted via a double labyrinthotomy technique. Inset shows fascia sealing both labyrinthotomies. (D) Postoperative CT scan shows the position of the electrode array within the common cavity. (Published with permission, copyright © 2007 P.A. Wackym, MD.)

of the Med-El Insertion Test Device (ITD) can be helpful to determine which of their various electrode options should be used. If the ITD can be inserted to the small flanges present 17.8 mm from the tip, the standard array should be used; if less than that, the medium or compressed array should be used. The medium electrode array (Pulsar$_{CI}^{100}$M) has all 12 pairs of electrodes distributed over 21 mm-spaced 1.9 mm apart. The Pulsar$_{CI}^{100}$ compressed electrode (Pulsar$_{CI}^{100}$S) is designed with the same number of electrode contacts ($n = 12$ pairs) but arranged closer together on the apical end of the array and spaced over 12.1 mm. With ossification present, the ITD is advanced through the cochleostomy and the depth of insertion is determined. If it is apparent that insertion of the standard electrode array would result in electrodes being extracochlear in location, the compressed or medium electrode array should be used and fully inserted.

For more severely ossified cochleas, the Med-El split electrode design (Pulsar$_{CI}^{100}$GB) has 2 compressed electrode arrays with five and 7 pairs of electrode contacts, respectively (Figure 16). These electrode arrays are inserted via 2 cochleostomies, which will be described in the surgical techniques section. They have a constant 0.5×0.6 mm diameter up to the fixation rings that are located 8.3 mm (on the longer array) and 6.1 mm (on the shorter array) from the apex. When the 2 arrays are in place, the electrode

contacts provide more sites of potential stimulation than a single standard array incompletely inserted into the cochlea. The sixth electrode design is for applications in patients who have a common cochlear cavity (Figures 16 and 17). This electrode uses the basic Pulsar$_{CI}^{100}$S array with 3 to 5 mm of silastic and a distal nonfunctional platinum ball. This array uses a double labyrinotomy approach that will be discussed later.

External Speech Processors

Each manufacturer offers a BW and behind-the-ear (BTE) processor. The BW processors were the first wearable devices for each implant type, followed by the introduction of BTE processors, which are generally preferred by adults and some children/parents. Both BW and BTE processors have program switches, volume and/or sensitivity controls, batteries (rechargeable or alkaline), and accessories. External processor wear options vary from one device to another, but may include, for example, a remote battery pack worn off the ear or a rechargeable battery pack worn on the processor at the ear. A variety of mechanisms exist (eg, earhooks, indicator lights) that perform functions such as alerting parents to a low battery or a disconnected headpiece. External auditory input sources can be connected to the processors, such as auxiliary microphones, telephone adaptors, tape recorders, television audio amplifiers, or FM systems. Other cosmetic considerations include a variety of processor and transmission coil colors, decorative caps, processor belt clips and harnesses, or hip packs for daily wear. Since the external equipment changes regularly, the specifics for each manufacturer are reviewed at the time of device discussion and selection, which occurs once cochlear implantation has been recommended.

Current Speech Processing Strategies

Specific aspects of current speech processing strategies are discussed in Chapter 33, "Cochlear Implant Coding Strategies and Device Programming," and the purpose of this section is to present the relevance of speech processing strategies to device selection.

Speech processing strategies used in auditory prostheses have evolved over the years to enhance presentation of the acoustic signal by electric stimulation. Early on, the primary goal for cochlear implant signal processing was to maximize encoding of the speech signal, which was a prudent and necessary starting place since the devices were designed to restore aural communication abilities to otherwise deaf individuals. The subsequent strides in development of speech processing strategies and the changes in cochlear implant candidacy have raised the bar beyond encoding speech in quiet to now including goals for understanding speech in noise and for appreciation of nonspeech acoustic stimuli such as music.

In general, signal processing improvements across all devices have addressed issues with electrical field interaction, extraction of temporal and spectral characteristics, and stimulation rate. Current strategies available tend to have faster sampling and stimulation rates, and new strategies are being developed to increase the number of perceived stimulus delivery channels, all of which allow for a higher resolution representation of an acoustic signal. Regardless of how ideal a signal processing strategy may be, however, there are always patient-based limitations due to physiologic or anatomic issues that affect the accurate neural encoding of the electrical signal. Many investigations are currently being undertaken to address both stimulation and patient-based limitations.

With respect to device selection, all devices offer several different speech processing strategies, with some strategies potentially more appropriate for an individual patient than others. For example, a person who has a relatively short-term hearing loss of cochlear origin likely to have a large number of auditory nerve fibers available for stimulation.[104] A high-resolution strategy would likely be appropriate for this individual, and this would be particularly desirable if the listening needs included various challenging listening environments and music appreciation. In some cases, however, it may be beneficial to employ a low-rate strategy, particularly in cases of reduced neural integrity such as demyelination or other neuropathies in which rapid stimulation

of nerve fibers can result in slowing or even blockage of action potential conduction along the nerve.[105,106] Although these are general guidelines, care must be taken to avoid underestimating a cochlear implant user's potential based on these factors alone.

Regardless of device choice, it is common clinical practice to allow patients to try various signal processing strategies or different parameter settings within a strategy (ie, pulse width, pulse rate, and paired versus simultaneous stimulation) in different listening situations and determine which results in the best speech perception performance and sound quality. Therefore, implementation of a speech processing strategy requires consideration of the cochlear implant user's cause of hearing loss, interests, performance, subjective judgments, and communication and listening needs.

Factors that Affect Device Choice

In our center, we currently implant over 100 patients per year. We approach device choice as a personal decision that the patient or the child's parents should make. Extensive counseling and education regarding the devices, operation and rehabilitation, which are important aspects of caring for patients with profound hearing loss who choose to receive a cochlear implant, help to prepare patients or a child's parents to make an informed decision. Below we have outlined several factors that are important for consideration preoperatively.

Need for Special Electrode Arrays. When individuals have hearing loss that is appropriate for cochlear implantation, it is possible that the cochlea may be malformed, depending on the etiology of the hearing loss. This includes varying degrees of Mondini malformation, in which there may be fewer cochlear turns or dehiscent cochleae. The cochlea may be ossified, to varying degrees, which may occur with meningitis, Paget disease, or otosclerosis. In addition, there are types of hearing loss that may necessitate preservation of hearing with implantation. In any of these cases, it may be necessary to have special electrode arrays available, such as short, compressed, split or custom arrays, all of which were described earlier.

Technology Differences in Speech Coding Strategy and Electrode Configuration. Device selection is also influenced by changes in technology that may make one device more appealing than another for a given individual. For example, a speech coding strategy that emphasizes both temporal and spectral cues may be desirable for a patient who has a great love of music. Depending on an individual's work or other daily life environment, certain noise reduction features may become relevant. As discussed previously, in some cases, a patient may be limited to selecting a given device based on his or her cochlear anatomy or hearing status that requires the use of a particular electrode array design.

Magnetic Resonance Imaging Compatibility. MRI is a powerful noninvasive diagnostic tool that uses magnetic fields and pulses of radio waves to generate images. The components of a MRI unit include: a static magnetic field (0.5 to 4 T); magnetic fields due to switched gradients (0 to 20 T/s at ~15 Hz); and radiofrequency energy (0 to 6 kW peak at 64 MHz [for 1.5 T]).[107,108] It is an imaging modality with an already wide range of clinical applications that continues to expand. Ideally, this diagnostic tool should be available for the benefit of cochlear implant (CI) recipients. The Cochlear Corporation's CI24M, CI24R(CA), and CI24ABI devices, as well as the Advanced Bionics Corporation's HiRes 90K device were all designed so that the internal magnet can be removed and replaced to complete a MRI study.

Studies with the Med-El Combi 40/40+ and Clarion 1.2 (Advanced Bionics) cochlear implants have delineated many of the factors in CI/MRI interactions.[109,110] The factors that have been studied include: demagnetization, artifacts, induced voltages, temperature increases, torque, and force. These investigations have utilized both the 0.3 and 1.5 T MRI units. The force and torque exerted by the MRI unit on the internal magnet of the cochlear implant receiver are of particular concern. The potential for a catastrophic force on the implant to fracture the inner table of skull and exert pressure on the brain demands full investigation of cochlear implant/MRI compatibility. Previous studies concluded that a 0.2 T MRI evaluation force and torque remained within "acceptable limits."[109,110] There have been several in vivo studies performed in Europe using 1.0 T MRI.[103] In this largest series of 30 patients with Med-El cochlear implants who underwent 1.0 T MRI evaluations with a variety of MRI sequences, none suffered pain, burning, auditory sensation, deterioration of their auditory abilities, or other adverse sequelae. Presently patients with the Med-El C40+, $Pulsar_{CI}$,[100] or $Sonata_{TI}$[100] devices in place greater than 6 months are approved by the FDA to undergo MRI studies with a 0.2 T scanner, provided the company approves the protocol for the radiologist.

We have completed studies to determine the magnitude of force required to fracture the floor of a cochlear implant receiver bed.[111] The testing protocol was designed to create a physical worst-case scenario, yet approximate the in vivo condition. Several considerations went into attaining this dual goal. Each recessed cochlear implant bed was drilled to a maximum uniform thinness rather than drilling just deep enough to accommodate the cochlear implant. A stainless steel template was chosen for impacting the specimens because the arc of its edge would closely approximate that of the cochlear implant impacting the skull in vivo. In addition, a line load system more realistically approximated the in vivo condition than a point load system. The center of the specimen was chosen for contact with the template. This placement minimized the risk of the template touching any surface other than the floor of the recessed cochlear implant bed. It also facilitated identical placement of the template for each specimen. Finally, this placement allowed the template to impact the specimen at its least reinforced site, thereby providing a worst-case scenario. Since the in vivo system had the thinned bone in continuity with the native skull and it is this region that receives the force vector during the cochlear implant magnet/MRI magnet interaction, it is anticipated that the biomechanical forces required to produce failure at this interface would be much greater than those measured in the study referenced above.[111] In an earlier investigation of cochlear implant/MRI compatibility, 0.3 to 1.0 N was used as an acceptable level of force exerted on a cochlear implant during MRI evaluation.[109] They recommended this range because it represents the magnitude of force that a cochlear implant may experience during a regular day in the life of a cochlear implant recipient. More specifically, this is the magnitude of the force exerted on the internal magnet of a cochlear implant when the external transmitter and magnet is removed. In these prior studies, the measured force vectors ranged from 0.17 to 0.42 N. Calculations using these measured forces vectors and appropriate geometry resulted in maximum forces of ~8 N exerted on the cochlear implant during 1.5 T MRI evaluation in a worst-case scenario. The results of our biophysics studies showed that the load carrying capacity of a recessed cochlear implant bed drilled into fresh frozen human calvaria specimens, with bone thickness of 0.3 to 0.6 mm (SD 0.11 mm), is more than an order of magnitude greater than this force (mean = 134.13 N).[111] When a bone island with exposed dura is necessary to inset the internal device, titanium or resorbable mesh has been shown in vitro to provide even greater mechanical support beneath a cochlear implant and this approach also has the advantage of providing immediate support.[112] Moreover, we have demonstrated that no demagnetization of the internal device magnet occurs after 15 successive MRI scans in a 1.5 T unit.[113] Further studies in patients will be necessary to demonstrate the safety of this practice using cochlear implants with the internal magnet remaining in place. However, for all candidates, and particularly those who are in need of frequent MRI scans, the options and limitations of each device should be discussed so that the patient can make an informed decision.

External Speech Processor Size, Weight, and Esthetics. Often, the design and esthetics of the external components, specifically the speech processor, has a great deal of influence on device selection (Figures 18 to 20). Individuals tend to prefer a BTE processor because it is lighter, smaller, and does not have a cord that runs down the back of the neck. For young children, it may be desirable to use a BW processor that can be worn on the child's back and out of reach. In addition, some BTE processors may be too large or heavy to stay on a child's ear. However, some manufacturers have introduced smaller, lighter BTE wear options designed specifically for children.

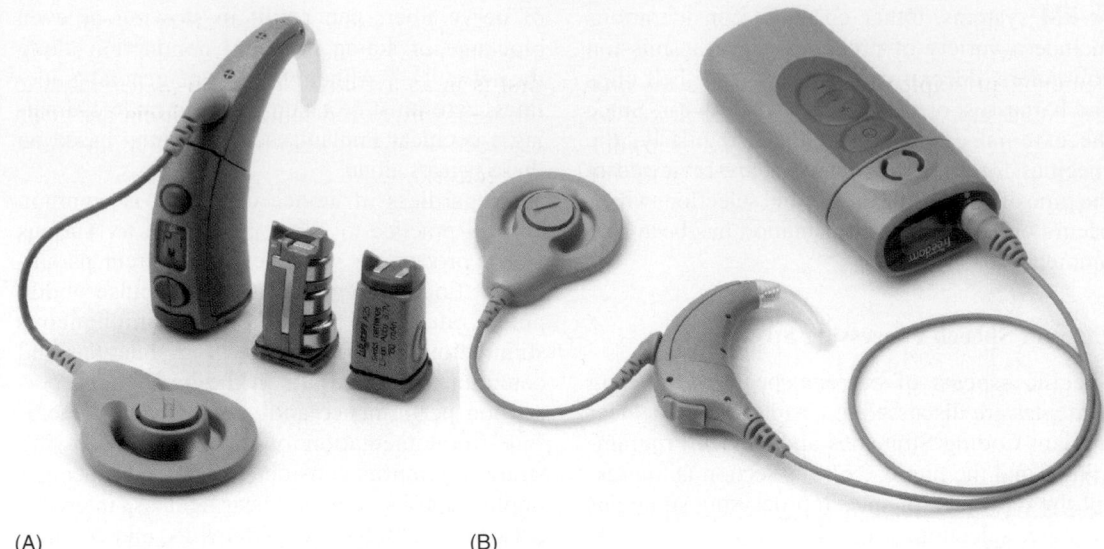

(A)   (B)

Figure 18 Ear-level and BW speech processors for the Nucleus Freedom System. (A) Freedom BTE speech processor. Multiple colors are also available. Disposable or rechargeable batteries are used. (B) Freedom BW speech processor. Note the ear hook, which contains the microphone and the magnet/transmitter coil. (Published with permission, copyright © 2007 Cochlear Americas.)

Patients with dexterity or vision problems often select a processor with larger, more accessible controls. Color choice of the external components is also relevant. Some prefer to match hair and/or skin tone, and others like interesting designs or colors they can change to match their clothing.

Batteries. The type, cost, and lifespan of batteries are important to some patients when choosing a device. BW speech processors can use either disposable alkaline or rechargeable batteries. BTE processors use either disposable high-power 675 hearing aid batteries or proprietary rechargeable batteries, depending on the manufacturer of the device. The specific processor, battery type, speech-coding strategy, and patient programming needs each affect battery life. However, the generally expected battery life and ease of changing the batteries may cause a patient or family to choose one implant design over another.

OPERATIVE TECHNIQUES IN COCHLEAR IMPLANTATION

The details of cochlear and brainstem implantation have recently been reviewed.[114]

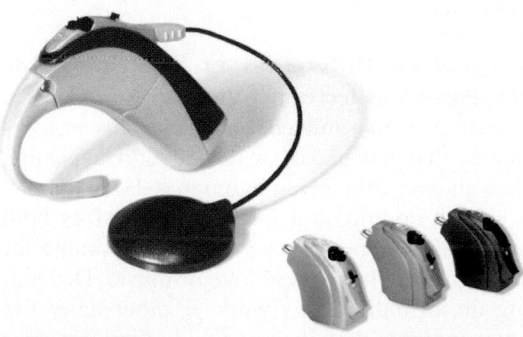

Figure 19 Harmony ear-level speech processor. Multiple colors are available, lower right, and multiple colored accent strips are also available. A separate BW battery pack is also available for infants with cochlear implants. (Published with permission, copyright © 2007 Advanced Bionics Corporation.)

Patient Positioning and Preparation

For both children and adult patients, the standard otologic position is used, supine with the head placed on a foam doughnut and turned away from the operated ear. Surgical preparation should always include review of the CT and/or MRI to determine the cochlear anatomy and whether the cochlea is filled with fluid, fibrous tissue, or neo-ossification. With the wide array of available cochlear implant electrode designs, this is particularly important to be certain that the appropriate electrode array has been ordered and is available in the operating room.

Soft Tissue Incisions and Approach

Over the years, several variations of scalp and skin incisions have been utilized in cochlear

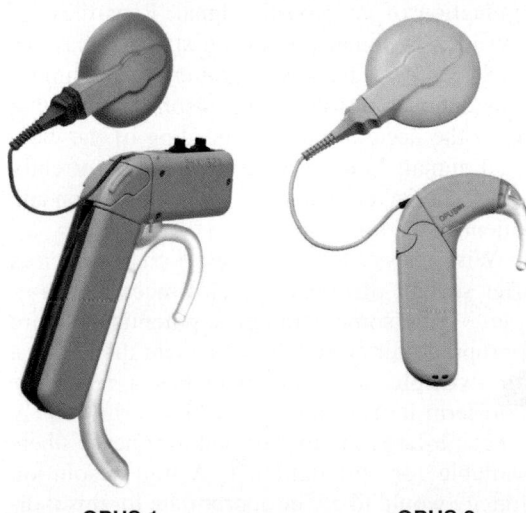

OPUS 1   **OPUS 2**

Figure 20 Ear-level speech processors for the Med-El cochlear implant systems. The OPUS 1 has a modular design with 2 small switches, whereas the OPUS 2 has a more ergonomic switch-free design. Multiple colors are available. A separate BW battery pack is also available for infants with cochlear implants. (Published with permission, © 2007 Med-El Corporation.)

implant surgery. While several flaps have been utilized with consistently good results, 2 fundamental principles must be adhered to: first, the blood supply of the flap must be ample for survival of the flap; and second, the skin incisions must not overlie the cochlear implant itself. With this evolution in flap design have also come changes in philosophy regarding the amount of hair that must be shaved. Figure 21 shows the commonly utilized skin and scalp incision designs that are currently used by most cochlear implant surgeons. The only hair shaved is that necessary to allow draping of the field around the incisions. The postauricular incision is designed to be at the hairline and is thereby camouflaged. The posterior scalp extension length can be varied depending on the implant design. Because the internal magnet and receiving coil can be placed lateral to the skull for the Nucleus Freedom device (Cochlear), the HiRes 90K device (Advanced Bionics) and the Sonata$_{TI}$^{100} device (Med-El), shorter scalp incisions are required for these devices, thereby permitting a "minimally invasive" approach. A pocket can be developed beneath the existing scalp flap to receive these portions of the device. For the Pulsar$_{CI}$^{100} (Med-El) device the entire ceramic receiver portion of the device must be inset into the skull; and, therefore, the scalp incision must be somewhat longer. This issue is of no functional consequence and does not produce additional morbidity in patients. Moreover, this scalp incision is placed within the patient's hair and is not seen once it is healed and the hair has regrown.

There are differences in the soft tissue approach between adults and children. For young children the incisions are carried through the skin, temporalis muscle and pericranium (periosteum), directly down to the bone. The soft tissue flaps are elevated en bloc, and subperiosteal elevation is completed to expose the sites of bone work necessary to accomplish cochlear implantation. An important point to consider and accomplish during this aspect of the operation is adequate exposure of the external auditory canal and zygomatic root. Ample elevation of the soft tissue necessary to protect the soft tissue from the surgical drill is also an important point.

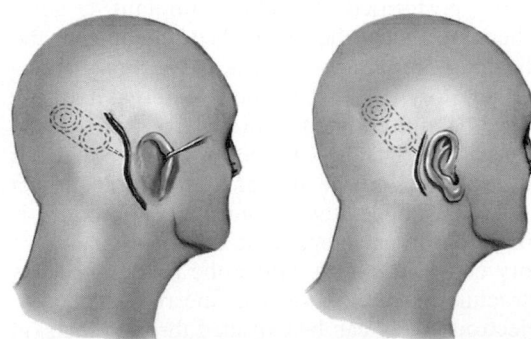

Figure 21 Cochlear implant surgery skin incision designs. This style is commonly referred to as a lazy S or traditional postauricular and scalp skin incision (*left*). This style is used with the minimally invasive cochlear implant surgery technique (*right*). (Published with permission, copyright © 2007 P.A. Wackym, MD.)

With adults and older children, it is possible and desirable to develop 2 tissue planes. The first is in an avascular subgaleal plane lateral to the pericranium and temporalis fascia and mastoid periosteum superiorly and anteroinferiorly, respectively. Once these flaps are elevated, incisions through the periosteum are made, first along the temporal line superiorly with a perpendicular extension down to the mastoid tip. The superior limb of this incision is carried posteriorly over the skull, and a periosteal flap is then elevated. These flaps are used to close the wound in 2 layers that further help in protecting the receiver portion of the cochlear implant and, thereby, minimize the risk of extrusion.

Several pieces of temporalis fascia or pericranium are harvested and kept sterile in the moist gauze sponge on the back table and are used for sealing the cochleostomy, for placing it between the facial nerve and electrode array, and in helping to retain the electrode array at the juncture of the trough housing the electrode array and the mastoid cavity. Once hemostasis has been achieved either with the bipolar or monopolar electrocautery, the monopolar cautery is taken off of the operative field and turned off. Once the cochlear implant has been opened and placed on the operative field, it is necessary to remove the monopolar cautery to prevent current-induced damage to the internal device.[115]

For both adults and children the elevated soft tissue flaps are protected with 1″ × 3″ cottonoids or moistened gauze sponges (Kendall Vistec sponges, TYCO Healthcare Group LP, Mansfield, MA) and retracted from the bone with dural fish hooks (DermaHooks, Weck Closure Systems, Research Triangle Park, NC) and rubber bands. Alternatively, after placement of the cottonoids and/or moist Vistec sponges, self-retaining retractors can be used.

Receiver Bed and Electrode Array Trough

Preparation of the receiver bed begins by selection and design of the placement. It is important to place the receiver bed posterior enough to accommodate the ear level hook or BTE speech processor. Placement of the receiver bed in a position that is too far anterior is a common mistake made by inexperienced cochlear implant surgeons. As is shown in Figure 22, the consequence of this is extrusion of the receiver following skin erosion due to the ear hook or BTE speech processor placing pressure on the skin overlying the receiver. Another consideration in designing the position of the receiver bed is the anticipated position of a hat band, should the patient frequently wear hats or wish to wear hats. Each device manufacturer provides templates that are used in designing the shape of the receiver bed, and these accurately represent the size of the receiver. There are specific differences in how the receiver bed is designed and these will be described in separate subsections of this portion of the chapter; however, general techniques are described first (Figure 23). Whereas it is possible

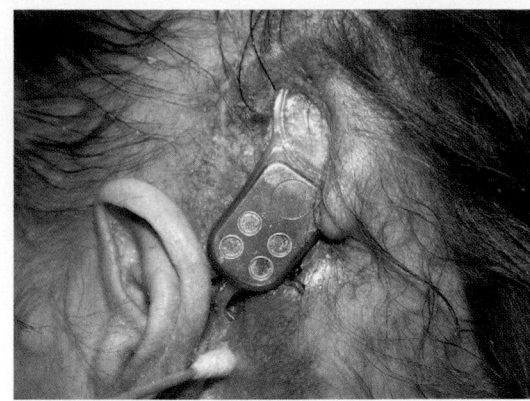

Figure 22 Placement at another institution of this Nucleus CI24M device too close to the posterior aspect of the pinna resulted in skin erosion and device extrusion. Pressure from the behind-the-ear hook/microphone rubbing against the skin above the internal receiver/stimulator contributed to the skin breakdown and device extrusion. (Published with permission, copyright © 2007 P.A. Wackym, MD.)

to inset the receiver in some adult patients, virtually all young children and the majority of older children and adults require a craniotomy that extends down to the dura and allows the in seting of the receiver. The technique for accomplishing this includes completing a craniectomy of the dimensions necessary for accommodating the receiver. The outer cortex and diploic layers are removed, and the inner cortex of the skull is thinned until the dura is visible through the bone. Next, the craniotomy is performed using a 2 mm coarse diamond bur, which is carried down to the dura without violating this layer. The surrounding bony edges are smoothed, and conformation of the craniotomy to the template is completed to be certain that the receiver will fit in the created space. It is estimated that 6 months are required for the bone to regrow across this gap and provide stable bone beneath the cochlear implant receiver; however, this important issue has not been systematically studied using CT imaging.[111,112] This is an important consideration in making a decision for a patient with a cochlear implant in place to undergo an MRI. For young

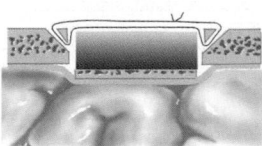 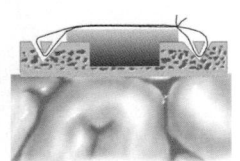

Figure 23 Craniotomy for placement of the internal receiver/stimulator using the bone island technique (*left*). A thin plate of bone together with the Med-El Pulsar$_{CI}$^{100} receiver/stimulator is displaced toward the brain. Tie-down sutures can be placed through channels created at an angle across the calvaria as shown or across the entire calvaria as shown in Figure 24. Craniectomy for placement of the Nucleus Freedom, HiRes 90K or Sonata$_{TI}$^{100} internal receiver/stimulator (*right*). With small children, the skull is too thin to accommodate the internal receiver/stimulator without performance of a craniotomy. In which case, a bone island technique is used with the remainder of the device remaining on the surface of the skull. (Published with permission, copyright © 2007 P.A. Wackym, MD.)

children a small cutting bur, usually 2.5 or 3 mm in diameter is used to remove the outer cortex and diploic layer while for older children and adults, a 6 mm cylinder bur is helpful because it allows perpendicular walls to be created around the receiver site while simultaneously, removing bone with the coarse diamond surface located on the tip of this type of bur. During the creation of the craniotomy and bone island necessary to accommodate the receiver–stimulator, inadvertent dural injury may occur. If this violation is small and fascia is placed through the opening, so that the fascia remains both medial to and lateral to the dura in a dumbbell-shaped manner the dura is easily sealed. It is also important to determine that no brain parenchymal injury has occurred.

Figure 24 shows the two methods available to create the tie-down suture holes through the bone, as well as the relative position of the internal device and the mastoidectomy. Two to 4 sites for suture tie-downs are created so that 3-0 nylon sutures can be used to secure the cochlear implant receiver.

Bone wax is useful for hemostasis; and, if there is epidural bleeding, strips of Surgicel (Ethicon, Inc., Somerville, NJ) are placed into the epidural space to achieve hemostasis and prevent postoperative epidural hematoma formation.

In the following subsections, specific details necessary to create the receiver beds for the currently available devices are described.

Nucleus Freedom. The Nucleus Contour device has two options regarding creation of the receiver bed. The first is to create the cylindrical well

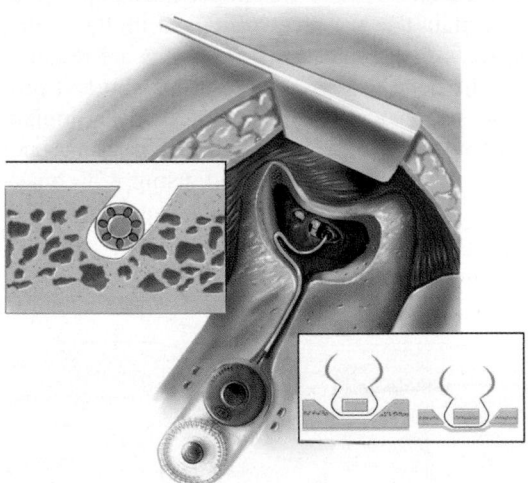

Figure 24 General relationships among the limited mastoidectomy, bony trough for the electrode array, the receiver/stimulator and the tie-down holes used for securing the device. When the skull is thick enough, a trough is created between the bone bed and the mastoidectomy site that is cantilevered to facilitate retention of the array beneath the surface of the skull (*left inset*). The bone dissection for the securing sutures varies according to skull thickness (*bottom right inset*). With thicker skulls, creation of a bony channel through the diploic layer and beneath the cortical layer is possible (*left*). For thinner skulls including most children, full thickness holes are drilled, and the suture is passed between the skull and the dura (*right*). (Published with permission, copyright © 2007 P.A. Wackym, MD.)

to receive the deepest portion of this cochlear implant. It is common in young children to require craniotomy down to dura and creation of the bony island as described above. For the majority of adults and older children, this is not necessary and a craniectomy is all that is required. The remaining portion of the internal device is placed lateral to the skull and in particular, the magnet and loop antenna have a low profile and are barely palpable beneath the scalp flap (see Figures 9 and 10). The remaining rectangular portion of the internal device/receiver is palpable; and, for this reason, it is especially important for this device to be placed well posterior to the position that will be occupied by the BTE speech processor. Another option for this device is to create a receiver bed that will accommodate most of the volume of the Nucleus Freedom receiver. This is done in the same manner as described above, and the advantage of this is that it allows a more integrated placement of the internal device but does require creation of a complex bony island and craniotomy, which requires additional surgical time.

The Nucleus Freedom device has a separate ground electrode that is placed beneath the temporalis muscle, which is located lateral to the principal electrode array. A trough is created between the internal receiver and the area of the mastoidectomy. A 2 mm cutting bur is used to create this trough, and an important point is that the dissection is completed so that one of the bony margins is cantilevered over the tract created in the bone. This further helps in securing and protecting the electrode array.

HiRes 90K. The HiRes 90K device has 2 ground electrodes, 1 built into the primary electrode array, just distal to the internal device, and the second built into the titanium internal case (see Figure 13). Therefore, a second electrode carrier containing the ground electrode is not used with these devices. The trough utilizes a cantilevered segment of the bone either on the superior or inferior aspect of this trough that is helpful in keeping the electrode array from becoming exteriorized on the lateral aspect of the skull (see Figure 24).

The HiRes 90K Bionic Ear has a silastic carrier surrounding the components and has a position for a replaceable internal magnet within the center of the loop antenna (see Figure 13). The issues specific to the HiRes 90K receiver bed are similar to those described in the Nucleus Freedom device. The design of the HiRes 90K differs from the Nucleus Freedom device principally in the mid-portion of the internal device between the magnet and loop antenna and the electrode array. The design allows for a more tapered device that will theoretically result in less frequent problems with extrusion and skin erosion than that experienced with the Nucleus devices. Thus, it is possible to create a small internal well to accommodate the most medial aspects of this device while allowing the remainder of the device to be positioned lateral to the skull. It is also possible to create a larger complex receiver bed

that would accommodate this entire component as has been described in the Nucleus Freedom device subsection. The trough to accommodate the electrode array is the same as is necessary to accommodate any of the available electrode arrays.

Med-El Pulsar$_{CI}$^{100} and Sonata$_{TI}$^{100}. The biggest difference in the receiver bed for the Med-El Pulsar$_{CI}$^{100} is that the electrode array and ground electrode emanate from the side of the cochlear implant instead of from the proximal end of the cochlear implant, as is the case with the other available devices (see Figure 15). Accommodation for this design feature requires that the bony trough begins at the side of the implant internal device and must be positioned so that 1 of the holes necessary to secure the implant can be placed. This is shown in Figures 17 and 25 and illustrates the relative distance between the electrode trough and the internal device necessary to accommodate this specific tie-down hole.

Because the depth of the Pulsar$_{CI}$^{100} is approximately 4 mm (3.9 mm) some of the adult patients do not require a craniotomy down to the level of the dura and creation of a bone island. This however, is necessary in virtually all children and many adults. The same principles described in earlier sections apply with this device, both in terms of creation of the bony island and the trough necessary to accommodate the electrode array. The ground electrode is separate and is placed beneath the temporalis muscle, as is the case with the Nucleus Freedom device. Regarding the titanium and silicone Med-El Sonata$_{TI}$^{100} device, 1 design goal for this new housing is to allow a minimal incision and, therefore, faster recovery. The surgical approach recommended for the Sonata$_{TI}$^{100} is similar to that used for the Nucleus Freedom and HiRes 90K devices.

Mastoidectomy, Facial Recess Approach, and Cochleostomy Techniques

Mastoidectomy. The important point in considering the mastoidectomy for placement of a cochlear implant is that the defect is much smaller than that utilized for chronic otitis media (Figures 24 and 26). In contrast to the standard method of saucerizing the mastoid cavity, this is not performed in cochlear implant surgery. There are 2 areas that should be skeletonized, and the most important of these is the bony external auditory canal. If the bony external auditory canal is not thinned appropriately, the angle through the facial recess becomes more difficult to negotiate and the size of the posterior aspect of the mastoidectomy becomes much larger. It is important to skeletonize the bony external auditory canal but not to violate the integrity of this structure. Should this occur, the risk is that the electrode array can be extruded through the skin of the external auditory canal. Consequently, it is necessary to reinforce this area either with a graft comprised of thick AlloDerm (LifeCell Corporation, Branchburg, NJ) or a bone graft harvested from the cortex of the skull. The second area that needs to be skeletonized is that

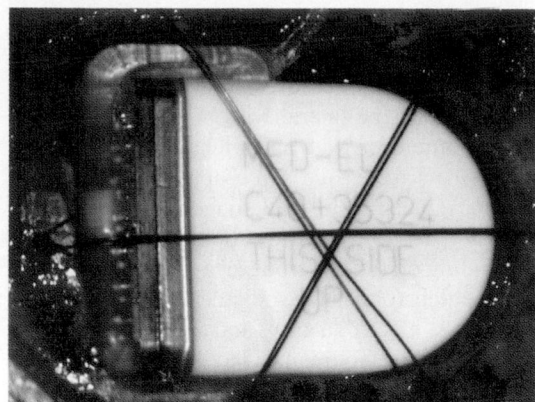

Figure 25 Six-month-old infant undergoing right cochlear implantation after completion of the craniotomy. The craniotomy and bone island were designed to conform to the receiver/stimulator device and allow the electrodes to remain in situ without compression. The bone island is inset approximately 4 mm for the Med-El C40+ receiver/stimulator to be placed so that the lateral aspect of the device is flush with the surface of the skull. Six holes were created through the skull to allow 3 3-0 nylon sutures to be used for securing the internal device. This was necessary due to the small head size, and this helps to avoid tilting or rolling of the device during healing and reformation of the bone beneath the receiver/stimulator. (Published with permission, copyright © 2007 P.A. Wackym, MD.)

of the tegmen mastoideum. This allows greater ease in completing the facial recess and approach and developing the cochleostomy. An additional advantage is providing better exposure and consequently better light delivery that results in better visualization within the facial recess and middle ear. It is also important to continue the skeletonization forward into the zygomatic root for the same reasons (Figures 27 and 28). In contrast, the posterior as well as inferior aspects of the mastoidectomy are not saucerized. It is also important to create bony overhangs in these posterior and inferior aspects of the mastoidectomy cavity that are helpful in retaining the electrode array, which is ultimately coiled into the mastoid cavity (Figure 29). These differences in the mastoidectomy technique also facilitate performance of cochlear implantation in children 6 to 12 months of age.

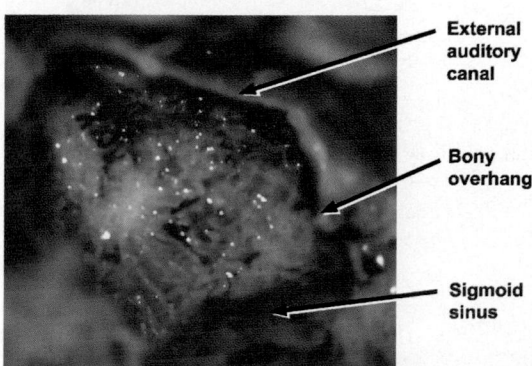

Figure 26 Six-month-old infant undergoing right cochlear implantation with mastoidectomy completed. Unlike an older child or an adult, it should be noted that the bony external auditory canal is extremely thin and the sigmoid sinus is dehiscent. Bony overhangs are designed to help retain the coiled electrode array. (Published with permission, copyright © 2007 P.A. Wackym, MD.)

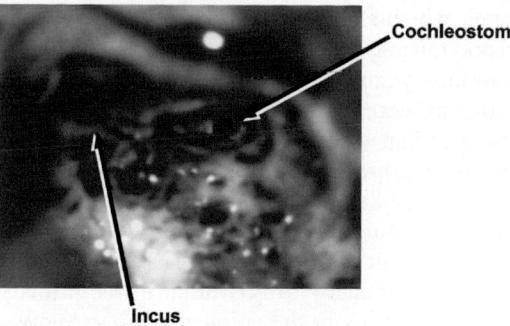

Figure 27 Six-month-old infant undergoing right cochlear implantation with completion of the facial recess approach and cochleostomy. Note the size of the facial recess is no different than in an adult; however, increased precision in thinning the bony external auditory canal is required. The relationship between the short process of the incus and the facial recess is shown. The lateral semicircular canal, facial nerve and round window niche are seen. (Published with permission, copyright © 2007 P.A. Wackym, MD.)

For those individuals who have undergone a canal wall down mastoidectomy procedure in the past and require cochlear implantation, a two-stage procedure is required. First, mastoid obliteration with removal of all epithelium, oversewing the external auditory canal, and filling the resulting dead space with abdominal fat is performed. Three to 6 months later, cochlear implantation can be undertaken. If no active disease is present, consideration of a one-stage procedure may be entertained; however, this is not recommended due to the risk of bacterial contamination.

Facial Recess Approach. Once the mastoidectomy has been completed the facial recess dissection is performed (Figures 27 and 28). The size of the facial recess is the same for individuals of any age, and based on the anatomic measurements

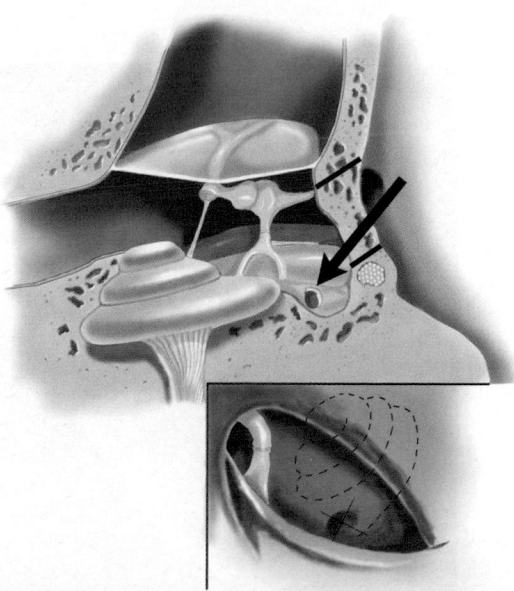

Figure 28 Facial recess approach to the round window niche and membrane, as viewed from the hypotympanic perspective (*top*). Bottom, round window niche as visualized through the facial recess. If the round window niche is divided into quadrants, the cochleostomy should be performed in the anterior inferior quadrant. (Published with permission, copyright © 2007 P.A. Wackym, MD.)

of human temporal bones, the facial recess is of adult size at by at least 2 weeks of age.[116] Facial nerve electromyography is appropriate during this portion of the operation, and this cochlear implant surgeon always uses facial nerve electromyography during the dissection of the facial recess, creation of the cochleostomy, and insertion of the electrode array (NIM-2, Xomed, Jacksonville, FL). A general guideline for determining the position of the facial recess is a direct inferior extension of the short process of the incus. Because there is no mechanical function of the incus in an ear receiving a cochlear implant, there is no adverse consequence of removing the incus buttress, which normally is preserved to maintain the suspensory ligament, attached to the incus. This has the advantage of delivering additional light into the middle ear and allows direct extension in an inferior direction below the short process of the incus. The vertical segment of the facial nerve is skeletonized, and a 1.5 mm diamond bur with a long shaft is helpful during this portion of the dissection. The dissection is carried inferiorly to the level of the chorda tympani nerve and in some of the patients undergoing cochlear implantation surgery; the chorda tympani nerve is divided to provide adequate access and visualization of the round window niche. Preoperative counseling of the parents or the patient is necessary so that they understand the consequences of dividing the chorda tympani nerve. The lateral limit of the facial recess is the tympanic annulus; and, for the majority of patients, this should be partially skeletonized to maximize the size of the facial recess.

While it is possible to create a small facial recess, most experienced cochlear implant surgeons do not do this and prefer opening the facial

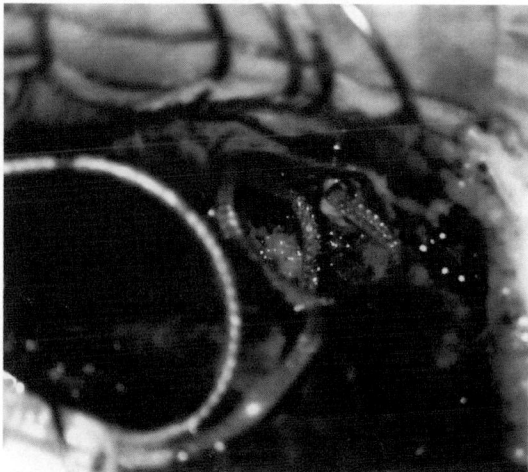

Figure 29 Six-month-old infant undergoing right cochlear implantation. The separate ground electrode of the Med-El C40+ device can be seen passing upward across the skull and has been placed beneath the temporalis muscle (*left center*). Due to the relative size of the skull and the resulting shorter distance between the cochleostomy and the internal receiver–stimulator, a larger amount of electrode array can be seen coiled within the mastoid cavity. Note the bony overhangs created by undercutting the mastoid cortex that were designed to facilitate retention of the electrode array. In this infant, a shallow trough was created because of her thin skull. (Published with permission, copyright © 2007 P.A. Wackym, MD.)

recess widely. This provides much better visualization of the round window niche and delivers additional light from the microscope into the middle ear. These factors facilitate completion of the cochleostomy and insertion of the electrode array. Figure 27 shows an intraoperative photograph that illustrates this point. The tympanic annulus can be well visualized with exposure of the promontory, and epithelium of the middle ear is also readily apparent.

During the facial recess dissection, violation of the tympanic annulus and tympanic membrane will result in contamination and direct communication with the external auditory canal. This raises the possibilities of postoperative infection and cholesteatoma formation. If this occurs, the area should be repaired; and the cochlear implantation should be performed as a staged procedure.

Cochleostomy. Placement of the electrode array within the scala tympani is accomplished through a cochleostomy. This cochleostomy is positioned relative to the round window membrane, and the most important factor in being able to place the electrode array within the scala tympani appropriately is visualization of the round window niche. The electrode inserted within the scala tympani is shown in Figure 30, and the specific electrode insertion techniques will be described later. This landmark is critical to determine the relative position of the basal portion of the scala tympani. In completing the facial recess approach, there is a temptation to begin preparing the cochleostomy when only the promontory is visualized. A cochleostomy into the scala vestibuli will likely result; however, this can also lead to the most common reason for failure to place the electrode

array, which is the inadvertent opening into the hypotympanic air cell tract and the extracochlear insertion of the electrode array (Figure 31).[117] If the drilling begins too inferiorly, dissection in this area can resemble an ossified basal turn of the cochlea. Often the hypotympanic air cell tract will appear like the open scala tympani following successful completion of a cochleostomy. The obvious result is an incomplete electrode insertion and ultimately no activation of the primary afferent neurons in the spiral ganglion. Another important anatomic landmark to keep in mind when experiencing difficulty in identifying the scala tympani is the position of the intratemporal internal carotid artery. With anterior dissection, when the scala tympani has not been adequately identified, the posterior aspect of the intratemporal carotid artery can be exposed and this is an especially important consideration when performing cochlear implant surgery in children between 6 and 12 months of age. A high index of suspicion must be maintained during the surgical dissection if the round window membrane and round window niche are not visualized at the beginning of the creation of the cochleostomy. This also underscores the importance of identifying this key landmark before beginning the cochleostomy. Those factors that help in the visualization of the round window niche include a wide facial recess and skeletonization of the bony external auditory canal.

Once the round window niche has been visualized, the use of a 1 mm diamond bur with a long shaft allows dissection of the niche until the round window membrane is directly seen. It is important to position the cochleostomy anterior and slightly inferior to the round window membrane as utilizing this position facilitates the angle of insertion of the electrode array (see Figure 28). If the round window is opened and

the electrode array inserted through the round window, the angle of insertion is too acute and results in excessive pressure on the electrode array against the lateral wall of the cochlea during the attempted advancement of the electrode array. This excessive force applied to the electrode array can result in damage.

The design of the cochleostomy varies depending on the electrode array used. The smallest cochleostomy is associated with the Med-El $Pulsar_{CI}^{100}$ electrode array and the diameter of the cochleostomy should only be 1.3 mm in diameter. For the Med-El $Pulsar_{CI}^{100}$ or $Sonata_{TI}^{100}$ with the standard array, the diameter of the electrode array increases from $\approx 0.5 \times 0.6$ mm at the apex (distal tip) to ≈ 1.3 mm at the proximal, thicker part of the array just before the marker ring. The marker ring is ≈ 1.5 mm in diameter. Thus, the cochleostomy can be as small as 1.3 mm and should be no larger than 1.5 mm to allow proper sealing of the cochleostomy with the marker ring. Small strips of fascia should be placed around the cochleostomy to seal the perilymphatic space from the middle ear (Figure 32). The cochleostomy required for placement of the Nucleus Freedom with the Contour Advance electrode is typically 1.5 to 2 mm. The electrode array itself has a diameter at the tip of $\approx 0.5 \times 0.6$ mm and the diameter at the basal portion of the array is 0.8 mm.

The present HiFocus 1j or Helix electrode utilizes a round cochleostomy, 1.6 mm in diameter, or an oval cochleostomy measuring 1.2×1.6 mm. The electrode array itself has a diameter at the tip of 0.6 mm, and the diameter at the basal contact is 0.8 mm (1j electrode) or 1.1 mm (Helix electrode).

With all 3 devices, once the cochleostomy has been created, it is important to irrigate the scala tympani via the cochleostomy to remove air bubbles and to wash bone debris from the

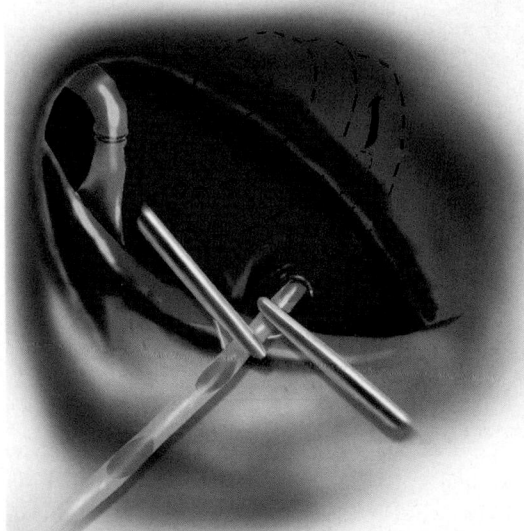

Figure 30 Bimanual insertion of a cochlear implant electrode array. After completion of the cochleostomy, the electrode array is introduced into the scala tympani. Incremental insertion of the electrode array using opposing claw instruments near the cochleostomy helps to avoid buckling of the array. Rotation of the electrode array in the direction opposite that of the ear being implanted, in this case to the left for a right cochlear implantation facilitates atraumatic insertion. (Published with permission, copyright © 2007 P.A. Wackym, MD.)

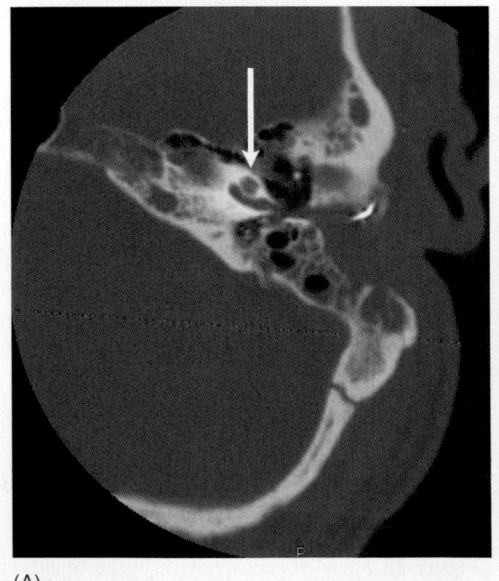
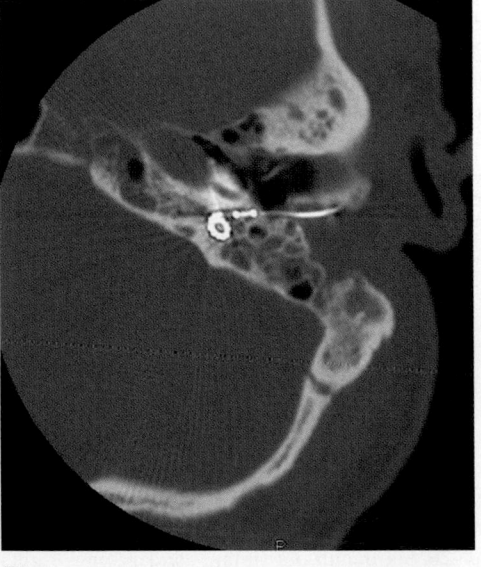

(A)   (B)

Figure 31 Hypotympanic air cell tract insertion of a cochlear implant electrode array by another surgeon. (A) Axial CT scan shows the position of the cochlea (*long arrow*) in relationship to the hypotympanic air cell tract (*short arrow*). Note the adjacency of the entrance to the hypotympanic air cell tract and the round window. (B) The coiled electrode can be seen within the hypotympanic air cell tract and outside of the cochlea. (Published with permission, copyright © 2007 P.A. Wackym, MD.)

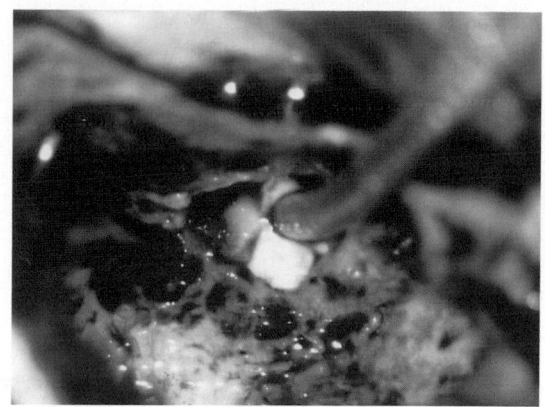

Figure 32 Six-month-old infant undergoing right cochlear implantation. After full insertion of the 31 mm Med-El C40+ electrode array into the cochlea, the cochleostomy is sealed with multiple small strips of temporalis fascia or pericranium. This is an important step to reduce the risk of meningitis should otitis media develop. (Published with permission, copyright © 2007 P.A. Wackym, MD.)

scala tympani. This bone debris, if left in place, will induce ossification, and it is important to minimize this because of the potential need for reimplantation in the future should a device fail. This is particularly important in young children being implanted between the ages of 6 months to 12 months, as there is a higher likelihood that they will encounter a device failure during their life span than an adult patient receiving a cochlear implant. Lactated Ringers solution with a 5 mL syringe and a 24 gauge suction tip is ideal for the irrigation and refilling of the scala tympani.

Securing the Receiver

Once the bone work has been completed and the cochleostomy opened, the internal device is secured in position with the retaining sutures. One to 3 nylon sutures are used for this purpose (see Figure 25). It is important during this process to be cognizant of the position of the electrode array so that excessive force or kinking is not encountered during the tightening of these sutures. It is also important that hemostats or other instruments not be used along any portion of the suture that will remain in the patient, as this weakens the material. Using a single throw in the first portion of the knot allows the second throw of the suture to slide along the monofilament nylon to achieve the appropriate level of tension and position of the internal device relative to the lateral aspect of the skull. It is also important that the knots be placed overlying the bone and not overlying the internal device. A total of 8 knots are placed into each suture and a medium length tail to the suture is created when cutting the suture. After both of these retaining sutures are placed, the ground electrode is placed beneath the temporalis muscle for the Med-El Pulsar$_{CI}$,[100] Sonata$_{TI}$,[100] and Nucleus Freedom devices. To accomplish this, a Freer elevator is used to elevate the periosteum and temporalis muscle, and the ground electrode is placed medial to the muscle. The Nucleus

Freedom device has a second extracochlear electrode that is attached to the receiver–stimulator device.

Electrode Insertion

The electrode insertion is specific for each device and subsections describe the technique used for each electrode insertion. Several different detailed descriptions of electrode insertion techniques have been published recently.[114] The standard electrodes are described below, and descriptions of special electrode designs are provided in the section dealing with ossification of the cochlea.

Nucleus Freedom Contour Advance. The Nucleus Contour Advance electrode is shown in Figure 11. This electrode design is a perimodiolar electrode and is preformed to conform to the modiolus. There is a stylet that is positioned within this electrode array that maintains the electrode in a straight configuration. In addition to the electrodes, there are 10 support bands that, together with the stylet, stiffen the electrode array. Of all available electrodes, this is the stiffest one and, consequently, is relatively easy to insert. The greatest disadvantage of this current electrode design is that once the stylet has been removed, it cannot be replaced. This is problematic should the electrode insertion be difficult because of anatomic variations. Manual positioning of the electrode tip within the opening of the cochleostomy is performed, and guiding the tip into this position is facilitated by the use of a claw-shaped instrument held in the dominant hand. Once the electrode tip is retained within the opening of the cochleostomy, bimanual advancement of the electrode array using 2 claw-shaped instruments held opposing each other, as close to the cochleostomy as possible, facilitates advancement of the electrode array within the scala tympani. The Nucleus Freedom with the Contour Advance electrode array has 3 silastic bands outside of the electrode array that represent the proximal limit, and these should remain outside of the cochleostomy. The electrode has a white marker that indicates that the electrode should not be advanced into the cochlea once this marker is positioned at the cochleostomy. After complete insertion has been achieved, fascia grafts are placed around the cochleostomy site to seal it, and fascia grafts are also placed between the electrode array and the facial nerve within the facial recess. In addition, fascia is placed between the electrode array and the tympanic annulus.

HiRes 90K. There are 2 electrode array systems available for the HiRes 90K, the 1j and the Helix electrodes (see Figure 14). For the 1j electrode, both a metal (outer diameter of 1.5 mm) and a Teflon (outer diameter of 2 mm) insertion tube are included and selection is based on surgeon preference. Gentle pressure along a thumb-driven advancement mechanism is required to insert the electrode. Should errors occur in electrode insertion, the electrode is easily reloaded into the insertion tube/insertion instrument and additional

attempts at electrode insertion can be made. The major advantage of this method is that uniform pressure during insertion can be made. The Helix electrode is a perimodiolar electrode; however, unlike the Nucleus Contour Advance perimodiolar electrode, the Helix has been designed so that it can be reloaded onto the stylet using a specially designed tool for that purpose. Subsequent to insertion, fascia grafts are placed around the cochleostomy site to seal it. Fascia grafts are also placed between the electrode array and the facial nerve within the facial recess as well as between the electrode array and the tympanic annulus.

Med-El Pulsar$_{CI}$[100] and Sonata$_{TI}$[100]. The Med-El Pulsar$_{CI}$[100] and Sonata$_{TI}$[100] systems each have 6 separate electrode designs (see Figure 16) including a design used for common cavity applications, which is custom made for each individual patient (see Figure 17). Once the internal receiver is secured and the cochleostomy is complete, the electrode array is held in the nondominant hand. A claw-shaped instrument is used to help guide the tip of the electrode into the cochleostomy, and once this is retained at the edge of the cochleostomy, two claw-shaped instruments are used to advance the electrode array (see Figure 30). The advancement is facilitated if small segments of the electrode array are inserted with each subsequent movement, as close to the edge of the cochleostomy as possible. There is a circumferential ring that represents the limit of the electrode array to be inserted; and, for the standard array, this is located 31.5 mm from the distal tip. Once this is sealed at the cochleostomy, the manufacturer states that an adequate seal will be obtained if the cochleostomy is created at the optimal size. In addition, it is advisable to place strips of fascia around the electrode array within the cochleostomy site, and free fascia grafts are placed between the facial nerve and the electrode array as well as between the electrode array and the tympanic annulus.

Ossification of the Cochlea and Common Cavity Malformations

There is a range of ossification that can occur within the cochlea; and, depending on the extent of the ossification, there are different solutions that can be employed (Figure 33). Scala tympani or scala vestibuli insertions may be necessary, depending on the degree of ossification (see Figure 33B and C). During the opening of the cochleostomy, if some ossification of the cochlea is encountered, and once drilling past 1 to 4 mm of the basal cochlea, a normal scala tympani is encountered, the compressed electrode array may be the appropriate array for insertion. The Pulsar$_{CI}$[100]S and the Pulsar$_{CI}$[100]M are designed with the same number of electrode contacts ($n = 12$ pairs), but the total lengths of the electrode arrays are 13 or 21 mm, respectively, as compared to the standard electrode array of 31.5 mm. The ITD can be used to determine which array is the appropriate electrode to be inserted before opening an individual cochlear implant. With this, ITD

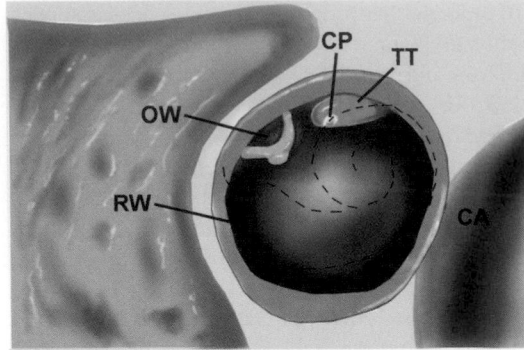

(A)

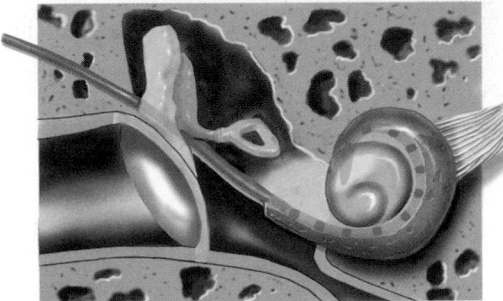

(B)

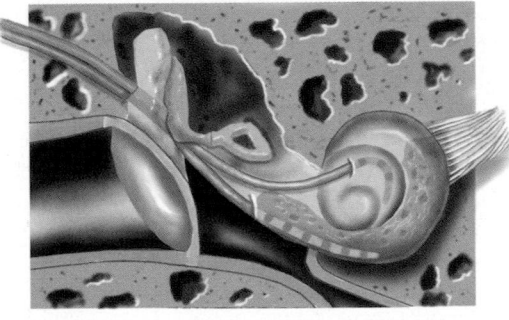

(C)

Figure 33 Cochlear implantation in the ossified cochlea. (A) The cochlea is shown ghosted in deep to the middle ear. The internal carotid artery (CA) is anterior to the basal turn of the cochlea. The round window (RW), is the most posterior aspect of the cochlea within the middle ear, and it can be found 1.5 mm inferior to the stapedial tendon. The tensor tympani (TT) tendon enters the middle ear at the cochleariform process (CP), which represents the level of the pars ascendens of the cochlea. This landmark is the limit of the dissection, thereby, avoiding injury to the facial nerve. The anterior edge of the oval window (OW) is the posterior limit of drilling. (B) Ossification of the scala tympani without ossification of the scala vestibuli allows placement of the cochleostomy and full electrode insertion in the scala vestibuli. Note the more superior position of the cochleostomy. (C) With more severe ossification of the cochlea, the use of a split electrode array allows placement of some electrode contacts into the ossified basal turn of the cochlea and other electrode contacts into the middle turn of the cochlea via a second cochleostomy. (Published with permission, copyright © 2007 P.A. Wackym, MD.)

is advanced through the cochleostomy, and the depth of insertion is determined. If it is apparent that the standard electrode array would result in electrodes being extracochlear, the compressed electrode array should be used and fully inserted.

For more severely ossified cochleas, both the Cochlear Corporation and the Med-El Corporation manufacture split electrode arrays

(see Figures 12 and 16). The Med-El split electrode design (Pulsar$_{CI}$^{100} GB) has 2 compressed electrode arrays with 5 and 7 pairs of electrode contacts, respectively. These electrode arrays are inserted via 2 cochleostomies (see Figure 33C).

Cochlear implantation with severe cochlear malformations, such as a common cavity, has been challenging.[118] Among these problems are CSF gushers and a need for frequent reprogramming due to migrating electrodes. One solution that targets the migrating electrode problem is the sixth electrode design available with the Pulsar$_{CI}$^{100} device. For children with this malformation, the surgeon provides the dimensions of the common cavity to the manufacturer, and a Pulsar$_{CI}$^{100}S electrode is custom made so that the distal end is lengthened with a nonactive segment of silicone ending with a small platinum ball at the tip (see Figure 16). Using the double posterior labyrinthotomy technique (see Figure 17C), the nonactive part of the implant is pushed into the superior labyrinthotomy until it is seen through the inferior labyrinthotomy. The small terminal ball is hooked through the inferior labyrinthotomy, and the terminal nonactive part of the array is pulled out, leaving a loop within the common cavity. Next the two arms are advanced together positioning the array along the inner wall of the cavity (see Figure 17D). Resistance is felt when the loop covers the internal circumference of the cavity. The surgical technique and early outcomes have been reported in a few small series of patients.[119,120]

Special Considerations Regarding Securing the Electrode Array

For all 3 devices manufactured for the United States marketplace, securing of the electrode array at the cochleostomy site and at the facial recess is important. The cochlea and facial recess are the same size at birth as they are throughout adulthood; and, therefore, it is important to secure the electrode array at the cochleostomy with the fascia graft, which will scar in place and bridge the surrounding promontory to the electrode array. Second sites of stabilization at the facial recess, with fascia grafts between the facial nerve and the electrode array as well as between the tympanic annulus and the electrode array, will further stabilize the relationship of the electrode array to the cochlea and facial recess. This is important in children because of their head growth. The sites of stabilization at the cochleostomy and facial recess will secure the distal electrode array anteriorly while the sutures and fibrous capsule that will form around the internal receiver as well as the electrode within the trough created at the time of the operation, will stabilize the proximal portion of the electrode array. The remainder of the electrode array is coiled within the mastoid and this air-filled space will allow the uncoiling of this electrode array during development as the child's head grows. This mechanism allows the

accomplishment of natural growth and development while maintaining the integrity and position of the cochlear implant and its electrode array within the cochlea.

Intraoperative Electrophysiologic Testing

Intraoperative testing of the cochlear implant is a critical portion of the operation. First, impedance measurements are conducted to determine if the electrode array has been damaged during insertion and that all of the available electrodes are functional. Intraoperative neural response telemetry (NRT) is available for the Nucleus Freedom device, and this allows direct recording from the eighth nerve distally following proximal stimulation. A similar system termed neural response imaging (NRI) is available for the HiRes 90K system. Med-El developed auditory response telemetry (ART); however, while it is available elsewhere in the world, it currently is not available in the United States pending FDA approval. NRT, NRI, and ART function in a similar manner.

For some of our patients, we perform intraoperative electrically evoked auditory brainstem response (EABR) testing. We do this with distal, intermediate and proximal electrodes and determine thresholds and maximum amplitudes of wave V. Beginning with the advent of perimodiolar electrodes, we performed this before placing the electrode array in the perimodiolar position and after placing the electrode array in the perimodiolar position.[102,121] The details of the performance of this are described below; however, the utility of performing EABR testing is most apparent with the management of young children. While it is possible to determine behavioral thresholds in young children as young as 6 months old, we have found that it is valuable in the initial programming of these devices to have having objective information regarding thresholds for 3 of the active electrodes. In addition, there is tremendous value to the families and to the patients receiving cochlear implants when we can state immediately postoperatively that not only is the electrode array fully inserted within the cochlea, but also that we have objective evidence of central auditory responses of the electrical stimulation delivered through these electrodes. This technique, together with NRT, NRI and ART, has obviated the need for intraoperative radiographic studies to confirm the position of the electrode array within the cochlea.

Procedures to record electrically evoked auditory potentials intraoperatively reliably from pediatric and adult patients are described in the following paragraphs. During the surgical preparation of the patient, subdermal needle electrodes are placed on the forehead, nape of the neck, vertex, and ear contralateral to the implant. Markers that identify the electrode location are placed on the electrode leads, which are then draped under the operating table until they are needed. A subdermal needle electrode is placed on the sterile table and is inserted in the ipsilateral earlobe prior to the beginning of the surgical procedure. The electrode leads are attached to the amplifier of the evoked potential average that is externally triggered by the stimulus output of the software for the respective implant.

After the surgeon has positioned the internal receiver/stimulator and the electrode array, a sterile sheath is opened and the transmission coil is placed inside. The surgeon places the transmission coil covered by the sterile sheath over the internal device with a sterile, moistened gauze sponge separating them. In this way, the external and internal devices are in communication with one another but separated, and the ground electrodes are not in direct contact with the air. The transmission coil is connected via a long cable to an external speech processor that is connected to the programming interface unit. When the programming interface unit is coupled to a computer, stimuli can be generated and delivered to the internal implant electrodes. Software programs provided by each of the cochlear implant manufacturers allow confirmation that the transmission coil is communicating with the internal system and that the electrodes are being activated with electrical stimuli.

From our intraoperative experience recording EABRs from patients receiving various implants, that is, Advanced Bionics, Nucleus, and Med-El, we have developed protocols for stimulation and recording that take into consideration the parameters of each device. Generally, stimulation occurs on 3 individual electrodes that represent apical, middle, and basal locations along the electrode array and within the cochlea. The initial stimulus levels used are those that typically generate a well-formed EABR. Stimulation begins on the most apical electrode, since responses from an apical position result in the best morphology, largest amplitude, and lowest EABR Wave V threshold.[122] Electrical stimulation is decreased until the Wave V threshold is determined. The absolute level of current varies depending on the particular cochlear implant device. The procedure is repeated for medial and basal electrodes. Waveform morphology, amplitude, and threshold are determined for all recording sets. Typically Waves II, III, and V are present at higher stimulus levels, and Wave V can be followed down to threshold as seen in Figure 34. Wave I is never observable due to the overlap with the stimulus artifact in the early portion of the time window (less than 1 ms). We have found, as have others, that the EABR threshold represents a stimulus level that falls somewhere within the electrical dynamic range for a given electrode. This corresponds to a current level that should be audible for the patient and can be approached from a minimum current level at the time of initial stimulation. The EABR threshold also provides prior knowledge of whether low, normal, or high current levels are expected at the initial stimulation, which can be quite helpful when presenting electrical stimuli to young children for the first time.

EABR tracings and threshold information for each tested electrode are provided to the programming audiologist prior to the initial activation of the implant. In addition, the operative outcome and any unusual circumstances that can affect performance, for example, partial electrode insertion, ossified cochlea, or unusual anatomy, are shared with the programming audiologist. This information assists in planning for the initial activation and avoids stimulation of electrodes that could generate unpleasant sensations, such as electrodes that may be outside the cochlea. Finally, as mentioned previously, the electrophysiologic test results are shared with the patient's family and assure that the electrode is properly placed and that electrical stimulation will successfully activate the auditory system. The EABR results can also reflect the degree of central auditory system maturation as seen in children implanted as young as 6 months of age (see Figure 34).

Closure and Postoperative Management

The closure of the soft tissue varies depending on the initial soft tissue approach utilized. For young children, since the periosteum, scalp, and skin are all raised together in 1 layer, these are closed in 2 layers. The first layer is closed with inverted interrupted 4-0 Vicryl sutures (Johnson & Johnson Co., Ethicon Inc., Arlington, TX) and includes the periosteum, galea, and subcutaneous tissues. Once this layer has been closed, the skin is closed with a running locked 5-0 plain gut fast-absorbing suture (Johnson & Johnson Co., Ethicon Inc., Arlington, TX). The advantage of using all absorbable sutures in young children is that the skin sutures do not need to be removed.

For adult patients and children large enough to have the soft tissue approach completed in 2 layers, the periosteum is closed over the implant with simple interrupted 3-0 Vicryl or 3-0 Monocryl suture (Johnson & Johnson Co., Ethicon Inc., Arlington, TX). Another important consideration, when thick scalp or unusually well-developed temporalis and scalp musculature is found, debulking of the muscle can be required. Also, defatting the scalp is possible; however, the vascular supply to the scalp runs with the galea and care should be taken to avoid compromising this. Maintaining a scalp, which is thin enough to allow the magnetic attraction of the transmitter coil to the internal cochlear stimulator device magnet, will allow the transmitter coil to be secured to the scalp without falling off; however, if the scalp is too thick, this will not be possible. An alternate strategy is to thin the scalp flap. Surgical judgment in thinning the scalp is essential. The galea and subcutaneous layers are then closed with inverted interrupted 3-0 (adults) or 4-0 (children) Monocryl or Vicryl pop-off sutures and the skin is closed with a running locked 5-0 fast-absorbing gut suture or 4-0 nylon for the postauricular and scalp incisions.

For adults and children, care is taken to protect the incision with antibiotic ointment and strips of Telfa, and a pressure dressing is applied. A small sheet of cotton is trimmed to conform to the pinna, which helps protect the pinna from pressure-induced necrosis. Fluffs are placed

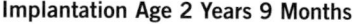

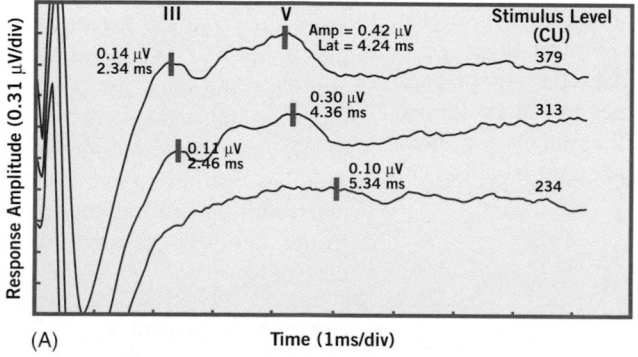

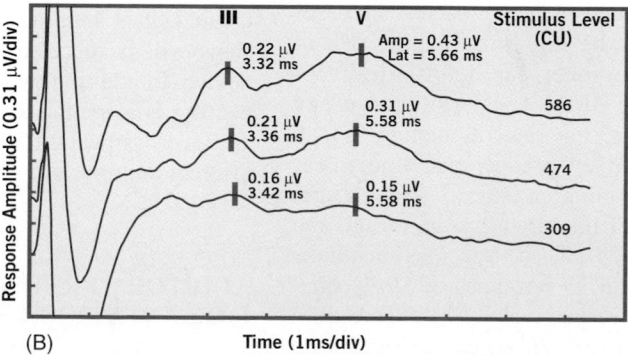

Figure 34 Intraoperative EABR growth functions from an older child aged 2 years 9 months (A) and the child's younger sibling, aged 6 months (B). Both children were implanted with Med-El C40+ (Med-El Corporation) devices, and both sets of recordings are from stimulation of apical electrode 1. Stimulation levels for the older child were 379, 313, and 234 clinical units (top to bottom tracings, respectively), and 586, 474, and 309 clinical units for the young child (top to bottom tracings, respectively). Comparison of the high, medium, and low stimulation-level tracings indicate similar Wave V response amplitudes between children; however, differences are apparent in Wave V latency. The widths of the Wave V peaks are larger for the younger child. (Published with permission, copyright © 2007 P.A. Wackym, MD.)

over the scalp and elevated flaps, and one Ker-lix (Kendall Healthcare Products Co., Mansfield, MA) and one Kling (Johnson & Johnson Co., Ethicon Inc., Arlington, TX) are wrapped around the patient's head. Umbilical tape (Johnson & Johnson Co., Ethicon Inc., Arlington, TX) is used over the forehead to secure the dressing and to lift this dressing away from the patient's eyes. The pressure dressing is left in place for the first postoperative night and is removed the following morning.

Virtually all cochlear implant operations are done on an outpatient basis with children being observed for less than 23 hours, principally to control postoperative pain. Adults are typically operated in an ambulatory manner unless their operation occurs late in the afternoon, as is the case when three cochlear implant operations are performed in one day.

Complications

The most common complications occurring after cochlear implantation are wound and flap related.[123,124] Wound breakdown is most often associated with placement of the internal device too close to the pinna (see Figure 22) or at the site of the skin incision. Injury to the intratemporal internal carotid artery is extremely rare; however, as discussed earlier in this chapter, in young children in whom the round window niche is not clearly seen, it is possible to follow the hypotympanic air cell tract to the carotid artery.[125] In such clinical situations, it is therefore important to maintain a high index of suspicion to identify the carotid artery prior to injury. Other risks of the cochlear implant procedure are similar to, and as rare as, those seen in operations for chronic ear otitis media: infection, facial paralysis, vertigo, CSF leakage, meningitis, and anesthesia-related complications.[58,123,126–128] Of these, the risk of meningitis most deserves further comment due to the recent heightened awareness of this complication. Early cases of meningitis are due to otitis media in the context of an unsealed cochleostomy. As discussed earlier, it is important to seal the cochleostomy with fascia. However, until the subsequent fibrosis has been completed, the inner ear is vulnerable to the passage of bacteria into the perilymphatic space and then the CSF space. Late cases of meningitis may be due to the higher risk of meningitis due to inner ear deformities[126] or inadequate sealing of the cochleostomy. In any of these situations, the risk of meningitis can be further reduced by preoperative immunization with Prevnar (children under 2 years of age) and Pneumovax 23 (children 2 years of age and all other individuals). These vaccines recognize seven serotypes and 23 serotypes of *Streptococcus pneumoniae*, respectively. Children should also be vaccinated with *Haemophilus influenzae* type b conjugate (Hib) and quadrivalent A, C, Y, W-135 meningococcal polysaccharide (Menomune). Our cochlear implant program requires vaccination with the age appropriate vaccine prior to implantation.

Facial nerve stimulation can occur after cochlear implantation due to electrical activation of the nerve by the active electrodes.[127] Placement of the fascia between the electrode array and the facial nerve as well as sealing the cochleostomy is designed to limit current spread. Certain primary bone diseases such as otosclerosis and Paget disease will increase the porosity of the bone, and this may allow extracochlear current spread and activation of the facial nerve. Similarly, placement of the electrode array within the IAC can result in facial nerve activation (see Figure 8). Programming the external speech processor can deactivate specific electrodes found to be stimulating the facial nerve, thereby eliminating this problem.

The final complication that should be mentioned is device failure. While this is uncommon, these failed devices are routinely removed, and the cochlea reimplanted.[129] This is uncomplicated in most cases and results in comparable performance or even enhanced performance if the failed device is replaced with a later generation device.

Special Considerations Regarding Bilateral Cochlear Implantation

For patients who have never received a cochlear implant and who choose to receive bilateral cochlear implants, the operation can be performed in a sequential or simultaneous manner.[130] For young children, the operations should be performed sequentially, primarily due to the small head size and because of the desire to avoid a longer anesthetic time. For older children and adults, the operations can be performed safely simultaneously.

Future Considerations

Multiple institutions and corporations are actively pursuing the development of a fully implantable cochlear implant. Reduced power requirements, improved battery life, and the ability to recharge the internal battery via a transcutaneous route are engineering issues that are being addressed. Likewise, the development of a microphone/transducer placed on the ossicular chain within the middle ear remains a technical challenge, which must be resolved before a fully implantable cochlear auditory prosthesis can be created. It is anticipated that additional surgical steps will be necessary to implant this type of device. In addition, work focused on tissue engineering is targeting strategies to reduce fibrosis and neo-ossification as well as increase primary afferent dendrite growth and spiral ganglion cell survival.

AUDITORY BRAINSTEM IMPLANTATION

The restoration of hearing in individuals with hearing loss of a wide range of causes has made dramatic strides over the past decades. At present, surgical intervention in the form of cochlear implants can provide useful auditory perception in individuals deriving little or no benefit from hearing aids; however, these auditory prostheses require an intact auditory nerve to conduct electrical signals to the brainstem. The restoration of auditory perception in individuals deafened by loss of the vestibulocochlear nerves is currently being provided by auditory brainstem implants (ABI).

The ABI is a device consisting of several electrodes placed on the brainstem surface to stimulate the cochlear nuclei directly.[131,132] Externally, it is coupled with a digital speech processor similar to that of a cochlear implant. Current studies have shown that such stimulation can provide individuals with NF2 useful perception of environmental sounds and even open-set speech comprehension.[131,132] However, there is also evidence that non-NF2 patients receiving an ABI, such as temporal bone fracture patients without a functional cochlear nerve, perform at a much higher level as measured by open-set speech discrimination testing.[50]

There is only one ABI available in the United States, and the Cochlear Americas' (Englewood, CO) ABI is approved by the FDA for use in individuals 17 years or older with NF2 undergoing resection of a vestibular schwannoma or in patients undergoing resection of a vestibular schwannoma in an only-hearing ear.[133] Patients with NF2 are often left with complete sensorineural deafness due to the sacrifice of both auditory nerves during resection of bilateral tumors.[134] Cochlear Americas' array is a 21-electrode device with the electrodes embedded in a silastic paddle backed with Dacron mesh. This device is also used intraoperatively as a stimulating electrode for the EABR to help identify optimal positioning of the electrode paddle.[131] The recommended protocol with this device utilizes a translabyrinthine approach to the tumor and subsequent implantation of the ABI.[131] An FDA clinical trial of a new electrode array utilizing a penetrating electrode is underway, and several patients have received this device to date.

Optimal placement of the electrode paddle onto the cochlear nucleus is difficult because it is not possible to visualize this complex directly with the operating microscope via the surgical approaches used to reach these tumors. However, the use of the endoscope in placement of an ABI electrode array has been explored to accomplish this goal.[135,136] Our team has taken a multidisciplinary approach in ABI electrode placement utilizing endoscopic guidance and electrophysiologic mapping to optimize electrode placement. This has resulted in increased numbers of active electrodes, as well as reduced numbers of electrodes producing side effects and nonactive electrodes.

Surgical Approaches

Translabyrinthine Approach. The translabyrinthine dissection should be performed in the standard fashion with an operating microscope and basic otologic instruments. In brief, a complete mastoidectomy is performed, and the facial

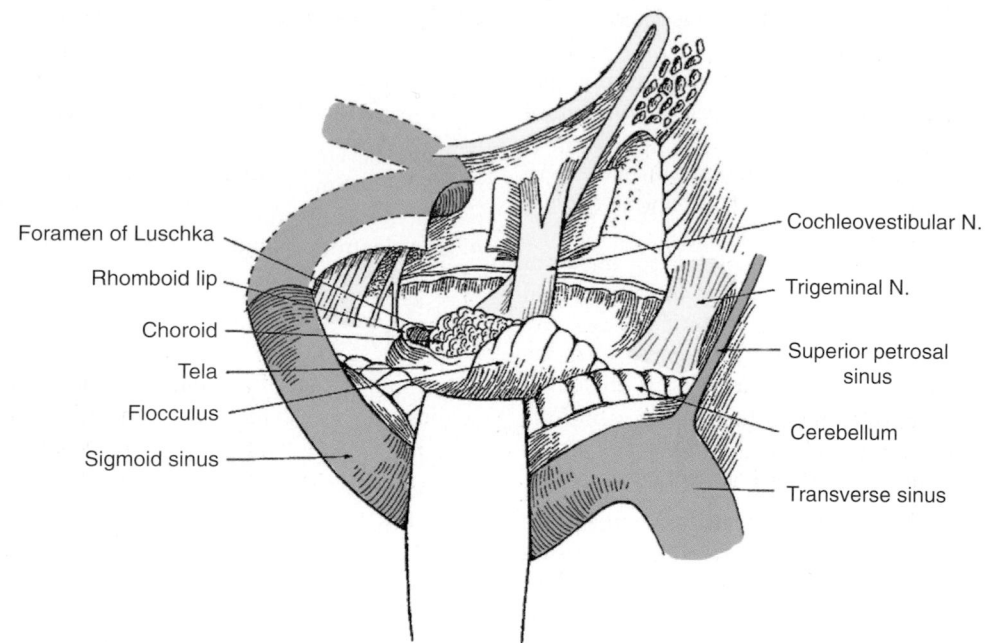

Figure 35 Detail of the landmarks visible near the cochlear nucleus via the translabyrinthine approach for placement of an auditory brainstem implant N-nerve. (Published with permission, copyright © 2007 P.A. Wackym, MD.)

nerve and semicircular canals are identified. The vestibular labyrinth is removed, and the posterior and middle fossa dura is exposed. Working from the superior canal ampulla, the IAC is skeletonized. The jugular bulb is identified and should be thoroughly decompressed to provide direct visualization of the rostral fibers of the glossopharyngeal nerve. This allows identification of an important landmark and provides access for the endoscope during implantation. The posterior fossa dura is then incised and reflected exposing the cerebellum and flocculus.

At this point the tumor is removed, and the following describes the ABI placement. Additional intraoperative challenges encountered result from the distortion of landmarks produced by tumor compression or by tumor extirpation. The use of the landmarks described is even more critical in such cases as a step-wise approach may allow identification of the implant site in a grossly distorted cerebellopontine angle.

A 0° endoscope is advanced into the operative field and used to identify the flocculus, vestibulocochlear, and glossopharyngeal nerves (Figure 35). In some individuals, the choroid plexus may be visible over or just inferior to the flocculus. The vestibulocochlear and glossopharyngeal nerves will appear to converge behind the flocculus with the imaginary point of convergence near the dorsal cochlear nucleus. A 30° or 45° endoscope can now be passed over, that is, lateral, to the flocculus allowing visualization of

the choroid plexus which can be traced medially to the rhomboid lip and foramen of Luschka. Use of the angled endoscope allows this to be accomplished with minimal retraction on the flocculus and thus helps to preserve the taenia chordae. The McCabe flap knife can now be used under endoscopic visualization to retract the choroid gently and expose the surface of the brainstem and lateral recess of the fourth ventricle. The surface of the brainstem within the recess has a characteristic glistening appearance due to the overlying ependyma.

The endoscope should be stabilized at the periphery of the operative field to allow introduction and manipulation of the electrode and instruments. It can be positioned superiorly against the tegmen or inferiorly against the bony ridge remaining over the tympanic and mastoid facial nerve. Decompression of the jugular bulb will allow adequate space for the distal aspect of the endoscope to be maneuvered. Positioning of the endoscope will be determined by the side of the patient being operated upon and the handedness of the surgeon. There is a tendency for the temperature of the distal endoscope to increase, which can cause neural stimulation and potentially neural damage. Care must be taken in positioning the endoscope near the facial nerve, and attention, must be paid to intraoperative neurophysiologic monitoring.

The implant is introduced into the site with a Rosen needle or a number 11 Rhoton dissector, and the paddle is directed into the foramen of Luschka. The angled endoscope allows visualization of the entire length of the electrode array insuring full contact with the brainstem. In addition, the position of the implant can be recorded with digital image capture and digital video. This can help to correlate anatomy with the results of electrophysiologic testing.

The distal portion of the electrode extends through the surgical defect to the receiver/stimulator. This is similar to that of a cochlear implant and is implanted identically. The defect is closed in standard translabyrinthine fashion, and routine postoperative management is followed.

Retrosigmoid Approach. The retrosigmoid or suboccipital approach is performed in the standard manner and should be of a size adequate for safe tumor extirpation or smaller when performing ABI placement for non-NF2 applications. The use of the endoscope actually allows for a smaller craniotomy than would be needed with the operating microscope, but the optical modality used for tumor removal should take precedence and determine the surgical approach. The dura is incised and reflected to expose the cerebellum. A cerebellar retractor is placed to provide access to the cerebellopontine angle. It is assumed here that decompression by opening the lateral medullary cistern and drilling of bone over the IAC is done in the course of exposing the tumor.

The principal criticism of the retrosigmoid approach for ABI placement is the perceived need for extensive cerebellar retraction to expose the implant site. However, for endoscopic

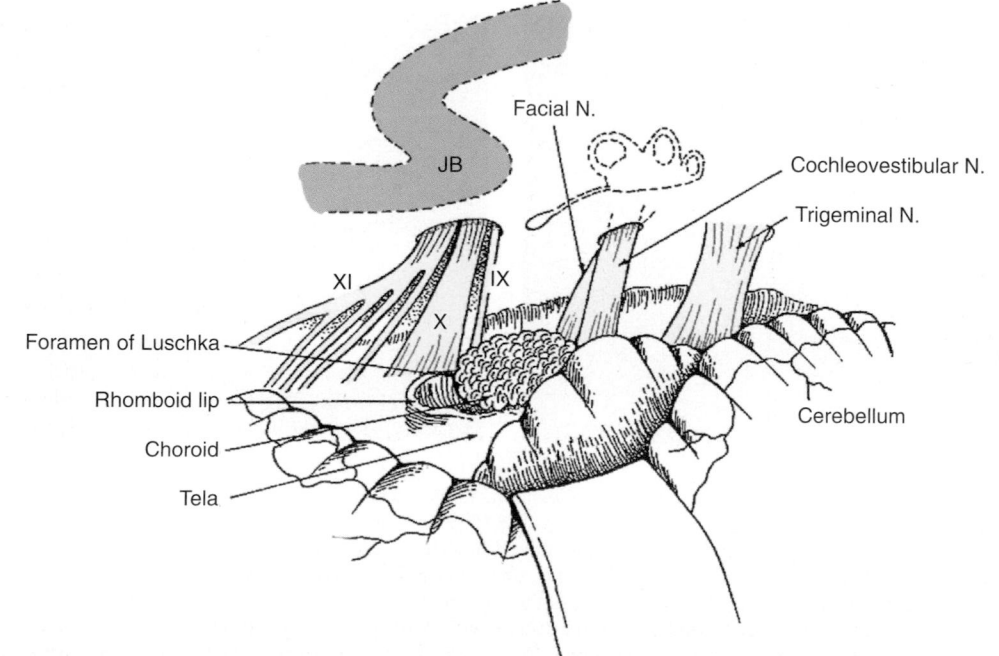

Figure 36 Detail of the landmarks visible near the cochlear nucleus via the retrosigmoid approach for placement of an auditory brainstem implant. IX = glossopharyngeal nerve fibers; X = vagal nerve fibers; XI = spinal accessory nerve fibers; JB = jugular bulb (ghosted in position) ; N-nerve. (Published with permission, copyright © 2007 P.A. Wackym, MD.)

visualization of the lateral recess of the fourth ventricle, less retraction is actually necessary relative to the translabyrinthine approach. The 30° or 45° endoscope can be passed along the cerebellar retractor and "look" medially into the implant site even though it may not be directly visible through the craniotomy.

The landmarks for the dorsal cochlear nucleus in the retrosigmoid approach are identical to those used in the translabyrinthine approach. The perspective is shifted in a slightly caudal direction; however, and visualization of the surface of the brainstem within the recess is less oblique and consequently easier to identify the ABI electrode contact site (Figure 36). As in the translabyrinthine approach, the operating microscope is introduced first to identify the flocculus and vestibulocochlear and glossopharyngeal nerves. The root entry zone of the eighth nerve will be hidden behind the flocculus, but the entry of the glossopharyngeal rootlets may be apparent.

Once the gross anatomy is identified, the 30° or 45° endoscope can be introduced to look "around" the flocculus. The root entry zones should be clearly visible as will the choroid plexus emerging from the foramen of Luschka. The flocculus can now be retracted with the McCabe flap knife exposing the rhomboid lip, lateral recess, and glistening brainstem surface overlying the dorsal cochlear nucleus. A small amount of teniae choroideae may be visualized helping to define the cochlear nuclear complex further.

The endoscope should be stabilized against the cerebellar retractor at either the superior or inferior aspect of the field. Side of operation and handedness of the surgeon will determine this. The ABI is advanced to the implant site with a Rosen needle and maneuvered into the foramen of Luschka. We found that this instrument combined with the less oblique approach to the brainstem makes placement of the implant relatively easy. The position of the implant can be confirmed with the endoscope.

Auditory Brainstem Implantation Highlights. A systematic approach to finding the dorsal cochlear nucleus is necessary to position the ABI appropriately on the brainstem surface. This is particularly important in situations in which tumor or surgical extirpation has altered the normal appearance of the cerebellopontine angle. The 0° and 30° endoscopes provide high-resolution views of these landmarks and allow examination of the cerebellopontine angle with minimal retraction or manipulation. This examination enables preservation of delicate structures, which can further delineate the dorsal cochlear nucleus.

In the translabyrinthine and retrosigmoid approaches identical landmarks are used and followed to localize the implant site:

- the flocculus and eighth and ninth cranial nerves are identified;
- the region between the root entry zones of these nerves and rostral to the flocculus will contain the choroid plexus;
- the choroid plexus can be followed into the foramen of Luschka and thus the lateral recess of the fourth ventricle;
- the fold of the tela choroidea forming the rhomboid lip further delineates the foramen of Luschka;
- the root entry zone of the eighth nerve will "point" to the region of the cochlear nuclear complex;
- the teniae choroideae, if preserved, attach at the junction of the dorsal and inferior ventral cochlear nuclei;
- the brainstem surface in the recess over the cochlear nuclear complex has a glistening ependymal layer; and
- the brainstem overlying the dorsal cochlear nucleus may demonstrate a slight bulge.

After initial placement using endoscopic guidance, electrophysiologic testing using EABR is performed. Repositioning the electrode array using endoscopic-control and retesting the EABR allow optimization of electrode placement. This process typically takes between 30 and 60 minutes; however, in one patient this process required 3 hours.

Clinical Experience and Discussion

To date our team has placed 7 ABIs in 6 patients, 5 with NF2 and 1 with a nonfunctional auditory nerve following temporal bone fracture (Figure 37). The same multidisciplinary approach to ABI electrode placement has been used in all patients. Intraoperative endoscopic placement of the electrode paddle was performed by the same surgeon (PAW) as we have described previously.[135,136] In addition, intraoperative EABR was performed using the paradigm suggested by Cochlear Americas, with the exception that repeated mapping was not completed until optimal placement, as defined by maximum number of active auditory electrodes using EABR, was achieved.

It has been stated that localization of the brainstem surface overlying the dorsal cochlear nucleus is difficult. Brackmann and colleagues noted that the dorsal nucleus in lower mammals forms a characteristic "bulge" on the brainstem surface which they have not observed in humans.[137] We have intermittently seen this surface bulge in both cadaveric specimens and our

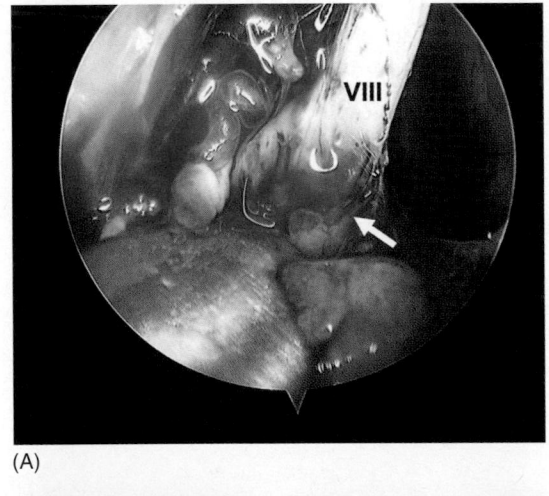
(A)

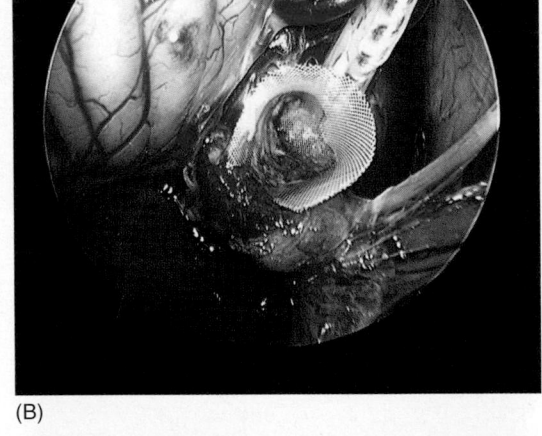
(B)

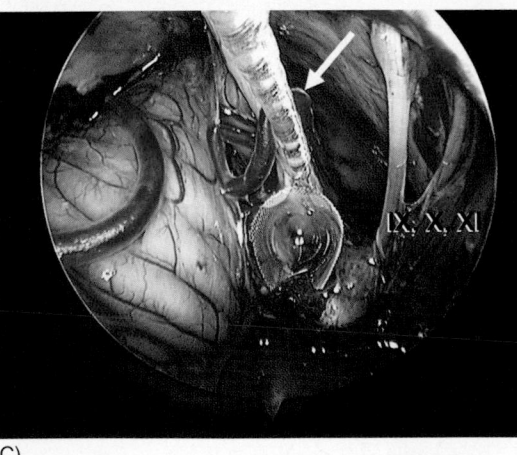
(C)

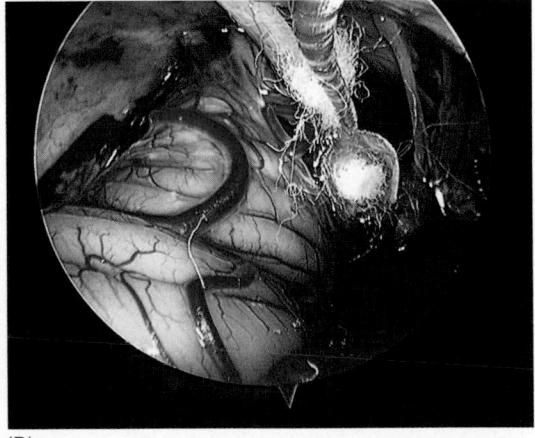
(D)

Figure 37 A 52-year-old man with bilateral temporal bone fractures and nonfunctional right auditory nerve. Right retrosigmoid approach and ABI placement December 2006 using 45° endoscope and electrically EABR guidance. (A) View of cochlear nucleus before placement of ABI. The rhomboid lip can be seen (*short arrow*) in relationship to the lateral recess and the vestibulocochlear nerve (VIII). Flocculus, bottom center. (B) ABI in position over the cochlear nucleus. The Dacron mesh wings are bowed around the inside of the rhomboid lip. A loop of the anterior inferior cerebellar artery (AICA) can be seen between the electrode array and cranial nerve VIII (*long arrow*). (C) CSF can be seen welling up through the foramen of Luschka, center. Cranial nerves IX, X, and XI are seen in relationship to the ABI electrode paddle. The extent of the AICA loop can be seen (*long arrow*). (D) Polytetrafluoroethylene (Teflon) felt placed between the vestibulocochlear nerve and the loop of AICA as well as within the lateral recess. (Published with permission, copyright © 2007 P.A. Wackym, MD.)

patients undergoing endoscopic placement of an ABI which may reflect the fact that such a landmark is, at best, inconsistent.[135,136] Further complicating localization of the dorsal cochlear nucleus is its position within the lateral recess of the fourth ventricle, an area reported to be *not* directly visible within the standard trans-labyrinthine surgical field.[138] Additional reports have likewise noted that the site of implantation may be obscured in a translabyrinthine dissection.[137] As such, this region is difficult to locate in a clinical setting, and the importance of surgical landmarks to guide the surgeon has been stressed.[135,136] We have found that the retrosigmoid approach provides a better view of the cochlear nucleus complex via the operating microscope.

While others have also utilized EABR to facilitate optimal placement of the electrode array, we have typically spent 30 to 60 minutes in mapping out this ideal location. However, we have taken up to 3 hours to accomplish this task. This multidisciplinary approach has resulted in excellent outcomes as measured by number of active electrodes and number of electrodes that are nonresponsive or produce side effects. As this series expands, generalization of these principles may be possible.

SUMMARY AND CONCLUSIONS

Cochlear implants and ABIs have advanced dramatically over half of a century. These auditory prostheses now are available in a wide range of transduction strategies and electrode designs allowing focused and effective solutions to the clinical problems of patients with hearing impairment who cannot be rehabilitated with hearing aids. These applications and outcomes will no doubt continue to expand and improve as the results of clinical trials and new innovations are incorporated into clinical practice.

REFERENCES

1. Van Camp G, Smith RJH. Hereditary Hearing Loss Homepage. http://dnalab-www.uia.ac.be/dnalab/hhh/
2. Morton NE. Genetic epidemiology of hearing impairment. Ann N Y Acad Sci 1991;630:16–31.
3. McGuirt WT, Smith RJ. Connexin 26 as a cause of hereditary hearing loss. Am J Audiol 1999;8:93–100.
4. Cohn ES, Kelley PM, Fowler TW, et al. Clinical studies of families with hearing loss attributable to mutations in the connexin 26 gene (GJB2/DFNB1). Pediatrics 1999; 103:546–50.
5. Kelsell DP, Dunlop J, Stevens HP, et al. Connexin 26 mutations in hereditary non-syndromic sensorineural deafness. Nature 1997;387:80–3.
6. Bruzzone R, White TW, Paul DL. Connections with connexins: The molecular basis of direct intercellular signaling. Eur J Biochem 1996;238:1–27.
7. Paul DL. New functions for gap junctions. Curr Opin Cell Biol 1995;7:665–72.
8. Bruzzone R, Veronesi V, Gomes D, et al. Loss-of-function and residual channel activity of connexin26 mutations associated with non-syndromic deafness. FEBS Lett 2003; 533:79–88.
9. Karp G. Cell and Molecular Biology, 4th edition. New York: John Wiley & Sons, Inc.; 2005.
10. Dahl E, Manthey D, Chen Y, et al. Molecular cloning and functional expression of mouse connexin-30, a gap junction gene highly expressed in adult brain and skin. J Biol Chem 1996;271:17903–10.
11. del Castillo I, Villamar M, Moreno-Pelayo MA, et al. A deletion involving the connexin 30 gene in non-syndromic hearing impairment. N Engl J Med 2002;346:243–9.
12. Kenneson A, Van Naarden Braun K, Boyle C. GJB2 (connexin 26) variants and non-syndromic sensorineural hearing loss: A HuGE review. Genet Med 2002;4:258–74.
13. Zelante L, Gasparini P, Estivill X, et al. Connexin26 mutations associated with the most common form of non-syndromic neurosensory autosomal recessive deafness (DFNB1) in Mediterraneans. Hum Mol Genet 1997; 6:1605–9.
14. Green GE, Scott DA, McDonald JM, et al. Carrier rates in the midwestern United States for GJB2 mutations causing inherited deafness. JAMA 1999;281:2211–6.
15. Lerer I, Sagi M, Malamud E, et al. Contribution of connexin 26 mutations to non-syndromic deafness in Ashkenazi patients and the variable phenotypic effect of the mutation 167delT. Am J Med Genet 2000;95:53–6.
16. Denoyelle F, Weil D, Maw MA, et al. Prelingual deafness: High prevalence of a 30delG mutation in the connexin 26 gene. Hum Mol Genet 1997;6:2173–7.
17. Fuse Y, Doi K, Hasegawa T, et al. Three novel connexin26 gene mutations in autosomal recessive non-syndromic deafness. Neuroreport 1999;10:1853–7.
18. Kudo T, Ikeda K, Kure S, et al. Novel mutations in the connexin 26 gene (GJB2) responsible for childhood deafness in the Japanese population. Am J Med Genet 2000;90:141–5.
19. Park HJ, Hahn SH, Chun YM, et al. Connexin26 mutations associated with non-syndromic hearing loss. Laryngoscope 2000;110:1535–8.
20. Harris KC, Erbe CB, Firszt JB, et al. A novel connexin 26 compound heterozygous mutation results in deafness. Laryngoscope 2002;112:1159–62.
21. Green GE, Scott DA, McDonald JM, et al. Performance of cochlear implant recipients with GJB2-related deafness. Am J Med Genet 2002;109:167–70.
22. Gorlin RJ, Toriello HV, Cohen MM. Hereditary Hearing Loss and its Syndromes. New York: Oxford University Press; 1995.
23. Benhorin J, Merri M, Alberti M, et al. Long QT syndrome. New electrocardiographic characteristics. Circulation 1990; 82:521–7.
24. Online Mendelian Inheritance in Man, OMIM (TM). McKusick-Nathans Institute of Genetic Medicine, Johns Hopkins University (Baltimore, MD) and National Center for Biotechnology Information, National Library of Medicine (Bethesda, MD) July 4, 2007. URL: http://www.ncbi.nlm.nih.gov/omim/
25. Starr A, Picton TW, Sininger Y, et al. Auditory neuropathy. Brain 1996;119:741–53.
26. Davis H, Hirsh SK. A slow brainstem response for low-frequency audiometry. Audiology 1979;18:445–61.
27. Kraus N, Özdamar Ö, Stein L, Reed N. Absent auditory brain stem response: Peripheral hearing loss of brain stem dysfunction? Laryngoscope 1984;94:400–6.
28. Starr A. The neurology of auditory neuropathy. In: Sininger Y, Starr A, editors. Auditory Neuropathy. San Diego, CA: Singular; 2001. p. 37–49.
29. Wang Q, Gu R, Han D, Yang W. Familial auditory neuropathy. Laryngoscope 2003;113:1623–9.
30. Kim TB, Isaacson B, Sivakumaran TA, et al. A gene responsible for autosomal dominant auditory neuropathy (AUNA1) maps to 13q14-21. J Med Genet 2004; 41:872–6.
31. Starr A, Isaacson B, Michalewski HJ, et al. A dominantly inherited progressive deafness affecting distal auditory nerve and hair cells. J Assoc Res Otolaryngol 2004;5:411–26.
32. Varga R, Kelley PM, Keats BJ, et al. Non-syndromic recessive auditory neuropathy is the result of mutations in the otoferlin (OTOF) gene (Letter). J Med Genet 2003; 40:45–50.
33. Rodriguez-Ballesteros M, del Castillo FJ, Martin Y, et al. Auditory neuropathy in patients carrying mutations in the otoferlin gene (OTOF). Hum Mutat 2003;22:451–6.
34. Wang Q, Li R, Zhao H, et al. Clinical and molecular characterization of a Chinese patient with auditory neuropathy associated with mitochondrial 12S rRNA T1095C mutation. Am J Med Genet A 2005;133:27–30.
35. Chaib H, Place C, Salem N, et al. A gene responsible for a sensorineural nonsyndromic recessive deafness maps to chromosome 2p22-23. Hum Molec Genet 1996;5:155–8.
36. Yasunaga S, Grati M, Cohen-Salmon M, et al. A mutation in OTOF, encoding otoferlin, a FER-1-like protein, causes DFNB9, a nonsyndromic form of deafness. Nature Genet 1999;21:363–9.
37. Leal SM, Apaydin F, Barnwell C, et al. A second middle eastern kindred with autosomal recessive non-syndromic hearing loss segregates DFNB9. Eur J Hum Gene 1998; 6:341–4.
38. Houseman MJ, Jackson AP, Al-Gazali LI, et al. A novel mutation in a family with non-syndromic sensorineural hearing loss that disrupts the newly characterized OTOF long isoforms (Letter). J Med Genet 2001;38:e25.
39. Mirghomizadeh F, Pfister M, Apaydin F, et al. Substitutions in the conserved C2C domain of otoferlin cause DFNB9, a form of nonsyndromic autosomal recessive deafness. Neurobiol Dis 2002;10:157–64.
40. Varga R, Avenarius MR, Kelley PM, et al. OTOF mutations revealed by genetic analysis of hearing loss families including a potential temperature-sensitive auditory neuropathy allele. J Med Genet 2006;43:576–81.
41. Migliosi V, Modamino-Hoybjor S, Moreno-Pelayo MA, et al. Q829X, a novel mutation in the gene encoding otoferlin (OTOF), is frequently found in Spanish patients with prelingual non-syndromic hearing loss (Letter). J Med Genet 2002;39:502–6.
42. Loundon N, Marcolla A, Roux I, et al. Auditory neuropathy or endocochlear hearing loss? Otol Neurotol 2005; 26:748–54.
43. Tekin M, Akcayoz D, Incesulu A. A novel missense mutation in a C2 domain of OTOF results in autosomal recessive auditory neuropathy. Am J Med Genet 2005;138A:6–10.
44. Yasunaga S, Grati M, Chardenoux S, et al. OTOF encodes multiple long and short isoforms: Genetic evidence that the long ones underlie recessive deafness DFNB9. Am J Hum Genet 2000;67:591–600.
45. Starr A, Sininger Y, Winter M, et al. Transient deafness due to temperature-sensitive auditory neuropathy. Ear Hear 1998;19:169–79.
46. Rouillon I, Marcolla A, Roux I, et al. Results of cochlear implantation in two children with mutations in the OTOF gene. Int J Ped Otorhinol 2006;70:689–96.
47. Wilson BS, Lawson DT, Müller JM, et al. Cochlear implants: Some likely next steps. Ann Rev Biomed Eng 2003; 5,207–49.
48. Robbins AM, Renshaw JJ, Berry SW. Evaluating meaningful auditory integration in profoundly hearing-impaired children. Am J Otol 1991;12:151–64.
49. Friedland DR, Wackym PA, Rhee JS, Finn MS. Cochlear implantation for auditory rehabilitation in Camurati-Engelmann disease (hereditary diaphyseal dysplasia). Ann Otol Rhinol Laryngol 2000;109/2:160–2.
50. Colletti V, Shannon RV. Open set speech perception with auditory brainstem implant? Laryngoscope 2005; 115:1974–8.
51. Belal A, Jr. Contraindications to cochlear implantation. Am J Otol 1986;7:172–5.
52. House WF, Luxford WM, Courtney B. Otitis media in children following the cochlear implant. Ear Hear 1985; 6:24S–6S.
53. Luntz M, Hodges AV, Balkany T, et al. Otitis media in children with cochlear implants. Laryngoscope 1996; 106:1403–5.
54. Gray RF, Irving RM. Cochlear implants in chronic suppurative otitis media. Am J Otol 1995;16:682–6.
55. Axon PR, Mawman DJ, Upile T, Ramsden RT. Cochlear implantation in the presence of chronic suppurative otitis media. J Laryngol Otol 1997;111:228–32.
56. El-Kashlan HK, Arts HA, Telian SA. Cochlear implantation in chronic suppurative otitis media. Otol Neurotol 2002; 23:53–5.
57. Hamzavi J, Baumgartner W, Franz P, Plenk H. Radical cavities and cochlear implantation. Acta Otolaryngol 2001; 121:607–9.
58. Luntz M, Teszler CB, Shpak T, et al. Cochlear implantation in healthy and otitis-prone children: A prospective study. Laryngoscope 2001;111:1614–8.
59. Lindsay D, von Holy A. Bacterial biofilms within the clinical setting: What healthcare professionals should know. J Hosp Infect 2006;64:313–25.
60. Dunn AK, Stabb EV. Beyond quorum sensing: The complexities of prokaryotic parliamentary procedures. Anal Bioanal Chem 2007;387:391–8.
61. Bachmann SP, VandeWalle K, Ramage G, et al. In vitro activity of caspofungin against Candida albicans biofilms. Antimicrob Agents Chemother 2002;46:3591–6.
62. Chandra J, Kuhn DM, Mukherjee PK, et al. Biofilm formation by the fungal pathogen Candida albicans: Development, architecture, and drug resistance. J Bacteriol 2001;183:5385–94.
63. Ramage G, Wickes BL, Lopez-Ribot JL. Biofilms of Candida albicans and their associated resistance to antifungal agents. Am Clin Lab 2001;20:42–4.
64. Rex JH, Walsh TJ, Sobel JD, et al. Practice guidelines for the treatment of candidiasis. Infectious Diseases Society of America. Clin Infect Dis 2000;30:662–78.
65. Seelig MS. The role of antibiotics in the pathogenesis of Candida infections. Am J Med 1966;40:887–917.

66. Fradis M, Brodsky A, Ben-David J, et al. Chronic otitis media treated topically with ciprofloxacin or tobramycin. Arch Otolaryngol Head Neck Surg 1997;123:1057–60.

67. Goldblatt EL. Efficacy of ofloxacin and other otic preparations for acute otitis media in patients with tympanostomy tubes. Pediatr Infect Dis J 2001;20:116–9.

68. Goldblatt EL, Dohar J, Nozza RJ, et al. Topical ofloxacin versus systemic amoxicillin/clavulanate in purulent otorrhea in children with tympanostomy tubes. Int J Pediatr Otorhinolaryngol 1998;46:91–101.

69. Cristobal R, Edmiston, CE, Jr, Runge-Samuelson CL, et al. Fungal biofilm formation on cochlear implant hardware after prophylactic antibiotic-induced fungal overgrowth within the middle ear. Ped Infect Dis J 2004;23:774–8.

70. Arnold W, Bredberg G, Gstottner W, et al. Meningitis following cochlear implantation: Pathomechanisms, clinical symptoms, conservative and surgical treatments. ORL J Otorhinolaryngol Relat Spec 2002;64:382–9.

71. Hall-Stoodley L, Hu FZ, Gieseke A, et al. Direct detection of bacterial biofilms on the middle-ear mucosa of children with chronic otitis media. JAMA 2006;296:202–11.

72. Antonelli PJ, Lee JC, Burne RA. Bacterial biofilms may contribute to persistent cochlear implant infection. Otol Neurotol 2004;25:953–7.

73. Jackler R, Luxford W, House W. Congenital malformations of the inner ear: A classification based on embryogenesis. Laryngoscope 1987;97:2–14.

74. Rothschild MA, Wackym PA, Som PM, Silvers AR. Isolated primary unilateral stenosis of the internal auditory canal. Int J Pediatr Otorhinolaryngol 1999;50:219–24.

75. Buchman CA, Roush PA, Teagle HF, et al. Auditory neuropathy characteristics in children with cochlear nerve deficiency. Ear Hear 2006;27:399–408.

76. Nabili V, Brodie HA, Neverov NI, Tinling SP. Chronology of labyrinthitis ossificans induced by Streptococcus pneumoniae meningitis. Laryngoscope 1999;109:931–5.

77. Pearsons KS, Bennett RL, Fidell S. Speech Levels in Various Environments. Bolt Beranek and Newman Report No. 321. Canoga Park, CA; 1976.

78. Tillman T, Carhart R, Wilbur L. A test for speech discrimination composed of CNC monosyllabic words (NU auditory test No. 6). USAF School of Aerospace Medicine, Report 55–66; 1966.

79. Nilsson M, Soli S, Sullivan JA. Development of the Hearing in Noise Test for measurement of speech reception thresholds in quiet and in noise. J Acoust Soc Am 1994; 95:1085–99.

80. Bamford J, Wilson I. Methodological considerations and practical aspects of the BKB sentence lists. In: Bench J, Bamford JM, editors. Speech-Hearing Tests and the Spoken Language of Hearing-Impaired Children. London: Academic Press; 1979.

81. Skinner MW, Holden LK, Holden TA, et al. Speech recognition at simulated soft, conversational, and raised-to-loud vocal efforts by adults with cochlear implants. J Acoust Soc Am 1997;101:3766–82.

82. Firszt JB, Holden LK, Skinner MW, et al. Recognition of speech presented at soft to loud levels by adult cochlear implant recipients of three cochlear implant systems. Ear Hear 2004;25:375–87.

83. Zierhofer CM, Hochmair IJ, Hochmair ES. The advance Combi 40+ cochlear implant. Am J Otol 1997;18:S37–8.

84. Kelsall DC, Shallop JK, Burnelli T. Cochlear implantation in the elderly. Am J Otol 1995;16:609–15.

85. Waltzman S, Cohen N, Shapiro W. The benefits of cochlear implantation in the geriatric population. Otolaryngol Head Neck Surg 1995;108:329–33.

86. Kiefer J, Pok M, Adunka O, et al. Combined electric and acoustic stimulation of the auditory system: Results of a clinical study. Otol Neurotol 2005;10:134–44.

87. Gantz BJ, Turner C, Gfeller KE. Acoustic plus electric speech processing: Preliminary results of a multicenter clinical trial of the Iowa/Nucleus hybrid implant. Audiol Neurotol 2006;11:63–8.

88. Syms CA, III, Wickesberg J. Concurrent use of cochlear implants and hearing aids. In: Kubo T, Takahashi Y, Iwaki T, editors. Cochlear Implants—An Update. The Hague, The Netherlands: Kugler Publications; 2002:p. 535–9.

89. Müller J, Schon F, Helms J. Speech understanding in quiet and noise in bilateral users of the Med-El Combi 40/40+ cochlear implant system. Ear Hear 2002;23:198–206.

90. Schleich P, Nopp P, D'Haese P. Head shadow, squelch and summation effects in bilateral users of the Med-El Combi 40/40+ cochlear implant system. Ear Hear 2004; 25:197–204.

91. Wackym PA, Runge-Samuelson CL, Firszt JB, et al. More challenging speech perception tasks demonstrate binaural benefit in bilateral cochlear implant users. Ear Hear 2007;28:80S–5S.

92. Sininger Y, Oba S. Patients with auditory neuropathy: Who are they and what can they hear? In: Sininger Y, Starr A, editors. Auditory Neuropathy. San Diego, CA: Singular; 2001. p. 15–36.

93. Peterson A, Shallop JK, Driscoll C, et al. Outcomes of cochlear implantation in children with auditory neuropathy. J Am Acad Audiol 2003;14:188–201.

94. Moog JS, Geers AE. Early Speech Perception Test. St. Louis, MO: Central Institute for the Deaf; 1990.

95. Kirk KI, Pisoni DB, Osberger MJ. Lexical effects of spoken word recognition by pediatric cochlear implant users. Ear Hear 1995;16:470–81.

96. Haskins HA. A phonetically balanced test of speech discrimination for children. Unpublished Master's thesis, Northwestern University, Evanston, Illinois; 1949.

97. Geers A, Brenner C, Davidson L. Factors associated with development of speech perception skills in children implanted by age five. Ear Hear 2003;24:24–35.

98. Fryauf-Bertschy H, Tyler R, Kelsay D, et al. Cochlear implant use by prelingually deafened: The influences of age at implant and length of device use. J Sp Lang Hear Res 1997; 40:183–99.

99. Zwolan TA, Zimmerman-Phillips S, Ashbaugh CJ, et al. Cochlear implantation of children with minimal open-set speech recognition. Ear Hear 1997;18:240–51.

100. Miyamoto RT, Houston DM, Bergeson T. Cochlear implantation in deaf infants. Laryngoscope 2005;115:1376–80.

101. Geshwind N, Levitsky W. Human brain: Left-right asymmetries in temporal speech region. Science 1968; 161:186–7.

102. Wackym PA, Firszt JB, Gaggl W, et al. Electrophysiological effects of placing cochlear implant electrodes in a perimodiolar position in young children. Laryngoscope 2004;114:71–6.

103. Baumgartner W, Youssefzadeh S, Franz P, Gstöttner W. MRI in 30 cochlear implanted patients. Otol Neurotol 2001;22:818–22.

104. Nadol JB, Young Y-S, Glynn RJ. Survival of spiral ganglion cells in profound sensorineural hearing loss: Implications for cochlear implantation. Ann Otol Rhinol Laryngol 1989; 98;411–6.

105. McDonald WI, Sears TA. The effects of experimental demyelination on conduction in the central nervous system. Brain 1970;93:583–98.

106. Rasminsky M, Sears TA. Internodal conduction in undissected demyelinated nerve fibres. J Physiol 1972; 227,323–50.

107. Heller J, Brackmann D, Tucci D, et al. Evaluation of MRI compatibility of the modified Nucleus multichannel auditory brainstem and cochlear implants. Am J Otol 1996; 17:724–9.

108. Portnoy WM, Mattucci K. Cochlear implants as a contraindication to magnetic resonance imaging. Ann Otol Rhinol Laryngol 1991;100:195–7.

109. Teissl C, Kremser C, Hochmair ES, Hochmair-Desoyer IJ. Magnetic resonance imaging and cochlear implants: Compatibility and safety aspects. J Magnet Reson Imag 1999;9:26–38.

110. Weber BP, Goldring JE, Santogrossi T, et al. Magnetic resonance imaging compatibility testing of the Clarion 1.2 cochlear implant. Am J Otol 1998;19:584–90.

111. Sonnenburg RE, Wackym PA, Yoganandan N, et al. Biophysics of cochlear implant/MRI interaction emphasizing bone biomechanical properties. Laryngoscope 2002;112:1720–5.

112. Poetker DM, Wackym PA, Yoganandan N, et al. Biomechanical strength of reconstruction plates when used for medial support of Med-El cochlear implants: Implications for diagnostic MRI. ORL J Otorhinolaryngol Relat Spec 2006;68:77–82.

113. Wackym PA, Smith MM, Banks KL, et al. Effect of MRI on internal magnet strength in Med-El C40+ cochlear implants. Laryngoscope 2004;114:1355–61.

114. Wackym PA, guest editor. Cochlear and brainstem implantation. Oper Tech Otolaryngol Head Neck Surg 2005; 16:73–163.

115. Poetker DM, Runge-Samuelson CL, Firszt JB, Wackym PA. Electrosurgery following cochlear implantation: Eighth nerve electrophysiology. Laryngoscope 2004; 114:2252–4.

116. Eby TL. Development of the facial recess: Implications for cochlear implantation. Laryngoscope 1996;106:1–7.

117. Hoffman RA, Cohen NL. Surgical pitfalls in cochlear implantation. Laryngoscope 1993;103:741–4.

118. McElveen JT, Carrasco VN, Miyamoto RT, Linthicum FH. Cochlear implantation in common cavity malformations using a transmastoid labyrinthotomy approach. Laryngoscope 1997;107:1032–6.

119. Beltrame MA, Frau GN, Shanks M, et al. Double posterior labyrinthotomy technique: Results in three Med-El patients with common cavity. Otol Neurotol 2005;26:177–82.

120. Manolidis S, Tonini R, Spitzer J. Endoscopically guided placement of prefabricated cochlear implant electrodes in a common cavity malformation. Int J Pediatr Otorhinolaryngol 2006;70:591–6.

121. Runge-Samuelson CL, Firszt JB, Gaggl W, Wackym PA. Electrically-evoked auditory brainstem responses in adults and children: Effects of lateral to medial placement of the Nucleus 24 Contour electrode array. Audiol Neurotol (in press).

122. Firszt JB, Chambers RD, Kraus N, Reeder RM. Neurophysiology of cochlear implant users I: Effects of stimulus current level and electrode site on the electrical ABR, MLR and N1-P2 response. Ear Hear 2002;23:502–15.

123. Waldman EH, Niparko JK. The avoidance and treatment of scalp flap complications in cochlear implant surgery. Oper Tech Otolaryngol Head Neck Surg 2005;16:149–53.

124. Kubo T, Matsuura S, Iwaki T. Complications of cochlear implant surgery. Oper Tech Otolaryngol Head Neck Surg 2005;16:154–58.

125. Gastman GR, Hirsch BE, Sando I, et al. The potential risk of carotid injury in cochlear implant surgery. Laryngoscope 2002;112:262–6.

126. Page EL, Eby TL. Meningitis after cochlear implantation in Mondini malformation. Otolaryngol Head Neck Surg 1997;116:104–6.

127. Kelsall DC, Shallop JK, Brammeier TG, Prenger EC. Facial nerve stimulation after Nucleus 22-channel cochlear implantation. Am J Otol 1997;18:336–41.

128. Steenerson RL, Cronin GW, Gary LB. Vertigo after cochlear implantation. Otol Neurotol 2001;22:842–3.

129. Alexiades G, Roland JT, Fishman AJ, et al. Cochlear reimplantation: Surgical techniques and functional results. Laryngoscope 2001;111:1608–13.

130. Lustig LR, Wackym PA. Bilateral cochlear implantation. Oper Tech Otolaryngol Head Neck Surg 2005; 16:125–30.

131. Otto SR, Shannon RV, Brackmann DE, et al. The multichannel auditory brain stem implant: Performance in twenty patients. Otolaryngol Head Neck Surg 1998; 118:291–303.

132. Laszig R, Sollmann WP, Marangos N. The restoration of hearing in neurofibromatosis type 2. J Laryngol Otol 1995;109:385–9.

133. Otto SR, Brackmann DE, Staller S, Menapace CM. The multichannel auditory brainstem implant: 6-month coinvestigator results. Adv Otorhinolaryngol 1997; 52:1–7.

134. Miyamoto RT, Campbell RL, Fritsch M, Lochmueller G. Preservation of hearing in neurofibromatosis 2. Otolaryngol Head Neck Surg 1990;103:619–24.

135. Friedland DR, Wackym PA. Evaluation of surgical approaches to endoscopic auditory brainstem implantation. Laryngoscope 1999;109:175–80.

136. Wackym PA, Firszt JB, Runge-Samuelson CL. Auditory brainstem implantation. Oper Tech Otolaryngol Head Neck Surg 2005;16:159–63.

137. Brackmann DE, Hitselberger WE, Nelson RA, et al. Auditory brainstem implant: I. Issues in surgical implantation. Otolaryngol Head Neck Surg 1993;108:624–33.

138. Kuroki A, Moller AR. Microsurgical anatomy around the foramen of Luschka in relation to intraoperative recording of auditory evoked potentials from the cochlear nuclei. J Neurosurg 1995;82:933–9.

33

Cochlear Implant Coding Strategies and Device Programming

Kaibao Nie, PhD

Ward Drennan, PhD

Jay Rubinstein, MD, PhD

Cochlear implants are designed to stimulate surviving auditory neurons with weak electric currents, generating neural spikes that the brain can interpret as sounds. To achieve this function, sounds are converted to safe electric currents. In most cochlear implant devices, this conversion is implemented with a sound processor running various coding strategies that take acoustic inputs, extract acoustic features, and then generate patterned electric outputs. Over 40 years of cochlear implant research and development, a variety of coding strategies have been developed. Associated with them are some fitting parameters, such as electric threshold level, electric most comfortable level, stimulation rate, pulse width, stimulation mode, and filter table. After the operation of implantation, each coding strategy is customized to take into account differences among patients such as the cause of the hearing loss, neural survival, electrode placement, and loudness perception. To optimally fit a patient with a specific coding strategy and its associated parameter set, it is necessary to understand thoroughly how each strategy processes sounds and converts them into electric stimulation signals. Throughout this chapter, a number of abbreviations are used and these have been summarized in Table 1.

Clinical programming of a cochlear implant with various coding strategies is not a simple task, given that it involves basic engineering concepts of digital signal processing (DSP), speech processing, electronics, and psychoacoustics. This chapter aims at facilitating the task by assisting in the understanding of the engineering structure of a cochlear implant, the history of implant coding strategies, the mechanisms of current sound coding strategies, as well as the practical procedures in clinical fittings.

ENGINEERING STRUCTURE OF A COCHLEAR IMPLANT

To build a cochlear implant, 1 major issue encountered is the safe transmission of electrical currents to the implanted electrodes through human skin. Earlier cochlear implants used a percutaneous link (wires directly pass through the human skin) between an external processor and an internal electrode array. The percutaneous link can efficiently send currents directly to the electrodes, but it has drawbacks. Patients with this type of implant have an exposed socket close to the implanted ear. Such exposure can cause infection, and it is therefore less than desirable. Modern commercial cochlear implants abandon this design, except for research purposes.

Currently, all 3 cochlear implant manufacturers (Cochlear Corporation, Advanced Bionics Corporation, and Med-El Corporation) utilize the transcutaneous wireless link, with one magnet coil placed underneath the skin and another matched externally on top of the implanted coil. Instead of delivering currents through a plug socket in the case of a percutaneous connection, the wireless link conveys binary codes of stimulating currents over a high frequency radio wave, and real stimulation currents are produced internally by one or more current generators.

Figure 1 presents the schematic diagram of a contemporary cochlear implant. The 5 essential components of a transcutaneous implant are:

1. *A microphone.* Normally, it is omnidirectional, picking up sounds from all directions. To improve the wearer's speech understanding in background noise, some devices now make use of a directional microphone, selectively picking up sounds from the front while attenuating others. Additionally, sound sources, such as TV, MP3 player, and FM (frequency modulation) assistive listening device, can also be directly connected as audio inputs.

2. *A sound processor.* It is responsible for digitizing the microphone's analog output, splitting the digital sound into frequency bands, extracting acoustic features, and generating current-related binary codes for transmission. Speech coding strategies run on the processor's digital signal processor chip, which is capable of performing millions of instructions per second.

3. *A wireless communication link.* A pair of magnet coils sitting on each side of the skin establishes a wireless communication link between the external sound processor and the internal implant. In the case of a transcutaneous link, stimulation currents are produced by controlled current sources inside an implantable electronic package without batteries. This requires that both control binary codes and electric power should be sent to the implant via the link. Most devices transmit both with a high voltage (eg, 5 to 10 V) and high frequency (eg, >10 MHz) radio wave as the carrier. The alternating carrier is transformed to a DC voltage for providing power to the internal electronic circuits. The wireless transmission can be bidirectional, from the external sound processor to the internal implant or vice versa. The inward data path is referred to as forward telemetry (FT). Reversely, an outward path, termed backward telemetry (BT), can also be

Abbreviation	Word or Phrase
ACE	Advanced combined encoder
AGC	Automatic gain controller
ART	Auditory response telemetry
BP	Bipolar
BT	Backward telemetry
CA	Compressed analog
CG	Common ground
CIS	Continuous interleaved sampling
DSP	Digital signal processing
EAS	Electric and acoustic stimulation
F0	Fundamental frequency
F1	First formant
F2	Second formant
FT	Forward telemetry
HiRes-P	Hi-Resolution-Paired
HiRes-S	Hi-Resolution-Sequential
MCL	Most comfortable level
MP	Monopolar
MPEAK	Multi-PEAK
NRI	Neural response imaging
NRT	Neural response telemetry
PPS	Paired pulsatile sampler
QPS	Quadruple pulsatile sampler
SAS	Simultaneous analog stimulator
SPEAK	Spectral PEAK
T level	Threshold level
pps	Pulses per second

Table 1 Abbreviations Used in This Chapter

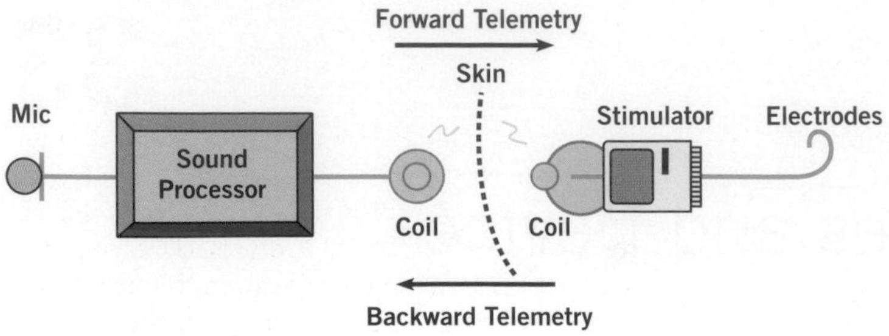

Figure 1 The engineering structure of a cochlear implant. A transcutaneous cochlear implant is composed of a microphone, a sound processor, a wireless link, a stimulator and an electrode array. The data transmission can be bidirectional, with forward telemetry and backward telemetry.

built on the same coil pair but at another radio-frequency band. The function of BT is to send back to the speech processor some implant diagnostic data, such as electrode impedance for monitoring electrode connectivity and neural responses for collecting neural evoked potentials as well as stimulation artifacts induced by current stimulations. The neural response collection is referred to as neural response telemetry (NRT) for Cochlear Corporation's implants, neural response imaging (NRI) for Advanced Bionics' implants, and auditory response telemetry (ART) for Med-El's implants.

4. *A stimulator*. It unloads data from the wireless transmission link to control current generators. A stimulator is composed of some digital control units and 1 or more constant current sources. The stimulator is sealed in a ceramic or titanium case placed at the temporal bone.

5. *An electrode array*. The electrode bundle is surgically inserted into the cochlea. The number of stimulation electrodes varies from 12 to 24 among current clinical devices.

CODING STRATEGIES IN COCHLEAR IMPLANTS

Having discussed the hardware of a cochlear implant, we shall consider what electrical signals are to be delivered to the electrode array. The stimulation pattern is crucial to restoring hearing, in that it fundamentally determines how auditory neurons will fire in response to current excitation. For better electric hearing, we assume that it is desirable that a cochlear implant mimics the neural encoding mechanisms by normal ears in response to acoustic excitation.

Psychoacoustic studies and neurophysiological experiments both have demonstrated the unique sensitivity and specificity of the normal inner ear. The snail-like cochlea functions as a tonotopic frequency analyzer, evenly spanning the audible frequency range of 20 Hz (apex) to 20,000 Hz (base) on a logarithmic scale. The frequency selectivity of the basilar membrane is also referred to as the "place theory" of hearing. Beyond the spectral coding, the temporal firing pattern of neurons also conveys speech information, according to 2 assumptions: volley theory (frequencies being represented by interlaced firing of neuron ensembles) and phase-locking theory (frequencies being coded by the neural

firing in synchronization with positive cycles of a sound).[1] Taken together, the auditory neurons can encode sounds both spectrally and temporally in the form of all-or-none spikes.

In light of these findings in normal auditory systems, scientists and engineers have conceived of numerous coding strategies throughout the history of cochlear implants to mimic the function of a normal cochlea.

The Past: Exploring the Nature of Electrical Stimulation

The idea of curing deafness with electrical stimulation was inspired by the discovery of eighteenth-century Italian scientist Alessandro Volta, the inventor of the electric battery. Out of curiosity, he inserted 2 metal rods into each of his ears and connected them to a circuit of roughly 50 V. Immediately he perceived a boiling sound. Volta's experiment on his own ears eventually led to the modern cochlear implants' worldwide use by over 100,000 deaf people to regain hearing.

The first trial of direct auditory nerve stimulation in a human was reported in the 1950s by two French investigators, André Djourno and Charles Eyriés.[2] During an operation for cholesteatoma, they placed wires in the modiolus and then applied currents. The patient heard a sound like "a roulette wheel" and could even discern a few words.

In hopes of reproducing hearing with an artificial apparatus, Dr. Willam House and his colleagues in the early 1970s built an experimental single-channel cochlear implant (House/3M).[3] In 1984, it became the world's first US Food and Drug Administration (FDA) approved device for implantation in adults. The device had a speech processor, a transcutaneous link, and 1 single electrode. The sound processor amplified speech and filtered it with a band-pass filter from 340 to 2,700 Hz. For the purpose of wireless transmission, the filtered speech was amplitude modulated with a carrier of 16 kHz. A pair of coils coupled the speech-carrying radio wave to the implanted single electrode. In this way, the stimulation current on the House/3M electrode was analog, and it varied at a rate of 16 kHz. Patients who received the House/3M implants were able to recognize some environmental sounds and discern some vowels but not open-set (choosing from among all possibilities in the language as opposed to selecting from a multiple-choice format) speech. The single-channel implants assisted lip reading, since the onsets and offsets of speech were reflected in

the temporal pattern of the 1-channel analog stimulation.

The advent of single-channel implants marked the beginning of conquering deafness with the help of a manmade prosthesis. But the simple device failed to produce good speech recognition, partially due to its poor spectral representation of speech.

At the time when the single-channel implants were under clinical trials, the design of experimental cochlear implants that can stimulate multiple cochlear sites was being conducted at other locations. One remarkable device was the four-channel Ineraid implant manufactured by the Symbion, Inc. (University of Utah) in 1980s.[4] The Ineraid implant increased the number of electrodes to 4, using the compressed analog (CA) speech processor. In the CA strategy, an automatic gain controller (AGC) compressed a sound's dynamic range. The compressed sound was then parsed into 4 subbands: 100 to 700 Hz, 700 to 1,400 Hz, 1,400 to 2,300 Hz, and 2,300 to 5,000 Hz. At the last stage, the 4 narrow-band analog signals were equalized in gain and directly delivered to the 4 intracochlear electrodes via a percutaneous connection. In assigning the stimulating electrodes, the higher frequency bands were toward the basal electrodes while the lower bands toward the apical electrodes, to mimic the place coding of speech. Experimental results showed that Ineraid patients benefited from the improvement in coding strategy, since they could achieve better open-set speech recognition than those using the single-channel device. Although the CA strategy provided patients with fine temporal and course spectral cues in speech, analog current stimulation of multiple sites could excite a large group of neurons simultaneously resulting in channel-to-channel interaction and loudness summation. These side effects could be detrimental to speech understanding.

The University of Melbourne group led by Dr. Graeme Clark and the Cochlear Corporation in Australia were also among the pioneers in cochlear implant coding strategy development. A series of specific coding strategies have been successfully designed for the Cochlear Corporation's Nucleus implants, and they are described in the following section.

The Present: Restoring Speech Perception

Continuous Interleaved Sampling (CIS). To address the channel interaction and loudness summation issues, Blake Wilson and colleagues at the Research Triangle Institute in North Carolina proposed in 1991 to use interleaved pulses instead of analog currents.[5] The CIS strategy is presented as a functional block diagram in Figure 2: a sound picked up by a microphone is preemphasized with a high-pass filter at 1,200 Hz to equalize its spectrum. A bank of band-pass filters then splits the sound into several narrow-band signals. Unlike the CA strategy, each subband signal further goes through an envelope detector, consisting of a rectifier and a low-pass filter typically at a 400 Hz cut-off frequency. The

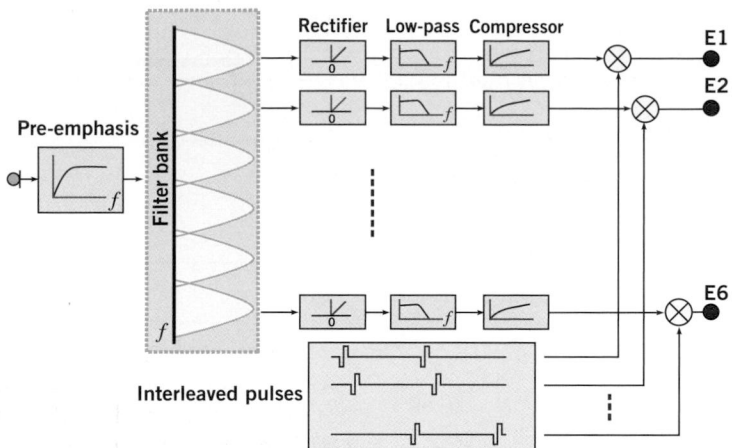

Figure 2 The block diagram of a 6-channel continuous interleaved sampling (CIS) coding strategy. The spectrum of input speech is first equalized with a preemphasis high-pass filter. A filter bank then splits the speech into 6 subband signals, vibrating around carrier frequencies from low to high, respectively. Each signal's slowly varying envelope is extracted with a rectifier followed by a low-pass filter whereas its fast-changing fine structure is discarded. The acoustic envelope is further compressed nonlinearly to match the narrow electric dynamic range. Finally, all six envelopes are sampled and modulated with interleaved biphasic pulses that are sent to stimulation electrodes (E1–E6).

envelope detector converts each subband signal into a slowly varying envelope signal no matter what center frequency it lies in. Finally, a nonlinear compressor matches the wide acoustic dynamic range of 60 dB to a narrow electric dynamic range of 3 to 5 dB. The most significant improvement of the CIS strategy over the CA strategy is that the compressed envelopes are further sampled with interleaved biphasic pulses, repeated at a rate of 833 pulses per second (pps). The sequential, nonoverlapping pulse pattern avoids simultaneous current stimulation.

Turning from simultaneous analog to interleaved pulsatile stimulation yielded remarkable progress in open-set speech perception. In a letter published in *Nature* in 1995, Wilson and colleagues reported that after being fitted with the new CIS strategy all 7 patients who had excellent performance with the CA processors showed significant improvement in speech recognition scores.[5]

The breakthrough in cochlear implant coding strategies brought cochlear implants into a new era, as DSP chips and integrated circuits became smaller and more powerful. All 3 commercial cochlear implant devices implement the CIS strategy or its variants. For example, the Nucleus implants by Cochlear Corporation can be programmed with a standard 4-, 6-, or 8-channel CIS. The Med-El implants implement the CIS+ strategy, at a higher stimulation pulse rate and with envelopes extracted through the Hilbert Transform instead of a rectifier followed by a low-pass filter. The Clarion devices by Advanced Bionics implement strategies with completely nonsimultaneous or partially simultaneous stimulation, such as the paired pulsatile sampler (PPS) or quadruple pulsatile sampler (QPS) strategies. In comparison with the CISs sequential stimulation ("Solo," eg, channel 1–2–3–4–5–6–7–8...), the PPS activates 1 pair of channels at the same time ("Duo," eg, [1, 5]–[2, 6]–[3, 7]–[4, 8] ...), while the QPS enables 4 channels simultaneously ("Quartet," for example [1, 5, 9, 13]–[2, 6,

10, 14]–[3, 7, 11, 15]–[4, 8, 12, 16] ...). Even though simultaneous stimulation exists in PPS and QPS, the chance of channel interaction is reduced by activating widely separated channels in Advanced Bionics' Clarion devices. Studies showed that some patients can benefit from the PPS and QPS strategies on consonant and word recognition.[6]

Spectral PEAK (SPEAK) and Advanced Combined Encoder (ACE). The Nucleus implants can be programmed with two proprietary coding strategies SPEAK and ACE. Both strategies are evolved from the earlier F0/F2 (fundamental frequency/the second formant), F0/F1/F2, and the multiple spectral peaks or multi-PEAK (MPEAK) strategies.[7,8]

At the time when the first-generation Nucleus implants were designed in 1980s, the objective was initially to restore speech understanding ability. Formants or resonating frequencies were known to be important for vowel identification. In the source-filter model of speech production from the 1960s, a voiced sound like a vowel was generated as periodic glottal pulses passing through a vocal tract filter at the rate of F0, whereas an unvoiced sound like a consonant was produced with random glottal pulses as the excitation source. Energy peaks in the vocal tract filter corresponded to formant frequencies. Possibly influenced by this model, the first Nucleus implant coding strategy F0/F2 attempted to encode the second formant F2, and the fundamental frequency F0 in a similar way. During stimulation, 1 of 20 electrodes in a Nucleus implant was stimulated with 1 pulse at a time according to the frequency of F2. The amplitude of the pulse was proportional to the energy height of F2 and the pulse's repetition rate was either proportional to F0 for periodic sounds or random for aperiodic sounds. A subsequent F0/F1/F2 strategy added the first formant F1 to the F0/F2 strategy. The basal 15 electrodes were assigned to F2 and the apical 5 electrodes were allocated

to F1. The F0/F1/F2 strategy provided superior open-set speech recognition.

Frequencies being encoded in F0/F2 or F0/F1/F2 are highly limited to 2,500 Hz and below, because the frequency ranges of F1 and F2 are 300 to 1,000 Hz and 1,000 to 2,500 Hz, respectively, for English vowels. This might be sufficient for vowel identification, but it is insufficient for identifying consonants, the energies of which mainly concentrate in frequency bands well above 2,500 Hz.

The MPEAK strategy was developed in the late 1980s to transmit more high frequency information. In MPEAK, the coding of F1 and F2 remained the same and 3 additional envelope detectors, that is, 2 to 2.8 kHz, 2.8 to 4 kHz, and 4 to 6 kHz, were added to the speech processor. During vowel-like sounds, not only 2 electrodes were stimulated in a way similar to F0/F1/F2, but 2 additional apical electrodes were also stimulated according to the outputs of the first 2 envelope detectors. All 4 electrodes being stimulated had a pulse rate at F0; during consonant-like sounds, F1 was not considered. In addition to the electrode being stimulated by F2, 3 basal electrodes were activated by the outputs of all 3 envelope detectors. The pulse rate was set randomly for consonants. The MPEAK strategy was shown to produce better speech recognition than the previous strategies encoding the first and the second formants only.[9]

The SPEAK strategy was introduced in the 1990s to overcome problems of inaccurately extracting formants and fundamental frequency in realistic listening environments. In SPEAK, a sound was divided into 20 bands followed by 20 envelope detectors. Rather than sending all envelopes to 20 electrodes, only 5 to 10 maxima among them were selected for activating corresponding electrodes from 1 cycle to another. The average stimulation cycle was 4 ms, or a pulse rate of 250 pps, which was lower than a typical CIS strategy. An advanced version that combines the SPEAK and the CIS strategies is the currently used ACE strategy with a stimulation rate of 900 pps up to 3,500 pps per channel. ACE represents the more general class of the "*n* of *m*" strategies, which select *n* maxima from a total of *m* processing bands for stimulation.

Simultaneous Analog Stimulator (SAS). The presence of channel interaction and loudness summation prevents the CA strategy from being programmed for most cochlear implant users. Analog stimulation preserves good temporal cues, which could potentially provide benefits to patients who can be fitted with the simultaneous settings. One strategy that can be programmed is the SAS strategy, used in Clarion devices by Advanced Bionics. The SAS uses high rate monophasic pulses to sample the analog waveform. This strategy has been successfully used by a small number of patients who have little or no issues with simultaneous stimulation. Good performance has been reported, particularly for music perception.[10]

Hi-Resolution Strategy. The standard CIS strategy offers 6-channel stimulation at a rate of 833 pps, which is capable of encoding temporal information below 400 Hz (roughly half of the stimulation rate). To deliver more spectral and temporal information, Advanced Bionics developed the high resolution (HiRes) strategy that stimulates 16 channels at a rate of up to 5,156 pps per channel.

In clinical fitting, the HiRes strategy can be either set as sequential stimulation (HiRes-S) or paired stimulation (HiRes-P), similar to the CIS or the PPS strategy described above. When the pulse width is 10.8 μs, for instance, the HiRes-S sequentially sends pulses to 16 monopolar channels at a maximum rate of 2,900 pps per channel. At the same setting, the HiRes-P can perform a duo of stimulation with 1 pair of channels being activated simultaneously, increasing the stimulation rate up to 5,156 pps. The HiRes strategy is now available in Advanced Bionics' HiRes90K and CII implants.

For comparison, Figure 3 shows a set of stimulation patterns illustrating the CA, SAS CIS, PPS, and ACE strategy's outputs in response to a short segment of speech stimuli. The CA strategy sends each individual channel the raw analog currents, oscillating around a specific center frequency. However, the SAS strategy samples each analog waveform, creating a series of stair waves. In contrast, discrete biphasic pulse trains are being used in the CIS, PPS, and ACE strategies. The black bars on top of panel (C), (D), and (E) indicate 1 stimulation cycle, respectively. Within 1 cycle, the CIS strategy sequentially stimulates each electrode. Instead, the PPS strategy simultaneously stimulates one pair of electrodes. In ACE, 6 of 20 electrodes are activated in this example within 1 cycle. Similar patterns can be found in the *n* of *m* and the SPEAK strategy.

The Future: Combination for Better Speech Understanding and Music Appreciation

Although only crude spectral and temporal cues are being encoded in all speech coding strategies, cochlear implants have been successful in restoring speech understanding abilities to deaf patients. Adults and children with monaural cochlear implants can achieve high levels of phoneme and sentence recognition under relatively quiet listening conditions.[11,12] Nonetheless, problems still remain under adverse listening conditions: multitalker speech or speech in background noise poses challenges to implant users; most implantees are unable to appreciate music normally[13]; they may understand what is being said but not who says it; and tone and pitch perception are poor compared to normal hearing listeners.[14]

One major cause for these existing problems is that current auditory prosthetic technologies are limited in their representation of sounds with high spectral and temporal resolutions. For the spectral resolution, even though 12 to 22 channels are being stimulated in implants, the number of

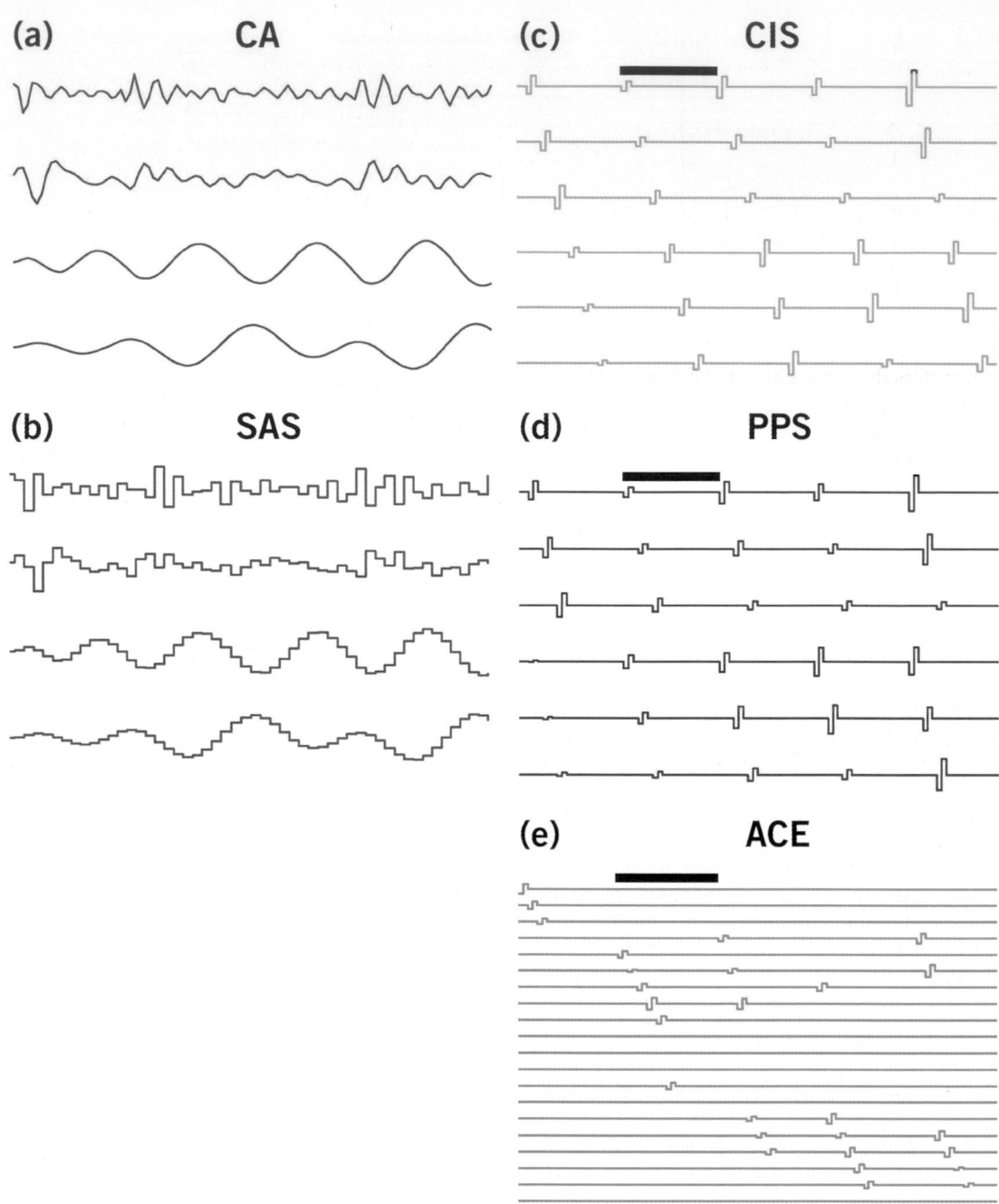

Figure 3 From (A) to (E), simulated outputs of the CA, SAS, CIS, PPS, and ACE strategies, respectively. The acoustic input is a short segment of speech. The black bars on (C), (D), or (E) indicate one stimulation cycle. Note: This figure is for illustration purpose only. Stimulation patterns in real cochlear implant devices may vary.

functional channel is from 4 to 8 as demonstrated by a variety of psychoacoustic experiments.[15] For the temporal resolution, only the temporal envelope cues are being coded in most strategies, and the fine structure cues are mostly discarded as a result of envelope extraction. Implant users can only detect temporal pitch change below 300 to 500 Hz (maximum 1,000 Hz).[16] Higher stimulation rate and analog strategies may provide more temporal cues, but to what extent a patient can utilize them remains a debatable issue.

Several novel technologies of improving coding strategies are under investigation or in clinical trial. One approach for patients with residual hearing is the combination of electric and acoustic stimulation (EAS) by inserting a short electrode array that provides high frequency information while preserving the residual low frequency hearing in the same ear, or by combining a cochlear

implant with a hearing aid in the opposite ear.[17,18] In addition, a hybrid coding strategy that combines the analog or digitized waveform stimulation at lower frequency bands with envelope stimulation at higher frequency bands could provide sufficient cues for tone, music and pitch perceptions. Another promising strategy is the utilization of "virtual channel" stimulation to improve spectral resolution. Balancing the weights of 2 adjacent simultaneously active electrodes can create intermediate channels. To improve temporal resolution further, a conditioning stimulation strategy is also under study.[19] In this experimental strategy, high rate pulse trains barely below the electric threshold levels are running in addition to a specific speech coding strategy. The conditioners can randomize the firing of auditory neurons to mimic the stochastic neural firing characteristics found in normal hearing. All these emerging new technologies hold the hope of restoring speech and music perception closer to normal hearing.[10,17–19]

PROGRAMMING A COCHLEAR IMPLANT

After implantation, a patient would not be able to hear any sounds until his/her speech processor is programmed with one of the aforementioned coding strategies. We have covered the theoretical aspects of a speech coding strategy. In practice, each strategy has various adjustable parameters that need either to be measured objectively through psychoacoustic experiments or to be determined subjectively by a clinician. The careful adjustment of these parameters is required to ensure the safety, audibility, and efficacy of electric stimulation.

Taking the CIS strategy as an example, we can group the fitting parameters into 2 categories: acoustic and electric. For example, acoustic parameters include: volume and sensitivity settings for auditory inputs, automatic gain control, number of channels, frequency table, and mapping function; electric parameters include: pulse width and rate, electric threshold and comfortable levels, and stimulation mode. We will start with the discussion on the fundamental electric settings, followed by an in-depth discussion of acoustic signal adjustment.

Setting Stimulation Mode

To stimulate auditory neurons, at least 1 pair of electrodes should provide a start-to-end path for the current flow. Each pair of electrodes forms 1 stimulation channel. Depending on the configuration of the returning electrode, stimulation mode in cochlear implants can be monopolar (MP), bipolar (BP), or common ground (CG) (Figure 4).

No matter which mode is selected, the active electrode is always an intracochlear electrode. In the MP mode, the returning ground electrode can be either one or two remote extracochlear electrodes, or the metal shell of an implant stimulator at the temporal bone. Due to a large distance between the paired electrodes, the monopolar mode generates wide spread of current field. In the BP mode, the returning electrode is one of the neighboring intracochlear electrodes. When the number of electrodes between the bipolar pair is N (eg, 0 to 3), it is referred to as BP ($N = 0$) or BP + N (eg, BP + 1, BP + 2, or BP + 3). In the CG mode, all of the intracochlear electrodes are connected to ground except the active electrode(s).

In selecting the stimulation mode, current spread and its associated loudness perception should be taken into consideration. Some strategies only allow a certain stimulation mode setting. In general, the BP mode produces less current spread, and the MP mode generates wide current spread. The CG mode is intermediate.[20] Most cochlear implant users prefer the MP stimulation mode. For certain coding strategies, the other 2 modes might provide benefits by focusing current stimulation.

Configuring Pulses

Biphasic pulse trains are the primary waveforms used in cochlear implants to keep charge-balance. A biphasic pulse consists of a leading negative pulse and a delayed positive pulse at equal amplitudes (see Figure 4). An interphase gap can be added between 2 phases. To define a pulse train, 3 parameters are needed: pulse width, interphase gap, and pulse rate. Pulse amplitude varies with the subband envelope as shown in a CIS strategy, and it is not a fitting parameter. The pulse width refers to the duration of 1 single phase, usually from 10 to 100 μs. The pulse gap can be 0 or up to several microseconds. Pulse or stimulation rate could affect temporal resolution. The higher the pulse rate is, the more temporal cues could possibly be encoded, but greater channel interaction may occur. The pulse rate can be as low as 100 Hz or as high as 10,000 Hz per channel among implant devices.

Measuring Threshold and Most Comfortable Level

Once the pulse pattern and stimulation mode are selected, the next step is to measure the minimal pulse amplitude that induces a just noticeable sound at the threshold (T) level, and the pulse amplitude that is at the most comfortable level (MCL). The T and MCL determine the dynamic range of electric stimulation. For some devices, the T and MCL are usually expressed in specific clinical units rather than the current units, microampere (μA).

Measuring the T and MCL is the main task in the clinical fitting of a cochlear implant, since these measurements are performed subjectively on each channel or on a set of preselected channels. Any change in the pulse configuration or stimulation mode setting could significantly affect T and MCL and they must be readjusted based on the new settings.

During measurement, bursts of a 300 to 500 ms long pulse train are presented to 1 selected channel and the subject is asked to rank its loudness. The ranking can be based on a loudness chart labeled as "off," "just noticeable," "soft," "medium loud," "loud," "comfortable loud," and "too loud," or on a rating scale between 0 ("off") and 10 ("too loud"). The T level is usually measured prior to the MCL. Starting from a level of no sound, the pulse train amplitude is gradually increased until the patient reports that a barely noticeable tone. Alternatively, the measurement can begin with the presentation of a pulse train at a suprathreshold level, and its amplitude is decreased until the subject reports no sound is heard. To avoid overestimation or underestimation, the T level should be set after several runs of decreasing or increasing pulse train presentations. To set the MCL levels, a medium loud pulse train is presented at the beginning, and its amplitude is thereafter increased slowly until the subject perceives a tone at the most comfortable level. One caveat for the MCL measurement is to avoid overstimulation because it could cause an extremely loud sound and hurt the patient.

After setting each individual channel's T and MCL, loudness balancing across all channels is recommended. A tone burst at either T or MCL can be played to all enabled channels sequentially. The T or MCL profile is adjusted for balancing loudness. For further confirming the tentative MCL setting, a sound processor can be activated for allowing the patient to listen to live speech sounds and judge the MCL setting. This functionality is known as "going live." To avoid sudden loud sounds, sound volume should be turned down before going to live speech. Final adjustments of MCL are made according to the patient's feedback.

The T and MCL can vary over time, particularly soon after the activation of a patient's speech processor. During this period, adjustments of T and MCL should be done regularly to maximize clinical benefit. Besides the behavioral measurement of T and MCL as discussed above, another way of setting them is by collecting neural response data via the BT. Such an approach can be useful for babies and young children. In data collection, 1 intracochlear electrode is activated, and 2 surrounding intracochlear electrodes are set as recording electrodes to collect evoked potentials. Neural responses are amplified, averaged and then sent back to the speech processor. The strength of stimulation current on the activating electrode is gradually increased, and the amplitude of neural responses on neighboring electrodes can be used to predict the T level.

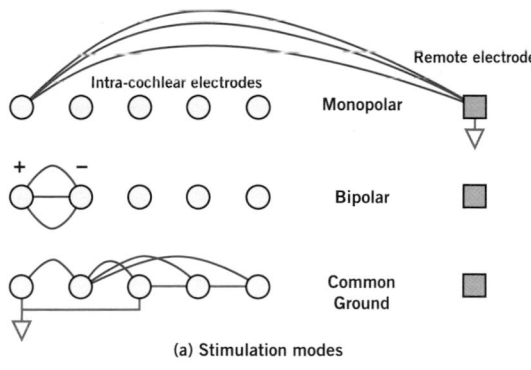

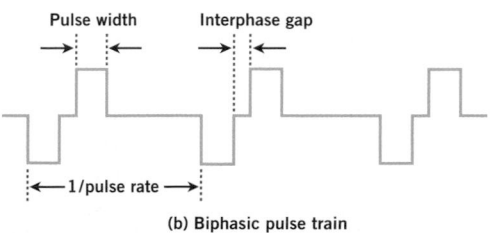

Figure 4 Illustration of stimulation modes and pulse train configuration. (A) Illustrates current flows of the monopolar (MP), bipolar (BP), and common ground (CG) settings, respectively. (B) Shows a biphasic pulse train defined with 3 parameters: pulse width, interphase gap, and pulse rate.

Adjusting Acoustic Parameters

Normal human hearing has a wide dynamic range of about 120 dB, whereas the input dynamic range of a sound processor usually is only 40 to 60 dB. Thus, an AGC is normally utilized to compress acoustic sounds, avoiding clipping of loud sounds and soft sounds. An AGC can apply higher gains to soft sounds, intermediate gains to medium-loud sounds, and lower gains to loud sounds. The sound levels of initiating gain changes are referred to as knee points. In clinical fitting, varying the knee points can benefit a patient wearing the implant in a variety of listening environments.

In acoustic signal processing, the most frequently used fitting parameters are the number of channels and their associated frequency allocation table. The channel number depends on the number of electrodes enabled, stimulation mode and the choice of coding strategy. When some electrodes are ineffective or disabled, the number of channels will be less. A filter bank relies on the frequency table to analyze input sounds. Most cochlear implants use a frequency table equally distributed on a logarithmic scale. For example, the corner frequencies of a 6-channel CIS strategy's table are 300, 460, 800, 1,385, 2,057, 2,800, 3,900, 4,500, and 5,500 Hz. The change of frequency table settings might depend on a patient's listening preference, for example, speech or music.

Changing Sensitivity and Volume

Sensitivity setting changes the minimal sound level that a patient can hear and volume sets the loudness of a sound. A patient might wear the speech processor in quiet or loud listening envi-

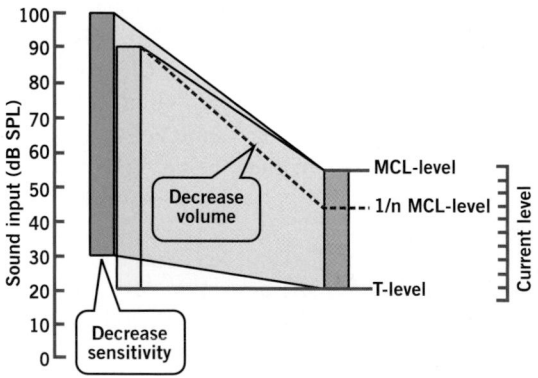

Figure 5 Illustration of how a volume or sensitivity decrease changes the acoustic input to electric output mapping.

ronments. Proper setting of sensitivity provides benefits to a patient when listening to speech at different background noise levels. Figure 5 shows how the sensitivity and volume settings can affect the acoustic input and the electric output dynamic range. In this example, the maximal acoustic input of 90 dB SPL is mapped to the electric MCL, and the minimal acoustic input of 20 dB SPL is mapped to the electric T level. When sensitivity is decreased, the acoustic input range is moved upward, thus, in this example the T level is mapped to 30 dB SPL. When the sound volume is decreased, the maximal acoustic input at 90 dB SPL is mapped to a fraction ($1/n$) of the MCL. The loudness of the input sound is reduced by decreasing the electric output.

Mapping from acoustic sounds to electric currents is implemented by a nonlinear function, such as a logarithmic mapping curve. Some devices allow the choice of the mapping curve shape by changing 1 parameter related to the compression function.

All parameters or settings associated with a specific coding strategy are assembled and stored into 1 map. It lists the designated value of each parameter, as well as the patient's identity and implant information. A map can also be customized to different listening environments, such as quiet or noise. Finally, a map is loaded to the patient's speech processor via a programming cable between a computer and the speech processor. A speech processor can hold at least 3 maps tailored for different coding strategies, stimulation modes, or listening environments. A patient can switch among maps to obtain optimal listening performance with a cochlear implant.

SUMMARY

Following the surgical placement of a cochlear implant, intensive programming of the auditory prosthetic device is required to optimally send electric sounds to the brain. Speech coding strategies have been developed over 40 years to map acoustic sounds to electric currents. This chapter reviews most coding strategies in clinical use along with the history of cochlear implant design, development, and manufacture. The chapter focuses on the strategies that are currently being programmed in commercial devices as well as on how to perform cochlear implant programming in a clinical setting. Even though there is no best solution to program an implant, fitting a patient with a suitable coding strategy and

optimal parameters can usually maximize patient performance.

REFERENCES

1. Moore BJ. Coding of sounds in the auditory system and its relevance to signal processing and coding in cochlear implants. Otol Neurotol 2003;24:243–54.
2. Djourno A, Eyriès C. Prosthese auditive par excitation electrique a distance du nerf sensoriel al'aid d' un bobinage inclus a demeure. [Auditory prosthesis by means of a distant electrical stimulation of the sensory nerve with the use of an indwelling coil]. Presse Med 1957;65:1417.
3. House WF, Urban J. Long term results of electrode implantation and electronic stimulation of the cochlea in man. Ann Otol Rhinol Laryngol 1973;82:504–17.
4. Eddington DK. Speech discrimination in deaf subjects with cochlear implants. J Acoust Soc Am 1980;68:885–91.
5. Wilson BS, Finley CC, Lawson DT, et al. Better speech recognition with cochlear implants. Nature 1991;352:236 8.
6. Loizou PC, Stickney GS, Mishra L, Assmann P. Comparison of speech processing strategies used in the Clarion implant processor. Ear Hear 2003;24:12–9.
7. Clark GM. The multiple-channel cochlear implant: The interface between sound and the central nervous system for hearing, speech, and language in deaf people—a personal perspective. Philos Trans R Soc Lond Biol Sci 2006;361:791–810.
8. Loizou PC. Mimicking the human ear: An overview of signal processing techniques used for cochlear implants. IEEE Sig Proc Mag 1998;15:101–30.
9. Skinner MW, Holden LK, Holden TA, et al. Performance of postlinguistically deaf adults with the Wearable Speech Processor (WSP) and Mini Speech Processor (MSP) of the Nucleus multi-electrode cochlear implant. Ear Hear 1991;12:3–22.
10. Wilson BS, Lawson DT, Muller JM, et al. Cochlear implants: Some likely next steps. Ann Rev Biomed Eng 2003;5:207–49.
11. Shannon RV, Zeng FG, Wygonski J, et al. Speech recognition with primarily temporal cues. Science 1995;270:303–4.
12. Smith ZM, Delgutte B, Oxenham AJ. Chimaeric sounds reveal dichotomies in auditory perception. Nature 2002; 416:87–90.
13. Gfeller K, Olszewski C, Rychener M, et al. Recognition of "real-world" musical excerpts by cochlear implant recipients and normal-hearing adults. Ear Hear 2005;26: 237–50.
14. Zeng FG, Nie K, Stickney GS, et al. Speech recognition with amplitude and frequency modulations. Proc Natl Acad Sci 2005;102:2293–8.
15. Fishman KE, Shannon RV, Slattery WH. Speech recognition as a function of the number of electrodes used in the SPEAK cochlear implant speech processor. J Speech Lang Hear Res 1997;40:1201–15.
16. Zeng FG. Temporal pitch in electric hearing. Hear Res 2002;174:101–6.
17. Zeng FG. Trends in cochlear implants. Trends Amplif 2004;8:1–34.
18. Dorman MF, Spahr AJ, Loizou PC, et al. Acoustic simulations of combined electric and acoustic hearing (EAS). Ear Hear 2005;26:371–80.
19. Rubinstein JT, Wilson BS, Finley CC, Abbas PJ. Pseudo-spontaneous activity: Stochastic independence of auditory nerve fibers with electrical stimulation. Hear Res 1999;127:108–18.
20. Zwolan TA, Kileny PR, Ashbaugh C, Telian SA. Patient performance with the Cochlear Corporation "20 + 2" implant: Bipolar versus monopolar activation. Am J Otol 1996;17:717–23.

34

Facial Paralysis

P. Ashley Wackym, MD
John S. Rhee, MD, MPH

Facial nerve abnormalities represent a broad spectrum of lesions, including numerous congenital and acquired causes.[1] The patient who suffers with facial paralysis experiences not only functional consequences but also the psychological impact of a change in self-image and impaired communicative ability. In fact, a 1991 poll revealed that the level of discomfort that Americans felt on meeting those with facial abnormalities was second only to that associated with interacting with the mentally ill, and this discomfort far exceeded anxiety about encountering the senile, mentally retarded, deaf, blind, and those confined to a wheelchair.[2]

FACIAL NERVE ABNORMALITIES

Table 1 summarizes the various causes of facial paralysis.

Congenital

MÖBIUS SYNDROME (CONGENITAL FACIAL DIPLEGIA). Möbius syndrome is a rare congenital disorder, which usually includes bilateral seventh nerve paralysis and unilateral or bilateral sixth nerve paralysis. Since the disorder was described, many authors have studied families with the syndrome.[3] It is considered to have an autosomal dominant inheritance pattern with variable expressivity. The inheritance pattern is thought to be no higher than 1 in 50 in families in whom myopathies or other extremity anomalies such as clubfoot, arthrogryposis, or digital anomalies are not present.

The etiology of Möbius syndrome is unclear. Neuropathologic studies have noted that the nuclei of cranial nerves (CNs) VI, VII, and XII are abnormal, with lesser abnormalities being found in the nuclei of CNs III and XI.[4] Other authors have reported that the facial nerves are smaller or absent at autopsy.[5] Pitner and colleagues advanced yet another hypothesis based on their observation that normal facial nuclei were present on postmortem analysis; they suggested that there was a primary failure of facial muscle development.[6] More recently, Cattaneo and colleagues characterized 2 groups of patients with Möbius syndrome.[7] The first group was characterized by increased facial distal motor latencies and poor recruitment of small and polyphasic motor unit action potentials. The second group

Table 1 Causes of Facial Paralysis

Birth and Congenital
  Aplasia of the facial nerve
  Molding
  Forceps delivery
  Myotonic dystrophy
  Möbius syndrome
Trauma
  Barotrauma
  Brainstem injuries
  Cortical injuries
  Facial (soft tissue injuries)
  Penetrating injury to middle ear
  Temporal bone fractures
Neurogenic
  Millard-Gubler syndrome (abducens palsy with contralateral hemiplegia owing to lesion in base of pons involving corticospinal tract)
  Opercular syndrome (cortical lesion in facial motor area)
Infection
  Bell palsy
  Acute or chronic otitis media
  Cholesteatoma, acquired and congenital
  Herpes zoster oticus (Ramsay Hunt syndrome)
  Mastoiditis
  Malignant otitis externa
  Meningitis
  Parotitis
  Chickenpox
  Encephalitis
  Poliomyelitis
  Mumps
  Mononucleosis
  Leprosy
  HIV (human immunodeficiency virus)
  Influenza
  Coxsackie virus
  Malaria
  Syphilis
  Tuberculosis
  Botulism
  Mucormycosis
  Lyme disease
Vascular
  Endovascular embolization (external carotid artery branches)
  Intratemporal aneurysm of internal carotid artery
  Anomalous sigmoid sinus
Neoplastic
  Facial neuroma
  Acoustic neuroma (rapid expansion or post resection)
  Paraganglioma (glomus jugulare)
  Leukemia
  Meningioma
  Hemangiopericytoma
  Hemangioma
  Hemangioblastoma
  Pontine glioma
  Sarcoma
  Hydradenoma (external auditory canal)
  Teratoma
  Fibrous dysplasia
  von Recklinghausen disease
  Carcinomatous encephalitis
  Cholesterol granuloma
  Carcinoma (invasive or metastatic)
Genetic and metabolic
  Diabetes mellitus
  Hyperthyroidism
  Pregnancy
  Hypertension
  Alcoholic neuropathy
  Sickle cell disease
  Bulbopontine paralysis
  Oculopharyngeal muscular dystrophy
  Camurati-Engelmann disease (hereditary diaphyseal dysplasia)
Toxic
  Thalidomide (cranial nerves VI and VII with atretic external ears [Miehlke syndrome])
  Tetanus
  Diphtheria
  Carbon monoxide
  Lead intoxication
Iatrogenic
  Anesthesia, local (mandibular block, face, mastoid)
  Tetanus vaccination
  Vaccine treatment for rabies exposure
  Otologic and neurotologic skull base surgery, parotid surgery
  Interventional neuroradiology (embolization)
Idiopathic
  Bell palsy
  Melkersson-Rosenthal syndrome
  Hereditary hypertrophic neuropathy
  Autoimmune syndromes
  Thrombotic thrombocytopenia purpura
  Guillain-Barré syndrome
  Multiple sclerosis
  Myasthenia gravis
  Sarcoidosis
  Wegener granulomatosis
  Eosinophilic granuloma
  Histiocytosis X
  Amyloidosis
  Paget disease
  Osteopetrosis
  Kawasaki disease

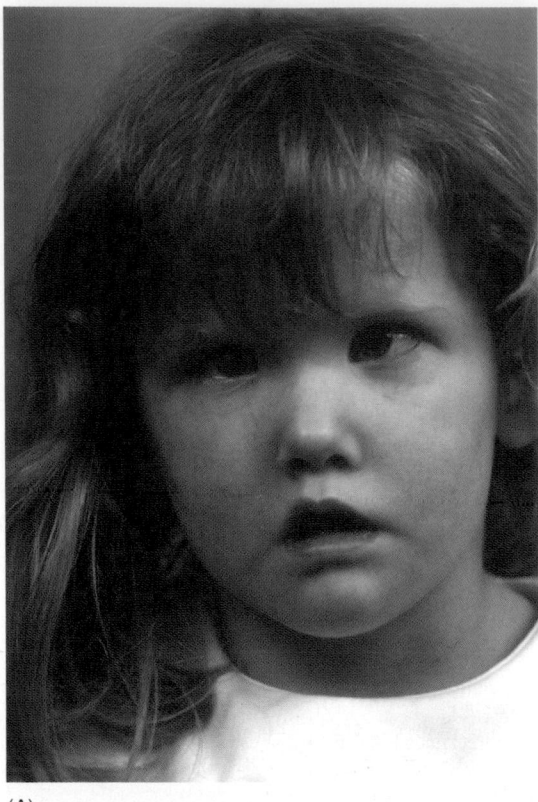

(A)

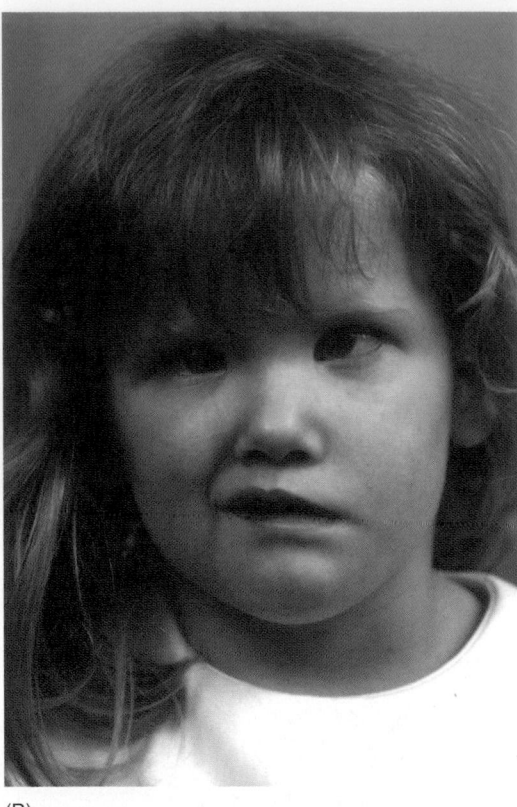

(B)

Figure 1 Möbius syndrome. (A) Left facial paralysis and right facial paresis photographed at rest. (B) With smiling and leftward gaze, the left facial paralysis, right facial paresis and left sixth nerve paralysis are apparent. (Reproduced with permission; copyright © 2007 P. A. Wackym.)

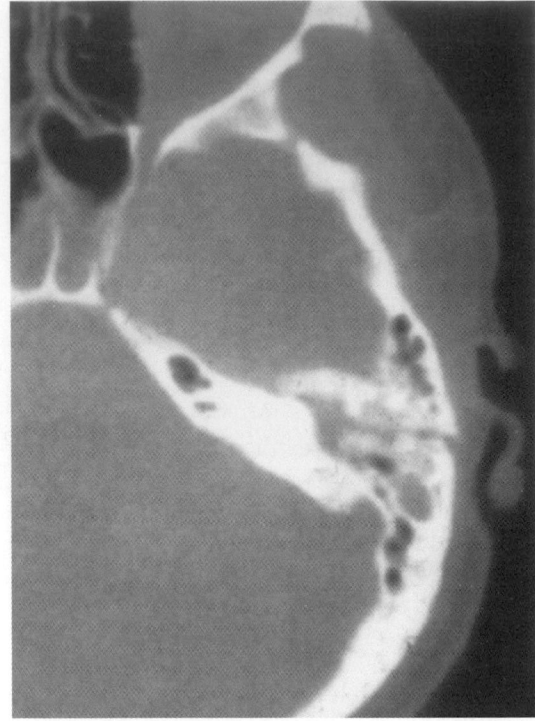

Figure 2 Axial computed tomographic scan with bone windows demonstrates a left longitudinal temporal bone fracture. (Reproduced with permission; copyright © 2007 P. A. Wackym.)

was characterized by normal facial distal motor latencies and neuropathic motor unit action potentials. They hypothesized that in the first group, the disorder is due to a rhombencephalic maldevelopment with selective sparing of small-size motor units, and in the second group, the disorder is related to an acquired nervous injury during intrauterine life, with subsequent neurogenic remodeling of motor units. The authors speculated that these 2 different neurophysiologically defined phenotypes could be used to distinguish sporadic from inherited Möbius syndrome.

The clinical observation of congenital extra-ocular muscle paralysis and facial paralysis is the typical presentation of this disorder (Figure 1). No mass lesions will be found on magnetic resonance imaging (MRI). Ophthalmologic consultation and management are mandatory. Reinnervation procedures such as crossfacial grafts or hypoglossal–facial nerve anastomosis yield poor results, either owing to the paucity of motor end plates or the atrophic seventh nerves. Significant improvements of resting tone and voluntary animation can result from temporalis muscle transposition, which brings in a new neuromuscular system.

Hemifacial Microsomia. The term hemifacial microsomia refers to patients with unilateral microtia, macrostomia, and mandibular hypoplasia. Goldenhar syndrome (oculoauriculovertebral dysplasia) is considered to be a variant of this complex and is characterized by vertebral anomalies and epibulbar dermoids. Although approximately 25% of patients with hemifacial microsomia have facial nerve weakness, 1 patient

with Goldenhar syndrome has been reported to have aplasia of the facial nerve.[8]

Osteopetrosis. Osteopetrosis is a generalized dysplasia of bone that may have an autosomal dominant or recessive inheritance pattern. The recessive form is more rapidly progressive and causes hepatosplenomegaly and severe neural atrophy secondary to bony overgrowth at neural foramina. Optic atrophy, facial paralysis, sensorineural hearing loss, and mental retardation are common in the recessive form, and death usually occurs by the second decade. However, in these severe cases of osteopetrosis, which were previously fatal, bone marrow transplantation has been reported to be of value.[9]

The dominant form causes progressive enlargements of the cranium and mandible and clubbing of the long bones. Increased bone density is seen radiographically. Progressive optic atrophy, trigeminal hypesthesia, recurrent facial paralysis, and sensorineural hearing loss are common. Complete decompression of the intratemporal facial nerve should be performed in patients with recurrent facial paralysis and radiographic evidence of osteopetrosis.

Acquired

Trauma. Approximately 90% of all congenital peripheral facial nerve paralysis spontaneously improves, and most can be attributed to difficult deliveries, cephalopelvic disproportion, high forceps delivery, or intrauterine trauma. These types of congenital facial paralysis are often unilateral and partial, especially involving the lower division

of the facial nerve. Since these causes involve extratemporal compression, surgical exploration or bony decompression is not indicated.[10]

Blunt trauma resulting in temporal bone fracture is best evaluated with high resolution temporal bone computed tomographic (CT) scans (Figures 2 and 3). Temporal and parietal blows to the head may occur anywhere along a coronal arc, from the vertex to the cranial base. When the vector of force is directed toward the base, it classically passes toward the external auditory canal, deflects off the otic capsule, and extends antero-

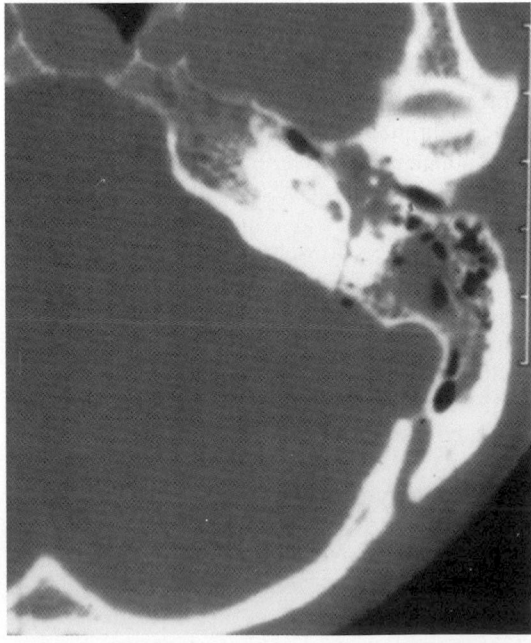

Figure 3 Axial computed tomographic scan with bone windows demonstrates a left transverse temporal bone fracture extending through the otic capsule. (Reproduced with permission; copyright © 2007 P. A. Wackym.)

medially along the anterior edge of the petrous bone to the foramen lacerum and foramen ovale. The resulting fracture is described as a longitudinal temporal bone fracture. This is the most common type of temporal bone fracture ($\approx$ 90%) and is also the most common type of fracture associated with facial nerve injury. The geniculate ganglion region of the facial nerve is most frequently injured. The indications for facial nerve decompression and exploration are the same as those discussed in detail under the Bell palsy section of this chapter.

Frontal and particularly occipital blows to the head tend to result in transverse fractures of the temporal bone. More severe head injury is usually required to cause these fractures.[11] Since they often extend through the internal auditory canal (IAC) or across the otic capsule, hearing loss and vertigo commonly result. Although only 10 to 20% of temporal bone fractures are transverse in orientation, they cause facial nerve injury in approximately 50% of patients. The anatomic region of the facial nerve most commonly injured is the labyrinthine segment. Ishman and Friedland recently compared traditional temporal bone classification systems with an expanded classification scheme.[12] They found that traditional temporal bone fracture descriptions correlate poorly with clinical findings. However, they found that distinguishing petrous from nonpetrous involvement demonstrated significant correlation with the occurrence of serious sequelae of temporal bone fractures. They also found that radiographically based subcategories of mastoid and middle ear involvement further refined this classification schema to correlate with minor complications and concluded that this scheme better focused clinical resources and attention toward more likely sequelae.

Penetrating injuries to the extratemporal facial nerve should be explored urgently to facilitate identification of the transected distal branches using a facial nerve stimulator. If primary repair is not possible, the principles of facial nerve repair using cable grafts, described later in this chapter, should be followed. In infected wounds, urgent exploration and tagging of identified distal branches should precede control of the infection and granulation. Subsequent repair usually requires the use of cable grafts.

Facial nerve injury may occur with otologic surgery. The risk of injury of the facial nerve is particularly high in children with congenital ear malformations.[13,14] Additional groups at higher risk for injury to the facial nerve include infants who are undergoing mastoid surgery since the mastoid tip has not become pneumatized and the facial nerve exits the stylomastoid foramen laterally. In these young children, a semihorizontal, curvilinear skin incision should be used, and, as is the case with all otologic surgery, a facial nerve monitoring system should be used.

Infection

Bacterial. Facial paralysis as a complication of otitis media has become rare in children owing to the ready access to medical care and antibiotics. Takahashi and colleagues published their series of over 1,600 patients with facial paralysis and found that only 11 of these patients were younger than 20 years old and had facial paralysis owing to otitis media (0.67%).[15] They described the facial paralysis in this group of patients to have a slower progression and less complete paralysis than that seen in Bell palsy. Temporal bone CT should be performed in all patients to eliminate the diagnosis of coalescent mastoiditis. Intravenous antibiotics in combination with myringotomy and tympanostomy tube placement remain our initial management algorithms for bacterial otitis media complicated by facial paralysis. Bacterial cultures should always be obtained at the time of myringotomy, and antibiotic selection should be tailored to the culture results.

Facial paralysis complicating mastoiditis or cholesteatoma is also rare. In Sheehy's series of over 180 children undergoing surgery for cholesteatoma, only 1 patient (0.5%) had facial nerve weakness.[16] The surgical management of these patients includes mastoidectomy, excision of the cholesteatoma, and appropriate antibiotic therapy.

Infection with the spirochete *Borrelia burgdorferi* (Lyme disease) can result in facial paralysis. This tick-borne infection is endemic to the northeastern United States and is named for the town of Lyme, Connecticut. Widespread infections have been reported from the west coast, midwest, and east coast, as well as throughout Europe and Australia. As is the case with other spirochete infections, the clinical manifestations of Lyme disease are protean. Facial diplegia has been reported in Lyme disease[17] and should be considered in children presenting with facial paralysis. Serologic diagnosis should be followed by antibiotic therapy. Tetracycline is considered to be the agent of choice; however, erythromycin and penicillin have been successfully used.

Viral. *Ramsay Hunt Syndrome (Herpes Zoster Oticus).* James Ramsay Hunt (1872–1937), an American neurologist, published his seminal article associating the clinical syndrome that now bears his name with herpetic inflammation of the geniculate ganglion.[18] Critical to the development of this hypothesis was the publication of the pathologic studies of Head and Campbell in 1900, which advanced a new hypothesis regarding the etiology of herpes zoster.[19] This work inspired Hunt to first postulate that the etiology of herpes zoster oticus was recrudescence of herpes varicella-zoster virus (VZV) in the geniculate ganglion.[18] Clinically, Ramsay Hunt syndrome may have a variety of manifestations. However, the original 4 classifications of the disease by Hunt included (1) disease affecting the sensory portion of the CN VII, (2) disease affecting the sensory and motor divisions of the CN VII, (3) disease affecting the sensory and motor divisions of the CN VII with auditory symptoms, and (4) disease affecting the sensory and motor divisions of the CN VII with both auditory and vestibular symptoms.

Herpes zoster oticus is the cause of 2 to 10% of all cases of facial paralysis, including 3 to 12% of adults and approximately 5% of children.[1,20–25] Patients may experience paresis or complete paralysis, with the poorest prognosis for recovery in the latter group. Approximately half of patients with Ramsay Hunt syndrome retain some facial motor disturbance; only a few maintain a complete paralysis.[20–23]

Based on the sensory distributions reflected by the VZV recrudescence observed by Hunt over his career,[18,26,27] the most common site of vesicular eruption is in the concha of the auricle (Figure 4). In addition, he described 3 other areas where vesicles can be found during herpes zoster oticus: a small strip of skin on the posteromesial surface of the auricle, the mucosa on the palate, and the anterior two-thirds of the tongue.[26] In his final publication, he detailed the sensory distributions of the facial nerve associated with the geniculate ganglion that subserve the axonal transport of the recrudescent VZV to form the vesicles visible during Ramsay Hunt syndrome.

With the advent of gadolinium diethylenetriamine pentaacetic acid (Gd-DTPA)-enhanced MRI, acute imaging of the facial nerve is possible throughout the clinical course of Ramsay Hunt syndrome.[28] Despite histopathologic reports of diffuse inflammation along the entire intratemporal facial nerve in the disorder,[20,29–32] Korzec and colleagues found that in 3 of the 6 patients with Ramsay Hunt syndrome who were studied with Gd-DTPA MRI, enhancement of the involved nerve was localized to the geniculate ganglion, labyrinthine segment, and the premeatal regions of the affected facial nerve, whereas three was no enhancement at all in the remaining 3 patients.[28] Likewise, in none of their 6 patients did they find enhancement of the vertical or tympanic segments of the facial nerve. These findings suggest that in the early stages of the clinical syndrome, the majority of the inflammation is found near the geniculate ganglion, whereas in the later stages, as examined postmortem, the inflammation has extended

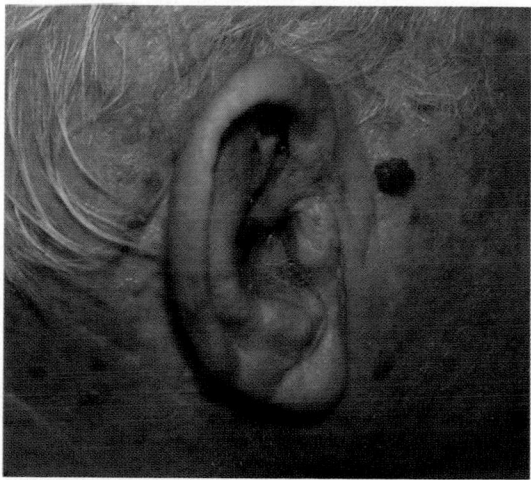

Figure 4 Vesicles in the concha of a patient with Ramsay Hunt syndrome (herpes zoster oticus) of the right facial nerve. (Reproduced with permission; copyright © 2007 P. A. Wackym.)

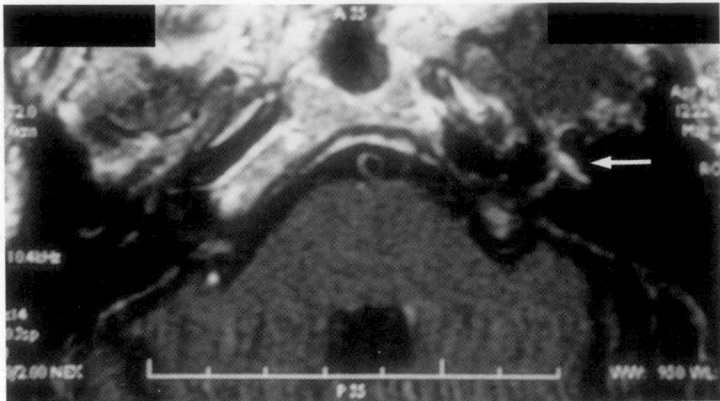

Figure 5 Magnetic resonance image (MRI) of a facial nerve in Ramsay Hunt syndrome (herpes zoster oticus). Gadolinium-enhanced axial MRI shows inflammation of the facial nerve within the internal auditory canal (IAC) labyrinthine segment, geniculate ganglion, tympanic segment, and greater superficial petrosal nerve (*arrow*). (Reproduced with permission; copyright © 2000 P. A. Wackym.)

throughout the intratemporal facial nerve. However, the senior author has seen diffuse enhancement of the facial nerve on MRI examination of patients with Ramsay Hunt syndrome (Figure 5).

Blackley and colleagues reviewed the histopathology associated with Ramsay Hunt syndrome in their 1 case and 5 others.[29] Aleksic and colleagues added another histologic case.[33] Payten and Dawes reviewed the pathologic studies of herpes zoster oticus with facial paralysis for a 60-year interval.[34] Wackym and colleagues used a molecular approach to demonstrate the presence of VZV deoxyribonucleic acid (DNA) combined with traditional histopathologic techniques to the study of the temporal bones from 2 patients with Ramsay Hunt syndrome.[32,35] The most consistent observation was diffuse inflammatory infiltration throughout the involved facial nerve; in addition, several investigators have shown lymphocytic infiltration of the geniculate ganglion, alteration of the geniculate ganglion somata, or both conditions.[20,29,31–33] Based on the models of VZV and herpes simplex virus (HSV) latency and reactivation,[36] these findings are expected. Unlike HSV, which remains dormant directly within sensory neuronal somata, VZV remains latent within the nonneuronal satellite cells surrounding each sensory neuronal somata. With recrudescence, the replication VZV virions are released from satellite cells into the extracellular matrix, where some are taken up by the sensory cell body and transported via the axons back to the skin or mucosa. This release of VZV into the extracellular matrix within the geniculate ganglion would cause an immune response that could result in inflammatory infiltrates throughout the intratemporal facial nerve. Therefore, the diffuse lymphocytic infiltration of the entire facial nerve remains consistent with Hunt's hypothesis.[31,32,34] Furuta and colleagues reported the distribution of VZV DNA in 11 (79%) of 14 trigeminal ganglia and in 9 (69%) of 13 geniculate ganglia collected at autopsy of adults.[37] These data suggest that latent VZV in the geniculate ganglion is a common biologic phenomenon; however, the small sample size and the lack of clinical history regarding whether the patients experienced herpes zoster oticus during their lifetime necessitate confirmation of these observations with a much larger sample size of

well-characterized patients. They have expanded this series recently.[38]

Other authors have suggested that Ramsay Hunt syndrome represents a cranial polyneuropathy.[30,39,40] Care must be taken in interpreting the histopathologic findings in each case as some may represent cephalic zoster with neuritis of multiple CNs.[30,40] Severe central neurologic deficits or multiple cranial motor neuropathies are well recognized in cephalic zoster.[41,42]

Surgical management with decompression of the facial nerve in Ramsay Hunt syndrome has been advocated by some authors (reviewed by Crabtree).[21] Although the advent of facial electroneuronography (ENoG) has resulted in a better idea about which patients with facial paralysis have severe facial nerve injuries requiring surgical decompression,[43] the diffuse inflammatory edema common in Ramsay Hunt syndrome has led most clinicians to avoid undertaking facial nerve decompression.

Experience with the use of intravenous acyclovir (Zovirax) during the acute presentation of Ramsay Hunt syndrome suggests that antiviral medications may facilitate recovery and minimize the morbidity associated with facial paralysis.[25,44–46] This intravenous route has more inherent expenses than an oral route of administration. However, tissue levels of acyclovir delivered by an oral route are not high enough to treat varicella-zoster infections. Alternate antiviral agents such as valacyclovir (Valtrex) (1 g orally 3 times a day for 10 to 14 days) or famciclovir (Famvir) (500 mg orally 3 times a day for 10 days), which achieve adequate levels by an oral route, are now available as an alternative to intravenous acyclovir for the treatment of patients with Ramsay Hunt syndrome.[47] Because the oral route is much more cost effective, this route is preferred. Likewise, oral corticosteroids have been advocated in patients with Ramsay Hunt syndrome.[48]

Bell Palsy. Bell palsy is responsible for 60 to 75% of all cases of facial paralysis. In the past, Bell palsy was defined as an "idiopathic facial paralysis" or as a mononeuropathy of undetermined origin. Recent observations have linked the cause to HSV 1.[49,50] Burgess and colleagues, using polymerase chain reaction amplification, identified HSV 1 DNA in paraffin-embedded sections of the geniculate ganglion from a patient

who died 6 days after the onset of Bell palsy.[49] Furuta and colleagues found HSV DNA in 71% of geniculate ganglia and in 81% of trigeminal ganglia in 8 random autopsy specimens taken from adult cadavers.[51] These data suggest that latent HSV in the geniculate ganglion may be a common biologic phenomenon; however, the small sample size and the lack of clinical history regarding whether the patients experienced Bell palsy during their lifetime necessitate confirmation of these observations with a much larger sample size of well-characterized patients. However, genetic, immunologic, vascular, entrapment, and other infectious causes have all been advanced in the etiology of Bell palsy.[52]

Bell palsy is an acute, unilateral paresis or paralysis of the facial nerve in a pattern consistent with peripheral nerve dysfunction (Figure 6). The onset and evolution are typically rapid, less than 48 hours, and the onset of paralysis may be preceded by a viral prodrome. The symptoms during the early phase of facial paralysis include facial numbness, epiphora, pain, dysgeusia, hyperacusis (dysacusis), and decreased tearing. The pain is usually retroauricular and sometimes radiates to the face, pharynx, or shoulder. Physical findings of this subtle polyneuritis include hypesthesia or dysesthesia of the CNs V and IX and of the second cervical nerve.[53] Motor paralysis of branches of the CN X is seen as a unilateral shift of the palate or vocal cord paresis/paralysis.

Recurrence of Bell palsy occurs in 7 to 12%[1,51] of patients. In the series of 140 patients with recurrent Bell palsy reported by Pitts and colleagues, ipsilateral recurrences were as common as development of contralateral Bell palsy.[54] Also of note in this series was the observation that the incidence of diabetes mellitus was 2.5-fold greater than nonrecurrent cases.

Gadolinium-enhanced MRI has been advocated as a diagnostic tool in assessing Bell palsy. Gadolinium enhancement of the normal facial nerve does not occur. Therefore, enhancement of this structure would be due to increased extracellular fluid from edema, inflammation, or neoplasm. Our observations with gadolinium-enhanced MRI in Bell palsy, as well as those of others,[28] are supportive of Fisch's hypothesis of axoplasmic damming at the meatal segment with subsequent edema and nerve conduction impairment (Figure 7).[55] However, 1 study demonstrated that there was no prognostic significance of gadolinium enhancement of the facial nerve on MRI in patients with Bell palsy.[28] Therefore, gadolinium-enhanced MRI is not indicated in every patient with facial paralysis. In patients suspected of having a tumor from clinical or electrodiagnostic data, gadolinium-enhanced MRI, along with high resolution CT of the IAC, fallopian canal, skull base, and parotid, should be performed.

Adour and colleagues examined the outcome of treating patients with Bell palsy with both acyclovir and corticosteroids in a prospective, randomized, double-blind trial.[56] Half of the patients received a 10-day course of

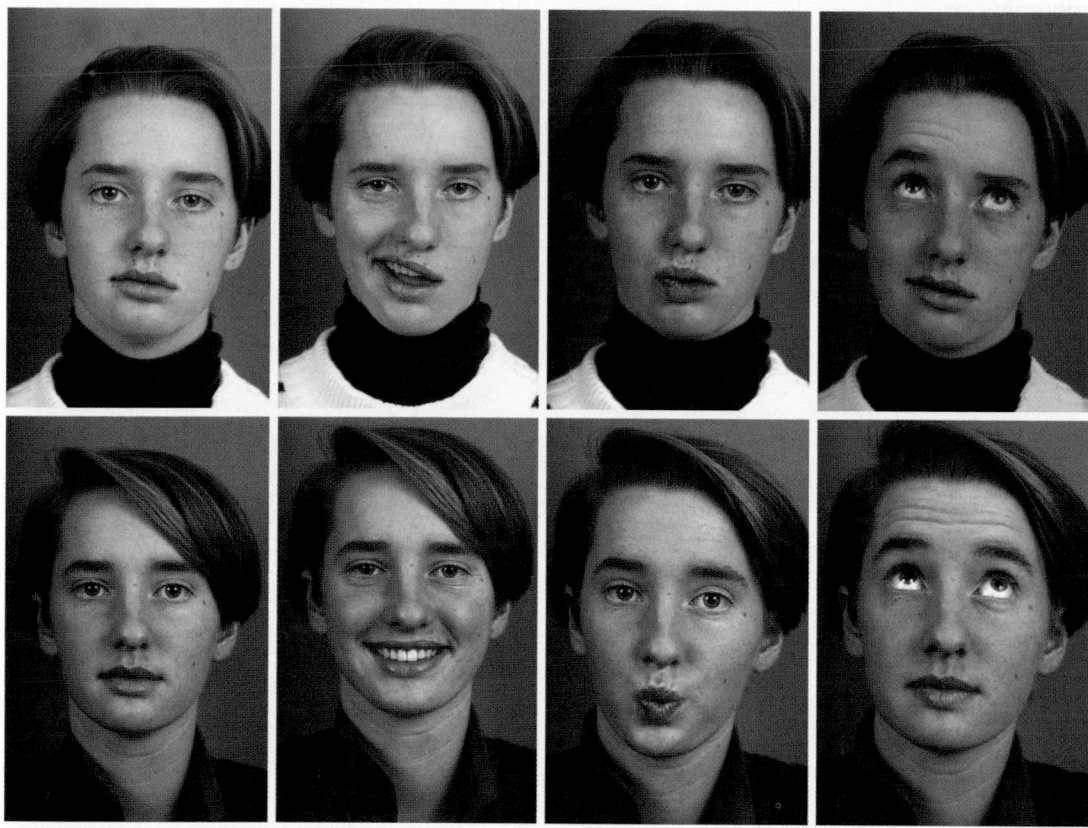

Figure 6 Preoperative facial photographs of a child with complete facial paralysis due to Bell palsy (*top row*). House-Brackmann grade I result 2 months after middle cranial fossa decompression of the labyrinthine segment and geniculate ganglion of the facial nerve (*bottom row*). (Reproduced with permission; copyright © 2007 P. A. Wackym.)

oral acyclovir (400 mg five times per day) and prednisone. The control group received prednisone and a placebo. All study patients began treatment within 3 days of the onset of facial paralysis. The placebo–prednisone group had lower facial function recovery scores (House-Brackmann grade III or IV in 23%) and was almost 3 times as likely to have an unsatisfactory result as the acyclovir–prednisone group (only 7% of the acyclovir–prednisonegroup had a House-Brackmann grade III or IV). A more contemporary review concluded that the current evidence favors the combination of acyclovir

and prednisone, if commenced within the first 72 hours of symptom onset.[57]

ENoG provides a quantitative assessment of facial nerve function and allows a relative comparison between the normal and affected sides and will be discussed in more detail later in this chapter. Our criteria for surgical decompression include ENoG degeneration greater than 90% relative to the unaffected side, no voluntary facial nerve electromyographic (EMG) activity on the affected side, and the operation within 14 days of onset.[43,58,59] Decompression is limited to the meatal and labyrinthine segments through

a middle cranial fossa approach.[59–61] Fisch and Esslen, in 1972, were the first to propose that the most likely site for neural compression and conduction block in Bell palsy was at the entrance to the meatal foramen, the narrowest bony point through which the facial nerve passes.[62] Interestingly, intraoperative evoked EMG documented the conduction block at this area in 94% of decompressed cases, and marked swelling proximal to this point was the typical observation.[62,63] Gantz and colleagues published a prospective study in which a well-defined surgical decompression of the facial nerve was performed in a population of patients with Bell palsy who exhibited the electrophysiologic features associated with poor outcomes (ENoG degeneration greater than 90% relative to the unaffected side, no voluntary facial nerve EMG activity on the affected side).[59] Subjects who did not reach 90% degeneration on ENoG within 14 days of paralysis all returned to House-Brackmann grade I ($n = 48$) or II ($n = 6$) at 7 months after onset of the paralysis. Control subjects self-selecting not to undergo surgical decompression when >90% degeneration on ENoG and no motor unit potentials on EMG were identified had a 58% chance of having a poor outcome at 7 months after onset of paralysis (House-Brackmann grade III or IV [$n = 19$]). A group with similar ENoG and EMG findings undergoing middle fossa facial nerve decompression exhibited House-Brackmann grade I ($n = 14$) or II ($n = 17$) in 91% of the cases. It is recommended that these criteria and this surgical algorithm be followed.

Other Viral Infections. Other viral infections such as primary chickenpox, mononucleosis, mumps, and poliomyelitis can result in facial paralysis that may or may not resolve spontaneously. For these specific viral infections, immunization, when available, is the most effective preventive measure, and supportive care is required during the active infection. Facial reanimation procedures are sometimes required after adequate follow-up suggests that spontaneous recovery will not occur.

Benign or Malignant Neoplasms

Tumor involvement of the facial nerve should be considered in facial paralysis if 1 or more of the following clinical features are present: facial paralysis that progresses slowly over 3 weeks, recurrent ipsilateral facial paralysis, facial weakness associated with muscle twitching, long-standing facial paralysis (greater than 6 months), facial paralysis associated with other CN deficits, or evidence of malignancy elsewhere in the body.

Several benign and malignant tumors can involve the facial nerve along its intracranial, intratemporal, or extracranial course (Table 1). Schwannoma is the most common primary tumor of the facial nerve. It is benign and usually involves the labyrinthine, tympanic, and mastoid segments of the facial nerve. Nerve resection and interpositional nerve grafting may initially

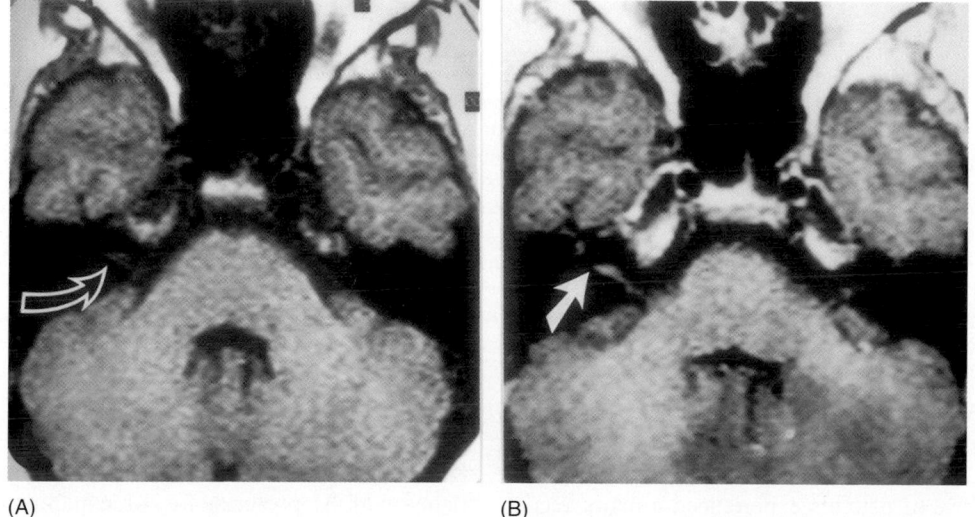

(A)   (B)

Figure 7 Magnetic resonance image (MRI) of facial nerve in Bell palsy. (A) Non–gadolinium-enhanced axial MRI shows normal-appearing seventh and eighth nerves within the right IAC (*open arrow*). (B) Gadolinium-enhanced axial MRI shows axoplasmic damming of the right facial nerve at the meatal foramen (*solid arrow*). This MRI finding was confirmed at surgical decompression. (Reproduced with permission; copyright © 2000 P. A. Wackym.)

be necessary for restoration of continuity[64,65]; however, decompression will often give patients many years of facial nerve function before resection and grafting must be completed.

The use of radiographic imaging is indicated if the characteristics of the facial paralysis are suggestive of a neoplasm. Radiographic studies should include visualization of the entire course of the facial nerve, from the brainstem to the facial musculature. Gadolinium-enhanced MRI (Figure 8) is extremely useful in imaging solid tumors involving the facial nerve, and high resolution CT scans are useful in identifying bony erosion of the fallopian canal. Tumors may arise in the vicinity of the facial nerve and cause facial weakness either by compression or direct invasion. When the tumor is benign, the continuity of the facial nerve should be preserved at all costs by sharp dissection and mobilization techniques. This is appropriate management, whether the nerve is compromised in the IAC by an acoustic neuroma or in the parotid gland by a pleomorphic adenoma. A malignant process with direct invasion of the nerve usually mandates resection of the involved portion of the nerve with immediate interpositional nerve grafting. If the management of the disorder involves chemotherapy or radiation therapy rather than surgical intervention, facial reanimation procedures may be indicated if there is persistent facial nerve dysfunction. As shown in Figure 8, there are many regions of the facial nerve from which facial neuromas may arise. Likewise, the phenotypes can vary between solid, cystic, and linear. These factors underscore the need for individualized treatment plans, which may include surgical decompression, partial resection, resection and nerve grafting, and/or stereotactic radiosurgery.

Hemifacial Spasm

Hemifacial spasm is typically a disorder of the fourth and fifth decades of life and occurs twice as often in women as it does in men. Electrophysiologic and surgical observations indicate that the facial nerve hyperactivity in hemifacial spasm is caused by vascular compression of the facial nerve.[66] Trigeminal neuralgia, hemifacial spasm, glossopharyngeal neuralgia, tinnitus, and disabling positional vertigo have all been associated with vascular compression.[67] Microvascular decompression operations involve separating the compressive vessel from its point of contact with the CN root entry or exit zone and interposition of a prosthesis (usually Teflon felt) to prevent further nerve compression.[66] Drawing from the experience with the more common microvascular compression syndrome of the trigeminal nerve, large series have reported that 62 to 64% of trigeminal neuralgia patients have a compressive artery, 12 to 24% have a compressive vein, 13 to 14% have both an artery and a vein, and 8% have either a tumor or vascular malformation pressing on the trigeminal nerve.[68] The initial failure rate for microvascular decompression for trigeminal neuralgia is 2 to 7%, with a 3.5% per year incidence of a major recurrence.[69–71] In the series of 1,185 patients who underwent

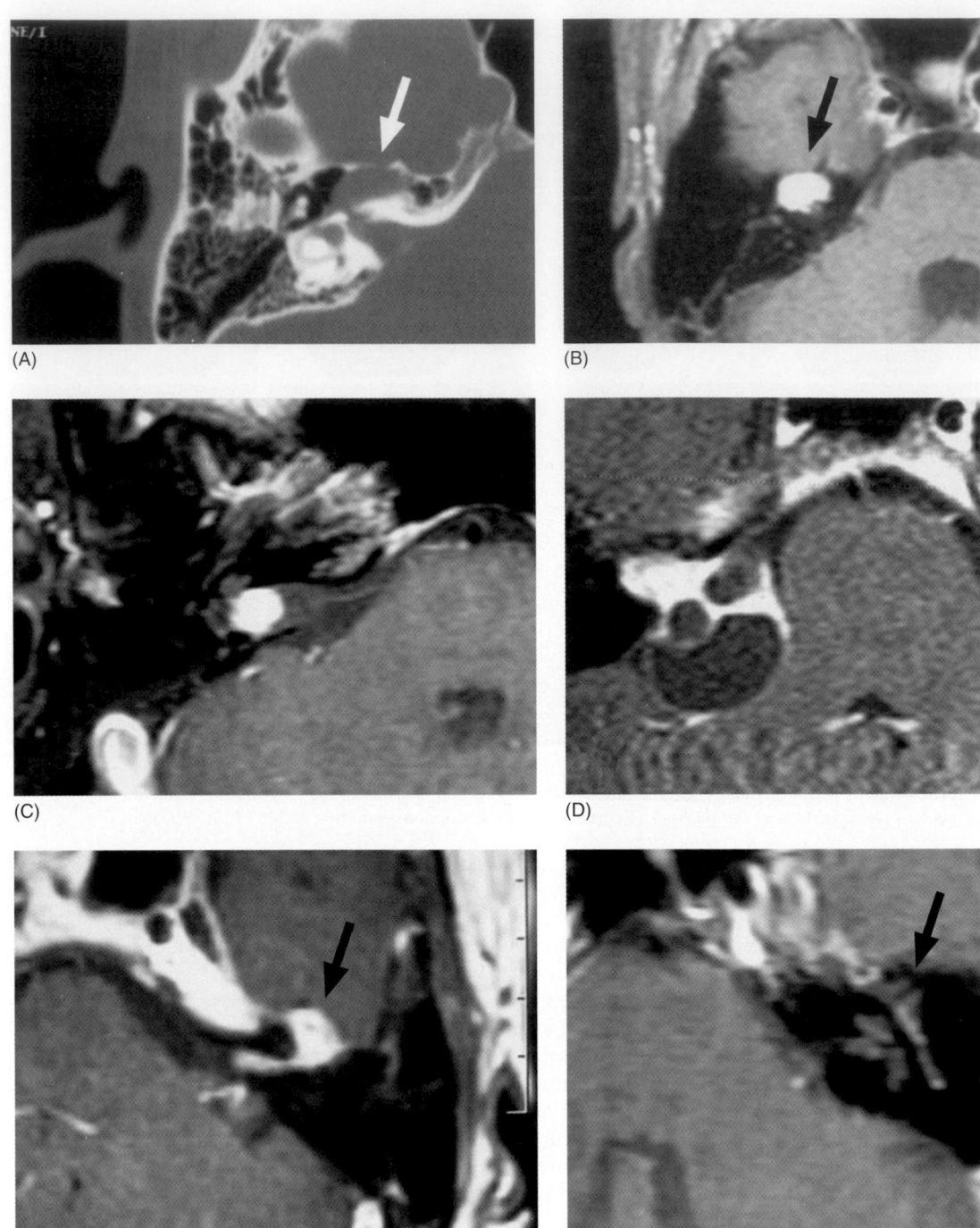

Figure 8 Imaging studies of 5 different facial neuromas. (A and B) Solid right facial neuroma confined to the region of the geniculate ganglion. (A) Axial computed tomographic scan with bone windows demonstrates soft-tissue mass in the region of the geniculate ganglion, resorption and expansion of surrounding bone, and extension into the middle ear (*white arrow*). (B) Gadolinium-enhanced axial magnetic resonance image (MRI) shows the solid facial neuroma in the region of the geniculate ganglion without extension into the labyrinthine segment or internal auditory canal (IAC) (*black arrow*). (C) Gadolinium-enhanced axial MRI shows a solid right facial neuroma within the distal aspect of the IAC. (D) Gadolinium-enhanced axial MRI shows a solid and cystic right facial neuroma filling the entire IAC and extending into the cerebellopontine angle. (E) Gadolinium-enhanced axial MRI shows a solid and linear left facial neuroma in the region of the geniculate ganglion and extending along the facial nerve within the entire length of the IAC (*black arrow*). (F) Gadolinium-enhanced axial MRI shows a linear left facial neuroma extending from the geniculate ganglion region along the tympanic segment of the facial nerve (*black arrow*). (Reproduced with permission; copyright © 2007 P. A. Wackym.)

microvascular decompression for trigeminal neuralgia reported by Barker and colleagues in 1996, there was a mean follow-up of 6.2 years, and 30% of patients experienced a major recurrence, with 11% requiring a second microvascular decompression.[72] The absence of a clear site of arterial compression has been associated with high recurrence rates.[72,73] Patients found to have

only venous compression and no arterial compression are more likely to suffer a recurrence.[72] Kureshi and Wilkins reported their surgical experience with 31 posterior fossa reexplorations for recurrent or persistent trigeminal neuralgia and hemifacial spasm.[74] They discovered 3 (10%) cases in which there was new or previously unrealized arterial compression of neural structures.

Similarly, in a series of 116 patients with microvascular compression syndrome reoperated on after failure, Wilkins reported the identification of previously unseen arterial compression in 65.5%.[75] Liao and colleagues discovered persistent vascular compression in 3 of 5 patients undergoing repeat microvascular decompression.[76]

Although some have doubted that microvascular compression of a CN can represent the cause of hemifacial spasm, the literature indicates that the identification of an arterial vessel compressing the facial nerve in hemifacial spasm and subsequent decompression results in higher cure rates and decreased recurrences than when a specific artery is not identified. We believe that some microvascular decompression procedures fail because the offending vessel has not been identified at the primary operation.[66] Some of these failures occur because the microscope provides incomplete information about the anatomic relationship between the nerves and vessels. The zero-degree endoscope provides a panoramic view of the cerebellopontine angle, and with angled endoscopes, provision for "looking around corners" is made. Magnan and colleagues used an endoscope in 60 patients with hemifacial spasm and demonstrated that with the operating microscope the offending vessel could be visualized in 28% of patients, whereas the endoscope was effectively employed in 93% of the same patients.[77] We have advocated the adjunctive use of the endoscope in microvascular decompression surgery and believe that this will improve surgical outcomes.[66]

Miscellaneous Disorders

The onset of simultaneous bilateral facial paralysis suggests Guillain-Barré syndrome, sarcoidosis, sickle cell disease, or some other systemic disorder.[6] Guillain-Barré syndrome is a relatively common neurologic disorder and is an acute inflammatory polyradiculoneuropathy that progresses to varying degrees of paralysis. The etiology remains unknown; however, autoimmune or viral mechanisms have been considered. Classic histopathologic features of the syndrome include a lymphocytic cellular infiltration of peripheral nerves and destruction of myelin. The facial paralysis is typically bilateral and often resolves spontaneously after a prolonged course of paralysis. Although there is no role for surgical decompression of the facial nerve in this disorder, reanimation is only considered late in the course of the disease.

Melkersson-Rosenthal Syndrome. Melkersson-Rosenthal syndrome is a neuromucocutaneous disease with a classic triad of recurrent facial (labial) edema and recurrent facial paralysis associated with a fissured tongue. Patients with Melkersson-Rosenthal syndrome may not present with the complete triad, and although facial paralysis is the most commonly recognized neurologic symptom, it is not mandatory for the diagnosis. Headache, granular cheilitis, trigeminal neuralgiform attacks, dysphagia, laryngospasm, and a variety of CN and cervical autonomic dysfunctions may also occur. The patient with Melkersson-Rosenthal syndrome may present at any age and with any variety of classic and associated features, which may wax and wane. Approximately one-third of the patients have recurrent facial paralysis as part of their syndrome. The underlying etiologic factor has been thought to be a neurotropic edema causing compression and paralysis of the facial nerve as it passes through the fallopian canal. Since the anatomically most constricted area of the fallopian canal is the meatal foramen and because most prior reports observed recurrence after transmastoid decompression, Graham and Kemink elected to decompress the proximal segment in addition to the mastoid segment of the facial nerve in all such cases by performing a combined transmastoid and middle cranial fossa facial nerve decompression and neurolysis of the nerve sheath.[78] The preliminary data presented by Graham and Kemink suggest that edematous involvement of the facial nerve in recurrent facial paralysis does occur intratemporally and that the recurrent paralysis can be prevented by transmastoid and middle cranial fossa total facial nerve decompression with neurolysis of the facial nerve sheath.[78] Recurrent paralysis over a prolonged period of time usually results in increasing residual dysfunction. If evidence of residual paresis exists, facial nerve decompression of the labyrinthine segment and geniculate ganglion through a middle cranial fossa exposure is recommended at the time of the next episode of paralysis.

SURGICAL ANATOMY OF THE FACIAL NERVE

Detailed knowledge and familiarity with the complex course of the facial nerve and its anatomic relationship to other vital structures are essential to the surgeon who plans to operate in this area. The facial nerve (CN VII) exits the brainstem at the pontomedullary junction approximately 1.5 mm anterior to the vestibulocochlear nerve (CN VIII). The facial nerve is smaller in diameter (approximately 1.8 mm) than the oval CN VIII (approximately 3 mm in the largest diameter). A third smaller nerve, the nervus intermedius, emerges between CN VII and CN VIII and eventually becomes incorporated within the sheath of CN VII. After leaving the brainstem, CN VII follows a rostrolateral course through the cerebellopontine cistern for 15 to 17 mm, entering the porus of the IAC of the temporal bone (Figure 9). Other important structures in the cerebellopontine cistern include the anterior inferior cerebellar artery (AICA) and the veins of the middle cerebellar peduncle. The AICA passes near or between CN VII and CN VIII; the veins are more variable in position and number. On entering the IAC, the facial nerve occupies the anterosuperior quadrant of this channel for 8 to 10 mm. Then it enters the fallopian canal at the fundus of the IAC. The IAC is anterior to the plane of the superior semicircular canal (SSC). Superiorly, the bone overlying the IAC is within a 60° angle, whose vertex is the SSC ampulla. At the entrance of the fallopian canal (meatal foramen), CN VII narrows to its smallest diameter, 0.61 to 0.68 mm.[79,80] Only the pia and arachnoid membranes form a sheath around the nerve at this point since the dural investment terminates at the fundus of the IAC. Many authors believe that the small diameter of the meatal foramen is an important factor contributing to the etiology of facial paralysis in certain diseases such as Bell palsy and Ramsay Hunt syndrome.[55,63,79,81]

The intratemporal course of the facial nerve has three distinct anatomic regions: the labyrinthine, tympanic, and mastoid segments. The labyrinthine segment is shortest ($\approx$ 4 mm),

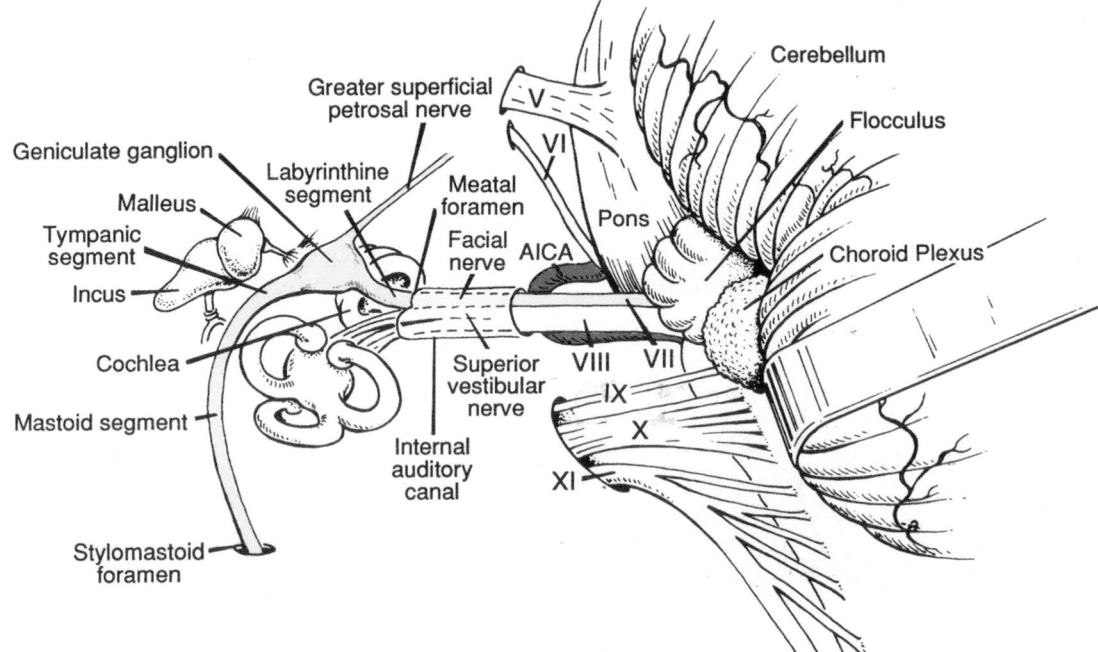

Figure 9 Course and relationships of the left facial nerve from the pontomedullary junction to the stylomastoid foramen. AICA = anterior inferior cerebellar artery. (Reproduced with permission; copyright © 2007 P. A. Wackym.)

extending from the meatal foramen to the geniculate ganglion. This segment travels anterior, superior, and lateral, forming an anteromedial angle of 120° with the IAC portion. The basal turn of the cochlea is closely related to the fallopian canal and lays anteroinferior to the labyrinthine segment of the facial nerve. At the lateral end of the labyrinthine segment, the geniculate ganglion is found, and the nerve makes an abrupt posterior change in direction, forming an acute angle of approximately 75°. Anterior to the geniculate ganglion, the greater superficial petrosal nerve exits the temporal bone through the hiatus of the facial canal. The hiatus of the facial canal is quite variable in its distance from the geniculate ganglion. The hiatus of the facial canal also contains the vascular supply to the geniculate ganglion region. The tympanic, or horizontal, segment of the nerve is approximately 11 mm long, running between the lateral semicircular canal superiorly and the stapes inferiorly, forming the superior margin of the fossa ovale. Between the tympanic and mastoid segments, the nerve gently curves inferiorly for about 2 to 3 mm. The mastoid, or vertical, segment is the longest intratemporal portion of the nerve, measuring approximately 13 mm. As the nerve exits the stylomastoid foramen at the anterior margin of the digastric groove, an adherent fibrous sheath of dense vascularized connective tissue surrounds it. The stylomastoid artery and veins are within this dense sheath.

NERVE INJURY AND NEURODIAGNOSTIC TESTS

Facial Nerve Histology

A connective tissue layer, the endoneurium, surrounds each myelinated axon (Figure 10). This layer is closely adherent to the Schwann cell layer of each axon. The importance of the endoneurial sheath, in the context of nerve injury and repair, is that it provides a continuous tube through which a regenerating axon can grow. The second layer of the nerve sheath is the perineurium. The perineurium provides tensile strength to the nerve. The perineurium is also the primary barrier to the spread of infection. The outermost layer is the

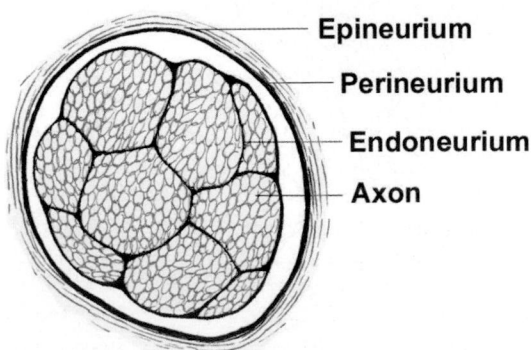

Figure 10 Schematic illustration of a cross-section of the facial nerve demonstrating the relationships among endoneurium, perineurium, and epineurium. (Reproduced with permission; copyright © 2007 P. A. Wackym.)

Table 2 Sunderland and Seddon Classifications of Nerve Injuries

Pathology	Sunderland[82]	Seddon[83]
Conduction block, damming of axoplasm	First degree	Neurapraxia
Transection of the axon with intact endoneurium	Second degree	Axonotmesis
Transection of nerve fiber (axon and endoneurium) inside intact perineurium	Third degree	Neurotmesis
Above plus disruption of perineurium (epineurium remains intact)	Fourth degree	Neurotmesis
	Fifth degree	Neurotmesis

epineurium. This layer contains the vasa nervorum, providing the blood supply as well as the lymphatic vessels.

Facial Nerve Injury

It is necessary to review the types of nerve damage to understand better electrodiagnostic testing of the facial nerve, prognosis for recovery, and the development of synkinesis, as well as the rationale for facial nerve decompression. Table 2 summarizes the Sunderland and Seddon classifications of nerve injuries.[82,83] A facial nerve grading system has been established by the American Academy of Otolaryngology–Head and Neck Surgery (Table 3).[84] The House-Brackmann scoring system was developed as a means of reporting facial recovery after facial nerve paralysis caused by idiopathic facial nerve paralysis or recovery after removal of an acoustic neuroma when an injury to the facial nerve had been sustained.[84] Although this scale is useful when measuring facial nerve function in patients who have suffered an incomplete nerve injury (Sunderland degree I to IV (see Table 2)), it is inappropriate for assessing patients who have suffered Sunderland degree V injury and have undergone facial nerve repair or grafting.

Gidley and colleagues identified 3 reasons why it is difficult to apply the House-Brackmann grading system to a repaired facial nerve: (1) all repairs result in mass movement, (2) most patients regain complete eye closure and competent oral sphincter function, and (3) almost none have the ability to raise their forehead.[85] Consequently, they have proposed a grading system that more accurately grades the outcome from facial nerve grafting or repair procedure (Table 4). A letter grading system was chosen to avoid confusion with the House-Brackmann classification.

Electroneuronography and Electromyography

The 2 most useful objective electrodiagnostic tests of facial nerve function are ENoG and EMG.

Facial Electroneuronography. ENoG uses supramaximal electrical stimulation of the facial nerve at the level of the stylomastoid foramen to produce a compound muscle action potential. This evoked electromyogenic response is recorded with surface electrodes placed over the perioral (nasolabial) muscles since a large representative

Table 3 House-Brackmann Facial Nerve Grading System

Grade	Description	Characteristics
I	Normal	Normal facial function in all areas
II	Mild dysfunction	*Gross:* slight weakness noticeable on close inspection; may have very slight synkinesis
		At rest: normal symmetry and tone
		Motion: forehead—moderate to good function; eye—complete closure with minimal effort; mouth—slight asymmetry
III	Moderate dysfunction	*Gross:* obvious but not disfiguring difference between the two sides; noticable but not severe synkinesis; contracture and/or hemifacial spasm
		At rest: normal symmetry and tone
		Motion: forehead—slight to moderate movement; eye—complete closure with effort; mouth—slightly weak with maximal effort
IV	Moderately severe dysfunction	*Gross:* obvious weakness and/or disfiguring asymmetry
		At rest: normal symmetry and tone
		Motion: forehead—none; eye—incomplete closure; mouth—asymmetric with maximum effort
V	Severe dysfunction	*Gross:* only barely perceptible motion
		At rest: asymmetry
		Motion: forehead—none; eye—incomplete closure; mouth—slight movement
VI	Total paralysis	No movement

Adapted from reference 84.

Table 4 Repaired Facial Nerve Recovery Scale	
Score	Function
A	Normal facial function
B	Independent movement of eyelids and mouth, slight mass motion, slight movement of forehead
C	Strong closure of eyelids and oral sphincter, some mass motion, no forehead movement
D	Incomplete closure of eyelids, significant mass motion, good tone
E	Minimal movement in any branch, poor tone
F	No movement

Adapted from reference 85.

population of facial nerve fibers would be sampled by recording the evoked response from this group of muscles. Needle electrodes are not used because intramuscular needle electrodes would not sample a sufficient number of motor units to yield the representative maximal amplitude. A supramaximal bipolar stimulation (galvanic) is provided to saturate the nerve and produce a complete and synchronous depolarization. The galvanic stimulation is typically delivered as rectangular pulses, with a pulse duration of 200 μs and an interpulse interval of 1 second. The amplitude of the evoked response is plotted as a function of time after stimulation. Both the normal and affected sides are tested, and the amplitude of the responses is compared. The percentage of degenerated fibers is calculated arithmetically, as follows:

$$\text{Percentage of degenerated fibers} = 100 - \left(\frac{\text{Amplitude of evoked response (in μV) Affected side}}{\text{Amplitude of evoked response (in μV) Normal side}} \times 100 \right).$$

This electrodiagnostic test depends on the physiologic premise of neural injury proposed by both Seddon and Sunderland (see Table 2). Injuries that are limited to producing a conduction block within the nerve (neurapraxia) do not disrupt axoplasmic continuity and will continue to conduct a neural discharge if the electrical stimulus is presented distal to the conduction block. With more severe injuries, axoplasmic disruption (axonotmesis) or neural tubule disruption (neurotmesis) will result in wallerian degeneration distal to the site of injury. Nerve fibers that undergo wallerian degeneration cannot propagate electrically evoked potentials distal to the injury. Axonotmesis, in contrast to neurotmesis, has a better prognostic outcome. With resolution of the neural injury, in a nerve that has undergone axonotmesis, the axon will regenerate through the intact neural tubule, potentially allowing complete return of motor function to the muscle fiber innervated by that nerve fiber. The more severely disrupted neural tubule injury of neurotmesis has the potential to regenerate in an unsuccessful manner and can thereby result in misdirection of fibers, clinically

causing synkinesis and incomplete return of motor function. ENoG can be used to differentiate nerve fibers that have minor conduction blocks (neurapraxia) from those that have undergone wallerian degeneration; however, ENoG cannot differentiate the type of wallerian degeneration (axonotmesis versus neurotmesis). The severity of the injury can be inferred from the rate of degeneration after injury. More rapid wallerian degeneration is associated with neurotmesis, whereas nerves that degenerate more slowly are more likely to exhibit axonotmesis.[43,58,59]

The timing for performing ENoG should take into consideration the time course of wallerian degeneration. With a known complete transection of the facial nerve (eg, traumatic injury), 100% wallerian degeneration occurs over 3 to 5 days as the distal axon slowly degenerates. Therefore, early testing, within 3 days of paralysis, may not be representative of the degree of injury, and as outlined above, the time course of degeneration may reflect the degree of injury. An important technical detail to be attentive to is the need to stimulate the nerve at the stylomastoid foramen 10 to 20 times before making an amplitude measurement. The initial stimulation will improve the synchronization within the nerve and therefore improve the reliability of the test.

As discussed earlier in this chapter, our criteria for surgical decompression include ENoG degeneration greater than 90% relative to the unaffected side, no voluntary facial nerve EMG activity on the affected side, and the operation within 14 days of onset.[43,58,59] Decompression is limited to the meatal and labyrinthine segments through a middle cranial fossa approach.[59–61]

Gantz and colleagues published a prospective study in which a well-defined surgical decompression of the facial nerve was performed in a population of patients with Bell palsy who exhibited the electrophysiologic features associated with poor outcomes (ENoG degeneration greater than 90% relative to the unaffected side, no voluntary facial nerve EMG activity on the affected side).[59] Subjects who did not reach 90% degeneration on ENoG within 14 days of paralysis all returned to House-Brackmann grade I (n = 48) or II (n = 6) at 7 months after onset of the paralysis. Control subjects self-selecting not to undergo surgical decompression when >90% degeneration on ENoG and no motor unit potentials on EMG were identified had a 58% chance of having a poor outcome at 7 months after onset of paralysis (House-Brackmann grade III or IV (n = 19)). A group with similar ENoG and EMG findings undergoing middle fossa facial nerve decompression exhibited House-Brackmann grade I (n = 14) or II (n = 17) in 91% of the cases. It is recommended that these criteria and this surgical algorithm be followed.

Electromyography. Facial nerve EMG is important to use as an adjunctive tool when making decisions regarding surgery. Early in the time course of recovery, regenerating nerve fibers conduct at differing rates, producing dyssynchrony, and, therefore, overestimate the degree of wallerian degeneration based on ENoG testing. In fact, it is possible to record "100% degeneration" with ENoG in patients with early recovery from Bell palsy while voluntary movement is observed. It is for this reason that a voluntary EMG is performed when the ENoG shows greater than 90% degeneration within 14 days of injury and surgical decompression is being considered. Needle electrodes are placed into the orbicularis oculi and orbicularis oris muscles, and the patient is asked to make voluntary contractions. If voluntary contractions occur during the first 2 weeks after the onset of paralysis, early deblocking of the neural conduction block has taken place, and a good recovery of facial function will most likely follow. It is also important to keep in mind that ENoG is useful only during the acute phase of the injury, between days 3 and 21, and after complete loss of voluntary function. EMG is the more useful single diagnostic study after 3 weeks of facial paralysis. As will be discussed later in the chapter, EMG testing is also important when deciding whether to perform nerve substitution procedures and other reanimation procedures.

GENERAL PRINCIPLES IN FACIAL NERVE SURGERY

Whenever the facial nerve is to be surgically exposed, several technical points must be observed. First, a system for monitoring facial nerve function during the operation should be employed.[86] Historically, visual observation during critical stages of the operation was performed. However, the standard practice for essentially all otologists is to use intraoperative facial nerve EMG with placement of needle electrodes into the orbicularis oculi and orbicularis oris muscles.

Instrumentation is crucial to successful exposure of the facial nerve. The largest diamond bur that the operative site can safely accommodate should be used when the surgeon is near the fallopian canal. Cutting burs have the potential to catch and skip in an unpredictable way and can consequently cause severe injury to the nerve. Continuous suction-irrigation keeps the burs clean and also dissipates heat, which can induce neural damage.

Blunt elevators, such as the Fisch raspatory (Leibinger, Dallas, Texas), should be used to remove the final layer of bone over the nerve. These instruments are thin but strong enough to remove a thin layer of bone. Stapes curettes are too large and can cause compression injury to the nerve. If a neurolysis is to be performed, disposable micro-blades are available (Beaver No. 5910, BD Medical—Ophthalmic Systems, New Jersey). Sharp dissection is less traumatic than blunt elevation when the nerve must be lifted out of the fallopian canal. The medial surface of the nerve usually adheres to the bone and contains a rich vascular supply. Cauterization near the nerve should be performed only with an irrigating bipolar electrocautery, low current, and insulated microforceps.

Middle Cranial Fossa (Transtemporal) Approach: Internal Auditory Canal Porus to Tympanic Segment

The middle cranial fossa exposure is used to expose the IAC and labyrinthine segment of the facial nerve when hearing preservation is a goal.[61,87] The geniculate ganglion and tympanic portion of the nerve can also be decompressed from this approach.

Technique. The patient is placed supine on the operating table with the head turned so that the involved temporal bone is upward (Figure 11A). The hair is shaved 6 to 8 cm above and anterior to the ear and 2 cm posterior to it. The surgeon is seated at the head of the table with the instrument nurse at the anterior side of the patient's head. A 6 cm × 8 cm posteriorly based trapdoor incision, or a preauricular incision, is marked in the hairline above the ear (Figure 11B). If exposure of the mastoid is necessary, the inferior limb of the incision can be carried postauricularly (Figure 11B, dashed line). The skin flap is elevated to expose the temporalis muscle and fascia. A 4 cm × 4 cm temporalis fascia graft is harvested for use during closure of the IAC dural defect. Alternatively, Alloderm (LifeCell Corp., Woodlands, TX) can be used. An anteriorly based trapdoor incision is used to elevate the temporalis muscle and periosteum (see Figure 11B, thin line). Staggering the levels of the muscle and skin incisions provides for a double-layer, watertight closure at the completion of the procedure. If exposure of the mastoid is not necessary, a preauricular incision is often used (Figure 11C).

The temporal root of the zygoma is exposed during elevation of the temporalis muscle. This landmark represents the level of the floor of the middle fossa. Dural fishhooks are placed in the skin and temporalis muscle flaps for retraction. A 3 cm × 5 cm bone flap for facial nerve decompression, or a 4 cm × 5 cm bone flap for tumor excisions, centered above the temporal root of the zygoma is fashioned with a medium-cutting bur (3 mm). It is important to keep the anterior and posterior margins of the craniotomy parallel to facilitate placement of the self-retaining retractor.

Branches of the middle meningeal artery are occasionally embedded within the inner table of the skull; therefore, elevation of the bone flap must be performed in a controlled manner. Bipolar coagulation and bone wax may be necessary to control bleeding. Elevation of the dura from the floor of the middle fossa can be one of the most difficult steps. Blunt dissection and magnification greatly facilitate dural elevation. The dura is elevated from the posterior to anterior direction to prevent accidental injury to an exposed geniculate ganglion and greater superficial petrosal nerve. Bipolar coagulation is used to cauterize dural reflections within the petrosquamous suture before transection with scissors.

The elevation proceeds until the petrous ridge is identified medially and the arcuate eminence, meatal plane, and greater superficial petrosal nerve are exposed anteriorly. No attempt is made to identify the middle meningeal artery and accompanying troublesome bleeding veins. The tip of a self-retaining retractor (Fisch, Leibinger) is placed at the petrous ridge anterior to the arcuate eminence and medial to the meatal plane (Figure 12). A medium diamond bur (2 to 3 mm) and a suction irrigation apparatus are used to identify the blue line of the SSC. A preoperative Stenvers projection radiograph helps to determine the level of the SSC in relation to the floor of the middle fossa and the degree of pneumatization above the SSC (Figure 13).

Drilling begins posterior to the arcuate eminence over the mastoid air cells until the dense yellow bone of the otic capsule is identified. Otic capsule bone is slowly removed until the blue outline of the SSC is seen. The IAC is located by removing bone with a 60° angle anterior to the blue line of the SSC and with the vertex based at the SSC ampulla. This dissection is continued until approximately 180° of the IAC are exposed for facial nerve decompressions (see Figure 12) or 270° of the IAC are exposed for schwannomas. Because of the close proximity of the SSC and the basal turn of the cochlea, only approximately 120° of the circumference of the IAC can be safely removed in its lateral 5 mm or so. The facial nerve occupies the anterosuperior portion of the IAC. Laterally, the vertical crest (Bill bar) marks the division between the superior vestibular nerve and the meatal foramen containing the facial nerve.

The entrance to the fallopian canal is the narrowest, most delicate portion of the facial nerve and consequently the most challenging portion of the dissection. At the meatal foramen, the facial nerve turns anterior and slightly superior. The basal turn of the cochlea can be within 1 mm inferiorly, and the ampulla of the SSC can be directly posterior to the nerve. The labyrinthine segment is followed to the geniculate ganglion. If the facial nerve needs to be exposed distal to the geniculate ganglion (eg, as with facial neuromas or with some traumatic injuries to the facial nerve), the tegmen tympani is removed with care to avoid injury to the head of the malleus and incus. The tympanic segment is easily seen to turn abruptly posterior; it is followed to where it courses inferior to the lateral semicircular canal. It is advisable to leave a thin shell of bone covering the nerve until its entire course is identified. Small blunt elevators are used to remove the final layer of bone. The nerve is tightly confined within the labyrinthine segment of the fallopian canal; larger curettes should be avoided to prevent compression injury. If the nerve is to be decompressed, a neurolysis is the final step. A disposable microscalpel (Beaver No. 5910) is used to slit the periosteum and epineural sheath.

Alternative methods to locate the facial nerve may be necessary, especially in traumatic cases. The greater superficial petrosal nerve can be traced posteriorly to the geniculate ganglion, or the tegmen tympani may be fractured and the tympanic segment visible through the fracture. The tympanic segment is then used to locate the geniculate ganglion and labyrinthine segments.

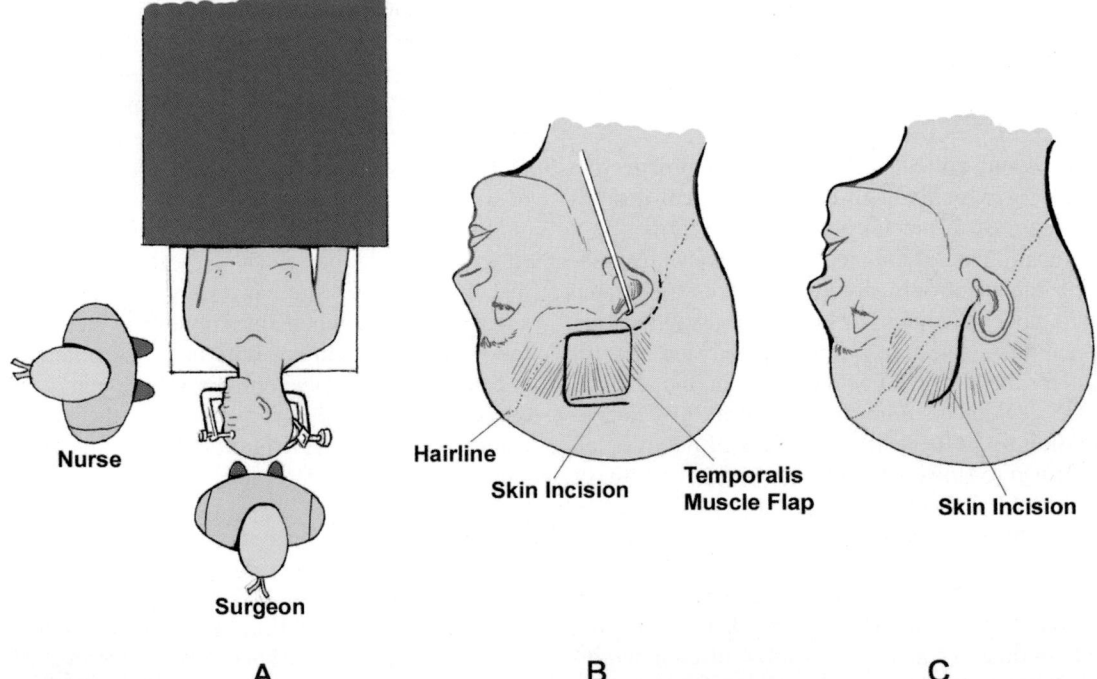

Nurse

Surgeon

Hairline

Skin Incision

Temporalis Muscle Flap

Skin Incision

A **B** **C**

Figure 11 Patient positioning and incision design for the middle cranial fossa approach. (A) Patient is in the supine position with the operated ear upward. Surgeon is seated at the vertex of the head. (B) Posteriorly based trap-door scalp incision (*bold line*). Surgical position illustrating the skin incision (*solid line*) for the middle cranial fossa approach. The dashed line shows the extension of the scalp incision that is required to reach the mastoid area for total facial nerve exposure. Design of anteriorly based temporalis muscle, fascia, and periosteal flap (*thin line*). (C) Alternative preauricular incision for the middle cranial fossa approach if mastoid exposure is not necessary. (Reproduced with permission; copyright © 2007 P. A. Wackym.)

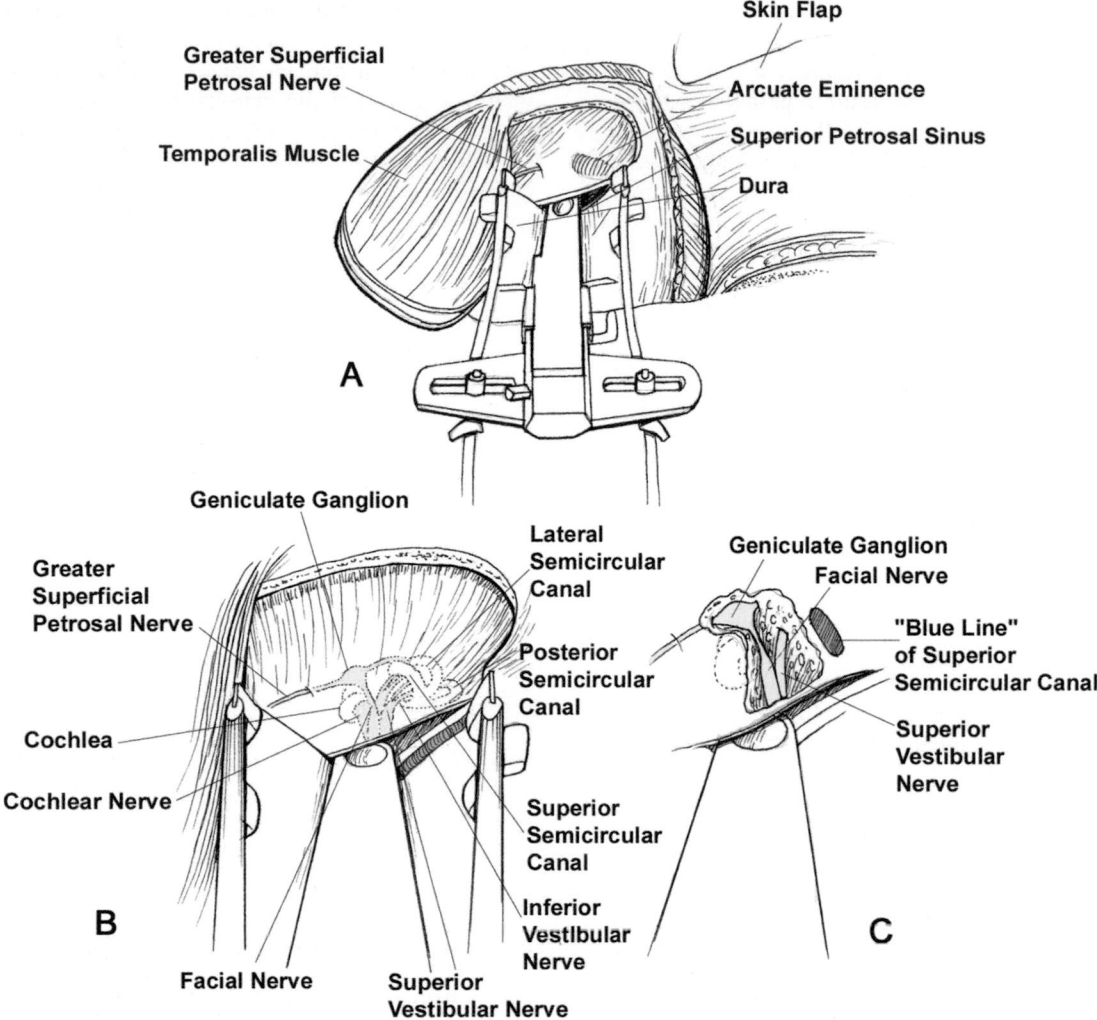

Figure 12 Surgical view of the right middle cranial fossa exposure after craniotomy, temporal lobe retraction, and bony exposure are complete. (A) Placement of the retractor with exposure of the arcuate eminence and greater superficial petrosal nerve. (B) The facial nerve, cochlea, and labyrinth within the temporal bone are shown ghosted beneath the bone as viewed through the middle cranial fossa approach. (C) Drilling of the IAC for facial nerve decompression. (Reproduced with permission; copyright © 2007 P. A. Wackym.)

temporalis fascia previously harvested is placed over the free bone graft to help seal the dural defect at the IAC. The craniotomy defect is then repaired using titanium mesh (Synthes Maxillofacial) and hydroxyapatite cement (Norian CRS, Synthes, Inc., West Chester, PA), and the temporalis muscle is closed with interrupted absorbable sutures. The skin is closed in layers with particular care in closing the galea. No drain is placed. A mastoid-type pressure dressing is applied.

Advantages and Uses. The middle cranial fossa route is the only method that can be used to expose the entire IAC and labyrinthine segment with preservation of hearing. This, in combination with the retrolabyrinthine and transmastoid approaches, enables visualization of the entire course of the facial nerve and still preserves function of the inner ear. The middle cranial fossa technique is the most commonly used for decompression of the facial nerve in Bell palsy[55,61] and longitudinal temporal bone fractures. However, as described earlier in this chapter, this approach may be useful in the management of patients with schwannomas of CN VII or CN VIII, as well as with patients with Melkersson-Rosenthal syndrome.

Postoperative Care/Complications and their Management. The anatomy of the floor of the middle cranial fossa is quite variable and presents some difficulty in identification of landmarks. The Stenvers projection radiograph provides important anatomic information regarding the degree of pneumatization above the SSC and should be performed in all cases to minimize the risk of surgical injury to the SSC. In addition, the surgeon must have a precise knowledge of 3-dimensional anatomy of the temporal bone. Many hours in a temporal bone dissection laboratory are required to attain the delicate microsurgical skills that are necessary for this type of surgery.

Middle cranial fossa facial nerve decompression can result in conductive and/or sensorineural hearing loss. Conductive hearing loss can be secondary to temporal lobe herniation or ossicular disruption during dissection in the attic.

At the end of the procedure, a free temporalis muscle graft is placed within the IAC and a corner piece of the bone flap is fashioned to cover the defects in the tegmen tympani and IAC (Figure 14). Alternatively, titanium mesh (Synthes Maxillofacial, Paoli, PA) between layers of Alloderm can be used. This prevents herniation of the temporal lobe into the middle ear or IAC. The

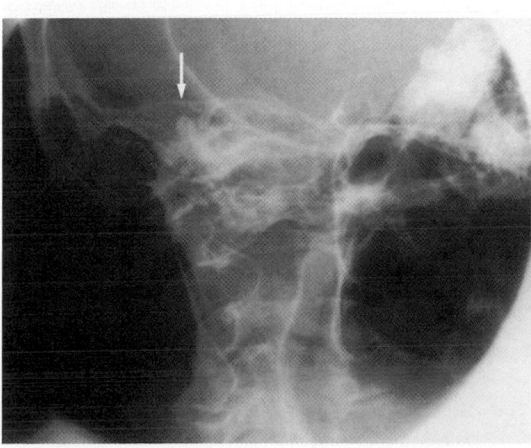

Figure 13 Stenvers projection radiograph demonstrating the anatomic variation of pneumatized air cells beneath the floor of the middle cranial fossa and the superior semicircular canal (*arrow*). (Reproduced with permission; copyright © 1995 P. A. Wackym.)

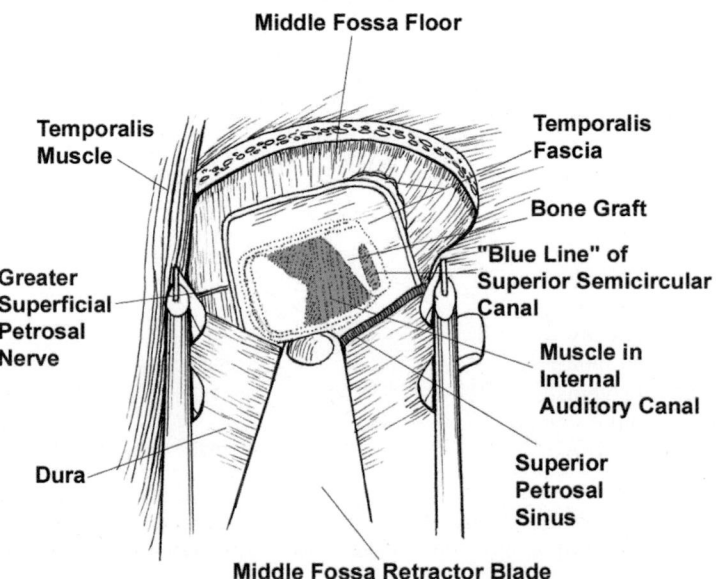

Figure 14 Reconstruction following right middle cranial fossa facial nerve decompression. Temporalis muscle is placed within the internal auditory canal (IAC) surgical defect to fill the dural and bony defect at the conclusion of the facial nerve surgical decompression. Temporalis fascia or Alloderm (LifeCell Corp., Woodlands, TX) is placed over the floor of the middle cranial fossa and muscle graft. A free bone graft or titanium mesh (Synthes Maxillofacial, Paoli, PA) is placed perpendicular to the axis of the IAC to prevent herniation of the temporal lobe onto the facial, cochlear, and vestibular nerves. Temporalis fascia or Alloderm is then used to seal the temporal lobe dura and cover the bone graft or titanium mesh. (Reproduced with permission; copyright © 2007 P. A. Wackym.)

A free bone graft, as already described, prevents temporal lobe herniation. Sensorineural hearing loss can result from direct injury to the inner ear by the drill exposing the cochlea or semicircular canals or from translational injury by the drill striking an ossicle. Should the SSC be entered during the surgical dissection, the fenestration should be immediately occluded with bone wax. Injury to the internal auditory vessels within the IAC can also result in loss of inner ear function. Loss of vestibular function can occur by the same mechanisms.

Postoperative intracranial complications including meningitis, temporal lobe edema, and epidural hematoma formation are possible. Perioperative antibiotics administered over 48 hours are recommended. Fluid restriction and dexamethasone (Decadron) are used for the first 3 days postoperatively to minimize temporal lobe edema following intraoperative retraction. In addition, our longer craniotomy flap decreases the amount of temporal lobe retraction required for complete exposure of the IAC and fallopian canal. With adequate intraoperative hemostasis using the bipolar cautery, oxidized cellulose (Oxycel or Surgicel, Ethicon, Inc., Somerville, NJ), and dural tacking sutures, we have never had a clinically significant postoperative epidural hematoma develop.

Leakage of cerebrospinal fluid (CSF) must be avoided to prevent meningitis. All exposed mastoid air cells must be obstructed with bone wax. A temporalis muscle-free graft is placed into the superior aspect of the IAC to separate the posterior fossa from the extradural floor of the middle cranial fossa. Temporalis fascia or Alloderm is then used to provide a second layer of closure between the posterior fossa and the extradural middle fossa. Meticulous care must be taken to ensure that there are no dural dehiscences overlying the temporal lobe through which CSF may drain. If these are identified, a temporalis fascia, muscle, or Alloderm patch must be used to repair the dural tears to prevent CSF leaks. After a three-layer watertight closure of the temporalis muscle, galea, and scalp, a mastoid-type dressing is applied daily for 5 days postoperatively. Should CSF leakage persist, a temporary lumbar drain is placed, and the patient is kept at bed rest. If the CSF leakage does not resolve within 5 to 7 days after placement of the lumbar drain, reexploration of the surgical field is indicated to identify and seal the area of CSF egress.

Uncontrolled bleeding or injury to the AICA poses the most serious complication during the operation; however, this is extraordinarily rare. The middle cranial fossa approach does not provide adequate access to the entire cerebellopontine angle. The AICA and accompanying veins can loop into the IAC. Control of bleeding of these vessels may require a suboccipital exposure. Injury to the AICA results in brainstem and cerebellar infarction of a variable degree, depending on its size and the area of its terminal arterial supply.

NERVE REPAIR

Whenever the continuity of the facial nerve has been disrupted by trauma, iatrogenic injury, or tumor invasion, every effort should be made to restore its continuity. In some instances, an end-to-end reapproximation can be accomplished, but if any tension occurs at the anastomotic site, an interposition nerve graft has a better chance of providing facial movement. All nerve repair techniques produce synkinesis, but sphincteric function of the mouth and eye is usually restored. Newer microsuture techniques and instrumentation should be employed to enhance return of function.

In general, the injured ends of the nerve should be freshened at a 45° angle. Experimental evidence has shown that cutting the nerve at this angle exposes more neural tubules and improves regrowth of the nerve.[85,88] In addition, a fresh razor blade induces less crush injury to the nerve than a scalpel blade or scissors does. We have found that the perineurium of CN VII does not hold 9-0 sutures, and attempting to suture it increases trauma to the neural tubules. Removing a portion of the epineurium before suturing prevents connective tissue growth at the anastomotic site. If the epineurium is cleaned from the end of the nerve for approximately only 0.5 mm, sutures can still be placed in the epineurium for reapproximating the nerve segments. Three or 4 9-0 nylon sutures are placed with jeweler's forceps or longer instruments (19 cm microforceps) for anastomosis in the cerebellopontine angle. At the brainstem, 2 or 3 sutures are placed (Figure 15).

When an interposition graft is required, the greater auricular and sural nerves are the preferred graft donor sources. The greater auricular nerve is readily available near the operative field if it is not involved in resection of a neoplasm and has approximately the same diameter as that of the facial nerve. It is easily located midway, perpendicular to a line drawn between the mastoid tip and the angle of the mandible. If a graft of greater than 8 to 10 cm is required, the sural nerve should be used. The sural nerve has another advantage in that the peripheral portion of the nerve has many branches that can be used to reconstruct the branching pattern of the facial nerve. There is little discomfort from removing the sural nerve since it provides only a small area of sensation to the lateral lower leg and foot. The sural nerve is found immediately posterior to the lateral malleolus, along the saphenous vein. The nerve graft should be 10 to 20% larger in diameter than the facial nerve and long enough to ensure a tension-free anastomosis.

FACIAL REANIMATION PROCEDURES

Contemporary strategies for management of patients with facial paralysis have been a product of a gradual evolution of past clinical successes and failures over the past century. The surgeon must consider the functional and cosmetic goals of reconstructive surgery, as well as the patient's desires, expectations, and motivations. Functional deficits include incomplete eye closure, speech difficulties, oral incompetence, and nasal airway obstruction. The cosmetic deficiencies of facial asymmetry and dysmorphism can be emotionally devastating for some patients. It is the achievement of facial balance and muscle coordination that continues to be the more challenging and elusive goal.

Management of Upper Third of the Face

Eye Care. Protection of the eye is paramount (Figure 16). It is necessary to protect the cornea from foreign bodies and drying. Dark glasses should be worn during the day, artificial tears instilled at the slightest evidence of drying, and a bland eye ointment used during sleep. Patients who demonstrate a poor Bell phenomenon or have trigeminal nerve deficits are particularly at risk for corneal damage. Taping of the eye closed is not usually recommended, but early-exposure keratitis may require patching or, rarely, a tarsorrhaphy. A formal ophthalmologic examination is recommended prior to any surgical intervention.

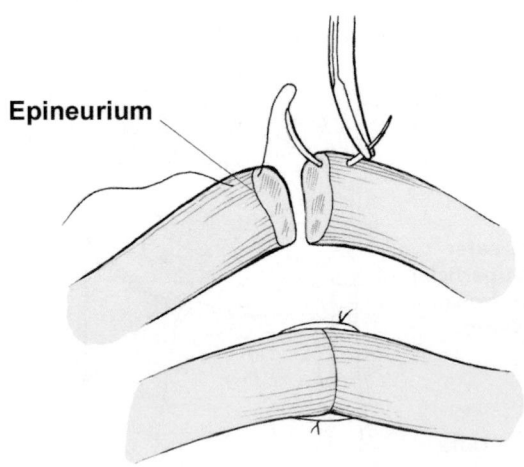

Figure 15 Epineurial end-to-end nerve repair using 9-0 nylon sutures. (Reproduced with permission; copyright © 2007 P. A. Wackym.)

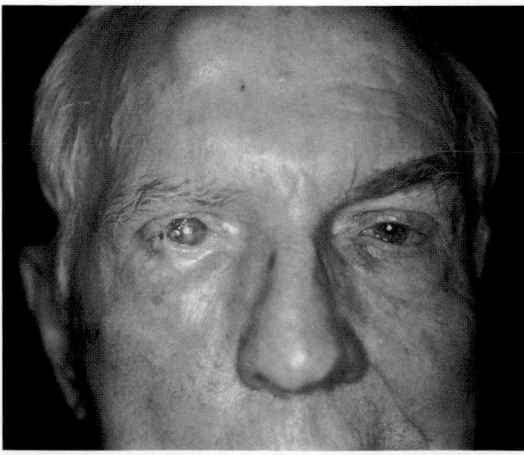

Figure 16 Inadequate eye care following a complete facial paralysis resulting from acoustic neuroma resection at another institution resulted in corneal opacification. (Reproduced with permission; copyright © 2000 P. A. Wackym.)

Eyebrow. Ptosis of the eyebrow can have functional and cosmetic consequences. In the elderly patient, the functional loss of the frontalis and orbicularis oculi muscles is compounded by the loss of tissue elasticity and decrease in the bulk of the subcutaneous tissue. This can lead to significant brow ptosis and hooding of the upper eyelid, which may cause lateral visual field compromise.

The 2 most commonly used procedures to correct brow ptosis are the midforehead lift and the direct brow lift. Both procedures require direct skin and subcutaneous tissue excision, followed by suspension of the orbicularis oculi muscle to the frontal bone periosteum. Slight overcorrection is needed as the brow position will settle during the next few weeks. The endoscopic approach for cosmetic browlifting is not commonly used owing to the severity of the brow ptosis associated with the complete loss of frontalis muscle function. However, there have been some recent reports of successful outcomes using a modified endoscopic browlift technique.[1,89] These techniques are sometimes combined with the use of a biodegradable brow stabilization device (ENDOTINE Forehead; Coapt Systems Inc. Palo Alto, CA).[90]

Upper Eye Lid. Historically, tarsorrhaphy had been the standard of care in patients with facial paralysis. Today, this procedure should be reserved for only those patients with a severe risk for exposure keratitis or those who have failed upper eyelid reanimation procedures. The most commonly used procedure is the insertion of a prosthetic, specifically a gold weight implant or a palpebral wire spring.

In experienced hands, the palpebral wire spring can produce excellent results, affording the capability of mimicking, to some extent, the spontaneous blink. However, the insertion of the palpebral wire spring is technically more difficult, with a higher reported extrusion and infection rate. In addition, these springs often need postoperative adjustment for optimal function.[1]

Gold weight implantation is a relatively simple procedure that is highly successful, well tolerated by patients, and easily reversible if facial muscle function returns (Figure 17). The ideal candidates for gold weight placement are those with the following factors: some existing ability to lower the upper lid, good Bell phenomenon, normal corneal sensation and tearing, prominent supratarsal lid crease, and nonprotruding eyes.

Prefabricated gold weight implants come in weights ranging from 0.8 to 1.6 g. Custom weighting can be requested, if needed. All patients should be correctly sized by taping different size weights to the eyelid in an upright position. The largest weight allowing eyelid closure without causing more than slight lid ptosis should be chosen; the most common weights are 1.0 and 1.2 g. The patient should be informed that the weights are often not helpful when lying supine. In fact, eyelid closure may be worse in some cases owing to the weight of the implant pulling the eyelid open when supine. Eye care, as described above,

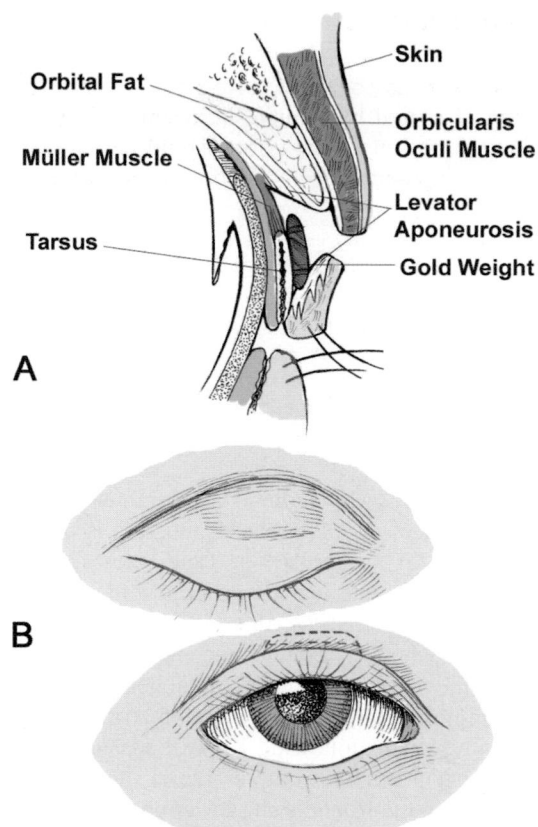

Figure 17 (A) Gold weight implant in position, superficial to the tarsal plate, deep to the levator aponeurosis. (B) Correct gold weight position in relation to the lid margin and pupil. (Reproduced with permission; copyright © 2007 P. A. Wackym.)

should be continued following the reanimation procedure.

After selecting the proper size implant, the procedure is performed under local anesthesia. An incision is made along the supratarsal fold down to the orbicularis oculi muscle. Sharp scissor dissection is carried down through the muscle to the tarsal plate. Dissection is continued inferiorly over the surface of the tarsal plate to within 3 mm of the lash line. An exact pocket is made for the implant to be placed just slightly medial to the center of the pupil. The gold weight is then inserted and suture fixated to the tarsus using 6-0 clear prolene sutures. The incision is closed in layers, 6-0 chromic suture for the levator aponeurosis/orbicularis muscle layer and 6-0 fast gut suture for the skin.

The most common problems associated with gold weight implantation are lid underclosure, excessive lid ptosis, and implant extrusion. The reported extrusion rate in the literature is greatly varied, from as low as 1% to as high as 43%.[1,91,92] The risk of implant extrusion can be minimized by meticulous surgical technique and proper patient selection. Removal of the implant is performed once facial nerve function has returned; however, the gold weight can also be used as a permanent means to achieve eye closure.

Lower Eye Lid. The goals for lower lid management are to improve lower lid margin approximation to the globe, correct ectropion, and

maximize the efficiency of the tear drainage system. Lid-tightening procedures must not disturb the delicate inter-face between the lacrimal punctum and the globe. A lateral traction test, simulating a lid-tightening procedure, will demonstrate the effect of the procedure on lid position and the displacement of the punctum. As a general rule, up to one-eighth of the lid can be resected without disturbing the relationship of the inferior punctum to the globe. If the lateral traction test indicates excessive punctum displacement (greater than 2 mm) or does not provide proper lid support, then alternative or adjunctive surgical procedures are indicated. Excessive punctum lateralization indicates medial canthal tendon laxity, thus indicating the necessity for a medial canthoplasty. If further elevation of the lower lid is needed, then "spacer" grafts (palate mucosa, conchal cartilage) are used to provide vertical height to the eyelid.

Lower lid-tightening procedures include the Bick procedure, tarsal strip, and midlid wedge resection. The Bick procedure is our procedure of choice for lower lid tightening. The procedure involves resecting a lateral wedge of the lower lid, developing a tongue of tarsus, and resuturing the lateral edge of the lid to the lateral orbital rim (Figure 18). The procedure allows for fine adjustment of the tension on the lower lid by resecting a precise amount of tissue. Care must be taken not to overshorten the lower lid, creating a hammock effect, with the lower lid actually bowing down under the globe.

Management of Lower Two-Thirds of the Face

The ultimate goal in treatment of the lower two-thirds of the face is to create symmetric, mimetic movement of the facial musculature. The best chance for this outcome is with primary repair of the facial nerve, with or without nerve interposition grafting. However, primary nerve repair is

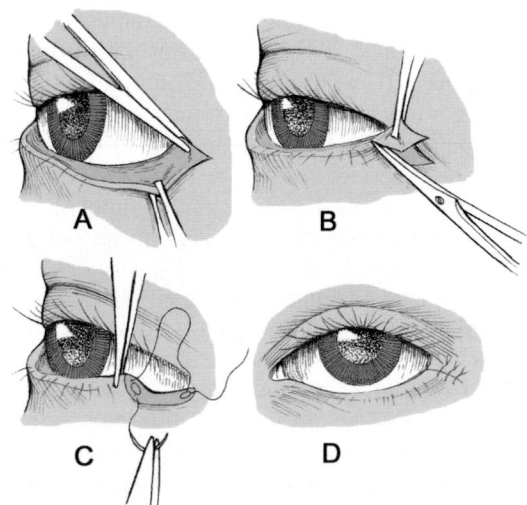

Figure 18 Bick procedure for lower lid ectropion repair. (A) Lower lid is grasped and canthotomy and cantholysis are performed. (B) Appropriate amount of lax lower lid (skin, muscle, conjunctiva, and tarsus) is sectioned. (C) Lateral margin of tarsus is sutured to canthal tendon and orbital periosteum. (D) Canthotomy is closed with absorbable sutures. (Reproduced with permission; copyright © 2007 P. A. Wackym.)

not always possible, and alternative procedures must be entertained. The choice of procedure is dictated by a number of factors including duration of paralysis, prognosis of the underlying illness, concomitant CN deficits, comorbid medical conditions, and the patient's wishes and motivations.

Role of Electromyography in Planning Facial Reanimation Procedures. The degree of motor end-plate degeneration and prognosis for spontaneous recovery of the facial nerve can be assessed with EMG. The presence of normal or polyphasic action potentials at 1 year following facial nerve injury portends a favorable outcome, and no reanimation procedures are indicated. If fibrillation potentials are found, this indicates intact motor end plates but no evidence of reinnervation. This finding supports the use of a nerve substitution procedure to take advantage of the potential neurotized tone and movement of the intrinsic facial musculature. Electrical silence obtained from EMG indicates complete denervation and atrophy of the motor end plates. Neurotized reanimation procedures are contraindicated, and other reanimation procedures should be entertained.

Nerve Substitution Procedures. Nerve substitution procedures are indicated when primary facial nerve repair is not possible. In addition, the following conditions are required for these procedures: intact proximal donor nerve, intact distal facial nerve, and viable motor end-plate function. Although these procedures provide facial tone and resting symmetry, they do not restore involuntary, independent mimetic facial expression. However, the majority of patients do achieve some voluntary facial movement with rehabilitation. The most commonly described nerve substitution procedures are the XI–VII crossover, VII–VII crossfacial, XII–VII crossover, and XII–VII jump graft.

The XI–VII procedure (accessory to distal facial nerve) has largely been abandoned owing to the morbidity of loss of trapezius muscle function. The VII–VII crossfacial grafting involves linking a functional branch of the facial nerve on the nonparalyzed side to a division of the facial nerve on the paralyzed side by using a long interposition nerve graft (sural, medial antebrachial cutaneous) (Figure 19). The disadvantages of this procedure include the sacrifice of a portion of the normal facial function on the contralateral side, a long interval for innervation (9 to 12 months), and a lack of substantial neural "firepower" owing to the relatively few number of axons grafted. Theoretically, the advantage of this technique is the possibility of symmetric, mimetic movement. Disappointing results from several investigators[1,93] have made this procedure less appealing.

Hypoglossal–facial (XII–VII) crossover is most appropriately performed for complete and permanent facial paralysis up to 2 years after injury (Figure 20). This situation may arise following radical parotidectomy, temporal bone resection, skull base surgery, severe temporal bone trauma, or cerebellopontine angle tumor

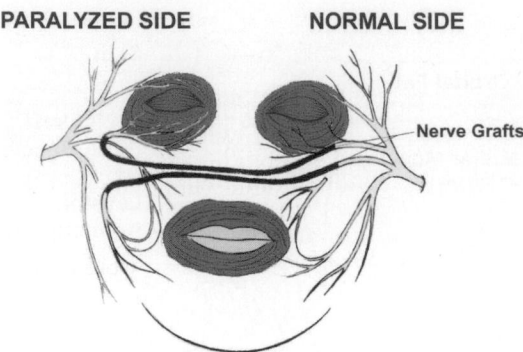

Figure 19 Facial-crossfacial nerve substitution technique. (Reproduced with permission; copyright © 2007 P. A. Wackym.)

resection. An EMG finding consistent with viable motor end plates of the facial muscles is a prerequisite for surgery. Poor candidates for the XII–VII crossover include patients with multiple lower CN deficits. Sacrifice of the hypoglossal nerve may not be well tolerated and compensated for in the presence of other cranial neuropathies.

Improved facial tone and symmetry occur in 90% of patients following XII–VII anastomosis.[1] The results are more impressive in the midface and less in the frontalis and lower portions of the face. The return of muscle tone is seen within 4 to 6 months following neurorrhaphy, with better results seen in earlier repairs.[94] Voluntary facial movements follow with progressive improvements over the next 1 to 2 years. True spontaneous facial expressions are rare, although through motor sensory reeducation, patients may develop spontaneous animation with speech.

Pensak and colleagues, in their series of 61 cases of XII–VII crossover, rated their results as excellent in 3%, good in 39%, fair in 49%, and poor in 10% of patients.[95] Conley and Baker, in their series of 122 cases, reported good or excellent results in 65%, fair in 18%, and poor in 17%.[94] They also noted better results in those patients who underwent "immediate" repair (<2 years) than in those who were "delayed" (>2 years).

Synkinesis, hypertonia, and hemilingual atrophy are all noted deficiencies of the classic XII–VII crossover. Most studies report minimal

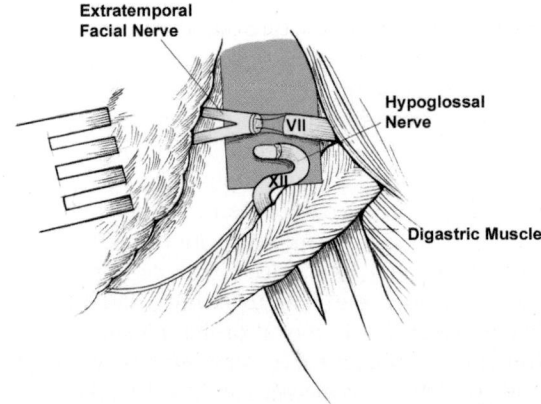

Figure 20 Hypoglossal–facial nerve crossover technique. Hypoglossal nerve is brought medial to digastric muscle to gain additional length and decrease tension at the suture line. (Reproduced with permission; copyright © 2007 P. A. Wackym.)

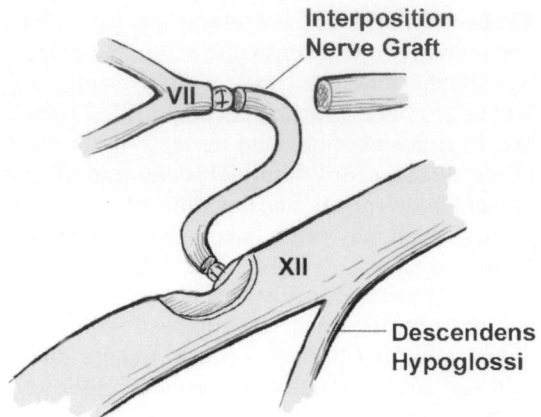

Figure 21 Hypoglossal–facial interpositional nerve graft technique. Approximately one-third of the hypoglossal nerve (XII) is sectioned, distal to the hypoglossal descendens. The nerve graft is sewn end to side with the hypoglossal nerve and end to end with the facial nerve (VII). (Reproduced with permission; copyright © 2007 P. A. Wackym.)

disabling sequelae owing to loss of unilateral hypoglossal function unless concomitant ipsilateral CN deficits exist.

The XII–VII jump graft technique was devised by May and colleagues to offset some of the above noted disadvantages of the classic XII–VII crossover.[96] The procedure entails placing an interpositional nerve graft between a partially transected hypoglossal nerve trunk, distal to the hypoglossal descendens, and the distal facial nerve trunk (Figure 21). Several authors have reported functional results comparable to the XII–VII crossover; however, the problems of hypertonia and mass facial movements have not been encountered.[96,97] Kartush and Lundy further modified this approach with anastomosis to only the lower division of the facial nerve, thereby reducing potential synkinesis.[98] Figure 22 represents an example of an excellent outcome of a patient who underwent a XII–VII jump graft technique 3 months after a large facial neuroma resection with facial nerve sacrifice at the skull base. The patient was able to obtain symmetric resting tone of the facial muscles with some voluntary motion of the lower two-thirds of the face with subtle tongue movement.

Muscle Transposition Procedures (Dynamic). Regional muscle transposition can provide dynamic reanimation of the mouth in patients with long-standing facial paralysis (over 2 years). It is indicated for patients with congenital facial paralysis (Möbius syndrome) or when facial nerve grafting or nerve substitution techniques are contraindicated. It can also be performed in conjunction with facial nerve grafting or nerve substitution procedure in select cases to augment results. The temporalis muscle is most commonly used because of its length, contractility, and favorable vector of pull. Masseter muscle transposition can be useful following radical parotid surgery or when the temporalis muscle is not available.

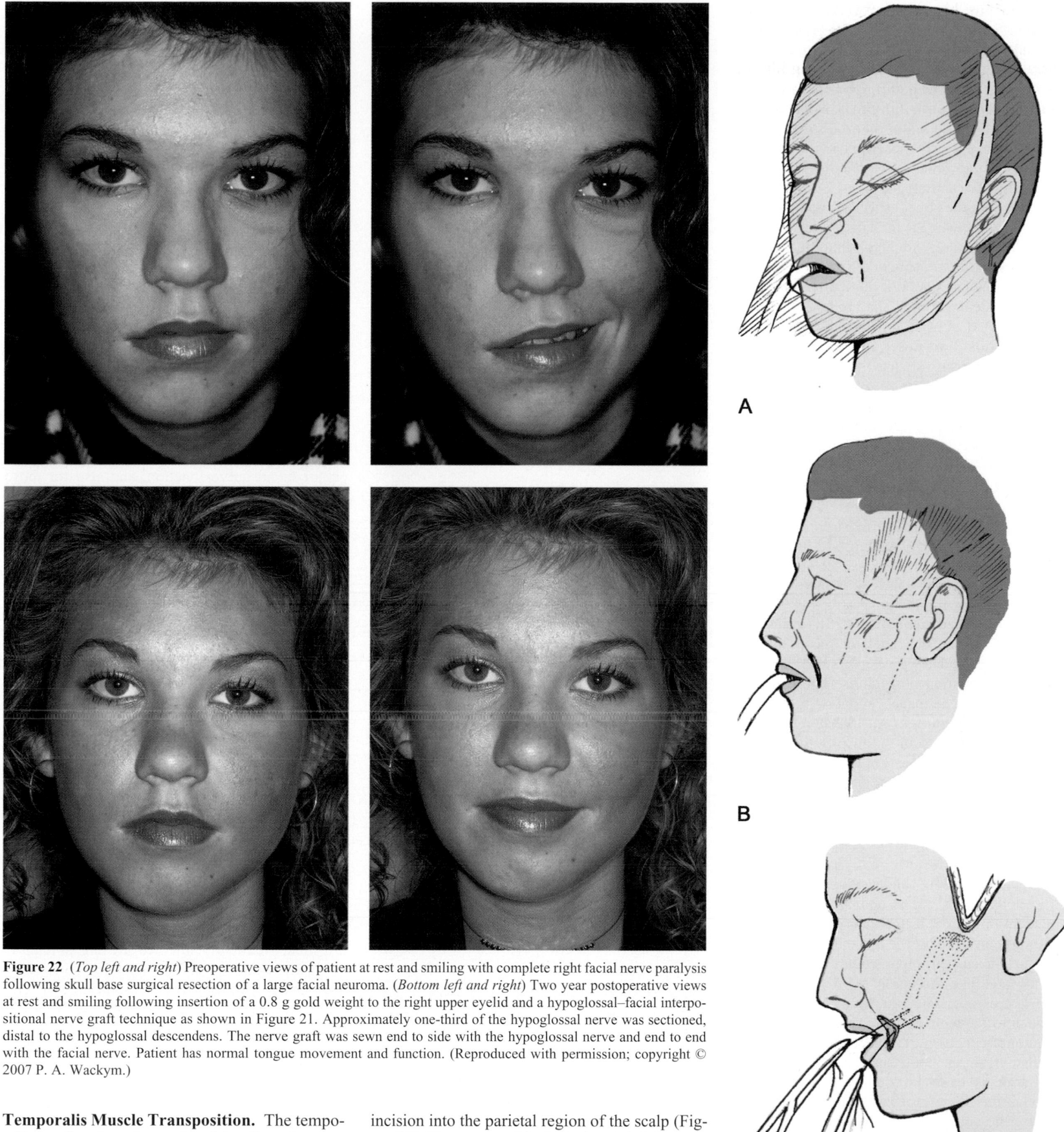

Figure 22 (*Top left and right*) Preoperative views of patient at rest and smiling with complete right facial nerve paralysis following skull base surgical resection of a large facial neuroma. (*Bottom left and right*) Two year postoperative views at rest and smiling following insertion of a 0.8 g gold weight to the right upper eyelid and a hypoglossal–facial interpositional nerve graft technique as shown in Figure 21. Approximately one-third of the hypoglossal nerve was sectioned, distal to the hypoglossal descendens. The nerve graft was sewn end to side with the hypoglossal nerve and end to end with the facial nerve. Patient has normal tongue movement and function. (Reproduced with permission; copyright © 2007 P. A. Wackym.)

Figure 23 Temporalis muscle transfer for lower face reanimation. (A) Dotted lines indicate the lip–cheek and temporal incisions. (B) Midportion of the temporalis muscle is harvested. (C) Temporalis muscle pulled through subcutaneous cheek tunnel into the lip–cheek incision. (Reproduced with permission; copyright © 2007 P. A. Wackym.)

Temporalis Muscle Transposition. The temporalis is a fan-shaped muscle arising from the temporal fossa. The motor branch of the trigeminal nerve innervates it, and branches off the internal maxillary artery provide its blood supply. Preoperative evaluation includes the assessment of the function and strength of the temporalis muscle.

To perform a temporalis muscle transposition procedure, the temporalis muscle and fascia are both exposed by extending a modified facelift incision into the parietal region of the scalp (Figure 23). The pretragal incision is carried down to the subdermal region, above the superficial musculoaponeurotic system of the face. A tunnel is created from the zygomatic arch in a subdermal plane between the temporal fossa and the cheek-lip crease incision (adult) or the oral commissure incision (children). The lateral portions of the zygomatic arch can be burred down to reduce the bulging appearance of the muscle at this fulcrum point. Only the midportion of the temporalis muscle is used. A portion of the pericranium is dissected with the muscle and its fascia to create additional length. The muscle is then transposed over the zygomatic arch, through the subcutaneous tunnel, and into the lip–cheek incision. The muscle–fascia–pericranium complex is sutured to the orbicularis oris muscle near the submucous layer of the corner of the mouth. Additional sutures are placed from the muscle to the subdermal layer of the upper aspect of the lip–cheek incision to accentuate the lip–cheek crease. Overcorrection is necessary for an optimal final result. The depression in the temporal area is corrected by rotating the remainder of the temporalis muscle into the deficient area. The redundant facial skin is resected as in a facelift, and wounds are closed in layers. Two closed suction drains and a compressive dressing are used for 48 hours postoperatively.

Ideally, the overcorrection of the lateral oral commissure and lip–cheek crease will resolve by 3 to 6 weeks. The results of the transposition should be evident by 4 to 6 weeks, with the patient able to produce a broad smile by tensing the temporalis muscle. Complications include infection, hematoma, and seroma. The most common reasons for failure of the procedure are inadequate overcorrection and suture dehiscence at the orbicularis oris–temporalis muscle interface.[99]

Suspension Procedures (Static). Static suspension procedures are indicated for those patients who are not candidates for nerve substitution or dynamic reanimation procedures. These procedures can provide permanent support, or, in cases in which reinnervation of the facial muscles is expected, static procedures can provide temporary or additional support until reinnervation of the facial muscles is complete. A variety of materials are available for static suspension procedures, ranging from autografts (palmaris longus tendon, fascia lata tendon) to alloplasts, such as Gore-Tex (GORE S.A.M., WL Gore & Associates Inc., Flagstaff, AZ) and acellular human dermis (Alloderm).[100,101] The choice of material is dependent on patient factors and desires, as well as the surgeon's preference and experience.

The static suspension procedure is most often used to lateralize the corner of the mouth and lip–cheek crease. The procedure is similar in approach to the temporalis muscle transposition. The autograft or allograft is placed in a subcutaneous tunnel from the lip–cheek crease to the zygomatic arch. In cases in which reinnervation of the facial muscles is expected, it is important not to injure the deeper facial nerve branches when creating the tunnel. Sutures are used to secure the graft to the orbicularis oris muscle and lip–cheek incision, whereas wires or screws are used for anchoring at the zygomatic arch (Figure 24).

A separate local suspension can also be performed to lateralize the nose in cases of alar valve compromise. The nasal base is exposed with incisions along the alar–facial and nasolabial creases. An allograft or autograft is then sutured to the

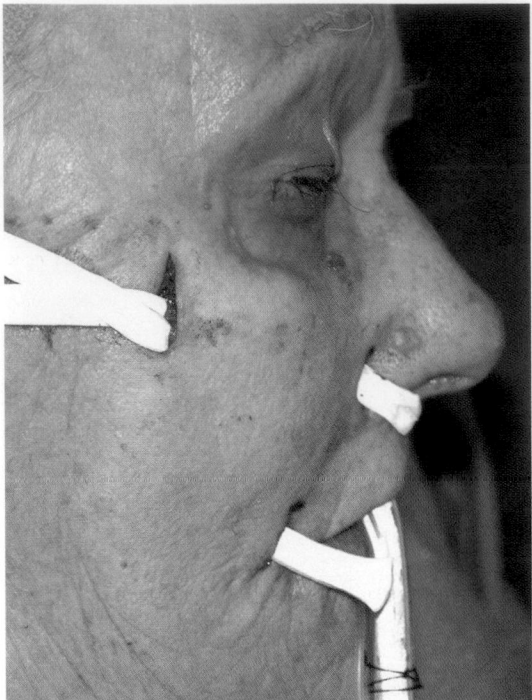

(A)

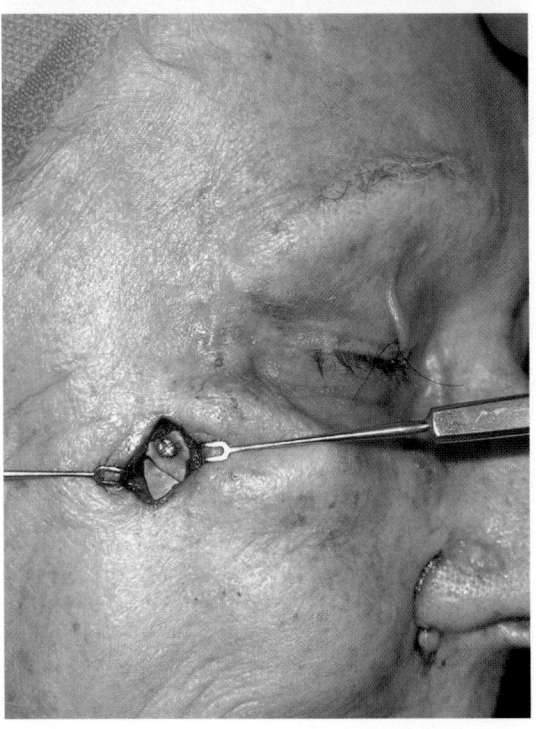

(B)

Figure 24 Static suspension procedure using allograft (Gore 2 mm nonreinforced sheet, W. L. Gore & Associates, Inc., Flagstaff, Arizona). (A) Strips of allograft placed in the subcutaneous cheek tunnel. (B) Allograft anchored to the malar eminence with a single titanium screw. (Reproduced with permission; copyright © 2007 P. A. Wackym.)

deep aspect of the nasal base. The nasal base is then pulled laterally to its desired position. After the periosteum of zygomaticomaxillary buttress is exposed, the other end of the graft is fixated to the bone with a screw.

Innervated Free Muscle Transfer

The ideal indication for innervated free muscle transfer is in the patient with Möbius syndrome,

for whom both facial nerve and musculature are not available. It is also indicated as an alternative to regional muscle transfers or static procedures in patients with long-standing facial paralysis (>2 years). It is usually performed as a two-stage procedure in which an initial cross-facial nerve graft is combined with a subsequent free muscle transfer (most commonly, gracilis or serratus anterior).[102] Alternatively, the innervated free flap may be grafted to the hypoglossal nerve, performed as a single-stage procedure.[103]

In select patients, this procedure provides the possibility for dynamic, mimetic movement that cannot be achieved by static procedures. The disadvantages, however, are manifold, including donor site morbidity, risk of vascular thrombosis, lengthy operative time, long interval for reinnervation, and muscle bulkiness.

NEUROMUSCULAR FACIAL RETRAINING TECHNIQUES

For patients who have experienced some recovery of facial nerve function, and also for those patients who experience synkinesis, neuromuscular facial retraining therapy is an important treatment modality. These techniques can be applied before and after reanimation procedures to optimize outcome. In general, these techniques can be used to address loss of strength, loss of isolated motor control, muscle tension hypertonicity, and/or synkinesis. This method combines techniques such as patient education in basic facial anatomy, physiology, and kinesiology; relaxation training; sensory stimulation; EMG biofeedback; voluntary facial exercises with mirror feedback; and spontaneously elicited facial movements.[104–106]

CHEMODENERVATION

The use of botulinum toxin for chemodenervation of synkinetic muscles has greatly aided in the treatment of patients who suffer from hypertonicity, spasms, and symptomatic fasiculations due to facial nerve regeneration.[107] The muscles that are most frequently injected are the obicularis oculi, zygomaticus major, mentalis, corrugator, and platysma. In some instances, the contralateral unaffected facial muscles are selectively weakened in order to achieve better facial symmetry. Dosages average 2.5 to 5 units per injection with Botulinum toxin Type A (Botox, Allergan, Irvine, CA).

SUMMARY

The etiology and pathogenesis of several disorders that produce facial paralysis have been reviewed.

Likewise, the diagnostic methods and algorithms that are used to make decisions regarding medical versus surgical management in acute facial paralysis have been summarized. Anatomy and surgical principles were highlighted and treatment alternatives for reanimation or neuromuscular facial retraining outlined.

REFERENCES

1. May M, Schaitkin BM, editors. The Facial Nerve, 2nd edition. New York: Thieme Medical Publishers; 2000.
2. Harris L. Public Attitudes Toward People with Disabilities. Report of a U.S. Survey to the National Organization on Disability. Washington (DC); 1991.
3. McKusick VA. Mendelian Inheritance in Man. A Catalog of Human Genes and Genetic Disorders, 12th edition. Baltimore MD: The Johns Hopkins University Press; 1998.
4. Huebner O. Ober angeborenen Kernmangel (infantiler Kernschwund, Möbius). Charite Ann 1900;25:211–43.
5. Hanissian AS, Fuste F, Hayes WT, Duncan JM. Moebius syndrome in twins. Am J Dis Child 1970;120:472–5.
6. Pitner SE, Edwards JE, McCormick WF. Observations on the pathology of the Möbius syndrome. J Neurol Neurosurg Psychiatry 1965;28:362–74.
7. Cattaneo L, Chierici E, Bianchi B, et al. The localization of facial motor impairment in sporadic Mobius syndrome. Neurology 2006;66:1907–12.
8. Ebbesen F, Petersen W. Goldenhar's syndrome: Discordance in monozygotic twins and unusual anomalies. Acta Paediatr Scand 1982;71:685–7.
9. Sieff CA, Chessells, Levinsky RJ, et al. Allogenic bone-marrow transplantation in infantile malignant osteopetrosis. Lancet 1983;1:437–41.
10. Toh EHY, Wackym PA. Injury to the temporal bone and facial nerve in children. Facial Plast Surg Clin North Am 1999;7:223–9.
11. Feuerman T, Wackym PA, Gade GF, Becker DP. Value of skull radiography, head computed tomographic scanning, and admission for observation in cases of minor head injury. Neurosurgery 1988;22:449–53.
12. Ishman SL, Friedland DR. Temporal bone fractures: Traditional classification and clinical relevance. Laryngoscope 2004;114:1734–41.
13. Glasscock ME, Schwaber MK, Nissen AJ, Jackson CG. Management of congenital ear malformations. Ann Otol Rhinol Laryngol 1983;92:504–9.
14. Lambert PR. Major congenital ear malformations: Surgical management and results. Ann Otol Rhinol Laryngol 1988;97:641–9.
15. Takahashi H, Nakamura H, Yui M, Mori H. Analysis of fifty cases of facial palsy due to otitis media. Arch Otorhinolaryngol 1985;241:163–8.
16. Sheehy JL. Cholesteatoma surgery in children. Acta Otorhinolaryngol Belg 1980;34:98–106.
17. Glasscock ME, Pensak ML, Gulya AJ, Baker DC. Lyme disease. A cause of bilateral facial paralysis. Arch Otolaryngol Head Neck Surg 1985;111:47–9.
18. Hunt JR. On herpetic inflammations of the geniculate ganglion. A new syndrome and its complications. J Nerv Ment Dis 1907;34:73–96.
19. Head H, Campbell AW. Pathology of herpes zoster and its bearing on sensory localization. Brain 1900;23:353–523.
20. Devriese PP. Facial paralysis in cephalic herpes zoster. Ann Otol Rhinol Laryngol 1968;77:1101–19.
21. Crabtree JA. Herpes zoster oticus. Laryngoscope 1968; 78:1853–78.
22. Byl FM, Adour KK. Auditory symptoms associated with herpes zoster or idiopathic facial paralysis. Laryngoscope 1977;87:372–9.
23. Robillard RB, Hilsinger RL, Adour KK. Ramsay Hunt facial paralysis: Clinical analysis of 185 patients. Otolaryngol Head Neck Surg 1986;95:292–7.
24. May M, Fria TJ, Blumenthal F, Curtin H. Facial paralysis in children: Differential diagnosis. Otolaryngol Head Neck Surg 1981;89:841–8.
25. Uri N, Greenberg E, Meyer W, Kitzes-Cohen R. Herpes zoster oticus: Treatment with acyclovir. Ann Otol Rhinol Laryngol 1992;101:161–2.
26. Hunt JR. The sensory field of the facial nerve. A further contribution to the symptomatology of the geniculate ganglion. Brain 1915;38:415–45.
27. Hunt JR. Geniculate neuralgia (neuralgia of the nervus facialis). A further contribution to the sensory system of the seventh nerve and its neuralgic conditions. Arch Neurol Psychiatry 1937;37:253–85.
28. Korzec K, Sobol SM, Kubal W, et al. Gadolinium-enhanced magnetic resonance imaging of the facial nerve in herpes zoster oticus and Bell palsy: Clinical implications. Am J Otol 1991;12:163–8.
29. Blackley B, Friedmann I, Wright I. Herpes zoster auris associated with facial nerve palsy and auditory nerve symptoms: A case report with histopathological findings. Acta Otolaryngol (Stockh) 1967;63:533–50.
30. Etholm B, Schuknecht HF. Pathological findings and surgical implications in herpes zoster oticus. Adv Otorhinolaryngol 1983;31:184–90.
31. Guldberg-Moller J, Olsen S, Kettel K. Histopathology of the facial nerve in herpes zoster oticus. Arch Otolaryngol 1959;69:266–75.
32. Wackym PA. Molecular temporal bone pathology: II. Ramsay Hunt syndrome (herpes zoster oticus). Laryngoscope 1997;107:1165–75.
33. Aleksic SN, Budzilovich GN, Lieberman AN. Herpes zoster oticus and facial paralysis (Ramsay Hunt syndrome): Clinico-pathologic study and review of literature. J Neurol Sci 1973;20:149–59.
34. Payten RJ, Dawes DDK. Herpes zoster of the head and neck. J Laryngol Otol 1972;86:1031–55.
35. Wackym PA, Popper P, Kerner MM, et al. Varicella zoster DNA in temporal bones of patients with Ramsay Hunt syndrome. Lancet 1993;342:1555.
36. Meier JL, Straus SE. Comparative biology of latent varicella-zoster virus and herpes simplex virus infections. J Infect Dis 1992;166:S13–23.
37. Furuta Y, Takasu T, Fukuda S, et al. Detection of varicella-zoster virus DNA in human geniculate ganglia by polymerase chain reaction. J Infect Dis 1992;166:1157–9.
38. Ohtani F, Furuta Y, Aizawa H, Fukuda S. Varicella-zoster virus load and cochleovestibular symptoms in Ramsay Hunt syndrome. Ann Otol Rhinol Laryngol 2006; 115:233–8.
39. Aviel A, Marshak G. Ramsay Hunt syndrome: A cranial polyneuropathy. Am J Otolaryngol 1982;3:61–6.
40. Schuknecht HF. Pathology of the Ear, 2nd edition. Philadelphia: Lea & Febiger; 1993.
41. Gilbert GJ. Herpes zoster ophthalmicus and delayed contralateral hemiparesis: Relationship of the syndrome to central nervous system granulomatous angiitis. JAMA 1974;229:302–4.
42. Pratesi R, Freemon FR, Lowry JL. Herpes zoster ophthalmicus with contralateral hemiplegia. Arch Neurol 1977;34:640–1.
43. Coker NJ. Facial electroneurography: Analysis of techniques and correlation with degenerating motoneurons. Laryngoscope 1992;102:747–59.
44. Inamura H, Aoyagi M, Tojima H, et al. Effects of aciclovir in Ramsay Hunt syndrome. Acta Otolaryngol Suppl (Stockh) 1988;446:111–3.
45. Dickins JRE, Smith JT, Graham SS. Herpes zoster oticus: Treatment with intravenous acyclovir. Laryngoscope 1988;98:776–9.
46. Stafford FW, Welch AR. The use of acyclovir in Ramsay Hunt syndrome. J Laryngol Otol 1986;100:337–40.
47. Beutner KR, Friedman DJ, Forszpaniak C, et al. Valaciclovir compared with acyclovir for improved therapy for herpes zoster in immunocompetent adults. Antimicrob Agents Chemother 1995;39:1546–53.
48. Harner SG, Heiny BA, Newell RC. Herpes zoster oticus. Arch Otolaryngol 1970;92:632–6.
49. Burgess RC, Michaels L, Bale JF, et al. Polymerase chain reaction amplification of herpes simplex viral DNA from the geniculate ganglion of a patient with Bell palsy. Ann Otol Rhinol Laryngol 1994;103:775–9.
50. Murakami S, Mizobuchi M, Nakashiro Y, et al. Bell palsy and herpes simplex virus: Identification of viral DNA in endoneural fluid and muscle. Ann Intern Med 1996; 124:27–30.
51. Furuta Y, Takasu T, Sato KC, et al. Latent herpes simplex virus type 1 in human geniculate ganglia. Acta Neuropathol (Berl) 1992;84:39–44.
52. Bauer CA, Coker NJ. Update on facial nerve disorders. Otolaryngol Clin North Am 1996;29:445–54.
53. Adour KK, Byl FM, Hilsinger RL, Jr, et al. The true nature of Bell palsy: Analysis of 1000 consecutive cases. Laryngoscope 1978;88:787–811.
54. Pitts DB, Adour KK, Hilsinger RL,. Recurrent Bell palsy: Analysis of 140 patients. Laryngoscope 1988;98:535–40.
55. Fisch U. Surgery for Bell palsy. Arch Otolaryngol 1981;107:1–11.
56. Adour KK, Ruboyianes JM, Von Doersten PG, et al. Bell palsy treatment with acyclovir and prednisone compared with prednisone alone: A double-blinded, randomized controlled trial. Ann Otol Rhinol Laryngol 1996;105:371–8.
57. Alberton DL, Zed PJ. Bell palsy: A review of treatment using antiviral agents. Ann Pharmacother 2006;40:1838–42.
58. Dennis JM, Coker NJ. Electroneuronography. Adv Otorhinolaryngol 1997;53:112–31.
59. Gantz BJ, Rubinstein JT, Gidley P, Woodworth GG. Surgical management of Bell palsy. Laryngoscope 1999;109:1177–88.
60. Gantz BJ, Wackym PA. Facial nerve abnormalities. In: Bumstead RM, Smith JD, editors. Pediatric Facial Plastic and Reconstructive Surgery. New York: Raven Press; 1993. p. 337–47.
61. Wackym PA, Andrews JC. Middle cranial fossa approach. In: Samii M, Cheatham M, Becker D, editors. Atlas of Cranial Base Surgery. Philadelphia: WB Saunders; 1995. p. 26–31.
62. Fisch U. Prognostic value of electrical tests in acute facial paralysis. Am J Otol 1984;5:494–8.
63. Gantz BJ, Gmur A, Fisch U. Intraoperative evoked electromyography in Bell palsy. Am J Otolaryngol 1982; 3:273–8.
64. Bergman I, May M, Wessle HB, Stool SE. Management of facial palsy caused by birth trauma. Laryngoscope 1986;96:381–4.
65. Lipkin AF, Coker NJ, Jenkins HA, Alford BR. Intracranial and intratemporal facial neuroma. Otolaryngol Head Neck Surg 1987;96:71–9.
66. Wackym PA, King WA, Meyer GA, et al. Endoscope assisted surgery of the trigeminal, facial, cochlear or vestibular nerve. In: Wackym PA, Rice DH, Schaefer SD, editors. Minimally Invasive Surgery of the Head, Neck, and Cranial Base. Philadelphia: Lippincott Williams & Wilkins; 2002. p. 101–16.
67. Schwaber MK. Vascular compression syndromes. In: Jackler RK, Brackmann DE, editors. Neurotology. St. Louis: Mosby-Year Book; 1994. p. 881–903.
68. Rohrer D, Burchiel K. Trigeminal neuralgia and other trigeminal dysfunction syndromes. In: Barrow D, editor. Surgery of the Cranial Nerves of the Posterior Fossa. Park Ridge (IL): American Association of Neurological Surgeons; 1993. p. 201–17.
69. Apfelbaum R. Surgery for tic doloreux. Clin Neurosurg 1984;31:346–50.
70. Burchiel K, Clarke H, Haglund M. Long-term efficacy of microvascular decompression in trigeminal neuralgia. J Neurosurg 1988;69:35–8.
71. Sweet W. Trigeminal neuralgia: Problems as to cause and consequent conclusions regarding treatment. In: Wilkins RH, Rengachary S, editors. Neurosurgery Update II. New York: McGraw-Hill; 1991. p. 366–72.
72. Barker FG, Jannetta PJ, Bissonette DJ, et al. The long-term outcome of microvascular decompression for trigeminal neuralgia. N Engl J Med 1996;334:1077–83.
73. Mendoza N, Illingworth RD. Trigeminal neuralgia treated by microvascular decompression: A long-term follow-up study. Br J Neurosurg 1995;9:13–9.
74. Kureshi SA, Wilkins RH. Posterior fossa reexploration for persistent or recurrent trigeminal neuralgia or hemifacial spasm: Surgical findings and therapeutic implications. Neurosurgery 1998;43:1111–7.
75. Wilkins RH. Cranial nerve dysfunction syndromes: Evidence for microvascular compression. In: Barrow D, editor. Surgery of the Cranial Nerves of the Posterior Fossa. Park Ridge (IL): American Association of Neurological Surgeons; 1993. p. 155–63.
76. Liao JJ, Cheng WC, Chang CN, et al. Reoperation for recurrent trigeminal neuralgia after microvascular decompression. Surg Neurol 1997;47:562–70.
77. Magnan J, Caces F, Locatelli P, Chays A. Hemifacial spasm: Endoscopic vascular decompression. Otolaryngol Head Neck Surg 1997;117:308–14.
78. Graham MD, Kemink JL. Total facial nerve decompression in recurrent facial paralysis and the Melkersson–Rosenthal syndrome: A preliminary report. Am J Otol 1986; 7:34–7.
79. Eicher SA, Coker NJ, Alford BR, et al. A comparative study of the fallopian canal at the meatal foramen and labyrinthine segment in young children and adults. Arch Otolaryngol Head Neck Surg 1990;116:1030–5.
80. Ge XX, Spector GJ. Labyrinthine segment and geniculate ganglion of the facial nerve in fetal and adult temporal bones. Ann Otol Rhino Laryngol 1981;90:1–12.
81. Jackson CG, Johnson GD, Hyams VJ, Poe DS. Pathologic findings in the labyrinthine segment of the facial nerve in a case of facial paralysis. Ann Otol Rhinol Laryngol 1990;99:327–9.
82. Sunderland S. Nerves and Nerve Injuries, 2nd edition. New York: Churchill Livingstone;1978. p. 258–9.
83. Seddon HJ. Three types of nerve injury. Brain 1943; 66:237–88.
84. House JW, Brackmann DE. Facial nerve grading system. Otolaryngol Head Neck Surg 1985;93:146–7.
85. Gidley PW, Gantz BJ, Rubinstein JT. Facial nerve grafts: From cerebellopontine angle and beyond. Am J Otol 1999;20:781–8.
86. Gantz BJ. Intraoperative facial nerve monitoring. Am J Otol 1985;6:58–61.
87. House W. Surgical exposure of the internal auditory canal and its contents through the middle cranial fossa. Laryngoscope 1961;71:1363–85.

88. Yamamoto E, Fisch U. Experiments on facial nerve suturing. ORL J Otorhinolaryngol Relat Spec 1974;36:193–204.

89. Rhee J, Gallo JF, Costantino PD. Endoscopic facial rejuvenation. In: Wackym PA, Rice DH, Schaefer SD, editors. Minimally Invasive Surgery of the Head, Neck, and Cranial Base. Philadelphia: Lippincott Williams & Wilkins;2002. p. 355–66.

90. Hadlock TA, Greenfield LJ, Wernick-Robinson M, Cheney ML. Multimodality approach to management of the paralyzed face. Laryngoscope 2006;116:1385–89.

91. May M. Gold weight and wire spring implants as alternatives to tarsorraphy. Arch Otolaryngol Head Neck 1987;113:656–60.

92. Kelly SA, Sharpe DT. Gold eyelid weights in patients with facial palsy: A patient review. Plast Reconstr Surg 1992;89:436–40.

93. Samii M. Rehabilitation of the face by facial nerve substitution. In: Fisch U, editor. Facial Nerve Surgery. Birmingham, AL: Aesculapius Publishing;1977. p. 224–45.

94. Conley J, Baker D. Hypoglossal-facial nerve anastomosis for reinnervation of the paralyzed face. Plast Reconstr Surg 1979;63:63–72.

95. Pensak ML, Jackson GG, Glasscock ME, Gulya AJ. Facial reanimation with the XII-VII anastomosis: Analysis of the functional and psychological results. Otolaryngol Head Neck Surg 1986;94:305–10.

96. May M, Sobel SM, Mester SJ. Hypoglossal-facial nerve interpositional jump graft for facial reanimation without tongue atrophy. Otolaryngol Head Neck Surg 1991; 204:818–26.

97. Hammerschlag PE. Facial reanimation with jump interpositional graft hypoglossal facial anastomosis and hypoglossal facial anastomosis: Evolution in management of facial paralysis. Laryngoscope 1999;109:1–23.

98. Kartush JM, Lundy LB. Facial nerve outcome in acoustic neuroma surgery. Otolaryngol Clin North Am 1992; 25:623–47.

99. May M, Drucker C. Temporalis muscle for facial reanimation: A 13-year experience with 224 procedures. Arch Otolaryngol Head Neck Surg 1993;119:378–82.

100. Fisher E, Froedel JL. Facial suspension with acellular human dermal allograft. Arch Facial Plast Surg 1999;1:195–9.

101. Konior RJ. Facial paralysis reconstruction with Gore-Tex Soft Tissue Patch. Arch Otolaryngol Head Neck Surg 1992;118:1188–94.

102. Ueda K, Harii K, Yaruada A. Long-term follow-up of nerve conduction velocity in cross-face nerve grafting for the treatment of facial paralysis. Plast Reconstr Surg 1994;93:1146–9.

103. Ueda K, Harii K, Yaruada A. Free neurovascular muscle transposition for the treatment of facial paralysis using the hypoglossal nerve as a recipient motor source. Plast Reconstr Surg 1994;94:808–17.

104. Beurskens CH, Heymans PG. Physiotherapy in patients with facial nerve paresis: Description of outcomes. Am J Otolaryngol 2004;25:394–400.

105. Segal B, Zompa I, Danys I, et al. Symmetry and synkinesis during rehabilitation of unilateral facial paralysis. J Otolaryngol 1995;24:143–8.

106. Brach JS, VanSwearingen JM, Lenert J, et al. Facial neuromuscular retraining for oral synkinesis. Plast Reconstr Surg 1997;99:1922–33.

107. Bikhazi NB, Maas CS. Refinement in the rehabilitation of the paralyzed face using botulinum toxin. Otolaryngol Head Neck Surg 1997;117:303–7.

35

Vestibular Schwannomas and Other Skull Base Neoplasms

Sumit K. Agrawal, MD

Nikolas H. Blevins, MD

Robert K. Jackler, MD

HISTORY OF NEUROTOLOGIC SKULL BASE SURGERY

Skull base anatomy is complex and may be affected by a wide variety of pathology. Historically, surgical access posed a challenge; and, therefore, the earliest surgical efforts did not take place until the later part of the nineteenth century, after the introduction of anesthesia. It became obvious that the most direct approach to certain inaccessible intracranial tumors was through the skull base rather than through the calvarium. The transtemporal approach to the cerebellopontine angle (CPA) was initially proposed by Panse in 1904[1]; and attempted by Borchardt in 1905[2] and Quix in 1911.[3] At the time, the absence of effective imaging modalities allowed considerable growth of the lesions prior to diagnosis, rendering initial surgical approaches too deep and narrow to resect large tumors effectively. In addition, effective closure against cerebrospinal fluid (CSF) leakage and atraumatic removal of bone surrounding neural and vascular structures had yet to be achieved. Therefore, in the first half of the twentieth century, surgeons avoided the complexity of the skull base and preferred the simpler solution of working through the thin calvaria, despite the fact that injurious degrees of brain retraction were often required.

In the 1960s, William House and others utilized modern operating microscopes and high-speed drills to resurrect a number of skull-base approaches that had previously been abandoned as impractical.[4] Contemporary skull-base surgery defined itself during the 1980s, with the advent of high-resolution multiplanar imaging (computed tomography (CT) and magnetic resonance imaging (MRI)), improved microsurgical instruments and optical systems, and neurophysiologic monitoring.

The term *skull base surgery* is somewhat of a misnomer, as very few surgical procedures are actually carried out to treat pathology intrinsic to the skull base. In reality, the majority of neurotologic skull base procedures are performed for lesions located beneath the cerebral cortex or adjacent to the brainstem, and the removal of bone allows exposure while minimizing cerebral and cerebellar retraction.

The majority of this chapter will focus on the pathology, diagnosis, and management of vestibular schwannonas. An overview of other, less common skull base neoplasms will also be presented.

RELEVANT ANATOMY

The *skull base* refers to the floor of the cranial cavity and is composed of the ethmoid, sphenoid, and occipital bones, as well as the paired frontal and temporal bones. It is divided into anterior, middle, and posterior fossae. This chapter will focus on the posterior fossa which is bordered by the clivus anteriorly, the posterior surface of the petrous portion of the temporal bone laterally, and the occipital bone posteriorly. An axial view of the skull identifying the mastoid, petrous apex, CPA, and clivus is shown in Figure 1.

The CPA is a fluid-filled space of the lateral cistern. It is bordered by the posterior surface of the temporal bone anteriorly, the anterior surface of the cerebellum posteriorly, the inferior olive medially, the inferior border of the pons and cerebellum superiorly, and the cerebellar tonsil inferiorly.[5] The facial (VII) and vestibulocochlear (VIII) nerves course laterally through the CPA toward the porus acousticus and internal auditory canal (IAC). The trigeminal nerve (V) is located superiorly and the lower cranial nerves (IX, X, XI) are located inferiorly (Figure 2). The vascular anatomy in the area includes the anterior inferior cerebellar artery (AICA), posterior inferior cerebellar artery (PICA), internal auditory artery, and superior cerebellar artery (Figure 3). The IAC contains the facial nerve anterosuperiorly, cochlear nerve anteroinferiorly, and the vestibular nerves posteriorly. These are separated by the vertical crest and transverse crest as shown in Figure 4.

The petrous portion of the temporal bone is pyramidal in shape, with anterior, posterior, and inferior surfaces. The petrous apex is the most medially located portion of the temporal bone. The anterior surface forms a portion of the middle cranial fossa, and the posterior surface marks

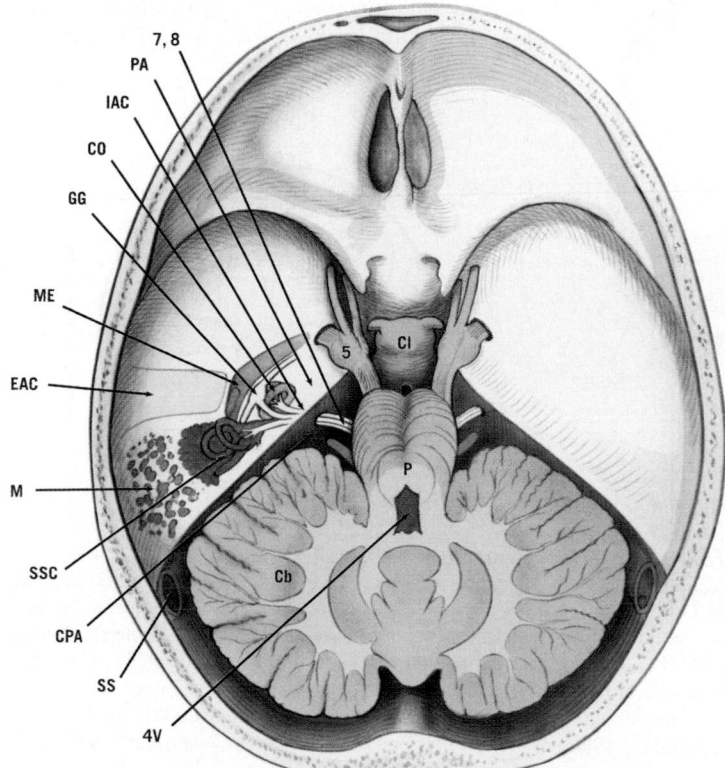

Figure 1 An axial view of the skull through the level of the internal auditory canal and cerebellopontine angle. 5 = trigeminal nerve; 7 = facial nerve; 8 = vestibulocochlear nerve; PA = petrous apex; IAC = internal auditory canal; CO = cochlea; GG = geniculate ganglion of the facial nerve; ME = middle ear; EAC = external auditory canal; M = mastoid air cell system; SCC = semicircular canals; CPA = cerebellopontine angle; SS = sigmoid sinus; 4V = fourth ventricle; Cl = clivus; P = pons; Cb = cerebellum. (Published with permission, copyright © 1996 R.K. Jackler, MD.)

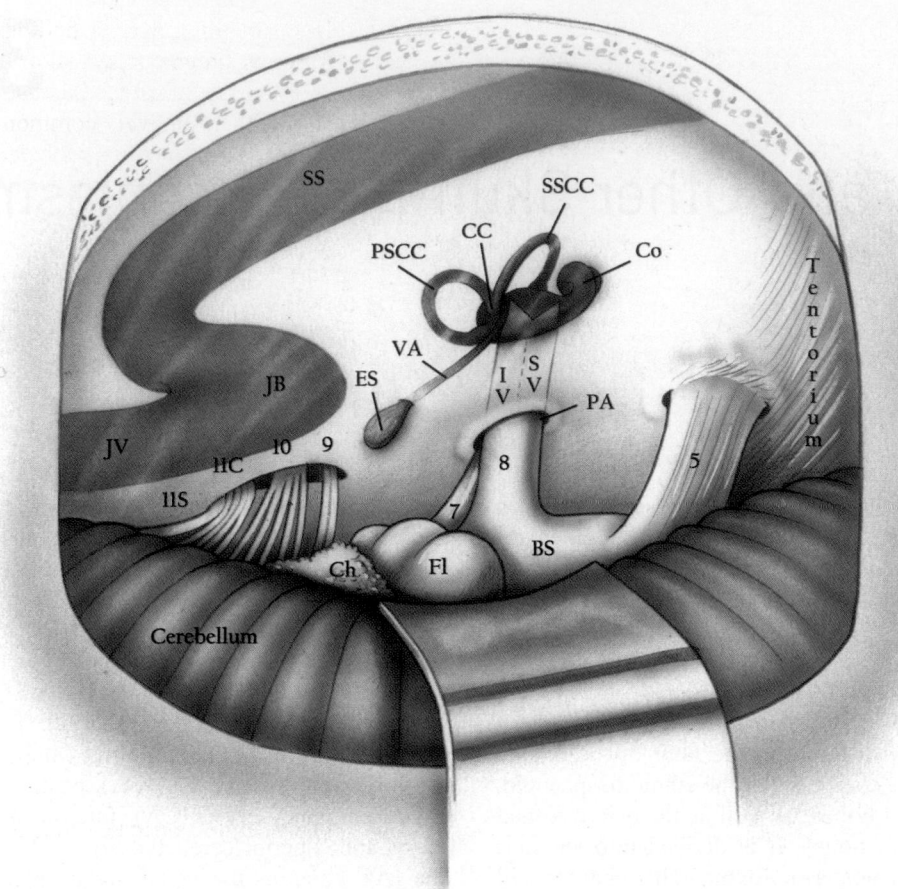

Figure 2 Anatomical relationships of the cerebellopontine angle shown through a retrosigmoid posterior fossa craniotomy. JV = jugular vein; JB = jugular bulb; SS = sigmoid sinus; 11s = spinal component of the accessory nerve; 11C = cranial component of the accessory nerve; 10 = vagus nerve; 9 = glossopharyngeal nerve; Ch = choroid plexus emanating from the lateral recess of the fourth ventricle; Fl = flocculus; BS = brainstem surface (pons); 5 = trigeminal nerve; 7 = facial nerve; 8 = vestibulocochlear nerve; PA = porus acousticus; IV = inferior vestibular nerve; SV = superior vestibular nerve; ES = endolymphatic sac; VA = vestibular aqueduct; PSCC = posterior semicircular canal; CC = common crus; SSCC = superior semicircular canal; Co = cochlea. (Published with permission, copyright © 1996 R.K. Jackler, MD.)

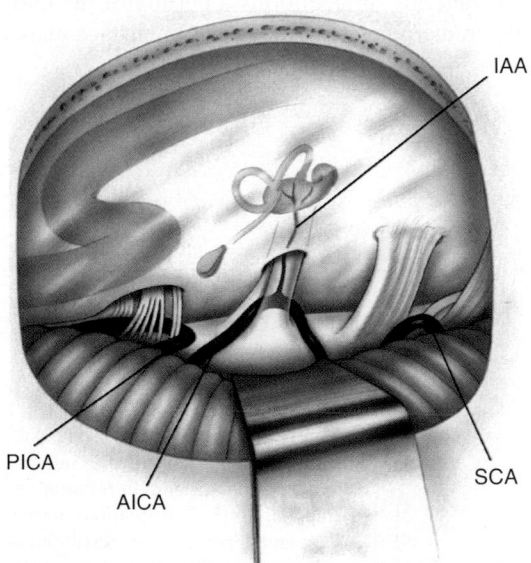

Figure 3 Arteries that traverse the cerebellopontine angle are shown through a retrosigmoid posterior fossa craniotomy. Note that a loop of the anterior inferior cerebellar artery often traverses between the facial and vestibulocochlear nerves at their brainstem entry site. This loop typically gives off a branch that enters the internal auditory canal and supplies the inner ear. PICA = posterior inferior cerebellar artery; AICA = anterior inferior cerebellar artery; SCA = superior cerebellar artery; IAA = internal auditory artery. (Published with permission, copyright © 1996 R.K. Jackler, MD.)

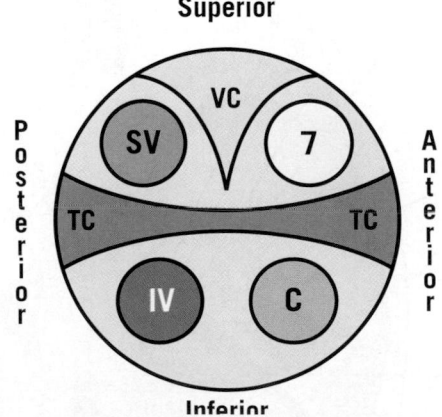

Figure 4 At the lateral extremity of the IAC the relationships of the superior vestibular (SV), inferior vestibular (IV), facial (7), and cochlear (C) nerves are highly predictable. In this location, the canal is completely divided in the horizontal plane by the transverse crest (TC), and its upper compartment is partitioned by a vertical bony crest (VC) also known as Bill bar (after William F. House, MD). (Published with permission, copyright © 1996 R.K. Jackler, MD.)

the petroclival and petrooccipital synchondroses, where it abuts the clivus. The clivus is located in the midline and is formed from the basal portion of the occipital bone (basiocciput) and the basisphenoid (Figure 5).

The jugular foramen lies inferiorly at the junction of the petrous portion and the occipital bone. Traditionally, the jugular foramen is described as having a posterior vascular compartment, *pars venosa*, and an anterior neural compartment, *pars nervosa*, which are separated by a fibrous or bony bridge connected to the jugular spine. In reality, each of these compartments has both neural and vascular elements. The pars venosa contains the vagus (X), spinal accessory (XI), and jugular bulb, while the pars nervosa contains the glossopharyngeal nerve (IX) and the inferior petrosal sinus (Figures 6 and 7).[6]

DIFFERENTIAL DIAGNOSIS

Skull base tumors may be classified either by pathology or according to anatomic location. These tumors involve the skull base either through primary growth, direct extension from adjacent sites, or by metastatic spread. They may be derived from endoderm, ectoderm, mesoderm, or neuroectoderm. Table 1 lists the most common skull base lesions by anatomic location.

EVALUATION

Signs and Symptoms

Skull base neoplasms may affect numerous anatomic subsites resulting in diverse clinical presentations. A general overview of symptoms and signs are presented in Table 2. These clinical signs can be organized based upon cranial nerves affected, brainstem and cerebellar compression, hydrocephalus, and direct invasion of structures. Symptoms specific to each disorder will be discussed in their individual sections throughout the chapter.

Audiologic and Vestibular Testing

All patients with a suspected skull base lesion should undergo pure tone and speech audiometry to establish the level of auditory function. Audiometry is a cost-effective screening tool to guide the acquisition of further studies, such as auditory brainstem responses (ABR) or imaging. Preoperative hearing levels are useful in guiding surgical approach (hearing conservation versus nonconservation) and can have prognostic value when a hearing conservation approach is being considered. ABR testing can also be used as a screening tool to facilitate a diagnosis and to estimate the probability of hearing preservation.

Vestibular testing, including electronystagmography (ENG) test battery, rotary chair testing, and dynamic posturography, may be useful in evaluating patients with balance distubance. However, such testing does not have the specificity to diagnose skull base lesions, therefore it is

the anterolateral extent of the posterior fossa. The lateral extent of the petrous portion is demarcated by the inner ear and intratemporal carotid artery. Medially, the posterior surface ends at

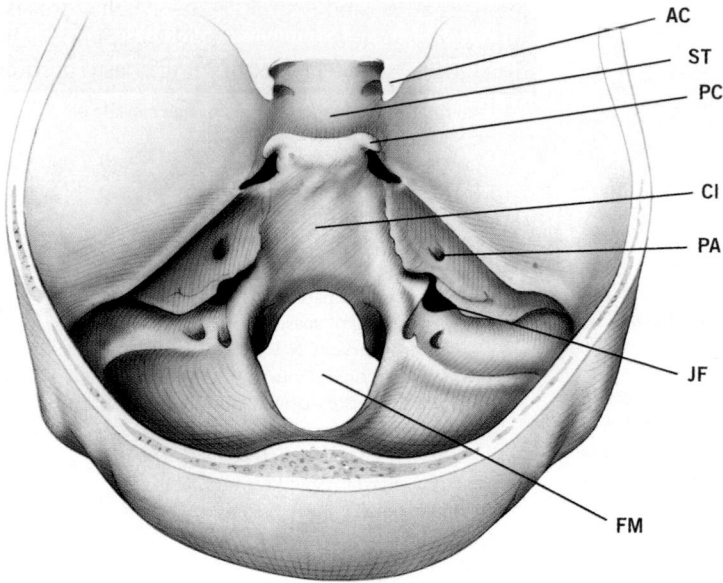

Figure 5 View of the cranial base as shown from above. The clivus is a portion of the occipital bone that extends from the anterior margin of foramen magnum to the dorsum sellae. Cl = clivus; AC = anterior clinoid; ST = sella turcica; PC = posterior clinoid; PA = porus acousticus; JF = jugular foramen; FM = foramen magnum. (Published with permission, copyright © 1996 R.K. Jackler, MD.)

not routinely ordered in our practice. The prognostic role of ENG in vestibular schwannoma management will be discussed below.

Imaging

Advances in skull-base surgery have evolved in parallel with modern imaging modalities, namely CT and MRI. In the skull base, MRI scanning has the advantage of soft tissue contrast and lack of ionizing radiation when compared to high-resolution CT. The combination of pre- and postgadolinium-enhanced T1-weighted images, T2-weighted images, diffusion scanning, and fat suppression techniques help to differentiate between various disorders (Table 3). CT scanning is useful to identify intralesional calcifications and surrounding bony changes or destruction. Angiography and endovascular techniques can be used in the evaluation of vascular lesions, such as aneurysms, arteriovenous malformations, dural arteriovenous fistulas, and jugulotympanic glomus tumors.

Cerebellopontine Angle. Approximately 10% of all intracranial tumors arise in the CPA. In a

series of 1,354 CPA tumors treated in a neurotologic practice, the following accounted for 98% of lesions: vestibular schwannomas (91.3%), meningiomas (3.1%), epidermoids (2.4%), non-vestibular schwannomas (1.4%), and arachnoid cysts (0.5%).[8] Vestibular schwannomas (VS) usually arise within the IAC and appear as ovoid or cylindrical structures filling the canal. These lesions enlarge into the CPA as rounded masses giving a typical "ice-cream cone" appearance, where the ice cream represents the CPA component and the cone the IAC and enlarged porus acousticus. As the VS enlarges, the CPA component often takes an ovoid configuration with the long axis parallel to the posterior petrous wall.[9] Schwannomas are typically isointense to brain on T1-weighted images, display intense enhancement with gadolinium, and constitute a "filling defect" in surrounding hyperintense CSF on T2-weighted images (Figure 8). These lesions may have heterogeneous enhancement secondary to nonenhancing microcystic and macrocystic components within the tumor. They are occasionally associated with adjacent arachnoid cysts (0.5%).[10] They may also rarely exhibit enhancement of

immediately surrounding dura, a finding termed a "dural tail," or pseudomeningeal sign.[11] Meningioma is the lesion most likely to be mistaken for a VS (Table 4). Other relatively common lesions of the CPA that can mimic VS include epidermoid cysts, arachnoid cysts, and facial nerve schwannomas (FNS). Epidermoid and arachnoid cysts can easily be differentiated from VS as they do not demonstrate solid enhancement. FNS confined to the CPA and IAC may be indistinguishable from VS. However, tumor extension into the labyrinthine segment of the Fallopian canal, as manifested by enlargement or enhancement, can be a helpful distinguishing factor between the two entities.

Meningiomas have 3 morphological growth patterns: (1) hemispherical or "mushroom cap" appearance, with a broad-base parallel to the petrous bone (75%); (2) plaque-like (*enplaque*) with bone invasion or hyperostosis (20%); and (3) ovoid or globular, mimicking VS (5%).[10] Meningiomas are usually eccentric to the porus acousticus, rarely penetrate or erode the IAC, and often extend superiorly into the middle cranial fossa. On MRI, they are typically isointense to gray matter on T1W and T2W images; however, relative hypo- or hyperintensity of the lesion to gray matter on T2 may signify internal fibrous or vascular composition, respectively. Meningiomas demonstrate avid enhancement with gadolinium (Figure 9). Adjacent dural thickening, known as the *dural tail* or *meningeal sign*, is found in 60% of cases and usually represents reactive thickening rather than neoplastic change.[12] CT may reveal internal calcifications in 25% of cases. Hyperostosis of adjacent osseous structures, although rare, can be a reliable indicator of meningioma.[13,14]

Epidermoid cysts commonly occur in the posterior fossa and tend to expand into areas of low resistance. Therefore, they often insinuate into various cisterns and have irregular margins that are scalloped or "cauliflower-like."[15] They tend to engulf cranial nerves and cisternal vessels. On MRI, they tend to be hypointense on T1-weighted and hyperintense on T2-weighted images (usually isointense to CSF). Rarely, "white epidermoids" may display reversed signal characteristics with a high T1 and low T2 signal. Epidermoids do not demonstrate solid enhancement; slight rim-enhancement can occasionally be seen. Arachnoid cysts are similar to epidermoids in terms of their T1 and T2 signal characteristics, however they have smooth borders, do not insinuate, and tend to displace surrounding nerves and vessels rather than engulf them.[10] Diffusion-weighted MR imaging is beneficial in the differentiation of epidermoid cysts (high signal) from arachnoid cysts (low signal).[16]

Mastoid and Petrous Apex. Petrous pyramid effusions, mucoceles, and cholesterol granulomas are the most commonly encountered radiographic abnormalities in the petrous apex and are thought to represent points along a continuum of pathology. Incidental petrous apex effusions are

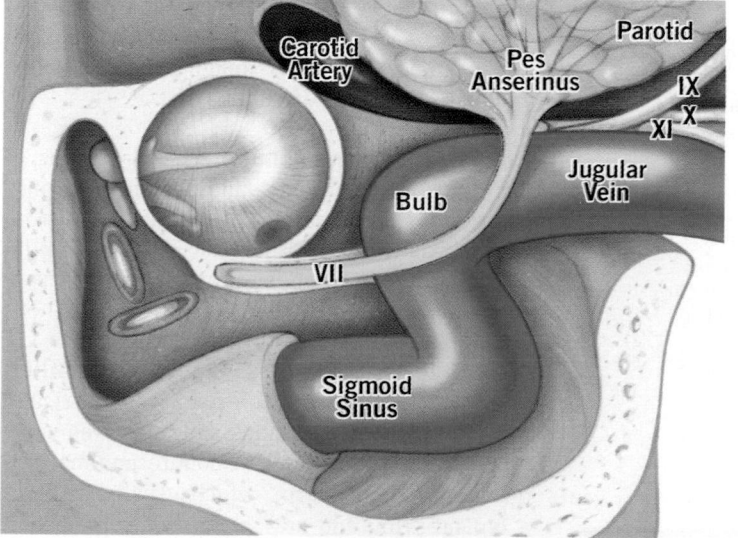

Figure 6 Lateral view of the jugular foramen region. VII = facial nerve; IX = glossopharyngeal nerve; X = vagus nerve; XI = spinal accessory nerve. (Published with permission, copyright © 2000 R.K. Jackler, MD.)

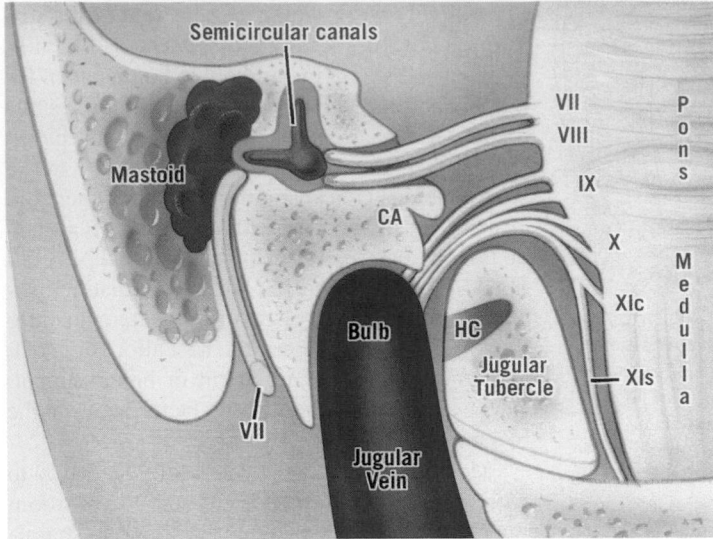

Figure 7 Coronal view of the jugular foramen region. VII = facial nerve; VIII = vestibulocochlear nerve; IX = glossopharyngeal nerve; X = vagus nerve; XIc = cranial root of spinal accessory nerve; XIs = spinal root of spinal accessory nerve; CA = cochlear aqueduct; HC = hypoglossal canal. (Published with permission, copyright © 2000 R.K. Jackler, MD.)

Table 2 Signs and Symptoms of Skull Base Neoplasms

1. Audiovestibular (involvement of otic capsule or CN VIII)
   (a) Hearing loss
   (b) Tinnitus
   (c) Vertigo/disequilibrium
   (d) Nystagmus
2. Facial nerve (CN VII)
   (a) Paralysis or paresis
   (b) Twitching or spasm
3. Trigeminal nerve (CN V)
   (a) Dysfunction of muscles of mastication
   (b) Facial sensory dysfunction
   (c) Trigeminal neuralgia
4. Lower cranial neuropathies (CN IX–XII)
   (a) Dysphagia/Aspiration
   (b) Dysphonia
   (c) Shoulder weakness
   (d) Tongue weakness
   (e) Glossopharyngeal neuralgia
5. Central ± hydrocephalus
   (a) Cerebellar signs
   (b) Headaches
   (c) Papilledema
   (d) Diplopia
   (e) Anosmia
   (f) Seizures
   (g) Long-tract sensory and/or motor dysfunction

Modified after reference 7.

often mistaken for disease with a variable T1-weighted signal and a high T2-weighted signal. They are easily distinguished from pathology on CT scan as the air-cell opacification is nonexpansile and lacks bone destruction. Mucoceles are typically dark on T1-weighted images, bright on T2-weighted images, and have peripheral rim enhancement.[17] Due to their predominantly hemorrhagic content, cholesterol granulomas are typically bright on both T1-weighted and T2-weighted images, although the T2-weighted images may demonstrate dark areas corresponding to hemosiderin.[18] Epidermoid cyst, termed cholesteatoma when originating from the middle ear, also occurs in the petrous apex and imaging characteristics are similar to their appearance in the CPA as discussed above. On CT, all 3 lesions demonstrate expansile growth, with remodelling of surrounding bone. Irregular "scalloped margins" are more suggestive of epidermoid cysts, while smooth margins are more characteristic of mucoceles or cholesterol granulomas. It should be noted that mucoceles, cholesterol granulomas, and epidermoids do not enhance centrally and should be differentiated from solid tumors, which demonstrate central enhancement.[19]

Less common lesions of the petrous apex include solid neoplasms, infectious processes, and osseous entities. Solid lesions of the petrous apex include metastasis, plasmacytoma, and endolymphatic sac tumors. These lesions often cause bone destruction and demonstrate variable degrees of central enhancement on postcontrast imaging. A unique feature of endolymphatic sac tumors is the presence of intralesional calcifications in the retrolabyrinthine area along the posterior semicircular canal.[20] Petrous apicitis is also destructive and reveals coalescence of the air cells on CT scan; on gadolinium-enhanced MRI, there is often enhancement of the petrous apex, surrounding dura, Meckel cave, and affected cranial nerves. Bony lesions including fibrous dysplasia, Paget disease, and osteoradionecrosis should also be considered in the differential diagnosis of temporal bone lesions.

Occasionally, asymmetric pneumatization of the petrous apex can be mistaken for pathology. The medullary fat from the nonpneumatized side has a high signal on T1-weighted MRI, and the air on the pneumatized side appears dark. This situation can be clarified using fat suppression sequences in which the marrow appears dark on T1-weighted MRI or CT imaging to define bone and marrow anatomy better.

Clivus. The most common primary lesions of the clivus are chordomas and chondrosarcomas. Chordomas are midline lesions that arise from notochordal remnants near the sphenooccipital synchondrosis. Chondrosarcomas arise from cartilage, commonly the petroclival synchondrosis, and are usually off the midline. On CT scan, both lesions are associated with infiltrative bony destruction with irregular margins, and many contain calcifications and bony fragments ("popcorn calcification"). Chondrosarcoma produces chondoid matrix, which usually displays a typical "ring and arc" pattern of calcification

Table 1 Common Skull Base Lesions by Anatomic Location

Site	Nonneoplastic	Benign	Malignant
Middle ear	Cholesteatoma	Glomus tympanicum Adenoma Schwannoma (VII) Meningioma	Squamous cell carcinoma (rare) Rhabdomyosarcoma
Internal auditory canal and cerebellopontine angle	Epidermoid cyst Arachnoid cyst Vascular lesions (aneurysm, arteriovenous malformation)	Vestibular schwannoma (VIII) Meningioma Nonvestibular schwannomas (V, VII, IX, X, and XI) Lipoma	Exophytic intra-axial lesions Metastasis
Mastoid and petrous pyramid	Mucocele Cholesterol granuloma Cholesteatoma Petrous apicitis Osseous lesions (fibrous dysplasia, Paget disease)	Chondroma	Chondrosarcoma Metastasis Endolymphatic sac tumor Squamous cell carcinoma (rare)
Clivus		Meningioma	Chordoma Chondrosarcoma Direct extension (eg, nasopharyngeal carcinoma) Metastasis
Jugular foramen		Glomus jugulare Schwannomas (IX–XII) Meningiomas	
Facial nerve		Schwannoma Geniculate ganglion hemangioma	

Table 3 Imaging Characteristics of Common Skull-Base Lesions

Pathology	CT Characteristics	CT Scan + Contrast	MRI T1-Weighted	MRI T1 + Gad	MRI T2-Weighted	Miscellaneous Features
Vestibular schwannoma	Heterogeneous in density	Heterogeneous enhancement	Iso- to hypointense to gray matter	Intense enhancement	Hyperintense to gray matter; hypointense to CSF: "filling defect"	See Table 4
Meningioma	Homogeneously hyperdense	Homogeneous enhancement	Isointense to gray matter	Intense enhancement	Variable; iso- to hypointense	See Table 4
Epidermoid cyst	Homogeneously hypodense	No enhancement	Hypointense (not necessarily identical to CSF)	No enhancement	Hyperintense	Irregular margins, engulfs structures, bright on diffusion-weighted MR
Arachnoid cyst	Homogeneously hypodense	No enhancement	Hypointense (identical to CSF)	No enhancement	Hyperintense (identical to CSF)	Smooth margins, displaces structures, dark on diffusion-weighted MR
Facial schwannoma	Widening of facial canal, smooth margins	Enhancement	Iso-/hypointense to gray matter	Intense enhancement	Hyperintense to gray matter; hypointense to CSF: "filling defect"	CPA/IAC—labyrinthine "tail"
Facial hemangioma	Irregular margins, "honeycomb" bony changes	Enhancement	Heterogeneously hypointense with low signal foci	Intense enhancement	Heterogeneously hyperintense with low signal foci	
Mucocele	Smooth, expansile	Rim enhancement	Hypointense	No internal enhancement	Hyperintense	
Cholesterol granuloma	Smooth, expansile	No enhancement	Hyperintense	No internal enhancement	Hyperintense	
Metastasis	Osseous destruction	Enhancement	Iso-/hypointense	Enhancement	Variable—typically hypointense to marrow	
Chordoma	Heterogeneous, destructive, calcifications	Heterogeneous enhancement	Hypo-/isointense	Heterogeneous enhancement	Strongly hyperintense	Located in midline
Chondrosarcoma	Heterogeneous, destructive, chondroid matrix	Heterogenous enhancement	Hypo-/isointense	Heterogeneous enhancement	Hyperintense	Located off midline
Paraganglioma	Destructive, irregular margins	Homogeneous enhancement	"Salt and pepper"—hypointense with punctate hyperintense areas (slow flow)	Intense enhancement	"Salt and pepper"—hyperintense with punctuate hypointense areas (flow voids)	
Jugular foramen schwannoma (IX, X, XI)	Fusiform shape, smooth margins	Homogeneous enhancement	Hypointense	Homogeneous enhancement	Hyperintense	

Adapted from reference 7.

on CT. On MRI, both lesions are classically dark on T1-weighted images, bright on T2-weighted images, and have heterogeneous enhancement with gadolinium. As the imaging characteristics of chordomas and chondrosarcomas are so similar, their location is the main differentiating feature with chordomas located in the midline and chondrosarcomas located off the midline (Figure 10). These lesions can be differentiated from osseous metastases, which often cause a decrease in normally hyperintense T1 and T2 marrow signal.

Meningiomas of the clivus may demonstrate a sessile configuration or have an *en plaque* growth pattern; their imaging characteristics have been discussed above. Pituitary macroadenomas can cause expansion of the sella with typically smooth bony expansion. However, once the tumor has transgressed the bone, the lesion may mimic a clival malignancy.[10] Nasopharyngeal carcinomas can also invade the clivus via the petroclival and petrosphenoidal fissures, and evidence of radiologic abnormalities of the nasopharynx must be diligently sought when evaluating a lesion involving the clivus.[19]

Jugular Foramen. Paragangliomas (glomus tumors) are common lesions affecting the jugular foramen (glomus jugulare) and the middle ear (glomus tympanicum). The radiographic differentiation of these subtypes is straightforward when the lesions are small and remain confined to their site of origin. However, differentiation can be more complex in larger tumors. Erosion of the lateral bony plate of the jugular fossa favors the diagnosis of a glomus jugulare.[19] CT imaging of glomus jugulare tumors reveals destructive changes to the lateral part of the jugular foramen with possible involvement of the carotid artery and descending facial nerve. The vascular nature of these tumors results in a "salt and pepper" appearance on T1-weighted MRI images: bright foci represent slow blood flow and dark foci represent high velocity flow voids (Figure 11). There is intense enhancement with contrast on both CT and MRI scans. Magnetic resonance venography (MRV) is useful to determine the patency and involvement of the sigmoid sinus.

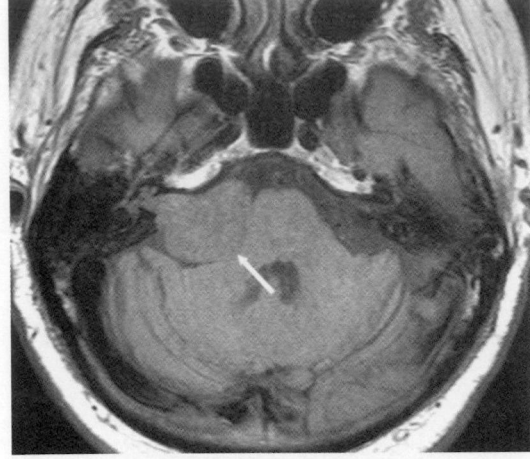

(A)

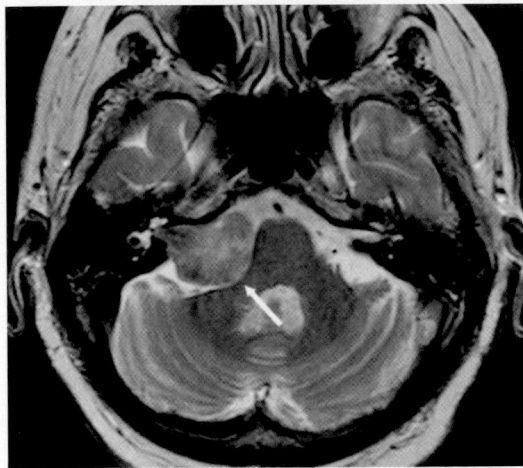

(B)

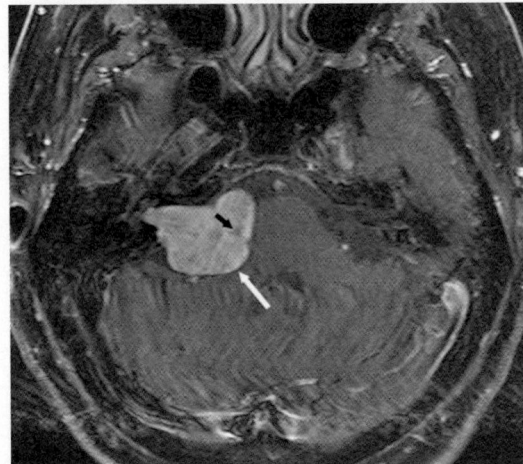

(C)

Figure 8 Vestibular schwannoma. Large lesion penetrating the IAC, eroding the porus acousticus, and extending into the CPA with moderate brainstem compression (*white arrows*). (A) T1-weighted image. Tumor is isointense to brain and hyperintense to CSF. (B) T2-weighted image. Tumor is slightly hyperintense to brain and hypointense to surrounding CSF. (C) Gadolinium enhanced. Marked enhancement of solid tumor. Central hypointense areas represent cystic change (*black arrow*). (Published with permission, copyright © 2007 R.K. Jackler, MD.)

Jugular foramen schwannomas (JFS) arise from cranial nerves IX, X, and XI. These lesions involve the medial portion of the jugular foramen, grow vertically along the course of the affected cranial nerves, and assume a fusiform or

Table 4 Key Differentiating Imaging Features between Vestibular Schwannoma and Meningioma of the Cerebellopontine Angle

Vestibular Schwannoma	Meningioma
Globular in shape	Broad-based (sessile)
Pseudomeningeal sign (rare)	Meningeal sign
Centered on internal auditory canal (IAC)	Extrinsic to IAC
Pentrates the IAC	Eccentric to long axis of IAC
IAC often eroded	IAC seldom eroded
Often cystic	Usually solid
No calcifications or hyperostosis	Calcifications and hyperostosis
Middle fossa penetration rare	Middle fossa penetration

dumbbell shape. In contrast to paragangliomas, there is a smooth, sharply marginated enlargement of the jugular foramen on CT scan. These lesions are hypointense on T1-weighted images and bright on T2-weighted images and enhance homogenously with gadolinium.

Jugular foramen meningiomas have imaging characteristics discussed above. They may be differentiated from paragangliomas by the presence of calcifications, hyperostosis, and dural tails.

Facial Nerve. FNS commonly affect the geniculate ganglion and may affect multiple segments of the nerve. They are typically fusiform, tubular masses with smooth bony margins on CT. On MRI, they are hypointense on T1-weighted images, hyperintense on T2-weighted images, and display homogeneous enhancement. Facial nerve hemangiomas, also known as ossifying hemangiomas, most commonly occur at the geniculate ganglion. In contrast to schwannomas, they have irregular bony margins on CT and display a "honeycomb" bone matrix. The MRI signal characteristics are similar between these two lesions, however hemangiomas tend to be more heterogeneous with low signal foci secondary to the ossified matrix. Further discussion regarding facial nerve tumors is found in Chapter 34, "Facial Paralysis."

CEREBELLOPONTINE ANGLE

Vestibular Schwannoma

Introduction. In neurotologic practice, VS represents the most common skull base neoplasm and a substantial amount of time is spent in both its diagnosis and treatment. These tumors have a wide range of clinical presentations and may be managed with a diverse array of treatment options. As the care for VS has evolved, patients may expect increasingly favorable outcomes.

Epidemiology. Vestibular schwannomas represent approximately 6% of all intracranial tumors and up to 90% of all lesions in the CPA.[8,21] There is no significant racial or gender predilection. The overall incidence of VS based on population studies from Denmark, Canada, and a US HMO appears to be between 10 and 13 per million people.[22–24] Occult VS has also been a topic of interest, with an autopsy series in 1936 suggesting that the prevalence may be as high as

2.5% in the general population.[25] Further studies, however, have revealed that this estimate is likely several orders of magnitude too high, as this prevalence would suggest that millions of Americans have occult VS, and the incidental finding of a VS on MRI would be quite common. In the era of gadolinium-enhanced MRI scans, less than 2% of VS patients were found to be completely asymptomatic[26] and a retrospective review of 46,414 patients found only nine with incidentally discovered VS.[27] The prevalence of occult VS is, therefore, approximately 2 in 10,000 adults.

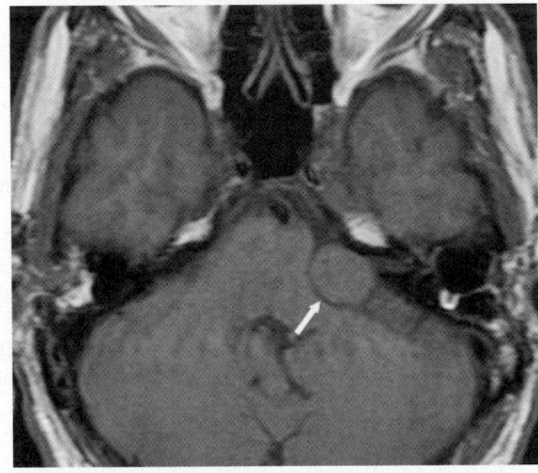

(A)

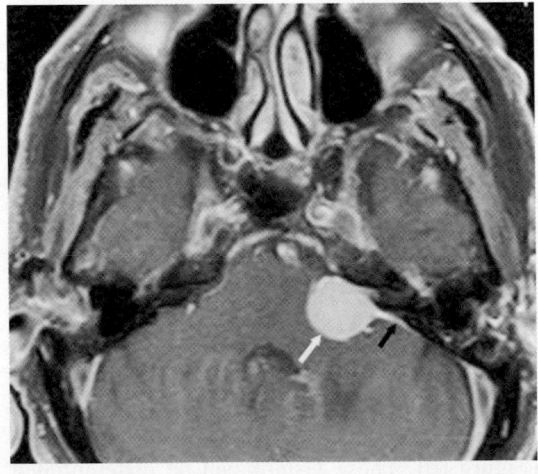

(B)

Figure 9 Meningioma (*white arrows*). (A) T1-weighted. Tumor is isointense to brain with minimal penetration of the IAC. There is no appreciable erosion of the porus acousticus. (B) Gadolinium enhanced. Avid enhancement of the tumor with a small dural tail (*black arrow*). (Published with permission, copyright © 2007 R.K. Jackler, MD.)

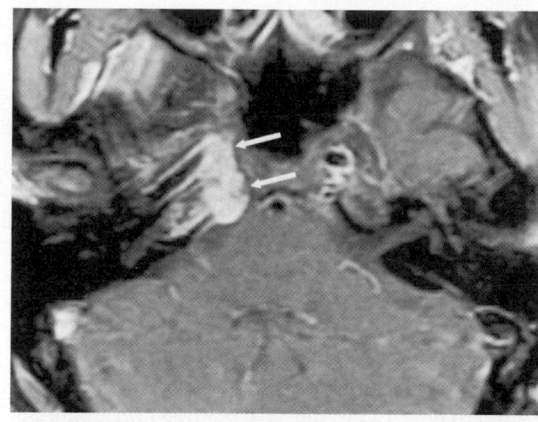

(A)

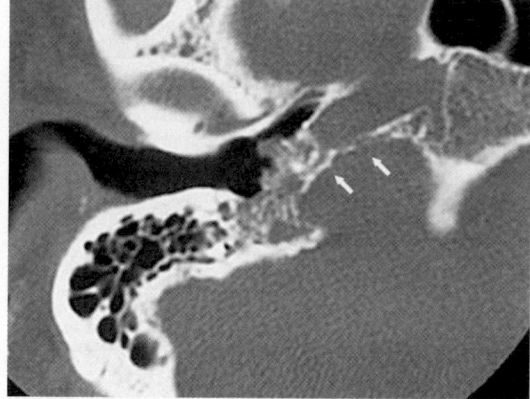

(A)

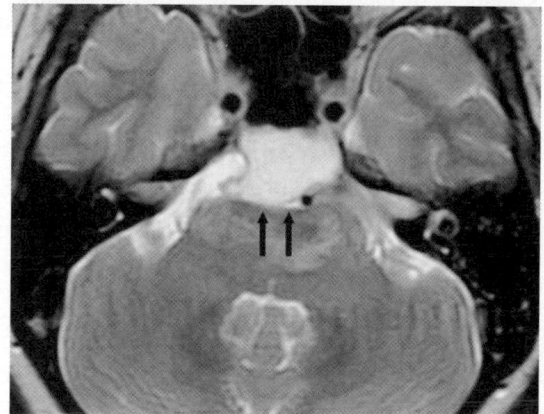

(B)

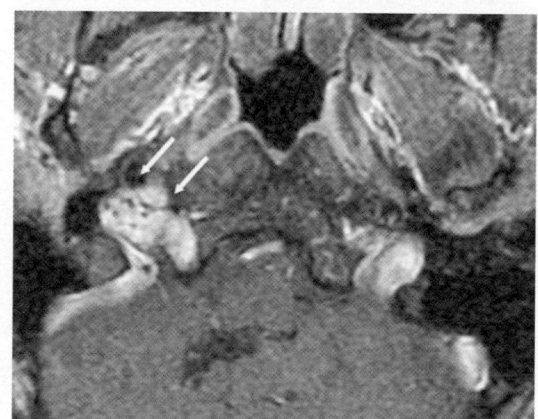

(B)

Figure 10 (A) Chondrosarcoma. Tumor located off midline at the petroclival junction, with avid postgadolinium enhancement (*white arrows*). (B) Chordoma. Tumor located in the midline and demonstrates marked hyperintensity on T2-weighted image (*black arrows*). (Published with permission, copyright © 2007 R.K. Jackler, MD.)

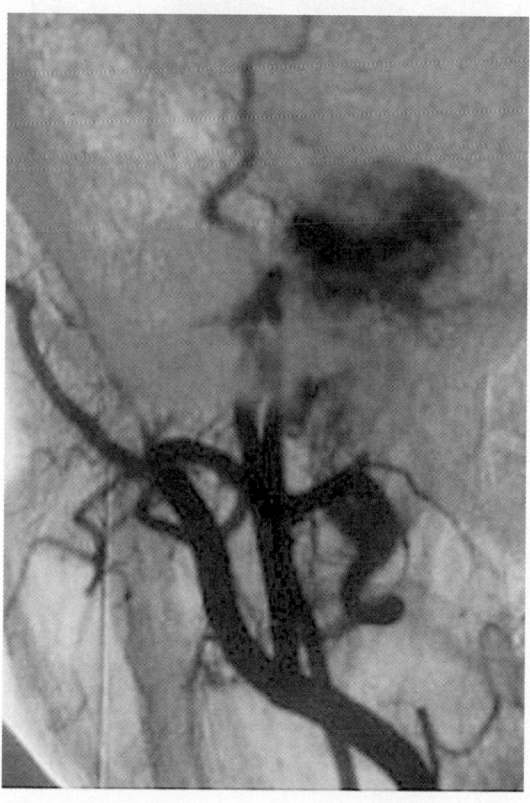

(C)

Figure 11 Glomus jugulare. (A) CT scan of right jugular foramen displaying bony erosion (*white arrows*). (B) Gadolinium-enhanced MRI in same patient demonstrates hypervascular lesion (*white arrows*) with typical "salt and pepper" pattern. (C) Angiogram in another patient demonstrates a tumor blush at the jugular foramen. (Published with permission, copyright © 2007 R.K. Jackler, MD.)

In terms of the affected patient population, there are 2 forms of VS: (a) sporadic; and (b) those associated with neurofibromatosis type 2 (NF2). Sporadic tumors comprise 95% of all VS, are unilateral, and typically present in the fifth to sixth decades of life. Neurofibromatosis is a rare disease, with a prevalence of 1 in 30,000 to 50,000. Patients with NF2 have 5% of VS, eventually develop bilateral tumors, and tend to present at a younger age. In contrast, the peripheral variant of neurofibromatosis (NF1) is much more common with a prevalence of 30 to 40 in 100,000. Although the exact incidence of VS in this population is not known, likely fewer than 2% of patients with NF1 develop unilateral VS and almost none develop bilateral tumors.[28]

Tumor Pathogenesis. In the past, vestibular schwannomas have traditionally been termed "acoustic neuromas," however these lesions are neither neuromas nor of acoustic origin. Rather, they are schwannomas which arise from the vestibular division of the eighth cranial nerve. In 1992, an NIH Consensus Development conference recommended that *vestibular schwannoma* be adopted as standard terminology.

The vast majority of VS arise within the IAC, which may be related to eighth nerve anatomy and myelin production. As it exits the brainstem,

the proximal eighth nerve is histologically more similar to central rather than peripheral nervous tissue. Therefore, its myelin is produced by oligodendroglial cells. Distally, its composition is more typical of peripheral nerves, with its myelin being produced by Schwann cells. The transition zone between this "central" and "peripheral" myelin, or the glial-schwannian junction, is known as the Obersteiner-Redlich zone. Traditionally, it has been proposed that VS arise from this region,[29] possibly due to a higher density of Schwann cells in this location. Recent literature, however, has suggested that VS actually occur *lateral* to this transition zone and not from Schwann cells at the transition zone itself.[30] The location of this transition zone varies considerably, but it is thought to occur in the vicinity of the vestibular (Scarpa) ganglion. There have been contradicting studies as to whether the superior or inferior vestibular nerve is more commonly the nerve of origin. Current opinion favors equal incidence from the superior and inferior divisions of the vestibular nerve.[31]

The genetic basis of VS has been derived from NF2 patients and the specific defect has been mapped to chromosome 22. This gene is believed to be a tumor-suppressor gene, and both copies of the gene are required to be dysfunctional to develop a tumor. NF2 patients are born with 1 defective copy and only require 1 more mutation for tumorigenesis. Sporadic cases, however, require 2 spontaneous mutations which is a rare event; this is also known as the "double hit" mechanism for tumor production. The role of the gene product, known as *merlin*, is unclear, but recent studies indicate that it may exert its activity by inhibiting phosphatidylinositol 3-kinase.[32,33]

Tumor Pathology. Grossly, the surface of a VS is typically smooth, regular, and has pronounced vascularity. The color ranges from yellow-tan to pale gray (particularly when cystic components are present). Internally, the tumor is quite heterogeneous with textures that range from soft and friable to firm and rubbery. Traditionally, these tumors have been described as encapsulated, but recent evidence reveals that they are surrounded by a very thin layer of connective tissue rather than a true capsule and that neoplastic Schwann cells extend to the tumor's margin.[34]

The histopathology of VS reveals 2 distinct morphologic patterns. Antoni type A describes densely packed cells with small, spindle-shaped, densely staining nuclei. Antoni type B refers to a loose arrangement of vacuolated, pleomorphic cells, which seem to occur predominantly in larger tumors with cyst formation. A whorled or palisading appearance of Antoni A cells is known as a *Verocay body*. A summary of the key pathologic features of VS are given in Table 5.

Nearly all VS are benign, and although malignant degeneration of benign VS has been described, it is exceedingly rare.[35]

Growth Characteristics. VS are benign slow-growing tumors. They enlarge primarily through

Table 5 Key Pathologic Features of Vestibular Schwannoma

Gross	Surface smooth and bright yellow to gray color
	Larger tumors are often cystic
	Unencapsulated
Microscopic	Antoni A—densely packed cells with small spindle-shaped nuclei
	Antoni B—loosely arranged vacuolated, pleomorphic cells
	Verocay body—whorled or palisading appearance of Antoni A cells
Immunohistochemistry	Positive S-100 immunoperoxidase stain
	Positive neuron-specific enolase
	Positive vimentin

From reference 7.

cellular proliferation although cellular hypertrophy may play a small role. Rapid expansion can occasionally occur secondary to cystic degeneration or intratumoral hemorrhage and lead to acute neurological deterioration. Tumor involution can also be seen when cystic areas spontaneously decompress or tumors outgrow their blood supply. Caution should be taken when comparing lesion size on serial imaging studies, as apparent tumor involution may be due to variations in technique and quality.

The growth of VS may be considered to occur in 4 anatomic stages: intracanalicular, cisternal, brainstem compressive, and hydrocephalic (Figure 12). VS typically originate in the IAC and are considered to be intracanalicular until they protrude into the CPA cistern. At this point, they enter the cisternal stage, in which they progressively displace CSF, AICA, and cranial nerves VII and VIII. The brainstem compressive stage begins when the tumor contacts the lateral pontine surface. At this point, cranial nerve V can become affected. The hydrocephalic stage begins when the fourth ventricle is effaced secondary to brainstem compression. Table 6 summarizes the various stages and their associated symptoms.

Improved measurement of the growth rate of VS has recently been made possible with the advent of serial imaging with high-resolution MRI and CT scans. In a meta-analysis of 13 studies and 571 tumors, the mean growth rate was found to be 0.18 cm per year, with 54% of patients showing radiologic growth over an average of 3 years.[37] In the patients with growing tumors, the average growth rate was 0.4 cm per year, and in those requiring intervention, the rate was 0.59 cm per year. Approximately 10 to 15% of lesions are considered fast-growing with a growth rate greater than 1 cm per year.[38,39] One must be cautious before assuming that a large percentage of VS will remain stable over the long term. First, the patients being chosen for observation in these studies may represent those with a more indolent course, thereby introducing a selection bias. Second, these slow-growing tumors may not show significant growth when followed for only 3 years, whereas their growth may become apparent if they were followed over the long term, for example, 10 or 20 years. Finally, methods used to measure tumor size remain somewhat inexact, making comparison difficult.

Unfortunately, there is still no universally accepted method of measuring VS. Most authors advocate measuring the maximal CPA component of the tumor in 3 axes: (1) parallel to the petrous ridge on an axial image, (2) perpendicular to the petrous ridge on an axial image, and (3) vertically on a coronal image. Many have simplified this to the single largest measurement in the axial plane. Unfortunately, due to the irregular geometry of VS, these measurements do not necessarily reflect tumor size, and computerized volumetric measurements are likely to replace diameter-based measurements in the future.

Clinical Presentation. Although the classic presentation of VS includes progressive unilateral sensorineural hearing loss, tinnitus, and disequilibrium, clinicians must be aware that these lesions can present with a variable array of symptoms. The natural progression of these symptoms based on tumor size is summarized in Table 6. Historically, the relative frequencies of various symptoms have changed with the evolution of improved of imaging modalities, which has allowed earlier diagnosis. This evolution of symptom frequencies is outlined in Table 7.

Hearing Loss. Hearing loss is the most common symptom of VS, occurring in over 85% in cases, and is also the most frequent initial symptoms for which patients seek medical attention.[26] It is typically unilateral and, in its initial stages, involves the high frequencies. Patients will often complain of poor clarity as word recognition is affected out

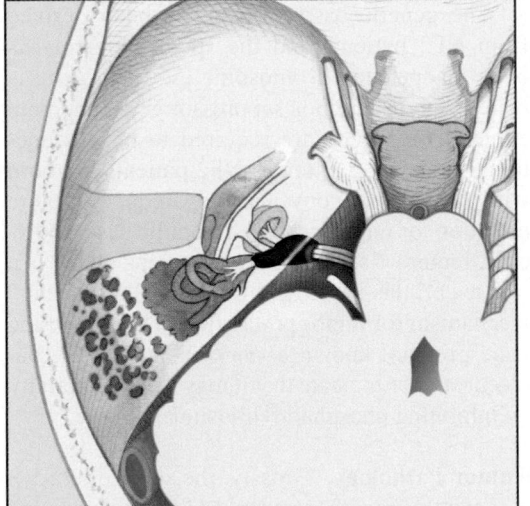
A

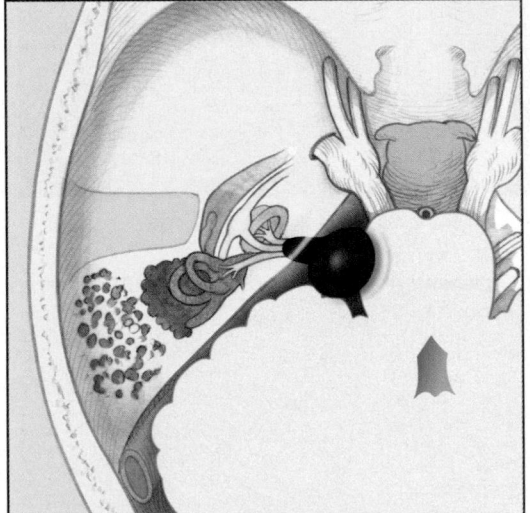
B

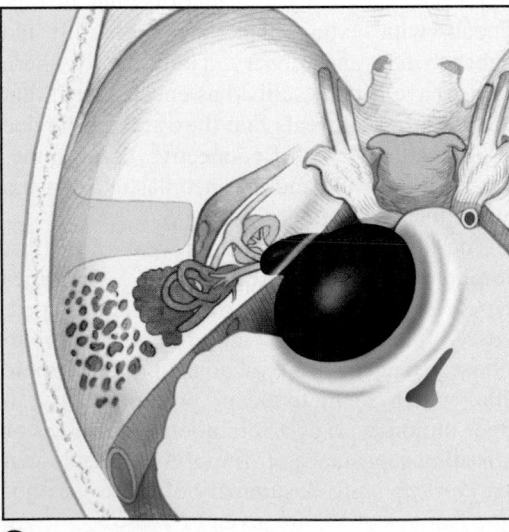
C

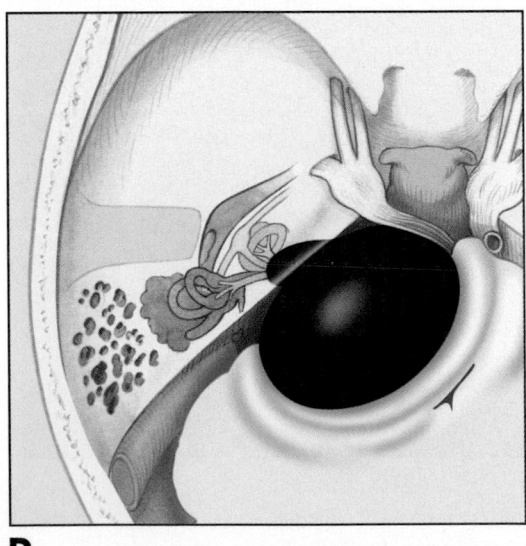
D

Figure 12 Vestibular schwannoma. (A) Intracanalicular stage. (B) Cisternal stage. The tumor has a 1 cm CPA component with no significant brainstem compression or trigeminal nerve displacement. (C) Brainstem compressive stage. Note the compression of the lateral aspect of the pons, indentation of the cerebellar peduncle, and displacement of the trigeminal nerve. (D) Hydrocephalic stage. Note the collapse of the fourth ventricle and resultant hydrocephalus. (Published with permission, copyright © 2000 R.K. Jackler, MD)

Table 6 Symptomatic Progression of Vestibular Schwannoma with Tumor Growth

Intracanalicular	Hearing loss
	Tinnitus
	Vertigo
Cisternal	Hearing loss worsens
	Vertigo diminishes
	Disequilibrium increases
Brainstem compressive	Midfacial and corneal hypesthesia (V)
	Occipital headache (occasionally)
	Ataxia begins
Hydrocephalic	Worsening of trigeminal symptoms
	Gait deteriorates
	Headache becomes generalized
	Visual loss due to increased intracranial pressure
	Lower cranial nerve dysfunction (hoarseness, dysphagia, aspiration, shoulder, and tongue weakness)
	Long tract signs
	Death due to tonsillar herniation

From reference 36.

of proportion to pure tone hearing loss. Clinicians must be aware that in the MRI era, recent series have reported up to 15% of patients had subjectively normal hearing, although only 4% were audiometrically normal.[26] In addition, asymmetry was not always present as 7% of patients had an audiometrically symmetric hearing loss.[26]

Complicating the clinical diagnosis even further, up to 26% of patients with VS complain of one or more episodes of sudden hearing loss which is typically ascribed to different causes.[26,42] As 1 to 2% of patients with sudden hearing loss will ultimately have a VS, we recommend imaging in all patients with a sudden hearing loss to rule out this possibility.

Tinnitus. Tinnitus is a frequent symptom of VS occurring in over half of patients. The tinnitus is typically constant, high pitched, and localized to the affected ear, however it may have variable qualities and be nonlocalizing. Patients with VS may also have unilateral tinnitus in the absence of subjective hearing loss, therefore further evaluation for VS should be considered in these individuals.

Vertigo, Disequilibrium, or Dysmetria. VS can affect both the peripheral and central vestibular system, therefore patients may present with a variety of complaints relating to their balance. Vertigo, defined as the illusion of motion, is surprisingly infrequent in VS. This is likely due to the slow destruction of vestibular function, which allows central adaptation to occur. When present, vertigo typically occurs from small tumors, affecting ears in which considerable vestibular function remains. The sensation of motion often resolves within several days to weeks. Disequilibrium is the continuous sense of instability, which is often secondary to an uncompensated peripheral vestibular disturbance and/or cerebellar compression. Unlike vertigo, this symptom is quite common in VS, often progressive, and associated with larger tumors (>3 cm) in the brainstem compression stage. Large tumors can present with dysmetria and truncal ataxia from significant cerebellar compression; they can also cause long-tract dysfunction from brainstem compression, clinically manifested by ipsilateral hyperactive deep tendon reflexes, hemiplegia, or hemiparesis.

Trigeminal Nerve Dysfunction. Trigeminal dysfunction typically presents as midface hypesthesia or parathesia and eventually progresses to involve other divisions of the face. As the tumor enlarges, anesthesia also occurs. Trigeminal

symptoms typically occur in the brainstem compressive stage when the trigeminal nerve becomes stretched and compressed superiorly. The corneal reflex is nearly always decreased or absent in these patients, and this sign may precede any sensory facial disturbance. Facial pain from VS has been described in larger tumors and is treated in the same manner as its idiopathic form (tic douloureux).[43]

The motor portions of the trigeminal nerve are much more resistant to compressive effects, therefore motor dysfunction is limited to a small percentage of advanced cases of VS. When present, it often manifests as unilateral temporal wasting, masseter atrophy, and secondary malocclusion.

Facial Nerve Dysfunction. The facial nerve is resistant to gradual compression and stretching from VS, therefore dysfunction of this nerve is quite rare. Facial nerve dysfunction may present as either hypofunction (weakness or paralysis) or hyperfunction (twitch, spasm). Clinically detectable weakness of the nerve may occur in large tumors, but the incidence is less than 2%. Facial hyperfunction is independent of tumor size and can coexist with facial weakness. Minor twitching of the face, commonly seen in the orbicularis oculi muscle, can occur in up to 10% of patients.[26] It is important to consider the diagnosis of facial nerve schwannoma in these patients.

The facial nerve has a sensory component distributed over the posterior ear canal and conchal bowl. Sensory dysfunction in this area secondary to VS, known as Hitselberger sign, is of little clinical significance.

Ophthalmologic Manifestations. The most common ophthalmologic findings in VS are (a) horizontal nystagmus from vestibular hypofunction, and (b) decreased corneal reflex from trigeminal dysfunction. The nystagmus in the horizontal plane typically beats away from the tumor side indicative of ipsilateral vestibular hypofunction. However, with larger tumors, a vertical plane nystagmus may be seen due to brainstem compression. Hydrocephalus is rarely seen today, however this can lead to papilledema and secondary visual loss. Chronic elevated intracranial pressure may also cause optic atrophy which is characterized by a progressive loss of peripheral vision and eventual blindness.

Lower Cranial Nerves. Lower cranial nerve dysfunction (IX through XII) clinically presents with hoarseness, aspiration, dysphagia, and/or ipsilateral shoulder and tongue weakness. These finding are extremely rare in VS regardless of tumor size. When present, such dysfunction should prompt the reevaluation of the diagnosis, and a jugular foramen schwannoma should be considered to be more likely.

Investigations

Audiometry. Conventional pure tone and speech audiometry are the most cost-effective screening tools to determine which patients should

Table 7 Clinical Manifestations of Vestibular Schwannoma

Symptoms	Cushing[40] (%)	Selesnick and colleagues[41] (%)	Matthies and Samii[42] (%)
Hearing loss	100	85	95
Tinnitus		56	63
Disequilibrium		48	61*
Vertigo		19	61*
Trigeminal nerve	63	20	16.5
Facial nerve	77	10	17
Headache	100	19	12
Visual symptoms	87	3	1.8
Lower cranial nerves		0	2.7–3.5
Dysphagia	53	0	
Papilledema			
Asymptomatic		1.6	

Adapted from reference 7.

*No distinction made between vertigo and other balance disturbances.

have further testing such as ABR or imaging. Patients with VS typically present with an asymmetric, high frequency, down-sloping hearing loss with a word recognition score (WRS) lower than expected based upon the pure-tone thresholds. The audiogram configurations are variable, and one study revealed a down-slope in 68%, a trough in 9%, flat in 9%, low frequency in 8%, a peak shape in 5%, and normal in 1%.[44] Historically, a battery of special audiologic tests was used to diagnose VS. However, these have largely been abandoned and only performance intensity function for phonetically balanced words test for rollover and acoustic reflex decay remain in widespread use. Although the sensitivity and specificity of these tests is poor, abnormal results may be an indication for further investigations.

In addition to screening for VS, audiometry can help determine the utility and prognosis for a hearing conservation microsurgical approach. In 1995, the Committee on Hearing and Equilibrium of the American Academy of Otolaryngology—Head and Neck Surgery established a classification system based upon the pure tone average (PTA) and WRS (Figure 13).[45] This classification is currently used for reporting the preoperative and postoperative hearing results when hearing conservation surgery is being considered. In general, better preoperative hearing is associated with higher rates of hearing preservation. A meta-analysis of 16 studies with 1,993 patients revealed preserved hearing (postoperative AAO-HNS Class A, B, or C) in 56.1% of patients with preoperative Class A, 43.4% with Class B, and 32.2% with Class C.[46]

Auditory Brainstem Responses. ABRs are the most sensitive and specific of all the audiologic tests for VS diagnosis. Prior to the advent of enhanced MRI scanning, ABR testing was used as a key diagnostic tool, and its diagnostic efficiency has been extensively studied. Among patients with documented VS, approximately

Word Recognition Score (%)

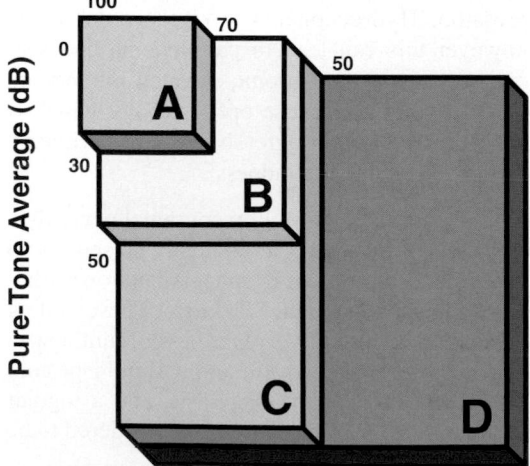

Figure 13 The American Academy of Otolaryngology–Head and Neck Surgery classification system for hearing following acoustic neuroma surgery.[45] The vertical axis represents the pure tone average (at 500, 1,000, 2,000, and 3,000 Hz), and the horizontal axis represents the word recognition score (%).

20 to 30% have no waves, 10 to 20% have only wave I and nothing thereafter, 40 to 60% have all waves but a wave V latency delay, and 10 to 15% have normal traces.[47] Although the rate of false-negatives (normal ABR with an acoustic neuroma) in the literature is approximately 15%,[47–49] it ranges from 33% for intracanalicular tumors to 4% for larger lesions. False-positive rates (abnormal ABR without an acoustic neuroma) are much higher and exceed 80% in a number of series.[50–52] Because of these limitations and the narrowing cost differential of ABR compared to MRI, the indication for ABR as part of the diagnosis of VS has diminished significantly. ABR testing may be considered in patients clinically at low risk for VS with a minimal pure-tone asymmetry, those with a decades-long history of stable asymmetric loss, or those with unilateral tinnitus and symmetric hearing. Any patient considered to be at high risk for VS based upon history, physical examination, or audiometry should proceed directly to a gadolinium-enhanced MRI scan.

ABR may also provide prognostic information for hearing preservation after microsurgical management. Good ABR morphology, lower wave V latencies, and the preservation of wave III have all been associated with an increased rate of hearing preservation.[53–55]

Vestibular Testing. The ENG test battery is abnormal in up to 90% of VS patients, and typically a reduced ipsilateral response with horizontal nystagmus is seen. Unfortunately, ENG has poor specificity for the diagnosis of VS, therefore it is not routinely ordered in our practice. However, arguments for ENG testing in patients with VS surround its potential prognostic value in predicting postoperative vertigo and the potential for hearing conservation. Patients with absent caloric responses tend to have less disabling vertigo in the postoperative period because they have already had the opportunity to compensate to the vestibular loss. This information may be used to counsel patients, but does not ultimately affect the choice in management.

In hearing conservation, it has been suggested that a VS originating from the superior vestibular nerve carries a favorable prognosis, since such tumors are farther away from the cochlear nerve and internal auditory artery.[56] The caloric response results from stimulation of the lateral semicircular canal which is innervated by the superior vestibular nerve. Therefore, an absent caloric response indicates injury to the superior vestibular nerve and occurs more frequently from tumors originating from the superior vestibular nerve itself. Three recent studies, however, have failed to demonstrate ENG as a significant prognostic factor in hearing conservation.[53,57,58]

Imaging. The imaging of VS has been discussed in the CPA imaging section of this chapter above.

Management. There are 3 treatment options for patients with VS: (1) observation with serial imaging, (2) microsurgery, and (3) stereotactic

radiation. The goals in management are: first, the preservation of life, second, the preservation of facial function, and third, the preservation of hearing. Of course, the risks and benefits of each of the treatment options should be discussed with the patient in this collaborative decision-making process.

Observation. The decision to choose observation with serial imaging is based upon the probability of needing treatment within the predicted lifespan of the patient. Therefore, unfavorable patient lifespan factors (advanced age, infirm health) and favorable tumor factors (small size, stable, or slow-growing) are considered indications for conservative management. Patients who are poor surgical candidates can be treated expectantly at first, with subsequent stereotactic radiotherapy as warranted by progressive tumor growth or clinical symptoms.

Since the growth rate cannot be established on the initial imaging study, the second study should be performed at 6 months with yearly studies thereafter if no significant growth is seen. VS will often fall into 2 categories based upon their growth rate. Patients with tumors growing at rates >0.2 cm/yr or with progressive clinical symptoms will likely require additional therapy in the form of stereotactic radiotherapy or microsurgery. Patients with tumors with slower growth rates over 3 years often do not require treatment and can be followed for extended periods with serial imaging.

Disadvantages to choosing observation include (1) patients may require treatment at a more advanced age thereby raising the risk of complications; (2) some patients may require treatment for larger tumors thereby compromising results; (3) the opportunity for hearing conservation may be lost with tumor growth or hearing deterioration; (4) tumor growth could exceed the limits amenable to stereotactic radiation (>3 cm); (5) some patients may have significant anxiety about having an "untreated" tumor; and (6) the time and expense associated with periodic radiologic follow-up.[59]

Microsurgical Management. There are 3 primary surgical approaches used in VS microsurgery: (1) translabyrinthine (TL), (2) retrosigmoid (RS), and (3) middle fossa (MF). The exposure afforded by each of these approaches is illustrated in Figure 14 (TL), Figure 15 (MF), and Figure 2 (RS). The advantages and disadvantages of these 3 approaches have been summarized in Table 8.

The amount of tumor removal can be classified as *total* removal, *near-total* removal, or *subtotal* removal. Near-total removal refers to a small thin capsule (<2 mm thick) being left behind, typically along the facial nerve in the CPA.[59] In a subtotal removal, larger amounts of tumor are left behind (>2 mm), and the residual can be quantified as a percentage of the total tumor volume.[59] Although total removal is normally achieved, partial resection can be considered for neural preservation, advanced patient age, decreased hearing status

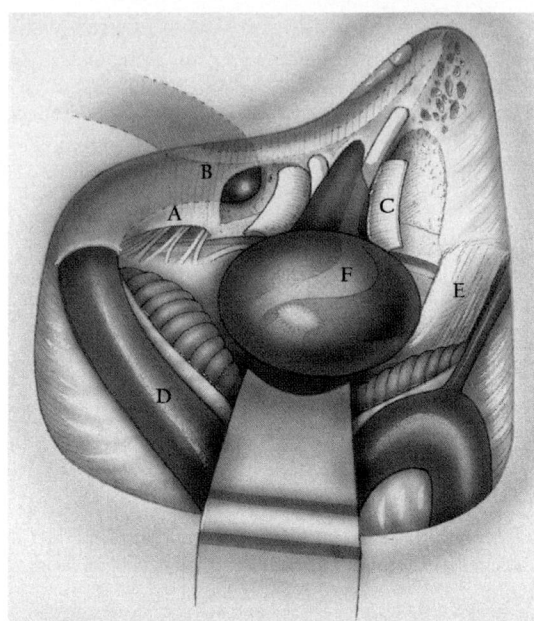

Figure 14 Typical left translabyrinthine posterior fossa craniotomy exposure of a medium-sized tumor. Infereiorly, the lower cranial nerves (A) are visible, and the jugular bulb (B) has been identified. Troughs have been drilled above and below the IAC, and the dura (C) has been reflected off the tumor surface. The sigmoid sinus (D) and cerebellum are gently retracted posteriorly. The trigeminal nerve (E) is located superiorly. The facial nerve (F) takes a variable and often serpentine course across the medial side of the tumor. (Published with permission, copyright © 1996 R.K. Jackler, MD.)

in the contralateral ear, or intraoperative events necessitating premature termination of the procedure.[59]

Although VS surgery can be performed by either a neurotologist or neurosurgeon alone, a team approach minimizes surgeon fatigue and allows specialized skills to be combined. The experience and skill of the surgeon and perioperative team play a significant role in the choice of surgical approach. Ideally, the surgical team should be comfortable with all approaches so that the choice can be based upon the attributes of the specific patient and tumor.

Factors Influencing Operative Approach

1. Hearing. In patients with nonserviceable hearing (AAO-HNS Class D) or in patients where the chance of hearing conservation is quite small, we advocate the TL approach regardless of tumor size, location, or nerve of origin. If hearing conservation is a viable option, either MF or RS is chosen based on the factors listed below.

2. Tumor Size. Tumor size is a major consideration in the choice of surgical approach. Intracanalicular tumors can be managed via either the MF or RS approaches. The MF approach probably provides the best chance of hearing conservation, but there is a greater need to manipulate the facial nerve as it often lies between the surgeon and the tumor. In tumors with a CPA component of less than 10 mm in diameter, the MF approach has been shown to have higher transient facial nerve dysfunction, but similar long-terms results compared to the RS approach.[60] In tumors with CPA

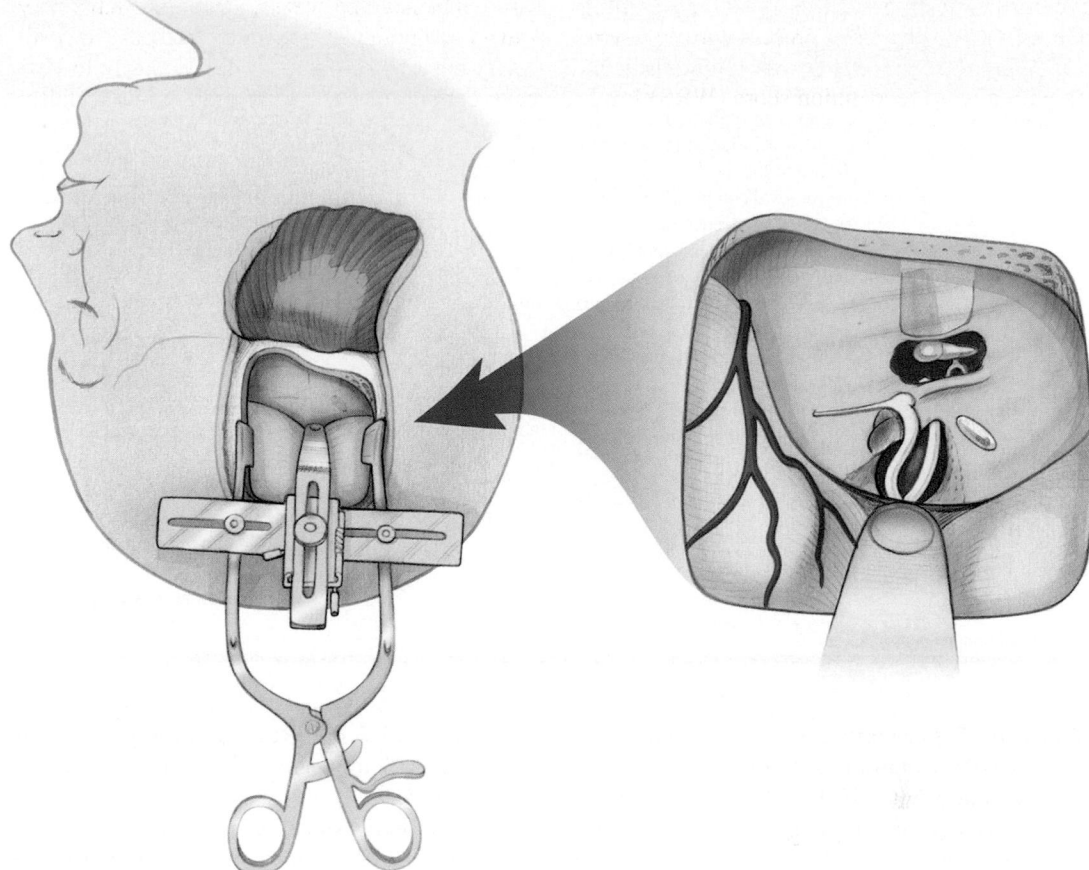

Figure 15 Middle fossa exposure of a small right-sided tumor. The retractor is engaged over the posterior lip of the petrous bone and retracts the temporal lobe. Bone has been removed around the IAC, and the dura has been opened to expose the tumor. The facial nerve typically courses across the superior aspect of the tumor surface. (Published with permission, copyright © 1996 R.K. Jackler, MD.)

components 10 to 18 mm in diameter, long-term facial nerve outcomes are worse with the MF approach than with a TL approach.[61] Informed patient participation in the choice of approach is essential since patients may differ in the relative importance given to hearing and facial function.

In patients with serviceable hearing and tumors with between 10 and 25 mm diameter extensions into the CPA, an RS approach is preferred provided that the lateral third of the IAC is free of tumor. Although hearing preservation rates are low in tumors with CPA extension greater than 25 mm,[62] it is still reasonable to attempt hearing conservation via the RS approach in these patients, particularly if there is excellent preoperative hearing and limited extension into the IAC.

3. Tumor Extension and Erosion. The depth of lateral extension in the IAC on gadolinium-enhanced MRI scans helps guide the selection of surgical approach. In the RS approach, only the medial two-thirds of the IAC can be directly exposed without sacrificing a portion of the otic capsule, thereby reducing the chances at hearing preservation.[63–65] Even in the MF approach, dissection in the lateral 25% of the IAC is often blinded by the overhang of the transverse crest.[66] In our experience, the presence of a "modiolar spike" of the lateral part of the tumor inferior to the transverse crest and deep into the fundus is a particularly poor prognostic sign for hearing conservation.

Erosion of the bony walls of the IAC has been shown to decrease the probability of hearing conservation.[61] Extensive erosion of the IAC, particularly of its anterior wall, is likely an indication of significant tumor pressure on the cochlear nerve and is an adverse prognostic sign. Similarly, if the tumor prolapses laterally into the cochlear modiolus, the possibility of hearing conservation is eliminated, and a TL approach is advocated.

4. Nerve of Origin. The origin of the tumor from either the superior or inferior vestibular nerve is of significance for preservation of both hearing and the facial nerve. Inferior vestibular nerve tumors tend to a more intimate relationship with the cochlear nerve and internal auditory artery, resulting in less hearing conservation. They also deflect the facial nerve superiorly, leaving it in a less favorable position for an MF approach. The utility of caloric vestibular testing to determine the nerve of origin has been discussed above. Instead, we routinely use coronal MRI scans to determine the tumor's location in relation to the transverse crest since this has practical implications in selecting a surgical approach.

5. Complications. Facial nerve transection is uncommon in modern acoustic neuroma surgery, and overall rates of permanent severe or total paralysis are well under 10%.[61] Facial nerve outcomes are similar between TL and RS approaches,[67] but the MF approach has a higher

Table 8 Comparison of Microsurgical Approaches for Vestibular Schwannoma

	Translabyrinthine	Middle Fossa	Retrosigmoid
Advantages	No tumor size limitation	Best hearing preservation rates	No tumor size limitation
	Early identification of facial nerve in IAC lateral to the tumor	Bone removal completed prior to dural opening	Hearing preservation possible
	Bone removal completed prior to dural opening	Low incidence of postoperative headache	No abdominal fat graft required
	Low tumor recurrence rate	Low incidence of CSF leak	
	Low incidence of persistent postoperative headache	Better exposure of lateral IAC than the RS approach	
	Low incidence of CSF leak requiring surgical management		
	Possibility of "mastoid-meatal" rerouting for VII injury		
Disadvantages	Complete sensorineural hearing loss	Tumor size limitation	Poor access to lateral one-third of IAC without violating labyrinth
	Requires large abdominal fat graft	Limited access to posterior fossa	Requires skull fixation (Mayfield head frame)
		Higher risk of transient postoperative facial nerve weakness	Higher risk of CSF leak requiring surgical management
		Requires small abdominal fat graft	Higher risk of persistent postoperative headache
		Occasional transient memory disturbance or aphasia	Bone removal completed after dural opening
		Risk of recurrence similar to RS approach	Higher risk of recurrence compared to TL

Modified from reference 7.

incidence of transient weakness in tumors with <10 mm CPA extension and of permanent weakness in tumors with 10 to 18 mm CPA extension.[60,61] Therefore, if a hearing conservation approach is being considered, we prefer the RS approach for all tumors with greater than 10 mm CPA extension.

Persistent postoperative headaches can cause significant morbidity. This is particularly problematic with the RS approach, although its incidence can be reduced by limiting spillage of bone dust in the CPA during drilling of the IAC, which can incite aseptic meningitis. In addition, replacing the bone plate at the conclusion of the resection can assist in reducing headaches, presumably by limiting traction of cervical musculature on the dura.[68–71] Nonetheless, the risk of postoperative headaches is 3.8 times greater with an RS than a TL approach even if the bone plate is replaced, and this difference has been shown to remain significant up to 6 months postoperatively.[72,73]

Retraction injuries can occur to the cerebellum during the RS approach and to the temporal lobe during the MF approach. After an RS approach, encephalomalacia involving the lateral 1 to 2 cm of the cerebellar hemisphere is sometimes seen on T2-weighted MRI scans. Most patients recover uneventfully; but, on occasion, the injury may extend deeply toward the midline, and prolonged ataxia may result. Retraction of the dominant temporal lobe during an MF approach can cause dysphasia, but this is quite rare. Rarely, transient short-term memory loss, seizure, and odd dreams can occur. Postoperative encephalomalacia is less common with the MF approach than with the RS approach because the retraction of the temporal lobe is extradural rather than intradural.

In a recent study, the incidence of CSF leak was equal (approximately 10%) following the TL, MF, and RS approaches.[74] However, some have maintained the CSF leak may be more common following RS craniotomy and may be more difficult to manage with conservative measures.[75,76]

In our experience, efforts to preserve the cochlear nerve in hearing conservation approaches lead to prolonged operative time, increased postoperative vestibular dysfunction, and a slightly greater risk of tumor recurrence. These observations have yet to be studied formally. The vestibular disturbance likely reflects abnormal signals from preserved vestibular nerve remnants which may slow vestibular compensation. Tumors can recur from a small fragment left in the fundus.[77] The chances of this are higher in the MF and RS approaches than in the TL approach because dissection of the lateral one-third of the IAC is often blinded by the preserved otic capsule.[63–66] Some have advocated the use of endoscopes to visualize the fundus for any residual tumor.[78] However, in our experience, it is often difficult to use angled endoscopes in such a small area, avoid injury to the facial nerve, and discern tumor from surrounding tissue.

Microsurgical Management Algorithm. A generalized algorithm used at Stanford University is shown in Figure 16. Individualized treatment depends on numerous factors discussed above including hearing status, radiologic characteristics (including tumor size and geometry), and the potential complications inherent in each approach.

Hearing Results. Hearing results from a number of major centers are presented in Table 9. The success rates in the literature vary widely, and one must consider the numerous variables that have not been controlled among series. Relevant confounding factors include tumor size, tumor location, preoperative hearing levels, surgical approach, reporting of hearing results, and the definition of success.

The highest rates of hearing preservation have been reported with small tumors treated via the MF approach.[60,61,81,83] In these most favorable conditions, the rate of preservation of "useful" hearing surpasses 50%. The MF approach, however, has 3 disadvantages: exposure of the CPA component of the tumor is limited; in contrast to the TL approach, the lateral IAC may require blind dissection; and in comparison with the other approaches, the facial nerve is at increased risk of permanent palsy if the cisternal component is >1.0 cm.[61,66]

Overall hearing preservation rates via the RS approach tend to be lower than for the MF approach, but direct comparison controlling for tumor size and preoperative hearing status is difficult. In our series, up to 25% of patients retained serviceable hearing after the RS approach for tumors less than 2 cm in CPA diameter.[60] Hearing preservation rates are diminished when the cisternal component is greater than 2 cm in diameter.[84,85,87,88]

When choosing a hearing conservation approach for a particular patient, overall success rates are not as important as individual prognostic factors. For example, a patient with a small tumor, minimal IAC involvement, excellent preoperative hearing, and a normal ABR will likely have a

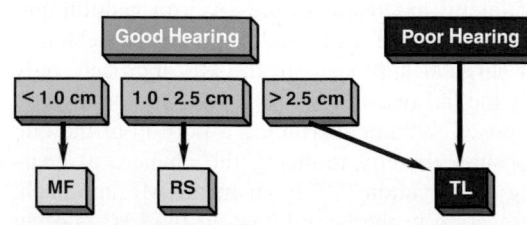

Figure 16 Vestibular schwannoma microsurgical management algorithm used at Stanford University. This scheme represents a general guideline only. Individualized treatment selection depends on numerous factors. Size is expressed in diameter of the CPA component. MF = middle fossa; RS = retrosigmoid; TL = translabyrinthine. (Published with permission, copyright © 2007 R.K. Jackler, MD.)

Table 9 Results of Hearing Preservation Studies

Study	Number (n)	Approach*	Tumor Size (cm)†	AAO-HNS Class A + B‡
Glasscock and colleagues[79]	136	38 MF, 98 RS	<1.5	37 (27%)
Brookes and Woo[80]	13	RS	<1.0	6 (46%)
Arriaga and colleagues[81]	26	RS	Mean = 1.66	14 (54%)
	34	MF	Mean = 0.72	24 (71%)
Slattery[57]	143	MF	Mean = 1.2	74 (52%)
Irving[60]	25	MF	Intracanalicular	11 (44%)
	20	MF	0.1–1.0	12 (60%)
	5	MF	1.1–2.0	1 (20%)
	17	RS	Intracanalicular	2 (12%)
	12	RS	0.1–1.0	3 (25%)
	21	RS	1.1–2.0	3 (14%)
Satar and colleagues[61]	104	MF	IC–0.9	57 (62%)
	47	MF	1–1.8	15 (33%)
Rohit and colleagues[82]	107	59 MF, 48 RS	<1.5	34 (32%)
Arts and colleagues[83]	62	MF	0.3–1.8	45 (73%)

				Hannover Class§ (H1 + H2)
Samii and Matthies[84]	29	RS	T1‖	6 (21%)
	96	RS	T2‖	25 (26%)
	249	RS	T3‖	39 (16%)

				Gardner–Robertson Class I + II
Cohen and colleagues[85]	128	RS	<0.5	32 (37%)††
			0.6–1.0	32 (34%)††
			1.1–1.5	38 (24%)††
			>1.5	26 (11%)††
Dornhoffer and colleagues[58]	65	MF	<0.5	39 (60%)††
	11	MF	0.5–1.0	7 (64%)††
	17	MF	1.0–1.5	8 (47%)††
Betchen and colleagues[86]	142	RS	0.4–4.0**	43 (30%)††
Rowed and Nedzelski[87]	26	RS	IC	13 (50%)‡‡
	68	RS	0.4–1.5	20 (29%‡‡

Modified after reference 7.

*MF = middle fossa; RS = retrosigmoid.

†Tumor size includes posterior fossa component except when indicated. IC = intracanalicular.

‡AAO-HNS classification system.

§New Hannover classification system.

‖T1 = intrameatal; T2 = intrameatal and extrameatal; T3 = filling the cerebellopontine angle.

**Size range of those tumors with preserved hearing.

††Pure-tone average <50 dB and word recognition >50%.

‡‡Pure-tone average <50 dB and word recognition >60%.

50% chance of preserving hearing regardless of whether the MF or RS approach is used. Conversely, patients lacking these favorable characteristics will likely have poor results. Taking into account that only a small fraction of patients with VS are candidates and the probability of success is limited, one can estimate that only 5% of all patients with VS will have useful hearing in the tumor ear following surgical excision.

Stereotactic Radiosurgery and Radiotherapy. Stereotactic radiosurgery and radiotherapy are discussed in Chapter 36, "Stereotactic Radiosurgery and Radiotherapy." There has been significant controversy regarding the relative roles of microsurgery and stereotactic radiotherapy in the primary treatment of VS. As these tumors are slow-growing, intervention can be typically withheld until tumor growth can be shown on serial imaging. In general, radiotherapy is recommended for smaller tumors in older individuals, whereas younger individuals are recommended microsurgery regardless of tumor size. The rationale is that younger patients will have more time to develop the potential adverse long-term complications of radiation such as secondary neoplasms. Microsurgery is recommended for patients with larger tumors (>3 cm) as radiotherapy carries the risk of edema and secondary brainstem compressive symptoms. Finally, tumors treated with radiotherapy require indefinite monitoring with MRI scans which can be cumbersome for patients and create difficulties when seeking to change health insurance plans.

Stereotactic radiosurgery or radiotherapy is commonly used for VS recurrence following microsurgery. In our experience, the recurrence rate following near-total removal is only 3%, however the rate rises to over 30% following subtotal resection.[89] In all cases of partial removal, the tumor should be carefully monitored for recurrence with serial imaging. Outcome for stereotactic radiation of tumor recurrence is similar to that of unoperated cases.[36]

Meningioma

Epidemiology. Meningiomas are the second most common tumor found in the CPA (<10%), the second most common intracranial tumor (<20%), and the second most common central nervous system tumor after gliomas.[90,91] Unlike vestibular schwannoma, there is a 2:1 female sex predilection, with the tumor being diagnosed most commonly in the fifth to sixth decades of life.[92]

Pathogenesis. Risk factors for meningioma include NF2, and it has been estimated that one-fifth of adolescents with meningioma have NF2. Radiation has been shown to increase the risk of meningioma fourfold.[93] There is also an association between meningioma and sex hormones; the tumor is more common in women, has been associated with breast cancer, and has been shown to have binding sites for estrogen and progesterone.[94]

The genetics of meningioma have revealed that monosomy 22 is a common early molecular event in tumorigenesis and cytogenetic losses in chromosomes 1, 7, 10, and 14 and telomerase activation are observed in clinically aggressive meningiomas. Genes associated with meningiomas include *S6-kinase*, *p53/MDM2*, protein 4.1B, *merlin* (NF2 gene), and *TSLC1*.[91]

Pathology. The gross and microscopic characteristics of meningiomas have been summarized in Table 10. Meningiomas arise from arachnoidal cap cells, pial cells, and dural fibroblasts. Histologically, meningiomas have been classified into 4 categories: *syncytial* or *meningotheliomatous* lesions (55%), *fibroblastic* lesions (15%), *transitional* lesions (30%), and *angioblastic* lesions (5%).[96,97] In 2000, the World Health Organization (WHO) updated the classification for meningiomas based upon aggressiveness, risk of recurrence, grade, and histologic subtype (Table 11).[98,99]

Meningiomas have a proclivity to arise either along the course of venous sinuses or in relation to neural foramina (Figure 17). Extratemporal meningiomas are the most common and usually originate at the CPA attached to the posterior surface of the petrous pyramid or adjacent to the superior petrosal sinus.[92] Other locations, in decreasing frequency, include the tentorium, clivus, cerebellar convexity, and foramen magnum. Although invasion of the temporal bone is usually secondary from extratemporal meningiomas, primary involvement can occur from the IAC, the jugular foramen, the geniculate ganglion, and the sulcus of the greater and lesser superificial petrosal nerves.[92–94,100–102] Rarely, a meningioma can be entirely within the IAC and mimic an intracanalicular VS.[96]

Diagnosis. Clinically, the symptoms at presentation in decreasing frequency are progressive hearing loss, headaches, vertigo, tinnitus, otorrhea, otalgia, facial weakness or loss of taste, diplopia or visual disturbance, dysphagia, dysarthria, dysphonia, nausea and vomiting, facial pain or

Table 10 Key Pathologic Features of Meningioma

Gross	Well-circumscribed, nodular, uneven pink-gray surface
	Cut surface "gritty"
	En plaque or globular
	Hyperostosis
Microscopic	Arachnoidal cap cell origin
	Psammoma bodies (calcospherites)
	Papillary formation—"whorls"
Immunohistochemistry	95% positive epithelial membrane antigen
	33% positive to antibodies to cytokeratins
	30% S-100 positive

From reference 95.

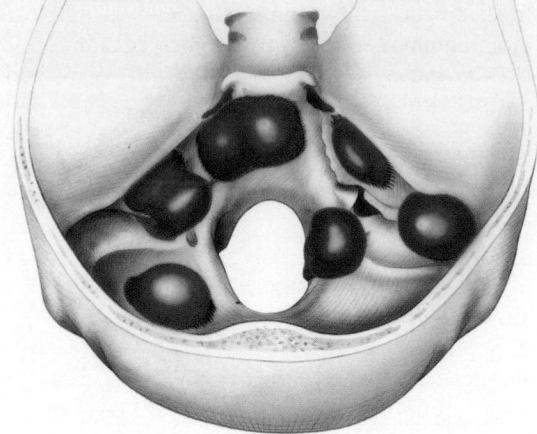

Figure 17 Meningiomas have a proclivity to arise either along the course of venous sinuses or in relation to neural foramina. Meningimoas of the posterior fossa may be classified according to their predominant location including cerebellopontine angle, superior petrosal sinus, tentorium cerebellar convexity, petroclival, jugular foramen, and foramen magnum. (Published with permission, copyright © 1996 R.K. Jackler, MD.)

paresthesias, exophthalmos, lower limb hemiparesis or paraparesis, and periauricular swelling or neck mass.[92,102] Although hearing loss, vertigo, and tinnitus are the most common presenting symptoms of both CPA meningiomas and VS, it has been suggested that only 60% of meningiomas present with hearing loss compared with 98% of VS.[103] Meningiomas extending to the middle ear may present with a hyperemic tympanic membrane, conductive hearing loss, and facial nerve involvement. Jugular foramen meningiomas present with pulsatile tinnitus, a middle ear mass, and lower cranial nerve dysfunction.[104]

Audiometric and vestibular testing reveals similar findings to other CPA lesions; therefore, their role in diagnosis is limited. Baseline audiometry is, however, useful in deciding upon various treatment strategies and counseling patients. MRI with gadolinium is the most effective imaging modality for the diagnosis of meningioma. The imaging characteristics of meningiomas and their differentiation from those of VS have been discussed in the imaging section previously.

Treatment Meningiomas are benign tumors, but are locally destructive with the ability to invade cranial nerves. The treatment options are similar to those of VS, but the variations in tumor location and symptoms make it difficult to create a standardized management algorithm. In general, the patient's age and estimated life expectancy,

the morbidity of tumor removal, and the natural history of an untreated tumor must be taken into consideration. Conservative management with serial imaging should be considered in tumors unlikely to cause symptoms within the patients expected life and tumors where excision would result in unacceptable morbidity.

Surgical excision is the treatment of choice when possible. In general, patients have better outcomes when surgery is performed prior to the onset to neurological signs. Therefore, tumors being followed conservatively should be carefully monitored for growth and symptoms. Young patients with large tumors or progressive neurological signs should be treated surgically. The surgical approach is dictated by the tumor size, location relative to neural and vascular structures, and the status of hearing. Adjacent bone involved with tumor should be resected due to the propensity of meningiomas to spread within osseous haversian canals. A wide variety of surgical approaches can be used based upon the tumor characteristics; these include middle fossa, retrosigmoid, tranlabyrinthine, transcochlear, and combined translabyrinthine-suboccipital approaches.[99] Hearing preservation is much more likely with meningiomas than with VS, therefore labyrinth-sparing approaches are used whenever possible regardless of tumor size. Simpson classified the extent of tumor removal (Grades I to IV), and this classification has been

correlated to outcome following surgery.[105] Complete tumor resection can often be difficult due to location and involvement of neural and vascular structures, therefore recurrence rates have been reported to be as high as 30% even following apparently complete removal. As clinical recurrence rates have been shown to increase over time, long-term follow-up with radiologic examination is recommended.[106]

The role of stereotacic radiosurgery or radiotherapy in meningiomas is controversial. Although stereotactic radiosurgery or radiotherapy can be used primarily for inaccessible tumors or patients unfit for surgery, it is being used increasingly as an adjunct following subtotal resection.[107–109]

MIDDLE EAR AND MASTOID

Squamous Cell Carcinoma

Squamous cell carcinoma is the most common primary malignant tumor of the temporal bone and represents 60 to 80% of all malignancies from the skin of the external auditory canal (EAC) and middle ear cleft.[110,111] Squamous cell carcinoma of the EAC is discussed in Chapter 14, "Diseases of the External Ear."

Adenomatous Tumors

Adenomatous tumors involving the middle ear and temporal bone are rare. Historically, it became clear that these "adenomas" could have either a benign or aggressive clinical course. It was not until 1990, however, that these tumors were classified into two distinct subtypes based upon clinical course and histopathology: *mixed pleomorphic cell* pattern and *papillary* pattern.[112] The mixed pleomorphic cell pattern will be discussed in this section on tumors of the middle ear and mastoid, however the papillary pattern will be discussed in the following section on inner ear tumors due to their origin from the endolymphatic sac.

Table 11 World Health Organization (WHO) Classification of Meningiomas[98,99]

WHO Grade	Histologic Subtypes	Recurrence/Aggressiveness
Grade I—Typical	Meningothelial	Low
	Fibrous (fibroblastic)	
	Transitional (mixed)	
	Psammomatous	
	Angiomatous	
	Microcystic	
	Secretory	
	Lymphoplasmacyte-rich	
	Metaplastic	
Grade II—Atypical	Chordoid	Low
	Clear cell (intracranial)	
	Atypical	
Grade III—Anaplastic	Papillary	High
	Rhabdoid	
	Anaplastic (malignant)	
	Any subtype or grade with high proliferation index and/or brain invasion	

Mixed Pleomorphic Adenoma. Mixed pleomorphic cell tumors (mucosal adenomas) are the more common of the two subtypes, remain localized to the middle ear and mastoid cavity, and rarely involve the facial nerve or otic capsule. They are believed to arise from poorly differentiated basement membrane cells within the normal middle ear mucosa. These tumors have a male sex predeliction and usually present between the ages of 20 and 60 years. The most common presenting symptom is conductive hearing loss, however otorrhea, tinnitus, and facial nerve weakness may be present. Physical examination reveals a middle ear mass, and CT scans often confirm a soft tissue mass confined to the middle ear and mastoid in the absence of bone destruction.

Because of the tumor location, presenting symptoms, and imaging characteristics, these lesions are commonly mistaken for chronic otitis media with cholesteatoma, and the diagnosis is often made during mastoidectomy. Mixed pleomorphic tumors are benign and less aggressive than their papillary counterpart, however there is still a high recurrence rate after excision. Therefore, complete resection with long-term follow-up is recommended as the treatment of choice.[113]

INNER EAR

Papillary Adenoma (Endolymphatic Sac Tumor)

In contrast to mixed pleomorphic adenomas, papillary tumors occur less frequently, often extend to the petrous apex and intracranially, and occur more commonly in women. These tumors have historically been termed Heffner tumors, low-grade papillary adenocarcinoma, and aggressive papillary middle ear tumors. Histologically, these tumors demonstrate papillary and cystic components, a single- to double-layered epithelial lining, and adjacent bony infiltration. The glandular features suggest that the origin of these tumors is the endolymphatic sac.[112,113] There is an association with von-Hippel-Lindau disease (VHL) and approximately 11% of patients with this disease have endolymphatic sac tumors.[114] Clinically, these tumors usually present with hearing loss, vertigo, tinnitus, and facial nerve paralysis. CT scans typically reveal a mass located near the vestibular aqueduct (between the sigmoid sinus and IAC), bony destruction, and erosion toward the vestibule (Figure 18).

Treatment for these tumors is surgical excision with adequate margins. Resection is often accomplished via the TL approach, however more extensive approaches may be necessary for medial or intracranial extension. These tumors are quite vascular, therefore preoperative angiography and embolization may play a role in larger tumors. There is a 90% cure rate after gross total surgical removal, and radiation therapy has been used after incomplete removal. It has been estimated that 50% of tumors respond favorably to radiation, however the small number of patients makes interpretation of the results difficult.[112,113,115,116]

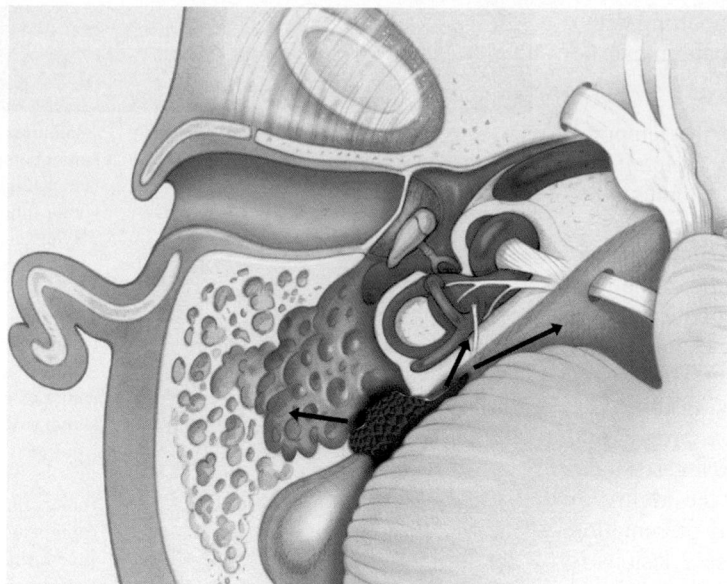

Figure 18 An early papillary adenomatous lesion (endolymphatic sac tumor) that may grow laterally into the mastoid, posteriorly into the posterior cranial fossa, or along the vestibular aqueduct to the inner ear (*arrows*). (Published with permission, copyright © 2000 R.K. Jackler, MD.)

Intralabyrinthine Schwannoma

Intralabyrinthine schwannomas originate within the inner ear and are differentiated from the more common VS which can secondarily invade the labyrinth. They can occur in a wide variety of locations within the labyrinth including the scala tympani within the basal turn of the cochlea, modiolus, ampulla of the lateral semicircular canal, and utricle.[117] Clinical manifestations depend on the location of the tumor and can include cochlear symptoms (hearing loss, tinnitus) or vestibular symptoms (vertigo, disequilibrium). Physical examination is often normal, but may reveal nystagmus during a vertiginous episode or a middle ear mass in large lesions. CT scans are usually normal, but MRI may reveal the absence of fluid density on T2-weighted sequences and an enhancing lesion postgadolinium within the cochlea and/or vestibule. Asymptomatic patients are often monitored with serial imaging as operative management universally results in a complete hearing loss. Surgical approaches include a standard TL approach for lesions within the vestibule and a transotic approach for lesions involving the cochlea.

JUGULAR FORAMEN

Paragangliomas (Glomus Tumor)

Paragangliomas, also known as glomus tumors, are the most common tumor of the middle ear and the second most common tumor of the temporal bone. Jugulotympanic paragangliomas have a clear female predilection, and they typically occur in the fifth decade of life.

Pathogenesis. Paraganglia are a part of the neuroendocrine system, and they migrate in association with the ganglia of the autonomic nervous system.[118] Extra-adrenal paraganglia, with the exception of the carotid bodies which serve a chemoreceptive function, normally undergo progressive involution until puberty. Tumors of these paraganglia are divided into 2 groups: (1) *adrenal* paragangliomas known as pheochromocytomas and (2) *extra-adrenal* paragangliomas located in the abdomen, chest, and head and neck regions. Head and neck paragangliomas are classified based on anatomic location and include the carotid body, jugulotympanic, vagal, laryngeal, nasal, and orbital paragangliomas.[119] Interestingly, the terms *glomus* was mistakenly attached to these tumors when it was believed their origin was similar to true glomus (arteriovenous) complexes.

The majority of glomus tumors appear sporadically, but a small proportion of these tumors (<10%) may be hereditary and associated with tumor syndromes including multiple endocrine neoplasia type II (MEN2), VHL, neurofibromatosis type 1 (NF1), and familial paraganglioma.[120] Familial paraganglioma is linked to 3 of the 4 mitochondrial complex II peptides namely the succinate dehydrogenase subunit B (SDHB), subunit C (SDHC) and subunit D (SDHD), and may have either maternal or paternal modes of mitochondrial inheritance.[121] Multicentricity occurs in approximately 10% of spontaneous tumors and increases to 30% in familial tumors.[122] Glomus tumors contain chief cells, which are part of the diffuse neuroendocrine system (DNES), and have the potential to produce catecholamines creating a physiologic response similar to pheochromocytomas. This is quite rare in head and neck paragangliomas (<3%) but may occur more frequently in familial syndromes. Finally, these tumors are histologically benign, although up to 4% may become metastatic.[122]

Pathology. Glomus tumors are typically reddish-purple, vascular, and lobulated masses. Histologically, a characteristic *zellballen* pattern in which nests of chief cells (type I) are surrounded by sustenacular cells (type II or supporting cells) in a highly vascular stroma. The pattern can be enhanced with silver staining.

Classification. Paragangliomas in the temporal bone can be divided into *glomus tympanicum* and *glomus jugulare* (Figure 19). Glomus tympanicum primarily involve the tympanic cavity and arise along the course of Jacobson nerve. Glomus jugulare arise from the dome of the jugular bulb and involve structures of the jugular foramen. These tumors are further characterized according to either the Fisch[123] or Glasscock-Jackson[124] classification systems (Table 12). Glomus tumors typically have slow, progressive growth spreading via paths of least resistance; however, advanced lesions have the ability to invade cranial nerves. The clinical presentation and operative management of these 2 lesions is quite different, therefore they will be discussed individually below. Another variant, the *glomus vagale*, arises beneath the skull base in proximity to the vagus nerve (X) and may involve the temporal bone via retrograde spread through the jugular foramen.

Investigations. The imaging characteristics of both glomus tympanicum and glomus jugulare on CT, MRI, and angiography have been discussed above. Angiography is used in glomus jugulare and should be deferred until the preoperative period so that both diagnostic and therapeutic (embolization) measures can occur in the single study. Angiography can reveal arterial supply, degree of vascularity, degree of arteriovenous shunting, evidence of major venous sinus occlusion, and identify multicentric lesions. Magnetic resonance angiography (MRA) and MRV are flow-sensitive MRI scans that can also be used. MRV in particular can reveal occlusion of the venous system and identify involvement of the jugular bulb.

Patients presenting at a young age, family history of paragangliomas, multicentric tumors, secreting tumors (symptoms of catecholamine release), or malignant tumors are all suggestive of possible hereditary disease.[121] In these cases,

Table 12 Classification of Jugulotympanic Paragangliomas			
Classification System	Type	Description
Glassock-Jackson[124]	Type I	Small mass limited to the promontory
Glomus tympanicum	Type II	Tumor completely filling the middle ear space
	Type III	Tumor filling the middle ear and extending into the mastoid
	Type IV	Tumor filling the middle ear, extending into the mastoid or through the tympanic membrane to fill the external auditory canal; may also extend anterior to the internal carotid artery
Glasscock-Jackson[125]	Type I	Small tumor involving the jugular bulb, middle ear, and mastoid
Glomus jugulare	Type II	Tumor extending under the internal auditory canal; may have intracranial extension
	Type III	Tumor extending into the petrous apex; may have intracranial extension
	Type IV	Tumor extending beyond the petrous apex into the clivus or infratemporal fossa; may have intracranial extension
Fisch[123]	Type A	Tumors limited to the middle ear cleft
Glomus tumors	Type B	Tumors limited to the tympanomastoid area with no infralabyrinthine compartment involvement
	Type C	Tumors involving the infralabyrinthine compartment of the temporal bone and extending into the petrous apex
	Type D1	Tumors with an intracranial extension less than 2 cm in diameter
	Type D2	Tumors with an intracranial extension greater than 2 cm in diameter

a detailed physical examination including fundoscopic examination for retinal angiomas (seen in VHL) and skin examination for café au lait spots (associated with NF1) should be performed. Urinalysis for hematuria, urine catecholamines, serum calcium, and serum calcitonin can also be measured for occult functioning tumors, VHL, and MEN2. Multcentricity can be screened with a CT scan (extending from mandible to bladder) and I[123] meta-iodobenzylguanidine (MIBG) scintigraphy.[121] Finally, specific genetic testing can also be ordered for the various familial syndromes.

Glomus Tympanicum The clinical presentation of glomus tympanicum includes pulsatile tinnitus (76%), hearing loss (conductive 52%, mixed 17%, sensorineural 5%), aural pressure/fullness (18%), vertigo/dizziness (9%), external canal bleeding (7%), and headache (4%).[125] Brown sign is seen clinically when a pulsatile, purple-red middle ear mass blanches with positive pneumatic otos-

copy.[126] Although frequently mentioned in the literature, it is of little clinical value.

Glomus tymanicum tumors are primarily treated with surgical excision. Small lesions that are limited to the mesotympanum on otoscopy and CT scan can be approached transcanal. A tympanomeatal flap is used to expose the middle ear, and the EAC can be drilled inferiorly to gain access to the hypotympanum. Larger lesions are exposed with a postauricular incision and an extended facial-recess approach. As these tumors are quite vascular, lasers and bipolar cautery are often used during resection for hemostasis. Complete tumor removal is achieved in >90% of cases and closure of the air-bone gap is normally achieved.[125] A small percentage of patients may experience some sensorineural hearing loss after resection.

Glomus Jugulare In contrast to glomus tympanicum tumors, which produce early symptoms as they grow in the confines of the middle ear, glomus jugulare tumors can often remain asymptomatic for years. Growth into the middle ear occurs in 70% of patients and causes the most common symptoms of pulsatile tinnitus, hearing loss, otalgia, and aural fullness.[125] Growth in the jugular foramen causes dysfunction of the lower cranial nerves and presents as hoarseness, dysphagia, and shoulder weakness. Vertigo, facial weakness, and headache can also occur. The hypoglossal nerve (XII) is unlikely to be involved, however its dysfunction is indicative of extensive disease.[6]

The imaging characteristics have already been discussed. On angiography, the primary arterial supply is from the ascending pharyngeal artery, although larger tumors may also have supply from other branches of the external carotid artery, the internal carotid artery, and the vertebral-basilar system.

Treatment of glomus jugulare tumors is more complicated than that for glomus tympanicum

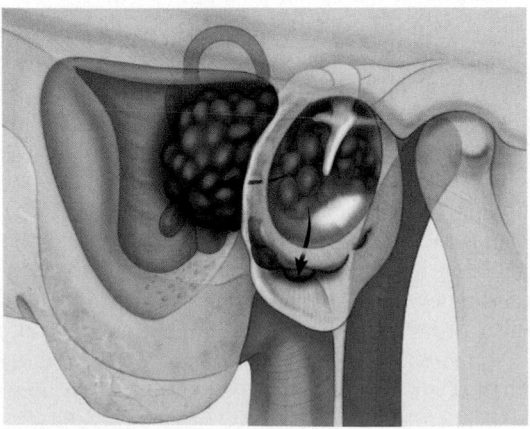

(A)

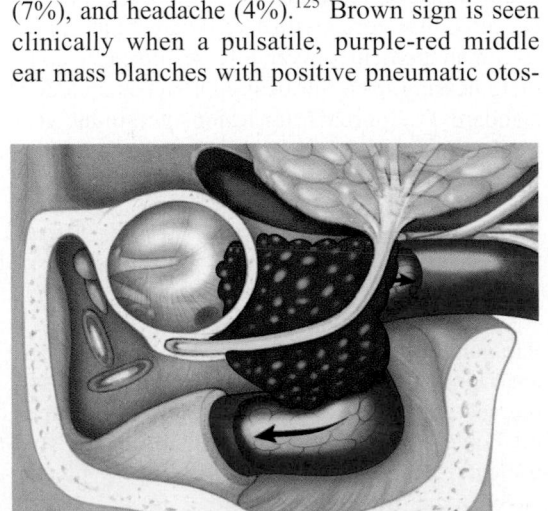

(B)

Figure 19 Paragangliomas. (A) Glomus tympanicum with extension superiorly into epitympanum, posteriorly through the aditus ad antrum, and adjacent to the facial nerve. The dome of the jugular bulb and caroticojugular spine are still intact. (B) Glomus jugulare with extension into the posterior cranial fossa and upward erosion into the hypotympanum. (Published with permission, copyright © 2000 R.K. Jackler, MD.)

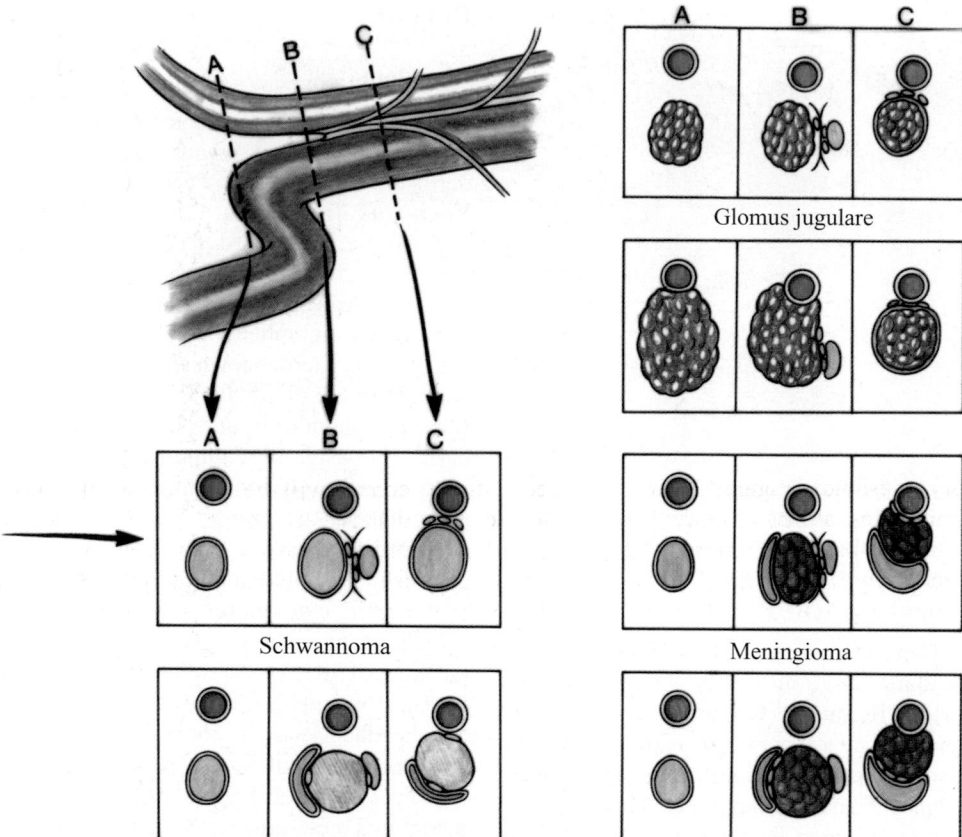

Figure 20 The relation of the ninth, tenth, and eleventh cranial nerves to the carotid artery and jugular vein vary in their course through the skull base and into the upper neck, as illustrated in this axial schematic. The surgical angle of view is indicated by the arrow. At the level of the apex of the jugular bulb (A), the internal carotid artery and internal jugular vein are widely separated. The lower cranial nerves lie entirely below this plane. At the mid-jugular foramen level (B), the carotid and jugular are separated by a tapering osseous spine (thicker superiorly), and the nerves are lined up on a fibroosseous septum, which partitions the jugular (pars venosa) from the channel for the inferior petrosal sinus (pars nervosa). At the extracranial orifice of the jugular foramen (C), the carotid and jugular lie in close approximation, with the lower nerves sandwiched between them. In schwannomas, the nerve of origin determines the tumor's relation to the uninvolved nerves. In meningiomas, the site of origin determines the tumor's relation to the lower cranial nerves. Clival meningiomas penetrate the medial aspect of the jugular foramen, whereas most petrous lesions enter laterally. (Published with permission, copyright © 1996 R.K. Jackler, MD.)

tumors because of the proximity to critical neural and vascular structures (Figure 20). Depending on the size and location of the tumor, surgical techniques include a canal-wall up or canal-wall down mastoidectomy, a translabyrinthine approach, an infratemporal fossa approach, a transcochlear approach, or a combination of the above. In our practice, we prefer the transjugular approach which involves a lateral craniotomy traversing the jugular fossa combined with resection of the sigmoid sinus and jugular bulb, which have often been occluded by disease.[127] Gaining control of the vessels above and below the lesion is a key surgical principle to have vascular control during tumor removal. Facial rerouting may be required in large tumors with erosion of the carotid canal in which additional anterior exposure is necessary. However, the Fallopian bridge technique, in which bone is removed circumferentially around the descending facial nerve while leaving it in situ, can often be used to provide sufficient exposure to the tumor and adjacent structures in these cases.[128] New postoperative cranial nerve deficits occur in 25 to 50% of cases, with larger lesions having a higher incidence of neuropathy. Rehabilitation with speech therapy, vocal cord medialization, and facial nerve reanimation are often effective. Patients must be counseled on the risks of surgery as well as the risks of functional deficits if the tumor is left untreated. Using contemporary techniques, surgical resection has a low recurrence rate, a low disability rate, and good functional outcomes.[125,128–130]

Stereotacic radiosurgery or radiotherapy is indicated in incompletely resected tumors or those with positive surgical margins. Certain centers also advocate radiation therapy as first-line therapy for advanced tumors or for elderly patients. Two large review articles found similar control rates, recurrence rates, and morbidity between surgery and radiation.[131,132] However, the lack of long-term follow-up and the tendency to include unresectable tumors in the radiation group may bias these results. The risk of radiation-induced malignancies must be considered, especially when treating younger patients with a long expected lifespan.[133]

Jugular Foramen Schwannoma

JFS are the second most common jugular foramen tumor, but are relatively rare with only 200 cases in the world's literature.[134] JFS represent 3% of all intracranial schwannomas and 1 of the larg-

est series in the literature only had 14 patients.[135] JFS can arise from cranial nerves IX to XI and determining the nerve of origin is often quite difficult. The anatomy of the surrounding structures in the jugular foramen region can vary, as is represented in Figure 20. Three growth patterns of JFS have been described: (1) distal jugular foramen tumors can expand inferiorly out of the skull base, (2) proximal jugular foramen tumors can expand into the posterior fossa, and (3) middle jugular foramen tumors can expand into bone or become bilobed.[136] Symptoms and signs related to lower cranial neuropathies predominate with cranial nerve X (63%), IX (55%), XI (41%), and XII (36%) being most commonly affected.[6] Other less common and signs symptoms include cranial nerve V and VII dysfunction, hemifacial spasm, nystagmus, ataxia, and papilledema.[135]

The imaging characteristics of schwannomas have been discussed, and JFS can be differentiated from paragangliomas by the absence of irregular bony destruction and flow voids. The treatment options include surgery and radiation. The surgical approaches, complications, and rationale are similar to those used for glomus jugulare tumors.

FACIAL NERVE

Facial Nerve Schwannoma

FNS are rare and can occur along the entire course of the facial nerve. Intratemporal FNS are more common than either intracranial or extratemporal (parotid) FNS. The presenting symptoms for intracranial FNS are similar to VS and include sensorineural hearing loss (100%), tinnitus (80%), and vestibular dysfunction (60%).[137] Extratemporal FNS typically present as a parotid mass.

Intratemporal FNS can originate from the geniculate ganglion and horizontal and vertical segments, in the IAC, and from the labyrinthine segment in descending frequency (Figure 21). Contiguous portions can be involved and, uncommonly, FNS may display multicentricity described as a "string of pearls."[138] In a large review of over 200 cases, the most common presenting symptoms and signs were facial paralysis (73%), hearing loss (50%), tinnitus (13%), ear canal mass (13%), and pain (11%).[139] Facial paralysis most commonly presents as a slow, progressive palsy with accompanying hyperfunction (facial twitch or hemifacial spasm). Although 14% of FNS can mimic Bell palsy and present with a sudden paralysis, patients with FNS will usually have progressively more severe episodes of palsy that is characteristic of these tumors.[139] Any patient with a suspected Bell palsy without functional recovery after 3 months should undergo an MRI scan to rule out a tumor. Hearing loss resulting from FNS is often conductive due to prolapse of the tumor onto the ossicles. These tumors can be seen on otoscopy in one-third of cases and may be found incidentally during an exploratory tympanotomy for conductive hearing loss. As a

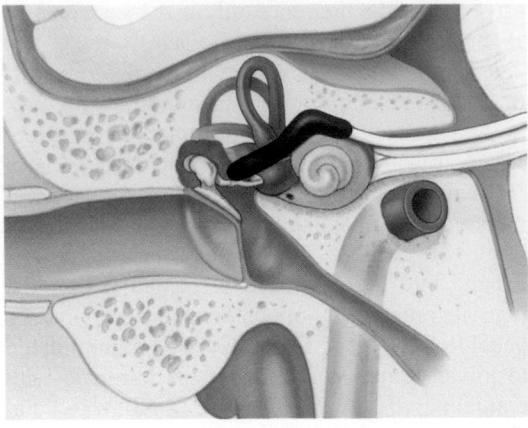

(A)

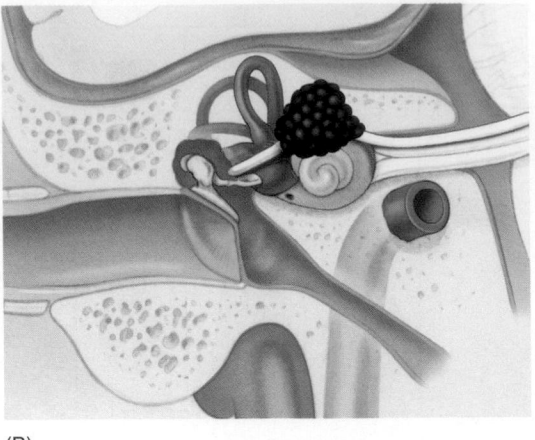

(B)

Figure 21 Facial nerve tumors. (A) Facial nerve schwannoma with proximal margin at the geniculate ganglion and distal extension through the tympanic segment of the facial nerve. There is impingement upon the ossicular chain. (B) Geniculate hemangioma with extension into the tympanic segment of the facial nerve but not distal to the cochleariform process. The middle cranial fossa floor is virtually always dehiscent overlying the tumor. (Published with permission, copyright © 2000 R.K. Jackler, MD.)

biopsy of FNS often results in facial paralysis, imaging should be undertaken in suspected cases to establish the diagnosis. Sensorineural hearing loss can also occur secondary to cochlear invasion, and vertigo can result from a labyrinthine fistula. The imaging characteristics of FNS have been discussed above.

The treatment of FNS focuses on preserving or restoring facial function. The best outcome after excision and replacement with an interposition graft is a House-Brackmann Grade 3 or 4, with good eye closure, but severe synkinesis. Therefore, with normal or near-normal facial function, observation with serial physical examination, MRI scans, and electroneuronography (ENOG) is recommended. There is no consensus as to when operative management should be undertaken. Some authors feel that if significant degeneration occurs (>50%), further observation may result in the inability to recover useful function with an interposition graft, and surgical intervention should be performed.[140] In our practice, we routinely wait until the facial function is worse than would be expected with an interposition graft (House-Brackmann Grade III) before operating. In small series, wide decompression of the FNS in certain cases may achieve a postoperative House-Brackmann Grade I or II with lasting preservation over time, however further data are needed to evaluate this procedure.[141]

It is rarely possible to resect an intratemporal FNS while preserving the facial nerve. More commonly, an interposition graft from either the greater auricular nerve or sural nerve is needed. A tympanomastoid approach is used to access FNS in the horizontal and descending portions of the nerve. Involvement of the IAC, labyrinthine segment, or geniculate ganglion requires the addition of an MF approach to expose these regions while preserving the integrity of the inner ear.

Geniculate Ganglion Hemangioma

Hemangiomas of the temporal bone are extremely rare, and when present, they most commonly occur at the geniculate ganglion or within the

IAC.[142] There are approximately 50 case reports of geniculate ganglion hemangioma to date in the world's literature. On gross examination, hemangiomas are rubbery red or purple masses with vascular spaces. The histologic appearance of geniculate hemangiomas is not characteristic of the more common hemangiomas found elsewhere in the body. In 1 report, geniculate ganglion hemangiomas with thin-walled vascular spaces were classified as hemangiomas and those with thick-walled vascular spaces as hamartomas or vascular malformations.[143] Osseous hemangiomas contain spicules of bone, and this has been variably seen within geniculate hemangiomas. The most common clinical manifestations of 17 reported cases were facial paralysis/paresis (100%), facial spasm/twitching (18%), tinnitus (18%), and pain (11%).[142] Anatomically, these lesions arise from the geniculate ganglion with limited extension into the middle ear and middle cranial fossa (Figure 21). Imaging characteristics have been discussed previously, and, unless bony changes typical for an "ossifying hemangioma" are seen, differentiation from an FNS on preoperative imaging can be difficult.

Management of geniculate hemangiomas is similar to that of FNS. Geniculate hemangiomas can produce symptoms when small, compared to FNS which are usually much larger when dysfunction becomes apparent. Therefore, early operative intervention is recommended when a geniculate hemangioma begins to cause facial dysfunction. An MF approach is usually required due to the anatomic location of these lesions. As geniculate hemangiomas were initially felt to cause symptoms through extraneural compression, early reports suggested resection was possible while leaving the facial nerve intact and recommended early surgical intervention to preserve facial nerve continuity.[144,145] A recent report of 6 cases, however, has revealed cases of facial nerve infiltration and encasement on pathologic examination.[146] Therefore, conservative management using the guidelines outlined for FNS have been recommended.

CLIVUS

Chordoma

Chordomas are neoplasms that arise from the primitive notochord, which is formed from ectoderm during the third week of development.[147] Remnants from both the cranial and sacral end of the notochord frequently persist after the period of regression; however, they rarely become a true neoplasm. The 3 major sites for chordomas are sphenooccipital (35%), vertebral (15%), and sacrococcygeal (50%).[148] Pathologically, they are divided into 3 types: conventional (classic), chondroid, and dedifferentiated (atypical).[149] Grossly, these tumors are gray and gelatinous with no obvious capsule. On microscopic examination, the primary cell types are stellate, intermediate, and physaliphorous. Immunohistochemistry reveals that these tumors are reactive to vimentin, cytokeratin, and S-100 protein.[150]

Chordomas are rare, occur in the fourth to fifth decades of life, preferentially affect males, and have a slow, insidious growth pattern.[151] Diplopia and headache are the most common presenting symptoms, and abducens nerve (VI) palsy was the most common deficit.[151] A number of other symptoms including lower cranial nerve dysfunction, cerebellar symptoms, and nasopharyngeal obstruction can occur. Imaging characteristics of chordomas have been discussed, however conventional angiography and MRA can be useful for preoperative planning and embolization.

The treatment of choice for chordoma is total or near-total surgical resection, although this is difficult given the tumor's location and surrounding neurovascular anatomy (Figure 22). Radical removal is associated with better long-term survival and decreased recurrence rates.[147] The surgical approach is chosen based on the particular tumor and often several different approaches may be necessary. Midline approaches can be used for lesions located medial to both hypoglossal canals and options include transoral-transpalatal, transmaxillary-transnasal, transphenoidal, and endoscopic transphenoidal.[147] Lateral approaches for tumors primarily on one side include the Fisch infratemporal fossa type B, frontal-temporal/lateral facial, extended lateral transcondylar, and transcervical-transmandibular.[147] An overview of the Fisch infratemporal fossa approaches in given in Figure 23.

Radiation is typically used for palliation or recurrence, however some have advocated high-dose irradiation immediately following radical surgery.[152] Recent reports examining both conventional radiotherapy and photon-beam radiotherapy as adjuvant treatment have shown palliation of pain, but no significant increase in survival.[153,154] Long-term prognosis is poor with 10-year progression-free survival rates of 15 to 55%, despite the manner of treatment.[147]

Chondrosarcoma

Chondrosarcoma is a rare primary malignancy of bone, potentially arising from any bone

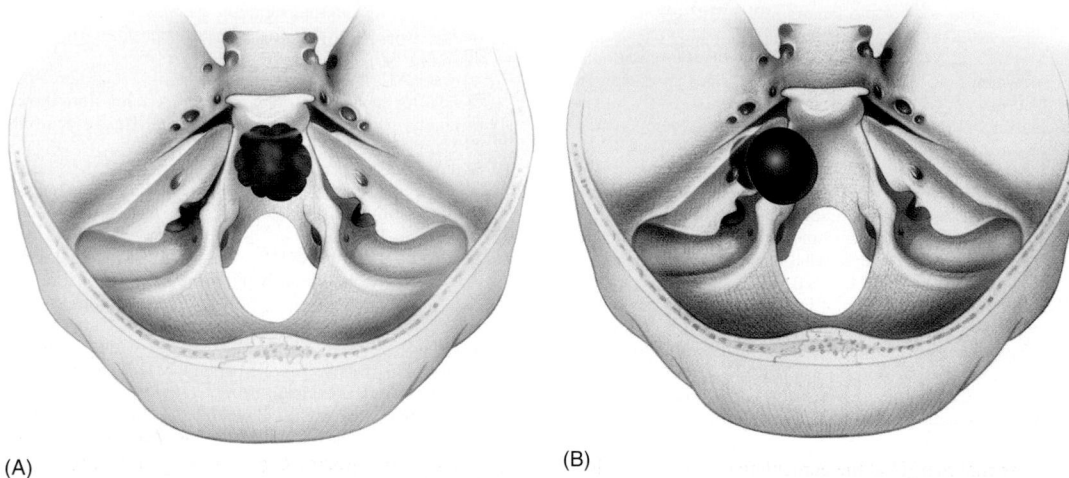

(A)   (B)

Figure 22 (A) Chordoma of the mid-clivus. The tumor is entirely contained within the clivus and symmetrically straddles the midline. (B) Chondrosarcoma of the petroclival junction. Origination from the fibrocartilage of foramen lacerum explains this classic location for these paramedian chondrasarcomas of the skull base. (Published with permission, copyright © 2000 R.K. Jackler, MD.)

developing from endochondral ossification, accounting for approximately one-third of all primary malignancies of bone.[155] Intracranial chondrosarcomas account for less than 0.2% of all intracranial tumors.[156] The cell of origin for chondrosarcomas has yet to be definitively proven, but it has long been suggested that chondrosarcomas arise from persistent chondrocytes at the petroclival junction. The development of chondrosarcoma from these embryologic rests of cartilage helps to explain the characteristic site of origin off the midline in contrast to skull base chordomas (see Figure 22B).

Grossly, chondrosarcomas tend to be gray, avascular, and gelatinous similar to chordomas. Chondrosarcomas can be divided into 5 histologic subtypes: conventional, myxoid, mesenchymal, clear cell, and dedifferentiated.[149] The expected natural history is correlated with histologic grade and well-differentiated tumors have better overall prognosis than poorly differentiated ones. Immunohistochemistry is important to differentiate chordoma from chondrosarcoma; whereas both lesions test positive to S100 and vimentin staining, only chordomas test positive for cytokeratin and epithelial membrane antigen.[157]

These tumors are slow growing, have an insidious onset, occur in the fourth to fifth decades of life, and have no sex predilection.[151,158] The most common symptoms include diplopia, headache, hearing loss, imbalance, visual field loss, and facial numbness.[159] The overall incidence of metastases is approximately 15%, with the rate increasing to 70% for poorly differentiated (Grade III) tumors.[151,158,160] The imaging characteristics of chondrosarcoma and the differentiation from chordoma have already been discussed above.

Surgical excision is the cornerstone of treatment. A variety of skull base approaches outlined above can be used to gain access to the petrous apex and clivus for tumor resection, depending on the size of the lesion, its location, and the existence of preexisting cranial nerve deficits.[161] Although the soft nature of these tumors facilitates dissection, complete resection is still difficult due to vital neural and vascular structures in the vicinity. Tumor recurrence has been associated with larger tumors, residual disease on postoperative imaging, younger patients, and lack of adjuvant radiotherapy.[159] The role of radiotherapy in chondrosarcoma remains to be fully defined, but it appears to be beneficial in many cases.[159,162] When surgical resection is not possible, stereotactic radiation has been advocated as the sole treatment in patients with small tumors.[163] The overall expected 5-year control rate with multimodality therapy is approximately 95%.[162]

CONCLUSIONS

The differential diagnosis of skull base neoplasms is broad, and a systematic approach is needed for the accurate diagnosis and management of patients with these tumors. Modern imaging modalities have allowed early identification of these tumors that may produce minimal signs until they are far advanced. A multidisciplinary skull base team is needed to manage patients with these tumors effectively with various microsurgical approaches. A thorough knowledge of alternate treatment options is essential to counsel these patients effectively.

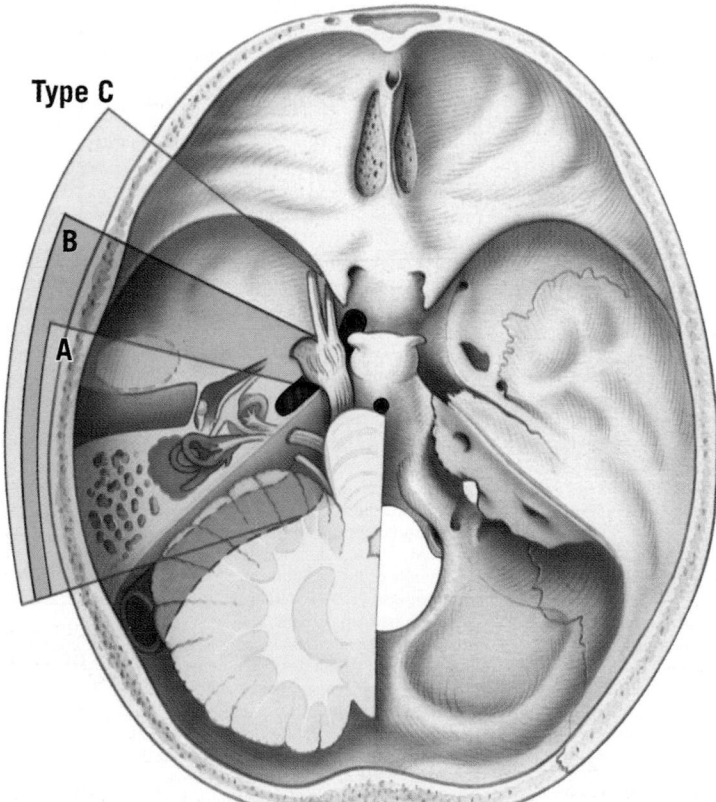

Figure 23 The infratemporal fossa approach, as described by Fisch, has 3 primary varieties. Type A is for access to the jugular foramen region, mandibular fossa, and posterior part of the infratemporal fossa. Type B is for the apical petrous bone and clivus, including the intrapetrous course of the internal carotid artery. Type C is an anterior extension used for exposure of the infratemporal fossa, pterygopalatine fossa, parasellar regions, and nasopharynx. (Published with permission, copyright © 1996 R.K. Jackler, MD.)

REFERENCES

1. Panse R. Glioms des Akustikus. Arch f Ohrenh 1904;61: 251–5.
2. Borchardt M. Uber operationen in der hinteren schadelgrube incl. der operationen der tumoren am kleinhirnbruckenwinkel. Arch f klin Chir 1906;81:386–432.
3. Quix F. Ein Acusticustumor. Arch f Ohrenh 1911;84:252–3.
4. House WF. Surgical exposure of the internal auditory canal and its contents through the middle cranial fossa. Laryngoscope 1961;71:1363–85.
5. Brackmann DE, Green JD. Cerebellopontine angle tumors. In: Bailey BJ, editor. Head & Neck Surgery—Otolaryngology. Philadelphia: Lippincott Williams & Wilkins; 2001. p. 1899–917.
6. Lustig LR, Jackler RK. The variable relationship between the lower cranial nerves and jugular foramen tumors: Implications for neural preservation. Am J Otol 1996;17:658–68.
7. Jackler RK, Driscoll CLW, editors. Tumors of the Ear and Temporal Bone. Philadelphia, Lippincott Williams & Wilkins; 2000.
8. Brackmann DE, Bartels LJ. Rare tumors of the cerebellopontine angle. Otolaryngol Head Neck Surg 1980;88: 555–9.
9. Lo W, Hovsepian M. Imaging of the cerebellopontine angle. In: Jackler RK, Brackmann DE, editors. Neurotology. Philadelphia: Elsevier-Mosby; 2005. p. 349–82.
10. Harnsberger HR. Diagnostic Imaging—Head & Neck. Salt Lake City: Amirsys; 2004.
11. Paz-Fumagalli R, Daniels DL, Millen SJ, et al. Dural "tail" associated with an acoustic schwannoma in MR imaging with gadopentetate dimeglumine. AJNR 1991;12:1206.

12. Wilms G, Lammens M, Marchal G, et al. Prominent dural enhancement adjacent to nonmeningiomatous malignant lesions on contrast-enhanced MR images. AJNR 1991; 12:761–4.
13. Lalwani AK, Jackler RK. Preoperative differentiation between meningioma of the cerebellopontine angle and acoustic neuroma using MRI. Otolaryngol Head Neck Surg 1993;109:88–95.
14. Valavanis A, Schubiger O, Hayek J, Pouliadis G. CT of meningiomas on the posterior surface of the petrous bone. Neuroradiology 1981;22:111–21.
15. Steffey DJ, De Filipp GJ, Spera T, Gabrielsen TO. MR imaging of primary epidermoid tumors. J Comp Assist Tomogr 1988;12:438–40.
16. Tsuruda JS, Chew WM, Moseley ME, Norman D. Diffusion-weighted MR imaging of the brain: Value of differentiating between extraaxial cysts and epidermoid tumors. AJR 1990;155:1059–65; discussion 1066–8.
17. Larson TL, Wong ML. Primary mucocele of the petrous apex: MR appearance. AJNR 1992;13:203–4.
18. Rosenberg RA, Hammerschlag PE, Cohen NL, et al. Cholesteatoma vs. cholesterol granuloma of the petrous apex. Otolaryngol Head Neck Surg 1986;94:322–7.
19. Fan G, Curtin HD. Imaging of the lateral skull base. In: Jackler RK, Brackmann DE, editors. Neurotology. Philadelphia: Elsevier Mosby; 2005. p. 383–418.
20. Mukherji SK, Albernaz VS, Lo WW, et al. Papillary endolymphatic sac tumors: CT, MR imaging, and angiographic findings in 20 patients. Radiology 1997;202:801–8.
21. Mahaley MS, Jr, Mettlin C, Natarajan N, et al. Analysis of patterns of care of brain tumor patients in the United States: A study of the Brain Tumor Section of the AANS and the CNS and the Commission on Cancer of the ACS. Clin Neurosurg 1990;36:347–52.
22. Frohlich AM, Sutherland GR. Epidemiology and clinical features of vestibular schwannoma in Manitoba, Canada. Canadian J Neurol Sci 1993;20:126–30.
23. Nestor JJ, Korol HW, Nutik SL, Smith R. The incidence of acoustic neuromas. Arch Otolaryngol Head Neck Surg 1988;114:680.
24. Tos M, Stangerup SE, Caye-Thomasen P, et al. What is the real incidence of vestibular schwannoma? Arch Otolaryngol Head Neck Surg 2004;130:216–20.
25. Hardy M, Crowe SJ. Early asymptomatic acoustic tumor. Report of six cases. Arch Surg 1936;32:292–301.
26. Selesnick SH, Jackler RK. Atypical hearing loss in acoustic neuroma patients. Laryngoscope 1993;103:437–41.
27. Lin D, Hegarty JL, Fischbein NJ, Jackler RK. The prevalence of "incidental" acoustic neuroma. Arch Otolaryngol Head Neck Surg 2005;131:241–4.
28. Rubenstein AE. Neurofibromatosis. A review of the clinical problem. Ann NY Acad Sci 1986;486:1–13.
29. Sterkers JM, Perre J, Viala P, Foncin JF. The origin of acoustic neuromas. Acta Otolaryngol 1987;103:427–31.
30. Xenellis JE, Linthicum FH, Jr. On the myth of the glial/schwann junction (Obersteiner-Redlich zone): Origin of vestibular nerve schwannomas. Otol Neurotol 2003;24:1.
31. Clemis JD, Ballad WJ, Baggot PJ, Lyon ST. Relative frequency of inferior vestibular schwannoma. Arch Otolaryngol Head Neck Surg 1986;112:190–4.
32. Gronholm M, Teesalu T, Tyynela J, et al. Characterization of the NF2 protein merlin and the ERM protein ezrin in human, rat, and mouse central nervous system. Mol Cell Neurosci 2005;28:683–93.
33. Rong R, Tang X, Gutmann DH, Ye K. Neurofibromatosis 2 (NF2) tumor suppressor merlin inhibits phosphatidylinositol 3-kinase through binding to PIKE-L. Proc Natl Acad Sci USA 2004;101:18200–5.
34. Kuo TC, Jackler RK, Wong K, et al. Are acoustic neuromas encapsulated tumors? Otolaryngol Head Neck Surg 1997;117:606–9.
35. Wilkinson JS, Reid H, Armstrong GR. Malignant transformation of a recurrent vestibular schwannoma. J Clin Pathol 2004;57:109–10.
36. Jackler RK, Pfister MHF. Acoustic neuroma (vestibular schwannoma). In: Jackler RK, Brackmann DE, editors. Neurotology. Philadelphia: Elsevier Mosby; 2005. p. 727–82.
37. Selesnick SH, Johnson G. Radiologic surveillance of acoustic neuromas. Am J Otol 1998;19:846–9.
38. Bederson JB, von Ammon K, Wichmann WW, Yasargil MG. Conservative treatment of patients with acoustic tumors. Neurosurgery 1991;28:646–50; discussion 650–1.
39. Nedzelski JM, Schessel DA, Pfleiderer A, et al. Conservative management of acoustic neuromas. Otolaryngol Clin N Am 1992;25:691–705.
40. Cushing H. Tumors of the Nervus Acusticus and the Syndrome of the Cerebellopontine Angle. Philadelphia: W. B. Saunders; 1917.
41. Selesnick SH, Jackler RK, Pitts LW. The changing clinical presentation of acoustic tumors in the MRI era. Laryngoscope 1993;103:431–6.
42. Matthies C, Samii M. Management of 1000 vestibular schwannomas (acoustic neuromas): Clinical presentation. Neurosurgery 1997;40:1–9; discussion 9–10.
43. Hoffman RA, Brookler KH, Reich EJ. Trigeminal neuralgia symptomatic of acoustic neuroma. NY State J Med 1979;79:1436–8.
44. Neary WJ, Newton VE, Laoide-Kemp SN, et al. A clinical, genetic and audiological study of patients and families with unilateral vestibular schwannomas. II. Audiological findings in 93 patients with unilateral vestibular schwannomas. J Laryngol Otol 1996;110:1120–8.
45. Committee on Hearing and Equilibrium guidelines for the evaluation of hearing preservation in acoustic neuroma (vestibular schwannoma). Otolaryngol Head Neck Surg 1995;113:179–80.
46. Khrais T, Sanna M. Hearing preservation surgery in vestibular schwannoma. J Laryngol Otol 2006;120: 366–70.
47. Fraysse B, Fraysse MJE, Bounaix MJ. Acoustic neuroma with normal ABR. In: Tos M, Thomsen J, editors. Proceedings of the First International Conference on Acoustic Neuroma. Amsterdam: Kugler; 1992. p. 91–5.
48. Ruckenstein MJ, Cueva RA, Morrison DH, Press G. A prospective study of ABR and MRI in the screening for vestibular schwannomas. Am J Otol 1996;17:317–20.
49. Wilson DF, Hodgson RS, Gustafson MF, et al. The sensitivity of auditory brainstem response testing in small acoustic neuromas. Laryngoscope 1992;102:961–4.
50. Weiss MH, Kisiel DL, Bhatia P. Predictive value of brainstem evoked response in the diagnosis of acoustic neuroma. Otolaryngol Head Neck Surg 1990;103:583–5.
51. Walsted A, Neilsen KB, Salomon G, et al. Auditory brainstem response in the diagnosis of acoustic neuroma. In: Tos M, Thomsen J, editors. Proceedings of the First International Conference on Acoustic Neuroma. Amsterdam: Kugler; 1992. p. 87–90.
52. Olsson JE, Barrs DM, Krueger WO, Gibbons DR. Use of receiver operating curves in the design of diagnostic strategies for retrocochlear lesions. In: Tos M, Thomsen J, editors. Proceedings of the First International Conference on Acoustic Neuroma. Amsterdam: Kugler; 1992. p. 77–81.
53. Brackmann DE, Owens RM, Friedman RA, et al. Prognostic factors for hearing preservation in vestibular schwannoma surgery. Am J Otol 2000;21:417–24.
54. Ferber-Viart C, Laoust L, Boulud B, et al. Acuteness of preoperative factors to predict hearing preservation in acoustic neuroma surgery. Laryngoscope 2000;110:145–50.
55. Matthies C, Samii M. Management of vestibular schwannomas (acoustic neuromas): The value of neurophysiology for evaluation and prediction of auditory function in 420 cases. Neurosurgery 1997;40:919–29; discussion 929–30.
56. Shelton C, Brackmann DE, House WF, Hitselberger WE. Acoustic tumor surgery. Prognostic factors in hearing conservation. Arch Otolaryngol Head Neck Surg 1989; 115:1213–6.
57. Slattery WH, III, Brackmann DE, Hitselberger W. Middle fossa approach for hearing preservation with acoustic neuromas. Am J Otol 1997;18:596–601.
58. Dornhoffer JL, Helms J, Hoehmann DH. Hearing preservation in acoustic tumor surgery: Results and prognostic factors. Laryngoscope 1995;105:184–7.
59. Driscoll CLW. Vestibular schwannoma (acoustic neuroma). In: Jackler RK, Driscoll CLW, editors. Tumors of the Ear and Temporal Bone. Philadelphia: Lippincott Williams and Wilkins; 2000. p. 172–218.
60. Irving RM, Jackler RK, Pitts LH. Hearing preservation in patients undergoing vestibular schwannoma surgery: Comparison of middle fossa and retrosigmoid approaches. J Neurosurg 1998;88:840–5.
61. Satar B, Jackler RK, Oghalai J, et al. Risk-benefit analysis of using the middle fossa approach for acoustic neuromas with >10 mm cerebellopontine angle component. Laryngoscope 2002;112:1500–6.
62. Yates PD, Jackler RK, Satar B, et al. Is it worthwhile to attempt hearing preservation in larger acoustic neuromas? Otol Neurotol 2003;24:460–4.
63. Domb GH, Chole RA. Anatomical studies of the posterior petrous apex with regard to hearing preservation in acoustic neuroma removal. Laryngoscope 1980;90:1769–76.
64. Kartush JM, Telian SA, Graham MD, Kemink JL. Anatomic basis for labyrinthine preservation during posterior fossa acoustic tumor surgery. Laryngoscope 1986;96: 1024–8.
65. Laine T, Johnsson LG, Palva T. Surgical anatomy of the internal auditory canal. A temporal bone dissection study. Acta Otolaryngol 1990;110:78–84.
66. Driscoll CL, Jackler RK, Pitts LH, Banthia V. Is the entire fundus of the internal auditory canal visible during the middle fossa approach for acoustic neuroma? Am J Otol 2000;21:382–8.
67. Lalwani AK, Butt FY, Jackler RK, et al. Facial nerve outcome after acoustic neuroma surgery: A study from the era of cranial nerve monitoring. Otolaryngol Head Neck Surg 1994;111:561–70.
68. Soumekh B, Levine SC, Haines SJ, Wulf JA. Retrospective study of postcraniotomy headaches in suboccipital approach: Diagnosis and management. Am J Otol 1996;17:617–9.
69. Schessel DA, Rowed DW, Nedzelski JM, Feghali JG. Postoperative pain following excision of acoustic neuroma by the suboccipital approach: Observations on possible cause and potential amelioration. Am J Otol 1993;14: 491–4.
70. Harner SG, Beatty CW, Ebersold MJ. Headache after acoustic neuroma excision. Am J Otol 1993;14:552–5.
71. Harner SG, Beatty CW, Ebersold MJ. Impact of cranioplasty on headache after acoustic neuroma removal. Neurosurgery 1995;36:1097–9; discussion 1099–100.
72. Levo H, Pyykko I, Blomstedt G. Postoperative headache after surgery for vestibular schwannoma. Ann Otol Rhinol Laryngol 2000;109:853–8.
73. Ruckenstein MJ, Harris JP, Cueva RA, et al. Pain subsequent to resection of acoustic neuromas via suboccipital and translabyrinthine approaches. Am J Otol 1996;17:620–4.
74. Becker SS, Jackler RK, Pitts LH. Cerebrospinal fluid leak after acoustic neuroma surgery: A comparison of the translabyrinthine, middle fossa, and retrosigmoid approaches. Otol Neurotol 2003;24:107–12.
75. Mangham CA. Complications of translabyrinthine vs. suboccipital approach for acoustic tumor surgery. Otolaryngol Head Neck Surg 1988;99:396–400.
76. Smith PG, Leonetti JP, Grubb RL. Management of cerebrospinal fluid otorhinorrhea complicating the retrosigmoid approach to the cerebellopontine angle. Am J Otol 1990; 11:178–80.
77. Roberson JB, Jr, Brackmann DE, Hitselberger WE. Acoustic neuroma recurrence after suboccipital resection: Management with translabyrinthine resection. Am J Otol 1996;17:307–11.
78. Wackym PA, King WA, Poe DS, et al. Adjunctive use of endoscopy during acoustic neuroma surgery. Laryngoscope 1999;109:1193–201.
79. Glasscock ME, III, Hays JW, Minor LB, et al. Preservation of hearing in surgery for acoustic neuromas. J Neurosurg 1993;78:864–70.
80. Brookes GB, Woo J. Hearing preservation in acoustic neuroma surgery. Clin Otolaryngol Allied Sci 1994;19: 204–14.
81. Arriaga MA, Luxford WM, Berliner KI. Facial nerve function following middle fossa and translabyrinthine acoustic tumor surgery: A comparison. Am J Otol 1994;15: 620–4.
82. Rohit, Piccirillo E, Jain Y, et al. Preoperative predictive factors for hearing preservation in vestibular schwannoma surgery. Ann Otol Rhinol Laryngol 2006;115:41–6.
83. Arts HA, Telian SA, El-Kashlan H, Thompson BG. Hearing preservation and facial nerve outcomes in vestibular schwannoma surgery: Results using the middle cranial fossa approach. Otol Neurotol 2006;27:234–41.
84. Samii M, Matthies C. Management of 1000 vestibular schwannomas (acoustic neuromas): Hearing function in 1000 tumor resections. Neurosurgery 1997;40:248–60; discussion 260–2.
85. Cohen NL, Lewis WS, Ransohoff J. Hearing preservation in cerebellopontine angle tumor surgery: The NYU experience 1974–1991. Am J Otol 1993;14:423–33.
86. Betchen SA, Walsh J, Post KD. Long-term hearing preservation after surgery for vestibular schwannoma. J Neurosurg 2005;102:6–9.
87. Rowed DW, Nedzelski JM. Hearing preservation in the removal of intracanalicular acoustic neuromas via the retrosigmoid approach. J Neurosurg 1997;86:456–61.
88. Sanna M, Zini C, Gamoletti R. Hearing preservation: A critical review of the literature. In: Tos M, Thomsen J, editors. Proceedings of the First International Conference on Acoustic Neuroma. Amsterdam: Kugler; 1992. p. 631–8.
89. Bloch DC, Oghalai JS, Jackler RK, et al. The fate of the tumor remnant after less-than-complete acoustic neuroma resection. Otolaryngol Head Neck Surg 2004;130:104–12.
90. Ferlito A, Devaney KO, Rinaldo A. Primary extracranial meningioma in the vicinity of the temporal bone: A benign lesion which is rarely recognized clinically. Acta Otolaryngol 2004;124:5–7.
91. Lusis E, Gutmann DH. Meningioma: An update. Curr Opin Neurol 2004;17:687–92.

92. Nager GT, Heroy J, Hoeplinger M. Meningiomas invading the temporal bone with extension to the neck. Am J Otolaryngol 1983;4:297–324.

93. Modan B, Baidatz D, Mart H, et al. Radiation-induced head and neck tumours. Lancet 1974;1:277–9.

94. Lesch KP, Gross S. Estrogen receptor immunoreactivity in meningiomas. Comparison with the binding activity of estrogen, progesterone, and androgen receptors. J Neurosurg 1987;67:237–43.

95. Irving RM. Meningiomas of the internal auditory canal and cerebellopontine angle. In: Jackler RK, Driscoll CLW, editors. Tumors of the Ear and Temporal Bone. Philadelphia: Lippincott Williams & Wilkins; 2000.

96. Langman AW, Jackler RK, Althaus SR. Meningioma of the internal auditory canal. Am J Otol 1990;11:201–4.

97. Morris JWS. The nervous system. In: Robbins S, Cotran R, Kumar V, editors. Pathologic Basis of Disease. Philadelphia: WB Saunders; 1984. p. 1370–436.

98. Kleihues P, Louis DN, Scheithauer BW, et al. The WHO classification of tumors of the nervous system. J Neuropathol Exp Neurol 2002;61:215–25; discussion 226–9.

99. Singh A, Selesnick SH. Meningiomas of the posterior fossa and skull base. In: Jackler RK, Brackmann DE, editors. Neurotology. Philadelphia: Elsevier Mosby; 2005. p. 792–840.

100. Roberti F, Sekhar LN, Kalavakonda C, Wright DC. Posterior fossa meningiomas: Surgical experience in 161 cases. Surg Neurol 2001;56:8–20; discussion 20–1.

101. Selesnick SH, Nguyen TD, Gutin PH, Lavyne MH. Posterior petrous face meningiomas. Otolaryngol Head Neck Surg 2001;124:408–13.

102. Thompson LD, Bouffard JP, Sandberg GD, Mena H. Primary ear and temporal bone meningiomas: A clinicopathologic study of 36 cases with a review of the literature. Mod Pathol 2003;16:236–45.

103. Laird FJ, Harner SG, Laws ER, Jr, Reese DF. Meningiomas of the cerebellopontine angle. Otolaryngol Head Neck Surg 1985;93:163–7.

104. Molony TB, Brackmann DE, Lo WW. Meningiomas of the jugular foramen. Otolaryngol Head Neck Surg 1992;106:128–36.

105. Simpson D. The recurrence of intracranial meningiomas after surgical treatment. J Neurol Neurosurg Psychiatry 1959;20:22–39.

106. Mirimanoff RO, Dosoretz DE, Linggood RM, et al. Meningioma: Analysis of recurrence and progression following neurosurgical resection. J Neurosurg 1985;62:18–24.

107. Liscak R, Kollova A, Vladyka V, et al. Gamma knife radiosurgery of skull base meningiomas. Acta Neurochir 2004;91:65–74.

108. Milker-Zabel S, Zabel A, Schulz Ertner D, et al. Fractionated stereotactic radiotherapy in patients with benign or atypical intracranial meningioma: Long-term experience and prognostic factors. Int J Rad Oncol Biol Phys 2005;61:809–16.

109. Tonn JC. Microneurosurgery and radiosurgery—An attractive combination. Acta Neurochir 2004;91:103–8.

110. Moffat DA, Chiossone-Kerdel JA, Da Crus M. Squamous cell carcinoma. In: Jackler RK, Driscoll CLW, editors. Tumors of the Ear and Temporal Bone. Philadelphia: Lippincott Williams and Wilkins; 2000. p. 67–83.

111. Morton RP, Stell PM, Derrick PP. Epidemiology of cancer of the middle ear cleft. Cancer 1984;53:1612–7.

112. Benecke JE, Jr, Noel FL, Carberry JN, et al. Adenomatous tumors of the middle ear and mastoid. Am J Otol 1990;11:20–6.

113. Batsakis JG. Adenomatous tumors of the middle ear. Ann Otol Rhinol Laryngol 1989;98:749–52.

114. Manski TJ, Heffner DK, Glenn GM, et al. Endolymphatic sac tumors. A source of morbid hearing loss in von Hippel-Lindau disease. JAMA 1997;277:1461–6.

115. Heffner DK. Low-grade adenocarcinoma of probable endolymphatic sac origin A clinicopathologic study of 20 cases. Cancer 1989;64:2292–302.

116. Li JC, Brackmann DE, Lo WW, et al. Reclassification of aggressive adenomatous mastoid neoplasms as endolymphatic sac tumors. Laryngoscope 1993;103:1342–8.

117. Green JD. Intralabyrinthine schwannomas. In: Jackler RK, Driscoll CLW, editors. Tumors of the Ear and Temporal Bone. Philadelphia: Lippincott Williams and Wilkins; 2000. p. 146–55.

118. Gulya AJ. The glomus tumor and its biology. Laryngoscope 1993;103:7–15.

119. Friedman RA, Brackmann DE. Jugulotympanic paragangliomas. In: Jackler RK, Driscoll CLW, editors. Tumors of the Ear and Temporal Bone. Philadelphia: Lippincott Williams and Wilkins; 2000. p. 343–60.

120. Bertherat J, Gimenez-Roqueplo AP. New insights in the genetics of adrenocortical tumors, pheochromocytomas and paragangliomas. Hormone and metabolic research. Hormonund Stoffwechselforschung 2005;37:384–90.

121. Benn DE, Richardson AL, Marsh DJ, Robinson BG. Genetic testing in pheochromocytoma- and paraganglioma-associated syndromes. Ann NY Acad Sci 2006;1073: 104–11.

122. Arriaga MA. Paraganglioma (glomus tympanicum). In: Jackler RK, Driscoll CLW, editors. Tumors of the Ear and Temporal Bone. Philadelphia: Lippincott Williams and Wilkins; 2000. p. 112–27.

123. Oldring D, Fisch U. Glomus tumors of the temporal region: Surgical therapy. Am J Otol 1979;1:7–18.

124. Jackson CG. Skull base surgery. Am J Otol 1981;3:161–71.

125. Woods CI, Strasnick B, Jackson CG. Surgery for glomus tumors: The Otology Group experience. Laryngoscope 1993;103:65–70.

126. Brown L. Glomus jugulare tumor of the middle ear: Clinical aspects. Laryngoscope 1953;63:281–92.

127. Oghalai JS, Leung MK, Jackler RK, McDermott MW. Transjugular craniotomy for the management of jugular foramen tumors with intracranial extension. Otol Neurotol 2004;25:570–9; discussion 579.

128. Pensak ML, Jackler RK. Removal of jugular foramen tumors: The fallopian bridge technique. Otolaryngol Head Neck Surg 1997;117:586–91.

129. House JW, Fayad JN. Glomus jugulare. Ear Nose Throat J 2004;83:800.

130. Jackson CG, Kaylie DM, Coppit G, Gardner EK. Glomus jugulare tumors with intracranial extension. Neurosurg Focus 2004;17:E7.

131. Carrasco V, Rosenman J. Radiation therapy of glomus jugulare tumors. Laryngoscope 1993;103:23–7.

132. Gottfried ON, Liu JK, Couldwell WT. Comparison of radiosurgery and conventional surgery for the treatment of glomus jugulare tumors. Neurosurg Focus 2004;17:E4.

133. Lustig LR, Jackler RK, Lanser MJ. Radiation-induced tumors of the temporal bone. Am J Otol 1997;18:230–5.

134. Doersten PG. Jugular foramen schwannoma. In: Jackler RK, Driscoll CLW, editors. Tumors of the Ear and Temporal Bone. Philadelphia: Lippincott Williams and Wilkins; 2000. p. 374–87.

135. Tan LC, Bordi L, Symon L, Cheesman AD. Jugular foramen neuromas: A review of 14 cases. Surg Neurol 1990;34:205–11.

136. Kaye AH, Hahn JF, Kinney SE, et al. Jugular foramen schwannomas. J Neurosurg 1984;60:1045–53.

137. Dort JC, Fisch U. Facial nerve schwannomas. Skull Base Surg 1991;1:51–6.

138. Janecka IP, Conley J. Primary neoplasms of the facial nerve. Plast Reconstr Surg 1987;79:177–85.

139. Lipkin AF, Coker NJ, Jenkins HA, Alford BR. Intracranial and intratemporal facial neuroma. Otolaryngol Head Neck Surg 1987;96:71–9.

140. Schaitkin BM. Facial nerve schwannoma. In: Jackler RK, Driscoll CLW, editors. Tumors of the Ear and Temporal Bone. Philadelphia: Lippincott Williams and Wilkins; 2000. p. 276–89.

141. Angeli SI, Brackmann DE. Is surgical excision of facial nerve schwannomas always indicated? Otolaryngol Head Neck Surg 1997;117:S144–7.

142. Arts HA. Geniculate hemangioma. In: Jackler RK, Driscoll CLW, editors. Tumors of the Ear and Temporal Bone. Philadelphia: Lippincott Williams and Wilkins; 2000. p. 290–302.

143. Mangham CA, Carberry JN, Brackmann DE. Management of intratemporal vascular tumors. Laryngoscope 1981;91:867–76.

144. Friedman O, Neff BA, Willcox TO, et al. Temporal bone hemangiomas involving the facial nerve. Otol Neurotol 2002;23:760–6.

145. Shelton C, Brackmann DE, Lo WW, Carberry JN. Intratemporal facial nerve hemangiomas. Otolaryngol Head Neck Surg 1991;104:116–21.

146. Isaacson B, Telian SA, McKeever PE, Arts HA. Hemangiomas of the geniculate ganglion. Otol Neurotol 2005;26:796–802.

147. Gantz BJ, Perry BP. Skull base chordoma. In: Jackler RK, Driscoll CLW, editors. Tumors of the Ear and Temporal Bone. Philadelphia: Lippincott Williams and Wilkins; 2000. p. 332–42.

148. Mabrey R. Chordoma: A study of 150 cases. Am J Cancer 1935;25:501–17.

149. Barnes L, Kapadia SB. The biology and pathology of selected skull base tumors. J Neuro-Oncol 1994;20:213–40.

150. Coffin CM, Swanson PE, Wick MR, Dehner LP. An immunohistochemical comparison of chordoma with renal cell carcinoma, colorectal adenocarcinoma, and myxopapillary ependymoma: A potential diagnostic dilemma in the diminutive biopsy. Mod Pathol 1993;6:531–8.

151. Volpe NJ, Liebsch NJ, Munzenrider JE, Lessell S. Neuroophthalmologic findings in chordoma and chondrosarcoma of the skull base. Am J Ophthalmol 1993;115:97–104.

152. al-Mefty O, Borba LA. Skull base chordomas: A management challenge. J Neurosurg 1997;86:182–9.

153. Catton C, O'Sullivan B, Bell R, et al. Chordoma: Long-term follow-up after radical photon irradiation. Radiother Oncol 1996;41:67–72.

154. Keisch ME, Garcia DM, Shibuya RB. Retrospective long-term follow-up analysis in 21 patients with chordomas of various sites treated at a single institution. J Neurosurg 1991;75:374–7.

155. Blevins NH, Heilman CB. Lesions of the petrous apex. In: Jackler RK, Brackmann DE, editors. Neurotology. Philadelphia: Elsevier Mosby; 2005. p. 1107–24.

156. Berkmen YM, Blatt ES. Cranial and intracranial cartilaginous tumours. Clin Radiol 1968;19:327–33.

157. Wojno KJ, Hruban RH, Garin-Chesa P, Huvos AG. Chondroid chordomas and low-grade chondrosarcomas of the craniospinal axis. An immunohistochemical analysis of 17 cases. Am J Surg Pathol 1992;16:1144–52.

158. Coltrera MD, Googe PB, Harrist TJ, et al. Chondrosarcoma of the temporal bone. Diagnosis and treatment of 13 cases and review of the literature. Cancer 1986;58:2689–96.

159. Oghalai JS, Buxbaum JL, Jackler RK, McDermott MW. Skull base chondrosarcoma originating from the petroclival junction. Otol Neurotol 2005;26:1052–60.

160. Lau DP, Wharton SB, Antoun NM, et al. Chondrosarcoma of the petrous apex. Dilemmas in diagnosis and treatment. J Laryngol Otol 1997;111:368–71.

161. Blevins NH, Jackler RK, Kaplan MJ, Gutin PH. Combined transpetrosal-subtemporal craniotomy for clival tumors with extension into the posterior fossa. Laryngoscope 1995;105:975–82.

162. Castro JR, Linstadt DE, Bahary JP, et al. Experience in charged particle irradiation of tumors of the skull base: 1977–1992. Int J Rad Oncol Biol Phys 1994;29: 647–55.

163. Muthukumar N, Kondziolka D, Lunsford LD, Flickinger JC. Stereotactic radiosurgery for chordoma and chondrosarcoma: Further experiences. Int J Rad Oncol Biol Phys 1998;41:387–92.

36

Stereotactic Radiosurgery and Radiotherapy

P. Ashley Wackym, MD
Christina L. Runge-Samuelson, PhD
Linda Grossheim, MD

It was in 1951 that Dr Lars Leksell first conceived of what is now known as gamma knife radiosurgery. As articulated, he envisioned "the delivery of a single, high dose of radiation to a small and critically located intracranial volume through the intact skull." He first thought that this would be accomplished via a center of arc principle; and, in fact, the early attempts at accomplishing this utilized a single arc across which radiation was delivered to the intracranial target. The first gamma knife unit (Elekta Instrument AB, Stockholm, Sweden) was installed in Stockholm, Sweden in 1968, and it was not until 1987 that the first gamma knife (model U) was installed at the University of Pittsburgh. The gamma knife model B was first introduced in 1996, and this is the unit which is most used throughout the United States. The gamma knife model C was introduced in 1999, and the biggest change associated with this unit was that there is an automatic positioning system (APS). Other than this, the unit is quite similar to the model B, and both contain 201 radioactive isotope cobalt 60 (^{60}Co) sources and beam channels. When the collimator helmet is locked into position, the 201 openings of the collimator helmet coincide with the cobalt sources. There is a shielded chamber within which the ^{60}Co sources are contained, and stainless steel shielding doors protect the treatment room from the ^{60}Co sources. There is a treatment couch with an adjustable mattress that slides into the gamma knife unit together with the collimator helmet and the patient. Figure 1 schematically shows the orientation of the components of the gamma knife model 4C, while Figure 2 shows the overall appearance of the gamma knife model 4C unit. During 2008, a completely redesigned gamma knife unit, named Perfexion, is being introduced (Figure 3). It uses 192 ^{60}Co sources, has a single collimator helmet with variable diameters, and can treat lesions within the entire head and neck, down to the level of the clavicles (Figure 4).

Whereas stereotactic radiosurgery can be applied to a wide range of skull base diseases, patients with vestibular schwannomas are most frequently treated with this modality. This form of treatment, just as is the case with microsurgery, has advantages and disadvantages, which must be thoroughly discussed with the patient.[1,2] For the patient, it is appealing to undergo an

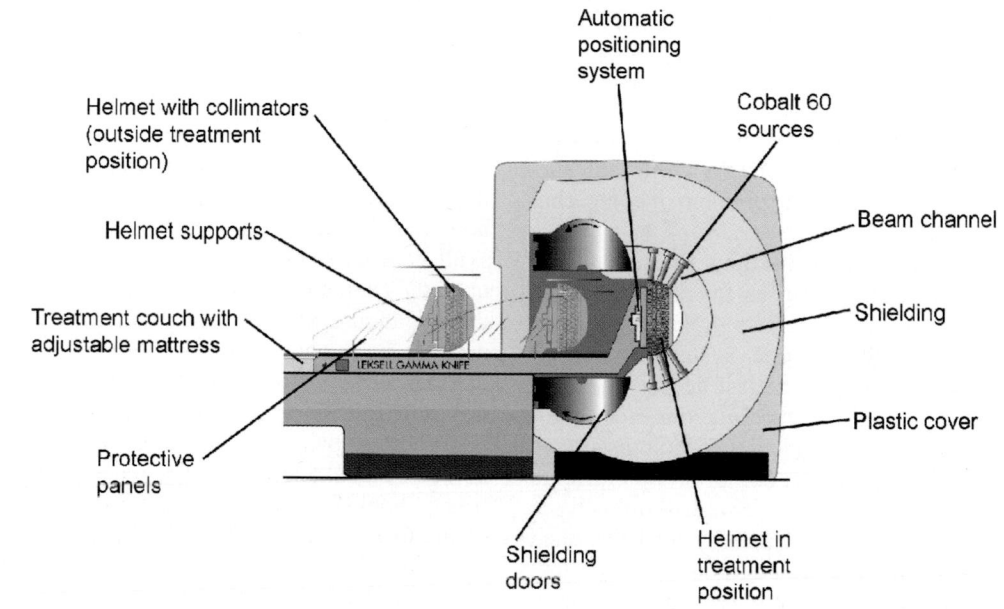

Figure 1 Gamma knife radiosurgery. Schematic illustration of the gamma knife model 4C which utilizes the automatic positioning system. (Published with permission, copyright © 2007, Elekta Instrument AB, Stockholm, Sweden.)

outpatient procedure rather than microsurgical management that requires a much longer period of care (Figure 5). As an example, with a typical vestibular schwannoma managed via microsurgery, surgery takes place on the day of admission, and an overnight stay in the intensive care unit is customary. This is subsequently followed by 5 to 7 days of hospitalization and a post discharge recovery of 2 to 4 weeks. This is in sharp contrast to gamma knife radiosurgery, which is performed on an outpatient basis. Clear demonstration of tumor control and, with current methods, low cranial nerve morbidity have been published. Unfortunately, there are sometimes advertised claims that are misleading to patients. It should be noted that magnetic resonance images (MRIs) at different levels artificially change the apparent size of a tumor. There is a critical need for accurate measurement and reporting of tumor volume over time. Competing therapeutic systems have made available to the public images in which the size of the tumor following treatments has been misrepresented. In fact, the MRI used to illustrate

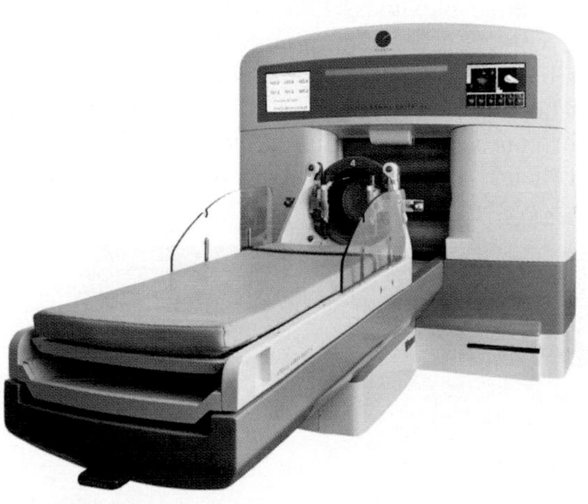

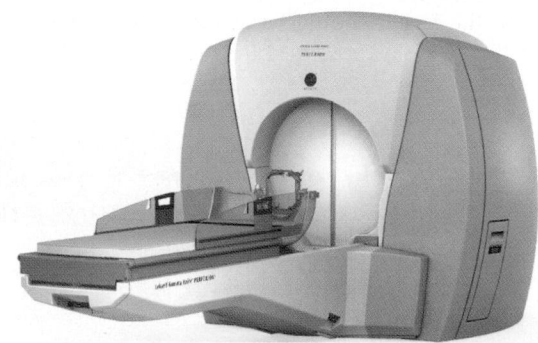

Figure 2 Gamma knife model 4C. (Published with permission, copyright © 2007, Elekta Instrument AB, Stockholm, Sweden.)

Figure 3 Gamma knife Perfexion. (Published with permission, copyright © 2007, Elekta Instrument AB, Stockholm, Sweden.)

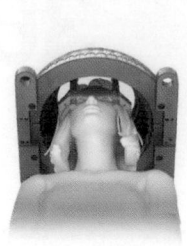 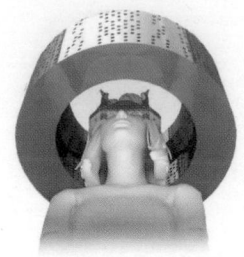

Gamma Knife 4C   **Gamma Knife Perfexion**

Figure 4 Comparison of the collimator helmets used with the gamma knife model 4C and the Perfexion. Note the increased diameter and length of the perfexion helmet which allows treatment down to the level of the clavicles and treatment of patients with large heads or laterally located lesions. (Published with permission, copyright © 2007, P.A. Wackym, MD.)

"tumor shrinkage" in the *New England Journal Medicine* article reporting outcomes of a cohort of patients treated with gamma knife radiosurgery suffers from the same problem of comparing different levels.[1]

Several medical institutions throughout the world offer training courses for physicians and radiation physicists at centers that have invested in the Leksell Stereotactic System or Leksell Gamma Knife. During the last decade and one-half, more than 1,500 neurosurgeons, neurotologists, physicists, and radiation oncologists have attended these educational programs. Elekta Instrument AB (Stockholm, Sweden) offers basic training courses as well as advanced technical workshops. The courses consist of didactic lectures, observation of patient treatment, and practical hands-on training. Additionally, all new installations of Leksell Gamma Knife are accompanied by a 1-week on-site start-up training, in which the neurotologists, neurosurgeons, radiation oncologists, and physicists constituting the gamma knife treatment team are responsible to participate.

FRAME ATTACHMENT

General Principles

The procedure used for the attachment of the stereotactic head frame is in sterotactic radiosurgery is of utmost importance. Two general principles been developed for gamma knife radiosurgery. When attaching the frame to the patient's head, first, the target should be as close to the center of the frame as possible, and, second, the frame

attachment should be stable. These principles should be addressed from the beginning of the frame attachment. In lateral targets, such as vestibular schwannomas, there is a potential risk for collisions between the collimator helmet of the gamma knife unit and the opposite lateral side of the frame, the posts, or the fixation screws. Similarly, other targets that are located in the posterior fossa can result in frame collisions with the anterior post. It is due to these factors that the target should ideally be located in the center of the frame.

The method of anesthesia used during frame placement is surgeon and patient dependent. In our program, either sedation with versed and fentanyl or monitored anesthesia with propofol, followed by injection of local anesthetic at the pin sites, is used.

Tools and Orientation

Absolute stability of the frame is required, including the necessity of avoiding screw fixation in bone flaps, cranioplasty materials, burr holes, or skull defects, since treatment accuracy is based upon the geometry of the stereotactic frame coordinates. Figure 6A shows the usual array of tools used for the frame attachment, including a variety of screw lengths, to be able to choose those ideally suited for the individual location of the post along with a pair of screwdrivers and generally 20 mL of local anesthesia. The placement of the frame should begin with an accurate orientation of the location of the target within the patient's head. Ideally, the target should be located within the fiducial range and placed centrally within the frame, thereby avoiding later collisions with the collimator helmet and granting sufficient accuracy for the stereotactic target definition.

Localization and Placement

After the surgeon is oriented regarding the location of the target, the stereotactic frame is preliminarily attached by using external auditory canal support pins, a Velcro band, or a stereotactic fiducial box. When using a fiducial box to facilitate frame placement, it is important to use the MRI fiducial box, rather than the CT or angiography fiducial box, since this is the smallest of the three plexiglass fiducial boxes (Figure 6B). Complete asymmetric frame placements are possible and do not impair the accuracy of imaging. The frame can either be shifted from side to side or can be moved as far as possible to the front or back. When the frame is successfully placed,

meaning that the position of the target is as close as possible to the center of the frame, the nurse or assistant holds and stabilizes the stereotactic frame with two hands. The frame is stabilized against the patient, thereby providing a constant position in the optimal localization. The surgeon can now adjust the length of the posts to suit the patient's head as well as to give stability to the frame while being careful to avoid bone flaps, cranioplasty materials, burr holes, or skull defects.

Post and Screw Attachment and Measurements

For targets in the posterior fossa, a low position of the anterior posts can sometimes help avoid anterior collisions with the collimator helmet, particularly if the patient has a large head. After the posts are adjusted and firmly fixed to the frame, local anesthesia is injected by inserting the needles through the holes provided for the screws. The screws can now be inserted. The goal of this step is to attain a preliminary frame fixation in the desired position. Fixation with diagonally opposing screws provides the best stability without changing the desired frame position. If the frame has to be shifted to 1 side, apply the longest screws first, thereby defining the desired distance of the target to the frame. The frame is now preliminarily stabilized with the screws on the patient's head (Figure 6C). The length of the screws is considered to be ideal if the tips do not extend more than 8 to 10 mm off the posts; however, this surgeon prefers to limit this projection to 4 to 6 mm. If the screw extends further, exchange the existing screw with a screw that has the ideal length for the position of the head. The length of the 4 posts is determined by measuring from the base of the frame to the tip of each post. In addition to that, the length of the screws that extend over the posts is measured. These measurements are required for the frame and skull section in Leksell GammaPlan treatment planning software. The stereotactic frame attachment is completed once the volume of the head has been measured using the plastic bubble, simulating the relationship of the frame to the collimator helmet (Figure 6D). In critical positions, collisions can sometimes be avoided by using the curved posts in the anterior position in certain patients with posterior fossa tumors.

RADIATION PHYSICS

Introduction

Small and well-delineated cerebral targets can under certain circumstances be treated selectively with narrow, high energy radiation beams. In the Leksell Gamma Knife, this radiation is emitted by 201 sources of ^{60}Co. Healthy brain tissue located between skull and target can be relatively spared provided that a suitable irradiation technique has been chosen and the target is small. Depending on the histologic type of target and

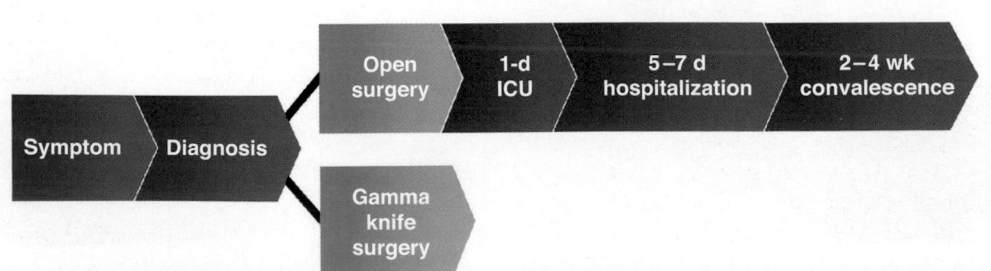

Figure 5 Schematic outline of treatment timelines of microsurgical resection compared to gamma knife radiosurgery of a vestibular schwannoma. (Published with permission, copyright © 2007, P.A. Wackym, MD.)

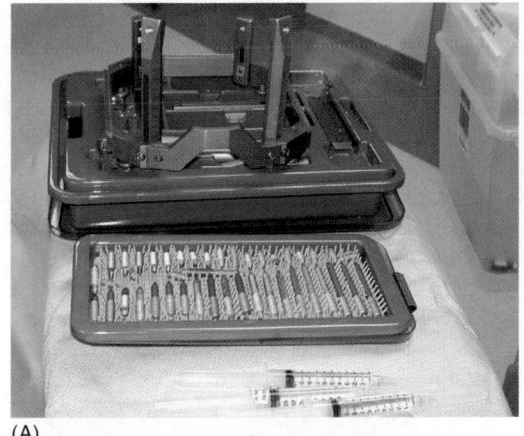
(A)

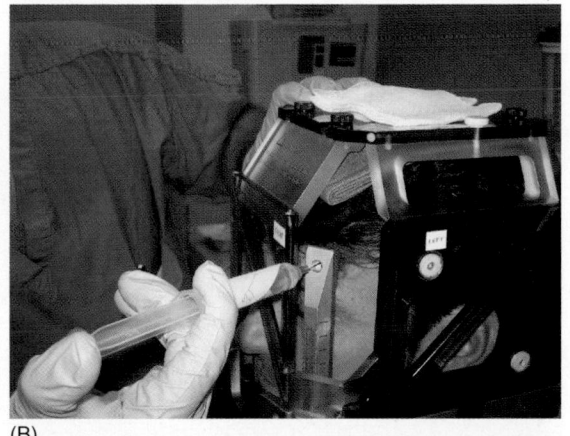
(B)

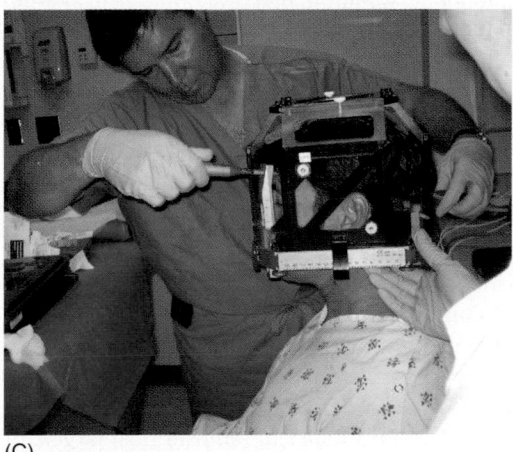
(C)

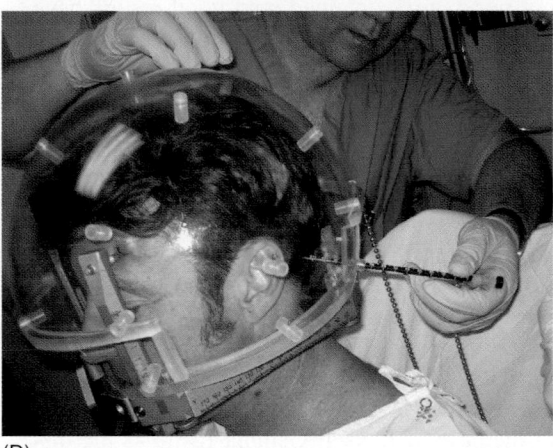
(D)

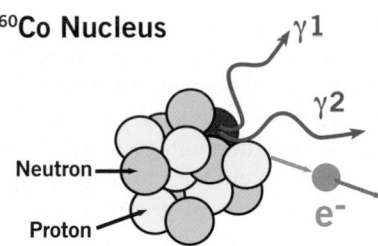

Figure 7 Gamma knife radiosurgery. The ^{60}Co-nucleus transforms spontaneously into a proton and an electron. Through this process it is transformed into a new element, ^{60}Ni, the nucleus of which instantly emits 2 gamma (γ) photons. (Published with permission, copyright © 2007, P.A. Wackym, MD.)

Figure 6 (A) Stereotactic headframe at the time of assembly. Pins used for fixation prior to imaging, treatment planning, and gamma knife radiosurgery are seen in the foreground. (B) With a towel placed on the vertex of the head, the magnetic resonance imaging (MRI) fiducial box is balanced on the head while topical anesthetic is infiltrated at the pin sites. (C) While the headframe and attached plastic MRI fiducial box is secured to the skull using the pins, an assistant stabilizes the assembly in place. Note the tightening of pins in opposing vectors. (D) After the frame has been secured to the skull, measurements are taken through defined entrance points in a plastic dome representing the size and position of the collimator helmet relative to the frame, head and face. These values are incorporated into the treatment planning software to create a wire grid representing the patient's head. The post height and pin length are also measured and are inputted into the treatment planning software. These values are used in the calculations used to predict collisions between the collimator helmet and the stereotactic headframe. (Published with permission, copyright © 2007, P.A. Wackym, MD.)

the size, a single maximum dose of 20 to 160 gray (Gy) is prescribed (10 to 80 Gy delivered to the 50% isodose line). Currently, for vestibular schwannomas, the routine prescription is 12 to 14 Gy delivered to the 50% isodose line, which will be defined later. The actual irradiation procedure is carefully planned for each individual patient by means of calculated dose distributions overlaid on images of the brain, cranial nerves, and surrounding structures. The quality of the resultant treatment plan, which is tailored using virtual reality within the Leksell GammaPlan treatment planning software, must then be assessed using tools described later.

Basic Concepts of Radiation Physics

"Radiation" is defined as the emission and propagation of energy through matter or space by means of electromagnetic disturbances that display both wave-like and particle-like behavior.[3] The particles are known as "photons." "Radioactivity" is a property of all unstable elements that regularly decay to an altered state by releasing energy in the form of photons or particles, such as electrons. In essence, then, radiation and radioactivity describe the release of energy to a medium. In addition, for clarification purposes, "X-ray" is the term used to describe energy that is emitted from a machine such as a linear accelerator; "gamma ray" is the term used to describe energy emitted from a radioactive source. Essentially, X-ray and gamma rays have the same properties; the only difference is that gamma rays have a much narrower range of energies, for example, 10 kilo-electron volts (keV) to 10 mega-electron volts (MeV), than X-rays.[4]

In the case of gamma knife, the source of radioactivity is cobalt 60. Cobalt 60 decays to a more stable element, nickel (Ni 60) when 1 of the neutrons of the ^{60}Co nucleus transforms spontaneously into a proton and an electron (Figure 7). The proton stays in the nucleus, but the electron, which is of low energy, is emitted, but is of such low energy that it has no biologic effect. Also during this process, gamma rays of 2 different energies are emitted by the nucleus: 1.17 and 1.33 MeV. The gamma rays are of high energy and are highly penetrating; this energy is absorbed in tissue and can cause a biologic effect. Thus the name is "*gamma knife*." The half-life

of a radioactive sample is the time required for half of the atoms in the sample to decay to its stable form.[5] The half-life of cobalt 60 is 5.27 years. In practice, this means that after little more than 5 years, the treatment time for the same prescribed dose is doubled because there are only half as many atoms decaying now, and therefore half as many gamma rays are being given off in a given period of time. In turn, it takes more time to get the prescribed dose to the target. Finally, the treatment time becomes too long, and the sources must be replaced.

Radiation can be ionizing or nonionizing. Types of nonionizing radiation include heat, microwaves, visible light, and radio waves. These types of energy have longer wavelengths than X- and gamma rays and therefore are of lower energy; usually the nonionizing types of energy are absorbed more uniformly and evenly and much greater amounts of energy in these forms are needed to produce damage in living things. On the other hand, ionizing radiation, such as X- and gamma rays, are of high energy; the important characteristic of ionizing radiation is the localized release of large amounts of energy, for example, enough energy to break chemical bonds and produce biologic effects. The biologic effects of radiation are caused mainly from damage to DNA. The process whereby this happens is described below.

The gamma rays from ^{60}Co are absorbed in tissue via the Compton effect. In this process, the gamma ray photon interacts with a loosely bound electron of an atom in the tissue. Part of the energy of the photon is given to the electron as kinetic energy. The photon, in turn, is deflected in its path, and has a reduced energy. The electron, now called a "fast" electron, is freed from its bond to the atom (therefore, the atom has been "ionized") and can go on to ionize other atoms of the tissue or break chemical bonds. The net result is the production of a large number of fast electrons in the tissue. These fast electrons, then, can cause damage to tissue in 2 ways: indirect action and direct action.

Direct action results when a fast electron interacts directly with DNA to cause damage, such as a single or double strand break. Indirect action occurs when a fast electron interacts with a water molecule to produce a hydroxyl radical, which is highly reactive; the hydroxyl radical can then produce DNA damage by breaking chemical bonds in the DNA. Eighty percent of a cell is composed of water; and, for gamma rays, indirect action dominates. Once the damage to DNA has been done; however, a cell does not die until it tries to reproduce. This is called mitotic cell death. The most common form of cell death is mitotic death: cells die attempting to divide because of damage to chromosomes.[6] Therefore, it may take days, months or even years for a biologic effect, such as tumor shrinkage, to be seen from radiation, depending on how fast the cells are replicating. There is, however, another type of cell death: apoptosis. Apoptosis is programmed cell death and is common in embryonic development as certain cells become obsolete, for example, when tadpoles lose their tales. However, radiation can induce apoptosis in certain cell types, such as lymphoid cells. Therefore, although mitotic death is the predominant mechanism of cell killing, apoptosis can also contribute, especially in lymphoid and hematopoietic cells.

Absorbed dose, or "dose," of radiation is the energy imparted per unit mass by ionizing radiation to matter at a specific point.[7] The International System of Units (SI) unit of absorbed dose is joules per kilogram, otherwise known as Gy. The previously used special unit of absorbed dose, the rad, was defined to be an energy absorption of 100 erg/g. Rad, however, is an older, outdated term and has been replaced by Gy; 1 Gy is equivalent to 100 rad.

Therapeutic radiation can be prescribed in many different ways. For example, it is frequently prescribed to a point, for example, "isocenter," the point at which the gantry of a linear accelerator rotates around, which ideally corresponds to somewhere inside the target, and sometimes to an "isodose line." Isodose lines are a way of describing the dose distribution: for example, the 100% isodose line shows the distribution of 100% of the prescribed dose, which is usually overlaid on the computed tomography (CT) or magnetic resonance (MR) images so one can visualize how much dose the target and surrounding tissue would be receiving from a particular treatment plan; the 90% isodose line shows the distribution of 90% of the prescribed dose, and so forth. The 50% isodose line shows where 50% of the prescribed dose lies. In the case of gamma knife treatments, the dose is frequently prescribed to the 50% isodose line, which ideally conforms tightly around the tumor. Therefore, this ensures that the periphery of the tumor will receive at least the prescribed dose, but the dose will be higher than the prescribed dose inside the tumor as discussed below.

There are 2 reasons for prescribing the dose in this way. The first reason is that for stereotactic treatments, 1 of the goals is to minimize the dose to the normal, surrounding tissue. If the dose is prescribed to the 50% isodose line, the fall-off of dose outside the target area is the most rapid. Therefore, the surrounding tissues are spared the most, when the treatment is prescribed in this way.

The second reason is that there are many clinicians who believe that a large hot spot of dose in the center of the tumor is critical for successfully treating with the gamma knife. When one prescribes to the 50% isodose line, the maximum dose in the tumor is actually double the prescribed dose; for instance, if one prescribes 12 Gy to the 50% isodose line, there is a hot spot of 24 Gy inside the tumor. Care is also taken in the treatment planning phase to avoid overlap of the hot spot with the course of the facial nerve or the cochlea.[8,9] Traditionally, this is the way gamma knife treatments have been prescribed and good results have been obtained. With linear accelerator stereotactic treatments, a hot spot in the center of the tumor is not necessarily obtained, and good results have also occurred with this type of treatment. Therefore, whether or not the hot spot in the center of the tumor is critical to the treatment is unknown, but there are many ardent believers that this is the reason why gamma knife is so effective.

The radiation dose decreases with depth in tissue due to 2 phenomena. First, the number of energy transporting photons decreases with depth as they are absorbed by the tissue. Second, the dose decreases with depth due to the inverse square law, which states that when the distance to the radiation source is doubled, the dose is decreased by a factor of 4. This effect dominates in the case of Leksell Gamma Knife as the distance from source to target is short; however, a single beam delivers most of its radiation dose to the region of its entrance. In the following section, the strategy developed by the gamma knife system to overcome this issue is outlined.

Irradiation Technique

To overcome the problem that single photon beams deliver most of their energy at the beam entrance, we need to cross fire the target with radiation from many directions. A large number of beams can be directed so that they converge toward 1 single region where the target resides during treatment. At the beam intersection, energy from all beams is delivered to the cells. Outside that region, the radiation dose decreases rapidly so that tissue between the beam entrance and target is spared of significant amounts of radiation.

There are several technical solutions for achieving a convergent beam irradiation technique. A single radiation source can be moved relative to the patient's head or vice versa. Naturally, a combination of patient and source movements can also be used. The safest and most reliable converging irradiation technique is the 1 with irradiation emitting sources moving and the patient remains stationary during treatment. This stationary procedure requires that the patient's head is surrounded by a large number of sources during treatment and all the beams are aiming at a common region where the radiosurgical target resides. This is the technique utilized in the Leksell Gamma Knife. Radiophysical and technical tolerances of all components that affect dose delivery are so narrow that all 201 beams of 1 unit are identical from a radiophysical perspective. This fact holds true not only for each unit but also for all units of the same design, facilitating comparison of clinical results published by different Leksell Gamma Knife centers. As the beam characteristics are identical, they do not need to be measured at each individual Leksell Gamma Knife installation. They are therefore prestored in the treatment planning software, Leksell GammaPlan, greatly simplifying commissioning of a new Leksell Gamma Knife.

When treatment is initiated, the treatment couch is automatically moved from its idle position into the treatment unit together with patient and helmet. Once the couch is docked in its treatment position, the helmet collimator and corresponding collimators in the unit form a beam channel, allowing the radiation that is continuously emitted by the sources to reach the patient (see Figure 1). At the end of each irradiation "shot," the couch is automatically withdrawn, either to its idle position or to a position outside the radiation focus to reposition the patient for the next irradiation "shot." There are 4 interchangeable helmets by means of which the size of the collimator (that part of the treatment unit that shapes the beam) can be changed between 4, 8, 14, and 18 mm (Figure 8). The combination of 4 different sized collimators and repositioning the patient in the 3-dimensional (3D) space defined by the stereotactic headframe are effective to deliver the radiation dose selectively and conformally to radiosurgical targets of any shape (Figure 9).

The use of convergent, narrow beams poses some strict technical and radiophysical requirements on the radiation delivering apparatus. The axis of all beams must intercept at 1 single point, and its exact location and space must be known precisely. The radiophysical character of the radiation beams must be well known, be stable in time, and optimize to the sharp beam edges. Figure 10 illustrates these basic requirements in principle, which are important for selective and reproducible dose delivery. Four beams are shown intersecting the center of a 2-dimensional (2D) target. It is important that the beam axes are precisely aligned. Any intersection of the beam axes that deviates from the ideal will affect the dose distribution. Imperfections inherent in all equipment, regardless of manufacturer, must be kept small enough not to have any clinical significance during the lifetime of the treatment unit. Consequently, technical and radiophysical characteristics of the system and their consistency limit the smallest collimator that safely and reproducibly can be used. Figure 11 illustrates the real narrow beam situation of Leksell Gamma Knife discussed previously on a hypothetical level with the combined dose distribution of all 201 beams. This also illustrates the beam size effect and the penumbra (the region near the edge of the field where the dose falls rapidly) associated with each of the 4 collimator helmet sizes. With wider beams, alignment is less critical. On the other hand, their edges begin to overlap farther from the target periphery (Figures 10 and 11). The distance at which the beams begin to overlap depends on beam size for a given irradiation technique, meaning that the dose outside the

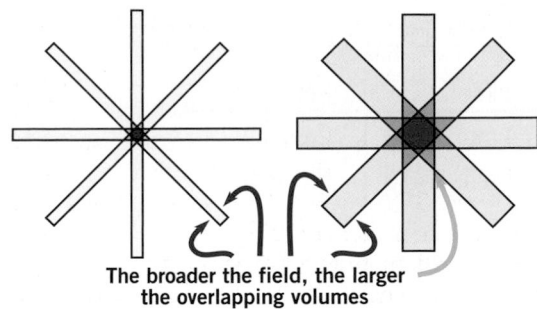

The broader the field, the larger the overlapping volumes

Figure 10 Gamma knife radiosurgery. Four overlapping beams of 2 different widths demonstrate the difference in additive radiation effects around a central target. (Published with permission, copyright © 2007, P.A. Wackym, MD.)

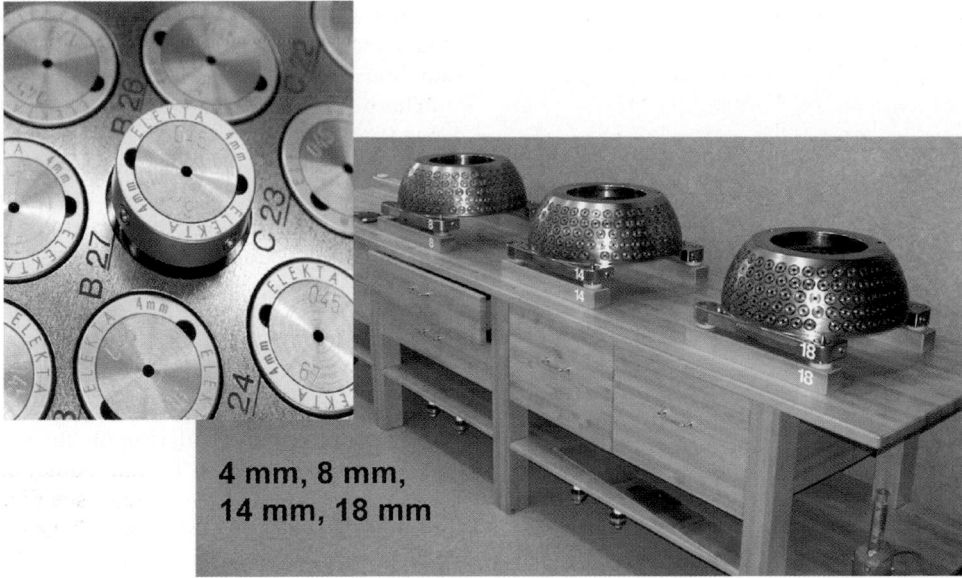

4 mm, 8 mm, 14 mm, 18 mm

Figure 8 Four different sized collimator helmets are used in gamma knife radiosurgery. The diameter of each opening determines the diameter of the sphere of radiation delivered with each shot (4, 8, 14, or 18 mm). (Published with permission, copyright © 2007, P.A. Wackym, MD.)

target periphery depends on the beam size. Figures 10 and 11 also show that an increasing number of beam edges overlap when the beams approach the target periphery. This theoretically means that a relatively high dose can be delivered outside the target to a large volume of normal tissue. Thus, as the beam size increases, at some point one can no longer claim that the treatment is selective, and one must find an alternative irradiation technique. The dose absorbed in normal tissue adjacent to the target periphery is the most significant factor limiting the largest volume that can be treated radiosurgically. The widest beam of Leksell Gamma Knife is 18 mm in diameter at isocenter, here shown as an off-axis distance (Figure 11).

Quality Assurance

When the radiophysical characteristics of a Leksell Gamma Knife are investigated for quality assurance purposes, measured and calculated dose profiles are compared. At present, experimental profiles are obtained by means of chromatographic film dosimetry. The special dose distribution is verified by means of 2 films. The films are consecutively exposed in Elekta's spherical head phantom and rotated 90° relative

to each other. The calculated profile is used as a template. Optical density (OD) profiles are measured from the films along the 3 main axes of the stereotactic coordinate system. The OD profiles are converted into dose profiles by means of an OD dose calibration procedure. The measured profiles are compared with corresponding profiles that are calculated using the Leksell GammaPlan software. The calculations are made assuming the same irradiation conditions as the experimental ones. These hypothetical profiles are used as reference. The distribution of the dose in a volume surrounding the radiation focus is investigated in this way. The stereotactic spherical volume used to expose films for evaluating dose distribution of Leksell Gamma Knife does not have the narrow geometrical tolerances required to determine the location of the radiation focus in the irradiation unit. For this purpose, an aluminum bar that is machined to narrow tolerances is used. It has a spring-loaded needle and a space for a small film. When the tool is aligned exactly between the trunnions of the helmet, the sharp tip of the needle is located in the exact mechanical isocenter. Just prior to the exposure of the film, it is pierced by the needle. The location of the OD distribution

is compared with the location of the narrow hole in the film. The two films are exposed consecutively with their planes rotated 90°. The deviation between the center of the OD and the needle hole is measured in the direction of the three main axes of the stereotactic coordinate system. The deviation between the mechanically defined isocenter and the location of the radiation focus is measured in this way.

Biologic Effects of Radiation

Radiation dose is the single most important factor that determines the outcome of a radiosurgical procedure, but it is far from being the only factor. The type of radiation is important. Earlier the treatment with gamma (photon) irradiation was described; however, protons, neutrons, and electrons are also used to treat certain tumors. This is called "particle radiation," and the different particles interact with tissue in different ways; however, the end result is still DNA damage that causes a biologic effect.

Fractionation is extremely important in radiation therapy. In stereotactic radiosurgery, there is typically 1 fraction; however, with traditional external beam radiation therapy, the fraction size (number of treatments) can be anywhere from 2 to 40 or more. Fractionation is important in terms of reducing normal tissue complications; and, in certain situations (such as optic nerve tumors), fractionated stereotactic radiotherapy (rather than radiosurgery) is preferred. The concept behind this is sublethal damage repair. Radiation causes a variety of injuries to DNA, the majority of which are repaired by cells. However, the capacity for DNA repair is diminished in cancer cells. Therefore, by breaking up the radiation into relatively small dose fractions (usually 1.8 to 2 Gy per day), normal cells tend to be marginally spared from permanent damage as compared to cancer cells after a given day of treatment. This increment in benefit is cumulative over a 30 to 40 day course of therapy that results in the net sparing of normal tissue. Note that this effect is lost if all the radiation is given in 1 day. Absence of sublethal damage repair is also the reason why lower doses are needed with radiosurgery to control the disease.

Radiosurgery does have the potential to cause significant toxicity. Therefore, it is important in radiosurgery to keep the high dose areas away

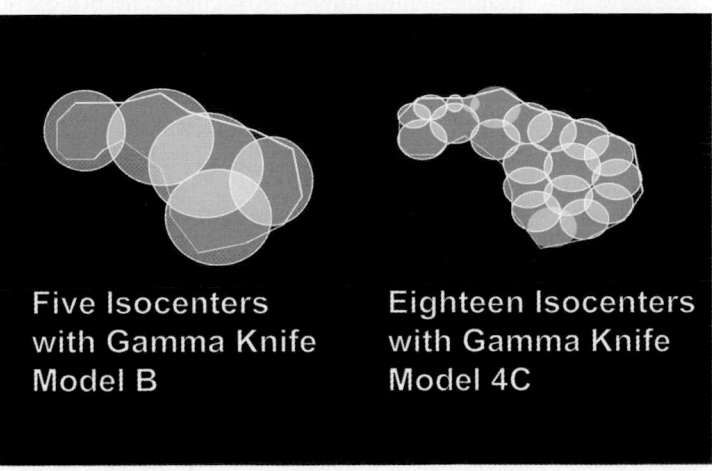

Five Isocenters with Gamma Knife Model B

Eighteen Isocenters with Gamma Knife Model 4C

Figure 9 Gamma knife radiosurgery. In this example, the tumor target can be filled with five shots using a larger collimator helmet, or 18 shots with a smaller collimator helmet. In contrast to the model U and model B, the model 4C utilizes an APS and can therefore complete a large number of shots in a timely manner. (Published with permission, copyright © 2007, P.A. Wackym, MD.)

The Beam Size Effect

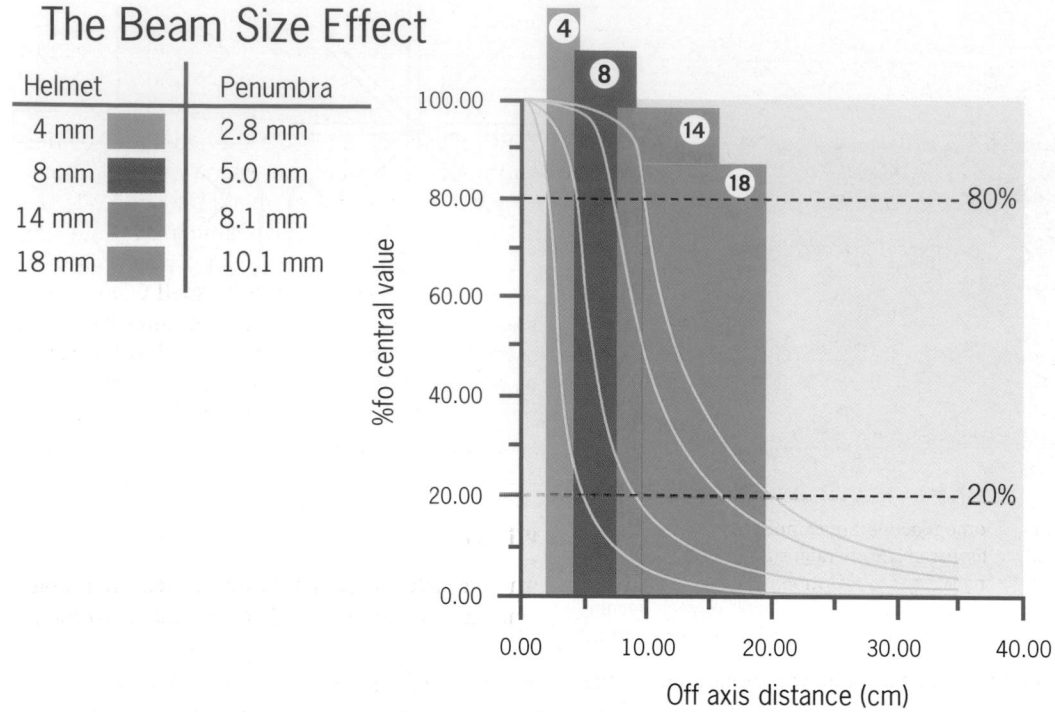

Helmet	Penumbra
4 mm	2.8 mm
8 mm	5.0 mm
14 mm	8.1 mm
18 mm	10.1 mm

Figure 11 Gamma knife radiosurgery. The beam size effect is shown graphically and numerically. The right-hand side of the figure shows the isodose curves for the 4, 8, 14, and 18 mm collimator helmets. (Published with permission, copyright © 2007, P.A. Wackym, MD.)

from normal tissue, especially radiation sensitive tissue, such as the optic nerves, optic chiasm, brainstem, and spinal cord. As an example, it has been found that approximately 8 Gy is the maximum tolerated dose of the optic chiasm when using a single fraction of radiation, such as in radiosurgery. However, if using fractionated treatment, the normal tissue tolerance of the chiasm is approximately 54 Gy. This same concept holds true for tumor control doses: higher total doses are needed in fractionated treatment to get the same tumor control as a lower dose in 1, single treatment, due to sublethal damage repair by the tumor cells between fractions. Therefore, considering the patient with a meningioma encasing the optic nerve, if the tumor was treated with stereotactic radiosurgery, a dose of approximately 12 Gy would be needed; however, the optic nerve can only tolerate approximately 8 Gy without risking serious vision compromise. With fractionated treatment, a dose of 54 Gy to the tumor would be adequate to control the tumor, and the optic nerve can tolerate 54 Gy if given in 1.8 Gy daily fractions; for this patient, then, one could treat the tumor adequately with fractionated radiotherapy while still respecting the tolerance of the optic nerve. However, the accuracy of radiation delivery via a fixed headframe in a single session compared to multiple sessions without a fixed headframe also should be considered. Therefore, each patient should be evaluated to determine whether radiosurgery or fractionated radiotherapy is the most appropriate treatment. The radiation tolerance of the cochlea is unknown.

Dose rate is also important in radiation therapy. Dose rate is defined as the radiation dose delivered per unit time; it is measured in Gy/h.[10] In general, as the dose rate decreases, the biologic

effect of a given dose is reduced. This is because sublethal damage repair can occur during a long radiation exposure, if the dose rate is low enough. There has been some concern regarding the aging sources in gamma knife units, and whether the lower dose rate affects tumor control rates. Kondziolka and colleagues, reviewing the University of Pittsburgh treatment outcomes, found no clinical difference in tumor control rates during the first 9 years of use of their first gamma knife unit, prior to reloading.[11] However, they did notice that cranial-nerve morbidity was higher than expected during the first year. It was felt that this may have been due to the higher dose rate during the first year of operation of their gamma knife unit. However, there has been no study to date to show a detrimental effect on tumor control due to decreasing dose rate from aging gamma knife sources. If there is an effect, it is most likely small and not clinically important.

In addition to dose, dose rate and fractionation, the volume of the radiated field is important. With vestibular schwannomas, treating with a plan in which the dose tightly conforms around the tumor is important, as the goal is also to spare as much normal tissue as possible. However, for brain metastases, for example, the actual borders of the target may be difficult to define and treating the target with some margin of surrounding normal tissue may be more effective in eradicating the tumor than a tight dose around the target. Also, certain tumors may be located in more critical areas, and it may be more important to have a rapid dose fall-off to spare normal tissues (such as the brainstem) rather than a high dose to the tumor. In certain patients, compromises may be made. In addition, the clinical result of the treatment (including late side effects) may

not occur for months or even years following the irradiation. The time interval between irradiating and observation is, therefore, important.

The biological response to radiation is also dependent on the type of cells that are irradiated. Some cell types are more radiosensitive than others; and, therefore, a lower dose may be needed to control 1 type of tumor versus another. Also, with the example of benign skull base tumors such as vestibular schwannomas, meningiomas, or paragangliomas, few cells are actively dividing at the time of treatment. Therefore, the primary effect may not be in destroying these more radiosensitive dividing cells, but rather a longer-term decrease in the vascular supply to the tumor. Radiosurgery appears to cause endothelial cell injury in the blood vessels; in turn, the vessels become hyalinized and thickened and eventually close. This takes many months to occur. Eventually, fibroblasts replace much of the vessel. In addition, it is believed that the blood vessels in tumors are abnormal and, therefore, are more sensitive to radiation injury than blood vessels outside of the tumor. Therefore, this may also explain, in part, why the tumor is destroyed while the surrounding tissue is spared. As will be discussed later, this was a hard lesson learned in the initial application of gamma knife radiosurgery to these types of benign tumors. The use of radiation doses appropriate for malignancy resulted in excellent tumor control; however, unacceptably high levels of hearing loss and trigeminal and nerve dysfunction occurred.[1] It has been pointed out by Pitts and Jackler,[12] however, that there has been no evidence presented that decreased vascularity occurs after gamma knife therapy and in the animal studies performed by Linskey and colleagues[13] there was no reduction of vascularity in xenograft vestibular schwannomas after treatment with 10 Gy. Using regional cerebral blood flow studies in patients with vestibular schwannomas before and after gamma knife radiosurgery, we have found a reduction in blood flow with the tumors. Figure 12 shows the pretreatment MRI and the typical appearance 6 months after gamma knife radiosurgery. This patient received 12 Gy at the 50% isodose line, which means that the maximum tumor dose was 24 Gy focused where the reduced gadolinium enhancement within the center of the tumor was found. It is thought that higher central doses in addition to a delayed decreased vascularity at the tumor periphery are most likely the reasons for the loss of contrast in the center of the tumor after radiosurgery.[11] In summary, although the radiation dose is a critical factor in tumor control, it is not the only factor that should be considered.

TREATMENT PLANNING

Placing Shots

Leksell GammaPlan is the dedicated software treatment planning system for Leksell Gamma Knife. Dose planning for gamma knife surgery means precisely conforming the isodose

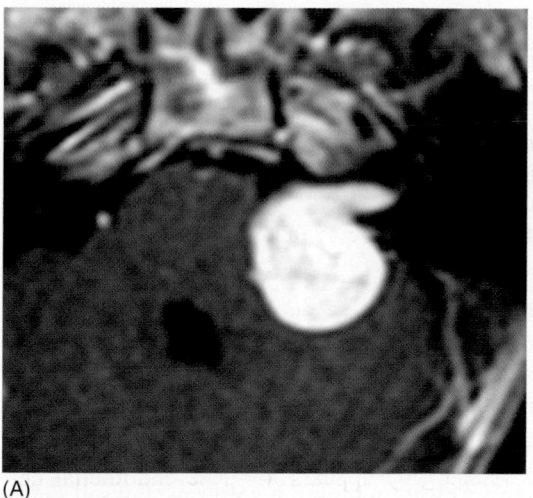 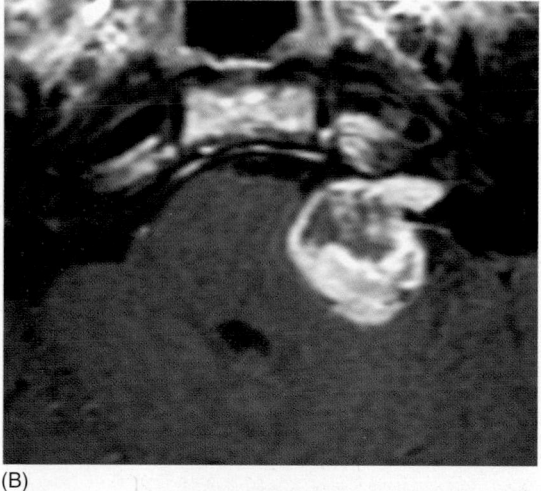

(A) (B)

Figure 12 (A) Gadolinium-enhanced T1-weighted axial MRI shows homogeneous appearance of left vestibular schwannoma at the time of gamma knife radiosurgery. (B) MRI 6 months after gamma knife radiosurgery shows reduced gadolinium enhancement within the center of the tumor, suggestive of decreased vascularization. (Published with permission, copyright © 2007, P.A. Wackym, MD.)

and additional shots with low weight quickly lead to a conformal dose plan. The dose plan can be checked using Leksell GammaPlan with the 3D image or the measurement tools, such as dose volume histograms. While the subject of conformity index is beyond the scope of this chapter, an excellent review of available methods has been published.[14] Leksell GammaPlan indicates the point in the stereotactic space where a global maximal dose can be found. Leksell GammaPlan also calculates the individual shot times. Once the treatment plan has been determined to be appropriate by the team (surgeon, radiation oncologist, and radiation physicist), the stereotactic coordinates and irradiation times are printed and used during the gamma knife treatment.

Wizard

An automated approach to initial treatment planning has been developed by Elekta Instruments AB. This software assists the treatment planner in generating a good initial dose plan quickly and is termed "the Wizard." This is an interactive tool that helps the operator develop the dose plan. The operator first selects the shot size and the degree of density with which the Wizard should fill the target. A mouse click instructs the Wizard to fill the target with shots. If the initial dose distribution is not sufficient, a mouse click on the run button instructs the Wizard to optimize the plan by moving and weighting the shots. This interaction results in a better dose plan, and after a few more changes a satisfactory dose plan can be created. However, in this surgeon's experience, manual placement of the shots, particularly for vestibular schwannomas, has always resulted in a better treatment plan.

Fine-Tuning

Fine-tuning is made with small adjustments, allowing optimization of the dose plan. Leksell GammaPlan simplifies this. For example, if the 3D image shows missed dose to part or parts of the target, shots can be moved, weighted, or added to produce a more conformal plan. As shown in Figure 14, high isodose lines show the dose distribution inside the target, making homogeneity and hot spots easily visible. Low isodose lines show the dose in the surroundings of the target. The purpose of this step is to show the dose distribution at risk structures, such as the facial nerve, to minimize the risk of complications after treatment. Leksell GammaPlan also allows the creation of different plans for the same target. This allows the operator to follow different strategies and later compare plans and select the best plan for the actual treatment. Treatment plans can utilize as few as 1 or 2 shots, such as when treating trigeminal neuralgia, or as many as 10 to 12 shots when treating a 2 cm vestibular schwannoma (maximum axial dimension within the cerebellopontine angle) plus filling the internal auditory canal. With the enhanced capabilities of Leksell Gamma Knife C, plans with 20 shots or more can easily be implemented

distribution to the target. The isodose distribution is built-up by a number of individual shots or isocenters. The Leksell GammaPlan software is designed to help the operator as much as possible to perform this procedure and is quite straightforward to use (Figures 13 and 19).

Dose planning using Leksell GammaPlan involves composing shots to develop a conformal isodose. By definition, this includes the whole target but spares the surrounding healthy tissue. Figure 13 shows an example of vestibular schwannoma. The target is well positioned on the screen and magnified for good visibility. When the shot menu is opened, one can select the size of the collimators. Selecting 14 mm would be too large for the target and would not give an effective treatment plan. The shots are placed sequentially, and the size of the collimator is selected based on the tumor shape and the gaps in coverage of the 50% isodose line displayed over the tumor. Shots are placed to cover the target as effectively as possible. Changing the position of the shots

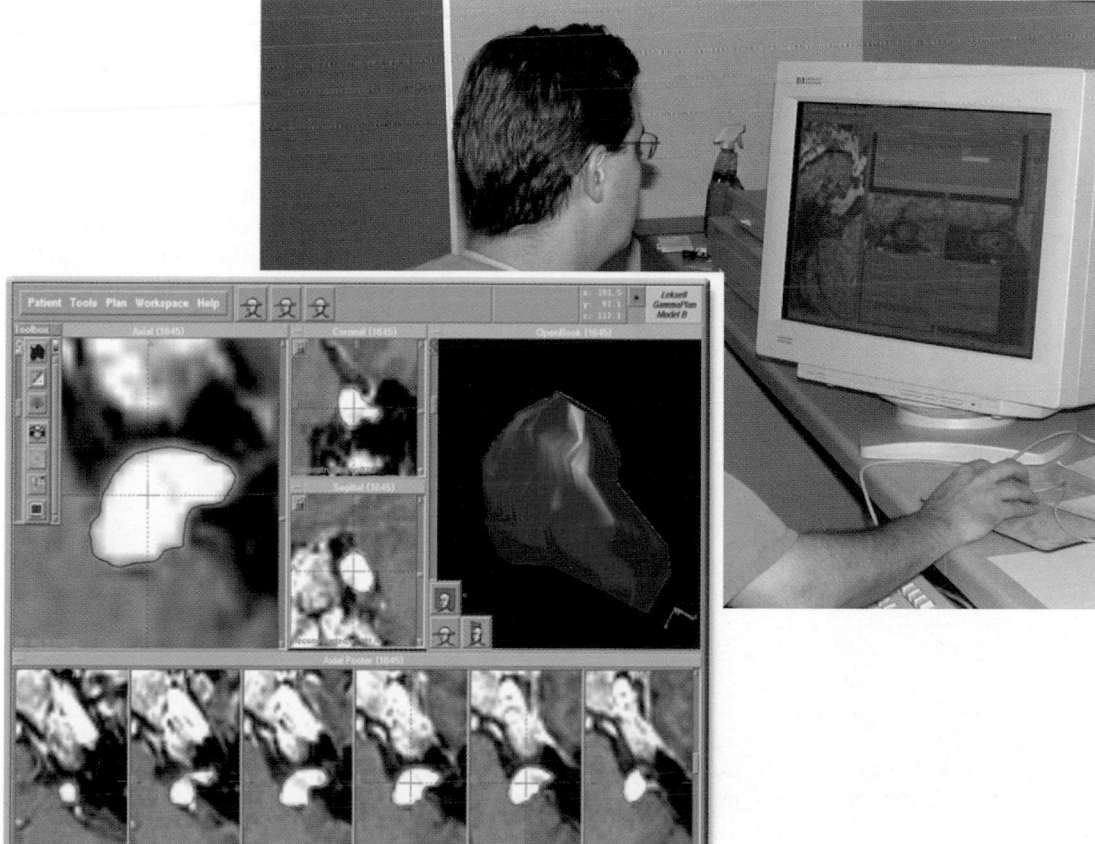

Figure 13 Initial treatment planning at the gamma knife workstation involves building a 3D model of the tumor. Determination of the conformation of the treatment plan follows placement of the shots and assignment of the radiation dose delivered to the specified isodose line. (Published with permission, copyright © 2007, P.A. Wackym, MD.)

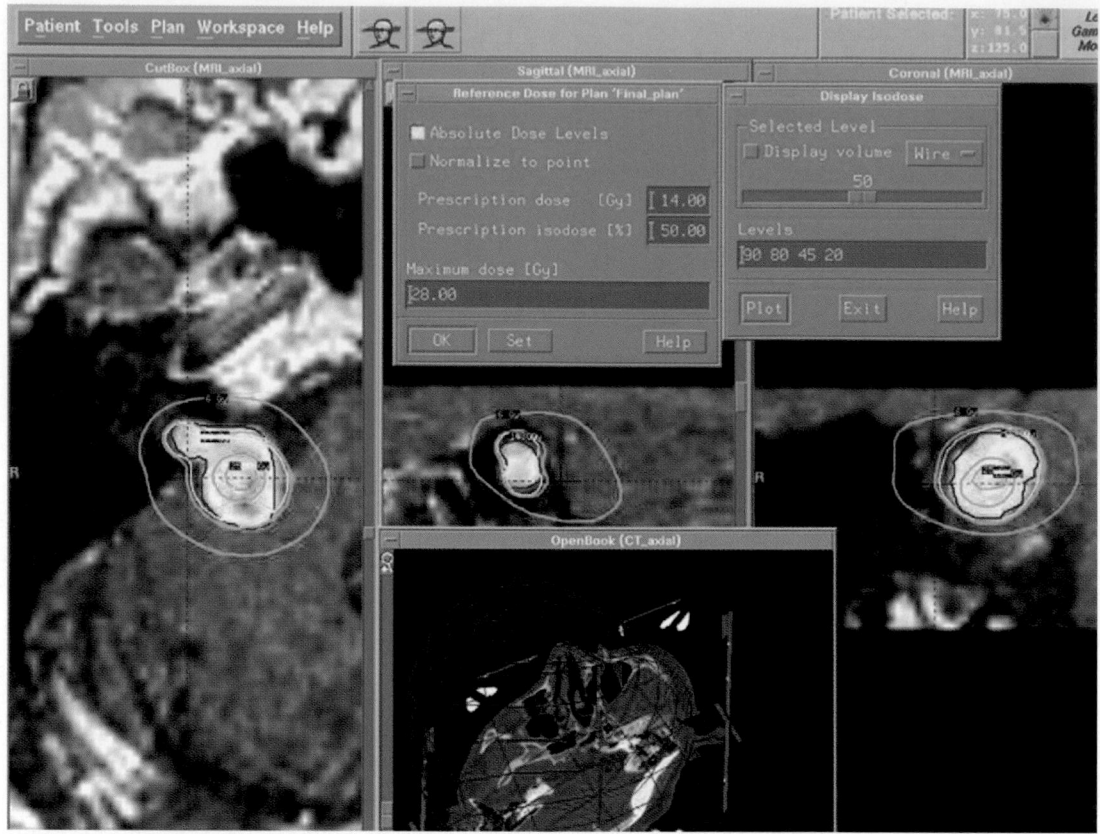

Figure 14 Gamma knife radiosurgery. Selecting the Absolute Dose Level and Display Isodose options allows verification that the maximal radiation dose is not delivered near critical structures, such as the facial nerve. In this example, 14 Gy delivered to the 50% isodose line was prescribed. As shown, the maximum dose (28 Gy) is delivered to the center of the tumor (*smallest circle*). The largest circle represents the 20% isodose line where 6 Gy of radiation is delivered. (Published with permission, copyright © 2007, P.A. Wackym, MD.)

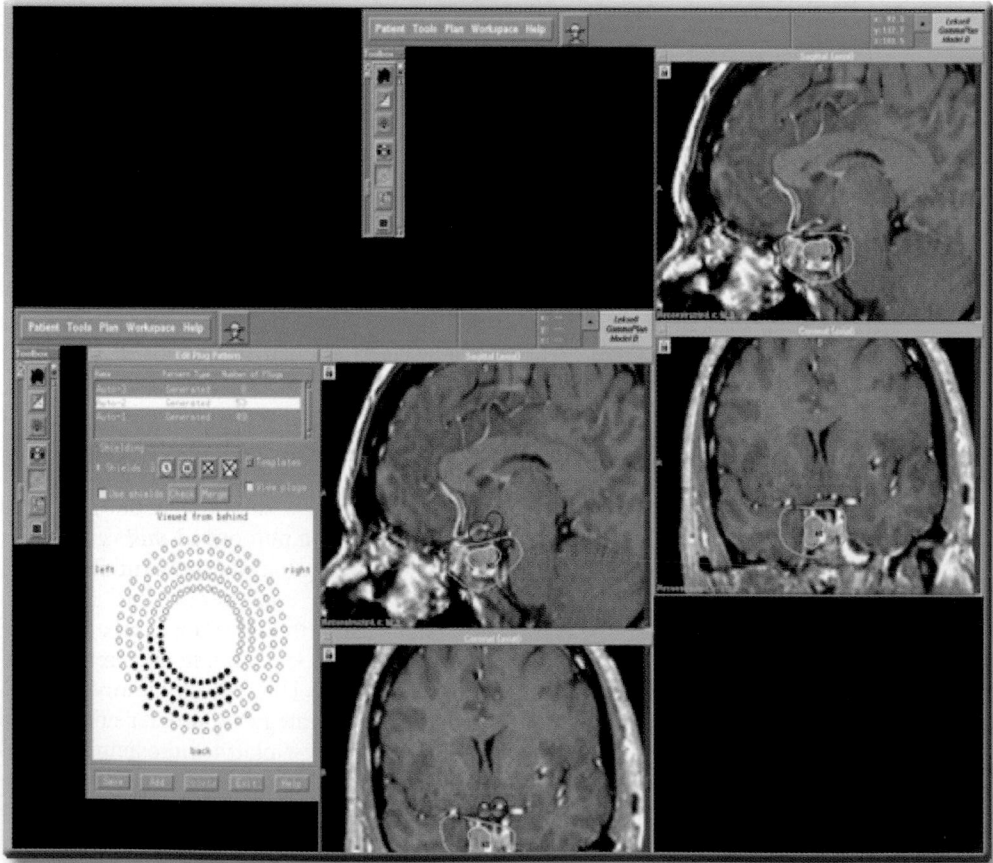

Figure 15 Gamma knife radiosurgery. Another strategy to avoid excessive radiation to critical structures, in this example the optic chiasm, is to use plugging. The treatment planning software determines which paths of the collimator helmet should be replaced with a solid plug to eliminate radiation from passing through the collimator helmet and contributing to the radiation delivered to the critical structure. (Published with permission, copyright © 2006, P.A. Wackym, MD.)

in a timely manner, since the model C does not require manual adjustments of the X, Y, and Z coordinates by the gamma knife treatment team. This allows improved conformity and selectivity of gamma knife surgery, potentially reducing the risk of complications.

Plugging

To shape the dose distribution for the low isodose lines in one direction in particular, one or more of the 201 collimators can be replaced with a closed shield, called a plug. One can select spherical areas called shields with different diameters and place them over risk centers in the brain, cranial nerves, or lens of the eyes. Once the shields are put in place, within the software, Leksell GammaPlan closes off all beams that would irradiate through the shielded area. The result is a modified dose plan in the low isodose lines with only little affect on the target peripheral isodose. The beam channels that need to be plugged can be seen in the plug pattern (Figure 15). The plug patterns can be merged for all shots of the same size so that the operator only has to plug the helmets for the treatment once.

Peripheral Isodose

In the final plan, the peripheral dose is set to a value, which is assessed as optimal for a particular patient. Indication, size, and location of the target are taken into account, as well as clinical experience. The peripheral isodose is usually set to the 50% isodose line. This is exactly half the maximum dose in the target, referred to as the hot spot (see Figures 12 and 14). Along the 50% isodose line the dose gradient is usually the steepest ensuring sufficient dose within the target, while the dose level outside falls steeply, sparing the surrounding healthy tissue. Leksell Gamma Plan can also display the absolute dose values if desired. It will show the point in the stereotactic space where the global maximum dose can be found. With vestibular schwannoma it is valuable to complete this exercise, as the maximal dose at the "hot spot" should be positioned well away from the facial nerve and cochlea. In addition, plotting the absolute dose lines will help in determining the actual level of radiation delivered to surrounding structures.

Grouping Shots

When the dose planning is completed, Leksell GammaPlan has to check and sort the shots. Assume for example, that the treatment consists of two shots with 8 mm collimators and five shots with 4 mm collimators. Leksell GammaPlan will group all shots and use the same collimators during each series of shots of a given size. For the model C unit, the operator does not have to enter the treatment room during a run. However, with the model B the treatment team reenters the treatment room after each shot is delivered and manually adjusts the X, Y, and Z coordinates, as well as the gamma angle, that is, the pitch of the head, if necessary. With both the model B and model C, the team has to change the collimator helmet manually when necessary, as dictated by the treatment plan.

Protocols

Detailed treatment and physics protocols can be viewed and printed out. All relevant data can be documented including details of the treatment plan, targets, dose volume histograms, snap shots, and images.

Export

When the treatment setup has been completed, the treatment protocol has to be exported to Leksell Gamma Knife. This is via a special secured direct serial connection. Leksell GammaPlan only accepts valid and verified treatment plans for export. An addition, a protective design limits the transfer of a treatment plan to the Leksell Gamma Knife to 1 patient at a time. Once the data have been transferred to the operator's console, it is verified, and the patient can be treated.

TREATMENT PROCEDURE

Manually Setting Coordinates

Treatment can be performed automatically using the APS or manually using trunnions. As described above, for the model B, manual setting of the X, Y, and Z coordinates as well as the gamma angle if necessary is accomplished by the treatment team. The Y and Z coordinates are set with the Y, Z slides on the coordinate frame, whereas the X coordinate and the gamma angle are set with the trunnions. Another check and balance that is in place is the visual verification of each coordinate by a different team member.

Automatic Positioning System

With the APS, the treatment is controlled from the operator console. Once the treatment starts, the selected run is carried out automatically. Before repositioning, the couch will move out a short distance to bring the patient out of treatment focus. At this point, the APS will move the patient's head to the next target position. When the first run is completed, the remaining runs, with different sized collimator helmets, are selected and performed in the same manner after manually changing the collimator helmet.

NEW GAMMA KNIFE TECHNOLOGY: PERFEXION

In 2002, a group of international experts were asked by Elekta Instrument AB to define the requirement specifications for a new gamma knife. The group concluded that the basic principle of multiple converging fixed beams and patient immobilization with the stereotactic frame provided the most reliably precise and accurate radiosurgical solution. The group agreed on 5 critical features: best dosimetry performance, best radiation protection for patient and staff, unlimited cranial reach, full automation and outstanding patient, and staff comfort. Based on these specifications, Elekta Instrument AB developed a completely new radiosurgical instrument which they named the Leksell Gamma Knife Perfexion. Interestingly, this instrument is capable of treating lesions of the head and neck using radiosurgery. Consequently, it is likely that this technology will play a much greater role in the practice of otolaryngology—head and neck surgery.

In contrast to earlier gamma knife units, the Perfexion has a single integrated permanent collimator system that incorporates openings for collimators of 3 different diameters. The new collimator design incorporates computer-controlled movements that vary the size and position of the openings, and these can be individually varied among 4, 8, and 16 mm or be blocked off. This provides a virtually unlimited ability for sculpting the dose distribution, enabling dynamic shaping with the same degree of accuracy inherent in a framed-based system.

Although the new Leksell GammaPlan PFX treatment planning software is more sophisticated than the current GammaPlan software, it was designed to have full backward compatibility to existing gamma knife radiosurgery protocols and methods. One major new feature is that the institution-based treatment planning system can be accessed remotely, providing access to all patient data in the online database. To increase the seamless access, Leksell GammaPlan PFX is now hosted on a personal computer platform with a Linux operating system rather than the dedicated proprietary workstation used in the past.

The first Perfexion unit was installed at Timone University Hospital of Marseille in July 2006. To evaluate the capabilities, advantages, disadvantages, and limits of this new technology, 83 patients were included in a prospective trial.[15] Among these, 59 patients were eligible for the comparative prospective study based on inclusion criteria of informed consent signed, tumor or vascular indication, and no previous radiosurgery or radiotherapy. In accordance with the blinded, randomization process, 29 patients were treated with Leksell Gamma Knife 4C, and 30 patients with Leksell Gamma Knife Perfexion. Dose planning parameters, dosimetry measurements on the patients' bodies, workflow, patient comfort, quality assurance procedure, and a series of other treatment-related parameters were prospectively evaluated in both arms. The analysis of their data indicated that procedures with Perfexion were collision-free even with extreme location of the lesion, for example, multiple metastases. The duration of the radiosurgical procedure, duration of nurse, physicist and physician intervention on the unit, and the duration of the quality assurance procedure were all reduced with the Perfexion unit. Radiation protection, already good with the Leksell Gamma Knife 4C, was improved with the Perfexion unit.

Collision risk reflects the relationship between the head, frame and collimator helmet, and the findings regarding this issue in the Régis and colleagues study are among the most important in this report.[15] Collision risk is determined before starting the procedure with both the model 4C and the Perfexion. Through a "dummy run," it is possible to assess whether any parts of the stereotactic frame will hit the inside of the collimator body during the automated treatment. A risk for collision was predicted by GammaPlan for at least 1 shot in 48.3% of the patients treated with the model 4C and in only 1 patient (3.3%) with the Perfexion. In this single patient, a direct check of the absence of collision was required by the system. Collision risk requiring technical adjustments was not required with Perfexion. With the 4C, collision risk forced a change in the frame angle for at least 1 shot in 27.6% of the patients and the use of manual (trunnion) mode for at least 1 shot in the treatment of 20.7% of the patients.

With the capability of reaching all areas within the head and neck region, the Leksell Gamma Knife Perfexion will no doubt contribute to future progress in head and neck radiosurgery. It is anticipated that this unit will be available in the United States in 2008.

GAMMA KNIFE RADIOSURGERY APPLICATIONS AND OUTCOMES

In this section, attention will be focused on remaining questions that should be answered as well as examples of good and poor outcome with hearing following gamma knife radiosurgery. Comparision to surgical outcomes[16,17] is addressed in Chapter 35, "Vestibular Schwannomas and Other Skull-Base Neoplasms." Application of the technology in areas which are inappropriate will be discussed.

Just as is the case with other forms of medical and surgical therapy, the techniques and outcomes of gamma knife radiosurgery for vestibular schwannomas have evolved and improved over time. These changes in methodology have been based on patient outcome. However, now that the tumor control and facial nerve preservation (motor function) occurs with virtually all patients treated with gamma knife, it is appropriate to focus attention on further improving the techniques so that optimal hearing and balance preservation can be achieved. In addition, better assessment of hearing and balance outcomes are necessary to provide adequate informed consent to patients deciding among expectant management, microsurgery, and stereotactic radiosurgery.[2]

In the Medical College of Wisconsin Acoustic Neuroma and Skull Base Surgery Program, we have established a clinical pathway for all of our patients undergoing gamma knife radiosurgery for primary or secondary treatment of their tumors. Following completion of their stereotactic radiosurgery, at 6-month intervals, each patient undergoes a gadolinium-enhanced MRI as well as an audiologic test battery and caloric testing to assess peripheral vestibular function. Pretreatment they undergo a complete electronystagmography test battery, a complete audiologic assessment, and facial nerve electromyography. We have published data regarding the early outcomes of a cohort of patients undergoing primary ($n = 24$) and secondary ($n = 5$) treatment of sporadic unilateral vestibular schwannomas using gamma knife radiosurgery,[8] and the data to be presented next extend this series both in number of patients undergoing primary ($n = 35$) and secondary ($n = 8$) treatment, as well as in duration, with some patients having more than 5-year follow-up data. First, the objective auditory thresholds (Figures 16 and 17), speech discrimination ability (Figure 18), and degree of vestibular paresis (Figure 19) are presented longitudinally, as are the classification of hearing using the AAO-HNS[18] (Table 1 and Figure 20) and Gardner-Robertson[19] (Table 2 and Figure 21) systems.

According to the subsection termed "Healthcare Professionals, Treatment Statistics" on the Elekta AB web site, there have been 32,482 vestibular schwannomas treated with gamma knife radiosurgery as of December 2005.[20] Numerous reports of the treatment outcomes of cohorts of these patients have been published in the literature; however, the literature has been relatively silent regarding the reporting of balance function before and after gamma knife radiosurgery. A recent technology assessment report from the Alberta Hertitage Foundation for Medical Research focused on reviewing the efficacy and costs of radiosurgery.[21] Similarly, the Acoustic Neuroma Patient Archive has a summary of patient outcomes and treatment methods for 3 series of patients treated with gamma knife radiosurgery, 4 series of patients treated with fractionated stereotactic radiosurgery, and 1 series of patients treated with proton beam radiation.[22] However, because the University of Pittsburgh group has the longest and largest clinical experience in treating vestibular schwannomas with gamma knife radiosurgery, their hearing outcomes will be outlined in this portion of the discussion. There have been several reports of this large series; however, the Lunsford and colleagues publication from 2005 summarizes their experience with 829 vestibular schwannomas treated between 1987 and 2002.[23] The evolution of treatment dose based on patient outcome is well described; however, there are several points regarding the reporting of hearing outcomes which deserve discussion.

This extensive clinical experience included an average tumor volume of 2.5 cm[3] and a median margin dose to tumor of 13 Gy. They reported what is currently felt to be the standard of tumor control in 97% of patients at 10 years, and facial nerve (motor) dysfunction in <1% of patients. Trigeminal nerve symptoms occurred in <3% of patients, and they reported that, in general, these post-gamma knife symptoms occurred when the tumors reached the level of the trigeminal nerve. No reporting of balance function has been included in the analysis of their series. Unfortunately, the reporting of their hearing preservation has limited representation of the entire 829 patients. Although the 15-year experience included 829 patients, "5-year actuarial rates of hearing level preservation and speech preservation" were reported in 103 patients, and hearing outcomes data were presented in only 267 patients. They reported "unchanged hearing preservation" in 50 to 77% of these patients, and this method of reporting auditory performance points to the difficulty in interpreting the outcome of most of the studies reporting hearing outcome in patients with vestibular schwannoma who have been treated with gamma knife radiosurgery. They also stated that "for patients with intracanalicular tumors, hearing preservation rates in those treated with 12.5 to 14 Gy at the margin showed 90% preservation of servicable hearing."[24] Unfortunately, pretreatment and longitudinal data are not available in these reports.

In an earlier series of 190 patients with vestibular schwannomas, Flickinger and colleagues. reviewed the University of Pittsburgh experience from 1992 to 1997.[25] The average dose to the tumor margin was reduced to 13 Gy, and excellent tumor control was achieved at 97.1%. In this study, issues highlighted earlier with reporting of hearing outcome are equally apparent. They reported "hearing-level preservation" in 71 ± 4.7% of patients. They also reported a "preservation of testable speech discrimination ability" in 91 ± 2.6% of subjects. Obviously, testable speech discrimination ability is far different than useful hearing, and it is unfortunate that these authors did not report the actual auditory thresholds or speech discrimination ability. Most importantly, these were not reported as a function of time post-gamma knife radiosurgery. In addition, they reported that "hearing levels improved" in 10 (7%) of 141 patients who exhibited decreased hearing defined as Gardner-Robertson grades II to V before undergoing gamma knife radiosurgery. Based on our clinical observations and those of other centers, this picture is far more complex over time than is represented in these publications.

Prasad and colleagues from the University of Virginia reported their series of 200 vestibular schwannomas treated with gamma knife radiosurgery over a 10-year interval in 2000.[26] Of these patients, 153 patients had follow-up data including 96 with primary treatment and 57 with secondary treatment. They reported no hearing pre-gamma knife in 105 patients, including 53 of 96 primary treatment and 52 of 57 secondary treatment patients. The Gardner-Robertson grading system and subjective assessment of hearing was used; however, no pure-tone average (PTA) or speech discrimination data were reported. Unfortunately, their data set included audiometric data from

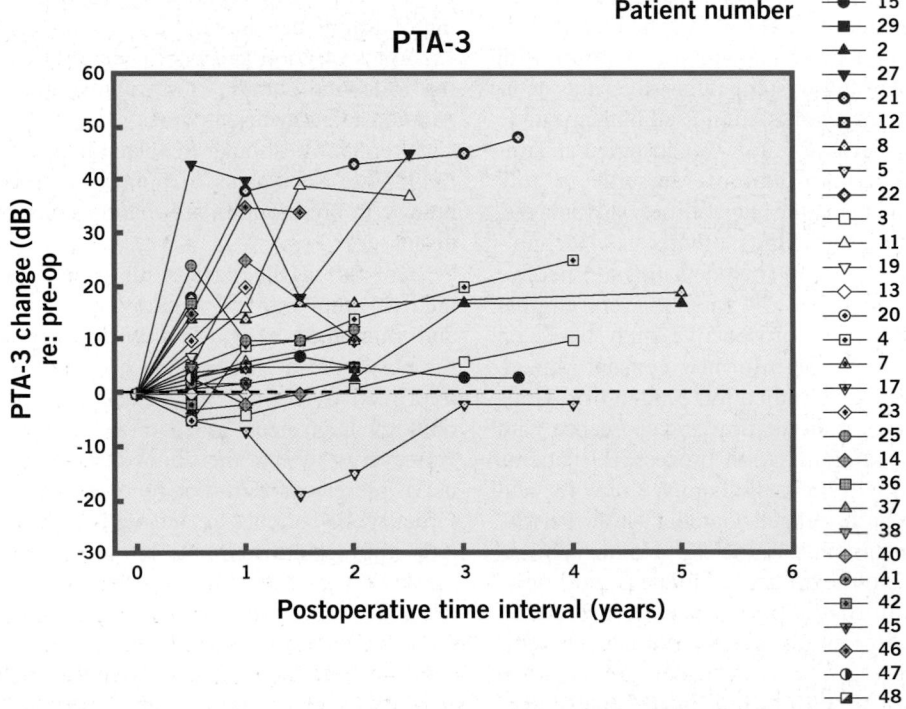

Figure 16 Auditory function over time after gamma knife radiosurgery treatment of unilateral vestibular schwannomas. Three-frequency averages of pure-tone thresholds (PTA-3) in dB HL at 0.5, 1, and 2 kHz were determined for all patients with measures at the preoperative time and at least 1 postoperative interval. The PTA-3 difference was calculated for each time interval relative to the preoperative PTA-3. The differences are plotted as a function of postoperative time interval, with 0 representing the preoperative time. A positive difference value indicates a higher or poorer, postoperative PTA-3. In general, over time, the vast majority of patients were found to have PTA-3s that were poorer or similar to preoperative PTA-3s, although a few individuals showed some initial improvement (eg, subject 5). The greatest changes in PTA-3 were measured at 6 months posttreatment although continued changes were observed up to 5 years posttreatment. (Published with permission, copyright © 2007, P.A. Wackym, MD.)

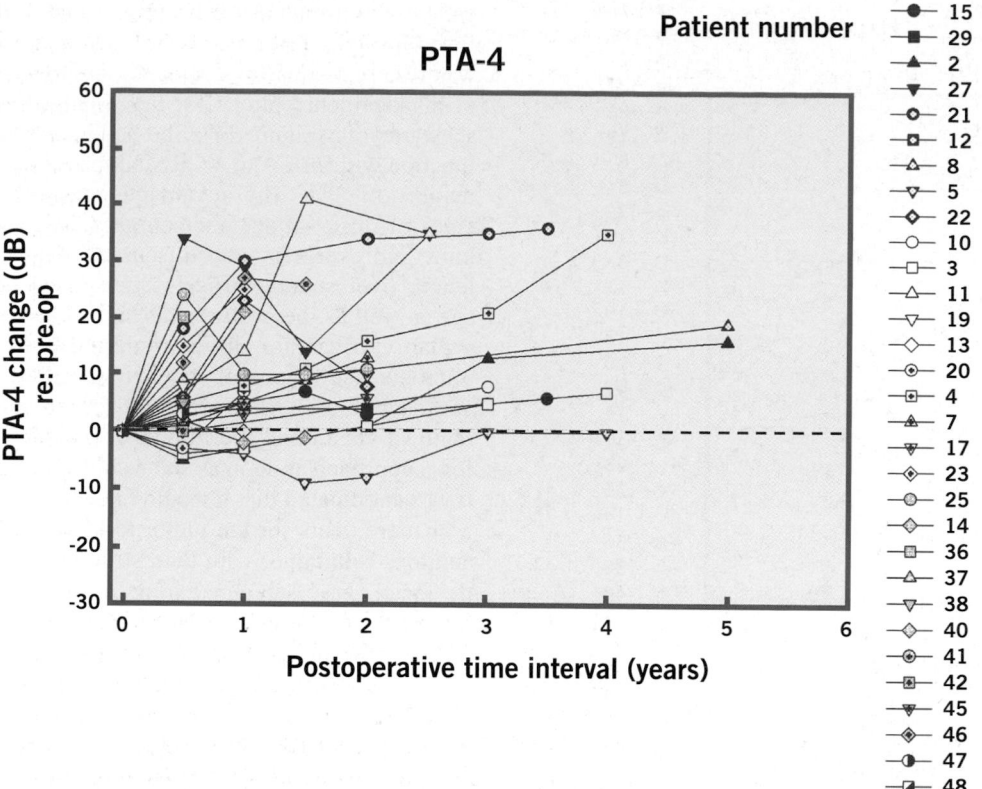

Figure 17 Auditory function over time after gamma knife radiosurgery treatment of unilateral vestibular schwannomas. Four-frequency averages of pure-tone thresholds (PTA-4) in dB HL at 0.5, 1, 2, and 4 kHz were determined for all patients with measures at the preoperative time and at least 1 postoperative interval. The PTA-4 difference was calculated for each time interval relative to the preoperative PTA-4. The differences are plotted as a function of postoperative time interval, with 0 representing the preoperative time. A positive difference value indicates a higher or poorer, postoperative PTA-4. In general, over time, the vast majority of patients were found to have PTA-4s that were poorer or similar to preoperative PTA-4s, even though a few individuals showed some initial improvement. The greatest changes in PTA-4 were measured at 6 months posttreatment although continued changes were observed up to 5 years posttreatment. (Published with permission, copyright © 2007, P.A. Wackym, MD.)

only 48 patients, and the intervals of audiometric testing were not reported. Despite these limitations, they found that, except for one patient, no change in hearing was observed in the first 2 years after gamma knife radiosurgery. Their data also showed that the greatest change in Gardner-Robertson grade occurred between years 2 and 4 post-gamma knife; however, without understanding the assessment intervals, the precise onset of the hearing loss is unknown. No outcomes regarding balance function were reported.

Kim's group at the Seoul National University reported the hearing outcomes in 25 patients with vestibular schwannomas with serviceable hearing.[27] The median tumor volume was 3.0 cm^3 (0.16 to 9.1 cm^3), and the dose used was 12 ± 0.7 Gy at the 49.8 ± 1.1% isodose line. They reported the hearing outcomes using the Gardner-Robertson grading system, PTAs, and speech discrimination scores. Pre-gamma knife, interim post-gamma knife, and last post-gamma knife data were reported. Similar to our data, they found that in 16 patients the hearing deteriorated >20 dB 3 to 6 months post-gamma knife and that this hearing loss continued for 24 months. The only prognostic factor for hearing deterioration that they identified was the maximum dose to the cochlear nucleus.

Based on the unpublished data of 43 patients with up to 60 months of follow-up (shown in Figures 16 to 21), it is clear that most of the

change in hearing and balance function occurs during the first 6 months after gamma knife radiosurgery; however, continued but less rapid worsening of function can occur up to 12 months. These objective measurements correspond well to the transient facial nerve dysfunction, trigeminal nerve dysfunction, tinnitus, and disequilibrium occurring in our patients with vestibular schwannomas undergoing gamma knife radiosurgery.[8,9] Upon reflection on the possible mechanisms underlying these changes, it is important to appreciate that there is an increased size of the tumor after radiosurgery. Typically this posttreatment edema persists for 6 months; however, this may remain for up to 1 year, as demonstrated by the longitudinal measurement data of our patients with vestibular schwannomas.[8,9] Since the labyrinthine artery, a branch of the anterior inferior cerebellar artery which follows the course of the cochlear and vestibular nerves, provides essentially all of the blood supply to the cochlea and vestibule, it is likely that the postradiation edema compromises the blood supply to the inner ear. The resulting inner ear devascularization could certainly explain the rapid change in hearing and balance function seen at the 6-month posttreatment assessment in our patients.

Considering causes that are important in clinical hearing and balance outcomes, the radiation dose is an important factor. Although

experimental studies of the alpha–beta ratio of the facial nerve and brainstem have been performed, to our knowledge, the radiation tolerance of cochlear inner and outer hair cells and the vestibular types I and II hair cells remains unknown. Based on review of our vestibular schwannoma dosimetry, the mean percent of cochlear volume exposed to 11.9 Gy was 5.3%[9]; however, it is unknown if this dose is capable of injuring auditory and/or vestibular hair cells.

With longitudinal assessment, several of our patients have had tumor control or regression and improvement of hearing and vestibular function. This is clearly divergent from the natural history of vestibular schwannomas. In contrast, worsening of auditory and vestibular function and the development of disequilibrium have occurred in a number of our patients. Continued systematic studies of these patients and expansion of the cohort of patients studied are important to determine the efficacy of gamma knife radiosurgery and to compare to other forms of radiosurgery and radiotherapy, as well as microsurgery. Recognition of symptoms such as disequilibrium and knowledge regarding the expected time course of vestibular paresis progression are important not only for patient counseling, but provide the opportunity to intervene with vestibular rehabilitation or nonspecific vestibular suppression until compensation has been completed, should this be needed clinically.

In addition to reporting hearing and balance function outcomes, it is important to provide a detailed reporting of tumor dimensions as a function of time and compare these data statistically to gain a better understanding of the tumor biology after gamma knife radiosurgery. It is also important that physical findings such as facial nerve and trigeminal nerve function be presented longitudinally, as have subjective symptoms such as tinnitus, disequilibrium, vertigo, and headache. The advantage of this approach is that a clear understanding of outcome over time will emerge. Analysis of these data will also provide the opportunity to identify critical time intervals during which additional interventions may be undertaken to optimize outcomes.

Based on longitudinal observations of hearing and balance function, and the statistical analysis of tumor size over time in patients with vestibular schwannomas treated with gamma knife radiosurgery and hypotheses of the mechanisms of injury, it may be possible to intervene to avoid the large changes in hearing and balance function found at the 6-month assessment. One potential method to optimize hearing and balance outcomes would include the use of oral corticosteroids. Critical questions would include dosage, duration of use, and when should the corticosteroids be started relative to the radiotherapy? The use of intratympanic steroids or intratympanic antioxidant compounds may be an alternative therapeutic strategy that would minimize systemic effects of high dose corticosteroids, provided that the primary mechanism of hearing and balance functional loss was due to hair-cell injury rather than vascular

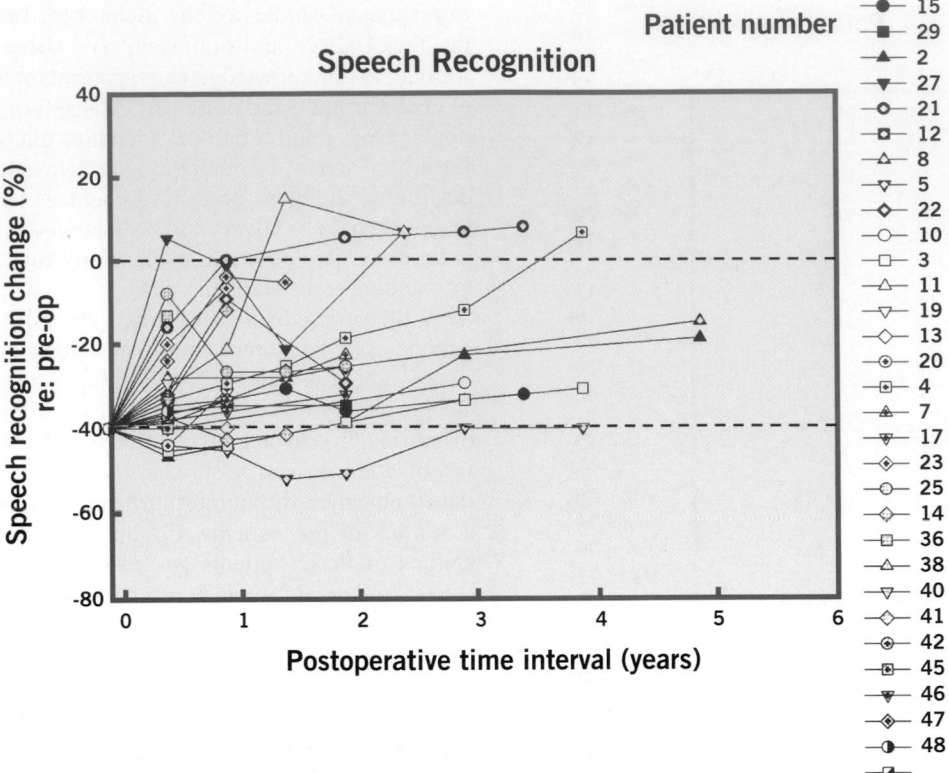

Figure 18 Speech recognition testing was performed using the Northwestern University Auditory Test No. 6 (NU-6) monosyllabic words. The stimuli were presented at 40 dB sensation level, that is, above speech recognition threshold, or if this was too loud, at the patient's most comfortable listening level. Speech recognition was scored in percent correct. As with PTA, the differences between pre- and postoperative speech recognition were calculated and plotted as a function of postoperative time interval. Positive values are consistent with an improvement in speech recognition. Approximately half of the patients showed improvement in speech recognition at 6 months posttreatment, while the other half showed a decrease in performance. Of those patients who experienced a reduction in speech discrimination ability, there was a greater range of change than that observed in the patients who enjoyed an improvement in speech discrimination ability. It should be noted that the greatest changes in speech discrimination ability occurred at 6 months post-gamma knife treatment. However, over time, the patients generally demonstrate speech recognition performance similar to or poorer than pretreatment performance. (Published with permission, copyright © 2007, P.A. Wackym, MD.)

compromise of the labyrinthine artery during the initial tumor swelling within the internal auditory canal. Until a detailed understanding of the pathophysiologic basis of late hearing loss and disequilibrium, such as the development of labyrinthine fistulas, progressive inner ear devascularization, or progressive loss of outer versus inner cochlear and vestibular hair cells, appropriate clinical interventions that will allow maximal preservation of hearing and balance function while maintaining the excellent tumor control and motor facial nerve function outcomes that our patients currently experience after gamma knife radiosurgery for vestibular schwannomas.

Anecdotal Cases

There are also anecdotal cases that are worthy of discussion to illustrate a few specific points about stereotactic radiosurgery and the outcomes associated with fractionated stereotactic radiosurgery or gamma knife radiosurgery. First, we have found that there is a distortion in the MRI data set produced by the stereotactic headframe used in gamma knife radiosurgery.[9] As shown in Figure 22, the treatment plan and outline of the tumor, based on MRI treatment planning, is approximately 1 mm more anterior than the position of the internal auditory canal as visualized with CT imaging. It is especially important to recognize that several

gamma knife centers utilize MRI exclusively to build the 3D work space and complete the treatment planning, raising questions about long-term treatment outcomes if regions of the tumor are undertreated, and adjacent structures, such as the facial nerve are overtreated.

An anecdotal case that points out the need to assess critically terms such as "tumor control" is a woman from my practice who decided to travel to a large center with a strong experience with fractionated stereotactic radiosurgery for treatment of a small vestibular schwannoma. As seen in Figure 23, the patient has had excellent tumor control when considering the medial portion of the tumor. However, it can be seen that she had progressive growth of the tumor laterally, until her fundus was completely filled with tumor. Office notes and direct conversations with the treating radiosurgeon indicated that he considered this complete tumor control. Unfortunately, as shown in Figures 24 and 25, her thresholds and speech recognition continued to worsen until she was ultimately left with no useful hearing on the side of the tumor. At 3.5 years postfractionated stereotactic radiotherapy, her PTA fell to 84 dB from 15 dB, and her speech discrimination fell to 8 from 92%, clearly a poor hearing outcome.

While also anecdotal, another case illustrates a dilemma that arises when counseling a

patient about management options and is, therefore, worthy of brief discussion. A young woman was referred to us for evaluation and discussion of management options for her small vestibular schwannoma (Figure 26). She had poor auditory function with a PTA of 52 dB and speech discrimination of 60%. The advantages and disadvantages of observation, microsurgery, and gamma knife radiosurgery were discussed with her at length over several office visits. Based on her age as well as the position and size of her tumor, a plan evolved for observation and ultimately microsurgical removal via a translabyrinthine approach or, alternatively, with microsurgical removal via a translabyrinthine or middle cranial fossa approach as soon as she would want to this. It was anticipated that it would likely take at least 5 or more years for the tumor to fill the internal auditory canal and, with that, still not to change the facial nerve outcome during translabyrinthine resection of the tumor. Despite this, she decided to undergo gamma knife radiosurgery. As shown in Figure 26, the tumor initially increased and later decreased in size. There was also a surprising improvement in both her auditory thresholds and speech recognition ability (Figures 27 and 28). At 3.5 years post gamma knife radiosurgery, her PTA had increased to 25 dB and her speech discrimination had improved to 90%. Longerterm follow-up is certainly necessary and will be completed; however, this outcome was not anticipated, and she continues to be extremely pleased with her management decision.

One statistic, which is particularly alarming to patients considering gamma knife radiosurgery for their vestibular schwannoma, and also often quoted by individuals who are biased against gamma knife radiosurgery, is that there have been 8 cases of malignancy within vestibular schwannomas reported to date. These have been summarized by Bari and colleagues in 2002.[28] Four of these patients had been previously treated with radiosurgery and 4 others cases did not receive radiation. Whereas it remains possible that these 4 malignancies developed after the radiation treatment, it is more likely that these malignant tumors were misdiagnosed as benign at the outset of evaluation and treatment. The concept of delayed development of radiation-induced neoplasms was addressed by Pollock and colleagues in 1998.[29] They reviewed the 26-year experience with radiosurgery in more than 20,000 patients worldwide, and they found no increased incidence of new neoplasm development. They defined neoplasm as a new growth of tissue serving no physiologic function, and this would include both benign and malignant disease. Rowe and colleagues recently published a retrospective cohort study comparing the Sheffield, England radiosurgery patient database with their national mortality and cancer registries.[30] These data comprised approximately 5,000 patients and 30,000 patient-years of follow-up, with more than 1,200 patients having a follow-up period longer than 10 years. Among all these patients treated with radiosurgery, a single new

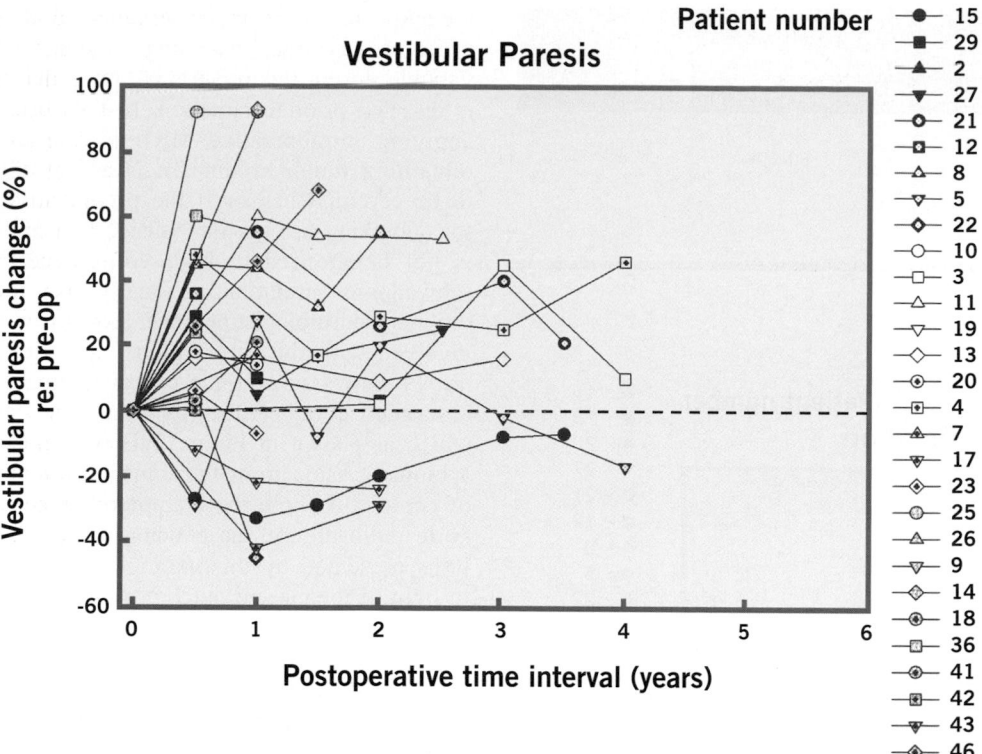

Figure 19 Vestibular paresis was determined with bithermal caloric testing. A positive difference value indicates greater vestibular paresis post-gamma knife radiosurgery. Both degradation and improvement in vestibular paresis are observed across patients. Within a patient, the postoperative degree of vestibular paresis generally tends to remain stable over time after the relatively large initial change observed at the 6 month posttreatment assessment. In those patients who had continued reduction in their vestibular function, there was continued difficulty with disequilibrium until vestibular compensation was complete and the vestibular paresis stabilized. (Published with permission, copyright © 2007, P.A. Wackym, MD.)

important to examine 4 major points: (1) the second neoplasm must arise in the irradiated field; (2) a latent period of at least several years must have elapsed between the radiation exposure and the development of the second neoplasm; (3) there must be histologic and radiographic evidence of the preexisting condition, in addition to microscopic proof of the second neoplasm; and (4) the second neoplasm must be of a different histologic type from that previously irradiated, to eliminate the possibility of recurrence of the original tumor or a missed diagnosis of the original tumor. With these criteria in mind, Lustig and colleagues in 1997 reported the development of a squamous cell carcinoma following radiation treatment of vestibular schwannoma.[32] In addition, Hanabusa and colleagues reported the malignant transformation of a vestibular schwannoma following gamma knife radiosurgery.[33] There was histologic evidence of vestibular schwannoma following a retrosigmoid resection. Four years after this resection, recidivistic tumor was identified, and the patient was subsequently treated with gamma knife radiosurgery. Six months posttreatment, the tumor had grown, and the patient underwent surgical resection via a combined retrosigmoid-translabyrinthine approach. Abnormal mitotic figures were observed on histologic sections, and the diagnosis of malignancy was assigned. The patient subsequently died 6.5 years after the initial treatment of the malignant disease.

A concerning early trend in stereotactic radiosurgery was the concept of "debulking" the tumor and subsequently radiating the tumor for

astrocytoma was diagnosed, whereas, based on their national incidence figures, 2.47 cases would have been predicted. Finally, to assess the risk of radiosurgery inducing malignancy in patients with neurofibromatosis type 2 (NF2) and von Hippel-Lindau disease, Rowe and colleagues completed a retrospective cohort study of 118 NF2 and 19 von Hippel-Lindau disease patients, totaling 906 and 62 patient-years of follow-up data, respectively.[31] They reported 2 cases of intracranial malignancy, both of which occurred in NF2 patients. One of these was thought to have arisen before the radiosurgery; the other was a glioblastoma diagnosed 3 years after radiosurgery. They concluded that because gliomas may occur in as many as 4% of NF2 patients, the single case may not represent an increased risk. Furthermore, they suggested that the late risk of malignancy arising after irradiation must be put in the context of the condition being treated, the treatment options available to these individuals, and their life expectancy.

Despite the limitations of the studies just reviewed, it is important to counsel patients about this possibility. It is likewise appropriate to

counsel them about the possible causes of these malignant schwannomas. Considering the possibility of radiation-induced malignancies, it is

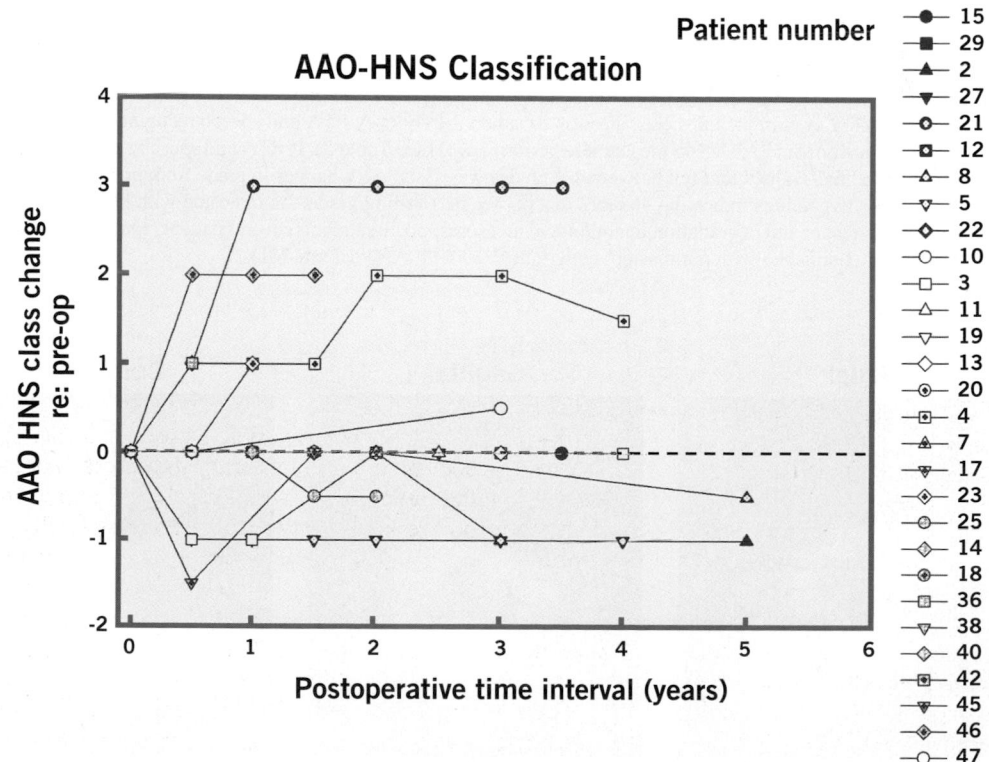

Figure 20 Hearing outcome data were also classified using the American Academy of Otolaryngology – Head and Neck Surgery (AAO-HNS) system (see Table 1). Incorporating pure-tone thresholds and speech recognition score, the classes range from A to D, or best performance to worst performance, respectively. For analysis purposes numerical values of 1 through 4 were assigned (ie, $A = 1$). Positive values denote a postoperative decrement in class. Postoperatively, the majority of patients remained within the same preoperative AAO-HNS class, although some individuals showed either better or poorer hearing outcomes. (Published with permission, copyright © 2007, P.A. Wackym, MD.)

Table 1 AAO-HNS Hearing Classification System[18]

Class	Pure-Tone Thresholds	Speech Discrimination Score (%)
A	≤30 dB	≥70 to 100
B	>30, ≤50 dB	≥50
C	>50 dB	≤50
D	Any level	<50

Table 2 Gardner–Robertson Hearing Grading System[19]

Auditory Grade	Hearing Levels	Pure-Tone Average (dB)	Speech Discrimination Score (%)
I	Good	0–30	70–100
II	Serviceable	31–50	50–69
III	Nonserviceable	50–90	5–49
IV	Poor	91 max	1–4
V	None	Nontestable	0

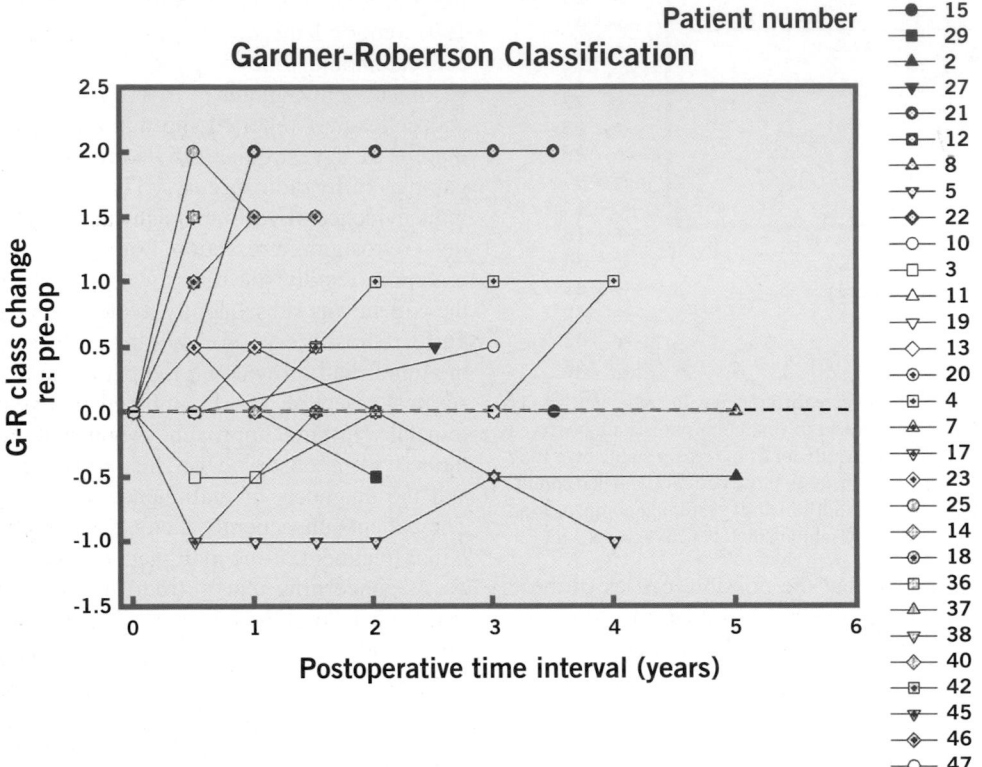

Figure 21 The Gardner-Robertson classification system was used to characterize audiometric outcome after gamma knife radiosurgery. The system includes classification based on 3-frequency PTA and speech recognition scores. Grades range from I (best performance) to V (no measurable performance) (see Table 2). If PTA and speech recognition fell into 2 different grades, a "half-value" that fell between the grades was assigned. Changes in grade from pre- to posttreatment are shown, with positive values indicating changes to a poorer-performing grade. As indicated with the other measures, there is both improvement and degradation in audiologic measures; posttreatment, several patients remained within their pretreatment grade. (Published with permission, copyright © 2007, P.A. Wackym, MD.)

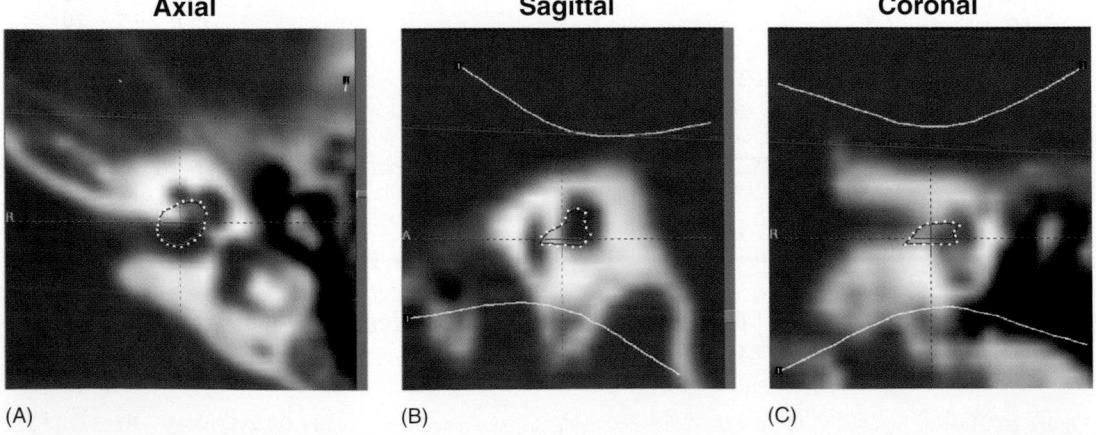

Axial	Sagittal	Coronal
(A)	(B)	(C)

Figure 22 Gamma knife radiosurgery. This example illustrates the distortion introduced by MRI relative to CT during the data acquisition for treatment planning. As shown, the tumor volume and 45% isodose line (*second circle*) as defined on the MRI data set are approximately 1 mm more anterior than the internal auditory canal as seen with CT. This has implications for the delivery of excessive radiation to the facial nerve and/or cochlea during treatment. (Published with permission, copyright © 2007, P.A. Wackym, MD.)

the purpose of "hearing preservation" and "facial nerve preservation." The single most important variable during this process is how much tumor is resected prior to radiation. In the absence of applying intraoperative MRI to visualize the remaining tumor volume, it is a difficult task to be certain when or if the preoperative goal for debulking has been achieved. This approach is not being used in high volume vestibular schwannoma programs nationally, and the traditional neurotologist/neurosurgeon team is not involved with this "innovative" approach. Figure 29 shows an example of a patient in whom a surgeon completed a "debulking procedure" which as shown in Figure 29B was essentially a biopsy. Aside from the unnecessary expense of completing both the craniotomy and gamma knife radiosurgery, the ethical and moral questions presented by this example are troubling. In light of the current outcomes in microsurgery or stereotactic radiosurgery,[16] there is no justification for this type of management algorithm. Figure 30 shows the treatment plan that the patient described above received. This is also an excellent example of a poor conformation to the tumor volume. As shown, the brightest (yellow) line seen outside of the tumor outline (best seen in the axial section) represents the 50% isodose line to which a prescription of 13 Gy was given. It should be noted that there is a significant amount of radiation that was delivered to the brainstem based on this plan. In contrast, Iwai and colleagues applied this concept in a more appropriate way.[34] They reported a series of 14 patients managed over a 6-year interval with vestibular schwannomas too large (range 3.0 to 5.8 cm) to treat primarily with radiosurgery. Subtotal resection was achieved in 13 and partial resection due to hypervascularity was performed in one patient. After recovery, radiosurgery was performed to treat the persistent tumor.

One final issue to consider is tumor growth after radiosurgery. It is important to appreciate that there is an increased size of the tumor after radiosurgery. In fact, we observed a statistically significant increase in tumor size for patients whose tumors extended outside of the internal auditory canal 6 months after gamma knife radiosurgery and a statistically significant decrease at 1 year posttreatment.[8,9] Typically, posttreatment edema persists for 6 months; however, this may remain for up to 1 year. Consequently pretreatment counseling should include this information. There have been anecdotal cases discussed and occasionally reported that describe increased tumor size early after radiosurgery. The challenge is in making a decision about whether to resect these tumors and when.[2,12,29,35–38] Pollock and colleagues emphasized the need to demonstrate sustained tumor growth by serial MRI before making the decision to operate and also to review the case with the surgeon who performed the radiosurgery before a surgical decision is made.[29] The other related controversy is whether the facial nerve dissection and preservation are more difficult during microsurgical resection

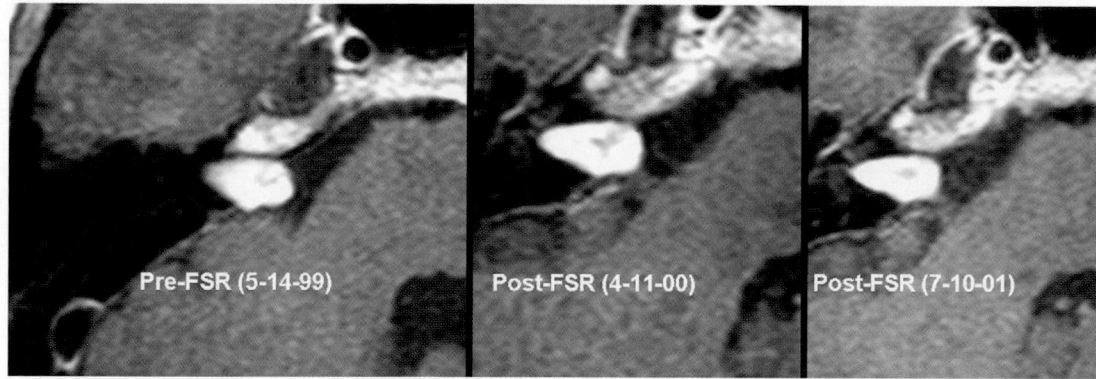

Figure 23 Fractionated stereotactic radiotherapy. Example of serial MRI studies of a small right vestibular schwannoma. Note excellent tumor control at medial aspect; however, continued growth laterally ultimately fills the fundus entirely. (Published with permission, copyright © 2007, P.A. Wackym, MD.)

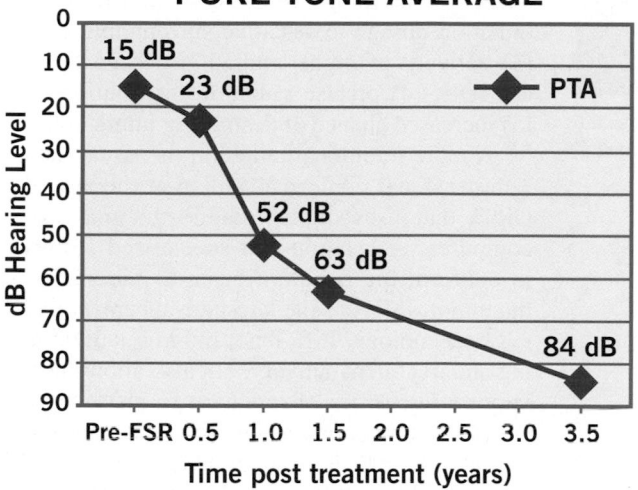

Figure 24 Fractionated stereotactic radiotherapy. As the tumor shown in Figure 23 grew laterally, the auditory performance in that ear progressively worsened. Over a 3.5-year interval, this patient's PTA fell from 15 to 84 dB. (Published with permission, copyright © 2007, P.A. Wackym, MD.)

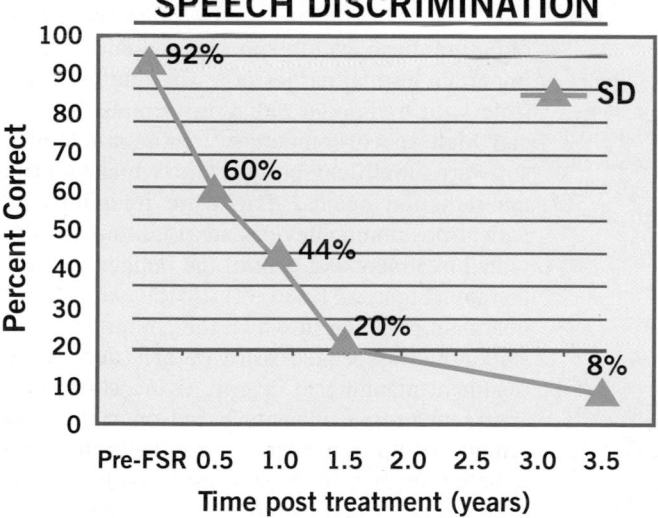

Figure 25 Fractionated stereotactic radiosurgery. As the tumor shown in Figure 23 grew laterally, the auditory performance in that ear progressively worsened. Over a 3.5-year interval, this patient's speech recognition fell from 92 to 8%. (Published with permission, copyright © 2007, P.A. Wackym, MD.)

if the neurotologist and the patient have made a decision to resect a tumor previously treated with radiosurgery, it is important to review the treatment plan to determine the amount of radiation delivered to the facial nerve to counsel the patient appropriately preoperatively.

OTHER STEREOTACTIC RADIOSURGERY AND RADIOTHERAPY TECHNIQUES

Fractionated Stereotactic Radiotherapy

In the preceding sections of this chapter, much attention was focused on gamma knife radiosurgery. This was intentional, as many principles of radiation biology and stereotactic surgery were illustrated. Many of these principles hold true for fractionated stereotactic radiotherapy. Historically, the maximum radiation dose that could be given to a tumor site has been restricted by the tolerance and sensitivity of the surrounding nearby healthy tissues. One-session gamma knife systems and other one-session linear accelerator (LINAC) technologies are available. In addition, several manufacturers currently offer conformal radiation treatment systems that can involve multiple, fractionated, treatments. The most well-recognized systems by trade name at this time are the Peacock (NOMOS Inc., Cranberry Township, PA), the SmartBeam IMRT (Varian Medical Systems Inc., Palo Alto, CA), The Precise (Elekta Inc., Stockholm, Sweden), and the CyberKnife (Accuray, Sunnyvale, CA). The CyberKnife is different in that it is an "image guided" technology as will be discussed below.

Conformal radiation is different from conventional radiation therapy in that radiation therapy targets a uniform shape to a total area to cover the tumor. Thus with conventional radiation therapy, some healthy tissue is always irradiated and the target area receives a homogeneous or even dose of radiation across the entire target area. Conformal radiation treatments have the ability to deliver a higher dose within the tumor and thus can cause more damage to the tumor target without as much damage to the surrounding healthy tissue as conventional external beam radiation treatment.

With the various methods of accomplishing fractionated stereotactic radiosurgery, the patient will be fitted with some type of reusable localization device, which may be a mask or a body frame. This assists in targeting with reproducibility and consequently greater accuracy. Typically, with skull base tumors including vestibular schwannomas, the localization device is molded to fit the precise contours of the individual patient. This molded device is placed on the patient each time they receive a treatment. Multiple treatments are usually required with conformal radiation as with conventional radiation therapy. These treatments may range from 1 to 28 treatments, which is lesser than usual conventional radiation treatments. Treatment time itself for each session is typically longer than with conventional radiation therapy because of the complexity of the treatment.

after radiosurgery. On 1 end of the spectrum, descriptions of no increased difficulty have been reported[29]; and, on the other end of the spectrum,[35–38] markedly increased difficulty in separating the tumor from the facial nerve and poorer facial nerve function outcome have also been reported. The report of Watanabe and colleagues included a histopathologic analysis of the resected facial nerve.[36] They found microvasculitis of the facial nerve, axonal degeneration, loss of axons, and proliferation of Schwann cells. In light of the

mechanism of delayed effects following radiosurgery, these findings are not surprising. Moreover, these findings emphasize the need for the neurotologist to be certain that the treatment plan avoids high radiation doses to the facial nerve. Recall as described earlier that a dose of 12 Gy delivered to the 50% isodose line means that the maximum tumor dose is 24 Gy. If the treatment plan delivers this maximal dose to the area of the facial nerve, it should be expected that greater radiation effects will be observed. For this reason,

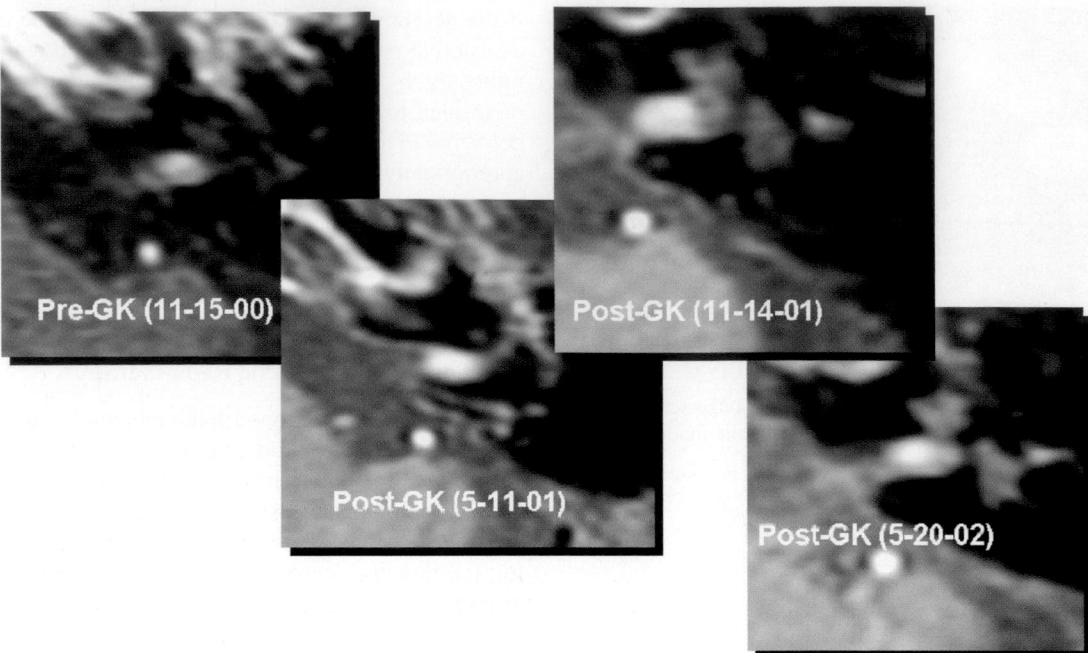

Figure 26 Gamma knife radiosurgery. Example of serial MRI studies of a small left vestibular schwannoma. Note at 6 and 12 months post-gamma knife radiosurgery the tumor is larger than pretreatment. By 18 months the tumor is smaller. (Reproduced with permission, copyright © 2007, P.A. Wackym, MD.)

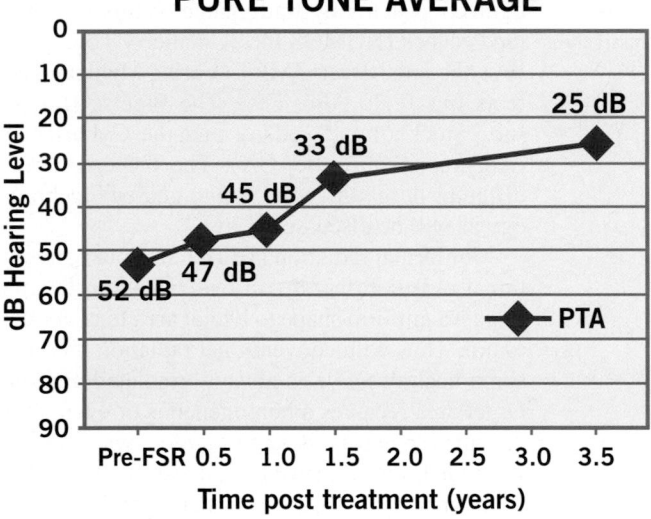

Figure 27 Gamma knife radiosurgery. Hearing outcome of the tumor shown in Figure 26. Over a 3.5-year interval, this patient's PTA improved from 52 to 25 dB. (Published with permission, copyright © 2007, P.A. Wackym, MD.)

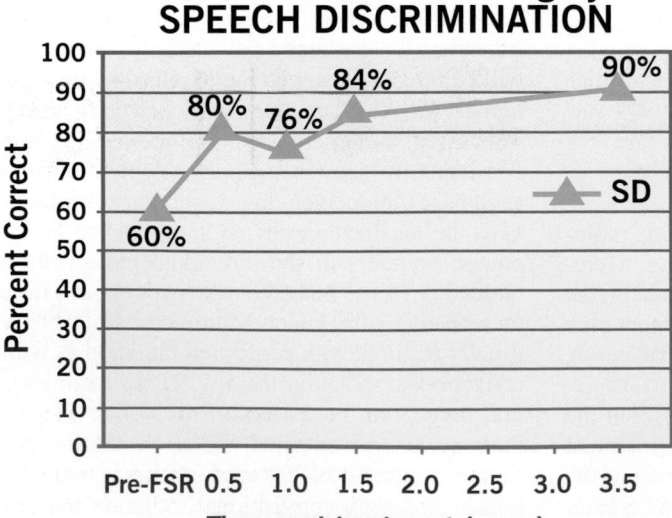

Figure 28 Gamma knife radiosurgery. Hearing outcome of the tumor shown in Figure 26. Over a 3.5-year interval, this patient's speech recognition improved from 60 to 90%. (Published with permission, copyright © 2007, P.A. Wackym, MD.)

The outcomes after treatment of vestibular schwannomas with fractionated stereotactic radiotherapy are being reported; however, fewer patients to date have been treated with these types of modalities than have been treated with gamma knife radiosurgery.[39–41]

Intensity Modulated Radiation Therapy

Intensity modulated radiation therapy (IMRT) is a powerful, relatively new technology. This therapy can be used to target skull base tumor cells while limiting radiation to important normal tissues such as the eyes, optic nerves, brain, brainstem, adjacent cranial nerves, inner ear, salivary glands, and spinal cord. There are 5 principal advantages of IMRT compared to traditional radiation therapy. These are: (1) decreased chance of harming normal cells; (2) decreased radiation dosage to sensitive surrounding tissue; (3) delivery of higher radiation dosage to cancer cells; (4) precise radiation distribution; and (5) increased chance of destroying tumor cells.

A more traditional radiation therapy is called 3-dimensional conformal radiation therapy (3D CRT) that uses digital diagnostic imaging, a computer workstation and specialized software to conform the radiation beam to the shape of the tumor. IMRT is the latest advancement in 3D CRT technology. IMRT not only uses 3D imaging and treatment delivery, but also allows use of varying intensities of radiation to produce dosage distributions that are more conformal to the tumor volume than those possible with 3D CRT.

In IMRT, small beams, sometimes referred to as beamlets, with varying intensities can be aimed at a tumor from many angles. The intensity of each beamlet can be controlled. The radiation dose can be made to bend around important normal tissues in a way that is impossible with traditional radiation techniques. Special high speed computers, treatment-planning software, multileaf collimators which control the radiation beams, diagnostic imaging, and patient-positioning devices are used to plan individual treatment and control the radiation during therapy (Figures 31 and 32). IMRT uses inverse treatment planning in which the computer workstation and associated software are used during treatment planning to determine the ideal beam arrangement and intensity based on the desired dosage. IMRT can improve the effectiveness of radiation therapy by delivering a larger radiation dose to tumor cells while reducing the dose to surrounding normal cells. The anatomical position of the tumor and surrounding normal tissues must be accurately defined for IMRT to be effective. CT and MRI scans provide the necessary 3D anatomical information which is used within the software platform during the treatment planning.

In contrast to gamma knife radiosurgery, but similar to fractionated stereotactic radiotherapy, a regimen of IMRT is usually given over several weeks. The total dose of radiation and the number of treatments needed depend on the size,

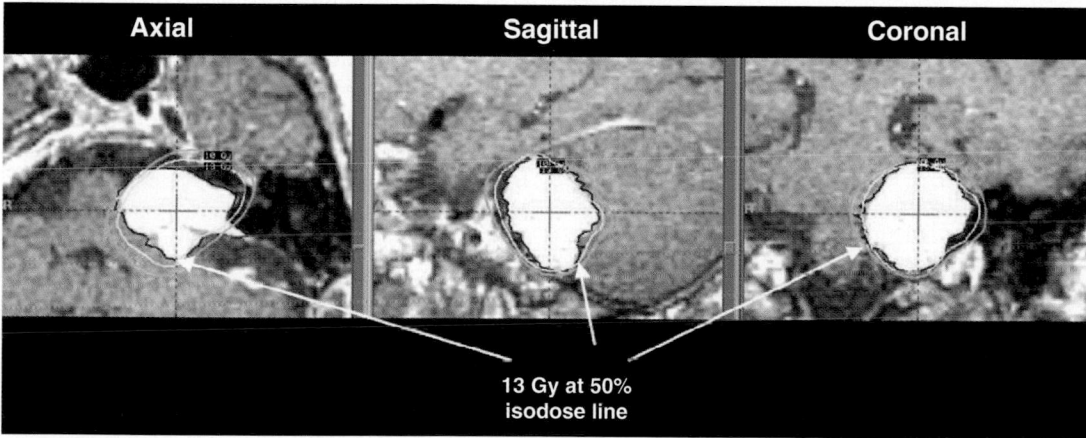

Figure 29 Gamma knife radiosurgery. An example of what is being described as an "innovative" combined microsurgery and radiosurgery approach to the management of acoustic neuromas. Advocates of this method anecdotally assert that better hearing preservation and facial nerve outcome can be achieved. With this example, essentially a biopsy of the tumor was performed, followed by gamma knife radiosurgery. Ethical and cost-effectiveness issues are raised. (Published with permission, copyright © 2007, P.A. Wackym, MD.)

Figure 30 Gamma knife radiosurgery. Poor treatment plan including poor conformation of radiation dose to tumor margin (brightest circle, yellow, represents 13 Gy at the 50% isodose line). Note excessive radiation delivered to brainstem (a portion receives 13 Gy at the 50% isodose line) and inadequate treatment of internal auditory canal portion of tumor (portion outside of the 50% isodose line). (Published with permission, copyright © 2007, P.A. Wackym, MD.)

location, and type of tumor, the patient's general health, and other medical therapy the patient is receiving.

TomoTherapy

In the same way that IMRT has improved on 3D techniques to allow more precise treatment to a specific target, TomoTherapy takes it 1 step farther. The TomoTherapy machine (TomoTherapy Inc., Madison, WI), has an appearance similar to a traditional diagnostic CT scanner (Figure 33). However, it is really a CT scanner and a linear accelerator combined. The linear accelerator delivers high energy radiation to treat a target, and the CT scanner is used to ensure that the patient is positioned properly on a daily basis. The CT is not of diagnostic quality, as high energy radiation is used (vs low energy used for diagnostic scans); but the scans are clear enough to detect bony anatomy and most soft tissue anatomy well enough, and small positioning changes can be made (within a few millimeters) to ensure as accurate a treatment as possible.

With IMRT, there are a specific number of stationary beams, usually 7 or 9, which are directed at the target from various angles. With TomoTherapy, however, radiation is delivered in a circular motion around the patient; and, after approximately every 7° of rotation, radiation is

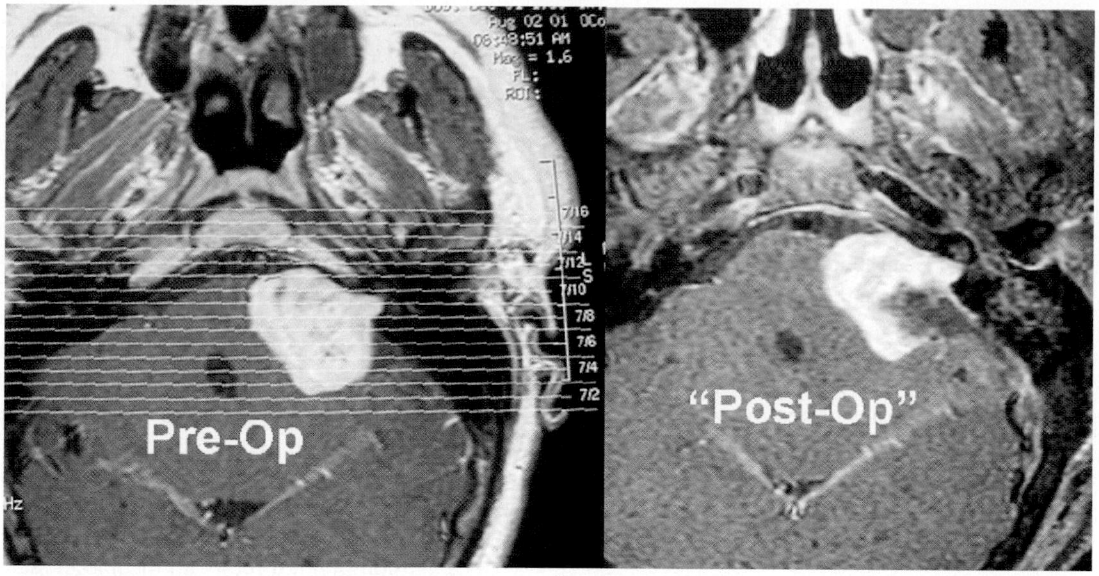

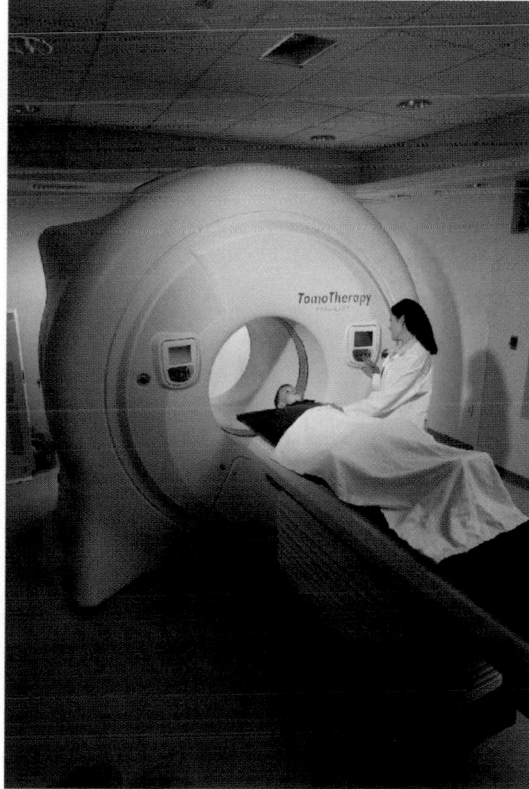

Figure 33 The TomoTherapy machine has an appearance similar to a traditional diagnostic CT scanner; however, it is really a CT scanner and a linear accelerator combined. The linear accelerator delivers high energy radiation to treat a target, and the CT scanner is used to ensure that the patient is positioned properly on a daily basis. The CT scans are able to detect bony anatomy and most soft tissue anatomy and therefore positioning changes within a few millimeters ensures treatment accuracy. (Published with permission, copyright © 2007, TomoTherapy, Inc., Madison, WI.)

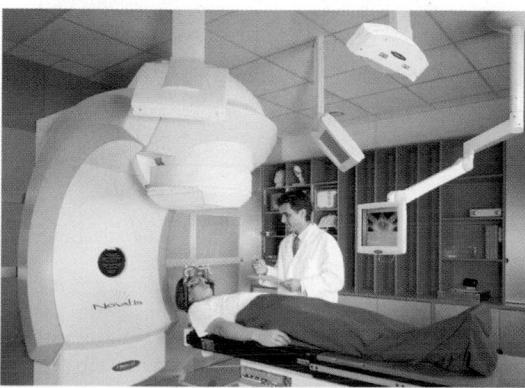

Figure 31 Stereotactic radiotherapy using intensity modulated radiosurgery. The Novalis Shaped Beam Surgery system is shown. This system is described as a high resolution intensity modulated radiotherapy instrument and technique. (Published with permission, copyright © 2007, BrainLAB AG, Munich, Germany.)

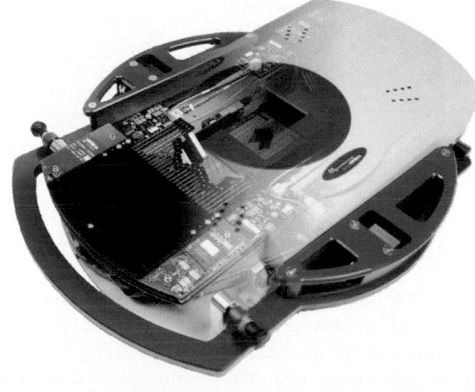

Figure 32 Multileaf collimator. Intensity modulated radiotherapy (IMRT) systems use multileaf collimators that shape the radiation fields that are delivered to the tumor. The Novalis Beam Shaper uses 3 mm fine leaves for high resolution IMRT. (Published with permission, copyright © 2007, BrainLAB AG, Munich, Germany.)

delivered to the patient. Therefore, instead of 7 or 9 beams, this is like having approximately 51 beams encircling a target. The result is a conformal treatment around a specific target, while sparing normal structures nearby. TomoTherapy is a new technology and has been available only since the mid- to late-1990s; therefore, new applications for its use are still being developed and at this point in time, there are no published studies using TomoTherapy for stereotactic radiotherapy. However, it is estimated that the accuracy of TomoTherapy is approximately within 1 mm, using an aquaplast mask for immobilization of the head (compared to 0.5 mm with the stereotactic head frame used with gamma knife), and there may be a role for treating certain tumors, such as brain metastases, in the future with TomoTherapy, either with fractionated treatment or a single fraction. One dosimetric difference between TomoTherapy and IMRT is that with TomoTherapy, the patient tends to have more low dose radiation to a larger area (since the beams are coming from 360°); with traditional IMRT, the low dose region is smaller, but the hot spots in and around the target tend to be higher. The clinical implications of having a larger low dose region are not known at this time. Therefore, based on these differences, the radiation oncologist and surgeon may choose 1 technology over the other for certain clinical cases.

CyberKnife Stereotactic Radiosurgery

Overview of Treatment Planning. The CyberKnife system's LINAC maneuverability offers the radiosurgery team several treatment options. The treatment planning system is designed to support the radiosurgery team in determining the optimal plan, including beam weight, targeting positions, dose distributions, and other factors for each patient's treatment. The CyberKnife stereotactic radiosurgery system permits the following planning and delivery options: (1) inverse planning; (2) nonisocentric delivery; and (3) hypofractionation. The system is based on CT scanning. MR images can be fused with the CT to provide optimal information on soft tissue as well as skeletal anatomy. CT angiography can be used when vascular skull base lesions, such as arteriovenous malformations or extensive glomus jugulare tumors are to be treated with this technique.

Additionally, the CyberKnife system provides a range of treatment options, including the ability to use either forward or inverse treatment planning, allowing the radiosurgery team to customize each patient's treatment plan. With forward treatment planning, the radiation oncologist determines what dose to deliver from a particular targeting position. Subsequently, the planning software calculates the total dose within the lesion for the user. With inverse treatment planning, the radiation oncologist specifies total dose to be delivered to the tumor, and the surgeon and radiation oncologist set boundaries to protect adjacent critical structures. The software

determines targeting positions and dose to be delivered from a particular targeting position. While other stereotactic radiosurgery systems offer the inverse planning option, the number of possible plans is somewhat limited by the constraints of the delivery system. The flexibility of the robotic arm supporting the linear accelerator potentially allows the CyberKnife to implement a wider range of treatment plans than other systems. Furthermore, because the system does not require the use of a stereotactic head frame temporarily attached to the patient's head, it allows scanning, treatment planning, and quality assurance to take place at any time prior to treatment itself.

Dose Distribution. The CyberKnife system offers a choice of a nonisocentric or an isocentric treatment approach. With other stereotactic radiosurgery systems, a fixed calculated isocenter is used. Isocentric treatment, or multiisocentric treatment, involves filling the lesion with a single or multiple, overlapping spherically shaped dose distributions. Isocentric treatment is effective for spherical lesions. However, with irregularly shaped lesions, isocentric delivery can produce significant dose heterogeneity (Figure 34). Clinically, this is not a significant issue, provided that the treatment plan accounts for the relationship of the maximuim dose to the critical structure to be considered. For example, if a gamma knife radiosurgery treatment plan for a vestibular schwannoma uses 12 Gy at the 50% isodose line, the maximal radiation dose at the "hot spot" will 24 Gy. During the treatment planning, assessment of the plan quality would include visualizing where this maximal dose would be located and during this assessment, determination that this maximal dose was adjacent to the facial nerve or brainstem. Similarly, it is important to determine the conformation of the treatment plan to the tumor volume to determine regions which may be undertreated by delivery of inadequate doses, resulting in areas that would allow continued tumor growth.

Nonisocentric treatment plans are also possible with the CyberKnife system. The delivery of these treatment plans is possible because of the robotic arm which, because of the 6 degrees of freedom (discussed below) enables the delivery of radiation to complex treatment volumes. The beams originate from arbitrary points in the workspace and are delivered into the lesion. The result is a nonisocentric concentration of beams within the lesion (Figure 35). Nonisocentric treatment allows nonsymmetrical irradiation.

With the CyberKnife system, the treatment plan can utilize fractionated or hypofractionated approaches. Fractionated treatment is possible because localization of the lesion is achieved using image guidance technology. Dose delivery over 2 to 5 treatment sessions, termed hypofractionation, is another option with the CyberKnife system. Although not directly applicable in managing tumors within the posterior fossa, it has been suggested to be particularly useful in the treatment of large tumors. The argument for fractionation is that lowering the dose for each of a number of treatments, as opposed to a single, larger dose, allows healthy tissue to rejuvenate between treatments. The advantage of fractionated or a single radiation dose remains an active area of investigation and debate. Because of the rigid fixation that occurs with securing the stereotacic headframe in gamma knife radiosurgery, fractionated, or hypofractionated delivery of radiation is not possible. Furthermore, it remains to be determined if equal accuracy can be achieved by these 2 systems or if there is an advantage of fractionation or hypofractionation in the treatment of skull base tumors.

Localization. The CyberKnife system's use of stereotactic principles for tumor localization differs from other stereotactic radiosurgery systems in 1 specific way. It uses an image guidance technology that depends on the skeletal structure of

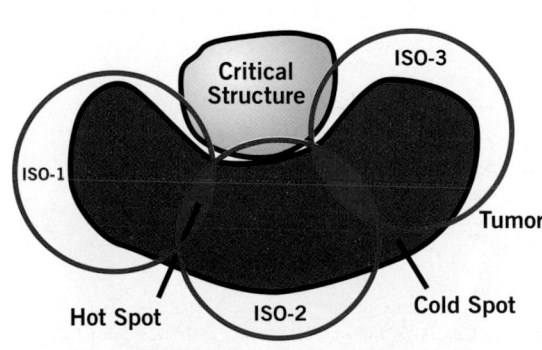

Figure 34 Isocentric treatment planning using the CyberKnife radiosurgery system. Isocentric treatment, or multiisocentric treatment, involves filling the lesion with a single or multiple, overlapping spherically shaped dose distributions (ISO-1, ISO-2, and ISO-3). Isocentric treatment is effective for spherical lesions; however, with irregularly shaped lesions, isocentric delivery can produce significant dose heterogeneity. Note radiation overlap with critical structure (eg, brainstem). (Published with permission, copyright © 2007, P.A. Wackym, MD.)

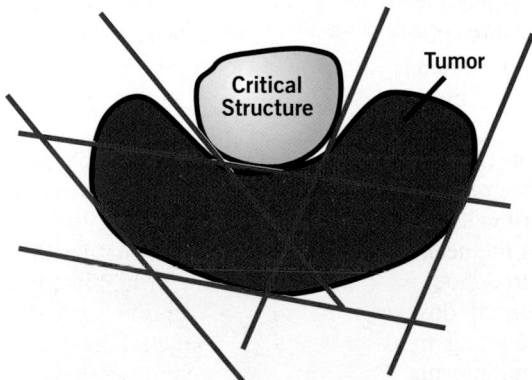

Figure 35 Nonisocentric treatment planning using the CyberKnife radiosurgery system. Nonisocentric treatment plans are possible because of the robotic arm which, because of the 6 degrees of freedom, enables the delivery of radiation to complex treatment volumes. The beams originate from arbitrary points in the workspace and are delivered into the lesion. The result is a nonisocentric concentration of beams within the lesion, avoiding critical structures such as the brainstem while maintaining tumor conformation. (Published with permission, copyright © 2007, P.A. Wackym, MD.)

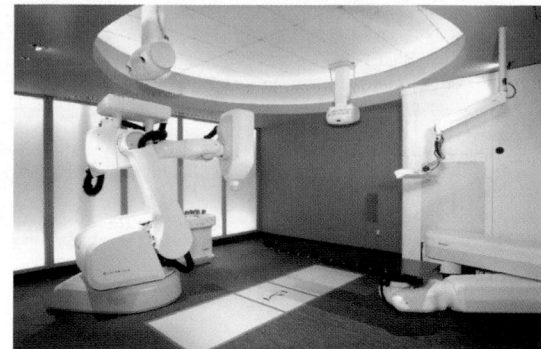

Figure 36 Ceiling-mounted diagnostic-energy X-ray sources emit low-dose X-rays through the patient's tumor treatment area. Amorphous silicon image detectors capture X-ray images from ceiling-mounted diagnostic-energy X-ray sources to produce live radiographs. The operating system (typically located adjacent to the treatment room) correlates patient location detected by image guidance system with reconstructed CT scan and directs the robot to adjust position accordingly. The compact linear accelerator mounted on a computer-controlled robotic arm which adjusts position to maintain alignment with the target, compensating for any patient movement and uses X-band technology for mobility. (Published with permission, copyright © 2007, Accuray Incorporated, Sunnyvale, CA.)

the body as a reference frame (Figure 36). In addition, it continually monitors and tracks patient position during treatment. The CyberKnife's operating system correlates live radiographic images with preoperative CT scans to determine patient and tumor position repeatedly over the course of treatment. The imaging information is transferred from the computer's operating system to the robot so that it may compensate for any changes in patient position by repositioning the LINAC.

Treatment Delivery. The CyberKnife stereotactic radiosurgery system utilizes a compact 6-MeV linear accelerator, a computer-controlled robotic arm with 6 degrees of freedom, and an image-guidance technology that does not depend on a rigid stereotactic frame and thereby enables treatment of extracranial sites. Potential benefits of this approach include: (1) increased access to and coverage of any target volume including the ability to treat lesions in and around the cranium that are unreachable with other systems, for example, in the lower posterior fossa and foramen magnum; (2) enhanced ability to avoid critical structures; (3) capability to treat lesions in the neck and spine; (4) ability to treat lesions throughout the body; (5) delivery of highly conformal dose distributions; (6) option of fractionating treatment; and (7) potential to target multiple tumors at different locations during a single treatment, for example, skull base and neck.

The CyberKnife system's computer-controlled robotic arm has 6 degrees of freedom. The robot can position the LINAC to more than 100 specific locations or nodes. Each node has 12 possible approach angles, translating to over 1,200 possible beam positions. The treatment planning system determines a set sequence of approach angles, beam weights, and dose distributions. The

calculated plan can be incrementally improved by the physicist and physicians. The actual delivery follows a step-and-shoot sequence. The patient is placed in a position approximating that of the CT scan. Image detectors acquire radiographs of the tumor region. The image guidance system software then compares the real time radiographs with the CT information to determine location of the tumor. This information is transmitted to the robot to initialize the pointing of the LINAC beam. The robotic arm then moves the LINAC through the sequence of preset nodes surrounding the patient. At each node, the LINAC stops, and a new pair of images are acquired from which the position is redetermined. Corrected position is transmitted to the robot which adapts beam pointing to compensate for any movement. LINAC delivers the preplanned dose of radiation for that position. The entire process is repeated at each node. The total time from imaging to robot compensation is about 7 to 10 seconds. The total treatment time depends on the complexity of the plan and delivery paths, but is comparable to standard LINAC treatments. Each treatment session ranges from 30 to 90 minutes. Physicians may elect to treat with a single dose, a hypofractionated dose typically two to five sessions, or a more traditional fractionated regimen. Outcomes following CyberKnife treatment of vestibular schwannomas are emerging at this time.[42]

SUMMARY

There is diversity in the techniques and instrumentation used to perform stereotactic radiosurgery and radiotherapy. The field continues to evolve rapidly, and advances are being made in improving accuracy, effective radiation dose, and parameters necessary to maximize patient outcome. Stereotactic radiosurgery and radiotherapy, just as any other treatment modality, have advantages and disadvantages that must be discussed with a patient who has a vestibular schwannoma or other skull base tumor. An informed decision to pursue observation, microsurgery, or stereotactic radiosurgery or radiotherapy, or a combination of these methods must be made, and it remains the responsibility of the surgeon to provide a balanced view as to the relative advantages and disadvantages of each method.

FINANCIAL DISCLOSURE

None of the authors have a financial interest in any of the companies discussed in this chapter.

REFERENCES

1. Kondziolka D, Lunsford LD, McLaughlin MR, Flickinger JC. Long-term outcomes after radiosurgery for acoustic neuroma. N Engl J Med 1998;339:1426–33.
2. Wackym PA. Stereotactic radiosurgery, microsurgery, and expectant management of acoustic neuroma: Basis of informed consent. Otolaryngol Clin North Am 2005; 38:653–70.
3. Hall E. Radiobiology for the Radiologist, 5th edition. Philadelphia: Lippincott, Williams & Wilkins; 2000. p. 544–45.
4. Shrieve DC. Basic principles of radiobiology applied to radiotherapy of benign intracranial tumors. Neurosurg Clin North Am 2006;17:67–78.
5. Hendee W, Ibbott G. Radiation Therapy Physics, 2nd edition. St. Louis: Mosby; 1996. p. 11.
6. Hall E. Radiobiology for the Radiologist, 6th edition. Philadelphia: Lippincott, Williams & Wilkins; 2006. p. 36.
7. Hall E. Radiobiology for the Radiologist, 5th edition. Philadelphia: Lippincott, Williams & Wilkins; 2000. p. 521.
8. Wackym PA, Runge-Samuelson CL, Poetker DM, et al. Gamma knife radiosurgery for acoustic neuromas performed by a neurotologist: Early experiences and outcomes. Otol Neurol 2004;25:752–61.
9. Poetker DM, Jursinic PA, Runge-Samuelson CL, Wackym PA. Distortion of magnetic resonance images used in gamma knife radiosurgery treatment planning: Implications for acoustic neuroma outcomes. Otol Neurotol 2005;26:1220–8.
10. Hall E. Radiobiology for the Radiologist, 5th edition. Philadelphia: Lippincott, Williams & Wilkins; 2000. p. 74.
11. Kondziolka D, Lunsford L, Flickinger J. The radiobiology of radiosurgery. Neurosurg Clin North Am 1999;10:157–66.
12. Pitts LA, Jackler RK. Treatment of acoustic neuromas. N Engl J Med 1998;339:1471–73.
13. Linskey ME, Martinez AJ, Kondziolka D, et al. The radiobiology of human acoustic schwannoma xenografts after stereotactic radiosurgery evaluated in the subrenal capsule of athymic mice. J Neurosurg 1993;78:645–53.
14. Paddick I. A simple scoring ratio to index the conformity of radiosurgical treatment plans. Technical note. J Neurosurg 2000;93:219–22.
15. Régis J, Tamura M, Guillot C, et al. Radiosurgery of the head and neck with the world's first fully robotized 192 cobalt-60 source Leksell Gamma Knife Perfexion in clinical use. J Neurosurg (in press).
16. Kaylie DM, McMenomey SO. Microsurgery vs gamma knife radiosurgery for the treatment of vestibular schwannomas. Arch Otolaryngol Head Neck Surg 2003;129:903–6.
17. Yamakami I, Uchino Y, Kobayashi E, Yamaura A. Conservative management, gamma-knife radiosurgery, and microsurgery for acoustic neurinomas: A systematic review of outcome and risk of three therapeutic options. Neurol Res 2003;25:682–90.
18. Committee on Hearing and Equilibrium guidelines for the evaluation of hearing preservation in acoustic neuroma (vestibular schwannoma). Otolaryngol Head Neck Surg 1995;113:179 80.
19. Gardner G, Robertson JH. Hearing preservation in unilateral acoustic neuroma surgery. Ann Otol Rhinol Laryngol 1998;97:55–66.
20. Healthcare professionals. Treatment statistics. Available at: http://www.elekta.com/assets/gammaknife/treat_stats/ww05.pdf. Accessed June 8, 2007.
21. Alberta Heritage Foundation for Medical Research. Health technology assessment report IP 14. Cost estimation of stereotactic radiosurgery: Application to Alberta. Ohinmaa A, May 2003. Available at: http://www.ihe.ca/hta/publications.html. Accessed June 8, 2007.
22. Acoustic Neuroma Patient Archive International. Gamma knife, LINAC, and proton beam: Comparison of recent radiosurgery outcomes. Available at: http://www.anarchive.org/spread.htm. Accessed June 8, 2007.
23. Lunsford LD, Niranjan A, Flickinger JC, et al. Radiosurgery of vestibular schwannomas: Summary of experience in 829 cases. J Neurosurg 2005; 102:195–9.
24. Niranjan A, Lunsford LD, Flickinger JC, et al. Dose reduction improves hearing preservation rates after intracanalicular acoustic tumor radiosurgery. Neurosurgery 1999;45:753–62.
25. Flickinger JC, Kondziolka D, Niranjan A, Lunsford LD. Results of acoustic neuroma radiosurgery: An analysis of 5 years' experience using current methods. J Neurosurg 2001;94:1–6.
26. Prasad D, Steiner M, Steiner L. Gamma surgery for vestibular schwannoma. J Neurosurg 2000;92:745–59.
27. Paek SH, Chung H-T, Jeong SS, et al. Hearing preservation after gamma knife radiosurgery of vestibular schwannoma. Cancer 2005;104:580–90.
28. Bari ME, Forster DM, Kemeny AA, et al. Malignancy in a vestibular schwannoma. Report of a case with central neurofibromatosis, treated by both stereotactic radiosurgery and surgical excision, with a review of the literature. Br J Neurosurg 2002;16:284–9.
29. Pollock BE, Lunsford LD, Kondziolka D, et al. Vestibular schwannoma management. Part II. Failed radiosurgery and the role of delayed microsurgery. J Neurosurg 1998; 89:949–55.
30. Rowe J, Grainger A, Walton L, et al. Risk of malignancy after gamma knife stereotactic radiosurgery. Neurosurgery 2007;60:60–5.

31. Rowe J, Grainger A, Walton L, et al. Safety of radiosurgery applied to conditions with abnormal tumor suppressor genes. Neurosurgery 2007;60:860–4.

32. Lustig LR, Jackler RK, Lanser MJ. Radiation-induced tumors of the temporal bone. Am J Otol 1997;18:230–5.

33. Hanabusa K, Morikawa A, Murata T, Taki W. Acoustic neuroma with malignant transformation. Case report. J Neurosurg 2001;95:518–21.

34. Iwai Y, Yamanaka K, Ishiguro T. Surgery combined with radiosurgery o f large acoustic neuromas. Surg Neurol 2003; 59:283–9.

35. Ho SY, Kveton JF. Rapid growth of acoustic neuromas after stereotactic radiotherapy in type 2 neurofibromatosis. Ear Nose Throat J 2002;81:831–3.

36. Watanabe T, Saito N, Hirato J, et al. Facial neuropathy due to axonal degeneration and microvasculitis following gamma knife surgery for vestibular schwannoma: A histological analysis. J Neurosurg 2003;99:916–20.

37. Lee DJ, Westra WH, Staecker H, et al. Clinical and histopathologic features of recurrent vestibular schwannoma (acoustic neuroma) after stereotactic radiosurgery. Otol Neurol 2003;24:650–60.

38. Friedman RA, Brackmann DE, Hitselberger WE, et al. Surgical salvage after failed irradiation for vestibular schwannoma. Laryngoscope 2005;115:1827–32.

39. Andrews DW, Suarez O, Goldman HW, et al. Stereotactic radiosurgery and fractionated stereotactic radiotherapy for the treatment of acoustic schwannomas: Comparative observations of 125 patients treated at one institution. Int J Radiat Oncol Biol Phys 2001;50:1265–78.

40. Koh ES, Millar BA, Ménard C, et al. Fractionated stereotactic radiotherapy for acoustic neuromas: Single-institution experience at The Princess Margaret Hospital. Cancer 2007;109:1203–10.

41. Likhterov I, Allbright RM, Selesnick SH. LINAC radiotherapy treatment of acoustic neuromas. Otolaryngol Clin North Am 2007;40:541–70.

42. Chang SD, Gibbs IC, Sakamoto GT, et al. Staged stereotactic irradiation for acoustic neuroma. Neurosurgery 2005;56:1254–61.

Embryology, Anatomy and Physiology of the Nose and Paranasal Sinuses

Peter H. Hwang, MD
Arman Abdalkhani, MD

The nasal cavity and paranasal sinuses comprise an anatomically complex aggregate of mucosa-lined airspaces within the bones of the face and skull. These airspaces contribute to a variety of functions, including: the warming and humidification of air; olfaction; lightening the skull; giving resonance to the voice; absorbing traumatic forces; and aiding in immune defense. Familiarity with the nuances of sinonasal anatomy is critical to understanding function and to mastering safe surgical technique.

EMBRYOLOGY

Nose

External Aspect of the Nose. The nose develops from the frontonasal process which, along with the maxillary and mandibular processes, is one of the 3 facial outgrowths visible in the fourth fetal week. In the fifth fetal week, ectodermal plaques develop on the lateral aspects of the frontonasal process and become paired nasal placodes, which are early precursors of the nares. By day 34, these convex placodes develop into concave nasal grooves, and the medial and lateral sides of the placodes begin to protrude forward to become medial and lateral nasal processes (Figure 1).

The nasal placodes develop into nasal grooves, eventually become blind-ending nasal pits by the seventh fetal week as the maxillary process grows forward and downward. It is at this time in fetal life that forward growth of both the medial and lateral ridges of the nasal placodes leads to development of the medial and lateral nasal processes, which ultimately contribute to formation of the nares and septum. The ultimate contributions of the facial processes to mature soft tissue and skeletal structures are summarized in Table 1.

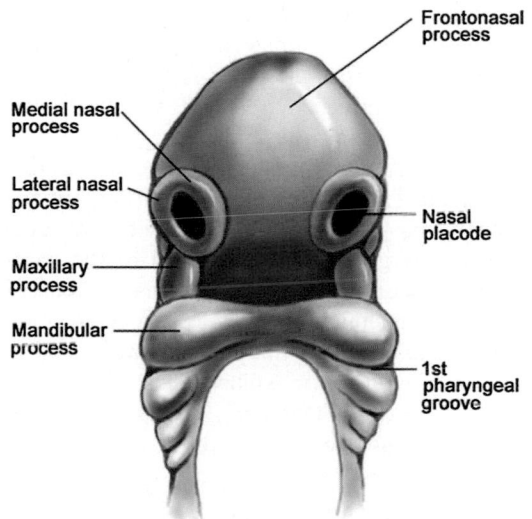

Figure 1 The frontonasal, maxillary, and mandibular processes can be appreciated. The nasal placode, which later develops into the nasal pit can be seen within the medial and lateral nasal processes. (Published with permission, copyright © 2007 P.A. Wackym, MD.)

Nasal Cavity. From fetal weeks 5 to 7, the nasal pit deepens and forms the nasal sac, which is a precursor to the nasal cavity. At the posterior border of the nasal sac, an epithelial lining called the oronasal membrane abuts the nascent oropharyngeal cavity. At day 42 to 44, this membrane ruptures, thus creating a communication between the nasal and oral cavities. Failure of rupture leads to choanal atresia. The nasal capsule, which is a cartilaginous envelope that encases the nasal cavity, forms a boundary to nasal and paranasal sinus development. This mesodermal structure begins to form in third fetal month, and chondrification and ossification of the nasal capsule begins shortly thereafter. There are several sites of ossification; but, prior to bone formation, a rudimentary nasal cavity can be seen.[1]

Lateral Nasal Wall. During the seventh and eighth gestational weeks, the lateral wall of the nasal capsule begins to form a series of ridges of mesenchymal tissue just superior to the palatal shelves. This first ridge, the maxilloturbinal, develops in the seventh week and gives rise to the inferior turbinate. During the eighth gestational week, a series of 5 to 6 ridges appear superior to the maxilloturbinal; through regression and fusion, these ridges form 3 to 5 ethmoturbinals. The first ethmoturbinal (sometimes referred to as the nasoturbinal) gives rise to the agger nasi from its ascending portion, and to the uncinate process from its descending portion.[2] The remainder of the first ethmoturbinal regresses.

Table 1 Summary of the Embryonic Precursors to the Facial Structures

Embryonic Precursor	Soft Tissue Correlate	Skeletal Correlate
Frontonasal process	Bridge of nose	Nasal bones
Median nasal process	Columella and philtrum	Perpendicular plate of ethmoid and vomer
Lateral nasal process	Nasal sidewall and ala	–
Maxillary process	Upper lip and cheek	Maxilla, zygoma, secondary palate
Mandibular process	Lower lip and cheek	Mandible
Nasal pit	–	Nasal cavity

Adapted from reference 1.

The second ethmoturbinal forms the middle turbinate while the third ethmoturbinal forms the superior turbinate. The fourth and fifth ethmoturbinals typically regress, but in some individuals persist and fuse to form the supreme turbinate (Figure 2).

The anatomic correlates of these ethmoturbinals, namely the uncinate process, middle turbinate and superior turbinate, in addition to the ethmoid bulla, have lamellar attachments to the lateral nasal wall that are used as important landmarks during sinus surgery (Table 2). The development of the ethmoturbinals is followed by the development of the paranasal sinuses.

Paranasal Sinuses

The frontal, maxillary, and ethmoid sinuses arise from evaginations of the lateral nasal wall, whereas the sphenoid sinus arises from a posterior evagination of the nasal capsule. The sinuses begin to develop in the third fetal month and only 2, the ethmoid and maxillary sinus, are present at birth. The development, vascular supply and innervation of each sinus are summarized in Table 3.

The arteries supplying the sinuses originate from either the internal or external carotid artery, or both. The sensory innervation of the sinuses derives from either the first branch of the trigeminal nerve, the second branch, or both. Where sensory innervation is supplied by V1, the corresponding arterial supply originates from the ophthalmic artery (internal carotid), and where innervation is supplied by V2, the arterial supply is derived from the internal maxillary artery (external carotid). The correlation between carotid blood supply and trigeminal nerve supply may relate to the course of fetal stapedial artery, a derivative of the second branchial arch. Its 2 major divisions, the dorsal (supraorbital) and ventral (maxillomandibular), run parallel to V1 and V2, respectively. Before the stapedial artery regresses, the dorsal division anastomoses with the ophthalmic artery and the ventral division anastomoses with the internal maxillary artery,

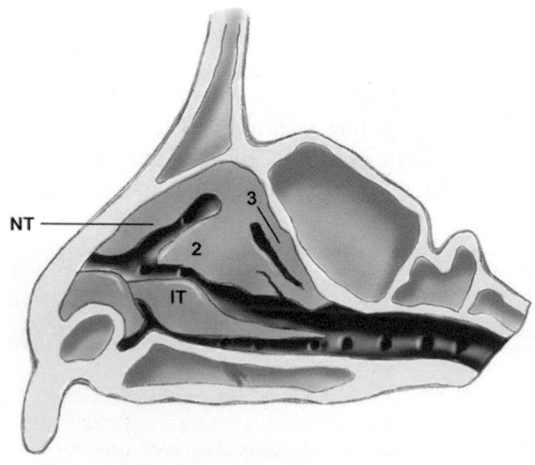

Figure 2 Sagittal diagram of the developing lateral nasal cavity. The fourth and fifth ethmoturbinal have regressed. IT = inferior turbinate; NT = nasoturbinal. (Published with permission, copyright © 2007 P.A. Wackym, MD.)

Table 2 Naming of the Lamellar Attachments to the Lateral Nasal Wall*

Lamella	Anatomic Correlate
First	Lateral extension of the uncinate process
Second	Lateral extension of the ethmoid bulla
Third	Middle turbinate attachment
Fourth	Superior turbinate attachment
Fifth	Supreme turbinate attachment (if present)

*The lamellae are named as they are encountered sequentially from an anterior to posterior direction.

bringing V1 and V2 into proximity with the internal and external carotid blood supplies, respectively.[3]

Maxillary Sinuses. The maxillary sinus begins as an outpouching of the lateral nasal wall at the tenth fetal week. It begins posterior to the descending portion of the first ethmoturbinal (the developing uncinate) and superior to the maxilloturbinal (the developing inferior turbinate). Nasal capsule resorption allows the maxillary sinus to enter into the developing maxillary process. The sinus is present at birth and expands in early childhood with the development of the maxilla and teeth. The floor of the maxillary sinus gradually descends through childhood. Until the age of 9, the floor of the sinus is above that of the nasal cavity. By age 9 the floor is generally at the level of the nasal floor and continues to descend as the maxillary sinus pneumatizes further. Pneumatization often brings the maxillary dentition into close proximity with the maxillary sinus; thus dental disease can cause maxillary sinusitis, and tooth extraction can occasionally result in oral-antral fistulae.

Ethmoid Sinuses. The ethmoid sinuses begin as evaginations of the lateral nasal wall at the third month of fetal life. The anterior ethmoid cells begin their development anterior to the second ethmoturbinal, while the posterior ethmoid cells originate posterior to the second ethmoturbinal, thus explaining why the basal lamella of the middle turbinate (second ethmoturbinal) ultimately defines the functional drainage paths of the anterior and posterior ethmoid sinuses. The anterior ethmoid drains through the middle meatus, anterior to the basal lamella of the middle turbinate through the middle meatus, whereas the posterior ethmoid drains through the superior meatus, posterior to the basal lamella. The ethmoid cells are present at birth and pneumatize further between years 0 to 3 and 7 to 12.

Frontal Sinuses. An outpouching medial to the most superior aspect of the uncinate process develops during the fourth fetal month. This frontal recess expands and grows cephalad after birth to form the frontal sinus which becomes radiologically apparent at years 7 to 12. The left and

right frontal sinuses develop independently, thus accounting for their asymmetry.

Sphenoid Sinuses. The sphenoid sinuses are unique in that they do not arise from outpouchings of the lateral nasal wall, but arise from within the nasal capsule of the embryonic nose. They remain undeveloped until age three. By age 7 the pneumatization has typically reached the sella turcica; and, by age 9 to 12, pneumatization is generally complete. The posterior pneumatization can be arrested in certain individuals giving rise to 3 configurations of the mature sphenoid sinus: conchal (fetal), presellar (juvenile), and sellar (adult) (Figure 3). The sellar type is the most common, representing 86% of adult sinuses, whereas the presellar (11%) and conchal (3%) variants are less common. A well-pneumatized sphenoid sinus is advantageous for transphenoidal surgical approaches to the sella and clivus, since critical structures such as the sella, optic nerve, and carotid artery are skeletonized and well visualized. Hypopneumatized sphenoid variants require drilling of sphenoid bone to access the skull base and thus make transphenoidal approaches more difficult.[4]

PHYSIOLOGY AND MICROSCOPIC ANATOMY

Air Flow

The nasal airway serves important physiologic functions, including filtration, humidification, and olfaction; these functions are dependent upon unrestricted airflow through the nasal cavity. Air which passes from the nares to the lungs encounters its greatest resistance at the internal nasal valve. Bounded medially by the antero-superior aspect of the nasal septum and laterally by the upper lateral cartilage, the triangular internal nasal valve has a cross-sectional area of 20 to 40 mm^2 on each side. The internal nasal valve is the narrowest part of the upper respiratory tract, and it provides about 50% of the total airway resistance.[5] The velocity of inspired air increases through the small cross-sectional area of the internal nasal valve and creates a Venturi effect (Figure 4). If the structural integrity of the nasal valve is compromised, the soft tissue structures may collapse in these high flow areas due to the Venturi effect, resulting in nasal obstruction.

Nasal resistance is also affected by the nasal cycle. Present in roughly 80% of individuals, the nasal cycle is an autonomic variance of blood flow to the erectile tissue of the nasal airway that results in alternating engorgement of the nasal airway from side to side.[6] The periodicity of the nasal cycle varies from 2 and 1/2 to 4 hours. The nasal cycle may be abolished by exogenous stimuli such as topical oxymetazoline. Postural changes may also affect nasal resistance; when an individual lies on their side, the nasal mucosa on the gravity-dependent side will engorge and cause increased resistance.

Table 3 Summary of the Development, Vascular Supply, Innervation, and Volume of the Paranasal Sinuses

Sinus	Fetal Appearance	Postnatal Appearance	Arterial Supply	Venous Drainage	Innervation
Maxillary Adult volume: 15 mL	Day 65 as bud along inferolateral surface of nasal capsule	Present at birth with two growth spurts between 1 to 4 years and 4 to 8 years	E: Internal maxillary artery branches—infraorbital, lateral nasal branch of sphenopalatine, descending palatine, posterior and anterior superior alveolar arteries	E: Facial vein to jugular system (anterior) and I/E: maxillary vein to jugular system or pterygoid plexus to dural sinuses	V2 to greater palatine, superior alveolar branch of infraorbital nerve, posterolateral nasal branches
Ethmoid Adult volume: 14 mL	Third fetal month as evaginations of the lateral nasal wall	Present at birth with two growth spurts between 0 to 3 years and 7 to 12 years	I: Ophthalmic artery to anterior and posterior ethmoid branches E: Sphenoplatine to nasal branches	I: Ethmoidal veins to ophthalmic veins to cavernous sinus E: Nasal veins to maxillary veins to jugular system	V1 to nasociliary nerve to anterior and posterior ethmoidal nerves V2 to posterolateral nasal branches
Frontal Adult volume: 6 to 7 mL	Fourth fetal month of upward extensions of the nasal capsule in frontal recess area	Seen radiologically at 7 to 12 years and adult size by age 20	I: Ophthalmic to supraorbital and supratrochlear arteries	I: Superior ophthalmic vein to cavernous sinus, Small venules through foramina of Breschet to dural sinuses	V1 to frontal nerve to suprorbital and supratrochlear arteries
Sphenoid Adult volume: 7.5 mL	Third fetal month as evagination in posterior capsule in the sphenoethmoid recess	Seen radiologically at 3 to 4 years and further posterior extension begins by seventh year	I: Posterior ethmoid to sphenoid roof E: Branches of sphenopalatine to the sphenoid floor	I/E: Maxillary vein to jugular system or to pterygoid plexus	V1 to nasociliary nerve to posterior ethmoid (roof) V2 to sphenopalatine branches (floor)

E = external; I = internal.

Warming and Humidification

As air passes through the nose, it is warmed and humidified. The increase of nasal airway temperature is logarithmic as it passes from anterior to posterior. In typical ambient conditions, air is quickly heated in the anterior segment of the nose and is more slowly heated posteriorly. The total increase in air temperature, as air leaves the nasopharynx, is approximately 8°C. Inspired air is also dramatically humidified by the nose, with an increase in ambient humidity from 40 to 98% between the nasal vestibule and the glottis.[7,8]

Olfaction

Olfaction is another important physiologic function of the nasal cavity. The olfactory bulb sends filae through the cribriform plate to from the olfactory neuroepithelium. The olfactory neuroepithelium is distributed in 3 major areas: the superior septum; the superior aspect of the superior turbinate; and to a slightly lesser degree the superior aspect of the middle turbinate. These structures define the olfactory cleft. Olfactory physiology is discussed in Chapter 38, "Olfaction and Gustation."

Microscopic Anatomy

The sinonasal cavities are lined with pseudostratified ciliated columnar epithelium composed of 4 basic cell types: ciliated columnar epithelial cells, nonciliated columnar cells, basal cells, and goblet cells (Figure 5).

Ciliated respiratory epithelial cells are found throughout the respiratory tract except for the nasal vestibule, the posterior oropharyngeal wall, portions of the larynx, and terminal rami of the bronchial tree. The ciliated cells have 50 to 200 cilia per cell, and each cilium has a 9 plus 2 microtubular structure with dynein arms. Experimental data indicate a typical ciliary beat frequency of 700 to 800 times a minute, with mucociliary transport occurring at a rate of 1 cm/minute (although the normal range can vary widely).

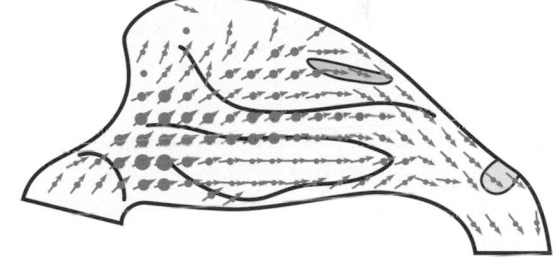

Figure 4 Diagram of the nasal airway and air speed, the size of the dot indicating the velocity.

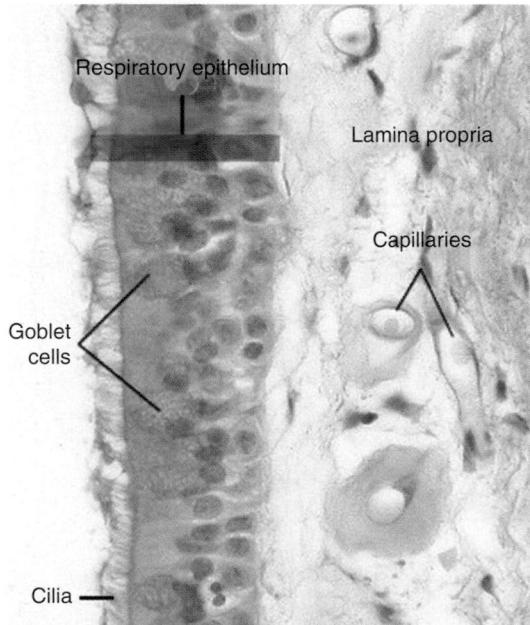

Figure 5 The microscopic structure of respiratory epithelium can be seen in this tissue sample of inferior turbinate stained with Alcian blue and van Gieson. The ciliated cells, goblet cells, and basal cells are apparent. (Reproduced with permission from: http://www.lab.anhb.uwa.edu.au/mb140/CorePages/Respiratory/respir.htm.)

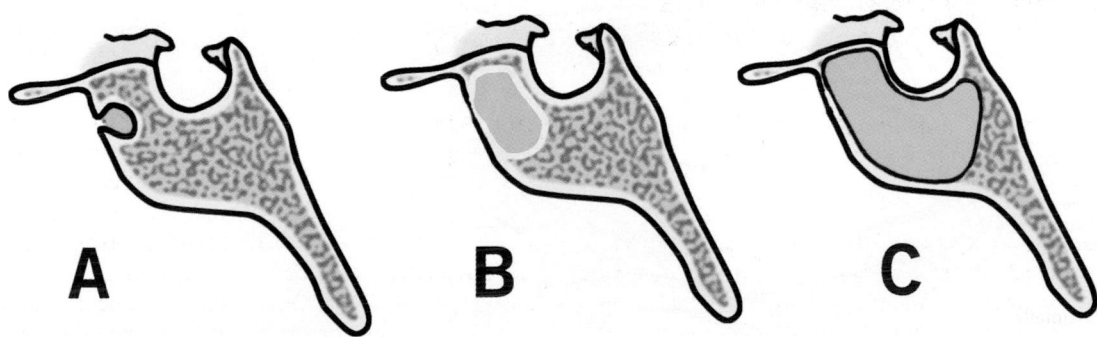

Figure 3 The sphenoid sinus can have varying configurations based on degree of pneumatization: (A) conchal, (B) presellar and (C) sellar types. (Adapted from reference 4.)

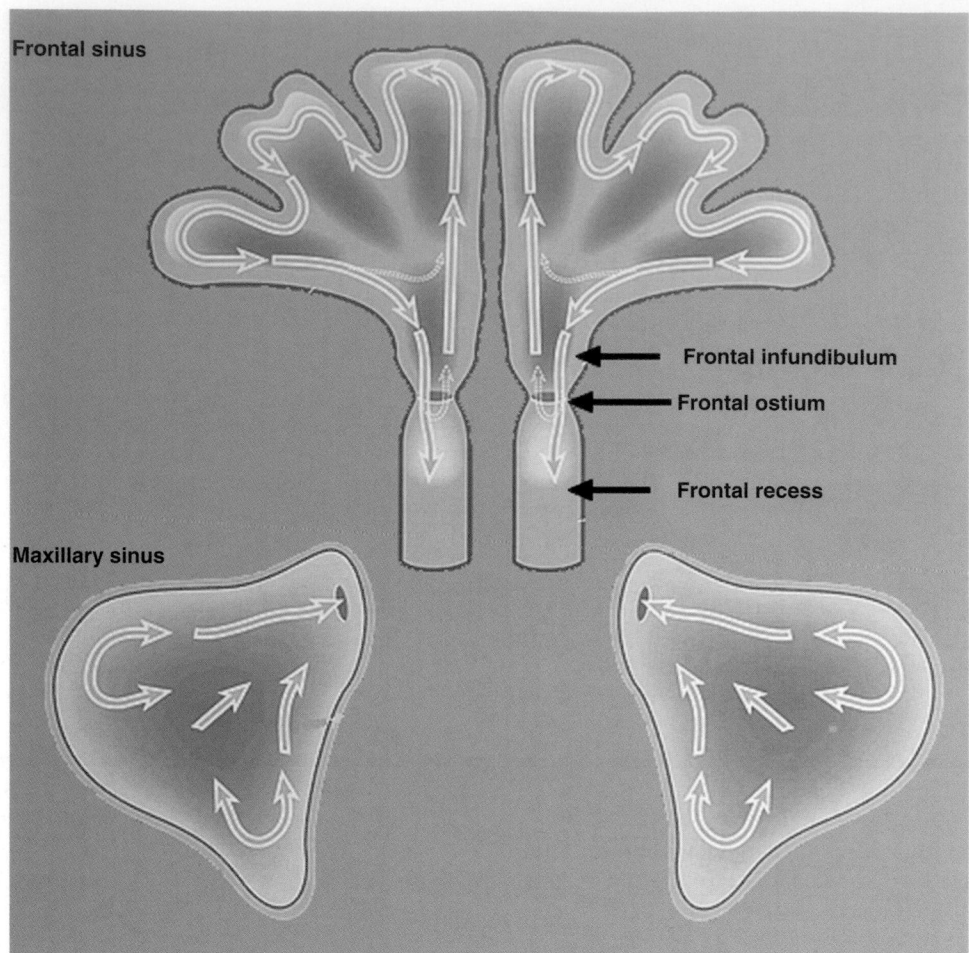

Frontal sinus

Frontal infundibulum

Frontal ostium

Frontal recess

Maxillary sinus

Figure 6 Mucociliary flow in the frontal and maxillary sinuses. Note that the mucociliary flow is not gravity-dependent. (Adapted with permission by Lanza, D. from http://www.sniflmd.com/nasal_functions.htm.)

layer. The outer, more viscous mucus layer, is termed the gel layer. The gel layer provides a confluent lining for the nasal cavity onto which inhaled particles can impact. Eighty percent of particles larger than 12.5 µg are filtered from the air before they reach the pharynx.[9]

Mucociliary Clearance

The ciliated cells of the respiratory epithelium move mucus through the sinonasal cavity in an organized, directional fashion toward the nasopharynx and pharynx, where the mucus is swallowed or expectorated. Mucociliary clearance serves a hygienic function to clear the nose of particulate debris and potential by-products of infection or inflammation. A pattern of mucus flow can be mapped for each sinus, as seen in the examples of the frontal and maxillary sinus in Figure 6.

Ostiomeatal Complex. The ostiomeatal complex represents a common central pathway of mucociliary clearance for the anterior ethmoid, maxillary, and frontal sinuses. The ostiomeatal complex is not a true anatomic designation, rather a functional area. It encompasses several structures that drain into the middle meatus: the maxillary ostium, ethmoid infundibulum, anterior ethmoid cells, and the frontal recess (Figure 7). Focal inflammation or mass obstruction in the ostiomeatal unit can disrupt mucociliary flow in multiple sites "upstream," potentially propagating rhinosinusitis.[10]

ANATOMY OF THE NASAL CAVITY

Nasal Septum

The mature nasal cavity is divided in the midline by a parting wall, the nasal septum. The nasal septum is derived from both bony and cartilaginous sources. The septum is formed anteriorly by the quadrilateral cartilage and premaxilla; posteriorly by the perpendicular plate of the ethmoid bone and the sphenoidal crest; and inferiorly by the crests of the vomer, maxillary, and palatine bones (Figure 8).

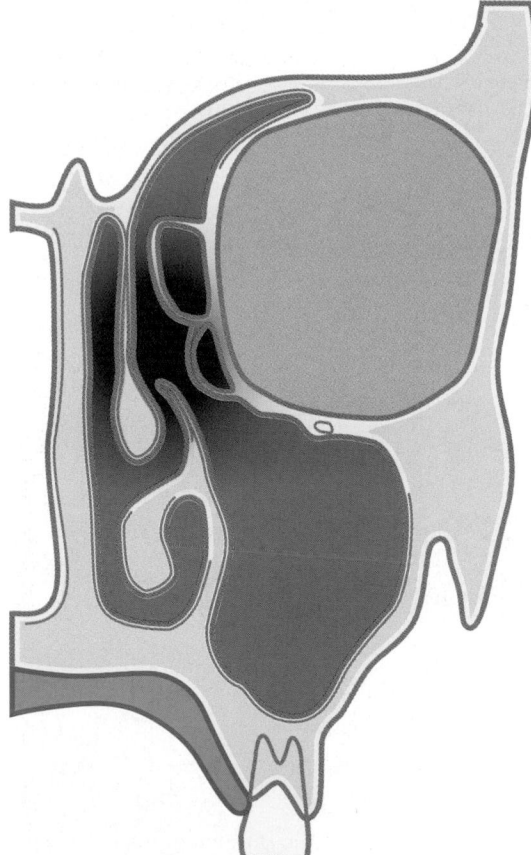

Nonciliated cells are characterized by microvilli which cover the apical aspect of the cell and serve to increase surface area. The function of basal cells is unknown, but it is theorized that they may serve as pluripotent stem cells. Goblet cells produce glycoproteins which are responsible for the viscosity and elasticity of mucus and respond to parasympathetic and sympathetic neural inputs. Between 20 and 40 mL of mucus are secreted from the normal nose daily from 160 cm² of nasal mucosa. The cilia beat within the lubricating periciliary layer fluid, termed the sol

Figure 7 The ostiomeatal complex is shown shaded in gray. It is not a distinct anatomical landmark, but an important region in the sinuses defined by multiple landmarks. (Adapted from reference 10.)

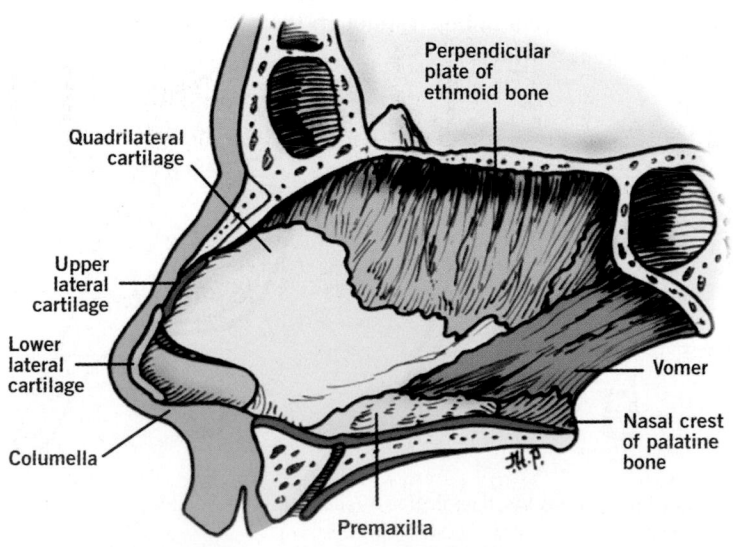

Perpendicular plate of ethmoid bone

Quadrilateral cartilage

Upper lateral cartilage

Lower lateral cartilage

Columella

Premaxilla

Vomer

Nasal crest of palatine bone

Figure 8 The bony and cartilaginous components of the nasal septum.

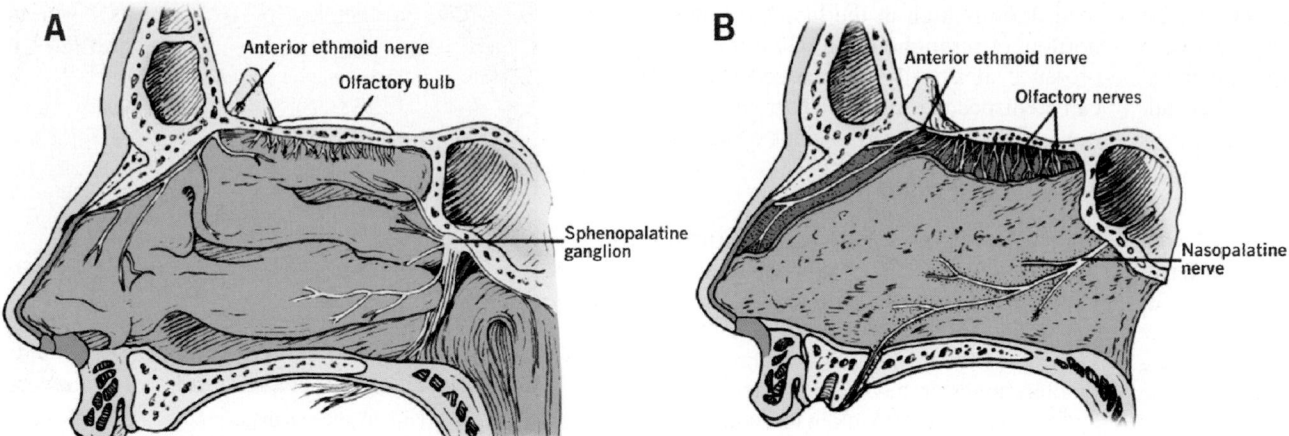

Figure 9 (A) Innervation of the lateral nasal wall. (B) Innervation of the nasal septum.

Nasal Mucous Membrane

The epithelial lining of the nasal cavity changes as one moves from anterior to posterior. The skin within the nasal vestibule is a keratinized, squamous cell epithelium containing vibrissae and sebaceous glands. At the leading edge of the inferior turbinate, the epithelium transitions into a cuboidal cell type and then into pseudostratified ciliated columnar respiratory epithelium. At the most posterior aspect of the nasopharynx, the mucosa returns to a nonkeratinized, squamous cell epithelium.

Nasal Innervation

Sensation to the nose is supplied mainly by the ophthalmic and maxillary divisions of cranial nerve V. The ophthalmic division gives rise to the nasociliary nerve, which divides into the anterior and posterior ethmoid and infratrochlear branches. The anterior ethmoid nerve passes over the cribriform plate and enters with the anterior ethmoid artery by way of the anterior ethmoid foramen, subsequently dividing into medial and lateral branches. The medial branch passes onto the nasal septum and the lateral branch over the lateral nasal wall. An external branch exits distally at the end of the nasal bone to supply the external surface of the nose. The posterior ethmoid nerve crosses the cribriform plate to enter the nose with the posterior ethmoid artery through the posterior

ethmoid foramen to supply the nasal septum as well as the olfactory region. The maxillary division of cranial nerve V gives rise to the posterior superior nasal nerves that enter the nose by way of the sphenopalatine foramen and pass over the anterior face of the sphenoid bone to reach the nasal septum as the nasopalatine nerve and then course through the incisive canal. A lateral branch, the posterior inferior nasal nerve, passes downward and forward to supply the middle and inferior turbinates (Figure 9).

Blood Supply

The blood supply of the nasal cavity is derived primarily from the anterior and posterior ethmoid arteries, (branches of the ophthalmic artery) and the sphenopalatine artery (a terminal branch of the internal maxillary artery). The anterior ethmoid artery crosses the medial rectus and penetrates the lamina papyracea. The artery then courses across the roof of the ethmoid sinus within a thin bony covering, eventually supplying the cribriform plate and anterior part of the septum. This artery, when identified, is the most posterior landmark for a frontal recess dissection (Figure 10). The posterior ethmoid artery emerges

from the orbit, approximately 12 mm posterior to the anterior ethmoid artery. It supplies a smaller posterior region, including the olfactory cleft.

The internal maxillary artery enters the pterygomaxillary fossa and emerges into the nasal cavity through the sphenopalatine foramen as the sphenopalatine artery. The sphenopalatine foramen is located just lateral to the posterior end of the middle turbinate. Upon entering the nose, the sphenopalatine artery divides into posterior lateral nasal and posterior septal branches.

Venous drainage follows a course parallel to that of the sphenopalatine artery and its branches, draining into the ophthalmic plexus and partly into the cavernous sinus. This valveless venous system predisposes the spread of infection from the nose upward to the cavernous sinus.

There are 2 areas of arterial anastomoses that are often implicated in epistaxis: Kiesselbach plexus, which gives rise to anterior bleeding, and Woodruff plexus, which gives rise to posterior bleeding. Kiesselbach plexus is located over the anterior nasal septum and is formed by anastamoses between the sphenopalatine, greater palatine, superior labial, and anterior ethmoid arteries. Woodruff plexus is located over the

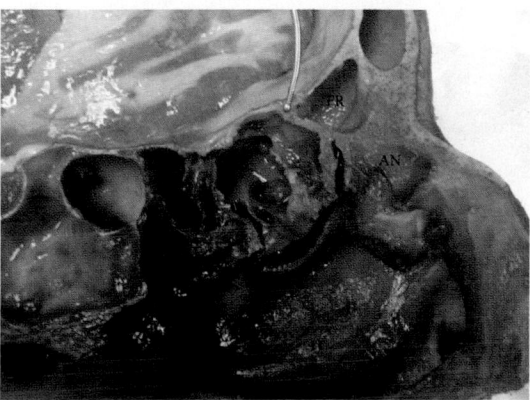

Figure 10 The anterior ethmoid artery location delineated by the probe. The frontal recess (FR), agger nasi (AN), uncinate process (UP), and inferior turbinate (IT) are also labeled.

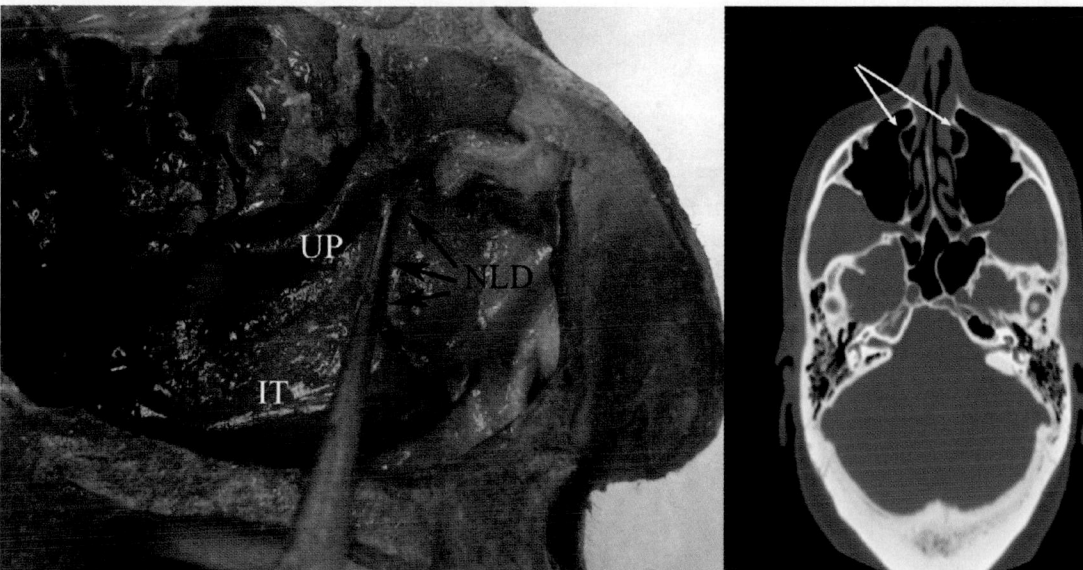

Figure 11 Probe running through the NLD in sagittal section. Its course anterior to the uncinate process (UP) and outflow below the inferior turbinate (IT) can be appreciated. An axial computed tomography scan (*right*) demonstrates the NLD bilaterally (*white arrows*).

posterior part of the middle turbinate and inferior meatus and is made up of anastamoses between branches of the internal maxillary artery, namely, the posterior nasal, sphenopalatine, and ascending pharyngeal arteries.

Inferior Turbinate

The most conspicuous of the lateral nasal wall structures on anterior rhinoscopy is the inferior turbinate. The inferior turbinate is composed of bone covered by mucoperiosteum, soft tissue embodying a cavernous plexus, and an overlying respiratory mucosa. The inferior turbinate bone articulates with the lacrimal bone anteriorly, and attaches to the medial process of the maxilla and palatine bone laterally. The cavernous plexus can become engorged with blood in response to the nasal cycle or to various environmental triggers.

Middle Turbinate

The middle turbinate forms the medial boundary of the middle meatus and serves as an important central landmark in sinus surgery (see Figure 7). The orientation of the middle turbinate runs along 3 different planes in its course from anterior to posterior and can be conceived schematically in thirds. The anterior third of the middle turbinate runs along a sagittal plane. This portion of the middle turbinate is most readily observed on anterior rhinoscopy, and it is attached superiorly to the lateral nasal wall and cribriform plate.

At the middle third, the turbinate reflects from a sagittal to a coronal orientation, forming the basal lamella of the middle turbinate as it traverses to insert on the lateral nasal wall. It is this transverse portion of the middle turbinate that separates the anterior ethmoid cells from the posterior ethmoid cells. Anterior to the basal lamella of the middle turbinate, the cells drain through the middle meatus. Posterior to the basal lamella, the cells drain through the superior meatus.

The posterior third of the turbinate runs in an axial plane with its attachment continuing along the lateral nasal wall. The posterior end of the middle turbinate inserts adjacent to the sphenopalatine foramen and to the emergence of the sphenopalatine artery into the nose.

Superior Turbinate

The superior turbinate is the most posterior of the 3 turbinates. It shares a common superior insertion onto the skull base with the middle turbinate and helps define the medial boundary of the posterior ethmoid cells. Medial to the superior turbinate and lateral to the septum is the area of the sphenoethmoidal recess, where the sphenoid ostium can be found.

Concha Bullosa

Any of the turbinates may pneumatize to form a concha bullosa, considered a normal variant of nasal anatomy. The middle turbinate is most commonly involved. Bolger has classified the pneumatization depending on whether the pneu-

matization is high in the lamella, in the bulbous portion, or throughout the whole structure.[11] The presence of a well-pneumatized concha bullosa can predispose to anatomic narrowing of the sinus outflow tracts and lead to sinus obstruction.

Nasolacrimal Duct (NLD)

The NLD drains tears from the lacrimal sac into the nasal cavity. It originates in the lacrimal fossa in the inferomedial part of the orbit and runs along the posterior aspect of the maxillary vertical buttress. The duct courses several millimeters anterior to the maxillary sinus ostium, and thus care must be taken to avoid injury to this structure during maxillary antrostomy. The duct empties through Hasner valve, below the bony attachment of the inferior turbinate, into the inferior meatus (Figure 11).

ANATOMY OF THE PARANASAL SINUSES

Maxillary Sinus

The maxillary sinus has a pyramidal shape defined by 4 major boundaries: the maxillary face anteriorly; the ascending process of the palatine bone medially; the orbital floor superiorly, and the pterygomaxillary space posteriorly. The infraorbital nerve traverses along the roof of the maxillary sinus and exits through the infraorbital foramen roughly 6 to 7 mm below the inferior orbital rim. The nerve can be dehiscent within the maxillary sinus up to 14% of the time (Figure 12).

Behind the posterior wall of the maxillary sinus lies the pterygomaxillary fossa, which contains the internal maxillary artery, sphenopala-

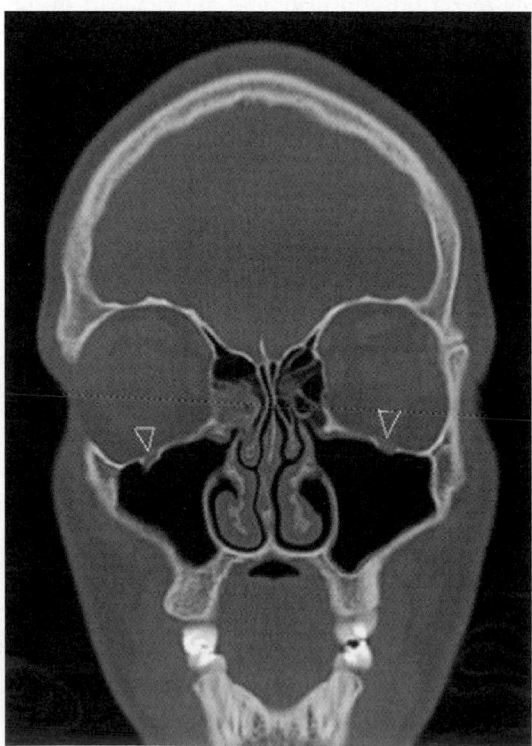

Figure 12 The course of the infraorbital nerve can be seen in the roof of the maxillary sinus (*arrowheads*).

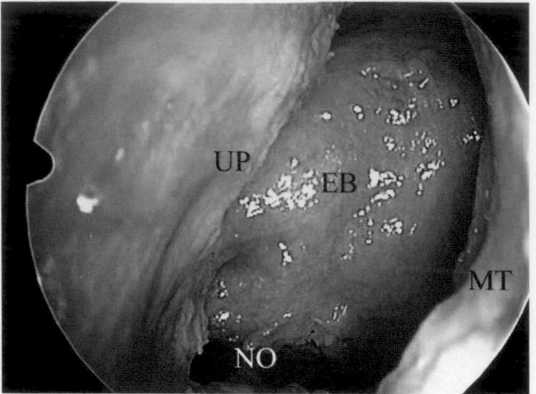

Figure 13 Part of the uncinate process (UP) has been removed in the right nasal cavity to show the natural ostium (NO) of the maxillary sinus. The middle turbinate (MT) and ethmoid bulla (EB) can also be seen.

tine ganglion, the vidian canal, the greater palatine nerve, and the foramen rotundum. The floor of the maxillary sinus is formed by the alveolar process of the maxilla. Roots of the molar teeth may occasionally be dehiscent through the floor of the sinus.

Maxillary Ostium. The natural maxillary ostium is the anatomic merging point for mucociliary flow in the maxillary sinus. The maxillary ostium is located at the anteromedial aspect of the sinus near the roof of the sinus. The maxillary ostium drains into the ethmoid infundibulum, lateral to the lower one-third of the uncinate process. The natural ostium is typically elliptical in shape, and rests about 2 mm posterior to the anterior most insertion of the uncinate process (Figure 13). The ostium size averages 2.4 mm in diameter, but can vary widely among individuals.

Two bony dehiscences, or anterior and posterior fontanelles, may exist along the medial wall of the maxillary sinus. These fontanelles are usually covered by mucosa but in some individuals may be patent, thereby forming an "accessory ostium." Endoscopic examinations of the nasal cavity reveal an accessory opening in the posterior fontanelle of the maxillary sinus in roughly 25% of patients.[12] Because mucociliary clearance moves mucus to the natural ostium and

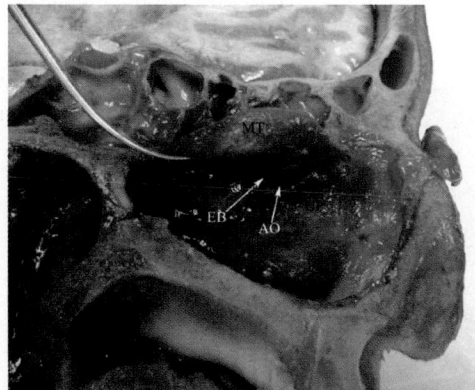

Figure 14 An accessory ostium (AO) can be seen tucked between the uncinate process (UP) and the ethmoid bulla (EB). The true ostium of the maxillary sinus is positioned anterior to the accessory ostium and is out of view, obscured by the intact uncinate process. The middle turbinate (MT) has been reflected upward for visualization.

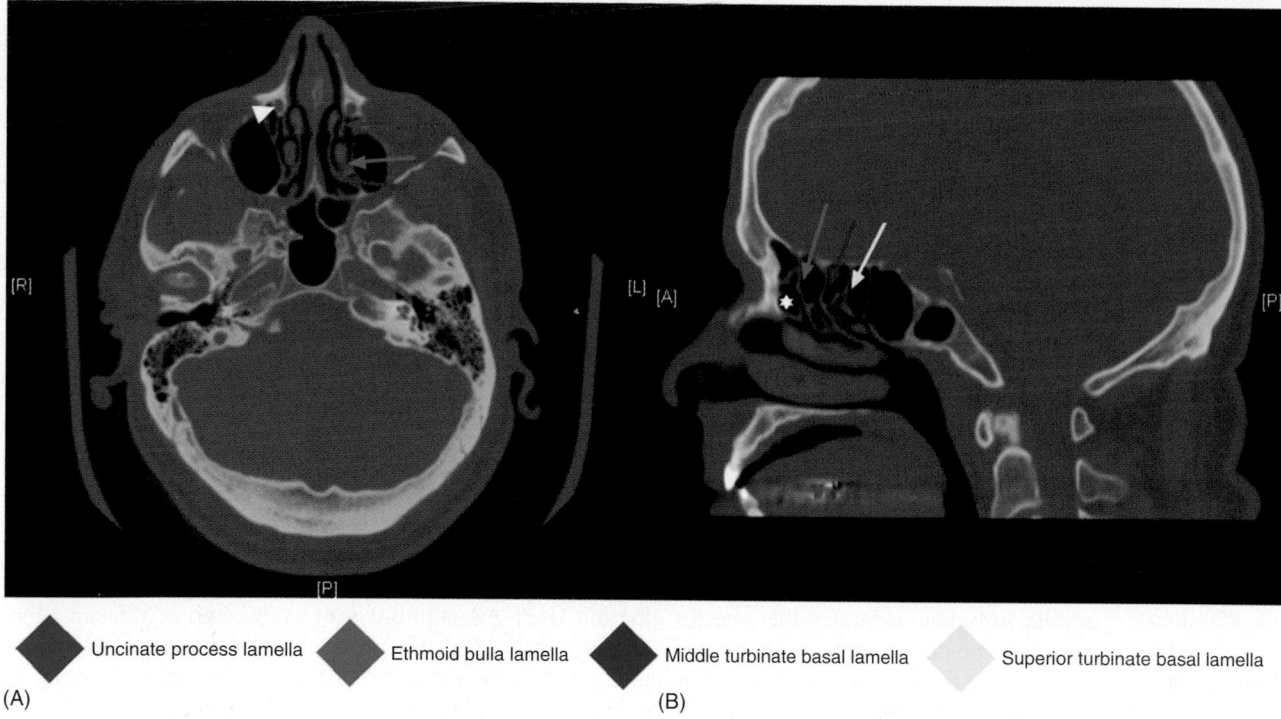

Figure 15 (A) Axial computed tomography (CT) image that reveals the uncinate process lamella, ethmoid bulla lamella, and middle turbinate lamella as well as the nasolacrimal duct (*white arrowhead*). (B) The sagittal CT scan reveals the ethmoid bulla lamella, middle turbinate lamella, superior turbinate lamella, and an agger nasi cell (*star*).

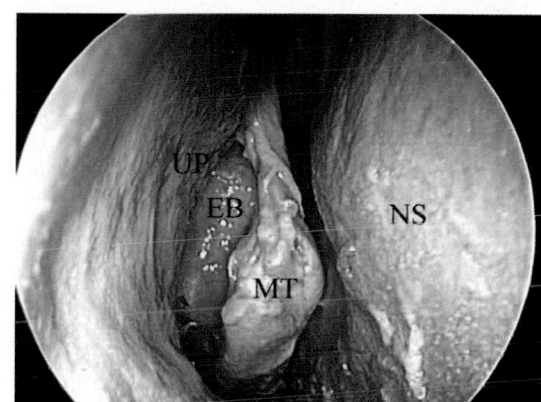

Figure 16 An endoscopic view of the right nasal cavity shows the nasal septum (NS), middle turbinate (MT), ethmoid bulla (EB), and uncinate process (UP). The hiatus semilunaris can be appreciated as the cleft between the ethmoid bulla and uncinate process.

not to the accessory ostia, these patent fontanelles are considered nonfunctional ostia and should not be confused for the native natural ostium during maxillary sinus surgery (Figure 14).

Infraorbital Ethmoid (Haller) Cell. Occasionally, an anterior ethmoid cell may pneumatize along the orbital floor inferior and lateral to the ethmoid bulla. When extensively pneumatized, this infraorbital ethmoid cell may narrow the ethmoid infundibulum and predispose patients to maxillary sinus obstruction. This entity was described by Haller in 1765, and the cell was given his name; but it is generally agreed that the term infraorbital ethmoid cell is more descriptive and is preferred.[13]

Ethmoid Sinus

The ethmoid sinus is composed of multiple individual cells, separated into anterior and posterior compartments by the basal lamella of the middle turbinate. The lateral boundary of the ethmoid is the medial wall (lamina papyracea) of the orbit. The medial boundary is formed by the middle turbinate in the anterior ethmoid and by the superior turbinate in the posterior ethmoid. The posterior border is the face of the sphenoid sinus. Superiorly, the ethmoid roof separates the ethmoid sinus from the intracranial cavity.

Superomedially the ethmoid roof thins considerably in the area of the cribriform plate, through which olfactory filae enter the cranial cavity. Depending on the pneumatization pattern of the ethmoid sinus, additional ethmoid air cells can be found outside the usual confines of the ethmoid labyrinth, extending to the maxillary, frontal, and sphenoid sinuses.

The Ethmoid Lamellae. A series of ethmoid lamellae, with attachments to the lateral nasal wall, develops from the ethmoturbinals and the ethmoid bulla. These 5 lamellae are encountered sequentially during ethmoid sinus surgery and can be important orienting landmarks for the surgeon. Listed from anterior to posterior, the lamellae are summarized in Table 2.

The uncinate process, ethmoid bulla, middle turbinate, and superior turbinate attachments can be appreciated radiologically (Figure 15).

First Lamella: Uncinate Process. The uncinate process is a crescent shaped operculum that overlies the ostium of the maxillary sinus. The uncinate process typically must be removed during endoscopic maxillary antrostomy to reveal the natural ostium of the maxillary sinus. Oriented sagittally, it forms the anterior and medial boundary of the ethmoid infundibulum. Anteriorly, the uncinate process inserts on the ethmoidal

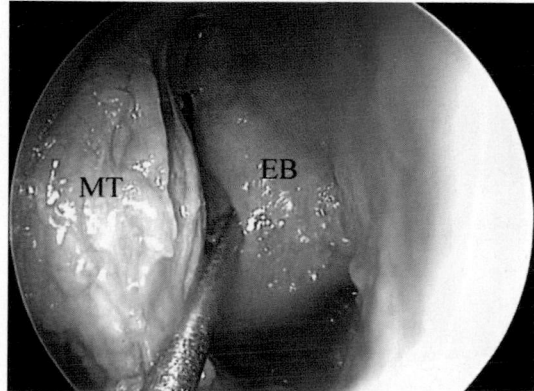

Figure 17 Endoscopic view of the left middle meatus with instrument placed behind the ethmoid bulla in the retrobullar space.

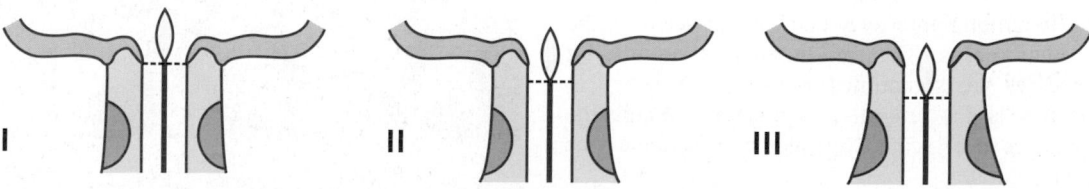

Figure 18 The 3 Keros subtypes characterize varying depths of the olfactory groove, defined by the length of the lateral lamellae of the cribriform plate. Type I: 1 to 3 mm in length; Type II: 4 to 7 mm; and Type III: greater than 8 mm. (Adapted from reference 7)

crest of the maxilla and the lacrimal bone; inferiorly, the uncinate attaches to the inferior turbinate. The posterior border of the uncinate has no attachment. Its free edge serves as a defining boundary of the hiatus semilunaris, which is the space between the crescentic border of the uncinate and the bulla ethmoidalis (see Figure 16). The superior most aspect of the uncinate process has a variable insertion that may fall under 1 of 3 main patterns: to the lamina papyracea laterally (70%), to the middle turbinate medially (19%), to the roof of the ethmoid superiorly (11%).[11] The pattern of uncinate insertion dictates the direction of frontal sinus outflow.

Ethmoid Infundibulum and Hiatus Semilunaris. The ethmoid infundibulum and the hiatus semilunaris are contiguous with each other. The ethmoid infundibulum develops as a space prior to the development of the sinuses. This recess, into which the anterior ethmoid sinus, maxillary sinus and frontal sinus drain, is formed by multiple structures. The anterior and lateral wall is formed by the uncinate process, the medial wall is the frontal process of the maxilla and the lamina papyracea and the posterior wall is the ethmoid bulla. The cleft between the free posterior edge of the uncinate and the ethmoid bulla is known as the hiatus semilunaris. Contiguous with the ethmoid infundibulum, the hiatus semilunaris can be appreciated on endoscopic evaluation of the nasal cavity.

Second Lamella: Ethmoid Bulla. The ethmoid bulla is typically the largest of the anterior ethmoid cells. Because it is readily visible within the middle meatus, the ethmoid bulla serves as a consistent landmark for sinus surgery. The ethmoid bulla drains medially via the retrobullar space. The ethmoid bulla may pneumatize superiorly to the ethmoid roof or it may extend a nonpneumatized lamella to the roof (bulla lamella). The anterior ethmoid artery courses along the ethmoid roof near the junction of the bulla lamella.

The retrobullar and suprabullar recesses are defined by the space between the bulla and the basal lamella of the middle turbinate. The dimensions of these contiguous air spaces are dependent upon the degree of pneumatization of the bulla ethmoidalis. The retrobullar recess is defined by the cleft between the basal lamella and ethmoid bulla (Figure 17). When the ethmoid bulla does not pneumatize to the skull base and a bulla lamella is present instead, the retrobullar recess may extend superiorly behind the bulla lamella to form the suprabullar recess. Enlargement of the suprabullar recess can advance the bulla lamella anteriorly and can encroach on the frontal recess. The retrobullar and suprabullar recesses are sometimes collectively referred to as the "sinus lateralis," a misnomer since the space is not located laterally and is not a true sinus.

Third Lamella: Basal Lamella (Ground Lamella) of the Middle Turbinate. The basal lamella of the

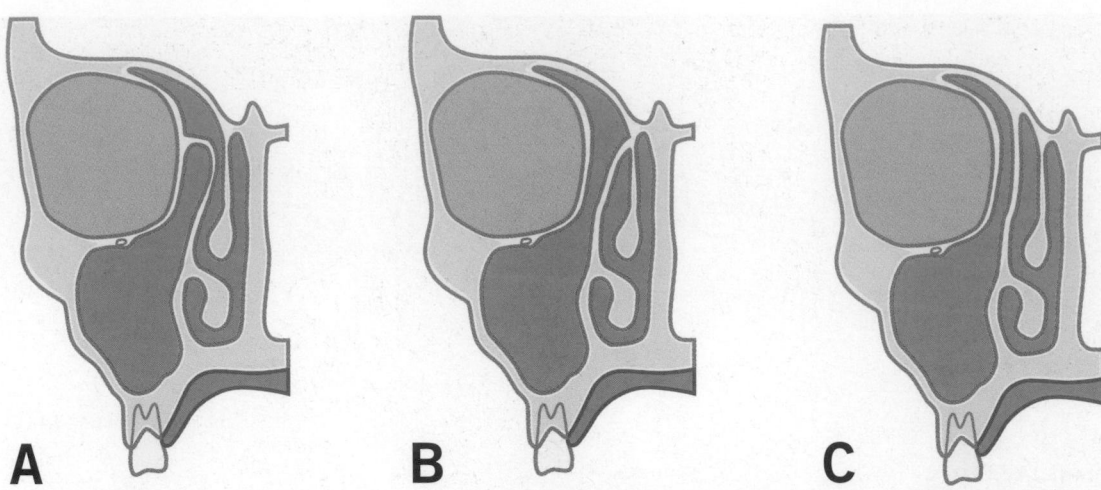

Figure 19 The variable attachment of the uncinate process can either be to: (A) the lamina papyracea; (B) the middle turbinate; or (C) the ethmoid roof. The first scenario leads to frontal sinus outflow that is medial to the unicinate, the other 2 lead to lateral outflow. (Adapted from reference 5.)

middle turbinate separates the anterior ethmoid cells from posterior ethmoid cells (see Figure 7). It represents the coronally oriented attachment of the middle turbinate to the lateral nasal wall. The basal lamella of the middle turbinate is traversed during ethmoid sinus surgery to enter the posterior ethmoid cavity.

Fourth Lamellae: Basal Lamella of the Superior Turbinate. The superior turbinate defines the medial border of the posterior ethmoid sinus. The posterior ethmoid cells drain into the superior meatus which is the space between the basal lamella of the superior turbinate and the basal lamella of the middle turbinate. The ostium of the sphenoid sinus lies medial to the superior turbinate within the sphenoethmoidal recess.

Fifth Lamella: Basal Lamella of the Supreme Turbinate. The supreme turbinate basal lamella is present in roughly 15% of the population.[14] Due to its rarity, it does not serve as a helpful anatomic landmark during sinus surgery.

Ethmoid Roof. The ethmoid roof is a critical landmark for surgical dissection. The slope of the ethmoid roof is steeper in the anterior ethmoid compared to the posterior ethmoid. The thickness

of the ethmoid roof varies and is thicker laterally and thinner medially. The thinnest portion of the ethmoid roof lies at the lateral lamella of the cribriform plate, adjacent to the superior part of the attachment of the middle turbinate. Thus at the lateral lamella of the cribiform plate, there is the portion of the ethmoid roof that is most susceptible to injury during sinus surgery. When the olfactory groove is deep, the lateral lamella of the cribriform plate can be elongated, thus placing a larger area of skull base at risk for surgical injury.[15] The 3 Keros subtypes that distinguish those patients at higher risk for damage to the lateral lamella of the cribriform plate based on the depth of the olfactory groove (Figure 18).

Frontal Sinus

The frontal sinus is formed by an outgrowth of the ethmoid labyrinth that pneumatizes superiorly into the frontal bone. The drainage of this sinus occurs at its inferior and medial extent. The frontal sinus outflow tract begins at the frontal infundibulum, then descends through the frontal ostium to the middle meatus via the frontal recess. The term "nasofrontal duct" should be avoided when referring to the drainage pathway below the frontal

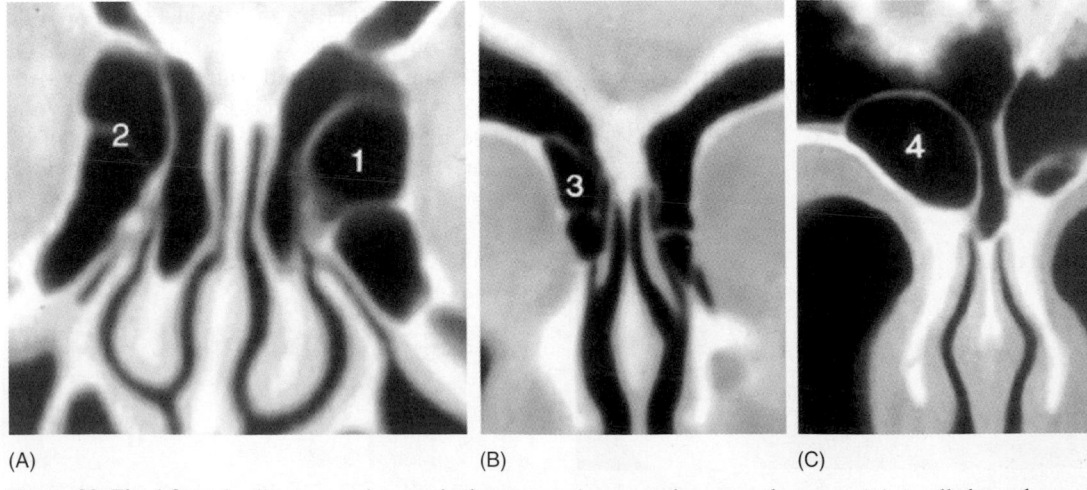

(A)   (B)   (C)

Figure 20 The 4 frontal cell types can be seen in these coronal computed tomography scans. (A) A cell above the agger (1); More than 1 cell above the agger (2). (B) A cell extending from the ethmoid into the frontal sinus (3). (C) A cell completely within the frontal sinus (4). (Adapted from reference 10.)

ostium, as it is not a tubular structure or true duct. It is instead a recess that has a variable shape depending on what cells have pneumatized at its base.[16] Specifically, the configuration of the recess will change based on the orientation of the uncinate process, ethmoid bulla, agger nasi, frontal cells, and supraorbital ethmoid cells. The boundaries of the frontal recess are the lamina papyracea laterally, the middle turbinate medially, the posterosuperior wall of the agger nasi anteriorly, and the ethmoid bulla posteriorly. Suprabullar cells or the suprabullar recess may alternatively define the posterior border of the frontal recess.

Agger Nasi. The agger nasi, which means "nasal eminence," is the portion of the lateral nasal wall located just anterior to the middle turbinate insertion. It is the remnant of the ascending portion of the first ethmoturbinal. The agger nasi is often pneumatized, and the resulting agger nasi cell is considered part of the anterior ethmoid labyrinth. The agger nasi is bordered anteriorly by the frontal process of the maxilla, posterosuperiorly by the frontal recess, anterolaterally by the nasal bones, inferomedially by the uncinate process of the ethmoid bone, and inferolaterally by the lacrimal bone. The agger nasi forms the anterior border of the frontal recess; when extensively pneumatized, the agger nasi cell can obstruct frontal sinus outflow and can predispose to frontal sinusitis. Dissection of the agger nasi may thus be critical to establishing adequate surgical patency of the frontal sinus.

Uncinate Process. The superior most aspect of the uncinate process is an important determinant of frontal sinus outflow. The insertion site of the uncinate process is variable and may fall under one of 3 main patterns: to the lamina papyracea laterally, to the roof of the ethmoid superiorly, or to the middle turbinate medially.[13] A lateral attachment to the lamina papyracea is the most common arrangement (70%) and results in frontal sinus outflow medial to the uncinate and ethmoid infundibulum. The other 2 configurations (middle turbinate 19%, ethmoid roof 11%)

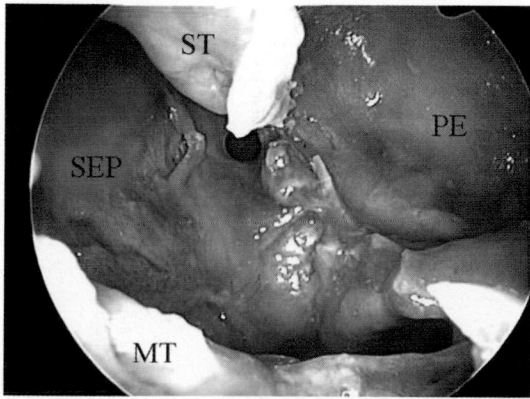

Figure 21 Left nasal cavity. The sphenoid ostium is found within the sphenoethmoid recess, which is bounded by the septum (SEP) medially and the superior turbinate (ST) laterally (inferior edge transected). The posterior ethmoid sinus is located lateral to the superior turbinate. The cut edge of the middle turbinate (MT) basal lamella can be seen anterior to the sphenoethmoid recess.

lead to outflow lateral to the uncinate, through the ethmoid infundibulum (Figure 19).

Frontal Cells and Supraorbital Ethmoid Cells. Frontal cells and supraorbital ethmoid cells are properly categorized as part of the anterior ethmoid labyrinth; however, because of their proximity to the frontal ostium, they can functionally affect frontal sinus outflow and are considered part of the frontal recess anatomy. Frontal cells are anterior ethmoid cells layered superior to the agger nasi. Frontal cells can be classified into 4 main types, depending on the number of cells and the superior extension of the cells into the frontal sinus (Figure 20).

Supraorbital ethmoid cells are the result of pneumatization of the ethmoid cells into the orbital plate of the frontal bone. When present, these cells are located lateral and inferior to the frontal sinus proper. These cells can be capacious and can be mistaken for the frontal sinus during endoscopic surgery.

Sphenoid Sinus

The sphenoid sinus can pneumatize as far as the clivus, the sphenoid wings, and the foramen magnum but typically takes the form of the sellar, presellar, and conchal pneumatizations as described earlier (see Figure 3). The walls of the sphenoid vary in thickness, with the anterosuperior wall and roof being the thinnest (<2 mm thick). The sphenoid sinus lies adjacent to vital structures such as the internal carotid artery, optic nerve, the Vidian nerve, the cavernous sinus, and foramen rotundum. Many of these structures can be identified as indentations on the roof and walls of the sinus in an extensively pneumatized sphenoid sinus. A small percentage may have dehiscence of bone over such vital structures as the optic nerve (4 to 6%) and carotid arteries (25%).[17] The ostium of the sphenoid sinus can be found in the sphenoethmoidal recess, between the posterior part of the septum and the superior turbinate (Figure 21).

Sphenoethmoidal (Onodi) Cell. A posterior ethmoid cell that pneumatizes posteriorly into the region of the sphenoid sinus is termed a sphenoethmoidal, or Onodi, cell. Because

sphenoethmoidal cells are positioned superior to the native sphenoid sinus, the optic nerve and carotid artery may often course through the lateral aspect of the sphenoethmoid cell instead of the sphenoid sinus proper (Figure 22). Failure to recognize the presence of a sphenoethmoidal cell could result in inadvertent damage to the optic nerve or carotid artery. The term sphenoethmoidal cell is a more descriptive and anatomically accurate term and is preferred to the eponym.[11]

REFERENCES

1. Levine HL, Clemente MP. Sinus Surgery—Endoscopic and Microscopic Approaches. New York: Thieme; 2004.
2. Rice DH, Schaefer SH. Endoscopic Paranasal Sinus Surgery, 3rd edition. Philadelphia: Lippincott Williams & Wilkins; 2003.
3. Tien HC, Linthicum FH Jr. Persistent stapedial artery. Otol Neurotol 2001;22:975–6.
4. Weiss RL, Bailey BJ. Approaches to the sphenoidal sinus. In: Bailey BJ, editor. Head and Neck Surgery—Otolaryngology, Vol 1. 3rd edition. New York: Lippincott Williams & Wilkins; 2001. p. 383–92.
5. Ballenger JJ. Anatomy and physiology of the nose and paranasal sinuses. In: Snow JB, Ballenger JJ, editors. Ballenger's Otorhinolaryngology Head and Neck Surgery, 16th edition. Hamilton, Ontario: BC Decker; 2002. p. 547–60.
6. Kim JK, Cho JH, Jang HJ, et al. The effect of allergen provocation on the nasal cycle estimated by acoustic rhinometry. Acta Otolaryngol 2006;126:390–5.
7. Keck T, Leiacker R, Riechelmann H, Rettinger G. Temperature profile in the nasal cavity. Laryngoscope 2000;110:651–4.
8. Wolf M, Naftali S, Schroter RC, Elad D. Air-conditioning characteristics of the human nose. J Laryngol Otol 2004; 118:87–92.
9. Boatsman JE, Calhoun KH, Ryan MW. Relationship between rhinosinusitis symptoms and mucociliary clearance time. Otolaryngol Head Neck Surg 2006;134:491–3.
10. Kennedy DW. Pathogenesis of chronic rhinosinusitis. Ann Otol Rhinol Laryngol 2004;113;S193:6–9.
11. Bolger WE. Anatomy of the paranasal sinuses. In: Kennedy DW, Bolger WE, Zinreich JS, editors. Diseases of the Sinuses. Hamilton, Ontario: BC Decker; 2000. p. 1–11.
12. Stammberger H. Functional Endoscopic Sinus Surgery. Philadelphia: BC Decker; 1991; p. 17–41.
13. Stammberger HR, Kennedy DW. Paranasal sinuses: Anatomic terminology and nomenclature. Ann Otol Rhinol Laryngol 1995;104:7–15.
14. Kim SS, Lee JG, Kim KS, et al. Computed tomographic and anatomical analysis of the basal lamellas in the ethmoid sinus. Laryngoscope 2001;111:424–9.
15. Ohnishi T, Tachibana T, Kanekyo Y, et al. High risk areas in endoscopic sinus surgery and prevention of complications. Laryngoscope 1993;103:1181–5.
16. McLaughlin RB, Jr, Rehl RM, Lanza DC. Clinically relevant frontal sinus anatomy and physiology. Otolaryngol Clin North Am 2001;34:1–22.
17. Yanagisawa E. The optic nerve and the internal carotid artery in the sphenoid sinus. Ear Nose Throat J 2002;81:611–2.

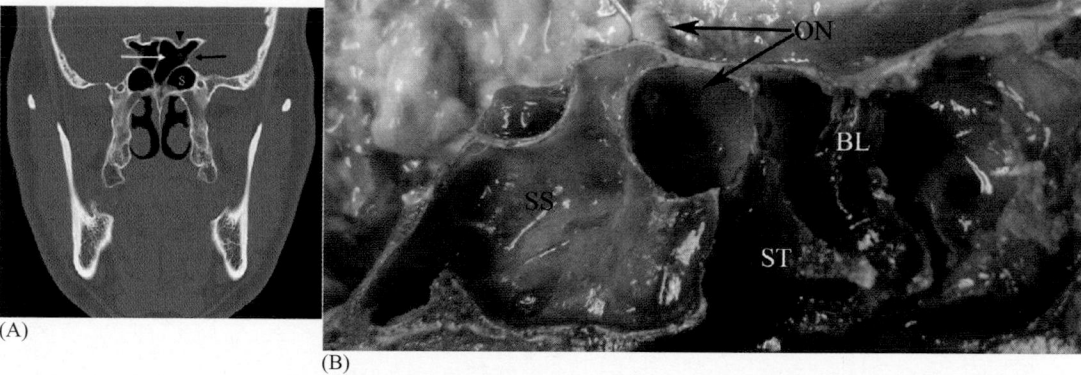

(A)　　　(B)

Figure 22 (A) In the coronal CT scan, an Onodi cell (*white arrow*) lies above the sphenoid sinus (S) and sits below the optic nerve (*black arrowhead*) and medial to the carotid artery (*black arrow*). (B) In the sagittally cut cadaveric specimen, an Onodi cell (OC) can be seen with the optic nerve (ON, over probe) running in the roof of the cell. The bulla lamella of the middle turbinate (BL) and the superior turbinate (ST) are also noted.

38

Olfaction and Gustation

Richard L. Doty, PhD
Alexis H. Jackman, MD

The chemical senses determine the flavor of foods and beverages and provide a sensitive and early means for detecting dangerous environmental situations, including the presence of fire, spoiled food, and leaking natural gas. These senses are important to otorhinolaryngologists as (a) their stewardship falls within the purview of their specialty, (b) some otolaryngologic operative procedures compromise the functioning of these senses, (c) alterations in chemosensory function can be an early sign of a number of other diseases, including Alzheimer's disease and idiopathic Parkinson disease, and (d) losses or distortions of chemosensation are of considerable personal and practical significance to the patient. The latter should not be underestimated and is particularly acute for patients whose lifestyle, livelihood, or immediate safety depend upon smelling and tasting (eg, cooks, firemen, homemakers, plumbers, professional food and beverage tasters, employees of natural gas works, chemists, and numerous industrial workers).

This chapter provides an overview of the anatomy and physiology of the smell and taste systems, describes basic chemosensory pathology, and discusses means for quantitatively assessing, managing, and treating disorders of these sensory systems.

THE OLFACTORY SYSTEM

Anatomy and Physiology

Olfactory Neuroepithelium. The olfactory neuroepithelium contains the olfactory receptors of cranial nerve I (CN I), as well as free nerve endings from CN V, and lines the cribriform plate and sectors of the superior turbinate, middle turbinate, and septum. Although it reportedly comprises approximately 2 cm^2 of the upper recesses of each nasal chamber, it is not a homogenous structure, at least in the adult, as metaplastic islands of respiratory-like epithelium accumulate within its borders beginning early in life, presumably as a result of insults from viruses, bacterial agents, and toxins.[1] On the basis of immunohistochemical and anatomical criteria,[2] at least 6 major classes of cells can be identified in this neuroepithelium: bipolar sensory receptor cells, supporting or sustentacular cells, microvillar cells, Bowman gland and duct cells, globose basal cells, and horizontal

basal cells. The approximately 6 million *receptor cells* are derived embryologically from the olfactory placode and, thus, are of central nervous system (CNS) origin. The cilia of these cells, which extend into the mucus of the nasal lumen, harbor the 7 domain transmembrane olfactory receptors. The axons of these cells ultimately unite into bundles of 50 or so "fila" ensheathed by glial cells that traverse the cribriform plate to form the outermost layer of the olfactory bulb. The *sustentacular cells* insulate the receptor cells from one another and extend microvilli, rather than cilia, into the mucus. These cells contribute to the mucus of the region and may be involved to some degree in deactivating odorants and xenobiotic agents. The function of the approximately 600,000 *microvillar cells* located at the epithelial surface is unknown.[3] The *Bowman glands* are a major source of the mucus in the olfactory region, whereas the *globose and horizontal basal cells* are the progenitor cells of the other cell types (Figure 1).[2]

Olfactory Bulb and Olfactory Cortex. The first processing station in the olfactory system, the olfactory bulb, is located directly over the cribriform plate. Its neural components are arranged in 6 concentric layers: the olfactory nerve layer, the glomerular layer, the external plexiform layer, the mitral cell layer, the internal plexiform layer, and the granule cell layer (Figure 2). The receptor cell axons of the olfactory nerve layer enter the glomeruli within the second layer of the bulb, where they synapse with the dendrites of the mitral and tufted cells within the spherical glomeruli. These second-order cells, in turn, send collaterals that synapse within the periglomerular and external plexiform layers, resulting in "reverberating" circuits in which negative and positive feedback occur. Indeed, mitral cells modulate their own output by activating granule cells (which are inhibitory to them). Whereas the olfactory bulbs of younger persons have thousands of glomeruli arranged in single or double layers within the glomerular layer, older persons typically have far fewer numbers of glomeruli, reflecting the decrease in olfactory receptor cell numbers within the neuroepithelium. After the age of 80 years, such structures are nearly absent.[6] Both endogenous and exogenous factors influence olfactory bulb structure, including early malnutrition.[7]

The mitral and tufted cell axons project ipsilaterally to the primary olfactory cortex via the

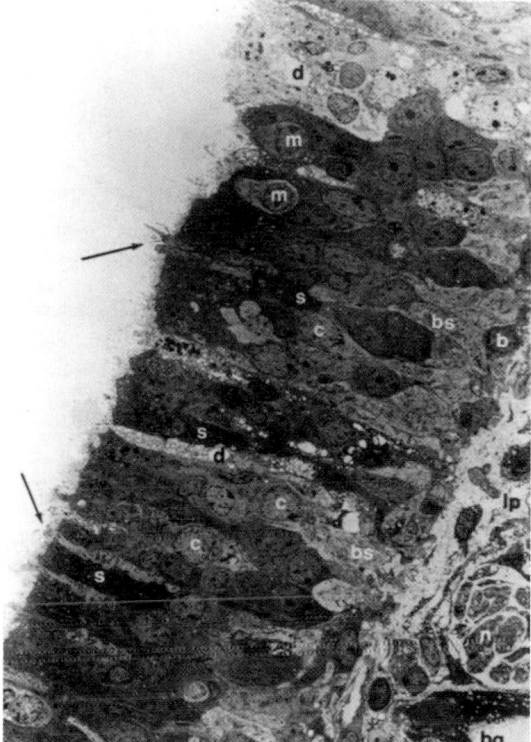

Figure 1 Low power electron micrograph (×670) of a longitudinal section through a biopsy specimen of human olfactory mucosa taken from the nasal septum. Four cell types are indicated: ciliated olfactory receptors (c), microvillar cells (m), supporting cells (s), and basal cells (b). The arrows point to ciliated olfactory knobs of the bipolar receptor cells. bg = Bowman gland; bs = base of the supporting cells; d = degenerating cells; lp = lamina propria; n = nerve bundle. (From reference 4 with permission. Copyright © 1982, Chapman & Hall.)

olfactory tract without an intervening thalamic synapse. The primary olfactory cortex is comprised of the anterior olfactory nucleus (AON), the piriform cortex, the olfactory tubercle, the entorhinal area, the periamygdaloid cortex, and the corticomedial amygdala. Some projections occur, via the anterior commissure, from pyramidal cells of the AON to contralateral elements of the primary olfactory cortex. A number of projections from primary to secondary (ie, orbitofrontal) cortex are direct, whereas others relay within the thalamus. Odor memories are stored not only in the hippocampus, but also within the piriform cortex.[8] Interestingly, functional imaging studies have found that odors reliably and significantly activate, in a concentration-dependent manner, posterior lateral areas of the cerebellum,

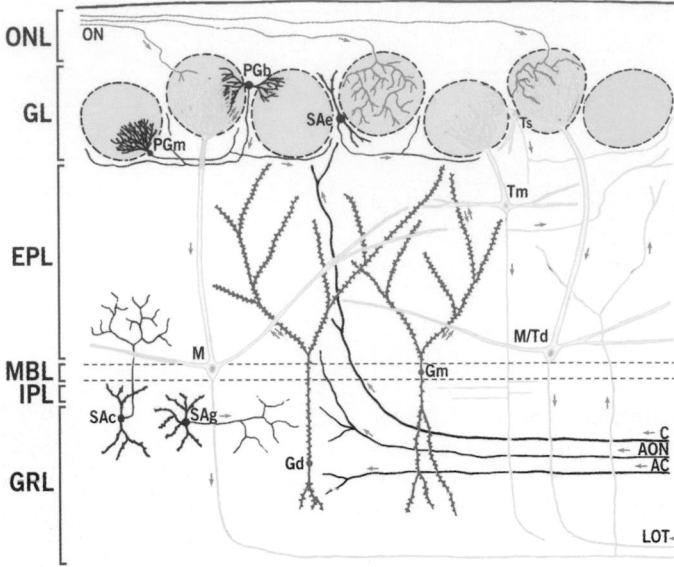

Figure 2 Diagram of major layers and types of olfactory bulb neurons in the mammalian olfactory bulb, as based on stained Golgi material. Main layers are indicated on the left as follows: AC = fibers from anterior commissure; AON = fibers from anterior olfactory nucleus; C = centrifugal fibers; EPL = external plexiform layer; Gd = granule cell with cell body in deep layers; GL = glomerular layer; Gm = granule cell with cell body in mitral cell body layer; GRL = granule cell layer; IPL = internal plexiform layer; LOT = lateral olfactory tract; M = mitral cell; M/Td = displaced mitral or deep tufted cell; MBL = mitral cell body layer; ON = olfactory nerves; ONL = olfactory nerve layer; PGb = periglomerular cells with biglomerular dendrites; PGm = periglomerular cell with monoglomerular dendrites; SAc = short-axon cell of Cajal; SAe = short-axon cell with extraglomerular dendrites; SAg = short-axon cell of Golgi; Tm = middle tufted cell; Ts = superficial tufted cell. (From reference 5 with permission. Copyright © 1972, American Physiological Society.)

whereas sniffing alone tends to active mainly anterior central cerebellar regions.[9] The cerebellar activity may reflect the circuits involved in modulating sniff size relative to the intensity of an odor or other movement-related behaviors.

Olfactory Transduction. Humans can detect and discriminate among thousands of airborne odorants. A total of 10 to 15% of the incoming airstream is shunted toward the olfactory cleft during inhalation (Figure 3). Some of the odorant molecules within this deflected airstream move from the air to the largely aqueous phase of the olfactory mucus, where they diffuse or are actively transported via "odorant binding proteins" to the olfactory receptors. Receptor activation then leads to transduction cascades that produce action potentials within the olfactory receptor neurons.

Most olfactory receptors are representatives of a large (~1,000) multigene family of G-protein-coupled 7 transmembrane receptors.[11] Each olfactory receptor neuron seems to express only 1 type of receptor, and neurons expressing the same

gene appear randomly distributed within a few segregated strip-like "spatial zones" of the neuroepithelium, at least in the rodent. Each receptor binds a number of odorant molecules, although not all odorant molecules activate all receptors. Since the olfactory neurons that express a given receptor gene project to the same glomeruli of the olfactory bulb,[12] the glomeruli can be considered functional units. Data from a variety of sources suggest that it is the pattern across the activated receptors or glomeruli that serves as the proximal code for odorant quality.

The stimulatory guanine nucleotide-binding protein, G_{olf}, is activated by most olfactory receptor proteins.[13] In turn, G_{olf} induces production of the second messenger adenosine monophosphate (cAMP) by activating the enzyme adenyl cyclase. cAMP then diffuses through the cytoplasm, producing cellular depolarization by opening cyclic-nucleotide-gated ionic channels and Ca^{2+}-dependent Cl^- or K^+ channels. Cyclic guanosine monophosphate (cGMP) is also activated by some odorants. cGMP appears, among other things, to modulate the sensitivity of olfactory receptor neurons during adaptation.[14] G proteins other than G_{olf} (eg, G_{i2} and G_o) are present in olfactory receptor cells and aid in axonal signal propagation, axon sorting, target innervation, and other such processes.[15]

Receptor Cell Regeneration. The olfactory neuroepithelium has the ability to regenerate, although in cases where significant damage to the basement membrane has occurred, regeneration is nonexistent or incomplete. While, under normal circumstances, relatively continuous neurogenesis occurs within basal segments of the neuroepithelium,

many receptor cells are relatively long lived and appear to be replaced only after they are damaged.[16] Receptor cell death, as well as replenishment from progenitor cells, is determined by both endogenous and exogenous factors.[17] For example, differentiated neurons send regulatory signals that program the numbers of new neurons that need to be produced by the stem cells so as to maintain equilibrium in the cell population.[18] Apoptotic cell death occurs in cells representing all stages of regeneration, implying that biochemical regulation of neuronal numbers occurs at multiple stages of the neuronal lineage.[19]

Classification of Olfactory Disorders

Smell dysfunction can be reliably classified as follows: *anosmia*: inability to detect olfactory sensations, that is, absence of smell function; *partial anosmia*: ability to perceive some, but not all, such sensations; *hyposmia or microsmia*: decreased sensitivity to odors; *hyperosmia*: abnormally acute smell function; *dysosmia*: distorted or perverted smell perception to odor stimulation (sometimes termed cacosmia or parosmia, depending upon the nature of the perversion); *phantosmia*: a dysosmic sensation perceived in the absence of an odor stimulus, for example, an olfactory hallucination; and *olfactory agnosia*: inability to recognize an odor sensation, even though olfactory processing, language, and general intellectual functions are essentially intact, as in some stroke patients. Olfactory dysfunction can be either bilateral (binasal) or unilateral (uninasal), although most commonly such dysfunction is bilateral. Although presbyosmia is sometimes used to describe smell loss due to aging, this term is less specific than those noted above (ie, it does not distinguish between anosmia and hyposmia) and is laden, by definition, with the notion that it is age per se that is causing the age-related deficit.

Clinical Evaluation of Olfactory Function

Three steps are involved in assessing a patient with chemosensory dysfunction: (a) obtaining a detailed clinical history; (b) testing olfactory function quantitatively; and (c) physically examining the head and neck.[20,21]

History. To determine the cause of olfactory loss, it is important to determine antedecent events such as head trauma, upper respiratory tract infections, toxic exposures, or iatrogenic interventions, for example, surgical procedures, although in some patients a determination of the basis of the problem is complicated. It is also valuable to note whether the olfactory loss has changed in its severity over time. Specifics concerning the nature, timing of onset, duration and pattern of fluctuations, if any, of the patient's chemosensory symptoms should be obtained. For example, *sudden olfactory loss* suggests the possibility of head trauma, infection, ischemia, or a psychogenic condition. *Gradual loss* can reflect the development of degenerative processes or progressive obstructive lesions within

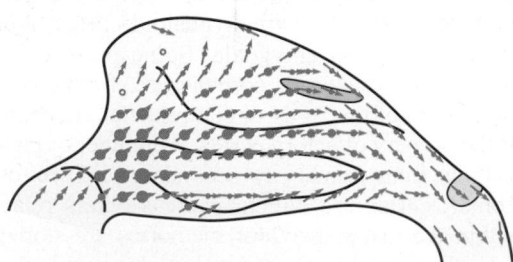

Figure 3 Pattern of the inspiratory nasal airflow as derived from studies in models. The external naris is to the left. Arrows indicate the direction of airflow and dot size indicates the velocity. (From reference 10 with permission. Copyright © 1977 Marcel Dekker, Inc.)

the olfactory receptor region or degeneration of more central neural structures. *Intermittent loss* can be indicative of an intranasal inflammatory process.[21]

Questions regarding sinonasal symptoms such as epistaxis, discharge (clear, purulent or bloody), nasal obstruction, allergies, and somatic symptoms, including headache or irritation, may have localizing value. When a clear-cut cause is not apparent, the clinician must explore a number of potential avenues to ascertain likely causal events or combinations of causal events. It is essential that potential underlying medical conditions known to have chemosensory consequences (eg, renal failure, liver disease, hypothyroidism, diabetes, or dementia) be identified or ruled out. A detailed assessment of the medications being used prior to and during the onset of the dysfunction is important, as many common medications (eg, antihypertensive and antilipid agents, and antibiotics) can produce smell or taste disturbances. Importantly, medication-induced deficits may take some time to appear, so simply because a patient has been taking a drug for some time does not rule out its possible causative involvement. Likewise, some medication-induced alterations do not disappear immediately upon drug cessation.

A review of the patient's social history, including past and current employment as well as tobacco, alcohol, or recreational drug use, may also provide clues to etiology (eg, chronic alcoholism or Wernicke Korsakoff syndromes). A family history of smell dysfunction may suggest a genetic cause. Delayed puberty in association with anosmia (with or without midline craniofacial abnormalities, deafness, and renal anomalies) suggests the possibility of Kallmann syndrome or some variant thereof. Subtle signs of central tumors, dementia, parkinsonism, and seizure activity (eg, automatisms, occurrence of black-outs, auras, and déjà vu experiences) should be sought in both the history and physical examination.

Quantitative Olfactory Testing. Many patients are inaccurate in describing their chemosensory function; some are unaware of a chemosensory deficit, whereas others overstate the nature of their problem. Hence, the otolaryngologist should employ modern means for quantitatively assessing olfactory function in the office setting. Reliable quantitative testing is needed to (a) verify the validity of the patient's complaint, (b) characterize the exact nature and degree of the problem, (c) monitor accurately changes in function over time (including those resulting from therapeutic interventions), (d) detect malingering, and (e) obtain an objective basis for determining compensation for disability. In the past, many physicians have tested olfaction by simply asking the patient to identify several crude odorants, such as licorice, coffee grounds, or tobacco, placed under the nose. Unfortunately, such qualitative testing can lead to false positives (eg, patients have difficulty identifying odors without response alternatives),

lacks reliability, has no normative reference, and is easily faked by malingerers.

During the last quarter century, a number of standardized and practical psychophysical tests have been developed.[22] The most widely used test is the 40-item University of Pennsylvania Smell Identification Test or UPSIT (commercially known as the Smell Identification Test; Figure 4).[23] This reliable (test–retest $r = .94$) test employs microencapsulated ("scratch and sniff") odorants and is available in 7 languages. It can be self-administered in 10 to 15 minutes in the waiting room by most patients and scored in less than a minute by nonmedical personnel. In addition to providing a percentile rank of a patient's performance relative to age- and sex-matched controls, an absolute determination of normosmia, mild microsmia, moderate microsmia, severe microsmia, anosmia, or probable malingering can be made.

In some cases, unilateral testing is warranted, although usually olfactory problems are bilateral. To assess olfaction unilaterally, the naris contralateral to the tested side should be occluded without distorting the nasal valve region. This can be easily accomplished by sealing the contralateral naris using a piece of Microfoam tape (3M Corporation, Minneapolis, MN) cut to fit the naris borders (Figure 5). The patient is instructed to sniff the stimulus normally and to exhale through the mouth. Such occlusion not only prevents air from entering the olfactory cleft from the contralateral naris (orthonasal stimulation), but also prevents active movement of odor-laden air into the occluded side from the rear of the nasopharynx (retronasal stimulation).

The measurement of olfactory event-related potentials (OERPs) is available in only a handful of specialized centers. In essence, synchronized brain electroencephalographic (EEG) activity induced by repeated pulsatile presentations of an odorant is isolated from overall EEG activity. Averaging of responses from repetitive stimulation increases the signal-to-noise ratio. Although OERPs are relatively sensitive and useful in detecting malingering, they presently are unable to localize where in the olfactory pathway an anomaly exists, unlike their visual and auditory counterparts. Unfortunately, OERP testing requires specialized and expensive equipment capable of delivering odorant pulses with rapid rise times (~30 to 40 ms) to the olfactory neuroepithelium within a background of continuously flowing warmed and humidified air without inducing confounding somatosensory sensations.[24]

The electro-olfactogram (EOG) is another electrophysiological measure of the olfactory system.[25] This surface potential, detected via an electrode placed on the surface of the olfactory mucosa, reflects summated generator potentials mainly from olfactory receptor neurons. The recording of the EOG is, from a practical perspective, more difficult than that of the OERP, and far fewer patients are amenable to such recording.

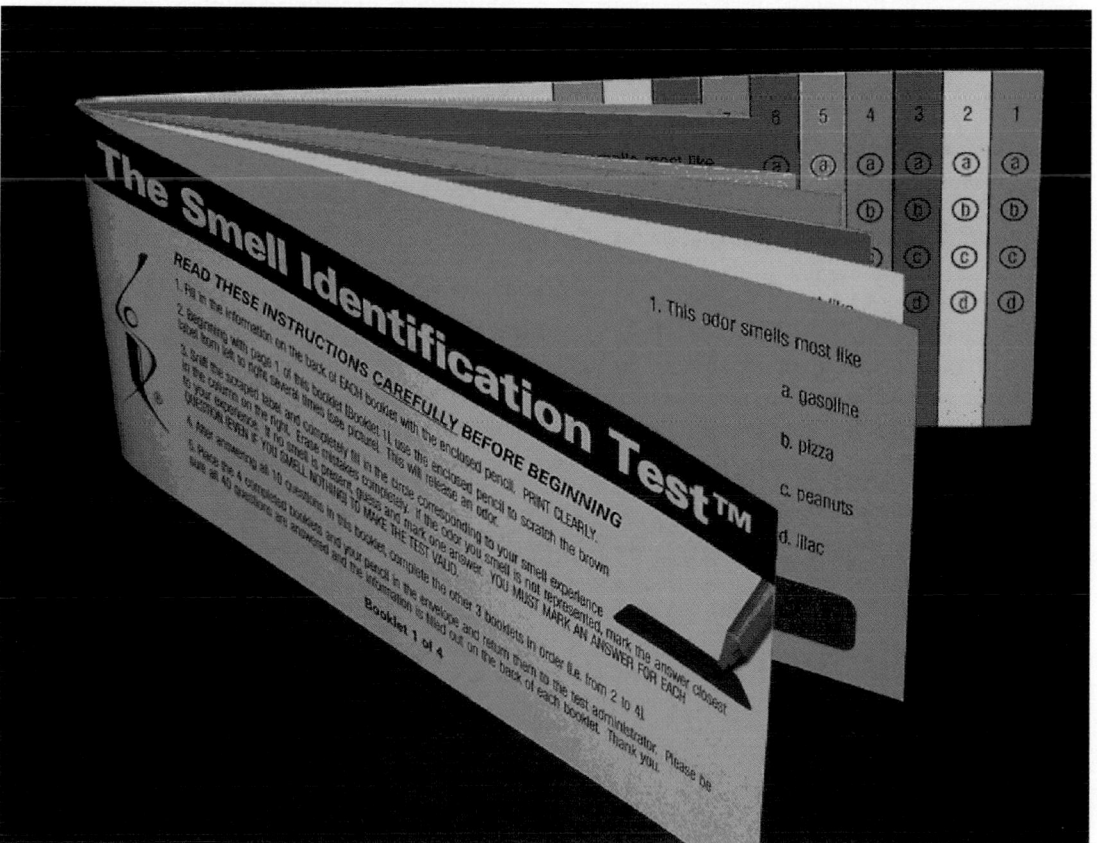

Figure 4 Booklet 1 of the 40-odorant University of Pennsylvania Smell Identification Test (UPSIT; commercially known as the Smell Identification Test). Each page of 4 10-page booklets contains a microencapsulated odorant that is released by means of a pencil tip, and a multiple-choice question as to which of 4 possibilities smells most like the odorant. Forced-choice answers are recorded on columns on the last page of the test. (Photograph courtesy of Sensonics, Inc., Haddon Hts., NJ. Copyright © 2005, Sensonics, Inc.)

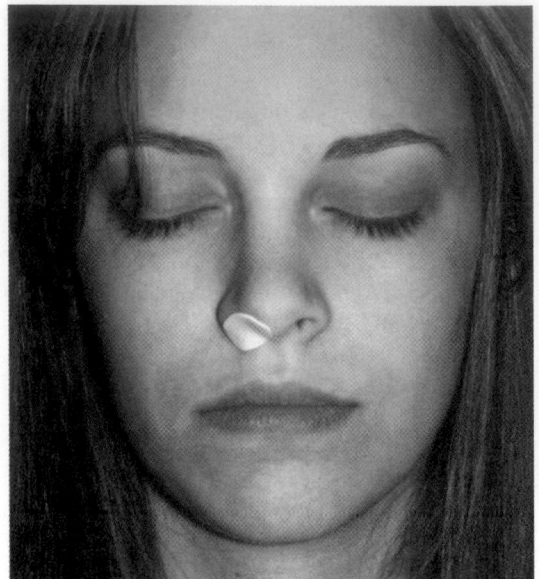

Figure 5 Picture of naris properly sealed for contralateral side testing with Microfoam tape. (Photograph courtesy of Sensonics, Inc., Haddon Hts., NJ. Copyright © 2000, Sensonics, Inc.)

The placement of the recording electrode is preformed under endoscopic guidance. Since local anesthesia must be avoided, this can be quite unpleasant. Importantly, even after the electrode has been placed correctly placed on mucus membrane containing olfactory neuroepithelium, an electricial potential cannot be readily detected in some patients. This may reflect the topographical distribution of specific olfactory receptors in combination with the relatively few number of odorants used, or the presence of metaplasia of respiratory-like epithelium within the olfactory neuroepithelium.

Physical Examination, Laboratory Tests, and Medical Imaging. Careful otolaryngologic and neurologic assessment is warranted in patients complaining of olfactory dysfunction.[20,21] Nasal endoscopy, employing flexible or rigid endoscopes, should be performed, with specific attention being paid to the area of the olfactory cleft. The nasal cavity should be inspected for the presence of pathologic masses, polyps, or mucosal lesions. In addition, any mucosal adhesions between the turbinates and the septum should be noted, as they may compromise airflow to the olfactory receptor region. The nasal mucosa should be assessed for evidence of inflammation such as the erythema, edema, nodularity, as well as erosion or ulceration. Futhermore, nasal secretions should be carefully examined. Mucopus below the eustachian tube orifice suggests involvement of the osteomeatal complex, whereas mucopus above this orifice suggests posterior ethmoid and/or sphenoid sinus disease. Unusual spaciousness, dryness, and crusting, as is seen in atrophic rhinitis, suggests atrophy of the lamina propria. A pale mucous membrane can be indicative of allergy, usually resulting from edema within the lamina propria. Industrial or environmental pollutants as well as tobacco smoking can produce metaplasia within the

epithelium in addition to swelling, inflammation, exudates, erosion, and ulceration.

Visual field and acuity tests, as well as optic disc examinations, should be performed to determine whether intracranial mass lesions that produce increased intracranial pressure (papillodema) and optic atrophy are present (eg, the Foster Kennedy syndrome, which consists of ipsilateral anosmia, ipsilateral optic atrophy, and contralateral papilledema caused by a meningioma of the ipsilateral optic nerve).

Blood serum or other laboratory tests may help to identify or confirm underlying medical conditions that may relate to the dysfunction, including infection, inflammatory diseases, nutritional deficiencies, for example, B6, B12, allergy, diabetes mellitus, and thyroid, liver, and kidney disease. Although biopsies of the olfactory neuroepithelium can be made, their interpretation is hindered by sampling issues and the fact that metaplasia of respiratory-like epithelium occurs throughout the olfactory neuroepithelia of even persons with normal olfactory function.

Medical imaging can be invaluable in understanding the basis of a number of smell and taste disturbances. Magnetic resonance imaging (MRI) is the method of choice for evaluating soft tissue, for example, olfactory bulbs, tracts, and cortical parenchyma. Computed tomography (CT) is the most useful and cost-effective technique to assess sinonasal tract inflammatory disorders and is superior to MRI in the evaluation of bony structures adjacent to the olfactory pathways, for example, ethmoid and cribriform plate. Coronal CT scans are particularly useful in evaluating paranasal anatomy. Plain radiographs have substantial limitations, and are rarely useful. Positron emission tomography (PET), functional MRI (fMRI), and single-proton emission computed tomography (SPECT) have limited usefulness at the present time.

Detection of Malingering

Traditionally, it has been suggested that malingering can be detected reliably by having a patient inhale a strong CN V stimulant, such as ammonia, and asking whether a smell is perceived. If denial occurs, the assumption is made that malingering is present. Unfortunately, this procedure is unreliable, since usually CN V stimulants produce reflexive coughing, secretion from nasal membranes, or other rejection reactions which the patient obviously cannot deny. Furthermore, CN V thresholds vary considerably, such that some patients experience little reaction to the ammonia and truthfully report perceiving no sensations. Indeed, anosmia is associated with heightened CN V thresholds.[26]

A preferred method of the detection of malingering is to employ forced-choice psychophysical tests, such as the UPSIT. On such tests, malingering appears as the reporting of fewer incorrect responses than expected on the basis of chance (as would be expected in an anosmic). Since, in the case of the UPSIT, there are 4 response

alternatives for each item and the patient must provide an answer even if no smell is perceived, 25% of the items, on average, should be correctly identified by chance alone, that is, 10 out of 40. A sampling distribution exists around this expected probability, and empirical data are available on this point.[23] The theoretical probability of a true anosmic having an UPSIT score 5 or less is less than 5 in 100. The theoretical probability of a true anosmic scoring 0 on the UPSIT is lesser than 1 in 100,000.[23] In general, if a patient scores within the probable malingering region of UPSIT scores, the UPSIT should be administered again to confirm the apparent avoidance of correct responses. Multiplication of the 2 probabilities is then used to establish the statistical likelihood of malingering. Malingering is also suspected if patient reports smell loss in the presence of a clear OERP, although olfactory agnosia in such cases cannot be ruled out.

It is noteworthy that malingering is sometimes discovered in head injury patients by their scores on forced-choice taste tests, rather than their scores on forced-choice smell tests, since bonafide smell loss is, in fact, present (negating the ability to avoid correct answers on the olfactory element of the examination). Such malingering implies relatively normal taste function, and reflects the patient's naïve attempt to embellish the "taste loss" which, in fact, results from lack of retronasal stimulation of the olfactory receptors.

Evidence for a general tendency to malinger can also be obtained using neuropsychological tests specifically designed for this purpose, for example, tests sensitive to head trauma patients trying to feign memory disturbances. Among those that are widely used is Rey Memory Test (RMT), also known as the Rey 3 × 5 Test and the Rey 15-item Memory Test.[27] The rationale behind this test is that malingerers typically fail at a memory task that all but the most developmentally disabled or severely brain injured persons perform easily.

Causes of Olfactory Dysfunction

Olfactory dysfunction can result from 3 general causes: (a) *conductive or transport impairments* from nasal passage obstruction (eg, by chronic rhinosinusitis, polyposis, excessive mucus secretion), (b) *sensorineural impairment* from injury to the olfactory neuroepithelium, for example, by viruses, airborne toxins, and (c) *central olfactory neural impairment* from injury to CNS structures, for example, tumors, masses impinging on the olfactory tract. These categories, however, are not mutually exclusive. For example, both blockage of airflow to the receptors and damage to the receptors and/or more central elements of the olfactory system can be simultaneously present or occur in stages. Thus, chronic rhinosinusitis can produce damage to the olfactory neuroepithelium in addition to blocking airflow, and altered neuroepithelial function can, over time, lead to degeneration within the olfactory bulb, a central structure.

There are numerous causes of olfactory disturbance (Table 1). Most cases of chronic

Table 1 Reported Agents, Diseases, Drugs, Interventions and Other Etiologic Categories Associated in the Medical or Toxicological Literature with Olfactory Dysfunction

Air pollutants and industrial dusts
  Acetone
  Acids, eg, sulfuric
  Ashes
  Benzene
  Benzol
  Butyl acetate
  Cadmium
  Carbon disulfide
  Cement
  Chalk
  Chlorine
  Chromium
  Coke/coal
  Cotton
  Cresol
  Ethyl acetate
  Ethyl and methyl acrylate
  Flour
  Formaldehyde
  Grain
  Hydrazine
  Hydrogen selenide
  Hydrogen sulfide
  Iron carboxyl
  Lead
  Nickel
  Nitrous gases
  Paint solvents
  Paper
  Pepper
  Peppermint oil
  Phosphorus oxychloride
  Potash
  Silicone dioxide
  Spices
  Trichloroethylene

Drugs
  Adrenal corticosteroids (chronic use)
  Amino acids (excess)
    Cysteine
    Histidine
  Analgesics
    Antipyrine
  Anesthetics, local
    Cocaine HCl
    Procaine HCl
    Tetracaine HCl
  Anticancer agents, eg, methotrexate
  Antihistamines, eg, chlorpheniramine maleate
  Antimicrobials
    Griseofulvin
    Lincomycin
    Macrolides
    Neomycin
    Pencillins
    Streptomycin
    Tetracyclines
    Tyrothricin
  Antirheumatics
    Mercury/gold salts
    D-Penicillamine
  Antithyroids
    Methimazole
    Propylthiouracil
    Thiouracil
  Antivirals
  Cardiovascular/antihypertensives
  Gastric medications

  Cimetidine
  Hyperlipoproteinemia medications
    Atorvastatin calcium (Lipitor)
    Cholestyramine
    Clofibrate
  Intranasal saline solutions with:
    Acetylcholine
    Acetyl, β-methylcholine
    Menthol
    Strychnine
    Zinc sulfate
  Local vasoconstrictors
  Opiates
    Codeine
    Hydromophone HCl
    Morphine
  Psychopharmaceuticals (eg, LSD, psilocybin)
  Sympathomimetics
    Amphetamine sulfate
    Fenbutrazate HCl
    Phenmetrazine theoclate

Endocrine/metabolic disorders
  Addison disease
  Congenital adrenal hyperplasia
  Cushing syndrome
  Diabetes mellitus
  Froelich syndrome
  Gigantism
  Hypergonadotropic hypogonadism
  Hypothyroidism
  Kallmann syndrome
  Pregnancy
  Panhypopituitarism
  Pseudohypoparathyroidism
  Sjögren syndrome
  Turner syndrome

Infections—viral/bacterial
  Acquired immunodeficiency syndrome (AIDS)
  Acute viral rhinitis
  Bacterial rhinosinusitis
  Bronchiectasis
  Fungal
  Influenza
  Rickettsial
  Microfilarial

Lesions of the nose/airway blockage
  Adenoid hypertrophy
  Allergic rhinitis
    Perennial
    Seasonal
  Atrophic rhinitis
  Chronic inflammatory rhinitis
  Hypertrophic rhinitis
  Nasal polyposis
  Rhinitis medicamentosa
  Structural abnormality
    Deviated septum
    Weakness of alae nasi
  Vasomotor rhinitis

Medical/surgical interventions
  Adrenalectomy
  Anesthesia
  Anterior craniotomy
  Arteriography
  Chemotherapy
  Frontal lobe resection
  Gastrectomy
  Hemodialysis
  Hypophysectomy
  Influenza vaccination
  Laryngectomy
  Oophorectomy

  Paranasal sinus exenteration
  Radiation therapy
  Rhinoplasty
  Temporal lobe resection
  Thyroidectomy

Neoplasms—intracranial
  Frontal lobe gliomas and other tumers
  Midline cranial tumors
    Parasagital meningiomas
    Tumors of the corpus callosum
  Olfactory groove/cribriform plate meningiomas
  Osteomas
  Paraoptic chiasma tumors
    Aneurysms
    Craniopharyngioma
    Pituitary tumors (esp. adenomas)
    Suprasellar cholesteatoma
    Suprasellar meningioma
  Temporal lobe tumors

Neoplasms—intranasal
  Neuro-olfactory tumors
    Esthesioepithelioma
    Esthesioneuroblastoma
    Esthesioneurocytoma
    Esthesioneuroepithelioma
  Other benign or malignant nasal tumors
    Adenocarcinoma
    Leukemic infiltration
    Nasopharyngeal tumors with extension
    Neurofibroma
    Paranasal tumors with extension
    Schwannoma

Neoplasms—extranasal and extracranial
  Breast
  Gastrointestinal tract
  Laryngeal
  Lung
  Ovary
  Testicular

Neurologic disorders
  Amyotrophic lateral sclerosis
  Alzheimer disease
  Cerebral abscess (esp. frontal or ethmoidal regions)
  Down syndrome
  Familial dysautonomia
  Guam amyotrophic lateral sclerosis/Parkinson
    disease/dementia
  Head trauma
  Huntington disease
  Hydrocephalus
  Korsakoff psychosis
  Migraine
  Meningitis
  Multiple sclerosis
  Myesthenia gravis
  Paget disease
  Parkinson disease
  Refsum syndrome
  Restless leg syndrome
  Syphilis
  Syringomyelia
  Temporal lobe epilepsy
    Hamartomas
    Mesial temporal sclerosis
    Scars/previous infarcts
  Vascular insufficiency/anoxia
    Small multiple cerebrovascular accidents
    Subclavian steal syndrome
    Transient ischemic attacks
Nutritional/metabolic disorders
  Abetalipoproteinemia

Continued

Table 1 Reported Agents, Diseases, Drugs, Interventions and Other Etiologic Categories Associated in the Medical or Toxicological Literature with Olfactory Dysfunction—Continued

Chronic alcoholism
Chronic renal failure
Cirrhosis of liver
Gout
Morbid obesity
Protein calorie malnutrition
Total parenteral nutrition without adequate
    replacement
Trace metal deficiencies
    Copper
    Zinc
Whipple disease
Vitamin deficiency
    Vitamin A
    Vitamin B6
    Vitamin B12

Pulmonary disorders
    Chronic obstructive pulmonary disease

Psychiatric disorders
    Anorexia nervosa (severe stage)
    Attention deficit disorder
    Depressive disorders
    Hysteria
    Malingering
    Olfactory reference syndrome
    Schizophrenia
    Schizotypy
    Seasonal affective disorder

Modified from reference 28.
Note that categories are not mutually exclusive.

anosmia or hyposmia are due to prior upper respiratory infections, head trauma, and nasal and paranasal sinus disease, reflecting long-lasting or permanent damage to the olfactory neuroepithelium.[29] Other causes include intranasal neoplasms (eg, inverting papillomas, hemangiomas, and esthesioneuroblastomas), intracranial tumors or lesions (eg, olfactory groove meningiomas, frontal lobe gliomas), neurological diseases (eg, Alzheimer disease, idiopathic Parkinson disease, multiple sclerosis, and schizophrenia), exposure to airborne toxins (including cigarette smoke), iatrogenic interventions (eg, septoplasty, rhinoplasty, turbinectomy, radiation therapy, and medications), epilepsy, psychiatric disorders, and various endocrine and metabolic disorders. The more common disorders or entities associated with smell loss are described in detail later in this section.

Most dysosmias reflect dynamic changes in the olfactory epithelium and remit over time.[29,30] Some anosmic patients report that prior to onset of their anosmia they experienced a period of weeks or months when dysosmia was present. Usually some smell function is present during the period of dysosmia. In rare instances, dysosmias present as aura-like hallucinations presumably associated with central, for example, temporal lobe, dysfunction. In many such cases, no seizure activity can be documented, and no evidence of CNS lesions or tumors is apparent. Nonetheless, low doses of anticonvulsant medication may be

effective in mitigating the frequency and severity of some of these dysosmias. Dysosmias can also occur in a number of neurological or psychiatric disturbances which usually are diagnosed on other grounds, for example, psychosis, multiple sclerosis. Infrequently, dysosmia may be due to the perception of foul odors produced by the body, such as those from purulent nasal secretions in sinusitis or from exhalations in halitosis or uremia. Other disorders which may present as dysosmia include trimethylaminuria (fish odor syndrome) and cat odor syndrome—a pediatric neurologic disorder associated with a β-methyl-crotonyl-CoA carboxylase deficiency. Such rare disorders usually exist in the presence of a normally functioning olfactory system.

In contrast to cases of anosmia, hyposmia, and dysosmia, cases of hyperosmia are rare. Although untreated adrenal cortical insufficiency has been reported to produce hyperosmia in humans, this finding has yet to be confirmed; and in animal studies, no evidence has been found for hypersensitivity following adrenalectomy.[31] There have been suggestions of hyperosmia in syndromes such as multiple chemical sensitivity, but the limited data available also fail to support this notion.[32] Hyperosmia reportedly occurs in some cases of epilepsy during the interictal period, although most patients with long-term epilepsy and intractable seizure activity, such as candidates for temporal lobe resection, are hyposmic.[33]

Viral Upper Respiratory Infections. Upper respiratory system viruses, for example, influenza and colds, are the most common cause of *permanent* smell loss in adulthood.[29] Factors that predispose individuals to viral-induced smell dysfunction or the mechanisms underlying it remain unclear although direct insult to an already compromised neuroepithelium is most likely. In rare cases, central structures may also become involved. If neural damage is present, topical or systemic corticosteroid treatment is ineffective. Reduced numbers of olfactory receptor cells and other epithelial abnormalities are commonly found in biopsies taken from the olfactory neuroepithelia of patients with postviral anosmia or hyposmia.

Head Trauma. Smell loss or distortion occurs in approximately 15% of patients with significant head trauma but can be present even in mild cases where rapid acceleration/deceleration of the brain has occurred (coup contra coup injury) (Figure 6). In general, the severity of trauma is roughly correlated with the degree of loss. Occipital blows tend to produce more frequent and more severe olfactory deficits than frontal blows.[35] The physiological mechanisms involved include shearing of the olfactory fila and contusions of the olfactory bulb and frontal and temporal poles.[36] Although the cribriform plate may become fractured in some cases, such fractures are not a prerequisite for smell loss.[35] In a study of 268 patients evaluated at the University of Pennsylvania Smell and Taste

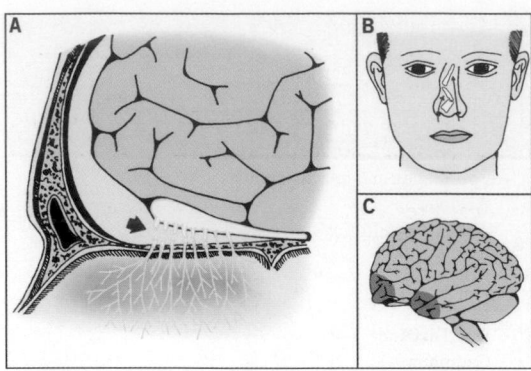

Figure 6 Mechanisms of posttraumatic olfactory dysfunction. (A) Tearing of the olfactory fila, (B) injury to the sinonasal tract, and (C) cortical contusions and brain hemorrhage. (From reference 34. Copyright © 1995, Marcel Dekker, Inc.)

Center who had experienced head trauma, 66.8% had anosmia and 20.5% hyposmia. Of 66 patients retested 1 month to 13 years later, only three, none of whom initially had anosmia, regained normal olfactory function. Dysosmia prevalence decreased from 41.1 to 15.4% over posttrauma periods averaging several years.[35]

Even though the loss of smell following head trauma is usually immediate, this is not always the case, and it may take the patient a while to recognize the presence of the loss. In some cases delayed loss reflects delayed receptor cell death. Rodent research shows that intracranial hemorrhage and ischemia can lead to degeneration of the olfactory neuroepithelium without transection of the olfactory nerves.[37]

Paranasal Sinus Disease. It is now apparent that the olfactory loss associated with nasal or sinus disease is not due solely to decreased conduction of airflow to the olfactory receptors. Although medical, for example, administration of topical or systemic steroids, or surgical, for example, excision of polyps, treatment can improve olfactory function in some cases, return to normal levels is not the norm.[38] In the case of rhinosinusitis, for example, factors other than, or in addition to, nasal airflow blockage are responsible for the loss. Chronic inflammation is likely toxic to olfactory neurons. Hence, many cases of rhinosinusitis have a significant sensorineural component. The severity of histopathology within the olfactory neuroepithelium of chronic rhinosinusitis patients is correlated with the degree of smell loss, as measured by the UPSIT.[39] Olfactory biopsies from patients with nasal disease are less likely to yield olfactory neuroepithelial tissue than biopsies from controls.[40] The same is true for anosmic versus nonanosmic rhinosinusitis patients.[41]

Systemic Diseases. Olfactory disturbances may be due to pathologic manifestations of systemic disease. Ciliary dysfunction syndromes, such as Kartagener syndrome and immotile cilia syndrome, are accompanied by chronic rhinosinusitis and often associated with olfactory loss. Granulomatous diseases causing nasal lesions include both infections, such as leprosy and tuberculosis, and connective tissue disorders, such Wegener granulomatosis and lupus erythematosus. Olfactory loss in these diseases may be due to direct damage to the olfactory neuroepithelium, obstruction of the nasal airway secondary to nasal secretions, or obstruction of airflow to the olfactory cleft resulting from the collapse of the cartilaginous and bony framework. Wegener granulomatosis is a systemic disease characterized by necrotizing vasculitis affecting small arteries of the repiratory tract and kidney. In the upper airway, nasal ulcerations are frequently observed. In addition to mucosal damage, septal perforation and collapse can contribute to olfactory loss by altering nasal airflow. Nasal sarcoidosis, a noncaseating granulomatous disease associated with olfactory loss, typically presents with small yellowish excrescences of the septal mucus membrane, atrophy of submucosal glands, and abundant crusting.

CNS Neoplasms. Olfactory disturbances can arise from tumors impinging on the olfactory bulbs or tracts, such as frontal lobe gliomas, olfactory groove meningiomas, and suprasellar ridge meningiomas arising from the dura mater of the cribriform plate. Other tumors located on the floor of the third ventricle, pituitary tumors extending above the sella turcica, and tumors in the temporal lobe or uncinate convolution can also be implicated.[20] The Foster Kennedy syndrome can result from tumors impinging on the bulb or tract.[42] *Pseudo* Foster Kennedy syndrome has been found in patients with increased intracranial pressure who had previous unilateral optic atrophy.[43]

Aging. Age-related smell loss is well documented and occurs in most older people, including those who are healthy and taking no medications (Figure 7).[44] Such loss clearly impacts on the quality of life of the elderly, influencing nutrition, appetite, and, possibly in some cases, even general immunity and defensive responses to illnesses.[45] About half of the population between 65 and 80 years of age experiences significant decrements in the ability to smell. Over the age of 80, this figure rises to nearly 75%. This is in

marked contrast to persons under the age of 65 years, of whom only 1 to 2% suffers from major difficulty smelling.[44]

Despite the association with age, smell loss in the later years should not be attributed simply to age, per se, as often an accumulation of damage over the years is the culprit and a single event, such as a bad cold, can be the precipitating factor. In general, age-related changes in smell function reflect decrements in both olfactory receptors and the number of olfactory bulb glomeruli.[8] Interestingly, age-related closure of cribriform plate formina by ossification is common in skulls from older persons.[46] Other age-related factors, such as the development of pathology related to Alzheimer disease (see below), may also contribute to the age-related losses in smell function.[47]

Neurodegenerative and Other Neurological Diseases. An exciting chapter in the study of olfaction has been the discovery that a number of neurological disorders are commonly accompanied by olfactory deficits, including Alzheimer disease, idiopathic Parkinson disease, Huntington disease, alcoholic Korsakoff syndrome, Pick disease, the Parkinsonism dementia complex of Guam, amyotrophic lateral sclerosis, schizophrenia, and multiple sclerosis.[48–51] Indeed, olfactory dysfunction appears to be the first clinical sign of Alzheimer disease and idiopathic Parkinson disease.[52,53] Although usually considered a neurodevelopmental disorder, smell loss is present in patients with schizophrenia and appears to be correlated with disease duration, suggesting a possible degenerative component in olfaction-related pathways.[51] Interestingly, patients with schizophrenia have much smaller olfactory bulbs and tracts than those of matched controls.[54]

Several studies provide data suggesting that smell testing is useful in identifying persons at risk for later significant cognitive decline and Alzheimer disease. Graves and colleagues administered a 12-item abbreviated version of the UPSIT (termed the Brief-Smell Identification Test or B-SIT) and several cognitive tests to 1,985 Japanese–American people around the age of 60, and then retested these people 2 years later.[55] Sixty-nine percent of the follow-up participants

were genotyped for apolipoprotein E (apoE). Low B-SIT scores in the presence of one or more APOE-e4 alleles were associated with a very high risk of subsequent cognitive decline. The B-SIT identified persons who came to exhibit later cognitive decline better than did a global cognitive test.

More recently, the UPSIT was administered by Devanand and colleagues to 90 outpatients with mild cognitive impairment and to matched healthy controls at 6-month intervals over a 5-year period.[56] Patients with mild cognitive impairment had lower UPSIT scores than did controls. Most importantly, patients with low UPSIT scores (<34) were more likely to develop Alzheimer disease than the other patients. Low UPSIT scores, combined with lack of awareness of olfactory deficits on the part of the patients, predicted the time to development of Alzheimer disease. UPSIT scores from 30 to 35 showed moderate to strong sensitivity and specificity for diagnosis of Alzheimer disease at follow-up.

The underlying cause for the olfactory deficit of Alzheimer disease is not yet clear, even though Alzheimer disease is associated with loss of neurons in the AON, olfactory bulb, and layer II of the entorhinal cortex.[49] Disproportionate numbers of neuritic plaques and neurofibrillary tangles are found within limbic brain regions which receive olfactory bulb projections. Several lines of evidence suggest that neurofibrillary tangles, rather than neuritic plaques, are most closely associated with the smell loss.[57] Central cholinergic deficits may also be involved, since (a) individuals with no history of cognitive loss that are in the early histopathologic stages of Alzheimer disease exhibit a cholinergic deficit within the inferior temporal lobe and (b) drugs that alter cholinergic function alter the ability to smell. For example, the cholinesterase inhibitor physostigmine improves odor discrimination performance, at least in rats,[58] whereas scopolamine, a muscarinic cholinergic antagonist, reportedly decreases olfactory sensitivity in humans.[59]

In idiopathic Parkinson disease, bilateral olfactory deficits are present early on in the disease, perhaps even during the preclinical period and occur at a higher frequency than some cardinal signs of this disorder, for example, tremor.[53] The olfactory impairment is unrelated to use of anti-parkinson medications, duration of illness, and severity of the symptoms, such as tremor, rigidity, bradykinesia, or gait disturbance.[60] Since smell loss is absent or infrequent in a number of other neurological disorders that exhibit similar motoric signs, smell testing can aid in differential diagnosis in some cases.[49] For example, patients with essential tremor, progressive supranuclear palsy, multiple system atrophy and parkinsonism induced by the proneurotoxin 1-methyl-4-phenyl-1,2,3,6-tetrahydropyridine (MPTP) exhibit little or no olfactory dysfunction.[61] It is of interest that familial Parkinson disease is also associated with olfactory impairment that occurs independently of the Parkinsonian phenotype.[62]

It has been generally assumed that olfactory function in multiple sclerosis is normal, since

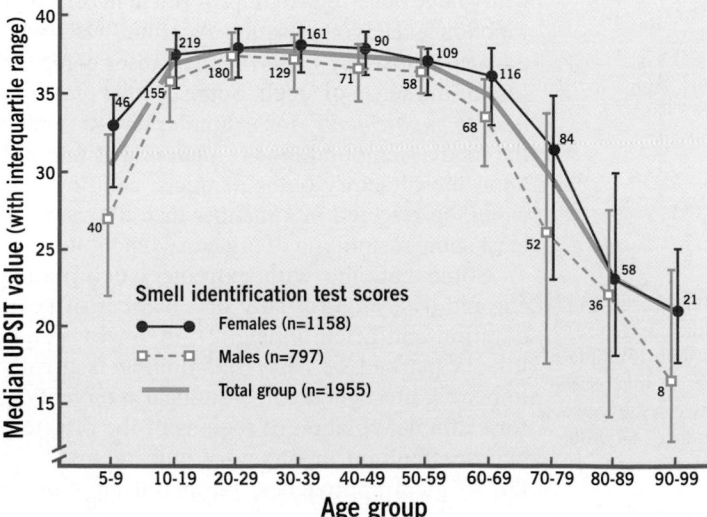

Figure 7 Scores on the University of Pennsylvania Smell Identification Test (UPSIT) as a function of age and gender in a large heterogeneous group of subjects. Numbers by data points indicate sample sizes. (From reference 44 with permission. Copyright © 1984, American Association for the Advancement of Science.)

the axons of the primary olfactory receptors are unmyelinated. However, myelin is present in other segments of the olfactory pathway, and at any one time, about a third of multiple sclerosis patients exhibit some degree of smell loss.[63] Furthermore, the degree of olfactory loss is directly related to the number of MRI-determined plaques in central brain regions associated with olfactory processing, for example, inferior middle temporal lobe and periorbital frontal cortex (Figure 8).[50,63] Indeed, a seemingly 1:1 longitudinal association is present between UPSIT scores and changes in plaque load over time (Figure 9),[64] implying that olfactory function waxes and wanes as the plaque numbers increase and decrease. In effect, knowledge of a patient's UPSIT score accurately predicts the plaque load in the olfaction-related regions, and vice versa.

Exposure to Neurotoxic Agents. A number of environmental and industrial chemicals have been linked to olfactory dysfunction, including acrylates, benzene, cadmium, cigarette smoke, formaldehyde, manganese, solvents, and nickel dust, among others, although few well-controlled studies exist in this area and most reports are largely anecdotal.[65] The best documented cases are those related to exposure to aerosolized heavy and transitional metals, such as present in welding fumes.[66] In many cases, the decrements are specific to the exposed compounds and reflect long-term adaptation rather than damage to the olfactory receptors, being reversed after the worker is away from the workplace for a relatively short period of time. In the case of cigarette smoking, olfactory ability decreases as a function of cumulative smoking dose. Long-term cessation of smoking leads to a gradual improvement of olfactory function that is inversely related to the amount and duration of prior smoking activity.[67]

Other Causes. As noted earlier in this chapter, medications commonly affect smell function and should be considered early in an evaluation, especially in the context of a new drug therapy (see Table 1). Olfactory hallucinations occur in mesial temporal lobe seizures and migraine, as well as in some other central brain lesion disorders. In epilepsy, the hallucinations are usually unpleasant and are rarely isolated events.[33] Recent work suggests that olfaction is compromised in the morbidly obese, although the basis for this dysfunction is unclear.[68]

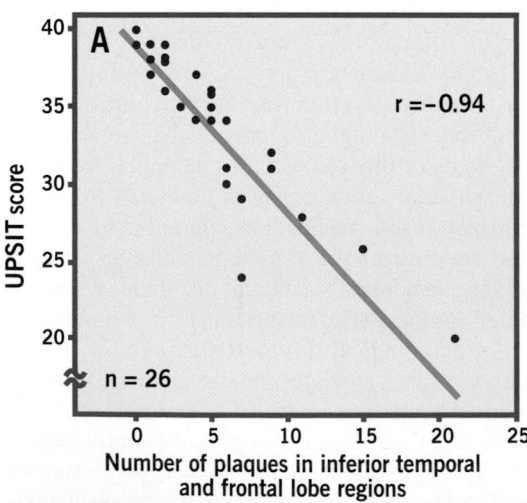

Figure 8 Relationship between number of multiple sclerosis-related plaques in subtemporal and subfrontal lobes and scores on the University of Pennsylvania Smell Identification Test (UPSIT). No such relationship was present between UPSIT scores and plaques in brain regions outside of the primary olfactory cortical areas (r = –.08). (From reference 63 with permission. Copyright © 1997 Massachusetts Medical Society.)

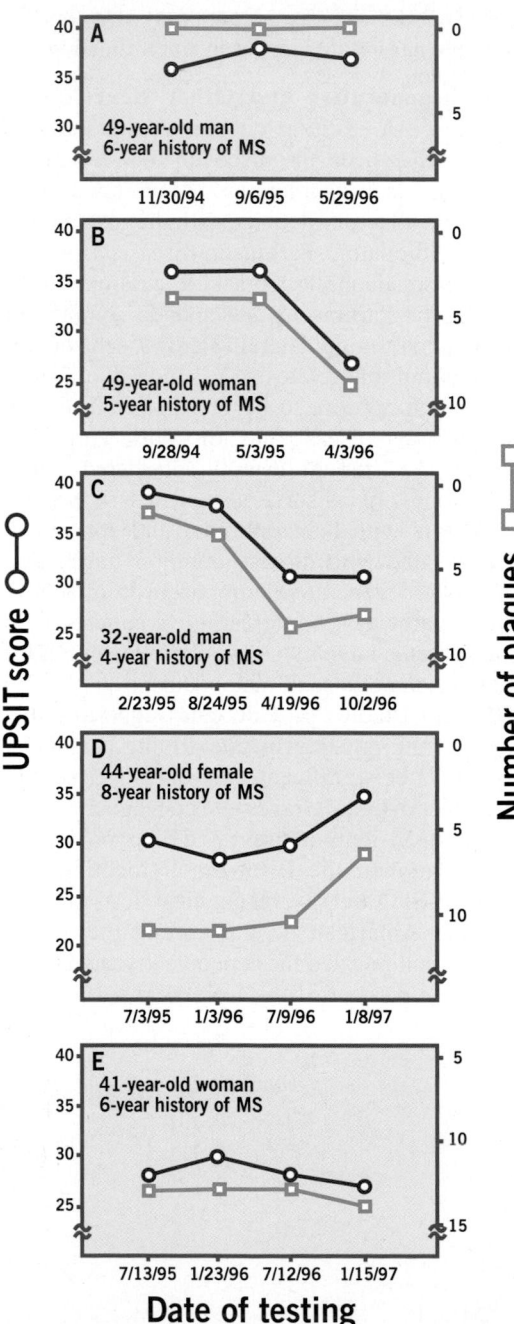

Figure 9 Longitudinal changes in UPSIT scores and plaque numbers within the inferior frontal and inferior temporal lobe regions of 5 patients with multiple sclerosis (A–E). Note that plaque number is inversely plotted. Also note the close association between the measures across time in all cases. (From reference 64 with permission. Copyright © 1999, American Academy of Neurology.)

Prognosis and Treatment of Olfactory Disorders

Prognosis is better for patients when smell loss is less severe, that is, for patients with UPSIT scores >25. This likely reflects, in cases having sensorineural damage, less extensive necrosis within the basal cell layer of the neuroepithelia and possibly less fibrosis around the foramina of the cribriform plate that can prevent regeneration or appropriate migration of receptor axons to the bulb. It is important for many patients to know the true degree of olfactory loss, given that prognosis relates to the magnitude of the loss. Quantitative testing places the patient's problem into perspective; it can be therapeutic for an older person to learn that, while his or her smell function is not what it used to be, it still falls above average for his or her peer group.

Mechanical obstruction secondary to distorted intranasal architecture or intranasal tumors can often be addressed surgically. However, inflammatory causes of sinonasal disease are more likely to be treated medically or in combination with surgery. Quantitative olfactory testing is advised before and after treatment to ensure an accurate assessment of the intervention and to assess long-term outcomes. Examples of treatments that have restored olfactory function in some patients include allergic management, topical and systemic corticosteroids, antibiotics, and functional endoscopic sinus surgery. A brief course of systemic steroid therapy can be useful in distinguishing between conductive and sensorineural olfactory loss as patients with the former will often respond positively to the treatment. Longer-term systemic corticosteroid therapy, however, is not advised. Topical nasal corticosteroids may be ineffectual in altering smell dysfunction because the corticosteroid fails to penetrate the higher recesses of the nose. Administering nasal drops or sprays in the head-down Moffett position can sometimes increase efficacy.

Sensorineural causes of olfactory dysfunction are more difficult to manage. When spontaneous recovery occurs in head trauma patients whose loss reflects damage to the olfactory receptor cell axons, it typically does so within 3 or 4 months of the injury. Patients who quit smoking tobacco typically have dose-related improvement in olfactory function and flavor sensation over time,[67] although tobacco smoking by itself rarely causes complete loss of the sense of smell. Some *central olfactory neural impairments*, for example, tumors within the medial temporal lobe or tumors that impinge upon the olfactory bulbs or tracts, can, in some cases, be resected in a manner that allows for at least some restoration of olfactory function.

Some patients with extremely debilitating chronic dysosmia (usually of a number of years duration and often unilateral), in whom weight loss is marked or daily functioning is greatly impaired, are benefited by surgical intervention, for example, ablation of regions of the olfactory neuroepithelium or olfactory bulb removal. Of the surgical approaches, intranasal ablation or stripping of tissue from the olfactory neuroepithelium on the affected side is more conservative and less invasive than removal of the olfactory bulb and/or tract via a craniotomy.[69] Should the dysosmia reappear after intranasal intervention, additional or repeat ablations can be performed. In the majority of individuals, demonstrable smell loss does not accompany the dysosmic condition. In general, at least some degree of olfactory system function is required for the dysosmia to occur.

When olfactory disturbances are attributed to a particular medication, discontinuance, dose changes, or substitution of other modes of therapy can be effective, although rapid reversal of the problem rarely occurs. Even though there are advocates for zinc and vitamin therapies, there is no compelling evidence that these therapies work except in rare cases where frank zinc or vitamin deficiencies are present.

THE GUSTATORY SYSTEM

Anatomy and Physiology

Such sensations as sweet, sour, bitter, and salty, as well as possibly "metallic" (iron salts), "umami" (monosodium glutamate, disodium gluanylate, and disodium inosinate), and "chalky" (calcium salts), are mediated via the taste buds of the gustatory system. Unlike olfaction, taste sensations are carried by several cranial nerves, ie, CNs VII, IX, and X, as discussed below. Because of this fact, complete loss of taste function is rare from peripheral insults or trauma (since all nerves would have to be involved) and is more likely due to systemic or central causes. Intraoral CN V free nerve endings are also stimulated by some foods and beverages, for example, carbonated or spicy foods, contributing to the overall gestalt of flavor. Hence, a piece of milk chocolate in the mouth is not only sweet but has texture and temperature. The sensation of "chocolate," however, is dependent upon retronasal stimulation of the olfactory receptors. Unfortunately, many patients and their physicians fail to distinguish between "taste" sensations mediated by the taste buds from CN I-mediated "taste" sensations, for example, strawberry, chocolate, meat sauce.

Taste Buds. The goblet-shaped taste buds are distributed over the dorsal surface of the tongue, the margin of the tongue, the base of the tongue, the soft palate, pharynx, larynx, epiglottis, uvula, and the first third of the esophagus.[70] The majority of taste buds are found on the lingual surface within the protruding papillae. Of the four types of papillae—fungiform, foliate, circumvallate, and filiform—only the first three harbor taste buds. Taste buds are continually bathed in secretions from the salivary glands and nearby lingual glands. von Ebner glands discharge into the troughs surrounding the circumvallate papillae, and lingual glands empty into the long fissures between the folds of the elongated foliate papillae on the posterior aspect of the margin of the tongue. The saliva contains not only such proteins as amylase (which initiates starch breakdown of foodstuffs), but also growth factors important for wound healing and the maintenance of taste buds. Indeed, removal of the submandibular and sublingual salivary glands leads to taste bud loss that can be prevented by supplying epidermal growth factor in the drinking water.[71]

The human tongue contains, on average, around 4,600 taste buds.[70] Each taste bud comprises 50 to 150 thin epithelial cells arranged much like the segments of an orange or grapefruit (Figure 10). The opening to the taste bud is termed the taste pore, and the excavation below the pore is termed the taste pit. Several types of cells are found within the taste bud, including cells that project microvilli into the taste pit and basal cells from which other cell types arise. On the basis of granule density in their apical regions, *light cells*, *dark cells*, and *intermediate cells* can be identified within each bud. Like the cells of the olfactory neuroepithelium, taste bud cells have the propensity to replace themselves periodically, with the time course for at least some of this "turnover" apparently being between 2 and 3 weeks.[73]

Gustatory Neural Transduction. A tastant must be in solution to enter the taste pore. Hence placing sugar or salt crystals on a dry lingual surface does not immediately lead to sweet or salty sensations, a common mistake made by some practitioners in attempting to assess taste function. After entering the taste pore, the tastant initiates the transduction process via 1 of 2 mechanisms: (a) activating receptors coupled to G-proteins that, in turn, activate second messenger systems (a process that occurs with sweet and bitter tasting stimuli); and (b) directly gating apical ion channels on the microvilli within the taste bud pit (a process that occurs with sour and salty tasting stimuli). Gustducin, a G-protein for taste reception, has been identified in taste receptor cells of fungiform, foliate, and circumvallate papillae.[74]

Taste threshold sensitivity is directly related to the number of taste papillae and hence taste buds that are actively stimulated.[75] Furthermore, taste thresholds are inversely correlated with stimulus duration.[76] Interestingly, there are agents, when swished in the mouth, that selectively alter the quality of taste sensations. For example, miraculin, a gylcoprotein from the berry of the African shrub *Syncepalum dilcificum*, temporarily changes most sour-like sensations to sweet sensations. Gymnemic acid, an extract from the leaves of the Indian plant *Gymnema sylvestre*, can mitigate the perception of sweet sensation (and the corresponding electrophysiologic activity) without significantly changing the perception of the other taste qualities.[77]

Taste Afferent Nerves. Different taste buds are innervated by different cranial nerves, depending upon the region of the oral cavity in which they are located. Unlike CN I, such nerves are mixed motor and sensory nerves that transmit multiple forms of information. An understanding of this fact can be important when clinical syndromes that involve taste dysfunction are considered. The nerve fibers from each of the taste nerves enter the brainstem and synapse within the nucleus of the tractus solitarius (NTS), which extends from the rosterolateral medulla caudally along the ventral border of the vestibular nuclei (Figure 11).[79]

Taste sensations from (a) the taste buds of the fungiform papillae on the anterior two-thirds of the tongue and (b) the taste buds of the soft palate are conveyed by two divisions of the facial nerve (CN VII): the chorda tympani nerve and the greater petrosal nerve (via the lesser palatine nerve). CN VII also supplies the salivary and lacrimal glands, the mucous membranes of the oral and nasal cavities, the muscles of facial expression, and the stapedius muscle. CN VII taste fibers, the cell bodies of which are located within the geniculate ganglion, share a common path with the lingual nerve (CN V_3) proximal to the tongue (see Figure 11). CN VII exits the skull via the stylomastoid foramen.

All circumvallate and most, if not all, foliate taste buds within the posterior third of the tongue are innervated by the lingual-tonsillar

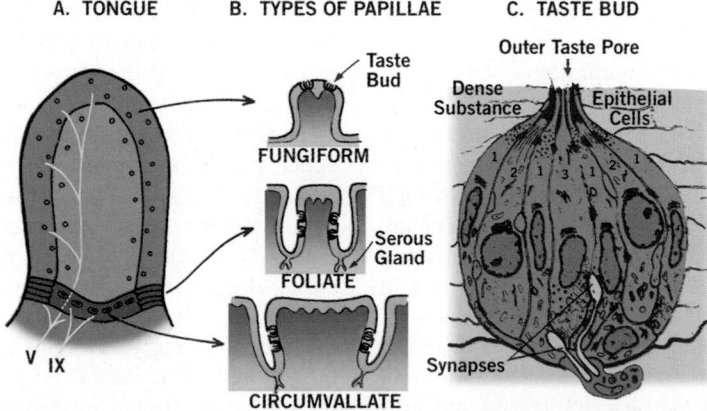

Figure 10 Schematic of tongue showing the three major types of taste bud-containing papillae (B) and their general lingual location (A). Structure of taste bud is shown in C. Although rough distribution of the trigeminal (CN V) and glossopharngeal (CN IX) cranial nerves is shown in A, CN IX likely projects more anteriorly than depicted. Not depicted is the chorda tympani branch of the facial nerve (CN VII) that innervates taste buds on the anterior tongue (see Figure 11). In C, 1 and 2 are supporting cells, which secrete materials into the lumen of the taste bud. 3 is a sensory receptor cell, whereas 4 is a basal cell from which the other types of cells arise. (Modified from reference 72 with permission. Copyright © 1983, Oxford University Press).

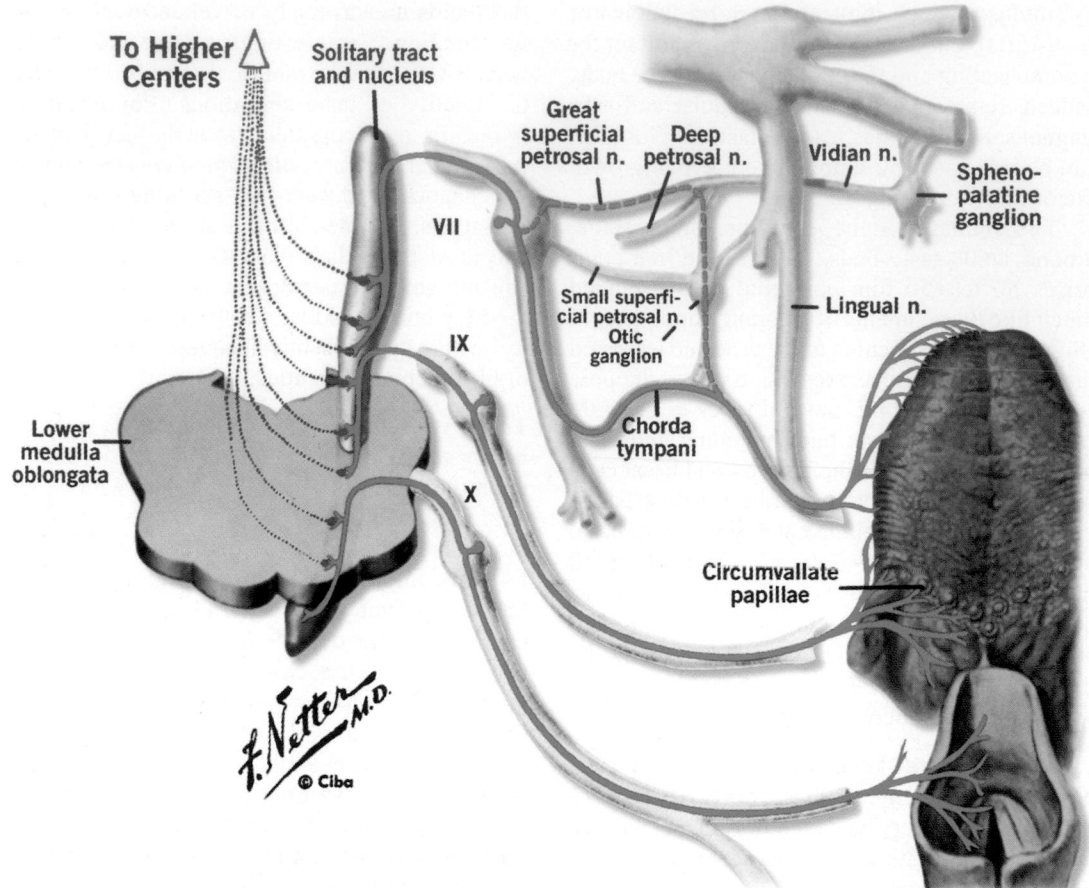

Figure 11 Distribution of cranial nerves to gustatory regions. CN VIII fibers from the geniculate ganglion innervate taste buds on the anterior portion of the tongue and on the soft palate. CN IX fibers from cell bodies within the petrosal ganglion innervate taste buds on foliate and circumvallate papillae of the tongue, as well as pharyngeal taste buds. CN X fibers from cell bodies in the nodose ganglion innervate taste buds of the epiglottis, larynx and esophagus. (Adapted from reference 78 with permission. Copyright © Ciba Pharmaceutical Corporation, New York, 1964.)

branch of the glossopharyngeal nerve (CN IX). The taste buds in the region of the nasopharynx are supplied by the pharyngeal branch of this nerve. The nerve cell bodies of these gustatory afferent fibers are found within the petrosal ganglion immediately outside the jugular foramen, where the fibers eventually pass to enter the cranium. CN IX also innervates the stylopharyngeus muscle, the parotid gland, the baroreceptors of the carotid sinus, and the pharyngeal mucus membrane.

The taste buds on the epiglottis, aryepiglottal folds, and esophagus are innervated by the vagus nerve (CN X) via the internal portion of its superior laryngeal branch.[80] Nontaste sensory functions are mediated by this nerve in such areas as the external ear, external auditory canal, external surface of the tympanic membrane, and the vocal cords. CN X also mediates (a) visceral sensation from the larynx and the gut, (b) motor function to the smooth muscle of the pharynx, larynx, and viscera, and (c) motor function to all striated muscles of the pharynx, larynx, and palate except stylopharyngeus (CN IX) and tensor veli palatini (CN V_3). Afferent fibers from the superior laryngeal nerve have their cell bodies in the inferior nodose ganglion. Like the glossopharyngeal nerve, the vagus passes through the skull base through the jugular foramen.

Central Gustatory Regions: Functional Anatomy. The first central relay station of the taste system is the NTS in the medulla.[80] The afferents from CN VII, IX, and X synapse within the NTS in descending (and overlapping) order. Cells from the NTS also make reflexive connections, via the reticular formation, with cranial motor nuclei that control such taste-related behaviors as chewing, licking, salivation, swallowing, and preabsorptive insulin release, as well as the muscles of facial expression.[81] The major gustatory projections from the NTS, however, are the tertiary ones that ultimately lead to activation of cortical gustatory structures. These occur via the thalamic taste nucleus (TTN) in primates, that is, the parvicellular division of the ventroposteromedial thalamic nucleus.[82] From the TTN, fibers project to the primary taste cortex deep in the parietal operculum and adjacent parainsular cortex.[83] PET and fMRI studies have found taste stimulus-induced activation largely within the insula and perisylvian regions, including the frontal operculum, superior temporal gyrus (opercular part), and inferior sectors of the pre- and postcentral gyrus.[84,85] A secondary cortical taste region is present within the caudomedial/caudolateral orbitofrontal cortex, several millimeters anterior to the primary taste cortex.[79]

The specific role of the gustatory cortical regions in the processing of taste information is not clear. These regions contain multimodal neurons responsive to touch and temperature as well as taste.[86] Some structures within the right hemisphere may play a more important role in taste perception than their left hemisphere counterparts. For example, citric acid presented to the whole mouth increases regional cerebral blood flow (rCBF) more in the right than in the left anteromedial temporal lobe and more in the right than in the left caudomedial orbitofrontal cortex although bilateral activation is observed in the caudolateral orbitofrontal cortex.[87] Also, patients who have had right anterior temporal lobe resection for intractable seizure activity have higher citric acid recognition thresholds than both controls and left anterior temporal lobe resection patients. There is some evidence, however, that handedness may need to be controlled in such studies. Thus, whereas fMRI data suggest that the superior part of the insula is activated by tastants similarly in left- and right-handed subjects, this is not the case for the inferior insulae, where the left is relatively more activated in right-handed subjects, and the right is relatively more activated in left-handed subjects.[84]

Classification of Gustatory Disorders

Gustatory disorders can be classified in a manner similar to olfactory disorders: *ageusia*: inability to detect qualitative gustatory sensations from all (total ageusia) or some (partial ageusia) tastants; *hypogeusia*: decreased sensitivity to tastants; *dysgeusia*: distortion in the perception of a normal taste, for example, an unpleasant taste induced by a stimulus that is normally associated with pleasant sensations or the presence of a taste in the absence of a stimulus (sometimes termed phantogeusia); *gustatory agnosia*: inability to recognize a taste sensation, even though gustatory processing, language, and general intellectual functions are essentially intact. Some patients complain of oral sensations of burning or numbness which may or may not have their genesis in gustatory afferents, for example, *burning mouth syndrome* (BMS) in which the sensation of "burning" occurs within the mouth without obvious physical cause.

Total ageusia is rare and, when present, is usually produced by central, for example, ischemic or medication, events since regeneration of taste buds can occur and peripheral damage would have to involve multiple pathways to induce taste loss. Thus, while 433 of 585 patients (74%) studied at the University of Pennsylvania Smell and Taste Center who exhibited olfactory loss complained of both smell and taste disturbance, fewer than 4% had verifiable whole-mouth gustatory dysfunction, and even that was limited.[29] Regional deficits are much more common. For example, in one study, sensitivity to 3 concentrations of NaCl was measured on the tongue tip and 3 cm posterior to the tongue tip in 12 young (20 to 29 years of age) and 12 elderly (70 to 79 years of age) subjects. On average, the young subjects were more sensitive to NaCl on the tongue tip than on the more posterior stimulation site and exhibited, at both tongue loci, in increase in detection performance as the stimulus concentration increased. The elderly subjects, who would be expected to exhibit, at worse, moderate deficits on whole-mouth testing, performed at chance levels.[88]

The majority of patients are unaware of regional taste deficits. In fact, most patients can sustain loss of taste sensation on half of the anterior part of the tongue following unilateral sectioning of the chorda tympani in middle ear surgery without noticing the problem. Such lack of awareness stems, in part, from the redundancy of the multiple taste nerves, as well as compensatory mechanisms.

Clinical Evaluation of Gustatory Function

History. A history similar to that described earlier for patients complaining of olfactory disturbance should be obtained from patients complaining of gustatory disturbance. Specific consideration as to the type of stimuli that can or cannot be detected by the patient is essential to distinguish between retronasal CN I flavor loss and true taste-bud mediated gustatory loss. One should specifically inquire whether the patient can detect the saltiness of potato chips, pretzels, or salted nuts, the sourness of vinegar, pickles or lemons, the sweetness of sugar, soda, cookies or ice cream, and the bitterness of coffee, beer, or tonic water. If the patient indicates that there is a problem in such detection, the possibility of a true taste bud-mediated dysfunction exists.

Previous or current problems with salivation, chewing, swallowing, oral pain or burning, dryness of the mouth, periodontal disease, speech articulation, bruxism, or foul breath odor should be ascertained. Inquiry as to diet, oral habits, stomach problems, and possible problems with acid reflux is relevant, given that acid reflux into the oral cavity can irritate or damage taste buds. Recent dental work or exposure to radiation should be noted. Documentation of hearing or balance problems should be made, since past or current ear infections or surgery can result in altered chorda tympani function and produce taste loss or distortions. A careful assessment of medication usage is critical. As described in detail later in this chapter, many drugs, including lipid-reducing agents, antibiotics, and antihypertensives, can produce significant distortions or other alterations in taste function.

Physical Examination. A thorough head and neck examination is essential for ascertaining the potential cause of a gustatory disorder.[21] Nongustatory deficits in CN VII, IX, and X can shed light on whether gustatory dysfunction may be present, for example, abnormal facial musculature, swallowing, salivation, gag reflex, or voice production. Changes in epithelial color, or visual signs of scarring, inflammation, or atrophy of lingual papillae should be noted. Neoplastic lesions in the tongue's musculature should be ruled out by pal-

pation. Specific attention to the condition of the teeth and gums is important since exudates produced by gingivitis may produce or contribute to dysgeusic symptoms. An inspection of the nature and integrity of the fillings, bridges and other dental work should also be made, for example, dissimilar metals can induce small electrical currents that, in turn, produce abnormal oral sensations. In individuals in whom an explanation of the taste problem is not clear, neuroimaging to rule out CNS tumors or lesions should be performed.

In some instances, it may be useful to evaluate biopsies of circumvallate or fungiform papillae to determine the presence of pathology. The tongue can also be stained with a dark food dye and photographed under high illumination and low power magnification to allow for counting or better visualizing selected classes of papillae. In general, there is a high correlation between the number of fungiform papillae and the number of taste buds.[75]

Quantitative Gustatory Testing. Quantitative taste testing is rarely performed in the clinic, largely because of issues of practicality, for example, time and expense of presenting and preparing limited shelf-life taste stimuli. While a number of whole-mouth taste tests have been described in the literature,[89] regional taste testing is needed to establish the function of each of the nerves innervating different taste bud fields. As noted above, whole-mouth tests are insensitive to even complete dysfunction of one or several of the nerves that innervate the tongue.

Regional taste testing can be made using either chemical or electrical stimuli. The former requires applying known concentrations of liquid stimuli (eg, sucrose, citric acid, caffeine, and sodium chloride as prototypical representatives of sweet, sour, bitter, and salty taste qualities) to the tongue or oral cavity (in some cases in comparison with blank trials), rinsing the stimuli off between trials, and expectorating after each presentation. Such testing can be quite time consuming. For example, if responsiveness to each of the 4 basic taste qualities is to be made on left and right anterior (CN VII) and posterior (CN IX) tongue regions, 16 trials (4 tastants × 4 tongue regions) would be needed to present a single stimulus for each quality. Since multiple stimuli are required to produce reliable responses, the number of trials increases considerably.

In the regional chemical test employed at our centre, a single suprathreshold concentration of each of 4 stimuli (sucrose, citric acid, sodium chloride, and caffeine) is used. The stimuli are equated for perceived intensity (using a magnitude matching procedure) and are presented at the same volume (15 µL from an Eppendorff pipette; Brinkman Instruments, Westbury, NY) and kinematic viscosity ($1.53 \text{ mm}^2/\text{s}^2$ using tasteless cellulose gum). Equating viscosity eliminates context effects and tactile cues and increases control of solution spread when placed on the tongue in microliter quantities. The stimuli are presented 6 times to each tongue region, resulting

in a test consisting of 96 stimulus trials and 96 rinses. Testing time is between 1 and 1½ hours. The task of the subject is to report the presence of a sweet, sour, bitter, or salty sensation using a forced-choice procedure with these 4 alternatives available and to rate the perceived intensity of the stimulus on a standardized rating scale with logarithmic visual properties.

A more practical approach to taste testing is to employ an electrogustometer, a device that presents brief µA currents to small regions of the tongue for known durations (Figure 12).[90] No stimulus preparation or rinsing is required. Electrogustometric thresholds can be obtained easily, although their relationship to chemical thresholds is still not clear and extreme care must be taken to apply the stimulator to the exact same region of the tongue on each trial, as considerable regional variation in sensitivity is present. At low current ranges electrogustometry has been demonstrated to activate only taste afferents, not trigeminal (CN V) afferents. In general, electrical thresholds are correlated with the number of taste papillae and buds in the regions evaluated.[90] Unfortunately, sound normative data based upon forced-choice testing paradigms are still generally lacking for such devices.

Imaging Studies. Imaging studies of the gustatory pathways can be useful in explaining the gustatory symptoms of some patients. In addition to detecting large central lesions and tumors, modern MRI techniques can detect discrete lesions, for example, infarcts, within brain structures that correlate both with patient complaints and with the results of sensory testing. As noted in detail in the next section, MRI-determined infarcts in the pons have been repeatedly associated with ageusia and dysgeusia.[91,92]

Causes of Gustatory Dysfunction

Although central or systemic factors are the most likely causes of ageusia, local factors can significantly alter taste perception. Proximal mechanisms include: (a) the release of foul-tasting materials from oral medical conditions,

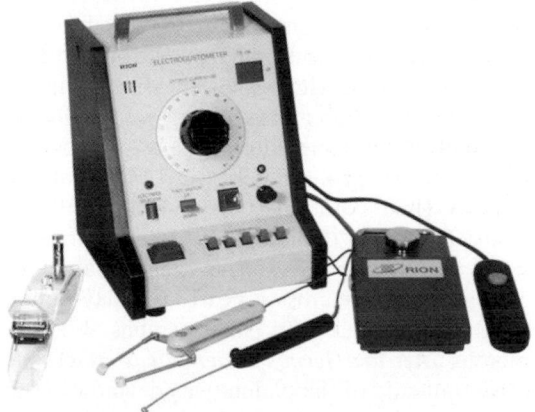

Figure 12 The Rion TR-06 electrogustometer, a practical device for quantitatively assessing regional taste function. This device stimulates the taste system using microamp level pulses of constant current of known duration. (Photograph courtesy of Sensonics, Inc., Haddon Hts., NJ. Copyright © 2000, Sensonics, Inc.)

for example, gingivitis, sialadenitis, (b) problems in movement of tastants to the taste buds, for example, damage to taste pores from a burn, (c) damage to the taste buds proper, as from caustic or allergic reactions to toxins or oral products, (d) damage to taste nerves, for example, Bell palsy, dental or surgical procedures, and (e) CNS damage, for example, from tumors, epilepsy, or infarcts. One cause of dysgeusia can be the use of different metals in the mouth that set up subtle electrical currents within the oral cavity. The more common causes of taste disorders are discussed below.

Aging. Although whole-mouth taste acuity declines with age, the perceptual decrease is not as marked as that seen for olfaction.[93] Compared to younger persons, the elderly tend to perceive tastes as being less intense. In conjunction with the loss seen with the sense of smell, decrements in taste function can be harmful to some of the elderly, leading to anorexia, weight loss, malnutrition, impaired immunity, and worsening of a medical illness.[45,94] Whole-mouth testing reveals moderate degrees of age-related taste loss, whereas regional taste testing reveals marked age-related decrements.[88]

Viral Infection. Bell palsy is the most frequent cause of facial nerve damage. Usually of viral origin, for example, Herpes simplex, this disease affects both sexes of all ages. This disorder typically begins with pain in or behind the ipsilateral ear, followed by symptoms of unilateral facial weakness over the course of a few days. Hyperacusis occurs in many cases, due to a weakening of the stapedius muscle. Although commonly accompanied by ipsilateral taste loss over the anterior two-thirds of the tongue, patients are often unaware of the taste problem without formal testing. There is suggestion that return of taste function by 2 weeks after onset is a positive prognostic indicator for complete and relatively rapid recovery from facial paresis, whereas longer lasting taste impairment is associated with poor prognosis. The taste-salivary reflex arc, which extends from the taste nerves via the NTS to the parasympathetic fibers innervating the salivary glands, can also be compromised in this disorder.

Ramsay Hunt syndrome results from a recrudescence of latent Herpes zoster virus within the geniculate ganglion and results in pain and vesicles in the external auditory canal or soft palate. Bartoshuk and Miller describe a patient with the Ramsay Hunt syndrome that involved both CN V and CN IX on the left side.[95] Intensity ratings were obtained for each of the 4 taste qualities at regular intervals across a nearly 600-day period for the front, back, and palate regions. About 3 months after the *Herpes zoster oticus* attack, the entire left side of the patient was devoid of taste function. After 400 days, all taste qualities were perceived on the left back and palate regions, but only sweetness could be perceived on the left front. Full taste recovery of the anterior part of the tongue was not present even by the end of the nearly 600-day-long testing period.

Burning Mouth Syndrome. In some cases, BMS, also termed glossodynia or glossalgia, is associated with salty or bitter dysgeusias. This poorly understood syndrome is characterized by idiopathic intense "burning" pain within the mouth without obvious physical cause. To what extent this disorder is mediated via gustatory or CN V afferents is not known. BMS typically begins by late morning and is continues throughout the day.[96] Suggested causes include: (a) diabetes mellitus (possibly predisposing to oral candidiasis), (b) nutritional and hormonal deficiencies, for example, iron, folic acid, B vitamins, zinc, and estrogen, (c) denture allergy (including reactions to amalgam fillings), (d) mechanical irritation from dentures or oral devices, (e) parafunctional habits of the mouth, for example, tongue thrusting, teeth grinding, or jaw clenching, (f) tongue ischemia as a result of temporal arteritis, (g) oral candidiasis, (h) periodontal disease, (i) reflux esophagitis, and (j) geographic tongue.[97] Anxiety and depression are common in the BMS population.

Central Lesions and Tumors. Taste dysfunction has been attributed to a variety of tumors and lesions, including vestibular schwannomas, tumors of the hypophysis with marked extrasellar growth, facial nerve schwannomas extending into the middle cranial fossa, and cerebellopontile angle lesions. Contralateral dysgeusia has been observed in patients with lateralized infarcts of the thalamus and in patients with infarcts in the corona radiata (reflecting the crossed taste pathways at this level of the nervous system).[98] Unilateral lesions above the brainstem do not usually cause complete loss of function because of the multiple areas involved in processing taste information.

Gustatory problems can arise from damage to the brainstem structures related to taste, often in conjunction with impairment of other cranial nerves or long tracts. Regions susceptible to damage include the NTS and the pontine tegmentum, which involves both gustatory lemnisci. Hemiageusia from an ipsilateral multiple sclerosis plaque at the midpontine tegmentum has been reported.[91] Similarly, ageusia to all taste qualities on the right side of the tongue was noted in a patient who had a small hemorrhage in the right tegmentum of the middle pons.[99] Three cases of ipsilateral hemiageusia due to focal ischemic lesions in the brainstem have been described.[100]

An example of unilateral hypogeusia resulting from a brainstem infarct is shown in Figure 13. In this case, ischemic activity is evident in a region of the upper medulla near the right NTS. Note that, in this image, the patient's right side is on the left side of the picture. This individual complained of dysgeusia on the right side of the tongue and, upon testing had a decrement in the ability to discern sweet, sour, bitter, and salty sensations that was greater on the right than on the left. Both CN VII and CN IX seemed to be involved.

Head and Neck Trauma. Trauma-related taste loss is much less common than trauma-related smell loss, with fewer than 1% of persons

with major head injury exhibiting ageusia to sweet, sour, salty, or bitter taste qualities.[29,101] Nonetheless, taste loss as well as dysgeusia can occur in some types of head trauma. For example, basilar temporal bone fractures and other injuries that impinge upon the middle ear have the potential for impairing chorda tympani nerve-mediated taste function unilaterally, as well as for altering salivary secretion. Injury to the lingual nerve in and around the mouth and tongue can also occur in some traumas. This nerve, a branch of the mandibular division of CN V, is the most proximal pathway to the tongue for general somatic sensation (touch) and special visceral sensation of taste (owning to concurrent facial nerve fibers).

Iatrogenic Injury. Numerous surgical interventions can induce taste dysfunction.[102] The glossopharyngeal nerve is susceptible to damage during tonsillectomy, bronchoscopy, or laryngoscopy,[103–105] reflecting the close proximity of the lingual branch of this nerve to the muscle layer of the palatine tonsillar bed.[106] Surgical treatment for snoring, for example, uvulopalatoplasty,[107] as well as such surgery-related procedures as endotracheal intubation,[108] and the employment of a laryngeal mask,[109] have all been associated with taste loss or alteration.

The chorda tympani nerve is at particular risk from surgical procedures that involve the middle ear, given its course between the malleus and the incus. The nerve is often stretched or sectioned during tympanoplasty, mastoidectomy, and stapedectomy, in some cases producing long-lasting symptoms. Bull, for example, found that 78% of patients with bilateral section and 32% of patients with unilateral section of the chorda tympani had persistent adverse gustatory symptoms.[110]

Shafer and colleagues evaluated gustatory function in 17 patients before third molar extraction and at 1 and 7 months thereafter.[111] On average, an approximately 15% reduction of perceived intensity was observed 1 month after extraction for NaCl, citric acid, and quinine hydrochloride. The taste quality of NaCl was identified correctly less often after than before third molar extraction. Citric acid intensity perception had not recovered by 6 months after the surgery. These data suggest that not only do gustatory deficits commonly occur after third molar extraction, but they can persist for at least 6 months after surgery. Furthermore, they seem to be associated with the depth of impaction.

Frey syndrome, a well-described complication of parotidectomy, also referred to as gustatory stimulated facial sweating, results from a misdirected growth of regenerating parasympathetic nerve fibers. Instead of innervating the parotid gland, regenerated nerve fibers innervate sweat glands in the overlying skin. Although usually provoked by taste stimuli, there is suggestion that such responses can come, in some cases, from the smell of food or even emotional excitement. Damage to the auriculotemporal nerve can produce a rare clinical syndrome of posttraumatic

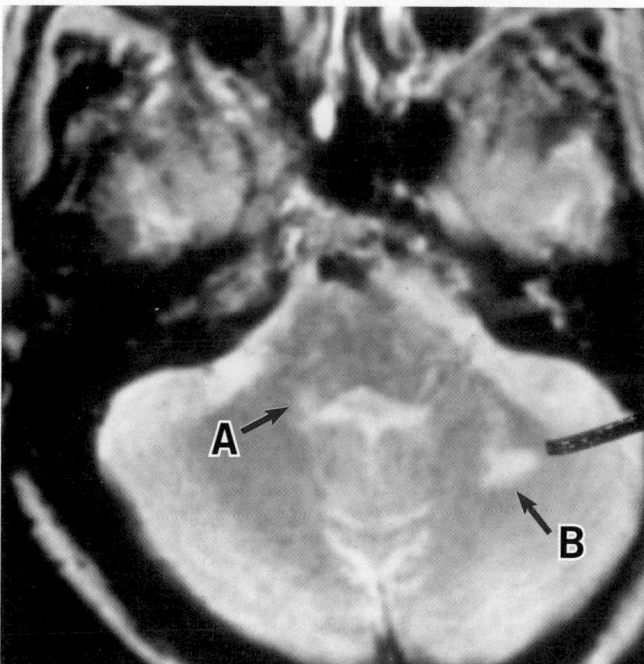
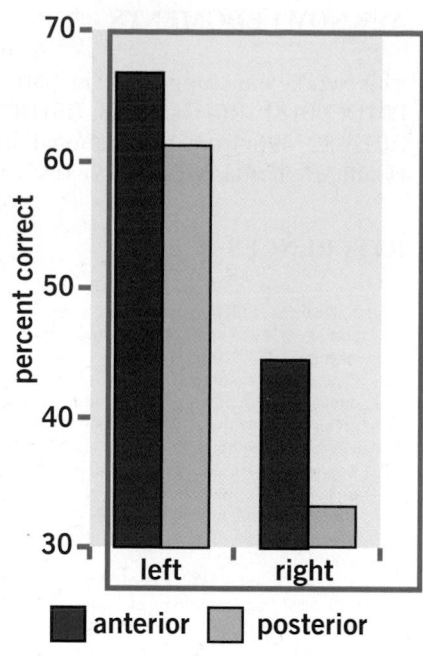

Figure 13 *Left*: Axial T2 (2500/90) MR scan through the upper brainstem reveals a hyperintensive infarct (4 × 3 mm) in the right side of the medulla (*Arrow A*). Note also large infarct (15 × 8 mm) inside the white matter of the left side of the cerebellum (*Arrow B*). *Right*: Taste identification scores showing relative decrement on the right side of the tongue. From a 65-year-old woman with a history of ministrokes who developed a persistent salty/metallic dysgeusia and soreness on the right side of the tongue following a severe 2-day bout of emesis accompanied by marked dehydration and increased blood pressure but unaccompanied by fever. (Reproduced with permission, copyright © 2001 Richard L. Doty.)

gustatory neuralgia, defined as a paroxysmal, lancinating facial pain in the cutaneous distribution of the auriculotemporal nerve following gustatory stimulation.[102,112] This condition can result from iatrogenic injury, for example, parotid gland surgery, temporomandibular joint surgery, carotid endarterectomy, orthognathic surgery, and oncologic surgery, as well as by viral induced damage and is characterized by episodic, transient, electric shock-like pain in the preauricular region.[102]

Medications. Medications produce taste disturbances more frequently than olfactory disturbances. Such side effects can be very debilitating and, in rare instances, have contributed to extreme weight loss and even suicide. Among offending agents are antiproliferative drugs, lipid-reducing drugs, antihypertensive agents, diuretics, antifungal agents, antirheumatic drugs, antibiotics, and drugs with sulfahydryl groups, such as penicillamine and Captopril.[28] For example, 0.6 to 2.8% of patients taking the antifungal agent terbinafine (Lamisil) report taste loss. The loss is more generalized across tongue regions for sucrose, citric acid, and quinine than for sodium chloride, whose loss is most pronounced at the back of the tongue.[113] Onset of taste dysfunction following terbinifine and some agents can take weeks or even months. For example, in a study of 87 patients experiencing terbinafine-related taste loss, the average time period from the first intake of the drug to the experience of taste loss was 35 days.[114] In most individuals, recovery after drug cessation took several months.

Taste function is reportedly altered by repetitive use of some oral topical agents, including hydrogen peroxide or corticosteroids. Some medications, for example, anticholinergics, anti-depressants, antihistamines, dry the oral cavity and result in the production of hyperviscous saliva, physical conditions which, in time, can result in lessened taste acuity. It is noteworthy that approximately one-fourth of all cardiac medicines (including antilipemic agents, adrenergic blockers, angiotensin-converting enzyme inhibitors, angiotensin II antagonists, calcium channel blockers, vasodilators, anticoagulants, antiarrhymics, and various diuretics) employed in the United States are listed in the *Physicians' Desk Reference* as having potential side effects of either "altered taste," "bad taste," "bitter taste," or "metallic taste."

Radiation Therapy. Radiotherapy for head and neck cancer can induce taste loss and dysgeusia, salivary dysfunction, and conditioned taste aversions. Such problems can alter quality of life and, on occasion, appetite to the degree that nutrition is compromised. Symptoms usually begin early in the course of treatment and posttreatment recovery can take months and, in rare instances, years.[115] The cause of such disturbances can be quite varied, including direct radiation-induced damage to taste cells and buds, salivary glands, and taste nerve fibers (which normally provide trophic factors that maintain the integrity of the taste bud). The xerostomia secondary to salivary gland damage can influence food transport, protection from bacterial invasion, and salivary proteins potentially involved in taste transduction[116] and can aid in the promotion of opportunistic oral infections, for example, oral candidiasis.[117] Although typically idiosyncratic and transient, some taste aversions can be long lasting and can produce generalized anorexia and cachexia. A means for mitigating such aversions is to have the patient consume a novel food immediately before the first course of chemotherapy or radiotherapy. This simple maneuver somehow focuses the aversion primarily on the novel food and interferes with the formation of conditioned aversions to preferred dietary items.[118]

Other Causes. Among other reported causes of taste dysfunction are hypothyroidism, renal disease, liver disease, myasthenia gravis, Guillain–Barre syndrome, numerous neoplasms, and familial dysautonomia (a genetic disorder with lack of taste buds and papillae). Idiopathic dysgeusia has been associated with blood transfusion.[119] Complaints of taste loss or distortion are reported in many carcinomas and mass lesions. For instance, while squamous cell carcinoma of the mucous membranes of the upper aerodigestive tract can interfere with taste by direct destruction of receptors, mass lesions along the course of CN VII, IX, and X may cause impairment through neural compression. Carcinoma-related malnutrition may also lead to ageusia.

A persistent and unpleasant sweet dysgeusia has been described in 3 patients with small cell carcinoma of the lung.[120] The dysgeusia was the presenting symptom in all 3 individuals, and hyponatremia secondary to the syndrome of inappropriate secretion of antidiuretic hormone was present in each case. Resolution of the dysgeusia paralleled an increase in serum sodium concentration after water restriction alone. The close association between the dysgeusia and the low serum sodium concentration suggests that hyponatremia was the causative factor, rather than the carcinoma, antidiuretic factor, medications, or chemotherapy.

Gustatory symptoms have been reported in association with epileptic seizures. Examples of taste sensations that have been reported in such cases include "peculiar," "rotten," "sweet," "like a cigarette," "like rotten apples," and "like vomitus."[33] Some of these "tastes," however, likely represent smell sensations that are miscategorized as tastes by both the patients and their physicians.

Selective taste nerve damage or alterations may produce some forms of *hyper*geusia and dysgeusia. For example, anesthetizing 1 chorda tympani nerve reportedly increases the perceived intensity of bitter substances, such as quinine, applied to taste fields innervated by the contralateral glossopharyngeal nerve.[121] In contrast, perceived intensity of NaCl applied to an area innervated by the ipsilateral glossopharyngeal nerve appears decreased. When both chorda tympani nerves are anesthetized, the taste of quinine is intensified and the taste of NaCl diminished in areas innervated by the glossopharyngeal on both sides of the tongue. In about 40% of their subjects, a phantom taste, usually localized to the posterior part of the tongue contralateral to the anesthesia, appeared in the absence of stimulation. This phantom taste was eliminated when the region of origin was anesthetized. These authors suggest that such phantoms arise because of release of inhibition normally present between the central projection areas of the different taste nerves.

Treatment of Taste Dysfunction

As in the case with other sensory systems, prognosis in cases of taste dysfunction is likely inversely related to the degree of neural or structural damage, although clinically such damage can rarely be assessed. Fortunately, the taste nerves and buds appear to be relatively resilient, as many cases of taste loss or distortion spontaneously resolve over time.[30] In some dysgeusic cases, antifungal and antibiotic treatments have been reported to be useful, although double blind studies of the efficacy of such treatments are lacking, and some of these agents themselves can produce taste disturbance. Chlorhexidine employed in a mouth wash has been suggested as having possible efficacy for some salty or bitter dysgeusias, possibly as a result of its strong positive charge.[122] In the case of neural damage from viruses or other agents, presumably the damaged taste afferents regenerate. Thyroid replacement therapy reportedly brings back taste sensitivity to normal levels in cases of taste loss secondary to hypothyroidism.[123] Taste disorders caused by medications can, in some instances, be reversed by discontinuing the offending drug, by employing alternative medications, or by changing drug dosage. It should be kept in mind, however, that a number of pharmacologic agents appear to induce long-term alterations in taste that may take months to disappear after drug discontinuance.

Since most BMS patients are postmenopausal, dysgeusias associated with this disorder may, in some cases, respond to estrogen replacement therapy. Topical capsaicin may also be helpful in some cases. Given that BMS is often associated with anxiety and depression, tricyclic antidepressants, for example, amitriptyline, desipramine, nortriptyline, and benzodiazepines appear, in selected instances, to have some therapeutic efficacy.[124]

CONCLUSIONS

Disorders of the chemical senses of taste and smell are relatively common, particularly in the elderly, and can result from a broad array of causes. Such causes range from simple irritation of the receptive elements to serious neurological disorders, including Alzheimer disease and idiopathic Parkinson disease. In this chapter, a succinct overview of the anatomy and physiology of the chemical senses, as well as of the primary causes of chemosensory dysfunction, has been provided. Approaches to therapy have been discussed, with an emphasis on the need for quantitative evaluation of patients before initiating surgical or medical interventions. Clearly, a number of disorders of the chemical senses can be approached with optimism, so long as the physician establishes the exact nature of the problem and is aware of the available avenues of treatment and objective assessments of efficacy.

ACKNOWLEDGMENTS

This work was supported, in part, by Grants P01DC00161, R01DC04278, R01DC02974, and R01AG27496 from the National Institutes of Health, Bethesda, MD.

REFERENCES

1. Nakashima T, Kimmelman CP, Snow JB, Jr. Structure of human fetal and adult olfactory neuroepithelium. Arch Otolaryngol 1984;110:641–6.
2. Huard JM, Youngentob SL, Goldstein BL, et al. Adult olfactory epithelium contains multipotent progenitors that give rise to neurons and non-neural cells. J Comp Neurol 1998;400:469–86.
3. Rowley JC, III, Moran DT, Jafek BW. Peroxidase backfills suggest the mammalian olfactory epithelium contains a second morphologically distinct class of bipolar sensory neuron: The olfactory microvillar cell. Brain Res 1989;502:387–400.
4. Moran DT, Jafek BW, Eller PM, Rowley JC, III. The ultrastructural histopathology of human olfactory dysfunction. Microsc Res Tech 1992;23:103–10.
5. Shepherd GM. Synaptic organization of the mammalian olfactory bulb. Physiol Rev 1972;52:864–917.
6. Meisami E, Mikhail L, Baim D, Bhatnagar KP. Human olfactory bulb: Aging of glomeruli and mitral cells and a search for the accessory olfactory bulb. Ann N Y Acad Sci 1998;855:708–15.
7. Frias C, Torrero C, Regalado M, Salas M. Organization of olfactory glomeruli in neonatally undernourished rats. Nutrit Neurosci 2006;9:49–55.
8. Gottfried JA, Smith AP, Rugg MD, Dolan RJ. Remembrance of odors past: Human olfactory cortex in cross-modal recognition memory. Neuron 2004;27:687–95.
9. Sobel N, Prabhakaran V, Desmond JE, et al. Sniffing and smelling: Separate subsystems in the human olfactory cortex. Nature 1998;392:282–6.
10. Swift DL, Proctor DF. Access of air to the respiratory tract. In: Brain JD, Proctor DF, Reid LM, editors. Respiratory Defense Mechanisms. New York: Marcel Dekker, 1977:63–93.
11. Buck L, Axel R. A novel multigene family may encode odorant receptors: A molecular basis for odor recognition. Cell 1991;65:175–87.
12. Ngai J, Chess A, Dowling MM, et al. Coding of olfactory information: Topography of odorant receptor expression in the catfish olfactory epithelium. Cell 1993;72:667–80.
13. Jones DT, Reed RR. G_{olf}: An olfactory neuron specific-G protein involved in odorant signal transduction. Science 1989;244:790–5.
14. Leinders-Zufall T, Shepherd GM, Zufall F. Modulation by cyclic GMP of the odour sensitivity of vertebrate olfactory receptor cells. Proc Roy Soc Lond B 1996;263:803–11.
15. Wekesa KS, Anholt RRH. Differential expression of G proteins in the mouse olfactory system. Brain Res 1999;837:117–26.
16. Hinds JW, Hinds PL, McNelly NA. An autoradiographic study of the mouse olfactory epithelium: Evidence for long-lived receptors. Anat Rec 1984;210:375–83.
17. Mackay-Sim A, Kittel PW. On the life span of olfactory receptor neurons. Eur J Neurosci 1990;3:209–15.
18. Calof AL, Rim PC, Askins KJ, et al. Factors regulating neurogenesis and programmed cell death in mouse olfactory epithelium. Ann N Y Acad Sci 1998;30:226–9.
19. Holcomb JD, Mumm JS, Calof AL. Apoptosis in the neuronal lineage of the mouse olfactory epithelium: Regulation in vivo and in vitro. Dev Biol 1995;172:307–23.
20. Murphy C, Doty RL, Duncan HJ. Clinical disorders of olfaction. In: Doty RL, editor. Handbook of Olfaction and Gustation, 2nd edition, New York: Marcel Dekker; 2003. p. 461–78.
21. Bromley SM. Smell and taste disorders: A primary care approach. Am Fam Physician 2000;61:427–36.
22. Doty RL. Olfaction. Ann Rev Psychol 2001;52:423–52.
23. Doty RL. The Smell Identification Test ™ Administration Manual, 3rd edition. Haddon Hts., NJ: Sensonics, Inc.; 1995. p. 1–57.
24. Doty RL, Kobal G. Current trends in the measurement of olfactory function. In: Doty RL. editor. Handbook of Olfaction and Gustation. New York: Marcel Dekker; 1995. p. 191–225.
25. Ottoson D. Analysis of the electrical activity of the olfactory epithelium. Acta Physiol Scand 1956;35:1–83.
26. Hummel T, Barz S, Lotsch J, et al. Loss of olfactory function leads to a decrease of trigeminal sensitivity. Chem Senses 1996;21:75–9.
27. Lezak MD. Neuropsychological Assessment. 3rd edition. New York: Oxford University Press; 1995.
28. Doty RL, Bromley SM. Effects of drugs on olfaction and taste. Otolaryngol Clin N Am 2004;37:1229–54.
29. Deems DA, Doty RL, Settle RG, et al. Smell and taste disorders, a study of 750 patients from the University of Pennsylvania Smell and Taste Center. Arch Otolaryngol Head Neck Surg 1991;117:519–28.
30. Deems DA, Yen DM, Kreshak A, Doty RL. Spontaneous resolution of dysgeusia. Arch Otolaryngol Head Neck Surg 1996;122:961–3.
31. Doty RL, Risser JM, Brosvic GM. Influence of adrenalectomy on the odor detection performance of rats. Physiol Behav 1991;49:1273–7.
32. Doty RL, Deems DA, Frye RE, et al. Olfactory sensitivity, nasal resistance, and autonomic function in patients with multiple chemical sensitivities. Arch Otolaryngol Head Neck Surg 1988;114:1422–7.
33. West SE, Doty RL. Influence of epilepsy and temporal lobe resection on olfactory function. Epilepsia 1995;36:531–42.
34. Costanzo RM, DiNardo LJ, Reiter ER. Head injury and olfaction. In: Doty RL, editor. Handbook of Olfaction and Gustation, 2nd edition. New York: Marcel Dekker; 2003. p. 629–38.
35. Doty RL, Yousem DM, Pham LT, et al. Olfactory dysfunction in patients with head trauma. Arch Neurol 1997;54:1131–40.
36. Yousem DM, Geckle RJ, Bilker WB, et al. Posttraumatic olfactory dysfunction: MR and clinical evaluation. AJNR 1996;17:1171–9.
37. Nakashima T, Kimmelman CP, Snow JB Jr. Progressive olfactory degeneration due to ischemia. Surg Forum 1983;34:566–8.
38. Doty RL, Mishra A. Influences of nasal obstruction, rhinitis, and rhinosinusitis on the ability to smell. Laryngoscope 2000;111:409–23.
39. Kern RC. Chronic sinusitis and anosmia: Pathologic changes in the olfactory mucosa. Laryngoscope 2000;110:1071–7.
40. Feron F, Perry C, McGrath JJ, Mackay S. New techniques for biopsy and culture of human olfactory epithelial neurons. Arch Otolaryngol Head Neck Surg 1998;124:861–6.
41. Lee SH, Lim HH, Lee HM, et al. Olfactory mucosal findings in patients with persistent anosmia after endoscopic sinus surgery. Ann Otol Rhinol Laryngol 2000;109:720–5.
42. Watnick RL, Trobe JD. Bilateral optic nerve compression as a mechanism for the Foster-Kennedy sydrome. Ophthalmology 1989;96:1793–8.
43. Schatz NJ, Smith JL. Non-tumor causes of the Foster Kennedy syndrome. J Neurosurg 1967;27:37–44.
44. Doty RL, Shaman P, Applebaum SL, et al. Smell identification ability: Changes with age. Science 1984;226:1441–3.
45. Schiffman SS. Taste and smell losses in normal aging and disease. JAMA 1997;278:1357–62.
46. Kalmey JK, Thewissen JG, Dluzen DE. Age-related size reduction of foramina in the cribriform plate. Anat Rec 1998;251:326–9.
47. Wilson RS, Arnold SE, Schneider JA, et al. The relation of cerebral Alzheimer's disease pathology to odor identification in old age. J Neurol Neurosurg Psychiatr 2007;78:30–5.
48. Mesholam RI, Moberg PJ, Mahr RN, Doty RL. Olfaction in neurodegenerative disease: A meta-analysis of olfactory functioning in Alzheimer's and Parkinson's diseases. Arch Neurol 1998;55:84–90.
49. Doty RL. Odor perception in neurodegenerative diseases. In: Doty RL, editor. Handbook of Olfaction and Gustation. New York: Marcel Dekker; 2003. p. 479–501.
50. Doty RL, Li C, Mannon LJ, Yousem DM. Olfactory dysfunction in multiple sclerosis: Relation to plaque load in inferior frontal and temporal lobes. Ann N Y Acad Sci 1998;855:781–6.
51. Moberg PJ, Doty RL, Turetsky BI, et al. Olfactory identification deficits in schizophrenia: Correlation with duration of illness. Am J Psychiatry 1997;154:1016–8.
52. Doty RL, Reyes PF, Gregor T. Presence of both odor identification and detection deficits in Alzheimer's disease. Brain Res Bull 1987;18:597–600.
53. Doty RL, Deems DA, Stellar S. Olfactory dysfunction in parkinsonism: A general deficit unrelated to neurologic signs, disease stage, or disease duration. Neurology 1988;38:1237–44.
54. Turetsky BI, Moberg PJ, Yousem DM, et al. Reduced olfactory bulb volume in patients with schizophrenia. Am J Psychiatry 2000;157:828–30.
55. Graves AB, Bowen JD, Rajaram L, et al. Impaired olfaction as a marker for cognitive decline: Interaction with apolipoprotein E epsilon4 status. Neurology 1999;53:1480–7.
56. Devanand DP, Michaels-Marston KS, Liu X, et al. Olfactory deficits in patients with mild cognitive impairment

predict Alzheimer's disease at follow-up. Am J Psychiatry 2000;157:1399–1405.

57. Doty RL, Bagla R, Kim N. Physostigmine enhances performance on an odor mixture discrimination test. Physiol Behav 1999;65:801–4.

58. Serby M, Flicker C, Rypma B, et al. Scopolamine and olfactory function. Biol Psychiat 1990;28:79–82.

59. Doty RL, Stern MB, Pfeiffer C, et al. Bilateral olfactory dysfunction in early stage treated and untreated idiopathic Parkinson's disease. J Neurol Neurosurg Psychiat 1992;55:138–42.

60. Macknin JB, Higuchi M, Lee VM-Y, et al. Olfactory dysfunction occurs in transgenic mice overexpressing human tau protein. Brain Res 2004;1000:174–8.

61. Doty RL, Singh A, Tetrude J, Langston JW. Lack of olfactory dysfunction in MPTP-induced parkinsonism. Ann Neurol 1992;32:97–100.

62. Markopoulou K, Larsen KW, Wszolek EK, et al. Olfactory dysfunction in familial parkinsonism. Neurology 1997;49:1262–7.

63. Doty RL, Li C, Mannon LJ, Yousem DM. Olfactory dysfunction in multiple sclerosis. New Engl J Med 1997;336:1918–9.

64. Doty RL, Li C, Mannon LJ, Yousem DM. Olfactory dysfunction in multiple sclerosis: Relation to longitudinal changes in plaque numbers in central olfactory structures. Neurology 1999;53:880–2.

65. Doty RL, Hastings L. Neurotoxic exposure and olfactory impairment. Clin Occup Environ Med 2001;1:547–75.

66. Antunes M, Bowler RM, Doty RL. San Francisco/Oakland Bay Brudge Welder Study: Olfactory function. Neurology 2007;69:1278–84.

67. Frye RE, Schwartz BS, Doty RL. Dose-related effects of cigarette smoking on olfactory function. JAMA 1990;263:1233–6.

68. Richardson BE, Vander Woude EA, Sudan R, et al. Altered olfactory acuity in the morbidly obese. Obesity Surg 2004;14:967–9

69. Leopold DA, Schwob JE, Youngentob SL, et al. Successful treatment of phantosmia with preservation of olfaction. Arch Otolaryngol Head Neck Surg 1991;117:1402–6.

70. Witt M, Reutter K, Miller IJ, Jr. Morphology of the peripheral taste system. In: Doty RL, editor, Handbook of Olfaction and Gustation. New York: Marcel Dekker, 2003; p. 651–77.

71. Morris-Witman J, Sego R, Brinkley L, Dolce C. The effects of sialoadenectomy and exogenous EGF on taste bud morphology and maintenance. Chem Senses 2000;25:9–19.

72. Shepherd GM. Neurobiology. New York: Oxford University Press; 1983.

73. Beidler LM, Smullman RL. Renewal of cells within taste buds. J Cell Biol 1965;27:263–72.

74. Takami S, Getchell TV, McLaughlin SK, et al. Human taste cells express the G protein alpha-gustducin and neuron-specific enolase. Brain Res Mol Brain Res 1994;193–203.

75. Doty RL, Bagla R, Morgenson M, Mirza N. NaCl thresholds: Relationship to anterior tongue locus, area of stimulation, and number of fungiform papillae. Physiol Behav 2001;72:373–8.

76. Bagla R, Klasky B, Doty RL. Influence of stimulus duration on a regional measure of NaCl taste sensitivity. Chem Senses 1997;22:171–5.

77. Kurihara K, Kurihara Y, Beidler LM. Isolation and mechanism of taste modifiers; taste modifying protein and gymnemic acids. In: Pfaffman C, editor. Olfaction and Taste. New York: Rockefeller University Press, 1969; p. 450–62.

78. Netter FH. The CIBA Collection of Medical Illustrations, Volume 1. Nervous System. New York: Ciba Pharmaceutical Corporation; 1964.

79. Rolls ET. Central taste anatomy and neurophysiology. In: Doty RL, editor. Handbook of Olfaction and Gustation, 2nd edition. New York: Marcel Dekker, 2003; p. 679–706.

80. Brodal A. Neurological Anatomy. New York: Oxford University Press; 1881.

81. Smith DV, Shipley MT. Anatomy and physiology of taste and smell. J Head Trauma Rehabil 1992;7:1–14.

82. Beckstead RM, Morse JR, Norgren R. The nucleus of the solitary tract in the monkey: Projections to the thalamus and brain stem nuclei. J Comp Neurol 1980;190:259–82.

83. Pritchard TC, Hamilton RB, Morse JR, Norgren R. Projections of thalamic gustatory and lingual areas in the monkey, Macaca fascicularis. J Comp Neurol 1986;244:213–28.

84. Cerf B, Lebihan D, Van De Moortele PF, et al. Functional lateralization of human gustatory cortex related to handedness disclosed by fMRI study. Ann N Y Acad Sci 1998;855:575–8.

85. Faurion A, Cerf B, Le BD, Pillias AM. fMRI study of taste cortical areas in humans. Ann N Y Acad Sci 1998;855:535–45.

86. Pritchard TC. The primate gustatory system. In: Getchell TV, Doty RL, Bartoshuk LM, Snow JB, Jr, editors. Smell and Taste in Health and Disease. New York: Raven Press, 1991; p. 109–25.

87. Small DM, Jones-Gotman M, Zatorre RJ, et al. A role for the right anterior temporal lobe in taste quality recognition. J Neurosci 1997;17:5136–42.

88. Matsuda T, Doty RL. Regional taste sensitivity to NaCl: Relationship to subject age, tongue locus and area of stimulation. Chem Senses 1995;20:283–90.

89. Frank ME, Hettinger TP, Barry MA, et al. Contemporary measurement of human gustatory function. In: Doty RL, editor. Handbook of Olfaction and Gustation, 2nd edition. New York: Marcel Dekker, 2003; p. 783–804.

90. Miller SL, Mirza N, Doty RL. Electrogustometric thresholds: Relation to anterior tongue locus, area of stimulation, and number of fungiform papillae. Physiol Behav 2002;75:753–7.

91. Combarros O, Sanchez-Juan P, Berciano J, De Pablos C. Hemiageusia from an ipsilateral multiple sclerosis plaque at the midpontine tegmentum. J Neurol Neurosurg Psychiatry 2000;68:796.

92. Fujikane M, Nakazawa M, Ogasawara M, et al. Unilateral gustatory disturbance by pontine infarction [Japanese]. Rinsho Shinkeigaku—Clin Neurol 1998;38:342–3.

93. Weiffenbach JM. Taste and smell perception in aging. Gerodontology 1984;3:137–46.

94. Schiffman SS. Taste and smell losses in normal aging and disease. JAMA 1997;278:1357–62.

95. Bartoshuk LM, Miller IJ, Jr. Taste perception, taste bud distribution, and spatial relationships. In: Getchell TV, Doty RL, Bartoshuk LM, Snow JB, Jr, editors. Taste Perception and Taste Bud Distribution. New York: Raven Press, 1991; p. 205–33.

96. Gorsky M, Silverman SJ, Chinn H. Clinical characteristics and management outcome in the burning mouth syndrome. An open study of 130 patients. Oral Surg Oral Med Oral Pathol 1991;72:192–5.

97. Tourne LP, Fricton JR. Burning mouth syndrome. Critical review and proposed clinical management. Oral Surg Oral Med Oral Pathol 1992;74:158–67.

98. Fujikane M, Itoh M, Nakazawa M, et al. Cerebral infarction accompanied by dysgeusia—A clinical study on the gustatory pathway in the CNS [Japanese]. Rinsho Shinkeigaku—Clin Neurol 1999;39:771–4.

99. Kojima Y, Hirano T. A case of gustatory disturbance caused by ipsilateral pontine hemorrhage [Japanese]. Rinsho Shinkeigaku—Clin Neurol 1999;39:979–81.

100. Lee BC, Hwang SH, Rison R, Chang GY. Central pathway of taste: Clinical and MRI study. Eur Neurol 1998;39:200–3.

101. Sumner D. Post-traumatic ageusia. Brain 1967;90:187–202.

102. Scrivani SJ, Keith DA, Kulich R, et al. Posttraumatic gustatory neuralgia: A clinical model of trigeminal neuropathic pain. J Orofacial Pain 1998;12:287–92.

103. Ohtuka K, Tomita H, Yamauchi Y, Kitagoh H. Taste disturbance after tonsillectomy [Japanese]. Nippon Jibiinkoka Gakkai Kaiho—J Oto-Rhino-Laryngol Soc Jpn 1994;97:1079–88.

104. Donati F, Pfammatter JP, Mauderli M, Vassella F. Neurologische Komplikationen nach Tonsillektomie. Schweizerische Medizinische Wochenschrift 1991;121:1612–7.

105. Arnhold-Schneider M, Bernemann D. Uber die Haufigkeit von Geschmacksstorungen nach Tonsillektomie. HNO 1987;35:195–8.

106. Ohtsuka K, Tomita H, Murakami G. Anatomical study of the tonsillar bed: The topographical relationship between the palatine tonsil and the lingual branch of the glossopharyngeal nerve [Japanese]. Nippon Jibiinkoka Gakkai Kaiho—J Oto-Rhino—Laryngol Soc Jpn 1994;97:1481–93.

107. Walker RP, Gopalsami C. Laser-assisted uvulopalatoplasty: Postoperative complications. Laryngoscope 1996;106:834–8.

108. Evers KA, Eindhoven GB, Wierda JM. Transient nerve damage following intubation for trans-sphenoidal hypophysectomy. Can J Anesth 1999;46:1143–6.

109. Ostergaard M, Kristensen BB, Mogensen TS. Reduced sense of taste as a complication of the laryngeal mask use [Danish]. Ugeskrift for Laeger 1997;159:6835–6.

110. Bull TR. Taste and the chorda tympani. J Laryngol Otol 1965;79:479–93.

111. Shafer DM, Frank ME, Gent JF, Fischer ME. Gustatory function after third molar extraction. Oral Surg Oral Med Oral Pathol Oral Radiol Endodont 1999;87:419–28.

112. Helcer M, Schnarch A, Benoliel R, Sharav Y. Trigeminal neuralgic-type pain and vascular-type headache due to gustatory stimulus. Headache 1998;38:129–31.

113. Doty RL, Haxel BR. Objective assessment of terbinafine-induced taste loss. Laryngoscope 2005;115:2035–7.

114. Stricker BH, Van RM, Sturkenboom MC, Ottervanger JP. Taste loss to terbinafine: A case-control study of potential risk factors. Brit J Clin Pharmacol 1996;42:313–8.

115. Bartoshuk LM. Chemosensory alterations and cancer therapies. NCI Monogr 1990;179–84.

116. Della Fera MA, Mott AE, Frank ME. Iatrogenic causes of taste disorders: Radiation therapy, surgery, and medication. In: Doty RL, editor. Handbook of Olfaction and Gustation. New York: Marcel Dekker, 1995; p. 785–91.

117. Conger AD. Loss and recovery of taste acuity in patients irradiated to the oral cavity. Radiat Res 1973;53:338–47.

118. Chambers KC, Bernstein IL. Conditioned flavor aversions. In: Doty RL, editor. Handbook of Olfaction and Gustation. New York: Marcel Dekker, 1995; p. 745–73.

119. Erick M. Idiopathic dysgeusia associated with blood transfusion: A case report. J Am Diet Assoc 1996;96:450.

120. Panayiotou H, Small SC, Hunter JH, Culpepper RM. Sweet taste (dysgeusia). The first symptom of hyponatremia in small cell carcinoma of the lung. Arch Intern Med 1995;155:1325–8.

121. Yanagisawa K, Bartoshuk LM, Catalanotto FA, et al. Anesthesia of the chorda tympani nerve and taste phantoms. Physiol Behav 1998;63:329–35.

122. Helms JA, Della-Fera MA, Mott AE, Frank ME. Effects of chlorhexidine on human taste perception. Arch Oral Biol 1995;40:913–20.

123. Mattes RD, Kare MR. Gustatory sequelae of alimentary disorders. Digest Dis 1986;4:129–38.

124. Grushka M, Epstein J, Mott A. An open-label, dose escalation pilot study of the effect of clonazepam in burning mouth syndrome. Oral Surg Oral Med Oral Pathol Oral Radiol Endodont 1998;86:557–61.

FURTHER READING

Doty RL, editor. Handbook of Olfaction and Gustation, 2nd edition. New York: Marcel Dekker; 2003. p. 1–2000.
A comprehensive overview of olfaction and gustation, including anatomy, physiology, and behavior in humans and other mammals.

Finger TE, Silver WL, Restrepo D, editors. The neurobiology of Taste and Smell. New York: John Wiley & Sons; 2000. p. 1–479.
A basic overview of neurobiological research in mainly nonhuman organisms, including nonvertebrates.

Mombaerts P. Genes and ligands for odorant, vomeronasal, and taste receptors. Nat Rev Neurosci 2004:5:263–78.
A masterful review of molecular mechanisms in olfactory coding and the early elements of transduction in the three major sensory systems of mammals.

Wilson DA, Stevenson RJ. Learning to Smell. Baltimore: Johns Hopkins University; 2006.
A comprehensive overview of how the brain is critically important for olfactory perception, demonstrating that olfaction is not a simple physiochemical process but a plastic synthetic process that is intimately tied to memory and other central nervous system processes.

39

Cellular Biology of the Immune System

Bradley F. Marple, MD
Raghu S. Athré, MD

The questions of how man acquires and fends off disease have plagued humanity since the beginning of time. The ancients saw disease as a manifestation of god's will and performed sacrifices to prevent angering the gods and becoming ill. In 1796, Edward Jenner showed that smallpox could be prevented by inoculation of cowpox, a less virulent virus. He initially made the observation that women who milked cows were somehow immune to smallpox after they contracted cowpox, which was similar to smallpox, but never fatal.[1] To further the knowledge base of the immune system and its workings, Louis Pasteur presented his landmark paper on germ theory in 1878 to the French Academy of Sciences.[2] He is credited with linking disease with microorganisms and thereby set the stage for all future research in the field of immunology.

THE HUMAN IMMUNE SYSTEM

The human immune system is a remarkable collection of many different cell types that work in synchronized orchestration to protect the host against a seemingly infinite number of possible environmental pathogens, while still not reacting against itself. Any entity capable of eliciting an immunologic response is termed an *antigen*.

The human immune system can distinguish between very similar antigens, even antigens that may differ by a single amino acid. This characteristic is termed specificity. Immune system responses are highly specific and are tailored to an individual antigen. For example, exposure to varicella may afford the host lifelong immunity to varicella, but not to paramyxovirus.

The immune system deals with many invading microorganisms by releasing cytotoxic chemicals that are deadly to the invading microorganism and to cells infected by the invading microorganism. Therefore, it is imperative that such responses are targeted only to foreign microorganisms and infected cells and not to normal host cells. The immune system has an intrinsic property in recognizing self from nonself; and, when this regulation pathway is disturbed, *autoimmunity* results. Autoimmunity is when the immune system starts attacking normal cells. An example of such a disease condition is myasthenia gravis. In myasthenia gravis, the immune system produces an immune response against the acetylcholine receptor in the neuromuscular junction producing progressive muscular weakness with repetitive muscular contraction.[3]

The immune system can be broken down into 2 large divisions: the innate immune system and the acquired immune system. Innate immunity is a nonspecific, genetically derived system that is present in each individual at birth. Examples of tissues and substances involved in the innate immune system include the skin, mucous membranes, saliva, tears, perspiration, and gastric acid.[4] Each one of these acts to retard the growth of pathogenic microorganisms and inhibit their infective capability. Acquired immunity is specific and adaptive in that it reacts with antigens to produce a specific immune response to that particular antigen. Furthermore, the acquired immune system learns which antigen it has been exposed to so that future exposure to the same antigen produces responses that are faster and more robust. This type of immunity will be discussed in this chapter.

Acquired immune responses can be divided into 2 subgroups: antibody-mediated and cell-mediated responses. Antibodies, also known as immunoglobulins (Igs), are proteins that circulate in the blood and are produced by specialized cells named B cells. Antibodies bind to antigen in a specific manner and can initiate several types of responses such as binding to and killing bacterial cells or binding and inactivating a bacterial toxin. On the other hand, cell-mediated responses involve the production of specialized cells that react with antigens on the surface of cells. An example of this is a viral-infected cell presenting foreign, viral antigens on its surface. The cell-mediated immune response would bind the foreign antigen and initiate a sequence of events that would result in the death of the infected cell before the virus could replicate.

What Are Lymphocytes?

Immune system cells are also known as white blood cells.[5] The category of white blood cells includes such cell types as macrophages and lymphocytes. Lymphocytes are the specialized cells that react in a specific manner to antigens and elicit and propagate immune responses. Lymphocytes can be further characterized as either B cells or T cells. B cells are responsible for antibody-mediated immune response, and T cells are responsible for cell-mediated immune responses.[5] There exist 2 types of T cells: helper T cells and cytotoxic T cells. Cytotoxic T cells kill infected cells that exhibit foreign antigens, whereas helper T cells modulate and enhance the immune response to antigens.[6]

Lymphocytes represent 1 of the most numerous cell types in the body. The combined total mass of all lymphocytes is equivalent to the mass of the brain! Lymphocytes develop from pluripotent stem cells that give rise to all blood cells including lymphocytes, red blood cells, and platelets. This maturation from pluripotent stem cells occurs in the bone marrow in adults and in the liver in fetuses. Also, T cells are "sensitized" in the thymus gland. Since the adult bone marrow, fetal liver, and thymus gland are involved in the production of lymphocytes, they are referred to as the primary lymphoid organs.

All leukocytes are derived from a common progenitor cell. The first division in the schema of differentiation is between the myeloid cell line and the lymphoid cell line. The myeloid cell line gives rise to monocytes, neutrophils, eosinophils, basophils, erythrocytes, and platelets.[7] On the other hand, the lymphoid cell line gives rise to T cells, B cells, and natural killer ((NK) or large granular lymphocytes) cells. Differentiation of a pluripotent stem cell into either the myeloid line or the lymphoid line is mediated through receptors on the stem cell surface and interaction with various soluble chemicals (cytokines) and through stem cell surface receptors. Presence of different cytokines and expression of different cell surface receptors guide the pluripotent cell down either the myeloid or lymphoid cell pathway. Stromal support cells in the bone marrow also control cell proliferation and maintenance via the release of cytokines such as interleukin-4 (IL-4), IL-6, IL-7, IL-11, and granulocyte-macrophage colony-stimulating factor (GM-CSF) (Figure 1).[7]

Other than B cells and T cells, NK cells are the last major subtype of lymphoid line. NK cells are also called large granular lymphocytes. NK cells are larger than B and T cells and do not have antibody or T cell receptors on their surface. The role of NK cells is to kill virally infected cells and tumor cells. NK cells do this in a nonspecific manner. Furthermore, activation of NK cells can cause secretion on interferon-gamma (IFN-γ), which subsequently causes proliferation of other cell types. T cells that have been activated can

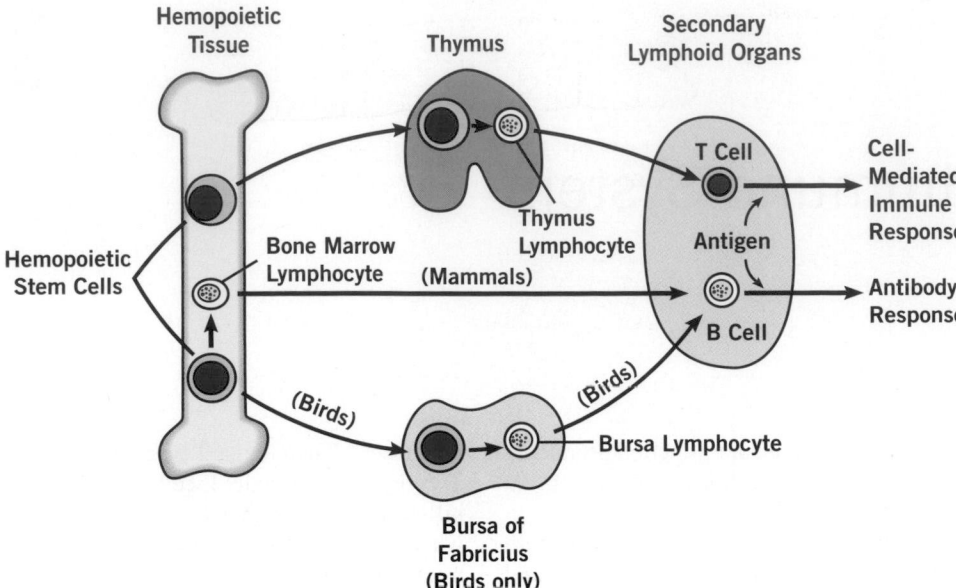

Figure 1 Schematic of hematopoiesis. All myeloid and lymphoid stem cells except for T-cell precursor cells mature in the bone marrow. T cell precursor cells leave the bone marrow and mature in the thymus gland. Mature lymphocytes then enter the circulation and are exposed to potential antigens in the secondary lymphoid organs.

secrete IL-2, which can cause proliferation of NK cells.[8,9] These mechanisms work in concert to amplify the immune response to foreign antigens.

Precursor T cells leave the marrow and travel to the thymus gland, where the rest of their maturation occurs.[10] B cells and other hematopoietic cells mature in the marrow itself.[11] Once the B cells and T cells have matured, they are released into the blood, where they travel to the secondary lymphoid organs. Secondary lymphoid organs include the lymph nodes, tonsils, adenoid, spleen, and epithelial-associated lymph tissue in the skin, gastrointestinal tract, and respiratory tract (Figure 2). In the secondary lymphoid organs, mature lymphocytes are exposed to antigens. The blood is essentially filtered, and some of the lymphocytes become activated as they are exposed to their specific antigen. Activated lymphocytes

initiate downstream immune responses. The other lymphocytes percolate through the lymph node and end up in the lymph fluid system. The lymph fluid system collects into various ducts and finally empties into the thoracic duct, which in turn empties into the subclavian vein. Thus, the entire system recirculates.

Differentiating between B cells and T cells is difficult. Prior to activation, both types of cells appear morphologically the same. Following activation, B cells secrete antibodies, and therefore develop extensive networks of rough endoplasmic reticulum in the cytosol. This way, B cells and T cells can be differentiated since T cells do not have a significant amount of rough endoplasmic reticulum. However, B cells and T cells can also be differentiated because of their cell markers. Different cells have different proteins on their cell surface. For example, T cells

have either the CD4 or CD8 protein on their cell surface. By using antibodies to these proteins, the cells can be sorted in the laboratory.

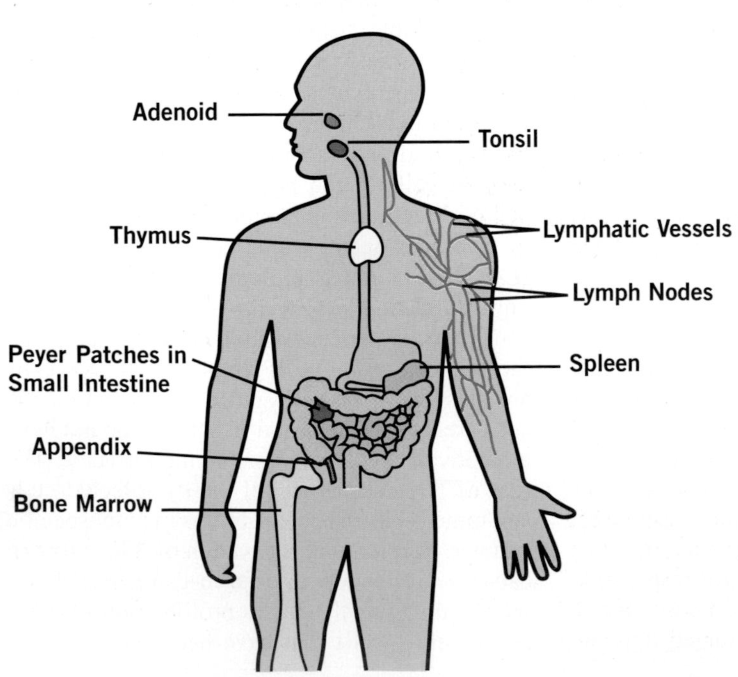

Pluripotent stem cells differentiate into 2 main classes, the myeloid line and the lymphoid line. The myeloid line subdivides into 5 categories of precursor cells: CFU-GM, CFU-Eo, CFU-BM, BFU-MEG,[12] and BFU-E.[13] CFU-GM cells give rise to monocytes, macrophages, and neutrophils. Monocytes mature in the bone marrow and are released into the circulation. In the circulation, they travel to various tissues, penetrate the tissue and become tissue macrophages. Examples of tissue macrophages include Kupffer cells and microglial cells. Cytokines such as stem cell factor (SCF), IL-3, IL-6, IL-11, and GM-CSF stimulate the proliferation of the myeloid line of stem cells.[14] Further differentiation is guided by other cytokines such as macrophage colony stimulating factor (MCSF) to induce end-line differentiation into monocytes and macrophages. The other postmyeloid differentiated ones give rise to the following cells: CFU-Eo → eosinophils, CFU-BM → basophils, BFU-MEG → platelets, and BFU-E → erythrocytes. Similar to the example given above with monocytes and macrophages, other interleukins and cytokines govern the differentiation of precursor cells to the aforementioned cell types.[14]

SPECIFICITY, CLONAL SELECTION, AND HOMING

As alluded to earlier, binding of an antigen to its receptor is a specific event. This gave rise to the lock and key hypothesis. Each receptor on a T cell or B cell can be viewed as locks, and their corresponding antigen as the key. Activation of a T cell or B cell requires binding its specific antigen to its receptor. The exact 3-dimensional portion of an antigen molecule that reacts with a receptor is called the epitope.[4] A particular antigen may have multiple epitopes, though 1 of those epitopes may induce a more robust immune response. That epitope is deemed to be the immunodominant epitope. Any 1 antigen may activate multiple lymphocytes. However, even activation of multiple lymphocytes will only represent a small portion of the overall lymphocyte pool.

The lock and key hypothesis presented above logically leads us to the next question: How does the body respond to the seemingly infinite number of antigens if each antigen requires a separate receptor? The method by which the immune system produces such a diversity of receptors is by a process called clonal selection.[15] This theory states that each host randomly generates a set of lymphocytes with specific receptors to antigens that have never been encountered by the host organism. The immune system is composed of numerous families of ancestral lymphocytes. Each ancestral lymphocyte is predetermined to produce a lymphocyte with a particular antigenic specificity. These lymphocytes are produced despite the fact that the host has not been exposed

Figure 2 Diagram of secondary lymphoid organs.

to that specific antigen. Each mature lymphocyte that is derived from 1 particular ancestral lymphocyte is a clone with the exact same receptor configuration. Once the host organism is exposed to an antigen, those lymphocytes with receptors for that particular antigen are chosen to multiply and mature.

Thus far, it has been established that lymphocytes start off in the primary lymphoid organs, circulate through the body to the secondary lymphoid organs, and return back to the circulatory system. Lymphocytes have certain homing receptors on their surface that guide them toward secondary lymphoid organs. Secondary lymphoid organs such as lymph nodes have special venules leading to the lymph node called high endothelial venules. These high endothelial venules have specialized mucin-like glycoproteins that are expressed solely on the surface of high endothelial venules. This specialized glycoprotein binds to an E-selectin molecule that is expressed on the surface of most lymphocytes. As the lymphocyte nears the lymph node, interactions between the E-selectin molecule on the surface of the lymphocyte and the specialized glycoprotein on the surface of the high endothelial venule cause the lymphocyte to slow down and start rolling along the surface of the high endothelial venule. Subsequently, a different molecule on the surface of the lymphocyte belonging to the integrin family of proteins binds to a counter-molecule on the surface of the high endothelial venule causing adhesion of the lymphocyte and extravasation of the lymphocyte into the lymph node (Figure 3). Similar types of homing cell surface receptors and counter-molecules guide individual lymphocytes to their respective locations within a lymph node.[16–18] For example, T cells and B cells are segregated into different locations within a lymph node. In various disease states, the numbers of homing receptors may be upregulated. An example of this occurs in nasal polyposis. In patients with nasal polyposis, there is an upregulation of cell surface integrin, very late activation antigen 4 (VLA-4), on eosinophils and vascular cell adhesion molecule 1 (VCAM-1) on the blood vessels of nasal polyps.[19] VLA-4 and VCAM-1 are a receptor/counter-receptor pair that allows homing of eosinophils to nasal polyps.[16,20,21] Such homing mechanisms are important in recruiting specific types of leukocytes to areas of inflammation or areas where immune responses are needed.

PRIMARY AND SECONDARY IMMUNE RESPONSES

One of the characteristics of the immune system is memory. This characteristic is the reason we retain lifelong immunity to common viral pathogens encountered as children, and the reason why vaccinations work. The primary immune response is the resultant response when the immune system is exposed to an antigen for the first time. Once the immune system is triggered with antigen, antibody, and cell-mediated

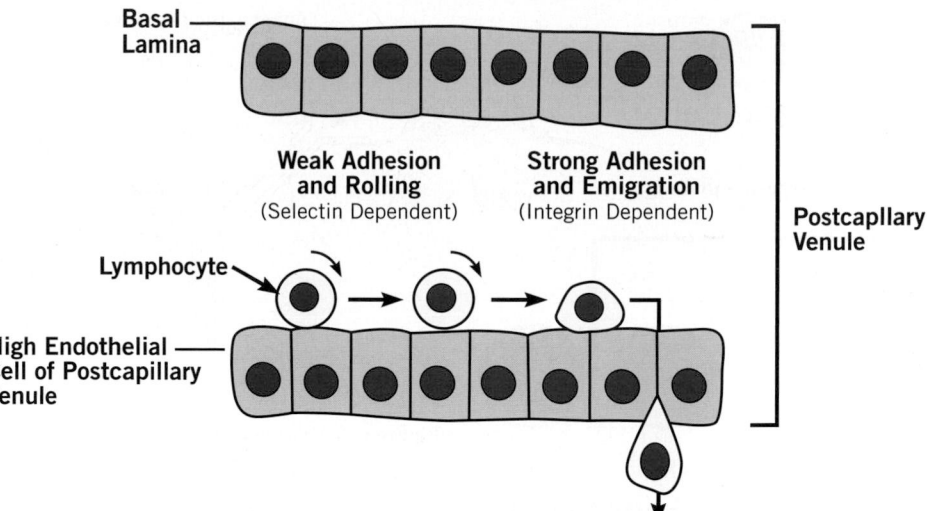

Figure 3 Pictorial representation of lymphocytes rolling and migrating through the high endothelial cell venules into the lymph node. Adhesion, rolling, and transmigration are based on the linking of cell surface molecules on the surface of the lymphocyte and their corresponding protein on the surface of the endothelial cell. These marker molecules can be upregulated in certain inflammatory disease states.

responses lag for several days, rise exponentially, and then taper off slowly. The secondary immune response results if the immune system is challenged with antigen following several weeks, months, or even years. The secondary immune response differs from the primary response in that the initial lag period is essentially nonexistent and the height of the response is more robust than in the primary response. Therefore, the immune system has essentially remembered its exposure to the initial antigen and responded to the invading antigen (Figure 4).

The theory of clonal selection presented above allows us to explain conceptually immune memory. T cells and B cells in the secondary lymphoid organs can be characterized into 3 stages of maturation: virgin cells, activated cells, and memory cells. Virgin cells are those lymphocytes that have never been exposed to antigen. As virgin cells are exposed to antigen, some become activated cells and others become memory cells. Activated cells carry out immune responses; activated B cells secrete antibodies, and activated T cells carry out cell-mediated responses.[15] Memory cells are not actively involved in carrying out immune responses. Rather, they multiply and

await a repeat exposure to the same antigen. If the immune system encounters the same antigen again, the memory cells are triggered. Memory cells bind antigen more tightly than virgin cells, have higher affinity receptors, adhere more strongly to other cells, and transduce intracellular messages more effectively. When memory cells are triggered, some memory cells become activated cells, and others are induced to become more memory cells for subsequent exposures to the same antigen (Figure 5).

ANTIBODIES

Antibodies are Igs synthesized exclusively by B cells. Antibodies are 1 of the most abundant protein components in the blood. All antibody molecules synthesized by an individual B cell are identical. Virgin B cells do not secrete antibodies. They synthesize antibodies and insert them onto their cell surface. These antibody molecules on the surface of the B cell serve as receptors for antigens. When the specific antigen for a particular antibody is encountered and binds an antibody receptor on the surface of a virgin B cell, the B cell is either activated or becomes a memory B cell.

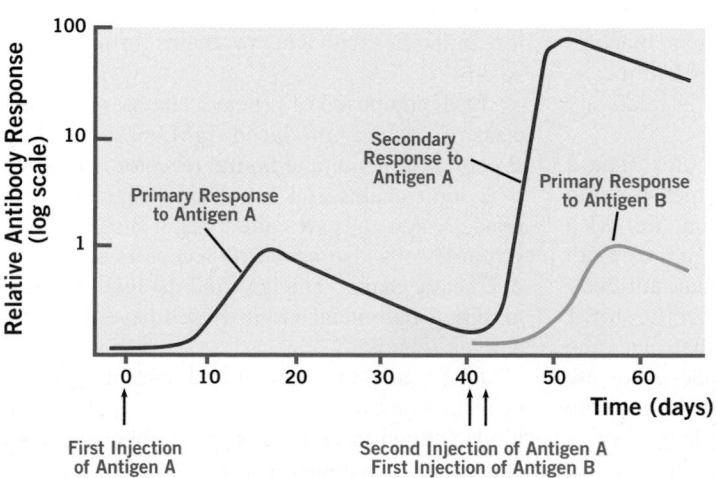

Figure 4 Graph of antibody response with the first exposure to antigen contrasted against antibody response with subsequent exposure to the same antigen.

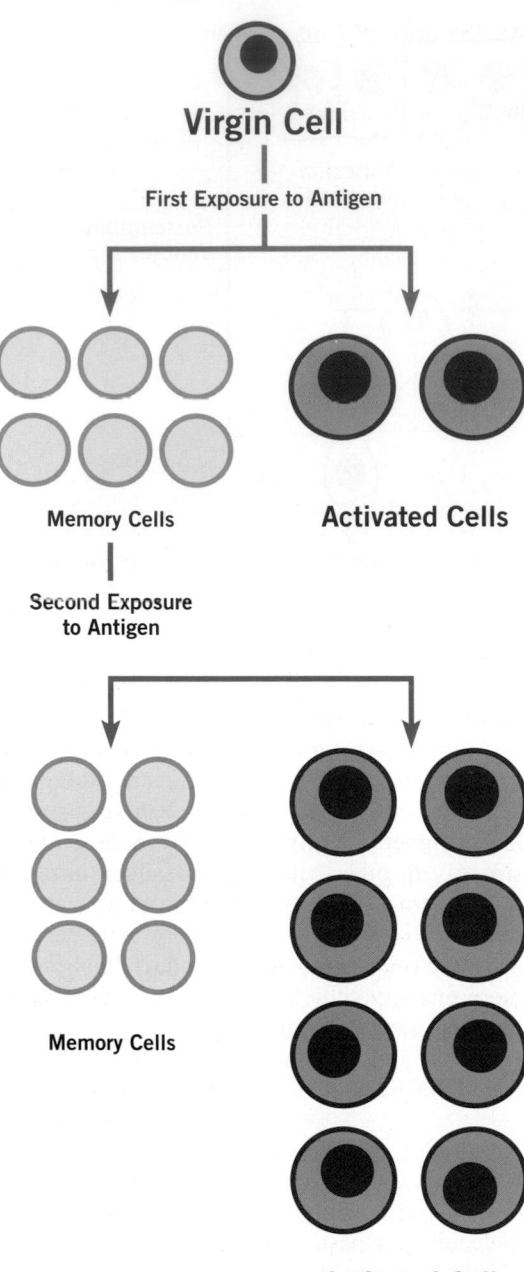

Virgin Cell

First Exposure to Antigen

Memory Cells

Activated Cells

Second Exposure to Antigen

Memory Cells

Activated Cells

Figure 5 Pictorial representation of clonal selection theory.

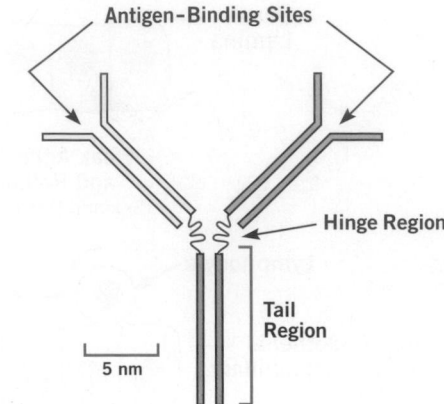

Antigen-Binding Sites

Hinge Region

Tail Region

5 nm

Figure 6 Schematic of an antibody molecule.

contributes to the efficiency of antigen binding and lattice formation by affording flexibility in the distance between the 2 antigen-binding sites within the antibody molecule.

The role of antibodies in the schema of the immune system is not solely to bind antigen and form lattice networks. The F_c region of the antibody molecule can confer additional functional properties to the antibody molecule. To understand this concept, a more in depth understanding of antibody structure and types of antibodies is necessary.

Each Y-shaped antibody molecule is composed of 2 light chains and 2 heavy chains. In any particular antibody molecule, the 2 light chains are identical and the 2 heavy chains are identical. The 2 light chains are involved in the antigen-binding portion of the antibody molecule.[22] The 2 types of light chains are κ and λ light chains. A particular antibody molecule may have κ or λ light chains, but not both. No biologic difference between the 2 types of light chains has been shown. The heavy chains have a component that is associated with the antigen-binding portion, and a component that forms the tail region. The 4 chains are held together with noncovalent and disulfide interactions.[23]

Antibody Classes

There are 5 main classes of antibodies: IgA, IgE, IgG, IgD, and IgM. Each class has a distinctive type of heavy chain. The 5 types of heavy chains are α, ε, γ, δ, and μ. Antibodies composed of α heavy chains fall within the IgA class of antibodies, antibodies with ε heavy chains form IgE, and so on.[23]

IgM, composed of μ heavy chains, is the first class of antibody produced. IgM is produced by B cells as a membrane-bound receptor composed of 2 light chains and 2 μ heavy chains. These nonactivated cells are called virgin B cells. Some virgin B cells also have IgD receptors composed of δ heavy chains. The IgM and the IgD receptors on any 1 individual virgin B cell have the same antigen specificity.[9]

IgM is also the first antibody produced in the primary immune response. Once a virgin B cell binds antigen in its F_{ab} region, it either becomes activated or becomes a memory B cell. If the

cell becomes activated, it starts to secrete IgM molecules with the same receptor specificity as the original membrane-bound IgM receptor. IgM is secreted as a pentamer of 5 four-chain units to form a macromolecule capable of binding 10 total epitopes (Figure 7). Each individual IgM molecule in the pentamer is linked to its adjacent partner via a special protein chain called a J chain (joining chain). The J chain binds 2 adjacent F_c regions. The binding of antigen by pentameric, secreted IgM causes the F_c region to bind and activate complement proteins, which in turn can unleash a cytotoxic biochemical attack on the surface of an invading microorganism. IgD is present within the body only in small amounts. The exact role of IgD other than serving as a membrane-bound receptor is unknown.[9]

The second major class of antibodies is the IgG family composed of γ heavy chains. The IgG family is subdivided into 4 subclasses: IgG_1, IgG_2, IgG_3, and IgG_4. IgG antibodies are important in the secondary immune response and the primary antibodies produced during the secondary or memory immune response. In addition to binding and activating complement proteins, the F_c portion

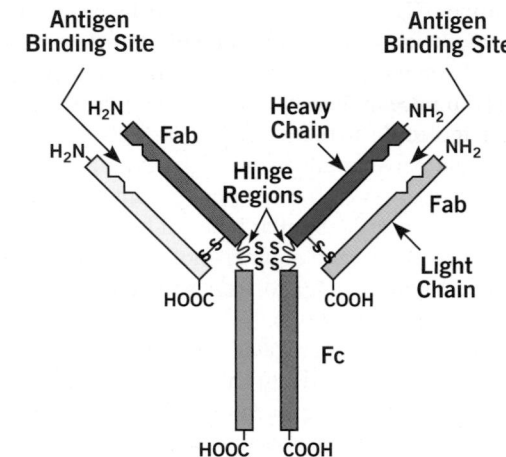

Antigen Binding Site

Antigen Binding Site

H_2N

Fab

Heavy Chain

NH_2

H_2N

NH_2

Hinge Regions

Fab

Light Chain

HOOC

COOH

Fc

HOOC   COOH

A

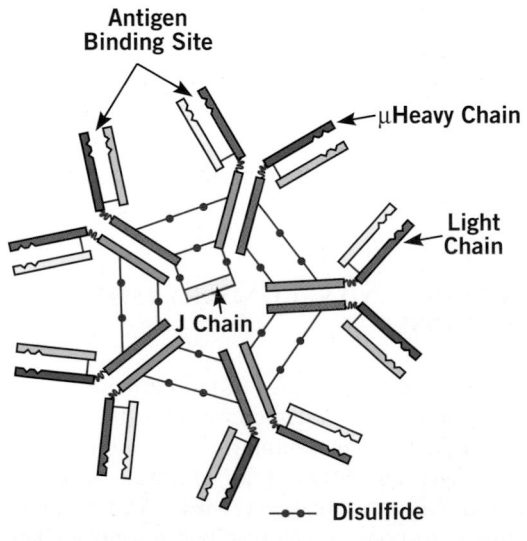

Antigen Binding Site

μHeavy Chain

Light Chain

J Chain

Disulfide

B

Figure 7 Schematic of an IgM molecule. IgM exists as a pentamer.

If the B cell is activated, it becomes a plasma cell and secretes soluble, rather than membrane-bound, antibody with the same antigen specificity as the original virgin B-cell antibody receptor. Activated B cells that secrete antibodies are termed plasma cells. Plasma cells have dedicated a great proportion of their intracellular machinery to the production and secretion of antibodies. Hence, the lifespan of plasma cells is relatively short.[22]

Antibodies are Y-shaped molecules. The 2 arms of the "Y" each have an antigen-binding site (F_{ab}) and are linked to a common "tail" (F_c) region via a flexible hinge region (Figure 6). Both antigen-binding sites on a particular antibody molecule are identical and are specific for 1 particular antigen. Because of the fact that each antibody molecule can bind 2 epitopes, they are said to be bivalent. Antigens with 3 or more epitopes can cross-link and form large lattice structures. The hinge region described earlier of antigen bound IgG molecules can activate and trigger macrophages and other phagocytic cells (Figure 8). Subsequently, the phagocytic cells engulf and destroy the invading microorganism. IgG antibodies are the only class of antibody that can traverse the placenta; also, IgG molecules are secreted in breast milk and subsequently taken up by the neonatal gut.[23]

IgA is the principal class of antibodies present in secretions such as tears, saliva, and mucus. IgA molecules exist in a dimeric state with a J chain joining the 2 individual F_c regions (Figure 9). This macromolecule binds to a specific receptor complex on the basal surface of epithelial cells. The entire IgA macromolecule/receptor complex is engulfed into a vesicle and transported across the breadth of the cell. The vesicle subsequently fuses with the luminal membrane to release the IgA dimeric macromolecule into the lumen of the secretory duct (Figure 10).

IgE is the final class of antibodies.[23] The F_c portion of the IgE molecule binds to a F_c receptor on the surface of mast cells and basophils with an extremely high affinity. The binding of antigen to this complex triggers the basophil or mast cell to release a variety of preformed, biologically active amines. The most important of these amines is histamine, which causes vasodilation, increase vas-

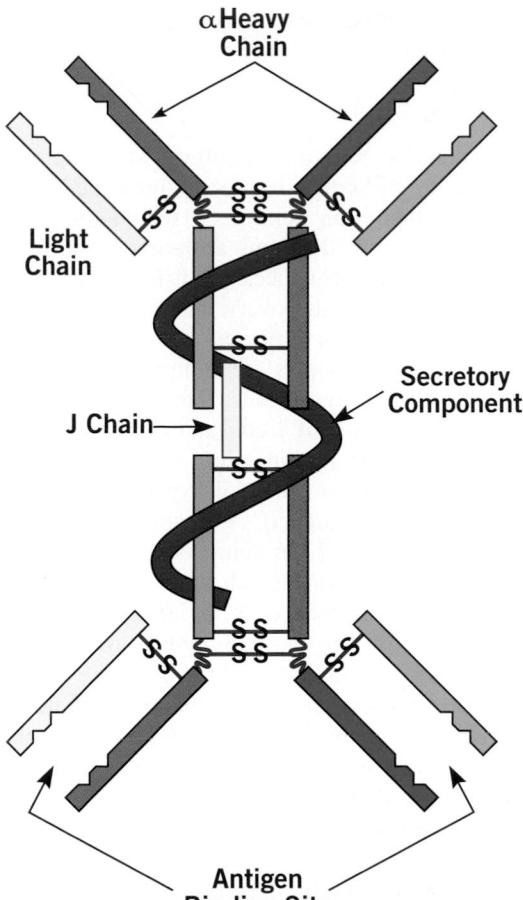

Figure 9 Schematic of an IgA molecule.

cular permeability, and bronchoconstriction.[4,24] This forms the basis of allergic reactions, such as hay fever, allergic rhinitis, and food allergies. Mast cells can also activate a specialized type of white blood cell called eosinophils. Eosinophils are important in immunity against parasites and can kill various types of parasites if they are coated with IgE or IgA antibodies.

Antibodies and Complement

The complement system is a family of approximately 20 soluble proteins that are mostly synthesized by the liver. The complement system *complements* the antibody response and protects the body against bacterial infections. Individuals with deficiencies in the production of complement proteins have increased susceptibility to bacterial infections, as do individuals with antibody deficiencies. Complement proteins are produced in the inactive form and are triggered by antigens on the surface of invading bacterial organisms by immune mediators secreted during an immune response or by antibodies bound to the cell surface of an invading microorganism. Once complement proteins are activated, they in turn activate downstream proteins, which in turn work in concert to kill the invading bacterium.[25,26]

The early components of the complement cascade belong to 2 pathways: the classical pathway and the alternate pathway (Figure 11). The classic pathway is activated by IgG or IgM antibodies bound to the surface of invading bacteria. The alternate pathway is directly activated by polysaccharides on the surface of invading bacteria. Therefore, the alternate pathway represents 1 of the initial lines of defense against invading bacteria before the entire immune system has responded.

The early complement proteins are proenzymes. Once the first enzyme in the series is activated, it generates a serine protease that cleaves and activates the next component in the pathway. The cascade also amplifies the response such that activation of a few early complement proteins triggers a large response. Furthermore, cleavage of the complement proenzyme reveals an active enzyme and a small membrane binding site. This causes the activated complement proteins to

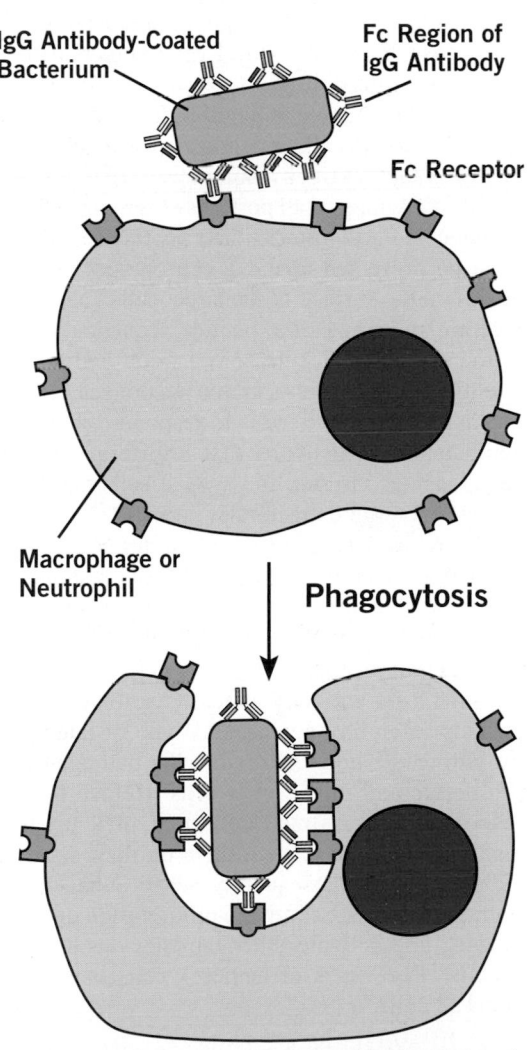

Figure 8 IgG molecules can coat bacteria with their antigen-binding epitopes. Subsequently receptors on macrophages for the F_c portion of IgG molecules can trigger phagocystosis of the coated, invading bacterium.

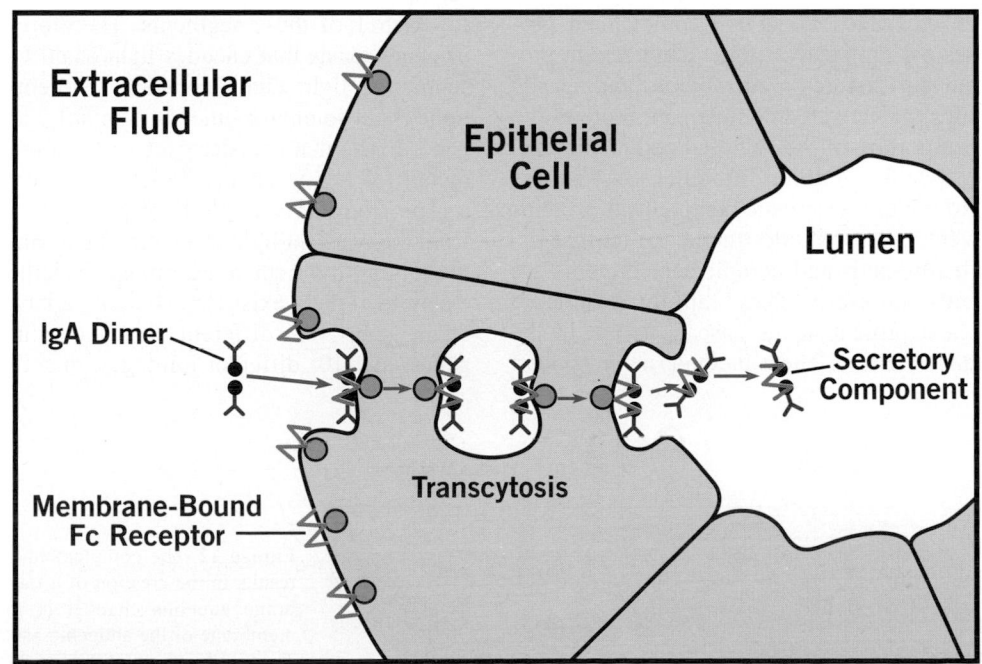

Figure 10 Diagram of trancytosis of IgA dimers across luminal epithelial cells prior to being secreted. IgA is the type of antibody present in secretions such as tears and saliva.

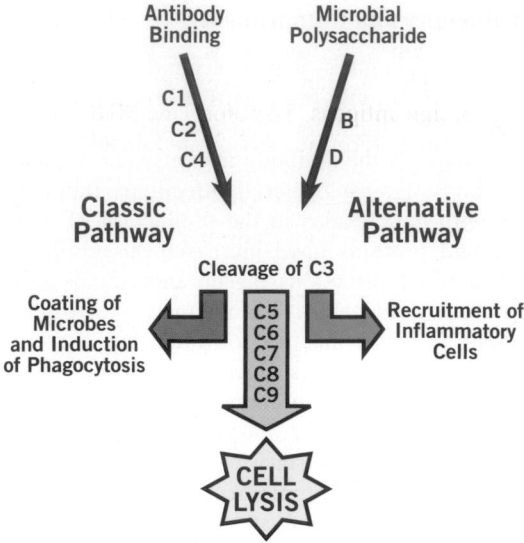

Figure 11 Schematic of the complement cascade.

adhere to the membrane of the invading bacterium, rather than diffusing into the bloodstream.

The classical and alternate pathways both merge at the cleavage of C3 into C3a and C3b. C3b acts as a protease bound to the bacterial membrane to cleave and activate the remainder of the late-stage complement proteins. The end result of activation of these complement proteins is that a macromolecule composed of these activated complement proteins is formed. This macromolecule acts as a transmembrane channel and perforates the bacterial cell wall causing bacterial death (Figure 12).

C3a acts as a diffusible signal that promotes inflammation and recruits white blood cells. The destructive properties of complement proteins make it essential that their activity is regulated and localized to prevent destruction of normal tissues. We have already discussed two methods in the regulation of complement proteins. First, complement proteins are secreted in inactive form and have to be activated by antigen. Second, cleavage of inactive complement proenzymes not only activates the complement protein, but also creates a membrane binding site that holds the activated complement protein to a localized portion of the bacterial cell membrane. Third, specific inhibitor proteins exist in the blood to rapidly deactivate complement proteins to prevent widespread destruction of normal tissue. Finally, activated complement proteins are inherently unstable. They rapidly deactivate if the next protein in the cascade is not in the immediate vicinity. These methods act in concert to control the potency and action of the complement system.[25]

Antibody Diversity

A discussion regarding antibody structure and types of antibodies has been presented thus far. The body can generate a seemingly limitless number of different antibodies. Scrutiny of amino acid sequences of different antibodies has led to the discovery that antibody diversity is achieved via hypervariable regions within each chain. Antibodies are composed of 2 light chains and 2 heavy chains. Each light chain (κ or λ) is composed of 1 constant region (C_L) and 1 hypervariable region (V_L). Similarly, heavy chains are also composed of hypervariable (V_H) and constant regions (C_H) (Figure 13). Heavy chains α, δ, and γ are composed of 1 variable and 3 constant domains; whereas, μ and ε heavy chains are composed of 1 variable and 4 constant domains. The variable segment of the light chain and the variable segment of the heavy chain together form the antigen-binding site or F_{ab} segment of the antibody molecule. The constant regions of the heavy chain (C_H) combine to form the F_C region of the antibody molecule, which confers the biologic properties of the antibody molecule.

The human body makes approximately 10^{15} different antibody molecules without previous immune stimulation. Just as other proteins, antibodies are encoded by genes, which are transcribed and translated. The human genome contains less than 10^5 genes, yet makes more than 10^{15} antibodies. This paradox lends itself to the question: "How can the body make more antibodies than it has genes?" The human body has a unique, compact method of dealing with this problem.

Antibodies are composed of heavy and light chains. Each chain is composed of (V) variable segments, (C) constant segments, and (J) joining segments. There exists a set of genes that codes for each 1 of these segments. Therefore, a set of genes exists that encodes light chain variable segments, light chain constant segments, and light chain joining segments. Similarly, a set of genes exists that encodes each of the above segments for heavy chains. Prior to transcription, a gene from the variable light chain set, a gene from the constant light chain set, and a gene from the joining light chain are brought together. For example, if there exist 10^2 different variable light chain genes, 10^2 different constant light chain genes, and 10^2 different joining segment genes,

there exist 10^6 different light chains that can be formed. A similar algorithm can be performed for heavy chains, giving 10^6 different heavy chains. If any light chain can combine with any heavy chain, 10^{12} different antibody combinations can be produced.[15,22] The numbers presented above are given for illustration purposes only. An additional factor that aids in antibody diversity is the high frequency of somatic mutations that occurs at the site of gene segment joining. In sum, it is easy to see how a virtually endless number of antibodies can be produced from a relatively small number of gene segments.

T LYMPHOCYTES

Thus far, we have focused our discussion on B cells. T cells form the other major class of lymphocytes. T cell responses fall into the category of cell-mediated responses.[27] Similar to B-cell responses, T-cell responses share the characteristic of specificity. T cell responses, however, act only in short range and interact with other cells. In contrast, B cells can secrete antibodies that act at great distances away from the original B cell. T cells interact with other cells in 1 of 2 fashions. They can either kill the interacting cell or use the interacting cell in a signaling cascade to recruit other cells and enhance the immune response. In either case, the cell that the T cell interacts with is called the target cell.

T cells recognize antigen in different fashion from B cells. B cells recognize specific epitopes on an intact antigen molecule.[10] In contrast, T cells recognize small portions of foreign peptide sequences. Furthermore, these peptide sequences must be presented to the T cell on special molecules on the surface of the target cell. The T-cell receptor recognizes the peptide sequence bound to the special molecule combination and subsequently initiates downstream responses. These mechanisms allow T cells to respond effectively against microorganisms that proliferate within cells, such as viruses, and against cells that have ingested foreign extracellular peptides.[28]

There are 2 types of T cells, cytotoxic T cells and helper T cells. Cytotoxic T cells respond to kill cells that present foreign antigen on their surface. Many times viruses and intracellular bacteria can proliferate within a cell, where they are safe from antibody attack. Cytotoxic T cells provide immunity against this type of pathogen by killing the host cell before the pathogen can proliferate and infect other cells. Helper T cells respond to specialized cells that pick up foreign peptides and present them on their surface. Helper T cells subsequently act to enhance the immune response, stimulate proliferation of other T cells, and activate other lymphocytes such as B cells. Two types of helper T cells exist, T_H1 and T_H2 cells.[6]

T-Cell Receptors

T-cell receptors are heterodimers similar to antibody molecules. Unlike antibody molecules,

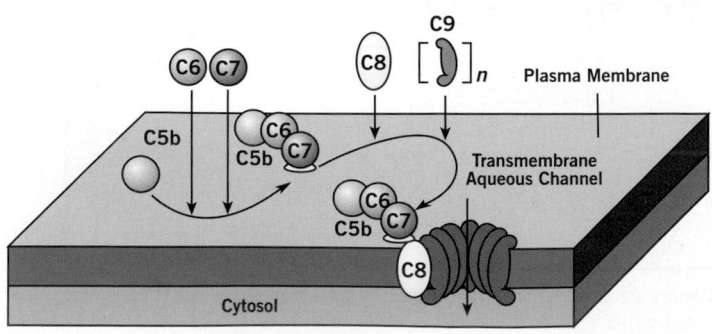

Figure 12 The complement cascade results in the creation of a transmembrane aqueous channel in the cell membrane of the antigenic bacterium. The result is death of the invading bacterium secondary to the influx of extracellular fluid into the bacterium.

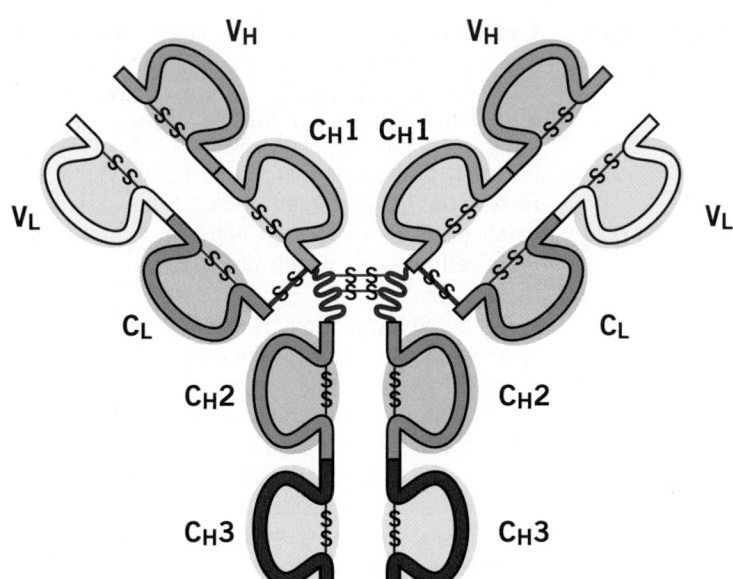

Figure 13 Diagram of the constant and hypervariable domains in the light and heavy chains of an antibody molecule.

T-cell receptors only exist in the membrane-bound form. T-cell receptors are composed of an α chain and a β chain dimer. The 2 chains are held together with disulfide bridges (Figure 14). Each chain has a variable segment and a constant segment. The variable segment extends into the extracellular space, while the constant segment inserts into the cell membrane. The constant segment allows transduction of signals upon binding and activation of the receptor to the intracellular space. A small minority of T cells have receptors composed of γδ dimers. These cells are primarily found in epithelial tissue, such as skin and gut, and in nasal mucosa.[6]

Diversity in T-cell receptors is created in the same fashion as diversity in B-cell antibodies. Each chain, α or β, is composed of a variable (V) and a constant (C) segment. Numerous genes encode for each of these segments. These genes are joined before transcription in a random manner to give an almost limitless diversity of T-cell receptors.[28]

MAJOR HISTOCOMPATIBILITY COMPLEX PROTEINS

As mentioned above, T-cell receptors can only bind antigen bound to a presenting molecule on the surface of a cell. This specialized presenting molecule is part of the major histocompatibility complex (MHC). MHC proteins were discovered far before their role was identified. It was first noted that MHC proteins serve as the target protein for attack in graft versus host reactions among transplant recipients. The immune system of the transplant recipient attacks the transplanted tissue, which it sees as "foreign." From such observations, it has been shown the MHC proteins, or their analog, are expressed on the cell surface of all higher vertebrates.

The loci coding for the MHC molecule are present in humans on chromosome 6, one of the most polymorphic areas in the human genome. This means that there exist a large number of different alleles in the population coding for different MHC proteins. Therefore, it is unlikely that any 2 individuals except identical twins will have the exact same MHC protein. It is therefore difficult to match transplant donors and appropriate recipients to minimize the recipient immune reaction against the transplanted organ. The main role of the MHC system is to target T cells to cells expressing foreign antigens. T cells respond to cells expressing foreign MHC proteins in the same fashion as they do to native cells expressing foreign antigens. Therefore, the MHC system serves to determine self from nonself in the immune system.

Two categories of MHC proteins exist in every individual; MHC class 1 (MHC1) and MHC class 2 (MHC2). MHC1 proteins present antigen to cytotoxic T cells, and MHC2 proteins present antigen to helper T cells (Figure 15).[29] These 2 classes of MHC proteins are functionally and structurally different. However, they both have a peptide-binding groove that holds small peptide segments of degraded foreign proteins. They present this degraded protein segment to their respective T cell, MHC1 to cytotoxic T cells and MHC2 to helper T cells. The T cell receptor can only bind its respective target peptide segment if it is bound to an MHC complex protein. The interaction of the T-cell receptor and the foreign peptide/MHC complex activates the T cell and triggers downstream responses.[30]

MHC1 and MHC2 proteins differ in their structure. MHC1 proteins consist of 1 long α chain with 3 domains (α_1, α_2, and α_3). The α_1 and α_2 domains are furthest from the cell membrane and contain the variable amino acid sequences that bind the degraded peptide fragment. The α_3 chain is close to the cell membrane. The MHC1 protein is associated with another protein, β_2 microglobulin. This protein is a small, extracellular protein that sits adjacent to the α_3 subunit. It is not encoded by the MHC locus and is not polymorphic. MHC2 proteins are heterodimers composed of an α chain and a β chain. The α chain is composed of an α_1 and an α_2 subunit, whereas the β chain is composed of a β_1 and a β_2 subunit. The α_1 and β_1 subunits are furthest from the cell membrane and represent the portion of the MHC2 protein that binds the degraded protein fragment for presentation to helper T cells (Figure 16).

MHC1 proteins are expressed on all somatic cells. All cells have the possibility of being infected and being destroyed. MHC2 proteins are only expressed on specialized antigen presenting cells (APC). Examples of APCs include B cells, macrophages, and dendritic cells. These cells take

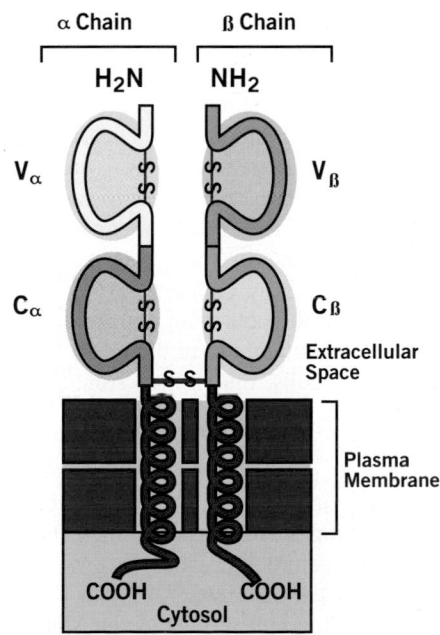

Figure 14 Diagram of a T-cell receptor.

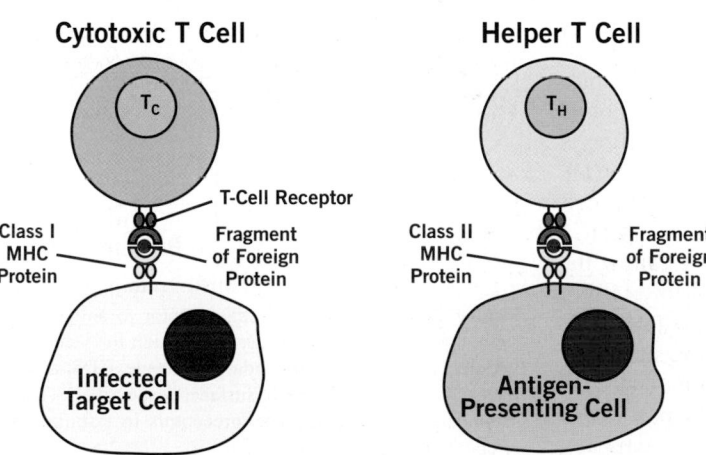

Figure 15 Cytotoxic T cells can only "see" antigen when it is presented on an MHC1 protein. Similarly, helper T cells are MHC2 restricted.

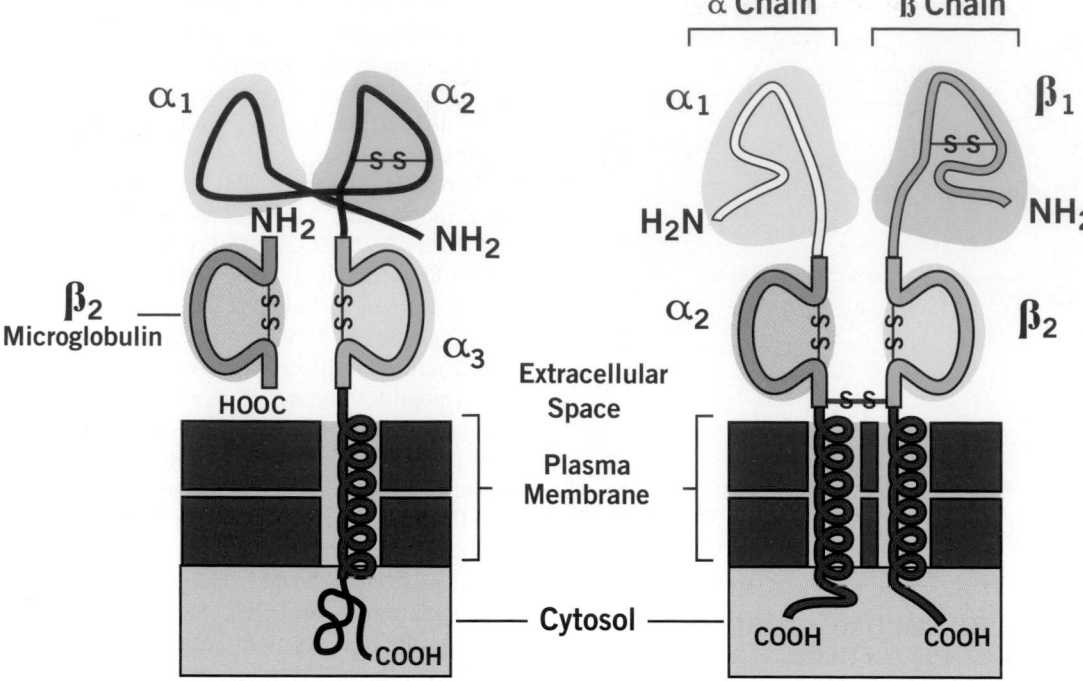

Figure 16 Schematic representations of an MHC1 and an MHC2 protein, respectively.

up antigen from the extracellular environment and present degraded portions of the antigen on MHC2 proteins to T_H cells. Examples of antigens that APCs can take up include botulinus toxin and tetanus toxin. Once taken up and presented to T_H cells, T_H cells stimulate B cells to produce antibodies against such toxins and stimulate macrophages to destroy ingested pathogens.[31]

The Major Histocompatibility Complex—Coreceptor Concept

The schema presented above of cytotoxic T (T_C) cells binding with MHC1 and helper T (T_H) cells binding with MHC2 is somewhat of a simplification. T_C cells have another protein on their surface called CD8. Therefore, cytotoxic T cells are also referred to as CD8+ cells. Similarly, T_H cells express a protein on their surface, CD4. The CD8 and CD4 proteins serve not only to differentiate T_C cells from T_H cells, but also to stabilize interactions with each cell type's respective MHC protein. Under normal conditions, the interaction between a T cell receptor and an antigen/MHC complex is not strong enough to initiate a downstream immune reaction. Therefore, the MHC1 molecule has a binding site for CD8, and the MHC2 protein has a binding site for the CD4 protein (Figure 17). For example, a T_C-cell receptor would bind an MHC1 protein with antigen bound in its peptide-binding groove. This interaction is not strong enough to activate the T cell. The CD8 molecule present on the surface of the T_C cell binds to the nonvariable portion of the MHC1 protein to stabilize the interaction and allow the T_C cell to become activated. The same is true for T_H cells. However, T_H cells bind to MHC2 proteins, and the CD4 molecule on the surface of the T_H cell stabilizes this interaction. The CD4 molecule binds to the nonvariable portion of the MHC2 protein. CD4 and CD8 proteins are,

therefore, necessary to stabilize T cell binding and to activate T cell responses. However, CD4 and CD8 molecules are also important in T cell development. Genetic mutations in the CD4 or CD8 genes will subsequently not allow T_C cells or T_H cells, respectively, to develop.[32]

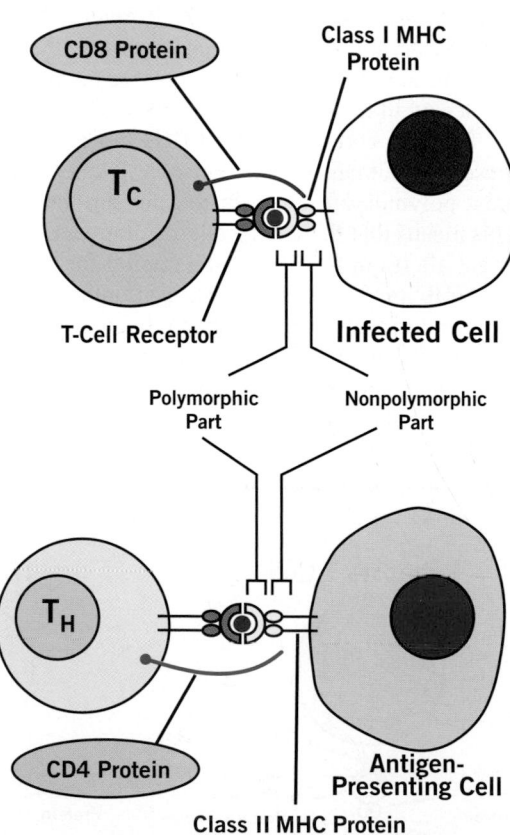

Figure 17 Binding of a T cell receptor to antigen presented on an MHC molecule is not enough for T cell activation. T_C cells have a secondary molecule, CD8, and T_H have CD4 present on their surface, respectively. These secondary molecules act as coreceptors to stabilize and strengthen the interaction.

Cytotoxic T Cells

As mentioned above, T_C cells bind with MHC1 proteins, and T_C cells primarily react to cells that have been infected with intracellular viruses or bacteria. Pathogens that reside within a cell are resistant to attack by antibodies. Such cells have small portions of foreign peptides exhibited on their cell surface, which targets them for attack by T_C cells.[10]

Intracellular pathogens take over the host cellular machinery and produce peptides and proteins. These proteins are manufactured in the rough endoplasmic reticulum (RER). Inside the RER, these proteins bind to MHC1 proteins that are present inside the RER. The protein/MHC1 complex is then transported to the cell surface.

When a T_C cell with a receptor specific for the presented protein binds to the protein/MHC1 complex, the T_C cell gets activated. In response to activation, the T_C cell secretes IFN-γ. IFN-γ is a signaling molecule that triggers upregulation of translation of MHC1 and MHC2 proteins, enhanced antiviral responses by the immune system, upregulation of manufacture of peptide pumps in the RER, and upregulation of specialized proteasome units. In sum, activation upregulates all of the machinery needed to present foreign antigen on the surface of the infected cell.

T_C cells act by killing the infected target cell by utilizing 2 mechanisms. The first mechanism utilizes a perforin. A perforin is a pore-forming protein that is secreted by the T cell. This protein punches a hole in the infected cell and causes cell death. In the second mechanism, the T_C cell activates a receptor on the infected target cell that causes the infected cell to undergo programmed cell death, apoptosis.[32]

Helper T Cells

T_H cells form the other major category of T cells. T_H cells do not directly kill infected cells like T_C cells. Also, T_H cells do not respond to MHC1 proteins. In these ways, T_H cells differ from T_C cells. T_H cells activate macrophages to become more effective at engulfing and destroying infected cells and activate other cells to respond to antigen and initiate an immune response.

T_C cells are activated by cells bearing foreign antigen being presented on MHC1 proteins. T_H cells respond to antigens bound to MHC2 proteins. A schema of how this happens is presented below. An APC takes up foreign antigen from the extracellular space by endocytosis. The antigen is stored within the cell in an endosome. MHC2 proteins are manufactured in the RER. Unlike in the case of T_C cells, the antigen stored in endosome does not enter the RER to combine with the MHC2 protein. MHC2 proteins are packaged in endosomal compartments, also. The endosomal units containing the foreign antigen and those containing MHC2 proteins fuse and create a larger endosomal compartment. Within this compartment, the antigen is trapped and binds to the peptide-binding groove of the MHC2 protein. Once this happens, the endosome travels toward the cellular membrane and fuses with the cell membrane. This effectively places the MHC2 protein/foreign antigenic peptide complex on the cell surface. A T_H cell with the appropriate receptor can bind to this complex and become activated.[33]

Few cells in the body express MHC2 proteins on their surface. Examples of cells that express MHC2 proteins include B cells, macrophages, Langerhans cells in skin, thymic epithelial cells, and interdigitating dendritic cells in lymphoid organs. These cells have MHC2 proteins on their surface and are capable of activating T_H cells.[28]

The process of activating a T_H cell is slightly more complicated than solely binding to an MHC2/peptide complex. T_H cells need 2 signals to be activated. The first signal is the binding of the T_H receptor to the peptide/MHC2 complex. The second signal is derived from chemical mediators. APC not only have MHC2 proteins on their surface, but also have a specialized signaling molecule termed B7 on their surface. This B7 molecule binds to a countermolecule, CD28, on the surface of the helper T cell. This mechanism can serve as the second signal for activation (Figure 18). Another option exists. In some cases, T_H cells are activated by the combination of binding the MHC2/peptide complex and receiving a secreted signal such as IL-1.[34]

Once a T_H cell is activated, the cell secretes IL-2 as well as increases production of surface IL-2 receptors. IL-2 causes the cell to proliferate and increase the immune response (Figure 19). This activation and secretion of IL-2 can continue after the T_H cell has left the surface of the APC. T_C cells also have IL-2 receptors and can become activated by T_H cell secretion of IL-2. IL-2 secretion is triggered by antigen-based activation of a T_H cell. Furthermore, IL-2 only allows proliferation of a population of T cells that have encountered the same antigen that triggered initially

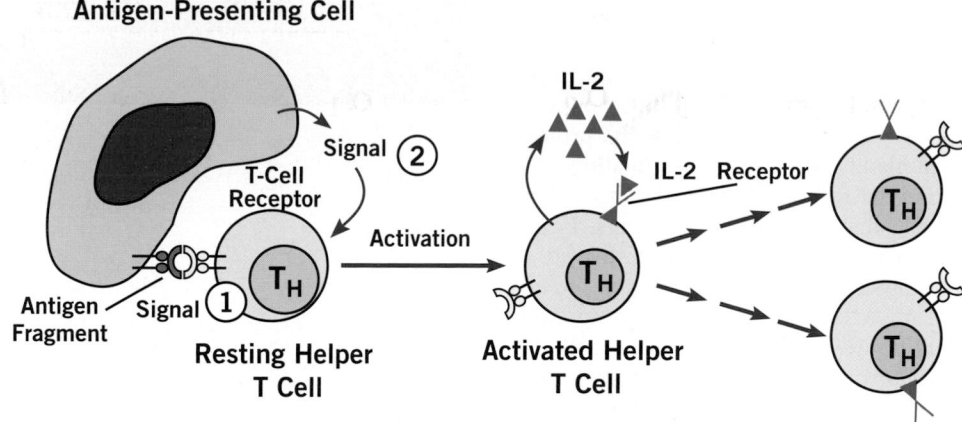

Figure 19 Once a T_H is activated, it can secrete IL2 that further amplifies the immune response.

T cell activation. This allows a controlled mode of attack within the spectrum of the immune system.[27]

INTERRELATIONSHIPS BETWEEN B CELLS AND HELPER T CELLS

In an earlier section, the activation process for B cells was explained. B cells can also be activated by helper T cells. A recurring pattern that has been shown in this chapter is that each cell type cannot function in isolation from others. Rather, the entire system is intertwined with each cell type being able to be activated in multiple interrelated fashions. It has been explained that B cells contain membrane-bound antibodies, which act as receptors, on their surface. These receptors are in continuous flux. Some of these antibody receptors will be recycled, removed from the cell surface, and ingested. The peptide fragments that result from proteolytic degradation of these receptors bind to MHC2 proteins, and are presented on the surface of the B cell as a peptide/MHC2 complex.[22,35]

If a T_H cell becomes activated, it can activate B cells with the same antigen specificity. T_H cells recognize peptide fragments bound to MHC2 proteins. If a B cell has degraded some of its surface antibody receptors and presents them on an MHC2 protein, a T_H cell can recognize those proteins from degraded antibody receptors. Therefore, an activated T cell can bind to B cells that present peptide fragments complexed with MHC2 proteins if the peptide fragment corresponds to a degraded antibody with the same antigen specificity as the T_H cell. In other words, if an antigen activates a T_H cell, the T_H cell subsequently activates B cells that hold the same antigen specificity to mount a more robust immune attack against that 1 specific antigen. B cells also act as APCs and can activate T_H cells. Interactions between T_H cells and B cells are not limited to the MHC2 protein complex. B cells have a protein on their surface called CD40.[9] Likewise, activated T_H cells have a counterprotein called CD 40 ligand.[36,37] The interaction between these 2 proteins acts as a second signal to stimulate B cells to mature, proliferate, and be able to switch the class of antibodies they produce.[38]

Interrelationships between B and T cells allow the immune system to work in concert and mount a robust response that is highly specific and controlled. Without such safeguards, the immune system could wreak havoc in the body and mount responses against normal tissue as well. Another example of such an interrelationship is the secretion of IL-4 by T_H cells. IL-4 causes B cells to mature and promotes the switching of antibody production from IgM to IgE and IgG_1. Genetic mutations in the CD40 ligand protein or in the ability to produce IL-4 result in individuals exhibiting severe immune deficiency with susceptibility to many opportunistic infections.

POSITIVE AND NEGATIVE SELECTION IN THE THYMUS

T cells develop in the thymus. T cells are released from the thymus and circulate through the entire body. It is important for T cells to react to foreign antigens and not react against normal body tissue. The thymus acts as a selection machine and

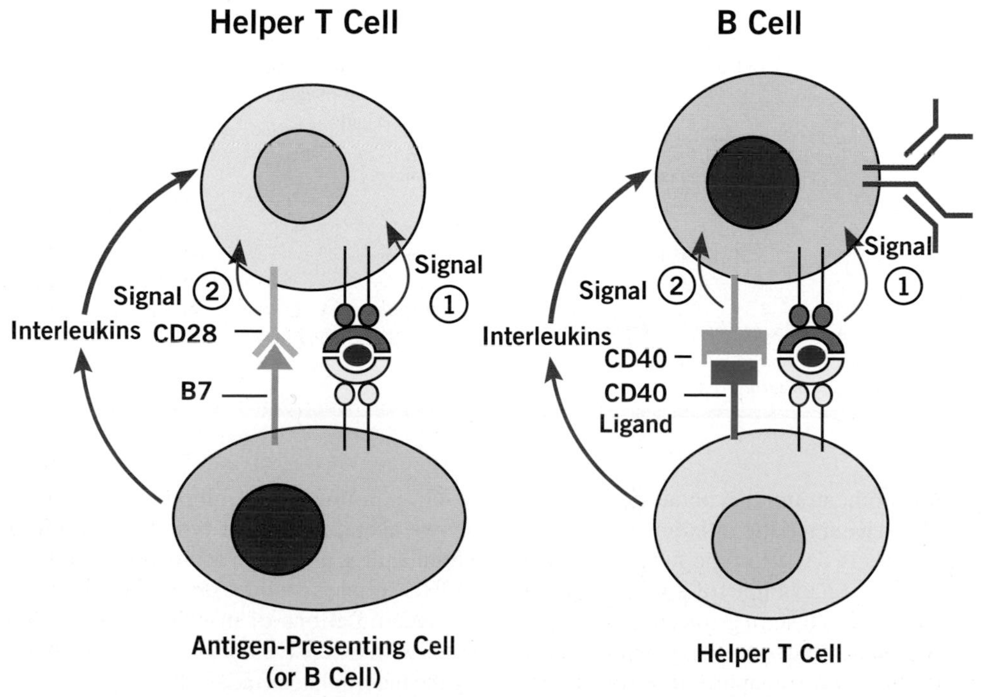

Helper T Cell

Signal ② Interleukins CD28

B7

Signal ①

Antigen-Presenting Cell (or B Cell)

B Cell

Signal ② Interleukins

CD40 CD40 Ligand

Signal ①

Helper T Cell

Figure 18 Comparison of the signals required for activating a helper T cell versus a B cell.

institutes a policy of positive selection and negative selection.[10]

T cells are exposed to MHC proteins with a variety of peptides, foreign and self, bound to the peptide-binding groove of the MHC protein. T cells that bind to MHC proteins are allowed to survive, and the rest are destroyed. This selects for the T cells that bind to MHC proteins. T cells that do not bind MHC proteins are destroyed. In the second process of negative selection, T cells that bind to MHC proteins exhibiting self-antigen are destroyed. This eliminates cells that would possibly initiate an autoimmune attack. These mechanisms allow the maturation of only those T cells that can recognize self from nonself and can initiate an immune attack against foreign antigens.

CYTOKINES

A comprehensive description of the ever-expanding universe of inflammatory mediators and cytokines would be immense. Cytokines are signaling molecules that have effect over short distances. Cytokines are released by cells and stimulate or inhibit other cells. Two examples of cytokines are TNFα and IL-1β.[24,39] Both of these chemicals are proinflammatory mediators. They are released by various cells in the immune system, and they act to upregulate the immune response. Their effect can be far reaching and include bone resorption by triggering osteoclasts, enhancement of B-cell proliferation, increased blood flow by triggering endothelial cells, and upregulation of cell adhesion molecules on the surface of endothelial lined vessels that attract other inflammatory cells such as eosinophils. Cytokines influence proliferation and differentiation of leukocytes, immunoglobulin class switching, inflammation induction, immune response modulation, lymphocyte chemotaxis, and lymphocyte adhesion molecule upregulation to mention a few examples (Table 1).

IMMUNE RESPONSES

Cell-mediated and humoral responses represent the 2 major categories of immune responses. Cell-mediated responses include T_H responses, T_C responses, and NK cell responses. T_H cells only recognize antigen bound to an MHC2 protein complex. After recognizing the antigen/MHC2 complex and becoming activated, the T_H secretes IL-2. IL-2 causes proliferation of sensitized T cells, B cells, and NK cells by acting as a positive feedback loop. The end result is that multiple types of cells, all with the same antigen specificity, are triggered and stimulated to create a lethal augmented, yet specific, attack on the offending antigen. T_H cells primarily secrete IFN-γ and IL-2, both of which induce inflammation.[27] A subset of T_H cells secretes IL-4 and IL-13 which act as modulators of B-cell antibody responses.[40]

Table 1 Selected Immune Cytokines and Their Activities*

Cytokine	Producing Cell	Target Cell	Function**
GM-CSF	T_H cells	progenitor cells	growth and differentiation of monocytes and DC
IL-1α IL-1β	monocytes macrophages B cells DC	T_H cells	co-stimulation
		B cells	maturation and proliferation
		NK cells	activation
		various	inflammation, acute phase response, fever
IL-2	T_H1 cells	activated T and B cells, NK cells	growth, proliferation, activation
IL-3	T_H cells NK cells	stem cells	growth and differentiation
		mast cells	growth and histamine release
IL-4	T_H2 cells	activated B cells	proliferation and differentiation IgG$_1$ and IgE synthesis
		macrophages	MHC Class II
		T cells	proliferation
IL-5	T_H2 cells	activated B cells	proliferation and differentiation IgA synthesis
IL-6	monocytes macrophages T_H2 cells stromal cells	activated B cells	differentiation into plasma cells
		plasma cells	antibody secretion
		stem cells	differentiation
		various	acute phase response
IL-7	marrow stroma thymus stroma	stem cells	differentiation into progenitor B and T cells
IL-8	macrophages endothelial cells	neutrophils	chemotaxis
IL-10	T_H2 cells	macrophages	*cytokine production*
		B cells	activation
IL-12	macrophages B cells	activated T_C cells	differentiation into CTL (with IL-2)
		NK cells	activation
IFN-α	leukocytes	various	*viral replication*
			MHC I expression
IFN-β	fibroblasts	various	*viral replication*
			MHC I expression
IFN-γ	T_H1 cells, T_C cells, NK cells	various	*viral replication*
		macrophages	MHC expression
		activated B cells	Ig class switch to IgG$_{2a}$
		T_H2 cells	*proliferation*
		macrophages	pathogen elimination
MIP-1α	macrophages	monocytes, T cells	chemotaxis
MIP-1β	lymphocytes	monocytes, T cells	chemotaxis
TGF-β	T cells, monocytes	monocytes, macrophages	chemotaxis
		activated macrophages	IL-1 synthesis
		activated B cells	IgA synthesis
		various	*proliferation*
TNFα	macrophages, mast cells, NK cells	macrophages	CAM and cytokine expression
		tumor cells	cell death
TNF-β	T_H1 and T_C cells	phagocytes	phagocytosis, NO production
		tumor cells	cell death

* CTL: cytotoxic T lymphocytes; DC: dendritic cells; GM-CSF: Granulocyte-Monocyte Colony Stimulating Factor; IL: interleukin; IFN: Interferon; TGF: Tumor Growth Factor; TNF: Tumor Necrosis Factor.

** Italicized activities are inhibited.

T_H cells orchestrate the acquired immune response. The characteristic inflammation caused by T_H responses is delayed type hypersensitivity (DTH) response. An example of a DTH response is the tuberculin skin test. In gross clinical appearance, DTH is manifested by local erythema, edema, induration, and warmth at approximately 24 to 48 hours after antigen challenge. On a microscopic level, examination of blood vessels in the area shows accumulation of lymphocyes in the perivascular area and fibrin deposition. Long-standing DTH responses produce granulomas characterized by accumulations of macrophages and lymphocytes with extensive fibrosis. Interleukins secreted by the macrophages induce fibroblast proliferation with deposition of fibrin, resulting in fibrosis.

The steps of the DTH response are as follows. An antigen challenge is given to a previously sensitized individual. Memory T_H cells are activated by portions of the antigen that are presented on APCs. As a result, proinflammatory cytokines are secreted that result in upregulation of cellular adhesion molecules [intercellular adhesion molecule-1 (ICAM-1) and VCAM-1] on the endothelium of blood vessels in the local area. More memory T_H cells are recruited to the area since these cells have ligands for the cell adhesion molecules presented on the surface of the endothelium. These cells become activated as they are presented with degraded portions of antigen complexed with MHC2 proteins on the surface of APCs. Activated T cells secrete IL-2, IFN-γ, and TNF.[41] These cytokines cause the proliferation of T cells, increased expression of cellular adhesion molecules on the endothelium, and recruitment of other cells such as neutrophils and macrophages. The recruited cells all act to phagocytose antigen and secrete various antimicrobial chemicals, which add to the tissue injury. The result is an enhanced immune attack against a specific antigen.

In stark contrast to T_H cells that orchestrate the immune attack, T_C cells act as cytotoxic effector cells. Once the T_C cell recognizes its specific antigen complexed to an MHC1 protein, transmembrane signaling is initiated. The transmembrane signaling occurs via lymphocyte-function-assisted antigen-1 (LFA-1) on the T_C cell with ICAM-1 on the target cell or CD2 on the T_C cell with LFA-3 on the target cell. Following the intercellular signaling phase, the T_C cell releases cytotoxic granules into the space between the 2 cells. In the cytoxic granules is a protein called perforin. This protein perforates the cell membrane of the target cell and causes death of the cell. A second method of killing affected cells is via the Fas system. Binding of the Fas molecule on the surface of the target cell with the Fas ligand on the surface of the T_C cell causes apoptosis of the target cell. The Fas method appears to be important in elimination of T cells during differentiation and tolerance.

NK cells also contribute to cell-mediated responses.[8] Unlike T cells that are MHC restricted, NK cells do not need to have antigen presented to them only via MHC proteins. NK cells are a discrete entity separate from T cells and B cells and can secrete cytokines independently. They have certain receptors on their cell surface that are unique to NK cells such as CD16, which is a receptor for the Fc portion of immunoglobulins. NK cells also have some receptors common to other lymphocytes such as CD2. NK cells are present in the peripheral circulation, in the liver and in the spleen; their cytotoxic mechanisms are similar to those of T_C cells with perforin-mediated and cell induced apoptosis mechanisms. NK cells can lyse tumor cells and play an important defense mechanism against proliferation of tumor and virally infected cells.[42]

The other major category of immune responses is humoral responses. Humoral responses involve B cells and can be subdivided into T cell dependent responses, T-cell independent responses and antibody dependent cellular cytotoxicity. B-cell responses that are T-cell independent involve B-cell responses to large carbohydrate-based antigens such as bacterial cell wall antigens. These large antigens can bridge several antibodies receptor molecules on a B-cell surface and activate the B cell. Subsequently, The B cell secretes antibodies in response to activation that can opsonize or coat the antigen.[9]

T-cell dependent responses are initiated by B cells that bind antigen on cell surface antibody molecules. This receptor/antigen complex is endocytosed, and protein fragments are created. These protein fragments are presented on surface MHC2 proteins, which subsequently bind T_H cells and activate them. Stabilization of the complex between the T_H and the B cell is mediated by the coreceptor interaction between CD4 on the surface of the T_H cell and MHC2 on the surface of the B cell. Activation of the T cell subsequently induces the expression of a molecule on the surface of the T cell that binds CD40 on the surface of the B cell and induces B-cell proliferation, activation, and secretion of antibodies. Multiple cytokines produced by the interaction of T_H cells and B cells such as Il-1, IL-2, Il-10, TGF-β, etc are important in regulation of immunoglobulin class switching and immunoglobulin production.[32,37,43]

HYPERSENSITIVITY REACTIONS

The cell-mediated and the humoral pathways of immune responses have been described above. The result of these pathways is an immune response that is specific, yet efficient, killing foreign antigens as well as native cells that are infected. These same mechanisms can cause injury to normal tissue as well. When these mechanisms cause such injury, it is termed hypersensitivity responses.

These hypersentivity responses are characterized into 4 main categories. These categories were originally described by Gell and Coombs in 1963.[44] Although the categorization into 4 categories and the presumed pathophysiology of each subtype are an oversimplification, it does allow the establishment of a basic scheme in which to understand hypersensitivity reactions. Hypersensitivity reactions rarely consist of 1 type only and involve all components of the immune system.

Type 1 hypersensitivity reactions are usually mast cell-mediated reactions that usually manifest within minutes to hours after antigen challenge. These reactions can be IgE dependant or IgE independent. The offending antigen essentially triggers the release of vasoactive and bronchoactive mediators from mast cells and basophils. An IgE-dependent response involves the binding of IgE antibodies to the offending antigen. The IgE antibodies then bind to receptors on mast cells and basophils, which causes these cells to release preformed vasoactive and bronchoactive mediators. Some antigens such as contrast media can cause activation of mast cells in an IgE independent fashion. The end result can cause bronchospasm and hypotension in anaphylactoid reaction.[45]

Type 2 hypersensitivity reactions involve IgG and IgM antibodies that bind to antigens on eythrocytes, platelets, epithelial cells on mucosal surfaces, and antigens on basement membranes. The triggering antigen can be self-antigens, modified self-antigens, or antigenic haptens complexed with self-antigens. When IgG or IgM molecules interface with these antigens, the result is destruction of the target cell causing tissue damage. The target cell can be opsonized, lysed, or killed by antibody-dependent, cell-mediated cytotoxicity. Examples of this type of reaction are seen in penicillin-induced hemolytic anemia and in quinine-induced autoimmune thrombocytopenia. In each of these examples, the drug in question coats normal cells. The complex of normal cell antigens complexed with the drug is recognized as a foreign antigen and induces an IgG/IgM attack. The attack kills the cell causing the anemia or the thrombocytopenia.[46]

Type 3 hypersensitivity reactions involve complexes of IgG or IgM bound to antigen. These immune complexes are deposited in basement membranes and other normal tissues due to their reduced solubility and initiate an immune attack. This type of reaction was widespread in the early part of the twentieth century when equine antisera to treat bacterial infections were used. Antibodies from horses would be injected into the patient in an attempt to cure an infection. The antibody and antigen would form insoluble complexes that deposited in the basement membrane of high flow blood vessels. The immune complex deposits initiated a vigorous complement cascade attack, which resulted in a vasculitis and tissue injury. This condition became known as scrum sickness.[6,47]

Type 4 hypersensitivity or DTH reactions are described above. An example of a DTH response is the tuberculin skin test. DTH reactions result when antigen is administered to a previously sensitized patient with memory T cells. Memory T_H cells are activated by portions of the antigen that are on APCs. As a result, proinflammatory cytokines are secreted that cause upregulation of cellular adhesion molecules on the endothelium of blood vessels in the local area recruiting more memory T_H cells to the area. These cells become activated as they are presented with degraded portions of antigen complexed with MHC2 proteins on the surface of APCs. Activated T cells secrete IL-2, IFN-γ, and TNF. These cytokines cause the proliferation of T cells, increased expression of cellular adhesion molecules on the endothelium, and recruitment of other cells such as neutrophils and macrophages. The recruited cells all act to phagocytose antigen and secrete various antimicrobial chemicals, which add to the tissue injury.[29]

CONCLUSIONS

The immune system is an elegant yet lethal system that specifically can recognize and react to a seemingly limitless number of foreign antigens. Small genetic alterations in receptors or in the structure of interleukins can wreak havoc on the host by predisposing the patient to numerous opportunistic infections. At the same time, the immune system recognizes self from nonself. Alteration in this fine balance can also lead to a host of disorders such as systemic lupus erythematosus and Wegener granulomatosis to name 2 examples.

REFERENCES

1. Jenner, E. An Inquiry Into the Causes of Variolae Vaccinae, a Disease Discovered in Some of the Western Counties of England, particularly Gloucestershire, and Known by the Name of Cow-Pox. London: D. N. Shoury; 1801.
2. Pasteur L. Speech at the French Academy of Sciences, 1878.
3. Lindstrom J. Immunobiology of myasthenia gravis, and Lambert-Eaton syndrome. Annu Rev Immunol 1985; 3:109–32.
4. Baumann H, Gauldie J. The acute phase response. Immunol Today 1994;15:74–80.
5. Gowans JL, McGregor, DD. The immunological activities of lymphocytes. Prog Allergy 1965;9:1–78.
6. Krensky AM, Weiss A, Crabtree G, et al. T-lymphocyte-antigen interactions in transplant rejection, N Engl J Med 1990;322:510–7.
7. Dorshkind K. Regulation of hemopoiesis by bone marrow stromal cells and their products. Annu Rev Immunol 1990; 8:111–37.
8. Storkus WJ, Alexander J, Payne JA, et al. Reversal of natural killing susceptibility in target cells expressing transfected class I HLA genes. Proc Natl Acad Sci U S A 1989; 86:2361–4.
9. Tony H, Phillips NE, Parker DC. Role of membrane immunoglobulin (Ig) crosslinking in membrane Ig-mediated, major histocompatibility-restricted T cell-B cell cooperation. J Exp Med 1985;162:1695–708.
10. Dalloul AH, Fourcade C, Debre P, Mossalayi MD. Thymic epithelial cell-derived supernatants sustain the maturation of human prothymocytes: Involvement of interleukin 1 and CD23. Eur J Immunol 1991;21:2633–6.
11. DeFrance T, Banchereau J. Role of Cytokines in the Ontogeny, Activation and Proliferation of B Lymphocytes. London: Academic Press; 1990.
12. Neben TY, Loebelenz J, Hayes L, et al. Recombinant human interleukin-11 stimulates megakaryocytopoiesis and increases peripheral platelets in normal and splenectomized mice. Blood 1993;81:901–8.
13. Erickson N, Quesenberry PJ. Regulation of erythropoiesis. The role of growth factors. Med Clin North Am 1992; 76:745–55.
14. Saito H, Hatake K, Dvorak AM, et al. Selective differentiation and proliferation of hematopoietic cells induced by recombinant human interleukins. Proc Natl Acad Sci U S A 1988;85:2288–92.
15. Ada GL, Nossal G. The clonal-selection theory. Sci Am 1987;257:62–9.
16. Bevilacqua MP, Pober JS, Wheeler ME, et al. Interleukin 1 acts on cultured human vascular endothelium to increase the adhesion of polymorphonuclear leukocytes, monocytes and related leukocytic cell lines. J Clin Invest 1985; 76:2003–11.
17. Bevilacqua MP, Nelson RM. Selectins. J Clin Invest 1993;91:379–87.
18. Bochner BS, Luscinskas FW, Gimbrone MA, Jr, et al. Adhesion of human basophils, eosinophils, and neutrophils to interleukin 1-activated human vascular endothelial cells: Contribution of endothelial cell adhesion molecules. J Exp Med 1991;173:1553–7.
19. Dobrina A, et al.: Mechanisms of eosinophil adherence to cultured vascular endothelial cells: eosinophils bind to the cyłokine-induced endothelial ligand VCAM-1 via the VLA-4 integrin receptor. J Chin Invest 1991;88:20.
20. Beck L, Stellato C, Beall LD, et al. Detection of the chemokine RANTES and endothelial adhesion molecules in nasal polyps. J Allergy Clin Immunol. 1996;98:766–80.
21. Bentley AM, Jacobson MR, Cumberworth V, et al. Immunohistology of the nasal mucosa in seasonal allergic rhinitis: Increase in activated eosinophils and epithelial mast cells. J Allergy Clin Immunol 1992;89:877–83.
22. Banchereau J, Rousset F. Human B lymphocytes: Phenotype, proliferation, and differentiation. Adv Immunol 1992;52:125–262.
23. Gascan H, Gauchat JF, de Waal Malefyt R, et al. Regulation of human IgE synthesis. Clin Exp Allergy 1991; 21Suppl:162–16.
24. Ackerman SJ. Eosinophils: Biologic and clinical aspects in allergy and inflammation. In: Rich RR, Fleisher TA, Shearer WT, et al, editors. Clinical Immunology: Principles and Practice, Volume 1. St Louis, MO: Mosby-Year Book; 1996. p. 431–48.
25. Reid KB. Activation and control of the complement system. Biochemistry 1986;22:26–68.
26. Reid KB. Structure-function relationships of the complement components. Immunol Today 1989;10:177–80.
27. Barcena A, Toribio ML, Gutierrez-Ramos JC, et al. Interplay between IL-2 and IL-4 in human thymocyte differentiation: Antagonism or agonism. Int Immunol 1991;3:419–25.
28. Goodman T, Lefrancois L. Intraepithelial lymphocytes. Anatomical site, not T cell receptor form, dictates phenotype and function. J Exp Med 1989;170:1569–81.
29. Mosmann TR, Coffman RL. TH1 and TH2 cells: Different patterns of lymphokine secretion lead to different functional properties. Annu Rev Immunol 1989;7:145–73.
30. Gomez E, Corrado OJ, Baldwin DL, et al. Direct in vivo evidence for mast cell degranulation during allergen-induced reactions in man. J Allergy Clin Immunol 1986;78:637–45.
31. Rappolee DA, Werb A. Macrophage-derived growth factors. In: Russell SW, Gordon S, editors. Macrophage Biology and Activation. Berlin: Springer-Verlag; 1992. p. 87–140.
32. Lanier LL, Le AM, Civin CI, et al. The relationship of CD16 (Leu-11) and Leu-19 (NKH-1) antigen expression on human peripheral blood NK cells and cytotoxic T lymphocytes. J Immunol 1986;136:4480–6.
33. Parronchi P, De Carli M, Manetti R, et al. IL-4 and IFN (alpha and gamma) exert opposite regulatory effects on the development of cytolytic potential by Th1 or Th2 human T cell clones. J Immunol 1992;149:2977–83.
34. Linsley PS, Brady W, Grosmaire L, et al. Binding of the B cell activation antigen B7 to CD28 costimulates T cell proliferation and interleukin 2 mRNA accumulation. J Exp Med 1991;173:721–30.
35. DeFrance T, Vanbervliet B, Briere F, et al. Interleukin 10 and transforming growth factor beta cooperate to induce anti-CD40-activated naive human B cells to secrete immunoglobulin A. J Exp Med 1992;175:671–82.
36. Jabara HH, Fu SM, Geha RS, Varcelli D. CD40 and IgE: Synergism between anti-CD40 monoclonal antibody and interleukin 4 in the induction of IgE synthesis by highly purified human B cells. J Exp Med 1990;172:1861–4.
37. Noelle RJ, Ledbetter JA, Aruffo A. CD40 and its ligand, an essential ligand-receptor pair for thymus-dependent B cell activation. Immunol Today 1992;13:431–3.
38. Lanzavecchia A. Antigen-specific interaction between T and B cells. Nature 1985;314:537–9.
39. Bradding P, Feather IH, Wilson S, et al. Immunolocalization of cytokines in the nasal mucosa of normal and perennial rhinitic subjects. The mast cell as a source of IL-4, IL-5, and IL-6 in human allergic mucosal inflammation. J Immunol 1993;151:3853–65.
40. Clutterbuck EJ, Hirst EM, Sanderson CJ. Human interleukin-5 (IL-5) regulates the production of eosinophils in human bone marrow cultures: Comparison and interaction with IL-1, IL-3, IL-6 and GM-CSF. Blood 1989; 73:1504–12.
41. Lefrancois L, Goodman T. In vivo modulation of cytolytic activity and Thy-1 expression in TCR-gamma delta+ intraepithelial lymphocytes. Science 1989;243:1716–8.
42. Timonen T, Ortaldo JR, Herberman RB. Characteristics of human large granular lymphocytes and relationship to natural killer and K cells. J Exp Med 1981;153:569–82.
43. Linden M, Greiff L, Andersson M, et al. Nasal cytokines in common cold and allergic rhinitis. Clin Exp Allergy 1995;25:166–72.
44. Gell PGH, Coombs RRA. Clinical Aspects of Immunology. Oxford: Blackwell; 1963.
45. Klementsson H and others: Eosinophils, secretory responsiveness and glucocorticoid induced effects on the nasal mucosa during a weak pollen season, Clin EXP Allergy 1991;21:705.
46. Petz LD, Branch DR. Drug induced immune hemolytic anemia. In: Chaplin H, editor. Methods in Hematology, Volume 12, New York: Churchill Livingstone; 1985. p. 47–94.
47. Kojis FG. Serum sickness and anaphylaxis: Analysis of 6,211 patients treated with horse serum for various infections. Am J Dis Child 1942;64:93.

40

Assessment of Nasal Function

Jacquelynne P. Corey, MD
Asli Sahin-Yilmaz, MD

The nasal cavity consists of a rigid framework that includes the bony lateral walls, the cartilaginous septum, and bony portions of the turbinates. There is also a highly vascular mucosal component which is the first contact area between the air and the respiratory tract. The functions of the nasal mucosa, besides being the air passage, include warming and humidifying the inspired air, cleaning and filtering the inspired air, sensing odors in the environment, and contributing to the resonance of speech. A person's well-being and quality of life are also affected by his or her ability to breathe through the nose.

Alterations in the functions of the nose can be induced by environmental changes in temperature, humidity, and posture, as well as by many pathologic conditions, including structural abnormalities, hyperreactivity of the mucosa, polyps or neoplasms, endocrine or metabolic diseases, drug-induced reactions, and systemic inflammatory or granulomatous conditions.[1] Traditionally, the clinician relies mostly on the history and physical examination to make a diagnosis. However, various subjective or objective tests have been developed that aid the physician. These tests can provide documentation in a standardized fashion, allowing intrapatient, interpatient, and interinstitutional comparisons. They may help decide the type of medical or surgical therapy, as well as monitor the effectiveness of therapy. They may also be helpful in medicolegal cases, especially concerning cosmetic septorhinoplasty.

This chapter gives brief information about the functions of the nose and outlines the methods available for evaluating these functions.

THE NOSE AS THE AIR PASSAGE TO THE LOWER RESPIRATORY TRACT

The nasal airway plays an important role in the normal homeostasis of the body. During normal breathing through the nose, approximately half of the resistance of the airways is located in the nasal airway.[2] Therefore, even small changes in nasal resistance affect the total airway resistance and influence the total respiratory function.

The nose is lined by a highly vascular mucosa containing arterioles, arteriovenous anastomoses, and venous sinusoids. Given a normal anatomy of the septum, nasal congestion is caused by swelling of the venous sinusoids, referred to as venous erectile tissue. Venous erectile tissue is most dense in the inferior and middle turbinates. The capacitance of these vessels is under the control of the autonomic nervous system. It may also be influenced by humoral factors, allowing for direct action on the vasculature, or indirectly by sensory-neural stimulation.[3]

Nasal Cycle

The nasal cycle has been recognized as a physiologic phenomenon that may cause a periodic change in the patency of the nasal airway associated with congestion and decongestion of the nasal venous sinuses. There is no agreement on a definition as to which changes in nasal airflow constitute a nasal cycle. In the ideal cycle, the left and right sides of the nose have identical periods, are 180° out of phase, and have similar airflow, resistance, amplitude, and volume changes. However, wide variations may occur in nasal air volume, with some subjects exhibiting spontaneous and reciprocal changes in unilateral airflow and others exhibiting irregular changes in airflow.[4,5] These changes range from 21 to 80%.[6,7] There is an increased amplitude of nasal patency fluctuation in subjects with allergic rhinitis; nasal patency fluctuates spontaneously in both healthy subjects and those with allergic rhinitis at intervals as short as 10 minutes.[8] Commonly, however, the nasal cycle lasts about 4 to 6 hours.

Causes of Nasal Obstruction

Nasal obstruction may be due to irreversible (structural) causes or reversible (mucosal) congestion. Structural causes include bony/cartilaginous deformities of the nasal septum or the nasal valves and chronic (bony) turbinate hypertrophy. Common conditions that cause mucosal (generally reversible) congestion include allergies, infection, nonallergic rhinitis, rhinitis medicamentosa, hormones, and drugs.[1]

Subjective Measurement of Nasal Congestion

Nasal congestion is a subjective complaint of discomfort. The patient's perception of congestion can be influenced by factors such as temperature, posture, emotions, or congestion in other parts of the cavity that the physician is unlikely to detect by an anterior examination of the nose with a speculum.[9]

Subjective scoring of nasal obstruction can be performed by use of ordinal 10-point or a 100 mm visual analog scale (VAS)[10] or a four-step symptom severity score.[11] Seventy-seven percent of patients who have cold symptoms are able to discriminate between high flow and low flow nasal passages by using a 100 mm VAS. However, if the differences in unilateral flow are smaller than 100 cm³/s, the percentage of correct responses declines to 50%.[12]

The physician's assessment of nasal obstruction following anterior rhinoscopy is another subjective method of evaluating the nasal airway. Different scales for the physician's estimate of the severity of nasal airflow limitation have been used by different investigators. A three-point scale of severity of nasal deviation (Boyce/Eccles three-point scale), employing the otolaryngologist's assessment of nasal obstruction, correlates with objective measurement by rhinospirometry ($r = .87$). The specificity of detecting nasal obstruction with this method is low; it cannot detect "zig-zag" obstructions or the location of the obstruction.[10]

Objective Measurement of Nasal Obstruction

Testing for nasal airflow should be convenient, reliable, and repeatable to aid in treatment planning. A test for nasal blockage should be able to document the location of the blockage as well as the effect of interventions, such as surgery on nasal airflow, volume, and physiology.

Since the late nineteenth century, researchers have tried to develop an accurate method for measuring nasal resistance and nasal patency. Initially, a simple mirror was placed under the nares for detecting nasal airflow. In time, rhinomanometric techniques evolved that measured pressure and flow simultaneously. More recently, we have seen the development of acoustic rhinometry. Other techniques used for objective measurement of the nasal airflow include nasal inspiratory peak flow (NIPF), rhinostereometry, radiographic techniques, and videoendoscopic documentation.

Acoustic Rhinometry

Acoustic rhinometry was first described by Hilberg and colleagues in 1989.[13] This technique uses reflected sound waves for measurement of nasal volume and the cross-sectional areas of the nose. It provides a topographic map of the nasal airway by converting the reflected sound wave to an area–distance graph (Figure 1).

The validity of acoustic rhinometry has been proved by comparison of measures obtained by this technique with those obtained by nasal endoscopy,[15] or by imaging methods such as computerized tomography (CT)[16] and magnetic resonance imaging (MRI).[17]

Principles. Acoustic rhinometry is based on the principle of analyzing changes in the reflected wave when an incident sound wave passes into the nasal cavity. Variations in the size and contour of the nasal airway cause distortions in the reflected sound wave. The time at which these reflected changes occur gives an estimate of the distance in the nasal cavity to the entity that causes the distortions, and the magnitude of the distortions is a measure of the change in the cross-sectional area.

Equipment. A trigger module generates an acoustic pulse that is conducted to the nasal cavity by means of a hollow plastic tube. The nasal end of this tube is fitted with a nosepiece that is placed against the anterior naris. The nosepiece is contoured and is available in different sizes. The sound wave passes through this tube and enters the nasal cavity. An analog-to-digital converter converts these waves into digital impulses that are fed into a computer. The computer uses these data to generate an area–distance graph by using mathematical algorithms. These graphs can be read on screen or printed, providing a topographic map of the nasal passage.

Technique. A major advantage of acoustic rhinometry over other methods is that it is very simple to perform and requires minimal patient cooperation. The test is done in a quiet room. The patient is seated comfortably and is allowed to relax for a few minutes before testing. The equipment is first calibrated by use of a test acoustic impulse. The tester stands in front of the patient

or sits to the side. The patient is steadied by fixing of gaze. Studies have evaluated the use of a head frame that fixes the head rigidly in a set position, but this approach has not been found to provide any better results.[18] The tester aligns the nasal tube in the same axis as the nose (Figure 2A and B). The nosepiece is held against the naris on the side to be tested first. A repeated acoustic pulse click is generated for 10 seconds and stopped as soon as a satisfactory curve is displayed on the computer screen. The nosepiece should be held against the naris in such a way as to ensure a seal without causing distortion of the anatomy. This seal can be facilitated by use of a jelly on the outer edge of the nosepiece. The procedure is repeated on the other side. Next, a nasal decongestant is applied, with two sprays of 50 µg each, in each nostril. The test is repeated after 10 minutes. By decongesting the nasal mucosa with a topical spray, the clinician eliminates or minimizes the reversible component. When the test is repeated, it gives a measure of the structural, or irreversible, causes of nasal obstruction. The amount of mucosal decongestion also gives an estimate of whether the mucosa is normal or diseased.

The computer generates a curve that shows the distance in centimeters on the *x*-axis and the cross-sectional area in square centimeters on the *y*-axis (Figure 1). The position of the anterior naris is at 0 cm. Only the first 6 cm is used for interpretation because the test loses accuracy in the posterior areas of the nasal cavity.[2] An anterior obstruction at the nasal valve region may cause a distortion of the posterior portion of the curve.[19]

The graph shows three "valleys" or "notches." These correspond to the nasal valve, the anterior head of the inferior/and/or middle turbinate, and the middle of the middle turbinate, respectively.[20]

In 2005, the European Rhinologic Society formed a committee that issued a consensus report on acoustic rhinometry (and rhinomanometry).[21] This comprehensive document provides recommended standards for objective assessment

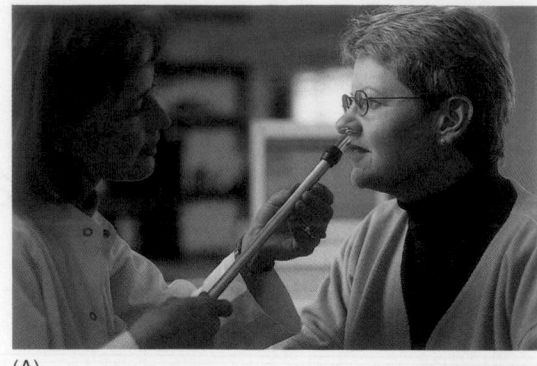

(A)

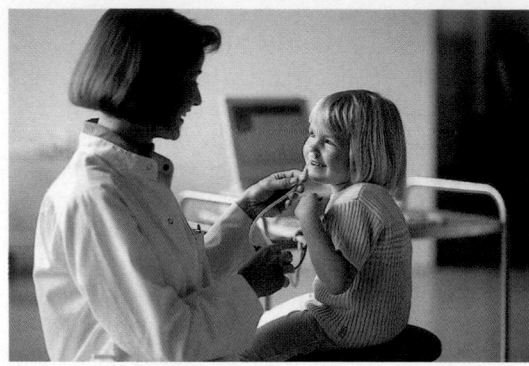

(B)

Figure 2 (A) Interacoustics (Interacoustics A/S, Assens, Denmark) RhinoScan Adult Acoustic Rhinometry. The patient is steadied by fixing of gaze and the tester stands in front of the patient or sits to the side. The tester aligns the nasal tube in the same axis as the nose. The nosepiece should be held against the anterior naris in such a way as to ensure a seal without causing distortion of the anatomy. (B) Interacoustics (Interacoustics A/S, Assens, Denmark) RhinoScan pediatric acoustic rhinometry.

of the nasal airway. In the American terminology, the waves produced by acoustic rhinometry are labeled "valleys" which encompass the three that are commonly seen. These are labeled minimal Cross-Sectional Area 1 (mCSA 1), mCSA 2, and mCSA 3. In the European terminology, the wave patterns are referred to as a "rising W" and the first notch is labeled the "I-notch" for the isthmus.[21]

Interpretation. Acoustic rhinometry allows an objective nasal assessment of whether an obstruction is structural, mucosal, or mixed with an objective grading of the disease according to standardized normal values. For grading of mucosal congestion, baseline mCSA 1, 2, and 3 values and total volume before and after the use of a nasal decongestant are noted. The congestion factor (CF) is calculated as follows:

$$CF = [CSA2 \text{ (decongested value)} - CSA2 \text{ (baseline value)}]/CSA2 \text{ (baseline value)}.$$

The CSA2 value for the side that shows the largest difference in the decongested state is used. The CF is then categorized as normal, mild, moderate, severe, or marked.[14] This scale uses normative values obtained from previously published data.[22] The severity of blockage can be calculated by comparison. A difference of greater than two standard deviations from nasal values of CSA2 in the baseline and the decongested state is considered to indicate an abnormality.[14]

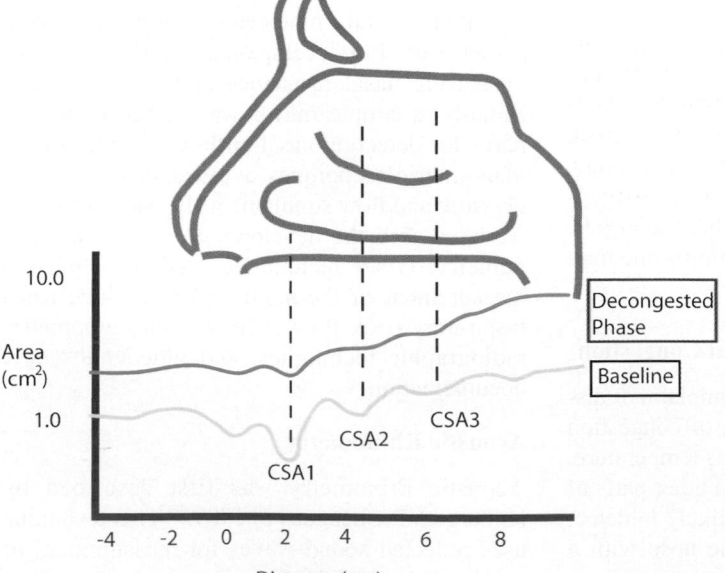

Figure 1 Acoustic rhinometry area–distance graph. The cross-sectional area 1 (CSA1) is thought to represent the anterior end of the inferior turbinate and nasal valve area. The CSA2 is usually identified at approximately 4 cm posteriorly and corresponds to the anterior half of inferior turbinate and nasal valve area. The CSA3 is usually identified at approximately 6 cm posteriorly and corresponds to middle portion of middle turbinate. The negative values are created by the acoustic rhinometry probe (Adapted from reference 14.)

Limitations. There may be small variations in measurements performed by different operators, or by the same operator in different sessions. External noise, changes in environmental temperature and humidity, changes in the position of the sound tube, sound leaks around the naris, and pressure changes due to swallowing and breathing are the main factors that influence the reproducibility and accuracy of acoustic rhinometry.[21] These variations are generally lesser than 10% and can be minimized by allowing the subject to acclimatize to room temperature (normally for 10 minutes), visually matching up the new with the previous, correct waveform, and performing the testing in a quiet room.

The body surface of an individual may influence the minimal cross-sectional area of the nose. Sex, height, weight, and race may influence the cross-sectional area, but only to a small extent.[22,23] Standardization of acoustic rhinometry is currently available for both sexes and all races and ages. Although height and weight may influence the readings, they do not do so in a consistent fashion. Therefore, most standardized reading scales omit this information. Acoustic rhinometry measurements correlate well with other objective measurements, but less so with subjective patient scoring.[24,25]

Clinical Applications. The last decade has seen the clinical uses of acoustic rhinometry expand; clinically relevant studies are now available for normal and diseased nasal passages. Acoustic rhinometry provides a topographic map that can be used for characterizing and localizing the deviations of the nasal septum. It can also identify the relative locations of valve stenosis and turbinate hypertrophy. Acoustic rhinometry is an effective method for comparing preoperative and postoperative values for patients undergoing operations such as septoplasty, turbinate reduction, facial cosmetic procedures (nasal valve reduction, rhinoplasty, osteotomies), cleft lip, palate repairs, and nose surgery, antrochoanal atresia and maxillofacial expansion procedures) and tonsillectomy for pediatric obstructive sleep apnea.[25–29] Acoustic rhinometry after sinus surgery with large antrostomies and ethmoid cavities or with a septal perforation will have different patterns or waves that should be carefully monitored with endoscopic anatomy.

Another use for acoustic rhinometry has been as an aid for the diagnosis and treatment of sleep apnea. Acoustic rhinometry can predict the tolerance of nasal continuous positive airway pressure (CPAP) in patients with sleep apnea.[30–32] Subjects whose cross-sectional area is less than 0.6 cm^2 at the head of the inferior turbinate are not able to tolerate nasal CPAP.[32]

Rhinomanometry

Rhinomanometry is the measurement of nasal airflow and nasal pressure required to achieve that flow. Rhinomanometry provides an objective, sensitive, and functional measure of nasal patency.

Objective measurements of nasal resistance with rhinomanometry do not correlate well with subjective measurements.[33,34] The nasal valve region is the primary determinant of nasal resistance, but the sensation of nasal obstruction may be related to congestion in other parts of the airway or perhaps to other factors such as somatization.[9,34]

Principles. For a better understanding of the principles of rhinomanometry, it is useful to have some basic knowledge of the ventilation mechanisms of the nose. Fluid-dynamic experiments performed on anatomically exact models of the human nose showed that the flow in the nose can be laminar or turbulent.[35] Laminar flow is the simplest type of airflow, in which there is no mixing within the air stream. Pure laminar flow occurs in very low velocity. As the velocity of the airflow increases, turbulent flow is observed. Turbulent air flow is characterized by mixing within the air stream, which is a precondition for an exchange between the flowing air and the mucosa.[21] Turbulent air corresponds to an airflow of 250 to 500 cm^3 in the nose. Decongestants give rise to increased turbulent airflow.

Nasal resistance is defined as the relationship between transnasal pressure and nasal airflow. During laminar flow, nasal resistance is constant and the relationship between pressure and airflow is linear. However, throughout turbulent flow, a nonlinear relationship is observed. Rhinomanometry measures the transnasal pressure and airflow, and it provides a nasal resistance value and a graph of the relationship between pressure and airflow.

Equipment. There are various techniques of measuring nasal airflow and pressure. These techniques may be combined in any manner to yield a value for resistance.

Airflow is measured by means of a pneumotachometer and a pressure transducer. The pneumotachometer is a resistor which induces laminar flow across it so that the pressure drop across it varies linearly with the flow. The pressure transducer converts the pressure differential to an electrical equivalent of flow that is measured by electronic means.[36]

The pneumotachometer may be attached to a nozzle which is inserted into the nasal vestibule. This has the disadvantage of deforming the compliant portion of the nasal valve. The pneumotachometer may also be attached to a face mask. However, this technique has the disadvantage of displacing the facial tissues.

The pneumotachometer may be connected to a head out displacement-type body plethysmograph. This leaves the face unrestricted for manipulation during the procedure. The disadvantage is that this apparatus is bulky and that considerable patient cooperation is required.

Transnasal pressure can be measured by three different techniques.

The *anterior* method of measurement places a tube at the nasal vestibule of one side, which is

occluded while the patient breathes through the other nasal cavity. The *posterior* method of measurement involves placement of the tube in the oropharynx, passed through closed lips between the tongue and the palate. In this method, the measurement result can differ to a great extent because the measured pressure difference may easily be affected by the position of the soft palate.[21] In the *postnasal* method of pressure measurement, a pediatric feeding tube is lubricated and passed along the floor of the wider nasal cavity to the nasopharynx.

The pressure and flow signals are transferred to a computer, and the data can be analyzed, displayed, saved, and printed.

Technique. In *active* rhinomanometry, the patient actively breathes through one nasal cavity while the narinochoanal (naris to choana) pressure difference is assessed in the contralateral nasal cavity. This is the most commonly used method of rhinomanometry.[21] In *passive* rhinomanometry, the pressure is measured for each nasal cavity separately at an airflow of 250 cm^3/s. This method is rapid but less accurate than the active technique.

New equipment has to be calibrated by the manufacturer, and also by the operator before measurements are taken on a given day. A standard preformed resistor should be used by the operator before and after studies. Rhinomanometric measurements are obtained with the patient in a sitting position after an adaptation period of 20 minutes. During measurement, the patient breathes spontaneously at rest. The mask that is used should not leak and should not result in deformation of the nose. The nasal connections of the pressure tube should not influence the shape of the nasal entrance and should not limit its mobility during testing (Figure 3). As the measurements are taken, the data points for each breath that are displayed on the monitor screen form a sigmoid pressure-flow curve in real time. When a series of breaths display regular repetition of the curve, data acquisition is activated to sample two consecutive breaths. If there

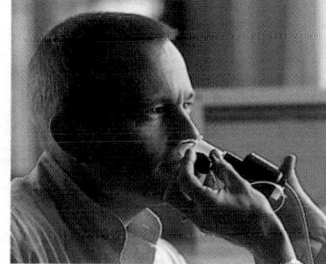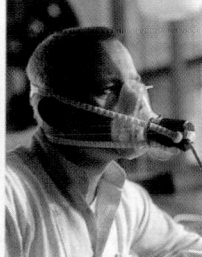

Figure 3 Rhinomanometry equipment. The anterior method of measurement involves placement of a tube at the nasal vestibule of one side, which is occluded while the patient breathes through the other nasal cavity. In *active* rhinomanometry, the patient actively breathes through one nasal cavity while the narinochoanal pressure difference is assessed in the contralateral nasal cavity. The nasal connections of the pressure tube should not influence the shape of the nasal entrance and should not limit its mobility during testing. The pressure and flow signals are transferred to a computer to be analyzed, displayed, saved, and printed.

is irregularity in the curve, the measurement must be repeated.

In the standard pressure and airflow graph obtained from modern rhinomanometry devices, airflow is recorded on the "*y*"-axis and pressure on the "*x*"-axis. The "mirror" image using four quadrants of the graph is accepted as the standard representation in active anterior rhinomanometry.[21] In this graph, the curve on the right of the flow axis represents the change in inspiration, and the curve on the left is the change in expiration. The right nasal cavity is represented on the upper part of the pressure axis, and the left nasal cavity on the lower part of the pressure axis. The greater the nasal resistance (the ratio of transnasal pressure to airflow), the closer the curve will be to the pressure axis. In other words, if the nose is obstructed, the curve will be closer to the *x*-axis (Figure 4).

The current standardized technique is called four-phase rhinomanometry. It involves studying separately, the ascending and descending parts of the curves during inspiration and expiration (Figure 5).[21]

Interpretation. Nasal congestion can be quantified in terms of total or unilateral nasal airway resistance. Resistance can be reported at a designated flow or a designated pressure. According to international standards, resistance should be given at a fixed pressure of 150 Pa, or according to Broms' model, at radius 2. In pathologic conditions, if, for whatever reason, a pressure level of 150 Pa cannot be reached, lower nasal pressures of 75 or 100 Pa can be used, but should be taken into account in the interpretation of results. For four-phase rhinomanometry, resistance is determined for phase 1 (ascending inhibitory phase) and phase 4 (descending expiratory phase) by use of the highest possible flow at a pressure of 150 Pa.[21]

In subjects free from signs of nasal disease, the mean total resistance has been reported to

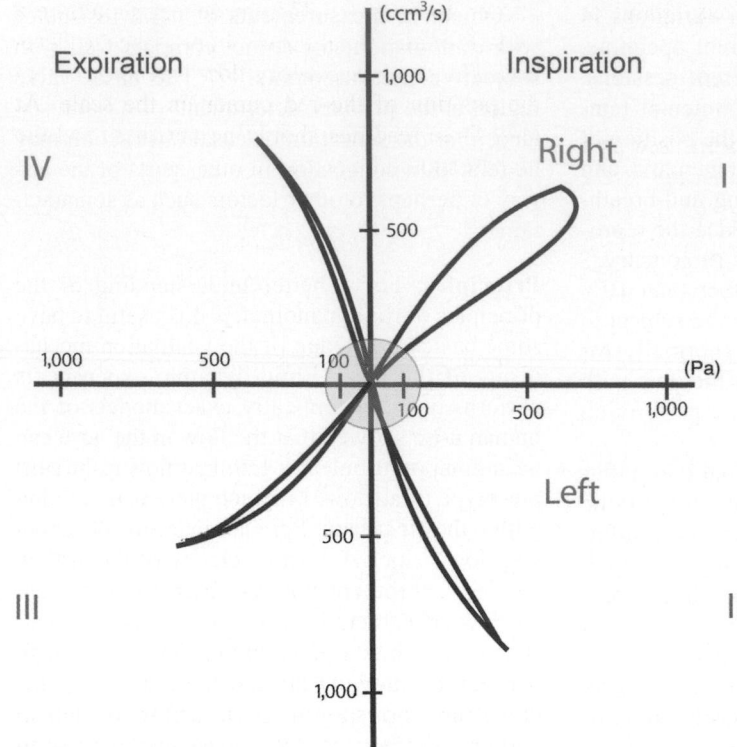

Figure 5 Four-phase rhinomanometry. This technique provides supplementary information; the ascending and descending parts of the curves during inspiration and expiration are also displayed (Adapted from reference 21.)

be around 0.23 Pa/cm³/s, ranging between 0.15 and 0.39 Pa/cm³/s.[37] A total nasal airway resistance of 0.3 Pa/cm³/s is generally accepted as the upper limit of normal.[7] The range of unilateral nasal airway resistance in healthy volunteers, when recorded over 6 to 8 hours, has been shown to have a fourfold fluctuation over time due to nasal cycling.[7] Therefore, it is not informative to quote a normal value for unilateral nasal airway resistance.[9]

Limitations. Factors that affect nasal resistance include postural changes, exercise, and temperature of the air.[38] There is also the possibility of an air leak around the face mask. The presence

of mucus inside the nasal cavity may increase the nasal resistance, therefore, it is suggested that subjects blow their nose gently before a resistance measurement.[38]

Rhinomanometry may take at least 20 to 30 minutes. Anterior rhinomanometry is easy to perform. However, it measures one side of the nose at a time, and it cannot be used if a septal perforation exists. Posterior rhinomanometry overcomes this problem. However, it has the disadvantages that it requires training of the operator, and the possibility of variation in results due to movement of the soft palate and due to bulky equipment. Postnasal measurements also require a trained operator. In addition, manipulation of the nasal mucosa with a catheter may be a confounding factor.

Clinical Applications. The clinical use of rhinomanometry has been limited, but it is an excellent tool for research. It is relatively easy to do the measurements, and if anterior active rhinomanometry is performed, it does not take a long time.

Rhinomanometry can be used for measuring the change in resistance before and after the use of a decongestant in disease states such as allergic or nonallergic rhinitis. If the decongestant causes less than a 35% decrease in resistance, a structural cause may be considered as the reason for nasal blockage.

Rhinomanometry is commonly used in nasal challenge studies.[39,40] Evidence suggests that rhinomanometry is able to demonstrate the efficacy of treatment with medications such as intranasal corticosteroids or antihistamines.[41,42] Rhinomanometry may be used for detecting correlations between nasal resistance and sleep apnea,[43] the effect of nose dilators on nasal resistance,[44]

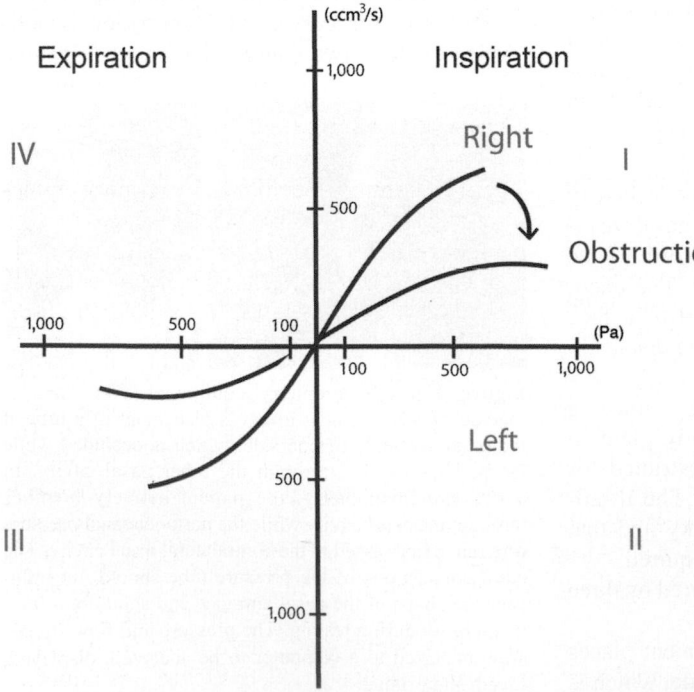

Figure 4 The pressure-flow graph of rhinomanometry. The airflow is recorded on the *y*-axis and pressure on the *x*-axis. In this graph, the curve on the right of the flow axis represents the change in inspiration, and the curve on the left is the change in expiration. The right nasal cavity is represented on the upper part of the pressure axis, and the left nasal cavity on the lower part of the pressure axis. The greater the nasal resistance (the ratio of transnasal pressure to airflow), the closer the curve will be to the pressure axis.

and the efficacy of surgery on the nasal valve or for septal deviation.[45]

Nasal Peak Flowmetry

Just as expiratory peak flow has been used as a measure of disease control in asthma, investigators have used nasal peak flow to assess upper airway function. The nasal peak flow rate provides a simple, cost-effective, reliable, and objective measure of airflow obstruction.

Several studies have evaluated the validity of this method in assessing nasal function. This test has high sensitivity and a variable correlation with patient symptoms and other objective measures of nasal blockage.[46–50] Nasal peak inspiratory flow appears to correlate better than does expiratory peak flow.

Equipment and Technique. Nasal peak flow may be measured as either inspiratory or expiratory. Nasal peak expiratory flow (NPEF) can be measured by use of a mini-Wright peak flow meter, which is equipped with an airtight face mask instead of a mouthpiece. The equipment is portable and useful for repeated examinations. During the procedure, the patient is told to hold the device horizontally and to ensure that the face mask forms an air-tight seal around the nose. The patient is instructed to inspire to maximal capacity while keeping the lips closed and to expire with maximal effort through the nose. The maximal flow rate is read from a scale in liters per minute. At least three readings should be obtained, and the highest should be recorded.

NIPF can be measured by use of Youlten peak nasal inspiratory flow meter attached to a face mask. During the procedure, the device is reset by returning the red cursor to its start position, and the patient is asked to exhale fully. The device is held horizontally. The face mask should form an air-tight seal around the nose (Figure 6). Different masks are available in a variety of sizes to suit different facial shapes. The patient is instructed to close the mouth and inhale forcefully through

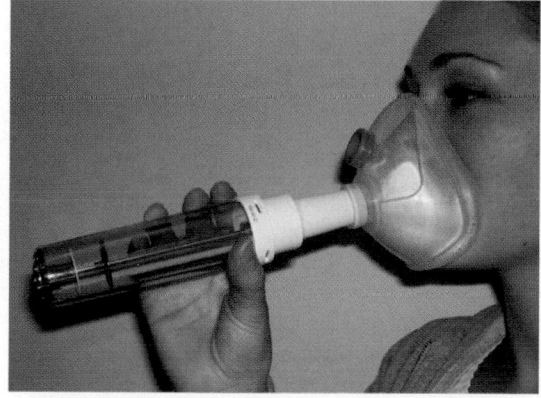

Figure 6 Nasal peak inspiratory peak flowmeter. This is a noninvasive, inexpensive method of measuring nasal patency. The device is held horizontally, and the mask should form an air-tight seal around the nose. The patient is instructed to close the mouth and inhale forcefully through the nose. This maneuver should be a short inspiratory action of about 1-second duration. The nasal inspiratory flow is recorded from the position of the red cursor on the scale.

his/her nose (sniff). This maneuver should be a short inspiratory action of about 1-second duration. The nasal inspiratory flow is recorded from the position of the red cursor on the scale. At least three readings should be obtained, and the highest should be recorded.

Interpretation. No standard limits have been defined for airflow measured by NPIF or NPEF. In a study of healthy subjects, participants who had no nasal symptoms had peak inspiratory nasal flows greater than 2.5 L/s.[51] NPIF and NPEF can be used as relative measurement in the same individual over time.[38]

Limitations. The major disadvantage of NPIF occurs when alar collapse is observed on forced inspiration. The disadvantage of NPEF is the possible expulsion of secretions in the mask on expiration. The limitation of both methods is that they are effort-dependent and assume normal function of the lower airways.[52] It has also been shown that, during NPIF testing in patients with partially blocked noses, the eustachian tube can be opened during maximal expiration, which results in discomfort and a decrease in expiratory effort.[53]

Furthermore, with NPIF, no information is obtained regarding the structure of the nose or the location of a nasal obstruction, as is the case with acoustic rhinometry. NPIF is not as sensitive as other objective methods of assessing nasal function. Small changes in airway resistance with low dose histamine challenge can be detected with rhinomanometry but not with NPIF.[50] At very low flow rates (<30 L/min), NPIF may not be possible, and an assessment should be made by means of other objective testing methods. Also, multiple repetitions of the testing procedure may cause a change in the blood content of nasal erectile tissue and result in changes in airway resistance over time.[9]

Clinical Applications. NPIF has better reproducibility than does NPEF, and it is the best-validated and best-studied peak flowmetry method. NPIF can be used in children, assuming adequate cooperation. A linear increase in NPIF occurs with age, height, and weight.[54]

There is a good correlation between NPIF and rhinomanometry when nasal patency is altered with allergen or histamine nasal challenge in the laboratory.[55,56] NPIF has been used in the evaluation of medical therapy for seasonal allergic rhinitis,[57,58] assessment of occupationally induced rhinitis,[59] evaluation of objective measures of septal or alar surgery[60,61] or as an outcome measure in nasal challenge testing.[62]

Rhinostereometry

Rhinostereometry is a noninvasive method of evaluation of the changes in the thickness of the nasal mucosa of the inferior turbinate. The method is relatively new and has been used in only a few centers.

Rhinostereometry has been used for correlating the subjective sensation of nasal stuffiness with measurements during histamine challenge in healthy subjects. The method has a high correlation with subjective symptom scores during a challenge,[63] but there is no significant correlation between acoustic rhinometry and rhinostereometry results during nasal cycling,[64] or in subjects who have vasomotor rhinitis.[65]

Equipment and Technique. The equipment consists of a surgical microscope placed on a micrometer table. The patient is seated and fixed to the measuring apparatus by a plastic tooth splint. The microscope has a small depth of focus, so that changes in the position of the mucosal surface on the medial side of the inferior turbinate are registered along a millimeter scale. Changes of 0.18 mm can be detected.

Limitations. Because it takes some time to fix the subject exactly to the measuring apparatus, rhinostereometry is a time-consuming method. Another limitation of the technique is that it is based on visual assessment by the investigator.

Applications. Rhinostereometry findings have been used as an outcome measure in studies evaluating the effect of nasal decongestants,[66] intranasal corticosteroids,[67] and nasal hyperreactivity.[68] This technique remains principally an experimental tool.[52]

Videoendoscopic Documentation

Videoendoscopic photodocumentation equipment is widely available in the practice of otolaryngology. A rigid or flexible endoscope is connected to a color camera (analog or digital). The operator passes the telescope, and a recording or print is made of the area of interest. This can be analyzed at a later date. The color and view may vary from visit to visit due to lighting, positioning, and the camera used.

The results compare favorably with other objective methods for nasal patency.[69] Digital image analysis of videoendoscopic images can be used in patients before and after nasal valve surgery.[70]

THE NOSE AS A FILTER

The pseudostratified columnar respiratory epithelium of the nasal mucosa is constantly exposed to pathogens and toxins. Mucociliary clearance is a crucial part of the defense against these agents and relies on the characteristics and dynamics of the cilia. These include the number of cells; the frequency, effectiveness, and coordination of ciliary beating the periciliary fluid and mucus.[71]

The nasal mucus blanket has two layers. The outer layer (gel phase) is relatively viscous and moves over the surface of the cilia, which are surrounded by a serous periciliary fluid layer (sol phase). The cilia beat in a coordinated fashion, but their beat frequency varies with physiologic and experimental conditions. In man, the frequency is normally about 15 to 20 Hz, which is equivalent to about 1,000 strokes per minute.[72]

The coordinated strokes of the cilia result in forward movement of the mucus layer at an average flow rate of 5 mm/min (with a range of 0.5 to 23.6 mm/min).[73]

Measurement of Mucociliary Clearance

The determination of nasal mucociliary clearance (NMCC) provides an integrated measure of ciliary function. The NMCC can be measured by use of traceable particles that may be soluble, such as saccharine, or insoluble, such as charcoal, or by use of radioisotopes.

Technique. The saccharin test is the most widely used method for in vivo assessment of NMCC. Before the beginning of the test, the patient is asked to blow the nose to remove excess secretions. A saccharin particle is placed on the medial surface of the inferior turbinate, at least 7 mm behind the anterior end to avoid the area of the mucosa where the cilia beat in an anterior direction.[74] The time from particle placement until the subject reports the first sensation of a sweet taste is measured and expressed as a clearance time. The same method can be utilized with substances like charcoal powder, which can be visualized in the nasopharynx and recorded with videoendoscopic photo documentation, if needed.

Another method for testing NMCC is by use of a radioisotope method. An insoluble radioisotope such as Tc99 is placed in the anterior part of the inferior turbinate and is followed and recorded with a gamma camera during its course to the nasopharynx. This method can provide an exact mucociliary transport rate in millimeters per minute. The NMCC in healthy adults is about 13 minutes (±3 minutes) for charcoal powder and 17 minutes (±5 minutes) for saccharine.[75] In healthy children, the times are 11 minutes (±3 minutes) for saccharine and 5 minutes (±6 minutes) for charcoal.

Limitations. Studies on cilial function in vitro have shown that the performance of cilia can be affected by factors, such as humidity, temperature, and pH. However, the confounding effect of these factors in vivo is unlikely to be very significant.[38]

The major limitation of NMCC is the fact that there is great interindividual and intraindividual variability in the values obtained, which may be due to normal physiologic factors or differences in testing methods. Evidence suggests that the rate in one nostril may be totally different from that in the other, possibly attributable to the nasal cycle.[76]

Clinical Applications. Studies on NMCC began in the 1880s. The radioisotope technique was described in 1964. Subsequently, several studies have been performed on the relationship of NMCC with physiologic and pathologic conditions of the nasal mucosa.

The effect of environmental pollutants on NMCC was also studied. Available data revealed no effect of ozone on NMCC,[77] but other pollutants such as cigarette smoke and sulfur oxides were found to impair NMCC.[78] The NMCC

changes in the presence of allergic rhinitis and rhinosinusitis[79] and after application of intranasal topical corticosteroids.[80,81]

THE NOSE AS A CONTRIBUTOR TO SUBJECTIVE WELL-BEING

Rhinitis has detrimental effects on the physiologic, physical, and social aspects of patients' lives and can decrease the quality of life.[82] For obtaining a complete measure of the health status of patients with rhinitis, health-related disease-specific quality of life assessments should be made in addition to clinical measurements.

Health-related quality of life (HRQOL) is defined as the functional effect of a disease and its management upon a patient, as perceived by the patient.[82] Health-related quality of life can be measured directly by use of generic or disease-specific instruments. To be useful, HRQOL instruments should have good psychometric performance characteristics.[83] These performance characteristics include validity, reliability, and responsiveness to change.

Generic questionnaires are designed to measure the burden of illness experienced by patients and can be used for comparison of the functional impairments caused by different health states. For example, quality of life in patients with allergic rhinitis can be compared to that of patients with asthma or other diseases. The disadvantage of generic questionnaires is that they lack sufficient depth to capture small but important changes that may occur in a particular disease either spontaneously or as the result of an intervention.[84] The most commonly used generic questionnaire for allergic rhinitis is the Medical Outcomes Survey Short Form-36 (SF-36).[85] This questionnaire includes a multiitem scale which assesses nine health concepts that can be combined into two primary functions, mental and physical. SF-36 is used extensively in a wide range of medical conditions including allergic rhinitis, acute rhinosinusitis, and nasal polyposis.[86–88]

Disease-specific questionnaires have developed because of the lack of depth of focus of the generic instruments.[82] They measure the extent of subjective disturbance of the particular disease symptoms and their emotional and practical effects.[85] Although several measures of HRQOL have been developed specifically for rhinitis and sinusitis, few have undergone psychometric testing. Psychometrically validated questionnaires include: the Rhinitis Quality of Life Questionnaire (RQLQ), the Sino-Nasal Outcome Test (SNOT-20), and the RhinoSinusitis Disability Index (RSDI). The RQLQ and SNOT-20 are the most commonly cited.

The RQLQ, developed by Juniper and Guyatt,[84] is one of the most frequently used disease-specific questionnaires validated to measure HRQOL. It has been shown to have strong measurement properties and has been translated into 28 languages and is used extensively throughout the world in clinical studies

and clinical practice. It has 28 items in seven domains (activity limitations, sleep impairment, nonnasal/eye symptoms, practical problems, nasal symptoms, eye symptoms, and emotional problems). The evaluation ranges from 0 (not troubled) to 6 (extremely troubled), and the overall quality of life is calculated from the mean values for the 28 items. Several versions of the RQLQ have been developed in an effort to increase its efficiency. These include but are not limited to an RQLQ with standardized activities, mini-RQLQ, RQLQ for children and adolescents, and RQLQ for nocturnal allergic rhinoconjunctivitis symptoms.[89]

The SNOT-20, developed by Piccirillo and colleagues,[90] is a valid outcome measure for patients with rhinosinusitis. It is a modification of the 31-item Rhinosinusitis Outcome Measure, and it contains 20 nose, sinus, and general items. To complete the questionnaire, patients indicate how much they are affected in each area in a five-point scale, and they identify the five most important items.

The RSDI, another measure of HRQOL, has been used both for patients with allergic disease and those with chronic nasal obstruction. The questionnaire has 30 items comprising three domains: physical, functional, and emotional. Each item is rated on a five-point Likert scale ranging from 0 (never) to 4 (always).[91]

All of these HRQOL questionnaires have limitations and are still being improved. Future developments will focus on shorter questionnaires and introduction of specific scales for specific purposes.[85,92]

THE NOSE AS SOURCE OF RESONANCE FOR THE VOICE

Resonance is the quality of voice that results from vibrations in the pharynx, oral cavity, and nasal cavity. The balance of sound vibration in these cavities determines whether the quality of speech and voice is perceived as normal or as abnormal. Speech resonance can be affected by several conditions related to the nose. Hypernasality is the presence of excessive nasal resonance during production of oral sounds and is due to velopharyngeal insufficiency. Hyponasality is the minimization or elimination of the nasal feature during production of nasal sounds due to obstruction in the nasal cavity or nasopharynx.

Nasometry is a method used for the clinical diagnosis of resonance disorders. It is available for use in a variety of languages. Nasometry uses a headset device worn by the patient which separates the oral and nasal cavities with a baffle plate. Acoustic energy during speech is collected by two microphones, one on the top and one on the bottom of the plate. The signal from each of the microphones is filtered and digitized by custom electronic modules. The instrument computes a ratio of the acoustic data acquired by the microphones.[93] This ratio is termed "nasalance" (the acoustic correlate of perceived nasality) and is displayed as percent, with higher percentages representing increased nasalance and lower percentages representing decreased nasalance.

Nasalance measures are commonly used in speech evaluation of patients. Acceptable levels of agreement between the measures provided by the nasometer (the nasalance score) and the auditory perceptual measure of hypernasality or hyponasality have been demonstrated in numerous studies.[94,95]

Although nasometry was originally designed to assess nasality of speech, it has been used in different studies for objective assessment of nasal obstruction. Nasal airway measurements with rhinomanometry do not allow for a distinction between contributions of the anterior and posterior components of the nasal airway resistance. Nasometry can be used for assessment of the effect of posterior nasal airway obstruction on speech resonance,[96] and for identifying patients who require adenoidectomy.[97] Active anterior rhinomanometry and nasometry show a significant association between the total nasal resistance and nasality measurements.[97] Nasal congestion and the action of nasal decongestant sprays affect the nasalance scores. Nasometry with and without a nasal decongestant may be used as a useful clinical tool for differentiating the localization of nasal obstruction.[96]

THE NOSE AS AIR CONDITIONER

Nasal inspiration is of significant importance for maintaining the internal milieu of the lungs. The air-conditioning capacity of the nose protects the lower airways from ambient conditions that can range in temperature from −42° to 48°C and from 0 to 100% relative humidity.[98,99] A healthy person may consume up to 350 kcal of heat and 400 mL of water per day to condition the inspired air under moderate environmental conditions.[100] In vivo measurements of nasally inspired air showed that most heating and humidification is accomplished in the space between the nasal valve and the middle turbinate.[101]

Evaluation of the conditioning capacity of the nose has been only investigational. A commonly performed technique for such evaluation is to insert a probe in the nasopharynx which is equipped with temperature and humidity sensors that continuously sample the air stream. The nasal air-conditioning capacity is calculated from measurements of the air stream temperature and of its relative humidity as it enters the nose and exits into the nasopharynx.[102] The conditioning capacity has been investigated in healthy noses as well as in those affected with inflammation and in patients undergoing surgical interventions. Natural and induced allergic challenges have been shown to increase the ability of the nose to condition inspired air.[103] Septal surgery improves nasal air conditioning.[104] Numerical simulation of nasal airflow and temperature in models of the human nose demonstrates disturbed air conditioning after septal perforation and turbinate resection.[105,106]

THE NOSE AS OLFACTORY ORGAN

The sense of smell is important for safety functions such as early detection of smoke, gas leaks, and numerous toxic agents as well as hedonic functions such as tasting foods and beverages and detecting of fragrances or aromas. Patients reporting olfactory impairment indicate that they have a high level of disability and have been found to have low quality-of-life measures.[107] Accurate assessment of olfactory dysfunction is of vital importance for management of this disability. Information on olfactory dysfunction and its assessment is available in Chapter 38, "Olfaction and Gustation."

CONCLUSIONS

Objective evaluation of nasal function can aid evidence-based medical treatment and research on disorders of the nasal airway. All of the tools for upper-airway evaluation, including objective airway measurement and validated patient questionnaires, have unique strengths and weaknesses that allow each technique to make a distinct contribution to the evaluation and ultimate treatment of patients with upper-airway diseases.

REFERENCES

1. Corey JP, Houser SM, Ng BA. Nasal congestion: A review of its etiology, evaluation and treatment. Ear Nose Throat J 2000;79:690–702.
2. Hilberg O. Objective measurement of nasal airway dimensions using acoustic rhinometry: Methodological and clinical aspects. Allergy 2002;57:5–39.
3. Patou J, De Smedt H, van Cauwenberge P, Bachert C. Pathophysiology of nasal obstruction and meta-analysis of early and late effects of levocetirizine. Clin Exp Allergy 2006;36:972–81.
4. Gungor A, Moinuddin R, Nelson RH, Corey JP. Detection of the nasal cycle with acoustic rhinometry: Techniques and applications. Otolaryngol Head Neck Surg 1999;120:238–47.
5. Flanagan P, Eccles R. Spontaneous changes of unilateral nasal airflow in man. A re-examination of the 'nasal cycle'. Acta Otolaryngol 1997;117:590–5.
6. Hasegawa M, Kern EB. The human nasal cycle. Mayo Clin Proc 1977;52:28–34.
7. Eccles R. Nasal airflow in health and disease. Acta Otolaryngol 2000;120:580–95.
8. Huang ZL, Ong KL, Goh SY, et al. Assessment of nasal cycle by acoustic rhinometry and rhinomanometry. Otolaryngol Head Neck Surg 2003;128:510–6.
9. Davis SS, Eccles R. Nasal congestion: Mechanisms, measurement and medications. Core information for the clinician. Clin Otolaryngol Allied Sci 2004;29:659–66.
10. Boyce JM, Eccles R. Assessment of subjective scales for selection of patients for nasal septal surgery. Clin Otolaryngol 2006;31:297–302.
11. Wang DY, Raza MT, Gordon BR. Control of nasal obstruction in perennial allergic rhinitis. Curr Opin Allergy Clin Immunol 2004;4:165–70.
12. Clarke JD, Hopkins ML, Eccles R. How good are patients at determining which side of the nose is more obstructed? A study on the limits of discrimination of the subjective assessment of unilateral nasal obstruction. Am J Rhinol 2006;20:20–4.
13. Hilberg O, Jackson AC, Swift DL, Pedersen OF. Acoustic rhinometry: Evaluation of nasal cavity geometry by acoustic reflection. J Appl Physiol 1989;66:295–303.
14. Mamikoglu B, Houser SM, Corey JP. An interpretation method for objective assessment of nasal congestion with acoustic rhinometry. Laryngoscope 2002;112:926–9.
15. Corey JP, Nalbone VP, Ng BA. Anatomic correlates of acoustic rhinometry as measured by rigid nasal endoscopy. Otolaryngol Head Neck Surg 1999;121:572–6.
16. Mamikoglu B, Houser S, Akbar I, et al. Acoustic rhinometry and computed tomography scans for the diagnosis of nasal septal deviation, with clinical correlation. Otolaryngol Head Neck Surg 2000;123:61–8.
17. Corey JP, Gungor A, Nelson R, et al. A comparison of the nasal cross-sectional areas and volumes obtained with acoustic rhinometry and magnetic resonance imaging. Otolaryngol Head Neck Surg 1997;117:349–54.
18. Wilson AM, Fowler SJ, Martin SW, et al. Evaluation of the importance of head and probe stabilisation in acoustic rhinometry. Rhinology 2001;39:93–7.
19. Cakmak O, Tarhan E, Coskun M, et al. Acoustic rhinometry: Accuracy and ability to detect changes in passage area at different locations in the nasal cavity. Ann Otol Rhinol Laryngol 2005;114:949–57.
20. Corey JP. Acoustic rhinometry: Should we be using it? Curr Opin Otolaryngol Head Neck Surg 2006;14:29–34.
21. Clement PA, Gordts F. Standardisation Committee on Objective Assessment of the Nasal Airway, IRS, and ERS. Consensus report on acoustic rhinometry and rhinomanometry. Rhinology 2005;43:169–79.
22. Corey JP, Gungor A, Nelson R, et al. Normative standards for nasal cross-sectional areas by race as measured by acoustic rhinometry. Otolaryngol Head Neck Surg 1998;119:389–93.
23. Jurlina M, Mladina R, Dawidowsky K, et al. Correlation between the minimal cross-sectional area of the nasal cavity and body surface area: Preliminary results in normal patients. Am J Rhinol 2002;16:209–13.
24. Tomkinson A, Eccles R. Comparison of the relative abilities of acoustic rhinometry, rhinomanometry and the visual analog scale in detecting change in the nasal cavity in a healthy adult population. Am J Rhinol 1996;10:161–5.
25. Larsson C, Millqvist E, Bende M. Relationship between subjective nasal stuffiness and nasal patency measured by acoustic rhinometry. Am J Rhinol 2001;15:403–5.
26. Grymer LF, Hilberg O, Elbrond O, Pederson OF. Acoustic rhinometry: Evaluation of the nasal cavity with septal deviations, before and after septoplasty. Laryngoscope 1989;99:1180–7.
27. Kemker B, Liu X, Gungor A, et al. Effect of nasal surgery on the nasal cavity as determined by acoustic rhinometry. Otolaryngol Head Neck Surg 1999;121:567–71.
28. Lueg EA, Irish JC, Roth Y, et al. An objective analysis of the impact of lateral rhinotomy and medial maxillectomy on nasal airway function. Laryngoscope 1998;108:1320–4.
29. Djupesland P, Kaastad E, Franzen G. Acoustic rhinometry in the evaluation of congenital choanal malformations. Int J Pediatr Otorhinolaryngol 1997;41:319–37.
30. Houser SM, Mamikoglu B, Aquino BF, et al. Acoustic rhinometry findings in patients with mild sleep apnea. Otolaryngol Head Neck Surg 2002;126:475–80.
31. Morris LG, Burschtin O, Lebowitz RA, et al. Nasal obstruction and sleep-disordered breathing: A study using acoustic rhinometry. Am J Rhinol 2005;19:33–9.
32. Morris LG, Setlur J, Burschtin OE, et al Acoustic rhinometry predicts tolerance of nasal continuous positive airway pressure: A pilot study. Am J Rhinol 2006;20:133–7.
33. Eccles R. Nasal airway resistance and nasal sensation of airflow. Rhinol Suppl 1992;14:86–90.
34. Passali D, Mezzedimi C, Passali GC, et al. The role of rhinomanometry, acoustic rhinometry, and mucociliary transport time in the assessment of nasal patency. Ear Nose Throat J 2000;79:397–400.
35. Kelly JT, Prasad AK, Wexler AS. Detailed flow patterns in the nasal cavity. J Appl Physiol 2000;89:323 37.
36. Cole P, Roithmann R, Roth Y, Chapnik JS. Measurement of airway patency. A manual for users of the Toronto systems and others interested in nasal patency measurement. Ann Otol Rhinol Laryngol Suppl 1997;171:1–23.
37. Morris S, Jawad MS, Eccles R. Relationships between vital capacity, height and nasal airway resistance in asymptomatic volunteers. Rhinology 1992;30:259–64.
38. Nathan RA, Eccles R, Howarth PH, et al. Objective monitoring of nasal patency and nasal physiology in rhinitis. J Allergy Clin Immunol 2005;115:S442–59.
39. Schwindt CD, Hutcheson PS, Leu SY, Dykewicz MS. Role of intradermal skin tests in the evaluation of clinically relevant respiratory allergy assessed using patient history and nasal challenges. Ann Allergy Asthma Immunol 2005;94:627–33.
40. Gosepath J, Amedee RG, Mann WJ. Nasal provocation testing as an international standard for evaluation of allergic and nonallergic rhinitis. Laryngoscope 2005;115:512–6.
41. Wilson AM, Sims EJ, Orr LC, et al. Effects of topical corticosteroid and combined mediator blockade on domiciliary and laboratory measurements of nasal function in seasonal allergic rhinitis. Ann Allergy Asthma Immunol 2001;87:344–9.
42. Bronsky EA, Dockhorn RJ, Meltzer EO, et al. Fluticasone propionate aqueous nasal spray compared with terfenadine

tablets in the treatment of seasonal allergic rhinitis. J Allergy Clin Immunol 1996;97:915–21.

43. Virkkula P, Maasilta P, Hytonen M, et al. Nasal obstruction and sleep-disordered breathing: The effect of supine body position on nasal measurements in snorers. Acta Otolaryngol 2003;123:648–54.

44. Peltonen LI, Vento SI, Simola M, Malmberg H. Effects of the nasal strip and dilator on nasal breathing—A study with healthy subjects. Rhinology 2004;42:122–5.

45. Calderon-Cuellar LT, Trujillo-Hernandez B, Vasquez C, et al. Modified mattress suture technique to correct anterior septal deviation. Plast Reconstr Surg 2004;114:1436–41.

46. Jose J, Ell SR. The association of subjective nasal patency with peak inspiratory nasal flow in a large healthy population. Clin Otolaryngol Allied Sci 2003;28:352–4.

47. Fairley JW, Durham LH, Ell SR. Correlation of subjective sensation of nasal patency with nasal inspiratory peak flow rate. Clin Otolaryngol Allied Sci 1993;18:19–22.

48. Panagou P, Loukides S, Tsipra S, et al. Evaluation of nasal patency: Comparison of patient and clinician assessments with rhinomanometry. Acta Otolaryngol 1998;118:847–51.

49. Sipila J, Suonpaa J, Silvoniemi P, Laippala P. Correlations between subjective sensation of nasal patency and rhinomanometry in both unilateral and total nasal assessment. ORL J Otorhinolaryngol Relat Spec 1995;57:260–3.

50. Clarke RW, Jones AS. The limitations of peak nasal flow measurement. Clin Otolaryngol Allied Sci. 1994;19:502–4.

51. Hooper RG. Forced inspiratory nasal flow-volume curves: A simple test of nasal airflow. Mayo Clin Proc 2001;76:990–4.

52. Lund VJ. Objective assessment of nasal obstruction. Otolaryngol Clin North Am 1989;22:279–90.

53. Wihl JA, Malm L. Rhinomanometry and nasal peak expiratory and inspiratory flow rate. Ann Allergy. 1988;61:50–5.

54. Prescott CA, Prescott KE. Peak nasal inspiratory flow measurement: An investigation in children. Int J Pediatr Otorhinolaryngol 1995;32:137–41.

55. Jones AS, Viani L, Phillips D, Charters P. The objective assessment of nasal patency. Clin Otolaryngol Allied Sci 1991;16:206–11.

56. Holmstrom M, Scadding GK, Lund VJ, Darby YC. Assessment of nasal obstruction. A comparison between rhinomanometry and nasal inspiratory peak flow. Rhinology 1990;28:191–6.

57. Fokkens WJ, Cserhati E, dos Santos JM, et al. Budesonide aqueous nasal spray is an effective treatment in children with perennial allergic rhinitis, with an onset of action within 12 hours. Ann Allergy Asthma Immunol 2002;89:279–84.

58. Jordana G, Dolovich J, Briscoe MP, et al. Intranasal fluticasone propionate versus loratadine in the treatment of adolescent patients with seasonal allergic rhinitis. J Allergy Clin Immunol 1996;97:588–95.

59. Miralles JC, Negro JM, Alonso JM, et al. Occupational rhinitis and bronchial asthma due to TBTU and HBTU sensitization. J Investig Allergol Clin Immunol 2003;13:133–4.

60. Marais J, Murray JA, Marshall I, et al. Minimal cross-sectional areas, nasal peak flow and patients' satisfaction in septoplasty and inferior turbinectomy. Rhinology 1994;32:145–7.

61. Di Somma EM, West SN, Wheatley JR, Amis TC. Nasal dilator strips increase maximum inspiratory flow via nasal wall stabilization. Laryngoscope 1999;109:780–4.

62. Terrien MH, Rahm F, Fellrath JM, Spertini F. Comparison of the effects of terfenadine with fexofenadine on nasal provocation tests with allergen. J Allergy Clin Immunol 1999;103:1025–30.

63. Graf P, Hallen H. Clinical and rhinostereometric assessment of nasal mucosal swelling during histamine challenge. Clin Otolaryngol Allied Sci 1996;21:72–5.

64. Moinuddin R, Mamikoglu B, Barkatullah S, Corey JP. Detection of the nasal cycle. Am J Rhinol 2001;15:35–9.

65. Hallen H, Graf P. Evaluation of rhinostereometry compared with acoustic rhinometry. Acta Otolaryngol 1999;119:921–4.

66. Grudemo H, Juto JE. Studies of spontaneous fluctuations in congestion and nasal mucosal microcirculation and the effects of oxymetazoline using rhinostereometry and micromanipulator guided laser Doppler flowmetry. Am J Rhinol 1999;13:1–6.

67. Hallen H, Enerdal J, Graf P. Fluticasone propionate nasal spray is more effective and has a faster onset of action than placebo in treatment of rhinitis medicamentosa. Clin Exp Allergy 1997;27:552–8.

68. Hallen H, Juto JE. A test for objective diagnosis of nasal hyperreactivity. Rhinology 1993;31:23–5.

69. Bellussi L, Ferrara Gorga A, Mezzedimi C. A new method for endoscopic evaluation in rhinology: Videocapture. Rhinology 2000;38:13–6.

70. Keck T, Leiacker R, Kuhnemann S, et al. Video-endoscopy and digital image analysis of the nasal valve area. Eur Arch Otorhinolaryngol 2006;263:675–9.

71. Stannard W, O'Callaghan C. Ciliary function and the role of cilia in clearance. J Aerosol Med 2006;19:110–5.

72. Illum L. Nasal clearance in health and disease. J Aerosol Med 2006;19:92–9.

73. Proctor DF, Andersen I. Nasal mucociliary function in normal man. Rhinology 1976;14:11–7.

74. Rusznak C, Devalia JL, Sapsford RJ, Davies RJ. Circadian rhythms in ciliary beat frequency of human bronchial epithelial cells, in vitro. Respir Med 1994;88:461–3.

75. Passali D, Bellussi L, Bianchini Ciampoli M, De Seta E. Experiences in the determination of nasal mucociliary transport time. Acta Otolaryngol 1984;97:319–23.

76. Nuutinen J. Asymmetry in the nasal mucociliary transport rate. Laryngoscope 1996;106:1424–8.

77. Gerrity TR, Bennett WD, Kehrl H, DeWitt PJ. Mucociliary clearance of inhaled particles measured at 2 h after ozone exposure in humans. J Appl Physiol 1993;74:2984–9.

78. Wolff RK. Effects of airborne pollutants on mucociliary clearance. Environ Health Perspect 1986;66:223–37.

79. Alho OP. Nasal airflow, mucociliary clearance, and sinus functioning during viral colds: Effects of allergic rhinitis and susceptibility to recurrent sinusitis. Am J Rhinol 2004;18:349–55.

80. Verret DJ, Marple BF. Effect of topical nasal steroid sprays on nasal mucosa and ciliary function. Curr Opin Otolaryngol Head Neck Surg 2005;13:14–8.

81. Naclerio RM, Baroody FM, Bidani N, et al. A comparison of nasal clearance after treatment of perennial allergic rhinitis with budesonide and mometasone. Otolaryngol Head Neck Surg 2003;128:220–7.

82. Juniper EF. Measuring health-related quality of life in rhinitis. J Allergy Clin Immunol 1997;99:S742–9.

83. Linder JA, Singer DE, Ancker M, Atlas SJ. Measures of health-related quality of life for adults with acute sinusitis. A systematic review. J Gen Intern Med 2003;18:390–401.

84. Juniper EF, Guyatt GH. Development and testing of a new measure of health status for clinical trials in rhinoconjunctivitis. Clin Exp Allergy 1991;21:77–83.

85. Kremer B. Quality of life scales in allergic rhinitis. Curr Opin Allergy Clin Immunol 2004;4:171–6.

86. Pasquali M, Baiardini I, Rogkakou A, et al. Levocetirizine in persistent allergic rhinitis and asthma: Effects on symptoms, quality of life and inflammatory parameters. Clin Exp Allergy 2006;36:1161–7.

87. Rechtweg JS, Moinuddin R, Houser SM, et al. Quality of life in treatment of acute rhinosinusitis with clarithromycin and amoxicillin/clavulanate. Laryngoscope 2004;114:806–10.

88. Radenne F, Lamblin C, Vandezande LM, et al. Quality of life in nasal polyposis. J Allergy Clin Immunol 1999;104:79–84.

89. Thompson AK, Juniper E, Meltzer EO. Quality of life in patients with allergic rhinitis. Ann Allergy Asthma Immunol 2000;85:338–47.

90. Piccirillo JF, Merritt MG, Jr, Richards ML. Psychometric and clinimetric validity of the 20-Item Sino-Nasal Outcome Test (SNOT-20). Otolaryngol Head Neck Surg 2002;126:41–7.

91. Benninger MS, Senior BA. The development of the Rhinosinusitis Disability Index. Arch Otolaryngol Head Neck Surg 1997;123:1175–9.

92. Gliklich RE, Metson R. Techniques for outcomes research in chronic sinusitis. Laryngoscope 1995;105:387–90.

93. Dalston RM. Acoustic assessment of the nasal airway. Cleft Palate Craniofac J 1992;29:520–6.

94. Dalston RM, Neiman GS, Gonzalez-Landa G. Nasometric sensitivity and specificity: A cross-dialect and cross-culture study. Cleft Palate Craniofac J 1993;30:285–91.

95. Dalston RM, Warren DW, Dalston ET. A preliminary investigation concerning the use of nasometry in identifying patients with hyponasality and/or nasal airway impairment. J Speech Hear Res 1991;34:11–8.

96. Pegoraro-Krook MI, Dutka-Souza JC, Williams WN, et al. Effect of nasal decongestion on nasalance measures. Cleft Palate Craniofac J 2006;43:289–94.

97. Parker AJ, Clarke PM, Dawes PJ, Maw AR. A comparison of active anterior rhinomanometry and nasometry in the objective assessment of nasal obstruction. Rhinology 1990;28:47–53.

98. Mercke U, Hakansson CH, Toremalm NG. The influence of temperature on mucociliary activity. Temperature range 20 degrees C-40 degrees C. Acta Otolaryngol 1974;78:444–50.

99. Wolf M, Naftali S, Schroter RC, Elad D. Air-conditioning characteristics of the human nose. J Laryngol Otol 2004;118:87–92.

100. Naftali S, Rosenfeld M, Wolf M, Elad D. The air-conditioning capacity of the human nose. Ann Biomed Eng 2005;33:545–53.

101. Keck T, Leiacker R, Riechelmann H, Rettinger G. Temperature profile in the nasal cavity. Laryngoscope 2000;110:651–4.

102. Rouadi P, Baroody FM, Abbott D, et al. A technique to measure the ability of the human nose to warm and humidify air. J Appl Physiol 1999;87:400–6.

103. Assanasen P, Baroody FM, Abbott DJ, et al. Natural and induced allergic responses increase the ability of the nose to warm and humidify air. J Allergy Clin Immunol 2000;106:1045–52.

104. Wiesmiller K, Keck T, Rettinger G, et al. Nasal air conditioning in patients before and after septoplasty with bilateral turbinoplasty. Laryngoscope 2006;116:890–4.

105. Lindemann J, Keck T, Wiesmiller KM, et al. Numerical simulation of intranasal air flow and temperature after resection of the turbinates. Rhinology 2005;43:24–8.

106. Pless D, Keck T, Wiesmiller KM, et al. Numerical simulation of airflow patterns and air temperature distribution during inspiration in a nose model with septal perforation. Am J Rhinol 2004;18:357–62.

107. Miwa T, Furukawa M, Tsukatani T, et al. Impact of olfactory impairment on quality of life and disability. Arch Otolaryngol Head Neck Surg 2001;127:497–503.

Imaging of the Nasal Cavities, Paranasal Sinuses, Nasopharynx, Orbits, Infratemporal Fossa, Pterygomaxillary Fissure and Base of Skull

Nafi Aygun, MD
David M. Yousem, MD, MBA

NASAL CAVITY, PARANASAL SINUSES, AND ANTERIOR SKULL BASE

Plain radiographs for the evaluation of the paranasal sinuses are infrequently used in modern practices largely due to the lack of detail they afford and the vast availability of computerized tomography (CT). CT, due to its exquisite ability to display and differentiate hypertrophic mucosa, bone, and air, is the current imaging standard for the evaluation of rhinosinusitis. CT data also serve to guide surgical navigation and planning. For the neoplastic diseases of the nasal cavity and paranasal sinuses, enhanced magnetic resonance imaging (MRI) is the preferred modality since it better resolves tumor from inflammatory changes and normal anatomic structures, although both CT and MRI are often required to determine the resectability of a particular tumor.

Multidetector (multislice) CT scanners are readily available in many imaging centers and provide a quick and comprehensive evaluation of the head and neck anatomy with thin slices that can be used to reconstruct images in any desired plane in two- and three-dimensional formats (Figure 1). CT uses ionizing radiation, which is a significant concern for the young and for patients who require repeated examinations. Various dose lowering strategies are employed by different manufacturers and radiologists, though the referring physicians should also bear responsibility since elimination of unnecessary CT examinations will have the greatest impact on radiation dose received by the patient. Iodinated contrast material administration is not necessary for rhinosinusitis and is reserved to assess neoplastic diseases and complications of acute sinusitis. High quality MRI examinations performed at 1.5 tesla and higher magnets are generally needed to demonstrate the intricate anatomy of the sinuses and skull base. In most cases gadolinium-based contrast material is required. T1 and T2 refer to nuclear magnetic resonance tissue relaxation times. Fat saturated postcontrast T1 weighted (T1W) images are of utmost importance in the evaluation of skull base and paranasal sinuses. Even T2 weighted (T2W) scans benefit from the

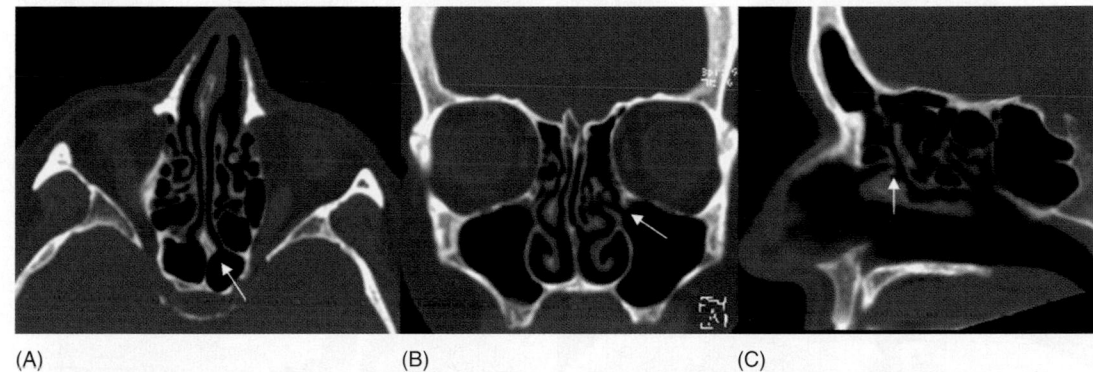

Figure 1 Paranasal sinus drainage pathways. Sphenoid ostium (A), maxillary infundibulum (B), and frontal recess (C) are demonstrated on the same patient. This study was obtained in the axial plane and multiplanar images were reconstructed without loss of image quality due to isotropic imaging afforded by multichannel CT scanner.

(A)   (B)   (C)

application of fat suppression technique, because otherwise inflammation (bright) and fat (bright) on fast spin echo T2 weighted images (T2WI) may be difficult to differentiate, particularly at the skull base or in the setting of abundant marrow fat, for example, petrous apex.

Rhinosinusitis

Rhinosinusitis refers to a continuum of inflammatory changes in the sinuses and nose regardless of etiology. Using a set of clinical criteria based on the type and duration of symptoms, five forms of rhinosinusitis are described; acute, subacute, chronic, recurrent acute, and acute exacerbation of chronic rhinosinusitis (CRS).[1] There is a large overlap of the imaging findings of these clinical entities, though certain findings such as air-fluid levels and osteitis are quite characteristic for acute and (CRS), respectively (Figure 2). Air-fluid levels are easily recognized on CT and their specificity in the appropriate clinical setting (absent recent instrumentation or irrigation) is 100% for acute inflammation of the sinus mucosa, though, the sensitivity of this finding is not known. In general, acute sinusitis is a clinical diagnosis, and imaging is not required unless there is a suspicion of a complication of acute sinusitis, which targets the orbit and/or the brain.

Through the natural dehiscences of the bony orbit and/or venous drainage, infection can gain access from the paranasal sinuses to the orbit; subperiosteal phlegmon and abscess may occur when the infection is limited by the periorbita which is a stout layer of connective tissue that lines the entire orbit and also contributes to the periosteum (Figure 3). Orbital cellulitis is a more advanced form of orbital infection and implies that the process has breached the periorbita. Orbital cellulitis can lead to permanent loss of vision due to increased intraorbital pressure and/or vascular thrombosis. Since the cavernous sinus receives venous drainage from the orbit, life-threatening complications, cavernous sinus thrombophlebitis and carotid artery vasculitis, may develop (Figure 4). Extension of infection to the intracranial compartment is the most feared complication of acute sinusitis and can present in the form of meningitis, epidural abscess, subdural empyema, sinus thrombosis, and brain abscess (Figure 5). Although contrast enhanced CT is appropriate for the evaluation of these complications, MRI is superior to CT, particularly for the intracranial extension of infection. Diffusion weighted imaging, a sequence well known for the ability to detect acute arterial or venous infarctions, is also relatively specific to infected collections and abscesses because of the limited water diffusivity within such lesions.

Pott puffy tumor consists of a subperiosteal abscess and osteomyelitis of the frontal bone secondary to direct spread of infection from the

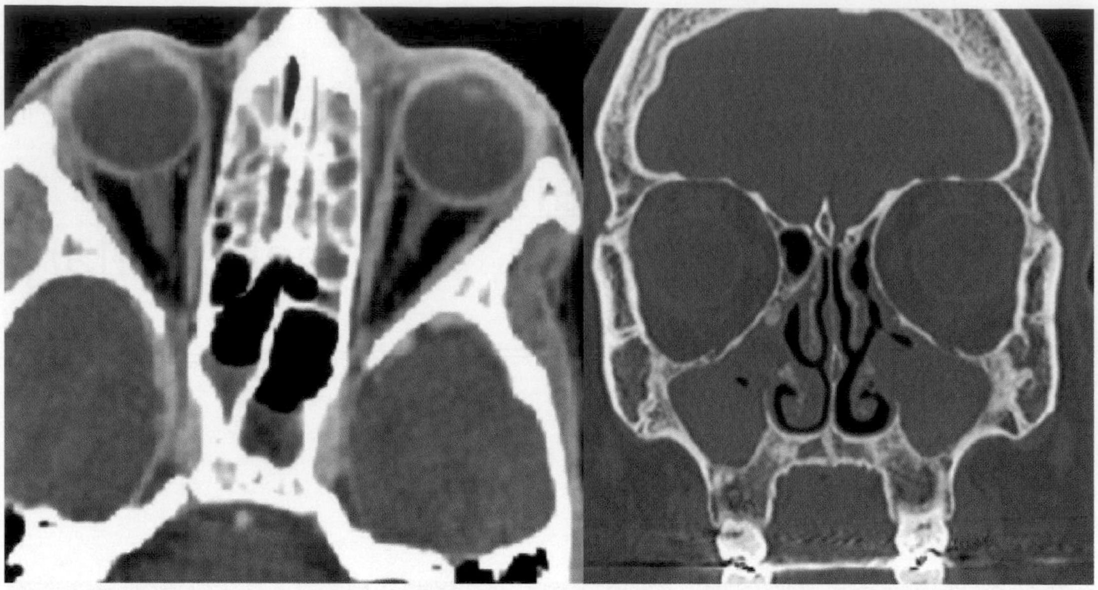

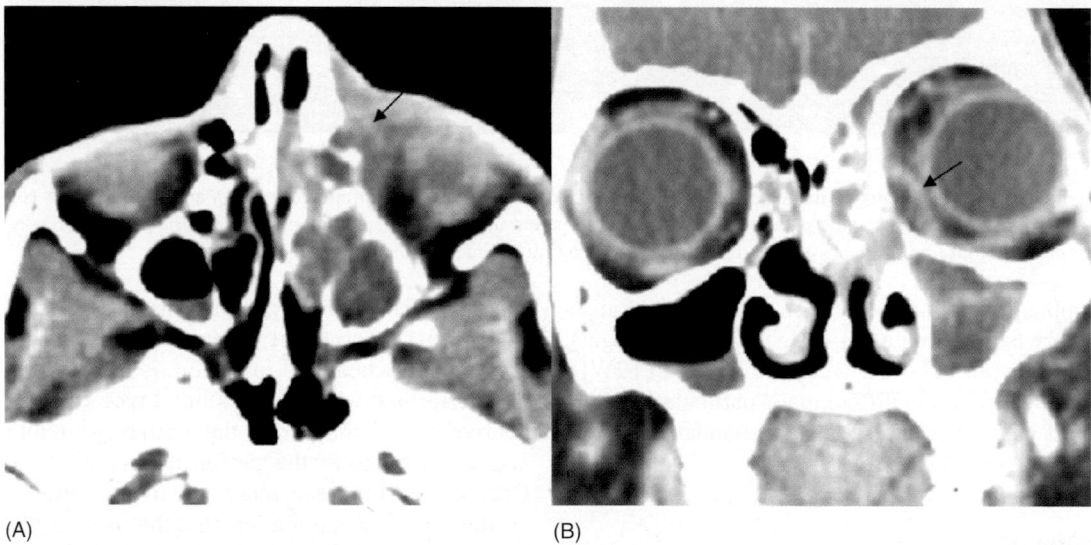

Figure 2 Acute and chronic sinusitis. (A) Acute sinusitis with air-fluid level is the hallmark of acute sinusitis. Note enhancing inflamed mucosa a nonenhancing central fluid in the ethmoid sinuses on this contrast-enhanced axial CT. (B) Chronic sinusitis. Coronal CT in a different patient shows marked bone thickening and opacification of the sinuses, characteristic for chronic sinusitis.

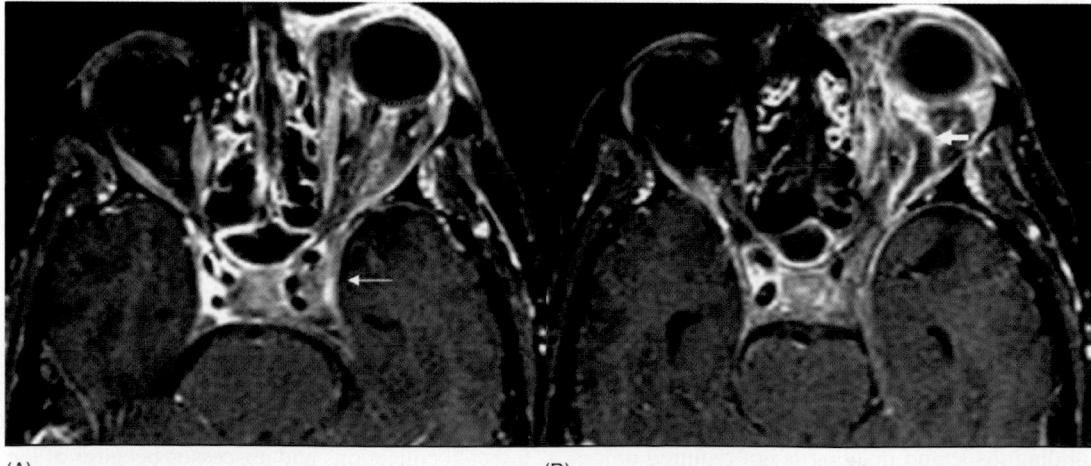

Figure 3 Subperiosteal abscess. Axial (A) and coronal (B) contrast enhanced CT demonstrates left ethmoid and maxillary opacification with a periorbital fluid collection that has an enhancing wall.

Figure 4 Cavernous sinus thrombophlebitis. Postcontrast, fat-suppressed axial MRI images (A and B) show a lack of enhancement in the left cavernous sinus (*arrow*) compared to the right. Lack of enhancement is also noted in the superior ophthalmic vein (*thick arrow*). There is proptosis and enhancement of the retrobulbar structures indicating edema and inflammation. This patient had a dental infection, which led to facial cellulitis and sinusitis (not shown).

frontal sinus to bone and adjacent soft tissue (Figure 6).

In the era of effective antibiotics these complications are quite uncommon and typically afflict young children and immunocompromised individuals.

Surveillance CT scans are often obtained in patients before bone marrow transplantation due to risk of aggressive transformation as they receive immunosuppressive medications. Surveillance scans are also performed in patients who are immune compromised in the setting of unexplained fevers. Careful evaluation of the orbits and soft tissues about the paranasal sinuses using both bone and soft tissue windows is crucial in these patients as mild soft tissue induration may be the only sign of early aggressive infection.

Chronic Rhinosinusitis. Mucosal thickening is the most common imaging finding of CRS, followed closely by mucus retention cysts. Polyp formation or polypoid mucosal thickening is found in approximately half of the patients with CRS and may indicate a different underlying pathological mechanism. Osteitis, presenting as thickening and/or sclerosis of the sinus walls on CT examinations, is indistinguishable from chronic osteomyelitis in histopathological examination but no microorganism has been demonstrated in humans in association with this condition. CT is an excellent modality to show the presence and extent of these changes in the mucosa and bone. Evaluation of the sinus drainage pathways and the ostiomeatal complex is crucial and best accomplished on either directly scanned or reconstructed (from axial) coronal CT images.

Although the majority of patients with CRS will present with a distribution of mucosal thickening that does not follow a blueprint, certain patterns can be delineated in CT examinations of some of the patients with CRS[2]: (1) opacification of the ostiomeatal complex is commonly associated with ipsilateral maxillary, frontal and anterior ethmoid disease (Figure 7), (2) opacification of the sphenoethmoid recess predicts ipsilateral sphenoid and posterior ethmoid sinus disease, (3) infundibular opacification is associated with ipsilateral maxillary sinus disease, (4) obliteration of the frontal recess leads to anterior ethmoid and frontal backfill sinusitis, and (5) sinonasal polyposis can be separated both clinically and radiographically from the ordinary mucosal thickening due to its mass effect and erosiveness and is associated with asthma, aspirin sensitivity, and eosinophilia.

The role of anatomic variations of the sinonasal cavity such as nasal septum deviation, concha bullosa, paradoxical middle turbinate, and Haller cells in the pathogenesis of CRS is debatable, but it is important to note these variations on imaging studies because of their potential implications on surgical management (Figure 8). The asymmetry of the ethmoid roof (fovea ethmoidalis), dehiscence of the lamina papyracea, Onodi cells, and position and integrity of the optic and carotid

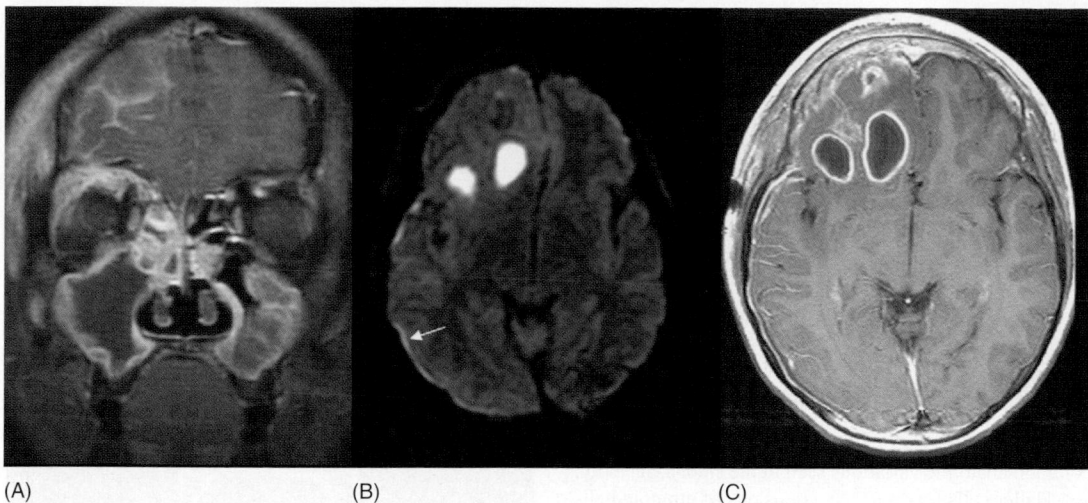

(A)   (B)   (C)

Figure 5 Complications of acute sinusitis. Bilateral maxillary and ethmoid sinusitis with extension of disease to the right extraconal orbit. Also note meningeal contrast enhancement in the right frontal lobe compatible with meningitis (A). In a different patient intraparenchymal abscesses and subdural empyema are seen. Diffusion weighted image (B) is very specific for infected collections. T1W postcontrast image (C) shows ring-enhancing abscesses, subdural empyema, and meningitis.

canals are particularly important since they are implicated in surgical complications.

Sinonasal secretions are relatively hypodense (10 to 25 Hounsfield unit [HU]) when they are acute and become hyperdense (30 to 60 HU) in the chronic stage due to increased protein content of the concentrated and desiccated secretions. At times the density may simulate that of acute blood. The varying protein content of sinus secretions in different stages of disease can be identified in CT based on density although this is rarely helpful from a diagnostic standpoint. Most secretions on MRI show low signal on T1 weighted image (T1WI) and high signal on T2WI similar to cerebrospinal fluid (CSF). However, the T1 signal increases and T2 signal decreases with increasing protein content of secretions up to 30% which can create confusing appearances mimicking soft tissue masses[3] (Figure 9). Sinus secretions with a protein concentration above 30% will show very dark signal on both T1WIs and T2WIs that resemble a normally pneumatized sinus.

Mucoceles are epithelium-lined mucus filled cavities arising from the paranasal sinuses that typically cause significant expansion of the sinus with thinning of the sinus walls. Obstruction of sinus drainage is responsible from mucocele formation. Bone thinning may be so severe that the wall of the sinus may not be perceptible on CT (Figure 10). Although generally benign, mucoceles can have serious complications when they extend to the brain and orbits. Mucoceles are most commonly seen in the frontal and ethmoid sinuses. The signal intensity of the mucocele on MRI will vary with the protein concentration but is frequently bright on T1WIs (Figure 11).

Retention cysts are generally asymptomatic and present as well-circumscribed cysts in the maxillary sinus, although they can occur in any of the paranasal sinuses.

It is presumed that the amount of mucosal hypertrophy demonstrated by CT is a good indicator of disease severity. Unfortunately, the correlation between symptom scores and CT scores is only modest.[4] The Lund-MacKay method (Table 1) is the most commonly used CT scoring system; a score of 0, 1, or 2 is given to each of the five anatomic sites on both sides for normal aeration, partial opacification and complete opacification, respectively.[5] The ostiomeatal unit receives 0 or 2, yielding a maximum score of 12 for one side.

Sinonasal polyposis is a distinct form of CRS. It is much more frequently associated with eosinophilia.[6] On CT and MRI, one can see expansion of the nasal cavity with smooth bony remodeling (Figure 12). In severe cases, expansion of the sinonasal cavity may involve the skull-base and orbits, mimicking a malignant tumor. The MRI signal characteristics of polyposis are quite variable due to varying protein concentration of the polyps and obstructed secretions. When the protein content is too high, polyposis may show no signal mimicking a normally pneumatized sinus, which may lead to underestimation of the extent of disease on MRI. CT, in these cases, is better able to demonstrate the extent of disease and bony changes.

Antrochoanal polyp is an inflammatory mass that arises from the maxillary sinus mucosa and emerges from the sinus via the natural or accessory ostium and extends into the nasopharynx through the choana. The imaging appearance is characteristic[7] (Figure 13). A well-defined mass with smooth remodeling of the maxillary ostium projecting into the nasal cavity or into the nasopharynx is seen.

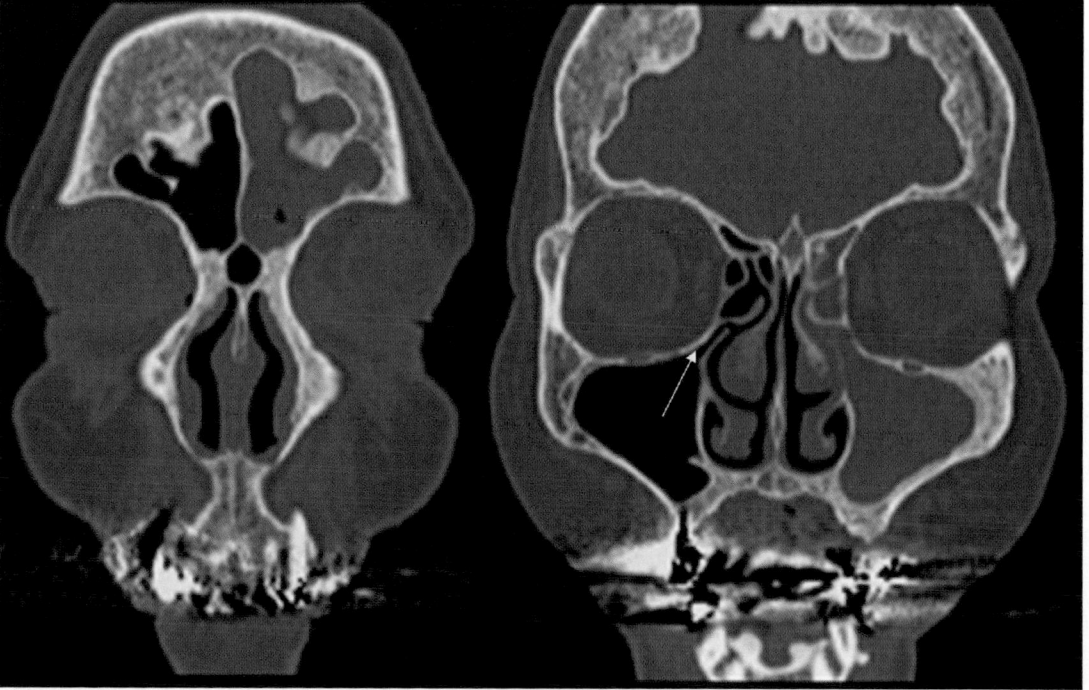

(A)   (B)

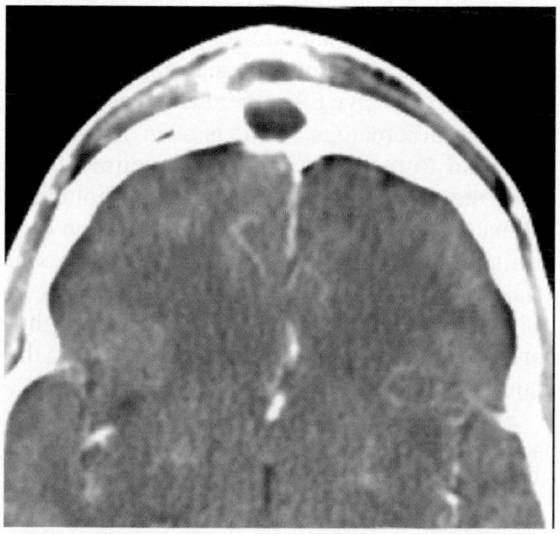

Figure 6 Pott puffy tumor. There is a ring-enhancing abscess in the frontal scalp with opacification of the adjacent frontal sinus on this axial contrast enhanced CT image.

Figure 7 Ostiomeatal unit obstruction. Coronal CT images (A and B) show opacification of the left OMU and ipsilateral maxillary, ethmoid, and frontal sinuses. The arrow points to the right maxillary infundibulum.

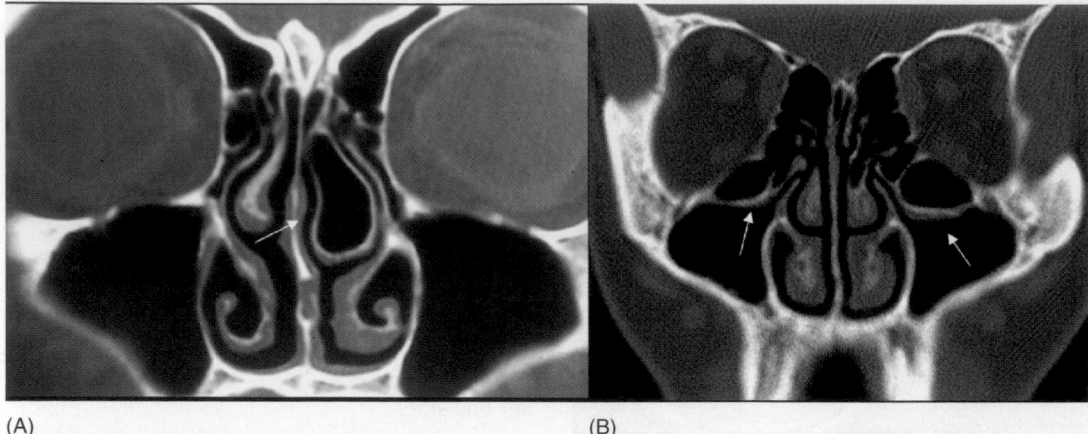

(A) (B)

Figure 8 (A) Concha bullosa and (B) Haller cells. Two of the common anatomic variations seen in the sinonasal cavity. Concha bullosa (*arrow*) refers to a pneumatized middle turbinate. Haller cells (*arrows*) are extensions of ethmoid cells into the maxillary sinuses.

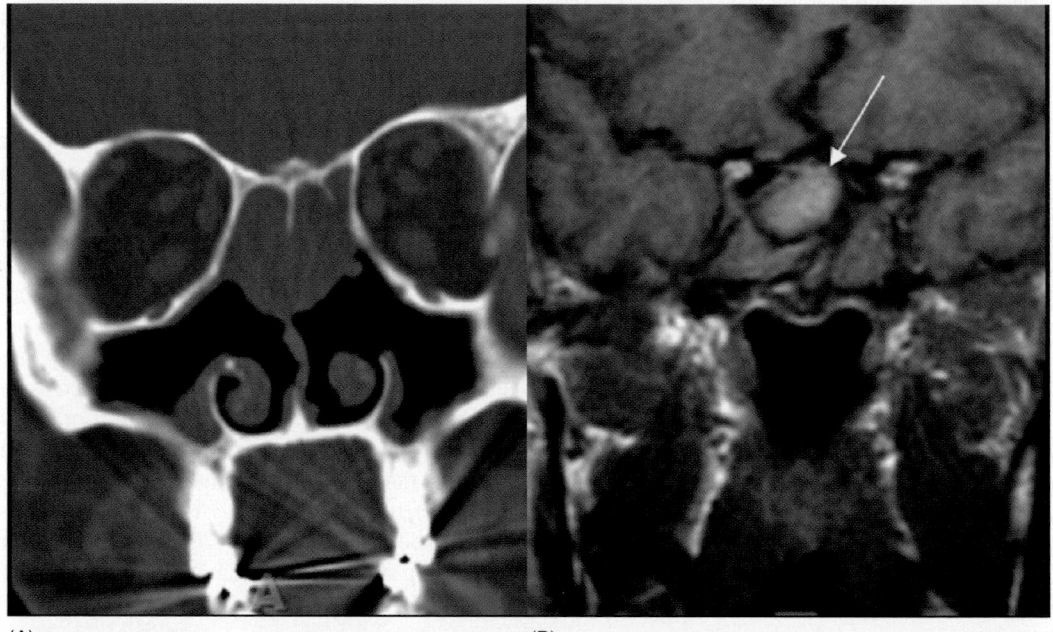

(A) (B)

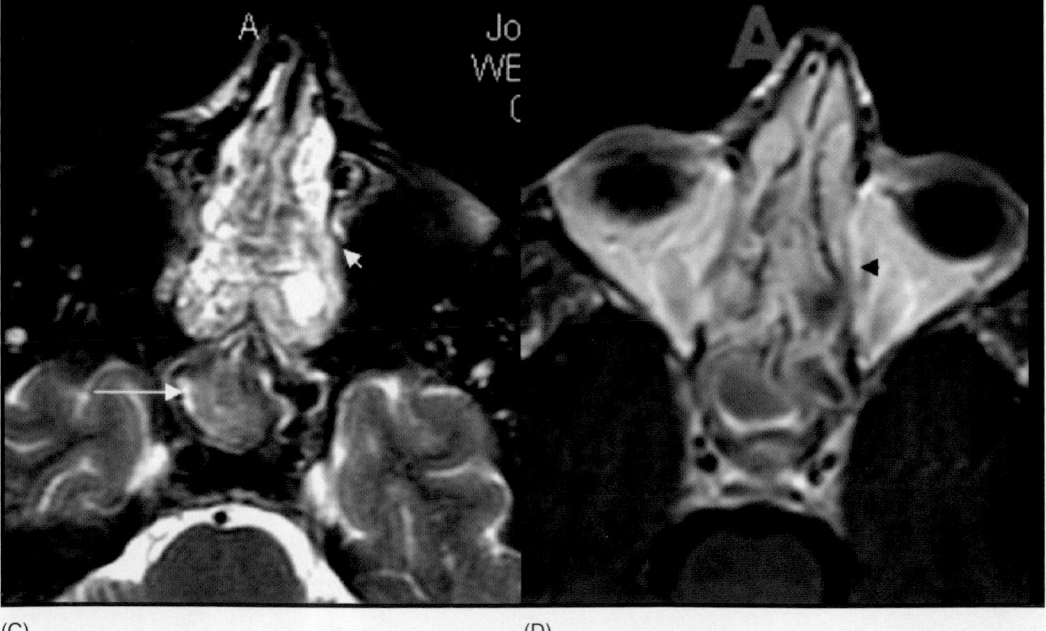

(C) (D)

Figure 9 Chronic sinusitis. (A) Coronal CT, (B) coronal T1W, (C) axial T2W, and (D) axial postcontrast T1W MRI. Mucosal hypertrophy in the bilateral ethmoid sinuses (*short arrows*) shows typical bright signal on T2WI and avid enhancement on postcontrast image. In the sphenoid sinus there is bright T1 signal, relatively dark T2 signal, and a lesser degree of enhancement indicating a high protein content of the obstructed secretions (*long arrows*). Patient had prior surgery.

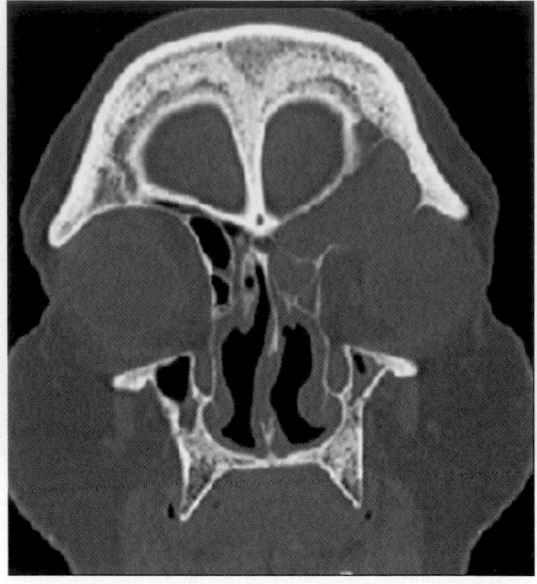

Figure 10 Mucocele of the left frontal sinus. Coronal CT image shows marked expansion of the left frontal sinus with thinning of the sinus walls. Mucocele extends into the orbit and displaces the globe. Along the inferolateral margin of the mucocele an ossified bone could not be seen.

Fungal Sinusitis

The role of fungi in the pathogenesis of CRS is under active investigation, and it is believed that at least some forms of fungal sinusitis (FS) and CRS may be within the same spectrum.[8] Nonetheless, there are five clinicopathologically distinct forms of FS in which the direct role of fungi has been established[9] (Table 2). It is important to note that saprophytic colonization of the sinonasal mucosa with fungi is very common in normal populations, and microbiological isolation of fungi from the mucosa is not enough to diagnose FS.

Acute invasive FS targets severely immuno-compromised patients and is often fatal despite treatment. Early CT findings are indistinguishable from ordinary rhinosinusitis and consist of mucosal thickening typically involving the nasal cavity.[10] Later, one can see edema in the soft tissues outside the sinuses. Intracranial and intraorbital extension of this process is often catastrophic (Figure 14). A high index of suspicion and biopsy of the middle turbinate are required to diagnose acute invasive FS in the treatable stage.

Chronic invasive FS, either the granulomatous or nongranulomatous form, is seen in patients with mild to moderate immune impairment and has a more protracted course. The radiological hallmarks of chronic invasive FS are bone erosion and intracranial extension of the process in a fashion similar to neoplasms and other mass lesions. Areas of increased CT attenuation within chronic invasive FS are demonstrated in the majority of patients.

Fungus ball, a benign form of FS, is a sinus mass packed with fungal hyphae that afflicts immunocompetent patients. On CT, it is seen as an opacified sinus with multiple foci of increased attenuation in the center of the sinus mass (Figure 15). Bone erosion is rare but expansion of the sinus can occur.

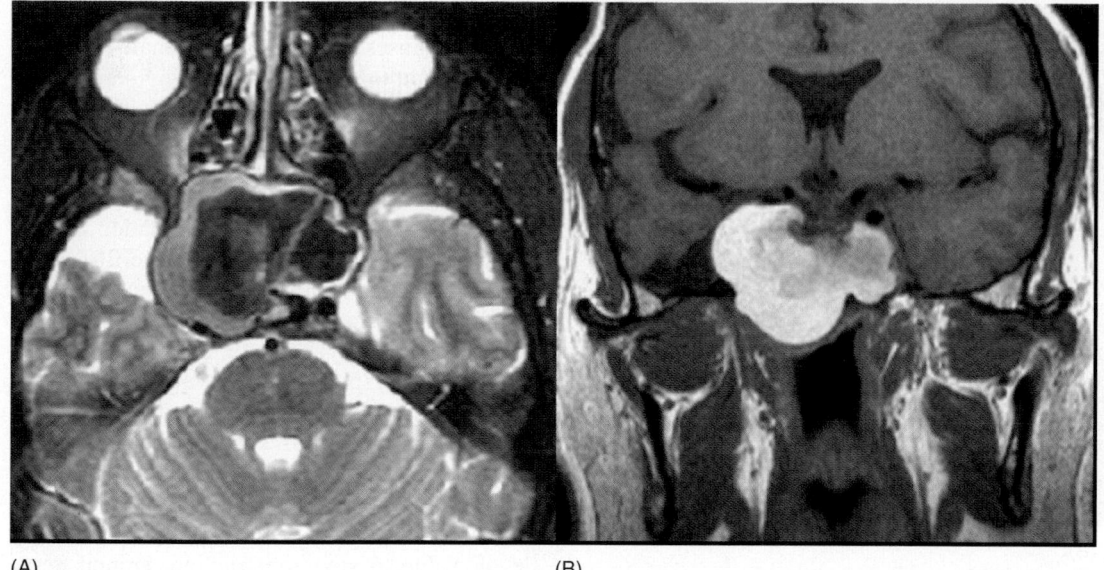

(A) (B)

Figure 11 Sphenoid mucocele. Axial T2W (A) and coronal T1W (B) images of the sphenoid sinus show marked expansion of the sinus on this patient with prior history of transsphenoidal pituitary surgery. Characteristic signal changes are seen due to desiccated secretions.

Allergic FS, an immunologically mediated hypersensitivity reaction, is perhaps a subgroup of CRS. The histopathological hallmark of this entity is infiltration of eosinophiles.[11] On CT, a central area of hyperattenuation is almost always seen within the sinus and corresponds to markedly decreased T2 signal on MRI (Figure 16). Expansion of the sinuses with bone remodeling or erosion is common in which case sinonasal tumors would be considered in the differential diagnosis.

Granulomatous Rhinosinusitis

Granulomatous inflammation of the paranasal mucosa is relatively rare, but it must be suspected in cases that are not responsive to therapy for CRS. Wegener granulomatosis (WG) is a systemic vasculitis that affects the kidneys, lungs, and upper respiratory system. It very commonly involves the upper respiratory tract, and approximately half of the patients present with rhinosinusitis before other systemic manifestations are apparent.[12] The radiologic manifestation of WG closely mimics that of CRS in the early stages since small granulomas in the mucosa are not resolved in imaging studies. Extensive osteitis,

diffuse mucosal thickening, nasal septum perforation, and erosion of the nasal turbinates are seen in the late stages of WG (Figure 17). Sarcoidosis is another systemic granulomatous disease that can involve the sinonasal cavity and erode the nasal septum. The radiographic appearance is more benign compared to WG and often indistinguishable from CRS since sarcoidosis rarely causes destructive changes. In previous generations, leprosy, tuberculosis, and syphilis would have been more commonly seen causes of granulomatous sinusitis and "saddle nose deformity."

Exposure to environmental toxins such as beryllium and chromate salts has been implicated in granulomatous sinusitis. Cocaine use may also lead to an erosive nasal septum process.

Cephaloceles and Cerebrospinal Fluid Leaks

Cephaloceles are meningeal or brain hernias that occur through a bony defect present at the skull base. Depending on the location of the defect and cephalocele sac, occipital cephaloceles, frontoethmoid cephaloceles (FECs), and basal cephaloceles (BCs) are defined. The congenital occipital cephaloceles are much more common but they are associated with neural tube closure defects and pathogenetically different from the FEC and BC. FECs are divided into nasofrontal, nasoethmoid, and nasoorbital varieties based on their morphology. Likewise, BCs are described in terms of its relationship to the sphenoid and ethmoid bones. Most FECs are apparent at birth and associated with a myriad of craniofacial deformities. BCs and some FECs may stay asymptomatic for years and present as a sinonasal or nasopharyngeal mass in adulthood. Meningoceles contain only meninges and CSF, whereas, encephaloceles contain brain tissue in addition to dural covering and CSF. Identification of the contents of a cephalocele is critically important since some, particularly BCs, can contain functioning brain tissue such as the optic chiasm and pituitary. In rare cases, vessels can be found in or near the vicinity of the cephalocele sac. The contents of the sac can be best evaluated with MRI, whereas, CT may permit better

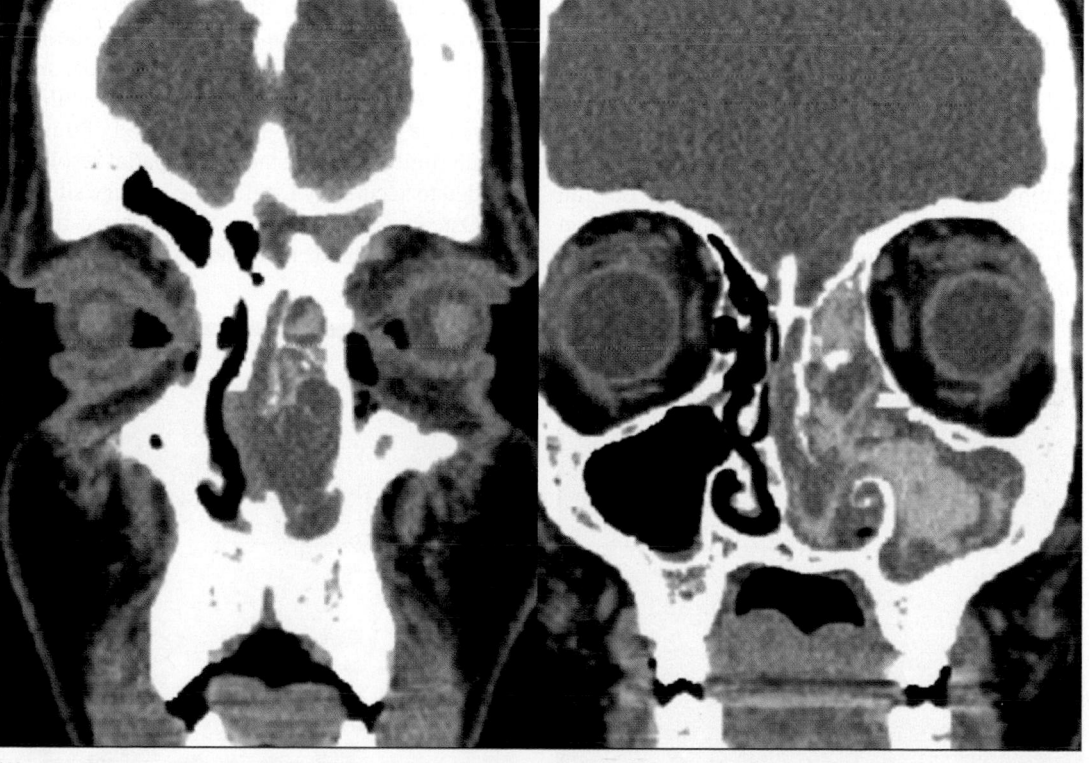

(A) (B)

Figure 12 Sinonasal polyposis. Coronal CT images (A and B) show soft tissue attenuation masses in the nasal cavity representing inflammatory polyps. Remodeling of the nasal septum and medial wall of the left maxillary sinus is noted. High attenuation in the central parts of the ethmoid and maxillary sinuses is due to desiccated secretions. This type of high attenuation may be seen in allergic fungal sinusitis but this was histopathologically ruled out.

Table 1 Lund-McKay Radiologic Sinusitis Grading System			
	Clear	Partial Opacification	Complete Opacification
Maxillary	0	1	2
Anterior ethmoid	0	1	2
Posterior ethmoid	0	1	2
Sphenoid	0	1	2
Frontal	0	1	2
Ostiomeatal complex	0	—	2

Total possible score for one side is 12.

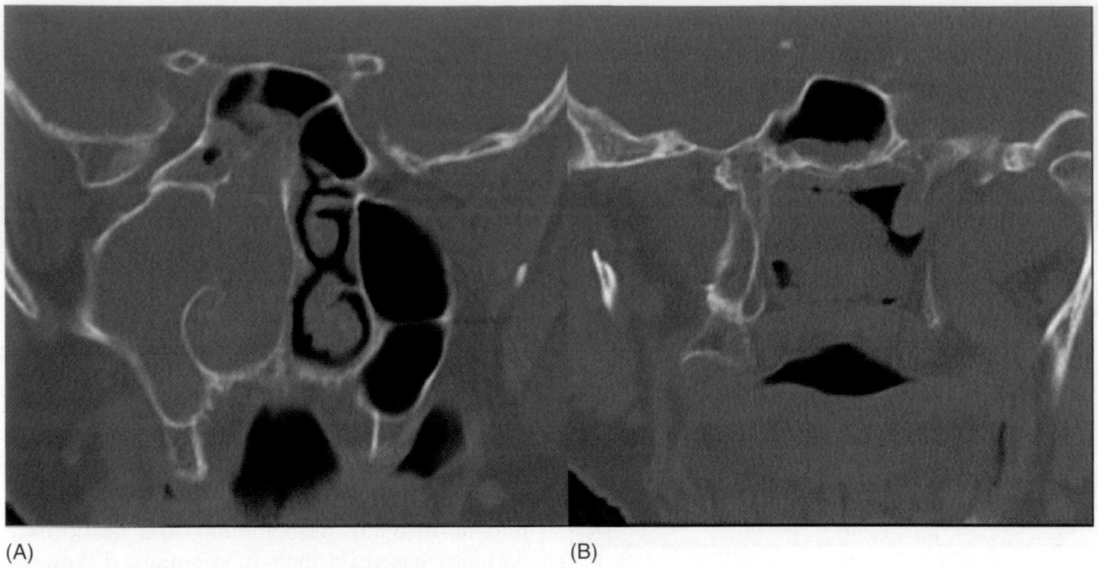

Figure 13 and Figure 14 CT images

Figure 13 Antrochoanal polyp. Coronal CT images through the paranasal sinuses (A) and nasopharynx (B) demonstrate expansion and remodeling of the maxillary infundibulum due to a large inflammatory polyp that fills the maxillary sinus and nasal cavity and extends the nasopharynx.

Table 2 Types of Fungal Rhinosinusitis

Invasive
  Acute
  Chronic granulomatous
  Chronic nongranulomatous
Noninvasive
  Fungus ball
  Allergic fungal sinusitis

anatomic classification due to its exquisite ability to demonstrate the three-dimensional anatomy of the skull base (Figure 18).

Acquired cephaloceles can occur as a result of head trauma and surgery. They are now more common than congenital ones because of the marked increase in functional endoscopic sinus surgery and prevalence of head injuries in motor vehicular collisions. These patients typically present with symptoms related to CSF leak and recurrent meningitis. Actual sac formation is rare but the bony defect is demonstrated with high-resolution CT in the majority of patients. CSF leak may be observed during endoscopic evaluation and is augmented if fluorescein is placed intrathecally,

although the use of intrathecal fluorescein is not approved in the United States by the Food and Drug Administration. Positive demonstration of a CSF leak from a skull base defect can be accomplished with CT-cisternogram, which involves intrathecal administration of iohexol followed by high resolution CT in the prone position (Figure 19). In nuclear medicine departments, CSF leak can be demonstrated by intrathecal administration of a radionuclide (usually indium diethylenetriamine pentaacetic acid (DTPA)) and imaging of the skull with a gamma camera. As an adjunct, several pledgets are placed in the nasal cavity before administration of radionuclide and several hours later, radioactivity on these pledgets is counted to predict the approximate location of the leak. While the nuclear medicine method is more sensitive than CT-cisternogram because of its ability to survey the patient over a longer period of time for an intermittent leak, it lacks the spatial resolution needed to accurately localize the leakage site.

Osteomas are common benign bone tumors and are often found incidentally in the paranasal

sinuses. They are more frequent in the frontal and ethmoid sinuses and are usually small. They can become symptomatic by obstructing sinus drainage or indenting the extraocular muscles in which case surgical treatment may be warranted and can be accomplished endoscopically in the majority of the cases. Osteomas appear as rounded, bone density mass lesions on CT examination and the diagnosis is straightforward (Figure 20). They appear as signal voids on MRI scans and may simulate an aerated sinus, leading to under diagnosis with MR.[13]

Fibrous dysplasia is a relatively common tumor-like condition characterized by abnormal proliferation of fibrous tissue and disorganized bone. It most commonly affects the craniofacial bones and is seen as an incidental finding on CT examinations of the sinuses. Symptoms may develop due to sinus obstruction, cranial nerve compromise, and mass effect. CT shows characteristic ground-glass appearance and local bone expansion allowing differentiation from osteoblastic metastasis in most cases (Figure 20). On MRI, fibrous dysplasia may have heterogeneous appearance and show enhancement with gadolinium based contrast material.

Ossifying fibroma can present in the nasal cavity and sinuses as a large soft tissue mass with mature bone formation within. Bone remodeling due to expansion of the sinonasal cavity is common.

Papillomas develop from the ectodermally derived Schneiderian mucosa of the sinonasal tract. Three patterns of Schneiderian papilloma are recognized microscopically: fungiform papilloma, cylindrical-cell papilloma, and inverted papilloma (IP). IPs typically arise from the lateral nasal wall, nasal septum, or the maxillary sinus and grow into the nasal cavity. Extension to the skull base and intracranial compartment is not uncommon. High rate of recurrence and malignant transformation or coexistent squamous cell carcinoma are the hallmarks of this tumor and necessitate a total surgical excision. The incidence of malignant transformation is a matter

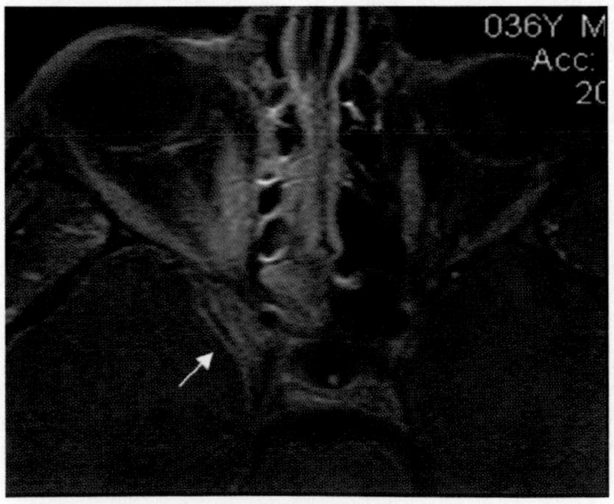

Figure 14 Acute invasive fungal sinusitis. Axial T1W fat suppressed contrast enhanced image shows right ethmoid sinusitis with orbital and intracranial (*arrow*) extension on this patient with leukemia who is severely neutropenic.

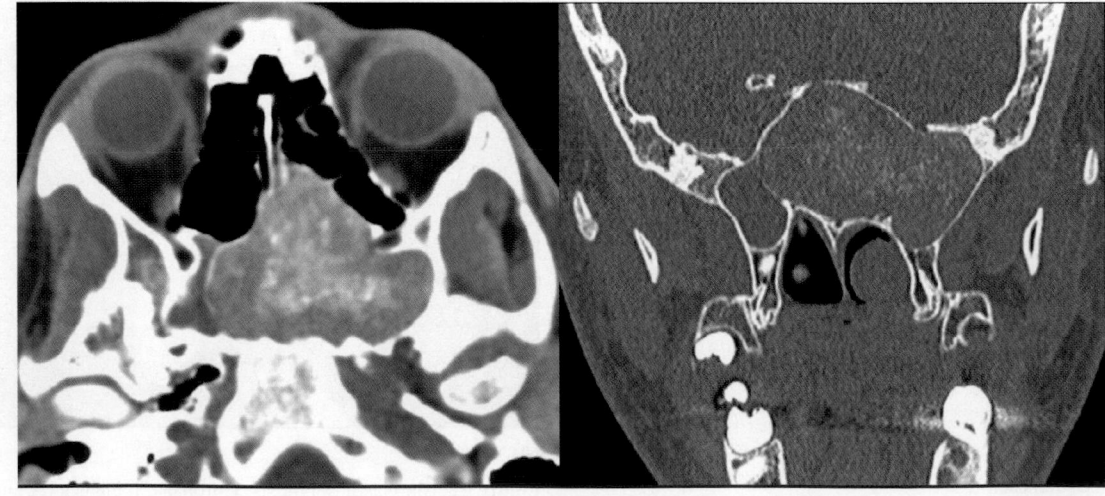

(A)   (B)

Figure 15 Fungus ball. Axial (A) and coronal (B) CT shows an expansile mass in the sphenoid sinus with small calcifications, characteristic of fungus ball.

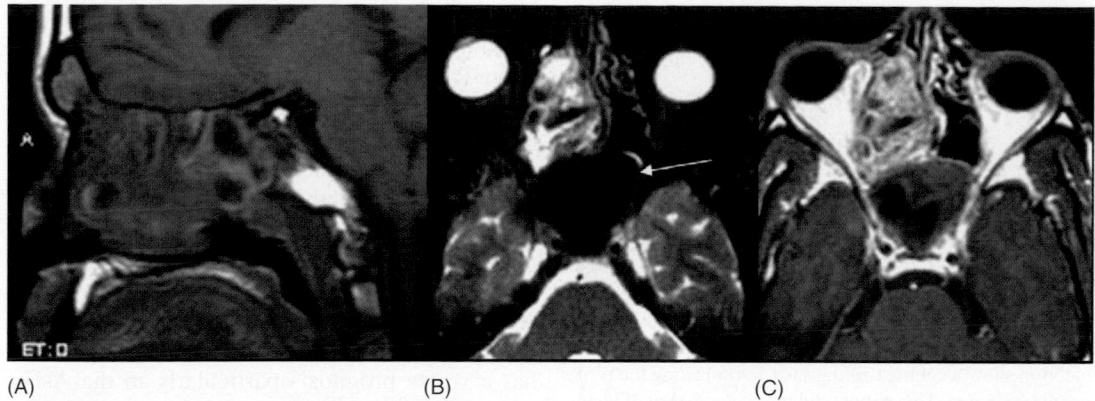

(A)   (B)   (C)

Figure 16 Allergic fungal sinusitis. On the sagittal T1WI (A) there is opacification of the right ethmoid air cells and the sphenoid sinus with a heterogenous signal material. Axial T2WI (B) shows expansion of the sphenoid and ethmoid sinuses. Note lack of signal in the sphenoid sinus resembling a normally pneumatized sinus. (C) Contrast enhanced axial T1WI demonstrates heterogenous enhancement of the sinus contents. Large amount of eosinophilic mucus was aspirated from the sphenoid sinus.

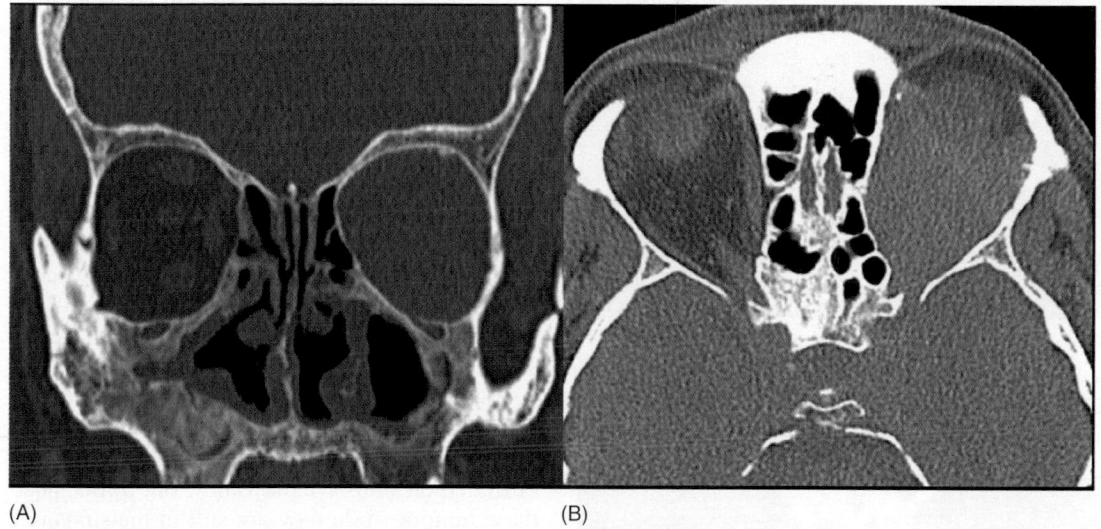

(A)   (B)

Figure 17 Wegener granulomatosis. Coronal CT (A) of the sinuses shows marked thickening of the sinus wall with destruction of the lateral nasal walls and mucosal thickening, typical for WG, although these findings can be secondary to ordinary chronic rhinosinusitis as well. Axial CT image of the orbit on the same patient (B) demonstrates a large intraconal mass engulfing the optic chiasm, an uncommon manifestation of Wegener granulomatosis.

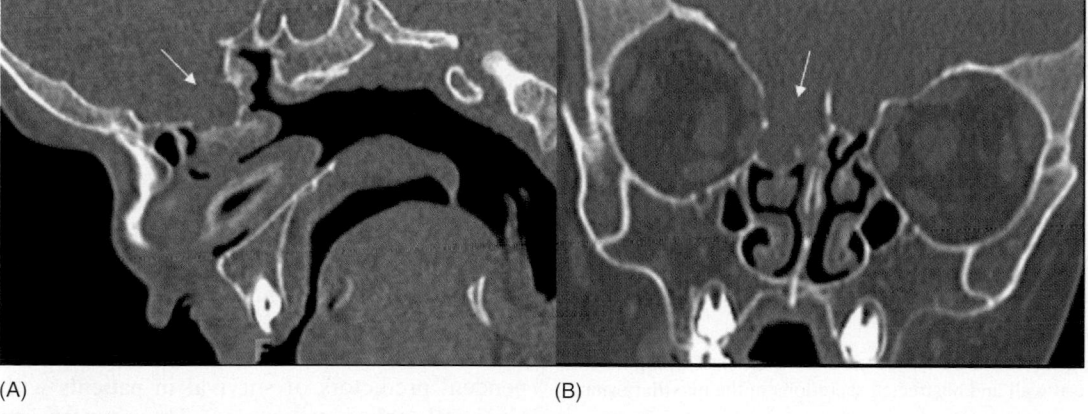

(A)   (B)

Figure 18 Nasoethmoid encephalocele. Sagittal (A) and coronal (B) CT images generated from axially obtained images reveal a defect of the cribriform plate and a cephalocele sac (*arrow*). MRI is better able to show the contents of the encephalocele.

of debate, but it is apparent that a substantial group of these patients harbor malignancy at first presentation, which escapes diagnosis. Elevated levels of epidermal growth factor receptor and transforming growth factor-alpha have been demonstrated in tumors with IP and squamous cell cancer (SCC) compared to IP.[14] In addition certain histopathologic features such as increase

in hyperkeratosis, presence of squamous epithelial hyperplasia, and increase in mitotic index are predictive of recurrence.[15] The presurgical imaging evaluation is crucial and requires both CT and MRI if the tumor is outside the sinonasal cavity.[16] CT, in addition to a sinonasal soft tissue mass, may show calcifications within the tumor and remodeling of the adjacent bones (Figure 21).

On MR this tumor will show low signal on T2WI and enhancement. Solid "fungiform" and "cerebriform" patterns of enhancement have been described with this entity and may suggest the diagnosis.[17] Due to high rate of recurrence and malignant transformation, careful follow-up is essential and often requires imaging for areas not amenable to endoscopic evaluation.[18]

A myriad of benign tumors including but not limited to schwannoma, neurofibroma, hemangioma, pleomorphic adenoma, plasmocytoma, meningioma, chordoma, giant cell tumor, and giant cell reparative granuloma has been reported to arise from the sinonasal tract. Meningiomas of the olfactory groove and planum sphenoidale involve the anterior skull base. These tumors are usually confined to the intracranial compartment. Extension into the sinuses is not common but occurs (Figure 22). Some of these tumors may be amenable to endoscopic surgery. Meningiomas often cause thickening or blistering or osteolysis of the adjacent bone, which may be reactive in nature or due to intraosseous extension.

Primary malignant tumors of the sinonasal cavity usually present late in the disease course since they do not elicit symptoms in the early stages. Serendipitous diagnosis of an asymptomatic sinonasal cancer is rare. Presenting symptoms are generally secondary to invasion of the skull base, orbit, pterygopalatine fossa (PPF), masticator space, and perineural spread (PNS) and include diplopia, epiphora, malocclusion, trismus, neck mass, and facial numbness.

SCC arising from the sinonasal epithelium accounts for the majority of malignant tumors. Most SCCs of the sinonasal tract arise from the nasal cavity and ethmoid sinuses with frequent secondary involvement of the maxillary sinus. Adenocarcinomas arising from the seromucinous glands interspersed in the sinonasal mucosa are the second most common and make up 10 to 30% of the malignant tumors of this region. They favor the ethmoid sinuses and have been associated with wood dust exposure. Adenoid cystic carcinoma and mucoepidermoid carcinoma are the two most common types of minor salivary gland (MSG) carcinomas. The feature most characteristic of adenoid cystic carcinoma is perineural growth. Melanomas are responsible for approximately 5% of the sinonasal malignant tumors and usually develop in the nasal septum, lateral nasal wall, or less frequently in the turbinates. They are readily diagnosed clinically because of their discoloration, but may have a wide variety of signal intensities on MRI scans depending upon the content of melanin (which leads to bright signal on T1WI) and/or hemorrhage.

Olfactory neuroblastoma (ONB) (esthesioneuroblastoma) and sinonasal undifferentiated carcinoma (SNUC) are rare tumors of the sinonasal cavity. SNUCs generally have a dismal prognosis and show a very rapid rate of growth and invade the orbit and skull base whereas ONBs have a much more favorable prognosis.[19,20] ONBs may be associated with intracranial cysts and preferentially involve the anterior ethmoid/nasal cavity

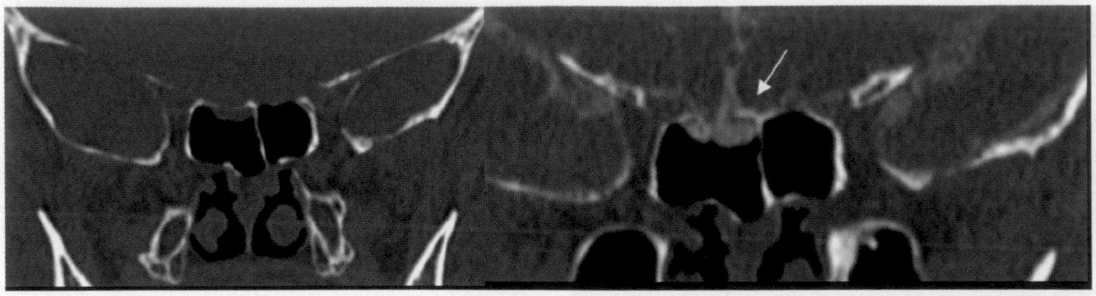

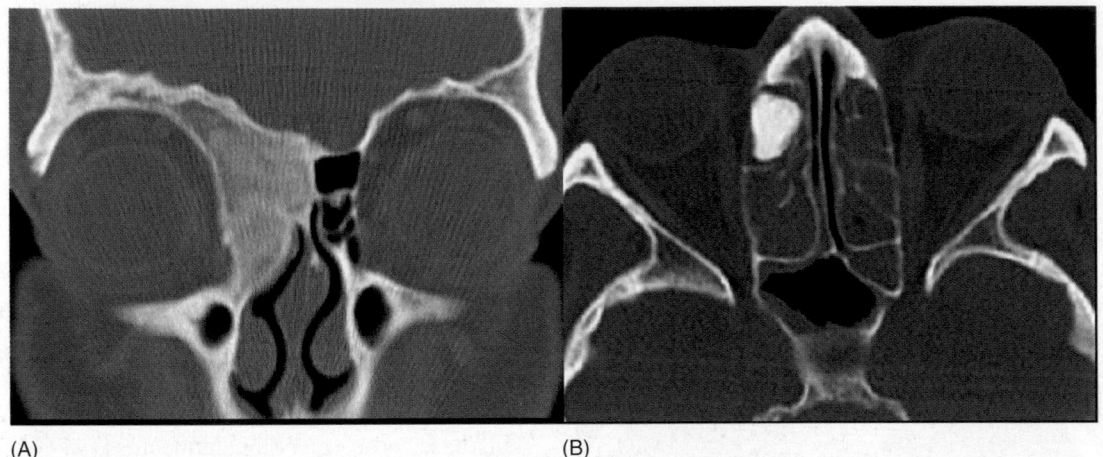

Figure 19 Spontaneous CSF leak demonstrated by CT-cisternogram. Coronal CT images through the sphenoid sinus before (A) and after (B) intrathecal iodinated contrast material injection show a contrast-filling sac (*arrow*) along the roof of the sinus, which appears as a focal mucosal thickening on noncontrast image. This patient did not have history of head trauma or surgery.

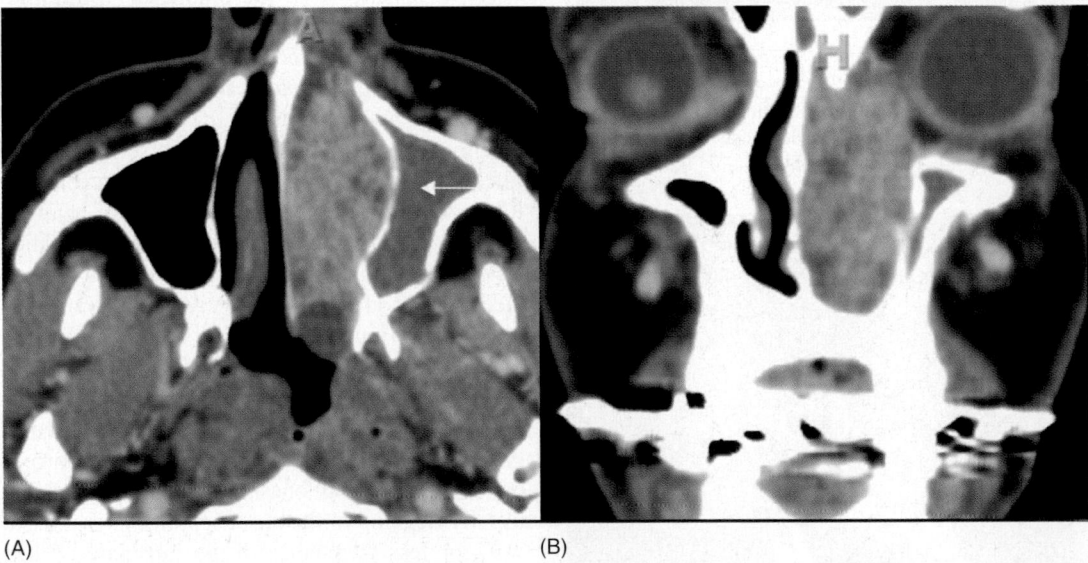

Figure 20 (A) Fibrous dysplasia and (B) osteoma. Bony expansion and ground glass appearance in the right frontal and ethmoid region; typical features of fibrous dysplasia. A right ethmoid osteoma and ethmoid sinusitis is seen on part (B). Note the lack of bone expansion and much higher attenuation due to osteoid formation.

Figure 21 Inverted papilloma. Contrast-enhanced axial (A) and coronal (B) CT show an enhancing mass filling the left nasal cavity with smooth remodeling (*arrow*) of the lateral nasal wall and obstructed secretions in the maxillary sinus. Mass marginally extends into the lacrimal fossa.

region. SNUCs have been reported to have the highest rate of dural/subarachnoid dissemination of sinonasal malignancies. Sarcomas may vary in imaging characteristics depending upon their osseous (osteosarcoma), chondroid (chondrosarcoma), or soft tissue (rhabdomyosarcoma or fibrosarcoma) matrix.

Malignant tumors of the sinonasal cavity with undifferentiated small round blue cells are rare and pose a significant challenge for the pathologist since defining the histological origin of these tumors may not be possible with light microscopy. Recent developments in immunohistochemical methods and electron microscopy allowed identification of entities such as ONB (esthesioneuroblastoma), SNUC, small cell undifferentiated (neuroendocrine) carcinoma, undifferentiated (lymphoepithelioma-like) carcinoma, malignant melanoma, Ewing sarcoma, peripheral neuroectodermal tumor, rhabdomyosarcoma,

mesenchymal chondrosarcoma, small cell osteosarcoma, synovial sarcoma, extranodal natural killer/T-cell lymphoma, and extramedullary plasmacytoma within the category of small round blue cell tumors.[21] Regardless of their specific origin, these tumors show very aggressive features in imaging studies.

Extranodal lymphomas of the nasal cavity and paranasal sinuses are rare in western populations.[22] The paranasal sinuses tend to harbor B-cell lymphoma whereas the nasal cavity lymphomas are usually of NK/T-cell variety which has a worse prognosis particularly in the Asian populations.[23]

Metastasis to the sinonasal cavity is a rare occurrence. Typical primary tumors are renal cell carcinoma, and adenocarcinoma of the gastrointestinal tract. The former may show hemorrhagic features whereas mucinous varieties of the latter may show stippled calcification. In children, neuroblastoma metastases favor the walls of the sinuses near suture lines and may be blastic or lytic.

In the early stages of the malignant tumors, CT findings may be indistinguishable from inflammatory disease. In fact, inflammatory changes are almost always present in association with a neoplasm due to retained secretions. MRI is better able to differentiate inflammatory disease from neoplasm due to the lower signal on T2WI of tumor tissue versus nonhyperproteinaceous secretions and due to the solid enhancement of neoplasms as opposed to the rim enhancement of inflammatory lesions (Figure 23). Detection of erosion and destruction of the thin bones as demonstrated on sinus CT may allow one to diagnose these tumors while they are still in the sinonasal cavity, which requires careful examination of all sinus CT examinations with the possibility of a malignancy in mind. In the late stages of the disease process, there is usually some degree of bone erosion and destruction, which appears different than the bone remodeling secondary to benign processes such as polyposis, mucocele, allergic FS, schwannoma, and papilloma. Differentiation of bone remodeling from more aggressive bone destruction allows the radiologist to offer a reasonable differential diagnosis. It is important to note that some malignant tumors such as melanoma and lymphoma tend to remodel the bone rather than destroying it.

In addition to the histology of the primary tumor, the status of surgical margins and presence/absence of intracranial extent are independent predictors of survival in patients with sinonasal malignant tumors.[24] Thus, appropriate treatment of sinonasal tumors requires an accurate depiction of tumor extent preoperatively. Knowledge of pathways of disease spread is important when interpreting these images. In general, CT is more accurate for the evaluation of bone integrity, whereas MRI is much superior to CT in assessing the extent of disease, perineural or meningeal spread, and differentiating the tumor from secondary inflammatory changes (Figure 24). In our practice, most patients are imaged with both MRI and CT before the surgery.

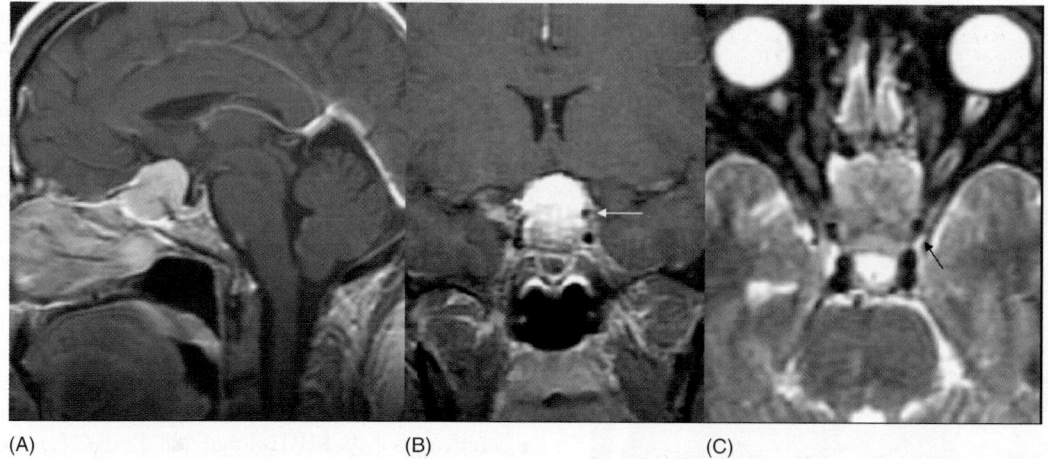

(A)   (B)   (C)

Figure 22 Meningioma of the planum sphenoidale. Sagittal T1W (A) and coronal T1W (B) postcontrast images of the sella show a homogenously enhancing mass in the sphenoid sinus, sella turcica, and suprasellar cistern. Mass is in contact with the internal carotid artery (*arrows*). The pituitary gland is separate from the mass. Mass shows intermediate T2 signal (C).

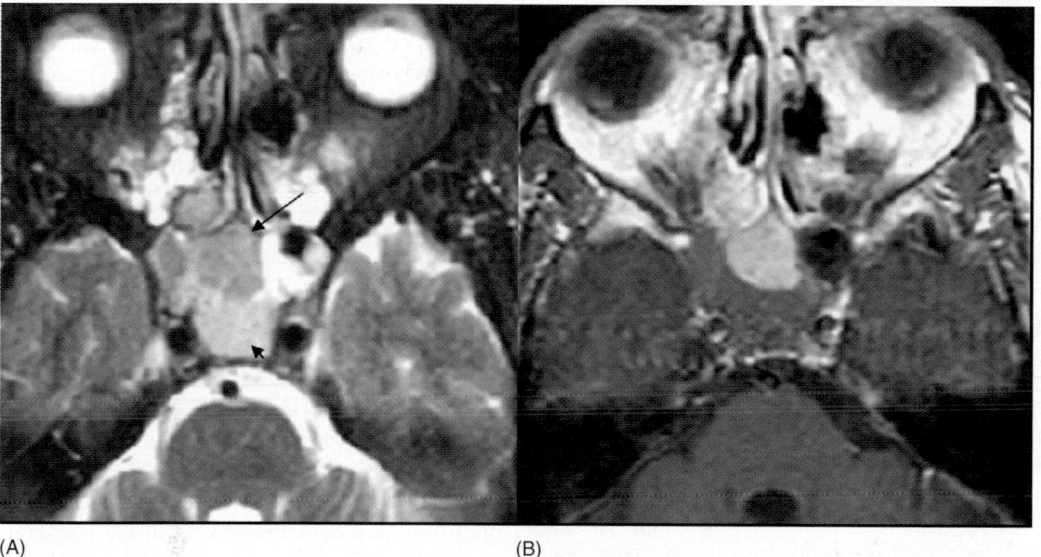

(A)   (B)

Figure 23 Squamous cell cancer of the ethmoid and sphenoid sinuses. Axial T2W (A) and axial postcontrast T1W (B) MRI shows a mass (*arrow*) in the right posterior ethmoid and sphenoid sinuses with surrounding inflammatory changes (*short arrow*) which could not be separated from the tumor on CT examination. MRI allows better delineation of tumor extent.

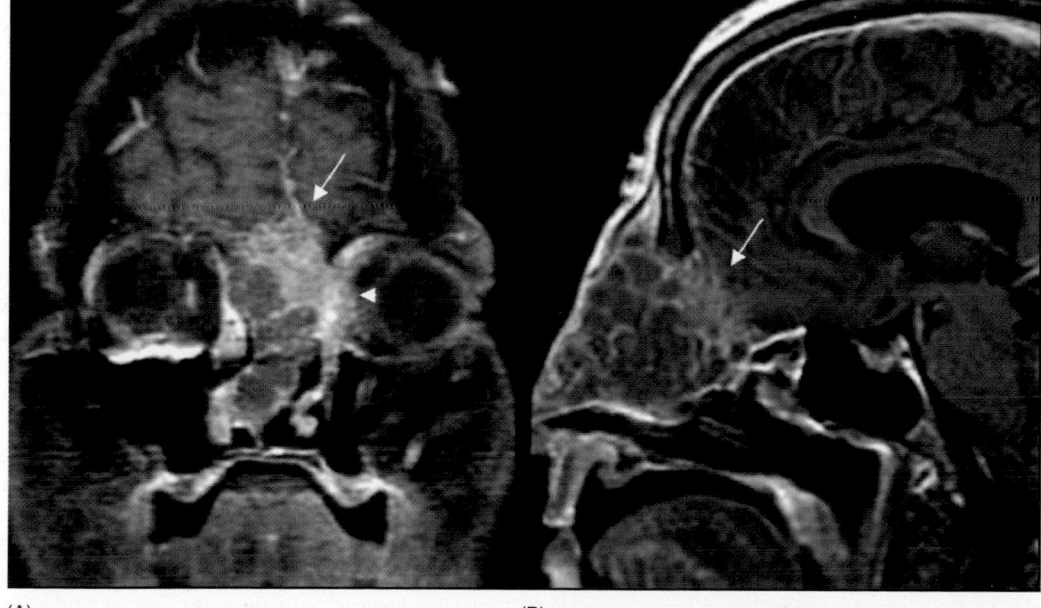

(A)   (B)

Figure 24 Nasoethmoid squamous cell cancer. A large and heterogeneous mass seen in the nasoethmoid region on coronal (A) and sagittal (B) postcontrast T1W MRI. Note the irregular margin of the tumor adjacent to the brain (*arrow*), compatible with brain invasion, confirmed surgically. Mass enters the orbit with thickening and enhancement of the medial rectus muscle compatible with periorbital infiltration.

There are two very important questions to answer in preoperative evaluation[25]: (1) Is the periorbita infiltrated?; and (2) Is the dura invaded? Most surgeons believe that tumor invasion of the orbital fat requires orbital exenteration. Preoperative determination of invasion of the periorbita is difficult due to the fact that tumor can destroy the bone and indent on the periorbita without infiltrating it (Figure 25). Therefore destruction of the bony orbit does not necessarily imply the need for orbital exenteration for orbital spread. Conversely, subtle invasion of the periorbita may not be apparent on imaging. Infiltration or stranding of the periorbital fat tissue and nodularity of the interface between the tumor and orbital tissue, enlargement and enhancement of the extraocular muscles are reliable signs of periorbital invasion but absence of these findings cannot always rule out tumor involvement[26] (Figure 24). High-resolution fat-saturated T2W and enhanced T1-weighted images are particularly helpful in this assessment. The overall accuracy of imaging for determination of presence or absence of periorbital invasion is about 60 to 70%. It is important to note that this modest accuracy is mainly a reflection of low negative predictive value. Thus, the presence of periorbital invasion is more accurately predicted than the absence of invasion.

Intracranial extension of tumor and dura/brain invasion is important to identify because of their impact on treatment and prognosis. MRI is the modality of choice in this scenario. When there is irregular/nodular thickening and enhancement of the dura or smooth thickening of the dura more than 5 mm, the diagnosis of dural invasion can be made with a 100% positive predictive value[27] (Figures 24 and 25). Difficulty arises when the thickening and enhancement are smooth and thin which can be seen both with dural invasion and reactive changes. As in the periorbital invasion, it is easier to confirm presence of invasion than absence of it.

Lymph node metastasis occurs in 25% of the malignant sinonasal cancers and signifies a poor prognosis. The ipsilateral submandibular and submental level I and high jugular level II chains are the most common sites of nodal metastasis.

PNS is another way by which sinonasal tumors can invade intracranial structures. Imaging can demonstrate PNS of disease before the patient becomes symptomatic, dramatically changing the course of treatment. Detection of perineural metastasis requires detailed knowledge of the skull base anatomy and good quality images. MRI is far superior to CT in this respect. Effacement of the fat pads surrounding the nerves outside the skull is an important clue to PNS of tumor and can be identified with high-resolution T1-weighted images. The authors find contrast enhanced fat-suppressed T1-weighted images extremely helpful for this diagnosis since the enhancing tumor is easily identified against the suppressed background. PNS mostly occurs along the fifth and seventh cranial nerves. The auriculotemporal, vidian, and greater superficial petrosal nerves provide anastomosis between the

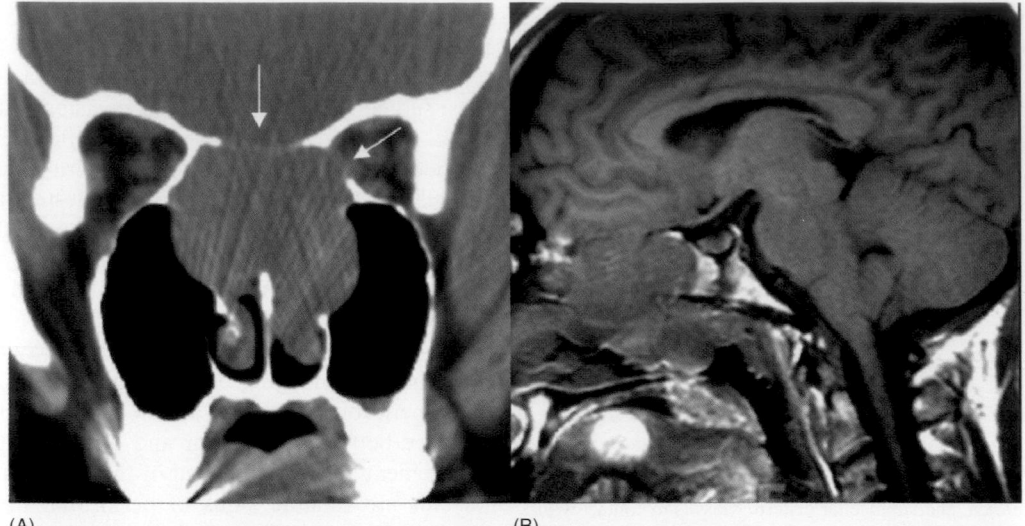

(A)

(B)

(C)

(D)

Figure 25 Esthesioneuroblastoma. (A) Coronal CT, (B) sagittal T1W, (C) coronal contrast enhanced T1W, and (D) coronal T2W MRI. There is a prominently enhancing soft tissue mass in the nasal cavity and ethmoid sinuses with destruction of the bony septa of the ethmoid and cribriform plate and the medial orbital wall. Note the irregular, nodular enhancement of the brain-tumor interface; tumor was found to be infiltrating the dura but not the brain. The periorbita was pushed but not grossly infiltrated by the tumor.

seventh and fifth cranial nerves and can act as conduits through which tumor spreads from the fifth to seventh nerve and vice versa. PNS mostly occurs in a centrifugal (from the periphery towards the skull base and brain) fashion but the opposite is also possible. The evaluation of the PPF is particularly important since the tumor, in most cases, first involves the PPF before it infiltrates the inferior orbital fissure, foramen rotundum, foramen ovale, vidian canal, and finally, cavernous sinus and Meckel cave (Figure 26). This region should show only speckles of soft tissue representing vessels and the pterygopalatine ganglion amidst a bright fat background on

T1WI. If this fat is obliterated or completely replaced with soft tissue on CT or T1WI, suspect neoplastic infiltration!

Positron emission tomography (PET) is a very robust tool in oncologic imaging in general. Unfortunately, PET and PET-CT have important shortcomings in the evaluation of skull base and sinonasal tumors. Lower resolution compared to CT and MRI is a major disadvantage in this anatomic area where the normal as well as abnormal structures of interest are often very small. PET performs worse than MRI in T staging of untreated patients. Identification of nodal metastasis is slightly more accurate with PET-CT compared to CT or MRI alone, but PET-CT is not sufficiently accurate to direct treatment decisions. For the detection of distant metastases PET has a clear advantage over the other modalities. The most significant advantage of PET-CT is seen in the follow-up of patients who had been treated with surgery or radiotherapy where granulation tissue may obscure "nonphysiologic" imaging.

NASOPHARYNX AND CENTRAL SKULL BASE

External examination of the central skull base and nasopharyngeal lesions is either limited or impossible, highlighting the importance of imaging. A high level of anatomic knowledge is a prerequisite to interpretation of imaging studies. The sphenoid bone is the central piece in the central skull base and forms the floor and anterior wall of the middle cranial fossa, houses the sella turcica, supports the cavernous sinuses and separates the orbits and nasopharynx from the intracranial structures. Through a number of bony channels and dehiscences, the nasopharynx and intracranial compartment are contiguous and these channels may serve as a path for disease spread. The nasopharynx is a fibromuscular tube attached to the sphenoid bone. The pharyngeal mucosal space is defined by the pharyngobasilar fascia, which surrounds the mucosa and the superior constrictor muscle and fills the gap between the muscle and the skull base. The eustachian tube pierces through the pharyngobasilar fascia at the sinus of Morgagni, which may allow nasopharyngeal cancer access to the skull base. The fossa of Rosenmuller, torus tubarius, and the orifice of the eustachian canal are on the lateral wall of the nasopharynx. The buccopharyngeal fascia, a part of the middle layer of the deep cervical fascia, separates the pharyngeal mucosal space from the retropharyngeal space. The alar fascia makes the posterior border of the retropharyngeal space and anterior border of the danger space, a potential space between retropharyngeal and perivertebral fascia. The prevertebral fascia separates the danger space from the prevertebral space, which contains the longus colli muscles and extends from the skull base to coccyx.

Nasopharyngeal adenoids can be very prominent and make it difficult to differentiate them from mass lesions particularly in young individuals.

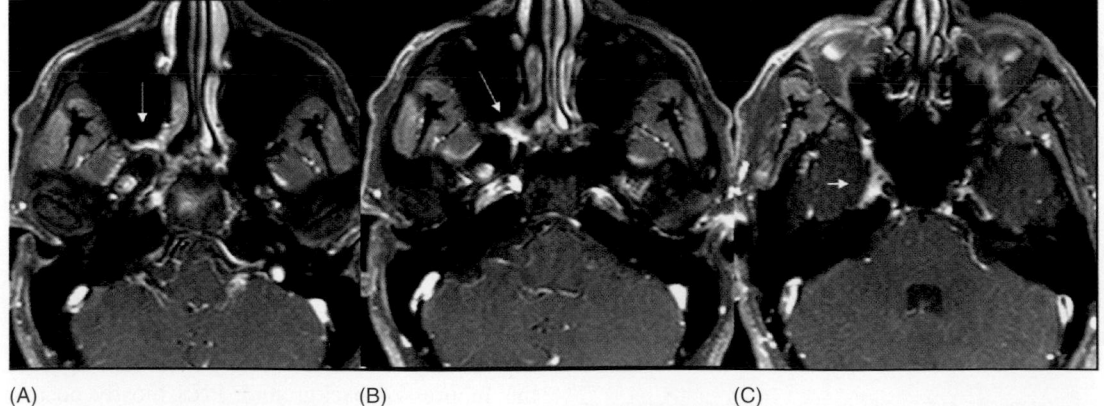

(A)

(B)

(C)

Figure 26 Perineural spread of tumor. High-resolution postcontrast fat-suppressed T1W images show enhancing tissue in the pterygopalatine fossa (A), vidian canal (B) and cavernous sinus, and Meckel cave (C) due to perineural spread of adenoid cystic cancer of the maxillary floor/hard palate.

By the third decade of life, most individuals have only a small residual amount of adenoid tissue in the nasopharynx. Asymmetric prominence of the adenoids should be regarded with suspicion for an underlying neoplastic process. Immune compromised individuals may show enlargement of this lymphoid tissue.

Tornwaldt, or Thornwaldt, cyst is an embryonic remnant of the pharyngeal bursa occurring at the posterior wall of the nasopharynx in midline and seen in approximately 3% of the population. These submucosal cysts are usually smaller than 1 cm and asymptomatic. They show very bright signal on T2WIs and can be bright or dark on T1WIs depending on the protein content of the fluid. A mild enhancement of the wall is usually seen.

Retention cysts of the nasopharyngeal mucosa are also generally asymptomatic. They can be uni- or multilocular and show similar signal characteristics on MRI to Tornwaldt cysts but occur off midline (Figure 27). Most pathologies of the nasopharynx arise from the pharyngeal mucosal space and extend to the neighboring spaces and skull base.

Most mass lesions in the nasopharynx are malignant. Nasopharyngeal carcinoma (NPC) makes about 70% of the mass lesions in this site and can be seen in a wide range of ages. The incidence begins to rise in the second decade and peaks in the fourth and fifth decades in the United States of America. In Asia, where the prevalence of NPC is 25 times higher in some parts, the peak age of presentation is in the third decade. NPC has three histologic subtypes: squamous cell, nonkeratinizing, and undifferentiated. NPC typically arises in the fossa of Rosenmuller and grows anteriorly to the nasal cavity and orbit, laterally to the parapharyngeal space and infratemporal fossa (ITF) (masticator space), posterosuperiorly to the skull base and intracranial space and anteroinferiorly to the PPF. Once in the ITF and PPF it can extend intracranially via perineural trigeminal neurotropic spread. Imaging is an essential part of staging since parapharyngeal and intracranial extension can only be reliably evaluated by radiologic means. MRI is superior to CT because of the exquisite soft tissue contrast it provides.[28] An added advantage of MRI is its ability to separate tumor from obstructed secretions in the sinuses and to track perineural or meningeal disease intracranially. Involvement of the skull base is also better evaluated with MRI than CT due to the fact that the cancellous part of the bone is "involved" earlier than the cortical bone. Fat in the cancellous part of the bone and signal changes due to replacement of fat are readily visualized on T1WI MRI whereas CT provides a better evaluation of the cortical integrity. It is not known whether these changes in the cancellous part identified on MRI in the absence of cortical erosion truly represent tumor infiltration or merely reactive changes (Figure 28). Regardless, simple bone involvement diagnosed by CT or MRI in the absence of intracranial extension of tumor and cranial nerve palsy does not seem to have an adverse effect on the prognosis.[29]

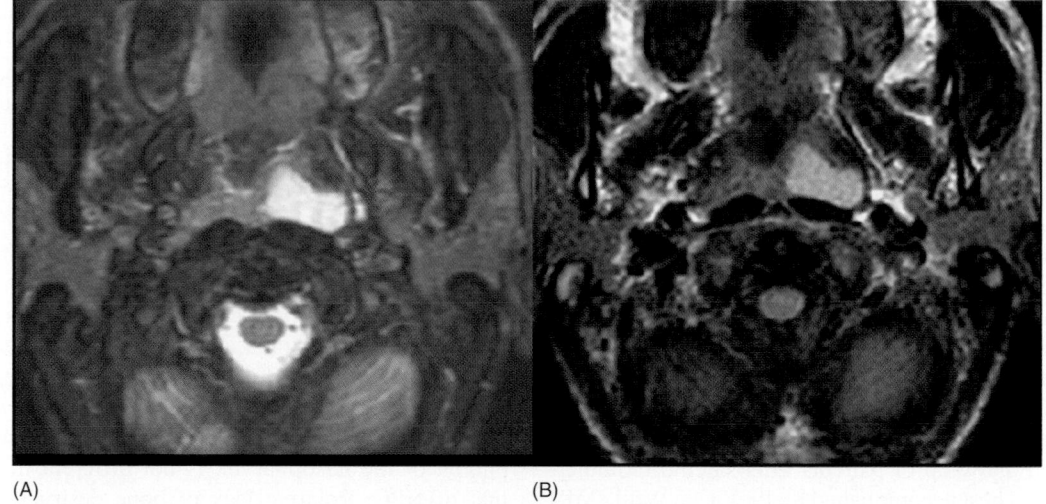

(A)   (B)

Figure 27 Nasopharyngeal retention cyst. A very well defined submucosal cyst is seen in the left fossa of Rosenmüller. Cyst shows a very bright signal on T2W (A) and bright signal on T1WI (B) due to slightly increased protein content.

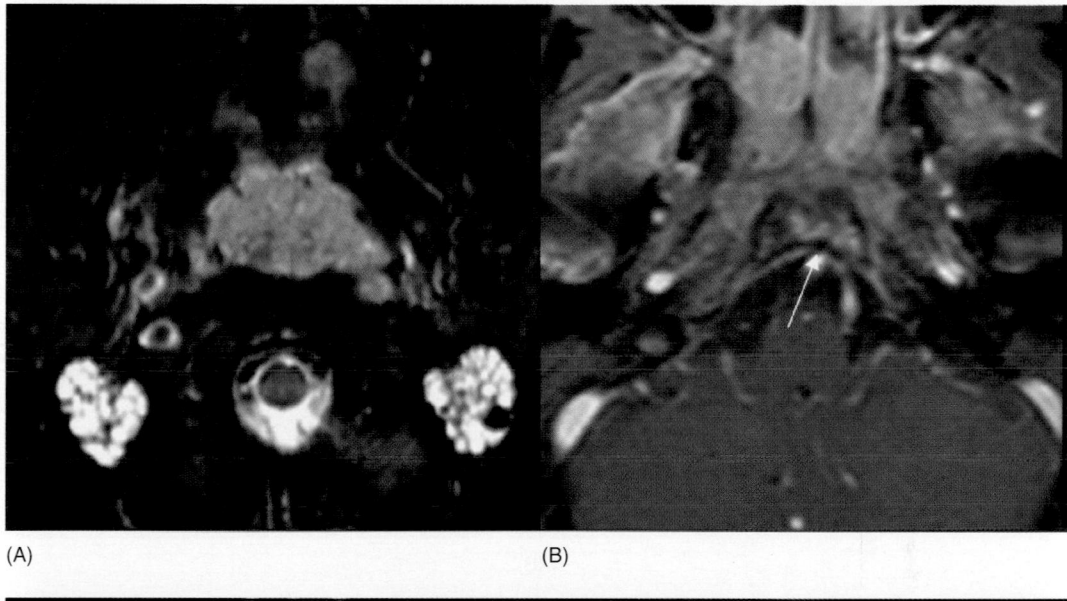

(A)   (B)

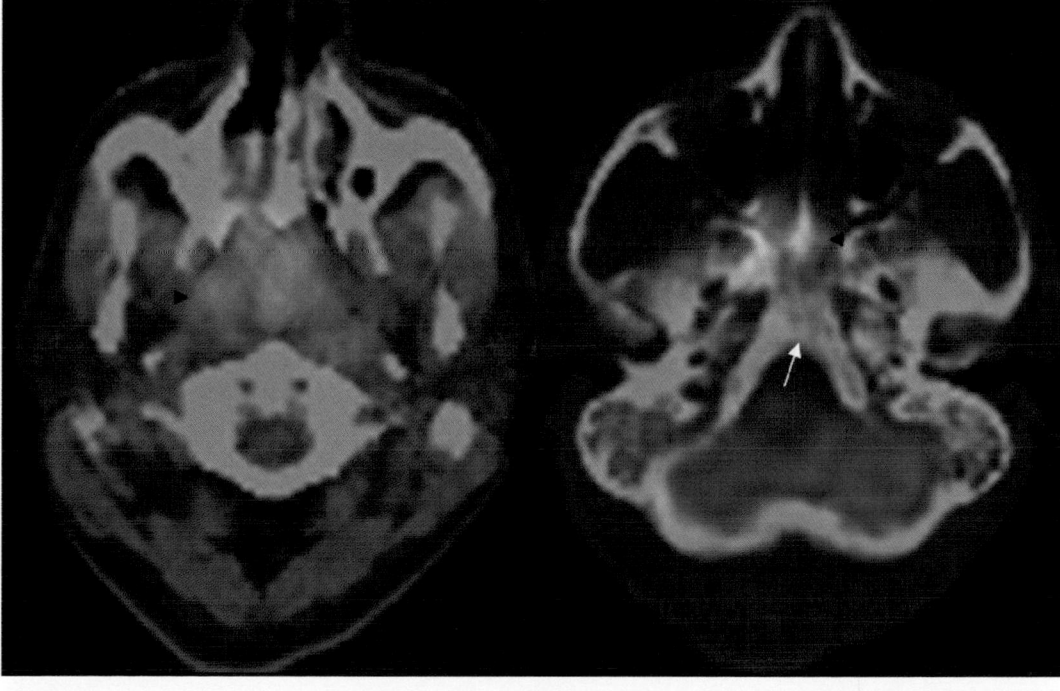

(C)   (D)

Figure 28 Nasopharyngeal cancer. A large nasopharyngeal mass is seen with obstruction of the eustachian canals (A). A focal area of abnormal enhancement is present in the clivus (*arrow*) (B), suspicious for clivus infiltration. PET-CT (C and D) shows FDG activity corresponding to the nasopharyngeal mass (*arrowheads*) but no uptake is seen in the clivus.

Lymph node metastasis from NPC can be evaluated by CT or MRI. MRI provides better differentiation of the primary mass from adjacent retropharyngeal nodal metastasis, which may appear as a single mass on CT. Due to abundant lymphatic drainage present in the nasopharynx, nodal metastasis occurs to bilateral retropharyngeal, parapharyngeal, and jugular chain nodes. Five percent of NPC patients will have systemic metastases at the time of diagnosis. Bones, lungs, and liver are the primary targets for hematogenic metastasis. PET-CT is beneficial in staging of patients with T4 disease since these patients have a distinctly higher propensity to have systemic metastases.[30]

Follow-up of patients after chemo/radiotherapy is best accomplished by PET-CT. While MRI and CT are also very informative, differentiation of viable tumor from posttherapy fibrosis is not consistently possible. Serial cross-sectional imaging is the most useful surveillance technique short of PET.

Lymphoma of the nasopharynx arises from the adenoids and is most commonly of non-Hodgkin variety. B-cell lymphoma is the most frequent type in the western world whereas T-cell lymphoma is more prevalent in Asian populations. Mucosa associated lymphoid tissue, a low-grade non-Hodgkin lymphoma, is rare in the nasopharynx. In half of the patients with nasopharyngeal lymphoma there is systemic involvement.

The imaging appearance of non-Hodgkin lymphoma of the nasopharynx is not different than that of NPC. Relative lack of bone destruction may be a useful hint for differentiating lymphoma from NPC (Figure 29).

Rare tumors of the nasopharynx include adenocarcinomas, rhabdomyosarcoma, plasmocytoma, and melanoma.

The central skull base mass lesions are much more diverse than the anterior skull base lesions. By far the most common mass lesions in this site are pituitary adenomas. Microadenomas, measuring less than 10 mm, are confined to the sella turcica and pose no diagnostic difficulty when they are visualized on MRI. Macroadenomas, on the other hand, can attain very large sizes and invade the suprasellar region and brain, cavernous sinuses, the sphenoid sinus, and skull base, making it very difficult to differentiate them from other tumors seen in this region. Two imaging findings can help make this distinction: (1) expansion of the sella turcica and (2) visualization of the pituitary gland. Macroadenomas invariably expand the sella whereas most tumors secondarily invading the sella do not expand it to the degree expected from their overall size and extent. Visualization of even a small remnant of the normal pituitary gland implies tumors other than macroadenomas, which typically leave no visible normal pituitary tissue (Figure 30). Macroadenomas may demonstrate variable signal since they can contain varying amounts of cystic and solid areas, hemorrhage, and calcification. Determination of whether a pituitary macroadenoma invades the cavernous sinus is crucial in treatment planning. High-resolution coronal MRI with and without contrast is helpful in this distinction. The likelihood of cavernous sinus (CS) involvement is very high if the tumor extends beyond the line drawn along the lateral margins of the turns of the cavernous carotid artery.[31]

Rathke cleft cyst arises from remnants of craniopharyngeal canal squamous epithelium in the sella turcica. They are often asymptomatic and found incidentally. The signal intensity on MRI, although usually bright on T1W, may vary depending on the protein content of the cyst but they do not demonstrate any enhancement other than perhaps minimal enhancement of its wall[32] (Figure 31). Large Rathke cleft cyst can extend into the suprasellar cistern and become symptomatic by compressing the optic chiasm or the pituitary.

Suprasellar tumors can grow into the sella turcica, sphenoid sinus, and skull base. The most common primary suprasellar tumor is craniopharyngioma, but suprasellar extension of a pituitary adenoma is the most common lesion in this space. Craniopharyngiomas are epithelium derived tumors seen in all age groups but the majority of the cases present at childhood and teens. More than half of the craniopharyngiomas are of adamantinomatous type and present as cystic masses with enhancing solid mural nodules. The amount of cholesterol crystals present in the cyst determines the MRI appearance. Calcification is one of the hallmarks of craniopharyngiomas. The less common papillary type craniopharyngiomas are solid enhancing tumors and typically seen in adults.

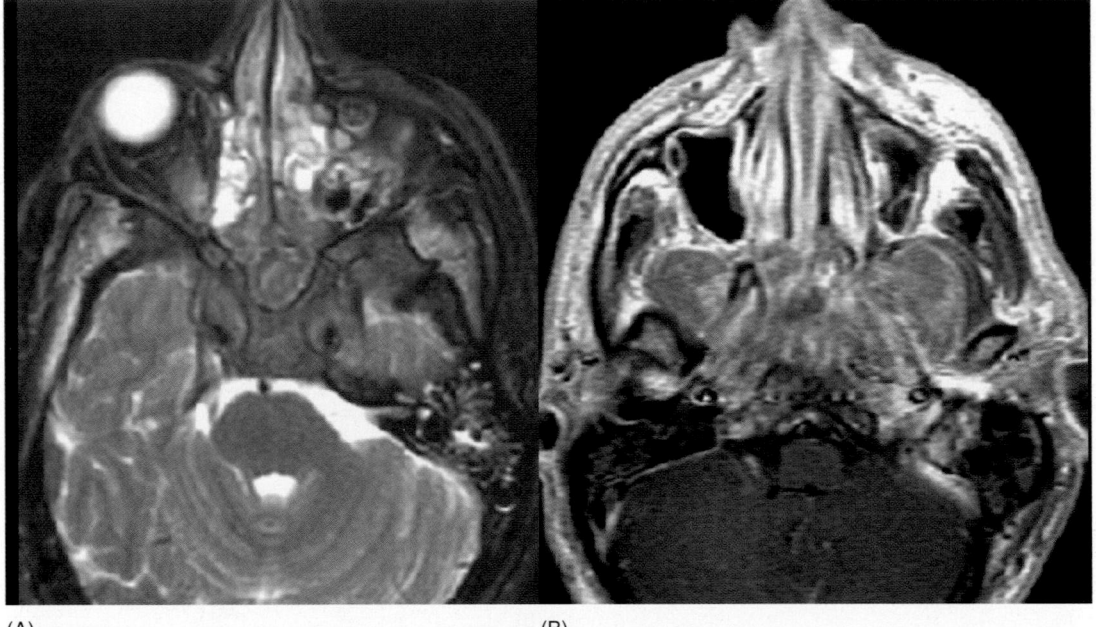

(A)　　　　　　　　　(B)

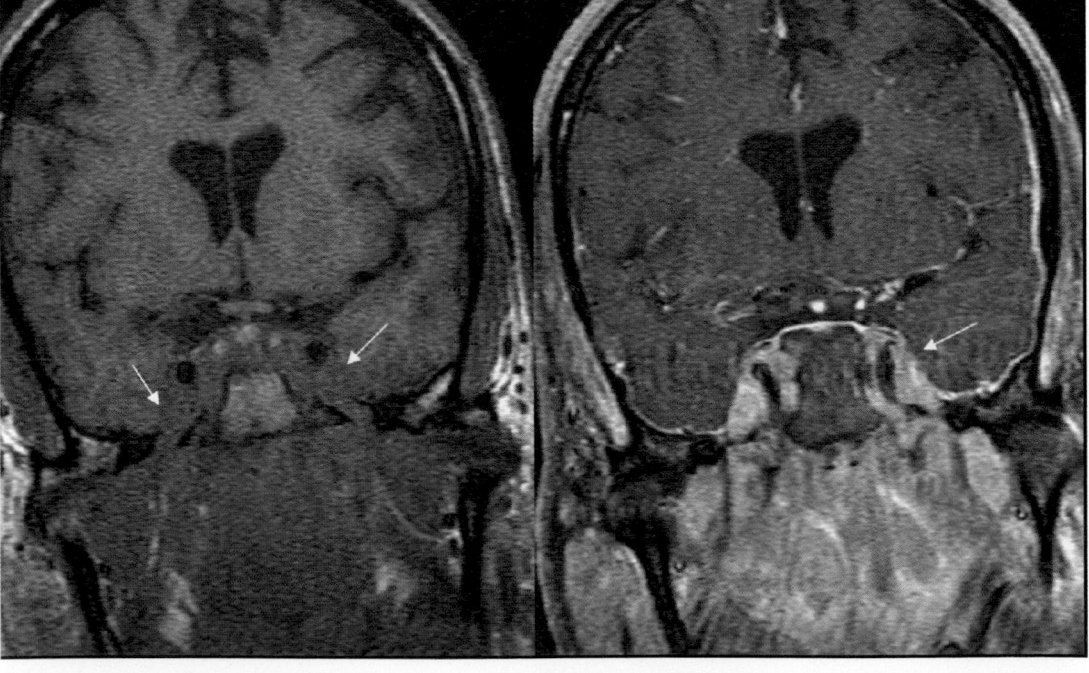

(C)　　　　　　　　　(D)

Figure 29 Lymphoma. A large nasopharyngeal mass is seen to extend through the foramen ovale (*arrows*, C) to the cavernous sinuses (*arrow*, D). Mass shows a relatively dark signal on T2WI (A) and prominent contrast enhancement on T1WI (B and D), typical of lymphoma.

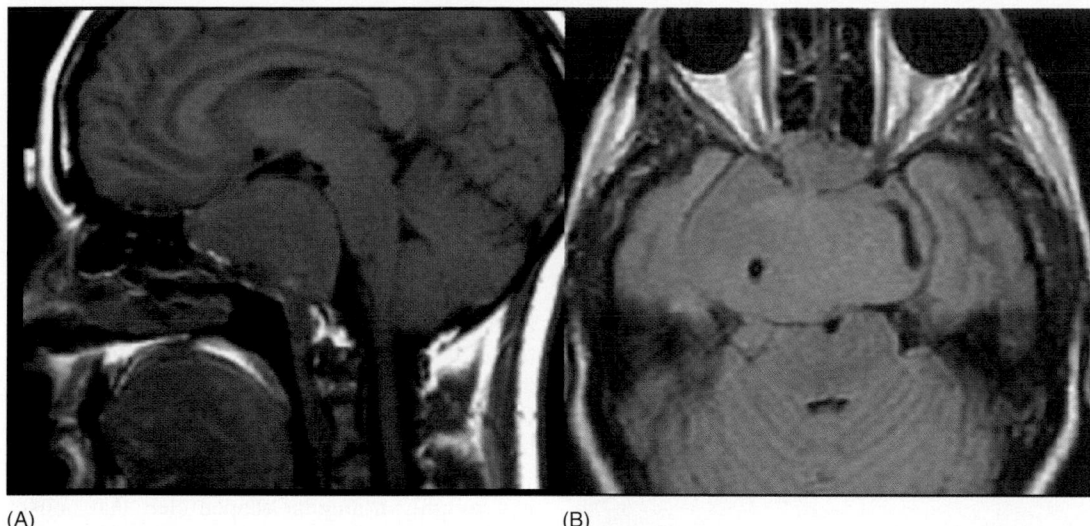

(A) (B)

Figure 30 Pituitary macroadenoma. Sagittal (A) and axial (B) T1W MRI shows a soft tissue mass in the clivus and sphenoid sinus that extends to the suprasellar and prepontine cistern. Inability to see the pituitary gland makes the diagnosis of macroadenoma very likely.

Meningiomas of the planum sphenoidale, sulcus chiasmaticus, and diaphragma sella can involve the sella and suprasellar region. Most meningiomas are seen in adults. They are more common in women than men. Meningiomas are typically solid and homogenous masses and show diffuse, intense enhancement with contrast material (Figure 22). They can have calcifications and occasional cysts. "Dural tail" refers to a smooth and tapered thickening of the dura adjacent to meningioma and is either reactive or due to tumor infiltration. Most meningiomas exhibit this finding, although other dural-based tumors can have a similar dural tail. Hyperostosis, thickening, and sclerosis, of the adjacent bone, are helpful in the differential diagnosis, when present.

Tumors of glial origin such as optic/hypothalamic glioma can present as suprasellar mass lesions and involve the sella and skull base. These are generally low-grade astrocytomas, although occasionally one may find a glioblastoma multiforme in the mix. The majority of the optic gliomas are pilocytic astrocytomas and seen in children. Gliomas of the chiasm tend to be more aggressive than optic nerve gliomas and adult presentation is associated with higher grade astrocytomas.

Other less common suprasellar masses include germinoma/teratomas and dermoid/epidermoid tumors. Suprasellar germinomas can represent metastasis from other sites such as the pineal region.

The sphenoid sinus may give rise to many central skull base lesions. Because of its proximity to the intracranial compartment acute sphenoid sinusitis should be treated aggressively. Invasive and allergic FS can easily extend from the sphenoid sinus into the intracranial compartment and mimic neoplastic lesions. Mucoceles of the sphenoid sinus are uncommon but they can substantially expand the sphenoid sinus (Figure 11). Primary benign and malignant epithelial tumors of the sphenoid sinus are much less common than the inflammatory/infectious lesions. Juvenile nasopharyngeal angiofibroma (JNA) is a disease of male children and teens. It arises from the posterior nasal cavity in the region of the sphenopalatine foramen and grows rather insidiously, invading the PPF, ethmoid and sphenoid sinuses, skull base and orbit. These are very vascular tumors and preoperative embolization is helpful in achieving a comprehensive resection (Figure 32). The most common malignant epithelial tumor of the sphenoid sinus is squamous cell carcinoma.

The sphenoid bone can give rise to a variety of bone tumors. The most frequent mass lesion of the sphenoid bone in adults is metastasis from a remote site (Figure 33). Chordomas derive from remnants of the primitive notochord associated with the sphenooccipital synchondrosis and therefore affect the clivus although some will arise from the petrous apex region. They can be seen at any age group but most patients are young adults. It is more common in men. Clival chordomas are histologically benign tumors but they are locally destructive and have a very high rate of recurrence. High signal on T2WIs is a common feature unless they have a calcified matrix. Chondrosarcomas usually arise from the petroclival fissure and are seen in younger ages than chordomas. Chondrosarcomas tend to invade the skull base through the foramen lacerum and petroclival fissure, reaching to the cavernous sinus, middle cranial fossa and posterior fossa (Figure 34).

Histologically, many chordomas and chondrosarcomas feature areas of hemorrhage, collections of mucin, necrotic regions, calcification, and entrapped bone trabeculae. Both chordomas and chondrosarcomas present as soft tissue masses with lytic destruction of the adjacent bone on CT exams. Due to the varied composition of these tumors MRI shows heterogenous signal intensity, which is predominantly hyperintense on T2W and iso- to hypointense on T1WIs. Enhancement is variable. Both tumors tend to have a lobulated appearance. Although chordomas favor midline and chondrosarcomas favor off-midline location, there is a significant overlap of the site of origin. Furthermore, it becomes impossible to determine the epicenter of a particular skull base mass when it attains a large size. Thus, the CT and MRI appearance of chondrosarcomas is very similar to chordomas rendering a preoperative diagnosis impossible in most cases unless the classic "popcorn-like" calcification of a chondrosarcoma is apparent.[33]

The relationship of the carotid arteries and the optic nerves to a skull base mass is of utmost importance to the surgeon. Any central skull base mass, regardless of its histology, can come in contact with or invade the carotid artery and preoperative documentation of this is critical in determining the extent of resection and avoiding catastrophic complications. Most benign tumors merely displace or occasionally compress the carotid artery without invading the adventitia, whereas malignant tumors

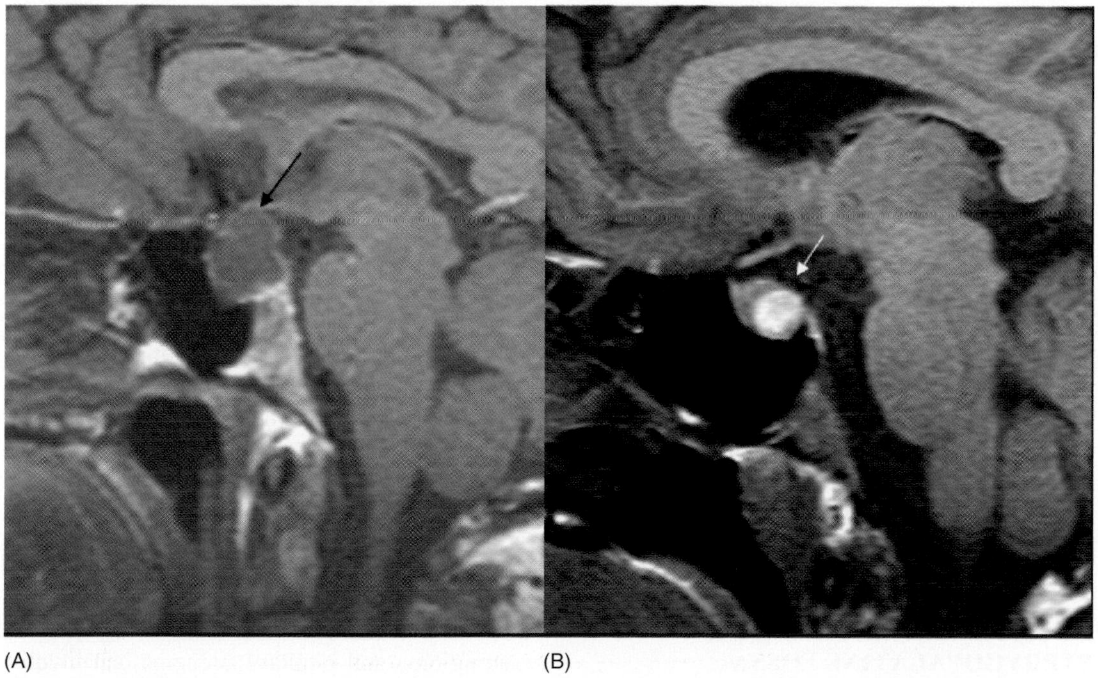

(A) (B)

Figure 31 Rathke cleft cyst. Sagittal T1W images on two different patients show Rathke cleft cysts with different signal characteristics. The cystic nature of the lesion is easily appreciated in part (A). High protein content of the cyst makes it appear bright in part (B).

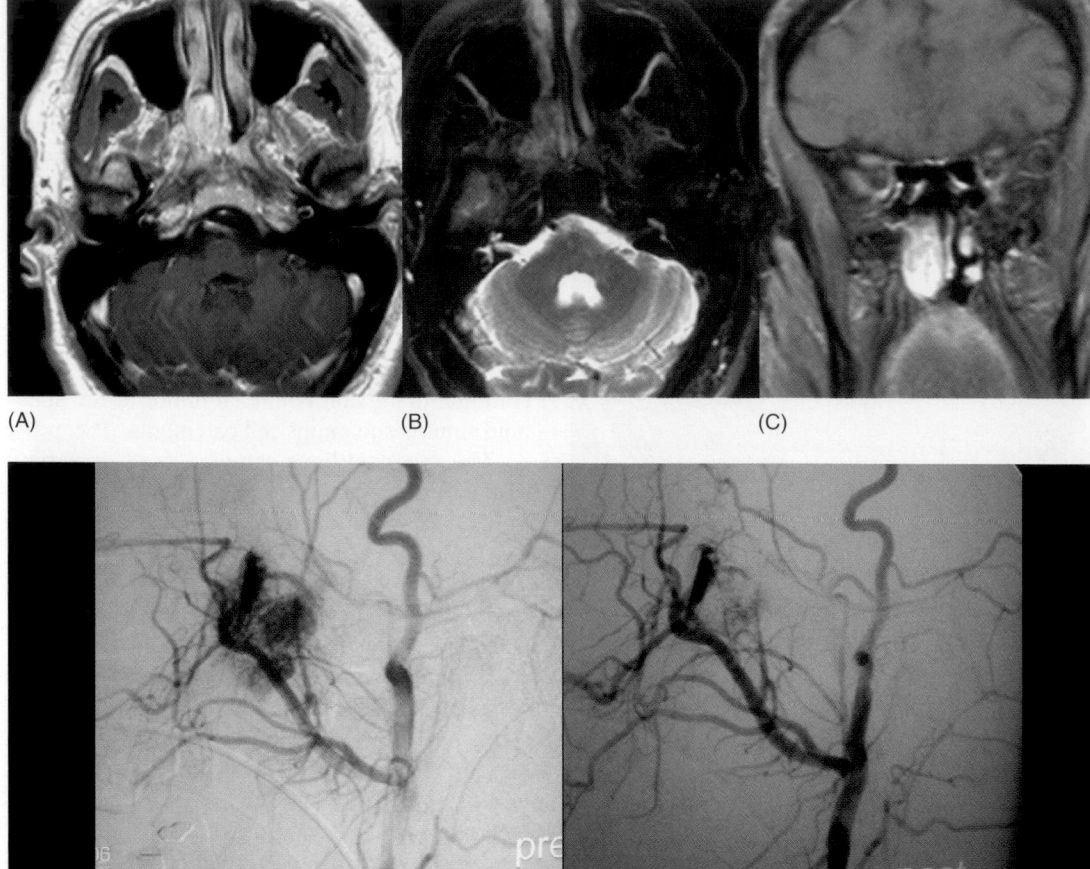

(A)   (B)   (C)

(D)   (E)

Figure 32 Juvenile nasopharyngeal angiofibroma. Axial (A) and coronal (C) postcontrast T1W and axial (B) T2W MRI show a well defined mass in the posterior nasal cavity which avidly enhances with contrast and has a relatively low T2 signal due to its fibrous content. Lateral angiographic projection (D) demonstrates the very vascular nature of the tumor. Same angiographic view after successful embolization (E).

tend to invade the adventitia. Meningiomas that completely encase the vessel are also invasive to the adventitia unlike pituitary adenomas. Complete encasement or narrowing of the carotid artery would render surgical resection impossible in most cases unless the vessel is sacrificed.[34] If the tumor does not encircle the vessel completely gross total resection may be possible but with significant morbidity. This assessment is best accomplished in T2W and postcontrast T1WIs. Computed tomography angiography (CTA) and magnetic resonance angiography (MRA) may be helpful in certain cases. Corollary to this, one has to make sure that the "mass" which is about to be resected or biopsied is not an aneurysm. Aneurysms of the internal carotid artery can grow into the sella turcica, suprasellar region, sphenoid sinus, and petrous apex and erode the skull base in a similar fashion with tumors (Figure 35). Most small aneurysms are easily recognized on MRI and MRA studies. Giant aneurysms, on the other hand, can very closely mimic mass lesions due to slow flow and partial thrombosis, which may render them very difficult to diagnose. Careful evaluation of the individual partitions of MRA generally allows identification of such aneurysms. Phase ghosting artifacts might also suggest the diagnosis. It is important to emphasize that, in most practices the individual partitions of MRA are not available to the clinicians as printed films. Active participation

of radiologists in the care of these patients is crucial. Perhaps the most important clue to the diagnosis of a giant aneurysm mimicking a mass lesion is the failure to identify the tissue of origin of the "mass." In other words, if one is unable to tell the anatomic and/or tissue origin of a particular tumor, an aneurysm must be suspected.

While the choice of imaging study is determined on an individual basis; however, MRA is generally the most practical and fruitful test in this scenario despite its limited sensitivity for slow flow. CTA has a much superior spatial resolution and affords superb contrast between the vessels and adjacent soft tissues but, sometimes, it may be difficult to differentiate enhancing vessel lumen from other enhancing structures and adjacent bone. An added advantage of CTA is that it can be used to guide surgical navigation.[35] Digital subtraction angiography may be necessary in rare occasions.

Dehiscences of the sphenoid sinus wall can allow protrusion of the internal carotid artery or the optic nerve into the sinus lumen, which can pose a surgical hazard if not recognized preoperatively.

INFRATEMPORAL FOSSA AND PTERYGOPALATINE FOSSA

The ITF contains the muscles of mastication, the mandibular nerve and its branches. The outer and

inner membranes of the superficial layer of the deep cervical fascia separate this space from the adjacent parapharyngeal space. The outer membrane of the superficial layer of the deep cervical fascia is continuous above the zygomatic process and invests the temporalis muscle. Thus, the prefix infra is unsuitable. Yet the term ITF has been used so extensively in the surgical literature that replacing it would not be advisable.

The PPF is bounded by the body of the sphenoid bone superiorly, the pterygoid process posteriorly, the posterior wall of maxillary sinus anteriorly, the inferior orbital fissure superoanteriorly, and the perpendicular plate of the palatine bone medially. Laterally, it is contiguous with the ITF through the pterygomaxillary fissure, which is a roughly triangular shaped cleft that houses the maxillary artery, alveolar arteries, veins, and nerves. The posterior openings of the PPF consist of the foramen rotundum superolaterally and the vidian (pterygoid) canal superomedially. The sphenopalatine foramen, situated on the medial wall of the PPF allows communication between the PPF and nasal cavity. Anteriorly, the PPF is in contiguity with the inferior orbital fissure. The greater and lesser palatine canals connect the palate/oral cavity to the PPF. The PPF contains the pterygopalatine ganglion and its branches, the maxillary nerve and the terminal branches of the internal maxillary artery, which are embedded in fat tissue. Due to its unique CT attenuation and MRI signal fat tissue is easily recognized in imaging studies and replacement of fat tissue by disease process is, thus, relatively easy to diagnose. Nonetheless, the small size of the involved structures and the intricate anatomy of the region pose significant challenges to imagers.

Imaging is essential in assessment of the ITF and PPF. MRI affords excellent visualization of the disease processes in the ITF and PPF. Extension of the disease process into the intracranial compartment and adjacent spaces can best be evaluated by MRI as well. While the involvement of cancellous bone is recognized much earlier with MRI compared to CT, the assessment of the bone cortex is better accomplished with CT.

Biopsy of ITF mass lesions is done using imaging guidance. CT is well suited for this purpose and allows access to virtually all ITF masses. Despite the proximity to vital structures, fine needle aspiration biopsy of ITF mass lesions is performed without significant complication in good hands and with small gauge needles.[36] MR-guided biopsy may be needed for lesions that are not visible on CT and requires special MR-compatible equipment.

Most tumors found in the ITF arise from the mucosal lining of the adjacent spaces such as the nasopharynx, nasal cavity, and paranasal sinuses and represent advanced cancer. Skull base lesions such as chordoma and chondrosarcoma and primarily intracranial tumors such as meningioma and pituitary adenoma can involve the ITF when they are large. SCCs and adenocarcinomas arising from the aerodigestive tract and skin can spread along the nerves to a considerable

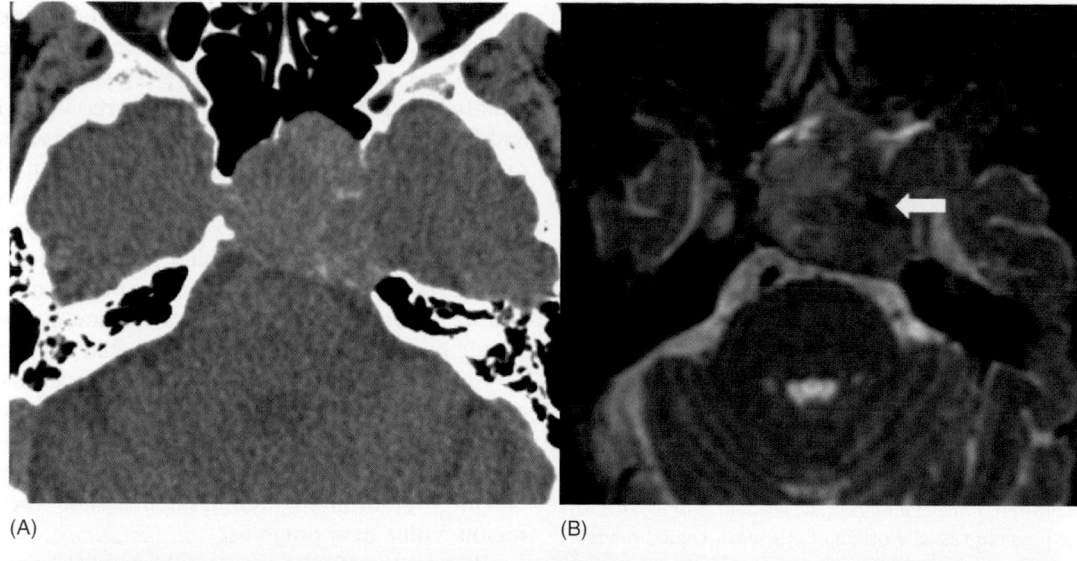

(A)   (B)

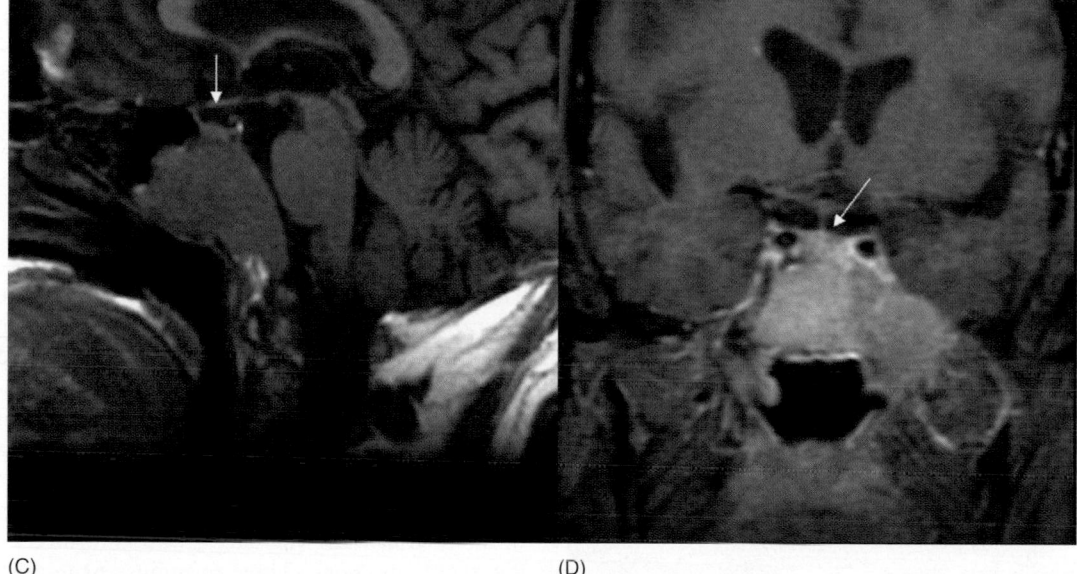

(C)   (D)

Figure 33 Clivus metastasis. Axial CT (A), axial T2W (B), sagittal T1W (C), and postcontrast coronal T1W (D) MRI show a lytic and destructive mass involving the clivus with encasement of the left carotid artery (*thick arrow*). Pituitary adenomas are by far the most common masses in this region but demonstration of a normal pituitary gland (*arrows*) eliminates that possibility. This was the only metastasis of a thyroid papillary carcinoma.

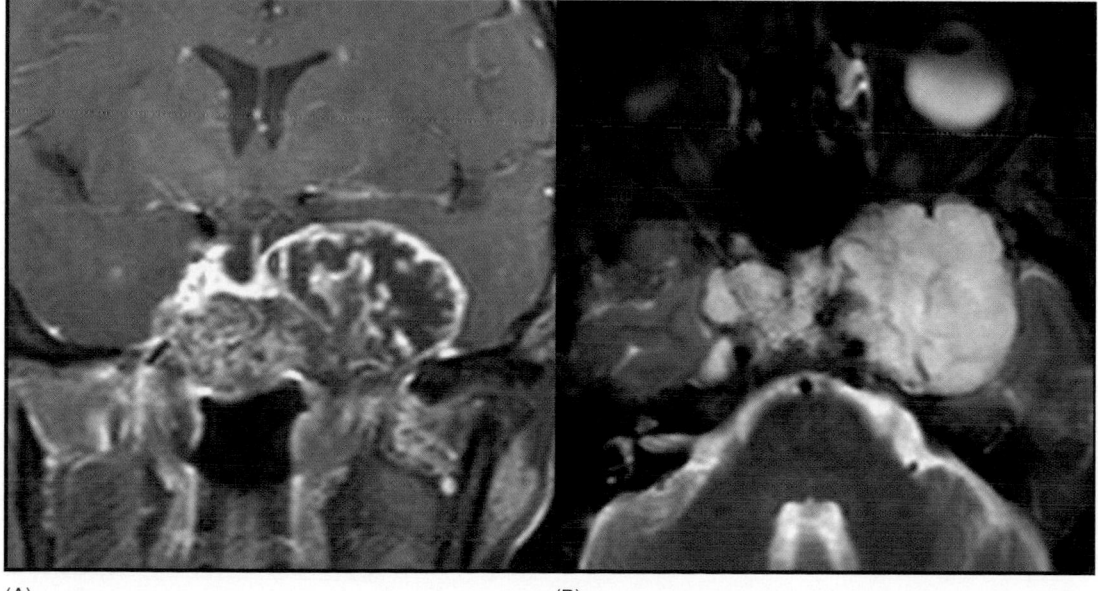

(A)   (B)

Figure 34 Chondrosarcoma. A large lobulated mass with very bright T2 signal (B) and curvilinear areas of enhancement on postcontrast T1W (A) image is seen to involve the clivus and grow into the left middle cranial fossa. This is a quite characteristic appearance for chondrosarcoma, although chordoma looks alike.

distance from the primary site. Because of its extensive distribution the trigeminal nerve is the most commonly affected cranial nerve by PNS. Involvement of the PPF is usually a turning point in PNS after which, tumor can extend intracranially via the foramen rotundum (maxillary nerve) and vidian canal (vidian nerve), intraorbitally via the infraorbital fissure and along the infraorbital nerve and into the ITF via the pterygomaxillary fissure (Figure 26). Similarly, PNS can occur via the mandibular nerve, which travels through the ITF and foramen ovale. Once reaching the trigeminal ganglion, PNS can occur towards the periphery via the maxillary, mandibular, and V-1 ophthalmic nerve, the latter of which can serve as a source for orbital invasion. PNS signifies a worse prognosis and sometimes can be diagnosed on imaging studies before it becomes symptomatic.

Primary tumors of the ITF are relatively uncommon and include vascular malformations, lipoma, juvenile angiofibroma, salivary gland tumors arising from ectopic salivary tissue, schwannoma, hemangiopericytoma, sarcomas, and lymphoma. The pterygoid venous plexus can be quite prominent and asymmetric mimicking vascular tumors on imaging studies. Pterygoid muscles can have various signal changes on MRI in postoperative patients or in patients with muscle denervation, which may simulate other pathologies. Since most tumors of the ITF originate outside the ITF, it is imperative to carefully evaluate the borders of a mass and its relationship with the surrounding structures before entertaining a primary ITF mass as the diagnosis.

JNA is a rare benign tumor of the PPF and ITF that originates from the superior posterior margin of the sphenopalatine foramen. It is usually very large at presentation and involves the nasopharynx, skull base, and intracranial compartment. JNA almost exclusively afflicts young males. Although histologically benign, JNA is very aggressive locally. Surgical resection and radiotherapy for the residual tumor when present is the standard approach for treatment. Because JNA is very vascular, presurgical embolization is routinely employed to help achieve a comprehensive resection, which is the most important step in curing the disease. Careful evaluation of the extent of disease before surgery and the residual tumor after surgery is critical in planning the surgery and radiotherapy.

Schwannomas limited to the ITF is rare. They appear similar on imaging studies to schwannomas seen elsewhere in the body (Figure 36). Surgical resection is the treatment of choice.

Bone tumors arising from the sphenoid bone, mandible, maxilla, or zygoma can present as ITF mass lesions. The level of aggressivity of a bone lesion can usually be predicted in imaging studies by looking at the bone expansion, remodeling and destruction, soft tissue component if present, and transition zone of the tumor. Osteoid and chondroid matrix can occasionally be identified on CT and MRI studies allowing a preoperative diagnosis. Needle biopsy of certain bone lesions,

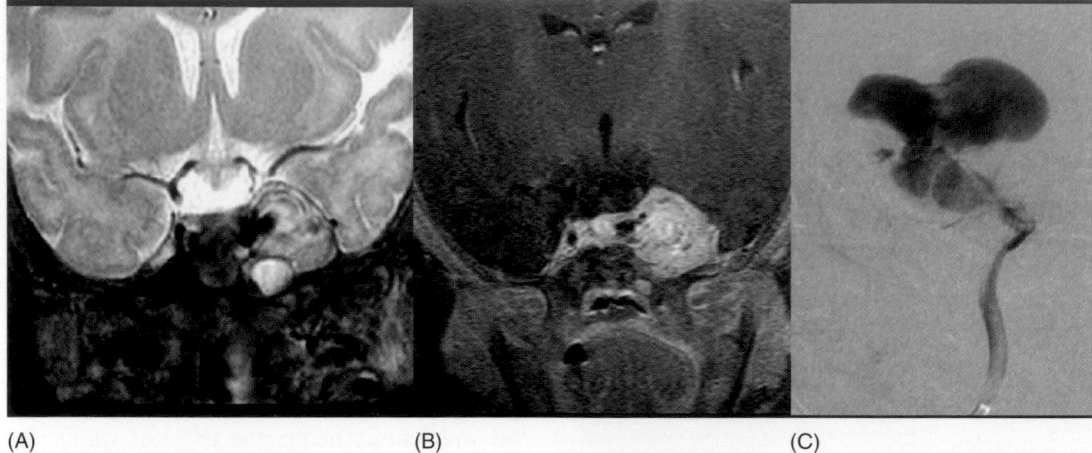

(A) (B) (C)

Figure 35 Giant aneurysm of the internal carotid artery. Coronal T2W (A) and postcontrast T1W (B) images demonstrate a large, heterogenous mass in the left cavernous sinus with erosion of the skull base. The small area of dark signal ("flow void") in the medial aspect of the mass (A) is a clue to the possible vascular origin of this mass. Digital subtraction angiography (C) reveals that the entire mass represents a giant internal carotid artery aneurysm with very slow flow accounting for the heterogeneity and enhancement.

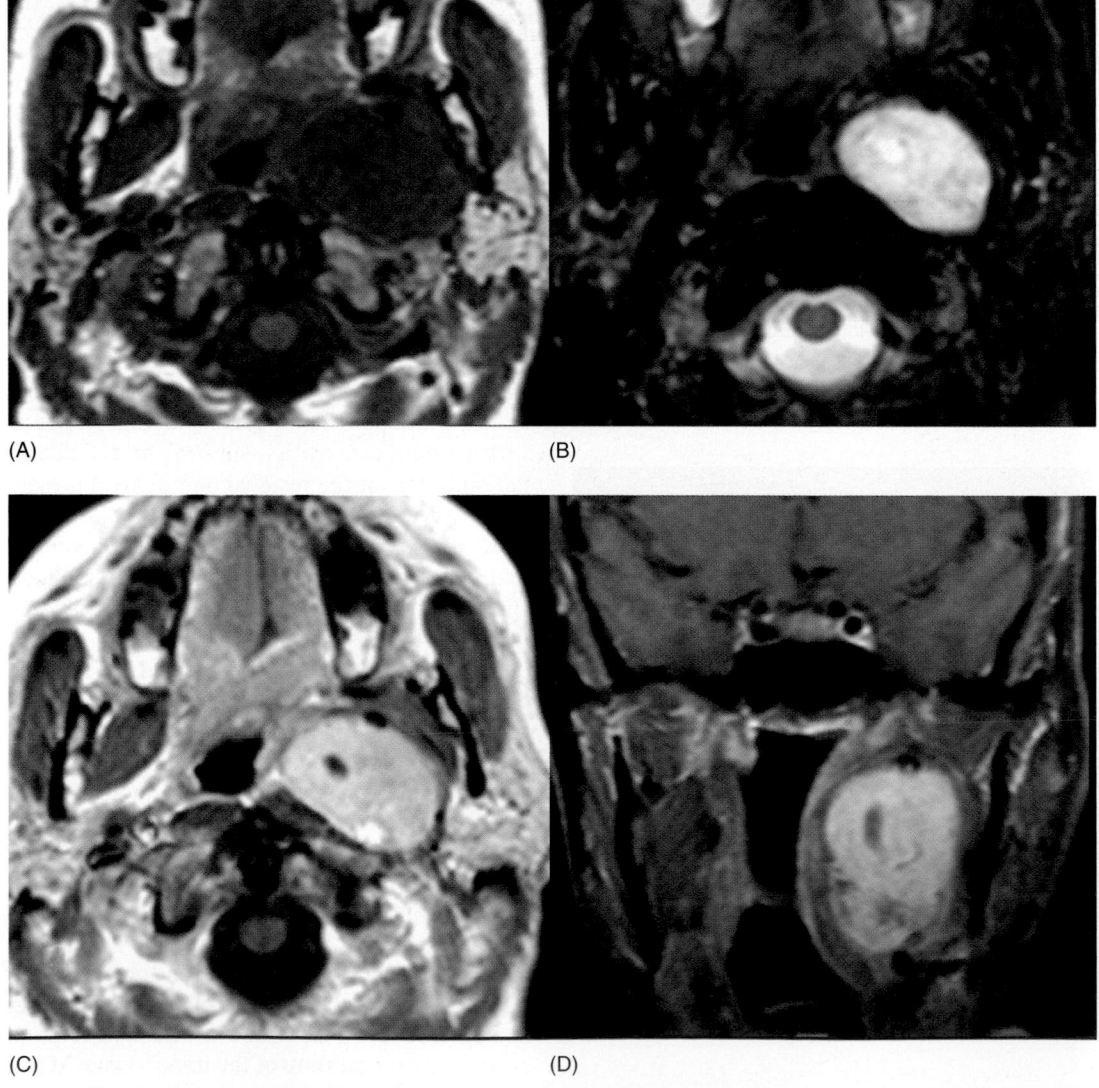

(A) (B)

(C) (D)

Figure 36 Schwannoma. A very well defined mass with very bright T2 signal (B) and prominent enhancement (C and D) with contrast is seen in the left infratemporal fossa. Typical appearance for schwannoma. A benign salivary gland tumor arising from the deep lobe of the parotid or minor salivary gland would be in the differential diagnosis.

while technically feasible, may be misleading due to presence of varying tissues. The age of the patient has a very significant bearing in the differential diagnosis of bone lesions. Osteosarcoma and Ewing sarcoma should be considered in the differential diagnosis of aggressive sphenoid bone lesions in children and teenagers. Chondrosarcoma is typically seen in young adults. A lytic and expansile lesion in an adult should prompt the diagnosis of giant cell tumor while aneurysmal bone cyst or giant cell reparative granuloma should be considered in children.

Soft tissue sarcomas, including hemangiopericytoma, synovial sarcoma, leiomyosarcoma, and spindle cell sarcoma can arise in the ITF (Figure 37). Rhabdomyosarcoma is a relatively common tumor in children in the head and neck region with a poor prognosis.

Primary tumors of the parapharyngeal space are usually either of MSG origin or schwannomas. Pleomorphic adenomas are most common. Nonetheless, the most common neoplastic processes in this space are spread from pharyngeal squamous cell carcinomas or deep lobe parotid masses (again pleomorphic adenomas or carcinomas).

ORBITS

The orbital roof is made by the frontal bone. The floor of the orbit is formed by contributions from the orbital plate of maxilla, the palatine bone, and the zygomatic bone. The frontal process of the maxilla and lacrimal bone make the anterior aspect of the medial wall of the orbit. The lamina papyracea forms the mid portion of the medial wall whereas the sphenoid bone contributes to the posterior part of the medial wall. The lateral wall is formed by the zygomatic bone. Three openings at the apex of the orbit allow entry/exit of the neurovascular structures. The superior orbital fissure is between the greater and lesser wings of the sphenoid and houses the oculomotor nerve (III), trochlear nerve (IV), abducens nerve (VI), ophthalmic division of the trigeminal nerve (V-1), and the superior ophthalmic vein. The optic canal is immediately medial to the superior orbital fissure and separated from it by a tiny bone called the optic strut, which is a projection of the anterior clinoid process. The optic nerve and the ophthalmic artery, which are covered by a dural sheet, travel through the optic canal. The inferior orbital fissure carries the inferior ophthalmic vein, infraorbital and zygomatic nerves (both V-2 branches), and branches of the pterygopalatine ganglion and allows communication between the orbit and ITF and PPF.

The bony orbit is lined by a tough fibrous sheath named the periorbita, which serves as a mechanical barrier between the intra- and extra-orbital structures. The medial, lateral, superior, and inferior rectus muscles arise from a common tendon, annulus of Zinn, and attach to the globe. The rectus muscles are enveloped by a fibrous membrane that forms the muscle cone and defines the intra-and extraconal spaces. The extraconal space is in between the periorbita and muscle cone and contains fat and the lacrimal

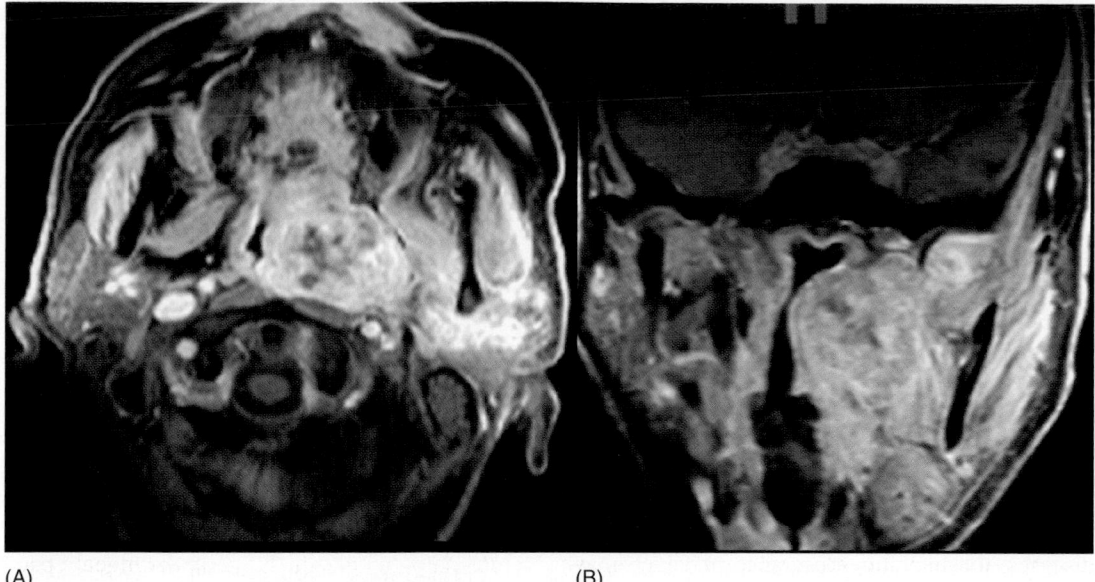

(A)   (B)

Figure 37 Leiomyosarcoma. Post contrast T1W axial (A) and coronal (B) images show a large and infiltrative mass in the left infratemporal fossa. The muscles of mastication are engulfed by the tumor. The pharyngeal mucosa is intact indicating the submucosal location of the mass.

gland superolaterally. The intraconal space contains the extraocular muscles, the optic nerve sheath complex, and other neurovascular structures in addition to fat.

When dealing with an orbital lesion, one should try to identify the anatomic site that the lesion originates from to narrow down the differential diagnosis. Most lesions respect these ana-tomic boundaries although transspatial involvement is not infrequently seen.

Optic nerve sheath complex mass lesions are meningiomas or gliomas in most cases. Optic nerve meningiomas arise from the dura around the optic nerve and tend to concentrically enlarge about the nerve. On MRI one can generally identify the optic nerve in the central aspect of the

mass.[37] Optic nerve meningiomas are generally confined to the orbit but extension to the optic canal and intracranial compartment is possible. The MR signal features of optic meningiomas resemble those of the intracranial meningiomas; isointense to the brain parenchyma on T1 and T2-weighted images with intense and homogenous enhancement with contrast material (Figure 38). The "sandwich sign" refers to enhancement of the optic nerve sheath on either side of the non-enhancing optic nerve in meningiomas of this region. Optic nerve sheath meningiomas arising in the optic canal may become symptomatic when they are very small. The optic canals should be investigated with good quality high resolution MRI to identify such small lesions in patients with unexplained progressive optic neuropathy.[38]

Optic nerve gliomas are usually of low-grade pilocytic astrocytomas and seen in children. One third of patients with optic glioma have neuro-fibromatosis I. Optic gliomas expand the optic nerve and it is not possible to identify the nerve separate from the tumor (Figure 38). MRI is the imaging study of choice and shows increased signal on T2 and isointense signal on T1-weighted images with variable enhancement on postcontrast images. Lymphoma and leukemia can rarely involve the optic nerve sheath and present as diffuse thickening of the nerve with enhancement on the postcontrast images.

Optic neuritis may show subtle enlargement of the nerve-sheath complex and may affect any part of the nerve. The majority of optic neuropathy in adults is ischemic in nature and can be diagnosed on clinical grounds. Multiple sclerosis is the leading cause of nonischemic optic neuropathy but optic neuritis may also occur in isolation. Eighty percent of patients with multiple sclerosis will have a bout of optic neuritis at some stage in their disease. Scanning the brain may reveal characteristic periventricular plaques. High signal on T2WI and enhancement in the acute setting are characteristic (Figure 38). In the chronic phase, optic atrophy may be present.

A variety of inflammatory and infectious diseases can present with optic neuritis with similar imaging findings. Idiopathic pseudotumor of the orbit is a nongranulomatous inflammatory process involving the orbit. It may present as a mass lesion, hence the name pseudotumor, or as an infiltrative process. It may involve a single structure or the entire orbit. The clinical presentation may be in acute, subacute or chronic form. The acute form is clinically characterized by abrupt onset of pain, redness and swelling of the eyelid. There is generally a quick and lasting response to steroid therapy. Since pseudotumor can involve any structure in the orbit in isolation or combination and present as a mass lesion or infiltrative process, the imaging differential diagnosis includes a number of possibilities from tumors and infection to thyroid ophthalmopathy. The combination of imaging feature and clinical presentation often obviate the need for biopsy, however. The myositic form of idiopathic pseudotumor mimics thyroid ophthalmopathy, whereas the tumoral form

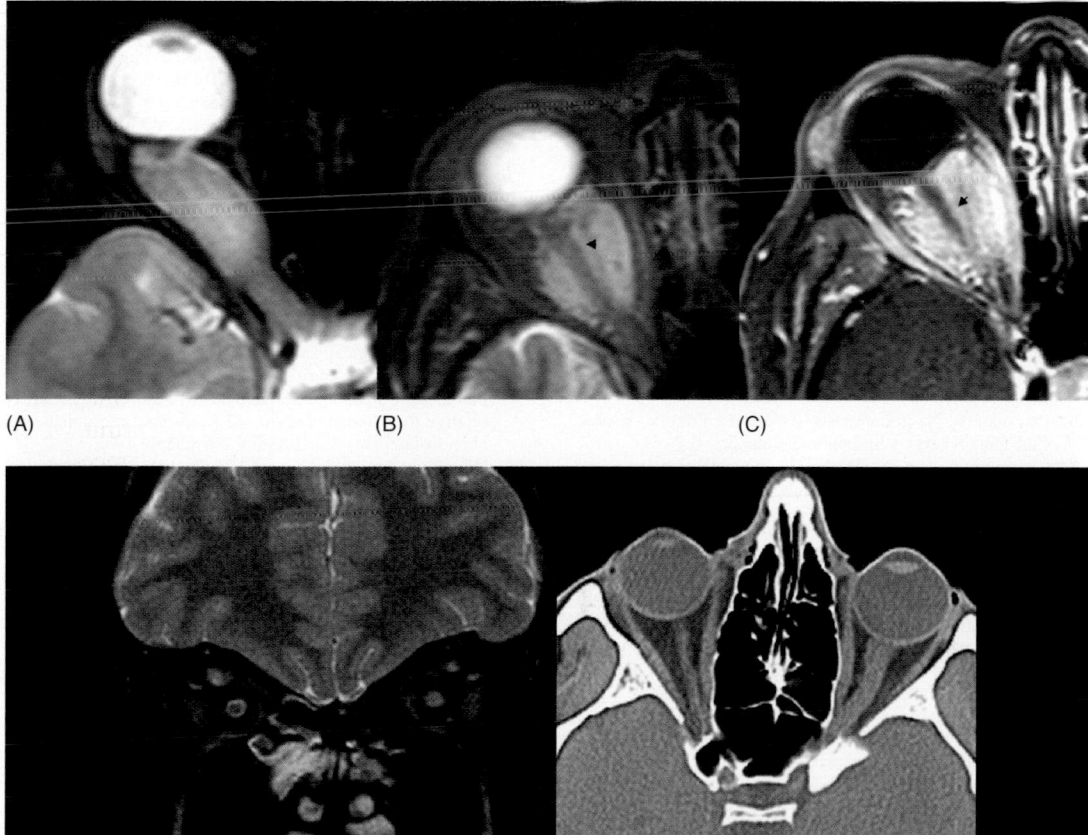

(A)   (B)   (C)

(D)   (E)

Figure 38 Optic nerve sheath tumors. (A) Glioma, (B and C) meningioma, (D) optic neuritis, and (E) pseudotumor. Glioma presents as a mass expanding the optic nerve. The optic nerve is seen within the meningioma (*arrowheads* in part B and C). Mild swelling of the nerve is seen with increased T2 signal in optic neuritis. Isolated optic nerve pseudotumor is rare. In this patient it presented with diffuse swelling of the nerve sheath complex.

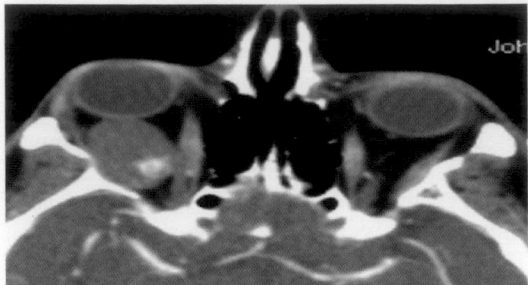

Figure 39 Orbital cavernous hemangioma. Axial CT image shows a very well defined intraconal mass with small calcification.

resembles benign and malignant neoplasms. The infiltrative form is usually mistaken for infectious and lymphoproliferative diseases.

A number of benign and malignant tumors can arise in the intraconal space outside the optic nerve sheath complex. Hemangioma, lymphangioma, lymphoma, and metastasis are the most common masses. Schwannoma, neurofibroma, and meningioma are relatively uncommon. Cavernous hemangiomas are the most common intraconal tumors of the adults. They usually present with painless and progressive proptosis. On MRI and CT they appear as very well-defined mass lesions with hyperintense signal on T2WI, patchy or homogeneous contrast enhancement, and small calcifications[39] (Figure 39). In children, dermoid tumor, capillary hemangioma, lymphangioma, and rhabdomyosarcoma are the most common mass lesions. Rhabdomyosarcomas are most frequently seen in the orbit. Other sites in the head and neck region include facial soft tissues, paranasal sinuses, skull base (perimeningeal) and ITF.[40] Encephaloceles of the anterior skull base can present as orbital mass lesion, typically in children, and this possibility must be considered when dealing with cystic lesions before any surgical procedure.

Vascular lesions of the orbit include caroticocavernous fistula, superior ophthalmic vein thrombosis, cavernous sinus thrombosis, venous varix, and arteriovenous malformations. They are usually easy to recognize because of their characteristic clinical presentation and imaging appearance, which includes increase in size of the lesion

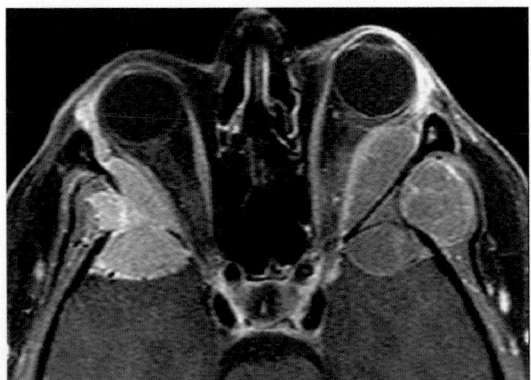

Figure 40 Multiple myeloma of the orbit. Bilateral sphenoid bone masses with extraosseous extension are seen.

with Valsalva maneuver. Flow voids or pulsation artifacts are typical features on MR. Enhancement is predictable with CT. Thrombi may be variable in signal intensity.

The extraconal lesions of the orbit most commonly include the lacrimal gland diseases and direct extension of sinonasal diseases. Infection arising from the sinonasal cavity can gain access to the orbit through the natural bony dehiscences or veins. Such extension is usually limited by the periorbita and results in subperiosteal abscess, although extension to the intraconal orbit can cause orbital cellulitis that may be catastrophic. Orbital or periorbital infection can spread to the intracranial compartment and cavernous sinus via direct contiguity or venous flow.

The lacrimal gland can be afflicted by infectious, inflammatory, neoplastic, and autoimmune diseases, the imaging appearance of which may be quite similar and consist of diffuse enlargement of the gland. The primary tumors of the lacrimal gland can often be differentiated from other entities; however. They include epithelial (MSG), lymphoid, and congenital (dermoid/epidermoid) origins.

Tumors arising from the bony orbit may present as extraconal mass lesions. Among these metastases and plasmocytoma/multiple myeloma are the most common (Figure 40).

REFERENCES

1. Benninger MS, Ferguson BJ, Hadley JA, et al. Adult chronic rhinosinusitis: Definitions, diagnosis, epidemiology, and pathophysiology. Otolaryngol Head Neck Surg 2003;129: S1–32.
2. Babbel RW, Harnsberger HR, Sonkens J, Hunt S. Recurring patterns of inflammatory sinonasal disease demonstrated on screening sinus CT. AJNR Am J Neuroradiol 1992;13:903–12.
3. Som PM, Dillon WP, Fullerton GD, et al. Chronically obstructed sinonasal secretions: Observations on T1 and T2 shortening. Radiology 1989;172:515–20.
4. Bhattacharyya T, Piccirillo J, Wippold FJ, IInd. Relationship between patient-based descriptions of sinusitis and paranasal sinus computed tomographic findings. Arch Otolaryngol Head Neck Surg 1997;123:1189–92.
5. Lund VJ, Kennedy DW. Quantification for staging sinusitis. The Staging and Therapy Group. Ann Otol Rhinol Laryngol Suppl 1995;167:17–21.
6. Pawankar R. Nasal polyposis: An update: Editorial review. Curr Opin Allergy Clin Immunol 2003;3:1–6.
7. Chung SK, Chang BC, Dhong HJ. Surgical, radiologic, and histologic findings of the antrochoanal polyp. Am J Rhinol 2002;16:71–6.
8. Lanza DC, Dhong HJ, Tantilipikorn P, et al. Fungus and chronic rhinosinusitis: From bench to clinical understanding. Ann Otol Rhinol Laryngol Suppl 2006;196:27–34.
9. Fatterpekar G, Mukherji S, Arbealez A, et al. Fungal diseases of the paranasal sinuses. Semin Ultrasound CT MR 1999;20:391–401.
10. DelGaudio JM, Swain RE, Jr, Kingdom TT, et al. Computed tomographic findings in patients with invasive fungal sinusitis. Arch Otolaryngol Head Neck Surg 2003; 129:236–40.
11. Schubert MS. Allergic fungal sinusitis: Pathogenesis and management strategies. Drugs 2004;64:363–74.
12. Llompart X, Aumaitre O, Kemeny JL, et al. Early otorhinolaryngological manifestations of Wegener's granulomatosis. Analysis of 21 patients. Ann Otolaryngol Chir Cervicofac 2002;119:330–6.
13. Som PM, Dillon WP, Curtin HD, et al. Hypointense paranasal sinus foci: Differential diagnosis with MR imaging and relation to CT findings. Radiology 1990;176:777–81.
14. Katori H, Nozawa A, Tsukuda M. Markers of malignant transformation of sinonasal inverted papilloma. Eur J Surg Oncol 2005;31:905–11.
15. Katori H, Nozawa A, Tsukuda M. Histopathological parameters of recurrence and malignant transformation in sinonasal inverted papilloma. Acta Otolaryngol 2006;126:214–8.
16. Oikawa K, Furuta Y, Oridate N, et al. Preoperative staging of sinonasal inverted papilloma by magnetic resonance imaging. Laryngoscope 2003;113:1983–7.
17. Maroldi R, Farina D, Palvarini L, et al. Magnetic resonance imaging findings of inverted papilloma: Differential diagnosis with malignant sinonasal tumors. Am J Rhinol 2004;18:305–10.
18. Minovi A, Kollert M, Draf W, Bockmuhl U. Inverted papilloma: Feasibility of endonasal surgery and long-term results of 87 cases. Rhinology 2006;44:205–10.
19. Loy AH, Reibel JF, Read PW, et al. Esthesioneuroblastoma: Continued follow-up of a single institution's experience. Arch Otolaryngol Head Neck Surg 2006;132:134–8.
20. Mendenhall WM, Mendenhall CM, Riggs CE, Jr, et al. Sinonasal undifferentiated carcinoma. Am J Clin Oncol 2006;29:27–31.
21. Iezzoni JC, Mills SE. "Undifferentiated" small round cell tumors of the sinonasal tract: Differential diagnosis update. Am J Clin Pathol 2005;124:S110–21.
22. Cuadra-Garcia I, Proulx GM, Wu CL, et al. Sinonasal lymphoma: A clinicopathologic analysis of 58 cases from the Massachusetts General Hospital. Am J Surg Pathol 1999;23:1356–69.
23. Vidal RW, Devaney K, Ferlito A, et al. Sinonasal malignant lymphomas: A distinct clinicopathological category. Ann Otol Rhinol Laryngol 1999;108:411–9.
24. Ganly I, Patel SG, Singh B, et al. Craniofacial resection for malignant paranasal sinus tumors: Report of an International Collaborative Study. Head Neck 2005;27:575–84.
25. Suarez C, Llorente JL, Fernandez De Leon R, et al. Prognostic factors in sinonasal tumors involving the anterior skull base. Head Neck 2004;26:136–44.
26. Eisen MD, Yousem DM, Loevner LA, et al. Preoperative imaging to predict orbital invasion by tumor. Head Neck 2000;22:456–62.
27. Eisen MD, Yousem DM, Montone KT, et al. Use of preoperative MR to predict dural, perineural, and venous sinus invasion of skull base tumors. AJNR Am J Neuroradiol 1996;17:1937–45.
28. King AD, Vlantis AC, Tsang RK, et al. Magnetic resonance imaging for the detection of nasopharyngeal carcinoma. AJNR Am J Neuroradiol 2006;27:1288–91.
29. Lu JC, Wei BQ, Chen WZ, et al. Staging of nasopharyngeal carcinoma investigated by magnetic resonance imaging. Radiother Oncol 2006;79:21–6.
30. Chen YK, Su CT, Ding HJ, et al. Clinical usefulness of fused PET/CT compared with PET alone or CT alone in nasopharyngeal carcinoma patients. Anticancer Res 2006;26:1471–7.
31. Vieira JO, Jr, Cukiert A, Liberman B. Magnetic resonance imaging of cavernous sinus invasion by pituitary adenoma diagnostic criteria and surgical findings. Arq Neuropsiquiatr 2004;62:437–43.
32. Kleinschmidt-DeMasters BK, Lillehei KO, Stears JC. The pathologic, surgical, and MR spectrum of Rathke cleft cysts [discussion 26–7]. Surg Neurol 1995;44:19–26.
33. Pamir MN, Ozduman K. Analysis of radiological features relative to histopathology in 42 skull-base chordomas and chondrosarcomas. Eur J Radiol 2006;58:461–70.
34. O'Sullivan MG, van Loveren HR, Tew JM, Jr. The surgical resectability of meningiomas of the cavernous sinus [discussion 245–7]. Neurosurgery 1997;40:238–44.
35. Leong JL, Batra PS, Citardi MJ. Three-dimensional computed tomography angiography of the internal carotid artery for preoperative evaluation of sinonasal lesions and intraoperative surgical navigation. Laryngoscope 2005;115:1618–23.
36. Sherman PM, Yousem DM, Loevner LA. CT-guided aspirations in the head and neck: Assessment of the first 216 cases. AJNR Am J Neuroradiol 2004;25:1603–7.
37. Miller NR. Primary tumours of the optic nerve and its sheath. Eye 2004;18:1026–37.
38. Jackson A, Patankar T, Laitt RD. Intracanalicular optic nerve meningioma: A serious diagnostic pitfall. AJNR Am J Neuroradiol 2003;24:1167–70.
39. Thorn-Kany M, Arrue P, Delisle MB, et al. Cavernous hemangiomas of the orbit: MR imaging. J Neuroradiol 1999;26:79–86.
40. Hicks J, Flaitz C. Rhabdomyosarcoma of the head and neck in children. Oral Oncol 2002;38:450–9.

42

Etiology of Infectious Diseases of the Upper Respiratory Tract

David M. Poetker, MD, MA
Timothy L. Smith, MD, MPH

Infectious diseases of the upper respiratory tract represent a broad topic, involving many different pathogens and targeting many different sites. Many of these result in multiple infections, with overlapping manifestations. In this chapter, we attempt to present an extensive, although not exhaustive, list of the various infectious agents affecting the upper respiratory tract. We have included the bacteria, viruses, fungi, and other pathogens specific to a given anatomical location. In addition, we have included special interest topics related to the upper respiratory tract.

OTITIS MEDIA

Otitis media is one of the most commonly diagnosed childhood illnesses.[1] It is estimated that there are about 2.2 million diagnosed episodes per year, at a total cost of about $4.0 billion.[2] It affects more than 90% of children in the preschool years and as many as 60% within the first two years of life.[2] There are several risk factors associated with otitis media. They fall into two categories, the preventable, and the nonpreventable. The preventable include daycare, tobacco smoke exposure, extended pacifier use, and lack of breast-feeding.[3] The nonpreventable risk factors include such things as gender, ethnicity, family history, older siblings, low socioeconomic status, and other health conditions.[3]

Common pathogens isolated from middle ear effusions (MEE) have been well documented.[4-6] Bluestone and colleagues reported their experience and the pathogens isolated from over 7,000 MEE over a 10 year period.[4] They found the three most common pathogens identified in acute otitis media (AOM) were *Streptococcus pneumoniae* (40% of isolates), nontypeable *Haemophilus influenzae* (25%), and *Moraxella catarrhalis* (12%) (Table 1).

They were able to isolate bacteria from only two-thirds of the effusions obtained from patients with chronic otitis media with effusion, and of the bacteria isolated, only one-third were considered pathogenic. The three most commonly isolated bacteria were the same as in AOM, however the ratios were slightly different. *H. influenzae* was the most commonly isolated at 15%, followed by *M. catarrhalis*, isolated from 10% of the cultured effusions, and *S. pneumoniae* was isolated from 7% of the effusions.[4] Studies have shown much higher identification rates of pathogenic bacteria using more sensitive methods of bacterial identification such as polymerase chain reaction (PCR) techniques. Other explanations for the low rates of bacterial isolation, include the presence of bacterial biofilms[7,8] (see Chapter 16, "Otitis Media and Middle-Ear Effusions," and Chapter 17, "Chronic Otitis Media and Cholesteatoma," on otitis media and cholesteatoma and Chapter 71, "Biofilms and Their Role in Ear and Respiratory Infections," on bacterial biofilms for more information).

More recent reports of MEE isolates in chronic otitis media with effusion have shown a decrease in the percent of *S. pneumoniae* positive cultures. The introduction of Prevnar heptavalent pneumococcal vaccine has been reported to have had a decrease in overall AOM incidence and has been reported to have contributed to a decrease in specific pneumococcal AOM episodes.[9,10]

Identification of the offending microorganism requires culture of the middle ear fluid. This is relatively straight forward in the case of a perforated tympanic membrane with purulent otorrhea. In the case of an intact tympanic membrane, a tympanocentesis is required. Given the impracticality of performing a tympanocentesis on every child with an intact tympanic membrane, empiric coverage is appropriate. If however the patient fails multiple antibiotic courses, one should consider tympanocentesis to confirm the diagnosis and direct therapy with culture and sensitivity results.[3]

The most recent set of treatment guidelines are from the American Academy of Pediatrics and the American Academy of Family Physicians from 2004. They recommend amoxicillin as the first line therapy for AOM. In those patients with a penicillin allergy, a cephalosporin, azithromycin, or clarithromycin is recommended. Patients that present with a temperature of greater than 39°C, or severe otalgia, amoxicillin/clavulanate is recommended with ceftriaxone for those allergic to penicillin. Those patients that fail the first line therapy should be given amoxicillin/clavulanate with the allergic alternative of ceftriaxone or clindamycin. Patients that present having failed first line therapy and have a temperature of greater than 39°C should be given ceftriaxone or clindamycin. A tympanocentesis should be considered.[3] Please see Chapters 16, "Otitis Media and Middle-Ear Effusions" and 17, "Chronic Otitis Media and Cholesteatoma" for a more complete discussion of otitis media.

A viral cause for AOM has been linked to such pathogens as the respiratory syncytial virus, influenza viruses, and adenoviruses. Since attempts at culture or identification of these are rarely performed, the incidence of these pathogens is not known. An association is logical, given that many episodes of otitis media follow a viral upper respiratory tract infection. In addition, viral upper respiratory tract infections have similar seasonal patterns as otitis media.[3]

THE COMMON COLD

The common cold represents a syndrome caused by a wide variety of infectious agents. It is usually a benign, self-limited illness of the upper respiratory tract. Despite this, the economic burden caused by the common cold is substantial. It accounts for approximately 20 million days of missed work, and 22 million days of missed school.[11]

Symptoms may present hours to days after inoculation. The most common initial symptom is a sore throat. This is followed by nasal congestion, rhinorrhea, sneezing, and cough. In addition, some patients experience fever, especially children, hoarseness, headache, malaise, lethargy, and myalgia, especially with the influenza virus infection. These symptoms usually last between 7 and 10 days.[11]

The cause of the common cold is almost exclusively viral, although there is overlap with the clinical experience with of many bacterial infections (Table 2). The most common of the viral infections is the rhinovirus, estimated to be responsible for 30 to 50% of cases.[11] More

Table 1 Common Causes of Otitis Media

Streptococcus pneumoniae
Nontypeable *Haemophilus influenzae*
Moraxella catarrhalis

than 100 different serotypes of rhinovirus have been identified. The corona viruses account for between 10 and 15% of colds. Influenza viruses are the third most common cause, responsible for 5 to 15% of colds. Although influenza infections can be much more severe than the average cold, there is enough overlap to include influenza. The respiratory syncytial virus and parainfluenza viruses each account for 5%, while adenoviruses and enteroviruses each account for less than 5% of all colds.[11] Twenty to thirty percent of the cases of the common cold go without identification of the specific agent, although this is likely due to technical issues. The human metapneumovirus is a relatively new respiratory virus identified in children. The percentage of infections due to the metapneumovirus has not yet been established.[11]

The incidence of infections varies, with the incidence decreasing with increased age. Younger children have between six and eight colds per year, while adults have between two and four. Risk factors include daycare attendance, psychological stress, and heavy physical training. Transmission routes include direct contact with viral particles, as well as small-particle and large-particle aerosols. The routes of transmission depend on the specific virus.[11]

The infectious process begins with the viruses entering the nose. The mucociliary clearance carries them to the adenoid area of the nasopharynx where they enter the epithelial cells via cell receptors such as the intercellular adhesion molecule-1. Once the virus is inside the epithelial cell, replication can occur as quickly as eight hours. Approximately 75% of patients infected will develop symptoms. Virus shedding usually peaks by the second day, but virus can be detected for several weeks.[11]

The pathophysiology of the manifestations of infection is not clearly understood. Viral infection has been shown to result in vasodilatation and increased vascular permeability. Mucous glands increase secretion due to the cholinergic stimulation. Certain viruses like influenza and adenovirus have been shown to cause extensive damage to the respiratory epithelium, however rhinovirus cause no histopathologic changes to the epithelium. This has led to the belief that inflammatory response to the infection and release of inflammatory mediators cause the symptoms.[11] Recent studies have shown that several viruses can infect and replicate in the lower respiratory tract, contributing to the pulmonary symptoms of the common cold, although the exact mechanism of cough development has not been clearly established.[11,12]

The gold standard for viral identification involves virus isolation in cell culture. Other identification techniques include antigen detection and PCR. These techniques are of little clinical significance, since most cases can be diagnosed based on patient symptoms. Obviously, patients that are not able to articulate their symptoms make the diagnosis more challenging.[11]

Many different therapies have been reported for the treatment of the common cold, though few have data to support their use. There are data to support the use of first-generation, however not second-generation, antihistamine/decongestants. These have been shown to help with the nasal congestion and discharge.[12] This is thought to be due to their anticholinergic properties, rather than the antihistamine effect. In addition, naproxen was shown to decrease cough, likely due to its anti-inflammatory properties. Other medications such as zinc, echinacea, and vitamin C have had mixed results in clinical trials evaluating efficacy.[13]

Antiviral medications targeted against influenza viruses have shown that they help to reduce the duration of symptoms by 1 to 2 days if taken within the first 48 hours of symptoms. Amantadine and rimantadine were first introduced for the treatment of influenza A; however, they showed poor efficacy against influenza B, resulted in the development of resistant strains, and had an unfavorable side effect profile. Newer anti-influenza drugs include zanamivir and oseltamivir. These have fewer side effects and are able to treat both influenza A and B. Antirhinoviral drugs ruprintrivir and pleconaril, have been shown to reduce the duration of symptoms by 1 to 1.5 days if started within 24 to 36 hours of the onset of symptoms.[11]

SINUSITIS

Acute and chronic rhinosinusitis are discussed in Chapters 46, "Acute Rhinosinusitis and Its Complications" and 47, "Chronic Rhinosinusitis and Polyposis." It is believed that most acute episodes of sinusitis are caused by viral infections, which lead to mucosal edema and potential obstruction of the paranasal sinuses. These viruses are the same as those that cause the common cold, as outlined above. When the mucosal edema occurs, this provides a favorable environment for the overgrowth of bacteria in the paranasal sinuses leading to acute bacterial sinusitis.[14] There exists a progression of infectious agents from acute sinusitis to chronic sinusitis. The aerobic bacteria commonly associated with acute sinusitis are the same as those associated with otitis media, *S. pneumoniae*, *H. influenzae*, and *M. catarrhalis* (Table 3). As the acute infection continues, the bacteria consume the available oxygen, thus decreasing the oxygen tension in the sinuses and increasing the acidity, making the environment more hospitable for anaerobic bacteria. The common anaerobic bacteria associated with chronic sinusitis include *Fusobacterium nucleatum*, *Prevotella*, *Porphyromonas,* and *Peptostreptococcus* species. In addition to the anaerobic bacteria, gram-negative bacteria have been associated with

Table 3 Common Causes of Sinusitis and Rhinitis
Bacterial
Sinusitis
Streptococcus pneumoniae
Haemophilus influenzae
Moraxella catarrhalis
Rhinitis
Klebsiella rhinoscleromatis
Actinomycosis israelii
Treponema pallidum
Mycobacterium tuberculosis
Mycobacterium leprae
Fungal
Blastomyces dermatitidis
Coccidioides immitis
Rhinosporidium seeberi
Mucormycosis
Aspergillosis
Parasitic
Leishmaniasis
Myiasis

chronic sinusitis.[14] These include *Pseudomonas aeruginosa*, *Klebsiella pneumoniae*, *Proteus mirabilis*, *Escherichia coli*, and *Enterobacter* species.

The role of fungus in rhinosinusitis is poorly understood. The three major groups of potential pathogens are Zygomycetes, *Aspergillus* species, and dematiaceous fungi. It has been shown that if looked for carefully enough, fungus can be isolated from almost everyone regardless of sinus disease.[15] What is not well understood is why certain individuals may react to the presence of fungi, while others do not. It is also unclear what the precise mechanism is that underlies the pathophysiology of the reaction to the fungi. One theory holds that when individuals are exposed to the fungus, the antigenic trigger, there are type I and III immune reactions and stimulation of an intense eosinophilic response. This response leads to mucosal edema, which then provides an environment that perpetuates the fungal growth. The increased fungal load leads to increased antigenic exposure, thus creating a continuous cycle. Other hypotheses include a nonallergic response to the presence of fungus, due to direct fungal stimulation of peripheral monocytes, which results in specific cytokine secretion that promotes eosinophilic response.[15] Further investigation will be required to understand this complex interaction fully.

RHINITIS

Bacterial

Rhinoscleroma is caused by the gram-negative, encapsulated bacterium *K. rhinoscleromatis*. Infection universally involves the nose, and initial infections are believed to occur at mucosal junctions, such as that found in the nasal vestibule. Disease can also involve the nasopharynx, larynx, and trachea.[16]

Infection is characterized by three distinct and successive phases. Patients typically show rather slow progression through each of the phases. The initial phase, the catarrhal or rhinitic phase, is characterized by symptoms consistent with the common cold. This includes a "honeycomb" colored discharge with a fetid odor. The second phase is the granulomatous phase, characterized by large, friable, granulomatous masses in the nasal cavity. These granulomas can cause epistaxis, nasal obstruction, and even bony remodeling of the turbinates and the medial maxillary wall. The final phase is the fibrotic or sclerotic phase, during which the cicatrization of the lesions leads to the anatomic distortion of the involved structures with nasal obstruction.[16]

The disease is endemic in areas of Central and South America, Central Europe, East Africa, and the Indian subcontinent and is associated with poor hygiene and overcrowded conditions. An increase in the incidence in the United States is most likely the result of immigration from endemic areas.[16]

When histiocytes, or Mikulicz cells, are stained with Warthin-Starry or Gram, they can show the gram-negative bacilli within the cytoplasm, thus suggesting the diagnosis. Cultures positive for *K. rhinoscleromatis* are diagnostic; however they are only positive in 50 to 60% of cases. Computed tomography characteristically shows homogenous, nonenhancing nasal masses with well-defined borders. Bone and cartilage involvement may be seen in advanced cases.[16]

Treatment involves long courses of antibiotics for at least 3 months. There is a high relapse rate, requiring multiple antibiotic courses. Tetracycline has been used traditionally; however, given the contraindications in children, other antibiotics including cephaloridine, chloramphenicol, chlortetracycline, rifampin, and trimethoprim–sulfamethoxazole have all been used.[16]

Actinomycosis is caused by a gram-positive, anaerobic, or microaerophilic bacterium of the genus *Actinomyces*. *A. israelii* is the most common species associated with human disease. Other species include *A. naeslundii*, *A. viscous*, and *A. odontolyticus*. The bacterium is part of the normal flora of the oral cavity, as well as the respiratory and the digestive tracts. It grows as a hyphae or a filamentous organism, with the initial infection producing microcolonies composed of branching filaments. These develop into tight clusters commonly referred to as sulfur granules.[17]

Actinomycosis has been identified throughout the head and neck, including the oral cavity, pharynx, dental plaques, tonsillar crypts, skin of the face, mastoid bone, skull, nasopharynx and paranasal sinuses, and the temporomandibular joint. The clinical course of disease can vary widely, with a typical presentation involving a slowly, progressively enlarging mass in the neck or at the angle of the jaw. Up to 40% of patients have sinuses or fistulas.[17] Involvement in the nasal cavity is relatively rare; however, it has been reported as a slowly enlarging nasal mass.[18]

Diagnosis is based upon clinical examination, culture results, and microscopic analysis of tissue samples including Gram stain, acid-fast staining, and histology, although cultures are difficult to obtain, with only 10 to 20% being positive. The bacterium will be acid-fast negative, and Gram staining demonstrates gram-positive, branching, thin, filamentous-like organisms with the characteristic sulfur granules.

Treatment is both medical and surgical with aggressive surgical debridement followed by a long course of antibiotic therapy to eradicate the infection. Penicillin therapy for up to 12 months is considered first line. Alternatives include doxycycline, ceftriaxone, erythromycin, and chloramphenicol.[19] If the infection recurs, longer courses of antibiotic therapy are required.[17] Some advocate the use of adjunctive hyperbaric oxygen therapy.[18]

Syphilis is caused by the spirochete *Treponema pallidum*. Involvement of the nose and paranasal sinuses varies, depending on the phase of the infection. Primary syphilis occurs 10 to 90 days after the initial infection and is characterized by the presence of a painless chancre at the site of initial inoculation. Primary syphilis is rarely associated with the nasal cavity, although can involve the mucocutaneous junction of the nasal vestibule. Secondary syphilis involves the hematogenous spread of the spirochete, coinciding with regression of the primary chancre. Nasal symptoms of secondary syphilis include irritation of the anterior nares and acute rhinitis with a scant, thick discharge. Mucosal surfaces of the upper aerodigestive tract may develop painless ulcers that are similar in appearance to aphthous ulcers. The disease then enters a latent phase, with approximately one-third of patients maintaining the latent infection, one-third spontaneously clearing the infection, and the final third developing tertiary syphilis. Tertiary syphilis may be manifested by benign, destructive lesions, called gummata, believed to be the result of a robust inflammatory response to spirochetes. These gummata often involve the nasal septum, causing destruction of the cartilage and ultimately a saddle-nose deformity. The gummata have been reported to cause stenosis of the nasopharynx from scarring. Congenital syphilis may be symptomatic in 10 to 75% of infected infants. They most commonly present with watery nasal discharge, which progresses to a thick and purulent, and ultimately bloody discharge. Nasal obstruction leading to feeding difficulties may occur, as well as erosion of the septal cartilage.[20]

There are two types of serologic tests for *T. pallidum*, the first is the nontreponemal tests. These include the venereal disease research laboratory test slide, the unheated serum reagin, the rapid plasma reagin (RPR) test and the toluidine red untreated serum test. They measure the antibody response to cellular antigens that are released as a result of treponemal infection and are not specific for *T. pallidum*. They are useful for following the progression of the disease. The RPR is approximately 80% sensitive in primary syphilis, and an RPR titer above 1:32 establishes the diagnosis in secondary syphilis. The second type is the treponemal tests, which detect the antibody response to *T. pallidum*. These include the fluorescent treponemal antibody absorption and the microhemagglutination-*T. pallidum* tests. These tests are qualitative not quantitative, remaining positive for life, and are not be used to follow disease progression.[20]

Microscopic identification of *T. pallidum* spirochetes using dark field examination confirms the diagnosis in all phases; however, the spirochetes are abundant only in primary, secondary, and congenital syphilis. Due to maternal antibodies, identification of spirochetes in nasal secretions is the only way to confirm the diagnosis of congenital syphilis. Histological examination of a primary syphilitic chancre reveals central necrotic debris with chronic inflammation at the distal zones. Secondary syphilis demonstrates plasma cells and lymphocytic infiltration of the epithelial lesions.[20]

Penicillin is the treatment of choice for syphilis, based on current Centers for Disease Control and Prevention guidelines.[19] Initial therapy can result in myalgias, fevers, headaches, and other constitutional symptoms; anti-pyretics may help minimize these side effects.[20]

Nasal tuberculosis, caused by the acid- and alcohol-fast bacilli *Mycobacterium tuberculosis,* is rare. It is speculated to be the result of either inhalation of infectious particles or direct inoculation from a contaminated finger. Atypical mycobacterial infections involving the nose or paranasal sinuses are exceedingly rare, although reports of *M. kansasii* causing a granulomatous infection and perforation of the nasal septum exist.[21]

Nasal tuberculosis infections present with nasal obstruction, anterior and posterior nasal discharge, nasal discomfort, epistaxis, crusting, epiphora, recurrent nasal polyps, and ulceration. The most commonly involved sites are the cartilaginous septum, turbinates, and nasal floor. On anterior rhinoscopy, the mass appears as a bright red, friable mass or as a nodular thickening of the mucosa and may have shallow ulcers. The mass can cause nasal obstruction by mechanical obstruction and/or from crusting around the mass. As the disease progresses, scaring may cause distortion of the nasal tip and vestibule.[21]

The diagnosis is confirmed by microscopic identification of acid-fast bacilli with Ziehl-Neelsen or auramine–rhodamine fluorescent staining. Histology demonstrates both caseating and noncaseating granulomas, with a greater number of epithelioid cells and Langhans giant cells than is seen in other granulomas. Tests, such as PCR, DNA probes, and high-performance liquid chromatography, may become more widely useful in the future.[21]

Nasal tuberculosis treatment follows the same guidelines established for extrapulmonary tuberculosis including rifampin, ethambutol, isoniazid, pyrazinamide, and streptomycin. Therapeutic courses are approximately 6 months, with an initial 2-month course of four antituberculosis drugs, followed by 4 months of a two-drug antibiotic course. In addition, nasal flushes have been advocated to clean away crusts and discharge.[21]

Leprosy is caused by *M. leprae*, an obligate intracellular, acid-fast bacillus that leads to a chronic granulomatous condition. *M. leprae* is highly infective, but demonstrates low pathogenicity, low virulence, and has an incubation time that ranges from 3 to 10 years. The most common route of spread is believed to be from nasal discharge.[22] Lepromatous leprosy involves the nasal mucosa in approximately 95% of cases. The earliest signs of the disease include a pale nodular or plaque-like thickening of the mucosa of the anterior end of the inferior turbinate and the anterior part of the nasal septum. This progresses to mechanical obstruction from the tissue mass, ulceration of the mucosa, neural involvement leading to a decrease in sensation, and cartilage involvement leading to septal perforation and saddle nose deformity.[22]

Diagnosis is made by biopsy, which demonstrates scattered neutrophils and a dense infiltrate of lipid-laden histiocytes with intracellular bacilli grouped in clumps as seen on modified acid-fast stains. Treatment involves a multidrug regimen of rifampin, dapsone, and clofazimine for 6 to 24 months.[22]

Viral

Viral causes of rhinitis are the same as those that are associated with the common cold. Those include, in order of frequency, rhinoviruses, coronaviruses, and influenza viruses. Other viral causes include the adenoviruses, respiratory syncytial viruses, and parainfluenza viruses.

Fungal

North American blastomycosis is caused by the fungus *Blastomyces dermatitidis*. Nasal and paranasal sinus involvement is rare, with most cases involving the cutaneous nasal vestibule. There have been relatively few cases of paranasal sinus involvement or cases of blastomycosis as a noncutaneous intranasal mass.[23] The histological appearance shows pseudoepitheliomatous hyperplasia, acanthosis, microabscesses, or giant cells. The use of specific stains, such as periodic acid-Schiff, Gomori silver methenamine, or mucicarmine, identify spherical, thick-walled, broad-based yeast. Cultures confirm the diagnosis but require Sabouraud agarose as a growth medium, and may take up to 4 weeks for sufficient growth for positive identification.[23]

Treatment of blastomycosis involves surgical drainage of any abscess if present, followed by systemic antifungals. Amphotericin B therapy is well-established. Although it requires long-term intravenous access and has an extensive side effect profile, it remains the treatment of choice in immunocompromised patients, or in complicated cases. Itraconazole has a lower side effect profile and a high therapeutic efficacy and is the preferred therapy for a 3 to 6 months course.[23]

Coccidioidomycosis is caused by disseminated infections of *Coccidioides immitis*. Diagnosis is made through serological testing, microbiologic cultures, and tissue staining revealing the fungal agent. Tissue specimens demonstrate double-walled spherules of *C. immitis* filled with endospores. Fungal cultures can confirm the diagnosis.[24] Treatment includes amphotericin B for severe pulmonary or rapidly progressing disease. Itraconazole and fluconazole are used for most other forms given their lower side effect profile, and good efficacy against *C. immitis*. Surgery is reserved for cases that require tissue diagnosis, or debridement.[24]

Rhinosporidium seeberi is a fungus, based on morphologic and histologic characteristics, and is believed to be the causative agent of rhinosporidiosis. It is most commonly found in the nose and nasopharynx, and presents with nasal obstruction, epistaxis, and nasal discharge. It is usually a pedunculated, friable, vascular mass that is studded with subepithelial spores, resembling a strawberry.[25] Histologically, the microorganisms are characterized by round or oval cells with thick walls, containing multiple sporangia, seen in a fibrovascular stroma with chronic inflammatory cells. Surgical excision with cauterization at the base of the lesion is the mainstay of treatment. Recurrence is common, and requires reexcision. Adjuvant antimicrobials have had limited success.[25]

Ubiquitous fungi of the genera *Rhizopus*, *Mucor*, *Rhizomucor*, and *Absidia* can lead to the opportunistic fungal infections referred to as mucormycosis. Mucormycosis is most commonly seen in poorly controlled diabetics, as well as individuals with a compromised immune system.[26]

Fungal spores are inhaled by the human host; when the host is unable to phagocytize the spores, germination and hyphae formation occur, leading to invasion of the mucosal tissues. Most patients present with fever, nasal ulcerations with black necrotic tissue in the nose, periorbital or facial edema, visual changes, headache, and facial pain. Computed tomography of the sinuses can demonstrate mucoperiosteal edema with bony destruction. Magnetic resonance imaging is useful to identify intracranial or intraorbital extension.[26]

Diagnosis of mucormycosis is made by the clinical examination and, the presence of nonseptate hyphae on histology and is confirmed by fungal culture. Treatment has included amphotericin B and extensive surgical debridement using frozen-section guidance, allowing for a more thorough debridement of the infected tissues. Hyperbaric oxygen therapy has been used for the beneficial effects of the increased oxygen tension on the host phagocytic cells, the direct fungicidal effects of the hyperbaric oxygen, and the decrease of the local acidosis, which decreases fungal growth.[26]

A. fumigatus and *A. flavus* cause both the noninvasive form as well as the invasive form of aspergillosis. The noninvasive infections, which do not involve destruction of the surrounding tissues, include allergic fungal sinusitis and aspergilloma. Invasive infections are most commonly found in immunocompromised patients and are characterized by destruction of the sinus mucosa and bony expansion.[27]

Most patients with invasive aspergillosis present with progressive facial pain or headaches. Computed tomography initially shows a focal soft tissue lesion and may show subtle, focal bony destruction, with focal hypodense areas appearing, which correspond to abscess formation. Diagnosis is based on microscopic analysis and fungal culture from tissue biopsy. On microscopy, *Aspergillus* characteristically shows haemotoxophilic organisms with 45° branching septate hyphae and can also be demonstrated with methenamine silver and periodic acid Schiff stains. *Aspergillus* cultures will show growth in 2 to 6 days. It is recommended, that if the initial biopsy is negative, and aspergillosis is suspected, a second biopsy be taken, especially before starting corticosteroids.[27] Treatment involves surgical debridement and amphotericin B, for initial disease control, followed by an oral ketoconazole or itraconazole to ensure eradication. Prolonged treatment is recommended, especially if the patient continues to be immunosuppressed.[27]

Parasitic

Leishmaniasis is caused by the parasites of the *Leishmania* genus, following a bite from an infected sand fly. Leishmaniasis is seen throughout the world. *L. braziliensis* or *L. panamensis* cause the mucocutaneous form of the disease, up to 10 years after the appearance of cutaneous lesions. The mucocutaneous form begins in the nasal septal mucosa, which can become inflamed, ulcerated, and ultimately perforated. The mucosal lesions can spread to involve the oral mucous membranes as well. Malnutrition and pneumonia are the leading causes of death in patients with the mucocutaneous variant of the disease.[28] The diagnosis of leishmaniasis is mostly clinical; however, histology and culture remain the gold standards. Biopsies show a predominant mononuclear infiltrate consisting of lymphocytes and histiocytes, as well as an abundance of plasma cells, especially in the mucocutaneous form. The histiocytes may be filled with small, oval, encapsulated protozoa with large peripheral nuclei and small, rod-shaped kinetoplast, known as Leishman-Donovan bodies. Biopsies can be cultured on blood agar, with promastigote growth apparent within 2 days to 2 weeks.[28]

Unlike the cutaneous form of the disease, the mucocutaneous lesions will not heal spontaneously and require medical treatment. Amphotericin B has only limited efficacy against the mucocutaneous form of the disease. Antimonials such as sodium stibogluconate and meglumine antimoniate, which seem to inhibit amastigote glycolytic activity and fatty acid oxidation, are the drugs of choice. Both medications must be given parenterally. Currently, there are no effective, oral medications for leishmaniasis.[28]

Infestation of the skin or mucous membranes by developing fly larvae is referred to as myiasis. Most cases of cutaneous myiasis are caused by the human botfly, *Dermatobia hominis*, whereas the majority of nasal myiasis have been reportedly caused by the green blowfly, *Phaenicia sericata*.[29,30] Cutaneous myiasis occurs when the fly eggs are deposited on the mammalian host skin, allowing for the hatched larvae to descend into the skin to mature. A pruritic papule develops and matures into a boil-like lesion that can become painful, crusted, and purulent. A characteristic feature of the papule is the opening at the top of the boil, allowing oxygen passage. The larvae secure themselves in place with large spines on their torsos and can remain in place for 2 to 3 months. When mature, they leave the skin, drop to the ground and pupate.[29] This can cause extensive necrosis and destruction of tissue, which may be very disfiguring if involving the nose, face, or orbit.[29] Myiasis can usually be distinguished from leishmaniasis by the complaints of pain at the site of the wound, a "crawling" sensation, and the ability to visualize the larvae within the lesion.[29,31]

Nasal myiasis differs in that it involves the flies depositing their larvae in the nasal discharge of patients and does not cause mucosal damage. Treatment involves only nasal lavage and eliminating the fly vector.[30] Most cases of myiasis are self-limiting; however, certain types of larvae are able to invade paranasal sinuses, orbital structures, and even into the cranial vault and brain tissue, thus prompt treatment is indicated.[29] Larvae should not be forcibly removed from the wound due to the spines on the body of the larvae. If parts of the larvae remain, a foreign body reaction may occur. Surgical debridement with wide local excision of the larvae is recommended, allowing the wound to granulate. Antiseptic dressings are recommended after removal, with an oral antibiotic to help prevent a secondary infection. Occlusion of the central punctum to cause suffocation and spontaneous emergence of the larvae has been described. Vaccination for *Clostridium tetani* should be considered with infestation.[29]

STOMATITIS

Bacterial

Stomatitis can result from a wide assortment of bacteria, viruses, fungi, and parasitic infections (Table 4). Most are directly or indirectly the result of poor oral hygiene, either through personal practices or environmental circumstances. Acute necrotizing ulcerative gingivitis is an acute infection of the gingiva that causes gingival bleeding, gingival ulceration, and pain.[32] It has been given many names including necrotizing gingivostomatitis, necrotizing ulcerative gingivitis, trench mouth, and Vincent infection. Vincent angina is an extension of acute necrotizing ulcerative gingivitis, or Vincent infection to involve the tonsils and pharynx. Gangrenous stomatitis, also known as noma and cancrum oris, is also an extension of acute necrotizing ulcerative gingivitis, once it involves the surrounding tissues. The infection has been reportedly caused by a mixture of bacteria, including spirochetes (*Treponema* species), fusobacteria (*F. nucleatum*), *P. intermedia*, *Veillonella* species, and streptococci. It is found most often in underdeveloped countries in Africa, Asia, and South America and has been associated with stress, smoking, and malnutrition,

Table 4 Common Causes of Stomatitis or Oral Lesions
Bacterial
Acute necrotizing ulcerative gingivitis (polymicrobial)
Actinomycosis israelii
Bartonella quintana, B. henselae
Neisseria gonorrhoeae
Mycobacterium tuberculosis
Mycobacterium. leprae
Treponema pallidum
Francisella tularensis
Streptococcus viridans
Viral
Measles virus
Coxsackie virus
Human papillomavirus
Herpes simplex virus
Fungal
Candida albicans
Aspergillosis
Histoplasma capsulatum
Blastomyces dermatitidis
Paracoccidioides brasiliensis
Mucormycosis
Cryptococcus neoformans
Coccidioides immitis
Fusarium species
Geotrichum candidum
Parasitic
Taenia sagenata, Taenia solium
Myiasis
Leishmaniasis

in addition to poor oral hygiene. Patients can develop severe, deep aching pain, along with rapid bone loss from the periodontitis. Treatment depends on antibiotics along with thorough debridement of involved soft tissues. Antibiotics alone will not cure the infection.[32]

Actinomycosis is caused by bacteria in the genus *Actinomyces*, which are normal flora of the oropharyngeal cavity. They are characterized as slow-growing, firm, nontender lesions that may develop multiple abscesses and form sinus tracts. Diagnosis is made by culture of the bacteria and indirect immunofluorescence microscopy. Treatment has been previously discussed.

Bacillary angiomatosis results from a *Bartonella quintana* or *henselae* infection and can occur in the oral cavities of severely immunocompromised individuals. It poses a diagnostic dilemma due to its gross appearance similar to Kaposi sarcoma, which is also seen in the immunocompromised.[32] The lesions are described as bluish or purple macules, pale bluish patches, and erythematous lesions on the gingival, palate, and buccal mucosa. Histologically, they appear as a lobular proliferation of small, round blood vessels with plump endothelial cells protruding into the vascular lumen. Warthin-Starry stains reveal the bacteria.[32] Treatment includes antibiotic therapy with a macrolide or doxycycline.[19]

Neisseria gonorrhoeae is a nonmotile, aerobic, gram-negative, spherical diplococcus. Gonorrhea remains one of the most common sexually transmitted diseases, and oral-genital contact can result in oral, tonsillar, and pharyngeal infections.

The oral and tonsillar manifestations include tonsils that are edematous and erythematous with a grayish exudate. Oral mucosal lesions may be ulcerated, painful, and may be diffusely erythematous and edematous. Diagnosis is by culture and identification, and current treatment guidelines include a third generation cephalosporin.[19,32]

Oral manifestations of tuberculosis are rare, occurring in less than 1% of all pulmonary cases of tuberculosis. Caused by *M. tuberculosis*, they present as a chronic, painless, irregular ulcer, with a vegetating surface, and a gray or yellow exudate. Primary oral lesions have been reported in the past, as transmission by infected dentists to patients, prior to the implementation of universal precautions.[32] Diagnosis is based on a delayed type reaction to a purified protein derivative skin test or a positive culture demonstrating acid-fast mycobacteria.

Leprosy, caused by *M. leprae*, may demonstrate oral lesions, depending on the stage of leprosy. The four stages of leprosy are, in increasing severity, indeterminate, tuberculoid, borderline, and lepromatous. Oral lesions are seen in up to 60% of patients with lepromatous leprosy.[32] The lesions start as nodules or lepromas that are filled with *M. leprae*, and progress to necrosis and ulceration. These ulcers may heal, forming scar tissue, or progress to further tissue destruction. These lesions are seen through the oral cavity. Diagnosis is based on the identification of acid-fast bacilli in smears of the oral lesions. Current treatment guidelines are based on the stage. Intermediate and tuberculoid are treated with dapsone and rifampin for approximately 6 months. Patients with the lepromatous and borderline stages are treated with dapsone, clofazimine, and rifampin.[19]

Syphilis may also manifest itself with oral lesions. The primary infection, caused by the spirochete *T. pallidum*, causes asymptomatic chancres, most commonly on the hard palate, although the soft palate, lips, and tongue may also be involved.[32] These chancres are often ulcerated centrally, with a raised indurated border. These usually heal spontaneously within weeks. These are followed by secondary syphilis, which is characterized by generalized symptoms such as fever, malaise, and headache, as well as oral lesions described as a grayish-white, glistening patch on the mucosa of the soft palate, buccal area, or tongue. If left untreated, 30 to 40% of patients will develop tertiary syphilis with oral manifestations of a localized granuloma, or gumma, on the hard palate, soft palate, lips, or tongue.[32] Diagnosis and treatment have been discussed above.

Tularemia is caused by *Francisella tularensis*, a noncapsulated, gram-negative coccobacillus. It can be found in various mammals, as well as blood sucking arthropods and insects. It has been reported to occur in the oral cavities of humans following direct contact with infected animals or animal tissue, ingestion of contaminated water, or inhalation of dust contaminated with infected arthropod feces.[33] There are two different biotypes, with varying clinical severities. The *F. tularensis biovar tularensis* (Jellison type A) is a more serious infection and is more dominant in North America. The *F. tularensis biovar palaearctica* (Jellison Type B) causes milder symptoms and is found in Europe, Asia, and North America. They cannot be differentiated by serological reactions, however the *biovar tularensis* is able to ferment glycerol, whereas the *palaearctica* is not.[33]

The incubation period for the disease ranges from 2 to 6 days, with the onset of generalized symptoms including fever, headache, sore throat, malaise, myalgias, cough, and cutaneous lesions. Imaging features are nonspecific, with enlarged lymph nodes, and lymph nodes with central necrosis. The microorganism is poorly grown on culture media, and the diagnosis is largely based on serological tests. These include seroagglutination and microagglutination. Patients will usually develop an antibody titer within 2 weeks of the onset of the disease.[33] The bacteria are resistant to beta-lactam antibiotics, however they respond well to aminoglycosides, macrolides, and fluoroquinolones.[33]

Stomatitis may also be the result of a streptococcal infection. *S. viridans*, as well as beta-hemolytic streptococci have been implicated. The infection can lead to an acutely inflamed, edematous, and erythematous mucosa and gingiva, with pain, fever, and malaise. It is often preceded by tonsillitis, and the patient is treated with first line penicillins.[32]

Viral

Viral infections of the oral cavity are numerous, and there exists overlap in the viruses responsible for the common cold, pharyngitis, and stomatitis. The first family of viruses that can cause oral manifestations is the Paramyxoviridae, to which the genus *Morbillivirus*, the cause of measles (rubeola), belongs. Although vaccinations have greatly reduced the incidence of measles, they remain a cause of childhood mortality in developing countries. They are highly infectious, transmitted through aerosolized droplets, and have an incubation period of approximately 2 weeks. The oral manifestation is known as Koplik spots, which are bluish-gray specks on an erythematous base near the molar teeth. These are pathognomonic for measles and appear up to 48 hours before cutaneous lesions. Diagnosis can be confirmed with measles-specific immunoglobulin M identified in oral secretions.[32] Treatment is supportive.

There have been important investigations over the years of regarding the roles that the measles virus, as well as another member of the Paramyxoviridae family, the mumps virus, play in sensorineural hearing loss. A serious complication of the measles virus infection, measles encephalitis, occurs in approximately 1 in 1,000 cases. These patients have a mortality rate of approximately 25%, and half of those who survive will have permanent neurological sequelae including deafness.[34] In addition, it is been shown that the virus can cause destruction or degeneration of the organ of Corti, the stria, and the cochlear neurons.[34] The measles virus has further been linked to otosclerosis, with viral RNA being identified in the foot plates of otosclerosis patients.[35] It was estimated that the measles virus was responsible for 5 to 10% of all profound bilateral sensorineural hearing loss before the widespread use of the vaccine.[34] Since the vaccination was instituted, the number of cases in the United States has decreased 99%.[36] Although the exact reduction in sensorineural hearing loss associated with measles is not yet known, the importance of worldwide vaccinations has been stressed.

The mumps virus has also been linked to sensorineural hearing loss, either through a direct viral invasion of the cochlea and/or the eighth cranial nerve, or an autoimmune reaction against inner ear structures.[37] The deafness associated with the mumps virus can often be unilateral, which may go undetected for some time, thus making a correlation to the infection more difficult. It is because of this, and the fact that individuals can still get clinical and subclinical mumps virus infections, that the reduction in hearing loss due to the vaccine is not clearly established.[34] The vaccine is believed to have played an important role, and is strongly encouraged.

The rubella (German measles) virus, a member of the *Rubivirus* genus of the Togaviridae family, can lead to sensorineural hearing loss through infection during pregnancy, leading to the congenital rubella syndrome of which deafness is a major component. Vaccination for rubella where used has virtually eliminated the problem. The measles, mumps, and rubella live virus vaccine is recommended for individuals 12 to 15 months of age or older with revaccination at 4 to 6 years of age.

The family of viruses called Picornaviridae are small RNA viruses, and include the genus *Enterovirus*. Coxsackievirus A and B are included in the genus *Enterovirus*. Coxsackieviruses are responsible for various ulcerative lesions differentiated based on gross appearance and location. Hand, foot, and mouth disease is caused by coxsackievirus A5, A10, and A16, and is manifested by ulceration on the buccal mucosa and soft palate, as well as the hands and feet. These are described as rhomboidal vesicles, or square blisters. Although the disease is benign and self-limited, acyclovir has been reported to be effective in the treatment.[32]

Herpangina is also caused by the coxsackieviruses and leads to clustered petechiae in the soft palate that become shallow ulcers that heal relatively quickly. Patients also experience high fevers, myalgia, and sore throat. Treatment is palliative. Coxsackieviruses are responsible for lymphonodular pharyngitis, which causes orange painful papules on the soft palate, and ulcerative pharyngitis, causing ulcerations on the palate, lips, and tongue.[32]

The human papillomavirus (HPV) belongs to the genus *Papillomavirus*, which is a member of the family of DNA viruses Papovaviridae. There are many identified types of the HPV, several of the types have been associated with intraoral lesions. Squamous cell papilloma appears as a small, pink, exophytic, cauliflower-like lesion with a narrow base on the oral mucosa. Condyloma acuminatum is similar, with multiple lesions on the mucosa. Both are associated with HPV types 6 and 11.[32] These lesions are managed with surgical excision. Verruca vulgaris is associated with HPV types 2 and 57 and can be seen on the gingiva, labial mucosa, oral commissure, hard palate, or tongue. These lesions are firm, sessile, exophytic growths with wide bases. These too are treated surgically. Focal epithelial hyperplasia presents as multiple, plaque-like or papular lesions, of the mucosa, usually in children. They are red to gray to white in color and are found on the oral mucosa exclusively. Other oral lesions have been associated with HPV, including erythroplakia, proliferative verrucous leukoplakia, candidal leukoplakia, squamous cell carcinoma, and lichen planus.[32]

Herpes simplex viruses are associated with intraoral lesions as well. They belong to the family Herpesviridae and the genus *Herpesvirus*. The intraoral lesions can present as a cluster of small, painful ulcers on the gingiva. They are initially discrete lesions but may coalesce to form a larger lesion. They are self-limiting and usually heal in less than 2 weeks. Acyclovir may speed the healing and prevent further outbreaks.[32]

Fungal

Fungal infections of the oral cavity are common among the immunocompromised, however, can occur in the immunocompetent as well. The most common oral fungal infection is oral candidiasis, caused by the genus *Candida*. Although there are more than 100 species of *Candida*, *C. albicans* is the most common cause of stomatitis.[38] The differentiating feature of *Candida* is the pseudo-hypha formation found in most of the species. Different types of oral candidiasis exist, the two most common forms are erythematous candidiasis and pseudomembranous candidiasis. The erythematous candidiasis presents as red, macular areas most commonly found on the palate. These can be acute or chronic. Histopathologic analysis reveals epithelial atrophy with loss of rete ridges, connective tissue papillae with epithelial cover of only a few cell layers, an inflammatory infiltrate of lymphocytes in the submucosa with hyperemia, and little or no penetration of hyphae into the epithelium. This responds well to topical antifungals such as nystatin. Pseudomembranous candidiasis is also referred to as thrush and is the most commonly identified form of the disease. The clinical appearance, which is usually diagnostic, includes white or whitish-yellow, curd-like patches that leave a red, bleeding surface when wiped or scraped off. Diagnosis can be confirmed by a wet-preparation of a smear using potassium hydroxide, demonstrating hyphae and mycelia. Histopathologic analysis shows a superficial infection with intraepithelial pseudomycelia which do not penetrate the spinous layer, thickened parakeratin, lymphocytes in the subepithelial region with fewer lymphocytes than in the erythematous form. Treatment consists of topical antifungals.[38]

Other forms of oral candidiasis include the hyperplastic, nodular or leukoplakia, and the plaque-like forms. These are chronic lesions that cannot be rubbed off. They can appear translucent to opaque or whitish and are found on the buccal mucosa, the angles of the mouth, and the dorsum of the tongue. Diagnosis is usually clinical. The hyperplastic form can have candidal hyphae invading the parakeratotic layer but not extending into the spinous layer.[38]

Aspergillosis is a fungal infection caused by the members of the class Ascomycetes, genus *Aspergillus*. Several species can cause infections including *A. fumigatus*, the most common, *A. niger*, *A. glaucis*, *A. terrus*, and *A. flavus*, which seems to be the most virulent.[38] It can present in three different forms, the saprophytic form without invasion, the allergic, and the invasive form which demonstrates extension into viable tissues. The disease is contracted through inhalation of the spores, which tend to germinate in mucus. The invasive form is found almost entirely in immunocompromised individuals. Lesions have been described as yellow to gray to black, necrotic ulcers. Diagnosis and treatment have been discussed under the Section on Rhinitis.

Histoplasmosis is caused by the soil saprophyte *Histoplasma capsulatum*, which exists in a mycelial form in the environment and a yeast form at body temperature. It is endemic to the Ohio and Mississippi river valleys, as well as Central and South America, Africa, India, East Asia, and Australia. It is the most commonly diagnosed systemic mycosis in the United States.[38] Oral lesions have been reported in up to 60% of patients with disseminated disease and occur throughout the oral cavity. The lesions are nontender, dusky, erythematous granulomas that can appear flat and plaque-like and may ulcerate and be painful. Therapy includes itraconazole for several months. Patients with severe infections or who are immunocompromised are treated with amphotericin B and itraconazole.[19]

North American blastomycosis is caused by the fungus *B. dermatitidis*, which is found endemically in the soils of northern Ontario as well as the watershed areas of the Mississippi and Ohio Rivers. It is a thermally dimorphic fungus that exists as a mycelial or mold form in the soil where it produces spores. These spores are inhaled by the host, where it transforms to the yeast form, stimulating a very aggressive inflammatory reaction. South American blastomycosis is caused by *Paracoccidioides brasiliensis*. It is rarely seen outside of the endemic area in South America, and has been reported to present orally as painful, chronic, irregular ulcers with a granulomatous or vegetating surface. They can occur on the palate, tongue, lips, and gingiva.[38,39]

Most presentations of South American blastomycosis are nonspecific with cough, weight loss, fevers, and hemoptysis. Oral lesions are reported as single or multiple ulcerations. Sessile projections and granulomatous or verrucous lesions have been described.[38]

The epidemiologic profile of South American blastomycosis is largely based on sporadic cases but is believed to have an average age of onset of 30 to 50 years with a male predominance ranging from 2:1 to 15:1 over females. Diagnosis can be made histologically and confirmed with positive fungal cultures. Fine needle aspiration has been shown as a reliable diagnostic tool in the hands of a talented cytopathologist. Histological appearance shows pseudoepitheliomatous hyperplasia, acanthosis, microabscesses, or giant cells. The intense inflammatory reaction may make identification of the microorganisms difficult. The use of specific stains, such as periodic acid-Schiff, Gomori silver methenamine, or mucicarmine, helps to identify spherical, thick-walled, broad–based yeast. Cultures confirm this diagnosis but may take up to 4 weeks to become positive and require Sabouraud agarose as a growth medium.[39,40]

Treatment of blastomycosis involves surgical drainage if an abscess is present, followed by systemic antifungals. Amphotericin B has been the standard therapy, however requires long-term intravenous access and has an extensive side effect profile. Amphotericin B remains the treatment of choice in immunocompromised patients, or in complicated cases. Ketoconazole is an effective oral agent, but has been shown to have high liver toxicity and multiple drug interactions. Itraconazole has a lower side effect profile and a high therapeutic efficacy, and is the preferred therapy for a 3- to 6-month course.[39,40]

Mucormycosis, caused by members of the order *Mucorales*, can have oral lesions as well. The microorganisms have broad, nonseptate hyphae, ranging from 6 to 15 µm in width and 100 to 200 µm in length, and the diagnosis can be confirmed by identification of the hyphae histopathologically or by culture on Sabouraud glucose agar.[38] The oral lesions have been described as palatal ulcerations or black, necrotic masses. The palate is the most common site for the original infection. Without proper treatment, the infection can extend, as outlined in the Section on Rhinitis.

Cryptococcosis is an infection that is caused by one of two forms of the fungus *Cryptococcus neoformans*. The first type is the *neoformans* variety and is associated with avian sources and causes the majority of human infections. The second type, the *gattii* variety, is associated with eucalyptus trees. The majority of infections are pulmonary; however, disseminated disease can be associated with oral cavity lesions. These lesions are described as red, ulcerated areas that have been reported to occur on the palate and tongue. The diagnosis is based on tissue biopsy with identification of the microorganism using Grocott and mucicarmine stains.[38] Therapy includes fluconazole or itraconazole. More severe infections require amphotericin B with or without fluconazole.[19]

Coccidioidomycosis, caused by *C. immitis*, is a fungal infection endemic to arid regions of the southwestern United States, and Latin America. Oral lesions have been reported, described as verrucous and necrotic ulcers. Diagnosis is confirmed by histology showing spherules containing endospores, serology, and cultures. Systemic antifungals are used for treatment.[38]

The filamentous fungi *fusarium* species are responsible for fusariosis. This infection can be a local, invasive, or disseminated form. The disseminated form can cause a secondary oral infection. These lesions, found in immunocompromised individuals, are described as black, necrotic ulcers occurring on the palate. The diagnosis is based on histology and culture. The histologic appearance of the microorganism is similar to that of *Aspergillus*; however, the cultured microorganisms, when grown on medium not containing cyclohexamide, demonstrate distinguishing fusoid macroconidia or microconidia. Superficial infections respond well to local therapy.[38]

The microorganism *Geotrichum candidum* has been associated with oral geotrichosis in immunocompromised patients. Clinically, the lesions are a sharply defined, with ulceration. Histologically, the tissue will demonstrate hyphae that segment into rectangular arthrospores with spherical blastospores budding from the hyphae. The fungus will grow flat, white or creamy colonies on Sabouraud glucose agar. Lesions have reportedly responded to 5-fluorocytosine and itraconazole.[38]

Trichosporonosis, caused by fungi of the genus *Trichosporon*, and sporotrichosis, caused by *Sporothrix schenckii* have each been reported to involve the oral cavity. However, the number of cases that have been reported are extremely small.[38]

Parasites

Parasitic infections of the oral cavity are not common, however must be considered when dealing with patients in developing countries. It is also important to be familiar with these types of infections when treating immigrants from developing countries or world travelers recently returned from endemic areas.

Parasitic tapeworms are commonly found in the intestinal lumen of vertebrate hosts, however they have been known to involve the oral cavity. These parasites belong to the phylum *Platyhelminthes*, class *Cestoidea*. Teniasis and cysticercosis are two different diseases that can have oral manifestations and are caused by the tapeworms *Taenia sagenata* and *T. solium*, which are found in beef and pork, respectively. Teniasis occurs when either of the above mentioned tapeworms infests the human small intestine following ingestion of infested and poorly cooked beef or pork. Oral manifestations of teniasis include erythematous, edematous, hyperplastic mucosa with bleeding gingiva and pain. Teniasis is diagnosed by the detection of the worms in the stool. Cysticercosis results from extraintestinal manifestations of the tapeworm cysts. The human hosts ingest either the cysts or the worms themselves, and penetration of the gastric mucosa by the embryos occurs, giving access to the circulation. The embryos are then distributed throughout the body. In the oral cavity, they can involve the tongue, lips, and buccal mucosa. They have been identified in all age ranges and present as discrete, firm, nontender nodules just deep to the mucosa. Diagnosis is made by microscopic examination of the excised cysts.[38] Treatment for both infections includes a single dose of either praziquantel or niclosamide.[19]

Oral or dental myiasis is larval infection of tissues of the oral cavity. Although rare, it continues to be a health concern in developing countries, particularly in Asia. It affects patients of both genders, and of all ages. Risk factors include oral wounds such as extraction sites, severe gingivitis or periodontitis, and a history of mouth breathing. The infection is presumed to occur while the patient is sleeping. Patients present with pain, swelling, bleeding, and an "itchy" feeling at the infection site. Intraoral examination usually reveals an orifice with the presence of active larvae. Treatment involves debridement of the larvae and copious irrigation, followed by treatment of the risk factors.[38]

Leishmaniasis, as described above, is a protozoan parasite which belongs to the genus *Leishmania*. The sand fly vector can infect the human host and cause either a visceral, cutaneous, or a mucosal disease. Oral leishmaniasis can be a manifestation of both the visceral and the mucosal forms. The lesions of the uvula and palate can appear edematous, red in color, and fissured. Although very rare, oral leishmaniasis must be considered in the differential for oral infections in endemic areas, such as the Mediterranean basin.[38] Diagnosis and treatment are as outlined above.

Other parasitic organisms such as echinococcosis, nematodes, trichinosis, gongylonema, and ascaris have all been reported to have oral manifestations; however, there have been few case reports of each in the literature.

PHARYNGITIS

Acute pharyngitis is an extremely common inflammation of the pharynx and tonsils. The exact incidence is not known and is not impacted by the presence or absence of the palatine tonsils.[41]

Bacterial

Several different types of bacteria are associated with pharyngitis (Table 5). The most important of these is the group A β-hemolytic *Streptococcus* (GABHS), the most common microorganism in this group is *S. pyogenes*. It is responsible for 15 to 30% of cases of pharyngitis in children, and 5 to 10% of cases in adults.[42] It results from direct contact with a person infected. The incubation period is between 2 and 5 days. Antibiotic therapy is indicated for the suppurative complications including peritonsillar and retropharyngeal abscesses, cervical lymphadenitis, sinusitis, otitis media, and the nonsuppurative complications including rheumatic fever.[42] Acute rheumatic fever has been reported to follow 0.5 to 3.0% of

Table 5 Common Causes of Pharyngitis
Bacterial
Group A beta-hemolytic *Streptococcus*
Groups C and G beta-hemolytic *Streptococcus*
Arcanobacterium hemolyticum
Neisseria gonorrhoeae
Mycoplasma pneumoniae
Chlamydia pneumoniae
Corynebacterium diphtheriae
Viral
Rhinovirus
Corona virus
Influenza virus
Respiratory syncytial virus
Parainfluenza virus
Epstein–Barr virus
Human immunodeficiency virus
Fungal
Candida albicans

ineffectively treated GABHS cases, and occurs because of a rise in streptococcal antibodies.[43] There is no evidence to suggest that treatment will prevent the development of acute glomerulonephritis, also known as poststreptococcal glomerulonephritis, often seen following streptococcal infections.[41,42] The clinical presentation includes fever, though it may be low grade, sore throat, headache, erythematous pharynx with tonsillar hypertrophy and possibly exudates, submandibular lymphadenopathy, and palatine petechiae. Rhinitis and cough are characteristically absent.[41] A scarlatiniform rash, described as an erythematous, fine, sandpaper-like exanthema is frequently seen. The rash often begins in the axilla and inguinal folds, then spreads.[41]

Diagnosis of GABHS pharyngitis is based on rapid antigen testing and throat cultures. The rapid antigen testing detects the presence of group A streptococcal carbohydrate on a throat swab. The results are available within minutes. The specificity is reportedly greater than 95%; however, the sensitivity varies from 80 to 97%.[44] Given the variability of the sensitivity, it is recommended to perform rapid antigen testing in conjunction with throat cultures.[41] Throat cultures grown on sheep-blood agar provide results within 24 to 48 hours. The throat culture is considered the gold standard, with a reported specificity of 99% and sensitivity of 97%. The sensitivity varies depending on the adequacy of specimen collection, which may be difficult in the case of small children.[41] First line therapy for GABHS pharyngitis is penicillin or any β-lactam antibiotic. Alternatives include macrolides, although resistance to macrolides is reportedly increasing.[19]

Additional bacterial causes of pharyngitis include the nongroup A β-hemolytic streptococci, *Arcanobacterium hemolyticum*, *N. gonorrhoeae*, *Mycoplasma pneumoniae*, *Chlamydia pneumoniae*, and *Corynebacterium diphtheriae*. Nongroup A β-hemolytic streptococci include groups C and G β-hemolytic streptococci and have many similar features to GABHS. They have been associated with epidemic outbreaks of pharyngitis. Although groups C and G are not associated

with the rheumatic fever, they have been linked to glomerulonephritis following infections. The majority of C and G streptococci are sensitive to penicillins, cephalosporins, and erythromycin.[41]

A. hemolyticum is an uncommon cause of pharyngitis and is most commonly seen in adolescents and young adults.[41] It can lead to lymphadenopathy, erythema of the pharyngeal tissue, exudates and a scarlatiniform rash. It is difficult to culture, and erythromycin is the drug of choice. Pharyngitis caused by *N. gonorrhoeae*, though rare, should be considered in sexually active adolescents. The presentation ranges from asymptomatic to sore throat, to ulcerative pharyngotonsillitis.[41] Diagnosis is based on a positive culture.[44] Gonococcus can be cultured on Thayer-Martin medium, and is treated with either ceftriaxone, or a combination of an oral quinolone and a macrolide or doxycycline. The latter two are given for possible chlamydial coinfections.[42] Both *M. pneumoniae* and *C. pneumoniae* can cause pharyngitis, but the frequency is unknown. The diagnosis is largely clinical. Both microorganisms respond to tetracycline or erythromycin.[42]

Diphtheria has become a rare cause of pharyngitis, although cases continue to be reported. Fatality rates for noncutaneous diphtheria have remained constant for the past five decades at 5 to 10%.[44] Currently, it is a disease of the unimmunized or poorly immunized members of disadvantaged socioeconomic groups. Examination reveals a grayish-white membrane extending from the tonsils to the soft palate, and even to the nares, larynx, and tracheobronchial tree.[42] This membrane in the tracheobronchial tree can cause life threatening obstruction. Removal of the membrane reveals bleeding, edematous tissue.[42] Soft tissue edema and lymphadenopathy also occur. The toxin from the bacterium can cause cardiac and neural toxicity. Diagnosis is suspected on clinical examination, and confirmed by culture. Treatment involves equine hyperimmune diphtheria antitoxin and penicillin or erythromycin.[42]

Kawasaki disease is most likely an infectious disease, however the agent is currently not known.[44] Clinical manifestations of the disease include a sore throat, fever, bilateral nonpurulent conjunctivitis, anterior cervical node enlargement, erythematous oral mucosa, and an inflamed pharynx with a strawberry tongue. Additional findings include cracked lips, a generalized rash, edema and erythema of the palms and soles, followed by periungual desquamation, and peeling of the palms.[44] Coronary artery damage resulting from Kawasaki disease is the leading cause of acquired heart disease in children in the developed world. Treatment includes supportive measures, high dose aspirin, corticosteroids, and high dose intravenous immunoglobulin.[45]

Viral

The most common cause of pharyngitis is viral. The viral causes overlap substantially with those associated with the common cold. There are two clinical presentations associated with viral infection; the first is a rather mild illness consisting of a low-grade fever, acute rhinitis, cough, and mild erythema of the pharynx. In this first group, cervical lymphadenopathy and sore throat may or may not be present. Viruses commonly associated with this presentation include rhinoviruses, coronaviruses, respiratory syncytial viruses, and parainfluenza viruses.[41]

A second clinical presentation pattern includes viruses such as the adenoviruses, influenza virus A or B, enteroviruses, Epstein-Barr virus, herpes simplex viruses type 1 and 2, and primary infection with the human immunodeficiency virus. The patients infected with one of these viruses present with more severe symptoms including fever, sore throat, malaise, pharyngitis, and cervical adenopathy. Adenovirus is the most common cause of this second group, accounting for 15 to 23% of cases. The coxsackievirus A can cause a pharyngitis, which is referred to as herpangina. When ulcers are present on the soft palate, palms, and soles, the disease is called "hand, foot, and mouth disease."[41]

Patients infected with the Epstein-Barr virus develop the constellation of symptoms known as infectious mononucleosis. This can also be seen, though much more rarely, with cytomegalovirus infection. Patients develop a viral tonsillitis and pharyngitis, with high fevers and lymphadenopathy. The pharynx becomes erythematous with a thick continuous exudate and palatal petechiae. This usually follows a prodrome of chills, sweats, fevers, and malaise.[42] It is commonly seen in patients between 15 and 24 years of age. Up to 50% of cases can develop splenomegaly, and 10 to 15% develop hepatomegaly. Approximately 5% will have a rash of variable form, and approximately 90% will develop a pruritic maculopapular rash if given ampicillin or amoxicillin.[42,44] Diagnosis of infectious mononucleosis can be confirmed by the monospot test, as well as by the presence of atypical lymphocytes on a white blood cell count differential. The monospot is a rapid slide agglutination test with an overall sensitivity of 86% and specificity of 99%. The sensitivity and specificity of the test improves as the disease progresses, with the first week of the illness having the lowest sensitivity and specificity of 69 and 88%, respectively.[44] The presence of at least 10% atypical lymphocytes on a differential is 92% specific for infectious mononucleosis.[44] Treatment is largely supportive. Corticosteroids provide symptomatic improvement, though their use should be reserved for tonsillar hypertrophy threatening airway obstruction, severe thrombocytopenia, or hemolytic anemia.[42]

Primary infections with the human immunodeficiency virus (HIV) can lead to an acute retroviral syndrome. This syndrome usually presents, after an incubation period of several weeks, with fever, nonexudative pharyngitis, lymphadenopathy, arthralgia, myalgia, and lethargy. Maculopapular rash can be present in 40 to 80% of patients. It can be differentiated from infectious mononucleosis by the more sudden onset, a higher percentage of patients with a rash, and the lack of pharyngeal exudates.[42] HIV can be diagnosed with assays for HIV RNA. The test for HIV antibodies is often negative during the acute syndrome.

Fungal

Fungal pharyngitis is caused by *C. albicans* and is often the result of medications that affect the normal oral flora such as antibiotics or corticosteroids. It is also seen in patients with immunosuppression. Examination reveals a diffusely erythematous and edematous pharynx. White plaques of various size are seen throughout the oral cavity and pharyngeal mucosa. Microscopic examination of smears can demonstrate pseudohyphae and fungal spores. Treatment is usually a topical antifungal such as nystatin or itraconazole for several days.[19]

EPIGLOTTITIS/SUPRAGLOTTITIS

Epiglottitis, or more appropriately supraglottitis, is a rare disease affecting both children and adults. There are many pathogenic microorganisms that can cause supraglottitis, however the most famous is *H. influenzae* type b (Table 6). This is the microorganism that was most frequently associated with pediatric supraglottitis until the introduction of the *H. influenzae* type b vaccination.[46] The vaccination program has dramatically decreased the pediatric incidence of supraglottitis, however, it has not impacted the incidence of adult supraglottitis; and the disease is now

Table 6 Common Causes of Supraglottitis

Bacterial
  Haemophilus influenzae type b
  Nontypeable *H. influenzae*
  H. parainfluenzae
  Staphylococcus aureus
  β-Hemolytic *Streptococcus*
  Groups A, B, and C *Streptococcus*
  Streptococcus pneumoniae (pneumococcus)
  Streptococcus pyogenes
  Streptococcus milleri
  Streptococcus viridans
  Escherichia coli
  Bacteroides melanogenicus
  Klebsiella pneumoniae
  Neisseria meningitides
  Pseudomonas aeruginosa
  Kingella kingae
  Vibrio vulnificus
  Serratia marcescens
  Pasteurella multocida
  Citrobacter diversus
  Moraxella catarrhalis
  Mycobacterium tuberculosis
Viral
  Herpes simplex virus
  Varicella zoster virus
  Cytomegalovirus
  Parainfluenza virus
  Influenza virus type B
Fungal
  Aspergillus
  Mucormycosis
  Candida albicans

seen more in adults than children.[46] The mortality rates associated with the disease have steadily declined since the 1970s for the pediatric population and are now less than 1%. This is largely due to aggressive treatment algorithms for children that present with supraglottitis. The mortality rate in the adult population has held steady for many decades around 6 to 7%, with reports up to 20%. This is believed to be in part related to delays in diagnosis.[46] In both pediatrics and adults, there seems to be a male predominance, ranging from 1.9:1 to 4:1.[46,47] The incidence of otitis media has not been influenced by the *H. influenzae* type b vaccine because it is caused by the nontypeable *H. influenzae*.

An extensive list of pathogens associated with supraglottitis include: *H. influenzae* type b, nontypeable *H. influenzae*, *H. parainfluenzae*, *Staphylococcus aureus*, β-hemolytic *Streptococcus*, groups A, B, and C *Streptococcus*, *S. pneumoniae* (pneumoccus), *S. pyogenes*, *S. milleri*, *S. viridans*, *E. coli*, *Bacteroides melanogenicus*, *K. pneumoniae*, *N. meningitidis*, *P. aeruginosa*, *Kingella kingae*, *Vibrio vulnificus*, *Serratia marcescens*, *Pasteurella multocida*, *Citrobacter diversus*, *M. catarrhalis*, *Aspergillus*, Mucormycosis, *C. albicans*, Herpes simplex virus, varicella zoster virus, cytomegalovirus, parainfluenza virus, influenza virus type B, and *M. tuberculosis*.[46] Although this is an exhaustive list, many cases of supraglottitis go without identification of the pathologic microorganism.[46]

Children and adults present similarly with a sore throat, fever, and respiratory distress. Many patients are unable to manage their secretions due to the severe dysphagia and odynophagia. Children will often assume the tripod position, sitting upright with their chins up, mouth open, and bracing themselves on their hands.[46,48] The voice is often muffled or hoarse, with stridor being a late sign.[48] Progression of the disease and the respiratory distress can occur remarkably fast, with patient usually seeking care within 24 hours of onset of symptoms, although there are reports of onset of symptoms to fatal respiratory arrest in less than 4 hours.[47,49]

The workup differs between adults and children, with care being taken to avoid unnecessary anxiety in children. The workup includes radiographic imaging in children, if stable, and a direct laryngoscopy using a flexible nasopharyngoscope in adults. The imaging studies will help rule out foreign bodies, retropharyngeal abscess, or croup.[48] A lateral neck film shows an enlarged epiglottis with thickening and rounding, referred to as the "thumb sign," with obliteration of the vallecular air space.[48] Direct laryngoscopy will show varying degrees of epiglottic, aryepiglottic fold, and arytenoid edema. The swelling of the epiglottis can be graded based on the amount of the vocal folds visualized, as well as whether or not the extent of the edema involves the arytenoids.[47] Blood work, including complete blood counts and blood cultures, should be performed as should bacterial cultures of epiglottic swabs. This may be achieved in the awake adult but is best done during direct laryngoscopy under anesthesia in the child.

In the pediatric patient, once supraglottitis is suspected, the child should be taken for a direct laryngoscopic and tracheobronchoscopic examination. Once the airway is stabilized, cultures may be taken. The preferred route of airway stabilization is the nasotracheal intubation. Extubation may be considered upon repeat endoscopic examination with improvement or resolution of the edema, and/or development of an air leak. Often times, a flexible endoscopic examination will provide information as to the progress.[48]

The need for airway intervention in the adult is less certain than in the child. This is due to the larger anatomy of the adult, and the belief that the larger anatomy affords the patient a larger degree of edema before airway compromise.[47] A recent report from Japan outlined a series of 96 adults with supraglottitis. Only 8 (8%) of the 96 patients required airway intervention. They elected to perform tracheostomies on the patients requiring intervention due to the concern that failed attempts at intubation would cause more laryngeal edema and risk for further airway compromise. They found that the patients that required airway intervention had a higher rate of stridor and muffled voice, edema involving the arytenoids, and epiglottic swelling that obstructed the view of at least one-half of the true vocal folds.[47]

Broad spectrum antibiotics are usually started immediately, then the coverage may be tailored to the results of the culture and sensitivities. Coverage should take into account *Haemophilus*, *S. aureus*, and *Streptococcus* species.[47,48] The use of corticosteroids in the treatment of epiglottitis is debated, and no controlled trials exist to support or refute their use.[46] The study discussed above by Katori and colleagues reported the use of corticosteroids in 83% of their patients.[47] They reported no change in duration of hospitalization in those that received the corticosteroids.[47] The use of prophylactic antibiotics has been described for contacts of patients with diagnosed *Haemophilus* supraglottitis. Reports of transmission from both children to adults and adults to children exist. Rifampin therapy for 4 days can eradicate carrier states in 86%.[46]

LARYNGITIS/TRACHEITIS/BRONCHITIS

Bacterial

Many of the bacteria associated with pharyngitis and supraglottitis can also cause bacterial laryngitis, especially *Staphylococcus*, and *Streptococcus* (Table 7). These are managed in the same manner with antibiotics, supportive care, and airway observation. The use of corticosteroids is debated, with the proponents of their use arguing for the anti-inflammatory effect and the decreased airway edema. There are also many other bacterial pathogens that can target the larynx and trachea. One such pathogen is the spirochete *T. pallidum*. Since the near eradication of syphilis in the 1950s, there continue to be sporadic outbreaks. The

Table 7 Common Causes of Laryngotracheobronchitis

Bacterial
  Treponema pallidum
  Klebsiella rhinoscleromatis
  Corynebacterium diphtheriae
  Staphylococcus aureus
  Moraxella catarrhalis
  Haemophilus influenzae
  Alpha-hemolytic *Streptococcus*
  Group A *Streptoccocus*
  Mycoplasma pneumoniae
Viral
  Herpes simplex virus
  Varicella zoster virus
  Cytomegalovirus
  Parainfluenza virus
  Influenza virus types A and B
  Respiratory syncytial virus
  Measles
  Adenovirus
Fungal
  Candida albicans
  Histoplasma capsulatum
  Blastomyces dermatitidis
  Cryptococcus neoformans
  Coccidioides immitis

current estimates of the disease are approximately 2.5 cases per 100,000 people in the United States, with the majority of cases occurring in the southeastern region of the country.[20] Primary syphilis has been associated with laryngeal chancres. Secondary syphilis manifests itself with laryngitis and hoarseness as it involves the laryngeal mucosa. Tertiary syphilis can lead to gummata of the larynx causing hoarseness or even cicatrix formation in the form of adhesions between the vocal folds, interarytenoid scar, or subglottic stenosis. Recurrent laryngeal nerve dysfunction can occur in neurosyphilis by direct involvement of the nerve or with cardiovascular syphilis in which aortic aneurysms compress the nerve.[20] Diagnosis and treatment are as outlined above.

Laryngeal manifestations of *K. rhinoscleromatis* have also been reported to occur in 15 to 80% of the cases of rhinoscleroma.[16,50] These manifestations include hoarseness, exudates, and vocal fold edema in the early, catarrhal-atrophic stage. The second, or granulomatous stage, can lead to airway narrowing with vocal fold motion impairment. The sclerotic stage, is the final stage, and can lead to progressive scarring of the larynx and subglottis, contributing to stridor and airway obstruction.[16] Please see the Section on Rhinitis for the diagnosis and treatment of rhinosclerosis.

As mentioned previously, diphtheria can extend inferiorly to involve the larynx and even the trachea with the thick exudates, causing airway obstruction in the extreme cases.[51] In addition to the diphtheria caused by *C. diphtheriae*, a second microorganism of the same genus, *C. ulcerans* can cause a similar disease. *C. ulcerans* is associated with bovine mastitis and can be transmitted to humans with ingestion of nonpasteurized dairy products. It causes a similar disease process with most of the infections being mild although deaths

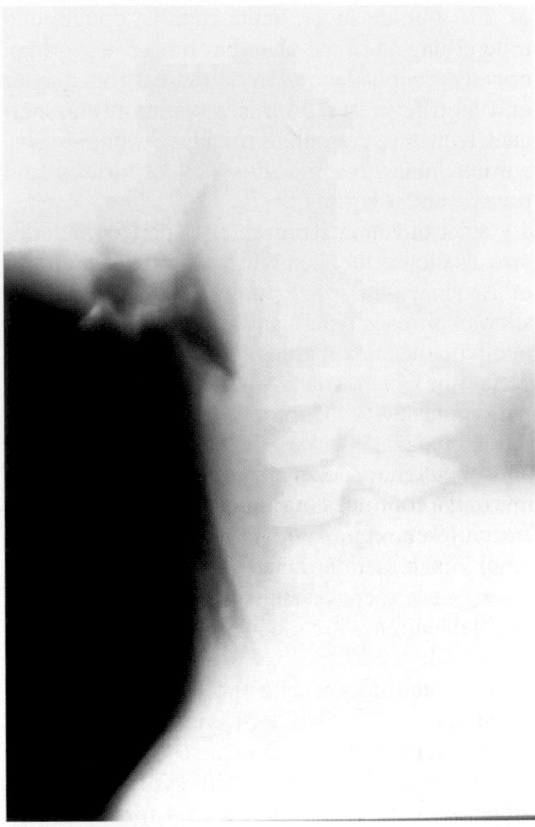

Figure 1 Lateral neck radiograph of a child with bacterial tracheitis. Note hazy pseudomembranes in the tracheal air column. (Courtesy of Stephen F. Conley, MD.)

have been reported. Treatment is the same as with classic diphtheria, antitoxin is administered immediately followed by antibiotics.[51]

Bacterial tracheitis is a complication of a viral laryngotracheobronchitis, which produces a thick, membranous material in the trachea and can lead to airway obstruction. The disease process affects children from 6 months to 8 years, with a peak incidence in fall and winter months. Microorganisms most commonly associated with bacterial tracheitis include *S. aureus*, *M. catarrhalis*, *H. influenzae*, alpha-hemolytic *Streptococcus*, group A *Streptococcus* and *M. pneumoniae*. Gram-negative microorganisms are rarely reported.[48]

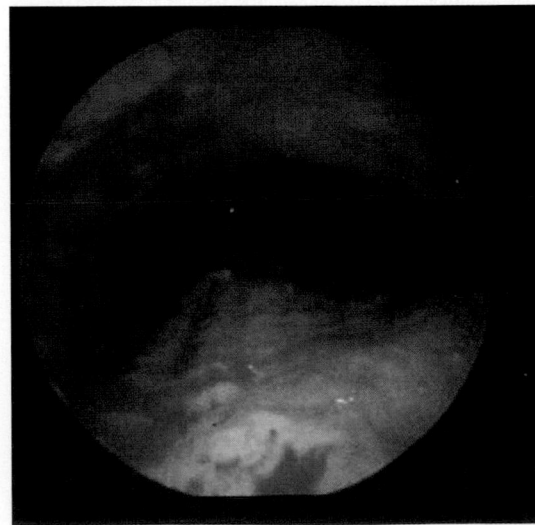

Figure 2 Endoscopic photo of a child with bacterial tracheitis. Note the pseudomembrane on the posterior wall of the trachea. (Courtesy of Stephen F. Conley, MD.)

The clinical presentation usually involves a several-day history of a viral upper respiratory tract infection. This can then lead to a rapid onset of a high fever and a toxic appearance although usually without drooling or odynophagia. Upon workup, an elevated white cell count is often found, and patients frequently have secondary sites of infection, most commonly pneumonia. Radiographic evaluation usually involves a lateral neck plain radiograph. This will often show a diffusely hazy air column, with areas of luminal soft tissue irregularities consistent with pseudomembrane detachment (Figure 1).[48]

Patients that are cooperative enough to tolerate a flexible nasopharyngeal endoscopic examination, should have it performed. If frank pus is visible or if a continued high level of suspicion exists, the children should undergo an open bronchoscopic examination. During the open bronchoscopy, a specimen of the pseudomembrane should be obtained for Gram stain, culture and sensitivity (Figure 2). The pseudomembrane itself should be removed as extensively as possible with suction or forceps. Most patients are then intubated, and left intubated for several days, until the patient has defervesced and tracheal secretions have decreased. Often times, repeat open bronchoscopy is required to debride the pseudomembrane further. Most patients are extubated within 3 to 7 days. Broad spectrum antibiotics are required initially, such as a third generation cephalosporin or ampicillin/sulbactam. Once the culture and sensitivity results are available, antibiotics should be appropriately tailored, for a total of 2 weeks.[48]

Viral

Most of the viruses associated with viral pharyngitis can cause a viral laryngitis and/or tracheitis (Table 7). One infection of particular concern is laryngotracheobronchitis, or croup. It is most commonly caused by the parainfluenza virus, types 1 and 2, although it has been associated with the influenza A and B viruses, the respiratory syncytial virus, herpes simplex virus, measles, adenovirus, and varicella. It is most commonly seen in children between 6 months and 3 years of age, and accounts for 90% of infectious airway obstructions. Approximately 5% of children have one episode, of whom 5% will have recurrent episodes. Children with recurrent episodes of croup should be taken, when healthy, for endoscopic evaluation of the subglottic airway for stenosis.[48]

Children often present with a several-day history of upper respiratory tract symptoms, which progress to a barking cough, hoarseness, and stridor. Patients often have a low-grade fever, and an elevated white blood cell count may be present. The stridor may progress from inspiratory to biphasic. This, along with retractions, tachypnea, and oxygen desaturations, strongly suggests impending airway collapse. Hospitalization and intubation are infrequently necessary, with respective rates ranging from 1.5 to 15% and 1 to 5%.[48]

The diagnostic evaluation most commonly includes an anterior–posterior radiographic view

of the soft tissues of the neck. This will show the classic "steeple sign," which is narrowing of the subglottic area. This narrowing is often dynamic, being more prominent on inspiration, thus distinguishing it from a fixed subglottic lesion such as stenosis or hemangioma. The anterior–posterior film may be falsely negative in as many as 50% of the patients with laryngotracheobronchitis. A flexible nasopharyngoscopic examination will show edema of the larynx and subglottis; however, it is not commonly performed given the airway instability.[48]

Laryngotracheobronchitis usually resolves on its own. As mentioned, it infrequently requires hospitalization or intubation. Most argue that mist helps soothe the inflamed mucosa and hydrates the secretions, making them easier to clear. Although there is no objective data to support cool or warm mist, enough anecdotal data exist to support its use. Racemic epinephrine is a combination of the epinephrine rotatory isomers dextro (D) and levo (L). They act to reduce airway edema by their alpha-adrenergic effect on mucosal vasculature and are given as a nebulized solution. Although both isomers have this alpha-adrenergic effect on the mucosa, the D-isomer is more potent and can thus lead to more systemic side effects than the L-isomer, which is why a mixture of the two is used. Of great concern are the cardiovascular side effects of high blood pressure and cardiac arrhythmias. Because of these side effects, caution must be used when administering epinephrine, and it should not be used in children with cardiac abnormalities or tachycardia. In addition, the potential for rebound edema exists with the use of epinephrine. Children should be monitored closely for at least 3 hours, although some still advocate hospital admission after the use of racemic epinephrine.[48]

The use of corticosteroids in cases of laryngotracheobronchitis is controversial. The reduced edema seen with corticosteroids, as well as the studies that have shown their efficacy are arguments for their use. However, the lack of complete understanding of their mechanism of action and their potential systemic side effects as well as the risk of bacterial and fungal superinfections argues against their use.[48]

A mixture of helium and oxygen, heliox, is commonly used for airway narrowing such as laryngotracheobronchitis or severe asthma.[48] It decreases the work of breathing by decreasing the airway turbulence and promoting laminar flow. The helium decreases the density of the gas mixture and increases the viscosity, thus increasing the laminar flow.[52] The mixture is approximately a 70% helium and 30% oxygen mixture, although exact percentages vary. This is used in addition to medical therapy to help stabilize a patient. It must be used cautiously, for if a patient fails heliox, there is usually little reserve, and the patient will likely require urgent intubation.

When intubation is required, nasotracheal intubation is the favored route. An endotracheal tube that is smaller than the expected size should

be used, given the reason for intubation. Patients should remain intubated until an air leak develops around the endotracheal tube, which is usually within 5 to 7 days.[48]

Although very rare, herpetic laryngitis has also been reported. It can be caused by both the varicella zoster virus and the herpes simplex virus.[53,54] The appearance can simulate a laryngeal neoplasm, fungal infection, abscess, or granulomatous disease. A mucosal biopsy is required for the diagnosis. If the histology is consistent with a herpes virus infection, antiherpes medications, such as acyclovir, should be used to treat the patient.[53,54]

Fungal

Fungal infections of the larynx are commonly seen in the immunocompromised patient, but also occur in the immunocompetent, likely at a rate higher than realized. The most common cause of fungal laryngitis is *Candida* species, however many other fungi can be the cause, including *Blastomyces*, *Histoplasma*, *Cryptococcus*, and *Coccidioides* (Table 7).[55,56] These most commonly appear secondary to an oral, pharyngeal, or pulmonary infection. In addition to immunocompromise, they are more common when the mucosal barrier is impaired, such as the case with smoking, radiation therapy, or corticosteroid use.[55]

Histopathologic analysis is required for diagnosis; however many argue that empirical treatment is reasonable initially. This point of view is based on the gross appearance similar to epithelial dysplasia of the larynx as well as the similarities seen in fungal colonization. Fungal spores, hyphae, and pseudohyphae are found within the upper layers of the epithelium in fungal infections. Hematoxylin and eosin stains will demonstrate what is known as pseudoepitheliomatosis hyperplasia. This specifically refers to epithelial hyperplasia with hyperkeratosis, neutrophils within the upper epithelial layers, lymphocytes, plasma cells, and scarring in the submucosal stroma. Fungal infection may also predispose to dysplasia; therefore, both elements may be present. Fungal colonization differs in that the fungal elements lie on top of the epithelial layer, with no penetration, and no associated hyperkeratosis or neutrophil infiltration.[55]

First line therapy for fungal laryngitis varies among authors, but a topical nystatin is a reasonable first option. An oral conazole for 3 to 4 weeks may be used if the topical is unsuccessful. Refractory cases may be treated with intravenous amphotericin B. If the fungal laryngitis continues to fail to respond, especially when dysplasia is present, a fungal infection secondary to a neoplasia must be considered.

REFERENCES

1. Rosenfeld RM, Bluestone CD. Evidence Based Otitis Media, 2nd edition. Hamilton, Ontario: BC Decker Inc; 2003.
2. Rosenfeld RM, Culpepper L, Doyle KJ, et al. Clinical practice guideline: Otitis media with effusion. Otolaryngol Head Neck Surg 2004;130:S95–118.

3. Cober MP, Johnson CE. Otitis media: Review of the 2004 treatment guidelines. Ann Pharmacother 2005;39:1879–87.

4. Bluestone CD, Stephenson JS, Martin LM. Ten-year review of otitis media pathogens. Pediatr Infect Dis J 1992;11:S7–11.

5. Berman S. Otitis media in children. N Engl J Med 1995;332:1560–5.

6. Pichichero ME, McLinn S, Aronovitz G, et al. Cefprozil treatment of persistent and recurrent acute otitis media. Pediatr Infect Dis J 1997;16:471–8.

7. Palmu AA, Saukkoriipi PA, Lahdenkari MI, et al. Does the presence of pneumococcal DNA in middle-ear fluid indicate pneumococcal etiology in acute otitis media? J Infect Dis 2004;189:775–84.

8. Ehrlich GD, Veeh R, Wang X, et al. Mucosal biofilm formation on middle-ear mucosa in the chinchilla model of otitis media. JAMA 2002;287:1710–5.

9. Poetker DM, Lindstrom DR, Edmiston CE, et al. Microbiology of middle ear effusions from 292 patients undergoing tympanostomy tube placement for middle ear disease. Int J Pediatr Otorhinolaryngol 2005;69:799–804.

10. Brunton S. Current face of acute otitis media: Microbiology and prevalence resulting from widespread use of heptavalent pneumococcal conjugate vaccine. Clin Ther 2006;28:118–23.

11. HeikkinenT, Järvinen A. The common cold. Lancet 2003;361:51–9.

12. Pratter MR. Cough and the common cold. ACCP Evidence-based clinical practice guidelines. Chest 2006;129:72S–4S.

13. Arroll B. Common cold. Clin Evid 2005;13:1853–61.

14. Brook I. The role of bacteria in chronic rhinosinusitis. Otolaryngol Clin North Am 2005;38:1171–92.

15. Luong A, Marple B. The role of fungi in chronic rhinosinusitis. Otolaryngol Clin North Am 2005;38:1203–13.

16. Ammar MEM, Rosen A. Rhinoscleroma mimicking nasal polyposis. Ann Otol Rhinol Laryngol 2001;110:290–2.

17. Cevera JJ, Butehorn HF III, Shapiro J, Setzen G. Actinomycosis abscess of the thyroid gland. Laryngoscope 2003;113:2108–10.

18. Özcan C, Talas D, Görür K, et al. Actinomycosis of the middle turbinate: An unusual case of nasal obstruction. Eur Arch Otorhinolaryngol 2005;262:412–5.

19. Gilbert DN, Moellering RC, Eliopoulous GM, Sande MA. The Sanford Guide to Antimicrobial Therapy 2006, 36th edition. Sperryville, VA: Antimicrobial Therapy, Inc; 2006.

20. Pletcher SD, Cheung SW. Syphilis and otolaryngology. Otolaryngol Clin North Am 2003;36:595–605.

21. Nayar RC, Al Kaabi J, Ghorpade K. Primary nasal tuberculosis: A case report. Ear Nose Throat J 2004;83:188–91.

22. Gupta A, Seiden AM. Nasal leprosy: Case study. Otolaryngol Head Neck Surg 2003;129:608–10.

23. Ling FTK, Wang D, Gerin-Lajoie J. Blastomycosis presenting as a locally invasive intranasal mass: Case report and literature review. J Otolaryngol 2003;32:405–9.

24. Arnold MG, Arnold JC, Bloom DC, et al. Head and neck manifestations of disseminated coccidiodomycosis. Laryngoscope 2004;114:747–52.

25. Chao SS, Loh KS. Rhinosporidiosis: An unusual cause of nasal masses gains prominence. Singapore Med J 2004;45:224–6.

26. Pelton RW, Peterson EA, Patel BCK, Davis K. Successful treatment of rhino-orbital mucormycosis without exenteration. Ophthal Plast Reconstr Surg 2001;17:62–6.

27. Sivak-Callcott JA, Livesley N, Nugent RA, et al. Localized invasive sino-orbital aspergillosis: Characteristic features. Br J Ophthalmol 2004;88:681–7.

28. Choi CM, Lerner EA. Leishmaniasis as an emerging infection. J Investig Dermatol Symp Proc 2001;6:175–82.

29. Meinking TL, Burkhart CN, Burkhart CG. Changing paradigms in parasitic infections: Common dermatological helminthic infections and cutaneous myiasis. Clin Dermatol 2003;21:407–16.

30. Beckendorf R, Klotz SA, Hinkle N, Bartholomew W. Nasal myiasis in an intensive care unit linked to hospital-wide mouse infestation. Arch Intern Med 2002; 162:638–40.

31. Sampson CE, MaGuire J, Eriksson E. Botfly myiasis: Case report and brief review. Ann Plast Surg 2001;46:150–2.

32. Rivera-Hidalgo F, Stanford TW. Oral mucosal lesions caused by infective mircroorganisms I. Viruses and bacteria. Periodontology 2000 1999;21:106–24.

33. Arikan OK, Koç C, Bozdo an Ö. Tularemia presenting as tonsillopharyngitis and cervical lymphadenitis: A case report and review of the literature. Eur Arch Otorhinolaryngol 2003;260:298–300.

34. McKenna MJ. Measles, mumps, and sensorineural hearing loss. Ann N Y Acad Sci 1997;830:291–8.

35. Karosi T, Kónya J, Petkó M, et al. Antimeasles immunoglobulin G for serologic diagnosis of otosclerotic hearing loss. Laryngoscope 2006;116:488–93.

36. Bento RF, Castilho AM, Sakae FA, et al. Auditory brainstem response and otoacoustic emission assessment of hearing-impaired children of mothers who contracted rubella during pregnancy. Acta Otolaryngol 2005;125:492–4.

37. Salvinelli F, Firrisi L, Greco F, et al. Preserved otoacoustic emissions in postparotitis profound unilateral hearing loss: A case report. Ann Otol Rhinol Laryngol 2004;113:887–90.

38. Stanford TW, Rivera-Hidalgo F. Oral mucosal lesions caused by infective microorganisms II. Fungi and parasites. Periodontology 2000 1999;21:125–44.

39. Ling FTK, Wang D, Gérin-Lajoie J. Blastomycosis presenting as a locally invasive intranasal mass: Case report and literature review. J Otolaryngol 2003;32:405–9.

40. Schweinfurth JM, Powitzky E. Cervical manifestation of blastomycosis. Am J Otolaryngol 2001;22:157–9.

41. Attia MW, Bennett JE. Pediatric pharyngitis. Pediatr Case Rev 2003;3:203–10.

42. Bisno AL. Acute pharyngitis. N Engl J Med 2001;344:205–11.

43. Stephenson KN. Acute and chronic pharyngitis across the lifespan. Lippincotts Prim Care Pract 2000;4:471–89.

44. Vincent MT, Celestin N, Hussain AN. Pharyngitis. Am Fam Physician 2004;69:1465–70.

45. Yeung RSV. Pathogenesis and treatment of Kawasaki's disease. Curr Opin Rheumatol 2005;17:617–23.

46. Carey MJ. Epiglottitis in Adults. Am J Emerg Med 1996;14:421–4.

47. Katori H, Tsukada M. Acute epiglottitis: Analysis of factors associated with airway intervention. J Laryngol Otol 2005;119:967–72.

48. Stroud RH, Friedman NR. An update on inflammatory disorders of the pediatric airway: Epiglottitis, croup, and tracheitis. Am J Otolaryngol 2001;22:268–75.

49. Deeb ZE. Acute supraglottitis in adults: Early indicators of airway obstruction. Am J Otolaryngol 1997;18:112–5.

50. El-Sherif M, Rosen A. Rhinoscleroma mimicking nasal polyposis. Ann Otol Rhinol Laryngol 2001;110:290–2.

51. Kaufmann D, Ott P, Zbinden R. Laryngopharyngitis by *Corynebacterium ulcerans*. Infection 2002;30:168–170.

52. Haynes JM, Sargent RJ, Sweeney EL. Use of heliox to avoid intubation in a child with acute severe asthma and hypercapnia. Am J Crit Care 2003;12:28–30.

53. Pinto JA, Pinto HCF, da Rosa Oiticica Ramalho J. Laryngeal herpes: A case report. J Voice 2002;16:560–3.

54. Wackym PA, Gray GF, Jr, Avant GR. Herpes zoster of the larynx after intubational trauma. J Laryngol Otol 1986;100:839–41.

55. Mehanna HM, Kuo T, Chaplin J, et al. Fungal laryngitis in immunocompetent patients. J Laryngol Otol 2004;118:379–81.

56. Nadrous HF, Ryu JH, Lewis JE, Sabri AN. Cryptococcal laryngitis: Case report and review of the literature. Ann Otol Rhinol Laryngol 2004;113:121–3.

43

Allergic Rhinitis

Robert M. Naclerio, MD
Asli Sahin-Yilmaz, MD

Allergic rhinitis is defined as a symptomatic disorder of the nose induced by immunoglobulin E (IgE)-mediated inflammation due to exposure to foreign substances, referred to as allergens. It is characterized by 1 or more nasal symptoms of pruritus, sneeze, discharge, and stuffiness. Additionally, the sense of smell and ability to taste can be altered. More than creating symptoms, the disease affects the individual's quality of life and is associated with comorbidities like asthma, eustachian tube dysfunction, sinusitis, and conjunctivitis.

EPIDEMIOLOGY

It is estimated that more than 20% of the world population suffers from IgE-mediated allergic diseases. In the Western world, allergic diseases have increased two- to threefold over the last 40 years and have reached epidemic proportions.[1] Allergic rhinitis is the most common allergic disease. The prevalence of allergic rhinitis varies throughout the world. The prevalence of seasonal allergic rhinitis ranges from 1 to 40%, and the prevalence of perennial allergic rhinitis varies from 1 to 18%.[2] Overall, allergic rhinitis affects 20 to 40 million people in the United States.[3] In an otolaryngologist's practice, the prevalence of allergic rhinitis in patients coming to the office exceeds that of the general population and is in the range of 50%.

Although it is a benign but chronic disease of the upper airway, quality-of-life studies demonstrate that allergic rhinitis has a great impact on the patients' well-being. It causes a significant decrease in energy, general health perception, and social function.[4] In the United States, the estimates of the annual cost of allergic rhinitis range from 2 to 5 billion dollars.[5] The decreased quality of life not only leads to absenteeism but also contributes to "presenteeism" or decreased productivity at work. The economic impact of work productivity losses due to allergic rhinitis was found to be $593 per year per employee, higher than that due to other common conditions like stress, migraine, depression, and respiratory infections.[6]

Allergic rhinitis in children results in a variety of problems that may affect their quality of life, such as learning impairment, inability to integrate with peers, anxiety, and family dysfunction. Diminished functional capacity in children due to allergic rhinitis alone causes the loss of 2 million school days each year.[4] These numbers are augmented when one considers related disorders such as asthma and sinusitis, which are thought to be affected by allergic rhinitis. Treatment-related side effects, such as sedation, can increase the negative impact of allergic rhinitis.

Evidence suggests that there has been an increase in the incidence of allergic rhinitis. The prevalence of self-reported allergic rhinitis was 16.5% in Norwegian school children in 1985 and increased to 24.7% by 1995, and to 29.6% by 2000.[7] Similar trends have been observed in other studies.[8,9] In a study from US-population-based National Health and Nutrition Examination Survey, data of the years 1976 to 1980 were compared to the data of 1988 to 1994. The prevalence of a positive test response to 6 common allergens observed in the latter survey was 2.1 to 5.5 times higher than in the former.[10] The cause of the increasing prevalence of allergic rhinitis is not clear.

Risk Factors Associated with the Disease

Genetics and Family History. A study of twins confirmed the hereditary transmission of allergic rhinitis. The concordance of allergic rhinitis in identical twins was higher than that in fraternal twins.[11] Several investigators have conducted genome-wide screens in a variety of populations in the search for susceptibility genes involved in allergic diseases, primarily asthma.[12–14] Evidence of linkage to allergic rhinitis and/or asthma for 2 chromosome regions (1p31 and 2q32) was shown in a genome screen from France. No region detected had evidence for linkage to asthma without also being linked to allergic rhinitis.[14] In another study from Denmark, significant evidence for linkage to chromosome segment 3q13.31 for allergic rhinitis was shown.[12] Heterogeneity of phenotype, gene environment interaction, complexity of molecular mechanisms, an unknown mode of inheritance, and the possibility of small effects of a number of genes complicate these approaches. This remains an area of intense interest and will likely accelerate in the near future.

Early Life Exposures. According to the hygiene hypothesis, infections in early life protect from the development of allergic diseases later in life. This hypothesis is based on observations that show a higher prevalence of allergic diseases in individuals brought up in smaller and wealthier families, particularly in children and young adults in developed nations. The lower prevalence of early childhood infections can be explained by a lowered risk of exposure to infectious agents early in life as a result of improved sanitary conditions and smaller family size. High exposure to acute respiratory infection between pregnancy and age 1 year has also been found to be associated with overall reduced odds for allergic diseases, the most effective period for protection being the first 9 months of life.[15]

It has been suggested that a decrease in exposure to infectious agents results in a skew in the balance between T-cell subpopulations from T helper 1 (Th1)-cell responses toward atopic Th2-cell responses, including increased production of IgE (Figure 1). Supporting the hygiene theory are studies demonstrating an inverse relationship between the frequency of allergic disorders and serologic evidence for acquisition of certain infections, mainly food-borne and orofecal infections.[16,17] Recently, it has become clear that innate responses to microbes are mediated in large part by the toll-like receptors (TLRs), a series of 13 cell surface receptors located on epithelial cells, and various cells of the immune system.[18] These receptors are known to recognize the ligands produced by viruses, bacteria, and fungi. Stimulation of the innate immune system causes the release of chemokines, cytokines, and growth factors that can drive the adaptive immune system in a specific direction that may decrease the likelihood of the individual being atopic. More studies are required for developing an understanding of the influence of TLR exposures on the maturation of the immune system and the risk for allergies.

Exposure to allergen is suggested to be a risk factor for the development and persistence of allergic rhinitis. Outdoor allergens appear to constitute a greater risk for seasonal allergic rhinitis than do indoor allergens.[2] New hypotheses on the effect of allergenic exposure on allergic rhinitis are controversial. It is suggested that early exposures to indoor allergens like pet dander may have a protective effect on the development of allergic rhinitis.[19] In primary intervention studies, in children of atopic parents, avoidance of house dust mites or similar indoor allergens resulted in a reduction of the incidence of sensitization during the first year of life.[20] However, continuing mite avoidance measures did not make any difference for allergy development in children at 4 years of age.[21]

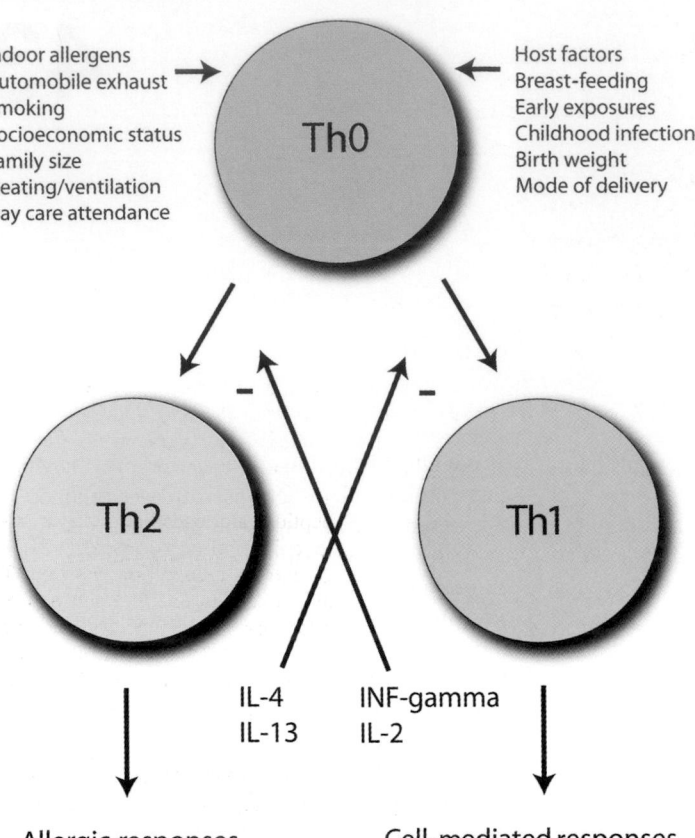

Figure 1 Current possible theory on development of allergic disease. Various factors have been suggested to influence predisposition to allergies. Cytokines produced in Th1 and Th2 responses inhibit the expression of the counterpart response. The Th1 pathway is primarily responsible for cell mediated immunity, whereas the Th2 pathway is important in the production of allergic responses.

In developing nations, rural locales were found to have lower rates of allergic diseases than did urban locales.[22] Close animal contact and exclusive breast-feeding in the families living in rural areas are shown to be associated with lower atopic sensitization. The beneficial effect of growing up on a farm against sensitization and development of allergic diseases in childhood has been reported in several other studies.[23,24] Most consistently, the "protective" farm effect was related to livestock farming and most likely was due to microbial exposure. A dose-dependent inverse relationship between exposure of children to endotoxin in the mattress dust and the occurrence of atopic diseases was shown in rural environments in Europe.[25] In addition, the blood cells of farmers' children were shown to express higher amounts of innate-immunity receptors. Toll-like receptor 4 (TLR4) is the principal receptor for bacterial endotoxin recognition and plays a critical role in the innate immune response to gram-negative pathogens and respiratory syncytial viruses. The evidence that exposure to endotoxin during early life is protective against development of atopy resulted in studies searching for a relationship between the genetic variations in the TLR4 locus and susceptibility to atopy. No evidence was found for an association between the TLR4 variants and atopy-related phenotypes.[26,27] This suggests that additional genetic determinants perhaps involving other important genes in the endotoxin signaling pathway contribute to the endotoxin responsiveness phenotype. This also suggests that gene-environment interactions play an important role in the development of atopy.

Previous data suggested that early introduction of solid foods, in the first year of life, is positively associated with development of allergic rhinitis.[28] A systematic review of available evidence demonstrated that early feeding of solids may increase the risk of eczema, however, the data supporting an association between early solid feeding and other allergic conditions, including allergic rhinitis, are limited.[29] Many other factors have been implicated in hypotheses and speculations on the possible cause–effect relationship in the development of allergic rhinitis. Some of these factors seem to be significant, such as mode of delivery, birth weight, day care outside the home, and socioeconomic status, but more prospective studies are needed for confirmation of the results.[30–32]

Pollution. The impact of pollution on allergic rhinitis is controversial. Pollution is suggested to cause an increase in nasal responsiveness to environmental allergens. Common outdoor pollutants include sulfur dioxide (SO_2), nitrogen dioxide (NO_2), and ozone, whereas indoor pollutants include side-stream cigarette smoke.

Persistent exposure to outdoor pollution, especially particulate matter from motor vehicles, has been suggested as one of the factors responsible for the increase in the prevalence of allergic rhinitis. Some studies have shown that exposure to diesel exhaust particles alter the nasal immunology by increasing IgE production, directing cytokine gene expression toward a Th2 profile as well as altering responses to allergen challenge.[33] However, results of other research provided a more complex picture. Outdoor pollution was found to be a poor predictor of physician visits for allergic rhinitis among adult patients.[34] A study on a different chemical content of diesel exhaust particles failed to show any differences in nasal total cell numbers or mediators compared to placebo.[35] The evidence for the effect of pollution on nasal allergies remains an area of further investigation.

Studies in children showed positive associations between lifetime allergic rhinitis and passive smoking.[36,37] A birth cohort study showed that infants exposed to 20 or more cigarettes per day compared with nonexposed infants are 3 times more likely to have allergic rhinitis at age 1.[38] Estimates of daily exposure of children to environmental tobacco smoke in the home range as high as 40 to 60%.[39] Environmental tobacco smoke is known to exacerbate allergic responses by promoting the production of allergen-specific IgE, the induction of a Th2 cytokine nasal milieu, and an increase in histamine after nasal allergen challenge.[40]

NATURAL HISTORY

Symptoms of allergic rhinitis can begin at any age, but are most frequently first reported in adolescence or young adulthood.[41] The prevalence in females was found to be slightly higher than that in males, but no racial or ethnic variations have been reported.[42] The incidence of developing an allergic diathesis is higher in children whose parents suffer from allergic rhinitis. If 1 parent has allergies, the chances of the child having rhinitis are 20 to 30% and increase to 40 to 50% when both parents have the disease.[28] The cumulative decrease in the rate of loss of allergic rhinitis symptoms has been estimated to be about 10%, and this occurs mostly in patients with the mildest form of the disease.[43]

Allergic rhinitis is highly related to asthma. The Tucson Epidemiologic Study of Obstructive Lung Diseases confirmed that rhinitis is a significant risk factor for adult-onset asthma. Allergic rhinitis or asthma or both are related to a combination of environmental and genetic factors, some of which affect either the upper or lower airways.[44]

CLINICAL SIGNIFICANCE

A part of the clinical importance of allergic rhinitis lies in its association with complications related to chronic nasal obstruction. Total nasal obstruction, regardless of etiology, can cause sleep disturbances. Whether interference with sleep or the effects of systemically released mediators contribute to the fatigue associated with the disease is unknown. Evidence for a role of the nervous system is a new and exciting area of investigation.[45] The prevalence of smell and taste problems in patients with allergic rhinitis is 21.4 and 31.2%, respectively.[46] Studies report a high prevalence of sensitization to inhalant allergens both in acute and chronic rhinosinusitis.[47,48] In animal studies, it has been shown that an ongoing allergic response in the nose augments acute bacterial sinus infection.[49]

Whether nasal polyps result from allergic rhinitis remains an open question. In an allergy practice setting, nasal polyps were present in 1.7% of patients with allergic rhinitis without asthma.[50]

Allergic rhinitis may contribute to middleear disease. Evidence suggests that an induced allergic reaction can cause eustachian tube dysfunction.[51,52] Expression of Th2 cytokines and inflammatory cells has been documented in the middleear mucosa of allergic patients.[53]

Rhinitis is linked to asthma by epidemiologic, pathologic, and physiologic characteristics and by a common therapeutic approach.[2] A large population-based follow-up study has shown that all subjects with allergic asthma had allergic rhinitis first.[54] In another study, allergic rhinitis was detected in 74 to 81% of asthmatic subjects, and 40% of allergicrhinitis patients had asthma, suggesting a close link between the two diseases.[55]

PATHOPHYSIOLOGY

Sensitization and IgE

The distinguishing characteristic of allergic rhinitis is the involvement of IgE immunoglobulins. IgE itself constitutes a small fraction of the human serum; however, the biological activities of IgE are enhanced by the activities of specific cell surface receptors to which it binds.[2] The impact of anti-IgE antibody on the symptoms of allergic rhinitis has proven the role of IgE in the pathophysiology of allergic rhinitis.[56]

In an individual with a susceptibility for developing allergic disease, an initial contact with allergen leads to the production of specific IgE molecules, a process termed sensitization. This begins when macrophages and other antigen-presenting cells process the allergen before presenting it to T-helper cells, which then interact with B lymphocytes, leading to their differentiation (isotype switching) into IgE-producing plasma cells, a process involving Th2 cytokines [interleukin (IL)-4 and IL-13] and accessory molecules such as cluster of differentiation molecule 40 (CD40)[57] (Figure 2). The newly formed antigen-specific IgE molecules are secreted and bind to high-affinity receptors (FcεRI) located on mast cells and basophils, platelets, activated eosinophils, and Langerhans cells and to low-affinity receptors (FcεRII/CD23) located on a variety of cells including B cells, macrophages, monocytes, follicular dendritic cells, and eosinophils.[58] The high-affinity IgE receptors on mast cells mediate the initial allergic response. The low-affinity receptors are thought to play a role in antigen presentation to T cells and in B-cell differentiation.[57]

In biopsy specimens obtained from symptomatic patients in season and also in specimens from asymptomatic patients with seasonal allergic rhinitis and exposed to allergen ex vivo, showed that class switching of B cells to IgE occurs locally in the nasal mucosa.[59,60]

Early Response

In a sensitized individual, another encounter with the same allergen initiates the second step of the allergic response process, an immediate (early) allergic reaction, which is characterized by rhinorrhea, obstruction, sneezing, and pruritus. Within seconds of entering the nasal cavity, antigens interact with specific IgE molecules on the surface of mast cells. Cross-linking of 2 adjacent IgE molecules by antigen initiates a sequence of intracellular events that resulting in mast-cell degranulation. Release of both preformed mediators (histamine and proteases [chymase and tryptase]) and newly synthesized mediators (prostaglandins [PGDs], cysteinyl leukotrienes [CysLTs], platelet activating factor, bradykinin, ILs, tumor necrosis factor-α [TNF-α], and granulocyte-macrophage colony-stimulating factor) follows. Plasma exudation results in edema and swelling in the nasal mucosa. The exudate also allows additional mediators and enzymes including kinins, albumin, proinflammatory mediators, and activated complement fractions to appear in nasal secretions.[2] The early-phase reaction also includes the activation of epithelial cells and release of neuropeptides like substance P (SP).

For ascertaining the importance of any mediator in the pathophysiology of allergic rhinitis, 3 criteria should be satisfied: (1) the mediator should be present during the allergic reaction; (2) instilling the mediator in the nasal cavity should mimic part of the pathophysiology or symptoms of the disease; and (3) a mediator antagonist must at least partially attenuate disease expression. To establish the importance of different mediators in allergic rhinitis, several investigators have attempted to satisfy 1 or more of these criteria. Multiple mediators have been recovered at increased levels in nasal secretions after allergen challenge; these include histamine,[61] kinins,[62] plasma and glandular kallikrein,[63] mast cell tryptase,[64] PGD_2,[61] LTC_4,[65] LTB_4,[66] and major basic protein (MBP).[67] Furthermore, several of these mediators have been used to challenge the nasal mucosa and observe resultant responses. Histamine provocation, for example, produces rhinorrhea, congestion, pruritus, and sneezing by stimulating receptors on sensory nerves and blood vessels.[68] Instillation of serotonin produces sneezing, whereas prostaglandin D_2 and kinins all produce nasal congestion.[69–71] The other approach to establishing the importance of a mediator involves the use of antagonists; the best example of these is H_1 antihistamines: the clinical utility of H_1 receptor antagonists serves to demonstrate the importance of this inflammatory mediator.

Whereas mast-cell degranulation and the released inflammatory mediators mimic most of the symptoms of allergic disease, the short duration of these events, as opposed to the prolonged symptoms of clinical disease, suggests that additional inflammatory processes are probably important in clinical disease. Furthermore, increased responsiveness and mucosal cellular changes that accompany chronic exposure to allergen cannot be explained by this mechanism alone. Many of these phenomena relate to the cellular infiltration that is a hallmark of the inflammatory response.[72]

Late Response

Various techniques of experimental nasal allergen provocation, in addition to being useful for an understanding of the early response, assist investigators in understanding subsequent inflammatory events. Following challenge, there is an increase in symptoms and mediator levels characteristic of the early allergic reaction, which soon return toward baseline. If one continues to monitor the response for several hours, symptoms recur, associated with an elevation of levels of inflammatory mediators in approximately 50% of the patients, referred to as the late-phase response.[73,74] During the late-phase response, subjects have a recurrence of sneezing, rhinorrhea, and congestion, with congestion predominating.[75]

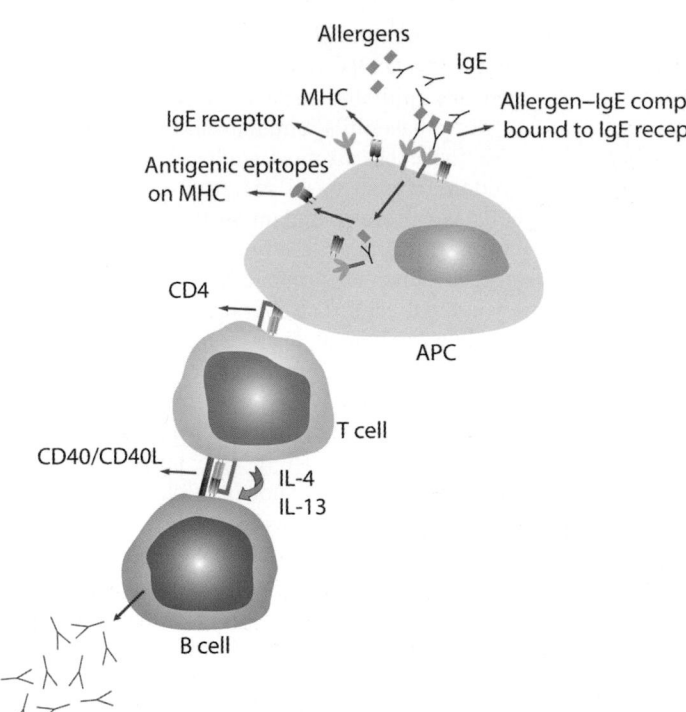

Figure 2 Production of allergen-specific IgE. Allergen and IgE complexes bind to IgE receptors on allergen presenting cell (APC) surface. This complex is internalized. Antigenic peptides are loaded onto major histocompatibility complex (MHC). Cognitive recognition between T and B cells results in production of allergen-specific IgE. This process involves IL-4, IL-13 and accessory molecules such as CD40. (Borrowed in part from reference 57.)

As in clinical disease, a striking characteristic of the late-phase response is cellular inflammation (Figure 3). Mediators released during the early phase reaction stimulate the production, maturation, and infiltration of inflammatory cells, including basophils, eosinophils, neutrophils, and mononuclear cells in nasal secretions, as recovered by nasal lavage. Nasal mucosal biopsies, performed 24 hours after topical allergen provocation, also show increases in the number of inflammatory cells, but, in contrast to the nasal secretions, in which eosinophils and neutrophils account for the majority of recovered cells, mononuclear cells predominate.[76] These are mostly of the T-helper category, as evidenced by positive staining with antibodies against CD4, and a portion of them are activated, as documented by IL2 receptor expression (CD25[+]).[77] These T lymphocytes have been shown to express messenger RNA for Th2-type cytokines.

The cellular changes observed after allergen provocation are similar to observations of nasal cytology during seasonal disease. In separately conducted studies, Bryan and Bryan, and Okuda and Otsuka observed basophilic cells in nasal secretions during seasonal exposure of allergic individuals to pollen.[79,80] In contrast to nasal secretions, which represent the most superficial compartment of the nasal mucosa, examination of nasal mucosal scrapings,[81] or biopsies[82] which sample deeper layers, showed that the majority of metachromatic cells in these compartments were mast cells. Enerbäck and colleagues, using biopsies and cytologic imprints to examine the cellular content of the nasal mucosa during the birch pollen season in Sweden, showed a seasonal increase in the number of mast cells on the surface of the

nasal epithelium after 4 or 5 days of pollen exposure.[83] Mast cells are found in high concentrations beneath epithelial surfaces, whereas their counterparts, basophils, circulate in the bloodstream. The consensus in most studies is that basophils predominate in nasal secretions, whereas mast cells are more abundant in the epithelium and lamina propria of allergic subjects exposed to antigen either experimentally or naturally. Bentley and colleagues also reported a significant seasonal increase in total MBP[+] and activated (EG2[+]) eosinophils in the submucosa of allergic patients when compared with preseasonal biopsies or biopsies from nonallergic control subjects.[84]

The late reaction is also accompanied by increases in some, but not all, of the inflammatory mediators associated with the early reaction and the presence of mediators not seen in the early response.[85] The mediators recovered in the nasal secretions during the late phase include histamine, CysLTs such as LTC$_4$, eosinophil-derived mediators like eosinophilic cationic protein, and kinins. It is now well known that cytokines and chemokines, more than any proinflammatory mediators, are involved in the recruitment and activation of inflammatory cells of the late phase.

Cytokines and Chemokines

In addition to the role of inflammatory mediators in allergic disease, cytokines are increasingly being recognized as important mediators of allergic inflammation and have been shown to have proinflammatory effects in vitro. The proinflammatory cytokines include IL-1, TNF, IL-6, and IL-18. These cytokines are involved in accumulation of inflammatory cells and induce expression of E-selectin, activation of T and B lymphocytes,

and induction of the arachidonic-acid mechanism. The Th2-related cytokines include IL-3, IL-4, IL-5, IL-10, and IL-13. IL-4 and IL-13 induce the synthesis of IgE and IgG4 and the expression of surface antigens on B cells.[2] IL-5 has been shown to be an important factor for eosinophilia that is observed in the late-phase reaction.[86]

Chemokines are chemoattractant cytokines which play an important role in the function and expression of leukocyte and endothelial adhesion molecules. Approximately 50 chemokines have been described to date. Many chemokines and their receptors are highly expressed in allergic patients.[87] These include RANTES [regulated on activation, normal T expressed and secreted chemokine L5, (CCL5)], eotaxin (CCL11), and monocyte chemoattractant protein-4 (CCL13).[88] Important sources of chemokines aside from inflammatory cells are epithelial cells. Both epithelial and inflammatory cells in the nasal submucosa of patients allergic to ragweed have been shown to be positive for eotaxin mRNA and protein.[88] The chemokine receptor CCR3 is expressed on the cell surface of eosinophils, Th2 lymphocytes, basophils, and mast cells and binds the eotaxin family of chemokines, whose production is upregulated after nasal challenge.[87] Therapeutic strategies with use of antibodies to chemokines or their receptors are currently under investigation as an alternative treatment for allergic rhinitis and asthma.[89]

Adhesion Molecules

Cellular adhesion molecules play an important role in recruiting circulating leukocytes to the vascular endothelium at sites of inflammation. Studies have demonstrated increases in

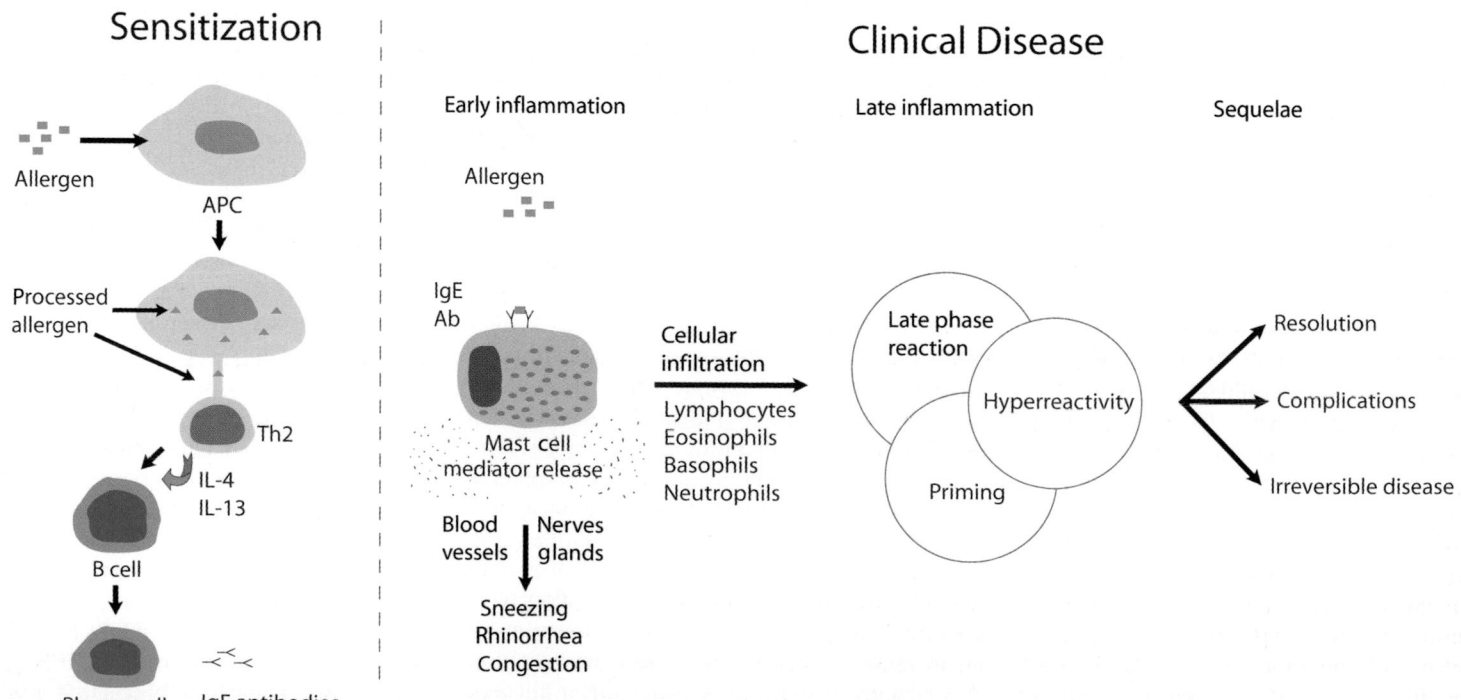

Figure 3 Pathophysiology of allergic rhinitis. On the left side of the figure, sensitization to allergen is depicted and involves the production of specific IgE antibodies to certain allergens. On subsequent exposure to the allergen, depicted on the right, there is a cross linking of specific IgE receptors with resultant degranulation of mast cells and the release of inflammatory mediators. Subsequent to the early reaction, inflammatory cells infiltrate the nasal mucosa and the late phase response develops. This is accompanied by a state of increased reactivity that renders the nasal mucosa more responsive to subsequent exposure to allergen (priming) or other stimuli (hyperreactivity). Finally, natural allergic disease might resolve or lead to complications. (Borrowed in part from reference 78.)

endothelial adhesion molecules, namely, vascular cell adhesion molecule-1 (VCAM-1) in nasal biopsies obtained from allergic subjects 24 hours after nasal allergen challenge.[90] This molecule is expressed on the surface of vascular endothelial cells and interacts with a counterligand, very late antigen-4 (VLA-4), which is present on the surface of several leukocytes, including lymphocytes, monocytes, eosinophils, and basophils, but not neutrophils.[91] The VLA-4/VCAM-1 adhesion pathway has been suggested as a mechanism for specific eosinophil, as opposed to neutrophil, migration from the circulation into allergic inflammatory sites.[92] However, in asthmatic patients, studies using an inhaled VLA antagonist did not result in any protection against allergen-induced airway responses.[93,94]

Other adhesion molecules thought to be important in the recruitment of inflammatory cells from the intravascular compartment into tissue sites of allergic inflammation are intercellular adhesion molecule 1 (ICAM-1), which is constitutively expressed in the nasal mucosa, and E-selectin, which is modestly upregulated 24 hours after allergen provocation.[90] ICAM-1, a ligand for the β_2 integrin molecules CD11a/CD18 (leukocyte function assisted antigen-1) and CD11b/CD18 (Mac-1), which are present on the surface of leukocytes, mediates the attachment of all classes of leukocytes to endothelial cells,[95] and E-selectin binds to sialyl Lewis X expressed on the surface of leukocytes.[96] The expression of the adhesion molecules VCAM-1 and E-selectin[90] was shown to be enhanced 24 hours after local allergen challenge. Similarly, ICAM-1 and leukocyte function assisted antigen-1 are increased in nasal epithelial cells of patients with seasonal[97] and perennial[98] rhinitis. It has recently been shown that the expression of adhesion molecules correlates with the severity of airway diseases.[99] ICAM expression has been shown to be suppressed by H_1 antihistamines and topical glucocorticosteroids.[100]

Cysteinyl Leukotrienes

CysLTs are synthesized by mast cells during the early-phase response and by eosinophils, basophils, and macrophages during the late-phase response of allergic rhinitis. The cysLTs include LTC_4, LTD_4, and LTE_4. The enzymes for the production and release of cysLTs are already present in inflammatory cells, unlike cytokines which require transcription and synthesis.[101] CysLTs stimulate mucous glands, which results in rhinorrhea, and they also have the ability to increase microvascular permeability and blood flow, which results in tissue edema. In addition to these local responses, cysLTs participate in the systemic immune response to allergens.[85] The use of leukotriene modifiers is an important therapeutic advance in the management of allergic diseases. Even though the role of leukotriene receptor antagonists has been more extensively established in asthma, studies on the effects of these drugs on the upper airways have shown that these drugs represent a useful approach to the treatment of seasonal and perennial allergic rhinitis.[102,103]

Nasal Reactivity

Besides the development of recurrent symptoms within hours after a nasal challenge, the inflammatory cellular influx is accompanied by increased nasal reactivity. In the 1960s, John Connell coined the term "priming" to refer to increased antigen responsiveness. Priming may explain why patients become more symptomatic to the same amounts of pollen in the environment later during the allergy season. Nonspecific reactivity implies increased responsiveness to nonantigenic substances and has been studied by provocation of individuals with methacholine, histamine, cold, dry air, or bradykinin. Like priming, nonspecific reactivity is not obligatorily linked to the appearance of a late reaction. Walden and colleagues found increased sensitivity to histamine 24 hours after antigen challenge.[104] The response to histamine challenge returned to baseline 10 days later, suggesting that increased responsiveness to histamine was reversible. Other studies showed a positive correlation between the number of eosinophils 24 hours after antigen challenge and the magnitude of the responsiveness to histamine, and this hyperresponsiveness was inhibited by pretreatment with topical corticosteroids.[105,106]

Majchel and colleagues examined the effect of seasonal exposure on nasal responsiveness to histamine by challenging allergic subjects with histamine before, at the peak of, near the end of, and 2 weeks after the end of the ragweed pollen season.[107] These investigators observed a significant increase in symptoms at the peak of the pollen season that returned to baseline with the disappearance of pollen. There was no significant increase above baseline at the peak of the season for any of the parameters measured. However, they suggested that increased reactivity to histamine with seasonal exposure appeared to represent a change in baseline rather than an increased sensitivity to histamine itself. This change in baseline reactivity was inhibited in subjects who were receiving immunotherapy. Similar studies have demonstrated nasal hyperresponsiveness to methacholine.[108]

Klementsson and colleagues measured the volume of nasal secretions after intranasal administration of 6 mg of methacholine before and after antigen challenge of allergic subjects out of allergy season and observed significant increases in methacholine-induced secretions at 2, 4, 6, 8, 10, and 24 hours after antigen challenge, compared to baseline.[109]

Although eosinophils in nasal secretions increased significantly after antigen challenge, no correlation was seen between their numbers and the increase in nonspecific hyperresponsiveness to methacholine. Klementsson and colleagues also showed that premedication with 2 different H_1 antihistamines (terfenadine and cetirizine) resulted in inhibition of both the acute allergic response and the allergen-induced increase in responsiveness to methacholine without affecting the eosinophil influx after antigen exposure.[110] This observation was confirmed by Baroody and colleagues for the H_1 antihistamines, terfenadine, and loratadine.[111]

In contrast, corticosteroids, given topically or orally, have dramatic inhibitory effects on cellular infiltration and both specific and nonspecific hyperresponsiveness.[105,106] An important consequence of nonspecific hyperactivity is the increase in symptoms upon exposure to irritants, such as gasoline odors, reported by patients during their allergy season.

Neural Reflexes

Neural reflexes are involved in the pathophysiology of allergic rhinitis. For example, sneezing and itching clearly involve the nervous system. Konno and Togawa and others demonstrated the importance of neural reflexes in patients with allergic rhinitis by showing that stimulating 1 nasal cavity with histamine led to bilateral nasal secretions.[112] Unilateral intranasal challenge with antigen in subjects with allergic rhinitis led to an increase in sneezes, rhinorrhea, nasal secretions, histamine, nasal airway resistance,[113] and PGD_2[114,115] on the side of the challenge. Contralateral to the challenge, rhinorrhea and secretion weights increased significantly, as did PGD_2.[115] The contralateral secretory response was rich in the glandular markers, lactoferrin and lysozyme,[114] and was inhibited by atropine, an anticholinergic, suggesting that the efferent limb was cholinergically mediated.[113] The muscarinic receptors that mediate the actions of acetylcholine in the human nasal mucosa are of both the M_1 and M_3 receptor subtypes and coexist at high densities in the submucosal glands.[116]

Immunohistochemical studies have established the presence of several neuropeptides in addition to sympathetic and parasympathetic nerves and their transmitters in the nasal mucosa. These neuropeptides are secreted by unmyelinated nociceptive C fibers (tachykinins, calcitonin gene-related peptide [CGRP], neurokinin A, and gastrin-releasing peptide), parasympathetic nerve endings (vasoactive intestinal peptide, peptide histidine methionine), and sympathetic nerve endings (neuropeptide Y). SP, a member of the tachykinin family, is often found as a cotransmitter with neurokinin A and CGRP and has been found in high density in arterial vessels and, to some extent, in veins, gland acini, and the epithelium of the nasal mucosa.[117] In addition to the identification of these neuropeptides in the nasal mucosa, Okamoto showed that incubation of nasal biopsy specimens of perennial rhinitic subjects and nonallergic rhinitic subjects with SP or mite allergen resulted in significant increases in mRNA for IL-1, IL-2, IL-3, IL-4, IL-5, IL-6, TNF-α, and interferon gamma (IFN-γ) in specimens from allergic subjects but not in those from nonallergic controls.[118] In nasal challenge studies in allergic subjects, Mosimann and colleagues showed that levels of SP, CGRP, and vasoactive intestinal peptide all increased significantly immediately after antigen challenge, with significant but modest increases in SP during the late response.[119] These experiments suggest that neuropeptides are released in vivo in man after allergen challenge and might be partly responsible for the symptoms of the allergic reaction. Repetitive application of capsaicin, the essence of chili peppers, depletes sensory nerves of their content of SP and CGRP and initiates both central and axonal reflexes. Unlike its effects in rodents, the capsaicin-induced nasal secretory response in man is primarily glandular and not due to increased vascular permeability.[120] In support of its proinflammatory effects, capsaicin nasal challenge caused significant increases in neutrophils, eosinophils, and mononuclear cells from the prechallenge baseline, with no difference between rhinitic and normal subjects.[121] Furthermore, capsaicin desensitization reduced nasal symptoms recorded for 24 hours after allergen challenge, and this reduction persisted for up to 2 months.[122]

Therefore, several experimental findings highlight the importance of neurogenic control of the allergic response. These include the presence of nasonasal reflexes after nasal antigen provocation, the presence of neuropeptides in nasal tissues and their recovery in nasal secretions after antigen challenge, the ability of these peptides to produce symptoms and inflammatory responses similar to those obtained after exposure to antigen, and the clinical efficacy of capsaicin, which depletes the stores of these substances.

Regulatory T Cells

In addition to Th cells, a further subtype of T cells with immunosuppressive function and cytokine profiles distinct from those of Th1 and Th2 cells has been identified[123] (Figure 4). These regulators of peripheral immunologic tolerance to allergens are called T regulatory (T_{reg}) cells. The identification of T_{reg} cells has opened an important era in the pathophysiology, prevention, and treatment of allergic disorders. The balance between the allergen-specific T_{reg} cells and Th2 cells appears to be involved in the development of allergic and healthy immune responses against allergens. Subsets of these cells include the naturally occurring $CD4^+$ $CD25^+FoxP3^+$ T_{reg} cells and the inducible *type 1* T_{reg} cells.[124] Evidence suggests that these *type 1* T_{reg} cells control the allergen-specific immune responses by: (1) suppressing antigen-presenting cells that support the generation of effector Th2 and Th1 cells, (2) suppressing Th2 and Th1 cells, (3) regulating B cells by suppression of allergen-specific IgE and induction of IgG4 or IgA or both, (4) suppressing mast cells, basophils, and eosinophils, and (5) interacting with resident cells and remodeling.[124]

Allergen-specific T_{reg} cell responses are shown to contribute to the control of allergic inflammation in several ways. Skewing of allergen-specific T cells to T_{reg} cells is probably a crucial event in the development of a healthy immune response. Future studies on T_{reg} cells and their suppressive cytokines are likely to have an enormous effect on the prevention and treatment of allergy.

Summary of Pathophysiology

One can summarize the pathophysiology of allergic rhinitis as follows: after sensitization of the nasal mucosa to an allergen, subsequent exposure to that same allergen leads to crosslinking of specific IgE receptors on mast cells and their resultant degranulation, with the release of a host of inflammatory mediators that are responsible for allergic nasal symptoms (Figure 3). Proinflammatory substances produced by other inflammatory cells are also generated after antigen exposure, most prominent among them eosinophil products and cytokines. Cytokines are thought to be generated, in part, by lymphocytes, which are found in abundance in both resting and stimulated nasal mucosa. Recent evidence also points to an important role for mast cells in the storage and probable production and secretion of cytokines. Cytokines can upregulate adhesion molecules on the vascular endothelium and possibly on marginating leukocytes, leading to the migration of these cells into tissues. Other cytokines also promote chemotaxis and survival of recruited inflammatory cells. Another important player is the nervous system, which amplifies the allergic reaction by both central and peripheral reflexes that result in changes at sites distant from those of antigen deposition. All of these changes lower the threshold of mucosal responsiveness and amplify it to a variety of specific and nonspecific stimuli, making allergic individuals more responsive than nonallergic individuals to stimuli to which they are exposed in daily life.

COMORBIDITIES OF ALLERGIC RHINITIS

Multiple lines of evidence support the observation that allergic rhinitis and sinusitis are closely associated disease entities; however, controlled studies of the incidence of rhinosinusitis in patients with allergic rhinitis have not been conducted. In a retrospective review of 200 chronic sinusitis patients who underwent endoscopic sinus surgery, Emanuel and Shah have shown that 84% of the patients tested positive for allergies, with a predominance of perennial allergens.[125] Friedman reported an incidence of atopy in 94% of patients undergoing sphenoethmoidectomies.[126] Holzmann and colleagues reported an increased prevalence of allergic rhinitis in children who had orbital complications of acute rhinosinusitis, and these complications occurred especially during pollinating seasons.[127] In a study involving 8,723 children, Chen and colleagues found the prevalence of sinusitis to be significantly higher in children with allergic rhinosinusitis than in children without allergies.[128] Comparison of otolaryngologic disqualifying events in naval flight personnel with and without allergic rhinitis revealed a significantly increased risk of having chronic sinusitis and the need for sinus surgery in the personnel with allergic rhinitis. The risk for the development of barotraumas and nasal polyps was also higher in this group.[129]

Complementing the above data that allergic rhinitis occurs frequently in patients with chronic sinusitis are data showing a high prevalence of sinus disease in patients with allergic rhinitis. Sinus radiographs are abnormal in more than 60% of adults who have perennial allergic rhinitis.[130] MRI scans demonstrate increased evidence of sinus mucosal abnormalities during major pollinating seasons.[131] A study of subjects with ragweed rhinitis during the pollen season showed that 60% of the subjects had sinus mucosal abnormalities on computed tomography (CT) imaging.[132] Subjects with allergic rhinitis were also shown to have more severe paranasal sinus changes in CT scans than did nonallergic subjects during viral colds.[133]

Multiple mechanisms are postulated to explain these relationships. In 1 study of subjects with seasonal allergic rhinitis outside their season, the nose was challenged with allergen, and nasal and ipsilateral maxillary-sinus responses were monitored by use of lavage.[134] There was a late increase in total cell count (the percentage of eosinophils and total eosinophils) within the sinus cavity in the allergen-challenged subjects but not in the control experiments. There were

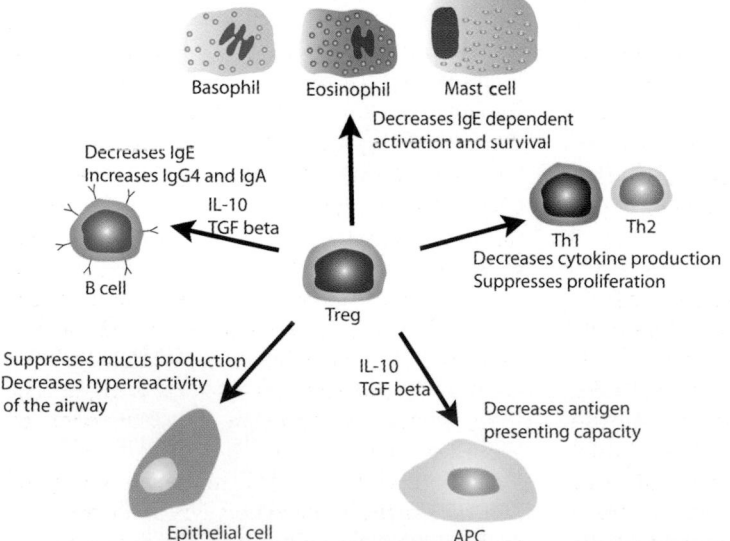

Figure 4 Mechanism of action of regulatory T cells (T_{reg}). (Borrowed in part from reference 124.)

significantly more total cells after allergen challenge than in controls, as well as a higher number of total eosinophils. This study highlights that important relationships exist between the nose and sinus in the response to allergen, possibly through axonal or central neural reflexes.

There are important relationships between the nose and other organs. A relationship between pulmonary disease such as asthma and allergic rhinitis has long been observed. Allergic rhinitis is present in up to 75% of patients with asthma; and, in a longitudinal follow-up study, patients with allergic rhinitis were 3 times more likely to develop asthma than were subjects without allergic rhinitis.[135] A beneficial influence of treatment with intranasal corticosteroids on bronchial hyperresponsiveness in patients with seasonal allergic rhinitis has been observed,[136] although other studies have failed to confirm this finding.[137] Treatment with orally inhaled corticosteroids not only prevented development of increased bronchial hyperresponsiveness to methacholine but also reduced nasal symptoms, eosinophils from nasal brushings, markers of eosinophil activation in nasal lavage fluid, and peripheral-blood eosinophilia.[138] A study by Braunstahl and colleagues demonstrated that segmental provocation with allergen in the lungs produced allergic inflammation in the nose in atopic patients.[139] In a study on the ability of the nose to condition cold, dry air, asthmatics had a reduced ability to warm and humidify cold, dry air as compared to normal subjects; subjects with seasonal allergic rhinitis also had a reduced ability to condition air, with possible adverse implications for the lower airways.[140] In a follow-up study, treatment of nasal inflammation with intranasal corticosteroids further decreased the ability of subjects with asthma to condition the inspired air,[141] suggesting that allergic inflammation has a beneficial effect on nasal air conditioning. This was supported by other studies which showed an increase in nasal conditioning by either seasonal exposure or allergen challenge.[142]

Studies on the effect of nasal challenge on bronchi in adults and children with allergic rhinitis have shown correlations between allergen induced nasal changes and bronchial hyperreactivity.[143,144] Cochrane analysis of the use of intranasal corticosteroids on asthma control showed that it tends to improve asthma symptoms and forced expiratory volume in 1 second; however, these results did not reach statistical significance.[145] Pathophysiologic connections between the nose and lungs are still not entirely understood and remain an active area of investigation. The above data, however, support the presence of important physiologic and pathophysiologic connections between contiguous areas of the respiratory tract.

Nasal inflammation with an allergic or infectious cause may be a factor involved in the development of otitis media and eustachian tube dysfunction.[146] Studies of the pathogenesis of otitis media have identified interactions among infection, allergic reactions, and eustachian tube dysfunction. Nguyen and colleagues demonstrated

that middle-ear fluid of atopic patients who had otitis media with effusion contained more eosinophils and IL-4 and IL-5 mRNA-positive cells than those in nonatopic patients with otitis media with effusion.[147] In the presence of allergic rhinitis, treatment may improve symptom resolution and therapeutic response. The inflammation found in allergic rhinitis is thought to promote eustachian tube dysfunction and supports the development of otitis through mediators and cytokines.

Studies on adults and adolescents with allergic rhinitis have shown disrupted sleep, difficulty concentrating, daytime fatigue, and a related significant decrease in quality of life parameters.[3,148] Ocular symptoms are observed in a large percentage of patients with seasonal allergies.[149]

ALLERGENS

Allergens are foreign substances capable of provoking an IgE-mediated response. Most allergens are between 5 and 20 μm in diameter, a size that permits their complete removal by the nose. They are proteins with molecular weights between 10 and 40 kDa. No distinguishing surface characteristics appear to differentiate allergens from non-antigenic substances.

According to the third National Health and Nutrition Examination Survey, the prevalences of positive skin test responses in the US population were as follows: 54.3% of the population had positive test responses to one or more allergens. Prevalences were 27.5% for dust mite, 26.9% for perennial rye, 26.2% for short ragweed, 26.1% for German cockroach, 18.1% for Bermuda grass, 17.0% for cat, 15.2% for Russian thistle, 13.2% for white oak, 12.9% for Alternaria alternata, and 8.6% for peanut.[10]

We often categorize allergens into indoor and outdoor types. In general, outdoor allergens are responsible for seasonal allergic rhinitis, whereas indoor allergens usually cause perennial rhinitis. Pollens causing allergy in temperate climates are released into the air from plants, trees, weeds, and grasses and are carried over great distances. Thus, cutting down trees around a suburban home in an effort to reduce the amount of pollen has little effect. Trees clearly have geographic variations; for example, Western red cedar is limited to the Northwest. Grasses are diverse and include timothy grass, often used for feeding horses, Kentucky bluegrass, widely used in lawn grass mixtures, orchard grass, rye grass, and English plantain. Common short ragweed is found throughout North America, with the exception of Newfoundland, and is just beginning to slow in the European continent.

Pollination, and hence the allergy season, occurs in a predictable annual pattern for different regions of the country. The pattern, however, varies throughout the country. In the Northeast, trees pollinate in mid-March to late April, grasses follow in May and June, and ragweed flowers from mid-August until the first frost. In the South, tree blooming begins in early February. In contrast to the sharply demarcated grass season that occurs

in the north, in the south, grasses may pollinate from March through September, and in some areas, pollination may be a year-round process. The pattern in the central United States resembles the patterns seen on the east coast. In the California lowlands, grass pollen is present from early March through November, and trees and short ragweed are present as in other regions. In the Northwest coastal region, trees and grass pollen are present, but the region is ragweed-free. In the traditionally arid Southwest, previously a haven for allergy sufferers, increased urbanization and irrigation have contributed to increasing the pollen load because humans tends to bring their allergens with them.

Global climate changes, driven by the increased concentrations of gases such as carbon dioxide, have been shown to stimulate opportunistic weeds and trees including ragweed, maples, birches, and poplars to produce more pollens. The increase in temperature also encourages growth of molds and fungi, which may result in important allergen loads for individuals who have asthma and allergic rhinitis.[150] Recent studies have shown that pollen grains, apart from their function as allergen carriers, are also a rich source of lipid mediators, which may contribute to the generation of local inflammation.[151]

The most frequent perennial allergens are animal danders, dust mites, cockroaches, and molds. Dust mites are microscopic, eight-legged organisms of the genus *Dermatophagoides*, including *D. pteronyssinus*, *D. farinae*, and *Euroglyphus maynei*. They are the major allergens in "house dust." Dust mites are found throughout the world, with the exception of regions with extremely dry climates such as northern Sweden, central Canada, and areas at elevations above 10,000 feet. These mites feed on human epithelial scales and thrive in warm, humid environments (60 to 70% relative humidity, temperature 65 to 80°F). Bedding provides an ideal environment for proliferation of dust mites. Other sites for mite accumulation are upholstered furniture, carpets, and stuffed toys. Dust mite feces, the source of the allergen, are relatively large particles that remain airborne for short periods, unlike outdoor pollen. When an individual sits on a bed, the particles become airborne and are inhaled. Because these particles are large, they settle from the air rapidly, and air filtration systems cannot effectively remove them. Lowering the indoor relative humidity to less than 50% during the summer months had a profound effect on the mite population and the antigen load throughout the year, suggesting a role for dehumidifiers even in homes with central air conditioning.[152] Although use of dust mite control measures such as impermeable covers has become an internationally accepted method for environmental control, a meta-analysis of recently published studies revealed no significant effect of these measures on symptom scores of allergic patients.[153]

Animal danders are an important source of indoor allergens. Cat and dog dander are the most frequent, but mice, guinea pigs, and horses can all be responsible for allergic symptoms. Laboratory workers can become allergic to animals at work. In most cases, the allergen is found in secretions. In cats, *Fel d I* is the principal allergen secreted in saliva. It dries on fur and is spread to furniture, bedding, and carpets. When these reservoirs are disturbed, the allergen becomes airborne and can provoke symptoms. Cat dander is "sticky," and children with cats can carry enough of it to school to cause symptoms in cat-allergic children who have no cats in their homes.[154]

Cockroaches are an important source of allergen in inner-city populations. Both the American (*Periplaneta americana*) and German cockroach (*Blatella germanica*) have been identified as important allergens in asthma. Allergenicity occurs to body parts and to feces. Molds, although less well-studied, are sources of allergens, particularly in warm, humid environments. They tend to be found inside older homes in areas of decreased ventilation or increased dampness. Although a phenomenal variety of molds exists, alternaria and cladosporium are principally responsible for symptoms due to outdoor exposure, and aspergillus and penicillium are most prevalent indoors.

The patient's work environment may be a source of allergens. Symptoms occurring only at work and subsiding on days off may reflect an occupational disorder. At risk are flour handlers, workers in paint and plastic industries, woodworkers, fish and shellfish processors, and animal handlers. Unfortunately, few specific tests exist for the diagnosis of these disorders.

Allergic reactions to natural-rubber latex have increased, especially in health-care workers who have high exposure by direct skin contact and inhalation of latex particles from powdered gloves. Latex allergy is observed in about 4% of health-care workers and is significantly associated with asthma and allergic rhinitis.[155] Eliminating powdered natural rubber latex from the work place and using latex-free material resulted in a decrease in markers of sensitization and symptoms in health-care workers.[156]

CLASSIFICATION OF ALLERGIC RHINITIS

Allergic rhinitis has always been subdivided, based on the time of occurrence during the year, into seasonal and perennial disease. Seasonal allergy is related to outdoor allergens such as pollens or molds. Perennial allergic rhinitis is related to indoor allergens such as dust mites, molds, cockroaches, and animal danders. This subdivision is not entirely satisfactory for the following reasons: (1) seasonal allergens in one region can occur throughout the year and cause perennial symptoms, and (2) patients with perennial allergies could present symptoms only during a short time of the year.

For these reasons, the allergic rhinitis and its impact on asthma workshop has changed the definition of the chronology of allergic rhinitis and subdivided the disease into "intermittent" and "persistent" categories. This classification has been validated.[157] The new classification of allergic rhinitis is shown in Table 1. It is designed as a system to initiate treatment guidelines, whereas "seasonal" and "perennial" is a system for identifying the allergens. Recently, a modification of this method of assessment was suggested. The questions used for assessing the severity of allergic rhinitis have been decreased to 2, 1 of them addressing sleep disturbance and the other, impairment of daily personal and/or professional life. If the answer to both questions is "no," the disease would be classified as mild, if the answer to 1 of the questions is "yes," as moderate, and if the answer is "yes" to both questions, the disease would be classified as severe.[158] This proposed modification has not yet been validated.

CLINICAL PRESENTATION

History

Antigen exposure causes itching within seconds, which is soon followed by sneezing. Rhinorrhea ensues, and within about 15 minutes nasal congestion peaks. Besides nasal symptoms, patients often complain about ocular pruritus, tearing, pharyngeal itching, throat clearing, cough, and ear popping. Other commonly reported symptoms include postnasal drip, increased lacrimation, dry cough, red eyes, headaches (pressure) over the paranasal sinus areas, and loss of smell or taste. These symptoms are nonspecific and have significant clinical overlap with other disorders. Itching of mucous membranes and repetitive sneezing, however, are the symptoms most suggestive of allergic disease. The relative importance of each symptom may vary among individuals, but nasal congestion tends to be the most bothersome. Each symptom is usually present, at least to some degree.

When obtaining the history, the physician should attempt to link exposure to allergens temporally with the occurrence of symptoms. This temporal correlation is the hallmark of allergic rhinitis. Patients with seasonal allergies complain of recurrent symptoms only at specific times of each year that coincide with pollination periods. In contrast, a history of year-around symptoms may indicate sensitivity to a perennial allergen or to multiple seasonal allergens. Symptoms immediately following exposure to a potential source of allergen, such as a cat, strongly suggest an allergy to that source. Exposures to perennial allergens tend to be accentuated in winter in colder climates, where ventilation is reduced. Symptoms occurring only at work or during the workweek and subsiding on weekends may reflect an occupation-related disorder. The presence of domestic pets (including birds) and whether these sleep in the patient's bedroom must be determined.

Additional considerations in history-taking include the response to prior therapy and evidence of complications. For example, nasal obstruction may lead to mouth breathing. In children, this may be manifested as adenoid facies with a high palatal arch, and abnormal dental development. In adults, nasal obstruction may contribute to snoring and sleep-disordered breathing. Sinusitis may be present and contributing to symptoms. A contribution of allergic rhinitis to middle ear disease has also been shown.

Obtaining a general medical history remains important. The medical history may document systemic disorders that affect the nose, such as hypothyroidism. Pregnancy can produce nasal congestion and may require modification of treatment strategies. The presence of pulmonary disease such as asthma should be sought. Indeed, a significant percentage of patients with allergic rhinitis have asthma. Between 5 and 10% of asthmatic subjects may have intolerance to aspirin and nonsteroidal anti-inflammatory drugs. The frequency of aspirin tolerance in patients with nasal polyposis is about 23%.[159] A family history of allergic rhinitis increases the chances of the patient having an allergic disorder. Nasal symptoms might also be due to intake of medications such as ß blockers, which may contribute to nasal congestion through interference with the adrenergic mechanism. Tricyclic antidepressants may produce dryness of the nasal mucosa by virtue of their anticholinergic effects. Angiotensin-converting enzyme inhibitors can produce a chronic cough. Birth control pills can cause nasal congestion, and topical eye drops can induce nasal symptoms. Overuse of topical decongestants may result in rhinitis medicamentosa.

Examination

Attentive history-taking and physical examination, combined with appropriate diagnostic tests, are required for establishing the correct diagnosis, because allergic rhinitis shares features of other nasal disease entities. The classical description of allergic facies includes mouth breathing, allergic "shiners" (resulting from periorbital venous stasis from chronic nasal obstruction), and a transverse supratip nasal crease from long-term rubbing of the nose upward to relieve itching. These classic

Table 1 Classification of Allergic Rhinitis[2]

"Intermittent" means that the symptoms are present:
  Less than 4 d a week
  Or for less than 4 wk
"Persistent" means that the symptoms are present:
  More than 4 d a week
  And for more than 4 wk
"Mild" means that none of the following items are present:
  Sleep disturbance
  Impairment of daily activities, leisure and/or sport
  Sleep disturbance
  Impairment of daily activities, leisure and/or sport
  Impairment of school or work
  Troublesome symptoms
"Moderate–severe" means that 1 or more of the following items are present:
  Sleep disturbance
  Impairment of daily activities, leisure and/or sport
  Impairment of school or work
  Troublesome symptoms

presentations occur especially often in children, but absence of these signs does not exclude the disease.

Physical examination must be complete. Ocular examination may demonstrate injection of the conjunctiva or swelling of the eyelids. Examination of the nose begins with observing the external appearance for gross deformities such as a deviation suggesting previous trauma, or expansion of the nasal bridge suggestive of nasal polyps. A nasal speculum permits evaluation of the anterior third of the internal nasal architecture and the character of the nasal mucosa. Structural anomalies providing an anatomic basis for obstruction or recurrent infections such as septal deviations or spurs should be sought. The character and consistency of nasal secretions should be noted. These can vary from thin and clear to thick and whitish. The nasal mucosa may be swollen and pale-bluish, although these signs are not pathognomonic of the disease as previously thought. The results of examination of allergic individuals often appear normal, and the primary importance of the physical examination is to rule out other causes of or contributors to the symptoms.

Decongestion of a swollen nasal mucosa with a topical decongestant improves visualization and allows the differentiation of reversible from irreversible changes. Combining the vasoconstrictor with a topical anesthetic allows complete examination with an endoscope. The choanae and the nasopharynx can be visualized in this manner. The region of the middle meatus should also be examined carefully because secretions there might be suggestive of acute or chronic sinusitis. Nasal polyps that were not visualized by anterior rhinoscopy may be seen during a careful endoscopic examination. Nasal polyps are infrequent in allergic rhinitis (<2%),[50] but are found in up to 20% of patients with cystic fibrosis. The presence of nasal polyps in children suggests a diagnosis of cystic fibrosis. Children with polyps should undergo sweat or genetic testing for cystic fibrosis.

DIAGNOSIS

The identification of allergen(s) responsible for the patient's symptoms is important both for establishing the diagnosis and for the institution of avoidance measures. Symptoms occurring in temporal relation to allergen exposure suggest sensitization but are not diagnostic. Sensitization implies the presence of elevated levels of IgE directed against a specific allergen and can be demonstrated by a wheal and flare response to skin testing with allergen extracts or by measurement of the level of antigen-specific IgE antibodies in the serum. However, individuals can show evidence of sensitization by a positive skin test or elevated specific antibody levels in the serum without having evidence of clinical disease. This emphasizes the importance of obtaining a good history in the evaluation of patients with suspected allergic disorders. In patients with a positive history, the magnitude of skin responses often corresponds to the severity of symptoms.

Skin Testing

Skin testing furnishes an excellent in vivo method for demonstrating sensitivity to a given allergen. This test evaluates the presence of specific IgE antibodies on skin mast cells, the reactivity of these cells, and the reaction of the end organ to released mediators. Its advantages include great sensitivity, the rapidity with which results can be obtained, and low cost. Like all diagnostic tests, skin testing also has disadvantages, which include the inability to perform the test in patients with dermatologic problems such as dermatographism and extensive eczema, poor tolerance of many children for multiple needle pricks, the inhibitory effect of certain ingested drugs such as antihistamines on skin test reactivity, the need to maintain the potency of the allergen extracts, and the possibility of systemic reactions.

Skin testing often begins with puncture testing, which provides a low-dose allergen exposure. A small drop of concentrated allergen is placed on the skin (usually on the volar surface of the forearm or on the back), and a minute quantity is introduced into the dermis with a sharp object. Skin puncture tests with various devices have been introduced that decrease the variability in the tests.[160] Positive responses occur within 10 to 15 minutes and produce a characteristic raised central area of induration (wheal), with a surrounding zone of erythema (flare). The response is graded in comparison with a positive histamine or codeine response, and a negative control with the diluent for the allergen extracts is included as control for nonspecific reactivity to the vehicle. The positive control ensures that the patient can mount a cutaneous reaction to histamine, and the absence of a reaction can unmask interference by medications, decreased skin reactivity, or technical problems with the procedure. Skin testing is valid in infants and young children, but here the criteria for a positive reaction need to be adjusted because the reactions are smaller.[161] Measurement of serum-specific IgE levels is also valid in this younger age group.[162] It is important, however, to test with only relevant antigens. Infants are more likely than adults to be allergic to foods, and children are more likely to be allergic to perennial rather than to seasonal allergens.

Negative puncture tests are usually confirmed by intradermal tests, which are more sensitive. In an intradermal test, a small (0.01 to 0.05 mL) quantity of dilute allergen is injected into the superficial dermis, and the same wheal and flare responses are observed and graded in comparison with a positive histamine or codeine control. Because antihistamines can interfere with the results of skin testing, most H_1 receptor antagonists are withheld for 2 days before the test. Tricyclic antidepressants suppress responses for several weeks, as can tranquilizers and antiemetics of the phenothiazine class through intrinsic anti-H_1 activity. Short-term oral corticosteroid and antileukotriene treatment has no effect on skin test reactivity. Testing with extracts that are standardized (ragweed, grass pollens) is more reliable than testing for nonstandardized antigens such as foods and molds.

In Vitro IgE Measurements

Drawing blood for the measurement of specific IgE can circumvent some of the disadvantages of skin testing. False-positive results may occur if patients have elevated IgE levels in their sera because of nonspecific binding. False-negative results may also occur from inhibition by IgG antibodies with affinities similar to those in patients receiving immunotherapy. Data from clinical studies comparing results of skin testing and in vitro tests for specific IgE determination in allergic subjects suggest a good correlation between the 2, with a higher sensitivity for skin testing.[163] Therefore, both determinations of specific IgE levels and skin testing are useful in the diagnosis of allergic disorders, but their results should always be interpreted in the context of clinical symptoms. Disadvantages in vitro testing include cost, slightly lower sensitivity, and the time delay between drawing blood and obtaining the results.

Other Diagnostic Tests

Peripheral eosinophilia, although nonspecific, may indicate the presence of atopic diseases. Nasal cytologic examination allows the identification of eosinophils and other inflammatory cells in nasal secretions and may be helpful in differentiating an infectious from an allergic cause during a clinical exacerbation of symptoms. In normal individuals, smears show the presence of epithelial cells, including some ciliated and goblet cells, with few eosinophils, neutrophils, basophils, or bacteria. In subjects with an infection, neutrophils increase in nasal secretions, and in symptomatic allergic subjects, the percentage of eosinophils increases. A value greater than 10% for eosinophils is suggestive of allergic disease[164]; however, they may also be present in the absence of IgE-mediated disease. Approximately 25% of patients with chronic rhinitis and negative skin tests demonstrate eosinophilia on nasal cytologic study, and this entity is known as the nonallergic rhinitis with eosinophilia syndrome.[165]

Soft-tissue radiography of the neck can be used for evaluating adenoid size, a major consideration in the differential diagnosis of rhinitis in children, especially when the predominant symptom is nasal obstruction. Sinus disease often complicates perennial allergic rhinitis and may need to be considered in the differential diagnosis. CT is now standard for evaluation of the presence and extent of sinus abnormalities. The common association of upper and lower airway disease makes tests of pulmonary function a useful adjuvant. This statement applies to such diverse disorders as cystic fibrosis, asthma, and bronchopulmonary aspergillosis.

THERAPY

Environmental Modifications

The increase in the prevalence of asthma and allergic diseases highlights the need for developing effective preventive strategies. The large number of potential environmental risk factors and the inability accurately to predict the development of asthma and allergy resulted in conflicting data from recent prevention studies. Environmental modifications consist of removal of specific antigen and the removal of irritants. The most important example of the latter is tobacco smoke. Avoidance of exposure to environmental tobacco smoke can be recommended safely for the whole population, not only for prevention of allergy but also for other known benefits. Although perfectly logical, the advantage of other avoidance measurements in the presence of good pharmacotherapy has been questioned.[166]

The most potent treatments cannot eliminate symptoms in the face of an overwhelming allergen load. Complete avoidance of the allergen(s) to which the patient is sensitive eliminates symptoms of the disease. Thus, measures aimed at reducing the allergen load from the patient's environment are effective in reducing symptoms. Although many methods of environmental control (removal of a pet, restriction of activities, home renovations) are difficult to execute, particularly with children, simple measures can be very effective. In seasonal allergic rhinitis, patients can reduce exposure by keeping windows closed on days when pollen counts are high and limiting physical activity outdoors in the early morning and evening when pollen counts are at their peak. Air conditioning can help, and the addition of special filters can prevent pollen grains and mold spores from entering the home. Pollen counts are often given during daily weather reports, and the previous day's pollen counts are the best predictor of the next day's counts. Rain, however, profoundly reduces the levels of outdoor pollens.

Measures to reduce exposure to dust mites concentrate on bedding. These include replacing feather pillows and bedspreads with synthetic ones that can be washed in hot water (hotter than 130°F) and covering mattresses with commercially available impermeable covers (pores <10 μm). A study showed that washing clothing with detergent plus bleach removes a significant portion of mites, and repeated washing is suggested to reduce the mites further.[167] Removing carpets and frequent vacuuming with a vacuum cleaner designed to trap allergen particles also help. Where carpets cannot be removed, acaricidal products can directly kill mites. Stuffed toys can be placed in the freezer for 2 days for reducing the number of dust mites. Mite-proof covers significantly reduce the level of exposure to mite allergens. Despite a decrease in mite exposure, intervention studies failed to show a clinical benefit of this single avoidance measure.[168]

In subjects with allergies to animal dander, removal of a domestic pet is the best step. Reduc-tion in the allergen load after pet removal may take up to 6 months, however, and thus symptoms may persist. Furthermore, complete removal of a pet may be difficult, but eliminating the animal from the bedroom, where we spend an average of 8 hours per day, is considered a helpful alternative. In the case of cats, regular washing of the animal may decrease the allergen load; however, this decrease is short-lived, and it is unlikely that one will obtain a meaningful symptomatic improvement with this measure.[169] Studies show that cat allergens are ubiquitous in the environment, including schools. This "secondhand" exposure to cats in the school environment increases the risk of cat sensitization in school children who have no regular contact with cats and can trigger symptoms in cat-sensitive subjects. It is most likely that cat dander is carried into classrooms on the clothes of a cat owner.[170]

Humidifiers must be cleaned regularly so that they do not become a source of mold allergens, which thrive in moist environments. The humidity should not exceed 40 to 45% because higher levels encourage the growth of dust mites and molds. The use of high-efficiency particulate air filters and of electrostatic filters effectively removes particulates larger than 1 μm in diameter. Particles, however, must be airborne for removal, for example pollens, whereas heavy particles that settle from the air rapidly, such as dust mites, are not eliminated by these measures.[171] High-efficiency particulate air filters are preferred to electrostatic ones, as they filter out particulate matter without generating ozone, an irritant.

General household changes may also be helpful. Repair of any plumbing or drainage problem areas in the house must be undertaken for eliminating mold. Decontamination of surfaces contaminated with mold by use of diluted bleach and elimination of soiled organic materials are useful. Appropriate packaging of garbage, as well as pesticide application, are necessary for eliminating cockroaches. Use of well-fitting, semirigid masks when vacuuming or using vacuum cleaners designed to trap allergens offers useful protection from airborne allergens such as dust mites.

Pharmacologic Therapy

Management of allergic rhinitis should encompass educating the patient to increase adherence to the treatment plan. Pharmacologic management should take into account efficacy, safety, the severity of the disease, patient's preference, and cost effectiveness.[172] Interestingly, increasing the co-pay by $10 of antihistamines decreases the number of refills, suggesting financial considerations are important to patients. This type of change in drug benefits has resulted in the decreased use of antihistamines. This reduction may cause short- or long-term clinical consequences in patients with allergic rhinitis.[173]

Antihistamines. Four receptors exist for histamine. H_1 receptors are found on blood vessels, on sensory nerves, on smooth muscles of the respiratory and digestive tracts, and in the central ner-vous system. Stimulation of these receptors leads to vasodilatation, increased vascular permeability, sneezing, pruritus, glandular secretion, and increased intestinal motility. H_2 receptors have a distribution similar to that of H_1 receptors but are principally involved in the regulation of gastric acid secretion. H_3 receptors are located primarily in the brain and seem to be involved in the regulation of histamine synthesis and release. H_4 receptors are expressed in various cells of the immune system, including mast cells, T lymphocytes, dendritic cells, and basophils. It has been suggested that H_4 receptors are involved in inducing chemotaxis of eosinophils and mast cells and in the control of IL-16 release from lymphocytes.[174] The contribution of histamine to the early allergic response, largely mediated by the H_1 receptor, has long been recognized and is the rationale for the large number of H_1 antagonists in clinical use.

H_1 antihistamines have been classified as first-generation, or sedating, and second-generation, or nonsedating, antihistamines. The first-generation antihistamines are effective in the relief of symptoms of allergic rhinitis. Some studies showed a better improvement in symptoms with diphenhydramine compared to the second-generation antihistamine desloratadine.[175,176] However, first-generation antihistamines have some undesirable side effects because of their lack of selectivity and the resulting nonspecific stimulation of other receptors. Among these side effects are sedation, anticholinergic effects, functional and performance impairment, and gastrointestinal distress. When applied topically, some act as local anesthetics. The most important of the side effects is sedation. In 1 study, diphenhydramine caused worse impairment to driving than does consuming alcohol to the level of being legally drunk.[177] In this study, the performance after a second-generation agent was similar to that after a placebo. Meta-analysis of other performance impairment trials failed to show a clear and consistent distinction between the sedating antihistamine diphenhydramine and nonsedating antihistamines including acrivastine, astemizole, cetirizine, fexofenadine, loratadine, and terfenadine.[178] Although the results of the analyzed studies varied in sample size, most of them tended toward more cognitive dysfunction with diphenhydramine than with placebo and second-generation antihistamines.[175,178]

Second-generation antihistamines are less lipophilic than first-generation H_1 antihistamines and do not penetrate the blood–brain barrier. Therefore, they produce no more somnolence than does placebo. Their greater receptor selectivity also reduces the incidence of anticholinergic side effects. In addition to antagonizing histamine at the H_1 receptor, some antihistamines, such as azatadine, of the piperidine class, and terfenadine, a non-sedating antihistamine, inhibit histamine release after intranasal antigen challenge.[179,180] Treatment with some antihistamines also reduces the production of leukotrienes and kinins, which are mediators with proinflammatory effects, as well as the allergen-induced increased responsiveness to methacholine.[181] Similarly, the topical antihistamine antagonist azelastine has shown a significant inhibitory effect on the methacholine response, whereas it failed to affect the early-and late-phase mediators.[182] Other described effects of antihistamines are reduction of soluble ICAM-1 levels in nasal secretions (loratadine and cetirizine),[183] modulation of the cytokine pattern by reducing IL-4 and IL-8 levels (levocetirizine),[184] and reduction of nasal neurogenic inflammation by modulating the release of SP (cetirizine).[185]

Oral antihistamines are readily absorbed. Their onset of action is rapid, usually within 60 minutes, and the maximum benefit occurs within hours. Metabolism of most antihistamines occurs primarily through the hepatic cytochrome P-450 system. Drugs that interfere with this system, such as antifungal agents, can lead to the accumulation of antihistamines to toxic levels. One exception is cetirizine, which is primarily excreted in the urine and does not depend on the cytochrome P-450 system. The clinical effectiveness of antihistamines exceeds the duration of measurable serum levels, perhaps due to the presence of active metabolites. Another explanation for the prolonged efficacy of H_1 receptor antagonists beyond their measurable serum levels relates to extended tissue levels. P-glycoprotein (a multidrug resistance 1 [MDR1] gene product) is a drug transporter that has been shown to contribute to the disposition of some drugs, including fexofenadine. Polymorphisms of the MDR1 gene have been reported to be associated with alterations in the disposition kinetics of fexofenadine.[186] Further studies on genetic variations of P-glycoprotein will be important for explaining the factors affecting the peripheral response to antihistamine.

In the United States, the following second-generation antihistamines are in clinical use: azelastine, cetirizine, fexofenadine, loratadine, and desloratadine. Levocetirizine has been approved for use in allergic rhinitis in Europe. This drug has been shown to have a duration of action exceeding 24 hours in adults.[187] Loratadine, one of the major second-generation antihistamines, has taken on a non-prescription status in the United States.

Azelastine, a phthalazinone derivative, is an intranasal preparation with efficacy comparable to that of other antihistamines.[182] It can be effective within 20 minutes of administration. Although it does not cause somnolence, a sensation of altered taste immediately after use is observed in 10% of patients.[188] Another H_1 antihistamine under development in a nasal spray formulation is olopatadine hydrochloride. It has been shown to elicit significant improvements in allergic rhinitis symptoms compared to placebo.[189]

Cardiac arrhythmias, fatal ventricular tachycardia, or prolongation of the QT interval associated with concomitant administration of agents that interfere with the cytochrome P-450 system have been reported with two older second-generation antihistamines, terfenadine and astemizole. These agents are no longer available in the United States. Fexofenadine, a metabolite of terfenadine, does not possess these cardiac risks. Second-generation agents have been shown to be effective. Cetirizine, fexofenadine, and desloratadine have been demonstrated to improve quality of life, as measured by generic and disease-specific tools.[190-192] They cause little or no somnolence, do not affect performance, and have no anticholinergic effects. Azelastine and fexofenadine are approved for children older than 5 and 6 years, respectively. Loratadine and cetirizine are approved for children older than 2 years, and desloratadine is approved for children older than 6 months.

All antihistamines are effective in the treatment of allergic rhinitis and differ principally in their side effects, duration of action, and cost. In equipotent doses, they are equally effective in suppressing histamine-induced skin wheals. H_1 receptor antagonists are most effective in treating sneezing, nasal and ocular pruritus, and rhinorrhea associated with allergic rhinitis but have little or no effect on nasal congestion. Thus, they are often combined with an oral decongestant. Some clinicians have tried to circumvent the sedation caused by first-generation antihistamines by directing that they be taken before bedtime, when somnolence is not a problem. The next day, prolonged tissue levels provide continued efficacy without the undesirable side effect of drowsiness.[193] Some studies, however, suggest that performance is impaired despite the lack of drowsiness. It is therefore important to warn patients receiving these drugs about their effect on daily activities, such as driving or operating heavy machinery. Patients who lack medical insurance or formulary coverage often use first-generation agents despite their significant side effects. This poses considerable public-health concerns, given recent studies demonstrating the marked performance impairment associated with their use.

Decongestants. Decongestants exert their effect through stimulation of α_1 or α_2 adrenergic receptors. These receptors are present on resistance vessels, where they control blood flow, and on capacitance vessels, where they control blood volume. In capacitance vessels, α_2 outnumber α_1 receptors. In resting conditions, sympathetic nervous activity regulates nasal patency by maintaining the sinusoids contracted to approximately half their maximal capacity. The resting state is affected by the nasal cycle, a periodic, reciprocal alteration of nasal-cavity congestion and decongestion that affects about 80% of normal individuals. Increased sympathetic stimulation, such as occurs during exercise, reduces nasal congestion.

Oral decongestants exert their effects directly and by stimulating release of norepinephrine. The 2 major decongestants are pseudoephedrine and phenylephrine, which can be prescribed separately or in combination with antihistamines. Oral medications including pseudoephedrine are now placed behind the counter because of their illegal use in the manufacture of methamphetamine.

Use of phenylpropanolamine in diet medication has been associated with rare hemorrhagic stroke and has been withdrawn from the US marketplace. Because oral decongestants also stimulate adrenergic receptors other than those in the nasal vasculature, overdosage has been associated with hypertensive crisis. When given in prescribed doses, however, they do not induce hypertension in normotensive patients, nor do they alter the pharmacologic control of blood pressure in stable hypertensive patients. Current recommendations suggest that decongestants should not be used in patients with uncontrolled hypertension, in those with severe coronary artery disease, or in patients receiving monoamine oxidase inhibitors. Decongestants should be prescribed with caution in patients with diabetes, hyperthyroidism, closed-angle glaucoma, coronary artery disease, cardiac insufficiency, prostatic hypertrophy, or urinary retention. Their major side effect is insomnia, which occurs in approximately 25% of patients.

Topical decongestants are effective in reducing nasal congestion, regardless of the cause. These include catecholamines (such as phenylephrine) and imidazoline derivatives (such as xylometazoline or oxymetazoline). Prolonged use can bring about rhinitis medicamentosa, which is characterized by a reduced duration of action and rebound nasal congestion after cessation of therapy. Because this phenomenon can appear even after a short period, use of these agents should be limited to a few days. These agents are reserved for patients in whom nasal congestion is so severe that it precludes the use of other topical preparations such as intranasal corticosteroids or restful sleep during acute exacerbations of disease. Seizures have occurred in children given these medications intranasally.

Topical Intranasal Corticosteroids. Topical intranasal glucocorticosteroids are potent medications for the treatment of allergic rhinitis. These agents profoundly reduce multiple aspects of the inflammatory response to allergen. Corticosteroids pass into the interior of the cell, where they are bound by a glucocorticoid receptor in the cytoplasm. The glucocorticoid receptor inhibits inflammation by genomic or nongenomic mechanisms (Figure 5). A genomic mechanism occurs within the nucleus and involves direct (induction of annexin I and mitogen-activated protein kinases) or indirect effects (nuclear factor-KB) on gene expression. The nongenomic pathway involves rapid effects on inflammation by second-messenger cascades (endothelial nitric oxide synthetase and phosphatidylinositol-3-hydroxykinase) which do not require changes in gene expression.[194] Many of the anti-inflammatory effects of glucocorticoids occur by suppression of a host of proinflammatory proteins with potential anti-inflammatory activity (such as annexin-1, IL-10, mitogen protein kinase) and proteins with potential proinflammatory activity (such as chemokine receptors, complements, IL-1 and IL-8 receptors, IFN-γ receptors, TNF, and TLR 2 and 4).[195]

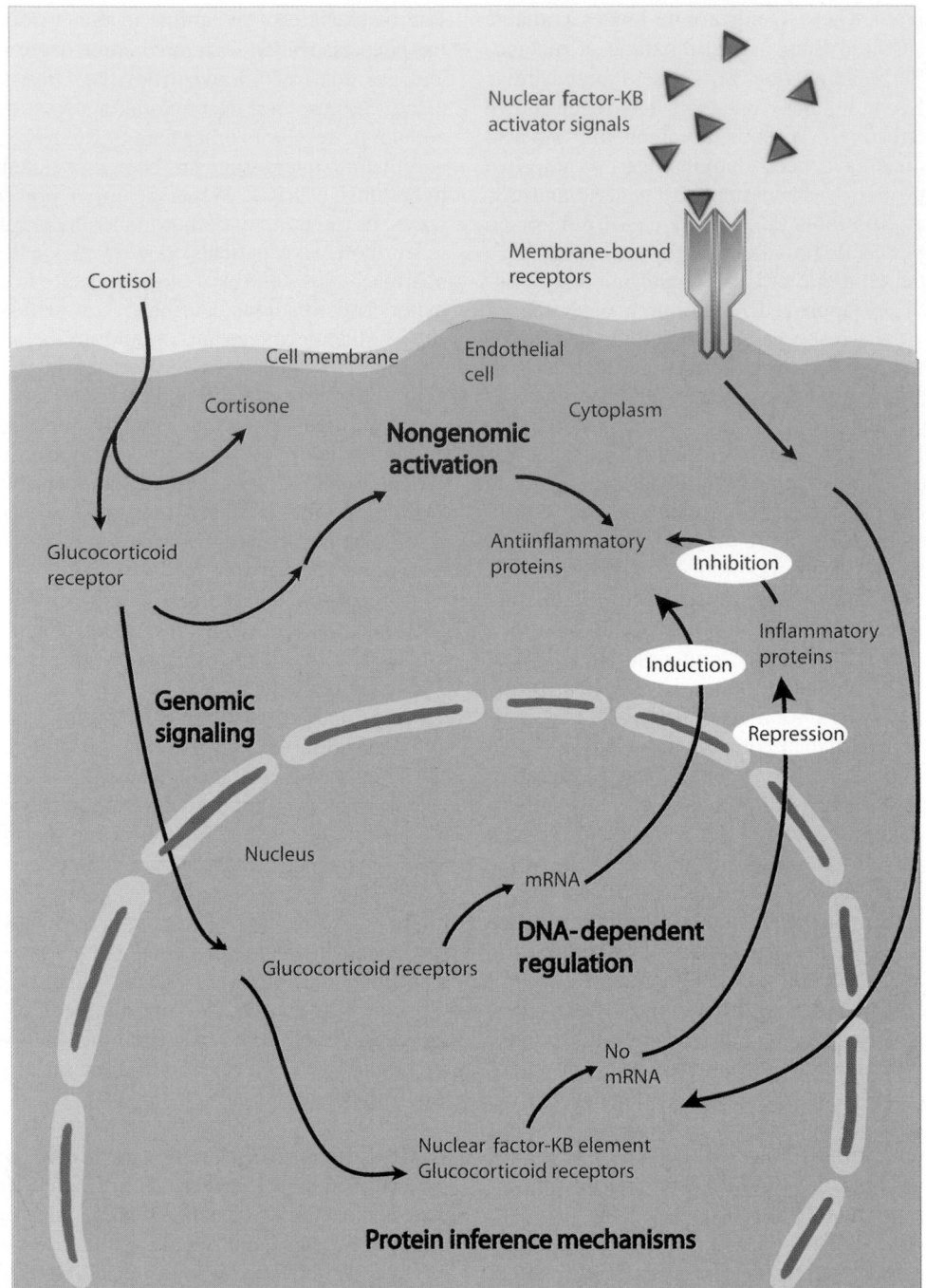

Cortisol

Cell membrane

Endothelial
cell

Membrane-bound
receptors

Nuclear factor-KB
activator signals

Cortisone

Cytoplasm

Glucocorticoid
receptor

**Nongenomic
activation**

Antiinflammatory
proteins

Inhibition

Induction

Inflammatory
proteins

Repression

**Genomic
signaling**

Nucleus

mRNA

**DNA-dependent
regulation**

Glucocorticoid receptors

No
mRNA

Nuclear factor-KB element
Glucocorticoid receptors

Protein inference mechanisms

Figure 5 Mechanism of action of intranasal corticosteroids. Glucocorticoid receptor inhibits the inflammation by genomic or nongenomic pathways. (Borrowed in part from reference 194.)

Studies on the unchallenged nasal mucosa showed that 4 weeks of intranasal corticosteroid administration leads to a significant reduction in epithelial Langerhans cells, macrophages, mast cells, T cells, and eosinophils.[196] Pretreatment with topical corticosteroids effectively suppresses the response to allergen provocation (Figure 6). In contrast to treatment with systemic corticosteroids, pretreatment with topical corticosteroids reduces the acute nasal response to allergen challenge, as shown by a reduction in symptoms and in levels of recovered inflammatory mediators in nasal secretions.[197] Treatment with topical corticosteroids also reduces symptoms, the levels of mediators, cellular infiltration during the late-phase reaction to allergen challenge, and the priming response to antigen.[76,197] Nasal allergen challenge following treatment with topical fluticasone propionate for 7 days resulted in significant decreases in the Th2 cytokines IL-4, -5, -6, and -13 and the chemokines eotaxin, RANTES, monocyte chemoattractant protein-1, MIP-1α (macrophage inflammatory protein 1α), IL-8, and IL-10. No significant changes have been shown in levels of Th1 cytokines such as IFN-γ, TNF-α, granulocyte-macrophage colony-stimulating factor, or IL-2, -3, -7, -12, and -15.[198,199] These beneficial anti-inflammatory effects of intranasal corticosteroids support the findings in several placebo-controlled clinical trials of a variety of these agents that demonstrated their efficacy in the reduction of nasal symptoms in both seasonal and perennial allergic rhinitis.[200,201] These agents inhibit hyperresponsiveness to nonantigenic stimuli such as histamine.[106] Topical corticosteroids also prevent the increase in mast cells and inflammatory cells seen during seasonal exposure to allergen. Furthermore, they result in suppression of the seasonal increase in specific IgE antibodies during the ragweed season.[202]

Currently used topical forms of corticosteroids include flunisolide, beclomethasone dipropionate, triamcinolone, budesonide, mometasone, and fluticasone. Although differences in the potency and strength of receptor binding among these molecules can be demonstrated in vitro and in certain in vivo models, none of these variations has been shown to translate into major clinical differences. Their onset of action has been reported to be as short as 7 to 8 hours after dosing, with most preparations having a peak effect between 3 days and 2 weeks. Previous studies suggested that these medications work best with continued usage, as opposed to intermittent, as-needed use.[203] However, they are also effective when used intermittently.[204] A large clinical trial compared the efficacy of intranasal fluticasone and placebo nasal sprays used as needed in patients with seasonal allergic rhinitis and showed that as-needed use of the intranasal corticosteroid led to significant improvement in symptoms and quality of life scores compared to placebo.[205] Additionally, data indicate that the as-needed use of intranasal corticosteroids is more effective for perennial allergic rhinitis than is a second-generation antihistamine.[206]

Side effects of intranasal corticosteroids are relatively rare. The most frequent is nasal irritation, which occurs in approximately 10% of patients. This is manifested as a nasal burning sensation or sneezing. Two percent of patients have blood-tinged secretions either because of the medication or because of the delivery system. Although septal perforations have been reported, they are extremely rare.[207] Nasal biopsies after prolonged use of these agents have not shown thinning of the nasal epithelium or abnormalities in the nasal mucosa.[208] Mucosal superinfection with *Candida albicans*, occasionally found with the use of topical, orally inhaled corticosteroids in the treatment of asthma, has not been a significant problem in the nose.[209]

Systemic side effects have long been a matter of concern. Preparations now available on the market have lower systemic absorption than did older preparations; and, at the standard doses used for the treatment of allergic rhinitis, no detectable effects on the hypothalamic-pituitary-adrenal axis have been found. A reduction in bone growth in children has concerned pediatricians. This problem has been studied best in asthmatic children, in whom the majority of studies suggest no effect and in whom they are confounded by the effect of asthma itself on growth.[210] Therefore, for long-term use, a topical corticosteroid with low bioavailability, administered in the lowest dose necessary to provide relief of symptoms, seems advisable and safe. In children, the rate of growth was reduced slightly in those regularly treated twice a day with intranasal beclomethasone over 1 year.[211] However, no such effect was observed in 1-year follow-up studies of children

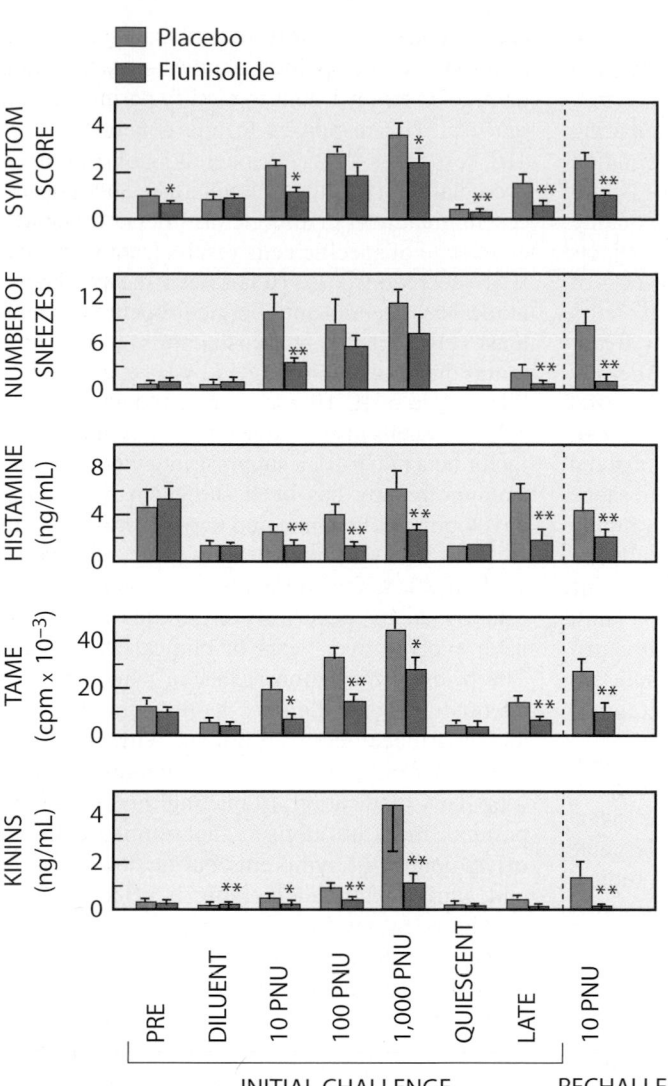

Figure 6 Effect of intranasal corticosteroid (flunisolide) on the nasal response to allergen. The protocol of challenge is seen on the abscissa: pre = prewash at the initiation of the allergen challenge protocol; diluent = challenge with the diluent for the allergen extract to control for nonspecific reactivity; 10, 100, and 1,000 protein nitrogen units (PNU) = increasing doses of allergen used for challenge; quiescent = the initial hours after allergen provocation; late = the late phase response; 10 PNU = rechallenge with the lowest dose of allergen 10 hours after the initial challenge. As can be seen from the response with subjects on placebo (*open bars*), there was a significant increase over diluent in all of the parameters measured both during the early and late responses. There was also an increase in responsiveness to the lowest dose of allergen (10 PNU) as assessed by levels of histamine, tosyl-L-argininemethyl-lester (TAME)-esterase, and kinins in nasal lavages, indicative of the priming response. Pretreatment with flunisolide (*closed bars*) resulted in inhibition of the early, late, and rechallenge responses to allergen. (Adapted from reference 197.)

treated with fluticasone,[212] mometasone,[213,214] or budesonide.[215]

The long-term effects of the reduction in growth velocity, including the final impact on adult height and the ability to catch up in growth after discontinuation of treatment, has not been adequately studied. Recent recommendations state that the growth of pediatric patients receiving intranasal corticosteroids should be monitored regularly (every 3 to 6 months) with an accurate instrument (stadiometer) by trained staff in a consistent way. Furthermore, it seems wise to use the newer agents with lower systemic bioavailability, such as mometasone and fluticasone, for the treatment of children. These agents have been approved by the FDA starting at the ages of 3 (mometasone) and 4 years (fluticasone), the recommended dose being half that used for adults. Mometasone and fluticasone are poorly absorbed from the gastrointestinal tract, with the remaining fraction of absorbed drug rapidly metabolized by the liver. The use of intranasal corticosteroids has not been associated with either an increased risk of fractures in the elderly[216] or an increased risk of cataracts.[217] However, a recently published position statement by the Joint Task Force of the American Academy of Allergy, Asthma and Immunology and the American College of Allergy, Asthma and Immunology recommends that intranasal corticosteroids should remain available by prescription and not be sold over the counter. This conclusion was reached based on the evidence that corticosteroids administered by any route, including the intranasal route, have the potential to cause adverse effects on growth, ocular structures, bones, the hypothalamic axis, and locally.[218]

In comparative trials, topical corticosteroids were more potent in relieving nasal symptoms and increasing nasal airflow than were second-generation antihistamines.[219] Comparison of the effectiveness of intranasal corticosteroid treatment with that of the combination of an antihistamine and leukotriene inhibitor in the treatment of seasonal allergic rhinitis showed that symptom improvement was better in the intranasal-corticosteroid group.[220]

Evidence suggests that intranasal corticosteroids help reduce ocular symptoms of allergic rhinitis. This approach may have advantages regarding compliance and cost.[221,222]

Studies on intranasal corticosteroids have shown that the properties of individual product may influence the preference of the patients. A multicenter study has shown that, compared with fluticasone and mometasone (original formulation), triamcinolone acetonide aqueous was associated with better product attributes, higher preference, and better compliance.[223] Meltzer and colleagues reported that scent-free mometasone

furoate nasal spray (current formulation) was preferred over fluticasone propionate nasal spray by patients based on the sensory attributes that were tested.[224]

Systemic Corticosteroids. Clinical practice suggests that oral corticosteroids reduce symptoms during seasonal allergies, but this has not been documented in patients with allergic rhinitis in placebo-controlled trials.[225] In a placebo controlled trial of patients with nasal polyposis and atopy, clinically significant improvement was observed in patients who received oral corticosteroids for 2 weeks and no significant adverse events were observed.[226]

These agents are usually administered to patients during severe exacerbations of allergic symptoms, when total nasal obstruction prevents the introduction of a topical intranasal corticosteroid. Furthermore, these agents are used successfully in combination with antibiotics for treatment of sinus infections complicating allergic rhinitis. Depot injections of corticosteroids have efficacy comparable with that of short-term oral prednisone therapy but have a longer duration of action and enjoy some popularity in Europe, including Scandinavia.[227]

Cromolyn Sodium. Cromolyn, which is available over the counter as a 4% solution for intranasal use, has been shown to be clinically effective in the treatment of allergic rhinitis. It exerts a protective effect on the allergic response when given 4 to 6 times daily beginning before the development of symptoms. Although it was initially thought to prevent mast cell degranulation, the exact mechanism of action of this agent is unknown. Like antihistamines, cromolyn is more helpful for sneezing, rhinorrhea, and nasal itching than for nasal congestion. Its safety profile, however, makes it an attractive treatment, especially in children and pregnant women.[228] When effective, the potency of this agent parallels that of antihistamines but is less than that of intranasal corticosteroids.[229]

Anticholinergics. Ipratropium bromide is the only anticholinergic agent available for topical use in the United States. Anticholinergic agents inhibit parasympathetic stimulation of glandular secretion by competing for muscarinic receptors on glands. They are highly effective in reducing rhinorrhea, but they have no effect on the other symptoms of allergic rhinitis. The clinical benefit of anticholinergic agents is primarily limited to the treatment of patients with rhinitis in whom rhinorrhea is the predominant complaint. This could occur in a variety of nasal conditions such as allergic and nonallergic rhinitis, as well as the rhinorrhea precipitated by exposure to cold, windy environments, often referred to as "skiers' nose."[230] The dosage should be titrated to avoid excessive drying of the nasal mucosa and epistaxis, which are the most frequent side effects. This agent serves as a useful adjuvant therapy in combination with topical corticosteroids and antihistamines for control of rhinorrhea. It is also safe and effective in children with rhinorrhea due to the common cold or allergies.[231]

Leukotriene Modifiers. Recognition of the importance of leukotrienes in the pathogenesis of asthma has led to the development of leukotriene modifiers. Controlled clinical trials with the 4 currently used leukotriene modifiers (montelukast, zafirlukast, and zileuton in the United States and pranlukast in Japan) have established their efficacy in improving pulmonary function, reducing symptoms, decreasing night-time awakenings, and decreasing the need for rescue medications in patients with asthma.

Among the many mediators in the nose, leukotrienes were detected both in the early and late phase of an allergic reaction. Leukotrienes stimulate mucous glands, which results in rhinorrhea, and they also have the ability to increase microvascular permeability and blood flow that result in tissue edema and subsequent congestion. Introduction of leukotriene modifiers increased the therapeutic options for patients who have allergic rhinitis with/without asthma.

Montelukast is the only leukotriene modifier that has been approved in the United States to be used for the symptoms of seasonal and perennial allergic rhinitis.[103] Montelukast is a cysLT1 receptor antagonist that inhibits the physiologic actions of LTD_4. It is rapidly absorbed after oral administration. The mean plasma concentration is achieved in 3 hours. The drug dose should be 10 mg, taken once daily. Montelukast is a safe and well-tolerated drug with adverse effect profiles similar to those of placebo.[232]

The efficacy of montelukast for the treatment of allergic rhinitis has been evaluated in several randomized double-blind trials. Montelukast significantly improved night-time symptoms (difficulty going to sleep, night-time awakenings, and congestion on awakening), as well as daytime symptoms (congestion, rhinorrhea, pruritus, and sneezing), compared with placebo in patients with allergies.[102] A meta-analysis of randomized controlled trials revealed that leukotriene receptor antagonists are modestly better than placebo, as effective as antihistamines, but less effective than nasal corticosteroids in improving symptoms and quality of life in patients with seasonal allergic rhinitis.[233]

In a comparative study, pseudoephedrine showed an efficacy equivalent to that of montelukast in decreasing symptom scores and increasing nasal airflow in subjects with seasonal allergic rhinitis.[234] A recent study in children between 2 and 6 years of age revealed that montelukast is as effective as cetirizine in quality of life symptom scores. For night sleep quality, montelukast was superior to cetirizine.[235]

Combined montelukast and cetirizine treatment started 6 weeks before the pollen season was effective in preventing symptoms of allergic rhinitis, and it reduced the allergic inflammation in the nasal mucosa during allergen exposure.[236] Comparison of the effectiveness of intranasal corticosteroid treatment with that of the combination of an antihistamine and leukotriene inhibitor in the treatment of seasonal allergic rhinitis showed that in the intranasal-corticosteroid group, symptom relief was better.[220] Another study comparing the fexofenadine–pseudoephedrine combination with that of loratadine-montelukast showed comparable efficacy in improving symptoms, quality of life scores, and nasal obstruction in subjects with seasonal allergic rhinitis.[237] The effects of fexofenadine alone or a combination of fexofenadine with montelukast were significantly better than placebo; however, combination therapy conferred no additional benefit.[238] A randomized clinical trial comparing the clinical efficacy of fluticasone proprionate nasal spray administered alone with fluticasone plus cetirizine or fluticasone plus montelukast showed that fluticasone is highly effective in the treatment of patients with allergic rhinitis, with efficacy exceeding that of cetirizine plus montelukast in combined therapy.[239] Thus, the combined therapy of fluticasone with cetirizine or montelukast has not offered any substantial advantage over fluticasone in monotherapy.

Ophthalmic Preparations. Treatment of ocular symptoms of allergy employs a regimen of medications similar to those used for nasal manifestations. After avoidance of allergens, pharmacotherapy includes the use of topical decongestants, antihistamines, mast-cell stabilizing agents, and anti-inflammatory preparations. Topical decongestants such as phenylephrine and tetrathydrozoline decrease vascular congestion and eyelid edema through α-adrenergic receptors. Several over-the-counter topical antihistamines are available, some in combination with a decongestant. Recently, second-generation topical antihistamines have become available. Levocabastine is a long-lasting topical antihistamine with rapid onset of action that has been shown to be effective for ocular allergies. Azelastine is approved for the treatment of allergic conjunctivitis. Emedastine and olopatadine are topical agents which have also been shown to be effective. Ophthalmic formulations of ketotifen fumarate, pemirolast potassium, olapatadine, and nedocromil sodium are agents with mast-cell-stabilizing properties. Ketorolac, a nonsteroidal antiinflammatory agent, diminishes ocular itching and hyperemia and is the only agent in this class approved by the FDA for treatment of allergic conjunctivitis. Mild topical corticosteroids can be utilized in patients who continue to have symptoms despite treatment with the aforementioned agents, but these can cause local complications.

Immunotherapy. Allergen-specific immunotherapy is a very effective method of treatment in carefully selected patients with allergic rhinitis. It is the only treatment that can lead to a life-long tolerance. The mechanisms underlying the success of immunotherapy are slowly being elucidated (Figure 7). In early research into immunotherapy mechanisms, circulating-antibody responses were examined. Immunotherapy with inhalant allergens is associated with increases in serum allergen-specific IgG1, IgG4, and IgA levels.[240] More recently, the focus has been on T-cell responses. Studies show that this treatment acts on T cells to modify peripheral and mucosal Th2 responses to allergen in favor of Th1 responses.[241,242] Peripheral-T-cell tolerance is crucial for a healthy immune response and successful treatment of allergic disorders.[240] The tolerant state of specific cells results from increased IL-10 secretion.[241] IL-10 has been shown to have numerous potential antiallergic properties against mast cells, T cells, and eosinophils. It also promotes the production of IgG4 by B cells. The cellular origin of IL-10 was demonstrated to be T_{reg} cells. T_{reg} cells also produce transforming growth factor beta (TGF-β), a suppressant cytokine.[241,242] Immunotherapy has been shown to reduce the development of asthma and new sensitizations in children with seasonal allergies.[243]

Indications for immunotherapy have not been established by experimental studies but rather have evolved over years of clinical experience. The primary indication is that of symptoms not adequately controlled by avoidance measures and pharmacotherapy. Patients with perennial symptoms may prefer immunotherapy to yearlong daily medication. In making their selection, patients must be advised that immunotherapy offers control of symptoms but is slow in onset and, unlike pharmacotherapy, is effective only for the allergens for which the patient is being treated. Whether years of successful therapy cure the patient of the disease after discontinuation of immunotherapy is an important but unanswered question. However, 1 study suggested that improvement in rhinitis symptoms persists for several years after the end of treatment.[245] The same effect was shown in children 6 years after discontinuation of specific immunotherapy.[246]

Immunotherapy begins with low-dose injections of allergen extracts and builds to a maintenance dose. Injections usually begin at weekly intervals and are reduced in frequency when maintenance doses are reached. The choice of allergens for treatment must be made after a careful diagnostic workup so that the probability of treatment being started with extracts from all of the allergens responsible for symptoms is high. Treatment should not be given if skin or serum testing cannot confirm evidence of an IgE-mediated mechanism. Whereas excellent relief can be expected with pollen allergens, dust mites, and some animal danders, treatment with molds is less reliable. Immunotherapy with too many allergens is impractical; usually, treatment with no more than six to ten allergens is attempted. Enzymes from some allergens can destroy other antigens, reducing the expected potency of the treatment. Furthermore, combining allergens of different clinical sensitivities may interfere with reaching adequate maintenance doses for all allergens. Patients who are taking β blockers should not receive immunotherapy because, if anaphylaxis occurs, patients cannot be resuscitated. Immunotherapy of symptomatic asthmatic patients should be administered with extreme caution because these patients have the greatest

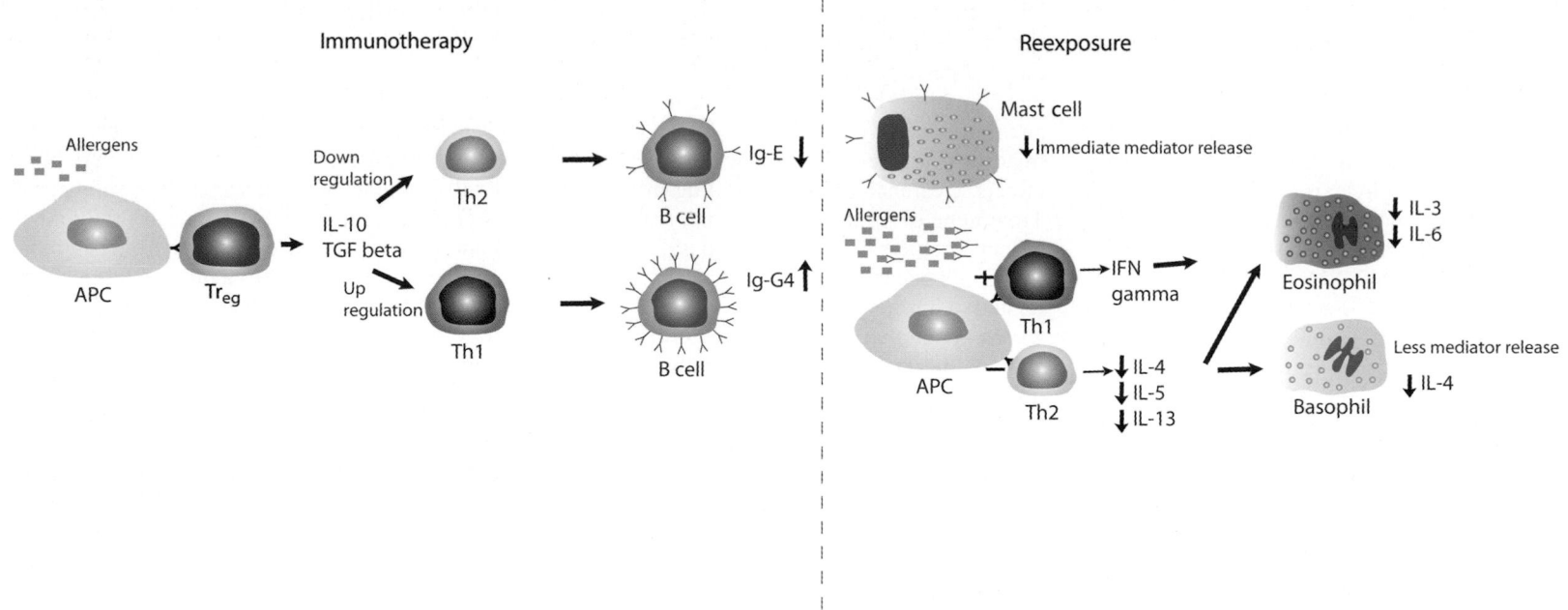

Figure 7 Mechanism of allergen-specific immunotherapy. Specific immunotherapy results in suppression of Th2 responses and induction of Th1 responses. The allergic inflammatory response to allergen exposure is down-regulated by several mechanisms which include the production of blocking antibodies (IgG4) and release of cytokines involved in allergen-specific hyporesponsiveness (IL-10 and transforming growth factor beta [TGF-β]). (Borrowed in part from reference 244.)

morbidity. Immunotherapy should not be started in pregnant women because of the risk of anaphylaxis and the resultant effect of hypotension on the fetus.

Lessening of symptoms may begin as soon as 12 weeks after initiation of treatment, but an optimal effect usually takes 1 year to attain. Effectiveness of immunotherapy requires administration of sufficient amounts of allergen. For ragweed, this has been shown to be between 6 and 12 μg of *Amb a 1* (the major antigen in ragweed) per injection. The effect is antigen-specific; thus, selection of relevant antigens for treatment is paramount. Patients who do not achieve symptomatic improvement after 1 year of immunotherapy should have it discontinued. No information is available on the length of time over which effective immunotherapy should be pursued, but most physicians treat for 2 to 5 years.

Allergen injections should be administered under the supervision of a qualified medical practitioner, and patients should be observed for at least 30 minutes after every injection. Local reactions at the site of injection are frequent with effective dosages and require no therapy. Repeated strong reactions (ie, swelling greater than 4 cm in diameter) persisting for 24 hours should lead to consideration of dose reduction. Proper resuscitative equipment should be present because anaphylactic reactions can occur at any time during treatment, even in patients receiving maintenance doses. Factors that seem to contribute to increased complications, including fatalities, seem to be labile, corticosteroid-dependent asthma that has required prior hospitalizations, high sensitivity to allergen (as demonstrated by serum-specific IgE tests or skin test), and a history of prior systemic reactions.[247] Therefore, although death from immunotherapy is uncommon, special precautions need to be taken with asthma, and a waiting period of at least 20 min-

utes after administration of the injection is recommended for all patients, with longer intervals (30 minutes) appropriate for high-risk patients. Results of a survey from the United States showed that fatal reactions occurred with 1 per 2.5 million injections, with an average of 3.4 deaths per year. Sixty percent of fatal reactions occurred during maintenance. The vast majority of patients were asthmatics. Twenty percent of fatal reactions occurred in a medically unsupervised setting. None of the fatal cases were receiving β-blockers.[248] An e-mail survey of allergists regarding incorrect allergy injections (wrong patient or wrong dose) revealed that 58% of allergists observed an event in which a patient received an injection meant for another patient, and 74% of allergists reported that patients had received an incorrect amount of vaccine. The effect of these mistakes on patients resulted in 1 fatality and underscores the need for care while using this form of treatment.

Sublingual Immunotherapy. Sublingual administration of allergen extracts has been shown to be a well-tolerated and efficacious approach to treatment of allergic rhinitis. In the last few years, reports on the safety and efficacy of this treatment have grown enormously. In a recent meta-analysis encompassing 22 clinical studies evaluating sublingual immunotherapy (SLIT), it was concluded that this method reduces both symptoms and medication requirements.[249]

The immunologic mechanisms of SLIT are less well established. An increase in IgG4 and induction of allergen-specific IgA without a change in IgE values has been reported with SLIT.[250] The evidence on the changes in Th1/Th2/T$_{reg}$ activity induced by SLIT should be confirmed.[241]

SLIT requires more allergen (at least 50 to 100 times) than does subcutaneous immunotherapy. It is rather unclear whether a dose-response

relationship exists. The allergen is kept under the tongue for one to two minutes and then swallowed. If the vaccine is swallowed immediately, the clinical efficacy decreases substantially.[251] It is now widely accepted that SLIT is much safer than subcutaneous immunotherapy, with no evidence of anaphylactic shock recorded after more than 500 million doses administered to human subjects.[252] Adverse events are reported to be local (oral itching, swelling, and irritation) and self-resolving.[253] Immunotherapy has to be continued for at least 3 years.

SLIT has the advantage of affecting both the patient's quality of life and the socioeconomic impact of allergic rhinitis. Whereas the first generation of sublingual vaccines used today are based on natural biological extracts, new vaccines that rely upon selected recombinant allergens are being developed.[254]

Anti-IgE. Omalizumab is a recombinant humanized monoclonal antibody that binds selectively to IgE. It lowers free IgE levels in the circulation. Several studies have shown that omalizumab, in addition to reducing the free IgE level in serum, is associated with an anti-inflammatory effect on cellular markers in blood and nasal tissue.[255] It inhibits allergen-induced seasonal increases in circulating and tissue eosinophils,[256] and it reduces the expression of FcεR1 on the mast cells and dendritic cells.[257]

This medication is currently available in the United States. It is indicated for patients older than 12 years who have moderate to severe asthma, who have a positive skin or in vitro test to a perennial allergen, and whose symptoms are inadequately controlled with inhaled corticosteroids. It is not approved for use in patients with allergic rhinitis.

Omalizumab is administered subcutaneously every 2 to 4 weeks. The doses and dosing frequency are determined by the patient's body weight and the pretreatment serum IgE level. It has a low incidence of side effects, such as reaction at the injection site, viral infection, headache, and upper respiratory tract infection. The most serious adverse reactions reported are malignancies (0.5%) and anaphylaxis (0.1%). Omalizumab reaches a peak concentration within 7 to 8 days after subcutaneous administration and has a half-life of approximately 26 days.

In a large clinical trial on subjects with seasonal allergic rhinitis, omalizumab decreased serum-free IgE levels and provided clinical benefit in a dose-dependent fashion.[56] It has been shown to decrease nasal symptoms and quality-of-life scores in adolescents and adults who have outdoor allergies.[258] The efficiency of this drug compared to H_1 antihistamines and intranasal corticosteroids remains to be established.

A recent study suggested that pretreatment with omalizumab increases the safety of rush immunotherapy in patients with allergic rhinitis.[259] Co-seasonal application of omalizumab after preseasonal specific immunotherapy resulted in decreases in nasal and ocular symptoms of children who had seasonal allergies.[260]

Future Therapies. As understanding of the complex immunologic pathophysiology of allergic rhinitis has developed, new targets have been surfacing for pharmacologic development. Drugs targeting several cytokines and chemokines known to play a role in the inflammatory process are being developed and tested. Classes of investigational agents that target other molecules thought to be important in the inflammatory processes of allergic rhinitis include tryptase inhibitors, phosphodiesterase-4 inhibitors, chemokine inhibitors, and adhesion receptor antagonists. A perhaps more elegant therapeutic strategy would be to effect long-lasting changes in immune responses away from an allergic phenotype. Such a strategy might alter the natural course of the disease and allow discontinuation of medication. The identification of T_{reg} cells as key regulators of the immunologic processes involved in the peripheral tolerance to allergens has opened an important era in this regard. A crucial area for future studies is the identification of drugs, cytokines, or costimulatory molecules that induce in vivo growth of T_{reg} cells while preserving their suppressing function.[124]

Recombinant DNA technology has enabled the cloning of many allergens, thus facilitating investigations aimed at improving the efficacy and safety of immunotherapy. Future prospects for allergen-specific immunotherapy include reconstitution of extracts by use of recombinant allergens, reconstitution of several major allergens in 1 protein as a T-cell-directed vaccine, and peptide immunotherapy.[242] These therapies will require further study, but ultimately may prove useful in expanding the armamentarium available against allergic rhinitis.

Special Considerations. Several patient populations require careful attention in the treatment of allergic rhinitis. In the case of elite athletes, preventive therapy must be initiated so that effects on peak performance can be avoided. The Olympic Committee bans pseudoephedrine-containing agents. Similarly, care must be taken in the treatment of elderly patients with respect to side effects, clearance of drug, and drug interactions. Treatment of rhinitis during pregnancy poses special problems. Rhinitis and nasal congestion frequently occur during pregnancy (30%) and are related to hormonal changes.

Pregnant patients require careful consideration in the choice of therapy. Ideally, no medication should be used, particularly during the first trimester. Avoidance measures should be implemented first. If symptoms of rhinitis interfere with maternal well-being, pharmacologic management is considered. The patient must be advised that no drug can be regarded as absolutely safe, because most drugs cross the placenta and can be measured in fetal blood.

The American College of Obstetricians and Gynecologists and The American College of Allergy, Asthma and Immunology make the following recommendations: medical treatment of allergic rhinitis should start with first-generation antihistamines. In patients who do not tolerate chlorpheniramine and tripelennamine and who fail other therapies, use of cetirizine and loratadine could be considered.[261] Sodium cromoglycate is a safe drug during pregnancy and should be considered in the treatment of allergic rhinitis

before corticosteroids. Maternal exposure to orally inhaled budesonide during pregnancy was not associated with an increased risk of congenital malformations or other adverse fetal outcomes. Data on pregnancy outcomes after maternal exposure to intranasal budesonide are limited, but the totality of evidence indicates that its safety profile is at least comparable with that of orally inhaled budesonide.[262] Budesonide is the only intranasal corticosteroid that carries a pregnancy category B rating. Other agents such as leukotriene modifiers may be considered in women who exhibited a good response to these agents before pregnancy. Maintenance immunotherapy may be continued safely during pregnancy for patients who are not prone to systemic reactions. However, because of the increased risk of systemic reactions, immunotherapy should not be initiated during pregnancy.

TOWARD A RATIONAL CHOICE OF THERAPY

Pharmacotherapy remains the mainstay of the treatment of allergic rhinitis (Figure 8). If allergen exposure can be reduced, this should be a part of any long-term management. Short-term avoidance does not result in an instant resolution of symptoms and is rarely completely achievable.

Pharmacotherapy provides the fastest relief. Oral antihistamines begin to take effect within 1 hour and traditionally constitute the first line of intervention. Topical antihistamines have an even

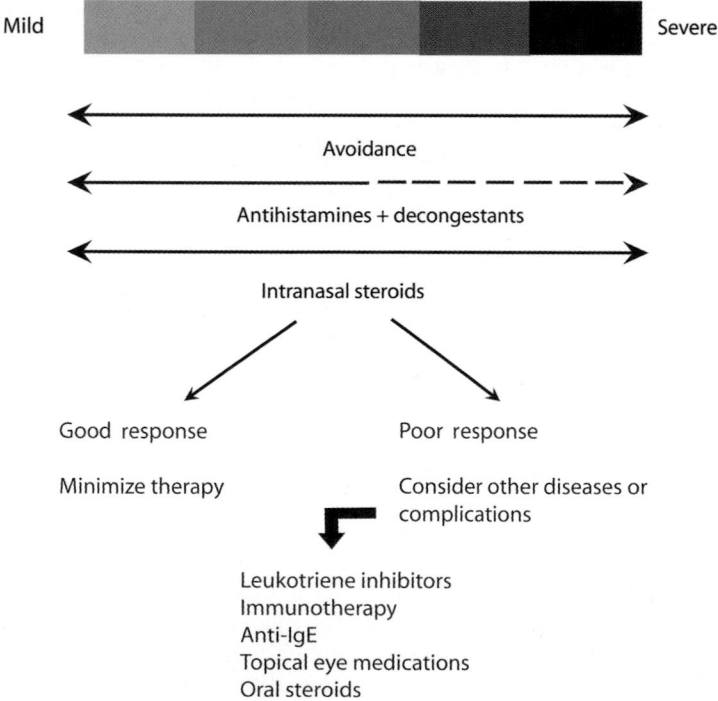

Figure 8 Approach to the treatment of allergic rhinitis. This schematic depicts the different treatments available for allergic rhinitis and establishes some guidelines for the use of these therapies in different stages of severity of the disease. Avoidance should be used in all stages. Antihistamines and/or decongestants are commonly used for allergic rhinitis of mild to moderate severity. Topical intranasal corticosteroids are also effective against a range of symptoms, including on an as-needed basis. Severe disease usually warrants more aggressive treatment. This may require combination and adjuvant therapy. Anticholinergics play a limited role in the control of rhinorrhea. Leukotriene modifiers are useful in the treatment of congestion, especially in asthmatic patients. Systemic corticosteroids are reserved for severe allergic rhinitis leading to complete nasal obstruction. Immunotherapy can be offered to patients who fail medical therapy. Clearly, these guidelines need to be varied in the context of different clinical settings, as some patients with mild disease might benefit from intranasal corticosteroids whereas some other patients with more severe disease might respond well to antihistamine/decongestant combinations.

faster onset of action. They are excellent for the treatment of sneezing and watery rhinorrhea. When cost is not an issue, nonsedating antihistamines should always be prescribed. Decongestants can be added to antihistamines in fixed combinations or as separate agents for relief of nasal congestion. Cromolyn sodium is an alternative to antihistamines as an initial treatment, but the need for frequent dosing, with the resultant reduction in compliance, should be kept in mind. Leukotriene modifiers may be utilized for effects against congestion in asthmatic or refractory patients and may be used in combination with antihistamines for patients who do not tolerate other therapies.

According to recent guidelines, intranasal glucocorticoids are regarded as a highly effective first line treatment for patients suffering from allergic rhinitis with moderate to severe and/or persistent symptoms.[2] They are highly effective in reducing all of the nasal symptoms of allergic rhinitis, including congestion. They are nonsedating, have few side effects, and are well-tolerated by patients. Topical corticosteroids are given initially at the dose recommended in the *Physicians' Desk Reference*. Patients should be seen 2 weeks after initiation of therapy for monitoring for the development of local side effects. Superficial septal erosions can occur secondary to trauma from the nozzle, and the application technique should be reviewed carefully with these patients. The dose is adjusted depending on the response: if a patient is doing better, but continues to have breakthrough symptoms, the frequency of administration is increased; if excellent control is achieved, the frequency or the dose should be reduced. In those doing better, but still having symptoms, other agents can be added to the intranasal corticosteroids.

Furthermore, periods of exacerbations can be predicted, based on a patient's pattern of allergies; and, therefore, the medication dosage can be varied accordingly. Ocular symptoms may be controlled only minimally by intranasal corticosteroids and thus adding an ophthalmic preparation or an oral antihistamine may be necessary.

As to children, the long-term use of certain topical corticosteroids is approved in patients as young as age 2 years or older. For most topical corticosteroids, it is recommended to give half the adult dose in young children. Because of the slight possibility that intranasal corticosteroids could interfere with growth, these medications should always be given in the lowest effective dose. Growth should be monitored carefully and regularly.

Treatment with topical corticosteroids requires patient education. The physician must often reassure patients as to the safety of intranasal corticosteroids, compared with oral preparations.

Initiation of immunotherapy depends on patient preference and the response to pharmacotherapy. It has the potential to alter the natural history of the disease.

Surgical management of nasal obstruction is presented in Chapter 45, "Acute and Chronic Nasal Disorders," and Chapter 53, "Rhinoplasty and Septoplasty." Septal deviations may need to be corrected because they may interfere with the delivery of intranasal medications or contribute to symptoms. Similarly, turbinate reduction by means of submucous resection, resurfacing with the laser, electrocautery, or radiofrequency ablation may be adjuvant procedures in patients with allergic rhinitis but more often find use in the management of nonallergic rhinitis. Functional endoscopic sinus surgery, covered in Chapter 49, "Primary Paranasal Sinus Surgery" can be used for the treatment of chronic rhinosinusitis, which frequently complicates perennial rhinitis.

REFERENCES

1. Johansson SG, Haahtela T. World allergy organization guidelines for prevention of allergy and allergic asthma. condensed version. Int Arch Allergy Immunol 2004; 135:83–92.
2. Bousquet J, Van Cauwenberge P, Khaltaev N. Aria Workshop Group; World Health Organization. Allergic rhinitis and its impact on asthma. J Allergy Clin Immunol 2001;108: S147–334.
3. Meltzer EO. The prevalence and medical and economic impact of allergic rhinitis in the United States. J Allergy Clin Immunol 1997;99:S805–28.
4. Meltzer EO. Quality of life in adults and children with allergic rhinitis. J Allergy Clin Immunol 2001;108:S45–53.
5. Reed SD, Lee TA, McCrory DC. The economic burden of allergic rhinitis: A critical evaluation of the literature. Pharmacoeconomics 2004;22:345–61.
6. Lamb CE, Ratner PH, Johnson CE, et al. Economic impact of workplace productivity losses due to allergic rhinitis compared with select medical conditions in the United States from an employer perspective. Curr Med Res Opin 2006;22:1203–10.
7. Selnes A, Nystad W, Bolle R, Lund E. Diverging prevalence trends of atopic disorders in Norwegian children. Results from three cross-sectional studies. Allergy 2005;60:894–9.
8. Galassi C, De Sario M, Biggeri A, et al. Changes in prevalence of asthma and allergies among children and adolescents in Italy: 1994–2002. Pediatrics 2006;117:34–42.
9. Lee SL, Wong W, Lau YL. Increasing prevalence of allergic rhinitis but not asthma among children in Hong Kong from 1995 to 2001 (Phase 3 International Study of Asthma and Allergies in Childhood). Pediatr Allergy Immunol 2004;15:72–8.
10. Arbes SJ, Jr, Gergen PJ, Elliott L, Zeldin DC. Prevalences of positive skin test responses to 10 common allergens in the US population: Results from the third National Health and Nutrition Examination Survey. J Allergy Clin Immunol 2005;116:377–83.
11. Thomsen SF, Ulrik CS, Kyvik KO, et al. Genetic and environmental contributions to hay fever among young adult twins. Respir Med 2006;100:2177–82.
12. Brasch-Andersen C, Haagerup A, Borglum AD, et al. Highly significant linkage to chromosome 3q13.31 for rhinitis and related allergic diseases. J Med Genet 2006;43:e10.
13. Brasch-Andersen C, Tan Q, Borglum AD, et al. Significant linkage to chromosome 12q24.32–q24.33 and identification of SFRS8 as a possible asthma susceptibility gene. Thorax 2006;61:874–9.
14. Dizier MH, Bouzigon E, Guilloud-Bataille M, et al. Genome screen in the French EGEA study: Detection of linked regions shared or not shared by allergic rhinitis and asthma. Genes Immun 2005;6:95–102.
15. Zutavern A, von Klot S, Gehring U, et al. Pre-natal and post-natal exposure to respiratory infection and atopic diseases development: A historical cohort study. Respir Res 2006;7:81. Available at http://respiratory-research.com/content/7/1/81.
16. Matricardi PM, Rosmini F, Panetta V, et al. Hay fever and asthma in relation to markers of infection in the United States. J Allergy Clin Immunol 2002;110:381–7.
17. Kinra S, Davey Smith G, Jeffreys M, et al. Association between sibship size and allergic diseases in the Glasgow Alumni Study. Thorax 2006;61:48–53.
18. Horner AA. Toll-like receptor ligands and atopy: A coin with at least two sides. J Allergy Clin Immunol 2006; 117:1133–40.
19. Ownby DR, Johnson CC, Peterson EL. Exposure to dogs and cats in the first year of life and risk of allergic sensitization at 6 to 7 years of age. JAMA 2002;288:963–72.
20. van Strien RT, Koopman LP, Kerkhof M, et al. Prevention and incidence of asthma and mite allergy study. Mattress encasings and mite allergen levels in the prevention and incidence of asthma and mite allergy study. Clin Exp Allergy 2003;33:490–5.
21. Corver K, Kerkhof M, Brussee JE, et al. House dust mite allergen reduction and allergy at 4 yr: Follow up of the PIAMA-study. Pediatr Allergy Immunol 2006;17:329–36.
22. Vedanthan PK, Mahesh PA, Vedanthan R, et al. Effect of animal contact and microbial exposures on the prevalence of atopy and asthma in urban vs rural children in India. Ann Allergy Asthma Immunol 2006;96:571–8.
23. Alfven T, Braun-Fahrlander C, Brunekreef B, et al. PARSIFAL study group. Allergic diseases and atopic sensitization in children related to farming and anthroposophic lifestyle– the PARSIFAL study. Allergy 2006;61:414–21.
24. Klintberg B, Berglund N, Lilja G, et al. Fewer allergic respiratory disorders among farmers' children in a closed birth cohort from Sweden. Eur Respir J 2001;17:1151–7.
25. Braun-Fahrlander C. Environmental exposure to endotoxin and other microbial products and the decreased risk of childhood atopy: Evaluating developments since April 2002. Curr Opin Allergy Clin Immunol 2003;3:325–9.
26. Raby BA, Klimecki WT, Laprise C, et al. Polymorphisms in toll-like receptor 4 are not associated with asthma or atopy-related phenotypes. Am J Respir Crit Care Med 2002;166:1449–56.
27. Yang IA, Barton SJ, Rorke S, et al. Toll-like receptor 4 polymorphism and severity of atopy in asthmatics. Genes Immun 2004;5:41–5.
28. Halken S. Prevention of allergic disease in childhood: Clinical and epidemiological aspects of primary and secondary allergy prevention. Pediatr Allergy Immunol 2004;15:4–5, 9–32.
29. Tarini BA, Carroll AE, Sox CM, Christakis DA. Systematic review of the relationship between early introduction of solid foods to infants and the development of allergic disease. Arch Pediatr Adolesc Med 2006;160:502–7.
30. Savilahti E, Siltanen M, Pekkanen J, Kajosaari M. Mothers of very low birth weight infants have less atopy than mothers of full-term infants. Clin Exp Allergy 2004; 34:1851–4.
31. Braback L, Hjern A, Rasmussen F. Social class in asthma and allergic rhinitis: A national cohort study over three decades. Eur Respir J 2005;26:1064–8.
32. Renz-Polster H, David MR, Buist AS, et al. Caesarean section delivery and the risk of allergic disorders in childhood. Clin Exp Allergy 2005;35:1466–72.
33. Diaz-Sanchez D, Garcia MP, Wang M, et al. Nasal challenge with diesel exhaust particles can induce sensitization to a neoallergen in the human mucosa. J Allergy Clin Immunol 1999;104:1183–8.
34. Villeneuve PJ, Doiron MS, Stieb D, et al. Is outdoor air pollution associated with physician visits for allergic rhinitis among the elderly in Toronto, Canada. Allergy 2006; 61:750–8.
35. Kongerud J, Madden MC, Hazucha M, Peden D. Nasal responses in asthmatic and nonasthmatic subjects following exposure to diesel exhaust particles. Inhal Toxicol 2006;18:589–94.
36. Penard-Morand C, Charpin D, Raherison C, et al. Long-term exposure to background air pollution related to respiratory and allergic health in schoolchildren. Clin Exp Allergy 2005;35:1279–87.
37. De S, Fenton JE, Jones AS, Clarke RW. Passive smoking, allergic rhinitis and nasal obstruction in children. J Laryngol Otol 2005;119:955–7.
38. Biagini JM, LeMasters GK, Ryan PH, et al. Environmental risk factors of rhinitis in early infancy. Pediatr Allergy Immunol 2006;17:278–84.
39. Thaqi A, Franke K, Merkel G, et al. Biomarkers of exposure to passive smoking of school children: Frequency and determinants. Indoor Air 2005;15:302–10.
40. Diaz-Sanchez D, Rumold R, Gong H, Jr. Challenge with environmental tobacco smoke exacerbates allergic airway disease in human beings. J Allergy Clin Immunol 2006;118:441–6.
41. Huurre TM, Aro HM, Jaakkola JJ. Incidence and prevalence of asthma and allergic rhinitis: A cohort study of Finnish adolescents. J Asthma 2004;41:311–7.
42. Fagan JK, Scheff PA, Hryhorczuk D, et al. Prevalence of asthma and other allergic diseases in an adolescent population: Association with gender and race. Ann Allergy Asthma Immunol 2001;86:177–84.
43. Aberg N, Engstrom I. Natural history of allergic diseases in children. Acta Paediatr Scand 1990;79:206–11.
44. Guerra S, Sherrill DL, Martinez FD, Barbee RA. Rhinitis as an independent risk factor for adult-onset asthma. J Allergy Clin Immunol 2002;109:419–25.

45. Togias A. Systemic effects of local allergic disease. J Allergy Clin Immunol 2004;113:S8–14.
46. Rydzewski B, Pruszewicz A, Sulkowski WJ. Assessment of smell and taste in patients with allergic rhinitis. Acta Otolaryngol 2000;120:323–6.
47. Savolainen S. Allergy in patients with acute maxillary sinusitis. Allergy 1989;44:116–22.
48. Emanuel IA, Shah SB. Chronic rhinosinusitis: Allergy and sinus computed tomography relationships. Otolaryngol Head Neck Surg 2000;123:687–91.
49. Blair C, Nelson M, Thompson K, et al. Allergic inflammation enhances bacterial sinusitis in mice. J Allergy Clin Immunol 2001;108:424–9.
50. Grigoreas C, Vourdas D, Petalas K, et al. Nasal polyps in patients with rhinitis and asthma. Allergy Asthma Proc 2002;23:169–74.
51. Lazo-Saenz JG, Galvan-Aguilera AA, Martinez-Ordaz VA, et al. Eustachian tube dysfunction in allergic rhinitis. Otolaryngol Head Neck Surg 2005;132:626–9.
52. Ohrui N, Takeuchi A, Tong A, et al. Allergic rhinitis and ear pain in flight. Ann Allergy Asthma Immunol 2005; 95:350–3.
53. Wright ED, Hurst D, Miotto D, et al. Increased expression of major basic protein (MBP) and interleukin-5 (IL-5) in middle ear biopsy specimens from atopic patients with persistent otitis media with effusion. Otolaryngol Head Neck Surg 2000;123:533–8.
54. Linneberg A, Henrik Nielsen N, Frolund L, et al. The link between allergic rhinitis and allergic asthma: A prospective population-based study. The Copenhagen Allergy Study. Allergy 2002;57:1048–52.
55. Leynaert B, Neukirch C, Kony S, et al. Association between asthma and rhinitis according to atopic sensitization in a population-based study. J Allergy Clin Immunol 2004;113:86–93.
56. Casale TB, Condemi J, LaForce C, et al. Omalizumab Seasonal Allergic Rhinitis Trail Group. Effect of omalizumab on symptoms of seasonal allergic rhinitis: A randomized controlled trial. JAMA 2001;286:2956–67.
57. Wilcock LK, Francis JN, Durham SR. IgE-facilitated antigen presentation: Role in allergy and the influence of allergen immunotherapy. Immunol Allergy Clin North Am 2006;26:333–47.
58. Gould HJ, Sutton BJ, Beavil AJ, et al. The biology of IGE and the basis of allergic disease. Ann Rev Immunol 2003;21:579–628.
59. Takhar P, Smurthwaite L, Coker HA, et al. Allergen drives class switching to IgE in the nasal mucosa in allergic rhinitis. J Immunol 2005;174:5024–32.
60. Fiset PO, Cameron L, Hamid Q. Local isotype switching to IgE in airway mucosa. J Allergy Clin Immunol 2005;116:233–6.
61. Naclerio RM, Creticos PS, Norman PS, Lichtenstein LM. Mediator release after nasal airway challenge with allergen. Am Rev Respir Dis 1986;134:1102.
62. Proud D, Naclerio RM, Togias AG, et al. Kinins as mediators of human allergic reactions. Adv Exp Med Biol 1986;198:181–7.
63. Baumgarten CR, Nichols RC, Naclerio RM, Proud D. Concentrations of glandular kallikrein in human nasal secretions increase during experimentally induced allergic rhinitis. J Immunol 1986;137:1323–8.
64. Castells M. Mast cell mediators in allergic inflammation and mastocytosis. Immunol Allergy Clin North Am 2006;26:465–85.
65. Creticos PS, Peters SP, Adkinson NF, Jr, et al. Peptide leukotriene release after antigen challenge in patients sensitive to ragweed. N Engl J Med 1984;310:1626–30.
66. Peters SP, Freeland HS, Kelly SJ, et al. Is leukotriene B4 an important mediator in human IgE-mediated allergic reactions? Am Rev Respir Dis 1987;135:S42–5.
67. Bascom R, Pipkorn U, Proud D, et al. Major basic protein and eosinophil-derived neurotoxin concentrations in nasal-lavage fluid after antigen challenge: Effect of systemic corticosteroids and relationship to eosinophil influx. J Allergy Clin Immunol 1989;84:338–46.
68. Togias A, Lykens K, Kagey-Sobotka A, et al. Studies on the relationships between sensitivity to cold, dry air, hyperosmolal solutions, and histamine in the adult nose. Am Rev Respir Dis 1990;141:1428–33.
69. Tønnesen P, Mygind N. Nasal challenge with serotonin and histamine in normal persons. Allergy 1985;40:350–3.
70. Bisgaard H, Olsson P, Bende M. Effect of Leukotriene D4 on nasal mucosal blood flow, nasal airway resistance and nasal secretions in humans. Clin Allergy 1986; 16:289–97.
71. Proud D, Reynolds CJ, Lacapra S, et al. Nasal provocation with bradykinin induces symptoms of rhinitis and a sore throat. Am Rev Respir Dis 1988;137:613–6.
72. Doyle WJ, Boehm S, Skoner DP. Physiologic responses to intranasal dose-response challenges with histamine, methacholine, bradykinin, and prostaglandin in adult volunteers with and without nasal allergy. J Allergy Clin Immunol 1990;86:924–6.
73. Gleich G. The late phase of the immunoglobulin E-mediated reaction: A link between anaphylaxis and common allergic disease? J Allergy Clin Immunol 1982;70:160–9.
74. Naclerio RM, Proud D, Togias AG, et al. Inflammatory mediators in late antigen-induced rhinitis. N Engl J Med 1985;313:65–70.
75. Iliopoulos O, Proud D, Adkinson NF, Jr, et al. Relationship between the early, late, and rechallenge reaction to nasal challenge with antigen: Observations on the role of inflammatory mediators and cells. J Allergy Clin Immunol 1990;86:851–61.
76. Bascom R, Wachs M, Naclerio RM, et al. Basophil influx occurs after nasal antigen challenge: Effects of topical corticosteroid pretreatment. J Allergy Clin Immunol 1988;81:580–9.
77. Varney VA, Jacobson MR, Sudderick RM, et al. Immunohistology of the nasal mucosa following allergen-induced rhinitis. Identification of activated T lymphocytes, eosinophils, and neutrophils. Am Rev Respir Dis 1992;146:170–6.
78. Naclerio RM. Allergic rhinitis. N Engl J Med 1991;325:860–9.
79. Bryan WTK, Bryan MP. Significance of mast cells in nasal secretions. Trans Am Acad Ophthalmol Otolaryngol 1959;63:613.
80. Okuda M, Otsuka M. Basophilic cells in allergic nasal secretions. Arch Otorhinolaryngol 1977;214:283–9.
81. Okuda M, Otsuka H, Kawabori S. Basophil leukocytes and mast cells in the nose. Eur J Respir Dis 1983;64:7–11.
82. Otsuka H, Denburg J, Dolovich J, et al. Heterogeneity of metachromatic cells in human nose: Significance of mucosal mast cells. J Allergy Clin Immunol 1985;76:695–702.
83. Enerback L, Pipkorn U, Granerus G. Intraepithelial migration of nasal mucosal mast cells in hay fever. Int Arch Allergy Appl Immunol 1986;80:44–51.
84. Bentley AM, Jacobson MR, Cumberworth V, et al. Immunohistology of the nasal mucosa in seasonal allergic rhinitis: Increases in activated eosinophils and epithelial mast cells. J Allergy Clin Immunol 1992;89:877–83.
85. Peters-Golden M, Henderson WR, Jr. The role of leukotrienes in allergic rhinitis. Ann Allergy Asthma Immunol 2005;94:609–18.
86. Kramer MF, Jordan TR, Klemens C, et al. Factors contributing to nasal allergic late phase eosinophilia. Am J Otolaryngol 2006;27:190–9.
87. Pease JE, Williams TJ. Chemokines and their receptors in allergic disease. J Allergy Clin Immunol 2006;118:305–18.
88. Fiset PO, Hamid Q. Chemokine expression in allergic diseases. J Allergy Clin Immunol 2006;118:536–8.
89. Pease JE. Asthma, allergy and chemokines. Curr Drug Targets 2006;7:3–12.
90. Lee BJ, Naclerio RM, Bochner BS, et al. Nasal challenge with allergen upregulates the local expression of vascular endothelial adhesion molecules. J Allergy Clin Immunol 1994;94:1006–16.
91. Walsh GM, Mermod JJ, Hartnell A, et al. Human eosinophil, but not neutrophil, adherence to IL-1-stimulated human umbilical vascular endothelial cells is alpha 4 beta 1 (very late antigen-4) dependent. J Immunol 1991;146:3419–23.
92. Schleimer RP, Sterbinsky SA, Kaiser J, et al. IL-4 induces adherence of human eosinophils and basophils but not neutrophils to endothelium. Association with expression of VCAM-1. J Immunol 1992;148:1086–92.
93. Ravensberg AJ, Luijk B, Westers P, et al. The effect of a single inhaled dose of a VLA-4 antagonist on allergen-induced airway responses and airway inflammation in patients with asthma. Allergy 2006;61:1097–103.
94. Diamant Z, Kuperus J, Baan R, et al. Effect of a very late antigen-4 receptor antagonist on allergen-induced airway responses and inflammation in asthma. Clin Exp Allergy 2005;35:1080–7.
95. Roebuck KA, Finnegan A. Regulation of intercellular adhesion molecule-1 (CD54) gene expression. J Leukoc Biol 1999;66:876–88.
96. Phillips ML, Nudelman E, Gaeta FC, et al. ELAM-1 mediates cell adhesion by recognition of a carbohydrate ligand, sialyl-Lex. Science 1990;250:1130–2
97. Ciprandi G, Pronzato C, Ricca V, et al. Allergen-specific challenge induces intercellular adhesion molecule 1 (ICAM-1 or CD54) on nasal epithelial cells in allergic subjects. Relationships with early and late inflammatory phenomena. Am J Respir Crit Care Med 1994;150:1653–9.
98. Ciprandi G, Buscaglia S, Pesce G, et al. Minimal persistent inflammation is present at mucosal level in patients with asymptomatic rhinitis and mite allergy. J Allergy Clin Immunol 1995;96:971–9.
99. Gorska-Ciebiada M, Ciebiada M, Gorska MM, et al. Intercellular adhesion molecule 1 and tumor necrosis factor alpha in asthma and persistent allergic rhinitis: Relationship with disease severity. Ann Allergy Asthma Immunol 2006;97:66–72.
100. Ciprandi G, Pronzato C, Passalacqua G, et al. Topical azelastine reduces eosinophil activation and intercellular adhesion molecule-1 expression on nasal epithelial cells: An antiallergic activity. J Allergy Clin Immunol 1996; 98:1088–96.
101. Figueroa DJ, Borish L, Baramki D, et al. Expression of cysteinyl leukotriene synthetic and signalling proteins in inflammatory cells in active seasonal allergic rhinitis. Clin Exp Allergy 2003;33:1380–8.
102. van Adelsberg J, Philip G, LaForce CF, et al. Montelukast Spring Rhinitis Investigator Group. Randomized controlled trial evaluating the clinical benefit of montelukast for treating spring seasonal allergic rhinitis. Ann Allergy Asthma Immunol 2003;90:214–22.
103. Patel P, Philip G, Yang W, et al. Randomized, double-blind, placebo-controlled study of montelukast for treating perennial allergic rhinitis. Ann Allergy Asthma Immunol 2005;95:551–7.
104. Walden SM, Proud D, Lichtenstein LM, et al. Antigen-provoked increase in histamine reactivity. Observations on mechanisms. Am Rev Respir Dis 1991;144:642–8.
105. Andersson M, Andersson P, Pipkorn U. Allergen-induced specific and non-specific nasal reactions: Reciprocal relationship and inhibition by topical glucocorticosteroids. Acta Otolaryngol (Stockh) 1989;107:270–7.
106. Baroody FM, Cruz AA, Lichtenstein LM, et al. Intranasal beclomethasone inhibits antigen-induced nasal hyperresponsiveness to histamine. J Allergy Clin Immunol 1992;90:373–6.
107. Majchel AM, Proud D, Freidhoff L, et al. The nasal response to histamine challenge: Effect of the pollen season and immunotherapy. J Allergy Clin Immunol 1992;90:85–91.
108. Druce HM, Wright RH, Kossoff D, Kaliner MA. Cholinergic nasal hyperreactivity in atopic subjects. J Allergy Clin Immunol 1985;76:445–52.
109. Klementsson H, Andersson M, Baumgarten CR, et al. Changes in non-specific nasal reactivity and eosinophil influx and activation after allergen challenge. Clin Exp Allergy 1990;20:539–47.
110. Klementsson H, Andersson M, Pipkorn U. Allergen-induced increase in nonspecific nasal reactivity is blocked by antihistamines without a clear-cut relationship to eosinophil influx. J Allergy Clin Immunol 1990;86:466–69.
111. Baroody FM, Lim MC, Proud D, et al. Effects of loratadine and terfenadine on the induced nasal allergic reaction. Arch Otolaryngol Head Neck Surg 1996;122:309–16.
112. Konno A, Togawa K. Role of the vidian nerve in nasal allergy. Ann Otol 1979;88:258.
113. Baroody FM, Ford S, Lichtenstein LM, et al. Physiologic responses and histamine release after nasal antigen challenge: Effect of atropine. Am J Respir Crit Care Med 1994;149:1457–65.
114. Raphael GD, Igarashi Y, White MV, Kaliner MA. The pathophysiology of rhinitis. V. Sources of protein in allergen-induced nasal secretions. J Allergy Clin Immunol 1991;88:33–37.
115. Wagenmann M, Baroody FM, Desrosiers M, et al. Unilateral nasal allergen challenge leads to bilateral release of prostaglandin D2. Clin Exp Allergy 1996;26:371–8.
116. Okayama M, Mullol J, Baraniuk JN, et al. Muscarinic receptor subtypes in human nasal mucosa: Characterization, autoradiographic localization, and function in vitro. Am J Respir Cell Mol Biol 1993;8:176–87.
117. Baraniuk JN, Lundgren JD, Mullol J, et al. Substance P and neurokinin A in human nasal mucosa. Am J Respir Cell Mol Biol 1991;4:228–36.
118. Okamoto Y, Shirotori K, Kudo K, et al. Cytokine expression after the topical administration of substance P to human nasal mucosa. The role of substance P in nasal allergy. J Immunol 1993;151:4391–8.
119. Mosimann BL, White MV, Hohman RJ, et al. Substance P, calcitonin gene-related peptide, and vasoactive intestinal peptide increase in nasal secretions after allergen challenge in atopic patients. J Allergy Clin Immunol 1993;92:95–04.
120. Philip G, Sanico AM, Togias A. Inflammatory cellular influx follows capsaicin nasal challenge. Am J Respir Crit Care Med 1996;153:1222–9.
121. Philip G, Baroody FM, Proud D, et al. The human nasal response to capsaicin. J Allergy Clin Immunol 1994;94:1035–45.
122. Stjarne P, Rinder J, Heden-Blomquist E, et al. Capsaicin desensitization of the nasal mucosa reduces symptoms upon

allergen challenge in patients with allergic rhinitis. Acta Otolaryngol 1998;118:235–9.

123. Chen Y, Kuchroo VK, Inobe J, et al. Regulatory T cell clones induced by oral tolerance: Suppression of autoimmune encephalomyelitis. Science 1994;265:1237–40.

124. Akdis M, Blaser K, Akdis CA. T regulatory cells in allergy: Novel concepts in the pathogenesis, prevention, and treatment of allergic diseases. J Allergy Clin Immunol 2005;116:961–8.

125. Emanuel IA, Shah SB. Chronic rhinosinusitis: Allergy and sinus computed tomography relationships. Otolaryngol Head Neck Surg 2000;123:687–91.

126. Friedman WH. Surgery for chronic hyperplastic rhinosinusitis. Laryngoscope 1975;85:1999–2011.

127. Holzmann D, Willi U, Nadal D. Allergic rhinitis as a risk factor for orbital complication of acute rhinosinusitis in children. Am J Rhinol 2001;15:387–90.

128. Chen CF, Wu KG, Hsu MC, Tang RB. Prevalence and relationship between allergic diseases and infectious diseases. J Microbiol Immunol Infect 2001;34:57–62.

129. Walker C, Williams H, Phelan J. Allergic rhinitis history as a predictor of other future disqualifying otorhinolaryngological defects. Aviat Space Environ Med 1998;69:952–6.

130. Berrettini S, Carabelli A, Sellari-Franceschini S, et al. Perennial allergic rhinitis and chronic sinusitis: Correlation with rhinologic risk factors. Allergy 1999;54:242–8.

131. Conner BL, Roach ES, Laster WS, Georgitis JW. Magnetic resonance imaging of the paranasal sinuses: Frequency and type of abnormalities. Ann Allergy 1989;62:457–60.

132. Naclerio RM, DeTineo ML, Baroody FM. Ragweed allergic rhinitis and the paranasal sinuses: A computed tomographic study. Arch Otolaryngol Head Neck Surg 1997;123:193–6.

133. Alho OP, Karttunen TJ, Karttunen R. Subjects with allergic rhinitis show signs of more severely impaired paranasal sinus functioning during viral colds than nonallergic subjects. Allergy 2003;58:767–71.

134. Baroody FM, DeTineo M, Haney L, et al. Influx of eosinophils into the maxillary sinus after nasal challenge with allergen. J Allergy Clin Immunol 2000;105:S70.

135. Greenberger PA. Interactions between rhinitis and asthma. Allergy Asthma Proc 2004;25:89–93.

136. Corren JAD, Adinoff AD, Buchmeier AD, Irvin CG. Nasal beclomethasone prevents the seasonal increase in bronchial hyperresponsiveness in patients with allergic rhinitis and asthma. J Allergy Clin Immunol 1992;90:250–6.

137. Thio BJ, Slingerland GL, Fredriks AM, et al. Influence of intranasal steroids during the grass pollen season on bronchial responsiveness in children and young adults with asthma and hay fever. Thorax 2000;55:826–32.

138. Greiff L, Andersson M, Svensson C, et al. Effects of orally inhaled budesonide in seasonal allergic rhinitis. Eur Respir J 1998;11:1268–73.

139. Braunstahl GJ, Kleinjan A, Overbeek SE, et al. Segmental bronchial provocation induces nasal inflammation in allergic rhinitis patients. Am J Respir Crit Care Med 2000;161:2051–7.

140. Assanasen P, Baroody FM, Naureckas E, et al. The nasal passage of subjects with asthma has a decreased ability to warm and humidify inspired air. Am J Respir Crit Care Med 2001;164:1640–6.

141. Pinto JM, Assanasen P, Baroody FM, et al. Treatment of nasal inflammation decreases the ability of subjects with asthma to condition inspired air. Am J Respir Crit Care Med 2004;170:863–9.

142. Assanasen P, Baroody FM, Abbott DJ, et al. Natural and induced allergic responses increase the ability of the nose to warm and humidify air. J Allergy Clin Immunol 2000;106:1045–52.

143. Bonay M, Neukirch C, Grandsaigne M, et al. Changes in airway inflammation following nasal allergic challenge in patients with seasonal rhinitis. Allergy 2006;61:111–8.

144. Silvestri M, Battistini E, Defilippi AC, et al. Early decrease in nasal eosinophil proportion after nasal allergen challenge correlates with baseline bronchial reactivity to methacholine in children sensitized to house dust mites. J Investig Allergol Clin Immunol 2005;15:266–76.

145. Taramarcaz P, Gibson PG. Intranasal corticosteroids for asthma control in people with coexisting asthma and rhinitis. Cochrane Database Syst Rev 2003;CD003570.

146. Doyle WJ, Friedman R, Fireman P, Bluestone CD. Eustachian tube obstruction after provocative nasal antigen challenge. Arch Otolaryngol 1984;110:508–11.

147. Nguyen LH, Manoukian JJ, Sobol SE, et al. Similar allergic inflammation in the middle ear and the upper airway: Evidence linking otitis media with effusion to the united airways concept. J Allergy Clin Immunol 2004;114:1110–5.

148. Stuck BA, Czajkowski J, Hagner AE, et al. Changes in daytime sleepiness, quality of life, and objective sleep patterns

in seasonal allergic rhinitis: A controlled clinical trial. J Allergy Clin Immunol 2004;113:663–8.

149. Bonini S. Allergic conjunctivitis: The forgotten disease. Chem Immunol Allergy 2006;91:110–20.

150. Rogers CA, Wayne PM, Macklin EA, et al. Interaction of the onset of spring and elevated atmospheric CO_2 on ragweed (*Ambrosia artemisiifolia* L.) pollen production. Environ Health Perspect 2006;114:865–9.

151. Plotz SG, Traidl-Hoffmann C, Feussner I, et al. Chemotaxis and activation of human peripheral blood eosinophils induced by pollen-associated lipid mediators. J Allergy Clin Immunol 2004;113:1152–60.

152. Arlian LG, Neal JS, Morgan MS, et al. Reducing relative humidity is a practical way to control dust mites and their allergens in homes in temperate climates. J Allergy Clin Immunol 2001;107:99–104.

153. Gotzsche PC, Johansen HK, Schmidt LM, Burr ML. House dust mite control measures for asthma. Cochrane Database Syst Rev. 2004:CD001187.

154. Almqvist C, Larsson PH, Egmar AC, et al. School as a risk environment for children allergic to cats and a site for transfer of cat allergen to homes. J Allergy Clin Immunol 1999;103:1012–7.

155. Bousquet J, Flahault A, Vandenplas O, et al. Natural rubber latex allergy among health care workers: A systematic review of the evidence. J Allergy Clin Immunol 2006;118:447–54.

156. Rueff F, Schopf P, Putz K, Przybilla B. Effect of reduced exposure on natural rubber latex sensitization in health care workers. Ann Allergy Asthma Immunol 2004;92:530–7.

157. Demoly P, Allaert FA, Lecasble M, Bousquet J. PRAGMA. Validation of the classification of ARIA (allergic rhinitis and its impact on asthma). Allergy 2003;58:672–5.

158. Van Hoecke H, Vastesaeger N, Dewulf L, et al. Is the allergic rhinitis and its impact on asthma classification useful in daily primary care practice? J Allergy Clin Immunol 2006;118:758–9.

159. Settipane GA. Aspirin and allergic diseases: A review. Am J Med 1983;74:102–9.

160. Carr WW, Martin B, Howard RS, et al. Immunotherapy Committee of the American Academy of Allergy, Asthma and Immunology. Comparison of test devices for skin prick testing. J Allergy Clin Immunol 2005;116:341–6.

161. Menardo JL et al. Skin test reactivity in infancy. J Allergy Clin Immunol 1985;75:646–51.

162. Ownby DR. Allergy testing: In vivo versus in vitro. Pediatr Clin North Am 1988;35:995–09.

163. Corey JP, Mamikoglu B, Akbar I, et al. ImmunoCAP and HY*TEC enzyme immunoassays in the detection of allergen-specific IgE compared with serial skin end-point titration by receiver operating characteristic analysis. Otolaryngol Head Neck Surg 2000;122:64–70.

164. Meltzer E, Orgel HA, Jalowayski A. Nasal cytology. In: Naclerio RM, Durham SR, Mygind N, editors. Rhinitis Mechanisms and Management. New York: Marcel Dekker; 1999. p. 175–202.

165. Bachert C. Persistent rhinitis—allergic or nonallergic? Allergy 2004;59:11–5.

166. Arshad SH. Primary prevention of asthma and allergy. J Allergy Clin Immunol 2005;116:3–14.

167. Arlian LG, Vyszenski-Moher DL, Morgan MS. Mite and mite allergen removal during machine washing of laundry. J Allergy Clin Immunol 2003;111:1269–73.

168. Terreehorst I, Hak E, Oosting AJ, et al. Evaluation of impermeable covers for bedding in patients with allergic rhinitis. N Engl J Med 2003;349:237–46.

169. Nageotte C, Park M, Havstad S, et al. Duration of airborne Fel d 1 reduction after cat washing. J Allergy Clin Immunol 2006;118:521–2.

170. Ritz BR, Hoelscher B, Frye C, et al. Allergic sensitization owing to 'second-hand' cat exposure in schools. Allergy 2002;57:357–61.

171. Reisman RE, Mauriello PM, Davis GB, et al. A double-blind study of the effectiveness of a high-efficiency particulate air (HEPA) filter in the treatment of patients with perennial allergic rhinitis and asthma. J Allergy Clin Immunol 1990;85:1050–7.

172. Bousquet J, van Cauwenberge P, Ait Khaled N, et al. Pharmacologic and anti-IgE treatment of allergic rhinitis ARIA update (in collaboration with GALEN).Allergy 2006;61:1086–96.

173. Goldman DP, Joyce GF, Escarce JJ, et al. Pharmacy benefits and the use of drugs by the chronically ill. JAMA 2004;291:2344–50.

174. Parsons ME, Ganellin CR. Histamine and its receptors. Br J Pharmacol 2006;147:S127–35.

175. Wilken JA, Kane RL, Ellis AK, et al. A comparison of the effect of diphenhydramine and desloratadine on vigilance and cognitive function during treatment of ragweed-induced

allergic rhinitis. Ann Allergy Asthma Immunol 2003; 91:375–85.

176. Raphael GD, Angello JT, Wu MM, Druce HM. Efficacy of diphenhydramine vs desloratadine and placebo in patients with moderate-to-severe seasonal allergic rhinitis. Ann Allergy Asthma Immunol 2006;96:606–14.

177. Weiler JM, Bloomfield JR, Woodworth GG, et al. Effects of fexofenadine, diphenhydramine, and alcohol on driving performance. A randomized, placebo-controlled trial in the Iowa driving simulator. Ann Intern Med 2000;312:354–63.

178. Bender BG, Berning S, Dudden R, et al. Sedation and performance impairment of diphenhydramine and second-generation antihistamines: A meta-analysis. J Allergy Clin Immunol 2003;111:770–6.

179. Togias AG, Naclerio RM, Warner J, et al. Demonstration of inhibition of mediator release from human mast cells by azatadine base. In vivo and in vitro evaluation. JAMA 1986;255:225–9.

180. Naclerio RM, Kagey-Sobotka A, Lichtenstein LM, et al. Terfenadine, an H_1 antihistamine, inhibits histamine release in vivo in the human. Am Rev Respir Dis 1990;142:167–71.

181. Naclerio RM, Proud D, Kagey-Sobotka A, et al. The effect of cetirizine on early allergic response. Laryngoscope 1989;99:596–9.

182. Saengpanich S, Assanasen P, deTineo M, et al. Effects of intranasal azelastine on the response to nasal allergen challenge. Laryngoscope 2002;112:47–52.

183. Campbell A, Chanal I, Czarlewski W, et al. Reduction of soluble ICAM-1 levels in nasal secretion by H1-blockers in seasonal allergic rhinitis. Allergy 1997;52:1022–5.

184. Ciprandi G, Cirillo I, Vizzaccaro A, Tosca MA. Levocetirizine improves nasal obstruction and modulates cytokine pattern in patients with seasonal allergic rhinitis: A pilot study. Clin Exp Allergy 2004;34:958–64.

185. Shirasaki H, Watanabe K, Kanaizumi E, et al. Effects of cetirizine on substance P release in patients with perennial allergic rhinitis. Ann Otol Rhinol Laryngol 2004; 113:941–5.

186. Shon JH, Yoon YR, Hong WS, et al. Effect of itraconazole on the pharmacokinetics and pharmacodynamics of fexofenadine in relation to the MDR1 genetic polymorphism. Clin Pharmacol Ther 2005;78:191–201.

187. Nelson HS. Advances in upper airway diseases and allergen immunotherapy. J Allergy Clin Immunol 2006; 117:1047–53.

188. McNeely W, Wiseman LR. Intranasal azelastine. A review of its efficacy in the management of allergic rhinitis. Drugs 1998;56:91–114.

189. Meltzer EO, Hampel FC, Ratner PH, et al. Safety and efficacy of olopatadine hydrochloride nasal spray for the treatment of seasonal allergic rhinitis. Ann Allergy Asthma Immunol 2005;95:600–6.

190. Bousquet J, Duchateau J, Pignat JC, et al. Improvement of quality of life by treatment with cetirizine in patients with perennial allergic rhinitis as determined by a French version of the SF-36 questionnaire. J Allergy Clin Immunol 1996;98:309–16.

191. Meltzer EO, Casale TB, Nathan RA, Thompson AK. Once-daily fexofenadine HCl improves quality of life and reduces work and activity impairment in patients with seasonal allergic rhinitis. Ann Allergy Asthma Immunol 1999;83:311–7.

192. Meltzer EO, Jalowayski AA, Vogt K, et al. Effect of desloratadine therapy on symptom scores and measures of nasal patency in seasonal allergic rhinitis: Results of a single-center, placebo-controlled trial. Ann Allergy Asthma Immunol 2006;96:363–8.

193. Majchel AM, Proud D, Kagey-Sobotka A, et al. Evaluation of a bedtime dose of a combination antihistamine/analgesic/decongestant product on antigen challenge the next morning. Laryngoscope 1992;102:330–4.

194. Rhen T, Cidlowski JA. Antiinflammatory action of glucocorticoids–new mechanisms for old drugs. N Engl J Med 2005;353:1711–23.

195. Goulding NJ. The molecular complexity of glucocorticoid actions in inflammation—a four-ring circus. Curr Opin Pharmacol 2004;4:629–36.

196. Holm A, Dijkstra M, Kleinjan A, et al. Fluticasone propionate aqueous nasal spray reduces inflammatory cells in unchallenged allergic nasal mucosa: Effects of single allergen challenge. J Allergy Clin Immunol 2001;107:627–33.

197. Pipkorn U, Proud D, Lichtenstein LM, et al. Inhibition of mediator release in allergic rhinitis by pretreatment with topical glucocorticosteroids. N Engl J Med 1987; 316:1506–10.

198. Benson M, Strannegard IL, Strannegard O, Wennergren G. Topical steroid treatment of allergic rhinitis decreases nasal fluid TH2 cytokines, eosinophils, eosinophil cationic protein, and IgE but has no significant effect on IFN-gamma,

IL-1beta, TNF-alpha, or neutrophils. J Allergy Clin Immunol 2000;106:307–12.
199. Erin EM, Zacharasiewicz AS, Nicholson GC, et al. Topical corticosteroid inhibits interleukin-4, -5 and -13 in nasal secretions following allergen challenge. Clin Exp Allergy 2005;35:1608–14.
200. Kaiser HB, Liao Y, Diener P, et al. Triamcinolone acetonide and fluticasone propionate nasal sprays provide comparable relief of seasonal allergic rhinitis symptoms regardless of disease severity. Allergy Asthma Proc 2004;25:423–8.
201. Gurevich F, Glass C, Davies M, et al. The effect of intranasal steroid budesonide on the congestion-related sleep disturbance and daytime somnolence in patients with perennial allergic rhinitis. Allergy Asthma Proc 2005;26:268–74.
202. Naclerio RM, Adkinson NF, Jr, Creticos PS, et al. Intranasal steroids inhibit seasonal increases in ragweed-specific immunoglobulin E antibodies. J Allergy Clin Immunol 1993;92:717–21.
203. Juniper EF, Guyatt GH, O'Byrne PM, Viveiros M. Aqueous beclomethasone diproprionate nasal spray: Regular versus "as required" use in the treatment of seasonal allergic rhinitis. J Allergy Clin Immunol 1990;86:380–6.
204. Jen A, Baroody F, de Tineo M, et al. As-needed use of fluticasone propionate nasal spray reduces symptoms of seasonal allergic rhinitis. J Allergy Clin Immunol 2000;105:732–8.
205. Dykewicz MS, Kaiser HB, Nathan RA, et al. Fluticasone propionate aqueous nasal spray improves nasal symptoms of seasonal allergic rhinitis when used as needed (prn). Ann Allergy Asthma Immunol 2003;91:44–8.
206. Kaszuba SM, Baroody FM, deTineo M, et al. Superiority of an intranasal corticosteroid compared with an oral antihistamine in the as-needed treatment of seasonal allergic rhinitis. Arch Intern Med 2001;161:2581–7.
207. Sahay JN, Ibrahim NB, Chatterjee SS, et al. Long-term study of flunisolide treatment in perennial rhinitis with special reference to nasal mucosal histology and morphology. Clin Allergy 1980;10:451–7.
208. Orgel HA, Meltzer EO, Bierman CW. Intranasal fluorocortin butyl in patients with perennial rhinitis: A 12 month efficacy and safety study including nasal biopsy. J Allergy Clin Immunol 1991;88:257–64.
209. Sorenson H, Mygind N, Pedersen C, Prytz S. Long term treatment of nasal polyps with beclomethasone dipropionate aerosol. III. Morphological studies and conclusions. Acta Otolaryngol (Stockh) 1976;182:260–2.
210. Agertoft L, Pedersen S. Effect of long-term treatment with inhaled budesonide on adult height in children with asthma. N Engl J Med 2000;343:1064–9.
211. Skoner DP, Rachelefsky GS, Meltzer EO, et al. Detection of growth suppression in children during treatment with intranasal beclomethasone dipropionate. Pediatrics 2000;105: E23. Available at http://www.pediatrics.org/cgi/content/full/105/2/e23.
212. Allen DB, Meltzer EO, Lemanske RF, Jr, et al. No growth suppression in children treated with the maximum recommended dose of fluticasone propionate aqueous nasal spray for one year. Allergy Asthma Proc 2002;23:407–13.
213. Schenkel EJ, Skoner DP, Bronsky EA, et al. Absence of growth retardation in children with perennial allergic rhinitis after one year of treatment with mometasone furoate aqueous nasal spray. Pediatrics 2000;105:E22. Available at http://www.pediatrics.org/cgi/content/full/105/2/e22.
214. Daley-Yates PT, Richards DH. Relationship between systemic corticosteroid exposure and growth velocity: Development and validation of a pharmacokinetic/pharmacodynamic model. Clin Ther 2004;26:1905–19.
215. Murphy K, Uryniak T, Simpson B, O'Dowd L. Growth velocity in children with perennial allergic rhinitis treated with budesonide aqueous nasal spray. Ann Allergy Asthma Immunol 2006;96:723–30.
216. Suissa S, Baltzan M, Kremer R, Ernst P. Inhaled and nasal corticosteroid use and the risk of fracture. Am J Respir Crit Care Med 2004;169:83–8.
217. Derby L, Maier WC. Risk of cataract among users of intranasal corticosteroids. J Allergy Clin Immunol 2000; 105:912–6.
218. Bielory L, Blaiss M, Fineman SM, et al. Joint Task Force of the American Academy of Allergy, Asthma and Immunology; American College of Allergy, Asthma and Immunology. Concerns about intranasal corticosteroids for over-the-counter use: Position statement of the Joint Task Force for the American Academy of Allergy, Asthma and Immunology and the American College of Allergy, Asthma and Immunology. Ann Allergy Asthma Immunol 2006;96:514–25.
219. Bhatia S, Baroody FM, deTineo M, Naclerio RM. Increased nasal airflow with budesonide compared with desloratadine during the allergy season. Arch Otolaryngol Head Neck Surg 2005;131:223–8.
220. Saengpanich S, deTineo M, Naclerio RM, Baroody FM. Fluticasone nasal spray and the combination of loratadine and montelukast in seasonal allergic rhinitis. Arch Otolaryngol Head Neck Surg 2003;129:557–62.
221. Bernstein DI, Levy AL, Hampel FC, et al. Treatment with intranasal fluticasone propionate significantly improves ocular symptoms in patients with seasonal allergic rhinitis. Clin Exp Allergy 2004;34:952–7.
222. DeWester J, Philpot EE, Westlund RE, et al. The efficacy of intranasal fluticasone propionate in the relief of ocular symptoms associated with seasonal allergic rhinitis. Allergy Asthma Proc 2003;24:331–7.
223. Stokes M, Amorosi SL, Thompson D, et al. Evaluation of patients' preferences for triamcinolone acetonide aqueous, fluticasone propionate, and mometasone furoate nasal sprays in patients with allergic rhinitis. Otolaryngol Head Neck Surg 2004;131:225–31.
224. Meltzer EO, Bardelas J, Goldsobel A, Kaiser H. A preference evaluation study comparing the sensory attributes of mometasone furoate and fluticasone propionate nasal sprays by patients with allergic rhinitis. Treat Respir Med 2005;4:289–96.
225. Mygind N. Glucocorticosteroids and rhinitis. Allergy 1993;48:476–90.
226. Hissaria P, Smith W, Wormald PJ, et al. Short course of systemic corticosteroids in sinonasal polyposis: A double-blind, randomized, placebo-controlled trial with evaluation of outcome measures. J Allergy Clin Immunol 2006;118:128–33.
227. Ostergaard MS, Ostrem A, Soderstrom M. Hay fever and a single intramuscular injection of corticosteroid: A systematic review. Prim Care Respir J 2005;14:124–30.
228. Keles N. Treatment of allergic rhinitis during pregnancy. Am J Rhinol 2004;18:23–8.
229. Lange B, Lukat KF, Rettig K, et al. Efficacy, cost-effectiveness, and tolerability of mometasone furoate, levocabastine, and disodium cromoglycate nasal sprays in the treatment of seasonal allergic rhinitis. Ann Allergy Asthma Immunol 2005;95:272–82.
230. Bonadonna P, Senna G, Zanon P, et al. Cold-induced rhinitis in skiers–clinical aspects and treatment with ipratropium bromide nasal spray: A randomized controlled trial. Am J Rhinol 2001;15:297–301.
231. Kim KT, Kerwin E, Landwehr L, et al. Pediatric Atrovent Nasal Spray Study Group. Use of 0.06% ipratropium bromide nasal spray in children aged 2–5 years with rhinorrhea due to a common cold or allergies. Ann Allergy Asthma Immunol 2005;94:73–9.
232. Kemp JP. Recent advances in the management of asthma using leukotriene modifiers. Am J Respir Med 2003;2:139–56.
233. Wilson AM, O'Byrne PM, Parameswaran K. Leukotriene receptor antagonists for allergic rhinitis: A systematic review and meta-analysis. Am J Med 2004;116:338–44.
234. Mucha SM, deTineo M, Naclerio RM, Baroody FM. Comparison of montelukast and pseudoephedrine in the treatment of allergic rhinitis. Arch Otolaryngol Head Neck Surg 2006;132:164–72.
235. Chen ST, Lu KH, Sun HL, et al. Randomized placebo-controlled trial comparing montelukast and cetirizine for treating perennial allergic rhinitis in children aged 2–6 yr. Pediatr Allergy Immunol 2006;17:49–54.
236. Kurowski M, Kuna P, Gorski P. Montelukast plus cetirizine in the prophylactic treatment of seasonal allergic rhinitis: Influence on clinical symptoms and nasal allergic inflammation. Allergy 2004;59:280–8.
237. Moinuddin R, deTineo M, Maleckar B, et al. Comparison of the combinations of fexofenadine–pseudoephedrine and loratadine-montelukast in the treatment of seasonal allergic rhinitis. Ann Allergy Asthma Immunol 2004;92:73–9.
238. Lee DK, Jackson CM, Soutar PC, et al. Effects of single or combined histamine H1-receptor and leukotriene CysLT1-receptor antagonism on nasal adenosine monophosphate challenge in persistent allergic rhinitis. Br J Clin Pharmacol 2004;57:714–9.
239. Di Lorenzo G, Pacor ML, Pellitteri ME, et al. Randomized placebo-controlled trial comparing fluticasone aqueous nasal spray in mono-therapy, fluticasone plus cetirizine, fluticasone plus montelukast and cetirizine plus montelukast for seasonal allergic rhinitis. Clin Exp Allergy 2004; 34:259–67. Erratum in: Clin Exp Allergy 2004;34:1329.
240. Till SJ, Francis JN, Nouri-Aria K, Durham SR. Mechanisms of immunotherapy. J Allergy Clin Immunol 2004;113:1025–34.
241. Akdis CA, Barlan IB, Bahceciler N, Akdis M. Immunological mechanisms of sublingual immunotherapy. Allergy 2006;61:11–4.
242. Jutel M, Akdis M, Blaser K, Akdis CA. Mechanisms of allergen specific immunotherapy–T-cell tolerance and more. Allergy 2006;61:796–807.
243. Moller C, Dreborg S, Ferdousi HA, et al. Pollen immunotherapy reduces the development of asthma in children with seasonal rhinoconjunctivitis (the PAT-study). J Allergy Clin Immunol 2002;109:251–6.
244. Norman PS. Immunotherapy: 1999–2004. J Allergy Clin Immunol 2004;113:1013–23.
245. Durham SR, Walker SM, Varga EM, et al. Long-term clinical efficacy of grass-pollen immunotherapy. N Engl J Med 1999;341:468–75.
246. Eng PA, Reinhold M, Gnehm HP. Long-term efficacy of preseasonal grass pollen immunotherapy in children. Allergy 2002;57:306–12.
247. Reid MJ, Lockey RF, Turkeltaub PC, Platts-Mills TA. Survey of fatalities from skin testing and immunotherapy 1985–1989. J Allergy Clin Immunol 1993;92:6–15.
248. Bernstein DI, Wanner M, Borish L, Liss GM. Immunotherapy Committee, American Academy of Allergy, Asthma and Immunology. Twelve-year survey of fatal reactions to allergen injections and skin testing: 1990–2001. J Allergy Clin Immunol 2004;113:1129–36.
249. Wilson DR, Lima MT, Durham SR. Sublingual immunotherapy for allergic rhinitis: Systematic review and meta-analysis. Allergy 2005;60:4–12.
250. Bahceciler NN, Arikan C, Taylor A, et al. Impact of sublingual immunotherapy on specific antibody levels in asthmatic children allergic to house dust mites. Int Arch Allergy Immunol 2005;136:287–94.
251. Passalacqua G, Villa G, Altrinetti V, et al. Sublingual swallow or spit? Allergy 2001;56:578.
252. Moingeon P, Batard T, Fadel R, et al. Immune mechanisms of allergen-specific sublingual immunotherapy. Allergy 2006;61:151–65.
253. Burastero SE. Sublingual immunotherapy for allergic rhinitis: An update. Curr Opin Otolaryngol Head Neck Surg 2006;14:197–201.
254. Mahler V, Vrtala S, Kuss O, et al. Vaccines for birch pollen allergy based on genetically engineered hypoallergenic derivatives of the major birch pollen allergen, Bet v 1. Clin Exp Allergy 2004;34:115–22.
255. Bez C, Schubert R, Kopp M, et al. Effect of anti-immunoglobulin E on nasal inflammation in patients with seasonal allergic rhinoconjunctivitis. Clin Exp Allergy 2004; 34:1079–85.
256. Holgate S, Casale T, Wenzel S, et al. The anti-inflammatory effects of omalizumab confirm the central role of IgE in allergic inflammation. J Allergy Clin Immunol 2005; 115:459–65.
257. Beck LA, Marcotte GV, MacGlashan D, et al. Omalizumab-induced reductions in mast cell Fce psilon RI expression and function. J Allergy Clin Immunol 2004;114:527–30.
258. Chervinsky P, Casale T, Townley R, et al. Omalizumab, an anti-IgE antibody, in the treatment of adults and adolescents with perennial allergic rhinitis. Ann Allergy Asthma Immunol 2003;91:160–7.
259. Casale TB, Busse WW, Kline JN, et al. Immune Tolerance Network Group. Omalizumab pretreatment decreases acute reactions after rush immunotherapy for ragweed-induced seasonal allergic rhinitis. J Allergy Clin Immunol 2006;117:134–40.
260. Rolinck-Werninghaus C, Wolf H, Liebke C, et al. A prospective, randomized, double-blind, placebo-controlled multi-centre study on the efficacy and safety of sublingual immunotherapy (SLIT) in children with seasonal allergic rhinoconjunctivitis to grass pollen. Allergy 2004; 59:1285–93.
261. Blaiss MS. Food and Drug Administration (US); ACAAI-ACOG (American College of Allergy, Asthma, and Immunology and American College of Obstetricians and Gynecologists). Management of rhinitis and asthma in pregnancy. Ann Allergy Asthma Immunol 2003;90:16–22.
262. Gluck PA, Gluck JC. A review of pregnancy outcomes after exposure to orally inhaled or intranasal budesonide. Curr Med Res Opin 2005;21:1075–84.

44

Epistaxis

Thomas A. Tami, MD
James A. Merrell, MD

Epistaxis is one of the most common otolaryngologic emergencies. Although the lifetime incidence of epistaxis is approximately 60%, only about 6% require formal medical intervention. Of these episodes of epistaxis, 10% can be serious and even life threatening. The nature and causes of the epistaxis vary with age. Since epistaxis may be a symptom of systemic disorders, all patients with epistaxis should undergo a careful medical evaluation.

ETIOLOGY

The causes of epistaxis are varied (Table 1), and both local and systemic factors may contribute. Several factors which have been shown to correlate strongly with epistaxis include: the season of year (winter being most common); sex (more common in males); age (epistaxis in the younger patient tends to be anterior and more minor

Table 1 Factors Contributing to Epistaxis

Local
  Desiccation
    Low ambient humidity
    Decreased nasal secretions (drug effects, systemic
      illnesses such as Sjögren disease)
  Trauma
    External
    Internal (digital)
  Neoplasms
    Juvenile nasopharyngeal angiofibroma
    Inverted papilloma
    Carcinoma
  Foreign body
  Chronic inflammation
    Infections
    Septal perforation
    Atrophic rhinitis
Systemic
  Coagulopathy
    Anticoagulation (aspirin, warfarin, antiplatelet
      drugs)
    Hepatic disease
    Thrombocytopenia
    Liver disease
    Hemophilia
  Hereditary hemorrhagic telangiectasia
  Systemic inflammatory disorders
    Wegener granulomatosis
    Sarcoidosis
    Churg-Strauss syndrome

whereas the more severe posterior epistaxis tends to be seen in those greater than 50 years of age). Hypertension is common in the older population, and while it has been associated with epistaxis, no causal relationship has been proven.[1]

RELEVANT ANATOMY

The nasal cavity is supplied by several arteries with extensive anastomotic connections. The primary sources include the external carotid artery with the branches being the facial artery giving off the lateral nasal and septal branches and the internal maxillary artery (IMA) giving off the sphenopalatine and lateral nasal and septal branches. There are also contributions from the posterior pharyngeal and greater palatine arteries of the external carotid system. The internal carotid artery supplies much of the superior portion of the nasal cavity via the anterior and posterior ethmoid arteries, which most often are terminal branches of the ophthalmic artery. There are 2 main areas in the nose where there are well-recognized confluences of anastomotic connections. These include the area on the anteroinferior part of the septum, "Little area" or "Kiesselbach plexus," and "Woodruff plexus" in the posterior part of the nasal cavity.

Little was an American physician who, in 1879, described 4 cases of epistaxis in which there was "an ulcer on the septum half an inch from the lower edge of the middle of the columella." Subsequent anatomical studies have clarified the anatomic detail of the anterior part of the nasal septum, clearly demonstrating that in most cases there were 3 dominant arteries supplying this region forming an anastomotic triangle of large thin-walled vessels as a dominant arterial arcade in the anterior part of the septum. The feeding arteries were found to be the middle septal branch of the sphenopalatine artery (SPA) posteriorly, the anterior ethmoidal artery from above and the superior labial branch of the facial artery anteriorly. The anastomotic vessels of the anterior septal triangle also seemed to be thinner-walled compared to the feeding arteries[2] (Figure 1).

Posteriorly on the lateral nasal wall is the area known as Woodruff plexus at the posterior end of the inferior turbinate where the sphenopalatine

and posterior pharyngeal arteries anastomose. Ninety percent of the nasal mucosa receives its blood supply via the SPA.[3] The SPA enters the nasal cavity through the sphenopalatine foramen located on the lateral nasal wall within the superior meatus, usually, between the middle turbinate and the posterior horizontal end of the lamella of the superior turbinate (Figure 2). Generally this is just above the posterior end of the horizontal lamella of the middle turbinate and just posterior to the ethmoidal crest off the perpendicular plate of the palatine bone. The sphenopalatine foramen is bounded superiorly by the body of the sphenoid, the anterior border is the orbital process of the palatine bone, the sphenoidal process of the palatine bone forms the posterior border, and the inferior border is the perpendicular plate of the palatine bone. In most cases the SPA divides into 2 major branches. These 2 major branches are the nasal septal branch and the posterior lateral nasal artery. The nasal septal artery crosses the lower portion of the anterior wall of the sphenoid sinus and runs toward the septum within the mucosa. It then supplies most of the posterior septum. This artery may cause profuse arterial bleeding if it is damaged when performing a sphenoidotomy since it usually lies just inferior to the sphenoid ostium. The posterior lateral nasal artery supplies the majority of the mucosa of the lateral nasal wall. It courses downward on the perpendicular plate of the palatine bone giving off major branches to the inferior and middle turbinates. Occasionally, the branch to the superior turbinate arises from the septal artery.[4,5]

The nasal cavity also receives blood supply via the anterior and posterior ethmoid arteries. These are branches of the ophthalmic artery of the internal carotid system. The anterior ethmoid supplies much of the anterior portion of the nasal cavity including both the septum as well as the anterior part of the lateral nasal wall. The posterior ethmoid supplies part of the superior turbinate as well as portions of the septum. Both arteries anastamose with end branches of the SPA and with the sublabial artery arising from the facial artery. The anterior and posterior ethmoid arteries are terminal branches of the ophthalmic artery. They exit the orbit medially at the superior portion of the lamina papyracea at the level of the cribriform plate through foramina in the frontoethmoid suture. There is

Nasal septal vasculature

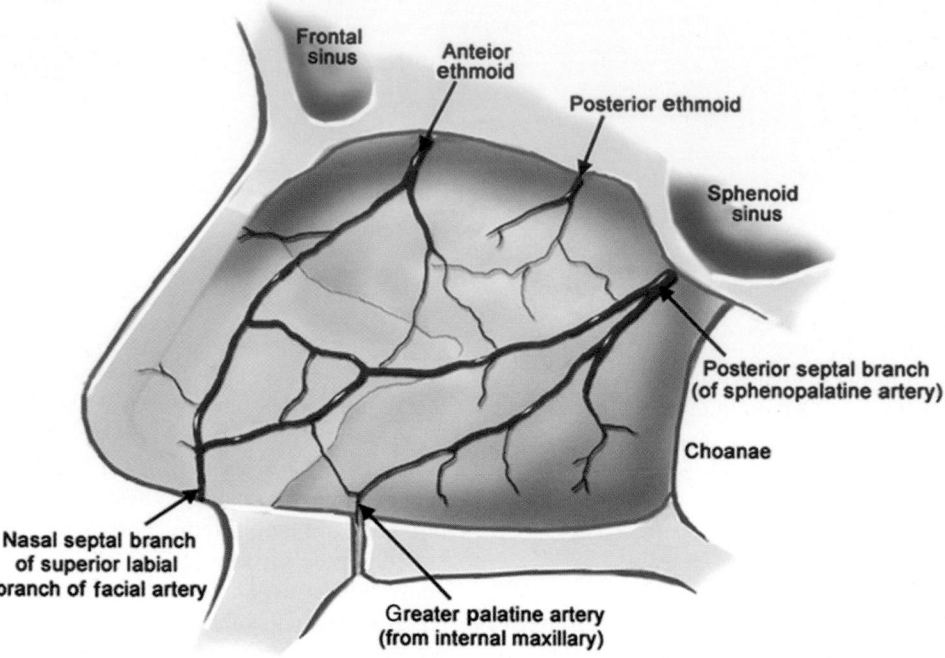

Figure 1 Vasculature of the medial (septal) wall of the nasal cavity.

variation in the exact locations of the foramina; however, the anterior ethmoid artery is generally found approximately 13 to 18 mm posterior to the frontomaxillolacrimal suture, and the posterior ethmoid artery is another 10 to 13 mm posterior to the anterior and is only about 4 to 7 mm anterior to the optic nerve. The ethmoid arteries then traverse the superior portion of the ethmoid

air cells along the roof and supply the superior portion of the nasal cavity.

CLINICAL AND LABORATORY EVALUATIONS

The approach to the patient with epistaxis begins with the initial evaluation. If bleeding has been

Lateral nasal wall vasculature

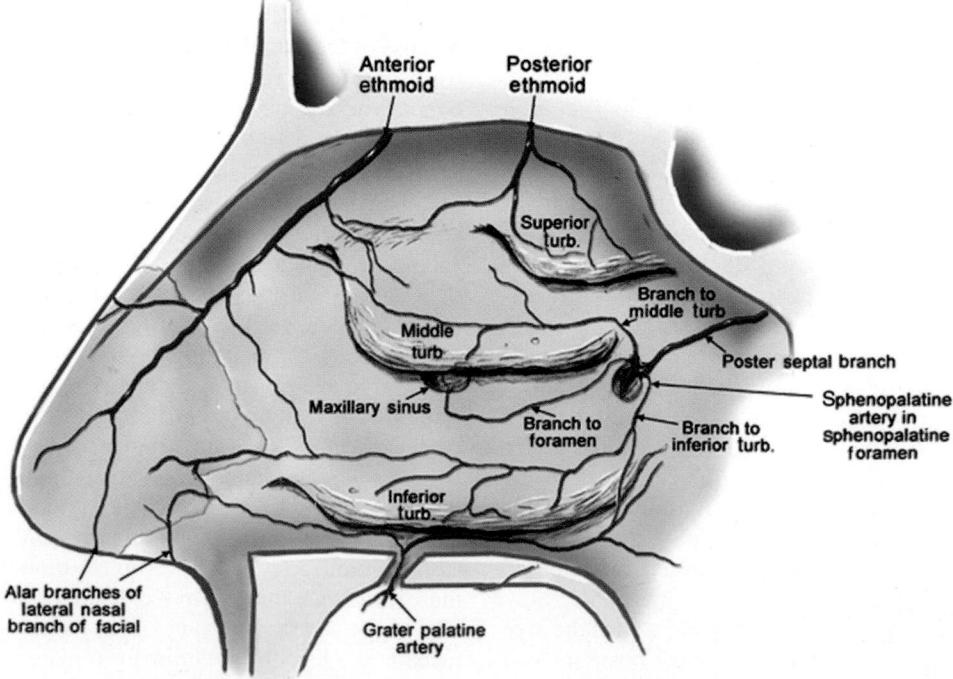

Figure 2 Vasculature of the lateral wall of the nasal cavity.

profuse, the patient may present in a state of shock and will require resuscitation according to well-established principles for the treatment of hemorrhagic shock. With the patient stable, it is important to first elicit the nature and history of the epistaxis. Essential historical information includes: when it began, duration of bleeding, frequency, inciting factors, and previous attempts, whether successful or not, at control of the bleeding. A thorough history should be obtained to detect the presence of comorbid conditions such as coronary artery disease, diabetes, and hypertension. Patient medications can also have an impact on the etiology and successful epistaxis management. Not only prescribed medications, for example, coumadin, nonsteroidal anti-inflammatory agents, or antiplatelet drugs, but some over-the-counter and herbal preparations can also impact clotting, for example, ginkgo, garlic, ginseng, high-dose vitamins A and E, and high doses of fish oil and flaxseed oil.[6,7] It is also essential to obtain a family history as certain inheritable conditions may predispose to epistaxis such as the hemophilias and related coagulopathies, and hereditary hemorrhagic telangiectasia (HHT). A social history may lead to important clues, especially such findings as alcohol or intranasal drug usage.

Once a thorough history as been obtained, a full head and neck examination is essential as it would be unwise to be so focused on the nasal examination as to miss such things as a neck mass or a unilateral tympanic membrane retraction or hemotympanum. The nasal examination should be undertaken with prior preparation. It would be wise to be prepared to intervene prior to beginning the examination. Table 2 provides a list of supplies which might be useful (Figure 3).

Nasal evaluation should begin by observing the external nose. Important signs found here might include evidence of trauma and side of anterior bleeding. Anterior rhinoscopy with a nasal speculum and headlight will commonly reveal a bleeding source on the anterior nasal septum, evidence of anterior septal trauma (as after digital manipulation), an eschar, a nasal septal perforation, or dilated vessels. Many studies recently have highlighted and demonstrated the importance of endoscopy in accurate diagnosis since the most important factor in determining and effectively treating epistaxis is visualization of the offending vessels. Thorough intranasal endoscopic evaluation is best performed following adequate local anesthesia and the topical application of a vasoconstrictive agent such as oxymetazoline. An additional maneuver which assists to anesthetize the nasal cavity and may also be therapeutic is transoral greater palatine nerve block by injecting 1 to 2 mL of local anesthetic containing epinephrine through the greater palatine foramen in the roof of the hard palate into the pterygopalatine fossa. In addition to providing anesthesia to the posterior nasal cavity and septum, it also serves to tamponade the IMA. As many as 20% of nosebleeds are from a posterior origin where the use of nasal endoscopy is particularly important. Epistaxis from a posterior source is more likely

Table 2 Supplies for Epistaxis Kit
Headlight
Nasal speculum
Suction
Tubing
Canister
Frazier tip
Oxymetazoline-lidocaine spray
Silver nitrate
Bayonet forceps
Nasal packing supplies
Inflatable nasal packs (epistat, rapid rhino, etc)
Petroleum gauze strip
Absorbable packing material
Surgicel (oxidised regenerated cellulose)
Gelfoam (processed gelatin)
Hemostatic sealants (Floseal, Surgiflo)
Foley catheters
Endoscopes
Flexible fiberoptic
Variety of rigid (0° and 30°)
Endoscopic cautery equipment (in operating suite)
Bipolar
Suction cautery
Saline irrigation

to be arterial than those that are from an anterior source. Bleeding from this region is also more likely to be serious and generally more difficult to control. Posterior nasal bleeding is much less accessible to direct intervention, especially in the office or emergency room setting, making it much more difficult to gain local control.

Laboratory studies are always helpful, if the situation allows. Determining the hemoglobin level is an indicator of chronic blood loss, although it may be normal in the setting of sudden acute blood loss. Also, coagulation studies and platelet counts are helpful when available. However, obtaining these studies must not interfere with the management of the patient who is acutely bleeding.

CLINICAL MANAGEMENT AND PROGNOSIS

Treatment has traditionally been divided into conservative (medical) management, or surgical treatment. This paradigm of considering all nonsurgical treatments as "conservative" has recently been challenged. However, for purposes of classifying forms of treatments, this approach is still somewhat useful.

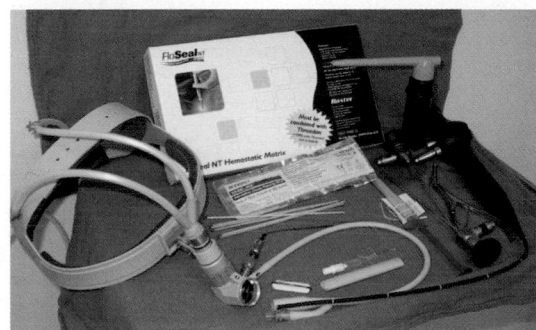

Figure 3 A sample epistaxis kit.

Treatment can be classified from least invasive to most invasive. As a part of the physical examination, the source of the bleeding should have been identified. This step is clearly the most important aspect of determining the most proper treatment.

Medical management consists of nasal pressure initially, having the patient hold the nose putting pressure on the anterior septum. A frequently useful adjunct procedure is to add oxymetazoline or phenylephrine as a vasoconstricting agent. By the time they have come to the attention of an otolaryngologist this has usually already failed to stop the acute hemorrhagic process or the problem has become recurrent or chronic in nature.

Medical Management

For the chronic recurrent epistaxis, the most commonly used medical management is the application of a moisturizing or humidifying agent to prevent desiccation. A recent study in the pediatric population showed that when patients were treated with nasal emollients alone, 61% of those who used the emollients had resolution by the first follow-up appointment.[8] Commonly used agents include nasal saline mist, nasal saline gels, irrigation, foam, petrolatum-based ointments, use of room humidifiers, and essential oil emollients. By definition, when these conservative measures fail, a patient is said to have intractable epistaxis. At this point, it is likely that another, more invasive step will need to be undertaken.

For the acute hemorrhagic process, the initial step will be to identify the bleeding vessel as described above. If the bleeding cannot be controlled adequately to identify the source of bleeding, measures will be needed to tamponade the bleeding. This generally means some form of nasal packing. Traditional methods of nasal packing include use of an inflated foley catheter or gauze roll in the nasopharynx for a posterior pack with layered petroleum, based ointment, coated gauze packed anteriorly. Other methods of anterior-posterior packing include inflatable premanufactured balloon devices with separate anterior and posterior inflation chambers. The Merocel nasal pack (Medtronic ENT, Jacksonville, FL) is a hydroxylate polyvinyl acetate material which expands when it comes in contact with water. Merocel has become quite popular as an easy to use, readily available product and has become readily available in most emergency departments.

While nasal packing has traditionally been considered noninvasive, conservative therapy, this has recently been challenged. Anterior-posterior packing carries significant risks and a high failure rate. Risks have been well-documented in the literature. First of all, the procedure itself is extremely uncomfortable and is accompanied by nasal obstruction, gagging, pain, and dysphagia. Nasal packs have traditionally been felt to be associated with the nasal pulmonary reflex which decreases pulmonary ventilation causing hypoxia as well as possibly arrhythmia, hypoxemia, and death. While most otolaryngologists still consider

this to be a risk of posterior nasal packing, recent evidence questions the validity of this phenomenon.[9] Another major risk is septicemia, and minor risks include alar necrosis, serous otitis media, local infections, acute sinusitis, and septal perforation. Aside from the risks, the success rate is generally poorer than for the more invasive techniques, with a failure rate approaching 40%. When the cost of keeping a patient in the hospital for several days in a monitored bed is compared to surgery or embolization, it has also been found to not be cost effective.[10,11]

Another potential complication of nasal packing is toxic shock syndrome (TSS). TSS is caused by a toxin which is released by either coagulase-positive staphlococci (*Staphylococcus aureus*) or group A beta-hemolytic streptococci (*Streptococcus pyogenes*). Although TSS has traditionally been associated with use of super-absorbent tampons in menstruating women, it has also been described with nasal packing The typical presentation for TSS includes: fever and chills, profuse watery diarrhea with abdominal pain, light-headedness and syncope, myalgias and arthralgias, pharyngitis, headache, and confusion. Physical findings may include: fever (>102°F), hypotension (systolic BP <90 mmHg), diffuse rash appearing on trunk, spreading to arms and legs involving palms and soles with subsequent desquamation 1 to 2 weeks later. Multiorgan involvement may include ventricular arrhythmias, renal or hepatic failure, disseminated intravascular coagulation, and acute respiratory distress syndrome.

Treatment includes parenteral antistaphylococcal and antistreptococcal antibiotics, removal of offending packing and intensive supportive care, often in a critical care setting so that aggressive fluid resuscitation, monitoring, and specific treatment for affected organ systems can be provided.

Hemostatic Agents. Various hemostatic compounds have also been used in an attempt to avoid the discomfort and morbidity associated with nasal packing. Antifibrinolytic agents such as epsilon amino caproic acid and tranexamic acid have both been shown to be somewhat effective, especially in HHT; however, their use (both systemically and topically) has not been widespread.[12] More recently, biodegradable hemostatic sealant compounds have been introduced as hemostatics. One of these, Floseal (Baster Health Care Corp., Deerfield, IL) is composed of collagen particles and topical bovine thrombin applied as a high viscosity gel. This easy to apply material has recently been shown to compare quite favorably with nasal packing in terms of efficacy and was much better tolerated by the patients. Treatment using this agent was, however, much more expensive than either merocel or petroleum gauze.

Surgical Treatment and Embolization

When conservative measures fail to control epistaxis, more invasive means are then usually undertaken. Where available, embolization of the offending arteries by means of interventional radiology can be effective. Comparisons of embolization versus surgery show success rates of embolization to be 71 to 100% with an average of 88%[13] and for surgical treatment approximately 87 to 100% averaging about 90% in various reports.[11,14–16] However, this expertise and associated equipment is not universally available. In one study, only 11% of otolaryngologists in nonurban regions in Ohio had access to interventional radiology.[16]

Cost effectiveness has also been looked at and seems to vary by institution. The cost of embolization has been found to be higher in some institutions than surgery, whereas it is lower in others.

While embolization may be both efficacious and cost effective, serious complications have been reported during these endovascular procedures. These include internal carotid artery intimal injury requiring anticoagulation, soft tissue necrosis, facial paralysis, myocardial infarction, blindness, and stroke.[16]

Traditionally, surgical treatment has consisted of ligation of the ethmoid, internal maxillary or the external carotid arteries. More recently endoscopic approaches have been added, most particularly the SPA. In fact, this technique is now often recommended as the first-line surgical treatment when more conservative measures have been unsuccessful. Even before ligation of the SPA is considered, endoscopic examination of the nasal cavity, usually under general anesthesia, can allow the surgeon to locate the exact site of bleeding (usually the lateral nasal wall or posterior nasal septum) and selectively cauterize these areas (bipolar diathermy or monopolar suction cautery). This can be a highly effective approach and essentially applies the same principles previously available for anterior epistaxis to the otherwise more challenging and refractory posterior bleeding.

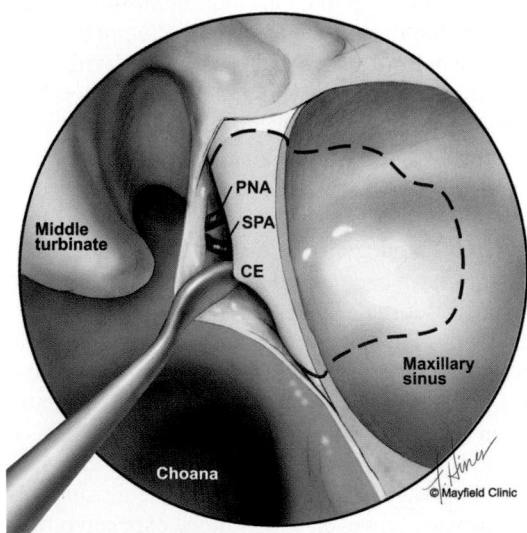

Figure 4 Endoscopic view of sphenopalatine artery (SPA) as viewed during endoscopic SPA ligation. A freer elevator is retracting the mucoperiosteum medially, and the SPA is seen being tented posterior to the crista ethmoidalis (CE) as it emerges from the sphenopalatine foramen. PNA = posterior nasal artery. (Published with permission, copyright © 2007, the Mayfield Clinic, OH.)

When the bleeding continues despite conservative measures, more invasive surgical approaches may be necessary. The traditional surgical approach is ligation of the internal maxillary and the anterior and posterior ethmoid arteries. The IMA is traditionally managed via a sublabial transantral approach. By accessing the pterygomaxillary space through the posterior wall of the maxillary sinus, the IMA can be identified, dissected and ligated with vascular clips. Recurrent bleeding following IMA ligation is usually attributed to failure to ligate all of the distal branches of the IMA. The more proximally the vessel is ligated, the more likely there will be unrecognized collateral branches that can contribute to continued bleeding. Thus, arterial ligation closer to the actual site of bleeding will produce a better likelihood for success. This is 1 reason that SPA ligation has come to be favored as a surgical approach for refractory posterior epistaxis. The endoscopic approach to this vessel has become a preferred surgical technique and is quickly becoming the standard surgical treatment for recalcitrant posterior epistaxis.

The procedure begins with decongestion and local anesthetic as routinely performed prior to functional endoscopic sinus surgery. Next a middle-meatal antrostomy can be performed, but is usually not necessary. A mucosal incision is made on the lateral nasal wall beginning just above the posterior part of the attachment of the inferior turbinate and extending anterior and superior just anterior to the attachment of the middle turbinate. Using this incision, a mucoperiosteal flap is elevated on the lateral nasal wall and continued until the crista ethmoidalis is encountered. The SPA is immediately posterior to this landmark as it exits the pterygopalatine fossa through the sphenopalatine foramen (Figure 4). After carefully identifying and dissecting this vessel, it should be ligated using surgical clips and then divided. Dissection posterior to this vessel will often reveal a second branch of the SPA which may exit through a separate foramen. Since this usually gives rise to the posterior nasal artery, it should be bipolar cauterized. Mobilizing and surgically clipping this artery is often quite difficult.[17]

Ethmoid artery ligation may also be necessary, particularly for those with continued bleeding despite IMA or SPA ligation, or those with a bleeding site identified in the superior nasal cavity, whether on the septum or lateral nasal wall superior to the middle turbinate. This is usually performed through a standard external medial canthal Lynch incision. The anterior ethmoid artery is difficult to access safely through an endoscopic approach.

HEREDITARY HEMORRHAGIC TELANGIECTASIA

HHT, also known as Osler-Weber-Rendu syndrome is an autosomal dominant disease characterized by localized angiodysplasia,

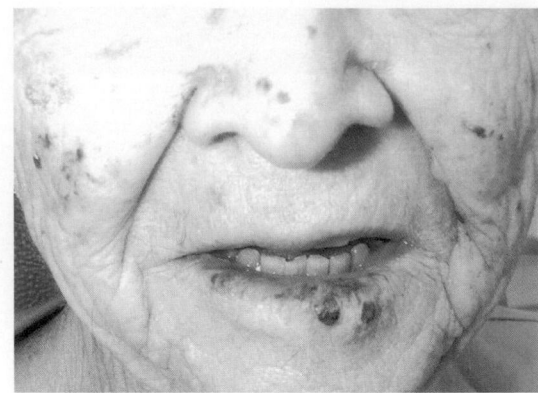

Figure 5 A patient with hereditary hemorrhagic telangiectasia. Note the cutaneous telangiectasias and arteriovenous malformations.

often manifested as dermal, mucosal, visceral, pulmonary, and cerebral arteriovenous malformations (AVMs). The prevalence has been found to be from 1 in 5,000 to 1 in 10,000. The penetrance also increases with age with more than ninety percent being symptomatic by the age of 21 years. It is incurable and progressive. Epistaxis is the most common presenting symptom, and it occurs in over 90% of individuals with HHT and becomes more frequent with increasing age. The vessels affected by this disorder are characterized as being thin-walled, dilated, postcapillary venules in the submucosa. They are frequently 1 to 2 mm in diameter and are characterized by a loss of elastic membrane in arterioles without a complete muscular layer. As the disease progresses, the capillaries become dilated and as the arterioles become involved, arteriovenous shunts develop (Figures 5 and 6).

Genes which have been found to be mutated in HHT include *Endoglin (ENG)* and *Alk1*, which have been localized to chromosomal loci 9q33 and 12q11 respectively. Other genes which have also associated with HHT include *MADH4* on 18q21, *BMPRII* on 2q33, and a third locus on 5q31. A common feature of HHT mutations is an endoglin deficiency in endothelial cells. These genes appear to play a role in transforming growth factor-beta signaling pathways which affect endothelial cell proliferation and migration

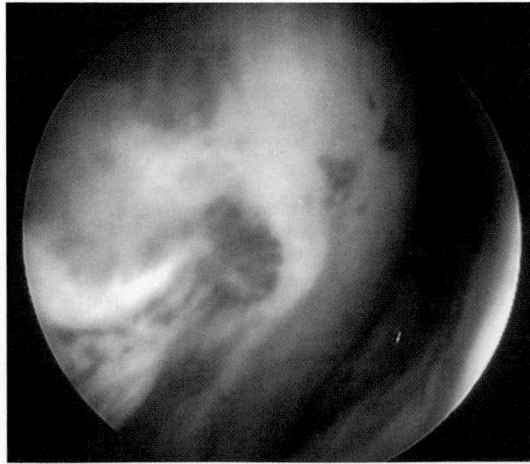

Figure 6 Endoscopic view of mucosal arteriovenous malformations on the nasal septum of a patient with hereditary hemorrhagic telangiectasia.

Table 3   Clinical Diagnostic Criteria for Hereditary Hemorrhagic Telangiectasia

I.	Nosebleeds, spontaneous and recurrent
II.	Telangiectases, multiple, at characteristic sites including lips, oral cavity, fingers and nose
III.	Internal lesions such as:
	Gastrointestinal telangiectasia (with or without bleeding)
	Pulmonary arteriovenous malformations (AVM)
	Hepatic AVMs
	Cerebral AVMs
	Spinal AVM
IV.	Family history—a first-degree relative with hereditary hemorrhagic telangiectasia according to these criteria

Diagnosis is definite if three criteria are present

Diagnosis is possible or suspected if two criteria are present

Diagnosis is unlikely if fewer than two criteria are present

leading to dysregulation in the organization of the capillary network, disorganized cytoskeletons which are prone to cell breaking with changes in shear stress and blood pressure.[18]

Currently, the clinical diagnosis of HHT is made by the Curação criteria (Table 3). A definitive diagnosis requires at least 3 of these 4 criteria. A suspected diagnosis based on having at least 2 of the 4 symptoms of the Curação criteria, should prompt further investigation searching for pulmonary, cerebral, and gastrointestinal vascular malformations.[19] Pulmonary AVMs may occur in up to 33% of patients and cerebral AVMs in 11%. Although any AVM can present with hemorrhage, the presentation for most pulmonary AVMs results from blood shunting through these abnormal vessels and causing transient ischemic attacks, embolic strokes, or cerebral hemorrhage. Cerebral AVMs may present with anything from seizure to cerebral hemorrhage.[20] All patients with HHT, as well as their first-degree relatives, should be routinely screened for pulmonary AVMs using chest computed tomography scans, and for intracranial

AVMs using brain magnetic resonance imaging with and without gadolinium.

Treatment is primarily focused on prevention and treatment of the recurrent epistaxis. Conservative measures begin with regular nasal mucosal care using nasal saline and emollient preparations. The second line and mainstay of treatment is endonasal Nd:YAG or KTP laser treatments at regular intervals as needed based on bleeding frequency. A regular schedule of laser treatments along with meticulous nasal care can dramatically reduce the frequency of epistaxis. Kuhnel and colleagues were able to improve their patients in this manner from at least daily epistaxis to an average of every 7 to 14 days.[21]

When these treatments fail, there are a number of surgical options. Septodermoplasty has previously been the treatment of choice. This was first described in 1960 by Saunders as a method for permanent control of epistaxis.[22] This involves removal of nasal mucosa, usually including the inferior turbinates, and replacing it with epidermal grafts. While this generally works well, vascular ingrowth and nasal drying can often result in recurrence of bleeding. The ultimate procedure for control of epistaxis is to permanently close the nasal cavities, the so called Young, or modified Young procedure.[23] This procedure does appear to be effective; however, it has the obvious disadvantage of loss of the nasal pathway, which is especially problematic during sleep. An interesting recent study examining quality of life following various treatment protocols for HHT suggested that the modified Young procedure has a high degree of acceptance by patients so treated.[24]

REFERENCES

1. Weiss NS. Relation of high blood pressure to headache, epistaxis, and selected other symptoms. The United States Health Examination Survey of Adults. N Engl J Med 1972;287:631–3.
2. Chiu T, Dunn JS. An anatomical study of the arteries of the anterior nasal septum. Otolaryngol Head Neck Surg 2006;134:33–6.
3. Loughran S, Hilmi O, McGarry GW. Endoscopic sphenopalatine artery ligation—when, why and how to do it. An on-line video tutorial. Clin Otolaryngol 2005;30:539–43.
4. Lee HY, Kim HU, Kim SS, et al. Surgical anatomy of the sphenopalatine artery in lateral nasal wall. Laryngoscope 2002;112:1813–8.
5. Schwartzbauer HR, Shete M, Tami TA. Endoscopic anatomy of the sphenopalatine and posterior nasal arteries: Implications for the endoscopic management of epistaxis. Am J Rhinol 2003;17:63–6.
6. Hodges PJ, Kam PC. The peri-operative implications of herbal medicines. Anaesthesia 2002;57:889–99.
7. Samuels N. Herbal remedies and anticoagulant therapy. Thromb Haemost 2005;93:3–7.
8. Damrose JF, Maddalozzo J. Pediatric epistaxis. Laryngoscope 2006;116:387–93.
9. Loftus BC, Blitzer A, Cozine K. Epistaxis, medical history, and the nasopulmonary reflex: What is clinically relevant? Otolaryngol Head Neck Surg 1994;110:363–9.
10. Wormald PJ, Wee DT, van Hasselt CA. Endoscopic ligation of the sphenopalatine artery for refractory posterior epistaxis. Am J Rhinol 2000;14:261–4.
11. Klotz DA, Winkle MR, Richmon J, Hengerer AS. Surgical management of posterior epistaxis: A changing paradigm. Laryngoscope 2002;112:1577–82.
12. Lozano M. Tranexamic acid in hereditary hemorrhagic telangiectasia. N Engl J Med 2002;346:457.
13. Christensen NP, Smith DS, Barnwell SL, Wax MK. Arterial embolization in the management of posterior epistaxis. Otolaryngol Head Neck Surg 2005;133:748–53.
14. Strong EB, Bell DA, Johnson LP, Jacobs JM. Intractable epistaxis: Transantral ligation vs. embolization: Efficacy review and cost analysis. Otolaryngol Head Neck Surg 1995;113:674–8.
15. Feusi B, Holzmann D, Steurer J. Posterior epistaxis: Systematic review on the effectiveness of surgical therapies. Rhinology 2005;43:300–4.
16. Cullen MM, Tami TA. Comparison of internal maxillary artery ligation versus embolization for refractory posterior epistaxis. Otolaryngol Head Neck Surg 1998;118:636–42.
17. Pothier DD, Mackeith S, Youngs R. Sphenopalatine artery ligation: Technical note. J Laryngol Otol 2005;119:810–2.
18. Fernandez-L A, Sanz-Rodriguez F, Blanco FJ, et al. Hereditary hemorrhagic telangiectasia, a vascular dysplasia affecting the TGF-{beta} signaling pathway. Clin Med Res 2006;4:66–78.
19. Shovlin CL, Guttmacher AE, Buscarini E, et al. Diagnostic criteria for hereditary hemorrhagic telangiectasia (Rendu-Osler-Weber syndrome). Am J Med Genet 2000;91:66–7.
20. Guttmacher AE, Marchuk DA, White RI, Jr. Hereditary hemorrhagic telangiectasia. N Engl J Med 1995;333:918–24.
21. Kuhnel TS, Wagner BH, Schurr CP, Strutz J. Clinical strategy in hereditary hemorrhagic telangiectasia. Am J Rhinol 2005;19:508–13.
22. Saunders WH. Permanent control of nosebleeds in patients with hereditary hemorrhagic telangiectasia. Ann Intern Med 1960;53:147–52.
23. Gluckman JL, Portugal LG. Modified Young's procedure for refractory epistaxis due to hereditary hemorrhagic telangiectasia. Laryngoscope 1994;104:1174–7.
24. Hitchings AE, Lennox PA, Lund VJ, Howard DJ. The effect of treatment for epistaxis secondary to hereditary hemorrhagic telangiectasia. Am J Rhinol 2005;19:75–8.

45

Acute and Chronic Nasal Disorders

Valerie J. Lund, MS, FRCS, FRCS(Ed)

There is a wide range of acute and chronic conditions which may affect the nose, either arising locally or occurring as part of systemic disease. These may broadly be divided into allergic and nonallergic,[1] and there are a number of etiologic factors and differential diagnoses which should be considered (Tables 1 and 2).[2] This chapter will consider some of the infectious conditions, the nonallergic, noninfectious diseases, and a number of other conditions which enter into the differential diagnosis of patients presenting with nasal symptoms. From an anatomical and physiological perspective, the nose is rarely affected in isolation, and the majority of conditions impact on the adjacent paranasal sinuses to a greater or lesser extent. Thus the term "rhinosinusitis" has been agreed upon in a number of international consensus documents primarily relating to infection; although in reality probably applicable to most disease processes in this region.[1–4] Similarly the upper and lower respiratory tract should be considered as one organ with many conditions manifesting themselves in both areas, sometimes in subtly different ways, for example, asthma and nasal polyps.[5]

INVESTIGATION

A considerable number of tests and procedures are now available for the investigation

Table 1 Classification of Rhinitis

Infectious
  Viral
  Bacterial
  Other infective agents
Allergic
  Intermittent
  Persistent
Occupational (allergic or nonallergic)
  Intermittent
  Persistent
Drug-induced
  Aspirin
  Other medications
Hormonal
Other causes
  Nonallergic rhinitis with eosinophilia syndrome
  Irritants
  Food
  Emotional
  Atrophic
  Gastroesophageal reflux
Idiopathic

After reference 2.

Table 2 Differential Diagnosis of Rhinitis

Polyps
Mechanical factors
  Deviated septum
  Adenoidal hypertrophy
  Foreign bodies
  Choanal atresia
Tumors
  Benign
  Malignant
Granulomas
  Wegener granulomatosis
  Sarcoid
  Infectious
  Malignant—midline destructive granuloma (T cell lymphoma)
Ciliary defects
Cerebrospinal fluid rhinorrhea

After reference 20.

of sinonasal disease (Table 3).[6] However, not all are routinely available nor indeed applicable to each individual patient, and their selection will depend upon clinical indicators and local factors.

HISTORY AND EXAMINATION

In practical terms, the nose has a limited repertoire of responses in any given condition, that is, nasal congestion, discharge, sneezing, itching, and epistaxis with associated symptoms of headache and/or facial pain. However, a careful history will usually suggest the diagnosis. A thorough general medical history should be followed by questions specific to rhinologic symptoms including information on environmental and occupational factors and family history. The frequency, duration, and severity of symptoms should also be discussed and a visual analogue score can be used to semiquantify severity by simply asking the patients to mark on a 10 cm line where they feel they lie for a particular symptom during the last week.[6] This method can be repeated on each subsequent visit with the patients acting as their own controls. Consistent obstruction on the same side suggests a polyp, structural problem or more rarely a tumor or even a congenital unilateral choanal atresia. Hyposmia and anosmia are most often associated with nasal polyps or more severe disease such as Wegener granulomatosis or sarcoid. Secondary symptoms related to

Table 3 Diagnostic Techniques[6]

Subjective assessment of symptoms
  Visual analogue score (VAS)
General otorhinolaryngology examination
Allergy tests
  Skin tests
  Total serum IgE
  Serum specific IgE
Endoscopy
  Rigid
  Flexible
Nasal smear
  Cytology
Nasal swab
  Bacteriology
Radiology
  CT
  MRI
  Chest X-ray
Mucociliary function
  Nasal mucociliary clearance (NMCC)
  Ciliary beat frequency (CBF)
  Electron microscopy
  Nitric oxide
Nasal airway assessment
  Nasal inspiratory peak flow (NIPF)
  Rhinomanometry (anterior and posterior)
  Acoustic rhinometry
Olfaction
  Threshold testing
  "Scratch and sniff" tests
Blood tests
  Full blood count and white blood cell differential
  Erythrocyte sedimentation rate
  Thyroid function tests
  Antineutrophil cytoplasmic antibody (ANCA)
  Immunoglobulins and IgG subclasses
  Antibody response to immunization with protein and carbohydrate antigens
Quality of life
  General health status
  Disease specific health status

blockage of the airways include frequent sore throats, dryness of the mouth, and oropharynx, a hyponasal quality to the voice and snoring. A full drug history may also give a clue to the source of the problem. Symptoms specific to particular conditions are discussed in the relevant sections.

Examination of the nose should be performed in all cases of rhinologic complaint and should include anterior rhinoscopy using a nasal speculum and head light, rigid endoscopy combined with flexible nasendoscopy in selected cases to ensure a full evaluation of the nasal cavity and nasopharynx.

The quantity and quality of secretion should be noted, both the viscosity and color and specimens may be taken for a nasal smear. Similarly under endoscopic control, a swab may be taken from the middle meatus which provides a reasonable correlation with the bacteriology of the dependent sinuses.[7]

The appearance of the mucosa rarely alters in a way that is pathognomonic for a particular disease. However, it is usually reddened in acute infections and overuse of topical medications, whereas a typical allergic mucosa appears pale and swollen. In granulomatous conditions such as Wegener granulomatosis and sarcoid, the mucosa is generally reddened, friable, and associated with crusting and evidence of previous epistaxis. A careful examination of the nasal cavity should reveal polyps, tumor, foreign bodies, or septal deflections, although it is important that the unwary examine beyond the deflection wherever possible as secondary pathology may be present and go unnoticed. The presence of a septal perforation should raise the possibility of cocaine abuse, previous surgery, or one of the systemic granulomatous diseases, although most often is "idiopathic" resulting from minor or repeated trauma.

Physical examination should not be confined to the nose alone and should be accompanied by a full otorhinolaryngologic examination, posterior rhinoscopy, indirect laryngoscopy, and palpation of the neck in selected cases. It should also be remembered that many conditions affecting the nose and sinuses also affect the lower respiratory tract which may be revealed by appropriate examination. Detailed information regarding imaging can be found in Chapter 41, "Imaging of the Nasal Cavities, Paranasal Sinuses, Nasopharynx, Orbits, Infratemporal Fossa, Pterygomaxillary Fissure, and Base of Skull," and allergy in Chapter 43, "Allergic Rhinitis."

MUCOCILIARY FUNCTION

Nasal Mucociliary Clearance

A simple test of mucociliary function can be performed by placing a 0.5 mm piece of saccharin on the anterior end of the inferior turbinate approximately 1 cm from the end to avoid areas of squamous metaplasia. The time taken to taste something sweet in the mouth is measured which normally takes 30 minutes or less. If longer than an hour has elapsed, it is worth repeating the test in case the particle has fallen out and checking that the patient is capable of tasting saccharin.

Ciliary Beat Frequency

When the saccharin test is prolonged or if specific ciliary abnormalities are suspected, it is possible to examine the cilia directly by taking a sample with a small disposable cupped spatula (Rhinoprobe, Arlington Scientific, Arlington, TX) and observing cilia activity under a phase-contrast microscope with photometric cell.[8] The frequency can be measured with a real time analyzer and expressed in hertz, the normal range from the inferior turbinate being 12 to 15 Hz. However, this technique is not available in every center.

Electron Microscopy

If the nasomucociliary clearance time and ciliary beat frequency are abnormal, samples may be obtained with the spatula or via biopsy for electron microscopy studies to diagnose conditions such as primary ciliary dyskinesia (PCD).

Nitric Oxide

Nitric oxide (NO) is found in the upper and lower respiratory tract and is a sensitive indicator of inflammation and ciliary function.[9] The majority of NO is made in the sinuses (chest <20 ppb [parts per billion], nose 400 to 900 ppb, sinuses 20 to 25 ppm [parts per million]). In PCD the NO is much reduced to double figures or less in the nose and to single figures from the chest. However, as NO is predominantly produced in the sinuses, conditions such as nasal polyposis which obstruct gas exchange from these areas can also result in a low reading from the nasal gases. The level is commensurately elevated in the presence of inflammation and may be improved by medical and surgical therapy.[10]

NASAL AIRWAY ASSESSMENT

Nasal Expiratory or Inspiratory Peak Flow

Nasal expiratory or inspiratory peak flow (NIPF) is a technique which uses a peak flow meter and has the advantage of being inexpensive, quick and easy to perform. It is useful for repeated examinations and compares well with active anterior rhinomanometry.[11] Of the two methods, forced inspiration is preferred although it can produce significant vestibular collapse in some individuals. Forced expiration inflates the eustachian tube, which may be uncomfortable and may also produce an unpleasant quantity of mucus in the mask.

Rhinomanometry

Rhinomanometry attempts to measure nasal airway resistance by making quantitative measurement of nasal flow and pressure.[12] It employs the principle that air will only flow through a tube when there is a pressure differential passing from areas of high to low air pressure. When the nasal mucosa is decongested, the reproducibility of rhinomanometry is good, but it requires some expertise to produce consistent results and has therefore remained primarily a research tool. Active anterior rhinomanometry is more commonly used as the posterior technique cannot be used in 20 to 25% of individuals due to an inability to relax the soft palate.

Acoustic Rhinometry. With the acoustic rhinometry technique an audible sound pulse is electronically generated and is passed into the nose where it is altered by variations in the cross-sectional area. The reflected signal is picked up by a microphone and analyzed allowing determination of the area within the nasal cavity as a function of distance. From this, volumes may be derived, thus providing topographical information rather than a measure of airflow.[12] It appears to be more reproducible and to have greater applicability than rhinomanometry but is still being evaluated as a clinical tool. Nasal airflow measurements are discussed in greater detail in Chapter 40, "Assessment of Nasal Function."

OLFACTION

Olfactory Thresholds

Estimation of olfactory thresholds may be established by presentation of serial dilutions of pure odorants such as PM-carbinol (phenylethyl methyl ethyl carbinol, Olfacto-Labs, El Cerrito, CA).[13] The patient is presented with two bottles, one containing only the diluent solution as the control, the other the odorant in progressively increasing or decreasing concentrations. Each is sniffed in turn until a point is reached when the patient cannot distinguish between the control and test bottle. This indicates the minimum detectable odor.

Scratch and Sniff Tests. The scratch and sniff tests use patches impregnated with microencapsulated odorants.[13] The patient is forced to choose between a number of options after scratching the patch to release the odor. The results are well validated for age and sex and take into account answers guessed correctly as well as giving an indication of malingering.

Alternative identification tests include the Zurich Smell Test in which eight odorants must be correctly identified. The test choices are offered pictorially as well as in English. The "Sniff 'n' Sticks" combine both a qualitative and quantitative assessment of olfaction. Testing of the sense of smell is discussed in greater detail in Chapter 38, "Olfaction and Gustation."

BLOOD TESTS

A wide range of haematological investigations may be appropriate given the suspected differential diagnosis, for example, thyroid dysfunction, Wegener granulomatosis, sarcoid, and immune deficiency.

INFECTIOUS RHINITIS

The separation of infections in the nose from those in the paranasal sinuses is now recognized as incorrect, and it is generally accepted that the term "rhinosinusitis" better encompasses infections in this region, although one area may be affected to a greater or lesser extent. This was supported by the work of Gwaltney and colleagues[14] who have demonstrated with computed tomography (CT) scanning that during a simple

Table 4 Infective Rhinitis: Causative Agents	
Viruses	
Common cold	Picornavirus
	Rhinovirus
	Coxsackie virus
	Reovirus
	Echovirus
	Parainfluenza
	Adenovirus
	Respiratory syncytial virus
Influenza	Influenza virus
Mucocutaneous herpes	Herpes simplex
Chicken pox, herpes zoster	Varicella zoster
Bacteria	
Furuncle	*Staphylococcus aureus*
Secondary infection	Various aerobes, anaerobes, bacteroides
Actinomycosis	*Actinomyces israelii*
Diphtheria	*Corynebacterium diphtheriae*
Rhinoscleroma	*Klebsiella rhinoscleromatis*
Leprosy	*Mycobacterium leprae*
Glanders	*Pseudomonas mallei*
Tuberculosis	*Mycobacterium. tuberculosis*
Syphilis	*Treponema pallidum*
Fungal	
Aspergillosis	*Aspergillus* species
Mucormycosis	*Mucor* or *Rhizopus oryzae*
Rhinosporidiosis	*Rhinosporidium seeberi*
Blastomycosis	*Blastomyces dermatidis*
Cryptococcosis	*Cryptococcus neoformans*
Histoplasmosis	*Histoplasma capsulatum*
Sporotrichosis	*Sporothrix schenkii*
Candidiasis	*Candida* species
Protozoa	
Leishmaniasis	*Leishmania* species
Parasites	
Myiasis	*Chrysomyia*

uncomplicated viral cold, the majority of subjects have some involvement of the paranasal sinuses. A long list of causative agents can produce infection in this region (Table 4) (see Chapter 42, "Etiology of Infectious Diseases of the Upper Respiratory Tract," for more information on infectious agents).

Etiologic Factors

A number of congenital conditions may predispose patients to infection of the respiratory tract.

Primary Ciliary Dyskinesia. Some individuals are born with a congenital abnormality of the cilia which affects their motility, and this is termed PCD. Electron microscopic examination reveals disorganized microtubules and the absence of dynein arms. In addition to nasal problems, patients usually exhibit lower respiratory tract infection, serous otitis media, and infertility problems. In the full blown Kartagener syndrome patients have bronchiectasis, sinus infection, and situs inversus in approximately 50% of cases.

Cystic Fibrosis. Cystic fibrosis is an autosomal recessive disease, the most common inherited fatal disease of Caucasian children, caused by a defective mucosal chloride transport gene. In its most severe form, it presents with malabsorption and progressive obstructive pulmonary disease; and approximately one-third of children and one-half of adults suffer from multiple bilateral nasal polyps and the majority of patients have a chronic pansinusitis (Figure 1). The polyps have been attributed to an abnormality of sodium and water transport across membranes, and the histology of the polyps differ significantly from those in other conditions having less eosinophils and more lymphocytes and plasma cells. *Pseudomonas aeruginosa* is commonly found in association with the sinus disease and may be targeted specifically with appropriate antibiotics such as the quinolones. The majority of patients are managed by a combination of medical therapies with intranasal corticosteroids and surgery. The results of surgery are compromised by the condition but are still regarded as worthwhile by patients. Other medical therapies have included intranasal furosemide and/or amiloride.

Viral Infections

The most obvious and frequently occurring example of infection is the common cold. A number of viruses are associated with upper respiratory tract infections of varying degrees of severity including over 100 different types of rhinovirus. This combined with the ability of viruses for mutation has so far confounded attempts at prophylactic immunization. Most young adults suffer from 2 to 3 colds each year, and it is estimated that 0.5 to 2% of these become bacterially infected. Predisposing factors such as climatic and environmental changes, fatigue, and stress have all been implicated but, the huge variety of viruses make it unlikely that there is preexisting immunity and as a consequence most individuals are susceptible most of the time. The virus is normally transported into the nose by direct

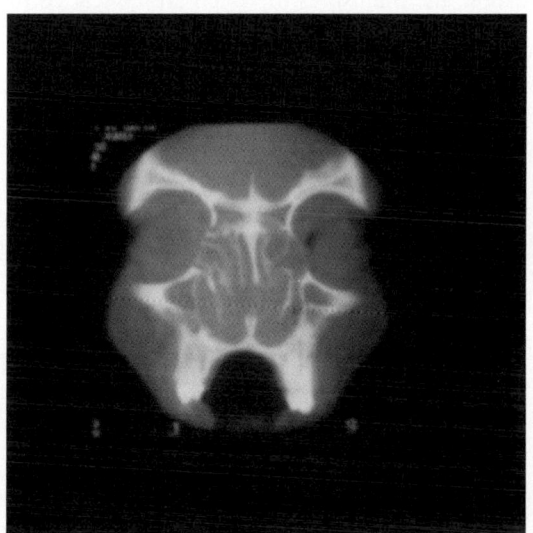

Figure 1 Coronal computed tomography scan showing massive nasal polyposis with expansion of the nasal cavity and ethmoid complexes in a patient with cystic fibrosis.

contact with the fingers rather than by air-borne contamination; and, once the virus gains access to the respiratory epithelium, it will produce ciliary stasis and damage to the cilia. The condition is characterized by edema, increased secretion and desquamation of respiratory epithelium. Clinically after 1 to 3 days incubation, a prodromal or "dry" phase follows. The subject feels unwell and shivery with a headache, myalgias, and loss of appetite while the nose feels irritated and sneezing occurs. The catarrhal phase follows after a few hours accompanied by profuse watery secretion, nasal obstruction, reduced sense of smell, and an increase in constitutional symptoms. The infection then enters a mucous phase in which symptoms improve or may continue after 5 days due to secondary bacterial infection with a progressively mucopurulent discharge. Other areas of the upper respiratory tract may be affected including the pharynx, middle ear, and tonsils.

From a practical point of view, symptomatic relief with decongestants and antipyretics are generally the mainstay of treatment. However, studies have suggested that a combination of oral chlorpheniramine and intranasal ipratropium bromide (Atrovent, Boehringer-Ingelheim) may be effective in reducing symptoms, if taken early in the prodromal phase. Antibiotics should be reserved for secondary bacterial infection although there are several trials supporting the use of topical nasal corticosteroids in acute rhinosinusitis prior to bacterial infection.[15] Decreasing symptoms after 5 days or near resolution of symptoms by 10 days suggests a viral "common" cold in contrast to those patients with increasing symptoms after 5 days or persistent problems after 10 days, which suggests progression to bacterial infection.[3]

Influenza in its many forms constitutes a more specific and potentially serious viral upper respiratory tract infection resulting in pandemics with significant morbidity and mortality in susceptible populations. Damage to the ciliated epithelium is more profound, facilitating secondary bacterial colonization, and the olfactory epithelium may be permanently damaged leading to anosmia. Vaccines have been developed and are increasingly used as prophylactics in vulnerable populations but their usefulness is again limited by the potential for viral mutation.

Bacterial Infections

Folliculitis and Vestibulitis. Specific bacterial infections can occur in the nasal vestibule when *Staphylococcus aureus* invades a pilosebaceous follicle to produce an extremely painful indurated area known as folliculitis. This will spontaneously burst and discharge its purulent contents after 4 to 5 days. The condition is exquisitely painful as the vestibular skin is tightly bound to the underlying cartilages providing little room for swelling. Local cleaning and systemic antibiotics which including flucloxacillin should be given, taking into account local bacterial resistance patterns. If the abscess is localized and fluctuant it may be incised, but the condition should always be treated seriously as it is associated with the potential complication of cavernous sinus thrombosis caused by retrograde spread of infection along the angular and superior ophthalmic veins.

The cavernous sinuses lie on either side of the sphenoid bone. Each cavernous sinus is broken up by trabeculae into many venous cavernous spaces through which the third and fourth cranial nerves and the first two divisions of the fifth cranial nerve, sixth cranial nerve, and internal carotid artery pass. It is connected by an extensive valveless venous system to the nose, adjacent face, nasopharynx, pharynx, orbit, and paranasal sinuses allowing retrograde spread of infection from any of these areas. Cavernous sinus thrombosis carries a serious morbidity, often with bilateral blindness and mortality. It is a complication predominantly of the young with two-thirds being under 20 years of age.[16] The patient complains of headache and painful paraesthesia in the distribution of the trigeminal nerve following which other cranial nerves related to the cavernous sinus become involved affecting extraocular movement and resulting in ophthalmoplegia. The sudden development of bilateral orbital signs should alert the clinician to this complication. Prior to antibiotics, cavernous sinus thrombosis carried a 50% mortality which nevertheless still stands at a significant 10 to 27%.[17] CT and magnetic resonance imaging confirm the diagnosis and high dose broad spectrum intravenous systemic antibiotic therapy should be given, together with anticoagulation in selected cases.

The increase of asymptomatic carriage of methicillin resistant *S. aureus* in the nasal vestibule is a source of considerable concern as it is implicated in nosocomial infection with serious consequences for debilitated patients. Despite vigorous eradication programs the incidence of methicillin resistant *S. aureus* appears to be increasing worldwide.

A mild form of nonspecific infective vestibulitis is often encountered producing mild irritation, small fissures, or pustules. The application of white petroleum jelly, triamcinolone acetonide 0.1%, or antibiotic ointments such as chlortetracycline hydrochloride 3% may be used.

Erysipelas. Erysipelas is an acute beta hemolytic streptococcus intradermal infection following a cut or surgical incision. The onset is usually abrupt with fever, redness, tenderness, and induration of the involved skin. On the face the infection frequently displays a butterfly pattern across the nose, adjacent cheeks, and upper lip. The infection generally responds well to penicillin or erythromycin and should be distinguished from cellulitis which is a more generalized deep infection of the skin and subcutaneous tissues also caused by *Staphylococcus* or *Streptococcus*.

A variety of other specific infections may occur in this region including diphtheria, rhinoscleroma, leprosy, tuberculosis, and syphilis (see Chapter 42, "Etiology of Infectious Diseases of the Upper Respiratory Tract").

NONALLERGIC, NONINFECTIOUS RHINITIS

Idiopathic (Vasomotor) Rhinitis

The term idiopathic rhinitis relates to any inflammation of the nose where the etiology is unknown. It is the diagnosis of exclusion as underlying causative or contributory factors can often be found if carefully sought. Patients are generally manifesting an upper respiratory hyperresponsiveness or reactivity which is simply an exaggeration of normal defense mechanisms to nonspecific environmental triggers such as changes in temperature and humidity or exposure to irritants, for example, cigarette smoke or strong odors. An extreme example of a normal physiologic response can be seen in "skier's nose" in reaction to cold dry air.[18] The commonly used term "vasomotor rhinitis" is less satisfactory as it suggests a known pathophysiological mechanism for the condition which is far from proven.[1]

Cigarette smoke is known to affect mucociliary clearance[19] and has been shown to cause an eosinophilic inflammation in the nasal mucosa of nonatopic children.[20] Challenge of smoke-sensitive individuals produces rhinorrhea and obstruction; and, in smokers, eye irritation and hyposmia are more common than in nonsmokers. It has also been shown that the more people smoke, the more they experience the symptoms of chronic rhinitis.[21]

In nonallergic, noninfectious rhinitis, symptoms vary in intensity but consist of nasal blockage, anterior rhinorrhea, and postnasal discharge, sometimes with sneezing. There is no characteristic seasonal variation and ocular symptoms are almost always missing. Skin prick tests are negative or do not correlate with the symptoms, that is, may be positive to grass pollen.

Therapy may encompass avoidance of obvious triggers, but most patients require medication, the mainstays of which are topical corticosteroids, which are safe for long-term usage. If watery rhinorrhea is the most significant or only symptom, a topical anticholinergic agent such as ipratropium bromide (Atrovent) may be helpful. Topical decongestants are best avoided because of their long-term side effects; and although oral decongestants are popular, their effect is variable and not without systemic cardiovascular and neurologic effects. Topical capsaicin has been investigated for intractable nonallergic rhinitis[22] as it produces a short-term neuronal defunctionalization but the effects are short-lived and accompanied by an unpleasant burning sensation so its role remains undetermined.

Surgery has a limited role to play in vasomotor rhinitis. Vidian neurectomy has had a vogue but has been largely abandoned as the effects are unpredictable and at best short-lived. Correction of septal deformity and/or turbinate hypertrophy is occasionally indicated if medication fails.

Occupational/Environmental Rhinitis

Airborne agents present in the workplace may affect the upper respiratory tract, producing either an allergic reaction or a nonallergic hyperresponsiveness. Chemicals such as acid anhydrides, platinum salts, glues, and solvents as well as dusts from grain and wood may act as irritants.[23] Considerable controversy now surrounds the adverse effect of environmental pollutants such as ozone, sulphur dioxide, nitric dioxide, particulate matter, volatile organic compounds, and formaldehyde. Some contradictory evidence should be clarified by carefully constructed epidemiological studies which may ultimately support present concerns. Healthcare workers exposed to latex on gloves not infrequently develop rhinoconjunctivitis which can progress to asthma and anaphylaxis.

A careful history will usually indicate the cause, confirmed by improvement once the patient is removed from the suspected irritant. However, there may be a reluctance to complain if a worker's job is jeopardized and prolonged exposure may produce chronic symptoms which do not abate for a week or more after exposure ceases.

The nasal symptoms of blockage and watery discharge may be accompanied by occupational asthma, conjunctivitis, and dermatitis. Clinical findings are usually nonspecific, and confirmation may require direct nasal challenge evaluated with symptom scores and assessment of nasal patency. Carefully graded exposure to increasing doses of the suspected agent in specialized ventilated environmental chambers may be necessary, especially if there are medicolegal consequences of the diagnosis.

Separation of patient and irritant, either by change of job, improved ventilation or use of masks may suffice complemented by conventional pharmacotherapy, for example, topical corticosteroids.

Hormonal Rhinitis

A range of physiological and pathological endocrine conditions can affect the nose. Changes are known to occur in the nose during puberty, the menstrual cycle, and pregnancy[24] with some women experiencing blockage, watery discharge, and sometimes severe epistaxis. The symptoms are worst during the last trimester of pregnancy, relating to the blood estrogen level and resolve with delivery. In women with preexisting perennial rhinitis, the nasal symptoms may improve or deteriorate during pregnancy. Hormonal change may also be responsible for the mucosal atrophy which occurs after the menopause. In specific endocrine disorders such as hypothyroidism[25] and acromegaly, nasal stuffiness, and discharge may occur.

From a therapeutic perspective, if the symptoms during pregnancy are sufficiently debilitating, medication must be considered but always taking the risk/benefit ratio into consideration. In the first instance saline douche may be of benefit but if ineffective, topical nasal corticosteroids have been used for many years without any evidence of a teratogenic effect or other adverse consequences. Certainly, extensive studies in asthmatics using inhaled corticosteroids have failed to show any abnormalities.[26] Oral decongestants theoretically could cause vascular disturbance in the placenta and fetus, but oral pseudoephedrine given within the recommended dosage is approved for use in pregnancy and has been widely prescribed in the United States.

Drug-Induced Rhinitis

A number of medications are known to produce nasal symptoms. These include:

- Aspirin and other nonsteroidal anti-inflammatory drugs. Aspirin intolerance typically increases nasal congestion and secretion and is associated with nasal polyposis and nonallergic asthma (see Chapter 47, "Chronic Rhinosinusitis and Polyposis"). Avoidance of aspirin and nonsteroidal anti-inflammatory drugs is clearly important though there is some controversy as to whether avoidance of salicylate-like substances in the diet is beneficial or not. Some have argued that complete avoidance may render individuals more susceptible to inadvertent challenge while others believe a complete salicylate-free diet to be worse than the disease. Other strategies have included salicylate desensitization which must be performed with great care in hospital to manage any severe respiratory reactions. The use of topical lysine aspirin is an alternative approach which has been shown to be of benefit.[27]
- Cardiovascular preparations such as reserpine, guanethidine, phentolamine, methyldopa, angiotensin converting enzyme inhibitors and alpha-adrenoceptor antagonists are all known to affect the nose, typically producing nasal stuffiness.
- Topical ophthalmic beta-blockers.
- Chlorpromazine.
- Oral contraceptives, by hormonal modulation.
- Cocaine, more often used recreationally than medically, is a significant irritant producing frequent rhinorrhea and resultant sniffing, hyposmia, and septal perforation.[28] In extreme cases a midline destruction of the nose may result which has proved difficult to distinguish from T cell lymphoma or Wegener granulomatosis.[29]

Rhinitis Medicamentosa. Rhinitis medicamentosa is a well-described condition classically resulting from long-term abuse of topical decongestants.[30] The patient initially suffers a rebound congestion which leads to further use of the decongestant and ultimately develops significant mucosal atrophy. Consequently these preparations are not recommended for longer than 7 to 10 days. Once the condition is established it can prove difficult to wean a patient off the medication. The reason for originally starting the drug should be considered and in mild cases it may be possible to substitute a topical nasal corticosteroid. However, if there are no contraindications, an initial short course of oral prednisolone (30 mg/d for 5 day) may be necessary.[1]

Food-Induced Rhinitis

Food can produce nasal symptoms in a variety of ways. While allergy is a rare cause of isolated rhinitis, food-induced hypersensitivity may result in reaction to the foods themselves or colorants and preservatives.[31] Alcoholic beverages can produce a physiologic vasodilatation with associated nasal blockage as well as allergic and nonallergic reactions to their many components.

Gustatory rhinorrhea may result from spicy hot foods, probably due to the capsaicin content of red pepper. This substance is known to stimulate sensory nerves inducing release of neuropeptides such as tachykinins.[22]

Emotion

Sexual arousal and stress are known to have an effect on the nose, hence "honeymoon rhinitis," probably due to autonomic stimulation, although therapeutic intervention is rarely sought.

Atrophic Rhinitis

Primary atrophic rhinitis has been attributed to infection, most notably to *Klebsiella ozaenae*[32] (from the word "ozaena" meaning "stench") but may also relate to environmental factors and general health. The condition is characterized by progressive atrophy of the mucosa with loss of the turbinate bone and resulting in a capacious cavity full of foul-smelling crust. This should be distinguished from secondary atrophy following excessive surgery, trauma, radiotherapy, and chronic granulomatous conditions.

Primary atrophic rhinitis has become less common in countries where social conditions and health have generally improved. It affects both sides of the nose, occurs after puberty and is more common in women. Because of this, an endocrine imbalance has been postulated as a cause while others believe it has an autoimmune basis, possibly initiated by a virus or due to vitamin or iron deficiencies.

The most unpleasant symptom is the foul smell of which the patient is often unaware. The copious crusts often bleed when they detach and may extend into the nasopharynx, producing an unpleasant choking sensation and snorting. The nose paradoxically feels blocked, due to the drying effect in the abnormally patent airway.

Having eliminated other possible underlying conditions by appropriate hematologic studies and imaging, local treatment with saline or alkaline douching, emollients and lubricants such as 25% glucose and glycerine drops and regular decrusting may suffice. Antibiotics directed at *Klebsiella* are rarely successful in the long term though the fluoroquinolones and metronidazole have been used. A wide range of surgical procedures have been suggested, largely aimed at reduction of the size of the cavity, all with limited success. Closure of the nostrils with small skin flaps as advocated by Young[33] can be helpful, but relapse often occurs on reopening. It was suggested that reduction of airflow inhibited growth of the microorganisms, but this is unproven.

Nonallergic Rhinitis with Eosinophilia/ Eosinophilic Rhinitis Syndrome

Nonallergic rhinitis with eosinophilia syndrome was described 20 years ago although its existence as a separate entity is disputed. It should probably be regarded as a subgroup of idiopathic rhinitis characterized by nasal eosinophilia and perennial symptoms of sneezing, itching, rhinorrhea, blockage, and sometimes hyposmia in the absence of demonstrable allergy. It is possible that it represents an early stage of aspirin sensitivity and may be associated with asthma and nasal polyposis or may be a form of localized nasal allergy without systemic involvement. Intranasal corticosteroids are the mainstay of medical treatment combined with surgery for the polyps.[34]

Gastroesophageal Reflux

Reflux is increasingly thought to play a role in nonallergic rhinitis, particularly in children.[35]

MECHANICAL NASAL OBSTRUCTION

A common nasal complaint is one of nasal blockage, congestion, or obstruction. This may arise for a variety of reasons, be it a genuine mechanical obstruction to airflow, a response to autonomic or sensory changes in the nose, inflammation within the ostiomeatal complex, allergic changes or even a perception paradoxically in the presence of a patent or overly patent airway. It is important to investigate carefully this complaint to elucidate the cause since in the past there has been a tendency to offer surgery for the septum and/or turbinates without consideration or treatment of other contributory factors, inevitably compromising a successful symptomatic outcome.

Septal Deviation

Causes of Septal Deviation. Septal deformity can be congenital or acquired, although it should be recognized that a completely straight septum is the exception rather than the rule. This may be due to prenatal or perinatal factors in utero or during delivery. A true dislocation of the septum is rare, more often a horizontal fracture above the maxillary crest occurs which can be relocated immediately. Small microfractures may go unnoticed, presenting in later life or be exacerbated by falls during the "toddler" stage. In adolescence and as young adults, sports injuries, assault, and traffic accidents may all have their effect.

Effects. Any part of the nasal internal and external structure may be damaged, leading to deflections and deformities of the cartilages and bones. These may not be immediately obvious to the individual until infection or allergy intervenes. With age, loss of tensile strength in collagen may lead to collapse of the nasal valve region, uncovering preexisting nasal asymmetry. The sensation of nasal obstruction may alternate with the nasal cycle or be apparent when lying on that side. Disordered airflow may result in crusting and epistaxis on the deflected area. "As goes the septum, so goes the nose" correctly indicates that septal deviation can be associated with cosmetic deformity of the bridge and columella (see Chapter 53, "Rhinoplasty and Septoplasty").

Assessment of the external and internal nose, including anterior rhinoscopy and rigid endoscopy is important to assess the septal position and spurs, turbinates and exclude other abnormalities, particularly in the middle meatus and nasopharynx. Instillation of a topical decongestant may help determine the degree of mucosal swelling, particularly of the anterior nasal septum and inferior turbinates. Where available, objective measures of airway can be helpful.

Treatment. Septal manipulation is only of value in neonates when trauma has occurred during delivery. Septoplasty or submucous resection has been described to formally correct septal deviation. The distinction between these two techniques relates primarily to the incision and in practice most surgeons perform a combination of the two. The anterior approach used for septoplasty via a transfixion incision gives excellent access to the whole septum, while the lateral approach used for submucous resection denies access to the caudal septum. Theoretically, there is also a difference in the amount of cartilage resected, but in practice this will vary from individual to individual.

Complications

Septal Hematoma. The septal cartilage relies upon the perichondrium and overlying mucosa for its blood supply. A hematoma may form between the cartilage and perichondrium or between the perichondrium and the septal mucosa (Figure 2). In the former case the blood supply to the cartilage will be damaged and unless the hematoma is drained, cartilage death may ensue. This situation is further exacerbated by secondary

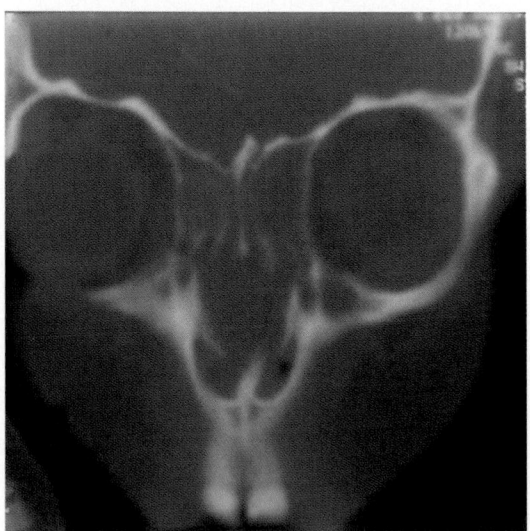

Figure 2 A coronal computed tomography scan showing expansion of the anterior nasal septum in a septal hematoma with opacification of the anterior ethmoid cells.

infection leading to a septal abscess associated with absorption of the cartilage and saddling of the nose. Consequently the hematoma should be drained, and the nose packed combined with giving broad-spectrum antibiotics.

Septal Perforation. There are many causes of septal perforation, the most common of which is some form of trauma, whether iatrogenic or self-inflicted (Figure 3 and Table 5). The most common site following septal surgery is in the region of the chondro-vomerine suture. Consequently, if a mucoperichondrial tear occurs during the surgery it is advisable to insert a piece of free cartilage at this point, ideally sutured in position.

Fortunately, many septal perforations are asymptomatic, but those of small diameter may make a whistling sound and the larger ones may be associated with crusting, spotting of blood and the sensation of nasal obstruction due to turbulence of airflow. The more anterior the perforation is, the more likely it is to cause symptoms. Although they will never heal spontaneously, only a minority of perforations require active treatment. In the first instance a trial of nasal douching with or without a topical corticosteroid may be given.

Many operations have been described to effect closure of septal perforations, the number being inversely proportional to the overall success of such interventions. These have included rotation and advancement of local tissue flaps, in particular "drop down" techniques, free grafts including fascia, split skin, and composites of, for example, pinna cartilage and skin. Bilateral labial flaps from the gingivolabial sulcus tunneled through into the nose have also been used; but, even if successful all these procedures suffer from the essential disadvantages of not providing a ciliated columnar epithelium and from being rather bulky. Alternatively the perforation may be quickly and easily filled with a commercially available button which can be customized to the individual perforation and left in place long term.

Infection/Toxic Shock Syndrome. Infection after nasal surgery is uncommon but is very painful and may cause an elevation of body temperature when it occurs. Cases of toxic shock syndrome have been described as a result of nasal packing. The condition is caused by the

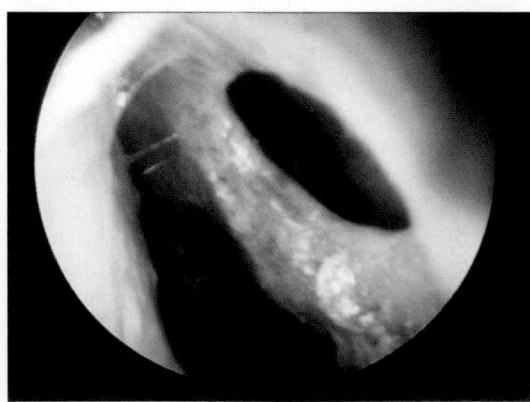

Figure 3 An endoscopic view of an anterior septal perforation.

Table 5 Causes of Septal Perforation
Traumatic
Septal surgery
Cauterization
Packing
Nasotracheal intubation
Foreign bodies, rhinolith
Inflammatory and infectious
Septal abscess or hematoma
Diphtheria
Typhoid
Syphilis
Tuberculosis
Serum lupus erythematosus
Sarcoid
Wegener granulomatosis
Toxic
Cocaine
Snuff-taking
Chromic acid fumes
Sulfuric acid fumes
Arsenicals
Mercurials
Phosphorus
Neoplasia
Carcinoma
Lymphoma
Midfacial necrotizing lesions
Leukemia
Idiopathic

toxin produced by a *Staphylococcus* that when absorbed produces headache, myalgia, nausea, and vomiting secondary to the pyrexia. Tachycardia, hypertension then hypotension, erythema of the skin are followed sometime later by desquamation of the skin of the hands. Toxic shock must be dealt with promptly and definitively. Cultures for *S. aureus* must be taken, a beta-lactamase-resistant antistaphylococcal antibiotic given systemically, and all packs and stitches removed.

Turbinate Enlargement

Causes. The inferior turbinates, and to a lesser extent, the adjacent septum and middle turbinates, have a complex submucosal structure, composed of vascular sinusoids under autonomic control. Under normal physiologic conditions, the inferior turbinates change in size with the nasal cycle throughout the day. This may be overridden by a number of factors such as exercise, posture, emotion, environmental temperature, and humidity. Generally one is unaware of these changes unless one side of the nose is narrower. A compensatory hypertrophy of the inferior turbinate is often seen on the wider side. A wide range of pathological processes including allergy, inflammation, and infection can produce symptomatic swelling of the turbinates.

Effects. Resistance to airflow primarily occurs in the valve region at the anterior ends of the inferior turbinates. To a lesser extent, the middle turbinate changes, obstructing the middle meatus and abutting the septum.

Treatment. *Medical.* Although topical decongestant sprays can significantly shrink the mucosa, long-term use will lead to rebound congestion and *rhinitis medicamentosa*. Topical nasal corticosteroids by contrast can be used over long periods of time for most forms of perennial rhinitis or rhinosinusitis.

Surgical. Surgery should only be considered after careful consideration of the cause of the patient's symptoms and after failure of adequate medication. Most of the techniques can be performed under local or general anesthesia and using headlight, microscope, or endoscopic visualization.[36] As no randomized controlled prospective trial has been performed to determine which of the many techniques is superior in the short or long term, choice devolves to personal preference and all may be accompanied by hemorrhage and crusting.

Lateral Out-Fracture. Single or multiple fractures of the inferior turbinate bone can be done with or without a submucous incision. The turbinate is pushed closer to the medial wall of the maxilla and may even be pressed into the maxilla (antroconchopexy), but the long-term results are debatable as the turbinate may resume its original position and the procedure does not deal with any soft tissue swelling or its cause. A modification, the submucosal out-fracture may be more effective in that it produces multiple small fractures of the turbinate bone through a small mucosal incision.

Submucous Diathermy. This technique has been popular since the early 1900s. A pointed electrode, insulated except for the terminal 3 to 5 mm is introduced into the anterior end of the inferior turbinate and passed along the whole length. The probe is then withdrawn slowly, over 20 seconds with the current on, and the procedure repeated at two or three points. Hemorrhage and adhesions can occur and the patient should be warned that there will be blockage due to reactionary swelling for some weeks after the surgery.

Linear Electrocautery. Linear electrocautery using a red-hot wire electrode to produce a thermal burn or a high-frequency coagulating current using a ball-tip electrode has enjoyed some popularity in the past. The technique has been largely superceded by more precise laser therapy, radiofrequency coblation, and reduction with powered microdebrider instrumentation.

Turbinectomy. Partial or subtotal removal of the turbinate offers a permanent solution to hypertrophy (the attachment of the inferior turbinate precludes genuine total turbinectomy unless a portion of the lateral nasal wall is removed). Apart from the occasional mulberry enlargement of the posterior end of the inferior turbinate, it should be remembered that it is the anterior end of the turbinate which offers the greatest resistance to airflow. As with all inferior turbinate surgery, patients must be warned about postoperative hemorrhage which can be profuse. A secondary hemorrhage rate of 8% is quoted, which will be severe in 1%.

Submucous Resection. Dissection of the mucoperiosteum of the turbinate is described though is difficult to perform in practice due to the

irregularities of the bone. It is best achieved by taking off an anterior sliver and then nibbling back the exposed bone so the mucosal edges fall together. A more elegant technique is the use of a powered microdebrider.

Laser Turbinectomy. A variety of cutting and coagulating lasers have been used to "cauterize" and reduce the inferior turbinate, including CO_2, argon, KTP, and neodymium YAG. A cross-hatching of the mucosa is thought to optimize shrinkage while preserving mucosa.

Cryosurgery. Cryosurgery with liquid nitrogen was popular in the past and has been largely superceded by other techniques.

Intraturbinal Corticosteroid Injection. Enthusiasm for the technique of intraturbinal corticosteroid injection diminished after reports of temporary and permanent blindness appeared. These may have occurred due to retrograde flow of particulate matter into the ophthalmic circulation, possibly associated with inadequate vasoconstriction.

Foreign Bodies

Types and Effects. A wide range of objects including metal, plastic, organic substances, and live insects find their way into the nose, either accidentally or deliberately with size being the only limiting factor. The result is a unilateral chronic purulent nasal discharge, which in a young child should be attributed to a foreign body until proved otherwise. If the foreign material has been present for some time it may form the nidus for deposition of calcium and magnesium salts, producing a rhinolith which is usually radiopaque (Figure 4).

Management. The history may be misleading and examination difficult, especially if the patient is uncooperative and the nose swollen. Imaging may be helpful but is not exclusive if negative. It is therefore, often necessary to examine the nose and remove the foreign body under a short general anesthetic, which should include a throat pack to avoid aspiration of the object.

GRANULOMATOUS CONDITIONS

A range of systemic conditions, including granulomas, vasculitides, connective tissue disorders such as systemic lupus erythematosus, relapsing polychondritis, eosinophilic angiocentric fibrosis, and skin conditions such as pemphigus, pemphigoid, and scleroderma can all manifest in the nose. Consequently, one should have a low-threshold of suspicion as one may have the first opportunity to make the diagnosis.

Sarcoidosis

Cause and Effects. Sarcoidosis is a systemic condition of unknown etiology characterized by noncaseating epithelioid granulomas. It rarely occurs in isolation in the upper respiratory tract, usually being found in association with lower

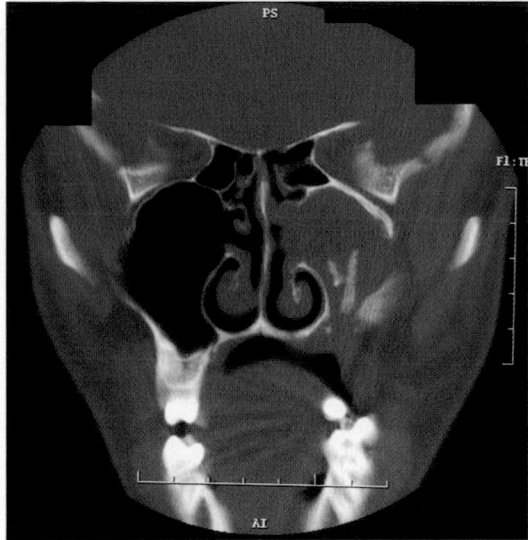

(A)

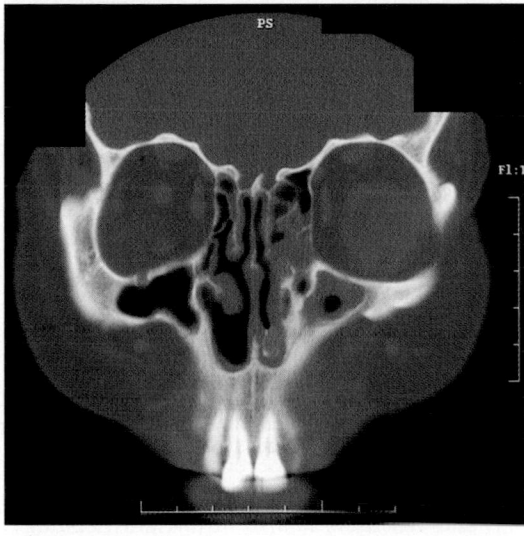

(B)

Figure 4 (A) Coronal computed tomography scan showing bone fragments in left maxillary sinus after facial trauma acting as foreign body with surrounding swelling of mucosa. (B) Coronal computed tomography scan showing silastic implant in left nasal cavity acting as a foreign body.

respiratory involvement. The condition has a predilection for certain geographical areas such as the rural southeast United States and Scandinavia, and certain ethnic groups such as West Indians, and is more common in women.

Nasal symptoms include obstruction, mucopurulent blood-stained discharge, and crusting.[37] There may be associated sinus infection, septal perforation with saddling of the nasal bridge, and violaceous lesions of lupus pernio on the nasal skin. The mucosa is inflamed with crust and old blood and a "strawberry skin" effect may be seen of the yellowish granulomas against the reddened lining.

Diagnosis includes erythrocyte sedimentation rate, serum calcium, and angiotensin converting enzyme, although there is no one absolute test for this condition. The Kveim test which was hitherto the most accurate has been withdrawn in the UK due to concerns over slow-viruses. Radiology of the chest is mandatory, plain radiographs may show punched-out erosion of the nasal bones

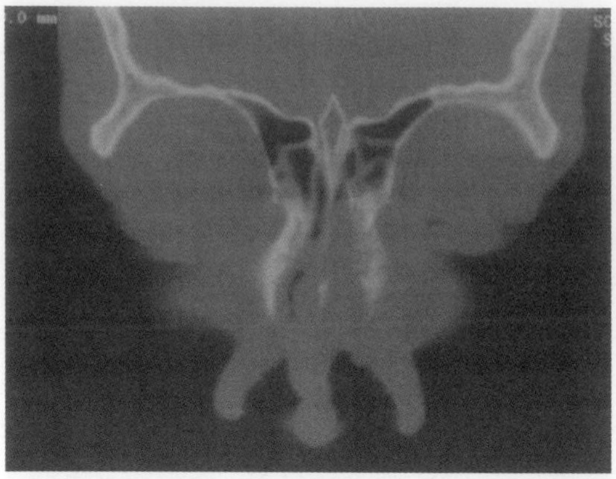

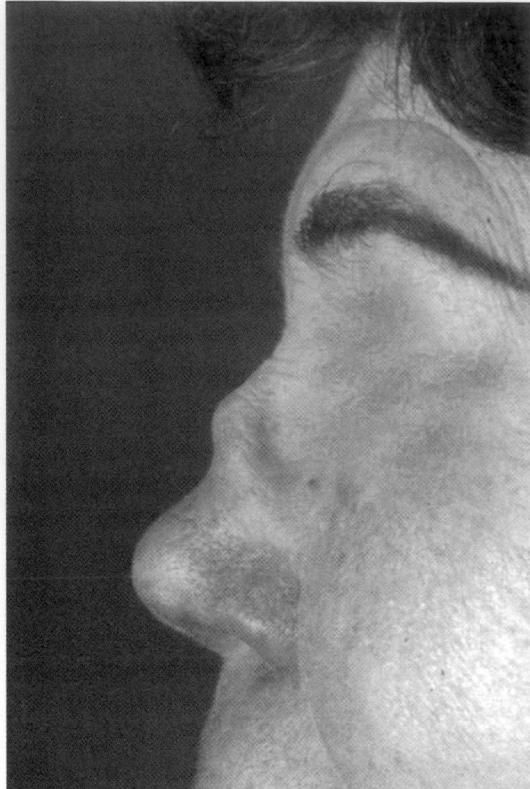

Figure 5 Coronal computed tomography scan showing osteitis of the nasal bones in a patient with sarcoidosis.

similar to that seen in dactylitis and CT may show a superficial nasal mass (Figure 5). Nasal biopsy can be useful when mucosal change is present but is only positive in 7% when the nose appears normal.[37] The condition must be distinguished from other granulomatous diseases such as tuberculosis, leprosy, berylliosis, Wegener granulomatosis, and acquired immunodeficiency syndrome.

Treatment. Local treatment with saline douche and topical corticosteroids are helpful, and the nose may improve with systemic treatment which usually includes oral corticosteroids, methotrexate, and hydroxychloroquine. Surgery, except for sinus infection, should be avoided as this can exacerbate collapse of the nose.

Wegener Granulomatosis

Cause and Effects. Wegener granulomatosis is a systemic condition characterized by granulomas and vasculitis is also of unknown etiology. An autoimmune basis or infection have been suggested but remain unproven.[38] It was originally described affecting the upper and lower respiratory tracts, together with a focal glomerulonephritis which rapidly led to renal failure and death. It is now known to affect any part of the body ab initio and to have a variable natural history, progressing inexorably in some individuals over a few weeks or months to a more insidious limited form in others, which may continue for some years before affecting other organs. Whether all of the latter ultimately progress to the full-blown disease is unknown.

Patients often present with a short history of progressive malaise, pyrexia, weight loss, and a disproportionate feeling of "unwellnesss" in comparison to what are often fairly nonspecific findings. In the nose the swollen inflamed mucosa produces blockage and blood-stained crusting. There may be destruction of the septum with a characteristic implosion of the nasal bridge (Figure 6). The nasopharynx, ears, mouth, larynx, trachea, cranial nerves, and orbit may all be involved. Unfortunately, the upper airway symptoms may be overlooked, and the diagnosis only made when other systems are affected.[39]

Diagnosis of the condition relied in the past on clinical acumen supported by a high erythrocyte sedimentation rate, C-reactive protein

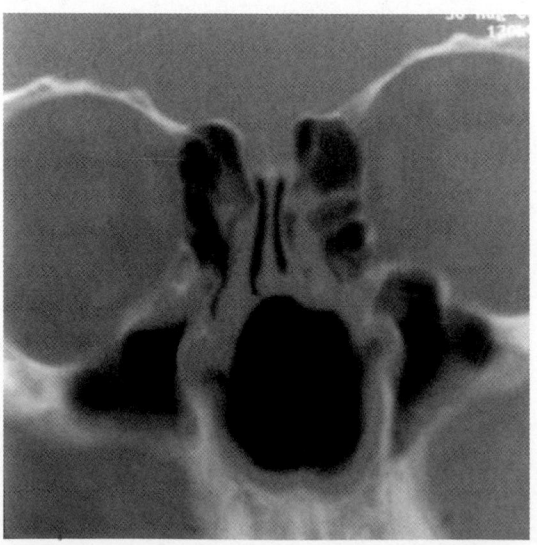

Figure 6 Clinical photograph showing typical collapse of the nasal bridge in a patient with Wegener granulomatosis.

and evidence of pulmonary and renal damage. The advent of the c-antineutrophil cytoplasmic antibodies greatly assisted diagnosis being highly specific and sensitive for the condition. However, a negative c-antineutrophil cytoplasmic antibody does not absolutely exclude the condition, particularly in the limited form and/or when oral corticosteroids have been given. CT of the nose and paranasal sinuses may show some midline destruction and often shows opacification of the sinuses[40] (Figure 7). This may be due to active granulomatous infiltration, burnt-out disease with fibrotic change or secondary infection.

Unfortunately, biopsy is not diagnostic, at best being described as "consistent with" Wegener granulomatosis but is helpful to exclude other pathology such as T-cell lymphoma.

Treatment. Medical therapy for Wegener granulomatosis includes systemic corticosteroids, a range of cytotoxic drugs, for example, cyclophosphamide, azathioprine and mycophenolate mofetil, immunoglobulin infusions, co-trimoxazole, and plasma exchange. Earlier diagnosis and careful monitoring has significantly improved the outcome for these patients, but the condition remains life-threatening in its more severe forms. The nose is again managed with douching and topical corticosteroids. Surgery may be required for secondary infection, but attempts to reconstruct the nose should be resisted until the disease has been quiescent for some years.

AMYLOIDOSIS

Apart from amyloid deposits in the skin of the vestibule in generalized amyloidosis, involvement of the nose and sinus is extremely rare. In contrast to the upper respiratory tract as a whole, only a handful of isolated amyloid deposits have been reported, whereas in generalized plasmacytic malignant lymphoma 20% of the patients may have sinonasal amyloid deposits. The diagnosis may be confirmed histologically by the presence of Congo red reactivity and green birefringence in polarized light. Colchicine has been used in the treatment of the condition.

RHINOPHYMA

In rhinophyma a disfiguring enlargement of the nose develops due to an overgrowth of sebaceous tissue and blood vessels. Tissue overgrowth begins at the tip of the nose and progresses to involve the ala nasae and the columella and is associated with a florid discoloration. The affected tissue may be pared down using a simple knife, electrodissection or laser therapy producing good cosmetic results.

NASAL GLIOMAS AND ENCEPHALOCELE

Nasal encephaloceles are protrusions of brain content through a congenital defect in the skull. If no defect is present then the mass is termed a glioma. These lesions are relatively uncommon and while many are diagnosed at birth some may not become apparent until adulthood when associated with a cerebrospinal fluid leak and meningitis. 60% of gliomas are extranasal, 30% intranasal, and the remainder have both intra- and extranasal components. The external lesions are found over the dorsum or to one side. There is a general agreement that nasal encephaloceles and gliomas are developmental rather than neoplasms probably due to a failure of the foramen caecum to close thus permitting the brain to

Figure 7 Coronal computed tomography scan in patient with Wegener granulomatosis showing midline destruction of the septum and loss of the inferior turbinates.

extrude. The intracranial connection may persist as in an encephalocele or be interrupted as in a glioma.

Clinical Features

Nasofrontal encephaloceles are compressible, fluctuant, and pulsatile. Swelling may increase in size on crying or straining. Intranasal encephaloceles protrude through the defect into the upper nasal cavity where they can be mistaken for a nasal polyp. By contrast gliomas do not change with crying or straining. Imaging is mandatory in any patient with a swelling in the frontonasal region or a unilateral nasal polyp[41] (Figure 8).

Treatment

The majority of these intranasal lesions can be managed endoscopically using an underlay, onlay or combination repair with a variety of homografts including cartilage, fascia and nasal mucosa.[42] External and more extensive lesions may require external approaches including a craniofacial approach.

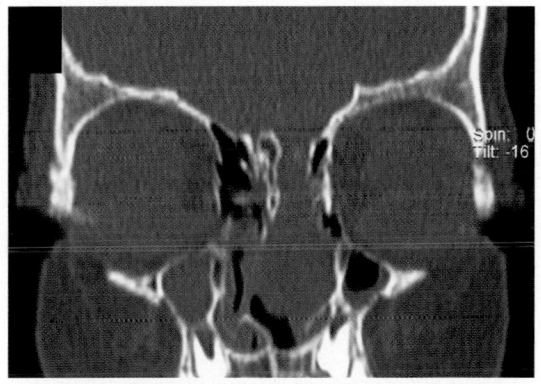

(A)

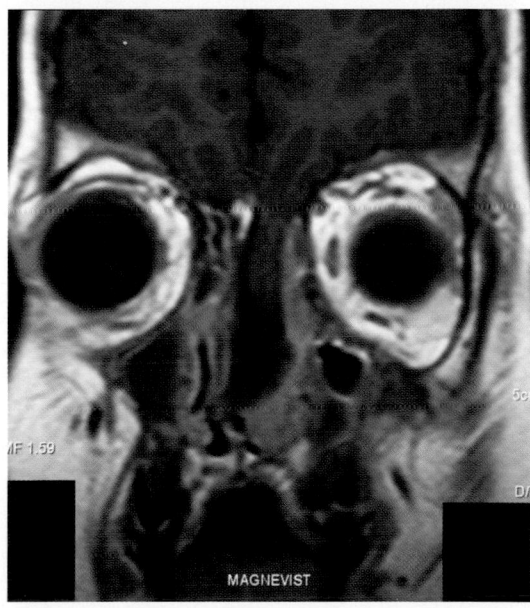

(B)

Figure 8 (A) Coronal computed tomography scan showing meningoencephalocoele presenting in nasal cavity. (B) Coronal magnetic resonance imaging scan of same patient.

MALIGNANT NEOPLASMS OF THE SKIN OF THE NOSE

Basal Cell Carcinoma

The skin of the nose is the most common site for basal cell carcinoma in the head and neck. It is considerably more common than squamous cell carcinoma with a peak incidence in the sixth to eighth decades. The most common areas are the side, dorsum, and tip of the nose, and the lesion may be a small nodular growth or form a chronic ulcer with a rolled edge. Although many behave in an indolent fashion, unless treated appropriately, they have a tendency to recur which may lead to considerable destruction of the face. The side of the nose adjacent to the medial canthal area can prove particularly problematic.

Basal cell carcinomas are usually very sensitive to radiotherapy but may require surgical excision particularly for recurrence. A variety of local rotation flaps or full thickness skin grafts are available and are discussed in Chapter 54, "Nasal Reconstruction."

Squamous cell carcinoma though less common may also affect the skin of the nose again in the sixth to eighth decades. The lesion is generally nodular, resembling a keratoacanthoma but can ulcerate. Differentiation from a basal cell carcinoma may be difficult without biopsy (Figure 9). Treatment again relies on radiotherapy and/or surgery. Squamous cell carcinoma has a higher propensity for metastatic spread than basal cell carcinoma, and lesions in the midline particularly on the columella may disseminate bilaterally. In-continuity lymphatic resection is not possible, leading to a potentially poor prognosis.

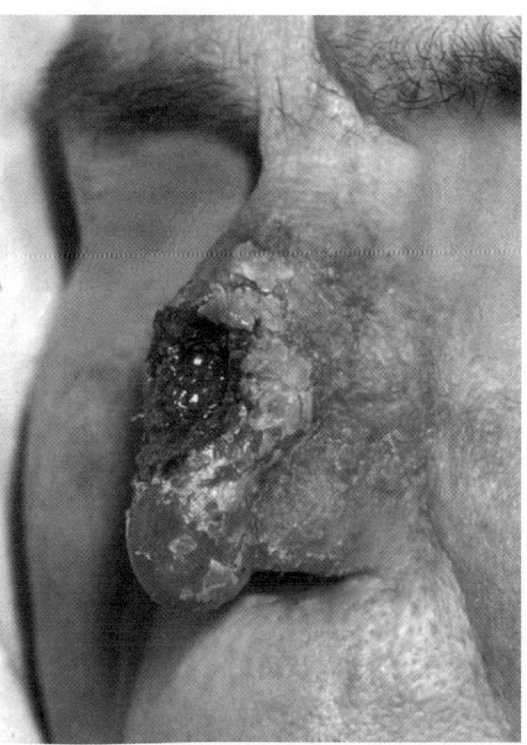

Figure 9 Clinical photograph showing a squamous cell carcinoma of the bridge of the nose.

REFERENCES

1. Lund VJ, Aaronsen D, Bousquet J, et al. International Rhinitis Management Working Group. The international consensus report on the diagnosis and management of rhinitis. Allergy 1994;49:1–34.
2. Bousquet J, Van Cauwenberge P, Khaltaev N, et al. World Health Organization. Allergic rhinitis and its impact on asthma. J Allergy Clin Immunol 2001;108:S147–334.
3. Fokkens W, Lund VJ, Bachert C, et al. Position paper on rhinosinusitis and nasal polyps. EAACI task force. Allergy 2005;60:583–601.
4. Meltzer EO, Hamilos DL, Hadley JA, et al. Rhinosinusitis: Establishing definitions for clinical research and patient care. Otolaryngol Head Neck Surg 2004;131:S1–62.
5. Hens G, Hellings PW. The nose: Gatekeeper and trigger of bronchial disease. Rhinology 2006;44:179–87.
6. Lund VJ, Scadding GK. Objective assessment of endoscopic sinus surgery in the management of chronic rhinosinusitis. J Laryngol Otol 1994;108:749–53.
7. Casiano RR, Cohn S, Villasuso E, III, et al. Comparison of antral tap with endoscopically directed nasal culture. Laryngoscope 2001;111:1333–7.
8. Rutland J, Dewar A, Cox T, Cole P. Nasal brushing for the study of ciliary ultrastructure. J Clin Pathol 1982;35:357–9.
9. Lindberg S, Cervin A, Runer T. Nitric oxide (NO) production in the upper airways is decreased in chronic sinusitis. Acta Otolaryngol 1997;117:113–7.
10. Ragab SM, Lund VJ, Saleh HA, Scadding G. Nasal nitric oxide in objective evaluation of chronic rhinosinusitis therapy. Allergy 2006;61:717–24.
11. Holmstrom M, Scadding GK, Lund VJ. The assessment of nasal obstruction—a comparison between rhinomanometry and nasal inspiratory peak flow. Rhinology 1990;28:191–6.
12. Clement PAR, Gordts F. Consensus report on acoustic rhinometry and rhinomanometry. Rhinology 2005;43:169–79.
13. Simmen D, Briner HR. Olfaction in rhinology—methods of assessing the sense of smell. Rhinology 2006;44:98–101.
14. Gwaltney JM, Phillips CD, Miller RD, et al. Computer tomographic study of the common cold. N Engl J Med 1994;330:25–30.
15. Meltzer EO, Bachert C, Staudinger H. Treating acute rhinosinusitis: Comparing efficacy and safety of mometasone furoate nasal spray, amoxicillin and placebo. J Allergy Clin Immunol 2005;116:1289–95.
16. Shahin J, Gullane PJ, Dayal VS. Orbital complications of acute sinusitis. J Otolaryngol 1987;16:23–7.
17. Lund VJ. Complications of sinusitis. In: Mackay IS, Bull TR, editors. Scott-Brown's Otolaryngology, Volume 4: Rhinology, 6th edition. Oxford: Butterworth-Heineman; 1997. p. 4/13/1–11.
18. Silvers WS. The skier's nose: A model of cold-induced rhinoohea. Ann Allergy 1991;67:32–6.
19. Bascom R, Kesavanathan J, Fitzgerald TK, et al. Sidestream tobacco smoke exposure acutely alters human nasal mucociliary clearance. Environ Health Perspect 1995;103: 1026–30.
20. Vinke J, KleinJan A, Severijnen LW, Fokkens W. Passive smoking causes an "allergic" cell infiltrate in the nasal mucosa of non-atopic children. Int J Ped Otorhinol 1999;51:73–81.
21. Annesi-Maesano I, Oryszczyn MP, Neukirch F, Kauffmann F. Relationship of upper airway disease to tobacco smoking and allergic markers: A cohort study of men followed up for 5 years. Int Arch Allergy Immunol 1997;114:193–201.
22. Lacroix JS, Buvelot JM, Polla BS, Lundberg JM. Improvement of symptoms of non-allergic chronic rhinitis by local treatment with capsaicin. Clin Exp Allergery 1991;21:595–600.
23. Schiffman SS, Nagle HT. Effect of environmental pollutants on taste and smell. Otolaryngol Head Neck Surg 1992;106:693–700.
24. Ellegard E, Karlsson G. Nasal congestion during pregnancy. Clin Otolaryngol 1999;24:307–11.
25. Schatz M. Special considerations for the pregnant woman and senior citizen with airway disease. J Allergy Clin Immunol 1998;101:S373–8.
26. Mazzotta P, Loebstein R, Koren G. Treating allergic rhinitis in pregnancy. Safety considerations. Drug Saf 1999;20:361–75.
27. Parikh AA, Scadding GK. Intranasal lysine-aspirin in aspirin sensitive nasal polyposis: A controlled trial. Laryngoscope 2005;115:1385–90.
28. Schwartz RH, Estroff T, Fairbanks DN, Hoffmann NG. Nasal symptoms associated with cocaine abuse during adolescence. Arch Otolaryngol Head Neck Surg 1989;115:63–4.
29. Seyer BA, Grist W, Muller S. Aggressive destructive midfacial lesion from cocaine abuse. Oral Surg Oral Med Oral Pathol Oral Radiol Endod 2002;94:465–70.

30. Graf P. Rhinitis medicamentosa: Aspects of pathophysiology and treatment. Allergy 1997;52:28–34.

31. Bousquet J, Metcalfe D. Warner J. Food allergy. Report of the Codex alimentarius. ACI International 1997;9:10–21.

32. Henriksen S, Gundersen W. The aetiology of ozaena. Acta Pathol Microbiol Scand 1959;47:380–6.

33. Young A. Closure of the nostrils in atrophic rhinitis. J Laryngol Otol 1967;81:515–24.

34. Blom HM, Godthelp T, Fokkens WJ, et al. The effect of nasal steroid aqueous spray on nasal complaint scores and cellular infiltrates in the nasal mucosa of patients with non-allergic, non-infectious perennial rhinitis. J Allergy Clin Immunol 1997;100:739–47.

35. Euler AR. Upper respiratory tract complications of gastro-esophageal reflux in adult and pediatric-age patients. Dig Dis 1998;16:111–7.

36. Lund VJ. Surgery of the inferior turbinate. Facial Plast Surg (Rhinoplasty and Airways) 1986;3:227–80.

37. Wilson R, Lund VJ, Sweatman M, et al. Upper respiratory tract involvement in sarcoidosis and its management. Eur J Resp Med 1988;1:269–72.

38. Lund VJ, Cambridge G. Immunologicals aspects of Wegener's granulomatosis. In: Veldman JE, Passali D, Lim DJ, editors. Immuno and Molecular Biology in ORL—State of the Art. Amsterdam, The Netherlands: Kugler Publications; 2000. p. 195–207.

39. Srouji IA, Andrews P, Edwards C, Lund VJ. General and rhinosinusitis related quality of life in patients with Wegener's granulomatosis. Laryngoscope 2006;116: 1621–5.

40. Lloyd G, Lund VJ, Beale T, Howard D. Rhinologic changes in Wegener's granulomatosis. J Laryngol Otol 2002;116:565–9.

41. Lund VJ, Savy L, Lloyd G, Howard D. Optimum imaging and diagnosis of cerebrospinal fluid rhinorrhoea. J Laryngol Otol 2000;114: 988–92.

42. Lund VJ. Endoscopic management of CSF leaks. Am J Rhinol 2002;16:17–23.

46

Acute Rhinosinusitis and Its Complications

Todd A. Loehrl, MD
Timothy Wells, MD
Grant Su, MD

Rhinosinusitis simply defined is an inflammatory and/or infectious condition of 1 or more of the paranasal sinus cavities. Acute rhinosinusitis (ARS) implies that the duration of the condition is less than 1 month. Most cases of ARS are community acquired and are associated with viral upper respiratory tract infections (URI), although other causes may be responsible. It is estimated that 0.5 to 2% of colds result in ARS, and up to 1 in 20 URI lead to acute bacterial rhinosinusitis (ABRS).[1,2] Acute infectious rhinosinusitis can be broken down into several different categories based on several characteristics including location of occurrence (hospital- or community-acquired), immune status of the patient, and offending microorganism (viral, bacterial, and/or fungal).

The diagnosis of ABRS can be challenging due to inaccessibility of the paranasal sinuses to direct examination. Thus, traditionally clinicians have relied upon relatively insensitive or nonspecific signs and symptoms to arrive at a diagnosis. Furthermore, the fact that paranasal sinus mucosal thickening and fluid is frequently associated with the common cold (acute viral rhinosinusitis) has led to further confusion.[3] Therefore, without culture confirmation, differentiation between acute viral rhinosinusitis and ABRS is difficult. This has lead to growing concern regarding the emergence of antimicrobial resistance as a result of the inappropriate prescription of antibiotics for viral URI. In addition, the excessive use of antibiotics for this condition can have a major impact on healthcare costs.

Although the complications of ABRS are less common in recent years, they are still associated with significant short- and long-term morbidity as well as mortality. Thus, although many of these cases are managed in a multidisciplinary manner, it is important that the otolaryngologist-head and neck surgeon have a thorough knowledge of the pathophysiology, evaluation, and medical/surgical treatment of these patients.

EPIDEMIOLOGY

Rhinosinusitis reportedly affects 32 million US adults annually and resulted in 11.7 million office visits as well as 1.2 million hospital outpatient unit visits. This generated direct annual costs in excess of $3.4 billion in that same year.[4] In addition, quality of life and productivity may be adversely affected. Epidemiologic studies suggest that one billion cases of acute viral rhinosinusitis can be anticipated annually. Therefore 20 million cases of ABRS are expected annually, given that approximately 2% of people with acute viral rhinosinusitis go on to develop ABRS. Thus the diagnosis of ABRS accounted for 21% and 9% of all adult and pediatric antibiotic prescriptions, respectively, written in 2002.[5]

The average adult and child in the United States experience 2 to 3 and 6 to 8 episodes of the common cold (viral upper respiratory tract infection) per year, respectively.[6] Viral upper respiratory tract infection rates have a predictable pattern with annual epidemics in the fall, winter, and spring periods, while summer rates are relatively low. As noted previously, 0.5 to 2.0% of the general population with acute viral sinusitis develop ABRS as opposed to the pediatric population where 5 to 13% of these viral infections result in ABRS. As one would expect, the seasonal trends in presumed ABRS have been correlated with those of viral URI.[7] Many other risk factors must be considered in addition to viral causes including allergy, swimming, sinus ostial obstruction due to anatomic abnormalities, tumors or foreign bodies, and polypoid disease. In addition, in some patients, immune deficiency and disorders of mucociliary clearance may predispose to ABRS.

PATHOGENESIS

Viral

The upper airway provides little in the way of defense to rhinovirus as >90% of nonimmunocompromised subjects inoculated go on to become infected.[8] Approximately 50% of common colds are caused by the human rhinovirus. Other viral offenders include influenza A and B viruses, parainfluenza virus, respiratory syncytial virus, adenovirus, and enterovirus. Influenza and adenovirus are known to injure the nasal epithelium while rhinovirus and coronavirus induce minimal damage.[9] Of the patients who are infected, about 75% go on to develop symptoms of an upper respiratory tract infection. After initial nasal exposure, the virus is transported posteriorly to the nasopharynx and attaches to intracellular adhesion molecule 1, resulting in the activation of several inflammatory pathways. In addition, the autonomic nervous system reaction, characterized by parasympathetic nervous system predominance, results in engorgement of the turbinate vasculature, intercellular leakage of plasma, seromucinous discharge, and stimulation of pain nerves as well as cough reflexes.[10]

Previous investigators have noted reversible computed tomography (CT) or magnetic resonance imaging (MRI) mucosal/fluid abnormalities in 87 and 88% of adults and children, respectively, with early community acquired URI (Figure 1). After 2 weeks, in the adult population, approximately 80% of these findings were found to resolve without antibiotic treatment.[11]

Bacterial

ABRS is most frequently preceded by a viral URI. The causes of secondary bacterial infection are unknown but probably depend upon several factors involving both the host and the offending microorganism. It is known that the passages of the paranasal sinuses and nasopharynx

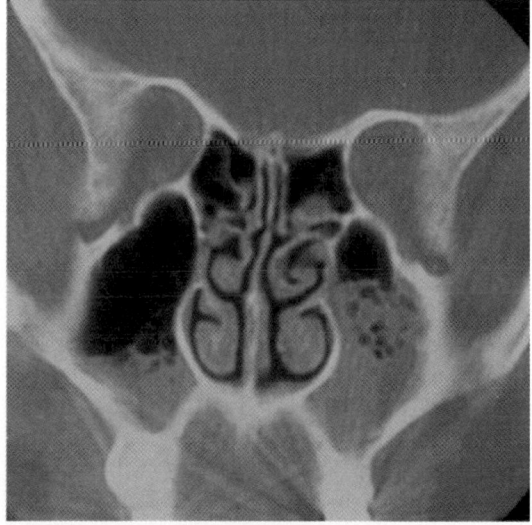

Figure 1 Coronal computed tomography scan of the sinuses demonstrating findings of acute rhinosinusitis based on bilateral maxillary sinus air/fluid levels. Note that acute bacterial rhinosinusitis cannot be differentiated from an acute viral rhinosinusitis based on this finding.

are colonized by the same bacterial species that cause ABRS. Frequently, as noted above, even in acute URIs air/fluid levels or air bubbles are noted on CT scanning; however, the composition of this material remains unknown. Gwaltney and colleagues demonstrated that nose blowing during an upper respiratory infection might propel mucous secretions into the paranasal sinuses. Specifically, they demonstrated that nose blowing (not sneezing or coughing) results in intranasal pressures that might be transiently elevated to 60 to 80 mm Hg. Furthermore, contrast material from the nasopharynx was propelled into the paranasal sinuses by this mechanism.[12] Thus, vigorous nose blowing may provide one explanation for the viscous exudates associated with colds. In addition, the exudates in these patients may be harder to clear both due to increased viscosity and mucociliary dysfunction.[13] Given the mucosal edema and compromised ventilation of the paranasal sinuses, conditions are favorable for bacterial overgrowth. In addition, viruses also have a substantial impact on neutrophil, macrophage, and lymphocyte function resulting in vulnerability to bacterial overgrowth by pathogens know to reside in the nose and nasopharynx as noted above.

Bacterial Pathogens. Most commonly, the pathogens in ABRS include *Streptococcus pneumoniae, Haemophilus influenzae,* and *Moraxella catarrhalis* (more common in the pediatric population).[14] In addition, other streptococcal species including *Streptococcus intermedius, Streptococcus pyogenes,* and other α-hemolytic streptococci may be involved as well as *Staphylococcus aureus* and anaerobic bacteria.

While the bacteria involved in ABRS have not changed over the last half century, their antimicrobial susceptibilities have changed dramatically. Penicillin resistance first appeared in *S. aureus* followed by β-lactam resistance in *H. influenzae* and *M. catarrhalis.* Finally, multiantibiotic resistant *S. pneumoniae* have emerged in recent years.

DIAGNOSIS

Viral

Viral URI's symptoms typically consist of rhinorrhea, sneezing, nasal airway obstruction, facial congestion, hyposmia, sore throat, cough, eustachian tube dysfunction, fevers, and myalgias. Purulent nasal drainage is not necessarily consistent with the development of ABRS as this may also occur due to an influx of neutrophils.[15]

Bacterial

The clinical signs and symptoms typically associated with ABRS lack sensitivity (69%) and specificity (64%).[16] Radiographically, the diagnosis of ABRS is difficult as well, given that approximately 87% of patients with early community acquired acute URI will have mucosal edema and/or fluid (with or without air bubbles) on CT

scan. Further complicating the accurate diagnosis of ABRS is the finding that duration of symptoms does not reliably distinguish prolonged viral infection from ABRS.[17] Thus, the clinician must rely on clinical judgment when making the decision regarding the diagnosis of ABRS. In general, ABRS can be considered when a viral URI does not resolve after 10 days or is worsening at 5 to 7 days. Some or all of the following signs and symptoms may be present: nasal drainage, facial pressure/pain, decreased/absent olfaction, fever, cough, fatigue, dental pain, and/or ear pressure.[5]

TREATMENT RECOMMENDATIONS

Therapeutic antimicrobial recommendations for ABRS are based upon published evidence of known bacterial pathogens and clinical improvement. Studies have confirmed that appropriately prescribed (spectrum, dose, and duration) antimicrobials are effective in reducing sinus cavity bacterial titers as compared to antimicrobials with an inadequate activity spectrum, dose, or duration.[18] In fact, bacteriologic cure rates of >90% have been reported for appropriately selected antibiotics.[19] In the adult population with mild disease and no antibiotics in the prior 6 weeks, the following choices may be considered: amoxicillin/clavulanate (1.75 g/250 mg/d), amoxicillin (1.5 to 4 g/d), cefpodoxime proxetil, cefuroxime axetil, or cefdinir. In patients with β-lactam allergies, trimethoprim-sulfamethoxazole, docycline, azithromycin, clarithromycin, erythromycin, or telithromycin may be used, but bacteriologic failure rates range from 20 to 25%. In those patients who have received antimicrobials in the prior 6 weeks, fluoroquinolones (levofloxacin, moxifloxacin) or higher dose amoxicillin-clavulanate (4 g/250 mg/d) may be considered. Failure to respond to treatment within 72 hours requires a switch to another antimicrobial and/or reevaluation of the patient.[5] Further management options might include imaging (CT scan), nasal endoscopy with culture/sensitivity, and/or sinus aspiration.

In the pediatric population, the choices are similar to the adult population with 2 exceptions: (1) dosing is based upon weight, and (2) fluoroquinolones are not an option in the pediatric population. A 10-day treatment course with 1 of the above antimicrobials is recommended. Finally, an inappropriate antibiotic of insufficient duration may prolong infection and potentially morbidity of the disease. Antibiotic options for those patients with severe infections and/or complications of ABRS will be discussed in the following sections.

ORBITAL COMPLICATIONS

There are several major ophthalmic complications of ARS that may occur, including preseptal and orbital cellulitis, subperiosteal abscess (SPA), orbital abscess, cavernous sinus thrombosis, eyelid abscess, and vision loss. The most

widely accepted classification of the orbital complications is the modified five-tier system proposed by Chandler and colleagues,[20] which depicts the spectrum of orbital involvement as follows: Group I-inflammatory edema or preseptal cellulitis; Group II-orbital cellulitis, Group III-SPA; Group IV-orbital abscess; and Group V-cavernous sinus thrombosis. It is important to note that these groups do not necessarily represent a rigid chronology of disease progression since they may be present in combination or evolve from one another. This classification system does however explain the signs and symptoms and helps to organize treatment plans as well as stratify outcomes.

Group I-Preseptal Cellulitis

The first group is inflammatory edema or preseptal cellulitis, which is an infection of the soft tissue of the eyelids and periocular region anterior to the orbital septum. Underlying rhinosinusitis has been implicated in 14.5 to 81% of hospitalized children with preseptal cellulitis.[21] On clinical examination, the eyelid is typically edematous, erythematous, as well as warm and tender to touch. Signs of postseptal orbital involvement such as proptosis, visual impairment, and chemosis of the conjunctiva are not observed. Visual acuity, pupillary reaction, extraocular motility, and intraocular pressure are normal. Preseptal cellulitis is usually managed medically with systemic antibiotics and careful clinical observation. However, due to the valveless facial veins, preseptal cellulitis may spread posterior to the septum and produce subsequent intraorbital infections in Groups II to V.

Group II-Orbital Cellulitis

Orbital cellulitis is an infection of the orbital soft tissues posterior to the orbital septum without abscess formation. Sinusitis is the major cause of orbital cellulitis, with studies reporting 96 to 100% of hospitalized patients with orbital cellulitis having concurrent sinusitis.[21] Orbital cellulitis is also more common in patients younger than 9 years old, with 1 study reporting 68% in a series of 303 patients with orbital cellulitis.[22] With the administration of the *Hemophilus influenzae* type B vaccine, the average age of children with orbital cellulitis has risen with the changing microbiological spectrum.[23] Symptoms of orbital cellulitis may include eyelid edema, erythema, conjunctival chemosis, axial proptosis, limitation of extraocular movement, pain with eye movement, and increased intraocular pressure. In addition to these signs, patients with orbital cellulitis often have more systemic toxicity, such as fever, leukocytosis, and elevated levels of C-reactive protein than patients with preseptal cellulitis. All patients with suspected orbital cellulitis should be imaged and treated with intravenous antibiotic therapy and nasal decongestants. Visual acuity and pupil reflex must be closely monitored. Patients who develop a decrease in visual acuity, an afferent pupillary defect, worsening extraocular muscle

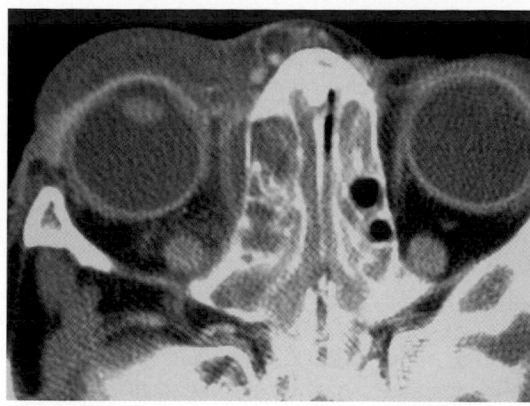

Figure 2 Axial computed tomography scan demonstrating ethmoid rhinosinusitis with adjacent right-sided medial subperiosteal abscess.

function, or failure to improve in 48 to 72 hours should undergo surgical sinus drainage with culture.

Group III-Subperiosteal Abscess

In SPA, there is an inflammatory fluid that collects in the potential space between the periorbita and the orbital wall. The diagnosis is confirmed by CT scan as a convex mass adjacent to the involved sinus (Figure 2). However, SPA can be suspected based on clinical examination. In addition to signs of orbital involvement, the eye may exhibit directional proptosis with the globe typically displaced away from the SPA (Figures 3 to 5). The patient may also have limited extraocular motility and pain on globe movement toward the abscess. The most common location of a SPA is along the medial orbital wall secondary to ethmoid rhinosinusitis. The abscess develops when infection breaks through the lamina papyracea or through the foramina of the anterior or posterior ethmoidal neurovascular bundles. The periorbita is loosely adherent along the medial orbital wall, which may permit abscess contents to migrate superiorly, inferiorly, or posteriorly within the subperiosteal space. Treatment recommendations for SPA include intravenous antibiotics alone in select cases with careful observation and surgical management in refractory cases. Several studies

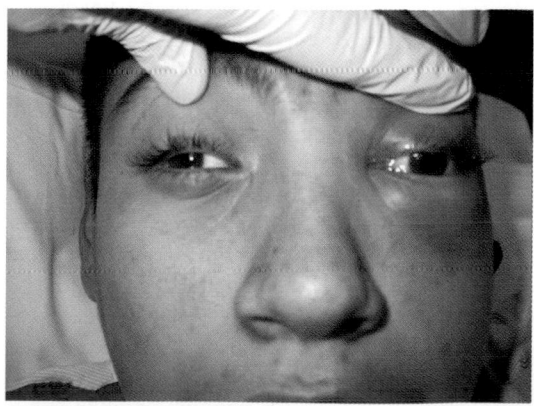

Figure 3 Fifteen-year-old patient with left maxillary, ethmoid, sphenoid, and frontal rhinosinusitis with a resultant left inferior and medial subperiosteal abscesses. The patient underwent left endoscopic sinus surgery and left anterior orbitotomy via inferior transconjunctival and medial transcaruncular approaches to drain the abscesses.

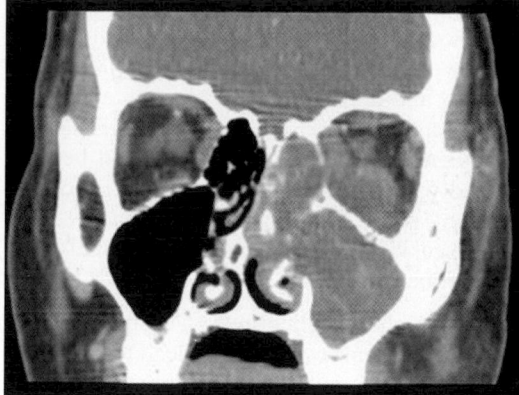

Figure 4 Coronal computed tomography scan of patient in Figure 3 demonstrating left pansinusitis and adjacent inferior and medial subperiosteal abscesses.

have reported good response to medical management alone in select cases. In a study by Garcia and Harris, 27 of 29 (93.1%) SPAs resolved with medical therapy in patients that satisfied the following inclusion criteria: (1) age of patients less than 9-years old; (2) absence of frontal sinusitis; (3) medial location of the SPA; (4) small size of the SPA; (5) absence of gas within the abscess space (visualized on CT scan to exclude anaerobic infection); (6) primary SPA; (7) absence of chronic sinusitis; (8) no evidence of optic nerve compromise; and (9) no history of infection of dental origin.[24] Failure of medical therapy is suggested by vision loss, afferent pupillary defect, persistent fever after 36 hours of antibiotic treatment, clinical deterioration after 48 hours of antibiotics, or failure to improve within 72 hours of antibiotic treatment.[24] In a more recent study, Oxford and McClay also showed that small medial SPAs without significant ophthalmic signs may be managed medically with favorable outcomes.[25] In their study, 18 of 43 (42%) SPAs resolved with medical management alone, including 5 children older than 9 years. The authors proposed several criteria for medical management of medial SPA including: (1) normal vision, pupil, and retina; (2) no ophthalmoplegia; (3) intraocular pressure <20 mm Hg; (4) proptosis of 5 mm or less; and (5) abscess width of 4 mm or less.[25] It is important to note that radiographic worsening of the SPA

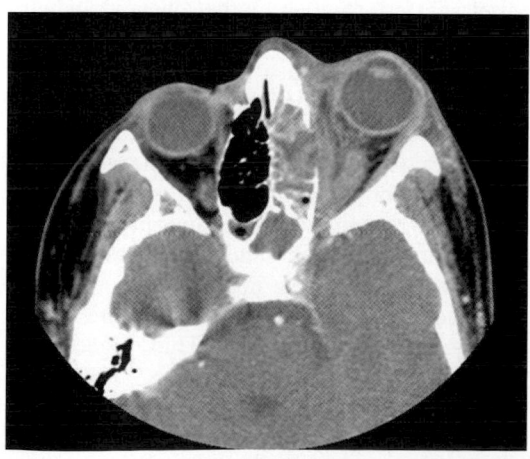

Figure 5 Axial computed tomography scan of patient in Figure 3 demonstrating lamina papyracea dehiscence as well as ethmoid and sphenoid rhinosinusitis.

should not be used as the only guide in the management strategy since the CT appearance may actually appear worse despite successful treatment with an antibiotic. In a study of 37 medial SPAs, the initial CT scans were not predictive of the clinical course.[26] Serial scans showed enlargement of abscesses during the first few days of intravenous antibiotic therapy regardless of the ultimate response to treatment. It was concluded that expansion of a SPA in serial CT scans during the first few days of treatment should not be considered antibiotic treatment failure. The time-dependent pharmacokinetics of antibiotic penetration into the SPA influences the resolution of the fluid collection. Given the temporal disparity between the clinical course and CT findings, the clinical course, not the radiographic appearance, should dictate management.

Group IV-Orbital Abscess

Orbital abscesses refer to the presence of pus within the orbital fat, which may occur within the muscle cone (intraconal) or outside the muscle cone (extraconal) as a consequence of coalescence of the infectious process. Diagnosis is confirmed by CT scan and corroborated by the signs of eyelid edema, conjunctival chemosis, proptosis, limited ocular motility, afferent pupillary defect, visual impairment, and venous engorgement or papilledema on funduscopic examination. Orbital apex syndrome, consists of unilateral ptosis, proptosis, vision loss, internal and external ophthalmoplegia (ie, palsy of the pupillary and extraocular muscles), and cranial nerve V1 anesthesia, is also indicative of orbital abscess. The clinical presentation may vary depending upon the size and location of the orbital abscess, duration of the infection, virulence of the microorganisms, and host factors. Orbital abscess has the potential for serious complications. Therefore, any clinical sign or symptom suggestive of orbital abscess warrants immediate imaging and intensive antibiotic therapy. Early surgical intervention is necessary when the presence of an orbital abscess is confirmed.

Abscesses can also occur in other orbital structures such as the lacrimal gland. Patel and colleagues reported a 9-year-old boy with lacrimal gland abscess thought to be caused by spread of infection from the paranasal sinuses. Despite initial surgery to drain the paranasal sinuses, the patient failed to improve, and a repeat CT scan which showed a fluid collection in the left lacrimal gland region causing downward and outward proptosis. Further surgical exploration of the orbit revealed an abscess of the lacrimal gland, which was incised and drained, resulting in complete recovery.[27] In another case, Mirza and colleagues reported a 72-year-old woman with myelodysplasia who initially presented with a preseptal cellulitis secondary to rhinosinusitis. Despite antibiotic therapy and endoscopic drainage of the sinuses, the infection failed to resolve completely, and repeated CT imaging revealed an abscess of the lacrimal gland. Subsequent incision and drainage of the lacrimal gland abscess led to a complete resolution of the infection. Although abscess formation of the lacrimal gland rarely complicates rhinosinusitis, it should be included in the differential diagnosis when the symptoms fail to resolve after appropriate therapy, especially when there is associated enlargement and tenderness of the lacrimal gland and predominate swelling of the lateral part of the upper eyelid.[28]

Group V-Cavernous Sinus Thrombosis

Discussed in Chapter 45, "Acute and Chronic Nasal Disorders."

Surgical Treatment of Orbital Complications

The surgical technique for drainage of an abscess should be determined by the location of the abscess. Surgical options include the traditional external drainage of a SPA with or without external ethmoidectomy through a Lynch incision (Figure 5). More cosmetically superior procedures including the transcaruncular external approach and transnasal endoscopic approach have also been described. The advantages of endoscopic ethmoidectomy drainage over external ethmoidectomy include the avoidance of external facial scar, less postoperative edema, and shorter hospital stay.[29] Potential complications of surgical drainage may include seeding of an intracranial abscess or epidural abscess.

Loss of Vision. Visual loss secondary to ARS may occur by several mechanisms including: (1) damage to the ocular surface from exposure keratopathy or neurotrophic keratitis; (2) sustained elevated intraocular pressure; (3) thrombophlebitis of the ocular vasculature; (4) optic neuritis caused by extension of infection; (5) mass effect of an abscess causing direct optic nerve compression or obstruction to the vessels supplying the ocular structures; and (6) severe proptosis causing a "stretch" optic neuropathy or ischemic optic neuropathy due to stretching of nutrient vessels.[30] Despite prompt treatment, frequent blindness has been reported in SPA (14 to 33%) and in orbital cellulitis (2.5 to 26%).[30,31] Some authors suggest that patients with acute sphenoethmoiditis are at a relatively higher risk of permanent vision loss due to the close anatomic relationship between the sphenoid and posterior ethmoid sinuses and the optic nerve.[32] In contrast, patients with anterior ethmoidal rhinosinusitis may have vision improvement 2 to 6 weeks after treatment.[33]

Eyelid Abscess. Abscesses of the eyelid have also been described as a complication of rhinosinusitis. Remulla and colleagues reported 2 patients with lower eyelid abscesses that were believed to have spread from the adjacent infected ethmoidal sinuses.[34] Casady and colleagues described 5 patients presenting with eyelid abscesses whose subsequent workup revealed occult sinusitis.[35] All abscesses were located in the upper eyelid and all patients had ipsilateral rhinosinusitis, including the overlying frontal sinus. In 2 cases, there was radiographic evidence of bony defects

between the infected frontal sinuses and the eyelid abscesses. All patients improved after treatment with intravenous antibiotics followed by incision and drainage of the abscess and endoscopic sinus surgery. The authors conclude that the diagnosis of eyelid abscess should be considered when the symptoms are associated with purulent nasal discharge and headache since decreased vision, fever, pain, and orbital signs may not be present.

Intracranial Complications. The infections in the paranasal sinuses frequently lead to the development of intracranial bacterial infections due to their anatomic proximity as well as the venous network that traverses the 2 areas. All of these infectious complications are associated with important morbidity and represent true emergencies. However, the incidence, which ranges from 3.7 to 10%, has improved over time.[36,37] This is felt to be a result of the widespread use of oral antibiotics, improved imaging, recognition of the paranasal sinuses as the source of the infection, expeditious medical and surgical treatment of the underlying rhinosinusitis, and improvements in intensive care medicine.[38]

Excluding meningitis, the development of intracranial complications of rhinosinusitis occurs more frequently in males and children older than 9 years.[39] The development of the frontal and sphenoid sinuses as well as the increased susceptibility to upper respiratory infections in this population may account for the association.

The intracranial complications of rhinosinusitis can be classified as follows: (1) meningitis, (2) epidural abscess, (3) subdural abscess, (4) intracerebral abscess, and (5) venous sinus thrombosis. It should be noted that multiple complications can occur in the same patient concurrently or sequentially. All these entities represent true medical emergencies with high morbidity and mortality warranting thoughtful, urgent medical and frequently surgical therapy.

Meningitis. Meningitis remains 1 of the most common intracranial complications of rhinosinusitis.[40] That being said, most cases of meningitis are not associated with rhinosinusitis. When the 2 are related, the most commonly involved paranasal sinus cavities are the sphenoid and ethmoid sinuses. It goes without saying that patients with anterior skull base defects (cerebrospinal fluid leaks, encephaloceles, etc) are at increased risk of developing meningitis. In addition, diving into water with an acute sinus infection has been associated with increased risk of meningitis and is felt to be related to the infectious process being forced intracranially through the olfactory neuroepithelium.[41] Permanent neurologic sequelae are not uncommon and may include seizures, focal deficits, and cognitive deficits. Thus, urgent evaluation and treatment are imperative.

Symptomatically, these patients may present with fever, headache, photophobia, nuchal rigidity, delirium, somnolence, as well as cranial nerve deficits. It is important to have the patient undergo MRI before the lumbar puncture to

determine if hydrocephalus is present, which would contraindicate performance of the lumbar puncture since uncal herniation could result. The diagnosis of meningitis is confirmed by lumbar puncture. Pertinent findings on lumbar puncture include increased intracranial pressure, elevated protein, decreased glucose, leukocytosis, and frequently the offending microorganism on gram stain study. Evidence for the origin of the meningitis in the paranasal sinuses should be sought on the MRI, and the MRI may demonstrate the relationship between the sinusitis and the meningitis as evidenced in part by the adjacent meningeal enhancement. A coronal CT scan of the sinuses should be performed to assess further the degree and location of the paranasal sinus infection. In a cooperative patient, nasal endoscopy should be considered to obtain specimen for culture and sensitivity.

The management of these patients is typically multidisciplinary and may include pediatricians, internists, critical care specialists, neurologists, infectious disease experts, as well as otolaryngologists and head and neck surgeons. The most common bacteria involved in acute bacterial meningitis include *H. influenzae, Neisseria meningitides,* and *S. pneumoniae.*[42] Initial therapy includes appropriate antibiotics which cross the blood–brain barrier and effectively treat the most common microorganisms. Further adjustment of antibiotic therapy is based on culture and sensitivity findings. If medical management is failing, endoscopic drainage of the involved paranasal sinuses is indicated to facilitate medical therapy as well as to obtain further material for culture and sensitivity. The decision to proceed with surgical intervention should be made in coordination with all of the consulting services.

Epidural Abscess. Epidural abscesses most commonly occur as a complication of frontal sinusitis and may occur in association with osteomyelitis. The relationship to the frontal sinus is felt to result from the interregional venous communications and the loosely adherent dura.[43]

Symptomatically, epidural abscesses tend to be more subtle in their presentation. Presenting symptoms might include frontal headache, drowsiness, and fevers. These symptoms may progress in severity to include focal neurologic deficits, seizures, and/or altered mental status. The diagnosis is dependent on the CT or MRI scan revealing findings consistent with a fluid collection in the epidural space. The treatment of epidural abscess again involves appropriately chosen antibiotics and thoughtful surgical intervention. Again, surgical intervention should be coordinated with the involved consultants, especially neurosurgery. The surgical procedure can be performed simultaneously with any necessary neurosurgical procedures and may include endoscopic ventilation/drainage, frontal sinus trephination, osteoplastic flap obliteration of the frontal sinus, or cranialization. Antibiotic therapy should be coordinated with infectious disease specialists and is typically culture directed.

Subdural Abscess. Subdural abscess, also known as subdural empyema, is usually unilateral and involves the space between the dura mater and subarachnoid space. In contrast to the other intracranial complications of rhinosinusitis, bacterial sinusitis is the source of infection for the majority, 50 to 70% of cases, while otitis media accounts for a relative minority, 10 to 20%, of cases.[44] Subdural abscesses are associated with relatively high morbidity, mortality, and permanent neurologic sequelae. Aggressive intervention with early craniotomy and direct management of the otorhinolaryngologic origin of the infection has been advocated.[45] These patients most commonly present with fevers, headache, altered mental status, hemiparesis, nausea and vomiting, seizures, and nuchal rigidity.[45,46] In addition to presenting with relatively severe symptoms, these patients can deteriorate quickly. These symptoms result from thrombosis of meningeal veins, inflammation of the pia mater, and subsequent spread of the infection through the subdural space to other areas.

Diagnosis is generally based upon CT scan and/or MRI (Figure 6).[45] MRI generally reveals a low signal on T1-weighted images while T2-weighted images are of high signal intensity. Post-gadolinium images demonstrate peripheral enhancement. CT scans may be falsely negative in 20% of cases.[47] Given that most of these infections are associated with rhinogenic or otogenic sources, these areas should be included on imaging as well.[45] Lumbar puncture is recommended only if hydrocephalus is not present, due to the high risk of uncal herniation.

Antibiotic therapy includes broad-spectrum antimicrobials that are capable of crossing the blood–brain barrier. They are further directed by culture and sensitivity results when they become available. Subdural abscesses are usually polymicrobial, most commonly including anaerobes, *H. influenzae*, an/aerobic streptococci, and staphylococci. Anticonvulsants and corticosteroids are frequently required for the associated seizures and cerebral edema, respectively. Surgical therapy is coordinated with other specialists and usually involves drainage of the abscess and diseased paranasal sinus region at the same setting.[45]

Intracerebral Abscess. Intracerebral abscesses are most frequently located in the frontal and frontoparietal lobes. Most commonly they result as a complication of frontal sinusitis, but ethmoid and sphenoid sinusitis may also be the source. Temporal lobe abscesses may occur secondary to sphenoid sinusitis but an otogenic origin is more common. The abscesses may be multiple in about 13% of cases.[48]

Early symptoms are due to cerebritis and typically consist of fever, lethargy, agitation, and headache. A quiescent period may occur as liquefaction necrosis occurs and the abscess is walled off. Finally as the abscess wall thickens, focal neurologic deficits and seizures may occur as a result of increasing cerebral edema. Subsequent rupture of the abscess or brain herniation can result in death.[49] Diagnosis is with MRI or CT scan. Lumbar puncture is especially dangerous due to potential uncal herniation and thus should be avoided.

Treatment is once again multidisciplinary in nature. Antibiotics can be started immediately, although if the patient is stable, can wait until after culture material is obtained. Surgical therapy is coordinated with other surgical disciplines such as neurosurgery, but consists of drainage either by craniotomy or by stereotactic aspiration. Any involved paranasal sinus cavities can be surgically ventilated as well at the same time.

Frontal Bone Osteomyelitis. Osteomyelitis of the frontal bone is an increasingly rare complication of frontal rhinosinusitis. The term "Pott puffy tumor" is commonly used and is defined as a SPA of the frontal bone associated with osteomyelitis.[50] The subperiosteal collection of pus in the forehead results in a "puffy" fluctuant swelling. In addition, osteomyelitis of the frontal bone may present with a discharging fistula. Both of these extracranial manifestations may occur

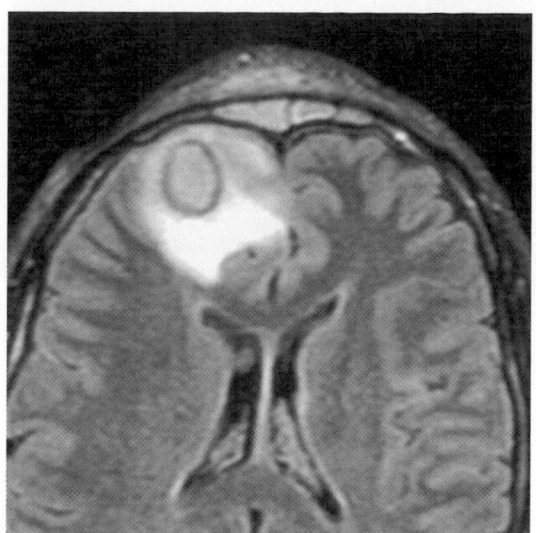

Figure 8 Axial T2 magnetic resonance image of patient with Pott puffy tumor and frontal abscess.

alone or in combination with the previously discussed intracranial complications.[51] Because of the venous drainage of the frontal sinus, infection of the frontal sinus can extend to the overlying bone by either propagation of septic thrombi or by direct extension.

Diagnosis is based on clinical suspicion in those patients presenting with forehead swelling, that is, puffiness or a fistula. A high degree of suspicion must be maintained for underlying intracranial complications. Appropriate imaging studies usually involving both CT and MRI scanning to assess for intracranial involvement is indicated (Figures 7 and 8).

Treatment again tends to be multidisciplinary in nature, especially in those patients with associated intracranial complications. In patients without associated intracranial complications, frontal trephination is helpful to obtain culture material and to drain the underlying infection. Culture directed intravenous antibiotics are initiated as well. If appropriate clinical improvement does not occur after trephination and intravenous antibiotics, debridement of nonviable bone is indicated. Intravenous antibiotics for 6 weeks duration are generally recommended. If the frontal rhinosinusitis does not resolve with antibiotics, the frontal sinus should be surgically ventilated or obliterated to prevent further complications. In the patient with associated intracranial complications, aggressive bony debridement is carried out in conjunction with any necessary neurosurgical procedures. Long-term culture directed antibiotics are indicated in this situation as well.

REFERENCES

1. Dingle JH, Badger GF, Jordan WS, Jr. Illness in the Home. A Study of 25,000 Illnesses in a Group of Cleveland Families. Cleveland: Western Reserve University Press; 1964. p. 66–88.
2. Berg O, Carenfelt C, Rystedt G, Anggaard A. Occurrence of asymptomatic sinusitis in common cold and other acute ENT-infections. Rhinology 1986;24:223–5.
3. Gwaltney JM, Phillips CD, Miller RD, Riker DK. Computed tomographic study of the common cold. N Engl J Med 1994;330:25–30.
4. National Disease and Therapeutic Index. Plymouth Meeting, PA: IMS Inc; 1994. p. 963–76.

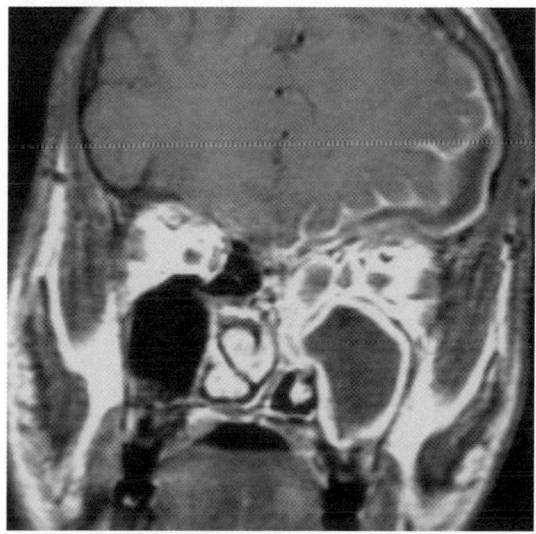

Figure 6 Coronal magnetic resonance image of patient with left ethmoid and maxillary sinusitis with resultant subdural empyema.

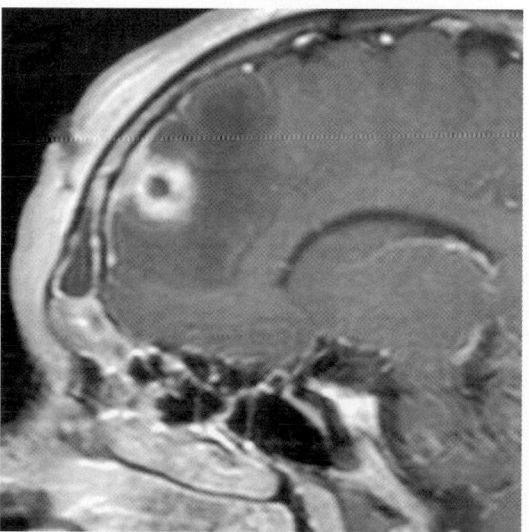

Figure 7 Sagittal T1 gadolinium enhanced magnetic resonance image of patient with Pott puffy tumor and frontal abscess.

5. Sinus and Allergy Health Partnership. Antimicrobial treatment guidelines for acute bacterial rhinosinusitis. Otolaryngol Head Neck Surg 2004;130:1–50.

6. Gwaltney JM, Jr. Rhinoviruses. In: Evans AS, Kaslow RA, editors. Viral Infections of Humans: Epidemiology and Control, 4th edition. New York: Plenum; 1997. p. 815–38.

7. Gable CB, Jones JK, Lian JF, et al. Chronic sinusitis: Temporal occurrence and relationship to medical claims for upper respiratory infections and allergic rhinitis. Pharmacoepidemiol Drug Saf 1994;3:337–49.

8. Gwaltney JM, Jr, Hayden FG. Response to psychological stress and susceptibility to the common cold. N Eng J Med 1992;326:644–5.

9. Makela MJ, Puhakka T, Ruuskanen O, et al. Viruses and bacteria in the etiology of the common cold. J Clin Microbiol 1998;36:539–42.

10. Gwaltney JM, Jr, Heainz BA. Rhinovirus. In: Richman DD, Whitley RJ, Hayden FG, editors. Clinical Virology. Washington DC: ASM Press; 2002. p. 995–1018.

11. Gwaltney JM, Phillips CD, Miller RD, Riker DK. Computed tomographic study of the common cold. N Engl J Med 1994;330:25–30.

12. Gwaltney JM, Jr, Hendley JO, Phillips CD, et al. Nose blowing propels nasal fluid into the paranasal sinuses. Clin Infect Dis 2000;30:387–91.

13. Winther B, Gwaltney JM, Jr, Humphries JE, Hendley JO. Cross-linked fibrin in the nasal fluid of patients with the common cold. Clin Infect Dis 2002;34:708–10.

14. Wald ER, Milmoe GJ, Bowen A, et al. Acute maxillary sinusitis in children. N Engl J Med 1981;304:749–54.

15. Winther B, Brofeldt S, Gronborg H, et al. Study of bacteria in the nasal cavity and nasopharynx during naturally acquired common colds. Acta Otolaryngol 1984; 98: 315–20.

16. Lacroix JS, Ricchetti A, Lew D, et al. Symptoms and clinical and radiological signs predicting the presence of pathogenic bacteria in acute rhinosinusitis. Acta Otolaryngol 2002;122:192–6.

17. Hickner JM, Bartlett JG, Besser RE, et al. Principles of appropriate antibiotic use for acute rhinosinusitis in adults: Background. Ann Int Med 2001;134:498–505.

18. Hamory BH, Sande MA, Sydnor A, Jr, et al. Etiology and antimicrobial therapy of acute maxillary sinusitis. J Infect Dis 1979;139:197–202.

19. Gwaltney JM, Jr, Scheld WN, Sande MA, Sydnor A. The microbial etiology and antimicrobial therapy of adults with acute community-acquired sinusitis. A fifteen-year experience at the University of Virginia and review of other selected studies. J Allergy Clin Immunol 1992; 90:457–62.

20. Chandler JR, Langenbrunner DJ, Stevens ER. The pathogenesis of orbital complications in acute sinusitis. Laryngoscope 1970;80:1414–28.

21. Ambati BK, Ambati J, Azar N, et al. Periorbital and orbital cellulitis before and after the advent of *Haemophilus influenzae* type B vaccination. Ophthalmology 2000; 107:1450–3.

22. Schramm VL, Curtin HD, Kennerdell JS. Evaluation of orbital cellulitis and results of treatment. Laryngoscope 1982;92:732–8.

23. Donahue SP, Schwartz G. Preseptal and orbital cellulitis in childhood: A changing microbiologic spectrum. Ophthalmology 1998;105:1902–5.

24. Garcia GH, Harris GJ. Criteria for nonsurgical management of subperiosteal abscess of the orbit: Analysis of outcomes. Ophthalmology 2000;107:1454–6.

25. Oxford LE, McClay J. Medical and surgical management of subperiosteal orbital abscess secondary to acute sinusitis in children. Int J Pediatr Otorhinolaryngol 2006;70:1853–61.

26. Harris GJ. Subperiosteal abscess of the orbit: Computed tomography and the clinical course. Ophthal Plast Reconstr Surg 1996;12:1–8.

27. Patel N, Khalil HM, Amirfeyz R, Kaddour HS. Lacrimal gland abscess complicating acute sinusitis. Int J Pediatr Otorhinolaryngol 2003;67:917–9.

28. Mirza S, Lobo CJ, Counter P, Farrington WT. Lacrimal gland abscess: An unusual complication of rhinosinusitis. ORL 2001;63:379–81.

29. Bhargava D, Sankhla D, Ganesan A, Chand P. Endoscopic sinus surgery for orbital subperiosteal abscess secondary to sinusitis. Rhinology 2001;39:151–5.

30. Hornblass A, Herschorn BJ, Stern K, et al. Orbital abscess: Review. Surv Ophthalmol 1984;29:169–78.

31. Wane AM, Ba EA, Ndoye-Roth PA, et al. Senegalese experience of orbital cellulitis. J Fr Ophtalmol 2005; 28:1089–94.

32. Tarazi AE, Shikani AH. Irreversible unilateral visual loss due to acute sinusitis. Arch Otolaryngol Head Neck Surg 1991;117:1400–1.

33. Kron TK, Johnson CM, 3rd. Diagnosis and management of the opacified sphenoid sinus. Laryngoscope 1983; 93:1319–27.

34. Remulla HD, Rubin PAD, Shore JW, Cunningham MJ. Pseudodacryocystitis arising from anterior ethmoiditis. Ophthal Plast Reconstr Surg 1995;11:165–8.

35. Casady DR, Zobal-Ratner JL, Meyer DR. Eyelid abscess as a presenting sign of occult sinusitis. Ophthal Plast Reconstr Surg 2005;21:368–70.

36. Bluestone C, Yang S. Brain abscess. A review of 400 cases. J Neurosurg 1981;55:794–9.

37. Bradley PJ, Manning KP, Shaw MDM. Brain abscess secondary to paranasal sinusitis. J Larngol Otol 1984;98:19–25.

38. Gallagher RM, Gross CW, Phillips CD. Suppurative intracranial complications of sinusitis. Laryngoscope 1998;108:1635–42.

39. Rosenfeld EA, Rowley AH. Infectious intracranial complications of sinusitis, other than meningitis, in children: 12-year review. Clin Infect Dis 1994;18:750–4.

40. Giannoni CM, Sulek M, Friedman EM. Intracranial complications of sinusitis: A pediatric series. Am J Rhinol 1998;12:173–8.

41. Donald PJ, Gluckman JL, Rise DH. The Sinuses. New York: Raven Press; 1995. p. 194.

42. Schlech WF III, Ward JI, Band JD, et al. Bacterial meningitis surveillance study. JAMA 1985;253:1749–54.

43. Giannoni CM, Stewart MG, Alford EL. Intracranial complications of sinusitis. Laryngoscope 1997;107:863–7.

44. Maniglia AJ, Goodwin WJ, Arnold JE, et al. Intracranial abscesses secondary to nasal, sinus and orbital infections in adults and children. Arch Otolaryngol Head Neck Surg 1989:114:1424–9.

45. Wackym PA, Canalis RF, Feuerman T. Subdural empyema of otorhinologic origin. J Laryngol Otol 1990;104:118–22.

46. Johnson JT, Yu VL. Infectious Disease and Antimicrobial Therapy of the Ears, Nose, and Throat. Philadelphia: WB Saunders Co; 1997.

47. Hoyt DJ, Fisher SR. Otolaryngologic management of patients with subdural empyema. Laryngoscope 1991;101:20–4.

48. Clayman GL, Adams GL, Paugh DR, et al. Intracranial complications of paranasal sinusitis: A combined institutional review. Laryngoscope 1991;101:234–9.

49. Zeidman SM, Geisler FH, Olivi A. Intraventricular rupture of a purulent brain abscess. Case report. Neurosurgery 1995;36:189–93.

50. Babu RP, Otdor R, Kasoff SS. Pott's puffy tumour: The forgotten entity. J Neurosurg 1996;84:110–2.

51. Marshall AH, Jones NS. Osteomyelitis of the frontal bone secondary to frontal sinusitis. J Laryngol Otol 2000;114:944–6.

47

Chronic Rhinosinusitis and Polyposis

Rodney J. Schlosser, MD
Bradford A. Woodworth, MD

Chronic rhinosinusitis (CRS) is a clinical disorder that encompasses a heterogeneous group of infectious and inflammatory conditions affecting the paranasal sinuses. Its definition continues to evolve as we increase our understanding of the various pathophysiologies that may result in a common clinical picture.

EPIDEMIOLOGY

CRS is an extremely widespread inflammatory disorder that is one of the most common health complaints in the United States. CRS and CRS with nasal polyps (NPs) comprise a variety of disorders that cause inflammation of the sinonasal mucosa. Estimates of the prevalence of CRS vary due to differences in the definition of rhinosinusitis and methods of diagnosis. In 2001, there were 18.3 million patient office visits for CRS despite many patients not seeking medical attention.[1] CRS with NPs is a subset of this disease which is also a prevalent condition affecting between 1 and 4% of the general US population.[2] CRS affects men and women equally, but subtypes of CRS appear to have different gender distributions. For example, CRS with NPs associated with aspirin-sensitivity has a female predominance of 2:1.[3] Sinus disease is more common in the Midwest and South than in the northeast and western United States and the incidence is lower during the summer months compared to the other seasons. CRS causes significant physical symptoms, decreases quality of life, and impairs daily functioning resulting in millions of days of lost productivity with an important impact on US economy. The total medical and economic impact of these disorders is unclear due to heterogeneous disease processes, imprecise diagnoses, and overlap with other conditions that produce similar symptoms. Nevertheless, the calculated direct health care expenditures from the primary diagnosis of CRS are approximately $3.39 billion in the United States. In 1996, the total direct and indirect costs were estimated at $5.8 billion annually.[4]

DIAGNOSIS

Historically, *sinusitis* was the commonly accepted terminology for inflammation of the paranasal sinuses. This terminology has gradually been phased out in favor of *rhinosinusitis* because nasal inflammation almost always coincides with inflammatory paranasal sinus involvement.[5] Clearly this terminology is more descriptive. This highlights only one of the many changes that have occurred in defining and categorizing CRS over the past several decades. There are still controversies regarding the definitions and diagnoses of all forms of rhinosinusitis. This is likely due to the fact that CRS encompasses a spectrum of diseases that have numerous causes and a range of appropriate treatments. The 1996 multidisciplinary rhinosinusitis task force of the American Academy of Otolaryngology–Head and Neck Surgery (AAO-HNS) proposed definitions of rhinosinusitis based on the duration of clinical signs and symptoms.[6] These were divided into acute (up to 4 weeks), subacute (4 to 12 weeks), chronic (>12 weeks), recurrent acute (≥4 episodes/yr plus each episode lasting ≥7 to 10 days plus no intervening signs of CRS), and acute exacerbation of chronic (sudden worsening of CRS, return to baseline after treatment). Temporal separations furnish the practitioner with a concrete way to define nasal and sinus inflammation and have since become widely accepted definitions of rhinosinusitis, but they are far from ideal.

For practical purposes, most practitioners refer to two general categories, acute and CRS. Since CRS encompasses a broad range of different disease processes, epidemiologic studies unfortunately lump many different disorders into this common category. While acute rhinosinusitis is discussed thoroughly in Chapter 46, "Acute Rhinosinusitis and Its Complications," it is important to note that acute rhinosinusitis may develop into CRS in some cases. However, acute rhinosinusitis is usually infectious in nature, whereas chronic disease might result from a wide range of inflammatory processes. CRS is less frequently bacterial in causation and is most broadly subdivided into categories of patients with hyperplastic mucosal changes with polyps and those without polyps.

The clinical diagnosis of CRS has always been somewhat difficult, due to the difficulty defining the disease and the variety of presenting signs and symptoms. The consensus opinion of leading experts in the field of rhinology was pivotal in creating a unifying diagnostic model based on the most common presenting signs and symptoms in patients with all forms of rhinosinusitis.[6] These signs and symptoms were divided into major and minor factors (Table 1). According to this report, a clinical diagnosis of CRS could be made if patients had two or more major factors or one major and two minor factors and these signs and symptoms lasted for >12 weeks. Numerous reports since this consensus opinion have shown a lack of close correlation between subjective measures established by the task force and objective measures commonly applied to CRS. This symptom-based definition of CRS also did not take into consideration the numerous causes of this heterogeneous disease process. In 2003, the Sinus and Allergy Health Partnership (SAHP) convened to help better define and diagnose CRS.[1] The SAHP criteria include the prior definition proposed by the 1996 AAO-HNS task force qualifying the duration of disease with continuous symptoms for >12 consecutive weeks or >12 weeks of physical findings. However, objective evidence of inflammation must be present and identified in association with the ongoing symptoms to establish the diagnosis (Table 2). Importantly, the SAHP also incorporates computed tomographic (CT) imaging of the sinuses or Water view plain sinus radiograph as a means of confirming the diagnosis. The SAHP task force also emphasizes the importance of CT scan and photoendoscopy for confirming the diagnosis for research purposes.

Table 1 Major and Minor Factors Associated with the Diagnosis of Chronic Rhinosinusitis Identified by the 1996 AAO-HNS Task Force

Major Factors	Minor Factors
Facial pain/pressure*	Headache
Nasal obstruction/blockage	Fever
Nasal discharge/purulence/ discolored postnasal drainage	Halitosis
Hyposmia/anosmia	Dental pain
Purulence in nasal cavity on examination	Cough
	Ear pain/pressure/ fullness

*Facial pain or pressure does not constitute a suggestive history in the absence of another major nasal symptom or sign.

Table 2 Additional Measures for Diagnosing Adult Chronic Rhinosinusitis as Proposed by the Sinus and Allergy Health Partnership*

Discolored nasal drainage arising from the nasal passages, nasal polyps, or polypoid swelling as identified by anterior rhinoscopy in the decongested state or nasal endoscopy.

Edema or erythema of the middle meatus or ethmoid bulla as identified by nasal endoscopy.

Generalized or localized erythema, edema, or granulation tissue. Radiologic imaging is required if it does not involve the middle meatus or ethmoid bulla.

CT scan demonstrating isolated or diffuse mucosal thickening, bone changes, or an air-fluid level. Plain sinus radiograph. Water view revealing mucous membrane thickening of >5 mm or complete opacification of one or more sinuses

*Chronic rhinosinusitis is present when signs and symptoms are continuous for >12 consecutive weeks, but one of the signs of inflammation in this table must be present and identified with the ongoing symptoms.

ETIOLOGY AND PATHOPHYSIOLOGY OF CHRONIC RHINOSINUSITIS WITHOUT NASAL POLYPS

CRS has multiple causes that include infectious (viral, bacterial, and fungal), anatomic, allergic, genetic or congenital mucociliary dysfunction, (eg, cystic fibrosis, primary or acquired ciliary dyskinesia), and systemic disorders (Table 3). The presence of bacteria within the nose and paranasal sinuses in the CRS population has been well documented,[7] and most practitioners believe bacteria play a role in the majority of cases. Whether the bacteria play a direct or indirect role in the development of CRS has not been adequately determined.

Progression of Acute Rhinosinusitis

The predisposing conditions for CRS parallel those for acute infections in terms of extrinsic, intrinsic, systemic, and local host factors. Furthermore, multiple episodes of acute rhinosinusitis may ultimately lead to mucosal dysfunction and chronic infections. Symptoms are more varied in CRS when compared to acute

Table 3 Intrinsic and Extrinsic Factors Associated with the Pathogenesis of Chronic Rhinosinusitis

Intrinsic Factors	Extrinsic Factors
Genetic and congenital conditions, eg, cystic fibrosis, primary ciliary dyskinesia	Infectious disease—viral, bacterial, and fungal microorganisms
Allergic conditions	Trauma and foreign bodies
Immunodeficiency	Noxious chemicals, pollutants, and smoke
Anatomic abnormalities	Medications
Endocrine	Surgery
Neuromechanism	
Neoplasms	
Acquired mucociliary dysfunction	

rhinosinusitis, especially when NPs are part of the disease process. CRS typically has extensive mucosal dysregulation and chronic inflammatory process that can be very difficult to treat. This disease is often recalcitrant to medical and surgical treatments that are currently available. Systemic corticosteroids are used more often in CRS, since this disease has a significant underlying chronic inflammatory component. Furthermore, acute rhinosinusitis is histologically an exudative process characterized by neutrophilic inflammation and necrosis, while CRS is a proliferative process that is most often characterized by thickened mucous membrane and lamina propria. Because acute rhinosinusitis is almost always infectious, it is marked by a normal T helper 1 (Th1)-type of inflammation that is associated with a recruitment of neutrophils as the predominant cell type to fight infection. While this type of infectious inflammation is certainly predominant in CRS secondary to cystic fibrosis, ciliary dyskinesia, and rhinosinusitis of dental origin, most CRS has an atopic (Th2)-type inflammatory response where eosinophils are the predominant inflammatory cells in both atopic and nonatopic individuals with CRS.

Anatomic Factors

In some cases, CRS develops from a chronic bacterial infection in a sinus cavity in the presence of an anatomically obstructed ostium. Anatomic abnormalities leading to narrow channels predispose individuals to developing CRS, especially in the presence of some sort of reversible inflammation. Certain anatomic variants may also predispose individuals to CRS, including Haller cells (infundibular), silent sinus syndrome or a narrow frontal sinus outflow tract from large agger nasi or frontal cells. Once the ostium becomes occluded, a local hypoxia develops in the sinus cavity and sinus secretions accumulate. This creates an environment suitable for rapid bacterial growth. Bacterial toxins and endogenous mediators subsequently damage the highly specialized ciliated respiratory epithelium resulting in a decrease in mucociliary clearance. A vicious cycle erupts with stasis of secretions and further infection.

Mucociliary Dysfunction

Mucociliary clearance is especially important in maintaining the homeostasis of the paranasal sinuses and deserves further mention. The ciliary beat of the epithelium removes allergens, bacteria, and pollutants trapped in the mucus or *gel* layer of the mucociliary blanket through natural drainage pathways. The mucus rests on a periciliary fluid or *sol* layer that enables the rapid elimination of viscous secretions. Mucociliary clearance can be disrupted by either defective ciliary function due to intrinsic or extrinsic factors or alterations in the viscosity and production of mucus. Intrinsic factors leading to ciliary dysfunction include primary ciliary dyskinesia or Kartagener syndrome. Extrinsic factors that

disrupt mucociliary clearance include injury by environmental irritants, endogenous mediators of inflammation, or surgical trauma. Patients with cystic fibrosis have high viscosity mucus secondary to alterations in water and electrolyte transport. The gel and sol layers of the mucus blanket are severely affected, thereby hindering bacterial removal. Airborne irritants, allergens, cold air exposure, or viral upper respiratory infections can increase the production of mucus and exceed the rate of mucociliary clearance. All of these factors may lead to the accumulation of mucus in the sinuses, decrease the removal of bacteria, and create a favorable environment for bacterial growth.

Bone Inflammation

Recent work suggests that the bone may play an active role in the disease process and that, at a minimum; the inflammation associated with CRS may spread through the Haversian system within the bone. The rate of bone turnover in CRS is similar to that seen in osteomyelitis. Furthermore, a surgically induced infection with either *Staphylococcus aureus* or *Pseudomonas aeruginosa* can induce all of the classic changes of osteomyelitis and induce chronic inflammatory changes in the overlying mucosa at a significant distance from the site of infection.[8] Therefore, the bone inflammation may be an important factor in the spread of chronic inflammatory changes and may explain the recalcitrance to medical therapy. It is still unclear, however, if the bone actually becomes infected with bacteria or if the observed changes are simply reactive.

Biofilms

Recent investigations have found that bacteria such as *P. aeruginosa* form biofilms in the sinuses that may lead to recalcitrant sinus disease.[9] Bacterial biofilms are a complex organization of bacteria anchored to a surface. They can evade host defenses and demonstrate decreased susceptibility to systemic and local antibiotic therapy. The persistence of biofilms is largely due to their method of growth. *P. aeruginosa* grows in microcolonies surrounded by an extracellular matrix of the exopolysaccharide alginate. Biofilms have now been implicated in many infectious processes, including dental caries, periodontitis, otitis media, musculoskeletal infections, necrotizing fasciitis, biliary tract infection, osteomyelitis, bacterial prostatitis, native valve endocarditis, and cystic fibrosis pneumonia. Furthermore, there is a long list of nosocomial-type infections in which biofilms are involved. These include ICU pneumonia, sutures, AV shunts, contact lenses, urinary catheter cystitis, endotracheal tubes, central venous catheters, and pressure equalization tubes.[10] Bacterial biofilms that have formed on mucosal surfaces have been referred to as *mucosal biofilms*, as they are bacterial biofilms that have formed in the special environment of ciliated mucosa, an area expected to have some protection from biofilm formation.

Dentigerous Sinusitis

Dental pathology can occasionally lead to sinusitis of the maxillary sinus with subsequent spread to adjacent sinuses. This pathology can include dental infections, tooth root abscesses, oral-antral fistulae and oral surgery procedures that incite a sinusitis. These patients typically require treatment of both the oral and the sinus pathology to eradicate the infection.

ETIOLOGY AND PATHOPHYSIOLOGY OF CHRONIC RHINOSINUSITIS WITH NASAL POLYPS

CRS may exist with or without NPs and these entities may represent two points along a spectrum of disease. For the purposes of this chapter, NP is not simply mucosal edema, but rather grape-shaped, soft, smooth, freely mobile mucosal swellings that are often visible on anterior rhinoscopy (Figure 1). Polyps arise from the lateral nasal wall and are best seen with nasal endoscopy when limited to the superior and middle meatus. Inflammatory polyps are most often bilateral but may have a unilateral predominance when existing in association with allergic fungal rhinosinusitis (AFRS). The detection of small polyps but no evidence of sinus disease is relatively common, reported as 32% in an endoscopic autopsy series.[11] Hence, NPs may be present without clinically significant sinus disease and vice-versa. This autopsy series also suggests that NPs are found mainly in the transition spaces between the nose and sinuses and often start in the narrow channels of the ostiomeatal complex. Because small NPs may be missed on anterior rhinoscopy, a diagnosis is more likely after nasal decongestion and nasal endoscopy.

Histologically, NPs are mucosal swellings that contain edema and an extensive fibrous stroma with vessels, glandular elements, and inflammatory cells covered by typical respiratory epithelium that may display benign squamous cell metaplasia. The epithelium has few nerve endings and submucosal glands, and the basement membrane is thickened. NPs are most often associated with a Th2-type cytokine profile and eosinophilic inflammation (85%). NPs that are associated with neutrophilic inflammation and

glandular hyperplasia are seen in bacterial infections of dentigerous origin, ciliary dyskinesias, cystic fibrosis, and Young syndrome. Naturally, the disparate inflammatory processes have led to a proposed histologic classification of CRS according to the predominant cellular inflammatory findings.[12]

The cause and effect relationship between NPs and bacterial CRS is a matter of debate. Polyps may form prior to infection from eosinophilic infiltration of the nasal mucosa in response to allergic or nonallergic inflammation. It is also plausible that enlargement of the polyps leads to blocked sinus ostia, stasis of secretions, and bacterial superinfection. However, polyps that arise from bacterial infection in the maxillary sinus of dental origin and those that develop secondary to cystic fibrosis lend support to the development of nasal polyposis secondary to different types of inflammation. The infectious component of chronic disease may ultimately result from the compromise of the normal mucosal barrier mechanisms by long-term inflammation. CRS with NPs should be considered a broad spectrum of disease processes with some individuals having a propensity to develop hyperplastic disease.

Although the etiology of CRS with NPs is largely not understood, there are a number of interesting theories that have been proposed over the last several years. Despite 85% of NPs having eosinophils as their predominating inflammatory cell, there is a dearth of epidemiologic evidence for allergy as the predominant cause. Patients with NPs do not have a higher incidence of allergy when compared to the non-CRS population, nor do patients with NPs have elevated rates of positive allergy skin tests.[1] Yet, in most cases, regardless of allergic status, patients with CRS with NPs have a mixed mucosal inflammatory infiltrate containing lymphocytes, plasma cells, and eosinophils, rather than neutrophilic inflammatory infiltrate consistent with infection. Furthermore, NPs are associated with a number of systemic diseases that include aspirin-sensitive asthma (Samter triad), intrinsic asthma, primary ciliary dyskinesia, and cystic fibrosis. Of note, the ability to form polyps in the presence of a purely infectious process, such as maxillary

sinusitis of dental origin, indicates the mechanisms behind polyp formation are multifactorial. We will discuss the current theories behind the development of CRS with NP as they relate to the two major subtypes, AFRS and eosinophilic CRS (ECRS).

Allergic Fungal Rhinosinusitis

AFRS is the most common form of fungal sinus disease, although the pathogenesis remains poorly understood. It was first recognized because of its histologic similarity to allergic bronchopulmonary aspergillosis (ABPA). Like ABPA, AFRS is recognized as an immunoglobulin E (IgE)-mediated response to a variety of fungi, typically from the dematiaceous family, growing in the eosinophilic mucin of the sinuses. The classic diagnosis of AFRS depends on five criteria: type I hypersensitivity, nasal polyposis, characteristic CT scan appearance (hyperdense material in the sinus cavity), positive fungal stain or culture, and the presence of thick, eosinophilic mucin[13] (Figure 2). Eosinophilic mucin is typically thick, tenacious, "peanut butter-like," brown-green mucus that contains eosinophils in sheets, Charcot-Leyden crystals, and fungal hyphae (Figure 3). Clinically, patients are usually younger, allergic, and mildly asthmatic (approximately one-third). They typically have increased total IgE, antigen-specific IgE, and increased peripheral eosinophil counts. The disease is often unilateral and can cause bony erosion and extension into the orbital or intracranial contents.

Fungal colonization of the nose and paranasal sinuses is a common finding in both normal and diseased sinuses due to the ubiquitous nature of the microorganisms. Taylor and colleagues showed that fungi can be isolated from nearly all sinuses as well as from patients without disease, given sufficiently sensitive culture techniques.[14] Furthermore, an elegant study by Lackner and colleagues showed that fungus could be cultured from the nasal mucus of 94% of neonates after only 4 months of life, proving that fungus colonizes the sinonasal cavities early in life.[15] Under some circumstances, fungal proliferation may lead to the development of fungus balls or saprophytic growth of fungus. In other cases, an intense inflammatory response to ubiquitous fungi

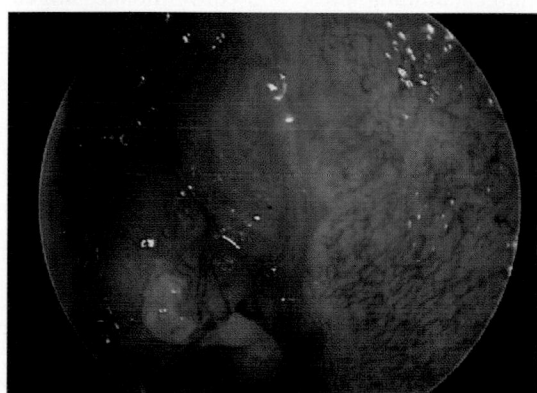

Figure 1 View of smooth, grape-shaped nasal polyp easily visible on anterior rhinoscopy.

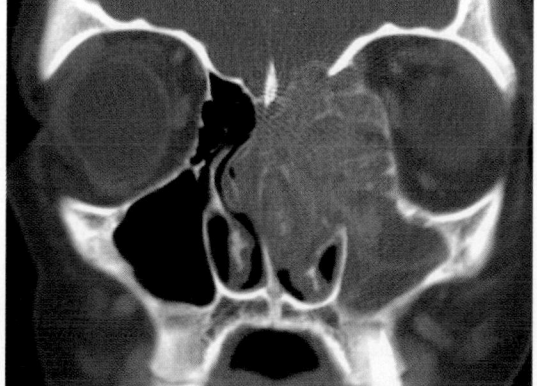
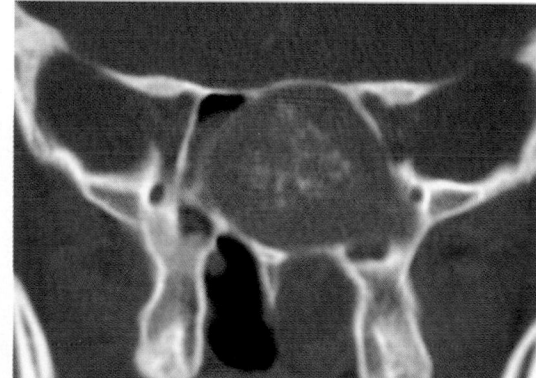

Figure 2 Coronal computed tomography of a patient with allergic fungal rhinosinusitis demonstrating bony erosion of the lamina papyracea (*left*) and the roof of the sphenoid (*right*). Note: Hyperdense secretions visible even on bone windows.

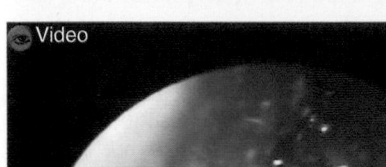

(A)

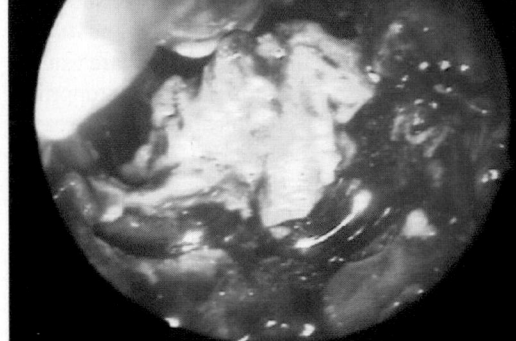

(B)

Figure 3 Nasal polyp (A) and fungal debris (B) seen in a patient with allergic fungal rhinosinusitis.

results in the disease process of AFRS. The most commonly proposed mechanism is that a patient with a tendency to develop allergies inhales a certain fungal spore that becomes adherent to the nasal or sinus epithelium long enough to germinate. This individual then secretes eosinophil-rich mucus in response to the fungi. The spores and germinated hyphae continue to grow in this eosinophilic mucin, thereby increasing antigenic stimulation and developing a vicious feedback cycle. The allergy to the germinated hyphae increases the secreted mucus, that allows further growth of the hyphae.[3] The presence of specific IgE to cultured fungus in a study by Manning and colleagues strongly supports this theory.[16] This study showed that 16 patients with histologically confirmed AFRS had uniformly elevated fungal-specific IgE and this corresponded with the results of fungal cultures. Fungal specific IgE was not elevated within the control group of patients with CRS. However, allergy to fungus alone does not explain the predominantly unilateral nature of the disease or that only a small minority of patients with fungal allergy develops AFRS. Therefore, other factors such as fungal antigen exposures, lymphocyte sensitization, anatomy, and genetics may all play a role in ultimately developing the disease.

Eosinophilic Chronic Rhinosinusitis

ECRS is a term that encompasses various forms of CRS with NPs which has an underlying eosinophilic inflammatory component and does not have all of the characteristic features of AFRS. While the polyps may appear similar to those of AFRS, CT scans typically demonstrate bilateral disease without characteristic hyperdense secretions and less bony invasion into the orbit or intracranially (Figure 4). In ECRS, a number of Th2 inflammatory cytokines and eosinophil-attracting chemokines are upregulated including vascular cell adhesion molecule-1, eosinophil cationic protein, interleukin-5 (IL-5), IL-13, monocyte chemoattractant protein-4 (MCP-4), eotaxin.[17] Two cytokines particularly important to the promotion of eosinophilic inflammation are IL-5 and IL-13. IL-5 is chemotactic for eosinophils and essential for activation and survival, whereas IL-13 induces expression of adhesion molecules necessary for eosinophil migration from the vasculature into the tissue. Eosinophils contain and release a variety of destructive proinflammatory mediators, including major basic protein, eosinophil cationic protein, and eosinophil-derived neurotoxin. These mediators are toxic to surrounding tissue and epithelium. Disruption of mucociliary clearance and the barrier function of the epithelium allows bacteria and fungi to propagate in the sinus cavities. However, other inflammatory cells besides eosinophils contribute to the pathogenesis of ECRS, including T cells, mast cells, and basophils. These cells also cause excess mucus secretion, vascular leak, and airway epithelial injury through the production of destructive inflammatory mediators. Corticosteroids interfere with the transcription of many proinflammatory mediators and cytokines. This halts the inflammatory process, and the sinus mucosa returns to normal function. Unfortunately, the reversal of inflammation is often temporary and recurs once the corticosteroids are withdrawn. The reasons for this persistent inflammation are poorly understood, but several of the theories are discussed.

IgE Independent Fungal Inflammation

Several recent studies point to fungus as a possible inflammatory trigger for CRS independent of a Type I IgE allergic mechanism as seen in AFRS. Ponikau and colleagues showed that 97 of 101 consecutive patients undergoing sinus surgery had eosinophils that were migrating through the epithelium into the mucus of the nasal and sinus lumen.[18] Furthermore, allergy in general or allergy to fungus was only present in half of these individuals. Because the observation was made that the eosinophils cluster around fungi, there is a possibility that eosinophils might target the fungi and trigger the inflammation in patients with CRS. With sensitive enough studies, 100% of patients will have fungus in their sinuses. Hence, eosinophils may be recruited and activated as a response to fungi in patients with CRS, but not in healthy controls. Furthermore, peripheral lymphocytes from patients with CRS will produce large quantities of the cytokines IL-5 and IL-13 when they are exposed to certain fungal antigens.[19] Thus, the fungi in the nasal and sinus mucus may activate and induce Th2 type cytokine production independent from allergy.

Aspirin-Sensitive Nasal Polyposis

If patients have NPs in association with asthma and aspirin-sensitivity, this form of ECRS is commonly referred to as Samter triad (Figure 5). Aspirin-sensitivity plays a definitive role in the development of ECRS due to an oversynthesis of leukotrienes. Leukotrienes, also known as the slow reacting substances of anaphylaxis, are a class of inflammatory mediators that increase vascular permeability, inflammatory cell chemotaxis, and smooth muscle constriction. They are produced by a number of cell types including eosinophils, mast cells, macrophages, and basophils and found in the nasal secretions of asthmatics. Arachidonic acid is cleaved from cellular membranes by phospholipase A2 and subsequently shunted to either the leukotriene pathway by the enzyme 5 lipoxygenase or the prostaglandin pathway by the enzyme cyclooxygenase. Prostaglandin E2, a product of the cyclooxygenase pathway, inhibits 5 lipoxygenase in a feedback loop. Aspirin and other nonsteroidal anti-inflammatories inhibit cyclooxygenase and decrease prostaglandin E2, resulting in a net increase in leukotrienes due to uninhibited production.[20] This manifests clinically as bronchospasm, increased mucus production, and inflammatory NPs.

Bacterial Superantigen

There is an emerging interest in the potential role of superantigens in the pathogenesis of ECRS. Bacteria possess the ability to produce pathogenic enterotoxins that can activate large subpopulations of the T-lymphocyte pool. These T-cell superantigens bind to human leukocyte antigen class II histocompatability complexes on antigen-presenting cells and the T-cell receptors of T lymphocytes that are separate from the antigen binding sites. The conventional antigen specificity is bypassed resulting in activation of up to 30% of the T-lymphocyte pool (normal <0.01%). Individuals with major histocompatibility class II molecules, which allow this binding, would be more at risk for this upregulation by a superantigen. The end result is that conventional antigen specificity is bypassed, and there is a subsequent massive cytokine release. An example of this process is seen with the secretion of toxic shock syndrome toxin-1 by *S. aureus* in toxic shock syndrome. This is the most well-known bacteria that produces superantigens, usually called enterotoxins, and is known to produce more than a dozen different forms. Superantigens are implicated in the pathogenesis

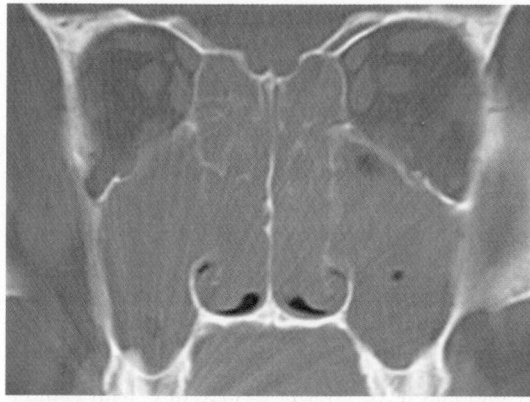

(A)

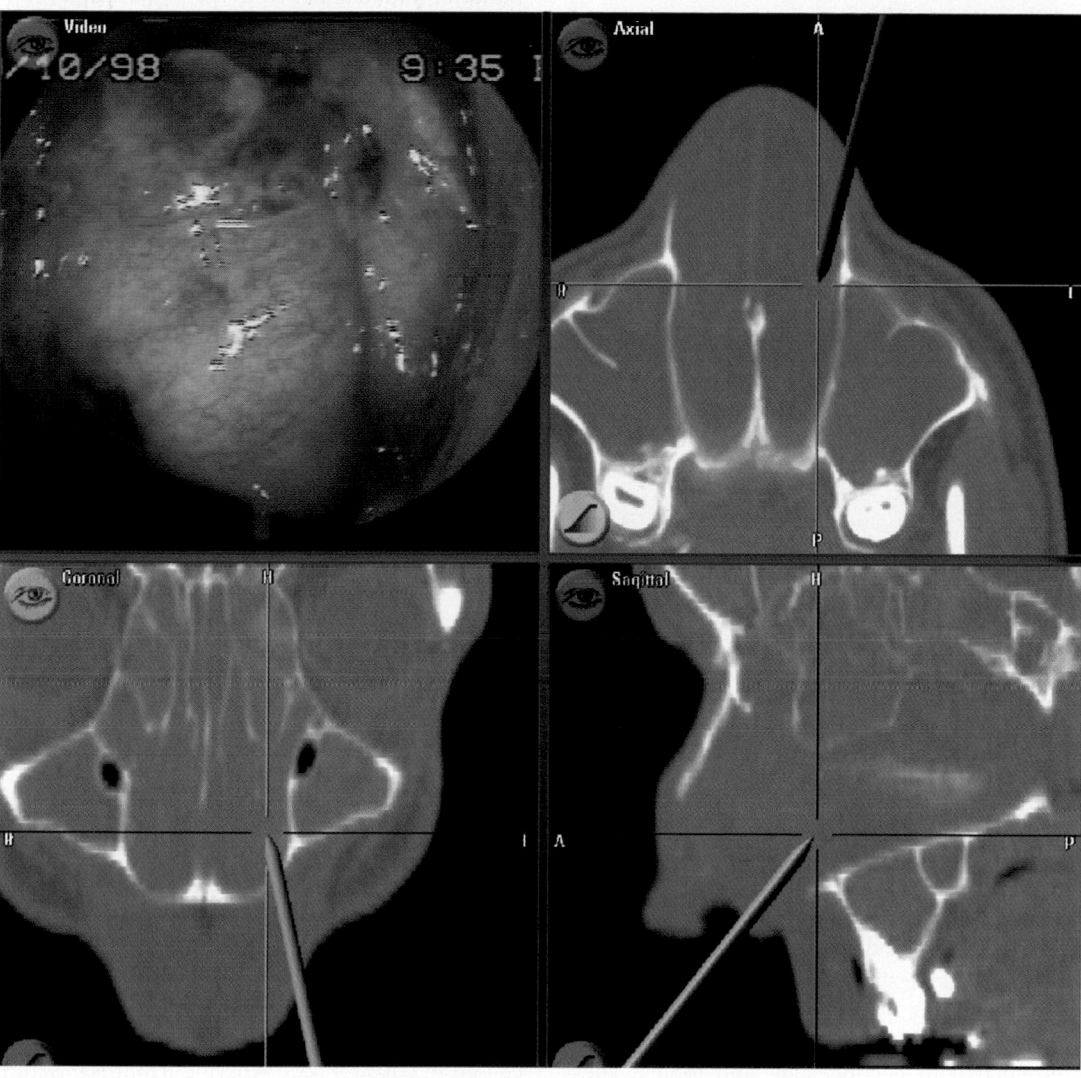

(B)

Figure 4 Computed tomographic scan of a patient with eosinophilic chronic rhinosinusitis (ECRS), asthma, and Churg-Strauss syndrome demonstrating severe bilateral disease without hyperdense secretions (A). ECRS can cause bony erosion, such as that seen in (B) with piriform aperture remodeling, but is less likely to extend intracranially or into the orbit.

pathogenesis of all types of ECRS. This theory proposes that microbial persistence, superantigen production, and host T-lymphocyte response are fundamental components unifying all common chronic eosinophilic respiratory mucosal disorders.[21] This helps explain how a number of coexisting immune responses, including type 1 hypersensitivity, cellular antigen-specific immune responses, and superantigen-induced T-lymphocyte activation, could contribute to the heterogeneity of the disease. Nevertheless, it is likely that there are additional mechanisms at work in ECRS.

CLINICAL AND LABORATORY EVALUATION

History and Physical Examination

Patients with CRS have a number of symptoms that may be similar to other nasal disorders. While nasal obstruction, nasal congestion, and postnasal discharge are the most common symptoms associated with CRS, the banality of these symptoms underscores the fact that these symptoms are also common in patients with allergic rhinitis or other nasal disorders. Thickening of the sinus and nasal mucosa and reactive swelling of the inferior and middle turbinates lead to these symptoms. In allergic rhinitis, a careful history may elicit a description of increasing symptoms with exposure to known allergens and assist with the correct diagnosis. Nasal congestion and rhinorrhea are also common in CRS with NPs, but olfactory dysfunction is far more common in this disorder. Generalized facial pain, pressure, or fullness is often described by patients with CRS and can be localized to an affected side. However, it is imperative the practitioner does not assign the diagnosis of CRS using facial pain or pressure in the absence of other signs and symptoms. Facial pain is not a specific finding, because there are many causes other than CRS. Furthermore, pain is much more common in the acute setting. Headache and dental pain are even less common and subject to the same scrutiny as facial pain/pressure. Other less common symptoms include halitosis, fatigue, cough, and ear pain/pressure. Completing a thorough history of concomitant disorders such as asthma, allergies, and aspirin-sensitivity, will assist with the establishment of an underlying pathophysiology in some cases.

Upon physical examination, CRS patients may have tenderness to palpation or percussion in the periorbital, forehead, or cheek areas. Transillumination of the maxillary and frontal sinuses can suggest the presence of fluid. Maxillary dentition should be inspected for pathology and the oropharynx inspected for postnasal discharge. Mucosal inflammation of the septum and inferior turbinate can be visualized with anterior rhinoscopy, but it should be performed in the decongested state. NPs, especially in children, can alert the physician to the possibility of a systemic disease, such as cystic fibrosis and ciliary dyskinesia.

of other inflammatory diseases, such as atopic dermatitis, Kawasaki disease, psoriasis, and rheumatoid arthiritis.[21]

In CRS, Bachert and colleagues demonstrated staphylococcal superantigen-specific IgE antibodies to the superantigens *S. aureus* enterotoxin A (SEA) and *S. aureus* enterotoxin B (SEB) in NP tissue.[22] In this study 7 of the 20 patients with nasal polyposis were nonallergic on skin prick testing, suggesting that a local

allergic response, may be more important than a systemic allergic response and provides evidence of a specific IgE-mediated response to the superantigen itself. Thus, superantigens appear to have the capacity to act as antigens in addition to stimulating nonspecific T-cell activation. Subsequently, Bernstein and colleagues[23] found evidence of SE production in 7 of 13 patients with NPs (55%). The bacterial superantigen hypothesis is a potential unifying theory for the

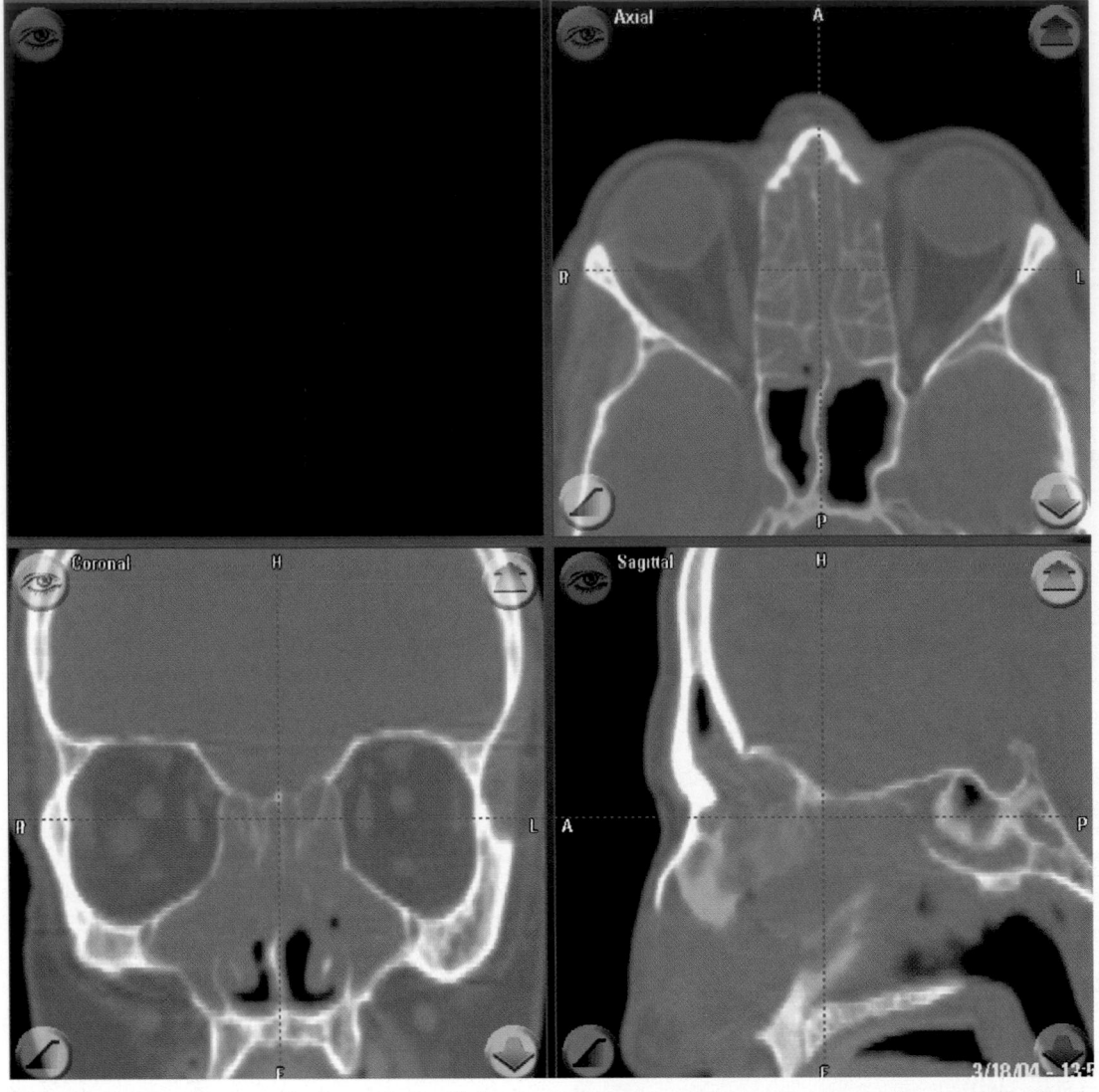

Figure 5 Computed tomography in a patient with Samter triad appears similar to other forms of eosinophilic chronic rhinosinusitis.

the presence of a probable bacterial infection, and thick, tenacious, "peanut butter" mucin is suggestive of AFRS or less commonly ECRS.

Establishing a differential diagnosis of nasal masses is an important part of the clinical evaluation when NPs are present. Sinonasal neoplasms should always be considered as part of the differential diagnosis with tissue sent for pathologic study on patients. "Polyps" may appear locally destructive and indicate the presence of such malignant neoplasms as esthesioneuroblastomas, sinonasal undifferentiated carcinomas, squamous cell carcinomas, and adenocarcinomas. Inverted papillomas are often mistaken for unilateral NPs and often found attached to the lateral nasal wall. Juvenile nasopharyngeal angiofibromas and hemangiopericytomas are extremely vascular tumors that reside in the sinus and nasal cavities. Severe epistaxis will ensue if these tumors are biopsied erroneously prior to an extensive evaluation. Intranasal encephaloceles also may present as a single polyp originating high in the nasal cavity. Further imaging should be performed prior to biopsy of unusual nasal masses. If the mass does not have the characteristic appearance of a polyp, bleeds easily, is unilateral or the site of attachment is not clearly identified, imaging studies are indicated before proceeding. In general, a high resolution CT scan is useful for bone imaging and can reveal dehiscences and erosions from a locally destructive neoplasm or the skull base defect of an encephalocele. Magnetic resonance imaging is complementary to CT scanning because of the ability to identify soft tissue and differentiate tumor from secondary mucosal disease and retained secretions.

Laboratory Studies

Generally, laboratory studies are ordered when the potential results will influence decision-making in the management of the patient. In addition, once a clinical impression is established, further laboratory studies may help confirm or refute that impression. Allergy testing is an example of further laboratory testing that can aid with a diagnosis, help explain the underlying etiology as in AFRS, and change medical decision-making based upon the results. Allergy testing is discussed in Chapter 43, "Allergic Rhinitis." Serum total and specific IgE and CBC with differential to assess for eosinophilia are useful in patients with CRS with NPs. Elevated IgE is a marker for atopic disease and can help differentiate a patient with AFRS from a patient with ECRS. Serum eosinophilia can be a marker for more extensive sinus disease and may help identify individuals more refractory to surgical therapy. In a retrospective comparative analysis of patients undergoing endoscopic sinus surgery, Zadeh and colleagues compared 34 patients with serum eosinophilia to 34 randomly selected CRS patients.[24] Patients with eosinophilia were more likely to have polyps (77% vs 15%), AFRS (39% vs 3%), asthma (35% vs 24%), multiple recurrent sinus infections (94% vs 32%), recurrent polyps (35% vs 3%),

Other important elements of the history and physical examination include eliciting signs and symptoms related to orbital or intracranial extension. Periorbital edema may indicate infection in the presence of a dehiscence of the lamina papyracea or periorbita. Changes in vision, orbital pain, or diplopia can occur with orbital extension of infection which is an emergent situation (see Chapter 46, "Acute Rhinosinusitis and Its Complications"). Gradual unilateral or bilateral orbital proptosis in the absence of orbital pain is often present in massive polyposis, as seen in AFRS. Changes in mental status or meningeal signs may indicate an extension of infection to the intracranial cavity in the form of meningitis or epidural or frontal lobe abscess. Clear rhinorrhea, especially in a previously operated patient, should be evaluated for cerebrospinal fluid leak as described in Chapter 51, "Endoscopic Surgery of the Skull Base, Orbits, and Benign Sinonasal Neoplasms."

Nasal Endoscopy

As discussed earlier in this chapter, groups of major and minor factors proposed by the rhinosinusitis task force of the AAO-HNS are

helpful, but the addition of a definitive sign of mucosal inflammation is the key to establishing a diagnosis. As such, a thorough nasal endoscopic examination is important for helping establish the diagnosis of CRS and CRS with NPs, and *indispensable* for following the course of the disease. Nasal endoscopes are either rigid or flexible fiberoptic designs and allow a very thorough inspection in the office setting with minimal discomfort to the patient if they are appropriately pretreated with decongestant and topical anesthetic. Nasal endoscopy allows the assessment of mucosal hyperemia, edema, the gross appearance and sites of origin of NPs, and septal deformities or other anatomic abnormalities impacting sinus drainage. In the postoperative patient, angled endoscopes enable the practitioner to evaluate the status of mucosal edema and inflammation within all the sinuses to assist with medical management decisions. Furthermore, the practitioner can obtain highly accurate sinus cultures under direct endoscopic visualization to help direct specific antibiotic therapy. The characteristics of the sinonasal discharge should be noted as part of the nasal endoscopic examination. Clear, thin secretions are typical of viral or allergic inflammation, mucopurulent discharge indicates and require revision surgery (84% vs 24%). An immunologic workup may be indicated with CRS, especially in children. Serum assays for total IgE, specific IgE, IgA, IgG, and IgG subclasses (IgG1, IgG2, IgG3, IgG4) and pneumococcal titers can help determine whether an immunoglobulin deficiency and a weak immune response contribute to refractory disease.

Radiology

Although CRS is primarily a clinical diagnosis, radiologic imaging can confirm the diagnosis in the presence of appropriate signs and symptoms. Plain X-ray films are fairly specific for acute maxillary sinusitis when air-fluid levels are seen, but not routinely useful as a screening study for CRS. The current imaging study of choice is a fine cut coronal CT (or axial with coronal reconstruction) of the sinuses. Imaging should include the entire ostiomeatal complex but also the sphenoid sinuses and the entire length of the anterior skull base. CT provides a road map for endoscopic sinus surgery, spots potential complications from bony dehiscences in the skull base or orbit, and identifies mucosal thickening and trapped secretions within the paranasal sinuses (Figures 6 to 9). Unfortunately, mucosal changes on CT scan are not specific for CRS and may be transient and not indicative of true disease. Approximately 40% of individuals without sinonasal complaints will have paranasal sinus mucosal abnormalities on CT scan.[25] This underscores the fact that nasal endoscopy is still the gold standard for identifying inflammatory mucosal disease. CT imaging is undoubtedly a standard next step when clinically diagnosed CRS fails to resolve to medical therapy or patients have persistent sinus symptoms without evidence of disease with nasal endoscopy.

As mentioned earlier, MRI is a complementary study that is helpful in differentiating inflammatory from neoplastic disease (Figure 10). MRI is also sensitive to detecting dural inflammation and the communications of encephaloceles with the intracranial space. However, MRI is limited in usefulness for the evaluation of bony anatomy and for its overly sensitive nature of detecting mucosal inflammation. For further details about MRI and radiologic imaging, please see Chapter 41, "Imaging of the Nasal Cavities, Paranasal Sinuses, Nasopharynx, Orbits, Infratemporal Fossa, Pterygomaxillary Fissure, and Base of Skull."

MEDICAL MANAGEMENT

Antimicrobial Therapy

Antibiotics are by far the most commonly prescribed drugs for CRS. There are few randomized, controlled studies evaluating antimicrobials in CRS. Therefore, antibiotic selection is typically inferred from studies evaluating efficacy in acute rhinosinusitis. *Streptococcus pneumoniae*, *Haemophilus influenzae*, and *Moraxella catarrhalis*

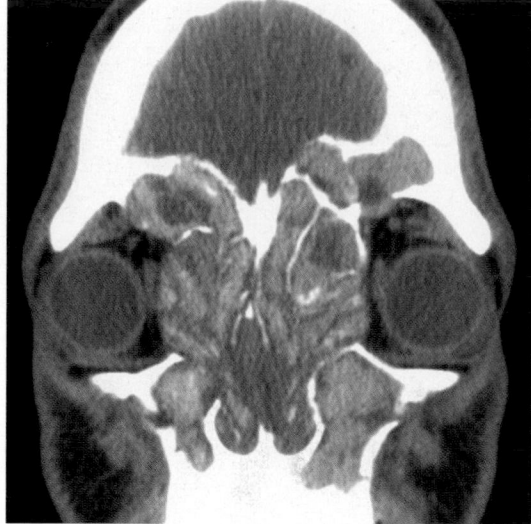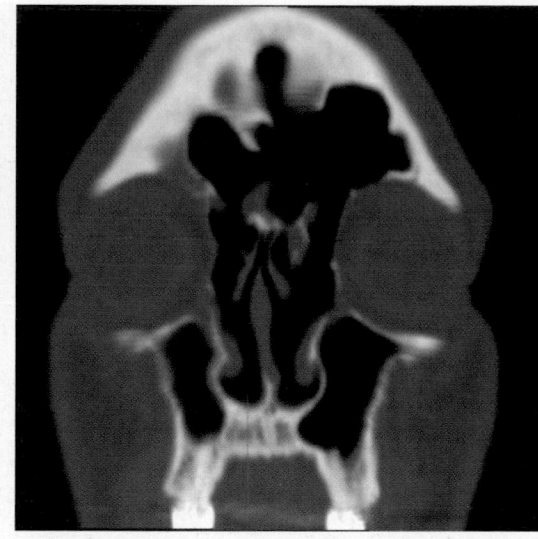

Figure 6 Coronal computed tomography (CT) with soft tissue windows demonstrates hyperdense secretions within the sinuses with bony expansion intracranially (*left*). Postoperative CT (*right*) demonstrates resolution of the nasal polyposis with surgical and medical therapy.

are the predominant microorganisms found in acute rhinosinusitis and pediatric CRS. Unfortunately, the causative microorganisms of CRS differ from those found in acute rhinosinusitis. Coagulase-negative staphylococcus is the most common microorganism in the majority of studies, but there is significant debate over the pathogenicity of this microorganism since it is frequently found colonized in asymptomatic individuals.[26] Other bacteria frequently cultured from

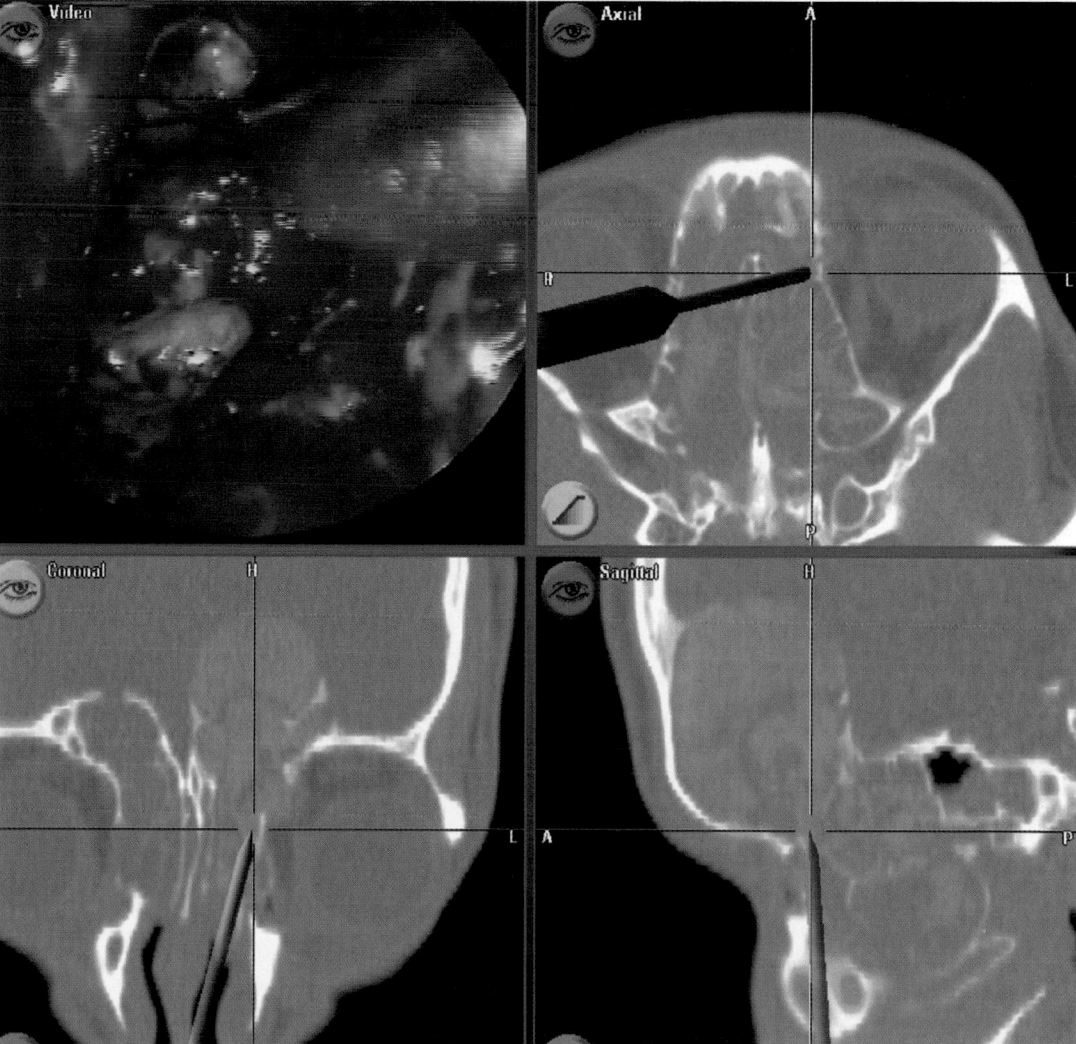

Figure 7 Triplanar computed tomography demonstrates massive extension of allergic fungal rhinosinusitis polyps and fungal debris compressing the frontal lobe.

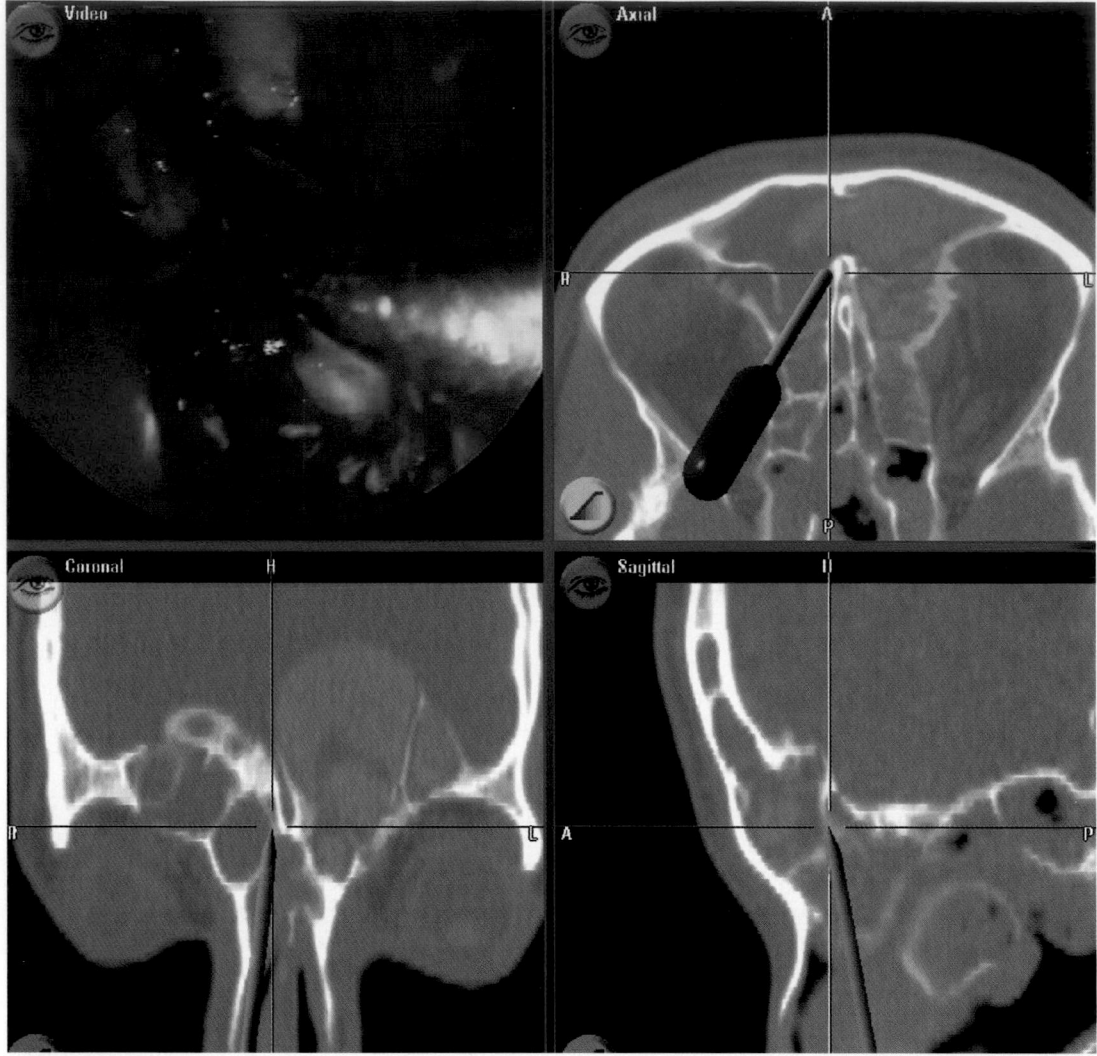

Figure 8 The crista galli is located with a frontal probe and triplanar imaging. Note the near complete bone erosion surrounding the crista galli.

the development of resistance of these valuable antibiotics. In fact, endoscopically directed cultures and sensitivity testing should generally be performed for all individuals with suspected or confirmed CRS if there is mucopurulent discharge present. The duration of antibiotic therapy is not clearly defined, but current recommendations include a 4-week course of first-line antibiotic in addition to a nasal anti-inflammatory medication such as a corticosteroid spray.[27] These recommendations are not based on hard data but extrapolated from several randomized controlled trials that showed inadequate treatment results in 30 to 40% of CRS patients taking antibiotics for 2 weeks or less.

When nasal mucopurulence is present, patients with CRS with NP typically will respond well to a 4-week course of a first-line antibiotic. However, prolonged courses of antibiotics rarely provide relief of nasal obstruction and decrease polyp size. Currently, there are no accepted guidelines for the use of antibiotics as a primary therapy in CRS with NPs, but they are often prescribed in conjunction with corticosteroid therapy in a manner consistent with CRS. On the other hand, the macrolide group of antibiotics may actually have beneficial effects on polyp size and symptoms in the treatment of CRS with NPs, albeit through an immunoregulatory rather than antimicrobial mechanism. Reports suggest a reduction in NP size and symptomatic relief in patients with CRS with NPs who have failed to respond to corticosteroids and surgery.[28] Macrolides are typically used in patients who have failed standard medical and surgical therapy.

Antimicrobial treatment may be used for refractory AFRS that has recurred in spite of standard therapy which should include surgical removal of the fungal eosinophilic mucin and polyps and systemic corticosteroids. Oral itraconazole has been shown to be efficacious for treating ABPA, the pulmonary form of the disease, and it has anti-inflammatory properties in addition to its antifungal actions.[29] Given the ubiquitous nature of fungi in our environment and the

patients with CRS include *S. aureus*, anaerobes, Group A *Streptococcus*, gram-negative rods, and *S. pneumoniae* with a tremendously wide variability among studies.[2] High-dose amoxicillin (2 g/d), amoxicillin/clavulanate, fluoroquinolones, later generation cephalosporins, and the newer ketolides are typical first-line antibiotics for CRS

in adults. These drugs have broad coverage and generally demonstrate adequate bactericidal activity against staphylococci and anaerobic species, although gram-negative coverage varies significantly. Many practitioners prefer to preserve fluoroquinolones for culture proven pseudomonas to reduce the potential for overuse and

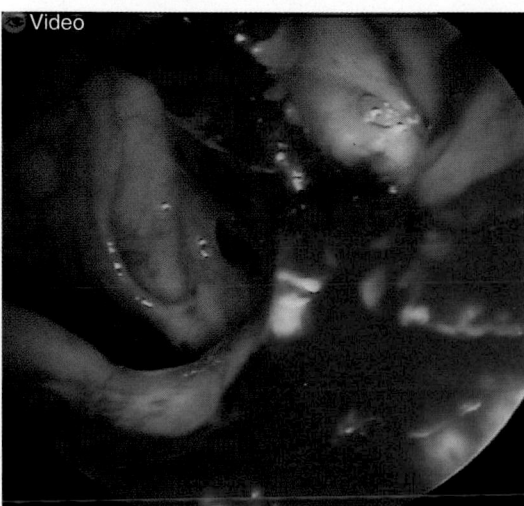

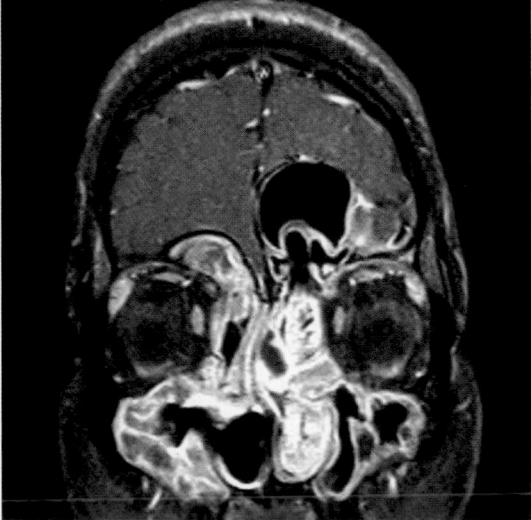

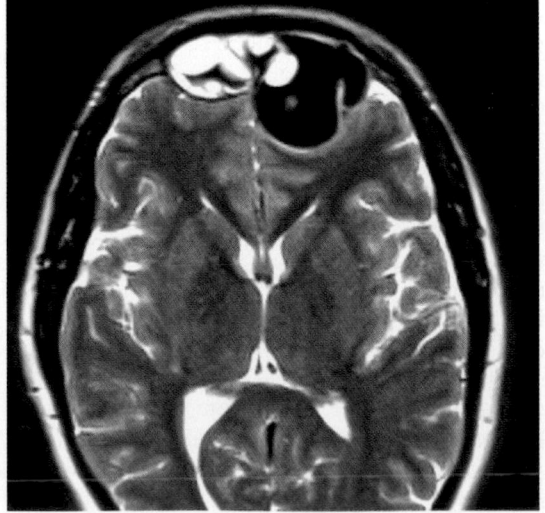

Figure 9 Endoscopic view of crista galli and skull base dehiscence with mucosalization over exposed dura.

Figure 10 Coronal T1 weighted magnetic resonance imaging (MRI) (*left*) and axial T2 weighted MRI (*right*) demonstrate the loss of signal intensity characteristic for AFRS pushing into the left frontal lobe.

colonization of even normal sinuses by multiple fungal species, the role of topical and systemic anti-fungal therapies is still unclear.

Therapy for bacterial superantigen-induced ECRS could theoretically attack the microorganism responsible. In many cases this could be *S. aureus*, because this colonizes one-third of individuals and was present in 55% of patients in the study by Bernstein and colleagues[23] Interestingly, all *S. aureus* produced an enterotoxin in that series. They advocated the use of a topical anti-staphylococcal medication, mupirocin, in these patients. In addition, vigorous saline nasal washes could wash away proinflammatory cytokines as well as bacteria from the nose. Enterotoxin-producing bacteria could also live in biofilms, thereby making them resistant to systemic antimicrobials. These bacteria would then be amenable to removal with vigorous nasal washings and cleansings, possibly augmented with topical antimicrobials. As in all the ECRS forms, either systemic corticosteroids or topical corticosteroids offer some therapeutic efficacy.

Systemic Corticosteroid Therapy

Oral corticosteroids are a mainstay of therapy for severe CRS and CRS with NPs. Systemic corticosteroids are potent anti-inflammatory agents with broad activity effective against almost all inflammatory conditions. Despite the lack of placebo-controlled trials to document efficacy in sinonasal inflammatory disorders, they are uniformly accepted as an efficacious treatment because clinical practice shows rapid relief of facial pressure and nasal blockage by reducing mucosal edema and polyp bulk. At the cellular level, corticosteroids inhibit the synthesis of multiple inflammatory mediators resulting in a decrease in vessel permeability and inflammatory cell influx. The effect on production of inflammatory mediators is especially profound in CRS with NPs since eosinophils require cytokines such as IL-5 for survival and function.[17]

There are no routine guidelines with regard to oral corticosteroid therapy for CRS or CRS with NPs. However, it is universally recommended to taper corticosteroids if administered for >2 weeks to prevent an Addisonian crisis. The dose of corticosteroids prescribed will typically depend upon the extent of disease. Therapy in otherwise healthy adults with moderate to severe polyposis typically starts at a mid-range dose (40 mg of prednisone per day for 3 to 4 days) that is tapered over an additional 5 to 14 days. If the patient has persistent disease, therapy may be maintained in preparation for surgery to maximize shrinkage of the NPs and reduce mucosal inflammation and vascularity or kept at lower doses following the procedure to help reduce the recurrence of NPs. Administration of oral corticosteroid therapy should not be taken lightly because of the myriad of potential disastrous side effects. These risks include hypothalamic–pituitary–adrenal axis suppression, gastric ulcers, psychiatric changes, and exacerbation of diabetes, as well as chronic side effects such as osteoporosis, weight gain, ocular problems, and hypertension. Avascular necrosis of the hip is a devastating complication that typically occurs following chronic oral corticosteroid use but can happen regardless of the route of administration (oral, topical, or injectable) or duration of administration. Separating corticosteroid treatment by 3-month intervals will reduce the risks of chronic corticosteroid use.

Topical Corticosteroid Therapy

Topical intranasal corticosteroids are a first-line therapy in almost all patients with CRS or CRS with NPs because they provide many of the benefits of systemic corticosteroid use without the side effects. Significantly elevated serum cortisol levels, or significant growth retardation in prepubescent children has not been detected.[30] Furthermore, clinical trials have confirmed intranasal corticosteroids as superior to placebo in reducing polyp size, improving nasal congestion and rhinorrhea, and increasing peak nasal airflow in patients with CRS with NPs.[31] Topical corticosteroid therapy also provides more rapid symptomatic relief during antibiotic therapy for CRS. Corticosteroid nasal sprays reduce proinflammatory cytokine production and decrease mucosal edema and inflammation through the same cellular mechanism as oral corticosteroids.

Topical intranasal corticosteroids should be administered once daily with a clinical follow-up in 8 to 12 weeks for mild CRS and CRS with NPs to determine the effect on symptoms and polyp size. For more advanced CRS and CRS with NPs, nasal corticosteroid sprays are almost never administered by themselves without initiating antibiotic and/or oral corticosteroid therapy as well. Head positioning is important during intranasal corticosteroid use, so patients should employ proper techniques by aiming the spray tip at the ipsilateral outer canthus or top of the auricle. Furthermore, an inverted head position is often necessary following surgery so that the corticosteroid spray will coat the frontal recess, an area of high polyp recurrence. Patients with massive polyposis secondary to AFRS, cystic fibrosis, or Churg-Strauss syndrome may have insufficient airspace in which to apply the drug even after a course of systemic corticosteroids. In this case, surgical debridement is necessary prior to the initiation of topical nasal corticosteroids. Should surgery eventually become necessary for CRS and CRS with NPs, topical corticosteroids and occasionally oral corticosteroids may be needed for long-term maintenance.

Antileukotriene Therapy

Currently, there are two classes of antileukotriene drugs approved in the United States for the treatment of asthma: leukotriene receptor blockers (montelukast and zafirlukast) and a 5-lipoxygenase inhibitor which blocks the enzyme that forms leukotrienes (zileuton). Montelukast has also been recently approved for treating inhalant allergies. Antileukotriene therapy is generally well-tolerated, with the most common side effects being headache and dyspepsia. Parnes and colleagues[32] showed in a prospective study that 72% of patients with CRS with NPs had a significant reduction in nasal symptoms, 50% had decreased polyp size, and 60% no longer required oral corticosteroids when they were treated with at least 1 month of antileukotriene therapy. Although further placebo controlled trials are indicated, antileukotrienes may provide at the least an alternative therapy in patients with CRS with NPs who are intolerant of chronic doses of corticosteroids. For obvious reasons, this drug class is likely to work best in patients with aspirin-sensitive ECRS.

Other Medical and Ancillary Therapies

Although debate exists over the percentage of patients with CRS who have coexisting seasonal or perennial allergic rhinitis, most agree that underlying allergic rhinitis is an important predisposing factor for CRS. Antihistamines reduce sneezing and rhinorrhea in patients with CRS with NPs, and are suitable in cases in whom allergy plays an important role. However, first generation antihistamines should generally be avoided since their anticholinergic activity can further desiccate already thickened mucus. Newer second-generation antihistamines have much less anticholinergic activity, and so they are frequently used as part of an overall treatment plan in patients who are suspected of having inhalant allergies. As mentioned previously, allergy testing should be considered in all patients with CRS with and without NPs, and those who test positive should be treated appropriately with antihistamines, topical corticosteroids, or immunotherapy.

Immunotherapy may play a role in patients with NPs, particularly those with IgE mediated disease, such as AFRS. We typically recommend immunotherapy for all fungi toward which a patient demonstrates atopy rather than basing it upon fungal cultures. A wide range of fungal species have been implicated in AFRS, and fungal cultures appear to change throughout the course of the disease. Bassichis and colleagues reported reoperation rates of 33% in patients with AFRS not receiving immunotherapy compared with 11.1% in those receiving immunotherapy (*n* = 36) in their series of 60 patients.[33]

Treatment for acid reflux can be useful in patients with refractory sinus disease.[34] We typically begin therapy using a proton pump inhibitor and/or H2 blockers and have found them useful in controlling symptoms of post nasal drip, globus sensation, and throat clearing. Certain populations, such as patients with cystic fibrosis or those less than 6 years old, seem to be more responsive.

A well-tolerated and inexpensive adjunctive therapy for both CRS and CRS with NPs is nasal saline irrigation. Randomized, controlled studies have demonstrated a reduction in sinus symptoms and an improved sinus-related quality of life in patients who used nasal saline irrigations.[35]

This therapy likely helps clear the nasal and sinus cavities of inspissated mucus, bacteria, allergens, and environmental irritants. Adding antimicrobials, such as tobramycin to nasal/sinus irrigations has been a routine part of management of patients with cystic fibrosis due to the heavy colonization and chronic infections of *Pseudomonas*. Mupirocin added to irrigations can help eradicate methicillin-resistant *S. aureus* infections. Some advocate this practice for patients with CRS with NPs in the hopes of eradicating any *Staphylococcus* eliciting enterotoxins functioning as superantigens.[27] Amphotericin B irrigations may also eliminate fungal elements that cause a local inflammatory response. Since staphylococcal or fungal microorganisms in this situation are not invasive and colonized on top of the nasal mucosa, they may be relatively protected from serum borne antimicrobial agents. For nearly all topical antimicrobial agents, the exact concentration, frequency, and duration of therapy have not been studied in a scientific fashion.

PEDIATRIC CHRONIC RHINOSINUSITIS

Pediatric CRS is discussed separately because of the unique issues involved in diagnosis, evaluation, and treatment. The clinical diagnosis of pediatric CRS is identical to the temporal, symptom-based criteria used for adult CRS diagnosis. However, the history and physical examination in a pediatric patient is challenging at best and often is unobtainable in young children. Nasal endoscopy is more difficult in younger children; and, in such cases, an otoscope can be used to examine the nose. However, nasal purulence is typically already present as anterior rhinorrhea. Nasal congestion, cough, and purulent rhinorrhea are the most common complaints in pediatric CRS. Sinus CTs may be helpful but are limited by the frequent presence of mucosal thickening secondary to viral respiratory infections in this population. The pathophysiology of pediatric CRS is similar to that of the adult population. However, unique issues in the pathogenesis of pediatric CRS include adenoid hypertrophy and gastroesophageal reflux disease. Adenoidectomy tends to be beneficial for pediatric CRS and is often considered the first-line surgical therapy. Some practitioners treat empirically with antireflux medication. The presence of CRS with NPs suggests cystic fibrosis in a child until proven otherwise, and the child should promptly be evaluated for this disease. Antibiotic therapy is the primary medical intervention and should be directed against *S. pneumoniae*, *H. influenzae*, and *M. catarrhalis*. Systemic corticosteroids must be used with extreme caution in the pediatric population to avoid severe side effects and possible growth retardation.

CONCLUSIONS

There are many scientific advances in the treatment and understanding of the pathophysiology of CRS that have occurred within the last decade. Advances in nasal endoscopy, radiologic imaging, medical treatments, and surgical technique have allowed for significant improvement in patient management. However, recalcitrant sinus disease is a particular problem and continues to await new therapeutic approaches. Hopefully, further research will lead to novel strategies of medical and surgical therapy that will decrease the need for systemic corticosteroids and their ill effects, while increasing the quality of life for patients stricken with this difficult disease.

REFERENCES

1. Benninger MS, Ferguson BJ, Hadley JA, et al. Adult chronic rhinosinusitis: Definitions, diagnosis, epidemiology, and pathophysiology. Otolaryngol Head Neck Surg 2003;129:S1–32.
2. Gillespie MB, Osguthorpe JD. Pharmacologic management of chronic rhinosinusitis, alone or with nasal polyposis. Curr Allergy Asthma Rep 2004;4:478–85.
3. Ferguson BJ. Categorization of eosinophilic chronic rhinosinusitis. Curr Opin Otolaryngol Head Neck Surg 2004;12:237–42.
4. Ray NF, Baraniuk JN, Thamer M, et al. Healthcare expenditures for sinusitis in 1996: Contributions of asthma, rhinitis, and other airway disorders. J Allergy Clin Immunol 1999;103:408–14.
5. Lanza DC, Kennedy DW. Adult rhinosinusitis defined. Otolaryngol Head Neck Surg 1997;117:S1–7.
6. Report of the Rhinosinusitis Task Force Committee Meeting. Alexandria, Virginia, August 17, 1996. Otolaryngol Head Neck Surg 1997;117:S1–68.
7. Wald ER. Microbiology of acute and chronic sinusitis in children and adults. Am J Med Sci 1998;316:13–20.
8. Perloff JR, Gannon FH, Bolger WE, et al. Bone involvement in sinusitis: An apparent pathway for the spread of disease. Laryngoscope 2000;110:2095–9.
9. Perloff JR, Palmer JN. Evidence of bacterial biofilms in a rabbit model of sinusitis. Am J Rhinol 2005;19:1–6.
10. Mah TF, O'Toole GA. Mechanisms of biofilm resistance to antimicrobial agents. Trends Microbiol 2001;9:34–9.
11. Larsen PL, Tos M. Origin of nasal polyps: An endoscopic autopsy study. Laryngoscope 2004;114:710–9.
12. Malekzadeh S, McGuire JF. The new histologic classification of chronic rhinosinusitis. Curr Allergy Asthma Rep 2003;3:221–6.
13. Bent JP, 3rd, Kuhn FA. Diagnosis of allergic fungal sinusitis. Otolaryngol Head Neck Surg 1994;111:580–8.
14. Taylor MJ, Ponikau JU, Sherris DA, et al. Detection of fungal organisms in eosinophilic mucin using a fluorescein-labeled chitin-specific binding protein. Otolaryngol Head Neck Surg 2002;127:377–83.
15. Lackner A, Stammberger H, Buzina W, et al. Fungi: A normal content of human nasal mucus. Am J Rhinol 2005; 19:125–9.
16. Manning SC, Mabry RL, Schaefer SD, Close LG. Evidence of IgE-mediated hypersensitivity in allergic fungal sinusitis. Laryngoscope 1993;103:717–21.
17. Woodworth BA, Joseph K, Kaplan AP, Schlosser RJ. Alterations in eotaxin, monocyte chemoattractant protein-4, interleukin-5, and interleukin-13 after systemic steroid treatment for nasal polyps. Otolaryngol Head Neck Surg 2004;131:585–9.
18. Ponikau JU, Sherris DA, Kern EB, et al. The diagnosis and incidence of allergic fungal sinusitis. Mayo Clin Proc 1999;74:877–84.
19. Shin SH, Ponikau JU, Sherris DA, et al. Chronic rhinosinusitis: An enhanced immune response to ubiquitous airborne fungi. J Allergy Clin Immunol 2004;114:1369–75.
20. Szczeklik A, Stevenson DD. Aspirin-induced asthma: Advances in pathogenesis, diagnosis, and management [quiz 922]. J Allergy Clin Immunol 2003;111:913–21.
21. Schubert MS. A superantigen hypothesis for the pathogenesis of chronic hypertrophic rhinosinusitis, allergic fungal sinusitis, and related disorders. Ann Allergy Asthma Immunol 2001;87:181–8.
22. Bachert C, Gevaert P, Holtappels G, et al. Total and specific IgE in nasal polyps is related to local eosinophilic inflammation. J Allergy Clin Immunol 2001;107:607–14.
23. Bernstein JM, Ballow M, Schlievert PM, et al. A superantigen hypothesis for the pathogenesis of chronic hyperplastic sinusitis with massive nasal polyposis. Am J Rhinol 2003;17:321–6.
24. Zadeh MH, Banthia V, Anand VK, Huang C. Significance of eosinophilia in chronic rhinosinusitis. Am J Rhinol 2002;16:313–7.
25. Havas TE, Motbey JA, Gullane PJ. Prevalence of incidental abnormalities on computed tomographic scans of the paranasal sinuses. Arch Otolaryngol Head Neck Surg 1988;114:856–9.
26. Newman LJ, Platts-Mills TA, Phillips CD, et al. Chronic sinusitis. Relationship of computed tomographic findings to allergy, asthma, and eosinophilia. JAMA 1994;271:363–7.
27. Anon JB, Jacobs MR, Poole MD, et al. Antimicrobial treatment guidelines for acute bacterial rhinosinusitis. Sinus and Allergy Health Partnership. Otolaryngol Head Neck Surg 2000;123:5–31.
28. Garey KW, Alwani A, Danziger LH, Rubinstein I. Tissue reparative effects of macrolide antibiotics in chronic inflammatory sinopulmonary diseases. Chest 2003;123:261–5.
29. Stevens DA, Schwartz HJ, Lee JY, et al. A randomized trial of itraconazole in allergic bronchopulmonary aspergillosis. N Engl J Med 2000;342:756–62.
30. Skoner DP, Gentile D, Angelini B, et al. The effects of intranasal triamcinolone acetonide and intranasal fluticasone propionate on short-term bone growth and HPA axis in children with allergic rhinitis. Ann Allergy Asthma Immunol 2003;90:56–62.
31. Jankowski R, Schrewelius C, Bonfils P, et al. Efficacy and tolerability of budesonide aqueous nasal spray treatment in patients with nasal polyps. Arch Otolaryngol Head Neck Surg 2001;127:447–52.
32. Parnes SM. The role of leukotriene inhibitors in patients with paranasal sinus disease. Curr Opin Otolaryngol Head Neck Surg 2003;11:184–91.
33. Bassichis BA, Marple BF, Mabry RL, et al. Use of immunotherapy in previously treated patients with allergic fungal sinusitis. Otolaryngol Head Neck Surg 2001;125:487–90.
34. DelGaudio JM. Direct nasopharyngeal reflux of gastric acid is a contributing factor in refractory chronic rhinosinusitis. Laryngoscope 2005;115:946–57.
35. Rabago D, Zgierska A, Mundt M, et al. Efficacy of daily hypertonic saline nasal irrigation among patients with sinusitis: A randomized controlled trial. J Fam Pract 2002;51:1049–55.

48

Headache and Facial Pain

James M. Hartman, MD
Jeffrey W. Yu, MD
Richard A. Chole, MD, PhD

The craniofacial region is the most common location in which pain drives patients to seek medical attention.[1] The wide diversity of causes and the extreme overlap of historical features coupled with nonspecific physical findings serve to challenge the physician's ability to diagnose and ultimately relieve or control patients' craniofacial pain. However, an understanding of the different types of craniofacial pain provides a powerful tool to meet the challenge.

INNERVATION FOR PAIN

Nociceptors serve as the sense organs in which noxious stimuli create a response that excites afferent nerve fibers that provide the brain with information about location, intensity, quality, and duration of the response.[2] Neurochemicals responsible for this excitation include serotonin and substance P as well as other neurotransmitters. These afferent fibers are carried to the central nervous system in cranial nerves V, VII, IX, and X and the first 3 cervical nerves.

Pain-sensitive innervation of facial structures is extensive, whereas intracranial pain sensation is limited to specific structures. The extracranial tissues innervated for pain sensation include the muscles of the head and neck, the scalp and facial skin, sinonasal mucosa and perichondrium, temporomandibular joint (TMJ) synovium and capsule, tooth pulp, the external and middle ear, orbital contents, salivary glands, cervical spine, and craniofacial periosteum. Intracranial structures with nociceptive neurons include major arteries, specifically the internal carotids, vertebrals, basilar, middle meningeals, ophthalmics, the circle of Willis, and the major venous sinuses. Nonvascular structures with pain nerve fibers are represented by cranial nerves V, VII, IX, and X and the upper 3 cervical nerves themselves, as well as the pituitary fossa and the base of skull dura mater. The remaining intracranial structures are insensate to pain, including the brain, most of the dura, the ventricles, and the cranium. The afferents converge on nuclei in the brainstem where multiple synaptic connections occur including transmission to the ipsi- and contralateral thalamus and the somatosensory cerebral cortex. The thalamic nuclei appear to play a role

in the affective response to pain, whereas the cortical centers' role is in localization and intensity recognition of noxious stimuli.[2] The extensive convergence of afferent neurons in brainstem nuclei, however, limits the brain's ability to distinguish between sources. The result is referral of pain to tissues with a past experience recognized as pain.[3] Specific patterns of pain referral are common, for example: from the TMJ and muscles of mastication, radiation is to the ear, cheek, and temple[4]; from the tonsillar fossa and supraglottic larynx to the middle ear; from the maxillary sinus to the maxillary teeth; from the sphenoid sinus to the vertex or occiput, and, of course, angina is sometimes referred to the jaw.

PATHOPHYSIOLOGY

Multiple mechanisms resulting in excitation of nociceptive neurons, that is, generating the perception of pain, are partially understood. One common mechanism is sustained muscle contraction resulting in tension headache. The exact source of excitation is unclear but may be the result of ischemic changes or the production of nitric oxide.[5] Another common scenario is vasodilation of intracranial arteries stimulating trigeminal sensory pathways, which release vasoactive peptides that increase the pain response.[6] The vasodilation seems linked to subtypes of serotonin 5-hydroxytryptamine (5-HT) receptors in vessel walls. Other subtypes of 5-HT receptors, such as 5-HT1B, yield vasoconstriction and inhibit the pain response.[7] It is this basis on which triptan antimigraine agents have their effect by selectively binding to 5-HT1B receptors. An inflammatory mechanism is thought to be responsible when neuropeptides such as substance P are released with mucosal inflammation. These result in neural excitation, resulting in the perception of pain.[8] Neural inflammation following injury or tumor invasion has an excitatory effect. Direct nerve pressure may induce nociceptor activity, as seen in foraminal stenosis. Many agents that result in vasodilation can trigger headache including hypoxia, carbon monoxide, caffeine withdrawal, acute alcohol withdrawal, oral contraceptives, hypoglycemia, and antihypertensives and other vasodilators such as nitroglycerin and

monosodium glutamate found in Chinese food.[9] Finally, cerebral mechanisms are also thought to play a role. For example, some migraineurs have been found to have defective release of endogenous opiates,[10] and lowered cortical pain thresholds occur in chronic tension headaches.[11]

CLASSIFICATION

Understanding headache and facial pain is essential to facilitate diagnosis and treatment. To this end, definitions and features of clinical syndromes were first organized by the International Headache Society (IHS) in 1988[12] and the second edition was released in 2004.[13] This classification, with inclusion of diagnostic criteria for headaches, cranial neuralgias, and facial pain, has facilitated the diagnostic approach and management of craniofacial pain across many medical fields. Table 1 lists the major classification of

---

Table 1 International Headache Society Classification of Headache and Facial Pain

Part I: The primary headaches

1. Migraine
2. Tension-type headache
3. Cluster headache and other trigeminal autonomic cephalalgias
4. Other primary headaches

Part II: The secondary headaches

5. Headache attributed to head and/or neck trauma
6. Headache attributed to cranial or cervical vascular disorder
7. Headache attributed to nonvascular intracranial disorder
8. Headache attributed to a substance or its withdrawal
9. Headache attributed to infection
10. Headache attributed to disorder of homeostasis
11. Headache or facial pain attributed to disorder of cranium, neck, eyes, ears, nose, sinuses, teeth, mouth, or other facial or cranial structures
12. Headache attributed to psychiatric disorder

Part III: Cranial neuralgias central and primary facial pain and other headaches

13. Cranial neuralgias and central causes of facial pain
14. Other headache, cranial neuralgia, central or primary facial pain

From reference 13.

headaches, neuralgias, and facial pains. Greater detail can be found in the IHS classification publication and website.

PATIENT EVALUATION

History is the essential tool to establish a diagnosis for headache or facial pain. It must be comprehensive to ensure accuracy of diagnosis. Once the features of the cephalalgia are discovered, one can refer to the IHS classification to determine which specific diagnostic criteria are fulfilled (Table 2).[14–16] In approaching a patient with headache, it is important to rule in or out a benign headache and to evaluate the patient for serious intracranial pathology.[17] For example, Figure 1 illustrates an algorithm for attempting to differentiate patients who have a migraine from patients who require neuroimaging.

Serious or even life-threatening conditions associated with headache usually will present with distinct characteristics of the headache, focal neurological signs, or systemic complaints (see Table 3 for specific serious conditions in which headache is a presenting symptom).[18] Warning features of the headache include sudden onset, highest severity, steady crescendo of intensity, awakening with headache, and exacerbation by coughing or straining. Dangerous associated systemic symptoms include fever, sudden vomiting, declining mental status, syncope, or seizures. Specific physical ailments such as neck rigidity, tender or enlarged temporal artery, unilateral rhinorrhea, skull percussion tenderness, or focal neurologic defects such as visual field loss, diplopia, hemiparesis, and facial nerve palsy may indicate serious underlying pathology. Finally, a history of preexisting malignancy or immunosuppression may herald a serious condition.[19]

The physical examination is guided by history and clinical suspicion. Routine measures should include a check of blood pressure and temperature; assessment of mental status and cranial nerve function; and a visual examination inclusive of pupil size, extraocular movement, visual fields, and funduscopy. Range of motion testing of the jaw and neck should be performed along with palpation of the TMJ, muscles of mastication, and paraspinal musculature searching for trigger points of neuritic or muscular pain. Abnormalities may be observed in the external or middle ear, the sinonasal passages, the mouth, and dentition, or herpetic lesions may be seen in dermatomes. Palpation of the temporal arteries should also be performed. Asymmetric skull percussion tenderness may suggest a subdural process. Laboratory testing, including lumbar puncture for cerebrospinal fluid (CSF) analysis, should be limited and guided by clinical impression. Radiologic imaging with computed tomography (CT), magnetic resonance imaging (MRI), or magnetic resonance angiography (MRA) may be indicated when organic pathology is suspected.

SPECIFIC CLINICAL SYNDROMES

The characteristic features of many craniofacial pain diagnoses are presented along with specific treatment recommendations (see Table 1 for the classification system).

Migraine-Type Headaches

Migraines comprise the second most common form of headache, with a prevalence of 18% in women and 6% in men and costing billions of dollars for treatment and lost productivity.[20] Its peak age of onset is in the second or third decade, but children and even infants may also be affected.[21] Migraine headaches usually occur as recurrent episodes of severe, throbbing, unilateral head pain of sudden onset lasting 4 to 72 hours. However, 40% of migraineurs have bilateral pain. The headache often strikes after awakening in the morning. In children, migraine headaches usually end between 2 and 48 hours. Routine activities of daily living may exacerbate the symptoms. Coexisting symptoms with the headache are common including nausea, vomiting, photophobia, and phonophobia. Stress is the usual precipitating factor. A family history of migraine is often present.

Migraine is divided into several types: those without aura (formerly *common migraine*) and those with aura (formerly *classic migraine*). They are the 2 most common by far. Migraine without aura is the most common type. It lacks

---

Table 2 Pertinent Elements of a Headache History[14–16]

Temporal Profile
  Course
    Duration of problem
    Frequency of headaches
  Duration of each headache
Location
  Unilateral or bilateral
  Focal or diffuse
  Radiates to other sites
Quality
  Intensity
  Characteristics
    Throbbing (vascular)
    Stabbing (neuritic)
    Pressure (viscus or chamber derived)
    Aching or burning (muscular)
Prodrome presence (hours to days prior to headache)
  Mood changes
  Fatigue
  Nausea
  Excessive yawning
  Chilling
  Anorexia or food craving
  Stiff neck
  Urinary frequency
  Diarrhea
  Fluid retention
Aura presence
  Visual disturbances
    Scotomata
    Photophobia
  Motor disturbances
    Ataxia
    Hemiparesis
    Aphasia or dysarthria
    Diplopia
  Sensory disturbances
    Hypo- or hypersensitivity to touch
    Paresthesias
    Phonophobia
    Tinnitus
    Vertigo
    Confusion
Family history of headache
  Migraine
  Tension type
  Temporomandibular joint disorders
  Subarachnoid hemorrhage
  Substance abuse
  Social history
  Smoking habits
  Alcohol intake
  Illicit drug use
  Occupation

Associated Symptoms
  Nausea and vomiting
  Lacrimation
  Nasal congestion
  Rhinorrhea
  Tender or pulsating scalp, vertigo, syncope, confusion
  Sweating
Precipitating factors
  Smell provocation
  Chewing head movement or sustained position
  Coughing
  Yawning
  Straining
  Position change
  Stress
  Sleep change
  Missed meals
  Menses
  Weather change
  Alcohol intake
  Specific food ingestion
  Medication use
Past medical and dental history
  Trauma to head or neck
  Surgery to head or neck
  Dental procedures
  Meningitis
  Hypertension
  Diabetes
  Glaucoma
  Rheumatoid arthritis
  Sinusitis
Medication use
  Over-the-counter analgesics
  Prescription analgesics
  Vasodilators
  Oral contraceptives
  Insulin
  Herbal remedies
Review of systems
  Fever
  Weight change
  Sleep habit change
  Appetite change
  Depression or anxiety
  Decreased range of motion
  Jaw
  Neck
  Bruxism
  Chest pain
Motivation (secondary gain)
  Disability
  School phobia

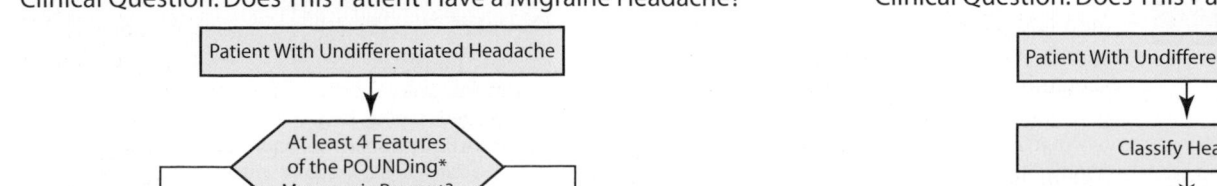

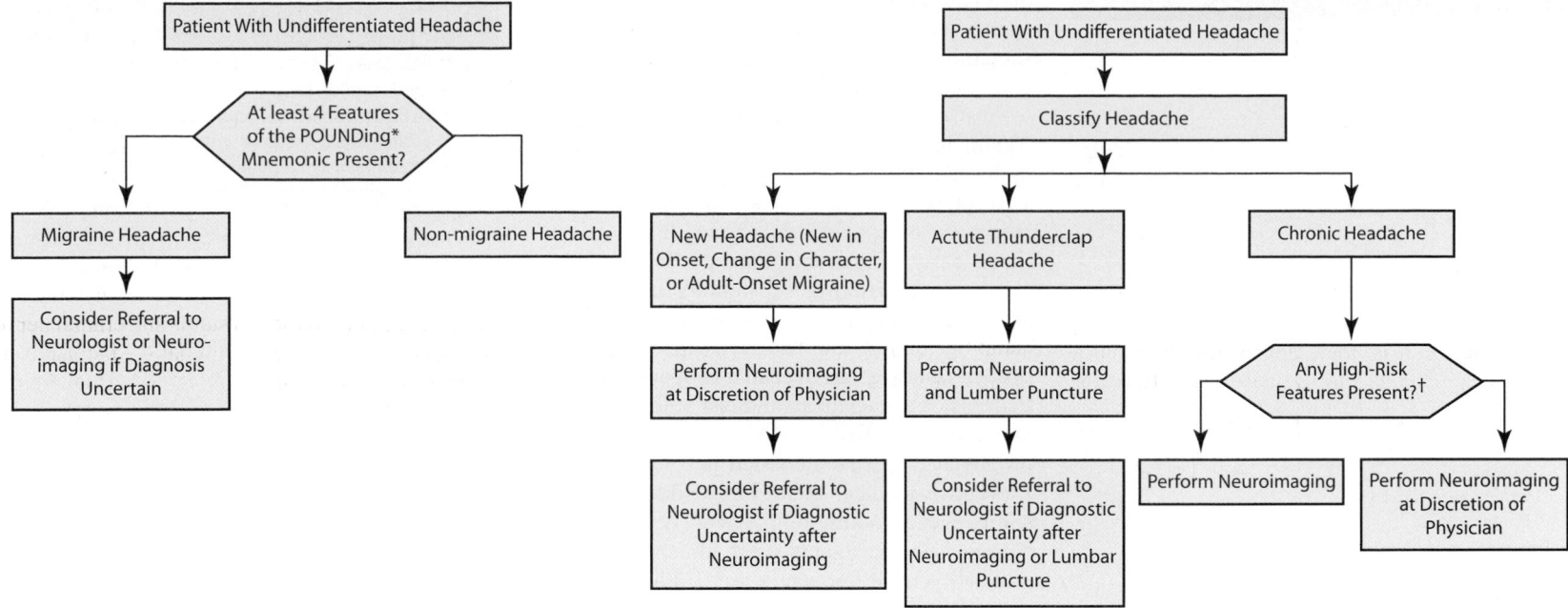

*POUNDing: Pulsatile quality; duration 4-72 hours; Unilateral location; Nausea and Vomiting; Disabling intensity.

†Cluster-type headache, abnormal findings on neurologic examination, undefined headache (ie, not cluster-, migraine-, or tension-type), headache with aura, headache aggravated by exertion of Valsalva-like maneuver, headache with vomiting.

Adapted with permission from Detsky ME, McDonald DR, Baerlocher MO, Tomlinson GA, McCrory DC, Booth CM, Does this patient with headache have a migaine or need neuroimaging? *JAMA.* Sep 13 2006:296(10):1274-1283.

Figure 1 Suggested algorithm for the approach to headache. (Adapted with permission from reference 17.)

any preheadache warning symptoms. Migraine with aura is also common, comprising 20% of migraine sufferers. The typical aura lasts <1 hour and immediately precedes the onset of cephalalgia. It may be precipitated by menses, pregnancy, oral contraceptives, certain foods, or bright lights. *Migraine with prolonged aura* has symptoms of the aura that last through and beyond the headache up to 7 days. Features of aura include focal neurologic symptoms including visual changes such as scotomata or sensory

Table 3 Life- or Organ-Threatening Causes of Headaches

Subarachnoid hemorrhage
Intracranial aneurysm
Meningitis
Encephalitis
Major artery dissection
Giant cell arteritis (temporal arteritis)
Acute glaucoma
Hypertensive encephalopathy
Carbon monoxide poisoning
Benign intracranial hypertension (pseudotumor cerebri)
Cerebral venous thrombosis
Preeclampsia and eclampsia
Cerebral vascular accident
Mass lesion
 Neoplasm
 Abscess
 Intracranial hematoma
Cerebrospinal fluid fistula

Adapted from reference 18.
Copyright © 2000 Massachusetts Medical Society.

and motor disturbances such as paresthesia, hemiparesis, or aphasia. Brainstem dysfunction may also occur, resulting in ataxia, lethargy, diplopia, tinnitus, vertigo, or dysarthria.[22]

Prodromes and postdromes are also common features, occurring in approximately 60% of migraine patients.[14] They experience premonition phenomena hours to days before the onset of head pain. Specific feelings include mood changes, fatigue, anorexia, or autonomic symptoms such as diarrhea or frequent urination. The postdrome essentially consists of general fatigue, irritability, and food cravings or anorexia. The IHS criteria for migraine without aura is as follows[13]:

1. at least 5 attacks;
2. headache attacks lasting 4 to 72 hours (untreated or unsuccessfully treated);
3. headache has at least 2 of the following characteristics:

    a. unilateral location
    b. pulsatile quality
    c. moderate or severe pain intensity
    d. aggravating by or causing avoidance of routine physical activity

4. during headache at least 1 of the following:

    a. nausea and/or vomiting
    b. photophobia and phonophobia

5. not attributed to any other disorder

For migraine with aura[13]:

1. at least 2 attacks;

2. headaches as described in migraine headache without aura;
3. aura (visual symptoms, sensory symptoms, dysphasic speech disturbance) which is fully reversible;
4. aural symptoms develops gradually over ≥5 minutes; and
5. each aural symptom lasts ≥5 minutes and ≤50 minutes

Nonpharmacologic treatment of migraine disorders includes avoidance of triggers and extremes of lifestyle patterns. Patients should be educated to aim for regularity in exercise, eating, drinking, and sleeping habits rather than a list of prohibitions.[23] Headache diaries are useful to decrease the frequency of attacks and monitor for the escalation in number of headaches and drug use. Medical therapy falls into 2 major categories: preventive and symptomatic treatment. The latter attempts to abort attacks at their onset and controls pain during the headache. Specific behavioral measures that are useful include the application of ice, isolation in a dark quiet room, use of biofeedback or acupuncture, and induction of sleep, as well as the avoidance of known triggers.[14,24] (Table 4).

Symptomatic treatment must be individualized to provide adequate relief with minimal risk and side effects. An approach of using stratified care has proven successful where the strength of the prescription is reflective of the severity of the headache.[25] Relief should not be limited to headache but also should address constitutional

Table 4 Triggers for Migraine[14]

Ingested food or drink
   Aged cheese
   Alcohol
   Artificial sweeteners
   Caffeine
   Chocolate
   Fermented foods
   Nitrites
   Red wine
Odor exposure
   Cigarette smoke
   Cleaning agents
   Exhaust
   Paints
   Perfumes
Hormonal variations
   Hormonal replacement therapy
   Menses
   Oral contraceptives
   Pregnancy
Irregular schedule
   Exercise
   Meals
   Sleep
Stress or anger
Flashing lights

Reproduced from reference 14, by permission of Blackwell Science, Inc.

symptoms such as nausea, vomiting, or insomnia. Factors influencing choice of drugs should include the frequency that medications will be required, contraindications, route of administration, prior medication successes and failures, or the need for breakthrough headache therapy.[14] The patient should be instructed to initiate treatment as soon as the headache component of the attack is recognized and at an adequate dose. Often antiemetics or metoclopramide should be given first to avoid worsening or triggering nausea; it facilitates the absorption of antimigraine medication.[23] Nonspecific migraine therapy includes analgesics and judicious use of opiates for only severe attacks. Specific therapy uses compounds that are known agonists of the 5-HT1 receptor and include ergot derivatives and synthetic triptan compounds. To avoid chronic ergotamine-induced headache, it should not be taken >2 d/wk.[26] In addition to nausea, angina may be induced by these compounds; thus, their use in patients with risk of coronary artery disease is contraindicated (see Table 5 for agents available for abortive therapy[14,24,26–30]). Triptan therapy can be used early in the course of treatment for patients with substantial disability in keeping with a stratified approach to care.[23]

The recurrence rate for headache in a 24-hour period is reported for some drugs: intranasal dihydroergotamine mesylate has a 14% relapse rate, whereas triptans relapse between 22 and 45% of the time,[28] and intranasal lidocaine relapse 40% of the time.[29] It is important to realize that severe attacks can be so disabling that occasional referral to the emergency department or admission for pain management is necessary. Finally, in difficult to treat cases, referral to a headache center

or neurologist is appropriate. For children, Annequin and associates reviewed the use of various agents and found good effectiveness for both acetaminophen and ibuprofen. Oral dihydroergotamine mesylate and sumatriptan in any form were also effective.[21] Opiates should be avoided. Again, abortive therapy should be initiated early in the attack.

Prophylactic therapy is indicated when the frequency of episodes is >5/mo. It can be initiated early in patients unresponsive to acute medication, suffering substantial disability, or showing accelerating frequency of either headache or medication use. Dosages should be titrated within recommended levels, and therapeutic trials of any agent should last at least 3 weeks given that the effects are often delayed. Specific prophylactic agents are listed in Table 6.[7,21,30–32] Preventive medical therapy in children has had some success, although fewer reports exist. Among specific agents used for children, propranolol is most frequently used. Other regimens make use of metoprolol, valproate, flunarizine, cyproheptadine, and pizotifen, a serotonin receptor antagonist.[21]

Tension-Type Headache

Tension-type headaches (TTHs) include a variety of previously described craniofacial pain conditions such as tension headache, stress headache, muscle contraction headache, fibromyalgia, chronic daily headache, myofascial pain syndrome, and temporomandibulor disorder (TMD). This category of headaches is by far the most common, afflicting approximately 80% of the adult population, but these headaches usually do not result in a physician evaluation. The IHS has delineated a spectrum of disorders based on frequency of headache episodes and the presence of palpable pericranial muscle tenderness. Clinically, it is not the intensity but the frequency that leads to the morbidity of the condition and dictates treatment decision making.[33] It is more likely to occur in women, and usually a family history of headaches is present. The headaches are characteristically bilateral, with a tightening or band-like sensation in the frontotemporal region around the head and spreading to the occipital region or trapezius muscles. The onset

Table 6 Prophylactic Medications for Migraine[7,21,30–32]

Antidepressants: amitriptyline, nortriptyline, doxepin, or trazodone
Ergotamine in a sustained-release form (bellergal)
Beta blockers: metoprolol, atenolol, or propanolol
Nonsteroidal anti-inflammatory drugs (NSAIDs): naproxen, ibuprofen, or aspirin
Calcium channel blockers: verapamil, nifedipine, nimodipine, or flunarizine
Anticonvulsants: divalproex, valproic acid, gabapentin, or topiramate
Others: methysergide, fluoxetine, cyproheptadine, pizotifen, riboflavin, or lithium

Table 5 Symptomatic Pharmacologic Treatment Options for Migraine[14,24,26–30]

Mild headaches
   Acetaminophen, oral, or rectal
   NSAIDs: naproxen or ibuprofen, oral butalbital and acetaminophen with or without caffeine, oral
   Acetaminophen and isometheptene and dichloralphenazone (Midrin), oral
Moderate headache
   Indomethacin, oral or rectal
   Ergotamine tartrate, oral, sublingual, or rectal
   Dihydroergotamine mesylate (Migranol), intranasal spray or subcutaneous
   Sumatriptan (Imitrex or Imigran), subcutaneous autoinjector, oral, or intranasal spray
   Naratriptan (Amerge), oral
   Rizatriptan (Maxalt), oral
   Zolmitriptan (Zomig), oral
   Lidocaine, intranasal spray
   Butorphanol, intranasal spray
   Butalbital and acetaminophen and codeine with or without caffeine, oral
Severe headache
   Dihydroergotamine mesylate, as for moderate, also intramuscular or intravenous
   Ketorolac, intramuscular
   Diphenhydramine, intravenous
   Prochlorperazine, intravenous
   Chlorpromazine, intravenous
   Haloperidol, intravenous
   Opiates: morphine sulfate, intramuscular or intravenous

Adapted from references 14, 24, 26 to 30.
NSAID = nonsteroidal anti-inflammatory drug.

is gradual, whereas the quality is dull, nonthrobbing, and constant, sometimes lasting for weeks. These headaches typically do not have associated autonomic symptoms as migraine headaches do, although it is possible when the headaches are severe. The headache by definition lasts from 30 minutes to 7 days and has 2 of the following characteristics: a tightening quality, mild to moderate intensity, bilateral location, and not aggravated by routine physical activity. The cephalalgia is triggered or exacerbated by stress or anxiety in most patients. Some evidence has discounted the idea that persistent muscle contraction is the cause of the pain. Instead, new theories suggest an abnormality in central pain control.[34] The subdivisions of infrequent episodic, frequent episodic and chronic differ by the following criteria[13]:

1. Infrequent episodic: at least 10 episodes occurring on <1 d/mo on average (<12 d/yr)
2. Frequent episodic: at least 10 episodes occurring on ≥1 but <15 d/mo for at least 3 months (≥12 and <180 d/yr)
3. Chronic: headache occurring on ≥15 d/mo on average for >3 months (≥180 d/yr)

The other category of TTHs is chronic and was previously labeled chronic daily headache. Some debate still exists as to whether all chronic daily headaches are tension type. The IHS also recognizes that migraine headaches can transform into a chronic daily headache with features more similar to TTHs. This may represent an evolution of the headache process which is often related to overuse of treating drugs. According to Silberstein and Lipton, chronic daily headache must be divided into both tension type and migrainous type, as well as other entities.[35] They note that the chronic tension type constitutes about 25% of all daily headache patients.

Treatment of TTHs uses nonpharmacologic and pharmacologic therapy. First, chronic medication overuse must be eliminated, a step that will improve many cephalalgia sufferers. Any psychiatric comorbid conditions should be identified and evaluated appropriately as a risk factor for treatment failure. Nonpharmacologic remedies include reassurance, muscle relaxation, simple muscle exercises, stress management, biofeedback, and physical therapy with thermal modulation, ultrasonography, or electrical stimulation. Pharmacologic therapy can be organized into abortive therapy in episodic and chronic TTHs and preventive therapy for chronic TTHs. Established abortive agents include: acetaminophen, acetylsalicylic acid, caffeine, and nonsteroidal anti-inflammatory drugs (NSAIDs). As a rule, immediate relief medication of any sort should not be taken >2 d/wk. Agents capable of fostering dependence are best avoided. These include caffeine, opiates, and benzodiazepines.

The use of medication in the management of chronic TTHs is more diverse. Injection of local anesthetics into trigger points may provide sustained relief.[36] Prophylactic therapy is indicated in patients with frequent headaches which is traditionally defined as ≥2/wk or detriment to quality of life.[37] TTHs characteristically are not severe, and the usual indication for prophylactic or preventative therapy is for frequency of headaches. Amitriptyline has been used most often, with proven success.[35] Sodium valproate, topiramate, protriptaline, venlafaxine XR, tizanidine, L-5-hydroxytryptophan, and the nitric oxide synthase inhibitor L-N^gmethyl arginine hydrochloride (L-NMMA) have also been used with reported success. Injection of botulinum toxin into pericranial muscles has recently been shown to be safe and effective although the mechanism of relieving pain is poorly understood.[35]

Cluster Headaches

Cluster headaches, previously known as Horton cephalalgia, are less common than tension-type or migraine-type headaches; however, the severity of the headaches is much greater. They affect men more often than women. They are unilateral, excruciating, and located around the eyes or in the maxilla and usually occur in middle age. The attacks typically last minutes to 3 hours. No aura or nausea occurs, but the cephalalgia is associated with unilateral lacrimation, rhinorrhea, and injected conjunctiva. Ptosis and miosis may also occur. The headaches often wake a patient at the same time each night. Typically, the patient "searches for relief" by pacing or rocking back and forth. A cluster period is the segment of time during which attacks tend to occur several times per day for several weeks. The cluster period ends with remission of attacks and start of a headache-free period, hence the attacks occur in "clusters." Triggers of attacks in a given cluster period include alcohol, histamine, nitroglycerine, rapid eye movement sleep and low oxygen saturation of obstructive sleep apnea (OSA). Rapid eye movement as a trigger causes sleep deprivation which in conjunction with the headache may lead to depression. Patients with strictly nocturnal attacks require an evaluation for OSA and an overnight polysomnography where indicated. Successful treatment of OSA using continuous positive airway pressure support may eliminate nocturnal cluster attacks.[38]

The IHS classification of cluster headaches requires meeting the diagnostic criteria[13] listed in Table 7.

Atypical features suggest a structural lesion influencing the cavernous sinus such as pituitary adenoma, impacted molar teeth, parasellar meningioma, and nasopharyngeal carcinoma. These features include absence of periodicity, low-grade background headache that does not subside, and neurological signs other than miosis and ptosis. Important disorders that require differentiation include giant cell (temporal) arteritis, acute closed angle glaucoma, cerebrovascular disorders, tumors, and trigeminal neuralgias (TGNs).[39,40]

The etiology of cluster headaches is unclear, but several mechanisms are suspected. Circadian hormonal fluctuation suggests a hypothalamic dysfunction, whereas excitation of a nerve plexus in the carotid sheath and adventitia may increase trigeminal discharge rates resulting in facial pain.[41] A subset of patients demonstrate an autosomal dominant transmission in their families.

Variants of cluster headache also occur. *Chronic paroxysmal hemicrania* (Sjaastad syndrome) is a variant with shorter, more frequent attacks, occurs more often in women, and is absolutely responsive to indomethacin.[13] *SUNCT syndrome* (an acronym for short-lasting unilateral neuralgiform headache attacks with conjunctival injection, tearing, sweating, and rhinorrhea) is a cluster-like headache, mostly in men, in which attacks last 10 to 60 seconds. It may be precipitated by touch to the nose or periorbital area, chewing, or ingestion of citrus fruits.[42]

Treatment of cluster headaches consists of abortive measures and prophylactic therapy. Along with providing reassurance for the patient, episodes can be ended with inhalation of 100% oxygen for 10 minutes. However, there are logistical challenges with this therapy. Sumatriptan is the most effective self-administered medication for the symptomatic relief of the cluster attack. Sumatriptan, 6 mg, administered subcutaneously will achieve relief in 15 minutes. Zolmitriptan is an effective oral medication that is effective in 30 minutes. Dihydroergotamine IM or IV may provide relief in 30 minutes or 10 minutes, respectively.[38] These 3 agents all work by inducing a central vasocontriction.[39] Intranasal 4% lidocaine may also be effective. At least 3 episodes of cephalalgia should be treated with any 1 agent before declaring it a failure and moving to another agent. Analgesics are too slow to be effective, and corticosteroids have not been proven to be beneficial in the acute setting.

Prophylactic medications are the mainstay of treatment. Short-term or transitional prophylaxis can be used during a cluster period to suppress attacks, while maintenance prophylaxis is used before and throughout the duration of the cluster period. In general, they should be used early in the cluster period until the patient has been headache free for at least 2 weeks and then followed by a tapering period.[38,41] Transitional prophylaxis includes short courses of prednisone, dexamethasone, and ergotamine tartrate or a greater occipital nerve blockade. Maintenance prophylaxis may be required when transitional prophylaxis and suppression therapy have been discontinued or in anticipation of seasons or months when attacks occur. Effective prophylaxis has been achieved with a variety of agents and is most often achieved using calcium channel blockers such as nifedipine or verapamil, low-dose ergotamine in sustained-release form, lithium carbonate, and methysergide for no greater than 4 months to avoid the rare complication of retroperitoneal fibrosis. Multidrug therapy may be necessary. Newer approaches have used valproate, topiramate, pizotifen, and phototherapy with bright light. Histamine desensitization may offer relief to patients with chronic cluster headaches refractory to treatment.[39] Invasive approaches for refractory cases include trigeminal nerve blockade and blockade of the sphenopalatine ganglion. The most effective procedure for typical cluster headache is radiofrequency ablation of the trigeminal ganglion.[41]

HEADACHE ATTRIBUTED TO HEAD AND/OR NECK TRAUMA AND POSTTRAUMATIC HEADACHE

Intracranial hematomas (intracerebral, subdural, or epidural) often have headache as a presenting symptom. It is moderate to severe and on the side of the hematoma. Ipsilateral skull tenderness

Table 7. IHS Criteria for the Diagnosis of Cluster Headache

Cluster headache	At least 5 attacks as described above
	Attacks last 15–180 min if untreated
	Frequency from 1 every other day to 8 per day
Episodic	Attacks as described and occurring at the frequency above
	At least 2 cluster periods lasting usually 2 wk to 3 mo and separated by pain-free remission periods of ≥1 mo
Chronic	Attacks as described and occurring at the frequency above
	Attacks over >1 yr without remission periods or with remission periods lasting <1 mo

to percussion is common. Hemotympanum or mastoid bruising may occur. Associated symptoms include altered level of consciousness and sometimes nausea and vomiting, as well as focal central nervous system changes. There is usually an antecedent history of head trauma, although the trauma may be temporally remote. Anticoagulated patients may report only minor head bumps. Diagnosis is confirmed by CT of the head. Treatment typically involves a craniotomy for drainage, but spontaneous resolution may occur over time. Once the hematoma is resolved, the headache ceases to occur.

Head and/or neck trauma has been associated with the onset of acute or chronic headaches. The headache may present with a head pain that is tension like, that is, a headache which is bilateral, nonthrobbing, with mild to moderate intensity. It can be aggravated by routine physical activities, and it may have associated symptoms of a migraine headache, usually sensitivity to light and noise.[43] These may be associated with postconcussive vertigo, decreased concentration, memory loss, and depression as part of the posttraumatic syndrome.[44] The pain is frontal, occipital, and constant, yet percussion of the skull is not painful as is sometimes seen in subdural hematomas.[30] The IHS classification requires the onset of headache to be <7 days after injury or regaining consciousness. After 3 months, the acute posttraumatic headache (PTH) is considered chronic. The patient should also be evaluated for psychiatric comorbidities or psychological changes. All patients should undergo repeat imaging, especially in cases of persistent headache or severe personality changes.[45,46] Treating migraine and tension type PTH follows the guidelines of acute and prophylactic medication described in the treatment of primary migraine and tension type headache. However, the clinician must have a lower threshold of suspicion for the use of preventative medication and the development of both medication overuse headache (MOH) and rebound headache. Furthermore, medication overuse may play a role in development or prolongation of chronic PTH.[43] Treatment includes reassurance, physical therapy and simple exercises, short courses of NSAIDs or over-the-counter analgesics, tricyclic antidepressants to modulate pain, injection of local anesthetic into trigger zones, carbamazepine for neuropathic pain, and avoiding recurrent head trauma.[44]

HEADACHE ASSOCIATED WITH VASCULAR DISORDERS

The IHS classifies 8 vascular disorders that are associated with headache. The diagnosis hinges on historical, physical, and radiographic data, as well as evaluation of the CSF when indicated. Also, the headache must occur in close temporal relation to the onset of the underlying disorder. Two of the 8 disorders, acute ischemic cerebrovascular disease and venous thrombosis, will not be reviewed here.

Subarachnoid Hemorrhage

Subarachnoid hemorrhage (SAH) accounts for 1 to 4% of all headaches evaluated in the emergency department.[18] It typically presents as the worst headache of the patient's life. Besides the severe intensity, the cephalalgia is sudden and may gradually worsen; it is bilateral and associated with neck stiffness, fever, transient loss of consciousness, diplopia, or seizures. A sentinel or warning headache that is severe occurs in as many as 50% of patients several days or weeks before the major hemorrhage. These headaches which abate within minutes to hours are called thunderclap headaches and may be difficult to distinguish from a benign headache. However, they do warrant evaluation.[47] Physical examination may reveal altered mental status, restlessness, nuchal rigidity, retinal hemorrhages, papilledema, and focal or general neurologic signs such as cranial nerve III or VI palsy, aphasia, hemiparesis, or ataxia. If aneurysmal bleeding is the source, onset is in minutes; with arteriovenous malformation leaking, the onset is often more insidious, occurring in less than 12 hours. Rupture of a moyamoya lesion may also produce SAH. The neurologic sequelae include devastating brain injury or death, but sometimes only minimal change occurs.

The diagnosis of SAH can be challenging, especially in a patient who loses consciousness and falls. Blood seen on CT may be incorrectly attributed to trauma rather than a ruptured aneurysm. Hypertension may occur with the hemorrhage and can be confused with hypertensive crisis. Even electrocardiogram findings are common after SAH and may incorrectly suggest cardiac disorders. Lastly, physicians must keep in mind that between one-third to half of patients will present atypically with symptoms that are mild, respond to analgesics or lack meningismus which results in a diagnosis of a benign headache.[18] The evaluation for SAH should include a noncontrast head CT with 3 mm cuts to find collections of blood. A lumbar puncture and evaluation of CSF should be performed next if the CT is negative for blood or mass effect. Abnormal findings include elevated CSF pressure and the presence of red blood cells that does not diminish from tubes 1 to 4. Red blood cells found only in the first tube are usually indicative of a traumatic tap. Xanthochromia is a much more specific finding for SAH but may require more than 12 hours to develop.[47] If any test indicates that a SAH has occurred, further diagnostic testing should be directed toward determining the cause using CT angiography, MRA, or angiography by direct intra-arterial catheterization, which is currently considered the gold standard. Radiographically detected unruptured aneurysms and vascular malformations should receive neurosurgical evaluation to prevent catastrophic hemorrhage.[48] Patients with SAH should be stabilized and transferred to centers with neurovascular expertise with a dedicated neurological critical care unit. The goals of therapy are twofold: prevention of rebleeding by either endovascular coiling or surgical clipping and prevention and management of vasospasm and other complications.[47]

Giant Cell Arteritis

Giant cell arteritis, often called temporal arteritis, is associated with polymyalgia rheumatica. Essentially, they are different manifestations of the same condition. The cause is unknown, but speculation relates immune responses, infectious triggers, and genetic susceptibility.[49] The condition mostly affects women over 50 years of age. It presents as a new-onset, daily, intermittent or continuous, temporal localized headache that is moderate to severe, burning sharp or throbbing, unilateral or bilateral and lasts months to years.[19]

Patients with giant cell arteritis complain of aching of the jaw during chewing, weight loss, generalized fatigue, and low-grade fever and often have extremity pain attributable to coexistent polymyalgia rheumatica. Visual symptoms include blurring, scotomata, and even sudden blindness. Physical findings consist of palpably thickened or tender scalp arteries that may have a diminished or absent pulse. Palpation of muscle does not reveal trigger points, and muscle strength is typically normal. An erythrocyte sedimentation rate (ESR) is almost always elevated over 50 mm/h in patients with giant cell arteritis. If the diagnosis is suspected, a temporal artery biopsy is essential to confirm the diagnosis. Inflammation in the artery is often segmental; therefore, a 5 cm long segment of artery should be excised; even then, false negatives may occur.[49] Histologic examination of involved vessels reveals necrosis in the vessel's media with infiltration of macrophages and giant cell formation. Color duplex ultrasonography is being investigated as a diagnostic tool potentially to replace biopsy. Treatment should begin immediately to avoid sudden blindness, a complication found in up to 30% of untreated patients. This is secondary to involvement of the ophthalmic artery. Prednisone is the drug of choice and should be administered at high daily doses of 60 mg. Pain reduces dramatically within days. Once headache has gone into remission and the ESR corrects, prednisone can be tapered over a period of weeks to a daily maintenance dose of 5 to 10 mg while continuing to check for a rise in the ESR.[49] Often treatment must be continued for several years to avoid the complication of blindness.[16] Sometimes the segmental excision of the temporal artery relieves the patient of localized tenderness. However, this does not preclude the need for treatment with corticosteroids.

Carotid Artery Pain

Carotid artery pain may occur secondary to *dissection* or *idiopathic carotidynia* or after endarterectomy. Carotid artery dissection is characterized by head and neck pain on the side of the condition following trivial trauma in a young or middle-aged patient. It may cause referred otalgia,[50] Horner syndrome, lower cranial nerve palsies, and pulsatile tinnitus. Hours later, signs of cerebral or retinal ischemia develop.[51] Dissection can be demonstrated by ultrasonography, MRI with MRA, intra-arterial angiography, or surgical findings. For treatment, early anticoagulation is essential to avoid the 15% risk of mortality. This is followed by warfarin for 6 months. If ischemic signs persist after acute heparinization, surgical intervention may be warranted.[51] Carotidynia is a self-limited inflammation of the carotid fascia or adventitia. It may be induced by viral infection. Physical findings include carotid tenderness, swelling, or intense pulsations. Structural evaluation of the artery is normal. Treatment with NSAIDs may alleviate the pain until spontaneous resolution occurs.

HEADACHE ASSOCIATED WITH NONVASCULAR INTRACRANIAL DISORDERS

The IHS classifies nonvascular intracranial causes of headache into 8 groups. The symptoms, signs, and diagnostic investigations of 3 important syndromes are presented below.

High CSF pressure associated headache may be caused by idiopathic intracranial hypertension (IIH), formerly known as pseudotumor cerebri or otitic hydrocephalus, and high-pressure hydrocephalus that sometimes follows head trauma. IIH is defined by the following criteria:

1. progressive headache with at least 1 of the following characteristics: daily occurrence, diffuse and/or constant (nonpulsating) pain, aggravated by coughing or straining;
2. intracranial hypertension fulfilling the following criteria:

   a. alert patient with otherwise normal neurological examination or has any of the following abnormalities: papilledema, enlarged blind spot, visual field defect, sixth nerve palsy, and increased CSF pressure (>200 mm H_2O in the nonobese, >250 mm H_2O in the obese) measured with lumbar puncture in the recumbent position or by epidural or intraventricular pressure monitoring;
   b. normal CSF chemistry and cellularity (low CSF protein is acceptable);
   c. intracranial disease (including venous sinus thrombosis) ruled out by appropriate investigations; and
   d. no metabolic, toxic, or hormonal cause of intracranial hypertension.

Associated symptoms include unilateral or bilateral pulsatile tinnitus,[52] visual dimming occurring for a minute or 2 at a time, eventual constriction of visual fields, and possible blindness. It may be triggered by otitis media or mastoiditis, irregular menses, recent rapid weight gain, corticosteroid withdrawal, or ingestion of vitamin A, tetracycline, or nalidixic acid. MRI and magnetic resonance venography have suc-

cessfully identified patients with sinus venous pathology who would have otherwise received a diagnosis of IIH. Magnetic resonance venography has become part of the routine work up as recognition of sinus thrombosis has a crucial therapeutic implication.[53] Treatment consists of weight reduction, a low-sodium diet, and diuretics, specifically acetazolamide or furosemide. In severe headache, lumbar puncture can be used to reduce CSF pressure acutely; however, repeated puncture is no longer advocated.[53] CSF diversion by a ventriculoperitoneal shunt may be necessary for refractory cases or when visual fields fail to improve.[30] Transnasal, transethmoidal optic nerve decompression with release of the optic nerve sheath and annulus of Zinn may also be necessary to correct chronic visual field disturbances. High-pressure hydrocephalus differs from benign intracranial hypertension by the identification of enlarged ventricles on head CT or MRI.

Low CSF pressure also commonly precipitates a headache. This may be in response to a lumbar puncture or CSF fistula. The headache appears or worsens when the head is upright and resolves after lying down. The pain is constant when the head is upright and is located in the occipital region or vertex. Nausea is common, and vomiting relieves the headache. Oculomotor or abducens palsies have been reported. Resolution is rapid (usually within several days) following lumbar puncture unless a persistent fistula occurs at the tap site. If this is suspected, a blood patch of the epidural space at the site of puncture is curative. This condition may occur without lumbar puncture and should raise suspicions of post-traumatic, iatrogenic, or spontaneous CSF fistula. If this occurs, site identification by intrathecal metrizamide/contrast CT or myelography should be performed and a surgical repair initiated.

Primary or metastatic *intracranial neoplasms* present with headache 40 to 50% of the time. The headache is usually bifrontal, but worse ipsilaterally and progressively worsens over time. It is exacerbated by Valsalva maneuver, rises in intrathoracic pressure, and bending over. However the classic early morning brain tumor headache is uncommon.[54] Sudden vomiting, cranial nerve dysfunction, and seizures may occur.[19,30] Control of pain may be initially achieved with nonnarcotic analgesics, but eventually, narcotics or neuralgia medications become necessary. Removal of the neoplasm, when feasible, is usually curative of the headache.

HEADACHE ASSOCIATED WITH SUBSTANCES OR THEIR WITHDRAWAL

Headaches are often caused by ingestion or withdrawal of specific substances. The IHS has 4 broad categories: headache induced by acute substance use or exposure, medication overuse headache as an adverse event attributed to chronic medication, and headache attributed to substance withdrawal.[13] The onset of a headache during carbon monoxide poisoning and the hang-

over after drinking alcohol serve as prime examples of *substance induced headache.* The IHS lists the following as causes of substance induced headache: phosphodiesterase inhibitors, carbon monoxide, alcohol, monosodium glutamate, food components/additives, cocaine, cannabis, histamine, calcitonin gene-related peptide, and others.

Patients with MOH typically have a history of prior episodic headache which is usually migraine. Escalating regular use of acute headache medication to >2 d/wk may "transform" migraine into a chronic daily headache.[55] The cephalalgia occurs daily (often early in the morning) and is generalized, bilateral, dull, and of moderate severity. It may be associated with nausea and be brought on with mild exertion. Tolerance to the offending analgesic seems to allow less and less relief to the patient, resulting in the use of increased dosages. Finally, headache-free intervals cease to exist. Both ergotamine and dihydroergotamine, nonnarcotic analgesics and narcotic analgesics have been implicated. Common examples include aspirin, acetaminophen, NSAIDs, barbiturates, codeine, hydrocodone, oxycodone, and propoxyphene. The IHS noted that use of ergot derivatives for 3 months puts the patient at risk, as does taking more than 50 g of aspirin or more than 100 tablets of an analgesic per month. Resolution within a month after discontinuing the substance is typical.

Although the IHS classification has separate criteria for chronic daily headache and MOH, both may be occurring in the same patient. Initially, therapy should be directed toward withdrawal of overuse medication and then toward the management of the underlying headache. The goals of therapy are to decrease the frequency, severity, and duration of headache by using both pharmacologic and nonpharmacologic measures. Nonpharmacologic measures include patient education, addressing psychosocial issues, and equipping the patient with behavior therapy skills like relaxation. Pharmacologic therapy involves the following: discontinuation of overused medication, initiation of bridge therapy, preventive therapy, and acute therapy in the postoveruse setting. Overuse medications such as barbiturates, opiates, and benzodiazepines should be tapered, whereas other medication such as NSAIDs can be withdrawn abruptly. With abrupt withdrawal, bridge therapy can include NSAIDs, for example, naproxen, prednisone 60 mg/d tapered over 2 weeks or subcutaneous dihydroergotamine. As medication is withdrawn, patients may revert back to their primary headache condition which should be evaluated for the appropriate acute therapy in the post-overuse setting. Medication should be used specifically for the primary headache. Relapse rates approach 45% so close follow-up is required.[56]

Headache from withdrawal of a chronically used substance may also occur. In general, the diagnostic criteria for withdrawal headache of a given drug is illustrated below[13]:

1. bilateral and/or pulsating headache;
2. daily intake of a substance for 3 months, which is interrupted;

3. headache develops in close temporal relation to withdrawal of the substance; and

4. headache resolves within 3 months after withdrawal.

For caffeine, opiates, and estrogen, there are specific time intervals for criteria B, C, and D.[13] The headache is diffuse, dull, and mild to moderate in severity. It may be associated with nervousness, restlessness, nausea and vomiting, insomnia, and tremor. Persistent abstinence is the mainstay of treatment but may require hospitalization to prevent the patient from consuming more of the offending medication.

HEADACHE ATTRIBUTED TO INFECTION

Intracranial infections include meningitis, encephalitis, brain abscess, or subdural empyema, which may present with a generalized, bilateral, severe, constant headache often with nuchal rigidity, positive Kernig and Brudzinski signs, and fever. The onset is rapid, usually over several hours.[19] Patients with meningitis will present with at least 2 of 4 symptoms: headache, fever, nuchal rigidity, and decreased level of consciousness.[57] Ambiguous presentations may occur in immunosuppressed patients, atypical infections such as tuberculosis, fungal meningitis, neurosyphilis, or epidural abscess. When evaluating a patient with suspected meningitis, CT scan before lumbar puncture is indicated in the following cases: immunocompromised state, history of central nervous system disease, new onset seizure (within 1 week), papilledema, abnormal level of consciousness and, focal neurological deficit. If lumbar puncture is delayed for neuroimaging, the patient should be given medical therapy including empirical antibiotics and dexamethasone.[58] Culture and antigenic studies from CSF from lumbar puncture are diagnostic.[30] Treatment requires appropriate intravenous antibiotic therapy and surgical drainage of abscesses.

HEADACHES ATTRIBUTED TO DISORDER OF HOMEOSTASIS

Hypoxia, as seen in high-altitude headache, is a known source of cephalalgia. Descent and oxygen therapy are the treatment. A more common cause of chronic hypoxia is found in sleep apnea syndrome, in which morning headache is common. It is diffuse, dull, and mild and may be associated with short-term memory loss and inability to concentrate. The diagnosis is suggested by more significant symptoms of the syndrome, specifically fatigue, daytime somnolence, and apneas witnessed by a bed partner. Resolution of the headache occurs quickly following correction of the hypoxia by continuous positive airway pressure or surgical intervention.

Headache is more likely to result from acute than chronic arterial hypertension. The acute rise in blood pressure can be secondary to administration of pressors, pheochromocytoma, malignant hypertension (including hypertensive encephalopathy), preeclampsia, and eclampsia. Typically, headache begins with diastolic pressures greater than 115 mm Hg. It is throbbing, associated with nausea, and does not respond to analgesics.[30]

Treatment involves controlling and correcting the source of the hypertension. Once this is achieved, the headache resolves within days to months.[13]

HEADACHE OR FACIAL PAIN ASSOCIATED WITH CRANIOFACIAL OR CERVICAL DISORDERS

This is a heterogeneous group of cephalalgias which encompasses a group of headaches attributed to a disorder of cranium, neck, eyes, ears, nose, sinuses, teeth, mouth, or other facial or cranial structure.

If disease involves any extracranial organ of the head or the skull itself, pain may ensue. Facial or head pain is localized to the affected structure but may radiate or be referred and develops in close temporal relationship with the pathological lesion. If the lesion is corrected, headache resolves in <1 month.[13] Examples affecting the cranial bones include osteomyelitis, multiple myeloma, and Paget's disease of bone.

Cervicogenic headache is a relatively common condition created by a disorder afflicting the cervical spine. Women are more frequently affected than men. It is characterized by headache that is unilateral, unchanging, dull, and nonpulsatile. It tends to start at the occiput and radiate to the frontal region where the pain is most intense. If it is bilateral, one side is usually of worse intensity. Pain may also radiate into the shoulder or arm. Attacks are precipitated by awkward positions, neck movement, or palpation of trigger points such as the greater occipital nerve or over the C2 vertebral body.[59] Associated symptoms of nausea and photophobia or phonophobia are present in 50% of patients. Neck examination reveals a reduced range of motion of the spine and possibly muscle tenderness, spasm, hypertrophy, or atrophy. Criteria for its diagnosis have been proposed by both the IHS and the Cervicogenic Headache International Study Group.[13,60] In the IHS criteria, currently established causes of cervicogenic headache include tumor, fracture, and rheumatoid arthritis but not cervical spondylosis and osteochondritis. One distinctive feature of cervicogenic headache is a positive response after an appropriate diagnostic nerve block, which is directed towards the structure suspected to be mediating or causing the headache. The objective of the diagnostic criteria is to assist the clinician to detect a lesion, which has been established as a cause of cervicogenic headache, then demonstrate the lesion to cause the headache, and finally abolish the headache consistently with a diagnostic blockade of the specific cervical structure or nerve supply.[61] The IHS criteria are described as follows[13]:

1. pain, referred from a source in the neck and perceived in one or more regions of the head and/or face;

2. clinical, laboratory and/or imaging evidence of a disorder or lesion within the cervical spine or soft tissues of the neck, known to be or generally accepted as a valid cause of headache;

3. evidence that the pain can be attributed to the neck disorder or lesion based on at least 1 of the following:

   a. demonstration of clinical signs that implicate a source of pain in the neck

   b. abolition of headache following diagnostic blockade of a cervical structure or its nerve supply using placebo or other adequate controls

4. pain resolves within 3 months after successful treatment of the causative disorder of the lesion.

Cervical radiographic data reveal either abnormalities on flexion and extension films, abnormal posture, or evidence of bone or joint pathology. Treatment centers around physical therapy and stretching exercises, use of NSAIDs, and chronic nerve blockade for refractory cases.

Sinonasal disorders are a frequent source of headaches but are probably over credited by the population as a whole. Frontal headache and facial pain are 2 of the 3 major symptoms suggesting the presence of sinusitis, the other being purulent nasal drainage. Acute sinusitis is a leading cause of facial pain, second only to dental disorders. The IHS classification for headache from rhinosinusitis is given below:

1. frontal headache accompanied by pain in one or more regions of the face, ears, or teeth;

2. clinical, nasal endoscopic, CT and/or MRI imaging and/or laboratory evidence of acute or acute-on-chronic rhinosinusitis;

3. headache and facial pain develop simultaneously with onset or acute exacerbation of rhinosinusitis; and

4. headache and/or facial pain resolve within 7 days after remission or successful treatment of acute or acute-on-chronic rhinosinusitis.

However, chronic sinusitis is not validated as a cause of headache or facial pain.[62] The cephalalgia feels like a dull pressure of moderate intensity and can be either unilateral, bilateral, or periorbital. It is worse in the morning and when bending or performing the Valsalva maneuver. Associated symptoms include purulent nasal drainage, nasal obstruction, altered sense of smell, asthma exacerbation, cough, malaise, and dizziness. Nausea and visual change are infrequent associated symptoms.[8,50,63]

Pain with the inflammatory process lasts days or weeks with fluctuating severity. The location and extent of the sinusitis do not correlate well with the severity or site of pain.[63] However, a few tendencies are common. The area overlying an infected sinus is often tender. Pain for sinusitis referred to upper maxillary teeth typically originates in the maxillary sinus. Occipital or vertex pain from sinusitis most likely represents sphenoid sinus disease. Any infected sinus can refer pain to the frontal, retro-orbital, and temporal regions. Physical examination finds tenderness to percussion over involved sinuses. Transillumination is not useful to delineate the presence of sinusitis. Other physical findings center around inflammatory changes in the nose. Radiographic imaging is helpful to confirm an uncertain diagnosis of sinusitis or to evaluate response to treatment. As plain films have poor sensitivity, a screening coronal sinus CT has become the imaging study of choice. Treatment requires medical therapy to reverse the inflammatory cause of the headache and includes antibiotics, decongestants, and possibly corticosteroids, with analgesics used in the interim for symptomatic relief until the sinusitis is resolved.

Rhinologic headaches other than those caused by sinusitis also occur, albeit much more rarely. Nasal anatomic abnormalities occasionally associated with facial pain include impacted septal deviation or spurs, hypertrophic turbinates, and even an occasional large maxillary retention cyst.[3] However, most sinonasal neoplasms do not cause pain. The cause of rhinogenic pain may be related to direct sensory stimulation from 2 mucosal surfaces contacting each other. The pain is usually dull and aching and unilateral. An anatomic abnormality can be seen on examination after decongesting the nose. If the cause is mucosal contact, topical lidocaine can be used as a diagnostic test as the pain should diminish or disappear after application. Medication may effectively control turbinate hypertrophy, but surgical approaches are effective in managing the anatomic defects.[50]

Elongated styloid process, better known as Eagle syndrome consists of recurrent throat and neck pain exacerbated by swallowing. Otalgia, dysphagia, and foreign body sensation are often present and are secondary to an elongated styloid process impinging on the carotid plexus or branches of cranial nerve IX. It may develop subsequent to tonsillectomy because of inflammatory changes. Palpation of the styloid process in the tonsillar fossa exacerbates the dull pain, whereas injection of a local anesthetic provides relief and is diagnostic. A lateral plain film of the head reveals a styloid process greater than 2.5 cm long.[64] Reassurance and medical therapy with NSAIDs or corticosteroid injection around the stylohyoid ligament may be successful. Otherwise, treatment involves surgical shortening of the calcified stylohyoid ligament (elongated styloid process) through the tonsillar fossa.[50]

TMJ disorders are frequent causes of facial pain and headache. These disorders are divided into 2 major groups: those with demonstrable organic disease, which is uncommon, and those of myofascial origin from masticatory muscles, which is common. The IHS has established the following diagnostic criteria for TMJ disease[13]:

1. Recurrent pain in 1 or more regions of the head and/or face;
2. X-ray, MRI, and/or bone scintigraphy demonstrate TMJ disorder;
3. Evidence that pain can be attributed to the TMJ disorder, based on at least 1 of the following:

   a. Pain is precipitated by jaw movements and/or chewing of hard or tough food;
   b. Reduced range of jaw opening or irregular jaw opening;
   c. Noise from one or both TMJs during jaw movements; and
   d. Tenderness of the joint capsule(s) of one or both TMJs.

4. Headache resolves with 3 months and does not recur, after successful treatment of the TMJ disorder.

Women are far more likely to suffer from TMJ pain. The pain is located preauricularly and in the temporal region of the head; is intermittent, lasting hours to days; is mild to moderate in intensity; can be unilateral or bilateral; and is exacerbated by jaw movement. Associated features include otalgia, bruxism, trismus, TMJ crepitus, and jaw locking. Usually, there are neither muscular trigger points nor symptoms of nausea or visual change. Etiology of the discomfort includes diseased joints that can occur on the basis of arthritis (the most common cause), traumatic causes such as fractures or dislocations, internal derangements of the intra-articular disk, or developmental defects.

Physical findings include audible joint clicking on one side or both and decreased range of motion. Normal vertical opening between central incisors ranges from 42 to 55 mm.[19] Palpation should cover the head and neck musculature and TMJs including intraoral pterygoid palpation, noting any asymmetry, tenderness, spasm, hypertrophy, atrophy, triggering of referred pain, or crepitus when opening or closing. If pathology is suspected, a TMJ radiographic series may reveal a joint abnormality. The usual indications for imaging include suspected fractures, degenerative joint disease, ankylosis, or tumors.

Management of TMJ disease includes reassurance, education, NSAIDs, restriction of jaw opening, a soft diet, and physical therapy. Occasionally, biofeedback or corticosteroid injection may be helpful. If pain is chronic, tricyclic antidepressants may be beneficial. Because of the potential for dependency in chronic conditions, narcotics are best avoided. Acute disk or condylar displacements may require manual reduction to relieve pain and restore range of motion or relieve a joint locked open or closed. Often sedation or general anesthesia is necessary to relax the muscles to facilitate the manual reduction. The use of a bite appliance may alleviate chronic headache or muscle pain secondary to bruxism or joint pain secondary to anterior disk displacement.[65] Arthrocentesis, sclerotic therapy, and arthroscopic surgery are reserved for chronic dislocations, disk derangements, or condylar anomalies.

Oromandibular dysfunction involves pain in the TMJ without organic disease. Other terms describing this condition include myofascial pain dysfunction syndrome and TMJ pain dysfunction syndrome. The etiology of pain seems to have its origin in myofascial tissues or central processes disinhibiting sensory pain pathways. The IHS system classified this as a TTH that does not purely meet the criteria of episodic or chronic TTHs. A diagnosis requires at least 3 of the following: the creation of noise with jaw movement, limited range of motion, pain during jaw use, locking of the jaw, or a history of clenching or grinding of the teeth.[12] The pain is typically a continuous, dull, aching, poorly localized, usually unilateral discomfort of mild to moderate degree involving the ear, angle of the jaw, and temple. The pain rarely wakes the patient, and the location of pain may shift. The patterns of referred pain often do not make neurologic sense. It may be associated with swelling, numbness, stiffness, or erythema. The hallmarks of this myalgia are the presence of trigger points that, when palpated, reproduce the referred pain.[66] Examination will reproduce the pain when masticatory and neck muscles are palpated. Full range of jaw motion may be lost with this disorder. A trigger point injection of an anesthetic (such as 1% procaine) can confirm that point's significance by relieving the pain.[66]

Therapy consists of reassurance, modification to a soft diet, physical therapy, trigger point local anesthetic injection, and medications. Amitriptyline for at least 2 months is an effective choice, whereas NSAIDs may or may not be. Occlusal splints relieving bruxism may help, as might attention to abnormal occlusal factors that can precipitate the disorder.[36] Because of the self-limited nature of the condition, invasive approaches should be avoided.

CRANIAL NEURALGIAS

Cranial neuralgias are conditions affecting nerves with sensory functions in the head and neck, resulting in severe stabbing or throbbing pain in the distribution of the involved nerve. They can involve any cranial nerve with sensory fibers or cervical roots 1, 2, or 3. The conditions are subdivided into persistent painful disorders and paroxysms of pain (tic-like) disorders.

Traumatic injury to a nerve or inflammatory changes can result in chronic neuralgia. Trauma or surgery to the cranium or face may result in entrapment neuritis or formation of a neuroma, typically 2 to 6 months later. The occurrence is greatest in the third branch of the trigeminal nerve because of the frequency of injury related to mandibular fracture or tooth extraction. Symptoms include hypersensitivity and pain to light touch, pain in an area of skin that has lost its sensory innervation, and aggravation of pain by cold or emotional duress. The pain is sharp and lancinating. A central cause of a neuritic pain can occur as anesthesia dolorosa following surgical ablation of the trigeminal ganglion. The condition is characterized by sharp pain and numbness in the distribution of any or all branches of the trigeminal nerve after trigeminal rhizotomy or trauma. Treatment uses anticonvulsant medications, in particular, carbamazepine, or sometimes baclofen or clonazepam. Amitriptyline has also been employed with success.[44] Injection of local anesthetics into trigger points or surgical resection or repair of neuromas is necessary for refractory cases.

Inflammatory conditions are also well known to cause neuralgia. A prime example is *acute herpes zoster* of a branch of the trigeminal nerve, the seventh cranial nerve, or cervical roots. The ophthalmic branch of cranial nerve V is the most commonly involved nerve. Acute herpes zoster is characterized by an intense burning or stabbing pain in the distribution of the involved nerve which is followed within 1 week by a herpetic eruption in the skin distribution of the same nerve. Motor divisions of involved nerves may be paretic. The pain subsides within 3 months of the onset, but the motor palsies have a poor prognosis for complete recovery. The goals of therapy during the acute phase is to minimize the duration of the attack, decrease the severity of pain, and prevent the development of postherpetic neuralgia. Treatment of the acute phase consists of a 7-to 10-day course of an antiviral agent. Prednisone or oral corticosteroid therapy has been demonstrated to accelerate healing of crusts and cessation of pain, but it has no effect on the prevention of postherpetic neuralgia. There is also a risk of disseminated herpes zoster, therefore it should be used only in patients with severe symptoms at initial presentation. Prednisone 40 mg can be started and tapered so that the last dose is given with the end of antiviral therapy.[67] Noncorticosteroidal anti-inflammatory drugs or opiates may be necessary to control pain. Acute herpes zoster is common in lymphoma patients, so a new outbreak should raise suspicions about that possible comorbidity.

Chronic postherpetic neuralgia exists when herpes zoster pain persists for >3 months. It remains in the distribution of the originally afflicted nerve. It is more likely to occur in patients who are over 60 years old when the acute infection starts, and in this group it is less likely to resolve spontaneously.[13,67] Noncorticosteroidal anti-inflammatory drugs and opiates fail to relieve the neuralgia. Instead, topical anesthetic in a self adhesive patch and anticonvulsants such as gabapentin are more effective and may be paired with tricyclic antidepressants to enhance their efficacy.[67]

Other inflammatory neuralgia syndromes include the following: (1) Tolosa-Hunt syndrome: episodic unilateral orbital pain with palsies in 1 or more of cranial nerves III, IV, and VI. Episodes last about 8 weeks untreated but generally resolve within 3 days after starting corticosteroids. It has been related to granulation tissue in the cavernous sinus, superior orbital fissure, or orbit and can be diagnosed on MRI or biopsy.[13] (2) Gradenigo's syndrome: progressive, intense, unilateral, retro-orbital pain with abducens palsy and otorrhea secondary to petrous apicitis of the temporal bone as a direct extension of middle ear and mastoid infection or an invasive tumor of the temporal bone.[68] (3) Raeder paratrigeminal neuralgia: retro-orbital pain with intact trigeminal sensation and an incomplete Horner syndrome, resulting in an ipsilateral dilated pupil. The paratrigeminal space housing the gasserian ganglion of cranial nerve V, cranial nerves III and IV, and the carotid artery may be encroached on by abnormal vascular structures and produce the syndrome.[9]

TGN, previously called tic douloureux, is the most common cranial neuralgia, and most often affects adults over 50 years old and women more than men. Typically, recurrent episodes of unilateral, excruciating, stabbing pain occur most often in the distribution of the maxillary and mandibular branches of the trigeminal nerve. During an episode, ipsilateral twitching may occur hence the name "painful tic." The episodes occur without warning, while patients are awake, and recur several to many times a day, with each episode lasting seconds to minutes. Numbness does not occur.

Light touching of the face may precipitate an attack, as can movement of the trigger zone by talking, chewing, or shaving. Physical findings include an intact neurologic examination and the presence of a trigger zone most often located in the nasolabial fold, lips, or gums. Diagnostic evaluation should include an MRI of the head and a lumbar puncture if the MRI is normal. The former is to rule out central causes including vascular anomalies or aneurysm, tumor, cholesteatoma, or multiple sclerosis (MS). Patients with MS are predisposed to TGN, and 2% of patients with TGN have MS.[19] The latter is to rule out MS, neurosyphilis, and cryptococcal or tuberculous meningitis. Treatment of idiopathic TGN includes patient education and reassurance with pharmacologic control. Carbamazepine will provide symptomatic relief acutely in the majority of patients.[19] Other agents shown to be effective include gabapentin, phenytoin, baclofen, sodium valproate, and chlorphenesin. Any drug should be employed for at least 2 weeks, and medications may be used in combination. Tricyclic antidepressants and NSAIDs may also be beneficial. Surgical radiofrequency ablation, specifically trigeminal rhizotomy, is recommended for patients refractory to medical therapy, whereas temporary blockade may be indicated for patients experiencing intense activation of the disease.

Glossopharyngeal neuralgia is a disorder similar to TGN but affecting cranial nerve IX. Men in their forties or fifties are more likely to have this disorder. The pain characteristics include repetitive, brief attacks of lancinating pain located in the soft palate, base of the tongue, pharynx, and ear. The trigger point is located in the tonsillar fossa and can be provoked by swallowing or yawning. Associated symptoms may include hiccoughing, nausea, vertigo, tinnitus, aural fullness, hearing loss, dysgeusia, bradycardia, and syncope. Evaluation and management are identical to those for TGN.[50]

Superior laryngeal neuralgia is characterized by unilateral lancinating attacks of pain at the side of the larynx over the thyrohyoid membrane. Pain radiates to the ear and submandibular region and is precipitated by swallowing, straining the voice, playing a musical instrument, or turning the head. The pain paroxysms last minutes to hours for days or weeks at a time. Dysphonia may be present secondary to involvement of the external branch of the superior laryngeal nerve affecting the cricothyroid muscle. Injection of local anesthetic as a nerve blockade confirms the diagnosis when pain is relieved.[50] The condition is managed with anticonvulsants as in TGN or with surgical sectioning of the superior laryngeal nerve.

Occipital neuralgia is a paroxysmal stabbing aching pain over the occiput in the distribution of the greater or lesser occipital nerve combined with reduced sensation in the same area. Associated symptoms include visual disturbances, dizziness, nausea, tinnitus, and scalp paresthesias. The physical findings include a positive Tinel sign or palpable tenderness of the involved occipital nerve.[69] Confirmation of the diagnosis is made by obtaining relief from pain after an injection of local anesthetic is performed to block the nerve. Management consists of heat, physical therapy, rest, transcutaneous electrical nerve stimulation units, NSAIDs, baclofen, or carbamazepine. Cervical collars are of questionable benefit. Invasive measures for refractory cases include local blockade with bupivacaine in combination with an injectable corticosteroid, alcohol blockade, or even nerve section.[69]

Sluder sphenopalatine neuralgia is currently classified as a cluster headache, though it is also considered a cranial neuralgia. When first described it was found to occur in episodes that recurred weekly to monthly. The pain is localized to the maxillary area with autonomic symptoms. On the affected side, there can also be diminished sensibility of the soft palate, a high arched palate, and diminished taste sensation. Treatment includes application of cocaine to the mucosa overlying the ganglion, removal of the precipitating septal spur, or ablation of the sphenopalatine ganglion.[41,70]

"Ophthalmoplegic migraine" is a syndrome with recurrent attacks of migraine-like headache accompanied by or followed by paresis of the third, fourth, or sixth cranial nerves which may be due to a recurrent dymyelination or ischemic neuropathy. It is a rare cause of monocular blindness.[13,22,71]

UNCLASSIFIABLE FACIAL PAIN (ATYPICAL FACIAL PAIN)

Atypical facial pain fails to fit the profile of any specific craniofacial condition. The prosopalgia (facial pain) is unilateral or bilateral, is located in the face and upper neck, and is a constant ache or burning with excruciating exacerbations. It does not localize to anatomic regions or have relation to specific structures as TMJ arthralgia or myofascial pain does. It lasts for years, is exacerbated by stress, and is associated with paresthesias of the face or mouth.[19] Comorbidities include chronic fatigue, depression, personality disorders, irritable bowel syndrome, and other idiopathic pain disorders. The cause is unknown, but theories propose central causes in which neuroregulation of pain input is disinhibited, systemic causes in which tyramine metabolism is deficient,[72] and psychogenic causes in which personality disorders are linked to the development of chronic pain conditions.

Treatment involves a multidisciplinary approach. Each patient should be reassured, receive only essential dentistry, and sparingly use analgesics. Tricyclic antidepressants are the mainstay of therapy; they should be taken at night and titrated up to a desired response. Other options include serotonin reuptake inhibitors, monoamine oxidase inhibitors, benzodiazepines, and phenothiazine. Once a good response has occurred, therapy should be maintained until the patient has been pain free for several months before it is discontinued.[72] Psychiatric evaluation may be beneficial. Refractory cases might respond to 1 of the several neurosurgical procedures.

REFERENCES

1. Dalessio DJ, Silberstein SD. Diagnosis and classification of headache. In: Dalessio D, Silberstein S, editors. Wolff's Headache and Other Head Pain, 6th edition. New York: Oxford University Press; 1993. p. 3.
2. Sessle BJ. Neural mechanisms and pathways in craniofacial pain. Can J Neurol Sci 1999;26:S7–11.
3. Chow J. Rhinologic headaches. Otolaryngol Head Neck Surg 1994;111:211–8.
4. Wright EF. Referred craniofacial pain patterns in patients with temporomandibular disorder. J Am Dent Assoc 2000; 131:1307–15.`
5. Jensen R, Olesen J. Tension-type headache: An update on mechanisms and treatment. Curr Opin Neurol 2000; 13:285–9.
6. Hargreaves RJ, Shepheard SL. Pathophysiology of migraine—new insights. Can J Neurol Sci 1999;26:S12–9.
7. Hamel E. The biology of serotonin receptors: Focus on migraine pathophysiology and treatment. Can J Neurol Sci 1999;26:S2–6.
8. Schor DI. Headache and facial pain-the role of the paranasal sinuses: A literature review. Cranio 1993;11:36–47.
9. Ballenger JJ. Headache and neuralgia of the face. In: Ballenger JJ, Snow JB, editors. Otorhinolaryngology: Head and Neck Surgery, 15th edition. Baltimore: Williams & Wilkins; 1996. p. 158–62.
10. Anselmi B, Baldi E, Casacci F, Salmon S. Endogenous opioids in cerebrospinal fluid and blood in idiopathic headache sufferers. Headache 1980;20:294–9.
11. Jensen R. Pathophysiological mechanisms of tension-type headache: A review of epidemiological and experimental studies. Cephalalgia 1999;19:602–21.
12. Headache Classification Committee of the International Headache Society. Classification and diagnostic criteria for headache disorders, cranial neuralgias and facial pain. Cephalalgia 1988;8:1–96.
13. Headache Classification Committee of the International Headache Society. The international classification of headache disorders, 2nd edition. Cephalalgia 2004;24: 23–136.
14. Saper JR. Diagnosis and symptomatic treatment of migraine. Headache 1997;37:S1–14.
15. Smetana GW. The diagnostic value of historical features in primary headache syndromes: A comprehensive review. Arch Intern Med 2000;160:2729–37.
16. Lance JW. Headache and face pain. Med J Aust 2000; 172:450–5.
17. Detsky ME, McDonald DR, Baerlocher MO, et al. Does this patient with headache have a migraine or need neuroimaging? JAMA 2006;296:1274–83.
18. Edlow JA, Caplan LR. Avoiding pitfalls in the diagnosis of subarachnoid hemorrhage. N Engl J Med 2000; 342:29–36.
19. Montgomery MT. Extraoral facial pain. Emerg Med Clin North Am 2000;18:577–600.
20. Stewart WF, Lipton RB, Celentano DD, Reed ML. Prevalence of migraine headache in the United States. Relation to age, income, race, and other sociodemographic factors. JAMA 1992;267:64–9.
21. Annequin D, Tourniaire B, Massiou H. Migraine and headache in childhood and adolescence. Pediatr Clin North Am 2000;47:617–31.
22. Solomon S. Migraine diagnosis and clinical symptomatology. Headache 1994;34:S8–12.
23. Goadsby PJ, Lipton RB, Ferrari MD. Migraine—current understanding and treatment. N Engl J Med 2002; 346:257–70.
24. Wilkinson M. Migraine treatment: The British perspective. Headache 1994;34:S13–16.
25. Lipton RB, Stewart WF, Stone AM, et al. Stratified care vs step care strategies for migraine: The disability in strategies of care (DISC) study: A randomized trial. JAMA 2000;284:2599–605.
26. Silberstein SD, Young WB. Safety and efficacy of ergotamine tartrate and dihydroergotamine in the treatment of migraine and status migrainosus. Working panel of the Headache and Facial Pain Section of the American Academy of Neurology. Neurology 1995;45:577–84.
27. Young WB. Appropriate use of ergotamine tartrate and dihydroergotamine in the treatment of migraine: Current perspectives. Headache 1997;37:S42–5.
28. Logemann CD, Rankin LM. Newer intranasal migraine medications. Am Fam Physician 2000;61:180–6.
29. Maizels M, Scott B, Cohen W, Chen W. Intranasal lidocaine for treatment of migraine: A randomized, double-blind, controlled trial. JAMA 1996;276:319–21.
30. Finkel AG, Mann JD, Lundeen TF. Headache and facial pain. In: Bailey BJ, editor. Head and Neck Surgery—Otolaryngology, 2nd edition. Philadelphia: Lippincott-Raven; 1998. p. 287–304.
31. Becker WJ. Evidence based migraine prophylactic drug therapy. Can J Neurol Sci 1999;26:S27–32.
32. Truelove EL. The chemotherapeutic management of chronic and persistent orofacial pain. Dent Clin North Am 1994;38:669–88.
33. Mathew NT. Tension-type headache. Curr Neurol Neurosci Rep 2006;6:100–5.
34. Silberstein SD. Tension-type headaches. Headache 1994;34: S2–7.
35. Silberstein SD, Lipton RB. Chronic daily headache. Curr Opin Neurol 2000;13:277–83.
36. Benoliel R, Sharav Y. Craniofacial pain of myofascial origin: Temporomandibular pain and tension-type headache. Compend Contin Educ Dent 1998;19:701–10.
37. Silberstein SD, Lipton RB, Goadsby PJ. Headache in Clinical Practice, 2nd edition. London: Martin Dunitz; 2002. p. 121.
38. Capobianco DJ, Dodick DW. Diagnosis and treatment of cluster headache. Semin Neurol 2006;26:242–59.
39. Mendizabal JE, Umana E, Zweifler RM. Cluster headache: Horton's cephalalgia revisited. South Med J 1998;91:606–17.
40. Carter DM. Cluster headache mimics. Curr Pain Headache Rep 2004;8:133–9.
41. Mathew NT. Cluster headache. Neurology 1992;42:22–31.
42. Pareja JA, Sjaastad O. SUNCT syndrome. A clinical review. Headache 1997;37:195–202.
43. Lew HL, Lin P-H, Fuh J-L, et al. Characteristics and treatment of headache after traumatic brain injury: A focused review. Am J Phys Med Rehabil 2006;85:619–27.
44. Benoliel R, Eliav E, Elishoov H, Sharav Y. Diagnosis and treatment of persistent pain after trauma to the head and neck. J Oral Maxillofac Surg 1994;52:1138–47.
45. Landy SH, Donovan TB, Laster RE. Repeat CT or MRI in posttraumatic headache. Headache 1996;36:44–7.
46. Saggese JA, Bruera OC. CT or MRI in posttraumatic headache. Headache 1998;38:554–5.
47. Suarez JI, Tarr RW, Selman WR. Aneurysmal subarachnoid hemorrhage. N Engl J Med 2006;354:387–96.
48. Raps EC, Rogers JD, Galetta SL, et al. The clinical spectrum of unruptured intracranial aneurysms. Arch Neurol 1993;50:265–8.
49. Meskimen S, Cook TD, Blake RL, Jr. Management of giant cell arteritis and polymyalgia rheumatica. Am Fam Physician 2000;61:2061–8.
50. Levine HL. Otorhinolaryngologic causes of headache. Med Clin North Am 1991;75:677–92.
51. Guillon B, Levy C, Bousser MG. Internal carotid artery dissection: An update. J Neurol Sci 1998;153:146–58.
52. Sismanis A. Pulsatile tinnitus. A 15-year experience. Am J Otol 1998;19:472–7.
53. Skau M, Brennum J, Gjerris F, Jensen R. What is new about idiopathic intracranial hypertension? An updated review of mechanism and treatment. Cephalalgia 2006;26:384–99.
54. Forsyth PA, Posner JB. Headaches in patients with brain tumors: A study of 111 patients. Neurology 1993;43:1678–83.
55. Mathew NT, Kurman R, Perez F. Drug induced refractory headache—clinical features and management. Headache 1990;30:634–8.
56. Boes CJ, Black DF, Dodick DW. Pathophysiology and management of transformed migraine and medication overuse headache. Semin Neurol 2006;26:232–41.
57. van de Beek D, de Gans J, Spanjaard L, et al. Clinical features and prognostic factors in adults with bacterial meningitis. N Engl J Med 2004;351:1849–59.
58. Tunkel AR, Hartman BJ, Kaplan SL, et al. Practice guidelines for the management of bacterial meningitis. Clin Infect Dis 2004;39:1267–84.
59. Vincent MB. Cervicogenic headache: Clinical aspects. Clin Exp Rheumatol 2000;18:S7–10.
60. Sjaastad O, Fredriksen TA. Cervicogenic headache: Criteria, classification and epidemiology. Clin Exp Rheumatol 2000;18:S3–6.
61. Göbel H. The classification and diagnosis of headache disorders. In: Olesen J, editor. Oxford Medical Publications; Frontiers in Headache Research Series, Volume 13. New York: Oxford University Press; 2005. p. 223–4.
62. Society HC, Cot IH. Introduction to the classification. Cephalalgia 2004;24:11–3.
63. Tarabichi M. Characteristics of sinus-related pain. Otolaryngol Head Neck Surg 2000;122:842–7.
64. Balbuena L, Jr, Hayes D, Ramirez SG, Johnson R. Eagle's syndrome (elongated styloid process). South Med J 1997; 90:331–4.
65. Major PW, Nebbe B. Use and effectiveness of splint appliance therapy: Review of literature. Cranio 1997;15:159–66.
66. Graff-Radford SB. Facial pain. Curr Opin Neurol 2000; 13:291–6.
67. Wareham D. Postherpetic neuralgia. Clin Evid 2005; 14:1017–25.
68. Lance J. The classification and diagnosis of headache disorders. In: Olesen J, editor. Oxford Medical Publications; Frontiers in Headache Research Series, Volume 13. New York: Oxford University Press; 2005. p. 235.
69. Kuhn WF, Kuhn SC, Gilberstadt H. Occipital neuralgias: Clinical recognition of a complicated headache. A case series and literature review. J Orofac Pain 1997;11:158–65.
70. Lance J. The classification and diagnosis of headache disorders. In: Olesen J, editor. Oxford Medical Publications; Frontiers in Headache Research Series, Volume 13. New York: Oxford University Press; 2005. p. 239.
71. Lance J. The classification and diagnosis of headache disorders. In: Olesen J, editor. Oxford Medical Publications; Frontiers in Headache Research Series, Volume 13. New York: Oxford University Press; 2005. p. 237.
72. Feinmann C, Peatfield R. Orofacial neuralgia. Diagnosis and treatment guidelines. Drugs 1993;46:263–8.

49

Primary Paranasal Sinus Surgery

James A. Stankiewicz, MD
Joseph M. Scianna, MD

The undertaking of primary paranasal sinus surgery requires a detailed familiarity of the relevant anatomy, a fundamental appreciation for the normal nasal physiology, a comprehensive understanding of the surgical indications, and a respect for the potential complications that may arise. The anatomy and physiology of the nose and paranasal sinuses are discussed in Chapter 37, "Embryology, Anatomy, and Physiology of the Nose and Paranasal Sinuses." Indications for primary paranasal sinus surgery can be divided into absolute and relative indications. Absolute indications include: orbital abscess secondary to acute infection, frontal lobe abscess/meningitis secondary to acute infection, mucocele, or fungal mycetoma. Relative indications include chronic rhinosinusitis failing medical therapy, headaches, facial pain, recurrent acute sinusitis, obstructive nasal polyposis, and asthma exacerbations in patients with Samter triad.

While the absolute indications for primary sinus surgery represent a relatively straightforward presentation and thought process, the relative indications for primary sinus surgery are hinged upon symptomatic rhinosinusitis with or without polyposis. The term rhinosinusitis to some degree has become an ambiguous term encompassing a plethora of disease processes that develop from both environmental and host factors. Rhinosinusitis can be acute, subacute (<3 months duration), chronic, or an acute exacerbation of chronic rhinosinusitis.[1] Rhinosinusitis may be accompanied by atopy and associated with polyps, asthma, and aspirin sensitivity (Samter triad).[2] Many theories exist regarding the formation of nasal polyps, although the exact mechanism is not yet understood.[3] Nasal polyps are present in 5% of nonatopic individuals and only 1.5% of people with allergic rhinitis.[4] No racial or sexual predilection is reported. The prevalence is increased in patients with cystic fibrosis and those with Samter triad.[5,6]

Controlling rhinosinusitis with medical therapy can be difficult. Currently, prolonged antibiotics, oral or topical antifungal agents, oral and nasal corticosteroids, nasal steroids, mucolytics, leukotriene inhibitors allergy evaluation, and immunotherapy—all represent medical measures aimed at controlling chronic rhinosinusitis. Clear documentation of medical intervention and failure is essential prior to advancing to surgery. Intervention requires a detailed preoperative evaluation including a radiographic evaluation,

concise surgical planning targeted at the specific disease areas, and most importantly a continued postoperative treatment period.

PREOPERATIVE EVALUATION

Preoperative evaluation of the patient with rhinosinusitis begins with a complete otolaryngologic history and physical examination.[7] For patients with absolute indications for surgery, the historical presentation is generally straightforward. Mental status alterations including obtundation, and visual changes can accompany meningitis or epidural or frontal lobe abscess. Acute progression of diplopia, visual loss, or ocular pain may accompany orbital cellulitis with abscess formation (Figure 1). Severe pressure and/or transcutaneous drainage may be presenting clues that a mucocele has developed. Lastly, fungal mycetoma may present innocuously, causing specific pain or symptoms related to the single sinus involved.

The typical presenting complaint of a patient with rhinosinusitis will be nasal obstruction and anosmia.[8] Repeated sinus infections, headache, and a medical history of asthma and aspirin sensitivity are commonplace.[9] History of hay fever or allergic symptoms may also be present.[10] A sinonasal questionnaire may aid in the evaluation of rhinosinusitis and nasal polyposis and can quantify the severity of subjective complaints. Although many different questionnaires exist in the literature, an effective questionnaire will focus on qualifying the baseline symptoms of the disease as well as the level of exacerbation of the disease process.[11]

Establishing the history of previous and current therapeutic measures and the relative effectiveness of these interventions provides an indication to the severity of the disease process.[12,13] In many instances, medical therapy including an oral corticosteroid and 4 to 8 weeks of antibiotics provided intermittent relief of symptoms, but rapid return to baseline upon cessation of therapy.[14] Besides the approved or recommended medical interventions that patients will disclose, questioning the patient with regards to nontraditional therapy especially over-the-counter remedies will provide additional insight. Over-the-counter topical decongestants, in particular, when used for prolonged periods can be exacerbating factors to

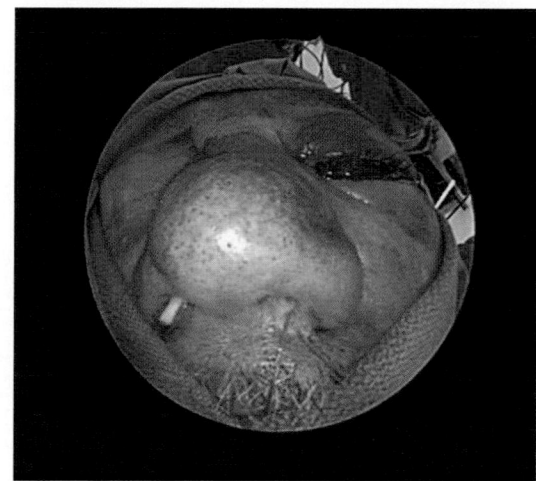

(A)

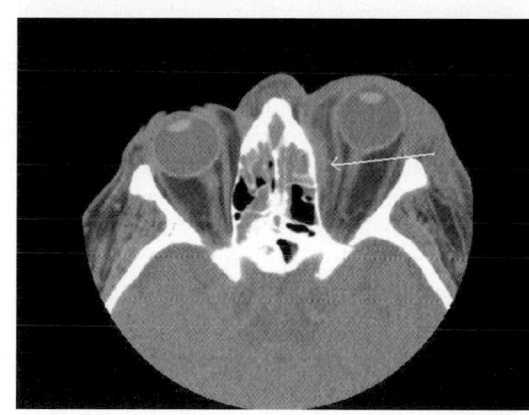

(B)

Figure 1 Orbital abscess. (A) External view swollen periorbital tissue and proptotic globe (B) Axial CT with arrow demonstrating subperiostial abscess collection.

rhinosinusitis. Herbal medications may increase the likelihood of intraoperative bleeding or postoperative difficulties.

Nasal or midface trauma or cosmetic intervention, including rhinoplasty and septoplasty, represents important historical information. Dehiscence of the lamina papyracea or intranasal anatomic alterations may occur in such injuries.[15] In addition, nasal trauma with severe septal deviation may necessitate septoplasty for visualization.[16] While most cosmetic interventions do not address the sinuses, occasionally intranasal scarring and synechiae may be associated with this type of surgery.

Assessing for risk of anesthesia, a propensity for bleeding or familial difficulties with coagulation or anesthesia will increase the safety of operative intervention.[17] A social history with emphasis on tobacco use, chemical exposure, and environmental exposures that may contribute to nasal irritation is important to establish. A complete review of systems with attention to endocrine disorders such as diabetes, immune disorders such as HIV infection and gamma globulin deficiencies as well as systemic disorders such as Wegener granulomatosis provides important diagnostic information.

A complete head and neck examination is routine in preoperative evaluation.[7] Obviously attention to the external and intranasal structures is important; however, documentation of extraocular muscle mobility, pupillary size and responsiveness, preexisting facial sensory deficits, and any facial deformity secondary to nasal polyposis is paramount.[18] Extensive nasal polyps may be visible on anterior rhinoscopy (Figure 2). Classification and documentation of the percentage of airway blockage provides pre- and posttherapy comparison. Evaluation of the turbinates, nasal septum, and the nasal valve helps determine potential causes for airway obstruction. Response of the nasal mucosa of the inferior turbinates to a vasoconstrictive agent such as neosynephrine may also aid in evaluating nasal obstruction.[19] This is important since it can be problematic to perform excellent sinus surgery but have the patient continue to complain of nasal obstruction due to large turbinates or septal deviation.

Flexible nasal endoscopy is highly important in the preoperative evaluation.[20] Determination of extent of disease and visibility of normal anatomic structures such as the uncinate process and middle turbinate will indicate the complexity of the surgical intervention. The presence of pus, indicative of active infection, or allergic or fungal mucin (a thick mucus with a peanut-butter like appearance and consistency) may be visible[21] (Figure 3). One must also be cognizant of the numerous intranasal tumors, such as esthesioneuroblastoma, sinonasal carcinoma, nasopharyngeal carcinoma, T-cell lymphoma (formerly known as midline destructive granuloma), and inverted papilloma, which may be causing sinonasal symptoms. If either a benign or malignant

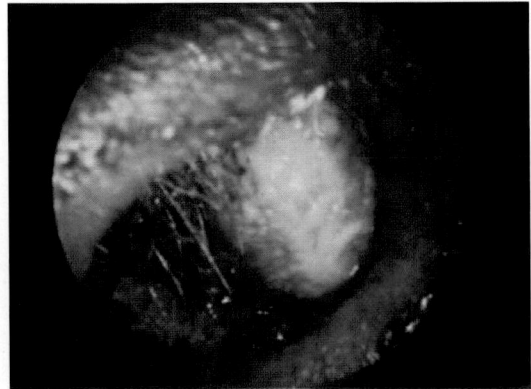

Figure 2 Endoscopic view of nasal polyp as seen during anterior rhinoscopy.

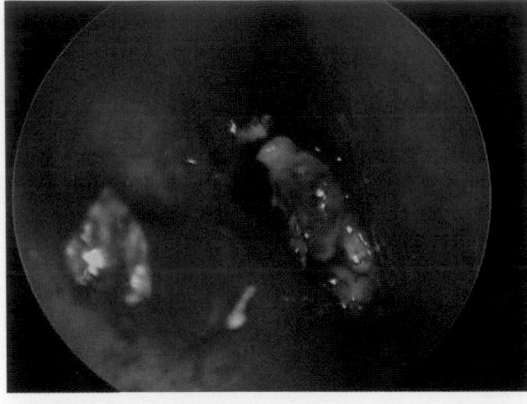

(A)

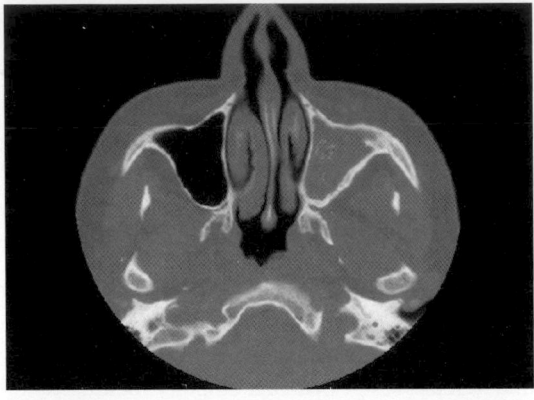

(B)

Figure 3 Fungal mucin. (A) Fungal debris on endoscopic examination with typical peanut butter consistency. (B) Axial computed tomography scan with calcification in left maxillary sinus typical of fungal debris.

neoplasm is suspected, proper radiographic and pathologic evaluation should be pursued.

Laboratory evaluation for the typical rhinosinusitis patient mandates an allergy screening.[22] The choice of allergy screening is based upon institutional and physician preference with the radioallergosorbent test and skin prick tests being the 2 most common forms of testing. Understanding the role that atopy plays in a patient's disease process will help to ensure a successful postoperative treatment strategy.[23] Obtaining a total IgE level is not essential, but this may be useful when allergic fungal sinus disease is suspected.[24] Expensive laboratory screenings that are more appropriate for the recalcitrant patient include evaluation for gamma globulin deficiencies.[25–27] The sweat chloride test is a necessary adjunct to the evaluation of the pediatric patient but is generally not necessary in the adult population.[28]

Computed tomography (CT) is a reliable and informative part of the preoperative evaluation. A screening coronal sinus CT (5 mm images) delineates the extent of disease as well as the relevant anatomy.[29] Identification of the level and integrity of the skull base, dehiscences of the lamina papyracea or the carotid canal, the frontal sinus drainage pattern, and anatomic variants, such as agger nasi, Haller, or Onodi cells, will aid in preventing operative complications.[30] The level of the skull base and its slant or slope can be measured by a variety of means. The medial rectus and superior

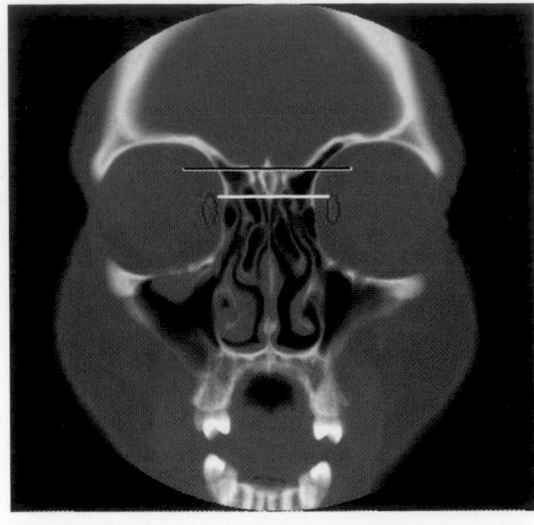

Figure 4 Normal coronal image from computed tomography scan. Level of normal skull base (*white line*) can be seen in relation to the medial rectus muscles (*red ovals*) and the superior most aspect of the orbit (*black line*).

aspect of the orbit can act as landmarks in the identification of a low-lying skull base (Figure 4). Other important information that can be obtained includes any deformity of the nasal septum, as well as the presence of a concha bullosa of the middle turbinate that may contribute to nasal or ostial obstruction. A heterogeneously opacified sinus may be indicative of fungal debris or inspissated secretions, and bowing of bony structures may suggest a chronic expansile process, such as mucocele formation.[31] Magnetic resonance imaging can differentiate a polypoid mass from inspissated secretions but is not an essential component of preoperative planning.[32]

While the screening sinus CT provides a cost-efficient evaluation of important bony anatomy, a 3-dimensional high-resolution CT such as those used for computerized guidance during surgery may provide additional information in significant detail.[33] The use of computer-assisted surgical navigation can be an effective adjunct to surgical intervention; but it is not standard of care for primary paranasal sinus surgery nor should it be used in lieu of an understanding of the sinonasal anatomy as viewed through an endoscope[34] (Table 1). The American Academy of Otolaryngology—Head and Neck Surgery (AAO-HNS) has endorsed the following statement regarding computer-aided surgery:

Table 1 Guidelines and Indications for Computer-Guided Sinus Surgery

Revision sinus surgery
Distorted sinus anatomy of developmental, postoperative or traumatic origin
Extensive sinonasal polyposis
Pathology involving the frontal, posterior ethmoid, and sphenoid sinuses
Disease abutting the skull base, orbit, optic nerve, or carotid artery
Cerebrospinal fluid rhinorrhea or condition in which there is a skull-base defect
Benign and malignant sinonasal neoplasms

Adapted from reference 35.

The AAO-HNS endorses the intraoperative use of computer-aided surgery in appropriately select cases to assist the surgeon in clarifying complex anatomy during sinus and skull base surgery. There is sufficient expert consensus opinion and literature evidence base to support this position. This technology is used at the discretion of the operating surgeon and is not experimental or investigational. Furthermore, the AAO-HNS is of the opinion that it is impossible to corroborate this with level 1 evidence. These appropriate, specialty specific, and surgically indicated procedural services should be reimbursed whether used by neurosurgeons or other qualified physicians regardless of the specialty. (AAO-HNS guidelines: http://www.entlink.net/practice/rules/image-guiding.cfm.)

PERIOPERATIVE CONSIDERATIONS

An important step in any sinonasal operative procedure is to obtain a detailed and comprehensive informed consent.[36] Explanation of risks of sinus surgery should include, at minimum: (1) entrance into the orbit resulting in hematoma, diplopia, or blindness, (2) violation of the skull base resulting in cerebrospinal fluid leak, meningitis, brain damage, or death, and (3) recurrent disease requiring repeat or revision surgery. These should be clearly understood by the patient.[37] An understanding that surgical resection of nasal polyps and maintenance of the sinonasal cavity will require continued postoperative medical therapy will alert the patient to the importance of follow-up and compliance.

After establishment of informed consent and prior to preparation in the operating room, an intranasal vasoconstrictive agent such as oxymetazolone begins the operative preparation. The choice of anesthetic depends on the preference of the surgeon, the degree of expertise of the anesthesiologist, and the patient. General anesthesia is favorable for the comfort of the patient, although local and sedative anesthesia can be used.[38]

After induction of anesthesia with the patient in a supine position, the operating table is placed in slight reverse Trendelenburg position and cantilevered to the patient's right. The patient's head is also turned slightly to the right and placed in a foam headrest to maintain this position. This provides comfortable positioning for the right-handed surgeon decreasing the potentially awkward endoscopic angle of working in the left nasal cavity. Administration of intravenous corticosteroids and antibiotics can ensue at this time.

Nasal preparation continues with injection of 1% lidocaine with 1:100,000 units of epinephrine along the lateral nasal wall in the region of the sphenopalatine foramen, the root of the middle turbinate (anterior and superior to the uncinate process), and into any visible polyps. After injection of both nasal cavities, insertion of 4% cocaine pledgets proceeds. Placement of a cocaine soaked pledget lateral to the middle turbinate in the middle meatus aids in vasoconstriction

of this area. This is not always possible depending on the extent and nature of the disease and other underlying patient factors. Several institutions employ pledgets soaked in topical epinephrine at strengths varying from 1:1,000 to 1:100,000 to aid hemostasis further.

After injection, an intraoral, obstructing throat pack may be placed to prevent ingestion of blood during the surgery and aspiration of resected sinonasal contents. During the positioning and preparation of the patient, care is taken to ensure that both eyes are clearly visible during the surgery. Taping of the lateral canthus will provide eye closure and protection from external abrasion, while providing the surgeon with the opportunity to visualize and palpate the eye during surgery.

Positioning of the bed, the patient, the anesthesia staff, the nursing staff, and the operative instrumentation should accentuate the surgeon's comfort while maintaining patient safety. While monitors are not essential for endoscopic sinus surgery, they allow the surgeon to operate in the upright position and avoid undue strain on the back and neck. A sitting or standing position is up to the surgeon's preference. If computer-guided imagery is being employed, proper registration and anatomical verification should proceed. Foot pedals for operating powered instrumentation should be positioned appropriately.

APPROACH TO PRIMARY PARANASAL SINUS OPERATIONS

Prior to beginning the operation, reverification of the site of disease and confirmation of the involved sinuses should take place both endoscopically and via review of available imaging. Identification of normal anatomic structures such as the uncinate process, the middle turbinate, the inferior turbinate, and the nasopharynx initiates the surgical procedure. If nasal polypoid disease is obstructing these structures, careful, conservative dissection of the polypoid tissues will allow visualization of important landmarks, anterior ethmoid sinuses, and maxillary antrostomy.

If a concha bullosa is identified on preoperative imaging or endoscopically, it may contribute to the obstruction of the natural ostium of the maxillary sinus and hinder surgical progress. The concha bullosa should be resected with maintenance of the structural integrity of the middle turbinate.[39] After injection of 1% lidocaine with epinephrine the anterior surface of the concha bullosa is incised with a sickle knife. A straight punch forceps can be used to remove the lateral wall of the concha bullosa while simultaneously preserving the mucosa of the medial wall of the middle turbinate (Figure 5). Loose fragments of bone can be trimmed with a punch forceps or carefully removed with a grasping forceps. Care should be taken to avoid tearing or shearing of normal sinus mucosa, particularly when using grasping forceps. In general, posterior- and inferior-directed movements after grasping bone fragments that may still have a

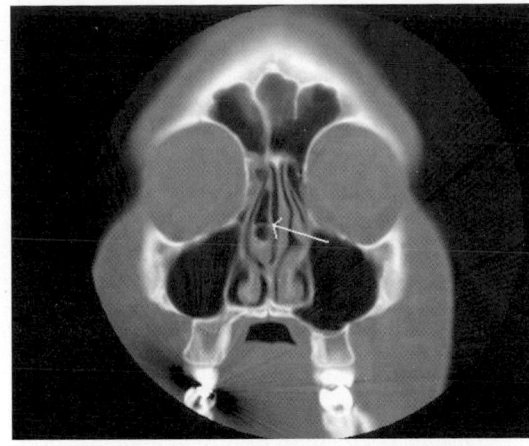

(A)

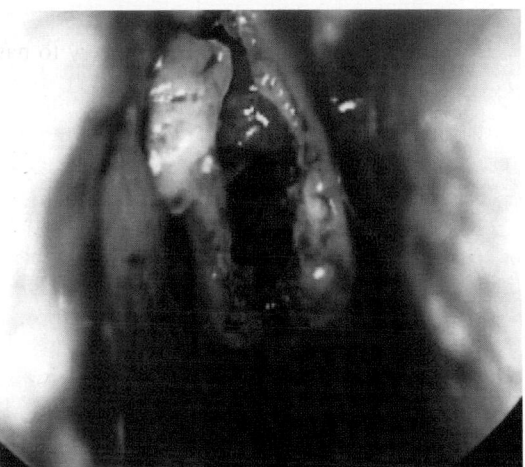

(B)

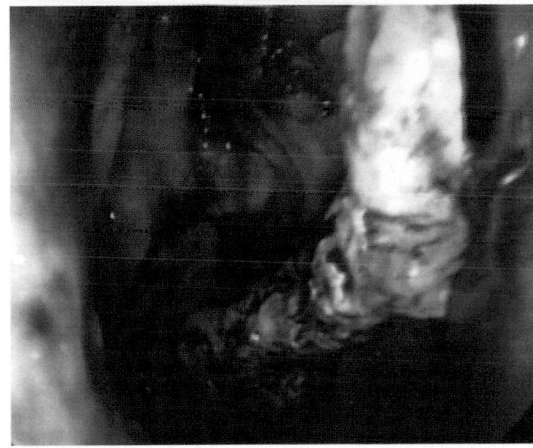

(C)

Figure 5 Computed tomography (CT) image and intraoperative images of a concha bullosa. (A) CT scan with right concha bullosa (*white arrow*). (B) Concha bullosa surgically opened. (C) Concha bullosa after resection of the lateral half.

mucosal attachment will help prevent tearing of the mucosa.

Maxillary Sinus

Once anatomic localization of structures occurs and clear visualization is available, manipulation of the maxillary sinus and its natural ostium represents a primary step in disease eradication. Anatomically, the uncinate process protects the natural ostium of the sinus and must be addressed to proceed. The uncinate process may be displaced anteriorly and medially secondary to polyposis or it may be lateralized and adherent to the lamina papyracea in conditions such as a hypoplastic maxillary sinus. A probe inserted in the hiatus semilunaris can be used to palpate the space between the uncinate process and the lamina papyracea (the ethmoid infundibulum), and this information will help prevent accidental puncture of the medial orbital wall. With the uncinate process identified, 1 technique for resection is to remove a portion of the inferior third in a retrograde fashion using a back-biting forceps. Opening this forceps to an acute angle will prevent inadvertent trauma to the lamina papyracea and violation of orbital contents. Retrograde uncinate resection should proceed to the hard lacrimal bone with avoidance of damage to the lacrimal duct. A probe can then be used to displace the superior and inferior uncinate remnants anteriorly for resection with the microdebrider. As with any maneuver in paranasal sinus surgery, care should be taken to avoid damage to the normal mucosa.

An angled telescope (30°, 45°, or 70°) can then be used to identify the natural ostium of the maxillary sinus. This may be obstructed by polyps, in which case visible polyps should be removed from the area. Positioning the microdebrider window vertically and not toward the lamina papyracea (medial orbital wall) will avoid inadvertent damage to orbital fat and its contents in situations in which either an iatrogenic or inherent dehiscence of the lamina is present.[40] If the natural ostium is open in nonpolypoid disease, no formal antrostomy is necessary. With careful identification of the diseased natural ostium of the maxillary sinus, a probe can be introduced and the ostium can be dilated posterior and inferiorly creating a wide maxillary antrostomy. The size of the maxillary antrostomy in nonpolyp disease is not nearly as important as ensuring that any antrostomy communicates with the natural ostium of the maxillary sinus. Inadvertent creation of a posterior fontanelle antrostomy may result in a recirculation phenomenon or persistent disease that will require revision surgery. In polypoid sinusitis, a large antrostomy is necessary. With the establishment of the maxillary antrostomy, the superior limit of the orbital floor and the lateral limit of the medial orbital wall can now be delineated. Disease adjacent to or within the maxillary sinus can then be safely removed with either a straight or a curved microdebrider. Avoidance of circumferential trauma around the antrostomy will help avoid postoperative cicatricial scarring.

Ethmoid Sinuses

If ethmoid disease is present, one should attempt to distinguish between anterior and posterior ethmoid disease. The anterior and posterior ethmoids are divided anatomically by the vertical portion of the basal lamella of the middle turbinate. However, the ethmoid bulla represents the most posterior of the anterior ethmoid cells

and should be removed to access the posterior ethmoid cells appropriately. Entrance into the bulla with resection of bone and polypoid disease should proceed with preservation of the mucosa overlying the lamina papyracea laterally. Clear identification of the maxillary ostium aids in clarifying the lateral extent of dissection. As the ethmoid bulla is removed, the vertical and horizontal portions of the basal lamella should be evident. Identifying the horizontal basal lamella and maintaining its integrity will avoid unnecessary damage to the sphenopalatine artery and maintain the stability of the middle turbinate. The suprabullar cells are removed to complete the anterior ethmoidectomy.

To enter the posterior ethmoid, the inferior and medial aspect of the vertical basal lamella must be removed. Preoperative identification on a CT scan of a posterior ethmoid cell lateral and superior to the sphenoid sinus (the Onodi cell) will ensure a complete posterior ethmoidectomy (Figure 6). Lack of recognition of an Onodi cell can result in inadvertent entrance through the skull base, potential optic nerve injury, and unaddressed sphenoid disease secondary to confusion of the Onodi cell with the sphenoid sinus.

Sphenoid Sinus

Once the inferior cells of the posterior ethmoids are adequately removed the natural ostium of the sphenoid sinus can be identified. Use of a calibrated probe can identify the anterior wall of the sphenoid at approximately 7 cm from the nasal sill at a 30° angle (Figure 7). Resection of the lower one-third of the superior turbinate may also be helpful to provide adequate visualization for the sphenoidotomy. In most cases, the natural ostium of the sphenoid lies just medial to or directly posterior to the lower one-third of the superior turbinate.[41] In the absence of an Onodi cell, visualization of the sphenoid os represents the termination of the posterior ethmoidectomy.

The sphenoid sinus can be approached via a posterior ethmoidectomy or transnasally medial to the middle and superior turbinates as previously described. Sphenoidotomy should proceed in an

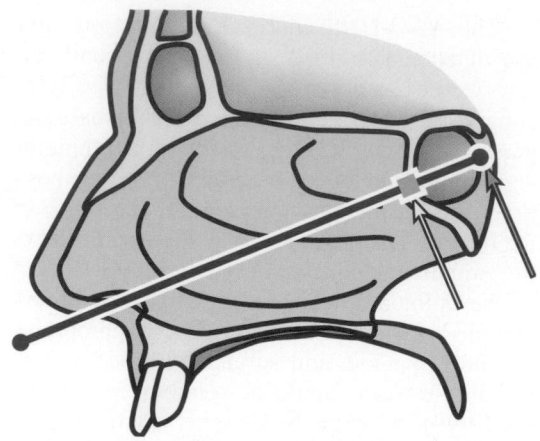

Figure 7 Measurements used to identify the skull base and guidelines to avoid violating the intracranial cavity. Anatomic drawing of calibration probe in relation to sphenoid ostium (7 cm [*yellow arrow*]) and posterior sphenoid wall (9 cm [*orange arrow*]).

inferior and medial direction with care taken not to disrupt the inner mucosa of the sphenoid sinus. The choice of instrument used for widening the sphenoid ostium is dependent upon surgeon preference. An optimal size of the sphenoidotomy should allow for adequate ventilation of the sinus and take into account the natural healing process, which will ultimately reduce the diameter of the surgically widened ostium (Figure 8). Circumferential damage to the os will potentiate cicatricial scarring.

Ethmoidectomy

Establishment of the posterior level of the skull base is dependent upon proper identification and visualization of the sphenoid sinus. A total ethmoidectomy may safely proceed beginning inferiorly and posteriorly and continuing in an anterior, superior direction after correct identification of the sphenoid sinus. Careful yet firm disruption of the ethmoid cell septations occurs tangentially along the skull base. While proceeding tangentially along the skull base, care must be taken to avoid cephalad movements that increase the likelihood of cranial base penetration. In addition, using instrumentation laterally in the

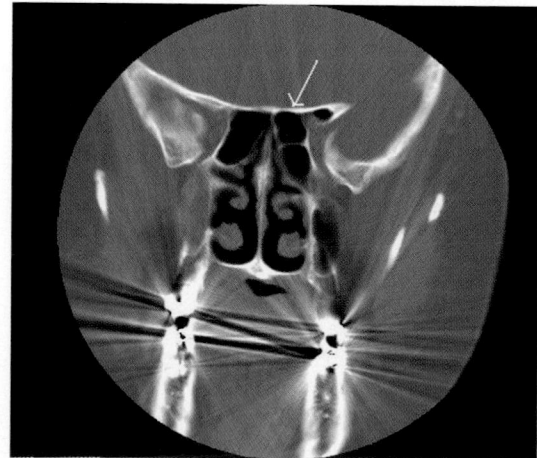

Figure 6 Computed tomography direct coronal image. Onodi cell can be seen (*arrow*). Note relationship to the skull base.

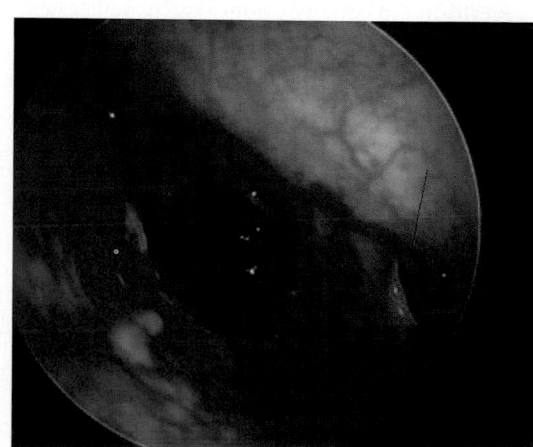

Figure 8 Endoscopic view of a wide sphenoidotomy. Note relationship between the sphenoid sinus and the accessory os of the maxillary sinus (*arrow*).

ethmoids will prevent injury of the lateral lamella (which lies medially) and decrease the likelihood of cerebrospinal fluid leak.

Anterior Ethmoid Sinus and Frontal Recess

Whether or not a posterior ethmoidectomy was completed, removal of the anterior ethmoid cells can provide eradication of disease sufficient to allow for drainage of the frontal sinus. Manipulation of the anterior ethmoid cells should be accomplished similarly to the posterior ethmoid cells. A blunt probe or curved dissecting curette angled laterally, away from the vertical lamella of the cribriform plate, will optimize safety while operating along the anterior skull base. Opening of the frontal recess at the termination of a total ethmoidectomy will avoid hemorrhage that tends to obstruct optimal visualization with the endoscope. Careful preoperative identification of an agger nasi cell and entrance into the cell in its most inferior medial extent or from a posterior to anterior direction is optimal. The frontal recess represents a difficult area to manipulate and sits posterior to the agger nasi cell and over the bulla ethmoidalis. Variable drainage of the frontal sinus into the middle meatus, the infundibulum or via a suprabullar tract provides distinct challenges. In general, a complete and thorough anterior ethmoidectomy will afford drainage of the frontal recess.

Patients with purely polypoid disease rarely complain of frontal sinus symptoms and often frontal sinusotomy is not necessary; however, persistent bacterial or fungal infection, complicated, refractory sinusitis, and frontal sinus pain that is uncontrolled with medical therapy represent indications for proceeding with frontal sinus surgery. Remember, the first place polyps return is generally in the area of the frontal recess. When the frontal recess requires manipulation, realize that the attachment and proximity of the anterior root of the middle turbinate increases the likelihood for obstructive scarring.[42] Careful identification with a curved probe or curette begins the process. Angled endoscopic viewing greatly assists the surgeon with manipulation in this area. Once identified, polypoid disease is removed with an up-biting forceps or a curved microdebrider. Again, careful avoidance of disruption of normal sinus mucosa will prevent scarring. Avoid circumferential tissue removal and concentrate on removing disease and bone anteriorly.

Whether a single sinus or multiple sinuses are addressed, careful cleaning of bony debris and residual mucosal disease at the termination of the procedure promotes controlled nasal healing and minimizes the debridement required at the first postoperative visit. Proper hemostasis can be achieved with minimal use of a suction electrocautery device. Many hemostatic topical agents are available; however, many result in the formation of granulation tissue, disrupting the optimal postoperative result.[43,44] Careful attention to the integrity of the middle turbinate will determine if there is a need for a medialization procedure. To obtain a controlled adhesion of the middle turbinate to the septum, a minor abrasion of the mucosa of the medial wall of the middle turbinate is created. A corresponding mucosal abrasion is created on the adjacent part of the nasal septum. To maintain the medialized position, a small pack is placed between the anterior aspect of the middle turbinate and the medial wall of the maxillary sinus for at least 1 week.[45]

In general, additional packing is not required.[46] Packing can be placed along the lateral aspect of the middle turbinate to control minor oozing.[47] In addition, lower packs along the floor of the nasal cavity can help control some immediate postoperative bleeding (common if a septoplasty was performed) but generally can be removed prior to discharge from the recovery area.[48] To aid the anesthesiologists and ensure an uneventful termination of anesthesia, removal of the previously placed throat pack and suctioning of the oral cavity pharynx and stomach should be carried out. Evaluation and documentation of mental status and vision should occur when the patient is awake and appropriate. Any abnormality should be taken seriously and appropriately investigated.

POSTOPERATIVE CARE

The postoperative care represents a key period in treatment of the patient with primary paranasal sinus surgery. Optimizing and controlling the healing process helps ensure that unwanted adhesions, scarring, and postoperative infections are minimized. In patients with severe polypoid disease, the use of a tapering dose of oral corticosteroids should be considered. In patients that demonstrated acute infections, a broad-spectrum antibiotic can be employed and altered appropriately based upon intraoperative cultures. Fungal disease may mandate corticosteroid tapers over a more prolonged, 3 to 4 weeks period. All patients with nasal packing require antibiotic coverage to prevent the development of toxic shock. Removal of nasal packing usually occurs within 3 to 5 days of the operation. Gentle endoscopic suctioning and debridement should occur at that time as well. Try to make sure all ostia are open but limit tissue trauma. A variety of nasal irrigation systems and solutions exist. Regardless of the type of nasal irrigation, flushing of the postoperative sinus cavity helps a clear and clean the nasal cavity. For most patients, continued use of a nasal inhaled corticosteroid is required for prevention of recurrent disease.[49] We feel that a topical corticosteroid drop (and not a spray), used postoperatively twice per day for patients with severe disease or once per day in limited disease for about 3 weeks, aids in the healing process.

COMPLICATIONS

While a variety of complications related to endoscopic sinus surgery can occur and include meningitis, blindness, and death. The use of applied anatomy and unobscured visualization will help minimize them.[47,50] Minor complications, such as persistent bleeding, postoperative infection, and unwanted adhesions, can be dealt with careful attention during the postoperative period. Intraoperative identification of violation of the lamina papyracea or damage of the skull base is an essential first step in prevention of major complications. Failure to recognize a complication will only result in magnification of the problem and potentiate recurrence of the complication in additional patients. Intraoperative management involves careful planning and open communication with anesthesia and nursing staff. Appropriate intraoperative consultations should be obtained. All parties involved should be aware of the necessity of adjunctive treatments, procedures, and hospitalizations. Documentation and communication with the patient, the patient's family, and the associated staff remain paramount.

SUMMARY

The first opportunity to eradicate disease surgically represents the best chance at therapeutic success. Understanding the proper indications for surgical intervention, and documentation of medical therapeutic failure are paramount. Sinonasal disease resulting in nasal obstruction, hyposmia, recurrent sinus infection, recalcitrant sinus infections, headache, and exacerbation of asthma represent the common symptoms of the patient with sinus disease. Allergy may play a prominent role and should be properly investigated and controlled. Surgical intervention requires careful planning and attentive surgical technique. Avoiding iatrogenic damage to nondiseased mucosa and sinuses, identification and preservation of normal anatomic structures, and early recognition of intraoperative complications are essential. An 85 to 90% success rate can be obtained with a single operation and adequate, attentive postoperative medical therapy.

REFERENCES

1. Lanza DC, Kennedy DW. Adult rhinosinusitis defined. Otolaryngol Head Neck Surg 1997;117:S1–7.

2. Steinke JW, Borish L. Clarification of terminology in patients with eosinophilic and noneosinophilic hyperplastic rhinosinusitis. J Allergy Clin Immunol 2003;112:222–3.

3. Pawliczak R, Lewandowska-Polak A, Kowalski ML. Pathogenesis of nasal polyps: An update. Curr Allergy Asthma Rep 2005;5:463–71.

4. Grigoreas C, Vourdas D, Petalas K, et al. Nasal polyps in patients with rhinitis and asthma. Allergy Asthma Proc 2002;23:169–74.

5. Hadfield PJ, Rowe-Jones JM, Mackay IS. The prevalence of nasal polyps in adults with cystic fibrosis. Clin Otolaryngol Allied Sci 2000;25:19–22.

6. Hedman J, Kaprio J, Poussa T, Nieminen MM. Prevalence of asthma, aspirin intolerance, nasal polyposis and chronic obstructive pulmonary disease in a population-based study. Int J Epidemiol 1999;28:717–22.

7. Hadley JA, Schaefer SD. Clinical evaluation of rhinosinusitis: History and physical examination. Otolaryngol Head Neck Surg 1997;117:S8–11.

8. Johansson L, Bramerson A, Holmberg K, et al. Clinical relevance of nasal polyps in individuals recruited from a general population-based study. Acta Otolaryngol 2004;124:77–81.

9. Deal RT, Kountakis SE. Significance of nasal polyps in chronic rhinosinusitis: Symptoms and surgical outcomes. Laryngoscope 2004;114:1932–5.

10. Asero R, Bottazzi G. Nasal polyposis: A study of its association with airborne allergen hypersensitivity. Ann Allergy Asthma Immunol 2001;86:283–5.

11. Fahmy FF, McCombe A, Mckiernan DC. Sino-nasal assessment questionnaire, a patient focused, rhinosinusitis specific outcome measure. Rhinology 2002;40:195–7.

12. Williams JW, Jr, Simel DL, Roberts L, Samsa GP. Clinical evaluation for sinusitis. Making the diagnosis by history and physical examination. Ann Intern Med 1992;117:705–10.

13. Damm M, Quante G, Jungehuelsing M, Stennert E. Impact of functional endoscopic sinus surgery on symptoms and quality of life in chronic rhinosinusitis. Laryngoscope 2002;112:310–5.

14. Fokkens W, Lund V, Bachert C, et al. EAACI position paper on rhinosinusitis and nasal polyps executive summary. Allergy 2005;60:583–601.

15. Polavaram R, Devaiah AK, Sakai O, Shapshay SM. Anatomic variants and pearls–functional endoscopic sinus surgery. Otolaryngol Clin N Am 2004;37:221–42.

16. Hwang PH, McLaughlin RB, Lanza DC, Kennedy DW. Endoscopic septoplasty: Indications, technique, and results. Otolaryngol Head Neck Surg 1999;120:678–82.

17. Thaler ER, Gottschalk A, Samaranayake R, et al. Anesthesia in endoscopic sinus surgery. Am J Rhinol 1997;11:409–13.

18. Liang EY, Lam WW, Woo JK, et al. Another CT sign of sinonasal polyposis: Truncation of the bony middle turbinate. Eur Radiol 1996;6:553–6.

19. Sipila J, Antila J, Suonpaa J. Pre- and postoperative evaluation of patients with nasal obstruction undergoing endoscopic sinus surgery. Eur Arch Otorhinolaryngol 1996;253:237–9.

20. Smith TL, Mendolia-Loffredo S, Loehrl TA, et al. Predictive factors and outcomes in endoscopic sinus surgery for chronic rhinosinusitis. Laryngoscope 2005;115:2199–205.

21. Thakar A, Sarkar C, Dhiwakar M, et al. Allergic fungal sinusitis: Expanding the clinicopathologic spectrum. Otolaryngol Head Neck Surg 2004;130:209–16.

22. Gutman M, Torres A, Keen KJ, Houser SM. Prevalence of allergy in patients with chronic rhinosinusitis. Otolaryngol Head Neck Surg 2004;130:545–52.

23. Dursun E, Korkmaz H, Eryilmaz A, et al. Clinical predictors of long-term success after endoscopic sinus surgery. Otolaryngol Head Neck Surg 2003;129:526–31.

24. Shin SH, Ponikau JU, Sherris DA, et al. Chronic rhinosinusitis: An enhanced immune response to ubiquitous airborne fungi. J Allergy Clin Immunol 2004;114:1369–75.

25. Van Kessel DA, Horikx PE, Van Houte AJ, et al. Clinical and immunological evaluation of patients with mild IgG1 deficiency. Clin Exp Immunol 1999;118:102–7.

26. Scadding GK, Lund VJ, Darby YC, et al. IgG subclass levels in chronic rhinosinusitis. Rhinology 1994;32:15–9.

27. Coste A, Girodon E, Louis S, et al. Atypical sinusitis in adults must lead to looking for cystic fibrosis and primary ciliary dyskinesia. Laryngoscope 2004;114:839–43.

28. Batsakis JG, El-Naggar AK. Cystic fibrosis and the sinonasal tract. Ann Otol Rhinol Laryngol 1996;105:329–30.

29. Kaluskar SK, Patil NP, Sharkey AN. The role of CT in functional endoscopic sinus surgery. Rhinology 1993;31:49–52.

30. Stankiewicz JA, Chow JM. The low skull base—is it important? Curr Opin Otolaryngol Head Neck Surg 2005;13:19–21.

31. Bhattacharyya N. Symptom and disease severity differences between nasal septal deviation and chronic rhinosinusitis. Otolaryngol Head Neck Surg 2005;133:173–7.

32. Okuyemi KS, Tsue TT. Radiologic imaging in the management of sinusitis. Am Fam Phys 2002;66:1882–6.

33. Tabaee A, Kacker A, Kassenoff TL, Anand V. Outcome of computer-assisted sinus surgery: A 5-year study. Am J Rhinol 2003;17:291–1.

34. Olson G, Citardi MJ. Image-guided functional endoscopic sinus surgery. Otolaryngol Head Neck Surg 2000;123:188–94.

35. AAO-HNS guidelines. Available at: http://www.entlink.net/practice/rules/image-guiding.cfm. Accessed September 2005.

36. Lynn-Macrae AG, Lynn-Macrae RA, Emani J, et al. Medicolegal analysis of injury during endoscopic sinus surgery. Laryngoscope 2004;114:1492–5.

37. Taylor RJ, Chiu AG, Palmer JN, et al. Informed consent in sinus surgery: Link between demographics and patient desires. Laryngoscope 2005;115:826–31.

38. Danielsen A, Gravningsbraten R, Olofsson J. Anaesthesia in endoscopic sinus surgery. Eur Arch Otorhinolaryngol 2003;260:481–6.

39. Bolger WE, Kuhn FA, Kennedy DW. Middle turbinate stabilization after functional endoscopic sinus surgery: The controlled synechiae technique. Laryngoscope 1999;109:1852–3.

40. Hackman TG, Ferguson BJ. Powered instrumentation and tissue effects in the nose and paranasal sinuses. Curr Opin Otolaryngol Head Neck Surg 2005;13:22–6.

41. Har-El G, Swanson RM. The superior turbinectomy approach to isolated sphenoid sinus disease and to the sella turcica. Am J Rhinol 2001;15:149–56.

42. Wormald PJ. Surgery of the frontal recess and frontal sinus. Rhinology 2005;43:82–5.

43. Chandra RK, Conley DB, Haines GK, III, Kern RC. Long-term effects of FloSeal packing after endoscopic sinus surgery. Am J Rhinol 2005;19:240–3.

44. Baumann A, Caversaccio M. Hemostasis in endoscopic sinus surgery using a specific gelatin-thrombin based agent (FloSeal). Rhinology 2003;41:244–9.

45. Friedman M, Landsberg R, Tanyeri H. Middle turbinate medialization and preservation in endoscopic sinus surgery. Otolaryngol Head Neck Surg 2000;123:76–80.

46. Orlandi RR, Lanza DC. Is nasal packing necessary following endoscopic sinus surgery? Laryngoscope 2004;114:1541–4.

47. Muluk NB, Oguzturk O, Ekici A, Koc C. Emotional effects of nasal packing measured by the hospital anxiety and depression scale in patients following nasal surgery. J Otolaryngol 2005;34:172–7.

48. Weber R, Hochapfel F, Draf W. Packing and stents in endonasal surgery. Rhinology 2000;38:49–62.

49. Mygind N, Dahl R, Nielsen LP, et al. Effect of corticosteroids on nasal blockage in rhinitis measured by objective methods. Allergy 1997;52:39–44.

50. Keerl R, Stankiewicz J, Weber R, et al. Surgical experience and complications during endonasal sinus surgery. Laryngoscope 1999;109:546–50.

50

Revision Paranasal Sinus Surgery and Surgery of the Frontal Sinus

Andrew P. Lane, MD
Marc G. Dubin, MD

Endoscopic sinus surgery has been utilized for the treatment of refractory chronic rhinosinusitis (CRS) for over 20 years. The goal of endoscopic sinus surgery is restoring normal sinus function with resultant subjective patient improvement.[1] However, there are some patients who fail to achieve lasting relief from sinus surgery. The management of these patients is challenging and medical management is the cornerstone of treatment. However, at times, additional surgery may be considered. Revision sinus surgery, which often necessitates primary or revision frontal recess surgery, is a technically challenging endeavor. Altered/complex anatomy, polyposis, infection, bleeding, and high patient anxiety all play a role.

ETIOLOGY OF PERSISTENT POSTOPERATIVE DISEASE

A primary consideration in the assessment of endoscopic sinus surgery failure is the presumed nature of the underlying disease process. CRS has been broadly defined into disease with and without polyps for the purposes of research.[2] In the majority of patients who do not have polypoid disease, the goal of an endoscopic sinus procedure is restoration of the normal sinus physiology that had been altered by chronic inflammation. These patients are, therefore, expected to achieve long-lasting relief from an endoscopic sinus procedure.

However, in patients with CRS with polyps it is recognized that there may be an underlying physiologic abnormality refractory to surgical cure. The surgical goal in these patients, therefore, is subjective quality of life improvement, decreased mechanical obstruction exacerbating inflammation, and improved access to the sinus cavities. In these patients, the source of the problem has been variably attributed to factors such as defective host immunity, IgE-mediated reaction to fungus, biofilms, osteitis, and superantigens, among others.[3–8] Whatever the cause, it is the mucosal inflammatory process that is the underlying pathology, with altered sinus drainage being a contributing or resultant factor. Taking this into consideration, there are carefully selected patients who have persistent polypoid disease after surgery that may receive benefit from revision procedures.

The reasons for surgical failure can be broadly classified into persistent mechanical obstruction, mucosal disease, or a combination of both. Mechanical obstruction can occur postoperatively from a failure to address successfully the initial disease or via the creation of iatrogenic obstruction. Mucosal preservation technique, appropriate instrumentation, computer navigation, and adequate postoperative debridement theoretically minimize these issues but cannot fully prevent them, even in the most skilled hands.

An early return of polyps and signs of persistent inflammation may, therefore, represent sequestered disease with persistent obstruction or evidence of refractory disease from mucous membrane abnormality. Additionally, clearly defined disease processes such as cystic fibrosis, Samter triad, and all of the granulomatous diseases can play a role.

EVALUATION OF THE PATIENT AFTER SINUS SURGERY

There are numerous reasons that sinus surgery may fail. Some of these are correctable, and most

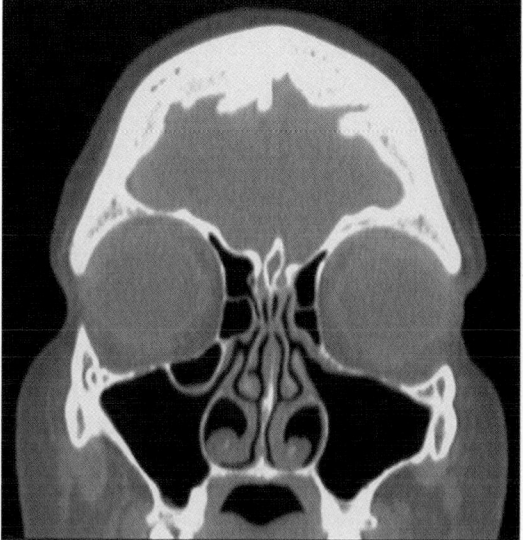

Figure 1 Large right-sided Haller (infraorbital) cell in a normal sinus computed tomography scan.

are treatable. Postoperative disease can manifest as an early return of symptoms, which must be carefully examined to determine any correctable reasons for failure.

Patients may complain of a recurrence of their symptoms or new symptoms. A careful history must be taken that compares the patient's symptoms before and after surgery. Questions must be focused on determining the benefit of the initial surgical or recent medical interventions. Are the symptoms the same as before surgery? Have the current symptoms replaced the old ones? Are the symptoms consistent with a recurrent acute or chronic process? Is the patient

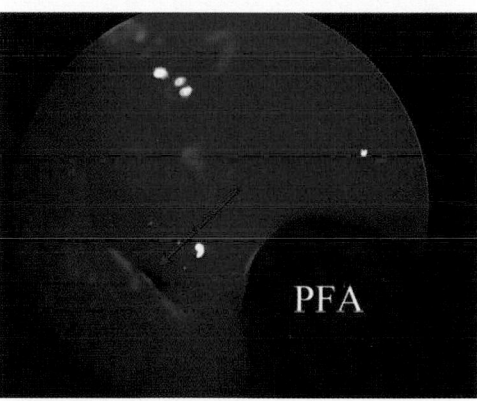

(A)

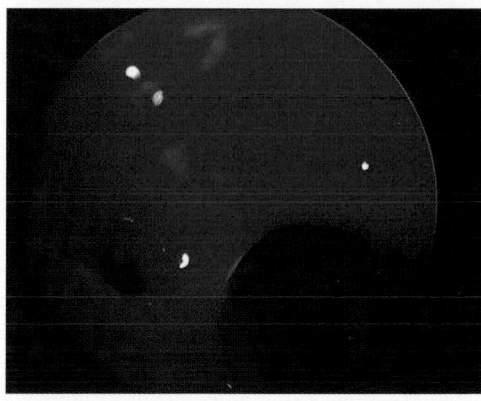

(B)

Figure 2 (A) View of the natural ostium of a right maxillary sinus (*arrow*) using 30° endoscopy. Notice the natural ostium's location anterior to the posterior fontanel antrostomy (PFA). (B) Same view with a 70° endoscope. The ostium is not visible with a 0° endoscope.

currently symptomatic? How often have they been treated with medical therapy, including prolonged courses of antibiotics and systemic corticosteroids? When was the most recent course of medical therapy?

The goal of the history is framing the current symptoms in light of a complex and prolonged sinus history. Knowledge of the current medical therapies is critical to an accurate assessment. Recurrent acute processes that improve with medical therapy are suspicious for disease that was not addressed at the initial surgery. If they are new compared to the preoperative condition, this is concerning for an iatrogenic process.

The routine use of nasal endoscopy in this setting is critical.[9] Nasal endoscopy assists in the accurate diagnosis of infection, early detection of polypoid disease and evaluation of the patency, and location of surgically created ostia. Furthermore, nasal endoscopy in the postoperative patient allows for an accurate culture of purulent debris and the determination of appropriate culture directed antibiotics.[10]

Any signs of inflammation, infection, or polyposis in the postoperative patient should prompt the practitioner to look for reasons for these changes. The postoperative cavity should be examined for signs of inflammation or infection, position, or resection of the middle turbinate or its remnant and visualization of the ostia. Typically a 30° or 45° endoscope is adequate. Examination with a 70° endoscope is often helpful. Attention to the position of the maxillary ostia with angled endoscopy and the visibility of the frontal recess and sinus are critical. Inflammation in the frontal recess may manifest as polyps or purulent drainage and may be the sign of an incomplete dissection or iatrogenic disease. This in turn may lead to downstream maxillary sinus disease. Again, a culture should be taken of any purulent secretions consistent with infection.[10]

With persistent symptoms, particularly with persistent disease on endoscopy, repeat computed tomography (CT) should be considered. Persistent symptoms with a normal endoscopic examination may also warrant a CT to look for radiographic areas of sequestration not visible on endoscopy or to rule out sinus disease as causing the patient's symptoms. The goal of CT, therefore, is to look for persistent bony partitions that may be contributing to areas of inflammation or to establish that the symptoms do not correlate with active sinus inflammation.

CT examination will reveal any evidence of a retained uncinate, persistent infraorbital cell or a posterior fontanel antrostomy. Residual ethmoid partitions and mucosal thickening in this area may be evident. Persistent or new disease in the frontal recess resulting from a residual uncinate, agger nasi cell, retained bullar lamella, and frontal sinus cells will also be evident. Image guidance scan with sagittal reconstructions is particularly useful in examining the frontal recess. Furthermore, magnetic resonance imaging may be necessary to evaluate patients in whom a bony dehiscence has been found on CT.

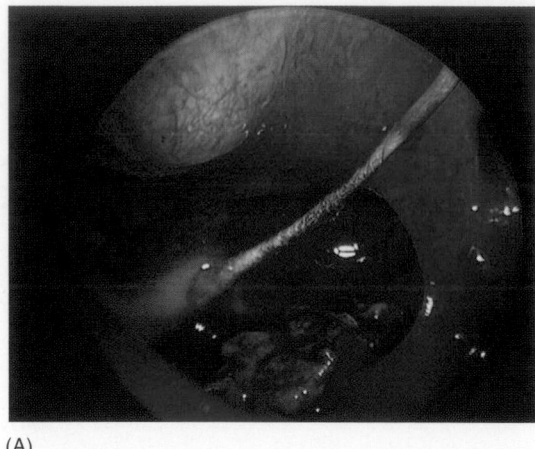 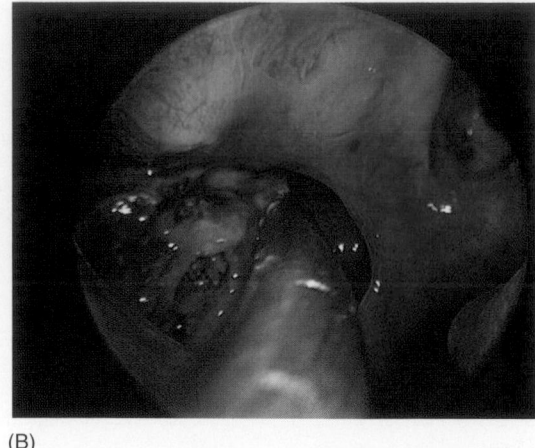

(A)　　　　　　　　　　　　　　　　(B)

Figure 3 Dehydrated debris at the base of a right maxillary sinus. (A) Culture swab of purulent debris in maxillary sinus. (B) 90° frontal curette being utilized to remove thick dehydrated debris from the base of the right maxillary sinus.

In the evaluation of the patient who has had sinus surgery, it is important to attempt to correlate symptoms with objective findings to prevent unnecessary surgical and medical interventions. For example, a patient who complains primarily of headache, but whose endoscopic examination and CT scan are normal, is unlikely to benefit from additional surgical procedures, and a careful headache evaluation is warranted. Alternatively, a patient who complains of recurrent infections but is currently asymptomatic with a normal endoscopic examination, is also uncertain to benefit from revision surgery and should be reevaluated during disease exacerbation. At the time of illness, it will then become apparent what contribution, if any, residual anatomic imperfections are playing in the disease complex. Only by attempting to tease out the nuances of the endoscopic appearance of the cavity, the radiographic appearance of the unseen portions of the cavity, and how the patient's symptoms correlate with changes in these objective measures will make an

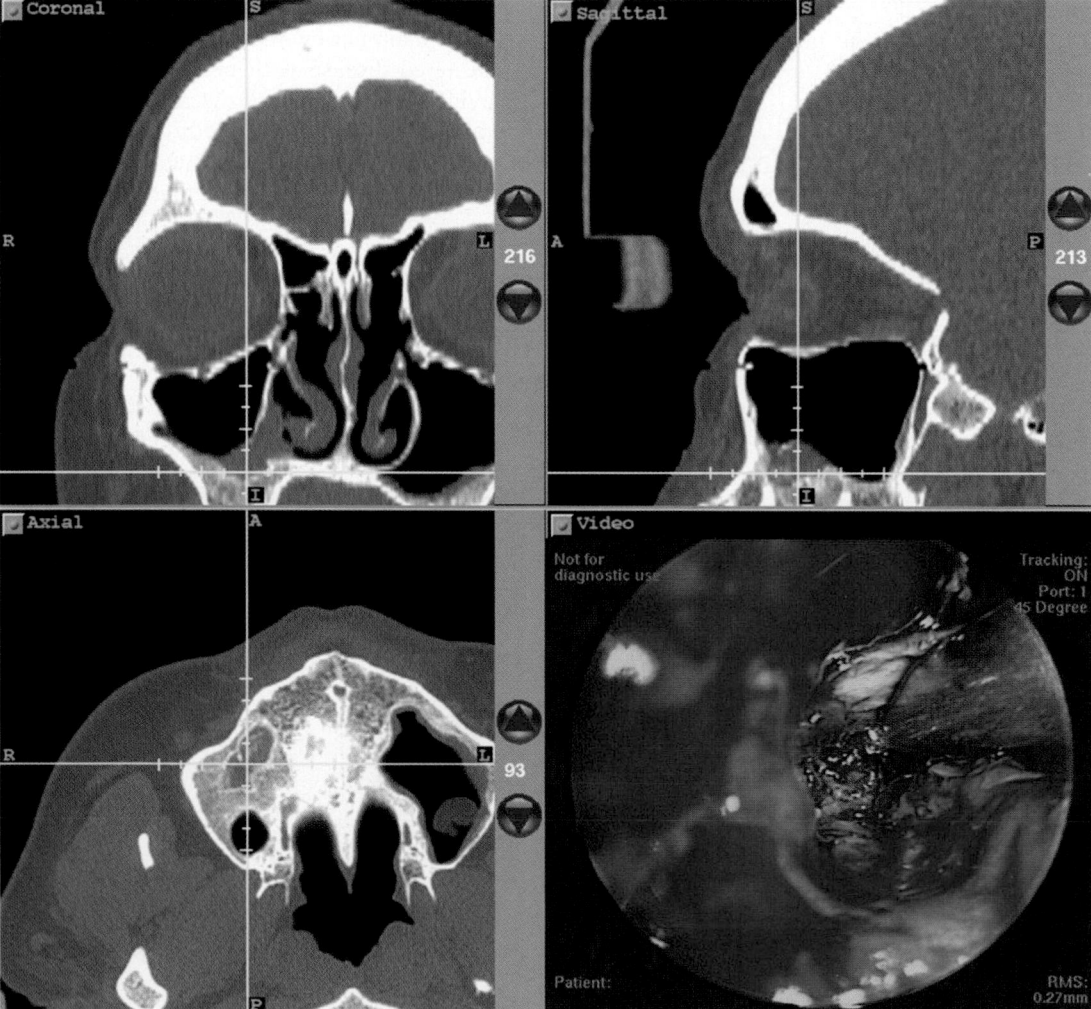

Figure 4 Computer guidance images of a patient with a previous Caldwell-Luc and inferior meatal window with persistent thickening of the base of the right maxillary sinus and recurrent acute maxillary infections. Exploration of this scar revealed debris trapped in the scar bed (*bottom right image*).

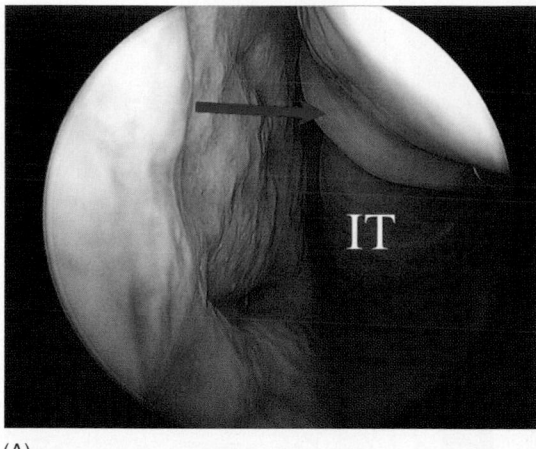
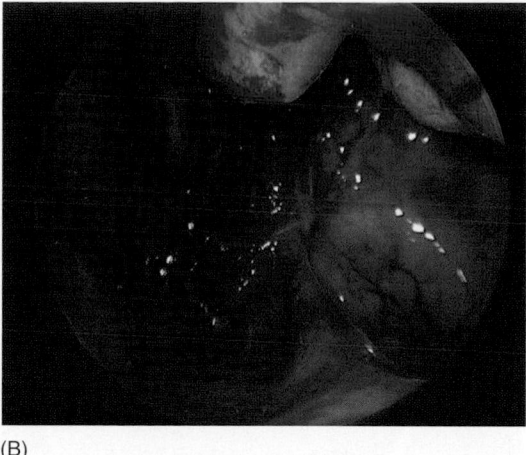

(A)   (B)

Figure 5 (A) Recirculation of mucus (*blue arrow*) from the middle meatus, over the left inferior turbinate (IT) into a large inferior meatal antrostomy. This recirculation resulted in recurrent acute sinusitis. (B) A large "mega-antrostomy" was created which resolved the recirculation and the recurrent acute infections.

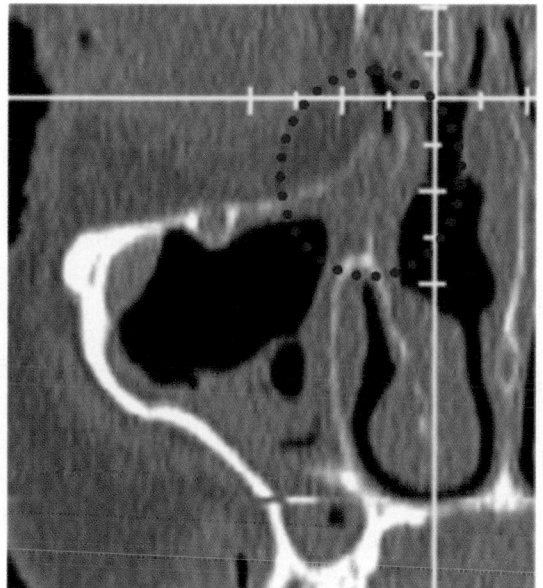

Figure 6 Computed tomographic scan of a maxillary sinus with a retained uncinate process (*red circle*). The retained uncinate resulted in persistent obstruction of the natural ostium of the maxillary sinus and continued chronic maxillary sinusitis.

appropriate determination for the need for future surgery.

GENERAL CONSIDERATION IN REVISION SINUS SURGERY

There is significant literature on the most common radiographic and anatomic findings necessitating revision surgery.[11–16] In one report, partial amputation of the middle turbinate with resultant lateralization was the most common finding.[12] In another, lateralization of the turbinate was followed by incomplete anterior ethmoidectomy and middle meatal antrostomy stenosis.[13] In a study on revision frontal sinus surgery, residual agger nasi cell, ethmoid bulla remnants, superior uncinate remnant, middle turbinate remnant, polyps, and unopened frontal recess cells were most commonly reported.[11] Regardless of the literature, however, each patient must be taken as an individual with careful evaluation of the unique anatomy that is factoring into his or her disease process.

The goals of a revision procedure must be carefully delineated. The endoscopic examination and

fine cut CT scan must be meticulously examined for the specific anatomic issues to be corrected. Focusing on what led to the initial failure, the revision surgery must attempt to accomplish its goals with different methods, that is, preoperative preparation with oral corticosteroids may alter the visualization, computer guidance may better delineate the anatomy, septoplasty may allow for increased access to the middle meatus, and more frequent postoperative debridements may prevent scarring. Simply performing the same procedure is less likely to result in long-term success than the initial procedure and is more likely to lead to negative long-term consequences, that is, intractable frontal recess scarring.

These clearly defined goals must be framed for a patient so that they have appropriate expectations. In the setting of a previous failure, it is unreasonable for a surgeon to assure a patient of cure with a revision sinus surgery. Expectations that include symptomatic improvement and increased ability to manage a difficult disease are more reasonable.

Operative Techniques

As previously stated, there are numerous challenges inherent to revision sinus surgery that make it orders of magnitude more challenging than primary surgery. Landmarks are often absent, polypoid change may obscure relevant anatomy and anatomic boundaries may have been removed, that is, dehiscent lamina papyracea, resected basal lamella, making the procedure more difficult and potentially more prone to complication.[12–16]

However, the basic principles of endoscopic sinus surgery still hold. Critical review of the CT scan at the time of the procedure is essential with emphasis on potential pitfalls and goals of the procedure.[17] Shape, slope, and symmetry of the skull base, location of the anterior ethmoid artery in relation to the skull base, dehiscence of the lamina papyracea or skull base, middle turbinate resection, and the presence or absence of Onodi cells are critical pieces of information to prevent potential complication.[18] Furthermore, both authors utilize image guidance for all but the most simple revision cases and all cases of frontal recess dissection.[19]

Osteitic bone, persistent inflammation, and polyps make revision sinus surgery bloodier with resultant decreased visualization. Adequate decongestion with injection of local anesthetic with epinephrine (1% lidocaine with 1:100,000 epinephrine) and topical oxymetazoline (or 4% cocaine) on pledgets can make the difference between success and failure.[18] An intraoral descending palatine block, an intranasal sphenopalatine block, injection of the residual uncinate, and insertion of the middle turbinate—all decrease intraoperative bleeding.[18] These injections can be done safely with a preinjection aspiration and slow infusion of small volumes. If polyps are present, injection of the polyps themselves can also minimize bleeding. Cotton pledgets soaked with decongestant should be placed

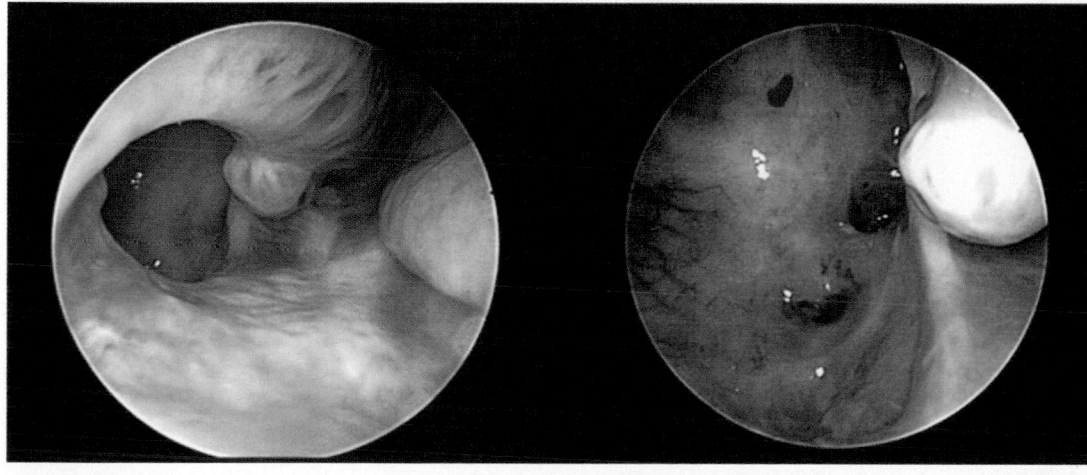

(A)   (B)

Figure 7 (A) Postoperative view with a 0° endoscope of an inferior meatal antrostomy made for postoperative access to the floor of the right maxillary sinus. (B) View through the inferior meatal antrostomy using a 30° endoscope turned upside down. The floor of the maxillary sinus is clearly seen and easily instrumented if necessary.

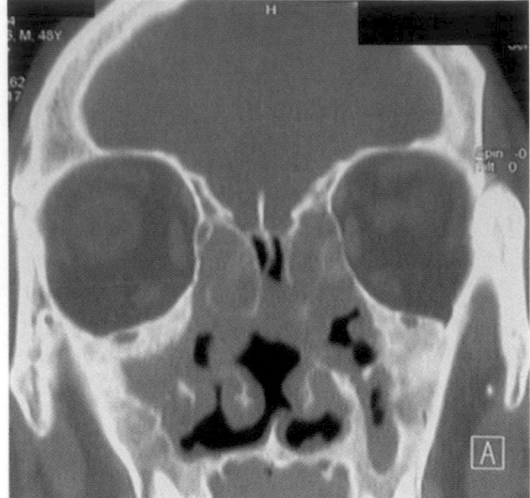

Figure 8 Thickened, osteitic bond in the maxillary sinuses due to mucosal stripping and chronic inflammation. Also note the residual partitions in the ethmoid cavity.

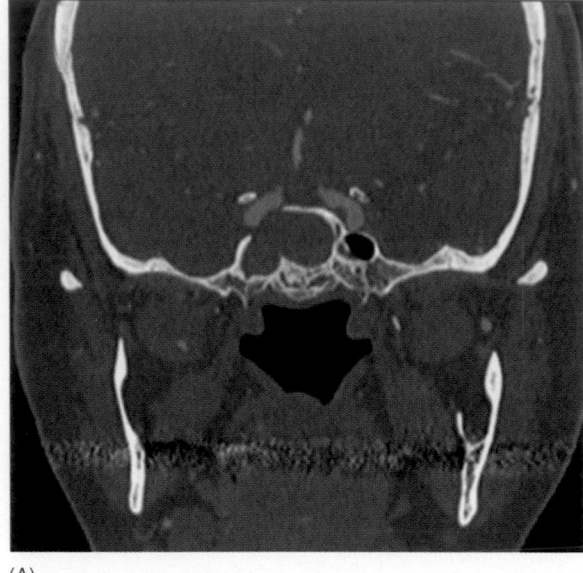
(A)

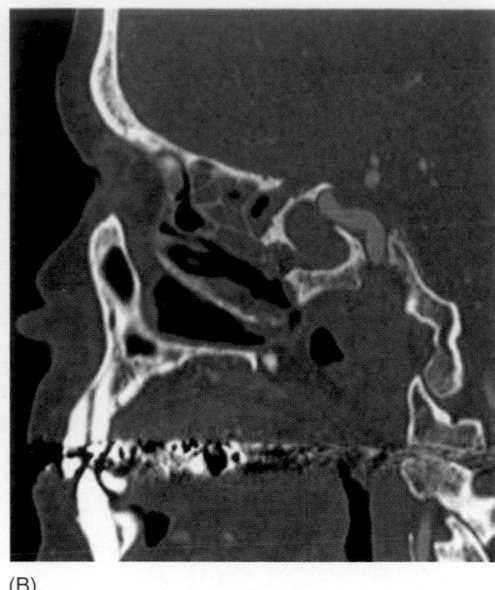
(B)

Figure 10 Coronal (A) and sagittal (B) computed tomographic scans with contrast of an opacified sphenoid sinus with a dehiscent right internal carotid artery.

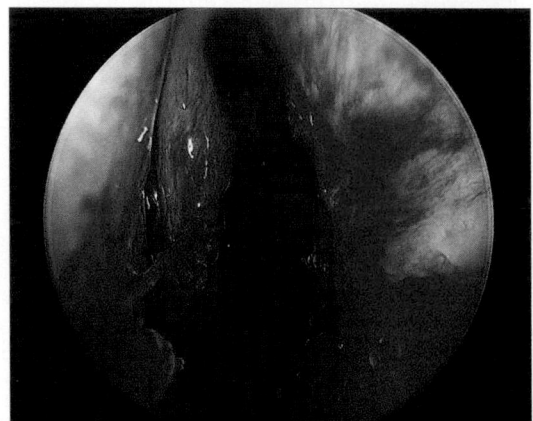

Figure 9 Example of a technique to avoid a destabilized middle turbinate. This can occur when the turbinate is medialized for middle meatal access. The destabilized turbinate may make intraoperative middle meatus access difficult, and it can scar laterally making postoperative access a challenge. Left middle turbinate is medialized with a transeptal stitch.

Revision Maxillary Sinus Surgery. Maxillary antrostomy is one of the most commonly performed endoscopic sinus procedures. When it fails to improve maxillary sinus inflammation, one should be prompted to look for the reason. Identification of the potential cause of the persistent disease is often more complicated than correcting it. The most common reasons for failed maxillary antrostomy are as follows:

1. retained uncinate and persistent inflammation in the area of the natural ostium;
2. persistent infra-orbital cell (Haller cell) with persistent obstruction (Figure 1);
3. posterior fontanel antrostomy with (Figure 2)
   a. persistent inflammation in the natural ostium and
   b. recirculation from the natural ostium into the posterior fontanel antrostomy;
4. trapped secretions including

a. dehydrated debris in maxillary sinus (Figure 3),
b. debris under scar at the base of the maxillary sinus after Caldwell-Luc or extensive mucosal stripping of the sinus (Figure 4); and
5. rarely, recirculation from a large middle meatal antrostomy over an inferior turbinate remnant into an inferior meatal antrostomy (Figure 5).

Identification of these factors requires a careful review of a CT scan and nasal endoscopy. Not infrequently, these processes manifest as recurrent acute infections with no objective measures in between. Therefore, serial examinations and CT may be necessary to observe the source of the inflammation.

Once identified, correction of persistent maxillary sinus disease requires comfort with angled

carefully, with endoscopic visualization to prevent mucosal trauma that exacerbates bleeding. It is beneficial to prevent trauma to the septum or turbinates from the start versus attempting to control it later.

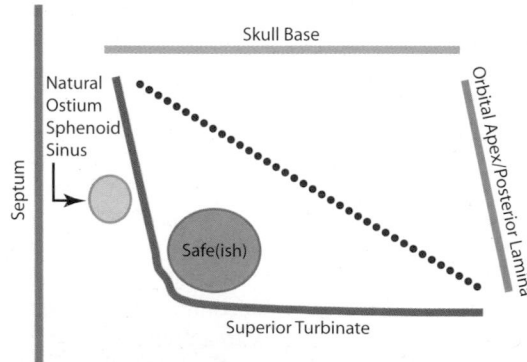

Figure 11 With preservation of the superior turbinate, the safe area to perform a sphenoidotomy is just lateral to the most inferior aspect of the vertical lamella of the superior turbinate.

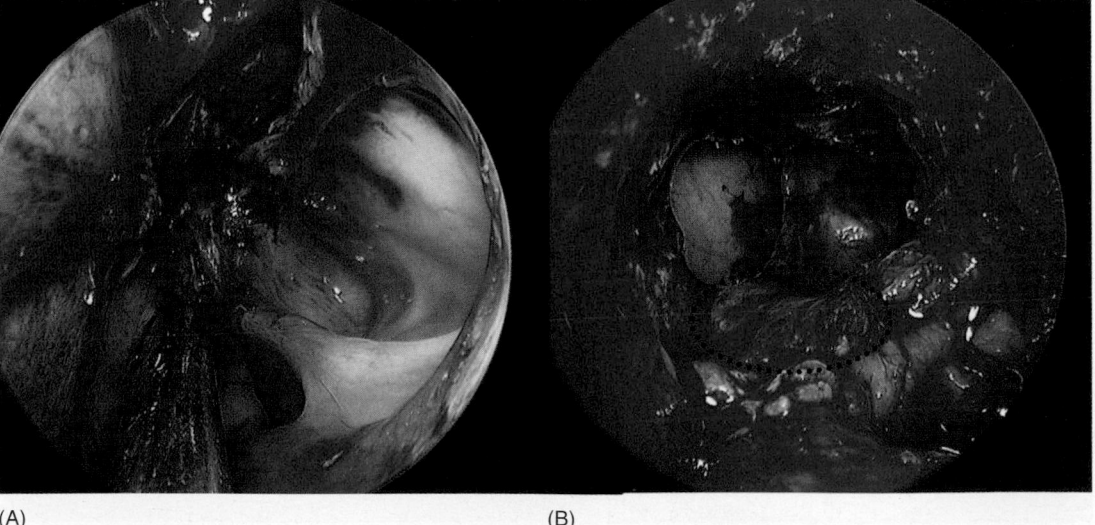
(A)   (B)

Figure 12 (A) Scarred sphenoidotomy with previous resection of the superior and middle turbinate. The patient had a large right sphenoid and a small left sphenoid. (B) Because of a previous failed attempt at a left sphenoidotomy, a common sphenoidotomy was created across a small posterior septectomy. A mucosal flap was retained from the sphenoid (black circle) and was reflected over the bare bone inferiorly.

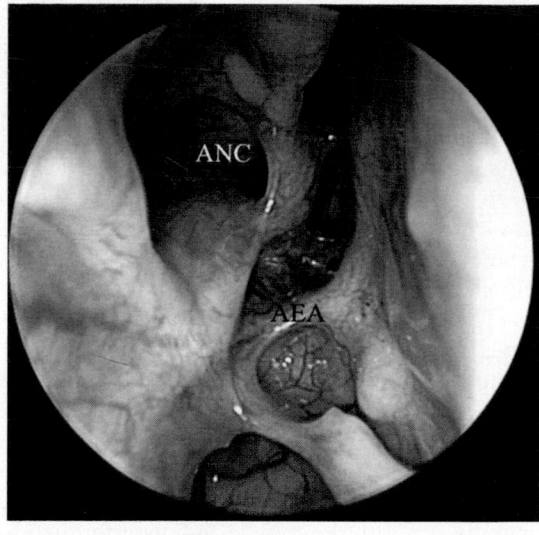

(A)

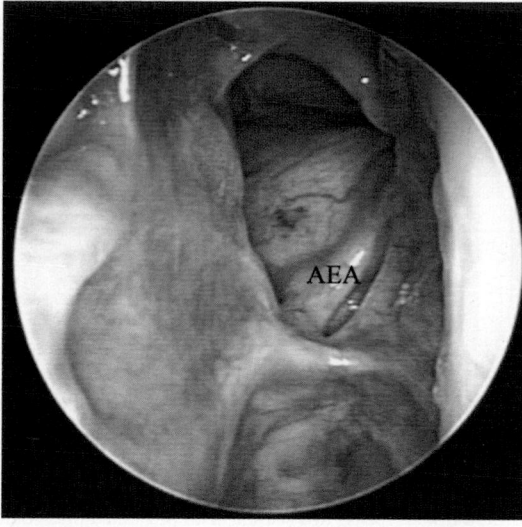

(B)

Figure 13 Endoscopic view of a right frontal sinus before (A) and 5 weeks after (B) completion of frontal recess dissection. The agger nasi cell (ANC) was carefully removed using a combination of frontal sinus seekers and punches. The anterior ethmoid artery (AEA) is clearly visible in both images. This patient had an opacified frontal sinus above this, which did not improve with medical therapy.

endoscopy. Often, the initial middle meatal procedure was performed with a straight endoscope, and the anatomic obstruction was not visible. Therefore, 30°, 45°, and often 70° endoscopy is necessary to examine carefully the maxillary sinus and anterolateral middle meatus. The natural ostium of the maxillary sinus is infrequently seen with a 0° endoscope (see Figure 2). Therefore, direct visualization of the natural ostium with an angled endoscope will assure its inclusion in the antrostomy. The natural ostium often lies directly posterior to the nasolacrimal duct, almost at the roof of the maxillary sinus, in a plane that is between axial and sagittal. With this knowledge, removal of the residual uncinate or Haller cell in this area may also necessitate angled frontal sinus instrumentation. In some instances image guidance is helpful, although it is rarely essential (Figure 6).

In a patient in whom there is significant mucosal thickening at the base of the maxillary sinus, particularly after a Caldwell Luc or nasal antral window, suspicion for trapped secretions at the base of the maxillary sinus must be high. The endoscopic appearance of this type of sinus may appear normal (but contracted), the sinus may collect mucopurulent debris or it may alternate between the two with antibiotics. Instrumentation down to the floor of the sinus is indicated in these cases. This will also require angled instrumentation and visualization. An inferior meatal antrostomy for access to the sinus may be helpful depending on the shape of the sinus. This antrostomy must be kept small and resection of the head of the inferior turbinate should be minimized. An inferior meatal antrostomy is not physiologic and will not function as a drainage pathway for the sinus. It will, however, allow access to the floor of the sinus both at the time of the procedure, and, if appropriately debrided, in the postoperative setting (Figure 7).

In these patients, instrumentation of the floor of the sinus will frequently identify areas of loculated secretions. The goal is to connect these loculations to the maxillary sinus proper. In patients in whom this fails, creation of a "mega-antrostomy" with removal of the inferior turbinate may be an alternative (see Figure 5). This "mega-antrostomy" is also a way to address recirculation between middle and inferior meatal antrostomies. It should be emphasized that this antrostomy is not routinely advocated and should be considered

only in these specific instances after failure of more conservative measures.

Occasionally, there are patients in whom there is persistent maxillary sinus disease from trapped dehydrated secretions or fungus at the base of the maxillary sinus. Simply removing this debris will likely solve the problem (see Figure 4).

Revision Ethmoid Sinus Surgery. The revision ethmoid cavity is often difficult to navigate due to altered landmarks, and image guidance is essential. Frequently, the loss of the middle and superior turbinates obscures the anatomy, and osteitic partitions complicate dissection (Figure 8). This osteitic bone is difficult to maneuver and leads to increased bleeding. Additionally, these osteitic partitions are often thicker than the adjacent lamina papyracea and skull base, making manipulation potentially disastrous. Furthermore, large segments of osteitic bone will recur, and it will not be possible to achieve mucosal normalcy.

Therefore, one of the primary goals of revision ethmoid surgery, as in primary surgery, is to prevent the development of osteitis. Meticulous mucosal preservation with removal of partitions with cutting instruments will minimize this problem. The goal is a single ethmoid cavity lined with normal mucosa so *all* partitions should be removed flush to the lamina papyracea and skull base if possible. It is common to find small loculations of mucopus trapped behind these partitions. Preservation of the residual middle turbinate is critical to maintain landmarks and prevent lateralization and iatrogenic frontal recess disease.

To maximize middle-meatal visualization and minimize ethmoid inflammation, any residual concha bullosa must be addressed. On CT, the concha may be completely opacified and may be difficult to identify, appearing like a thickened middle turbinate. Pneumatization may not involve the head of the turbinate and may involve only the vertical lamella. Therefore any middle turbinate that is thicker than several millimeters must be carefully analyzed. The lateral lamella should be carefully removed with cutting instrumentation. Image guidance is also helpful as a concha bullosa that was missed on the initial procedure can be challenging to locate.

One potential consequence of revision ethmoid surgery is a destabilized middle turbinate. This can occur when the turbinate is medialized for middle meatal access. The destabilized turbinate may make intraoperative middle meatus access difficult and it can scar laterally making postoperative access a challenge. Controlled synechiae of the turbinate to the septum, suture to the septum, or prolonged middle meatal packing should be considered in these patients to decrease the likelihood of this occurring[20] (Figure 9).

In revision ethmoid surgery, the skull base must be identified early, and the lateral cavity should be examined for undissected cells. These lateral cells are often the result of a retained uncinate that pushed initial dissection medially. If visualization and instrumentation in the lateral posterior ethmoid cavity is limited with

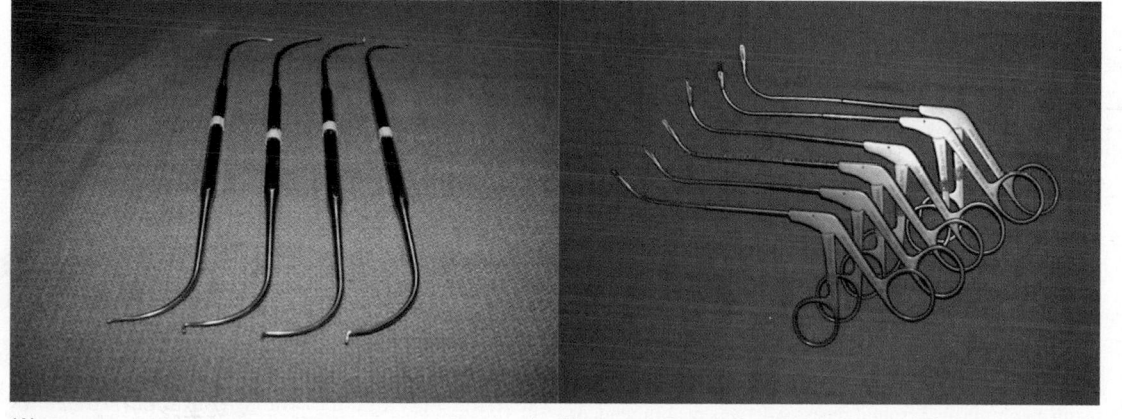

(A)

(B)

Figure 14 Frontal sinus instruments by Karl Storz. (A) Frontal sinus seekers, (B) Kuhn frontal sinus punches.

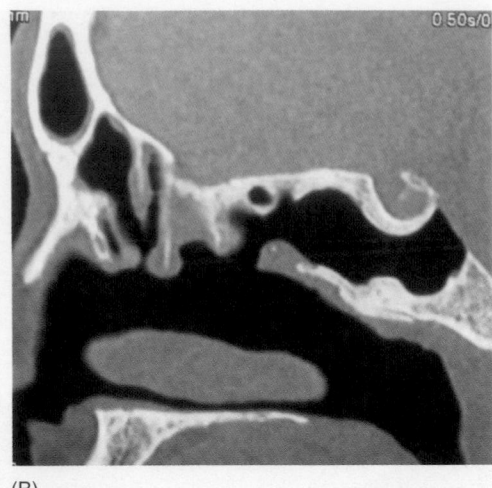

(A) (B)

Figure 15 (A) (coronal) and (B) (sagittal) CT scan of a complicated frontal recess in a patient with presumed polypoid chronic sinusitis. Due to the refractory nature of her disease, she was recommended a frontal sinus obliteration. One year after frontal recess dissection, she remains free of disease.

a 0° endoscope, there is likely to be residual uncinate.

The importance of delicate, mucosal-preservation technique with cutting instruments cannot be overemphasized. The microdebrider has revolutionized sinus surgery in this regard but must be used with caution as it can also strip mucosa and can violate both the lamina papyracea and the skull base.

As in primary sinus surgery, dissection should proceed from a posterior to anterior direction after

identification of the skull base. Partitions should be removed to the skull base with cutting instruments. Care must be taken to not twist partitions as they may be more robust than the skull base. In the revision case, the middle turbinate may be absent, and medial skull base dissection must proceed carefully to prevent inadvertent injury to the lateral lamella of the cribriform. When the limits of the 0° endoscope and/or the limits of 45° cutting instruments have been exhausted, an angled endoscope should then be used. Anterior

ethmoid dissection should then proceed and will be discussed in the section on frontal sinus surgery.

Revision Sphenoid Sinus Surgery. The reasons for sphenoidotomy failure can broadly be categorized into 2 groups. In the first, the sphenoid was not entered (intentionally or unintentionally); whereas in the second, it was entered, but it was closed by secondary scarring.

The revision sphenoidotomy, as is all revision sinus surgery, is often complicated by altered anatomy. The natural ostium of the sphenoid sinus always lies medial to the superior turbinate and is reliably identified in this position in primary sphenoidotomy.[21,22] However, after primary surgery, the superior turbinate may be missing, may be fused to the middle turbinate forming a "uniturbinate," or may be altered in appearance by resection of its basal lamella making reliable identification difficult. Additionally, the natural ostium may be scarred and osteitic and may not be easily penetrable. In fact, the face of the sphenoid may be thicker than the back wall of the sphenoid, making vigorous penetration of the sphenoid face potentially disastrous.

An opacified sphenoid sinus on CT poses a challenge when the lateral wall or roof is dehiscent and the contents of the sinus are unknown (Figure 10). Magnetic resonance imaging in these cases will help identify the contents of the sphenoid and will determine the location of the carotid artery, pituitary, optic nerve, and dura.

The 2 principal endoscopic approaches to the sphenoid are transnasal (medial to the middle turbinate) and transethmoid. The vast majority of revision sphenoidotomies utilize the transethmoid approach as there is often ethmoid surgery that should be revised. Additionally, in the setting of a failed transnasal sphenoidotomy, the transethmoid approach should be attempted.

In the transnasal approach, the middle turbinate is gently lateralized and the superior turbinate is identified. The natural ostium of the sphenoid sinus is identified medial to the superior turbinate and is enlarged with a J-curette, sphenoid mushroom punch, and/or Kerrison rongeur. The inferior aspect of the superior turbinate is often trimmed to allow for additional lateral enlargement. In this approach, lateral dissection is limited by the middle turbinate which may result in a smaller than adequate sphenoidotomy. Additionally, if work should be performed on the ethmoid or maxillary sinuses, the middle turbinate is at risk for becoming flail as work is done both medial and lateral to the turbinate. As stated previously, the flail turbinate can scar laterally, prevent postoperative access to the middle meatus and create iatrogenic frontal recess disease. Furthermore, the postoperative care of the transnasal sphenoidotomy is difficult due to discomfort from instrumentation medial to the middle turbinate, adjacent to the nasal septum. Postoperative scarring may occur if the sphenoidotomy cannot be adequately debrided. The transnasal sphenoidotomy may fail for all these reasons.

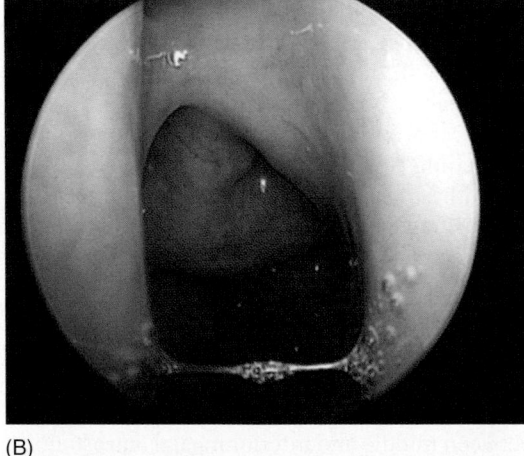

(A) (B)

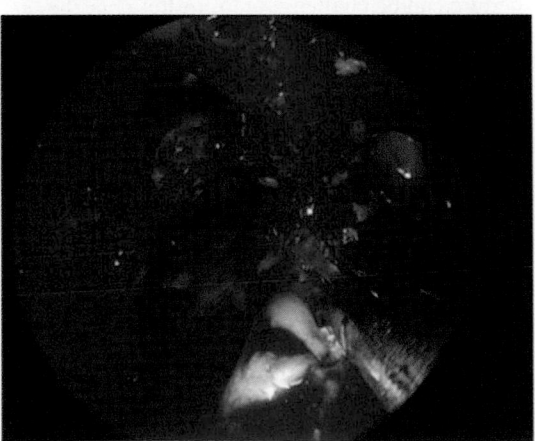

(C)

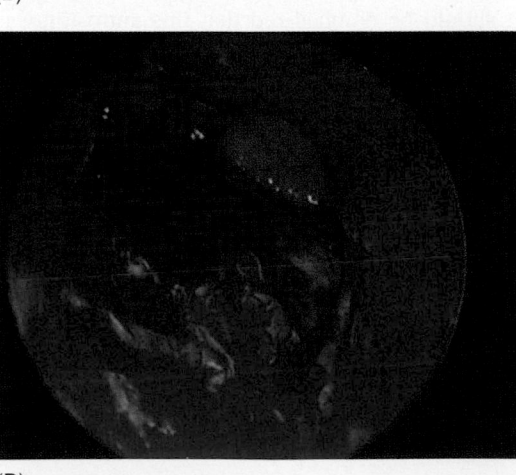

(D)

Figure 16 Preoperative [(A) right and (B) left] view of patient with a complicated frontal recess who was recommended frontal sinus obliteration due the refractory nature of her disease. Postoperative view after frontal recess dissection [(C) right, (D) left].

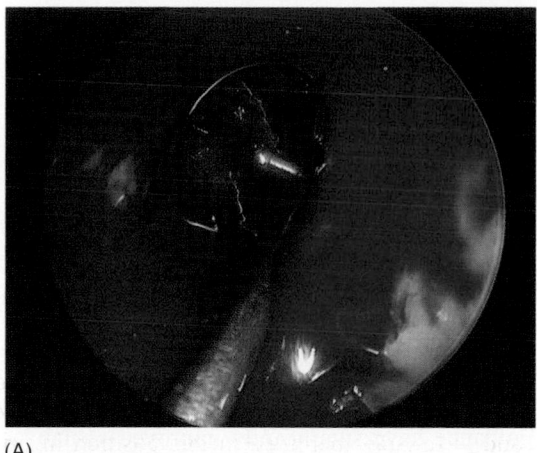
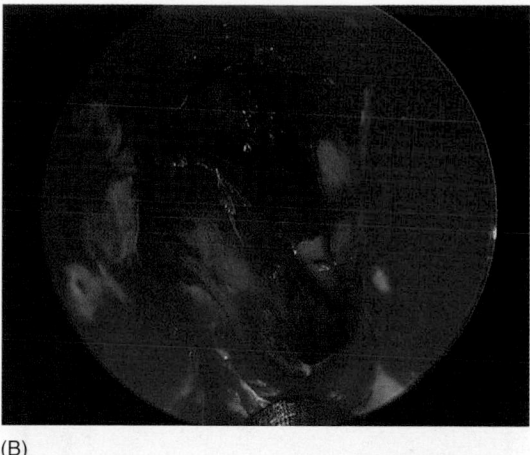

(A)   (B)

Figure 17 Seventy degree endoscopic view of frontal recess dissection. (A) Frontal sinus seeker is used to fracture the cap of the frontal bullar cell. Bone is then removed with a frontal sinus giraffe forceps. (B) Endoscopic view after removal of cap of frontal bullar cell.

One of the biggest reasons for failure of primary transethmoid sphenoid surgery is difficultly identifying the sphenoid or misidentifying an Onodi cell as the sphenoid sinus. This is even more challenging in revision cases, when the anterior edge of the superior turbinate may be difficult to identify. In these instances, critical review of the radiographic relationships among the superior turbinate remnant, Onodi cell, if present, and the location of the actual sphenoid sinus is paramount. Image guidance may be essential to performing a safe sphenoidotomy.[19]

Assuming the superior turbinate is still present, it can be preserved or the inferior aspect of it can be resected. When the superior turbinate is preserved, the sphenoidotomy is performed just lateral to the most inferior aspect of the vertical portion of the superior turbinate just above the superior turbinate horizontal lamella (Figure 11). This can be done with a straight probe or a J-curette and can be enlarged with a circular punch or Kerrison-type forceps.

Alternatively, the sphenoidotomy can be performed after identifying the natural ostium of the sphenoid sinus, which is always medial to the superior turbinate.[23] Some argue against this technique as it requires resecting the inferior portion of the superior turbinate and potential olfactory neuroepithelium loss. After identification of the natural ostium, it is enlarged as described above. One advantage of this approach is the large potential size of the ostium; from the septum medially to the orbital apex laterally.

In all sphenoidotomies, care must be taken inferiorly to avoid injury to the posterior septal branch of the sphenopalatine artery, which runs along the inferior face of the sphenoid. Injury can occur without intraoperative bleeding due to vasoconstriction from local anesthetic injection and may manifest as significant postoperative epistaxis. When injury occurs, cautery may be necessary to achieve hemostasis.

When approaching the revision sphenoidotomy, as in all revision surgery, considerations for the reason for initial failure must be made. One of the most common is misidentification of an Onodi cell for the sphenoid sinus. This is common when there is a large Onodi cell and a small sphenoid. In rare instances, the entire sphenoid may lie medial to the superior turbinate. Resection of the inferior aspect of the superior turbinate is necessary in these cases as the point of normal entry just lateral to the superior turbinate is the intracranial cavity.

When a large Onodi cell is present in a revision case, it is helpful to remove the common wall between the medially located sphenoid and the lateral Onodi cell. It is critical to remember that in these cases the optic nerve and carotid artery lie in the Onodi wall and may be dehiscent.[24] In the setting of a revision procedure with a small sphenoid, it is beneficial to create a large sphenoidotomy in continuity with the natural ostium.

In cases of a scarred ostium, the most likely initial insult is circumferential mucosal injury to the sphenoidotomy. In a large sphenoid, the creation of a large sphenoidotomy to the anatomic boundaries of the skull base, orbital apex, and septum may be adequate. In cases of a small sphenoid and a failed revision, creation of an inferior mucosal flap that is rolled over the edge of the raw bone may be helpful (Figure 12). Resection of the floor of the sphenoid has also been described. The sphenoid may also be connected to the contralateral sphenoid via a posterior septectomy with removal of the intersphenoid septum.

Frontal Sinus Surgery. Frontal sinus surgery is one of the most complex aspects of rhinology. It is included in a chapter on revision surgery for this reason and for the fact that the frontal sinus surgery is one of the most common causes of refractory or iatrogenic sinus disease requiring surgical revision.

One useful way to consider frontal sinus surgery is the "integrated approach" as described by Kuhn.[25] In this approach, frontal sinus disease is evaluated in a systematic, step-wise

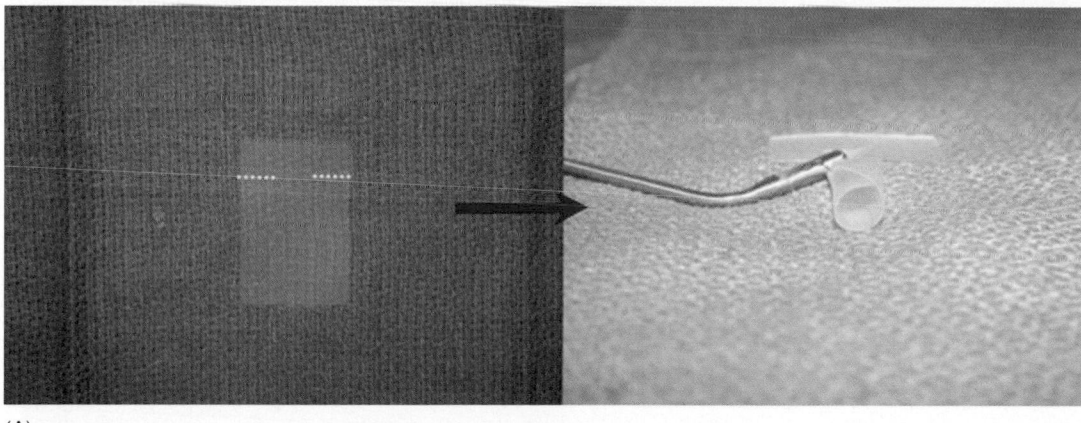

(A)

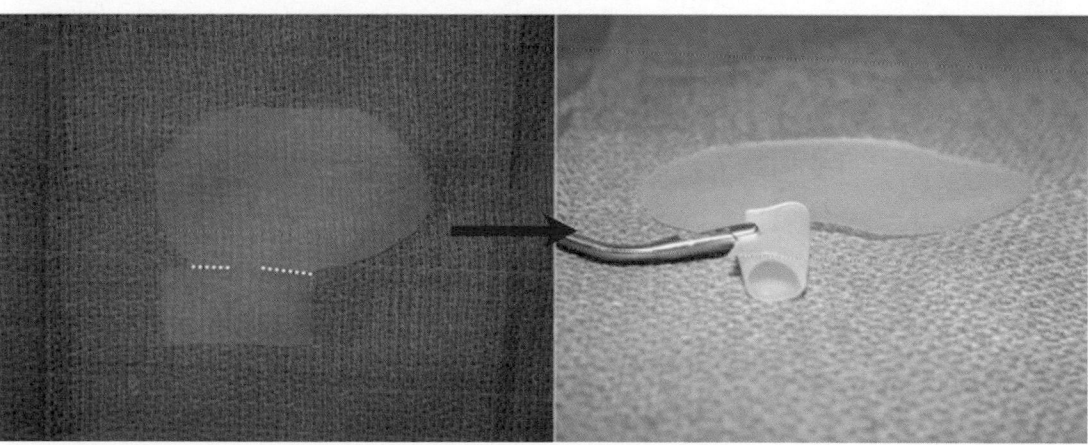

(B)

Figure 18 Silastic (0.01 in.) cut into frontal sinus stents for (A) endoscopic placement or (B) placement after an osteoplastic flap. In the case of an open procedure, the silastic can be cut to the shape of the frontal sinus with a segment fashioned to be rolled for placement into the frontal recess.

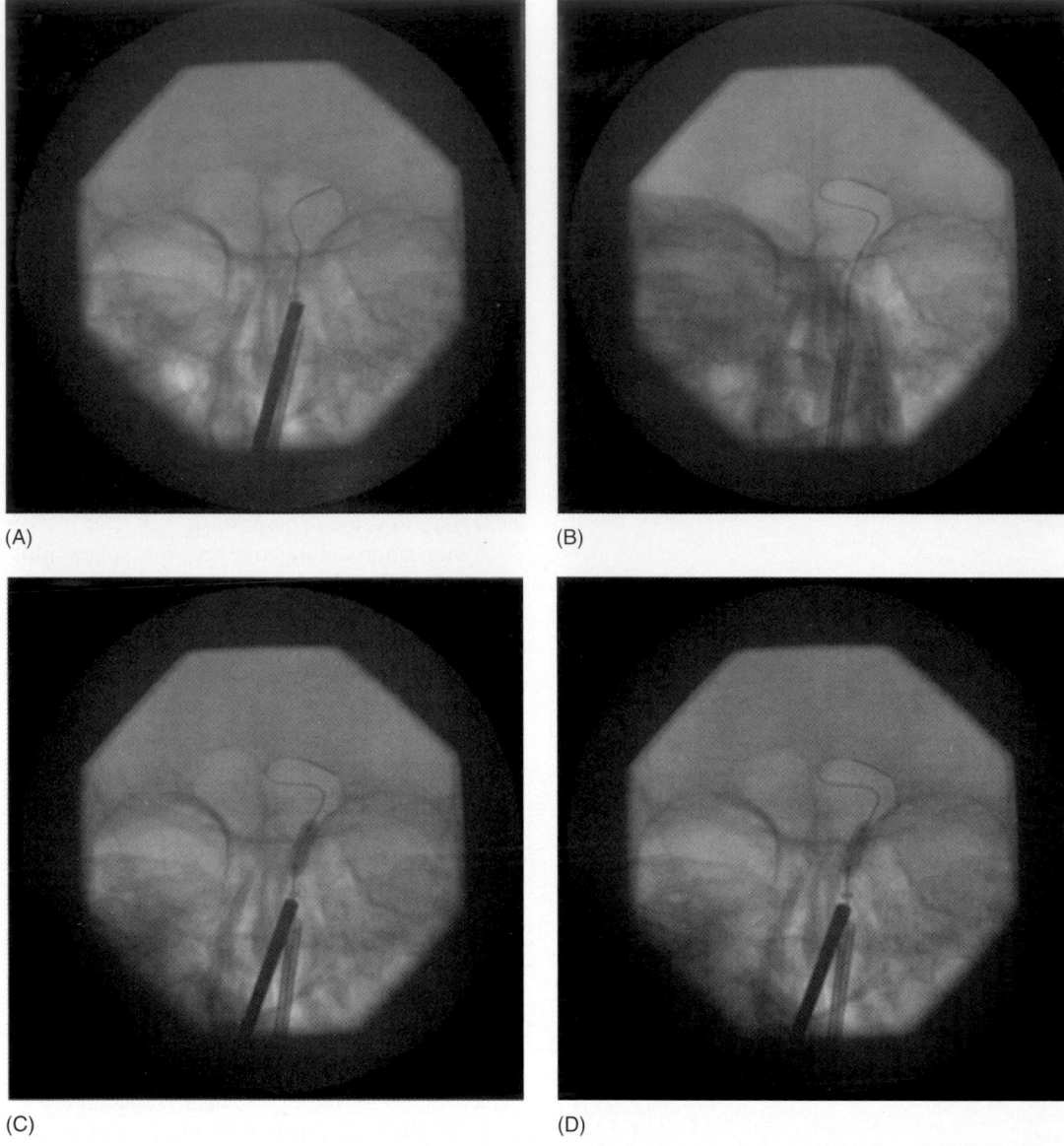

(A)   (B)

(C)   (D)

Figure 19 Fluoroscopy images of balloon dilation of a left frontal sinus. The guidewire is advanced into the frontal sinus (A) and a balloon is advanced over the guidewire (B). The balloon is then gradually inflated (C) and (D) and then deflated and withdrawn. The efficacy of this technique within the spectrum of frontal sinus disease remains to be demonstrated.

   c. modified intranasal endoscopic Lothrop (with or without drill) procedure;
3. open procedures:
   a. osteoplastic flap (without obliteration) combined with endoscopic frontal sinusotomy,
   b. osteoplastic flap with frontal sinus obliteration,
   c. frontal sinus unobliteration and
   d. frontal sinus cranialization.

Endoscopic Frontal Sinusotomy. Advances in frontal sinus instrumentation, angled endoscopy, fine cut CT scanning techniques, and image guidance have significantly improved visualization of and access to the frontal recess and sinus (Figure 14). However, the tenets of frontal sinus surgery remain unchanged from initial techniques described nearly one-quarter century ago. A fundamental understanding of frontal recess anatomy, which is highly variable from patient to patient, is the key to successfully performing and maintaining frontal sinusotomy patency (Table 1). The relationships between the uncinate insertion, middle turbinate, agger nasi cell, bullar lamella, supraorbital cells, and various Kuhn-type frontal cells must be completely understood preoperatively if frontal sinus surgery is to be attempted.[27] Often, harm is done by blunt instrumentation (ie, curved suction, curette) of the frontal recess without adequate resection of the partitions between these cells. Bluntly dissecting with large suctions or image guidance seekers in the frontal recess will increase the likelihood of postoperative scarring and iatrogenic frontal recess disease. Therefore, the frontal recess should be left alone and the superior aspect of the uncinate should be preserved if a surgeon is not comfortable using angled endoscopy and instrumentation. Furthermore, image guidance should be available for frontal sinus surgery.[19]

approach starting from the least invasive surgical procedure. Key to understanding this thought process is the knowledge that the cause of frontal sinus disease is obstruction of the drainage pathway (frontal recess) of the frontal sinus, rather than a problem with the frontal sinus itself. It must be emphasized that the term "frontal duct" has been abandoned because no such structure exists. The frontal recess is in fact an "inverted funnel" shaped space that connects the frontal sinus to the anterior ethmoid region.[26] Furthermore, the natural mucociliary clearance of the frontal sinus is down the lateral wall of the frontal recess, whereas the mucociliary clearance of the medial aspect of the recess and interfrontal sinus septum is in the superior direction.[26]

The "integrated approach" to the frontal sinus consists of the following procedures[25]:

1. endoscopic frontal sinusotomy (Figure 13);
2. extended endoscopic procedures:
   a. frontal sinus rescue (FSR) procedure,
   b. endoscopic frontal sinusotomy combined with trephination, and

Table 1 Frontal Sinus Cells	
Frontal Cell	Description
Agger nasi cell	"Most anterior ethmoid cell"
	Pneumatization of the agger nasi region
Type I frontal cell	Single anterior ethmoid cell above agger nasi cell
Type II frontal cell	Tier of two or more anterior ethmoid cells above the agger nasi cell
Type III frontal cell	Single large anterior ethmoid cell above the agger nasi cell
	Posterior wall is *not* the skull base, but is a free partition in the frontal recess
Type IV frontal cell	Isolated cell within the frontal sinus above the agger nasi cell
	Posterior boundary is a cell wall, not the skull base
Supraorbital cell	Ethmoid cell that extends over the orbit from the frontal recess
	Opens into the lateral frontal recess posterior to the frontal ostium
Frontal bullar cell	Ethmoid cell above the ethmoid bulla
	Posterior wall is the anterior cranial fossa
	Anterior border extends into the frontal sinus
	Located posterior to the true frontal outflow
Suprabullar cell	Ethmoid cell above ethmoid bulla
	Superior wall is anterior cranial fossa
	Anterior border does not extend into the frontal sinus
Interfrontal sinus septal cell	Pneumatization of the interfrontal sinus septum
	Drains into one frontal recess
Recessis terminalis	Recess created when the superior uncinate inserts onto the lamina papyracea, below the frontal ostium

Adapted from reference 27.

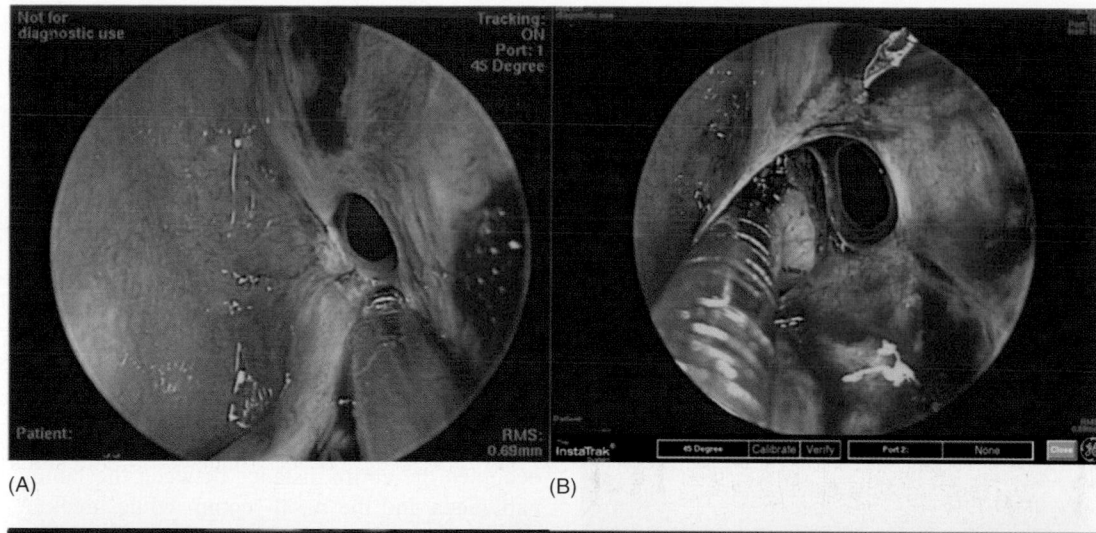

(A)   (B)

(C)   (D)

Figure 20 Left frontal sinus rescue (FSR). (A) Stenotic frontal ostium with a partially resected middle turbinate. (B) Incision is made over the middle turbinate remnant in order to remove the mucosa from the roof of the nose medial to the frontal ostium. (C) Mucosa was removed from the middle turbinate remnant medial to the frontal ostium. (D) Bone of the middle turbinate remnant is then removed using a combination of cutting instruments.

tion and will allow for dissection of the frontal recess if extensive high recess dissection is not necessary.

After switching to an angled endoscope, partitions are removed with a combination of frontal sinus punches and seekers (see Figure 14). Historically, the curette was used, and the fragments were removed with angled giraffe forceps. This technique is still valid; however, removal of the fragments with the giraffes may result in mucosal stripping if not done carefully. Judicious use of a microdebrider with an angled blade will separate these fragments from the bone and allow for safer removal. The position of the anterior ethmoid artery must be determined on the preoperative scan and can be noted by its indentation in the lamina. In a significant percentage of individuals, the artery will be in a partition below the skull base and is located in a position that makes it susceptible to injury during frontal recess instrumentation.

Dissection proceeds from a posterior to anterior direction. Care must be taken medially and posteriorly as the bone may be exceptionally thin in the areas of the lateral lamella of the cribriform and posterior frontal recess, respectively. Once the anterior ethmoid partitions have been removed, a 70° endoscope (or continued use of the 45° endoscope) can be utilized to visualize the frontal recess. Removal of the free walls of the agger nasi and frontal sinus cells can then proceed. The posterior and medial walls of the agger nasi cell are free, while the anterior wall is the frontal bone and the lateral wall is the lamina papyracea. The posterior and medial walls of the frontal sinus cells are also free-floating (except the frontal bullar cell, to be discussed separately and the suprabullar cell) (see Table 1). Dissection of the frontal recess and agger nasi cells must then proceed from a posterior to anterior and medial to lateral direction. The location and position of the uncinate insertion must also be determined. Lateral insertion onto the lamina papyracea will create a recessis terminalis, which may be mistaken for the agger nasi cell or perhaps the frontal recess. This can be determined by careful examination of the coronal CT scan and must be addressed from medial to lateral. These cells and the partitions between them are removed using a combination of frontal sinus punches, seekers, and judicious use of an angled microdebrider. (Figures 15 and 16).

A frontal cell that pnuematizes high into the recess warrants special note as it poses a particular challenge in frontal sinus surgery. These cells may have a free edge laterally, medially, and anteriorly. The cap of the cell may also be violated. They may be Type III frontal cells with a free posterior edge or a frontal bullar cell without posterior access. Frontal bullar cells cannot be approached from posterior to anterior as the posterior wall of the cell is the skull base. These cells are particularly difficult to manage when they pneumatize high into the frontal sinus, and the cap of the cell is difficult to reach from below. These well-pneumatized cells often have

The anterior ethmoidectomy and endoscopic frontal sinusotomy are performed after completion of the posterior ethmoidectomy. Angled endoscopes are used (initially 30° or 45°) when visualization with the 0° endoscope is limited. It is impossible to perform an appropriate, safe, functional frontal sinusotomy with a straight endoscope without unnecessary resection of structures, that is, middle turbinate, middle turbinate

insertion, so this should not be attempted. The advantage of a 30° endoscope is that it allows continued visualization of the posterior skull base and sphenoidotomy. However, complete frontal dissection is not possible with this endoscope. The 45° endoscope may provide better illumina-

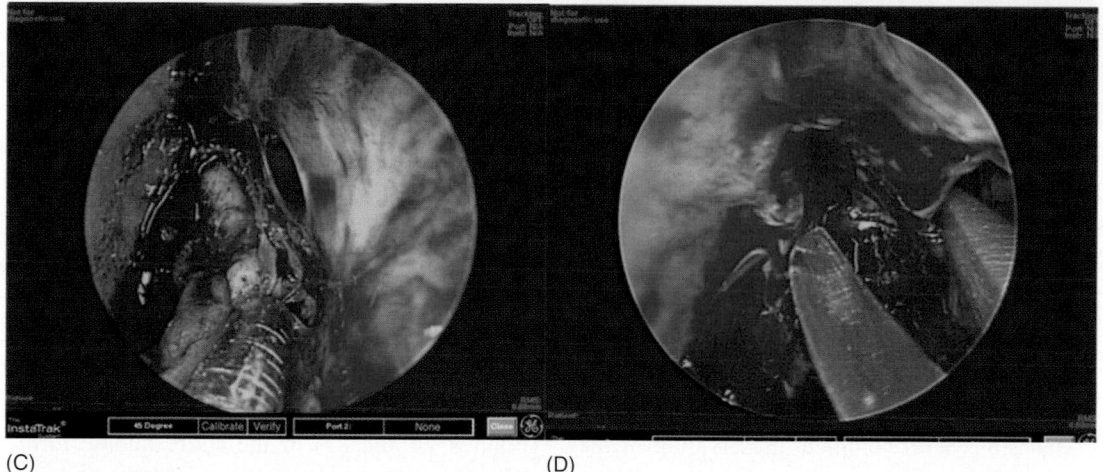

Figure 21 Frontal ostium after a frontal sinus rescue (FSR) as shown in Figure 20.

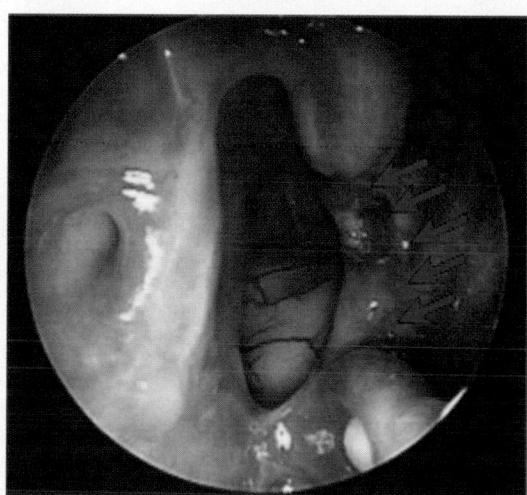

Figure 22 Extended frontal sinus rescue 5 weeks after surgery. Note the channel cut into the middle turbinate that had previously been lateralized. Mucosal flap (*blue arrows*) was reflected over the bare bone to facilitate healing and break up the circumferential scar.

Figure 23 (A) Complicated frontal recess with a interfrontal sinus septal cell (IFSS) and stenotic frontal recess (FS). (B) The scar was violated (*blue arrow*); and, due to previous failure, the decision to perform a trephine was made (C) and (D). When the trephination was visualized endoscopically (E), there was noted to be a pocket of pus lateral in the sinus, which was suctioned out of the sinus with direct visualization. A stent [*blue arrow* (E)] was then placed from below and visualized from above. (F) Final view of the stent visualized via the nose with a 70° endoscope.

Extended Endoscopic Frontal Sinus Procedures. Extended endoscopic frontal sinus procedures are considered in the setting of a failed primary endoscopic procedure and not as the primary mode of treating frontal sinus disease. They should be considered in order of presentation, as they result in progressively more destruction of normal anatomy. The least invasive procedure should be considered first, followed successively by more invasive procedures.

The FSR is a delicate procedure that potentially creates a large frontal sinusotomy.[30,31] The FSR addresses the lateralized middle turbinate or middle turbinate remnant. The goal of this procedure is to create a frontal sinusotomy that occupies the entire distance between the lamina papyracea and the nasal septum while breaking up the circumferential scar of the ostium with a mucosal flap (Draf IIb proceedure).[32]

The mucosa of the roof of the nose is removed medial to the existing frontal sinusotomy. If the middle turbinate remnant is adherent to the nasal sidewall, it is separated from it with a sharp knife. The bone of the middle turbinate remnant is removed carefully up to the roof of the nose, with care taken not to dissect too far posteriorly with resultant injury to the cribriform plate. Image guidance is essential. The remaining mucosal flap from the lateral aspect of the middle turbinate remnant is reflected to the roof of the nose, thereby breaking up the circumferential opening (Figures 20 and 21). If the entire middle turbinate is present, and the recess is narrow, this procedure can still be performed (extended frontal sinus rescue) by creating a "neo-middle turbinate remnant." A large straight-through cutting instrument can be used to cut a channel through from the insertion of the middle turbinate at the nasal sidewall to the skull base. The FSR can then be performed on the remnant of the middle turbinate anterior to the cut. Seventy-degree endoscopy is critical for both of these procedures (Figure 22).

lateral and medial walls that are opposed to the interfrontal sinus septum and lateral frontal sinus/frontal sinus floor, which makes access to the frontal sinus difficult without stripping mucosa. The technique for removing these cells involves careful manipulation of a frontal sinus seeker between the mucosa of the frontal sinus and the mucosa of the wall of the cell, fracture of the wall of the cell, and careful removal of the wall fragment with a giraffe. Often, all of the cell cannot be removed (Figure 17). If stenting of the frontal recess is considered, soft, flexible material should be used[28] (Figure 18).

The safety of a balloon system for dilating sinus ostia was introduced at the annual meeting of the American Academy of Otolaryngology in September of 2005.[29] Preliminary data on

intermediate length results were then presented in September of 2006. This instrument system allows for the dilation of the natural ostium of the frontal sinus with complete preservation of the mucosal lining of the frontal outflow tract. Bone is not removed and instrumentation of the narrow confines of the recess is limited. At the time of the writing of the chapter, this was performed utilizing fluoroscopy although the guides are able to be tracked with image guidance. The exact role that these instruments play in frontal sinus surgery is unclear. However, particularly in the case of an isolated frontal sinus process, they may be considered (Figure 19).

Figure 24 View of bilateral frontal recesses with a 30° endoscope after an endoscopic modified Lothrop. This one was performed utilizing frontal sinus punches and did not require a drill.

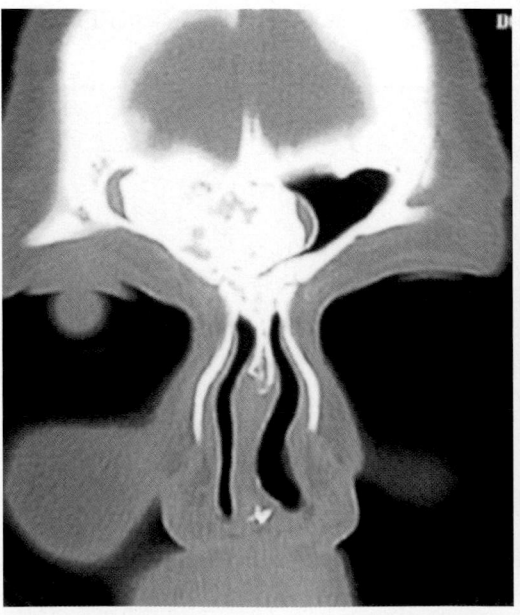

(A)

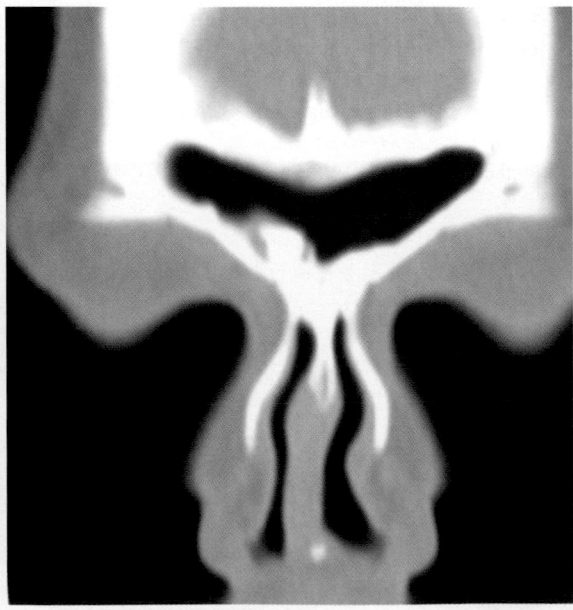

(B)

Figure 25 Computed tomography (CT) scans before (A) and after (B) an osteoplastic flap without obliteration for a frontal sinus osteoma. Postoperative CT was performed 6 months after the procedure.

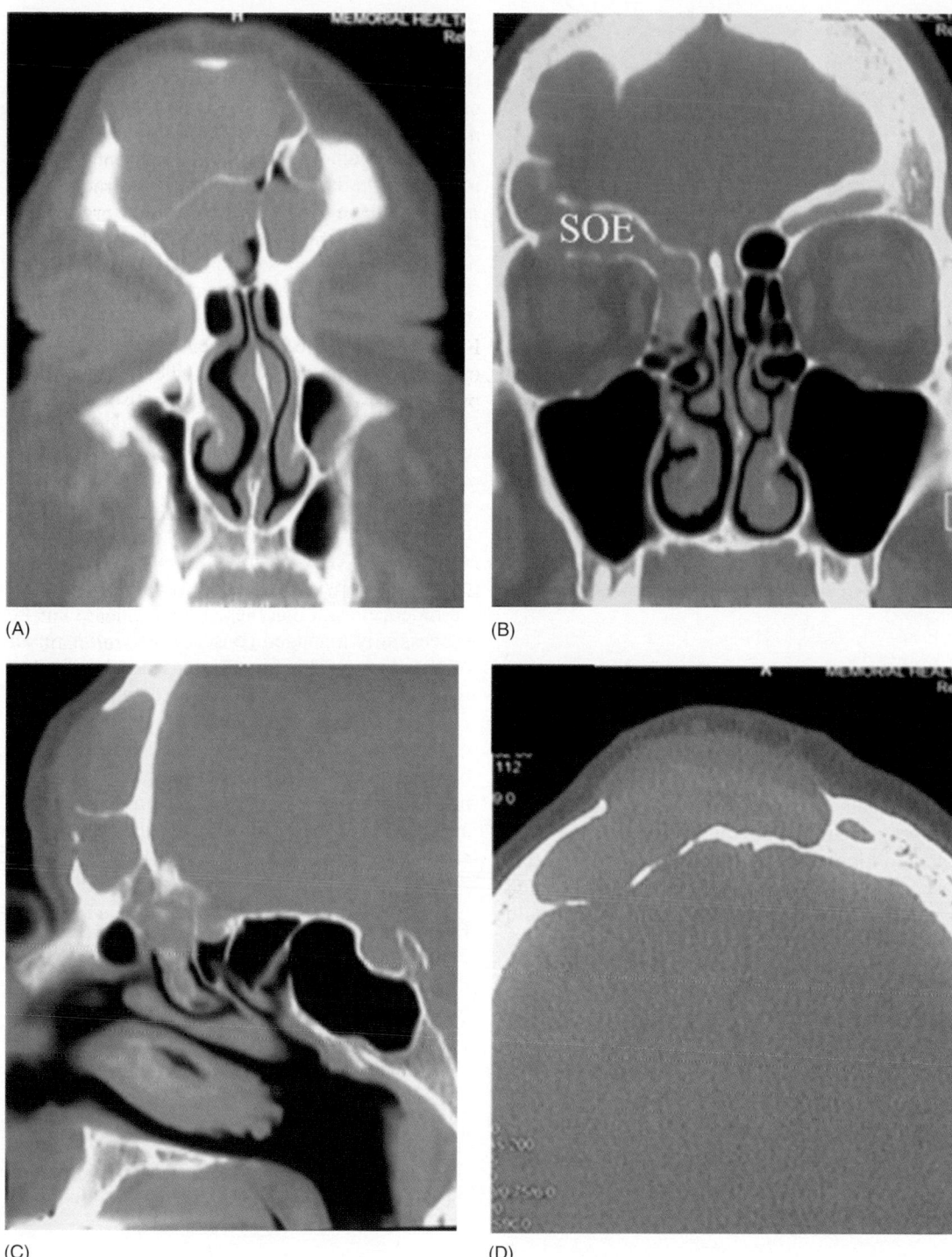

(A)

(B)

(C)

(D)

Figure 26 Coronal (A) and (B), sagittal (B) and axial (C) computed tomography scan of a patient with extensive supraorbital pneumatization with a failed frontal sinus obliteration. SOE = supraorbital ethmoid.

If the frontal sinus cannot be successfully instrumented with endoscopy alone, the addition of a frontal sinus trephine should be considered.[33] An incision is made in the eyebrow and deep dissection is made superiorly and medially to the area over the frontal sinus. The proper location of the trephine is through the anterior table of the frontal sinus, which allows visualization of the frontal sinus and frontal recess.

After incising the periostium and confirming the location with the CT scan, a 4 mm bur is used to drill a hole through the frontal sinus anterior table. The frontal recess can then be visualized from above after inserting the endoscope through the trephination. The recess can then be instrumented from below, and vice versa. This technique is particularly helpful when there is pneumatization of a cell into the frontal sinus that cannot be reached via standard instrumentation from below (Figure 23).

The Draf III is a procedure that creates a common outflow track for both frontal sinuses across a superior septectomy[32,34] (Figure 24). It is commonly performed with a drill (modified intranasal endoscopic Lothrop), which detractors have claimed creates a large circumferential area of denuded bone. McLaughlin and colleagues modified this technique by describing a transseptal approach, which protects the lateral frontal recess mucosa.[35] Additionally, it can also be performed with frontal sinus punches, which theoretically limit mucosal damage.[36] However, this technique is limited by the anterior to posterior dimensions of the frontal recess and frontal ostium.[37] Furthermore, due to the ease of drilling in the frontal recess, it is frequently performed prematurely before endoscopic maneuvers that directly address the anatomy causing frontal recess obstruction are attempted.

Open Procedures. Historically, the osteoplastic flap with frontal sinus obliteration has been championed as the "gold standard" for treatment of frontal sinus disease.[38] However, this approach is prone to late failure and is plagued by the inability to image the frontal sinus after obliteration. It is for this reason, that obliteration of the frontal sinus should be considered the absolute last resort when all other attempts to manage the sinus have failed.

However, the osteoplastic flap unequivocally provides the best visualization of the frontal sinus and frontal recess and should be considered without obliteration when endoscopic approaches have failed. It is the ideal approach for managing benign tumors of the frontal sinus, that is, inverted papilloma or bony tumors. A tumor that extends laterally into the frontal sinus can be addressed with direct visualization with preservation of the functional sinus[39] (Figure 25). The osteoplastic flap can also be used in the management of the previously obliterated frontal sinus.

The approach is via a standard coronal incision. Care is taken laterally over the temporalis muscle to remain deep to the superficial layer of the deep temporal fascia, remaining in the temporal fat pad to prevent injury to the frontal branch of the facial nerve. Subgaleal, that is, supraperiosteal, dissection then proceeds to the glabella. The periosteum is incised lateral and superior to the frontal sinus. A 6 ft Caldwell radiograph or image guidance may be used to determine roughly the size of the sinus. The outline of the sinus should then be made using the 6 ft Caldwell or image guidance, staying as close to the periphery as possible.[40] Transillumination should be avoided as a technique for frontal sinus size determination as it overestimates the size of the sinus.[40] A sagittal saw is used to make the bony cuts, and the anterior table is fractured forward, while remaining pedicled at the glabella region by the intact periosteum. The pathology of the sinus can then be directly addressed. The tumor can be removed, and any drilling is done under direct visualization. This is combined with an endoscopic frontal sinusotomy as described above.

In the case of tumor removal, frontal sinus function can be maintained by fashioning silastic sheeting to lay in the sinus with a portion that extends into the frontal recess (see Figure 18). This can be removed 6 months later, after the completion of wound healing. This has been shown to maintain frontal sinus aeration even in the setting of significant frontal sinus pathology.[39]

Patients who have had frontal sinus obliteration warrant specific consideration. It is common for these patients to have significant pain, pain for which the obliteration may have been the

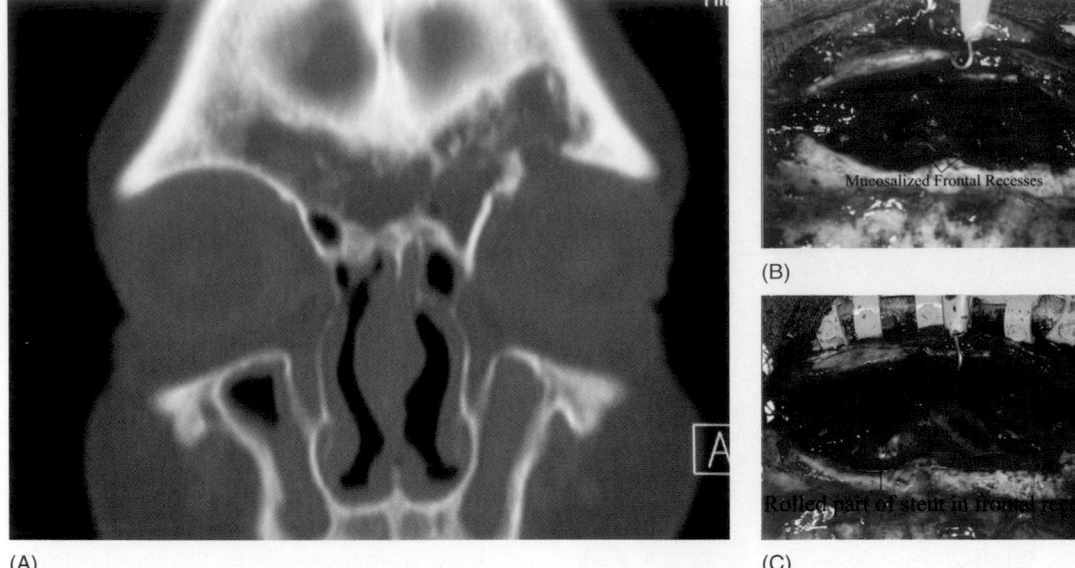

Figure 27 (A) CT scan of a patient with a previous frontal obliteration and significant forehead pain. (B) Osteoplastic flap was performed which revealed extensive areas of mucosa and mucopurulent debris in the frontal recesses and low in the frontal sinus as well as pockets of mucus in the periphery of the sinus. (C) Silastic was cut to the shape of the frontal sinus and rolled into each frontal recess to be removed endoscopically.

initial indication. In these patients it is difficult to determine if there are trapped areas of mucus or pus that are symptomatic but not expansile. This is a particular worry when there is extensive supraorbital pneumatization that would have been difficult or impossible to obliterate successfully at the initial procedure. Unfortunately, interpretation of imaging in these patients is difficult, and referral to a rhinologist should be considered. However, if there is clear radiographic evidence of an expansile process, a frontal mucopyocele will need to be addressed endoscopically or via an osteoplastic flap (Figure 26).

When these sinuses are addressed via an osteoplastic flap, it is common to find a large collection of mucopus in a mucosal lined portion of the frontal sinus, multiple pockets of mucopus throughout the sinus, mucopus in an obstructed supraorbital cell, and/or mucopurulent debris above scar in the frontal recess but below the frontal sinus. These mucosal lined spaces

should be connected to the nose utilizing silastic sheeting and stenting as the conduit (Figure 27). Reobliteration can also be considered but is realistically no more likely to result in a cure at a second attempt.

As stated, above, the frontal sinus obliteration has been championed for decades as the gold standard for the management of frontal sinus disease. At present, it should be used sparingly, and if considered a referral to a rhinologist should also be considered. Additionally, there are many situations in which frontal sinus obliteration should be avoided. The principle behind these contraindications is that an obliterated frontal sinus is impossible to image postobliteration and it is difficult, if not impossible, to remove all the mucosa of the frontal sinus.[25] Relative contraindications to frontal obliteration include: frontal sinus tumors, polypoid eosinophilic inflammatory disease of the frontal sinus, extensive supraorbital pnuematization, frontal sinus posterior

table dehiscence and orbital roof dehiscence.[25] In the setting of tumors, obliterating the site of the tumor is oncologically unsound as visualization and observation is not possible. Obliteration for inflammatory polypoid disease does not address the actual pathology. In cases of dehiscent frontal sinus walls, it is impossible to remove the mucosa that is adherent to the dura or periorbita. In these patients, it is better to maximize drainage into the nose and create a large frontal sinusotomy that allows for endoscopic visualization and radiographic imaging. There are limited circumstances, however, when obliteration of a small frontal sinus without extensive supraorbital pnuematization may be an option of last resort.

Lastly, frontal sinus cranialization is a procedure that has a limited role in the setting of frontal sinus management in certain craniofacial approaches to the skull base. It is used for comminuted frontal sinus fractures as well. There are some, however, who argue that the risk of intracranial mucopyoceles exceeds the risk of a frontal mucocele and that these frontal sinuses can be successfully managed conservatively after repair of the dura.[25] The frontal sinus can be drained into the nose at the initial setting or subsequently. However, the standard of care of the management of these complex frontal sinus issues has yet to be determined in the era of endoscopic management of sinus disease. At present, a conservative approach to anterior table fractures has been advocated by Smith, and colleagues[41] (Figure 28).

POSTOPERATIVE CARE

Postoperative care is crucial to the success of revision and frontal sinus surgery. In the revision cavity, areas of previous scarring are prone to scar again and must be attended carefully. Early suctioning of clot, removal of bone fragments and lyses of adhesions are critical. Furthermore, if frontal sinus surgery is going to be successful, comfort with frontal debridement and having the appropriate equipment for debridement are essential.

CONCLUSIONS

The field of rhinology is in its adolescence and continues to evolve. Technology is continuously advancing, as is the knowledge regarding the complexity of disease management. However, certain tenets of surgery remain unchanged: (1) operate from known to unknown; (2) maintain visualization and appropriate instrumentation at all times; and, above all else, (3) do no harm. These basics must be applied to all sinus surgery, particularly revision and frontal sinus surgery, within each individual practitioner's limitations.

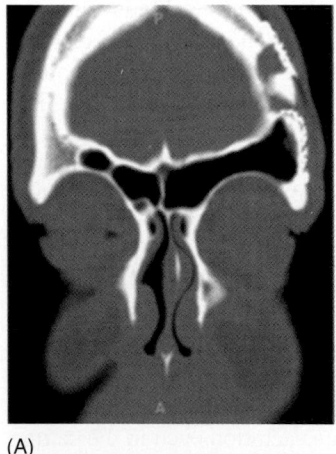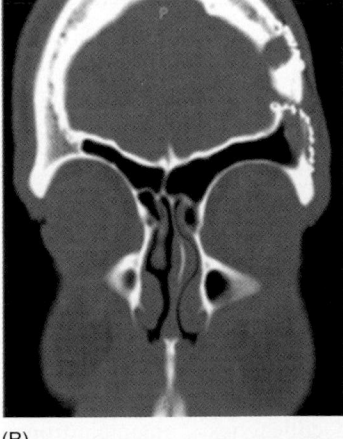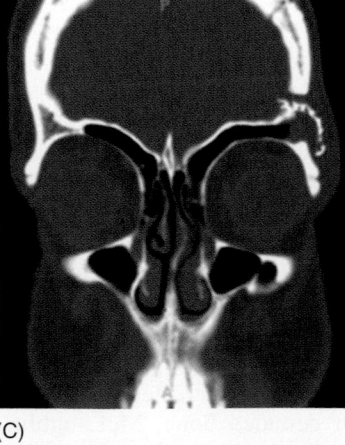

Figure 28 Computed tomographic scan of a patient 1 year after conservative management of iatrogenic trauma to the left frontal sinus from a craniotomy. The mucosa of the sinus was carefully preserved, and the communication to the intracranial cavity was plugged with fascia and reinforced with a titanium plate. A computed tomography scan was obtained 3 months after injury and 1 year after injury, which showed stable scarring of the lateral part of the frontal sinus with no evidence of an expansile process.

REFERENCES

1. Senior BA, Kennedy DW, Tanabodee J, et al. Long-term results of functional endoscopic sinus surgery. Laryngoscope 1998;108:151–7.

2. Meltzer EO, Hamilos DL, Hadley JA, et al. Rhinosinusitis: Establishing definitions for clinical research and patient care. Otolaryngol Head Neck Surg 2004;131:S1–62.

3. Bernstein JM, Kansal R. Superantigen hypothesis for the early development of chronic hyperplastic sinusitis with massive nasal polyposis. Curr Opin Otolaryngol Head Neck Surg 2005;13:39–44.

4. Cryer J, Schipor I, Perloff JR, et al. Evidence of bacterial biofilms in human chronic sinusitis. ORL J Otorhinolaryngol Relat Spec 2004;66:155–8.

5. Kennedy DW, Senior BA, Gannon FH, et al. Histology and histomorphometry of ethmoid bone in chronic rhinosinusitis. Laryngoscope 1998;108:502–7.

6. Lane AP, Truong-Tran QA, Schleimer RP. Altered expression of genes associated with innate immunity and inflammation in recalcitrant rhinosinusitis with polyps. Am J Rhinol 2006;20:138–44.

7. Perloff JR, Gannon FH, Bolger WE, et al. Bone involvement in sinusitis: An apparent pathway for the spread of disease. Laryngoscope 2000;110:2095–9.

8. Sherris DA, Ponikau JU, Kern EB. Eosinophilic mucin rhinosinusitis. Laryngoscope 2001;111:1670–2.

9. Kaplan BA, Kountakis SE. Role of nasal endoscopy in patients undergoing endoscopic sinus surgery. Am J Rhinol 2004;18:161–4.

10. Coffey CS, Sonnenburg RE, Melroy CT, et al. Endoscopically guided aerobic cultures in postsurgical patients with chronic rhinosinusitis. Am J Rhinol 2006;20:72–6.

11. Chiu AG, Vaughan WC. Revision endoscopic frontal sinus surgery with surgical navigation. Otolaryngol Head Neck Surg 2004;130:312–8.

12. Chu CT, Lebowitz RA, Jacobs JB. An analysis of sites of disease in revision endoscopic sinus surgery. Am J Rhinol 1997;11:287–91.

13. Musy PY, Kountakis SE. Anatomic findings in patients undergoing revision endoscopic sinus surgery. Am J Otolaryngol 2004;25:418–22.

14. Parsons DS, Stivers FE, Talbot AR. The missed ostium sequence and the surgical approach to revision functional endoscopic sinus surgery. Otolaryngol Clin North Am 1996;29:169–83.

15. Ramadan HH. Surgical causes of failure in endoscopic sinus surgery. Laryngoscope 1999;109:27–9.

16. Richtsmeier WJ. Top 10 reasons for endoscopic maxillary sinus surgery failure. Laryngoscope 2001;111:1952–6.

17. Zinreich SJ, Kennedy DW, Rosenbaum AE, et al. Paranasal sinuses: CT imaging requirements for endoscopic surgery. Radiology 1987;163:769–75.

18. Kennedy DW. Functional endoscopic sinus surgery: Anesthesia, technique and postoperative management. In: Kennedy DW, Bolger W, Zinreich J, editors. Diseases of the Sinuses. London: BC. Decker; 2001. p. 210–21.

19. Dubin MG, Kuhn FA. Stereotactic computer assisted navigation: State of the art for sinus surgery, not standard of care. Otolaryngol Clin North Am 2005;38:535–49.

20. Bolger WE, Kuhn FA, Kennedy DW. Middle turbinate stabilization after functional endoscopic sinus surgery: The controlled synechiae technique. Laryngoscope 1999;109:1852–3.

21. Bolger WE, Keyes AS, Lanza DC. Use of the superior meatus and superior turbinate in the endoscopic approach to the sphenoid sinus. Otolaryngol Head Neck Surg 1999;120:308–13.

22. Orlandi RR, Lanza DC, Bolger WE, et al. The forgotten turbinate: The role of the superior turbinate in endoscopic sinus surgery. Am J Rhinol 1999;13:251–9.

23. Millar DA, Orlandi RR. The sphenoid sinus natural ostium is consistently medial to the superior turbinate. Am J Rhinol 2006;20:180–1.

24. Kennedy DW, Zinreich J, Hassab M. The internal carotid artery as it relates to endonasal sphenoethmoidectomy. Am J Rhinol 1990;4:7.

25. Kuhn FA. An integrated approach to frontal sinus surgery. Otolaryngol Clin North Am 2006;39:437–61, viii.

26. Messerklinger W. On the drainage of the normal frontal sinus of man. Acta Otolaryngol 1967;63:176–81.

27. Lee WT, Kuhn FA, Citardi MJ. 3D computed tomographic analysis of frontal recess anatomy in patients without frontal sinusitis. Otolaryngol Head Neck Surg 2004;131:164–73.

28. Neel HB, Whicker JH, Lake CF. Thin rubber sheeting in frontal sinus surgery: Animal and clinical studies. Laryngoscope 1976;86:524–36.

29. Bolger WE, Vaughan WC. Catheter-based dilation of the sinus ostia: Initial safety and feasibility analysis in a cadaver model. Am J Rhinol 2006;20:290–4.

30. Kuhn FA, Javer AR, Nagpal K, et al. The frontal sinus rescue procedure: Early experience and three-year follow-up. Am J Rhinol 2000;14:211–6.

31. Citardi MJ, Javer AR, Kuhn FA. Revision endoscopic frontal sinusotomy with mucoperiosteal flap advancement: The frontal sinus rescue procedure. Otolaryngol Clin North Am 2001;34:123–32.

32. Draf W. Endonasal micro-endoscopic frontal sinus surgery: The Fulda concept. Oper Tech Otolaryngol Head Neck Surg 1991;2:234–40.

33. Bent JP, 3rd, Spears RA, Kuhn FA, et al. Combined endoscopic intranasal and external frontal sinusotomy. Am J Rhinol 1997;11:349–54.

34. Gross WE, Gross CW, Becker D, et al. Modified transnasal endoscopic Lothrop procedure as an alternative to frontal sinus obliteration. Otolaryngol Head Neck Surg 1995;113:427–34.

35. McLaughlin RB, Hwang PH, Lanza DC. Endoscopic transseptal frontal sinusotomy: The rationale and results of an alternative technique. Am J Rhinol 1999;13:279–87.

36. Dubin MG, Kuhn FA. Endoscopic modified Lothrop (Draf III) with frontal sinus punches. Laryngoscope 2005;115:1702–3.

37. Farhat FT, Figueroa RE, Kountakis SE. Anatomic measurements for the endoscopic modified Lothrop procedure. Am J Rhinol 2005;19:293–6.

38. Goodale RI, Montgomery WW. Technical advances in osteoplastic frontal sinusectomy. Arch Otolaryngol 1964:522–29.

39. Dubin MG, Kuhn FA. Preservation of natural frontal sinus outflow in the management of frontal sinus osteomas. Otolaryngol Head Neck Surg 2006;134:18–24.

40. Melroy CT, Dubin MG, Hardy SM, et al. Analysis of methods to assess frontal sinus extent in osteoplastic flap surgery: Transillumination versus 6-ft Caldwell versus image guidance. Am J Rhinol 2006;20:77–83.

41. Smith TL, Han JK, Loehrl TA, et al. Endoscopic management of the frontal recess in frontal sinus fractures: A shift in the paradigm? Laryngoscope 2002;112:784–90.

51

Endoscopic Surgery of the Skull Base, Orbits and Benign Sinonasal Neoplasms

Brent A. Senior, MD
John Alldredge, MD

As the experience and success of endoscopic sinus surgery for benign, inflammatory conditions have increased over the past two decades, so too have its applications. The indications for endoscopic sinus surgery have broadened to include the treatment of a variety of orbital conditions, repair of cerebrospinal fluid (CSF) leaks, and resection of sinonasal and skull base tumors. Endoscopic surgical techniques provide improved visualization and magnification over traditional open procedures and when combined with modern computed tomography (CT) scanning, magnetic resonance imaging (MRI), and image guidance, result in less morbidity and bleeding, no need for external incisions, and shorter hospital stays than external surgical approaches.[1,2]

ENDOSCOPIC CEREBROSPINAL FLUID LEAK REPAIR

Central to extended application of endoscopic surgery for skull base and orbital lesions is management of CSF leaks. The repair of CSF leaks has evolved tremendously over the past several decades. In 1926, Dandy first described intracranial repair of an anterior skull base CSF fistula via a frontal craniotomy. Advantages of the intracranial approach include the direct visualization of a dural tear and ability to treat an adjacent injury and to use a vascularized pericranial flap in repair of the defect. Among the disadvantages, however, are the need for a large external incision, high risk of anosmia, need for frontal lobe retraction, and the risk of intracranial hemorrhage.[3,4] This type of intracranial approach, with a quoted success rate of between 60 to 80% became the standard for many decades and is still frequently utilized today.[5,6] In 1948, Dohlman performed the first extracranial repair of a CSF fistula via a naso-orbital incision. This extracranial approach was taken a step further in 1952, when Hirsch performed the first transnasal approach. In 1981, Wigand reported the first endoscopic repair of a CSF leak.[7] Since that time, minimally invasive surgical approaches have been refined, and diagnostic tests and equipment improved. High success rates greater than 90% and low morbidity have led to the minimally invasive endoscopic approach becoming the standard of care for repair of CSF leaks.[8–10]

To ensure successful endoscopic repair and management of CSF leaks, one must have an understanding of normal CSF physiology. Most of CSF (70%) is formed from the choroid plexus in the lateral, third, and fourth ventricles, with the remaining 30% produced from a combination of capillary ultrafiltration and water metabolism.[11,12] CSF is produced at a rate of 20 mL/h or 350 to 500 mL/d; the total volume of CSF in a person at any one time is about 90 to 150 mL, as the volume is turned over approximately three to five times each day. Normally, the CSF flows from the lateral ventricles, to the third and fourth ventricles, and finally into the subarachnoid space surrounding the brain and spinal cord. CSF absorption occurs via the arachnoid villi which act as one-way valves for CSF flow into the connecting dural sinuses. A pressure gradient of 1.5 to 7 cm H_2O is required for anterograde flow; anything less causes closure of the valves, preventing retrograde flow. Normal CSF pressures measured in the lumbar cistern with the patient lying in the decubitus position vary with respiration but range from 5 to 15 cm H_2O. Reasons for variation include age, time of day, and activity level. Neurologic symptoms may develop with pressures exceeding 15 to 20 cm H_2O.[11,12]

The cause of a suspected CSF leak must also be taken into account before making any decisions regarding definitive treatment or management. CSF leaks occur in approximately 1 to 3% of all closed head injuries, usually presenting between 2 days and 3 months after the initial insult.[11,13] As an estimated 70% of these CSF leaks may close without surgical treatment, initial conservative management includes elevation of the head of bed, strict bed rest, stool softeners, and possibly a lumbar drain. Surprisingly, despite the high closure rate of posttraumatic CSF leaks with conservative therapy, long-term follow-up has shown a 30 to 40% incidence of ascending meningitis in these patients. This may be secondary to closure with only a thin layer of fibrous tissue or mucosa, as dura lacks the capacity to regenerate.[10,14]

The most common causes of iatrogenic CSF leaks are functional endoscopic sinus surgery and neurological surgery. In sinus surgery, iatrogenic injuries may result from bone resection with or without powered instrumentation, resulting in a variety of leaks ranging from pinpoint disruption of dural sheaths surrounding olfactory fila to large leaks greater than 2 cm in size; however, injuries that might have been minor or inconsequential with more traditional instruments, may prove to be major when created as a result of a misuse of powered instrumentation. The recent increased use of powered instrumentation has also led to devastating injuries of the orbit, optic nerve, and carotid artery.[15] These iatrogenic leaks created as a result of endoscopic sinus surgery usually occur at the lateral lamella of the cribriform or the posterior ethmoid roof. The lateral lamella of the cribriform plate is thin, and injuries usually occur when dissecting in the frontal recess or resecting the middle turbinate too close to the skull base. It is particularly susceptible to injury in the setting of a deep olfactory fossa resulting from a tall lateral lamella, a feature that should be sought out on preoperative computed tomographic scanning. It is similarly susceptible when asymmetry of the ethmoid roof is present with one side much higher than the other, potentially leading an operator to dissect too high.

Injury to the posterior ethmoid roof may occur in the presence of a low roof or a highly pneumatized maxillary sinus that extends superomedially, resulting in a relative decrease in the height of the posterior ethmoid roof.[10] Injury to the sella diaphragm during transsphenoidal pituitary surgery is the most common cause of iatrogenic CSF leak encountered during neurological surgery.[16]

Both intracranial and sinonasal tumors may lead to CSF leak directly or indirectly. Invasion of tumors across the skull base with resultant destruction can lead to large defects. Treatment of such tumors with surgery, radiation, and chemotherapy may also lead to devascularization of the adjacent tissue, resulting in a difficult to repair skull-base defect. Tumors may also obstruct CSF outflow causing an increased intracranial pressure (ICP), hydrocephalus, and a resultant CSF leak. Treatment of these leaks must first be directed toward the primary tumor to correct obstruction. Repairing a leak without first treating an obstructing lesion may elevate an already increased ICP by closing off the relief valve created by the CSF fistula.[10] In some situations, long-term shunting may be needed.

Congenital CSF leaks are somewhat rare. They usually result from defects at the foramen cecum or cribriform plate, presenting with a meningoencephalocele.[17] Any underlying congenital hydrocephalus must also be treated prior to repair of the skull-base defect.[10]

CSF leaks, for which no cause can be identified, are classified as being "spontaneous" CSF leaks. Over the past several years, studies have demonstrated that many of these patients may actually have a form of benign intracranial hypertension, with an ICP predisposing them to "spontaneous" CSF leaks.[11] These patients tend to be obese, middle-aged females with pulsatile tinnitus and pressure headaches. Imaging studies often reveal an expanded, empty sella, and multiple small defects along the skull base. The chronically elevated intracranial pressures lead to CSF leaks in the weakest areas of the skull base, mainly the ethmoid roof, cribriform plate, and lateral recess of the sphenoid sinus.[12,18,19] Multiple, small defects may be present in an often rather attenuated skull base. In addition to elevated intracranial pressures, these patients are also prone to large meningoencephaloceles protruding through the small bony defects. All of these factors contribute to the higher recurrence rates of "spontaneous" leaks as compared to other causes.[10]

Once a CSF leak is suspected, diagnosis and localization of the leak can be challenging. Several studies and tests can aid in these tasks. If a patient presents with a history of multiple episodes of meningitis, headache after blowing their nose, and obvious unilateral salty tasting clear rhinorrhea, the nasal secretions can be collected and sent for beta-2 transferrin analysis; this protein is only found in CSF, perilymph, and aqueous humor. Although this test will not reveal the location of the leak, only 0.17 mL is required, and false positives are rare.[10,20] Beta-trace protein, which is the second most abundant protein in CSF, may be an alternative to beta-2 transferrin, as it is a less costly and quicker test. Used mainly in Europe, its use in the United States has been mostly limited to research.[21,22]

High resolution thin-cut axial and coronal computed tomography scans are invaluable for locating suspected skull base defects. Although these scans cannot definitively diagnose a leak, they may reveal subtle skull base dehiscences suggestive of leak origin. Radioactive cisternograms may also be helpful in both diagnosis and localization of a CSF leak. In this study, pledgets are placed intranasally for several hours after intrathecal injection of a radioactive tracer. A diagnosis can be made and a rough location of the leak can be determined by the location of the pledgets positive for the radioactive tracer. Although not used often, this test may be particularly useful for slow or intermittent leaks as the pledgets stay in for several hours.

Another imaging modality, CT cisternography, requiring a lumbar puncture for the instillation of intrathecal contrast, may also be helpful in diagnosing and identifying CSF leaks. This modality may be particularly beneficial in identification of leaks in the frontal recess and sphenoid sinus where contrast pooling may occur over time. MRI and MRI cisternograms are noninvasive studies that do not require intrathecal contrast; they may be a helpful complement to high resolution thin-cut axial and coronal computed tomography in identifying CSF leaks, especially if an intracranial lesion or neoplasm is suspected.[10–12,23,24]

Preoperative injection of intrathecal fluorescein can be useful in the diagnosis and localization of a CSF leak prior to repair (Figure 1). This can, of course, be placed in conjunction with insertion of a lumbar catheter in selected cases for use in the perioperative period. Intrathecal fluorescein may be a sensitive study if adequate exposure of the skull base is obtained to ensure optimal visualization; the use of a blue light filter on the endoscopic light source may also increase accuracy in difficult cases. When utilizing this technique, it is important to use a minimal concentration of fluorescein so as to avoid seizures and other unwanted neurologic side effects. A solution of 0.1 mL of 10% fluorescein diluted in 10 mL of autologous CSF or injectable saline has been used safely and efficaciously around the world; however, it is not approved by the US Food and Drug Administration for this purpose.[10,12]

In some cases of CSF leak repair, particularly spontaneous and high pressure leaks, a lumbar drain may be utilized. Initial placement of the lumbar drain may prove somewhat difficult for patients with significant leaks. Placement in this situation can be assisted by either placing the drain before intubation with the patient in the upright sitting position or after intubation with the head of the bed elevated. Before graft placement, 10 to 15 mL of CSF drained from the lumbar catheter may facilitate graft positioning. Once the graft is placed, and the repair is complete, the drain should be kept open, draining 5 to 10 mL/h. Lumbar drains are usually left in for 48 to 72 hours postoperatively, with the first 24 hours being the most important. They can be clamped for approximately 24 hours to ensure that no leak is present with mobilization of the patient before removal. If a leak is present, they may be left in place for 2 to 4 more days or the patient can be taken back to the operating room for exploration of the persistent leak.[10] Surgeons must be aware of the complications associated with the use of lumbar drains including meningitis and air-siphoning with resultant pneumocephalus. Pneumocephalus is a greater risk in the setting of large skull base defects, seen frequently in the setting of trauma.

One must also avoid positive pressure ventilation when repairing CSF fistulas. Positive pressure ventilation carries the risk of pneumocephalus, which can be fatal.[10] A "deep-extubation" or extubation under deep anesthesia is also preferred so as to avoid any coughing and/ or straining that might occur during extubation; this may cause a sudden increase in ICP and displace grafting materials.[24] The use of antibiotics is somewhat controversial; the author chooses to use perioperative antibiotics, such as ceftriaxone or vancomycin, which have suitable penetration across the blood–brain barrier. Antibiotics are generally continued as long as nasal packing remains in place.

The specific approach to a CSF leak is determined by its proper identification and exact location. Transnasal endoscopic surgery for CSF leaks of the cribriform plate and ethmoid roof begins with adequate decongestion with topical oxymetazoline (0.05%) and injection of 1% lidocaine with epinephrine (1:100,000). Next, a standard endoscopic total ethmoidectomy and maxillary antrostomy are performed to maximize exposure. In addition, a sphenoidotomy, frontal sinusotomy, or middle turbinate resection may be performed for exposure purposes but more importantly to prevent postobstructive mucoceles.[10,12]

For sphenoid sinus lesions, location is of utmost importance (Figure 2). Centrally located leaks can usually be repaired with an endoscopic transethmoid or transsphenoid approach. After a wide sphenoidotomy is performed, resection of the posterior nasal septum and intersinus septum may further improve visualization. Lesions located in the lateral recess of the sphenoid can be more challenging. Although most can be reached with a combination of a transethmoid approach and various angled endoscopes and instruments, some may require a transpterygoid approach. In this approach, the posterior wall of the maxillary sinus is removed after endoscopic sphenoethmoidectomy and maxillary antrostomy are performed. Next, the pterygopalatine fossa is entered, and the main branches of the internal maxillary artery are identified, and clipped or cauterized. Great care is taken to preserve the vidian nerve, infraorbital nerve, and sphenopalatine ganglia. The periosteum of the commonly pneumatized pterygoid plates is then elevated. Finally, the bone of the anterior face of the sphenoid is drilled or curetted away to gain access to the lateral recess of the sphenoid sinus.[1,25]

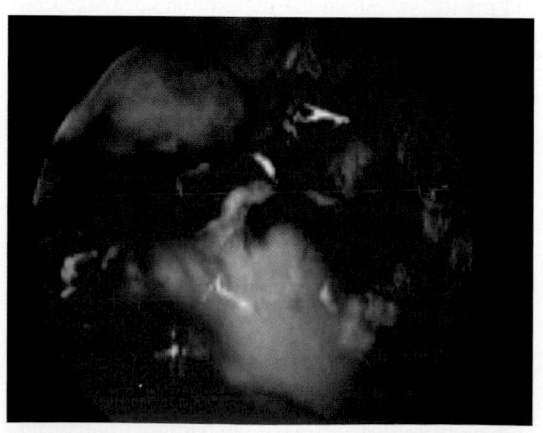

Figure 1 Intrathecal fluorescein is used to locate a cerebrospinal fluid leak located in the left sphenoid sinus.

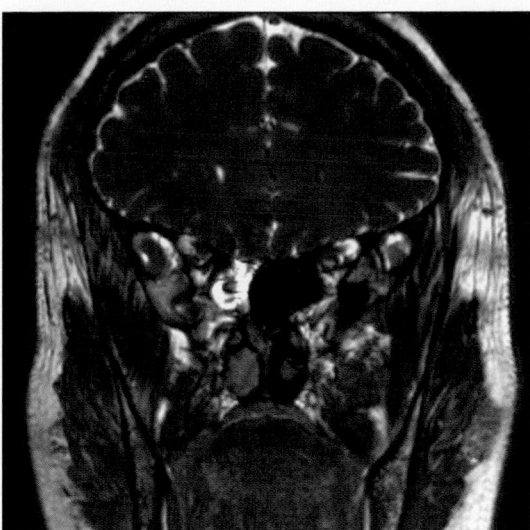

Figure 2 T2 weighted magnetic resonance imaging demonstrating a right sphenoid meningoencephalocele.

Frontal sinus leaks can be divided into those adjacent to the frontal recess, involving the frontal recess, or involving the frontal sinus proper. Leaks located just posterior to the frontal recess in the anterior ethmoid roof can usually be repaired endoscopically; a complete frontal sinus dissection should be performed in these cases to avoid a postobstructive mucocele. CSF leaks that involve the frontal recess itself can often be repaired with a combined endoscopic and open technique or "above-and-below" approach. Although endoscopic techniques and equipment are constantly evolving, CSF leaks that involve the frontal sinus proper, especially the lateral and superior walls, usually require an osteoplastic flap for adequate exposure. Endoscopic Draf 3 procedures or modified Lothrop procedures, which resect the floor of the frontal sinus combined with frontal trephination, are useful adjunctive procedures for lesions that extend into the frontal recess from the frontal sinus.[10,12]

Although repairs of CSF leaks and encephaloceles have an approximately 90% success rate when repaired endoscopically, open extracranial approaches involving a traditional craniotomy may be necessary in patients with multiple, large skull base defects or large tumors with extensive intracranial extension.[11]

In all cases of repair, after the leak has been identified and maximal exposure obtained, the surgical site is carefully prepared by removing several millimeters of mucosa surrounding the defect until the entire surrounding bone edges are exposed. At this point, if an encephalocele is present, it is reduced and fulgurated to the level of the skull base with a flexible bipolar-suction cautery (Figures 3 and 4). Great care is taken to achieve optimal hemostasis so as to avoid retraction and intracranial hemorrhage. After this is done, 10 to 15 mL of CSF may be drained from the lumbar drain before graft placement. The drain is then set to a continuous drainage of 5 to 10 mL/h.[10]

The decision of how to repair the actual defect depends on the size of the defect, the cause of the leak, and the ICP.[11] Smaller defects (1 to 3 mm)

can usually be repaired with a soft tissue overlay graft, whereas larger defects (>3 to 4 mm) may require multiple layers of repair. Large defects, and smaller defects with an accompanying elevated ICP (Figure 5) should be repaired with a more rigid underlay graft, followed by a soft tissue overlay graft.[10]

When using an underlay graft, adjacent dura is optimally elevated from the skull base. This, of course, is performed intracranially, and smaller otologic instruments are often useful. Once adequate elevation of the dura has been achieved, a rigid or soft tissue graft can be gently placed within the epidural space; this may be followed by an external overlay soft tissue graft. Once the tissue grafts are in place, a thin layer of fibrin glue or microfibrillar collagen may be applied to maximize graft adherence (Figure 6). Only a small amount of material is used; however, as too much may prevent remucosalization and actually impair healing of the repair. Multiple layers of absorbable packing follow graft placement.[4,10] Ultimately, a nonabsorbable packing, such as a Merocel sponge, is placed for added support of the repair site and allowed to remain for several days. These multi-layered types of closures are used to maximize grafting success, ensure a more watertight closure to prevent meningitis, and add rigid structural support to the repair site, thus preventing future herniation of intracranial contents. Studies have shown that free mucosal grafts act as a sort of scaffolding and adhere to overlying bone at 1 week; they are replaced by fibrous tissue by 3 weeks.[10,26]

Various free grafting materials can be used in the repair of skull base defects, as none has shown to be consistently superior to others. Common rigid grafts include septal bone, septal cartilage, turbinate bone, and mastoid cortex. Soft tissue grafting materials include septal mucosa, temporalis fascia, turbinate mucosa, abdominal fat, fascia lata, pericardium, alloplastic collagen, and cadaveric dermis. Composite grafts consisting of turbinate bone and mucosa have also been used successfully. One must remember that if a mucosal graft is used, the mucosal side of the graft must be directed extracranially, so as to avoid serious intracranial complications such

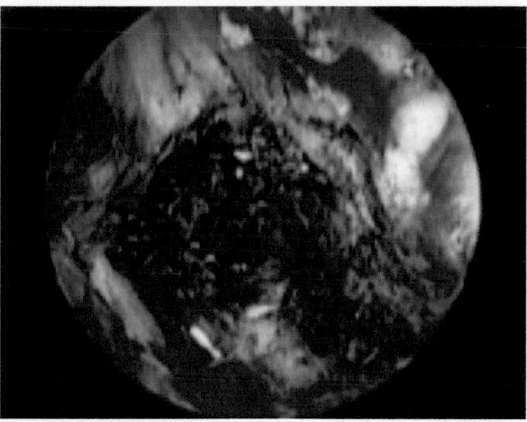

Figure 4 A flexible bipolar suction cautery was used to fulgurate a right frontoethmoid encephalocele to the level of the skull base.

as mucocele formation and meningitis.[4,10,23,27,28] For this reason, a surgical marking pen is used to make a blue dot on the mucosal surface of the graft so as to avoid any confusion when placing the graft into tight spaces.

As mentioned previously, "spontaneous" CSF leaks represent a difficult, distinct clinical entity and deserve additional discussion. In fact, while endoscopic repair of "nonspontaneous" CSF leaks may enjoy only a 10% recurrence rate, that is, 90% success rate, the rate of recurrence for "spontaneous" leaks can be anywhere from 25 to 87%.[16,29–31] So, although most patients who have undergone CSF leak repair do not require long-term CSF diversion, it should be considered in patients with "spontaneous leaks."[4,32–34] These "spontaneous" CSF leaks may be classified as being "high-pressure" leaks. Clinically, they may represent a form of benign intracranial hypertension, as patients are often middle-age obese females who present with pressure-type headaches, pulsatile tinnitus, balance problems, and visual disturbances.[11] Radiographically, these patients with increased ICP may have an empty sella syndrome, where the elevated ICP may lead to dural herniation through the sella diaphragm into the sella turcica, giving the appearance of an absent pituitary.[35] Dilated temporal horns and ventricles may also be noted on CT scans of the head in these patients.[4] This elevated ICP may

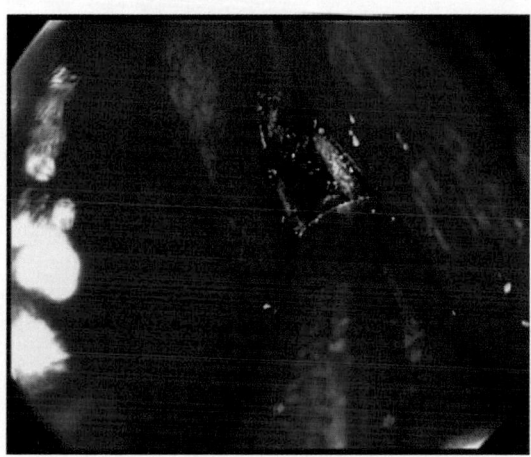

Figure 3 A flexible bipolar suction cautery is used to cauterize a meningocele of the left cribriform plate.

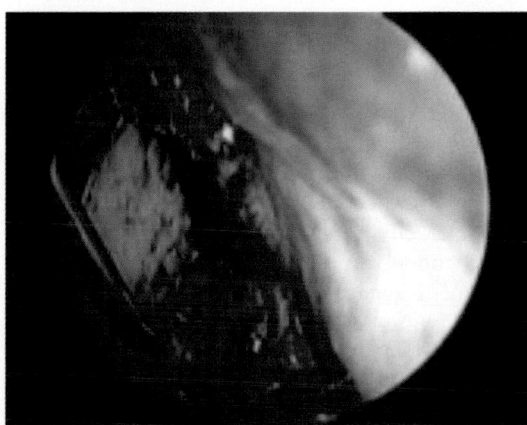

Figure 5 A cartilage underlay graft is placed to provide rigid support during repair of right frontoethmoid cerebrospinal fluid leak.

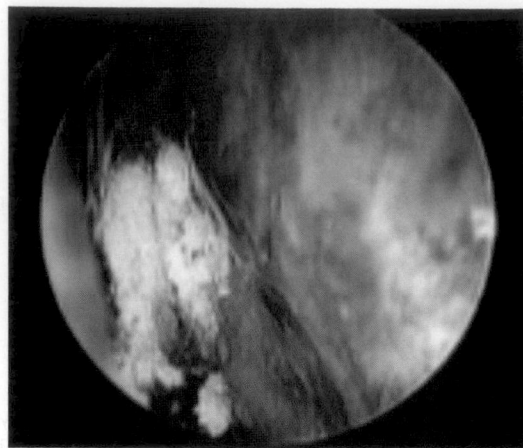

Figure 6 Microfibrillar collagen is packed over a mucosal underlay graft for additional support.

be transmitted by pulsatile hydrostatic forces to the weaker areas of the skull base such as the ethmoid roof, cribriform plate, and especially the lateral recess of the sphenoid sinus which is often extensively pneumatized.[1,12,27]

Schlosser and colleagues have recommended routinely placing lumbar drains in the setting of spontaneous CSF leaks at the time of surgery.[33] This approach facilitates removal of CSF immediately before repair, confirmation of a watertight seal after repair, CSF diversion in the immediate postoperative period, and making decisions regarding long-term management. By measuring CSF pressures on postoperative day 2 through the already indwelling lumbar drain, they confirmed that most patients with "spontaneous" leaks had an elevated ICP with the mean pressure being over twice the upper limit of normal; in addition, they recognized that patients with "traumatic" leaks had lower ICPs. Patients with "spontaneous" leaks noted to have elevated ICPs, can be given a challenge of intravenous acetazolamide. The lumbar drain can be reopened to monitor the effect of the diuretic on ICP. If the pressure is lowered appropriately (<10 cm H_2O), the lumbar drain can be removed, and the patient started on oral diuretic therapy. If the ICP is not lowered appropriately or remains elevated (>35 cm H_2O), neurosurgical consultation can be obtained for long-term diversion via placement of a ventriculoperitoneal shunt. In this way, lumbar drains and measurement of ICPs can aid in the long-term management of patients with "spontaneous" CSF leaks.[33]

Postoperatively, patients are kept on strict bed rest, especially when a lumbar drain is in place. The patient is placed on stool softeners with the head of the bed elevated approximately 30° to decrease CSF pressure at the repair site. After the lumbar drain is removed, they are instructed to continue to sneeze with an open mouth and avoid nose-blowing, Valsalva maneuvers, heavy lifting, and strenuous activity for up to 4 weeks. After this, they are restricted to only light activity for the next 4 weeks. Patients are seen 1 week postoperatively when any nonabsorbable packs are removed and minimal debridement is performed. Thereafter, they are then seen every 1 to 2 weeks

for debridement, suctioning, and routine postoperative management so as to avoid infection, mucus stasis, and crusting. Of course, great care is taken to avoid any manipulation of the repair site.

ENDOSCOPIC SURGERY OF THE ORBIT

Orbital Decompression

In 1990, Kennedy and colleagues described transnasal endoscopic orbital decompression for Graves orbitopathy, also known as dysthyroid orbitopathy.[36] Graves disease is an autoimmune disorder that can affect the thyroid gland, as well as the orbit. In Graves disease, autoantibodies to thyrotropin receptors in the thyroid gland result in over stimulation of the gland and subsequent hyperthyroidism. Orbital manifestations result from pronounced inflammation, migration of T-cells, and deposition of glycosaminoglycans. This can lead to enlargement of orbital fat content and extraocular muscles, resulting in increased orbital pressure, proptosis, and possible optic nerve compression (Figure 7). Symptoms of Graves orbitopathy may include tearing, proptosis, diplopia, and visual loss. Graves disease can also be classified as either acute or chronic. Active inflammation for 6 to 18 months marks the acute phase; symptoms are initially treated with local conservative measures such as taping and lubrication. In severe cases, systemic corticosteroids or radiation may be considered. The chronic phase involves severe fibrosis of orbital contents and may respond to surgical management.[37] Indications for endoscopic orbital decompression include visual changes as well as severe proptosis resulting in exposure keratitis or cosmetic deformity.

An orbital decompression is begun by performing a large endoscopic maxillary antrostomy to identify the infraorbital nerve coursing along the roof of the maxillary sinus. This is followed by a total sphenoethmoidectomy and possibly a frontal sinusotomy. Next, the lamina papyracea is gently removed with blunt dissection, taking care to avoid entering the periosteum of the orbit. After the entire medial orbital wall (lamina papyracea) is removed up to the skull base and down to the floor of the orbit, the dissection is taken to the posterior limit at the anulus of Zinn, just anterior to the face of the sphenoid sinus. Anteriorly, the dissection is continued to the nasal lacrimal apparatus. After this is completed, the orbital floor medial to the infraorbital nerve is removed through the maxillary antrostomy. A sickle knife is used to make several parallel incisions through the periorbita beginning posteriorly and superiorly, allowing the orbital contents to prolapse into the sinonasal cavities (Figure 8). Great care is taken to avoid injury to the extraocular muscles during this maneuver.[37] Success rates of these procedures range from 22 to 89%.[36,38,39] Ocular recession as a result of orbital decompression averages approximately 3.5 mm, with an additional 2 mm provided by the addition of lateral decompression.[39] Complications of this technique include diplopia, bleeding, epiphora, CSF leak, and blindness.[37] Of particular concern is chronic sinusitis, and specifically frontal

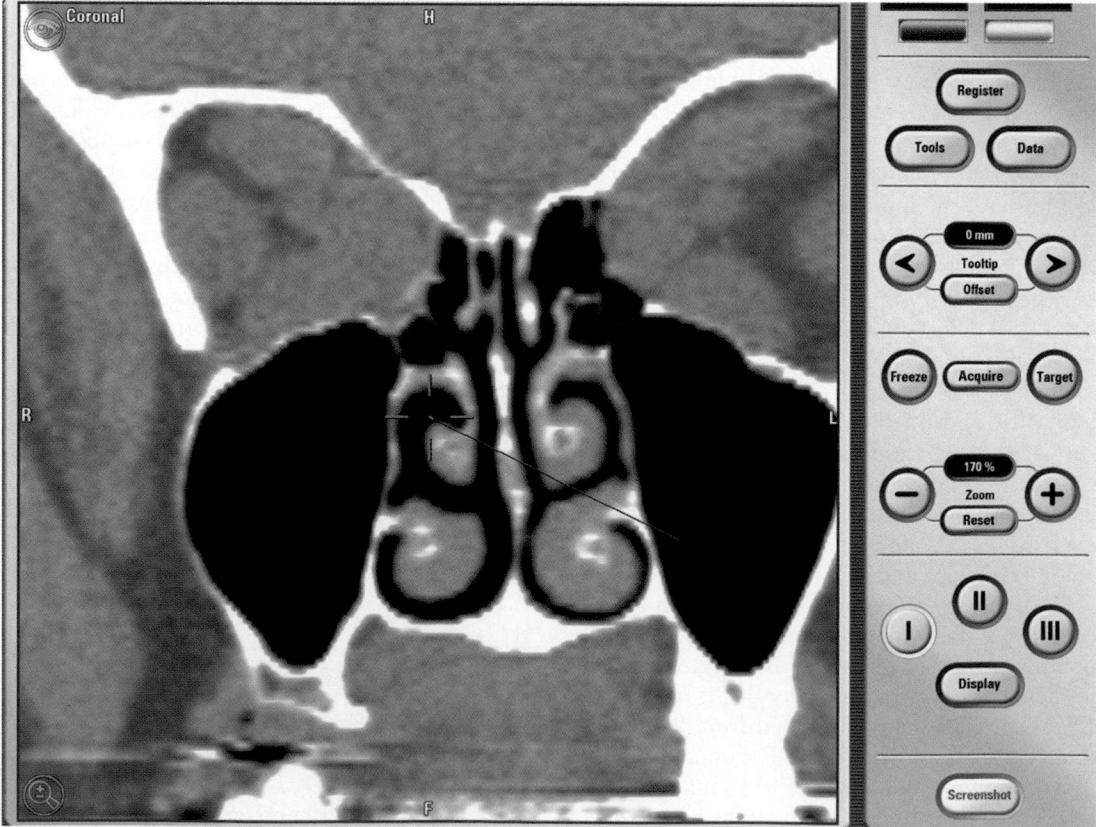

Figure 7 Computed tomography scan showing hypertrophy of extraocular muscles and orbital contents in a patient with Graves orbitopathy.

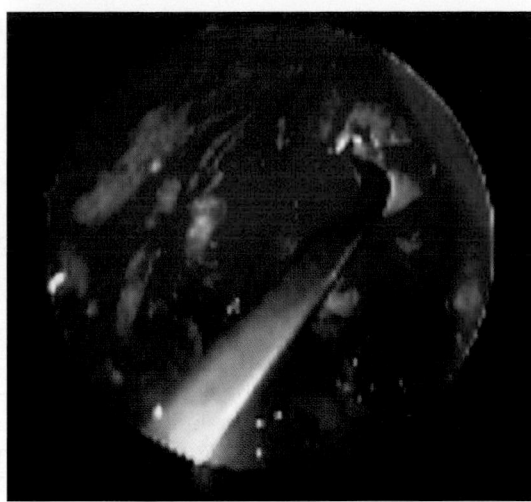

Figure 8 A sickle knife is used to make several posterior to anterior parallel incisions through the periorbita until a prolapse of orbital fat is visualized.

sinusitis, occurring in the presence of prolapsed orbital contents scarring to the middle turbinate. Postoperative debridements are essential to help reduce this risk.

Optic Nerve Decompression

Endoscopic optic nerve decompression can be performed for both traumatic optic neuropathy (TON), as well as for relieving compression from fibro-osseous lesions and various neoplasms. The optic nerve may be injured in 0.5 to 1.5% of all cases of closed head injury that often involve the optic canal[40,41] (Figure 9). The endoscopic approach offers several advantages over more traditional approaches, including decreased morbidity, preservation of olfaction, rapid recovery, no external scars, and less operative stress.[42]

The optic nerve can be divided into three segments: intraorbital, intracanalicular, and intracranial; the main goal in optic nerve decompression is to relieve compression of the intracanalicular portion. The optic canal, which carries both the

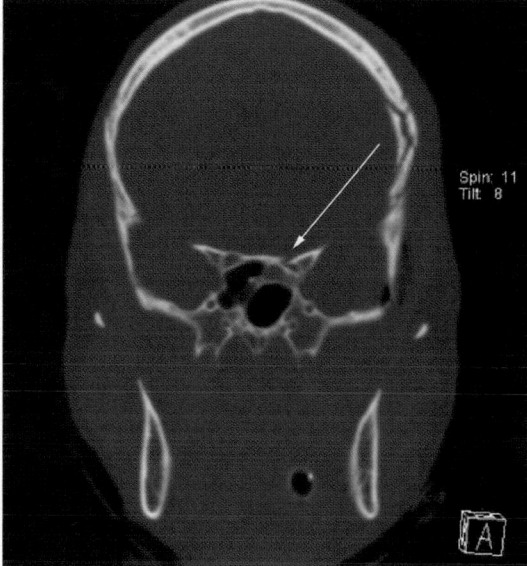

Figure 9 Coronal computed tomography scan showing injury and fracture of the left optic canal in a patient who sustained severe head trauma.

optic nerve and ophthalmic artery, is formed by the lesser wing of the sphenoid bone. The optic nerve is encased by the three meningeal layers within the canal. At the orbital apex, lies the fibrous anulus of Zinn, the most accessible site for nerve compression.[43] Trauma to this fixed intracanalicular segment can be attributed to primary and secondary ischemic injury resulting from shearing and swelling.[41,44] TON is a clinical diagnosis based on a thorough history and physical examination as well as a complete ophthalmologic examination. Once the diagnosis is suspected, high resolution CT scans of the orbit and sphenoid sinus are invaluable in evaluating the optic canal for injury and neural impingement.[41]

The treatment for TON is controversial; in fact, 20 to 38% of these patients will experience spontaneous recovery of vision.[45–48] The benefit of intervention of any kind is unclear. Many authors recommend conservative treatment with corticosteroids to reduce edema and inflammation, while others recommend surgical decompression alone or in combination with corticosteroids. Several reports show a 31 to 82% improvement in vision in patients undergoing surgical intervention with or without corticosteroid therapy.[41,49,50] McMains and Kountakis, however, found that endoscopic optic nerve decompression may be beneficial to patients who have not responded favorably to 48 hours of high-dose corticosteroids.[41] Regardless, the treatment options and management strategies should be individualized to specific patients.

After adequate decongestion and vasoconstriction are achieved, the procedure is begun by performing a standard sphenoethmoidectomy, opening the face of the sphenoid sinus widely. At this point, the bulge of the optic canal may be seen on the lateral wall of the sphenoid sinus, just superior to the internal carotid artery. Alternatively, the nerve may be identified in a posterior sphenoethmoid cell, that is, Onodi cell. At this point, once the optic canal bulge is identified, the lamina papyracea is fractured and removed in an anterior to posterior direction toward the anulus of Zinn. The optic tubercle is a thick buttress of bone formed at the junction of the posterior part of the lamina papyracea and the anterior and lateral walls of the sphenoid sinus; this marks the location of the optic nerve foramen and anulus of Zinn.[41] Once the thick lesser wing of the sphenoid bone of the optic canal is encountered, a diamond burr is used to thin the canal medially, after which a microcurette is used to fracture and remove the thinned bone. The nerve is usually decompressed approximately 1 cm posterior to the face of the sphenoid. Although much controversy exists, the optic nerve sheath can also be opened; this is carefully performed with a sickle knife starting just anterior to the anulus of Zinn in the superiomedial quadrant to avoid injury to the ophthalmic artery.[37] Fibrin glue can be applied to the incision site to prevent CSF leak.[37,42] Extensive packing is avoided so as to assure maximal decompression.[41] The true success rate of optic-nerve decompression is difficult to quantify, as randomized, prospective studies

are lacking; moreover, many patients have significant improvement in vision with observation. Complications of this procedure may include CSF leak, meningitis, and visual loss.[37] Of particular concern is the risk of internal carotid artery injury given the proximity of the vessel to the nerve, and the presence of bony fragments in injuries of this type.

Nasolacrimal Duct Surgery

Historically, surgery for nasolacrimal duct obstruction mainly involved external techniques. In 1989, endoscopic dacryocystorhinostomy (DCR) was described by McDonogh and Meiring.[51] Initially, however, endoscopic techniques yielded somewhat lower success rates than traditional approaches; attributed to an early limited understanding of the anatomy, poor visualization, and suboptimal instrumentation. However, due to continued improvement in these areas, many studies have shown that endoscopic DCR now yields results that are comparable to external procedures.[52–55]

Tearing epiphora results from either excess lacrimation or impairment of drainage. Epiphora can be unilateral, bilateral, constant, or intermittent. It can be associated with many conditions including, midfacial trauma, sinus disease or sinus surgery, as well as systemic disease. Several tests can be used for diagnosis of nasolacrimal duct obstruction: the dye disappearance test, lacrimal system irrigation/probing, scintigraphy, and contrast dacryocystography. The definitive treatment of this difficult problem is DCR.[56]

Knowledge of the anatomy of the nasolacrimal system is of utmost importance when performing surgery on the lacrimal system. The lacrimal sac rests in an oval shaped fossa measuring approximately 15 × 10 mm. The anterior crest of the fossa is formed by the thick frontal process of the maxilla, whereas the posterior crest is formed by the thinner lacrimal bone. The suture line formed by these two bones corresponds to the important maxillary line.[56] A landmark study by Wormald and colleagues in 2000 demonstrated that the lacrimal sac actually lies above the axilla of the middle turbinate rather than anteroinferior as previously believed.[57] This anatomical knowledge has aided in the development of newer techniques in endoscopic DCR that allow for more complete bone removal superiorly and the creation of the largest possible opening in the lacrimal sac, ensuring adequate drainage and avoiding restenosis.[58]

The endoscopic DCR technique begins with identification of the maxillary line, uncinate process, and middle turbinate as important landmarks. After adequate decongestion and infiltration with 1% lidocaine with epinephrine, a sickle knife or #15 blade is used to fashion a posteriorly based mucosal flap over the lacrimal fossa. The incision is started 5 to 6 mm above the insertion of the middle turbinate and continued anteriorly for approximately 8 mm. A vertical incision is carried inferiorly to the midpoint between the middle turbinate insertion and inferior turbinate, and finally posteriorly to the uncinate process. Next, a suction elevator is used to elevate the mucosal flap, identifying the important maxillary line. Once this is done, the thin lacrimal bone is removed with a curette, and the thicker frontal process of the maxilla is partially removed with a rongeur or punch. The remainder of the frontal process of the maxilla superior to the axilla of the middle turbinate may be removed with a powered diamond burr. After the lacrimal sac has been completely exposed, especially superiorly, the inferior or superior punctum is dilated and the sac is cannulated with a lacrimal probe. When the probe is visualized tenting the sac medially, a vertical incision is made along the length of the sac, followed by superior and inferior relaxing incisions horizontally. The redundant anterior and posterior lacrimal sac flaps can either be resected or reapproximated with the original flap of nasal mucosa. After this is done, silastic stents are placed within the lacrimal apparatus and secured intranasally.[56,58] Complications are rare but may include surgical failure, chronic sinusitis, epistaxis, CSF leak, and orbital injury. Success rates for endoscopic DCR versus external approaches are equivalent (93.5 vs 95%).[53] This can be attributed to a better understanding of the relevant anatomy ensuring adequate removal of bone superiorly, as well as advances in endoscopic equipment and instrumentation.[56]

ENDOSCOPIC SURGERY OF BENIGN SINONASAL NEOPLASMS

In the mid-1980s, Kennedy and Stammberger first introduced the concept of endoscopic sinus surgery for benign, inflammatory sinus disease.[59,60] Since then, "functional endoscopic sinus surgery" has become the standard of care for such disease processes. As expertise, instrumentation, and technology have advanced, so too have the applications of endoscopic sinus surgery. With the advent of tools such as powered instrumentation, angled burrs and curettes, and image-guided surgery, the endoscopic endonasal approach is now being used routinely for the resection of multiple types of benign sinonasal neoplasms. Inverted papillomas (IPs), fibro-osseous lesions, neural-related neoplasms, hamartomas, and vascular neoplasms have all been treated successfully with endoscopic resection. In selected patients, the endoscopic approach allows for complete tumor resection, shorter hospital stays, minimal blood loss, no external incision, and less overall morbidity as compared to more traditional open approaches. Endoscopes provide greater magnification and visualization of sinonasal lesions and enable a more precise resection as well as identification and preservation of certain vital structures.[61] Endoscopic approaches can also be combined with open approaches for resection of tumors when absolute visualization and total resection may be anatomically impossible with an endoscopic-only resection. In addition, imaging studies such as MRI and CT can be employed along with endoscopic examination, allowing for improved evaluation of sinonasal lesions and selection of optimal surgical approaches.[2] CT scans are used to evaluate bony involvement of lesions, while MRI is more useful in assessing the soft tissue characteristics of tumors, such as intracranial and intraorbital extension. Specifically, T2 weighted MRI images may differentiate brightly enhancing neuromas and minor salivary gland tumors from other more intermediate-enhancing sinonasal neoplasms. T1 weighted images can be used to differentiate between postobstructive secretions and soft tissue.[61,62] In addition, MRI can be used to differentiate between inflammatory and neoplastic lesions.

Benign sinonasal neoplasms are a diverse group that may have similar clinical presentations. Common presenting symptoms include nasal obstruction, epistaxis, epiphora, rhinorrhea, and recurrent sinusitis. Patients may also be asymptomatic, presenting with lesions discovered as incidental findings on imaging studies ordered for nonrhinologic purposes. Although several of these lesions may have characteristic presentations, as well as endoscopic and radiographic findings, final diagnosis rests on pathological analysis of a biopsy specimen. In general, benign sinonasal neoplasms can de divided into various categories: IPs, fibro-osseous lesions, neural-related neoplasms, hamartomas, and vascular neoplasms.[63]

Fibro-Osseous Lesions

Three distinct clinical entities exist that can be classified as fibro-osseous lesions of the paranasal sinuses: osteomas, fibrous dysplasia, and ossifying fibroma. Although their appearance and presentation may be somewhat similar, their clinical implications vary tremendously. Osteoma is the most common tumor of the paranasal sinuses. Most commonly located in the frontal sinuses, osteomas have been reported to have been identified on 1% of routine sinus radiographs, and on as many as 3% of routine CT scans of the head and sinuses.[64,65] Osteomas are slightly more common in men and usually present in the second and third decades of life. Most lesions are benign, but many exhibit a slow, steady progressive growth pattern with resultant local infiltration, cosmetic change, and/or postobstructive sinusitis. Recurrence after complete resection is very rare.[64,66–70] Gardner syndrome should also be considered when first evaluating patients suspected of having osteomas. Gardner syndrome is an autosomal dominant disorder characterized by multiple osteomas, soft tissue tumors (such as epidermal inclusion cysts or subcutaneous fibrous tumors), and colorectal polyposis. It is caused by a mutation in the *adenomatous polyposis coli* gene on chromosome 5q. Early diagnosis is crucial, as the colorectal polyps have a high incidence of malignant degeneration.[63,71]

Although the exact etiology of osteomas is unknown, three accepted theories exist. In the *developmental theory*, the apposition of endochondral and membranous tissues traps embryonic cells, leading to osseous proliferation.[72] This may explain osteomas occurring at the fronto-ethmoid suture line, as the ethmoid bone is endochondral bone and the frontal bone is membranous bone; however, this theory does not explain lesions located elsewhere in the body away from such sutures.[68] The *traumatic theory* states that osteomas may occur as a result of localized inflammation. Moretti and colleagues reported that approximately 20% of sinus osteomas occur as a result of trauma.[72] The resulting trauma may lead to an inflammatory response leading to the formation of osteomas. Similarly, Sayan and colleagues reported that osteomas of the mandible occur commonly in places where muscles insert into the bone; resultant muscle traction may incite minor trauma leading to inflammation and subsequent osteoma formation.[70] This theory, although explaining why males are more prone to developing osteomas, does not explain osteoma formation in older individuals who have not experienced traumatic injury.[66,68] The *infectious theory* is similar to the traumatic theory and indicates that inflammation from chronic infection leads to osteoma formation. This, however, does not explain lesions developing in patients without a history of infection or osteitis.[68]

On gross examination, osteomas may be sessile or pedunculated with their sinus mucosal covered surfaces being smooth and lobulated.[69] Histologically, there are three types. The eburnated type, also known as the compact type, consists of dense bone, and lacks Haversian canals. The mature type is composed of cancellous bone. The mixed type contains elements of both the eburnated and mature forms[67–69] (Figure 10).

Osteomas are most commonly located in the frontal sinus (80%), with the remainder occurring in the ethmoid (20%), maxillary (5%), and sphenoid (rare).[67,72–74] Symptoms from paranasal sinus osteomas commonly result from their "mass effect" on surrounding structures. Common symptoms include frontal pain and headache, as well as sinusitis and/or mucocele formation from obstruction of adjacent sinus ostia.[67,68,71–73,75]

Radiographically, osteomas appear as dense, homogeneous, well-circumscribed masses on both

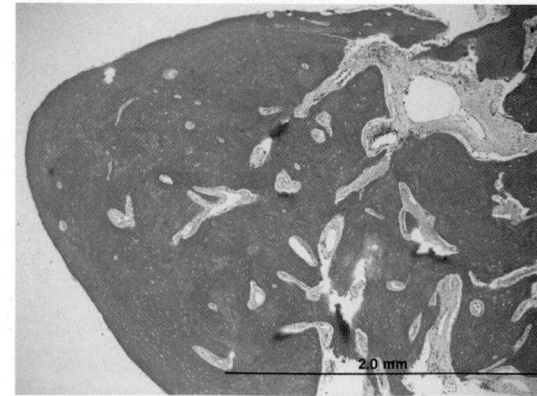

Figure 10 Photomicrograph of osteoma showing exuberant lamellar bone.

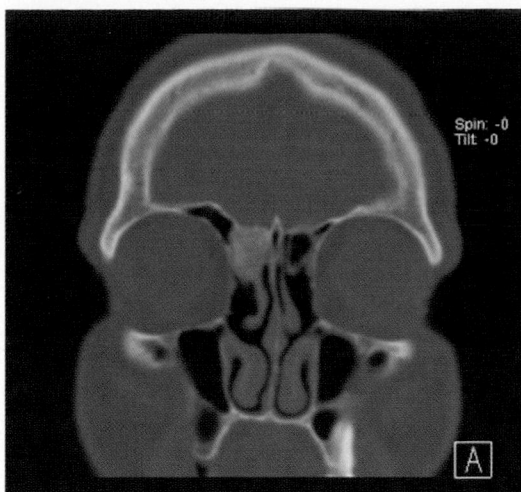

Figure 11 Coronal computed tomography scan showing a dense, homogeneous, well-circumscribed mass consistent with a right frontoethmoid osteoma.

CT and plain film radiographs (Figure 11). These lesions are usually found to be pedicled to relatively normal appearing adjacent bone although extensive lesions may cause some bone-thinning secondary to mass effect.[68] MRI is recommended to evaluate lesions suspected of having extrasinus or intracranial extension; MRI also allows for differentiation of sinus secretions from mass lesions, brain parenchyma, and orbital structures.[76]

The primary dilemma in the management of osteomas is determining whether or not surgical resection is necessary. Many surgeons advocate observation with periodic CT imaging at 6-month intervals in asymptomatic patients. This allows decision making and surgical intervention prior to the development of complications, should a lesion increase in size on serial imaging. While small, asymptomatic lesions may be observed, larger, symptomatic tumors should undergo surgical resection. Rapid growth, infection, compression of vital structures, severe pain, facial deformity, vision changes, mucocele formation, and intraorbital and/or intracranial complications are all indications for tumor resection.[68,72] Several recommendations have also been proposed as indications for tumor removal in asymptomatic patients. These include a tumor occupying greater than 50% of the frontal sinus,[73] having a posteriorly based frontal sinus lesion,[77] and any osteoma occupying the frontal recess or ethmoid sinus cavity.[78]

Multiple surgical techniques are available for resection of paranasal sinus osteomas. In general, approaches can be divided into three groups: endoscopic, open/external, or combined. Regardless of the approach chosen, the goals of surgery should include complete tumor removal with minimal damage to surrounding mucosa and vital structures.[68] While most surgeons agree that most ethmoid lesions can be treated with endoscopic resection, frontal sinus osteomas may require further evaluation and surgical planning.[68,72] Schick and colleagues recommend measuring the anterior–posterior dimension of the frontal sinus outflow tract to determine whether endoscopic

instrumentation is feasible; endoscopic resection usually then requires a Draf 2 or 3 procedure. They also recommend that most lesions that are either anteriorly based or located lateral to the sagittal plane of the lamina papyracea should undergo an open osteoplastic procedure.[78]

Traditional past surgical techniques involved open approaches, such as the Lynch frontoethmoidectomy; however, due to postoperative stenosis of the frontal recess and visible scarring, other procedures were soon developed. An osteoplastic flap approach via a coronal, brow, or midforehead incision, allows for optimal direct visualization of the frontal sinus and its outflow tract. This technique also allows the option for other adjunctive procedures, such as sinus obliteration, cranialization, or CSF leak repair if deemed necessary. Although such open procedures do have their advantages, the disadvantages are obvious including the increased morbidity of a surgical wound, postoperative pain, scalp paresthesias, visible scars, and possible mucocele formation.[68,79]

Many tumors may lend themselves to combined "above and below" type procedures. Combined endoscopic and osteoplastic flap approaches are often used to gain optimal access to large frontal sinus osteomas. In addition, small frontal trephines may be combined with endoscopic approaches for smaller lesions that do not require a full osteoplastic flap but cannot be managed solely endoscopically.[68,80] Chui and colleagues have proposed a grading system for frontal sinus ostcomas (Table 1).[79] They recommend endoscopic resection for grade 1 lesions; grade 2 lesions may require a trephine for an "above and below" type of approach. Lesions that are grade 3 and 4 usually require an external approach with or without endoscopic assistance.[79]

All of the various complications of sinus surgery may occur with resection of osteomas of the paranasal sinuses. This, of course, includes injury to the orbit, optic nerve, and skull base. Should a CSF leak be encountered, it should be repaired at the time of surgery. Reactive bony hyperplasia may also occur with mucosal injury, leading to obstruction of sinus ostia and subsequent

Table 1 Grading System for Frontal Sinus Osteoma[79]

Grade 1: Tumor base of attachment is posterior-inferior along the frontal recess; the tumor is medial to a virtual sagittal plane through the lamina papyracea; the anterior-posterior diameter of the lesion is <75% of the anterior–posterior dimension of the frontal recess

Grade 2: Tumor base of attachment is posterior-inferior along the frontal recess; the tumor is medial to a virtual sagittal plane through the lamina papyracea; the anterior–posterior diameter of the lesion is >75% of the anterior-posterior dimension of the frontal recess

Grade 3: Tumor base of attachment is anteriorly or superiorly located within the frontal sinus *and/or* the tumor extends lateral to a virtual plane through the lamina papyracea

Grade 4: The tumor fills the entire frontal sinus

sinusitis. Postoperatively, patients should be followed and managed appropriately. After mucosal healing has taken place, CT scans at 6 to 12 month intervals can be used to monitor for tumor recurrence.[68]

Fibrous dysplasia is another type of fibro-osseous lesion that can be found in the paranasal sinuses. Two forms of fibrous dysplasia exist: monostotic and polyostotic. Monostotic lesions (70 to 85%) involve only one bone, while the polyostotic form (15 to 30%) can affect multiple bones.[81] The monostotic form involves the facial skeleton approximately 25% of the time, with the mandible and maxilla being the most common locations in the head and neck.[81] Interestingly, the polyostotic form may present in patients with McCune–Albright syndrome; this syndrome also presents with precocious puberty in girls, abnormal skin pigmentations, and early skeletal bone maturation.[63,82] While risk of malignancy is somewhat low in patients with the polyostotic form of fibrous dysplasia (0.5%), patients with McCune–Albright syndrome have an approximately 4% risk of malignant degeneration.[68,81] Biopsy may not always be warranted as fibrous dysplasia has a characteristic "ground glass" appearance on CT scan (Figure 12). Fibrous dysplasia is usually present in younger patients, with growth actually decreasing around the age of puberty; because of this, treatment is usually conservative[63] with surgical intervention reserved for symptomatic patients or those with cosmetic deformity.[68]

Ossifying fibroma is the most concerning of the fibro-osseous lesions. Also known as cemento-ossifying fibroma, psammotoid ossifying fibroma, and juvenile-aggressive ossifying fibroma, differentiation from fibrous dysplasia is paramount as their management may differ.[63] Radiographically, ossifying fibroma appears as a well-circumscribed lesion with an eggshell rim and central lucency, whereas fibrous dysplasia takes on its characteristic "ground glass" appearance.[83] Ossifying fibroma presents as an expansile lesion with a definite demarcation from

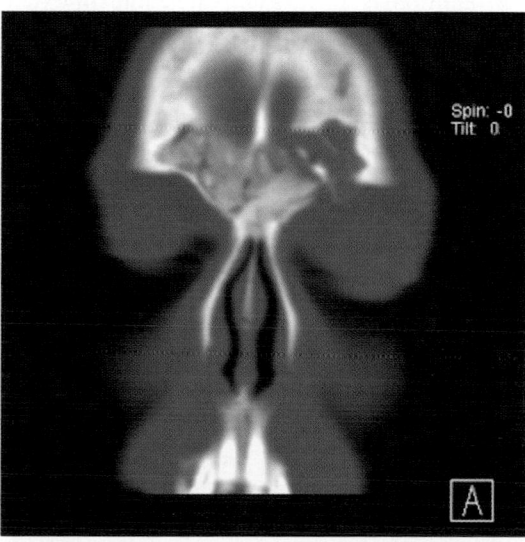

Figure 12 Coronal computed tomography scan demonstrating the characteristic "ground glass" appearance of fibrous dysplasia involving the frontal sinuses.

surrounding bone; fibrous dysplasia has more diffuse margins. Histologically, fibrous dysplasia lacks the peripheral osteoblasts and lamellar bone that ossifying fibroma possesses.[84] Most importantly, ossifying fibroma can be locally erosive and very destructive. While these lesions are most commonly found in the mandible, they are even more aggressive when located in other locations, such as the paranasal sinuses.[83,84] Due to the destructive nature of these lesions, early complete resection is recommended. While most lesions have been resected via external open approaches in the past, endoscopic surgery offers a viable alternative in selected cases. The well-defined borders may allow for a complete endoscopic resection with tumor-free margins. Endoscopy is also an invaluable tool for tumor surveillance.[84]

Inverted Papilloma

IP is a benign epithelial growth in the underlying stroma of the nasal cavity and paranasal sinuses that is best known for its invasiveness, tendency to recur, and association with malignancy.[63,85] IP has a long history which deserves discussion.

In 1854, Ward first documented the occurrence of IP in the sinonasal cavity.[86] However, in 1935, Reingertz histologically described the nature of the tumor and noted its classic inverted nature in underlying connective tissue stroma.[87] Since then, this tumor which is characterized by its epithelial inversion into underlying connective tissue, has taken on many names: IP, inverting papilloma, epithelial papilloma, papillary sinusitis, Schneiderian papilloma, inverted Schneiderian papilloma, soft papilloma, transitional cell papilloma, cylindrical cell papilloma, polyp with inverting metaplasia, and benign transitional cell growth.[88] Needless to say, there has been much confusion regarding the clinical and histological nature of this tumor. In 1971, Hymans reviewed several cases of this tumor at the Armed Forces Institute of Pathology; his report aided in solidifying the terminology and pathology of this distinct lesion. Here, sinonasal papillomas were subdivided into inverted, fungiform, and cylindrical cell types.[63,89,90]

Pathologically, this tumor is distinct. Grossly, it appears to be exophytic, polypoid, and vascular. It is pink to gray in color, with frond-like projections extending from the bulk of the lesion.[88] This benign tumor, which may fill the entire nasal cavity, usually emanates from a discrete pedicled site. It should also be noted that when the tumor rests on mucosa not intimately involved in the lesion, the native, uninvolved sinonasal mucosa remains normal.[63] Histologically, the epithelium is distinct from the surrounding mucosa; the epithelium can be squamous, respiratory, or transitional.[88] The epithelium of the tumor appears to be proliferative but different from surrounding tissues as it lacks mucus-secreting cells and eosinphils.[91] The nuclear to cytoplasmic ratio is normal with few mitotic figures. Squamous metaplasia can occur, and the cells can become hyperkeratotic. In addition, the

orderly maturation of the cells outward from the basal membrane is preserved. The epithelium rests on an intact basement membrane, with characteristic invaginations into the underlying connective tissue stroma (Figure 13). Diagnosis is established via biopsy.[63]

The exact cause of IP is uncertain. The Schneiderian membrane, the embryologic origin of the sinonasal mucous membranes, is at risk for developing this epithelial lesion; therefore the eponym has persisted.[92] The role of allergy has been discounted secondary to the lack of allergic history in many patients with IP. Chronic rhinosinusitis has also been proposed as a possible etiologic factor due to a temporal relationship and the increased incidence of sinusitis on the opposite side from the lesion; however, it has also been proposed that chronic sinusitis develops in these patients secondary to the obstructive nature of the neoplasm itself.[93] Additionally, there has not been any association found between IP and environmental chemical exposure. Due to the known relationship between common papillomas and human papilloma virus (HPV), a viral etiology has been sought.[94] Interestingly, in situ hybridization techniques have isolated HPV DNA in IP similar to HPV types 6 and 11.[63,95,96] The results and implications of these findings, however, are unfortunately still unclear.

The incidence of IP has been documented as approximately 0.6 cases per 100,000 people per year.[97] It comprises 0.5 to 4% of all primary nasal tumors,[91] usually affecting patients in the fifth and sixth decade of life.[85] Common symptoms include unilateral nasal obstruction, epistaxis, nasal drainage, bilateral nasal obstruction, nasal mass, and sinusitis.[63,90] IP affects males more commonly with a male to female ratio of 3:1. Cases are usually unilateral with no side predilection although bilateral lesions do occur in 4.9% of patients.[98] IP usually originates from the middle meatus or lateral nasal wall, involving at least one paranasal sinus 82% of the time: maxillary sinus (69%), ethmoid sinus (53 to 89%), sphenoid sinus (11 to 20%), and frontal sinus (11 to 16%).[85,99]

Radiographic studies are commonly used to evaluate IP with CT and MRI being the most

common. Bony changes, including a bowing of the bones located near the mass, are common CT findings (Figure 14). Tumors involving the maxillary sinus may lead to widening of the infundibulum on CT, making the uncinate process difficult to discern.[100] Although the term "bony erosion" is often used to describe CT changes seen with IP, this term is usually reserved for true malignant lesions that grossly invade adjacent normal structures. "Bony remodeling" may be a better term to describe the changes that occur secondary to the constant pressure and mass effect on surrounding bony structures from IP[101] commonly seen at the medial wall of the maxillary sinus and lamina papyracea.[63,91] IP affecting the skull base may also have characteristic findings; it is postulated that the bony skull base may have a limited response to pressure, leading to more erosive changes rather than remodeling.[63,101,102] In addition, contrasted CT may demonstrate slight enhancement and calcifications.[101] On MRI, IP is hypo- to isodense on T1-weighted images and iso- to hyperdense on T2 weighted. Additionally, and most importantly, MRI scans with T1-weighted images with contrast and T2-weighted images can be used to differentiate between tumor mass and postobstructive secretions[63,85,101,103,104] (Figure 15).

IP is a benign neoplasm with an association with squamous cell carcinoma. Krouse documents the occurrence of malignancy as 9.1% in all patients with IP.[98] Although this association is real, the exact relationship is unclear. Squamous cell carcinoma may present in the setting of IP in three different circumstances. First, patients may present with IP with a small foci of squamous call carcinoma within it. Patients may also present with malignancy as a separate synchronous lesion, with no evidence of malignancy present within the IP itself. Lastly, and thought to be least common, patients may present with metachronous carcinoma in areas of prior resection of benign IP.[63,88,105]

This association with malignancy, along with a propensity for invasion and recurrence, drives the treatment paradigm for IP.[63] Initially, IPs were excised via a transnasal closed approach with

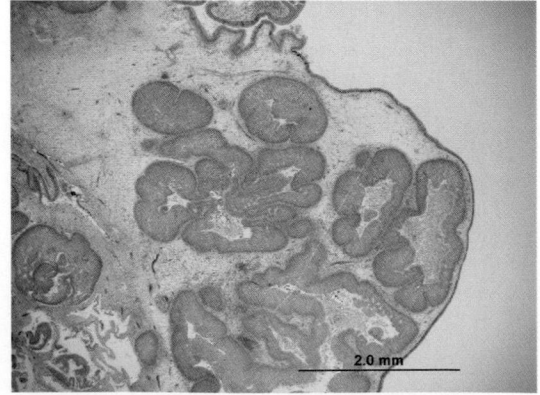

Figure 13 Inverted papilloma with characteristic epithelial invaginations into underlying connective tissue stroma.

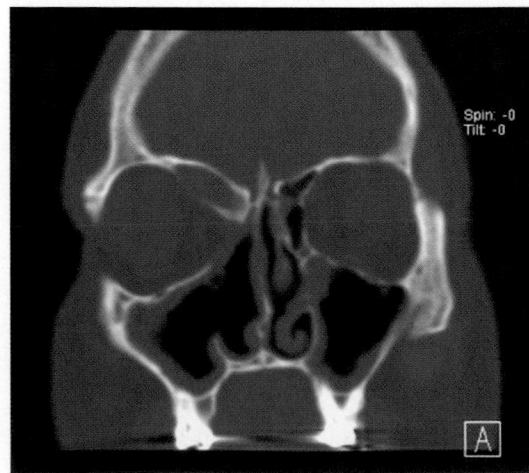

Figure 14 Coronal computed tomography scan of a right-sided supraorbital inverted papilloma.

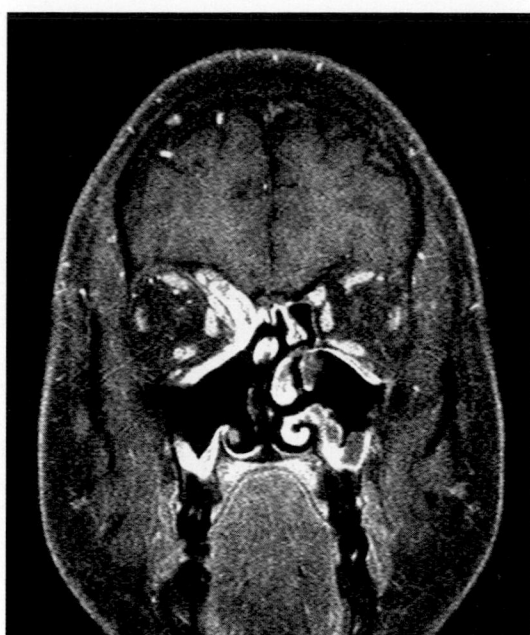

Figure 15 T1 weighted magnetic resonance imaging with gadolinium demonstrates an enhancing right-sided supraorbital inverted papilloma.

headlight illumination; in fact, these early procedures mimicked polypectomies.[63,106] Although the intent of these procedures was curative, recurrence rates of 40 to 80% were unacceptably high.[85,107] This, in turn, led to the use of external approaches, such as the Caldwell-Luc and external ethmoidectomy. Open approaches such as the lateral rhinotomy and midfacial degloving procedures allowed for increased tumor visualization and more complete resections with most of these resections usually involving some form of maxillectomy.[63] In the review written by Weissler and colleagues, a recurrence rate of 71% was noted for closed intranasal procedures compared to 29% for open procedures (lateral rhinotomy and midfacial degloving).[90] Open surgical resections such as lateral rhinotomy, were adopted as the standard of care for the treatment of IP.[63]

Since the advent of functional endoscopic sinus surgery in the 1980s, advanced endoscopic techniques have been utilized for the resection of benign sinonasal neoplasms. Waitz and Wigand were among the first to publish their results comparing endoscopic resection of IP to traditional open procedures; they noted similar recurrence rates of 17% versus 19%, respectively, in a series of selected patients.[108] Although several other studies have noted similar findings,[104,107] it has been revealed that selection bias does exist, with smaller, more limited tumors being managed endoscopically and larger, more extensive tumors managed with open approaches.[63]

The success of endoscopic resection of IPs has been facilitated by the numerous advances in radiologic imaging, image guidance, and instrumentation such as angled burrs and microdebriders.[109] As more extensive sinonasal tumors are being managed endoscopically, the confidence of surgeons has increased. Complete resection of the neoplasm requires identification of the site to where it is pedicled to native mucosa. By

debriding the bulk of the tumor first and retaining its pedicled attachment, the sinonasal cavities may be optimally visualized and inspected to allow for a more directed, complete tumor resection, while minimizing damage to surrounding structures and mucosa.[63,109] Once the tumor has been removed, many advocate that the adjacent mucosa and underlying bone be drilled away with a diamond burr or the bone itself resected when needed.[109,110] As endoscopic approaches are being used for resection of larger tumors, more advanced techniques and procedures are being developed, with the goal being adequate exposure for complete resection and postoperative endoscopic tumor surveillance.[63,109] Determining the exact location of the tumor using radiologic imaging studies and preoperative nasal endoscopy allows the optimal surgical approach and technique to be planned ahead of time.[85]

Adjunctive open procedures, such as Caldwell-Luc and maxillary canine fossa puncture, can also be added to endoscopic resection of IP of the maxillary sinus to maximize visualization and ensure complete tumor removal. Even with 45° and 70° angled telescopes, the entire sinus cavity is often difficult to visualize completely; these adjunctive open procedures may allow passage of both endoscopes and instruments transnasally and through the puncture site. Tumors of the posterior wall of the maxillary sinus may be best approached via a large middle meatal antrostomy, making sure that maximal bone is removed both posteriorly and superiorly to provide optimal visualization; a working port through a canine fossa puncture provides additional exposure.[63] Tumors of the inferior, anterior, lateral, or medial walls of the maxillary sinus may also be resected via endoscopic medial maxillectomy.[106,111] Here, the medial aspect of the maxillary sinus along with the lateral nasal wall is resected endoscopically. Sadeghi and colleagues have described an "en-bloc" tumor removal with this technique, and it appears to be more oncologically sound than piecemeal removal.[111] Tumors of the frontal sinus may present more of a challenge for endoscopic resection. While limited involvement of the frontal recess lends itself to endoscopic resection, tumors of the frontal sinus itself may require advanced techniques.[63,111] The endoscopic modified Lothrop procedure may be used in select cases where IP involves the frontal recess and frontal sinus;[104] frontal trephination may also be combined with endoscopic approaches to improve visualization and optimize tumor removal. For larger lesions involving the lateral part of the frontal sinus, an osteoplastic flap may be required for complete tumor extirpation; unless it is deemed absolutely necessary, obliteration is not carried out as an unobliterated sinus allows for easier clinical and radiographic tumor surveillance.[63] In addition, a wide frontal sinusotomy at the time of surgery helps with endoscopic tumor surveillance.[63,107]

As mentioned previously, selection bias exists when comparing recurrence rates of IP resected via open approaches versus endoscopically.[63] In

an attempt to standardize reporting and communication between investigators, Krouse has proposed a staging system for IP primarily based on disease extent, location, and presence of malignancy[112] (Table 2). T1 tumors may be resected endoscopically without much bone removal, while T2 lesions may require more bony excision. T3 tumors may be resected endoscopically, if adequate visualization can be achieved; an open medial maxillectomy may be required. T4 tumors usually necessitate an open approach for maximal visualization and complete resection.[63,98]

Other Benign Tumors

Numerous other less common benign sinonasal neoplasms occur. Neural neoplasms include meningiomas, schwannomas, and neurofibromas. Meningiomas arising from ectopic arachnoid tissue are rarely encountered in the nose and paranasal sinuses. Sometimes, sinonasal meningiomas can be difficult to differentiate from their intracranial counterparts; sinonasal tumors can have bowing of bone in the direction of an intact skull base.[63,113] Neurofibromas may present along peripheral nerves in the sinonasal cavity, whereas schwannomas may present both in the region of the nasal septum along branches of the trigeminal nerve, as well as along peripheral nerves.[63,114]

Hamartomas are nonmalignant lesions that represent congenital errors in development; they are extremely rare in the paranasal sinuses. While they are neither neoplastic nor inflammatory, they are chacterized by an abnormal proliferation of tissue elements indigenous to a specific area of the body.[115] Additionally, they do not have the capacity to metastasize and symptoms usually result from mass effect.[116] Although rare, extension outside of the sinuses may give rise to orbital complaints such as proptosis or symptoms of ICP such as headaches.[115] Differential diagnosis includes benign lesions such as IP as well as malignant lesions such as adenocarcinoma. Accurate diagnosis is paramount, as hamartomas are benign lesions that should undergo conservative resection.[115]

Juvenile nasopharyngeal angiofibroma is a benign, vascular lesion, most commonly seen in males during the second decade of life. Common presenting symptoms include nasal obstruction and epistaxsis. These neoplasms are firm, well-encapsulated lesions, usually arising from the region of the sphenopalatine foramen.[63]

Table 2 Krouse Staging System for Inverted Papilloma[112]
T1: Tumor isolated to one area of the nasal cavity without extension into the paranasal sinuses
T2: Tumor involves the medial wall of the maxillary sinus, ethmoid sinus, and/or the ostiomeatal complex
T3: Tumor involves the superior, inferior, posterior, anterior, or lateral walls of the maxillary sinus, frontal sinus, or sphenoid sinus
T4: Tumor with extrasinonasal extension or malignant tumor

Endoscopic techniques are commonly employed for resection of selected lesions; the endoscopic approach is advantageous for such lesions as external approaches with osteotomies may negatively impact facial growth in these young patients. In addition, preoperative embolization of the internal maxillary artery system may limit blood loss, aiding in endoscopic resection of these highly vascular tumors.[117] Other rare benign vascular neoplasms include hemangiomas and hemangiopericytomas.

Endoscopic Sphenopalatine Artery Ligation

In all cases of benign tumor removal, adequate hemostasis is essential and may be aided by control of the sphenopalatine artery posteriorly. Pioneered in 1992 by Budrovich and Saetti, endoscopic sphenopalatine artery ligation or diathermy is useful as both a primary method of controlling posterior epistaxis, as well as an adjunctive procedure prior to more extensive and involved endoscopic surgical procedures.[118] This procedure is performed by first decongesting the nasal cavity and injecting 1% lidocaine with epinephrine into the mucosa of the lateral nasal wall adjacent to the posterior aspect of the middle meatus. A small vertical incision is made through mucosa and periosteum 1 cm anterior to the posterior aspect of the middle turbinate. Alternatively, a middle meatal antrostomy is performed and carried posteriorly to the same location. Next, a suction elevator is used to raise a mucosal flap posterosuperiorly until the crista ethmoidalis is encountered just anterior to the sphenopalatine foramen (Figure 16). Once the sphenopalatine artery is identified, a vascular clip or bipolar cautery is applied to the vessel. Great care must be taken to ensure that all branches of the artery are identified exiting the foramen.[119] Kumar and colleagues demonstrated that the success rates of hemaclip and diathermy approach 96 and 100%, respectively.[119,120] Complications of this procedure are rare.

ENDOSCOPIC SURGERY OF THE SKULL BASE AND PITUITARY GLAND

The first transsphenoidal resection of a pituitary neoplasm via a lateral rhinotomy transethmoid approach was described by Schlofer in 1907.

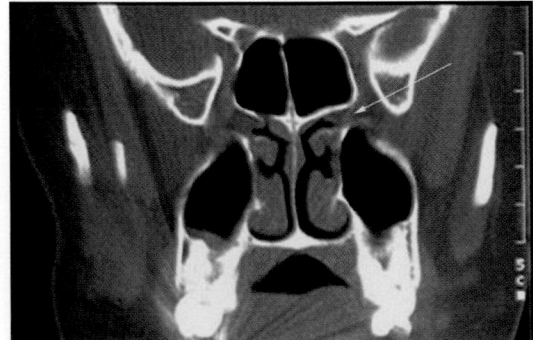

Figure 16 Axial computed tomography scan demonstrating the location of the sphenopalatine foramen.

A few years later in 1910, Cushing described the sublabial transeptal approach to the pituitary; with the advent of fluoroscopy, and more importantly, the operating microscope, the sublabial transseptal transsphenoidal approach soon became the standard approach for resection of pituitary tumors.[121] In the 1980s, surgeons were introduced to endoscopic sinus surgery and provided with optimal optical illumination, magnification, and understanding of the paranasal sinus anatomy.[59,60,121] In 1992, Jankowski described the first successful endonasal endoscopic resection of a pituitary tumor via a transsphenoidal approach. More recently, over the past decade, the endoscopic transsphenoidal approach has gained popularity and acceptance, with favorable complication rates as compared to traditional sublabial transseptal approaches.[122–126] Success of this procedure, however, requires close cooperation and coordination between otolaryngological and neurosurgical teams.[127]

The pituitary gland is approximately 1 cm in size and rests in the sella turcica in the dorsal aspect of the sphenoid bone. The gland is composed of anterior and posterior lobes and is connected to the brain via the infundibulum. The sella turcica is in close proximity to the optic chiasm anteriorly, the clivus posteriorly, the cavernous sinus laterally, and the hypothalamus superiorly. The lateral walls of the sphenoid are in fact the medial walls of the cavernous sinus, and the various neural and vascular structures in the cavernous sinus can be identified in the lateral walls of the sphenoid sinus. The sphenoid sinus begins developing around 5 to 7 years of age, and it is variably pneumatized in adults. An intersinus septum usually separates the two sides of the sphenoid sinus; however, it is off midline in 60 to 70% of cases.[127]

A team approach should be used when evaluating and treating patients with pituitary tumors. The multidisciplinary team should include an otolaryngologist, neurosurgeon, endocrinologist, ophthalmologist, and radiation oncologist. Indications for resection of adenomas may include compressive symptoms, pituitary apoplexy, or severe headaches. Patients with active prolactinomas (prolactin-producing adenomas) are offered surgery only after failure of medical treatment, whereas patients with acromegaly, hyperthyroidism, and Cushing disease are offered surgery primarily. The preoperative evaluation must include an otolaryngologic evaluation, with complete sinonasal endoscopy and review of CT scans for image guidance to understand the patient's individual anatomy. Ophthalmology evaluation is also encouraged before any surgical intervention.[127]

Minimally invasive pituitary surgery (MIPS) begins with the patient positioned in the "beach-chair" position with the head rotated 15° toward the surgeon. After registration of the image guidance scans, the face and abdomen are separately prepped and draped in sterile fashion, and the nasal cavities decongested. Hemostasis is achieved by injecting 1.5 mL of 1% lidocaine

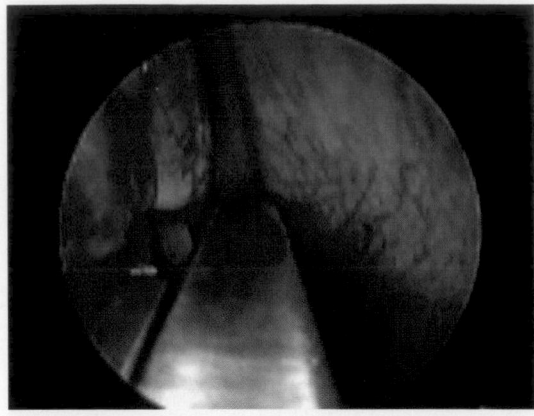

Figure 17 Resection of the posterior-inferior third of the superior turbinate allows for optimal visualization and identification of the natural sphenoid ostium.

with 1:100,000 epinephrine transorally into the greater palatine foramina bilaterally (Figure 16). Lidocaine with epinephrine is also injected endoscopically into the tissues adjacent to the sphenopalatine foramen bilaterally. At this point, the most patent nasal cavity is selected, and the middle turbinate slightly lateralized. Next, the natural sphenoid ostium is identified posteromedially to the superior turbinate. After the posterior-inferior third of the superior turbinate is resected, the ostium is clearly identified and enlarged (Figure 17). Various forceps, rongeurs, punches, and drills are used to resect the bone of the sphenoid rostrum. Resection of the posterior aspect of the septum allows entrance into the contralateral sinus, thereby facilitating further removal of the rostrum and intersinus septum for maximal exposure of the posterior wall of the sphenoid sinus and sella. At this point, the endoscope is placed in a holder allowing for two-handed dissection. The mucosa overlying the sella is cauterized and the sella itself is entered with either a 4 mm chisel or drill. Wide resection of bone between the internal carotid arteries is achieved with Kerrison-like forceps.[127]

The neurosurgical team takes over, cauterizing and entering the dura with a stellate incision (Figure 18). Once the tumor is identified usually bulging from the sella, a small piece is sent for both frozen and permanent pathologic diagnosis. At this time, suction-assisted resection

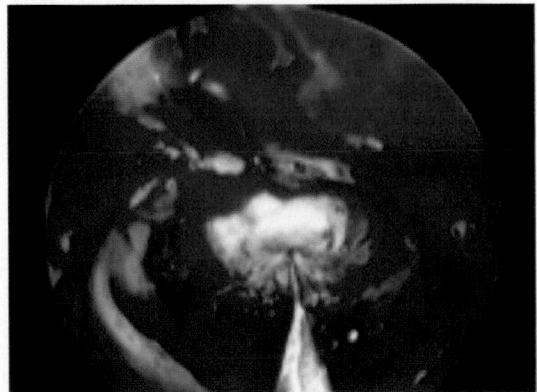

Figure 18 After adequate exposure is achieved, a dural incision is made overlying the pituitary tumor.

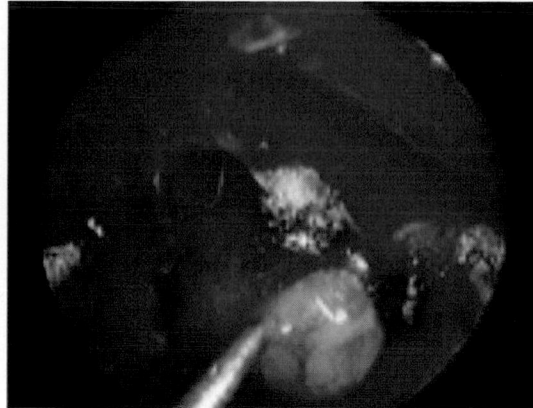

Figure 19 A suction-assisted curette resection of a pituitary adenoma is performed.

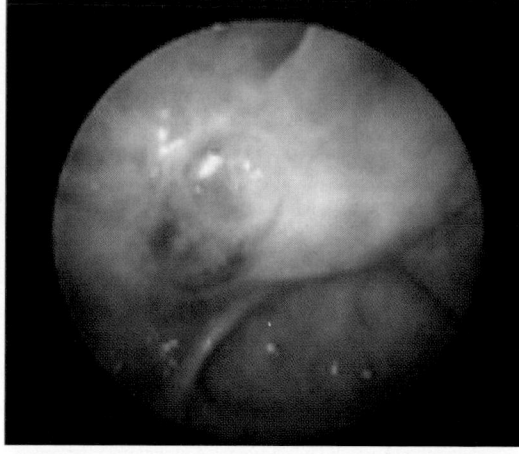

Figure 21 Posterior aspect of sphenoid sinus appears well-healed 6 weeks postoperative from a minimally invasive pituitary surgery procedure.

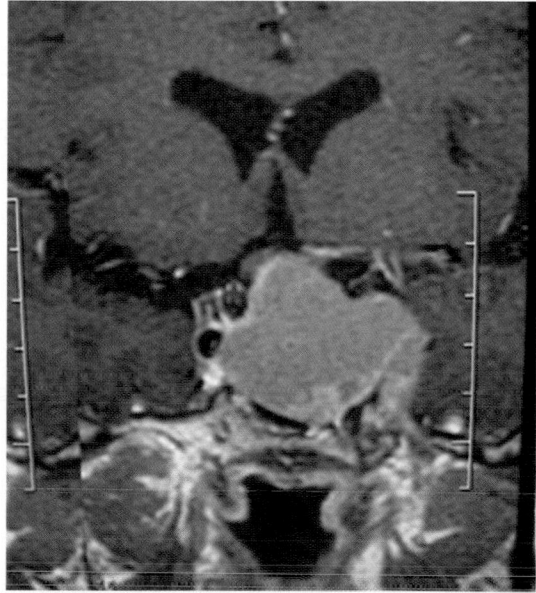

(A)

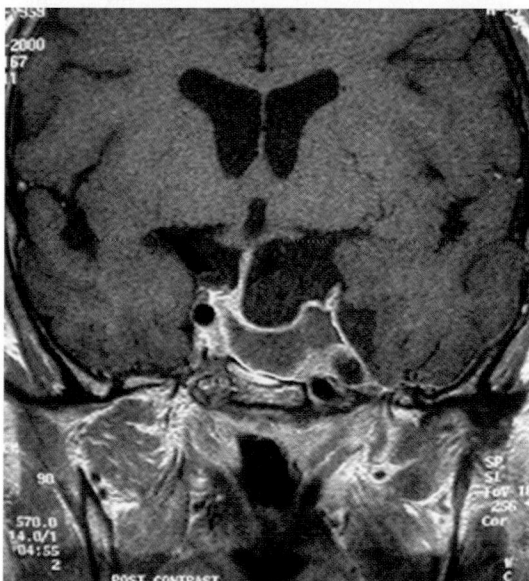

(B)

Figure 20 Preoperative (A) and postoperative (B) magnetic resonance imaging scans illustrate successful resection of pituitary adenoma via a minimally invasive procedure.

of the tumor is performed (Figure 19). Once the resection is complete, the sella is inspected via "hydroscopy," in which normal saline is instilled into the sella via a low-pressure system attached to the endoscope. When adequate tumor resection has been confirmed, hemostasis is achieved with microfibrillar collagen which is allowed to sit for a few minutes before being removed. If a CSF leak is suspected, abdominal fat is harvested from a periumbilical incision and packed into the sella; the sphenoid sinus is then packed with an absorbable hemostatic agent. Patients are admitted postoperatively and an MRI is obtained on the first postoperative day to evaluate the extent of resection (Figure 20). Patients are discharged on appropriate antibiotics and hormones as needed. In 3 weeks, patients return to clinic where sinonasal endoscopy is performed to evaluate surgical site wound healing[127] (Figure 21).

MIPS may provide improved complication rates when compared to more traditional pituitary surgery.[124] Major complications, such as meningitis, intracranial hemorrhage, internal carotid artery injury, optic nerve injury, and death, regardless of approach are rare. In one study, MIPS resulted in shorter hospital stays, as well as decreased use of lumbar drains and nasal packing, when compared to the standard sublabial transseptal approach.[124] Although immediate postoperative diabetes insipidus (DI) may occur 60% of the time, permanent DI is rare (0.4 to 3%) with few patients requiring long-term treatment.[124] The most common complication, CSF leak, usually manifests itself within the first 72 hours postoperatively. If the leak does not resolve with initial conservative management, either a lumbar drain is placed or the patient is taken back to surgery for definitive repair.[127]

REFERENCES

1. Bolger WE. Endoscopic transpterygoid approach to the lateral sphenoid recess: Surgical approach and clinical experience. Otolaryngol Head Neck Surg 2005;133:20–6.
2. Pasquini E, Sciarretta V, Frank G, et al. Endoscopic treatment of benign tumors of the nose and paranasal sinuses. Otolaryngol Head Neck Surg 2004;131:180–6.
3. Anand VK., Murali RK, Glasgold MJ. Surgical decisions in the management of cerebrospinal fluid rhinorrhoea. Rhinology 1995;33:212–8.
4. Zweig JL, Carrau RL, Celin SE, et al. Endoscopic repair of cerebrospinal fluid leaks to the sinonasal tract: Predictors of success. Otolaryngol Head Neck Surg 2000;123:195–201.
5. Aarabi B, Leibrock LG. Neurosurgical approaches to cerebrospinal fluid rhinorrhea. Ear Nose Throat J 1992;71:300–5.
6. Hughes RG, Jones NS, Robertson IJ. The endoscopic treatment of cerebrospinal fluid rhinorrhoea: The Nottingham experience. J Laryngol Otol 1997;111:125–8.
7. Wigand ME. Transnasal ethmoidectomy under endoscopical control. Rhinology 1981;19:7–15.
8. Lanza DC, O'Brien DA, Kennedy DW. Endoscopic repair of cerebrospinal fluid fistulae and encephaloceles. Laryngoscope 1996;106:1119–25.
9. Mattox DE, Kennedy DW. Endoscopic management of cerebrospinal fluid leaks and cephaloceles. Laryngoscope 1990;100:857–62.
10. Schlosser RJ, Bolger WE. Endoscopic management of cerebrospinal fluid rhinorrhea. Otolaryngol Clin North Am 2006;39:523–38.
11. Schlosser RJ, Bolger WE. Nasal cerebrospinal fluid leaks: Critical review and surgical considerations. Laryngoscope 2004;114:255–65.
12. Bleier B, Govindaraj S, Palmer J. State of the art cerebrospinal fluid leak and encephalocele repair. Oper Tech Otolaryngol 2006;17:49–57.
13. Zlab MK, Moore GF, Daly DT, et al. Cerebrospinal fluid rhinorrhea: A review of the literature. Ear Nose Throat J 1992;71:314–7.
14. Bernal-Sprekelsen M, Bleda-Vazquez C, Carrau RL. Ascending meningitis secondary to traumatic cerebrospinal fluid leaks. Am J Rhinol 2000;14:257–9.
15. Graham S. Complications of sinus surgery using powered instrumentation. Oper Tech Otolaryngol 2006;17:73–7.
16. Gassner HG, Ponikau JU, Sherris DA, et al. CSF rhinorrhea: 95 consecutive surgical cases with long term follow-up at the Mayo Clinic. Am J Rhinol 1999;13:439–47.
17. Woodworth BA, Schlosser RJ, Faust RA, et al. Evolutions in the management of congenital intranasal skull base defects. Arch Otolaryngol Head Neck Surg 2004;130:1283–8.
18. Schlosser RJ, Bolger WE. Management of multiple spontaneous nasal meningoencephaloceles. Laryngoscope 2002;112:980–5.
19. Schlosser RJ, Bolger WE. Significance of empty sella in cerebrospinal fluid leaks. Otolaryngol Head Neck Surg 2003;128:32–8.
20. Skedros DG, Cass SP, Hirsch BE, et al. Sources of error in use of beta-2 transferrin analysis for diagnosing perilymphatic and cerebral spinal fluid leaks. Otolaryngol Head Neck Surg 1993;109:861–4.
21. Sanders EL, Clark RJ, Katzmann JA. Cerebrospinal fluid leakage: Agarose gel electrophoresis detection of beta(2)-transferrin and nephelometric quantification of beta-trace protein. Clin Chem 2004;50:2401–3.
22. Risch L, Lisec I, Jutzi M, et al. Rapid, accurate and noninvasive detection of cerebrospinal fluid leakage using combined determination of beta-trace protein in secretion and serum. Clin Chim Acta 2005;351:169–76.
23. McMains KC, Gross CW, Kountakis SE. Endoscopic management of cerebrospinal fluid rhinorrhea. Laryngoscope 2004;114:1833–7.
24. Carrau RL, Snyderman CH, Kassam AB. The management of cerebrospinal fluid leaks in patients at risk for high-pressure hydrocephalus. Laryngoscope 2005;115:205–12.
25. Woodworth B, Neal J, Schlosser R. Sphenoid sinus cerebrospinal fluid leaks. Oper Tech Otolaryngol 2006;17:37–42.
26. Gjuric M, Goede U, Keimer H, et al. Endonasal endoscopic closure of cerebrospinal fluid fistulas at the anterior cranial base. Ann Otol Rhinol Laryngol 1996;105:620–3.
27. Tosun F, Gonul E, Yetiser S, et al. Endonasal endoscopic repair of cerebrospinal fluid leaks of the sphenoid sinus. Arch Otolaryngol Head Neck Surg 2003;129:576–80.
28. Lopatin AS, Kapitanov DN, Potapov AA. Endonasal endoscopic repair of spontaneous cerebrospinal fluid leaks. Arch Otolaryngol Head Neck Surg 2003;129:859–63.
29. Ommaya AK, Di Chiro G, Baldwin M, et al. Non-traumatic cerebrospinal fluid rhinorrhoea. J Neurol Neurosurg Psychiatry 1968;31:214–25.
30. Hubbard JL, McDonald TJ, Pearson BW, et al. Spontaneous cerebrospinal fluid rhinorrhea: Evolving concepts in diagnosis and surgical management based on the Mayo Clinic experience from 1970 through 1981. Neurosurgery 1985;16:314–21.
31. Schick B, Ibing R, Brors D, et al. Long-term study of endonasal duraplasty and review of the literature. Ann Otol Rhinol Laryngol 2001;110:142–7.

32. Casiano RR, Jassir D. Endoscopic cerebrospinal fluid rhinorrhea repair: Is a lumbar drain necessary? Otolaryngol Head Neck Surg 1999;121:745–50.

33. Schlosser RJ, Wilensky EM, Grady MS, et al. Cerebrospinal fluid pressure monitoring after repair of cerebrospinal fluid leaks. Otolaryngol Head Neck Surg 2004;130:443–8.

34. Komisar A, Weitz S, Ruben RJ, et al. Cerebrospinal fluid dynamics and rhinorrhea: The role of shunting in repair. Otolaryngol Head Neck Surg 1983;91:399–403.

35. Zagardo MT, Cail WS, Kelman SE, Rothman MI. Reversible empty sella in idiopathic intracranial hypertension: An indicator of successful therapy? AJNR Am J Neuroradiol 1996;17:1953–6.

36. Kennedy DW, Goodstein ML, Miller NR, Zinreich SJ. Endoscopic transnasal orbital decompression. Arch Otolaryngol Head Neck Surg 1990;116:275–82.

37. Metson R, Pletcher SD. Endoscopic orbital and optic nerve decompression. Otolaryngol Clin North Am 2006;39:551–61.

38. Schaefer SD, Soliemanzadeh P, Della Rocca DA, et al. Endoscopic and transconjunctival orbital decompression for thyroid-related orbital apex compression. Laryngoscope 2003;113:508–13.

39. Metson R, Dallow RL, Shore JW. Endoscopic orbital decompression. Laryngoscope 1994;104:950–7.

40. Obenchain TG, Killeffer FA, Stern WE. Indirect injury of the optic nerves and chiasm with closed head injury. Report of three cases. Bull Los Angeles Neurol Soc 1973;38:13–20.

41. McMains K, Kountakis S. Contemporary diagnosis and approaches toward optic nerve decompression. Oper Tech Otolaryngol 2006;17:178–83.

42. Luxenberger W, Stammberger H, Jebeles JA, et al. Endoscopic optic nerve decompression: The Graz experience. Laryngoscope 1998;108:873–82.

43. Anand V, Al-Mefty C. Optic nerve decompression via transethmoid and supraorbital approaches. Oper Tech Otolaryngol 1991;2:157–66.

44. Walsh FB. Pathological-clinical correlations. I. Indirect trauma to the optic nerves and chiasm. II. Certain cerebral involvements associated with defective blood supply. Invest Ophthalmol 1966;5:433–49.

45. Hughes B. Indirect injury of the optic nerves and chiasma. Bull Johns Hopkins Hos 1962;111:98–126.

46. Lessell S. Indirect optic nerve trauma. Arch Ophthalmol 1989;107:382–6.

47. Wolin MJ, Lavin PJ. Spontaneous visual recovery from traumatic optic neuropathy after blunt head injury. Am J Ophthalmol 1990;109:430–5.

48. Seiff SR. High dose corticosteroids for treatment of vision loss due to indirect injury to the optic nerve. Ophthalmic Surg 1990;21:389–95.

49. Kountakis SE, Maillard AA, El-Harazi SM, et al. Endoscopic optic nerve decompression for traumatic blindness. Otolaryngol Head Neck Surg 2000;123:34–7.

50. Cook MW, Levin LA, Joseph MP, et al. Traumatic optic neuropathy. A meta-analysis. Arch Otolaryngol Head Neck Surg 1996;122:389–92.

51. McDonogh M, Meiring JH. Endoscopic transnasal dacryocystorhinostomy. J Laryngol Otol 1989;103:585–7.

52. Wormald PJ. Powered endoscopic dacryocystorhinostomy. Laryngoscope 2002;112:69–72.

53. Tsirbas A, Davis G, Wormald PJ. Mechanical endonasal dacryocystorhinostomy versus external dacryocystorhinostomy. Ophthal Plast Reconstr Surg 2004;20:50–6.

54. Cokkeser Y, Evereklioglu C, Er H. Comparative external versus endoscopic dacryocystorhinostomy: Results in 115 patients (130 eyes). Otolaryngol Head Neck Surg 2000;123:488–91.

55. Ben Simon GJ, Joseph J, Lee S, et al. External versus endoscopic dacryocystorhinostomy for acquired nasolacrimal duct obstruction in a tertiary referral center. Ophthalmology 2005;112:1463–8.

56. Kingdom T, Durairaj V. Endoscopic dacryocystorhinostomy. Oper Tech Otolaryngol 2006;17:43–8.

57. Wormald PJ, Kew J, Van Hasselt A. Intranasal anatomy of the nasolacrimal sac in endoscopic dacryocystorhinostomy. Otolaryngol Head Neck Surg 2000;123:307–10.

58. Wormald PJ. Powered endoscopic dacryocystorhinostomy. Otolaryngol Clin North Am 2006;39:539–49.

59. Kennedy DW. Functional endoscopic sinus surgery. Technique. Arch Otolaryngol 1985;111:643–9.

60. Stammberger H. Endoscopic endonasal surgery—concepts in treatment of recurring rhinosinusitis. Part II. Surgical technique. Otolaryngol Head Neck Surg 1986;94:147–56.

61. Sciarretta V, Pasquini E, Frank G, et al. Endoscopic treatment of benign tumors of the nose and paranasal sinuses: A report of 33 cases. Am J Rhinol 2006;20:64–71.

62. Som PM, Brandwein MS, Maldjian C, et al. Sinonasal tumors and inflammatory tissues: Differentiation with MR imaging. Radiology 1988;167:803–8.

63. Melroy CT, Senior BA. Benign sinonasal neoplasms: A focus on inverting papilloma. Otolaryngol Clin North Am 2006;39:601–17.

64. Mehta BS, Grewal GS. Osteoma of the paranasal sinuses along with a case report of an orbito-ethmoidal osteoma. J Laryngol Otol 1963;77:601–10.

65. Earwaker J. Paranasal sinus osteomas: A review of 46 cases. Skeletal Radiol 1993;22:417–23.

66. Naraghi M, Kashfi A. Endonasal endoscopic resection of ethmoido-orbital osteoma compressing the optic nerve. Am J Otolaryngol 2003;24:408–12.

67. Osma U, Yaldiz M, Tekin M, Topcu I. Giant ethmoid osteoma with orbital extension presenting with epiphora. Rhinology 2003;41:122–4.

68. Eller R, Sillers M. Common fibro-osseous lesions of the paranasal sinuses. Otolaryngol Clin North Am 2006;39:585–600.

69. Chen C, Selva D, Wormald PJ. Endoscopic modified lothrop procedure: An alternative for frontal osteoma excision. Rhinology 2004;42:239–43.

70. Sayan NB, Ucok C, Karasu HA, et al. Peripheral osteoma of the oral and maxillofacial region: A study of 35 new cases. J Oral Maxillofac Surg 2002;60 1299–301.

71. Smith ME, Calcaterra TC. Frontal sinus osteoma. Ann Otol Rhinol Laryngol 1989;98:896–900.

72. Moretti A, Croce A, Leone O, et al. Osteoma of maxillary sinus: Case report. Acta Otorhinolaryngol Ital 2004;24:219–22.

73. Summers LE, Mascott CR, Tompkins JR, et al. Frontal sinus osteoma associated with cerebral abscess formation: A case report. Surg Neurol 2001;55:235–9.

74. Gezici AR, Okay O, Ergun R, et al. Rare intracranial manifestations of frontal osteomas. Acta Neurochir (Wien) 2004;146:393–6.

75. Atallah N, Jay MM. Osteomas of the paranasal sinuses. J Laryngol Otol 1981;95:291–304.

76. Aygun N, Zinreich SJ. Imaging for functional endoscopic sinus surgery. Otolaryngol Clin North Am 2006;39:403–16.

77. Rappaport JM, Attia EL. Pneumocephalus in frontal sinus osteoma: A case report. J Otolaryngol 1994;23:430–6.

78. Schick B, Steigerwald C, el Rahman el Tahan A, Draf W. The role of endonasal surgery in the management of fronto-ethmoidal osteomas. Rhinology 2001;39:66–70.

79. Chiu AG, Schipor I, Cohen NA, et al. Surgical decisions in the management of frontal sinus osteomas. Am J Rhinol 2005;19:191–7.

80. Lindman J, Sillers M. Operative trephination for non-acute frontal sinus disease. Oper Tech Otolaryngol 2004;15:67–70.

81. MacDonald-Jankowski DS. Fibro-osseous lesions of the face and jaws. Clin Radiol 2004;59:11–25.

82. Verdaguer JM, Lobo D, Garcia-Berrocal JR, et al. Radiology quiz case 4. McCune–Albright syndrome. Arch Otolaryngol Head Neck Surg 2005;131:181–5.

83. Vaidya AM, Chow JM, Goldberg K, et al. Juvenile aggressive ossifying fibroma presenting as an ethmoid sinus mucocele. Otolaryngol Head Neck Surg 1998;119:665–8.

84. Post G, Kountakis SE. Endoscopic resection of large sinonasal ossifying fibroma. Am J Otolaryngol 2005;26:54–6.

85. Han JK, Smith TL, Loehrl TA, et al. An evolution in the management of sinonasal inverting papilloma. Laryngoscope 2001;111:1395–400.

86. Ward N. A mirror of the practice of medicine and surgery in the hospitals of London. London Hospital Lancet 1854;2:87–99.

87. Ringertz N. Pathology of malignant tumors arising in the nasal and paranasal cavities and maxilla. Acta Otolaryngol 1938;27:31–42.

88. Lawson W, Le Benger J, Som P, et al. Inverted papilloma: An analysis of 87 cases. Laryngoscope 1989;99:1117–24.

89. Hyams VJ. Papillomas of the nasal cavity and paranasal sinuses. A clinicopathological study of 315 cases. Ann Otol Rhinol Laryngol 1971;80:192–206.

90. Weissler MC, Montgomery WW, Turner PA, et al. Inverted papilloma. Ann Otol Rhinol Laryngol 1986;95:215–21.

91. Vrabec DP. The inverted Schneiderian papilloma: A 25-year study. Laryngoscope 1994;104:582–605.

92. Stammberger H. New aspects in the genesis of inverted papillomas. Laryngol Rhinol Otol (Stuttg) 1983;62:249–55.

93. Kramer R, Som ML. True papilloma of the nasal cavity. Arch Otolaryngol 1935;22:22–43.

94. Frenkiel S, Mongiardo FD, Tewfik TL, et al. Viral implications in the formation of multicentric inverting papilloma. J Otolaryngol 1994;23:419–22.

95. Respler DS, Jahn A, Pater A, et al. Isolation and characterization of papillomavirus DNA from nasal inverting (schneiderian) papillomas. Ann Otol Rhinol Laryngol 1987;96:170–3.

96. Weber RS, Shillitoe EJ, Robbins KT, et al. Prevalence of human papillomavirus in inverted nasal papillomas. Arch Otolaryngol Head Neck Surg 1988;114:23–6.

97. Buchwald C, Nielsen LH, Nielsen PL, et al. Inverted papilloma: A follow-up study including primarily unacknowledged cases. Am J Otolaryngol 1989;10:273–81.

98. Krouse JH. Endoscopic treatment of inverted papilloma: Safety and efficacy. Am J Otolaryngol 2001;22:87–99.

99. Phillips PP, Gustafson RO, Facer GW. The clinical behavior of inverting papilloma of the nose and paranasal sinuses: Report of 112 cases and review of the literature. Laryngoscope 1990;100:463–9.

100. Lee JT, Bhuta S, Lufkin R, et al. Isolated inverting papilloma of the sphenoid sinus. Laryngoscope 2003;113:41–4.

101. Som PM, Lawson W, Lidov MW. Simulated aggressive skull base erosion in response to benign sinonasal disease. Radiology 1991;180:755–9.

102. Roobottom CA, Jewell FM, Kabala J. Primary and recurrent inverting papilloma: Appearances with magnetic resonance imaging. Clin Radiol 1995;50:472–5.

103. Yousem DM, Fellows DW, Kennedy DW, et al. Inverted papilloma: Evaluation with MR imaging. Radiology 1992;185:501–5.

104. Stankiewicz JA, Girgis SJ. Endoscopic surgical treatment of nasal and paranasal sinus inverted papilloma. Otolaryngol Head Neck Surg 1993;109:988–95.

105. Lawson W, Ho BT, Shaari CM, et al. Inverted papilloma: A report of 112 cases. Laryngoscope 1995;105:282–8.

106. Wormald PJ, Ooi E, van Hasselt CA, et al. Endoscopic removal of sinonasal inverted papilloma including endoscopic medial maxillectomy. Laryngoscope 2003;113:867–73.

107. McCary WS, Gross CW, Reibel JF, et al. Preliminary report: Endoscopic versus external surgery in the management of inverting papilloma. Laryngoscope 1994;104:415–9.

108. Waitz G, Wigand ME. Results of endoscopic sinus surgery for the treatment of inverted papillomas. Laryngoscope 1992;102:917–22.

109. Jameson MJ, Kountakis SE. Endoscopic management of extensive inverted papilloma. Am J Rhinol 2005;19:446–51.

110. Wolfe SG, Schlosser RJ, Bolger WE, et al. Endoscopic and endoscope-assisted resections of inverted sinonasal papillomas. Otolaryngol Head Neck Surg 2004;131:174–9.

111. Sadeghi N, Al-Dhahri A, Manoukian JJ. Transnasal endoscopic medial maxillectomy for inverting papilloma. Laryngoscope 2003;113:749–53.

112. Krouse JH. Development of a staging system for inverted papilloma. Laryngoscope 2000;110:965–8.

113. Daneshi A, Asghari A, Bahramy E. Primary meningioma of the ethmoid sinus: A case report. Ear Nose Throat J 2003;82:310–1.

114. Shinohara K, Hashimoto K, Yamashita M, et al. Schwannoma of the nasal septum removed with endoscopic surgery. Otolaryngol Head Neck Surg 2005;132:963–4.

115. Athre R, Ducic Y. Frontal sinus hamartomas. Am J Otolaryngol 2005;26:419–21.

116. Kapadia SB, Popek EJ, Barnes L. Pediatric otorhinolaryngic pathology: Diagnosis of selected lesions. Pathol Annu 1994;29:159–209.

117. Sciarretta V, Pasquini E, Farneti G, et al. Endoscopic sinus surgery for the treatment of vascular tumors. Am J Rhinol 2006;20:426–31.

118. Budrovich R, Saetti R. Microscopic and endoscopic ligature of the sphenopalatine artery. Laryngoscope 1992;102:1391–4.

119. Buchwald C, Tranum-Jenson J. Endoscopic sphenopalatine artery ligation or diathermy. Oper Tech Otolaryngol 2006;17:28–30.

120. Kumar S, Shetty A, Rockey J, et al. Contemporary surgical treatment of epistaxis. What is the evidence for sphenopalatine artery ligation? Clin Otolaryngol Allied Sci 2003;28:360–3.

121. Sethi DS, Leong JL. Endoscopic pituitary surgery. Otolaryngol Clin North Am 2006;39:563–83.

122. Sonnenburg RE, White D, Ewend MG, et al. Sellar reconstruction: Is it necessary? Am J Rhinol 2003;17:343–6.

123. Senior BA, Dubin MG, Sonnenburg RE, et al. Increased role of the otolaryngologist in endoscopic pituitary surgery: Endoscopic hydroscopy of the sella. Am J Rhinol 2005;19:181–4.

124. White DR, Sonnenburg RE, Ewend MG, et al. Safety of minimally invasive pituitary surgery (MIPS) compared with a traditional approach. Laryngoscope 2004;114:1945–8.

125. Jho HD, Carrau RL, Ko Y, et al. Endoscopic pituitary surgery: An early experience. Surg Neurol 1997;47:213–22.

126. Carrau RL, Jho HD, Ko Y. Transnasal-transsphenoidal endoscopic surgery of the pituitary gland. Laryngoscope 1996;106:914–8.

127. Bassim M, Senior B. Minimally invasive pituitary surgery. Oper Tech Otolaryngol 2006;17:31–6.

FACIAL PLASTIC AND RECONSTRUCTIVE SURGERY

52

Otoplasty for the Prominent Ear

John S. Rhee, MD, MPH

Jeffrey Tseng, MD

Otoplasty is a common surgical technique primarily used to establish the normal anatomical relationships of the ear. Achieving an optimal result begins with understanding the three-dimensional anatomic relationships of the auricle. Over the past century and a half, numerous surgical techniques have been described, but recent trends have pointed to more conservative approaches that minimize risk and unnatural appearing outcomes.

In this chapter, the embryology and surface anatomy of the ear will be reviewed, along with the ideal anatomical relationships of the ear. Furthermore, common definitions of auricular abnormalities will be described followed by preoperative considerations. Finally, the four essential steps necessary for correction of the protruding ear will be discussed along with postoperative management, common pitfalls, and complications.

EMBRYOLOGY AND SURFACE ANATOMY

Embryology

The auricle is formed from six mesenchymal proliferations (hillocks of His) that originate from the first and second branchial arches. These six hillocks are thought to be the precursors for the tragus, helical crus, helix, antihelix, scapha, and the lobule, respectively.[1] The first three hillocks are located anteriorly and they originate from the first branchial (mandibular) arch, whereas the last three hillocks are posterior and they originate from the second branchial (hyoid) arch. The hillocks first appear during the sixth week of gestational life and achieve final orientation by the twentieth week. By the end of development, the hillocks will have moved fro m their original position in the upper part of the future neck to a posterior cranial position at the level of the eyes.[2]

Surface Anatomy

The auricle is a complex structure of fibroelastic cartilage with a thin overlying layer of skin. On its anterior aspect, the skin directly overlies the perichondrium. On its posterior aspect, a layer of connective tissue and fat separates the perichondrium from the skin. The helix forms a fold at the superior edge of the auricle extending from the crus helicus to a posterior-inferior arc that enters the lobule inferiorly as the cauda helices (Figure 1). The antihelical fold, or antihelix, runs parallel to the helix along its medial edge. The superior portion of the antihelix forms the superior and inferior crura divided by an area termed the fossa triangularis. The scapha is the depression immediately posterior to the antihelix. Medial to the antihelical fold lies the concha, a cavity that forms the deep cup-like appearance of the ear. The helical crus separates the concha into the cymba conchae and the cavum conchae.

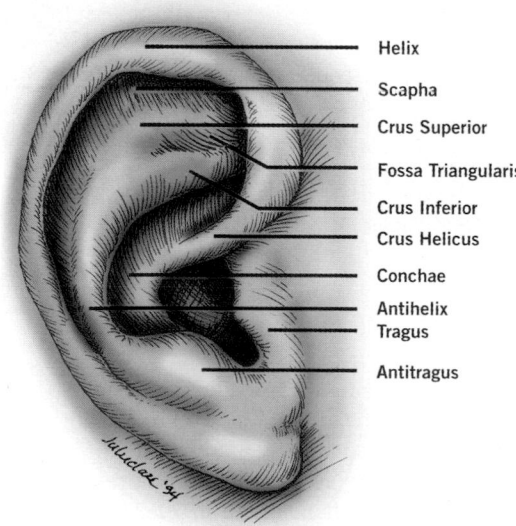

Helix
Scapha
Crus Superior
Fossa Triangularis
Crus Inferior
Crus Helicus
Conchae
Antihelix
Tragus
Antitragus

Figure 1 Auricular landmarks.

The tragus is a cartilaginous projection that lies anterior to the external opening of the external auditory canal. Finally, the lobule is primarily made of fat and skin and is at the most inferior edge of the auricle. Sensory innervation of the auricle is through C3 (greater auricular nerve), C2 and C3 (lesser occipital nerve), cranial nerve X (Arnold nerve), cranial nerve V_3 (auriculotemporal nerve), and cranial nerve VII. The predominant arterial blood supply of the auricle is through the posterior auricular and superficial temporal branch of the external carotid artery and a branch of the occipital artery.

Ideal surface anatomy of the ear can be defined in a series of five anatomical relationships. First, the "line of balance" is defined as an axis through the longest dimension of the ear and should recline 20° from the vertical plane.[3] Second, the typical ear has an average height of 63.5 mm.[4] Third, the auricular width should be approximately 55% of its height.[4] Fourth, the angle of protrusion (auriculomastoid angle) may vary in different individuals but should be between 15 and 30°.[5-7] Finally, the helical rim should be 15 to 20 mm from the temporomastoid surface of the skull at the point of maximum prominence.[7,8]

Categories and Definitions

Perhaps the most common defect that presents for surgical correction is the prominent ear (alternatively, the outstanding, or protruding ear). The most common cause of this appearance is the lack of development of the antihelical fold. However, other pathologic features, most commonly a deep conchal bowl and/or a malpositioned lobule, can also contribute to the pathogenesis of the protruding ear. The prominent ear can also be described as an auriculomastoid angle greater than 30°. Most patients with a prominent ear will have a positive family history, as the genetic transmission is autosomal dominant with variable penetrance.

Another defect is known as the lop ear and is characterized by a thin, flat auricle with the helix acutely folded downward at the superior pole. The most common causes of this appearance are a poorly developed antihelix, excessive conchal cartilage, and an overprojected lobule.

A third defect is the cup (or shell) ear and is characterized by a smaller than normal ear with weak cartilage resulting in a cupping or deepening of the conchal bowl (Figure 2). The cause of this appearance is poor development of the superior pole with a short, thickened helix and deformed antihelix.

PREOPERATIVE CONSIDERATIONS

The timing of otoplasty remains a subject of debate.[9] Typically, the optimal age for otoplasty is between 4 and 6 years of age. A study of 2,300 ears concluded that 85% of auricular development is complete at 4 years of age.[8] Furthermore, the onset of psychological distress regarding physical appearance is typically thought to begin at 4 to 6 years of age, and there is no data to indicate that the psychological effect of otoplasty performed at age 3 years or younger is different than that when the operation is performed after 5 years of age. Also, an older child will be more capable of participating in the postoperative care of the ear and hence decrease the risk of postoperative complications. Finally, at this young age, the cartilage remains soft and pliable and is amenable to surgical manipulation.

The physical examination should focus on the absence of an antihelical fold, a determination of the conchal bowl size and projection, an assessment of the lobule size and position, and the degree of asymmetry between the right and left ears.

Indications for surgery include the absence or poor development of the antihelical fold with greater than 20 mm projection of the helical rim from the mastoid skin, a deep conchal bowl with an auriculomastoid angle greater than 30°, asymmetrically projecting ears, and a desire for correction by the patient. Contraindications for surgery include a child younger than 4 years of age, a history of keloid formation, and unrealistic surgical expectations.

Photodocumentation is essential for preoperative planning with standard frontal, lateral, and oblique views captured for all patients. Posterior and closeup lateral views are optional.

HISTORICAL PERSPECTIVE

Although the first known reference to an otoplasty was published in a book by Dieffenbach, *Die Operativechirurgie*, in 1845, an otologist named Edward Ely is widely credited for the first published description of the otoplasty technique.[10] Early otoplasties described a multitude of techniques including skin excision, conchal cartilage remodeling, and manipulation of the angle between the auricle and the mastoid skin. In 1910, Luckett was the first to understand the connection between

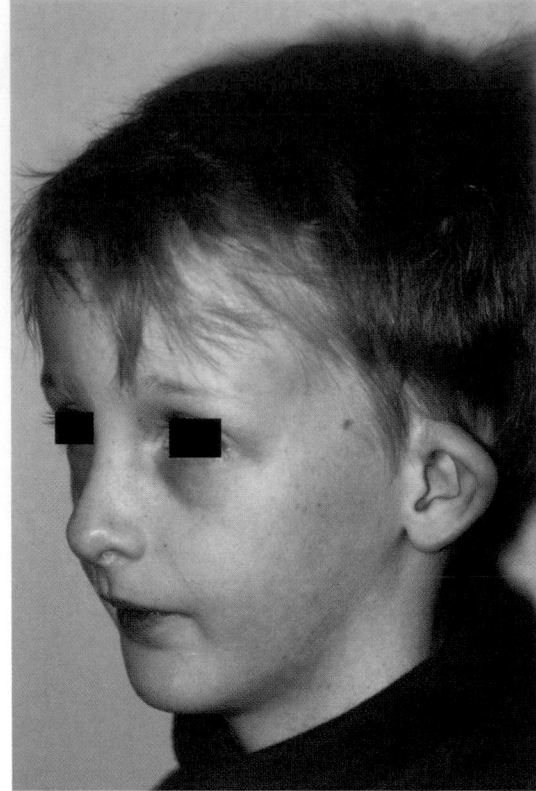

(A)

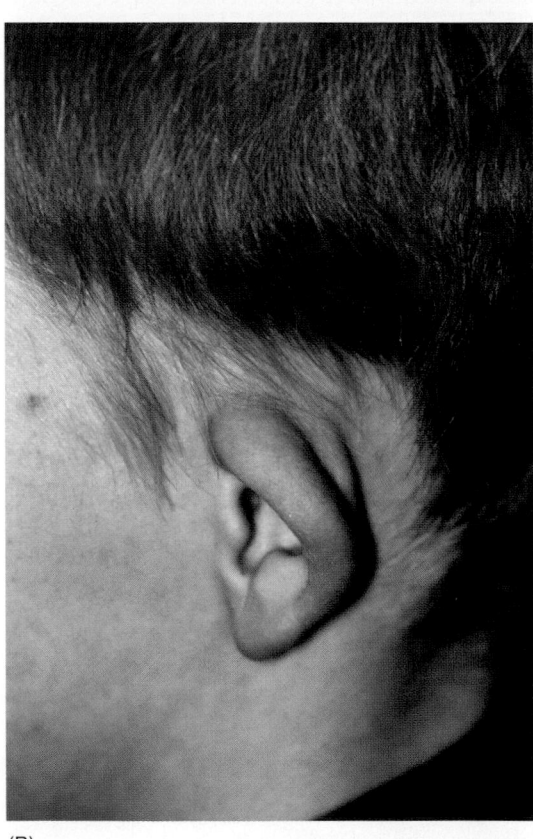

(B)

Figure 2 Five-year-old boy with cup ear deformity. (A) Oblique view. (B) Close-up lateral view.

an abnormal or absent antihelical fold and the protruding ear; he excised a portion of the auricular cartilage to create a new antihelical fold.[11] Mustarde was the first to use mattress sutures to establish a proper antihelical fold in 1963.[12] Mustarde avoided incising cartilage in an effort to prevent the creation of a surgically altered ear; he instead

placed sutures on the posterior surface of the ear cartilage to create a new antihelical fold. In 1968, Furnas introduced the conchal setback technique of placing sutures to fix the conchal cartilage to the mastoid periosteum in an effort to remodel a deeply cupped conchal bowl.[13]

CARTILAGE-INCISION VERSUS CARTILAGE-SPARING TECHNIQUES

The goal of all surgeons performing otoplasty is to establish normal anatomical relationships. However, the fibroelastic cartilage of the auricle is different in every individual. Subsequently, there are both cartilage-incision techniques useful for stiff and thick cartilage and cartilage-sparing techniques that can be utilized in more soft and pliable cartilage. When treating a diverse patient population, the surgeon must realize that increasing age tends to bring stiffer cartilage that may need partial or complete cartilage resection for the creation of normal anatomical relationships. Stucker and colleagues found that in the adult population, 98.9% of patients required use of lateral conchal cartilage resection combined with a mattress suture technique.[14] Alternatively, in the pediatric population, all patients required use of a mattress suture technique, and in 83.2% of selected cases, limited lateral conchal cartilage resection was required to obtain proper anatomical relationships. Cartilage-incision techniques either consist of a complete incision through the cartilage or a series of partial thickness incisions that cause the cartilage to bend away from the cut side. The drawback to the complete incision technique is that it may leave a sharp irregularity over the surface of the antihelical cartilage. Partial thickness incision techniques rely on several parallel incisions in the cartilage rather than one full thickness incision to minimize the risk of developing an irregular edge in the new antihelical fold. On the other hand, the partial thickness incision technique can lead to problems if the sutures used to establish normal anatomical relationships fail. Furthermore, any cartilage-incision technique can create unfavorable scarring.

Cartilage-sparing techniques were developed in part to minimize the risk of developing a sharp edge along the antihelix. Two other reasons were to avoid a technique that irreversibly changed anatomical landmarks and to minimize dissection of the ear. These techniques are most useful in patients with soft and pliable cartilage and utilize horizontal mattress sutures (Mustarde) to form the proper antihelical fold and create the appropriate conchomastoid angle (Furnas sutures) by bringing the conchal bowl to the mastoid periosteum. One potential drawback to utilizing the Mustarde sutures is that the technique may create an antihelical fold that is too prominent if the cartilage is too thick. Therefore, surgeons utilizing this cartilage-sparing technique may shave the medial aspect of the cartilage in an effort to decrease the extra bulk, most commonly at the level of the superior crus.

SURGICAL TECHNIQUE

The surgical considerations and techniques outlined below are most applicable to the prominent ear deformity. Correction of other auricular deformities is beyond the scope of this chapter, but certain portions of the outlined techniques can be used for other auricular malformations. The six major goals of a successful otoplasty outlined by McDowell include: (1) correct protrusion in the upper third of the ear; (2) ensure that the helices of both ears are lateral to the antihelices on antero-posterior view; (3) create a helix with a smooth and regular contour; (4) avoid a markedly decreased or disturbed postauricular sulcus; (5) realize that the ear should not be placed too close to the head (especially in males); and (6) achieve symmetry between the two ears with no more than 3 mm difference at any given point.[15]

In essence, there are four major steps to correction of the prominent ear. Depending on the deformity, not all four steps are necessary to achieve an optimal result.

Step 1: Skin and Soft Tissue Excision

After local anesthesia is injected subcutaneously, an eccentric fusiform incision is made around the postauricular sulcus to address the undeveloped antihelical fold (Figure 3). This is preferable in situations where a very deep conchal bowl is the primary cause of the protruding ear; the subsequent conchomastoid (Furnas) suture placement and soft tissue excision aids in conchal setback. As the incision is made, more tissues are removed from the auricle than the mastoid area and the fusiform area is 10 to 12 mm at its widest point. Dissection is taken down to the perichondrium of the auricle and periosteum of mastoid bone with subcutaneous tissue, fat, and postauricular muscle excised with the overlying skin. Care is taken to avoid injury to the greater auricular nerve, as tissues lateral to the mastoid fascia are dissected to expose the periosteum of the mastoid bone. An optional releasing incision may be necessary at the superior pole of the incision to facilitate exposure to the antihelical fold.

Alternatively, a dumbbell-shaped incision can be used, especially in cases in which conchal bowl reduction or repositioning is unnecessary

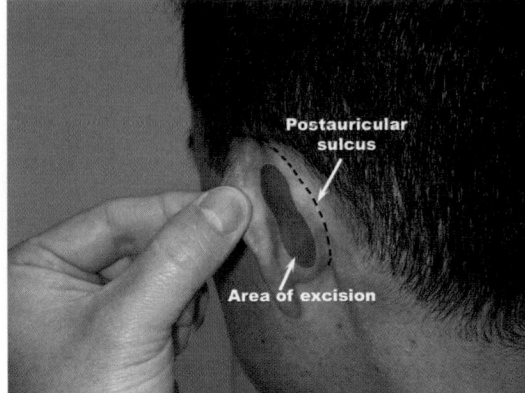

Figure 4 Dumbbell-shaped skin excision pattern.

(Figure 4). Although this dumbbell-shaped incision creates easier access to the antihelical fold for placement of Mustarde sutures, it does make conchomastoid suture placement more difficult. However, this pattern of incision aids in preventing the overcorrection of the middle portion of the auricle and the relative prominence of the superior and inferior poles known as the "telephone-ear" deformity which will be discussed below.

Step 2: Correction of the Deep Conchal Bowl

Once the dissection is at the level of perichondrium of the ear, the prominent posterior eminence of the conchal cartilage can be shaved off (in the shape of small disks) using a scalpel. This facilitates conchal setback and reduces cartilage bulk that prevents the auricle from lying closer to the head. It is important to remember that only a partial thickness excision is performed here to prevent overcorrection of the conchal bowl. Conchomastoid (Furnas) sutures are now placed in a horizontal mattress fashion using 4-0 mersilene (or clear nylon) suture in one or two locations to appose the conchal bowl to the mastoid periosteum (Figure 5). The purpose of the sutures is to reduce the auriculomastoid angle to between 15 and 30°. Incorrectly placed sutures can project the conchal cartilage anteriorly, which can subsequently result in stenosis of the external auditory canal. This complication can be avoided by placing the mastoid end of the conchomastoid suture as far posteriorly as possible without distorting the entrance of the external auditory canal.

Step 3: Creation of the Antihelical Fold

Once the auriculomastoid angle has been corrected, Mustarde sutures are used to create the antihelical fold. As discussed previously, in the adult patient or in those patients with thick, inelastic cartilages, cartilage incision techniques can be used in conjunction with the Mustarde sutures to help form the antihelical fold. Horizontal mattress sutures (4-0 mersilene or nylon sutures) are placed in the auricular cartilage along the scapha to recreate the antihelical fold (Figure 6). The sutures should pass through posterior perichondrium, cartilage, and anterior perichondrium. Care should be taken to include the full thickness of the cartilage and lateral perichondrium without involving the lateral skin. Four to five sutures are usually needed to establish the natural curve to the antihelical fold. Knots should be tied sequentially from top to bottom after placement of all the sutures; this allows the tension from superior sutures to secure the optimal fold and allows the surgeon to adjust sequentially as he or she moves inferiorly. Overtightening or undertightening of these sutures will result in a suboptimal outcome. These sutures are vital to maintain the repair until enough scar tissue forms to maintain the new antihelical fold. Special attention should be placed on the superior pole as this is the most likely area for unraveling to occur.[16,17]

Step 4: Lobule Repositioning or Reduction

Once the antihelical fold is created, it is important to examine the lobule. The helix, antihelix, and lobule should all be in the same plane. Proper orientation of the tail of the helical cartilage can restore correct lobule position. Abnormal lobule position can result in the "telephone-ear" and "reverse telephone ear" deformities. The conchal setback step may improve the lobule position without further intervention. However, overcorrection of the middle third of the ear via Mustarde sutures may accentuate a malpositioned lobule. Often, a protruding lobule results from a flared caudal helical cartilage. Alternatively, the lobule may be congenitally enlarged with excess fat and skin. If further lobule medialization is needed, incision of the cauda helicis or a horizontal

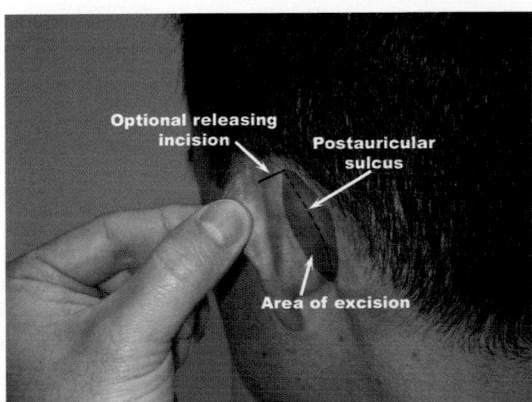

Figure 3 Eccentric fusiform skin excision pattern. Dashed line indicates optional releasing incision.

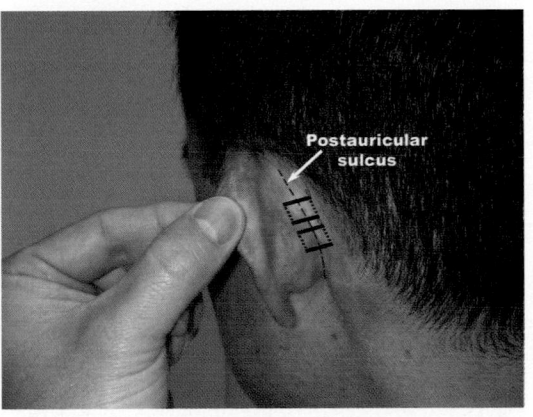

Figure 5 Conchomastoid suture placement.

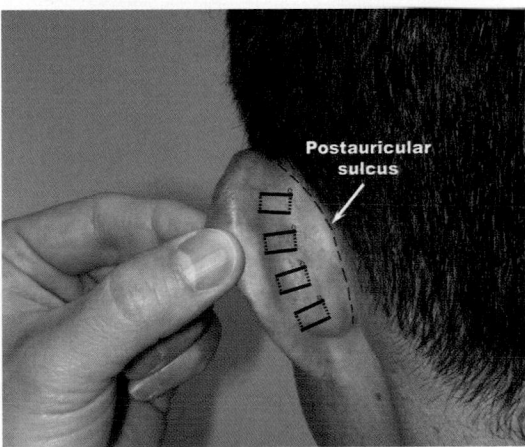

Figure 6 Mustarde suture placement.

mattress suture placed between the cauda helicis and the inferior conchal cavum may be necessary. Lobule reduction can be performed with a fusiform wedge excision at the posterior-inferior border of the lobule or a curvilinear excision along the inferior aspect of the lobule depending on the area of excess.

Once lobule repositioning is complete, hemostasis is obtained with cautery. The skin incision is closed in a single layer with interrupted 5-0 gut suture. The opposite ear is then addressed with the ultimate goal being to achieve proper symme-

try between ears. Antibiotic ointment is applied to the incisional line. Cotton, saturated in mineral oil, is molded to the lateral surface of the ear and a pressure dressing is applied to decrease the risk of developing a hematoma. A drain is not required.

Figure 7 demonstrates a typical patient with prominent ears with poor antihelical fold development. Conchal bowl excess, lobule malpositioning, or excess lobule size was not appreciated in the preoperative condition. In this case, a dumbbell-shaped skin excision was used to facilitate

the placement of the Mustarde sutures and to minimize the chances for a telephone-ear deformity. No conchal reduction or setback was necessary. The lobule-helix relationship was facilitated by the skin and soft tissue excision only.

In some instances, antihelical fold correction alone is insufficient. The patient in Figure 8 had some conchal bowl excess along with poor antihelical fold definition. An elliptical excision of soft tissue was performed along with conchal bowl shave, placement of conchomastoid and Mustarde sutures, and division of the cauda helices.

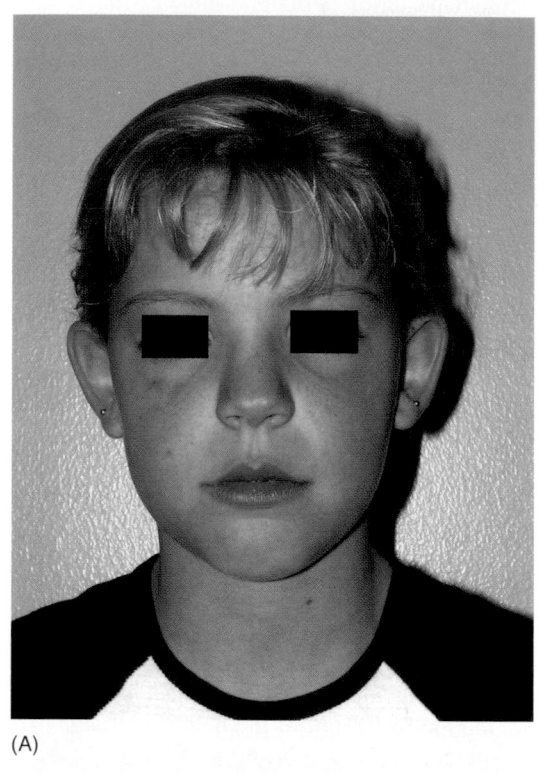

(A)

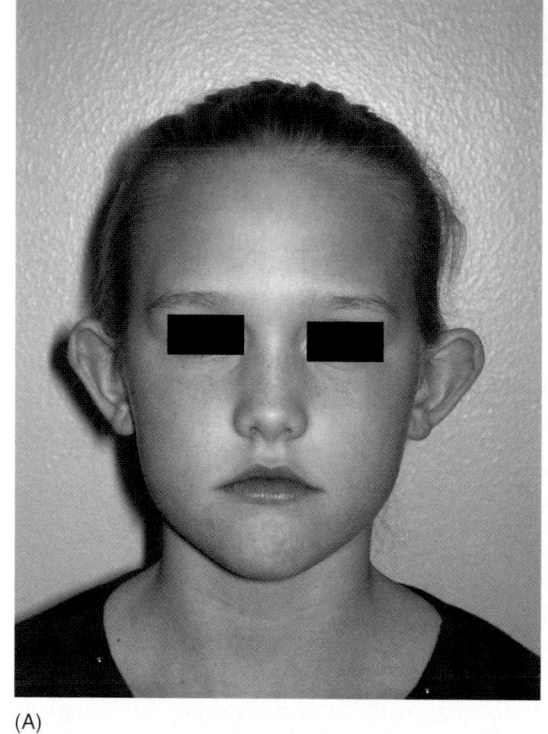

(A)

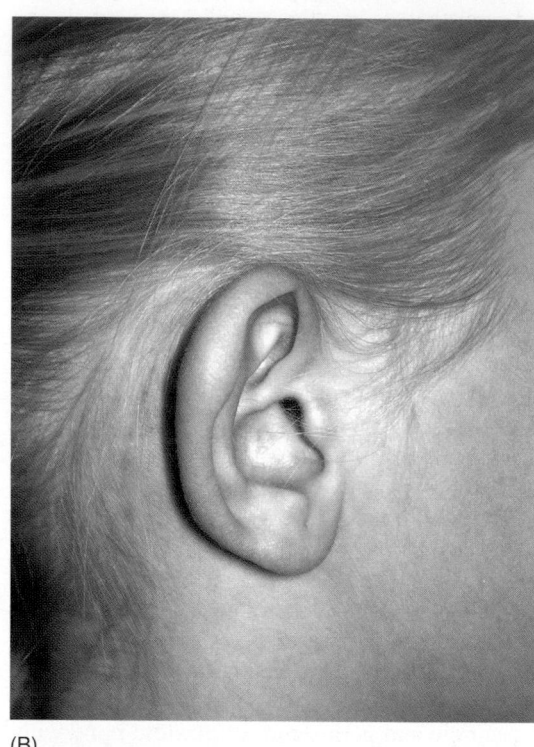

(B)

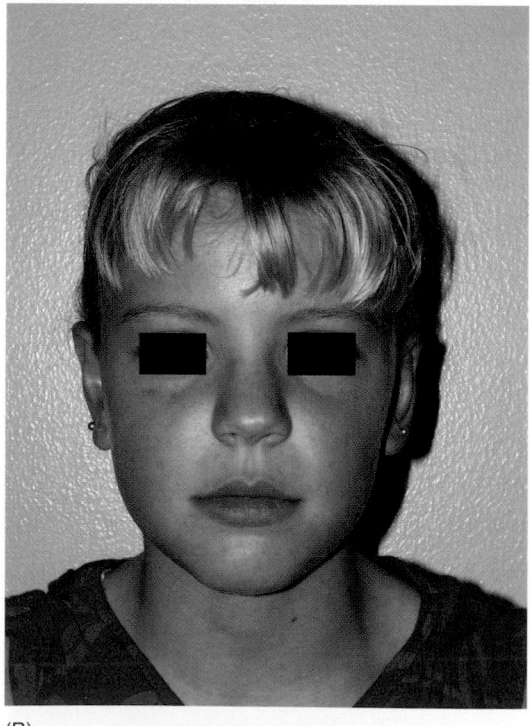

(B)

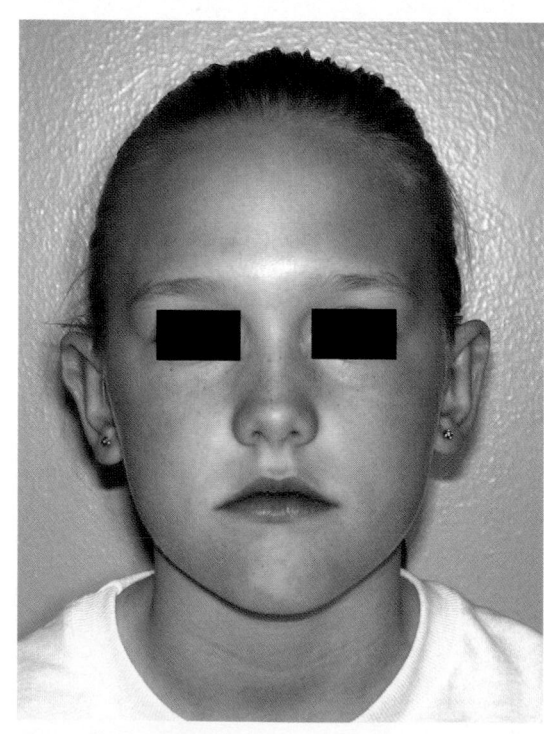

(C)

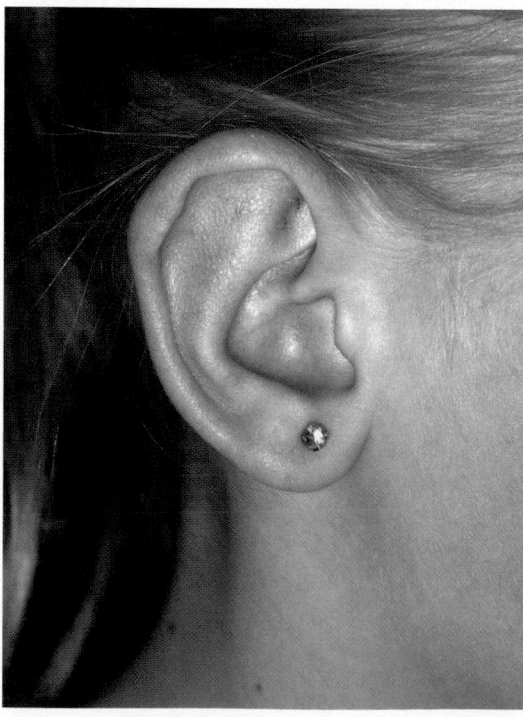

(D)

Figure 7 (A) Preoperative and (B) postoperative photographs of a 12-year-old girl who underwent bilateral otoplasty.

Figure 8 (A) and (B) Preoperative and (C) and (D) postoperative photographs of an 8-year-old girl who underwent bilateral otoplasty.

POSTOPERATIVE CARE

It is important to check for hematoma formation on the first postoperative day. The pressure dressing should be left on for 3 to 4 more days. After the pressure dressing is removed, a light head band should be worn at night for the next 4 to 6 weeks postoperatively.

PITFALLS AND COMPLICATIONS

Hematoma

Hematoma commonly presents with significant and persistent pain or "tightness." A tense swelling with or without ecchymosis is usually seen underneath the pressure dressing and necessitates immediate evacuation. The clot should be removed and the wound examined for any potential bleeding sources. If the hematoma is not removed quickly enough, the overlying cartilage and/or skin can necrose and chondritis may result.

Infection

Infection may result in permanent cosmetic deformity. Fortunately, it is rare because of the abundant blood supply to the head and neck region. Symptoms include fever, and the signs are erythema, swelling, and/or pus along the incision. Minor forms of cellulitis can be treated with broad-spectrum antibiotics that cover *Staphylococcus aureus* and *Pseudomonas aeruginosa*. If the infection fails to respond to oral antibiotics, the patient will need inpatient admission, wound irrigation, and parenteral antibiotics.

Hypertrophic Scar or Keloid Formation

Keloid formation more frequently develops in African-Americans than in Caucasians. One retrospective study involving 570 ears found keloid formation in 11% of African-American ears and 2.1% of Caucasian ears.[18] Intraoperative considerations for prevention of keloid formation include conservative skin excision, adequate tissue mobilization, and tension free closure. Most early keloids can be treated with intradermal Triamcinolone injections.

External Auditory Canal Stenosis

As noted previously, this may result if the conchomastoid suture is placed too far anteriorly on the mastoid region. This complication can be treated directly with trimming of the redundant cartilage at the ear canal. Alternatively, the conchomastoid sutures can be repositioned to the more appropriate posterior position.

Aesthetic Complications

The most common complications relate to a suboptimal aesthetic outcome. Although some loss of correction is to be expected, thick auricular cartilage placed under excessive tension with Mustarde sutures may be the source of recurrence of the deformity. This undercorrection may also result if too few Mustarde sutures are used when creating the antihelical fold. Rates of relapse of auricular projection range from 2 to 13%.[17]

Slight asymmetries in projection between the auricles are well tolerated and acceptable. However, greater than 2 mm difference between the helical rim projections from the temporomastoid surface of the skull will likely be noticeable and may warrant revision. Similarly, significant lobule position or size discrepancies should be revised.

The telephone-ear deformity results from either overcorrection of the middle third of the ear along with inadequate flexion at the superior and inferior auricular poles or excessive removal of postauricular skin or mastoid soft tissue. Prevention of this complication is best achieved by rechecking the suture tension immediately before wound closure. Treatment of this complication is problematic if it stems from overresection of conchal cartilage from the middle third of the ear. The upper third needs to be set closer to the mastoid and the lobule must be revised. The reverse telephone ear deformity results from overcorrection of the upper and lower poles of the ear and failure to address a deeply cupped conchal bowl.

REFERENCES

1. Gulya AJ. Developmental anatomy of the ear. In: Glasscock ME, III, Shambaugh GE, Jr, editors. Surgery of the Ear, 4th edition. Philadelphia: WB Saunders; 1990. p. 5–33.
2. Moore KL. The Developing Human, 4th edition. Philadelphia: WB Saunders; 1988.
3. Tolleth H. Artistic anatomy, dimensions, and proportions of the external ear. Clin Plast Surg 1978;5:337–45.
4. Farkas L. An thropometry of normal and anomalous ears. Clin Plast Surg 1978;5:401–12.
5. Rubin LR, Bromberg BE, Walden RH, Adams A. An anatomic approach to the obtrusive ear. Plast Reconstr Surg 1962;29:360–70.
6. Pitanguy I, Flemming I. Plastic operations on the auricle. In: Naumann HH, editor. Head and Neck Surgery. Philadelphia: WB Saunders; 1982. p. 1–18.
7. Gluckman JE, editor. Renewal of Certification IA Study Guide in Otolaryngology—Head Neck Surgery. Dubuque, Kendall/Hunt; 1998. p. 678–84.
8. Adamson JE, Horton CE, Crawford HH. The growth pattern of the external ear. Plast Reconstr Surg 1965;36:466–70.
9. Gosain AK, Kumar A, Huang G. Prominent ears in children younger than 4 years of age: What is the appropriate timing for otoplasty? Plast Reconstr Surg 2004;114:1042–54.
10. Ely ET. An operation for prominence of the auricles. Arch Ophthalmol Otol 1881;10:97.
11. Luckett WH. A new operation for prominent ears based on the anatomy of the deformity. Surg Gynecol Obstet 1910;10:635–7.
12. Mustarde JC. The correction of prominent ears by using simple mattress sutures. Br J Plast Surg 1963;16:170–8.
13. Furnas DW. Correction of prominent ears by concha-mastoid sutures. Plast Reconstr Surg 1968;42:189–92.
14. Stucker FJ, Vora NM, Lian TS. Otoplasty: An analysis of technique over a 33-year period. Laryngoscope 2003;113:952–6.
15. McDowell AJ. Goals in otoplasty for protruding ears. Plast Reconstr Surg 1968;41:17–27.
16. Adamson PA, McGraw BL, Tropper GJ. Otoplasty: Critical review of clinical results. Laryngoscope 1991;101:883–8.
17. Messner AH, Crysdale WS. Otoplasty clinical and long-term results. Arch Otolaryngol Head Neck Surg 1996; 122:773–7.
18. Baker DC, Converse JM. Otoplasty: A 20 year retrospective. Aesthetic Plast Surg 1979;3:29–39.

53

Rhinoplasty and Septoplasty

Richard E. Davis, MD

THE ART AND SCIENCE OF AESTHETIC RHINOPLASTY

Fueled by the timeless and universal quest for human beauty, cosmetic rhinoplasty has become a permanent fixture of American cultural life. For some patients, the impact of cosmetic rhinoplasty can be remarkable, transforming the face from a collection of disjointed anatomic features to a harmonious and captivating blend, in which the cosmetic whole exceeds the sum of its individual parts. Moreover, unlike many cosmetic procedures, the effects of rhinoplasty are permanent and largely immune to the effects of aging. Owing to its durable, predictable, and dramatic surgical results, cosmetic rhinoplasty enjoys enormous popularity and remains an extremely gratifying cosmetic procedure for both patient and surgeon alike.

However, cosmetic nasal surgery is also among the most challenging of all cosmetic surgical procedures. Considerable harm can result when rhinoplasty is performed improperly, and the adverse effects can dramatically alter both facial cosmesis and nasal physiology. Although rhinoplasty ranks among the most commonly performed cosmetic operations, few surgeons ever master its numerous subtleties and peculiar nuances. No doubt, the difficulty of cosmetic rhinoplasty is attributable to the unique cosmetic, functional, and anatomic characteristics of the nose. In addition to its prominent cosmetic location, the nose is a complex three-dimensional organ with delicate tissues of varying histologic type; including skin, bone, cartilage, muscle, and nasal mucosa. The surgeon must execute exacting and precise changes to this complicated anatomic structure; these changes must remain stable over time, and they must not occur at the expense of satisfactory nasal airway function. "Do no harm" remains the cardinal rule of elective cosmetic surgery.

In addition to understanding all the many technical aspects of cosmetic nasal surgery, the accomplished rhinoplasty surgeon must also possess a strong artistic eye. Indeed, without *accurate* cosmetic analysis of the nose, successful rhinoplasty is all but impossible. The ability to identify correctly aesthetic disharmony, define its component parts, and envision the cosmetic changes necessary to beautify the nose is the hallmark of the gifted rhinoplasty surgeon. Once the aesthetic analysis is complete, the surgeon must gently expose the misshapen nasal framework, finalize the anatomic diagnosis, and refine the preoperative surgical strategy to accommodate hidden surgical findings. The nose is then surgically reconfigured by assembling a mosaic of dissimilar tissues and creating an attractive surface contour that blends harmoniously with the surrounding face. Even when this challenging task is executed to perfection, the result remains at the mercy of wound healing and potential distortions therein. Hence, the truly insightful surgeon will also anticipate unfavorable wound healing characteristics and employ effective countermeasures to mitigate these adverse effects. It is the unique blend of an artistic eye, a gentle and precise hand, and an analytical mind that makes the master rhinoplasty surgeon a rarity in the medical profession.

In addition to surgical and artistic skills, the accomplished rhinoplasty surgeon must also prove adept at psychological assessment and emotional support. Each patient must be carefully evaluated in terms of their motivations, expectations, goals, and apprehensions. The ethical surgeon must also explain the operation, its limitations, and its associated risks in an honest and candid manner, providing full disclosure and a realistic assessment of the anticipated cosmetic outcome. Reassurance, patience, kindness, and empathy are all essential components of the surgical process as a compassionate and supportive surgeon is greatly appreciated during the sometimes disconcerting adjustment to a new self-image. Likewise, the rhinoplasty surgeon must also remain vigilant for unrealistic patient expectations, inappropriate patient motives, and/or a lack of sincere commitment to the surgical recovery process. While the overwhelming majority of properly executed rhinoplasties result in a satisfied patient, the individual with unrealistic expectations, inappropriate motives, or psychological disorders may never reach contentment no matter how favorable the surgical result. When unhealthy motives are suspected, surgery should be avoided to prevent baseless claims of failed surgery and potential conflicts therein.

Another potential reason for avoiding rhinoplasty is an unacceptably high risk of wound healing complications. Although the vast majority of rhinoplasty patients heal favorably with good end results, a small subset of patients may exhibit aberrant wound-healing characteristics despite appropriate surgical strategy and sound surgical technique. In rare but extreme cases, this aberrant healing may manifest as severe subcutaneous fibrosis, aggressive scar contracture, and/or dense hypertrophic scarring that may dramatically impair the cosmetic outcome and lead to potentially permanent nasal deformity. While it is impossible to screen accurately all such predisposed patients, the accomplished rhinoplasty surgeon is distinguished from the novice by the ability to predict and mitigate these unfavorable healing characteristics in a majority of circumstances. The knowledgeable and prudent surgeon will also temper the expectations of scar-prone patients and decline surgery in those patients with an inordinate level of surgical risk.

Although the challenges of cosmetic nasal surgery are formidable, the rewards of a well-executed rhinoplasty are a noticeably more attractive face, in which the eyes predominate and the newly shaped nose blends harmoniously and inconspicuously with the surrounding features. For the typical patient, modest cosmetic improvements produce a satisfied and more confident individual making rhinoplasty a rewarding and worthwhile endeavor. However, for the occasional patient, dramatic cosmetic improvements profoundly transform the self-image leading to equally dramatic increases in self-esteem, self-confidence, and sense of self-worth. For these rare patients, cosmetic rhinoplasty can represent a life-changing milestone in which a far more outgoing, self-assured, and confident individual results; and for the cosmetic surgeon, these patients can be especially gratifying.

ASSESSMENT AND HEALING

All human tissues are susceptible to the effects of aging and the nose is no exception. For individuals with naturally strong and stout nasal cartilage, age-related changes may be subtle or inconsequential since skeletal support is abundant. However, for individuals with naturally weak or flaccid nasal cartilage, the adverse effects of aging may be significant and premature. In severe cases, spontaneous age-related deterioration may even lead to progressive nasal tip ptosis, nasal sidewall collapse, and contour deformities of the alar cartilage. For these individuals, naturally weak nasal cartilage predisposes to loss of structural support ultimately leading to altered nasal contour and increased airway resistance. Indeed, the human nose is in a perpetual state of decay with gradual loss of structural support as the natural byproduct of aging, disease, and/or injury.

Even though aging changes typically require decades to manifest fully, overly aggressive nasal surgery can instantly erode even the most robust skeletal support leading to progressive nasal airway collapse and conspicuous nasal contour deformities. In susceptible individuals, such as those with frail cartilage and naturally weak skeletal support, the consequences of surgical cartilage reduction can be devastating, resulting in profound cosmetic and functional disability. Indeed, the large number of cosmetic rhinoplasty patients seeking treatment for surgically induced nasal contour deformities underscores the importance of tissue conservation and the preservation of adequate skeletal support.

Although the rhinoplasty community has been slow to recognize the risks and adverse effects of aggressive cartilage excision, mounting evidence has condemned the practice of excessive cartilage reduction. Reliable and aesthetically superior results are now achieved by conserving structural elements whenever possible and by trimming oversized elements judiciously. Misshapen tip cartilages are now reconfigured using suture techniques to retain intrinsic structural support, rather than by excising large portions of alar cartilage in a haphazard attempt to alter tip contour through partial collapse of the alar tripod. When cartilage reduction is unavoidable (as often occurs with nasal hump deformities), dorsal height is kept strong and augmentation grafts are often used, even in treatment of the oversized nose, to strengthen residual structural elements weakened by heredity, age, or surgical manipulation. It is this philosophical shift from "volume reduction" to "structural rhinoplasty" that has propelled contemporary cosmetic nasal surgery into a new era of enhanced precision, control, and efficacy.

Although the typical rhinoplasty patient desires immediate improvement following cosmetic nasal surgery, postoperative recovery is a slow and gradual process. Acute nasal swelling and inflammation typically persist for 4 to 6 weeks and complete recovery often requires up to 12 months, even in young healthy patients with favorable wound-healing characteristics. In most cases, gradual restoration of the lymphatic and capillary circulation leads to a progressive reduction in lymphedema and softening of the firm and contracted nasal soft tissues. This in turn gives rise to a thinner, more delicate, and more tightly adherent skin envelope, producing a more attractive and better defined nasal contour. While the speed and pattern of recovery varies widely even among healthy individuals, the recovery process is seldom complete in less than 1 year. Teenage patients with smooth healthy skin often recover faster than adults, but vigorous exercise, heavy sun exposure, prolonged dependent posture, excessive salt intake, or coexisting nasal allergies may prolong the presence of postoperative lymphedema. In contrast, older patients,

patients with thick sebaceous skin, or patients with previously operated (scarred) noses may require several additional months for complete healing even when the circumstances for recovery are optimized. Regardless of age, all patients should be counseled that a nose will seldom look perfect upon dressing removal due to the inevitable presence of edema. In fact, good rhinoplasty outcomes often look disappointing during the first few months following surgery since nasal contour is distorted by swelling; whereas noses that appear thin and delicate at the time of dressing removal may appear pinched, skeletonized, or overresected once all surgical edema has resolved.

Even though surgical edema typically resolves in the first year after surgery, for some rhinoplasty patients the inflammatory changes initiated by cosmetic nasal surgery may take much longer to manifest fully. Unlike patients with forgiving nasal skin, patients with contracture-prone skin may experience a slowly progressive distortion of the nasal framework which may continue for years, or even decades after cosmetic rhinoplasty. This unwanted complication, commonly called the "shrink-wrap phenomenon," develops in susceptible individuals who have both weak cartilage and aggressive contractile tendencies. Naturally weak cartilage or excessive reduction of the cartilage framework results in poor skeletal support and predisposes to twisting, buckling, or migration of the cartilage elements. Initially the skeletal distortion may be concealed by surgical swelling; but, as edema subsides and contracture progresses, the shrink-wrap deformities become increasingly obvious and gradually more det-

rimental to the cosmetic outcome. For affected patients, progressive distortion may take years, or even decades to manifest fully, and the true impact of surgery cannot be determined until all manifestations of scar contracture are complete. Because shrink-wrap deformities are a byproduct of poor skeletal support, long-term structural integrity is now commonly acknowledged as a fundamental requirement of good rhinoplasty technique. Similarly, the importance of long-term patient assessment to confirm the ultimate impact of cosmetic nasal surgery cannot be overemphasized.

Because rhinoplasty is only partially understood, all practitioners should continually strive to increase their understanding of this challenging and sometimes mysterious operation. Even the accomplished rhinoplasty surgeon lacks complete understanding of rhinoplasty and can benefit from an objective self-assessment of his or her long-term surgical results. To facilitate self-assessment, the specifics of each operation are carefully recorded using a hand-drawn schematic rhinoplasty worksheet (Figure 1).

The rhinoplasty worksheet provides an indispensable reference document, which can be used to assess the long-term effectiveness of each individual surgical maneuver. By comparing the surgical worksheet to standardized "before and after" patient photographs, each long-term follow-up visit provides an opportunity to critique the surgical methodology, identify shortcomings, and continually refine one's surgical technique and philosophy. It is only through continual and honest evaluation of the long-term cosmetic result that surgical excellence can be

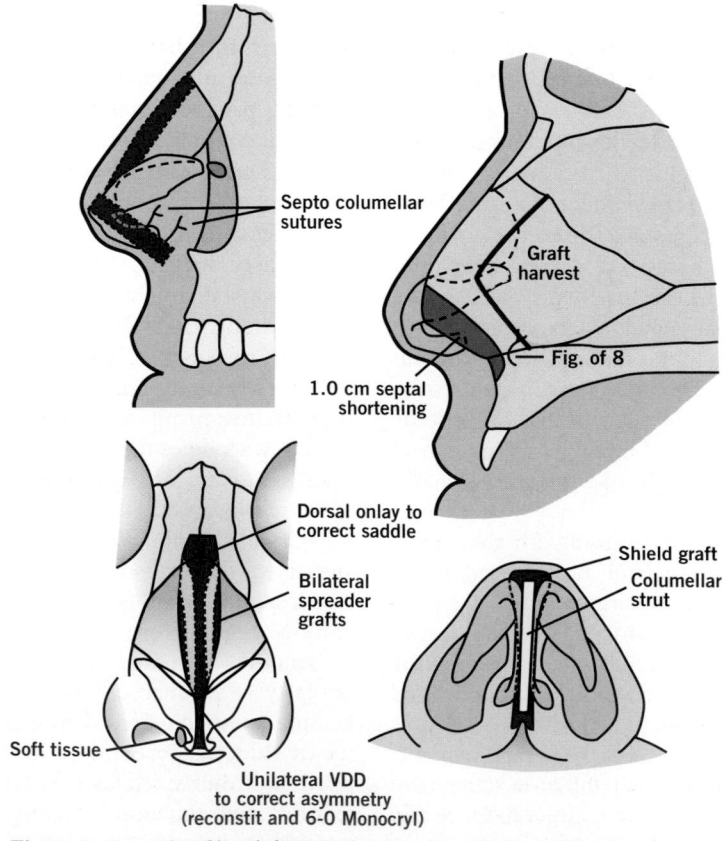

Figure 1 Example of hand-drawn schematic rhinoplasty worksheet.

achieved, and meticulous documentation of the surgical procedure is critical to the evaluation process.

Because rhinoplasty is a uniquely challenging and demanding operation, few surgeons can achieve consistent, state-of-the-art surgical results without specializing in this difficult procedure. For the surgeon who performs rhinoplasty only sporadically, consistently favorable results are seldom attained and complications are far more common. In contrast, the surgeon who restricts a large portion of his or her practice to the specialty of cosmetic nasal surgery will often develop a thriving practice based upon consistent and enviable surgical results. While devotion to this operation is necessary to achieve surgical mastery, no surgeon ever fully masters this complex and sometimes baffling procedure. Indeed, for the true devotee, rhinoplasty is a life-long quest for perfection which yields enhanced skill and improved outcomes, but only if diligently sought and studiously pursued.

THE NOMENCLATURE OF NASAL SURGERY

Cosmetic rhinoplasty has developed its own unique and somewhat unconventional medical nomenclature. Although this specialized nomenclature occasionally violates the traditional rules of anatomic classification, it is commonly accepted within the surgical community, and it appears throughout the medical literature. Any serious student of rhinoplasty must be familiar with the peculiarities of this unique terminology to comprehend fully the surgical concepts contained in this chapter and elsewhere. Hence a brief review of rhinoplasty nomenclature is in order. Terms fundamental to the nomenclature of rhinoplasty appear in italics throughout this chapter.

Owing to the atypical (oblique) alignment of the nose relative to the human body, the terminology used to describe the external nasal contour has been modified. For example, the outer nasal bridge, which protrudes from the ventral aspect of the human body, is commonly referred to as the nasal *dorsum*. Likewise, the superior (upper) aspect of the nasal framework is referred to as the *cephalic* aspect, whereas the inferior (lower) portion is commonly called the *caudal* aspect. Ironically, within the inferior (caudal) aspect of the nose, the nasal septum has both superior and inferior corners, known commonly as septal *angles* (Figure 2). The superior septal angle is known interchangeably as the *anterior septal angle*, and the inferior septal angle is also known interchangeably as the *posterior septal angle*. Owing to the unique anatomic references used to describe nasal anatomy, the nose has been said to have "its roots above, its wings below, and its front in back."

In Figure 3, key surface landmarks are shown from the frontal and profile perspectives. While some of these landmarks are derived from ceph-

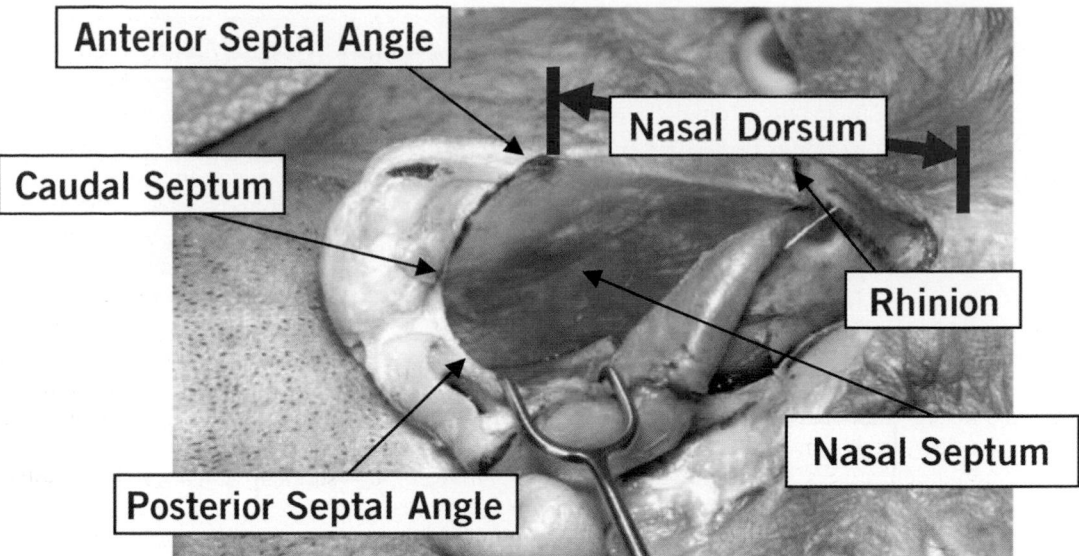

Figure 2 Cadaver specimen with the left nasal sidewall removed to reveal the cartilaginous nasal septum.

alometric nomenclature, most are soft tissue landmarks critical to nasal analysis and surgical modification. Familiarity with these terms is essential for any serious student of cosmetic rhinoplasty who wishes to master the art of facial aesthetic analysis.

NASAL ANALYSIS

Attractive noses are widely variable in shape and do not conform to a single aesthetic ideal. What may appear attractive and harmonious on one face may appear obtrusive and unattractive on another. Although cosmetically appealing noses all share a common base architecture, individual variations in contour must complement the patient's gender, bone structure, and ethnicity if the nose is to look natural and inconspicuous. Hence, a universal or "ideal" nasal contour does not exist.[1] While classic aesthetic norms of Western civilization, for example, Greco–Roman aesthetic ideals, have traditionally served as the template for cosmetic enhancement of the nose, these aesthetic standards may not be appropriate for every patient, particularly those of minority ethnic heritage. For that reason, cosmetic rhinoplasty requires individualized facial analysis, and surgical objectives must be tailored to suit both the patient's aesthetic preferences and the individual facial anatomy. Finally, the concept of nasal beauty varies widely among individuals, even those of the same gender and ethnicity, making the optimal nasal contour a highly personalized choice based upon widely varying individual tastes and preferences. Just as two people may have completely different tastes in clothing, jewelry, or hairstyle, so too the concept of nasal beauty is also widely variable among individuals. It is imperative that the rhinoplasty surgeon seeks to identify and respect the personal preferences of each patient to the greatest extent possible. Surgeons who habitually disregard the cosmetic desires of their patients will no doubt suffer the adverse consequences of these overbearing and paternalistic practices.

One of the most important components of a successful cosmetic rhinoplasty is accurate preoperative analysis. Almost any anatomic nasal deformity can be corrected by more than one surgical technique; and, while the choice of technique depends upon a host of different factors, all surgical techniques are predicated upon a proper understanding of the surface anatomy. In fact, correct aesthetic interpretation of the topographic anatomy is the first and, perhaps, the most critical step in planning cosmetic nasal surgery. In addition to shape, the surgeon must also evaluate the size and symmetry of each nasal component in relation to the surrounding facial features. Features that possess the proper shape and symmetry will appear unattractive if not in proper scale with the surrounding anatomy. Conversely, features with compatible size will also appear unattractive if lacking bilateral symmetry and a pleasing contour. Although virtually all humans can recognize an unattractive nose, few individuals can accurately identify the specific anatomic traits that are responsible for aesthetic disharmony. Although an "artistic eye" is an inherited talent that enables a surgeon to "see" aesthetic nasal disharmony, like any other natural talent, this unique skill must be actively cultivated to reach its full potential.

Once the surface deformities are properly identified, they must then be linked to the underlying skeletal anatomy to permit surgical modification of the nasal contour. Understanding how each surgical maneuver affects the surface topography, and faithfully executing these maneuvers, is the final piece of the surgical puzzle. Because the surgical game plan is entirely predicated upon the cosmetic analysis, a flawed analysis will inevitably result in surgical misjudgment, often leading to subsequent misjudgments and a domino effect of surgical errors. Perhaps the most common example of this phenomenon occurs when nasal hump size is misjudged, leading to overresection of the nasal dorsum. Because tip projection now appears to be excessive, the error is compounded when tip projection is aggressively reduced, further contributing to the

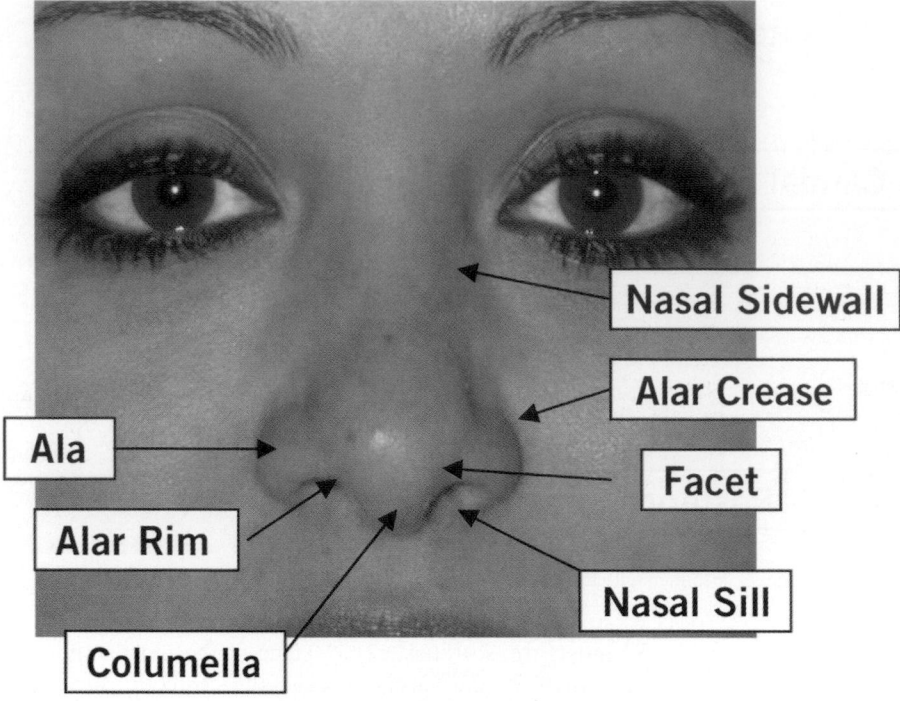

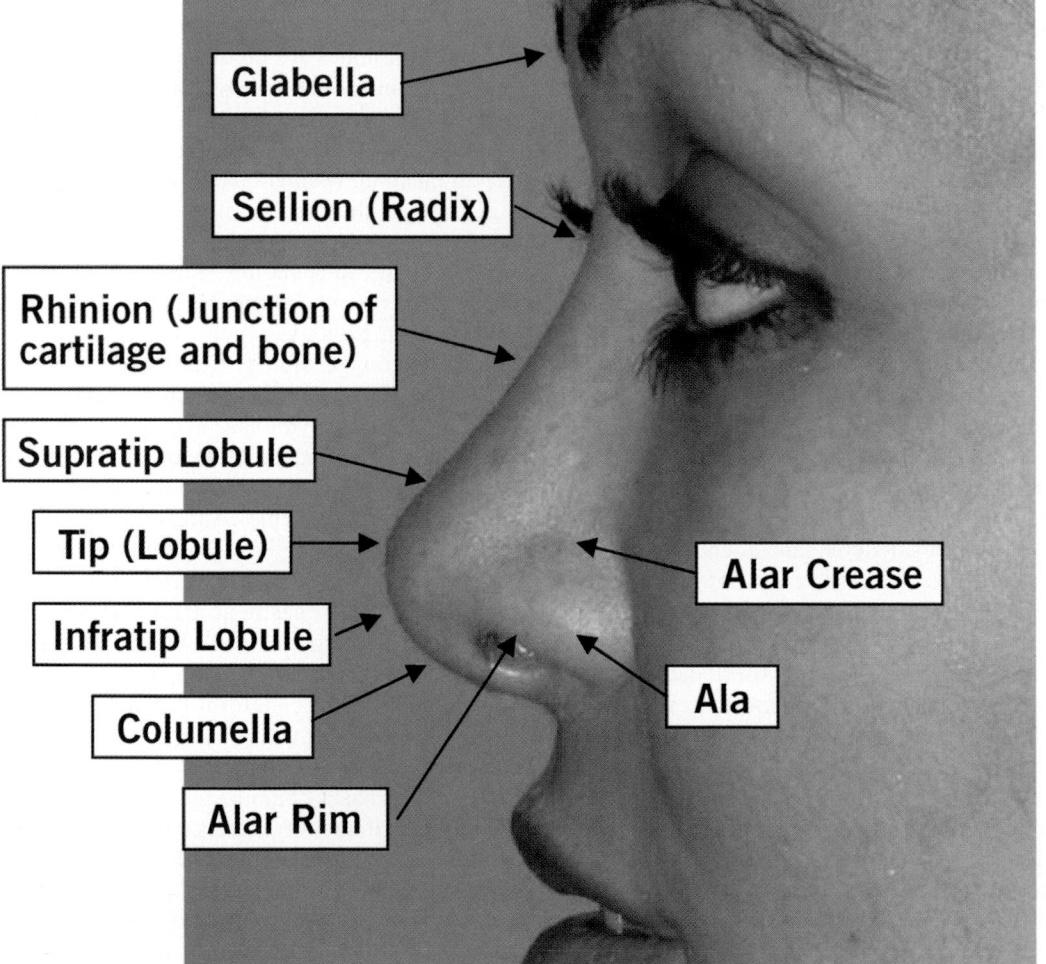

Figure 3 Key surface landmarks of the nose.

mon cause of surgical disappointment. Thus, the importance of preoperative nasal analysis cannot be overemphasized.

PATIENT PHOTOGRAPHY

Patient photographs are an essential part of cosmetic rhinoplasty and should be included in the official medical record of all rhinoplasty patients. In addition to documenting the presenting nasal contour, patient photographs provide an indispensable and mandatory tool for preoperative nasal analysis and surgical planning. Patient photographs are also the primary means by which a surgeon can evaluate the surgical outcome and perfect his or her surgical technique. A series of standardized and uniform photographs have been proven more informative than the most carefully detailed notes, both as a planning and self-instructional device and as a necessary medico-legal record.[2]

Color photographs of the face can be taken with a 35 mm single-lens reflex camera equipped with a lens-mounted flash attachment. A portrait lens is used to prevent parallax distortion; and frontal, bilateral profile, bilateral oblique, base, and optional (profile) smiling views are obtained (Figure 4). Although conventional format cameras are still acceptable, digital cameras offer numerous advantages including instantaneous review of picture quality with deletion of unsatisfactory photos, immediate image access, electronic storage, and the absence of developing delays or processing costs. Patients should be comfortably seated in front of a sky-blue background with feet firmly positioned on the floor. Soft overhead lighting is used for general illumination and should be augmented with flash photography. Although the optimal focal length will vary according to camera format and lens size, the face should fill nearly the entire frame when the camera is held in the vertical "portrait" orientation. Once the focal length has been established, it should remain constant for all subsequent views (except the closeup base view) so that image size remains constant. To keep focal length constant, focusing is achieved by moving the camera back and forth until the image appears in sharp focus, rather than by adjusting the focusing ring. On both the right and left profile views, the head should be positioned with the Frankfort Horizontal line parallel to the floor (the Frankfort Horizontal line extends from the upper tragus to the infraorbital rim). This alignment is maintained for all subsequent fullface views. Moreover, the patient should maintain a solemn facial expression for all views except for (optional) smiling profile views. For the oblique views, the patient is rotated approximately 45° from frontal plane until the inner canthus is vertically aligned with the ipsilateral oral commisure. On frontal view, the midsagittal plane is oriented perpendicularly to the floor, and the gaze is directed forward directly into the camera lens (primary gaze). Forward directed primary gaze should also

cosmetic deformity produced by dorsal overreduction. Historically, the overresected dorsum is one of the most common errors prompting patients to seek revision rhinoplasty, and while overresection of the nasal hump can also occur for technical reasons, failure of the surgeon to

assess hump size properly is an all too frequent cause of the unsatisfactory rhinoplasty outcome. Although the vagaries of wound healing may occasionally spoil a properly executed operation, a flawed nasal analysis condemns the operation to failure from the very start and is a far more com-

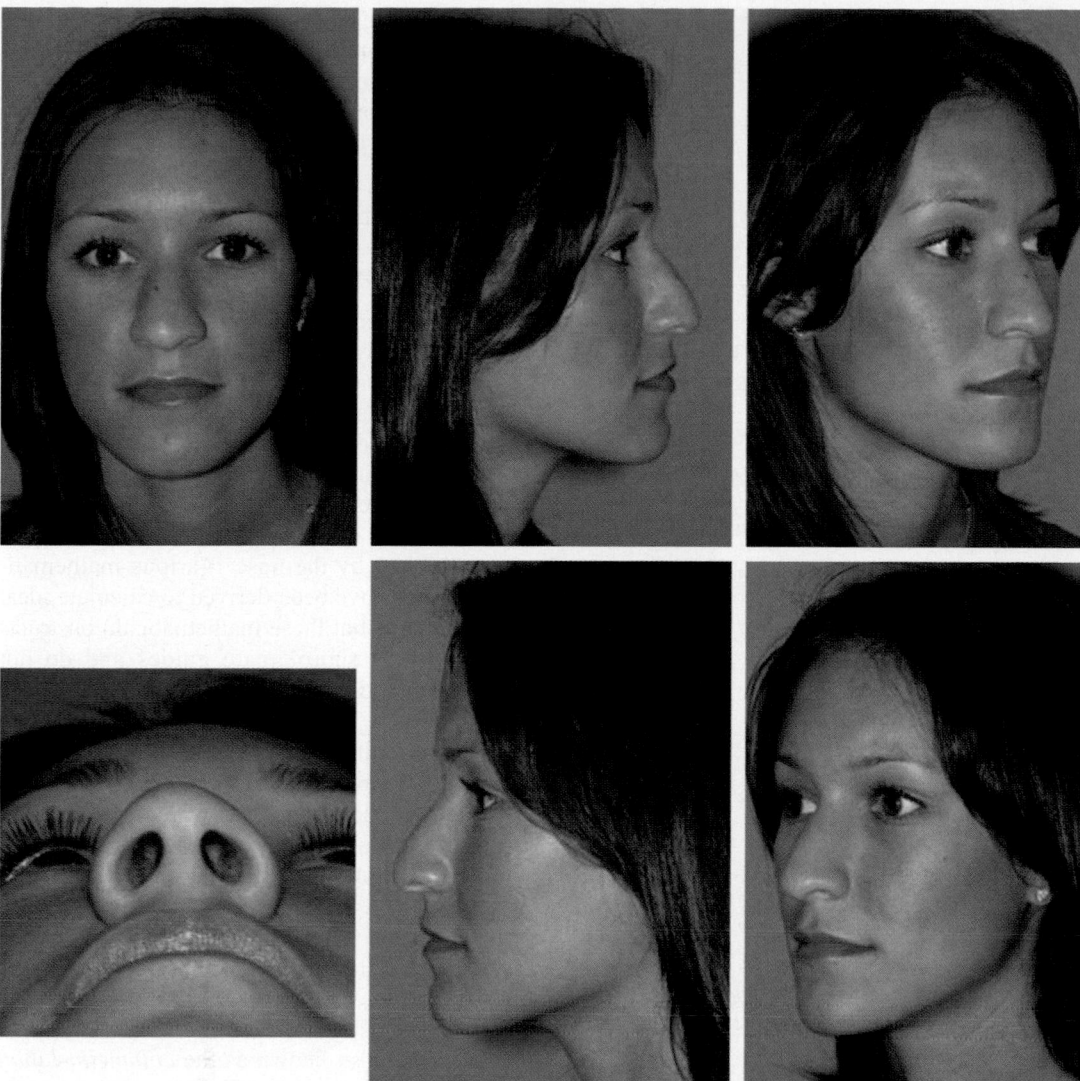

Figure 4 Preoperative rhinoplasty views for standard documentation.

allows the patient to "preview" the new look and to approve recommended cosmetic changes. Alterations to the nasal contour can be added sequentially until both patient and surgeon are pleased with the proposed nasal contour, and the impact of deleting specific modifications can also be assessed. Although the surgeon must restrict the "design" process to changes that are both surgically realistic and aesthetically compatible, the result is a mutually agreeable blueprint from which the surgical plan is ultimately derived. Moreover, the ability to fade electronically between images in real time, that is, to "morph" between the original image and the simulated new nose, greatly enhances the analytical power of the computer imaging software. For the surgeon, the morphed image becomes a powerful assessment and planning tool, which unambiguously demonstrates the anatomic flaws so that appropriate surgical treatment measures can be devised. Aesthetic analysis is simplified since the extent of nasal hump reduction, tip projection, lobular narrowing, or other contour changes can be more accurately quantified. For the patient, real-time transformation provides immediate intuitive understanding of the cosmetic deformity and the proposed surgical corrections. Even subtle deformities become obvious and the surgical plan becomes exacting and tailored to the desires of the patient. While patients must be counseled that exact replication of the simulated images is seldom possible, a skilled surgeon can usually produce surgical outcomes that closely resemble the computer-generated simulations. This technology has greatly expanded the capacity to analyze complex nasal morphology and it is rapidly becoming a requirement of the typical rhinoplasty consumer.

be maintained for all other photographic views. Finally, a closeup basal view is included in the standard perioperative photographic documentation. In this important view, the patient tilts the head back until the nasal tip eclipses the brow ridge. The camera frame is turned to the horizontal "landscape" orientation and focal length is reduced until the outer canthus appears slightly within frame. Postoperative photographs are best taken with the same equipment, lighting, focal length, and positioning at various intervals during the healing process.

COMPUTER-GUIDED NASAL ANALYSIS

Because nasal analysis is most accurate when applied to static images, the absence of patient photographs during the initial consultation was formerly a handicap in patient assessment. Fortunately, the traditional practice of analyzing color slides several days after the initial examination has become obsolete. With the advent of digital photography and computer imaging technology, standardized high-resolution digital photographs are now available at the onset of the rhinoplasty consultation. This not only permits the surgeon

to evaluate standardized photographs and nasal deformities in tandem, it also permits the patient to observe the evaluation process and better understand the cosmetic deformity. When subjected to computer-based analytical tools, even the slightest discrepancy in nasal symmetry, size, or shape becomes obvious, making digital photography a powerful tool in preoperative nasal analysis. Moreover, the contemporary rhinoplasty patient also participates in the evaluation process and bears witness to the anatomic deformities revealed by digital photography. Deformities that were previously unseen by the patient now become obvious, and the full scope of contour irregularities becomes evident to patient and surgeon alike.

In addition to static image analysis, the preoperative cosmetic evaluation is further enhanced by the use of computer morphing software. This technological innovation permits the skilled user to electronically edit digital photographs to produce life-like simulated images, which depict the effects of cosmetic nasal surgery (Figure 5). By incorporating input from the patient, morphing software permits the surgeon to electronically "design" a new nose, which reflects the patient's aesthetic tastes and preferences. It also

COSMETIC ANALYSIS OF THE NOSE

Profile and Upper Vault

The cosmetically pleasing nasal contour is characterized by a tall and straight dorsal *profile* terminating cephalically in a well-defined *nasofrontal* angle. Although the size of the nasofrontal angle varies widely in attractive people, the apex of this angle, the *sellion*, represents the *nasal starting point*, and should rest at or near the upper lid margin[3] (Figure 6).

Noses in which the nasal starting point is located inferior to this anatomic reference point possess a "deep" or "underprojected" *nasal root* (alternatively known as the nasal *radix*) forming an obtuse nasofrontal angle. Often, this deformity is accompanied by a weak underprojected rhinion, but a normal or overprojected bony dorsum may also be observed. The underprojected radix frequently results from a congenitally flat nasal dorsum, but a low nasal starting point may also result from acquired bone loss, such as occurs with overresection of a nasal hump deformity. Noses characterized by excessive width (the *platyrrhine* morphology) typically lack strong dorsal projection and are often associated with

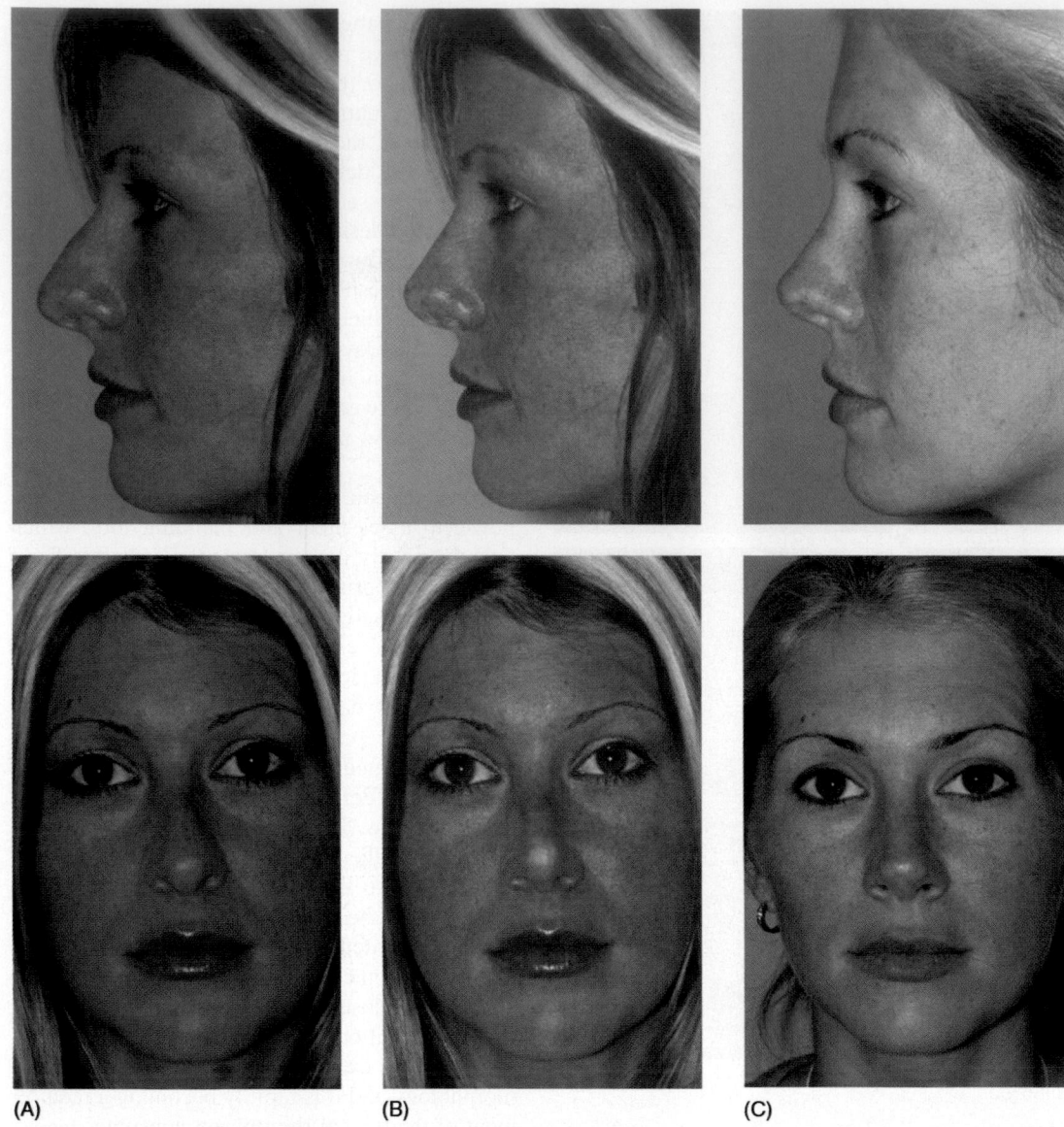

(A)   **(B)**   **(C)**

Figure 5 Profile and front views demonstrating: (A) preoperative nasal contour; (B) computer-simulated morphs depicting proposed cosmetic changes; and (C) actual postoperative nasal contour.

tour. Failure to recognize a malpositioned nasal starting point may significantly compromise the cosmetic outcome of profile surgery and may lead to overresection or underresection of the nasal dorsum and/or corresponding tip malformations.

NASAL ANALYSIS

Profile and Lower Vault

Profile analysis of the lower nasal vault is challenging and involves multiple aesthetic variables, including tip *projection*, tip *rotation*, *columella-alar harmony*, and the *nasolabial angle*. Tip *projection* refers to the extent of forward protrusion of the nose parallel to the Frankfort horizontal plane of the face. Patients may better understand this concept as the extent of "Pinocchio" elongation exhibited by the nose. Various mathematical formulas have been derived to calculate ideal tip projection, but these mathematical constructs serve only as approximate guides and do not supersede good aesthetic judgment. As a general rule of thumb, tip projection should be roughly equivalent to the vertical height of the upper lip. However, this rule does not apply in patients with the caudal excess deformity since lip height is artificially reduced. Fortunately, with the aid of modern computer imaging software, the aesthetics of tip projection are ultimately governed by the patient's cosmetic preference as long as the desired projection falls within the scope of surgical feasibility.

Like its analog the nasofrontal angle, the *nasolabial angle*, also known as the *columella-labial* junction, is an important parameter of profile aesthetics.[7] Ideally, the apex of the nasolabial angle should rest on a horizontal line drawn through the lowest portion of the *alar crease* (see Figure 6). The apex should also rest slightly posterior to the labial tubercle creating a gentle backward slope to the upper lip. In patients with the *caudal excess nasal deformity*, the nasolabial apex is shifted both anteriorly and caudally, creating an obtuse or "webbed" nasolabial angle and foreshortening the upper lip.

In contrast to tip projection, tip *rotation* describes a change in tip configuration produced by movement along a fixed arc of rotation (Figure 9). When nasal tip position shifts caudally along this arc of rotation, the tip becomes *counterrotated* or *ptotic*. From the front view, the nostril openings become less visible or may be hidden entirely, and the distance from the sellion to the tip defining points, known as the *dorsal line*, increases in length. In general, a long dorsal line and ptotic nasal tip are associated with an aged appearance as nasal elongation is a common manifestation of human aging. In contrast, when nasal tip position shifts cephalically along the same arc of rotation, the dorsal line is shortened and nostril show is increased from the front.

Typically, the youthful, feminine nose will exhibit a greater degree of tip rotation, but care must be taken to avoid the overrotated nose with prominent porcine-like nostril show. In women,

a nasal starting point positioned below the upper lid margin (Figure 7A). In patients with an underprojected radix and a normally projected rhinion, there is an illusion of a nasal hump, the so-called *pseudohump* deformity (Figure 7B). This unique anatomic combination, sometimes called *low radix disproportion*, can lead to inappropriate removal of the pseudohump resulting in an overresected nasal dorsum. To avoid this unwanted complication, augmentation of the radix is necessary to maintain position of the nasal starting point and eliminate the illusion of a nasal hump[4] (Figure 8).

In contrast to the underprojected sellion common to extremely wide noses, extremely narrow noses (the *leptorrhine* morphology) are often characterized by overprojection of the nasal dorsum, often with a cephalically displaced nasofrontal angle (Figure 7C). In this situation, profile aesthetics are restored by removing the dorsal hump and deprojecting the radix to lower or recess the nasal starting point. Typically, radix deprojection requires removal of dense frontal bone using powered instrumentation.[5,6]

While a properly positioned nasal starting point is appropriate for patients of either gender, the relationship of the nasal dorsum to the nasal tip often varies slightly between men and women. Even though a straight dorsal profile is universally acceptable, in the feminine nose the nasal tip often projects slightly above the dorsal line creating a subtle curvature at the supratip, known as *retroussé* or a *supratip break* (see Figure 6). In contrast, a masculine nasal contour may lack a supratip break, having a completely straight or even a slightly convex dorsal profile. While these profile characteristics represent commonly observed gender-based tendencies in the naturally attractive nose, there are also many attractive noses that defy these generalizations.

Surgery to alter the dorsal profile is a common objective of cosmetic rhinoplasty, making accurate cosmetic assessment of the nasal dorsum and nasofrontal angle a critical aspect of nasal aesthetic analysis. Moreover, dorsal profile analysis should precede analysis of the tip, since tip positioning must conform to proper dorsal height to achieve a natural-appearing nasal con-

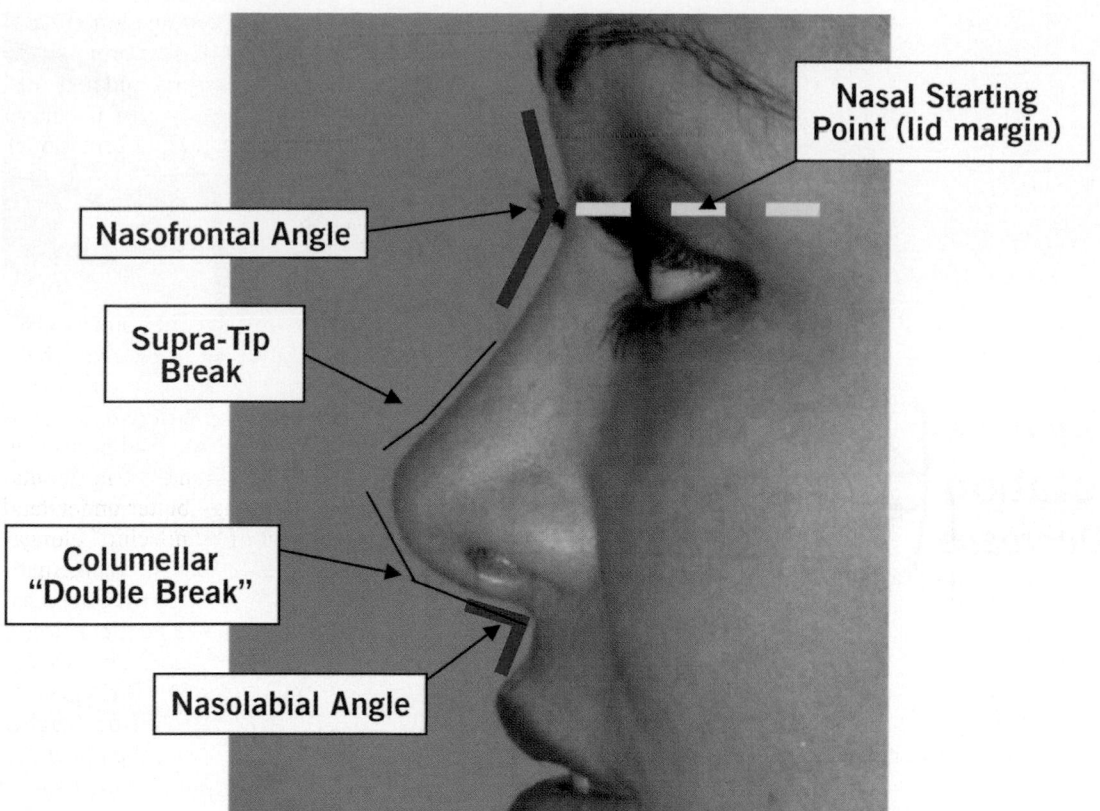

Figure 6 Cosmetic reference angles of the external nose.

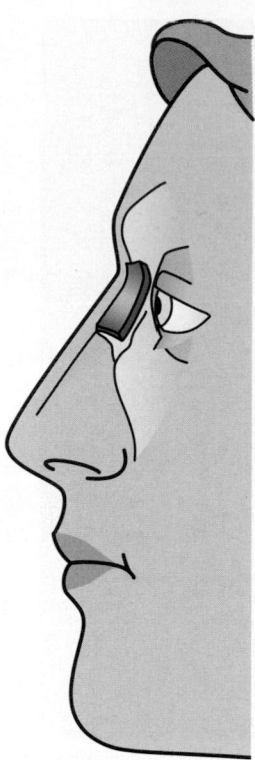

Figure 8 Schematic illustration demonstrating radix graft augmentation of "pseudohump" deformity.

a greater degree of tip rotation equates to a more obtuse nasolabial angle of approximately 95 to 110°, whereas in men a longer dorsal line with an acute nasolabial angle of 90° to 100° is typical. Although tip rotation can be gauged by nasolabial angle size, like tip projection, this method of assessment may prove unreliable in the presence of columellar retraction or nasolabial protrusion (webbing) as often occurs in the caudal excess nasal deformity.

Another aspect of profile aesthetics involving the nasal base is the *columella-alar relationship*. In the cosmetically appealing nose on profile view, the leading edge of the *columella* is visible as it protrudes slightly beyond the *alar rim* (see Figure 6). In women, and to a lesser degree in men, the columella has a gentle downward curvature, the so-called *double-break*, created by divergence of the underlying medial crura. In the cosmetically appealing nose, the alar rim possesses a reciprocal curvature resulting in 2 to 5 mm of columellar reveal, also known as *columellar show*. Disturbances in the columellar–alar relationship may result from a variety of deformities including excessive columellar show, *columellar retraction*, *alar retraction*, *alar rim ptosis*, or combinations therein (Figure 10). Both congenital anomalies and acquired deformities may account for disturbances in the columellar–alar relationship.

Frontal View and Upper Vault

In recent years, the cosmetic importance of the *brow-tip aesthetic lines* (BTALs) has been emphasized. These paired lines, formed by shadows of the nasal sidewall, should be parallel or slightly divergent as they extend inferiorly off the supraorbital rim (Figure 11). BTALs should also be smooth, symmetric, and unbroken, connecting the medial brow to the *alar crease*. For most patients, the optimal spacing between BTALs is approximately half of the intercanthal distance.

Width discrepancies between the upper bony vault, and the middle cartilaginous vault, are a common cause of disrupted BTALs. In severe cases, the pinched middle vault cartilages will produce a progressively narrow sidewall shadow that converges superiorly at the rhinion, the so-called *inverted-V* deformity (Figure 12A). Overresection of the nasal dorsum typically exacerbates width discrepancies and is commonly associated with formation of the inverted-V deformity. However, even a conservative hump reduction with a high residual profile can result in the inverted-V shadow if pinching of the upper lateral cartilages (ULCs) develops. Correction involves increasing separation of the pinched ULCs and/or reducing separation of the nasal bones (Figure 12B).

Frontal View and Lower Vault

The nasal tip, or *lobule*, is one of the most important cosmetic features of the nose. From the front, the lobule should be easily distinguished from the adjacent nostrils, separated by faint shadows that blend smoothly into the adjacent alar crease. The ideal lobular width varies considerably according to a host of aesthetic factors including personal preference, nostril size, and dorsal width; but as a rule, the lobule should be about 10 to 20% wider than the aesthetically pleasing nasal

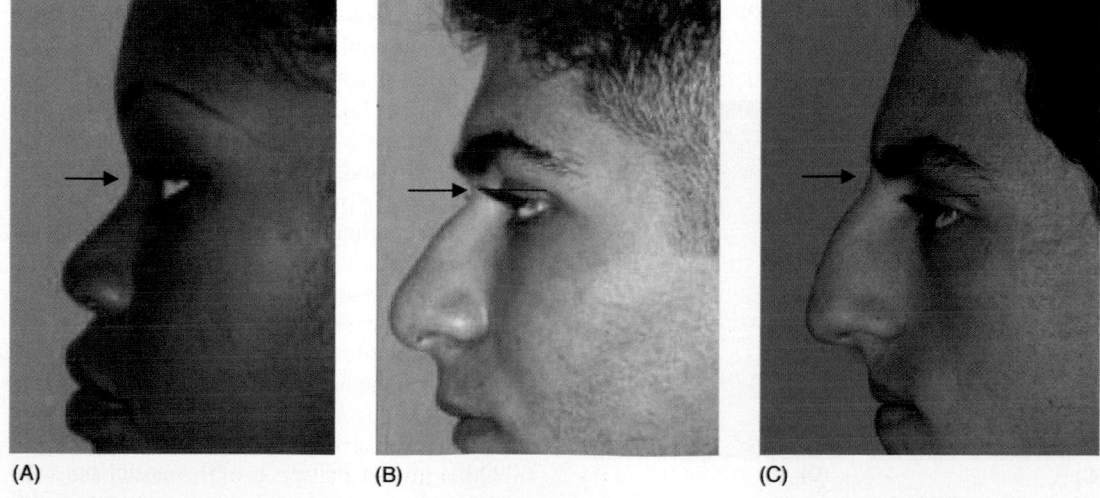

Figure 7 Variations in nasal starting point in: (A) platyrrhine; (B) deep radix; and (C) leptorrhine nasal morphologies. Note differences in location of the sellion (*black arrow*) relative to the upper eyelid margin (*red line*).

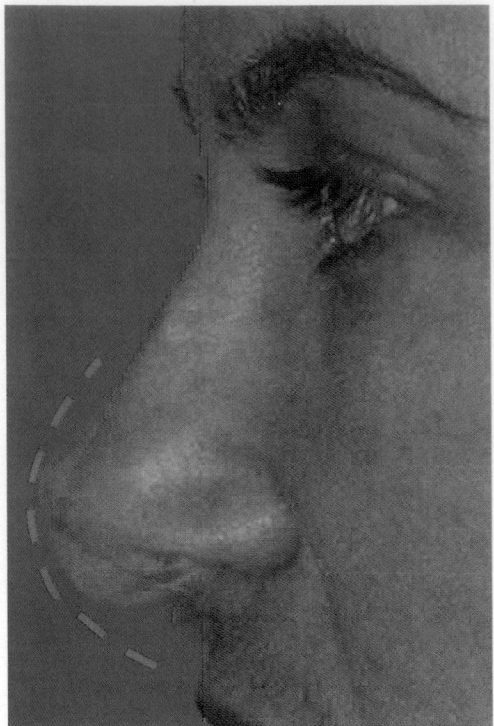

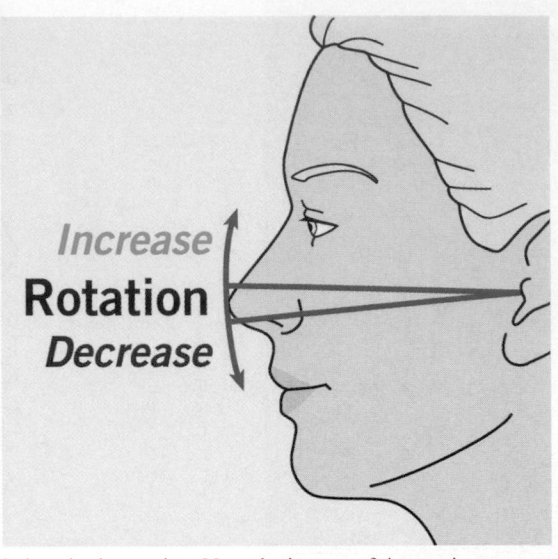

Figure 9 Computer-generated simulation depicting variations in tip rotation. Note the impact of tip rotation or counter-rotation upon length of the dorsum.

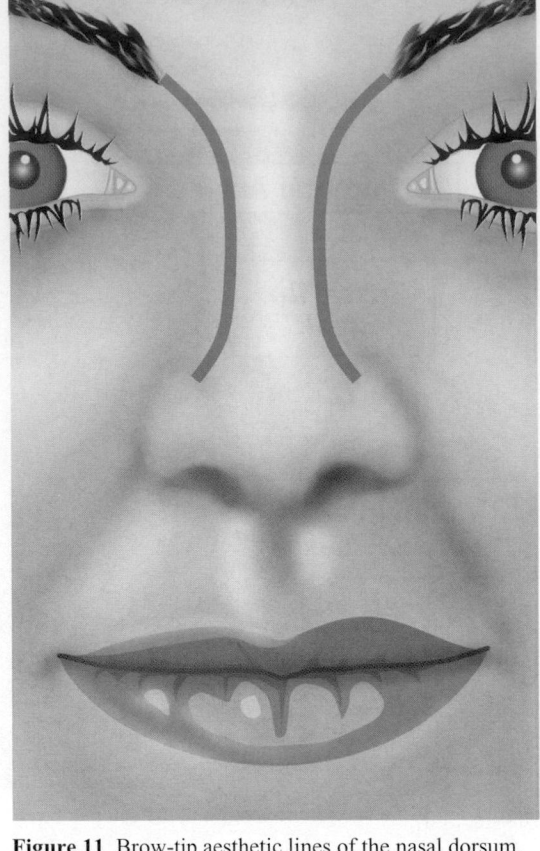

Figure 11 Brow-tip aesthetic lines of the nasal dorsum.

dorsum. Lobular shape also varies considerably, but the attractive nasal tip typically possesses a symmetric diamond shape created by flaring of the underlying alar domes (Figure 13).

Overly broad nasal domes, excessive convexity of the lateral crura, or absence of domal divergence, result in broad, bulbous, or "uni" tip deformities, respectively. Excessive grooving between the alar domes, a condition known as *bifidity*, is common in patients with thin skin and strong, round alar cartilage. A modest degree of bifidity within the infratip lobule is cosmetically desirable, but conspicuous bifidity within the lobule itself is generally considered cosmetically undesirable.

The *alae* and *nostril* openings, comprise the remainder of the nasal base. In addition to symmetry, the nostril openings should be oblong with a gentle "gull wing" configuration from the front view (Figure 14). In most patients, the outer alar margin should fall within a few millimeters of the medial canthal line, equating

nasal base width to the intercanthal distance. Although surgical narrowing of the nasal base is occasionally desirable, care must be taken to avoid nostril deformity by confining nasal skin excision to the nasal sill. Sagittally oriented fusiform excisions of the nasal sill effectively narrow the nasal base without distorting nostril shape. In contrast, skin excision from the lateral ala as with the so-called "Weir incision," often results in unsightly blunting of the nostril/cheek interface and should be avoided in most circumstances. Moreover, because excessive tip width is often mistakenly confused with excessive alar width, alar base reductions are often performed unnecessarily.

Although refinement of the oversized lobule is a frequent objective of cosmetic rhinoplasty, over-resection of the lateral crura in an ill-conceived attempt to narrow the lobule will frequently result in stigmatic deformity of the nasal tip. Typically, the overoperated tip is characterized by lobular pinching, excessive tip rotation, and cephalic

migration of the lateral crura (Figure 15). In addition to pinching of the diamond-shaped lobule, cephalic malposition of the lateral crus typically results in a conspicuous notching of the nostril rim leading to unwanted distortion of the ideal "gull wing" configuration. In general, these tip deformities are best prevented by limiting excision of alar cartilage and preserving adequate crural strength.

Base View

Examining the nose from the base view can greatly augment the nasal analysis and reveal problems not always seen on the frontal or profile views. Hence, the base view remains a key component of the nasal analysis and should not be neglected. Ideally, when viewed from the basal perspective, the nose should conform to an equilateral triangle (Figure 16). Assuming that the nasal base width is approximately equal to intercanthal width, the triangular base configuration will provide a cosmetically acceptable tip configuration and insures a cosmetically pleasing degree of tip projection. However, as with all aesthetic guidelines, allowances must be made for morphologic variants such as the patient with extremely wide-set eyes or extremely narrow-set eyes. In both cases, the ideal nasal base width may not coincide with the existing intercanthal distance, and the nasal width should be calibrated to the overall facial bone structure for optimal cosmetic results.

Other important aspects of the nasal base analysis include the width and alignment of the columella, the columella to lobule ratio, and the shape

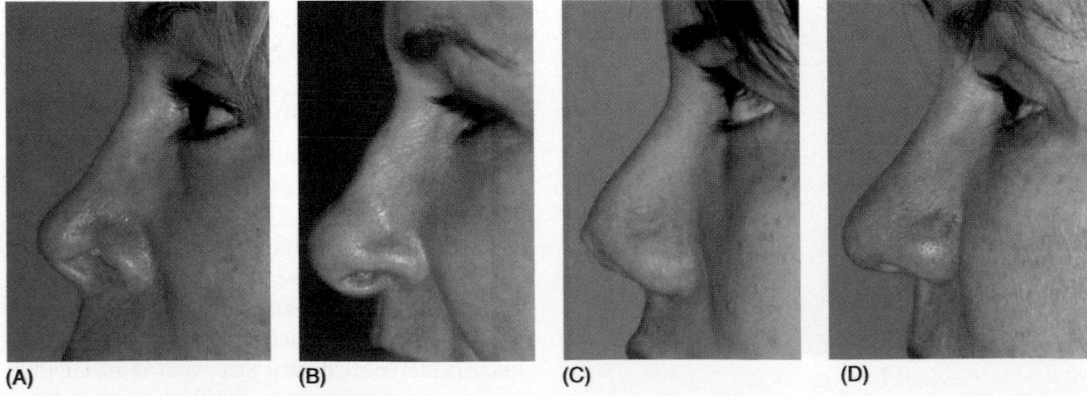

(A) (B) (C) (D)

Figure 10 Alar-columellar disharmony produced by (A) alar retraction; (B) excess columellar show; (C) alar rim ptosis; and (D) columellar retraction.

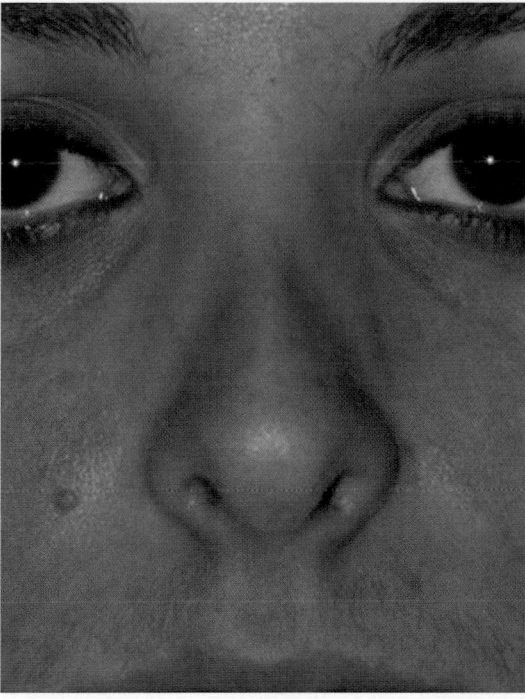 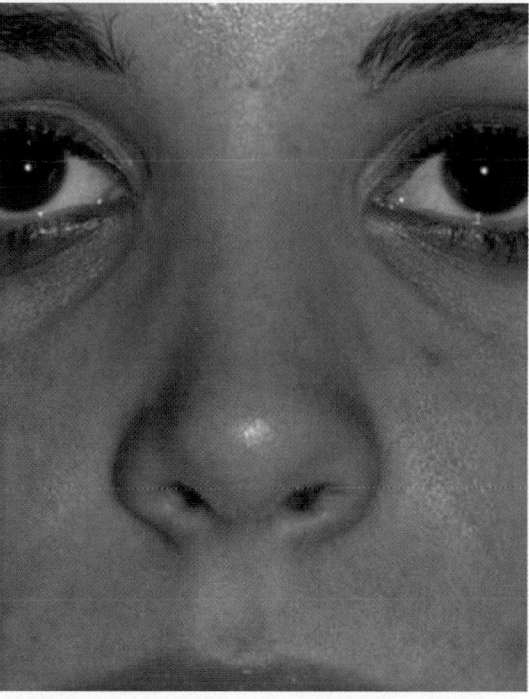

(A)　　　　　　　　　　　　　　　　(B)

Figure 12 Disruption of the brow-tip aesthetic lines (BTALs) secondary to the "inverted-V" nasal deformity. (A) Note pinching of the upper lateral cartilages caudal to the nasal bones producing inverted V-shaped shadows. (B) Improved continuity of BTAL following spreader graft placement.

of the alar sidewall. Ideally, the columella lies in the midline and widens gently at its base due to the flared footpods of the medial crura. Columellar height should also be approximately twice that of the lobule, and the nostril sidewall should appear straight or very slightly concave without pinching or significant indentation.

SURGICAL ANATOMY OF THE NOSE

Upper Vault

The *nasal bones* are paired membranous bones arranged in a crude "A-frame" configuration. Distally the nasal bones are thin and delicate,

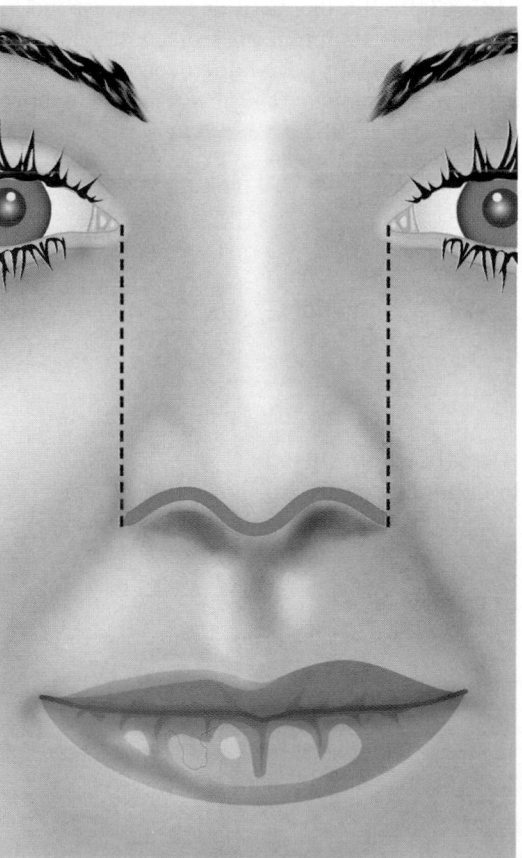

Figure 13 Schematic overlay of diamond-shaped lobule configuration.

Figure 14 Schematic overlay illustrating "gull-wing" nostril configuration and positioning of the medial canthal line.

whereas their dense cephalic union with the *nasal process of the frontal bone* is seldom prone to injury. Laterally, the nasal bones fuse with the *nasal process of the maxilla* at the *lateral nasal suture line* (Figure 17). Collectively, the nasal bones and the adjoining process of the maxilla comprise the *bony* (or *upper*) *nasal vault*. The nasal bones are supported in the midline, from beneath, by the *perpendicular plate of the ethmoid bone*; and they typically comprise approximately one-third of the nasal dorsum.

The union of the nasal bone with the maxilla lies medial to the *nasofacial groove*, which is formed by the anatomic junction of the nasal sidewall with the adjacent cheek. The misconception that the bony vault is composed entirely of nasal bone is dispelled by the presence of maxillary bone within the lateral most aspect of the nasal sidewall. Because optimal narrowing of the bony vault typically requires infracture of the entire nasal sidewall, the preferred placement for lateral osteotomy is typically within the nasofacial groove (Figure 17). Thus, lateral osteotomy bone cuts typically lie within the maxilla and only briefly traverse the nasal bone at its cephalic extent. During osteotomy of the nasofacial groove, dense bone of the anterior maxillary buttress located immediately lateral to the nasofacial groove, serves to help protect the adjacent lacrimal fossa from inadvertent injury.

Beyond the rhinion, the nasal bones give rise to the cartilaginous nasal dorsum, also known as the *middle nasal vault*. Similar to the A-frame configuration of the upper nasal vault (which is supported from beneath by the vertical ethmoid plate), the middle vault is formed by the *ULCs* which are supported from beneath by the *quadrangular* (cartilaginous) *septum*. Even though the right and left ULCs and quadrangular cartilage are individually named (inappropriately suggesting they are separate anatomic structures), in reality, these three plates of cartilage are a single anatomic structure. The cephalic margin of the ULC is tightly fused to the undersurface of the caudal aspect of the nasal bone, whereas the quadrangular cartilage and ethmoid bone are similarly fused. The resulting *osseocartilaginous pyramid* is a structurally uniform and anatomically contiguous vault, which constitutes the complete nasal dorsum.

The confluence of the nasal bones with the ULCs and the nasal septum occurs at the rhinion, which is sometimes referred to as the "*keystone*" or "*K-area.*" Complete disruption of the bony-cartilaginous union within the keystone area due to trauma or overaggressive surgery may lead to irreversible collapse of the nasal pyramid and should be avoided whenever possible. Nasal deformities affecting the keystone area are particularly challenging due to the increased potential for skeletal instability.

Internally, the junction of the paired ULCs with the midline dorsal septum, results in a critically important anatomic and physiologic feature: *the nasal valve* (Figure 18). The nasal valve is the narrowest segment of the human airway and it plays a vital role in creating sufficient airway

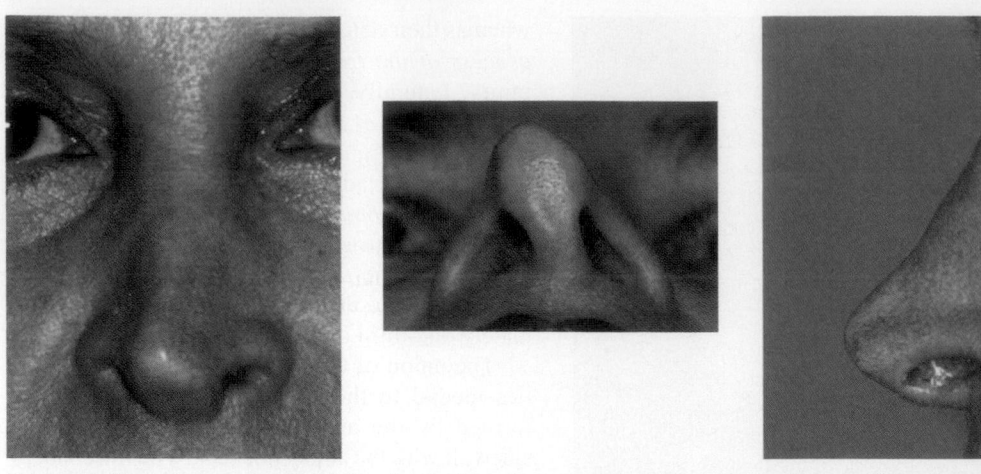

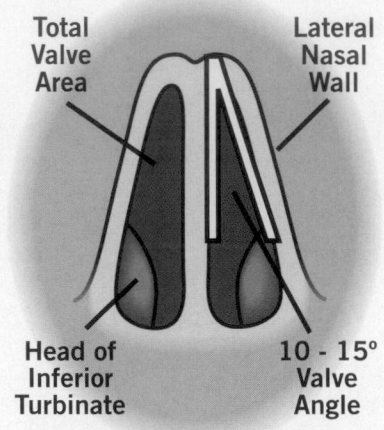

Figure 15 Typical stigmatic nasal deformity resulting from overaggressive excision of alar cartilage.

Figure 18 Schematic cross-sectional diagram of the nasal valve area indicating the typical nasal valve angle of 10 to 15°.

resistance to facilitate filtration, warming, and humidification of the inspired air. Typically, the ULCs attach to the dorsal septum at a 10° to 15° angle resulting in an internal cross-sectional airway dimension of only 55 to 73 mm^2.[8,9]

Of note, in nearly all healthy noses the quadrangular septum widens and flares at the junction with the ULCs. This anatomic widening of the dorsal septum increases the horizontal separation of the ULCs contributing to both improved nasal sidewall support and greater internal airway dimension. Because anatomic reductions in nasal valve cross-sectional area are associated with an exponential increase in nasal airway resistance, reductions in valve width as little as 1 mm can produce symptoms of nasal airway obstruction.[10] Consequently, medialization of the ULC from a nasal hump reduction that reduces septal flaring may result in symptomatic nasal valve dysfunction. Therefore, in patients with weak cartilage or narrow noses predisposed to nasal valve collapse, compensatory surgical measures such as spreader graft placement or flaring sutures are sometimes necessary to prevent nasal valve obstruction secondary to pinching of the middle vault.

The *lower lateral cartilages* (LLC) are the most anatomically complex, and perhaps the most

aesthetically important, skeletal structures of the nose (Figure 19). These paired, mirror-image cartilages are closely approximated within their medial (columellar) segment, but fold sharply at the nasal tip diverging in nearly opposite directions to span the lower nasal sidewall. Each LLC or *alar cartilage* is arbitrarily subdivided into smaller anatomic segments for greater clarity. Although the nomenclature varies slightly among different authors, the designations *lateral* and *medial crura* are used commonly throughout the medical literature. Moreover, certain descriptive terms are used consistently across all classification systems and these include the *nasal domes* and the *columellar footpods*. The nasal domes represent the acute angle formed by the junction of the medial and lateral crural segments of the LLC. Clinically, the nasal domes correspond to the point of maximum tip projection, and their shape and spacing govern the overall contour of the nasal tip or *lobule*. The *lateral crura* comprise

the "alar wings," which extend superolaterally, connecting the nasal domes medially to the pyriform aperture laterally, just above the alar crease. The strength and rigidity of the lateral crura are integral to the support and functional integrity of the nasal sidewall; and anatomic deformities, injuries, or improper surgical alterations can profoundly impair nasal breathing. Aesthetically, the lateral crura tend to be most pleasing when flat, and in large unsightly noses they often possess natural convex or concave curvatures in both their long and/or their short axes.

The anatomic junction of the lateral crus with the adjacent ULC forms a unique interlocking joint which amplifies strength of the nasal sidewall. This anatomic junction, commonly known as the *nasal scroll*, is formed by the cephalic margin of the lateral crus which curls internally to

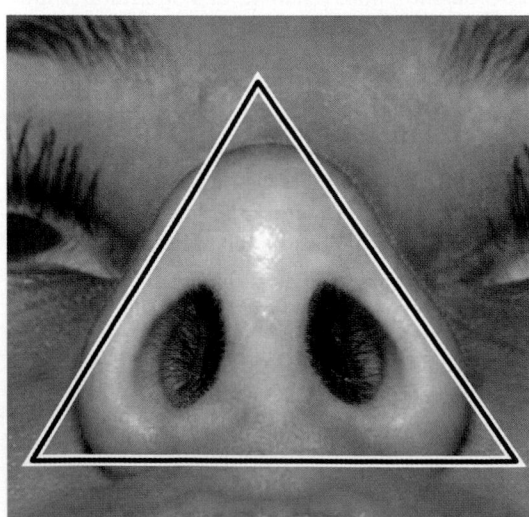

Figure 16 Base view demonstrating the ideal equilateral triangle configuration.

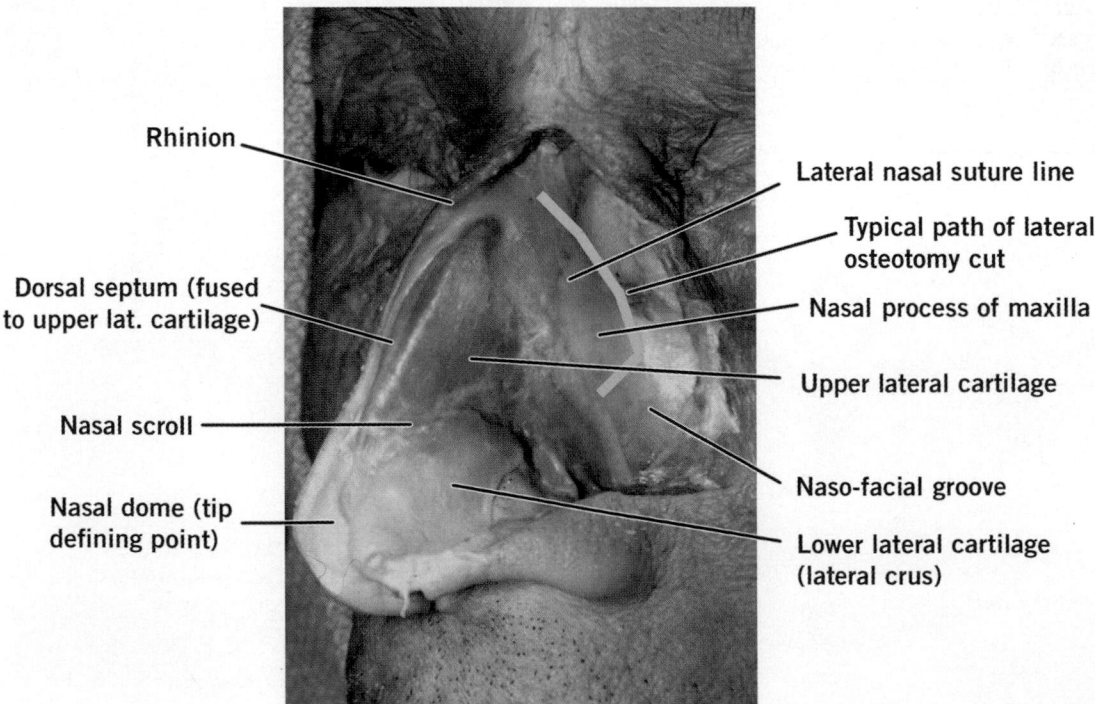

Figure 17 Cadaver specimen with skin removed revealing the nasal skeleton. Note typical placement of lateral osteotomy cut (*blue line*) for infracture of the nasal sidewall.

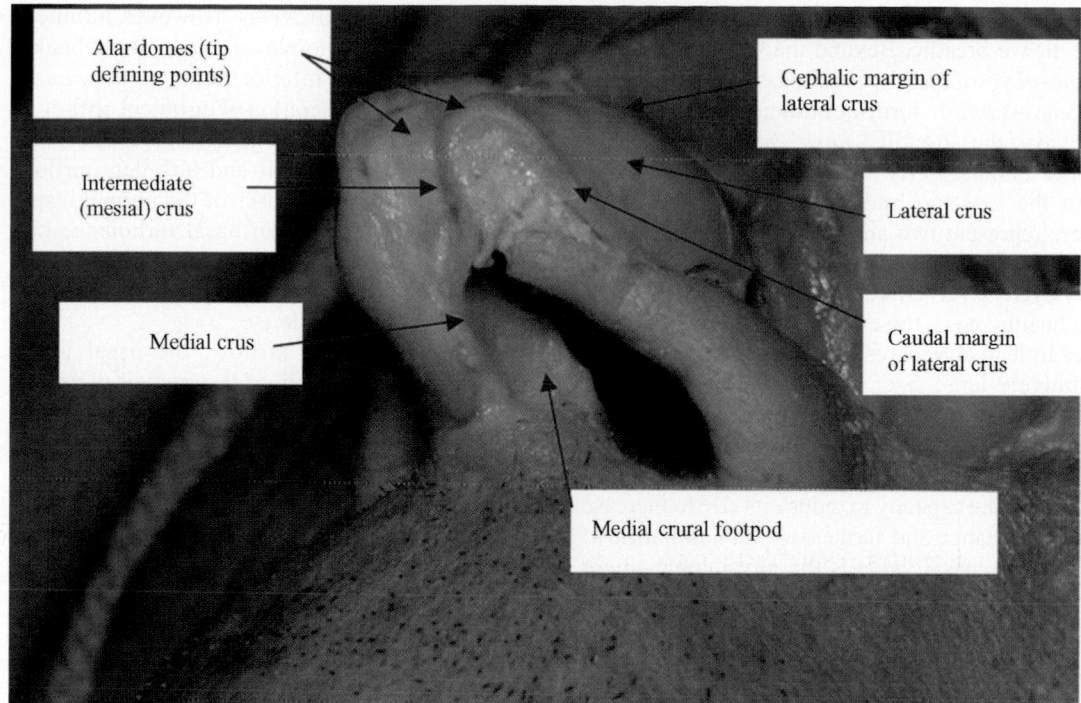

Figure 19 Cadaver specimen with skin partially removed revealing left alar cartilage.

slowly beginning to recognize the potential long-term implications of aggressive cephalic scroll resection, the practice remains widespread and the adverse consequences will no doubt manifest for decades to come. Fortunately, contemporary rhinoplasty techniques have since evolved which maintain lateral nasal sidewall support while permitting a cosmetically pleasing nasal contour.

At its medial end, the nasal scroll terminates 5 to 6 mm from the midline forming a small gap between the ULC, lateral crus, and anterior septal angle, known as the *weak triangle*. The inferior most aspect of the LLCs, the so-called *medial crural footpods,* are rounded (often flared) feet which rest on either side of the posterior septal angle and nasal spine (Figure 21). The anatomic complex formed by the footpods, nasal spine, and posterior septal angle is sometimes called the *nasal pedestal.* Undesirable widening of the nasal pedestal is commonly seen in the *tension nose deformity* in which excessive anterior septal projection causes tenting of the lower part of the nose and upper lip.[11]

Starting with the crural footpods below, extending to the nasal domes above, are the *medial crura.* The medial crura are the paired, conjoined, sagittally oriented segments of the LLC, which give rise to the *columella* and *infratip lobule.* For purposes of further differentiation, some authors have proposed subdividing the medial crura by renaming the infratip lobular segment as the *intermediate* or *mesial crus.* While the medial crura are nearly parallel in the columellar segment, they diverge just above the nostril, giving rise to a flared infratip lobule on front view and a columellar *double-break* on profile view.

fuse with the externally curled caudal margin of the ULC (Figure 20).

The unique configuration formed between the upper and LLCs creates a tube-like strut which confers additional rigidity to the nasal sidewall. Analogous to an automotive roll bar, the nasal scroll resists inward collapse from *transmural pressure* generated by gentle (resting) inspiration. Since the nasal scroll defines the anatomic outer border of the *nasal valve region* and since the scroll supports the only mobile section of the valve perimeter, it also governs the threshold for *dynamic nasal valve collapse* during more vigorous inspiration. If the nasal scroll is damaged, such as may occur with aggressive "cephalic resections" typical of traditional reduction rhinoplasty, the remaining cartilage may be too weak

to support the nasal sidewall. In addition to fixed anatomic narrowing of the nasal valve leading to an increase in airway resistance, a weakened nasal sidewall may lower the threshold for inspiratory collapse, permitting pathologic valve dysfunction, that is, dynamic collapse, even upon resting inspiration. External manifestations of static nasal valve dysfunction include lobular pinching, alar retraction, and dimpling of the alar crease. Although contemporary rhinoplasty surgeons are

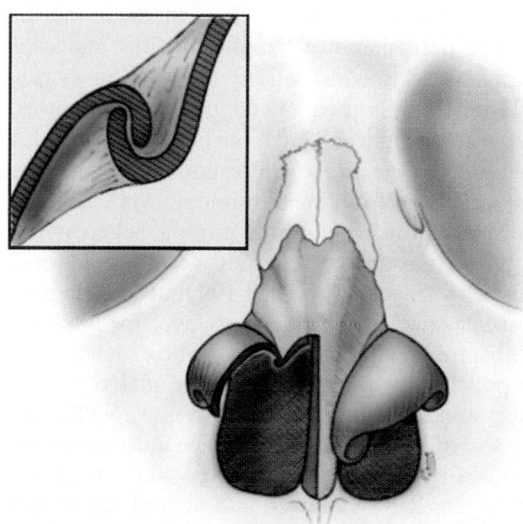

Figure 20 Schematic cross-section of the nasal scroll demonstrating interlocking configuration between the upper and lower lateral cartilages.

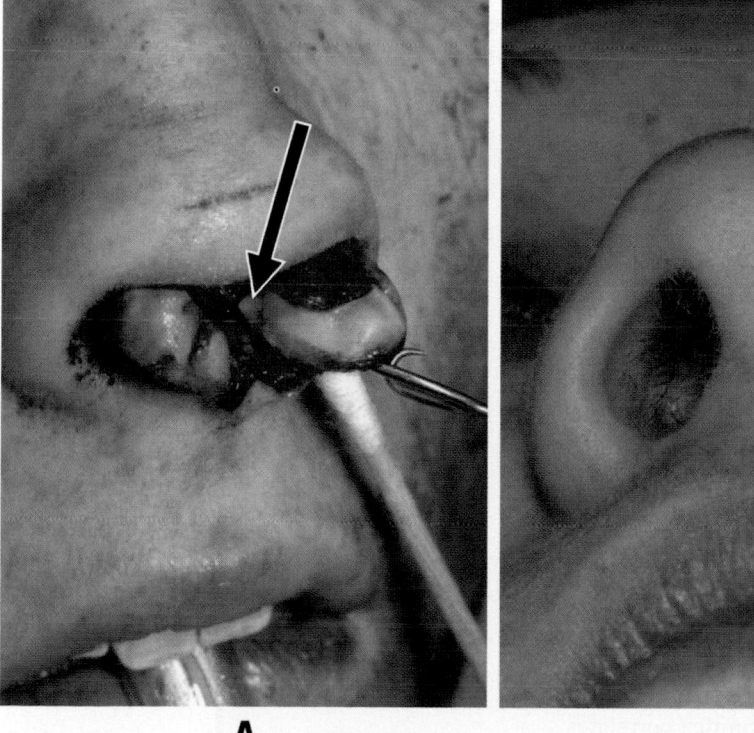

A

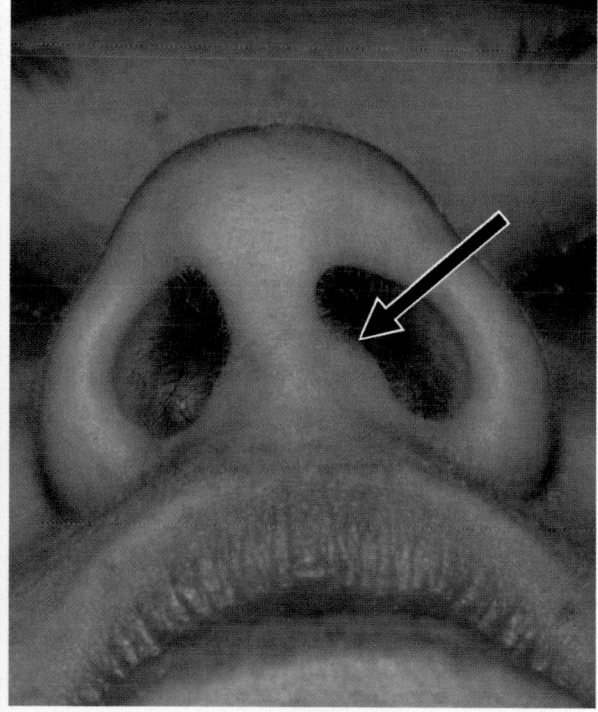

B

Figure 21 (A) Intraoperative and (B) preoperative view of left medial crural footpod (*arrow*). Note asymmetry of the nasal pedestal due to flaring of the left footpod.

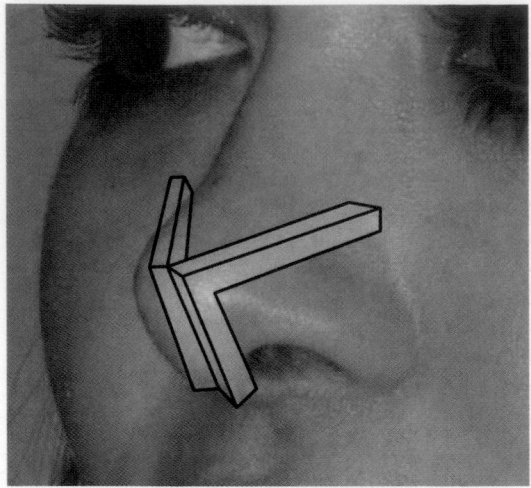

Figure 22 Schematic representation of the nasal tip tripod as conceived by Anderson.

In addition to their functional role in the nasal valve segment, the LLC also play a critical role in nasal aesthetics. Because the LLC are paired, mirror-image structures, they must be perfectly symmetric if a pleasing nasal contour is to be achieved. Any surgical intervention that seeks to alter the LLC must ultimately maintain bilateral symmetry while also producing a cosmetically pleasing tip configuration from all angles.

Owing to the complex three-dimensional relationships generated by the LLC, ULC, and nasal septum, it is useful to conceptualize the LLC using the *tripod theory* originally described by Anderson and coworkers.[12] This theory regards the paired conjoined medial crura as a single structural unit or "leg" within a three-legged structural framework. The remaining legs are composed of the divergent lateral crura, thereby forming a cartilaginous "tripod" (Figure 22). By lengthening or shortening various legs of this skeletal tripod, changes in tip projection, tip rotation, and/or tip alignment can be accomplished making this concept useful in nasal analysis and surgical planning.

NASAL PHYSIOLOGY

A meaningful discussion of contemporary rhinoplasty is not complete without a brief review of nasal respiratory physiology. The nasal airway is the body's preferred conduit for ordinary respiration. Inability to breathe through the nose is decidedly unpleasant, and chronic nasal obstruction may result in secondary side effects such as dry mouth, sore throat, snoring, anosmia, sinus dysfunction, or sleep disturbance. Other pathologic conditions such as mucosal contact headaches, epistaxis, or eustachian tube dysfunction may also result from anatomic deformities of the nasal airway.[13] Nasal valve dysfunction is also associated with corresponding reductions in disease-specific quality of life measures as determined by validated psychological assessment questionnaires, and surgical correction of nasal valve deformities correlates closely with improved quality of life measures.[14]

Much of the body's total airway resistance is generated by the nose as a consequence of spe-

cial adaptations which warm, humidify, and clean the air we breathe. Beyond the skin-lined nostril or *nasal vestibule*, the nasal passage tapers at the *limen vestibulé* to form the bottleneck of the human airway—the so-called *nasal valve* (Figure 23). Some authors prefer to subdivide the nasal valve into the *external* and *internal* segments since these represent two anatomic sites where airway dimensions fluctuate during the normal respiratory cycle, a valve-like phenomenon. However, in the healthy nose, the external nasal valve contributes little to airway resistance because of its comparatively large size; whereas the internal nasal valve constitutes the narrowest segment of the human airway and is responsible for nearly half of all airway resistance. Moreover, the internal valve has the capacity to reduce its size to increase nasal resistance and further restrict nasal airflow. Hence, the nasal valve is the physiologic spigot that controls the rate of airflow through the nasal cavity en route to the lungs.

Beyond the internal nasal valve, the nasal cavity, also known as the nasal *cavum*, is somewhat conical in shape, enlarging as it extends to join the nasopharynx. Mucosal-covered shelves of bone called *conchae*, protrude from the outer sidewall of the nasal cavum giving rise to the inferior, middle, and superior nasal *turbinates*. These unique anatomic structures serve to increase the mucosal surface area within the nasal cavity and enhance contact between inspired air and the sticky, moist nasal mucosa. In addition, the inferior turbinate impinges upon the lower nasal valve region where its specially adapted erectile tissues serve to regulate airflow within the nasal valve and facilitate heat and moisture exchange. Although airflow dynamics are critical to the physiology of a properly functioning nose, considerable controversy remains among experts regarding the precise nature of normal nasal airflow. The character of nasal airflow (turbulent versus laminar) and the principal path of airflow through the nasal cavity

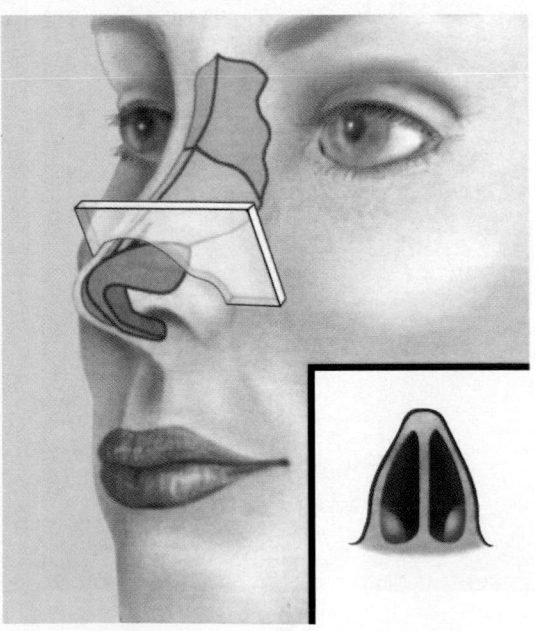

Figure 23 Schematic illustration demonstrating cross-sectional anatomy of the internal nasal valve and its orientation relative to the nasal skeleton.

remain topics of controversy. However, turbulent airflow does appear to play a role in normal nasal physiology and the inferior turbinate appears to participate in the generation of turbulent airflow.[15] Moreover, some investigators have observed a combination of laminar and turbulent airflow occurring at different phases of the normal inspiratory cycle.[16] Increase in nasal turbulence has also been observed in association with the nasal cycle[17] and with increased physiologic demand, such as occurs with exercise.[18]

To regulate nasal airflow, the nasal valve increases the transit time of inspired air to permit sufficient warming, humidification, and cleansing of the air destined for the sensitive lower airway. Shaped as a slit-like triangular opening, the internal nasal valve is bounded mostly by rigid skeletal structures including the quadrangular septum medially, the pyriform aperture inferiorly, and the head of the inferior turbinate bone inferolaterally. Although these skeletal structures are rigid and unyielding, the overlying mucosa of the anterior septum and inferior turbinate contain specially adapted erectile tissues composed of multiple venous sinusoids that can be quickly filled or drained to permit rapid variations in cross-sectional area of the nasal valve with corresponding variations in airway resistance and nasal airflow.[19] Because these unique vascular structures are also covered by only a thin layer of respiratory mucosa, they efficiently transfer both moisture and heat to the inspired air as it transits the nasal cavity. Hence, the nasal valve serves a dual purpose: the regulation of airflow through the nasal cavity and the transfer of moisture and heat to the inspired air.

While the regulatory mechanism of the nasal airway is only partially understood, it is predominantly under the domain of the sympathetic nervous system, with additional input from the parasympathetic nervous system and numerous vasoactive peptides.[20] Nasal airway resistance in healthy individuals is also influenced by a wide range of exogenous factors, such as posture, ambient temperature, ambient humidity, activity level, alcohol ingestion, and various medications. In a large percentage of healthy humans, mucosal shrinkage (vasoconstriction) and swelling (vasodilation) occur in a cyclic pattern alternating between the right and left nasal passages, a process known as the *nasal cycle*. Presumably this permits one side to perform the physiologic work of filtration, humidification, and warming, whereas the opposite side is protected from overdrying and permitted to self-cleanse. The nasal mucosa also possesses a specialized mucous bilayer for filtration of inspired particulate debris. Debris such as dust or pollen are entrapped within the sticky mucous layer and transported from the nose propelled by a wave of beating microcilia. The mucous stream eventually reaches the pharynx where entrapped pathogens are swallowed and neutralized by the harsh pH of the stomach. However, mucociliary dysfunction resulting from genetic disorders or toxic ingestion such as cigarette smoking may impair this natural cleansing mechanism.

While the medial and inferior borders of the nasal valve are rigid and stationary, the lateral border is composed of thin, flexible cartilage that is far less rigid and easily deflected by external compressive forces. When high inspiratory flow rates produce transmural pressures that exceed lateral sidewall support, inward collapse of the nasal sidewall results in dynamic nasal valve collapse. Although dynamic nasal valve collapse is normal in healthy individuals during periods of high ventilatory activity such as exercise, nasal valve collapse should not occur at rest with gentle inspiration. However, various abnormal conditions may compromise nasal sidewall support leading to pathologic valve collapse and symptomatic nasal airway obstruction. Anatomic alterations that weaken the nasal sidewall, such as those caused by overzealous cosmetic rhinoplasty, are a frequent cause of nasal valve dysfunction.

SURGICAL FUNDAMENTALS OF RHINOPLASTY

Anesthesia

Rhinoplasty may be performed comfortably under either general anesthesia or *conscious sedation*, alternatively known as "twilight anesthesia" or "intravenous sedation." Both options have advantages and disadvantages, and surgeon preference will usually dictate the anesthetic approach used. Regardless of the approach chosen, infiltration of the nasal soft tissues with epinephrine-containing local anesthetic is necessary to prevent excessive surgical bleeding. Premixed anesthetic solutions containing 1% lidocaine and epinephrine in a concentration of 1:100,000 are commercially available for soft tissue injection. For twilight anesthesia, infiltration of local anesthetic is preceded by topical anesthetization of the nasal mucosa, augmented by regional nerve blocks to enhance pain control; whereas for general anesthesia, regional nerve blocks are typically omitted. To prevent systemic side effects and limit unwanted hydrostatic tissue distortion, care must be taken to monitor vital signs during injection and restrict the volume of local anesthetic administered.

Surgical Approaches

Cosmetic rhinoplasty is accomplished via the artistic and structurally sound alteration of the nasal skeleton. To that end, surgical exposure must permit satisfactory access to the misshapen anatomy, while minimizing unwanted surgical morbidity. Two surgical approaches to the nasal skeleton are currently used for cosmetic rhinoplasty: the *open* (or *external*) approach and the *closed* (or *endonasal*) approach. In the closed rhinoplasty approach, all incisions are confined to the nasal vestibule and surgery is conducted entirely through the nostrils. The closed approach offers several advantages over open rhinoplasty, including the absence of visible incisions and limited disruption of the skin-soft tissue envelope. The absence of external incisions shortens closure time, while the

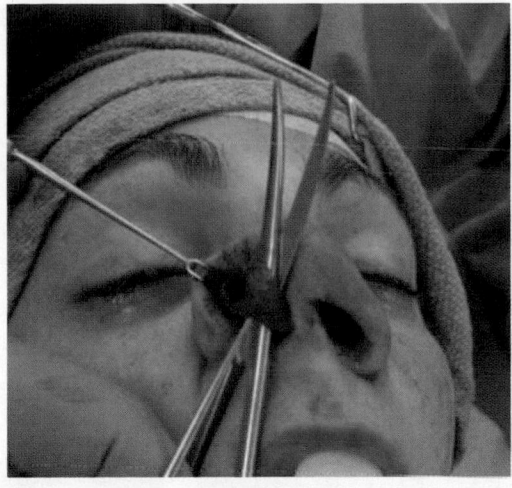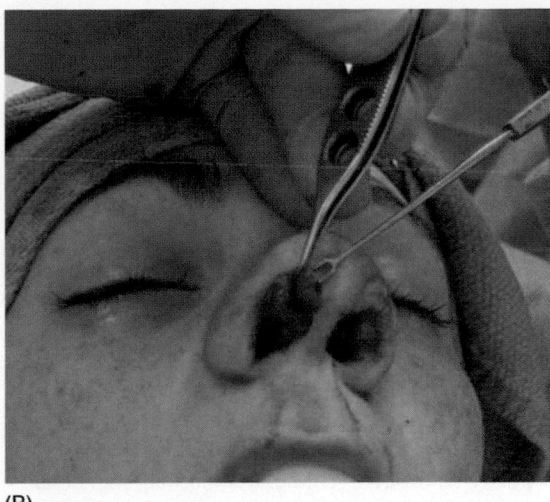

(A)   **(B)**

Figure 24 Intraoperative view of alar cartilage "delivery" technique. (A) Right alar cartilage delivered as chondrocutaneous flap via right nostril. (B) Both alar cartilages delivered via the right nostril for suture approximation.

limited tissue disruption not only minimizes acute swelling and ecchymosis but also proportionately limits the potential for scar contracture or subcutaneous fibrosis. Because the endonasal approach does not require elevation of a pedicled skin flap, distortion of the nasal skin is minimized, and cosmetic changes to the nasal skeleton are more easily appreciated. Although reduced access to the nasal skeleton does not facilitate suture fixation of grafts or implants, the closed approach does permit creation of "precise pockets" to stabilize onlay grafts and limit unwanted graft migration. Despite these many advantages, the limited surgical exposure typical of endonasal rhinoplasty prevents the application of many advanced operative techniques, making closed rhinoplasty poorly suited to complex revision procedures. Nevertheless, endonasal rhinoplasty remains the preferred approach for numerous cosmetic surgeons, particularly in the previously unoperated nose (primary rhinoplasty) or for limited revision ("touch-up") procedures.

Presently, most endonasal rhinoplasty is performed using the *delivery* method of alar cartilage exposure in which *intercartilaginous* (IC) and *marginal* incisions are combined to externalize or "deliver" the alar cartilage as a bipedicled chondrocutaneous flap (Figure 24). The IC incision divides the attachment of the upper and LLCs at the nasal scroll, then extends medially past the anterior septal angle where it continues along the leading edge of the caudal part of the septum (Figure 25A). In addition to permitting access to the nasal tip, the IC incision also permits surgical access to the nasal bridge for alterations of the dorsal profile (Figure 25B).

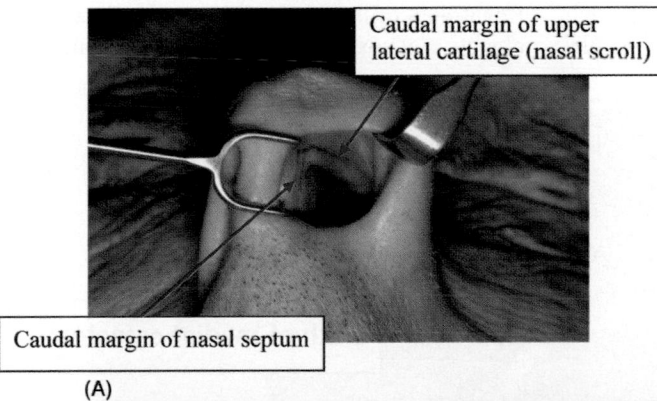

Caudal margin of upper lateral cartilage (nasal scroll)

Caudal margin of nasal septum

(A)

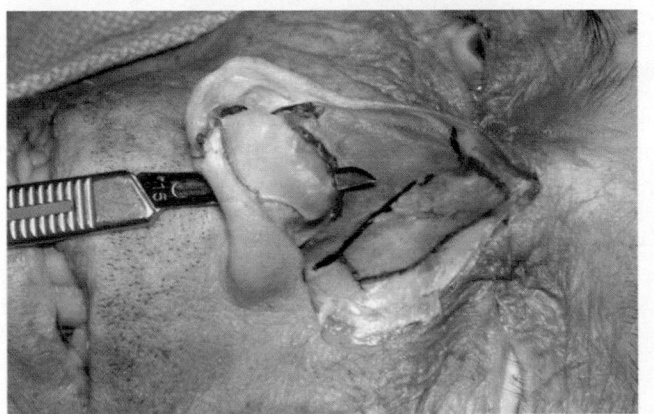

(B)

Figure 25 Cadaver specimen with skin partially removed. (A) Endonasal view of the intercartilaginous rhinoplasty incision. (B) "Intercartilaginous" knife cut dividing the lower lateral and upper lateral cartilages for access to the upper part of the nasal dorsum.

In contrast to the IC incision which follows the *cephalic border* of the alar cartilage, the *marginal* incision follows the caudal border (or "margin") of the alar cartilage giving rise to the name "marginal" incision (Figure 26). Since the caudal border of the alar cartilage runs oblique to the nostril rim, the marginal incision should not be confused with the seldom-used *rim* incision which runs parallel to the inner nostril rim. Use of the rim incision is discouraged owing to its characteristically conspicuous and unsightly appearance and the increased risk of nostril stenosis.

Although the marginal incision is mandatory for delivery of the tip cartilage, it is also the principal incision used in the *external* rhinoplasty approach. Bilateral marginal incisions are connected by a single bridging incision of the columellar skin, the so-called *transcolumellar* incision (Figure 27). Usually less than 5 to 7 mm long, the transcolumellar incision is typically located at the mid-columella and is often irregularized to improve camouflage and minimize scar contracture. While this incision results in a potentially visible scar, it also permits wide-field surgical *degloving* of the nasal framework for dramatically improved access to the nasal skeleton. Moreover, when repaired properly, the transcolumellar scar is frequently indiscernible.

Because the external approach obviates the need for IC incisions, both the mucosal envelope and nasal scroll remain intact. Thus, contamination from the underlying nasal cavity is minimized, and structural support to the nasal sidewall is preserved. The open approach also facilitates en bloc elevation of the skin-soft tissue envelope, thereby limiting disruption of the cutaneous capillary and lymphatic networks. Perhaps most importantly, the external approach offers vastly improved surgical exposure result-

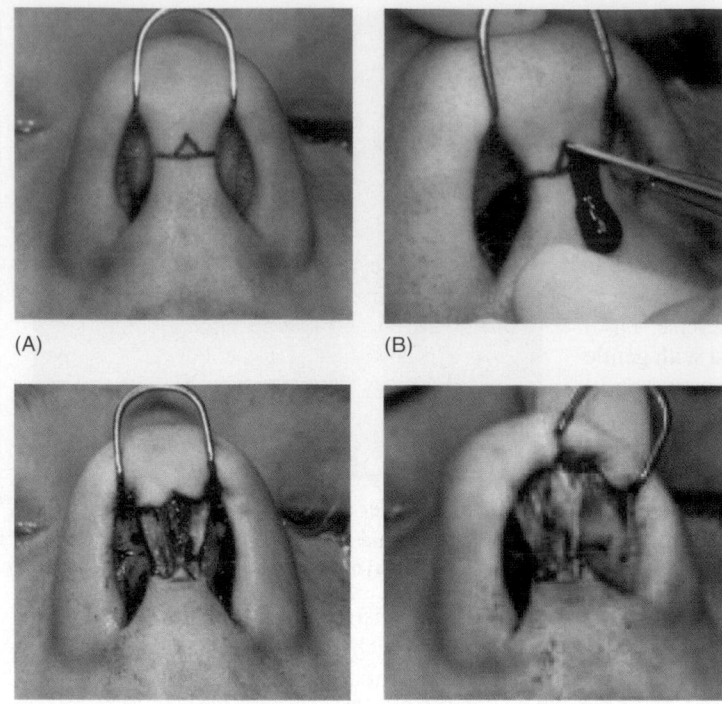

Figure 27 Intraoperative photos demonstrating: (A) location of the transcolumellar incision; (B) stab technique; (C) initial flap elevation; and (D) marginal incision.

ing in better diagnostic accuracy, diminished distortion of the exposed skeletal anatomy, and direct access for suture fixation of most grafts or implants (Figure 28). Although endonasal rhinoplasty is still in widespread use, the external approach has become the procedure of choice for complex *structural* reconstruction of the collapsed nasal framework. Owing to its greater diagnostic accuracy and therapeutic versatility, external rhinoplasty will no doubt remain the workhorse of revision nasal surgery.

Fundamentals of Tip Rhinoplasty

Regardless of the surgical approach selected, the objective of cosmetic rhinoplasty is the controlled and artistic reconfiguration of the nasal framework. For the nasal tip, a wide variety of techniques have been devised to modify the LLCs and improve tip contour, projection, and/or rotation. Because many of the early refinement techniques relied solely upon alar cartilage excision to partially collapse the alar tripod, cosmetic results were often unpredictable and frequently disappointing. Even satisfactory cosmetic results were too often prone to delayed shrink-wrap deformities and eventual nasal sidewall collapse. Despite the large number of tip refinement techniques described to date, few methods have withstood the test of time, and many have been abandoned or condemned due to consistently poor surgical results.

While considerable disagreement exists among accomplished surgeons regarding the optimal method of tip enhancement, all successful tip-plasty techniques share several common

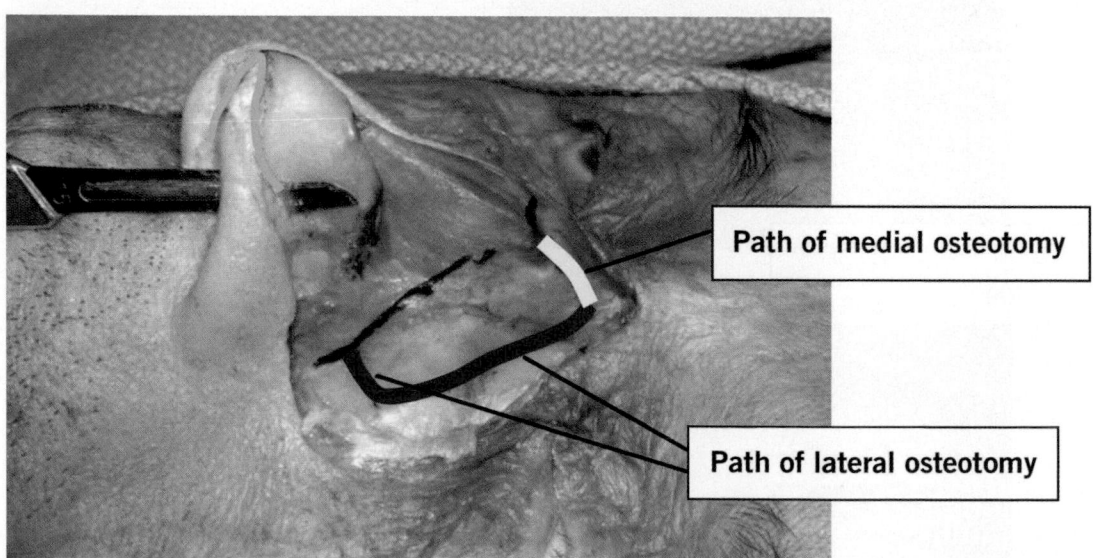

Figure 26 Cadaver specimen with skin partially removed showing the "marginal" incision at the inferior border of the lower lateral cartilage (*blue line*), lateral osteotomy cut (*red line*), and medial osteotomy cut (*yellow line*).

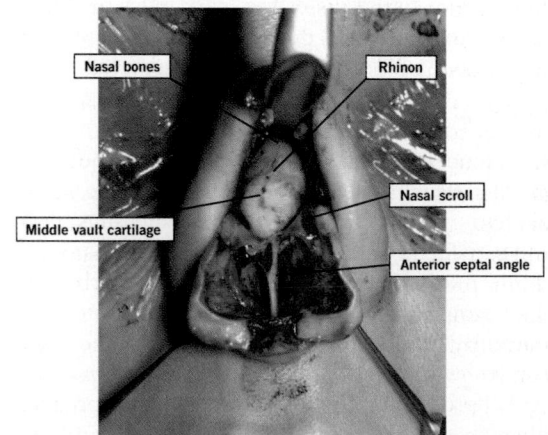

Figure 28 Intraoperative photograph demonstrating wide field exposure gained through the external rhinoplasty approach.

characteristics. Perhaps the most important universal element in a successful tip-plasty is adequate preservation of structural tip support. Without effective support of the nasal tip, the lobule eventually succumbs to the persistent forces of muscle movement, gravity, or aging; and an elongated, counterrotated, and/or underprojected nose ensues. Indeed, poor tip support is frequently a causative factor, not only in the failed rhinoplasty, but also in the naturally unattractive nose as well.

Another important characteristic of successful tip modification is an aesthetically pleasing separation of the nasal domes. Whether from congenital malformation or failed surgical intervention, tightly approximated nasal domes produce an objectionable "pinched" or "unitip" appearance. Moreover, noses with this appearance are frequently plagued by functional collapse of the nasal airway, making the combined aesthetic and functional deficits a common motive for seeking corrective surgery. Like the overly narrow nasal tip, excessive domal width is also highly disruptive to cosmetic harmony, and both a wide ball-like lobule or a bulbous tip are highly undesirable and conspicuous features that often prompt cosmetic rhinoplasty. Although a large nasal tip does not guarantee satisfactory nasal airway function (since it may also conceal functional deformities of the underlying nasal passages), progressive narrowing of the nasal tip is limited by continued patency of the nasal airway. Hence, all effective tip reduction techniques must precisely narrow tip width without invoking functional encroachment of the nasal airway. Since divergence of the medial crura and separation of the nasal domes are mandatory attributes of any attractive nasal tip, all effective tip modification techniques must also preserve these critically important aesthetic features.

Finally, the last element common to all effective tip-plasty techniques is versatility. Because virtually no two noses are alike, surgical alteration of the nasal tip must be able to accommodate individual variations in tip morphology including projection, rotation, symmetry, and width. Furthermore, because maneuvers which enhance nasal contour from one perspective, may disrupt nasal aesthetics from another, all effective tip-plasty techniques must be able to compensate for unwanted secondary or tertiary effects of cartilage reshaping. The result should be a stable, natural, and attractive tip contour when viewed from all angles. Although it has been stated that mastery of the tip equates to the mastery of rhinoplasty, this represents a gross oversimplification of the numerous challenges and complexities of cosmetic rhinoplasty. Nevertheless, no rhinoplasty can be considered truly successful if an attractive tip is lacking, and achieving a cosmetically pleasing tip contour can present one of the more daunting facets of cosmetic nasal surgery.

The Wide Tip. Refining the overly wide tip involves narrowing broad domal arches, reducing excessive interdomal space, and restoring domal symmetry. However, before the naturally

attractive nasal tip can be replicated, the surgeon must first understand the skeletal configuration which characterizes the naturally attractive nose.

The ideal nasal tip framework is typified by angular, V-shaped domal apices oriented slightly oblique to the sagittal midline (Figure 29). The caudal border of the domal apex is separated from its counterpart by several millimeters, whereas the cephalic margins are typically in close approximation. The resulting divergent configuration creates a diamond-shaped surface contour which surrounds a small interdomal cleft. Ordinarily the cleft is filled with supportive ligaments and other fibromuscular tissues, resulting in a smooth, slightly convex, external contour. When domal spacing is ideal, this configuration leads to a slender and elegant lobule with distinct, individual domal highlights.

However, domal spacing alone does not assure an attractive nasal tip. In addition to optimal domal spacing, the ideal tip configuration is also characterized by flat, straight, and symmetric lateral crura. Although modest convexity may be tolerable in the wide nose, a flat, uniplanar lateral crus typically provides the most appealing nasal shape.

While virtually no two noses are exactly alike, variations of this alar cartilage configuration are found in virtually all naturally attractive noses. While the angle of divergence will vary according to the desired tip width, the presence of a diamond-shaped lobule and smooth, flat lateral crura are essential to an attractive tip contour, and all tip-plasty techniques either mimic or recreate these crucial skeletal features.

In the broad nasal tip deformity, wide, rounded domal arches result in excessive separation of the alar domes (Figure 30). In the thick-skinned patient, the large interdomal space is typically filled with fibromuscular tissue, but lobular bifidity may also be observed in the absence of thick nasal skin. From below, the broad nasal tip appears trapezoidal in shape rather than the preferred equilateral triangle, and the lateral crura are generally flat or gently convex presenting a conspicuous bulbous appearance.

Refining the boxy tip involves creating a more angular domal arch to narrow the excessive interdomal space. Typically the lateral crura require very little modification other than modest cephalic resection at the "paradomal" region to eliminate supratip fullness in the nasal profile.

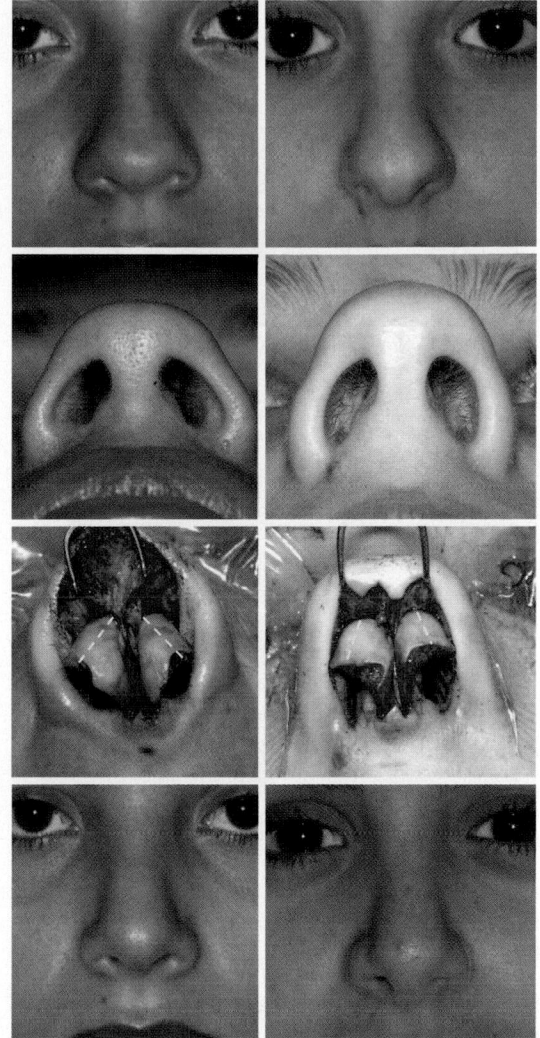

Figure 30 Examples of the broad nasal tip deformity. Note the wide interdomal spacing, linear alar sidewall, and trapezoidal tip configuration on base view. (Note postoperative views at the bottom)

In contrast to the broad tip, the classic *bulbous* nasal tip deformity is characterized by unusually broad and widely separated domal arches exacerbated by overly round, convex lateral crura (Figure 31). Refinement of the bulbous tip deformity involves narrowing the overly wide tip (as described above for the broad-tip deformity) followed by flattening of the convex lateral crura. Eliminating convexity in the cupped and bowed lateral crus without compromising nasal sidewall support can be extremely challenging and may require a combination of cartilage excision, suture modification, and/or cartilage grafting techniques.

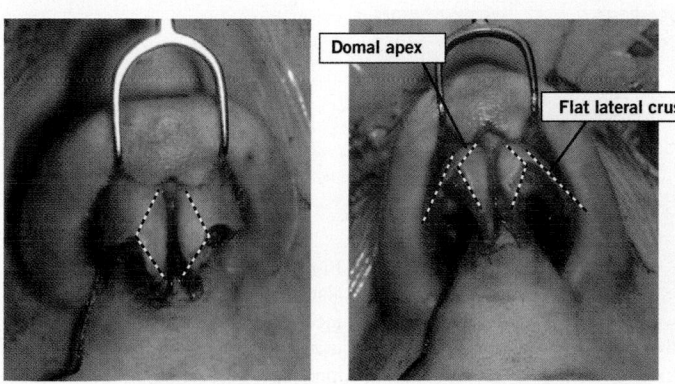

Figure 29 Natural configuration of tip cartilages in the aesthetically pleasing nose. Note the divergent mesial crura, diamond-shaped lobule, and flat lateral crura.

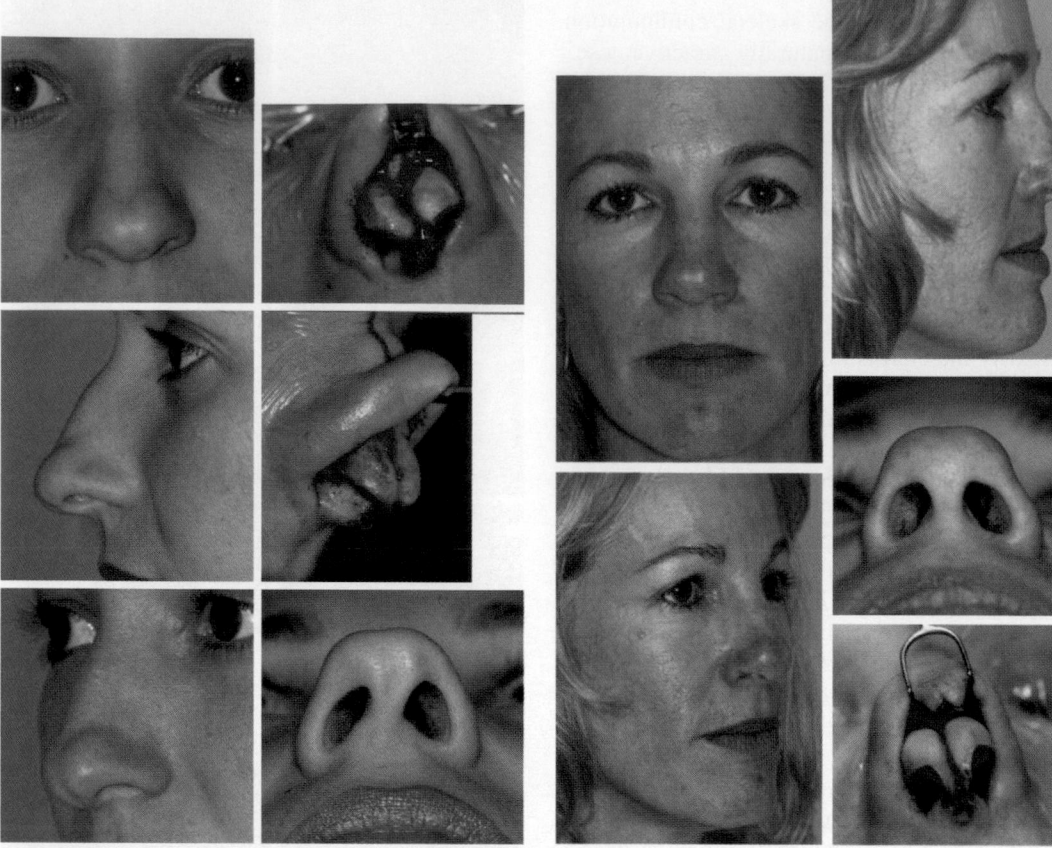

Figure 31 Examples of the bulbous nasal tip deformity. Note the broad convex lateral crura, pronounced interdomal bifidity, and exaggerated trapezoidal shape on base view.

Finally, in the *asymmetric* tip deformity, the domal arches lack mirror image symmetry due to inconsistencies in domal contour, projection, and/or rotation (Figure 32). Modest domal asymmetries are often evident in the misshapen lobule, and the deformities described above are commonly observed in combination. Although the malpositioned alar cartilage often responds favorably to repositioning, correction of congenital size discrepancies between LLCs is far more challenging and may require augmentation, unilateral cartilage excision, and/or camouflage grafts for correction.

Because excessive tip width is a common feature of the misshapen nose, a number of techniques have been described to address the wide lobule. Perhaps the most effective approach for tip refinement is suture modification of the alar tripod. Suture-based refinement techniques rely upon cartilage reshaping, rather than the traditional technique of cartilage excision, to

reconfigure the oversized lobule. These techniques permit narrowing of the domal arch, reduction of the interdomal space, or combinations therein, while simultaneously conserving structural support and minimizing the risk of contracture-mediated deformities.

Typically, suture-based techniques are performed as a two-step procedure. In the first step, each dome is individually narrowed using a horizontal mattress "*dome-unit*" or "*dome-binding*" suture (Figure 33). To create the desired V-shaped domal configuration, scoring of the domal apex is often necessary to break the "spring" of the alar arch. When simultaneous increases in tip projection and rotation are also needed, the hinge-point can be repositioned laterally, outside the existing dome, to increase length of the medial element. In the second step, the newly narrowed domal arches are then coapted with a third "*interdomal*" mattress suture, placed between the domes, to control precisely the extent

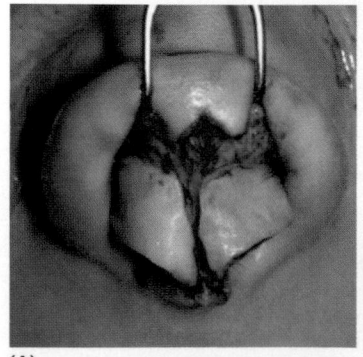
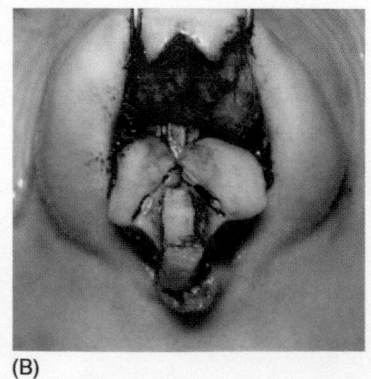

(A)   (B)

Figure 32 Intraoperative view of alar cartilages. (A) Congenital asymmetry. (B) Reconfigured alar tripod using suture modification and augmentation grafts.

of interdomal separation and diminish lobular width. As with the ideal (natural) dome configuration, the cephalic aspects of the domes are positioned in close approximation while the caudal ends remain separated by up to several millimeters (see Figure 32). This is accomplished by angling the interdomal suture with the caudal segment placed away from the domal apices. The result is a natural-appearing diamond-shaped lobule that avoids the pinched "unitip" deformity resulting from complete coaptation of the nasal domes.

While suture techniques provide an effective means of refining the wide nasal tip, the bulbous nasal tip deformity normally requires additional measures to address the broad, convex lateral crura. Typically, bulbous alar cartilages are strong and stiff as a consequence of their cupped, convex shape. Obtaining a smooth, flat crural contour is often challenging and various ancillary techniques such as curetting, augmentation grafting (eg, lateral crural strut grafts), or sculpting sutures may be required to achieve the desired nasal contour.[21,22] However, stubborn convexities may also require judicious excision of the cephalic part of the crus in order to sufficiently flatten the cupped alar cartilage. Since bulbous alar cartilages are generally more resistant to cartilage excision, the volume of excised tissue is typically greater than that necessary for the average nose. Nevertheless, the bulbous nose is also subject to the same requirements of adequate structural sidewall support, and overexcision is ill-advised.

Although conservative excision of the lateral crus is sometimes necessary to shape the unusually strong alar cartilage or to refine the supratip profile, the practice of subtotal lateral crural resection (eg, the "rim strip") is seldom justified and should be abandoned. While this technique has been taught as a reliable means of achieving tip rotation or tip narrowing, loss of crural rigidity is commonly associated with buckling of the residual cartilage producing a host of associated deformities including bossae, lobular pinching, alar dimples, and/or domal asymmetries (see Figure 15). Moreover, in contracture-prone patients, the skeletal void created by the missing cephalic segment leads to cephalic migration of the remnant cartilage producing a conspicuous retraction of the nostril rim. Because alar retraction is difficult to reverse, excision of the cephalic margin, particularly within the nasal scroll, should be avoided whenever possible. Fortunately, the traditional practice of subtotal crural excision has fallen into disfavor, and numerous, far more effective and reliable alternatives to "excisional" rhinoplasty, such as suture-based cartilage reshaping, have been developed.

The Ptotic Tip. Another frequent challenge of tip rhinoplasty is eliminating the *ptotic* nasal tip deformity. The ptotic tip deformity stems from compromised tip support and is characterized by a counterrotated and often underprojected lobule (Figure 34). Causes for inadequate tip

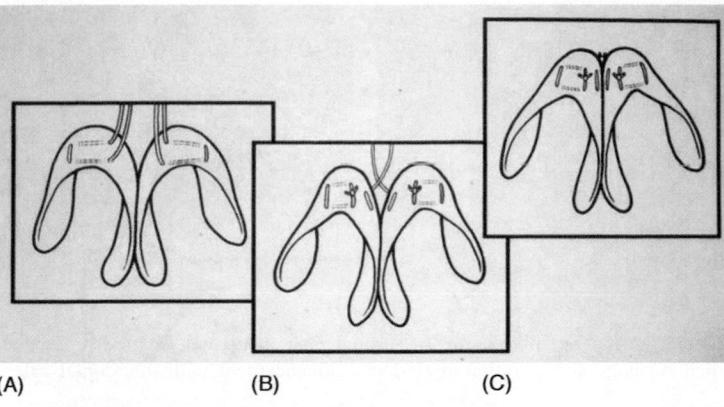

Figure 33 Schematic illustration of two-step suture modification of the wide nasal tip. (A) Placement of dome-unit sutures. (B) Placement of interdomal sutures. (C) Suture-based tip refinement.

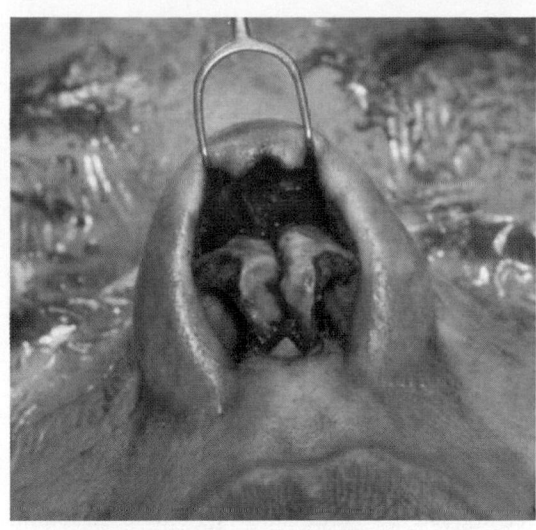

Figure 35 Intraoperative view of buckled medial crura in ptotic nasal tip.

support include widely spaced medial crura, buckled medial crura, short medial crura, and/or excessive activity of the depressor septi muscles (Figure 35).

Because the ptotic tip lacks adequate projection and sufficient rotation, treatment mandates correction of both deficiencies. As with tip narrowing, a wide range of procedures have been devised to rotate and project the ptotic nasal tip. Techniques include coaptation of the medial crura, augmentation of medial crural strength, extension of medial crural length, suspension of the alar cartilage, and/or reduction of the oversized alar arch.

Perhaps the most common technique for treatment of the ptotic tip is placement of a *columellar strut* graft (Figure 36). Fashioned from septal cartilage to create a long flat strip of rigid tissue, the columellar strut graft behaves as a structural pillar to enhance tip recoil and lengthen the central limb of the tripod. Although septal cartilage is often preferred, the graft may also be fashioned

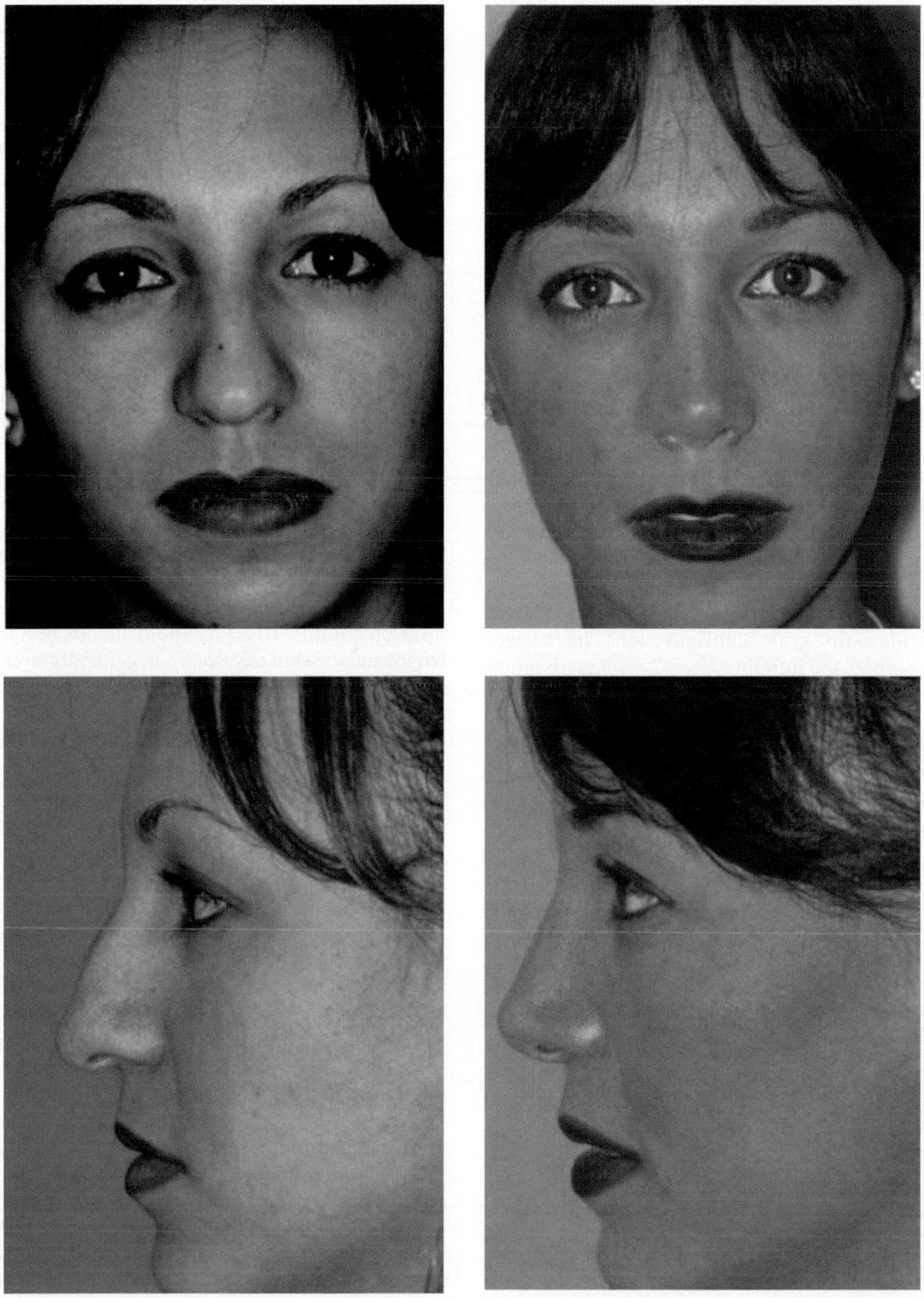

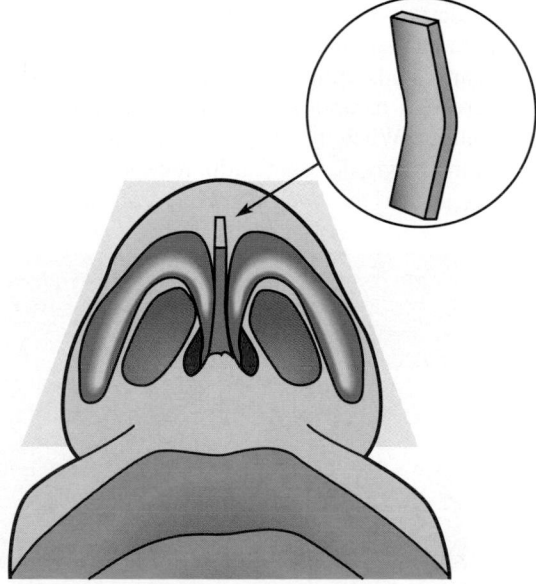

Figure 36 Schematic illustration demonstrating placement of a floating columellar strut. Note the angled configuration used to create a columellar double-break.

Figure 34 Front and profile view of ptotic tip deformity (A) before, and (B) after tip-plasty using a columellar strut and tip suture technique.

from conchal cartilage, rib cartilage, or irradiated rib cartilage when autologous septal tissue is unavailable. Sandwiched between the medial crura, the graft is coapted with multiple transfixion sutures, functionally uniting the three separate skeletal components into a single reinforced structural element. Normally the graft terminates above the crural footpods and is supported from below by a sling of intercrural ligamentous tissue which prevents direct articulation with the nasal spine. However, this type of "*floating*" strut design may lose projection when subjected to extreme loading forces typical of the severely underprojected nose. In contrast, the *articulated* columellar strut, which rests directly upon the nasal spine via a variety of complex fixation techniques, provides rigid unyielding structural support and is preferred for the severely underprojected or overrotated nose. However, maintaining secure midline fixation upon the nasal spine is challenging and muscle activity produced by smiling may displace the articulated strut from the nasal spine if secure fixation is lacking. Nevertheless, the extended columellar strut is often the only effective means of forcibly reprojecting the scarred or severely hypoplastic tip.

Regardless of strut design, the strut profile can be angled by 10° or 15° to simulate a columellar "double break" when a feminine profile is desired. Similarly, by adjusting the extent of caudal projection, columellar profile disturbances such as columellar retraction or an overly acute nasolabial angle can also be eliminated. Although either an open or closed rhinoplasty approach can be used to insert a columellar strut graft, secure fixation of the articulated strut usually necessitates the external approach. In both cases, the columellar strut graft is initially overprojected, then sequentially trimmed until the desired profile aesthetics are achieved (Figure 37). Because the residual strut protrudes beyond the underprojected alar domes, a unitip deformity is temporarily produced and additional measures are needed to restore tip fullness (Figure 38). Using the strut as a fulcrum, the alar cartilages are then pulled forward and sutured to the distal graft to project the alar tripod, camouflage the protruding graft, and create a natural and cosmetically appealing tip contour. When the alar domes are too short to reach the newly designated tip, recruitment techniques, such as the "*lateral crural steal*," are used

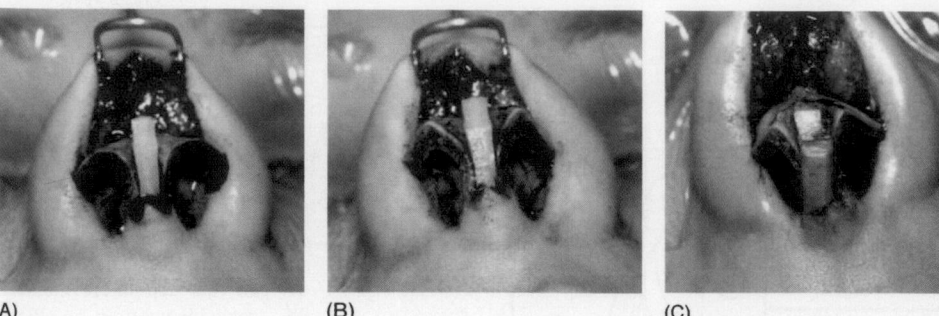

Figure 38 Intraoperative views of columellar strut graft placement. (A) Initial placement with desired projection. (B) Dome unit suture placement. (C) Final cartilage configuration after domal advancement with interdomal suture placement.

to relocate the alar domes and increase projection of the alar arch.[23] This technique increases tip projection and rotates the lobule by repositioning the dome apices laterally and "stealing" lateral crura to lengthen the medial element. When used in combination with a columellar strut graft, the wide, ptotic, and underprojected lobule can be narrowed, rotated, and projected simultaneously (Figure 39). Although placement of a columellar strut will result in palpable rigidity of the nasal tip, it also confers a potentially permanent increase in tip support to maintain appropriate rotation and projection of the ptotic lobule indefinitely.

Tip Grafts. Often, the severely underprojected nose is only partially corrected with the application of a columellar strut graft. Although recruitment techniques, such as the lateral crural steal, are capable of yielding additional tip projection, these increases may be prevented by overrotation of the lobule. Thus, when columellar struts and recruitment techniques fail to achieve the desired tip projection, *tip augmentation grafts* may be used to achieve additional projection. Although various tip graft configurations have been described, the infratip "*shield*" *graft* is by far the most popular option. Fashioned to mimic the diamond-shaped lobule and its divergent domes, the heart-shaped graft is secured to the infratip lobule for a simultaneous increase in nasal length and tip projection (Figure 40). Care must be taken to bevel the outer graft edges for satisfactory camouflage and to ensure that the lateral crura blend smoothly with the graft shoulders. When crafted properly, the shield graft provides a cosmetically pleasing lobular contour and a sizeable increase in tip projection. Moreover, graft shape can be

adjusted to suit the desired tip width, and graft length can be adjusted to modify the columellar profile. Since the shield graft also functions as a mechanical gusset plate, stability of the alar tripod is greatly enhanced with shield graft placement.

Another popular tip augmentation graft is the *cap* or *supradomal* augmentation graft. Like the shield graft, the cap graft is used to increase tip projection by lengthening the domal apices (see Figure 40). As with all onlay grafts, the edges are beveled to enhance camouflage and care is taken to ensure a smooth transition with the surrounding cartilage. However, unlike the more commonly used shield graft, the cap graft does not alter tip rotation since dorsal length remains constant. Hence the cap graft is a useful adjunct for the underprojected nose in which counterrotation is not desired.

Tip Extension Grafts. The successful application of a columellar strut graft requires an elastic skin-soft tissue envelope that can stretch to accommodate to the newly projected nasal framework. For the ptotic nasal tip deformity, the increase in tip projection is offset by the decrease in nasal length and the skin envelope can generally stretch to accommodate the reconFigured tip tripod. However, when attempting to increase tip projection in patients with scarred or contracted nasal skin, the absence of skin elasticity leads to excessive cephalic displacement of the strut, and tip projection gives way to an overrotated, underprojected lobule with excessive nostril show.

To prevent unwanted rotation of the lobule, the cephalic aspect of the graft may be extended into the membranous septum and overlapped with the caudal L-strut. This type of modified strut can be sutured to the caudal septum to stabilize the central tripod and prevent unwanted strut displacement. By using both the caudal septum and the nasal spine as a mechanical buttress, the extended columellar strut, also known as a *septal extension graft*, achieves maximum structural stability and permits forceful elongation of the nasal skin envelope to increase projection dramatically while simultaneously maintaining appropriate rotation of the lobule. Although the septal extension graft is a powerful tool in revision rhinoplasty, in severely inelastic noses, careful excision of subcutaneous fibrous tissue may be needed to enhance skin elasticity further and permit adequate tip lengthening.

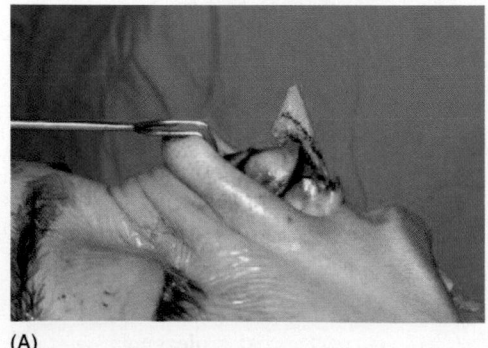
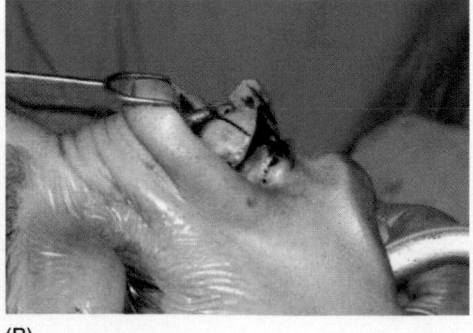

Figure 37 Intraoperative photographs showing (A) initial installation of a floating strut prior to final shaping, (B) final strut contour reflecting the desired profile aesthetics.

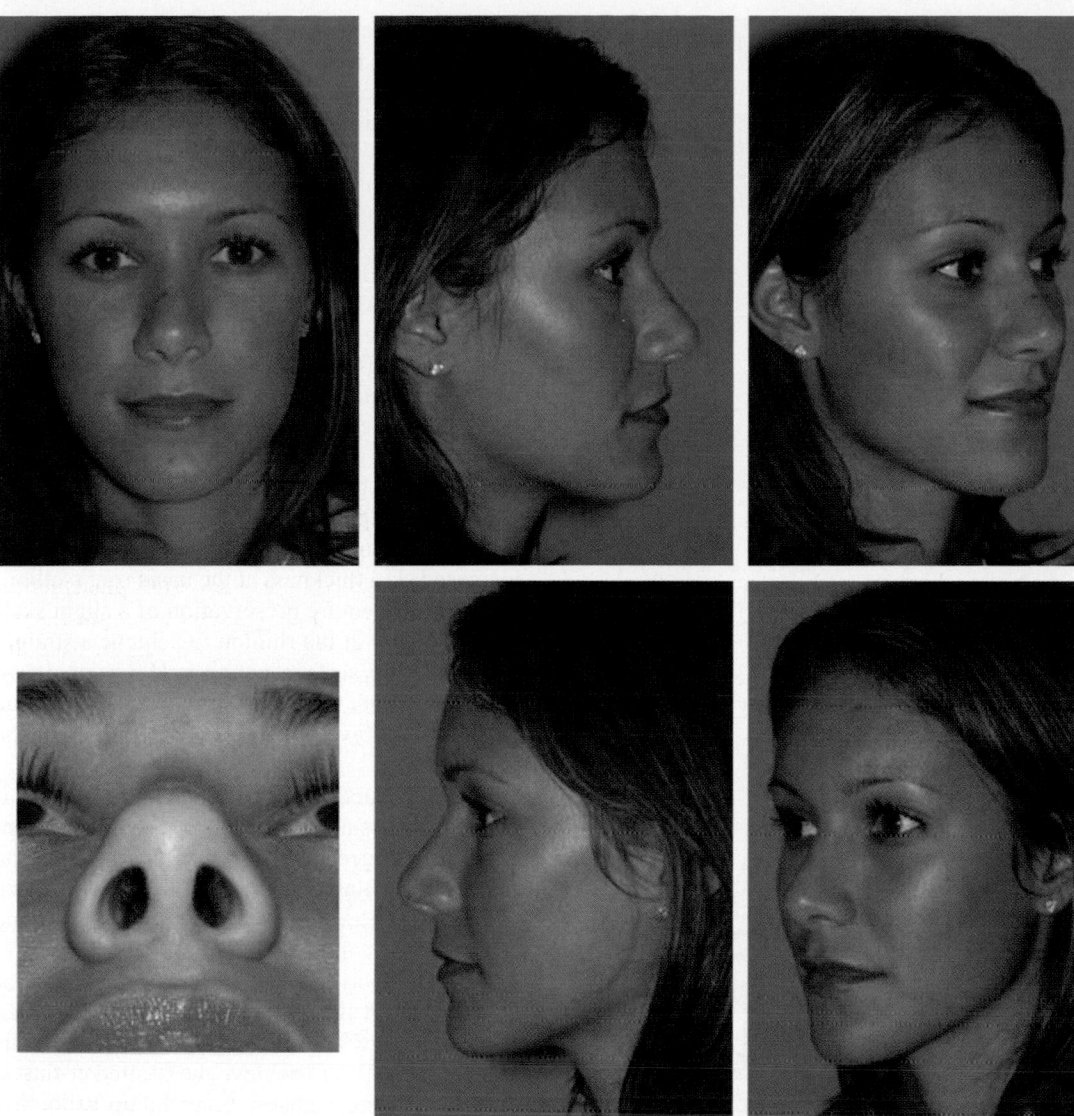

Figure 39 Postoperative views demonstrating lateral crural steal and columellar strut tip-plasty techniques. Preoperative views are shown in Figure 5, and intraoperative views are shown in Figures 32 and 38.

The technique requires surgical separation of the membranous septum and medial crura, followed by a "setback" repositioning and imbrication of the medial crura upon the caudal aspect of the septum to stabilize the repositioned tripod. In this manner, the caudal aspect of the septum functions as a columellar strut to support the newly projected tip and cephalically repositioned alar tripod. The result is a shortened nose with greater tip projection (Figure 45). In addition to increasing tip projection, the tongue-in-groove technique can also be used to decrease tip projection by altering juxtaposition of the alar tripod relative to the caudal aspect of the septum. Hence, the tongue-in-groove technique is a versatile method for cosmetic tip refinement in the overly long nose; and tip rotation, tip projection, or tip deprojection may all be accomplished with this technique.

Finally, the ptotic tip can also be addressed with the crural overlay technique in which the lateral crura are vertically divided, shortened or overlapped, and reconstituted with suture[28,29] (Figure 46). Typically, the lateral crura are divided well lateral to the nasal dome in the mid to lateral segments, although the precise location is often governed by the shape and strength of the alar cartilage. While the lateral crural overlay technique rotates the lobule effectively, unlike many of the aforementioned techniques, the lateral crural overlay does not increase tip projection. For this reason, the lateral crural overlay is often preferred for the *overprojected* ptotic nose. In cases of severe overprojection, medial crural overlap can also be used to optimize deprojection while avoiding overrotation.

Tip Surgery and Nasal Skin Thickness. Regardless of the craftsman's skill, the quality of the final product is only as good as the materials used in the construction process. In the case of cosmetic rhinoplasty, time-honored methods in the hands of a master surgeon cannot always overcome the constraints of unfavorable tissues. Perhaps the most daunting challenge is the wide nose with thick sebaceous skin and naturally weak cartilage. As a strong and rigid nasal framework is needed to shape forcefully the thick, amorphous skin, weak, flexible cartilage is ill-suited to a well-defined nasal contour. The problem is compounded by excessive nasal size since an oversized sebaceous skin envelope seldom conforms to a reduced skeletal framework in a favorable manner. Moreover, even when favorable results are achieved, the healing process usually takes much longer to conclude. Since a large, shapely nose is generally preferable to a small misshapen one and since the large thick-skinned nose may respond poorly to size reduction, contour enhancement should take priority over size reduction in the oversized nose with heavy nasal skin. If existing septal tissues lack sufficient rigidity or are in short supply, rib cartilage grafting may be necessary to achieve a strong and aesthetically pleasing skeletal framework and to stretch the thickened nasal skin forcibly for a well-defined nasal contour.

Several variations of the septal extension graft have been described in which tip support is augmented using various grafts anchored to the nasal septum.[24–26] Lengthening of the septum with cartilage grafts can be used to correct a host of nasal deformities including severe columellar retraction, septal overresection, or the congenitally short nose (Figure 41). While many of these techniques employ single or bilateral spreader grafts to stabilize the columellar strut, they all rely upon the nasal septum to buttress the nasal tip in a more projected or counterrotated configuration.

Another accepted method for addressing the ptotic tip deformity is the technique of *vertical dome division*.[27] This technique and its variations vertically divide the alar cartilage adjacent to the existing dome to increase medial crura length (Figure 42). A portion of the divided lateral crus is then recruited to lengthen the foreshortened medial crus, simultaneously increasing both tip rotation and tip projection. Tip support is further enhanced by coapting the medial crura with transfixion sutures, with or without an intervening columellar strut graft. Vertical division of the alar cartilage also serves to "break the spring" of the domal arch contributing to tip refinement from narrowing of the lobule. Although vertical dome division may be performed via the external rhinoplasty approach, it is most commonly performed using an endonasal (delivery) approach and can be embellished with the addition of onlay grafts or conservative alar cartilage excision.

While vertical dome division is commonly used to increase tip projection, segmental excision of the alar arch using "vertical" incisions can also provide a powerful means of reducing the overprojected nasal tip (Figure 43). By reducing all three limbs of the alar tripod simultaneously, segmental excision of the alar domes produces a controlled reduction in tip projection. Moreover, by simultaneously adjusting the relative length of the medial and lateral tripod legs, concomitant changes to tip rotation can also be achieved. Hence, vertical dome division is a versatile technique that may be used to alter tip projection and rotation in a variety of combinations.

Another method of simultaneously improving tip projection and tip rotation is the "*tongue-in-groove*" setback technique. This powerful technique, applicable only to overly long noses, achieves simultaneous tip projection and tip rotation by cephalically repositioning the alar tripod upon the caudal aspect of the septum (Figure 44).

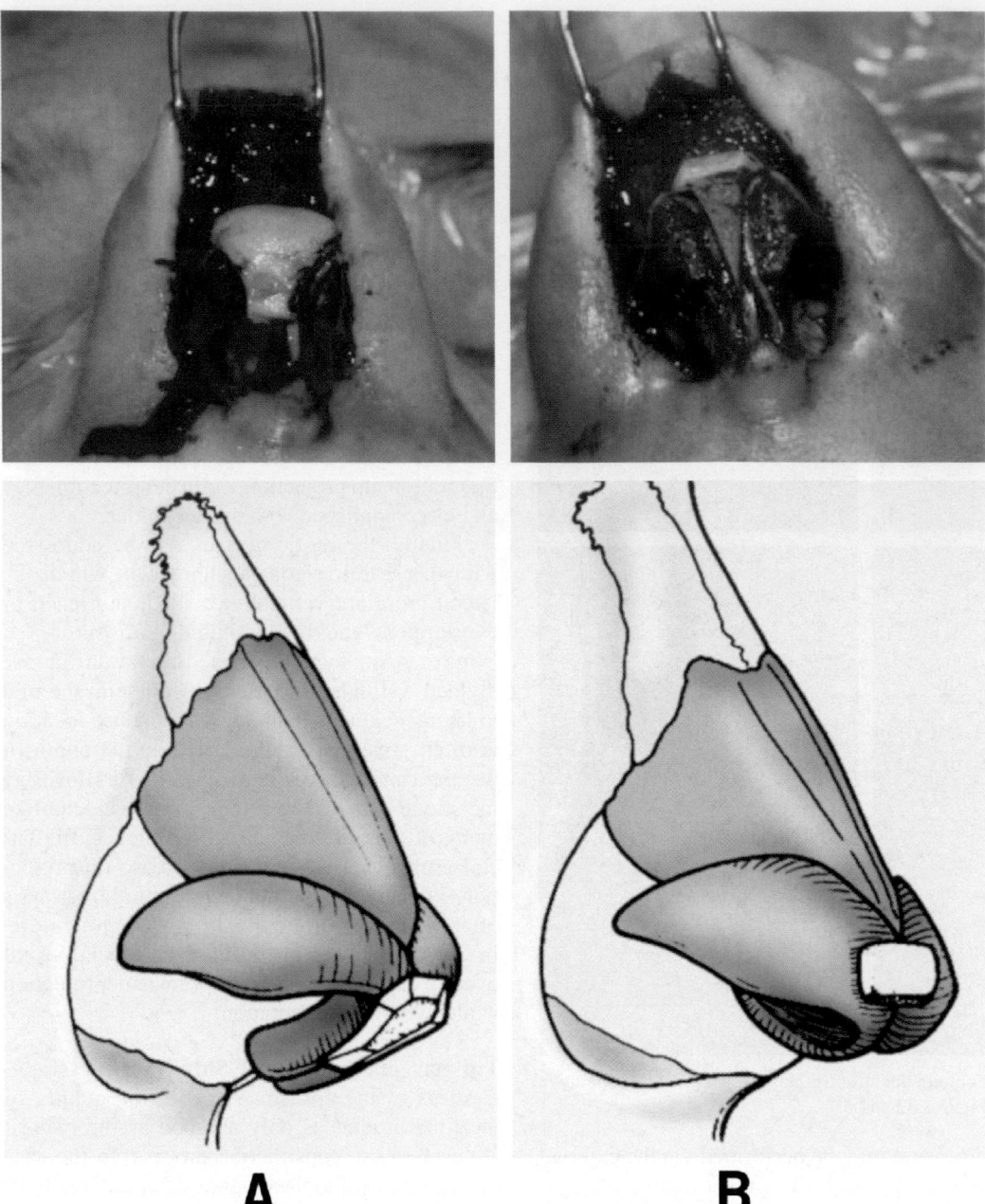

Figure 40 Intraoperative photographs revealing various tip graft configurations. (A) "Shield" graft. (B) "Cap" graft.

In contrast to the thick-skinned patient, patients with extremely thin skin lack the subcutaneous camouflage necessary to conceal minor topographic flaws in the nasal framework. Often the thin-skinned nose may appear skeletonized and vascular dyschromias are frequent after surgical intervention. For patients with pathologically thin nasal skin, subcutaneous augmentation grafts of dermis, perichondrium, superficial musculoaponeurotic system tissue, or fibrous tissue are necessary to achieve a smooth and even surface contour by increasing skin thickness.[30] Although graft viability is tenuous in the smoker or diabetic, in healthy young patients, permanent augmentation is typical. Intermediate skin thickness is generally preferred since it conceals minor skeletal imperfections, while adhering faithfully to the underlying skeletal anatomy to yield a well-defined and elegant nasal contour. However, even patients with optimal skin thickness may also experience cosmetic derangements

as a result of excessive subcutaneous fibrosis or scar contracture. Although healthy intermediate-thickness skin with a clear complexion and firm symmetric cartilage has the best prognosis for a favorable surgical outcome, no patient is immune from potential wound-healing derangements, and all prospective patients should be counseled accordingly.

Dorsal Hump Reduction

Perhaps the most common maneuver in cosmetic rhinoplasty is nasal hump reduction. Although realignment of the dorsal nasal profile is often regarded as a comparatively simple maneuver, in reality, the flawless execution of a dorsal hump reduction is a demanding and exacting surgical procedure that may take years to master fully. This is attributable to the complex and delicate anatomy of the nasal dorsum, comprised of widely dissimilar tissues, all of variable thickness and consistency. Moreover, because the nasal

bones are obscured by the overlying soft tissues, "blind" hump reduction adds to the challenge of precise profile alignment. Indeed, many expert rhinoplasty surgeons regard hump reduction as one of the most challenging maneuvers in cosmetic rhinoplasty.

In humans, the nasal bridge is seldom more than one-third bone, and the typical nasal hump is usually composed mostly of cartilage (Figure 47). Although most humps project only a few millimeters above the cosmetically ideal profile, overresection of the dorsum is an all too common tendency among novice rhinoplasty surgeons. Even extremely large nasal humps seldom require more than 3 to 4 mm of bony deprojection to achieve a satisfactory profile alignment. Although a straight dorsal profile is the goal in almost any hump reduction, naturally increased skin thickness at the nasal root (sellion) and supratip require preservation of a slight skeletal convexity at the rhinion to achieve a straight and attractive surface contour. However, in all noses, a smooth transition from cartilage to bone is essential to avoid step-off irregularities of the dorsal profile.

Hump reduction begins with composite elevation of soft tissues off the *dorsal crest*. Sufficient exposure is needed to visualize and remove the bony and cartilaginous humps, but care must be taken not to elevate all of the lateral nasal bone periosteum as these attachments are needed to maintain support following bony infracture. Prior to hump removal, the surgeon must carefully plan the height and angulation of the cartilaginous and bony profiles to achieve the desired cosmetic changes. In most noses, bony hump reduction requires only a triangular wedge resection, beginning at the rhinion and tapering at the radix (see Figure 47). While the length, width, and thickness of the bony wedge may vary, the overall shape is remarkably consistent in most noses. In contrast, the cartilage fragment will often vary in both size and shape since the dorsal septum has widely variable morphology. In patients with an overprojected rhinion and a normally projected anterior septal angle, the cartilage fragment will be tapered, thinnest at its caudal end. Alternatively, in patients with an overprojected anterior septal angle, the resulting fragment may have a more rectangular shape. Because the desired skeletal contour will determine the position and angulation of the tissue cuts and because there is a wide variation in size, shape, and composition of nasal humps, the parameters of hump reduction will vary significantly for almost every patient. Nevertheless, skeletal tissue should be conserved in all patients since a strong and prominent dorsum is both aesthetically pleasing and functionally advantageous. The novice surgeon should also remember that surprisingly little bone removal is usually sufficient to achieve a satisfactory cosmetic outcome. Clearly, the ability to properly judge and execute the tissue resection is fundamental to a successful surgical outcome and is typically far more challenging than many surgeons realize. Good aesthetic

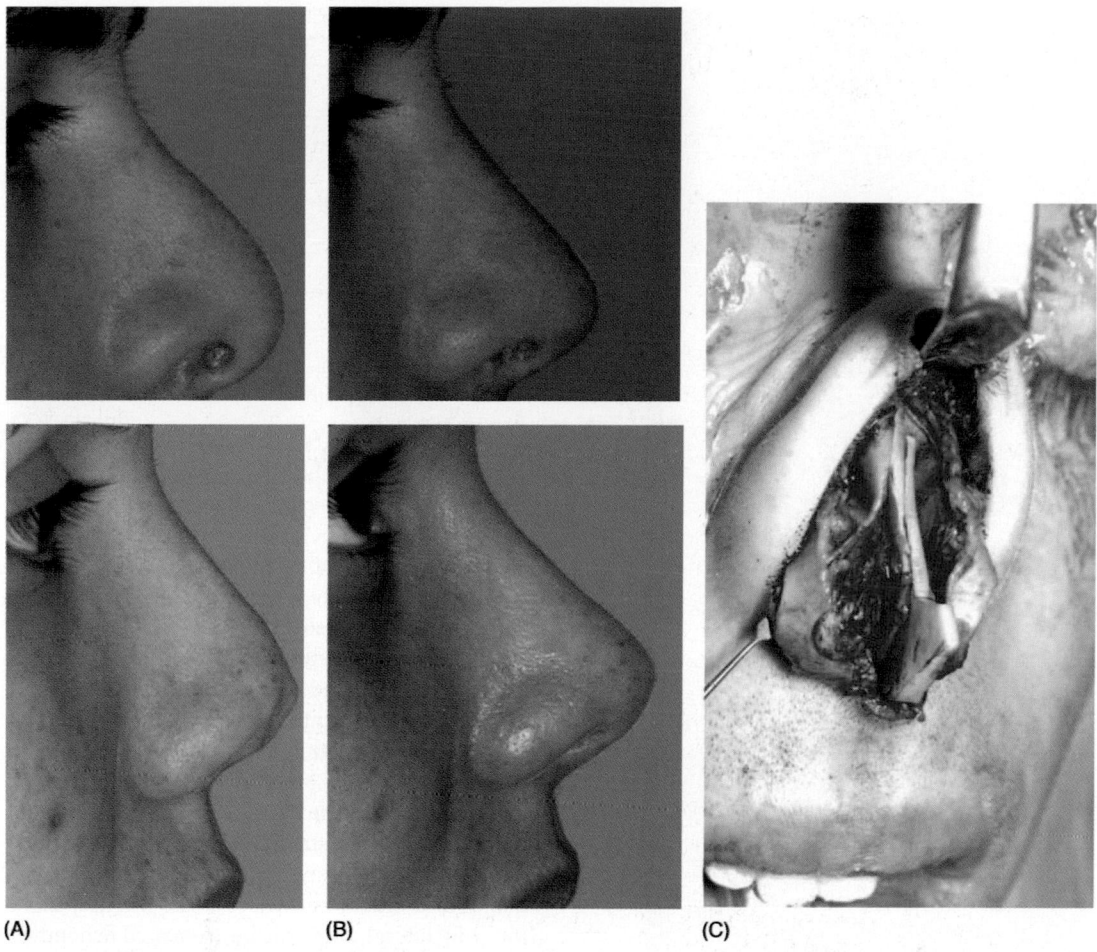

(A) **(B)** **(C)**

Figure 41 Increased tip projection and nasal length. (A) Preoperative views. (B) Postoperative views after septal extension graft placement for treatment of septal overresection. (C) Intraoperative view of left septal extension graft.

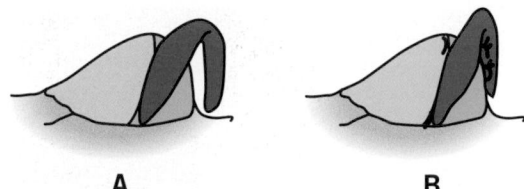

A **B**

Figure 44 Schematic illustration demonstrating a "tongue-in-groove" setback of the alar tripod upon the caudal aspect of the septum. (A) Long underprojected nose. (B) Foreshortened nose with increased tip projection.

bloc using a sharp osteotome, whereas smaller humps are reduced using manual rasps. Because the bony hump represents a U-shaped plate of membranous bone of varying density, guiding the osteotome in a perfectly straight path to cleave the overprojected bone is a formidable task. Not surprisingly, this method of blunt force bone reduction is fraught with numerous potential complications such as overresection, underresection, asymmetry, and/or bony comminution. Although minor residual bony abnormalities can be eliminated with the manual rasp, these defects must be addressed prior to lateral osteotomy which destabilizes the bony pyramid and prevents effective rasping.

Because blunt force bony hump removal is associated with a host of potential complications, the powered reciprocating rasp offers a less traumatic and more precise alternative to the traditional method. Using the reciprocating power rasp, bone is removed sequentially with minimal trauma to the overlying soft tissues. Small humps, minor asymmetries, and surface contour imperfections are all easily eliminated with the power-assisted rasp while blunt force trauma is avoided. The resulting bony pyramid can also be "sculpted" to create a more natural skeletal contour. Although lateral osteotomies are still required in most cases to narrow the widened vault, the power-assisted rasp facilitates a polished, smooth, and straight bony contour for more predictable cosmetic outcomes.[30]

Although a well-executed bony hump reduction immediately improves the nasal profile aesthetics, the realigned profile occurs at the expense of altered frontal aesthetics. Since lowering the nasal bridge leads to increased separation of the nasal bone remnants, the upper *BTALs* appear significantly wider following nasal hump removal. Typically the additional width is considered undesirable since humped noses are often too wide from the start. Moreover, the gap separating the cut edge of the nasal bone and the adjacent ethmoid complex, the so-called "*open roof deformity*," creates a flat and unnatural appearance, further contributing to the adverse cosmetic impact of hump removal. To compensate for the cosmetic deformity produced by hump reduction, dorsal ostetomy is usually followed by (bilateral) infracture of the nasal sidewall. This is accomplished by detaching and medializing the bony sidewall using curvilinear bone cuts positioned within the nasofacial groove, a procedure commonly known as a *lateral osteotomy*. Although osteotomy releases

judgment is predicated upon careful preoperative analysis that is well worth the time invested.

The sequence of cartilage and bone removal is at the discretion of the surgeon. Likewise, the use of scalpel or scissor to resect the cartilage hump is also a matter of surgeon preference. However, most surgeons prefer to reduce the cartilaginous dorsum first and then set the bony profile to complement the newly aligned middle vault. While some surgeons prefer to resect the ULC and dorsal septum in a single cut, in practice the middle vault cartilage often flexes making a precise cut difficult. As an alternative, many surgeons prefer first to separate the ULCs from the dorsal septum and then resect each element individually. Regardless of the method chosen, the final result should be a straight, smooth cartilaginous vault in which the cut upper edges of all three elements are equal in height.

Once the cartilage reduction is complete and the desired cartilaginous profile has been achieved, the bony hump is removed. Traditionally, a medium to large bony hump is resected en

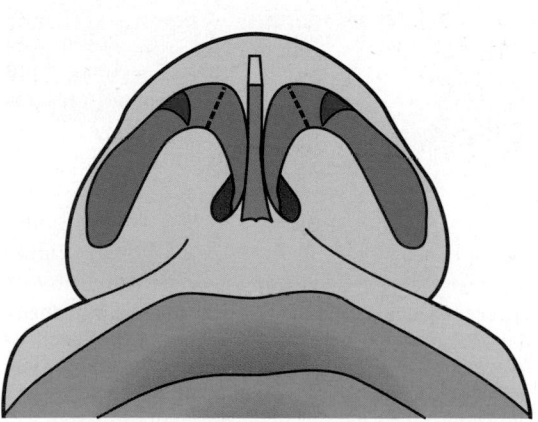

Figure 42 Schematic illustration showing location of vertical incisions lateral to alar domes (*dashed red lines*) used in the vertical dome division technique.

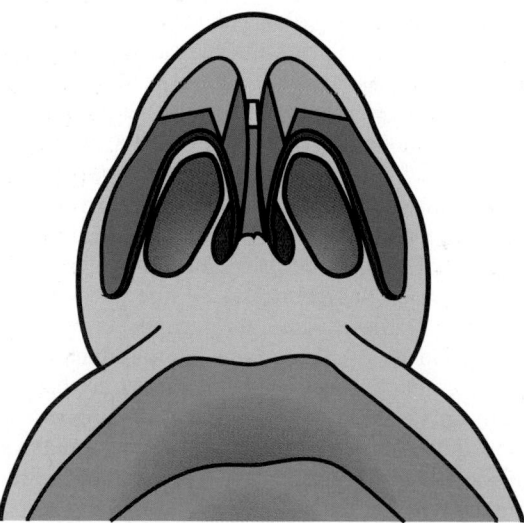

Figure 43 Schematic illustration demonstrating decreased tip projection with segmental excision using vertical dome division.

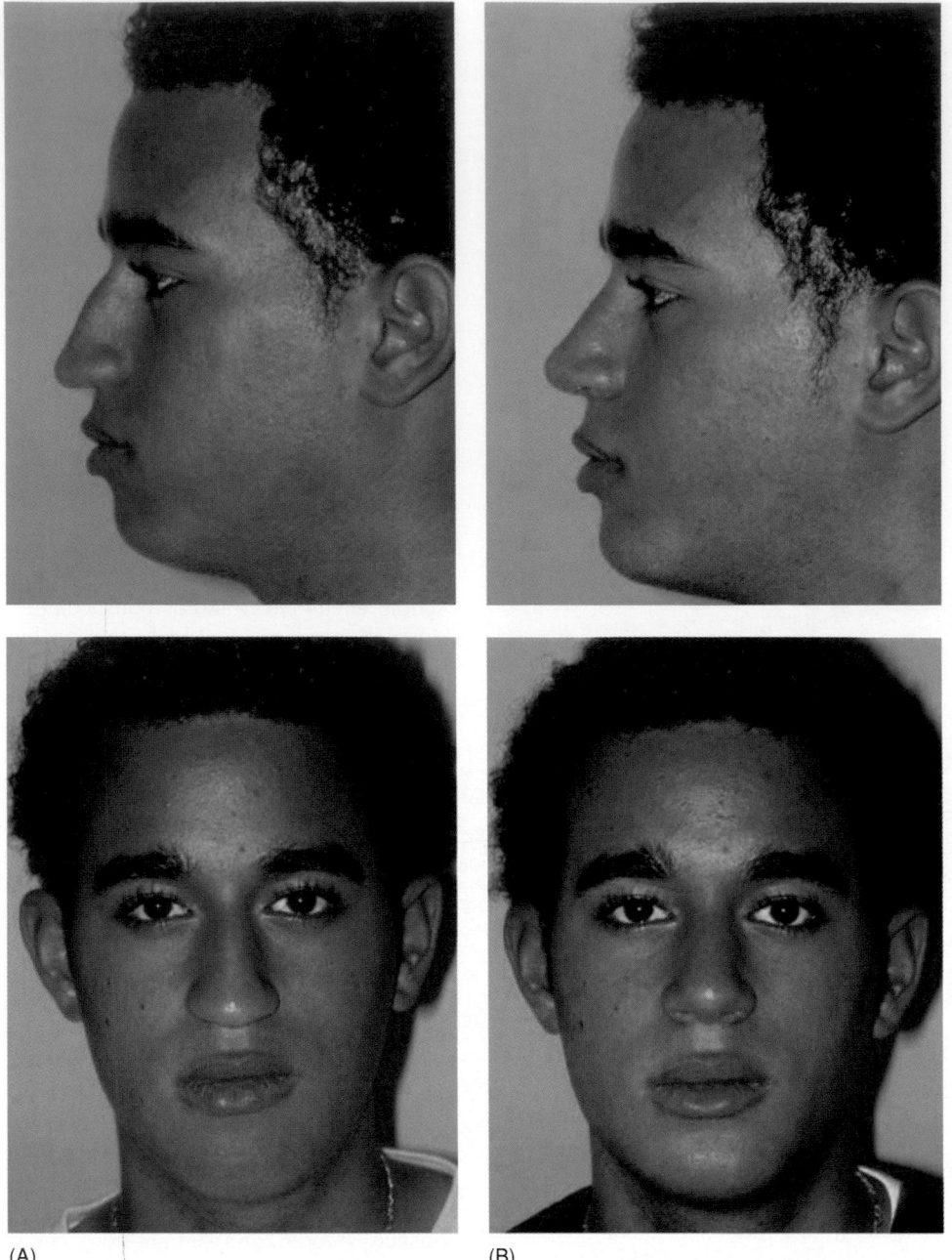

(A)   (B)

Figure 45 Front and profile view of ptotic tip deformity (A) before, and (B) after tip-plasty using the tongue-in-groove of tip rotation.

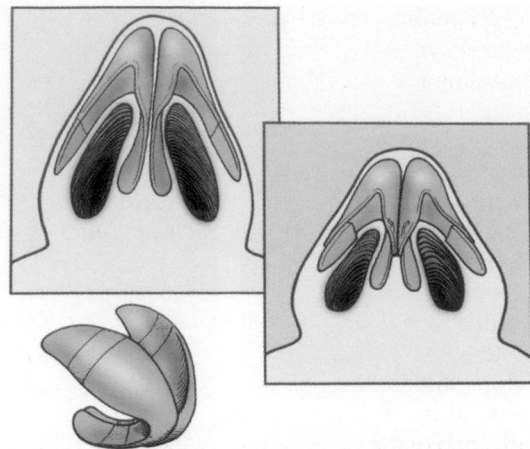

Figure 46 Schematic illustration of tip deprojection using the crural overlay technique.

from all adjacent bony attachments leaving the nasal bones suspended by the attached periosteum and overlying soft tissues. However, if upper vault narrowing is desired in the absence of a bony hump reduction, medial osteotomies are necessary to release the intact (medial) attachments of the nasal bones to the central ethmoid complex. Medial osteotomies are performed much like the lateral bone cuts using a narrow sharp osteotome directed along the lateral aspect of the central ethmoid complex (see Figure 26). Typically the medial and lateral cuts meet at the interpupillary line, but lateral cuts can be truncated whenever bony vault instability is a concern.

Like the dorsal osteotomy, the lateral osteotomy is also associated with potential complications. In addition to asymmetric cuts, comminution, or sidewall collapse, the mobilized bone fragments may heal unevenly leading to a crooked bony vault. Often this complication results from unrecognized deviation of the perpendicular ethmoid complex, emphasizing the importance of the bony septum to the symmetry of the bony vault. Skeletal irregularities resulting from untreated injuries to the bony vault may necessitate aggressive countermeasures including *intermediate osteotomies* to eliminate severe convex or concave deformities of the bony sidewall.

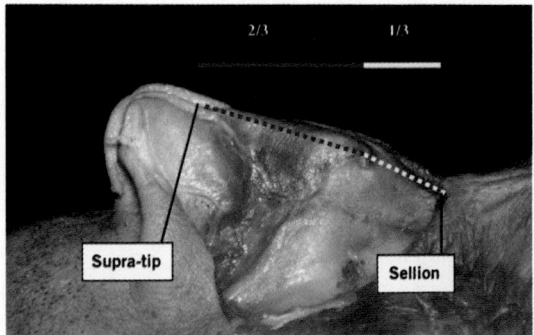

Figure 47 Cadaver specimen with nasal skin partially removed revealing relative distribution of cartilage (*red line*) and bone (*yellow line*) in a typical nasal bridge. Note characteristic thickening of skin at the sellion and supratip. Dashed lines indicate optimal path of cartilage resection (*red*) and bone resection (*yellow*) for a straight dorsal profile. Note slight residual rhinion hump and comparatively small amount of bone reduction.

more than just the nasal bone remnants (since the lateral nasal sidewall includes the nasal process of the maxilla), the upper nasal vault can be narrowed to compensate for iatrogenic widening of the BTALs. Traditionally, the lateral osteotomy is performed in a subcutaneous plane with a sharp narrow osteotome through a small endonasal incision. However, instead of a continuous subcutaneous osteotomy, some surgeons prefer interrupted "postage stamp" osteotomy cuts via a *percutaneous* approach. While both approaches have advantages and disadvantages, the traditional osteotomy is far more commonly used.

The traditional osteotomy begins at the pyriform aperture just above the attachment of the inferior turbinate bone. This starting point is approximately halfway along the pyriform aperture allowing effective narrowing of the bony vault without functional narrowing of the nasal airway. Osteotomy cuts that begin lower on the

pyriform aperture are ill-advised since medialization of the inferior turbinate will assuredly obstruct the nasal airway. Initially the osteotomy is directed superolaterally toward the pupil until the dense bone of the anterior maxillary buttress is reached (see Figure 26). The osteotomy cut is then redirected approximately 90° superomedially toward the nasion where the cut follows the nasofacial groove along the medial edge of the anterior maxillary buttress. As the cut extends cephalically its course curves gently toward the radix and terminates at the interpupillary line. Because the traditional lateral osteotomy begins high on the nasal sidewall, then continues low into the nasofacial groove and then terminates high on the nasal root, this type of lateral osteotomy is often termed a "*high-low-high*" lateral osteotomy. When performed in conjunction with a bony hump resection, the high-low-high osteotomy releases the bony sidewall remnants

As multiple osteotomies are employed to restore symmetry and produce a cosmetically appealing nasal contour, the stability of the nasal pyramid is diminished and the likelihood of collapse, asymmetry, or deviation increase as the extent of destabilization increases. Care must be taken to protect the union of the cartilage and the bony framework, particularly at the keystone area and the junction of the nasal bones with the ULCs. In both anatomic areas, the fused junction between cartilage and bone is difficult to restore once disrupted, and profound nasal collapse can ensue. While obtaining a straight and symmetric nasal pyramid is a worthwhile goal, aggressive destabilization of the skeletal framework with multiple blunt force osteotomies may not always produce reliable and predictable results. In the severely traumatized nose, alternative techniques such as camouflage (onlay) grafts and/or power-assisted rasp contouring offer a safer and equally effective means of achieving the desired nasal contour.

The Inverted-V Deformity

One of the most common cosmetic side effects of nasal hump reduction is the *inverted-V deformity*. The inverted-V deformity is a V-shaped shadow produced by a skeletal step-off formed between the wide bony nasal vault and the narrow middle nasal vault (see Figure 12). Formation of a bony-cartilaginous step-off results from either excessive width of the nasal bone remnants and/or pinching of the middle vault cartilage. Although the step-off deformity is a common complication of the overresected nasal hump (since overresected nasal bones can seldom be narrowed sufficiently), the deformity can also be seen in patients with a normal rhinion projection. Patients with normal rhinion projection develop the inverted-V step-off deformity when cartilage hump resection narrows the dorsal septum giving rise to medialization of the ULC remnants. In these patients, the stable bony vault remains wider than the pinched cartilaginous vault producing a disparity in nasal width. The resulting upside down V-shaped shadow disrupts the parallel BTALs producing a discontinuity of the normally continuous sidewall shadows.

Treatment of the inverted-V deformity involves restoration of dorsal height (when appropriate) and elimination of the nasal sidewall width discrepancy. This can be achieved by physically narrowing the bony vault if bony infracture is cosmetically acceptable. Alternatively, the cartilaginous sidewall can be repositioned using cartilage augmentation grafts to eliminate pinching of the middle vault.

Spreader Grafts

Perhaps one of the most versatile and important grafts in rhinoplasty is the *spreader graft*. In addition to restoring ULC width for elimination of the inverted-V deformity, spreader grafts can also be used to straighten a deviated dorsal septum, widen a pinched nasal valve, elongate the short nose,

and/or correct minor saddle nose deformities. Fashioned from autologous septal, conchal, or rib cartilage, speader grafts are long thin strips of cartilage placed in a submucosal pocket alongside the dorsal septum (Figure 48). When placed endonasally, spreader grafts are immobilized by creating a precise longitudinal pocket beneath the upper septal mucoperichondrium. When placed via the external rhinoplasty approach, spreader grafts can be sutured directly to the dorsal septum with mattress sutures at both ends. In patients with weak nasal cartilage who are susceptible to mid-vault pinching, "*prophylactic*" spreader grafts are used at the time of cartilage hump resection to prevent inverted-V deformities from scar-induced pinching of the ULCs. In revision rhinoplasty, depending upon the deformity at hand, grafts can be applied to one or both parasaggital spaces to provide increases in mid-vault width, improved rigidity or alignment of the dorsal septum, or small increases in height of the dorsal septum. When extended caudally, the spreader graft becomes a septal extension graft capable of elongating the foreshortened nose. Although spreader grafts have numerous cosmetic applications, placement of bilateral spreader grafts will do little to increase nasal valve patency in patients with lateral nasal sidewall collapse since only modest lateralization of the upper nasal sidewall is achieved. However, a variation of the conventional spreader graft, known as the *butterfly* spreader graft, uses an oval or trapezoid-shaped cartilage onlay graft to lift the collapsed lateral nasal sidewall using the inherent spring of the flexed cartilage graft. The butterfly spreader graft may also be used to augment the middle-vault profile in patients with modest saddle nose deformities.

Dressing

Once the various maneuvers of the surgical procedure are complete and wound closure has concluded, dressing of the nose is performed promptly to restrict swelling and maintain alignment of the delicate nasal framework. Sterile tape is applied across the dorsum and around the lobule followed by a molded plastic or contoured aluminum splint. Blood pressure control is closely maintained and anti-emetic precautions are continued. Ice packs are applied intermittently for 1 to 2 days, and elevation of the head is continued for 2 to 3 weeks. Vigorous exercise, heavy sun exposure, sunglasses, and platelet-inhibiting

medications are all avoided for several additional weeks until acute inflammation subsides.

Revision Rhinoplasty

Without doubt, some of the most vexing problems in nasal surgery result from the need for revision rhinoplasty. Severe collapse of the nasal skeleton, often accompanied by symptomatic nasal airway obstruction, can challenge even the most gifted rhinoplasty surgeon. However, even daunting anatomic deformities can be overshadowed by the turbulent emotional issues which attend the patient needing revision. Instead of the promised outcome of an attractive new nose, the patient must first cope with the initial shock and disappointment of a newly acquired physical deformity. Coupled with sizeable investments in time and money, the resulting emotional responses range from shame and embarrassment to anger and distrust of the medical community. Moreover, many patients report serial rhinoplasty failures, having undergone multiple unsuccessful revisions, each one more disfiguring and more disappointing than the last. Not surprisingly, most patients needing revision rhinoplasty are apprehensive and reluctant to risk further nasal surgery without sufficient justification, support, and encouragement.

Sadly, the overwhelming majority of failed rhinoplasties are the result of surgical error, whereas poor healing tendencies account for the remainder. Although an incomplete operative procedure is occasionally responsible for the unsatisfactory outcome, (for example, a residual hump,) overaggressive excision of the nasal skeleton is a far more common cause of the unsatisfactory rhinoplasty result. Indeed, badly misshapen cartilage, gross skeletal asymmetries, and overresected bony remnants are the usual findings in the multiply operated nose. In addition to a paucity of skeletal support, the patient needing revision may also present with severe soft tissue fibrosis, epithelial adhesions, and disfiguring scar contractures compounding the skeletal deficiencies. To make matters even worse, surplus septal or auricular cartilages necessary to graft the collapsed nose are often absent, having been depleted during previous attempts at surgical restoration.

Because misguided attempts at surgical repair only magnify the surgical challenge, complex revision surgery should be reserved for the accomplished rhinoplasty surgeon with abundant experience in revision rhinoplasty. For complex

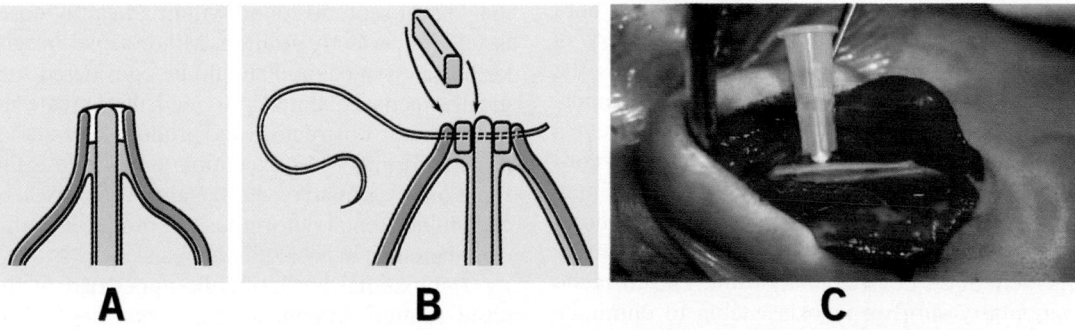

A **B** **C**

Figure 48 Conventional spreader graft placement. (A) Schematic cross-section of pinched middle vault. (B) Increased middle vault width after bilateral spread graft placement. (C) Intraoperative view of left spreader graft placement.

revision cases, the external rhinoplasty approach is mandatory; and slow, deliberate, and meticulous dissection are required to expose the skeletal remnants without causing further damage. Emphasis is placed upon first restoring the midline skeletal structures of the dorsal septum and columella. Once the central support structures are reconstituted, lateral skeletal elements of the middle and lower vault are then suspended from the central complex to restore width, symmetry, and airway patency. When necessary, missing or severely damaged skeletal components are reconstituted with replacement grafts of similar tissue type. Onlay augmentation grafts of cartilage and/or soft tissue are then used to perfect and refine the outer nasal contour.

Because augmentation grafts are associated with donor site morbidity and are typically in short supply, the experienced surgeon will use these materials in a creative and sensible manner to conserve tissue and optimize the surgical outcome. Moreover, the effects of preexisting scar tissue must be anticipated, and compensatory measures must be implemented whenever possible to prevent delayed skeletal distortion from shrink-wrap contracture. Although failed rhinoplasty appears to be a growing problem worldwide, the vast majority of revision patients can be restored to a normal, if not attractive nasal contour, when appropriate reconstructive techniques are undertaken. However, a "perfect" nose is all but impossible, and careful assessment of the deformity, tissue characteristics, healing capacity, and patient motivation are necessary to determine the prognosis for a successful outcome.

Of note, a small minority of revision rhinoplasty patients possesses unusually poor healing characteristics and may experience unfavorable results even when the operation is executed properly. Signs of unfavorable healing response, such as hypertrophic scarring, cicatricial stenoses, ischemic tissue loss, and so forth, should be diligently sought; and, when identified, these patients should be counseled accordingly. On the other hand, patients with favorable healing tendencies have an excellent prognosis when proper surgical technique is combined with abundant and quality graft materials. For this reason, surgical consent for all anticipated graft materials is essential.

SEPTAL SURGERY

Septal surgery is an integral component of both cosmetic rhinoplasty and functional nasal airway surgery. The time-honored adage "as goes the septum, so goes the nose" underscores the importance of correcting septal deformities to achieve a symmetric and cosmetically appealing nasal contour. Because a neglected septal deviation may prohibit proper realignment of the scoliotic nose, septal deformities are best corrected prior to management of the deviated bony vault. The cosmetic rhinoplasty surgeon who is unable to eliminate coexisting septal deformities is severely handicapped; and, because septal deformities often

contribute to the unattractive nose, this limitation will frequently compromise the cosmetic result. Septal surgery has been traditionally regarded as a functional discipline, but its mastery is equally important for the cosmetic surgeon.

Because the nasal septum supports both the internal nasal airway and the external nasal framework, deformities of the nasal septum may cause functional disturbances, cosmetic disturbances, or combinations therein. When confined to the internal nasal septum, functional disturbances are usually treated via septoplasty without alteration of the external nasal contour. In contrast, functional disturbances of the septum are frequently accompanied by visible deformities of the outer nose, and rhinoplasty techniques may be required to eliminate both the functional and aesthetic problems. In either case, care must be taken to preserve adequate septal support since an overaggressive septoplasty or an overzealous rhinoplasty can lead to symptomatic nasal obstruction from unsightly skeletal collapse.

Although cosmetic and functional disturbances of the septum may occur independently, they are frequently observed in tandem. Since joint cosmetic and functional disturbances are anatomically interrelated, combined treatment with septorhinoplasty typically provides the most effective means of evaluating and eliminating complex septal deformities. Moreover, because reduction rhinoplasty will inevitably diminish breathing space, correction of coexisting airway blockage is sometimes needed to prevent symptomatic nasal airway obstruction arising from a purely aesthetic procedure. Combined treatment is also preferable since it spares the patient from the additional discomfort, down-time, and expense of a second operation. Although the nasal septum is commonly regarded as a functional entity, complex septal deformities almost always affect nasal cosmesis; and correction of external septal deformities usually improves nasal contour. Clearly, septoplasty and rhinoplasty are permanently intertwined, and septal deformities should be regarded as an anatomic malformation with variable cosmetic and functional manifestations.

The nasal septum is a skeletal partition that bisects the nasal cavities in the midline sagittal plane. Composed of cartilage anteriorly and the fused vomer and ethmoid bones posteriorly, the nasal septum is an aesthetically prominent and functionally important nasal structure that is often subject to blunt force injury. However, the "normal" nasal septum, found within a healthy nose, is seldom perfectly straight. Minor septal irregularities are typical and should be considered surgically inconsequential provided they create no symptomatic obstruction and produce no external nasal deformity. The exception to this rule is the functionally sensitive nasal valve region where even minor septal deformites can produce significant increases in nasal airway resistance.

The external border of the upper part of the nasal septum, known as the *dorsal septum*, is the structural foundation for the nasal bridge. Deflections, scoliosis, or saddle deformities of

the dorsal septum may severely compromise aesthetics of the nasal bridge and/or patency of the nasal valve. Similarly, the caudal border of the external nasal septum, commonly called the *caudal septum*, is also prone to anatomic deformities resulting in columellar asymmetry, nostril deformity, or retraction of the columella. Typically, visible deformities of the outer aspects of the nasal septum are also linked to hidden internal septal deformities that severely constrict nasal airflow. Thus, a thorough endonasal examination is mandatory for all patients undergoing skeletal surgery of the nose.

Symptomatic internal deformities of the nasal septum are common and are known generically as a "deviated septum." Septal deformities comprise a wide range of anatomic irregularities, including deviations of the bony-cartilaginous junction, dislocation of the quadrangular cartilage from the nasal spine and/or maxillary crest, accordion-like folds within the quadrangular cartilage, cartilage duplications, or spurs anywhere within the septal partition (Figure 49). Complex obstructing septal deformities are frequently the result of trauma, but childhood growth disturbances, failed surgical manipulation, or combined causes, may also result in septal irregularities. Because septal deformities are sometimes congenital, and because the septum is prone to trauma in nearly all individuals, the exact cause of the deviated septum is often difficult to determine. While comparatively large deformities of the posterior part of the nasal septum are necessary to occlude airflow within the nasal cavum, a comparatively modest deformity of the anterior part of the nasal septum may cause severe nasal airway obstruction. Anterior septal deformities, particularly high septal deviations, obstruct the already narrow internal nasal valve, making the septal deformities the most common cause of nasal valve dysfunction.[31,32] Despite the importance of anterior septal deformities, their presence is often overlooked on endonasal examination since the obstruction is frequently bypassed upon insertion of the nasal speculum. While the diagnosis of a large posterior septal deformity is comparatively straightforward, the diagnosis of nasal valve narrowing requires

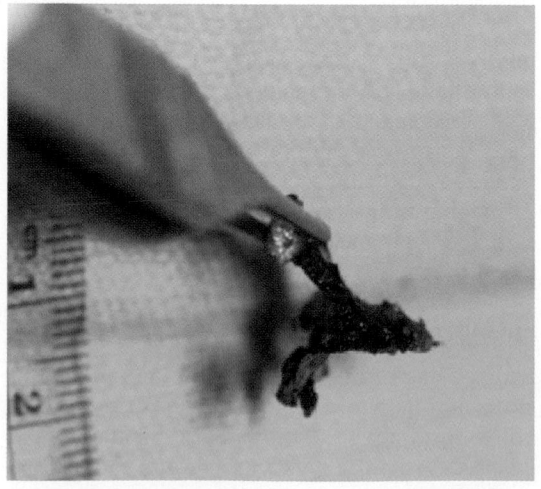

Figure 49 Photograph of vomerine spur removed during routine septoplasty.

(speculum-free) inspection of the valve inlet within the posterior part of the nasal vestibule. In addition to deflections of the anterior part of the nasal septum, the seasoned examiner routinely inspects the posterior part of the nasal vestibule for related signs of nasal valve dysfunction such as dynamic nasal sidewall collapse, lateral crural cartilage recurvature, or cicatricial stenosis of the vestibular epithelium.

Septoplasty

In general, septal surgery should conserve skeletal support via the strategic restructuring of deviated elements, rather than endanger skeletal support via the reckless excision of vital structural components. Complications of overaggressive septoplasty, such as saddle deformity, columellar retraction, compromised tip support, nasal airway collapse, and septal perforation, are all exceedingly rare when septal support is conserved, but the cavalier excision of essential structural elements is certain to invoke unwanted complications. Care must also be taken to protect blood supply to the septal cartilage by limiting mucosal elevation to a single side whenever possible and by coapting elevated flaps securely to facilitate rapid flap readherence. Nutrient blood supply to the septal cartilage can be temporarily interrupted in the healthy individual with minimal risk of ischemic injury; but the threshold for cartilage resorption is unpredictable, and limited mucosal elevation is a far safer practice.

Corrective septal surgery may be performed via a number of well-known surgical approaches including the direct (Killian) incision, the hemitransfixion incision, or even the external rhinoplasty approach. Each option has inherent pros and cons, and surgeon preference will generally dictate which approach is preferred. Regardless of which approach is selected, the successful septoplasty requires powerful fiberoptic illumination and effective vasoconstriction to facilitate direct visualization. Topical anesthetization and decongestion precedes injection of the septal mucosa with a standard solution of 1% lidocaine containing epinephrine. In addition to intensifying the vasoconstriction produced by topical decongestion, the injection serves to "hydro-dissect" (or hydraulically elevate) the injected mucoperichondrium to facilitate rapid and bloodless flap elevation. Once skeletal modifications are undertaken, the skeletal anatomy and the surrounding nasal airway are both repeatedly assessed, since septoplasty is a dynamic process in which each step will often dramatically influence the next.

The simplest technique for minor septal deformities is the direct (Killian) approach, in which an L-shaped mucosal incision is made immediately anterior to the septal deformity for direct access. The septal deviation is then exposed by elevating the overlying mucoperichondrium and/or mucoperiosteum behind and above the L-shaped access incision. Typically the skeletal malformation is then removed with care to preserve the opposite mucoperichondrium; however, shaving, curetting,

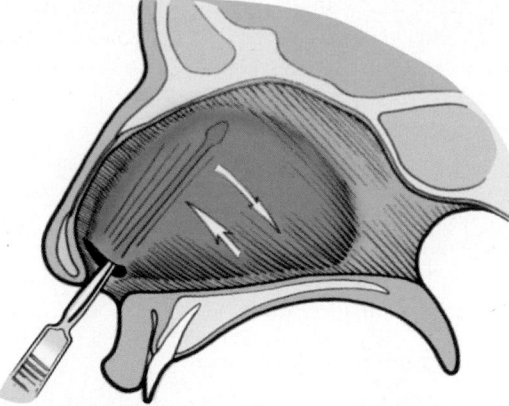

Figure 50 Schematic demonstrating creation of a broad-based septal flap elevation using a Cottle elevator

or morcelizing the deviated segment are acceptable alternatives as long as a flattened septal partition results. Recently, endoscopic elimination of septal spurs has been advocated using power assisted microdebriders (commonly used for sinus surgery) via a Killian-type incision.[33] While this "minimally invasive" approach to minor septal surgery has several advantages including limited dissection and improved visualization, copious instrumentation is required, rendering this method impractical unless concurrent sinus surgery is planned. Regardless of the method chosen for skeletal correction, care must be taken to avoid or repair opposing mucosal tears to prevent iatrogenic septal perforation. While the direct (Killian) septoplasty is still widely used today, it is only suitable for focal septal deformities involving the central nasal septum, thereby limiting its widespread use. However, for small protrusive spurs, such as those producing mucosal contact headaches or obstruction of the middle meatus, the Killian septoplasty remains an excellent technique.

Perhaps the most commonly used approach for nasal septoplasty is the *hemitransfixion* approach. This technique employs a unilateral mucosal incision spanning the caudal aspect of the septum for broad surgical exposure. For most surgeons, the hemitransfixion incision is placed within the left nasal vestibule to facilitate right-handed surgical dissection, although some surgeons prefer placing the incision on the concave

side of the septal deformity to facilitate easier flap elevation. Mucoperichondrial and/or mucoperiosteal flaps are then elevated until all of the deformities are exposed. Elevation is begun in the submucoperichondrial plane at the leading edge of the caudal aspect of the septum using a flat, semisharp elevator such as a Cottle or Freer. A nasal speculum is also used to keep the partially elevated flap under tension, thereby facilitating both dissection and visualization. A broad-based flap is recommended to enhance exposure and reduce perforation risk, but flap elevation is confined to essential areas to minimize disruption of the blood supply (Figure 50).

Once the correct subperichondrial plane is established, the healthy flap can be quickly elevated using a top to bottom sweeping action with a #10 Frasier suction tip. However, for complex deformities, the dissection is sometimes hindered by the presence of fracture adhesions, cartilage duplications, or severe scarring. In such cases, the stubborn area is encircled from above and below until retrograde dissection can complete the flap elevation. Again, care is taken to avoid mucosal tears during dissection to minimize perforation risk. The creation of fenesta during flap elevation is not unusual, especially at the apex of sharp deflections or with complicated septal deformities. Small unopposed fenestra can be ignored as they provide an escape route for submucosal blood accumulations, but large fenestrations must be repaired with small caliber absorbable suture to prevent iatrogenic septal perforation, especially if opposing tears are present.

Although a variety of published methods have been described for the elimination of skeletal deviations, excision of the deviated septal segment (known as a *submucous resection*) provides excellent long-term results as long as adequate structural support is preserved. Typically, this is accomplished by maintaining an outer rim of healthy residual cartilage containing the interconnected dorsal and caudal struts. Collectively, this outer rim forms an L-shaped truss, commonly called the "*L-strut*" (Figure 51).

As long as a sufficient L-strut is preserved, surplus cartilage can be removed from behind and

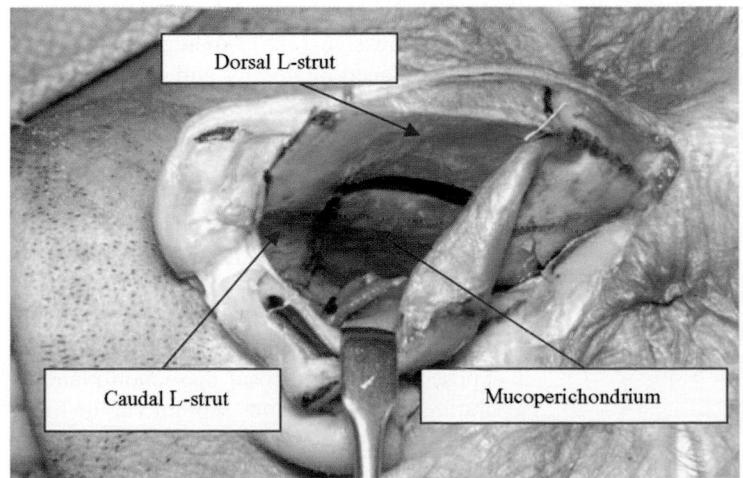
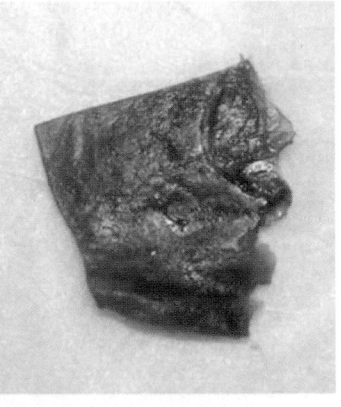

Dorsal L-strut

Caudal L-strut

Mucoperichondrium

Figure 51 Cadaver dissection demonstrating preservation of the L-strut. Note residual segments of interconnected caudal and dorsal septum and the plate of missing quadrangular cartilage (*insert*).

beneath the L-strut, whether for septal straightening, cartilage graft harvest, or combinations therein. Since structural integrity of the L-strut will vary according to intrinsic cartilage strength, the L-strut is always kept as wide as possible, particularly with naturally weak or flaccid cartilage, so that adequate long-term structural support is assured. However, in cases where L-strut augmentation grafts (eg, spreader grafts, septal extension grafts) are also used, the additional structural support gained through augmentation grafting may permit safe L-strut width reductions allowing more extensive cartilage removal.

Once septal straightening is complete, the mucosal leaflets must be coapted to prevent septal hematoma and ischemic insult to the exposed cartilage. Typically, this is accomplished with absorbable transseptal quilting sutures and/or with gentle compression using soft septal splints with or without temporary nasal packing material (Figure 52). When quilting sutures are used, nasal packing can usually be removed within 24 hours to restore comfortable nasal breathing.

Perhaps the most challenging septal deformities are those that involve malformations of the septal L-strut (Figure 53). Deformities involving the dorsal part of the septum, anterior septal angle, and/or caudal aspect of the septum are not amenable to submucous resection since structural support to the middle vault, nasal tip, and/or columella would be jeopardized, respectively. To maintain vital structural support provided by the L-strut, alternative techniques to realign and/or reinforce the deformed septum are necessary. For deformities affecting the caudal aspect of the septum, the cause is frequently a vertically overgrown caudal segment or a traumatic deviation of the caudal aspect of the septum. For the overgrown caudal segment, the elongated cartilage is frequently bowed and dislocated from the nasal spine. Treatment involves trimming the posterior septal angle to permit straightening and midline repositioning of the septum. Often a figure of eight suture is used to anchor the newly shortened caudal segment. This approach is commonly known as the "swinging door" technique since the septum is analogous to a swinging door that must be trimmed just enough to clear the metaphorical "door jam." The swinging door technique is also used when the quadrangular cartilage is displaced from the maxillary crest onto the nasal floor since a narrow strip of cartilage can be removed from

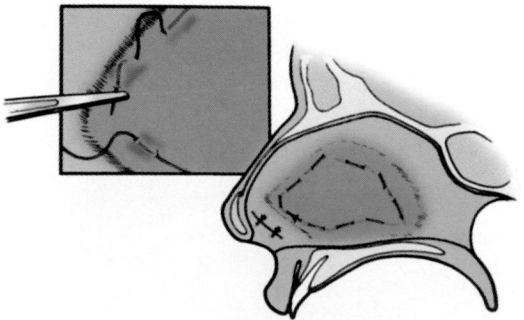

Figure 52 Schematic illustration of septal quilting suture placement.

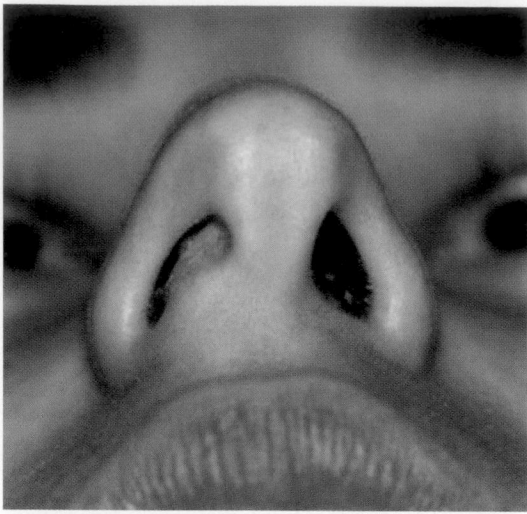

Figure 53 Base view demonstrating right-sided deflection of the caudal aspect of the septum with associated airway obstruction and nostril asymmetry.

the lower border of the quadrangular septum to realign the entire cartilaginous septum.

For traumatic deflections of the caudal part of the septum, a vertical accordion-like fracture posterior to the caudal strut results in a hinge-like deflection of the caudal part of the septum. Often the caudal deflections are associated with nasal base asymmetries and ipsilateral nasal airway obstruction.

Correction of the severely deviated caudal septum necessitates bilateral elevation of mucoperichondrium followed by release, repositioning, and fixation of the deviated segment. In rare cases the L-strut may require partial or even complete division at its junction with the dorsal part of the septum to eliminate stubborn angulations occurring at the anterior septal angle. However, complete division of the L-strut destabilizes support to both the dorsum and the columella, and suture reconstitution of the L-strut, with or without onlay graft reinforcement, is required to maintain adequate structural support. As an alternative technique, serial (incomplete) "picket fence" incisions along the deviated L-strut segments may be used to straighten a scoliotic L-strut. While this method can realign a warped or deviated L-strut, the use of multiple incisions may also destabilize the L-strut and lead to persistent deformity. In cases of aggressive L-strut manipulation, septal splints are placed bilaterally and secured with a temporary transfixion suture to serve as bookends and lend temporary support during the first week after the operation.

Although the hemitransfixion approach to the nasal septum can be safely used in conjunction with external rhinoplasty, the nasal septum can also be accessed through the external rhinoplasty approach without the need for a hemitransfixion incision. Instead, the caudal aspect of the septum is exposed in a submucosal dissection plane by separating the membranous septum via the transcolumellar incision. For removal of large septal cartilage grafts or bone fragments, the ULC must be divided from the dorsal septum to create satisfactory egress. Because this approach demands

considerable dissection within the columella and membranous septum, it is not suitable for all patients. Nevertheless, the external rhinoplasty approach is an excellent alternative for patients with complex deformities of the L-strut since exposure of the nasal base is optimized.

CONCLUSIONS

Rhinoplasty is a complex and demanding operation with many intriguing peculiarities. While the dedication required to achieve mastery in rhinoplasty is formidable, transformation of the human nose from a misshapen appendage to an attractive facial attribute is a uniquely gratifying experience. For the beginner, mastery of nasal analysis and relentless self-assessment will pave the way for a long and rewarding career in nasal surgery.

REFERENCES

1. Davis RE. Rhinoplasty and concepts of facial beauty. Facial Plast Surg 2006;22:198–203.
2. Tardy MD, Brown RJ, Childs C. Principles of Photography in Facial Plastic Surgery. New York: Thieme; 1992.
3. Johnson CM, Jr, Cheney ML, Toriumi DM. Nasal aesthetics. In: Johnson CM, Jr, Toriumi DM, editors. Open Structure Rhinoplasty. Philadelphia: WB Saunders; 1990. p. 23–9.
4. Molenaar A. The depressed nasofrontal angle in aesthetic rhinoplasty. Plast Reconstr Surg 1988;82:698–706.
5. Guyuron B. Guarded burr for deepening of nasofrontal junction. Plast Reconstr Surg 1989;84:513–6.
6. Davis RE, Raval J. Powered instrumentation for nasal bone reduction: Advantages and indications. Arch Facial Plast Surg 2003;5:384–91.
7. Davis RE. Diagnosis and surgical management of the caudal excess nasal deformity. ArchFacial Plast Surg 2005; 7:124–34.
8. Cole P, Roithmann R. The nasal valve and current technology. Am J Rhinol 1996;10:23–31.
9. Kasperbauer JL, Kern EB. Nasal valve physiology. Implications in nasal surgery. Otolaryngol Clin North Am 1987; 20:699–719.
10. Roithmann R, Cole P, Chapnik J, et al. Acoustic rhinometry, rhinomanometry, and the sensation of nasal patency: A correlative study. J Otolaryngol 1994;23:454–8.
11. Johnson CM, Godin MS. The tension nose: Open structure rhinoplasty approach. Plast Reconstr Surg 1995;95:43–51.
12. Anderson JR, Ries WR. Surgery of the nasal base: Setting tip projection and location. In: Smith JD, editor. Rhinoplasty: Emphasizing the External Approach. New York: Thieme; 1986:64.
13. McNicoll WD, Scanlan SG. Submucous resection. The treatment of choice in the nose-ear distress syndrome. J Laryngol Otol 1979;93:357–67.
14. Rhee JS, Poetker DM, Smith TL, et al. Nasal valve surgery improves disease-specific quality of life. Laryngoscope 2005;115:437–40.
15. Churchill SE, Shackelford LL, Georgi JN, Black MT. Morphological variation and airflow dynamics in the human nose. Am J Hum Biol 2004;16:625–38.
16. Simmen D, Scherrer JL, Moe K, Heinz B. A dynamic and direct visualization model for the study of nasal airflow. Arch Otolaryngol Head Neck Surg 1999;125:1015–21.
17. Lang C, Gratzenmacher S, Mlynski B, et al. Investigating the nasal cycle using endoscopy, rhinoresistometry, and acoustic rhinometry. Laryngoscope 2003;113:284–9.
18. Fregosi RF, Lansing RW. Neural drive to nasal dilator muscles: Influence of exercise intensity and oronasal flow partitioning. J Appl Physiol 1995;79:1330–7.
19. Wexler D, Braverman I, Amar M. Histology of the nasal septal swell body (septal turbinate). Otolaryngol Head Neck Surg 2006;134:596–600.
20. Davis RE. Nasal Airway Obstruction. Patient of the Month Program Monograph Series, American Academy of Otolaryngology–Head and Neck Surgery Foundation. Hamilton, Ontario: BC Decker; 2004.
21. Gruber RP, Friedman GD. Suture algorithm for the broad or bulbous nasal tip. Plast Reconstr Surg 2002;110:1752–64.

22. Baker SR. Suture contouring of the nasal tip. Arch Facial Plast Surg 2000;2:34–42.

23. Kridel RW, Konior RJ, Shumrick KA, Wright WK. Advances in nasal tip surgery. The lateral crural steal. Arch Otolaryngol Head Neck Surg 1989;115:1206–12.

24. Naficy S, Baker SR. Lengthening the short nose. Arch Otolaryngol Head Neck Surg 1998;124:809–13.

25. Guyuron B, Varghai A. Lengthening the nose with a tongue-and-groove technique. Plast Reconstr Surg 2003; 111:1533–9.

26. Byrd HS, Andochick S, Copit S, Walton KG. Septal extension grafts: A method of controlling tip projection shape. Plast Reconstr Surg 1997;100:999–1010.

27. Simons RL. Vertical dome division in rhinoplasty. Otolaryngol Clin North Am 1987;20:785–96.

28. Constantinides M, Liu ES, Miller PJ, Adamson PA. Vertical lobule division in rhinoplasty: Maintaining an intact strip. Arch Facial Plast Surg 2001;3:258–63.

29. Adamson PA, Morrow TA. The nasal hinge. Otolaryngol Head Neck Surg 1994;111:219–31.

30. Davis RE, Wayne I. Rhinoplasty and the nasal SMAS augmentation graft: Advantages and indications. Arch Facial Plast Surg 2004;5:124–132.

31. Elwany S, Thabet H. Obstruction of the nasal valve. J Laryngol Otol 1996;110:221–4.

32. Kasperbauer JL, Kern EB. Nasal valve physiology. Implications in nasal surgery. Otolaryngol Clin North Am 1987; 20:699–719.

33. Raynor EM. Powered endoscopic septoplasty for septal deviation and isolated spurs. Arch Facial Plast Surg 2005;7:410–2.

54

Nasal Reconstruction

Shan R. Baker, MD

Over the last decade, reconstruction of the nose has reached a high level of sophistication with enhancement of aesthetic results.[1–3] This has been achieved by emphasizing the need to replace surgically ablated tissue with like tissue. Skin is replaced with skin that matches in color and texture as closely as possible. Cartilage and bone are replaced and mucosa is used to replace any loss of the nasal lining. The concept of nasal aesthetic units has emerged with an emphasis on reconstructing an entire unit, if the majority of the unit is missing. Another important concept that has led to enhancement in the results of restorative surgery of the face has been the emphasis on the placement of incisions for local flaps along borders of aesthetic regions or units to maximize camouflage of scars. Whenever possible, local flaps are designed so that they are not transferred across the borders of aesthetic regions, particularly if the border has a concave topography. An example of such a border is the alar facial sulcus which represents a concave border between three aesthetic facial regions: the nose, the cheek, and the upper lip.[4,5]

FACIAL AESTHETIC REGIONS

The face can be divided into topographical regions, each with its individual intrinsic characteristics of skin color, texture, contour, and hair growth.[5,6] Each has an individual shape created by the underlying facial skeleton. The nose is one of the aesthetic regions of the face and can be divided into several aesthetic units (Figure 1). Each unit may be proportionally over- or under-developed relative to other noses, but there is a consistent general configuration from nose-to-nose.[3] There are nine aesthetic units of the nose identified by distinctive convex or concave surfaces, including the tip, dorsum, paired sidewalls, paired alae, paired nasal facets, and the columella. In general, the shape of the nasal tip is determined by the size and contour of the alar cartilages, and specifically by the domal portion of the alar cartilages. It is covered by relatively thick sebaceous skin. The skin of the dorsum tends to be less thick and sebaceous than the tip, becoming progressively thinner as it ascends to the rhinion and thickens again as it approaches the glabella. The nasal bones together with the upper lateral cartilages and cartilaginous septum provide skeletal support for the dorsum. The nasal

sidewalls are most often a combination of convex and concave elements extending laterally from the dorsum to the junction of the nose with the cheek. Structurally, the sidewalls are supported

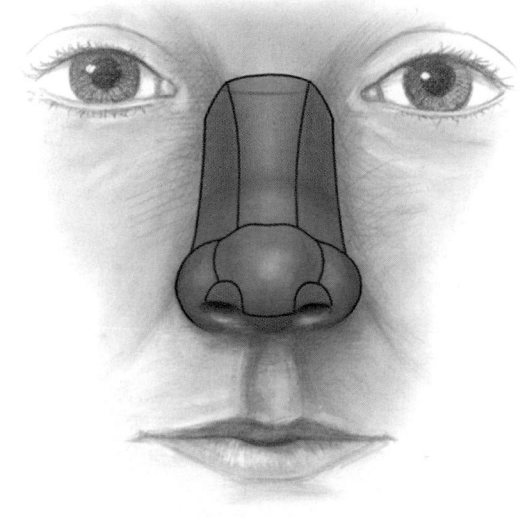

(A)

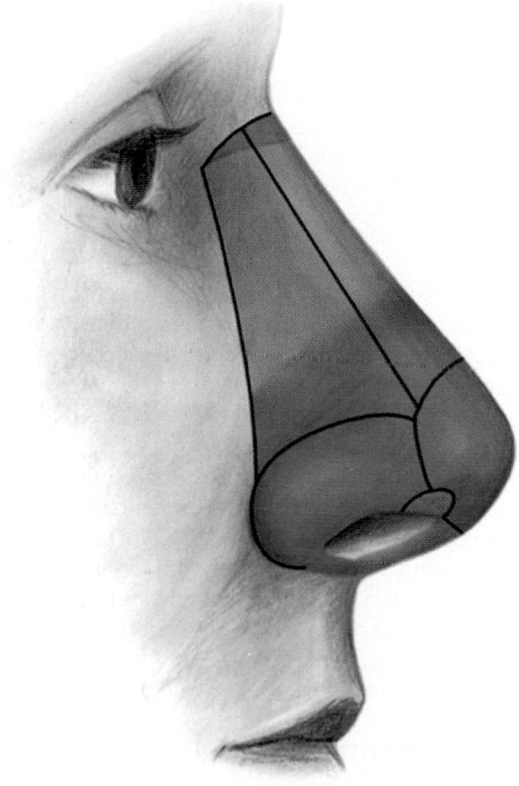

(B)

Figures 1 (A) and (B) Topographic aesthetic nasal units. (Reproduced with permission from reference 6.)

by the nasal bones, and upper lateral cartilages, and the medial extensions of the frontal processes of the maxillae. The skin of the sidewalls is thin and less sebaceous than that of the dorsum and tip. Inferiorly, the skin of the sidewall becomes progressively thicker. The alar unit is covered with thick sebaceous skin similar in texture and porosity to the skin of the tip and adjacent superior melolabial fold. The structural support of the ala is provided by thick fibrofatty tissue which does not contain cartilage.

The soft tissue facets contribute to a portion of the nostril margin and span the arch between intermediate and lateral crura of each lower lateral cartilage. They are covered by thin, nonsebaceous skin and have only a small amount of fibrous connective tissue for structural support. The columella, like the tip and dorsum, is a nonpaired aesthetic unit extending from the inferior aspect of the infratip to the upper lip. It is covered by the thinnest of nasal skin and structurally is supported by the medial crura. The lining for each of the nine aesthetic units of the nose is also distinctive.[3] Thin nonhairbearing skin lines the tip, while the nasal facets and alae are lined by thicker skin, the caudal aspect of which is hair bearing. The columella is backed by the membranous septum, which is covered by thin nonhairbearing skin. At the piriform aperture, the lining transitions to mucosa which lines the dorsum and sidewall units.

Menick has stressed that the goal of restorative nasal surgery is not simply to fill a defect.[2] Depending on the extent of the defect; wounds should be altered in size, configuration, and depth to allow reconstruction of an entire unit. If the majority of the surface skin of a unit is lost, resurfacing the entire unit is usually preferable. This is accomplished by discarding the remaining skin of the unit and designing the flap used to resurface the defect so it will compensate for the discarded skin. This arrangement places the scars in the junction between units where they will lie in depressions or along shadow lines, maximizing scar camouflage. By placing the scars in these junctions, they tend to blend with the normal contour lines of the nose and will not distract the viewing eye. Menick has noted that resurfacing the entire unit also takes advantage of the mild trap door scar contraction phenomenon, which causes the entire unit to bulge slightly, simulating the normal convexity of the tip, dorsum, and alae.[2] However, more important than resurfacing an entire nasal unit is the creation of the proper contour of the covering flap so that it exactly replicates the normal topography of the unit.

The surface area and pattern of each nasal aesthetic unit should be restored as accurately as possible. Because the nose is a three-dimensional structure, each reconstructed unit must duplicate normal contour. This is accomplished by concomitantly integrating structural support in each step of the repair. Reconstructed skeletal elements must be attached to a stable foundation such as remaining nasal cartilages or the bone of the maxilla. This will prevent collapse or distortion during the healing process.[2] When a nasal defect is full thickness; nasal lining is replaced with mucoperichondrium from the septum or mucosa of the turbinates when possible. Similar to surface defects, lining defects are repaired with tissue that has the same surface areas as the defect. Application of the nasal aesthetic unit principles provides a logical cognitive approach to nasal reconstruction. Missing tissue is replaced with like tissue in a quantity and quality that exactly replicates the pattern, surface area, and contour of the absent unit.

LINING FLAPS

Burget and Menick have described a bipedicle flap of vestibular skin and mucosa based medially on the septum and laterally on the floor of the nasal vestibule.[1] Such a flap can be elevated off of the undersurface of the lateral crus and mobilized inferiorly to reline full thickness alar defects limited in height to 1 cm.

Burget and Menick have studied the vascularity of the nasal septal mucosa and have documented that the entire ipsilateral septal mucoperichondrium can survive on a narrow pedicle containing the septal branch of the superior labial artery (Figure 2).[1] Likewise, the entire contralateral mucoperichondrium based on the anterior and posterior ethmoid arteries can be reflected laterally as a dorsally based hinge flap to line the cephalic sidewall of the nose (Figure 3).[1] Burget and Menick have also shown that if both right and left septal branches are included in the pedicle, the entire septum can be rotated out of the nasal passage as a composite flap containing a sandwich of cartilage between the two mucoperichondrial leaves (Figure 4).[1] Such flaps, whether they be composite or simple mucoperichondrial hinge flaps are designed to extend from the floor of the nose to within 1 cm of the junction of the upper lateral cartilage and cartilaginous septum. The flaps typically extend posteriorly well beyond the bony-cartilaginous junction of the septum producing a hinged mucoperichondrial flap measuring as much as 3 cm wide and 5 cm long.[1] Burget and Menick advocate a back cut of the mucosa at the anterior septal angle to facilitate flap transfer.[3] I prefer leaving the flap hinged on the entire length of caudal septum to maintain a wider pedicle and enhance the vascularity of the flap. The ipsilateral flap is reflected laterally to resurface the lining

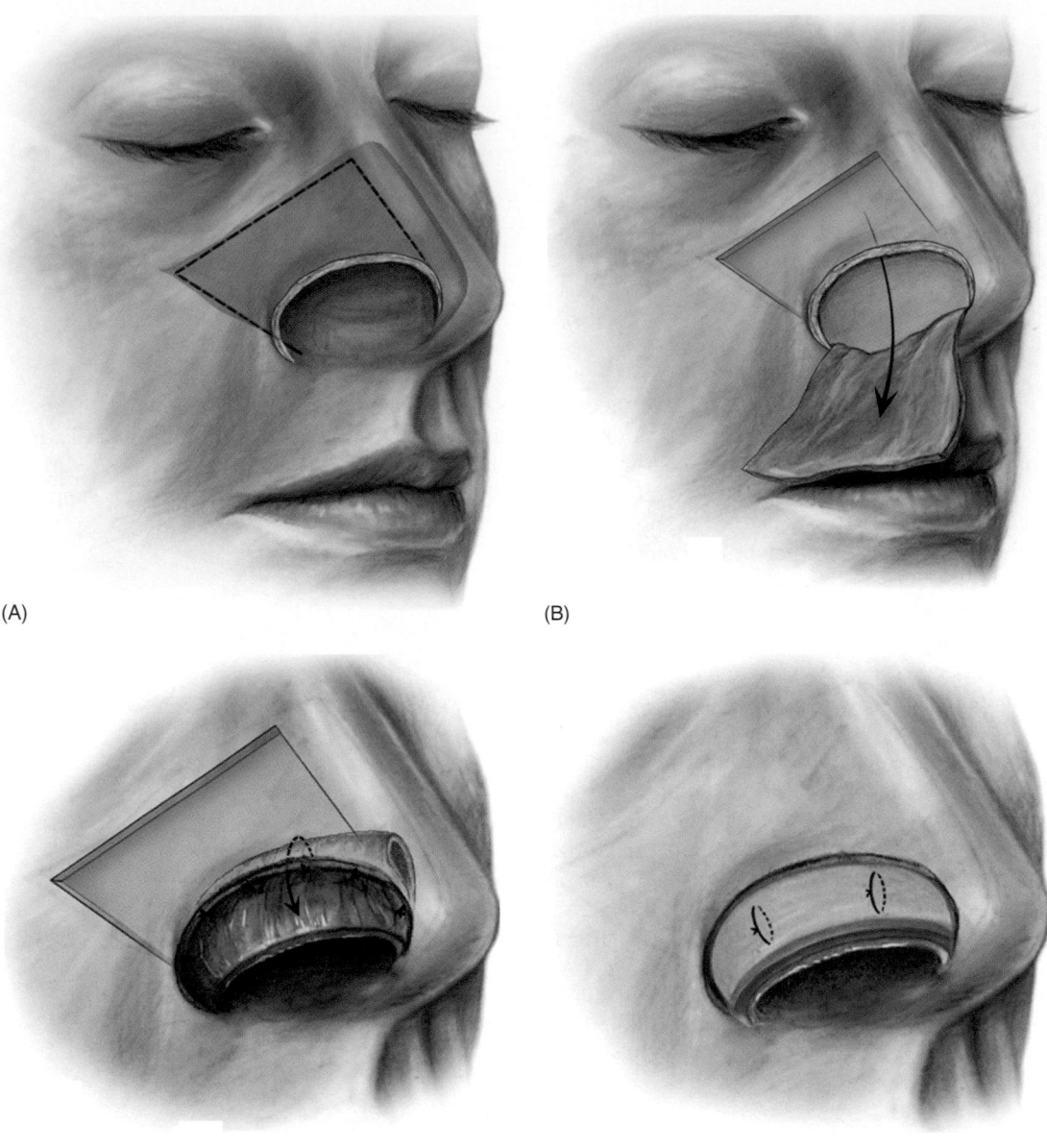

(A)   (B)

(C)   (D)

Figure 2 (A) Unilateral septal mucoperichondrial hinge flap developed by incising mucosa and perichondrium along floor of nose and 1.5 cm below and parallel to the cartilaginous dorsum. Parallel incisions are connected to the vertical posterior incision over the bony septum. (B) Flap is dissected from superior to inferior and from posterior to anterior. Anterior dissection remains 1 cm posterior to caudal border of septum and 1.5 cm posterior to nasal spine. (C) Hinged on the caudal septum, the flap is reflected laterally to line the caudal nasal vault. (D) Cartilage graft provides nasal framework. Lining flap secured to framework with a few mattress sutures. (Reproduced with permission from reference 6.)

defect. By necessity, the flap traverses the nasal passage and must be detached from the septum 3 weeks after transfer. This is usually performed at the same time as detachment of the interpolated skin flap used to cover the defect. Nasal lining flaps have a reliable vascularity and are thin and supple, providing natural physiological material for the interior of the nasal passage. They do not distort the external shape of the nose or compromise the nasal airway. Importantly, these well-vascularized lining flaps allow the concomitant use of cartilage grafts for restoring the nasal framework which when properly fashioned prevent nasal distortion from scar contraction.

FRAMEWORK

If missing, the absent portion of the nasal framework of each aesthetic unit is completely replaced. Cartilage grafts are used to replace the

missing framework of the dorsum, tip, and caudal sidewalls. Additionally, a strip of cartilage is placed along the reconstructed nostril margin whenever connective tissue framework is missing. In instances of alar reconstruction, this usually means employing a cartilaginous strip that spans the distance from junction of the alar base with the cheek to the region of the nasal facet, even though the alae do not normally contain cartilage. This is required in order to support the nostril rim and prevent migration upward of the nostril margin during wound healing (Figure 5).

The function of the grafted framework is to provide contour and maintain a patent airway. Framework grafts are used at the time of initial reconstruction and consist of grafts which, as nearly as possible, replicate the exact size, shape, and contour of the missing framework. When covered by a thin, conforming cutaneous flap, the contour of the framework is distinctively

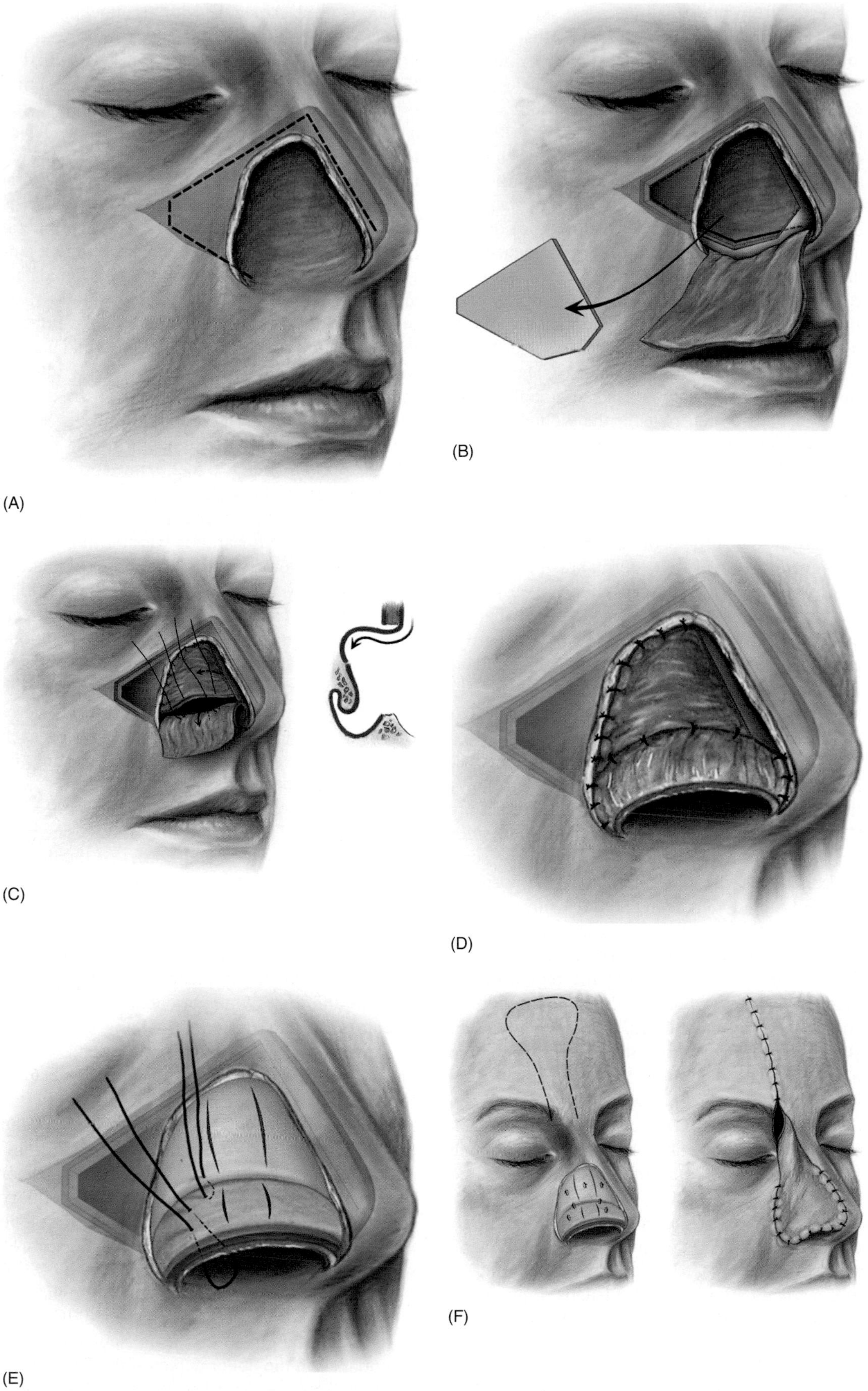

(A)

(B)

(C)

(D)

(E)

(F)

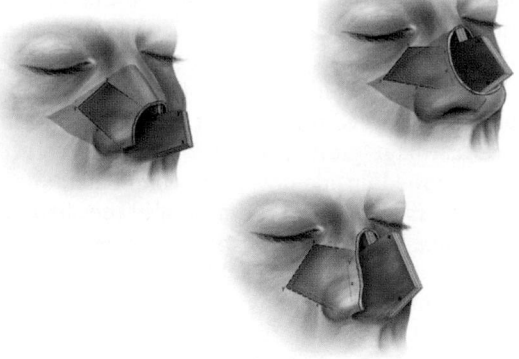

Figure 4 Composite flaps based on dual blood supply of septal branches of superior labial artery. Wedge of cartilage along floor of nose removed to allow flaps to turn outward to provide structure and lining to nose. Mucoperichondrial flaps reflected laterally from composite flaps to line nasal defect. (Reproduced with permission from reference 6.)

manifested and produces a normal appearing restoration of the missing part. Framework grafts fix in place the soft tissues used in nasal repair by virtue of providing skeletal support for both lining and cover.

Bone and cartilage are the tissue grafting materials available to the surgeon for replacing the framework of the nose. The framework of the nasal dorsum may be replaced with bone or cartilage. Cranial bone grafts are the preferred material for more cephalic skeletal defects and are anchored to the frontal bone with miniplates. Limited caudal dorsal skeletal defects are best replaced with septal or auricular cartilage when available. When the entire dorsum is absent, costal cartilage is the preferred grafting material. The dorsal framework prevents cephalic contraction and subsequent shortening of the nose. It also provides shape and projection to the bridge. The framework of the sidewalls can be replaced with septal bone and cartilage or cranial bone contoured into a trapezoid shape and fixed to the dorsum and maxilla. Costal cartilage may also be used. Sidewall skeletal grafts support the middle vault and prevent collapse. They also serve as a

Figure 3 (A) The septal branch of the superior labial artery can supply large ipsilateral mucoperichondrial flap hinged on caudal septum. (B) Exposed septal cartilage removed maintaining adequate dorsal and caudal strut. (C) Contralateral mucoperichondrial flap hinged on dorsum turned laterally to line cephalic portion of sidewall. Under surface of ipsilateral flap tacked to caudal margin of contralateral flap. (D) Ipsilateral flap used to line caudal portion of nasal sidewall and ala. Contralateral flap used to line cephalic portion of sidewall. (E) Septal cartilage used to replace missing upper lateral cartilage. Auricular cartilage replaces missing portions of alar cartilage and provides structural support to ala. Hinge mucosal flaps secured against under surface of cartilage grafts with mattress sutures. (F) Interpolated paramedian forehead flap used to cover exposed cartilage grafts. (Reproduced with permission from reference 6.)

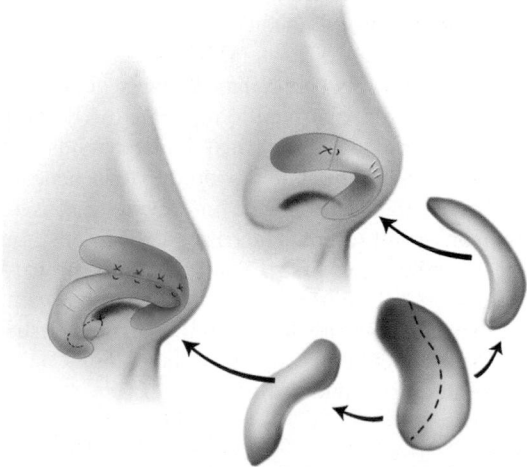

Figure 5 Auricular cartilage grafts are well suited for replacing missing segments of alar cartilage and for support of ala and nostril margin. (Reproduced with permission from reference 6.)

foundation for attaching the lower framework of the nose, specifically the alar cartilages or their replacements.

The nasal tip is shaped by the alar cartilages, and the preferred replacement framework is conchal cartilage grafts (Figure 5). By coincidence, when turned upside down, the contralateral conchal cymba often closely resembles the shape of the dome cartilage (intermediate crus) and the conchal cavum resembles the shape of the lateral crus. Grafts 5 to 8 mm wide from the auricle can be scored and bent to replace entirely the lower lateral cartilages. These grafts can be used bilaterally or unilaterally as required and are fixed to any residual stumps of the medial and lateral crura. They support the lower nasal vault and recreate the contour of the nasal tip. Additional projection and modification of the shape of the tip can be accomplished with Peck-type cartilage grafts anchored on top of the reconstructed alar cartilages[2] or by the fabrication of shield shaped septal cartilage tip grafts placed caudal to the reconstructed alar cartilages.

Structural support for the columella can be provided by conchal cartilage grafts as described for the tip, but placed in such a fashion to span any gaps of the medial crura. They may also extend all the way to the nasal spine if all medial crura are absent. Septal cartilage grafts are very effective for this purpose as well, but must be thinned, scored and bent so they replicate the diverging angle that naturally occurs at the junction of the medial and intermediate crura.

An alar batten of septal or conchal cartilage 0.5 to 1 cm wide is used for the framework of the ala and nasal facets. When available, the natural curvature of the conchal cartilage makes this material preferable to septal cartilage. When all, or portions of the lateral crus is missing in addition to the ala, the conchal cartilage graft is designed as a wider graft (0.75 to 1.0 cm) to concomitantly replace the lateral crus and simultaneously provide support to the ala. The graft is placed along the planned margin of the missing nostril from the alar base to the nostril apex. It is inserted into a deep tissue pocket in the alar facial sulcus and is attached medially to the framework of the nasal dome. The tissue pocket serves to stabilize the graft laterally. Similar to grafts used to replace missing alar cartilage, grafts are thinned, scored, and bent to replicate the bulging contour of the ala. If the nasal defect extends into the nasal facet, the batten should extend beneath the diverging angle of the intermediate crus to span any gap present. The batten fixes in position the reconstructed nostril rim preventing upward migration and subsequent notching of the rim. It also prevents inward migration of the nostril and subsequent constriction of the external nasal valve during wound healing.

COVERING FLAPS

Small defects of the nasal skin 2 cm or less in size can sometimes be repaired with local flaps harvested from the remaining nasal skin, if there is sufficient redundancy of the skin. Most notable of the local flaps is the bilobe flap as modified by Zitelli.[7,8] The bilobe flap was originally designed for repairing nasal tip defects. Each lobe of the flap and the defect were separated by 90° for a total transposition over a 180° arc. Whereas this recruited skin is at some distance from the defect, it also maximized the standing cutaneous deformities (SCDs) and the likelihood of development of a trap-door deformity or pincushioning of both the first and second lobe of the flap. Zitelli[7] emphasized the use of narrow angles (45° angles) between lobes so that the total arc of tissue transferred occurs over no more than 90 to 100°. This flap design reduces the SCD and pincushioning effects. Bilobe flaps are double transposition flaps which transfer the wound closure tension from the defect through a 90° arc to the donor site areas. A major disadvantage of using the bilobe flap to repair nasal skin defects is the formation of extensive incisional scar that does not fall along borders of nasal aesthetic units. However, postoperative dermabrasion is very helpful in obscuring the scar.

Whenever possible, the nasal bilobe flap is based laterally.[9] Medial-based flaps are hardy, although the vascular supply is not as abundant as those based laterally. Bilobe flaps are ideally suited for repairing defects less than 1.5 cm in maximum dimension, located on the central or lateral nasal tip and without extension to the ala. Ideally, the defect should be at least 0.5 cm superior to the margin of the nostril. The flap recruits skin from the mid and upper dorsum and sidewall, where more generous skin laxity is present. Defects of the cephalic one-half of the nose are not well suited for reconstruction with a bilobe flap unless they are 0.5 cm or less in size. This is because bilobe flaps harvested in this area necessitates use of skin from the region of the medial canthus, which is thin and immobile. Bilobe flaps are most useful in patients with thin skin and an ample degree of skin laxity along the nasal sidewall. The surgeon may estimate laxity by pinching the lateral nasal skin between the thumb and index finger. Patients with thick sebaceous skin have a higher risk of developing flap necrosis, trap-door deformity, and depressed scars.

Bilobe flaps of the nose must be geometrically precise and are designed using the following method (Figure 6).[9] The radius of the defect is measured. For laterally based flaps, a point lateral to the border of the defect is marked in the alar groove that is the distance of the length of the radius. This point is used for designing both lobes of the flap. Two arcs are drawn with their centers at the marked point. The first arc passes through the center of the defect, and the second makes a tangent with the border of the defect most distal to the point. Calipers and rulers are not used to draw the arcs because these devices measure straight-line distances. In contrast, the topography of the nose is convex in the area of the tip and dorsum. Therefore a flexible measuring device is used. A needle with an attached suture is passed full-thickness through the nose at the point marked in the alar groove. A knot is tied in the suture inside the nasal vestibule. The suture is draped from the point across the defect, and a clamp is applied to the suture at the center of the defect. The clamp with attached suture is then rotated about its pivotal point to indicate the first arc, which is marked with a pen. The clamp is advanced along the suture to the most peripheral point of the defect, and a second arc is drawn tangent to the peripheral border of the defect and parallel to the first arc. The base of the two lobes rests on the first arc. The height of the first lobe extends to the second arc so its height is equal to the distance between the two arcs. The width of the first lobe is equal to the width of the defect. The width of the second lobe is slightly less than the width of first lobe. The height of the second lobe is approximately 1.5 to 2.0 times greater than the height of the first lobe. The first lobe has the configuration of the defect, and the second lobe is triangular. The linear axis passing through the center of each lobe is positioned at approximately 45° from each other, with the axis of the first lobe positioned 45° from the central axis of the defect. This orientation of the lobes inevitably positions the axis of the second lobe along the center of the nasal sidewall or diagonally at the junction of the sidewall with the dorsum. The design also creates a triangular peninsula of skin between each lobe with a 45° angle. A triangle representing the eventual SCD resulting from the pivot of the first lobe is marked with its apex pointing laterally and one side parallel to or in the alar groove. The base of the triangle is the lateral border of the defect, and the height of the triangle is equal to the radius of the defect.

The flap is elevated after local anesthetic is injected. Like other nasal cutaneous flaps, it is dissected in the tissue plane between the nasal muscles and underlying perichondrium and periosteum. The flap and the remaining skin of the entire nose are completely undermined, sometimes extending the dissection into the cheek a short distance. Wide peripheral undermining of all the nasal skin is essential to reduce wound closure tension, facilitate flap transfer, and minimize trap-door deformity (Figure 7). The donor site for the second lobe is closed first by primary approximation of the muscle layer. The first lobe is then transposed to the nasal defect and secured with a few deep dermal sutures. Next, the SCD is removed in or cephalad and parallel to the alar groove. The second lobe is transposed, trimmed of its excess height so that it fits snugly without redundancy in the donor defect of the first lobe.

SUBCUTANEOUS TISSUE PEDICLE MELOLABIAL INTERPOLATED FLAP

The ala is best resurfaced with cheek skin from the area of the melolabial fold. The sebaceous quality of the skin of the fold closely resembles that of the ala. Menick has noted that as melolabial flaps contract, they become rounded resembling the

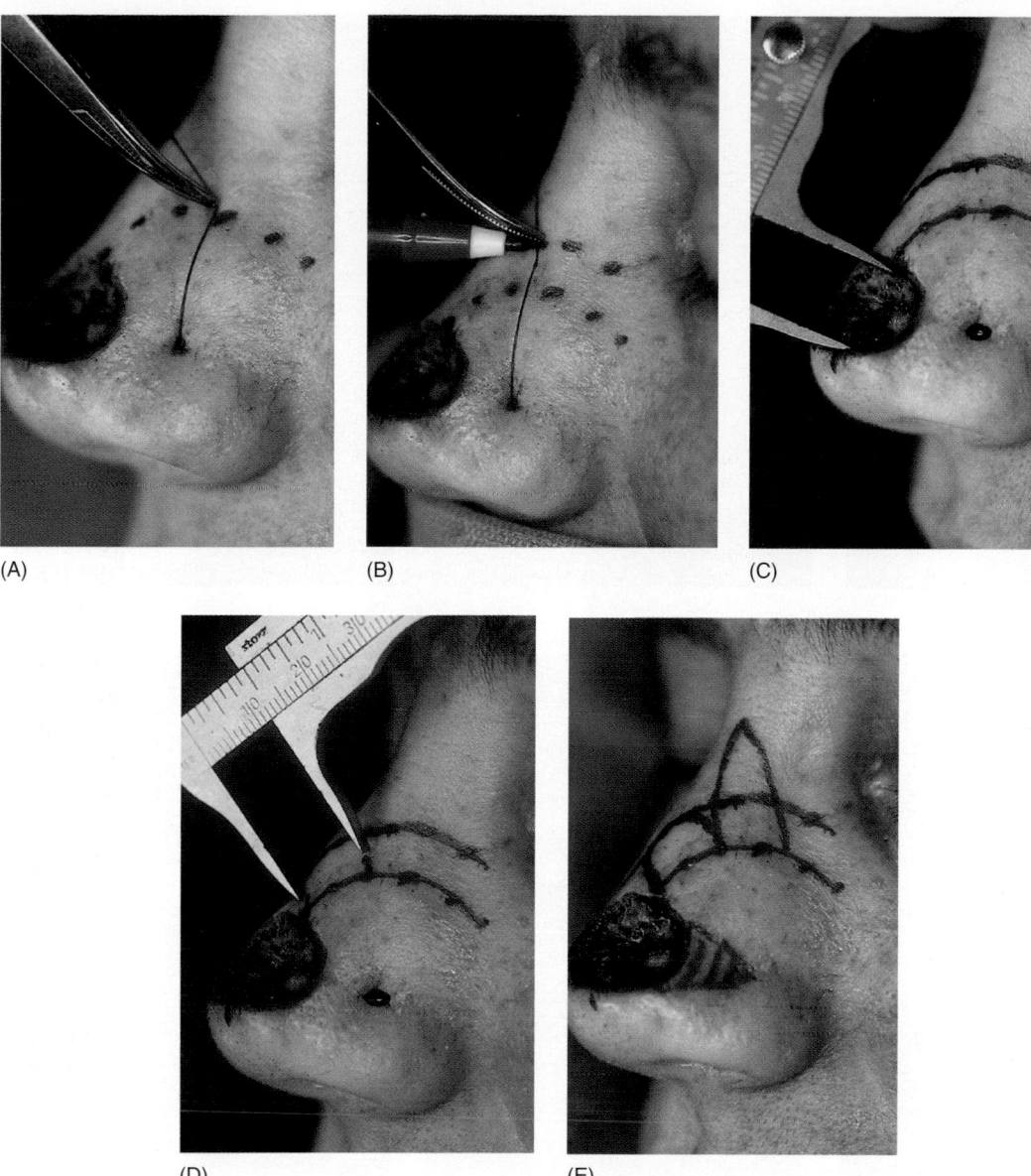

(A)   (B)   (C)

(D)   (E)

Figure 6 (A) and (B) Suture rotated about pivotal point used to mark two arcs for design of bilobe flap. (C) and (D) Width of defect equals width of first lobe. (E) Base of lobes arises from first arc. Height of first lobe extends to second arc. Height of second lobe is twice the height of first lobe. Standing cutaneous deformity marked in alar groove. (Reproduced with permission from reference 9.)

contour of the normal ala.[2] Skin of the melolabial fold is limited, and its use can flatten the fold causing marked asymmetry of the face. Nor can it easily be transferred to the nasal tip or dorsum. Skin of the melolabial fold is transferred to the ala as an interpolated flap, the pedicle of which crosses over but not through the alar facial sulcus. The pedicle is superiorly based and may consist of skin and subcutaneous fat or subcutaneous fat only (Figure 8). It is detached from the cheek 3 weeks after the initial transfer to the nose. Although 3 weeks is a lengthy period for the patient to endure the deformity caused by the flap, this interval allows the surgeon to defat aggressively and sculpture the flap both at the time of the flap transfer and at the time of pedicle detachment and flap inset.

When reconstructing the ala, the entire ala is resurfaced with the cheek flap, except for 1 mm of alar skin just anterior to the alar facial sulcus. This small skin tag preserves the alar facial sulcus and often provides a better scar than when the flap extends to the sulcus. This approach is simi-

lar to the method recommended by Sheen and Sheen[10] for performing a type II Weir excision to reduce the size of the nasal base. Maintaining the excision outside of the alar facial sulcus lessens the risk of developing a depressed scar. This approach also avoids the technically challenging requirements of integrating the flap into the nasal sill at the time of flap inset. When using cheek flaps for repair, I often delay excising the extreme lateral portions of the residual alar skin until the time of pedicle detachment and flap inset. This delay reduces the wound tension on the flap at the time of initial transfer.

A fashioned template of the ala or defect, if it extends beyond the ala, is placed on the melolabial fold so that the center of the template is positioned slightly above the horizontal plane of the oral commissure. The template is positioned so that the medial border of the designed flap lies in the melolabial crease. This arrangement insures that the flap is harvested from the cheek, not from the lip, and that the donor site wound closure

will lie within the melolabial crease, providing maximum scar camouflage. The flap is designed to pivot 90° toward the midline in a clockwise direction when harvested from the left cheek and counterclockwise when harvested from the right cheek. Thus, the template is positioned to design the flap with a specific orientation. As the flap is pivoted and transferred to the recipient site, the medial border of the in situ flap is sutured to the cephalic border of the nasal defect. This in turn causes the inferior border of the in situ flap to join the anterior border of the defect. The lateral border of the in situ flap becomes the inferior border of the reconstructed ala.

A tracing is made around the template. A triangle of skin is marked superior and inferior to the tracing in order to fashion a crescentic island of skin. The two triangles extending from the template tracing represent SCDs that will form when the cheek donor site is closed. The inferior triangle of skin is excised and discarded at the time of flap transfer, and the superior triangle of skin is transferred with the flap and is excised and discarded at the time of pedicle detachment and inset of the flap. The superior triangle of skin is minimized to reduce loss of tissue from the superior melolabial fold where the fold is well developed. Removing skin from the superior portion of the fold may result in considerable asymmetry of the medial aspects of the cheeks.

The flap is incised, and the distal portion is elevated in the subcutaneous plane. The distal third of the flap is thin, leaving 1 to 2 mm of subcutaneous fat attached to the undersurface. As the dissection proceeds superiorly, the plane of dissection extends deeper to facilitate development of the subcutaneous tissue pedicle. The pedicle of fat is freed from the surrounding cheek fat by incising through borders of the pedicle perpendicular to the surface of the skin. The depth of the incision is carried to the level of the superficial surface of the zygomatic major and levator labii muscles. On reaching the zygomatic major muscle, blunt dissection continues upward on the surface of the muscle, releasing the attachments of the pedicle to deeper structures until the flap can reach the recipient site without undue tension. To aid in reducing tension, it is sometimes helpful to place a 4-0 polypropylene suture between the superior skin edge of the donor incision and the alar base. This has the effect of pulling the pedicle upward toward the ala without the need to place additional traction on the subcutaneous tissue pedicle. The suture is released when the pedicle is divided at the time of flap inset.

To close the donor wound following transfer of an interpolated cheek flap, the skin adjacent to the incision is undermined peripherally for a distance 2 cm in the superficial subcutaneous tissue plane, and the SCD that develops inferiorly from advancement of wound margins is removed. Depending on the shape of the flap, the lateral border of the donor site may be considerably longer than the medial border. If this is the situation, it may be necessary to excise an additional SCD (Burow's equalizing triangle) at right angles to

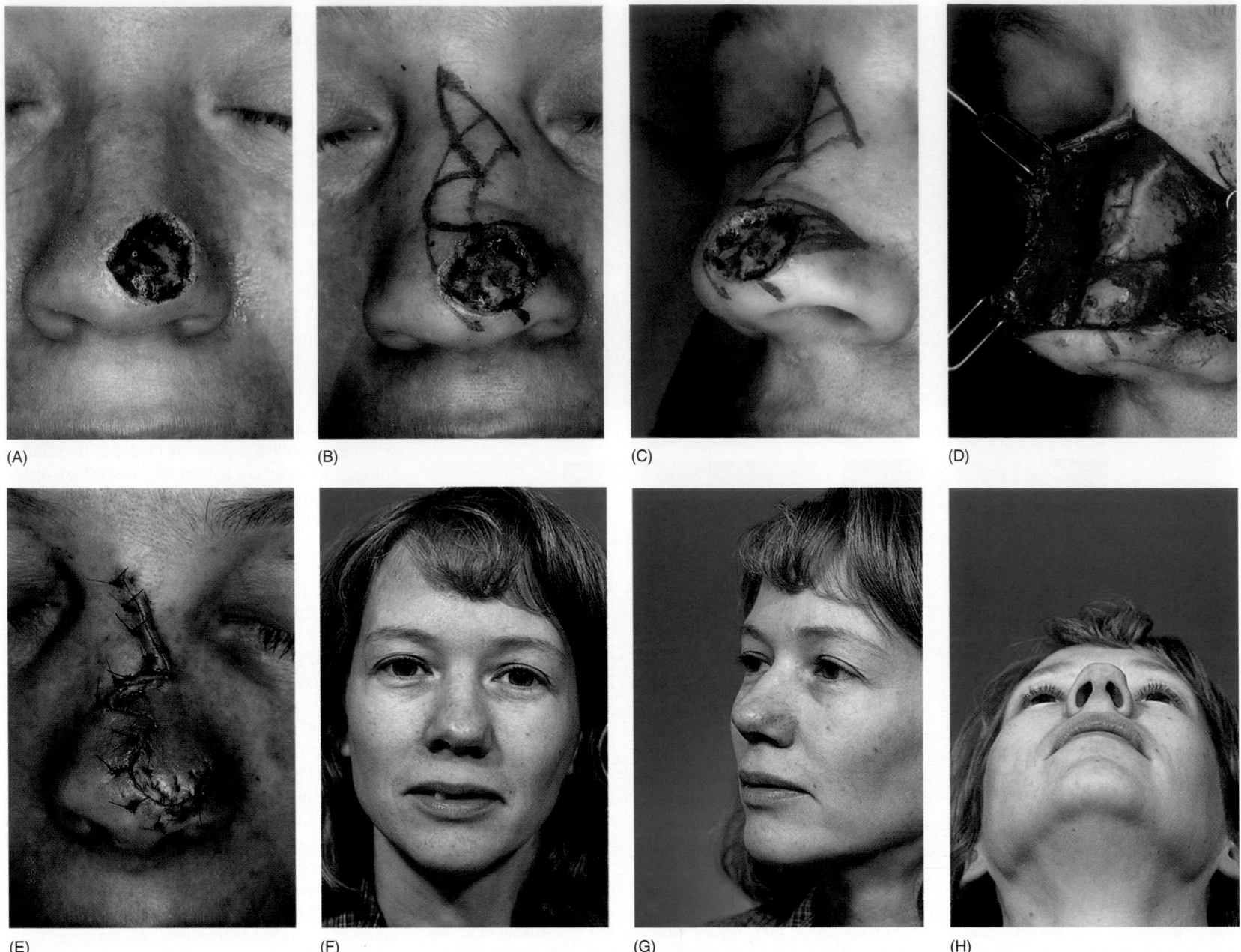

(A)　　　　　　　　(B)　　　　　　　　(C)　　　　　　　　(D)

(E)　　　　　　　　(F)　　　　　　　　(G)　　　　　　　　(H)

Figure 7 (A) 1.8 cm skin defect of nasal tip. (B) and (C) Bilobe flap designed. Standing cutaneous deformity marked laterally so scar from excision of deformity will lie in alar groove. (D) and (E) Wide undermining of flap and nasal skin necessary. (F to H) One year postoperative. Flap dermabraded 2 months after transfer. (Reproduced with permission from reference 9.)

the axis of the melolabial wound closure. This is accomplished at the inferior pole of the wound.

Cheek flaps are detached 3 weeks following transfer. For subcutaneous tissue pedicled flaps, the pedicle is transected at the base, and the cheek skin is undermined for a distance of 2 cm around the periphery of the amputated pedicle. After freshening the skin margins with a scalpel, the wound is closed by advancing the borders together. As this is accomplished, it is usually necessary to open the superior end of the donor site scar to facilitate excision of redundant subcutaneous tissue and a small SCD that often forms as the wound margins are approximated.

The lateral portion of the flap attached to the nose is released from attachments to the adjacent nasal skin for a distance of 0.5 to 1.0 cm to achieve sufficient freedom to unfurrow the flap. Release enables the surgeon to remove excessive subcutaneous fat not trimmed at the time of flap

transfer. The residual skin of the alar facial sulcus is preserved. The flap is precisely trimmed to fit the skin defect and sutured in place. When the alar base is absent, the flap is tailored to replace the missing base and is integrated with the nasal sill. When the sill requires reconstruction, the flap is trimmed so that it has a tapered end that may serve as the sill. The end is turned medially and sutured to the upper lip.

CUTANEOUS PEDICLE MELOLABIAL INTERPOLATED FLAP

In most of the cases, I prefer to design cheek flaps on a subcutaneous tissue pedicle because this design limits the quantity of skin in the superior aspect of the melolabial fold that is included in the flap or excised to facilitate closure of the donor site.[11] The island design has a greater free-

dom to pivot on its pedicle and may have a better blood supply by incorporating within the pedicle of the flap a greater number of perforating vessels arising from the angular artery. The pedicle of the island flap does not require tailoring and inset following detachment of the flap. The subcutaneous pedicle is simply excised, and the skin edges surrounding the pedicle are freshened and the wound closed primarily. However, harvesting the island flap is technically more difficult than harvesting a cutaneous pedicle flap because the plane of dissection is considerably deeper, placing the branches of the facial nerve supplying the zygomatic major and minor muscles at greater risk of injury.

A cutaneous pedicle interpolated melolabial flap is a peninsular flap with a linear axis centered on a cutaneous pedicle that connects the flap to the cheek. This is in contrast to the subcutaneous tissue pedicle (island) flap, which does not

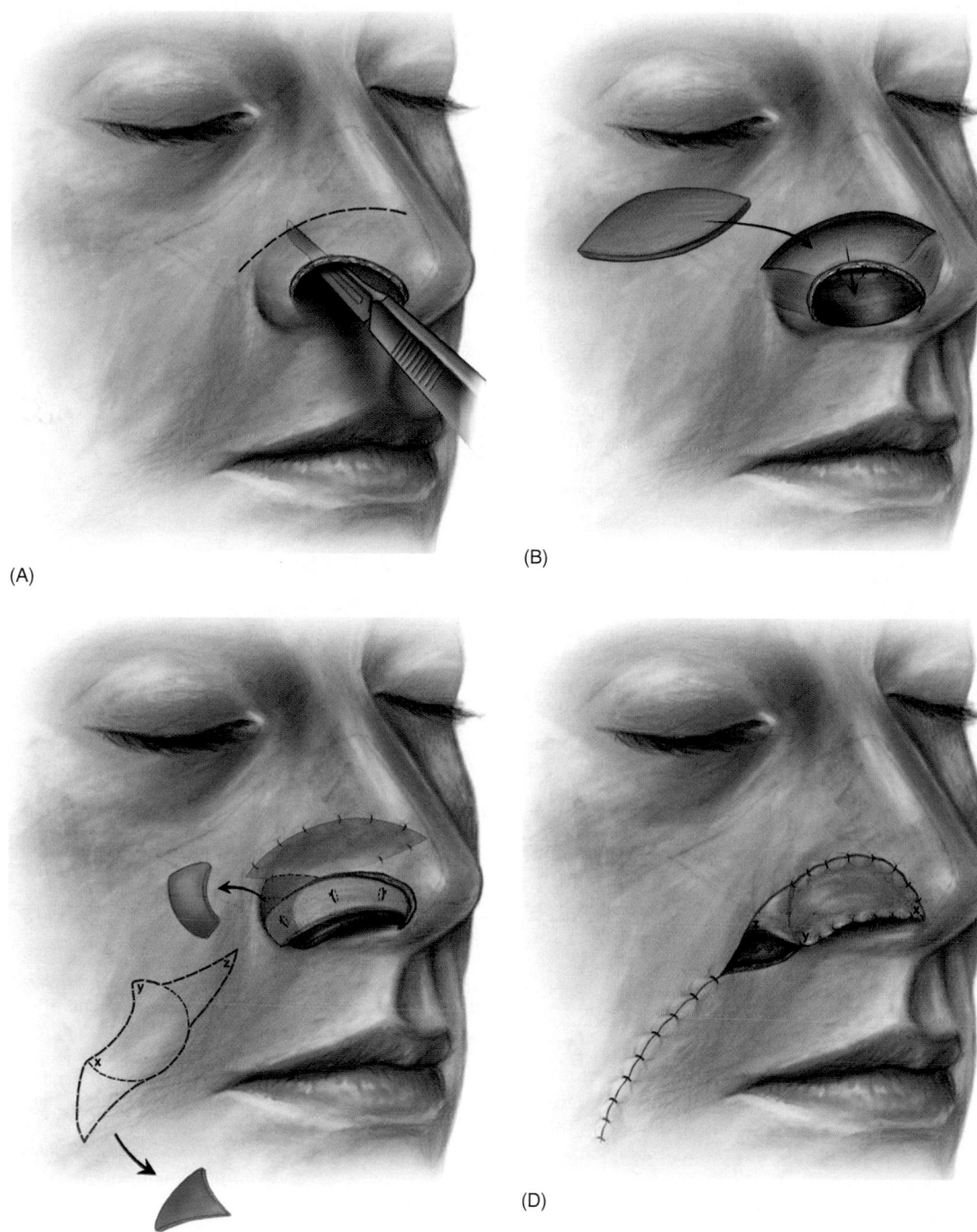

(A)

(B)

(C)

(D)

Figure 8 (A) Full thickness defect of ala that does not extend cephalically more than 1.5 cm may be lined by bipedicle advancement vestibular skin flap based medially on septum and laterally on floor of nasal vestibule. Extended intercartilagenous incision necessary to develop flap. (B) Bipedicle flap advanced caudally and donor site covered with thin full thickness skin graft. (C) Remaining skin of ala discarded (*arrow*). Auricular cartilage provides structural support to nostril margin. Superiorly based subcutaneous tissue pedicle interpolated cheek flap designed to cover cartilage graft. (D) Interpolated cheek flap sutured in place. Caudal border of cheek flap sutured to caudal border of bipedicle advancement flap. (Reproduced with permission from reference 6.)

flap, the distal half of the peninsular flap may be thinned as necessary to replicate the thickness of the recipient site. The proximal portion of the flap bridging between cheek and nose is not thinned to insure a sufficient vascular supply.

Similar to the island flap, the peninsular flap remains attached to the cheek for 3 weeks to enable the establishment of collateral vascularity. The pedicle is divided at a second stage, and the proximal portion of the pedicle is inset in the cheek by opening the superior portion of the donor site scar 1 to 2 cm. The wound edges are spread widely, creating a space to accommodate the proximal pedicle. The skin adjacent to the opened wound is undermined for 2 cm. This allows the cheek skin to retract, assisting in enlarging the wound.[11] The pedicle stump is then trimmed to fit the wound precisely and inset in the melolabial fold, creating a V-shaped wound closure. Returning most of the skin of the proximal pedicle to the cheek helps maintain the natural fullness observed in the upper portion of the melolabial fold. Alternatively, the proximal pedicle may be amputated in an elliptical configuration, and the cheek wound closed primarily. This has the advantage of a linear donor site scar within the melolabial crease. The distal portion of the flap left attached to the nose is thinned and inset using methods similar to those for the island flap. Less aggressive sculpturing of subcutaneous fat from the flap is recommended both at the time of flap transfer and at the time of flap inset for patients who use tobacco products.

PARAMEDIAN FOREHEAD FLAP

A number of studies of the vascular anatomy of the forehead have been reviewed by Baker and Alford.[12] These studies confirm that the supratrochlear artery is the primary axial blood supply of midforehead flaps, which include the median and paramedian vertically oriented flaps. Additionally, the studies have shown that in the medial canthal region a rich anastomotic network exists among the supratrochlear, supraorbital, and angular arteries. Identification of this vascular network and the surgical techniques of flap harvest that preserve this regional blood flow have allowed surgeons to harvest paramedian forehead flaps based on pedicles narrower than those used for medial forehead flaps.[13] The narrower pedicle enables the flap more freedom to rotate about its pivot point, and therefore provides more effective flap length. At the same time, this design reduces the donor site deformity in the glabellar area which results from the transfer of the flap. When the paramedian forehead flap is based on the supratrochlear artery and its anatomoses to surrounding vessels, the flap is an axial pivotal interpolated flap with an abundant blood supply that allows transfer without delay.

The paramedian forehead flap may be designed with the assistance of a Doppler probe to localize the supratrochlear artery, but the author has not found this to be necessary.[14] The base of the pedicle is usually centered over the supratrochlear

have a cutaneous pedicle and is connected to the cheek by subcutaneous fat. Whether a peninsular or island flap, the pedicle is developed at the superior aspect of the melolabial fold.

The peninsular flap depends on the dermal and subdermal vascular plexes of the cutaneous pedicle to provide vascularity to the distal flap. The cutaneous pedicle must have sufficient width and depth to ensure this vascularity. When designing a peninsular flap, the orientation of the template remains the same as for designing an island flap.[11] The width of the cutaneous pedicle is approximately the width of the template, although it may

be narrower than the template when a wide (more than 2 cm) flap design is required. The peninsular flap is elevated in a subcutaneous tissue plane, maintaining 3 mm of fat on the undersurface of the cutaneous pedicle. This is in contrast to the island design, based on a subcutaneous tissue pedicle that may be as much as 1.5 cm thick. Thus, the plane of dissection for the cutaneous pedicle flap is considerably more superficial. Like the island flap, the peninsular flap pivots 90° toward the midline and is sutured to the nose in a similar fashion. Care is taken not to kink the pedicle on transferring the flap. Like the island artery on the same side as the majority of the nasal defect for which the flap is intended for repair. The vertical axis of the supratrochlear artery is 2 cm lateral to the midline, which corresponds to the medial border of the eyebrow. Therefore, the base of the flap is centered over the medial border of the eyebrow. The width of the pedicle is designed 1.5 cm wide and is not flared as this restricts the pivotal movement of the flap.

The cutaneous defect is outlined by squaring off the corners of the defect with a skin marker. Giving the defect angular rather than curvilinear borders reduces the propensity for developing a trap-door deformity. If the defect occupies more than 50% of the surface area of a given nasal aesthetic unit, the remaining skin of the unit is marked for removal. When a unilateral cutaneous defect encompassed one-half or less of the surface area of the nasal tip, the defect is usually enlarged only to the degree that the enlargement creates a hemi-tip defect. This will limit the size of the forehead flap necessary for reconstruction which in turn, minimizes the deformity of the forehead. The aesthetic result of resurfacing a hemi-nasal defect with a paramedian forehead flap is equally pleasing as resurfacing the entire nasal tip.[14]

The nasal dorsum is an exception to the rule of resurfacing the entire nasal unit when the defect occupies one half or more of the surface area of the unit. When cutaneous defects occur on the dorsum, the thin skin of the rhinion is never removed unless required for tumor abla-tion.[14] In most patients; the intrinsic thickness of forehead skin is greater than that of the native skin covering the rhinion. Even with removal of all the subcutaneous tissue from a forehead flap, the thickness of the flap may not match the thin-ness of the in situ skin and muscle of the rhinion. In this region, contour outweighs the advantage of placing the borders of the flap along the junc-tion of aesthetic units. It is wise to leave this skin intact and resurface only the caudal dorsum than resurface the entire dorsal nasal aesthetic unit.

Similar to the rhinion, the skin of the nasal facets is delicate and thin. It is supported only by fibroconnective tissue. Forehead skin cannot replicate the delicate nostril margin in this area of the nose. Nasal tip defects requiring a forehead flap as a cover should be enlarged only to a line along the superior border of the facet. This line corresponds to the caudal border of the interme-diate crura of the lower lateral cartilages.

A three-dimensional template exactly dupli-cating the surface area and contour of the region to be resurfaced is fashioned from a foil or a thin sheet of foam rubber. The author prefers foam rubber because it has the flexible qualities of skin and easily conforms to the convex and concave contours of the nasal topography.[14] The final defect to be resurfaced is marked on the nasal skin, outlining additional skin removal to square off the defect or to remove the remaining cutane-ous portions of the aesthetic unit. The template is designed before the defect is enlarged because once the additional skin is removed the wound will spread and the defect will appear larger than

it is. For this reason, if the nasal defect involves an aesthetic unit that has an intact counterpart, the intact unit is used to design the template because it will give a more accurate measurement of sur-face area. The template is then reversed to design the flap. When the defect involves an aesthetic unit that is unpaired, the template is designed as an ideal size for the specific patient. When dealing with large surface defects, it is helpful to suture the rubber foam template to the margins of the defect to assist with fashioning the template more precisely. Cartilage grafts are required to replace missing framework, and the template is designed after the grafts are in place.

The template is used to design the flap on the forehead skin. The center of the template is posi-tioned approximately 2 cm lateral to the midline. At a minimum, the upper border of the template is positioned at the frontal hairline unless the patient has a receding hairline or frontal balding. The length of the flap is measured by a length of suture extending from the distal end of the positioned template to the level of the medial eyebrow. Hold-ing it at the eyebrow, the suture is rotated 180° in the coronal plane toward the midline to the most distal recipient site on the nose. If the suture does not reach this point, the template must be reposi-tioned higher on the forehead, or the pedicle must be lowered by extending it below the level of the eyebrow. By using this method of determining flap length, a decision can be made concerning the necessity of placing a portion of the template over hair-bearing scalp. The flap is then precisely outlined on the forehead with a skin marker, fol-lowing the exact shape of the template.

Paramedian forehead flaps are usually dissected using local anesthetic and intravenous sedation[14] (Figure 9). One percent lidocaine with 1:100,000 concentration of epinephrine is injected circum-ferentially and deeply about the surgical defect. The skin along the entire length of the supraorbital bony rims is infiltrated to the level of the perios-teum. Particular attention is given to a broad verti-cal band of skin in the axes of the supratrochlear and supraorbital nerves. The anesthetic is injected into the subcutaneous tissue plane because this is the location of the nerves and vessels supply-ing the forehead skin. The base of the flap and skin over the root of the nose are also injected. Intravenous dolasetron mesylate is adminis-tered to control postoperative nausea commonly associated with the procedure. To avoid oversiz-ing the flap, incisions are made inside the lines of the designed flap. The flap is incised through the skin, subcutaneous tissue, muscle, and fascia. The flap is elevated from superior to inferior in the subfascial plane, just superficial to the periosteum of the frontal bone. Rapid dissection may be per-formed in this plane until the corrugator supercilii muscle is encountered, at which point the muscle is dissected away from the underlying periosteum bluntly with scissors or a periosteal elevator. If it is necessary to extend incisions of the pedicle below eyebrow level, it is accomplished with a scalpel cutting through skin only. Blunt dissec-tion by spreading tissue with a hemostat is then

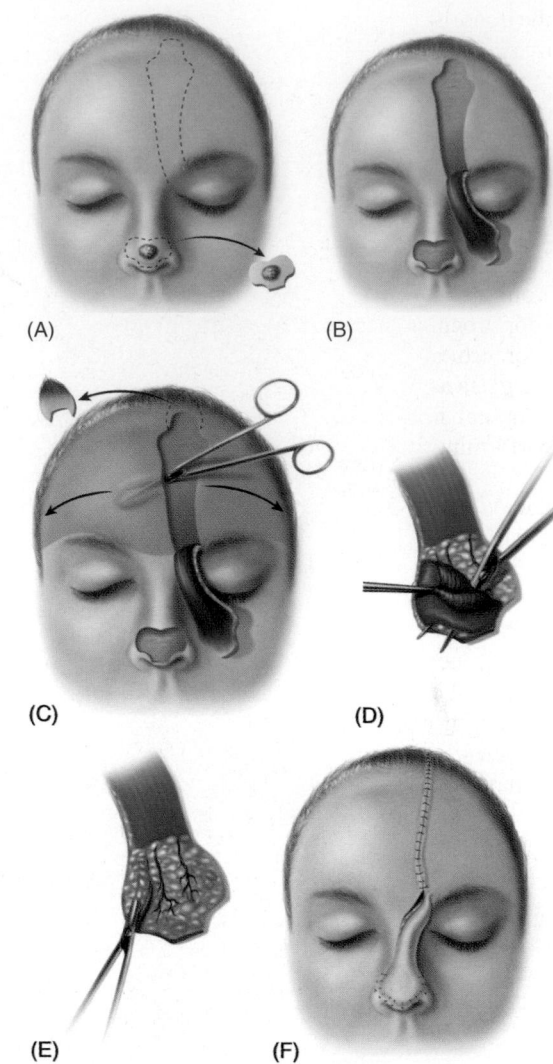

Figure 9 (A) Base of interpolated paramedian forehead flap is 1.5 cm wide centered over the medial end of the eyebrow. Axis of pedicle is vertical and 2 cm from mid-line. (B) Flap elevated from underlying periosteum. (C) Donor site closure achieved by undermining in subfas-cial plane from one temporalis muscle to other. Stand-ing cutaneous deformity of scalp from advancement of forehead skin removed vertically. (D) Galea and frontalis muscles completely removed from distal flap. (E) Major-ity of subcutaneous fat removed from distal flap. (F) Flap sutured at recipient site with vertical mattress cutaneous sutures. Forehead donor site closed in two layers: inter-rupted suture approximation of muscle and galea continu-ous cutaneous suture. (Reproduced with permission from reference 14.)

performed to mobilize the pedicle away from the medial bony orbit. The supratrochlear artery may sometimes be visually identified in the area on the deep surface of the frontalis muscle just as it exits over or through the corrugator supercilii muscle and before passing deep to the orbicularis oculi muscle to enter the orbit. Adequate flap mobiliza-tion usually requires complete sectioning of the corrugator muscle to achieve sufficient flap length. Blunt and sharp dissections are used to continue flap elevation downward into the root of the nose or until sufficient pedicle length and flap mobility have been attained to allow tension-free wound closure. Hemostasis along the border of the flap is achieved with electrocautery applied judiciously.

The forehead flap is covered with a damp sponge and reflected downward to allow repair of the donor site. Donor site closure is accomplished by extensive undermining of the forehead skin in the subfascial plane from the anterior border of one temporalis muscle to the other. A few parallel vertical galeatomies 2 to 3 cm apart may be made to facilitate primary repair of the superior portion of the donor site if the donor defect is large. Galeatomies should be made just through the galea to the level of the muscle and removed from the vertical corridor of the supraorbital and supratrochlear nerves. The deep branch of the supraorbital nerve can readily be seen through the galea as it travels superiorly just medial to the temporal line, and it should be protected when performing galeatomies.

Horizontal incisions along the hairline to facilitate closure of the donor site are not performed. This would increase anesthesia of the anterior scalp by cutting through the distal branches of the supraorbital nerves and create an additional visible scar on the forehead. As the wound edges are advanced, a SCD of scalp tissue occurs at the superior apex of the flap donor site defect. This is excised completely by extending an incision sufficiently superiorly in the scalp to enable excision of the tissue cone.

The forehead donor site wound is repaired before the flap is sutured in place. The thickness of the flap is tailored by thinning the distal portion. This usually requires removal of the muscle and most of the subcutaneous fat in order to match the depth of the nasal defect. When necessary, all but the subcutaneous fat immediately attached to

the dermis may be removed. If the vertical height of the nasal defect is less than 2 cm, the portion of the flap covering the entire defect may be thinned at the time of initial transfer. For larger defects, the proximal flap covering the more cephalic portion of the defect is left with all of its muscle and

subcutaneous fat intact and is thinned at the time of pedicle division. If necessary, the muscle and galea may be removed from the entire length of the flap beginning 1 cm superior to the point at which the supratrochlear artery pierces the frontalis muscle. Any hair follicles transferred with

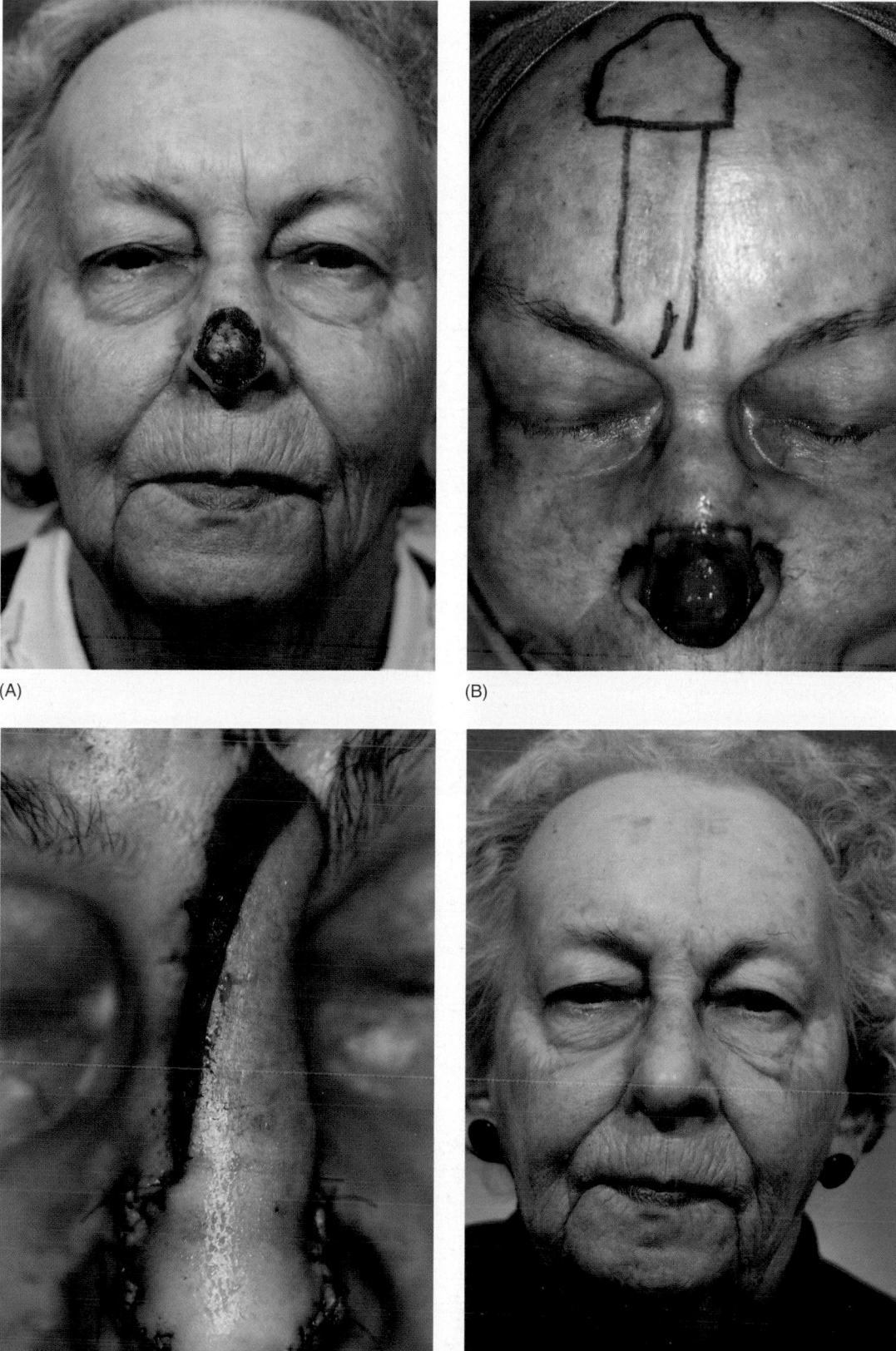

Figure 10 (A) Flap pedicle separated 3 weeks following flap transfer. (B) Donor site wound opened and area between eyebrows widely undermined to release wound contracture. (C) Proximal pedicle converted to small triangular flap which is advanced superiorly to restore original position of eyebrow. It is sometimes necessary to excise Burow triangle immediately above medial aspect of eyebrow. Flap inset in nose by trimming redundant tissue. (D) Wound repair accomplished with vertical cutaneous sutures. (Reproduced with permission from reference 14.)

Figure 11 (A) Patient with a 2 × 2 cm skin defect of nasal tip. (B) Interpolated paramedian forehead flap designed for repair. (C) Flap transferred. (D) Three months following flap inset.

the flap should be individually cauterized with a fine-pointed electric cautery or removed manually. The distal flap, appropriately thinned, will be sufficiently supple and thin to conform to the nasal framework and manifest its contour.

After thinning, the flap is pivoted either clockwise or counterclockwise in an arc toward the midline and reflected downward toward the nasal defect. The distal flap is sutured in position with interrupted vertical mattress cutaneous sutures. Deep dermal or subcuticular sutures are not used. Following placement of vertical mattress sutures, a single running 5-0 fast absorbing plain gut suture on a fine-tipped needle is used to precisely approximate the epidermis by placing the suture in the superficial plane of the skin.

Pedicle separation is accomplished under local anesthesia 3 weeks following initial flap transfer (Figure 10). One percent lidocaine containing epinephrine is injected into the base of the pedicle and circumferentially around the flap where it attaches to the nose followed by the usual sterile preparation and draping. The pedicle is separated with a scalpel at the superior margin of the defect

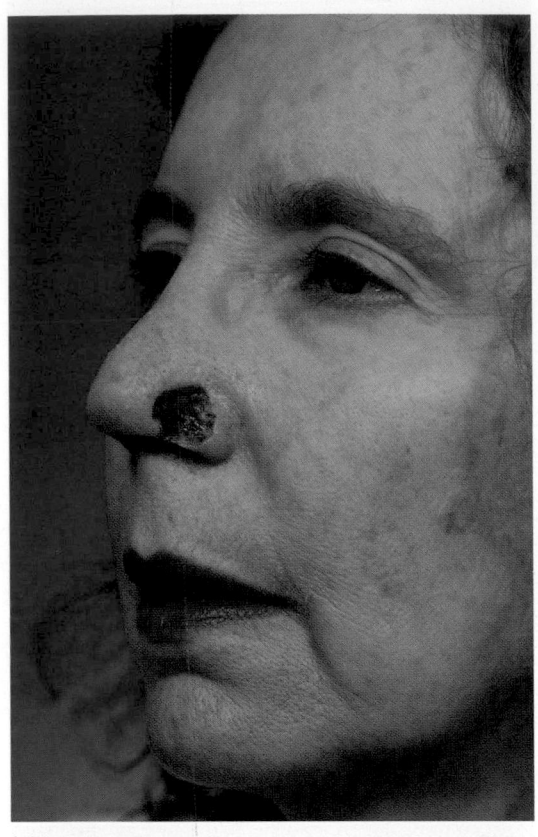

(A)

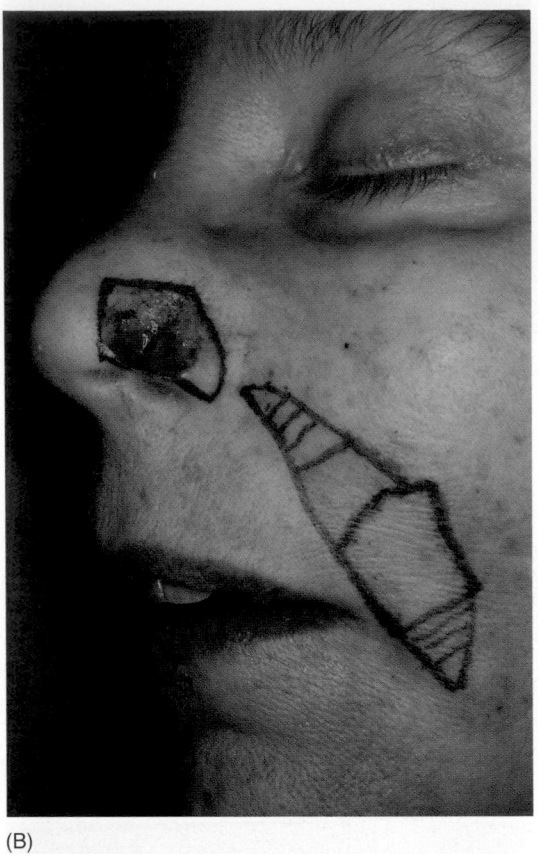

(B)

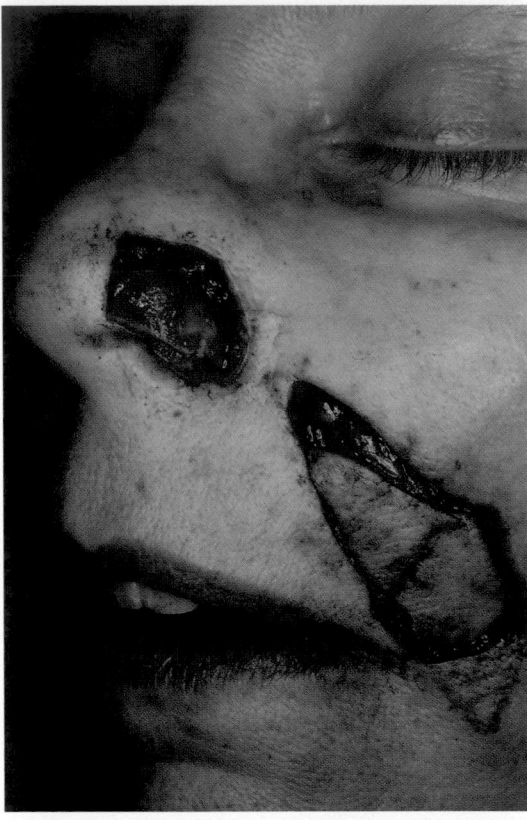

(C)

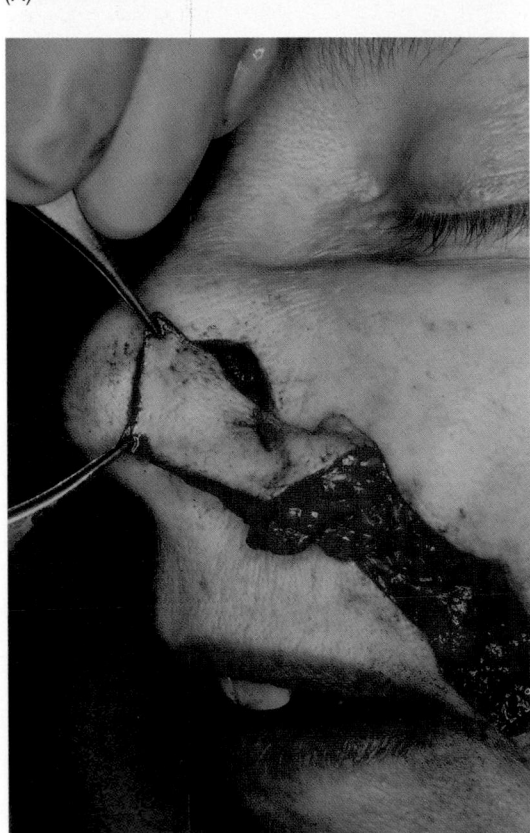

(D)

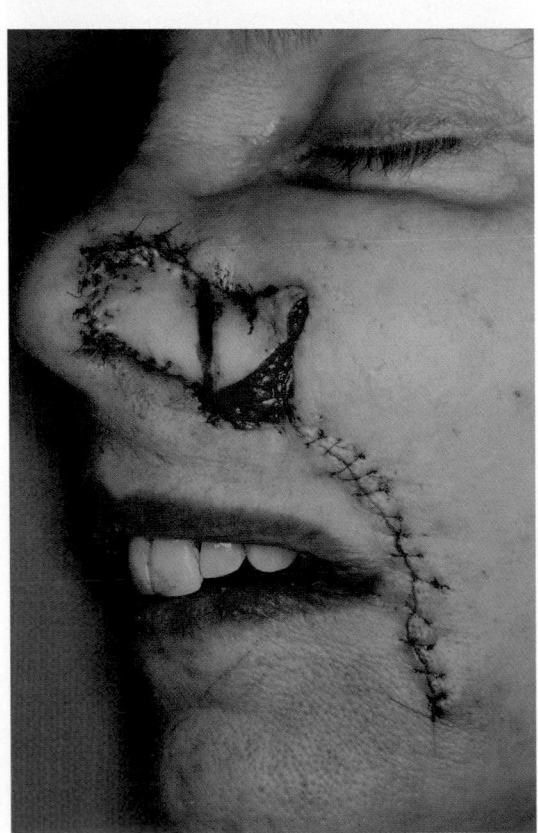

(E)

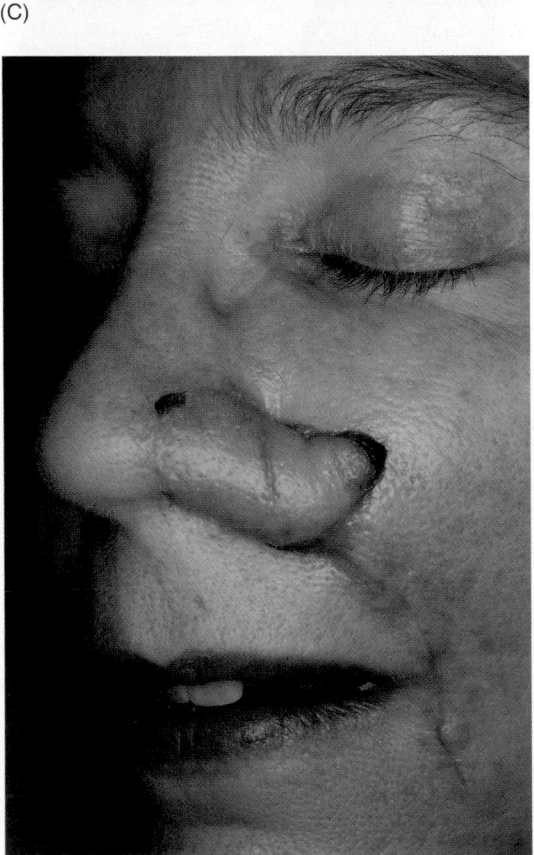

(F)

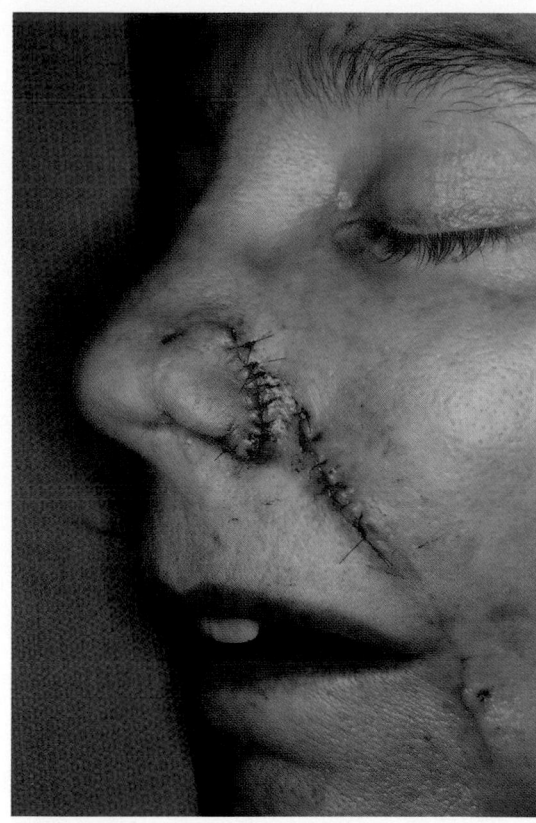

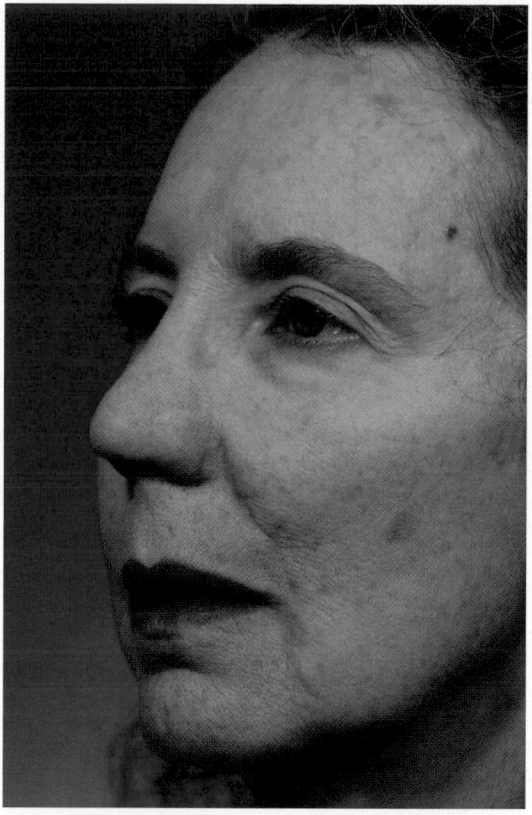

(G)   (H)

Figure 12 (A) Patient with a 1.5 × 1.5 cm deep skin and soft tissue defect of ala. (B) Remaining alar skin marked for resection. Interpolated subcutaneous tissue pedicle melolabial flap designed for external cover. Proximal and distal horizontal lines represent standing cutaneous deformities (SCDs) that will form as donor site is closed. Distal SCD excised at time of wound closure. Proximal SCD transferred with flap and discarded at time of flap inset. (C) Auricular cartilage graft positioned for structural support. Cheek flap incised. (D) Flap based on subcutaneous tissue pedicle. (E) Flap transferred. Donor site closed. (F) Three weeks following flap transfer. (G) Immediately following flap inset. (H) Seven months postoperative.

or higher if additional nasal skin is to be removed from the superior aspect of the aesthetic unit. An incision is made in the cephalic portion of the old scars between the flap and adjacent nasal skin on either side of the pedicle. The extent of this incision should be such that it releases the cephalic quarter of the flap from the nose. This is necessary to provide sufficient exposure for thinning and proper trimming and inset of the flap. The skin margins surrounding the skin defect created by the flap release are undermined 1 cm. Thinning is performed of any portion of the flap left attached to the recipient site that was not adequately thinned at the time of the initial flap transfer. It is often necessary to remove early scar tissue under the flap to facilitate proper tailoring. Deep-layer wound closure is unnecessary because there is no wound closure tension. The flap is inset using interrupted vertical mattress and simple 5-0 cutaneous sutures. An overnight compression dressing is applied.

The base of the pedicle is returned to its donor site to restore the normal distance between the medial aspect of the eyebrows. Just as with the inset of the flap at the recipient site, it is often necessary to remove early scar deposition in the donor area to enable the pedicle to lie flat between the eyebrows. The medial aspect of both eyebrows is undermined for several centimeters to release all contractions. This maneuver enables the surgeon to position the eyebrows in proper relationship to each other and to the superior bony orbital rims.

Typically, the medial aspect of the eyebrow on the flap side is displaced inferiorly as a result of secondary movement from flap transfer. The brow must be mobilized sufficiently to correct malposition. This is accomplished by converting the proximal pedicle of the flap into a small triangular flap incorporating in its base the medial aspect of the eyebrow on the donor side. To accommodate for scar contraction and inferior migration of the eyebrow during healing, the flap is mobilized upward until the level of the horizontal axis of the medial aspect of the eyebrow on the flap side is positioned 2 mm above the level of the horizontal axis of the opposite eyebrow. Pedicle tissue should not be returned to the forehead beyond what is required to position the donor side eyebrow properly. Excess pedicle tissue above the portion of the triangular flap necessary for securing the medial eyebrow in proper position is resected and discarded. To facilitate superior advancement of the triangular flap, and thus the medial aspect of the eyebrow on the donor side, it is sometimes necessary to excise a small crescent or triangular segment of skin just lateral to the base of the flap along the superior medial border of the eyebrow.

DEFECTS EXTENDING BEYOND THE NOSE

Cutaneous defects that involve the nose and significant portions of the medial cheek or upper

lip are reconstructed in stages. The first surgical stage is directed toward repair of the cheek and lip to provide a stable foundation for subsequent reconstruction of the nose. The surgical plan of first restoring the foundation on which to place the constructed nose, before initiating nasal reconstruction, is used whenever a sizeable full thickness defect of the cheek or lip is associated with a full thickness nasal defect.[15] For example, when there is a full thickness loss of the ala or columella and adjacent upper lip, it is prudent to delay reconstruction of the nose until the lip is repaired and scars have contracted to their maximum propensity.

In contrast to full thickness nasal defects, defects of the nose which are not full thickness and which extend into the lip or cheek can usually be reconstructed concurrently. This is because there is less scar contracture surrounding the nose during the healing stages compared with repair of full thickness nasal defects. Thus there are fewer problems with distortion of the constructed segments of the nose. Keeping with the principle of repairing each portion of a defect involving multiple facial aesthetic regions with an independent covering flap, individual flaps are used to reconstruct the cheek, nose, and lip if all three aesthetic regions are involved by the defect. The most common circumstance leading to defects involving the nose, lip, and cheek are skin malignancies arising from the ala and extending into the alar facial sulcus with subsequent growth into the medial cheek and upper lip. Another common circumstance is for the malignancy to arise from the nasal sidewall and extend across the nasal facial sulcus into the medial cheek. The cutaneous defect resulting from resection of this type of neoplasm should be reconstructed with two independent flaps.[16] In such instances; the cheek defect is typically reconstructed with a cheek advancement flap. The flap is advanced medially to the nasal-facial sulcus. The leading border of the flap is secured to the periosteum of the ascending process of the maxilla to prevent the flap from migrating laterally during the healing process. The cheek flap is secured in place first before designing a template for the paramedian forehead flap which is used to resurface the nasal sidewall. If periosteal sutures are inadequate to hold the advancement flap in place, holes are drilled in the exposed bone along the pyriform aperture. These holes are used for anchoring sutures placed along the advancing border of the cheek flap.

DEFECT CLASSIFICATION

Defects of the nose may be classified according to location, depth, and size. Skin only defects are repaired with full thickness skin grafts, local flaps (if the defect is small), or skin transferred form the cheek or forehead.[17] Defects involving loss of skeletal structure require replacement with like tissue. Full-thickness defects of the nose require replacement of the missing lining with flaps harvested from the interior of the nose whenever possible. These defects always require replacement of the missing skeletal framework and thus should be resurfaced with an interpolated paramedian forehead or melolabial flap.

The size of the nasal defect determines the source of the covering flap. In the case of defects greater than 2.0 cm in greatest dimension, there is rarely sufficient residual nasal skin for closure by a local flap of nasal skin without creating undue wound closure tension. Thus, the forehead or cheek is used as a donor site unless the defect is superficial and favorable for repair with a full thickness skin graft.

Reconstruction of Columella

The columella is the most difficult region of the nose to reconstruct. Small defects limited to 1.5 cm in greatest dimension can occasionally be repaired with composite grafts from the auricle in patients who do not use tobacco products or have peripheral vascular disease.[18] The grafts are chilled with ice compresses for 3 days following transfer and systemic steroids are administered for 1 week. It is preferable to allow the initial defect to heal by secondary intention and then

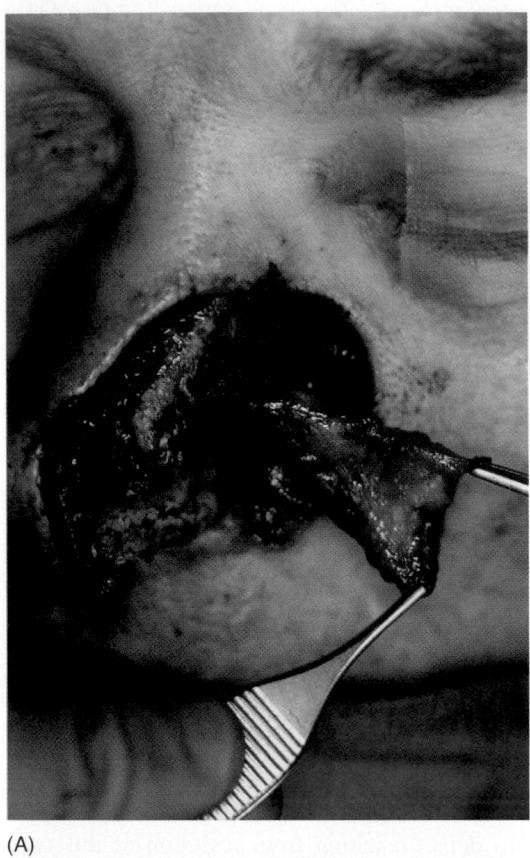

(A)

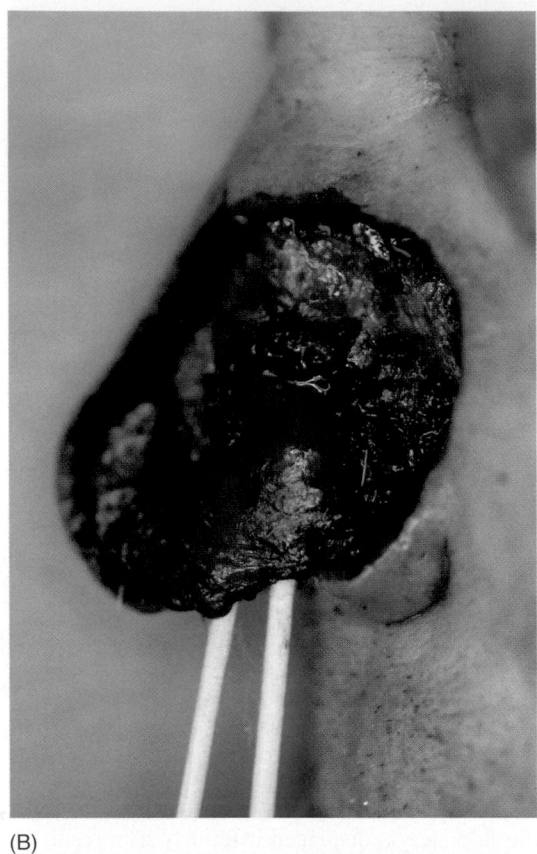

(B)

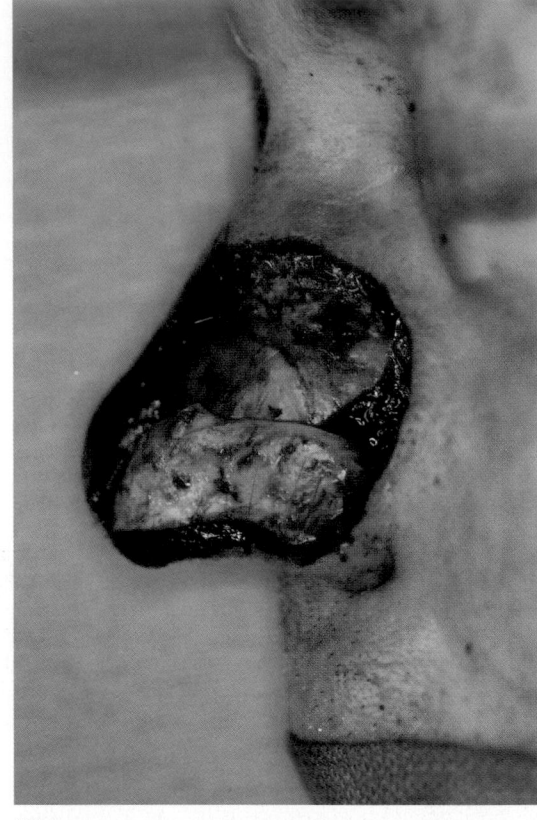

(C)

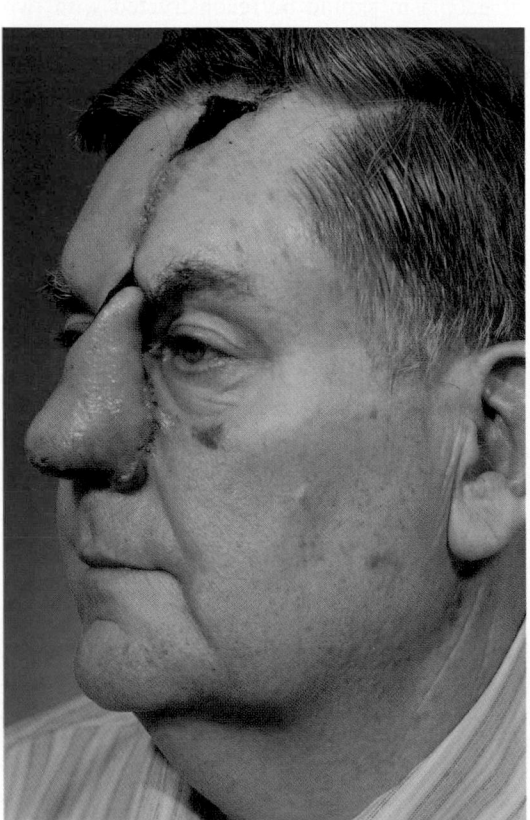

(D)

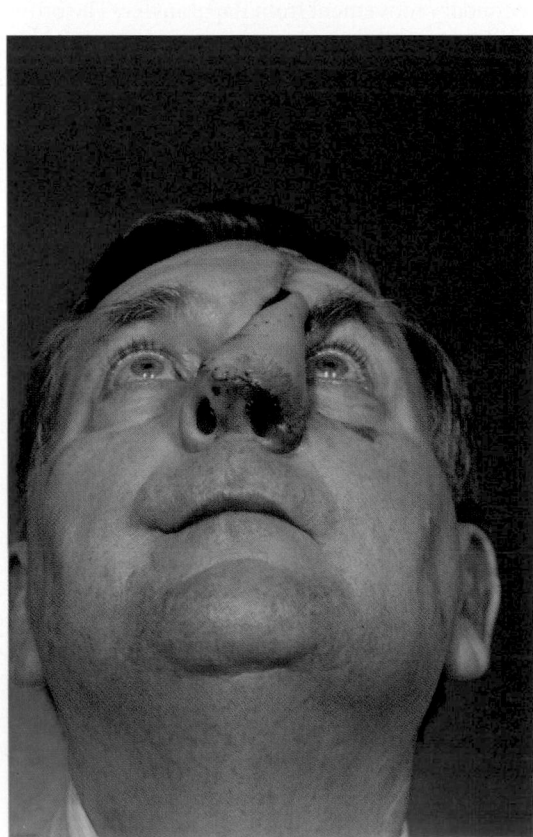

(E)

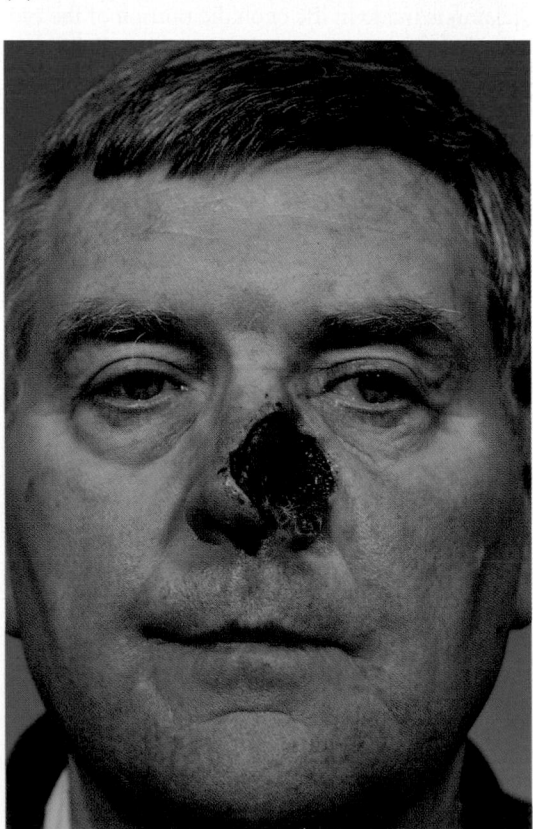

(F)

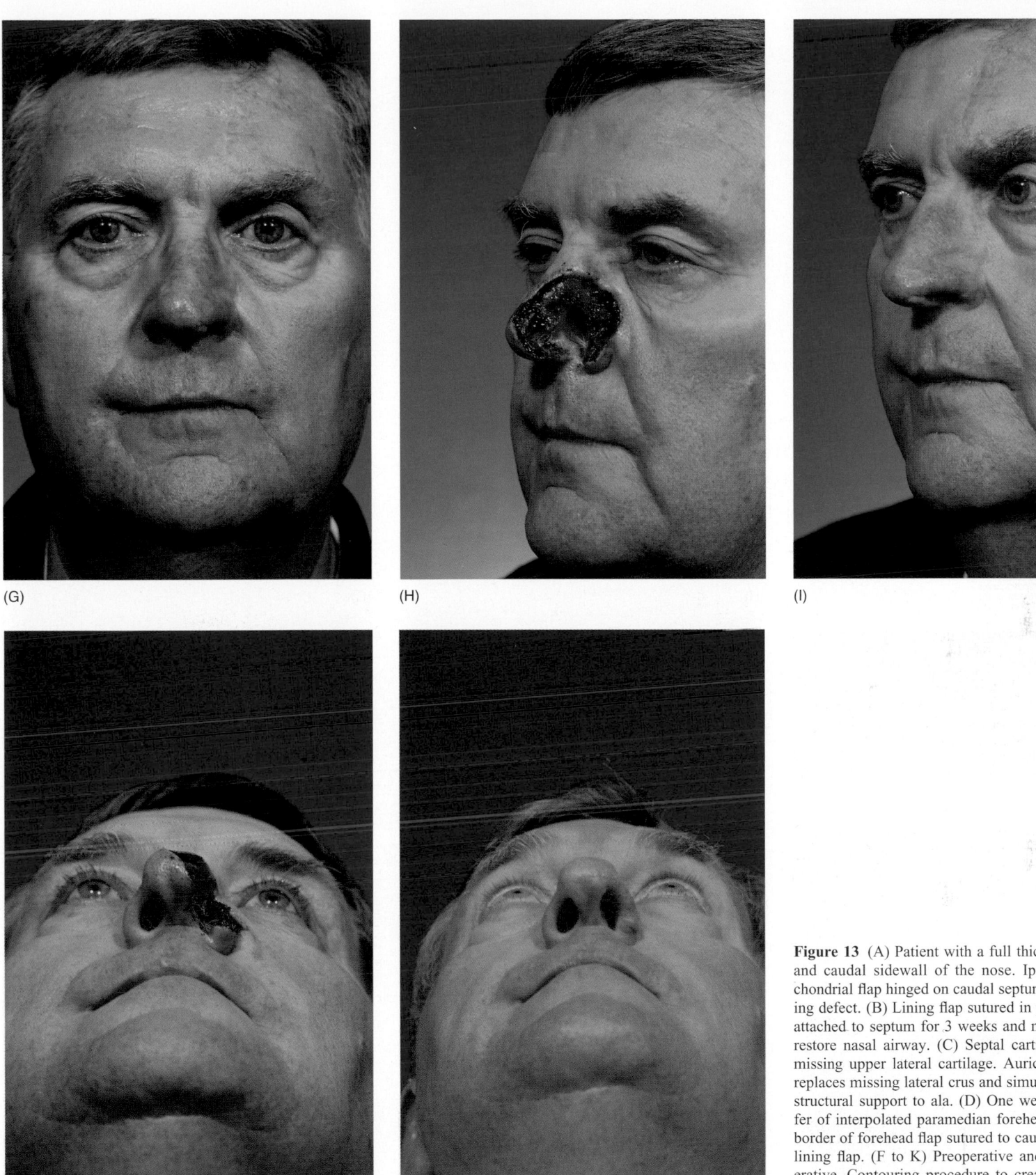

(G)

(H)

(I)

(J)

(K)

Figure 13 (A) Patient with a full thickness defect of ala and caudal sidewall of the nose. Ipsilateral mucoperichondrial flap hinged on caudal septum used to repair lining defect. (B) Lining flap sutured in place. Flap remains attached to septum for 3 weeks and must be detached to restore nasal airway. (C) Septal cartilage graft replaces missing upper lateral cartilage. Auricular cartilage graft replaces missing lateral crus and simultaneously provides structural support to ala. (D) One week following transfer of interpolated paramedian forehead flap. (E) Caudal border of forehead flap sutured to caudal border of septal lining flap. (F to K) Preoperative and 1.5 years postoperative. Contouring procedure to create alar groove and eliminate hair from flap performed 3 months following flap inset.

perform the composite graft after preparing a fresh recipient site by removing all scar and neoepithelialization. The graft is oversized by 2 mm to accommodate for wound contraction.

Depending on extent of tissue loss, larger defects of the columella are best repaired with unilateral or bilateral superiorly based interpolated melolabial flaps.[11] Septal cartilage grafts

are utilized for the framework. The initial flap transfer will create a thick columella, which will require a contouring procedure following inset of the flap. Defects that extend into the tip from the columella require structural support with cartilage grafts and an interpolated paramedian forehead flap for cover. By extending the incision for the forehead flap into or below the eye-

brow, the flap can be made to reach the upper lip without excessive wound closure tension.

Full thickness defects of the columella and tip are best reconstructed with a tilt out, hinge composite nasal septal flap.[19] Mucosa of the flap is peeled downward bilaterally to provide internal lining. Auricular cartilage grafts are attached to the composite flap to provide structural support

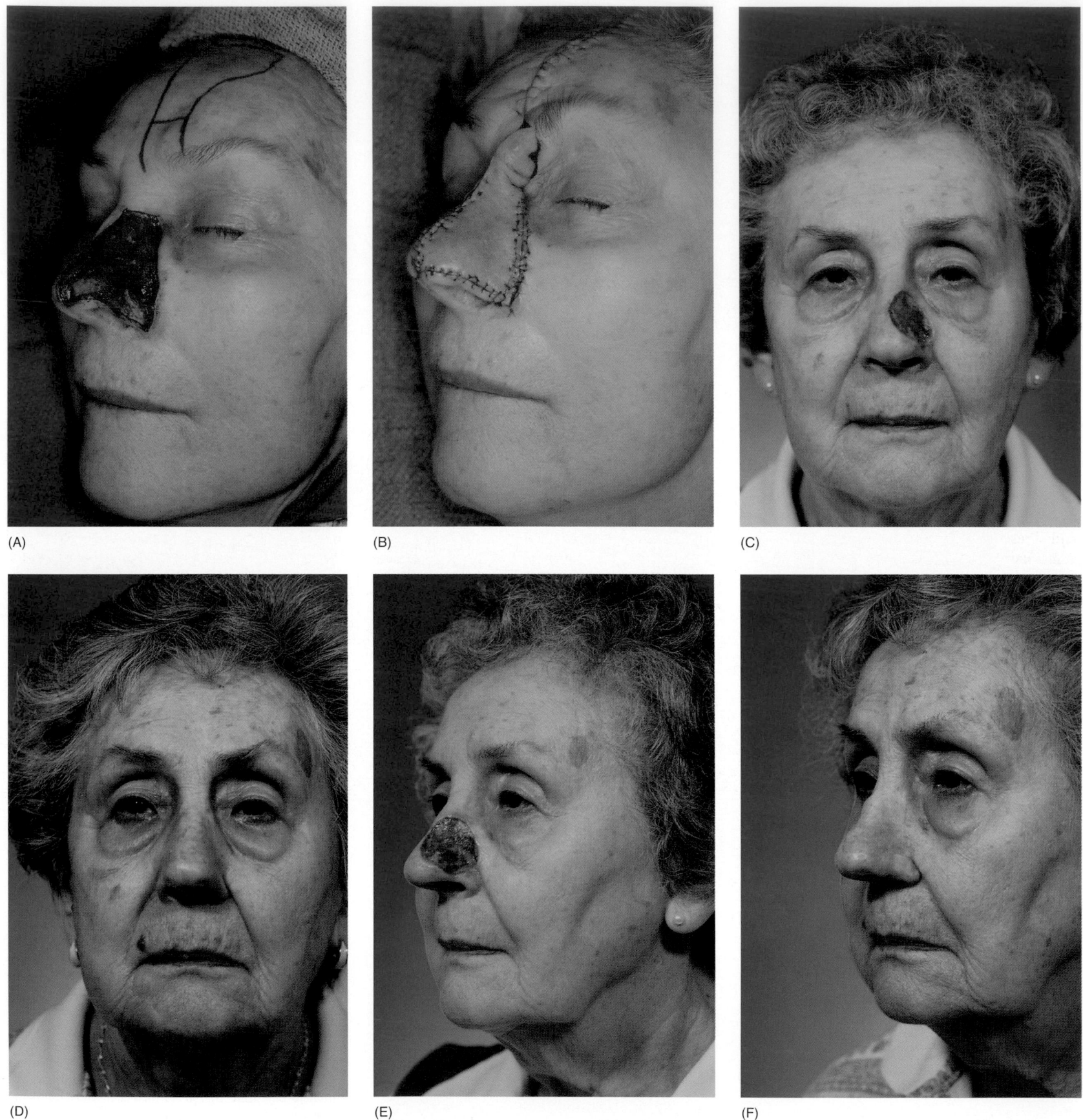

(A)

(B)

(C)

(D)

(E)

(F)

Figure 14 (A) Patient with a 3 × 3 cm skin defect of sidewall with extension to ala and dorsum. Skin of remaining ala and sidewall aesthetic units removed. Auricular cartilage graft in place along margin of nostril. Interpolated paramedian forehead flap designed for external cover. (B) Forehead flap transferred. (C to F) Preoperative and 5 years postoperative. Contouring procedure to create alar groove performed.

laterally. An interpolated paramedian forehead flap is best for exterior covering.

Reconstruction of Nasal Tip

Small skin-only superficial defects of the nasal tip may be repaired with a nasal bilobe flap as

described in detail earlier or a full thickness skin graft.[20] However, an interpolated paramedian forehead flap will usually give a more natural result, because the entire aesthetic unit can be covered by the flap, placing scars in borders of aesthetic units (Figure 11). Cartilage grafts are

used routinely along the margin of the nostril when the defect extends from the tip into the nasal facet. This is in addition to any missing lower lateral cartilage which is replaced as well.

Bilateral full thickness defects of the nasal tip are repaired with a tilt out hinged composite septal flap as discussed.[19] However, the lining of unilateral full thickness defects of the tip can be nicely reconstructed with an ipsilateral intranasal hinge mucoperichondrial flap. The lining flap spans the nasal passage on the affected side. Following restoration of the absent cartilaginous framework, an interpolated paramedian forehead flap provides an external cover replacement. In instances of hemi-tip defect, the author usually only resurfaces the hemi-tip rather than the entire tip. Concomitant with detachment of the forehead flap 3 weeks following transfer, the hinge mucosal flap is released from the septum restoring patency of the nasal airway.

Reconstruction of Ala

Defects confined to the ala with or without limited extension into the nasal tip or sidewall are best resurfaced with an interpolated superiorly based melolabial flap.[11] The author routinely resurfaces the entire ala regardle ss of the size of the alar defect if a cheek flap is utilized for resurfacing the ala[4] (Figure 12). The melolabial flap based on a subcutaneous pedicle is preferred, since this design minimizes the amount of skin that is disturbed in the superior melolabial fold. Preserving the superior fold is paramount in maintaining symmetry of the cheeks following reconstruction of the ala with a cheek flap. Cartilage grafts are used when repairing the majority of alar defects.[21] This is because most lesions involving resection of alar skin also require removal of the underlying firm fibrofatty subdermal tissue which provides the ala with form and structural support. This support is replaced by cartilage to prevent upward migration of the ala or medial constriction of the margin of the reconstructed nostril.

Internal lining for full thickness alar defects is provided by a bipedicle vestibular skin flap or unilateral hinge septal mucoperichondrial flap[19] (Figure 13). Occasionally an additional contralateral hinge mucoperichondrial flap, as discussed in the earlier portion of this chapter, may be necessary. This flap is required when the vertical height of the lining defect is such that an ipsilateral hinged mucoperichondrial flap will not provide sufficient tissue to replace the entire missing lining. When ipsilateral flaps are used to line defects of the ala or tip, they traverse the nasal passage and block the airway. To restore the airway, the pedicle is detached from the septum 3 weeks following transfer of the flap. Redundant tissue is trimmed and the distal portion of the flap is left in situ.

Reconstruction of Nasal Dorsum

The nasal dorsum is perhaps the least complex portion of the nose to reconstruct. Forehead skin in the form of an interpolated paramedian forehead flap is usually preferred for resurfacing skin only defects of the caudal dorsum. However, bilobe flaps or full thickness skin grafts may also be used. Likewise, skin defects of the cephalic dorsum can be repaired with glabellar flaps such as the dorsal nasal flap or full thickness skin grafts, but interpolated paramedian forehead flaps are preferred for extensive defects that involve cartilage or bone and for large defects with loss of most of the skin of the dorsum.[22] Small defects of the dorsal framework are replaced with septal cartilage grafts. More extensive defects of the nasal skeleton extending from the frontal bone to the tip are best replaced with calvarial bone grafts secured to the frontal bone or remaining nasal processes of the maxillae with plate and screw fixation.[23] Costal cartilage grafts may also be used for this purpose. To prevent medialization of the nasal sidewall during wound healing, structural defects that extend into the nasal sidewall require replacement concurrent with replacement of the dorsal framework. Septal cartilage or additional cranial bone grafts plated to the dorsal graft work well for this purpose. Internal lining for full thickness dorsal nasal defects can usually be provided by mucoperichondrial hinge flaps reflected laterally from the exposed dorsum so long as there is sufficient height to the remaining septum. Unilateral or bilateral hinge septal mucoperichondrial flaps based on the caudal septum and including the septal branch of the labial artery can sometimes be used for lining when there is considerable loss of septal height. A tilt out composite septal flap, as discussed earlier in this chapter, is used to provide lining and structural support for the nasal bridge in extensive bilateral full thickness dorsal nasal defects. In instances where this approach will not provide sufficient tissue, bilateral paramedian forehead flaps are recommended. One flap provides internal lining and the other provides external coverage.[24] A cranial bone graft is placed between the flaps for structural support.

Reconstruction of Nasal Sidewall

Reconstruction of the sidewall of the nose, is relatively uncomplicated. Small skin-only defects may be repaired with a bilobe flap harvested from the remaining nasal sidewall skin. Full thickness skin grafts harvested from the clavicular area of the anterior chest also provide a reasonable option for covering defects located in the superior portion of the sidewall, because of the thin skin in this location. Larger surface defects are best covered with an interpolated paramedian forehead flap (Figure 14). When structural support is absent from the cephalic one-third of the nasal sidewall, it is replaced with a calvarial bone graft, while the caudal two-thirds of the sidewall skeleton is best replaced with septal cartilage grafts. Unilateral full thickness sidewall defects can be lined using contralateral hinged septal mucoperichondrial flaps based on the nasal dorsum and delivered through a superiorly positioned nasal septal fenestrum. For more caudally located full thickness sidewall defects, a unilateral mucoperichondrial flap hinged on the caudal septum may provide sufficient lining. This arrangement, however, requires subsequent detachment of the pedicle. It is usually necessary to use both a contralateral dorsally based flap and an ipsilateral caudally based septal flap to provide lining for full thickness defects that involve the ala and extend cephalically to include the entire length of the nasal sidewall.

SUMMARY

Reconstruction of the nose has over the last decade progressed to a new level of finesse that allows the surgeon to restore near normal form and function to all but the most extensive defects of the nose. These advances are based on the contemporary concepts of respecting the borders of aesthetic units of the nose. The nose is reconstructed separately from any extension of a nasal defect into the cheek or lip, which in turn is repaired by tissue within their respective aesthetic region. The other concept that has contributed to this higher level of surgical achievement is the policy of replacing missing tissue with like tissue. Internal lining is replaced with intranasal mucoperichondrial flaps which because of their nature provide adequate vascularity to nourish and sustain the cartilage and bone grafts used in skeletal replacement. Missing bone and cartilage are replaced with similar tissue, which is carefully crafted to replicate the exact size, configuration, and contour of the missing nasal skeleton. Surface defects are covered with cheek or forehead skin transferred by interpolation so as not to violate the aesthetic boundary between nose and other aesthetic regions of the face. This surgical approach provides natural building material precisely fitted to reconstruct nasal deficits so that the restored nose is as near normal as possible.

REFERENCES

1. Burget GC, Menick FJ. Nasal support and lining: The marriage of beauty and blood supply. Plast Surg 1989; 84:189–203.
2. Menick FJ. Reconstruction of the nose. In: Swanson NA, Baker SR, editors. Local Flaps in Facial Reconstruction. St. Louis: Mosby; 1995. p. 305–37.
3. Burget GC, Menick FJ. Aesthetic Reconstruction of the Nose. St. Louis: Mosby; 1993.
4. Baker SR, Johnson TM, Nelson BR. The importance of maintaining the alar-facial sulcus in nasal reconstruction. Arch Otolaryngol Head Neck Surg 1995;121:617–22.
5. Baker SR. Contemporary aspects of nasal reconstruction. In: Myer E, Krause CJ, editors. Advances in Otolaryngology-Head and Neck Surgery, Volume 12. St. Louis: Mosby; 1998. p. 235–61.
6. Baker SR. Principles of Nasal Reconstruction. St. Louis: Mosby; 1995.
7. Zitelli JA. Bilobe flaps. In: Baker SR, Swanson NA, editors. Local Flaps in Facial Reconstruction. St. Louis: Mosby; 1995. p. 165–80.
8. Zitelli JA. The bilobe flap for nasal reconstruction. Arch Dermatol 1989;125:957–9.
9. Baker SR. Nasal cutaneous flaps. In: Baker SR, editor. Principles of Nasal Reconstruction. St. Louis: Mosby; 2002. p. 103–20.
10. Sheen JH, Sheen A, editors. Aesthetic Rhinoplasty, 2nd edition. St. Louis: Mosby; 2002. p. 255.
11. Baker SR. Interpolated cheek flaps: Reconstruction of the alar and columellar units. In: Baker SR, editor. Principles of Nasal Reconstruction. St. Louis: Mosby; 2002. p.153–70.
12. Baker SR, Alford EL. Mid-forehead flaps, operative technique. Otolaryngol Head Neck Surg 1993;4:24–30.

13. Menick FJ. Aesthetic refinements in use of the forehead flap for nasal reconstruction: The paramedian forehead flap. Clin Plast Surg 1990;17:607–22.

14. Baker SR. Interpolated paramedian forehead flaps. In: Baker SR, editor. Principles of Nasal Reconstruction. St. Louis: Mosby; 2002. p.171–95.

15. Baker SR. Reconstruction of ala, cheek, and upper lip. In: Baker SR, editor. Principles of Nasal Reconstruction. St. Louis: Mosby; 2002. p. 284–8.

16. Baker SR. Reconstruction of nasal dorsum, sidewall, cheek and medial orbit. In: Baker SR, editor. Principles of Nasal Reconstruction. St. Louis: Mosby; 2002. p. 289–95.

17. Naficy S. External covering. In: Baker SR, editor. Principles of Nasal Reconstruction. St. Louis: Mosby; 2002. p. 58–70.

18. Jewett BS. Skin and composite grafts. In: Baker SR, editor. Principles of Nasal Reconstruction. St. Louis: Mosby; 2002. p. 89–102.

19. Baker SR. Internal lining. In: Baker SR, editor. Principles of Nasal Reconstruction. St. Louis: Mosby; 2002. p. 31–46.

20. Baker SR. Reconstruction of lateral tip: Two methods of repair. In: Baker SR, editor. Principles of Nasal Reconstruction. St. Louis: Mosby; 2002. p. 224–30.

21. Naficy S. Structural support. In: Baker SR, editor. Principles of Nasal Reconstruction. St. Louis: Mosby; 2002. p. 47–57.

22. Baker SR. Reconstruction of nasal sidewall and dorsum. In: Baker SR, editor. Principles of Nasal Reconstruction. St. Louis: Mosby; 2002. p. 269–74.

23. Baker SR. Near-total nasal reconstruction. In: Baker SR, editor. Principles of Nasal Reconstruction. St. Louis: Mosby; 2002. p. 275–83.

24. Baker SR. Bilateral paramedian forehead flaps. In: Baker SR, editor. Principles of Nasal Reconstruction. St. Louis: Mosby; 2002. p. 263–8.

55

Facial Fractures

Paul J. Donald, MD

High-speed auto travel, increased sports participation by people of all ages and both genders, and the high incidence of violent crime continue to make facial fractures important injuries in our society. Contrary to the pattern of care in other countries, the management of facial fractures in the United States spreads across the disciplines of oral surgery, plastic surgery, and otolaryngology. Due to the comprehensive training in head and neck anatomy and physiology, the otolaryngologist is uniquely prepared to deal with these injuries. It is vitally important for the otolaryngologist to have a working knowledge of dental occlusion, facial esthetics, and an understanding of the healing of membranous bone.

The first encounter with the patient with a facial fracture is usually in the emergency department. Attention to the standard airway-breathing-circulation of emergency medical management must be invoked immediately. The patient is often the victim of an accident that involves many body systems, and almost always, attention to these injuries takes precedence. Addressing the impaired airway is preeminent. Extensive soft tissue contusion, bilateral mandibular body fractures, and Le Fort fractures of the maxilla can all result in airway obstruction. In mandibular fractures, a nasotracheal intubation is appropriate; however, in maxillary fractures there is always a risk of fracture to the cribriform plate or the fovea ethmoidalis. Since intubation by the nasal route presents the danger of intracranial passage of the tube, oral intubation, cricothyroidotomy, or tracheostomy should be used to secure the airway. Fractures of the facial skeleton rarely present with life-threatening hemorrhage. The only time in the author's experience, in which a problem of serious hemorrhage occurred, was in an instance of a Le Fort III fracture in which both internal maxillary arteries were severed. An associated fracture of the temporal bone rarely ruptures the petrous portion of the internal carotid artery and a fracture through the basisphenoid bone rarely tears the cavernous portion of the internal carotid artery.

A "C" collar is most often immediately placed on the patient to prevent displacement of a possible cervical spine fracture. After the patient's condition has been stabilized, careful physical and radiographic examination of the cervical spine must be performed to rule out cervical spine injury. At this point, a careful evaluation of the other important systems is performed.

Treatment of the patient with facial trauma should include a thorough history and physical examination to determine the location and extent of all injuries.[1] The goal of treatment of patients with craniomaxillofacial injuries should be reconstitution of all injured regions.[2] Both soft tissue and bony injuries should be assessed, and a treatment plan should be established. The goals of treatment should be the restoration of function and appearance. The premorbid form and function of dental, skeletal, and soft tissues should be reestablished as much as is possible. Recent photographs and dental records, if available, are most helpful to establish the pretraumatic appearance.

If the initial injury involves skin or mucosal lacerations, attempts should be made to utilize these lacerations when possible for the approach to fracture repair. If no epithelial injury is present, approaches to fractures should attempt to maximize exposure, while minimizing scarring and risk to adjacent neural and vascular structures.

As much as possible, a thorough history is taken. Often, these patients have suffered multiple injuries and may be either unconscious or intubated. Information may be gleaned from friends or relatives at the scene or the police or ambulance attendants. Physical examination includes a careful inspection of dental occlusion, examination of the facial contour, and palpation of the facial bones. A computed tomography (CT) scan of the facial skeleton is crucial in securing the correct diagnosis.

After fracture diagnosis is completed, a systematic treatment plan is established. Surgical treatment of facial fractures involves adequate exposure, meticulous reduction, and stable fracture fixation. Surgical approaches should utilize transmucosal incisions or incisions that are camouflaged in relaxed skin tension lines (RSTL) or at the junctions of facial aesthetic units.[3] The incision and approach chosen must not compromise the basic principle of providing adequate exposure for diagnosis and treatment of any fracture. After exposing the facial fracture, meticulous reduction must be performed and maintained until adequate fixation of the fracture can be done. Precise reduction is imperative when rigid fixation is utilized. Fixation techniques should allow for complete bone healing with reconstitution in three dimensions: height (superior–inferior), width (lateral–medial), and depth or projection (anterior–posterior).

Repair of soft tissue injuries is often as important as fracture treatment in the complete restoration of the patient with craniomaxillofacial injuries. This is especially true in the periorbital region, where injuries such as telecanthus, enophthalmos, and dysopsia often accompany the skeletal injury. Complete treatment of facial injuries requires attention to these soft tissue injuries and the accurate reattachment of soft tissue fascial layers after fracture repair.

The basic principles of diagnosis and initial treatment of patients with facial fractures are listed in Table 1. The principles of fracture repair are listed in Table 2. Adherence to these principles will maximize function and appearance.

DENTAL OCCLUSION

The key to proper fracture reduction is the restoration of the patient's premorbid occlusion. Understanding dental occlusion is an essential element in the management of facial fractures. Dental occlusion is the relationship of the maxillary to the mandibular teeth with regard to their cutting and grinding surfaces. This relationship largely depends on the relative position of the teeth and their angulation to one another. In 1899, Angle described three basic types of occlusion.[4] Certain subtypes of this system as well as other classifications of occlusion have been devised, sometimes adding to the confusion rather than clarifying the problem. In the Angle system, the

Table 1 Principles of Diagnosis and Initial Treatment of Facial Fractures

Establishment and securing airway
Control of bleeding
Detailed history
Careful physical examination

Table 2 Principles of Fracture Repair

Repair of both skeletal and soft tissue injuries
Use of lacerations when possible
Use of mucosal incisions when possible
Exposure of all fractures adequately for fracture reduction
Reduction of all fractures
Stabilization of fractures
Fixation of all fractures adequately to allow bone healing

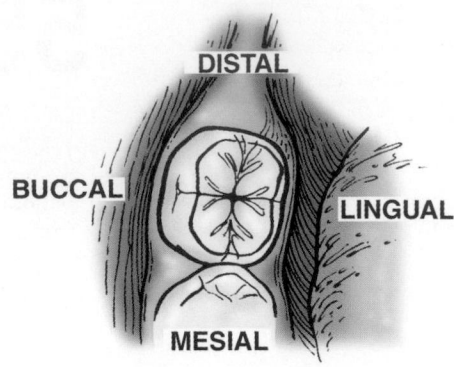

Figure 1 Orientation of molar cusps. (Reproduced with permission from reference 5.)

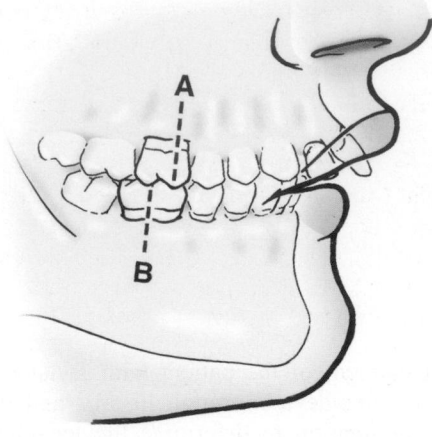

Figure 3 Class II occlusion. (A) Mesial buccal cusp of first maxillar molar. (B) Buccal intercuspal groove of mandibular first molar. (Reproduced with permission from reference 5.)

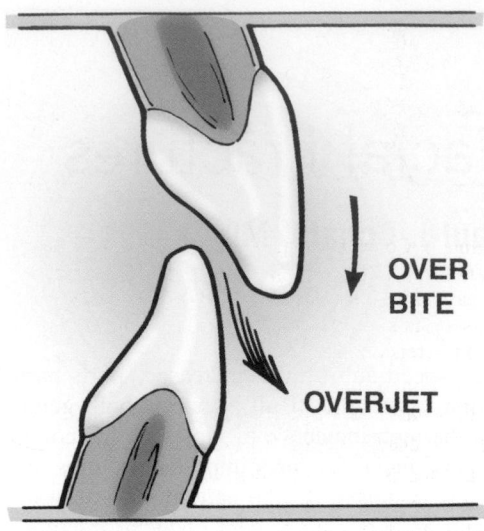

Figure 5 Cuspal relationships of central maxillary incisor with central mandibular incisor. Direction of overbite and overjet are indicated (*arrows*). (Reproduced with permission from reference 5.)

reference point is the relationship of the first maxillary molar tooth to the mandibular molar tooth below it. Each molar commonly has four grinding surfaces called cusps. The cusps adjacent to the tongue are called lingual and those adjacent to the cheek, buccal. Those cusps situated toward the oropharynx in the posterior aspect of the oral cavity are described as distal, and those located more anteriorly are mesial (Figure 1).

Class I occlusion is the ideal form (Figure 2). In this type, the mesial buccal cusp of the first maxillary molar fits in the groove on the lateral or buccal surface of the first mandibular molar tooth. The buccal cusps of the maxillary teeth overlap the buccal surfaces of the mandibular molars.

In Class II occlusion, the mesial buccal cusp of the first maxillary molar is mesial, in front of the buccal groove of the first mandibular molar (Figure 3). It may be over the first mandibular molar's mesial cusp or between it and the second premolar (bicuspid).

In Class III occlusion, the reverse of Class II is seen. The mesial buccal cusp of the first maxillary molar is distal to the corresponding mandibular molar's distal cusp or between it and the second molar (Figure 4).

Usually, these relationships are maintained in the remaining teeth as progression toward the

anterior aspect of the dental arches occurs. In Class II and III occlusion, this progression results in aberrations in the relationship of the incisor teeth as reflected in characteristic facial deformities.

In Class II, the mesial or anterior relationship of the maxillary teeth may result in a protrusion of the upper incisors beyond the lower. Not only is there a jutting forward of these upper central teeth, a condition called overjet, but often the lower incisors may bite more deeply toward the palate, a condition called overbite (Figure 5). This condition produces a profile described as "bucktooth" or "weak-chin." This look is caricatured in the cartoon characters "Andy Gump" and "Sad Sack." When the condition is due to a lack of mandibular development with a backward positioning of the lower jaw, it is called retrognathism. The setback chin often prevents the upper lip from completely covering the upper incisor teeth. This lack of lip protection, called lip procumbency, can render the incisors more

vulnerable to injury. Fractured incisors are often found in this group.

Often in Class III occlusion, an abnormally protrusive mandible causes maxillary incisors to sit behind or distal to the mandibular incisors. This produces a so-called bulldog or Dick Tracy profile. The overbite results in the upper incisors biting into the gingival lingual sulcus below. The malocclusion is often so severe the patient has an extremely difficult time chewing solid food. Often only two or three cuspal pairs are able to occlude. In edentulous patients, it is often exceedingly difficult to fit them with a denture.

The opposite of the closed bite of overbite deformities is the open bite. This may be seen in both class II and class III types of malocclusion. This open bite deformity produces a marked functional disturbance and is extremely unsightly. Even though the molar teeth are in some form of apposition, the anterior teeth never meet.

Class II malocclusions may arise from an underdeveloped mandible or an abnormally protuberant maxilla. Similarly, a Class III malocclusion may arise from a large overdeveloped mandible or a retruded or retroplaced maxilla. Retrognathia is classically used to describe a Class II bite, and prognathism to describe a Class III bite.

In addition to aberrations in the anteroposterior relationship of the dentition are deformities involving malposition in the medial and lateral direction, as well as abnormalities involving a lateral tilt of the occlusal plane. Instead of having their buccal cusps positioned lateral to the buccal face of the opposing mandibular molars, the maxillary molar teeth may be biting end to end or even over the lingual cusps of the mandibular teeth (Figure 6). This is called a lingual crossbite deformity. If both arches are symmetric, the maxillary molars of the opposing side will be put into a more buccal relationship with the opposing mandibular teeth, thereby creating a buccal crossbite

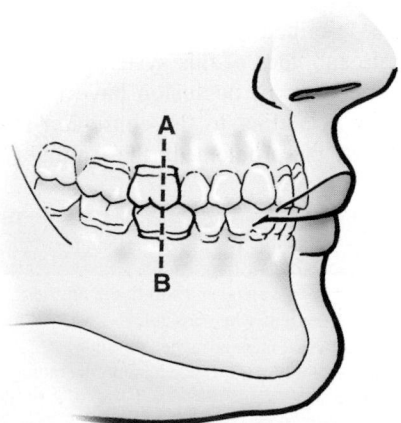

Figure 2 Class I occlusion. (A) Mesial buccal cusp of first maxillary molar. (B) Buccal intercuspal groove of mandibular first molar. (Reproduced with permission from reference 5.)

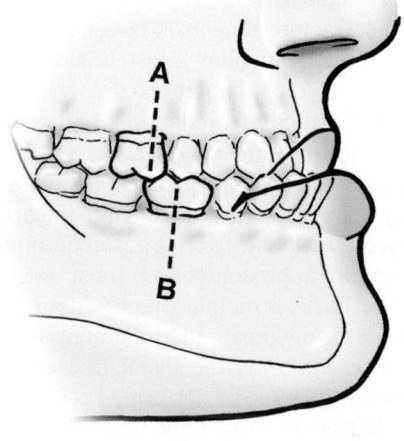

Figure 4 Class III occlusion. (A) Mesial buccal cusp of first maxillary molar. (B) Buccal intercuspal groove of mandibular first molar. (Reproduced with permission from reference 5.)

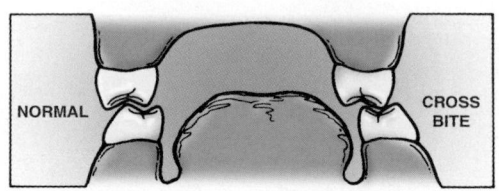

Figure 6 Coronal view of oral cavity showing normal relationship (*left*) with maxillary buccal cusp related to buccal surface of underlying molar. Example of lingual crossbite is shown (*right*). (Reproduced with permission from reference 5.)

on this particular side. Because an abnormality in the arch configuration of either or both of the dental arches is often present, it is not uncommon to have a crossbite on one side with a fairly normal occlusal relationship on the other. For instance, a narrow maxillary arch coupled with a fairly normal mandibular arch, as seen in hemimandibular hypoplasia, often produces a buccal crossbite on one side and normal occlusion on the other. In patients with hypoplasia, the plane of the bite is often abnormal as well. These patients normally have a diagonal bite. When they bite down on a tongue blade placed laterally across the teeth, the blade tilts at an angle that is oblique to the horizontal plane (Figure 7). It is not uncommon to see a combination of many of these occlusal abnormalities in any given patient.

FRACTURES OF THE MANDIBLE

Anatomy

The mandible, a horseshoe-shaped bone, is the largest bone of the face. It is divided into regions well described by Dingman and Natvig.[6] The condyle is the portion extending from the mandibular notch to the condylar head, which articulates in the glenoid fossa. The coronoid process is the anterior–superior extension of the mandibular ramus projecting above the mandibular notch into the infratemporal fossa. Below the mandibular notch is the ramus, which is composed of thin cortical bone. The angle is a non-tooth-bearing portion of the mandible between the ramus and the body. The parasymphyseal region is composed of the anterior arch of the mandible and is bounded by the two mental foramina. The body and the

parasymphyseal areas are where the teeth are found. The alveolar ridge or process is composed of thin cortical bone (lamina dura) that encompasses the teeth and atrophies when the teeth are gone.[6] In the edentulous mandible, the tooth-bearing bone resorbs, decreasing mandibular height.

The inferior alveolar nerve enters on the medial (lingual) aspect of the mandibular ramus and passes through its own canal to the mental foramen. While traversing this canal, it gives off sensory innervation to the dentition and gingival. The terminal portion of the inferior alveolar nerve is the mental nerve which exits the body of the mandible on the labial surface just below the second premolar tooth. It is important to remember that the nerve travels about 2 to 3 mm anteriorly beyond the foramen before it doubles back and exits the bone. It provides sensation to the lower lip and ipsilateral chin. After a fracture of the angle and body, the alveolar canal is often fractured. Unless there is a complete transection or avulsion of the nerve, full sensation often returns within 9 months to 1 year.

The muscles of mastication inserting on the mandible include the temporalis, internal pterygoid, external pterygoid, and masseter. These muscles contribute to the movement of the temporomandibular joint (TMJ), a synovial joint with both a hinge and a gliding action. This joint contains a capsule with a fibrocartilaginous disk. The capsule is densely innervated with proprioceptive and sensory fibers, which are extremely sensitive to subtle changes in movement of one or both joints. A slight alteration in occlusion from muscle spasm or a displaced fracture may alter the central perception of joint position. Feedback loops in the central nervous system force the contralateral muscles of mastication to compensate. This series of events may lead to chronic TMJ syndrome in an unrepaired or poorly repaired mandible fracture.

Understanding the various attachments of the aforementioned muscles of mastication, as well as the mylohyoid, geniohyoid, genioglossus, and digastric muscles, is important in understanding the forces of displacement in a mandible fracture. The floor of the mouth and extrinsic tongue muscles tend to displace fractures posteriorly and inferiorly. The medial pterygoid and masseter muscles act as a sling in the posterior part of the body and angle area and tend to elevate a displaced fragment of the angle or posterior part of the body. Condylar fractures are displaced by the pull of the lateral pterygoid muscle, which rotates and dislocates the fracture medially.[7]

Classification

Fractures of the mandible may be classified according to specific characteristics and anatomic location. A fracture is considered simple when both the external skin and oral mucosa are intact, or compound (open) when a laceration in the skin or intraoral mucosa is present. If the patient is dentulous and the fracture line passes into the tooth root, the fracture is theoretically compound because the periodontal pocket of that tooth often extends to the fracture site. If the fracture is incomplete and involves only one cortex, it is termed "greenstick." The comminuted mandible fracture is one with several fragments of bone. Mandibular fractures are most commonly characterized by anatomic location (Figure 8). The most frequent location of fractures of the mandible is the condylar-subcondylar region. Other common sites include the body and the angle. The coronoid process is rarely fractured. An alveolar ridge fracture involves the occlusal surface of a part of the mandible, but does not extend into the inferior cortical surface (Figure 9).

Mandibular fractures can also be classified as dentulous, edentulous, or pediatric. The last category is important because of the vulnerability of unerupted dentition and the conical shape of the teeth, which do not hold a wire ligature well. The accuracy in approximation of the edentulous mandible is not as critical in a jaw without teeth as is the exacting task of establishing the preinjury occlusion of the dentulous mandible. A denture can compensate for minor irregularities in the edentulous jaw.

The final classification may be made according to the stability of the fracture. Vertical instability is lent by virtue of the pull of the temporalis, masseter, and pterygoid muscles. The angle of pull of these muscles will tend to impact a jaw fracture that is obliquely inclined from distal to mesial, (posterior to anterior), rendering it stable. On the other hand, if the inclination is in the opposite direction, then the forces of these muscles will distract the distal segment in a superior and medial direction. An interesting situation presents itself regarding an unfavorably inclined fracture in the distal body, near the angle, just anterior to the third molar tooth. While the tooth is present, the fracture will not dislocate, but, if the tooth is then extracted, the fracture becomes unstable (Figure 10). A fracture becomes horizontally unstable by virtue of its obliquity in the occlusal plane. A fracture with an angulation running

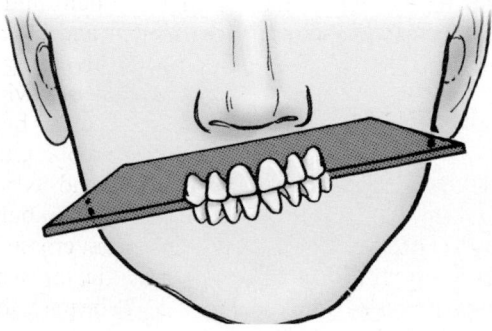

Figure 7 Obliquely oriented bite. (Reproduced with permission from reference 5.)

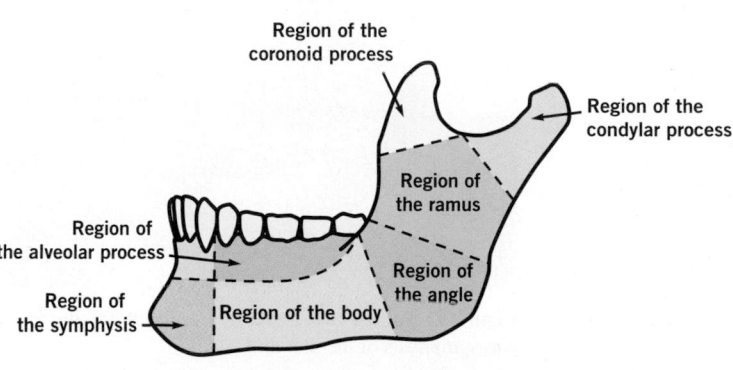

Figure 8 Schematic diagram of the regions of the mandible. The canine line can be seen to distinguish the parasymphyseal region from the body of the mandible. (Reproduced with permission from reference 6.)

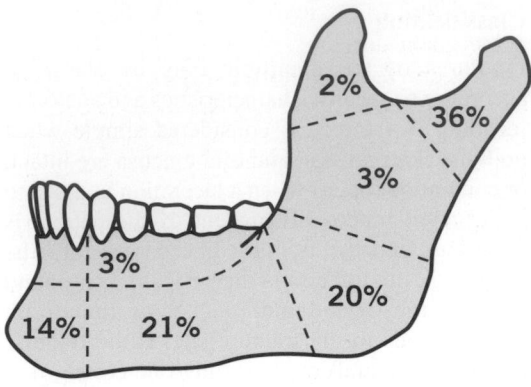

Figure 9 Schematic diagram of fractures of the mandible according to the incidence of fracture. (Reproduced with permission from reference 6.)

from the buccal to lingual surface in a posterior to anterior direction is favorably aligned, whereas the opposing obliquity is unstable by virtue of the pull of the mylohoid muscle (Figure 11).

Diagnosis of Mandibular Fractures

A good history and physical examination, along with plain radiographic films, fully delineate the large majority of fractures to the mandible. When obtaining the history, determine the nature of the injury, and the force with which it was applied. If the fracture is the result of a gunshot wound, then it is necessary to know the weapon's caliber and the nature of the bullet type. Previous orthodontic work should be noted. Any history of previous mandible or maxillary fractures should also be elicited. Questions should be directed toward establishing the neurologic status of the patient as well as the status of the cervical spine. Frequently, a patient presenting with a mandible fracture has other associated facial fractures. Questions regarding pain, hearing, vision, and facial disharmony involving areas other than the mandible are pertinent.

A mandible fracture may cause the patient to complain of malocclusion, for example, "My teeth don't come together right." Displacement of the maxillary or mandibular teeth of even less than 1 mm can cause severe patient complaints because of the proprioceptive fibers in the

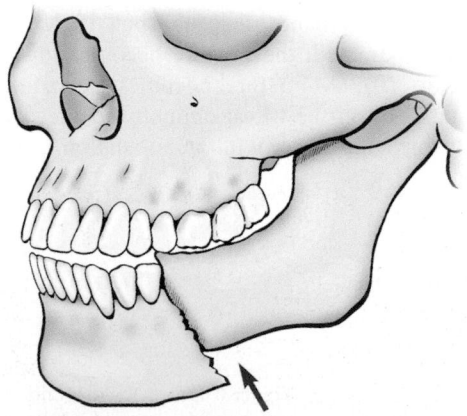

Figure 10 Diagram illustrating how absence of teeth in the distal segment of an unfavorably aligned mandibular fracture will result in displacement. (Reproduced with permission from reference 6.)

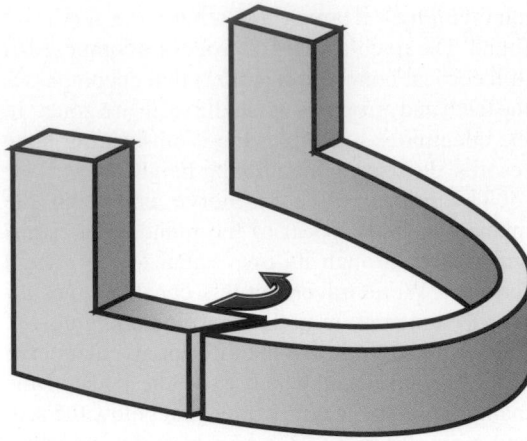

Figure 11 Horizontally unfavorable fracture. (Reproducedd with permission from reference 8.)

peridontal membranes of the dentition, as well as, in the TMJ. The patient often complains of pain in the region of the fracture, most often from the disrupted periosteum surrounding the bone. Muscle spasm (trismus) also plays a key role in contributing to the pain of mandible fractures. Difficult and painful opening of the jaw is a common complaint. Painful swallowing and sneezing may also occur. Numbness of the lower lip from an avulsed or badly contused inferior alveolar nerve in any part of its course from the ramus to the parasymphyseal area, is commonly encountered.

Physical examination confirms the patient's complaint of malocclusion. If the fracture is in a tooth-bearing area, loose or missing teeth may be noted. Ecchymosis of the gingiva also indicates the presence of a fracture. Gross displacement of the fragments may be obvious (Figure 12). There may be a foul odor in the patient's breath from a combination of stagnant food, blood, and frequently alcohol. Bony crepitus and tenderness are also elicited on palpation. A thorough dental examination should be undertaken, including assessment of the presence or absence of teeth and the fractures of dental crowns. Dentures, even if broken, are preserved. The maxillomandibular occlusal relationships are documented. Soft tissue swelling over the point of contact is often found. If there is a missing tooth that is unaccounted for, aspiration is a possibility. In the unconscious

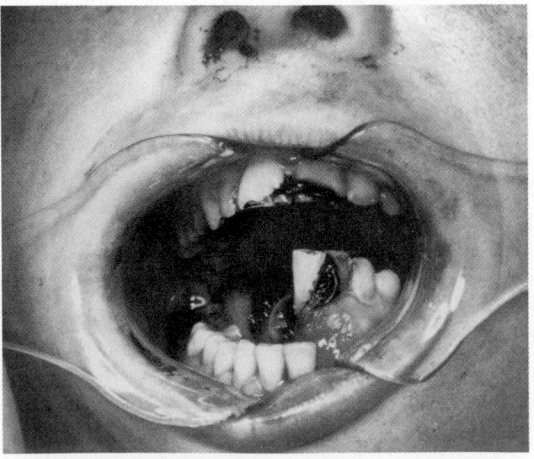

Figure 12 Patient with a grossly displaced fracture of the parasymphysis of the mandible.

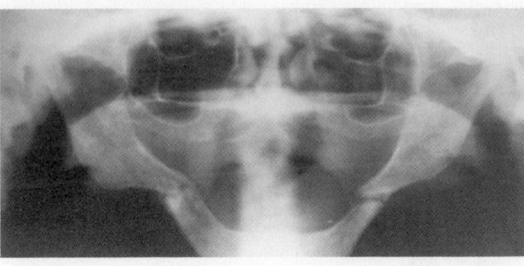

Figure 13 Panorex film showing bilateral body fractures.

patient, evidence of a recently lost unrecovered tooth necessitates a chest X-ray.

Radiographic evaluation can be used to confirm the physical findings and assess the severity of the fracture, including whether it is comminuted and whether there are actually fractured teeth involved. When there is one obvious fracture in the mandibular arch, one must always be aware that there may be an occult fracture in the contralateral ramus or condyle. The panoramic radiograph (Panorex film) is excellent for viewing fractures of the ramus, angle, and body[9] (Figure 13). This type of X-ray is limited, however, in visualizing the symphyseal area as well as telescoping fractures of the condylar area. A modified Townes view usually visualizes significant fractures of the condyles (Figure 14). If a strong suspicion of subcondylar fracture exists, a CT scan will delineate the degree of fragment overlap or displacement into the infratemporal fossa (Figure 15). CT scan reconstructions in three-dimension are often helpful in establishing site of fracture and particularly deformity (Figure 16). If a parasymphyseal or symphyseal fracture is suggested clinically, but not visualized on plain radiographs, then the CT scan will demonstrate it. Dental fractures are best diagnosed with dental occlusal films. If the patient sustains massive trauma as in a motor vehicle accident or other collision, CT scans of other pertinent anatomic areas should be taken, including full facial and cervical spine films.[10] The scan is usually extended superiorly to rule out any intracranial injury.

Treatment

After an adequate history and physical examination have been obtained, and a radiographic assessment has confirmed the physical findings, and ruled out any "occult" fracture, treatment is dictated by the following factors: (1) presence

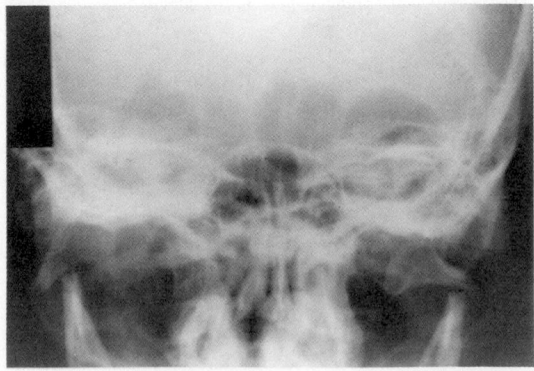

Figure 14 Modified Towne view showing bilateral displaced subcondylar fractures.

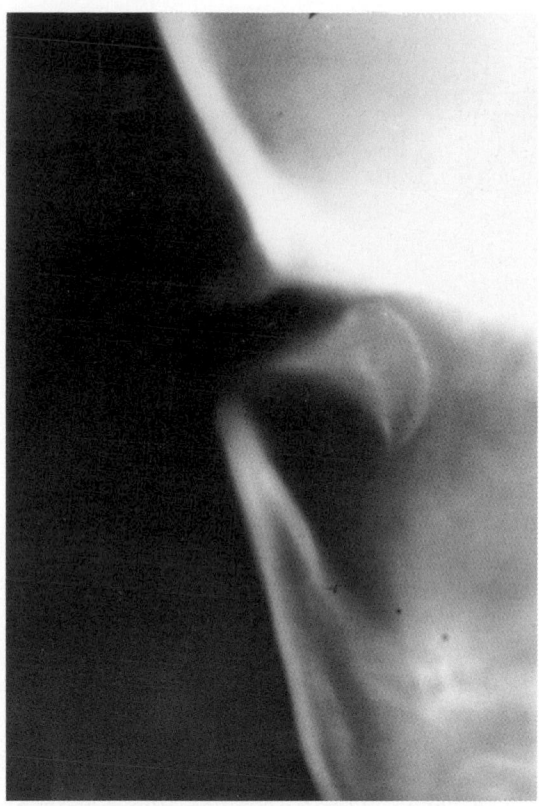

Figure 15 Linear tomogram demonstrating dislocation of the mandibular condyle into the infratemporal fossa.

of absence of other serious trauma, intracranial, intrathoracic, or intra-abdominal and clearance of the cervical spine by a qualified neurosurgeon or orthopedist; (2) adequate surgical consent from the patient; (3) a thorough dental evaluation, including preoperative documentation of occlusion; and (4) availability of bridgework or dentures that accompany the patient to the operating room.

Although many authorities recommended surgical intervention as early as possible to prevent infection, there is no conclusive evidence for this.[6,10–12] To decrease the incidence of infection, it is better to administer preoperative antibiotics. Surgery should be done as soon as possible with

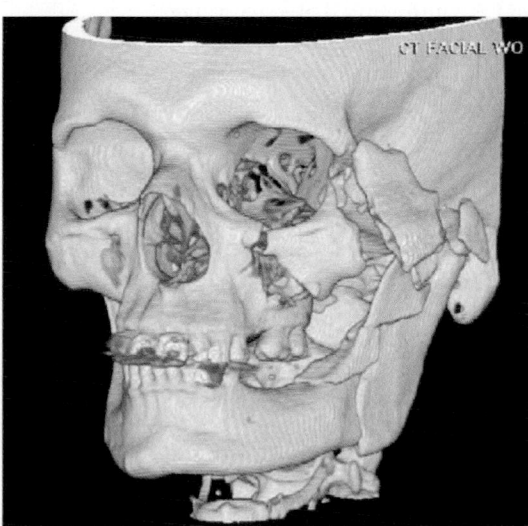

Figure 16 Three-dimensional reconstruction of multiple facial fractures. Note the comminution and displacement of the maxilla and zygoma as well as the displaced fracture of the right mandibular angle.

the previously mentioned factors taken into consideration. It must be emphasized that repairing a mandible fracture is not, in the true sense of the word, an emergency but rather should be done as soon as possible when safe. Some fractures of the mandible do not require surgical intervention. When there is no complaint of malocclusion, most commonly, nondisplaced ramus fractures as well as some subcondylar fractures should be treated with a soft diet. The remainder of mandible fractures,[6] especially when there is malocclusion, should be treated either by closed or open reduction, or in some cases, both.

The cornerstone of facial fracture repair is still intermaxillary fixation. This method of repair entails the ligation of the teeth of each arch to those that oppose it. According to Dingman and Natvig, ligation of teeth to each other dates back to the time of Hippocrates.[13] The ancients advised fixing the teeth to one another with gold wire or linen thread. The Greek physician, Soranos of Ephesus, first described the concept of support of the fractured jaw by a barrel-type bandage in the second century AD[14] These first methods appeared to rely on healing resulting from the wiring of adjacent teeth in the same arch. William of Saliceto, who practiced in Bologna and Verona, first suggested interarch fixation for mandibular fractures in the thirteenth century. He used waxed, twisted silk threads and bound "the injured to the uninjured jaw," It remained for Gilmer in 1887 to be the first to propose actual rigid interdental and intermaxillary fixation, which he accomplished with iron wire.[15]

Intermaxillary fixation began by separately wiring each individual tooth of the maxillary and mandibular arches and then connecting these wires one by one as the teeth were brought into occlusion. From this method, certain modifications were made and evolved into the method we know today. The most significant contribution was the development of the arch bar. Grunell Hammond in 1871 may have described the first arch bar, a firm wire that went around the lingual and buccal surfaces of the teeth. Sauer in 1882 used a circumferential gold wire with a spring attachment. These evolved into the Erich and Jelanko arch bars we recognize today. The Erich bar, the one most commonly used, is a malleable metal bar that easily adapts to the buccal surfaces of the teeth and has hooks to which intermaxillary wires or rubber bands can be attached. The Jelanko bar is rigid and difficult to accommodate to the dental arches. Only the application of eyelet wires and the Erich arch bar will be described.

Eyelet Wires. The eyelet wire is best used for subcondylar fractures, greenstick fractures, and favorably aligned noncomminuted mandibular fractures in patients who are cooperative and compliant. The eyelet wire may also be used as temporary fixation until definitive fixation is done. The wire is constructed by taking a half-length of no. 26 gauge wire, bending it in half, and twisting in a small loop.

The idea of the eyelet wire is to capture two independent teeth on each side of a mandibular fracture and then fix these to two adjacent pairs of maxillary teeth. The ends of the wire are directed from the buccal side through the interdental space below the contact point and close to the gum between the pair of mandibular teeth distal to the fracture. Each wire is brought around the neck of each tooth, and the end of one is passed through the loop and twisted to its mate at a comfortable distance from the loop. The wire ligature now captures the two teeth. Care is taken to be sure the wire is pushed below the embrasure of each tooth and cinched around the tooth neck. The pair of teeth mesial to the fracture line is now ligated in the same way. Similar wires are placed in the same fashion around the maxillary teeth that occlude with the opposing wired mandibular teeth. Pairs of mandibular and maxillary teeth are captured with eyelet wires on the opposite side of the arch for additional stabilization. The patient is placed in his/her premorbid occlusion, and each loop on the mandibular side is individually wired to the loop above. The fracture is now fixed, and the wires are checked on a weekly basis. Occasionally, the interloop wires may loosen or break and may need tightening or replacement. The wire eyelet itself may also come loose and require tightening. Wires are removed at 3 weeks for subcondylar fractures and 6 weeks for others.

Arch Bars. Erich arch bars generally come in a roll. The correct length of bar for each arch is measured by placing one end of the bar on the most distal tooth in the arch on which it is to be fixed. The bar is bent around to the space between the central incisors. This length is now doubled and the bar cut from the roll. Adjustments are made for missing molar teeth. If significant gaps of two or more teeth are present, the gap can be filled in with a pad of cold cure acrylic pressed into the bar.

Once trimmed to length, the bar is carefully contoured to the teeth by hand. Great care is taken to shape the distal ends to fit around the last teeth in the arch, so the bar will not dig into the cheek. Each bar is placed over the buccal surfaces of the teeth and wired into position with the hooks facing away from the occlusal surface (Figure 17).

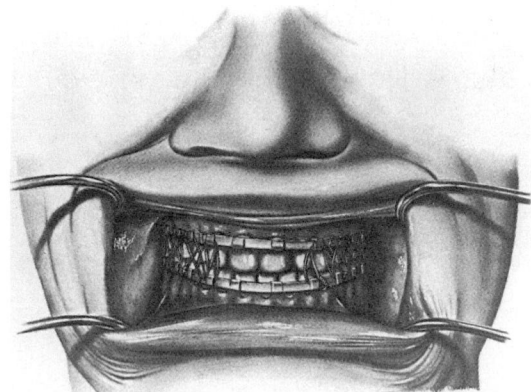

Figure 17 Maxillary and mandibular arch bars applied and intermaxillary wires in place. (Reproduced with permission from reference 6.)

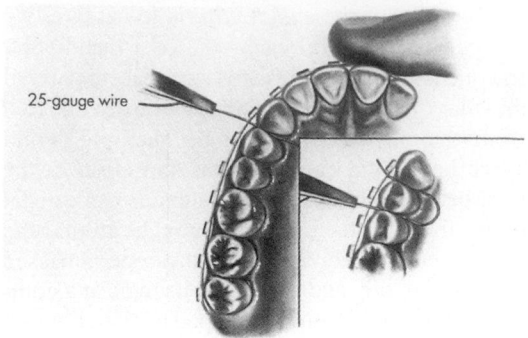

Figure 18 The wiring of an arch bar to the teeth (see text). (Reproduced with permission from reference 6.)

The best teeth for securing the bar are the molars and premolars. The canine has the longest root but has a shape that is not conducive to retention of a wire. The incisor teeth, because of their peg-like configuration, hold the wire even more poorly. If enough teeth are present in the arch, the four incisor teeth of each arch are left unligated. For purposes of orientation, the application of the arch bar to the maxillary teeth will be described first. A 6 in. piece of prestretched 25-gauge wire is passed through the interdental space below the bar (Figure 18). Care is taken to prevent injury to the interdental papillary; however, in patients with periodontal disease, this may be unavoidable. The wire is placed around the tooth adjacent to the interdental space. The two ends are twisted together with forceps while the wire is held at the level of the neck of the tooth with a periosteal elevator (Figure 19). The wire is twisted until tight. The resulting knot is turned into a tight loop and placed away from the lug on the arch bar. Its end is twisted away from the cheek. The molar and premolar teeth are all ligated to the arch bar using the anterior wire above the bar and the posterior below formulation. All the wires are twisted in a clockwise direction. This convention helps in tightening loose wires during follow-up.

Special attention is spent in securing the canine tooth. Its long root embedded in thick bone makes it the key anchor for the bar. Because of it unfavorable shape, adaptation of the wire ligature enhances its holding ability. The wire is placed above the bar, both anteriorly and poste-

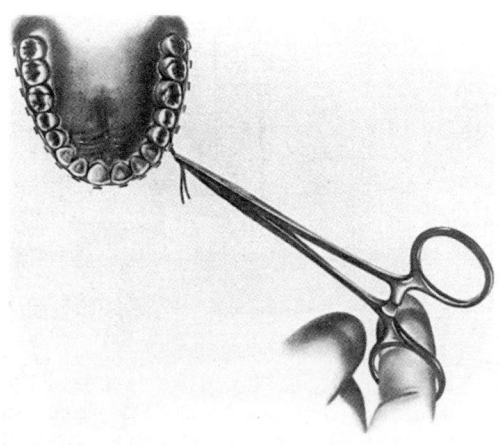

Figure 19 Wire twisting to lock arch bar into position. (Reproduced with permission from reference 6).

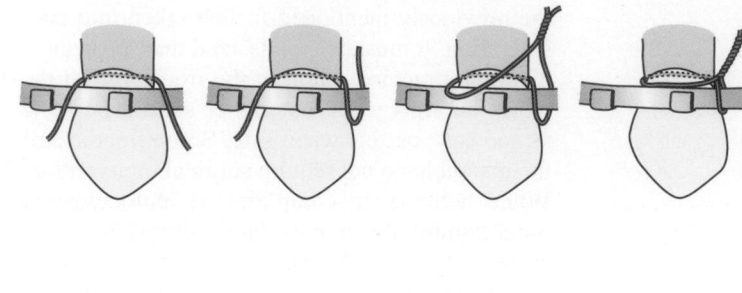

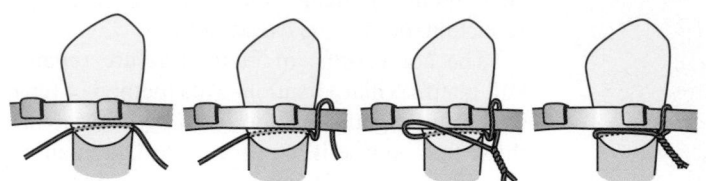

Figure 20 The special adaption for wiring a canine tooth. (Reproduced with permission from reference 9.)

riorly to the tooth, and then looped around the anterior aspect of the bar (Figure 20).

Once bars have been placed on both upper and lower teeth, they are secured to one another either with wire or elastics. Dental wax may be placed on a protrusive edge that irritates the soft tissues. The patient is also given a stick of wax and instructed how to apply it to irritating wire or lugs. All patients are followed on a weekly basis to check for bar stability and tightness of the inter-arch wires. Loose wires are tightened and broken wires replaced. Additionally, careful attention is paid to dental hygiene and nutrition. Already carious dentition, a condition not uncommon in patients with facial fractures, is usually the reflection of past neglect. Careful and insistent instructions in proper brushing technique and use of a "water pick" type of device are essential features in the follow-up regimen. Dental caries can lead to the formation of a dental abscess during the healing phase, which in turn, result in osteomyelitis of the jaw.

Nutritional advice is important. The average weight loss in our patient population following intermaxillary fixation is 15 lb. A booklet on dental hygiene and nutrition is supplied to each patient, with instruction on brushing technique and diets that can be employed while in fixation. Of course, only food with the consistency that can be sucked in the free space around the back of the teeth can be used. Balanced high-calorie supplements such as Ensure-plus and Sustacal can be used to augment caloric intake. These products come in both liquid and pudding forms and are quite palatable. When the patient is fixed into occlusion with either Erich arch bars or eyelet wires, it is important to supply the patient with wire cutters so that if he or she vomits, the interocclusal connection can be cut to prevent aspiration.

Gunning Splints. In the edentulous patient, the patient's reduced mandible can be maintained by the use of Gunning splints. In 1861 T.P. Gunning of New York was, according to Dingman and Natvig,[6] the first to describe the use of inter-maxillary splints, which he fabricated from vulcanite. To make the splint, a dental impression of the jaws are taken with an impression compound such as alginate and poured in stone. The stone model of the mandible is cut at the fracture line and realigned in the normal anatomical position and fixed with sticky wax. An impression of the realigned model is taken and a hot-cured acrylic stent is made. A stent is also made of the maxilla. A flange and corresponding groove are constructed so that the maxillary splint can fit into the mandibular splint in a lock and key type of articulation. Care is taken so that the normal pre-occlusal relationship is established between the mandible and maxilla. An arch bar is imbedded into the splint before hardening so that the splints can be ligated together.

At the time of surgery, the mandibular fracture is reduced and the splint fixed to the jaw by at least four circummandibular wires. A pair of drop wires suspends the upper splint from the bone of the piriform apertures and from the zygomata by wires which encircle the arches. Once the flanges on each side of one splint are fitted into the slots of the corresponding splint then the lugs of the maxillary and mandibular arch bars are wired together. Alternatively, the splint may be fixed with screws that pass through the splint and the unfractured alveolar ridge.

A cruder type of splint can be made in the operating room at the time of fracture reduction in the edentulous patient using cold cure acrylic. A lock and key arrangement is constructed and arch bars pressed into lateral surfaces of the acrylic before it cures. This is a less precise splint and less comfortable for the patient. Any denture, even one that is broken and once mended, will serve well as a Gunning splint. Even a loose fitting denture will provide adequate stabilization of the fracture.

Fractures of the Parasymphyseal Area. These fractures tend to occur in an oblique line, sometimes even approaching the midline from the mental foramen. The mental foramen is the most commonly involved site of a parasymphyseal fracture. A "pure" symphyseal fracture, a fracture through the central incisors, is rare. Either an ipsilateral or contralateral fracture of the angle, ramus, or condyle often accompanies unilateral parasymphyseal fractures. Parasymphyseal fractures may present with a crossbite on the involved side from the posterior pull of the mylohyoid. This is especially true when there is a concomitant ipsilateral fracture of the ascending portion of the mandible. Loose anterior dentition, ecchymotic mucosa, and grossly mobile fractured segments are the hallmarks of these fractures.

The presence of posteriorly displaced bilateral parasymphyseal fractures constitutes an airway emergency. An adequate airway should be established promptly by placing the fractured anterior mandibular segment in one's forefinger and thumb and projecting it anteriorly. Usually the airway can easily be secured by placing a towel clip in the anterior tongue and pulling the tongue and fractured mandible forward. Often an emergency tracheostomy or cricothyrotomy is indicated.

Treatment of a parasymphyseal fracture with only intermaxillary fixation is not usually adequate. However, it is often necessary to stabilize these fractures with interosseous wires, plates, or a lingual splint to prevent a permanent crossbite.[6,15–17] The approach to open reduction of these fractures can be either intraoral or external but is usually internal. Care must be taken to avoid avulsing the mental nerve by way of either approach.

Fractures of the Body and Angle of the Mandible.
Patients with fractures of the mandibular body with good dentition have a distinct advantage over the edentulous or partially dentulous patient. Intermaxillary fixation stabilizes many of these fractures sufficiently, alleviating the need for open reduction. The forces generated by the pterygoid-masseteric sling may distract these fractures, requiring open reduction. Once closed reduction is accomplished by means of Erich arch bars, a decision can be made whether the repair is stable. If it is not, an open reduction can be approached by means of a gingivabuccal incision intraorally.[18] Rarely an extraoral approach will be necessary, and if so a modified Risdon incision is made with care taken to preserve the marginal mandibular branch of the facial nerve. Angle fractures may be treated the same way as body fractures. If the oblique line of fracture is in a favorable direction, closed reduction is adequate. When there is an "unfavorable" fracture, open reduction is often necessary.[19]

Fractures of the Condylar Process and Ramus.
Fractures of the condylar process and condylar neck of the mandible are usually handled by closed reduction. Fractures of the mandibular ramus can be treated in a similar fashion to condylar fractures; even if there is displacement of the fractures and malocclusion results. The closed reduction may be all that is needed. If there is a massive comminution or severe telescoping or just displacement that is not adequately reduced by closed reduction, open reduction should be undertaken to avoid occlusal discrepancies. Severe condylar fractures are defined as (1) telescoping greater than 1.5 cm; (2) a condylar head displaced out of the condylar fossa;

or (3) bilateral subcondylar fractures associated with a Le Fort or maxillary fracture.[20]

The open approach begins with an incision in the preauricular area extending into the temporal hairline, going deep to the temporalis fascia superficial.[6,21] A flap of superficial temporalis fascia should be raised, and the root of the zygoma should be followed down to the fracture site. The trunk of the facial nerve is avoided by staying on the zygomatic process of the temporal bone, tracking down to the glenoid fossa. With a gentle retraction of the superior parotid tissues, the fossa can be exposed and the fracture reduced by means of either a wire or miniplate. Alternatives to repair of a condylar fracture include a Kirschner wire placed by way of the angle of the mandible projected superiorly toward the glenoid fossa.[20,21] External pin fixation with a Morris biphase and plating techniques have also been described.[22,23]

Open Reduction. Before performing open reduction of a mandible fracture, it is always advisable, if possible, to place the patient in closed reduction to establish the occlusal relationship of the teeth. It is folly to attempt an open reduction of any sort when the maxillomandibular dental relationships have not yet been established.

Surgical Approaches. Intraoral approaches have the advantages of scar camouflage and more direct approach to the fracture reduction and fixation. These approaches require more elaborate instrumentation to allow less direct visualization of fractures. Adequate exposure and accurate reduction through this approach requires an experienced surgeon. Extraoral approaches have the advantage of increased exposure and increased visualization in the region of the posterior part of the body, angle, and ramus. External exposure requires a cervical incision; however, this involves potential risk to the marginal mandibular branch of the facial nerve.

The incision and approach chosen for a given fracture of the mandible depend on several factors. These include the location and type of the fracture, as well as, the available instrumentation and technology and, most important, the surgeon's comfort with the given approach. The choice for simple fractures of the symphyseal and parasymphyseal region is intraoral. Simple, linear posterior fractures may be approached intraorally, whereas more comminuted fractures or fractures with significant bone loss usually require an extraoral approach. The approach chosen should allow adequate exposure to diagnose, reduce, and immobilize the given fracture.

The symphyseal and parasymphyseal regions of the mandible are easily approached through either an intraoral or an extraoral route. The intraoral incision is made from canine tooth to canine tooth, leaving an adequate mucosal cuff for closure of the incision (Figure 21). Subperiosteal dissection is made, identifying and preserving the mental nerves. The symphyseal and parasymphyseal regions are also easily approached through an external submental incision oriented in RSTL. Reapproximation of the mentalis muscle must be

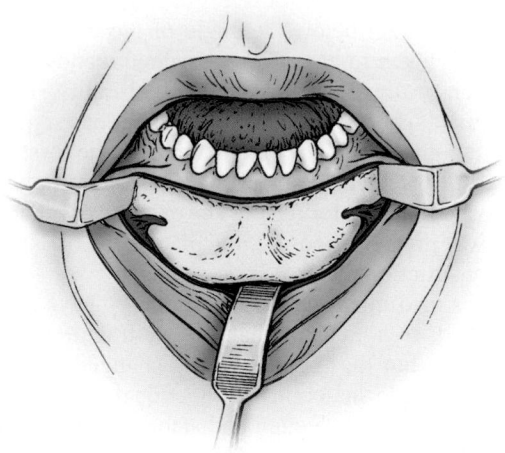

Figure 21 Schematic diagram of intraoral approach to symphyseal and parasymphyseal fractures. The dissection is subperiosteal and isolates and preserves the neurovascular pedicles from the mental foramina.

carefully performed to prevent postoperative ptosis of the soft tissues of the chin.

The approach to the mandibular fracture posterior to the mental foramen depends on the surgeon's experience and the extent and comminution of the fracture.[15] Intraoral approaches to the body and angle are best performed by making a gingivobuccal incision immediately adjacent to the fracture. Repair of posterior mandibular fractures requires surgical experience and advanced technology to achieve fracture reduction fixation. Fracture fixation is achieved with a transbuccal system placed through transcutaneous facial stab incisions (Figure 22). The extraoral approach to

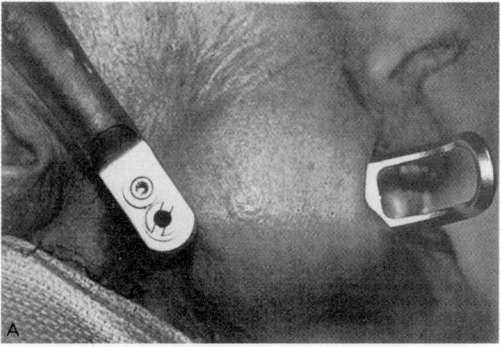

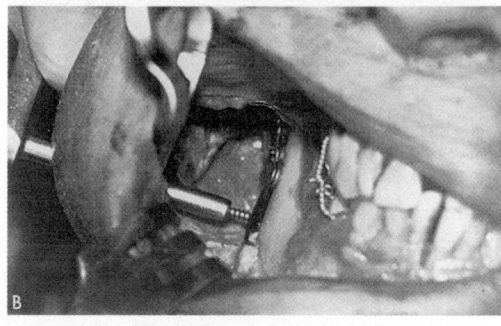

Figure 22 Lateral view of a cadaver showing the use of the transcutaneous-transbuccal system for approach for posterior fractures of the mandible. (A) Stab wound incision has been used to insert the transbuccal system. (B) Intraoral view showing utilization of the transbuccal system to place a plate and screws for fixation of a fracture of the angle of the mandible.

fractures of the mandibular body, angle or ramus is made through a transcervical incision two-finger-breadth below the angle of the mandible. Care is taken to elevate the marginal mandibular branch of the facial nerve to prevent injury. This approach is preferred when the patient has significant comminution of the fracture or bone loss. In each of these cases, a larger reconstruction plate may be required for repair. The external approach allows greater exposure for placement of large reconstruction plates.

As instrumentation and technology have progressed, treatment of mandibular fractures has evolved, but the goals have not changed. These goals include anatomic and functional stability of the mandible. Reduction and stabilization of any mandibular fracture should result in subsequent pain-free function of the mandible without any eventual changes in the TMJ.

The strength of any bony fixation must be adequate to overcome any forces that will act on the repaired bone during function.[24] As previously mentioned, former techniques used fixation with interosseous wiring.[15,25] This method allows the bone to heal indirectly. Wire fixation is rarely used today. The only theoretic advantage of wire fixation for repair of mandibular fractures is the possibility of increased flexibility in cases with significant bone loss or comminution. In these situations, if rigid fixation is applied without proper restoration of premorbid occlusion, the result can be either poor occlusion or eventual change in the TMJ. If interosseous wiring is used, intermaxillary fixation should also be used for approximately 6 weeks for stable bone repair.

The rationale for the use of rigid internal fixation for repair of mandibular fractures is well documented.[15,26] With interosseous wire fixation, there is a clinically proven decrease in mouth opening seen 6 months after release of intermaxillary fixation.[17–20] Additionally, experimental and clinical evidence against wire fixation includes muscle atrophy[20] and histologic changes in the TMJ[23] after prolonged periods of intermaxillary fixation. Although an increased rate of infection has not been conclusively shown with intermaxillary fixation and interosseous wiring, the increased bone movement with nonrigid fixation makes this a theoretic consideration. As knowledge and technology have progressed, rigid internal fixation has become the standard in most centers for treatment of mandibular fractures. This allows the direct form of bone healing. Use of this type of bone repair requires surgical experience, advanced technology, and patient compliance. Direct bone healing can only be achieved with rigid fixation.[27] If properly applied, stable rigid fixation of the mandible obviates the need for intermaxillary fixation.

Rigid fixation of the mandible can be performed by a variety of methods. The fracture is usually first reduced, and the teeth are put into premorbid occlusion by placing the patient in intermaxillary fixation. The fractures are then directly approached (with intermaxillary fixation in place), and anatomic fragment reduction is obtained. Rigid fixation is then performed. This

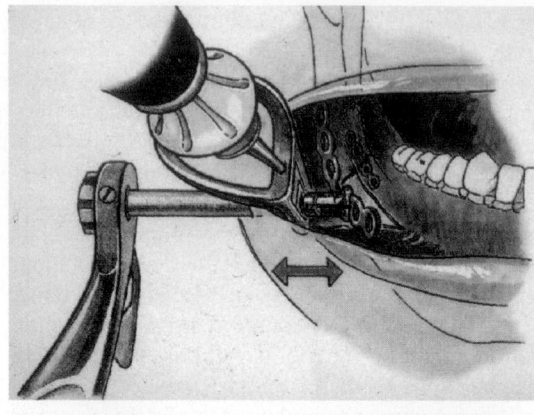

(A)

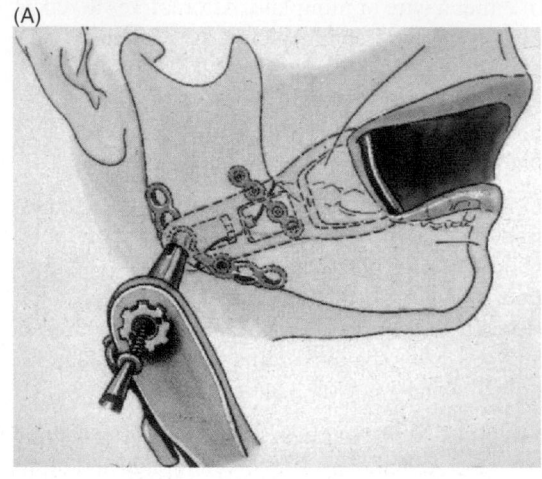

(B)

Figure 23 Transbuccal system for intraoral plating. (A) Plate holder passed through stab wound in cheek. The buccal retractor is being secured to plate holder. (B) The drill hole has been made through the plate holder, and now the screw will be placed to fix the plate to the mandible.

can be accomplished with an inferior mandibular fracture plate (2.4 to 2.7 mm) and a superior monocortical two-hole tension band.

The intraoral incision is retracted with a special intraoral retractor that is fitted to an extraoral device that will maintain a trochar passed through a stab incision in the cheek over the fracture site. Figure 23 illustrates the use of the device developed by Stryker-Leibinger for this purpose. The hollow trochar enables the passage of a plate-grasping device that itself is hollow and permits the passage of the drill bit. The plate is contoured to conform to the surface of the mandibular bone

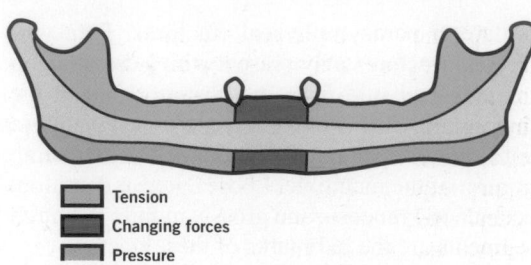

Figure 25 Forces of compression at inferior border of mandible and forces of tension at superior border with a mandibular fracture.

at the fracture site. With the plate in position, the screw holes are drilled, and the bicortical screws passed. Two screws, as a minimum, are placed at each side of the fracture line. Three screws on either side of the fracture are preferable and mandatory in complex fractures.

In 1973 Michelet and colleagues introduced the use of small monocortical plates for the fixation of mandibular fractures.[28] Champy and colleagues popularized the use of these plates and emphasized the importance of lines of osteosynthesis[29] (Figure 24). The line of natural compression forces at the angle and distal part of the body of the mandible are exerted at the inferior border of the mandible while the lines of tension or distraction occur at the superior border at the so-called lines of osteosynthesis (Figure 25). At the angle only one plate is needed, but two plates are required at the parasymphyseal area because of the two lines of osteosynthesis. The plates are 0.9 mm thick and have either 4 to 6 holes or 8 to 16 holes. The diameter of the screw holes is 2.1 mm, and the holes are beveled at 30°. Their rigidity and tensile strength are well within the normal forces of mastication and other forces normally encountered in mandibular activity. In angle fractures, the plate is placed at the external oblique line; and, in the symphyseal area of the jaw, one at the inferior line and one in the superior line of osteosynthesis (Figure 26). The plates are placed in such a fashion to avoid contact with the tooth roots although such contact is of no consequence in most instances. Care must be taken to avoid overtightening of the screws as this will produce microfractures and destabilize the fixation.

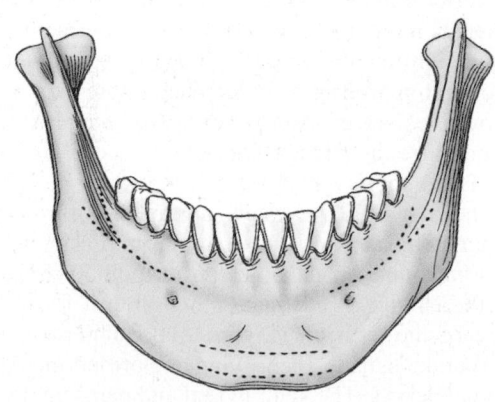

Figure 24 Lines of osteosynthesis on mandible. Plate holder passed through stab wound in cheek. (Reproduced with permission from reference 27.)

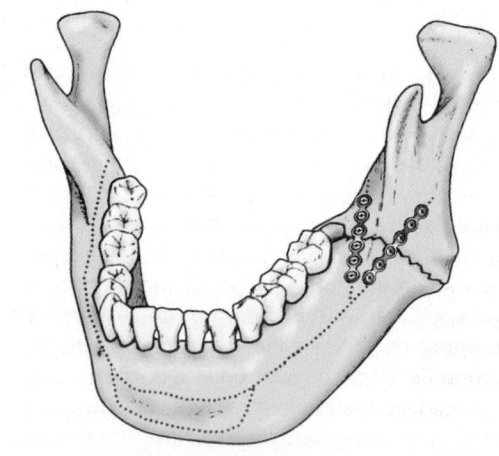

Figure 26 Champy miniplates placed on the mandible to secure an angle fracture of the mandible.

Another means to achieve stable rigid fixation is the placement of lag screw fixation.[24] This method employs a basic principle of woodworking and applies compression across the fracture line with minimal direct bone healing. This technique requires adequate exposure and subperiosteal undermining to allow placement of long screws that engage sufficient bone for fixation.

Lag screw fixation requires that there will be sufficient obliquity to the fracture line that allows at least two, preferably three, lag screws be placed at a significant distance from one another that will catch both mandibular cortices thus stabilizing the reduction. The exception to this is the mandibular angle where one screw is sufficient to achieve adequate fixation. This technique is not applicable to all mandibular fractures and takes a degree of understanding of the dynamics of mandibular function and skill in inserting the screws appropriately. Through an intraoral approach the fracture line is exposed, the fracture is reduced, and the reduction is maintained with arch bars or eyelet wires. For anteriorly located fractures in the parasymphyseal and mesial part of the body an intraoral approach can be used. For those fractures near the angle, the transbuccal approach is employed. A trochar is introduced through a stab incision in the cheek, and the penetrating point is removed prior to introducing the drill bit (Figure 27). A drill guide is placed that will produce the "glide hole" for the portion of the screw that will pass through the buccal cortex. Once the fracture line is encountered, a second guide is inserted through the hole just made to make the smaller guide hole in the lingual fragment. This screw hole must begin precisely in the center of the glide hole and carried through the lingual cortex. A countersink is made at the start of the glide hole to accommodate the head of the screw. The screw is slid through the glide hole, and the threads engage the thread hole. The fracture is compressed as the screw head enters the countersink.

In those fractures in the parasymphyseal area the exposure can be done intraorally. The elevation of the mucoperiosteal flap must be done with an eye to avoid injuring the mental nerves. The gliding hole and the threading hole are placed in the same fashion as those in the area of the angle. The countersink is made and the lag screw placed to ensure stability. Two or three screws are placed (Figure 28). Screws are now available with the screw flutes wider than the diameter of the glide portion of the screw. This then requires that only one screw hole is drilled and the passage of the thread portion of the screw pulls the gliding part through giving tighter grip to the latter while achieving the necessary compression.

If rigid fixation is stable, the patient may be taken out of intermaxillary fixation and allowed to function.[30] Of course, this decision is based on the stability of the rigid fixation and on the individual patient's compliance. If either the fixation stability or patient compliance is in question, the patient may be left in intermaxillary fixation for up to 6 weeks.

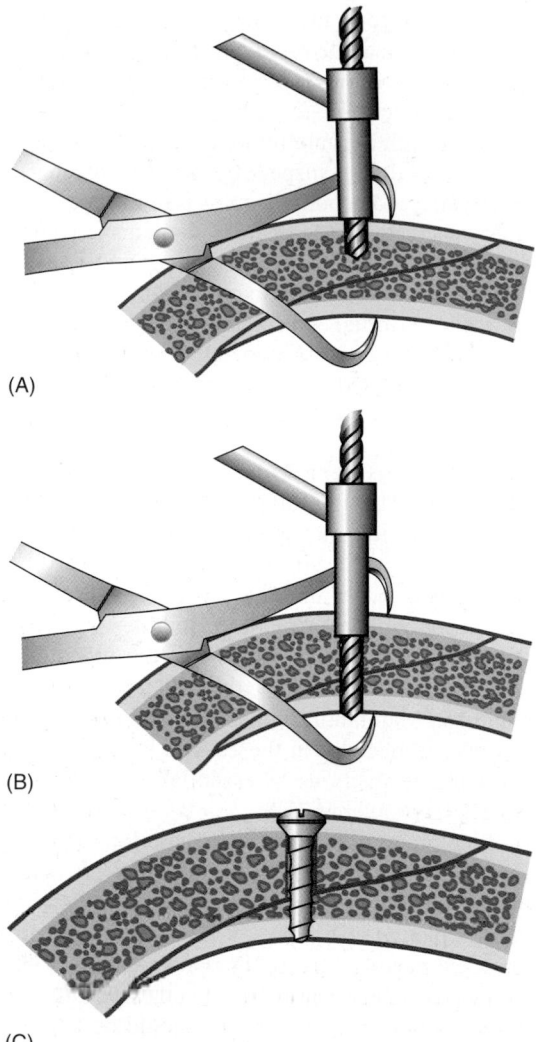

(A)

(B)

(C)

Figure 27 Steps in the insertion of a lag screw for mandibular fracture fixation. (A) A large glide hole is made in the lateral fragment using a drill guide. (B) A smaller gripping hole is made in the inner fragment using a drill guide of smaller diameter. (C) After a countersink is made in the lateral fragment, the screw is placed so that it glides through the outer hole, seats in the countersink, and the screw flutes grip the inner fragment. (Reproduced with permission from reference 25.)

Dental Injury. Injury to the dentition is a common accompaniment to fractures of the mandible and maxilla. A simple chipping of the teeth, which does not extend to the dentin, can be managed by the dentist by simply grinding the occlusal surface smooth. Such injuries are usually unaccompanied by pain. Larger fractures of the tooth substance expose the dentin or pulp and are painful. It is important to dress the tooth immediately

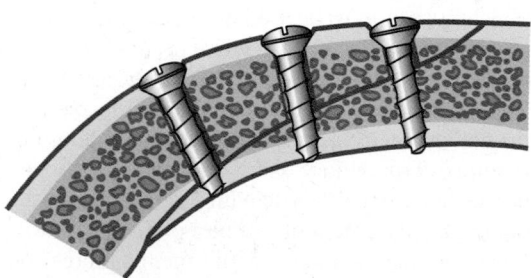

Figure 28 Illustration of the importance to place two or three lag screws to ensure rigid fixation. (Reproduced with permission from reference 25.)

with a dental compound that not only protects the tooth, but also alleviates discomfort. A simple mixture of zinc oxide and eugenol done with a metal spatula or a glass plate forms a sticky compound with the consistency of putty that hardens when wet by the saliva. Eugenol helps to soothe the pain. Other proprietary compounds such as Dycal may be used. Later, the dentist can restore the tooth with a crown. In the case of fracturing of a slab of tooth face in a vertical direction, especially from the incisors, the tooth can be repaired by bonding.

Avulsion of the crown at the gum line is managed either by the extraction of the root or by application of a dressing until the tooth can later be restored with a crown. If the dentition is neglected and carious, extraction is the best solution.

Dental fractures that occur through the root present a special problem. Root fractures seriously jeopardize the viability of the tooth. If the soft tissue of the pulp is sufficiently traumatized, the tooth will die. Once the pulp undergoes necrosis, the stage is set for the development of a root abscess. This may occur a short time after the injury or may be delayed for years. If such an abscess were to occur during intermaxillary fixation, an osteomyelitis and even a nonunion could occur.

The management of a tooth in the line of fracture is controversial. Some guidelines do exist that may be of help. If the tooth is carious and the root is fractured, the tooth should be removed. If a carious tooth has a fracture through the periodontal ligament, but the root is intact, extraction should be seriously entertained. If the tooth is healthy, the vital consideration is the importance of the tooth in the stability of the fracture. This is especially cogent in the circumstance of the erupted third molar tooth that lies in an unfavorably aligned fracture of the mandibular angle. In such a fracture, the line extends obliquely from anterior to posterior as it proceeds from the occlusal surface to the inferior border of the mandible. If the molar is in the distal fragment, its occlusion with the maxillary third molar above it will preclude its displacement. If the molar is extracted the pull of the medial pterygoid and masseter muscles will displace the distal fragment upward. The wisdom tooth, being the most poorly calcified in the mouth, is the most susceptible of all to caries. One should probably remove a carious or impacted third molar in such a circumstance and achieve fixation by an open technique.

Any dental trauma can cause pulp necrosis, even without a root fracture. It is important to follow-up patients after facial fractures with vitality testing of the teeth. Once viability is lost, a root canal procedure should be performed to prevent abscess and tooth loss.

The final consideration is that of avulsed teeth. Such teeth should be immediately replaced in the avulsion socket and fixed with wires to the adjacent teeth for splinting. Many such teeth later become nonvital and require a root canal procedure. Most are retained, however, and their preservation helps greatly in the maintenance of dental arch integrity. An avulsed tooth that remains out of its socket for longer than 1 or 2 hours will likely not survive if reimplanted. It is important to stabilize the tooth in the arch after reimplantation. Some type of bonding material is applied to the face of adjacent teeth and the fixation achieved by a form of banding.

Postoperative Care. Drains are usually placed in open reduction wounds of the body, angle, and ramus. These drains are usually removed on the first postoperative day. Local wound care to the suture line is best done with peroxide cleaning and antibiotic ointment to avoid infection. Intraoral care should begin as soon as possible and consist of a water pick to the dentition but not the suture line and gargle of a solution of mouthwash and peroxide. The lingual aspect of the dentition is inaccessible in the patient with closed reduction in intermaxillary fixation. The effervescence of the peroxide will help to debride the areas of the gingiva and teeth of the lingual surface.[18] Patients often complain of pain, especially in the first two postoperative weeks because of the spasm of the pterygoid and masseter muscles while the patient is in intermaxillary fixation. Codeine and acetaminophen with codeine syrup are useful analgesics during this immediate postoperative phase. Persistence of pain beyond 2 weeks requires nonsurgical examination of the operative site as well as a radiographic study to determine whether there has been a shift in the fracture site.

The increased metabolic demands of healing and the difficulty of eating while in intermaxillary fixation make adequate nutrition a common problem. Liquid diets must be supplemented with a protein powder as well as whole milk. It is not uncommon for patients to sustain severe weight loss during the ensuing 6 weeks of intermaxillary fixation. Dietary counseling is often helpful. If the patient remains in intermaxillary fixation, weekly checkups to tighten the intermaxillary wires are absolutely necessary. If the wire ligatures are used for intermaxillary fixation, the wire stretches loosening the fixation. If there is no close contact with the maxillary and mandibular teeth, a lingual version may develop. This results in a severe malunion if not corrected before fibroosseous union occurs. Tightening of the wires every week prevents this from happening. Dental checkups, when possible, are also necessary in the case of impending dental abscess.

Intermaxillary fixation may be removed 5 to 6 weeks postoperatively, providing that there is no evidence of a nonunion. Nonunion can best be assessed by palpation at the fracture site. If there is pain in the mandible and not the teeth at the operative site, a nonunion or fibrous union should be strongly suspected, especially when accompanied by mobility. Another technique is the "torque test," which involves placing a standard wooden tongue blade on the side of the fracture and having the patient bite down and break the tongue blade.[19] If there is no bone pain with this

procedure, a good union has been achieved and the arch bars may be removed. The patient is still cautioned to remain on a soft diet for two to three additional weeks.

When arch bars are removed, a dental consultation is needed to inspect the teeth for occlusal discrepancy. Orthodontia may provide the necessary correction. Major malunions may require osteotomy of the involved segment and repositioning with further intermaxillary fixation. With an accurate initial assessment, careful surgical technique and good postoperative care, the need for further adjustments of occlusion should be infrequent.

Special Considerations: The Edentulous Mandible. The fractured edentulous mandible presents specific management problems for the surgeon. With the absence of teeth, the alveolar cortical bone undergoes total resorption. The superior portion of the mandible is greatly attenuated. The overall height of the mandible, therefore, is much less than that of a tooth-bearing mandible. Maintaining correct mandibular height, however, especially in the case of angle, ramus, and condyle fractures, is essential to avoid possible TMJ problems.

Ideally, in a completely edentulous patient with mandible fractures, the dentures can simply be wired into place. In the maxilla, screws used in plating techniques or Kirschner wires are excellent means of fixing the upper denture to the palate. The lower denture is affixed using circummandibular wires. The patient should be kept in some form of intermaxillary fixation for at least 6 weeks.

Another form of fixation, although less acceptable, is a cap splint. This can be especially helpful in a fracture involving the body or symphyseal area. The cap splint is formed, by placing acrylic over the ridge of the mandible with the fracture, and affixing it to the mandible, using circummandibular wires. When dentures are not available or the fracture is in an area that cannot be splinted but intermaxillary fixation is necessary, dental impressions can be made as a template for Gunning splints. Gunning splints can be affixed to the edentulous upper and lower jaw by means of the same techniques used to affix dentures.

Open reduction is necessary in edentulous mandibles with unfavorable "fracture lines" and in severely comminuted fractures. Interosseous wiring can be accomplished in the same fashion as with tooth-bearing mandibles. Intermaxillary fixation, however, must be used in this situation. Compression plating is also convenient in these cases, by way of either the external or intraoral approach. The advantage of using a compression plate is the achievement of rigid fixation, which does not require intermaxillary fixation. In elderly patients, however, especially those with osteoporosis of the mandible, placement of a secure plate may be difficult and may be loosen with time. Compression plating, once the state of the art in mandibular fracture repair, has largely gone out of fashion and has been replaced by the titanium plating systems.

Pediatric Mandibular Fractures. A mandibular fracture in a patient younger than 15 years, requires a knowledge of the state of both permanent and deciduous dentition. The tooth buds of the permanent teeth are located below the roots of the deciduous teeth. Surgical trauma to the tooth buds may retard or completely negate the buds' ability to erupt later. Primary teeth are fully erupted usually by the second or third year of life. The central incisors are the first teeth to appear, followed by the lateral incisors, the first molars, cuspids, and second molars. The shedding of these teeth occurs in the same order and is usually complete by 12 years of age. Therefore, in the first 12 years of life, there are tooth buds of permanent teeth or partially erupted permanent teeth that may be endangered by surgery. The presence of these tooth buds also makes the tooth-bearing areas of the mandible in a child more prone to fracture than in an adult. They, in effect, create a more porous bony surface with less structural support.

In the tooth-bearing areas of a mandibular fracture in a pediatric patient, an overlapping cap splint provides adequate, stable reduction to promote anatomic bone healing. Because of the ability of children to heal rapidly, the splint is required only for approximately 4 weeks. In the angle area, if the fracture is in an unfavorable line, open reduction may be attempted. Radiographic documentation of the proximity of the erupting of the third molar bud and second molar tooth bud should always be confirmed. If the fracture line is close to a tooth bud, closed reduction may be necessary. Arch bars can be used in a pediatric patient with wire ligatures; however, they may cause premature shedding of the deciduous teeth. Generally, intermaxillary fixation is not necessary in a child for safe healing of a fracture of the symphysis or body. Condylar fractures in the pediatric population have been seen to remodel completely without surgical intervention; therefore, no treatment is recommended.

Complications in Pediatric Fractures. The tooth buds of an infant or young child are especially susceptible to damage that may cause deformities of the erupted mature tooth later.[31] A long-term follow-up study of 28 children with mandibular fractures was done by McGuirt and Salisbury.[32] The mean length of follow-up was 10.5 years. The children were divided into condylar only, noncondylar fractures, and condylar fractures with other facial fractures. Forty-six percent of the patients had TMJ compromise. Five patients were concerned about their external facial asymmetry, although a medical/dental team reviewed abnormalities in 47% of the patients radiographically. Sixteen percent of the overall group was thought to be both clinically and radiographically abnormal enough to require interventional therapy. Therefore, one can expect nearly one out of five children with a mandible fracture to have some sort of difficulty that may require later intervention. It is recommended that these patients be followed closely postoperatively by a dentist and/or orthodontist, and the use of braces

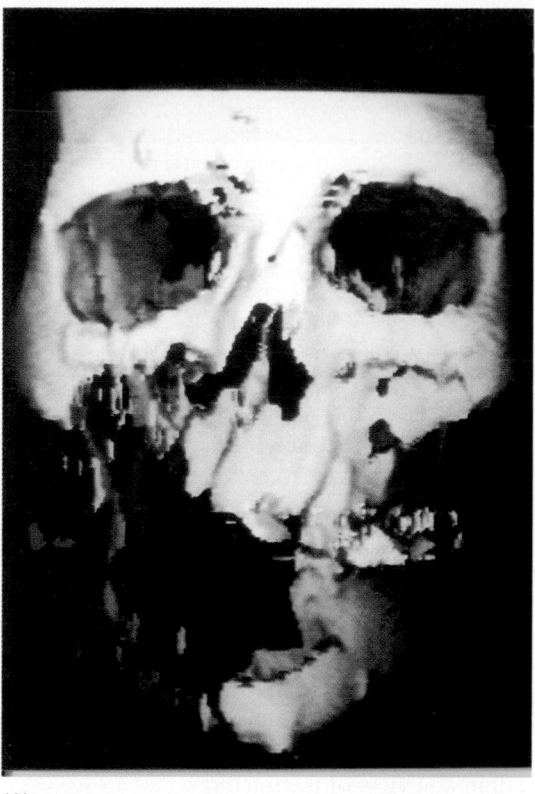

(A)

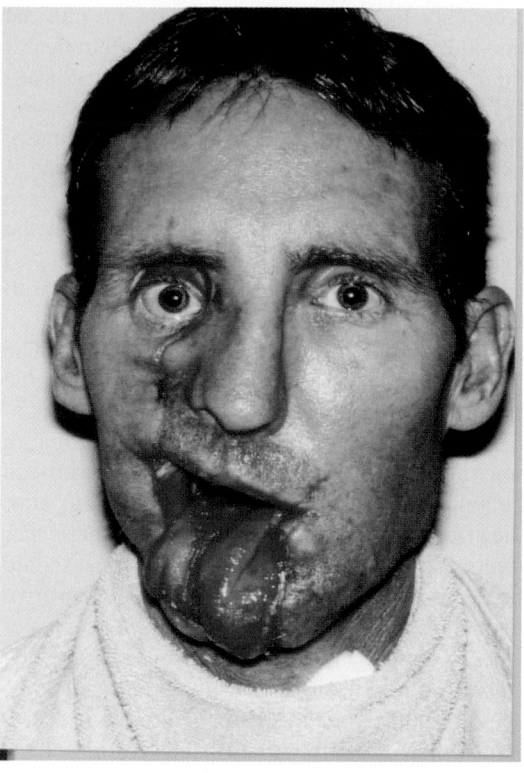

(B)

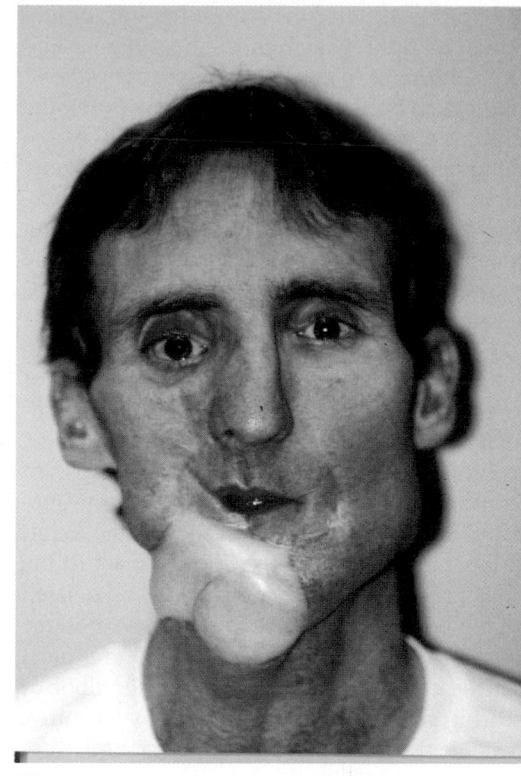

(C)

Figure 29 (A) Three-dimensional computed tomographic scan of patient with a large defect secondary to self-inflicted high power rifle wound to the face. (B) Preoperatively, the patient can be seen to have loss of mandible and soft tissue of chin and neck. (C) Reconstruction with a fibular free flap.

and elastics may be necessary to promote growth and development of the fracture area.[33] The remodeling of untreated subcondylar fractures is well documented.[33,34]

Severe Mandibular Fractures. If the trauma is from an explosion or a gunshot wound or if the blunt trauma is excessively severe, there can be multiple missing pieces of mandible.[35,36] In these cases, open reduction and exploration are mandatory if the patient's condition permits. The bony fragments that do not have periosteal attachments should be removed, and the area should be debrided and cleaned aggressively. Often in these fractures, there are portions of mandible that are pedicled on small pieces of periosteum. If less than 25% of the bone surface area is attached to periosteum, most surgeons would agree that debridement is necessary to prevent this from becoming a sequestrum.

Gunshot wounds require soft tissue debridement, especially high-velocity wounds in which there may be a large temporary cavity. High-velocity weapons cause extensive soft tissue damage from both the impact of the missile and the secondary-missile effect of fractured bone fragments through soft tissues. The utilization of external pin fixation and the application of the biphase appliance to the mandibular segments alleviate the possibility of infection that would otherwise be incurred by placement of a foreign body such as a plate in a potentially grossly infected wound.

If the wound can be cleaned adequately and soft tissue coverage achieved, a long mandibular plate can be used to approximate the (usually) multiple segments. Once healing has taken place

and infection is cleared, in 6 months to 1 year this area can be reconstructed using autogenous bone from a variety of sources or a free flap[34] (Figure 29).

ZYGOMATIC FRACTURES

The zygoma is the third most frequently fractured facial bone, with 85% of fractures occurring in men. Blunt trauma, caused by motor vehicle accidents or sports, make up the great majority of fractures. Fractures of this region are often called trimalar fractures, meaning fractures of the zygomaticotemporal, frontozygomatic, zygomaticomaxillary suture lines[37] (Figure 30). Indeed, the fracture of the zygomatic sphenoid suture makes these fractures quadramalar.[7] The zygoma can withstand severe force, but owing to the most lateral extension of the facial skeleton, it is prone to injury in both the anterior–posterior direction and the lateral and transverse directions. The attachments of the temporalis superiorly and the masseter muscle inferiorly tend to neutralize the action of each other. However, the movement of the jaw with the masseter muscle does tend to distract the segments downward and medially.

The arch of the zygoma, which has contributions from both the zygomatic bone and the temporal bone, lies over the coronoid process. A depressed fracture of the arch pushing into the temporal fossa often results in restriction in movement of the jaw because of impingement of the arch on the coronoid process. The fractures of the zygoma tend to occur at the articulations with the aforementioned bones. Although the

body of the zygoma, which makes up the inferolateral orbital wall, is often the point of impact from trauma, is rarely fractured because it is the thickest part of the bone. Comminuted fractures of the zygomatic body are a difficult problem in surgical management.

Surgical Anatomy

The zygoma has four suture lines connecting it with the temporal, frontal, maxillary, and sphenoid bones. In addition to the temporalis and masseter muscles, the lesser and greater zygomatic muscles are also inserted on its surface. The orbital process of the zygoma makes up the anterolateral portion of the infraorbital foramen in the floor of the orbit. It is not uncommon, with a severe zygoma fracture, for there to be a prolapse of orbital contents through the orbital floor due to fracture of the maxillary zygomatic suture line.

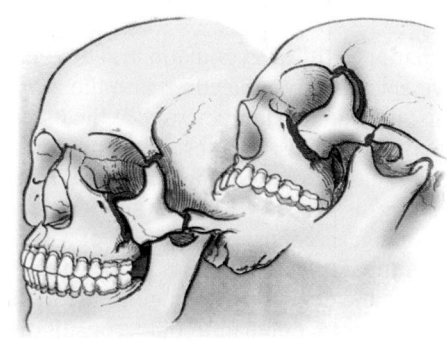

Figure 30 Tripod fracture of the zygoma. (Reproduced with permission from reference 38.)

The infraorbital nerve exits from the infraorbital foramen at the articulation of the zygoma and maxilla. Damage to this nerve causes hypesthesia of the cheek on the affected side as well as the lateral aspect of the nose. From the body of the zygoma exit two sensory nerves, the zygomatic frontal and zygomatic temporal, which generally are clinically insignificant. When discussing a fracture of the zygoma, one must realize the importance of the intimate association to the lateral canthal tendon and the suspensory ligaments of the globe. There is some downward displacement in many fractures of the zygoma because of the previously mentioned traction of the masseter, and therefore the globe position can change. The entire globe can be pulled down because of downward displacement of the suspensory ligament of Lockwood, which attaches to the Whitnall tubercle, located on the lateral aspect of the orbital process of the zygoma. Also associated with the floor of the orbit are the inferior oblique and inferior rectus muscles, which are most often the cause of entrapment when the floor of the orbit is badly fractured (blowout fracture). Impalement of the muscles on a fracture fragment puts the muscle into spasm, which limits upward gaze. True entrapment of these muscles, which is rare, must be corrected surgically.

Diagnosis

History and physical examination are of primary importance in evaluating a zygomatic fracture. The patient gives a history of having received a blow from a fist, a ball, or other blunt object or has been involved in a motor vehicle or motorcycle accident. He or she complains of localized pain and often has numbness over the ipsilateral cheek. If there is significant herniation of fat into the maxillary sinus, diplopia ensues from simple herniation of orbital fat or entrapment of the inferior rectus and/or inferior oblique muscles. With no herniation of fat or evidence of an orbital floor dehiscence, inferior displacement of the zygomatic complex inferiorly displaces the Whitnall tubercle and, therefore, the ligament of Lockwood, causing the same problem of diplopia.[7]

Trismus can result from impingement of the zygomatic arch on the coronoid process of the mandible. Often there is substantial masseter and temporalis spasm from contusion to that area, which may produce trismus even if the arch is intact.

The patient with a zygomatic fracture may also have epistaxis from bleeding into the maxillary sinus; the blood exiting by way of the ostium of the maxillary sinus and nose. On inspection, the patient has severe periorbital ecchymosis and swelling as well as a lateral subconjunctival hemorrhage secondary to tearing of vessels of the canthi. Blood in the anterior chamber (hyphema) indicates severe damage to the globe, and an emergency ophthalmologic consultation is mandatory.[39] Hemorrhage restricted to the subconjunctiva does not imply serious damage

secondary to fat and muscle herniation into the maxillary sinus. Because concomitant intraocular injury is so common, an ophthalmologic consultation should be obtained in all cases.

There is palpable facial skeletal asymmetry over the malar eminence and zygomatic arch if the swelling is not too severe. One may place a gloved finger into the oral cavity to feel the zygomatic buttress and appreciate crepitus and swelling. This movement is exquisitely tender to a patient with a fracture. There is trismus as well as difficult and painful opening of the jaws. The inability to open the mouth more than a 3 cm strongly suggests a fracture involving the zygomatic arch. In the absence of severe swelling, a fracture of the arch and the infraorbital rim can be palpated. The patient may be unable to raise the affected eye from the equator and experiences diplopia (Figure 31). A forced duction test should be done on all patients with diplopia. A positive test indicates entrapment of the inferior rectus or inferior oblique muscle. Table 3 provides a listing of symptoms and signs of zygomatic fractures.

Zygomatic fractures can be classified according to their severity. An isolated fracture of the zygomatic arch may occur with no orbital involvement. However, most fractures involve the four suture lines previously mentioned. Fracture of the zygomaticomaxillary suture line and orbital floor without involvement of the frontozygomatic or zygomaticotemporal suture line constitutes an impure blowout fracture. A pure blowout fracture refers to a dehiscence of the orbital floor with an intact orbital rim.[8] A severely comminuted body fracture requires extensive exposure and is managed differently than a tripod fracture. The treatment of these various fractures differs, and diagnosis should be confirmed with X-rays.

Standard facial films, including Waters, Caldwell, Townes, and submental vertex views are usually obtained. This battery of films helps rule out associated facial fractures. The Waters and submental vertex views are of greatest help in diagnosis. The Waters view can reveal an orbital floor dehiscence by the teardrop sign indicating herniation of orbital contents into the maxillary sinus. There is often blood in the maxillary sinus, however, which may obscure this

Table 3 Symptoms and Signs of Zygomatic Fractures	
Symptoms	Signs
Pain	Infraorbital tenderness
Double vision	Diplopia
Numbness	Hypoesthesia: cheek, upper teeth
Epistaxis	Malar flattening
Trismus	"Hypoophthalmos" and enophthalmos
Cosmetic deformity	Subconjunctival hemorrhage

finding. Also, the orbital rim frontozygomatic suture line and the body of the zygoma are well visualized with the Waters view. The submental vertex view is excellent for evaluating the zygomatic arch. Although, most zygoma fractures are readily diagnosed on plain radiographs, the CAT scan affords a more accurate rendition of the fracture details. It is especially good at depicting the degree and severity of orbital floor and in detecting fractures of the orbital apex. Subtle unilateral associated fractures of the palate will be detected as well. Three-dimensional CT scanning provides a dramatic view of the fracture.

Treatment

The decision to repair a zygomatic fracture should be based on the goals one hopes to attain by such surgical intervention. The only strict indications for surgery are relief of trismus and correction of diplopia from an inferior displacement and entrapment of the inferior rectus and inferior oblique muscles. Most often, the patient desires repair for cosmetic reasons. If there is ipsilateral numbness after a fracture, this improves, in the large majority of cases, with no surgical intervention. Therefore, numbness of the cheek should not be the indication for surgery. When obtaining the patient's consent for surgery, one must be careful to counsel about the proximity of the globe to the surgical site and alert the patient to the real risk of retrobulbar hematoma and retinal tear from retraction of the globe.[37] These complications are extremely rare with careful surgical technique. Also important in preoperative counseling, if an infraorbital rim approach is needed, is the need to inform the patient of the possibilities of prolonged lower lid edema and ectropion. The onset of visual field changes, diplopia, or a change in the patient's visual acuity required an ophthalmologic consultation.

One of the possible occult injuries of a zygomatico-orbital fracture is a retinal tear. Traction of the globe during surgery to repair a zygoma may extend a small, insignificant retinal tear, creating a large visual field defect. This can be avoided by limiting retraction of the globe to short periods of time and using extreme caution.

Serious intraocular injury mandates delay of repair until the globe has stabilized. Otherwise, the timing of the repair of a zygomatic fracture depends on the degree of soft tissue swelling. If swelling is severe, waiting for 5 to 10 days is acceptable and reducing the zygoma will not be

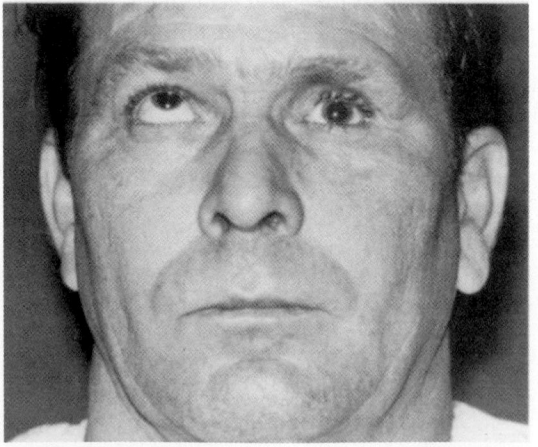

Figure 31 Patient with diplopia and restriction of upward gaze.

a significant problem during that time. After 10 to 14 days, the zygoma may form a fibrous union, making mobilization of the fracture difficult. A good rule of thumb is to reduce the fracture as soon as the swelling has subsided enough to compare both zygomas intraoperatively.

Surgical Technique. Multiple techniques have been used to repair a zygomatic fracture. The four fracture lines imply that there should be 4 points of fixation to stabilize the fracture, both laterally and inferiorly. The technique of placing a plate or wire in the frontozygomatic fracture line and the zygomaticomaxillary suture line at the infraorbital rim provides adequate stabilization for a large majority of fractures. Some fractures treated in this manner are not adequately stabilized and require antral packing or an intraoral approach to reduce the inferior aspect of the fracture. One-point fixation techniques have been described using, either a Kirschner wire[40] or more recently, a rigid miniplate.[41–43]

Fractures of the zygomatic arch (Figure 32) with a significant cosmetic defect or trismus can be elevated by means of a Gillies incision in the temporal hairline and reduced directly. The temporal branch of the facial nerve is avoided by placing the elevator deep to the superficial fascia of the temporalis muscle. The Boies elevator is placed under the arch, and the fragments are lifted into position. A plate is rarely required for fixation because of the splinting action of the underlying temporalis muscle. It is vitally important not to lever the arch into position. The point of the fulcrum becomes the lateral wall of the skull which can be fractured when a lot of force is required for arch reduction.

For the repair of the more commonly occurring trimalar fracture, two principal open approaches are used: the transfacial and the bicoronal scalp flap approach. In a few minimally displaced or noncomminuted zygomatic fractures, a closed approach may be performed using a towel clip or a small bone hook under the malar eminence, relocating the zygoma in an upward–outward direction.

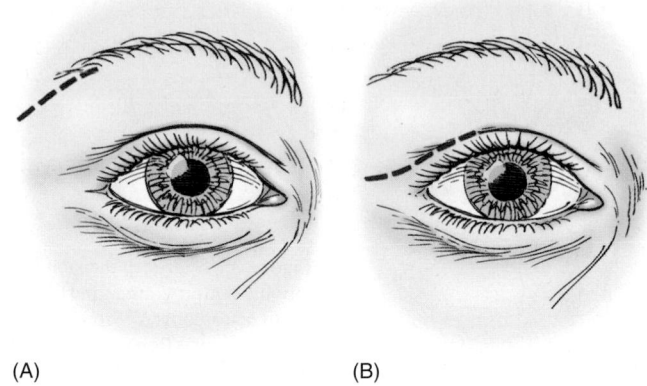

(A)　　　　　　　　　　(B)

Figure 33 (A) Schematic diagram of a right lateral brow incision for approach to the frontozygomatic suture line. (B) Schematic diagram of a right extended upper blepharoplasty incision for approach to the frontozygomatic suture line.

When performing the more commonly used open approaches, the transfacial approach begins with a supraorbital brow incision made within the brow line or as an extended upper blepharoplasty incision (Figure 33), and the frontozygomatic suture line is exposed. The approach to the infraorbital incision varies depending on the surgeon's discretion. Choices include a transconjunctival approach (Figure 34) or an approach through the skin of the lower lid at various distances from the grey line of the lower lid. The placement of the subciliary incision should be along the crease and should be at least 3 to 4 mm below the ciliary line to avoid ectropion and prevent lid edema. The author advocates the stair-step technique (Figure 35), in which a skin flap is elevated, leaving the orbicularis oculi muscle intact to prevent fat herniation from obstructing visualization of the fracture. Once the step incision of approximately 4 mm in length is made, an inferior skin flap is elevated over the orbicularis occuli muscle until the maxilla inferior to the infraorbital rim can be palpated. Using a pair of Steven scissors the muscle is split in the direction of its fibers and carried down to the maxilla below the infraorbital rim. The periosteum is entered below the infraorbital rim to avoid interruption of the orbital septum that may cause later scarring and ectropion. The orbicularis oculi muscle and orbital septum are retracted superiorly.

These approaches provide good visualization of the rim and orbital floor while, at the same time, decreasing the chance of trauma to the infraorbital nerve (Figure 36A). If there is a significant dehiscence of the orbital floor (>1.5 cm) or entrapment of the inferior rectus or inferior oblique muscle, a graft of malar bone, nasal septum, gel film, or suitable alloplast should be used to repair the defect. We recommend homografts to reconstruct the floor and feel the danger of migration or extrusion with silastic sheeting prohibits its use.[44–46] Titanium rigidly placed mesh has been added to the armamentarium of alloplasts to reconstruct the orbital floor. Initial results are encouraging, but the implant will need to stand the test of time.

A Boies elevator is placed into the infratemporal fossa from the brow incision, beneath the arch and the zygoma is elevated to align the infraorbital rim and elevate the arch. Once the fracture

has been put in proper position, a miniplate is bent to adapt to the reduced lateral orbital rim and held in position to drill the screw holes. Holes to accommodate the screws for the miniplate that will be used to fix the frontozygomatic fracture are drilled on each side of the fracture line. Usually two holes will be sufficient, but on occasion, three holes are placed. Most plating systems now have self-taping screws so that a tap is unnecessary. Some systems have self-drilling screws; however, a small amount of pressure is initially required to get the screw stated. This is not usually a problem in the lateral orbital wall but may be impossible in the infraorbital rim. A miniplate is adapted to the infraorbital rim, and two drill holes are placed on either side of the fracture line (Figure 36B). The screws are placed in the infraorbital and lateral orbital rims providing the necessary two-point fixation. It is not uncommon to have more than one fracture in the infraorbital rim and multiple fragments that require fixation. It is important to remember that the purpose of the reconstruction of the rim is aesthetic. Although the rim may look acceptable when the fragments are not properly aligned, when the periorbital edema resolves the irregularities in the rim will be visibly and palpably apparent. Some fragments are so small that

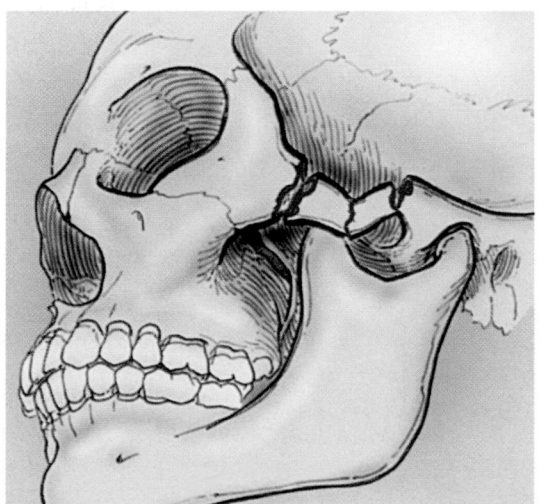

Figure 32 Depressed fracture of the zygomatic arch. (Reproduced with permission from reference 38.)

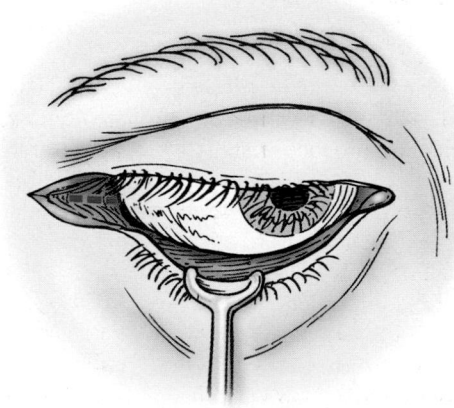

Figure 34 Schematic illustration of a transconjunctival approach to the infraorbital rim and orbital floor. It shows the transconjunctival incision and the lateral canthotomy already performed. The dotted line indicates the area for inferior cantholysis to improve exposure.

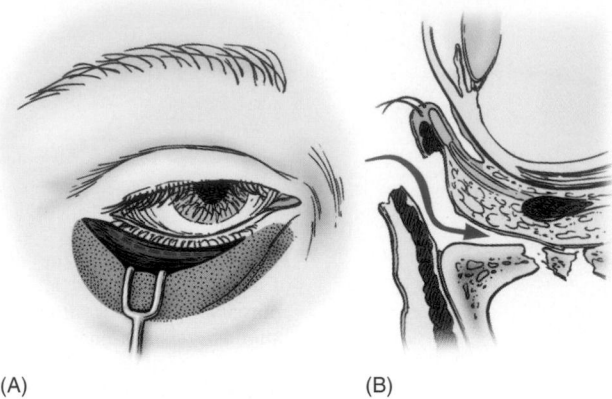

(A)   (B)

Figure 35 Stair-step incision through the infraciliary area, performed to avoid ectropion. (A) Frontal view. (B) Lateral view. (Reproduced with permission from reference 12.)

their approximation may need to be done with fine wire or suture material. Some surgeons add an additional plate at the inferior aspect of the zygomatic buttress. This will require an additional incision in the gingival buccal sulcus like an extended Caldwell-Luc incision. A subperiosteal elevation will expose the under side of the zygomatic buttress. In most trimalar fractures, this step is entirely unnecessary.

Compound comminuted fractures of the body (Figure 37) require a direct approach to the way of either a coronal scalp incision or extending the infraorbital incision superiorly and the upper brow incision laterally. Either a rigid miniplate or a multiple interosseous wires can be used to fix multiple comminuted body fractures. When interosseous wiring is used for the compound body fracture, it is sometimes necessary to maintain elevation of the zygoma as it tends to prolapse. This can be done with an external pin fixation device such as a Morris biphase appliance.

Postoperative Care. After surgery if the fracture is unstable, a head dressing should be applied to hold a zygoma guard in place (Figure 38). This guard will not necessarily protect the zygomatic arch from collapsing with some pressure, but it will remind the patient not to roll on that side of the face while sleeping. This protective device is best retained for at least 2 weeks but can be removed when the patient is not sleeping. The zygoma guard is necessary in patients who have had interosseus wiring of a trimalar fracture, a reduced but not rigidly fixed arch fracture or an unstable fracture with multiple comminution. Most fractures fixed with a rigid plating system will not need the guard.

Routine wound care is administered in the postoperative period and the sutures should be removed within 3 to 5 days. Diplopia from the operation surgery may not be resolved for up to 2 months. If there is postoperative diplopia and a thorough exploration of the orbital floor revealed

no significant blowout fracture, the patient may be managed expectantly with a good prognosis. Unrepaired zygoma fractures often lead to cosmetic deformity. Because of the pull of the masseter, the zygoma is distracted in a downward and medial direction. This type of deformity causes lack of cheekbone prominence and an increase in orbital volume.

Enophthalmos is the result of failure to reduce an orbital floor fracture properly, with subsequent atrophy of herniated orbital fat. The actual orbital volume is increased if the zygoma heals in a rotated position. If orbital volume is increased appreciably, the remaining orbital contents are insufficient to maintain normal anterior protrusion of the globe, resulting in the "sunken eye" appearance of enophthalmos.[45] In rare instances, posteromedial displacement creates a smaller orbital compartment and a concomitant exophthalmos.[46]

In the nonseeing eye, the problems of enophthalmos can be corrected with minimal risk. Allografts or autogenous material may be placed in the orbit to increase orbital volume. Bony deformities are treated with onlay grafts or osteotomies of the zygoma with interposed calvarial bone grafts. Enophthalmos in a person with vision can safely be corrected with calvarial bone grafts to the orbital floor. The use of other material such as titanium mesh or mesh covered in hydroxyapatite bone cement has also been advocated. Danger to the optic nerve and of extrusion or migration of alloplastic material[44] makes this procedure potentially hazardous.

An unreduced fracture of the zygomatic arch or one that is incompletely elevated into position may form a bony union with the coronoid process of the mandible. This is a rare complication but will produce severe trismus that can only be eliminated by an open osteotomy and rigid fixation of the arch. Removal of the bony connection between the arch and the coronoid is essential, and placement of a silastic sheet between the two bony structures may be necessary to prevent a relapse. The silastic may have to be removed at a future time; but, if it is not problematic, it may remain indefinitely.

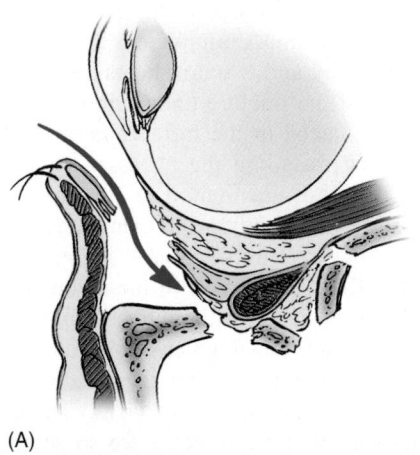

(A)

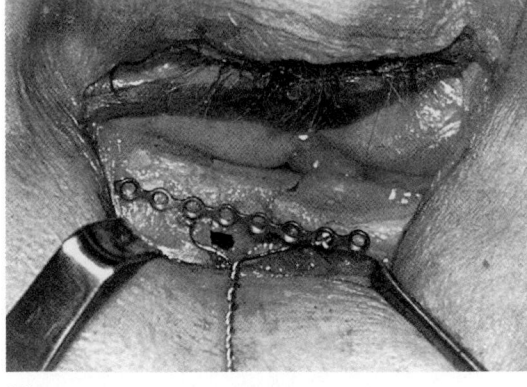

(B)

Figure 36 (A) Lateral view of the transconjunctival approach to the infraorbital rim and orbital floor. Note that the fracture in the infraorbital rim extends into the orbital floor where a defect is present in the bone with herniation of intraorbital contents. (B) Microplate fixation of a fracture of the infraorbital rim. Note that a single interosseous wire has been placed to assist in reduction of the fracture while plating is performed.

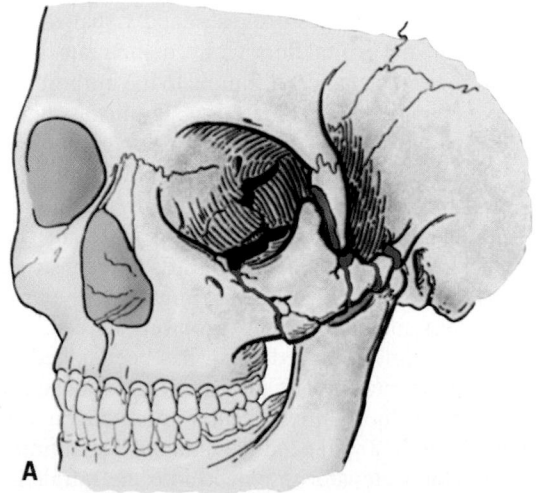

A

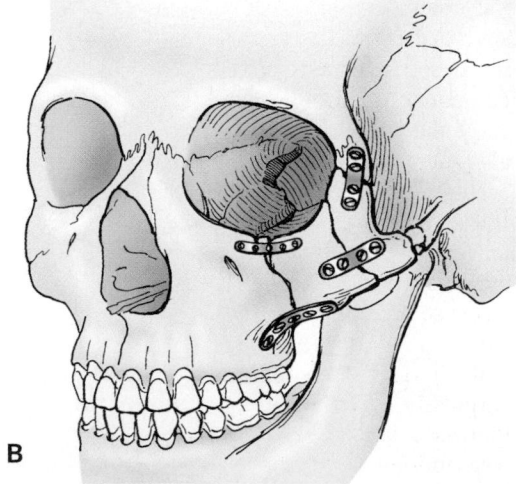

B

Figure 37 (A) Complex body fracture of zygoma. (B) At least three-point stabilization is required for adequate fixation. (Reproduced with permission from references 47.)

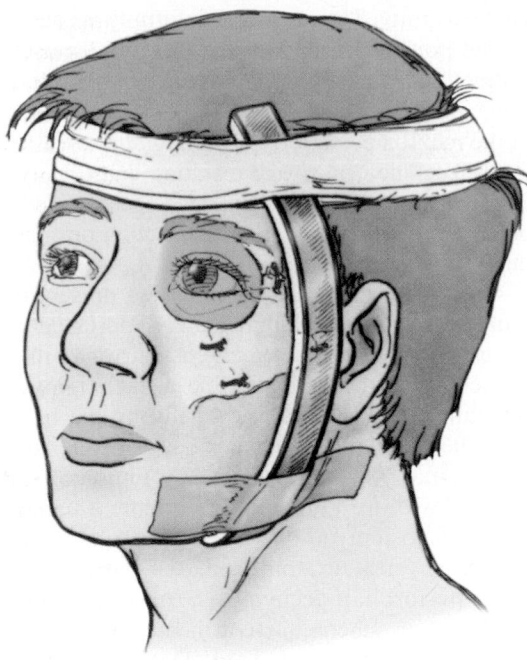

Figure 38 Guard placed to prevent displacement of the fracture reduction.

MAXILLARY (LE FORT) FRACTURES

Causes

Fractures of the midface, commonly referred to as Le Fort fractures, occur with much less frequency than fractures of the mandible, zygoma, or nose. Most often, they are the result of blunt trauma from accidents in automobiles, motorcycles, snowmobiles, or boats. The force required to fracture the maxilla and pterygoid plates of the sphenoid, which are the two fractured bones common to all Le Fort fractures, is considerable. Because of the alignment of the buttresses of the midface, which protect this area from vertical displacement, most of these fractures are caused by horizontal forces from the lateral, oblique, or anterior direction. The cranium and the orbit are intimately associated with these injuries and should be addressed with a high index of suspicion in all patients with midface injuries.

In the early 1900s, Rene Le Fort described the common lines of fractures associated with severe blunt trauma to cadaver heads.[48] Although his descriptions are not characteristic of many compound midfacial fractures, they do serve to stage the degree of severity of the fractures and also alert the physician to concomitant antecedent injuries that are peculiar to the three types of fractures. It is much more accurate to describe an injury in such terms as a compound palatal zygomaticomaxillary or maxillonasal fractures. Because of the number of bones in the face that can be associated with large compound midfacial injuries and because many of them are not surgically accessible by any means other than that associated with those injuries, the classic descriptions of Le Fort become useful indices for patient management and as the tools for communication between physicians of different specialties.

Anatomy

The maxillae are the large paired bones of the midface that are approximately box shaped and almost fully pneumatized by their own sinuses. The lateral wall is a part of the infratemporal fossa and articulates with the zygoma superiorly and the temporal bone posteriorly. The anterior wall has a medial articulation with the nasal bones by way of the frontal process of the maxilla, which extends along the pyriform aperture up toward the bony orbit to form the anterior crest of the lacrimal fossa. The medial wall is intimately associated with the ethmoid complex superiorly as well as the inferior turbinate. The posterior wall is relatively more substantial than the anterior wall "protecting" the pterygomaxillary fossa and its nerves and vessels. Posteriorly, the maxilla also communicates with the sphenoid bone, both superiorly with the inferior aspect of the greater wing of the sphenoid and posterolaterally with the pterygoid plates. The vomer, ethmoid complex, palatine bones, zygoma, and nasal bones should also be considered part of the midface. One or all of these bones are often fractured in Le Fort fractures, although they may not all need direct treatment.

Le Fort Classification. Le Fort classification refers to the lines of the three most common types of midface fractures (linae minores resistentiae) (Figure 39). The Le Fort I fracture is a lower palatal fracture also called the Guérin fracture. Le Fort II fractures are also referred to as pyramidal fractures. Le Fort III fractures are also known as craniofacial disjunctions.

The Le Fort I fracture involves the floor of the nose, lower third of the maxilla, palate, and pterygoid plates, usually in one segment. Le Fort II fracture occurs across the nasal bony superstructure and the frontal process of the maxilla, down across the face of the anterior wall of the maxilla, and orbital floor, including the infraorbital foramen. The fracture line goes through the lateral wall of the maxilla extending to the pterygoid plates, usually higher than the Le Fort I. Le Fort III fractures extend laterally across the orbital floor into the lateral orbit through the zygoma. They can include the frontal zygomatic suture line. If the zygoma moves during palpation of the palate with movement, a Le Fort II fracture is present.

Le Fort fractures are commonly found in combinations. A Le Fort I fracture may have an associated Le Fort II or III on the side of impact. A Le Fort II fracture may be a Le Fort III fracture on the side of the impact. The exact classification of the fractures on each side is important because of the differences of treatment associated with the various types. One should refer to the fractures based on the type of fracture on each side, for instance, left Le Fort III or right Le Fort I.

The Structural Pillars of the Midface. Le Fort's classification was surprisingly complete in its description of the midfacial fractures, although there are certain limitations to

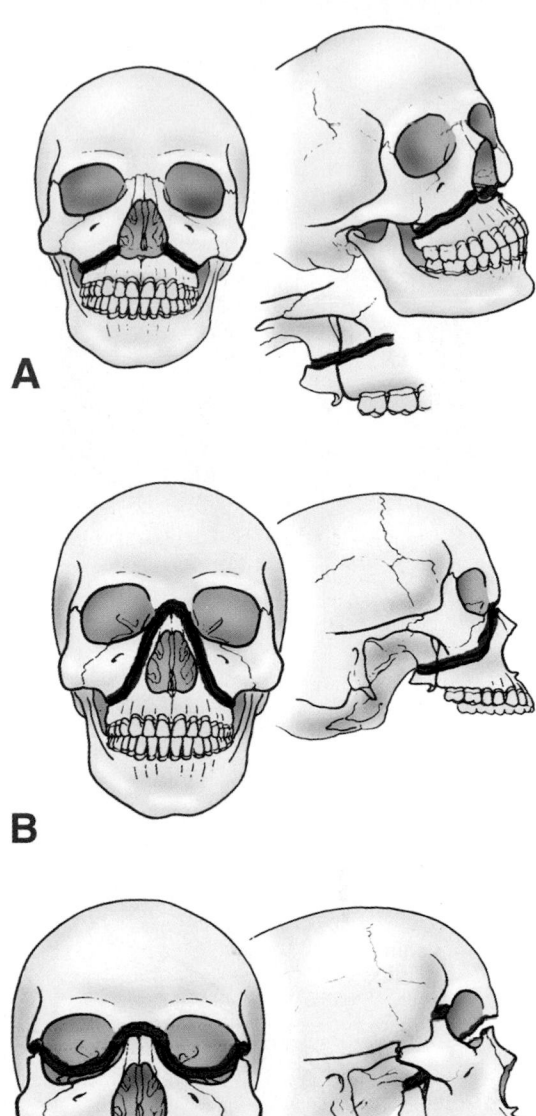

Figure 39 Le Fort fractures of the maxilla. (A) Le Fort I. (B) Le Fort II. (C) Le Fort III.

his original description. The classification of Le Fort fractures is based on the most superior fracture line involved in the fractures and does not take into account the facts that many of the fractures of the midface are comminuted and that within the confines of the midfacial skeleton these multiple fractures may take on many configurations.[48–50] The concept of the structural pillars of the midface (Figure 40) helps to elucidate the key areas of fracture and, therefore, the subsequent stabilization of the midface as it relates to both potential cosmetic deformities and functional problems. An understanding of these structural pillars not only aids in assessment of the severity of the fracture but also provides an excellent strategic framework for surgical intervention.

There are three main buttresses of the midface–cranial complex.[51] Going from anterior to posterior, the anteriormost buttress is the

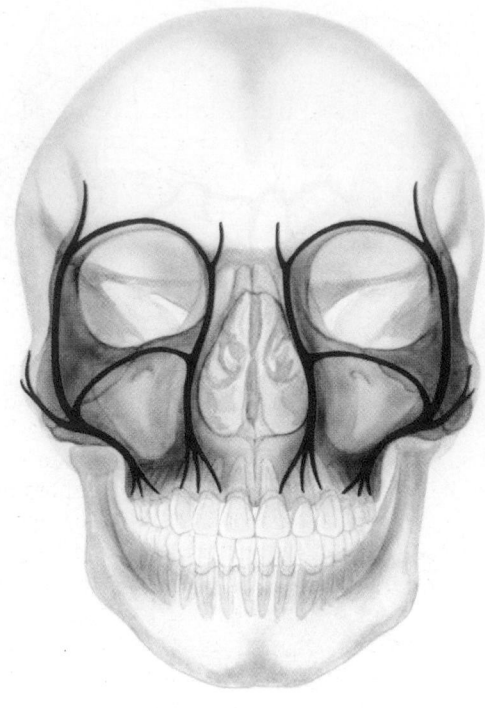

(A)

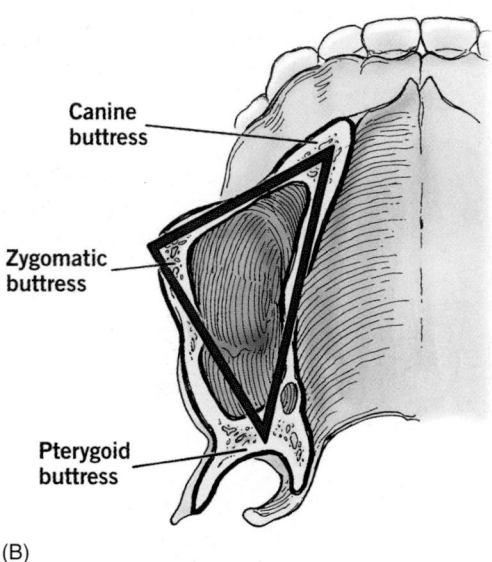

Canine
buttress

Zygomatic
buttress

Pterygoid
buttress

(B)

Figure 40 (A) and (B) Biomechanical stress curves of the middle one-third of the face.

nasomaxillary (canine) buttress extending from the maxillary alveolar ridge along the pyriform aperture up to the medial side of the orbit through the anterior lacrimal crest, the frontal process of the maxilla to the superior orbital rim and ending at the frontal bone of the cranium.

The zygomaticomaxillary buttress extends from the maxillary alveolar ridge above the anterior molar teeth to the zygomatic process of the frontal bone with a vertical component consisting of the zygomatic arch articulating with the zygomatic process of the temporal bone at the base of the skull.

The buttress of the pterygomaxillary alveolar ridge articulates with the base of the skull through the orbital process of the palatine bone and posteriorly with the sphenoid bone. The pterygoid portion of this vertical buttress consists of the

pterygoid plates extending inferiorly and anteriorly toward the maxilla. The horizontal system of buttresses divides the oral, nasal and orbital regions of the face.

If one considered these pillars in midfacial fractures, therapy should be directed toward the stabilization of as many of these buttresses as possible. Probably the two most important areas of stabilization are the nasomaxillary buttress and the zygomaticomaxillary buttress. The more posterior vertical pterygomaxillary buttress is more inaccessible surgically, although the most inferior portion of it can be stabilized if necessary. In severely comminuted Le Fort fractures, the surgeon must appreciate the advantage of open reduction and internal fixation of multiple fragments in their anatomic positions, especially those relating to this buttress complex. Without proper reduction of the midface fractures or proper stabilization of concomitant subcondylar mandible fractures, there is always the possibility of midfacial telescoping, which results in a shortened midface.[51–53]

Diagnosis

Eliciting an accurate history on a patient with severe midfacial injury is often difficult or impossible because of associated intercranial, abdominal, or intrathoracic injuries. The motor vehicle accident victim may also be inebriated. If the patient is conscious, however, and does not have any life-threatening injuries requiring emergency surgical intervention, a thorough history is helpful in ascertaining the extent and severity of facial injury.

Because the maxilla forms the anterior floor of the orbit, there may be herniation of the orbital soft tissues into the maxillary sinus, similar to that seen in a blowout fracture. Diplopia is a complaint in Le Fort II or Le Fort III fractures. Complaints of blurred vision or a change in visual acuity mandate an ophthalmologic evaluation. Epiphora may also be a component of compound fractures involving the lacrimal duct and/or the inferior medial orbital area. Difficulty in breathing is a common problem from congestion associated with edema from the fractures as well as physical derangement of the nasal bones and septal structures. The commonest cause of upper airway obstruction in these patients is the posterior inferior displacement of the maxillary segments by the pull of the medial pterygoid muscles, which pull the maxilla via the pterygoid plates toward their insertions at the lingual surface of the mandible. Bleeding from the maxillary or ethmoid ostia or from lacerations within the nasal cavity may cause severe nasal obstruction. Patient complaints of a salty taste in the mouth should alert the physician of the possibility of a cerebrospinal fluid leak. Most commonly these are found in the cribriform plate or the roof of the ethmoid sinuses.[6,7] Displacement of the maxilla causes the patient to complain of malocclusion. Although there may be either buccal or lingual version, the most common occlusal abnormality is an open-

bite deformity. The open-bite deformity is caused by the powerful forces of the pterygoid muscle distracting the posterior part of the maxilla inferiorly.[7] A blow from the front causes displacement of the maxilla posteriorly, resulting in a so-called "dish face" deformity and resulting in a Class III malocclusion. A more detailed discussion is of occlusal abnormalities is in the section on mandible fractures.

Airway compromise is often the presenting problem and must be immediately addressed by the establishment of an emergency airway, either a cricothyrotomy or if feasible a tracheostomy. Intubation is dangerous especially by the nasal route because of accidental passage of the tube intracranially. In the author's opinion, most patients with Le Fort fractures require a temporary tracheostomy.

On physical examination, the patient may have periorbital ecchymosis, massive tissue swelling, or subconjunctival hemorrhage if the infraorbital rim is involved. Dental examination confirms the previously mentioned findings relating to open bite, lingual/buccal version, and Class III malocclusion. Bony crepitus of the midface, especially in severely comminuted injuries, is common. Also, extensive fractures in the presence of a large communication with the anterior part of the antrum and the nose cause subcutaneous emphysema.

Nasal or pharyngeal hemorrhage may be massive. This is important because most patients are evaluated in the supine position. Nasal and pharyngeal bleeding drain toward the posterior part of the pharynx and may go unnoticed. Palpation reveals a mobile palate. If the palate does not move even though there appear to be gross occlusal differences and/or obvious fractures, it is because the midface has impacted into an immobile position.[54] To move the palate in these cases may require excessive force. Pain in the areas of the fractures are exacerbated by attempting to bite down. The patient may notice the mobility of his midface on moving his jaws. The complaint of amaurosis suggests either intraocular injury or damage to the optic nerve. Progressive blindness in the presence of a fracture of the optic canal constitutes the major indication for orbital decompression among those individuals who are proponents of this procedure. Despite years of controversy and discussion over the value of orbital decompression, definitive evidence as to its efficacy is still wanting. However, I think that in a patient with failing vision with an optic canal fracture not responding or worsening with a short course of large doses of corticosteroids, surgical decompression is indicated.

Imaging

Radiologic diagnosis of Le Fort fractures is an important adjunct to their treatment. Many midfacial fractures can be assessed with routine sinus X-rays, but the precision of the CT scan is a huge advantage in delineating the extent and severity of midfacial fractures. Central injuries can be

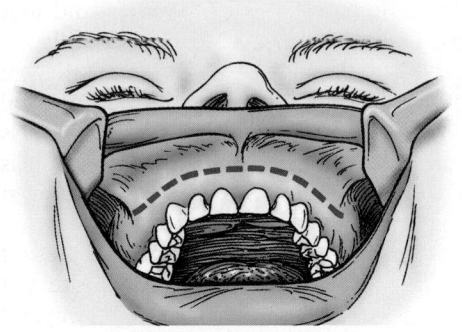

Figure 41 Schematic diagram of a sublabial incision for approach to midfacial fractures.

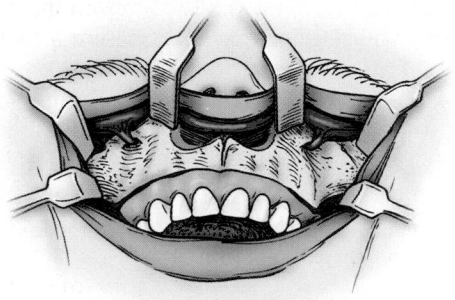

Figure 42 Schematic diagram of subperiosteal dissection through a sublabial incision exposing the infraorbital nerves.

ruled out by extending the scan through the head, any nasal-frontal or frontal sinus components can be delineated and fractures of the sphenoid and orbital apex are excellently portrayed. Scans in both the axial and coronal planes are necessary for the most complete analysis. MRI is of little added assistance except in the case of cerebral trauma or compromise of the optic nerves. Three-dimensional reconstruction, although spectacular to look at, offers little additional information that will guide therapy.

Treatment

As in all patients involved in trauma, the fundamental precepts of trauma care apply. The airway is of great importance in these patients. A displaced Le Fort fracture can compromise the airway, especially if it is associated with concomitant massive swelling of the tongue and oropharynx.[6,7] A cricothyrotomy may be required urgently. Endotracheal intubation should be avoided because of the problems of poor visualization, the possibility of aggravating a cervical spine injury, and possibly causing injury to the central nervous system from the endotracheal tube. Nasotracheal intubation is even worse because of the danger of intracranial intubation through a fracture line in the skull base. Tracheostomy preferably should not be done in the emergency room but performed electively in the operating room. All other injuries should be ruled out, including intra-abdominal, intrathoracic, and intracranial injuries. The cervical spine should undergo radiographic evaluation.

If the patient is to undergo immediate general anesthesia for a related injury and is hemodynamically stable, immediate repair can be undertaken if good radiographic documentation of the injury has been obtained. Often, if a patient is rushed to the operating room because of a life-threatening injury, proper radiographs may not have been obtained and, if a Le Fort fracture is suspected, the patient should be placed temporarily into intermaxillary fixation and undergo tracheostomy. In this emergency situation, the patient can be more fully evaluated radiographically at a later time to ascertain the extent of the midfacial fractures.

Definitive repair of all fractures may be delayed for up to 10 days before bony union may make reduction difficult. Thorough preoperative planning to repair these fractures includes ophthalmologic examination, dental evaluation, and clearance by neurosurgeons if there are concomitant intercranial injuries. Repair should also be delayed until the status of the cervical spine is determined.

Surgical Approaches. Incisions used to approach midfacial fractures vary according to the specific location of the fracture. Isolated Le Fort I fractures are usually approached by an extended sublabial incision (Figures 41 and 42). This incision allows exposure of the zygomaticomaxillary buttresses and pyriform apertures bilaterally. If the fracture involves the infraorbital rim (Le Fort II), a transconjunctival-lateral canthotomy or subciliary incision is usually used to expose these fracture sites. If a Le Fort II fracture is more extensive and greater exposure to the nasoethmoid complex is required, an external Lynch incision or extended coronal incision may be used. The frontozygomatic suture line may be approached with a coronal, brow, or extended upper blepharoplasty (supratarsal) incision. The coronal incision has the advantage of providing exposure to the zygomatic arch and the nasoethmoid region. This incision obviates the need for a Lynch incision for nasoethmoid exposure.

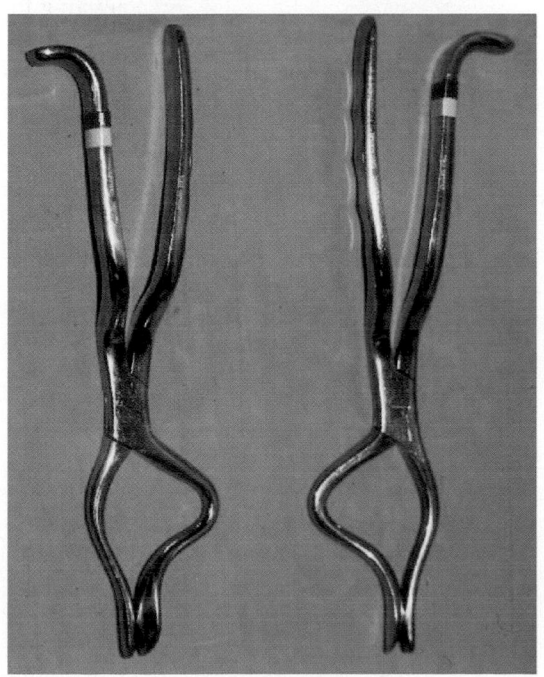

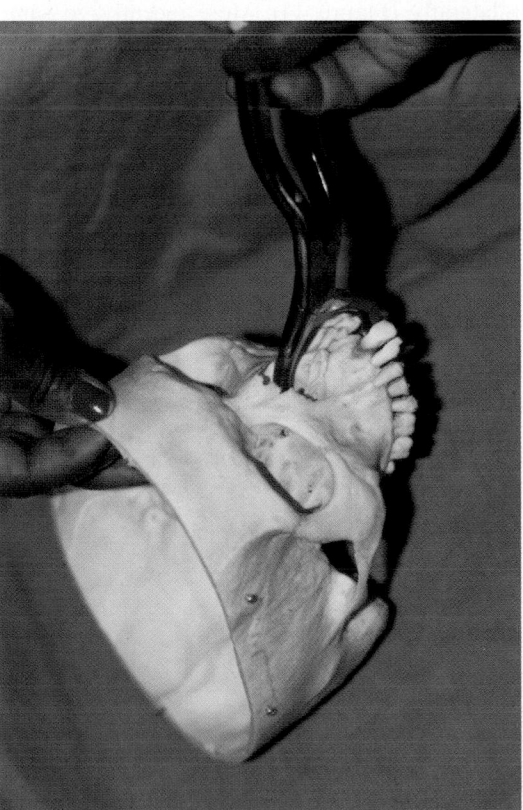

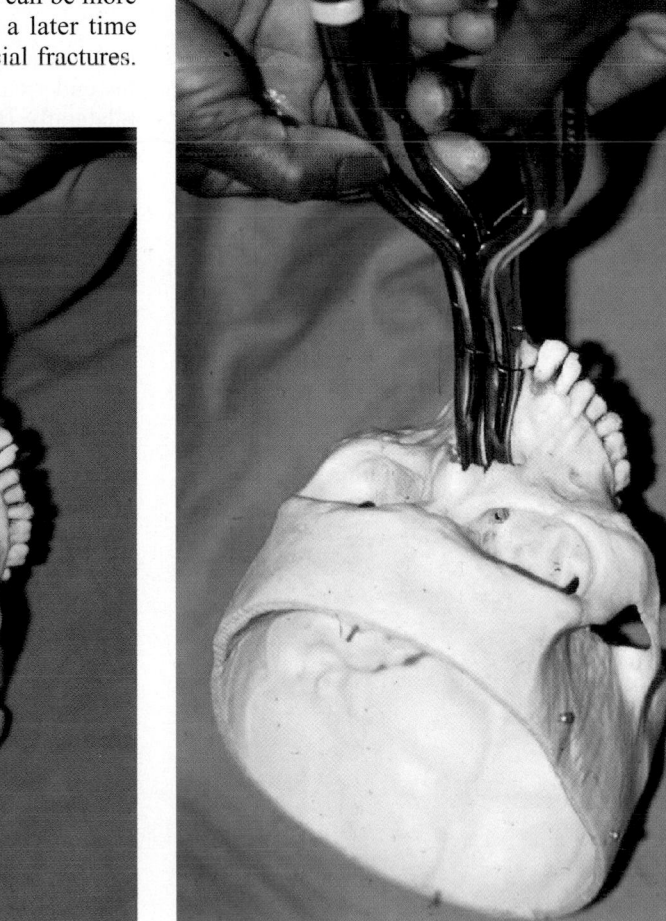

(A)   (B)   (C)

Figure 43 Maxillary disimpaction using Rowe-Killey forceps. (A) Pair of forceps. (B) Forceps applied on one side. (C) Forceps applied on both sides.

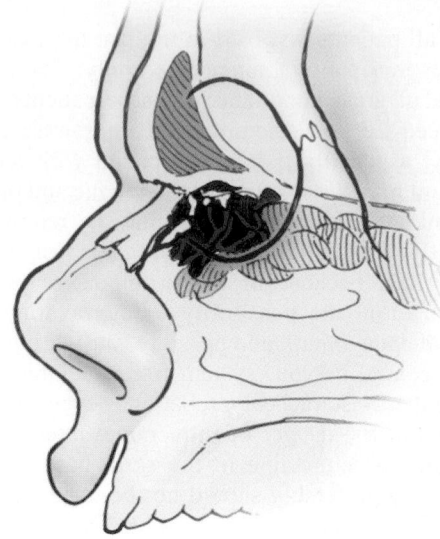

Figure 44 Miniplate fixation of a Le Fort I fracture. Note the stabilization of the nasomaxillary and zygomatico-maxillary buttresses.

The incisions used depend on the location and extent of the fractures. Most Le Fort fractures do not manifest as the original description, but these are combinations of complex fractures of the midface and require knowledge of multiple surgical approaches.

In patients with dentition, arch bars and intermaxillary fixation are initially applied to reestablish pretrauma occlusion. In edentulous patients, a splint or denture containing an arch bar is fixed to the mandible or maxilla to reestablish appropriate skeletal relationships. This is performed with circummandibular wires or drop wires from the pyriform rim or zygoma. The maxillary (palatal) splint may also be fixed to the palate with two transpalatal screws. In any case, splints or dentures are placed to reestablish the occlusal and skeletal relationship.

In patients whose midfacial fractures are displaced, disimpaction of fractures may be required before placement of intermaxillary fixation. Disimpaction is best achieved by use of the Rowe-Killey disimpaction forceps (Figure 43). The straight blade is placed in the nasal cavity along the nasal floor and the curved blade over the alveolar ridge and along the palate. Grasping the handles firmly a downward and anterior pull will disimpact the maxilla and restore it into its normal relationship with the mandible and skull base. After the occlusal relationship is reestablished, all fracture sites are fully exposed. The facial skeleton should then be reconstituted in three dimensions: height, width, and depth.[51,52] Careful attention should be paid to reestablishing

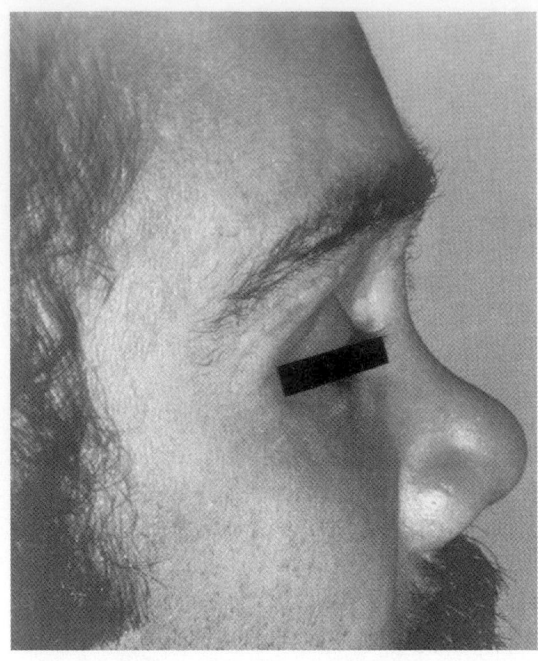

Figure 46 Nasofrontal complex fracture. Note nasal bones driven under the frontal bones. (Reproduced with permission reference 55.)

all important facial buttresses. In particular, the vertical zygomaticomaxillary and nasomaxillary buttresses should be carefully reduced and fixated to reestablish vertical facial height. All rigid fixation should be applied with sufficient stability to counteract any forces that could disrupt bone repair during healing.

For a Le Fort I fracture, a two-point stabilization at the nasomaxillary and zygomaticomaxillary buttresses is established on each side. Titanium low profile miniplates in an "L," "X" or square configuration are placed on the anterior buttresses and usually an "L" shaped plate on the under-curve of each zygoma onto the maxilla bilaterally (Figure 44). More recently, in same cases, low-profile absorbable plates of polymers comprising polyglycolic or polylactic acid or a combination have been employed in place of titanium plates. These plates are reputed to retain sufficient strength to maintain fixation over the critical period of healing and then are absorbed. This especially is an advantage in children in whom the metal plates may impede bony facial

Figure 48 "Pig snout" deformity characteristic of naso-frontal-ethmoidal complex fracture. (Reproduced with permission from reference 55.)

growth at suture lines. In adults, the principal advantages of absorbable plates are in preventing pain that occasionally occurs with the metal plates and eliminating the palpable plate at the lateral and infraorbital rims once they have been absorbed. The durability and utility of absorbable plating systems have yet to stand the test of time.

Le Fort II fractures require fixation at the infra-orbital rim and the zygomaticomaxillary buttress. If the nasal bones are comminuted, microplates

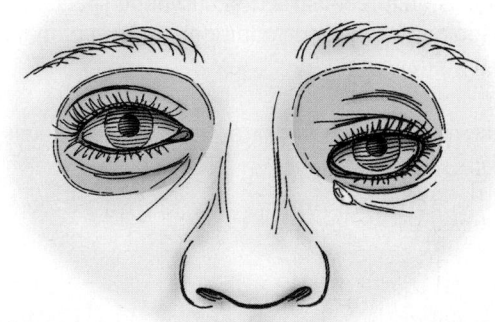

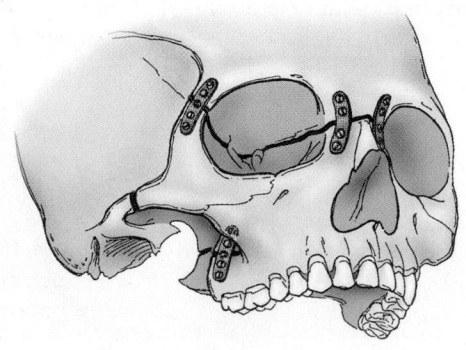

Figure 45 Three point rigid fixation of Le Fort III fracture.

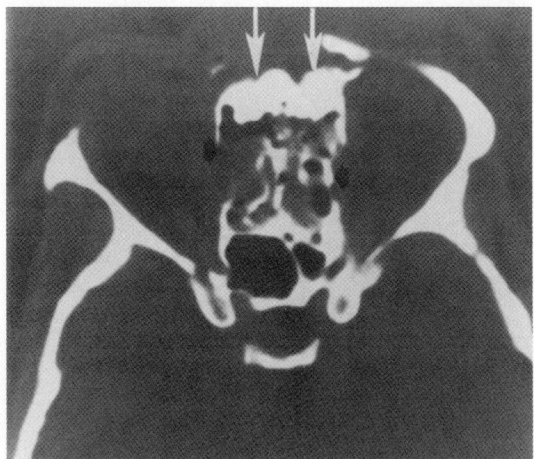

Figure 47 Computed tomographic scan showing naso-frontal-ethmoidal fracture. Arrows show direction of displacement. (Reproduced with permission from reference 55.)

(A)

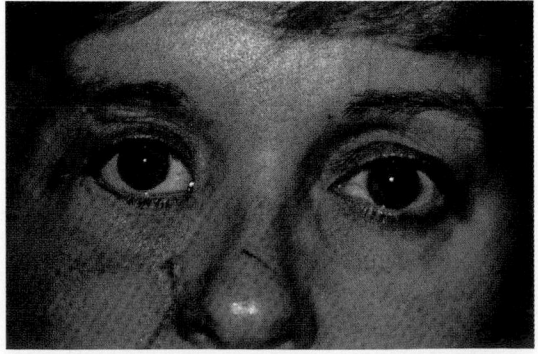

(B)

Figure 49 (A) Diagram showing telecanthus. (B) Patient with unilateral telecanthus.

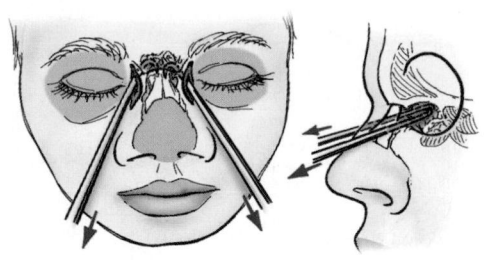

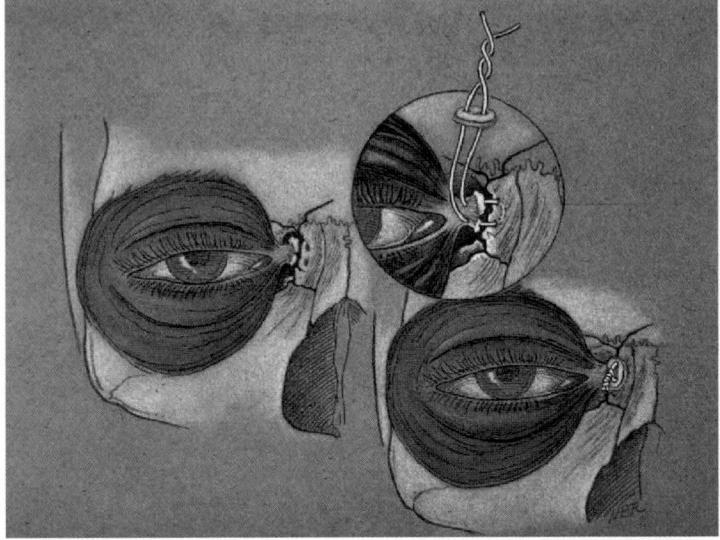

Figure 50 Reduction of frontal-ethmoidal fracture. Stout bone hooks are placed through lamina papyracea into the ethmoid fracture. Forward and downward traction is exerted until fracture is reduced. (Reproduced with permission from reference 55.)

Figure 52 Standard method of fixation of unilateral medial canthal tendon avulsion. (A) Fixation to medial orbital wall with wire. Two small holes are drilled in the lacrimal bone. (B) Wire is passed through the tendon and bone. Wire is passed through a small Dacron felt bolster to prevent wire tearing through the tendon. (C) Wire is gently twisted for the ligature. (Reproduced with permission from reference 55.)

are used on the nasal bones. The infraorbital rims will be fixed with microplates as well. As in most instances the miniplates have too high a profile and will be obvious through the skin.

The Le Fort III fracture is often a devastating injury usually accompanied by cerebral trauma. It is not uncommon to have a staged type of treatment in which the neurosurgeon controls the intracranial injury and the management of the facial component is limited to the performance of a tracheostomy and the application of arch bars and interdental elastic bands. The treatment of the maxillary fracture is delayed until the patient's neurological status has stabilized. The shattered maxilla must be fixed between two stable platforms. The cranium provides the superior stabilization point and the mandible the inferior. All displaced fractures of the cranial vault must be restored to their normal anatomical position. Similarly all fractures of the mandible must be rigidly fixed in a correct position to establish the occlusal template for the maxillary dentition to approximate accurately. Rigid fixation of all mandibular fractures is vital to ensure this relationship. Displaced subcondylar fractures must be fixed to provide the stable platform even when only unilateral. Undisplaced subcondylar fractures are usually sufficiently stable to avoid rigid fixation. The goals of reduction and fixation of the Le Fort III fracture must be clearly borne in mind as fixation proceeds. First, the supporting buttresses of the face must be reestablished. Second, the functional elements must be restored, such as the correct orbital volume, including an adequately restored orbital floor with orbital contents free of entrapment, a patent nasal airway bilaterally and maxillary sinuses that will adequately drain.[53] Third, all-important aesthetic landmarks must be restored, such as the orbital rims, nasal dorsum,

and malar eminencies.[54] It is not necessary and in some instances, is indeed impossible to approximate every small maxillary fragment. The lateral orbital rims and the buttresses are fixed with miniplates and the nasal dorsum and infraorbital rims with microplates (Figure 45). Occasionally small fragments in key positions may require fixation with fine wire or even suture material. The use of titanium wire will prevent interference in subsequent scans.

If rigid fixation is considered stable and if the patient is compliant, intermaxillary fixation may be removed at the conclusion of the operation or within the first 1 to 2 weeks after the operation. If the stability is in question, that is, with bone comminution or bone loss, intermaxillary fixation should be left in place for up to 6 to 8 weeks. This will help maintain the occlusion while bone healing occurs.

NASOFRONTAL-ETHMOIDAL FRACTURES AND TRAUMATIC TELECANTHUS

A central blow to the face created by a small diameter object, such as the head of a hammer, may not produce a Le Fort type maxillary fracture, but if of sufficient force, may cause a severely comminuted nasal fracture that shatters the medial orbital walls and telescopes into the ethmoid block lodging the fractured bones under the nasal process of the frontal bone (Figure 46). Not uncommonly this nasofrontal-ethmoidal fracture will be accompanied by telecanthus that result from either the shearing away of the medial canthal tendons or a displacement of the lacrimal and maxillary bone onto which the tendon or tendons insert. The nasal

dorsum is essentially displaced into the fractured anterior ethmoid sinuses (Figure 47). This injury produces a typical clinical picture of a patient with a "pig snout" deformity consisting of a flattened nasal dorsum with an exaggerated excessively superiorly rotated tip (Figure 48).

The telecanthus may be unilateral or bilateral. The natural contraction of the orbicularis oculi, whose tendonous extension comprises the bulk of the medial canthal tendon, pulls the medial canthus away from the midline. This produces a blunting of the medial canthus, with a widening of the medial canthal angle, a shortening of the width of the palpebral fissure, a slight ectropion and an inferior inclination of the medial canthus (Figure 49). The width of each palpebral fissure should normally be the width between both eyes, approximately 25.5 to 37.5 mm in adult women and 26.5 to 37.8 mm in men.[56] With this injury, there is usually the absence of the "bowstring" sign. If tension is created in the medial canthal tendon of the normal eye by pulling laterally on the lateral canthus of the eye, a taught bowstring-like sensation is felt by the palpating finger. If instead there is a soft, loose boggy feeling at the inner canthus, the presence of a ruptured tendon is highly likely. In addition, there may be injury to the lacrimal system with fracturing of the bony nasolacrimal duct. This will produce epiphora. Epiphora may also result from the loss of the effectiveness of the "lacrimal pump" mechanism. This is formed by the splitting of the medial canthal tendon into two slips of tendon which then insert onto the lacrimal bone both anteriorly and posteriorly to the lacrimal sac. With slackening of the tendon by displacement of the medial canthal tendon, the pump is unable to function effectively.

At times the nasal skeleton is so badly comminuted that the small fragments cannot even hold the small 0.8 mm screws required for microplate fixation. A solution to this is the use of suspension wires and lead plates.[55] The wires are driven from one side of the nose to the other with the nasal skeleton in the reduced position. The wires penetrate skin, the nasal bone, and ethmoid sinuses on one side then pass through the septum and the same structures of the other side (Figures 50 and 51). It

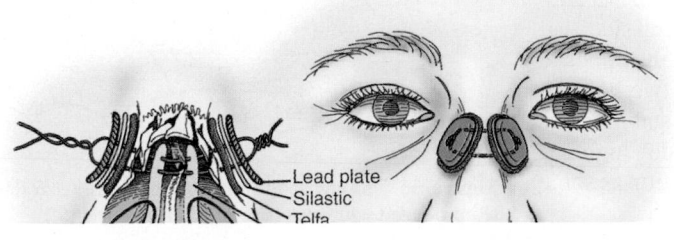

Figure 51 Nasal bones fixed with lead plates. (Reproduced with permission from reference 55.)

Lead plate
Silastic
Telfa

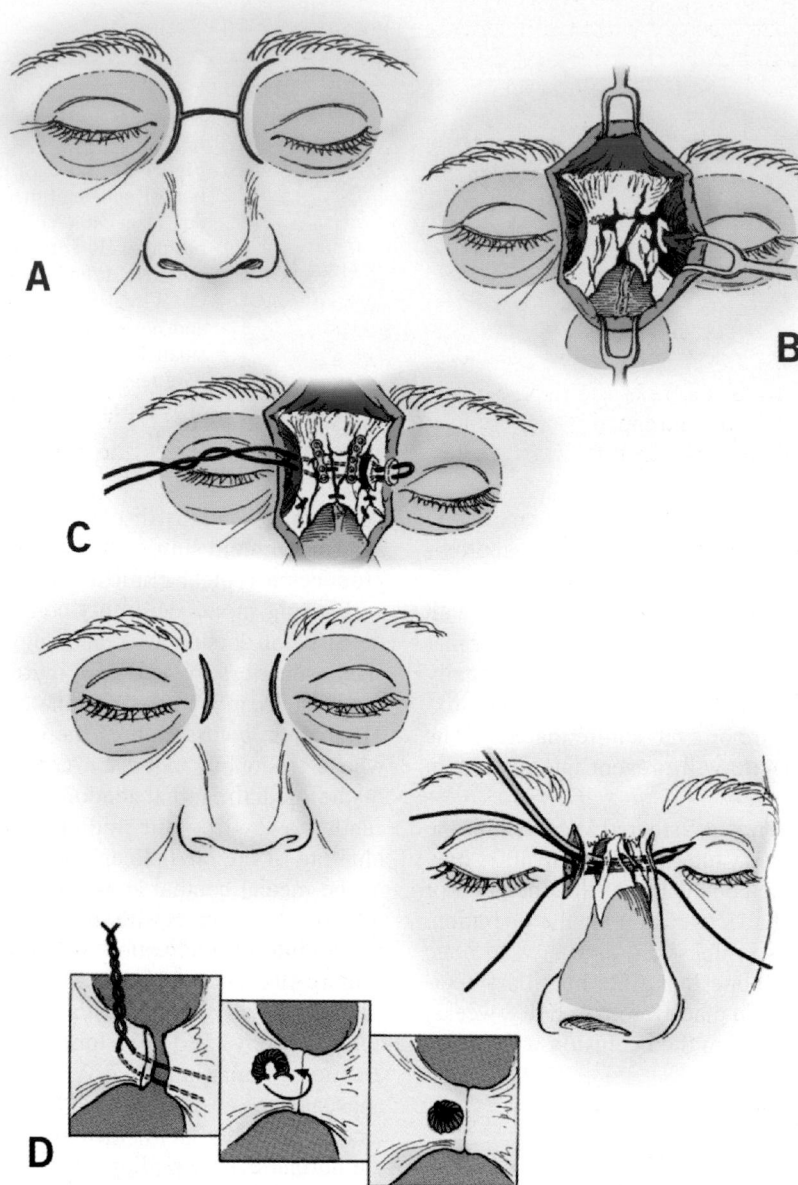

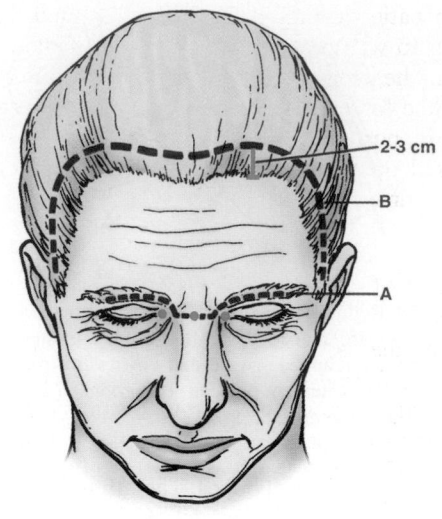

Figure 54 Incisions used for access for frontal sinus fracture repair. (A) Butterfly incision. (B) Coronal scalp incision.

The worse injury is the bilateral lateral canthal tendon avulsion. The Converse-Hogan open sky technique is probably the most effective[59] (Figure 53). This method wires one canthal tendon to that of the opposite side and supports the skin of the nasal area with lead plates.

Bone Grafting

In some patients with midfacial fractures, bone comminution or bone loss prevents proper reestablishment of facial buttresses. Loss of vertical height with midfacial shortening can result. When this condition is recognized, immediate bone grafting is indicated.[53] Grafting is usually performed by harvest of split calvarial bone grafts. These grafts have a good viability and stabilize fixation in cases with significant bone loss.

Figure 53 Bilateral medial canthal tendon avulsion repaired using the Converse-Hogan "open sky" technique. (A) Incisions opened. (B) Fractures are reduced. (C) Two pairs of wires inserted—one through the medial canthal tendons (*above*), the second through the adjacent nasal bones (*below*). (D) Wires are tightened, bringing canthal tendons into position. The wires are twisted together over each avulsed tendon, pulling the tendons together. Tendons are supported, and soft tissue is splinted by Tefla pad-Silastic-lead plate assembly (see Figure 51).

must be remembered that the plates act simply as anchoring sites for the wires and not as a means of narrowing the nose. Over-tightening of the wires can lead to underlying skin necrosis. The wires are removed after 3 weeks.

Obtaining an excellent cosmetic result in the reduction of dislocated medial canthal tendons is one of the most demanding tasks in the surgery of facial trauma. The repair is best done as soon as possible after the accident. Late repairs are notoriously noted for their less than optimal results. Often the tendon comes away with a fragment of attached lacrimal bone. In those instances, two small holes are placed in the bone that will serve as anchor points for the wire used in fixation. If no anchoring bone exists, some kind of stabilization

must be created to prevent the wire from pulling through. The Kazanjian button may be created by twisting the two wires passed through the tendon into the configuration of a rosette.[57] Another method is the use of a Dacron bolster (Figure 52) that is usually used to stabilize hemostatic sutures placed in the aorta.[58] In a unilateral canthal repair, the wire can be secured to the bone of the medial wall of the opposite orbit. If enough bone of adequate strength is present on the ipsilateral side, that would be preferable. A bone graft on the opposite side of the nose can be used or even two holes in a microplate that has been used to stabilize the nasal bones. It is vital to place the tendon high and posterior with some small overcorrection as some degree of relapse is almost inevitable.

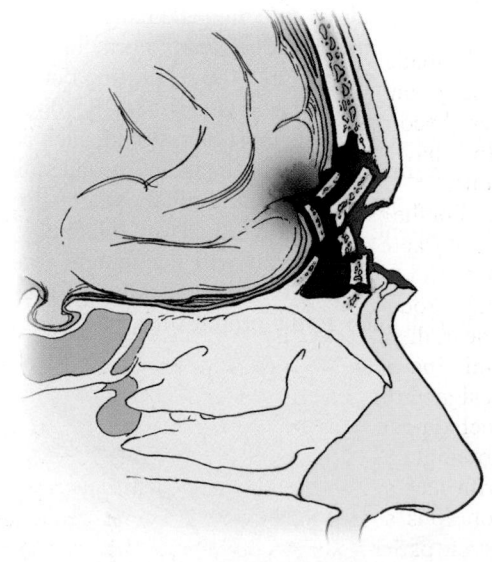

Figure 55 Through-and-through frontal sinus fracture. (Reproduced with permission from reference 55.)

In these patients, intermaxillary fixation usually should remain in place for at least 6 weeks.

In patients with severely comminuted nasal bones, in whom an aesthetically acceptable nose cannot be created, an onlay graft cantilevered from the forehead using a microplate can restore a more normal nasal dorsum. Small areas of avulsed or missing bone can also be replaced with hydroxyappetite bone cement.[60]

FRONTAL SINUS FRACTURES

Despite the use of the shoulder harness in automobiles, frontal sinus fractures still occur with regularity. The old-fashioned lap belt that restrained the passenger in the seat during the impact of a car crash unfortunately allowed the face to move forward, striking the dashboard with the frontal calvaria often fracturing the frontal sinus. A considerable amount of force is required to fracture the anterior wall of the frontal sinus because of its arch configuration and thickness. In Nahum's study, it was apparent that it took more foot-pounds of force to break the frontal sinus anterior wall than any other facial bone including the symphyseal area of the mandible and the zygomatic body.[61]

The problems of the frontal sinus center around the issues concerning the cavity, the duct and the mucosa. The cavity on each side has a thick anterior wall but thin posterior and inferior walls. It has only one point of egress; a funnel shaped structure at the anteromedial part of the frontal sinus floor that empties into the middle meatus of the nose. According to Lang, 77.3% of individuals have a frontonasal duct and 22.7% have a foramen.[62] A fractured or even damaged duct has a marked propensity to undergo stenosis. The mucosa of the sinus cavity acts in a uniquely pathologic manner when traumatized. It has a tendency not to reconstitute itself with normal-appearing and normal-behaving mucosa as the other paranasal sinuses do when they are injured. In the frontal sinus, damaged mucosa has a propensity for subepithelial fibrosis, especially in the area of the frontonasal ducts. Furthermore, it has a tendency to form cysts, some of which will enlarge and erode bone; the resulting mucocele may become infected and form a mucopyocoele. Both have the notable characteristic of eroding bone.[63,64]

For the sake of treatment considerations frontal sinus fractures can be classified as: anterior wall, posterior wall, nasofrontal duct, and "through and through." They can further be classified as: linear, displaced, compound, and compound with "missing bone." A treatment algorithm has been designed that specifically addresses each site and each type of fracture, bearing in mind that seldom do single fractures occur in isolation. However, with each site and each type, different therapeutic solutions should be invoked. Therefore, in any given patient, some combination of procedures should be employed to repair the fracture adequately and safely.

Linear fractures of the anterior frontal sinus wall require no operative intervention. Depressed fractures must be opened, the fragments elevated, and all mucosa entrapped between the fragments excised. The fragments are restored to their normal anatomic position and fixed with miniplates. Exposure is through a coronal scalp flap or the so-called "butterfly incision" (Figure 54). If the patient has a compound fracture the exposure can be gained by extending the laceration into a natural crease line in the forehead.[65]

Displaced posterior wall fractures are notoriously difficult to diagnose even with fine-cut CT scanning. In the author's opinion, all posterior wall frontal sinus fractures should be opened. Even when a small amount of displacement occurs, mucosa can be entrapped and grow into the anterior cranial fossa or form a mucocele. Because the victims of trauma are often hard to follow clinically, the first subsequent presentation of a patient that has been followed rather than operated upon may be in the emergency department with meningitis or a brain abscess. The treatment of choice is the osteoplastic flap and fat obliteration procedure.

The area of the frontal sinus that is the most difficult to visualize radiographically is the region of the frontonasal duct. The most important radiographic sign is the presence fluid in the sinus as demonstrated by sinus opacification. If this persists over a 3-week period, the index of suspicion regarding the possibility of a duct fracture should be high. If the patient has sustained an anterior wall fracture and early intervention for its repair is undertaken, at the same time, a sinus endoscope

can be placed through the site of the fracture and the duct visualized directly. If, however, there is a suspicion of an isolated duct fracture, a trephine hole in the orbital roof will provide access to wash the sinus out with saline, instill some cocaine and place a radiopaque dye within the sinus cavity. A subsequent radiograph will show presence of the dye in the nose if the duct is patent and absence of the contrast material if the duct is fractured. Surgical treatment of the fractured duct is somewhat controversial. The author prefers to do the osteoplastic flap and fat obliteration operation to eliminate the duct. Others prefer the Lynch procedure combined with a nasal septal or medially based lateral nasal wall flap; the so-called Sewall-Boyden flap.[66] Removal of the intersinus septum will allow egress of mucus from the fractured to the nonfractured side. More lately, the interest in functional endoscopic sinus surgery has prompted some to do a conservative removal of the duct through the nose. They have yet to stand the test of time.

The most serious of all the frontal sinus injuries is the "through-and-through fracture."[67] In this dramatic injury, the frontal skin is lacerated, both anterior and posterior walls of the sinus are fractured, often with extensive comminution, the dura is torn and the brain contused (Figure 55). The frontal sinus is often merely an inferior extension of a larger compound cranial fracture.

Approximately 50% of these patients afflicted by a through-and-through injury die at the scene of the accident. Often the first encounter with the patient by the otolaryngologist is during the craniotomy being done by the neurosurgeon to remedy the patient's intracranial injuries. Usually

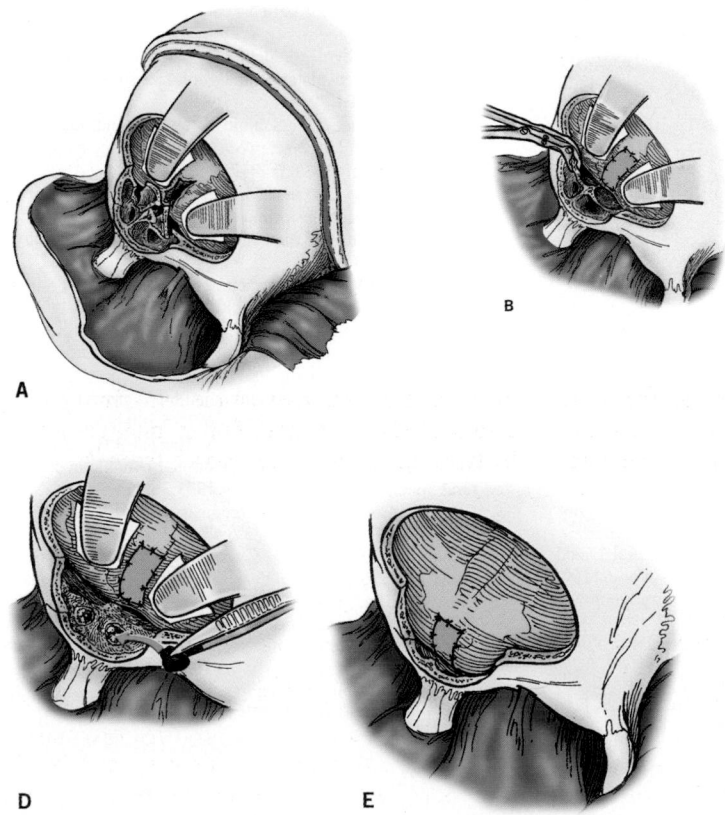

Figure 56 Repair of through-and-through fracture of the frontal sinus. (A) Anterior craniotomy completed. Anterior wall fragments are cleansed and stored. Fracture of both sinus walls, dural rent, and damaged brain exposed. (B) Brain debrided, dura patched, and posterior wall remnants removed with double-actioned rongeur. (C) Removal of remaining posterior wall of frontal sinus producing cranialization. (D) The mucosa of the sinus is removed from the sinus lumen, the nasofrontal duct mucosa is inverted on itself and the frontonasal ducts are plugged with temporals muscle. (E) Brain migrates forward to fill defect. (Reproduced with permission from reference 55.)

a large anterior craniotomy has been done. Once the neurosurgeon has controlled the central hemorrhage, removed the devitalized brain and repaired the dura, the otolaryngologist should manage the severely damaged frontal sinus. This is best done by the cranialization procedure[67] (Figure 56). The anterior wall fragments are removed, divested of mucosa, thoroughly irrigated, and debrided to ensure the removal of all the contaminants acquired at the trauma scene. The bone fragments are stored in Betadine until the end of the procedure. The posterior wall of the frontal sinus is completely removed with a rongeur and a cutting bur. The anterior cranial fossa is now entirely in continuity with the cavity of the frontal sinus. The cutting bur is used to remove thoroughly all vestiges of sinus mucosa including the small projections into the vascular pits in the frontal sinus anterior wall and floor. This is the most important step in the procedure. Any remaining mucosa provides the potential for its regrowth and subsequent infection. The mucosa of the nasofrontal duct is inverted on itself toward the anterior ethmoid sinuses. The duct is plugged with a block of temporalis muscle or bone dust. The anterior wall fragments are restored, and the dural graft will expand with time and fill the new space created in the anterior cranial fossa.

CONCLUSIONS

In summary, treatment of facial fractures requires a multisystem approach. All bony and soft tissue injuries should be diagnosed, and reconstitution of all tissue layers should be performed, if possible. The advancement of technology has enabled rigid fixation to become the standard care for the fixation of most facial fractures. More precise stability and fixation of fractures have become possible, and intermaxillary fixation is used less frequently. Well-planned incisions minimize scarring. Adequate exposure, precise reduction, and stable fixation remain the hallmarks of treatment of facial fractures.

REFERENCES

1. Dingman RO, Natvig P. Surgery of Facial Fractures. Philadelphia, WB Saunders; 1964.
2. Sykes JM, Donald PJ. In: Meyerhoff WL, Rice DH, editors. Reconstruction of the Head and Neck. Philadelphia: WB Saunders; 1992. p. 923.
3. Sykes JM, Murakami CS. Principles of local flaps in head and neck reconstruction. Oper Tech Otolaryngol Head Neck Surg 1993;4:2–10.
4. Angle EH. Classification of malocclusion. Dent Cosmos 1899;41:248.
5. Donald PJ. The Surgical Management of Structural Facial Disharmony: A Self-Instructional Package No. 85100. Washington, DC: American Academy of Otolaryngology—Head and Neck Surgery; 1985. p. 12–17.
6. Dingman RO, Natvig P. Surgery of Facial Fractures. Philadelphia: WB Saunders; 1969.
7. Mathog R. Maxillofacial Trauma. Baltimore: Williams & Wilkins; 1984.
8. Converse JM. Surgical Treatment of Facial Injuries, 3rd edition. Baltimore: Williams and Wilkins; 1974.
9. Chayra GA, Meador LR, Laskin DM. Comparison of panoramic and standard radiographs for the diagnosis of mandible fractures. J Oral Maxillofac Surg 1986;44:677–9.
10. Hemmings KW. Fracture of the cervical spine complicating bilateral fractures of the mandible. A case report. Br J Oral Macillofac Surg 1985;23:279–83.
11. Kruger E, Schilli W. Oral and Maxillofacial Traumatology, Volume 1. Chicago: Quintessence Publishing Co; 1982.
12. Foster CA, Sherman JE. Surgery of Facial Bone Fractures. New York: Churchill Livingston; 1987.
13. Dingman RO, Natvig P. Occlusion and intermaxillary fixation. In: Dingman RO, Natvig P, editors. Surgery of Facial Fractures. Philadelphia: WB Saunders; 1964. p. 114.
14. Hoffman-Axthelm W. The treatment of mandibular fractures and dislocations: A historical perspective. In: Kruger E, Schilli W, editors. Oral and Maxillofacial Traumatology, Volume 1. Chicago IL: Quintessence Books; 1982. p. 17.
15. Gilmer TL. A case of fracture of the lower jaw with remarks on treatment. Arch Dent 1887;4:388.
16. Kellman R. Repair of mandibular fractures via compression plating and more traditional techniques: A comparison of results. Laryngoscope 1984;94:1560–7.
17. Szabo G, Kovacs A, Pulay G. Champy plates in mandibular surgery. Int J Oral Surg 1984;13:290–3.
18. Gaynor R, Stephanak W. Prosthetic splinting as an alternative in the treatment of mandibular fractures. Ear Nose Throat J 1983;62:32–43.
19. Chuong R, Donoff R. Intraoral open reduction of mandible fractures. Int J Oral Surg 1985;14:22–8.
20. Donald PJ, Bernstein L. Open reduction for subcondylar fractures of the mandible. In: Bernstein L, editor. Plastic and Reconstructive Surgery of the Head and Neck: The 3rd International Symposium, Volume 2. New York: Grune and Stratton; 1981. p. 357–63.
21. Brown E, Obeid G. Simplified method for the internal fixation of fractures of the mandibular condyle. J Oral Maxillofac Surg 1984;22:145–50.
22. Wennogle C, Delo R. A pin in groove technique for reduction of displaced subcondylar fractures of the mandible. J Oral Maxillofac Surg 1985;43:659–65.
23. Fernandez J, Mathog R. Open treatment on condylar fractures with biphase technique. Arch Otolaryngol 1987;113:262–3.
24. Ikemura K. Treatment of condylar fractures with other mandible fractures. J Oral Maxillofac Surg 1985;43:810–3.
25. Kellman RM, Marenette LJ. Atlas of Craniofacial Fixation. New York: Raven Press; 1995.
26. Freihofer HM, Sailer HF. Experiences with intraoral wiring of mandibular fractures. J Maxillofac Surg 1973;1:248.
27. Larsen OD, Nielsen A. Mandibular fractures: II. A follow-up study of 229 patients. Scand J Plast Recontr Surg 1976:10:219–26.
28. Michelet FX, Deymes J, Dessus B. Osteosynthesis with miniaturized screwed plates in maxillofacial surgery. J Maxillofac Surg 1973;1:79–84.
29. Champy M, Lodde JP, Schmitt R, et al. Mandibular osteosynthesis by miniature screwed plates via a buccal approach. J Maxillofac Surg 1978;6:14–21.
30. Glineburg RW, Laskin DM, Blaustein DI. The effects of immobilization of the primate temporomandibular joint. A histological study and histochemical study. J Oral Maxillofac Surg 1982;40:3–8.
31. Mekubjian S. Mandibular fracture in a five week old infant. J Oral Maxillofac Surg 1985;43:814–5.
32. McGuirt WF, Salisburg P. Mandibular fractures: Their effect on growth and dentition. Arch Otolaryngol 1987;113:257–61.
33. Boyne PJ. Osseous repair and mandibular growth after subcondylar fractures. J Oral Surg 1967;25:300–9.
34. Leake DL, Leake RD, Davee JS, Hansen RW. Long term follow up of fractures of the mandibular condyle in children. Oral Surg Oral Med Oral Pathol 1973;36:164–9.
35. Close L, Lomba J. Facial reconstruction following blast injury. Head Neck Surg 1983;6:639–52.
36. Kellman R, Marenette L. Zygomatic "tripod" fractures. In Atlas of Craniomaxillofacial Fixation. New York: Raven Press; 1995. p. 288.
37. Shuker S. Management of comminuted mandibular war injuries with multiple circumferential wires. J Oral Maxillofac Surg 1986;44:152–5.
38. Donald PJ. Zygomatic fractures. In English GM, editor. Otolaryngology. Philadelphia: JB Lippincott; 1990.
39. Binder P. Evaluation of the eye following periorbital trauma. Head Neck Surg 1978;1:134–47.
40. Fryer MP, Brown JB, Davis G. Internal wire pin fixation for fracture dislocation of the zygoma: Twenty-year review. Plast Reconstr Surg 1969;44:576–81.
41. Luhr H. Vitallium Luhr systems for reconstructive surgery of the facial skeleton. Otolaryngol Clin North Am 1987;20:573–606.
42. Champy M, Lodde JP, Kahn JL, Kielwasser P. Attempt at systemization in the treatment of isolated fractures of the zygomatic bone: Technique and results. J Otolaryngol 1986;15:39–43.
43. Eisele D, Duckert L. Single point stabilization of zygomatic fractures with mini-compression plates. Arch Otolaryngol 1987;113:267–70.
44. Burres SA, Cohn AM, Mathog RH. Repair of orbital blow-out fractures with marlex mesh and gelfilm. Laryngoscope 1981;91:1881–6.
45. Weintraub B, Cucin RL, Jacobs M. Extrusion of an infected orbital floor prosthesis after 15 years. Plast Reconstr Surg 1981;68:506–7.
46. Kohn R, Romano P, Pulkin J. Lacrimal obstruction after migration of orbital floor implant. Am J Ophthamol 1976;82:934–6.
47. Donald PJ. Zygomatic fractures. In English GM, editor. Otolaryngology. Philadelphia: JB Lippincott; 2003.
48. Le Fort R. Etude experimentale sur les fractures de la machoire supèrieure. Rev Chir (Paris) 1901;23:208–360.
49. Fujii N, Yamshiro M. Classification of malar complex fractures using computed tomography. J Oral Maxillofac Surg 1983;41:562–7.
50. Godoy J, Mathog R. Malar fractures associated with exophthalmos. Arch Otolaryngol 1985;111:174–7.
51. Manson P, Hoopes J, Su C. Structural pillars of the facial skeleton: An approach to the management of Le Fort fractures. Plast Reconstr Surg 1980:66:54–62.
52. Stanley RB. Reconstruction of the midfacial vertical dimension following Le Fort fractures. Arch Otolaryngol 1984;110:571–5.
53. Manson P, Crawley W, Yaremchuk M. Midface fractures: Advantages of immediate extended open reduction and bone grafting. Plast Reconstr Surg 1985;76:1–12.
54. Close L. Fractures of the maxilla. Ear Nose Throat J 1983;62:42–53.
55. Donald PJ. Frontal and ethmoid complex fractures. In: Donald PJ, Gluckman JL, Rice DH, editors. The Sinuses. New York: Raven Press; 1995. p. 412.
56. Gunter H. Konstitutionelle Anomalien des Augenabstrandes und der Interorbitalbrilite. Virchows Arch A Pathol Anat 1933;290–373.
57. Converse JM. Kazanjian and Converse's Surgical Treatment of Facial Injuries, Volume 1, 3rd edition. Baltimore: William and Wilkins; 1974. p. 157.
58. Donald PJ. Frontal and ethmoid complex fractures. In: Donald PJ, Gluckman JL, Rice DH, editors. The Sinuses. New York: Raven Press; 1995. p. 415.
59. Converse JM, Hogan VM. Open-sky approach for reduction of naso-orbital fractures. Plast Reconstr Surg 1970;46: 396–8.
60. Friedman CD, Constantino PD, Tagaki S, Chow LC. BoneSource hydroxyapatite cement: A novel biomaterial for craniofacial reconstruction. J Biomed Mater Res 1998;43:428–32.
61. Nahum AM. The biomechanics of maxillofacial trauma. Clin Plast Surg 1975:2:59–64.
62. Lang J. Clinical Anatomy of the Nose, Nasal Cavity and Paranasal Sinuses. New York: G Thieme Verlag; 1989. p. 62–9.
63. Donald PJ. Tenacity of frontal sinus mucosa. Otolaryngol Head Neck Surg 1979;87:557–656.
64. Donald PJ, Ettin M. The Safety of frontal sinus fat obliteration when sinus walls are missing. Laryngoscope 1986;96:190–3.
65. Donald PJ, Gluckman JL, Rice DH. Frontal sinus fractures. In: Donald PJ, Gluckman JL, Rice DH, editors. The Sinuses. New York: Raven Press; 1995. p. 369–99.
66. Barron SH, Dedo HH, Henry CR. The mucoperiosteal flap in frontal sinus surgery (the Sewall-Boyden-McNaught operation). Laryngoscope 1973;83:1266–80.
67. Donald PJ. Frontal Sinus and Nasofrontoethmoidal Complex Fractures. Self-Instructional Package #804000. Alexandria, VA: American Academy of Otolaryngology–Head and Neck Surgery; 1980.

56

Wound Healing and Flap Physiology

John L. Frodel Jr, MD
Ian J. Alexander, MD

Wound healing is an essential part of any discussion of plastic and reconstructive surgery, and a general understanding of it is beneficial to aid in promoting the most favorable environment for minimal scar formation. Despite this, unwanted scars and poor healing may occur. It is helpful to have an understanding of the possible causes of poor wound healing as well as basic flap physiology to minimize iatrogenic causes for failure.

ANATOMY

The epidermis and dermis are the major components in a discussion of cutaneous wound healing (Figure 1). The outer layer, the epidermis, is the most apparent and also the most prone to scar formation that is readily visible. It is highly durable, waterproof, and serves to protect underlying tissue from dehydration and bacterial invasion.

The epidermis consists of four distinct cell types including keratinocytes, melanocytes, Langerhans cells, and Merkel cells. Merkel cells are of an unknown function and origin. The most numerous is the keratinocyte, and it comprises 80% of the cell composition. Keratinocytes form the major layers of squamous cell epithelium originating with the basal germinal layer (stratum germinativum), which is highly mitotic. As cells mature they migrate toward the surface and take on a more granular appearance (stratum granulosum) and then begin to dehydrate as they migrate away from the blood supply located nearest to the basal layer in the dermis. The next layer (stratum spinosum) retains cell-to-cell junctions but the cell decreases in size causing it to have angle sides or "spines." There is a translucent layer (stratum lucidum) comprised of flattened picnotic cells followed by a layer of cell bodies (stratum corneum), which is relatively inert and serves as a protective shield.[1] Langerhans cells are one of the most efficient antigen-presenting cells and essential in the immune response within the epidermis. Although they are found mostly in the epidermis, they are a bone marrow derived cell. Melanocytes are neural crest cells that produce melanin, a pigment that shields the nuclei of the squamous cell epithelium from ultraviolet radiation. Although the number of melanocytes does not vary with race, the activity of the pigment production does, causing the difference in skin color.

Injuries to the epidermis are relatively superficial and heal without scarring, as there is no collagen deposition. Rapid turnover and cell replication pushes new cells into the wound replacing lost tissue. This occurs in only a few hours. In addition, the basal cell layer migrates rapidly to replace and cover exposed dermis and regenerate lost skin. This is one of the reasons why skin resurfacing and skin grafts are successful. In exchange for rapid growth potential and quick response time, wound strength is minimal. Although there is no scarring with superficial wounds, melanocytes are located in this layer and may cause discoloration.

The dermis is deep to the epidermis and is tightly adherent to it as a result of its irregular border. There are two primary anatomical components to the dermis, the papillary and reticular layers. The papillary layer consists of outpouchings extending up into the epidermis and is vascular, supplying the metabolic needs of the basal layer. The dermis has great intrinsic strength secondary to its abundant collagen producing fibroblasts. As might be expected, repair and healing in this layer are not as rapid as in the epidermis, but the dermal layer provides tensile strength to the wound. In addition, the dermis contains epithelial lined skin appendages such as sweat glands, hair follicles, and sebaceous glands. Sebaceous glands are of particular importance as they are a reservoir for germinal cells for epidermal regeneration.

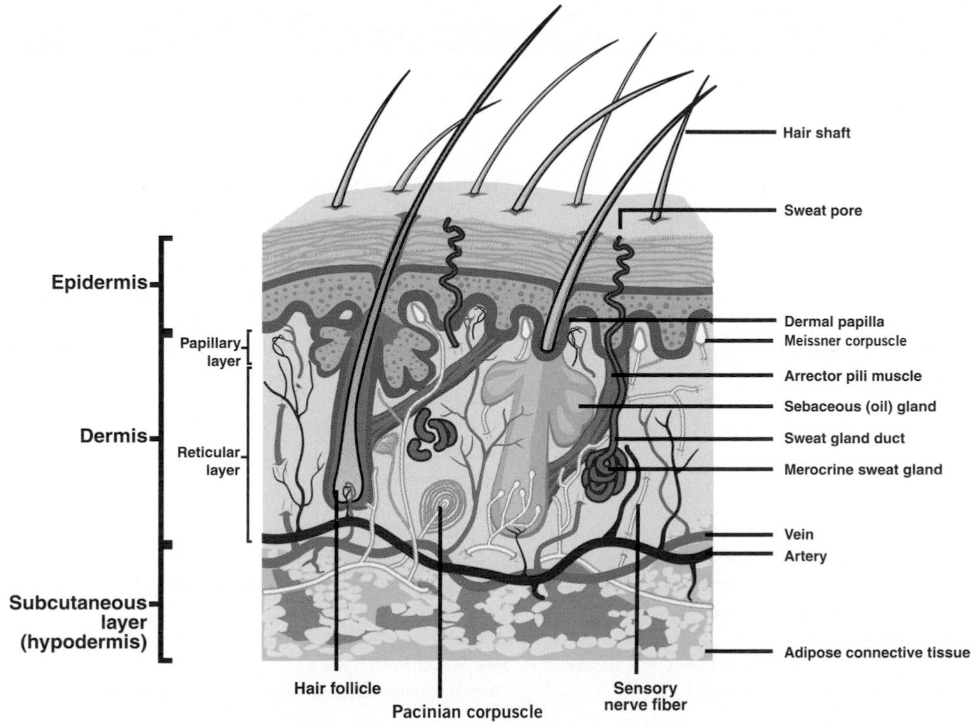

STEPS IN WOUND HEALING

After an injury, wound healing has been described as progressing in three major phases: (1) inflammatory, (2) proliferative, and (3) maturation or remodeling (Figure 2).[2] The entire process can take up to a year to complete and, thus, many plastic surgeons will wait until the scar has matured prior to revision.[3]

Inflammatory Phase

The inflammatory phase begins at the initial insult and is characterized by local vasoconstriction, which lasts for up to 10 minutes. If endothelial injury has occurred, the coagulation cascade is activated. Platelet adhesion and clot formation

Figure 1 Cross sectional illustration of skin and appendages. (Reproduced with permission from reference 1.)

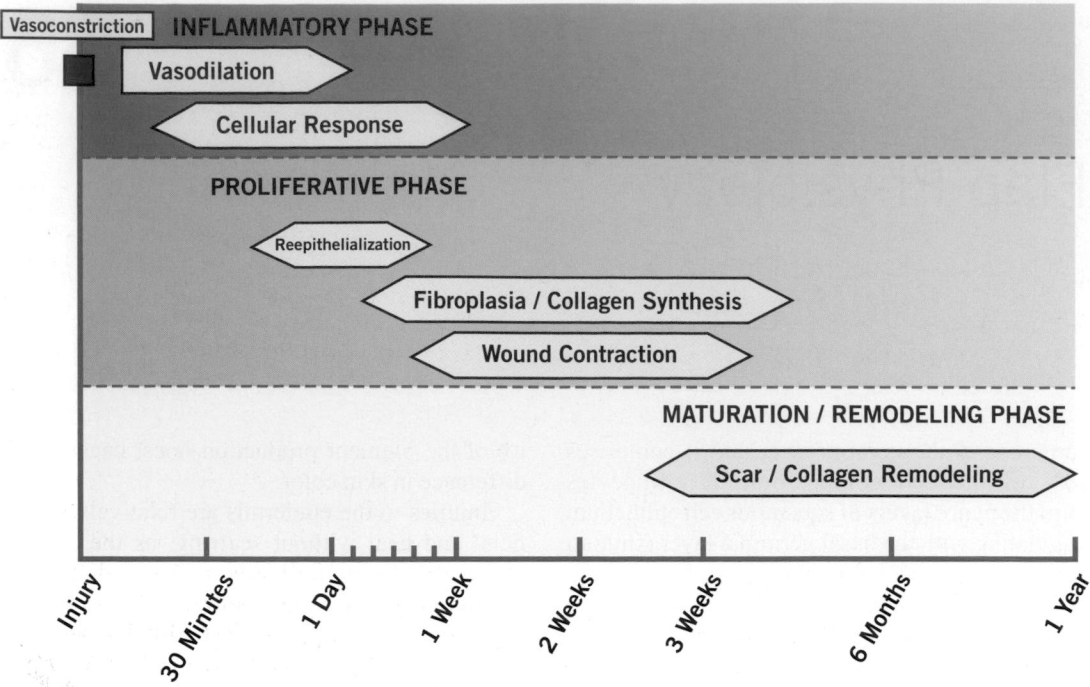

Figure 2 Phases of wound healing. (Reproduced with permission from reference 2.)

result from numerous cytokines released from the endothelium and activated platelets. Vasoactivators such as serotonin, histamine, proteases, and thromboxane as well as platelet derived growth factor (PDGF), insulin-like growth factor-1 (IGF-1), transforming growth factor-beta (TGF-ß), epidermal growth factor (EGF), and fibroblast growth factor (FGF) are secreted to aid in cell recruitment and scar formation[4,5] (Table 1).

Following vasoconstriction, vasodilatation is mediated by histamine release from local mast cells. Vascular permeability increases for the next 2 to 3 days with continuation of the inflammatory phase. This is mediated by proteolytic activation of kallikrein, and in turn the kinins, which induce endothelial-cell separation and permeability to inflammatory cells.[6]

As vascular permeability increases, the cell-mediated responses increase. Fibronectin-mediated migration of circulating cells, such as neutrophils, monocytes, fibroblasts and locally derived endothelial cells, forms granulation tissue. This conglomerate along with the clot formation and fibronectin forms a network for fibroblasts and migratory endothelial cells to proliferate[7] (Figures 3 and 4).

The primary action of the neutrophils and monocytes is phagocytosis of bacteria and wound debris. These cells are usually short lived unless the wound is contaminated, then they persist and continue to migrate until the wound is sufficiently clean. Prolongation of the inflammatory phase secondary to wound contamination is a significant contributor to increased scar formation. In a noncontaminated wound, collagen deposition begins, provided the macrophages, fibroblasts, and endothelial cells are functioning normally.[8]

Macrophages are extremely important for wound debridement but also have a significant role in days three to four of wound healing as they facilitate granulation tissue formation and collagen deposition through release of chemokines and growth factors essential in cell signaling.[9] Macrophages release PDGF, TGF-α, EGF, TGF-ß, and FGF, among many other cytokines, which activate endothelial cells to migrate into the wound and fibroblasts to produce collagen.[10,11] The important function of macrophages is readily apparent when they are dysfunctional and wound healing is hindered.[12]

Initial wound strength relies on the fibrin clot and rapid re-epithelialization of the wound and is relatively weak. Collagen deposition does not begin until the inflammatory phase has subsided. Although this model of wound healing would suggest three distinct phases, the process is much more fluid and overlapping.[1]

Proliferative Phase

The next recognized phase is the proliferative phase and is characterized by regeneration of the epithelium, collagen deposition, neovasculariza-

Table 1 Inflammatory Mediators Involved in Wound Healing			
Abbreviati on	Cytokine	Source	Function
BDNF	Brain-derived neurotrophic factor	CNS, skeletal muscle, heart, lung	Support motor neurons after axotomy
CNTF	Ciliary neurotrophic factor	Schwann cells	Promote survival, differentiation of nerve and glial cells in nervous system
CSF-1	Colony-stimulating factor I	Multiple cells	Macrophage activation, granulation formation
EGF	Epidermal growth factor	Platelets, saliva, milk, plasma, urine	Proliferation and migration of epithelium, fibroblasts; angiogenic
FGF (basic, acidic)	Fibroblast growth factor	Macrophages, brain, pituitary	Proliferation, migration of vascular endothelial cells; mitogenic, chemotactic for fibroblasts, keratinocytes
GH	Human growth hormone	Pituitary	Fibroblast proliferation; stimulates IGF-1
HB-EGF	Heparin-binding epidermal growth factor	Macrophages	Cell motility and proliferation
IFN	Interferon	Fibroblasts, lymphocytes	Inhibits fibroblast proliferation and collagen synthesis
IGF-1	Insulin-like growth factor-1	Fibroblasts, liver, plasma	Fibroblast proliferation, proteoglycan and collagen synthesis, reepithelialization
IL	Interleukins	Macrophages, lymphocytes, others	Fibroblast proliferation, neutrophil chemotaxis
KGF	Keratinocyte growth factor	Fibroblasts	Epithelial proliferation
NGF	nerve growth factor	Schwann and muscle cells	Promotes growth of motor neurons, Schwann, and muscle cells
PDGF	Platelet-derived growth factor	Platelets, macrophages, fibroblasts, endothelium, smooth muscle cells	Chemoattractan for neutrophils and macrophages; mitogenic for fibroblasts and smooth-muscle cells
TGF (beta1 and 2)	Transforming growth factor	Platelets, fibroblasts, neutrophils, macrophages, lymphocytes	Proliferation of epithelium and fibroblasts, fibrosis and increased tensile strength
TGF beta 3	Transforming growth factor	Macrophages	Antiscarring effects
TNF	Tumor necrosis factor	Macrophages, mast cells, lymphocytes, others	Fibroblast proliferation
VEGF	Vascular endothelial growth factor	Epidermal cells, macrophages	Angiogenesis, increase vascular permeability

Adapted with permission from reference 4.

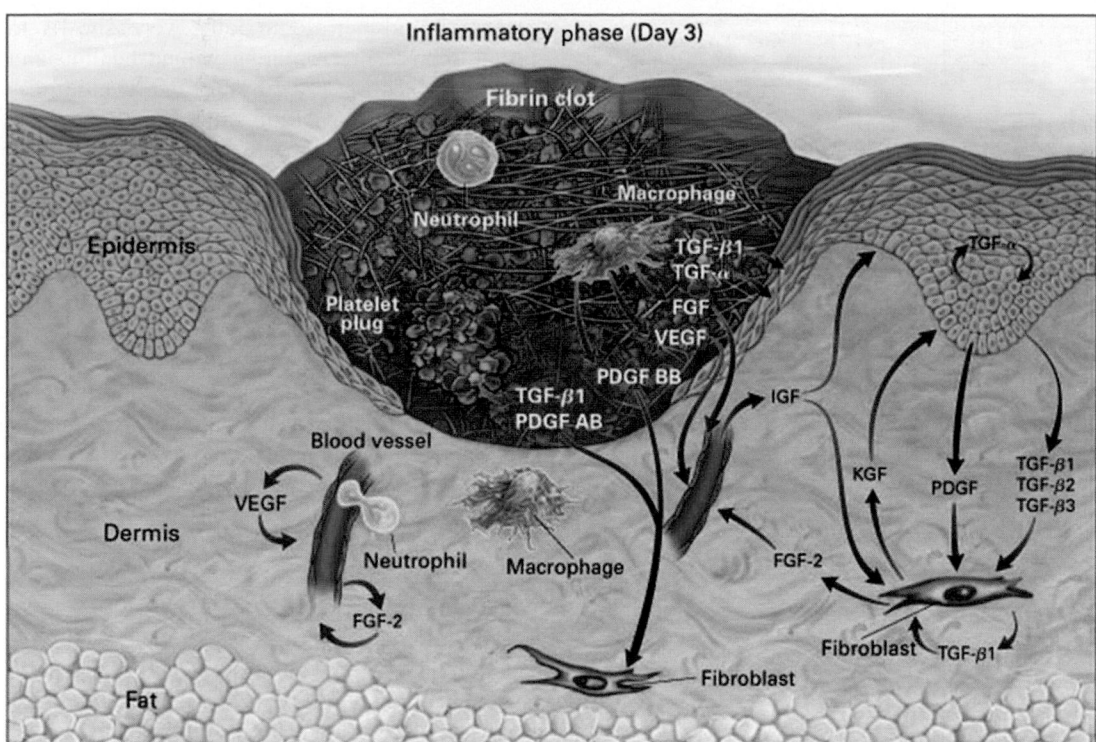

Figure 3 A cutaneous wound 3 days after injury. Growth factors thought to be necessary for cell movement into the wound are shown. TGF-ß1, TGF-ß2, and TGF-ß3 denote transforming growth factor-beta1, -beta2, and -beta3, respectively; TGF-α, transforming growth factor alpha; FGF, fibroblast growth factor; VEGF vascular endothelial growth factor; PDGF, PDGF AB, and PDGF BB, platelet-derived growth factor, platelet-derived growth factor AB, and platelet-derived growth factor BB, respectively; IGF, insulin-like growth factor; and KGF keratinocyte growth factor. (Reproduced with Permission from reference 3.)

tion, and wound contracture. This phase typically is thought to begin during the initial 24 hours and lasts for up to 3 weeks.

The initial part of this phase is characterized by epithelial migration into the wound and is activated by EGF and TGF-α. These polypeptides induce the germinal basal membrane to undergo rapid mitosis and subsequent migration cells into the wound both from the edges and from deep structures, for example, hair follicles and sebaceous glands, within the dermis. Cell-to-cell contact results in further cell messaging, increased mitotic activity, and stratification of the basal cell layer resulting in recreation of the stratified squamous cell epithelium.[11,12] This critical phase occurs relatively quickly and peaks in 48 to 72 hours thus laying down a protective layer to insulate underlying tissue from bacteria and foreign material.

This phase is much quicker in primary closed wounds taking as little as 24 hours to re-epithelialize. In large or full thickness injuries that are allowed to close by secondary intention, this process can be up to five times as long.

This knowledge of the basic cellular level of wound healing provides an apparent reason for keeping wounds clean and moist during early healing. Packing wet to dry dressings and meticulous cleansing of wounds to remove crusting and scabs allows for more rapid epithelial migration. Large scabs formed by early clots that become dehydrated may protect the wound initially, but adhere to the dermis and form a barrier to impede migrating basal cells thus prolonging the wound closure and increasing the size of the final scar[13] (Figure 5).

Besides macrophages, fibroblasts also have a critical role in wound healing. Mediators such as C5a from the coagulation cascade, fibronectin, PDGF, FGF, and TGF-ß attract fibroblasts and signal them to replicate and secrete collagen, elastin, glycosaminoglycan, fibronectin, and collagenase, the latter playing an important role in the final phase of wound healing. Wound contracture is accomplished through differentiated fibroblasts and perivascular mesenchymal cells. Glycosaminoglycan is a polysaccharide necessary for granulation formation. Collagen is formed through a complex intermolecular reaction.[14]

Initially, type III collagen is deposited, but this is replaced with type I as the scar matures. With the formation of collagen, wound strength increases to about 10% at the end of the inflammatory phase. Collagen deposition and fibroblast activity peaks at about 3 weeks after injury, and tensile strength peaks at 80% by 10 weeks.[3]

The final aspect of the proliferative phase is closing of the wound and revascularization, also termed neovascularization. Contracture maximizes at 10 to 15 days and is mediated by myofibroblasts. Neovascularization is stimulated by macrophages, platelets, mast cells, and lymphocytes. Cytokines, such as FGF, TGF-α and -ß, PDGF, vascular endothelial growth factor (VEGF), and low oxygen levels induce new vascular channel formation.[1]

Maturation or Remodeling Phase

The final stage in wound healing is marked by decrease in scar size and inflammation and is secondary to remodeling of the wound. This phase begins sometime between the second and third week and continues for up to a full year. It is characterized by dehydration of the surrounding area, change in collagen type, and parallel arrangement of previous randomly arranged collagen fibers. Vascularity is also decreased as scars are usually avascular.[3]

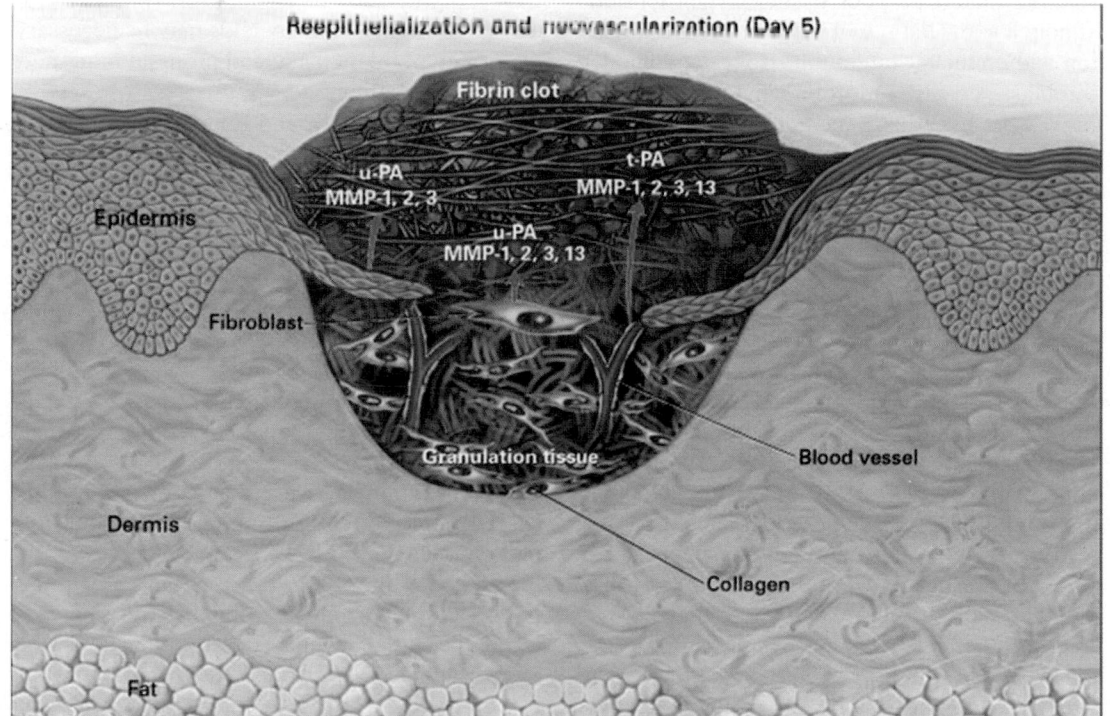

Figure 4 A cutaneous wound 5 days after injury. Blood vessels are seen sprouting into the fibrin clot as epidermal cells resurface the wound. Proteinases thought to be necessary for cell movement are shown. The abbreviation u-PA denotes urokinase-type plasminogen activator; MMP-1, 2, 3, and 13, matrix metalloproteinases 1, 2, 3, and 13 (collagenase 1, gelatinase A, stromelysin 1, and collagenase 3, respectively); and t-PA tissue plasminogen activator. (Reproduced with permission from reference 3.)

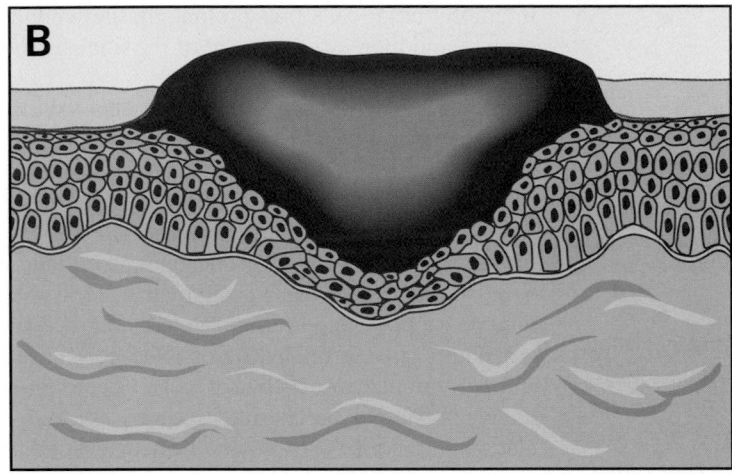

Figure 5 (A) Differentiated and dividing basal epithelial cells migrating beneath dried clot. (B) Contact inhibition and further differentiation with epithelial stratification. (Reproduced with permission from reference 2.)

FACTORS AFFECTING WOUND HEALING

Factors such as metabolic deficiencies, local environment, cellular deficiencies, and delayed wound closure can all have an affect on the timing and strength of wound healing. Many of these factors can be influenced by the physician and the educated patient.

Closure technique is one factor at the forefront of the surgeon's mind. Some of the more common mistakes include injury to wound edges while suturing, excessive cauterization, and ischemia induced by suture material or constriction. These factors play a part in increasing the length of the inflammatory phase by causing necrosis, inflammation, and increase the risk of infection thus prolonging healing.

As mentioned, tissue ischemia may prolong wound healing as well. Tying sutures too tightly may induce local tissue ischemia as well as local collections of blood and serum to cause hematoma or seroma formation. Good surgical technique, drain placement as necessary, and appropriate suture material and technique are recommendations to prevent the above-mentioned complications.

Systemic disease such as anemia and inadequate debridement of the wound are also contributing factors to poor tissue oxygen tension. Although a low PaO_2 will induce neovascularization and epithelial migration, it will also hinder fibroblast activity and collagen formation. For this reason, hyperbaric oxygen therapy has been thought to speed the healing process. Studies suggest it may increase the rate of epithelialization and improve long-term healing results.[15]

Wound healing is further retarded by desiccation. Large clots dehydrate and create a barrier to migrating epithelial cells. These cells require more energy as their course is deviated to migrate around a scab that penetrates into the dermis. In a closed system without a ready blood supply, this can prolong healing and use up necessary nutrients. Many dressings have also been studied to help prevent crusting and maintain a properly humidified environment to improve wound healing efficiency. As the literature suggests that little atmospheric oxygen is absorbed through a wound, either occlusive or semiocclusive dressings are beneficial. An occlusive dressing has the added benefit of fluid collecting under the impermeable membrane which can be rich in chemotactic factors and further promotes recruitment and decreases healing time.[4]

In addition to dressings, one study demonstrated a 28% increase in healing rate with the use of antibiotic ointment. Conversely, corticosteroid ointment and petroleum jelly were shown to be ineffective in promoting wound healing and decreased healing rates by 34 and 8%, respectively.[16] Topical bacteriostatic agents, such as Silvadene, may promote healing, but caution is advised because others, such as Provodine iodine, may actually inhibit healing.[17]

Despite excellent surgical technique, wound healing can be hindered by systemic diseases as well. Most common on this list is diabetes and hypertrophic scar formation. Although rarer, pseudoxanthoma elasticum, osteogenesis imperfecta, progeria, dermatochalasis, and Ehlers-Danlos syndrome are also a consideration in wound healing. Any congenital or acquired deficiency in the wound healing process or collagen formation has potential to slow the healing process.[18]

Diabetes deserves focused attention in discussing the biological pathways disrupted by this congenital and acquired disease. One well-known way is microangiopathy causing decreased oxygen delivery to the wound site. Another is insulin deficiency causing leukocyte dysfunction. Many of these effects have been linked to glycosylation of membrane proteins. For this reason, and probably several others, patients with diabetes are at increased risk for infections in addition to the slower wound healing. Collagen synthesis has also been found to be adversely affected by low or ineffective insulin levels. Studies suggest that insulin therapy and supplemental vitamin A (25,000 U/d) benefit diabetics in the healing process.

Although one would expect nutritional status to be a significant liability in wound closure and healing, it has only been observed in severe cases. Physicians should be cautious in patients with a malignancy or alcoholism. Building protein in the form of amino acids may be necessary to correct any deficiency and promote more normal wound healing.

Vitamins A, C, K, and E have been observed to be important cofactors in the healing process as well. Vitamin A deficiency manifests as poor epithelialization and wound closure. Deficiency causes decreased collagen cross-linking and formation. Deficiency of vitamin C causes scurvy. The body cannot synthesize this essential vitamin and can only store about 4 to 5 months worth. It is an important cofactor in the hydroxylation of lysine and proline in collagen synthesis. Vitamin C is also a reducing agent in neutrophil superoxide formation necessary for bacterial extermination. Vitamin K is a cofactor in the clotting cascade and is specifically implicated in the formation of factors II, VII, IX, and X. As a result, longer bleeding times and large hematomas inhibit collagen matrix formation and increase ischemia to the wound site. Vitamin E is well known as necessary for collagen formation and tensile strength, but its clinical importance has not been demonstrated.[7] Trace elements such as iron and zinc are also included in the healing pathway. Zinc is involved in collagenase activity and enzymes used to synthesize RNA and DNA. Other medical conditions that may cause nutritional deficiencies or immune dysfunction should also be considered. Although this list is extensive, several are worth mentioning here. Congestive heart failure, atherosclerosis, venous stasis, and lymphedema cause poor tissue delivery of oxygen and nutrients. Chronic renal failure, Cushing syndrome, and hyperthyroidism are other systemic diseases known to inhibit wound healing. Chronic liver disease, human immunodeficiency virus (HIV) or other immune deficiency states (chemotherapy, leukemia), thrombocytopenia, and previous radiation therapy have also been implicated as decreasing healing. Aging is associated with slower healing and decreased strength of scars. Medications such as chemotherapeutic agents and corticosteroids can have a clinically significant effect on wound healing by decreasing inflammatory agents and prolonging the inflammatory phase. Although the oral administration of vitamin A has been shown to reverse the effects of corticosteroids, the routine use of other vitamins does not seem to promote overall wound healing.

Abnormal Scar Formation

Hypertrophic scarring is a problem for surgeons. Keloids are an example of extreme hypertrophy of a scar and represent excessive collagen deposition without the normal degradation to shrink the scar. The difference between keloid scars and hypertrophic scarring is one of severity. Hypertrophic scars are along the wound line and may regress with time whereas keloid scars tend to invade surrounding tissue. Treatment for both is aimed at decreasing collagen formation by use of intralesional corticosteroids. Severe keloids may also require postoperative excision with direct pressure dressings, silicone gel sheeting, interferon-alpha 2b, or radiation to inhibit excessive collagen deposition. Recurrence is frequent, but one study showed promising results with only 8% recurrence of keloid scars with surgical excision combined with radiation or intralesional corticosteroids and interferon-alpha 2b.[19] Although no marketable therapy is currently available, TGF-ß1 has been shown to inhibit keloid growth. Further research into the science of cell-mediated cytokines and wound healing may lead to new and better treatments in the future for those prone to excessive scarring.

FLAP PHYSIOLOGY

In discussing the physiology of flaps, a basic understanding of the surgical anatomy of the skin and superficial tissues is necessary. The dermis (and epidermis) is supplied by two major vascular plexus (Figure 6). The deep vascular plexus, or subdermal plexus, exists at the junction of the reticular dermis and subcutaneous fat (hypodermis). Arterioles from the deep vascular plexus supply sweat glands and pilosebaceous units consisting of hair follicles and sebaceous glands. The superficial vascular plexus exists at the superior border of the reticular dermis and consists

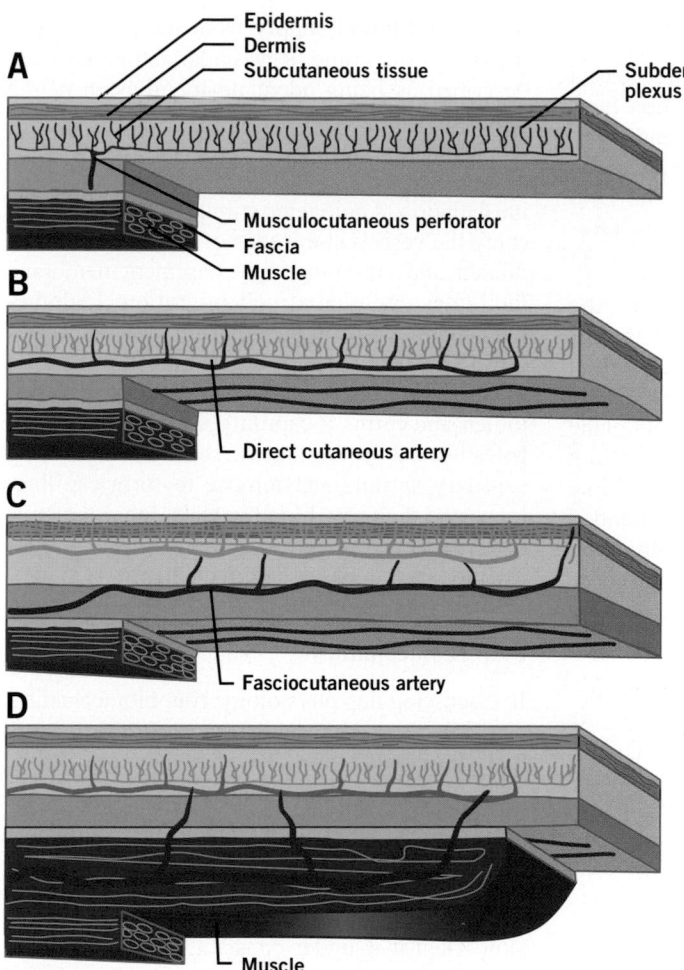

Figure 6 Classification of skin flaps based on vascular supply: (A) random, (B) axial, (C) fasciocutaneous, and (D) musculocutaneous. (Reproduced with permission from reference 1.)

of capillary loops within the dermal papilla. The superficial plexus provides the major blood supply to the epidermis through diffusion as it does not extend up into the epidermis. In the head and neck, especially the face, there may also be a large network of deep subcutaneous perforating vessels named according to the anatomical location, for example, transverse facial and submental. This network provides a rich source of blood supply to the skin.[20]

The arterial blood supply to the skin consists of two major categories, the musculocutaneous and cutaneous. Musculocutaneous vessels arise from segmental arteries, which are named branches of the aorta, and run deep to muscle groups. These musculocutaneous arteries permeate through underlying muscles before reaching the skin and supply blood to both muscle and skin. Musculocutaneous arteries run perpendicular to skin for much of their course and thus typically supply only a small area superficially.[19]

Direct cutaneous, also called septocutaneous or fasciocutaneous, arteries traverse within the fascial septa of the muscular bundles and course directly to the dermis. These vessels supply blood only to the skin and not to the adjacent muscle tissue. As opposed to musculocutaneous arteries, direct cutaneous arteries run parallel to skin and supply a large area of skin.[21]

Blood flow through the skin is one of the most variable in the body its thermoregulatory responses. Even at its baseline flow rate, the skin

receives 10 times the rate that is required for nutritional support. It is because of this abundant blood flow that random flaps are able to survive. An extensive network of capillaries supplies the skin with its blood volume and flow and is controlled by precapillary sphincters. These sphincters are induced to relax by local hypoxemia and an increased level of metabolic products. In addition, arteriovenous (AV) shunts further regulate flow through the capillary network. The AV shunts also have regulatory sphincters that control both thermoregulation and systemic blood pressure. An increase in core body temperature causes a decrease in norepinephrine release, which results in contracture of the AV shunt sphincters and increased blood flow to the skin. Increase in metabolic products may cause the same reaction. This control mechanism is of utmost importance in flap survivability.

The skin is innervated by both the sensory and sympathetic nervous systems. Sensory nerves are distributed in a predictable segmental fashion along the skin. The sympathetic nerves control the AV shunt sphincters by release of norepinephrine. Incisions at the flap edges interrupt the parallel superficial and deep cutaneous plexus causing decreased perfusion pressure to the skin. In addition, when sympathetic nerves are severed, norepinephrine is released from the nerve terminal and catecholamine reuptake is eliminated. This surgical sympathectomy contributes to decreased blood flow to the flap.

Flap Designs

The four basic types of flap designs are based on the vascular supply. The most common flaps used in the head and neck are random and axial. Fasciocutaneous and musculocutaneous flaps discussed in Chapter 97, "Neoplasms of the Oral Cavity" and Chapter 98, "Neoplasms of the Oropharynx and Hypopharynx."

Random Flaps. Random flaps represent the majority of local facial flaps. As the vascular supply to these flaps arises from the subdermal plexus through the base, which is supplied by musculocutaneous arteries, the appropriate plane of dissection for elevation of the flap is along the subcutaneous (hypodermal) adipose. Multiple length-to-width ratios have been recommended in the literature to increase flap survivability, but, practically speaking, survivability may be more related to the perfusion pressure of the feeding blood vessels.

Axial Flaps. Axial flaps derive their blood supply from the named direct cutaneous arteries. As a result, axial flaps are capable of a greater length-to-width ratio than are random flaps. The plane of dissection is, therefore, deeper and includes the fascia containing the relevant named artery. Some additional length is obtainable with axial flaps if more tissue at the distal tip is included with its corresponding blood supply derived from the random subdermal plexus. Examples of axial flaps and their corresponding direct cutaneous artery are the paramedian forehead (supratrochlear artery) and the nasolabial flap (angular artery). Axial flaps are discussed in Chapter 54, "Nasal Reconstruction."

Fasciocutaneous and Musculocutaneous Flaps.

Fasciocutaneous flaps contain associated skin, subcutaneous fascia, and deep fascia. One such example is the radial forearm flap. Musculocutaneous flaps include all the elements of the fasciocutaneous flap with the added underlying muscle. An example would be the latissimus dorsi flap.

Cellular Physiology of Flaps

Following transposition and insetting of a flap, the first 48 hours represent the most critical period with respect to determining flap survival. A surge in the level of catecholamines occurs locally with tissue damage and flap placement, resulting in vasoconstriction secondary to catecholamine release. The catecholamines released from traumatized nerves are exhausted after 48 hours. In addition, the inflammatory cascade releases increased levels of thromboxane A2 (also a powerful vasoconstrictor) and free radicals, with resulting edema. The combination of these factors can cause both ischemia and direct injury to the flap. During the inflammatory phase, a fibrin layer forms at the recipient site. Neovascularization is delayed until 3 to 7 days in the proliferative phase and thus the flap is depending on nutrient absorption from the surrounding tissues and blood supply from the pedicle during this critical time. Revascularization has been described as being adequate for division of the flap pedicle at 7 days.[22]

This revascularization occurs through two processes, direct in growth (neovascularization) and inosculation. Angiogenic stimuli such as ischemia cause the vessels at the edge of the flap to become dilated, and a thinning of the basement membrane facilitates endothelial cell migration. Endothelial cells move from the adjacent vascular lumen toward the vascular stimulus. Replication of endothelial cells is stimulated in the bordering vessel lumen and forms a capillary sprout which elongates toward the angiogenic source. Neighboring capillary sprouts anastomose to form capillary loops and then new blood vessels. Inosculation is direct ingrowth of surrounding recipient capillaries into preexisting vessels in the flap.

Flap Biomechanics

In discussing flap physiology, four biomechanical principles are emphasized: stress, strain, creep, and stress relaxation. The first concept, stress, refers to the force applied per cross-sectional area of the skin. Strain, the second principle, refers to the change in length divided by the original length of the given tissue to which a force is applied. Creep is the increase in strain applied to skin when it is under constant stress. Creep can occur over a brief amount of time (minutes) and is due to the extrusion of fluid from the dermis and breakdown of the dermal framework. The final principle, stress relaxation, is the decrease in stress on skin when it is held in tension at a constant strain for a given period of time. Stress relaxation occurs days to weeks after flap placement and is due to the increase in skin cellularity and permanent stretching of skin components with wound healing and contracture. The concept of serial excision is based upon the principles that skin closed under tension will display stress relaxation and creep over time.[1]

In forming a flap, the distal segment from the proximal end with the blood supply is referred to as the tip and is usually the most tenuous area with reference to survivability. The probability of tip necrosis has been directly related to both the length of the flap and distance from proximal vessels and the tension under which it is closed. In essence, longer flaps display a higher probability of tip necrosis when placed under the same closing tension as shorter flaps.

Undermining is the usual surgical technique for relieving tension in a flap but may not always represent the best means of correcting for excessive tension. Undermining has been shown to be of little benefit on tension beyond four centimeters. Other studies performed on animals demonstrated that excessive undermining actually increases flap necrosis probably by decreasing the vascular supply from both the superficial and deep vascular plexus.[23,24]

Many physiologic factors have been indicated to affect flap survival. The common denominator involves two basic factors. The first is the blood supply to the flap through its base, and the second is the formation of neovascularization between the flap and the recipient bed. It has been thought that the survivability of a flap depends entirely on the width of the base. However, the surviving length of random pattern flaps is determined by perfusion pressure within the arterioles and intravascular resistance. Widening the base of a flap does not affect either perfusion pressure nor intravascular resistance. Widening the base of a flap is necessary to a certain critical ratio, but more is not necessarily better when it comes to flaps; and there is no benefit to widening the base beyond that ratio. The literature suggests that a length to width ratio of 3:1 to 4:1 will result in a viable random pattern flap for the face or scalp.[1]

Historically, delaying of flaps was the generally accepted answer to tip necrosis and flap failure secondary to ischemia. In random flaps, this was performed by incising the long axis of the flap and undermining without dividing the ends of the flap. Axial flaps are incised around the margins excluding the base, or vascular pedicle, of the flap without undermining. In this way, the flaps are initially incised and then left in place at the donor site to be transposed and inset into the recipient bed after 1 to 2 weeks. Of note, any benefits gained from a delayed flap are lost if delayed beyond 3 weeks. There are several proposed reasons why delayed flaps seem to perform better. It is thought that delaying the flap improves blood flow after insetting by reorienting vascular channels and inducing the formation of new vascular collaterals. In addition, the flap itself is conditioned to withstand ischemia, and delaying causes diversion of blood from the AV shunts thus ensuring adequate flow to the tissue.

Management of Complications

The same complications to wound healing apply to skin and tissue flaps as well. The most common causes of complications are poor flap design and increased tension from closure. These concerns must be addressed prior to forming the flap and while in the operating room. Potential postoperative complications of local skin flaps also include infection, hematoma, ischemia, flap necrosis (distal flap or tip necrosis), dehiscence, and an undesirable cosmetic result.

Tension on a flap increases the risk of tissue necrosis. Some flaps, such as a transposition flap, tend to have decreased tension on the distal extension of the flap. Often times, a flap that is thicker will perform better than a flap with a wider base in the prevention of tip necrosis. Adequate perfusion is assured if, at the conclusion of the inset, the flap is pink with brisk capillary refill. The progression of ischemia to necrosis may be in a stepwise fashion with blanching and increasingly prolonged capillary refill until capillary refill is no longer evident with direct pressure. The natural consequence of poor perfusion without intervention follows a stepwise fashion as well. Tissue ischemia causes cell death, which is initially superficial, but may progress to full thickness. With tissue necrosis, eschar formation follows. Eschar formation leads to widening of the scar secondary to poor migration of epithelial cells and goes on to separation of the eschar with an exposed defect and healing by secondary intent.[23]

Cyanosis of flaps in the immediate postoperative period is most often attributed to insufficient venous drainage. Clinical symptoms include an edema, purplish or bluish hue to the flap with dark colored blood on pinprick. Initial management should include removal of tense sutures that are potentially compromising venous drainage. It may be necessary to explore the vascular pedicle to remove any kinking or compression caused by hematoma formation. In addition, multiple punctures may be made with a 22-gauge needle to relieve venous hypertension. Application of heparin-soaked gauze and even medicinal leeches have been used. Should medicinal leeches be utilized, antibiotic prophylaxis is recommended to prevent Aeromonas infection. Although medicinal leeches are raised in a sterile environment, their digestive tracts are colonized with this microorganism and it is transferred in the saliva.[25]

Clinical symptoms of ischemia secondary to arterial insufficiency include pallor, delayed capillary refill, decreased temperature, and decreased or absent bleeding with pinprick. Arterial insufficiency may be due to the same causes of venous congestion. Mechanical pressure from a wound dressing applied too tightly, hematoma, or a kinked pedicle is the most common cause that can be remedied initially. It is recommended that adequate perfusion be assured prior to leaving the operating room. Otherwise, the option of further delay of flap placement is lost, nevertheless, the outcome may be a necrotic flap in its original position with a remaining tissue deficiency. It is important to note that although a flap can survive arterial insufficiency for up to 13 hours, venous congestion will cause flap failure within 3 hours.[23]

In combating flap ischemia, hyperbaric oxygen (HBO) therapy should be considered although it is not a mainstay of therapy. Positive results have been demonstrated in studies involving animals and humans. Therapy is initiated through multiple "dives" in which 100% oxygen is administered at two to three times atmospheric pressure. This results in an increased amount of dissolved oxygen in plasma, which increases the oxygen level in the peripheral tissue by a reported 10- to 20-fold. HBO therapy is dependent on an efficient cardiopulmonary system to deliver the oxygen and may not be useful in individuals who are compromised such as those with congestive heart failure or emphysema. To determine if a patient is a good candidate for HBO therapy, transcutaneous oxygen measurements are made with the patient breathing room air and compared to the patient breathing 100% oxygen. An increase in the oxygen saturation while breathing 100% oxygen suggests that the patient has sufficient cardiopulmonary function to benefit from HBO therapy.[15]

HBO therapy has been discussed as benefiting tissue flaps for a number of reasons. First of all, it encourages capillary neovascularization within the flap thus increasing blood supply and oxygen delivery to the ischemic tissue. Secondly, HBO therapy is thought to decreases tissue reperfusion injury, a major cause of tissue damage after an ischemic event such as a tissue flap transfer. Thirdly, HBO therapy induces vasoconstriction in healthy tissue, but not ischemic tissue, which decreases edema and allows more blood to be diverted to tissue that needs it. Lastly, HBO therapy decreases hypoxia and helps prevent cellular death for the first 72 hours, which is the most critical time for ischemia and until revascularization has begun. HBO therapy has demonstrated a 90% salvage rate in ischemic flaps when performed one to two times per day for 3 to 5 days.[25,26]

HBO therapy is not without potential risks. Complications may be various and usually result from either barotraumas or oxygen toxicity. These complications can include pneumothorax, barotrauma to the middle ear with tympanic membrane perforation, seizure, pulmonary toxicity, myopia, and an increased rate of cataract formation, particularly in patients with preexisting cataracts. Myopia usually resolves within 6 months following treatment, but the other complications can be serious and longterm. Oxygen-induced seizures have been reported in one in 10,000 patients.[25]

Some authors have argued that aggressive debridement is contraindicated until the wound has marginated and the eschar has begun to separate. However, a wound may benefit from some debridement as it increases migration of epithelial cells. This is counterintuitive; as previously discussed, scabbing causes widening of the scar. Fortunately, the eschar acts as a biological dressing in protecting the defect. Local wound care is recommended even with partial distal tip necrosis. Although debridement is rarely necessary, failure of a flap may necessitate another reconstruction if more conservative measures fail to provide adequate coverage of the tissue defect.

Infection, another dreaded complication in surgery, is surprisingly uncommon in head and neck local flaps, although higher than in traditional facial surgery. The reasoning is multifactorial. Plausible reasons include delayed flaps becoming contaminated, higher colonization rates in the head and neck regions, for example, nose and oral cavity, and lastly, because those undergoing surgery for head and neck flaps usually have increased risk factors for infection including malignancy, diabetes, and malnutrition.[27]

Regardless of the cause, the results can be devastating. Infection may be as problematic as dehiscence with widening or thickening of scar or as devastating as flap necrosis or sepsis. For these reasons, prevention of infection is critical because of the potential for catastrophic consequences. Simple measures, such as observance of sterile technique, handling tissues gently, avoidance of aggressive hemostasis, closing and suturing with as little tension as possible, and postoperative irrigation with hydrogen peroxide to remove dried blood which increases local bacterial load, are recommended to prevent untoward events. Antibiotic prophylaxis has been proven effective for clean-contaminated operations such as with delayed wound closure, but not necessarily for clean wounds. As expected, *Staphylococcus aureus* as a skin contaminant is the most common pathogen isolated from infected wounds. An infection typically becomes manifest between postoperative days 3 to 6. Management usually includes opening up a small area of the incision to facilitate drainage of pus and decrease bacterial load as well as pressure on the flap. Any purulent fluid should be sent for culture and sensitivities for isolation of the microorganism, and the patient should be started on broad-spectrum antibiotics until a more specific antibiotic is indicated by the sensitivities. The wound may be packed open, or a wick placed to drain purulent fluid. When the drainage stops and the infection has resolved, the wound is allowed to close. Failure to pack the wound can result in further dehiscence and persistent infection with abscess formation.[23,28]

Another contributor to flap failure is hematoma formation. Hematomas cause flap failure by increasing tension on the wound closure thus increasing the likelihood of ischemia and dehiscence. Hematoma formation also increases both the risk of infection and the inflammatory response that directly interferes with flap circulation.

Two of the most common causes of bleeding that result in hematoma formation are preventable. Meticulous hemostasis at the time of the operation is essential to prevent a hematoma. Caution is advised as one cannot be too aggressive if electrocautery is used since it contributes to poor wound healing and can also contribute to flap ischemia and failure. The second major cause of hematoma formation is drug-induced coagulopathy. The most common medications associated with increased bleeding leading to hematoma formation are over-the-counter therapeutic agents including aspirin, nonsteroidal anti-inflammatory drugs (NSAIDs), vitamin E, and herbal remedies and garlic. Prior to the operation, the patient's medications should be reviewed for other medications, such as coumadin, low molecular weight heparins, and Plavix, which also cause increased bleeding. Typically, it is recommended that patients who are undergoing an operation with flap placement be instructed to stop these medications for 2 weeks prior and 1 week after the operation if medically feasible. Patients who are high risk for pulmonary embolism or other hypercoagulable states may require special consideration.[23]

Although prevention is the preferred course, several options are available for intraoperative control of bleeding. Specific and selective electrocautery is most often the first step. Other options include reverse Trendelenberg positioning of the patient, application of epinephrine soaked cotton pledgets, and direct pressure. Continued oozing of the tissue despite adequate efforts to control bleeding is often removed via a sterile rubber band drain or suction drain placed under the flap or adjacent to the oozing tissue overnight (or until output is decreased) to prevent hematoma formation. In such cases, the patient should be held for observation in case a return trip to the operating room is necessary.[29]

In the event a hematoma should form despite the best efforts at prevention, evacuation is easiest within the first 2 days. Persistent bleeding necessitates re-exploration of the wound. If the hematoma persists beyond 2 days, the clot organizes into a solid mass, and removal may require mechanical debridement. Although resorption of the hematoma begins after 10 to 14 days, this is long after the critical first few days.[30]

Another serious complication, dehiscence, usually is caused by hematoma formation, infection, tip necrosis, or from dynamic facial movement. Because the wound is weakest during the first week prior to collagen deposition, bolstering the wound after suture removal with steristrips can be beneficial to support the flap edges. A simple dehiscence can be repaired if recognized early (within 24 hours). After 24 hours or with a more complex breakdown, it may be better to allow the wound to heal by secondary intention.

Despite good wound care, an undesirable scar or poor cosmetic result will occur. Dermabrasion should be considered for smoothing height differences between the flap and surrounding skin and in areas with thick, sebaceous skin such as the nasal tip. Dermabrasion produces the best results at 6 to 9 weeks postoperatively when fibroblast activity is greatest. Operative scar revision should be delayed for at least 6 months, and more often 1 year, when the scar has matured. Widened scars that parallel relaxed skin tension lines can be simply excised. This is also a good option if the scar is within an aesthetic unit. However, longer linear scars may need to be excised and revised with either a W-plasty or geometric broken line closure. Contracted scars may require a Z-plasty to lengthen and change the direction of the scar if unfavorable.[23] Scar revision and skin resurfacing are discussed in Chapter 57, "Scar Revision and Skin Resurfacing."

CONCLUSIONS

A basic knowledge of wound healing and flap physiology is beneficial to the surgeon in preventing untoward events. Many of the causes of poor healing are preventable with the use of proper surgical technique, knowledge of patient risk factors, adequate patient education, and appropriate wound care. When complications arise, proper awareness of the practical treatment is essential in salvaging flaps and preventing undue scar formation. This may include drainage of a hematoma postoperatively, early infection control measures, and watchful waiting for demarcation of flap necrosis prior to debridement.

REFERENCES

1. Gaboriau HP, Murakami CS. Skin anatomy and flap physiology. Otolaryngol Clin North Am 2001;34:555–69.
2. Frodel JL, Fisher E. Wound healing. In: Papel ID, Frodel JL, Holt GR, et al, editors. Facial Plastic and Reconstructive Surgery, 2nd edition. New York: Thieme Medical Publishers, Inc; 2002. p. 16.
3. Singer AJ, Clark RA. Cutaneous wound healing. N Engl J Med 1999;341:738–46.
4. Goslen JB. Wound healing for the dermatologic surgeon. J Dermatol Surg Oncol 1988;14:959–72.
5. Heldin C-H, Westermark B. Role of platelet-derived growth factor in vivo. In: Clark RAF, editor. The Molecular and Cellular Biology of Wound Repair, 2nd edition. New York: Plenum Press; 1996. p. 249–73.
6. Koopman CF. Cutaneous wound healing: An overview. Otolaryngol Clin North Am 1995;28:835–45.
7. Grinnell F, Billingham RE, Burgess L. Distribution of fibronectin during wound healing in vivo. J Invest Dermatol 1981;76:181–9.
8. Simpson DM, Ross R. The neutrophilic leukocyte in wound repair: A study with antineutrophil serum. J Clin Invest 1972;51:2009–23.
9. Diegelmann RF, Cohen IK, Kaplan AM. The role of macrophages in wound repair: A review. Plast Reconstr Surg 1981;68:107–13.
10. Kanzler MH, Gorsulowsky DC, Swanson NA. Basic mechanisms in the healing cutaneous wound. J Dermatol Surg Oncol 1986;12:1156–64.
11. Pierce G. Macrophages: Important physiologic and pathologic resources of polypeptide growth factors. Am J Respir Cell Mol Bio 1990;2:233–4.
12. Leibovich SJ, Ross R. A macrophage-dependent factor that stimulates the proliferation of fibroblasts in vitro. Am J Pathol 1976;84:501–14.
13. Wheeland RG. The newer surgical dressings and wound healing. Dermatol Clin 1987;5:393–407.
14. Hom DB. A new era of discovery in facial plastic surgery. Arch Facial Plast Surg 2000;2:166–72.
15. Bill TJ, Hoard MA, Gampper TJ. Applications of hyperbaric oxygen in otolaryngology head and neck Surgery. Otolaryngol Clin North Am 2001;34:753–66.
16. Eaglstein WH, Mertz PM. "Inert" vehicles do affect wound healing. J Invest Dermatol 1980;74:90–1.
17. Li W, Dasgeb B, Phillips T, et al. Wound-healing perspectives. Dermatol Clin 2005;23:181–92.
18. Seifter E, Rettura G, Padawer J, et al. Impaired wound healing in streptozotocin diabetes. Prevention by supplemental vitamin A. Ann Surg 1981;194:42–50.
19. Berman B, Bieley HC. Adjunct therapies to surgical management of keloids. Dermatol Surg 1996;22:126–30.
20. Whetzel TP, Mathes SJ. Arterial anatomy of the face: An analysis of vascular territories and perforating cutaneous vessels. Plast Reconstr 1992;89:591–603.
21. Connor CD, Fosko SW. Anatomy and physiology of local skin flaps. Facial Plast Surg Clin N Am 1996;4:447–54.
22. Knight KR, Lepore DA, O'Brien BM. Interrelationship between prostanoids and skin flap survival: A review. Prostaglandins Leukot Essent Fatty Acids 1991;44:195–200.
23. Larrabee WF, Holloway GA, Sutton D. Wound tension and blood flow in skin flaps. Ann Otol Rhinol Laryngol 1984;93:112–5.
24. Larrabee WF, Sutton D. Variation of skin stress–strain curves with undermining. Surg Forum 1981;32:553–5.
25. Vural E, Key JM. Complications, salvage, and enhancement of local flaps in facial reconstruction. Otolaryngol Clin North Am 2001;34:739–51.
26. Pellitteri PK, Kennedy TL, Youn BA. The influence of intensive hyperbaric oxygen therapy on skin flap survival in a swine model. Arch Otolaryngol Head Neck Surg 1992;118:1050–4.
27. Sebben JE. Prophylactic antibiotics in cutaneous surgery. J Dermatol Surg Oncol 1985;11:901–6.
28. Sebben JE. Sterile technique and the prevention of wound infection in office surgery—Part II. J Dermatol Surg Oncol 1989;15:38–48.
29. Salache SJ, Grabski WJ. Complications of flaps. J Dermatol Surg Oncol 1991;17:132–40.
30. Mulliken JB, Healey NA. Pathogenesis of skin flap necrosis from an underlying hematoma. Plast Reconstr Surg 1979;63:540–5.

57

Scar Revision and Skin Resurfacing

Theda C. Kontis, MD

Scars can come in useful. I have one myself above my left knee which is a perfect map of the London Underground.
–Dumbledore: *Harry Potter and the Philosopher's Stone*

SCAR REVISION

Unlike the wizard's scar, most scars serve no useful purpose. Facial scars, in particular, can be emotionally devastating and may affect self-esteem in some patients. Facial plastic surgeons may be called upon to aid in correction of these defects. While not all facial scars require surgical intervention, scars are unacceptable when they are excessively long, not oriented along the relaxed skin tension lines (RSTLs) or when wound edges are of uneven heights.

Ideally, a scar should be parallel to the RSTLs, or hidden in the junction between facial subunits. Scar revision may be indicated when scars lie perpendicular to the RSTLs or are widened, depressed, elevated, or hypertrophic. The goal of scar revision is to reorient the scar for maximal camouflage, not to simply "remove" the scar. A long scar which is oriented across RSTLs can be camouflaged by breaking it up into multiple smaller units. A contracted scar can be lengthened by Z-plasty technique.

Most scar revision techniques require excision of tissue and repositioning of the scar. This is normally performed on mature scars at least 6 to 12 months after the initial injury. Scar revision techniques include excision, irregularization, or dermabrasion.

Simple Excision and Serial Excision

Simple fusiform excision of facial scars is performed on wide or hypertrophic scars, when the suture line can be oriented parallel to the RSTLs. The scar is excised sharply, undermined in the subdermal plane, and closed meticulously in a layered fashion. Occasionally, scar tissue is left in the deeper planes to prevent a concavity in the skin from soft tissue loss.

Serial excision may be performed for lesions which are extremely wide. A portion of the scar is removed in fusiform fashion, and the resultant scar is placed either in a RSTL or at a junction between facial subunits. After 6 to 8 weeks, the tissue has regained enough strength and elasticity to undergo another excision. These excisions are performed every 6 to 8 weeks until the scar is completely removed. The result of serial excisions is to produce one narrow scar which is cosmetically acceptable. Techniques to lessen tension on the closure, such as subcutaneous sutures or taping, can decrease the chance for postoperative widening of the new scar.

Z-Plasty

Scar excision with Z-plasty reconstruction is performed when scars are contracted and lie across the RSTLs.[1] The technique of Z-plasty both lengthens a contracted scar and changes the orientation of the scar. The Z-plasty technique consists of two triangular flaps of equal size which are transposed and sutured into place (Figure 1).

The design of the Z-plasty is critical. The limbs of the Z-plasty should be the same length as the excised scar. There are usually two ways to draw the flaps, mirror images of each other (Figure 2). The surgeon can draw out both options, then choose the design which best places the limbs of the Z in the RSTLs. Scar lengthening is dictated by the angle that the limbs extend from the scar. If the limbs are drawn at 30° angles, the scar will be lengthened 25%, 45° angles will lengthen the scar by 50%, and 60° angles will lengthen the wound by 75% (Figure 3).

Dissection should be carried out in the subdermal plane for ease in flap transposition. Wide undermining is necessary to achieve a tension-free closure. The wound may be closed in one or two layers.

Common areas on the face where Z-plasty scar revision is used include: medial canthal webs, postauricular webs after facelift or parotidectomy surgery (Figure 4), contracted scars of the neck

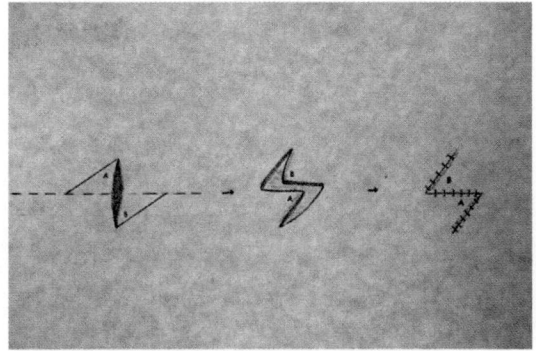

Figure 1 Z-plasty technique. Triangular flaps A and B are transposed to reorient and lengthen the scar.

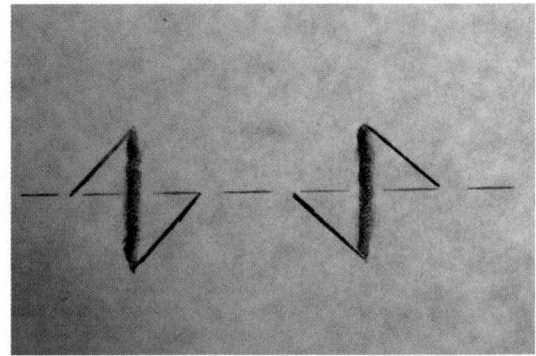

Figure 2 Two Z-plasty patterns are possible for every wound. The design selected is the one which best places the limbs of the Z-plasty in the relaxed skin tension lines (RSTLs).

(Figure 5), scars which are oriented perpendicular to the nasolabial fold, misaligned vermillion-cutaneous junctions, and occasionally for the repair of torn earlobes (Figure 6).

Z-plasty excisions may be single or multiple. When a multiple Z-plasty technique is performed, the final scar is lengthened, the scar is irregularized for maximal camouflage, and wound tension is more evenly distributed in the final scar. Multiple Z-plasty excisions can be used to improve pincushioned or trap-door deformities.

W-Plasty

Scar irregularization is a common technique for scar camouflage. Scars which cross the RSTLs at angles of 35° or more can be camouflaged by breaking up the scar into smaller, irregular segments. This irregularization of the scar makes it more difficult for an observer's eye to follow. The two most common techniques of scar irregularization are W-plasty and geometric broken line closure (GBLC).[2] Unlike Z-plasty, these techniques require removal of surrounding normal tissue and do not result in significant scar lengthening.

The W-plasty technique, or "running W-plasty" is a bilateral advancement flap that is relatively easy to diagram and to perform. The scar is excised by using a series of triangularly shaped segments (Figure 7). The limbs of these segments should be oriented along the RSTLs. Each limb of the triangle should be approximately 3 to 5 mm in length and the base of the triangle should be approximately 5 mm in width. The apex of the triangle is approximately 60°. The triangles become slightly smaller at the ends

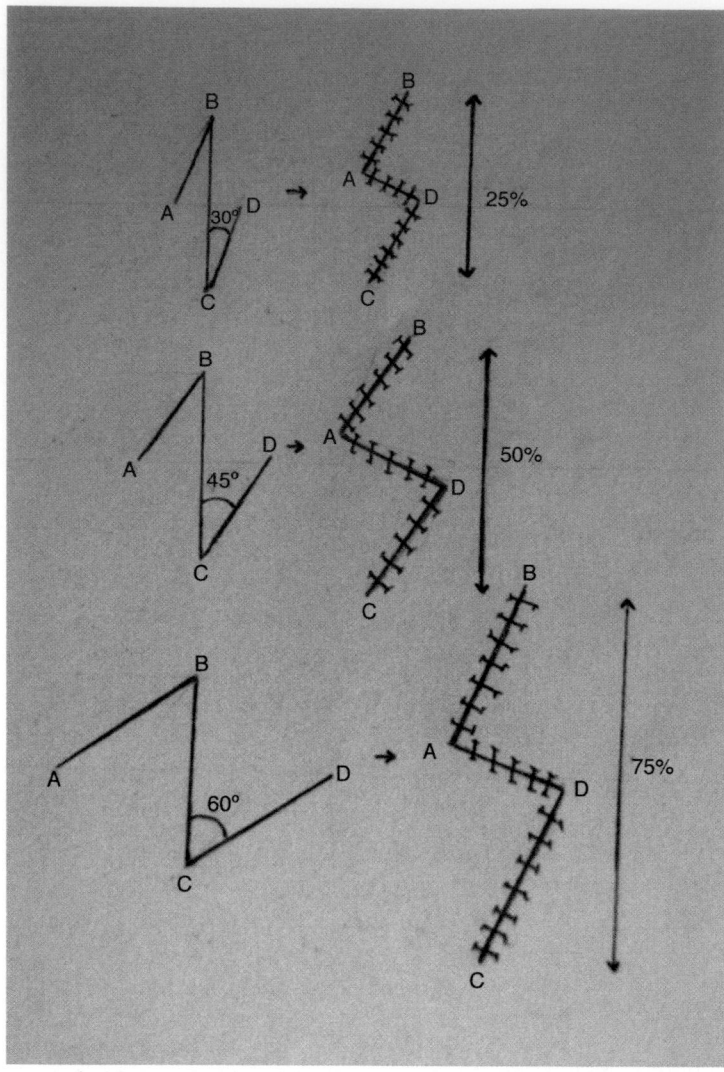

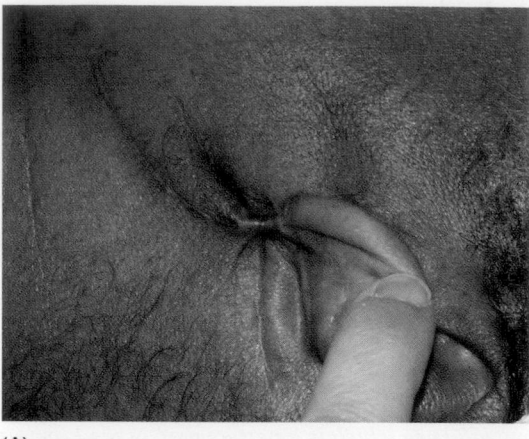

(A)

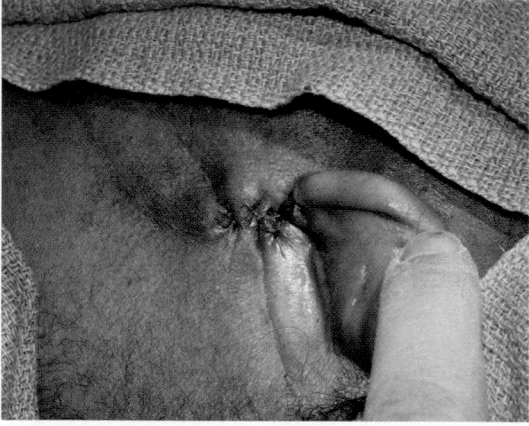

(B)

Figure 3 The angle of the Z-plasty limbs determines the amount of scar lengthening.

of the wound to allow closure without standing cone or "dog ear" formation. The scar itself can be excised with the W-plasty design or can be excised before the flaps are designed. Once the W-plasty flap is diagrammed on the skin, a No. 11 scalpel blade assists in the exact excision of the segments. The wound edges are undermined and closed in a layered fashion to minimize wound tension. The resultant scar is usually slightly longer than the original scar which aids in the prevention of standing cones.

Running W-plasty techniques have been used to camouflage coronal browlift incisions, especially in the frontal hairline. They are also used to improve the appearance of long linear facial scars, forehead vertical scars, and along concave facial areas which have formed a webbed scar.

Geometric Broken Line Closure

The GBLC technique is similar to the running W-plasty technique; however, in addition to triangularly shaped limbs, rectangles, semicircles and squares are used (Figure 8). The limbs are placed parallel to the RSTLs for maximal camouflage. Unlike W-plasty, this technique is more difficult to draw preoperatively. It is used primarily for long scars that are oriented 45° or more from the RSTLs. Each limb should be 3 to 7 mm in length because longer limbs become difficult

to camouflage and shorter limbs produce flaps which are difficult to close.

The scar is incorporated in the GBLC design. A straightforward technique to design the flaps is to outline the scar, then draw lines parallel to the RSTLs (Figure 9). Next the geometric shapes are drawn in each segment, along with its mirror image on the opposite side. The scar is excised with a No. 11 blade, the wound edges undermined and closed in a layered fashion.

Dermabrasion

Dermabrasion is a resurfacing technique which can be used to aid in camouflage of surgical or traumatic scars or scars with uneven contours (Figure 10). Dermabrasion may be performed on mature scars, such as acne scars or scars with elevated and uneven wound edges. It may also be used within the first 2 to 3 months postoperatively to improve scar camouflage (Figure 11).

The technique involves using a low speed powered sanding burr (either wire brush or diamond fraise) to plane down the scar. The endpoint of sanding is usually when pinpoint bleeding is noted from the capillary plexus of the dermal papillae. Scarring may be worsened if dermabrasion is carried out too deeply into the reticular dermis.

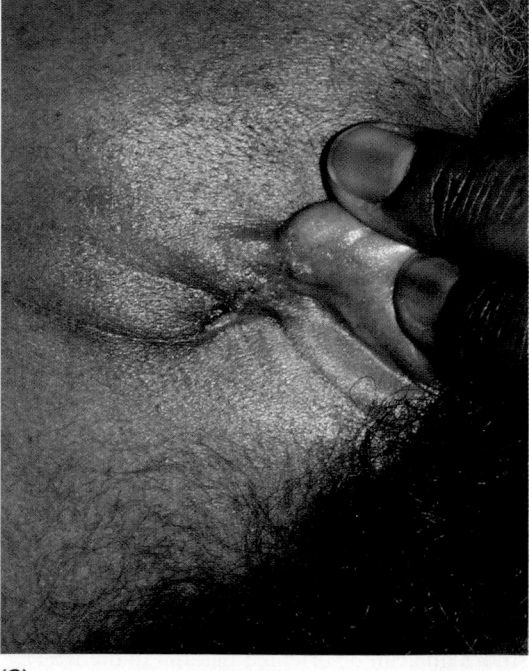

(C)

Figure 4 (A) Contracted scar after parotidectomy surgery. (B) Z-plasty performed to release the contracture. (C) Nine-month postoperative result showing scar contracture release.

Postoperative Wound Care

Poor postoperative wound care can contribute to a poor surgical result. Wound care may include local care with hydrogen peroxide and antibiotic ointment. The hydrogen peroxide is frequently

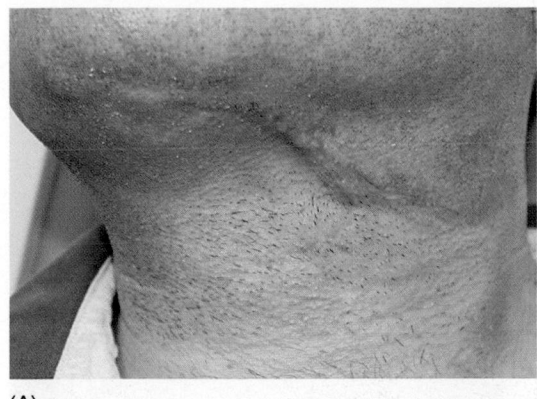

(A)

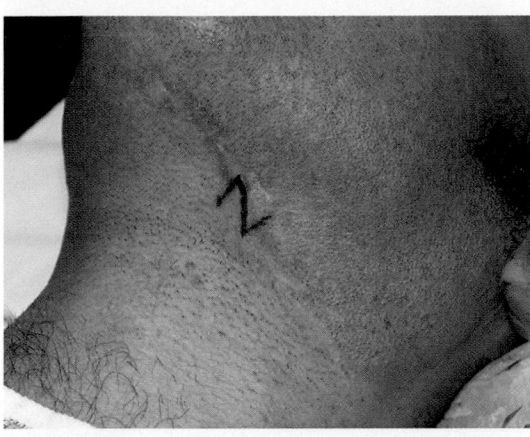

(B)

(C)

Figure 5 (A) Contracted neck scar from prior trauma. (B) Z-plasty design for scar contracture release. (C) Six-week postoperative result.

diluted 50:50 with saline to prevent burning the skin. Adhesive strips (Steri-strips) may be placed to minimize wound tension in the early postoperative period.

The patient is generally seen at 1 week, when the nonabsorbable skin sutures are removed. Although surgeons vary in their postoperative instructions for wound care, all agree that sun exposure should be minimized for 6 months to 1 year after scar revision surgery. If sunburned, scars may become hypertrophic, widened, or hyperpigmented. When the patient is outdoors, the wound should be covered with a bandage or a sunscreen lotion (SPF [sun protective factor] 30 or more) generously applied over the scar.

Complications

There are few complications for scar revision procedures when they have been well planned

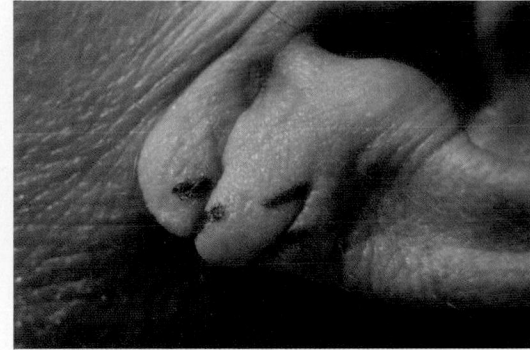

(A)

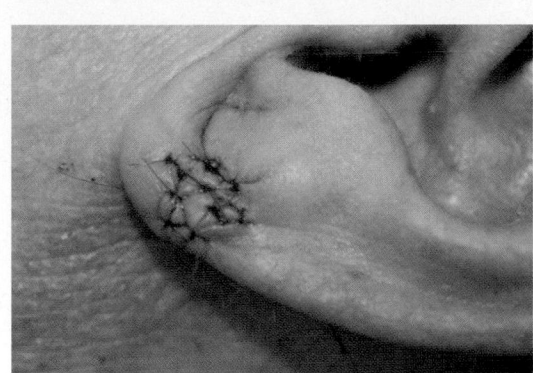

(B)

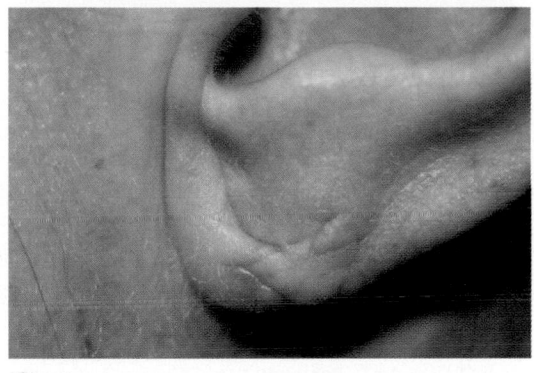

(C)

Figure 6 (A) Two Z-plasties designed to repair splits in the earlobe. (B) Meticulous closure of the Z-plasty flaps. (C) Six-week postoperative result.

preoperatively, performed meticulously, and cared for appropriately in the postoperative period. Wounds closed under tension can widen or necrose, so adequate undermining is necessary to prevent a closure under tension. Tension can also be reduced by the use of taping either at the time of the operation or after suture removal. Hypertrophic scars can be treated with silicone gel sheeting.

Nonsurgical Treatments for Scars

Depressed scars may be improved by the use of filler agents like collagen and hyaluronic acid. The use of filler agents in these scars removes the shadowing effect from the depressed scar and improves cosmesis. The surgeon can pull the skin taught and if the scar elevates, it likely will be improved by filling the dermis and subcutaneous tissues. Some scars do not elevate due to deep dermal adhesions. In this case, release of the dermal attachments by subcision techniques,

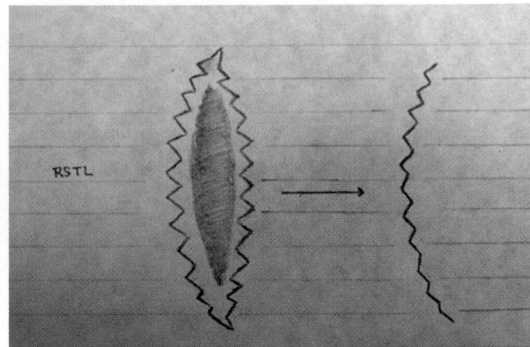

Figure 7 Running W-plasty technique for scar excision. The triangles at the ends of the design are drawn progressively smaller to prevent standing cone deformities.

that is, separating the skin tissue in the affected area from the deeper scar tissue, before the filler is placed, will aid in scar elevation.

Keloids and hypertrophic scars result from abnormal deposition of collagen and glycoprotein during wound healing. Keloids grow beyond the original wound boundaries, whereas hypertrophic scars do not (Figure 12). Interestingly, there is no animal model to study keloids because they only occur in humans after tissue injury.[3] Hypertrophic scars and keloids often respond to intralesional corticosteroid injections such as triamcinolone acetonide (Kenalog) and triamcinolone diacetate (Aristocort). Corticosteroids reduce blood vessel formation and decrease fibroblast proliferation and fibrosis in healing wounds. Mature hypertrophic scars and small keloid scars may respond to a series of corticosteroid injections given 4 to 6 weeks apart. Larger keloids should be excised, and corticosteroids injected either intraoperatively, or in the early postoperative period, as well as every 4 to 6 weeks. Low dose external beam radiation has also been used for the treatment of recurrent keloids. Mechanical compression may be used to flatten some hypertrophic scars and keloids. The mechanism by which compression improves scars currently is not known, but it is possible that the wounds exposed to silicone sheeting have less scar contraction, possibly by downregulating fibroblasts and decreasing fibrogenic cytokines such as transforming growth factor-beta 2 (TGF-β2).[4]

Hyperpigmented scars can occasionally occur in darker skinned patients. It is crucial these patients avoid sun exposure to the healing

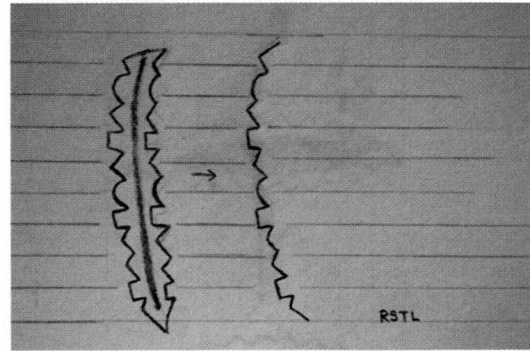

Figure 8 Geometric broken line closure design. The limbs of the geometric shapes should be parallel to the relaxed skin tension lines (RSTLs).

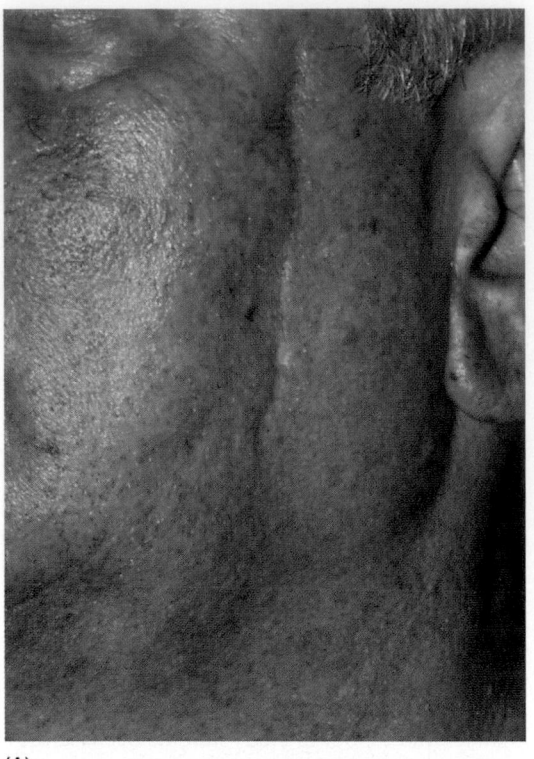 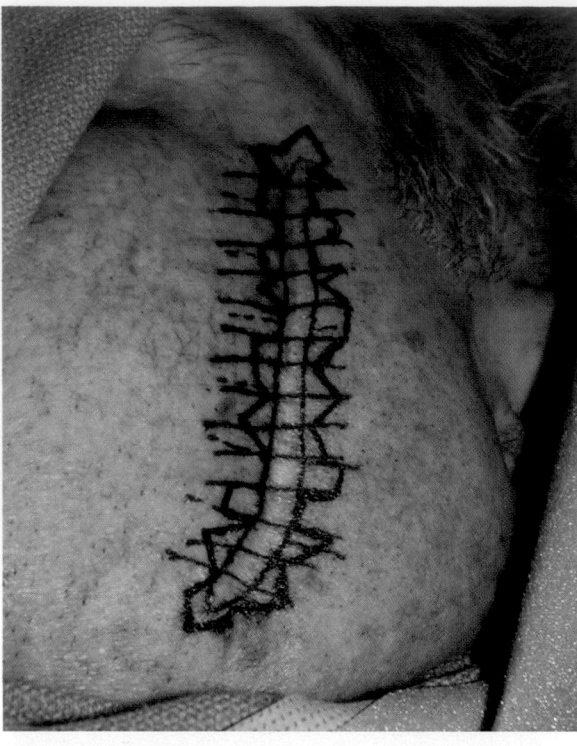 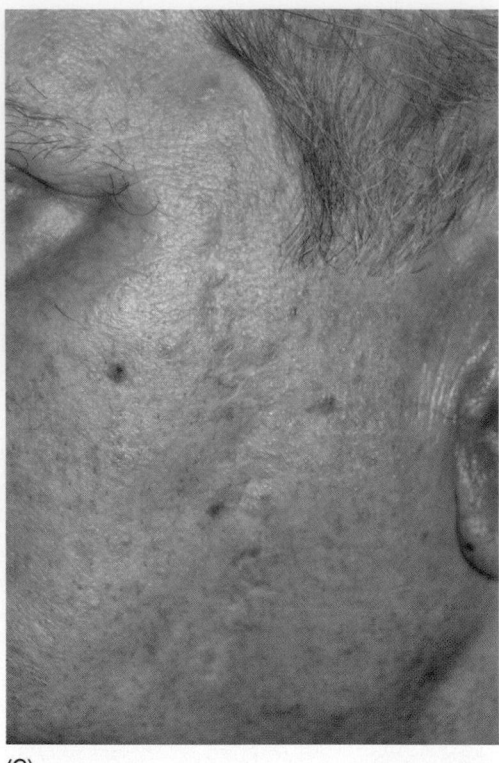

(A)   (B)   (C)

Figure 9 (A) Vertically oriented cheek scar. (B) Geometric broken line closure design. (C) Six-month postoperative result.

wound. Hyperpigmented scars can be treated with skin bleaching agents such as hydroquinone 4%; however, they occasionally improve with no treatment.

The flashlamp pulsed dye (FLPD) laser can be used to treat hypertrophic scars, especially those with erythema. Components of living tissue that absorb particular wavelengths of laser light are called chromophores. The FLPD laser is a "vascular" laser with a wavelength of 585 nm. At this wavelength, the laser energy is best absorbed by the chromophore hemoglobin. This principle of selective photothermolysis allows for treatment of vascular lesions without harming the surrounding tissues. Hypertrophic scars become more pliable and smaller when treated with the FLPD laser. The mechanism of action is not clearly understood, but it is believed that the laser energy breaks the disulfide bonds in collagen. The collagen fibers are then able to reorient, and the scar flattens. Treatment with the FLPD laser is relatively painless; the patients often describe the discomfort like a "rubber band snapping against the skin." Topical anesthetics are usually not used because the vasoconstrictive properties diminish the erythema, a necessary component for the laser. The patients may experience bruising after treatment, which may last 7 to 10 days and may be covered with camouflage makeup. Subsequent treatments also may be necessary. Occasionally hyperpigmentation can occur after FLPD laser treatment (Figure 13). This minor complication usually resolves without treatment.

Scarless Healing

Small fetal wounds induced early in gestation can heal with normal dermis and skin appendages, essentially without producing a scar. This observation had yielded vigorous research in the mechanism of "scarless healing." Initially it was believed that the intrauterine environment, bathed in amniotic fluid rich in growth factors and hyaluronic acid, was necessary for scarless healing to occur. However, studies have shown that fetuses which heal outside a uterus, for example, marsupials, are also capable of scarless fetal healing.[5] In humans, scarless repair is dependent on both the gestational age of the fetus and the size of the injury.[6] Scarless repair can occur when small wounds are induced in human fetuses before 24 weeks of gestation.

The normal wound healing process consists of four phases: hemostasis, inflammation, proliferation, and remodeling. Immediately after injury, the initial response is coagulation, mediated by platelets and fibrin. The inflammatory phase then occurs over the next 3 days, as neutrophils and macrophages phagocytize foreign material and bacteria. The macrophages also secrete growth factors: transforming growth factor alpha, TGF-β, epidermal growth factor, fibroblast growth factor, and platelet derived growth factor. Proliferation occurs from 3 to 12 days after injury, as fibroblasts synthesize collagen and neovascularization occurs. In the final phase, which occurs for several months after injury, remodeling takes place as the wound is re-epithelialized and collagen is remodeled. Myofibroblast activity is responsible for wound contraction. The final result is a mature scar, which histologically is noted to have disorganized dermal collagen and the absence of dermal appendages.

Quite different reactions occur after injury in scarless healing. Fetal wounds have no inflammatory infiltrate, partly due to the characteristics of fetal platelets. Unlike adult platelets, which aggregate when exposed to collagen, fetal platelets degranulate less and aggregate poorly. In addition, few neutrophils and macrophages are present in fetal wounds. This lack of inflammatory response is critical in fetal scarless healing. Manipulations which induce inflammation in fetal wounds result in scarring.[7] Myofibroblasts, which appear in adult wounds at 1 to 3 weeks postinjury and contribute to wound contracture, appear only briefly in fetal wounds.

Lorenz and colleagues have shown that the critical factor in scarless healing is the fetal fibroblast which is the major source of collagen in wound repair.[8] Fetal fibroblasts have more receptors for hyaluronic acid (HA) and synthesize more Type III and IV collagen than adult fibroblasts. In scarless wounds, the collagen is laid down in a fine, organized, reticular pattern, which is identical to uninjured skin. Scars, however, are characterized by disorganized bundles of thick collagen fibers. In addition, scarless fetal wounds manifest a more rapid and higher content of HA than do adult wounds. HA stimulates fetal fibroblast migration and may result in scarless healing. TGF-β1 inhibits fibroblast migration and is associated with scar formation.

Many of the differences in adult and fetal responses to injury originate at the gene expression level. Recently, homeobox genes, a group of genes which influence the expression of other genes early in physical development, have been implicated in fetal wound healing. As our knowledge of wound healing improves, we may one day be able to prevent the formation of scars.

Tissue Engineering

Another exciting area of genetic research involves the use of undifferentiated cells.

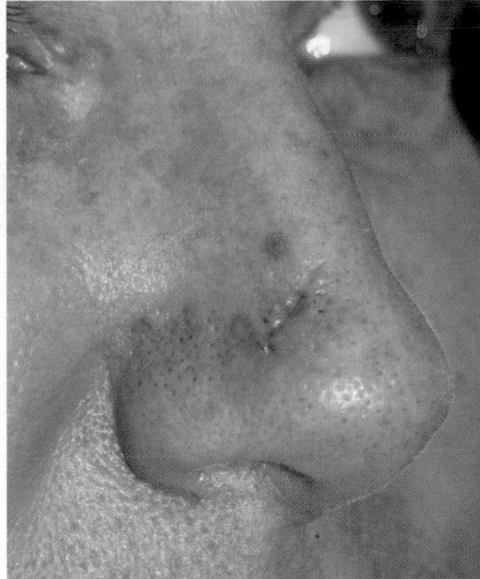

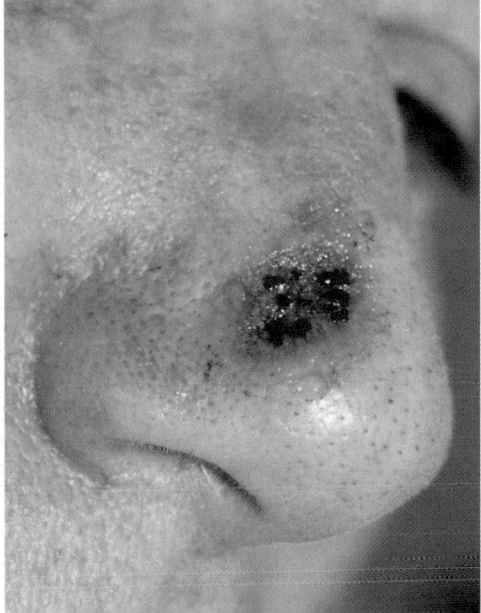

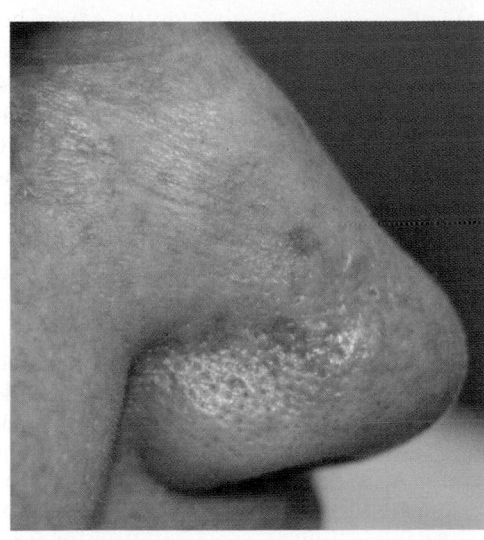

Figure 10 (A) Poorly healed nasal tip scar after basal cell carcinoma excision and linear closure. (B) Pinpoint bleeding from the dermal capillary plexus immediately post dermabrasion. (C) Postoperative scar improvement at 5 months.

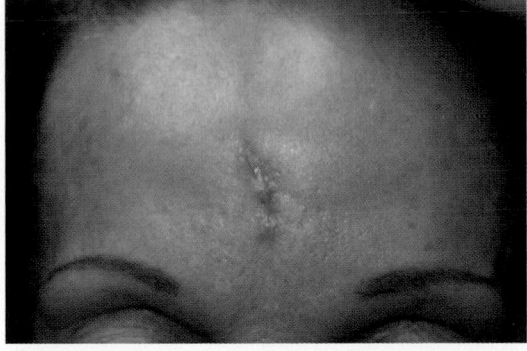

(A)

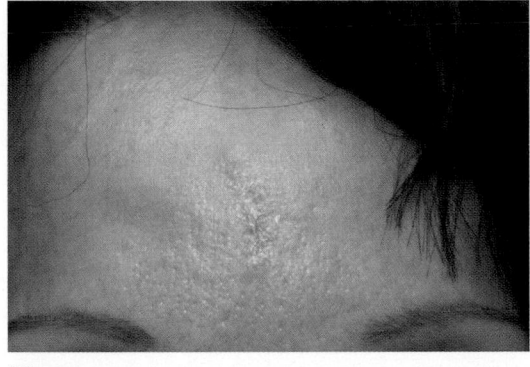

(B)

Figure 11 (A) Poorly healed traumatic forehead scar. (B) Four months following dermabrasion.

Embryonic stem cells can be propagated in vitro and maintain their pluripotent potential. In the murine model, embryonic stem cells have been cultured to produce a multilayered epidermis with underlying dermis which was similar to native skin.[9] This bioengineered skin is a powerful tool for studying skin development and has the potential in humans for production of bioengineered skin grafts.

In 1975, Rheinward and Green developed a cell culture technique by which keratinocytes could be cultured on a "feeder layer" of lethally irradiated mouse fibroblasts.[10] By using this technique, a small skin biopsy could, in just 3 to 4 weeks, produce enough sheets of epithelial cells to cover the entire body. This had dramatic potential for the treatment of burn victims. Subsequent developments in tissue engineering allowed the grafts to be grown serum free and without a feeder layer of fibroblasts.

However, controversies developed over the use of bioengineered grafts. The main disadvantage is the high cost, which has precluded widespread use. The cultured sheet grafts are usually three to five cell layers of epithelial cells and are delicate to handle and are easily injured. Even after graft "take" the grafts are susceptible to blistering as a response to sheering forces. Wound infection is also problematic because the tissue is more susceptible to bacterial infection from wound contamination. In addition, the uncertain "take" rates of grafts may be due to the lack of anchoring fibrils present in normal skin dermis. For these reasons, human allografts may be used early in burn wound coverage to produce a well-vascularized and clean wound bed. The use of

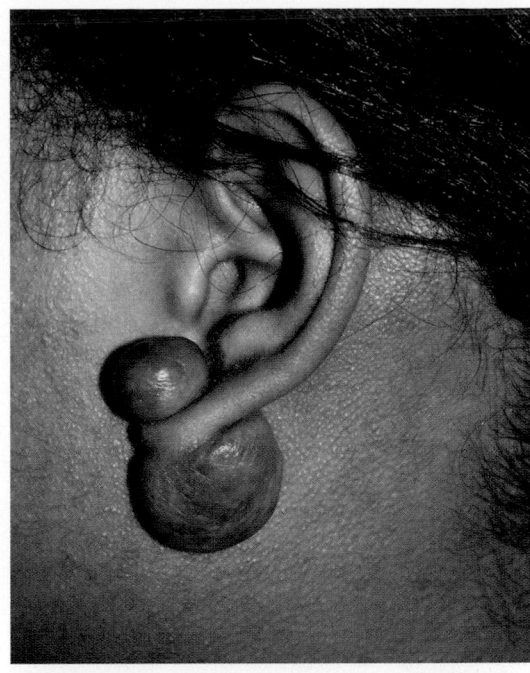

(A)

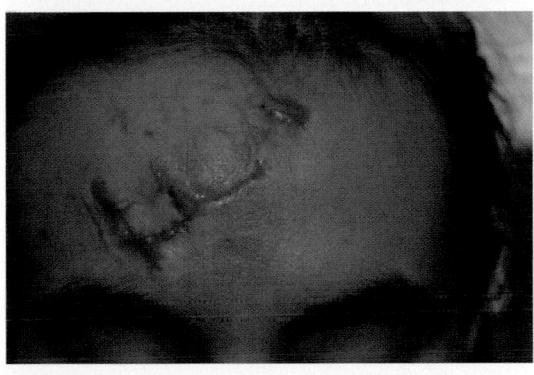

(B)

Figure 12 (A) Typical keloid of the earlobe as a complication of piercing. (B) Hypertrophic scarring of forehead following trauma.

temporary allograft placement can increase the chance for success of a subsequently placed epidermal sheet graft.

Cell suspensions are known to attach better to wound beds than skin grafts.[11] Cultured keratinocytes can be suspended with fibrin sealant and placed on a wound bed then covered with an allograft. As it heals, the allograft initially becomes revascularized, like an autologous graft, then after approximately 2 weeks, the epithelial components slough and the wound becomes stable as it is covered by epithelium produced from the cultured keratinocytes. Suspended keratinocytes with fibrin sealant can also be either sprayed onto the surface of the wound or placed as a gel. These methods result in more reliable cell delivery.

The combination of gene therapy and keratinocyte culture techniques has potential to both improve the performance of cultured skin substitutes as well as address healing and scar formation. The goals of future research will be to improve both cosmesis and function of healing tissues and one day to develop the ability for wounds to heal without scars.

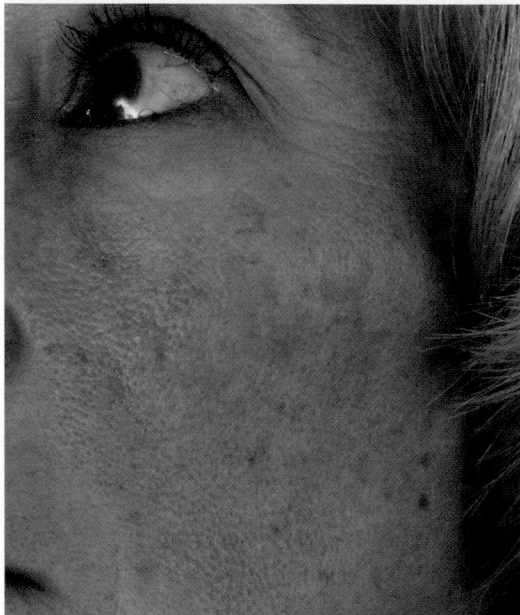

(A)

(B)

Figure 13 (A) Facial telangiectasias. (B) Hyperpigmented scarring 3 weeks after flashlamp pulsed dye laser treatment.

SKIN RESURFACING

Techniques of facial skin resurfacing have been known for thousands of years; the ancient Egyptians described treating the skin with ground rocks and chemicals. Hungarian gypsies were known to place chemicals on the face for skin rejuvenation, and these techniques were brought to the United States in the 1900s by European dermatologists. The classic methods of facial resurfacing have been chemical peels; however, newer laser technologies have been able to produce similar results.

Chemical Peel

Chemical peeling involves the application of chemicals which injure the epidermis and dermis to produce the stimulation of new growth of the epidermis and tightening of the dermis (Figure 14). The peels can be superficial, injuring only the

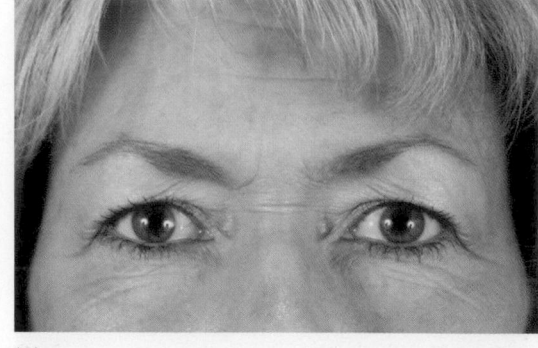

(A)

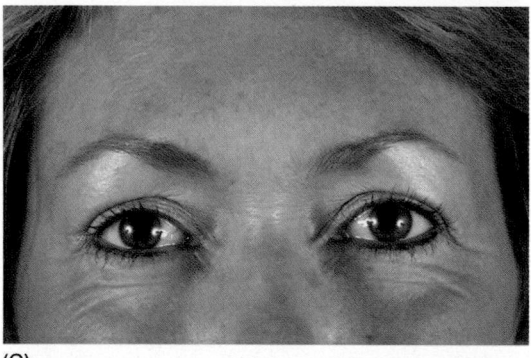

(B)

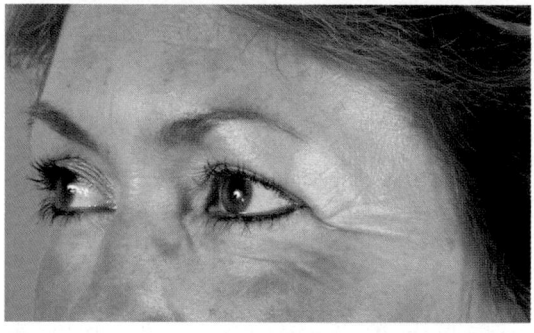

(C)

(D)

Figure 14 (A) and (B) Preoperative endoscopic forehead lift, upper blepharoplasty and phenol peel of lower lids. (C) and (D) Three-month postoperative result shows tightening of the lower lid skin from the chemical peel.

epidermis, medium-depth, injuring the papillary dermis, and deep causing a reaction in the deep reticular dermis and induction of collagen and ground substance.

Superficial chemical peels, such as glycolic acid, salicylic acid and 10% trichloroacetic acid (TCA), exfoliate the stratum corneum of the epidermis. These peels do not cause significant changes in rhytides but do improve the skin quality and texture.

Superficial peels such as 10 to 20% TCA, Jessner solution (combination of resorcinol, salicylic acid, lactic acid, and ethanol), and 40 to 70% glycolic acid remove the stratum corneum and damaged upper epidermis. These peels are performed without anesthesia, and patients can return to normal activities immediately after the procedure. Erythema and desquamation may persist for several days.

Medium-depth chemical peels injure tissue down to the papillary dermis. Classically 50% TCA has been used for these peels; but, because of increased risks of scarring at that concentration, 35% TCA is combined with either Jessner solution or 70% glycolic acid. The procedure is moderately uncomfortable, and patients are usually given a mild oral sedative preoperatively.

Deep chemical peels injure tissue into the deep reticular dermis. The Baker–Gordon chemical peel has been the standard method for skin resurfacing for nearly one half century. It consists of 88% phenol, water, Septisol, and croton oil. The soap acts as a surfactant which allows an even penetration of the solution. The croton oil is an epidermalytic agent that enhances phenol absorption. Phenol is cardiotoxic, so cardiac monitoring is crucial during its application. Intravenous fluids should be given because phenol is also hepatotoxic and nephrotoxic. Because of these toxicities, the chemical peel solution is placed on single cosmetic units of the face at 15-minute intervals.

The chemical peel solution is usually applied with a cotton-tipped applicator after the face has been vigorously cleansed and degreased. As the chemical is applied, frosting of the skin occurs, which indicates keratocoagluation. It is important to assure even peeling by producing an even frost. If the frosting is not even, the nontreated areas may be retreated. Care must be taken not to over treat areas because deeper penetration of the chemical increases the chance of scarring.

Immediately after placing the chemical, the peeled skin can be either occluded or left unoccluded. When occluded with a biosynthetic dressing (Vigilon or Flexan), the peel is absorbed deeper into the tissues into the mid-reticular dermis. As the peel penetrates deeper, the risk of post treatment scarring also increases. Re-epithelialization generally occurs from days 3 to 10; however, erythema can last for several months.

Complications can be minimized by adequate training in chemical peeling procedures as well as meticulous attention to details. The solutions must be mixed correctly and applied to the face appropriately. The novice surgeon should, after adequate training, proceed slowly with chemical peeling until a level of comfort is reached with the solutions and their effects.

The complications of chemical peels include hypopigmentation, hyperpigmentation, infection, and scarring. Pre- and postprocedure skin care and wound care are of the utmost importance. The skin should be kept moist with ointments during the healing phase. Sun exposure is contraindicated. Acetic acid soaks may be performed

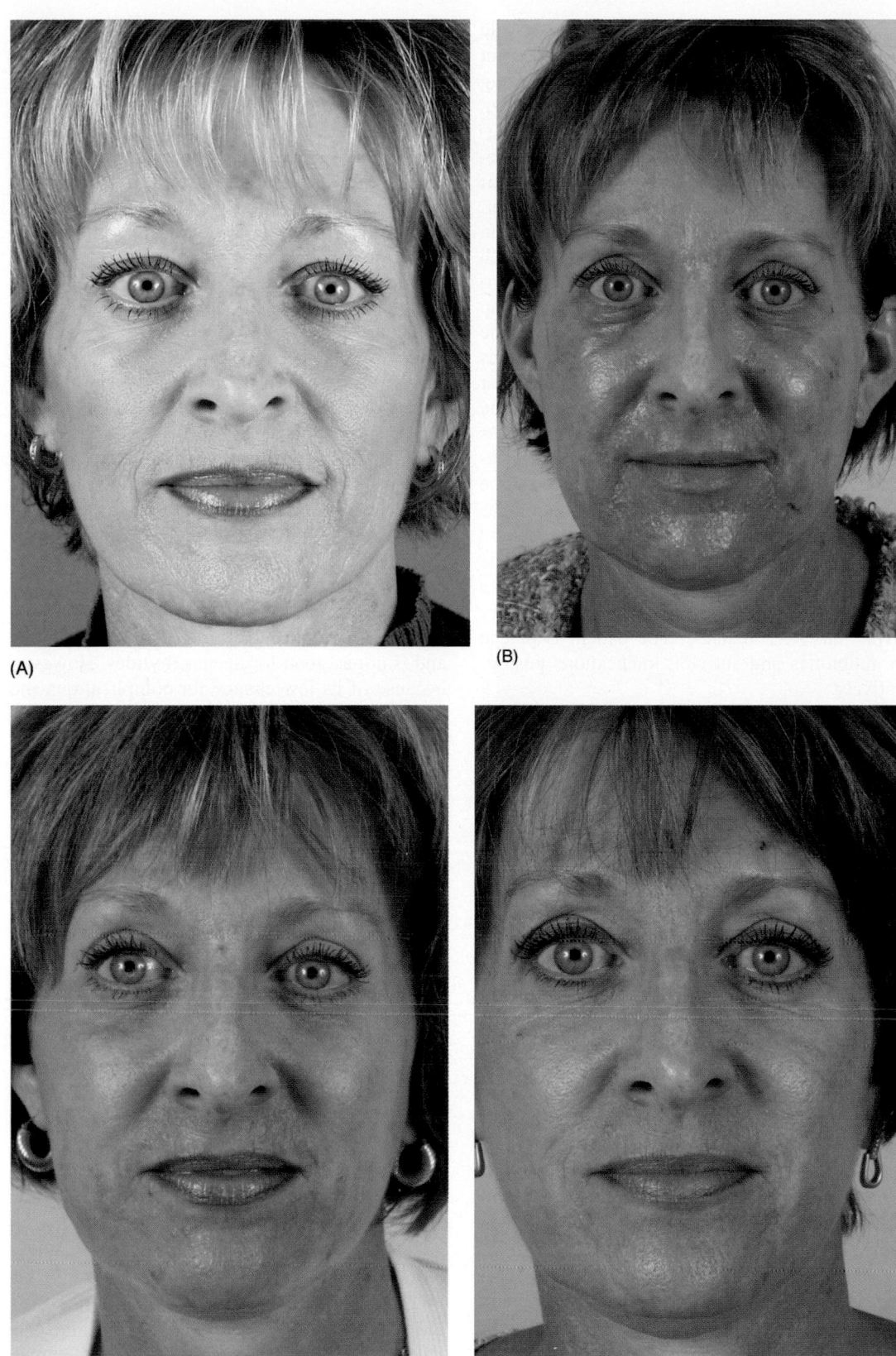

(A)

(B)

(C)

(D)

Figure 15 (A) Preoperative CO_2 laser resurfacing for acne scarring and mild facial aging. (B) One-week postoperative appearance with erythema and early skin regrowth. (C) Two-week postoperative with less erythema. (D) At two-month postoperative, the erythema and edema have subsided. The fine rhytides and acne scars are improved.

companies today are producing a myriad of lasers and pulsed light devices which are being used for cosmetic enhancement of the skin. When laser skin resurfacing was first introduced, many complications emerged due to physician inexperience with the new technology. Companies currently are striving to develop a device which produces the best cosmetic results with the least risk of complications.

Carbon Dioxide Laser. Many surgeons believe the carbon dioxide (CO_2) laser has become the gold standard for skin resurfacing and skin rejuvenation. CO_2 laser resurfacing can produce results analogous to deep chemical peels. It has been used to treat actinic keratoses, uneven scars, dyschromias, and rhytides (Figure 15). The laser removes the epidermis and part of the papillary dermis without damaging the dermis. Keeping the dermis intact is crucial because hair follicles are the source of skin epithelial regeneration after laser treatment.

The mechanism for skin tightening and wrinkle reduction is not fully understood. Laser treated tissue does show increased levels of Type I collagen and elastic tissue.[12] Most lasers destroy tissue by the process of photothermolysis, the destruction of tissue by the conversion of laser energy into heat. Laser energy can be absorbed by three cutaneous chromophores: hemoglobin, water, and melanin. At a wavelength of 10,600 nm, the CO_2 laser energy is absorbed by water and heats the tissue by vaporization. The heat energy is then released by the tissue. The period of time it takes for half of the energy generated to be released by the target tissue is called the thermal relaxation time. The thermal relaxation time for the skin is less than one millisecond. Not to cause heat damage to the skin, pulses of laser light are randomly placed in a pattern. By randomly pulsing the light, the pulse duration is decreased to less than the target tissue thermal relaxation time. Most CO_2 resurfacing lasers are equipped with at computerized pattern generator (CPG) hand piece that allows for the random placement of laser spots in a variety of geometric shapes. The amount of spot overlap, or density, can be varied.

Appropriate patient selection and the setting of realistic expectations are of paramount importance when performing laser resurfacing. The ideal candidates have facial wrinkles but not significantly loose skin. Because the laser cannot be used on neck skin, patients with significantly lax neck skin are counseled that they would be better treated by facelift or neck lift procedures.

A commonly used description of skin types is known as the Fitzpatrick skin type classification (Table 1). This classification denotes six different skin types, skin color, and reaction to sun exposure. Patients with Fitzpatrick skin types I and II generally are the most ideal candidates for laser resurfacing. Patients with Fitzpatrick skin types III and IV can be candidates, but may develop postoperative dyschromias. Patients with acne scarring are also ideal patients, and usually can

postoperatively to prevent infection. A history of herpes simplex also should be ascertained, because perioral resurfacing can stimulate the eruption of herpetic lesions or "fever blisters" that can spread to the resurfaced areas and may result in scarring. Because of the severe risk of disfigurement from herpetic infection, all resurfacing patients, no matter their history, are placed

on antiviral medication perioperatively. If scars develop from resurfacing, they may be treated with topical or injected corticosteroids.

Laser Resurfacing

Initially used for scar revision and tattoo removal, laser skin resurfacing has found its niche in wrinkle reduction and skin rejuvenation. Equipment

Table 1 Fitzpatrick Skin Type Classification

Fitzpatrick Skin Type	Description
I	Extremely fair skin, always burns, never tans
II	Fair skin, always burns, sometimes tans
III	Medium skin, sometimes burns, always tans
IV	Olive skin, rarely burns, always tans
V	Moderately pigmented brown skin, never burns, always tans
VI	Markedly pigmented black skin, never burns, always tans

expect approximately a 50% improvement in their skin quality postoperatively. It is important to document the prior use of isotretinoin (Accutane), which affects epidermal differentiation, especially at the follicular infundibulum. It is recommended that patients wait at least a year after Accutane use before undergoing laser resurfacing, so as to allow recovery of the dermal sebaceous elements necessary for skin regrowth.

Preoperative skin care is an important adjunct to surgery and usually is initiated at least 4 to 6 weeks preoperatively. Hydroquinones are used to decrease melanin production and lessen the chance for postoperative dyschromias, but do have some controversies associated with their use.[13,14] Although hydroquinones are called "bleaching" agents, they actually function to decrease the formation of melanosomes in the melanocytes and, therefore, stop the production of melanin. This works well with the concomitant use of tretinoins, which stimulate keratinocyte maturation and turnover.

The use of tretinoins or retinoids (Retin-A) is important preoperatively in skin resurfacing, although it can be controversial. Retin-A has been shown to increase dermal collagen synthesis, decrease the thickness of the stratum corneum, reduce epidermal dysplasia and atypia, increase angiogenesis, and reconstitute the papillary dermis. Benefits to its use include reduced postoperative milia formation, reduced hyperpigmentation, and accelerated epidermal regeneration with faster healing. Disadvantages include increased angiogenesis, which may contribute to prolonged postlaser erythema. Retin-A can be irritating to the skin, especially in the first few weeks of use, and can increase photosensitivity.

Alpha-hydroxy acids (AHAs), such as glycolic acid, are used as superficial peeling agents to both reduce keratinization and increase thickness of the epidermis and papillary dermis. The AHAs are less irritating than the retinoids and can be used in addition to retinoids in a prelaser skin treatment regimen.

Facial laser resurfacing is usually performed in the operating suite with the patient under intravenous sedation or general anesthesia. Laser safety precautions are performed at all times, both protecting the eyes of the patient and operating room staff, as well as taking precautions for fire prevention. If the patient is intubated, a laser-safe endotracheal tube must be utilized. Oxygen is not delivered to the patient at the time of laser firing when the procedure is performed under sedation. The patient's face is prepared with a nonflammable solution, and the face is draped with saline-soaked towels. If desired, the treatment areas of the face can be outlined with a surgical marker. The laser is then applied to resurface the face in the designated areas. Care is taken to place each pattern of the CPG directly adjacent to the previous one to prevent skip-areas and not to overlap the treated areas. Once the area is treated, the char is wiped away with a moist gauze. This is crucial so that the char does not absorb the laser heat and cause increased thermal injury to the tissue. Once the char is removed, a second pass can be performed. Collagen tightening demonstrated by tissue tightening and shrinkage can be observed during the second pass. Resistant areas of the face, such as the perioral lip lines, can be treated with three to six passes, if necessary. The endpoint of laser resurfacing is when a chamois color is noted; indicating the level of the papillary dermis has been reached. The patient is placed on antibiotics and antiviral medications postoperatively.

After the resurfacing has been completed, an occlusive or nonocclusive dressing may be applied to the face. Some surgeons prefer petrolatum ointments (Vaseline) or soybean emollient (Crisco) application due to the low incidence of sensitivity to these products, however, the use of petrolatum ointments is associated with milia formation postopertivley. Semi-occlusive dressings, such as polyurethane foam adhesive dressing (Flexzan), can be applied and left in place for several days. Occlusive dressings are associated with faster healing times but increased chance of wound infections.

Postoperative complications can include prolonged erythema that can last from 4 to 8 weeks and can be camouflaged with makeup, or treated with topical or systemic corticosteroids. Hyperpigmentation can be treated with hydroquinone postoperatively. Hypopigmentation is more difficult to treat and may resolve over time. Telangiectasias can be worsened after laser resurfacing and can be treated with the FLPD laser.

More serious complications include scarring and infection. Bacterial infection generally resolves with wound care and appropriate antibiotics (cultures usually show *Staphylococcus aureus* or *Pseudomonas aeruginosa*). Herpetic outbreaks must be treated aggressively to prevent scarring. Scarring itself can be a devastating complication of laser resurfacing. Areas of hypertrophic scarring can be treated with topical fluorinated corticosteroids, silicone gel sheeting, corticosteroid injections, and the FLPD laser.

Erbium:YAG Laser Resurfacing. The erbium:YAG (yttrium–aluminum–garnet) laser also uses water as its chromophore, but the absorption of erbium light by water is ten times that of the CO_2 laser. The laser wavelength of 2,940 nm corresponds to the optimal absorption peak of collagen and causes much less thermal damage than the CO_2 laser. The erbium:YAG laser thus produces a more superficial injury by vaporization. Both the CO_2 and erbium-YAG lasers are considered ablative lasers because they remove the epidermis and part of the papillary dermis.

The erbium laser is much less painful than the CO_2 laser and can be performed under topical or local anesthesia. Unlike the CO_2 laser, the pulses are placed with 10 to 12% overlap. Debris is minimal, and wiping is often not necessary between passes. The endpoint of treatment is when pinpoint capillary bleeding is observed. Unlike the CO_2 laser treatment, collagen tightening is not observed during erbium laser treatment. Ointment is applied postoperatively, erythema is minimal, and makeup may be applied in approximately 4 days. Erythema is generally gone by 2 weeks postoperatively. Dyschromias rarely occur postoperatively.

When the results with the erbium-YAG laser are compared to those of the CO_2 laser, they are not as dramatic. The erbium-YAG laser does not produce the same amount of collagen remodeling and is not as good for deeper rhytides. However, because of its low chance for complications and quick recovery, it does have a role in skin resurfacing of superficial rhytides and scars.

Newer Technologies. Fractional photothermolysis (Fraxel, Reliant Technologies, San Diego, CA) was introduced in 2004 as a nonablative laser, which selectively damages the dermis and spares the epidermis by cooling the skin during treatment. Like the CO_2 and erbium-YAG lasers, the Fraxel laser uses water as a chromophore. The Fraxel technology is a 1,550 nm diode-pumped erbium fiber laser which produces "microthermal treatment zones": thousands of small columns of thermal energy that penetrate the epidermis and dermis. This fractional energy does not injure the surrounding tissue, which allows for more rapid healing. Only about 20% of the surface area is affected, therefore, about four to five treatments are needed for complete effect. Fraxel laser treatments can be used on all skin types and can be used to treat the neck, chest, and hands.

Fraxel treatments are performed under topical anesthesia. A blue tint is applied to the face, to guide the laser, and is removed after the procedure. The patients may look pink and swollen for up to 4 days.

Newer lasers are combining both CO_2 and Fraxel technologies for the ultimate in flexibility for resurfacing. In addition, companies are continuing to produce skin resurfacing laser technology aimed at improving results and minimizing risk.

Skin resurfacing techniques should only be performed by surgeons with the proper training and experience. Complications of these procedures can be devastating when not performed properly. The novice surgeon is admonished to proceed with caution when employing these procedures.

REFERENCES

1. Hove CR, Williams EF, Rodgers BJ. Z-plasty: A concise review. Facial Plast Surg 2001;17:289–93.
2. Rodgers BJ, Williams EF, Hove CR. W-plasty and geometric broken line closure. Facial Plast Sur 2001;17:239–44.
3. Yang GP, Lim IJ, Toan-Thang P, et al. From scarless fetal wounds to keloids: Molecular studies in wound healing. Wound Repair Regen 2003;11:411–8.
4. Kuhn MA, Moffit MR, Smith PD, et al. Silicone sheeting decreases fibroblast activity and downregulates TGFbeta2 in hypertrophic scar model. Int J Surg Investig 2001;2: 467–74.
5. Dang C, Ting K, Soo C, et al. Fetal wound healing current perspectives. Clin Plastic Surg 2003;30:13–23.
6. Ferguson MWJ, Whitby DJ, Shah M, et al. Scar formation: The spectral nature of fetal and adult wound repair. Plast Reconstr Surg 1996;97:854–60.
7. Mackool RJ, Gittes GK, Longaker MT. Scarless healing: The fetal wound. Clin Plast Surg 1998;25:357–65.
8. Lorenz HP, Lin RY, Longaker MT, et al. The fetal fibroblast: The effector cell of scarless fetal skin repair. Plast Reconstr Surg 1995;96:1251–9.
9. Aberdam D. Derivation of keratinocyte progenitor cells and skin formation from embryonic stem cells. Int J Dev Biol 2004;48:203–6.
10. Rheinwald JG, Green H. Serial cultivation of strains of human epidermal keratinocytes: The formation of keratinizing colonies from single cells. Cell 1975;6:331–43.
11. Horch RE, Kopp J, Kneser U, et al. Tissue engineering of cultured skin substitutes. J Cell Mol Med 2005;9:592–608.
12. Keller GS, Rawnsley J, Cutcliffe B, Watson J. Erbium:YAG and carbon dioxide laser resurfacing. Facial Plast Surg Clin North Am 1998;6:167–81.
13. Kooyers TJ, Westerhof W. Toxicology and health risks of hydroquinone in skin lightening formulations. JEADV 2006;20:777–80.
14. Norlund J, Grimes P, Ortonne JP. The safety of hydroquinone. J Cosmetic Dermatol 2006;5:168–70.

58

Local Flaps in Facial Reconstruction

Peter A. Hilger, MD
Kofi O. Boahene, MD

The face is the central focus for one's identity, and any disfigurement of it draws undesirable attention. Even minor soft tissue defects can disrupt the delicate highlights and shadows of the face. To look normal minor, and major soft tissue defects of the face should be repaired with a carefully selected plan based on proper principles of cutaneous flaps and appreciation for the esthetic aspects of the face.

Soft tissue defects of the face most commonly result from resection of cutaneous malignancies or trauma. Unfortunately, the incidence of skin cancers of the face is on the rise with a particularly notable increase in younger patients. Esthetics standards for younger people are often high and during their lifetime they have the possibility of developing additional cancers and associated defects. This fact requires judicious use of available flaps as one anticipates numerous reconstructive interventions over many years. Basal cell carcinoma, squamous cell carcinoma and melanoma are the most common cutaneous malignancies. Surgical excision with confirmation of margins must be ensured before embarking on any reconstruction. Mohs excision should be considered in the surgical plan as it has the highest rate of cancer clearance. Facial avulsion injuries from vehicular accidents, human or animal bites, and burns also present complex and irregular defects that may require the use of local flaps. Dog bite injuries with tissue loss are often encountered in children, and their repair can be both emotionally and technically challenging.

While some facial soft tissue defects can be closed primarily by advancing adjacent tissue, others require skin grafting or healing by secondary intention. The disadvantages of the these methods are the limitation in scar placement, contour irregularities, color and texture mismatch, wound contracture, and distortion of mobile facial structures. Local flaps recruit tissue from adjacent local or regional facial subunits and can provide skin, fat, cartilage, or hair with appropriate color, contour, and texture matching. When properly executed, local flaps can be used to repair most small and intermediate sized defects with excellent esthetic results.

ANATOMY AND PHYSIOLOGY OF LOCAL FLAPS

Local flaps can be designed to recruit skin, fat, other subcutaneous tissue, cartilage, hair follicles, and accompanying adnexal tissue. The survival of all these recruited tissues depends primarily upon the adequacy of the blood supply. A thorough appreciation of vascular anatomy of the facial skin is, therefore, central to the successful execution of local flaps.

The face has an extensive vascular supply arising from branches of both the internal and external carotid systems with rich collateralization and defined vascular territories. Knowledge of these vascular territories and the extensive collateralization of these vessels allow the successful design of a variety of local flaps. The vascular territories of the face and scalp have been thoroughly investigated by dye injection techniques.[1] Eleven vascular territories each supplied by a distinct vessel have been described: the transverse facial, submental, zygomatico-orbital, anterior auricular, posterior auricular, occipital, supratrochlear, frontal and parietal branches of the superficial temporal, and superior and inferior labial arteries (Figure 1). Terminal perforators arise from these vessels

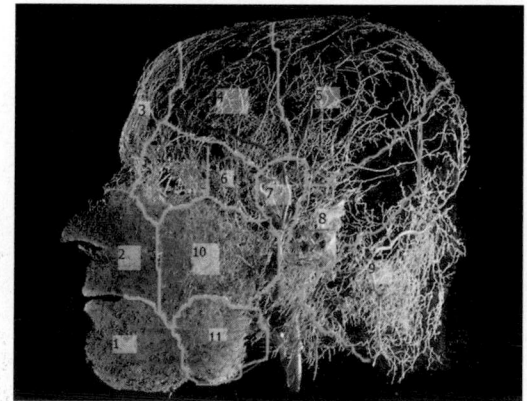

Figure 1 The vascular cutaneous territories of the face. The face is richly supplied by branches of the internal and external carotid arteries and their associated veins. Terminal vessels send perforators that form defined vascular territories: 1. inferior labial, 2. superior labial, 3. supratrochlear, 4. frontal branch of superficial temporal, 5. parietal branch of superficial temporal, 6. zygomatico-orbital, 7. anterior auricular, 8. posterior auricular, 9. occipital, 10. transverse facial, 11. and submental.

to form the subdermal plexus. The subdermal plexus resides at the junction of the deep dermis and the subcutaneous tissue. From the subdermal plexus, ascending vessels arise to form a more superficial subepidermal plexus between the papillary and reticular dermis. Angiographic studies of the head and neck have shown that the subdermal plexus exists in defined territories that tend to vary in size, pattern, and orientation among regions of the face.[2] Adjacent territories of subdermal plexuses are interconnected by reduced caliber vessels known as choke vessels. Choke vessels may dilate under certain physiologic circumstances such as when a flap is delayed allowing the inclusion of adjacent vascular territory in local flap design.

CLASSIFICATION OF LOCAL FLAPS

Local flaps of the face are commonly classified based on their vascular supply (axial vs random) or method of movement (sliding or lifting).

Classification of Flaps by their Vascular Supply

The blood supply of random flaps is primarily based on the subdermal plexus derived from fasciocutaneous, musculocutaneous, or direct cutaneous perforators. The distribution of these perforators and their associated vascular territories are well defined on the face (see Figure 1). Knowledge of these territories allows the safe design of random flaps. Examples of common random flaps are the rhomboid flap used in cheek reconstruction and the bilobe flap used in nasal reconstruction. It was long thought that the surviving length of a flap was entirely dependent upon the width of its base. Generally, a 3 to 1 ratio was felt to be optimal. This is now known to be inaccurate, but the length to width ratio should still serve as a rough guide. More important than the width of a flap is the perfusion pressure through the supplying vessels. When the perfusion pressure along the length of a flap drops below the critical closing pressure of the arterioles in the subdermal plexus, perfusion of the flap ceases. A wider random flap will only include additional subdermal arterioles that have the same perfusion pressure since they are all based on the same feeding vessel. Adding additional vessels at the same perfusion pressure, that is, widening the base of the flap, does allow for some increased collateral circulation which can be beneficial but does not affect the perfusion pressure at the distal portions of the flap. It is now recognized that the length to width ratio is only a rough guideline and varies with different flaps.

In contrast to random flaps, axial flaps receive their blood supply from named vessels which extend along the linear axis of the flap giving off perforators to form the subdermal plexus. The distal portion of axial flaps can be random. The forehead flap based on the supratrochlear vessels is an example of an axial pattern flap.

Classification of Flaps by Method of Movement

When characterized by their method of transfer, two basic local flap movements can be described: sliding or lifting. Advancement and rotation flaps slide adjacent tissue into a defect, whereas transposition and staged interpolation flaps move tissue into defects by lifting.

Flaps that Move Tissue by Sliding

Advancement Flaps. Advancement flaps are designed directly adjacent to a defect and slide in a linear vector into the primary defect. In advancement flaps, one border of the defect becomes the leading edge of the flap. Examples of advancement flaps are the V-Y advancement flaps (Figure 2A) and pedicle advancement flaps (Figure 2B).

V–Y Advancement Flaps. V–Y advancement flaps are versatile flaps based on an island subcutaneous pedicle. Movement of the V–Y flap depends on the mobility of the subcutaneous tissue. It is most suitable in regions of the face such as the cheek and melolabial (formerly known as the nasolabial) area where there is abundant subcutaneous tissue and rich vascularity (Figure 3). When designing a V–Y flap, one of the limbs of the V is placed along an anatomic boundary when possible. The incisions made through the subdermal plane are beveled outward and the surrounding skin is undermined in this plane. Deeper dissection of the subcutaneous tissue is carried out only at the distal end of the flap adjacent to the defect. Blunt dissection can be carried out lateral to the flap until the island of skin advances into the defect without tension. Variations to the classic V–Y island flap have been described in which a complementary transposition flap is added to one end of the flap to increase its length and versatility.[3]

Pedicle Advancement Flap. A single pedicled advancement flap is raised as a square or rectangle with one edge bordering the defect and two parallel incisions along the sides of the defect (see Figure 2B). The plane of flap elevation is deep to the subdermal plexus in the subcutaneous tissue. The tissue surrounding the defect is undermined to allow for secondary movement in a direction opposite to that of the stretched advancement

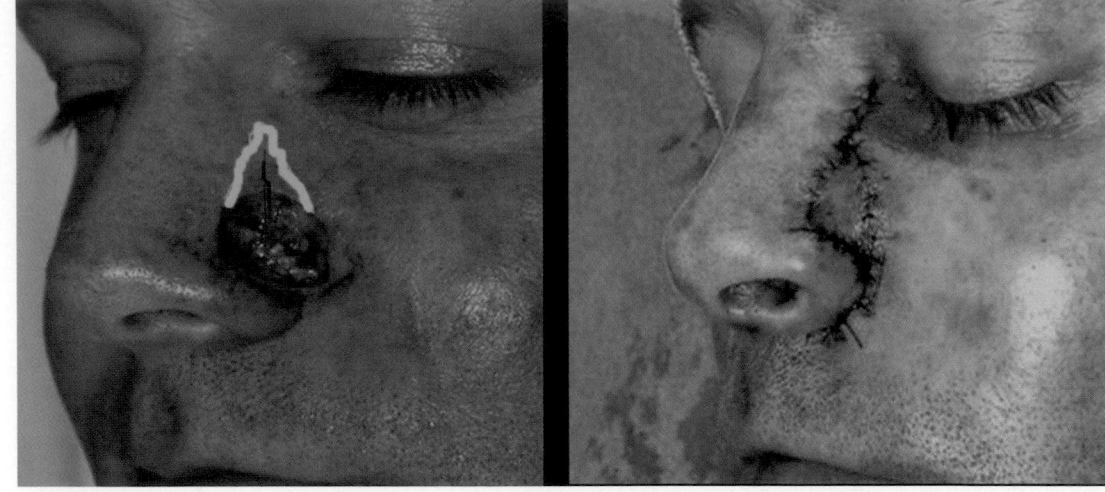

(A)

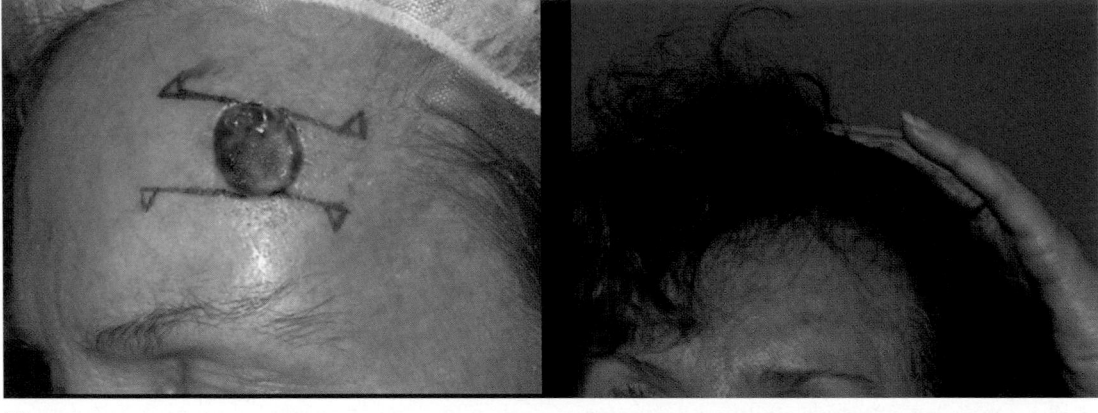

(B)

Figure 2 Advancement flaps move tissue by a sliding movement. (A) V–Y advancement flap. (B) Advancement flap with excision of Burow triangles.

flap. The pedicled advancement flap depends on the elasticity of the skin to stretch into the defect. A secondary defect primarily consisting of a wound of unequal length results. The closure of this secondary defect is facilitated by excising Burow triangles. A small Z-plasty may also be incorporated at the base of the flap to achieve greater advancement. Pedicled advancement

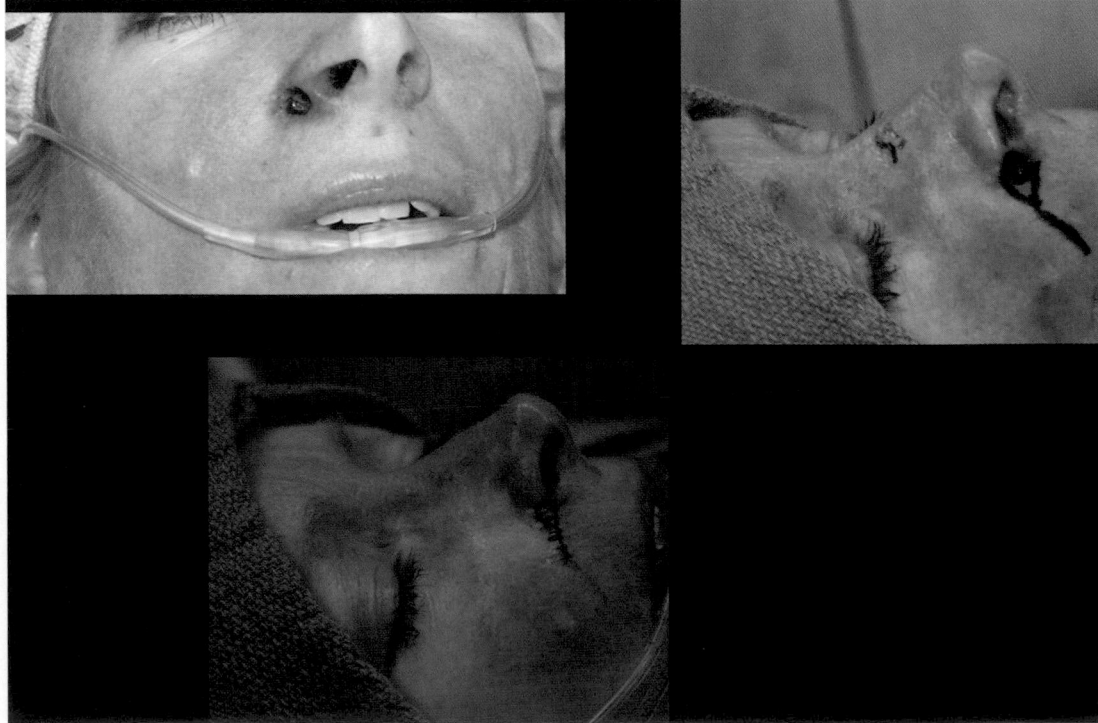

Figure 3 Repair of alar base defect with a V–Y advancement flap.

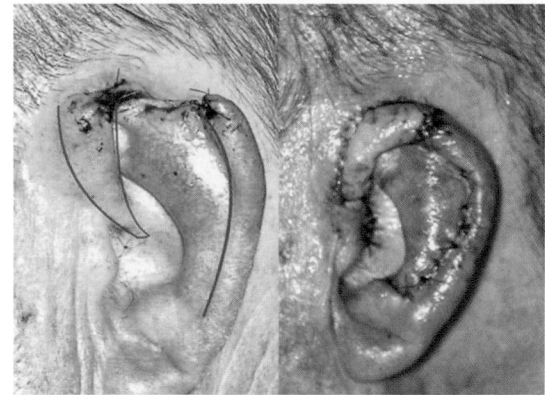

Figure 4 Repair of auricular defect with two pedicled advancement flaps. Incisions are made through the anterior helical skin and cartilage leaving the posterior auricular skin intact. A Burow triangle can be excised from the posterior auricular skin to facilitate closure of the secondary defect.

flaps are useful for reconstruction of defects of the forehead where the incisions can be placed parallel to the horizontal forehead rhytides. Two pedicled advancement flaps can be designed on opposite ends of a defect and each advanced over a shorter distance to close a defect such as helical defects on the ear (Figure 4).

Bipedicled Advancement Flaps. Advancement flaps pedicled on both ends are also useful in repairing longitudinal defects. They are designed by making two incisions that parallel the defect margin keeping the base and midsection of the flap wide. The flap is then elevated in the subcutaneous plane leaving the two ends attached (Figure 5). It can then be advanced sideways into the defect. Examples of bipedicled advancement flaps are the tubed postauricular flap for helical reconstruction and the bipedicled advancement scalp flap for hairline reconstruction.

Rotation Flaps. Rotation flaps move tissue by sliding a semicircular flap into a defect along an arc of rotation and a pivot point. They are usually random flaps and are commonly used for closing triangle defects. When the primary defect is circular, it is first converted into a triangular shape by excising a Burow triangle (Figure 6). A semicircular flap is then raised starting from the edge of the defect. The resulting secondary defect is mainly a wound of two unequal lengths. The greatest tension is along a line between the pivotal point and the most peripheral point of the flap. Closure is accomplished by distributing the extra length and tension along the arc or by including a Burow triangle or a Z-plasty adjacent to the pivot point. Rotation flaps are commonly used in closing scalp defects where tissue stretch necessary for advancement flaps is minimal. A cervicofacial rotation flap is also another common rotation

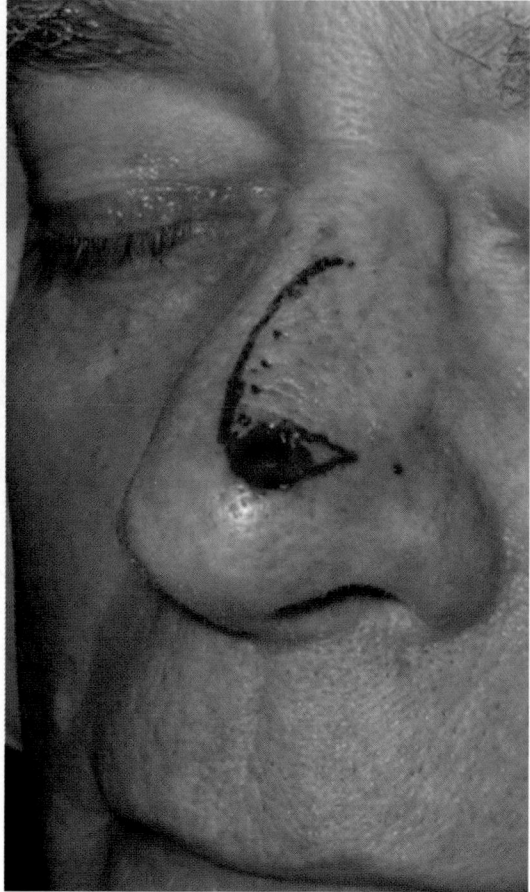

Figure 6 Rotation flap. A circular defect is first converted to a triangular defect by excising a Burow triangle. Wide undermining allows rotation of the flap into the defect.

flap useful for closing large cheek defects. A rotation flap may also be designed as a double flap (referred to as an O to Z flap) to recruit tissue

from both sides of the defect (Figure 7). These flaps are useful in locations where the arc of rotation may be less noticeable as in the lateral side of the face and scalp. Limitations of rotation flaps are tissue resistance to rotation and the noticeable dog ear that is created at the rotation pivot. The cheek and the scalp tend to rotate well while the tip of the nose, the nasal alar region and the auricle rotate poorly. In addition, any back-cut at the base of the flap to achieve lengthening or correct dog ears, compromises the blood supply to the flap. To circumvent this problem, dog ears may be left in place and allowed to settle over time. Alternatively, cuts placed at the base of the flap to improve rotation or to remove dog ears should be directed away from the pedicle and designed as a Z-plasty or Burow triangle, thus maintaining a wide pedicle base.

Flaps that Move Tissue by Lifting

Transposition Flaps. A transposition flap is usually a random flap that is incised on three sides and lifted laterally into an adjacent defect. It has a pivot point located at the base of the defect. Transposition flaps are versatile in that they can be designed with borders that are removed from the defect thus allowing flexibility in placing incisions. Examples of transposition flaps commonly used in head and neck reconstruction include the Limberg or rhomboid flap, note flap, bilobe flap, interpolation flap, and hinge flap.

Limberg (Rhomboid) Flap. The Limberg flap is an extremely versatile example of a transposition flap used in closing rhomboid-shaped defects. The flap is designed by extrapolating the short axis of the rhomboid defect onto the adjacent skin

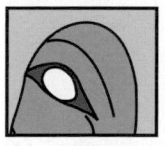 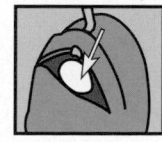 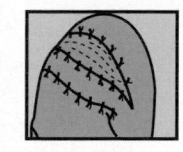

Figure 5 Diagram of a bipedicled advancement flap of the posterior aspect of the auricle.

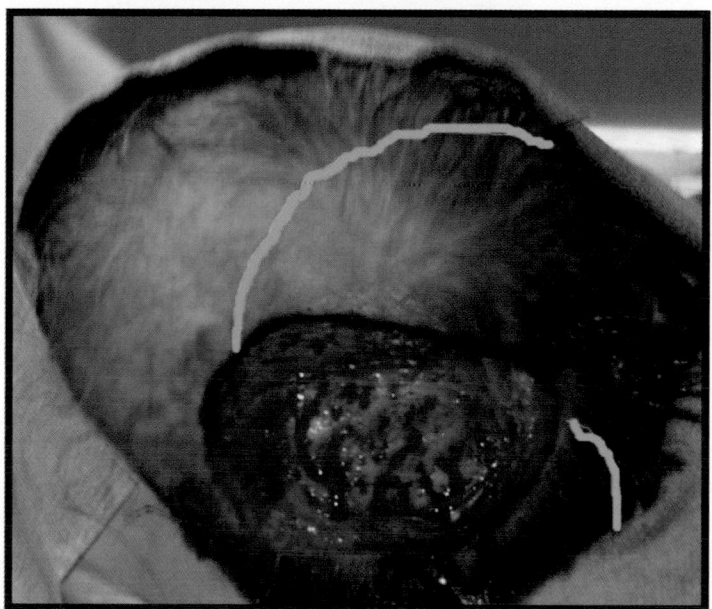 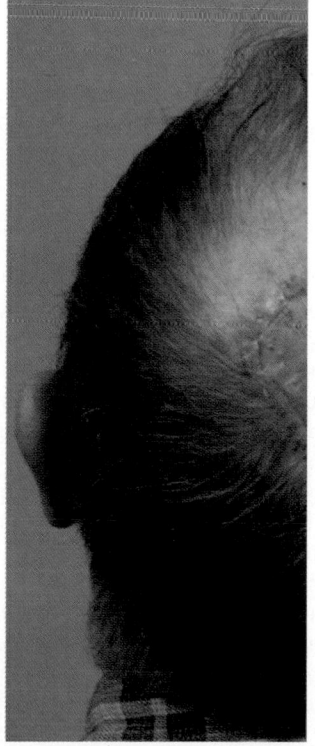

Figure 7 Double rotation flap (O to Z flap) reconstruction of a large scalp defect. The defect was initially closed with a split thickness skin graft and placement of two 100 cc tissue expanders. After tissue expansion, two broadly based rotation flaps were designed to recruit tissue from both sides of the defect.

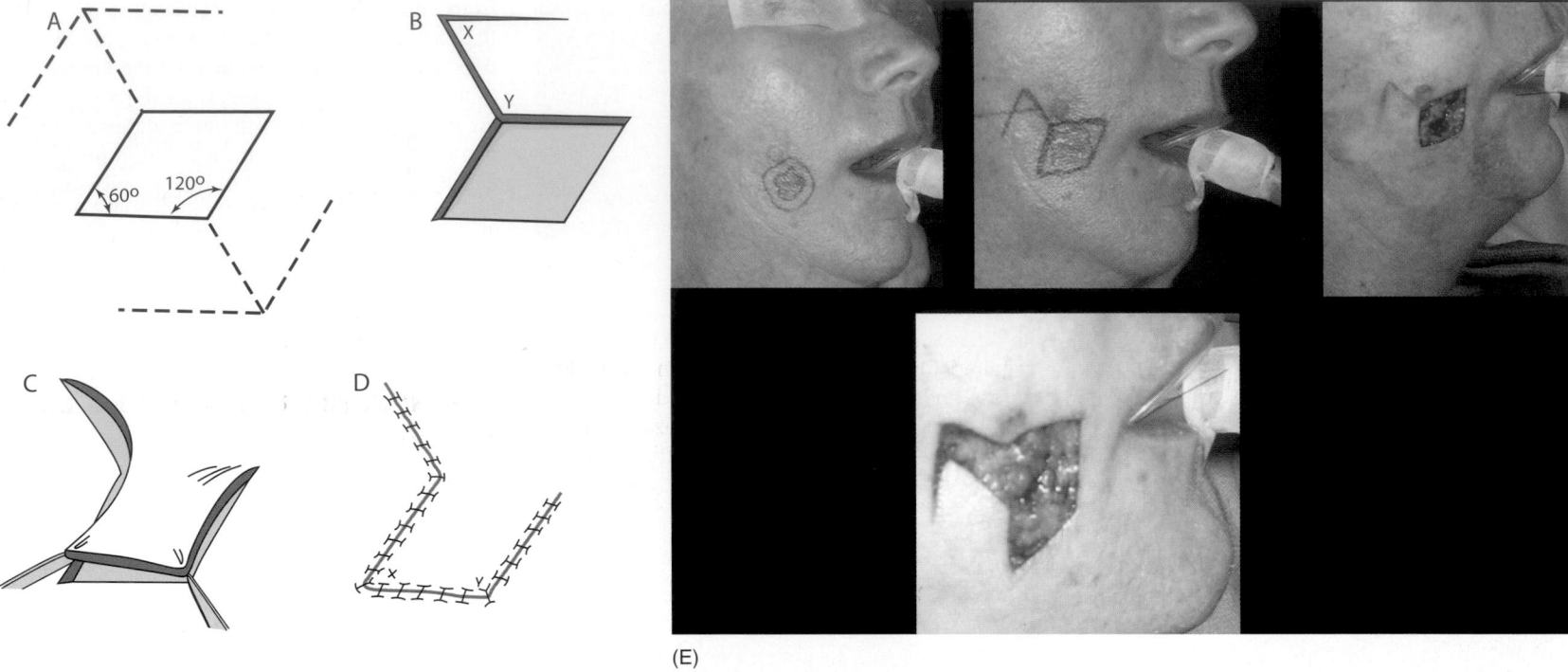

Figure 8 The classic Limberg (rhomboid) transposition flap design with 60° and 120° angles (A to E).

(Figure 8). Four options for placing the third limb of the flap can be selected and drawn parallel to the edge of the defect. Thus for a given rhomboid defect, four Limberg flaps can potentially be raised depending on where the third limb is placed. The third limb is selected to recruit the most mobile skin that allows for the best camouflage without distortion of surrounding structures. All limbs of the flap should be of equal length. The rhomboid-shaped flap is then incised and lifted into the primary defect. The resulting secondary defect is then closed primarily by undermining and advancing the surrounding tissue. The classic Limberg flap has 60 and 120° angles. For larger defects two or more Limberg flaps can be used.

One modification of the classic Limberg flap is the Dufourmentel flap (Figure 9). Like the Limberg flap, the Dufourmentel flap is also a transposition flap designed to close rhomboid defects. It differs from the Limberg flap by having angles that are not necessarily 60° and 120°. The flap is designed by extending one line from the short axis to a length equivalent to the side lengths, similar to a classic rhomboid flap, and another line is drawn by extending the side adjacent to the lower angle to a similar length. However, the incision is made along a line that bisects these two extended lines. A second incision is made along a line that is dropped from the end of the bisected line parallel to the long axis of the rhomboid defect to complete the flap. With this modification, the pedicle is wider and the leading angle more obtuse. This results in less vertical pull. Therefore, the Dufourmentel flap is useful in areas where lateral tension is acceptable but vertical pull is not.

One disadvantage of the rhomboid transposition flap is that more than half of the resulting scar does not fall within or parallel to the natural skin lines. It is therefore best suited for repair of defects of the lateral facial subunits: lateral cheek, mandible, and temple regions.

Z-Plasty. The classic Z-plasty is essentially two adjacent random triangular flaps that interchange position by being lifted into each others defect thereby lengthening and reorienting their common central limb. Z-plasties are used to lengthen tight, contracted scars or reorient tissue or scars into a more desirable location. In the classic Z-plasty, the adjacent triangles are equilateral triangles with 60° angles. Varying this angle alters the theoretical gain in scar lengthening. A 30°, 45°, and 60° Z-plasty can theoretically lengthen a scar by 25%, 50%, and 75% respectively. The actual gain in length is dependent on the elasticity of the surrounding tissues. Occasionally the best flap design requires that the two flap angles be of different sizes or angles. Other variants of the classic Z-plasty are the double opposing Z-plasty used in cleft palate and epicanthal fold repair, and the multiple running Z-plasty used in scar revisions.

Note Flap. Another common transposition flap is the "note flap," so called because the design is reminiscent of a musical eighth note. A note flap is useful for repairing small circular defects. To design the flap, a tangent is drawn from the edge of the circular defect parallel to a relaxed skin tension line for a distance of 1.5 diameters. A second line equal in length to the first is drawn at 50° to 60° to the first to create a triangular flap. The flap is then elevated with wide undermining of the tissue surrounding the defect. The note flap is then transposed into the defect. The secondary defect is closed primarily (Figure 10).

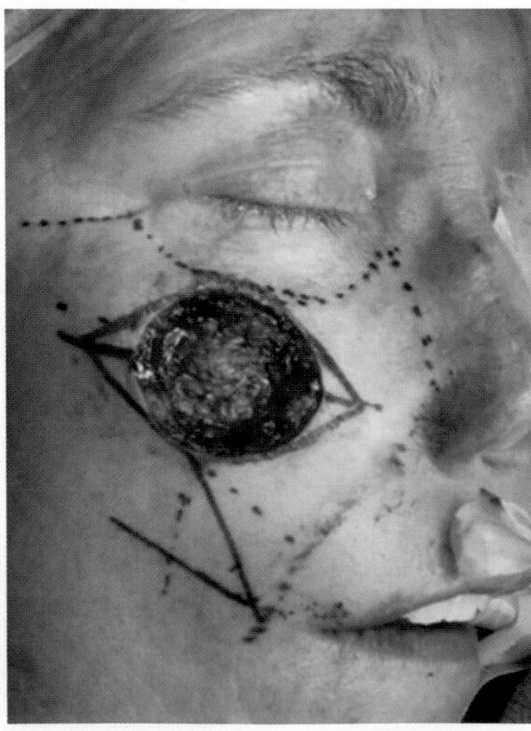

Figure 9 Dufourmentel modification of the rhomboid flap. Compared to the classic Limberg design, the pedicle base is broader and the leading angle is more obtuse.

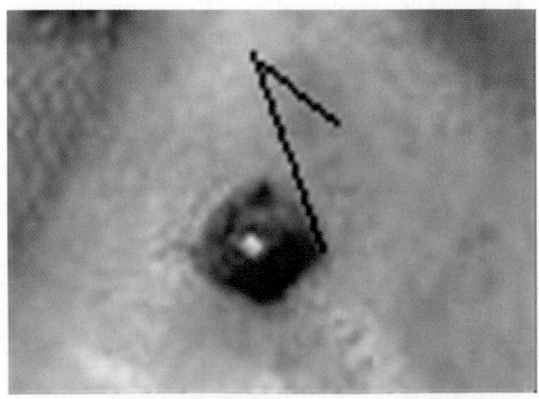

Figure 10 Note flap reconstruction of a nasal defect.

Bilobe Flap. Bilobe flaps are double transposition flaps that share a single base. They move tissue by lifting the first lobe into the primary defect. The resulting secondary defect is closed by transposing the second lobe. A tertiary defect results which is closed primarily. Invariably a standing cone deformity develops, the size of which is dependent upon the arc of rotation. In its original description, the two lobes of the bilobe flap were at 90° angles so that the final transposition was over an 180° arc. An increased arc of rotation leads to a more prominent standing cone deformity. Final arcs of transposition of 90° to 110° are more optimal with less resulting deformity. The bilobe flap is primarily used in closing defects of the lower third of the nose but can be used in other regions of the face such as the infraorbital region.[4] It has the distinct advantage of recruiting tissue farther away from the primary defect and therefore reducing the final tension of closure. A disadvantage of the flap is that the resulting scar is unable to follow skin tension lines in many cases. It is also more prone to pincushioning because the curvilinear scars and the wide bed of scar that contracts deep to the flap.

A simple way of designing a bilobe flap is to first pick out a pivot point one diameter away from the center of the defect (Figure 11). A needle is inserted at this pivot point and a suture is wrapped around a marking pen. Using this as a guide, the path of rotation is drawn out starting from the edge of the defect. The first lobe of the flap equaling the size of the defect can then be drawn adjacent to the defect. The second lobe is usually designed as a triangular flap to facilitate closure and can be made smaller than the secondary defect. The distal portion of the flap can be tailored to fill the depth of the primary defect, but the rest of the flap should be kept thick to optimize its vascularity. A Burow triangle centered on the pivot point is then excised at the base of the primary defect to facilitate transposition of the lobes.

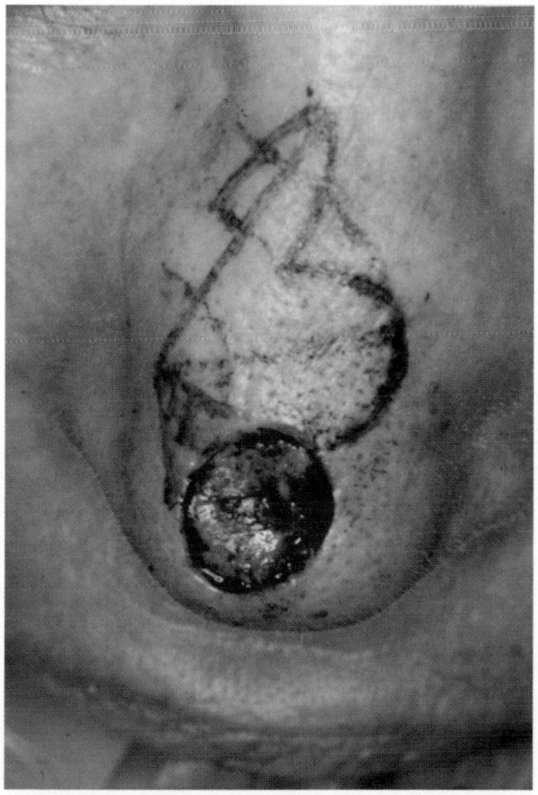

Interpolation Flaps. The interpolation flap is a random or axial flap designed and lifted into a nearby defect over or under an intervening bridge of normal skin. Common examples include the melolabial flap, the paramedian forehead flap, and Monk eyelid flap. When the flap passes over an intervening tissue, a second stage procedure is required for pedicle division. When the pedicle passes under a bridge of normal skin, a portion of the pedicle can be de-epithelialized to allow a one-stage procedure. The paramedian forehead flap is the flap of choice for reconstructing extensive nasal defects. It can also be use for reconstructing complex periorbital and medial cheek defects. A detailed discussion of the paramedian forehead flap is provided in Chapter 54, "Nasal Reconstruction."

The melolabial flap is another example of an interpolation flap that lifts tissues from the cheek and is often used in reconstructing defects of the lower part of the nose. It is often raised as a superiorly based axial pattern flap supplied by direct cutaneous perforators exiting from the angular branch of the facial artery. It is best suited for alar, nasal tip, or columellar defects. To facilitate flap mobilization, the flap can be designed as an elliptical island flap with a wide based subcutaneous pedicle. The melolabial crease is drawn on both sides to establish symmetry. Using a template of the defect, the necessary width of the flap is determined (Figure 12). The distal portion of the flap is raised in the subcutaneous plane but the base of the pedicle should be kept as a wide subcutaneous pedicle by blunt mobilization of the surrounding tissue. Closure of the secondary defect before flap insertion further improves the rotation of the flap. The melolabial incision should be closed in such a manner so as to mimic the contralateral melolabial fold, thus minimizing cheek asymmetry. Pedicle division can be performed in 3 to 4 weeks depending on individual patient factors.

Hinge Flap. The hinge or turn-in flap is a random flap that moves tissue by lifting tissue pivoted along the edge of a defect to fill the deep aspect of the defect. It is commonly used to provide closure of the inner layer of a full-thickness nasal or cheek defect. It is also useful in repairing full thickness central auricular defects. It is used in conjunction with a second flap that provides the external coverage (Figure 13).

PLANNING THE REPAIR OF A FACIAL DEFECT

Optimal repair of facial defects with local flaps requires thoughtful planning. The defect should be analyzed in the context of facial esthetics, function, and adjacent tissue characteristics. A systematic, rather than a "cookbook" approach fosters creativity and a consistently superior outcome. First, it is important to draw the esthetic units and define the defect size, depth, and location. The following questions and considerations should be contemplated in the planning process: How much of a facial subunit is involved and does it cross subunit boundaries? Next, consider potential donor sites by looking within the involved subunit as well as surrounding subunits. Where is tissue redundant? Assess tissue movement by sliding or pinching the adjacent tissue. Consider the secondary consequences of tissue movement from each of these potential donor sites. Where will the maximum tension vector be distributed and will it cause any distortion of free margins? Can incisions be placed along anatomic boundaries and in the direction of relaxed skin tension lines? Consider the vascularity of the surrounding tissue. Are there previous scars that may compromise blood supply to the flap? Are there any patient factors such as smoking, diabetes, previous radiation, or small vessel disease

Figure 11 Design of a bilobe flap in nasal reconstruction.

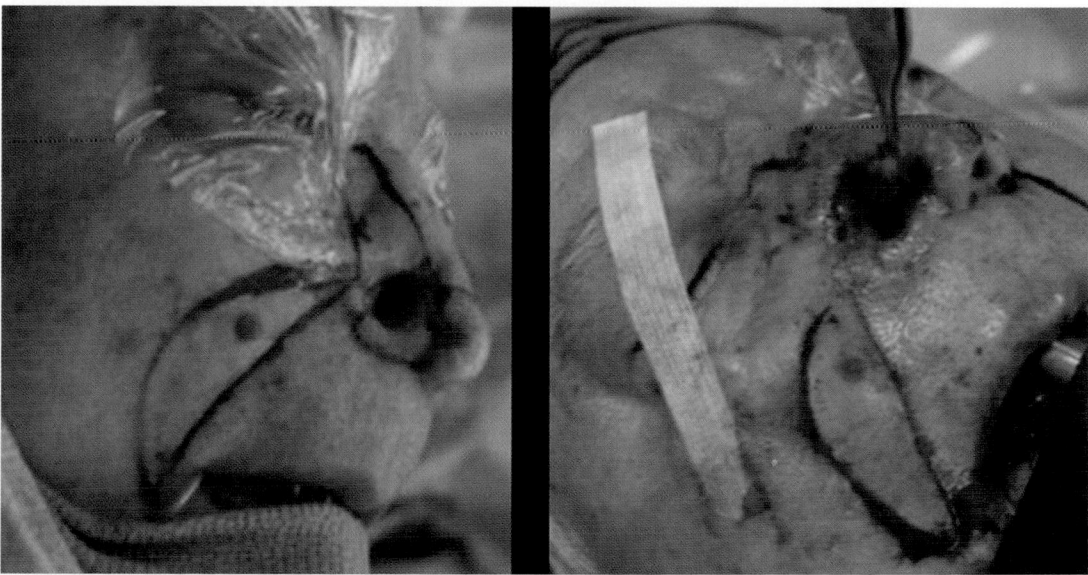

Figure 12 The melolabial flap can be designed as an island flap with an elliptical skin incision. This facilitates mobilization of the flap.

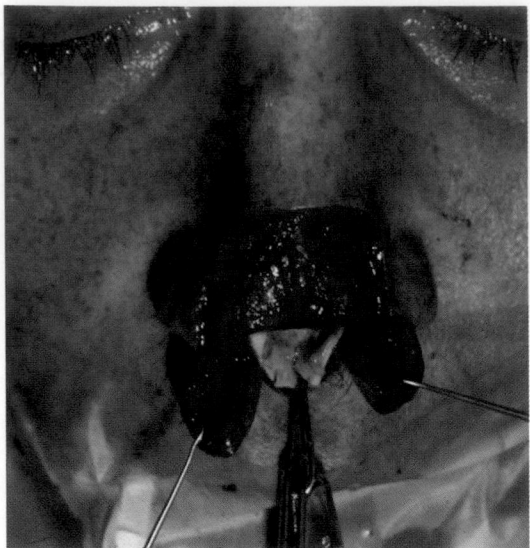

Figure 13 The hinge or turn-in flap provides lining for a full-thickness nasal tip defect.

that may be influence the vascularity of a chosen flap? Finally, consider patient factors such as esthetic expectations, ability to tolerate multistaged procedures, natural history of the underlying problem that resulted in the defect and impact on the patient's quality of life.

Pretransfer Flap Manipulation

With further understanding of flap physiology, various techniques have been used to manipulate local flaps prior to their transfer to improve their survival, extent, or structure. These techniques include flap delay, tissue expansion, and flap prelamination.

Flap Delay. Surgical delay of flaps before transfer has long been known to improve the vascularity and survival of cutaneous flaps. The phenomenon of flap delay first involves full-thickness incisions around portions of the flap to raise a bipedicled flap and later converting it to a singled pedicled flap after a "delay" period before transfer. The delay process improves the flap microcirculation and maximizes flap survival. Dhar and Taylor performed various animal studies with angiographic techniques and identified a consistent pattern of arterial vasodilatation after flap delay.[5] Further investigation revealed that this vasodilation is most obvious at the level of choke vessels of adjacent angiosomes and that the process continues for approximately 7 days.[5,6] The benefits of flap delay can be seen as early as 48 to 72 hours with maximal effect noted on the seventh day.[5] The delay of flaps may increase potential flap length up to 100%.[7] Several factors are believed to underlie the improved survival of delayed flaps. These include: a change in the sympathetic tone as a result of local sympathectomy, dilatation of choke vessels bridging adjacent vascular territories, ischemic conditioning of the flap by metabolic alteration, and reorientation of vessels in the flap as well as new vessel formation.

Today, surgical delay remains a reliable method for maximizing flap survival and has evolved to include tissue expansion and division

of large vessels supplying musculocutaneous territories. Flap delay should be considered in high-risk situations such as in smokers and in patients with postradiation or traumatized tissue. The delay of forehead flaps in nasal reconstruction is common in facial reconstruction and helps in extending the survival and reach of the flap for nasal tip and columellar repair.

Although surgery remains the first choice for delaying a flap, many have searched for alternative methods to create the same effect with less morbidity and reduced cost. The use of the potassium–titanyl–phosphate (KTP), pulsed-dye, and carbon dioxide lasers produces the effects of flap delay in animal studies.[8–10] The explanation forwarded for the delay effects of lasers are the inflammatory changes induced by laser injury as well as the partial vessel blockage that targets hemoglobin. Potential applications of laser flap delay include pretreatment of planned skin flaps in high-risk patients before surgery, for example, pretreatment of the preauricular skin with the pulse dye laser 1 or 2 weeks before large cervicofacial rotational flaps in smokers. Other potential uses include paramedian forehead flaps and Juri flaps in high-risk patients. Potentially, pretreatment with these lasers can be done in the office setting with minimal discomfort, bleeding, and cost. The clinical benefit of lasers as a delay tool awaits confirmation in clinical studies.

Tissue Expansion. The technique of tissue expansion has found a wide range of application in head and neck reconstruction. It provides local tissue of appropriate thickness, texture, color, and sensibility at a nominal donor-site cost. Expansion is achieved by inserting a silicone expander and gradually filling it with saline over time, often waiting 3 to 5 days between injections. The base of the expander selected should be at least 2 to 2.5 times the size of the defect. The incision made to insert the tissue expander should be placed with thoughtful consideration of the final flap design. When used in the neck, scalp, or forehead, massive amounts of expanded skin can be made available for reconstructing large defects.

Tissue expanders are most effective when there is a solid bony support. Hence the scalp and forehead are ideal sites for tissue expansion. In children, expansion of neck and cheek skin may allow single staged resurfacing of burn injuries and extensive hairy nevi. Stretching skin prior to transfer has some of the physiologic benefits of flap delay as there is increased flap vascularity. In expanded skin, angiogenesis is stimulated, and epidermal proliferation results in a thicker epidermis. Dermal thickness initially decreases but returns to normal. In hair bearing areas, new hair follicles do not arise but rather become separated. Fat cells do not tolerate prolonged expansion well. These cells flatten, lose their fat content and may become replaced with fibrous tissue. Nerves gradually lengthen in response to expansion. Invariably, expanded tissue generates a dense fibrous capsule around the implant. While the capsule improves the flap vascularity,

it also contributes to its contracture and makes it unsuitable for reconstruction in regions where thin skin is desirable. The molecular mechanisms by which the mechanical strain of tissue expansion affects skin biology remains unclear, but it appears to involve modulation of various cellular mechanisms including the cytoskeleton system, extracellular matrix, enzyme activity, second messengers, and ion channels. Mechanical stimulation is capable of activating a series of signal transduction pathways resulting in the production of new skin.[11]

Flap Prelamination. The concept of flap prelamination has recently been introduced into the reconstructive literature. This involves the insertion of other tissues such as cartilage in a preplanned portion of a flap to allow structural integration before the final flap transfer. Prelaminated local flaps have been used in nasal reconstruction in combination with a paramedian forehead flap where lining, structural support, and outer skin coverage is essential.[12]

CASE ILLUSTRATIONS: LOCAL FLAP RECONSTRUCTION BY FACIAL REGIONS

Defects of the Forehead-Brow-Temple

The forehead–brow–temple area is a particularly challenging area for reconstruction. The forehead skin is thick and lies in a broad convex plane that extends from the hairline superiorly to the brows inferiorly. It extends laterally to the temples and has skin of varying thickness. The eyebrow, scalp hairline, and lateral canthus comprise the esthetic boundaries of the temple and limit the available tissue for repair of defects. The goal of forehead reconstruction is to recreate the esthetic boundaries of the forehead and to regain symmetry with the contralateral side. Several cases are presented for illustration of local flaps used in this area.

Case 1. A 54-year-old male presented with two separate defects following Mohs excision of a basal cell carcinoma (Figure 14). The defects extended into the subcutaneous tissue. The superior defect is close to the hairline while the inferior defect involves the eyebrow. The patient preoperatively had a baseline asymmetric brow with the right side lower than the left. While various options exist for closing the defects, a simple linear closure in the direction of the forehead rhytides was chosen. The forehead skin was widely undermined. The defects were converted into an ellipse and closed primarily. Primary closure within relaxed skin tension lines by advancing surrounding skin often gives the best result and should always be considered before more complex local flaps. In this case, the expected temporary asymmetry of the eyebrow was discussed with the patient. Botulinum toxin was also injected for chemoimmobilization to improve the final scar result.

Case 2. A middle aged female presented with a forehead defect following Mohs excision of a basal cell carcinoma (Figure 2B). The defect

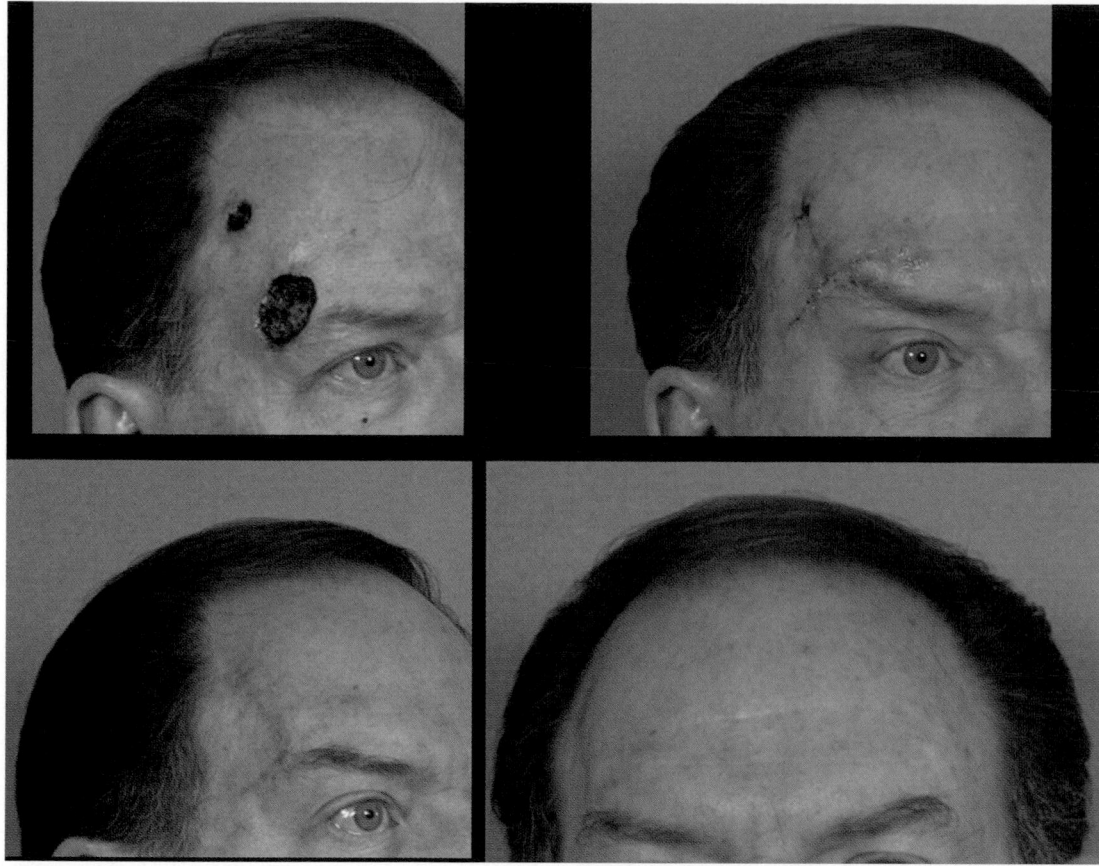

Figure 14 Primary closure reconstruction of two separate forehead defects following Mohs excision of basal cell carcinoma.

extends down to the frontalis muscle. She has dynamic forehead rhytides and a moderate degree of skin laxity. The defect was reconstructed with two pedicled advancement flaps. Small Burow triangles were included at the base of the flaps to facilitate tissue advancement. Incisions parallel to the relaxed skin tension lines were used to minimize visible scars.

Case 3. A 56-year-old male presented with a large defect of the temple following wide local excision of a fibrosarcoma (Figure 15). The defect extended down to the underlying temporalis muscle with partial excision of the muscle. The temporal branch of the facial nerve was excised. Multiple subunits were involved, including the cheek, temple, forehead, and lateral brow. The facial subunits were drawn. A template was taken from the uninvolved side and transposed to the involved side to help define the hairline as well as the extent of the various subunits involved. Reconstruction of the defect was accomplished with a combination of a large medially based cervicofacial rotational flap, rhomboid flap, and full thickness skin graft. In the future, the skin graft portion can be secondarily removed by serial excision or following scalp expansion.

Cheek Defects

The cheek unit of the face is defined laterally by the preauricular sulcus, superiorly by the lower lid-cheek boundary extending laterally across the zygomatic arch, medially by the nasofacial and melolabial groove, and inferiorly by the jaw line. The lateral cheek contour is relatively flat

while the medial cheek is soft and rounded. In primary gaze, the medial cheek is more visible hence distortions in this region are more apparent than in the lateral cheek. The reconstructive goals for cheek defects are uniform color and texture matching, preservation or restoration of the temporal hair tuft, and prevention of lower lid retraction. Unlike defects of the central part of the face, the rule of resurfacing an entire subunit takes on a lesser importance.

Cheek defects may be divided into lateral and medial defects. The site of defect influences the choice of flap, pedicle base, and direction of tissue movement. Small to medium defects located in the medial or lateral cheek may be closed in the direction of relaxed skin tension lines by wide undermining and bidirectional advancement of surrounding tissue. When possible, deep tension sutures should be placed around stable structures such as the nasal spine, nasal periosteum, or periorbital periosteum to minimize distortion of the alar or eyelid margins. Standing cone deformities are excised with incisions placed in natural rhytides.

Larger medial cheek defects may be closed with laterally based cervicofacial rotation advancement flaps that recruit skin from the inferior face, jowl, and neck. Incisions for this flap extend from the defect along the nasofacial groove, the alar crease, and the melolabial groove. This incision can be extended as needed across the mandible in which case the addition of a Z-plasty is helpful. If the medial cheek defect extends onto the nose or eyelid, these latter subunits should be reconstructed with a separate flap or graft. This flap is vascularized by branches from the superficial temporal artery and branches of the occipital artery in the neck. Flap elevation may include platysma or superficial musculoaponeurotic system to improve vascularity, especially in high-risk patients.

Larger lateral cheek defects may be closed with medially based cervicofacial rotation-advancement flaps. The flap is vascularized by branches of the facial and submental arteries. The incision extends from the edge of the defect, around or through the temporal hair tuft, inferiorly along the preauricular sulcus and then around the earlobe. In the temporal region, the incision is placed along the temporal hair tuft to prevent movement of the hair tuft. Beyond the earlobe, the extension and design of the incision depends on the amount of skin needed.

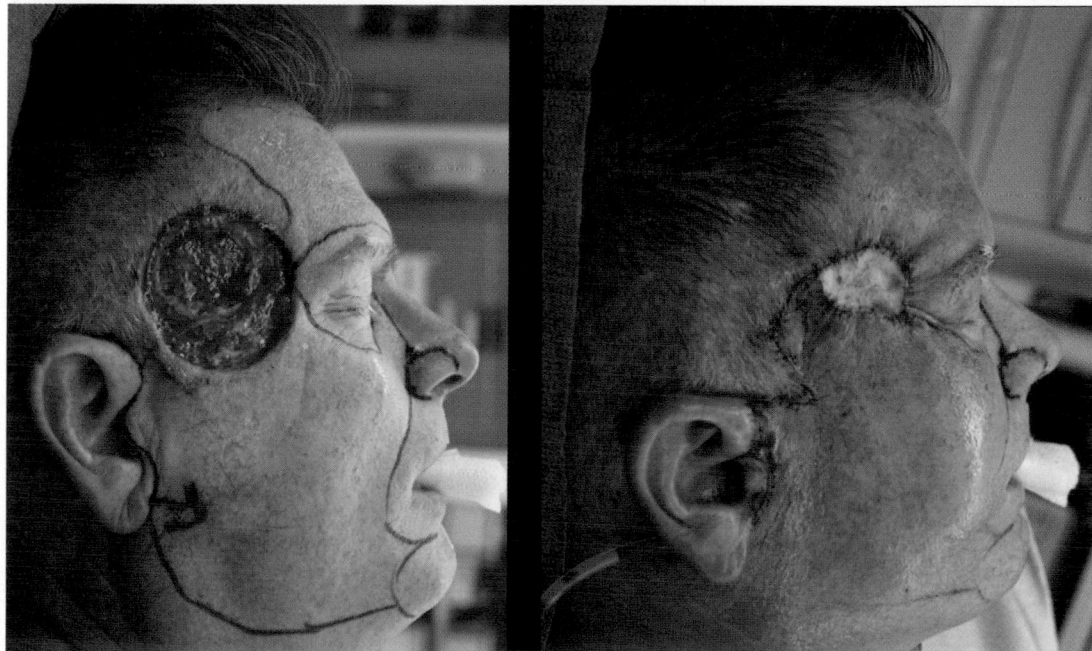

Figure 15 Large temple defect following wide local excision of a fibrosarcoma. Closure was accomplished with the combination of a cervicofacial rotation flap, rhomboid flap and full thickness skin graft.

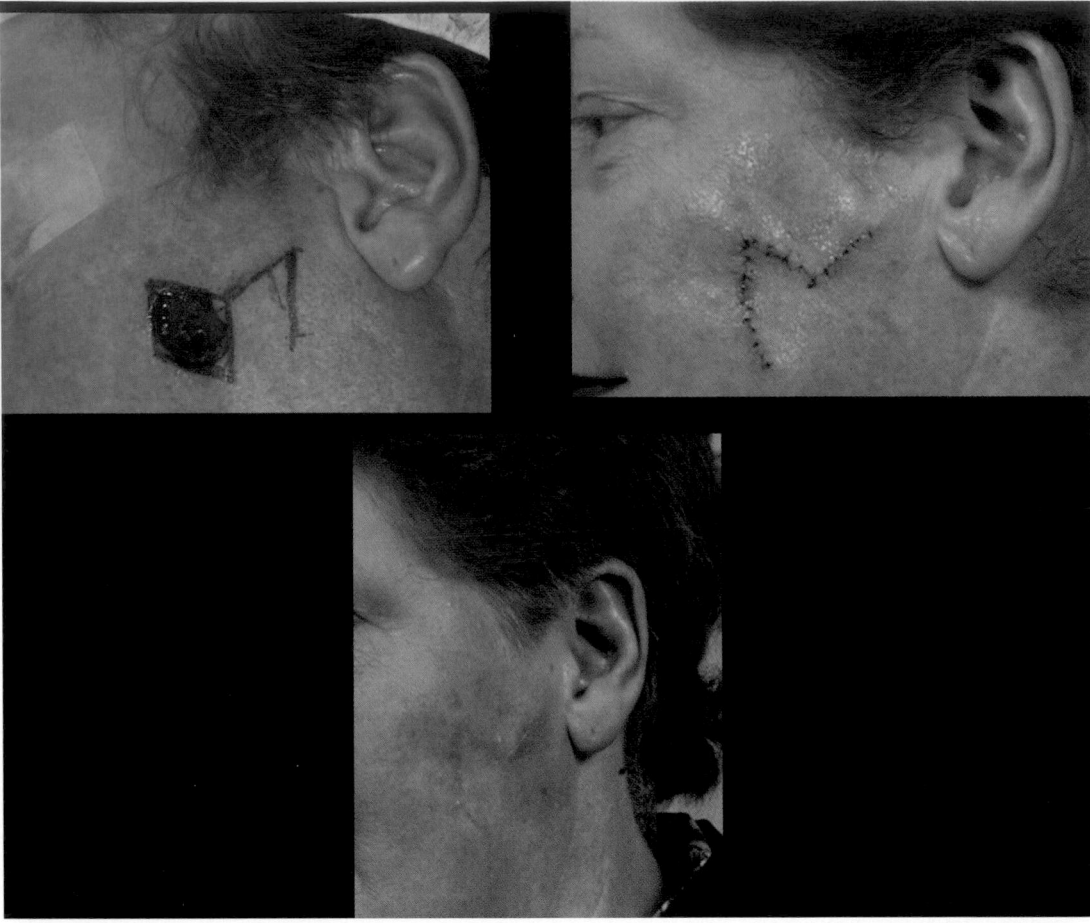

Figure 16 Reconstruction of a defect of the lateral aspect of the cheek with a rhomboid flap. The rhomboid flap on a lateral facial defect produces a less noticeable scar.

Case 4. A 47-year-old female presented with a lateral cheek defect following Mohs excision of basal cell carcinoma (Figure 16). The cheek defect was repaired with a classic rhomboid transposition flap. One disadvantage of the rhomboid flap is that the incisions do not follow relaxed skin tension lines. This drawback is better tolerated in the lateral facial subunits such as the lateral cheek and temple.

Case 5. A 49-year-old female presented with an intermediate size cheek defect following Mohs excision of a basal cell carcinoma (Figure 17). The defect is mainly confined to the lateral cheek subunit but extends slightly into the temple. The defect was reconstructed with a medially based cervicofacial rotation flap. In females incisions are placed in the preauricular skin crease and extended into the infralobular crease. In males, a similar incision may distort the preauricular hair tuft. Modifications should, therefore, be made in males to preserve the nonhair bearing skin in the pretragal region.

Scalp Reconstruction

Reconstruction of small and intermediate size defects of the scalp can be more challenging than similar size defects in other parts of the head and neck. This is mainly due to the inelasticity of the scalp. The primary goal of scalp reconstruction following tumor ablation is to provide soft tissue coverage of the skull in time to start radiation therapy when indicated. Some small and intermediate size defects are amenable to primary closure facilitated by external expansion or rapid intraoperative expansion. In the presence of periosteum, skin grafts can be placed. When the periosteum is absent, one can rotate a pericranial flap to provide bone coverage and then place a skin graft. Alternatively, the outer cortex of the exposed calvaria can be drilled down to bleeding bone which can adequately support split thickness skin grafts. Meticulous wound care can also allow healing by secondary intention. The application of vacuum assisted wound healing devices has been useful in speeding up the process of generating granulation tissue. When designing local flaps for scalp defects, the base and arc of rotation should be kept wide relative to the defect because of the inelasticity of the scalp. The scalp is an ideal region to consider tissue expansion. A principal advantage of tissue expansion of the scalp is the movement of hair-bearing skin into the defect. The primary disadvantage is the prolonged period involved in the expansion process. Animal studies have shown that the expansion process can be accelerated by the topical application of papaverine cream, but its clinical utility is yet to be proven.[13]

Case 6. A large scalp defect is reconstructed with a double rotation (O to Z) flap (see Figure 7). The defect was initially minimized with deep tension sutures, skin grafting, and tissue expansion. Tissue expansion preceded this double rotation flap closure (Figure 7).

Complex Defects Involving Multiple Subunits

Reconstruction of complex defects involving multiple facial subunits can be challenging. These may require an integrated technique that

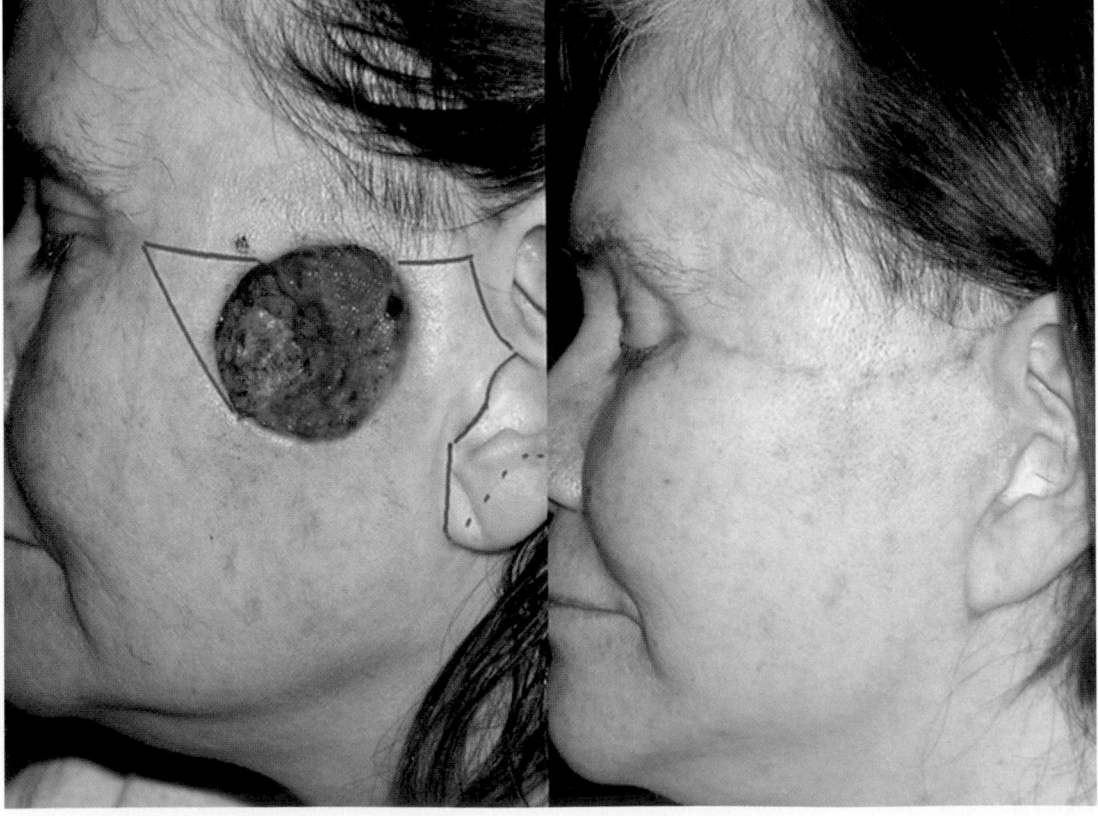

Figure 17 Medially based cervicofacial rotation flap.

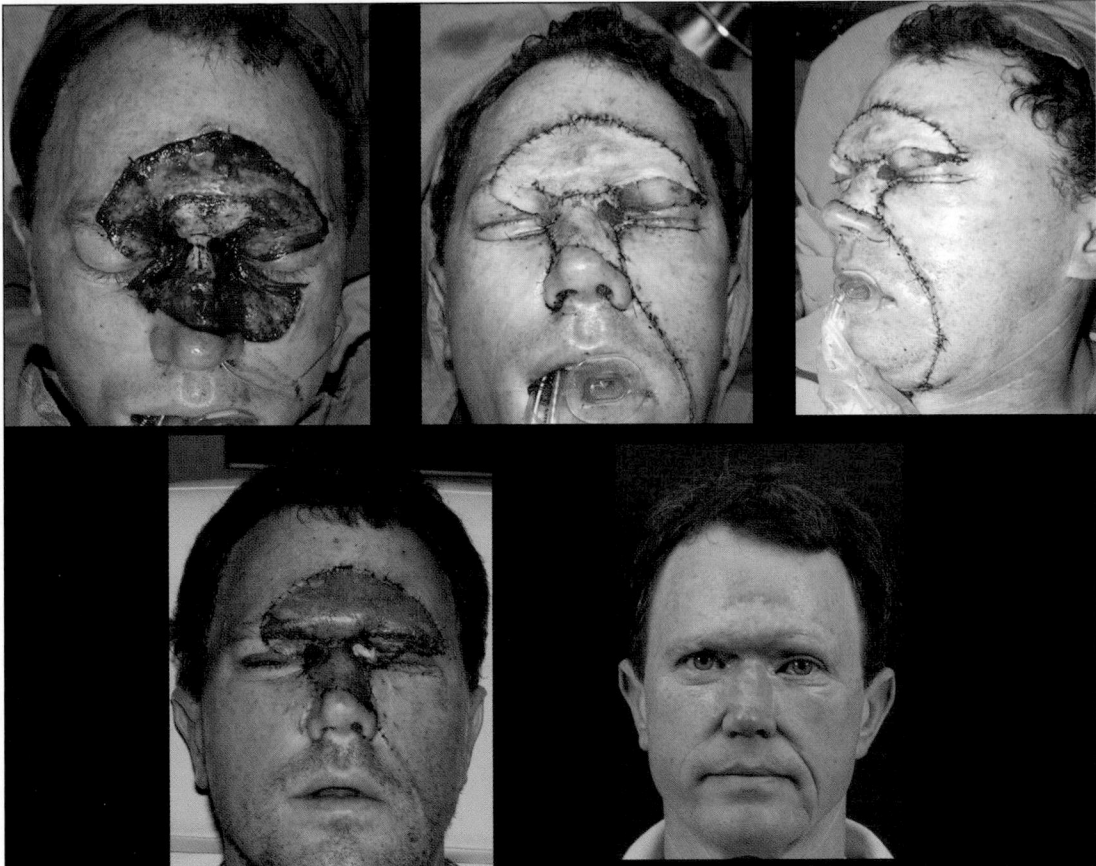

Figure 18 Reconstruction of a complex facial defect involving the forehead, nasal, eyelid, and cheek subunits. Closure was accomplished with a combination of split thickness skin grafting to the forehead and nose, full thickness skin grafting to the eyelids and cervicofacial rotation flap and z-plasty for the cheek defect.

employs a combination of local flaps and grafts to restore the esthetic contours, highlights, and shadows of the face. Frequently, normal tissue must be removed to allow placement of incisions at the junction of facial subunits. Conceptualizing the complex defect as a combination of smaller subunit defects helps to simplify an otherwise intimidating defect. The illustrative case below underscores this approach.

Case 7. This case is an example of a reconstruction of a complex defect involving multiple subunits following the excision of a malignant melanoma (Figure 18). In this patient, the forehead, nasal, eyelid, and cheek subunits are extensively involved. The forehead and nasal defects were full thickness down to bone with loss of periosteum. A retrograde elevation of the scalp was performed and a bipedicled pericranial flap was advanced to cover the bare bone. This allowed placement of a split thickness skin graft. The eyelid defects were then closed with skin grafts harvested from the postauricular region. A laterally based cervicofacial flap was rotated to close the medial cheek defect. Note that the incision for the cervicofacial flap was placed in the melolabial

crease and extended onto the mandibular margin. The portion of the incision overlying the mandible was broken up with a Z-plasty to minimize potential scar contracture and to align the incisions along skin tension lines.

ADJUVANT TREATMENT

Dermabrasion

To improve camouflage of scars resulting from local flaps, scar dermabrasion can be carried out as early as 6 weeks following flap reconstruction. Scar dermabrasion can often be done under local anesthesia on an outpatient basis.

Botulinum Toxin

An important factor determining the final cosmetic appearance of cutaneous scars is tension acting along wound edges during healing. Recently, the principle of chemoimmobilization to reduce wound tension and improve scar appearance was investigated in primates. Injection of botulinum toxin into the musculature underlying cutaneous

wounds resulted in significantly better cosmetic appearance of the wounds when compared to controls.[14] The beneficial role of botulinum toxin in wound healing has been confirmed in clinical studies and may be considered as an adjuvant treatment in local flap closure especially of the forehead.[15]

SUMMARY

Local flaps remain an effective method of reconstructing simple, intermediate, and complex defects of the head and neck. A fundamental understanding of the vascular territories of the face and the dynamics of soft tissue movement is necessary for the optimal selection and design of local flaps. Complex defects can be fragmented into smaller defects and reconstructed based on the principle of facial subunits. Flap prefabrication, tissue expansion and flap delay are important techniques that may be employed to expand the composition, vascularity, and survival of local flaps.

REFERENCES

1. Whetzel TP, Mathes SJ. Arterial anatomy of the face: An analysis of vascular territories and perforating cutaneous vessels. Plast Reconstr Surg 1992;84:591–605.
2. Chang H. Arterial anatomy of subdermal plexus of the face. Keio J Med 2001;50:31–4.
3. Pribaz JJ, Chester CH, Barrall DT. The extended V-Y advancement flap. Plast Reconstr Surg 1992;90:275–80.
4. Yenidunya MO, Demirseren ME, Ceran C. Bilobe flap reconstruction of infraorbital skin defects. Plast Reconstr Surg 2007;119:145–50.
5. Dhar SC, Taylor IG. The delay phenomenon: The story unfolds. Plast Reconstr Surg 1999;104:2079–91.
6. Morris SF, Taylor GI. The time sequence of the delay phenomenon: When is a surgical delay effective? An experimental study. Plast Reconstr Surg 1995;95:526–33.
7. Lopez JLA, Nieto CS, Garcia PB, Ortega LMR. Evaluation of angiogenesis in delayed skin flaps using monoclonal antibody for vascular endothelium. Br J Plast Surg 1995;48:479–86.
8. Aslan G, Karacal N, Gorgu M, Erdogan B. Nonsurgical delay of cutaneous flaps using the flash lamp pumped pulsed dye laser. Ann Plast Surg 2000;45:277–81.
9. Odland RM, Rice RD, Jr. Comparison of tunable dye and KTP lasers in nonsurgical delay of cutaneous flaps. Otolaryngol Head Neck Surg 1995;113:92–8.
10. Reichner DR, Scholz T, Vanderkam VM, et al. Laser flap delay: Comparison of Erbium:YAG and CO2 lasers. Am Surg 2003;69:69–72.
11. Takei T, Mills Ira, Arai K, Sumpio E. Molecular basis for tissue expansion: Clinical implications for the surgeon. Plast Reconstr Surg 1998;102:247–58.
12. Pribaz JJ, Fine N, Orgill DP. Flap prefabrication in the head and neck: A 10-year experience. Plast Reconstr Surg 1999;103:808–20.
13. Tang Y, Luan J, Zhang X. Accelerating tissue expansion by application of topical papaverine cream. Plast Reconstr Surg 2004;114:1166–9.
14. Gassner HG, Sherris DA, Otley CC. Treatment of facial wounds with botulinum toxin A improves cosmetic outcome in primates. Plast Reconstr Surg 2000;105:1948–54.
15. Gassner HG, Brissett A, Otley C, et al. Botulinum toxin to improve facial wound healing: A prospective, blinded, placebo controlled study. Mayo Clin Proc 2006;81:1023–8.

59

Regional Flaps and Free Tissue Transfer

Mark K. Wax, MD
Shri Nadig, MD

The majority of neoplasms involving the head and neck are easily treated by local resection and reconstruction. Cosmetic and functional outcomes have proven to be excellent whether this reconstruction involves letting the tissues granulate or the transfer of local regional flaps utilizing skin from the surrounding face or neck. Regional flaps and free tissue transfer are most often used in reconstruction of defects following ablation for neoplasms of the upper aerodigestive tract. They are occasionally used for congenital and traumatic defects. This chapter reviews the commonly used flaps in head and neck reconstruction with an emphasis on their indications in particular circumstances. Local and regional flaps for nasal reconstruction are discussed in Chapter 54, "Nasal Reconstruction."

Patients with head and neck cancers often have had multiple treatment modalities over a prolonged period of time. They present unique reconstructive problems. Oftentimes because of the previous resections with tissue rearrangement, a large composite defect is left (Figure 1). The area previously treated with radiation as well as a number of local tissue transfers is not able to support local tissue reconstruction with standard flap techniques. Adding to this reconstructive problem is the fact that resection of recurrent neoplasms involves more than single tissue subunits. The orbital contents, maxilla, mandible, auricle, nose, and lateral portion of the temporal bone often require resection. This problem is particularly prominent in primary neoplasms of the upper aerodigestive tract. The reconstruction after large primary and secondary resections can be challenging and requires composite tissue from a distant site.

TYPES OF FLAPS

Modern head and neck reconstruction relies heavily on the use of tissue flaps fed by a distinct vascular supply (pedicle). These flaps may consist of

1. skin and subcutaneous tissue;
2. skin, subcutaneous tissue, and bone;
3. bone alone; and
4. muscle and skin.

Flaps may be further subdivided into pedicled flaps and free tissue transfer flaps:

1. A pedicled flap consists of tissue with a dominant artery that can be transposed into the area of the defect.
2. A free tissue transfer flap is completely removed from its anatomic location, including division of its dominant vascular pedicle and is inset into the recipient location. Flap perfusion is reestablished by creation of vascular anastamosis from the flap pedicle to nearby native vessels with microsurgical techniques.

PEDICLED MYOCUTANEOUS FLAPS

Myocutaneous (musculocutaneous) flaps are composite flaps that include skin, subcutaneous fat, fascia, and muscle. The blood supply to this type of flap is based on a single dominant arterial trunk that provides adequate perfusion through an arborizing arterial network to a large volume of muscle, despite ligation of adjacent contributing vascular pedicles. Myocutaneous flaps are utilized in the reconstruction of large defects that require restoration of a cutaneous or mucosal surface and bulk to fill a voluminous defect following resection of the neoplasm. Examples in which a myocutaneous flap would be considered an option for reconstruction include large defects of the scalp, oropharynx, and skull base (these defects may include portions of the facial skeleton, paranasal sinuses, and palate).

Pectoralis Major Myocutaneous Flap

The pectoralis major myocutaneous (PMMC) flap has been one of the most versatile flaps for head and neck reconstruction. Its introduction in the 1970s revolutionized the care of these patients by allowing rapid healing and rehabilitation. In the 1970s and 1980s, it was the workhorse flap for regional reconstruction. The introduction of free tissue transfer with the ability to reconstruct composite tissue has relegated the PMMC flap to a secondary role. The four primary indications for this flap are protection of threatened great vessels or free flap vascular pedicles with wound dehiscence due to fistula or infection, prevention of potential wound breakdown in anticipation of compromised healing, coverage of small pharyngeal defects, and protection of the mandible following debridement for osteoradionecrosis.

The pectoralis major is a thick, triangular muscle that forms the anterior wall of the axilla. In the female, it is covered by the breast that is attached to the pectoral fascia. It originates as two heads. The clavicular head from the medial half of the clavicle inserts into the lateral lip of the intertubercular groove of the humerus, deltoid tuberosity, and deep fascia of the arm. The larger sternocostal head originates from the manubrium and body of the sternum, costal cartilages of upper five or six ribs, body of the sixth rib, and aponeurosis of the abdominal external oblique muscle, and it inserts as a bilaminar tendon deep to the insertion of the clavicular head's fibers. The large pectoral branch of the thoracoacromial artery is the axial vessel upon which the pectoralis major myocutaneous flap is based. The thoracoacromial artery arises from the second part of the axillary artery just behind the medial border of the pectoralis minor muscle. It runs anteriorly around the upper border of the pectoralis minor muscle, pierces the costocoracoid membrane, and divides into four branches: acromial, clavicular, deltoid, and pectoral. The deltoid branch accompanies the cephalic vein in the deltopectoral groove. The largest branch, the pectoral, runs inferomedially along the posterior surface of the pectoralis major muscle within the thin fatty layer between it and the pectoralis minor. There is a natural surgical plane deep to this vessel which allows blunt dissection to separate it and the overlying pectoralis major muscle from the underlying pectoralis minor muscle.

A perforator, branching from the pectoral branch immediately after its branching from the thoracoacromial trunk approximately 2 cm medial

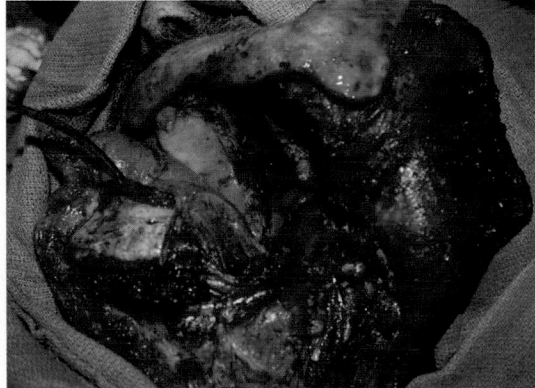

Figure 1 Photograph that illustrates the point that patients with head and neck cancer often have complex composite defects after surgical ablation.

to the cephalic vein and within 2 cm of the lower border of the clavicle, crosses directly anteriorly from the surface of the pectoralis major muscle to the overlying subcutaneous tissue. Recognition of this vessel accurately localizes the position of the proximal portion of the pectoral branch of the thoracoacromial artery before elevation of the pectoralis major muscle has been started.

This flap is reliable with predictable cutaneous survival. Success rates of over 90% are reported. This flap provides vascularity at the recipient site due to its excellent blood supply. It has sufficient bulk to fill cavities, augment contour, and to provide structural support (Figure 2). Elevated on a narrow muscle pedicle, it can replace the contour of the sternocleidomastoid muscle and restore symmetry to the neck after a radical neck dissection. In addition, if the muscle pedicle is elevated without the overlying skin as a myogenous flap, a skin "paddle" at the end of the muscle can be transported to the recipient site under the neck flaps in one stage without the need for a later division and inset of the flap. The donor site is usually closed primarily by undermining and advancing the adjacent skin.

One of the frequent criticisms of the PMMC flap is the difficulty in working with a thick skin paddle and a tenuous blood supply to the distal skin paddle. In women or obese patients, problems in working with a thick skin paddle may be severe. Combining this with the resultant deformity of the breast makes the authors reluctant to use this flap in women. If skin coverage is required for a portion of the PMMC flap, a split-thickness skin graft may be harvested and sutured to the muscle to provide either internal or external coverage. In some situations, it is preferable to allow the exposed muscle to "mucosalize" when used for internal lining.

Latissimus Dorsi Myocutaneous Flap

The latissimus dorsi muscle is a versatile myocutaneous flap that is commonly used in head and neck reconstruction.[1,2] It can be transferred either pedicled or as a free flap, depending on the intended position of the flap. Details of this flap as a free tissue transfer flap are covered later in this chapter. As a pedicled rotational flap for reconstruction of neck and inferior scalp defects,

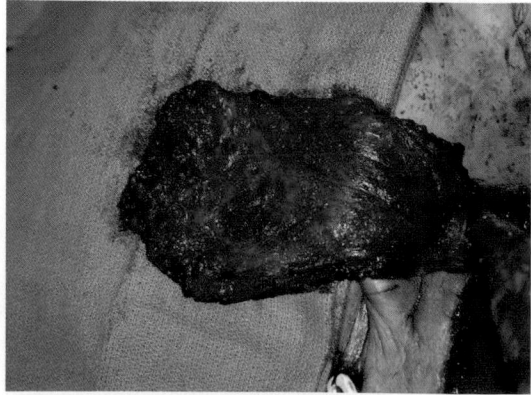

Figure 2 The pectoralis major myocutaneous muscle flap provides significant tissue bulk with both muscle and skin components. It is transferred as a pedicled flap.

the latissimus dorsi muscle has a wide range of rotational motion and can be employed even when the muscle remains attached at its insertion on the humerus. When reconstruction with a pedicled flap is possible, the requirement for microvascular anastomosis is eliminated, reducing operative time.

Fortunately, when the use of a pedicled flap is undesirable or when the defect is distant from the rotational limits of the muscle, the latissimus dorsi is hearty and tolerant of free tissue transfer. The large vessel caliber (1.5 to 4 mm diameter) and pedicle lengths of 6 to 10 cm allow for flexibility in positioning the flap and improves the likelihood that the pedicle will reach larger caliber recipient vessels in the neck. There is minimal donor-site morbidity as resection of the latissimus muscle results in no long-term postoperative functional limitation. The donor defect can generally be closed primarily, avoiding the need for a skin graft. One or two closed suction drains should always be placed at the site of muscle harvest to prevent the accumulation of serum.

As a pedicled flap the most significant disadvantage is the limitation in positioning of the flap in the recipient site. The position of a pedicled flap is limited by the arc of rotation of the muscle and the orientation of the vascular pedicle, so the final positioning of the pedicled flap is less versatile than when the flap is transferred as a free flap. Secondly, the cosmetic appearance of the pedicled latissimus dorsi flap is less acceptable as the bulk of the rotated muscle is visible throughout its course toward the recipient site.[1,2] Secondary revision operations are sometimes necessary to restore a more cosmetically acceptable contour. The thick skin of the cutaneous paddle (up to 4 mm) and its poor color match with the skin of the head and the neck, although acceptable, reduce the subtlety of this flap in the recipient site.

FREE TISSUE TRANSFER FLAPS

A salient advance in the complete treatment of the patient with a head or neck neoplasm is primary reconstruction. The use of free tissue from a distant site allows for reconstruction with similar tissues. In general, one can envision the three dimensional defect that will be created after resection of the neoplasm. Knowledge of various tissue components of various free tissue transfer flaps will allow the reconstructive surgeon to choose a flap that will best mimic the volume as well as the tissue composition of the resected tissue. Even with this ability, patients should be made aware that multiple revisions are often necessary to achieve the desired functional as well as cosmetic goals.

Although over 40 donor sites for free tissue transfer have been described and utilized, a smaller number have been consistently applied for routine reconstruction of large head and neck defects. The radial forearm fasciocutaneous, radial forearm osteocutaneous, and fibular osteocutaneous free flaps account for over 80% of head and neck microvascular reconstructions. This is due

in large part to the particular advantages of the characteristics of these flaps that include versatility, high success rate, and low donor-site morbidity. The arterial and venous supply of almost any area of the body can be isolated. However, donorsite selection must take into account characteristics of the defect, including location, volume, quality, and type of tissue required for reconstruction (ie, skin, muscle, and/or bone) and that the dissection of the flap will not be overly tedious or result in unacceptable donor-site morbidity. Function of the flap in the recipient site is also considered, as nerve anastomosis may be performed to reestablish sensation and mobility to transferred tissue. This is particularly relevant in reconstruction of the oral cavity, wherein sensation and mobility may be restored to a reconstructed tongue, significantly improving postoperative function. With all these factors considered, surgical flaps are divided into several categories based on the type of tissues included in the flap: fasciocutaneous, myocutaneous (musculocutaneous), myogenous, and osteocutaneous. Each of these categories will be discussed, with examples of reconstructive options available within each category.

Fasciocutaneous Flaps

The fasciocutaneous flap is a composite flap that includes skin, subcutaneous tissue, and fascia. The blood supply to the fasciocutaneous flap typically consists of perforating vessels arising from regional arteries coursing through fascial septa, known as septocutaneous perforators. Cadaveric studies have demonstrated that the fasciocutaneous perforators and their fascial plexus lie in the longitudinal axis, and therefore the length-to-breadth ratio is dictated by a longitudinally oriented pattern of blood flow. Fasciocutaneous flaps have the advantage of being thin and pliable and function well for reconstruction of low volume, moderate surface area defects. Many different areas of the body are suitable for harvesting of a fasciocutaneous free flap (Table 1).

Radial Forearm Fasciocutaneous Flap. The radical forearm fasciocutaneous flap is a "workhorse" flap that is the most commonly utilized free flap in of modern head and neck microvascular reconstruction. The radial forearm fasciocutaneous flap may also be elevated as an osteocutaneous flap, inclusive of a segment of vascularized radius bone.

This flap is based on the radial artery with its paired venae comitantes and/or the cephalic vein (Table 2). The vascular pedicle is long (up to 20 cm) and the vessels are of large caliber (2.5 to 3 mm). This allows a variety of orientations while maintaining adequate pedicle length for vascular anastomosis to the larger caliber external carotid branch vessels in the neck (facial, superior thyroid, or lingual arteries).

The radial artery, with its paired venae comitantes, courses in the lateral intermuscular septum and has several fascial branches in the forearm that supply the fascia and skin. The proximal extent of the pedicle is defined by the

Table 1 Similarities and Differences among the Various Fasciocutaneous Flaps Used in Reconstruction of Head and Neck Defects

Flap	Advantages	Disadvantages
Radial forearm	• Thin, pliable tissue paddle • Large caliber, long vascular pedicle • Consistent anatomy • Technically straightforward • Two-team approach possible	• Donor site visible • Requires skin graft • Potential for vascular compromise of hand
Ulnar flap	• Thin, pliable tissue paddle • Relatively hairless • Two-team approach possible	• Potential for ulnar nerve injury • Smaller, shorter vascular pedicle than radial forearm flap • Two venous anastamosis • Donor site visible • Requires skin graft
Anterolateral thigh	• Large skin paddle available • Versatile in volume • Primary closure usually possible • Low donor-site morbidity • Two-team approach possible	• Inconsistent vascular anatomy • Technically challenging • Poor color match • Lateral thigh numbness
Lateral arm	• Thin, pliable tissue paddle • Donor site easily hidden • Primary closure usually possible	• Small caliber, short vascular pedicle • Potential for radial nerve injury • Poor color match • Two-team approach difficult

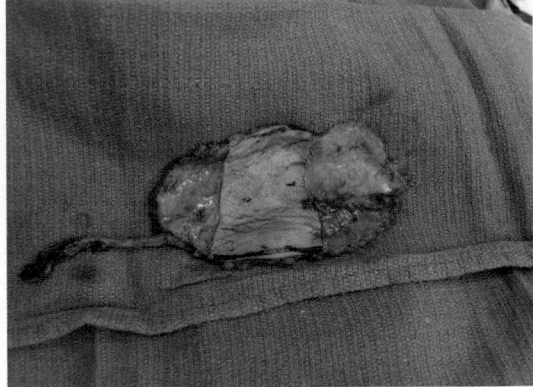

Figure 3 The radial forearm fasciocutaneous free flap is versatile soft tissue that is easily moldable in three dimensions.

radial recurrent artery and by the convergence of the two venae comitantes into a single vein, which occurs near the antecubital fossa in over 80% of patients. The skin paddle is incised in the distal forearm, and the dissection is taken to the subfascial level. The pedicle is followed proximally to the antecubital fossa, where it is divided distal to the radial recurrent artery and prepared for microvascular anastomosis. The cephalic vein may additionally be harvested to supplement superficial venous drainage of the flap. When a sensate flap is desired, for example, for tongue reconstruction, the lateral antebrachial cutaneous nerve is identified as it courses near the cephalic vein and is harvested along with the vascular pedicle for anastomosis at the recipient site. Some sensory recovery is also present in most patients when neural anastomosis is not performed, but recovery of sensation is greatly accelerated and enhanced by addition of nerve anastomosis. Once the flap is completely divided from the forearm, the flap is carefully inset into the recipient site and vascular anastomosis is performed under the microscope. The forearm donor site is covered with a split-thickness skin graft and a volar splint is left in place for 5 days postoperatively.

Its thinness, pliability, and low volume allow positioning in various three-dimensional orientations in the recipient site (Figure 3). It is used commonly for reconstruction of cutaneous defects of the face and scalp, as well as reconstruction of the oral cavity, tongue, and pharynx.[3,4] The consistent anatomy and predictable characteristics of its vascular pedicle make this the technically most straightforward flap to harvest. As a result, this flap may be elevated more quickly than do more technically challenging free flaps such as the anterolateral thigh flap. Elevation of the flap can generally be performed simultaneously with the resective procedure when a two-team approach is applied. These factors result in shorter operative times, reduced anesthetic time for the patient, and lower operating room costs.

The main disadvantage associated with use of the radial forearm free flap is unacceptable cosmetic appearance of the forearm following flap harvest and skin grafting. A recent study demonstrated the surface area of the forearm defect is reducible by up to 50% by the application of a purse-string suture circumferentially around the donor-site defect.[4] This additional maneuver results in a smaller, more cosmetically acceptable donor site and a reduced requirement for split-thickness skin graft. The postoperative incidence of functional deficits is not increased by this technique. Five to fifteen percent of patients may have at least partial loss of the skin graft. Functional deficits in the donor arm are uncommon, with a prospective study demonstrating some degree of functional deficit in the donor arm in 16% of patients at 1 year.[5] Despite attention to preservation of the superficial branch of the radial nerve during flap elevation, up to 30% of patients report transient paresthesias or dysesthesias in the anatomic snuffbox region, typically resolving within 12 months postoperatively. This may be attributable to operative trauma to the nerve, traction injury, or ischemia related to tense closure of the surgical site.

A devastating complication of radial forearm free flap elevation is the development of hand ischemia. Critical to the selection of donor site is the accurate performance of a preoperative Allen test. This test is an easily executed clinical examination that evaluates the perfusion of the hand by both the ulnar and the radial arterial systems. The radial artery may not be harvested safely in patients with an incomplete palmar arch or compromised perfusion by the ulnar artery,

Table 2 Fasciocutaneous Free Flaps

Flap	Artery	Artery Diameter	Vein(s)	Pedicle Length	Nerve
Radial forearm	Radial	2.5–3 mm	Paired venae comitantes (may converge into one) and/or cephalic vein	Up to 20 cm	Lateral antebrachial cutaneous
Ulna forearm	Ulnar	1.5–2.5 mm	Paired venae comitantes and/or cephalic vein	>10 cm	Medial antebrachial cutaneous
Anterolateral thigh	Lateral femoral circumflex — descending branch	1.5–3.5 mm	Paired venae comitantes	Up to 7 cm	Lateral femoral cutaneous
Lateral arm	Posterior radial collateral	1.25–1.75 mm	Paired venae comitantes and/or cephalic vein	Up to 10 cm	Posterior cutaneous nerve of the arm
Scapula	Circumflex scapular (may be followed to subscapular artery)	4 mm (6 mm if followed to subscapular artery)	Paired venae comitantes	7–10 cm (11–14 cm if followed to subscapular vessels)	Dorsal cutaneous rami of T1 and T2 (experimental)

and alternate reconstructive options must be explored.

Ulnar Fasciocutaneous Flap. The ulnar fasciocutaneous free flap shares many of the advantageous characteristics of the radial forearm fasciocutaneous flap (see Table 2). The ulnar flap may be selected when preoperative physical examination (Allen test) of the nondominant hand is suggestive of inadequate radial arterial perfusion. In this setting, reconstructive surgeons often elect to pursue harvest of a radial forearm free flap from the dominant side. In the setting of a complex head and neck reconstruction, which often includes temporary tracheostomy, a 5-week postoperative splinting of the dominant donor arm also limits the patient's ability to communicate in writing, which may be highly frustrating.

The ulnar flap is based on the ulnar artery and its two venae comitantes. In a 2002 review, the dimensions of the vascular pedicle proved to be quite consistent, with average ulnar artery diameter measuring 2.5 mm and average diameter of the two venae comitantes measuring 1.0 to 1.5 mm.[6] In contrast to the radial forearm flap pedicle, the two venae comitantes rarely converge into one larger vein, and therefore two venous anastamoses are generally required, slightly lengthening the operative time. Pedicle length is consistently greater than 10 cm, which allows for versatility in positioning the flap in its recipient location. The medial antebrachial cutaneous nerve provides sensation to the skin paddle, and it may be harvested as a sensate flap (Figure 4).

Advantages of the ulnar flap, like its radial counterpart, are its reliable, soft, pliable, and moldable in three dimensions characteristics and option of additional bulk with inclusion of the underlying palmaris longus tendon. Because the skin paddle is centered more medially than that of the radial forearm flap, it has the advantage of containing less hair-bearing tissue than does the radial forearm flap. This may be a consideration in hirsute patients undergoing oropharyngeal reconstruction. The location of the skin paddle at the distal part of the forearm allows for simultaneous elevation of the flap with the resective procedure when a two-team approach is employed. The ulnar fasciocutaneous flap can be used as an

alternative to the radial forearm free flap in certain settings and is suitable for reconstruction of cutaneous defects of the face and scalp, as well as for reconstruction of the oral cavity, tongue, and pharynx.[6]

There are several disadvantages of this flap that limit its use as a primary reconstructive option. The ulnar flap is technically more difficult to harvest than the radial forearm free flap. The ulnar artery is less superficial than the radial artery and runs adjacent to the ulnar nerve. Multiple small perforators travel from the ulnar artery to the ulnar nerve, and meticulous dissection is crucial to avoid functional morbidity associated with damage to the nearby nerve. Although uncommon, it is devastating when it occurs, as it results in functional limitation of the muscles of the hand and the forearm. A smaller disadvantage of the ulnar flap in comparison to the radial forearm flap is that the vascular pedicle is somewhat less favorable, as the ulnar artery averages 1 mm less than the diameter of the radial artery. In spite of this disadvantage, the arterial diameter of 2 to 2.5 mm is adequate to match reliable recipient vessels in the head and neck. More significantly, the paired venae comitantes are small and do not generally converge into one larger vein resulting in slightly longer operative times. Overall, in the presence of contraindications to the use of the radial forearm free flap, the ulnar flap is an excellent alternative when the desirable characteristics of the radial forearm flap are required.

Anterolateral Thigh Fasciocutaneous Flap. The anterolateral thigh fasciocutaneous flap is a versatile fasciocutaneous flap that is a potential source of a large skin paddle, making it ideal for reconstruction of large cutaneous and oropharyngeal defects. Topographically, the skin paddle of the anterolateral thigh flap lies on the middle third of the axis of the septum dividing the vastus lateralis and the rectus femoris muscles. This is conceptualized as an imaginary line connecting the anterior superior iliac spine and the lateral border of the patella. Arising from the profunda femoral trunk, the lateral femoral circumflex artery distributes both ascending and descending branches. This descending branch supplies the perforators coursing deep within the intramuscular septum, often deep in the septal plane, but on occasion within the substance of the rectus femoris muscle. This septal plane can be used to identify the artery and flap blood supply if the septum is accompanied by at least one septocutaneous perforating artery and vein. If no septocutaneous perforators are present, the superior portion of the septal plane that meets the tensor fascia lata muscle can be used to find the lateral femoral circumflex vessels of the descending branch. Because of the variability of arterial anatomy, in up to 80% of patients, the anterolateral thigh flap is not solely supplied by fasciocutaneous perforators and the surgeon must be prepared to dissect the musculocutaneous perforators traversing the rectus femoris muscle meticulously to maintain optimal flap perfusion. This can be difficult when the

entire course of the artery is in the substance of the rectus femoris muscle. The flap is innervated by a large branch of the lateral femoral cutaneous nerve and this nerve, can be dissected with the pedicle to create a sensate flap with neural anastomosis at the recipient site (see Table 2).

The descending branch of the lateral femoral circumflex artery is a large caliber pedicle (1.5 to 3.5 mm), with length up to 7 cm. In most instances, two veins accompany the artery. A skin paddle as large as 8 cm × 25 cm can be harvested with wider skin paddles (Figure 5). The use of a split-thickness skin graft to close the donor site is usually necessary.

The flap is innervated by a large branch of the lateral femoral cutaneous nerve. The nerve can be dissected with the pedicle at the superior aspect, and can be traced inferiorly to create a sensate flap with neural anastomosis at the recipient site (see Table 2).

Despite the potential for a technically challenging operation, the advantages of the anterolateral thigh flap include its high success rate, large skin paddle, the ability to perform flap elevation simultaneously with the resective procedure, resulting in reduced operative time. Donor-site morbidity following harvest of the anterolateral thigh flap is low, and patients recover function quickly postoperatively. A 2002 report of a series of 672 anterolateral thigh flaps reported a success rate of 95.7%, with complete flap loss occurring in 1.8% of patients.[7] Flap volume is quite versatile and can be easily tailored to the recipient site by either thinning subcutaneous tissues or by adding volume with inclusion of vastus lateralis, rectus femoris, or tensor fascia lata muscle to provide additional soft tissue bulk. For this reason, the anterolateral thigh flap is an excellent source of soft tissue for the reconstruction of medium- to large-volume defects, including those involving the lateral part of the temporal bone or maxilla. Success rates of the anterolateral thigh flap are similar to those of the widely used radial forearm free flap, and the anterolateral thigh flap is preferred when larger volume reconstruction is required or in the presence of contraindications to the use of the radial forearm free flap.

In addition to the technical challenge of anterolateral thigh flap elevation, several disadvantages

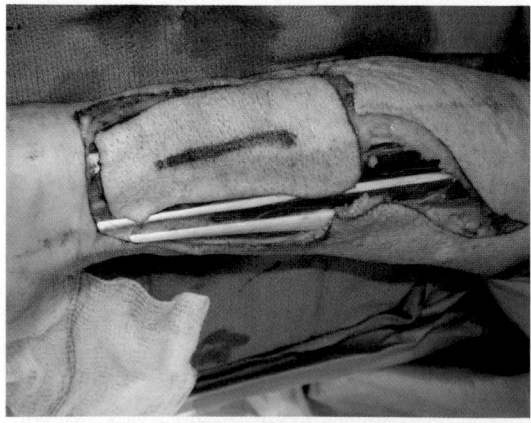

Figure 4 The ulnar free flap supplies the same soft tissue characteristics and components as the radial forearm.

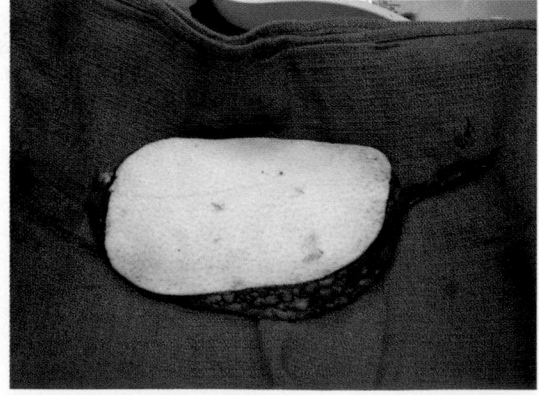

Figure 5 The anterolateral thigh flap provides significant soft tissue that can be tailored to reconstruct many soft tissue defects in the head and neck.

of this flap should be noted. Whereas the flap volume is versatile, the orientation of this flap in the recipient site is less flexible as the flap is dense and not amenable to complex molding in three dimensions. The cosmetic result of anterolateral thigh flap reconstruction of head and neck defects is acceptable, but not ideal. The color match to the skin of the head and neck is poor, and the pale appearance of the flap persists, reducing the subtlety of the reconstruction. Finally, some functional morbidity may result from division or resection of the regional nerves. When a sensate flap is elevated to include the lateral femoral cutaneous nerve, numbness involving the entirety of the lateral thigh is perceived by the patient and may be bothersome but does not typically limit the patient functionally. True functional morbidity is uncommon but generally is the result of mild to moderate lower extremity weakness. This postoperative complication may occur because the femoral nerve branch to the vastus lateralis muscle travels with the pedicle and, because of its intimate relationship to the supplying vessels, occasionally must be divided to dissect the full length of the pedicle.

Lateral Arm Fasciocutaneous Flap. The lateral arm fasciocutaneous flap was first described in 1982 by Song, and its application to head and neck reconstruction was reported by Sullivan and colleagues in 1992.[8] Similar to the radial forearm free flap, it provides thin, pliable tissue with skin quality well suited for the head and neck reconstruction. The volume of the lateral arm flap is intermediate between the volumes of the radial forearm flap and the anterolateral thigh flap, and thus, the lateral arm flap is suitable for reconstruction of low- to medium-volume defects (Figure 6).

The skin paddle topographically lies between the lateral epicondyle and the insertion of the deltoid on the humerus and is based on four to five septocutaneous perforators (see Table 2). The posterior radial collateral artery and its venae comitantes supply this flap. Division of the posterior radial collateral artery does not jeopardize forearm and hand perfusion, as it is a terminal branch of the profunda brachii artery supplying the upper arm. This vessel courses with the radial nerve in the lateral intermuscular septum between the triceps muscle and the brachialis and

brachioradialis muscles. This flap may be transferred as a sensate flap based on the posterior cutaneous nerve of the arm. If the size of the skin paddle is limited to 6 to 8 cm width, the donor site can generally be closed primarily after wide undermining of the adjacent soft tissue, avoiding the need for skin grafting.[8]

Several disadvantages of the lateral arm flap have resulted in its diminishing use in the present era of the head and neck reconstruction. First, dissection of the flap and pedicle proceeds in close proximity to the radial nerve.[8] There is, therefore, risk of injury to this important nerve during flap elevation. The morbidity of radial nerve injury is significant, resulting in loss of finger and wrist extensor function and loss of sensation over the dorsal arm and hand. Even incomplete injury of the radial nerve may result in temporary or permanent pain, paresthesias, and dysesthesias. Ultimately, the consequence of radial nerve injury is functional loss involving hand and wrist, which is poorly tolerated by patients. The second disadvantage of this flap is relatively small vessel caliber (1.25 to 1.75 mm) and short pedicle length (maximum of 8 to 10 cm). In practice, it is difficult to obtain more than 6 cm of pedicle length, as additional pedicle dissection requires detaching a large amount of the triceps muscle and increases the risk of injury to motor branches of the radial nerve. The two-team approach of simultaneous tumor resection and flap elevation may be possible, but it is more difficult than with the use of a forearm donor site, and limited by awkward patient positioning, prolonging operative time. Finally, color match is generally poor in head and neck reconstruction, and the flap maintains a pale appearance in comparison to its surroundings. Most reconstructive surgeons have abandoned this flap as a primary reconstructive modality, but it should still be considered an alternate reconstructive method when other options are unavailable or unsuitable.

Scapular Fasciocutaneous Flap. The scapular fasciocutaneous flap is used primarily as an osteocutaneous flap in head and neck reconstruction and is discussed in detail later in this chapter but may also be used as a fasciocutaneous flap for reconstruction of soft tissue defects (see Table 2).

The blood supply of the scapular fasciocutaneous flap is from the circumflex scapular artery a branch of the subscapular artery. Arterial diameter averages 4 mm and pedicle length of 7 to 10 cm; however, with dissecting along the subscapular artery proximally, an arterial diameter up to 6 mm and pedicle length up to 11 to 14 cm can be obtained. Although there has been success with the experimental use of the dorsal cutaneous rami of the T1 or T2 spinal nerves for flap nerve anastomosis, there is not a dominant segmental nerve supply to the skin of this region; and, therefore, this flap is not considered to have the potential for transfer as a sensate flap.

The skin paddle of this flap is soft and pliable and has a good color match to the surrounding

skin of the head and neck. Because the vascular pedicle is long, there is great versatility in positioning the flap in its recipient location. The branching vascular supply of the flap allows individual components of the flap to be positioned in various three-dimensional orientations relative to one another, resulting in great versatility in the reconstruction of large defects. The skin paddle can be designed horizontally (scapular-based on the transverse cutaneous arterial branch) or vertically (parascapular-based on the descending cutaneous arterial branch). Two separate skin paddles may even be elevated in continuity with the bulk of the flap, allowing ideal reconstruction of defects that require both intraoral mucosal and external skin coverage. For high-volume defects, the bulk of this flap may be expanded further by harvest of underlying muscle (latissimus dorsi and/or serratus anterior muscle), creating potential for use as a myocutaneous flap to fill maximal defect volume (Figure 7). The donor site can generally be closed primarily owing to the surrounding soft tissue pliability, avoiding a skin graft.

The main disadvantage of the use of this flap is the need to reposition the patient in the lateral decubitus position during the operation, which limits the two-team approach for simultaneous resection of the neoplasm and flap elevation. This may prolong operative and anesthetic times and increase hospital costs. There is also limited potential for a sensate flap although some success has been achieved with use of the dorsal cutaneous rami of T1 or T2 spinal nerves for nerve anastomoses.

Jejunal Free Flap

Jejunal free flap reconstruction is used to reconstruct circumferential defects of the upper aerodigestive tract, commonly after laryngopharyngectomy. It is a good replacement owing to its tubed nature and the presence of lubricating mucous glands.

Tube lengths of up to 30 cm can replace lost segments of the cervical esophagus from the

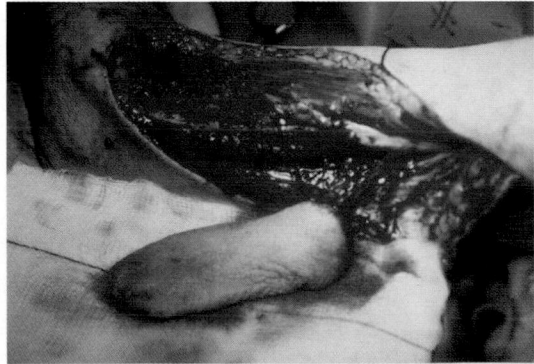

Figure 6 The lateral arm flap provides thicker subcutaneous tissue than the radial forearm but less than the anterolateral thigh.

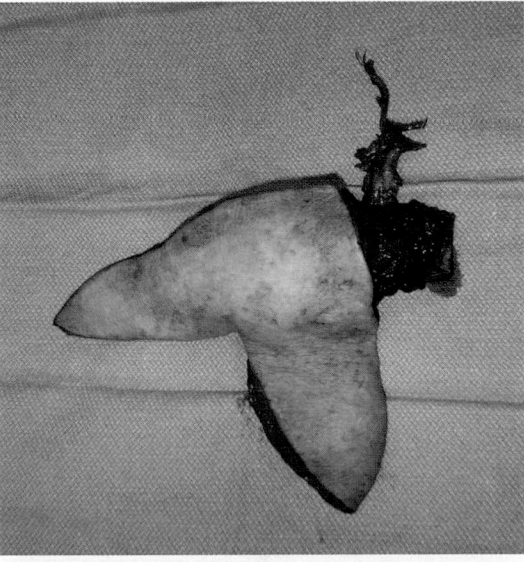

Figure 7 The scapula free flap can be harvested with multiple soft tissue components. The skin is the thickest of all the fasciocutaneous flaps. It remains very versatile.

nasopharynx to the thoracic inlet. Defects that extend into the chest, placing the anastomotic site in the chest, can potentially result in mediastinitis should a leak occur. A gastric pull-up or colonic interposition is performed in these cases. With an intact larynx, if the jejunal free flap is not below a functioning cricopharyngeus, the normal secretions from the jejunum may result in aspiration. An alternate tubed free flap may be needed in these situations.

The small bowel is composed of three distinct anatomic and physiologic segments. The jejunum, the second segment, begins at the ligament of Treitz and extends distally 6 to 8 ft. Its vascular supply is the superior mesenteric artery and vein; these pass over the mid duodenum and enter the mesentery of the jejunum. A single arcade is formed in this mesentery, which gives rise to the vasa recta supplying the jejunum.

This single arcade allows a closer relationship between the superior mesenteric jejunal artery and the vascular territory of the jejunum it perfuses. Distally in the small bowel, the number of vascular arcades increases in the ileum, and therefore, indistinct perfusion patterns of single arterial pedicles arise. Typically, the second jejunal branch is the pedicle of choice. When the dissection is carried right down to the superior mesenteric artery, arterial pedicles up to 3 to 4 mm in diameter and up to 10 cm in length can be obtained. Transilluminating the mesentery greatly aids harvest of the pedicle.

The desired length of jejunum is excised marking out the proximal or distal end. The flap is moved to the neck and inset into place under a little tension because when perfusion is reestablished with microvascular anastomosis, the jejunum tends to lengthen. Kinking or bowing of the jejunum impairs food passage. Avoiding kinking of vascular pedicle also decreases the chances of venous thrombosis. An end-to-end enteric anastomoses is performed, in an isoperistaltic fashion. The microvascular anastamoses are then completed. We usually design a sentinel-monitoring loop of jejunum that is left free and brought out through the skin incision as a postoperative monitor. This monitor loop is removed 1 week postoperatively (Figure 8).

Spatulation proximally of the enteric anastomosis may be necessary to allow the small-calibre

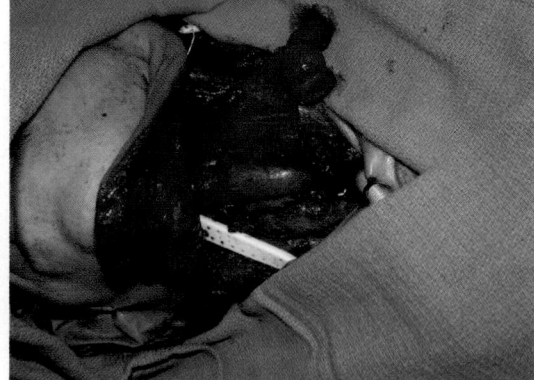

Figure 8 The jejunal free flap is a visceral flap that is useful in total pharyngeal defects.

jejunum to fit larger defects. Triangular interdigitation distally into the esophagus decreases the incidence of stricture formation. Excess mesentery available can be used to reinforce the enteric anastomosis.

Complications can occur in the donor area, the microvascular anastomoses, or at the enteric anastamoses. Each can compromise reconstructive efforts or the patient's life. This flap has poor ischemia tolerance. Regular monitoring of the external monitoring segment for signs of arterial or venous compromise, allows timely rapid vascular reanastomosis and salvage. Fistula formation and stricture formation can occur with any reconstructive technique and are more frequent with prior radiation. The rate of fistula formation is reported at 18%. Of these, over two-thirds close spontaneously. Larger, more persistent leaks may respond to pectoralis major myocutaneous flap reinforcement. There is a low rate (8%) of stricture formation.[9] Strictures may be due to fibrosis of the distal anastomosis or from kinking of the jejunal segment. Dysphagia due to strictures can be treated with endoscopic dilatation or exceptionally excision of the redundant segment may be needed. Dysphagia may also result from dyskinetic peristalsis due to delayed emptying of the jejunal segment particularly with solids. Flap success rates are around 98%.[10] Voicing with tracheal puncture provides acceptable speech, but one of the most significant problems with jejunal reconstruction is the "wet" and relatively poor quality of voice.

Myocutaneous Free Flaps

Myocutaneous flaps are composite flaps that include skin, subcutaneous fat, fascia, and muscle. The blood supply to this type of flap is based on a single dominant arterial trunk that provides adequate perfusion through an arborizing arterial network to a large volume of muscle, despite ligation of adjacent contributing vascular pedicles. The overlying skin and subcutaneous tissue

are supplied by secondary terminal perforating branches running vertically from the underlying muscular branches. It is the cutaneous portion of the myocutaneous flap that is most vulnerable to ischemia, as it relies on these small caliber perforators for perfusion. Because of this pattern of perfusion, it is the number of musculocutaneous perforators and their particular distribution that defines the limit of the skin paddle size, shape, and orientation. Vascular insufficiency to the skin paddle can result in partial flap loss, with necrosis of the skin and the subcutaneous tissue, but the muscle is preserved. Also as a consequence of this vascular pattern, the skin is anchored to the underlying muscle, and therefore, the flap is not pliable in three dimensions. Because a skin paddle is excised with the myocutaneous flap, donor-site complications resulting from excessive tension on the closure (eg, wound dehiscence, patient discomfort, or requirement for a skin graft) are slightly more common than seen with a myogenous flap without a skin paddle. Overall, donor-site morbidity following harvest of myocutaneous flaps is acceptably low as surrounding tissues are generally pliable and amenable to primary closure. A comparison of the common myocutaneous free flaps used in the head and neck are described in Table 3.

Myocutaneous flaps are utilized in the reconstruction of large defects that require restoration of a cutaneous or mucosal surface and also significant bulk to fill a voluminous defect following resection of the neoplasm. Examples wherein a myocutaneous flap would be considered an option for reconstruction include large defects of the scalp, oropharynx, and skull base (where defect may include portions of the facial skeleton, paranasal sinuses, and palate). The arteries and their diameters, veins, pedicle length, and nerves of the various myocutaneous free flaps used in the head and neck are compared in Table 4.

Latissimus Dorsi Myocutaneous Flap. The latissimus dorsi myocutaneous flap is versatile

Table 3 Differences and Similarities between the Common Myocutaneous Free Flaps Used in Head and Neck Reconstruction

Flap	Advantages	Disadvantages
Latissimus dorsi	• Large caliber, long vascular pedicle • Large surface area available • Versatile in volume • Transferred as free or pedicled flap • Low donor-site morbidity • Primary closure usually possible • Technically straightforward	• Repositioning patient in operating room • Two-team approach difficult • Unpredictable final volume after atrophy • Frequently requires revision • Poor color match
Rectus abdominis	• Large caliber, long vascular pedicle • Large surface area available • Versatile in volume • Consistent anatomy • Primary closure usually possible • Technically straightforward • Two-team approach possible	• Potential for ventral hernia • Requires abdominal wall reconstruction • Unpredictable final volume after atrophy • May require revision • Poor color match • Skin paddle less reliable with loose or thick subcutaneous tissue
Gracilis	• Low donor-site morbidity • Two-team approach possible • Suitable for facial reanimation procedures	• Small caliber, short vascular pedicle • Limited versatility in positioning

Table 4 Characteristics of the Vascular Pedicles of Myocutaneous Free Flaps Used in the Head and Neck

Flap	Artery	Artery Diameter	Vein(s)	Pedicle Length	Nerve
Latissimus dorsi	Thoracodorsal	1.5–4 mm	Single vein	6–10 cm	
Rectus abdominis	Inferior epigastric artery	3–4 mm	Paired inferior epigastric veins (usually converge into one)	Up to 10 cm	–
Gracilis	Adductor artery—terminal branch	1–2 mm	Paired venae comitantes	Up to 4 cm	Obturator nerve branch

and commonly used in the head and neck reconstruction.[1,2] It can be transferred either as a pedicled or a free flap, depending on the intended position of the flap.

The latissimus dorsi is a bulky muscle that arises from the lower six thoracic vertebrae, the thoracolumbar fascia, and the iliac crest. It inserts as a narrower apex onto the medial surface of the humerus. The muscle is supplied by the thoracodorsal artery, a branch of the subscapular system of the axillary artery. Several musculocutaneous perforators supply the overlying skin and are most abundant in the upper two-thirds of the muscle. Based on this pattern of cutaneous blood supply, the skin paddle is centered on the upper portion of the muscle. The remainder of the muscle may be utilized to provide bulk for the reconstruction of large-volume defects, such as large scalp defects and skull-base defects, and the tongue after glossectomy. Innervated latissimus dorsi myocutaneous flaps have been described for the reconstruction of tongue following glossectomy. In this case, the thoracodorsal nerve is preserved in continuity with the neurovascular pedicle, and a neural anastomosis to the lingual nerve is performed.

As a pedicled rotational flap for reconstruction of neck and inferior scalp defects, the latissimus dorsi muscle has a wide range of rotational motion and can be employed even when the muscle remains attached at its insertion on the humerus. When reconstruction with a pedicled flap is possible, the requirement for microvascular anastomoses is eliminated, reducing operative time.

Fortunately, when the use of a pedicled flap is undesirable or when the defect is distant from the rotational limits of the muscle, the latissimus dorsi is hearty and tolerant of free tissue transfer (Figure 9). The large vessel caliber (1.5 to 4 mm

diameter) and pedicle lengths of 6 to 10 cm allow for flexibility in positioning the flap and improves the likelihood that the pedicle will reach larger caliber recipient vessels in the neck. There is minimal donor-site morbidity as resection of the latissimus muscle results in no long-term postoperative functional limitation. The donor defect can generally be closed primarily, avoiding the need for a skin graft. One or two closed suction drains should always be placed at the site of muscle harvest to prevent the accumulation of serum.

Since the inception of free tissue transfer, the latissimus dorsi free flap has been recognized as an excellent option for scalp reconstruction because of its large surface area, long vascular pedicle, ease of harvest, and provision of well-vascularized tissue for compromised recipient beds. The length of the thoracodorsal vascular pedicle is usually sufficient to reach recipient vessels in the neck although reconstruction of defects of the scalp vertex may require use of the more superiorly located superficial temporal vessels as recipient vessels. Adding to its versatility, the latissimus dorsi can be transferred as either a myogenous or a myocutaneous flap, depending on the desired flap volume and the presence or absence of a cutaneous defect. The myogenous flap without overlying skin and soft tissue reduces bulk and improves contour on the scalp. Transfer of a myogenous flap requires coverage with a split-thickness skin graft. Cosmetic outcomes are acceptable, as the latissimus flap atrophies and appears much like normal scalp once the skin graft matures. The incidence of major complications in the setting of scalp reconstruction is low and flap loss is reported to occur in 3 to 5% of cases.

The major disadvantage of the latissimus dorsi flap is that the patient generally must be repositioned into the lateral decubitus position in the operating room for harvest of the flap. This lengthens operative time and often prohibits simultaneous resection and flap elevation. The large latissimus dorsi muscle is prone to a significant amount of atrophy and volume loss with deconditioning. When the bulky muscle is inset as a reconstructive flap, the ultimate flap volume that will remain after the muscle atrophies is unpredictable. For this reason, defects are generally overfilled with a large-volume flap, and it frequently requires subsequent revision to tailor volume and contour to the recipient site. The secondary revision rate has been reported to be as high as 20 to 32%. Because of the large surface area of the muscle, marginal flap necrosis may occur over the most distal aspects of the flap. In the event of marginal necrosis, local debridement

may be necessary to remove necrotic debris. When possible, the most proximal aspect of the muscle should be used for calvarial and cranioplasty coverage and the most distal (least reliable) aspect of the flap positioned distally so that morbidity is minimized in the event of partial flap loss.

As a pedicled flap the most significant disadvantage is the limitation in positioning of the flap in the recipient site. The position of a pedicled flap is limited by the arc of rotation of the muscle and the orientation of the vascular pedicle, so the final positioning of the pedicled flap is less versatile that it is when the flap is transferred as a free flap. Secondly, the cosmetic appearance of the pedicled latissimus dorsi flap is less acceptable as the bulk of the rotated muscle is visible throughout its course toward the recipient site.[1,2] Secondary revision operations are sometimes necessary to restore a more cosmetically acceptable contour. The thick skin of the cutaneous paddle (up to 4 mm) and its poor color match with the skin of the head and the neck, although acceptable, reduce the subtlety of this flap in the recipient site.

Rectus Abdominis Myocutaneous Flap. The rectus abdominis myocutaneous free flap is an excellent choice for reconstruction of medium- to large-sized head and neck defects. The rectus abdominis muscle is easy to harvest, has a long vascular pedicle, and may be transferred as a myocutaneous or a myogenous flap, depending on the amount of skin and soft tissue volume required (see Table 4).

The arterial supply is based on the deep inferior epigastric system of the external iliac vessels, and its takeoff defines the transition from external iliac to the common femoral vessels. After elevation of the flap, the pedicle is followed to its origin, that is, the external iliac vessels, and a pedicle length of 8 to 10 cm is attainable. The vessel caliber is also well suited for microvascular anastomosis, with an average diameter of 3 to 4 mm. Few variations of the vascular supply have been described, so the dissection of the pedicle is generally predictable because of the rich system of perforators in the periumbilical region.

This allows for the entire muscle or a large-sized skin paddle to be utilized to reconstruct large-volume defects such as large cutaneous ones those due to, total glossectomy or skull-base resections or medium-volume defects including cutaneous ones or those due to hemiglossectomy. The flap is highly reliable in the head and neck reconstruction, with published 0 to 2% failure rates.[11] The rectus abdominis flap can usually be

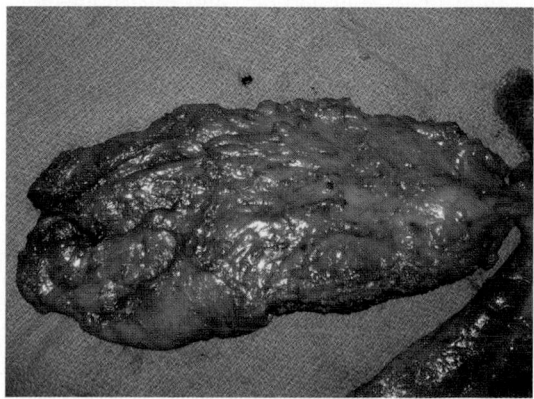

Figure 9 The latissimus dorsi free flap provides the greatest volume of free tissue that can be transferred. It may be transferred as a muscle only or with the overlying skin.

elevated simultaneously with the resective procedure; reducing operative times (Figure 10).

The potential morbidity of this operation is the development of a ventral hernia, and prevention of this complication is accomplished by conscientious repair of fascial layers after harvest of the muscle. The rectus abdominis muscle is invested by anterior and posterior fascial layers, the anterior and posterior rectus sheaths, that provide support to the ventral abdominal wall. When the muscle is resected without overlying tissue, that is, as a myogenous flap, the posterior rectus sheath is left intact and the vertical incision in the anterior rectus sheath is closed primarily to maintain the continuity of both the anterior and the posterior fascial layers. When a portion of the overlying fascia is resected, either for additional bulk or when the muscle is harvested to include subcutaneous tissue and skin, that is, as a myocutaneous flap, the anterior rectus sheath is repaired with prosthetic or biologic mesh. A 1995 review of 268 patients who had undergone rectus abdominis muscle harvest for breast reconstruction demonstrated a low incidence of abdominal wall complications, with a 2.6% rate of ventral hernia and a 3.8% rate of perceptible abdominal bulges.[4]

On an esthetic level, the disadvantage of the rectus abdominis flap is that the skin is a poor color match for the head and neck reconstruction. The skin of the abdomen contains a lower concentration of melanocytes, and therefore the flap appears pale in comparison to the surrounding skin of the head and neck. The flap may also be bulky until the muscle scars and atrophies in its recipient position and occasionally requires revision or liposuction to gain acceptable esthetic contour. Because of the wide variability in abdominal wall thickness among patients, body habitus is an important consideration when selecting the rectus abdominis muscle as a myocutaneous flap. A thick panniculus or loose, floppy abdominal wall (frequently present in multiparous women) may render a myocutaneous flap unacceptable for free tissue transfer, as the resultant flaps are highly bulky with unreliable cutaneous perforators.

Gracilis Myocutaneous Flap. The gracilis myocutaneous flap is a thin muscle flap utilizing

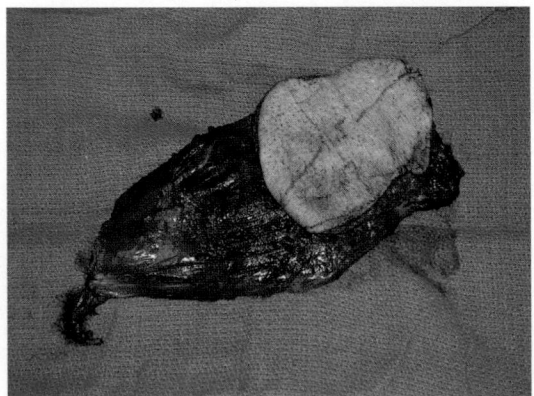

Figure 10 The rectus abdominis flap is a moderate volume flap that may be harvested with or with out a skin component.

this narrow adductor muscle of the medial aspect of the thigh. The dominant blood supply of the flap is the terminal branch of the adductor artery, which is a branch of the profunda femoris artery. The artery of the pedicle enters the muscle at a relatively constant 8 to 10 cm below the pubic tubercle, and is accompanied by paired venae comitantes. While blood supply to the muscle is relatively predictable, there is some variability of the blood supply to the skin. This supply may arise from musculocutaneous perforators, septocutaneous vessels, or from an inferior branch of the superior external pudendal artery. Motor innervation of this muscle is a branch of the obturator nerve. Since the gracilis muscle functions as one of the several hip adductors and knee flexors, patient mobility and strength are not diminished by harvest of this muscle (see Table 4).

The use of this flap became more common with the advent of its use as a myogenous flap in dynamic facial reanimation surgery, which is performed for permanent facial nerve paralysis. In this procedure, the thin muscle is transferred, revascularized, and nerve anastomosis is performed to the facial nerve directly or with a sural nerve graft. The dynamic facial reanimation operation has been demonstrated to restore facial movement and expression in long-term follow-up and is considered a reliable reconstructive and rehabilitative procedure. As a myocutaneous flap, however, the gracilis is mainly useful for reconstruction of small- to medium-sized cutaneous defects.

Disadvantages of this flap are a short pedicle length (up to 4 cm) and small caliber vessels (1 to 2 mm). This limits the versatility of positioning the flap and its use in the head and neck for facial reanimation in reconstruction of small- to moderate-sized cutaneous defects.

Myogenous Free Flaps

The myogenous flap is composed of muscle and fascia, but unlike the myocutaneous flap, it does not include the overlying subcutaneous tissue and skin. This flap, like the myocutaneous flap, is utilized for defects that require large volume for reconstruction but either do not require reconstruction of a cutaneous surface or include a cutaneous deficit in which the surface area is sufficiently large that it is best reconstructed with a split-thickness skin graft overlying the transferred muscle. Any muscle that can be used as a myocutaneous flap can also be transferred as a myogenous flap (see Table 4). The disadvantage of free transfer of a myogenous flap without overlying skin and subcutaneous tissue, however, is that muscle can be expected to undergo a significant amount of atrophy in its recipient environment. While the myogenous flap may initially fill a large volume, the ultimate volume of the flap after atrophy is unpredictable and atrophic degeneration may result in insufficient volume filling at long-term follow-up.

The region of the myocutaneous flap most vulnerable to ischemia is the skin paddle, as it relies on small caliber perforators for perfusion. In the myogenous flap, perfusion is dictated by the main pedicle and its branches, and the absence of a skin paddle reduces the likelihood of flap ischemia. In addition, donor-site morbidity is lower for myogenous flaps than for myocutaneous flaps. The main reason for this difference in morbidity is that the skin and subcutaneous tissue of the donor site after myogenous flap harvest can be reapproximated without tension and without the need to undermine the subcutaneous tissues widely, which is often required when closing the donor-site defect after elevation of a myocutaneous flap. The potential need for skin grafting at the donor site is also avoided, eliminating possible complications related to skin grafting. Myogenous flaps include the latissimus dorsi, rectus abdominis, and gracilis as well as many other muscles amenable to free tissue transfer.

Osteocutaneous Free Flaps

When treatment for the neoplasm requires resection of the underlying bone, particularly the mandible, an osteocutaneous flap may be utilized to reestablish mandibular continuity, allow dental rehabilitation and restore masticatory function. Resected calvaria and facial bone, most commonly the maxilla, also often require reconstruction at the time of resection. Modalities utilized for reconstruction of bony defects in this setting include nonvascularized bone grafts with plate and screw fixation, alloplastic materials (eg, methyl methacrylate and hydroxyapatite cement), and vascularized bone or osteocutaneous free tissue transfer. The osteocutaneous flap is the most histologically diverse of the flaps, and includes skin, subcutaneous tissue, bone, and generally a cuff of muscle. When a vascularized bone flap is utilized, the success rate is greater than 90%.[12] This success is attributable to the vascular supply of the transferred bone, allowing rapid healing and incorporation into the remaining mandible independent of the vascularity of the recipient bed. Vascularized bone is well suited for the previously irradiated oral cavity, where nonvascularized methods (such as bone grafts) are prone to failure, with failure rates as high as 75% in the acute setting. Bony healing and integration of osteocutaneous flaps are similar to fracture healing in its time course, and this more rapid healing allows patients the return of function earlier than with the use of nonvascularized bone grafts. Enosseous dental implants can be inserted into the bone graft at the time of primary reconstruction, and dental prostheses may be fitted 4 to 6 months postoperatively to allow resumption of normal masticatory function. A comparison of the common osteocutaneous flaps used in head and neck reconstruction is in Table 5.

Fibula Osteocutaneous Flap. The osteocutaneous fibula free flap is a reliable source of well-vascularized bone and soft tissue, and has become the mainstay of modern mandibular reconstruction. Up to 25 cm of bone is available for harvest, and because the fibula is not a load-bearing

Table 5 Similarities and Differences among Osteocutaneous Free Flaps that Are Commonly Used in Head and Neck Reconstruction

Flap	Advantages	Disadvantages
Fibula	• Up to 25 cm of bone available • Large caliber, long vascular pedicle • Ideal bone height • Multiple osteotomies possible • May be used for total mandibular recon-struction • Accepts enosseous dental implants • Two-team approach possible	• Usually requires skin graft • Potential for vascular compromise of lower extremity • Skin paddle fixed to bone • Moderate donor-site morbidity • May be difficult to fit with dental prostheses (dentures)
Radial forearm	• Thin, pliable tissue paddle • Large caliber, long vascular pedicle • Consistent anatomy • Versatile positioning in recipient site • Supports dental prostheses (dentures) • Two-team approach possible	• Limited bone length and height • Donor site visible • Requires skin graft • Potential for vascular compromise of hand • Plating of radius recommended
Scapular	• Large skin paddle available • Skin paddle may be oriented independent of bone axis • Versatile in volume • Multiple osteotomies possible • Primary closure usually possible • Minimal atrophy • Good color match	• Repositioning patient in operating room • Bulky, thick skin • Potential for long-term shoulder dysfunction • Low potential for transfer as sensate flap • Two-team approach difficult
Iliac crest	• Large skin paddle available • Contour similar to mandible • Donor site easily hidden • Primary closure usually possible • Supports enosseous dental implants • Two-team approach	• Bulky skin paddle • Short pedicle • Not pliable in three dimensions • Donor-site morbidity, pain, hernia • Requires abdominal wall reconstruction • Technically challenging • Small caliber, short vascular pedicle • Poor color match

bone, its resection has no functional consequence at the donor site once the wound has healed. With strategic placement of osteotomies and metallic plate fixation, the fibula can be curved to match the contour of the mandible, and both functional and cosmetic outcomes are good. The fibula is the only vascularized bone flap that is versatile and hearty enough to be used for total mandibular reconstruction, as its rich blood supply will allow for multiple shaping osteotomies without compromising perfusion of the bone (Table 6). The fibula will also support enosseous dental implants for future dental rehabilitation, allowing the patient to return to a regular diet eventually and improving perception of quality of life. When dental implants are not planned, however,

the "neomandible" can be a difficult surface to fit with dentures and plates, and in certain cases, this may limit the patient to a soft diet.

The fibula is a long, thin bone of the lateral lower leg whose arterial supply is derived from the most lateral of the three major perfusion trunks of the lower extremity, the peroneal artery. With its venae comitantes, this pedicle provides long and large caliber vessels (1.5 to 4 mm) for microvascular anastomoses at the recipient site. The peroneal artery is positioned close to the fibula and sends perforators laterally to the skin both through a septocutaneous route (through the lateral intermuscular septum) and via muscular perforators. The skin paddle is designed with its epicenter over an axis just posterior to the fibula,

where septocutaneous perforators are predicted to be centered and skin perfusion is maximal. The skin paddle is marked and dissection of the flap proceeds in an anterior to posterior direction, with identification of septal perforators. If no septal perforators are identified, then posteriorly based muscular perforators are preserved by including a cuff of soleus muscle. The appropriate length of fibula is then resected, with caution to preserve the distal 6 to 8 cm of fibula in order to spare the ankle mortise. When the paddle is less than 5 to 7 cm in width, the skin of the lower leg may be closed primarily after undermining of the soft tissues. If a wider skin paddle is required, or if there is tension in closure, a skin graft is used to close the donor site (Figure 11).

The peroneal artery that supplies the fibula flap is one of the three major arteries providing perfusion to the lower leg and foot. Since these vessels are prone to atherosclerotic disease, particularly in the elderly, smokers, and diabetics, it is crucial to confirm adequate three-vessel inflow to the distal part of the lower extremity prior to resection of the peroneal artery. Failure to confirm adequate arterial flow to the lower leg and foot preoperatively can result in devastating ischemic consequences if the peroneal arterial inflow is interrupted in already compromised vascular supply. Because of this risk, harvest of the fibula free flap is absolutely contraindicated in patients with significant arterial ischemic disease of the lower extremities and in patients with inadequate arterial inflow to the distal part of the lower extremity via the posterior tibial and anterior tibial arteries. Historically, routine preoperative arteriography was performed on patients being considered for fibula free flap, but arterial duplex ultrasonography has largely replaced angiography as an inexpensive, noninvasive imaging modality effectively utilized for this purpose.

The primary disadvantage of the fibula osteocutaneous flap is that the limits of the skin paddle are defined by the location of the septocutaneous perforators. To enhance cutaneous vascular supply, a cuff of soleus muscle may be included with the flap to preserve musculocutaneous perforators. Even when all identifiable perforators are preserved, the skin paddle may not be large enough to provide adequate cutaneous coverage

Table 6 Osteocutaneous Free Flaps

Flap	Artery	Artery Diameter	Vein(s)	Pedicle Length	Nerve	Bone
Fibula	Peroneal	1.5–4 mm	Paired peroneal veins (may converge into one)	Up to 8 cm	Lateral sural cutaneous nerve	Fibula (up to 25 cm length)
Radial forearm	Radial	2–2.5 mm	Paired venae comitantes (may converge into one) and/or cephalic vein	Up to 20 cm	Lateral antebrachial cutaneous nerve	Radius (up to 12 cm length)
Scapular	Circumflex scapular (may be followed to subscapular artery)	4 mm (6 mm if followed to subscapular artery)	Paired venae comitantes	7–10 cm (11–14 cm if followed to subscapular vessels)	Dorsal cutaneous rami of T1 and T2 (experimental)	Lateral border of scapula (up to 14 cm length)
Iliac crest	Deep circumflex iliac	2–3 mm	Deep circumflex iliac vein	Up to 6 cm	—	Iliac crest (up to 16 cm length)

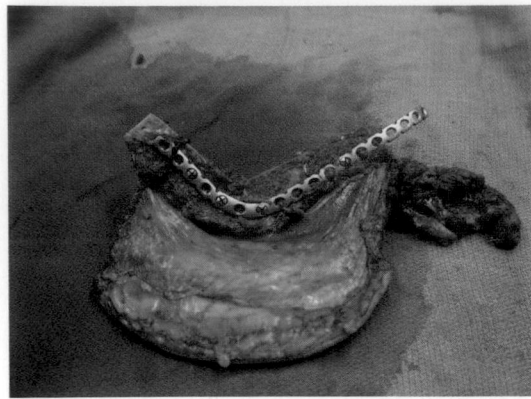

Figure 11 The fibula osteocutaneous flap is a versatile composite flap. The bone can be used to reconstruct a mandibular defect, while the skin is used to reconstruct the soft tissue defect.

and a split-thickness skin graft may be required as an adjunct to free flap reconstruction. An additional limitation of this flap is that the skin paddle is tethered to the underlying fibula, and therefore, positioning and orientation in the recipient site are limited by relatively fixed anatomic relationships within the flap.

Published reports of donor-site complications of fibula osteocutaneous flap harvest have been variable, ranging from 15 to 55%. A 2001 retrospective review of donor-site complications following fibula free flap reported a 39% complication rate with primary closure and a 19% complication rate when a skin graft was employed for closure of the donor site.[13] This difference was hypothesized to be the result of reduction in local ischemia in the setting of tension-free wound closure. Studies of postoperative functional deficits following fibula free flap harvest have generated similar variability in their results. Seventy-two percent were free of any donor pain, and the remainder 28% had only occasional mild discomfort.[14] Other complaints included ankle stiffness 41%, mild ankle instability 10%, and transient peroneal motor 7% or sensory 28% loss, which resolved in all patients. A majority of these patients reported satisfaction with their overall quality of life following surgery.

Radial Forearm Osteocutaneous Flap. The radial forearm is a versatile donor site that may be employed as a source of both soft tissue and bone. A portion of the radius with blood supply based on perforators in the intermuscular septum may be utilized for reconstruction of the mandible or maxilla. A segment of radius measuring 10 to 12 cm in length can be harvested without concern for significant forearm dysfunction. A radial forearm osteocutaneous flap can be raised with attention to preservation of the attachment of the lateral intramuscular septum to the periosteum of the radius, the tissue plane in which the radial-artery-based perforators to the radius travel (see Table 6). A small cuff of flexor pollicis longus muscle is taken to facilitate preservation of these small vessels. The volar (palmar) radial cortex is then incised with an oscillating saw, resulting in resection of a monocortical segment of radial

bone. When a segment of bone is resected from the radius, the bone is weakened, with increased vulnerability to torsional forces. Pathologic fractures may occur as a sequela of radial bone harvest; thus, most surgeons limit the thickness of bone harvest to 40% of the circumference of the radius. Even using this precaution, pathologic fracture rates averaging 8 to 43% may result.[15] A number of surgeons have adopted the practice of routine prophylactic internal plate fixation of the radius at the time of harvest, usually with the assistance of an orthopedic surgeon. The fracture rate has been reduced with keel-shaped osteotomies and prophylactic plating of the donor radius to 1.9% at our institution[16] (Figure 12).

The main advantage of the radial osteocutaneous flap is its association with a cutaneous paddle that is large, pliable, and potentially sensate for oral reconstruction. Because of its long pedicle with large caliber vessels, the flap is also versatile in terms of its position in the recipient site and easily reaches large caliber recipient vessels in the neck. With routine internal fixation of the radius, donor-site morbidity is equivalent to that of the radial forearm fasciocutaneous flap. These potential morbidities include partial necrosis and delayed healing of the skin graft, unappealing cosmetic appearance of the donor site, pain, paresthesias, and rarely, arterial insufficiency of the distal part of the upper extremity. Functional deficits in the donor arm have been reported to occur in 16 to 32% of patients undergoing radial forearm osteocutaneous free flap harvest, with these deficits ranging from subtle alterations in grip strength to marked reduction in range of motion.[17] Because the blood supply of the radius segment is entirely based on a small number of vertical perforators in the intermuscular septum, osteotomies created for establishment of contour must be limited to one or two. Additional disruption of the continuity of the bone is likely to create free-floating, avascular segments that are prone to fail in the recipient site.

Although a limitation of the osteocutaneous radial forearm flap is the length of the bone available, this flap has been utilized widely for oromandibular reconstruction in limited mandibular defects. The rate of postoperative complications of the osteocutaneous radial flap has been

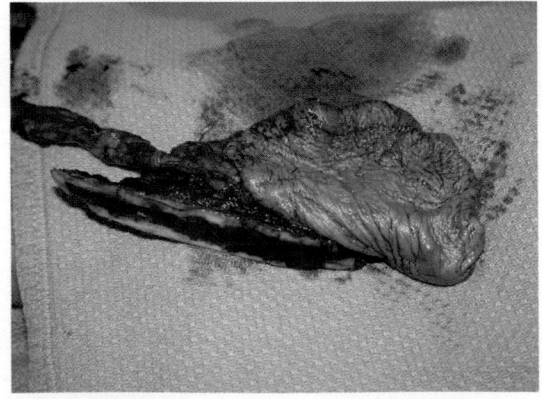

Figure 12 The radial forearm osteocutaneous flap supplies all the advantages of the radial fasciocutaneous flap along with a well-vascularized piece of bone.

demonstrated in several independent studies to be lower than that for the oromandibular reconstruction utilizing a radial fasciocutaneous flap reconstruction paired with plate reconstruction of the mandible. While radial bone is not considered to be hearty enough to support dental implants, a mandible reconstructed with radius will generally support a tissue-borne prosthesis (denture). This is in contrast to more widely utilized osteocutaneous flaps including fibula and scapula, which generally are more difficult to fit with dentures due to their breadth and contour. As most third-party insurers will not cover dental implants, dental rehabilitation is financially less burdensome when radial flap reconstruction is coupled with eventual fitting with dental prostheses.

Scapular Osteocutaneous Flap. The scapular osteocutaneous free flap is considered an extremely versatile flap. A large surface area of skin is available for harvest, and the availability of two underlying muscles (serratus anterior and latissimus dorsi muscles) creates versatility with regard to flap volume. In addition, the thick skin and subcutaneous tissue of the back contribute to the extensive soft tissue bulk that may be harvested from this site. Generally, the soft tissue bulk of this flap is quite durable and persists over years without significant atrophy. The skin, underlying muscles, and scapula are all supplied by one major vascular pedicle that has the advantage of favorable length and vessel caliber. The main arterial supply to the scapular osteocutaneous flap is the circumflex scapular artery. When the pedicle is dissected from its origin, that is, the subscapular artery, arterial diameter averages 4 mm and pedicle length of 7 to 10 cm can be obtained. If a larger caliber vessel or a longer pedicle is required, dissection can proceed proximally along the subscapular artery, where the arterial diameter is up to 6 mm and pedicle length is increased to 11 to 14 cm. There is not a dominant segmental nerve supply to the skin of this region, and therefore this flap is not considered to have the potential for transfer as a sensate flap. There have been reports, however, of use of the dorsal cutaneous rami of T1 or T2 spinal nerves for flap nerve anastomosis, creating the potential for a sensate flap[18] (see Table 6).

Bone harvest is performed at the lateral border of the scapula, with 10 to 14 cm of bone being available from this location. The blood supply to the bone is derived from the periosteal branch of the circumflex scapular artery; and, because the bone is well vascularized, several osteotomies may be performed to create desired contour as long as the highly vascular periosteum is preserved.

The scapular osteocutaneous flap is highly reliable for mandibular reconstruction as the bone of the lateral border of the scapula is well perfused and conforms well to the contour of the mandible (Figure 13). This flap is an excellent choice for reconstruction of complex oromandibular or oromaxillary defects, particularly in complex composite defects involving both the

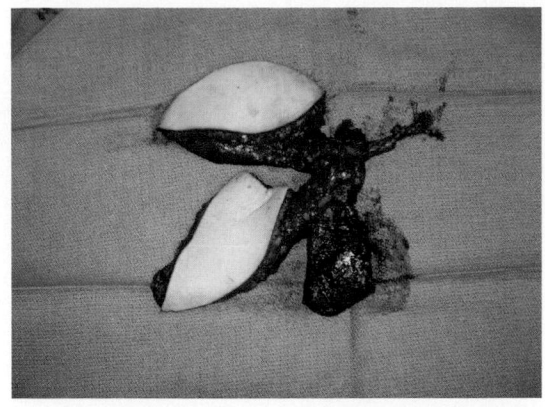

Figure 13 The scapula osteocutaneous free flap supplies a well-vascularized piece of bone that is well suited for bony reconstruction in the head and neck.

oral cavity and the skin of the face and neck. Cosmetically, the skin of the scapular flap is a good color match to the skin of the head and the neck. A unique advantage of this flap for use in mandibular reconstruction is that the skin paddle can be oriented independently from the axis of the bone, based on the circumflex scapular artery that arborizes into several fasciocutaneous branches. As a result of this property, the skin paddle can be designed horizontally (scapular-based on the transverse cutaneous arterial branch) or vertically (parascapular-based on the descending cutaneous arterial branch). Two separate skin paddles may even be elevated in continuity with the bulk of the flap, allowing ideal reconstruction of defects requiring both intraoral mucosal and external skin coverage. For the largest of defects, the bulk of this flap may be expanded by harvest of the scapular "mega flap." This flap includes scapular bone, extensive skin, and a large volume of latissimus dorsi and/or serratus anterior muscle to fill maximal defect volume. Despite the great bulk of this flap, the branching vascular supply of the flap allows the individual components of the flap to be positioned in various three-dimensional orientations relative to one another, resulting in great versatility in the reconstruction of large defects.

Although the scapular osteocutaneous flap is a versatile and durable flap, several disadvantages remain. The first is that the bone of the scapula quickly transitions from thick bone at the lateral border to a thin, flat bone within a distance of 1 to 2 cm medial to that free edge. This limited bone stock is not sufficient for achieving the height of bone required for enosseous dental implant placement into a reconstructed mandible. Secondly, long-term shoulder dysfunction has been reported following harvest of this flap, with postoperative deficits including winging of the scapula, decreased range of motion, and chronic pain. Aggressive physical therapy has demonstrated some benefit in reduction of postoperative functional morbidity, although clearly persistent functional limitations present a significant concern for patients. Finally, there is limited potential for creation of a sensate flap. As an additional consideration for the reconstructive surgeon, a logistical disadvantage of the use of this flap is the need to reposition the patient during the operation, which

limits the ability of surgical teams to perform simultaneous resection of the neoplasm and flap elevation. This results in prolongation of operative and anesthetic times.

Iliac Crest Osteocutaneous Flap. Iliac crest bone has long been used as a reliable source of bone for nonvascularized bone grafts. The vascularized iliac crest osteocutaneous flap is an excellent source of bone and soft tissue suitable for use in free tissue transfer reconstruction of mandibular defects. The iliac crest osteocutaneous flap is based on the deep iliac circumflex vessels, which perfuse the bone and provide cutaneous perforators supplying the skin and subcutaneous tissue. Arterial diameter averages 3 mm, and pedicle length is limited to around 6 cm. Up to 16 cm of bone may be harvested, and skin paddle dimensions up to 10 cm × 30 cm may be transferred on the basis of the arterial supply. Because the perforators of the deep iliac circumflex vessels traverse the abdominal oblique muscles, a cuff of muscle is generally taken with the flap to assure preservation of these vessels. Inclusion of a larger volume of internal oblique muscle with the paddle allows for versatility in the volume of soft tissue transferred (see Table 6).

The native curvature of the iliac crest bone lends itself to reconstruction of the ipsilateral mandible and overlying skin and soft tissue. When the periosteum of the iliac crest bone is preserved, several osteotomies can be made to create the mandibular contour without disrupting the blood supply to the bone. Studies comparing dental rehabilitation following various types of mandibular reconstruction have suggested that iliac crest bone provides the highest quality bone for the support of osseointegrated dental implants.[19] The skin paddle is bulky, and thus, the iliac crest osteocutaneous flap is not ideal for intraoral reconstruction but may be an appropriate choice for medium-volume defects requiring both mandibular and cutaneous reconstructions, such as cheek, neck, or chin defects. Because of the bulky soft tissue overlying the bone, the flap is not pliable in three dimensions, and the versatility of its positioning in the recipient site is limited. To reduce the soft tissue bulk, the flap may also be harvested without skin and covered with a split-thickness skin graft at the recipient site.

A disadvantage of the use of iliac crest osteocutaneous flap is postoperative morbidity related to the development of hernia at the donor site. To reduce this risk, attention must be given to meticulous closure of the layers of the abdominal wall. The transversus abdominis muscle and transversalis fascia are sutured to the iliacus muscle and iliac fascia. The closure of this deep layer may also be reinforced by anchoring the transversus abdominis muscle to drilled holes in the iliac bone. Next, the internal and external oblique muscles and their aponeurosis are sutured to the gluteus medius muscle and tensor muscle of fascia lata muscles. To decrease the likelihood of direct herniation, the internal oblique muscle is retained in a position inferior to the anterior superior iliac

spine and the muscle is secured to the lateral rectus sheath. The inguinal ligament is reattached and inguinal floor repaired. Careful attention to abdominal wall reconstruction reduces but does not completely eliminate the risk of postoperative incisional hernia, and therefore, patients are encouraged to avoid heavy lifting and strenuous activity for a period of 3 months postoperatively.

MIDFACE, MAXILLARY, AND MANDIBULAR RECONSTRUCTION

Variable losses of soft tissue and/or bone, following ablative surgery of the mid face structures can lead to a compromise of the lip, cheek, periorbital soft tissues, palate, and bite. The anatomical, physiological and resulting overall impact on oropharyngeal feeding, speech and esthetics present a challenging dilemma for reconstructive surgeons.

Midface Defects

The midface, including the palate, cheek, maxilla, upper lip, orbit, and nose is a functional and esthetic cornerstone of the facial unit. The maxilla is the structural support between the skull base and the occlusal plane, resisting the forces of mastication, anchoring the dentition, separating the oral and nasal cavities, supporting the globe, and supporting the face and its mimetic musculature. The bony and soft-tissue midface is supported by the maxilla and provides much of the facial appearance that is unique to each individual.

Neoplasms of the maxilla are rarely confined by the bony walls, and resection of adjoining tissues such as the velum, palate, midface, and orbits is frequently required. The associated functional and cosmetic morbidity from loss of these structures is therefore significant. Reconstruction of the midface mandates effective separation of the oral and nasal cavities, restoration of maxillary buttresses, dentition, globe position, and nasal airway as well as the esthetic and dynamic rehabilitation of facial and ocular structures.

Prostheses

The traditional method of rehabilitation of a palatal defect is the use of an obturator. The obturator allows for separation of the oronasal cavities and allows for dental rehabilitation. The surgical complexity and length of procedure are less with obturators than with tissue reconstruction. Other maxillary, nasal, orbital, and ocular prostheses can be employed.

Adequate function and fit of the prosthesis requires fixation of the prosthesis to a nonmobile oral structure. This is most commonly the canine and maxillary teeth. When these are missing, the prosthesis often fits poorly and has limited use. A further limitation of the prosthesis is that it should be removed and cleaned regularly. This may prove difficult for elderly people or those left with vision in only one eye.[5,20,21]

Poor retention of the prosthesis can be due to denture bulkiness, poor residual dentition (both quality and quantity), or poor retentive surfaces. This can create leakage and oronasal regurgitation.[4,6] Furthermore, as more of the zygomatic prominence is lost, the esthetic success and stability of the prosthesis is decreased. Radiotherapy also has a negative effect on the comfort and retention of the obturator and the underlying tissues that support it. Buildup of secretions on the prosthesis contribute to a foul odor that may make it unmanageable.

The theoretical advantage in detection of recurrent tumor with prostheses compared with flap coverage remains unproven, probably because of the accuracy and availability of modern imaging methods that allow accurate assessment of the resection bed without direct inspection.[6] Primary reconstruction is technically superior a secondary procedure although primary use of a prosthetic does not exclude later reconstruction with flaps. Primary reconstruction of a large defect avoids the substantial psychological and emotional distress due to disfigurement.[22] Attesting to the complexity of these anatomical defects, several classification schemes exist.[23]

Palate and Alveolar Ridge

The amount, location, and quality of residual bone of the midface and dentition or denture-bearing alveolar arch largely determine whether or not a bone-containing flap is necessary. Small defects involving the alveolar ridge, teeth, and surrounding mucosa with adequate dentition and no oroantral fistula can be allowed to heal by secondary intention or covered with a local flap such as the palatal-island flap (greater palatine vessel based).[24]

Soft tissue reconstruction, without bony reconstruction, with free flaps may be adequate for patients with dentition and those who do not or cannot undergo more complex reconstructive procedures.[25,26] Bony reconstruction partly preserves the three-dimensional ridge and allows use of osseointegrated implants for functional dentition when adequate bone stock is replaced [27–29] such as fibula, iliac crest, and scapula.[19,30]

Inferior Maxillectomy

Defects that leave an oroantral or oronasal fistula should be closed. In the presence of pre- or post-operative radiation, the radial forearm flap can be used for deep central palatal defects. The pedicled temporalis flap plus skin grafting with or without calvarial bone is another alternative.[31–33] The length and width of the bony component of the radial osteocutaneous free flap is limited to small anterior defects not requiring dental implantation.[26,33,34] Acceptable esthetic result without retraction of the upper lip and near-normal speech may be achieved. For larger defects fibular osteocutaneous[28] or scapular osteocutaneous flaps[35] iliac crest free flaps[29] with appropriate often multiple osteotomies to donor bone for contouring may be necessary. If the patient needs

a dental implant, it can be placed easily as early as 6 to 8 weeks after the reconstruction.

Total Maxillectomy with Orbital Preservation

When the inferior orbital wall is resected there is loss of support of the globe. Without adequate support of the orbit, enophthalmos, "hypophthalmos," and diplopia will result. Various reconstructive techniques range from a prosthetic device to free tissue transfer. Prosthetic reconstruction for orbital support is normally not a good option. Soft-tissue pedicled flaps, such as the temporalis flap, rotated through the osteotomies of the zygomatic arch, are useful in patients who cannot undergo free-tissue transfer.[36,37] The pedicled temporalis and vascularized calvarial bone flap offers appropriately thin and high-quality bone to support the orbit[32,38] and the important zygomaticomaxillary buttress in these patients. Thus, this flap might be used for patients who are not candidates for free-tissue transfer. Since total maxillectomy defects involve multiple soft tissue and bony components of the midface, this option can be combined with other soft-tissue flaps, which could provide bulk to refill the midface contour, for example, a latissimus dorsi flap or a rectus abdominis free flap. These soft-tissue reconstructions, however, do not include the maxillary bony skeleton, particularly the orbit, zygoma, and alveolar ridge which may require vascularized soft-tissue flaps with primary or secondary nonvascularized bone grafting. Rigid globe support may be maintained with cranial or rib bone grafts, whereas the remainder of the defect is filled with the fat and muscle free-tissue transfer. The palate is sealed with soft tissue only.[33,37] Then free tissue is used to reconstruct the maxillary defect, and alloplastic material is used for orbital reconstruction. Titanium mesh or porous polypropelene can be used.

Total Maxillectomy with Orbital Removal

Reconstructive options after total maxillectomy and orbital exenteration depend on the amount of remaining dentition. If enough teeth and alveolar arch remain, a prosthesis can be used although with poor cosmesis and all of the issues mentioned above. A better approach is to complete the palate and alveolar arch with a prosthetic device in conjunction with a bulky myocutaneous flap, such as the rectus abdominis to fill the midface volume, including the orbit.[39,40] The free flap obliterates the dead space and separates the remaining midface sinonasal structures from the oral cavity. Often it is problematic to set a prosthesis that fits.

The bony options described above can be used for both the infraorbital and zygomatic regions and the alveolar arch, but adequate soft tissue should be harvested to fill or line the orbital component of the defect. If the barrier between the brain and the sinuses has been removed with resection of the neoplasm, it must be replaced with vascularized tissue to seal the skull base.

In a study of 16 patients, those who had defects resulting from orbital removal and had less than

30% of the bony orbital rim received reconstruction with an osteocutaneous forearm flap.[41] By contrast, patients who only had cavities where the orbit had been removed received reconstruction with fasciocutaneous forearm flaps. Finally, for radical orbital exenteration cavities with resection of overlying skin and bony malar eminence, osteocutaneous scapula flaps were used. This study cited advantages of autologous tissue reconstruction of the orbit to include durability, defect size kept to a minimum, avoidance of potential accidental displacement of a patch or prosthesis, and the tendency for other peoples' attention to be drawn toward the functional eye instead of a static ocular prosthesis. Additionally, when the eyelids and orbicularis oculi muscles remain unresected, the lids could be sewn together, skin color matched, and facial expression, including the blink reflex, preserved.

Mandible

Segmental mandibulectomy defects after oral cancer resection are usually associated with composite bone and soft tissue defects. Although this discussion focuses on the bony aspects, it must be remembered that the ultimate reconstruction paradigm should factor in the following associated constructs. An ideal reconstruction should restore mandibular continuity, maintain dental occlusal relationships, and restore the contour of the lower third of the face.

The advent of osteocutaneous free flaps has greatly increased the reliability of bone graft for immediate reconstruction of segmental mandibular defects.[42] In the previous era of immediate mandibular reconstruction using nonvascularized bone grafts, the rate of successful restoration of mandibular continuity was only about 50%.[43] A considerable experience with vascularized bone containing free flaps has shown that the rate of successful immediate mandibular reconstruction exceeds 90%.[40,44] The fibular osteocutaneous, radial osteocutaneous, and scapular osteocutaneous flaps may be used depending on the defect and the osteocutaneous tissue available in an individual patient.

A combination of bridging mandibular reconstruction plates may be used to span lateral mandibulectomy defects, with a low volume and a short length of mandibular resection along with a soft tissue free flap. A titanium hollow screw reconstruction plate provides a mechanism for osseointegration at the bone-to-screw interface as well as a locking mechanism at the screw-to-plate interface, resulting in superior hardware stability.[45] Complex three-dimensional composite defects of the lateral parts of the mandible and oropharynx, when the soft tissue resection includes the base of the tongue, lateral oropharyngeal wall and tonsillar fossa, and the soft palate, can be reconstructed using a thin and pliable fasciocutaneous radial forearm free flap and bridging plate.[46] However, bridging plates are not suitable as permanent mandibular substitutes with anterior mandibular defects due to an unacceptably high incidence of intraoral plate extrusion. Further, in select cases, plates may be used with free cancellous iliac bone grafts.

CONCLUSIONS

The advent of free tissue transfer has widely expanded the capabilities of the reconstructive surgeon to recreate acceptable form and function following extensive tissue resection. Selection of a flap for reconstruction is dependent on the characteristics of both the donor and the recipient sites and should be individually tailored to suit each case. Advantages of each flap are weighed against potential morbidity; and, ultimately, a flap is chosen on the basis of its overall suitability for reconstruction of the recipient site. Detailed knowledge of reconstructive options enables the surgeon to select an appropriate reconstructive modality that will achieve an acceptable functional and esthetic outcome for each patient.

REFERENCES

1. Chen TM, Wang HJ, Chen SL, Lin FH. Reconstruction of posttraumatic frontal bone depression using hydroxyapatite cement. Ann Plast Surg 2004;52:303–8.

2. Dias FL, Sa GM, Kligerman J, et al. Prognostic factors and outcome in craniofacial surgery for malignant cutaneous tumors involving the anterior skull base. Arch Otolaryngol Head Neck Surg 1997;123:738–42.

3. Kane WJ, McCaffrey TV, Wang TD, et al. The effect of tissue expansion on previously irradiated skin. Arch Otolaryngol Head Neck Surg 1992;118:419–26.

4. Kroll SS, Schusterman MA, Reece GP, et al. Abdominal wall strength, bulging, and hernia after TRAM flap breast reconstruction. Plast Reconstr Surg 1995;96:616–9.

5. Kimata Y, Uchiyama K, Ebihara S, et al. Versatility of the free anterolateral thigh flap for reconstruction of head and neck defects. Arch Otolaryngol Head Neck Surg 1997;123:1325–31.

6. Levine H. Cutaneous carcinoma of the head and neck: Management of massive and previously uncontrolled lesions. Laryngoscope 1983;93:87–105.

7. Wei FC, Jain V, Celik N, et al. Have we found an ideal soft-tissue flap? An experience with 672 anterolateral thigh flaps. Plast Reconstr Surg 2002;109:2219–26; discussion 2227–30.

8. Sullivan MJ, Carroll WR, Kuriloff DB. Lateral arm free flap in head and neck reconstruction. Arch Otolaryngol Head Neck Surg 1992;118:1095–101.

9. Disa JJ, Pusic AL, Mehrara BJ. Reconstruction of the hypopharynx with the free jejunum transfer. J Surg Oncol 2006;94:466–70.

10. Disa J, Pusic A, Hidalgo DA, et al. Microvascular reconstruction of the hypopharynx: Defect classification, treatment algorithm, and functional outcome based on 165 consecutive cases. Plast Reconstr Surg 2003;111:652–60.

11. Thoma A, Veltri K, Khuthaila D, et al. Comparison of the deep inferior epigastric perforator flap and free transverse rectus abdominis myocutaneous flap in postmastectomy reconstruction: A cost-effectiveness analysis. Plast Reconstr Surg 2004;113:1650–61.

12. Wax MK, Burkey BB, Bascom D, et al. The role of free tissue transfer in the reconstruction of massive neglected skin cancers of the head and neck. Arch Facial Plast Surg 2003;5:479–83.

13. Zimmermann CE, Borner BI, Hasse A, Sieg P. Donor-site morbidity after microvascular fibula transfer. Clin Oral Investig 2001;5:214–9.

14. Anthony JP, Rawnsley JD, Benhaim P, et al. Donor-leg morbidity and function after fibula free flap mandible reconstruction. Plast Reconstr Surg 1995;96:146–52.

15. Hartman EH, Spauwen PH, Jansen JA. Donor-site complications in vascularized bone flap surgery. J Invest Surg 2002;15:185–97.

16. Kim JH, Rosenthal EL, Ellis T, Wax MK. Radial forearm osteocutaneous free flap in maxillofacial and oromandibular reconstructions. Laryngoscope 2005;115:1697–701.

17. Richardson D, Fisher SE, Vaughan ED, Brown JS. Radial forearm flap donor-site complications and morbidity: A prospective study [see comments]. Plast Reconstr Surg 1997;99:109–15.

18. Rhee JS, Weisz DJ, Hirigoyen MB, et al. Intraoperative mapping of sensate flaps. Electrophysiologic techniques and neurosomal boundaries. Arch Otolaryngol Head Neck Surg 1997;123:823–9.

19. Moscoso JF, Keller J, Genden E, et al. Vascularized bone flaps in oromandibular reconstruction: A comparative anatomic study of bone stock from various donor sites to assess suitability for enosseous dental implants. Arch Otolaryngol Head Neck Surg 1994;120:36–43.

20. Funk GF, Laurenzo JF, Valentino J, et al. Free tissue transfer reconstruction of midfacial and cranio-orbito-facial defects. Arch Otolaryngol Head Neck Surg 1995;121:293–303.

21. Kimata Y, Uchiyama K, Ebihara S, et al. Anatomic variations and technical problems of the anterolateral thigh flap: A report of 74 cases. Plast Reconstr Surg 1998;102:1517–23.

22. Lipa JE, Butler CE. Enhancing the outcome of free latissimus dorsi muscle flap reconstruction of scalp defects. Head Neck 2004;26:46–53.

23. Futran ND, Mendez E. Developments in reconstruction of midface and maxilla. Lancet Oncol 2006;7:249–58.

24. Moore BA, Magdy E, Netterville JL, Burkey BB. Palatal reconstruction with the palatal island flap. Laryngoscope 2003;113:946–51.

25. Futran ND. Improvements in the art of midface reconstruction. Curr Opin Otolaryngol Head Neck Surg 2001;9:214–9.

26. Futran ND. Retrospective case series of primary and secondary microvascular free tissue transfer reconstruction of midfacial defects. J Prosthet Dent 2001;86:369–76.

27. Funk GF, Arcuri MR, Frodel JL, Jr. Functional dental rehabilitation of massive palatomaxillary defects: Cases requiring free tissue transfer and osseointegrated implants. Head Neck 1998;20:38–48.

28. Futran ND, Wadsworth JT, Villaret D, Farwell DG. Midface reconstruction with the fibula free flap. Arch Otolaryngol Head Neck Surg 2002;128:161–6.

29. Brown JS. Deep circumflex iliac artery free flap with internal oblique muscle as a new method of immediate reconstruction of maxillectomy defect. Head Neck 1996;18:412–21.

30. Frodel JL, Jr, Funk GF, Capper DT, et al. Osseointegrated implants: A comparative study of bone thickness in four vascularized bone flaps. Plast Reconstr Surg 1993;92:449–55.

31. Colmenero C, Martorell V, Colmenero B, Sierra I. Temporalis myofascial flap for maxillofacial reconstruction. J Oral Maxillofac Surg 1991;49:1067–73.

32. Choung PH, Nam IW, Kim KS. Vascularized cranial bone grafts for mandibular and maxillary reconstruction: The parietal osteofascial flap. J Craniomaxillofac Surg 1991;19:235–42.

33. Villaret DB, Futran NA. The indications and outcomes in the use of osteocutaneous radial forearm free flap. Head Neck 2003;25:475–81.

34. Freije JE, Campbell B, Yousif NJ, Mathoub HS. Reconstruction after infrastructure maxillectomy using dual free flaps. Laryngoscope 1997;107:694–97.

35. Granick MS, Ramasastry SS, Newton ED, et al. Reconstruction of complex maxillectomy defects with the scapular-free flap. Head Neck 1990;12:377–85.

36. Muzaffar AR, Adams WP, Hartog JM, et al. Maxillary reconstruction: Functional and aesthetic considerations. Plast Reconstr Surg 1999;104:2172–83.

37. Coleman JJ, 3rd. Osseous reconstruction of the midface and orbits. Clin Plast Surg 1994;1:113–24.

38. Parhiscar A, Har-El G, Turk JB, Abramson DL. Temporoparietal osteofascial flap for head and neck reconstruction. J Oral Maxillofac Surg 2002;60:619–2

39. Cordeiro PG, Santamaria E. A classification system and algorithm for reconstruction of maxillectomy and midfacial defects plastic and reconstructive surgery. Plast Reconstr Surg 2000;105:2331–46.

40. Cordeiro PG, Disa JJ. Challenges in midface reconstruction. Semin Surg Oncol 2000;19:2135.

41. Chepeha DB, Moyer JS, Bradford CR, et al. Osteocutaneous radial forearm free tissue transfer for repair of complex midfacial defects. Arch Otolaryngol Head Neck Surg 2005;131:513–7.

42. Brown JS, Rogers SN, McNally DN, Boyle M. A modified classification for the maxillectomy defect. Head Neck 2000;22:17–26.

43. McGregor IA, McGregor FM. Cancer of the Face and Mouth: Pathology and Management for Surgeons, 1st edition. New York: Churchill Livingstone; 1986.

44. Wells MD, Luce EA. Reconstruction of midfacial defects after surgical resection of malignancies. Clin Plast Surg 1995;522:79–91.

45. Brown KE. Peripheral consideration in improving obturator retention. J Prosthet Dent 1968;20:176–81.

46. Edgerton MT, DeVito RV. Closure of palatal defects by means of a hinged nasal septum flap. Plast Reconstr Surg 1963;31–33:537–40.

60

Rejuvenation of the Upper Face and Midface

Theda C. Kontis, MD
John S. Rhee, MD, MPH

As the face ages, forehead horizontal rhytides develop and deepen, eventually followed by vertical lines in the glabella. The eyebrows begin to descend and flatten, resulting in lateral hooding of the upper eyelid region. Lax and redundant eyelid skin, along with the appearance of fat protrusion, is also a component of the aging upper third of the face. Ptosis and soft tissue hollowing of the malar complex are the key aging changes of the midface, which result in changes in the lower eyelid complex as well as the nasolabial fold (Figure 1).[1] Rejuvenation of the upper one-third of the face consists of treating the forehead, eyebrow, and periorbital complex. Rejuvenation of the midface consists of addressing the malar complex and its relationship to the lower eyelid and nasolabial fold.

The primary focus of the chapter is to provide an overview of the surgical techniques that are available for addressing the aged mid and upper thirds of the face.

APPLIED SURGICAL ANATOMY

Forehead

The central forehead and scalp is composed of five distinct layers, described by the mnemonic device SCALP: skin, subcutaneous tissue, galea aponeurosis, loose areolar tissue, and pericranium (Figure 2).[2] The skin is thick and densely adherent to the underlying subcutaneous tissue. The galea aponeurosis is a thin, mobile, fibromuscular sheet that envelops the entire skull and splits anteriorly to encase the frontalis and procerus muscles. The galea is an extension of the superficial musculoaponeurotic system (SMAS) in the face and the temporoparietal fascia of the temple. The loose areolar tissue plane is a relatively avascular plane and the traditional layer of dissection for coronal approaches. This layer is continuous with the loose connective tissue which separates the temporoparietal fascia and the deep temporal fascia. The pericranium is a thickened layer of connective tissue adherent to the skull and is continuous with the periorbita at the level of the supraorbital ridges.[3]

The sensory innervation of the forehead and scalp is supplied by the supraorbital and supratrochlear nerves, which are divisions of the ophthalmic branch of the trigeminal nerve. Both nerves exit the frontal bone through a notch or

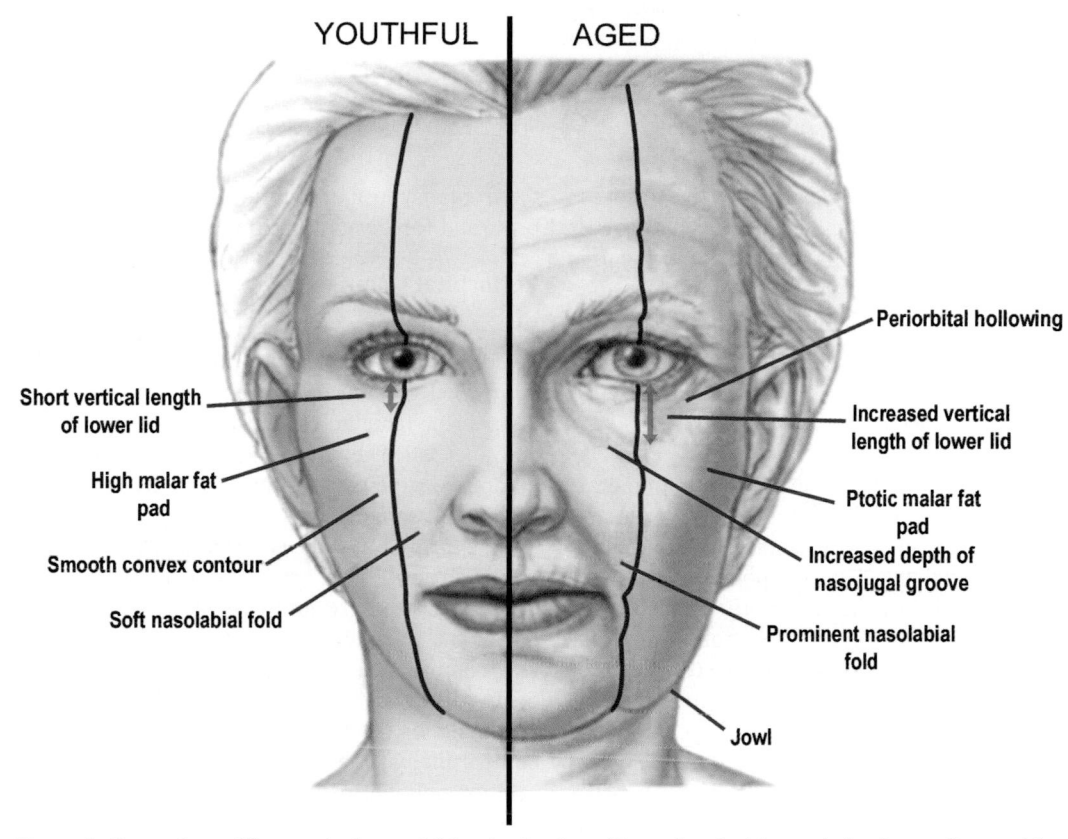

Figure 1 Comparison of features in the youthful and aging face. (Reproduced with permission from reference 1.)

foramen, pierce the orbital septum, turn upward to pierce the corrugator supercilii muscle, and travel on the superficial aspect of the frontalis muscle (Figure 3).

The actions of the muscles of the brow and forehead are listed in Table 1. The temporal branch of the facial nerve innervates all of these muscles. It is the mimetic actions of these muscles

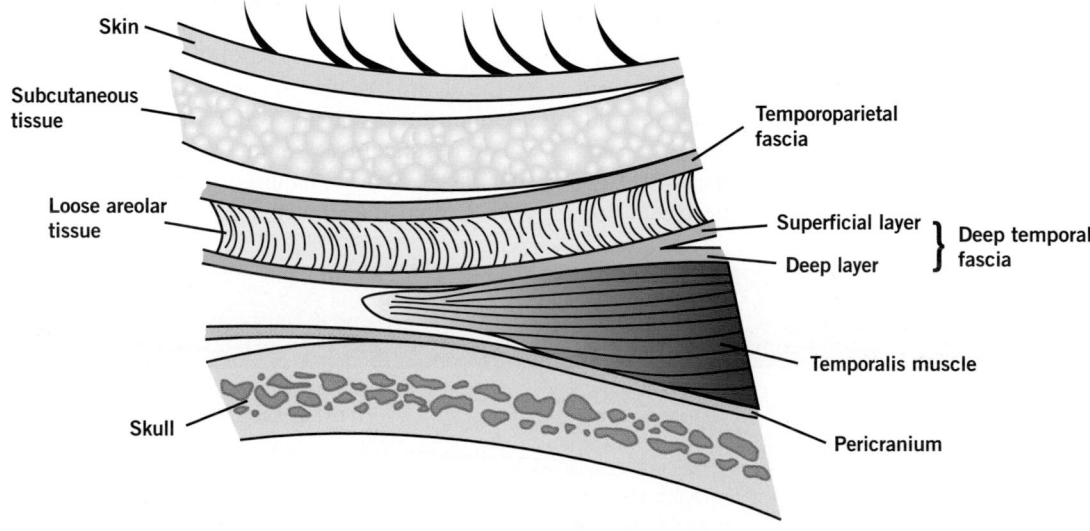

Figure 2 The layers of the scalp and temple. (Reproduced with permission from reference 2.)

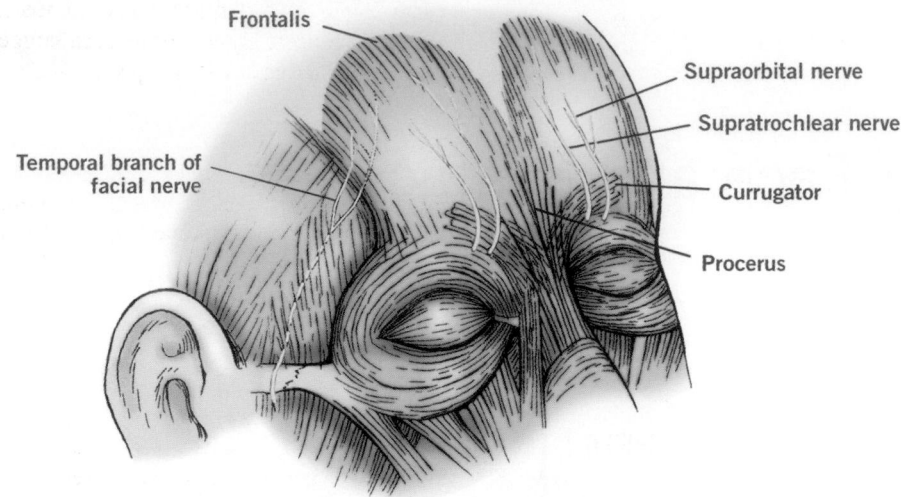

Figure 3 The nerves and expressive muscles of the forehead and temple. (Reproduced with permission from reference 2.)

that produce the wrinkles and furrows in the skin of the forehead and glabellar areas. The corrugator and procerus muscles are usually surgically weakened in the correction of the aging brow and forehead. These muscles are also the targets of temporary chemodenervation by the injection of botulinum toxin.

Temporal Fossa

The transition from the forehead to the temporal fossa occurs at the superior temporal line, demarcated by the conjoint fascia, a condensation of the pericranium and the deep temporal fascia. The temporal fossa is bounded inferiorly by the zygomatic arch and anteriorly by the frontal process of the zygomatic bone. The fascial layers of the temporal fossa have been prone to confusing and conflicting nomenclature (see Figure 2).

The temporoparietal fascia is a thin, vascular layer, densely adherent to the overlying subcutaneous tissue and skin. This layer is continuous with the galea aponeurosis of the scalp and SMAS of the face. The deep temporal fascia envelops the temporalis muscle and divides into a superficial and deep layer at approximately 2 cm above the zygomatic arch. The arch and the temporal fat pad are ensheathed by the superficial and deep layers of the deep temporal fascia.

Understanding the course of the temporal branch of the facial nerve is critical to safe dissection in this area. The nerve enters the temporal fossa by crossing superficially over the midportion of the zygomatic arch. It travels in the temporoparietal fascia layer and then exits the temporal fossa to course along the deep aspect of

the frontalis muscle, supplying the muscles of the brow and forehead (see Figure 3).

Periorbital Complex

The eyelids are formed by multiple soft tissue layers and are divided into an anterior lamella, composed of skin and orbicularis muscle, and a posterior lamella, composed of the tarsus and conjunctiva. The upper and lower eyelids are composed of analogous structures that are better defined in the upper lid (Figure 4).[4]

The orbital septum is a fibrous structure that lies superficial to the orbital fat pads. With aging, the septum weakens allowing prolapse of the fat pads. The preaponeurotic fat is subdivided into two compartments in the upper lid: medial and central. The lacrimal gland fills the lateral compartment. In the lower lid, the fat lies in three compartments: medial, central, and lateral. The inferior oblique muscle lies between the medial and central compartments. Relatively large blood vessels supply the fat pads.

The levator palpebrae superioris muscle is the primary elevator of the upper eyelid and is innervated by the oculomotor nerve. The levator muscle arises from the orbital apex and courses anteriorly where it thins to a broad aponeurosis that inserts onto the anterior surface of the tarsal plate. The supratarsal crease is created by anterior extension of some of the fibers to attach to the dermis of the eyelid skin. In the Asian lid, aponeurotic fibers do not attach to the skin, which results in a "single eyelid," without a supratarsal crease. Acquired ptosis of the upper eyelid often is a result of levator dehiscence

from the tarsal plate and must be identified preoperatively.

Midface

The midface is the triangular region bounded by the inferior orbital rim, nasolabial fold, and anterior border of the masseter muscle. The malar fat pad is a large fibrofatty subcutaneous pad which lies superficial to the zygomaticus major and minor muscles. The zygomatic branch of the facial nerve travels deep to the superior aspect of the zygomaticus muscles. In the youthful face, the subobicularis oculi fat (SOOF) pad lies between the orbicularis muscle and orbital rim periosteum at the level of the arcus marginalis[5] (Figure 5). The arcus marginalis is the attachment of the orbital septum to the periosteum of the inferior orbital rim. The orbital septum inserts into the inferior tarsal margin. Fat repositioning procedures target the arcus marginalis as the site of fat release.

The levator labii superioris muscle arises on the medial aspect of the inferior orbital rim, and the SOOF envelops it in youth. The infraorbital nerve foramen and nerve are located just deep to the origin of the levator labii superioris muscle. The SOOF in the aging face is often located below the origin of the levetor labii superioris muscle.[6] Midfacial rejuvenation techniques target resuspension of the SOOF and/or malar complex. In addition, blepharoplasty techniques now emphasize orbital fat preservation and repositioning to improve the tear trough deformity. The tear trough deformity, or nasojugal groove, is a depression of the soft tissue between the medial canthus and the lateral nasal sidewall (see Figure 1).

ESTHETIC CONSIDERATIONS

Brow and Forehead

The eyebrow is shaped as a graceful, gentle arch. The ideal position and shape of the eyebrow is quite subjective and varies according to gender, ethnicity, and current fashion trends. As a general rule, the medial brow has a clubhead configuration and begins at a point tangent to a vertical line drawn through the medial canthus and lateral nasal ala margin (Figure 6). The brow gradually tapers to a handle shape, with the lateral third of the brow coursing above the superior orbital rim in women and at the rim in men. It terminates laterally at a point tangent to an oblique line drawn from the lateral nasal ala to the lateral canthus.[7] Depending on one's esthetic sense, the apex of the brow arch should lie between the lateral limbus of the cornea and the lateral canthus.[8]

The upper third of the face is a focal point for expression and emotions. With the aging process, there is loss of tissue elasticity, decrease in the bulk of the subcutaneous tissue, and an increase in skull bone resorption. Excessive displacement of the medial portion of the eyebrows along with deep glabellar furrows may project expressions of anger or malice. A similar lateral hooding or drooping of the eyebrows suggests a fatigued or sad appearance.[9]

Table 1 Muscles of the Upper Third of the Face		
Muscle	Action	Result
Frontalis	Elevates brow	Forehead rhytides
Obicularis oculi	Depresses brow	Crows feet
	Closes eyelids	
Procerus	Depresses medial brow	Transverse glabellar rhytides
Corrugator	Depresses brow	Vertical glabellar rhytides
	Medializes brow	

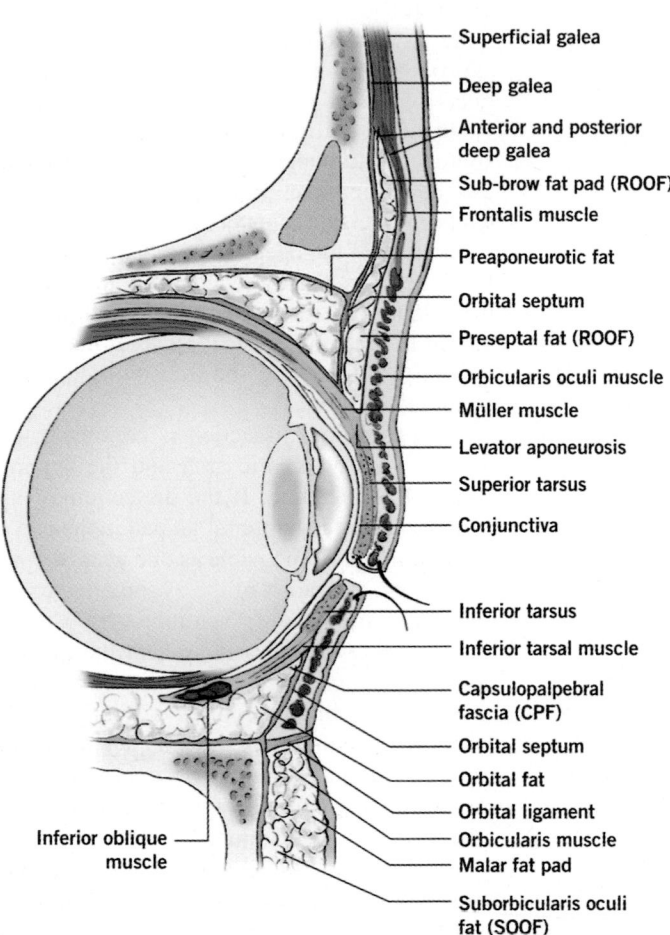

Superficial galea

Deep galea

Anterior and posterior deep galea

Sub-brow fat pad (ROOF)

Frontalis muscle

Preaponeurotic fat

Orbital septum

Preseptal fat (ROOF)

Orbicularis oculi muscle

Müller muscle

Levator aponeurosis

Superior tarsus

Conjunctiva

Inferior tarsus

Inferior tarsal muscle

Capsulopalpebral fascia (CPF)

Orbital septum

Orbital fat

Orbital ligament

Orbicularis muscle

Malar fat pad

Suborbicularis oculi fat (SOOF)

Inferior oblique muscle

Figure 4 Sagittal view of the upper and lower eyelid anatomy. (Reproduced with permission from reference 4.)

Some surgeons have turned to more objective parameters when assessing harmony of the upper third of the face. McKinney and colleagues described the existence of brow ptosis when the distance from the midpupil to the top of the brow was less than 2.5 cm[10] (see Figure 6). In addition, they noted that the female forehead should measure 4 to 6.2 cm (mean 4.8 cm). Farkas and Kolar found that the most attractive women had a relatively smaller upper third of the face compared to the middle and lower thirds of the face.[11] It is important to remember that certain browlifting techniques can raise the hairline which can significantly alter the harmony and balance of the horizontal facial thirds.

Periorbital Complex

The ideal esthetic appearance of the upper eyelid varies with gender and ethnicity. In Caucasian women, the tarsal crease lies 10 to 11 mm above the lash line. In men, the crease lies only 8 to 10 mm above the eyelid margin. Approximately 50% of Asians have an absent tarsal crease.

The upper eyelid should cover the corneal limbus by approximately 1 to 2 mm. If the sclera is visible between the lid margin and limbus, lid retraction is present and may be due to thyroid ophthalmopathy. Ptosis, or drooping of the upper eyelid, can be congenital or acquired and should be evaluated preoperatively.

The lower eyelid margin should just meet the limbus. Scleral show in this area suggests a weakening of the lower lid support.

Midface

A prominent malar complex is generally associated with youth and beauty. Because the midface ages as a result of both volume loss and the effects of gravity on the tissues, the goal of midface rejuvenation is the restoration of volume as well as repositioning the ptotic tissues.

As one ages, the soft tissues of the malar complex become ptotic, accentuating the infraorbital bony rim. The nasolabial fold deepens, and the lower eyelid becomes lax, increasing scleral show. The distance between the inferior lid and malar crescent widens,[12] and the nasojugal or "tear trough" deformity appears. Pseudoherniated fat lies above the orbital rim and the descended malar pad below, creating a double convexity deformity of the lower lid midface complex (see Figure 1).

SURGICAL APPROACHES

Brow and Forehead

Careful patient selection and appropriate surgical goals will help to ensure optimal results. In evaluating candidates for rejuvenation of the upper third of the face, it is important to keep in mind the esthetics of the brow and the upper third of the face. The need for an upper lid blepharoplasty may either be obviated by a brow lift or it may markedly reduce the requirements for skin excision. The entire orbital complex, brow position, frontal hairline, hair density,

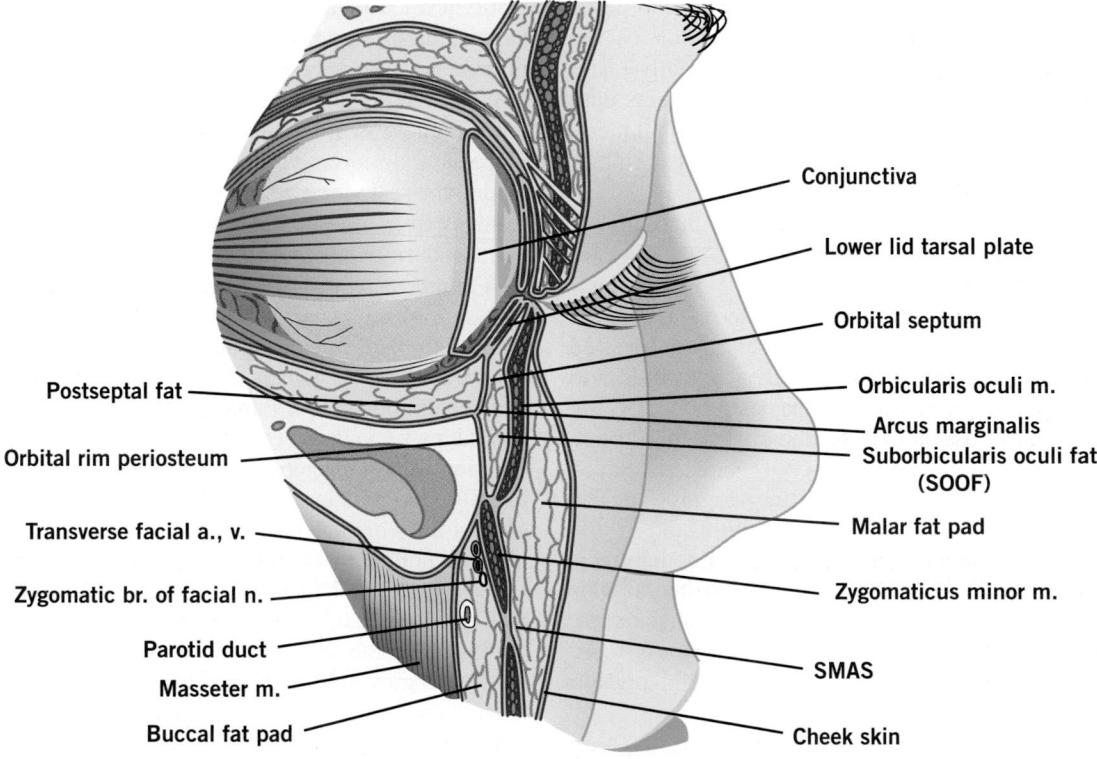

Conjunctiva

Lower lid tarsal plate

Orbital septum

Orbicularis oculi m.

Arcus marginalis

Suborbicularis oculi fat (SOOF)

Malar fat pad

Zygomaticus minor m.

SMAS

Cheek skin

Postseptal fat

Orbital rim periosteum

Transverse facial a., v.

Zygomatic br. of facial n.

Parotid duct

Masseter m.

Buccal fat pad

Figure 5 Sagittal view of midface anatomy. (Reproduced with permission from reference 1.)

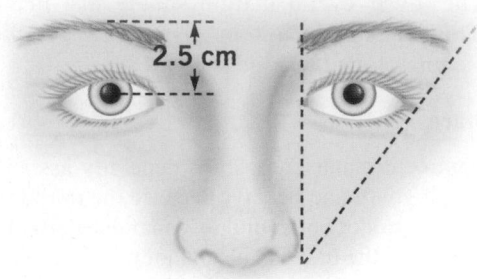

Figure 6 Ideal eyebrow position and proportion. The medial aspect of the brow begins at a point tangent to a vertical line drawn through the medial canthus and lateral nasal ala margin and terminates laterally at a point tangent to an oblique line drawn from the lateral nasal ala to the lateral canthus. The apex of the brow arch should lie between the lateral limbus of the cornea and the lateral canthus. Brow ptosis exists when the distance from the midpupil to the top of the brow is less than 2.5 cm. (Reproduced with permission from reference 2.)

forehead contour, forehead rhytides and furrows caused by the actions of the underlying musculature should all be considered in the preoperative assessment.

There are several surgical approaches, endoscopic, coronal, trichophytic, direct, and mid forehead. The latter two choices are less commonly used and more appropriate for facial paralysis patients or in men with thick and heavy skin with prominent forehead rhytides. The ideal candidate for the endoscopic approach has the following characteristics: female, low hairline, abundant hair, flat contour of the forehead, normal or thin skin, and moderate brow ptosis.

Patients requiring extensive bone recontouring may be better treated with an open procedure. Patients with thick, heavy sebaceous skin and severe brow ptosis are less favorable candidates and may be better served with conventional open skin excision techniques (coronal or trichophytic approaches). Also, surgical weakening of the brow depressor muscles is often technically easier using the open approaches. Finally, patients with high hairlines, sparse hair, male pattern baldness, and rounded foreheads are less ideal candidates for the endoscopic approach.

Regardless of the choice of incisions or approaches, there are basically four steps in executing the brow lift: (1) placement of precise incisions, (2) dissection and adequate release of the scalp and forehead, (3) myotomy of the desired facial expressive muscles, and (4) elevation and fixation of the forehead to the desired level.

The endoscopic forehead lift has been described using four, five, or six incisions placed 2 to 3 cm behind the hairline (Figure 7). The central incision marks the midline and is the main endoscopic port. The two paramedian incisions are placed at the level of the lateral limbus or canthus. The two temporal incisions are needed for dissection over the temporalis fossa and allow better positioning the lateral portion of the brow.

For the coronal brow lift approach, the skin excision is fusiform and placed 5 to 6 cm behind

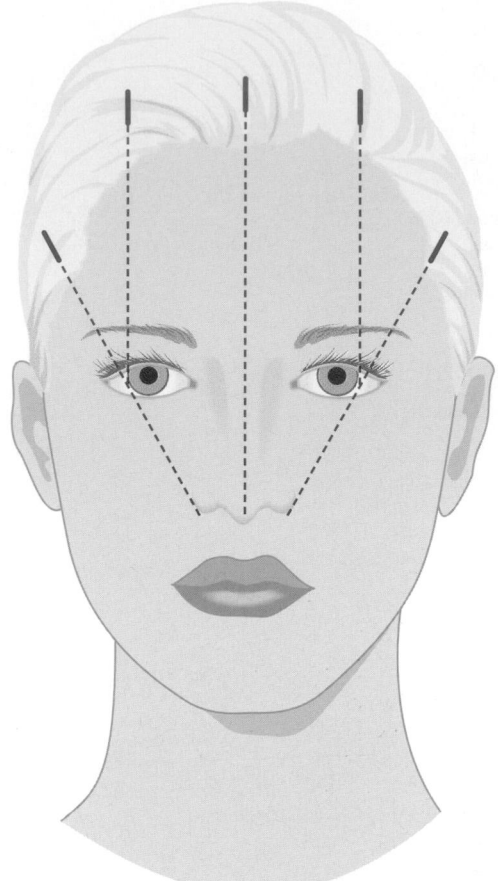

Figure 7 Placement of the incisions for the endoscopic brow lift. The paramedian incisions should be tangent to the lateral limbus of the cornea. The temporal incisions should be tangent to a line between the lateral limbus of the cornea and the lateral alar base. The temporal incisions may be placed made more laterally, depending on individual esthetic desires and goals. (Reproduced with permission from reference 2.)

the anterior aspect of the hairline. A curvilinear incision is drawn to parallel the hairline with the blade beveled parallel to the natural axis of the hair follicles. The amount of skin excised is determined preoperatively, generally about 1 to 2 cm. The main disadvantages of this approach include undesirable elevation of the hairline, potential alopecia and more visible scars, and paresthesia behind the scalp incision. Usually the paresthesia resolves over time, but it can be bothersome to patients during the recovery.

Candidates who have a high hairline may be best served with a trichophytic approach. The incision is made in the gradual transition zone between the thick hair of the scalp and the thin wispy hair at the true hairline. The incision parallels the natural curvature of the hairline, and the excision pattern resembles a gentle W-plasty. The lateral extensions proceed into the temporal hair about 4 to 5 cm bilaterally. The bevel of the blade is usually 60° to 90° to the natural axis of the hair follicle along the hairline and then becomes parallel to the natural hair follicle in the temple. The goal is allow the hair follicles along the anterior hairline to grow through the incision to help camouflage the scar. As in the coronal approach, usually about 1 to 2 cm of scalp is excised. Meticulous closure of the anterior hairline is essential

for a successful cosmetic outcome. The main disadvantages of this approach are potentially a more visible incision compared to the endoscopic approach and paresthesia behind the incision line.

In all browlifts, regardless of the surgical approach, the plane of dissection over the skull can be either subperiosteal or subgaleal. The temporal incision is extended down to the superficial layer of the deep temporalis fascia. Using a freer elevator, the dissection is continued along this plane and the temporal dissection is connected to the subperiosteal plane of the forehead by sharply dissecting the transition zone at the temporal crest line.

The temporal dissection is continued to the level of the zygomatic arch and the zygomaticofrontal suture line. If the dissection is in the correct plane, the temporal fat pad in the elevated flap should become visible as one nears the zygomatic arch. A branch of the zygomaticotemporal communicating vein ("sentinel vein") is often encountered when dissecting near the zygomaticofrontal suture line. The vein can either by cauterized with a bipolar cautery or gently dissected from the surrounding tissue. The temporal branch of the facial nerve runs in close proximity to the vein. Bleeding caused by injury to this vein can lead to poor visualization, and possibly inadvertent injury to the facial nerve from cauterization or further dissection. Overzealous upward retraction in the temporal area should be avoided as it may cause traction neuropraxia of the frontal branch of the facial nerve.

It is important to release fully the entire length of the superior arcus marginalis to achieve adequate brow elevation. The periosteum and galea are horizontally scored at this point, exposing the corrugator muscle, procerus muscle, supraorbital nerve, and supratrochlear nerve. In patients in whom glabellar muscle modification is desired, the supratrochlear and supraorbital nerves are dissected from the corrugator muscles by using a gentle vertical spreading motion with Takahashi forceps.

Once the nerves are safely separated from the corrugator muscle, the muscle is gently avulsed or transected. The procerus muscle can be approached in similar fashion. The subcutaneous fat will become visible upon removal of the muscle. Care should be taken not to remove any subcutaneous tissue, as dimpling or contour irregularities will occur. It is not necessary to remove all of the muscle fibers to achieve the desired result; the extent of the resection should be tailored to the preoperative assessment of the severity of the glabellar frown lines.

Surgeons differ in their use of fixation methods to reposition the forehead soft tissues. Central brow fixation techniques include the use of miniplates, screws, bone bars, bioabsorbable fixation devices (ENDOTINE Forehead device, Coapt Systems, Inc., Palo Alto, CA), and various suture techniques[13–16] (Figure 8). The temporal fixation determines the final position of the lateral brow. In the endoscopic approach, the anterior corner of

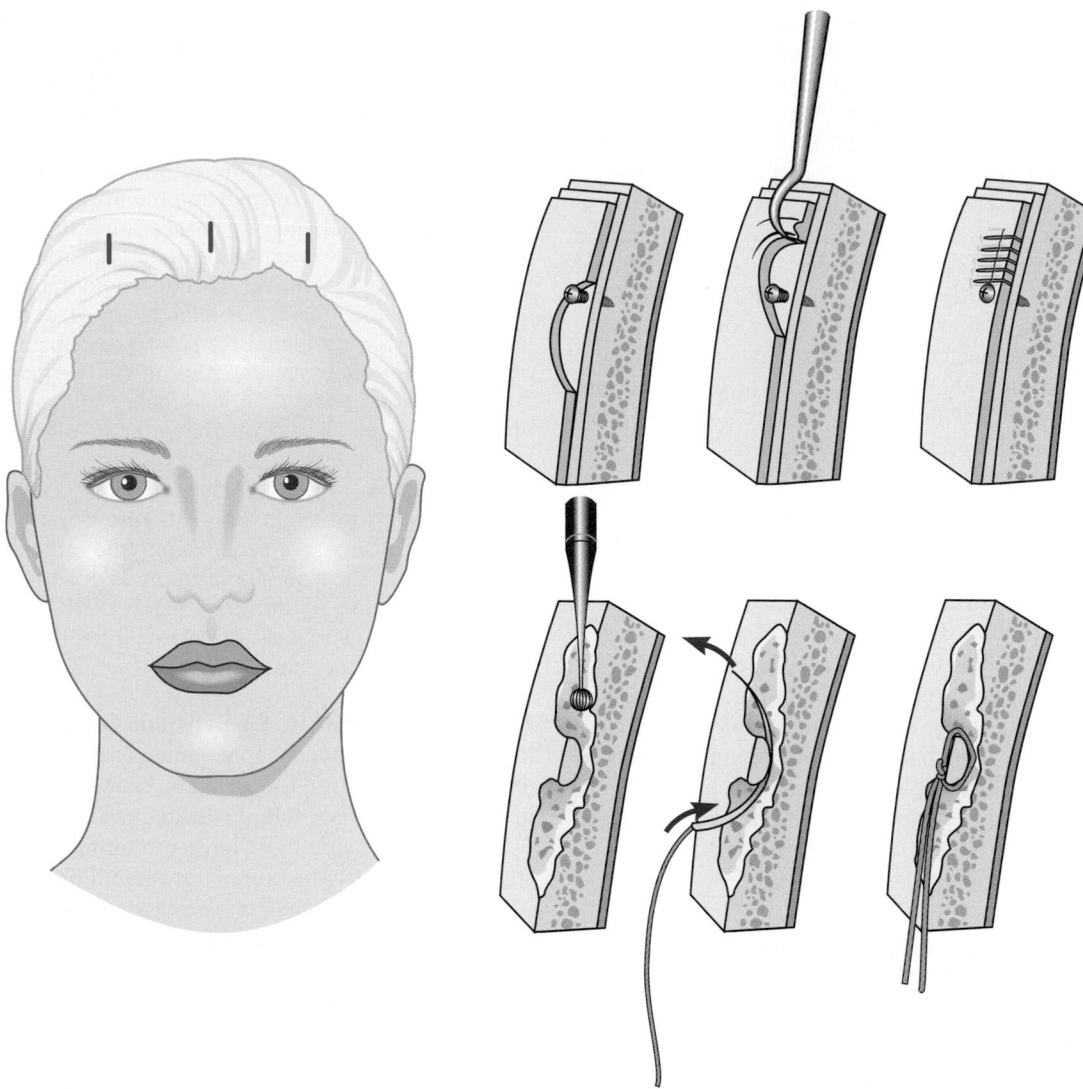

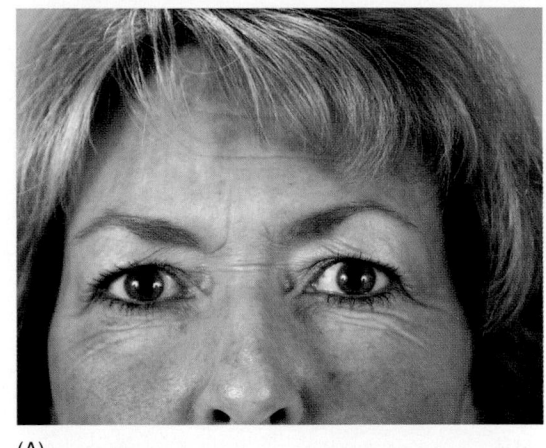

(A)

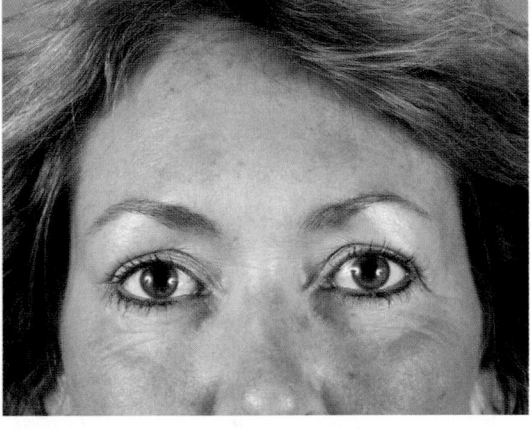

(B)

Figure 9 (A) Preoperative view. This patient underwent an endoscopic browlift with the ENDOTINE Forehead device used for fixation, upper blepharoplasty and chemical peel of the lower lid skin. (B) Six-week postoperative result.

Figure 8 Fixation techniques. Top row: Variation on the external screw technique. A screw is placed at the posterior extent of the vertical incision and the scalp complex is advanced posteriorly. Surgical staples are placed behind the protruding screw. Bottom row: Creation of an outer cortex bone bar with a cutting burr. Suture from the galeal-periosteal layer is secured to the bone bar. (Reproduced with permission from reference 2.)

the incision is engaged and secured to the desired point on the temporalis fascia, determined by the desired vector pull. Regardless of the method of fixation, adequate dissection and mobilization of the forehead tissue are paramount for successful brow elevation. In the skin excision techniques, deeper fixation is not necessary; but, as mentioned above, complete release and mobilization of the brow and forehead are necessary for a successful outcome.

Blepharoplasty

Upper Blepharoplasty. Surgery of the upper eyelids involves excision of an ellipse of skin, just superior to the tarsal crease. The lower limb of the incision is placed in the natural upper lid crease. In cases in which the natural crease is not well demarcated, then the lower incision is made 10 to 11 mm above the lash line in women and 8 to 10 mm above the lash line in men. The incision extends from the level of the punctum medially to a natural crow's feet crease laterally at the level of the lateral orbital rim. The shape of the excised skin is generally elliptical, with the incision tapered gently medially and wider

laterally to address lateral hooding. The incisions must be drawn symmetrically or in such a way to account for preoperative asymmetry. If a browlift is to be performed, it is performed first to prevent excessive removal of upper eyelid skin during blepharoplasty.

Once the skin and subcutaneous skin is removed, the orbicularis muscle is divided which reveals the fine connective tissue of the orbital septum. This area is carefully separated to expose the medial and central fat pads. In some cases, a strip of obicularis muscle can be removed paralleling the skin incision to accentuate the creation of the upper lid crease or to remove hypertrophic muscle. The orbital septum is opened to expose the two fat pads of the upper eyelid. The fat is conservatively removed from the medial and middle compartments, and hemostasis is meticulously obtained. The skin edges are then reapproximated (Figure 9).

Lower Blepharoplasty. Surgical approaches used to remove prolapsed fat from the lower eyelids can be performed through subciliary or transconjunctival incisions. The subciliary approach

is generally selected when excess lower lid skin must be excised. The plane of dissection is usually under the orbicularis muscle. When this approach is used, care must be taken to assess the laxity of the lower lid. By using a "snap" or "pinch" test, the resiliency of the lower lid can be ascertained. When a lower lid is pulled down and slowly returns to its original position or is pinched and slowly returns to touching the globe, a tarsal suspension procedure must be performed to prevent postoperative ectropion. The transconjunctival approach to the lower lids was developed mainly to prevent ectropion.

After performing the lower lid incision, the three orbital fat compartments (medial, central, lateral) are exposed. Each fat pad is dissected free, cauterized, and excised. Because the fat pads retract after manipulation, meticulous hemostasis is necessary to prevent an orbital hematoma. Increased pressure in the globe from a hematoma can cause a decrease in retinal artery flow and potentially result in blindness.

Because modern techniques of facial rejuvenation focus on volume restoration, often fat preservation rather than removal is performed on the lower lids, especially in the presence of a tear trough deformity (Figure 10). This area can be approached by either a subciliary or transconjunctival incision. Once the three fat

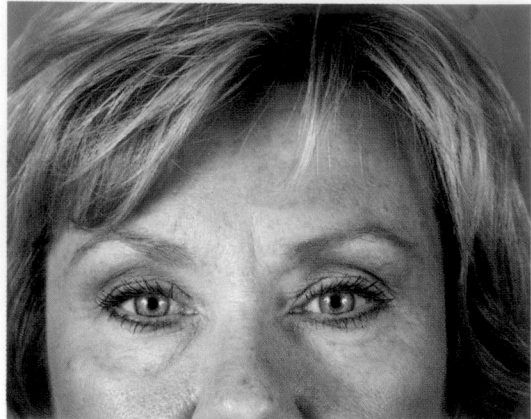

(A)

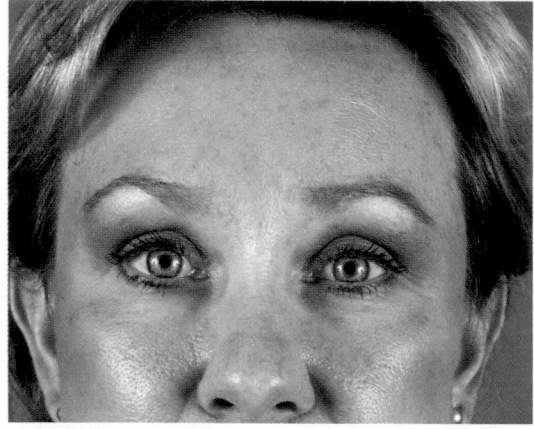

(B)

Figure 10 (A) Preoperative view. This patient underwent upper and lower blepharoplasty with lower lid fat preservation and transposition to improve the tear trough deformity, and endoscopic browlift with ENDOTINE Forehead Device fixation. (B) Six-week postoperative view.

pads are isolated, conservative removal of fat from the lateral compartment is performed. Fat from the central pocket may be removed conservatively, if required. The white band of the arcus marginalis is identified on the bony infraorbital rim and divided, exposing the anterior maxilla. The subperiosteal plane is dissected to allow insertion of the freed fat pad. Dissection can instead be performed in the supraperiosteal plane, but dissection through the orbicularis muscle makes this a bloodier plane. The fat pad is dissected to allow sufficient rotation and the pedicle thinned to a width of 0.5 to 1.0 cm. The pedicled fat pad is actually a random flap, despite the presence of somewhat large feeding vessels. Suture stabilization of the fat pad can be performed by suturing to the SOOF or by imbrication. Once the fat is positioned, a forced duction test of the globe is performed to ensure no restriction of extraocular movement with upward gaze. Patients may experience prolonged edema from subperiosteal dissection. The fat pedicle may become hardened for 3 to 6 months postoperatively. Long-term fat survival rate may vary, but most patients maintain improvement in the nasojugal region. This approach specifically targets the tear trough deformity and does not elevate the SOOF or malar pad.

Midface

Transblepharoplasty Midface Suspension. With the transblepharoplasty midface suspension, an extended subciliary approach allows elevation of the malar complex at the same time as softening of the nasojugal groove. The subciliary incision is extended 1.5 cm lateral to the lateral canthus. A skin-muscle flap is elevated in the plane between the orbicularis muscle and orbital septum. An incision is created along the arcus marginalis, and the subperiosteal dissection is performed along the anterior aspect of the maxilla. The dissection extends laterally to the zygomatic arch and medially to the nasolabial fold, with care to protect the infraorbital nerve. The orbital septum is opened and the infraorbital fat from the medial and/or central compartments is draped over the inferior orbital rim, softening the nasojugal groove. Through a temporal hairline incision, the superficial layer of deep temporal fascia is isolated for suture suspension of the malar soft tissue complex in the vertical direction. Alternatively, an absorbable Endotine implant may be placed on the inferior orbital rim by screw fixation and used to suspend the malar complex. A canthoplasty or canthopexy is usually performed to prevent postoperative ectropion. Conservative eyelid skin removal may be performed. The skin blood supply is not compromised because of the deep plane of dissection, and laser resurfacing or chemical peels can be performed at the same time.[17]

Endoscopic Midface Suspension. Since the introduction of endoscopic sinus techniques, the endoscope is used to perform browlifts and midface elevations. Multiple techniques for midface elevation exist, most have in common the approach and differ mainly in how the midface is suspended. These techniques provide significant elevation of the ptotic malar complex and can be easily combined with an endoscopic browlift.

Release of the midface tissues is accomplished by creating either a lower blepharoplasty incision or a gingival-buccal sulcus incision and a temporal incision. Through the intraoral or blepharoplasty incisions, soft tissue is freed from its attachments to the anterior maxilla via extensive

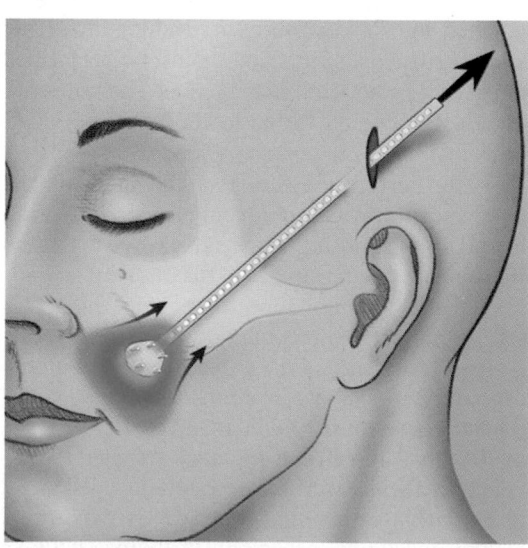

(A)

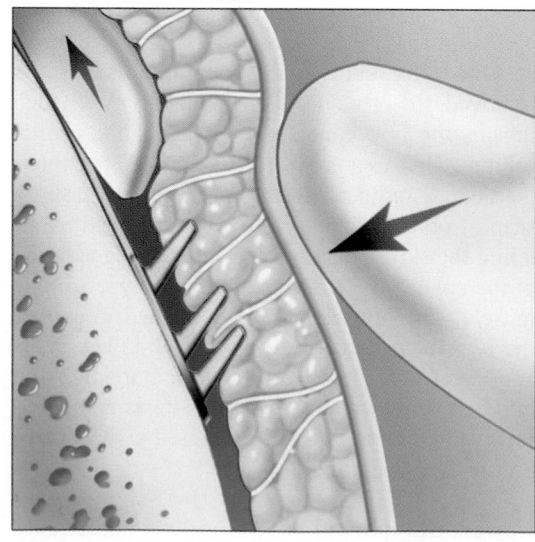

(B)

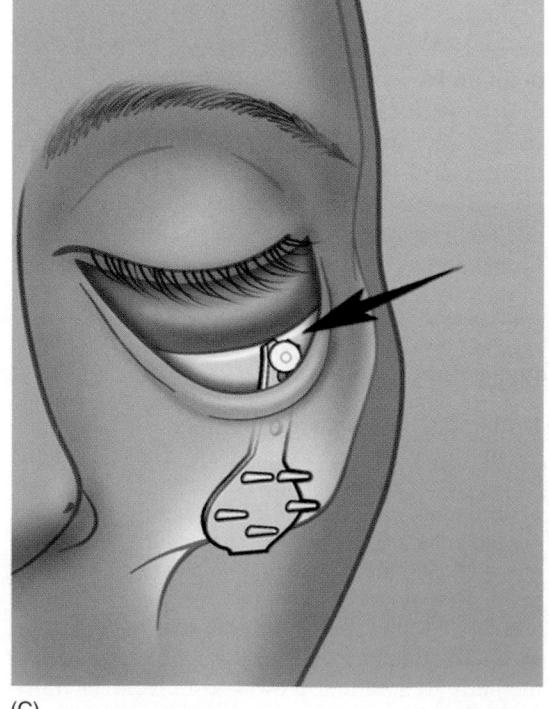

(C)

Figure 11 (A) Endotine Midface ST resorbable implant is used to suspend the soft tissues of the midface. (B) The five prongs atraumatically grip the soft tissue. (C) The ENDOTINE B implant can be used to suspend the malar soft tissues in the vertical direction. The superior aspect of the implant is secured to the inferior orbital rim by screw fixation.

subperiosteal dissection. Care is taken to preserve the infraorbital nerve as it exits from its foramen along the inferior orbital rim. The temporal incision is carried down to the superficial layer of the deep temporal fascia. This dissection is carried inferiorly to the zygomatic arch, where the two pockets are joined over the zygomatic arch. (see Figure 2). The endoscope may be used during the temporal dissection, or a lighted Aufrecht retractor may also be used. The temporal dissection follows the temporalis fascia to the zygomatic arch. The sentinel vein in identified and dissection proceeds lateral to the vein.

Once the temporal and malar dissections have been connected over the zygomatic arch, the tissue must be suspended. Many techniques for suspension exist. Sutures can be placed in the malar mound, passed through the tunnel, and sutured to the temporalis fascia. This technique is difficult to perform because the sutures can cause puckering of the cheek skin, and it is difficult to obtain symmetry.

In the past, endoscopic suspension techniques were technically difficult and often required special instrumentation. For these reasons, we prefer to use the ENDOTINE Midface ST implant for midface suspension (Figure 11). This implant, a copolymer made of 82/18 L-lactide/glycolide, is biodegradable 6 months after placement. The implant is placed in the midface through the tunnel created over the zygomatic arch. The five prongs are used to grasp the malar soft tissue, and the extension or "leash" is pulled superiolaterally and sutured to the temporalis fascia. This maneuver elevates the malar complex and slightly flattens the nasolabial fold (Figure 12). The implant is resorbed in approximately 6 months, after the tissue has become adherent to the maxilla.

COMPLICATIONS

Brow and Forehead Lift

The incidence of complications for this procedure is quite low. Hypesthesia over the forehead and scalp due to traction neuropraxia of the sensory nerves is usually temporary and returns to normal in 6 to 10 weeks. There have been some anecdotal reports of temporary weakness of the frontal branch of the facial nerve following the procedure. Permanent facial nerve paralysis has not been reported to date.

Imprecise surgical technique may result in asymmetrical brows, excessive brow elevation or, more commonly, recurrence of brow ptosis. Sufficient release of the brow at the level of the orbital rim and adequate fixation will prevent the recurrence of brow ptosis. There may be some temporary local alopecia at the incision sites, and bunching of the skin usually resolves in 2 months.

Blepharoplasty

Asymmetry of the upper eyelid tarsal creases is a risk of upper blepharoplasty. Failure to recognize a lid ptosis preoperatively can result in an

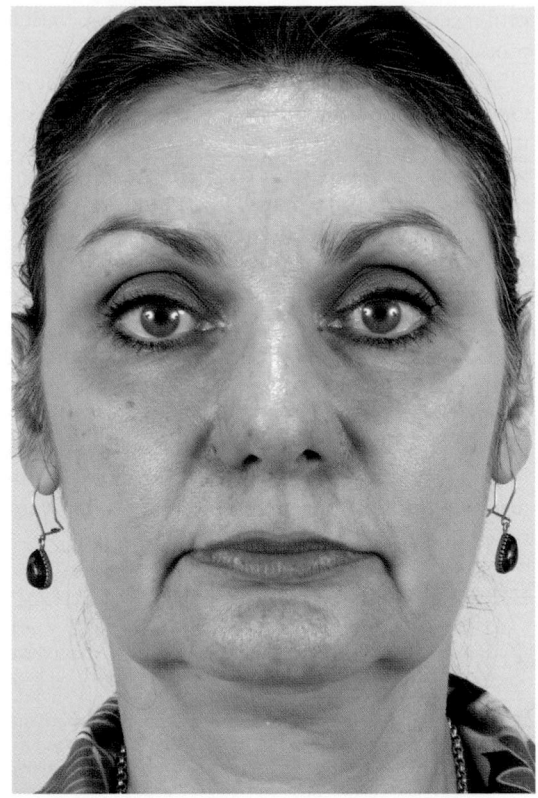

(A)

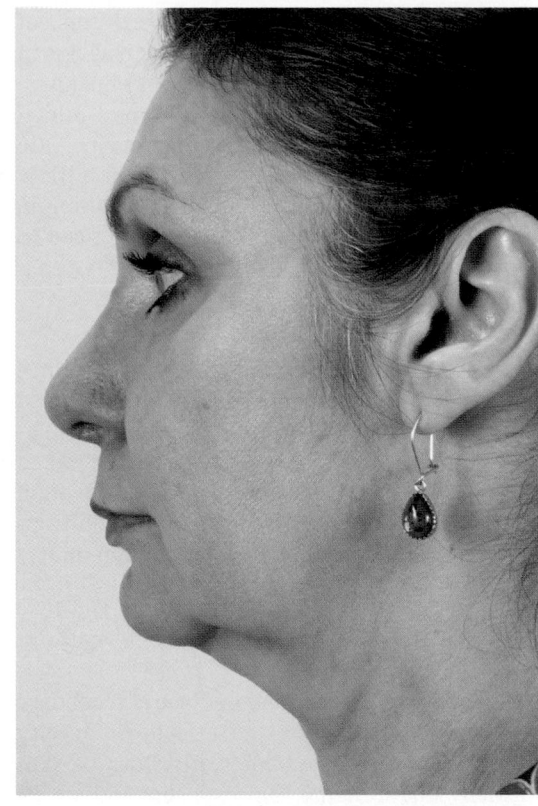

(B)

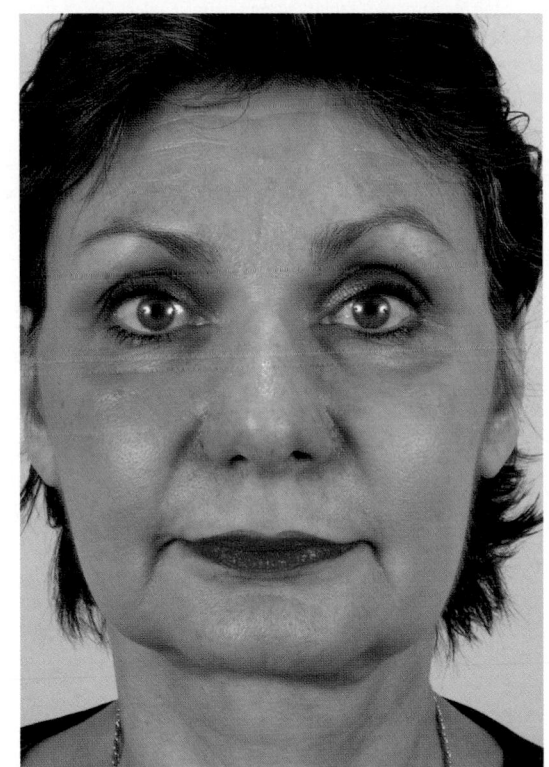

(C)

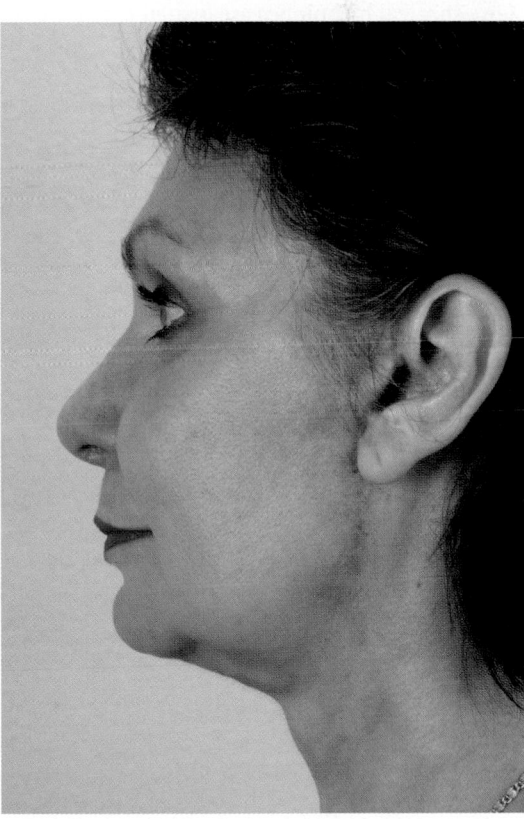

(D)

Figure 12 (A and B) Preoperative views. This patient underwent a rhytidectomy and midface lift using the ENDOTINE Midface ST implant. (C and D) Six-month postoperative photograph shows elevation of the malar tissue.

asymmetric result. Lagophthalmos, the inability to close the lid, can result from excessive upper lid skin excision. For that reason, the young surgeon is cautioned to remove conservative amounts of skin during upper lid blepharoplasty. If necessary, redundant skin may be removed after the patient has healed, but it is difficult to replace skin postoperatively if the lid is too short.

A retained fat pad is a common cause of revision surgery of the lower eyelids. Occasionally a fat pad is inadequately excised, and a noticeable prominence is present especially on upward gaze. These can usually be removed easily by the transconjunctival approach. Serious complications of blepharoplasty include injury to the ocular muscles and hematoma. Unlike the upper lid, the lower lid fat is associated with the globe. A hematoma of the upper lid is not as serious a problem as it is in the lower lid. Meticulous hemostasis is imperative in lower lid blepharoplasty to avoid retro-orbital hematomas. Hematomas of the globe can increase intraocular pressure and diminish bloodflow through the retinal artery, ultimately resulting in blindness. In addition, extraocular muscles can be injured during lower blepharoplasty.

Midface

The most common complication of midface surgery is asymmetry. There do not appear to be any significant complications from the fixation devices themselves. Care must be taken intraoperatively to ensure symmetric elevation of the malar complex. The infraorbital and frontal nerves must be protected from traction injury.

CONCLUSIONS

Aging of the upper face and midface is secondary to a variety of causes: the effects of gravity pulling the soft tissues inferiorly, loss of skin elasticity due to aging, sun exposure and smoking, and loss of volume of the facial soft tissues. Many surgical techniques are available to remove prolapsed fat, remove excess skin, and reposition ptotic soft tissues.

No one operation is right for every patient. Once the patient identifies the areas of concern, the surgeon may recommend several procedures which can be used to correct such areas. Minimally invasive procedures, like botulinium toxin and dermal filler injections, can be used for early signs of aging. Once the patient has lost tissue elasticity and support, rejuvenation of the upper face and midface may be necessary. Surgical techniques have progressed significantly in these areas in the past 15 years. Tissue preservation rather than complete removal is being practiced. We can predict that in the future even less invasive techniques will be developed with minimal morbidities and more rapid recovery times.

REFERENCES

1. Hester TR, Codner MA, McCord CD, Nahai F. Transorbital lower-lid midface rejuvenation. Op Tech Plast Reconstr Surg 1998;5:163–85.
2. Rhee JS, Gallo JF, Costantino PD. Endoscopic facial rejuvenation. In: Wackym PA, Rice DH, Schaefer SD, editors. Minimally Invasive Surgery of the Head, Neck, and Cranial Base. Philadelphia: Lippincott Williams & Wilkins; 2002. p. 355–66.
3. Larrabee W, Makielski K, Sykes J. Surgical anatomy for endoscopic facial surgery. In: Keller GS, editor. Endoscopic Facial Plastic Surgery. St. Louis: Mosby; 1997. p. 3–33.
4. Most SP, Mobley SR, Larrabee WF. Anatomy of the eyelids. Facial Plast Surg Clin N Am 2005;13:487–92.
5. Aiache AE, Ramirez OH. The suborbicularis oculi fat pads: An anatomic and clinical study. Plast Reconstr Surg 1995; 95:37–42.
6. Freeman MS. Transconjunctival sub-orbicularis oculi fat (SOOF) pad lift blepharoplasty. Arch Facial Plast Surg 2000;2:16–21.
7. Sullivan MJ. Brow and forehead aesthetics. Facial Plast Surg Clin North Am 1997;5:95–8.
8. Cook TA, Brownrigg AJ, Wang TD, et al. The versatile midforehead browlift. Arch Otolaryngol Head Neck Surg 1989;115:163–8.
9. Sullivan MJ. Endoscopic facial surgery. In: Cheney ML, editor. Facial Surgery: Plastic and Reconstructive. Baltimore: Williams & Wilkins; 1997. p. 913–26.
10. McKinney P, Mossie RD, Zubowsi ML. Criteria for the forehead lift. Aesthetic Plast Surg 1991;15:141–7.
11. Farkas LG, Kolar JC. Anthropometrics and art in the aesthetics of women's faces. Clin Past Surg 1987;14:559–616.
12. Hamra ST. Composite rhytidectomy. Plast Reconstr Surg 1992;90:1–13.
13. Graham HD. Methods of soft-tissue fixation in endoscopic surgery. Facial Plast Surg Clin North Am 1997;5:145–54.
14. Bostwick J, Eaves F, Nahai F. Forehead lift and glabellar frown lines. In: Bostwick J, editor. Endoscopic Plastic Surgery of the Head and Neck. St. Louis: Quality Medical Publishing; 1995. p. 166–230.
15. Berkowitz RL, Jacobs DI, Gorman PJ. Brow fixation with the Endotine Forehead device in endoscopic brow lift. Plast Reconstr Surg 2005;116:1761–7.
16. Guyuron B, Kopal C, Michelow BJ. Stability after endoscopic forehead surgery using single-point fascia fixation. Plast Reconstr Surg 2005;116:1988–94.
17. Patel BCK. Midface rejuvenation. Facial Plast Surg 1999; 15:231–42.

61

Rejuvenation of the Lower Face and Neck

Craig S. Murakami, MD
Bryan T. Ambro, MD, MS

Despite the ever-evolving standards of beauty, several classic characteristics of facial beauty have undoubtedly stood the test of time. The full, ovoid face highlighted by taut skin, high cheek bones, and an angular neck line remains the esthetic ideal for the youthful face and neck.

Aging of the lower face and neck is complex and varies from one individual to the next. Generally speaking, cervicofacial aging can be characterized by four changes: (1) ptosis of fat and soft tissue, (2) volumetric loss of facial adipose, (3) bony resorption, and (4) laxity of the overlying skin. It naturally follows that surgical strategies aimed at rejuvenation of the lower face and neck involve correction of these signs of aging.

The goal of this chapter is to provide an overview of the relevant anatomy of aging, appropriate analysis of aging, and, lastly, the corrective surgical options available. The reader is reminded that not all techniques for lower cervicofacial rejuvenation are covered in this chapter. Less invasive procedures such as soft tissue fillers and skin resurfacing, although effective in an adjunctive role, are presented in Chapter 57, "Scar Revision and Skin Resurfacing." Although much of this text reflects the philosophy of the authors, we have attempted to present a thorough review of the literature highlighting the many different surgical strategies available.

HISTORICAL PERSPECTIVE

In the early part of the twentieth century, European surgeons pioneered the surgical treatment of rhytides (*rhytidectomy*—Greek for removal of wrinkles). By simply undermining and removing the excess skin, the subcutaneous rhytidectomy was, for nearly a half century, the gold standard for aging face surgery. Unhappy with its limited duration of benefit, Skoog, in 1974, published improved, longer lasting results in the lower third of the face by dissecting in a "subfascial plane."[1] Two years later, Mitz and Peyronnie, described in detail this muscle and fascial plane of the face, naming it the superficial musculoaponeurotic system (SMAS).[2] With better, longer-lasting results in the neck and jowls, the sub-SMAS procedure emerged as the new standard in facelifting techniques.

The literature is replete with further modifications of the SMAS rhytidectomy technique (eg, deep plane,[3] composite,[4] triplane rhytidectomy[5]) as well as isolated procedures for the aging anterior part of the neck or midface, giving today's facelift surgeon many rejuvenation options. Particularly important, however, is the surgeon's ability to recognize the differing degrees of aging from one individual to the next and to tailor the surgical strategy accordingly.

SURGICAL ANATOMY AND ANALYSIS OF THE AGING FACE

A thorough understanding of the relevant anatomy is essential to achieving the optimal surgical result. Accurate preoperative analysis of the aging anatomy should include all tissue layers of the face and neck, beginning superficially with the skin and working deep through the subcutaneous adipose, fascia layers, cervicofacial musculature, and the underlying bony framework.

Skin and Adipose Tissue

The condition of the skin plays a significant role in the appearance of youth. With aging, the skin undergoes a progressive loss of elastic and collagen fibers and a decrease in the amount of ground substance (hyaluronic acid). This results in an overall decrease in thickness and loss of elasticity allowing for the formation of rhytides. Chronic sun exposure (photoaging) and habitual tobacco use greatly accelerate this process as well as contribute a coarse, leathery texture to the skin. Further "sagging" of the skin can also be attributed to laxity of underlying fasciocutaneous and osteocutaneous ligaments. These facial retaining ligaments allow the skin to resist downward effects of gravity by providing support from rigid underlying muscle and bone. Habitual facial expressions caused by underlying mimetic muscles can also lead to progressive recontouring of the skin and subsequent rhytide formation.

The subcutaneous fat layer also undergoes age-related changes, demonstrating atrophy in some areas (midface) and excess accumulation in other regions (submentum). Atrophy of subdermal adipose tissue can be quite pronounced in the cervicofacial region, contributing to a gaunt, hollowed appearance in thin-faced patients. With newer, more reliable methods of lipotransfer, fat can now be harvested from other areas of the body and used to augment the facial areas demonstrating atrophy.

Aging, as it relates to fat, can also be seen in certain facial areas where excessive accumulation occurs out of proportion to surrounding regions. This is especially true of the submental region, where some individuals have a genetic propensity for undesirable fat distribution even at a relatively young age, despite normal body weight. Other individuals may experience submental adipose accumulation as a direct result of progressive weight gain. Either way, the end result is premature blunting of the cervicomental angle and loss of an esthetic neckline. Isolated submental liposuction or open lipectomy can provide an excellent result in patients with this deformity.

The malar fat pad is a triangular-shaped fibro-fatty thickening of subcutaneous tissue in the midface. The fat pad lies immediately superficial to the SMAS, but firmly adherent to the skin and subcutaneous fat. In younger individuals, the superior border of triangular fat pad lies over the malar eminence and covers the infraorbital rim. Its medial border abuts the nasolabial fold, and the lateral border is approximated by a line drawn from the lateral canthus down to the corner of the mouth.

With advancing age and the extended effects of gravity, the malar fat pad descends by sliding over the SMAS in an inferomedial direction. This ptosis can contribute to the appearance of increased fullness in the nasolabial fold, hollowness in the submalar area, and skeletonization of the orbital rim. The vertical repositioning of the ptotic malar fat pad is key to restoring a youthful appearance in the aging midface.

Superficial Musculoaponeurotic System and Neurovascular Structures

The SMAS is a fibromuscular layer investing and interlinking the muscles of facial expression. As originally described, the SMAS is a facial layer superficial to and separate from the underlying parotid fascia. The term musculoaponeurotic was used due to occasional muscular fibers seen in the fascia overlying the parotid. Moreover, the SMAS contains fibrous septa that extend through the fat and attach to the overlying dermis. As a result, the SMAS acts as a network to distribute facial muscle contractions to the skin (Figure 1).[6]

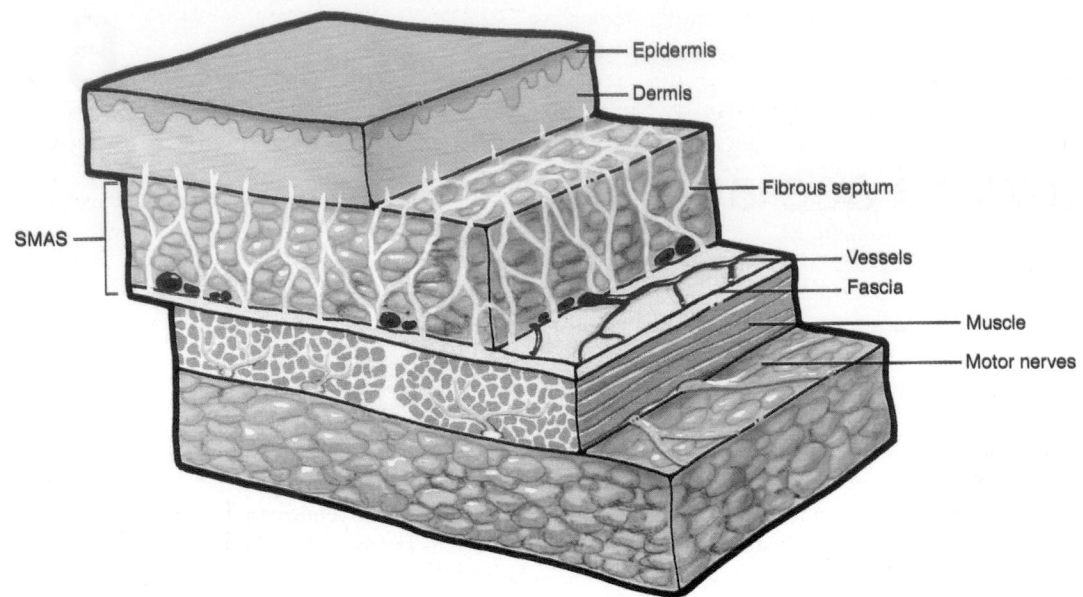

Figure 1 Cross section of superficial musculoaponeurotic system (SMAS). The SMAS fascial layer envelopes the muscles of facial expression. Fibrous septa extend through the fat and attach to the overlying dermis to distribute facial muscle contractions to the skin. (Reproduced with permission from reference 6.)

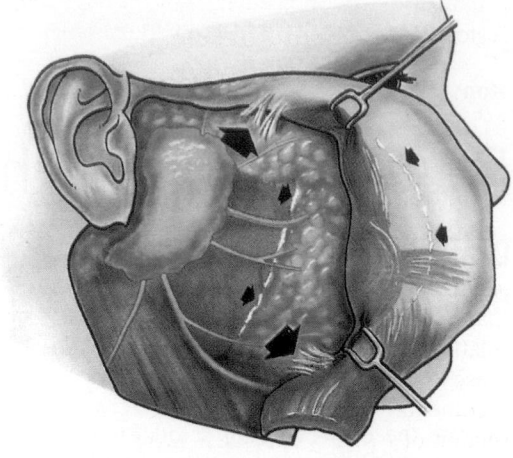

Figure 2 Retaining ligaments of the face. Stout osteocutaneous ligaments (*large arrows*) are found at the zygoma (McGregor patch) and the mandible. Weaker fasciocutaneous ligaments (*small arrows*) are seen at the anterior border of the masseter muscle. (Reproduced with permission from reference 7.)

Superiorly, there is a discontinuity of the SMAS at the level of the zygomatic arch because of various attachments of fascial layers at the bony arch. Above the arch in the temporal region, the SMAS becomes confluent with the temporoparietal fascia. Inferiorly in the neck, the SMAS represents the caudal extention of the deep layer of the superficial cervical fascia investing the platysma. It is here that the extended effects of gravity on the SMAS are most often noted. SMAS ptosis and age-related laxity contributes to inferiomedial platysmal migration and the development of jowls and anterior neck banding. Facelift techniques that resuspend the ptotic SMAS are the primary surgical options available to correct aging in this region.

There are important regional variations in the relationship of the SMAS to the key neurovascular structures. In the lower face and neck, the facial nerve branches are always deep to the SMAS and platysma and innervate the facial mimetic muscles through their undersurface. The exception to this rule is the deep facial muscles: the levator anguli oris, the buccinator, and the mentalis, which are all innervated through their surfaces. The vessels and sensory nerves in the lower part of the face similarly arise deep to the SMAS and remain at that level, except for their terminal branches. These structures are thus protected if dissection is superficial to the SMAS and platysma. The marginal mandiblar nerve lies deep to the platysma muscle and, therefore, is fairly well protected throughout its course along the mandible. As it approaches a point 2 cm lateral to the corner of the mouth, it becomes more superficial and dissection past this point should be avoided. In the midface, the facial nerve branches are protected if dissection is superficial to the facial muscles, for example, the zygomaticus major muscle.

The temporal branch of the facial nerve emerges from the parotid beneath the midpoint of the zygomatic arch. The nerve crosses over the periosteum in a superficial plane immediately beneath the subcutaneous fat and continues superiorly on the deep surface of the temporoparietal fascia before entering the undersurface of the frontalis muscle. To avoid injury to the temporal branch when elevating flaps, the dissection should be in the immediate subcutaneous plane or deep to the temporoparietal fascia.

The vascular supply of the lower face is, primarily, provided by branches of the external carotid artery. The anterior part of the face is supplied by musculocutaneous perforators from the facial and infraorbital arteries, while the posterior part of the face receives additional blood flow from the transverse facial and postauricular branches. Blood supply, as it relates to facelift surgery, is dependent on the surgical technique utilized. Methods that employ more extensive subcutaneous dissection create large subcutaneous skin flaps that rely on the subdermal plexus fed by the anteriorly located facial artery. Techniques, such as the deep-plane rhytidectomy, minimize subcutaneous dissection and create a composite flap of skin and SMAS that has a more robust blood supply; making it less likely to be compromised in suboptimal conditions, for example, increased wound tension and tobacco use.

In the cheek region, the skin and subcutaneous tissue is easily dissected free of the underlying SMAS. As one continues to dissect the skin flap anteriorly, several retaining ligaments of the face are encountered (Figure 2).[7] These fibrous bands are known as fasciocutaneous and osteocutaneous ligaments. The faciocutaneous ligaments, particularly dense at the anterior border of the masseter muscle, emanate from the SMAS and attach to the overlying dermis. The osteocutaneous ligaments are the strongest of the ligament attachments and exist between the periosteum and the overlying skin. These stout ligaments emanate from the periosteum of the zygoma and mandible and are termed the zygomatic cutaneous ligaments (McGregor patch) and the mandibular cutaneous ligaments. Release of these attachments is essential to gaining adequate mobilization of the overlying soft tissue structures such as the malar fat pad.

Mimetic Facial Muscles

The noteworthy facial muscles important in rejuvenation of the lower face and neck are the zygomaticus major and minor and the platysma.

Originating superiorly at the zygoma, the zygomatic muscles insert into the modiolus and act as elevators of the corner of the mouth and lip. They serve as important landmarks for deeper dissection plane techniques. The zygomatic branch of the facial nerve, which innervates these muscles from their undersurface, is protected from injury when a plane of dissection superficial to the muscle is undertaken.

The platysma is a broad, flat sheet of muscle arising inferiorly from the fascia of the pectoralis major and the deltoid muscles. Its fibers cross the clavicle and extend obliquely and upward along the side of the neck. Superiorly and laterally, the fibers extend across the angle of the jaw and insert into the skin and subcutaneous tissue of the lower face as well as blend into the SMAS layer. Medially, the platysmal fibers insert into muscles and subcutaneous tissue surrounding the lower part of the mouth as well as the mandibular periosteum. Below the mentum, the muscle fibers from each side interdigitate and form an inverted V. The apex of the inverted V is quite variable from one individual to the next, with its vertical position being at the mentum, 1 to 2 cm below the chin (most common) or at the level of the thyroid cartilage. The platysma muscle is innervated by the cervical branch of the facial nerve, and its primary action is to depress the lower lip.

With aging, the medial portion of the muscle becomes lax and separates to form two diverging vertical bands. Platysmaplasty is performed to correct this banding by reapproximating the muscular diastasis. When this is performed in conjunction with the posterior pull of facelift, a hammock-like muscular sling is recreated to restore cervicomental definition.

Bony Anatomy

Choosing the optimal strategy for correction of cervicofacial aging requires an understanding of not only the soft tissue structures but also the bony components of the region. An accurate analysis of key osseous elements should include: (1) assessment of projection and resorption of the chin/mandible and (2) the position of the hyoid bone relative to the mandible. The relationship between these two structures is key to determining the cervicomental angle, which is defined as an intersection of two cephalometric lines. In the lateral view, the first line is drawn from the menton to the hyoid and the second from the hyoid to the sternal notch. The ideal angle created by the intersection of these lines should approximate 90°. An underprojected chin or a low, anterior hyoid can cause the angle to become more obtuse and thus less attractive. Currently, there are no procedures to correct a malpositioned hyoid; therefore, patients with this configuration should be counseled on the limits this places on outcomes (Figure 3). If, however, the same patient has a small chin, surgical efforts should be directed toward chin projection as a means of improving the angle.

A well-defined mandibular line and chin with appropriate height and projection has certainly remained a constant esthetic ideal. Perhaps the simplest way to determine ideal chin projection is to drop a vertical line from the vermillion border of lower lip. If the line falls anterior to the soft tissue pogonion, then the chin is underprojected. Microgenia is a term used to describe a congenital small chin with normal dental occlusion. This must be distinguished from retrognathia (underprojected chin with Angle class II malocclusion) and mandibular hypoplasia (age related loss of bony projection), as the treatment options can differ between the three. Microgenia and mandibular hypoplasia are more likely to be corrected by alloplastic implantation or sliding genioplasty (if also vertically deficient), whereas retrognathia often requires mandibular osteotomies and advancement.

The aging process can lead to varying degrees of bony resorption of the mandible (mandibular hypoplasia). The presence or absence of dentition plays a signifcant role in the amount of bone loss, especially at the alveolar ridge. One specific area of age related resorption occurs between the chin and jowl that, when combined with overlying soft tissue atrophy, creates a vertical groove termed the prejowl sulcus (see Figure 3). This is of significance because although a facelift can correct jowling, it will leave the prejowl sulcus behind. Specific types of extended chin implants or soft tissue fillers are often utilized to augment this atrophic region.

Assessment of the Neck

With an understanding of the anatomy of cervicofacial aging, it is quite obvious that each individual's face ages differently. It naturally follows that the surgical approach to rejuvenation will vary from one patient to the next and that careful preoperative analysis is essential to achieve optimal results.

The Dedo classification system of the aging neck is a useful tool for evaluating patients for rhytidectomy[8] (Figure 4).[9] It identifies six classes of neck anatomy based upon the deepest affected tissue layer, that is, skin, fat, muscle, and bone. A Class I neck is typically seen in younger patients with a well-defined cervicomental angle, good skin and muscle tone, and absence of submental fat. A class II neck demonstrates mild skin laxity without underlying muscle or fat deformity. This class of neck is rare as even early signs of aging usually occur in all tissue layers. These patients are counseled that surgical correction will require wide skin undermining and some degree of lateral SMAS tightening. The class III patient shows evidence of submental and submandibular fat accumulation. This can either be congenital or age related. Rejuvenation begins with liposuction and can also require facelifting if there is concomitant SMAS and skin laxity. A class IV neck refers to anterior banding of the platysma muscle. Corset platysmaplasty (anterior platysma plication) with lateral lift and suspension is utilized to correct this type of neck. The class V neck reveals either a congenital microgenia of retrognathia or an age related chin hypoplasia. Corrective measures should include some type of chin augmentation as previously discussed. Lastly, a class VI neck is characterized by a low-lying hyoid bone with or without any of the others signs of aging. These patients are counseled that there is an anatomical limitation of the result that can be achieved in the neck.

PREOPERATIVE EVALUATION AND CONSIDERATIONS

The initial consultation should begin with the patient filling out a detailed medical history questionnaire. This is a quick method to ascertain important information regarding prior cosmetic procedures, medications, allergies, tobacco habits, and existing medical conditions. Emphasis is placed on medical conditions that would preclude facelift surgery. To maximize safety, complicated medical issues warrant appropriate preoperative clearance. All medications (including herbal) that affect the body's ability to clot, are discontinued 2 weeks prior to surgery. Because of the vasoconstrictive properties of nicotine, smokers are strongly encouraged to abstain from all forms of nicotine (including transdermal patches and chewing gum) 2 weeks prior to surgery until 2 weeks after. A less aggressive facelift technique may be recommended to prevent tissue ischemia in a patient with a smoking history.

The patient is positioned in front of a mirror and asked to describe the areas of facial aging that are of concern. After the patient has shared his or her concerns, the full face and neck should be examined. Although the patient's primary interest may be the lower face and neck, the upper half of the face, that is, brow and the eyelids, should also be assessed. It may need to be explained to the patient that the face ages as a whole and that isolated correction of the lower third only can yield an unbalanced, unnatural appearance. Working inferiorly, midfacial analysis should include bone structure as well as malar fat pad ptosis and its contribution to the nasolabial mound. Examination of the lower third should include the specific areas of aging previously discussed. Lastly, the quality of skin should be addressed. Patients often need to be educated that, although facelift surgery can remove excess skin, it does not improve the texture of the skin. Improvement of photoaged or dyschromic skin, can only be accomplished with medium to deep resurfacing techniques, topical therapy, and healthy skin care.

In addition to the physical examination, an accurate evaluation of the patient's psychological status is critical to determining patient candidacy for any cosmetic operation. Throughout the consultation process, the surgeon should assess the patient's concerns, motivations and expectations to determine if these are realistic and can be met. Ideally, the patient should be appropriately self-motivated and psychologically prepared for a facelift and the demands of its convalescence.

The consultation typically ends with the surgeon answering any questions that the patient may have. It is imperative that the procedure, its risks and, benefits as well as the alternatives be fully explained to the patient prior to making any final decisions.

Prior to surgery, standardized rhytidectomy photographic documentation is performed in the fullface frontal, left and right oblique, and left and right lateral views. An additional lateral view with the chin angled down at 30° to 45° emphasizes

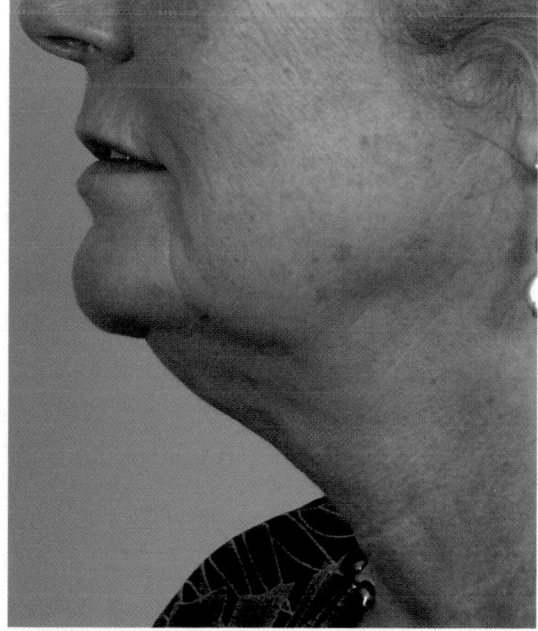

Figure 3 Lateral view of a patient with a poorly defined neckline. The jowling and submental lipoptosis can be improved by rhytidectomy and submental liposuction, however, the primary surgical limitation is due to the anteroinferior position of the hyoid bone. The prejowl sulcus is often not improved by rhytidectomy alone, and its effacement will require some form of soft tissue augmentation.

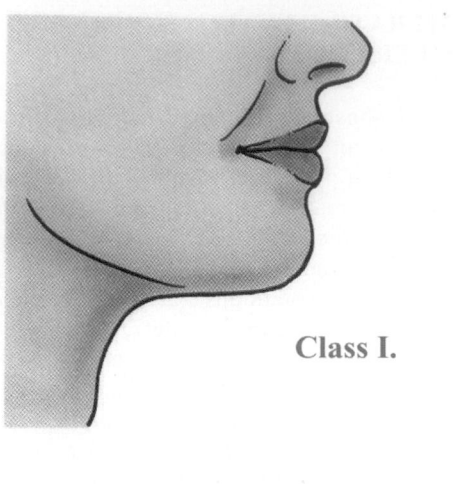

Class I.

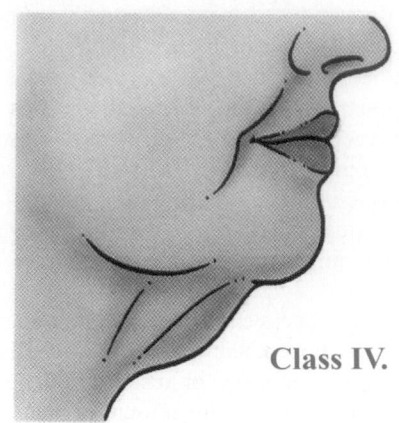

Class IV.

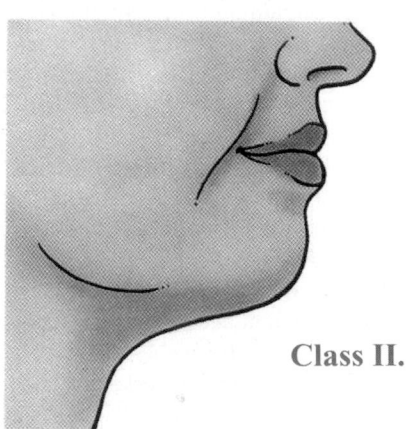

Class II.

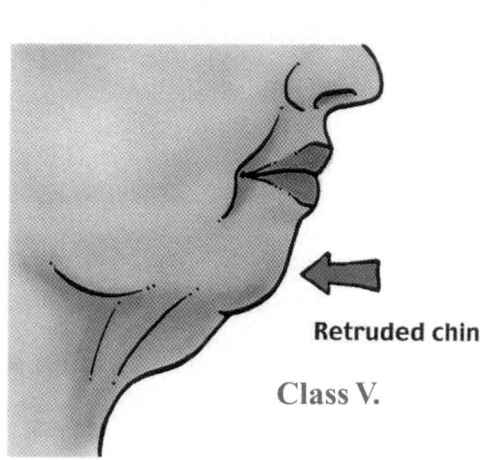

Retruded chin

Class V.

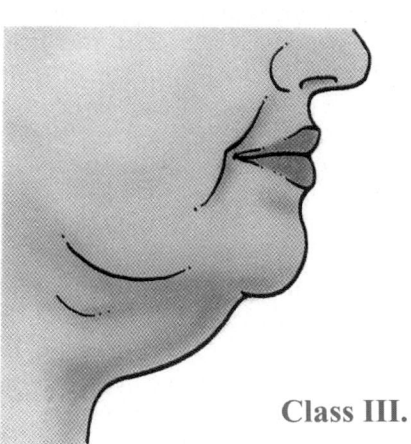

Class III.

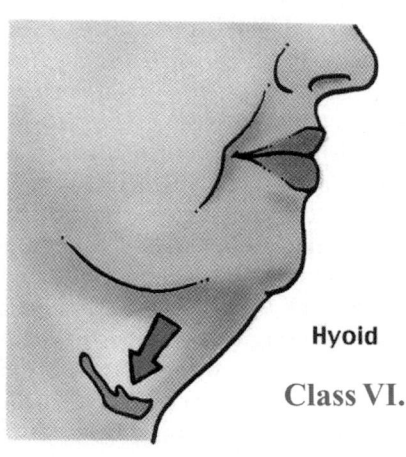

Hyoid

Class VI.

Figure 4 Dedo classification of the neck. (Reproduced with permission from reference 9.)

laxity in the submental region. Closeup photos taken to document specific areas are done on an individualized basis. We do not routinely offer digital image morphing in our consultations but do perform it upon patient request.

SURGICAL PLANNING

Anesthesia and Perioperative Medications

We typically perform cervicofacial rejuvenation procedures under general anesthesia, although intravenous sedation is acceptable. Prophylactic intravenous antibiotics (cefazolin 1 gm or clinda-mycin 600 mg if penicillin allergic) are routinely given preoperatively and are continued orally until the seventh postoperative day. Intravenous dexamethasone (10 mg) and odansetron (400 mg) are also given preoperatively

Facelift Incisions

There are several important considerations when planning the placement of facelift incisions. The preauricular tuft of hair is the key determinant of what type of temporal hair incision we make. If the tuft of hair is more than 2 cm below the superior helical attachment, then a curvilinear incision is carried into the temporal hair in a more vertical direction (Figure 5). This allows for a greater posterior-superior vector of pull in the temporal and lateral brow area, while maintaining a cosmetically acceptable temporal hair tuft position at or below the helical insertion. If the hairline is at or above the helical insertion point, the temporal incision made in a V-Y fashion above the helical root and then gently curved anteriorly just above the inferior border of the sideburn. This configuration avoids the unnaturally raised temporal hairline seen in the "facelift cripple" (Figure 6). and can actually lower a preexisting high hairline. All incisions in hair bearing skin are beveled in the direction of hair shafts to preserve follicles and allow growth of hair through the scar.

When planning the preauricular incision, we typically follow a retrotragal line in women and a pretragal incision in men. The posttragal incision in men will displace hair-bearing skin onto the tragus which can be problematic. If a scar from a prior facelift exists, this is excised; and an attempt is made to cosmetically position the new incision. Postauricularly, the incision is directed 5 mm up onto the posterior surface of the conchal cartilage, so that during healing contracture the scar ultimately falls in the sulcus and not onto the non–hair-bearing surface of the mastoid. The posterior limb of the incision is gently sloped into the occipital hair at the point of posterior most projection of the pinna to maximize incision coverage in the profile view.

SURGICAL TECHNIQUE

Because the face and neck age as a whole, many patients undergoing rhytidectomy elect to have additional facial procedures performed in combination. If procedures such as browlift or blepharoplasty are indicated, these are performed prior to the facelifting. Fat grafting and skin resurfacing are routinely performed after rhytidectomy. By performing the facelift at or near the end of the operative sequence, we minimize the time the patient is without a compressive cervicofacial dressing.

Neck and Chin

Submental Liposuction and Platysmaplasty (Submentoplasty). The submentoplasty can be performed alone or in combination with a facelift to achieve the optimal esthetic result in the lower face and neck. It is comprised of two separate procedures: submental liposuction and anterior platysmaplasty. Although they are commonly performed together in the patient with an aging face, isolated submental liposuction may be all that is required for younger patients (Dedo class III) with excess adipose tissue. Both liposuction and platysmaplasty are always performed before rhytidectomy, as the liposuction helps raise the neck skin flaps and the midline platyma plication is difficult if attempted after lateral SMAS/platysmal flap tightening.

Removal of excess submental fat has long been recognized as a relatively simple method to improve neck line esthetics. The excess adipose tissue is usually located in the subcutaneous

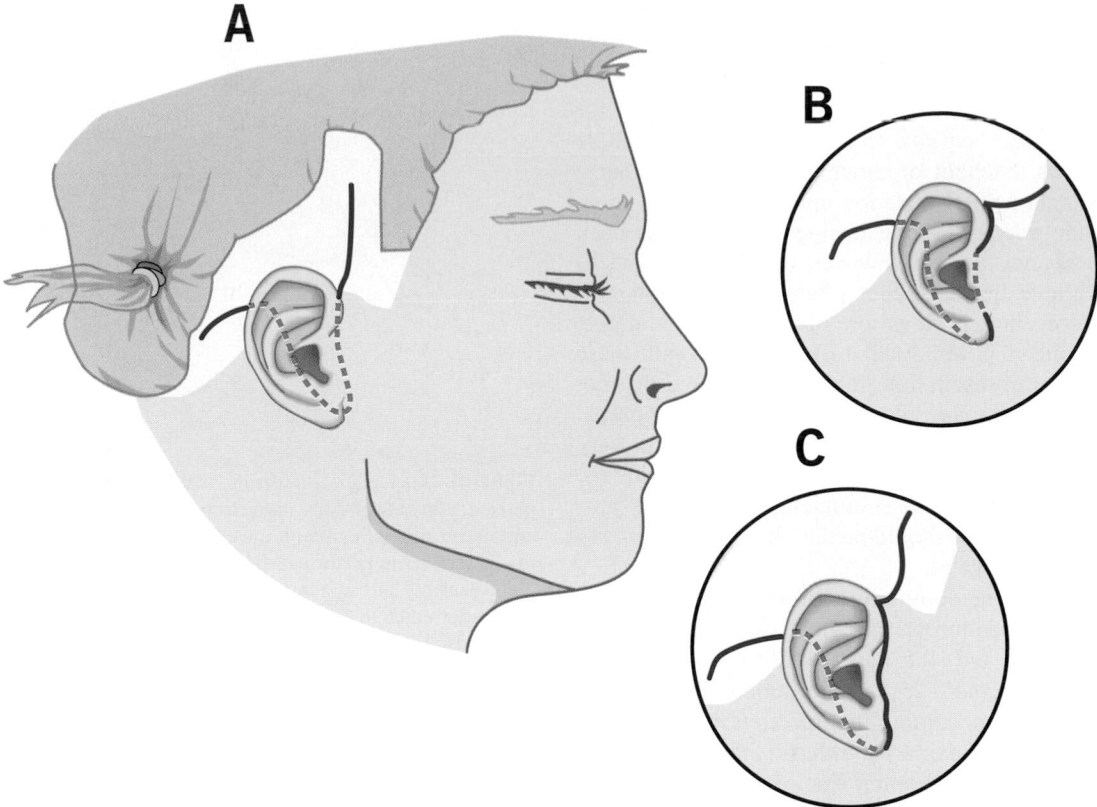

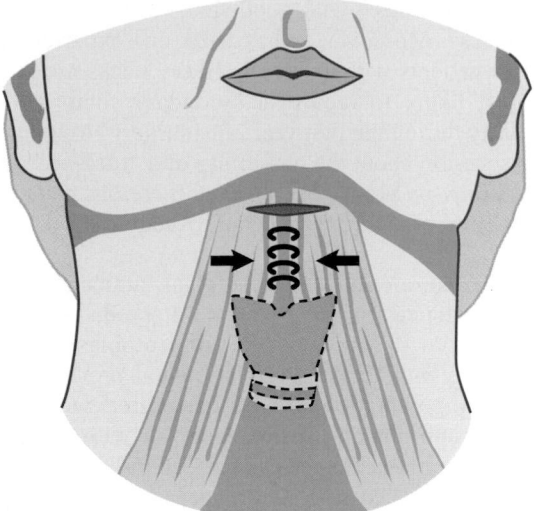

Figure 5 Variations of facelift incisions. (A) The standard retrotragal incision with temporal extension. (B) Incision used to maintain temporal tuft and sideburn in stable position. (C) Demonstrates the pretragal incision commonly used in male patients or patients with a deep preauricular crease.

Figure 7 Platysma plication sutures. Beginning at the thyroid notch, buried interrupted sutures are used to approximate the medial platysma muscle edges. This helps to redefine an esthetic cervicomental angle.

or supraplatysmal layer, however, it can also accumulate deep to the platysma. Numerous methods for fat removal have been described, for example, open lipectomy,[10] liposuction,[11] or lipo-shaving,[12] with liposuction being the most commonly employed technique.

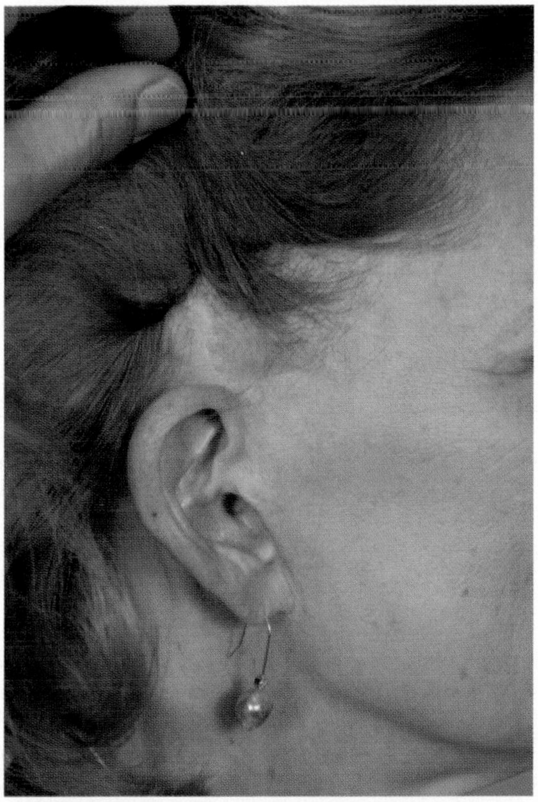

Preoperatively, it is important to mark the areas of fat removal with the patient sitting upright, as the appearance of submental fat changes in the supine position. After induction of general anesthesia, 0.5% lidocaine and 0.25% bupivicaine with 1:200,000 epinephrine are injected under the neck skin flaps to provide both anesthesia and vasoconstriction. The patient is prepped and draped, and a 15 blade is used to make 1 cm stab incision in the submental crease. A liposuction cannula (2 to 4 mm) is introduced into the subcutaneous layer, and dry tunnels, that is, no suction applied, are made in the fanlike fashion from one inferior mandibular border to the other. We recommend staying below the mandibular border as this minimizes the risk of injury to the marginal mandibular nerve. Great care is also always taken to position the cannula holes facing deep, away from the skin flap as trauma to the overlying dermis can result in scarring and contour irregularities. The nondominant, guide hand is used to tent up the skin as well as help advance to the tissue toward the cannula. The suction (1 atmosphere negative pressure) is then applied, and fat is aspirated until the desired contour is created. Some authors recommend two other stab incisions just posterior to the ear lobules to facilitate submandibular and posterior neck line contouring. In younger patients with good skin tone, the overlying skin flaps typically contract down favorably to the recreated neck line, where as older, inelastic skin often requires some degree of lateral re-draping and excision to prevent contour irregularities. In selected cases, where excessive submental fat deposition obscures the platysmal muscle edges or discrete subplatysmal fat pads remain after liposuction, a conservative open lipectomy with scissors may be performed. When performing submental lipectomy, great care must be taken to avoid uneven cervical contour or worse yet a "cobra" deformity caused by excessive removal of fat. To avoid this complication, conservative removal of fat is stressed, and the anterior platysmal borders are often suture approximated after central lipectomy is conducted.

In general, we perform a relatively aggressive posterior tightening of the platysma and do not routinely perform anterior platysmaplasty unless significant banding is noted during preoperative examination. If correction of platysmal banding is planned, the submental incision is extended to 3 cm. Using a lighted retractor and scissors, subcutaneous dissection under direct vision is performed until the medial borders of the dehiscent platysma muscle are identified. The anterior muscle edges are plicated with several buried 4-0 polydiaxone sutures beginning at the thyroid notch and working superiorly to create a midline corset (Figure 7). If severe platysmal laxity is noted, the redundant edges of muscle are grasped with a clamp and excised prior to placement of sutures. Meticulous hemostasis with bipolar cautery should be exercised, as even small collections of blood under the flaps during the healing phase can lead to irregular scarring and contour irregularies.

Despite the effectiveness of the submentoplasty, patients should be counseled about the rebound relaxation inherent to soft tissue that can lead to the reappearance of submental muscle or skin laxity. Revision submentoplasty rates ranging from 15 to 50% have been reported.[13,14] To combat this tissue relaxation, as well as improve neck contouring without the need for rhytidectomy, several authors have used suture techniques[15] and expanded polytetrafluoroethylene

Figure 6 Lateral view of a patient who had a prior rhytidectomy that resulted in an unnatural appearing elevation of the temporal hair tuft. There is also an area of alopecia surrounding the vertical incisional scar.

cervical slings[16] with good short- and long-term success. Moreover, it has been our experience that patients with extremely heavy necks are the most likely to require a secondary submentoplasty during the first year after surgery. An open discussion about the possibility of a "tuck-up" as a follow-up procedure certainly increases patient acceptance if such a procedure is required.

Chin Augmentation. If surgical augmentation of the deficient chin is planned it should be performed at this time, after submentoplasty and prior to rhytidectomy. As discussed previously, chin augmentation can be performed with an alloplastic implant (mentoplasty) or with a sliding genioplasty (which can correct horizontal and vertical deficiencies). As the focus of this chapter is on rejuvenation of age-related changes, we will concentrate our discussion on alloplastic mentoplasty which constitutes greater than 95% of the chin procedures in our aging face practice.

Decision as to what shape and size of chin implant to use should be made during the preoperative evaluation. Patients with congenital microgenia who require only several milimeters of anterior projection typically have a standard chin implant (thicker in the center) inserted. This type of implant, however, does not possess sufficient lateral bulk to correct the aging chin's characteristic prejowl sulcus—a vertical groove formed between the chin and jowl as the underlying bone and soft tissue of this region atrophies (see Figure 3). The patient with microgenia and significant prejowl sulci will require an implant designed with lateral extensions intended to augment this atrophic area.

Currently there are several commonly used alloplastic materials (silastic, polytetrafluoroethylene, mersilene) used to construct chin implants. The type of implant material chosen is ultimately dependent on the individual surgeon's experience and preference.

The submental incision utilized for submentoplasty is also used for insertion of the alloplastic implant. The chin is infiltrated with 5 mL of 1% lidocaine with 1:100,000 epinephrine, and a dissection pocket approximately 10% larger than the implant is made. The dissection plane is performed supraperiosteally centrally and a subperiosteally laterally, as this helps stabilize the implant and prevent migration during the healing period. A more detailed description of chin augmentation is beyond the scope of this chapter and we direct the reader to the suggested reading list for further intraoperative details. The submental incision is not closed until after the rhytidectomy flaps have been elevated and the lateral SMAS suspension is completed. We prefer a layered closure with 5.0 polydiaxone used to approximate the subcutaneous layer and interrupted 6.0 nylon for the skin.

Rhytidectomy

Cervicofacial rhytidectomy, or facelifting, remains the most powerful surgical procedure

to rejuvenate the aging lower face and neck. The literature is replete with various facelifting techniques, each with advantages and disadvantages that many surgeons have debated for years and continue to do so. For example, there exists a school of thought that contends that a simple SMAS plication/imbrication yields more than adequate, long lasting results in the neck and jowl region. However, others (we included) believe that a deeper plane of dissection produces better elevation of the ptotic midface. While it is important to be familiar with these points of discussion, it must be stressed that not all patients age the same and that the optimal technique for each individual patient can vary considerably. A surgical strategy that yields the best results, while minimizing unnecessary surgery and risk, should be the ultimate goal for any facelift surgeon.

Nearing completion of the submental and chin procedures, the right side rhytidectomy incisions and skin flap are infiltrated with 0.5% lidocaine and 0.25% bupivicaine with 1:200,000 epinephrine. Timing the injection in this fashion allows for maximal anesthesia and vasoconstriction. Similarly, the left side of the face should be injected prior to completion of the right side.

The previously delineated rhytidectomy incisions are made starting superiorly in the temporal area and continued inferiorly around the ear ending in the postauricular hairline. If a vertical oriented temporal incision is chosen to improve the temporal or lateral brow region, dissection is carried down through the scalp layers to identify the temporalis fascia. Undermining can be performed superficial to the deep temporal fascial layer all the way down to the lateral brow and superior border of the zygomatic arch. Utilization of the sideburn sparing incision requires the dissection to be in a subcutaneous plane, so as to avoid injury to the temporal branch of the facial nerve as it crosses over the zygomatic arch. Vertical retraction with skin hooks and countertraction on the flap allow for sharp facelift scissors easily to elevate the skin flap anteriorly into the cheek. Transillumination of the flap with an overhead light directed through the flap allows for the identification of the proper dissection plane and aids in maintaining the appropriate flap thickness. The cheek skin is typically elevated anteriorly to a line drawn between the malar eminence and the mid mandible (mandibular notch). Minimizing the extent of skin separation from the underlying SMAS creates a more vascular, composite flap that is less likely to be compromised. In the occipital area, care must be taken to stay deep to the hair follicles to avoid alopecia, while staying superficial to the sternocleidomastoid fascia to prevent inadvertent injury to the great auricular nerve. The cervical skin flap is elevated in the subcutaneous plane to the second major cervical rhytide and extended to the midline. The subcutaneous elevation avoids injury to the marginal mandibular and cervical nerves.

After subcutaneous dissection is complete, manipulation of the SMAS layer is performed.

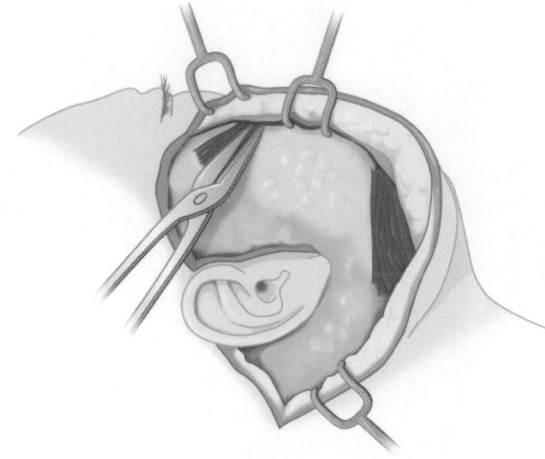

Figure 8 Deep plane dissection. The SMAS has been incised, the sub-SMAS dissection is carried anterior, and the zygomatic major muscle is identified. Careful dissection is performed on the surface of this muscle releasing the zygomatico-cutaneous ligaments of McGregor patch to release and mobilize the malar fat pad into a posterior superior position.

The SMAS can be suspended by several different techniques. SMAS plication is the most direct method and suspends by simply folding redundant SMAS onto itself and securing the fold with permanent sutures. Imbrication of the SMAS layer involves incision and resection of lax SMAS with reapproxiamtion of the cut edges. A variable amount of SMAS flap elevation can be performed prior to suture reapproximation. There are still many surgeons that utilize plication or imbrication as the cornerstone of their facelift operation. As stated before, we prefer a deep plane dissection that is described below.

Once the skin flap has been elevated, the SMAS is incised from the malar eminence to a point 1 cm below the ear lobule. Adson Brown forceps are used to grasp the anterior SMAS edge gently and a sub-SMAS dissection is continued over and anterior to the parotid by gentle, vertical spreading with scissors. The zygomatic major muscle is identified and blunt dissection is performed on the surface of this muscle releasing the zygomatico-cutaneous ligaments of the McGregor patch (Figure 8). The primary goal is to release and mobilize the malar fat pad into a posterior

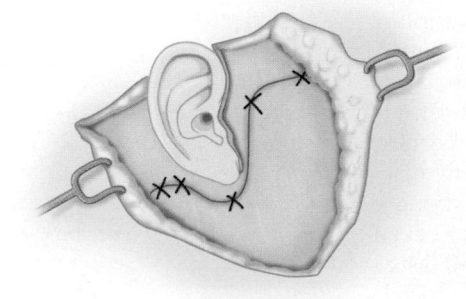

Figure 9 SMAS Closure. The SMAS-platysmal flap has been advanced and suspended with key sutures (Xs).

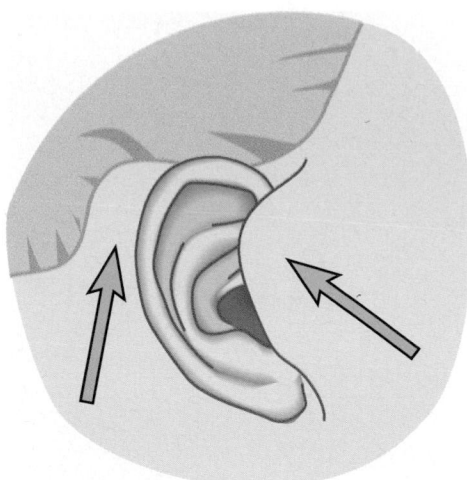

Figure 10 Redraping the skin. The anterior flap is advanced posteriorly and superiorly. The posterior flap is advanced superiorly and anteriorly to recreate, without notching, the posterior hairline.

superior position. Inferiorly the dissection is then carried deep to the platysmal muscle for approximately 3 or 4 cm. In this region, care is taken to avoid injury to the external jugular vein, greater auricular nerve, and cervical branch of the facial nerve. The SMAS-platysmal flap is then trimmed. Beginning at the superior margin, a strip of SMAS is incised down to a point 2 to 3 cm from the free edge of SMAS anterior to the lobule. This creates an inferiorly based SMAS flap that is rotated posterior to the pinna and suspended to the mastoid periosteum with interrupted 4-0 polydiaxone or 4-0 prolene sutures (Figure 9). The next suspension suture is placed from the postero-superior SMAS margin to the temporalis fascia anterior to the helical root. It is this suture that repositions the malar fat pad. A third fixation suture is placed at the level of the lobule. The last few interrupted suspension sutures are used to fixate the free edge of platysma to the mastoid periosteum. It should be stressed that a superior vector of pull on this tissue is critical to establishing a well-defined cervicomental angle. The preauricular skin flap is redraped with a similar vector of pull, while the postauricular skin is draped in a more superior fashion (Figure 10). The skin closure should be tension free, as the underlying SMAS closure should provide all the support necessary for the repositioned tissue.

The hair-bearing skin is reapproximated with staples, and the remaining preauricular and postauricular skin is closed under minimal tension with 4-0 polydiaxone sutures buried in the deep layer and interrupted 5-0 sutures superficially (nylon for preauricular skin and chromic in the postauricular skin). A 5-0 polydiaxone suture placed from the pretragal soft tissue to the overlying dermis recreates the pretragal crease. The skin advanced over the tragus is thinned, and a 6-0 fast absorbing gut suture is used to close the post-tragal incision.

We do not routinely use drains. At the conclusion of the procedure, white petrolatum is applied to the suture lines and petroleum smeared

cotton balls are placed in the conchal bowls. Nonadherent Telfa gauze is placed over the incisions, and a bulky cotton/kerlex compression dressing is applied.

An example of an excellent candidate for a deep plane facelift is depicted in Figure 11. Preoperatively, this surgical candidate would be categorized as a Class IV using the previously described Dedo classification: skin laxity, SMAS and platysmal laxity, mild excessive submental fat, anterior platysmal banding, adequate chin projection, and normal hyoid positioning. The patient underwent a deep plane facelift, submental liposuction, and platysmaplasty to address the above concerns. The deep plane approach was chosen in particular to elevate the ptotic malar fat pad and improve the midface and malar regions. The patient also underwent concomitant upper face rejuvenation including upper lid blepharoplasty and endoscopic browlift.

POSTOPERATIVE CARE

On postoperative day one, the dressing is removed and flap viability is assessed. If any small collections of serosanguinous fluid or clot are palpated these are gently expressed through the postauricular incision. A new lighter dressing is applied and left in place until the third postoperative day. The patient is then instructed to wear a commercial elastic dressing around the clock for the remainder of the first week after the operation. During this period, a regimen of cleaning the incision lines and reappyling white petrolatum is performed several times a day. The patient is allowed to shower and gently wash the hair starting the third day after surgery. For the first 72 hours after the operation, head of bed elevation is encouraged and cold compresses are applied to the face and neck at intervals of 20 minutes on and 20 minutes off. Oral antibiotics are continued for a total of 7 days.

The patient is seen for their second postoperative visit on day 6, at which time the submental sutures, preauricular sutures, and skin staples are removed. The postauricular chromic sutures are left in place to dissolve. The patient is asked to continue wearing the elastic facelift wrap at night for an additional 2 weeks. We routinely remind the patients that ecchymosis typically resolves in 2 weeks and that the majority of edema dissipates over 4 to 6 weeks. Routine follow-up visits are scheduled at 1, 3, 6, and 12 months after the operation. A consultation with our estheticians is also helpful for postoperative skin care and makeup recommendations.

COMPLICATIONS AND THEIR MANAGEMENT

Major complications following rhytidectomy are relatively uncommon. However, due to the elective nature of the procedure any complications, major or minor, are poorly tolerated by both patient and surgeon. All surgeons who per-

form rhytidectomy should preoperatively inform their patients of the potential risks, including hematoma, infection, skin flap necrosis, nerve injury, poor scarring, alopecia, ear lobe deformity, and parotid gland injury.

Hematoma

The most common complication after rhytidectomy is formation of hematoma, occurring in 2 to 15% of patients.[17] Risk factors for hematoma formation include hypertension and usage of products that inhibit platelet or clotting function, for example, aspirin, nonsteroidal anti-inflammatory drugs, and vitamin E. Postoperative vomiting and coughing can also predispose to bleeding. Male patients tend to have a higher incidence of hematoma formation, which is thought to be due to an increased blood supply to the hair follicles of the bearded skin.

The majority of reported hematomas are minor, small collections of fluid or clot that are identified in the first week after surgery. Often these can be managed by removing one or two of the postauricular sutures and gently expressing the clot. If the clot has already liquefied then an 18-gauge needle can be used to aspirate the collection. Unrecognized small collections can lead to infection, scarring, and skin discoloration.

Major hematomas requiring exploration and drainage usually occur within the first 12 hours after the operation. Clinical signs and symptoms include increasing unilateral pain, edema, skin flap ecchymosis, and bleeding from the incisions. In cases where treatment is delayed, pressure under the flaps can lead to skin necrosis. Treatment should include immediate clot evacuation, irrigation, and identification and cautery of bleeding vessel(s). In our experience, it is often difficult to identify one discrete vessel, rather there is a diffuse oozing that requires careful cautery of many suspicious sites in the dissection bed. A compressive dressing is reapplied, and the patient is reevaluted the following morning.

Infection

The rich facial blood supply and the routine use of prophylactic antibiotics are the principal reasons that postrhytidectomy infection is seldom seen. In the rare case of frank abscess formation, drainage, culture, and broad-spectrum oral or intravenous antibiotics should be implemented as indicated.

Skin Flap Necrosis

Rhytidectomy skin flaps receive their blood supply through the subdermal plexus in a random fashion. Compromise of this vascular supply can lead to necrosis and loss of skin, most commonly seen in the distal portion of the flaps, that is, periauricular skin. Risk factors include excessive thinning of the flap, excessive closure tension, hematoma, smoking, and systemic disorders, for example, diabetes mellitus. Techniques such as the deep-plane rhytidectomy theoretically should have less risk of flap complications

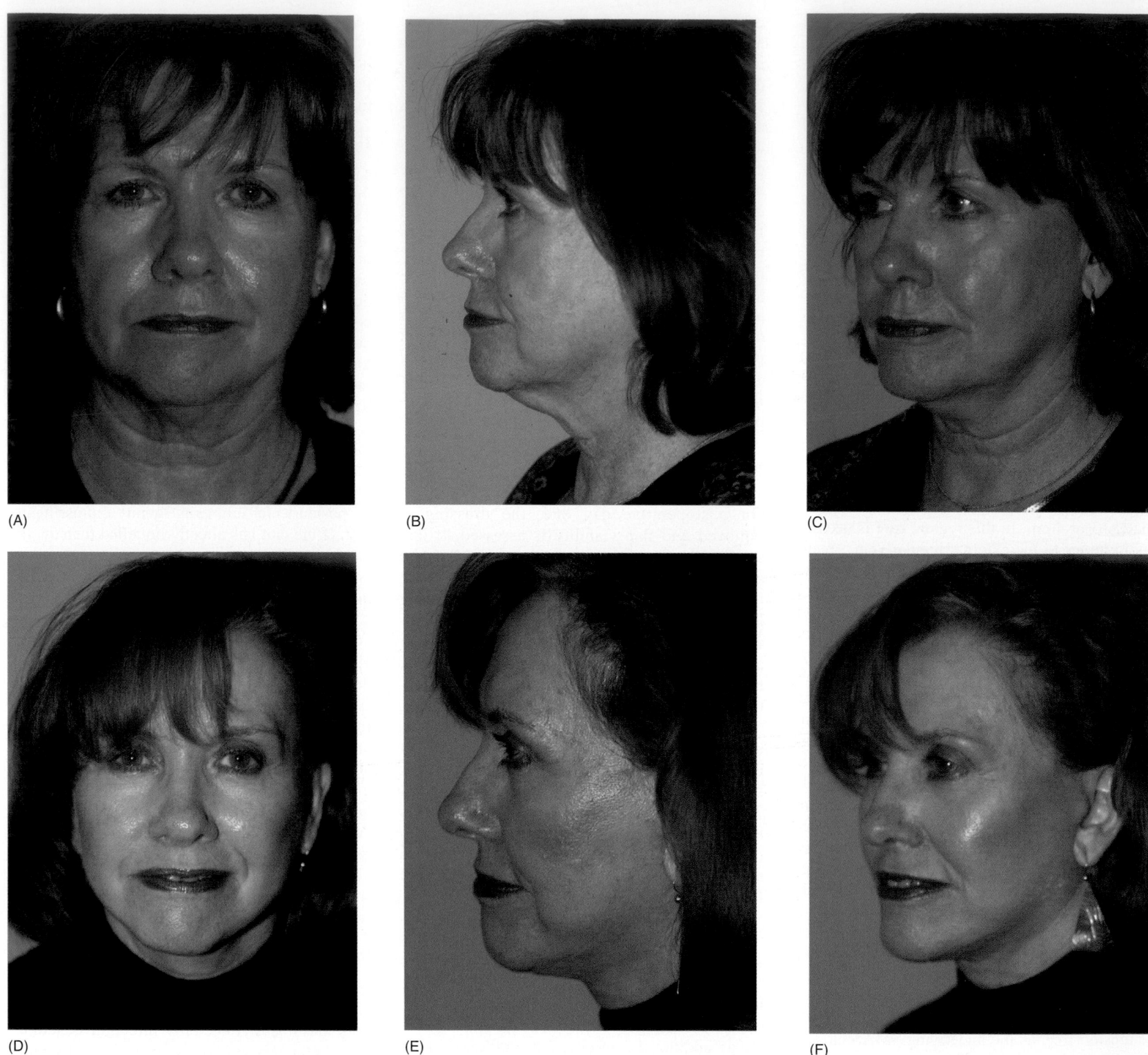

Figure 11 Preoperative (A, B, C) and postoperative (D, E, F) frontal, oblique and lateral views of a middle-aged woman who underwent deep plane rhytidectomy, plastysmaplasty, submental liposuction, endoscopic browlift, and upper lid blepharoplasty. The deep plane dissection has elevated the ptotic malar fat pad and produced improvement of the midface and malar region.

due to a better vascularized composite flap and closure tension placed on the deeper SMAS layer.

Cyanosis often precedes flap necrosis. If this is recognized early enough, it is potentially reversible. Partial-thickness skin loss can be treated conservatively with occlusive dressings or ointments. Full-thickness necrosis should be managed with limited debridement of devitalized tissue and local care to provide the best conditions for healing by secondary intention. These areas

often heal well but certainly carry an increased risk of undesirable scarring.

Nerve Damage

The most commonly injured sensory nerve is the great auricular nerve, occurring in up to 7% of cases.[18] The nerve, along with the external jugular vein, crosses the anterior border of the sternocleidomastoid muscle several centimeters below the angle of mandible. Injury to the nerve can occur when attempting to obtain hemostasis

from inadvertent injury to the vein. If the nerve is transected, an end-to-end anastomosis with epineural repair should be attempted. Failure to repair such as injury can result in formation of a painful neuroma. Injury to this nerve is often permanent, however, the affected sensory area usually decreases over time.

Injury to motor branches of the facial nerve is far less common, occurring in 0.5 to 2.6%.[17] Injuries of the temporal and marginal mandibular branches are the two most often reported. The buccal branches are also susceptible to injury when extended dissection techniques, for example, deep-plane lift, are used. The cervical branch can be injured while mobilizing the lateral edge of the platysma muscle resulting in a "pseudomarginal" nerve paresis. Damage to the cervical branch can be distinguished from marginal mandibular nerve injury by the fact that the patient will be able to evert the lower lip due to a functioning mentalis muscle. As mentioned earlier in this chapter, a thorough understanding of the facial nerve anatomy can help avoid these complications.

Fortunately, the majority of nerve injuries are neurapraxic in nature. This temporary paresis often resolves over the first few months after injury. In our experience, the majority of immediate postoperative paralysis or paresis is due to local anesthetic effects, which dissipate in several hours.

Hypertrophic Scarring

Excessive skin closure tension is commonly regarded as the primary cause of hypertrophic scars after rhytidectomy. Other predisposing factors include race, skin type, and prior history of abnormal scarring. Most commonly located in the postauricular region, these scars usually develop in the first 3 months after the operation. Initial treatment consists of intralesional corticosteroid injections (triamcinolone 5 to 10 mg/mL) at 3-week intervals. Excision of these scars should be delayed for 6 to 12 months, and potential recurrence of lesions can be lessened with judicious use of deep sutures.

Alopecia and Ear Lobe Deformity

Alopecia is usually due to excessive closure line tension causing transient shock of the hair follicles. Patients are reassured that recovery is usually within 3 to 6 months. If follicles do not fully recover, the hairless skin can be excised and closed primarily. The use of hair transplantation techniques can also be employed to fill in bare areas or restore loss of the temporal tuft.

Post-rhytidectomy ear lobe deformity (pixie ear) can be a sequela of poor incision placement, malpositioning of the lobule at closure, and tension on the closure. Correction of this complication can be challenging, often requiring an advancement flap technique with closure tension supported by deeper layers.

Parotid Injury

Inadvertent injury to the parotid gland can occur during SMAS flap or platysma elevation. The subsequent formation of a glandular pseudocyst (sialocele) or salivary fistula is seldom seen but is a potential concern. If parotid parenchyma is exposed during the dissection, the overlying fascia should be sewn over the defect. Postoperative seroma formation in the area of the mandibular angle should raise suspicion of sialocele formation. Conservative treatment with oral anticholinergics, serial aspirations, and pressure dressing are recommended. Recurrent collections may require surgical exploration and placement of a suction drain.

CONCLUSIONS

Performed alone or in combination, procedures such as submental liposuction, platysmaplasty, chin augmentation, and rhytidectomy can provide a dramatic rejuvenation of the lower face and neck. A thorough understanding of the relevant anatomy coupled with an accurate preoperative analysis of the aging anatomy is essential to determining which procedures are to be recommended as well as achieving the optimal surgical result.

REFERENCES

1. Skoog T. Plastic surgery: The aging face. In: Skoog TG, editor. Plastic Surgery: New Methods and Refinements. Philadelphia: WB Saunders; 1974. p. 300–30.
2. Mitz V, Peyronie M. The superficial musculoaponeurotic system (SMAS) in the parotid and cheek area. Plast Reconstr Surg 1976;58:80–8.
3. Hamra ST. The deep-plane rhytidectomy. Plast Reconstr Surg 1990;86:53–61.
4. Hamra ST. Composite rhytidectomy. Plast Reconstr Surg 1992;90:1–13.
5. Baker SR. Tri-plane rhytidectomy. Arch Otol Head Surg 1997;123:1167–72.
6. Larrabee WF, Makielski KH, Henderson JL. Surgical Anatomy of the Face, 2nd edition. Philadelphia: Lippincott Williams and Wilkins; 2004. p. 50.
7. Larrabee WF, Makielski KH, Sykes J. Surgical anatomy for endoscopic facial surgery. In: Keller GS, editor. Endoscopic Facial Plastic Surgery. St. Louis: Mosby; 1997. p. 28.
8. Dedo DD. A preoperative classification of the neck for cervicofacial rhytidectomy. Laryngoscope 1980;90:1894–6.
9. Larrabee WF, Makielski KH, Henderson JL. Surgical Anatomy of the Face, 2nd edition. Philadelphia Lippincott Williams and Wilkins; 2004. p. 26.
10. Millard DR, Jr, Garst WP, Beck RL, Thompson ID. Submental and submandibular lipectomy in conjunction with a facelift, in the male or female. Plast Reconstr Surg 1972;49:385–91.
11. Illouz Y-G. Body contouring by lipolysis: A 5-year experience with over 3000 cases. Plast Reconstr Surg 1983;72:591–7.
12. Becker DG, Cook TA, Wang TD, et al. A 3-year multi-institutional experience with the liposhaver. Arch Fac Plast Surg 1999;1:171–6.
13. Perkins SW, Gibson B. Use of submentoplasty to enhance cervical recontouring in face-lift surgery. Arch Otolaryngol Head Neck Surg 1993;119:179–83.
14. Kamer FM, Frankel AS. Isolated submentoplasty: A limited approach to the aging neck. Arch Otolaryngol Head Neck Surg 1997;123:66–70.
15. Giampapa VC, DiBernardo BE. Neck recontouring with suture suspension and liposuction: An alternative for the early rhytidectomy candidate. Aesthetic Plast Surg 1995;19:217–23.
16. Prabhat A, Dyer WK. Improving surgery on the aging neck with an adjustable expanded polytetrafluoroethylene cervical sling. Arch Fac Plast Surg 2003;5:491–501.
17. Sullivan CA, Masin J, Maniglia AJ, Stepnick DW. Complications of rhytidectomy in an otolaryngology training program. Laryngoscope 1999;109:198–203.
18. Pitanguy I, Cervello MP, Degand M. Nerve injuries during rhytidectomy: Considerations after 3,203 cases. Aesthetic Plast Surg 1980;4:257–65.

PEDIATRIC OTORHINOLARYNGOLOGY

62

Microtia, Canal Atresia, and Middle Ear Anomalies

Simon C. Parisier, MD

Jose N. Fayad, MD

Charles P. Kimmelman, MD

Anthony P. Sclafani, MD

George Alexiades MD

The child born with a malformed ear faces a lifelong hearing and communication impairment along with the social stigma of a facial deformity. Associated disturbances of the vestibular system may add the developmental hurdle of a motor delay. Frequently, there are additional anomalies, such as mandibular hypoplasia, as well as other facial and skeletal deformities. There may be dysfunction of associated neural pathways, including cranial nerves and intracranial structures. Additionally, there are psychological factors to be considered, including parental guilt, peer ridicule, and the shame of "being different." Educationally and economically, these hearing-impaired children face the prospect of limited opportunities. The appropriate management involves recognizing the problems and limitations of therapy, which need to be thoroughly understood by the parents and, when appropriate, the patient.

EMBRYOLOGY OF ATRESIA AND MICROTIA

In the 3 to 4 mm embryo (3 to 4 weeks), the first indications of aural ontogenesis are the first and second branchiomeric structures and the otic placode, an ectodermal thickening on the lateral surface of the head opposite the fourth ventricle. The placode invaginates to first form a pit and then a vesicle detached from its surface origin. This otocyst forms the inner ear membranous structures, with the endolymphatic duct developing first at the 6 mm stage, followed by the appearance of the semicircular ducts and the cochlear diverticulum at the 15 mm stage (6 weeks). By the end of the third month, the cochlea is fully coiled.

The cranial nerves entering the otocyst exert an inductive influence to produce neuroepithelium, for which retinoic acid is a potent morphogen. Retinoic acid receptors are uniquely expressed in the developing organ of Corti; medications that affect retinoic acid metabolism, such as isotretinoin (Accutane, Roche, Nutley, New Jersey), can lead to embryopathies, including inner ear malformation.[1]

The cochleovestibular ganglia develop from the otic placode epithelium. The nerve fibers themselves not only influence sensory cell development but are also directed to the developing inner ear by the sensory cells.[2]

As the membranous structures of the inner ear form, they become enveloped in a cartilaginous capsule, which eventually gives rise to the petrous portion of the temporal bone. Concurrently, the structures that originate from the first pharyngeal pouch develop separately but adjacent to the otic capsule derivatives. The pouch begins to form in the 3 to 4 mm embryo and expands into a tubotympanic recess, which will eventually give rise to the eustachian tube, middle ear space, and mastoid air cell system. The third branchial arch migrates superiorly to the level of the recess, and its artery (the internal carotid) comes to lie dorsal to the eustachian tube. Variations in this relationship may result in a lateralized displacement of the internal carotid artery into the middle ear space. In adults, an ectopic carotid artery can be mistaken for a middle ear mass, such as a glomus tumor.

As the pharyngeal pouches form in the 3 to 4 mm embryo, corresponding grooves develop on the external surface of the nascent cervical region. The first of these branchial clefts deepens until it approaches the tubotympanic recess, being separated only by the thin layer of mesoderm destined to become the middle fibrous layer of the tympanic membrane. Subsequently, in the 30 mm embryo (8 weeks), the primordial external canal becomes occluded by an ectodermal plug. By the twenty-first week, this begins to resorb to form the definitive external auditory canal, replete with its hair and glandular appendages. Aberrations in the canalization process can lead to stenosis, canal tortuosity, or fibrous or osseous obliteration. Since middle ear structures develop independently, the tympanic cavity and ossicles may be normal.

Defects in the canalization process may also be associated with faulty formation of the pinna, which arises in the 8 to 11 mm embryo from six mesodermal thickenings. These hillocks surround the entrance of the first branchial cleft. The first branchial arch cartilage (Meckel cartilage) forms the tragus and superior helical crus; the remainder of the pinna derives from the second arch cartilage (Reichert cartilage), although some authorities posit a hyoid arch derivation for all but the tragus. The developing auricular appendage migrates from its initial position in the lower face toward the temporal area. This movement occurs along the fusion plane of the first and second branchial arches. The auricle is initially located anteriorly in a horizontal axis; with development of the branchial structures it migrates from its original position in the lower face laterally, and as its axis rotates, it assumes a more vertical angulation. Branchial cleft dysmorphogenesis can impede this migration and leave the pinna in a low, transverse orientation (Figure 1).

As the middle ear forms, the separation between the first pharyngeal pouch and cleft is filled in by mesenchyme. In the 8 mm embryo (6 weeks), part of the connective tissue condenses to form the malleus handle; the subsequent expansion of the tympanic cavity

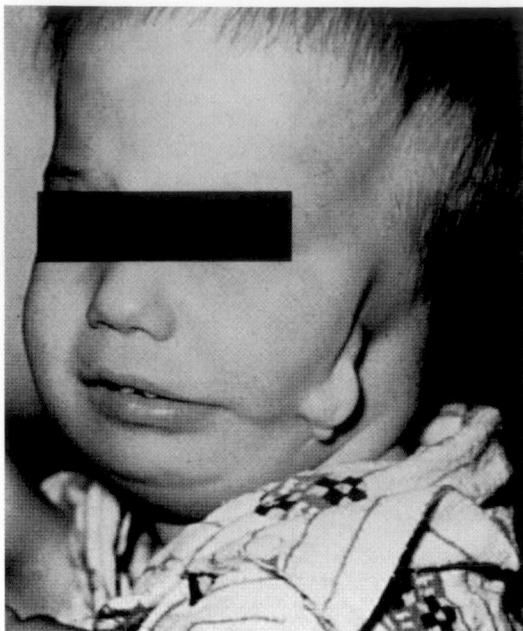

Figure 1 This child's auricle has not migrated from its embryonic low, transverse position.

superiorly is delayed until the cartilaginous otic capsule fully forms. The expansion of the first pharyngeal pouch results in the envelopment of the ossicles in an endodermal epithelium. The ossicles predominantly originate from mesenchymal visceral bars of the first and second arches. The first arch forms the head of the malleus and body of the incus, with the second arch giving rise to the manubrium, long process of the incus, stapes superstructure, and lateral portion of the footplate. The medial lamina of the footplate is derived from the otic capsule. The obturator foramen of the stapes forms around the stapedial artery, which usually remains diminutive while the stapes enlarges. If variations in vascular development cause enlargement of the artery, a conductive hearing loss may result from impairment of stapes motion. As the derivatives of the first pharyngeal pouch continue to extend into the developing temporal bone, the antrum, mastoid air cells, and petrous pyramid cells begin to form. Most mastoid development is postnatal; abnormalities that arrest middle ear formation result in a poorly pneumatized bone.

The facial nerve is intimately related to the development of the middle and inner ear structures outlined above. The blastema of the stapes is adjacent to the seventh nerve, which divides the second (hyoid) visceral mesenchymal bar into a laterohyale, stapes blastema, and interhyale. The interhyale forms the stapedius tendon, whereas the laterohyale forms part of the bony fallopian canal and pyramid. Thus, the development of the stapes is closely related to that of the facial nerve. Abnormalities in the development of the stapes are frequently associated with facial nerve anomalies. This relationship of facial nerve to developing middle ear structures increases the likelihood of an anomalous course of the nerve in the malformed middle ear.[3,4] Development of the ear is also discussed in Chapter 2, "Development of the Ear."

ETIOLOGY OF AURAL ATRESIA

Atresia and microtia are part of several known syndromes associated with inherited defects or acquired embryopathies owing to intrauterine infection (rubella, syphilis), ischemic injury (hemifacial microsomia), or toxin exposure (thalidomide, isotretinoin).

Although inner ear abnormalities, such as Usher syndrome, Waardenburg syndrome, and the neurofibromatoses, are becoming understood on a molecular biologic basis, the genetic basis of external and middle ear anomalies generally remains poorly characterized.[5] Aural atresia occurs in approximately 1 in 20,000 live births. Although the inner and middle ears develop separately, inner ear abnormalities coexist in 12 to 50% of cases. Atresia is bilateral in 30% of cases, occurring more commonly in males and in the right ear.[6]

Microtia occurs in 1 in 7,000 live births and can be associated with aural atresia. Microtia represents a failure of normal development of first and second branchial arch fusion. It is more common in males (two-thirds) and in the right ear (60%). Ten percent of cases are bilateral. Prenatal maternal history is not associated with the development of microtia.

Children with microtia should be screened for hemifacial microsomia and other first and second arch anomalies, and coordination of care with a maxillofacial surgeon beginning at an early age can be critical in optimizing facial symmetry.

It is not surprising that an embryonic insult severe enough to cause aural atresia would also affect other organ systems. The following organs or systems may be anomalous in patients with atresia: neurocranium defects (Crouzon disease or craniofacial dysostosis), central nervous system (mental retardation), oral cavity (first and second branchial arch syndromes), the eye (Goldenhar syndrome), the neck (branchial fistula), the CHARGE association (coloboma, heart defect, choanal atresia, retarded growth, genitourinary defects, and ear anomalies), Treacher Collins syndrome (mandibulofacial dysostosis), Duane syndrome (abducens palsy with retracted globe), VATER complex (probable disorganization of the primitive streak with impairment of early mesodermal migration causing vertebral defects, anal atresia, tracheoesophageal fistula, renal defects, and genital anomalies), and Pierre Robin syndrome. Chromosomal anomalies affecting the external and middle ears include Turner syndrome and trisomy 13 to 15, 18, 21, and 22 syndromes.[7]

Anomalies of the ear in the absence of syndromes are usually not familial. From the above information, it is obvious that other congenital anomalies should be assiduously sought; some, such as renal dysgenesis, may not be readily apparent. A chromosomal analysis may be indicated. As progress is made in the identification of genes and their products in the recently mapped human genome, the genetic basis for many of these disorders may provide a means of treatment or prevention.[8] The genetic and molecular

determinants of malformations of the ear are discussed in Chapter 2, "Development of the Ear."

DIAGNOSIS AND EVALUATION

In the more severe cases of microtia, the diagnosis is apparent on inspection of the external ear. Depending on the degree of the abnormality, the microtic ear may be classified into three grades. In grade I, the auricle is developed and, though misshapen, has a readily recognizable, characteristic anatomy (Figure 2). In grade II, the helix is rudimentary and the lobule developed (Figure 3). In grade III, an amorphous skin tag is present[9] (Figure 4). Grade III microtia can be further described as conchal remnant or lobular remnant. Lobular remnants typically present with a vertically oriented skin covered mass of deformed cartilage superiorly, extending into a soft tissue and skin portion inferiorly. Conchal remnant microtias present with all of the above, with additionally a blind pouch, which represents a primitive conchal bowl. In all stages, wide variations of morphology exist. The pinna may be fully formed with a transverse and low-set orientation. There may be accessory appendages of the pinna (pretragal tags with or without cartilage) and preauricular sinus tracts. The external canal may be stenotic or atretic to varying degrees[10] (Figure 5). In cases of stenosis, entrapped squamous cell epithelium may lead to a retention cholesteatoma with bone destruction.

Schuknecht observed that in 7 ears with congenital meatal stenosis, all had cholesteatomas, whereas 3 of 11 ears with partial atresia and narrowed canals had cholesteatoma.[11] In 50 ears with complete atresia, only 2 had cholesteatomas.

Abnormalities of the tympanic cavity alone may occur with a normal tympanic membrane and external ear. In ears with conductive hearing losses and normal otoscopic examinations, isolated ossicular anomalies should be suspected (Table 1). Ossicular fixation can be produced by a variety of abnormalities and may involve the stapes, incus, or malleus. Alternatively, there may be a failure of bone development producing an ossicular discontinuity, which generally involves the incus and/or stapes arch. Ossicular malformations caused by abnormalities related to first or second branchial cartilaginous derivatives can frequently be surgically repaired (see Table 1, groups I and II). However, ossicular fixations owing to cochlear capsule abnormalities, especially when associated with an aberrant facial nerve, may not be surgically correctable (see Table 1, group III). Otic capsule abnormalities producing stapedial fixation are frequently associated with abnormal communication between the inner ear and the subarachnoid space. In these instances, manipulation of the stapes results in a persistent gusher of cerebrospinal fluid. Vascular malformations also occur in the middle ear, such as high jugular bulb, persistent stapedial artery, and anomalous course of the carotid artery.[12]

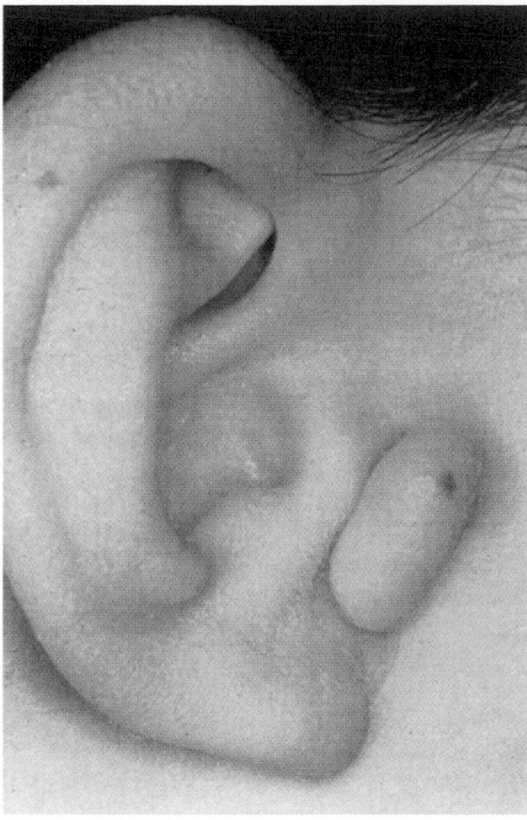

Figure 2 This pinna exhibits a grade I microtia with canal atresia. The size of the auricle and the characteristic anatomic landmarks are fairly normal. A pretragal skin tag is present.

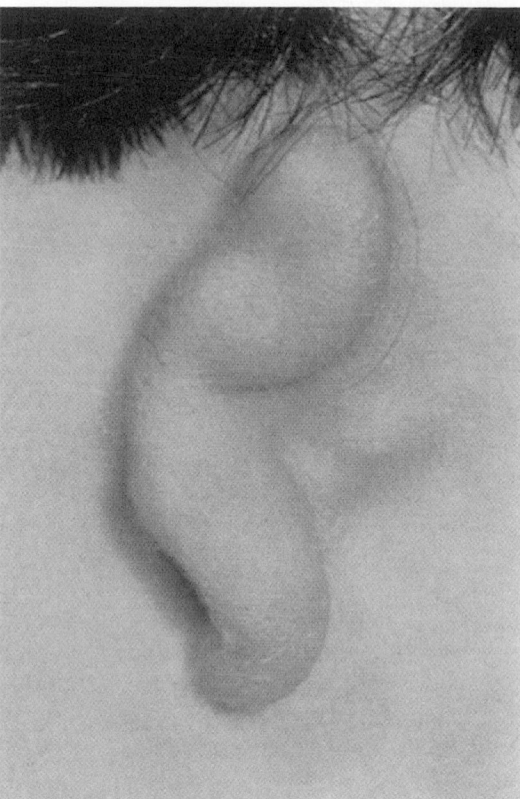

Figure 4 Auricle showing a grade III microtia. An amorphous ridge of skin and nubbins of cartilage are present in place of a recognizable, well-developed auricle.

Table 1 Congenital Middle Ear Abnormalities with Patent Ear Canal, Mobile Tympanic Membrane, and Conductive Loss
I. Ossicular fixation
a. Stapes fixation
1. Deficient annular ligament
2. Elongated pyramidal process, ossified stapedial tendon
b. Malleolar-incudal fixation
1. Lateral epitympanic ankylosis
2. Medial epitympanic ankylosis of body of incus, head of malleus
3. Ossified anterior malleolar ligament
II. Ossicular discontinuity
a. Absent stapes arch
b. Deficient lenticular process of incus
c. Deficient long process of incus
III. Cochlear capsule and facial nerve anomalies
a. Aplasia of oval or round window
b. Facial nerve anomaly occluding oval window
c. High jugular bulb occluding the round window niche

Further delineation of structural abnormalities requires computed tomography (CT).[13] Younger children may require sedation if they are unable to cooperate. The images are processed with a bone algorithm image enhancement using 1.5 mm slices

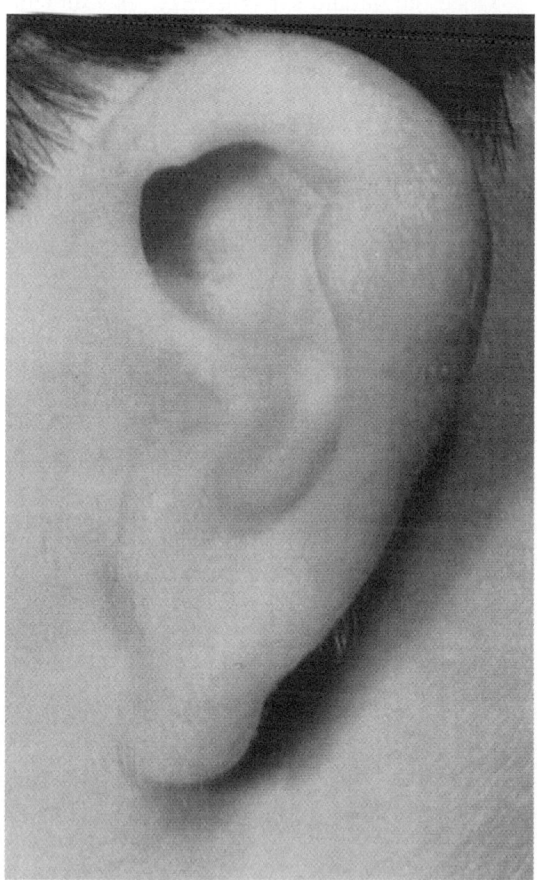

Figure 3 An example of a grade II microtia. The auricle is reduced in size and has a characteristic recognizable shape. The inferior and superior crura have not developed, although the helix is well preserved.

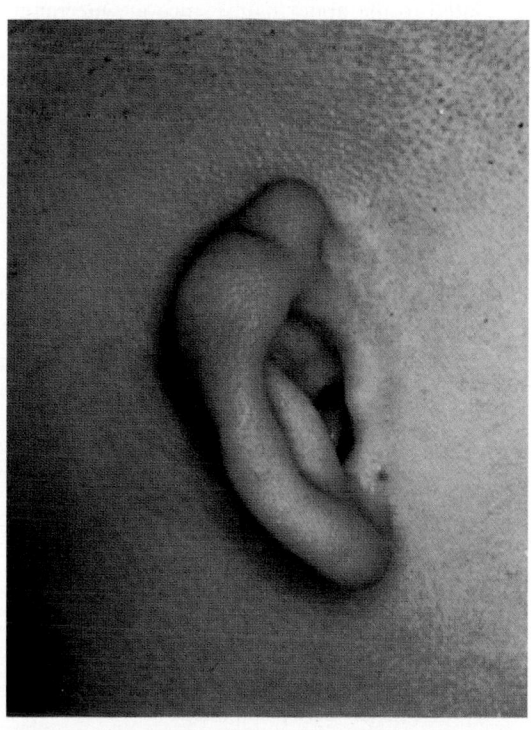

Figure 5 A grade II to III microtia with poor formation of the superior third of the auricle and a preauricular pit, possibly because of a first branchial arch dysmorphism. The lower portion of the ear, which is derived from the second branchial arch, has a relatively normal appearance. The canal is stenotic, leading to the subsequent development of a retention cholesteatoma.

at either 1.5 or 1 mm intervals. Optimally, both axial and coronal scans are obtained, although reformatted coronal or sagittal images may be adequate. Three-dimensional reconstruction may be useful in visualizing the temporal bone topography.[13,14] Auditory brainstem responses (ABRs) should be performed in all children born with either microtia or atresia as neonates. In cases of microtia with fairly normal canals, an ossicular malformation producing a conductive hearing loss may be present. In patients with unilateral atresia, it is not unusual for the seemingly normal contralateral ear to have a hearing loss. Bilateral involvement may cause masking dilemmas; such is the case when one ear has a conductive loss and the other a sensorineural loss. These dilemmas may be minimized by using multichannel analysis of ipsilateral versus contralateral responses to determine the laterality of wave I.[15] As the infant matures, behavioral audiometric evaluations must be obtained to confirm the neurophysiologic tests of hearing. In children older than 1 year, conditioned free field play audiometry should help to quantify the overall hearing levels. Eventually, pure-tone and speech testing with masking should be obtained in children with fairly normal canals. Impedance and stapedial reflex measures in a seemingly normal ear can provide valuable information as well as more extensive malformations occurring in Treacher Collins syndrome and hemifacial microsomia. CT studies allow determination of the degree of the canal atresia, the thickness of the atresia plate (Figure 6A), the extent of pneumatization of the middle ear and mastoid, the distance between the glenoid fossa and mastoid, the intratemporal course of the facial nerve, the status of the malleus and incus, and, in some instances, the presence or absence of the stapes and oval window (Figure 6B). However, subtleties of oval and round window anatomy are often not revealed. An unsuspected cholesteatoma may also be apparent. The normalcy of the osseous inner ear structures is also revealed by CT.

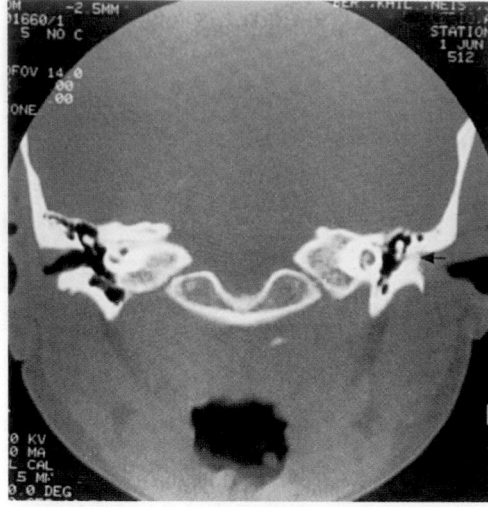

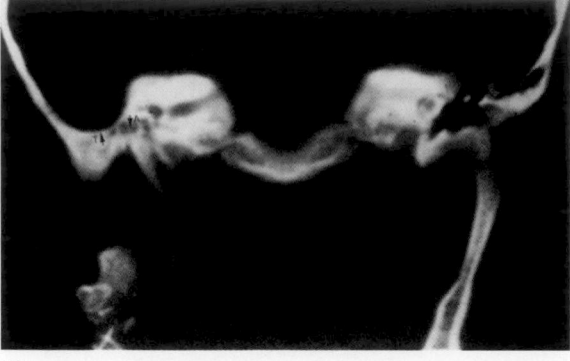

(B)

(A)

Figure 6 (A) A coronal computed tomographic (CT) scan showing a bony atresia plate (*arrow*). The middle ear space is normally pneumatized. (B) Coronal CT scan showing a low-lying tegmen (T), which precludes construction of an external canal. The middle ear cleft has not developed. A rudimentary antrum is unaerated (A). Atresia surgery is contraindicated in this case.

Evaluation of the function of other organ systems should be considered by the otologist. For example, some of the syndromal associations of atresia involve mandibular and laryngeal anomalies that can lead to airway obstruction; cardiac, renal, endocrine, and immune function should be ascertained in selected instances.

MANAGEMENT OF AURAL ATRESIA AND MICROTIA

Nonsurgical

The prime concern in the young child is the assessment and improvement of hearing. When ear deformities are present, the ABR techniques outlined above are helpful in determining the type and severity of hearing loss and should be performed as early in life as possible. Early amplification, auditory training, and speech therapy can improve speech and language skills. In children with bilateral atresia, amplification with bone-conduction aids should be provided as soon as possible, preferably within the first few months of life.[16–18] In infants with a unilateral atresia and conductive hearing loss in the seemingly normal ear, an air-conduction aid should be fitted to the ear with a canal.

Surgical

In the unilateral case with normal contralateral hearing, repair of either the microtia or the atresia is considered elective, and there is less urgency to intervene during childhood. When the atresia is bilateral with acceptable-appearing auricles, reconstructive surgery can be performed at a fairly young age. However, in cases of microtia that require reconstruction, atresia repair should be deferred until the initial stages of the auricular repair are completed. Generally, microtia surgery requires a cartilage graft that is obtained from the lower costochondral region. An adequate graft requires sufficient growth and fusion at the

donor site, which has usually occurred by 5 to 6 years of age. Additionally, in bilateral cases, many authorities recommend postponing surgery for the restoration of hearing until at least age five so that pneumatization can develop.[11] In children with frequent upper respiratory infections and suspected eustachian tube dysfunction, it may also be necessary to delay hearing reconstructive surgery.

Surgical Treatment of Congenital Conductive Hearing Loss. The success of the surgical correction of congenital conductive hearing losses is related to the abnormality since a wide range of malformations is possible.[10] Surgery in an ear that has an isolated ossicular malformation with an otherwise patent canal, intact tympanic membrane, aerated middle ear cleft, normal facial nerve, and mobile stapes has the potential for excellent hearing (Table 2, class I). Conversely, an ear with canal atresia, a narrowed and poorly aerated middle ear space, and an anomalously positioned facial nerve occluding the oval window is destined to have poor postoperative hearing (see Table 2, class III). Between these two extremes is an array of anomalies with variable surgical outcomes. Even with sophisticated

imaging techniques, the preoperative prediction of what awaits the otologist is not always accurate.[19]

Surgeons wishing to correct congenital conductive hearing losses are embarking on a procedure with significant potential complications. Generally, the initial attempt is the procedure most likely to improve the hearing. Unplanned revisions are often more complex and less successful. Additionally, if a significant sensorineural hearing loss occurs after surgery in a patient with bilateral malformations, the opposite ear is effectively excluded from surgical correction since it becomes the better hearing ear. Before assuming this responsibility, especially in children, the otologic surgeon must have sufficient experience to maximize the likelihood of a successful outcome.

The presence of a conductive hearing loss in an ear with a normal canal and mobile drumhead generally indicates that the ossicular chain is not transmitting sound energy to the cochlea. Isolated ossicular malformations involving the stapes arch and long process of the incus may not be appreciated on CT studies. In these cases, the middle ear can be explored by elevating a tympanomeatal flap and assessing the normalcy of the ossicular transduction mechanism. If the canal is small, a postauricular approach will improve operative exposure. Frequently, even the young child's ear canal has a sufficient diameter to admit an adequately sized ear speculum, even though the length of the canal is shorter.

Once the middle ear is entered, the surgeon needs to decide if the chain is fixed. If so, what is the cause of the fixation (see Table 1). First, the motility of the incus and malleus is ascertained. Is the fixation in the epitympanum and, if not, where (Figure 7)? Drilling away the bone over the malleus head and body of the incus provides the required exposure to explore this area. Is the stapedial tendon ossified? If the stapes is fixed, mobilization may produce a sustained improvement. Alternatively, a stapedectomy using a replacement prosthesis with an oval window tissue graft to

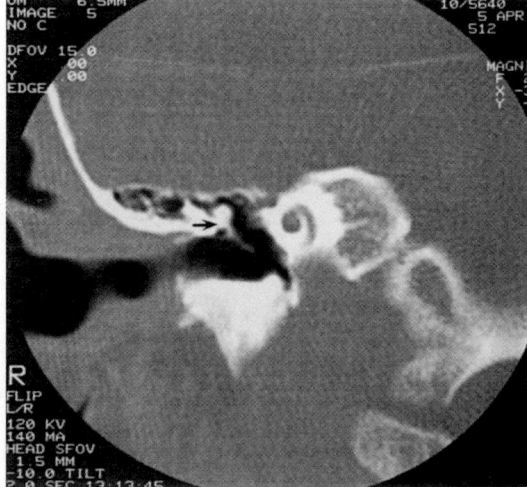

Figure 7 A coronal computed tomographic scan in a patient with a congenital conductive hearing loss caused by osseous fixation of the malleus head to the lateral epitympanic wall (*arrow*).

Table 2 Congenital Atresia Classification

Class I
    a. Aerated normal middle ear space
    b. Developed oval window with mobile stapes
    c. Oval window not obstructed by facial nerve
Class II
    a. Narrowed, but aerated, middle ear space
    b. Fixed stapes, oval window aplasia
    c. Oval window not obstructed by facial nerve
Class III
    a. Nonaerated, hypoplastic middle ear space
    b. Oval window obstructed by facial nerve
    c. Tegmen low hanging, obstructs access to middle ear space

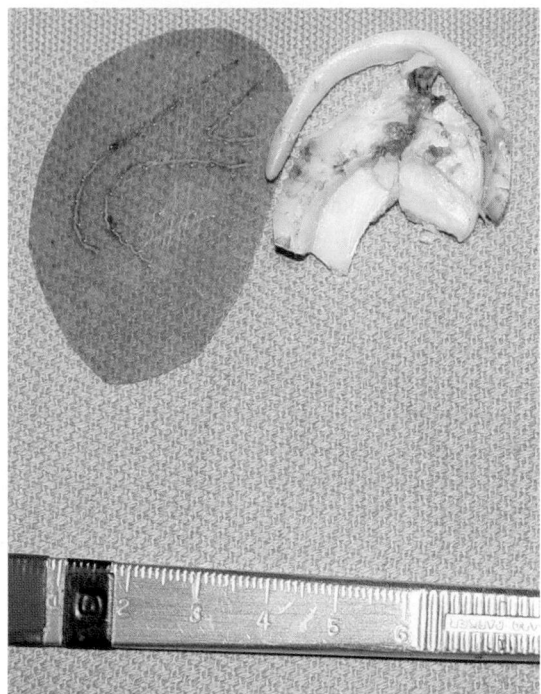

Figure 8 Costal cartilage framework for repair of right microtia. Sixth and seventh rib cartilage is used to recreate the antihelix and conchal bowl; eighth rib cartilage is thinned and sutured to sixth and seventh rib cartilage to serve as the helical rim.

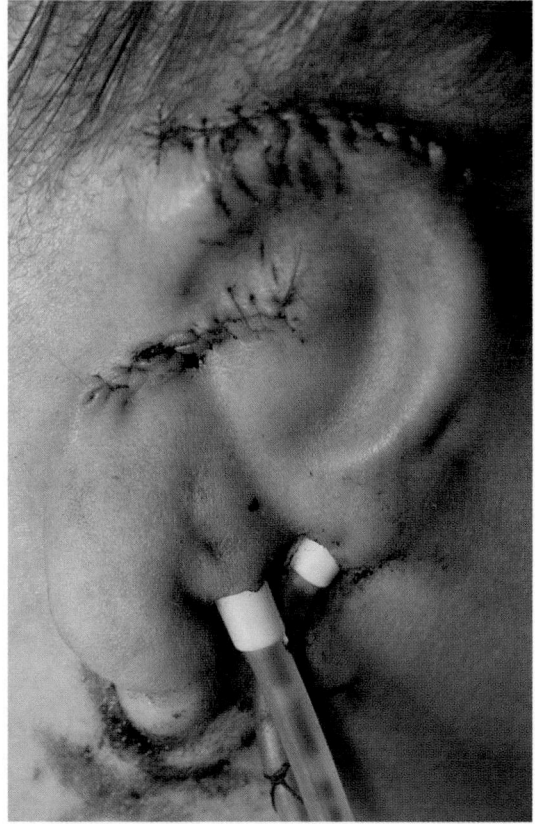

Figure 9 At the conclusion of the first stage, the framework has been placed and suction drains coapt skin to the framework.

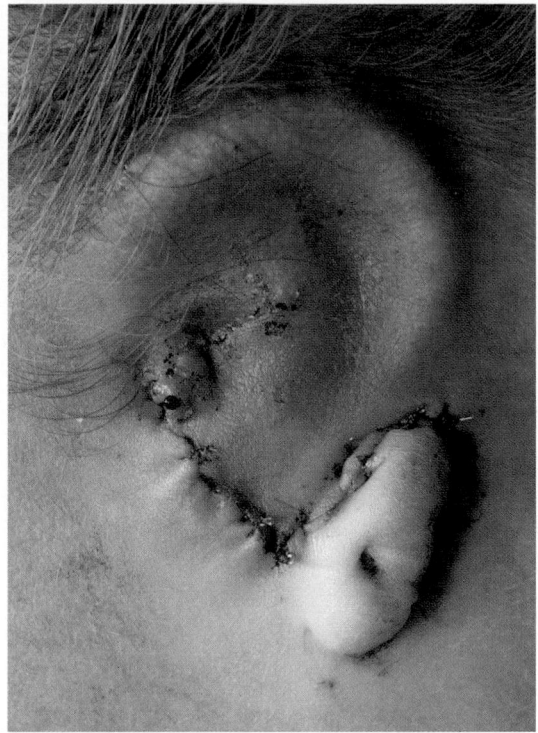

Figure 10 Prior to the second-stage procedure, the lobular remnant is displaced anteriorly and is separate from the tail of the neohelix.

prevent a perilymphatic leak may be performed. In some cases, the surgeon may elect to defer stapes surgery until the child is grown.

A gap interrupting the ossicular chain's continuity occurs most commonly at the incudostapedial joint, either owing to absence of the lenticular process or long process of the incus or the stapes arch. The presence of a mobile stapes facilitates the surgery and greatly improves the operative result. A variety of techniques have proven useful in the restoration of ossicular chain continuity by means of bridging an existing gap. If there is a small distance between the stapes capitulum and the long process of the incus, a tragal cartilage graft can successfully negotiate the gap. Deficiencies of the long process of the incus can be corrected by either interposing the reshaped incus between the mobile stapes and the malleus handle or using an alloplastic prosthesis designed for this purpose (type III tympanoplasty). When the stapes arch is absent, similar procedures can be performed to bridge the gap from either the malleus handle or the undersurface of the drumhead to the mobile footplate (type IV tympanoplasty). A coexisting fixation of the stapes or obstruction of the oval window by the facial nerve increases the technical difficulty, yields poorer hearing results, and increases the chance of complications, such as sensorineural hearing loss or facial nerve injury.[20]

Surgery for Microtia and Canal Stenosis or Atresia. Congenital malformations of the auricle, external canal, and middle ear may occur as isolated abnormalities or in various combinations. Reconstruction of the external ear is usually performed by a plastic surgeon, whereas external auditory canal and middle ear defects are

corrected by the otologist; both work as a team to achieve the optimal result.

Microtia surgery is technically difficult, and not infrequently, the results are somewhat disappointing. The surgery should be performed by individuals with special expertise.[21] Auricular reconstruction is an elective procedure. The deformity can usually be masked by a longer hair style. Generally, the slight deformity of a grade I microtia may be cosmetically acceptable. Reconstruction of a moderately deformed grade II microtia must be individualized. Correction of a severe grade III microtia requires several staged procedures.

Treatment of microtia must begin with a frank discussion of the surgical and nonsurgical options with the patient's parents, as well as surgical timing considerations. Generally, surgery is deferred until the child reaches 5 to 6 years of age. Prior to this, the contralateral ear is undersized and underdeveloped and available costal cartilage is limited; moreover, the child is not sufficiently mature to comply and assist with postoperative care. Significantly, children younger than 5 years of age generally have not been stigmatized because of their deformity by their peers.

The standard surgical technique for microtia reconstruction has been well-described by Tanzer[22] and subsequently refined by Brent.[23] During the first stage, costal cartilage is harvested from the contralateral sixth to eighth ribs using a curvilinear incision near the medial aspect of the costal margin. A template based on the contralateral ear is made from sterilized, exposed radiographic film and accurately copies the contour

and size of the pertinent structures of the normal auricle (Figure 8). Using the template as a guide, the appropriate sections of costal cartilage are harvested. The medial portion of the seventh rib will serve as the posterior rim of the conchal bowl and superior crus, and the synchondrosis between the sixth and seventh ribs is harvested en bloc with the seventh rib and is later sculpted to serve as the inferior crus. A segment of the eighth rib is harvested separately and is used to

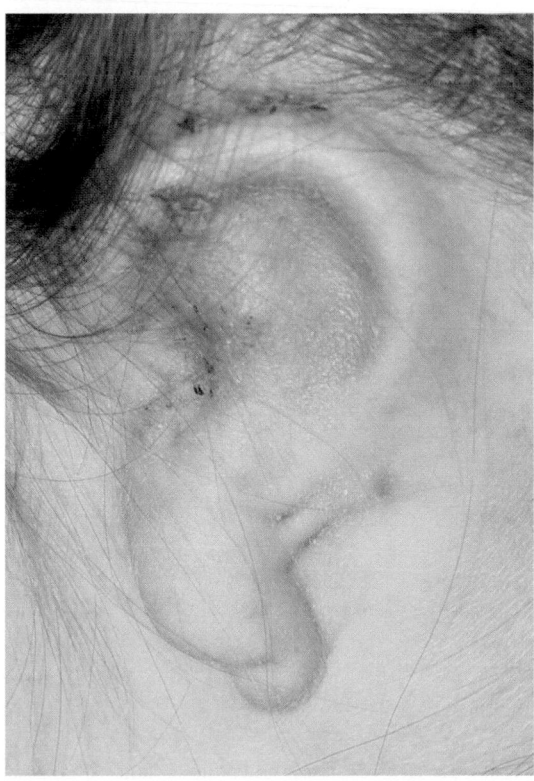

Figure 11 At the conclusion of the second stage, the lobule has been transposed using a Z-plasty technique.

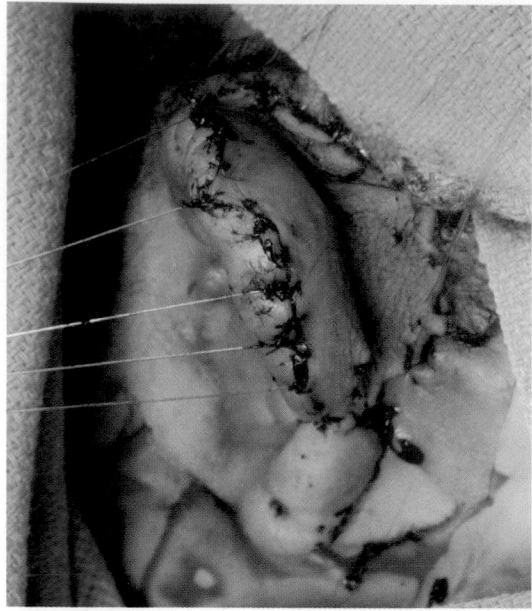

Figure 12 During the third stage of microtia repair, the framework is elevated from the temple, the posterior scalp is advanced into the postauricular sulcus and the bare areas of the auricle and sulcus covered with a skin graft.

construct the helical rim which generally requires at least an 8 cm long segment. Great care is taken to dissect in a subperichondrial plane on the deep side to avoid puncture of the parietal pleura and a pneumothorax. Once all cartilage is harvested, meticulous hemostasis is ensured. The wound is then filled with warm, sterile saline, and positive pressure ventilation manually applied and held by the anesthesiologist for 10 seconds. If no bubbles indicative of an air leak are observed, the wound is drained and closed in layers; however, if an air leak is identified, the site of pleural

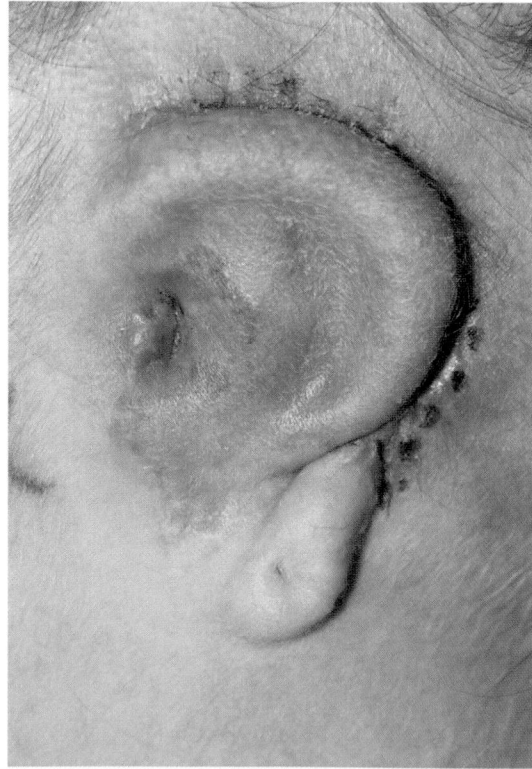

Figure 13 Healed auricle after three stages of repair, prior to atresia repair. Blue dotted line indicates incision that will be made for the atresia repair.

injury is identified. If small, a red rubber catheter is placed through the pleural tear, and a purse string suture is placed around the periphery of the tear. The suture is then tied as suction is applied through the catheter as it is withdrawn. Patients are followed by serial chest X-rays to ensure that a pneumothorax does not develop. Larger pleural injuries may require chest tube placement.

The individual pieces of cartilage are then carved using the template as a guide. Finally, the eighth rib is thinned to allow it to be curled around the conchal and antihelical framework, and the two pieces are sutured to each other with clear nylon sutures. It is important when constructing the framework to exaggerate features, as these will be blunted by the thicker temporal skin.

Next, the unusable portion of microtic appendage is removed, generally consisting of the superior "knot" of deformed cartilage; the inferior portion is retained for later reconstruction of the lobule. Using the contralateral ear as a guide, the ideal position of the reconstructed auricle is determined and marked. A 2 cm curvilinear incision is then made approximately 2 cm above the location of the superior part of the helix, and a subcutaneous dissection is performed under the markings for the auricle location and carried approximately 1 cm beyond these markings to allow for appropriate skin draping. The framework is then carefully positioned in the skin pocket, with care taken to ensure proper positioning and orientation. Residual cartilage is banked subcutaneously under hair bearing temporal skin. Two 4 mm drains are then positioned to coapt the skin to the framework and to evacuate any blood or serum and are left on gentle

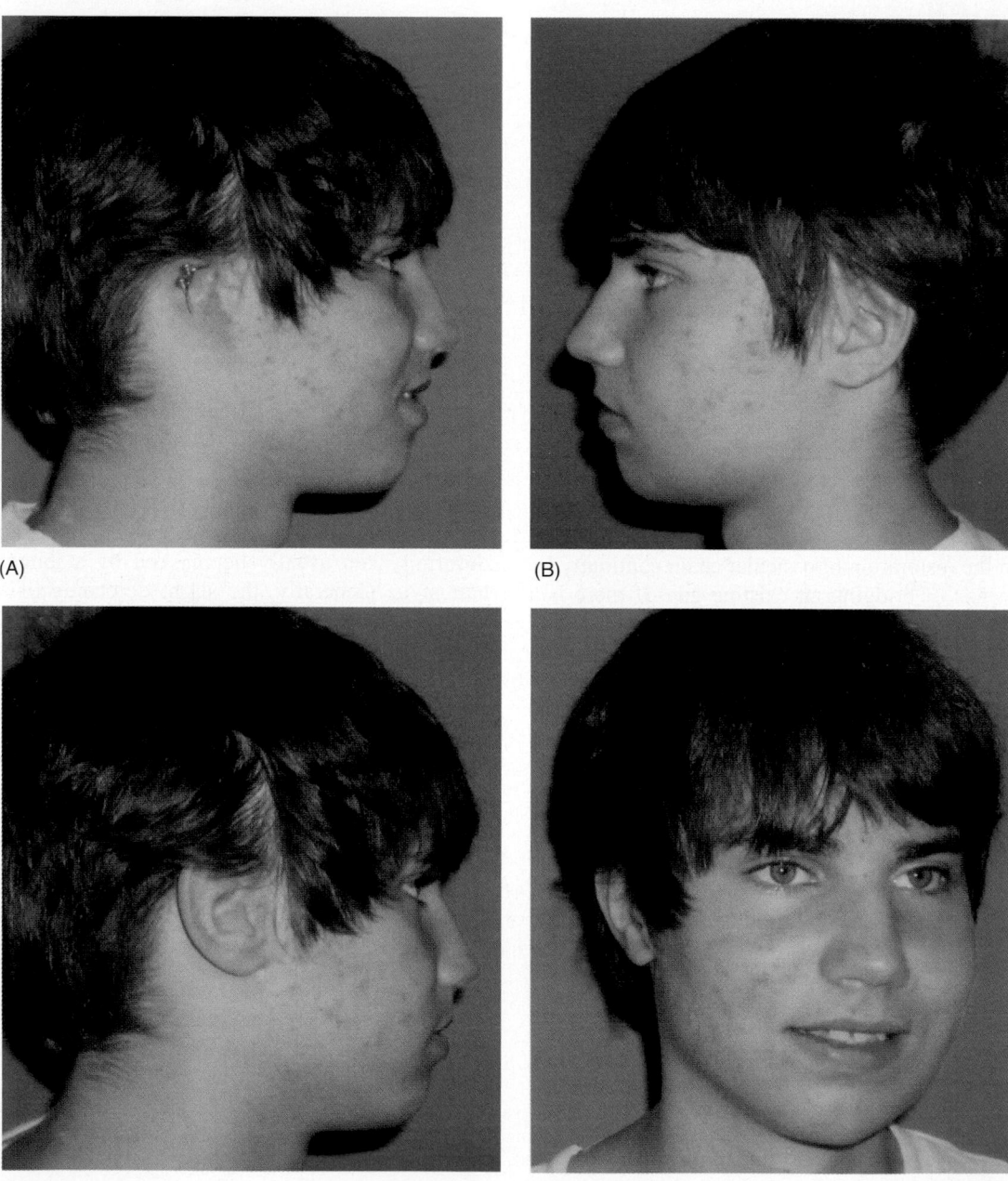

Figure 14 Placement of osseointegrated implants for attachment of a prosthetic pinna. (A) The percutaneous abutments and associated wire framework used to attach the right prosthetic pinna via clips. (B) The normal left pinna can be seen. (C) The right prosthetic pinna in place. It should be noted how similar the prosthesis appears compared to the normal pinna seen in B. (D) Oblique view of the prosthetic pinna. (Published with permission, copyright © 2007 P. A. Wackym, MD.)

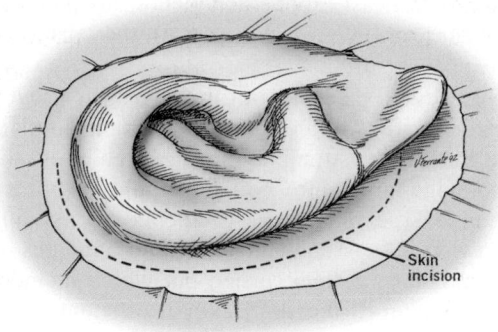

Figure 15 Surgery for canal atresia. A postauricular incision is made. While exposing the mastoid cortex and dysmorphic tympanic bone, the previously implanted cartilaginous auricular scaffold should be protected during retraction.

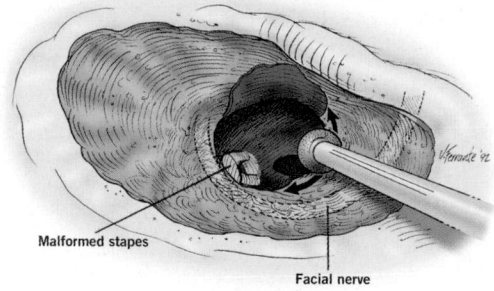

Figure 17 Drilling is continued until a normal-sized middle ear opening has been created. Great care is taken not to drill on a mobile, deformed, but intact ossicular chain. The anteriorly coursing facial nerve is identified.

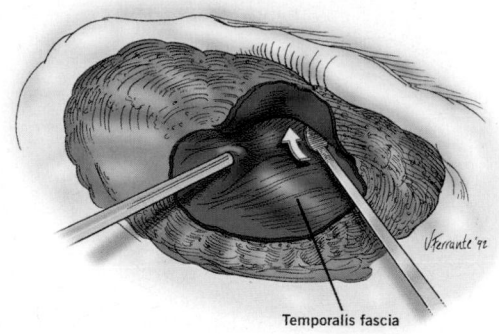

Figure 19 Temporalis fascia is used to construct a tympanic membrane.

suction for 3 to 4 days (Figure 9). The incision is closed with nylon suture.

Two to three months after the first stage, lobule creation can be performed. Essentially, Z-plasty double transposition flaps reorient the vertically positioned skin tag to align with the inferior part of the helical tail while the skin from this area is transposed anteriorly to close the donor site (Figures 10 and 11). In conchal remnant microtias, transposition of the remnant can construct an inferior conchal bowl, lobule and, occasionally, an antitragus.

Two to three months later, the third stage of reconstruction is performed. A split thickness skin graft (0.015 to 0.020 in. thick) is harvested from the posterior aspect of the thigh. An incision is then made approximately 8 to 10 mm peripheral to the buried framework, from the anterior part of the helix down to the repositioned lobule. The framework is then elevated, leaving a generous amount of scar and subcutaneous tissue on the medial aspect of the framework. The banked costal cartilage is retrieved and sutured to the anteromedial aspects of the framework to maintain lateralization. Posteriorly the scalp is undermined widely and advanced into the postauricular sulcus, and the portions of the sulcus and auricle still bare are covered with the skin graft. A bolster dressing is placed into the postauricular sulcus and left for 1 week (Figure 12). Atresia repair can be performed 3 to 4 months later (Figure 13). An additional stage can reconstruct the tragus using a portion

of the contralateral conchal bowl as a composite graft several months after atresia repair.

Alternatives to this standard approach for reconstruction exist. An externally mounted prosthesis can be modeled on the normal ear and can appear quite realistic. However, the prosthesis needs to be mounted onto the temporal skin with adhesives on a daily basis. Percutaneous osseointegrated implants can be placed into the temporal bone and used to anchor the prosthesis more securely. These prostheses need lifetime care. They may become dislodged at socially inconvenient times. Pediatric patients may find compliance difficult and socially unacceptable; however, the cosmetic result can be vastly superior compared to the multistage reconstruction approach (Figure 14). Nagata has described a two-stage procedure using autologous rib cartilage.[24] This is a technically challenging procedure, and results may not be as predictable as the Tanzer/Brent method. Finally, a single stage procedure has been described using a porous high density polyethylene custom implant covered by a temporoparietal fascia flap and split thickness skin graft.[25] While results can be good, if flap failure occurs early, salvage may be difficult. Additionally, trauma to the implant can lead to framework cracking, and even minor injuries can lead to skin loss, implant exposure, and chronic infection. Exposure of the synthetic framework to the mastoid cavity can lead to chronic implant infection and recurrent drainage, and the prior use of a temporoparietal fascia flap limits the tissue available for salvage.

The timing of the microtia and atresia repairs requires close communication between the surgeons. Because scarring interferes with the auricular repair, reconstruction of the atresia is deferred until the auricular cartilaginous scaffolding is completed. However, it is important to position the reconstructed auricle correctly so that it aligns with the meatal opening and the middle ear. The meatal, canal, and middle ear reconstruction is frequently performed as part of the second or third stage of the auricular reconstruction.[13,26]

A postauricular approach is used, with great care being taken to avoid exposing the scaffold (Figure 15). Temporalis fascia is harvested for reconstruction of the tympanic membrane. The periosteum of the lateral surface of the temporal bone is elevated. A bony circular canal is created by drilling between the glenoid fossa anteriorly and the tegmen plate superiorly while trying to avoid entering mastoid air cells posteriorly (Figure 16). Continuous suction irrigation cools the bone and clears away blood and bone dust while the water enhances the translucency of the wet bone. This permits visualization of structures such as dura, facial nerve, and glenoid fossa through the intact thinned bone. The surgeon should anticipate that the facial nerve will be located more anteriorly and more laterally than in the normal temporal bone. The nerve frequently follows a C-shaped path in its course between the geniculate ganglion and its point of emergence from the temporal bone. The purposeful identification of the facial nerve will prevent inadvertent injury. A facial nerve monitor may facilitate identification of the nerve in atretic ears.

Visualization of the facial nerve as a landmark permits the opening of the atresia plate to approximate the size of a normal middle ear opening. While drilling on this plate, it must be remembered that the malleus handle may be fused to it. Precautions must be taken to avoid drilling on the mobilized atresia remnant since this may transmit traumatic vibratory energy through the ossicular chain to the inner ear and result in a permanent sensorineural hearing loss (Figure 17).

The status of the ossicular chain is assessed. If the stapes is mobile, an appropriate ossicular reconstruction is performed (Figure 18). If it is fixed or the oval window is obscured by the facial nerve, the ossicular reconstruction should be deferred. Temporalis fascia is used to fabricate a

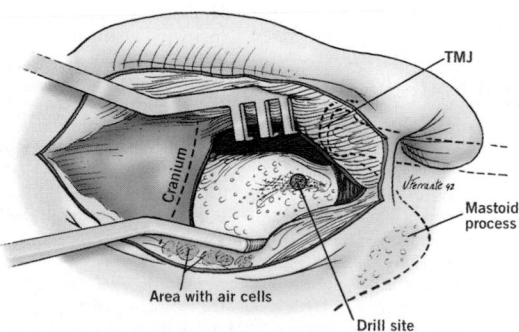

Figure 16 Construction of a canal is begun by drilling between the glenoid fossa anteriorly and the superior temporal line. The latter roughly corresponds to the tegmen (floor of the middle cranial fossa). When possible, entry into the mastoid air cells is avoided. TMJ = temporomandibular joint.

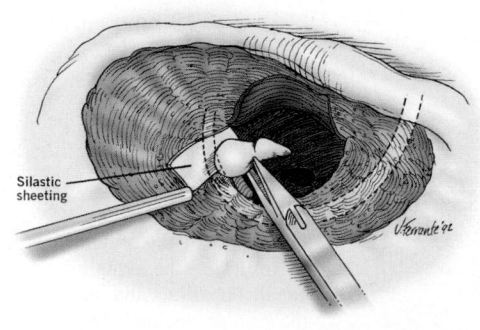

Figure 18 The ossicular chain is reconstructed by interposing the malformed, sculpted ossicle onto the stapes. Silastic sheeting, 0.005 in. thick, is positioned to prevent bony ankylosis.

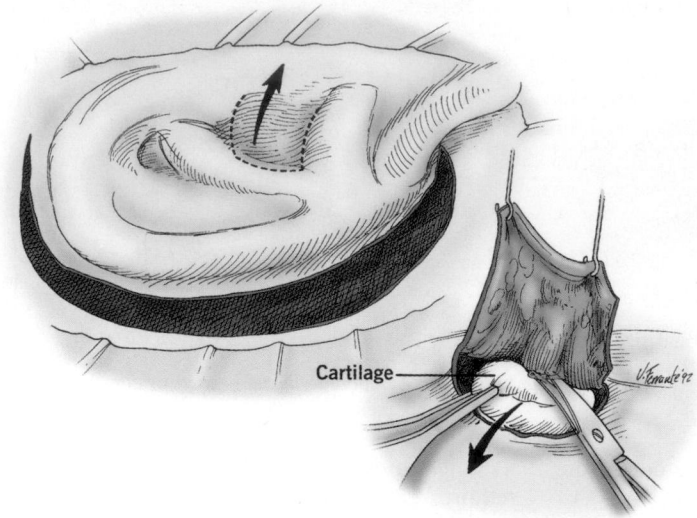

Figure 20 A meatal opening is made through the imperforate conchal skin. A rectangular, anteriorly based skin flap is debulked and rotated to line the anterior lateral third of the new canal.

new tympanic membrane (Figure 19). A meatal opening is made in the area of the imperforate concha, incising the skin to create a rectangularly shaped, anteriorly based conchal skin flap. The underlying cartilage and soft tissue are removed to debulk the flap and create an opening that communicates with the drilled out external canal (Figure 20). The conchal flap is rotated to resurface the anterior third of the external canal and is stabilized by suturing it to the adjacent soft tissues (Figure 21). A thin split-thickness skin graft is harvested from the lower part of the abdomen and is used to resurface the remaining ear canal. The canal is packed snugly with Gelfoam (Upjohn, Kalamazoo, Michigan) to compress the skin graft against the underlying bone and soft tissue. The postauricular incision is reapproximated using absorbable sutures.

Risks and Benefits of Atresia Surgery. Atresia surgery is technically demanding. The results achieved are directly related to the experience and skill of the operating surgeon. Generally, hearing improvement to a serviceable level can be achieved in approximately 65 to 75% of selected patients.[27,28] Complications of surgery include the small risk of facial paralysis, a severe to profound sensorineural hearing loss, stenosis requiring additional surgery, persistent otor-

rhea, and tympanic membrane graft failure with perforation.

In children with a unilateral atresia and a normal contralateral ear, surgery may not be routinely indicated.[19] The potential benefit of this sophisticated surgery, that is, achieving binaural hearing, may not justify the risk of complications. In binaural cases, the successful creation of an external canal, even when hearing cannot be improved, will allow the use of an ear-level air-conduction hearing aid to restore hearing without using a cumbersome bone-conduction aid. Thus, in bilateral cases in which the facial nerve obstructs the oval window or when a hearing improvement cannot be achieved, providing the patient with a stable, skin-lined canal is a worthy goal in and of itself.

Another hearing restorative technique for external auditory canal atresia is the placement of a bone anchored hearing aid (BAHA).[29] This procedure involves implanting a titanium post which becomes osseointegrated into the calvaria. A special hearing aid is attached to this post via a percutaneous abutment and uses bone conduction to stimulate the cochlea. The titanium post requires a 3-month period for osseointegration in an adult and a 4- to 6-month period for children, before the external appliance can be attached to the abutment. The use of the BAHA

requires at least a bone conduction threshold in one ear to be at a minimum of 40 to 45 dB to be effective.

In adults, placement of the BAHA is usually performed in a one-stage procedure to implant the titanium post and abutment. In children, the two-stage procedure can be employed which involves the placement of the post only and allowing it to osseointegrate for 3 to 6 months. A second stage is then carried out which includes the thinning of the skin flap for efficient transduction as well as placement of the percutaneous abutment. The external processor is fitted 3 to 4 weeks after the skin flap heals. Frequently, a second "sleeper" fixture is placed at the same time, which allows its immediate use in the future should the first fixture ever extrude or fail to osseointegrate.

The BAHA system has some distinct advantages which make this procedure a viable option for atresia patients. The hearing result with the BAHA is superior to an atresia repair which usually results in a mild conductive hearing loss in the best circumstances. Furthermore, this procedure poses no risk to the facial nerve and is not dependent on a patent external auditory canal. Succcesful atresia surgery involves a split-thickness skin graft to resurface the bony canal. This may require that the child take water precautions to keep the ear dry. This is not a problem with the BAHA. Drawbacks include failure to osseointegrate, loss of post fixation over time, and periodic infections around the abutment if daily cleaning is not performed. In addition, there are the cosmetic issues of a permanent percutaneous abutment and the depilated skin around the fixture. The cosmetic issue is usually more of a concern for boys or for girls with short hair as the abutment is more apparent in these situations.

REFERENCES

1. Lefebvre PP, Malgrange B, Staecker H, et al. Retinoic acid stimulates regeneration of mammalian auditory hair cells. Science 1993;260:692–5.
2. Anson BJ, Davies J, Duckert LG. Embryology of the ear. In: Paparella MM, Shumrick DA, Gluckman JL, et al, editors. Otolaryngology, 4th edition. Philadelphia: JB Lippincott; 1991. p. 3–21.
3. Williams GH. Developmental anatomy of the ear. In: English GM, editor. Otolaryngology. Philadelphia: JB Lippincott; 1990.
4. Nager GT, Proctor B. Anatomic variations and anomalies involving the facial canal. Otolaryngol Clin North Am 1991;24:531–53.
5. Snow JB. Preface. Otolaryngol Clin North Am 1992;25: xv–i.
6. Jafek BW, Nager GT, Strife J. Congenital aural atresia: Analysis of 311 cases. Trans Am Acad Ophthalmol Otolaryngol 1975;80:580–95.
7. Sando IS, Shibahara Y, Wood RP. Congenital anomalies of the external and middle ear. In: Bluestone CD, Stool SE, editors. Pediatric Otolaryngology. Philadelphia: WB Saunders; 1990. p. 271–302.
8. Bergstrom LB. Anomalies of the ear. In: English GM, editor. Otolaryngology. Philadelphia: JB Lippincott; 1990.
9. Teunissen EB, Cremers CWRJ. Classification of congenital middle ear anomalies. Report on 144 ears. Ann Otol Rhinol Laryngol 1993;102:606–12.
10. Jahrsdoerfer RA, Yeakley JW, Aguilar EA, et al. Grading system for the selection of patients with congenital aural atresia. Am J Otol 1992;13:6–12.
11. Schuknecht HF. Congenital aural atresia. Laryngoscope 1989;99:908–17.

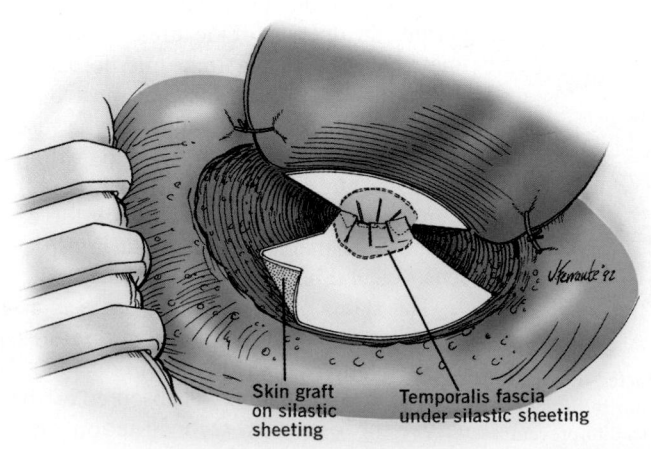

Skin graft on silastic sheeting

Temporalis fascia under silastic sheeting

Figure 21 A thin, split-thickness skin graft harvested from the lower part of the abdomen is used to resurface the remainder of the canal. Handling and placement of the graft are facilitated by gluing the epidermal surface to thin (0.005 in.) Silastic sheeting. The raw surface of the graft is compressed against the bone by filing the canal lumen with Gelfoam.

12. Curtin HD. Congential malformations of the ear. Otolaryngol Clin North Am 1988;21:317–36.

13. Jahrsdoerfer RA, Garcia ET, Yeakley JW, et al. Surface contour three-dimensional imaging in congenital aural atresia. Arch Otolaryngol Head Neck Surg 1993;119:95–9.

14. Andrews JC, Anzai Y, Mankovich NJ, et al. Three-dimensional CT scan reconstruction for the assessment of congenital aural atresia. Am J Otol 1992;13:236–40.

15. Jahrsdoerfer RA, Yeakley JW, Hall JW, et al. High-resolution CT scanning and auditory brain stem response in congenital aural atresia: Patient selection and surgical correlation. Otolaryngol Head Neck Surg 1985;93:292–8.

16. Granstrom G, Bergstrom K, Tjellstrom A. The bone-anchored hearing aid and bone-anchored epithesis for congenital ear malformations. Otolaryngol Head Neck Surg 1993;109:46–53.

17. van der Pouw KT, Snik AF, Cremers CW. Audiometric results of bilateral bone-anchored hearing aid application in patients with bilateral congenital aural atresia. Laryngoscope 1998;108:548–53.

18. Tjellstrom A, Hakansson B. The bone anchored hearing aid (BAHA) design principles, indications and long-term clinical results. Otolaryngol Clin North Am 1995; 115:1–20.

19. Trigg DJ, Applebaum EL. Indications for the surgical repair of unilateral aural atresia in children. Am J Otol 1998;19:679–84.

20. Jahrsdoerfer RA, Lambert PR. Facial nerve injury in congenital aural atresia surgery. Am J Otol 1998;19:283–7.

21. Chandrasekhar SS, De la Cruz A, Garrido E. Surgery of congenital aural atresia. Am J Otol 1995;16:713–7.

22. Tanzer RC. Microtia: A long-term follow-up of 44 reconstructed auricles. Plast Reconstr Surg 1978;61:161–4.

23. Brent B. Technical advances in ear reconstruction with autologous rib cartilage grafts: Personal experience with 1200 cases. Plast Reconstr Surg 1999;104:319–24.

24. Nagata S. A new method of total reconstruction of the auricle for microtia. Plast Reconstr Surg 1993;92:187–93.

25. Romo T, Fozo M, Sclafani AP. Microtia reconstruction using a porous polyethylene framework. Facial Plast Surg 2000;16:15–22.

26. Bellucci RJ. Congenital aural malformations: Diagnosis and treatment. Otolaryngol Clin North Am 1981;14: 95–124.

27. Shih L, Crabtree JA. Long-term surgical results for congenital aural atresia. Laryngoscope 1993;103:1097–102.

28. Lambert PR. Congenital aural atresia: Stability of surgical results. Laryngoscope 1998;108:1801–5.

29. Wazen JJ, Caruso M, Tjellstrom A. Related articles, Long-term results with the titanium bone-anchored hearing aid: The U. S. experience. Am J Otol 1998;19:737–41.

63

Anatomy and Physiology of the Oral Cavity

Margaret A. Kenna, MD, MPH
Manali Amin, MD

The oral cavity is important for many vital bodily functions including speech and swallowing. It is a complex space, bounded anteriorly by the lips and posteriorly by the oropharynx. Its two compartments are the vestibule, or external compartment, and the internal compartment. The vestibule is the space lateral to the alveolar ridges and medial to the lips and buccal mucosa. The oral cavity proper is bounded by the alveolar ridges laterally, the hard and soft palates superiorly and posteriorly and the floor of mouth caudally. Its primary contents are the teeth, the anterior two-thirds of the tongue, minor salivary glands, and the parotid and submandibular salivary ducts. The palatoglossus muscles form the anterior tonsillar pillars. All structures anterior to the anterior tonsillar pillars are contained within the oral cavity. All structures posterior to the pillars are part of the oropharynx. The oropharynx contains the posterior one-third of the tongue, the lingual and palatine tonsils, and the paired tonsillar pillars formed by the palatoglossus and palatopharyngeus muscles. It extends from the soft palate superiorly to the base of tongue inferiorly.

TONGUE

The tongue is a large muscular organ in the oral cavity. The anterior two-thirds of the tongue is mobile and has four surfaces: the dorsum, the ventral surface, and the lateral borders. The dorsal surface opposes the hard palate and has an irregular mucosal surface covered with multiple epithelial appendages known as papillae. The ventral surface faces the floor of mouth and is covered by a thin mucosal layer that meets in the midline to form a band of tissue known as the frenulum. The mucosa is continuous with the mucosa of the floor of mouth.

All tongue movements are accomplished by the anterior two-thirds of the tongue, also known as the mobile tongue. Tongue movement is accomplished through use of both intrinsic and extrinsic muscles. The tongue is divided into two halves by a median fibrous septum that is fixed to the body of the hyoid bone. Each half of the tongue contains two sets of muscles, extrinsic and intrinsic. The extrinsic muscles are the genioglossus, hyoglossus, and stylopharyngeus. The palatoglossus is sometimes considered an extrinsic muscle of the tongue and sometimes a muscle of the soft palate. The extrinsic muscles allow for tongue movement anteriorly, backward, upward, and downward. The genioglossus functions to protrude and retract the tongue as well as depress its tip. The styloglossus and hyoglossus aid in retracting the tongue and in raising and depressing its margins respectively. The intrinsic muscles are the superior and inferior longitudinal, transverse, and vertical. The intrinsic muscles function to change the shape of the tongue during speech and swallowing. The palatoglossus muscle within the anterior tonsillar pillar also elevates the tongue. Although it helps with tongue movement, the primary function is in the downward movement of the soft palate, and it may be an important regulator in the transition from the oral phase to the pharyngeal phase of swallowing.[1]

The posterior one-third of the tongue is divided from the anterior two-thirds by an inverted V-shaped groove known as the sulcus terminalis (Figure 1). The foramen cecum, the origin of the thyroglossal duct, is at the apex of the sulcus. The posterior one-third of the tongue is composed primarily of the lingual tonsil.

Motor innervation of the tongue is almost exclusively through the hypoglossal nerve, that is, CN XII. It innervates all of the extrinsic and intrinsic muscles except for the palatoglossus. The hypoglossal nerve enters the tongue on the lateral surface of the genioglossus muscle, anastomosing with fibers from the lingual nerve. The paired motion of the genioglossus allows for straight protrusion of the tongue. When one of the hypoglossal nerves is paralyzed, the tongue will deviate to the side of the paralysis upon protrusion. The palatoglossus is innervated by branches from the pharyngeal plexus which is derived from the vagus nerve, that is, CN X.

Sensory innervation of the tongue is somewhat more complex (Table 1) (Figure 2). General sensation (touch, pain, and temperature) of the anterior two-thirds of the tongue is carried by afferent fibers from the third or mandibular division of the trigeminal nerve (CN V3) in the form of the lingual nerve. Taste in the anterior two-thirds of the tongue is carried by afferent fibers of the seventh cranial nerve in the form of the chorda tympani nerve. By contrast, both general sensation and taste to the posterior one-third of the tongue are carried by afferent fibers of the glossopharyngeal nerve.

Taste Receptors

Taste is mediated through specialized receptors known as taste buds. Taste buds are located within epithelial appendages on the dorsal surface of the tongue known as papillae (Figure 3). In addition, taste buds are found in the epithelium of the soft palate, pharynx, larynx, epiglottis, and esophagus. Their distribution varies widely both within an individual and among individuals. In general, newborns and children have a higher number of extralingual taste buds than adults.[2]

Taste buds are oval sensory end organs composed of 50 to 150 spindle-shaped, epithelial cells with receptor properties.[2,3] They are involved in the perception of chemical stimuli and in taste transduction. A single taste bud is an almost ovoid structure, 70 μm in height with a diameter of approximately 40 μm and a central opening on its epithelial surface, known as the taste pore. The taste pore, approximately 2 to 10 μm in size, exposes the apical surface of receptor cells to molecular food particles dissolved in saliva.

Ultrastructurally, the taste bud is composed of three types of cells: basal cells, edge cells, and taste receptor cells. Basal cells are undifferentiated cells from which the other taste receptor cells are derived. Edge cells, as their name suggests, define the lateral aspect of the taste bud. Three different types of taste receptor cells have been identified: dark cells (type I cells), light cells (type II cells), and intermediate

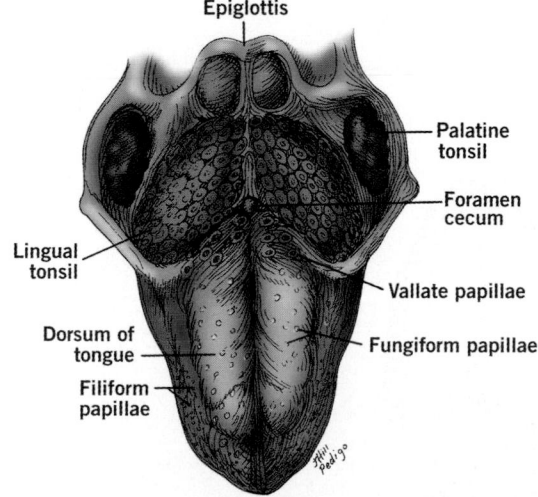

Figure 1 The dorsal surface of the tongue. Filiform papillae cover the dorsum. The lingual tonsil and palatine tonsils are part of Waldeyer ring.

Table 1 Relationship of the Branchial Arches and Their Nerves to the Sensation of the Tongue

Neural Branch	Cranial Nerve	Branchial Arch	Sensory Modality Served
Lingual nerve	V	First arch	Sensation to anterior two-thirds of tongue
Chorda tympani	VII	Second arch	Taste to anterior two-thirds of tongue
Glossopharyngeal	IX	Third arch	Taste and sensation to posterior one-third of tongue

cells (type III cells). Type I cells are known as dark cells because they contain dense granules near their apex. Type II cells are known as light cells because they lack these dense granules. Intermediate cells are felt to be intermediate between the other two types of cells. The function of these cells and how they differ from one another or whether they represent a progression, is not well understood.[2] All three of the receptor cell types contain microvilli at their apical end and synapse with afferent nerve endings at their basal end. The microvilli project into the taste pore and expose the taste receptors to gustatory stimuli.[2] The two primary classes of receptors are the seven-transmembrane G-protein coupled receptors (GPCRs) and ion channels.[4] The GPCR proteins consist of a second messenger cascade which is activated upon binding of the receptor. The ion channels allow passage of different cations or protons and modulate the membrane permeability. The final mechanism of taste transduction, irrespective of the receptor type stimulated, is an increase in intracellular Ca^{2+} and subsequent neurotransmitter release.

Gustatory Papillae. Taste buds are found in both extralingual sites as well as in lingual papillae. The dorsal surface of the tongue has four types of papillae: fungiform, circumvallate, foliate, and filiform. The papillae have a core of connective tissue covered with epithelium that expresses hair-like keratins. Filiform papillae are distributed throughout the dorsal surface of the anterior part of the tongue. They are the only form of papillae that do not contain taste buds.

Their primary function is to assist with tactile aspects of feeding.

The fungiform, circumvallate, and foliate papillae, collectively referred to as the gustatory papillae, differ from filiform papillae in that their epithelial covering contain sense organs capable of perceiving taste. The fungiform papillae, as their name suggests, are mushroom-shaped, raised structures found on the anterior two-thirds of the tongue surface. There are 200 to 300 fungiform papillae containing a total of nearly 1,600 taste buds on the human tongue.[3] The foliate papillae are found on the posterolateral surface of the tongue and contain approximately 1,000 taste buds.[3] Finally, the circumvallate papillae are found in an inverted V-shape along the anterior margin of the sulcus terminalis. Similar to the sulcus, it marks the division between anterior and posterior parts of the tongue. There are a total of 8 to 12 circumvallate papillae, containing approximately 250 taste buds each.[3] The circumvallate papillae are associated with deep lingual salivary glands also known as von Ebner glands. Von Ebner glands secrete serous saliva and open into the trenches around the circumvallate papillae and into mucous glands found in the posterior part of the tongue. Mucous glands are found within the crypts of the lingual tonsil.[5,6]

The exact function of the von Ebner glands remains debatable. One study has shown that they may have three possible functions.[5] First, they produce a digestive enzyme, lingual lipase, which may be important in the neonatal period when pancreatic function is limited and pancreatic lipase sparse. Secondly, they have been shown to

produce a small, soluble protein from the lipocalin family. Lipocalins assist in the transmission of pheromonal chemoreception. Finally, von Ebner gland proteins have been postulated to be involved in the transduction of taste.

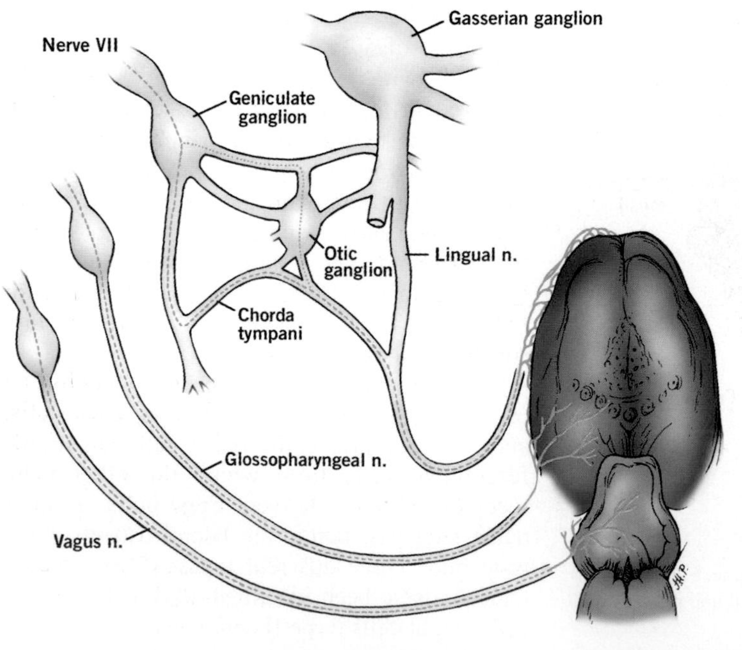

Taste. Chemosensory stimulation of these taste receptors occurs when saliva mixed with molecular food particles washes over the different taste buds within the papillae.[3] Humans are able to distinguish five taste qualities: sour, salty, bitter, sweet, and umami. Umami is the taste associated with monosodium glutamate and certain other 5′-ribonucleotides.[7] Recent studies have shown that the perception of bitter, sweet, and umami are mediated through stimulation of the GPCRs. Furthermore, the action potential produced by stimulation of these receptors may be modified by members of the transient receptor potential (TRP) family of ion channels. One study has shown that TRP channels may be stimulated by temperature. In fact, their results suggest that sweet foods are perceived as being sweeter when they are warm.[8]

Unlike bitter, sweet, and umami, sour and salty tastes are transmitted by stimulation of ion channels.[7] The action potentials produced by depolarization or hyperpolarization of these channels may be involved in the coding of taste.[7] For more information on gustatory physiology, the reader is referred to Chapter 38, "Olfaction and Gustation."

FLOOR OF THE MOUTH

The floor of the mouth is a muscular sling formed primarily by the paired mylohyoid muscles. The muscles arise from the medial surface of the mandible and extend toward the midline where they insert with muscle fibers from the opposite side, forming a midline raphe. The posterior most aspect of the mylohyoid musculature inserts into the body of the hyoid bone. The anterior belly of the paired digastric muscles bound the sling inferiorly. A majority of the submandibular gland also lies beneath the mylohyoid muscles. A smaller portion of the gland curves around the posterior border of the muscle and lies above it, along with the sublingual gland, the lingual and hypoglossal nerves and the tongue vasculature. Medial to the nerves and vessels lie the paired geniohyoid muscles. The geniohyoid muscles arise from the mental spine and internal surface of the mandible and insert onto the hyoid bone, lateral to the midline. Covering the structures superior to the mylohyoid is a layer of superficial cervical fascia. There is a potential space between the fascia and the mylohyoid muscle. An abscess in this potential space is known as Ludwig angina and is considered a potentially life threatening airway emergency.

All of the muscles that combine to form the floor of the mouth, including the digastric muscles, mylohyoid muscles, stylohyoid muscles, and the geniohyoid muscles elevate the hyoid bone and assist in swallowing.

Figure 2 Diagram of the nerves serving the sense of taste on the tongue and surrounding regions.

Oral Cavity

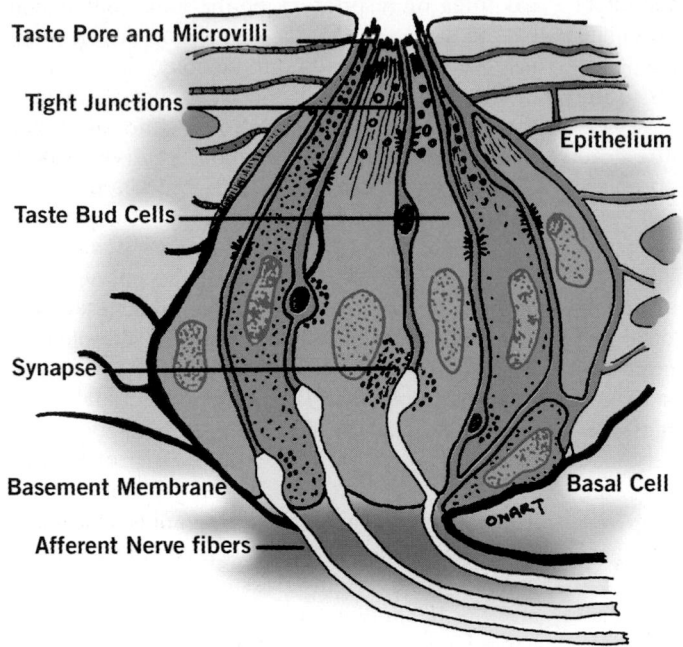

Figure 3 Taste bud demonstrating the relationship of the taste pore to the oral cavity. Afferent nerve fibers go to several different types of cells.

BONES AND DENTITION OF THE ORAL CAVITY

The oral cavity is surrounded by bone on its external surface as well as superiorly. The bony structures that compose a portion of the oral cavity include the mandible, the alveolar and palatine processes of the maxilla and the palatine bones.

The hard or osseous palate separates the nasal cavity from the oral cavity. It is a bony plate formed by the alveolar and palatine processes of the maxilla and the palatine bones (Figure 4). The alveolar process of the maxilla is the most inferior aspect of the maxilla and contains the maxillary dentition. The alveolar process articulates with the horizontal or palatine processes of the maxilla medially at the level of the second and third molars. The alveolar process is formed by the palatine processes of the maxilla anteriorly and the horizontal plates or horizontal lamina of the palatine bones posteriorly. The suture line that fuses these two bones lies approximately at the level of the second and third molar interspace. This suture line is in the transverse plane. There is also a longitudinal suture that fuses the respective horizontal lamina medially. Bony ridges or bulges sometimes develop along the longitudinal suture line and are known as torus palatinus. An additional suture is often visible in young people. This is the palatine raphe or suture between what was once the premaxillary part of the maxilla and the maxillary palatine processes. It is the site of fusion of the median and lateral palatine processes during embryonic development. The midline junction of these two sutures is marked by the incisive foramen, also known as the incisive fossa. The incisive foramen separates the primary palate anteriorly from the secondary palate posteriorly.

The incisive foramen is one of several openings in the hard palate. It is the opening of the incisive canal that transmits the nasopalatine nerve and the terminal branch of the sphenopalatine artery. Other openings in the hard palate include the greater and lesser palatine foramina. The greater palatine foramen is the opening of the greater palatine canal. It is located on the lateral border of the palate, at approximately the level of the upper third molar. The canal transmits the greater (anterior) palatine nerve and the greater palatine artery. After exiting the foramina, branches of the nerve and artery run anteriorly in two grooves on the palate. The lesser palatine foramina are situated posterior to the greater palatine foramina, at the edge of the hard palate. The foramina transmit the lesser palatine nerves and arteries.

The hard palate is covered by a layer of mucosa that is firmly adherent to the underlying periosteum. The mucosa contains numerous minor salivary glands. As is evident from patients with cleft palates, the palate is vital in the process of swallowing and in speech articulation.

As with the palate, the other skeletal component of the oral cavity, the mandible, is crucial to oral cavity function. The mandible is the most prominent bone surrounding the oral cavity and forms the inferior part of the face. It is the strongest and largest of the facial bones.

The different parts of the mandible are the body (horizontal part), the angle, and the ramus (vertical part). The two sides are fused embryologically at the midline, an area known as the symphysis. At the anterior most aspect of the symphysis is the mental protuberance, a triangular bony prominence. The ramus ends in two bony projections. The condylar process is on the posterior aspect of the ramus. The coronoid process is anterior to the condylar process and separated by the mandibular notch. The lateral pterygoid muscle inserts on the pterygoid fovea on the neck of the condylar process. A portion of the temporalis inserts on the coronoid process. Other muscles that attach to the mandible include the masseteric, medial pterygoid, genioglossus, geniohyoid, the mylohyoid, and the anterior bellies of the digastric muscles. The masseter attaches to the lateral aspect of the mandibular angle and ramus whereas the medial pterygoid inserts on the medial surface of the angle and ramus; together they form a muscular sling around the mandible. The bone of the mandibular angle may be slightly raised on either or both the lateral and medial aspect, known as the masseteric tuberosity and pterygoid tuberosity, respectively. The genioglossus and geniohyoid insert on the mental spinc (genial tubercle). The mylohyoid attaches to the mylohyoid line, a line that runs up and back from the sublingual fossa. The anterior belly of the digastric attaches at the digastric fossa.

The mandible has multiple other bony grooves, markings, and foramina. On the medial surface of the mandible, in addition to the mental spine, digastric fossa and mylohyoid line can be found the sublingual and submandibular fossae, the mylohyoid groove and the mandibular foramen. The mylohyoid groove carries the mylohyoid nerve and vessels anteriorly and inferiorly after they exit from the mandibular foramen. The sublingual and submandibular fossae shield the respective salivary glands. Externally on the body of the mandible is the oblique line, the mental foramen, and the mental protuberance. The mental foramen is the terminal aspect of the mandibular canal, a bony canal that starts at the mandibular

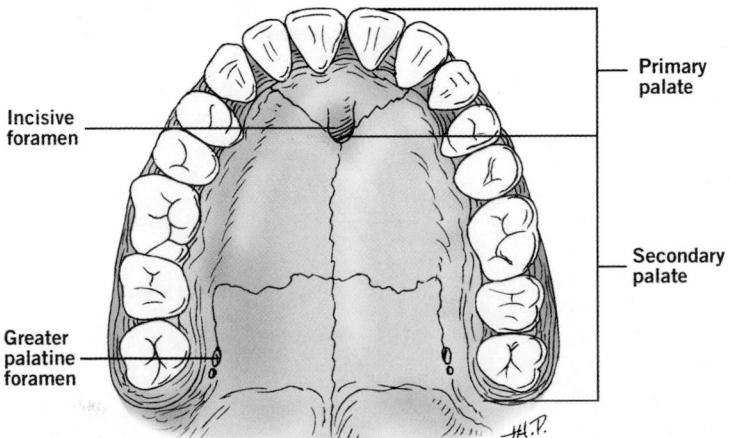

Figure 4 The hard palate and its divisions. Permanent teeth 1 through 16 are shown.

foramen and courses through the ramus and body carrying the inferior alveolar nerve and vessels. The mental foramen is located along a vertical line through the second and third premolar interspace. Upon exit through the foramen, the nerve is known as the mental nerve and provides sensory innervation to the chin and lower lip.

Similar to the maxilla, the mandible has a bony ridge known as the alveolar process. The maxillary and mandibular alveolar processes support dentition. Although teeth are not truly bone, they are formed from dentine, a modified bone, and will be included in this section for the sake of completeness.

Deciduous teeth generally begin eruption around 6 to 8 months of age and are complete by age 24 months. There are a total of 20 deciduous teeth (two medial incisors, two lateral incisors, two canines, two first molars, and two second molars on both the maxillary and mandibular arches.) The teeth are labeled from A to T, starting with the right maxillary second molar (A) across the maxilla to the left maxillary second molar (J) down to the left mandibular second molar (K) and across the mandible, ending at the right mandibular second molar (T). Deciduous dentition is generally shed and replaced by permanent dentition between the ages of 6 and 12 years. Permanent dentition consists of a total of 32 teeth (two medial incisors; two lateral incisors; two canines; two first and second premolars; and two first, second and third molars in both the maxilla and mandible). These teeth are labeled in similar fashion to the deciduous teeth, starting with the right maxillary third molar and ending with the right third mandibular molar. Unlike deciduous teeth, however, permanent teeth are labeled from # 1 to # 32.

BLOOD SUPPLY TO THE ORAL CAVITY, PHARYNX, AND TONSILS

The blood supply to the oral cavity, pharynx, and tonsils is derived primarily from the external carotid artery (ECA) and its many branches. The artery originates at the bifurcation of the common carotid, passing superiorly in the neck, deep to the posterior belly of the digastric and the stylohyoid muscle, paralleling the ramus of the mandible. The branches which primarily supply the oral cavity, pharynx, and Waldeyer ring include the ascending pharyngeal, lingual, facial (external maxillary), internal maxillary, and superficial temporal arteries. The ascending pharyngeal artery arises from the posterior surface of the ECA and supplies several branches to the pharynx, palate, and tonsils. The lingual and facial arteries arise from the anterior surface of the ECA. The lingual artery and its branches supply the tongue and floor of mouth. The facial artery has multiple branches including the ascending palatine, tonsillar branches, branches to the submandibular gland, the submental artery and branches to the masticator muscle. As the names of the branches imply, the external maxillary

supplies the palate, tonsils, submandibular gland, submental space, and masticator muscle. Finally, the two terminal branches of the ECA, the internal maxillary artery (IMAX) and the superficial temporal artery arise within the substance of the parotid gland and provide small branches to the pharynx and tonsils. The many blood vessels allow for collateral circulation to the entire head and neck area in the event that one or more vessels are injured or surgically ligated.

The blood supply of the tonsils is derived from multiple vessels: the ascending pharyngeal artery, tonsillar branches of the external maxillary artery, the tonsillar branch of the dorsal lingual artery, and the descending palatine artery from the IMAX (Figure 5). The tonsillar branch of the dorsal lingual artery, the ascending palatine branch of the external maxillary artery, and the tonsillar branch of the external maxillary are typically found at the inferior pole. The superior pole is supplied by the ascending pharyngeal artery and the descending palatine artery.

The venous drainage of the oral cavity, pharynx, and Waldeyer ring is through multiple smaller veins to the internal and anterior jugular veins.

WALDEYER RING

Waldeyer ring is a ring of lymphoid tissue found in the pharynx. It is composed of the adenoid superiorly in the nasopharynx, both palatine tonsils laterally in the oropharynx and the lingual tonsil inferiorly in the hypopharynx and posterior one-third of the tongue. In addition, it includes the lateral pharyngeal bands and scattered lymphoid follicles throughout the pharynx, particularly adjacent to the eustachian tubes. Lymphoid tissue in this ring provides the body's first line of defense against inhaled or ingested pathogens. Waldeyer ring is involved in the production of immunoglobulins and the development of both B and T cell lymphocytes.

Adenoid

The adenoid, also known as the pharyngeal tonsil, is on the posterior wall of the nasopharynx extending toward the eustachian tubes. Unlike

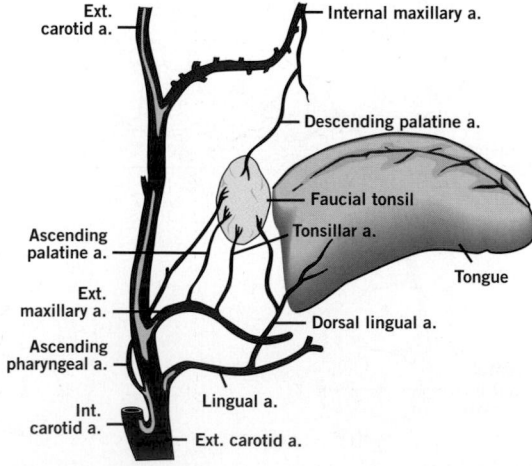

Figure 5 The blood supply of the palatine tonsil.

palatine and lingual tonsils, the pharyngeal tonsils does not contain crypts. It is formed by vertical folds of respiratory epithelium from which extend the Arey glands. There is no distinct capsule which surrounds the adenoid. Enlargement of the tissue can interfere with eustachian tube function and result in nasal obstruction with difficulty breathing. The adenoid is discussed in Chapter 64, "Diseases of the Oral Cavity, Oropharynx, and Nasopharynx," and Chapter 66, "Sleep Apnea in Children."

At the posterior midline of the pharynx just above the superior constrictor muscles lies a small sac-like depression known as the pharyngeal bursa. It is occasionally the site of a cystic formation known as Tornwaldt cyst.

Palatine Tonsils

The palatine tonsils are dense, compact bodies of lymphoid tissue. They are located within a fossa created by the palatoglossus muscle anteriorly and the palatopharyngeus muscle and superior constrictor muscles posteriorly and laterally. The tonsil has a thin but distinct capsule on its lateral surface which is formed from condensation of the pharyngobasilar fascia. The fascia extends into the tonsil itself forming septa which allow for passage of nerves and vessels. Whereas the capsule is densely adherent to the tonsillar tissue, it is readily separated from the underlying pharyngeal musculature. Continuous with the palatoglossal arch and the tonsillar capsule is a layer of mucosa and connective tissue known as the triangular fold. In rare instances a similar fold may be seen posteriorly. In approximately 40% of people, a fold of tissue known as a semilunar fold is found at the superior pole.[6]

The medial or free surface of the tonsil is covered by a thin layer of stratified squamous cell epithelium (mucosa). Epithelial tubules extend from the surface deep into the tonsil, forming tonsillar crypts. There is some evidence to suggest that the epithelium lining the crypts is semipermeable, allowing sampling of ingested material. Although they extend from the surface, the deepest parts of the crypts remain stable. The growing end is closest to the surface and is often narrower, preventing material from escaping once it has entered a crypt. There are a total of 8 to 10 crypts per tonsil.[9]

Tonsillectomy is one of the most common surgical procedures performed in children. They are generally removed for obstructive sleep apnea or chronic tonsillitis. In children, large palatine tonsils may occupy a significant portion of the oropharynx resulting in obstructed breathing and dysphagia. Some individuals have chronic colonization of the tonsillar crypts with streptococcus and other bacteria. These individuals may have frequent infections and halitosis. Others may have infections which result in the accumulation of pus between the tonsillar capsule and the pharyngeal musculature, referred to as a peritonsillar abscess or quinsy. This can lead to fibrosis of the capsule to the underlying pharyngeal musculature.

A surgeon removing a tonsil must be cognizant of the fact that the pharyngeal musculature is fairly thin and that there are numerous structures lateral to the fossa. For instance, the glossopharyngeal nerve lies on the lateral surface of the musculature. If it is injured, it can lead to a taste disturbance affecting the posterior one-third of the tongue. Indeed, it is not uncommon to see a transitory taste disturbance resulting from edema of CN IX following a tonsillectomy.[6] Other structures that may be in close proximity include the stylopharyngeus and styloglossus muscles, the stylohyoid ligament, the ascending pharyngeal artery, the ascending palatine branch of the facial artery and in rare instances, an aberrant vertebral or tortuous internal carotid artery.

Lingual Tonsil

The lingual tonsil is lymphoid tissue found in the base of the tongue. It extends from the foramen cecum to the epiglottis. Irregular folds of lymphoid tissue are covered by a thin layer of stratified squamous cell epithelium which invaginates to form small crypts. The lymphoid tissue lacks a distinct capsule or separation from the tongue musculature, preventing complete removal.

LYMPHATICS OF THE ORAL CAVITY

The oral cavity is drained by a dense network of lymphatic vessels. The most peripheral part of the lymphatic collecting system is a collection of avalvular capillaries with wide lumina, up to 100 μm in diameter.[10] These capillaries are surrounded by an elastic fiber network which helps to regulate fluid and cell transport into and out of the lymphatic channels. There are both superficial and deep networks which help to drain the tissues of the head and neck. The superficial network is composed of avalvular capillaries and drains into precollecting vessels found at the mucosa-submucosa junction. Multiple precollecting vessels join to drain into a lymph node. Another set of vessels, known as postcollecting vessels, carry the lymph from the nodes to the right and left lymphatic ducts and into the jugular veins. The lymphatic ducts drain into the jugular vein at its junction with the subclavian vein.

The highest concentration of lymph vessels in the oral cavity are found in the floor of the mouth (FOM).[10] Lymphatic vessels in the FOM drain lymph from the tongue, FOM, and mandibular gingival (Figure 6). Although several smaller collecting vessels in the anterior part of the FOM drain directly into submental lymph nodes, drainage in the FOM primarily occurs through collecting vessels in a direction along the mandibular axis and into both ipsilateral and contralateral submandibular lymph nodes. A portion of the ventral surface of the tongue also drains into the submandibular lymph nodes, similar to FOM drainage pathways. The remainder of the ventral surface of the tongue drains into the upper jugular nodes.

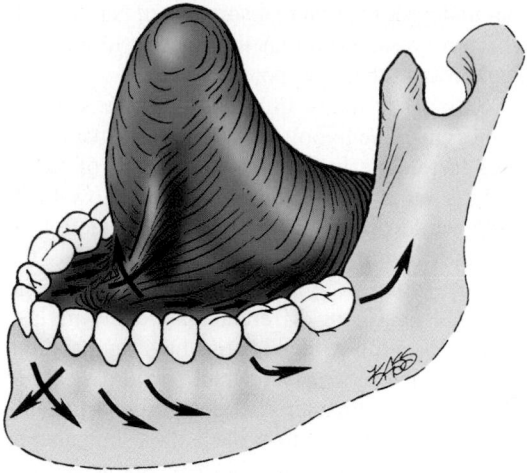

Figure 6 Superficial lymphatic drainage patterns of the floor of the mouth.

Understanding the lymphatic drainage of the tongue is of paramount importance in the treatment of patients with carcinoma of the tongue. Although all of the lymphatic channels in the tongue eventually drain to the deep cervical lymph nodes, the routes that these channels may take are extremely varied and can be somewhat unpredictable. Lymphatic drainage may be either ipsilateral or contralateral and may or may not involve regional nodes first. Indeed some of the drainage pathways will skip directly to the deep cervical nodes (Figure 7).

Although drainage can be somewhat unpredictable, there are some general rules for lymphatic drainage of the tongue (Figure 8). Lymph from the anterior two-thirds of the tongue, also known as the oral tongue, drains into the marginal and central lymphatic vessels. The marginal vessels drain the outer one-third of the dorsal surface of the tongue, the lateral margins of the tongue and a small portion of the edge of the ventral surface. The central vessels drain the central two-thirds of the dorsum of the tongue. The vessels generally run between

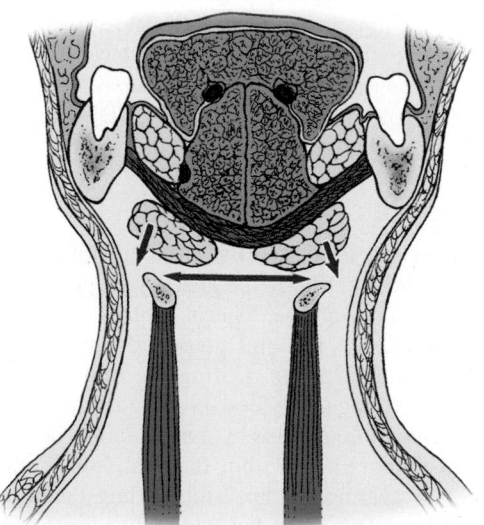

Figure 7 Drainage pattern of the upper jugular efferent lymphatics demonstrating a bypass of the submandibular nodes.

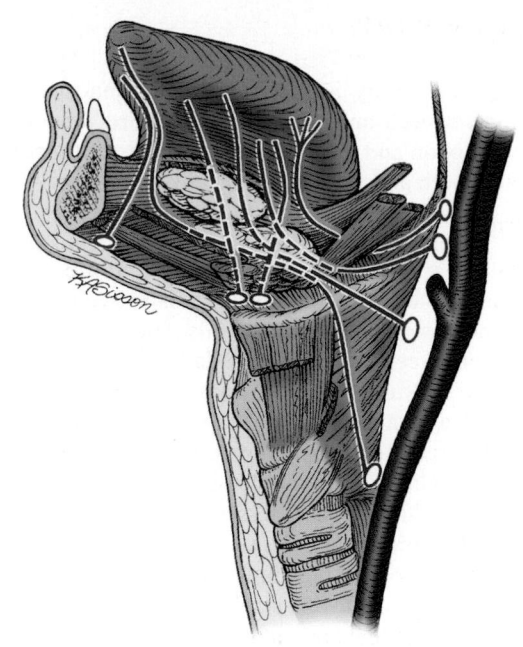

Figure 8 Lymphatic drainage routes from the tongue.

the two genioglossus muscles to the submental and submandibular lymph nodes. Anteriorly, the dorsal surface of the tongue drains primarily to submental and midjugular lymph nodes. The remainder of the tongue or the middle one-third of the tongue, drains primarily into submandibular lymph nodes. The vessels in the base of tongue, that area posterior to the circumvallate papilla drain into level II and III nodes in the neck. The tongue contains a particularly high concentration of lymphatic vessels in both its superficial and deep networks with the density progressively increasing from the tip to the base of the tongue. Overall, there is a higher density of lymphatic vessels in the mucosal layer than in the muscular portion of the tongue.

Vessels in the buccal mucosa and maxillary gingiva drain inferiorly toward the FOM and posteriorly to the oropharynx. A total of 8 to 10 collecting vessels drain lymph from these areas directly into the submandibular lymph nodes. Lymph vessels from the hard and soft palates also drain inferiorly toward the mandibular gingiva and oropharynx.

MINOR SALIVARY GLANDS

Between 600 and 1,000 minor salivary glands are found throughout the upper aerodigestive tract including the palate, buccal areas, and lips. These glands have excretory ducts. The highest concentration of minor salivary glands is found on the palate, with approximately 250 on the hard palate and 150 on the soft palate.[9] The glands on the palate receive parasympathetic innervation from the sphenopalatine ganglion while those in the remainder of the oral cavity and oropharynx are innervated by parasympathetic fibers from the lingual and glossopharyngeal nerves. These glands contribute to the overall production of saliva.

PHYSIOLOGY

The oral cavity is involved in two main functions: speech and swallowing. A third function, production and excretion of saliva, also occurs in the mouth and upper aerodigestive tract.

Salivary Production and Regulation

Saliva is produced by the paired parotid, submandibular and sublingual glands as well as the numerous minor salivary glands. The average person produces 1.5 L of saliva daily.[9] Unstimulated whole saliva flow is estimated to be 0.33 to 0.65 mL/min.[9] This can increase to 1.7 mL/min in the stimulated state. The major contributor to unstimulated salivary flow is the submandibular gland (69%). Although to a lesser degree, the parotid glands (26%) and sublingual glands (5%) also contribute to total unstimulated salivary flow. It is interesting to note that subjective sensation of dry mouth in patients on anticholinergic medications is not reported until resting salivary flow decreases by 40 to 50% of initial values.[11] Unstimulated and stimulated salivary flow may be altered by many factors including age, hormones, systemic disease states, circadian rhythms, diet, mastication, hydration, and drugs.[9,11] The largest volumes of saliva are secreted in response to cholinergic stimulation. Drugs, especially anticholinergic drugs, may therefore result in a decrease in salivary flow. Similarly, age has been shown to produce a decrease in salivary flow.[11] Disease states such as diabetes are associated with decreased salivary flow. However, it is unclear as to whether this is the result of the disease itself or of the medications used as treatment. By contrast, mastication has been associated with an increase in salivary flow. In fact, one study demonstrated that chewing four pieces of sugar-free gum daily for a total of 8 weeks resulted in an increase in basal flow of whole saliva.[11] Furthermore, chewing sugar-free gum has been shown to stimulate saliva and, thereby, enhance remineralization of teeth.[11]

The composition of the saliva secreted by the three major salivary glands varies somewhat in that the parotid glands produce a more serous saliva while the submandibular glands produce a higher mucin containing saliva. Hence, high mucin containing submandibular saliva makes up a greater proportion of resting saliva, whereas parotid saliva composes a greater percentage of stimulated saliva. The more serous, highly buffered saliva produced by the parotid protects the oral cavity from the detrimental effects of acid and is secreted principally upon stimulation by eating. Similarly, the unstimulated secretion of submandibular saliva has a higher mucin content to provide continual oral comfort through lubrication. The chemical composition of saliva is complex and contains a myriad of proteins and minerals including amylase, statherin, histatins, mucins, lysozyme, lactoferrin, peroxidases, secretory IgA, proline-rich proteins, thiocyanite, salts, gases, and other organic substances.[9,11] It initially begins as an isotonic plasma-like fluid secreted by acinar cells within the salivary gland that undergoes active reabsorption of Na^+ and Cl^- as it progresses through the duct resulting in a final product that is hypotonic.

Saliva has many important functions in the oral cavity. The hypotonic nature of saliva facilitates taste. The inorganic constituents of saliva such as bicarbonate and phosphate allow buffering while phosphate and calcium function to maintain the mineral integrity of teeth. Each of the salivary proteins contributes to overall oral and systemic health in different manners. Amylase aids in digestion while histatins have anticandidal effects. Lactoferrin, lysozyme, peroxidases, and IgA all have antibacterial effects. Mucins provide lubrication and help to protect the esophagus in gastroesophageal reflux disease. Statherins aid in the maintenance of dentition, and proline-rich proteins protect the teeth from the detrimental substances in the human diet. Indeed, saliva has been credited with numerous functions including lubrication of the oral cavity, taste, digestion, and protection against infection. Although commonly believed to prevent caries, quantitative studies of saliva's effect on caries have been inconclusive.[11] Saliva has, however, been shown to regulate the pH of plaque.

Speech

Speech is the production of meaningful sounds for the purpose of communication. It is the result of coordinated activity of the respiratory tract including the larynx as well as the pharynx and palate and related structures. Specifically, the soft palate frequently apposes the nasopharynx during speech allowing the passage of air through the oral cavity. While the production of the voice is unitiated at the glottis, modification of the voice and articulation of speech occurs throughout the upper aerodigestive tract and is mediated by many structures including the pharynx, palate, mandible, tongue, teeth, and lips. Alterations in any of these structures may be associated with alterations in speech, as is often seen in children with velopharyngeal insufficiency and in patients who have undergone surgical resection of any part of the upper aerodigestive tract for treatment of a malignancy or other lesion. Speech production is discussed in Chapter 73, "Assessment of Vocal Function," and Chapter 74, "Disorders of Speech and Language."

Swallowing

Swallowing is generally divided into three phases: the oral phase, the pharyngeal phase, and the esophageal phase. The oral phase is further subdivided into the oral preparatory phase and the oral transit phase. During the oral preparatory phase, ingested food is mixed with saliva and formed into a bolus by mastication. The food bolus is contained within the oral cavity anteriorly by sealing the lips and holding the cheek musculature close to the teeth. Posteriorly, the soft palate contacts the tongue preventing the bolus from entering the pharynx too soon. As a person chews, the food bolus is constantly repositioned within the oral cavity and held anterolaterally along the hard palate by the tongue. The food bolus must be the right size, consistency and temperature before initiating the oral transit phase. Once the bolus is ready to be swallowed, the tongue propels the entire bolus posteriorly into the oropharynx with sequential supero-posterior movements. The sequential tongue movements initiate the pharyngeal reflex and pharyngeal phase of swallowing.

The pharyngeal phase is characterized by multiple, simultaneous actions including velopharyngeal closure, laryngeal elevation, contraction of the pharyngeal constrictor muscles, and cricopharyngeal relaxation. These actions are reflexive and associated with a temporary apnea, which in adults may last anywhere from 0.5 to 10.02 seconds.[12] This is followed in rapid succession by superior and anterior movement of the hyoid bone and laryngeal elevation and closure. The arytenoids cartilages closely approximate the epiglottis. Once the bolus has passed, the arytenoids separate from the epiglottis and the hyoid returns to its resting position. Breathing is once again initiated. The bolus is propelled through the pharynx and into the esophagus by contraction of the three pharyngeal constrictor muscles and relaxation of the cricopharyngeal muscle. Relaxation of the cricopharyngeus allows for passage of the bolus into the esophagus and the start of the final stage of swallowing. The esophageal phase is also an involuntary phase. The bolus is transmitted to the stomach by peristalsis of the esophageal musculature. Additional information on swallowing is contained in Chapter 82, "Imaging of the Larynx, Trachea, and Esophagus," and Chapter 85, "Esophagology."

REFERENCES

1. Tachimura T, Ojima M, Nohara K, et al. Change in palatoglossus muscle activity in relation to swallowing volume during the transition from the oral phase to the pharyngeal phase. Dysphagia 2005;20:32–9.
2. Linden RWA. Taste. Br Dent J 1993;175:243–53.
3. Hadley K, Orlandi RR, Fong KJ. Basic anatomy and physiology of olfaction and taste. Otolaryngol Clin North Am 2004;37:1115–26.
4. Spector AC, Travers SP. The representation of taste quality in the mammalian nervous system. Behav Cogn Neurosci Rev 2005;4:143–91.
5. Sbarbati A, Crescimanno C, Osculati F. The anatomy and functional role of the circumvallate papilla/von Ebner gland complex. Med Hypotheses 1999;53:40–4.
6. Hollingshead WH. Anatomy for surgeons. The Head and Neck, 3rd edition. Philadelphia: JB Lippincott Co; 1982.
7. Huang L, Cao J, Wang H, et al. Identification and functional characterization of a voltage-gated chloride channel and its novel splice variant in taste bud cells. J Biol Chem 2005;280:36150–7.
8. Liman E. Thermal gating of TRP ion channels: Food for thought? Sci STKE 2006;326:pe12.
9. Lowry LD, Onart S. Anatomy and physiology of the oral cavity and pharynx. In: Snow JB, Ballenger JJ, editors. Ballenger's Otorhinolaryngology Head and Neck Surgery, 16th edition. Hamilton, Ontario: BC Decker, Inc; 2003. p. 1009–19.
10. Werner J, Dunne AA, Myers JN. Functional anatomy of the lymphatic drainage system of the upper aerodigestive tract and its role in metastasis of squamous cell carcinoma. Head Neck 2003;25:322–32.
11. Dodds MW, Johnson DA, Yeh CK. Health benefits of saliva: A review. J Dent 2005;33:223–33.
12. Martin-Harris B, Brodsky MB, Michel Y et al. Breathing and swallowing dynamics across the adult lifespan. Arch Otolaryngol Head Neck Surg 2005;131:762–70.

64

Diseases of the Oral Cavity, Oropharynx and Nasopharynx

Kenny H. Chan, MD
Vijay R. Ramakrishnan, MD

Diseases of the oral cavity, oropharynx, and nasopharynx are among the most commonly seen disorders in pediatric otolaryngology. Although each subunit is anatomically distinct, the entire area may be conceptualized as a single functional unit (Figures 1, 2, and 3). These areas have contiguous anatomy and are subjected to the same causative factors of disease. The oral cavity is defined anteriorly by the vermilion border and posteriorly by the circumvallate papillae and junction of the hard and soft palate. The oral cavity includes the lips, oral tongue, floor of mouth, maxillary and mandibular alveoli, hard palate, gingiva, and buccal mucosa. The oropharynx extends posteriorly from the oral cavity to the valleculae. Structures of the oropharynx include the tongue base, palatine and lingual tonsils, soft palate, and uvula. The nasopharynx is the space bounded by the posterior part of the nasal cavity and skull base to the level of the posterior surface of the soft palate. This includes the adenoid, eustachian tubes, and fossae of Rosenmuller. Functionally, these portions of the pharynx contribute to speech, swallowing, and respiration. This chapter will address common pediatric diseases of the oral cavity, oropharynx, and nasopharynx.

DISEASES OF THE TONSILS AND ADENOID

Lymphatic tissue of Waldeyer ring in the nasopharynx and oropharynx comprises the pharyngeal tonsil (adenoid), palatine tonsils, and lingual tonsil. There has been much historic debate regarding indications for and cost-effectiveness of adenotonsillectomy. Currently, much of the controversy exists in the field of pediatric obstructive sleep apnea (OSA) and sleep disordered breathing. Chapter 66, "Sleep Apnea in Children," contains a discussion of pediatric OSA. Indications for tonsillectomy with or without adenoidectomy are listed in Table 1.

Adenotonsillar Hypertrophy

Acute and chronic upper airway obstruction due to adenotonsillar hypertrophy is a common chief complaint faced by pediatricians and otolaryngologists. The relative overgrowth of lymphoid tissue to skeletal growth during ages 3 to 8 years may initiate symptoms such as snoring, mouth

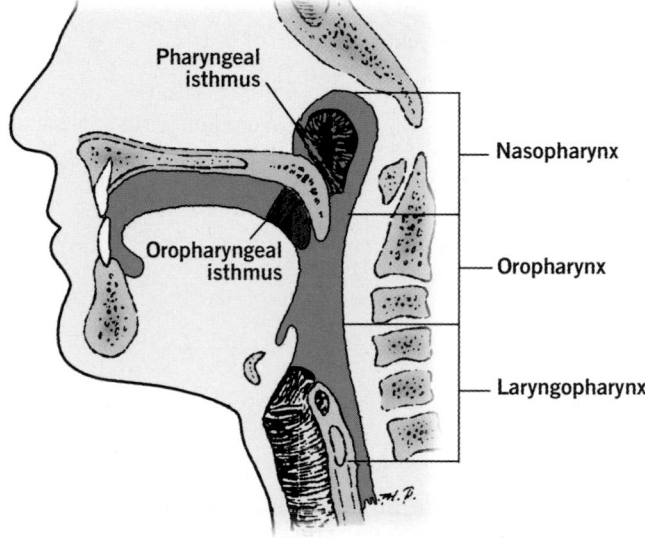

Figure 1 Anatomy of the pharynx.

breathing, apnea, and dysphagia. These symptoms may be chronic or may be acutely exacerbated by viral or bacterial pharyngitis. Further history may reveal snorting, gasping, hyponasal speech, restless sleep, enuresis, growth disturbance, and even failure to thrive. Physical examination may reveal tonsillar hypertrophy, and endoscopy or lateral soft tissue radiographs may

confirm adenoid hypertrophy. Lymphoid hypertrophy and relaxation of the pharyngeal musculature during sleep increases the obstruction. Children with craniofacial anomalies or neuromuscular disorders are more susceptible to this process. To confirm sleep apnea, polysomnography (PSG) must be performed. During PSG, the frequency of apneas, hypopneas, and arousals

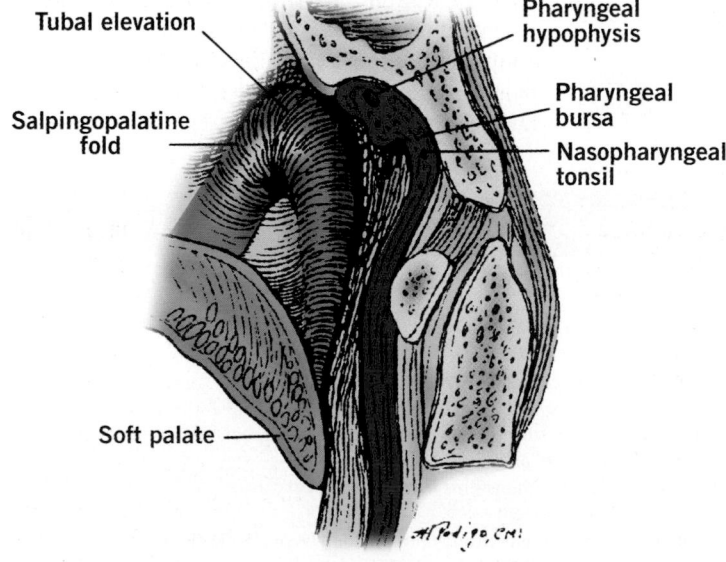

Figure 2 Anatomy of the nasopharynx.

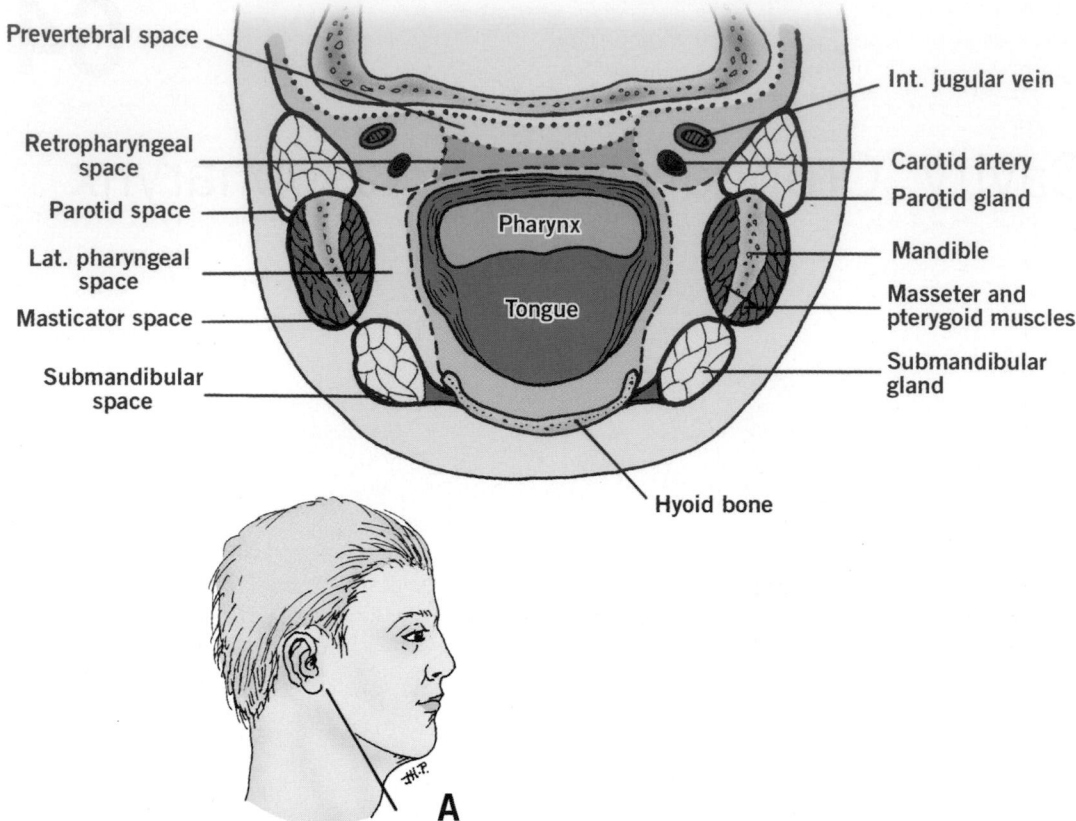

Figure 3 Anatomical spaces of the neck.

are measured. The number and degree of oxygen desaturations are also recorded. Other factors are monitored to determine the obstructive or central component of the respiratory disturbance and to document associated hypercapnia or cardiac arrhythmia. Most studies use a respiratory disturbance index (RDI) greater than one event per hour to diagnose pediatric OSA, although this remains a subject of controversy. However, clinical history and physical examination are often sufficient to infer sleep disordered breathing without the need of a PSG. Adenotonsillar hypertrophy and sleep disordered breathing have become one of the primary indications for adenotonsillectomy in children. Obstructive breathing in children may have detrimental long-term neuropsychologic and cardiovascular effects which can be reversed with surgery when appropriate.[1] In cases of isolated adenoid hypertrophy, a trial of nasal corticosteroids is indicated prior to surgical intervention.

Adenotonsillar Infection

Acute tonsillitis is an infectious process causing fever, sore throat, odynophagia, and malaise. Oropharyngeal erythema, edema, and exudates may be present. Associated rash or lymphadenopathy may be present. Group A beta-hemolytic streptococcal pharyngitis is discussed in further detail later in this chapter. Children who experience recurrent episodes of acute tonsillitis may be considered for surgical treatment. In 70% of patients, the core adenoid and tonsil tissue harbor the same pathogens, which are eradicated with adenotonsillectomy. Patients with three or more episodes of acute pharyngitis with significant associated symptoms per year may be candidates for tonsillectomy. Chronic tonsillitis, or persistent tonsillar infection, occurs in older children and young adults. Presenting complaints are constant throat pain, fatigue, halitosis, and expulsion of tonsillar debris. On examination, enlarged tonsillar

crypts filled with debris are often visualized. Tonsillectomy is indicated in chronic tonsillitis when symptoms are severe or quality of life is affected. The adenoid tissue may chronically harbor infection or become acutely infected during respiratory tract infections or sinusitis. Nasal obstruction, purulent secretions, hyponasal speech, postnasal drip, throat pain, or ear pain may be present. Indirect or direct examination may reveal inflamed, exudative adenoid tissue. Acute adenoiditis is treated similarly to acute tonsillitis. Clinically, adenoiditis may be difficult to distinguish from sinusitis. Chronic adenoiditis may be a causative factor in cases of recurrent sinusitis. It has been recommended that adenoidectomy be performed in the child with chronic sinusitis prior to pediatric endoscopic sinus surgery, but its efficacy is unknown. Regardless of size, adenoid tissue may cause extrinsic eustachian tube dysfunction in patients with chronic or recurrent otitis media with effusion. Bacterial colonization of the adenoid may also contribute to recurrent otitis media. Adenoidectomy is recommended for children undergoing repeat tympanostomy tube placement over the age of 3 years or those undergoing primary tube placement who have complaints of nasal obstruction due to adenoid hypertrophy.

Peritonsillar infection may occur in any age group but is most common in adolescents and young adults. It is the most common complication of acute tonsillitis. Infection is thought to spread through the tonsillar crypts and capsule into the peritonsillar space. The infection begins as a cellulitis and progresses to an abscess, most commonly near the superior pole of the tonsil. Patients will complain of fever, odynophagia, unilateral sore throat, and otalgia. Classic signs include a muffled voice, trismus, uvular deviation away from the affected side, and soft palate fullness or edema. The oral airway may be compromised, and the patient may have some difficulty with secretions. Diagnosis is usually

Table 1 Indications for Tonsillectomy +/– Adenoidectomy	
Absolute indications	Upper airway obstruction
	Severe dysphagia
	Cardiopulmonary complications
	Unresponsive or recurrent peritonsillar abscess
	Tonsillitis with febrile convulsions
	Biopsy needed for tissue pathology
Relative indications	Three or more tonsillar infections per year despite proper medical treatment
	Persistent foul taste or halitosis
	Chronic or recurrent tonsillitis in a streptococcal carrier unresponsive to medical management
	Unilateral tonsillar hypertrophy presumed to be of neoplastic origin

Adapted from the American Academy of Otolaryngology-Head and Neck Surgery Clinical Indicators Compendium 1995.

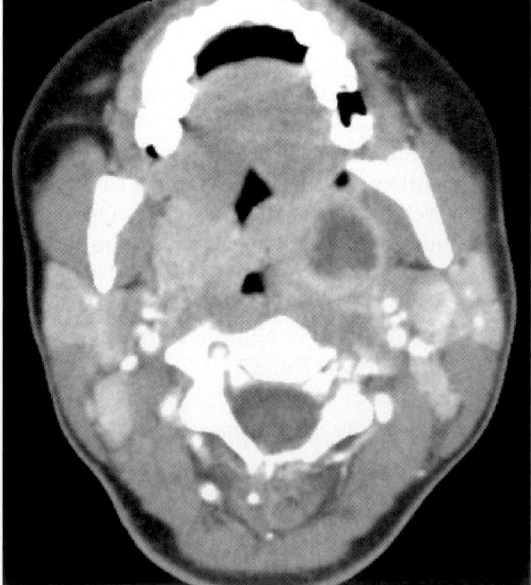

Figure 4 Postcontrast axial computed tomography (CT) scan, peritonsillar abscess.

made clinically, although it may be difficult to distinguish cellulitis from an abscess, as seen in Figure 4. Hydration, analgesics, and antibiotics are required. If abscess formation is suspected, needle aspiration or incision and drainage is indicated. Both have success rates greater than 90%. Tonsillectomy in the acute setting can be risky due to an increased chance for hemorrhage. Those patients who experience recurrent infections or abscesses are recommended to undergo tonsillectomy when not acutely infected.

Tonsilloliths

Tonsilloliths are collections of epithelial debris buried in the tonsillar crypts. Malodorous, granular, white or yellow calculi may be removed with irrigation or instrumentation. They generally tend to recur and can reach sizes up to 1 cm.

Unilateral Tonsillar Enlargement

In the routine examination, it is not uncommon for an asymptomatic patient to have the appearance of unilateral tonsillar hypertrophy. In most cases, the tonsil is situated medially in the tonsillar fossa, giving the illusion of a larger tonsil. In other cases, unilateral infection may cause an enlarged tonsil. Rarely is there in underlying malignancy causing unilateral tonsillar enlargement in the pediatric population.[2] Most studies recommend watchful waiting unless there is heightened suspicion for malignancy in the history or physical examination, particularly in the presence of constitutional symptoms.

Neoplasm

Nasopharyngeal carcinoma and non-Hodgkin lymphoma may present in the nasopharynx as a painless mass that causes nasal obstruction, rhinorrhea, epistaxis, or serous otitis media. Proper diagnosis and staging requires biopsy and complete radiographic evaluation. Hodgkin lymphoma rarely presents in Waldeyer ring but rather as cervical or supraclavicular adenopathy. Transplant-associated lymphoproliferative disorder is characterized by a spectrum of clinical and histologic entities including lymphomas. Head and neck manifestations include a mononucleosis-like syndrome characterized by constitutional symptoms, cervical lymphadenopathy, pharyngitis, and tonsillar enlargement with or without obstructive symptoms.

Rhabdomyosarcoma is the most common soft tissue malignancy of childhood. It is a highly aggressive, primitive mesenchymal tumor which presents with local symptoms. The head and neck is the most frequent site of origin, where it often presents in parameningeal regions. Although outcome is most closely tied with clinical staging, multimodality treatment using surgery, chemotherapy, and radiotherapy offers the best chance for survival in patients with rhabdomyosarcoma when the tumor presents in an operable location.[3]

The oral cavity and oropharynx contain up to 1,000 minor salivary glands. Salivary gland neo-plasms in children are rare. Most salivary gland neoplasms in children are hemangiomas or lymphangiomas. Benign tumors such as mixed tumors, Warthin tumor, oncocytoma, adenomatous tumors, and lymphoepithelial tumors are rare in children. Malignant salivary gland tumors include mucoepidermoid carcinoma, adenocarcinoma, adenoid cystic carcinoma, malignant mixed tumor, and acinic cell carcinoma. These are more likely to occur in the major salivary glands, that is, parotid and submandibular glands.

Juvenile nasopharyngeal angiofibroma (JNA) is a highly vascular, locally aggressive tumor of the nasopharynx. It accounts for only 0.05% of all tumors of the head and neck, and typically affects adolescent males. The tumor originates in the sphenopalatine foramen and expands locally, causing symptoms of nasal obstruction. Preoperative embolization and surgical excision are the appropriate treatment. Endoscopic approaches have proved equally effective to conventional open approaches in the majority of cases.[4] Figure 5 shows an axial view of an extensive, locally destructive JNA. JNAs are discussed in greater detail in Chapter 96, "Neoplasms of the Nasopharynx."

Surgical Technique: Adenotonsillectomy

Many techniques have been used over the years for removal of the tonsils and adenoid. The generally accepted technique for tonsillectomy consists of dissection in the subcapsular plane with a knife or electrocautery under general anesthesia. This dissection may also be achieved with a harmonic scalpel or laser. Hemostasis is achieved with electrocautery, suture ligation, and topical thrombin. The adenoid is most frequently removed with an adenoid curette or may be vaporized with electrocautery.

The patient is intubated and placed in the supine position with a roll under the shoulders. Perioperative corticosteroids are administered for antiemetic effect if not contraindicated. A mouth gag is inserted for proper exposure of the oropharynx. The palate is palpated to ensure an intact palate is present. Adenoidectomy is generally performed first unless tonsillar hypertro-

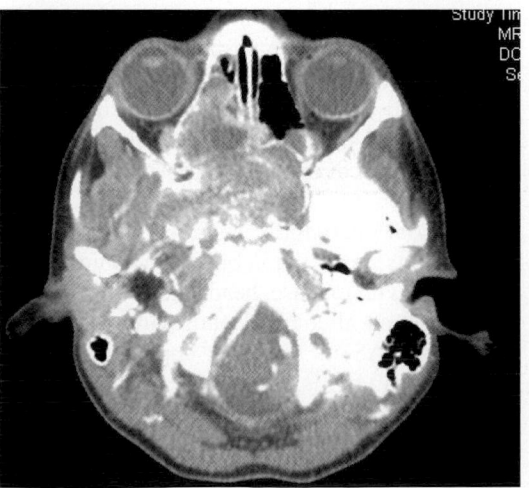

Figure 5 Postcontrast axial computed tomography (CT) scan, pediatric juvenile nasal angiofibroma.

phy prevents easy access to the nasopharynx. Adenoidectomy is contraindicated in the presence of a cleft palate or a submucous cleft. If obstructive sleep apnea occurs in a child with a submucous cleft, only the superior adenoid tissue should be removed accurately and the electrocautery method is preferred to assure velopharyngeal closure. One or two urinary catheters are used to retract the soft palate and the adenoid is visualized with a mirror. Adenoidectomy can be performed with an adenoid curette, suction electrocautery, or powered instrumentation. Care should be taken to stay away from the eustachian tube orifice and torus tubarius to prevent scarring and iatrogenic eustachian tube dysfunction.

Tonsillectomy is performed in the following fashion. The superior pole of the tonsil is grasped and retracted medially with an Allis clamp. The mucosa of the anterior tonsillar pillar is incised and the plane of the tonsillar capsule is identified. Dissection continues in this plane with electrocautery or using the cold technique, as the tonsil is retracted medially. The inferior attachment to the lingual tonsil is then divided with electrocautery. Care is taken to preserve normal mucosa of the anterior and posterior tonsillar pillars. A Hurd retractor may be used to aid in visualization of the tonsillar fossa. Hemostasis is achieved using electrocautery or suture ligature. The oropharynx and nasopharynx are irrigated and observed for hemostasis. An orogastric tube is passed and gastric contents are suctioned to limit postoperative nausea and emesis.

Recent trends in the surgical techniques for tonsillectomy include both new instrumentation and subtotal tonsillectomy. New instrumentations that have undergone rigorous clinical trials include the radiofrequency and microdebrider methods. The revival of subtotal tonsillectomy is partly driven by the improved postoperative pain profile of children who have undergone this procedure and is also driven by the easy adaptation of the newer surgical instruments. The radiofrequency instrumentation is utilized for both total and subtotal tonsillectomy. Although the pain profile is improved significantly using these instruments and the subtotal technique, continued studies are needed to monitor the cost benefit of such techniques and the long-term sequelae of performing subtotal tonsillectomy in terms of tissue regrowth and eradiation of streptococcal disease.

Dehydration, odynophagia, and otalgia are common in the postoperative period. Occasionally, children will need intravenous hydration until adequate oral intake can be maintained. Antibiotics in the postoperative period may aid marginally in return to normal activity, but recent metaanalyses show that their use does not appear to decrease postoperative pain.[5,6] Post-tonsillectomy hemorrhage is the most common complication, occurring in approximately 2 to 5%, and should be taken seriously. Some can be treated with observation; some will need to be controlled in the operating room. Risk of hemorrhage is higher in patients on aspirin therapy or those with bleeding disorders. Hypernasal speech is common in the postoperative period, but lasting velopharyngeal insufficiency following adenoidectomy is uncommon and estimated to occur in 1:2,000 cases. Treatment for this complication includes speech therapy, or surgical creation of a pharyngeal flap. Nasopharyngeal stenosis can occur with the use of extensive cautery with the KTP laser or with extensive resection of the posterior tonsillar pillars. Obstructing scar tissue forms from the soft palate to the posterior tonsillar pillars or posterior pharyngeal wall at times causing obstructive sleep apnea. Treatment consists of corticosteroid injection, lysis of scar bands, stent placement, and rotation or advancement flaps.

INFECTIOUS DISEASES OF THE ORAL CAVITY AND OROPHARYNX

Infections of the oral cavity and oropharynx are common. These infections may be isolated to the head and neck or may represent a part of a systemic disease process. Recognition of the clinical pattern of infections and distinction of these from other patterns of disease, are important clinical skills leading to proper treatment.

Viral infections of the oral cavity and oropharynx are among the most common reasons patients seek medical care. Viral pharyngitis is a syndrome of sore throat with a variety of other symptoms including fever, cough, and congestion. Many viruses can cause pharyngitis, for example, coxsackie virus, rhinovirus, adenovirus, influenza, parainfluenza, coronavirus, enterovirus, and respiratory syncitial virus. Viral studies are usually not necessary, and treatment is symptomatic. Mononucleosis caused by the Epstein-Barr virus is discussed in Chapter 42, "Etiology of Infectious Diseases of the Upper Respiratory Tract."

Herpangina is a common viral infection of young children that resembles bacterial pharyngitis. The etiologic agent is usually coxsackie A or B virus, but other enteric viruses may cause a similar clinical presentation. The peak incidence is during the summer and fall seasons. Symptoms usually consist of severe sore throat, fever, and malaise. Severe erythema, vesicles, and superficial ulcerations may be present in the posterior aspect of the oropharynx. The disease is usually self-limited, and treatment is aimed at symptomatic relief. Coxsackie A virus is also the pathogen in *hand-foot-and-mouth disease*. This syndrome is similar to herpangina, except that the oral cavity is more frequently involved than the oropharynx, and vesiculopapular lesions erupt on the palms and soles. *Herpes simplex* infections may present in one of two ways. Primary herpetic gingivostomatitis is common in the young child; it begins with a prodrome of fever and malaise, with subsequent onset of painful, erythematous oral vesicles. The vesicles rupture within 24 hours, leaving coalescent ulcerations that may form a gray pseudomembrane over the oral cavity. Diffuse lymphadenopathy is almost always present.

Diagnosis may be made by viral studies or biopsy. The virus may remain dormant in the patient's neuronal ganglia for life and may be activated to cause a secondary herpetic infection consisting a burning sensation and vesicular eruption in the oral cavity. It is termed herpes labialis when the lips are involved. Precipitating factors include stress, systemic illness, fever, sunlight, bacterial infection, and immunodeficiency. Treatment is symptomatic with spontaneous resolution occurring within 2 weeks. Some studies demonstrate a benefit from antiviral therapy.

Herpes zoster infection presents as a painful, vesicular eruption over the distribution of a branch of the trigeminal nerve. It usually occurs in older patients as a reactivation of dormant varicella virus in the neurosensory ganglia. Treatment consists of antiviral therapy.

The *German measles (rubella) virus* infection is uncommon in the immunized population but is a potentially serious systemic infection characterized by cough, coryza, conjunctivitis, and maculopapular rash. The *measles (rubeola)* virus produces a similar though more severe clinical course distinguished by the initial appearance before the rash of red spots with central bluish white specks on the buccal mucosa known as Koplik spots. Infectious complications such as otitis media or pneumonia can occur due to temporary immunosuppression following the disease. Treatment of measles involves vitamin A supplementation and human immunoglobulin in addition to supportive measures. *Cytomegalovirus*, also a member of the herpes family of viruses, infects immunocompromised patients. Infections are characterized by large mucosal ulcers, exudative pharyngitis, and cervical lymphadenopathy. The disease presents similarly to mononucleosis, and treatment is symptomatic. *Recurrent respiratory papillomatosis* is a disorder caused by the human papilloma virus and is characterized by the formation of exophytic, cauliflower-like masses. Papillomas may form in the airway or the oral cavity, specifically on the soft palate or tongue. Surgical excision by cold knife, electrocautery, powered instrumentation, or laser is the standard of care. Recurrences in the oral cavity and oropharynx are uncommon after excision, but the recurrence rate is substantially higher in the airway. Recent studies demonstrate an improvement in disease severity and regrowth with repeated intralesional injection of mitomycin or cidofovir in selected patients, although clear evidence from randomized, controlled, prospective studies is lacking.

Bacterial pharyngitis is similar to viral pharyngitis in its presentation but more commonly is associated with malaise, headache, chills, nausea, vomiting, and abdominal pain. Group A streptococcus (GAS) is the most common cause of bacterial pharyngitis.

Other causes of bacterial pharyngitis are addressed in Chapter 42, "Etiology of Infectious Diseases of the Upper Respiratory Tract." Physical findings consistent with, but not diagnostic for, GAS include pharyngeal erythema

and exudates, palatal petechiae, and tender cervical lymphadenopathy. Throat culture is considered the gold standard for detection of GAS, but there is a 5 to 10% false negative rate and there are many GAS carriers who will be falsely positive. The majority of rapid detection kits available have a high specificity (95%) and a sensitivity of between 70 and 90% compared with conventional culture on sheep blood agar. White blood cell count, erythrocyte sedimentation rate, and C-reactive protein have low positive predictive values and are not diagnostic of bacterial pharyngitis. Antibody titers do not have a role in acute streptococcal infection. Treatment consists of antibiotics and supportive care. Scarlet fever or scarlatina is an acute exanthematous disease caused by streptococcal pharyngeal infection and production of an erythrogenic toxin. The complications of streptococcal tonsillopharyngitis may be classified as suppurative and nonsuppurative. The nonsuppurative complications include acute rheumatic fever and poststreptococcal glomerulonephritis. Suppurative complications include peritonsillar, parapharyngeal, and retropharyngeal cellulitis or abscess formation.

Periodic fever, adenitis, pharygitis, and aphthous ulcer (PFAPA) syndrome is in the differential diagnosis for recurrent pharyngitis. These children are frequently seen in the pediatrician's office or the emergency room for high fever. Although cimetidine and corticosteroids purportedly are effective medical treatment, tonsillectomy is an alternative.

Fungal infection of the oral cavity is almost always the result of *Candida albicans*, an opportunistic microorganism that is part of the normal oral flora. Decrease in host immunity or alteration in the oral flora allows *Candida* overgrowth and infection. Predisposing conditions include long-term antibiotic use, diabetes, corticosteroid therapy, immunosuppression, and radiation to the oral cavity. Thrush, or pseudomembranous candidiasis, is the most common type of oral candidiasis. It occurs most commonly in infants but may affect any age group. It is characterized by dry, painful, white plaques covering the tongue, hard palate, and buccal mucosa. These lesions may be scraped off of the raw underlying mucosa. Invasive oropharyngeal or esophageal candidiasis is known to occur in children with diabetes or immunosuppression. Fungal smears may demonstrate hyphae, but fungal culture is needed for a definitive diagnosis. Acute atrophic candidiasis is less common and manifests as sore throat, burning of the mouth, and foul taste. Erythematous, ulcerated mucosa is the characteristic appearance. Angular chelitis, painful fissures at the oral commisure, may also be due to candida overgrowth. In children, a search for an underlying condition must be undertaken along with treatment of the acute fungal infection. Most can be treated with a topical antifungal agent, although recalcitrant infections may require intravenous antifungal therapy. Other fungal agents that can involve the oral cavity include histoplasmosis and mucormycosis, which typically affect the hard palate.

Odontogenic infections are common in children and may lead to abscess formation or Ludwig's angina, a potentially life-threatening floor of mouth cellulitis. This process is more commonly seen in adults with poor dentition than in children who have shorter deciduous dental roots. Anaerobic bacteria must be considered present in the odontogenic infection, and these often have B-lactamase resistance. Recent studies demonstrate that high doses of amoxillicin-clavulanate may overcome this resistance if penicillins are to be used. A recent study showed that greater than 50% of deep neck infections in adults were found to have an odontogenic source, with *Streptococcus viridans* and *Klebsiella pneumoniae* as the two most common pathogens.[7] In children, the odontogenic source of deep neck infection is second in likelihood to an oropharyngeal source. Antibiotic therapy, abscess drainage when present, and definitive treatment of the source of infection are crucial to patient care. In cases of Ludwig's angina, airway stability is the initial concern, and tracheostomy may be required. Deep neck infections are discussed in Chapter 65, "Deep Head and Neck Space Infections."

Oral manifestations of human immunodeficiency virus (HIV) infection occur in 30 to 80% of the infected population. The most common sites of involvement are the palate, tongue, lips, buccal mucosa, and gingiva. In children, the most common signs of HIV infection are oral candidiasis, diffuse parotitis, and oral ulcers. Other oral pathology that may suggest underlying HIV infection includes xerostomia, recurrent herpetic or aphthous ulcers, angular chelitis, hairy leukoplakia, gingivitis and periodontitis, and papillomas. Oral hairy leukoplakia presents as an asymtptomatic, corrugated lesion along the lateral margin of the tongue, caused by the Epstein-Barr virus. Kaposi sarcoma presents in the oral cavity as a pigmented macule, nodule, or hemorrhagic lesion. It may darken with age, ulcerate, necrose, or become lobulated.[8]

INFLAMMATORY AND SYSTEMIC DISEASES

Lesions of the oral cavity and oropharynx are often presenting signs of an underlying systemic disorder. These lesions are easily accessible, and many times are diagnostic. Systemic inflammatory diseases most commonly affect adults but may occur in children and adolescents; lasting sequelae may result from a delay in diagnosis.

Kawasaki disease, or mucocutaneous lymph node syndrome, is an acute onset, idiopathic, multisystem vasculitis. It occurs in children under 5 years of age, with a peak incidence in 1- to 2-year-olds. It is characterized by several days of high fever, conjunctivitis, rash, erythema and edema of the extremities, cervical lymphadenopathy, and multiple oropharyngeal signs. These include strawberry tongue, fissured lips, mucosal erythema, and necrotic pharyngitis. Up to 20% of untreated children will develop cardiac complications, with coronary artery aneurysm being the most dangerous. Kawasaki disease is the most common cause of acquired cardiac disease in children under 5 years of age. Treatment consists of intravenous gammaglobulin and aspirin.

Wegener granulomatosis commonly affects the oral cavity although it is more commonly seen in the nasal cavity and subglottic sites in teenagers. Gingival hyperplasia is common, but painful mucosal ulcerations surrounded by an erythematous margin may also be present. Behçet syndrome is a systemic inflammatory disorder characterized by recurrent oral and genital ulcers which resemble apthous ulcers. Ocular inflammation, such as uveitis or iridocyclitis, aids in diagnosis. Corticosteroids, chlorambucil and acyclovir have been used for treatment. Reiter syndrome classically presents as urethritis, uveitis, conjunctivitis, and arthritis in young men. Superficial, erythematous oral ulcers with a white rim are associated with this syndrome. Sjögren syndrome is a collagen vascular disease that causes xerostomia, keratoconjunctivitis, and arthritis. Labial biopsy confirms the diagnosis by demonstrating a lymphocytic infiltrate in the minor salivary glands. Approximately 25% of patients with systemic lupus erythematosus will have oral cavity manifestations including xerostomia, petechiae, hemorrhagic bullae, and white mucosal keratoses.

Primary macroglossia may occur in hypothyroidism, acromegaly, and Beckwith-Wiedemann syndrome. Secondary macroglossia may occur in angioneurotic edema, amyloidosis, glycogen storage diseases, neurofibromatosis, actinomycosis, syphilis, tuberculosis, and in neoplastic processes. Macroglossia occurs in 15 to 20% of patients with amyloidosis and can grow to massive proportions. Amyloidosis may also occur as nodules or polypoid lesions and can be located anywhere in the larynx or trachea. Burning mouth syndrome is a local neuropathy of the tip and lateral aspects of a normal appearing tongue. This disorder of peri- and postmenopausal women is treated with amitryptiline and clonazepam. Geographic tongue is an idiopathic benign migratory glossitis resulting from a loss of filiform papillae. In this process, there are central, red, atrophic lesions on the dorsum of the tongue with a margin of desquamating epithelium. Lesions may occur on the buccal mucosa, as well. This chronic condition may persist for years and does not require treatment. Fissured tongue is similar in that multiple lesions occur on the dorsum of the tongue and treatment is not necessary. However, these fissures may become irritated with food particles, bacteria, or fungi. Fissured tongue has been associated with Down syndrome and Melkersson-Rosenthal syndrome, a recurrent process of facial nerve palsy and facial edema. Hairy tongue is a benign disorder characterized by hypertrophy of the filiform papillae, which may then become colonized with pigmented bacteria. Poor hygiene, tobacco use, oral antibiotics, and radiation therapy are predisposing factors.

Aphthous stomatitis and recurrent aphthous ulcers are the most common condition affecting the oral cavity. Recent studies have demonstrated an alteration in cellular immune response as a predisposing factor. In the pediatric population, this disease occurs in older children and adolescents, with a gender predilection for females. There is a 48-hour prodrome of dysesthesia and erythema of the oral mucosa prior to appearance of an ulcer. There are three categories of aphthous ulcers. Minor aphthous ulcers account for approximately 80%; these are shallow, painful ulcers of the oral mucosa covered by a gray membrane and surrounded by an erythematous rim. These ulcers typically affect the buccal mucosa, lips, and tongue. They resolve spontaneously in approximately 2 weeks and may recur regularly in intervals. Major aphthous ulcers are characterized by painful ulcerations greater than 0.6 cm in size. These may occur on the soft palate, floor of mouth, and peritonsillar mucosa. Major ulcers may persist for up to 6 weeks and may also recur in regular intervals. Less common are herpetiform ulcers, crops of multiple painful, pinpoint lesions. These may coalesce into large, irregular ulcerations anywhere in the oral cavity. Treatment for all forms is symptomatic, with topical anesthetics or corticosteroids providing some degree of pain relief. In severe cases, intralesional or systemic corticosteroids and acyclovir may be of some benefit.

Lichen planus is a common immune-mediated, inflammatory disorder of the epithelial surface of the skin and mucous membrane. It may occur in children and adolescents, although it is considered a disease of adulthood. The disease process is a cell-mediated immune response that may be a part of a systemic disease. Lichen planus of the oral cavity is found on the tongue, buccal mucosa, and gingival margin. The reticular type is more common and appears as isolated or coalescent white papules or lines known as Wickham striae. This can be symmetric and is usually asymptomatic. An erosive type contains an ulcerative center with lines or papules at the periphery and may undergo malignant transformation. Biopsy of the periphery of a lesion provides a diagnosis. Symptomatic lesions may be treated with topical, injectable, or systemic corticosteroids.

The autoimmune disorders pemphigus vulgaris, pemphigoid, and cicatricial pemphigoid similarly affect adults more than children. These conditions may be distinguished by their clinical, histologic, and immune characteristics. All demonstrate a loss of cohesion among epidermal cells that results in accumulation of intradermal fluid and blisters. In pemphigus vulgaris, this loss of cohesion occurs in the epidermal layer, and in pemphigoid occurs at the basement membrane. Nikolsky sign, a loss of epidermis by rubbing skin or mucous membrane, occurs in pemphigus vulgaris. Most cases of pemphigus vulgaris in children begin in the oral cavity. Vesicles and bullae form and rupture, leaving painful ulcerations similar to erythema multiforme. Oral lesions in pemphigoid occur in approximately 40% of patients.

Erythema multiforme is an acute inflammatory disorder of the skin and mucous membranes that is associated with infections, autoimmune disease, stress, and certain antibiotics. It affects males more than females and occurs mostly in the second and third decades of life. Two forms exist. Erythema multiforme minor is a self-limited disease of minimal skin and mucosal injury, lasting 2 to 3 weeks. Erythema multiforme major, known as Stevens-Johnson syndrome, consists of hemorrhagic skin and mucosal lesions. Target lesions consisting of a central bulla and surrounding erythema usually begin on the palms and soles. They typically merge and spread symetrically. Oral lesions involve the lips, tongue, and floor of mouth but are absent in 25%. Erythema multiforme major is also associated with systemic symptoms and purulent conjunctivitis. It is more commonly associated etiologically with drug ingestion and can lead to death from pulmonary involvement. Diagnosis is made clinically, and treatment involves discontinuation of the causative agent, systemic corticosteroids, antihistamines, and supportive and local care.

THE NECK MASS

Pediatric patients commonly present with a chief complaint of a new neck mass. Although malignancy is a concern in the pediatric population, infectious and inflammatory causes are much more likely. To date, there is not an established guideline for the diagnosis of a new pediatric neck mass. The differential diagnosis is quite different than that of the adult population, in which the rate of malignancy may be as high as 50%.

A differential diagnosis may be generated based upon the age of the patient, the history, and the location and physical features of the neck mass. Table 2 illustrates the most common causes based upon age of the patient. In children, the most common cause of neck masses is inflammatory lymph nodes from viral or bacterial infections. Congenital neck masses are also common. Primary malignancy, such as lymphoma and leukemia, may occur but are less common. In older children and young adults, congenital or developmental lesions and salivary gland lesions are more common. For adults over 40, primary or metastatic malignancy must be the first consideration, with inflammatory and systemic disease being of second importance.

Workup consists of a thorough history and physical examination. A rapidly enlarging mass suggests an inflammatory or malignant cause. Temporal association with head and neck infection indicates an infectious or inflammatory origin. Constitutional symptoms of fever, sweats, weight loss, and fatigue are indicative of a systemic process such as lymphoma or mycobacterial infection. Neck masses should be assessed for size, multiplicity, character, surrounding tissue changes, and the presence of bruits or thrills. Lymph nodes greater than 2 cm in a child are considered abnormal, especially if enlarging, and warrant further investigation. There is no standard guideline for diagnosis or workup of the neck mass. Imaging is often undertaken even when a diagnosis is suggested by history and physical examination to establish the anatomy of the lesion and assist in surgical planning. Ultrasound is frequently used initially to determine if the lesion is cystic and unilocular or multilocular. CT and MR imaging provides essential information on the location that allows optimal preoperative planning. If a malignancy is suspected, chest radiography is indicated. When a diagnosis cannot be established, excisional biopsy is preferred over needle aspiration to provide adequate tissue for thorough pathologic analysis.

Midline neck masses include reactive lymphadenopathy, ranulas, thyroglossal duct cysts, and epidermoid, dermoid, teratoid, and thymic cysts. The thyroglossal duct cyst is the most common congenital neck mass, accounting for 70% of congenital neck anomalies. Approximately 50% of patients present before 20 years of age, with a second group of patients presenting in young adulthood. Treatment is surgical. Lateral neck masses are most commonly reactive lymphadenopathy, branchial arch anomalies, lymphatic malformations, major salivary gland tumors, and rarely, external laryngoceles. Lymphoma may present as a lateral, firm, fixed, neck mass. Branchial cleft anomalies may manifest as any combination of sinus tracts, fistulas, or cystic masses. Depending on the embryologic origin, these anomalies may present in the external auditory canal, the tonsillar fossa, periparotid area, or the anterior or posterior cervical triangles. Lymphatic malformations include lymphangiomas and cystic hygromas and may be either uni- or multilocular. Approximately, 75 to 80% of all cystic hygromas involve the neck and the lower portion of the face. Treatment historically has been surgical, but recent studies have demonstrated benefit with intralesional sclerotherapy in selected cases.[9] A laryngocele or dilated laryngeal saccule may present as an external neck mass in approximately 25% of cases. Congenital anomalies are discussed further in Chapter 70, "Congenital Anomalies of the Head and Neck." Discussion of diseases of the salivary glands is found in Chapter 100, "Salivary Glands."

Ranulas may occur in all age groups and present as one of two distinct types. The simple ranula is a cystic lesion of the floor of mouth representing either mucocele formation from obstruction or a mucus extravasation pseudocyst of the sublingual gland. It appears as a clear blue, superficial, fluctuant, nontender cystic mass in the lateral part of the floor of the mouth. A small simple ranula may be asymptomatic, whereas larger ones can cause dysphagia or impairment of speech. Simple ranulas may be treated with marsupialization or excision of the sublingual gland. Recurrence rates are markedly improved when excision of the sublingual gland is performed.[10] The plunging ranula is the less common of the two types, extending through the floor of the mouth into the submandibular space. It presents as a soft, painless, ballotable, submandibular mass which may or may not have an intraoral component. Surgical treatment of the plunging ranula includes sublingual gland excision and evacuation of the ranula. Intralesional sclerotherapy with a streptococcal preparation, OK-432, has shown promising short-term results although long-term outcomes are yet to be established.[12]

BENIGN LESIONS OF THE GINGIVA, MAXILLA, AND MANDIBLE

Several benign lesions are found in the newborn. The congenital epulis presents as a pink, lobulated, pedunculated mass of the anterior aspect of the maxillary gingiva. Treatment is local excision. The melanotic ectodermal tumor of infancy is a firm, well-circumscribed, often pigmented, mass arising at the junction of the globular and maxillary processes in the first 6 months of life. It may be associated with nasal obstruction and facial swelling, and the patient is treated with complete excision. Epstein pearls are small keratinous cysts found on the palate or alveolus. These cysts are transient and exfoliate within a few weeks.

The torus palatinus and torus mandibularis are not congenital lesions but arise after puberty.

Table 2 Differential Diagnosis of a Neck Mass*		
	Age (yrs)	
0–15	**16–40**	**>40**
Congenital/developmental		
Thyroglossal duct cyst	Branchial cleft cyst	Lymphangioma
Dermoid	Thymic cyst	
Laryngocele	Sialadenopathy	
	Pharyngeal diverticulum	
Inflammatory		
Lymphadenitis (viral, bacterial)	Lymphadenitis	Lymphadenitis
Granuloma	Granuloma	Granuloma
	Sialadenitis	
Neoplastic		
Thyroid	Lymphoma	Lymphoma
Lymphoma	Metastatic cancer	Metastatic cancer

*Does not include neurogenic or vascular masses.

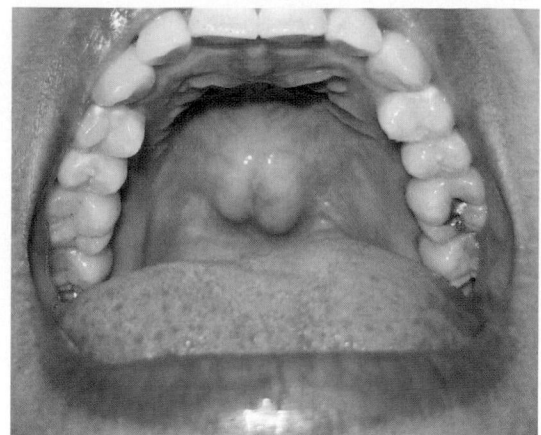

Figure 6 Torus palatinus.

These are asymptomatic bony growths occurring in 8 to 20% of the population and do not require treatment. A classic torus palatinus is seen in Figure 6. The pyogenic granuloma is a smooth, soft, red, friable, pedunculated lesion that arises as a response to trauma or chronic irritation. Treatment is local excision. Fibrous dysplasia of the monostotic type affects the maxilla more commonly than the mandible. This disease presents as a painless swelling in the zygoma or canine fossa that grows rapidly from childhood to early adolescence. The disease process tends to stabilize with puberty. When cosmesis or function is altered, conservative resection is recommended. The giant cell reparative granuloma occurs in older children and affects the mandible more frequently than the maxilla. This tender intraoral mass can be deforming, and the patient is treated with curettage or excision. Osteomas are slow growing lesions with a characteristic radiographic appearance; they are normally completely asymptomatic and treatment is not necessary. Eosinophilic granuloma is a benign variant of Langerhans cell histiocytosis that may present in the mandible or skull with fever, pain, swelling, and leukocytosis. They may occur in children or adolescents and regress spontaneously.

Benign lesions of the gingiva, maxilla, and mandible may arise from an odontogenic source. The most common odontogenic tumor is the odontoma, a hamartomatous tumor of dentin, enamel, and cementum. The odontoma rarely grows large enough to become symptomatic, and the patient is treated by enucleation of the lesion. The ameloblastoma is a deforming, locally aggressive tumor that arises from tissue evolved in enamel formation. It initially presents as a firm, painless mass but will eventually undergo cystic degeneration into an osteolytic, multicystic, expansile mass. Treatment is complete excision. The odontogenic myxoma is a painless mass in an older child that is associated with eruption of permanent dentition. It may be locally aggressive, and the patient is treated with wide excision of the lesion. There are a number of other rare odontogenic tumors, including the adenoameloblastoma, cementoma, and cementoblastoma.

PENETRATING TRAUMA TO THE ORAL CAVITY AND OROPHARYNX

Injuries to the soft palate and oropharynx are common in young children during the oral phase of childhood. Most of these injuries are relatively minor and will require no intervention. However, penetrating oropharyngeal injuries may rarely lead to devastating consequences such as airway compromise, retropharyngeal abscess, mediastinitis, and carotid injury leading to a cerebrovascular accident. There are fewer than thirty reported cases of isolated carotid injury from oropharyngeal trauma, but the mortality from this type of injury is 30 to 45%.[11] The mean age at presentation is 3 to 4 years of age, with some studies showing a slight male predominance.[12]

Penetrating injury to the oropharynx requires a more extensive evaluation than that of the oral cavity due to the intimate anatomic relationships of the carotid artery, jugular vein, vagus nerve, sympathetic plexus, and cranial nerves IX and XII. The posterolateral oropharynx is considered an area of low resistance, with only the palatine tonsil and superior constrictor muscle protecting the carotid sheath. Carotid injury is thus exclusively related to penetrating trauma of the lateral peritonsillar musculature.[11] The internal carotid artery (ICA) is compressed between the foreign object and the skull base or second or third vertebra, leading to intimal dissection or thrombus formation.

Lacerations anywhere in the oropharyngeal wall may violate fascial planes, allowing direct spread of salivary contents into deep neck spaces continuous with the mediastinum. Gravity and negative intrathoracic pressure with inspiration facilitate the flow of air and secretions into these spaces. The child may present with stridor, subcutaneous emphysema, pneumothorax, and airway compromise. Recommendations exist for operative repair of free hanging edges, although some authors have observed equivalent outcomes with observation and repair by secondary intention. Antibiotic prophylaxis is reserved for injuries greater than 1 cm.[13] Soft tissue plain radiographs or computed tomography may suggest abscess formation, in which case operative drainage and intravenous antibiotics are indicated.

A thorough history and physical examination is imperative to rule out these rare but devastating consequences. Examination of the injury for depth of penetration and laterality will direct the physician toward possible sequelae. The airway should be secured primarily, and then thorough physical examination should be completed, including a complete neural and vascular examination. Hematoma, Horner syndrome, and transient ischemic attacks are heralds of blunt ICA injury. One must remember that lucid intervals of up to 72 hours are common with blunt ICA injury, and delayed onset of progressive focal neurologic signs may arise after an initial normal examination. Soft tissue plain radiography is indicated in oropharyngeal injury.

Suspicion for carotid injury is raised with lateral oropharyngeal injury that penetrates muscle or a mechanism that provides sufficient compressive force without mucosal penetration. In children with a high suspicion of injury or noncompliant families, imaging is recommend. The gold standard has been angiography, but recent evidence shows that contrast-enhanced computed tomography may be sufficient.[14] Computed tomography (CT) angiogram has been studied in the adult population and appears to provide a high sensitivity but mediocre specificity for carotid injury. Thus, it may be a viable option as an initial radiographic study, with angiography reserved for abnormal findings on CT. Magnetic resonance angiogram (MRA) has also been shown to provide excellent detection of carotid injury.[15] An outpatient treatment protocol consisting of serial examination has been recommended in cases of an asymptomatic child greater than 1 year of age with reliable parents who lives in close proximity to medical care. Treatment for traumatic oropharyngeal lacerations is summarized in Table 3.[16] Interventional or conventional neurosurgical techniques have had mixed outcomes. Anticoagulation with aspirin, tissue-plasminogen activator, or heparin is controversial.

MISCELLANEOUS DISEASE OF THE ORAL CAVITY AND OROPHARYNX

Leukoplakia

The World Health Organization (WHO) defines oral leukoplakia as a predominantly white lesion of the oral mucosa that cannot be characterized as any other definable lesion. Leukoplakia may be idiopathic or associated with tobacco smoking. It is primarily a condition of the adult population, with a prevalence of 0.1 to 5%. It is less common in children but is often found in those with candidiasis or viral infections. Leukoplakia is considered a precancerous lesion; malignant transformation occurs in 2 to 6%, with an annual transformation rate of less than 1%. Histologic

Table 3 Assessment of Oropharyngeal Trauma	
Finding	**Recommendation**
Contaminated or greater than 1 to 2 cm	Antibiotics
Avulsed flap, foreign body, gross contamination	Exploration/repair + antibiotics
Suspicion for neural or vascular injury	Imaging
Unreliable social situation	Imaging

Adapted from reference 16.

features of keratosis, inflammation, and dysplasia are highly variable. Risk of malignancy increases in extremely adherent lesions with abundant keratosis. Small studies have shown that vitamin A, retinoids, and beta-carotene may completely resolve the oral lesions and that retinoic acid may prevent histological worsening. Routine follow-up and excision of the lesion in high-risk populations is recommended.[17]

Vitamin Deficiency

Iron deficiency is common in children, with oral manifestations consisting of burning tongue, mucosal pallor and atrophy, angular chelitis, and hyperkeratotic mucosal lesions. In adults, iron deficiency may be associated with esophageal ulcerations and webs in Plummer-Vinson syndrome. Vitamin C deficiency, or scurvy, presents as swollen red gingiva which progresses to hemorrhagic ulcerative gingivitis. Other findings include oral petechiae, stomatitis, and hemorrhagic mucosal lesions. Riboflavin deficiency manifests as glossitis, gingivolabial pallor, angular chelosis, and a burning sensation of the oral cavity. Folate and B12 deficiency both cause recurrent oral ulcers and painful atrophy of the tongue and oral mucosa. Niacin deficiency, or pellagra, causes painful erythema and edema of the oral mucosa and tongue, as well as angular chelitis and necrotizing ulcerative gingivitis. Examination findings may be mixed, as multiple deficiencies may occur simultaneously.

Elemental Heavy Metal Toxicity

It is quite common to have oral signs and symptoms of heavy metal toxicity, as many of these are often metabolized and secreted in saliva. Lead poisoning is considered the most important chronic environmental illness affecting children today. In the pediatric population, nearly every organ system is subject to lead toxicity. In children, lead sulfide precipitates or "lead lines" at the gingival margin are fairly specific for lead poisoning. Environmental mercury toxicity has become a major concern because of its industrial uses in fossil fuels and agriculture. It has been used historically in dental amalgams and many medical therapies. Recent widespread exposures have occurred in fish, grain, and beauty creams. Otolaryngic manifestations of toxicity include metallic taste, sialorrhea, and ashen-gray mucous membranes. Other elements known to cause similar discoloration of the tongue and oral mucosa include arsenic and bismuth.

Drooling

Sialorrhea is the inability to control oral secretions, usually due to dysfunction of the swallowing mechanism. Although most commonly due to chronic nervous system impairment, many chronic disease processes may lead to this entity. Drooling can lead to further medical ailments, such as impaired masticatory function, risk of aspiration, perioral infections, and loss of fluid, electrolytes, and proteins. Nonsurgical methods of treatment include oral motor therapy, behavioral modification, and oral appliances. When not contraindicated, medications including cholinergic muscarinic receptor antagonists, for example, atropine, scopolamine, or glycopyrronium bromide, appear to be effective in many cases. Radiotherapy is not recommended for children because of the risk of inducing malignancy, growth retardation, xerostomia, mucositis, radiation caries, and osteoradionecrosis; however, this may be a reasonable treatment modality in the elderly population. Surgical treatment includes parotid or submandibular duct relocation or ligation, sublingual duct ligation, submandibular or sublingual gland excision. Duct relocation may be effective in the initiation of the swallowing mechanism and has a role for certain patients. Bilateral sublingual and submandibular duct ligation has been effective in approximately 80% of cases.[18] This may be done surgically or with a Nd:YAG laser. When injected in the salivary gland, botulinum toxin inhibits acetylcholine release in the cholinergic nerve endings at neurosecretory junctions. Percutaneous injection under ultrasound guidance into the parotid and submandibular glands provides a safe, minimally invasive alternative that provides effect for 6 weeks to 6 months.

REFERENCES

1. Chervin RD, Ruzicka DL, Giordani BJ, et al. Sleep-disordered breathing, behavior, and cognition in children before and after adenotonsillectomy. Pediatrics 2006;117:769–78.
2. Cinar F. Significance of asymptomatic tonsil asymmetry. Arch Otolaryngol Head Neck Surg 2004;131:101–3.
3. Daya H, Chan HS, Sirkin W, Forte V. Pediatric rhabdomyosarcoma of the head and neck: Is there a place for surgical management? Arch Otolaryngol Head Neck Surg 2000;126:468–72.
4. Pryor SG, Moore EJ, Kasperbauer JL. Endoscopic versus traditional approaches for excision of juvenile nasopharyngeal angiofibroma. Laryngoscope 2005;115:1201–7.
5. Dhiwakar M, Eng CY, Selvaraj S, McKerrow WS. Antibiotics to improve recovery following tonsillectomy: A systematic review. Arch Otolaryngol Head Neck Surg 2006;134:357–64.
6. Burkart CM, Steward DL. Antibiotics for reduction of posttonsillectomy morbidity: A meta-analysis. Laryngoscope 2005;115:997–1002.
7. Huang TT, Liu TC, Chen PR, et al. Deep neck infection: Analysis of 185 cases. Head Neck 2004;26:854–60.
8. Reznik DA. Oral manifestations of HIV disease. Top HIV Med 2006;13:143–8.
9. Lee HM, Lim HW, Kang HJ, et al. Treatment of ranula in pediatric patients with intralesional injection of OK-432. Laryngoscope 2006;116:966–9.
10. Zhao YF, Jia Y, Chen XM, Zhang WF. Clinical review of 580 ranulas. Oral Surg Oral Med Oral Pathol Oral Radiol Endod 2004;98:281–7.
11. Hengerer A, DeGroot TR, Rivers RJ, Jr, Pettee DS. Internal carotid artery thrombosis following soft palate injuries: A case report and review of 16 cases. Laryngoscope 1984;94:1571–5.
12. Hellman J, Shott SR, Gootee MJ. Impalement injuries of the palate in children: Review of 131 cases. Int J Pediatr Otorhinolaryngol 1993;26:157–63.
13. Schoem SR, Choi SS, Zalzal GH, Grundfast KM. Management of oropharyngeal trauma in children. Arch Otolaryngol Head Neck Surg 1997;123:1267–70.
14. Brietzke S, Jones D. Pediatric oropharyngeal trauma: What is the role of CT scan? Int J Pediatr Otorhinolaryngol 2005;69:669–79.
15. Klufas R, Hsu L, Barnes PD, et al. Dissection of the carotid and vertebral arteries: Imaging with MRA. AJR 1995;164:673–7.
16. Randall DA, Kang DR. Current management of penetrating injuries of the soft palate. Otolaryngol Head Neck Surg 2006;135:356–60.
17. Lodi G, Sardella A, Bez C, et al. Interventions for treating oral leukoplakia. Cochrane Database Syst Rev 2004;3:CD001829.
18. Meningaud JP, Pitak-Arnnop P, Chikhani L, Bertrand JC. Drooling of saliva: A review of the etiology and management options. Oral Surg Oral Med Oral Pathol Oral Radiol Endod 2006;101:48–57.

65

Deep Head and Neck Space Infections

Robert F. Yellon, MD

Deep head and neck space infections continue to occur and may involve resistant microorganisms despite the use of broad-spectrum antimicrobial agents. Easy access to imaging studies such as computed tomography (CT) scans has improved our diagnostic abilities in differentiation of cellulitis versus abscesses of the fascial spaces of the head and neck in children. In general, patients with cellulitis and small early, uncomplicated abscesses may be treated with intravenous antimicrobials whereas larger abscesses will require incision and drainage or in selected patients needle aspiration.

ETIOLOGY OF DEEP HEAD AND NECK SPACE INFECTIONS

Deep head and neck space infections generally follow the lymphatic drainage pathways. Paranasal and nasopharyngeal infections generally precede retropharyngeal space infection. Tonsillar infections precede peritonsillar and parapharyngeal space infections. Dental and gingival infections may be the source of mandibular, submandibular, masticator, parotid, parapharyngeal, and buccal space infections. Abscess of the root of the canine teeth may lead to canine space infection. Trauma to the pharynx may provide a portal of entry for infection of the retropharyngeal, parapharyngeal, or visceral spaces. Sialoadenitis may lead to infection in the parotid or submandibular spaces. Congenital anomalies such as branchial cleft remnants, lymphangiomas, or dermoid cysts may become infected and cause infection of adjacent spaces. Hematogenous *Haemophilus influenzae* infection in the past often led to buccal space infection, but this is now rare in the H influenzae type b immunization era.

It is of critical importance to determine the original site of infection that led to the development of a deep head and neck space infection and to treat the patient adequately for both processes. This may include procedures such as mastoidectomy, sinus surgery, removal of a salivary gland, or dental surgery. For example, mastoiditis may be complicated by bone erosion and abscess below the mastoid cortex and into the upper neck (Bezold abscess) and be the source of an associated parapharyngeal space abscess (Figure 1). Both the mastoid and deep neck space infections must be surgically drained to adequately treat the child.

If deep neck space infection occurs repeatedly in the same anatomic site, the presence of

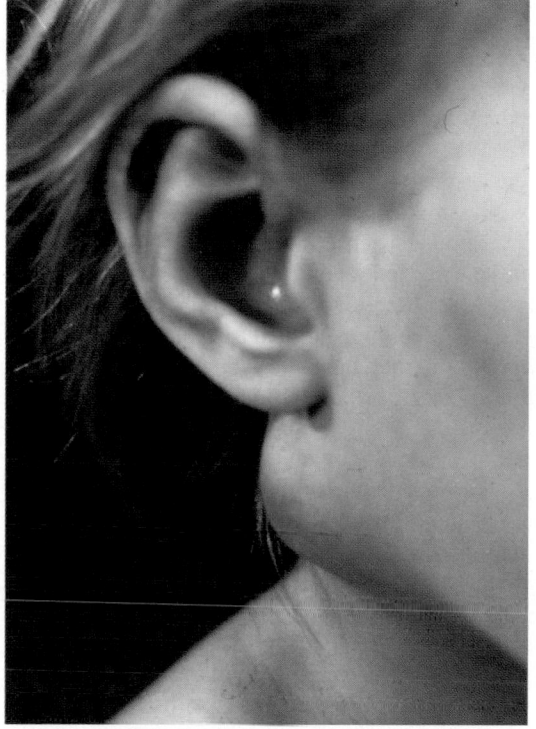

Figure 1 Bezold abscess. Mastoiditis with bone erosion of mastoid cortex and abscess cavity extending into the upper neck. There was an associated parapharyngeal space abscess. Both the ear and neck infections required surgical therapy for resolution.

a congenital anomaly such as a branchial cleft remnant should be considered. For example, a third branchial cleft sinus with an opening into the pyriform sinus may be the cause of recurrent infections in the neck (Figures 2 and 3). After incision and drainage and resolution of the infection, the branchial cleft anomaly should be completely excised for definitive cure.

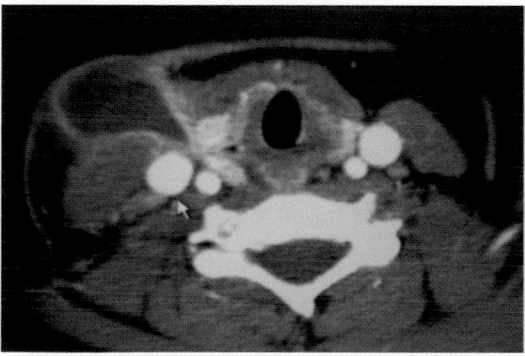

Figure 2 Computed tomography scan of the neck of a child with recurrent deep neck infections showing an infected third branchial cleft sinus.

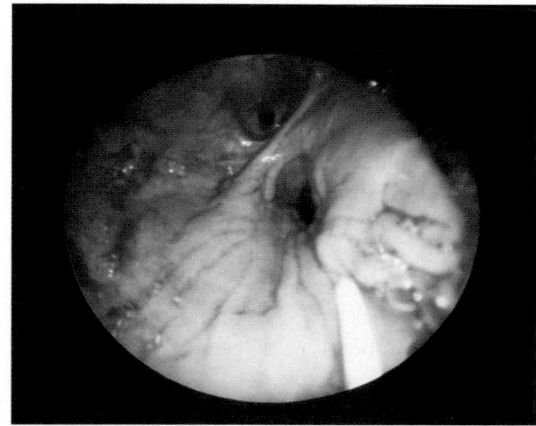

Figure 3 Endoscopic photograph from the child with recurrent deep neck infections whose computed tomography scan is shown in Figure 2. The third branchial cleft sinus is seen opening into the pyriform sinus adjacent to the esophageal inlet.

BACTERIOLOGY AND ANTIMICROBIAL THERAPY FOR DEEP HEAD AND NECK SPACE INFECTIONS

Infections of the fascial spaces of the head and neck are often polymicrobial and include gram-positive and anaerobic microorganisms. Studies have also shown a considerable percentage of gram-negative microorganisms in deep head and neck space infections in the pediatric population.[1–3] In view of the presence of gram-positive, gram-negative, and anaerobic microorganisms in these infections, ampicillin-sulbactam is a good choice. For patients allergic to penicillin, cefuroxime, or clindamycin plus an aminoglycoside are good alternatives. Additionally, methacillin resistant *Staphylococcus aureus* has become more prevalent as a cause of these infections. If a child has a serious infection and has been exposed to methacillin resistant *Staphylococcus aureus* or is very ill or toxic despite ampicillin-sulbactam, then vancomycin or linezolid may be considered. *Eikenella corrodens* infection may be associated with human bites. *E. corrodens* is resistant to clindamycin but sensitive to penicillin and cephalosporins.[4,5]

If incision and drainage, needle aspiration or blood or wound cultures detect a specific microorganism, the antimicrobial therapy may be narrowed based on susceptibility studies.

For deep head and neck space infections intravenous antimicrobial therapy is usually continued for approximately 5 days. Once a child has responded favorably to intravenous and/or surgical therapy, oral therapy may be continued for 7 to 10 days with amoxicillin-clavulanate, cefuroxime, cefdinir, or clindamycin.

DIAGNOSTIC STUDIES

Laboratory diagnostic studies include complete blood count with white blood cell differential, electrolytes, and urine specific gravity. Blood, throat, and wound cultures should be obtained when appropriate.

Radiographic studies include anteroposterior and lateral neck films. If the retropharyngeal soft tissues are wider than 7 mm or the retrotracheal soft tissues are wider than 13 mm, then infection in the retropharyngeal space is likely. However, unless the lateral neck film is taken with the neck in extension and during inspiration, there will be spurious thickening of the retropharyngeal tissues. Air in the retropharyngeal tissues usually indicates the presence of an abscess.

CT is an excellent diagnostic tool to differentiate deep neck space cellulitis versus abscess. An abscess appears as a lesion with a contrast enhancing rim and a lucent center. As can be seen from the studies listed in Table 1,[1,6–10] CT scan is accurate (positive predictive value) for the detection of deep neck space abscess approximately 76% of the time.

Although lateral neck radiography and computed tomography are the most often utilized diagnostic studies, magnetic resonance imaging and ultrasonography may also be useful for selected patients to determine the site of deep neck space infection and whether an abscess is present. Magnetic resonance imaging and ultrasound also have the advantage of no radiation exposure for the child.

PRESENTATION AND TREATMENT OF DEEP NECK SPACE INFECTIONS

Peritonsillar Space Infection

Peritonsillar space infection is the most common deep neck space infection. It is most often a complication of tonsillitis. Clinically, red, swollen tonsils are seen bilaterally, usually with exudate, and there is significant swelling lateral and superior to the tonsil on one side. In severe cases, the uvula is displaced by the mass effect. Although bilateral peritonsillar space infections have been reported, they are rare and unilateral peritonsillar

infections are seen in the vast majority of cases. Neck adenopathy is often present and more prominent on the side of the peritonsillar infection. Pain on opening the mouth occurs when infection and inflammation extend to the internal pterygoid muscle in the parapharyngeal space. It usually occurs in more serious peritonsillar space infections such as severe cellulitis and abscess. In most cases, if pain on opening the mouth is absent, abscess is not present. Pain on opening the mouth may limit adequate examination and treatment.

Peritonsillar cellulitis in an older child with adequate oral intake may be treated with oral antimicrobial agents such as those listed above whereas those with poor oral intake must be treated with intravenous antimicrobials.

When severe pain, fever, significant bulging of the peritonsillar area, pain on opening the mouth and displacement of the uvula are present, a peritonsillar abscess is likely. CT may be used in selected patients to determine whether peritonsillar abscess versus cellulitis is present when the examination is limited by pain on opening the mouth or when the child fails to improve after an initial trial of antimicrobials. CT is not needed for the majority of patients, and the diagnosis can usually be made by clinical examination.

Peritonsillar cellulitis usually responds to antimicrobial agents, however, peritonsillar abscess requires incision and drainage, tonsillectomy, or needle aspiration, in addition to antimicrobial therapy. The decision to perform incision and drainage, tonsillectomy, or needle aspiration is based on several factors. If a child with a peritonsillar abscess has had a history of prior peritonsillar abscess, numerous episodes of recurrent tonsillitis, or adenotonsillar hypertrophy with obstructive sleep apnea or if previous incision and drainage or needle aspiration were not effective, then tonsillectomy can be done immediately. Tonsillectomy performed at the time of peritonsillar abscess is called "Quinsy tonsillectomy," or "tonsillectomy à chaud." "Quinsy" is an obsolete term for peritonsillar abscess, and "tonsillectomy à chaud" is derived from the French for "hot tonsillectomy."

Review of the literature shows that recurrent peritonsillar abscess occurs in approximately 17% and recurrent tonsillitis occurs in approximately 28% of patients with peritonsillar abscess.[11–16] Tonsillectomy is usually not performed for patients with a single episode of peritonsillar abscess. Some surgeons have anecdotally

claimed that immediate tonsillectomy for peritonsillar abscess is associated with an increased risk of bleeding. However, pooled data from a total of 1,169 patients who underwent immediate tonsillectomy showed only a 3.5% incidence of excessive perioperative or delayed hemorrhage.[11–13,17–19] Only one of these studies showed an increased rate of secondary hemorrhage (22%) following immediate tonsillectomy.[19]

Tonsillectomy may therefore be performed immediately for some patients, whereas in other patients a decision may be made to perform tonsillectomy after an interval of approximately 6 weeks (interval tonsillectomy). Immediate tonsillectomy would be considered if there is acute severe airway obstruction or if incision and drainage has failed. Immediate tonsillectomy has the advantages of having only one period of hospitalization and morbidity and decreasing overall time and expense. Interval tonsillectomy should be considered if the general condition of the child is poor or the child has a coagulopathy or has taken anticoagulants.

Needle aspiration has also been advocated for drainage of peritonsillar abscess but is less reliable than incision and drainage, or immediate tonsillectomy. Repeat needle aspiration may be required.[20,21] Even when incision and drainage are performed for peritonsillar abscess, a needle aspiration is used to locate the abscess.

Retropharyngeal Space Infection

Retropharyngeal space infections usually present with fever, dysphagia, irritability, muffled cry or speech, torticollis, and stertor. Drooling and stridor may be present in severe cases. The retropharyngeal space consists of bilateral spaces separated by a midline raphe which is clinically important because infection in this space usually causes unilateral pharyngeal bulging. Occasionally, swelling from a retropharyngeal space infection may displace the tonsil in an anterior direction that mimics peritonsillar infection. CT can usually determine the correct space of the infection.

Infections in the retropharyngeal space can be severe and can spread from the base of skull to the mediastinum since the fascial planes are potentially contiguous (Figure 4). Retropharyngeal

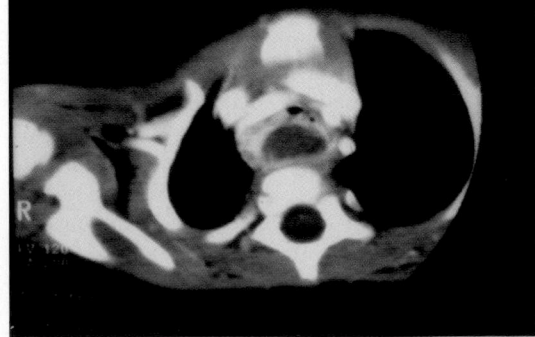

Figure 4 Computed tomography scan showing a rim enhancing mediastinal abscess with a lucent center (*center*). This abscess resulted from an inferior extension of a retropharyngeal abscess.

Table 1 Studies in Which Children Had Computed Tomography Scans Showing Abscesses and Had Incision and Drainage		
Authors	Number	Percentage Identified
Lazar and colleagues[6]	38 children	76% abscess at surgery
Unganont and colleagues[1]	16 children	91% abscess at surgery
Choi and colleagues[7]	45 children	75% abscess at surgery
Elden and colleagues[8]	95 children	76% abscess at surgery
Vural and colleagues[9]	41 children	63% abscess at surgery
Daya and colleagues[10]	27 children	81% abscess at surgery
Total	262 children	76% abscess at surgery

space infections occur between the prevertebral and buccopharyngeal fascial layers. Although the origin of retropharyngeal space infections is usually the nose, paranasal sinuses, or pharynx; foreign body ingestion with pharyngeal trauma can also lead to infection in this space, and some authors recommend routine esophagoscopy to rule out a foreign body.[2]

Retropharyngeal cellulitis is, of course, treated with intravenous antimicrobial agents. Retropharyngeal abscesses are usually treated with transoral incision and drainage plus intravenous antimicrobials. The abscess may first be located with a needle aspiration.

Prevertebral Space Infection

Prevertebral space infections usually arise from staphylococcal or tuberculous infections of the vertebral bodies. These infections occur between the vertebral bodies and the prevertebral fascia. In contrast to retropharyngeal space infections which are unilateral because of the attachment of the retropharyngeal midline raphe, prevertebral space infections cause a bulge in the midline. While retropharyngeal space abscesses are usually drained by transoral incision and drainage, prevertebral abscesses are drained externally. A prevertebral space abscess requires long-term drainage.

Parapharyngeal Space Infection

The parapharyngeal (lateral pharyngeal) space is shaped like an inverted pyramid and extends from the lateral part of the base of the skull to the hyoid bone. It is divided into prestyloid and poststyloid compartments. The styloid process and the attached fascia of the tensor veli palatini divide the parapharyngeal space into a prestyloid compartment that contains the internal maxillary artery, the maxillary nerve, and the tail of the parotid gland; and a poststyloid compartment that contains the carotid artery, internal jugular vein, cervical sympathetic chain, and cranial nerves IX, X, XI, and XII. Parapharyngeal space infections usually present with pain, fever, stiff neck, and occasionally pain on opening the mouth which is from involvement of the internal pterygoid muscle. Imaging studies are useful to differentiate abscess versus cellulitis. Similar to the other deep neck space infections, parapharyngeal space cellulitis may be treated with intravenous antimicrobials. Abscesses in this space are usually drained by the external surgical approach described below.

Submandibular Space Infection

The submandibular space is divided into supramylohyoid and inframylohyoid portions by the mylohyoid muscle. The supramylohyoid portion contains the sublingual glands and the submandibular gland ducts. The inframylohyoid portion contains the submandibular glands and the associated submandibular lymph nodes. These two portions of the submandibular space are in continuity at the posterior aspect of the mylohyoid

muscle. As the duct of the submandibular gland passes posterior to the mylohyoid muscle, it also connects the supramylohyoid and inframylohyoid portions of the submandibular space. The capsule surrounding the submandibular gland creates the space of the submandibular gland, which is also a potential site of abscesses. Bounded by the anterior bellies of the digastric muscles, the submental space contains lymph nodes and is a potential space for infection.

Visceral Space Infection

Containing the thyroid gland, trachea, and esophagus, the visceral space can be infected and result in quite serious laryngeal edema and airway obstruction. The retrovisceral compartment of the visceral space is in continuity with the retropharyngeal space. Early aggressive therapy is indicated to avoid airway obstruction.

OPEN SURGICAL APPROACH TO DEEP NECK SPACE INFECTIONS

The indications for the open external neck approach to deep neck space infections include larger abscess (>1 cm), multilocular abscesses, failure of needle aspiration, complications, no improvement following 24 to 72 hours of intravenous antimicrobials, and possibly when an unusual or resistant microorganism is suspected. This approach is useful for drainage of infections in the parapharyngeal, submandibular, visceral, retropharyngeal, and prevertebral spaces and the carotid sheath.

An incision is made approximately two fingerbreadths below the lower border of the mandible. The lower border of the submandibular gland is identified and retracted superiorly. If the infection is in the space of the submandibular gland, the fascial capsule of the gland is incised inferiorly and the fascial capsule is dissected superiorly and gently retracted superiorly along with the marginal mandibular branch of the facial nerve. Care should be taken to preserve this nerve and to avoid a crush injury to the nerve from using a retractor against the mandible.

Once the submandibular area has been addressed, the dissection continues deeply to identify the carotid sheath. Once the carotid sheath has been identified, if an abscess is present in the sheath it should be opened and drained. An abscess in the jugular vein may be drained by this approach, and the vein may also be ligated superior and inferior to the abscess. The carotid sheath is an excellent landmark and pathway for further dissection to other deep neck spaces such as the parapharyngeal, retropharyngeal, and visceral spaces. Blunt finger dissection is an excellent and safe method to drain these spaces. Once the abscess cavity or cavities have been entered, blunt finger dissection is also used to break up loculations and to make separate abscess cavities into contiguous cavities when feasible. Iodoform gauze packing is placed into the deep aspect of the wound and brought out through the skin

incision. The skin incision is only partially closed to allow drainage and removal of the packing. The packing is slowly advanced out of the wound in daily increments over 3 to 4 days.

AIRWAY MANAGEMENT FOR DEEP NECK SPACE INFECTIONS IN CHILDREN

If deep neck space infection results in partial airway compromise in a child, early establishment of an artificial airway is strongly advised before the airway obstruction results in an acute emergency. Elective establishment of an airway with a bronchoscope, endotracheal tube, nasopharyngeal airway, or tracheostomy is strongly advised prior to the need for emergent intervention which has a higher risk of complications. The artificial airway should be established in the operating room where equipment, good lighting, suction, and the most experienced airway personnel are available.

In small children, surgical manipulation and drainage of an abscess may result in edema and airway compromise. In such children, planning to leave the endotracheal tube in place until edema resolves following drainage of the deep neck space abscess should be considered. A plan to leave the endotracheal tube in place following drainage of a deep neck space abscess should be discussed with the parents prior to the operation to avoid parental anxiety.

Ludwig Angina

Ludwig angina is a severe and potentially lethal variant of submandibular space infection. It is a rapidly progressive, bilateral cellulitis of the supramylohyoid and inframylohyoid portions of the submandibular space. With Ludwig angina, there is "woody induration" of the floor of the mouth. Ludwig angina is by definition a bilateral cellulitis of the submandibular space, and an abscess may or may not be present.

Pain on opening the mouth occurs as the infection and inflammation spread to the internal pterygoid muscle in the parapharyngeal space. Laryngeal edema also occurs as the infection progresses. Thus the combination of edema of the floor of the mouth, elevation of the tongue, pain on opening the mouth, and laryngeal edema contribute to significant airway obstruction (Figure 5). All but the occasional, earliest, mildest cases of Ludwig angina should have an artificial airway established rapidly before the child progresses to complete airway obstruction. A rare, early, mild case, with minimal edema can be treated expectantly in the intensive care unit, without an artificial airway, with intravenous antimicrobials alone.

Although an abscess may not be present, Ludwig angina is the exceptional deep head and neck space infection in which incision and drainage is recommended even in the absence of an abscess. After the airway has been established by endotracheal intubation or tracheostomy, a horizontal

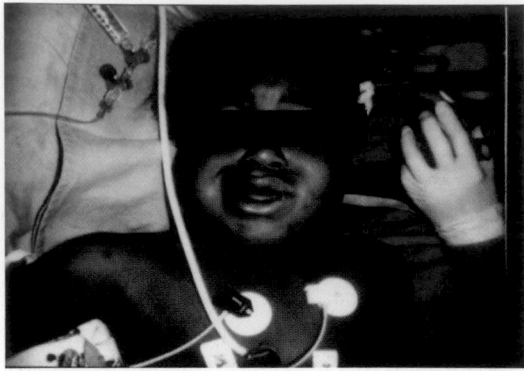

Figure 5 Ludwig angina. Photograph of a girl with rapidly progressive edema and airway obstruction from bilateral cellulitis of the submandibular spaces, woody induration of the floor of the mouth, elevation of the tongue, and laryngeal edema.

incision is made in the submental area and the fascial layers and muscles that are encountered are separated in the midline. Lateral dissection is also undertaken between the muscle layers to drain any abscesses that may or may not be present. The wound is packed with iodoform gauze which is advanced out over several days. The artificial airway is removed when the edema and infection have resolved.

OTHER HEAD AND NECK SPACE INFECTIONS

Masticator Space Infection

The masticator space is a potential space created by the splitting of the superficial layer of the deep cervical fascia around the masseter, internal pterygoid, and temporalis muscles. This space contains the ramus of the mandible and the temporalis muscle. The superior portion of the space is known as the temporalis portion of the masticator space. Abscesses may occur medial or lateral to the temporal muscle. Drainage of the lateral portion is accomplished by hairline incisions that extend through the temporalis fascia. When abscess occurs deep to the temporalis muscle in the infratemporal fossa, the incision must also extend through the temporalis muscle.

When infection occurs in the inferior portion of the masticator space, it may occur in a medial or lateral position. Infection in the lateral portion will involve the masseter muscle, and incision and drainage will require preservation of the facial nerve and its branches prior to detaching the fascia from the mandible. Infection in the medial compartment will involve the internal pterygoid muscle. Infections in the medial portion of the masticator space may be drained via intraoral incision. Infections in the masticator space often arise from extension of dental infection.

Parotid Space Infections

The parotid space is created by the splitting of the superficial layer of the deep cervical fascia around the parotid gland. Infections in this space usually arise from sialoadenitis. Even when an abscess is present, fluctuance is usually not palpated, since

the fascial capsule is so dense and thick. Imaging studies such as computed tomography are needed to demonstrate an abscess.

Superficial abscesses in the parotid space may be drained by small superficial skin incisions in the direction of the facial nerve branches with gentle deeper blunt dissection. Deep abscesses in the parotid space may only be drained after facial nerve identification and preservation.

Mandibular Space Infection

The superficial layer of deep cervical fascia splits to surround the mandible and thus forms the mandibular space. Infection in this space usually arises from dental infection. Intraoral pain and swelling are noted, and the abscess may be drained by intraoral incision.

Buccal Space Infection

Buccal space infection usually arises from dental infection. Infection in this space can also arise from hematogenous spread of *Haemophilus influenzae*, but this is now rare in the immunization era. Cheek swelling and pain on opening the mouth are present. The abscess may be drained via skin incisions in the direction of the facial nerve branches with gentle deep blunt dissection. Buccal space abscesses may also be drained via intraoral incision.

Canine Space Infection

Canine space infections are a result of root abscesses of the upper canine teeth. Toothache commonly precedes the facial swelling that occurs lateral to the nares. The abscess may drain spontaneously near the medial canthus. It is important not to mistake canine space infection for dacryocystitis. This abscess may be drained by incision in the labial sulcus with superior elevation of the facial soft tissues. The canine root abscess must also be addressed by the dentist.

TREATMENT OPTIONS: ANTIMICROBIALS ALONE, INCISION AND DRAINAGE OR NEEDLE ASPIRATION

For patients with deep head and neck space infections that are mild with cellulitis and/or lymphadenopathy but without abscess formation or complications, antimicrobial therapy is indicated. If there is no improvement after 48 to 72 hours, repeat imaging studies and open surgical therapy should be considered. In seriously ill children without abscess who do not respond rapidly to standard antimicrobial therapy, the presence of resistant microorganisms such as methacillin resistant *Staphylococcus aureus* should be considered and vancomycin should be added to the therapy.

Seriously ill children with large and multilocular abscesses or those with complications or Ludwig angina should be treated with aggressive incision and drainage. Needle aspiration may be useful for drainage of small unilocular

Table 2 Complications of Deep Head and Neck Space Infections
Airway obstruction
Septicemia
Neuropathy
Carotid artery rupture
Jugular vein thrombosis
Mediastinitis
Rupture into pharynx

abscesses.[22,23] Ultrasound or CT are useful to locate the abscess and guide needle aspiration.

Some authors have recommended treatment of patients with small (≤ 1 cm) uncomplicated abscesses with intravenous antimicrobials alone with good success.[24,25] However, this approach should not be used if the abscess lies in a critical location such as immediately adjacent to the great vessels. In such patients the abscess may erode into the great vessels with catastrophic consequences; and, therefore, aggressive incision and drainage is recommended.

COMPLICATIONS

Complications associated with deep neck space infections are an indication for incision and drainage. The complications are listed in Table 2. The complication of internal jugular vein thrombosis deserves special discussion. Patients with deep head and neck space infections that spike fevers repeatedly in the so called "picket fence" pattern may have internal jugular vein thrombosis which is releasing septic emboli. CT angiography and magnetic resonance angiography are excellent diagnostic studies for internal jugular vein thrombosis. Traditional angiography is also useful but is associated with increased risk of complications. Treatment of internal jugular vein thrombosis includes aggressive incision and drainage of the abscess. In addition, if the septic emboli continue, the internal jugular vein may be ligated or excised. Postoperative anticoagulation may help decrease the chances of propagation of the emboli.

CONCLUSIONS

Although deep head and neck space infections continue to be serious, with appropriate use of diagnostic tests, antimicrobial agents, surgical drainage, or needle aspiration, complications can be avoided and favorable outcomes can be achieved.

REFERENCES

1. Ungkanont K, Yellon R, Weissman J, et al. Head and neck space infections in infants and children. Otolaryngol Head Neck Surg 1995;112:375–82.
2. Sethi DS, Stanley RE. Deep neck abscesses—changing trends. J Laryngol Otol 1994;108:138–43.
3. Tan PT, Chang LY, Huang YC, et al. Deep neck infections in children. J Microbiol Immunol Infect 2001;34:287–92.
4. Knudsen TD, Simko EJ. Eikenella corrodens: An unexpected pathogen causing a persistent peritonsillar abscess. Ear Nose Throat J 1995;74:114–7.

5. Zgheib A, el Allaf D, Demonty J, Rorive G. Intrathoracic infections with bacteraemia due to Eikenella corrodens as a complication of peritonsillar abscesses: Report of a case and review of the literature. Acta Clin Belg 1992;47:124–8.

6. Lazor JB, Cunningham MJ, Eavey RD, et al. Comparison of computed tomography and surgical findings in deep neck infections. Otolaryngol Head Neck Surg 1994;111:746–50.

7. Choi SS, Vezina LG, Grundfast KM. Relative incidence and alternative approaches for surgical drainage of different types of deep neck abscesses in children. Arch Otolaryngol Head Neck Surg 1997;123:1271–5.

8. Elden LM, Grundfast KM, Vezina LG. Accuracy and usefulness of radiographic assessment of cervical neck infections in children. J Otolaryngol 2001;30:82–9.

9. Vural C, Gungor A, Comerci S. Accuracy of computerized tomography in deep neck infections in the pediatric population. Am J Otolaryngol 2003;24:143–8.

10. Daya H, Lo S, Papsin BC, et al. Retropharyngeal and paraphyaryngeal infections in children: The Toronto experience. Int J Pediatr Otorhinolaryngol 2005;69:81–6.

11. Beeden AG, Evans JNG. Quinsy tonsillectomy—a further report. J Laryngol Otol 1970;84:443–8.

12. McCurdy JA. Pertonsillar abscess: A comparison of treatment by immediate tonsillectomy and interval tonsillectomy. Arch Otolaryngol 1977;103:414–5.

13. Templer JW, Holinger LD, Wood RP, et al. Immediate tonsillectomy for the treatment of peritonsillar abscess. Am J Surg 1977;134:596–8.

14. Herbild O, Bonding P. Peritonsillar abscess: Recurrence rate and treatment. Arch Otolaryngol 1981;107:540–2.

15. Holt GR, Tinsley PP. Peritonsillar abscesses in children. Laryngoscope 1981;91:1226–30.

16. Nielsen VM, Greisen O. Peritonsillar abscess. I. Cases treated by incision and drainage: A follow-up investigation. J Laryngol Otol 1981;95:801–5.

17. Grahne B. Abscess tonsillectomy; seven hundred twenty-five cases. Arch Otolaryngol 1958;68:332–6.

18. Richardson KA, Birck H. Peritonsillar abscess in the pediatric population. Otolaryngol Head Neck Surg 1981;89:907–9.

19. Dunne AA, Granger O, Folz BJ, et al. Peritonsillar abscess—critical analysis of abscess tonsillectomy. Clin Otolaryngol Allied Sci 2003;28:420–4.

20. Herzon FS. Permucosal needle drainage of peritonsillar abscesses. Arch Otolaryngol 1984;110:104–5.

21. Schechter GL, Sly DE, Roper AL, Jackson RT. Changing face of treatment of peritonsillar abscess. Laryngoscope 1982;92:657–9.

22. Brodsky L, Belles W, Brody A, et al. Needle aspiration of neck abscesses in children. Clin Pediatr (Phila) 1992;31:71–6.

23. Herzon FS. Management of nonperitonsillar abscesses of the head and neck with needle aspiration. Laryngoscope 1985;95:780–1.

24. Broughton RA. Nonsurgical management of deep neck infections in children. Pediatr Infect Dis J 1992;11:14–8.

25. McClay JE, Murray AD, Booth T. Intravenous antibiotic therapy for deep neck abscesses defined by computed tomography. Arch Otolaryngol Head Neck Surg 2003;129:1207–12.

66

Sleep Apnea in Children

Nira A. Goldstein, MD

Pediatric sleep-disordered breathing (SDB) is viewed as a continuum of severity from partial obstruction of the upper airway producing snoring, to increased upper airway resistance to continuous episodes of complete upper airway obstruction or obstructive sleep apnea (OSA). Although the prevalence of primary snoring in children is 12%, the prevalence of OSA is 1 to 3%. SDB is an important cause of morbidity in children and may lead to growth failure, neurocognitive and behavioral abnormalities, cor pulmonale, and rarely death. Early recognition and treatment are important to prevent or treat these disorders.

HISTORICAL PERSPECTIVE

The earliest description of pediatric OSA is found in a novel by Charles Dickens, *The Posthumous Papers of the Pickwick Club*, which was published in 1837. Dickens described an obese, red-faced, hypersomnolent boy named Joe. In the medical literature, William Osler gave an extremely accurate description of pediatric OSA in his textbook in 1892. "At night the child's sleep is greatly disturbed; the respirations are loud and snoring, and there are sometimes prolonged pauses, followed by deep, noisy inspirations." He also coined the term "pickwickian" to describe morbidly obese, hypersomnolent patients. In 1956, Spector and Bautista associated pediatric respiratory distress with tonsillitis and adenoiditis. In 1965, both Noonan and Menashe described reversible cor pulmonale in children with adenotonsillar hypertrophy. Guilleminault and colleagues first described the clinical features of pediatric OSA in 1976.[1] Since then, additional case series and cohort studies have drastically increased our knowledge regarding the potential morbidities of SDB and potential therapies, although much is still unknown.

DEFINITIONS

Classically childhood OSA has been defined as partial or complete upper airway obstruction during sleep, usually associated with sleep disruption, hypoxemia, hypercapnia, or daytime symptoms (Figure 1).[2] The diagnosis of OSA has been based on threshold criteria on the overnight polysomnogram (PSG) such as apnea index or degree of oxygen desaturation. Children who

snored but did not meet the threshold criteria for OSA were considered to be primary snorers (see Figure 1B), a condition which was believed to be clinically insignificant. In recent years, upper airway resistance syndrome (UARS) has identified children with elevated upper airway resistance characterized by snoring, labored breathing, and paradoxical breathing without classic apnea or hypopnea (see Figure 1C). These children exhibit similar clinical features to children with classic OSA and improve after treatment.

ETIOLOGY AND PATHOGENESIS

Pediatric OSA is caused by fixed and dynamic narrowing of the airway which may occur at several sites. Most commonly, enlarged tonsils and adenoid are the source of nasopharyngeal and oropharyngeal narrowing. The tissues of Waldeyer ring (tonsils, adenoid, and lingual tonsil) progressively enlarge between ages 2 and 8 years and are largest in relation to the airway between 3 and 6 years of age. Craniofacial abnormalities such as micrognathia or maxillary hypoplasia can narrow the upper airway. Lower airway abnormalities such as laryngomalacia can also impact airway patency. Rapid air movement through a narrowed airway from any of these conditions induces further airway collapse and obstruction. The pharyngeal muscle hypotonia and muscle incoordination

found in children with neuromuscular conditions and cerebral palsy produce dynamic airway narrowing.

Given the multiple predisposing factors for pediatric SDB, no single factor accounts for all cases (Figure 2). Large tonsils and adenoid alone do not cause SDB. Numerous studies have been unable to find a relationship between tonsil and adenoid size and the development of OSA. Children with OSA do not exhibit obstruction when awake underscoring sleep-related dynamic airway collapse. Also, there have been reports of successful treatment by adenotonsillectomy in childhood with recurrence of SDB in the teenage years. The current view is that children with OSA have an underlying abnormality of upper airway motor control or tone which when combined with enlarged tonsils and adenoid results in dynamic airway obstruction during sleep.

The mechanisms underlying the development of the neurocognitive and behavioral deficits found in pediatric SDB are unknown. Proposed mechanisms include sleep disruption, sleep fragmentation, intermittent hypoxia, alterations in brain neurochemistry, brain inflammation, hormonal changes, changes in cerebral bloodflow, or altered cerebral perfusion pressure. Additional research is critically important in this area. Other consequences of pediatric SDB, including pulmonary hypertension (cor pulmonale), hypertension, and growth impairment, are likely caused in part by the effects of intermittent hypoxia during sleep. Hypoxemia or sleep fragmentation

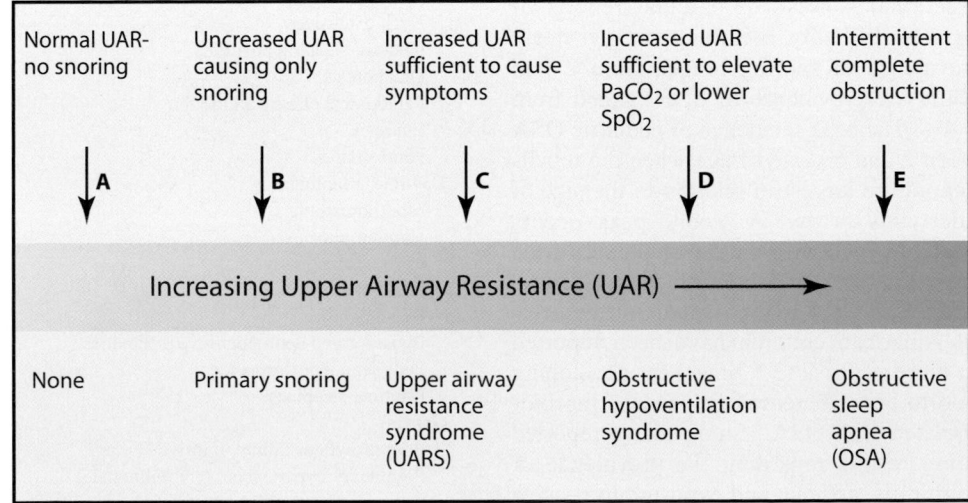

Figure 1 Spectrum of upper airway resistance and obstruction. (Adapted from reference 2.)

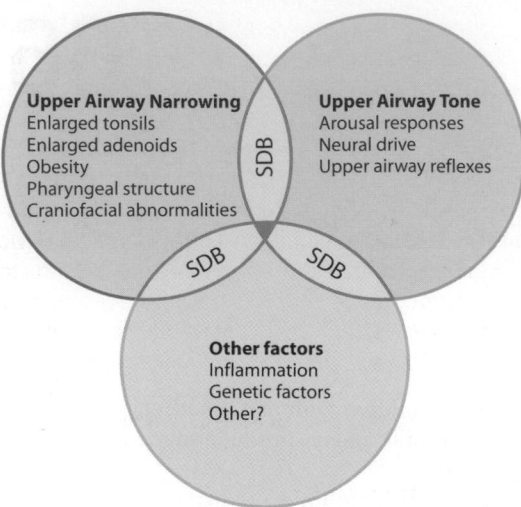

Figure 2 Pathophysiology of childhood sleep-disordered breathing (SDB). (Adapted from reference 2.)

may affect brain neurochemistry and growth hormone secretion. Increased work of breathing with fewer calories available for growth may lead to failure to thrive. Large swings in intrathoracic pressure may affect cardiac afterload directly. The etiology of enuresis is unclear but may be secondary to increased urine production due to OSA, abnormal secretion of antidiuretic hormone (ADH), or merely reflect increased awakenings and arousals.

There is mounting evidence that there is a familial predisposition to the development of OSA as genetic-epidemiologic surveys of families of index patients with OSA have demonstrated a higher prevalence of SDB in family members as compared to the general population.[3] Genes associated with obesity, craniofacial structure, and muscle development of the upper airway soft tissues are likely involved in the development of OSA, but further work is needed to identify specific loci.

EPIDEMIOLOGY

The prevalence of snoring and pediatric OSA have been estimated from community-based cross sectional surveys of parental reports of snoring and difficulty breathing during sleep. The prevalence of snoring ranged from 2.4 to 12% while the prevalence of SDB ranged from 0.69 to 4%. The peak incidence of pediatric OSA is between 2 and 6 years of age when the tonsils and adenoid are largest in relation to the size of the underlying airway. A second peak occurs during adolescence with the development of the adult body habitus and craniofacial structure. Most studies do not report gender differences. African American children have been reported to be at increased risk (3.5 times) for developing OSA and to be at increased risk for the morbidity associated with OSA.[3] Studies have reported conflicting results regarding the prevalence of allergic rhinitis, asthma, and exposure to passive cigarette smoking in children with SDB.

CLINICAL FEATURES

Nighttime Symptoms

Snoring is the most common symptom of SDB, and OSA is extremely unusual in children who do not snore (Table 1). Other nighttime symptoms include apneic pauses, snorting, gasping, restless sleep, frequent arousals, frequent awakenings, sleeping with the neck hyperextended, unusual sleeping positions, for example, sitting, propped up on pillows, fetal position, diaphoresis, enuresis, and other parasomnias. A resuscitative snort often follows the apneic episodes. Occasionally stridor is found. Children may exhibit paradoxical inward rib cage motion while cyanosis is rarely observed. In children, OSA occurs mainly in rapid eye movement (REM) sleep, therefore symptoms may be absent for a significant portion of the night.

Daytime Symptoms

Hypertrophy of the tissues of Waldeyer ring may lead to daytime obstructive symptoms including mouthbreathing, hyponasality, chronic rhinorrhea, nasal obstruction, and dysphagia (Table 1). A history of any of these symptoms should lead to an investigation of nighttime symptoms including snoring and possible apnea. During an acute upper respiratory infection, there may be enlargement of the lymphoid tissues of Waldeyer ring resulting in snoring and nighttime breathing difficulties. These symptoms may be temporary and resolve once the infection subsides but may signal the onset of chronic upper airway obstruction.

Failure to thrive has been reported to occur in approximately 10% of children and 42 to 56% of infants with OSA. There have been several

Table 1 Clinical Features of Pediatric Sleep-Disordered Breathing

Nighttime symptoms
  Snoring
  Apneic pauses
  Gasping
  Restless sleep
  Frequent arousals and awakenings
  Neck extension
  Unusual sleeping positions
  Diaphoresis
  Paradoxical chest wall motion
  Enuresis
  Parasomnias
Daytime symptoms
  Mouthbreathing
  Hyponasality
  Chronic rhinorrhea
  Nasal obstruction
  Dysphagia
  Behavior and neurocognitive difficulties
  Poor school performance
  Daytime sleepiness
General
  Poor growth or failure to thrive
  Pulmonary hypertension (cor pulmonale)
  Systemic hypertension

reports documenting improvement in growth for children with failure to thrive and OSA after adenotonsillectomy.[4]

Pulmonary hypertension is a rare complication of SDB. Goldstein and colleagues, in two prospective studies evaluating the clinical diagnosis of SDB performed echocardiograms on all study participants.[5] Pulmonary hypertension was found in 0/30 (0%) and 1/56 (2%) of patients and resolved in the one patient after adenotonsillectomy. Miman and colleagues identified 17 children with obstructive symptoms and adenotonsillar hypertrophy who had mild pulmonary hypertension by echocardiography.[6] The pulmonary hypertension resolved in all patients after surgery. In the studies by Goldstein and colleagues, systemic hypertension was also found in 5/30 (16.7%) and 8/59 (20%) of patients.[5] It resolved in all patients after adenotonsillectomy.

While daytime sleepiness is extremely common in adults with OSA, it is an uncommon finding in children. Behavioral and neurocognitive difficulties have been found in 8.5 to 63% of children with SDB. Children with primary snoring but otherwise normal sleep study indices have also been shown to have lower scores on measures of behavior and cognition using a battery of neurobehavioral tests as compared to control children, although the mean scores for both groups were still in the normal range.[7] Studies using standardized behavioral and neurocognitive assessments have documented significant improvements in test scores after adenotonsillectomy in children with SDB, suggesting that neurocognitive deficits are potentially reversible.

Poor academic performance has also been found in several studies of children with SDB. Only one study has evaluated improvement in academic performance after adenotonsillectomy. Gozal evaluated 297 first grade children in the lowest tenth percentile of their class by overnight pulse oximetry and transcutaneous CO_2 measurement.[8] Fifty-four children demonstrated sleep-associated gas exchange abnormalities and 24 of these children underwent adenotonsillectomy. The mean grades of the children who underwent surgery increased significantly during the following academic year as compared to the children whose parents refused surgery. There was no academic improvement in the children with primary snoring and the children without SDB. These finding also suggest that the neurocognitive difficulties found in children with SDB are reversible with treatment. To further evaluate the long-term impact of SDB in early childhood, Gozal and Pope mailed questionnaires to the parents of seventh and eighth graders whose school performance was in the top 25% of the class or the bottom 25% of the class, and who were matched for age, gender, race, school, and street of residence.[9] Snoring in early childhood was significantly more common in the low performance group than the high performance group, but there was no significant difference in current snoring. Significantly, more low performance children had a history of adenotonsillectomy than high performance children. These findings suggest that the neurocognitive impairments of pediatric SDB may not be fully reversible especially if they occur during a critical period of brain development.

CONDITIONS ASSOCIATED WITH PEDIATRIC SLEEP APNEA

A summary of conditions predisposing children to sleep apnea is provided in Table 2.[10]

Obesity

Although obesity is a risk factor for pediatric SDB, most children with SDB are not obese. However, the prevalence of SDB in obese children is 25 to 40%. Obesity predisposes children to SDB by decreasing the cross-sectional area of the upper airway by the deposition of adipose tissue adjacent to the pharynx as well as compression from subcutaneous fat deposits in the neck. Individual symptoms and PSG abnormalities do not correlate with the degree of obesity. Soultan and colleagues found that 10 of 17 children who were obese or morbidly obese with OSA had substantial weight gain after adenotonsillectomy.[11] Therefore treatment of the SDB will not help with weight reduction in obese children and might exacerbate the obesity. Diet, exercise, and behavior therapy are needed in addition to surgical therapy.

Down Syndrome

The anatomic and physiologic factors that predispose children with Down syndrome to OSA include midfacial and maxillary hypoplasia, macroglossia, a narrow nasopharynx, a shortened palate, generalized hypotonia, and a tendency to

Table 2 Predisposing Conditions
Obesity
Down syndrome
Craniofacial syndromes
Craniosynostoses (Apert, Crouzon, Pfeiffer, and Saethre-Chotzen syndromes)
Pierre Robin sequence
Stickler syndrome
CHARGE syndrome
Mandibulofacial dysostosis (Treacher Collins syndrome)
Craniofacial microsomia (hemifacial microsomia, Goldenhar syndrome, 1st and 2nd branchial arch syndrome)
Hallermann-Streiff syndrome
Mucopolysaccharidoses
Achondroplasia
Neuromuscular disease
Cerebral palsy
Beckwith-Wiedemann syndrome
Klippel-Feil syndrome
Prader-Willi syndrome
Arnold-Chiari malformation
Sickle cell disease
Postpharyngoplasty

Adapted from reference 10.

obesity. Shott and colleagues found the incidence of OSA to be 57% in a 5-year longitudinal study of 56 children with Down syndrome.[12] Of the children with abnormal sleep studies, 77% of the parents reported no sleep problems in their children. Since many of the manifestations of SDB including daytime sleepiness, behavioral problems, developmental delay, and pulmonary hypertension are also common in children with Down syndrome, there is often a delay in diagnosis.

Although adenotonsillectomy is usually the first-line treatment of SDB in children with Down syndrome, persistent significant PSG abnormalities have been reported in up to 60% of children. Additional therapies may include nasal continuous positive airway pressure (CPAP), uvulopalatopharyngoplasty (UPPP), tongue reduction, maxillomandibuloadvancement, or tracheostomy. The efficacy of these surgical procedures in this patient population is unknown.

Craniofacial Syndromes

The prevalence of SDB in children with craniofacial syndromes is estimated to be 40 to 50%. Abnormalities that predispose these children to OSA include midfacial and mandibular hypoplasia, increased nasal resistance, macroglossia, soft palate abnormalities, hypotonia, abnormal neural control of the airway, and structural defects. OSA has been found in children with Pierre Robin sequence, Treacher Collins syndrome, Apert syndrome, Pfeiffer syndrome, Larsen syndrome, Crouzon syndrome, Stickler syndrome, Goldenhar syndrome, velocardiofacial syndrome, and fragile X syndrome. Infants with Pierre Robin sequence (micrognathia, glossoptosis, and cleft palate) may present with severe upper airway obstruction, although appropriate management may prevent many of the complications. With growth of the mandible, the upper airway obstruction improves with age. PSG is important for the diagnosis of SDB in children with craniofacial abnormalities and to evaluate the children's response to therapy. Therapy includes adenotonsillectomy, UPPP, maxillary and mandibular advancement, mandibular distraction osteogenesis, nasal CPAP, and tracheostomy.

Achondroplasia

Achondroplasia is an autosomal dominant syndrome which is the most common form of dwarfism. Midfacial hypoplasia, dysplasia of the basiocciput, foramen magnum stenosis with compression of the cervical spinal cord, and thoracic cage restriction predispose these children to OSA. Surgical management may involve adenotonsillectomy, ventriculoperitoneal shunt, and foramen magnum decompression. PSG and neurological and respiratory assessments are important in the workup of these patients.

Mucopolysaccharide Storage Diseases

The mucopolysaccharidoses are genetic disorders in which enzyme deficiencies lead to defective

degradation of lysosomal glycosaminoglycans with accumulation of mucopolysaccharides in the soft tissues of the body, including the respiratory tract. The type of mucopolysaccaridosis is determined by the particular enzyme deficiency. Examples are Hurler and Scheie syndromes (α-L-iduronidase deficiency), Hunter syndrome (iduronate sulfatase deficiency), and Sly syndrome (β-glucuronidase deficiency). In addition to hypertrophy of the tonsils, adenoid, tongue, and oropharyngeal mucosa, deposits in the tracheobronchial tree often lead to chronic pulmonary disease. These children often develop scoliosis, spinal problems, and hepatosplenomegaly. OSA may be severe and a cause of death. Treatment options include adenotonsillectomy, nasal CPAP, and tracheostomy. These patients present complex airway management, and even tracheostomy may not insure control of the airway.

Neuromuscular Disease and Cerebral Palsy

Children with neuromuscular disease are a heterogeneous group and include children with neuropathies, congenital myopathies, muscular dystrophies, myotonias, and myasthenia gravis. These children have a loss of respiratory muscle function and a drop in central respiratory drive leading to both obstructive and central apnea. The symptoms of SDB may be underestimated as they may be difficult to distinguish from the underlying disease. Treatment options include adenotonsillectomy, UPPP, tracheostomy, or CPAP. Children with cerebral palsy have poor neuromuscular control, increased oropharyngeal secretions, seizures, and gastroesophageal reflux disease (GERD) which may predispose them to SDB. Adenotonsillar hypertrophy along with decreased pharyngeal tone contribute to upper airway collapse. Treatment options include adenotonsillectomy, UPPP, tongue hyoid advancement, mandibular advancement, tongue reduction, CPAP, and tracheostomy.

Miscellaneous Conditions

Children with Arnold-Chiari malformation present with central and obstructive apnea as a result of brainstem compression (see the central apnea discussion below). Treatment involves decompression of the malformation. Children with sickle cell disease are at risk for the development of SDB, and SDB may be a predisposing factor for the occurrence of cerebrovascular accidents. Adenotonsillectomy has been shown to be successful in the resolution of symptoms and improvement in alveolar hyperventilation. Children with Prader–Willi syndrome have severe infantile hypotonia, feeding difficulties, developmental delay, craniofacial abnormalities, and obesity which all contribute to the development of SDB. Early treatment of SDB may delay the development of cor pulmonale, a common cause of death in these children. Iatrogenic causes of SDB are possible, most commonly from velopharyngeal flap surgery.

PHYSICAL EXAMINATION

The child's general appearance should be assessed with measurement of height, weight, and blood pressure. The craniofacial structure should be assessed for midfacial hypoplasia, retrognathia, micrognathia, and adenoid facies (open mouth, long face, mandibular hypoplasia). The presence of mouthbreathing, stertor, and hyponasality should be assessed. The nose should be examined for the presence of structural abnormalities. The oropharyngeal examination should evaluate tonsil size, tongue size, position of the palate, dentition, and the presence of any structural abnormalities. The neck should be examined for any neck masses. The adenoid may be evaluated by flexible fiberoptic nasopharyngoscopy or by the use of a small rigid telescope. If laryngeal abnormalities are suspected, flexible fiberoptic laryngoscopy may also be performed. The chest should be examined for the presence of a pectus excavatum. Neurologic function and development should be assessed.

DIAGNOSTIC STUDIES

Ancillary Studies

A lateral neck X-ray may be obtained to assess adenoid size. Cephalometric studies and upper airway fluoroscopy may be useful in children with craniofacial abnormalities but are not routinely used for otherwise healthy children. An electrocardiogram, echocardiogram, and chest radiograph may be obtained in children with severe OSA or children with signs of congestive heart failure to evaluate for pulmonary hypertension.

A home audiotape recording of the child's breathing during sleep has a reported sensitivity of 71 to 88% and a specificity of 52 to 72% in predicting a positive result on PSG in otherwise healthy children.[5,13] A home videotape recording has been shown to have a sensitivity of 94% and specificity of 68% in predicting a positive PSG.[14] Although not specific enough to distinguish children with positive and negative sleep studies, these tapes are convenient, inexpensive methods to confirm the parents' description of the child's nighttime breathing difficulties and are useful in the clinical setting.

Pulse oximetry is not useful as a screening tool because of its low sensitivity but may prove useful if positive in a snoring child in whom there is a high index of suspicion for OSA. Nap polysomnograms also exhibit poor sensitivity and are only useful if they are positive. The difficulty with nap studies is that children over 4 years of age rarely nap, and REM sleep may be missed on a nap study. Ambulatory, unattended PSG performed in the child's home may have a role in the diagnosis of SDB although end tidal CO_2, EEG, and upper airway resistance are usually not measured.

Polysomnography

The PSG consists of electroencephalography and electromyography for sleep staging, chest and abdominal motion by strain gauges or respiratory inductive plethysmography, electrocardiography, pulse oximetry, nasal and oral airflow, and end-tidal or transcutaneous CO_2. UARS is best detected by esophageal pressure monitoring, but this is not routine in most centers. Ideally, pediatric sleep studies should be performed in a pediatric sleep laboratory with a technical staff trained to work with children.

Obstructive apnea or the cessation of airflow with continued respiratory effort is defined as lasting at least 10 seconds in adults (Figure 3). Since children have faster respiratory rates than adults, the duration of an obstructive apnea in a child is two times the typical breath interval. An obstructive hypopnea is the partial cessation of airflow with continued respiratory effort, although there is no uniform definition of hypopnea in children among sleep laboratories. A central apnea is the cessation of airflow due to lack of respiratory effort (see Figure 3). Sleep study findings are commonly reported as the apnea-hypopnea index (AHI) or the number of apneas plus hypopneas per hour of sleep or the respiratory disturbance index (RDI) or the number of all respiratory events including respiratory arousals per hour of sleep.

The PSG criteria commonly used to diagnose OSA in a child are presented in Table 3. Marcus performed sleep studies on 50 normal children and found the average apnea index (AI) to be 0.1 ± 0.5 events per hour, minimal O_2 saturation was 96 ± 2% and average maximal desaturation was 4 ± 2%. She concluded that apnea more frequent than one time per hour was abnormal. Obstructive hypoventilation can be identified when the end tidal CO_2 pressure is equal to or greater than 50 mm Hg for more than 8 to 10% of the total sleep time. Awake esophageal pressure is usually between –10 and –5 cm of water, and UARS is diagnosed on the PSG when a repetitive breathing pattern with increasingly more negative esophageal pressure culminating in an arousal is found. In the absence of esophageal pressure monitoring, some pediatric centers,

Table 3 Abnormal Values of Pediatric Polysomnography

Obstructive apnea index (AI) >1/h
Apnea-hypopnea index (AHI) >5/h
Peak end-tidal CO_2 >53 mm Hg
End-tidal CO_2 >50 mm Hg for
  >10% of total sleep time
Minimum oxyhemoglobin saturation (SpO_2) <92%

based on experience, will consider a study suggestive of UARS if the thresholds for nocturnal awakenings (<1/hr), arousal index (<10/hr), or sleep efficiency (>80%) are exceeded.

Limitations of Polysomnography. Standards for positive PSG in children have been based on studies of their normative values. However, few studies have documented the relationship between PSG abnormalities and daytime sleepiness, impaired neurocognitive function, behavioral abnormalities, or other adverse outcomes of pediatric SDB. It is unclear whether children with mild PSG abnormalities, although outside of the normative range, require therapy. PSG focuses heavily on breathing with minimal measures of sleep quality. Normative data are limited to classic OSA and are not available for UARS.

It is controversial whether an otherwise healthy child needs a PSG prior to adenotonsillectomy. Reports have documented the inaccuracy of predicting which children with histories and physical examinations suggestive of OSA will have positive PSG. In seven trials, the accuracy of clinical evaluation of OSA was poor, ranging from 30 to 85%. On the basis of the published studies and because only 20 to 30% of snoring children have positive PSG, the American Thoracic Society Consensus Committee recommended PSG be obtained before adenotonsillectomy to differentiate primary snoring from OSA.[15] Although the published studies suggest that clinical evaluation is inaccurate in diagnosing OSA in children, most of the studies used adult criteria for interpretation of the sleep studies, which are now recognized to be inappropriate for children. In addition, none of the studies considered the diagnosis of UARS in the evaluations. Weatherly and colleagues found that the accuracy of clinical assessment increased as the PSG criteria for a positive study became less stringent.[16] In a prospective, randomized, controlled trial of children with a positive clinical assessment for OSA but negative PSG, children who underwent adenotonsillectomy had significant improvement in clinical assessment scores compared to children who did not undergo surgery at 6-month follow-up.[5] In addition, recent research has suggested that primary snoring in children may not be benign.[7,9]

PSG has been most useful to confirm the diagnosis of OSA and document its severity in the following situations: children who are younger than 2 years; high-risk patients for which surgery is contraindicated; children with craniofacial abnormalities, morbid obesity, or cerebral palsy; when

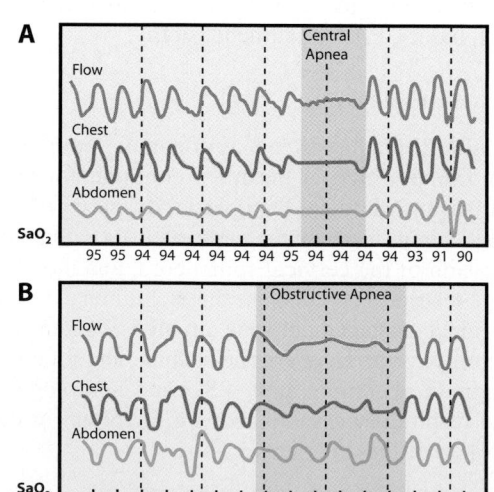

Figure 3 (A) Polysomnogram recording of a central apnea. (B) Polysomnogram recording of an obstructive apnea.

there is a discrepancy between the history and physical examination; and children who remain symptomatic after adenotonsillectomy. PSG is also a prerequisite to treatment with nasal CPAP or bilevel positive airway pressure (BIPAP) in high risk children or surgical failures.

NATURAL HISTORY

Little is known about the natural history of untreated SDB. As children with OSA and clinically significant SDB are routinely treated, there are no studies evaluating long-term effects or possible resolution of SDB. Two studies have evaluated children with untreated primary snoring and found that only 8 to 10% progressed to mild OSA at 1- to 3-year follow-up.[17] Although infantile and childhood OSA may predispose individuals to adult OSA because of anatomical and familial factors, there is no current evidence that adults with OSA had SDB during infancy and childhood.

TREATMENT

Medical

Topical nasal corticosteroids have been studied to determine their ability to improve nasal airflow and improve SDB. Brouillette and colleagues performed a randomized, triple-blind, placebo-controlled trial of 6 weeks of nasal fluticasone propionate in 25 children with SDB.[18] There was significant reduction in the mixed/obstructive apnea/hypopnea index in the study patients from 10.7 ± 2.6 to 5.8 ± 2.2 as compared to the placebo group, although there was no significant change in symptom score and tonsil and adenoid size between groups. Although the study demonstrated a moderate reduction in the AI, an index of 5.8 is still abnormal and the patients continued to have episodes of desaturation. In addition, patients with severe OSA, 4+ tonsils, and craniofacial conditions and infants were excluded. The study also did not address the duration of therapy, so it is unclear whether the topical nasal corticosteroids must be continued for a continued response.

Al-Ghamdi and colleagues performed an open-label pilot study of 5 days of oral prednisone on nine children with OSA.[19] There was no improvement in symptomatology, sleep study indices, or tonsil and adenoid size. There have been two studies evaluating oral antibiotics. Sclafani and colleagues performed a prospective, randomized, double blinded, placebo-controlled trial of 30 days of amoxicillin/clavulanate potassium in 168 children with obstructive symptoms.[20] Sleep studies were not performed. Treatment with the antibiotic significantly reduced the need for adenotonsillectomy at 1-month follow-up as compared to placebo (37.5% vs 62.7%). By 24 months, most of the children in both groups had undergone adenotonsillectomy (83.3% of the study group versus 98.0% of the placebo group). Don and colleagues performed a randomized,

double-blinded, placebo-controlled trial of 30 days of azithromycin in 22 children with OSA documented by PSG.[21] There were no significant differences in sleep study indices, tonsil size, or symptoms in the azithromycin group as compared to the placebo group. These preliminary studies suggest that the above therapies are not indicated for children with severe OSA but may have a role in the treatment of milder SDB or for temporary relief of symptoms.

Nasal CPAP or BIPAP is used in children with predisposing factors for OSA including craniofacial anomalies, neuromuscular weakness, or obesity in whom adenotonsillectomy is ineffective or not indicated and for children with idiopathic OSA after adenotonsillectomy. Studies have reported efficacies of 86 to 100% in normalizing PSG indices with long-term compliance rates of 80%. Supplemental oxygen has been used as a temporary measure to improve oxygenation in children with OSA, although end tidal CO_2 must be monitored as alveolar hypoventilation can occur. It is not recommended as the sole treatment modality for OSA. Weight loss is important in obese children to improve SDB and to reduce the risk for additional comorbidities related to obesity.

Children with a constricted maxillary arch and associated narrowing of the nasal airway may benefit from rapid maxillary expansion. An orthodontic appliance is fixed to anchor teeth and rapidly expanded over 3 weeks followed by a stabilization period of 6 to 12 months. Studies in selected children demonstrate improvements in SDB. It should be considered in older children who have failed other treatments.

Tonsillectomy and Adenoidectomy

The first-line therapy for the treatment of OSA or significant SDB in otherwise healthy children is adenotonsillectomy. It may also be the first line treatment in complex patients if the tonsils and adenoids are enlarged. Review of the published literature evaluating the success of adenotonsillectomy in otherwise healthy children reveals prospective observational, uncontrolled studies, and restrospective case series. Due to ethical concerns, there are no randomized, controlled trials comparing adenotonsillectomy to no treatment. Most studies report a success rate for resolution of PSG abnormalities of 75 to 100%. A meta-analysis by Lipton and Gozal reported a success rate of 80%.[22] Studies evaluating clinical resolution of obstructive symptoms after adenotonsillectomy report higher cure rates in the range of 90 to 100%, highlighting the need for further evaluation of the validity of PSG abnormalities in predicting future morbidity.

The postoperative pain associated with adenotonsillectomy as well as the small risk of postoperative hemorrhage has led the development of a number of different surgical techniques. Adenoidectomy may be performed using curettes, electrocautery, or the microdebrider. The classic technique of tonsillectomy was the "cold-dissection" in which the tonsil was grasped, the

anterior tonsillar pillar incised, and the capsule dissected off the pharyngeal constrictors using blunt and sharp dissection. Hemostasis was obtained by suture ligature or electrocautery. Monopolar electrocautery has become the most popular technique of tonsil dissection in the past quarter century as it affords greater hemostasis during the dissection. It may be associated with increased postoperative pain and longer healing times.

Newer techniques include bipolar cautery, harmonic scalpel, plasma excision (coblation), powered intracapsular tonsillectomy (PIT), and radiofrequency volume reduction. Bipolar cautery allows precise coagulation with less tissue injury and may be performed using a small bipolar bayonet forceps with the operating room microscope or bipolar electrosurgical scissors. The harmonic scalpel uses ultrasonic vibration to transfer mechanical energy sufficient to break hydrogen bonds. Its vibrating titanium blades cut at a frequency of 55.5 kHz, generating minimal heat and tissue damage. Coblation uses current that is conducted through normal saline fluid or gel. The radiofrequency energy excites the saline solution creating a field of active protons that break molecular bonds between tissues. There is potentially reduced thermal injury and postoperative pain because of the lower temperatures produced. Preliminary studies comparing the harmonic scalpel and coblation with the traditional techniques have not demonstrated a clear advantage in terms of postoperative pain and reduction of postoperative hemorrhage rates, but additional studies are needed.

PIT using the microdebrider allows removal of the bulk of the tonsil with preservation of the tonsillar capsule to act as a "biologic dressing" over the pharyngeal constrictor muscles. Due to decreased thermal injury to the tonsillar fossa musculature, there is potentially reduced postoperative pain and hemorrhage. However, there is potential regrowth and infection of the remaining tonsil tissue. Retrospective studies comparing PIT with monopolar electrocautery tonsillectomy have revealed significantly less postoperative pain, use of analgesics, and a quicker return to normal diet in the PIT group. The largest of the studies was able to show a significant reduction in delayed postoperative bleeding and readmission for dehydration in patients who had PIT; these patients had a low rate of tonsil regrowth (0.46%, 95% CI 0.009 to 0.9%).[23] Two recent prospective studies comparing PIT with monopolar electrocautery tonsillectomy show more modest benefits, and there were no differences in groups with respect to postoperative complications. Although the technique appears promising, more data are needed regarding its effectiveness and potential for recurrence of SDB secondary to tonsil regrowth.

Radiofrequency tonsil reduction involves inserting a temperature-controlled radiofrequency probe directly into the tonsillar tissue. The probe generates a current that creates a region of tissue destruction which contracts over time, reducing tonsil volume. In adults, the procedure may be performed in the office under local anesthesia. Because of their inability to cooperate and the need for concomitant adenoidectomy, children still require a general anesthetic. Preliminary results are promising but larger studies are still needed.

Children with OSA are at risk for postoperative respiratory complications. Although the risk of postoperative respiratory complications in the general pediatric population ranges from 0 to 1.3%, rates of 16 to 27% have been reported in children with OSA.[24] Risk factors are age under three, pulmonary hypertension or other cardiac abnormalities, craniofacial syndromes, failure to thrive, hypotonia, acute airway obstruction, morbid obesity, and severe sleep study indices. These high-risk children require inpatient monitoring of their cardiorespiratory status after adenotonsillectomy. Narcotic analgesics should be used judiciously. These children may require oxygen therapy, corticosteroids, a nasopharyngeal airway, CPAP or BIPAP, or endotracheal intubation if respiratory compromise develops. Postoperative pulmonary edema is a rare complication that may occur after the relief of chronic upper airway obstruction. Treatment includes oxygen therapy, possible mechanical respiratory support with positive end-expiratory pressure (PEEP), restriction of intravenous fluids, diuretics, and possibly corticosteroids.

After tonsillectomy, children experience throat pain that lasts 1 to 2 weeks, referred otalgia from the pharyngeal surgical site, and halitosis. Nausea and vomiting may develop from the anesthetic agents, the swallowing of bloody secretions, or adverse reactions to narcotic analgesics. Some children after adenoidectomy will develop neck pain especially with extension and neck stiffness secondary to prevertebral inflammation. If the neck pain persists longer than two weeks, C1–C2 subluxation should be suspected. A soft diet is recommended for 10 to 14 days with a gradual return to normal activities. Acetaminophen should be used liberally. Acetaminophen with codeine may also be used but with discretion in high-risk patients. Nonsteroidal anti-inflammatory agents are avoided due to the increased risk of postoperative hemorrhage. Postoperative antibiotics are usually prescribed because of their beneficial effects on pain, fever, and halitosis. Perioperative corticosteroid administration has been shown to reduce vomiting and pain in the first 24 hours.

Dehydration is a complication of adenotonsillectomy that may require readmission for intravenous hydration and pain management. Rehydration should be performed with isotonic solutions in appropriate volumes. Hyponatremia has been reported as a potential lethal complication after tonsillectomy caused by inappropriate administration of hypotonic solutions in children with intravascular depletion. In the surgical patient, free water is retained because there is an increase in antidiuretic hormone (ADH) secretion in response to decreased circulating blood volume. Administration of hypotonic solutions maintains these elevated ADH levels leading to the retention of free water with a resultant decrease in serum sodium and serum osmolality.

Postoperative hemorrhage is the most common severe complication of tonsillectomy, occurring in 2 to 4% of patients. Primary bleeding occurs within the first 24 hours and is considered to be related to surgical technique while delayed bleeding occurs within the first 10 days (most commonly on the sixth or seventh day) and is attributed to the slough of eschar. Bleeding may stop spontaneously, but children with significant bleeding should be admitted and observed. Attempts may be made to control bleeding in the emergency room, but many children require control in the operating room. A clot in the tonsillar fossa indicates recent bleeding and must be removed to determine if the bleeding has stopped. Repeated bleeding may indicate injury to a large vessel with pseudoaneurysm formation. Angiography and selective embolization may be required to diagnosis and treat this rare complication.

Preoperative coagulation studies are not performed routinely before adenotonsillectomy as they have limited predictive value and are not cost-effective. However, children with a history of abnormal bleeding or children with a family history of bleeding or coagulation disorders do warrant a preoperative workup. Children with sickle cell disease are at increased risk for complications after adenotonsillectomy. Protocols have been developed which include aggressive hydration and preoperative transfusions to reduce the percentage of hemoglobin S to less than 30 to 40%. Children with type 1 von Willebrand disease are successfully managed with preoperative administration of desmopressin acetate (DDAVP). Children with sickle cell disease, hemophilia, and other coagulopathies should be managed in conjunction with a pediatric hematologist.

Other Surgical Modalities

Surgical modalities other than adenotonsillectomy are considered for children who are not improved with it and children with other comorbid conditions. PSG is mandatory in this group of children to confirm the diagnosis and document the severity of SDB. The other surgical procedures for OSA are presented in Chapter 86, "Sleep Medicine and Surgery." Most studies on surgical modalities other than adenotonsillectomy have evaluated children with comorbid conditions. Four studies have evaluated UPPP in neurologically impaired patients. Success rates measured by clinical or PSG criteria ranged from 80 to 87%.[25] UPPP may be considered in children or adolescents with continued palatal obstruction after adenotonsillectomy. Concerns about midface growth have limited the use of septoplasty in the preadolescent, but it may be considered in older children with continued nasal obstruction. Although temperature-controlled radiofrequency reduction has been used for reduction of the inferior turbinates, soft palate, and base of tongue in adults, little has been published regarding its use in children.

Mandibular distraction osteogenesis has been described in children with micrognathia and respiratory distress from Pierre Robin sequence, Treacher Collins syndrome, Nager syndrome, and hemifacial microsomia. The procedure has been used successfully to prevent tracheostomy in affected infants, treat OSA in older children without tracheostomy, and allow decannulation. In the largest of the published series, 7 of 8 (88%) infants avoided tracheostomy and 5 of 6 (83%) older micrognathic children were cured of OSA, but only 2 of 12 (17%) children with tracheostomies and complex congenital syndromes were successfully decannulated.[26]

Cohen and Burstein have published several case series describing their use of skeletal expansion combined with soft-tissue reduction in their children with craniofacial syndromes or cerebral palsy and refractory OSA.[27] In addition to adenotonsillectomy and UPPP, soft-tissue procedures included septoplasty and turbinectomy, tongue reduction, and tongue hyoid suspension. Skeletal expansion procedures included mandibular advancement, costochondral grafts, mandibular distraction, temporomandibular joint arthroplasty, and LeFort procedures. Tracheostomy was avoided in 90% of their patients, whereas 80% of their patients with tracheostomies were successfully decannulated. Supplemental oxygen therapy or CPAP was still required by 8% of the patients. Mandibular osteotomy with genioglossus advancement, hyoid myotomy with suspension, and maxillary-mandibular advancement may also be considered in otherwise healthy children who do not improve with adenotonsillectomy if the facial skeleton and dentition are mature, although there are few studies addressing these procedures in this group of children. Tracheostomy is thought to be curative in children with refractory OSA and should be considered if the RDI is greater than 60 and oxygen desaturation is less than 70% if CPAP is not tolerated.

CENTRAL APNEA

Central apnea is abnormal if it lasts 20 seconds or longer or is of any duration but associated with 4% oxygen desaturation or bradycardia. Three or more events per hour are considered abnormal. Periodic breathing describes an alternating pattern of respirations followed by a central respiratory pause. Periodic breathing is commonly found in healthy neonates but should be considered abnormal in infants and children if it accounts for more than 5% of total sleep time. Diagnosis of central apnea and periodic breathing may be difficult as these children may appear perfectly healthy when awake. Premature infants may exhibit these breathing patterns in the neonatal intensive care unit or may be admitted after an acute life-threatening event. Older children may have daytime sleepiness, restless sleep, and cyanosis during sleep but usually not snoring. A PSG is required for diagnosis.

The differential diagnosis of central apnea and periodic breathing is large, and the workup should be tailored to the likely cause (Table 4).[28] Apnea of prematurity occurs in 84% of infants less than 1,000 g and 25% of infants less than 2,500 g and is commonly a pattern of mixed central and obstructive apnea. The most common cause is respiratory control immaturity, but central nervous system abnormalities, bacterial or viral infection, anemia, hypoglycemia, electrolyte imbalance, and sedating medications are also causative. The role of GERD is controversial. While chemical irritation of the larynx by a reflux episode may activate the laryngeal reflex and cause apnea, a clear causal relationship between GERD and apnea of prematurity has not been determined. Treatment options include CPAP, high-flow nasal cannula therapy, and methylxanthines such as theophylline and caffeine.

Congenital central hypoventilation syndrome (CCHS or Ondine curse) is an extremely rare entity in which affected children demonstrate severe hypoventilation particularly during sleep because they lack the normal ventilatory responses to hypercarbia and hypoxia. These children usually present shortly after birth with cyanosis upon falling asleep. CCHS is a diagnosis of exclusion as primary neuromuscular, cardiac, pulmonary, and metabolic diseases must be excluded. Most children will require placement of a tracheostomy and mechanical ventilation for treatment. Diaphragm pacing via phrenic nerve stimulation or BIPAP is another alternative. Approximately 15 to 20% of these children will present with Hirschsprung disease, but other autonomic nervous system abnormalities are common.

Disruption of the normal anatomical relationships within the brainstem can result in respiratory control abnormalities. This can occur in brainstem tumors or Chiari malformations. In Type I Chiari malformation (CM-I), there is herniation of the cerebellar tonsils through the foramen magnum often with an associated syrinx. CM-I usually presents in older children and adults. CM-I may be asymptomatic, but patients may present with occipital headaches, a wide variety of neurologic symptoms, and central apnea. In Chiari malformation Type II (CM-II), there is caudal displacement of the cerebellar vermis and brainstem. There is always an associated myelomeningocele and hydrocephalus is common. CM-II is usually diagnosed shortly after birth. Infants may present with prolonged expiratory apnea and cyanosis that can lead to bradycardia and death. Stridor may be indicative of vocal cord paralysis and can manifest as obstructive apnea. Children with suspected Chiari malformations require magnetic resonance imaging of the posterior fossa, brainstem, and spine and should be referred to a neurologist or neurosurgeon for management. Patients with CM-II and hydrocephalus require immediate shunting followed by decompression surgery. Asymptomatic patients with CM-I may be observed, but patients with apnea, syncope, vocal cord paralysis, and aspiration and those who fail medical management require decompression. Success rates for CM-I approach 80 to 90%, but the outcomes for CM-II are not as good, with up to 15% dying by age three and one-third having continued central nervous system deficits.

Table 4 Differential Diagnosis of Central Apnea

Congenital
  Apnea of prematurity
  Mild alveolar hypoventilation
  Congenital central hypoventilation syndrome
  Late-onset central hypoventilation with
    hypothalamic dysfunction
Congenital central nervous system anomalies
  Chiari malformation
  Myelomeningocele
  Prader-Willi syndrome
  Riley-Day syndrome
  Shy-Drager syndrome
Normal child
  High-altitude periodic breathing
Acquired
  Brainstem, cervical spinal cord, or phrenic nerve
    trauma
  Encephalitis
  Cervical transverse myelitis
  Brainstem or cervical spinal tumor
  Hydrocephalus
  Brainstem infarct
  Asphyxia
  Drug-induced (long-acting opiates)
Neuromuscular diseases
  Botulism
  Spinal muscular atrophy
  Guillain-Barré syndrome
  Amyotrophic lateral sclerosis
  Poliomyelitis
  Myasthenia gravis
  Muscular dystrophies
  Metabolic disorders (acid maltase deficiency,
    hypophosphatemia, hypermagnesemia, Leigh
    disease, pyruvate dehydrogenase deficiency,
    carnitine deficiency)

Adapted from reference 28.

REFERENCES

1. Guilleminault C, Eldridge FL, Simmons FB, Dement WC. Sleep apnea in eight children. Pediatrics 1976;58:23–30.
2. Carroll JL. Obstructive sleep-disordered breathing in children: New controversies, new directions. Clin Chest Med 2003;24:261–82.
3. Redline S, Tishler PV, Schluchter M, et al. Risk factors for sleep-disordered breathing in children: Associations with obesity, race, and respiratory problems. Am J Respir Crit Care Med 1999;159:1527–32.
4. Ahlqvist-Rastad J, Hultcrantz E, Melander H, Svanholm H. Body growth in relation to tonsillar enlargement and tonsillectomy. Int J Pediatr Otorhinolaryngol 1992; 24:55–61.
5. Goldstein NA, Pugazhendhi V, Rao SM, et al. Clinical assessment of pediatric obstructive sleep apnea. Pediatrics 2004;114:33–43.
6. Miman MC, Kirazli T, Ozyurek R. Doppler echocardiography in adenotonsillar hypertrophy. Int J Pediatr Otorhinolaryngol 2000;54:21–6.
7. O'Brien LM, Mervis CB, Holbrook CR, et al. Neurobehavioral implications of habitual snoring in children. Pediatrics 2004;114:44–9.
8. Gozal D. Sleep-disordered breathing and school performance in children. Pediatrics 1998;102:616–20.
9. Gozal D, Pope DW, Jr. Snoring during early childhood and academic performance at ages 13 to 14 years. Pediatrics 2001;107:1394–9.
10. Richardson MA. Sleep apnea in children: History and physical exam. In: Richardson MA, Friedman NR, editors. Clinician's Guide to Pediatric Sleep Disorders. New York: Informa Healthcare USA, Inc.; 2007. p. 65.
11. Soultan Z, Wadowski S, Rao M, Kravath RE. Effect of treating obstructive sleep apnea by tonsillectomy and/or adenoidectomy on obesity in children. Arch Pediatr Adolesc Med 1999;153:33–7.
12. Shott SR, Amin R, Chini B, et al. Obstructive sleep apnea: Should all children with Down syndrome be tested? Arch Otolaryngol Head Neck Surg 2006;132:432–6.
13. Lamm C, Mandeli J, Kattan M. Evaluation of home audiotapes as an abbreviated test for obstructive sleep apnea syndrome (OSAS) in children. Pediatr Pulmonol 1999;27:267–72.
14. Sivan Y, Komecki A, Schonfeld T. Screening obstructive sleep apnoae syndrome by home videotape recording in children. Eur Respir J 1996;9:2127–31.
15. American Thoracic Society. Standards and indications for cardiopulmonary sleep studies in children. Am J Respir Crit Care Med 1996;153:866–78.
16. Weatherly RA, Ruzicka DL, Marriott DJ, Chervin RD, Polysomnography in children scheduled for adenotonsillectomy. Otolaryngol Head Neck Surg 2004;131:727–31.
17. Marcus CL, Hamer A, Loughlin GM. Natural history of primary snoring in children. Pediatr Pulmonol 1998;26:6–11.
18. Brouillette RT, Manoukian JJ, Ducharme FM, et al. Efficacy of fluticasone nasal spray for pediatric obstructive sleep apnea. J Pediatr 2001;138:838–44.
19. Al-Ghamdi SA, Manoukian JJ, Morielli A, et al. Do systemic corticosteroids effectively treat obstructive sleep apnea secondary to adenotonsillar hypertrophy? J Pediatr Laryngoscope 1997;107:1382–7.
20. Sclafani AP, Ginsburg J, Shah MK, Dolitsky JN. Treatment of symptomatic chronic adenotonsillar hypertrophy with amoxicillin/clavulanate potassium: Short- and long-term results. Pediatrics 1998;101:675–81.
21. Don DM, Goldstein NA, Crockett DM, Davidson Ward S. Antimicrobial therapy for children with adenotonsillar hypertrophy and obstructive sleep apnea: A prospective randomized trial comparing azithromycin vs placebo. Otolaryngol Head Neck Surg 2005;133:562–8.
22. Lipton AJ, Gozal D. Treatment of obstructive sleep apnea in children: Do we really know how? Sleep Med Rev 2003;7:61–80.
23. Solares CA, Koempel JA, Hirose K, et al. Safety and efficacy of powered intracapsular tonsillectomy in children: A multi center retrospective case series. Int J Pediatr Otorhinolaryngol 2005;69:21–6.
24. McColley SA, April MM, Carroll JL, et al. Respiratory compromise after adenotonsillectomy in children with obstructive sleep apnea. Arch Otolaryngol Head Neck Surg 1992;118:940–3.
25. Kerschner JE, Lynch JB, Kleiner H, et al. Uvulopalatopharyngoplasty with tonsillectomy and adenoidectomy as a treatment for obstructive sleep apnea in neurologically impaired children. Int J Pediatr Otorhingolaryngol 2002;62:229–35.
26. Mandell DL, Yellon RF, Bradley JP, et al. Mandibular distraction for micrognathia and severe upper airway obstruction. Arch Otolaryngol Head Neck Surg 2004;130:344–8.
27. Cohen SR, Simms C, Burstein FD, Thomsen J. Alternatives to tracheostomy in infants and children with obstructive sleep apnea. J Pediatr Surg 1999;34:182–7.
28. Lee RL. Nonobstructive sleep patterns in children. In: Richardson MA, Friedman NR, editors. Clinician's Guide to Pediatric Sleep Disorders. New York: Informa Healthcare USA, Inc.; 2007. p. 35.

SUGGESTED READING

Carroll JL. Obstructive sleep-disordered breathing in children: New controversies, new directions. Clin Chest Med 2003;24:261–82.
This article is a comprehensive review of pediatric SDB highlighting new developments and controversies regarding definitions, diagnostic criteria, pathophysiology and treatment.
Messner AH. Evaluation of obstructive sleep apnea by polysomnography prior to pediatric adenotonsillectomy. Arch Otolaryngol Head Neck Surg 1999;125:353–6.
This paper discusses the pros and cons of obtaining a PSG prior to adenotonsillectomy in otherwise healthy children with suspected SDB.

67

Robotic Surgery, Navigational Systems and Surgical Simulators

Todd A. Loehrl, MD
Bert W. O'Malley, MD
Gregory S. Weinstein, MD
Aaron Sulman, MD

The development of image-guidance and robotic surgical systems has facilitated the expansion of minimally invasive approaches to complex surgical head and neck problems. In addition, the development of surgical simulators allows for alternative methods to develop surgical skills. This chapter reviews the roles of these technologies in otorhinolaryngology head and neck surgery.

IMAGE-GUIDANCE SYSTEMS

Image-guidance systems were initially developed for neurotological and neurosurgical procedures using a stereotactic frame that required fixation of the patient's head.[1] They have been subsequently adapted for use in endoscopic sinus surgery. These systems assist the surgeon with intraoperative stereotactic anatomic localization through the use of computerized tracking devices. The tracking devices can localize the position of endoscopic instruments within the sinonasal cavity and depict them on a real-time video display of the preoperative computed tomography (CT) scan using the digital data set of the imaging study.

At this time, there are four types of technology that allow intraoperative image guidance: electromechanical, electromagnetic, optical, and sonic. For practical purposes, electromagnetic and optical systems are the most useful for computer-guided endoscopic surgery (CGES). The sonic system is not widely available in the United States. An example of the electromechanical system was introduced by ISG Technologies (Mississauga, Ontario, Canada) and uses a mechanical arm ("wand") for anatomic localization. Anon and colleagues reviewed their experience with this system in 70 patients. No complications were reported; and, anecdotally, the authors felt the system was useful in revision surgery, massive disease, frontal recess or sphenoid surgery, and the presence of anatomic variants.[2] However, this system requires preoperative placement of fiducial markers, re-registration with intraoperative head movement, and a mechanical arm.[3] While these more complex systems are necessary for

use with neurotologic skull base surgery applications, the electromagnetic and optical systems are currently the most commonly used for paranasal sinus surgery.

There is only one electromagnetic system, represented by the InstaTrak (General Electric Medical Systems, Milwaukee, WI). This system relies on a radio frequency transmitter mounted to a patient headset and an electromagnetic sensor incorporated into a handpiece. The InstaTrak is a frameless, wandless system that uses preoperative CT images for triplanar real-time intraoperative localization of curved and straight surgical aspirators. The headset contains seven fiducial markers. Disadvantages of this system include the need to wear a headpiece during the preoperative CT scan and interference from metallic objects near the surgical field. Neumann and colleagues reported their experience using the electromagnetic InstaTrak system in 109 patients, 76 of whom had undergone previous surgery.[4] The estimated accuracy was <3 mm in 106 (97.2%) patients and in no patients did unacceptable intraoperative drift occur. Setup of the InstaTrak system, including headset placement, draping, calibration, and verification took less than 5 minutes in all cases. Orbital fat exposure occurred in two patients and was the only reported intraoperative complication. Two patients developed cerebrospinal fluid (CSF) leaks, but these were anticipated given the underlying pathology (osteoma and meningioma). Postoperative complications included persistent synechiae in four patients and epistaxis in one patient. These authors concluded that the technology was useful for all patients undergoing revision sinus surgery, patients with skull base defects or paranasal sinus neoplasms, and patients undergoing primary surgery with extensive disease.

The optical-based image-guidance system utilizes an infrared camera to monitor instrument and head position. Light emitting diodes (LEDs) are mounted on the surgical instrument and the headset worn by the patient, which are tracked by an infrared camera. The tracking data are processed by an optical digitizer which displays the

instrument location on reformatted and triplanar CT images. Several authors have evaluated the utility of this stereotactic system in neurotologic skull base surgery and in endoscopic sinus surgery.[2,5,6] Metson and colleagues reviewed 754 consecutive patients undergoing CGES by 34 physicians using the LandmarX system (Xomed, Inc., Jacksonville, FL). This is a wandless, frameless system that does not require fiducial or headset placement for the preoperative CT scan. The mean accuracy of anatomical localization at the beginning of surgery was 1.69 ± 0.38 mm when five anatomical fiducials were used in the registration process. The use of the image-guidance system was estimated to increase operating room time by 15 to 30 minutes for the first five cases each surgeon performed. With experience, surgeons required only 5 to 15 minutes setup time. There were no intraoperative complications although there were three patients experienced epistaxis that occurred within one week after the operation. The epistaxis was not thought to be related to CGES. The mean follow-up was 15 months. A questionnaire was also completed by the surgeons who used the system. The most common situation in which CGES was utilized was after revision sinus surgery. The major reported disadvantage was increased operating room time (71%), and the major advantage was an increased level of confidence during surgery (85%). The overall use of this system was rated either "easy" (31.8%) or "very easy" (50%) by the surgeons. In addition, most surgeons (92%) anticipated continued use at the same or increased frequency. The authors conclude that optical-based CGES can be successfully integrated into a busy operating room environment used by multiple sinus surgeons. In addition, when properly used, it may extend the limits of safe and effective sinus surgery, especially in patients with distorted landmarks.[7]

Computer-Guided Endoscopic Sinus Surgery: Indications

Endoscopic sinus surgery is a viable option for the management of medically refractory sinonasal inflammatory disease, neoplasms, and skull base defects. However, frequently, the anatomy has been distorted by previous surgery or the disease process. In addition, bleeding in severe sinonasal inflammation or some neoplasms, bleeding can obscure the surgeon's visualization. This can make thorough removal of diseased tissue difficult and potentially hazardous. Given the close proximity of vital structures including the intracranial contents and orbit, even minimal intraoperative disorientation can result in serious complications. In an attempt to improve the safety and efficacy of the endoscopic approach to sinonasal disease, image-guidance systems have been developed. Several authors have reviewed their experience with the different types of image-guidance systems; however, it is still unclear from the current published literature if computer-guided endoscopic sinus surgery (CGESS) accomplishes these goals.

The ideal image-guidance system allows for correlation of the patient's anatomy with the CT image to 2 mm or less. Additionally, intraoperative head movement should not affect the accuracy of the system. Other favorable characteristics include a frameless, wandless system, ease of setup and use, and lack of need for skin fiducial placement. There are several drawbacks to using the skin fiducial method, including the need for placement of the fiducials and the CT scan the day before the operation. In addition, the fiducials may fall off or may move after the patient is anesthetized and the facial musculature relaxes.

Metson and colleagues reviewed their experience with both optical- and electromagnetic-based systems in 79 patients.[8] Both systems provided an accuracy of <2 mm at the start of the operation. However, by the completion of the operation, accuracy had deteriorated by an average of 0.89 mm due to anatomical drift. Even at this accuracy level the authors thought both systems were useful. This is because, when properly used, image-guidance systems should be used to identify larger and not to distinguish margins of safety at a millimeter level. Disadvantages of the system include increased operating room time and expense. CGESS increased the mean total operating room time by 17.4 minutes. However, the actual operating time was not prolonged since the time required to set up, calibrate, and register the system was carried out before the start of the operation. In addition, the time represented a mean, and once operating room personnel became familiar with the system this value was reduced to less than 10 minutes. With regard to expense, the authors calculated that use of CGESS increased total charges by $496 per operation due to the increased operating room time. Because of the increased time and expense associated with CGESS, the authors do not recommend it for routine head and neck cases.

Current indications for image-guided sinus surgery (IGSS) are as follows:

1. Revision sinus surgery.
2. Distorted sinus anatomy of developmental, postoperative, or traumatic origin.
3. Extensive sinonasal polyposis.
4. Pathology involving the frontal, posterior ethmoid, or sphenoid sinuses.
5. Disease abutting the skull base, orbit, optic nerve, or carotid artery.
6. CSF rhinorrhea or conditions where there is a skull-base defect.
7. Benign and malignant sinonasal neoplasms.

("Intraoperative use of computer-aided surgery: AAO-HNS Policy on Intraoperative use of computer-aided surgery," American Academy of Otolaryngology—Head and Neck Surgery).

Several articles have been published since the introduction of the technology in the 1990s; however, to date, there is limited evidence that the intraoperative use of IGSS reduces complications and/or improves clinical outcomes. Recently, a systematic review of the evidence-based literature was performed to address these issues.[9] The authors concluded that randomized clinical trials of IGSS are not practical, ethical, or feasible and that clinical experience, expert opinion, and case series support the current indications for IGSS. In addition, studies designed to draw conclusions regarding the role of IGSS in decreasing major complications are not possible.

At the Medical College of Wisconsin, an optical-based, computerized image-guidance system (Stealth with LandmarX software) is set up, calibrated, and registered as follows.[10] The patient undergoes a preoperative image-guided CT scan without fiducials. During the induction of anesthesia, the system is set up and the CT data are loaded onto the computer. Once the patient is asleep, topical decongestants are placed in the sinonasal cavity. While waiting for decongestion to occur, the image-guided headset is placed. The patient is subsequently prepped and draped. The endoscopes and instrumentation is set up and local anesthetic (1% lidocaine, 1:100,000 epinephrine) is injected into the side to be operated on first. While allowing vasoconstriction to occur, the registration is carried out using the tracer contour technique which takes less than a minute.

Once accurate registration is obtained (<2 mm), CGESS commences. In most cases, this takes less than 2 minutes to accomplish, and we still wait another 3 to 5 minutes for vasoconstriction. Thus, although it could be argued this process adds to operating room time, it is substantially less than 5 minutes of net additional time.

We have found the system to be most useful in cases requiring frontal sinus ventilation, revision surgery, repair of skull base defects, and resection of sinonasal neoplasms.[10] The instrumentation, which can currently be integrated, is particularly useful in the endoscopic approach to the frontal sinus. CGESS should be viewed as a means to help identify spaces within the sinonasal cavity, not to measure millimeter increments (Figures 1 and 2). In addition, it is not a replacement for sound surgical technique, anatomic knowledge, and experience.

SURGICAL SIMULATORS

Simulation is becoming accepted in the surgical community as an alternative in surgical skill training. In large part, this trend evoked due to the large number of medical errors identified in the Institute of Medicine's report entitled *To Err Is Human: Building a Safer Health System.* This publication estimated that between 44,000 and 98,000 patients die as a result of medical errors annually. One of the mechanisms cited by the authors to reduce medical errors is to incorporate simulation into surgical training.[11]

In addition to "learning by doing," cadaveric and live animal dissections and procedures have been historically utilized to facilitate surgical development; however, limitations on the availability of these resources (as well as cost) limit these as long-term solutions. In addition, they may not represent the best models for many types of human surgery and techniques.[12] Computer simulation has been used successfully in other fields for pilot and astronaut training, in military exercises, and for nuclear power plant operations training. Although the initial costs may be larger, the long-term costs may be less than those associated with the more traditional training methods noted above. Advantages of simulation include the reality that there is no risk to patients, it is always available, tasks can be practiced repeatedly without concern for materials or cost, and the potential for objective monitoring of surgeon proficiency and progress exists.

Endoscopic sinus surgery has become the treatment of choice for those patients who fail medical therapy for chronic rhinosinusitis. While conceptually quite simple, performing endoscopic sinus surgery safely and effectively is quite challenging.[13] Successful completion of endoscopic sinus procedures depends on a detailed knowledge of the relevant anatomy, as well as the ability to effectively manipulate the endoscope and instruments within the tight confines of the nose and paranasal sinuses. Furthermore, the close proximity of several vital structures including the brain, orbit, and internal carotid artery adds to the difficulty. These procedures require coordination of the endoscopes with the surgical instruments in a three-dimensional (3-D) space which requires the development of complex ambidextrous perceptual, visuospatial, and psychomotor skills for which virtual reality simulators are gaining acceptance as means of training.[14] This skill set is quite different than that needed to perform open surgical procedures.

The endoscopic sinus surgery simulator (ES3) was developed by Lockheed Martin Corporation and has been investigated as an adjunctive training tool in otolaryngology residency programs. Glaser and colleagues demonstrated that the ES3 provided medical students with significant subjective training benefits as well as objectively measured performance benefits.[15] Thus, they concluded that the ES3 holds much promise as a training tool in the development of endoscopic sinus surgery skills. Further development

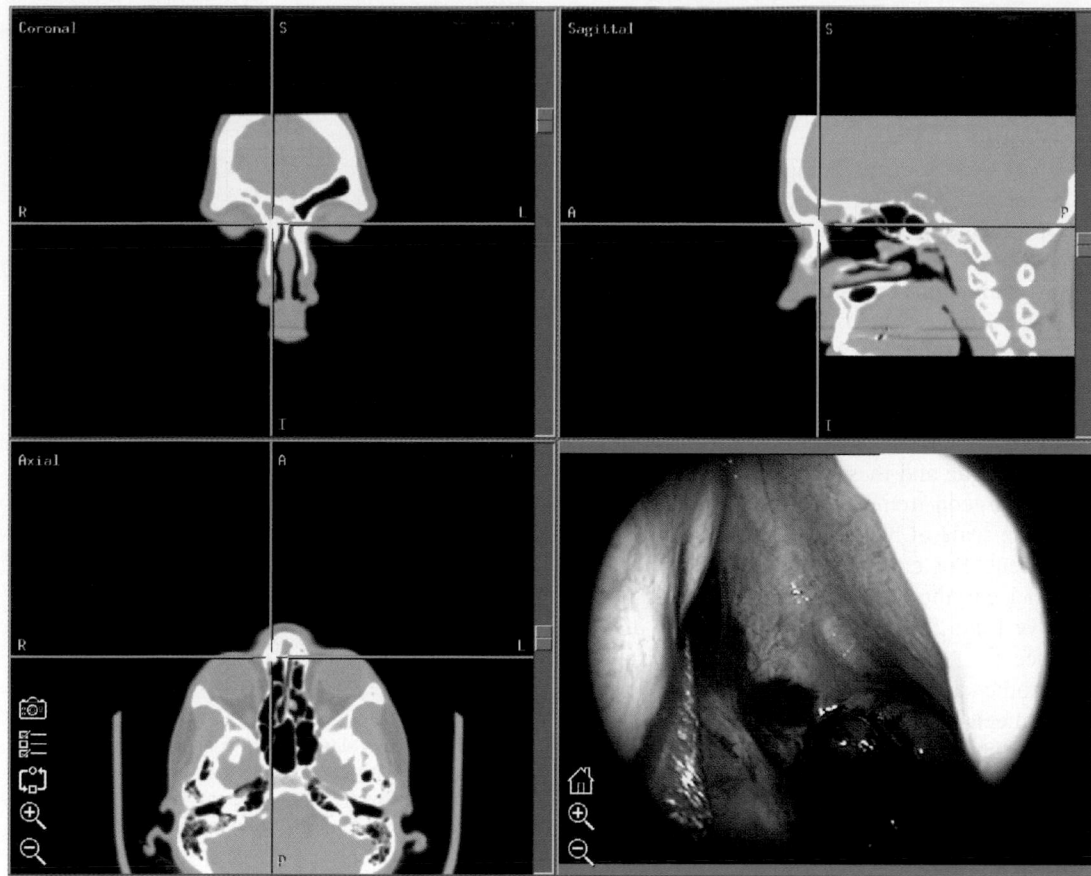

Figure 1 Patient with history of extensive endoscopic sinus surgery with resection of the middle turbinate and subsequent stenosis of right frontal sinus outflow tract. Note how image guidance is utilized to confirm the surgeon's location with regard to the skull base, orbit, and frontal sinus outflow. The image-guidance findings must be correlated with all available anatomic landmarks.

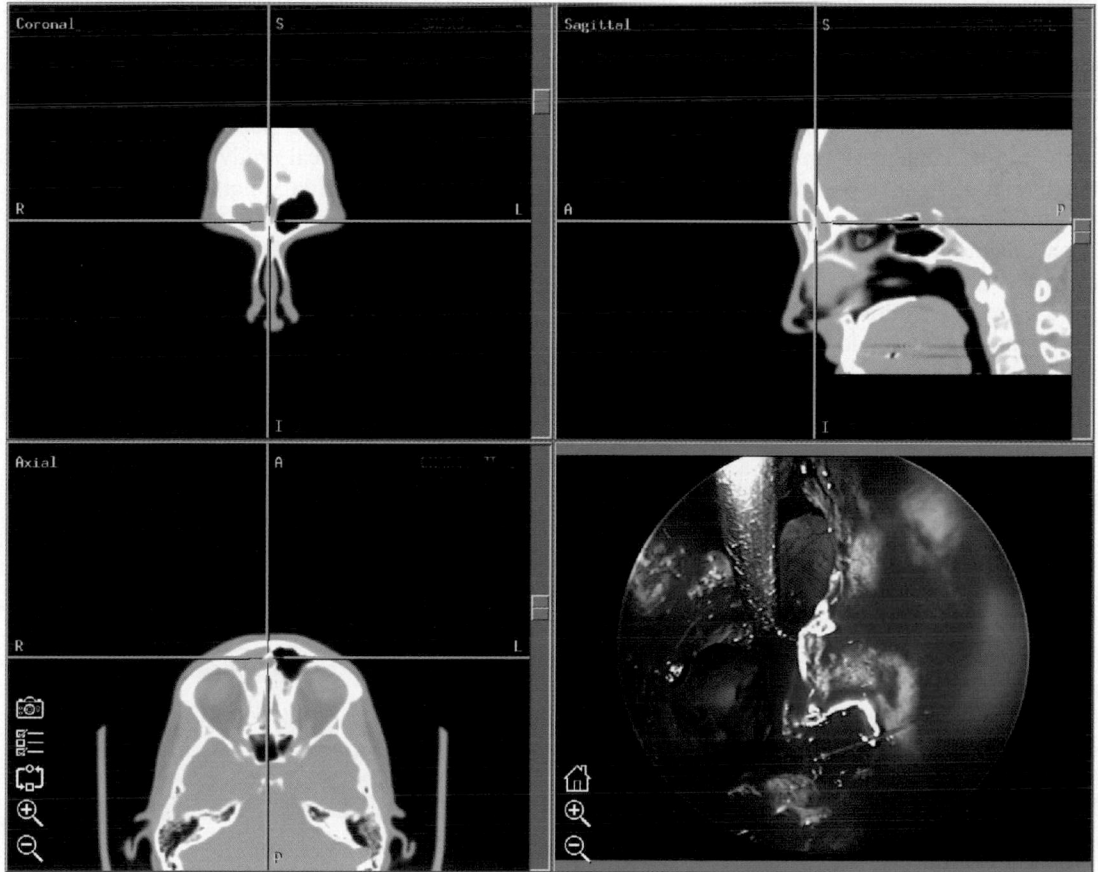

Figure 2 Same patient shown in Figure 1 after endoscopic frontal sinusotomy (Draf Type IIb) is completed. Note location of probe and correlation with anatomic landmarks.

of ES3s will hopefully decrease the initial costs as well as enhance the virtual reality experience necessary to develop endoscopic sinus surgery skills.

Simulators have also been developed for use in temporal bone dissection and airway management. A virtual temporal bone dissection environment has been developed utilizing high-resolution, multimodal, and multiscale data sets. These data sets are then used to create visual, haptic, and auditory interfaces. This system allows the development of an environment in which temporal bone surgery can be learned in a way similar to that experienced with cadaver material. Eventually such technology may be available over the Internet.[16] Simulators have also been developed as an assessment tool for resident airway management skills.[17] Utilizing manikins, the residents were asked to manage two pediatric airway emergency cases. The authors conclude that medical simulation is useful for assessing individuals' technical skills, that is, intubation, as well as related knowledge base.

ROBOTIC SURGERY

A robot can be defined as "a mechanical device that is controlled using a computer system."[18] Over the past decade, robotic surgery had transitioned from science fiction to common practice.[18] Recently, systems have been developed for use with laparoscopic, open, and percutaneous surgical procedures. This type of device overcomes limitations that occur with a human assistant such as fatigue, tremor, and miscommunications between the surgeon and assistant. In addition, robotic systems add precision and help to improve visualization. Finally, robotics allows for telesurgery, in which a surgeon can operate at a location remote from the patient.

There are multiple types of robotic systems which will be described. With continued engineering advancements, the devices continue to evolve, with different ones designed to achieve a variety of surgical goals. Some are intended for an assistant's role, some are designed to perform a procedure autonomously, and some are designed to be a conduit between the surgeon and the patient.

Although many robotic devices exist with a variety of intended applications, they can be separated into two general categories: offline and online systems. Offline robots are programmed to perform an entire procedure without using direct human interaction.[18] This includes an orthopedic device, RoboDoc (Integrated Surgical Systems, Davis, CA), which once calibrated, performs bone drilling necessary for insertion of knee and hip replacements. This has been shown to drill more accurately than manual drilling.[19,20] Another offline system is MrBot, a device created for transperineal MRI-guided placement of radioactive seeds for prostate brachytherapy (Johns Hopkins University, Baltimore, MD). Another offline system is a device called the PAKY-RCM (Percutaneous Access to Kidney-Remote Center of Motion) (Johns Hopkins University, Baltimore, MD) for obtaining intrarenal access for percutaneous stone treatment. A radiotherapeutic device being used with increasing prevalence is the Cyberknife (Sunnyvale CA), which allows a robotic arm to deliver radiation from a linear accelerator to a specific lesion in the body from numerous different vectors based upon image guidance.[19,21] With each of these described systems, the robot is calibrated with coordinates, usually employing image guidance. Once calibrated, the robotic system performs an autonomous task which is monitored by the surgeon and can be halted if there is concern of an untoward event.[20]

Online systems differ in that the surgeon has complete control over the device at all times.[1] One such device that has been in use for the past decade is the AESOP, an acronym for Automated Endoscopic System for Optimal Positioning (Computer Motion, Goleta, CA).[18] This is a remote controlled robotic arm which holds the camera during laparoscopic procedures. It can be manipulated by voice-activation, a foot pedal, or a handheld joystick. In the absence of surgeon commands, this device remains in a static position.

Recently, more complex online systems have been utilized with increasing frequency. These are "master/slave" telemanipulator systems. This consists of a "master" surgeon console where the operating surgeon sits and uses hand, foot, or voice controls to manipulate surgical instruments.[20] The slave is the apparatus docked to the patient. This portion consists of robotic arms that contain and manipulate surgical instruments and an endoscopic camera. Hand controls are present at the master console and are used to manipulate the instruments using remotes.

Two systems have been developed to accomplish this and both have received FDA approval for general surgical applications.[19,22] These systems, Zeus and da Vinci, were developed by separate companies which have since merged. Production of the Zeus system has been discontinued in favor of the da Vinci although existing machines are still in use. With Zeus (Computer Motion, Goleta, CA), the slave device consists of two robotic arms manipulated by the hand controls, containing the surgical instruments. The third arm is an AESOP device which controls the camera. Three-dimensional visualization is possible when polarizing glasses are used. All three of the arms are attached to the patient's bed; and, therefore, when the position of the bed is altered, all robotic arms remain in a constant location relative to the patient.

The second master/slave device is the da Vinci robot (Intuitive Surgical, Sunnyvale, CA). This consists of a master console and a bedside slave. With this system, there are three or four arms (depending upon the model) mounted on a central surgical cart. These consist of one arm which manipulates a 3-D camera and two or three arms which contain and manipulate interchange-

able instruments. All of these robotic arms are docked to the patient. Since the slave apparatus is separate from the bed, the bed position cannot be manipulated once the robotic arms are docked to the patient.

There are both advantages and limitations of currently available robotic systems. They are able to overcome constraints inherent to human surgery. For instance, offline robots allow for preprogrammed, accurately reproducible interventions. These systems can be highly precise. For instance, the MrBot, an MRI-compatible offline robot has been shown to place brachytherapy seeds to an accuracy of within 0.652 mm.[23] Online robots avoid loss of dexterity caused by human fatigue and they have the capacity to filter out surgeon tremor by allowing the surgeon to set the scale of hand movement to instrument movement. For example, if the hand control is moved 1 cm, the robot can scale the instruments to move 1 cm, 5 mm, or a smaller fraction of that distance.

Another advantage is the dexterity afforded by the mechanical properties of the robotic surgical instruments. Da Vinci instruments are currently manufactured in 5 and 8 mm diameter and they allow manipulation with 7° of freedom. This contrasts with the Zeus system which allows 5° of freedom.[19,22,24] Of great benefit is the fact that the distal ends of the instruments articulate and provide the instrument with the same motion as that of a human wrist. This enables the surgeon to articulate the instrument around corners in difficult-to-reach small spaces a long distance from the incision or port site. With regard to laparoscopic surgical procedures, this increases dexterity compared with traditional instruments because there are 7° of freedom as opposed to 4 with the traditional laparoscopic instruments. This accelerates the learning curve compared with traditional laparoscopic procedures since the instruments and the controls simulate the idea that the instruments are an extension of the surgeon's hands. The console is constructed in such a manner so that the surgeon is able to operate from a seated position with the hand controls in an optimal ergonomic location.[24,25]

Figures 3 through 6 illustrate the da Vinci Surgical System. Pictured are the surgeon console (master), the bedside robotic device (slave) with attached robotic arms, and a wristed instrument with 7° of freedom.

Visualization with online robotic systems is also advantageous. With the da Vinci surgical system, the camera is a high-resolution, 3-D system. This is made possible by having two cameras present in a single instrument. Feedback from these is routed through a binocular viewing screen present in the surgeon console. Additionally, the slave cart is constructed so that the camera is initially aligned in the center of the operative field so that proprioception regarding left/right and forward/backward is maintained. This allows the surgeon to have the operative field of view aligned directly with the instruments that are being manipulated.

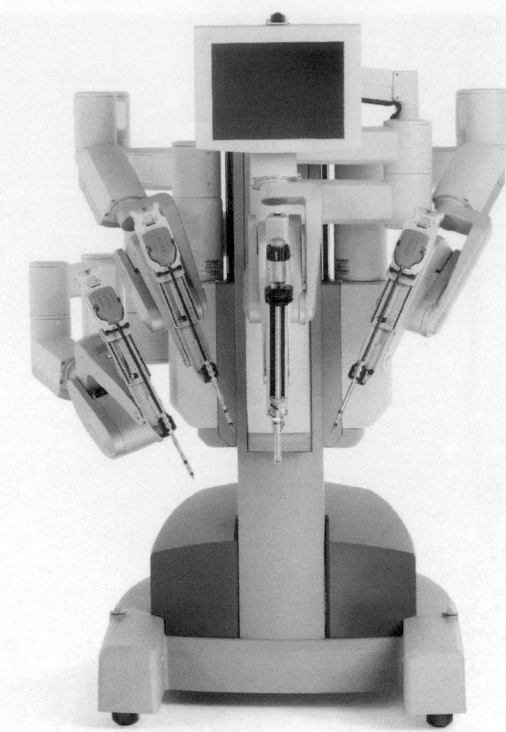

Figure 3 Da Vinci slave patient console with four robotic arms containing three surgical instruments in the three lateral arms as well as the camera in the central arm. (Reprinted with permission from Intuitive Surgical, Inc., Sunnyvale, CA.)

Many surgical procedures have been accomplished using the da Vinci robot. Radical prostatectomies, nephrectomies, pyeloplasties, coronary artery bypass, uterine fibroid excisions, mitral valve replacement, gastric bypass, cholecystectomies, and even supraglottic partial laryngectomies have been performed (www.intuitivesurgical.com).[20,24–26] Suturing with the da Vinci robot has a faster learning curve than with conventional laparoscopy.[16] Most of these procedures have shorter convalescence periods when compared with the open surgical equivalent. Blood loss is also less with some da Vinci surgical procedures

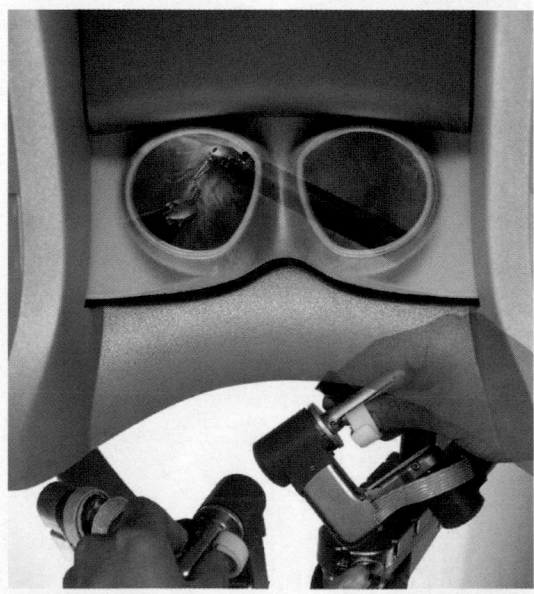

Figure 4 Da Vinci master console. Note hand controls and built in binocular monitor allowing 3-D visualization. (Reprinted with permission from Intuitive Surgical, Inc., Sunnyvale, CA.)

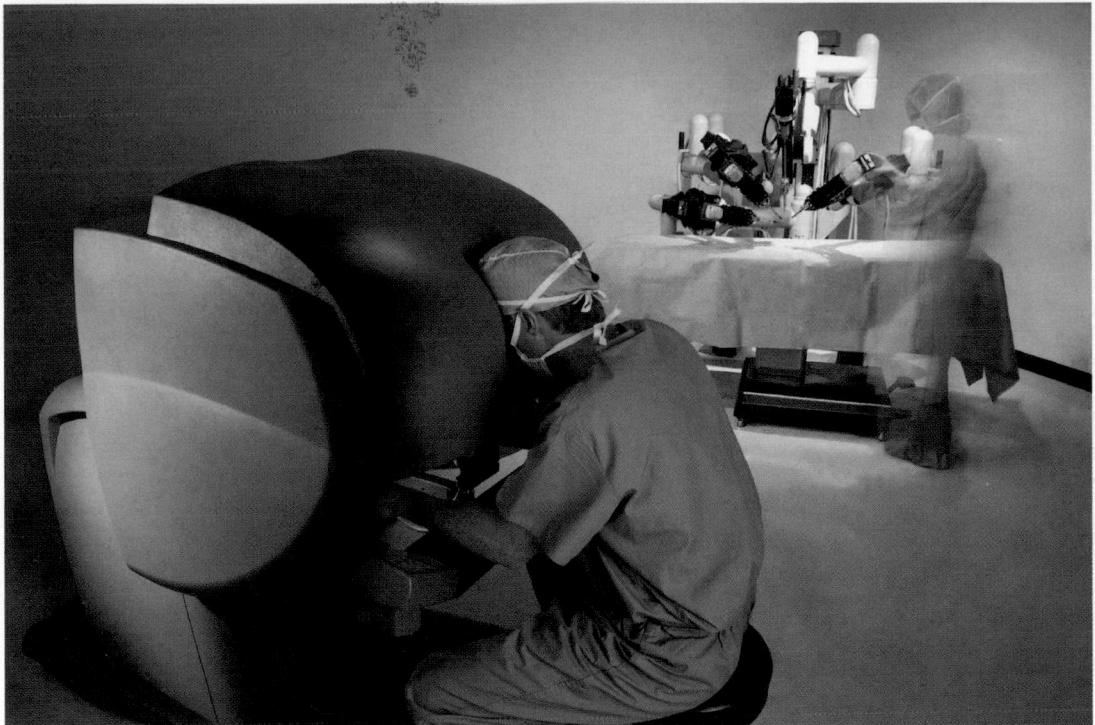

Figure 5 Da Vinci surgical system with the surgeon manipulating the robotic instruments at the slave cart by moving the hand and foot controls at the master console. (Reprinted with permission from Intuitive Surgical, Inc., Sunnyvale, CA.)

such as radical prostatectomies compared with traditional open surgical procedures.[27–29]

One of the original reasons why robotic surgery was developed was for telesurgery, where the surgeon is able to operate on a patient from a remote location. The intent at the time of the earliest research and development was for battle field applications so that injured soldiers could undergo emergent surgical intervention in an armored vehicle with the robotic instruments controlled by a surgeon at a more secure location.[30] Multiple transcontinental telesurgical procedures have indeed been performed including

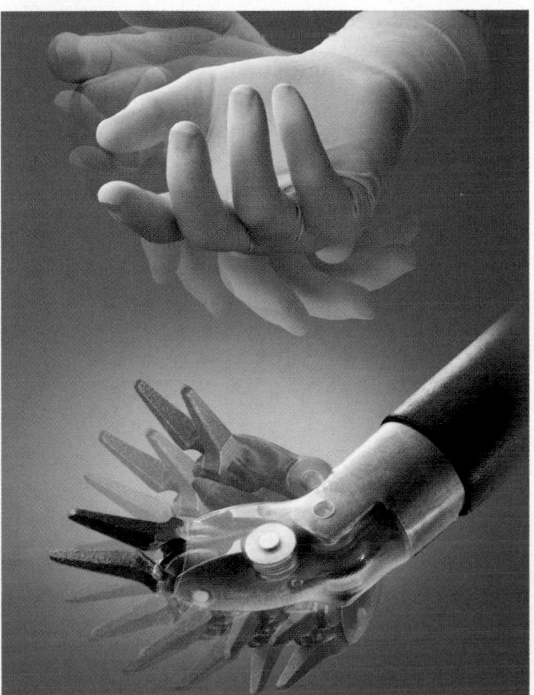

Figure 6 Note the wrist-like maneuverability of the da Vinci surgical instruments. (Reprinted with permission from Intuitive Surgical, Inc., Sunnyvale, CA.)

a laparoscopic cholecystectomy and obtaining percutaneous renal access for treatment of nephrolithiasis. This allows the potential for an experienced surgeon to mentor others or to prevent or repair surgical errors from a remote location. Also, robots allow surgeons to avoid or minimize exposure to radiation or other hazardous materials since they can often manipulate the robotic devices at a safe distance from the patient.[23]

There are several disadvantages of robotic surgery which bear discussion. Presently, the technology is expensive. The cost of the robot ranges from $1.12 to $1.65 million with an annual maintenance fee ranging from $109,000 to $165,000 depending upon the specific da Vinci model (Intuitive Surgical, February, 2007 price list). The instruments used have a limited number of uses, usually 10 uses before they need to be discarded. They generally cost from $200 to $320 per instrument per use (often five instruments per case are used). One likely contributing factor to the present high cost is the paucity of competition in the market place. Several competing companies are currently in the process of developing telerobotic systems, and it is possible that in the future this may lead to improved cost containment.

Extent of operating room time and space utilization are also potential considerations. Considering the different stages of procedures such as setting up the robot and docking it to the patient, operating room time increases. With master/slave robot systems, the setup time is substantial, and there is significant training involved for the operating room staff being able to set up the robot. Setup times and surgical times do, however, improve with experience. Also, often additional space in the operating room needs to be dedicated to storing the robot.

There are other logistical issues unique to robotic surgery that can add some adversity. For instance, the smallest instruments currently available for the da Vinci robot are 5 mm in diameter and additional miniaturization may be needed to facilitate microsurgical procedures within a confined space such as the oropharynx. Another disadvantage with the master/slave device is that the surgeon is not part of the sterile field and is therefore reliant upon the assistant to change instruments contained within the robotic arms. If there is a sudden and unexpected change within the operative field such as arterial bleeding which cannot be controlled robotically, the surgeon is dependent upon the assistant at the patient's bedside until he or she is able to scrub in for portions of the surgery which may be safest performed without using the robotic slave component.

Although there are currently ongoing projects to improve this, robotic devices currently also lack haptic feedback. Particularly with novice surgeons, it is possible to break sutures when tying knots or to crush or tear tissue because one must rely solely on visual cues to assess for how hard one is pulling on or pinching a suture or bit of tissue. With additional practice, surgeons are able to adapt to visual feedback as opposed to haptic feedback.

Robotic surgery may represent an ongoing paradigm shift in surgical practice. The available technology will continue to improve, making robotic surgery easier and likely more affordable in the future. This technology will continually broaden in its applicability. With respect to otorhinolaryngologic applications, progressive miniaturization will be advantageous for extirpative and reconstructive procedures which are presently difficult to accomplish with handheld instrumentation.

As has been described previously in this chapter, there are inherent advantages of robotic surgical technology including its tremendous 3-D visualization, the ability to finely scale instrument motion, its filtration of hand tremor, and the small and versatile end-effector instrumentation that allows one to operate in confined spaces in a manner similar to open surgery.

Transoral Robotic Surgery

The development and application of transoral robotic surgery (TORS) have followed transoral laser microsurgery which has gained limited popularity over the past 5 years. There are certain factors that may have hindered the widespread use of endoscopic laser microsurgery that may be overcome with TORS. One of the basic disadvantages is the well-recognized steep learning curve associated with transoral microsurgical procedures. The surgeon typically sits at arms length from the patient's oropharynx and larynx while looking through the microscope. This operative configuration requires the use of long instruments that have an inherent fulcrum effect. This fulcrum effect results in the tip of the instrument moving in the opposite direction

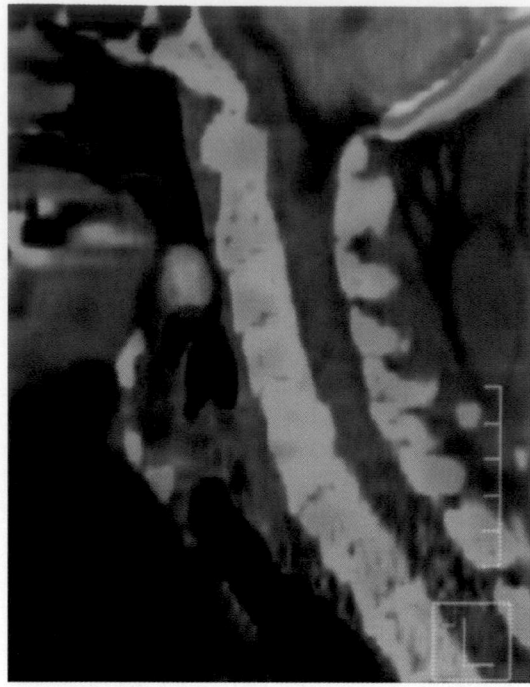

(A)

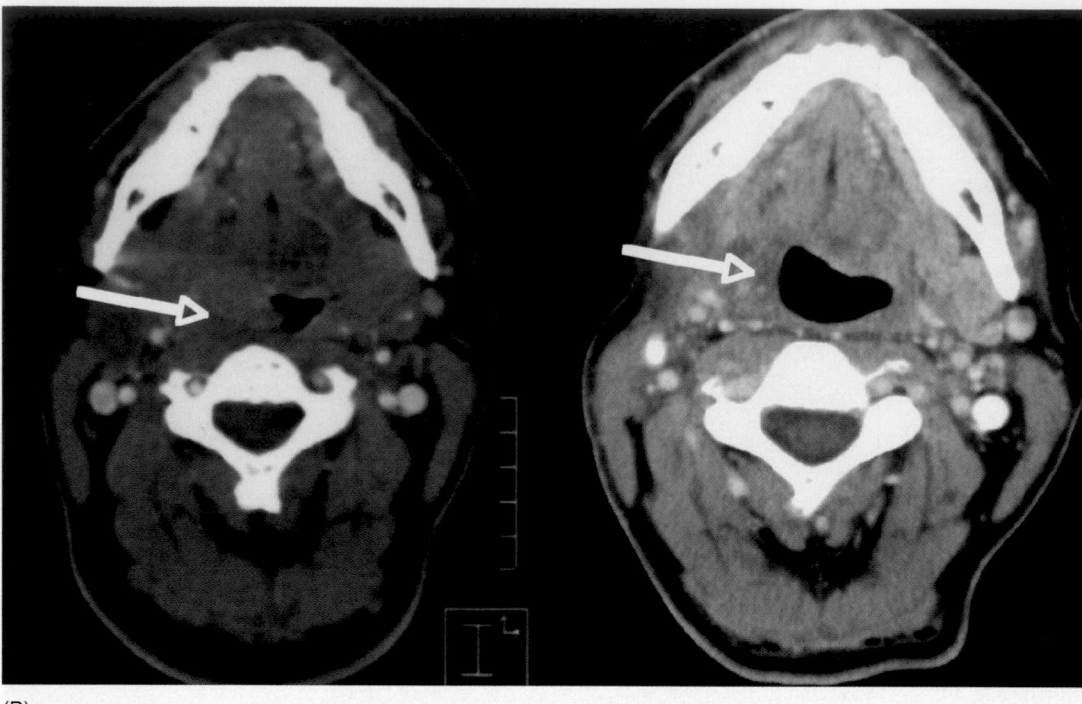

(B)

Figure 7 (A) Preoperative fused positron emission tomography/computed tomography (PET/CT) sagittal section of a T2 squamous cell carcinoma of the right side of the base of the tongue. (B) Preoperative CT with right T2 squamous cell carcinoma (left, *arrow*) and postoperative CT scan at approximately 6 months showing the surgical defect and no evidence of tumor (right, *arrow*). (Published with permission, copyright © 2007 B.W. O'Malley Jr, MD and G. Weinstein, MD).

of the hand movements, and small movements of the surgeon's hand translate into much larger movements at the instrument tip. In addition, small hand tremors are further magnified through the optics of the operating microscope. Also, the tips of the classic endoscopic oropharyngeal and laryngeal instruments are fixed, and this lack of rotation or wristed movement limits the actual surgery and does not allow more advanced techniques such as suturing. Overall, these disadvantages that are inherent to conventional transoral or endoscopic microsurgery are for the most part eliminated with the evolving robotic technology.

Pioneering work with TORS in preclinical and early human evaluation has established its feasibility for oropharynx and supraglottic procedures while providing principles for exposure and patient safety.[31–35] While it is still early in the human clinical trial experience with TORS, for base of tongue cancers, O'Malley and Weinstein (unpublished data) are successfully resecting T1 to T3 cancers to negative margins with excellent postoperative healing and speech and swallowing results (Figure 7). The following sections will discuss some key operating room setup and technical principles for TORS procedures ranging from the larynx to nasopharynx.

Basic Operating Room Setup. For TORS, the operating suite configuration and robot position varies significantly as compared to the typical abdominal and pelvic robotic procedures where the patient's head is situated toward the anesthesiologist and the robot is aligned perpendicular to the long axis of the patient. For transoral work, this setup would not allow access and robotic arm alignment. In TORS, the patient's head is rotated 180° away from the anesthesiologist and the robot is introduced at approximately 30 to 45° angle to

the long axis of the patient (Figure 8). The operating console is placed in the corner of the operating suite with a clear path for the surgeon to reach the patient's head should this be required.

Surgical Exposure. The surgical exposure for TORS differs from conventional endoscopic microsurgery of the larynx and pharynx in that the robotic instruments are not introduced through a standard closed tube or even a bivalved laryngoscope. Standard closed tube or even bivalved laryngoscopes do not provide sufficient space anterior to posterior and lateral to introduce the high-magnification, 3-D endoscopic camera and the two or even three end-effector robotic instruments. For TORS, either the standard Crowe–Davis retractor (Figure 9) or the FK retractor (Figure 10) are used to provide access to the tonsil, base of tongue, supraglottis,

glottis, and even the pyriform sinus. For the majority of procedures, once the Crowe–Davis or FK retractor is placed, further repositioning is not required. Upon adequate retractor positioning and exposure, a 0° or 30° endoscope can be used for excellent visualization depending on the particular operative site. A key advantage of the 30° endoscope is the ability to rotate the endoscope 360° to get angular exposure which significantly aids in anterior and lateral visualization of the anatomy and reduces the need for frequent retractor manipulation that may be required to gain visualization in conventional transoral endoscopic procedures.

Maintaining Hemostasis and Managing Secretions. An important principle to any surgical procedure, but in particular endoscopic procedures, is the maintenance of hemostasis. For

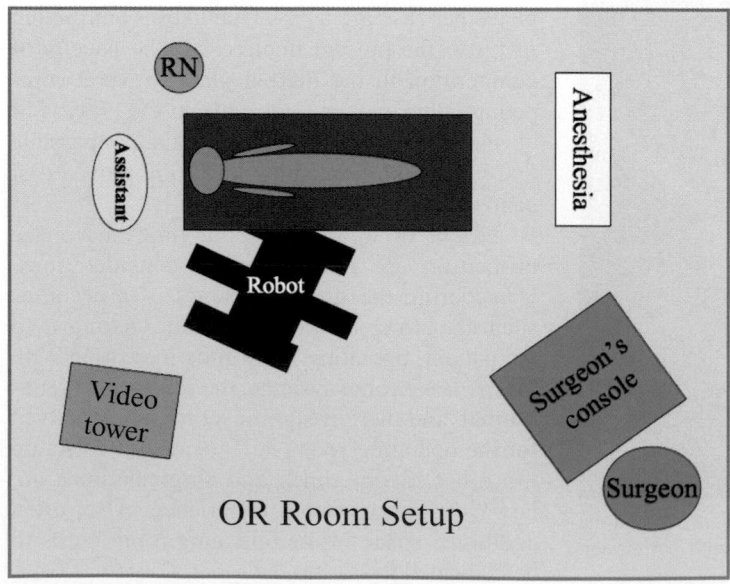

Figure 8 Schematic of the operating room setup for transoral robotic surgery with the operating table rotated 180° away from the anesthesiologist and the robot positioned at 30° relative to the long axis of the patient at the head of the bed. An assistant surgeon sits at the head of the bed as an added measure of safety and to suction smoke, blood, and secretions. (Published with permission, copyright © 2007 B.W. O'Malley Jr, MD and G. Weinstein, MD.)

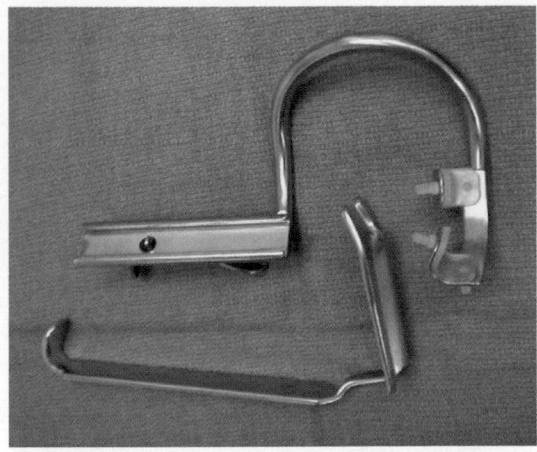

Figure 9 Crowe–Davis mouth retractor used for standard exposure to the tonsil and superior base of the tongue and lateral pharynx for transoral robotic surgery (TORS). (Published with permission, copyright © 2007 B.W. O'Malley Jr, MD and G. Weinstein, MD.)

TORS, one key factor in the ability to achieve hemostasis is the tremendous high magnification and 3-D optics that allow the surgeon to see very tiny tissue vessels prior to transecting them. Also, the typical robotic instruments used are a standard grasper or robotic forceps and a spatula tipped monopolar cautery (Figure 11). The robotic forceps can be used to grasp small vessels or bleeding areas and the spatula cautery used to coagulate the vessels or actual bleeding sites. Furthermore, tissue incision and dissection is performed using either coagulation setting or a blended cutting and coagulation setting on the bovie console. In addition, laryngeal clip appliers or robotic instrument clip appliers can be used to control larger vessels such as the lingual artery and superior thyroid artery. For those who are concerned about using bovie cautery for laryngeal or pharyngeal procedures, the CO_2 or thulium laser can be easily attached to the robotic end-effector instruments. However, there are reports that show electrocautery produces similar tissue injury to that of the carbon dioxide laser, and so this may prove to be an unnecessary concern.[36–39]

Another key factor in TORS is the need for suctioning of secretions, blood, and smoke from the bovie or laser cautery. At present, the da Vinci

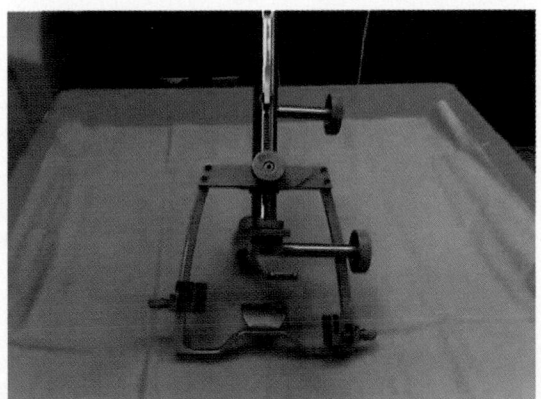

Figure 10 FK retractor used for inferior base of tongue, vallecula, pyriform sinus, supraglottic, and glottic exposure for transoral robotic surgery (TORS). (Published with permission, copyright © 2007 B.W. O'Malley Jr, MD and G. Weinstein, MD.)

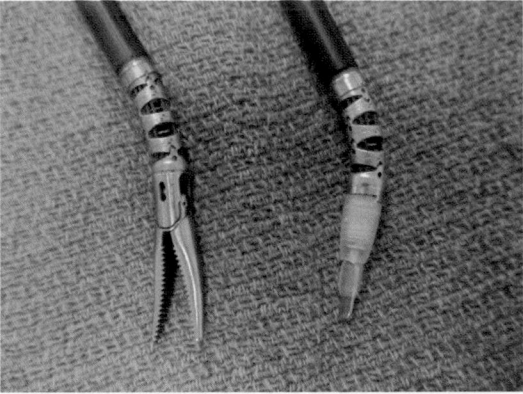

Figure 11 Photograph of the two most commonly used instruments for transoral robotic surgery (TORS), the Maryland 5 mm forceps and the spatula tipped monopolar cautery end effectors. (Published with permission, copyright © 2007 B.W. O'Malley Jr, MD and G. Weinstein, MD.)

surgical robot has no suctioning apparatus or instruments integrated into the system. Therefore, for TORS, a surgical assistant must sit at the head of the bed and use one or two suctioning devices to clear secretions, blood, and smoke. The surgical assistant typically views the anatomy from a flat-screened monitor and directions the suctions accordingly while keeping them out of the line of sight of the endoscopic camera. Although there is a learning curve to suctioning while keeping the suctioning instruments away from the robotic instruments and endoscopic camera, this has not posed an important problem in the clinical procedures performed to date (Weinstein and O'Malley, unpublished).

Safety Concerns. The use of robotic technology for transoral surgery exposes patients to certain risks that are inherent to either positioning of the robot or the manipulation of the instruments. While it is important to acknowledge the potential for patient injury, the safety record of the da Vinci system in thoracoscopic and laparoscopic procedures established a firm background of overall device safety.[40,41] For TORS, specific issues related to instrumentation positioning and transoral placement of the robotic arms include the potential for lip and tooth injuries, nose, face, and ocular injuries, mucosal injuries, and neck or spine injuries. These safety concerns have been addressed in preclinical models with TORS and from unpublished results to date in clinical experimentation (Weinstein and O'Malley, unpublished). Also, for human TORS procedures, safety goggles with malar cushioned safety shields are used for enhanced patient protection (Figure 12).

Future Applications of Transoral Robotic Surgery. It has been the experience of the authors that the excellent 3-D optics and wristed movements of the robotic instruments provide the surgeon with views of the anatomy including vascular and nerve structures that are not possible even with conventional endoscopic microscopy techniques. These key attributes of visualization and instrument mobility are prov-

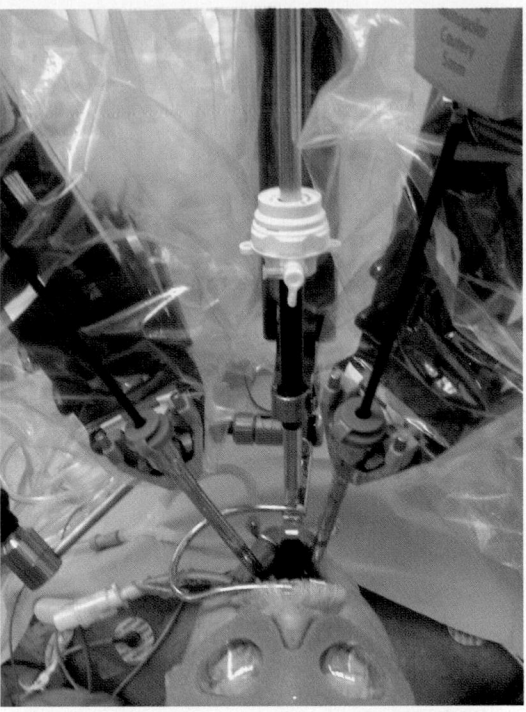

Figure 12 Photograph of a human patient with blue safety goggles that protect the cheeks and eyes during transoral robotic surgery (TORS). Note that the high magnification and 3-D robotic endoscope and two arms with end effector instruments are easily positioned via a transoral approach. (Published with permission, copyright © 2007 B.W. O'Malley Jr, MD and G. Weinstein, MD.)

ing invaluable for manipulating soft tissues and critical structures within the oral cavity, pharynx, and larynx. These key factors of vision and tissue manipulation should allow robotic head and neck surgery to extend well beyond the upper aerodigestive tract and into the retropharynx, parapharynx, neck, and even skull base.

As robotic surgery technology continues to advance and with the design and manufacturing of smaller instrumentation, integrated suctions, and drills, and even the addition of tactile feedback or haptic technology, the opportunities to apply robotic surgery to all aspects of otorhinolaryngology head and neck surgery will surely increase.

REFERENCES

1. Goerss SJ, Kelly PJ, Kall BA, Alker GJ, Jr. A computed tomographic stereotactic adaptation system. Neurosurgery 1982;10:375–9.
2. Anon JB, Lipman SP, Oppenheim D, Holt RA. Computed-assisted endoscopic sinus surgery. Laryngoscope 1994;104:901–5.
3. Casiano RR. Intraoperative image-guidance technology. Arch Otolaryngol Head Neck Surg 1999;125:1275–8.
4. Neumann AM, Pasquale-Niebles K, Bhuta T, Sillers MJ. Image-guided transnasal endoscopic surgery of the paranasal sinuses and anterior skull base. AJR 1999;13:449–54.
5. Sargent EW, Bucholz RD. Middle cranial fossa surgery with image-guided instrumentation. Otolaryngol Head Neck Surg 1997;117:372–9.
6. Goldsmith MM, Bucholz RD, Smith KR, Nitche N. Clinical applications of frameless stereotactic devices in neurotology: Preliminary report. Am J Otol 1995;16:475–9.
7. Metson RB, Cosenza MJ, Cunningham MJ, Randolph GW. Physician experience with an optical image guidance system for sinus surgery. Laryngoscope 2000;110:972–6.
8. Metson R, Cosenza M, Gliklich RE, Montgomery WW. The role of image-guidance in head and neck surgery. Arch Otolaryngol Head Neck Surg 1999;125:1100–4.

9. Smith TL, Stewart MG, Orlandi RR, et al. Indications for image-guided sinus surgery: The current evidence. Am J Rhinol 2007;21:80–3.

10. Loehrl T, Toohill RJ, Smith TL. The use of computer-aided surgery for frontal sinus ventilation. Laryngoscope 2000;110:1962–7.

11. Kohn LT, Corrigan JM, Donaldson MS. To Err is Human: Building a Safer Health System. Washington, DC: National Academy Press; 1999.

12. McCarthy MC, Raninger MR, Nolan DJ, et al. Accuracy of cricothyroidotomy performed in canine and human cadaver models during surgical skills training. J Am Coll Surg 2002;195:627–9.

13. Tendick F, Jennings RW, Tharp G, et al. Sensing and manipulation problems in endoscopic surgery: Experiment, analysis, and observation. Presence 1993;2:66–81.

14. Gallagher AG, McClure N, McGuigan J, et al. Virtual reality training in laparoscopic surgery: A preliminary assessment of minimally invasive surgical trainer virtual reality. Endoscopy 1999;31:310–3.

15. Glaser AY, Hall CB, Uribe JI, Fried MP. Medical students' attitudes toward the use of an endoscopic sinus surgery simulator as a training tool. Am J Rhinol 2006;20:177–9.

16. Wiet GJ, Stredney D, Sessanna D, et al. Virtual temporal bone dissection: An interactive surgical simulator. Otolaryngology Head Neck Surg 2002;127:79–83.

17. Overly FL, Sudikoff SN, Shapiro MJ. High-fidelity medical simulation as an assessment tool for pediatric residents' airway management skills. Pediatr Emerg Care 2007;23:11–15.

18. Kim HL, Schulam P. The PAKY, HERMES, AESOP, ZUES, and da Vinci robotic systems. Urol Clin North Am 2004;31:659–69.

19. Sim HG, Yip SKH, Cheng CWS. Equipment and technology in surgical robotics. World J Urol 2006;24:128–35.

20. Davies B. Robotic devices in surgery. Minim Invasive Ther Allied Technol 2003:12:5–13.

21. Adler JR, Jr, Chang SD, Murphy MJ, et al. The Cyberknife: A frameless robotic system for radiosurgery. Stereotact Funct Neurosurg 1997;69:124–8.

22. Ruurda JP, van Vroonhoven T, Broeders I. Robot-assisted surgical systems: A new era in laparoscopic surgery. Ann R Coll Surg Engl 2002;84:223–6.

23. Cleary K, Melzer A, Watson V, et al. Interventional robotic systems: Applications and technology state-of-the-art. Minim Invasive Ther 2006;15:2;101–13.

24. Sung GT, Gill IS. Robotic laparoscopic surgery: A comparison of the da Vinci and Zeus systems. Urology 2001;58:893–8.

25. Ballantyne GH. Telerobotic gastrointestinal surgery: Phase 2-safety and efficacy. Surg Endosc February 8, 2007.

26. Weinstein GS, O'Malley BW, Jr, Snyder W, Hockstein NG. Transoral robotic surgery: Supraglottic partial laryngectomy. Ann Otol Rhinol Laryngol 2007;116:19–23.

27. El-Hakim A, Leung RA, Tewari A. Robotyic prostatectgomy: A pooled analysis of published literature. Expert Rev Anti Cancer Ther 2006;6:11–20.

28. Farnham SB, Webster TM, Herrell SD, Smith JA, Jr. Intraoperative blood loss and transfusion requirements for robotic-assisted radical prostatectomy versus radical retropubic prostatectomy. Urology 2006;67:360–3.

29. Morgan JA, Peacock JC, Kohmoto T, et al. Robotic techniques improve quality of life in patients undergoing atrial septal defect repair. Ann Thorac Surg 2004;77:1328–33.

30. Satava RM. Robotic surgery: from past to future—a personal journey. Surg Clin N Am 2003;83:1491–1500.

31. Weinstein GS, O'Malley BW, Jr, Hockstein NG. Transoral robotic surgery (TORS): Supraglottic laryngectomy in a canine model. Laryngoscope 2005;115:1315–9.

32. O'Malley BW, Jr, Weinstein GS, Hockstein NG. Transoral robotic surgery (TORS): Glottic microsurgery in a canine model. J Voice 2006;20:263–8.

33. O'Malley BW, Jr, Weinstein GS, Snyder W, Hockstein NG. Transoral robotic surgery (TORS) for base of tongue neoplasms. Laryngoscope 2006;116:1465–72.

34. Hockstein NG, O'Malley BW, Jr, Weinstein GS. Assessment of intraoperative safety in transoral robotic surgery. Laryngoscope 2006;116:165–8.

35. Weinstein GS, O'Malley BW, Jr, Snyder W, Hockstein NG. Transoral robotic surgery: Supraglottic partial laryngectomy. Ann Otol Rhinol Laryngol 2007;116:19–23.

36. Carew JF, Ward RF, LaBruna A, et al. Effects of scalpel, electrocautery, and CO_2 and KTP lasers on wound healing in rat tongues. Laryngoscope 1998;108:373–80.

37. Liboon J, Funkhouser W, Terris DJ. A comparison of mucosal incisions made by scalpel, CO_2 laser, electrocautery, and constant-voltage electrocautery. Otolaryngol Head Neck Surg 1997;116:379–85.

38. Rudert HH, Werner JA, Hoft S. Transoral carbon dioxide laser resection of supraglottic carcinoma. Ann Otol Rhinol Laryngol 1999;108:819–27.

39. Steiner W, Ambrosch P. Endoscopic Laser Surgery of the Upper Aerodigestive Tract. 1 ed. Stuttgart, Germany: Gerg Thieme Verlag; 2000.

40. Menon M, Tewari A, Peabody JO, et al. Vattikuti institute prostatectomy, a technique of robotic radical prostatectomy for management of localized carcinoma of the prostate: Experience of over 1100 cases. Urol Clinics N Am 2004;31:701–17.

41. Tatooles AJ, Pappas PS, Gordon PJ, Slaughter MS. Minimally invasive mitral valve repair using the daVinci robotic system. Ann Thoracic Surg 2004;77:1978–82.

68

Airway Management in the Infant and Child

Michael J. Rutter, MBChB
Robin T. Cotton, MD

An infant or child presenting with acute airway obstruction is an emergency and potentially one of the most challenging patients to manage. However, the fundamentals of airway management, whether acute or chronic, child or adult, remain the same. Therefore, developing a mental algorithm for the management of airway compromise is highly desirable.

Management of neonatal and pediatric airway disease reflects in a large part the evolution in neonatal standards of care. Prolonged intubation of the neonate in the 1960s effectively gave rise to neonatology as we now know it but, as a consequence, resulted in many infants requiring tracheostomy for the "new" disease of pediatric acquired subglottic stenosis. This in turn led to the development of techniques to repair subglottic stenosis, such as laryngotracheal reconstruction. Historically, the majority of these children were normal children with an airway stenosis. Currently, the advent of neonatal nasopharyngeal continuous positive airway pressure (CPAP) has resulted in far fewer neonates requiring prolonged intubation but with this being balanced by the salvage of more infants with extreme prematurity and complex congenital disorders. As a consequence, children presenting to an otolaryngologist with subglottic stenosis increasingly have their airway obstruction as merely one of a list of complex problems.

PRENATAL AIRWAY COMPROMISE

Congenital causes of neonatal airway compromise are usually discovered at birth or in the first few days or weeks following delivery. However, the increasing sophistication of prenatal fetal imaging has resulted in both a greater appreciation and a rising rate of diagnosis of potential causes of neonatal airway obstruction. Sophisticated Doppler ultrasound and fetal magnetic resonance imaging (MRI) may reveal cervicofacial pathology with the potential to cause acute airway compromise on delivery or in the neonatal period. These may be divided into three main groups, namely massive cervical tumors such as lymphatic malformations or teratoma (Figure 1), severe mandibular hypoplasia, and atresia of the larynx or trachea with complete neonatal airway occlusion. This latter condition is known as the congenital high airway obstructive syndrome (CHAOS) and

occurs in association with polyhydramnios, lung hyperexpansion with everted diaphragms and prune-belly syndrome.[1] Frequently, fetal hydrops may be seen in association with this. In some rare cases, complete upper airway obstruction may not result in the secondary features of CHAOS because of airway decompression through a tracheoesophageal fistula, and in some of these cases esophageal intubation at the time of delivery may allow fetal oxygenation and ventilation through the tracheoesophageal fistula until such time as the airway can be secured.

In any of the above conditions, if the fetus has impaired swallowing due to the nature of the disease, polyhydramnios may also be noted with a predisposition to premature delivery.

In pregnancies, in which fetal airway compromise at delivery is anticipated, fetal salvage may be achievable through use of the ex-utero intrapartum treatment (EXIT) procedure as originally described by Harrison and colleagues[2] While there are differing techniques for achieving the same end, the intent is that the fetal airway is secured while the fetus is still oxygenated by the placental circulation. One of the two most commonly used techniques is the EXIT procedure with the mother and fetus fully anesthetized and with a caesarean section exposing the head and one arm of the fetus while maintaining the bulk of the fetus and as much amniotic fluid as possible within the uterus to prevent placental abruption.[3] This technique has the advantage of allowing time, up to 60 minutes of placental circulation, in which the airway may be secured. However, the disadvantages are that the fetus is fully anesthetized and, therefore, unable to maintain its own airway should this be an option and that access to

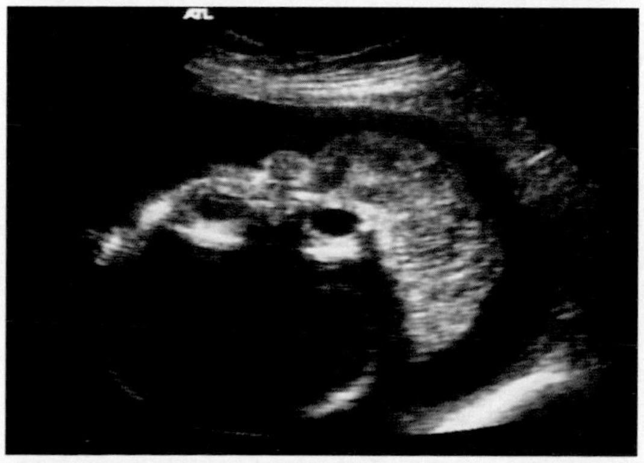

Figure 1 Prenatal ultrasound of a cervicofacial teratoma.

the fetus is suboptimal as only part of the fetus is exposed to the surgeon securing the airway.

The second technique is for the caesarean section to be performed under spinal anesthesia, so that both the mother and fetus are awake and, therefore, the fetus has the potential to maintain its own airway if this is possible.[4] The whole fetus is delivered through the caesarean section still attached to the umbilical cord and laid on a tray on the mother's thighs while the airway is secured. The advantages of this technique are that the fetus may be able to maintain its own airway and breathe spontaneously, and if the airway does need to be secured, access to the infant's airway is optimal. However, the significant disadvantage is that, as the uterus has effectively been evacuated, the placenta will abrupt usually within 5 minutes as the empty uterus contracts, limiting the available time to secure the airway. These interventions are complex, teamwork is essential to achieving a good outcome, and, therefore, the best results are usually obtained in the small number of institutes with a tertiary care fetal therapeutics unit. Needless to say, securing the airway is not the end point for management of the neonatal airway under these circumstances, but rather the commencement of a cascade of intervention designed to both maintain a safe and secure airway while managing the underlying disease process that necessitated an EXIT procedure. Often these children may be intubated at delivery, but this is usually an inherently unstable airway because of the difficulty of intubation; and, therefore, conversion to tracheostomy is usually required once the infant has been otherwise stabilized.

EVALUATION OF THE COMPROMISED NEONATAL AIRWAY

The signs and symptoms of airway compromise in the neonatal period reflect not only the severity of the obstruction but also the level of obstruction. Therefore, it is useful to subdivide the presenting signs of airway compromise into nasal, pharyngeal, laryngeal, and tracheal.

Neonatal Nasal Obstruction

The neonate is an obligate nasal breather for the first 6 weeks of life; and, therefore, nasal obstruction may present with life-threatening airway compromise. Presentation may be with life-threatening apnea, usually when sleeping or quietly resting. However, an excellent airway is maintained when upset and crying due to transoral respiration. Whereas traditionally evaluation of airway compromise in the neonate has involved evaluation of the ability to pass a 6 French suction catheter or seeing whether a mirror will mist on an expiratory breath through the nose, the cornerstone of evaluation currently is flexible nasopharyngoscopy and laryngoscopy using a small flexible endoscope placed through the nose. This is complemented by the use of computed tomography (CT) scanning which is the radiological study of choice.

Pharyngeal Airway Compromise

Compromise of the pharyngeal airway, whether due to tumor, pharyngomalacia, glossoptosis, or supralaryngeal cysts, usually presents with stertor rather than stridor (higher pitched) and with the compromise being most marked during sleep or when the child is supine. Dependent upon the pathology, symptoms may be markedly worse in certain positions, and presentation may include apnea, cyanosis, retractions, and "dying" spells. If there is significant mass effect in the supralaryngeal pharynx, the cry may be muffled.

Laryngeal Airway Compromise

Supraglottic, glottic, or subglottic laryngeal compromise of the neonatal airway classically presents with inspiratory stridor; and, if the pathology is fixed as opposed to dynamic, such as is seen with a subglottic stenosis, expiratory stridor will also be present. While stridor is the most noticeable manifestation of laryngeal airway compromise, the severity of retractions is a more accurate reflection of the severity of the airway compromise. Retractions usually occur in the supraclavicular and suprasternal regions, but intercostal, sternal, or substernal retractions may also be seen. The area of maximal retractions does not seem to have a direct bearing on the underlying obstruction causing the retractions. Infants with laryngeal airway compromise frequently also present with apnea and cyanosis and may have an abnormal cry if the vocal folds are involved.

Tracheal Involvement

Compromise of the tracheal airway may be from tracheomalacia, vascular compression, or congenital tracheal stenosis. These children may present with biphasic stridor with a fixed stenosis or inspiratory stridor and expiratory wheeze with a dynamic compromise. Retractions are common while apnea and cyanosis are comparably unusual; dying spells may be noted in severe cases. In dynamic tracheal obstruction there is often a characteristic "honking" cough, while lower tracheal narrowing is often characterized by a biphasic wet-sounding breathing pattern, sometimes termed "washing machine breathing" with retained tracheal secretions moving in and out

through an area of narrowing. Characteristically, these children will occasionally cough and clear the secretions and then sound markedly improved for 15 to 20 minutes until the secretions start building up again. The appropriate investigations for suspected tracheal compromise include bronchoscopic evaluation and contrast enhanced CT scan of both the trachea and surrounding vasculature. Before commencing these investigations, a plain airway (high kilovolt) X-ray will often provide valuable information warning the prospective bronchoscopist of tracheal narrowing or tracheal deviation.

EVALUATION OF THE INTUBATED NEONATAL AIRWAY

In neonates who present to the otolaryngologist already intubated, the first question is whether the airway is still compromised despite being intubated. If there is still airway compromise by implication, there is probably pathology distal to the tip of the endotracheal tube. If the airway is adequately maintained with an endotracheal tube, history should be sought on the indications, symptoms and signs that led to intubation; whether attempts at extubation have been made; and, if so, what was the reason for failure. It should also be established how straightforward the intubation was, as an infant known to be a difficult intubation should not be extubated lightly except under controlled conditions. If a child has had a previous failed extubation attempt but did not require immediate reintubation, evaluation of the child in the hours following extubation may provide the most valuable information in terms of the cause of airway compromise. However, if a child immediately failed extubation and required rapid reintubation, reevaluation in the operating room may be the most prudent approach with the child minimally sedated and with both flexible and rigid endoscopy on hand to evaluate the airway immediately following extubation.

In the infant, feeding is the most strenuous form of exercise bar crying. Whereas an older child with a compromised airway may present with exercise intolerance, an infant will present with feeding difficulty. This may be reflected in stridor, cyanosis, retractions, choking episodes, or failure to thrive. The more acute the onset of airway compromise is, the more severe the degree of feeding difficulties is likely to be.

Oxygenation and Ventilation

In infants with premature lungs, an ancillary oxygen requirement to maintain adequate oxygen saturations is common, and in extreme prematurity inevitable. However, term infants with a compromised airway frequently do not present with oxygen desaturations until the degree of airway compromise is extreme. Often the presentation is not with an inability to oxygenate but rather an inability to ventilate with this being reflected in the CO_2 level. Hypercapnia may be acute or chronic. Acute hypercapnia may result

in respiratory depression and with a relative respiratory acidosis. However, chronic hypercapnia may be reflected in a relative metabolic alkalosis. In these children airway compromise may be distal to the trachea with bronchomalacia or bronchopulmonary dysplasia being ultimately the greatest contributing factor.

ACUTE MANAGEMENT OF NEONATAL AIRWAY COMPROMISE

In a neonate presenting with acute airway compromise, be it at delivery or subsequent to delivery, intervention may be required. Following delivery this may occur in a neonate who is having an acute episode of stridor, an apneic event, a dying spell, or following extubation with an obvious need for the intubation. The fundamentals of resuscitation, namely airway, breathing, and circulation, are paramount to neonatal resuscitation. Securing the airway may be seen as a cascade of increasing levels of intervention. At the most basic level, providing a high concentration of oxygen whether by face mask, nasal cannula, high flow nasal cannula, or nasopharyngeal CPAP is desirable. If this is not adequate, a bag and mask will provide stability in an acute situation in the majority of infants. However, this does require an adequate mask fit and in some infants and children their underlying anatomy is not favorable to allow the face mask to seal the nose and oral cavity. In some of these patients an oral airway may be useful. If an adequate airway cannot be achieved or be maintained with a bag and mask, intubation is warranted. Intubation in the neonatal period does not mandate use of sedation or muscle relaxation. In a term infant, the age appropriate size of endotracheal tube is usually a 3.5 mm tube with an outer diameter of 4.8 mm. However, the age appropriate size of endotracheal tube is not necessarily the infant appropriate size of endotracheal tube. The ideal size of endotracheal tube for an individual infant or child is the smallest tube that will permit adequate ventilation, ideally maintaining a subglottic air leak pressure of less than 20 cm of water. In some infants, the requirement for adequate positive pressure ventilation takes precedence over the maintenance of the subglottic air leak, and a larger endotracheal tube may be tolerated for a period of time to permit more adequate ventilation of the infant. Infants are tolerant of prolonged intubation, but the longer the intubation and the tighter the fit of the endotracheal tube in the subglottis, the higher the relative probability of complications associated with intubation such as the development of subglottic granulation tissue, subglottic cyst formation, and subglottic stenosis will be. One alternative to the use of a snug endotracheal tube in children is the use of a smaller cuffed endotracheal tube[5] although cuffed pressure needs to be monitored carefully so there is not an equivalent lesion caused in the trachea from the endotracheal cuff. Tracheal stenosis is a more difficult problem to manage than subglottic stenosis.

While the size of endotracheal tube and the duration of intubation are the most significant factors influencing the risk of development of subglottic scarring, there are several other factors which may be synergistic, including the composition of the endotracheal tube, gastroesophageal reflux disease, and concurrent infection, especially with respiratory syncytial virus. The composition of the endotracheal tube is now almost universally silastic tubing which has low reactivity. Historically, red rubber catheters were used as endotracheal tubes and had a high associated stenosis rate. The other influencing factor is whether the intubation is transnasal or transoral. Transoral intubation is more easily accomplished but the endotracheal tube is less stable, more prone to movement, and the angle of the tube puts a relatively higher pressure on the posterior part of the subglottis. Meanwhile, transnasal intubation is slightly more technically challenging, requires an adequate nasal airway to allow passage of the tube, and places slightly more pressure in the posterior glottic area. However, the tube is more easily secured and, therefore, more stable. The true benefit of a nasal versus oral intubation is relatively small and, therefore, is a minor consideration with regard to neonatal intubation.

The Difficult Intubation

Neonatal intubation is normally straightforward; however, under some circumstances intubation may be challenging. Even in children in whom intubation is difficult, laryngeal exposure with an anesthetic laryngoscope blade and intubation with an endotracheal tube with an introducer placed transorally will permit intubation in the majority of children. Allowing some tip angulation with the bevel of the endotracheal tube facing posteriorly is also useful (Figure 2). The retrognathic and glossoptotic neonate may be particularly challenging to intubate, as laryngeal exposure is limited due to the anterior lying larynx and the larynx may be difficult to see permitting only a limited visualization of the arytenoid cartilages. In the neonate, laryngeal exposure may be optimized by pressure on the cricoid cartilage delivered by the little finger of the left hand that is holding the laryngoscope blade, while the endotracheal tube is manipulated with the right hand in the standard

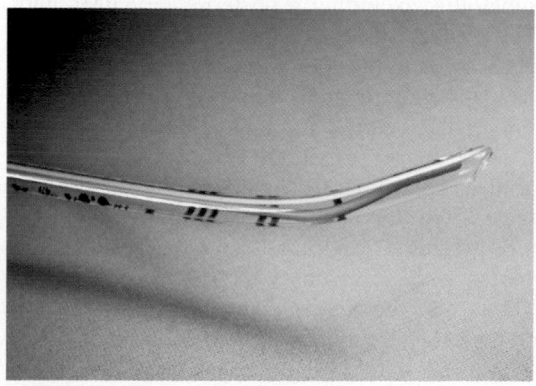

Figure 2 An endotracheal tube with a stylet allowing anterior angulation, and the bevel of the tube faces posteriorly.

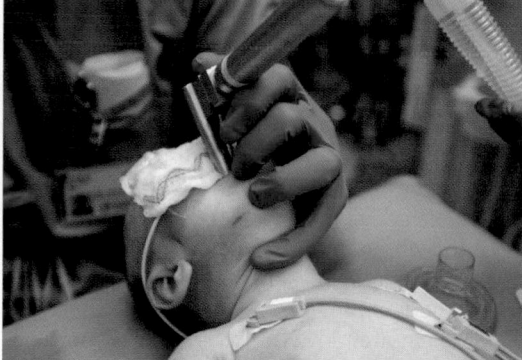

Figure 3 Intubation in the neonate, with the little finger of the left hand applying pressure to the cricoid cartilage.

fashion (Figure 3). Other special circumstances in which intubation may be challenging include children with oropharyngeal masses, laryngeal clefts, subglottic stenosis, and tracheal stenosis. The difficulty in children with laryngotracheoesophageal clefts is that the endotracheal tube will pass through the vocal folds but then falls through the cleft into the esophagus. In these children, and in children with oropharyngeal masses, a transnasal intubation flexible endoscope passed through an endotracheal tube may be useful to negotiate the anatomy and place the tip of the endotracheal tube in an appropriate position in the trachea.

Securing the airway with a ventilating bronchoscope is invaluable in the acute situation; however, it does not provide a long-term solution although it may facilitate airway stability until a tracheostomy can be performed. An alternative to securing the airway with a ventilating bronchoscope is to secure the airway with a Hopkins rod endoscope with an appropriate sized endotracheal tube placed over the rigid endoscope (Figure 4), so that once the endoscope is placed in the desired segment of trachea, the endotracheal tube can be advanced and secured. This, of course, can only be performed transorally.

Occasionally, intubation cannot be performed because the degree of subglottic stenosis is such that an endotracheal tube cannot pass the stenotic area. The smallest commercially available endotracheal tube has a 2.0 mm inner diameter with an outer diameter of 2.8 mm. In some forms of congenital subglottic stenosis, even this small tube cannot be passed. In these children, the airway is best managed temporarily with bag and mask ventilation or placement of a small laryngeal

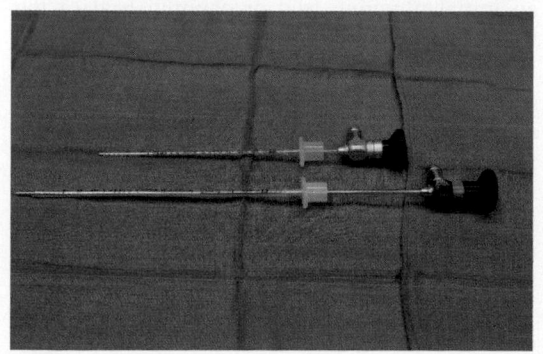

Figure 4 Endotracheal tubes placed over Hopkins rod lens telescopes.

mask airway. Tracheostomy is then required to secure the airway. In some children, the subglottis is of adequate size, but the trachea is stenotic and does not allow passage of an endotracheal tube through the area of stenosis. Under these circumstances, an endotracheal tube may need to be placed barely below the vocal folds down to the level of tracheal stenosis but not through the level of stenosis. These children similarly cannot have a tracheostomy placed as the smallest tracheostomy tube is considerably larger than the smallest endotracheal tube; and, under these circumstances, urgent tracheal reconstruction is required.

Extubation

In an infant who was difficult to intubate as occurs with severe retrognathia or an infant in whom extubation is not realistically achievable as in severe bronchopulmonary dysplasia, proceeding straight to tracheostomy is appropriate. However, if an infant has the potential to be successfully extubated, then optimizing the extubation is desirable. The infant should be weaned from sedation to permit maximal respiratory effort, and consideration should be given to treatment with coritcosteroids to try to minimize any laryngeal swelling at the time of extubation. Our routine is to deliver a single dose of dexamethasone, 0.5 mg/kg, 12 hours prior to extubation. In the 24 hours following extubation, there still may be some reactive glottic and subglottic edema, and the airway status may initially deteriorate before recovery. Over this time period, alternatives to reintubation include the use of racemic epinephrine, nasopharyngeal CPAP, or use of a high flow nasal cannula. If despite these measures, adequate oxygenation and ventilation cannot be maintained, the child will require reintubation. If the child repeatedly fails, attempts at extubation, tracheostomy is indicated. In certain children, an alternative to tracheostomy may be an anterior cricoid split operation which is discussed in Chapter 69, "Congenital Anomalies of the Larynx."

Tracheostomy

Elective tracheostomy in a stable neonate should be a controlled procedure. In an infant in whom a definitive decision has been made to proceed with tracheostomy, it is best to place the tracheostomy before removing the endotracheal tube and evaluating the airway. However, in an infant in whom it is desirable to evaluate the airway before proceeding to tracheostomy, the endotracheal tube may be removed and rigid or flexible bronchoscopic evaluation of the airway may be performed to exclude a correctable anatomical problem, such as glottic granulation tissue or laryngomalacia. In the child known to have had a difficult intubation, it is prudent to inspect the larynx prior to removal of the endotracheal tube; and, if the surgeon is not confident that he or she can reintubate, it is best to proceed directly to tracheostomy before removing the endotracheal tube.

When performing tracheostomy in a neonate, one should appreciate how soft and difficult to palpate structures in the infant neck may be, and, therefore, it is prudent to remove catheters from the esophagus, such as nasogastric tubes and temperature probes, to prevent confusion of the esophagus for the trachea. The initial incision may be vertical or horizontal; and, in the neonatal neck, defatting the area of the tracheostomy is advisable as it allows easier identification of the trachea and improves maturing of the stoma. An infant's neck is a surprisingly easy place to get lost, and frequent palpation of the trachea while separating the strap muscles and dividing the thyroid isthmus is useful. Once the trachea and specifically the tracheal rings have been identified, the location of the cricoid is established; and stay sutures are placed just lateral to the midline in the region of the second to fourth tracheal cartilages. During exposure of the trachea, blunt dissection is employed where possible, staying strictly in the midline as the lung apices in an infant may rise well above the level of the clavicles, particularly in a child who has been ventilated for a long period. The lung apices may cross the midline. In some patients, the innominate artery may be high above the level of the sternum. When placing the stay sutures and incising the trachea, it is best to start distally and work proximally with sharp instruments, be it knife or needle, to prevent injury to the pleura or the innominate artery. Once the airway is open, it is best to sew the skin edges to the trachea, particularly in the lower aspect of the wound, to minimize the risk of formation of a false passage anterior to the trachea should decannulation occur and require emergent replacement of a tracheostomy tube. Once the stoma has been created, the endotracheal tube can be slowly withdrawn until the tip of the endotracheal tube is seen to lie proximal to the incision, and the tracheostomy tube is inserted. Only once the tracheostomy tube has been inserted and both oxygenation and ventilation confirmed, should the endotracheal tube be removed. In a term infant, a 3.0 mm or 3.5 mm tracheostomy tube of neonatal length is chosen. In a child with a relatively expanded trachea due to long-term ventilation, a 4.0 mm tracheostomy tube may be required. If long-term ventilation is anticipated and there is a significant air leak around the sides of the tracheostomy tube prohibiting adequate ventilation, a cuffed tracheostomy tube may be required.

Once the tracheostomy tube is secured, its position in the trachea should be established with flexible endoscopy to ensure that the tip of the tube lies above the carina. At this point, formal bronchoscopic evaluation of the airway may be performed if desired.

Emergent tracheostomy in a neonate is something to be avoided whenever possible, and securing the airway with an endotracheal tube prior to tracheostomy is still the most desirable option. However, when a tracheostomy is truly emergent, the same principles apply whereby palpation of the trachea repeatedly with clear identification of tracheal rings is key before incising the trachea to ensure that an incision is not inadvertently attempted in the esophagus, cervical spine, or carotid artery. Once the tracheostomy is secured with twill ties, routine management includes tie changes on day three and the first tracheostomy tube change on day five with Velcro ties being acceptable at this time.

Whereas most children dependent on a tracheostomy require a reasonable amount of routine care, in certain groups, special considerations are required. In a child with severe tracheomalacia, a special length tracheostomy tube that extends close to the carina may allow the majority of the tracheomalacia to be bypassed and, therefore, may negate the need for positive pressure support. However, this is not effective if bronchomalacia is also present. Occasionally, children who have had a high tracheoesophageal fistula repair will have a mid-tracheal pouch on the back wall of the trachea comprising the remnant of the tracheoesophageal fistula. In these children, during tracheostomy tube changes, the tip of the tube may be placed into the pouch instead of the trachea resulting in an inability to ventilate. The key to management is recognizing the situation and pulling back on the tube and repositioning it. If this is a recurrent problem, marsupialization of the tracheal pouch effectively manages the problem.

LONGER TERM TRACHEOSTOMY CARE

In most children, conversion from a neonatal length tracheostomy tube to a longer pediatric length tracheostomy tube occurs around 9 months of age. Bronchoscopic airway evaluation should occur every several months to evaluate whether subglottic stenosis has developed and to evaluate whether it is time to consider decannulation. If the underlying airway problem that initially required tracheostomy either spontaneously resolves or is surgically repaired, the child may be decannulated. The airway should be evaluated prior to decannulation to ensure that there is no tracheostomy associated problem such as suprastomal collapse or suprastomal granulation that would preclude decannulation. This also allows evaluation of other pathology or secondary considerations that would counsel against decannulation, such as upcoming major surgery with anticipated prolonged intubation. If there is no anatomical reason against removing the tracheostomy tube, an initial plugging trial or capping trial of the tracheostomy is advisable to ensure that the child is able to breathe adequately without a tracheostomy prior to its removal. When possible, the narrowest diameter tracheostomy tube should be placed in the airway, and a cap placed over it for 24 to 48 hours with the child being observed and closely monitored. In young children, fenestrating the tracheostomy tube may be required to achieve this end. The child may be sent home for a period with the tracheostomy tube being capped to be quite sure that an adequate airway is maintained prior to removal of the tube. When the child is ultimately decannulated, close observation is recommended for 24 to 48 hours. Following decannulation, a final bronchoscopy is performed several weeks later to ensure that the trachea has healed on the inside without the formation of granulation tissue, which may occur in up to 2% of cases.

PEDIATRIC AIRWAY MANAGEMENT

In older children, airway evaluation is more nuanced with an increasing number of factors that should be considered. The role of the pediatric larynx is primarily as a conduit for air passage, secondarily, a guardian against aspiration, and finally as an organ of voice production. Any one of these roles may compromise the other functions of the larynx, and surgical intervention seeking to improve one of these functions may inadvertently compromise the others. Therefore, evaluation of the pediatric airway not only involves evaluation of these disparate laryngeal functions but also evaluation of the rest of the child. Laryngeal and tracheal airway obstruction in the child, similar to the neonate, is characterized by stridor and retractions. However, in the child, exercise intolerance, voice quality, and evaluation of aspiration risk are now considerations. In a child whose symptoms warrant further evaluation, initial evaluation should ideally include flexible laryngoscopy and high kilovolt airway films. Flexible laryngoscopy is an excellent method for evaluating airway pathology from the nose to the vocal folds but is poor at evaluating subglottic and tracheal pathology. If flexible laryngoscopic findings do not explain the symptoms, rigid bronchoscopy is indicated. This is also true in adequate evaluation of the child dependent on a tracheostomy.

Rigid bronchoscopy evaluation of the pediatric airway is performed under general anesthesia either with suspension laryngoscopy, or utilizing an anesthetic laryngoscope blade. The bronchoscopic evaluation may be performed with a hollow ventilating bronchoscope, a ventilating bronchoscope containing a Hopkins rod endoscope, or with a Hopkins rod endoscope alone. Comprehensive evaluation should also include the laryngeal structures and surrounding base of the tongue and pharynx, with special attention being paid to the posterior part of the glottis and the subglottis, excluding a posterior laryngeal cleft. The evaluation should then continue below the vocal folds to the subglottis, trachea and bronchi with any stenotic areas being carefully evaluated for length, severity, and inflammation.

The degree of subglottic stenosis may be graded according to the Myer-Cotton grading scale,[6] with the subglottic leak pressures of differing sizes of endotracheal tube being a convenient way to evaluate the degree of stenosis. The size of the airway is determined by the size of the largest endotracheal tube that still maintains a leak with a subglottic pressure of less than 20 cm of water pressure. Most children with a Grade 1 subglottic stenosis (<50% stenosis) will be asymptomatic, while Grade 4 stenosis means a complete occlusion of the subglottic lumen, with tracheostomy dependency and aphonia. The resistance to airflow through the area of stenosis is influenced by Poiseuille's law, namely, that flow is inversely proportional to the fourth power of the radius. This means that halving the radius will result in one-sixteenth of the airflow.

Thorough evaluation should also include consideration of flexible endoscopy looking at airway dynamics including pharyngomalacia, laryngomalacia, glossoptosis, vocal fold paralysis, and tracheomalacia. It should be noted that flexible bronchoscopy is a poor tool for evaluating the posterior part of the glottis and that posterior glottic stenosis and posterior laryngeal clefts are difficult to evaluate with flexible endoscopy.

COMPLEMENTARY EVALUATION

In a child in whom airway reconstructive surgery is a consideration, optimization of the patient is critical to ensure the best outcome of surgery. Factors that may strongly influence the outcome of surgery include gastroesophageal reflux disease, eosinophilic esophagitis, pulmonary disease, sleep apnea (whether central or obstructive), and aspiration. It is a disservice to a child to attempt to rid them of a tracheostomy while creating for the child a condition that predisposes to significant aspiration in the process. While not mandatory, it is prudent to consider whether esophagogastroduodenoscopy or pH probe evaluation (or more recently impedance probe evaluation) of the patient, anticipating airway reconstructive surgery, is warranted.[7] This is especially true in patients who have already had previous unsuccessful surgery. The outcome of surgical reconstruction of the airway is less favorable in children with poorly controlled gastroesophageal reflux disease or eosinophilic esophagitis.[8] Similarly sleep apnea, whether obstructive or central, may have a negative impact on the outcome of pediatric airway reconstruction, and a sleep study may be indicated in some children before or after surgical intervention.

Pediatric aspiration is also an important consideration during evaluation, not only to evaluate the current degree of aspiration, but also to evaluate the relative risk of aspiration following airway reconstructive surgery. Evaluation may include a video swallow study, functional endoscopic evaluation of swallowing, and pediatric dye testing. Pediatric dye testing involves using a green food dye to color food, drink, or the child's secretions, and then evaluating whether any green material is seen in the airway. This is only useful in a child with a tracheostomy who does not have a Grade 4 subglottic stenosis. Other complementary tests for aspiration include CT scanning of the lungs and flexible bronchoscopy with bronchoalveolar lavage looking for lipid-laden macrophages.

While an adequate airway is a greater consideration than voice in young children, pediatric voice disorders and the influence of airway surgery on a child's voice have become a greater

concern. Pediatric voice evaluation is becoming an increasingly important part of airway evaluation, both before and after surgical intervention. Voice preservation techniques, including avoidance of laryngofissure, balloon dilation of the airway, and endoscopic alternatives to open airway reconstruction are all playing an increasing role in the management of the pediatric airway.

SPECIFIC DISORDERS AFFECTING THE PEDIATRIC AIRWAY

Pediatric airway disease may be best considered in a proximal to distal fashion, as may causes of congenital stridor. Stridor is the sound produced by turbulent air flowing through a confined space, and in a child, is the result of laryngeal or tracheal pathology. With dynamic airway compromise, such as occurs with laryngomalacia or vocal fold paralysis, inspiratory stridor is noted with no expiratory component. However, with a fixed stenosis, such as subglottic stenosis or tracheal stenosis, the nature of the stridor is biphasic. The cause and anatomical location of congenital stridor reflect the frequency of the occurrence of the disorder, and a generalization is that the more proximal the location of the obstruction is, the more frequently the disorder is encountered. For example, laryngomalacia is more common than vocal fold paralysis which is more common than subglottic stenosis which is more common than congenital tracheal stenosis. Severe laryngeal webs and subglottic hemangiomas may also present with stridor, and these along with laryngomalacia, vocal fold paralysis, and subglottic stenosis are discussed in Chapter 69, "Congenital Anomalies of the Larynx."

COMMON CAUSES OF SUPRALARYNGEAL AIRWAY OBSTRUCTION

If obstruction of the supralaryngeal airway is considered in a proximal to distal fashion, starting at the nasal cavities, consideration should be given to piriform aperture stenosis, nasolacrimal duct cysts, choanal atresia, adenotonsillar hypertrophy, retrognathia, and glossoptosis. Choanal atresia is discussed in Chapter 70, "Congenital Anomalies of the Head and Neck," while adenotonsillar hypertrophy is discussed in Chapter 64, "Diseases of the Oral Cavity, Oropharynx, and Nasopharynx," and chapter 66, "Sleep Apnea in Children."

Piriform Aperture Stenosis

Piriform aperture stenosis is a comparatively rare developmental anomaly characterized by bony obstruction of the anterior nares by bony overgrowth of the lateral walls of the piriform aperture.[9] The presentation is in infancy and may mimic the symptoms and signs that occur with choanal atresia. Anterior rhinoscopy is diagnostic, with confirmation made on CT scan (Figure 5). This may also reveal the other midline anomalies

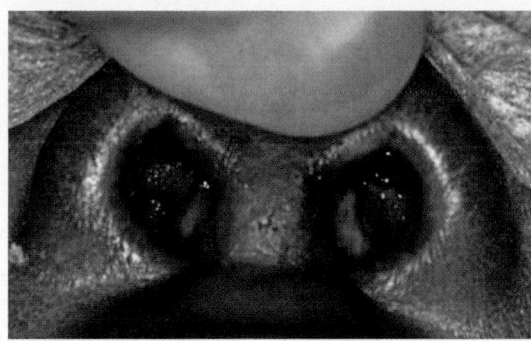

(A)

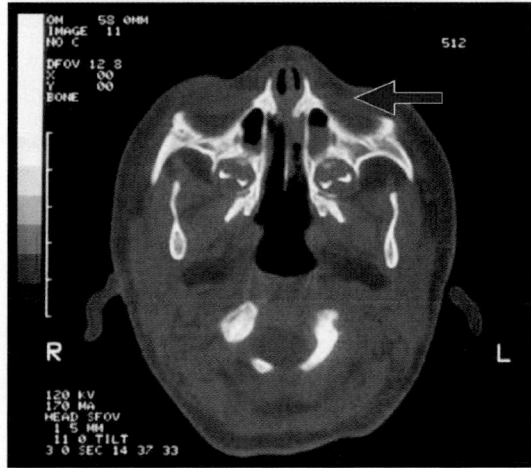

(B)

Figure 5 (A) Piriform aperture stenosis. (B) Computed tomographic scan showing a piriform aperture stenosis.

frequently seen with this condition, including a large single central upper incisor and midline anomalies of the central nervous system. Treatment requires drilling down of the bony overgrowth through a sublabial approach, with temporary placement of transnasal stents.

Nasolacrimal Duct Cysts

Nasolacrimal duct cysts occur as a consequence of failure of the nasolacrimal duct to recanalize during fetal development and may be unilateral or bilateral.[10] Presentation is with nasal obstruction due to a large cyst under the inferior turbinate occluding the anterior part of the nasal airway (Figure 6), and there may be swelling of the nasolacrimal sac in the medial canthal area. Epiphora is present as the tears cannot drain; and, if the cyst is infected, as is frequently the case, there may be abscess formation in the nasolacrimal sac region, and the neonate may be septic. Investigation is with anterior rhinoscopy and CT scanning of the nasal passages (Figure 7). Treatment is transnasal endoscopic removal or marseupialization of the cyst with placement of nasolacrimal duct catheters if required.

Retrognathia and Glossoptosis

Retrognathia is a descriptive term for mandibular hypoplasia and occurs in a variety of conditions, including Pierre Robin sequence, Treacher Collins syndrome, and Stickler syndrome. A consequence of the mandibular hypoplasia is crowding of the tongue posteriorly and superiorly, which

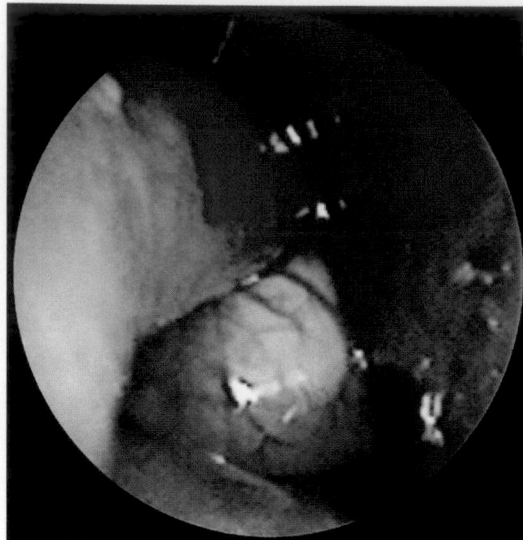

Figure 6 Endoscopic view of a nasolacrimal duct cyst under the right inferior turbinate.

may cause airway obstruction and a cleft of the secondary palate, as the palate anlagen are unable to close around the cephalically displaced tongue. The degree of retrognathia is not always a reliable indicator of the degree of obstruction or of the potential problems with intubation. Although obstructing retrognathia is usually a problem encountered in the neonatal nursery, problems may be encountered years later. While such problems are often triggered by seemingly trivial surgical procedures, the insidious onset of severe sleep apnea is the most notable presentation.

In the neonatal period, management includes prone positioning, the use of high-flow nasal cannula, and occasionally the use of a nasal trumpet (nasopharyngeal airway). CPAP is often not successful, as the mask tends to exacerbate the relative retrognathia. Because these infants struggle with feeding, nasogastric tube placement is often required. If the airway remains compromised, intubation is desirable, but as discussed previously, may be challenging.

In infants with significant obstructive symptoms or feeding problems, surgical intervention is desirable. Performing a tracheostomy is standard;

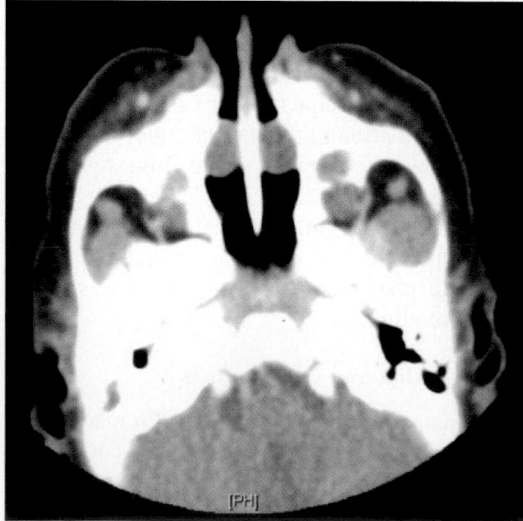

Figure 7 Computed tomographic scan of a nasolacrimal duct cyst.

and in most nonsyndromic children, catchup growth of the mandible will permit decannulation within 1 to 2 years. If catchup growth is not apparent by 1 year of age, consideration can be given to mandibular distraction. In some cases, neonatal mandibular distraction may be an alternative to tracheostomy; however, this remains controversial.[11,12]

Pharyngeal and Laryngeal Cysts

Supralaryngeal and laryngeal cyst formation may be life threatening in the neonatal age group. A significant number of case reports in this age group are of infants in whom the diagnosis was established at autopsy. Supralaryngeal cysts in this age group present with a muffled cry and intermittent positional apnea. In some cases, stridor and retractions may be presenting symptoms. Flexible laryngoscopy is ideal for diagnosis of supraglottic pathology and occasionally may permit evaluation of subglottic pathology. The most commonly encountered cysts are lingual thyroglossal duct cysts, vallecular cysts, laryngoceles and saccular cysts, and subglottic cysts. Laryngoceles and saccular cysts are discussed in Chapter 69, "Congenital Anomalies of the Larynx." Thyroglossal duct cysts tend to present in the midline of the tongue posterior to the foramen cecum and usually proximal to the glossoepiglottic ligament. They are midline and deeply placed with a thick layer of mucosa overlying them (Figure 8). Care should be taken upon induction of general anesthesia as an infant with a lingual thyroglossal duct cyst may have acute respiratory obstruction upon induction. This is not true in the older child. Treatment is complete excision through an endoscopic approach. This may be done with an elongated guarded tip needlepoint Bovi through a medium Lindholm suspension laryngoscope. The resultant raw area is left to heal by secondary intention. Marsupialization of the cyst may be effective, but complete excision is curative. Usually the hyoid bone is not involved; and, therefore, a Sistrunk operation is not required.

Vallecular cysts in contrast are thin walled and usually arise from the lingual surface of the epiglottis, and marsupialization is an effective treatment. In the subglottic region, cysts may occur and are often multiple. Subglottic cysts may be superficial and thin walled (Figure 9); but, if lying deep in the submucosal layer, they may be

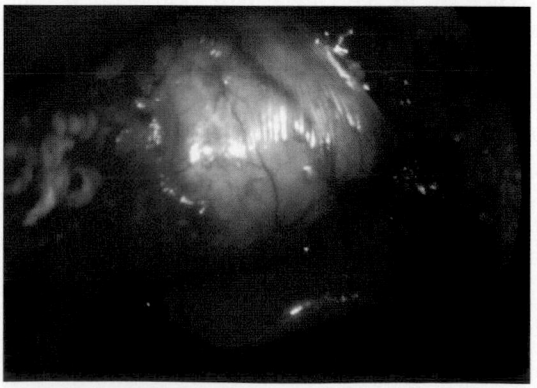

Figure 8 Lingual thyroglossal duct cyst.

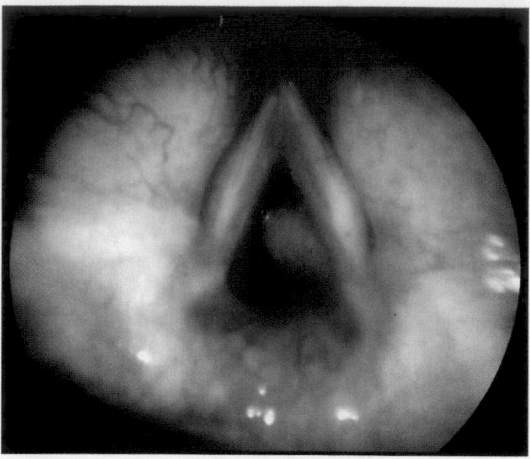

Figure 9 Subglottic cysts.

confused with a subglottic hemangioma or with subglottic stenosis. Invariably they are a consequence of prolonged intubation of a premature infant. They are readily treated by deroofing the cyst using either microlaryngeal instrumentation, powered instrumentation, CO_2 laser, or Bugbee electrocautery.[13] They have a tendency to recur and may need to be removed on several occasions before complete resolution. Therefore, follow-up bronchoscopy is mandatory. The pathogenesis for the development of subglottic cysts is not similar to the pathogenesis for the development of subglottic stenosis; both problems may coexist.

Tracheomalacia

Tracheomalacia describes any relative dynamic collapse of the trachea; it is more usually applied as a descriptive term for excessive movement of the posterior membranous tracheal wall, namely the trachealis muscle (Figure 10). Although tracheomalacia may occur with normally shaped tracheal cartilages, more frequently it is seen in conjunction with excessively wide and flattened tracheal cartilages. This is a problem that may occur in isolation without any other congenital anomalies but is more commonly seen in conjunction with other congenital anomalies, and tracheoesophageal fistula, esophageal atresia, and posterior laryngeal clefting are particularly common associations.[14] It is also more common in infants who have required prolonged ventilation and in children with Pierre Robin sequence. Tracheomalacia is a dynamic disorder, with the degree of malacia governed by the velocity of nonturbulent air flow, that is, the same Bernoulli principle that applies to airflow generating lift across an airplane's wing. Therefore, the maximal degree of tracheomalacia occurs in the area with the highest relative airflow and with this occurring at the narrowest point within the trachea. Tracheomalacia may present with a characteristic honking cough, may have symptoms of wheezing, airway obstruction, retractions, and occasionally dying spells and may get worse over the first few months of life before slowly and steadily improving. This is a problem that resolves with time in the majority of children. However, in severe cases interim intervention may be required. The standard for

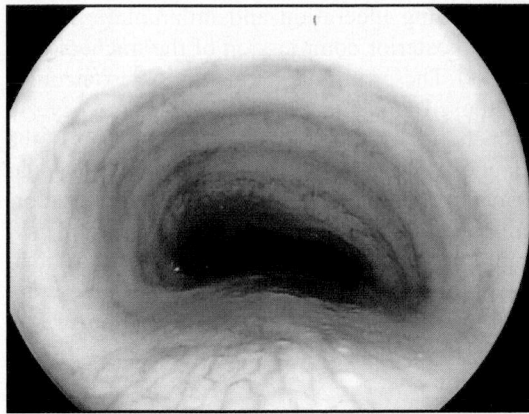

Figure 10 Tracheomalacia.

intervention in severe tracheomalacia is tracheostomy with the tip of the tracheostomy tube lying relatively close to the carina to bypass the most significant areas of malacia. In severe cases, positive pressure ventilation may also be required. An alternative to tracheostomy is aortopexy whereby the thymus gland is removed, and the aorta pexed forward to the posterior surface of the sternum, bringing the trachea anteriorly with it, thereby decreasing the relative flattening of the trachea and improving tracheomalacia. This is only required in a minority of patients. Another more controversial solution is placement of intratracheal stents, either hollow silicone stents, or expandable metal wire stents. There is a significant complication rate with these devices, and this approach is not recommended in a child with isolated tracheomalacia.[15]

In a child who has required tracheostomy for management of tracheomalacia, decannulation is usually achievable within 2 to 4 years as the tracheomalacia resolves, with the worse segment of malacia often occurring at the tracheostomy site where there is a relative narrowing of the trachea as a consequence of the tracheostomy. A significant number of children with tracheomalacia also have bronchomalacia. Whereas tracheomalacia may be bypassed by placement of a long endotracheal tube, this is not possible with bronchomalacia; and, if there is significant diffuse bronchomalacia, positive pressure support may be required through the tracheostomy tube until such time as the child slowly outgrows this problem.

Vascular Compression

Vascular compression of the pediatric airway encompasses several different disorders. The most common cause of vascular compression is due to anterior impingement of the innominate artery on the trachea as it crosses from the arch of the aorta to the right side of the body (Figure 11). Mild innominate artery compression is a comparatively common incidental finding on bronchoscopy, and is usually asymptomatic or mildly symptomatic with cough, retained secretions, and retractions being notable, and spontaneously improving with time. In severe cases, there may be marked airway compromise with stridor and retractions warranting surgical intervention with aortopexy or even innominate artery reimplantation. Placement of

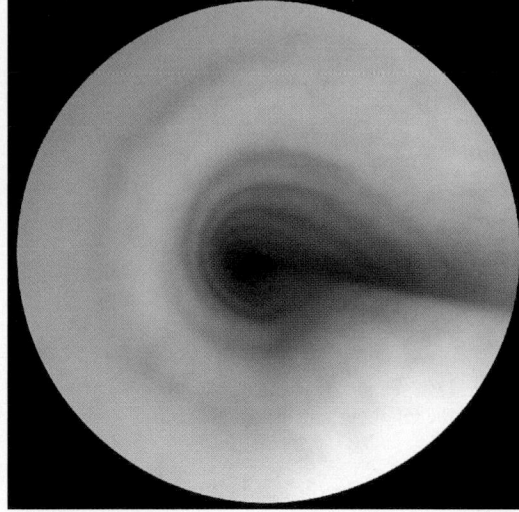

Figure 11 Innominate artery compression.

a tracheostomy tube in these children should be done with a certain degree of caution, as the tip of the endotracheal tube may rub against the pulsating anterior impression of the innominate artery, creating a small but real chance of formation of a tracheo-innominate artery fistula, an extremely life threatening condition.

Other forms of vascular compression are less common and include a right sided aortic arch, a double aortic arch compressing the trachea and esophagus, and a pulmonary artery sling compressing the distal part of the trachea.[16] A pulmonary artery sling describes the left pulmonary artery arising to the right of the trachea and passing back between the trachea and esophagus before coursing to the left lung. The characteristic radiographic finding is a barium swallow revealing an anterior filling defect in the anterior wall of the esophagus where the artery passes between the trachea and esophagus. However, all forms of vascular compression may be usefully imaged with MRI scanning or with contrast enhanced CT scanning of the chest. The right-sided aortic arch rarely requires treatment unless there is a complete vascular ring, in which case the ring may be divided, usually with division of the ligamentum arteriosum. With the double aortic arch, the least dominant of the arches is divided, this usually being the left. A pulmonary artery sling requires division and reimplantation into the main pulmonary artery trunk. However, the main consideration in evaluating a child with a pulmonary artery sling is not necessarily the tracheal compression but the high association, up to two-thirds of patients, in whom congenital tracheal stenosis due to complete tracheal rings is also present.

Complete Tracheal Rings

The most common cause of congenital tracheal stenosis is due to complete tracheal rings (Figure 12). The tracheal cartilages are normally in a horseshoe shape with a posterior membrane consisting of trachealis muscle. However, if the cartilages are circular and continuous, over varying lengths of the trachea, tracheal stenosis due to complete tracheal rings is present. While

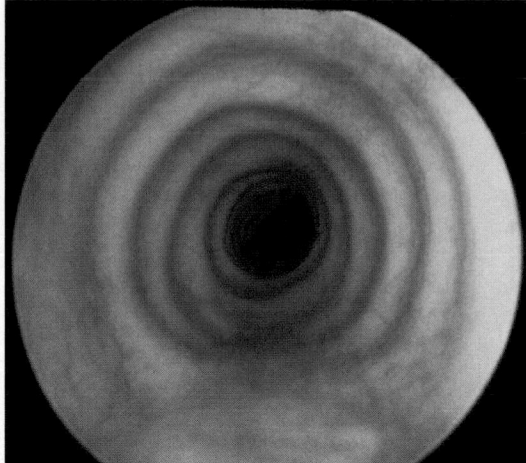

Figure 12 Complete tracheal rings.

rare, this is an important diagnosis as the initial management of these children may have a marked impact on the outcome both short term and long term. Complete tracheal rings are invariably smaller in diameter than a normal trachea, and over 90% of the patients have tracheal rings affecting either the majority of the trachea or the lower trachea. In a full 50% of patients upon presentation, the smallest tracheal ring is smaller than the smallest endotracheal tube. Therefore, these children cannot be intubated or have a tracheostomy tube placed through the segment of complete tracheal rings and as a consequence their care should be delivered with the utmost respect and circumspection. Historically, children with complete tracheal rings had a mortality rate in excess of 80% although currently a mortality rate of less than 10% is expected. Children with complete tracheal rings are usually noisy from birth with stridor and retractions and a characteristic wet sounding "washing machine" breathing pattern. As the child grows over the first few months of life, the trachea does not grow significantly; and, therefore, symptom progression is common, and often decompensation occurs around 4 months of age with the infant presenting in respiratory failure. In over 80% of children with complete tracheal rings there are other congenital anomalies present, sometimes multiple and severe. In approximately 50% of children with complete tracheal rings, the other anomalies are cardiovascular in origin. Initial evaluation should include plain airway films as this will provide a warning that congenital tracheal narrowing may be present. Definitive diagnosis is made with rigid bronchoscopy, and it is important to diagnose that complete rings are present even if the airway cannot be fully evaluated, as passing to large a telescope through a segment of complete tracheal rings may cause mucosal swelling and convert a compromised airway into a critical airway. If the airway has been traumatized and the child cannot be ventilated, the only alternative may be stabilization with extracorporeal membrane oxygenation (ECMO). If a small enough telescope is available, bronchoscopy will show congenital tracheal stenosis with cartilage rings that replace the posterior muscular trachealis, and frequently the tracheal rings extend down to the carina. Other appropriate investigations in these children include high resolution contrast enhanced CT scanning to evaluate not only the tracheal airway and bronchi but also the major blood vessels within the chest to see if there are any underlying vascular anomalies that also require repair, such as a pulmonary artery sling. Whereas two-thirds of children with a pulmonary artery sling have complete tracheal rings, approximately one-third of children with complete tracheal rings will also have a pulmonary artery sling. Other necessary investigations include echocardiogram to exclude any intracardiac anomalies. Whereas a small proportion of children do not need tracheal repair, 80% of patients require tracheal reconstruction, usually with a sternotomy and consideration of placement on cardiopulmonary bypass. The recommended method of repair of complete tracheal rings is a slide tracheoplasty.[17] Any cardiovascular anomalies that may also require repair may be undertaken at the same time.

ACQUIRED DISORDERS OF THE PEDIATRIC AIRWAY

Foreign Body

Foreign bodies of the pediatric aerodigestive tract have the potential to be life threatening and frequently require emergent management. Foreign bodies in the aerodigestive tract may be conveniently subdivided into glottic and tracheal, bronchial, and esophageal. Glottic and tracheal foreign bodies are true emergencies, and a significant proportion of children present at the emergency room are dead on arrival.[18] These are usually toddlers whose limited dentition does not allow effective chewing; and, therefore, smooth and rubbery consistencies of food may be aspirated and may lodge in the glottis or trachea. The classical foreign body causing glottic obstruction is a hot dog sausage with the presentation usually being abrupt and complete airway obstruction. Under these circumstances, a Heimlich maneuver may be life saving. If the child obtains limited air passage past the foreign body and survives transport to the hospital, emergent evaluation and stabilization of the airway is critical for survival, with attempted removal of the foreign body with an anesthetic laryngoscope blade and anesthetic McGill forceps if the child is in extremis. If the child is maintaining an airway, albeit tenuous, removal under general anesthetic in the operating room is still preferable with a slow induction with a volatile inhaled anesthetic being required due to the airway obstruction. There is a high risk on induction that the airway will be lost, and emergent bronchoscopy may then be required to remove the foreign body.

Modern foreign body forceps utilizing Hopkins rod endoscopes play a pivotal role in the current management of aerodigestive foreign bodies in children, and a variety of such foreign body forceps exists to aid in removal of particular foreign bodies (Figure 13). Once a laryngeal or

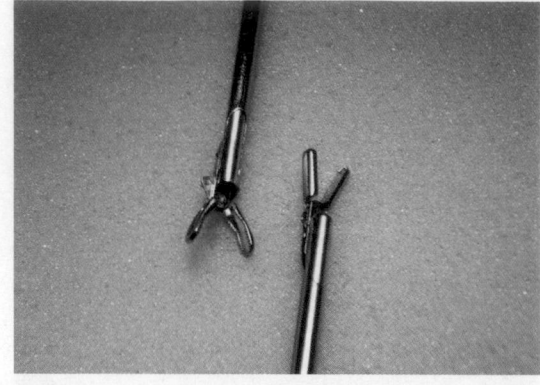

Figure 13 Specialized foreign body forceps. Peanut forceps on the left, coin forceps on the right.

tracheal foreign body has been removed, the rest of the tracheobronchial tree should be inspected to ensure that there are no remnants of the foreign body or second foreign body present. In the presence of a glottic foreign body without the equipment to remove the foreign body at hand, an alternative form of airway management is emergency tracheostomy with a vertical incision being placed directly down on the trachea below the cricoid cartilage and with insertion of an endotracheal tube through the neck into the trachea.

By contrast, bronchial foreign bodies present an urgent but not emergent problem in that even with one bronchus completely occluded by a foreign body, it is still possible to ventilate the contralateral lung. There is still the potential for an unstable airway in a child who has a foreign body ball-valving across the carina between the bronchi or in a child in whom a bronchial foreign body has been present for days or weeks as this will often induce bronchial granulation tissue and distal stasis of secretions with secondary infection. The most common bronchial foreign body in the United States is the peanut aspirated by a toddler who does not yet have erupted molars with which to crush the peanut. Peanuts, like most forms of vegetable aspirated matter, are extremely irritating to surrounding mucosa and may become buried within granulation tissue within a few days; and, therefore, removal should be performed on an urgent if not emergent basis. This is a frequent enough foreign body that optically guided peanut removing forceps are available to assist with removal (see Figure 13). Whereas a chest X-ray may either show consolidation of the lung distal to the foreign body or hyperinflation distal to the foreign body when air trapping has occurred, a normal chest X-ray does not exclude a bronchial foreign body. History alone is adequate indication for bronchoscopic evaluation, particularly in a child who has had a witnessed choking event. As with appendicitis, it is preferable that a few bronchoscopies are performed with no foreign body being found rather than potentially miss any foreign bodies that later present with sequelae.[19]

The final group of foreign bodies that deserve consideration are chronic esophageal foreign bodies. Acute esophageal foreign bodies rarely cause airway compromise, but if an esophageal foreign body has been present for weeks, it may cause

surrounding ulceration and inflammation leading to posterior compression of the trachea (Figure 14). These children frequently are erroneously diagnosed as being asthmatic, nonresponsive to bronchodilator therapy, and not infrequently the diagnosis is made following chest X-ray evaluation for recalcitrant asthma.[20] The classical foreign body in United States is a swallowed penny, and again, this is a frequent enough event that endoscopically guided coin removing forceps are available to assist with removal (see Figure 13).

Infection

Historically, the most frequent cause of fatal pediatric airway disease was diphtheria, and in the early part of the twentieth century, this was also the commonest cause for tracheostomy in the pediatric age group. The diphtheria toxin was responsible for even more deaths than the associated airway obstruction. This disease has essentially been eradicated by immunization against *Corynebacterium diphtheriae*. It is notable that immunization has also almost eradicated the commonest cause of infective life-threatening airway obstruction of the late twentieth century.[21] In much of the Western World, even as recently as the 1990s, epiglottitis or supraglottitis due to *Haemophilus influenzae Type b* (Hib) was a feared cause of acute airway obstruction in otherwise healthy children between the ages of 3 and 8 years. This was a disease characterized by rapidly progressive edema of the supraglottic structures, especially the epiglottis, with pain, fever, and severe stridor (Figure 15). Children would present sitting upright and leaning forward drooling as they could not swallow. The severe stridor and retractions would be exacerbated by the child being upset; and the supraglottits had the potential to precipitate complete loss of the airway, so the child was kept sitting on the parent's lap, and invasive evaluation (blood tests, intravenous line placement, X-ray, flexible laryngoscopy) was avoided. Emergent transfer to the operating room, for intubation or tracheostomy placement was advocated, with the child being anesthetized with

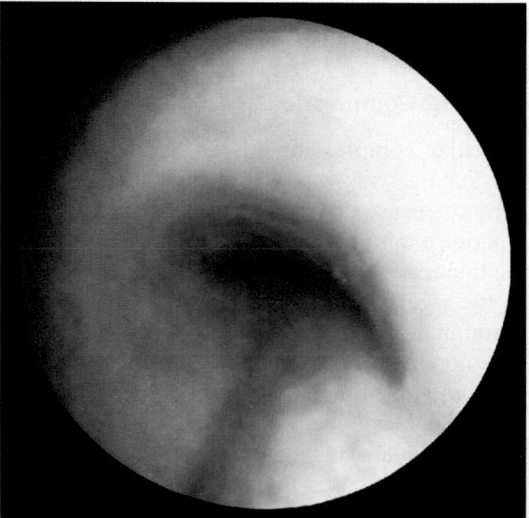

Figure 14 Posterior tracheal compression secondary to a chronic esophageal foreign body.

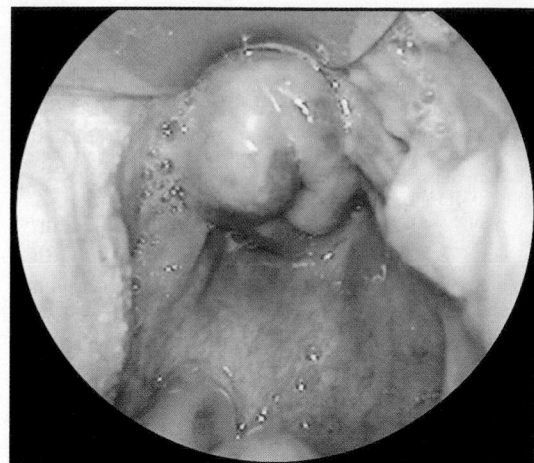

Figure 15 Epiglottitis.

an inhalational agent, still sitting on the parent's lap. Due to the airway obstruction, this was often a prolonged induction. Once anesthetized, the parents were ushered from the room, and intubation with a small endotracheal tube (with an introducer) was attempted, usually by whoever was available with the most intubation experience, whether otolaryngologist, intensivist, or anesthesiologist. The vocal folds could not be visualized due to the laryngeal edema, so the endotracheal tube was inserted where air bubbles could be seen emitting from the larynx. If the child could not be intubated, an attempt was made with a ventilating bronchoscope, and if that too failed, emergent tracheostomy was required. Resolution of the disease was usually rapid following administration of a beta-lactamase resistant penicillin. As with diphtheria, introduction of an effective immunization (Hib vaccine), has not only caused the virtual eradication of epiglottis but also of the other diseases caused by Hib, notably meningitis. This has had a secondary impact on the otolaryngologist in that the incidence of postmeningitic profound sensorineural hearing loss due to Hib meningitis has also plummeted. Supraglottis still occurs rarely, either in the unvaccinated, or with differing causative microorganisms, but generally is a milder disease and is seen in older children.

A more common and benign infection is that caused by parainfluenza virus, namely croup. This is a seasonal disease caused by edema of the subglottic tissues due to a viral infection (usually parainfluenza, but many viruses have been implicated), usually affecting children between 3 months and 5 years of age. There is a characteristic seal-like barking cough with accompanying inspiratory stridor and retractions, exacerbated when the child is upset. Although the child may have a mild fever and rhinorrhea, he or she usually looks otherwise well. In mild cases, investigations are not warranted; but, in more severe episodes, airway films will show characteristic "steepling" of the subglottis, and flexible laryngoscopy will confirm that no supraglottic pathology exists and that there is an edematous subglottic airway. Treatment is usually supportive, with humidity and cool air being useful in the home setting. Symptoms rarely last longer than 3 days. In more severe cases, systemic corticosteroids or

racemic epinephrine are effective, and, in rare cases, intubation may be required.[22] Bronchoscopy is not indicated unless croup is atypical, that is, very severe, occurring at an atypical age, or with crescendo croup (each episode is worse than the previous episode). In some children croup is more severe due to a mild underlying congenital subglottic stenosis.

A more regional disease is bacterial tracheitis, with no specific microorganism being responsible for the majority of cases, but a variety of bacteria may be responsible.[23] Children with it are usually otherwise healthy and between 6 and 14 years of age. There is a severe sore throat, exacerbated by coughing and swallowing, that restricts fluid intake, and the infection results in increasingly thick tenacious tracheal secretions. There is usually associated subglottic edema, and presentation is with stridor and retractions. In advanced cases, the child may be febrile and appear toxic. Airway films may demonstrate tracheal membranes (Figure 16), and flexible laryngoscopy shows thick subglottic secretions that are hard for the patient to cough out. In mild cases rehydration with intravenous fluids, analgesia, broad spectrum antibiotics, and encouragement to cough may be all that is required to manage

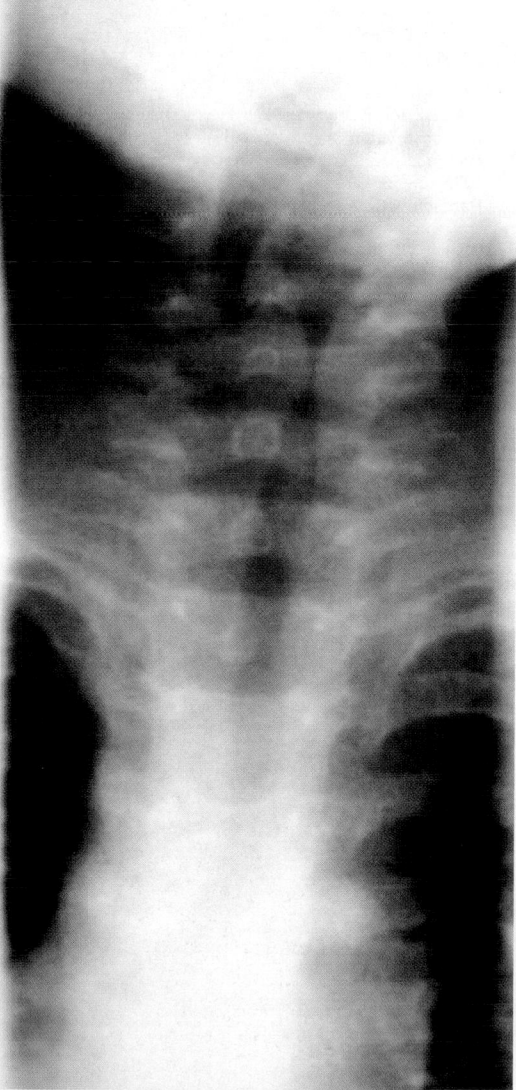

Figure 16 Airway films of a child with bacterial tracheitis and tracheal membranes.

the disease, but in most cases bronchoscopic airway clearance is required. Bronchoscopic findings are subglottic and tracheal edema, with thick tenacious secretions in the trachea but sparing the bronchi (Figure 17). Frequently, the secretions are so tenacious that they cannot be adequately suctioned, and removal with foreign body forceps may be required. Postoperative intubation for a few days is frequently required.

Other Causes of Pediatric Airway Obstruction

Other causes of pediatric airway obstruction are comparatively rare and include trauma, inflammatory diseases, and neoplasms. Inflammatory and neoplastic causes are discussed in Chapter 64, "Diseases of the Oral Cavity, Oropharynx, and Nasopharynx."

Traumatic causes of airway compromise are highly individualized; if intubation injury is excluded, the two main groups are airway burns and blunt trauma to the neck. Airway burns may be a consequence of a chemical or thermal injury, and the injury may affect the pharynx, larynx, trachea, or esophagus. In the acute situation, airway edema (and other injuries the patient has suffered) requires airway stabilization with intubation, and in severe injuries, prolonged intubation and ventilation may require tracheostomy. The longer-term degree of scarring depends upon the depth of injury, and even extensive mucosal damage may heal without scarring if the injury is only superficial. Chemical injuries are more severe with alkali exposure than acid exposure, as alkalis cause liquifactive necrosis, and therefore tend to penetrate deeply. Pharyngeal and esophageal stenosis may be a severe and long-term consequence of alkali injuries. As with all forms of aerodigestive burn injury, there may be skip lesions, and relative sparing of some areas, with severe injury to others. Inhalational thermal burns may result in supraglottic, subglottic or tracheal scarring, and scarring in these children may take months to years to mature fully; and, until mature, operative intervention is less

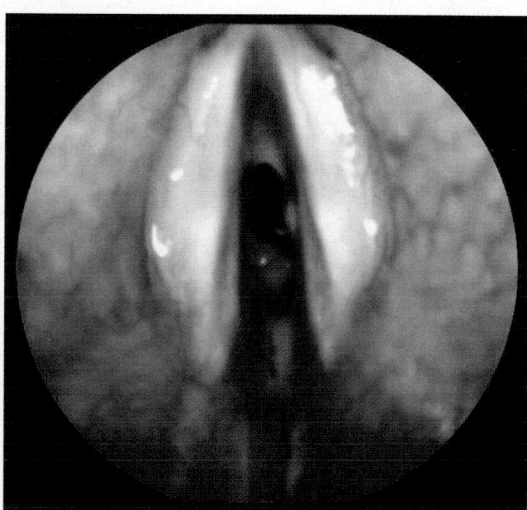

Figure 17 Endoscopic view of the tenacious secretions seen in bacterial tracheitis.

likely to have a successful outcome.[24] A particularly severe burn occurs with a laser fire, when an endotracheal tube is ignited with a CO_2 laser; the oxygen rich environment causes the end of the endotracheal tube to act like a blowtorch. Immediately removing the endotracheal tube and filling the pharynx with water may limit the depth of heat penetration; but severe scaring is still to be anticipated, and early tracheotomy is indicated.

Blunt trauma to the neck may cause two characteristic injuries, namely a fractured larynx and laryngotracheal separation. A patient with a fractured larynx usually presents with mild stridor, hoarseness, and sometimes with subcutaneous air. Investigation includes plain airway films, CT scan of the neck, flexible laryngoscopy, and rigid bronchoscopic evaluation of the larynx. Undisplaced fractures may require no intervention bar observation, but if the airway is compromised by swelling then intubation may be required, this being with a cuffed endotracheal tube if there is subcutaneous emphysema. In severe injuries with cartilage displacement, open repair of the fractures is indicated, using sutures since in children the larynx is not yet calcified and will not hold miniplates.

Laryngotracheal separation is a more severe injury due to blunt trauma as in a "clothesline" injury.[25] The trachea is ripped off the cricoid, often damaging both recurrent laryngeal nerves. Often there are other associated injuries, including cervical spine fracture and esophageal rupture. While many such injuries result in death at the scene of injury, a surprising number of children may maintain an airway despite quite a long gap between the larynx (which retracts up under the chin), and the trachea (which retracts into the chest). Apart from stridor, there is characteristic eccymosis of the anterior neck, a "flat" neck, and subcutaneous emphysema. Intubation should be approached with great caution as the cervical spine should be treated as though fractured until

proven otherwise, and hence neck extension is inadvisable. Induction of anesthesia risks collapse and loss of the airway, while intubation risks the endotracheal tube passing through the vocal folds and into the soft tissues of the neck, rather than into the distal trachea. Under these circumstances, flexible nasotracheal intubation in an awake patient may be the safest method of securing the airway. The alternative is tracheostomy, with the skin incision opening into a large cavity, with the end of the trachea found in the thoracic aspect of the space. When possible, immediate reconstruction with laryngotracheal anastomosis over a T-tube or suprastomal stent is recommended. If this is not possible, then an end-tracheostomy can be performed and later an extended cricotracheal resection may be considered.

Wegener granulomatosis, relapsing polychondritis, and idiopathic subglottic stenosis are rare in children, more commonly occur in females, and have a predilection for the subglottis. Whereas costal cartilage graft laryngotracheal reconstruction is an effective treatment for subglottic stenosis in most children, with inflammatory disorders affecting the subglottis, cricotracheal resection has a much better prognosis for maintaining a long-term adequate airway than laryngotracheal reconstruction.

REFERENCES

1. Hartnick CJ, Rutter M, Lang F, et al. Congenital high airway obstruction syndrome and airway reconstruction: An evolving paradigm. Arch Otolaryngol Head Neck Surg 2002;128:567–70.
2. Harrison MR, Adzick NS, Flake AW, et al. Correction of congenital diaphragmatic hernia in utero VIII: Response of the hypoplastic lung to tracheal occlusion. J Pediatr Surg 1996;31:1339–48.
3. Hirose S, Farmer DL, Lee H, et al. The ex-utero intrapartum treatment procedure: Looking back at the EXIT. J Pediatr Surg 2004;39:375–80; discussion 375–80.
4. Preciado DA, Rutter MJ, Greenberg JM, et al. Intrapartum management of severe fetal airway obstruction. J Otolaryngol 2004;33:283–8.
5. Newth CJ, Rachman B, Patel N, Hammer J. The use of cuffed versus uncuffed endotracheal tubes in pediatric intensive care. J Pediatr 2004;144:333–7.
6. Myer CM, III, O'Connor DM, Cotton RT. Proposed grading system for subglottic stenosis based on endotracheal tube sizes. Ann Otol Rhinol Laryngol 1994;103:319–23.
7. Strople J, Kaul A. Pediatric gastroesophageal reflux disease—current perspectives. Curr Opin Otolaryngol Head Neck Surg 2003;11:447–51.
8. White DR cotton RT, Bean JA, Rutter MJ. Pediatric cricotracheal resection. Surgical outcomes and risk factor analysis. Arch otolaryngol Head Neck surg 2005;131:896–9.
9. Van Den Abbeele T, Triglia JM, Francois M, et al. Congenital nasal pyriform aperture stenosis: Diagnosis and management of 20 cases. Ann Otol Rhinol Laryngol 2001;110:70–5.
10. Paoli C, Francois M, Triglia JM, et al. Nasal obstruction in the neonate secondary to nasolacrimal duct cysts. Laryngoscope 1995;105:86–9.
11. Mandell DL, Yellon RF, Bradley JP, et al. Mandibular distraction for micrognathia and severe upper airway obstruction. Arch Otolaryngol Head Neck Surg 2004;130:344–8.
12. Rhee ST, Buchman SR. Pediatric mandibular distraction osteogenesis: The present and the future. J Craniofac Surg 2003;14:803–8.
13. Johnson LB, Rutter MJ, Shott SR, Cotton RT. Acquired subglottic cysts in preterm infants. J Otolaryngol 2005;34:75–8.
14. McNamara VM, Crabbe DC. Tracheomalacia. Paediatr Respir Rev 2004;5:147–54.
15. Lim LH, Cotton RT, Azizkhan RG, et al. Complications of metallic stents in the pediatric airway. Otolaryngol Head Neck Surg 2004;131:355–61.
16. Wright CD. Pediatric tracheal surgery. Chest Surg Clin N Am 2003;13:305–14.
17. Rutter MJ, Cotton R, Azizkhan R, et al. Slide tracheoplasty for the management of complete tracheal rings. J Ped Surg 2003;38:928–34.
18. Lima JA. Laryngeal foreign bodies in children: A persistent, life-threatening problem. Laryngoscope 1989;99:415–20.
19. Tan HK, Brown K, McGill T, et al. Airway foreign bodies (FB): A 10-year review. Int J Pediatr Otorhinolaryngol 2000;56:91–9.
20. Miller RS, Willging JP, Rutter MJ, Rookkapan K. Chronic esophageal foreign bodies in pediatric patients: A retrospective review. Int J Pediatr Otorhinolaryngol 2004;68:265–72.
21. McEwan J, Giridharan W, Clarke RW, Shears P. Paediatric acute epiglottitis: Not a disappearing entity. Int J Pediatr Otorhinolaryngol 2003;67:317–21.
22. Leung AK, Kellner D, Johnson DW. Viral croup: A current perspective. J Pediatr Health Care 2004;18:297–301.
23. Salamone FN, Bobbitt DB, Myer CM, et al. Bacterial tracheitis reexamined: Is there a less severe manifestation? Otolaryngol Head Neck Surg 2004;131:871–6.
24. White DR, Preciado DA, Stamper B, et al. Airway reconstruction in pediatric burn patients. Otolaryngol Head Neck Surg 2005;113:362–5.
25. Granholm T, Farmer DL. The surgical airway. Respir Care Clin N Am 2001;7:13–23.

69

Congenital Anomalies of the Larynx

Rodney P. Lusk, MD

Congenital lesions of the larynx are relatively rare; however, in their laryngeal laboratory, Chen and Holinger found congenital laryngeal lesions in 33 of 115 specimens.[1] Of all the anomalies noted, the most common deformities are of the cricoid cartilage. The lesions develop during respiratory differentiation, which occurs during the fourth to tenth weeks of gestation. The clinical manifestations of laryngeal lesions fall into three broad categories:

1. Respiratory distress: which may range from complete obstruction with no air movement to minor types of stridor. The characteristics of the stridor are variable and depend on the site and degree of the obstruction. Most laryngeal lesions produce stridor during the inspiratory phase. The reason for this is found in the Bernoulli principle, which states that when a fluid or a gas is in motion, the pressure exerted on the wall of the airway decreases as the velocity of the gas increases. A well-known example is the wing of an airplane, shown in Figure 1. When the site of the obstruction is in an area not firmly fixed or supported, such as the supraglottis or larynx, as the air rushes into the airway, it produces a relatively negative pressure, which tends to close the airway (Figure 2). The harder the child breathes in, the faster the flow and the greater the created negative pressure, with the net effect of further decreasing the airway lumen. The negative pressure generated during inspiration may also cause supraclavicular and sternal retractions and nasal flare.
2. Dysphonia: which may be caused by laryngeal lesions that interfere with vocalization, with voice quality ranging from complete aphonia to hoarseness.
3. Failure of the larynx to close the airway during swallowing may cause feeding difficulties,

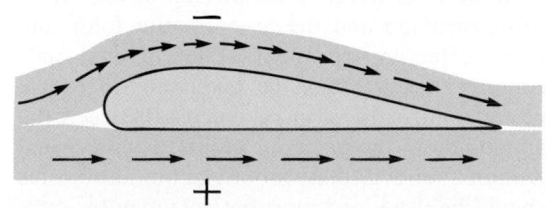

Figure 1 For a wing to produce lift, the air pressure on the top of the wing must be less than the pressure on the bottom. According to the Bernoulli principle, this can occur only when the velocity of the air is greater over the top of the wing, which is accomplished by increasing its upper curvature.

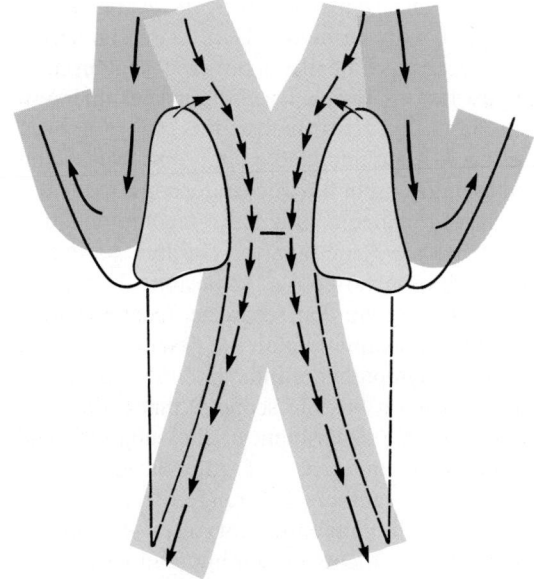

Figure 2 Demonstration of the arytenoid cartilages and the subglottis as compared to an airfoil. Note that as the velocity of the air increases in the glottis, it creates negative pressure in the airway, pulling the cuneiform cartilages and aryepiglottic folds into the airway.

with aspiration, cyanosis, or respiratory compromise.

Although this chapter deals only with laryngeal lesions and airway distress, any airway lesion may result in stridor, tachycardia, tachypnea, cyanosis, or restlessness. When evaluating patients with these signs, a history and examination of the entire airway should be performed. The history and physical examination are the most important diagnostic tools, Radiographic imaging (plain films, computed tomography [CT], and magnetic resonance imaging [MRI]) and laryngoscopy (direct and indirect) are important adjuncts and are discussed in each section.

LARYNGOMALACIA

Laryngomalacia is a condition in which the laryngeal inlet collapses on inspiration, causing stridor. The terminology is confusing, with congenital laryngeal stridor,[2] congenital laryngeal obstruction,[3] congenital stridor of infants,[4] and inspiratory laryngeal collapse[5] all used synonymously. The term laryngomalacia, introduced by Jackson and Jackson in 1942,[6] is most frequently used. Some physicians confuse this entity with tracheomalacia, which is altogether another disease.

Incidence

Laryngomalacia is the most common cause of stridor in the newborn. In some children, it may be an autosomal dominant lesion.[7] Hawkins and Clark evaluated 453 patients with the flexible fiberscope and found 84 with primary and 29 with secondary laryngomalacia.[8] Nussbaum and Maggi found that 68% of 297 children with laryngomalacia had other respiratory disorders, as noted with flexible bronchoscopy.[9] It is the most common diagnosis for airway obstruction in children with Down syndrome.[10,11]

Symptoms and Signs

The most common symptoms produced by laryngomalacia are inspiratory stridor, feeding problems, and gastric reflux. The inspiratory stridor worsens with increased respiratory effort, such as crying or feeding, and in the supine position. The symptoms begin shortly after birth in most patients,[12] increase in severity until 6 to 8 months of age, plateau at 9 months, and steadily improve thereafter.[5,13–15] No correlation exists between the duration of stridor and the severity or time of onset.[12] Manning and colleagues, however, have found a direct correlation between short aryepiglottic folds and severe apnea.[16]

Two theories have been proposed to account for the narrowing of the laryngeal inlet. The first is that a neuromuscular abnormality, by not allowing proper support of the supraglottis, causes increased flaccidity.[17] Kelemen suggested that the cause is ineffective dilators of the supraglottis,[18] but dissections by Belmont and Grundfast showed the dual insertion of the palatopharyngeus, lateral glossoepiglottic, and stylopharyngeal muscles, which could dilate the laryngeal inlet.[17] The incidence of neuromuscular disorders appears to be higher in children with laryngomalacia.[13] Reports of higher incidence of mental retardation in these patients[13] have not been substantiated.[12,17]

The other proposed mechanism is anatomic, with the narrowing resulting from (1) a flaccid epiglottis that folds against the posterior laryngeal wall or into the airway, (2) a long, tubular epiglottis that curls on itself, or (3) short and redundant aryepiglottic folds with varying sizes of cuneiform cartilage that rotate medially into the airway (Figures 3 and 4).[19] The W-shaped epiglottis is not thought to be a significant factor because it occurs in 30 to 50% of patients,[3,20–22] most of whom do not have stridor.

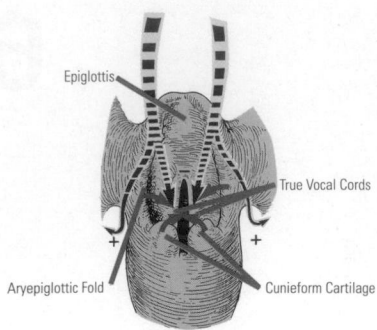

Figure 3 The airflow through the larynx creates a relative negative pressure and pulls the aryepiglottic folds and cuneiform cartilages into the airway.

Feeding problems are frequent with laryngomalacia. Radiographic evidence of gastric reflux occurs in 80% and regurgitation in 40% past 3 months of age.[17] In the study by Zalzal and colleagues, 5 of 21 patients presented with feeding problems.[23] Some investigators believe that feeding problems are secondary to the high negative pressures generated during inspiration. Aspiration pneumonitis has been reported in 7% of children with laryngomalacia.[17] The mechanism for this is unclear but may be associated with the negative pressure and feeding problems.

Obstructive sleep apnea (23%) and central apnea (10%) have also been noted.[24] Cor pulmonale can develop secondary to laryngomalacia.[23] If untreated, it may also be associated with increased pulmonary arterial pressures.[25]

Diagnosis

The diagnosis is most frequently based on the symptoms and signs, flexible laryngoscopy, and lateral radiographs of the neck and chest and rigid endoscopy to identify possible synchronous airway lesions such as subglottic stenosis. Hawkins and Clark have shown flexible laryngoscopy to be effective, even in neonates.[8] It is more accurate than using a general anesthetic

and rigid endoscopy.[26] The advantage of using the flexible scope in an awake patient is that the dynamics of the supraglottis can readily be appreciated. The disadvantage is that the milder forms of laryngomalacia may be missed if the child is crying. The flexible scope can also be used to diagnose other synchronous glottic lesions such as vocal cord paralysis and glottic cysts. Mancuso and colleagues retrospectively evaluated 233 patients with laryngomalacia to assess the necessity of performing a complete diagnostic workup in all patients.[27] Their conclusion was that rigid endoscopy in evaluation of an infant with laryngomalacia is rarely necessary because clinically significant synchronous airway lesions which require surgical intervention are rare. Historically, this has not been the case. Hawkins and Clark and Nussbaum and Maggi[9] used flexible endoscopy to evaluate laryngomalacia, but their recommendation was that "all symptomatic" children be evaluated with bronchoscopy.[8,9] Bluestone, Healy and Cotton have gone "on record as recommending a complete evaluation of the tracheobronchial tree in all symptomatic infants.[28]" The disadvantage of using a flexible scope is that it does not allow accurate assessment of the subglottis and trachea. The incidence of other lesions noted by additional authors has ranged from 18% in patients with congenital laryngeal lesions to 59.8% of all patients presenting with stridor.[29,30] The controversy lies in the likelihood of missing a clinically significant synchronous airway lesion that would have been otherwise treated if rigid endoscopy had been performed. Mancuso and colleagues concluded that rigid endoscopy was not necessary in otherwise asymptomatic children.[27] Bluestone and colleagues reached the opposite conclusion based on their "retrospective careers, we (they) have encountered countless number of infants who have had a clinically significant airway problem in whom the diagnosis of laryngomalacia was previously made by flexible fiberoptic laryngoscopy, but rigid endoscopy

was omitted.[28]" Deaths have been described in patients with severe disease.[31–33] This controversy is going to require additional data that are prospectively acquired. Currently, it would appear that if symptoms are not compatible with laryngomalacia alone or if the patient fails to thrive, direct laryngoscopy and rigid bronchoscopy should be performed to rule out secondary lesions. It is the surgeon's obligation to closely follow his or her patients until the symptoms resolve.

Treatment

Expectant observation is sufficient in most cases. The small percentage of patients (10 to 15%) with failure to thrive or more than one lesion may require surgical intervention. Iglauer, in 1922, was the first to alter the supraglottis surgically in laryngomalacia.[33] Schwartz, in 1944, removed a V-shaped wedge from an epiglottis with good results.[5] Fearon and Ellis, in 1971, successfully treated a patient by suturing the epiglottis to the base of the tongue.[34] In that same year, hyomandibulopexy was advocated in France.[35,36] Templer and colleagues, in 1981, performed a supraglottectomy in an adult for long-standing stridor and obstructive sleep apnea secondary to laryngomalacia.[37] Lane and colleagues, in 1984, excised the tips of the arytenoids, edematous mucosa, a portion of the corniculate cartilages, and a portion of the aryepiglottic fold with microcupped forceps and Bellucci scissors.[38] Seid and colleagues successfully treated three patients with the laser in 1985.[39] Since then, numerous case reports have appeared in the literature.[40] Zalzal and colleagues trimmed the lateral edges of the epiglottis, aryepiglottic folds, and the corniculate cartilages with microlaryngeal scissors.[23] Solomons and Prescott recommended trimming the supraglottis and performing an anterior epiglottopexy.[20] The trimming of the aryepiglottic folds may involve both sides or only one side. Kelly and Gray recommended unilateral removal of redundant supraglottic tissue (supraglottoplasty) and operation on the other side if the patient is not asymptomatic.[41] We have recommended doing both sides at one setting. Either appears to give satisfactory results.

Holinger and Konior prefer the term supraglottoplasty to describe the surgical procedures for removing the flaccid supraglottic tissues.[19] Whymark and colleagues, in a large study, used the laser to remove a portion of the cuneiform cartilage and the aryepiglottic folds and noted effective treatment of laryngomalacia[42] (Figure 5). Care must be taken not to excise or traumatize the strip of mucosa between the arytenoids in the posterior glottis. Holinger and Konior believe that prophylactic antibiotics should be used, and most patients may be extubated in the immediate postoperative period but should be observed overnight in the intensive care unit.[19] A supraglottoplasty may improve the gastroesophageal reflux, however, this remains controversial.[43,44]

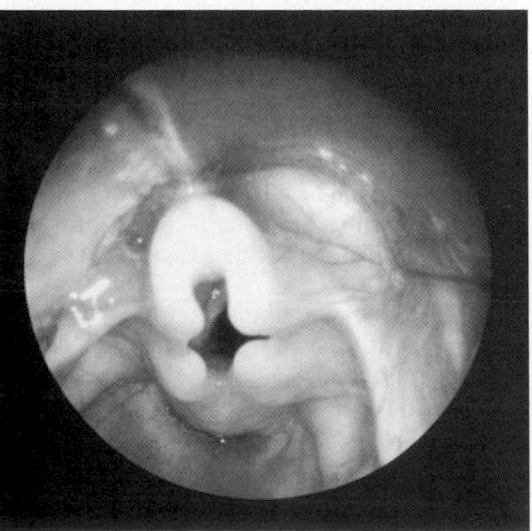

(A)

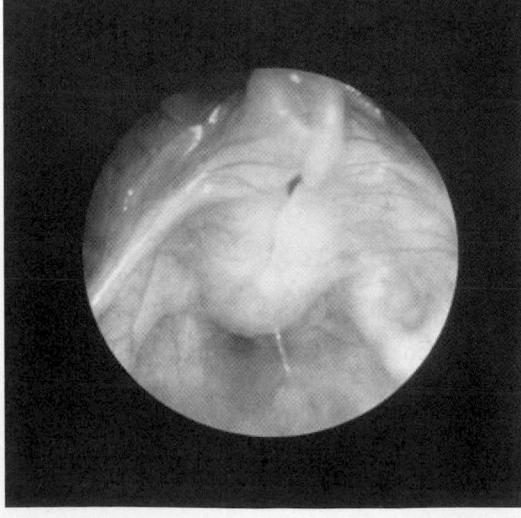

(B)

Figure 4 Example of laryngomalacia. (A) Supraglottis at beginning of inspiration. (B) Complete collapse of the supraglottis toward the end of inspiration. (Courtesy of Dr G.B. Healy, Boston's Children's Hospital, Boston, Massachusetts.)

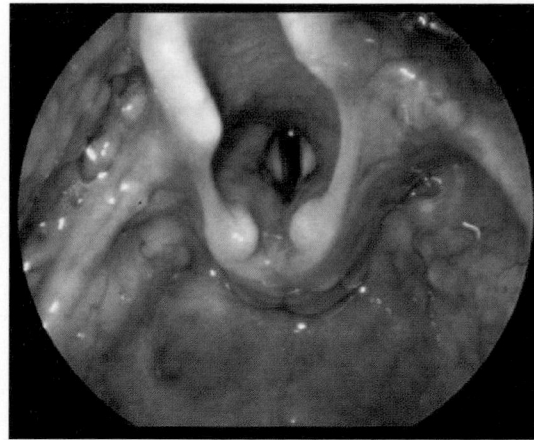

(A)

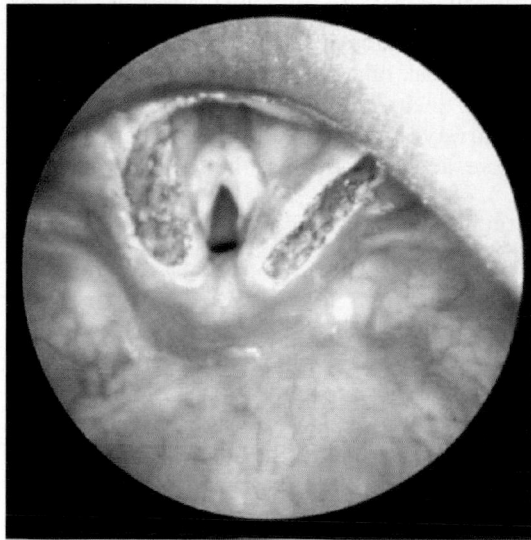

(B)

Figure 5 Laryngomalacia.

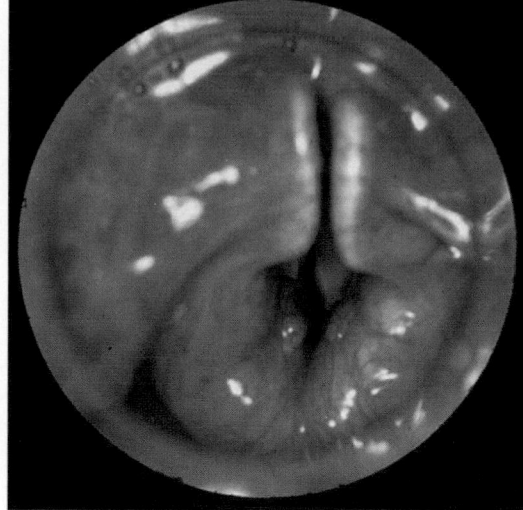

Figure 6 Bifid epiglottis.

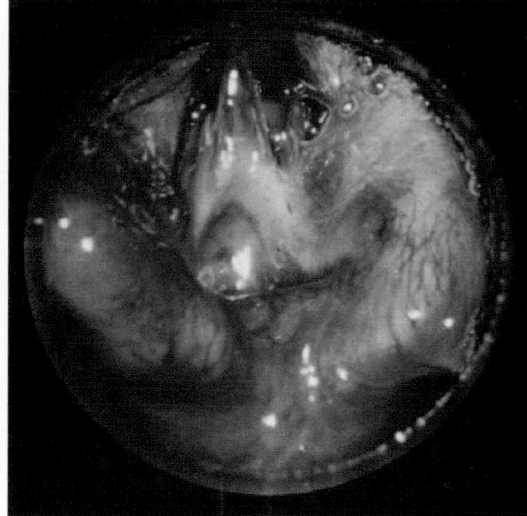

Figure 7 Laryngeal atresia.

ABSENT OR RUDIMENTRY EPIGLOTTIS

Incidence

These rare lesions can be associated with stridor and aspiration. In 1949, in the only thorough review of the world literature, Montreuil found only five clearly documented cases.[45] Since then, six additional cases have been reported.[46–48] Most of these patients had a bifid epiglottis.

Symptoms and Signs

Patients have presented with respiratory distress secondary to rotation of the two halves of the epiglottis into the airway. The incidence of multiple congenital anomalies is high. A 44% incidence of polydactyly has been reported.[49] Graham and colleagues have reported three cases of hypopituitarism.[47]

Diagnosis

The only means of diagnosing a bifid epiglottis is with flexible or direct laryngoscopy (Figure 6). Because of the high incidence of associated airway lesions, direct laryngoscopy is suggested for all patients.

Treatment

If the airway distress is significant, a tracheostomy is warranted. Montreuil amputated the epiglottis

with good results.[45] Healy and colleagues performed a tracheostomy in two patients, in time the epiglottis matured and both patients were decannulated without surgical intervention on the epiglottis.[49]

ATRESIA

Atresia occurs when the laryngeal opening fails to develop and an obstruction is created at or near the glottis. Tracheal agenesis may also occur but is thought to be a rarer lesion.[50]

Incidence and Etiology

Congenital laryngeal atresia is a rare lesion, with only 51 cases reported in the world literature in 1987.[51] It is thought to be the rarest laryngeal lesion, accounting for only 1 of 846 congenital lesions evaluated by Holinger and colleagues and none of 433 congenital lesions evaluated by Fearon and Ellis.[31,34,52] The lesion is thought to arise from the premature arrest of normal vigorous epithelial ingrowth into the larynx during the fourteenth to seventeenth stages of embryonic development.[53] In the embryonic larynx, a pharyngoglottic duct divides the larynx into an anterior (membranous) portion and a posterior (cartilaginous) portion.[54]

Symptoms and Signs

At delivery, the infant makes strong respiratory efforts but does not move air, cry, or manifest any stridor. The infant becomes markedly cyanotic when the umbilical cord is clamped. Most of these infants die at birth unless an emergency tracheostomy is performed. Some infants survive if they have a large tracheoesophageal fistula and if the esophagus is intubated. Not infrequently, a pharyngotracheal duct is present in the larynx. This should not be confused with a tracheoesophageal fistula, which is located much lower.

Diagnosis

The diagnosis is most frequently made at autopsy.[55] With the increased use of ultrasound,

the diagnosis of laryngeal atresia can be made before birth by noting enlarged edematous echogenic lungs, dilated airways, inverted diaphargms, compressed fetal heart, severe ascites, and fetal hydrops.[56–60] This is now termed congenital high airway obstruction syndrome (CHAOS) and can be diagnosed prenatally with ultrasound.[61,62] Smith and Bain outlined three types of laryngeal atresia deformities; these investigators indicated that these types are not absolute but are gradations of a continuous spectrum.[63] Type 1 involves the supraglottic and infraglottic larynx with fused arytenoids, an absent vestibule, and a deformed cricoid cartilage. Type 2 involves only the cricoid (subglottic area) with normal arytenoids, vestibule, and vocal cords. Type 3 involves a fused glottis with a normal vestibule and cricoid (Figure 7). The extent of the obstruction can be diagnosed with ultrasound.[64,65] The subglottic lesions have been found to be cartilaginous or membranous.[53]

Treatment

The patient will not survive unless an emergency tracheostomy is performed or the patient is ventilated through a tracheoesophageal fistula. Identifying laryngeal atresia prenatally with ultrasound dramatically improves the chance of survival by allowing caregivers with appropriate expertise to be present at delivery.[65] Treatment is a tracheostomy combined with exutero intrapartum treatment (EXIT) which is basically performing the tracheostomy prior to severing the umbilical cord.[61,66] Tracheoesophageal fistulas are frequently associated with this condition and usually arise at the tracheal bifurcation[63,67,68] (Figure 8). Most of the survivors had the membranous type 3 lesion or a type 2 lesion and a tracheoesophageal fistula which allowed ventilation until a tracheostomy could be performed.

WEBS

Laryngeal webs occur in the glottis. Rarely, webs extend from the epiglottis to the lateral or posterior aspects of the hypopharynx and can result in

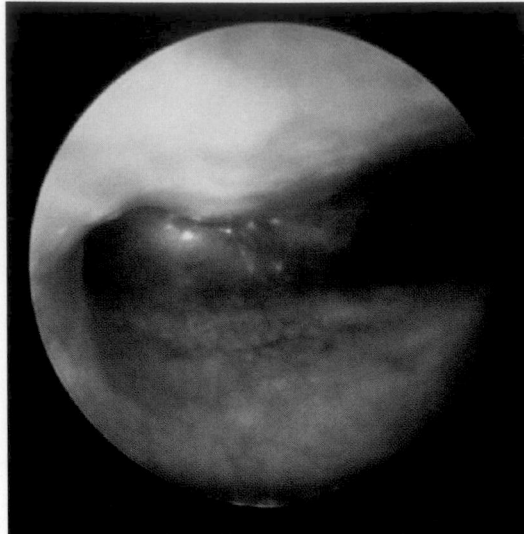

(A)

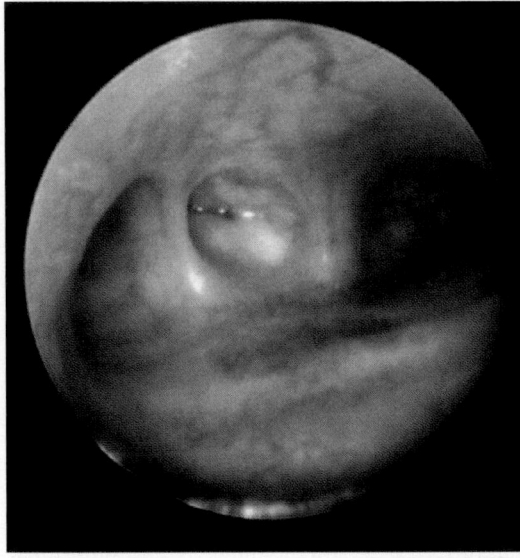

(B)

Figure 8 (A) Tracheal esophageal fistula. (B) Tracheal esophageal fistula.

significant airway compromise.[69] Holinger and colleagues described a patient with simultaneous supraglottic and glottic webs.[70] Most webs are located anteriorly and extend a varying length toward the arytenoids. The webs vary in thickness from a thin structure to one that is thicker and more difficult to eradicate. Benjamin and Mair described a rare type known as a congenital interarytenoid web, which limits the abduction of the arytenoids.[71]

Incidence

Congenital laryngeal webs are uncommon, occurring in 5% of all congenital laryngeal lesions.[53,72] Acquired lesions are more common than congenital lesions, in a 60:40 ratio.[73] Associated anomalies are frequently seen, especially higher in the airway.[72,74,75] Posterior glottic webs occur in only 1 to 4% of patients.[73]

Symptoms and Signs

Symptoms of laryngeal webs are present at birth in 75% of the patients and within 1 year in all patients.[75] The types of symptoms depend on the severity of the web. Many children are asymptomatic until they are stressed, have an infection, or are intubated for a surgical procedure. Vocal dysfunction is the most frequent symptom and was noted in 47 of 51 patients evaluated by Cohen.[74] The severity of the dysphonia is not necessarily indicative of the severity of the web. Cohen reported on 11 patients who complained of aphonia, 16 with weak or whispery voices, 7 with husky voices, and 4 with some hoarseness. The second most common symptom is airway obstruction, and the severity is directly proportional to the degree of obstruction. The compromise may be so severe that stridor cannot be produced because of limited air movement through the larynx. If stridor is present, it will occur in both inspiratory and expiratory phases, and if stridor is severe, the airway must be secured with intubation or a tracheostomy. Forty percent of Cohen's patients required a tracheostomy.[74] Croup rarely occurs in children younger than 6 months. Cohen reported 15 of 51 children with a significant history of recurrent croup, of whom 7 required tracheostomy, 9 presented with pneumonia, and 6 had tracheobronchitis.[74]

Diagnosis

The only way to diagnosis the extent of the web correctly is with direct laryngoscopy under general anesthesia.[76] The flexible scope may also have a role in the initial diagnosis, but experience in using it in patients with laryngeal webs is limited. Lateral radiographs of the neck may allow assessment of the width of the web.

Cohen has divided laryngeal webs into four types, based on their appearance and an estimation of the degree of airway obstruction.[74] Type 1 is uniform in thickness with no subglottic extension and with the true vocal folds clearly visible in the web and compromises less than 35% of the airway (Figure 9). Hoarseness is usually only slight. Type 2 is slightly thicker, with a significantly thicker anterior component that may extend into the subglottis. The web restricts the airway by 35 to 50% and usually causes little airway distress unless the patient has an acute infection or is traumatized during intubation (Figure 10). The voice is usually husky. Type 3 is a thick web that is solid anteriorly with the true vocal folds

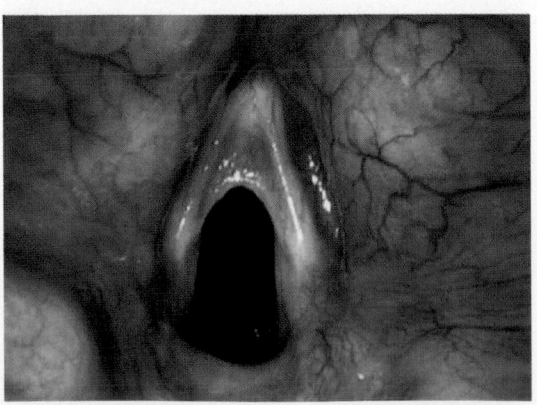

Figure 9 Type I laryngeal web.

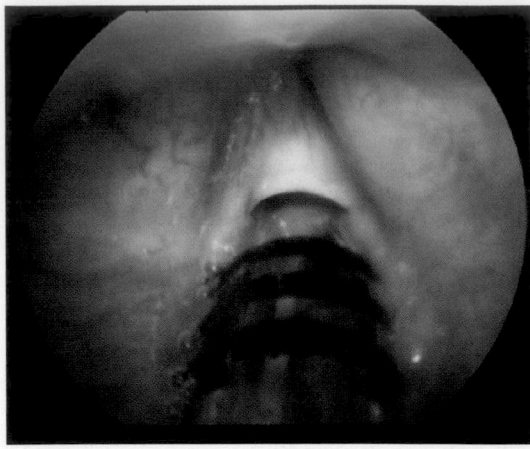

Figure 10 Type 2 laryngeal web that is intubated.

not well delineated. The web restricts the airway by 50 to 75%, creates marked vocal dysfunction, with a weak or whispery voice. Type 4 is a uniformly thick, solid web occluding 75 to 90% of the airway (Figure 11). Respiratory obstruction is severe, and the patient is almost always aphonic.

Treatment

Approximately 60% of patients require surgical intervention.[75] Some webs are not repaired because the patients succumb to other systemic complications. Of all patients with laryngeal webs, 30 to 40% require a tracheostomy.[74,75] The type of lesion dictates the surgical approach. In general, the thinner webs are easier to treat; the more severe webs are resistant to surgical management. It is difficult to obtain a crisp anterior commissure and, even if one is obtained, this does not ensure a good voice.

Type I lesions are not life-threatening. Many do not require surgery, but if surgery is performed, dilations or excisions with a knife, scissors, or laser are effective. Type 2 lesions require treatment, but not in childhood. Multiple procedures are necessary for excising small portions of the web in multiple steps. Corticosteroids and antibiotics decrease the amount of scarring, and speech therapy may be necessary to maximize phonation. Type 3 lesions frequently require

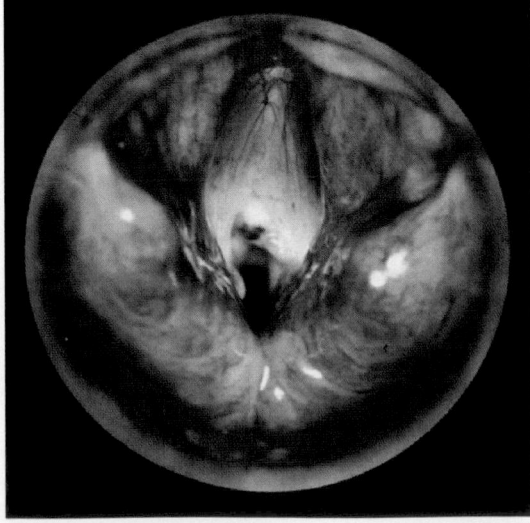

Figure 11 Type 4 laryngeal web.

tracheostomy to establish the airway. The child may develop progressive airway distress because of increased airway demands, trauma from intubation, or infection. These lesions may require multiple excisions and frequently necessitate the placement of a keel.[77,78] McGuirt and colleagues described a method using the laser to develop flaps of the web and reported near normal results in all patients.[73] Type 4 lesions all require a tracheostomy and excision of the web with placement of a keel. Because they are tracheostomy dependent, these patients should be monitored with apnea monitors. Most surgeons would resect the web and place the keel through a laryngofissure. The airway results are good, but the voice is poor.[74]

SACCULAR CYSTS AND LARYNGOCELES

Laryngoceles and laryngeal saccular cysts are thought to arise from the laryngeal ventricle or saccular appendage[79–83] or from retention cysts resulting from obstruction of mucus gland ducts.[84] Morgagni incompletely described the saccule, and Galen also had mentioned it previously.[85] The appendage arises from the anterior aspect of the ventricle, extends superiorly, and curves slightly posteriorly deep to the false vocal folds and aryepiglottic folds. The orifice opens into the ventricle and measures only 0.5 to 1 mm. The ventriculosaccular fold probably serves to help store mucus and direct it posteromedially to lubricate the vocal folds.[86] In the adult, the appendage extends as high as the superior border of the thyroid cartilage. Broyles found that 75% of the saccules measured 6 to 8 mm in length, 25% measured more than 10 mm, and 7% measured more than 15 mm.[87] In the fetus, 25% extend as high as the thyrohyoid membrane.[85] The type of lesion that develops is based on the size of the saccule, whether there is free communication with the laryngeal lumen, and whether there is inflammation within the sac. DeSanto and colleagues believe that the differentiating factor between the development of a cyst or a laryngocele is the patency of the ventricle.[85,88]

Saccular Cysts

Incidence. Laryngeal saccular cysts are most likely to become manifest in infancy.[85] Congenital laryngeal cysts are rare, but the awareness of their possibility is important because almost 50% of these cysts are diagnosed at autopsy after the infant has asphyxiated.[86] In 1967, Suehs and Powell found 27 reported cases of congenital laryngeal cysts.[89]

Symptoms and Signs. Forty percent of congenital laryngeal cysts are discovered within a few hours of birth, and 95% of the infants have symptoms before 6 months of age.[90] The most frequent symptom is stridor (90%), which is primarily inspiratory, although it may be biphasic.[86] The stridor improves in some infants during

extension of the neck. The cry has been reported as feeble, muffled, shrill, hoarse, or normal.[52,89] Dyspnea, apnea, and cyanosis have been noted in 55% of patients.[90] The associated feeding problems are similar to those in esophageal atresia, or tracheoesophageal fistula without atresia, and lead to failure to thrive in a large number of patients.[89,90]

Diagnosis. Chest and lateral neck radiographs, barium swallow, and computed tomographic scan are useful preoperative evaluations of the stridor, but they are not diagnostic.[86,91] Hemangiomas, for example, can cause identical findings, although these lesions appear most frequently in the subglottis. The only way to make the diagnosis definitively is with direct laryngoscopy.[90] Cotton and Richardson suggested that at the time of endoscopy one should have a large-bore needle, a tracheostomy tray, and an appropriate-size rigid bronchoscope available.[92] The cysts are typically divided into lateral wall saccular cysts and anterior saccular cysts. Lateral saccular cysts are most frequently located in the aryepiglottic fold, epiglottis, or lateral wall of the larynx[89,90] (Figure 12). Anterior saccular cysts extend medially and posteriorly between the true and false vocal folds and directly into the laryngeal lumen.[90,91] They are most frequently sessile but may be pedunculated. Mitchell and colleagues reported four subglottic cysts in patients who had previously been intubated and considered the cysts to be probably secondary to intubation.[90]

Treatment. Treatment of laryngeal cysts may require emergency tracheostomy.[86,93,94] Mitchell and colleagues noted that 20% of their patients required emergency intervention.[90] In the infant, the cysts should be treated primarily with endoscopic deroofing or aspiration. Suehs and Powell recommended endoscopic incision and drainage as needed.[89] Holinger and colleagues thought that smaller anterior saccular cysts could be effectively treated with cup forceps removal (excision biopsy) at the time of direct laryngoscopy.[86] These investigators would not attempt

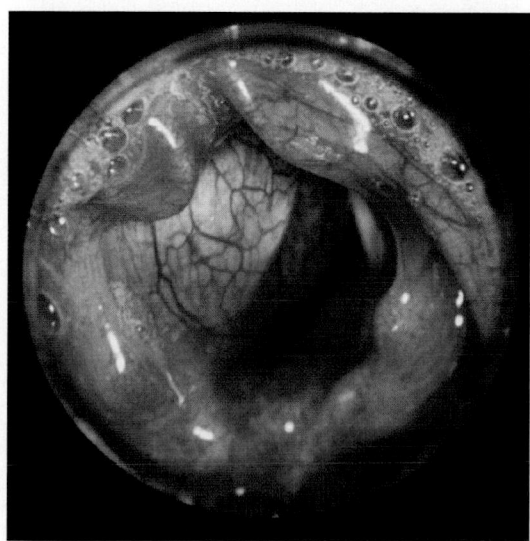

Figure 12 Anterior saccular cyst.

endoscopic dissection of the entire sac. Aspiration has also been recommended, but the incidence of recurrence is high.[80,95] Mitchell and colleagues reported successful treatment of 7 of 17 patients with deroofing or marsupialization.[90] A second deroofing was required in 6 of 7 recurrences. The remaining failure was treated with total excision through a laryngofissure.

Laryngoceles

Incidence. As of 1977, 300 laryngoceles had been recorded in the world literature.[96] They may occur in infants and children, and they cause airway obstruction.[97] The presence of laryngoceles in this age group appears to be rare, however. Laryngoceles are much more common in adults and appear most commonly in the fifth decade.[96] Holinger and Brown reported on 12 patients with congenital laryngocele in infancy.[52] Baker and colleagues found an increased incidence of laryngoceles in laryngeal cancer and suggested that obstruction of the saccule by the carcinoma was a factor in developing laryngoceles.[98]

Symptoms and Signs. Laryngoceles are symptomatic only when they are filled with air or fluid, so the symptoms may be intermittent. Because the laryngocele may rapidly inflate and deflate, several radiographs may be necessary to document the lesion (Figure 13). A fluid-filled laryngocele may be difficult to differentiate from a cyst. If it becomes infected, it fills with mucopus and is called a laryngopyocele.

Diagnosis. The definitive diagnosis is made with direct laryngoscopy but, because the symptoms are intermittent, more than one examination may be necessary. Laryngoceles originate from the ventricle and bulge out between the true and false vocal folds or dissect posteriorly into the arytenoid and aryepiglottic fold. In general, three types have been described: internal, external, and mixed[96]; however, this classification is artificial. The internal type is limited to the larynx, whereas the external type extends into the neck through the isthmus of the thyrohyoid membrane. The mixed type involves both internal and external cysts and is the most common. Laryngoceles should be diagnosed with direct laryngoscopy and radiographic findings when they are symptomatic. Trapnell has emphasized that the radiographic appearance of a large saccule does not warrant the diagnosis of a laryngocele.[98,99]

Treatment. Only symptomatic lesions require treatment. DeSanto preferred the external approach[85]; however, most of his experience was in adults. The procedure described by Yarington and Frazer provides adequate exposure for resection.[100] Holinger and colleagues emphasized that true laryngoceles are rare in children and should be treated endoscopically by deroofing with cup forceps.[86] On occasion, the laryngocele can be aspirated and a more orderly resection can be performed at a later date.[101] The laser is also an alternative.

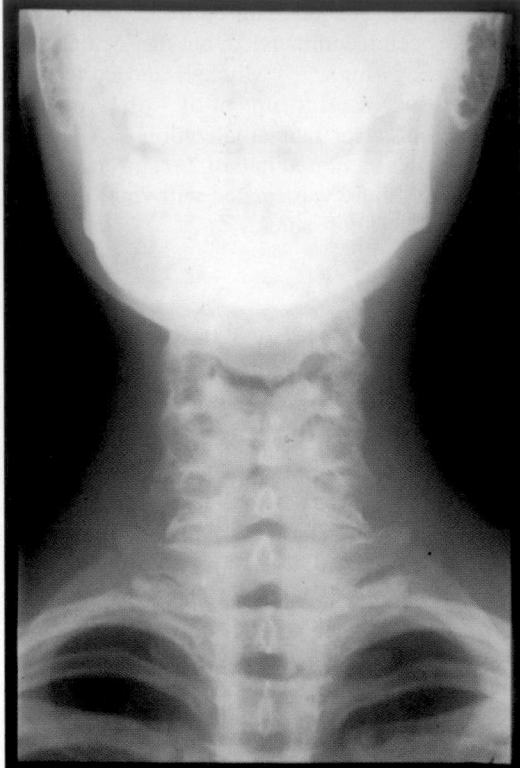

(A)

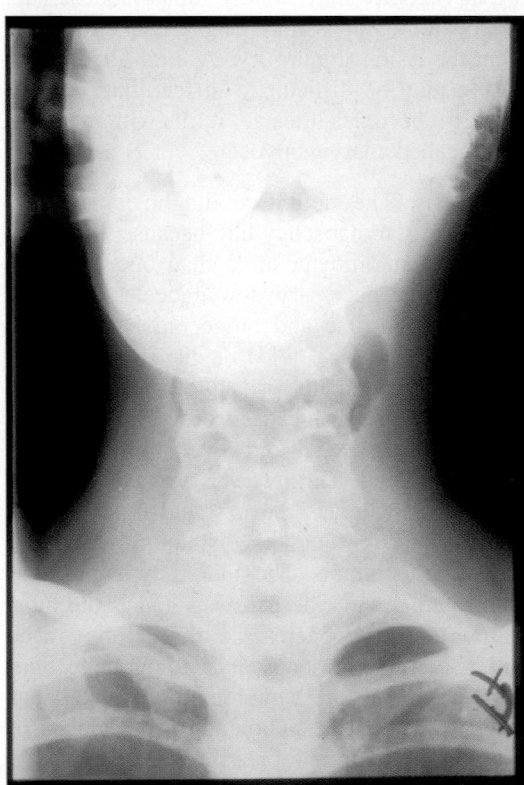

(B)

Figure 13 (A) Laryngocele preinflation, and (B) laryngocele postinflation.

LARYNGEAL CLEFTS

The congenital laryngotracheoesophageal cleft is characterized by a deficiency in the separation between the esophagus and the trachea or larynx. Type one clefts are recognized more frequently,[102,103] however, the true incidence is not yet known. Larger clefts are associated with a high mortality.[104] Early diagnosis is crucial to prevent permanent pulmonary damage.[105]

Incidence

Most clefts occur through the posterior part of the glottis; however, ventral or rare anterior clefts have been reported.[106] Clefts may be classified into three broad categories. Type I is called the laryngeal cleft and is found only in the posterior part of the glottis. Type II and type III involve the trachea in addition to the larynx (Figure 14).[107] Type II extends down to but not beyond the sixth tracheal ring, and type III can extend to the carina. As of 1983, 85 well-documented cases of clefts have been reported in the world literature.[108] Finlay observed a family in which two of five children developed a cleft larynx.[109] Other investigators have reported similar examples. The inheritance pattern is almost always autosomal dominant. Posterior glottic clefts have been associated with tracheal agenesis, as well as many other congenital anomalies.[108]

Symptoms and Signs

The following manifestations, in order of frequency, are associated with laryngotracheoesophageal clefts: aspiration and cyanosis (53%), postpartum asphyxia (33%), increased mucus production (23%), recurrent pneumonia (16%), voiceless crying (16%), stridor (10%), and impaired swallowing (5%).[109] Aspiration of thin liquids is the most common presenting sign for Type I clefts.[110] The simultaneous occurrence of increased saliva production, low, soundless, or hurried crying, and stridor should lead to the suspicion of a cleft. The inspiratory stridor is produced by the collapse of redundant mucosa around the cleft and from the intrusion of the arytenoid into the airway.[111,112] Cohen reported that the stridor may be expiratory because of aspirated secretions.[107] One sees a frequent combination of posterior laryngeal clefts and tracheoesophageal fistulas.

Diagnosis

Occult posterior laryngeal clefts have been diagnosed with magnetic resonance imaging.[113] A laryngeal cleft is frequently demonstrated by an esophagram with water-soluble contrast medium or is suggested by aspiration pneumonia on a chest radiograph.[114] A recent endoscopic diagnostic test, functional endoscopic evaluation of swallow (FEES) has been applied to the diagnosis of laryngeal clefts with some success.[110] The most important diagnostic test, however, remains direct laryngoscopy, and it should be combined with a high index of suspicion. If one does not specifically look for the entity, it frequently escapes detection.[115] When the larynx is examined, redundant mucosa in the posterior part of the glottis is usually the first clue to the defect (Figure 15). On inspiration, this redundant mucosa may rotate into the airway. The cleft can best be demonstrated by placing a laryngoscope, such as a Dedo or Jako, into the supraglottis and examining the posterior glottis. If a posterior laryngeal cleft is present, this maneuver will clearly demonstrate the lesion and its extent (Figure 16). The posterior part of the glottis can also be palpated with a spatula or a similar thin instrument to demonstrate the defect. Some authors find microlaryngoscopy helpful.[111] Some clefts are submucous, and diagnosis is made only on laryngeal sections.[116,117] The clinical significance of submucous clefts is unknown. There is a high incidence of associated esophageal lesions and tracheoesophageal fistulas, for which careful examination must be made.[107,111,116,118,119]

Treatment

The prognosis for a patient with this lesion is not favorable without early diagnosis to prevent pulmonary damage and associated morbidity or mortality.[105] In the review presented by Roth and colleagues, 24 patients died before surgical intervention; of patients with type III clefts, 13 of 14 died; of those with type II clefts, 13 of 31 died; and of those with type I, 13 of 30 died.[108] Almost two-thirds of the deceased patients had other severe malformations. Clefts were repaired in 48 patients, 13 of whom died. A tracheostomy was performed in 50% of all patients. The first

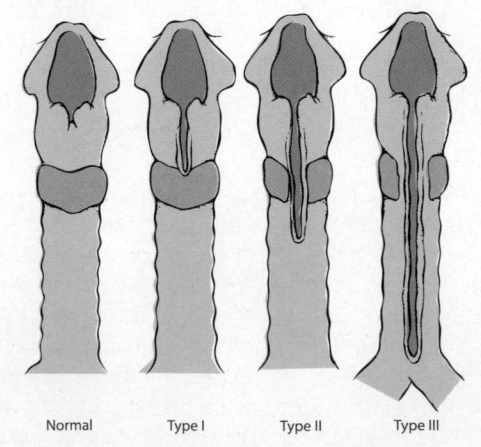

Normal   Type I   Type II   Type III

Figure 14 Classification of laryngeal and tracheoesophageal clefts as proposed by Evans.[107]

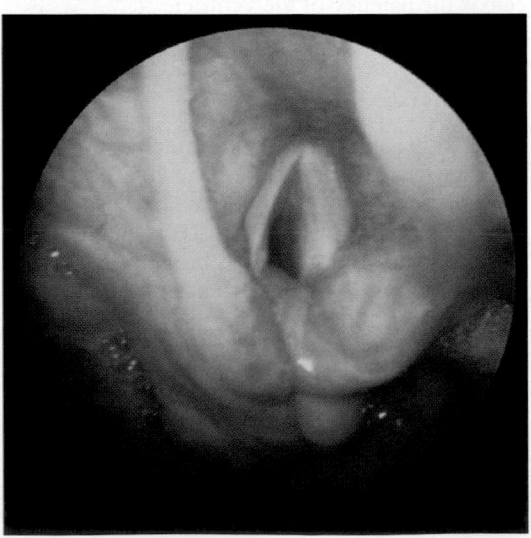

Figure 15 Laryngeal cleft.

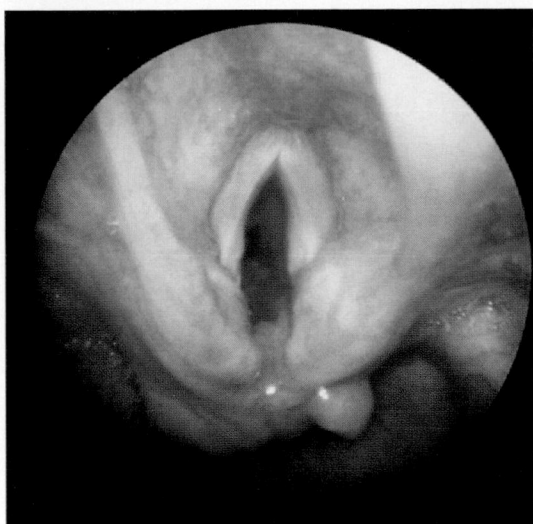

Figure 16 Laryngeal cleft.

successful operative correction of the defect in the larynx was achieved by Petterson.[120]

Three surgical approaches to the posterior aspect of the larynx have been described. Minor (type I clefts) can be repaired endoscopically.[121,122] Recent attempts to perform the repair utilizing robotics have met with some success, however, the application is limited by the exposure available in infants or neonates.[123] A lateral pharyngotomy has been used frequently, especially for the larger laryngeal clefts.[108,111] but the major disadvantage of this approach lies in the danger of injuring the recurrent laryngeal nerve. Also, the exposure is limited, and it is difficult to obtain a good layered closure. The anterior laryngofissure does not risk the recurrent laryngeal nerve and has been used in neonates.[107,108,112,124–126] Evans reported better exposure and a better two-layer closure in type II and III clefts with a laryngofissure[111] (Figure 17). Prescott[127] successfully repaired a cleft with a posterior rib graft through a laryngofissure. A disturbance of the laryngeal growth appears unlikely. Intraoperative airway management has been a problem in repairing these lesions. Ahmad and colleagues solved the problem by using a bifurcated endotracheal tube.[128] Geiduschek and colleagues reported the use of extracorporeal membrane oxygenation for

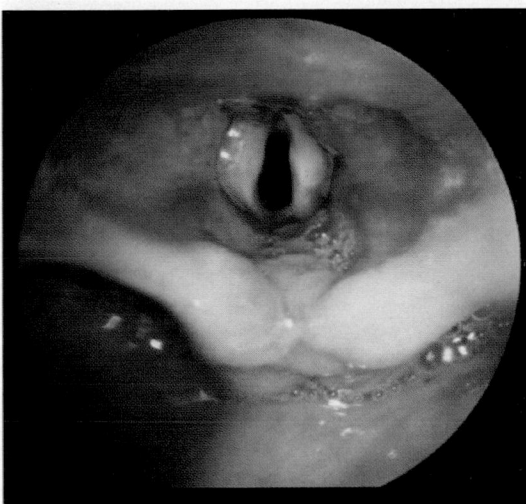

Figure 17 Type I cleft repaired through a laryngofissure.

extensive cleft repair.[129] We have used bypass to repair long-segment tracheal stenosis.

Cotton and Schreiber have noted that, after repair of posterior clefts, the patient may have continued esophageal reflux and aspiration of gastric contents.[130] There appears to be a significant decrease in successful repair if a tracheoesophageal fistula is present.[119] When this occurs, these investigators recommend a high gastric section with a double gastrostomy to minimize the chance of aspiration of gastric contents. Robie and colleagues reported that of 170 clefts repaired, 19 required revision surgery.[126]

VOCAL FOLD PARALYSIS

Vocal fold paralysis can be categorized into congenital and acquired lesions. One or both of the true vocal folds may be involved, and bilateral vocal fold paralysis is more frequent.[131–133] Apnea is frequently seen in bilateral vocal fold paralysis.[134–136] Congenital laryngeal paralysis is frequently associated with central nervous system lesions, including hydrocephalus, meningomyelocele, Arnold-Chiari malformation, meningocele, encephalocele, cerebral agenesis, nucleus ambiguus dysgenesis, neuromuscular disorders, and myasthenia gravis.[137,138] Arnold-Chiari is the most frequent malformation and is likely a contributing factor in most cases.[139,140] An underlying neurogenic cause for unilateral or bilateral vocal fold paralysis must be sought in the pediatric patient.

Incidence and Etiology

Estimates of the frequency of vocal fold paralysis range from 1.5 to 23%[133,141,142]; according to some authors, it ranks second in frequency among all congenital laryngeal lesions.[137] Holinger and colleagues found that congenital paralyses were more frequent than acquired.[138] The acquired group can be further categorized into traumatic, infectious, or neoplastic. Traumatic lesions are most frequent secondary to stretching of the recurrent laryngeal nerve during vaginal delivery or surgical trauma in management of bronchogenic cysts, tracheoesophageal fistulas, or patent ductus arteriosus.[137] Infectious diseases such as whooping cough, encephalitis, poliomyelitis, diphtheria, rabies, tetanus, syphilis, and botulism are now rarely seen but can cause vocal fold paralysis.[136] Tumors of the brain and spinal column are also rare but can cause unilateral or bilateral vocal fold paralysis.

The pathophysiology of bilateral vocal fold paralysis is unclear, but the condition may result from (1) compression of the vagus nerve in its course through the foramen magnum, (2) traction of the cervical rootlets of the vagus nerve by the caudal displacement of the brainstem, or (3) brainstem dysgenesis.[143,144] Most authors favor the compression theory because, with timely decompression of hydrocephalus or the Arnold-Chiari malformation, the vocal folds regain function. Familial bilateral vocal fold paralysis[145–147] and

persistent apnea after tracheostomy[134] appear to be most appropriately explained by the dysgenesis theory. Probably, more than one mechanism can cause vocal fold paralysis.

Laryngeal lesions such as subglottis stenosis, laryngomalacia, and posterior laryngeal clefts have also been associated with, but do not cause, vocal fold paralysis.[147,148]

Symptoms and Signs

Any of the three laryngeal functions of respiration, voice production, and deglutition can be affected by vocal fold paralysis. With unilateral vocal fold paralysis, the voice is breathy and weak, but the patient has an adequate airway unless stressed. Stridor, weak cry, and some degree of respiratory distress can be seen in all patients with bilateral vocal fold paralysis.[144] Children have more problems than adults with reflux, choking, and feeding difficulties.[149] Dedo noted that, if both the recurrent and superior laryngeal nerves are paralyzed, the vocal folds will be in the intermediate position and the airway will frequently be sufficient to allow adequate ventilation.[137,150] If the recurrent nerves only are paralyzed, the vocal folds will be in the paramedian position, resulting in an inadequate airway.

Stridor is the most frequent presenting symptom of bilateral vocal fold paralysis,[138] and its onset may be sudden.[144] Older children suppress laughing and coughing because of the increased respiratory demand. The airway becomes narrower, and there will be an increase in stridor, the development of nasal flaring, restlessness, and the use of accessory respiratory muscles, with an indrawing of the sternum and epigastrium. The stridor may progress to cyanosis, apnea, and respiratory and cardiac arrest if not recognized and treated.

Aspiration and dysphagia are frequently noted in patients with bilateral vocal cord paralysis.[143,151] Pneumonia may first be apparent when signs of increasing cranial pressure appear.

Diagnosis

The diagnosis is made by flexible laryngoscopy or direct laryngoscopy. Vocal fold mobility may be difficult to examine in an infant, and the intermediate versus paramedian position may be impossible to assess.

Treatment

Once the diagnosis of vocal fold paralysis is made, the airway should be secured if the patient has significant airway distress. The airway is best established with intubation, followed by a full workup to ascertain the cause of the vocal fold paralysis. One must look specifically for associated findings of meningomyelocele, Arnold-Chiari malformation, and hydrocephalus.[138] If the compression of the nerves is relieved within 24 hours, the vocal folds will regain function within 2 weeks[138,144]; otherwise, vocal fold function may not return for a year and a half, if at all. If intervention has been timely, the larynx should be examined periodically to assess vocal fold function. If the patient shows no evidence of function within 1 to 2 weeks, a tracheostomy should be performed to relieve the airway distress,[136] but central apnea may continue even with appropriate early decompression.[134] Once the tracheostomy is in place, periodic examinations will be necessary to assess vocal fold function.

Approximately 50% of children with bilateral vocal fold paralysis require tracheostomy.[131,138,144] Bluestone and colleagues noted a 50% mortality rate secondary to shunt failure or infection in patients with Arnold-Chiari malformation.[144] Of those who survive, 25 to 48% can be decannulated.[132,143]

Collagen augmentation has been advocated in children with unilateral vocal fold paralysis.[152] The long-term effects of collagen injections in the developing larynx still requires further evaluation.

SUBGLOTTIC LESIONS

The principal subglottic lesions are stenoses and hemangiomas.

Stenosis

Stenoses of the subglottic area can be divided into cartilaginous stenoses, which are usually congenital, and acquired membranous or soft tissue stenoses.

Incidence and Etiology. A stenosis is considered to be congenital when the patient has no history of endotracheal intubation or trauma. The normal subglottic lumen is 4.5 to 5.5 mm in a full-term neonate and 3.5 mm in a premature neonate. We do not know in how many infants' extubations fail because of congenitally small cricoid cartilages.

Congenital subglottic stenosis is the third most common congenital abnormality. Cricoid cartilage deformities are usually congenital and consist of abnormal shapes and sizes. The cricoid cartilage may have a normal shape but be small or hypoplastic. It may also be elliptical, flattened, or otherwise distorted. The first tracheal ring can also be trapped under the cricoid cartilage resulting in a narrowed subglottis. The primary causes of acquired or membranous subglottic stenosis (Figure 18) in children are (1) external injury from blunt trauma or a high tracheostomy and (2) internal injury from prolonged intubation and chemical or thermal burns. External injuries are rare in infants. Internal trauma, secondary to prolonged intubation, is thought to account for approximately 90% of acquired subglottic stenosis.[153,154] The incidence of stenoses after intubation ranges from 0.9 to 8.3%.[155–158] The stenoses most frequently occur in the subglottis because (1) the cricoid cartilage is a complete circular ring without any "give" for edema, (2) the edema can accumulate rapidly in the loose areolar tissue of the subglottis, (3) the pseudostratified, ciliated columnar respiratory epithelium is delicate and

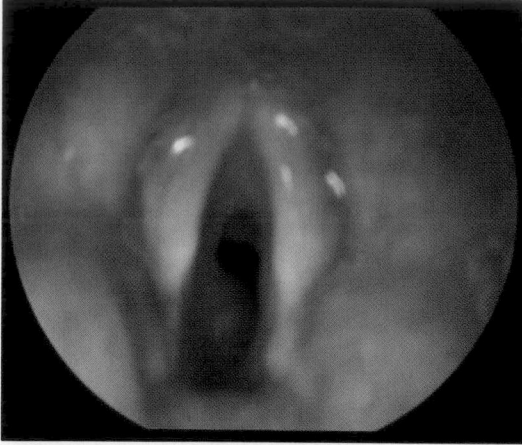

Figure 18 Membranous subglottic stenosis, cyst.

easily traumatized, and (4) the narrowest portion of the upper airway is the subglottis and is therefore the most likely to be traumatized.[154]

The pathophysiology of acquired subglottic stenoses is well described. The endotracheal tube causes pressure necrosis of the respiratory epithelium. Edema and superficial ulceration begin, and the normal ciliary flow is interrupted. As the ulcer deepens, secondary infection of the areolar tissue and perichondrium begin. Chondritis may eventually occur, with necrosis and collapse of the cricoid cartilage. Benjamin characterized the traumatic lesions formed in the larynx with prolonged intubation.[159] He noted that, in the acute phase, one sees formation of posterolateral ulcerations at the vocal processes ("ulcerated troughs") (Figure 19), and usually one sees an "intact median strip" of mucosa and an "annular ulceration" of mucosa in the subglottis. "Tongues of granulation tissue" (Figure 20) form anterior and posterior to the ulceration, and frequently one sees generalized inflammation and edema of the ventricle that results in ventricular protrusions. The long-term complications of these lesions are characterized as posterior glottic synechiae, "healed furrows," posterior subglottic and glottic stenoses (Figure 21), "healed fibrous nodules," submucosal mucous gland hyperplasia with ductal cysts, and submucosal fibrosis and stenosis.

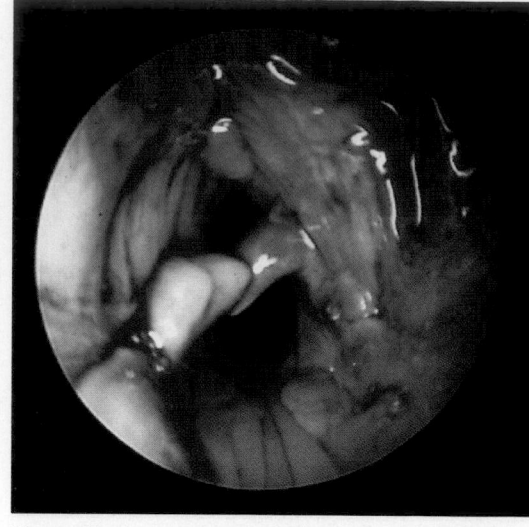

Figure 20 Tongues of granulation tissue.

The scar tissue forms in the subglottis and limits the airway.[160–164] Healing is inhibited in part by poor blood supply in the subglottis and constant motion of the larynx.

Neonates tolerate prolonged intubation better than adults. The reasons for this are unclear, but more pliable cartilage[160] and the higher position in the neck[162] have been suggested as considerations.

Certain factors can increase the chances of developing subglottic stenosis. An oversized endotracheal tube or a tube of appropriate size in a patient with a small cricoid cartilage can increase the mucosal pressure and result in a deep ulceration. Primary intubation can traumatize the subglottis. In children, an endotracheal tube that allows a leak at pressure less than 20 cm. H_2O should be chosen. Reintubation,[160,165,166] shearing motion of the tube on movement of the head,[167] and superimposed local or systemic bacterial infections[161] increase the risk. Gastroesophageal reflux can increase the inflammation and tissue trauma. Nasogastric tubes and endotracheal tubes have been noted to cause pressure necrosis of the cricoid cartilage[161] and increase the risk of reflux.

Systemic factors such as immunodeficiency, anemia, neutropenia, toxicity, hypoxia, dehy-

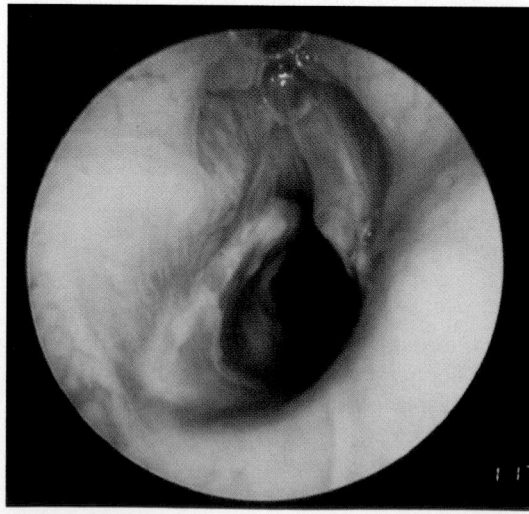

Figure 19 Ulceration of the mucous membrane over the right vocal process.

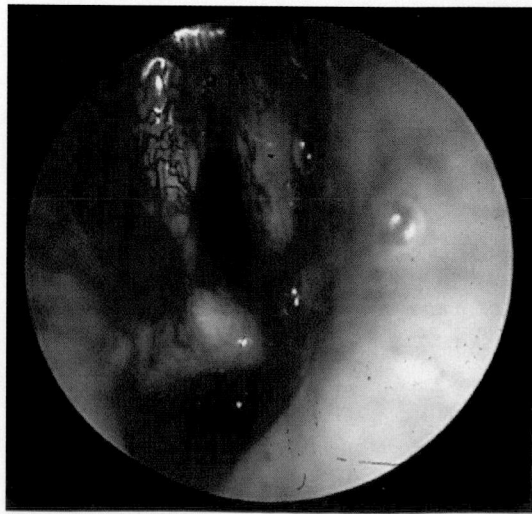

Figure 21 Posterior glottic web.

dration, and poor perfusion increase the risk of developing mucosal ulceration and subsequent scar formation.

Symptoms and Signs

In the intubated neonate, evidence of subglottic stenosis may not manifest until the patient is ready for extubation. If a subglottic ulcer is present, the airway may be compromised immediately or edema may accumulate over a few hours. In some patients, symptoms do not develop until 2 to 4 weeks after intubation. If the patient has mild to moderate congenital subglottic stenosis, symptoms may not appear until an infection of the upper respiratory tract causes additional narrowing and respiratory distress.

If the stenosis is congenital, the only manifestation may be prolonged or recurrent croup. A common dictum is that "there is no such thing as croup under 1 year of age." As respiratory demands increase, the infant may become symptomatic.[92]

The main symptoms and signs relate to airway, voice, and feeding. Stridor is the primary sign and is biphasic, with the inspiratory phase always louder. With progressive narrowing of the airway, respiratory distress ensues. If the vocal folds are affected, hoarseness, abnormal cry, and aphonia will indicate that an anterior web is present. Dysphagia and aspiration pneumonia can occur.

Diagnosis

Soft tissue radiographs of the lateral neck may demonstrate subglottic narrowing. Xeroradiography demonstrates the tissue–air interface better and is believed by many to be the best method for evaluating chronic airway problems.[167–169] Computed tomographic scans do not give adequate additional information.

Direct laryngoscopy is the most important diagnostic step in assessing the thickness and length of the stenosis and involvement of the larynx. Flexible fiberoptic laryngoscopy is most useful in assessing vocal fold function.[168] Because the flexible scope provides only a limited view of the posterior glottis and subglottis, rigid endoscopy is necessary to assess the size and patency of the lumen. The airway may be sized with the bronchoscope or endotracheal tubes. Storz Hopkins optical telescopes are especially important in visualizing the extent of the stenosis in the subglottis. Because of the wide-angle view, estimating the actual dimensions of the lumen is difficult. Often the narrowing is so great that only the telescope can be used.

Treatment

Congenital subglottic stenosis that is mild and causing mild symptoms and signs can be treated expectantly. Some patients outgrow their lesions and are unlikely to need surgical correction.[170] Treatment must be individualized.

Tracheostomy is required in fewer than half of patients with congenital subglottic stenosis.[160]

Normal growth and development may allow decannulation within 2 to 5 years.

The anterior cricoid split was initially devised to treat acquired subglottic stenosis,[171] and it was later applied to patients with the congenital form.[172,173] This procedure breaks the cartilaginous cricoid ring anteriorly to allow expansion of the subglottis. It is used in patients who have confirmed stenosis and failed extubation but do not require airway support and have mature lungs with oxygen concentration requirements less than 35%. The procedure involves making a vertical incision through the lower third of the thyroid cartilage, the cricoid cartilage, and the first two tracheal rings. Many of the cricoid rings spring open, and the endotracheal tubes are readily seen through the incision. Others do not open to any significant degree. Some surgeons have recommended placement of auricular or rib grafts at the time of the decompression.[174–176] The patient is left intubated with an endotracheal tube one size bigger for 5 to 7 days and reexamined at the time of extubation. Corticosteroids are usually administered 3 to 5 days before planned extubation.

In weighing the advantages of endoscopic and open procedures, the surgeon must take into account the extent of the scarring and the expertise required. The goal of any surgical procedure is to extubate or decannulate the patient by repairing the stenosis with minimal effect on the voice.

Dilatation is useful if the ulceration is still present and granulation tissue is forming. It is most appropriately used with immature scar or submucosal fibrosis. Gentle dilation is performed with a round, smooth instrument usually in conjunction with corticosteroid injection.[177] Aggressive dilatation with corticosteroid injection can induce additional trauma and cause significant necrosis of the cartilage.

The use of corticosteroids is controversial. They tend to decrease scar formation through their anti-inflammatory action and by delay of collagen synthesis. They may be used systemically or injected locally. Corticosteroids have not been successfully used to treat mature scar in the subglottis. Mitomycin C has been recommended as an agent to help maintain or decrease the amount of scarring in the subglottis after laser resection or dilatation of the stenosis.[178] It is thought to interfere with the fibroblasts ability to produce scar without preventing epithelialization.[179] Halofuginone is another agent that has been shown to decrease the amount of fibroblast growth of the trachea even more than mitomycin C.[180] Clinical trials have not yet begun.

A variety of methods for endoscopic correction of subglottic stenosis have been suggested, including microcauterization,[181] cryosurgery[182,183] serial electrosurgical resection,[184] and carbon dioxide laser.[185] The carbon dioxide laser appears to be the current modality of choice.[162,185–190] The laser can only be used to resect membranous stenosis, and the procedure has to be performed in stages. The more aggressively the laser is used, the less the likelihood of a successful outcome and the greater the risk of inducing additional

scarring. Cotton and Manoukian identified several factors associated with poor results: (1) circumferential scarring; (2) scar tissue greater than 1 cm in length; (3) scar in the posterior commissure; (4) severe bacterial infection of the trachea after a tracheostomy; (5) exposure of the perichondrium or cartilage with the laser; (6) combined laryngotracheal stenosis; (7) failure of previous endoscopic procedures; and (8) previous loss of cartilaginous framework.[191] Prophylactic systemic antibiotic therapy is recommended for endoscopic procedures. Adequate exposure of the subglottis is necessary. The subglottiscope designed by Healy is useful if the patient does not have a tracheostomy in place. Supraglottic jet ventilation provides the best exposure. Thin webs are most appropriately treated with the laser.

The open procedures have been traditionally used for the more severe lesions. Surgeons are increasingly using single-stage reconstruction.[175,192] This allows for more rapid correction of the problem and is perhaps more cost effective. The hyoid interposition was first reported by Looper.[193] Bennett also reported the use of a hyoid bone graft for the treatment of subglottic stenosis.[194] Bone resorption was a problem, which led to the development of pedicle hyoid–sternohyoid (myoosseous) flaps.[195–197]

The anterior cricoid split with endotracheal tube stenting has been recommended for treatment of milder forms of stenosis.[198] The standard reconstruction has been with autogenous costal cartilage.[199–201] Because of its abundance, costal cartilage is a better material to use than thyroid cartilage, hyoid bone, or muscle pedicle.

The costal cartilage reconstruction has been the standard method for subglottic reconstruction for the past several years. The fifth or sixth cartilaginous rib or costal margin cartilage is harvested. One incision can be used to harvest two ribs, but this is seldom necessary. The perichondrium is left on the lateral surface of the rib, with incisions through it along the superior and inferior borders, and stripped from the medial surface. Some surgeons use the rib stripper on small double prong hooks and a Freer elevator. The incision in the neck is usually a U-shaped flap through the tracheostoma or a horizontal incision over the cricoid cartilage if a tracheostomy is not in place. The larynx and trachea are exposed, and a midline incision is made through the length of the stenosis. If the stenosis is severe, the lumen can be first identified with a 25-gauge needle under endoscopic visualization. When only an anterior graft is used, the incision usually extends from the tracheal rings through the cricoid and the lower third of the larynx. If a posterior graft and stent are required, a full laryngofissure will be necessary. The intraluminal scar and mucosa are incised strictly in the midline. This is best performed by first marking the lumen transtracheally with a 25-gauge needle. Once the airway is open, the scar is not removed. The length of the trachea and larynx to be reconstructed is measured, and the rib graft is designed to fit the defect. The graft

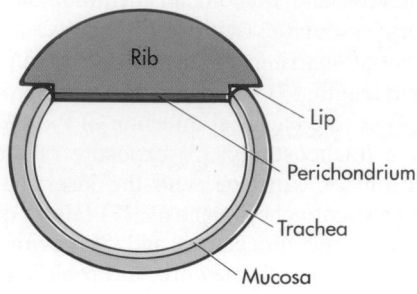

Figure 22 Drawing depicting the rib graft, which has not been thinned, and a lip to prevent collapse into the lumen.

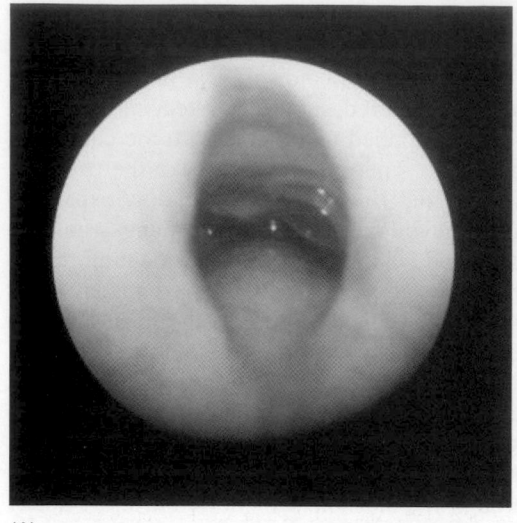

(A)

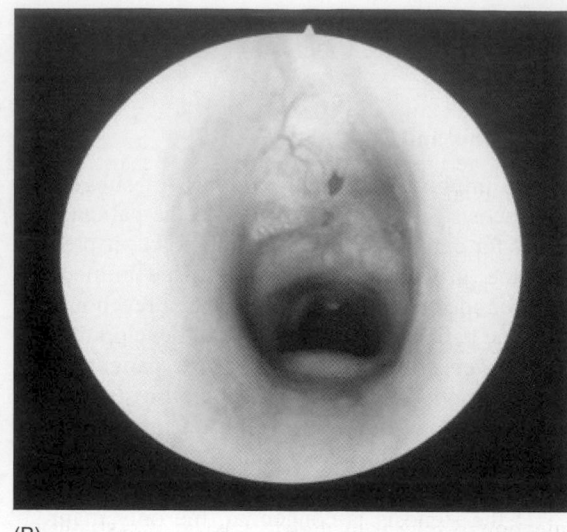

(B)

Figure 23 (A) Preoperative and (B) postoperative photographs of a laryngotracheoplasty with auricular cartilage.

is elliptical, with the perichondrium toward the lumen. The rib is not thinned, and care is taken to shape the cartilage to be as wide as possible, with a lip or shelf to prevent the graft from falling into the airway (Figure 22).

In patients with greater subglottic stenosis, a posterior graft is needed, and the posterior cricoid lamina is divided in the midline to but not through the hypopharyngeal mucosa. In complete stenosis, a four-quadrant split has been recommended. The cricoid is separated to a distance of approximately 1 mm per year of age up to 10 mm between the two halves.[191] An appropriate wedge of rib with the perichondrium facing the lumen is sutured into the posterior cricoid cleft. If a posterior graft has been performed, a stent will be required to maintain the lumen postoperatively. The current stent of choice is the Aboulker-styled Teflon stent, which is round. Unfortunately, it can cause significant blunting, trauma, and granulation tissue formation at the anterior commissure.

Once the posterior cricoid graft is positioned, the stent is placed and the anterior tracheal wall is closed. Usually, posterior and anterior grafts are used concomitantly. When a stent is used, it first must be positioned in the airway with the tracheostomy in place. The best method of securing the tracheostomy to the stent is with wire, as described by Cotton and Manoukian.[191] Placement must be checked endoscopically. The stent should come to the level of the false vocal folds. If necessary, the stent length should be revised to hold the proper position. The rib is sutured into place with 4-0 Vicryl or polydioxanone suture, taking care to go through the cartilage and not allowing the suture to be exposed intraluminally. If suture is located in the lumen, granulation tissue and chronic infection will result. The neck wound is closed in layers. The stent is left in place for a variable length of time based on the surgeon's judgment and the severity of the stenosis.

Auricular cartilage has been used as a graft material.[174,175] It is useful because it is malleable; its curved shape allows for greater (anterioposterior) dimensions than available with the rib graft (Figure 23). The auricular cartilage graft has not been used extensively with staged reconstructions.

Cricotracheal resection has been recommended for Cotton grade 3 or 4 stenosis with

success.[202,203] These are frequently performed as single staged procedures even in young children; however, granulation tissue formation and additional endoscopic procedures are frequently required.[204,205] This aggressive procedure has a high rate of success in these significant stenoses. Failure to decanulate the patient is usually secondary to unilateral or bilateral vocal fold paralysis.[202] The long-term effect of growth on the larynx and trachea are not clear.[206]

Results of successful decannulation depend in part on the severity of the stenosis. Viral infections such as respiratory syncytial virus, and bacterial infections such as pseudomonas, have been associated with an increased failure rate.[207] The ultimate outcome of grade 1 is 92% successful, that of grade 2 is 85% successful, that of grade 3 is 70% successful and, that of grade 4 is 36% successful.[208] The voice is frequently compromised in patients with repaired subglottic stenosis. Ettema and colleagues have noted significant dysphonia in children with repaired subglottic stenosis.[206]

SUBGLOTTIC HEMANGIOMA

Incidence and Etiology

Congenital subglottic hemangiomas are relatively rare lesions and develop primarily in the submucosa. Fifty percent are associated with cutaneous hemangiomas. No correlation exists between the size of the cutaneous lesion and the size of the laryngeal lesion.[209] A 2:1 female preponderance is recognized.

Symptoms and Signs

Subglottic hemangioma develops in a typical growth pattern, with increasing size usually causing symptoms in the first 8 weeks of life. Almost all these lesions will become manifest before 6 months of age. Some lesions extend into the perichondrium and tracheal rings and beyond the trachea. There is a predilection for the left side.[210] Variable and fluctuant respiratory distress usually progresses to persistent distress. The stridor is

more prominent on inspiration but is present during expiration. The voice is altered to a varying degree, depending on the involvement of the larynx. Altered cry, hoarseness, barking cough, and failure to thrive are the other frequently noted manifestations. Recurrent croup is the most frequent erroneous diagnosis.

Diagnosis

Lateral radiographic studies suggest a subglottic abnormality consistent with hemangioma. This is not diagnostic, however, and the diagnosis can only be made endoscopically (Figure 24). The appearance of these lesions is characteristic and can be made by the experienced endoscopist without a biopsy. The lesion is sessile, fairly firm but compressible; pink, red, or bluish; and poorly defined. The vessels are rarely, if ever, cavernous. If a biopsy is performed, the bleeding is usually not profuse, but the airway must be maintained, most frequently with a tracheostomy. The lesion is usually unilateral or asymmetric. Multiple hemangiomas of the airway have been reported.[211] A thorough workup of the possible extent of the hemangioma in the mediastinum is recommended.

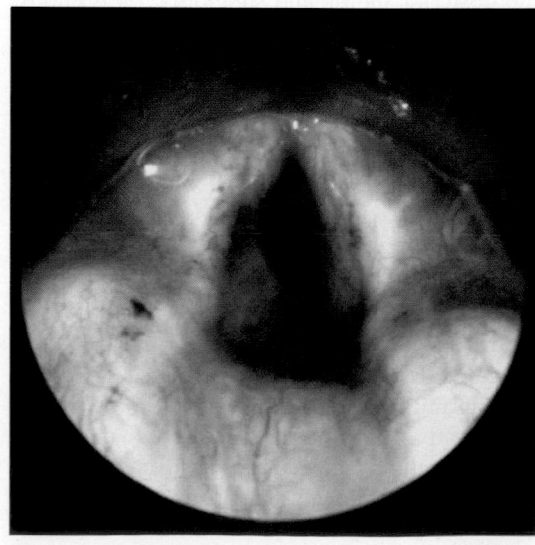

Figure 24 Subglottic hemangioma.

Treatment

If the airway distress is significant at the time of diagnosis, immediate airway control will be necessary. Endoscopy may compromise the airway. If necessary, the airway may be secured with intubation or a tracheostomy. The most significant factors are degree of subglottic narrowing, location of the hemangioma and presence of hemangioma extending outside of the trachea.[210] If the patient is intubated, tracheostomy is more likely to be required.

A wide range of treatments have been advocated. They include the following: tracheostomy with observation and awaiting spontaneous resolution; prolonged endotracheal intubation, with and without intralesional corticosteroid injection; injection of sclerosing agents; the use of systemic corticosteroids; cryosurgery; external beam irradiation; gold seed irradiation; and laser excision. The judicious use of a laser to excise the lesion in stages, with the patient's airway protected by a tracheostomy when necessary, appears to be the treatment favored by most surgeons. Bitar and colleagues noted a success rate of 88.9% with laser excision but if it is used too aggressively subglottic stenosis occurred in 5.5% of the patients.[212] External beam irradiation has been reported to have a cure rate of 93%, but the threat of radiation induced malignant tumors of the thyroid gland strictly limits its use. Gold seeds are the treatment favored by Benjamin.[209] Open resection of subglottic hemangiomas have recently been recommended with good results.[212–214] The microdebrider has also been recently recommended as an effective tool for subglottic hemangioma resection.[215] Unrecognized or improperly treated subglottic hemangiomas have a high mortality rate.

REFERENCES

1. Chen JC, Holinger LD. Congenital laryngeal lesions: Pathology study using serial macrosections and review of the literature. Pediatr Pathol 1994;14:301–25.
2. Thomson JM. On infantile respiratory spasm (congenital laryngeal stridor). Edinb Med J 1892;38:205–16.
3. Sutherland GA, Lack HM. Congenital laryngeal obstruction. Lancet 1897;2:653–5.
4. Thomson JM, Turner AL. On the causation of congenital stridor of infants. Br Med J 1900;2:1561–3.
5. Schwartz L. Congenital laryngeal stridor (inspiratory laryngeal collapse). New theory as to its underlying cause and the desirability of a change in terminology. Arch Otolaryngol 1944;39:403–12.
6. Jackson C, Jackson CL. Diseases and Injuries of the Larynx. New York: Macmillian; 1942.
7. Ford GR, Irving RM, Jones NS, Bailey CM. ENT manifestations of Fraser syndrome. J Laryngol Otol 1992;106:1–4.
8. Hawkins DB, Clark RW. Flexible laryngoscopy in neonates, infants, and young children. Ann Otol Rhinol Laryngol 1987;96:81–5.
9. Nussbaum E, Maggi JC. Laryngomalacia in children. Chest 1990;98:942–4.
10. Mitchell RB, Call E, Kelly J. Diagnosis and therapy for airway obstruction in children with Down syndrome. Arch Otolaryngol Head Neck Surg 2003;129:642–5.
11. Bertrand P, Navarro H, Caussade S, et al. Airway anomalies in children with Down syndrome: Endoscopic findings. Pediatr Pulmonol 2003;36:137–41.
12. McSwiney PF, Cavanagh NP, Languth P. Outcome in congenital stridor (laryngomalacia). Arch Dis Child 1977;52:215–8.
13. Apley J. The infant with stridor: A follow-up survey of 80 cases. Arch Dis Child 1953;28:423–35.

14. Holinger PH, Johnston KC. The infant with respiratory stridor. Pediatr Clin North Am 1955;2:403–11.
15. Daniel SJ. The upper airway: Congenital malformations. Paediatr Respir Rev 2006;7:S260–3.
16. Manning SC, Inglis AF, Mouzakes J, et al. Laryngeal anatomic differences in pediatric patients with severe laryngomalacia. Arch Otolaryngol Head Neck Surg 2005;131:340–3.
17. Belmont JR, Grundfast K. Congenital laryngeal stridor (laryngomalacia): Etiologic factors and associated disorders. Ann Otol Rhinol Laryngol 1984;93:430–7.
18. Kelemen G. Congenital laryngeal stridor. Arch Otolaryngol 1953;58:245–68.
19. Holinger LD, Konior RJ. Surgical management of severe laryngomalacia. Laryngoscope 1989;99:136–42.
20. Solomons NB, Prescott CA. Laryngomalacia. A review and the surgical management for severe cases. Int J Pediatr Otorhinolaryngol 1987;13:31–9.
21. Cotton RT, Richardson MA. Pediatric Otolaryngology. Philadelphia: WB Saunders; 1983.
22. Ferguson CF. Congenital abnormalities of the infant larynx. Otolaryngol Clin North Am 1970;3:185–200.
23. Zalzal GH, Anon JB, Cotton RT. Epiglottoplasty for the treatment of laryngomalacia. Ann Otol Rhinol Laryngol 1987;96:72–6.
24. McCaffrey TV, Cortese DA. Neodymium:YAG laser treatment of subglottic hemangioma. Otolaryngol Head Neck Surg 1986;94:382–4.
25. Unal E, Oran B, Baysal T, et al. Pulmonary arterial pressure in infants with laryngomalacia. Int J Pediatr Otorhinolaryngol 2006;70:2067–71.
26. Sivan Y, Ben-Ari J, Soferman R, Derowe A. Diagnosis of laryngomalacia by fiberoptic endoscopy: Awake compared with anesthesia-aided technique. Chest 2006;130:1412–8.
27. Mancuso RF, Choi SS, Zalzal GH, Grundfast KM. Laryngomalacia. The search for the second lesion. Arch Otolaryngol Head Neck Surg 1996;122:302–6.
28. Bluestone CD, Healy GB, Cotton RT. Diagnosis of laryngomalacia is not enough. Arch Otolaryngol Head Neck Surg 1996;122:1417–8.
29. Holinger LD. Etiology of stridor in the neonate, infant and child. Ann Otol Rhinol Laryngol 1980;89:397–400.
30. Holinger PH, Johnson KC, Schiller F. Congenital anomalies of the larynx. Ann Otol Rhinol Laryngol 1954;63:581–606.
31. Reardon TJ. Congenital laryngeal stridor. Am J Med Sci 1907;134:242–52.
32. Blackader AD, Muckleston HS. Inspiratory stridor and dyspnea in infants. Arch Pediatr 1909;26:401–16.
33. Iglauer S. Epiglottidectomy for the relief of congenital laryngeal stridor, with report of a case. Laryngoscope 1922;32:56–9.
34. Fearon B, Ellis D. The management of long term airway problems in infants and children. Ann Otol Rhinol Laryngol 1971;80:669–77.
35. Narcy P, Bobin S, Contencin P. Anomalies laryngies du Nouveau-ne apropos de 687 observations. Ann Otolaryngol Chir Cervicofac 1984;101:363–73.
36. Cagnol C, Garcin M, Unal D. Un Cas de Stridor Larynge Congenital Grave Laoite Pan Hyomandibulopexie. J Fr Otorhinolaryngol 1971;20:625–6.
37. Templer J, Hast M, Thomas JR, Davis WE. Congenital laryngeal stridor secondary to flaccid epiglottis, anomalous accessory cartilages and redundant aryepiglottic folds. Laryngoscope 1981;91:394–7.
38. Lane RW, Weider DJ, Steinem C, Marin-Padilla M. Laryngomalacia. A review and case report of surgical treatment with resolution of pectus excavatum. Arch Otolaryngol 1984;110:546–51.
39. Seid AB, Park SM, Kearns MJ, Gugenheim S. Laser division of the aryepiglottic folds for severe laryngomalacia. Int J Pediatr Otorhinolaryngol 1985;10:153–8.
40. Katin LI, Tucker JA. Laser supraarytenoidectomy for laryngomalacia with apnea. Trans Penn Acad Ophthal Otolaryngol 1990;42:985–8.
41. Kelly SM, Gray SD. Unilateral endoscopic supraglottoplasty for severe laryngomalacia. Arch Otolaryngol Head Neck Surg 1995;121:1351–4.
42. Whymark AD, Clement WA, Kubba H, Geddes NK. Laser epiglottopexy for laryngomalacia: 10 years' experience in the west of Scotland. Arch Otolaryngol Head Neck Surg 2006;132:978–82.
43. Hadfield PJ, Albert DM, Bailey CM, et al. The effect of aryepiglottoplasty for laryngomalacia on gastro-oesophageal reflux. Int J Pediatr Otorhinolaryngol 2003;67:11–4.
44. Stavroulaki P. Diagnostic and management problems of laryngopharyngeal reflux disease in children. Int J Pediatr Otorhinolaryngol 2006;70:579–90.
45. Montreuil F. Bifid epiglottis, report of a case. Laryngoscope 1949;59:194–9.

46. DelMonico ML, Haar JG. Bifid epiglottis. Report of a case. Arch Otolaryngol 1972;96:178–81.
47. Graham JM, Brown FE, Saunders RL, et al. Bifid epiglottis, hand anomalies, and congenital hypopituitarism (letter). Lancet 1985;2:443.
48. Tobeck A. Halbseitige Aplasie der Epiglottis. Z Laryng Rhinol Otol 1949;28:502–3.
49. Healy GB, Holt GP, Tucker JA. Bifid epiglottis: A rare laryngeal anomaly. Laryngoscope 1976;86:1459–68.
50. Mar S, Essex C. Type 2 tracheal agenesis without tracheoesophageal fistula. Int J Pediatr Otorhinolaryngol 1997;39:159–61.
51. Gatti WM, MacDonald E, Orfei E. Congenital laryngeal atresia. Laryngoscope 1987;97:966–9.
52. Holinger PH, Brown WT. Congenital webs, cysts, laryngoceles and other anomalies of the larynx. Ann Otol Rhinol Laryngol 1967;76:744–52.
53. Woo P, Karmody CS. Congenital laryngeal atresia. Histopathologic study of two cases. Ann Otol Rhinol Laryngol 1983;92:391–5.
54. McIlwain JC. The posterior glottis. J Otolaryngol 1991;20:1–24.
55. Asano S, Yamagiwa K, Konnai I. Congenital laryngeal atresia: Two autopsy cases, one describing the use of computed tomography. APMIS 2000;108:313–7.
56. Dolkart LA, Reimers FT, Wertheimer IS, Wilson BO. Prenatal diagnosis of laryngeal atresia. J Ultrasound Med 1992;11:496–8.
57. Watson WJ, Thorp JM, Jr, Miller RC, et al. Prenatal diagnosis of laryngeal atresia. Am J Obstet Gynecol 1990;163:1456–7.
58. Garel C, Legrand I, Elmaleh M, et al. Laryngeal ultrasonography in infants and children: Anatomical correlation with fetal preparations. Pediatr Radiol 1990;20:241–4.
59. Balci S, Altinok G, Ozaltin F, et al. Laryngeal atresia presenting as fetal ascites, olygohydramnios and lung appearance mimicking cystic adenomatoid malformation in a 25-week-old fetus with Fraser syndrome. Prenatal Diag 1999;19:856–8.
60. Morrison PJ, Macphail S, Williams D, et al. Laryngeal atresia or stenosis presenting as second-trimester fetal ascites—diagnosis and pathology in three independent cases. Prenatal Diagn 1998;18:963–7.
61. Lim FY, Crombleholme TM, Hedrick HL, et al. Congenital high airway obstruction syndrome: Natural history and management. J Pediatr Surg 2003;38:940–5.
62. Kanamori Y, Kitano Y, Hashizume K, et al. A case of laryngeal atresia (congenital high airway obstruction syndrome) with chromosome 5p deletion syndrome rescued by ex-utero intrapartum treatment. J Pediatr Surg 2004;39.E25–8.
63. Smith, II, Bain AD. Congenital atresia of the larynx. Ann Otol Rhinol Laryngol 1965;74:338–49.
64. Kalache KD, Chaoui R, Tennstedt C, Bollmann R. Prenatal diagnosis of laryngeal atresia in two cases of congenital high airway obstruction syndrome (CHAOS). Prenatal Diagn 1997;17:577–81.
65. Hedrick MH, Ferro MM, Filly RA, et al. Congenital high airway obstruction syndrome (CHAOS): A potential for perinatal intervention. J Pediatr Surg 1994;29:271–4.
66. Kohl T, Hering R, Bauriedel G, et al. Fetoscopic and ultrasound-guided decompression of the fetal trachea in a human fetus with Fraser syndrome and congenital high airway obstruction syndrome (CHAOS) from laryngeal atresia. Ultrasound Obstet Gynecol 2006;27:84–8.
67. Peison B, Levitzky E, Sprowls JJ. Tracheoesophageal fistula associated with tracheal atresia and malformation of the larynx. J Pediatr Surg 1970;5:464–7.
68. Cohen MS, Rothschild MA, Moscoso J, Shlasko E. Perinatal management of unanticipated congenital laryngeal atresia. Arch Otolaryngol Head Neck Surg 1998;124:1368–71.
69. Gerson CR, Tansek K, Tucker GF, Jr. Pharyngolaryngeal web. Report of a new anomaly. Ann Otol Rhinol Laryngol 1983;92:331–2.
70. Holinger LD, Wong HW, Hemenway WG. Simultaneous glottic and supraglottic laryngeal webs: Report of a case. Arch Otolaryngol Head Neck Surg 1975;101:496–7.
71. Benjamin B, Mair EA. Congenital interarytenoid web. Arch Otolaryngol Head Neck Surg 1991;117:1118–22.
72. McHugh HE, Loch WE. Congenital webs of the larynx. Laryngoscope 1942;52:43–65.
73. McGuirt WF, Salmon J, Blalock D. Normal speech for patients with laryngeal webs: An achievable goal. Laryngoscope 1984;94:1176–9.
74. Cohen SR. Congenital glottic webs in children. A retrospective review of 51 patients. Ann Otol Rhinol Laryngol Suppl 1985;121:2–16.
75. Benjamin B. Chevalier Jackson lecture. Congenital laryngeal webs. Ann Otol Rhinol Laryngol 1983;92:317–26.

76. Milczuk HA, Smith JD, Everts EC. Congenital laryngeal webs: Surgical management and clinical embryology. Int J Pediatr Otorhinolaryngol 2000;52:1–9.
77. Parker DA, Das Gupta AR. An endoscopic silastic keel for anterior glottic webs. J Laryngol Otol 1987;101:1055–61.
78. Mouney DF, Lyons GD. Fixation of laryngeal stents. Laryngoscope 1985;95:905–7.
79. Laff HI. Cysts in the ventricular area of the larynx. Laryngoscope 1953;63:227–40.
80. Davidson JI. Congenital cyst of the larynx. Lancet 1943;2:508–9.
81. Ahlen G, Ranstrom S. Congenital laryngeal cysts in early infancy. Acta Otolaryngol 1944;32:483–95.
82. Beautyman W, Haidak GL, Taylor M. Laryngopyocele: Report of a fatal case. N Engl J Med 1959;260:1025–7.
83. Horowitz S. Laryngoceles. J Laryngol Otol 1951;65:724–34.
84. Hockmuth LN, Martin SJ. An obstructing laryngeal cyst in a newborn. Conn Med 1962;26:691–700.
85. DeSanto LW. Laryngocele, laryngeal mucocele, large saccules, and laryngeal saccular cysts: A developmental spectrum. Laryngoscope 1974;84:1291–6.
86. Holinger LD, Barnes DR, Smid LJ, Holinger PH. Laryngocele and saccular cysts. Ann Otol Rhinol Laryngol 1978;87:675–85.
87. Broyles EN. Anatomical observations concerning the laryngeal appendix. Ann Otol Rhinol Laryngol 1959;68:461–70.
88. DeSanto LW, Devine KD, Weiland LH. Cysts of larynx: Classification. Laryngoscope 1970;80:145–76.
89. Suehs OW, Powell DB Jr. Congenital cyst of the larynx in infants. Laryngoscope 1967;77:654–62.
90. Mitchell DB, Irwin BC, Bailey CM, Evans JN. Cysts of the infant larynx. J Laryngol Otol 1987;101:833–7.
91. Shackelford GD, McAlister WH. Congenital laryngeal cyst. Am J Roentgenol Radium Ther Nucl Med 1972;114:289–92.
92. Cotton RT, Richardson MA. Congenital laryngeal anomalies. Otolaryngol Clin North Am 1981;14:203–18.
93. English GM, DeBlanc GB. Laryngocele: A case presenting with acute airway obstruction. Laryngoscope 1968;78:386–95.
94. Ferguson GB. Laryngocele. Laryngoscope 1967;77:1368–75.
95. Donegan JO, Strife JL, Seid AB, et al. Internal laryngocele and saccular cysts in children. Ann Otol Rhinol Laryngol 1980;89:409–13.
96. Canalis RF, Maxwell DS, Hemenway WG. Laryngocele—an updated review. J Otolaryngol 1977;6:191–9.
97. Chu L, Gussack GS, Orr JB, Hood D. Neonatal laryngoceles. A cause for airway obstruction. [Review]. Arch Otolaryngol Head Neck Surg 1994;120:454–8.
98. Baker HL, Baker SR, McClatchey KD. Manifestations and management of laryngoceles. Head Neck Surg 1982;4:450–6.
99. Trapnell DH. The radiological diagnosis of laryngoceles. Clin Radiol 1962;13:68–72.
100. Yarington CT, Frazer JP. An approach to the internal laryngocele and other submucosal lesions of the larynx. Ann Otol Rhinol Laryngol 1966;75:956–60.
101. Thomas DM, Madden GJ. Bilateral laryngoceles. Ear Nose Throat J 1993;72:819–21.
102. Parsons DS, Herr T. Delayed diagnosis of a laryngotracheoesophageal cleft. Int J Pediatr Otorhinolaryngol 1997;39:169–73.
103. Parsons DS, Stivers FE, Giovanetto DR, Phillips SE. Type I posterior laryngeal clefts. Laryngoscope 1998;108:403–10.
104. Samuel M, Burge DM, Griffiths DM. Prenatal diagnosis of laryngotracheoesophageal clefts. Fetal Diagn Ther 1997;12:260–5.
105. Rahbar R, Rouillon I, Roger G, et al. The presentation and management of laryngeal cleft: A 10-year experience. Arch Otolaryngol Head Neck Surg 2006;132:1335–41.
106. Cohen SR, Thompson JW. Ventral cleft of the larynx: A rare congenital laryngeal defect. Ann Otol Rhinol Laryngol 1990;99:281–5.
107. Cohen SR. Cleft larynx. A report of seven cases. Ann Otol Rhinol Laryngol 1975;84:747–56.
108. Roth B, Rose KG, Benz-Bohm G, Gunther H. Laryngotracheooesophageal cleft. Clinical features, diagnosis and therapy. Eur J Pediatr 1983;140:41–6.
109. Finlay HV. Familial congenital stridor. Arch Dis Child 1949;24:219–23.
110. Chien W, Ashland J, Haver K, et al. Type 1 laryngeal cleft: Establishing a functional diagnostic and management algorithm. Int J Pediatr Otorhinolaryngol 2006;70:2073–9.
111. Evans JN. Management of the cleft larynx and tracheoesophageal clefts. Ann Otol Rhinol Laryngol 1985;94:627–30.
112. Jahrsdoerfer RA, Kirchner JA, Thaler SU. Cleft larynx. Arch Otolaryngol 1967;86:108–13.
113. Garel C, Hassan M, Hertz-Pannier L, et al. Contribution of MR in the diagnosis of "occult" posterior laryngeal cleft. Int J Pediatr Otorhinolaryngol 1992;24:177–81.
114. Delahunty JE, Cherry J. Congenital laryngeal cleft. Ann Otol Rhinol Laryngol 1969;78:96–106.
115. Corbally MT. Laryngotracheooesophageal cleft. Arch Dis Child 1993;68:532–3.
116. Holinger LD, Tansek KM, Tucker GF, Jr. Cleft larynx with airway obstruction. Ann Otol Rhinol Laryngol 1985;94:622–6.
117. Tucker GF, Jr, Maddalozzo J. "Occult" posterior laryngeal cleft. Laryngoscope 1987;97:701–4.
118. Tyler DC. Laryngeal cleft: Report of eight patients and a review of the literature. Am J Med Genet 1985;21:61–75.
119. Walner DL, Stern Y, Collins M, et al. Does the presence of a tracheoesophageal fistula predict the outcome of laryngeal cleft repair? Arch Otolaryngol Head Neck Surg 1999;125:782–4.
120. Petterson G. Inhibited separation of larynx and the upper part of trachea from oesophagus in a newborn. Acta Chir Scand 1955;110:250–4.
121. Koltai PJ, Morgan D, Evans JN. Endoscopic repair of supraglottic laryngeal clefts. Arch Otolaryngol Head Neck Surg 1991;117:273–8.
122. Nuutinen J, Karja J, Karjalainen P. Measurements of impaired mucociliary activity in children. Eur J Respir Dis Suppl 1983;128:454–6.
123. Rahbar R, Ferrari LR, Borer JG, Peters CA. Robotic surgery in the pediatric airway: Application and safety. Arch Otolaryngol Head Neck Surg 2007;133:46–50.
124. Pettit PN, Butcher RB, Bethea MC, Danks DM. Surgical correction of complete tracheoesophageal cleft. Laryngoscope 1979;89:804–11.
125. Froehlich P, Truy E, Stamm D, et al. Cleft larynx: Management and one-stage surgical repair by anterior translaryngotracheal approach in two children. Int J Pediatr Otorhinolaryngol 1993;27:73–8.
126. Robie DK, Pearl RH, Gonsales C, et al. Operative strategy for recurrent laryngeal cleft: A case report and review of the literature. [Review]. J Pediatr Surg 1991;26:971–3.
127. Prescott CA. Cleft larynx: Repair with a posterior cartilage graft. Int J Pediatr Otorhinolaryngol 1995;31:91–4.
128. Ahmad R, Horwitz PE, Sami KA, Rabeeah A. A bifurcated endobronchial tube in the management of laryngotracheooesophageal cleft repair [published erratum appears in Br J Anaesth 1994;72:371]. Br J Anaesth 1993;70:696–8.
129. Geiduschek JM, Inglis AF, Jr, O'Rourke PP, et al. Repair of a laryngotracheoesophageal cleft in an infant by means of extracorporeal membrane oxygenation. Ann Otol Rhinol Laryngol 1993;102:827–33.
130. Cotton RT, Schreiber JT. Management of laryngotracheoesophageal cleft. Ann Otol Rhinol Laryngol 1981;90:401–5.
131. Cohen SR, Geller KA, Birns JW, Thompson JW. Laryngeal paralysis in children: A long-term retrospective study. Ann Otol Rhinol Laryngol 1982;91:417–24.
132. Swift AC, Rogers J. Vocal cord paralysis in children. J Laryngol Otol 1987;101:169–71.
133. Phelan PD. "Oscopy" in children: Laryngoscopy and bronchoscopy. Aust Fam Physician 1979;8:853–7.
134. Hoffman HJ, Hendrick EB, Humphreys RP. Manifestaions and management of Arnold-Chiari malformation in patients with myelomeningocele. Child Brain 1975;1:255–9.
135. Krieger AJ, Detwiler JS, Trooskin SZ. Respiratory function in infants with Arnold-Chiari malformation. Laryngoscope 1976;86:718–23.
136. Cavanagh F. Vocal palsies in children. J Laryngol Otol 1955;69:399–418.
137. Dedo DD. Pediatric vocal cord paralysis. Laryngoscope 1979;89:1378–84.
138. Holinger LD, Holinger PC, Holinger PH. Etiology of bilateral abductor vocal cord paralysis: A review of 389 cases. Ann Otol Rhinol Laryngol 1976;85:428–36.
139. Gardner E, O'Rahilly R, Prolo D. The Dandy-Walker and Arnold-Chiari malformations. Arch Neurol 1975;32:395–407.
140. Setz AC, De Boer HD, Driessen JJ, Scheffer GJ. Anesthetic management in a child with Arnold-Chiari malformation and bilateral vocal cord paralysis. Paediatr Anaesth 2005;15:1105–7.
141. Mackenzie IJ, Kerr AI, Cowan DL. A review of endoscopies of the respiratory tract and oesophagus in a children's hospital. Health Bulletin 1984;42:78–80.
142. Richardson MA, Cotton RT. Anatomic abnormalities of the pediatric airway. Ear Nose Throat J 1985;64:47–60.
143. Holinger PC, Holinger LD, Reichert TJ, Holinger PH. Respiratory obstruction and apnea in infants with bilateral abductor vocal cord paralysis, meningomyelocele, hydrocephalus, and Arnold-Chiari malformation. J Pediatr 1978;92:368–73.
144. Bluestone CD, Delerme AN, Samuelson GH. Airway obstrucion due to vocal cord paralysis in infants with hydrocephalus and meningomyelocele. Ann Otol Rhinol Laryngol 1972;81:778–84.
145. Gacek RR. Hereditary abductor vocal cord paralysis. Ann Otol Rhinol Laryngol 1976;85:90–3.
146. Watters GV, Fitch N. Familial laryngeal abductor paralysis and psychomotor retardation. Clin Genet 1973;4:429–33.
147. Plott D. Congenital laryngeal-abductor paralysis due to nucleus ambiguus dysgenesis in three brothers. N Engl J Med 1964;27:593–7.
148. Cohen SR, Geller KA, Birns JW, Thompson JW. Laryngeal paralysis in children: A long-term retrospective study. Ann Otol Rhinol Laryngol 1982;91:417–24.
149. Ishman SL, Halum SL, Patel NJ, et al. Management of vocal paralysis: A comparison of adult and pediatric practices. Otolaryngol Head Neck Surg 2006;135:590–4.
150. Holinger PC, Vuckovich DM, Holinger LD, Holinger PH. Bilateral abductor vocal cord paralysis in Charcot-Marie-Tooth disease. Ann Otol Rhinol Laryngol 1979;88:205–9.
151. Bressler KL, Kaiser PC, Dunham ME, Holinger LD. Primary closure of persistent tracheocutaneous fistula in children. Ann Otol Rhinol Laryngol 1994;103:835–7.
152. Patel NJ, Kerschner JE, Merati AL. The use of injectable collagen in the management of pediatric vocal unilateral fold paralysis. Int J Pediatr Otorhinolaryngol 2003;67:1355–60.
153. Cotton RT, Evans JN. Laryngotracheal reconstruction in children. 5-year follow-up. Ann Otol Rhinol Laryngol 1981;90:516–20.
154. Holinger LD. Treatment of severe subglottic stenosis without tracheotomy: A preliminary report. Ann Otol Rhinol Laryngol 1982;91:407–12.
155. Hawkins DB. Hyaline membrane disease of the neonate prolonged intubation in management: Effects on the larynx. Laryngoscope 1978;88:201–24.
156. Papsidero MJ, Pashley NR. Acquired Stenosis of the upper airway in neonates: An increasing problem. Ann Otol Rhinol Laryngol 1980;89:512–4.
157. Parkin JL, Stevens MH, Jung DL. Acquired and congenital subglottic stenosis in the infant. Ann Otol Rhinol Laryngol 1976;85:573–81.
158. Whited RE. A prospective study of laryngotracheal sequelae in long-term intubation. Laryngoscope 1984;94:367–77.
159. Benjamin B. Prolonged intubation injuries of the larynx: Endoscopic diagnosis, classification, and treatment. Ann Otol Rhinol Laryngol 1993;160:1–15.
160. Holinger PH, Kutnick SL, Schild JA, Holinger LD. Subglottic stenosis in infants and children. Ann Otol Rhinol Laryngol 1976;85:591–9.
161. Sasaki CT, Horiuchi M, Koss N. Traheostomy-related subglottic stenosis: Bacteriologic pathogenesis. Laryngoscope 1979;89:857–65.
162. Healy GB. An experimental model for the endoscopic correction of subglottic stenosis with clinical applications. Laryngoscope 1982;92:1103–15.
163. Cotton RT, Silver P, Nuwayhid NS. Chronic laryngeal and tracheal stenosis. In: Paparella MM, Shumrick DA, editors. Otolaryngology. 2nd edition. Philadelphia: WB Saunders Co; 1980. p. 2931–50.
164. Fee WE, Wilson GG. Tracheoesophageal space abscess. Laryngoscope 1979;89:377–84.
165. Lindholm CE. Prolonged endotracheal intubation, a valuable alternative to tracheostomy. Bronches 1968;18:398–408.
166. Pashley NR. Risk factors and prediction of outcome in acquired subglottic stenosis in children. Int J Pediatr Otorhinolaryngol 1982;4:1–6.
167. Noyek AM. Xeroradiography in the assessment of the pediatric larynx and trachea. J Otolaryngol 1976;5:468–74.
168. McMillan WG, Duvall AJ, III. Congenital subglottic stenosis. Arch Otolaryngol 1968;87:272–8.
169. Marshak G, Grundfast KM. Subglottic stenosis. Pediatr Clin North Am. 1981;28:941–8.
170. Cotton RT. Management of subglottic stenosis in infancy and childhood: Review of a consecutive series of cases managed by surgical reconstruction. Ann Otol Rhinol Laryngol 1978;87:649–57.
171. Cotton RT, Seid AB. Management of the extubation problem in the premature child. Anterior cricoid split as an alternative to tracheotomy. Ann Otol Rhinol Laryngol 1980;89:508–11.
172. Cotton RT. Prevention and management of laryngeal stenosis in infants and children. J Pediatr Surg 1985;20:845–51.
173. Holinger LD, Stankiewicz JA, Livingston GL. Anterior cricoid split: The Chicago experience with an alternative to tracheotomy. Laryngoscope 1987;97:19–24.

174. Lusk RP, Kang DR, Muntz HR. Auricular cartilage grafts in laryngotracheal reconstruction. Ann Otol Rhinol Laryngol 1993;102:247–54.

175. Lusk RP, Gray S, Muntz HR. Single-stage laryngotracheal reconstruction. Arch Otolaryngol Head Neck Surg 1991;117:171–3.

176. Richardson MA, Inglis AF. A comparison of anterior cricoid split with and without costal cartilage graft for acquired subglottic stenosis. Int J Pediatr Otorhinolaryngol 1991;22:187–93.

177. Othersen HB Jr. Steroid therapy for tracheal stenosis in children: Clinical experience in 4 children with severe strictures. Ann Thorac Surg 1974;17:254–9.

178. Hueman EM, Simpson CB. Airway complications from topical mitomycin C. Otolaryngol Head Neck Surg 2005;133:831–5.

179. Sanders KW, Gage-White L, Stucker FJ. Topical mitomycin C in the prevention of keloid scar recurrence. Arch Facial Plast Surg 2005;7:172–5.

180. Eliashar R, Ochana M, Maly B, et al. Halofuginone prevents subglottic stenosis in a canine model. Ann Otol Rhinol Laryngol 2006;115:382–6.

181. Kirchner FR, Toledo PS. Microcauterization in otolaryngology. Arch Otolaryngol 1974;99:198–202.

182. Rodgers BM, Talbert JL. Clinical applications of endotracheal cryotherapy. J Pediatr Surg 1978;13:662–8.

183. Strome M, Donahoe PK. Advances in management of laryngeal and subglottic stenosis. J Pediatr Surg 1982;17:591–6.

184. Downing TP, Johnson DG. Excision of subglottic stenosis with the urethral resectoscope. J Pediatr Surg 1979;14:252–7.

185. Simpson GT, Strong MS, Healy GB, et al. Predictive factors of success or failure in the endoscopic management of laryngeal and tracheal stenosis. Ann Otol Rhinol Laryngol 1982;91:384–8.

186. Friedman EM, Healy GB, McGill TJ. Carbon dioxide laser management of subglottic and tracheal stenosis. [Review]. Otolaryngol Clin North Am 1983;16:871–7.

187. Healy GB, McGill T, Simpson GT, Strong MS. The use of the carbon dioxide laser in the pediatric airway. J Pediatr Surg 1979;14:735–40.

188. Koufman JA, Thompson JN, Kohut RI. Endoscopic management of subglottic stenosis with the CO2 surgical laser. Otolaryngol Head Neck Surg 1981;89:215–20.

189. Lyons GD, Owens R, Lousteau RJ, Trail ML. Carbon dioxide laser treatment of laryngeal stenosis. Arch Otolaryngol 1980;106:255–6.

190. Strong MS, Healy GB, Vaughan CW, Fried MP. Endoscopic management of laryngeal stenosis. Otolaryngol Clin North Am 1979;12:797–805.

191. Cotton RT, Manoukian JJ. Glottic and subglottic stenosis. In: Cummings CW, Fredrickson JM, Harker LA, et al, editors. Otolaryngology-Head and Neck Surgery. 1st edition. St. Louis: CV Mosby Co; 1986. p. 2159–80.

192. Seid AB, Pransky SM, Kearns DB. One-stage laryngotracheoplasty. Arch Otolaryngol Head Neck Surg 1991;117:408–10.

193. Looper EA. The use of hyoid bone as graft in laryngeal stenosis. Arch Otolaryngol 1938;28:106.

194. Bennett T. Laryngeal strictures. South Med J 1960;53:1101–4.

195. Finnegan DA, Wong ML, Kashima HK. Hyoid autograft repair of chronic subglottic stenosis. Ann Otol Rhinol Laryngol 1975;84:643–9.

196. Thawley SE, Ogura JH. Panel discussion: The management of advanced laryngotracheal stenosis. Use of the hyoid graft for treatment of laryngotracheal stenosis. Laryngoscope 1981;91:226–32.

197. Ward PH, Canalis R, Fee W, Smith G. Composite hyoid sternohyoid muscle grafts in humans. Its use in reconstruction of subglottic stenosis and the anterior tracheal wall. Arch Otolaryngol 1977;103:531–4.

198. Eze NN, Wyatt ME, Hartley BE. The role of the anterior cricoid split in facilitating extubation in infants. Int J Pediatr Otorhinolaryngol 2005;69:843–6.

199. Cotton RT. Pediatric laryngotracheal stenosis. J Pediatr Surg 1984;19:699–704.

200. Fearon B, Cinnamond M. Surgical correction of subglottic stenosis of the larynx: Clinical results of the Fearon-Cotton operation. J Otolaryngol 1976;5:475–8.

201. Fearon B, Cotton R. Surgical correction of subglottic stenosis of the larynx in infants and children. Progress report. Ann Otol Rhinol Laryngol 1974;83:428–31.

202. White DR, Cotton RT, Bean JA, Rutter MJ. Pediatric cricotracheal resection: Surgical outcomes and risk factor analysis. Arch Otolaryngol Head Neck Surg 2005;131:896–9.

203. varez-Neri H, Penchyna-Grub J, Porras-Hernandez JD, et al. Primary cricotracheal resection with thyrotracheal anastomosis for the treatment of severe subglottic stenosis in children and adolescents. Ann Otol Rhinol Laryngol 2005;114:2–6.

204. Garabedian EN, Nicollas R, Roger G, et al. Cricotracheal resection in children weighing less than 10 kg. Arch Otolaryngol Head Neck Surg 2005;131:505–8.

205. Ciprandi G, Nicollas R, Triglia JM, Rivosecchi M. Fetal cricotracheal manipulation: Effects on airway healing, cricoid growth, and lung development. Pediatr Surg Int 2003;19:335–9.

206. Ettema SL, Tolejano CJ, Thielke RJ, et al. Perceptual voice analysis of patients with subglottic stenosis. Otolaryngol Head Neck Surg 2006;135:730–5.

207. Ludemann JP, Hughes CA, Noah Z, Holinger LD. Complications of pediatric laryngotracheal reconstruction: Prevention strategies. Ann Otol Rhinol Laryngol 1999;108:1019–26.

208. Cotton RT, Gray SD, Miller RP. Update of the Cincinnati experience in pediatric laryngotracheal reconstruction. Laryngoscope 1989;99:1111–6.

209. Benjamin B. Congenital disorders. In: Cummings CW, Fredrickson JM, Harker LA, et al, editors. Otolaryngology-Head and Neck Surgery. 1st edition. St. Louis: CV Mosby Co; 1986. p. 2329–38.

210. Rahbar R, Nicollas R, Roger G, et al. The biology and management of subglottic hemangioma: Past, present, future. Laryngoscope 2004;114:1880–91.

211. Wooley AL, Lusk RP. Multiple Vascular lesions of an infant's airway. Otolaryngol Head Neck Surg 1994;111:305–8.

212. Bitar MA, Moukarbel RV, Zalzal GH. Management of congenital subglottic hemangioma: Trends and success over the past 17 years. Otolaryngol Head Neck Surg 2005;132:226–31.

213. Vijayasekaran S, White DR, Hartley BE, et al. Open excision of subglottic hemangiomas to avoid tracheostomy. Arch Otolaryngol Head Neck Surg 2006;132:159–63.

214. Naiman AN, Ayari S, Froehlich P. Controlled risk of stenosis after surgical excision of laryngeal hemangioma. Arch Otolaryngol Head Neck Surg 2003;129:1291–5.

215. Pransky SM, Canto C. Management of subglottic hemangioma. Curr Opin Otolaryngol Head Neck Surg 2004;12:509–12.

70

Congenital Anomalies of the Head and Neck

Lee D. Rowe, MD

Congenital head and neck anomalies represent a diverse group of clinical disorders that are the result of errors in embryogenesis or the product of intrauterine events that affect embryonic and fetal growth. Frequently, these present as upper aerodigestive tract neoplasms and neck masses, with thyroglossal duct abnormalities most common, followed by branchial arch defects, lymphangiomas (cystic hygromas), and subcutaneous vascular anomalies (hemangiomas, arteriovenous malformations). Less common are teratomas, heterotopic neural tissue, and nasopharyngeal neoplasms. Additional disorders encountered include congenital disorders of the oral cavity including cleft lip and palate, Pierre Robin sequence (PRS), and other aberrations such as primary ciliary dyskinesia, Kartagener syndrome, and craniofacial anomalies.

CONGENITAL DISORDERS OF THE NECK

Branchial Cleft Anomalies

Lateral cervical lesions termed branchial cleft cysts are congenital developmental defects that arise from the primitive branchial apparatus (branchial arch, cleft, and pouches). First branchial cleft anomalies are discussed elsewhere in this chapter.

Embryogenesis. The branchial arches consist of five parallel mesodermal bars, each with its own nerve supply and blood vessel (primitive aortic arches that develop during the third and fourth embryonic weeks). The branchial arches are separated externally by branchial clefts consisting of ectoderm and internally by endodermally lined branchial (pharyngeal) pouches. A branchial plate is located between each arch separating pouch from cleft. The nerves are anterior to their respective arteries, except in the fifth arch, where the nerve is posterior to the artery. Caudal to all the arches is the twelfth nerve which arises from the epicardial ridge. The sternocleidomastoid muscle is derived from cervical somites posterior and inferior to the foregoing arches. In each arch, a central artery develops connecting the two ventral and two dorsal aortas. The two ventral aortas fuse completely, whereas the two dorsal aortas only fuse caudally. With continued development, the ventral aortas become the external and common carotid arteries, whereas the arteries of the first and second arch degenerate. Segments of the dorsal aorta persist as the internal carotid artery

along with the artery of the third arch. The left fourth arch artery becomes the arch of the aorta, and the right fourth arch artery becomes the proximal subclavian artery. The primitive clefts pass between the corresponding arteries. Development of the pharyngeal region and branchial arches depends on the integration of surface ectoderm, foregut endoderm, paraxial mesoderm, and the neural crest. It is believed that the regional development of the branchial arches is controlled by nested expression of related homeobox genes (*HOM-C/Hox*).[1] Studies in mutant mouse embryos lacking the homeobox gene (*Hoxa3*) demonstrate bilateral defects of the common carotid artery, a third branchial arch derivative. Mice homozygous for a hypomorphic allele of *Fgfr1* have craniofacial defects, some of which are due to the failure of entry of neural crest cells into the second branchial arch. In addition, hemizygous deletion of chromosome 22q11 in humans involves defects in pharyngeal arch and neural crest development.[2] The resulting branchial pouch anomalies are generally lined with stratified squamous cell epithelium containing subepithelial lymphoid follicles, keratin, hair follicles, sweat glands, cartilage, and sebaceous glands.

Clinical Presentation. Typically, branchial clefts present as smooth, round, fluctuant, non-tender masses along the anterior border of the sternocleidomastoid muscle, anywhere from the external auditory canal to the clavicle. During upper respiratory tract infections, a painful increase in size is common and occasionally may be associated with external drainage through an unrecognized fistula. Small cysts may not be recognized until the second decade in life. Male and female incidences are equal, and nearly all these lesions are recognized by the time the patient reaches 30 years of age.

Second Branchial Cleft Anomalies. Second branchial cleft lesions are the most common anomalies and are encountered most frequently in the anterior triangle of the neck along the anterior border of the sternocleidomastoid muscle inferior to the angle of the mandible. The fistula tract, if present, ascends along the carotid sheath, crosses over the hypoglossal and glossopharyngeal nerves, and courses between the internal and external carotid arteries. It ends in the tonsillar fossa, a second branchial pouch derivative. Second pouch remnants may form blind sinuses in the palatine tonsil and frequently cause recurrent unilateral tonsillitis. A tonsillectomy and excision of the sinus tract is necessary.

Third Branchial Cleft Anomalies. Third branchial cleft anomalies are unusual and constitute less than 1% of all branchial cleft anomalies. The external ostium occurs at the same position as the second branchial cleft anomaly, and the cyst may be located anywhere along the fistula. The fistula tract ascends along the carotid sheath behind the internal carotid artery and over the hypoglossal nerve, and it enters the pyriform sinus, piercing the middle constrictor muscle below the glossopharyngeal nerve. Clinically, the anomaly may mimic suppurative thyroiditis or symptoms of an external laryngocele and can cause recurrent infection, discharge, and rarely, stridor.

Fourth Branchial Cleft Anomalies. Fourth branchial cleft anomalies are extremely rare. As of 2004, only 60 cases have been reported. The fistula tract descends along the carotid sheath, enters the chest passing under either the aortic arch on the left or the subclavian artery on the right, and ascends in the neck to open at the apex of the pyriform sinus. The sinus tract or cyst may become clinically manifested by recurrent episodes of neck abscess or acute suppurative thyroiditis which may cause acute airway obstruction in infants. A left neck predominance has been confirmed.

Treatment. Complete surgical excision is the treatment of choice for branchial cleft anomalies and is indicated for recurrent infection, cosmetic deformity, and potential for malignant degeneration. Preoperative assessment with ultrasonography, computed tomography (CT) scanning, and/or magnetic resonance (MR) imaging is essential and may be combined with a fistulogram or pharyngoesophagram when indicated. A "stepladder" surgical approach with transverse incisions paralleling skin creases is used to avoid long, cosmetically unsatisfactory incisions, paralleling the sternocleidomastoid muscle. To avoid recurrence, combined endoscopic examination for a pharyngeal pouch and sinus tract with meticulous dissection of a sinus tract, if present, along with endoscopic cauterization of the sinus tract's internal opening will facilitate complete resection. It is essential to excise enbloc any portion of the thyroid involved in the sinus tract. Removal of fourth branchial pouch sinuses can be facilitated via a modified oblique thyrotomy above the cricothyroid joint after detaching the inferior constrictor.

Branchiogenic Carcinoma. The hypothesis that squamous cell carcinoma arises in a branchial cleft cyst (branchiogenic carcinoma) is controversial.

Cystic squamous cell carcinoma presenting in the neck without an apparent primary is almost universally secondary to metastasis from a neoplasm arising in the faucial or lingual tonsillar crypt epithelium or nasopharyngeal tissue.[3] Malignant transformation with in situ branchial cyst carcinoma is therefore a rarity. Management is wide excision of the tumor and ipsilateral radical neck dissection followed by adjuvant radiation therapy or chemoradiation.[4]

LYMPHANGIOMAS, HEMANGIOMAS, AND OTHER VASCULAR ANOMALIES

Congenital lymphangiomatous malformations of the head and neck represent a wide clinical spectrum. Lymphangiomas result from abnormal development of the lymphatic system at sites of lymphatic-venous connection, with obstruction of lymph drainage from the affected area causing multicystic endothelium-lined spaces. The neck is the most common site (25% of all cases). Over half these lesions are present at birth, with 90% manifesting by 2 years of age. Those lymphangiomas arising above the mylohyoid muscle are more infiltrative and tend to extend from skin to mucosa while those below the mylohyoid are more discreet and cystic.

Cystic Hygroma

Cystic hygromas are large lymphangiomas most commonly found in the posterior triangle of the neck and axilla in children. Cervical cystic hygromas commonly appear before 30 weeks' gestation and are usually associated with karyotypic abnormalities, various malformation syndromes and several teratogenic agents. The prognosis is poor for these types of hygromas. By contrast, cystic hygroma developing late in pregnancy has a more favorable outcome and is more likely to be encountered by the head and neck surgeon. Cystic hygromas are soft, painless, and compressible masses that may increase when the patient cries. Two-thirds are asymptomatic. After an upper respiratory tract infection, however, sudden enlargement with inflammation, infection, dysphagia, and stridor may develop. This is more commonly seen if the anterior triangle of the neck is involved or in patients with pharyngolaryngeal extension or intraoral involvement.

Vascular Anomalies

Other congenital vascular anomalies of the head and neck include hemangiomas and arteriovenous malformations or lymphovenous lesions. Diagnostic imaging of these anomalies is based on the need for surgical treatment. Only those lesions that cause functional impairment or developmental disturbance are surgically addressed. Angiography, combined with MR imaging, allows separation into low-flow lesions (hemangiomas, venous, and lymphatic malformations) and high-flow lesions (arteriovenous malformations and invasive, combined lymphovascular malformations). Treatment of small cystic hygromas that

have not regressed but have enlarged is with surgical excision with staged debulking of larger cystic hygromas. Neural structures such as the facial nerve, vagus nerve, and phrenic nerves should not be sacrificed. Recurrence is uncommon when gross neoplasm is removed. Hemangiomas are frequently multiple with the parotid gland, a common site of occurrence. They proliferate during the first year of life, then involute at a variable rate over several years. Subcutaneous recombinant interferon alpha 2 a or oral methylprednisolone administered over 6 to 12 months is effective treatment if initiated early in the proliferative phase. Alternatively, cyclophosphamide may induce fast regression in neonates with life threatening hemangiomas.[5] Surgical excision is reserved for severe cosmetic deformity or life-threatening aerodigestive tract impairment.

For low-flow, macrocystic-type lymphangiomas less than 5 cm, sclerosant therapy with the agent OK-432, a lyophilized mixture of low-virulence group A *Streptococcus pyogenes* with penicillin G potassium, is effective, either alone or combined with surgical resections or embolization (Figure 1).[6] Preoperative embolization at the time of selective angiography and surgical excision are the treatment of choice in high-flow malformations. Ultimately, biomolecular markers

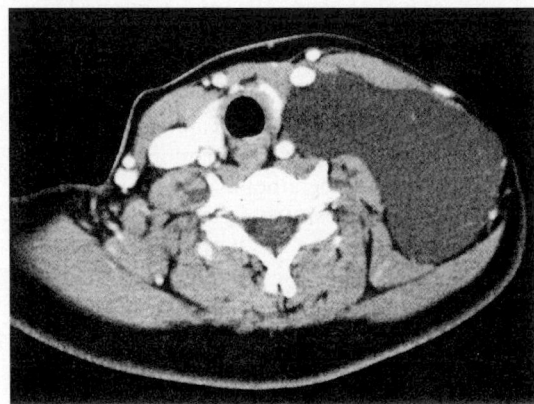

(A)

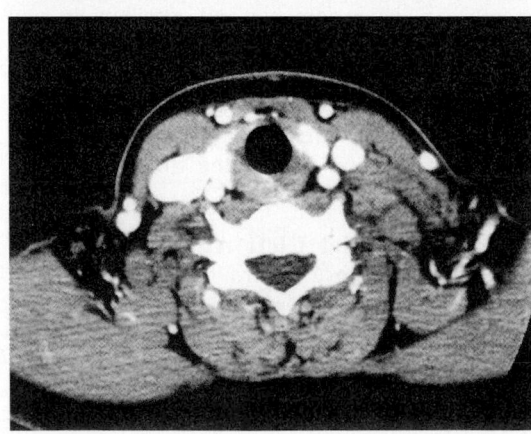

(B)

Figure 1 Computed tomography (CT) of pre- and postsclerotherapy with OK-432 in congenital lymphatic malformation. (A) Presclerotherapy CT of a 36-year-old female with a large cystic mass in the lower neck. (B) Postsclerotherapy CT after three treatments with OK-432 reveals complete resolution. (Used with permission from reference 6.)

will characterize vascular anomalies with specific clinical behaviors. Key cytokines driving angiogenesis include vascular endothelial growth factor (VEGF) family members and receptors (placental growth factor [PGF], VEGF-A, and VEFG-C) and angiopoietins. Distinct patterns of angiogenic factor expression, endothelial vascular mural cell status, and vessel architecture may eventually be used to predict which lesions will involute.[7]

ABERRANT THYROID TISSUE

Ectopic thyroid tissue can occur anywhere from the foramen cecum to the lower neck (Figure 2). Most frequently, it occurs as a thyroglossal duct cyst associated with a normal thyroid gland. Less common is total ectopia, manifesting as a lingual thyroid. True lateral neck thyroid ectopia lateral to the carotid artery and jugular vein cannot be confirmed based upon embryogenesis. As a result, the findings of aberrant thyroid tissue should direct attention to the ipsilateral thyroid lobe. If papillary carcinoma is found in an aberrant position, then total thyroidectomy with central lymph node dissection is performed. Because cervical metastases of papillary thyroid carcinoma (PTC) can mimic branchiogenic cysts clinically and histopathologically, it is difficult to distinguish between true PTC arising within a branchial cyst and metastatic disease. Immunohistochemical staining for thyroid transcription factor 1 (TTF-1) is not specific to thyroid tissue as it is positive in 10% of isolated branchial cleft cysts. However, detection of p63 expression in the nuclei of the lining epithelia of the branchial

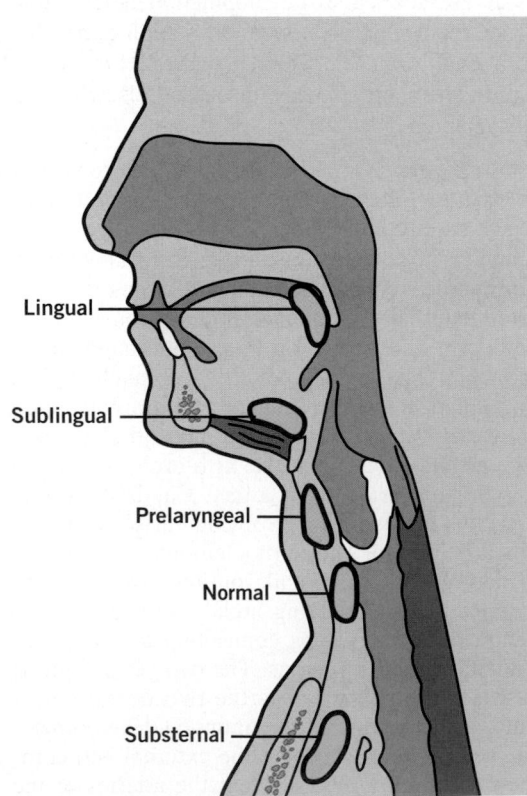

Figure 2 Most common locations of midline aberrant thyroid tissue schematically illustrated.

cleft cyst may suggest that p63 contributes to the development of PTC arising within the cyst.[8]

Embryology

In the 4-week-old embryo, the primitive thyroid gland begins as a ventral diverticulum of endodermal origin, arising in the floor of the pharynx between the tuberculum impar and the copula. Ultimately, it becomes the foramen cecum, and the copula becomes the posterior third of the tongue. The thyroid descends caudally through or adjacent to the primitive hyoid bone. The developing thyroglossal duct reaches its final position in the midline of the neck and develops into the median lobe of the thyroid. It normally persists as a hollow stalk for 6 weeks and then atrophies. Thyroglossal duct anomalies result from a failure of complete obliteration of the thyroglossal duct and are located anywhere along the descent of the gland.

Lingual Thyroid

A lingual thyroid presents in the midline as a sessile, nontender reddish mass in the base of the tongue, anterior to the valleculae. It is the most frequent benign mass encountered in the oropharynx and, unlike other aberrant thyroid anomalies, has a female preponderance of 7:1. Symptoms may include dysphagia, cough, dysphonia, dyspnea, and in extremely rare cases, symptoms of obstructive sleep apnea and hemorrhage. A lingual thyroid may become apparent during pregnancy because of increased thyroid function, and approximately 70% will have hypothyroidism.

A lingual thyroid is covered with squamous cell epithelium and often exhibits an abundant aberrant vascular supply. The mass consists of normal or immature thyroid tissue, which may be either functional or dysfunctional. Indications for surgical removal include uncontrollable hyperthyroidism, hemorrhage, symptomatic enlargement, or question of malignancy. Carcinoma arising in a lingual thyroid is rare with only 28 cases reported. Preoperatively, a thyroid uptake study and scan should be obtained to determine whether functioning thyroid tissue exists in its normal cervical location. MR imaging may also be of value because it allows multiplanar imaging and provides the best soft tissue definition. Excision is performed by the transcervical transhyoid route. Alternatively, iodine-131 ablation for benign lingual thyroid is a safe and effective treatment while transposition of the gland via a lateral pharyngotomy incision with random tongue muscle flap revascularization has been used to preserve thyroid function.[9]

Thyroglossal Duct Anomalies

Signs and Symptons. A thyroglossal duct cyst is the most common congenital neck mass and the second most common of all childhood cervical neck masses. Cysts, sinuses, and fistulas of the thyroglossal duct manifest as anterior midline neck masses from the foramen cecum to the thyroid gland, typically before 20 years of age (most

before 10 years). Thyroglossal ducts and fistulas are often asymptomatic. They may also become recurrently infected during upper respiratory tract infections, which can cause cyst enlargement, abscess development, and rupture with external sinus formation. Thyroglossal duct cysts most commonly are found below the hyoid bone and above the thyroid gland, displaying movement with anterior tongue protrusion and swallowing. Usually, the cysts are 1 to 3 cm in diameter and are smooth, round, and fluctuant. A precise pathogenesis of thyroglossal duct cysts has not been determined. However, a hereditary predisposition is suspected. Overall, a predominantly autosomal dominant pattern of inheritance in non-United States families has been reported in older patients (mean age 13.9 years) versus an autosomal recessive pattern in younger patients (mean age 6.2 years).

Histopathologic Features. Thyroglossal duct cysts and fistulas are lined with squamous, ciliated columnar, or transitional cell epithelium. They may be surrounded by fibrous tissue with infiltrating inflammatory cells lacking organized lymphoid tissue. Islands of ectopic thyroid tissue and mucus glands are not uncommonly identified. The cyst or sinus tract is filled with mucoid or mucopurulent material. The male-to-female ratio varies between 1.2:1 and 1.6:1.

Differential Diagnosis. The differential diagnosis includes dermoid cyst, pyramidal lobe hyperplasia or cyst, teratomas, hamartoma, lipomas, sebaceous cysts, cavernous hemangiomas, hyperplastic lymph nodes, and malignant primary or metastatic neoplasms.

Treatment. As with a lingual thyroid, a preoperative thyroid scan and uptake study are mandatory, even though concomitant agenesis of the thyroid is extremely rare. Malignant degeneration, recurrent infections, undesirable cosmetic appearance, and rarely, intermittent upper airway obstruction are indications for surgical excision of thyroglossal duct cysts and fistulas. Incision and drainage may be necessary in the interim if an abscess has developed. Because of the high recurrence rate after excision the Sistrunk procedure is recommended to prevent recurrence. This involves a transverse incision over the cyst or a fusiform incision over an external fistula opening. All abnormal tissue including the cyst, fistula, body of the hyoid bone (preferably more than 15 mm), and the fibrous cord extending to the foramen cecum should be resected. Recurrence develops in up to 20% of cases as a result of failure to removal all abnormal tissue including accessory ducts and is significantly increased by the presence of inflammation at the time of surgery and greater than two infections prior to surgery.[10] Malignant degeneration of the thyroglossal duct remnants occurs in 1 to 2%.[11] Approximately 173 cases of thyroglossal duct carcinoma, predominantly of the papillary type, have been reported. Additional cases of Hürthle cell adenoma have also been described. Most patients with papillary carcinoma are in their forties, although 20% are less than 20 years of age. Typically, the tumor is small and clinically unsuspected, and in rare

cases it may be associated with regional or distant metastasis. Rarely, squamous cell carcinoma arising directly from the lining epithelium in a thyroglossal duct remnant has been reported and, as a rule, has a poor prognosis. Treatment of thyroglossal duct remnant carcinoma consists of the Sistrunk procedure, total thyroidectomy, central lymph node dissection, ablative iodine-131 therapy for residual metastatic thyroid carcinoma subsequent thyroid suppression therapy and careful interval follow up with whole body thyroid scanning.

THYMIC CYST

Cervical ectopic thymus and thymic cysts are extremely rare. About 100 cases have been reported in the English language with most occurring asymptomatically in children and adults. Only 10% have involved patients younger than 1 year of age. Cysts can arise from nests of thymic tissue anywhere along the descent of the thymic primordia from the mandible to the mediastinum and are primarily located anterior and deep to the middle one-third of the sternocleidomastoid muscle. In up to 50% of the cervical thymic cysts there is a mediastinal connection possibly requiring a sternotomy. Thymic lesions are more common in males. Ectopic cervical thymus is best imaged by MRI whereas thymic cyst has a more consistent appearance on CT. Surgical resection provides definitive diagnosis and cure (Figure 3).[12,13]

NEUROGENIC NEOPLASMS

Congenital neurogenic lesions involving the head and neck include all neoplasms or anomalies originating in the neural tissue or its covering. Two groups have been recognized: (1) heterotopic brain lesions with developmental defects, which are discussed in the next section; and (2) neoplasms of neurogenic origin

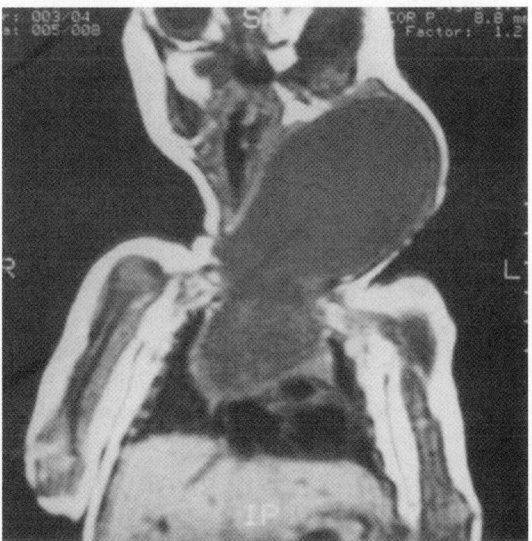

Figure 3 Coronal T1-weighted magnetic resonance image of a neonate with a cervical thymic cyst with mediastinal involvement. (Reproduced with permission from reference 13.)

including neuromas, neurofibromas, ganglioneuromas, and meningiomas. Neuromas originating from the connective tissue sheath of the nerve are termed schwannomas. They may appear as multiple neurofibromas arising from cutaneous, visceral, and cranial nerves in neurofibromatosis type 1 (NF1) or type 2 (NF2) and have a predilection to arise in deep planes of the neck. NF1 is a common autosomal dominant disease characterized by complex and multicellular neurofibromas arising from Schwann cells, pigmentation anomalies, and increased risk of low grade tumors undergoing high-grade malignant transformation. 95% of patients with NF1 exhibit a mutation in the NF1 gene on chromosome 17 whose product, neurofibromin, functions in Ras signal transduction and cell proliferation and differentiation. Allelic loss and/or basepair deletions in the NF1 gene are associated with malignant transformation.[14] NF1 is defined by the absence of bilateral vestibular schwannomas which are the main diagnostic criteria for NF2. Neurofibromatosis type 2 (NF2) is also an autosomal dominant disease with sporadic and familial forms. A mutation in the tumor suppressor gene, named merlin, on chromosome 22 occurs in approximately 1 in 40,000 live births. As in NF1, at least two mutations are required in which all patients develop bilateral vestibular schwannomas. Missense mutations in *CABIN 1* genes and rearrangements in the immunoglobulin lambda locus as well as merlin lead to alterations in gene transcript expression which includes oncogene products. The incidence of head and neck manifestations in patients with NF1 and NF2 varies between 14 and 37%. In NF1 (classic von Recklinghausen disease) functional deficits include speech and voice abnormalities, airway obstruction, dysphagia, facial paresis, lip incompetence, and impaired mastication. NF2 patients with bilateral vestibular schwannomas exhibit hearing loss. Typically, neuromas appear as solitary, encapsulated lesions with elongated spindle-shaped cells with an oval or flattened nucleus. Ganglioneuromas, rarely seen in the head or neck, are characterized by ganglion and glial cells. Meningiomas are usually benign and arise from embryonic arachnoid rests. They may appear extracranially at the nasal root or in the sinuses. Whorl-like fibroblastic nuclei with hyaline formations producing a sand-like appearance may be present (psammoma body). Pharyngeal neuromas are rare and appear as smooth, firm, rounded, and yellow masses. Symptoms depend on the size and location of the tumor. If multiple brown discolorations of the skin or café au lait spots are present, neurofibroma may be suggested. Treatment is surgical excision and must be complete because recurrence is common.

CONGENITAL DISORDERS OF THE NOSE AND PARANASAL SINUSES

Heterotopic Neural Tissue

Aberrant embryogenesis of the frontonasal and anterior neuropore leads to three main types of anomalies: heterotopic neural tissue (either nasal glioma or anterior cephalocele) and nasal dermal sinus. Heterotopic neural tissue or glioma may manifest as isolated ectopic brain tissue with only a fibrous band connecting it to the endocranium. A glioma may be of the external or endonasal type. The external nasal glioma is typically found in the nasion as a red, relatively firm, mobile mass located subcutaneously that does not increase in size when the patient cries. The endonasal glioma is less common and arises from the middle turbinate or the lateral nasal vault, where it may be mistaken for a polyp. By contrast, a meningiocele is a hernial protrusion of the meninges, and if it contains brain tissue, it is called an encephalocele. An encephalocele is caused by a defect of the fetal skull and contains an ependyma-lined cavity filled with cerebrospinal fluid. Two basic types of hernial protrusions are identified: (1) the sincipital type; and (2) the basal type. The sincipital type is uncommon and is associated with termination of the meninges near the base of the nose. This type has three different forms: (1) nasofrontal, in which the encephalocele extends between the nasal and frontal bones, resulting in a midline swelling at the base of the nose; (2) nasoethmoidal, in which a defect among the nasal, frontal, and ethmoid bones allows the encephalocele to appear as a mass beneath the skin of the bony-cartilaginous junction; and (3) naso-orbital protrusion of the encephalocele through the suture line among the lacrimal, frontal, and ethmoidal bones appearing as a conjunctival mass. The basal type, in which the hernia extends into the naso-orbital and pharyngeal region, is rarer than the sincipital. Three varieties have been identified: (1) sphenoid-pharyngeal, in which the encephalocele extends through the ethmoid or sphenoid bones or their sutures lines into the nasal or nasopharyngeal cavity; (2) sphenoid-orbital, in which the encephalocele extends through the spheno-orbital fissure into the posterior aspect of the orbit, resulting in pulsatile exophthalmos; and (3) sphenomaxillary, in which the encephalocele herniates through the spheno-orbital fissure into the orbit, with extension inferiorily through the inferior orbital fissure into the pterygopalatine fissure. This results in a mass bulging into the cheek or into the oropharynx, medial to the ramus of the mandible. In all cases, unlike with gliomas, pulsations and an increase in size of the mass can be observed when the patient coughs or strains. Thin cut axial and coronal CT and/or multiplanar MR imaging are necessary to determine the appropriate combined transfacial and intracranial approach for surgical resection. Three-dimensional CT is helpful in complex cases providing additional information for surgical planning.

Dermoid Cysts

Dermoid cysts occasionally occur in the neck, usually in the midline. Overall, fewer than 10% of all dermoid cysts occur in the head and neck. One-fourth of the head and neck dermoid cysts are found in the floor of the mouth, with the remainder in the nasal and periorbital region. The most common presentation is a midline nasoglabellar mass. These lesions are seen primarily in children and adolescents during the second decade of life, but they also may occur in infants. Cyst walls consist of squamous cell epithelium containing epidermal appendages. These cysts are thought to originate from displacement of epidermal elements during the intramembranous growth phase of the nasal bones in the embryo. Because of the variability in clinical presentation and contiguous structure involvement, segregation of periorbital lesions into three distinct subgroups is helpful: (1) frontotemporal region dermoid cysts; (2) orbital region dermoid cysts; and (3) nasoglabellar dermoid cysts. Midline nasoglabellar cysts may have associated sinus tracts or fistulae (10 to 45%) which, in rare cases, may have intracranial extensions. In those patients with intracranial extension, the sinus tract traverses either the cribriform plate or foramen cecum and is attached to the dura, falx cerebri, or other intracranial structures. The treatment of choice is surgical excision after CT and MR imaging to evaluate intracranial extension.[15] All tissue must be removed to prevent recurrences. In patients with intracranial extension, a coronal flap is employed to facilitate removal and to prevent postoperative meningitis and abscess formation. Transnasal endoscopic techniques have been advocated when the dermoid cyst is confined to the nasal cavity with no cutaneous involvement.

Other congenital midface cysts are those associated with the facial clefts, including the nasoethmoidal cleft cyst, nasolabial cyst, subalar cleft cyst, globulomaxillary cyst, cysts connected with cleft lip or palate, premaxillary cyst, nasopalatine cyst, foraminal incisor cyst, and Jacobson organ cysts.

Choanal Atresia

Bilateral atresia of the choanae is the most frequently encountered congenital nasal anomaly (1 in 7,000 to 8,000 live births) and is a common cause of neonatal respiratory distress. Approximately 50% of individuals with choanal artesia have the anomaly bilaterally. Analysis of CT scans and histopathologic sections demonstrates 29% pure bony, 71% mixed bony and membranous and no pure membranous atresia. A 2:1 female predisposition is seen in choanal atresia, and recent evidence points to an autosomal recessive mode of inheritance.

Failure of breakdown of the buccopharyngeal membrane on gestational day 45 is considered to be the cause of choanal atresia. Other theories include abnormalities in the migration of the cephalic neural crest following neural tube closure. Several craniofacial abnormalities including skull-base defects and systemic malformations have been described in association with choanal atresia, including the CHARGE association (Table 1). The CHARGE association is a nonrandom clustering of congenital anomalies which

Table 1 Congenital Anomalies Associated with Choanal Atresia

Branchial anomalies
CHARGE association
Humeroradial synostosis
Mandibular facial synostosis
Microcephaly
Micrognathia
Nasopharyngeal anomalies
Palatal defects

has an estimated prevalence of 1 in 10,000 births. It occurs with C, coloboma of the iris or retina; H, congenital heart disease; A, atresia choanae; R, retarded growth and development; G genital anomalies in males; E, ear abnormalities and deafness. Almost all patients have malformed pinnae and exhibit hypoplastic incudes, cochlear anomalies and ageneses or hypoplasias of the semicircular canals on CT scan (Figure 4).[16] The majority demonstrate severe conductive or mixed hearing loss and vestibular dysfunction. Other commonly associated anomalies are facial nerve palsy (50%), tracheoesophageal fistula (33%) and cleft lip/palate. Arhinencephaly is a constant feature which is being increasingly recognized antenatally. Chromodomain helicase DNA-binding protein gene (*CHD7*) mutations on chromosome 8q12.1 account for the majority of cases with CHARGE syndrome and exhibit broad clinical expression without obvious genotype-phenotype correlation.[17] The combination of malformations in the CHARGE association suggests that this syndrome is a polytopic developmental

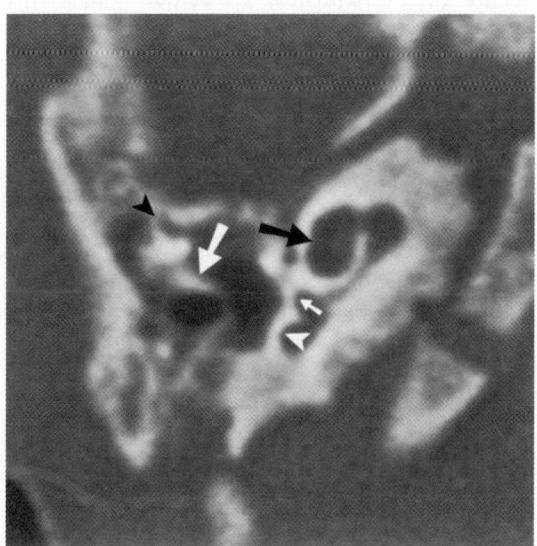

Figure 4 Axial 1mm thick computed tomographic section through right mesotympanum in patient with CHARGE association. Note fixation of the malleus head to the anterior tympanic wall (*black arrowhead*), malformation and narrow rotation of the incus (*large white arrow*), and absence of stapes. Also note absence of the oval window (*small white arrow*) and presence of a round window niche with bony obliteration (*white arrowhead*). Tympanic sinus, pyramidal eminence, and stapedius muscle are absent. Interscalar septum between middle and apical turns of the cochlea is missing, as well as a normal cochlear modiolus (*black arrow*). (Reproduced with permission from reference 16.)

field defect involving the neural tube and neural crest cells secondary to dysfunctional developmental gene expression as well as mesodermal patterning.

Symptoms. Respiratory distress at birth is the sine qua non of bilateral choanal atresia. In spite of vigorous attempts at respiration, effective air exchange does not occur until the neonate begins to cry, bypassing the nasal obstruction. Once the crying ceases, however, the neonate's mouth closes, and a pattern of cyclic obstruction gradually develops, resulting in increasing respiratory failure. Because neonates are obligatory nasal breathers, placement of an oral airway or McGovern nipple is lifesaving. By contrast, children with unilateral choanal atresia present later in life with unilateral rhinorrhea without respiratory distress.

Diagnosis. The diagnosis of bilateral choanal atresia is confirmed by the inability to pass a No. 5 or 6 French feeding catheter at least 3 cm through the nose into the nasopharynx. In addition, direct observation with nasofiberoptic endoscopy and CT scan is essential to determine the type of obstruction. Specifically, the CT scan demonstrates the thickness of the atretic plate as well as its medial encroachment of the posterior aspect of the medial maxilla.

Treatment. Multiple methods are available to repair choanal atresia. The appropriate method is determined by the age of the patient and whether the atresia is bilateral or unilateral. In all methods, the challenge is to provide adequate mucosal lining to the new choana and to prevent granulation tissue formation, osteoneogenesis, and subsequent stenosis. Treatment requires perforation of the atresia plate with either a curette or powered instrumentation and removal of lateral choanal bone and a portion of the vomer with preservation of mucosal flaps. The use of stenting, laser, mitomycin C or topical nasal corticosteroids is controversial, and no controlled studies have evaluated their true efficacy.[18]

Transnasal Approach. The most direct and simplest route for choanal atresia repair is transnasal, using a No. 2 Lempert or similar curette inserted 3 to 3.5 cm beyond the nares along the nasal floor, and exerting firm pressure against the bony atresia plate until it is perforated. The anterior nasal mucous membrane is sacrificed after satisfactory enlargement of the choana to permit placement of a 3.5 mm Silastic endotracheal tube as a stent. Posterior membranous flaps are developed in a stellate fashion to cover the denuded bone (Figures 5 and 6). Care must be taken to prevent injury to the roof of the choana and the skull base because reported complications of this approach have included meningitis, cerebrospinal fluid leaks, brain injuries, Gradenigo syndrome, and cervical vertebral subluxation. Reported laser techniques include the use of the carbon dioxide, KTP, or neodymium: yttrium–aluminum–garnet (Nd: YAG) lasers. An endoscopic approach with a 2.5 mm or 4 mm telescope and powered instrumentation using a microdebrider with continuous suction

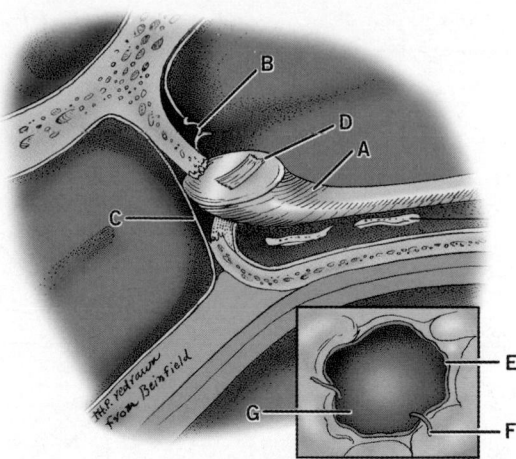

Figure 5 Choanal atresia repair. (A) curette; (B) posterior nasal mucous membrane elevated off of bony atresia plate; (C) intact nasopharyngeal mucous membrane; (D) spicule of bone removed from atresia plate; (E) subtotal removal of bony atresia plate; (F) shreds of posterior nasal mucous membrane; and (G) intact nasopharyngeal mucous membrane.

is effective, especially for neonates[19] (Figure 7). After effective removal of bone and stenting and the use of topical corticosteroids to diminish granulation tissue formation, stenosis may still occur, and dilatation may be necessary. If this fails, a transpalatal approach will be required. A transseptal approach, which is reserved for older children with unilateral atresia, offers better exposure of the posterior vomer without risk of palatal injury and impairment of growth. The transpalatal approach can be modified either via sublabial extension or by an external rhinoplasty approach to improve visualization.

Transpalatal Approach. The transpalatal approach provides superior visualization of membranous or bony atresia and may be useful for both bilateral and unilateral atresia. CHARGE patients with bilateral atresia should have primary transpalatal repair due to the high transnasal

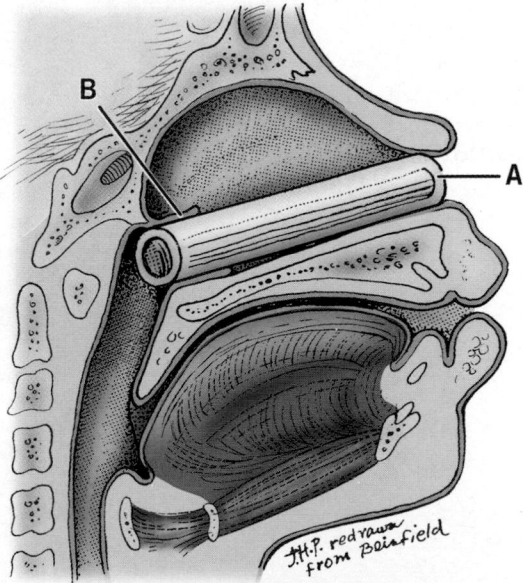

Figure 6 The tube in place. (A) The anterior end of the tube lying just within the nares. (B) Nasopharyngeal mucous membrane covering the raw bony surface.

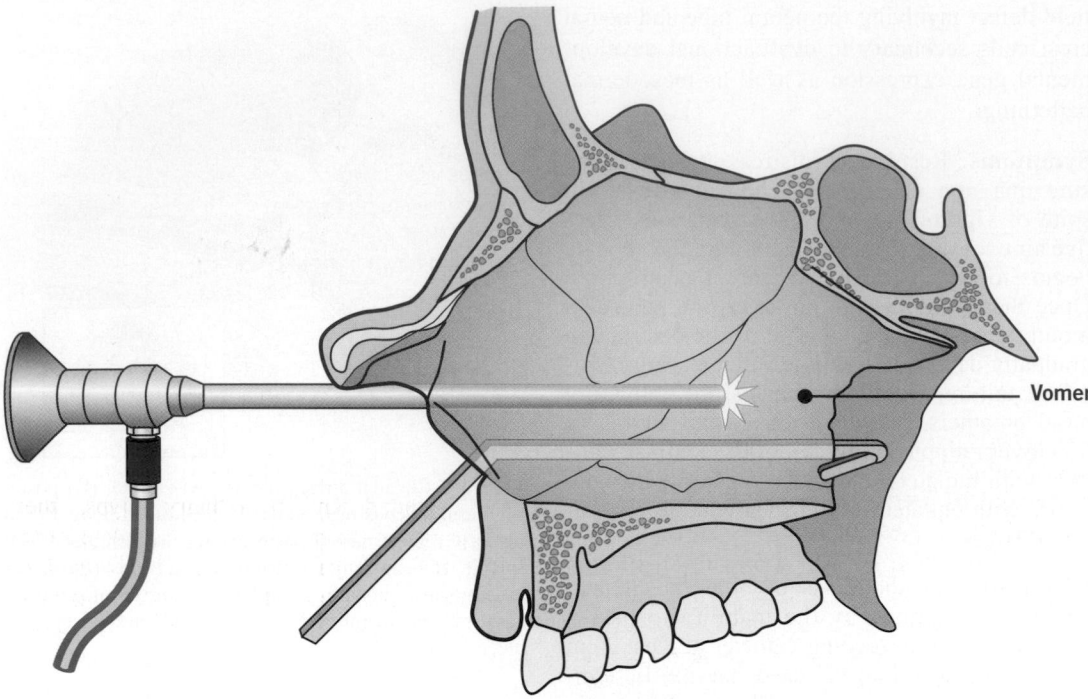

Figure 7 An endoscopic approach to choanal atresia repair with a backbiting instrument placed in the nasal cavity to resect a portion of the vomer. (Reproduced with permission from reference 19.)

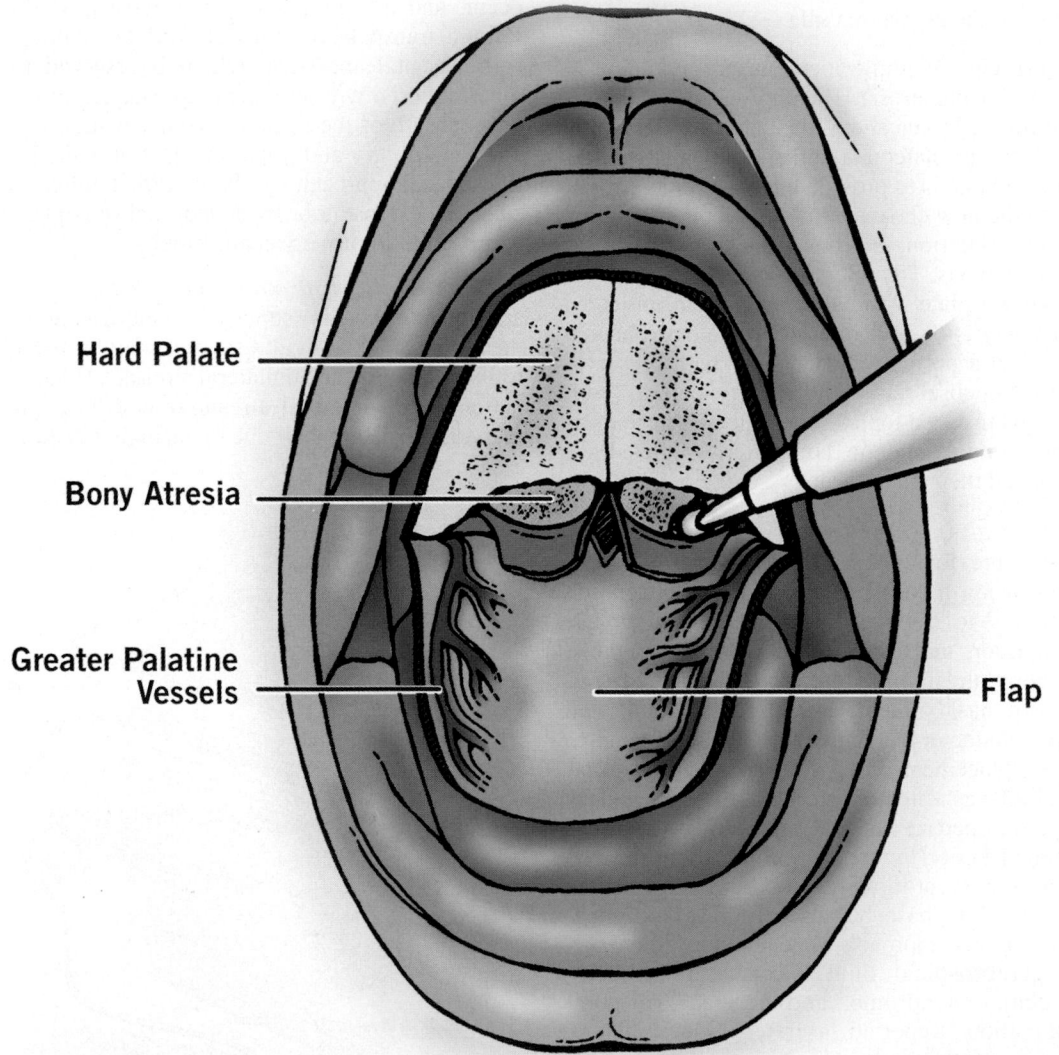

Figure 8 A transpalatal approach using a drill to remove the bony atretic plate; mucosa over the atretic plate has been preserved for reconstruction of the neochoana. (Reproduced with permission from reference 19.)

surgical failure rate in this population.[20] Although impaired palatal growth is a potential problem in the neonate, the procedure can be safely used in patients older than 5 years of age who are treatment failures, if one takes great care to avoid injury to the posterior palatine canals. The procedure is carried out with the patient in the supine position and the head hyperextended. After infiltration of local anesthesia, a horseshoe-type incision is developed several millimeters posterior to the alveolar ridge, and a mucoperiosteal flap is then raised based on the greater palatine vessels. Once the posterior edge of the hard palate is reached, the mucosa is divided, providing access to the atretic plate. An attempt is made to maintain mucosal flaps on both sides of the atretic plate. The atretic plate, posterior vomer, and medial aspect of the posterior maxilla are removed with a microdebrider, diamond bur, otologic curette, or rongeur (Figure 8). After removal of bone, mucosal flaps are transposed to cover the superior and inner surfaces of the choana, with stents placed as previously described. The palatal flap is reapproximated anteriorly with absorbable sutures. If stenosis occurs after surgical repair, patients generally slowly develop progressive respiratory difficulties. Revision surgery or dilatation may be necessary.

CONGENITAL DISORDERS OF THE NASOPHARYNX AND OROPHARYNX

Tornwaldt Cyst and Rathke Pouch Cyst

If the pharyngeal segments of the primitive notochord remain connected to the endoderm in the nasopharynx, a bursa or embryonic pouch occurs. In approximately 3% of individuals, this invaginated connection persists, and the resulting sac and canal, located in the posterior midline of the nasopharynx, extends posteriorally and cephalad toward the occipital bone. If the bursa is occluded by inflammation, a cyst will develop, and if the cyst becomes infected, an abscess will result. Anterior to the invagination and above the bursa is a small pharyngeal hypophysis developed from Rathke pouch, which sometimes persists as the craniopharyngeal canal running from the sella turcica through the body of the sphenoid.

Most Tornwaldt cysts appear clinically in the second and third decades of life, with males and females affected equally. Symptoms include intermittent or persistent postnasal discharge of tenacious mucus or purulent material, associated with odynophagia, halitosis, unpleasant taste, and occcasionally, a dull occipital headache exacerbated by head movement with associated stiffness of the posterior cervical muscles. Nasopharyngoscopy reveals a smooth, submucosal, 1 to 2 cm midline cystic mass, superior to the adenoidal pad. Frequently, a central dimple or fistula is identified. CT scan demonstrates a soft tissue mass located high on the posterior nasopharyngeal wall with sharp borders. MR studies of the nasopharynx reveal high signal intensity on T-1 weighted, T-2 weighted, and fluid attenuated inversion recovery image (FLAIR).

Microscopically, Tornwaldt cyst is lined by respiratory epithelium with minimal amounts of lymphoid tissue in the wall. Treatment requires either excision to the periosteum or wide marsupialization.

Rathke pouch cysts, on the other hand, are basically cysts lined by columnar or cuboidal, ciliated epithelium that may become secondarily infected or rupture intracranially and are most commonly associated with headache followed by galactorrhea, visual field loss, and hypopituitarism. Treatment is transsphenoidal drainage of the cyst with complete removal of the cyst wall. If no demarcation between normal and involved tissue is evident at operation, the cyst and residual pituitary are radically removed.[21] Radiation therapy is not indicated.

Chordomas

Chordomas are rare malignant neoplasms arising from primitive notochordal remnants, primarily in the fifth or sixth decade of life. Fifty percent occur in the spheno-occipital area with a mean patient age of 40 to 45 years. Males and females are approximately equally affected. Presenting signs and symptoms include an expanding nasopharyngeal mass, frontal headaches, cranial nerve palsies (sixth nerve involvement is seen in 60% of patients followed equally by ninth and tenth nerve involvement), and pituitary abnormalities.

Children under 5 years of age have a wider range of presenting symptoms, a greater prevalence of atypical histological findings with aggressive behavior and a higher incidence of metastases to lung and lymph nodes. A chondroid component (23%) has been identified in a series of children and adolescents. MR imaging with gadolinium is essential to evaluate the extent of the tumor, and it may be helpful in distinguishing classic chordoma from the chondroid variant. CT scanning frequently reveals extensive bone destruction at the skull base and is used to plan surgical resectability. Because patients with chordomas are rarely cured by surgery alone or combined with conventional radiation therapy, surgical resection via a skull base approach is combined with postoperative radiation therapy or proton–photon particle beam treatment. Particle beam therapy is beneficial for chordomas characterized by poor radiosensitivity and cortical location. Interestingly, skull base chordomas in children and adolescents treated with proton beam radiation have better survival than chordomas in adults.[22] The overall prognosis is directly related to the histologic pattern of the tumor: atypical and poorly differentiated chordomas carry a poor prognosis. There appears to be no significant difference for prognosis in patients older than 5 years of age with a classic or chondroid tumor. At a molecular level, alterations in adhesion proteins have been shown to participate in proliferation, invasiveness, and metastasis in epithelial tumors such as chordomas. Changes in the relative expression of the epithelial cadherin–catenin adhesion protein complex reflect chordoma aggressiveness: decreased expression of E-cadherin and increased expression of N-cadherin may underlie the transition from a less to more aggressive tumor phenotype.[23] For metastatic chordoma multiagent, systemic chemotherapy with intrathecal or intraventricular hydrocortisone, cytosine arabinoside (Ara-C) and methotrexate has been effective in controlling central nervous system disease due to chordoma.

Craniopharyngioma

Craniopharyngiomas arise from Rathke pouch epithelial remnants and are located in the sellar, parasellar and third ventricular regions. They are composed of well-differentiated epithelial elements including bone, cysts, and ameloblasts. Rarely, this lesion is first seen in the nasopharynx; and, most commonly, it occurs intracranially above the sella turcica. It accounts for approximately 10 to 15% of all childhood and adolescent intracranial neoplasms. Clinical manifestations include visual field defects, sudden blindness, extraocular motor paralysis, and hypopituitarism. The median age at presentation in children is 7.5 years, with an approximately equal female-to-male ratio. MR imaging with gadolinium or gadodiamide injection is mandatory for pretreatment assessment. Management of craniopharyngiomas has been controversial with two main surgical approaches advocated: macroscopic complete excision or a conservative subtotal resection.[24] Surgical resection followed by radiation therapy achieves long-term control with low morbidity for tumors smaller than 5 cm. 10-year actuarial overall survival rates are 90%. Despite major microsurgical advances, however, total removal of these tumors is associated with a high risk of visual and endocrinological complications, obesity, sleep disorders and behavioral dysfunction. Transsphenoidal removal of those craniopharynoingiomas located within an enlarged sella that are not adherent to parasella structures have a lower incidence of recurrence. The use of megavoltage linear accelerators and stereotactic radiosurgery (SRS), three-dimensional conformational radiation treatment (3D CRT), stereotactic radiotherapy (SRT) and intensity modulated radiation therapy (IMRT) should reduce complications and improve cure rates.[25]

Teratomas

Teratomas are true neoplasms that contain tissues foreign to the site in which they arise. The haphazard arrangement of tissue with asynchronous maturation is believed to escape the controlling influence of the primitive streak notochord or adjacent structures. Teratomas grow aggressively; and, in the head and neck, they most commonly occur in the cervical area, followed by the nasopharynx. Nasopharyngeal teratomas occur with a female-to-male ratio of 6:1. Overall, teratomas of the head and neck comprise approximately 2 to 9% of all teratomas. Teratomas of the nasopharynx typically arise on the lateral or superior wall. Four basic types are recognized: (1) dermoid cyst, the most common form, composed of ectoderm and mesoderm arising as an epithelial-lined cavity with variable numbers of skin appendages; (2) teratoid cyst, derived from all three germ layers but poorly differentiated; (3) true teratoma, composed of ectoderm, mesoderm, and endoderm, with specific tissue and organ differentiation; and (4) epignathus, in which well-developed fetal parts are recognizable; this type of teratoma arises from the soft or hard palate and is frequently incompatible with life.

Clinically, dermoids are more common than true teratomas, and in the nasopharynx, the dermoid cyst is the most common developmental anomaly found. Known as "hairy polyps," these lesions appear at birth as a pedunculated mass filling the nasopharynx, often with oropharyngeal extension. Patients with teratomas have nasal obstruction, dysphagia, and copious secretions. Infants with nasopharyngeal teratomas have a higher incidence of preterm birth, neonatal airway distress, and associated congenital anomalies along with polyhydramnios than do infants with dermoids. CT and MR imaging is critical to define the extent of the neoplasm and to exclude either a nasoencephalomeningocele or intracranial extension of a sphenoid-based teratoma through the craniopharyngeal canal. Most cervical teratomas occurring in the neonate are benign. The tumor can surround or encroach on the airway, thereby causing progressive dysphagia and airway obstruction.

Surgical removal must be carefully planned to ensure a controlled airway throughout the intraoperative and postoperative periods. Tracheostomy is generally not necessary if orotracheal intubation is combined with a transoral removal of pedunculated nasopharyngeal teratomas or with early excision of cervical teratomas. Operative and postoperative bleeding in patients with nasopharyngeal teratomas is usually only slight because these tumors are poorly vascularized; and, if removal is complete, recurrences are rare. Most sessile tumors arising in the nasopharynx require a transpalatal approach. Malignant metastasizing cervical teratoma is extremely rare. Epignathi, arising from the palate or pharynx that protrude from the mouth, result in life-threatening airway obstruction and commonly cause asphyxia at birth. Antenatal ultrasound diagnosis in these rare cases allows for preparation for an ex-utero intrapartum treatment (EXIT) procedure: intrapartum tracheostomy of the fetus at term while still connected to the placenta and subsequent debulking of the large extraoral portion of the tumor followed by complete intraoral resection.[26]

CONGENITAL DISORDERS OF THE ORAL CAVITY AND LIP

Numerous congenital defects of the oral cavity and related structures may occur. Common major anomalies, such as cleft lip and palate, are described in detail, whereas less common deformities are mentioned for completeness.

Congenital lesions of the tongue include aglossia, microglossia, and macroglossia (secondary to lymphangioma, hemangiomas, or as commonly found in Down syndrome). Ankyloglossia due to varying degrees of underdevelopment of the lingual frenulum is not uncommon. Indications for frenuloplasty with a four flap Z-plasty or traditional horizontal-to-vertical repair are notching of the protruding tongue tip, inability to contact the maxillary alveolus with the tongue, or restriction of protrusion of the tongue beyond the mandibular alveolus. Other glossal anomalies include dermoid cysts, hamartomas, lingual thyroid, fissured (scrotal) tongue, median rhomboid "glossitis," and enteric duplication cysts.

Nonodontogenic cysts derived from epithelial remnants trapped in embryonic fusion lines during the developmental stage include midline maxillary cysts (median alveolar, nasal palatal, median palatal) and lateral maxillary cysts (globomaxillary, nasolabial). Nasopalatine duct cysts are the most common cystic lesion of nonodontogenic origin of the maxilla. Treatment varies from marsupialization to enucleation from the palatal side, with or without adjacent teeth. Noncleft lip congenital anomalies encountered include microstomia, congenital pits, and "double lip," the latter which usually involves the upper lip.

Congenital epulis or gingival granular cell tumor arises exclusively from the alveolus and is a rare lesion of unknown origin found in newborn female infants 8 to 10 times more often than males. The tumor usually protrudes from the mouth at birth and may require an EXIT procedure with immediate surgical resection.[27]

Cleft Lip and Palate

Cleft lip and palate are the most common congenital malformations of the head and neck, occurring approximately once in every 700 births. The risk of additional siblings having a defect increases when an older sibling is affected. Both cleft lip with or without cleft palate and isolated cleft palate may be further classified into those classes associated with (syndromic) or without (nonsyndromic) a recognized malformation. The cause of syndromic clefting may be single gene transmission, chromosomal aberrations, teratogenicity, or environmental factors. Recent evidence points to multigenic inheritance with allelic variation at different loci. However, some pedigrees are monogenic with either autosomal dominance or recessive inheritance and exhibit mutations in the *p63* gene.[28] In nonsyndromic clefting, exposure to teratogens such as ethanol, retinoids, or folate antagonists during the first trimester are associated with an increased risk of cleft lip or cleft palate. In addition, a dose response relationship between maternal smoking and an increased risk of having a child with cleft lip or cleft palate has been demonstrated. Associated head and neck anomalies such as maxillary or malar hypoplasia, abnormal pinnae or atresia, facial nerve paresis or paralysis, and mandibular dysmorphism or

abnormal excursion may be identified in syndromic clefting. The etiology of nonsyndromic clefting is extremely complex and is associated with no obvious first or second arch anomalies or systemic organ malformation. Multifactorial inheritance is the cause of these clefts, and calculated risk rates are essential to provide genetic counseling to families. It has been shown that polymorphic variants of genes encoding key proteins of folate and methionine metabolism significantly increase the risk of nonsyndromic cleft lip with or without cleft palate.[29] However, to date, causal mutations with a specific functional effect have not yet been identified.

Anatomy. The lips are a movable muscular sphincter composed primarily of orbicularis oris muscle with motor supply from the seventh cranial nerve. The lips are covered by skin on the outer surface and mucosa on the inner. The vermillion or lip edge forms a junction with the skin (white line) that creates a gentle arching in the upper lip or "Cupid's bow." The cephalic extension from the handle of the Cupid's bow encloses a small depressed area at the base of the columella called the philtrum. These anatomic landmarks plus the protrusion of the vermillion below Cupid's bow or the tubercle are used for orientation in cleft lip repair.

The palate is composed of a hard anterior portion and a soft muscular posterior portion. The anterior primary palate is formed by the alveolar ridge and four incisor teeth plus the triangular premaxilla. The remaining hard palate is formed by the palatine processes of the maxillary and palatine bones, which, with the soft palate, comprise the secondary palate. The soft palate is a muscular curtain formed by the tensor veli palatini muscle innervated by the fifth cranial nerve and the levator veli palatini muscle, musculae uvulae, and glossopalatine and palatopharyngeus muscles innervated by the pharyngeal plexus.

Embryogenesis. Clefts of the lip, alveolus, or palate are midfacial soft tissue and skeletal fusion abnormalities. In the normally developing fetus, the median nasal process fuses with the maxillary processes to form the upper lip, the premaxilla, and the corresponding segments of the alveolar process. Together, the premaxilla and the alveolus form the primary palate. The palatal processes fuse with each other to form the secondary palate, along with the nasal septum and premaxilla in the vicinity of the incisive foramen between gestational weeks 8 and 10. Palatal growth proceeds posteriorly toward the uvula. Failure of ingrowth of mesodermal tissue at this point results in a lack of cohesion of the palatal segments, causing a cleft palate, which may be seen in conjunction with clefts of the lip or alveolar process or alone. Interruption in the migration of mesodermal tissue during the first 2 months of embryonic life results in cleft lip deformities. Ultimately, a lack of fusion of the median nasal processes with the maxillary processes causes a cleft of the upper lip, premaxilla, and alveolus. The incidence of cleft palate increases in the presence of a cleft lip, which occurs in an earlier stage than cleft pal-

ate. Moreover, the tongue is positioned higher in the oral cavity in cleft lip, further interfering with palatal fusion and leading to greater palatal clefting. Recent studies of craniofacial development in animal models have identified components of several major signaling pathways that are critical for proper midfacial development or lip fusion. It also appears that these signaling pathways cross-regulate genetically and cross talk intracellularly to control cell proliferation and tissue patterning.[30]

Management. The head and neck surgeon is part of a cleft palate or craniofacial team that includes pediatrics, ophthalmology, general plastic surgery, neurosurgery, audiology, speech and language pathology, orthodontics, prosthodontics, oral surgery, genetics, dentistry, cytology, psychiatry, social work, and nursing. The goals of this team are to restore normal anatomy and physiology, with an emphasis on muscular reconstruction of the lip and palate to allow normal facial development and to minimize growth disturbance.

The initial priority for infants with clefts is to establish adequate feeding and nutrition. Infants with a unilateral or bilateral cleft lip and alveolus feed generally well by either breast or bottle. Infants with bilateral cleft lip, alveolus, and palate have significant feeding problems and require modified nipples, with feeding in the upright position to minimize nasal regurgitation.

Although the timing of surgical repair is controversial, most experts perform cleft lip repair at 3 months of life and cleft palate repair at 12 months, to establish a competence velopharyngeal sphincter. Two schools of thought have evolved: one, advocating early closure of the lip and palate, a procedure imparting a high priority to early speech development; and the other, recommending delayed closure of the hard palate, thus according a high priority to maxillary growth. Surgical treatment is dictated by the anatomic defect, and a classification scheme is helpful in planning surgical repair: (1) cleft lip, unilateral or bilateral; (2) cleft palate, either with unilateral or bilateral cleft lip; and (3) isolated cleft palate.

Unilateral Cleft Lip. In the basic complete defect, the floor of the nose communicates with the oral cavity, and the alveolar defect passes through the developing dentition. One sees significant nasal deformity, including columellar displacement, nasal dome deformity, and alar flattening and retrodisplacement. The goals of surgical repair are restoration of orbicularis muscle function, alar base, and columellar height and creation of symmetry of philtral columns, tip height, Cupid's bow, and vermillion. This can be accomplished with a Millard rotation advancement procedure in concert with either preoperative orthodontic appliances or lip adhesion.

Bilateral Cleft Lip. The floor of the nose is absent bilaterally, and the nasal and oral cavities communicate freely. The central alveolar arch is displaced forward and superiorly, whereas the nasal tip is widened and the columella is short.

The goals of bilateral cleft lip repair are the same as for unilateral defects. Bilateral lip adhesion, if indicated is performed when the child is 2 to 4 weeks old, with definitive lip repair followed at 4 to 6 months of age. If no lip adhesion is necessary to align the underlying maxillary segments before definitive lip repair, bilateral lip repair is performed at 3 months.

Cleft Palate. The basic defect, absence of the nasal floor, may be complete or incomplete, with or without associated cleft lip. The goals of cleft palate repair are to close the defect without inhibiting maxillary arch growth, to achieve adequate velopharyngeal function, and to normalize oronasal resonance and speech patterns. Although the exact timing of the repair is controversial, the procedure is performed when the patient is 10 to 18 months old, and may require preoperative orthopedic devices used as an alternative to move the premaxilla posteriorly and to expand the lateral maxillary segments, facilitating surgical closure of the lip. Of the many techniques described for bilateral cleft palate repair, the two-flap palatoplasty by Bardach is commonly employed: (1) complete two-layer closure (oral and nasal sides); and (2) dissection, redirection, and suturing of the soft palatal musculature.

Secondary problems of cleft lip and palate that require subsequent treatment include correction of nasal airway impairment, cosmetic nasal defects, velopharyngeal insufficiency with associated hypernasality, and recurrent acute and chronic otitis media with effusion.

Pierre Robin Sequence

The patients with the Pierre Robin sequence (PRS) are a subgroup of the cleft palate population; and, as with the etiology of cleft lip and palate, the etiology of PRS is unknown. Candidate genes and their loci are on chromosomes 2, 11, and 17.[31] The classic PRS of glossoptosis, micrognathia, and cleft palate (50% of cases) may occur as an isolated, nonsyndromic congenital disorder or as part of a larger syndromic anomaly that may include facial dysmorphism, cardiac defects, mental retardation, and musculoskeletal anomalies. Möbius syndrome or nonprogressive congenital facial diplegia is such an example of PRS, with concomitant brachial and thoracic muscle aplasia along with cranial neuropathies (six and seven). PRS has no sex predilection, and it may be secondary to an intrauterine insult during the fourth month of gestation or due to polygenic mutations. Syndromic PRS is often associated with ocular anomalies (detached retina or glaucoma) or aural abnormalities (chronic otitis media, ossicular deformities, and low-set pinnae which can be traced to defects of the first and second branchial arches). The most frequent diagnoses in patients with syndromic PRS are Stickler syndrome and velocardiofacial syndrome. Ophthalmologic assessment and fluorescent in situ hybridization of chromosome 22 should be performed in all patients with PRS.[32] Heredity also appears to be a factor in isolated nonsyndromic PRS and usually

a complete U-shaped cleft palate is the primary determinator of the associated triad.

Infants with PRS are at increased risk of airway obstruction and resulting hypoxemia, cor pulmonale, failure to thrive, and cerebral anoxia. Obstructive sleep apnea and snoring are common. Aspiration is a primary cause of death. Aerophagia associated with vomiting frequently results in aspiration. When compared with normal infants, infants with PRS exhibit a shorter tongue and mandibular length, with a narrow airway and a posteroinferior position of the hyoid bone resulting in airway compromise. Patients are initially given a trial of prone positional management with high-calorie gavage feeding. Most infants (~70%) are effectively managed in this fashion. When continued respiratory distress and failure to thrive develop, a modified glossopexy, attaching the tongue at the mandibular alveolus and the lower lip, is performed. The genioglossus is also released to lengthen the tongue. Bedside polysomnography may help to identify those infants without clinically severe airway obstruction who may benefit from a modified tongue–lip adhesion. Tracheostomy is reserved for those patients following tongue–lip adhesion who have continued failure to thrive and respiratory embarrassment. Alternatively, early bilateral mandibular distraction osteoneogenesis is employed for failures of tongue–lip adhesion in which isolated tongue base obstruction is documented. This approach may also be used to avoid tracheostomy or allow earlier decannulation in severely affected infants.[33] Overall, patients with syndromic PRS have a higher rate of tracheostomy and gastrostomy tube placement and exhibit significantly lower Apgar scores and longer hospital stays.

CONGENITAL DISORDERS OF THE SALIVARY GLANDS

Congenital anomalies of the salivary glands are uncommon. Rarely, bilateral ageneses of the parotid glands in association with first and second branchial arch syndromes occur and are associated with severe xerostomia. Congenital sialoadenitis with cystic dilatation of the salivary ducts can occur, resulting in single or multiple cystic spaces. Sialography in the infant under sedation may help to demonstrate ductal ectasia. If obstruction and stasis develop, recurrent infections may result, necessitating parotidectomy with seventh nerve preservation. Heterotopic salivary gland tissue (HSGT) may also appear in or adjacent to the salivary glands, developing from a defect in the growth of the ductal system or in relation to first branchial cleft anomalies. Usually these congenital lesions present as a discharging sinus in the base of the neck. Embryogenesis of HSGT is probably related to ectodermal heteroplasia of the precervical sinus of His.[34]

First Branchial Cleft Anomalies

Altered embryogenesis of the first branchial cleft potentially produces a wide array of anomalies

affecting the external auditory canal. Maldevelopment results in either absence of a normally patent external auditory canal (atresia or stenosis) or a duplication anomaly (cyst, sinus, or fistula). First branchial cleft anomalies have been classified into two groups: type 1 and type 2. Type 1 anomalies are first cleft ectodermal defects or duplication anomalies of the membranous external auditory canal. Type 1 cysts are found anterior and inferior to the pinnae in association with the parotid gland. The fistulous tract extends superiorly along the facial nerve and parallel to the external auditory canal, where it terminates. Type 2 branchial cysts are primarily first cleft and arch defects (ectodermal and mesoderm) with duplication of the external canal and pinnae. Type 2 cysts are found below the angle of the mandible along the sternocleidomastoid muscle. The fistulous tract, like in type 1 anomalies, is variable and may run lateral to, medial to, or between the main branches of the facial nerve, ultimately ending in the external auditory canal.

Clinically, first branchial cleft cysts are associated with repeated infection and may require incision and drainage of an apparent neck abscess which is typically located above a horizontal plane passing through the hyoid bone. Occasionally, purulent otorrhea may occur in the absence of demonstrable middle ear disease. A third common clinical presentation is preauricular swelling in the parotid area. Microscopically, the cyst is lined with hair follicles, apocrine or sweat glands, and sebaceous glands. Treatment is surgical excision of the cyst, sinus tract, and skin surrounding the sinus tract orifice. Because of the intimate relationship between the seventh nerve and the sinus tract, it is critical to expose the seventh nerve as in a parotidectomy, using the bony landmarks (styloid process, mastoid tip, and tympanomastoid suture line) to help identify the nerve, instead of the tragal pointer. A nerve integrity monitoring system is essential in these difficult cases because of the variable relationship of the sinus tract to the facial nerve.[35] Hemangiomas and lymphangiomas are congenital lesions that may involve the salivary glands and are discussed earlier in this chapter.

PRIMARY CILIARY DYSKINESIA (KARTAGENER SYNDROME)

Primary ciliary dyskinesia (PCD) is primarily an antosomal recessive disease with extensive genetic heterogeneity characterized by recurrent upper and lower respiratory tract infections secondary to dyskinetic or completely absent ciliary motility. Only rarely other modes of inheritance such as x-linked transmission are observed.[36] Also termed immotile cilia syndrome, its most recognizable form is in Kartagener syndrome which occurs in 50% of patients with PCD and exhibits bronchiectasis, chronic sinusitis, situs inversus, and sterility. It has also been recognized in Usher syndrome type I, congenital heart disease, congenital esophageal dysfunction, and cutaneous abnormalities including folliculitis, nummular eczema, and pyoderma gangrenosum.

This disorder is characterized by defects in human axonemal dynein complexes in respiratory cilia, sperm tails and, cilia of the embryonic primitive or Hensen node. Currently three genes (*DNAI1, DNAH5, DNAH11*) that encode dynein proteins (cytoplasmic heavy chains from the outer arms of the axonemes) have been linked to recessive PCD. Dyneins are large multi–subunit ATPases that interact with microtubules in cilia to generate force. The resulting ultrastructural defect causes impaired mucociliary clearance throughout the pulmonary and sinonasal passages. Headache, a common complaint in PCD patients, has been associated with absence of cilia lining the brain ventricles, leading to decreased circulation of cerebrospinal fluid. As a screening test, nasal nitric oxide measurement (patients with PD have low levels of nasal nitric oxide), is widely used while transmission electron microscopy is the most commonly employed diagnostic tool for confirmation of this disorder.[37] Early recognition and treatment, with rigorous lung physiotherapy, prophylactic and microorganism-specific antibiotics and immunization against common pulmonary pathogens, could lead to reduction in irreversible sinus and pulmonary complications with improved survival.

REFERENCES

1. Depew MJ, Simpson CA, Morasso M, Rubenstein JL. Reassessing the Dlx code: The genetic regulation of branchial arch skeletal pattern and development. J Anat 2005;207:501–61.
2. Byrd NA, Meyers EN. Loss of Gbx2 results in neural crest cell patterning and pharyngeal arch artery defects in the mouse embryo. Dev Biol 2005;284:233–45.
3. Jereczek-Fossa BA, Casadio C, Jassem J, et al. Branchiogenic carcinoma-conceptual or true clinico-pathological entity? Cancer Treat Rev 2005;31:106–14.
4. Katori H, Nozawa A, Tsukuda M. Postoperative adjuvant chemoradiotherapy with carboplatin and 5-fluorouracil for primary branchiogenic carcinoma. J Laryngol Otol 2005;119:467–9.
5. Meyer S, Gottschling S, Schneider G, et al. Two infants with life-threatening diffuse neonatal hemangiomatosis treated with cyclophosphamide. Pediatr Blood Cancer 2006;46:239–42.
6. Kim KH, Sung MW, Roh JL, Han MH. Sclerotherapy for congenital lesions in the head and neck Otolaryngol Head Neck Surg 2004;131:307–16.
7. Frischer JS, Huang J, Serur A, et al. Biomolecular markers and involution of hemangiomas. J Pediatr Surg 2004;39:400–4.
8. Lanzafame S, Caltabiano R, Puzzo L, Cappellani A. Thyroid transcription factor 1 (TTF-1) and p63 expression in two primary thyroid papillary carcinomas of branchial cleft cysts. Virchows Arch 2006;449:129–33.
9. Danner C, Bodenner D, Breau R. Lingual thyroid: Iodine 131: A viable treatment modality revisited. Am J Otolaryngol 2001;22:276–81.
10. Kaselas Ch, Tsikopoulos G, Chortis Ch, Kaselas B. Thyroglossal duct cyst's inflammation. When do we operate? Pediatr Surg Int 2005;21:991–3.
11. Plaza CP, Lopez ME, Carrasco CE, et al. Management of well-differentiated thyroglossal remnant thyroid carcinoma: Time to close the debate? Report of five new cases and proposal of a definitive algorithm for treatment. Ann Surg Oncol 2006;13:745–52.
12. Khariwala SS, Nicollas R, Triglia JM, et al. Cervical presentations of thymic anomalies in children. Int J Pediatr Otorhinolaryngol 2004;68:909–14.
13. Nguyen Q de Tar M, Wells W, Crockett D. cervical thymis cyst: Case reports and review of the literature. Laryngoscope 1996;106:247–52.
14. Oguzkan S, Terzi YK, Cinbis M, et al. Molecular genetic analyses in neurofibromatosis type 1 patients with tumors. Cancer Genet Cytogenet 2006;165:167–71.
15. Hanikeri M, Waterhouse N, Kirkpatrick N, et al. The management of midline transcranial nasal dermoid sinus cysts. Br J Plast Surg 2005;58:1043–50.
16. Dhooge I, Lemmerling M, Lagache M, et al. Otological manifestations of CHARGE association. Ann Otol Rhinol Laryngol 1998;107:935–41.
17. Jongmans MC, Admiraal RJ, van der Donk KP, et al. CHARGE syndrome: The phenotypic spectrum of mutations in the CHD7 gene. J Med Genet 2006;43:306–14.
18. Kubba H, Bennett A, Bailey CM. An update on choanal atresia surgery at Great Ormond Street Hospital for Children: Preliminary results with mitomycin C and the KTP laser. Int J Pediatr Otorhinolaryngol 2004;68:939–45.
19. Park AH, Brockenbrough J, Stankiewicz J. Endoscopic versus traditional approaches to choanal atresia. Otolaryngol Clin North Am 2000;33:77–90.
20. Schraff SA, Vijayasekaran S, Meinzen-Derr J, Myer CM. Management of choanal atresia in CHARGE association patients: A retrospective review. Int J Pediatr Otorhinolaryngol 2006;70:1291–7.
21. Alfieri A, Schettino R, Tarfani A, et al. Endoscopic endonasal removal of an intra-supraseller Rathke's cleft cyst: Case report and surgical considerations. Minim Invasive Neurosurg 2002;45:47–51.
22. Hoch BL, Nielsen GP, Liebsch NJ, Rosenberg AE. Base of skull chordomas in children and adolescents: A clinicopathologic study of 73 cases. Am J Surg Pathol 2006;30:811–8.
23. Triana A, Sen C, Wolfe D, Hazan R. Cadherins and catenins in clival chordomas: Correlation of expression with tumor aggressiveness. Am J Surg Pathol 2005;29:1422–34.
24. Franzone P, Berretta L, Barra S. Review of the role of radiotherapy in craniopharyngiomas: How does patient age influence management decisions? J Pediatr Endocrinol Metab 2006;19:395–7.
25. Kalapurakal JA. Radiation therapy in the management of pediatric craniopharyngiomas—A review. Childs Nerv Syst 2005;21:808–16.
26. Izadi K, Smith M, Askari M, et al. A patient with an epignathus: Management of a large oropharyngeal teratoma in a newborn. J Craniofac Surg 2003;14:468–72.
27. Kumar P, Kim HH, Zahtz GD, et al, Obstructive congenital epulis: Prenatal diagnosis and perinatal management. Laryngoscope 2002;112:1935–9.
28. Leoyklang P, Siriwan P, Shotelersuk V. A mutation of the p63 gene in nonsyndromic cleft lip. J Med Genet 2006;43:e28.
29. Mostowska A, Hozyasz KK, Jagodzinski PP. Maternal MTR genotype contributes to the risk of nonsyndromic cleft lip and palate in the Polish population. Clin Genet 2006;69:512–7.
30. Jiang R, Bush JO, Lidral AC. Development of the upper lip: Morphogenetic and molecular mechanisms. Dev Dyn 2006;235:1152–66.
31. Jakobsen LP, Knudsen MA, Lespinasse J, et al. The genetic basis of the Pierre Robin sequence. Cleft Palate Craniofac J 2006;43:155–9.
32. van den Elzen AP, Semmekrot BA, Bongers EM, et al. Diagnosis and treatment of the Pierre Robin sequence: Results of a retrospective clinical study and review of the literature. Eur J Pediatr 2001;160:47–53.
33. Schaefer RB, Stadler JA, III, Gosain AK. To distract or not to distract: An algorithm for airway management in isolated Pierre Robin sequence. Plast Reconstr Surg 2004;113:1113–25.
34. Chang WY, Lee KW, Tsai KB, Chen GS. Heterotopic salivary gland tissue: A case report demonstrating evolution and association with the branchial apparatus. J Dermatol 2005;32:731–6.
35. Solares CA, Chan J, Koltai PJ. Anatomical variations of the facial nerve in first branchial cleft anomalies. Arch Otolaryngol Head Neck Surg 2003;129:351–5.
36. Van's Gravesande KS, Omran H. Primary ciliary dyskinesia: Clinical presentation, diagnosis, and genetics. Ann Med 2005;37:439–49.
37. Roomans GM, Ivanovs A, Shebani EB, Johannesson M. Transmission electron microscopy in the diagnosis of primary ciliary dyskinesia. Ups J Med Sci 2006;111:155–68.

SUGGESTED READINGS

Bloom DC, Perkins JA, Manning SC. Management of lymphatic malformations. Curr Opin Otolaryngol Head Neck Surg 2004;12:500–4.
The advances in the understanding of the etiology, diagnosis, and treatment of lymphatic malformations of the head and neck are reviewed.

Foley DS, Fallat ME. Thyroglossal duct and other congenital midline cervical anomalies. Semin Pediatr Surg 2006;15:70–5.
This discussion provides an overview of the embryology, pathophysiology, and diagnostic tests for congenital midline cervical anomalies.

Donald PJ. Vascular anomalies of the head and neck. Facial Plast Surg Clin North Am 2001;9:77–92.
This paper by an experienced head and neck surgeon presents treatment strategies based upon the pathogenesis and natural history of hemangiomas and vascular malformations of the head and neck.

Mandell DL. Head and neck anomalies related to the branchial apparatus. Otolaryngol Clin North Am 2000;33:1309–32.
A comprehensive review of the branchial apparatus serves as the basis for greater precision in clinical diagnosis and management of branchial arch anomalies.

Manning SC, et al. Diagnostic and surgical challenges in the pediatric skull base. Otolaryngol Clin North Am 2005;38:773–94.
This review paper covers advances in the diagnosis and surgical management of pediatric skull base lesions with an emphasis on improvements in skull base approaches.

Merritt L. Part 1. Understanding the embryology and genetics of cleft lip and palate. Adv Neonatal Care 2005;5:64–71.

Merritt L. Part 2. Physical assessment of the infant with cleft lip and/or palate. Adv Neonatal Care 2005;5:125–34.
As a two-part paper, this presentation focuses on the embryology and genetics of cleft lip and palate, and the systematic physical assessment of these infants with the most commonly occurring craniofacial birth defects.

71

Biofilms and Their Role in Ear and Respiratory Infections

J. Christopher Post, MD, PhD

Garth D. Ehrlich, PhD

To my great surprize perceived that the aforesaid matter [plaque] contained very many small living Animals, which moved themselves very extravagantly.
—Antony van Leeuwenhoek, 1684, writing to the *Royal Society of London* (Plaque is now known to be a complex multispecies bacterial biofilm)

WHAT IS A BIOFILM?

Bacterial biofilms are structurally complex, organized, sessile communities of attached bacteria embedded in an extracellular matrix or glycocalyx (Figure 1). The matrix is a dynamic structure that provides stability and protection for the embedded bacteria and is composed of water and a variety of macromolecules, including exopolysaccharides, proteins, and DNA.[1] The extracellular DNA provides much of the viscoelastic properties of the biofilm and is what allows for remodeling during environmental changes. Recent work has demonstrated the presence of extracellular DNA and protein in *Streptococcus pneumoniae* and *Haemophilus influenzae* biofilms.[2,3] Biofilms can form on any surface, either biotic or abiotic; and, shortly after attachment, the bacteria start elaborating the matrix and forming various types of three-dimensional (3-D) structures including mushroom-like towers, dense lawns with streamers that form above the canopy, and variegated surfaces. In some biofilms water channels deliver nutrients and remove waste products via convective flow.[4] Biofilms can be thought of as being analogous to the coral reef, with sessile polyps surrounded by a protective matrix, relatively impervious to environmental dangers. Just as the reef will produce free-swimming medusae, biofilms will release free-swimming (planktonic) bacteria to populate distant habitats.

Biofilms are dynamic systems that are much more analogous to multicellular organisms in terms of physiological sophistication and environmental homeostatic mechanisms than they are to simple accretions of unicellular organisms. Some of the organismal characteristics of biofilms include intercellular communication systems,[5] specialized phenotypes,[6] a primitive circulatory system, and differentiated metabolism.[7] A biofilm is composed of multiple ecosystems, each varying in pH, cellular density, and oxygen tension, with the base of the biofilm generally anoxic. These ecosystems are distinct microenvironments, thus biofilms can be composed of a single species or of multiple species. Biofilms are best thought of as symbiotic microbial communities, where the organisms are not simply clumped together, but rather are involved in a wide array of physical, metabolic, and genetic interactions. The communal nature of a mixed species microbial community is a much more sophisticated view of bacteria than we are accustomed to considering (Table 1).

Why Do Bacteria Form Biofilms?

Biofilm formation provides a multitude of advantages to the bacteria. Biofilms are a protected mode of growth that allows bacteria to survive in otherwise lethal environments and broadens the potential habitat range. The biofilm forms a persistent nidus from which the bacteria can populate new niches. The exchange of genetic material is facilitated in a biofilm, thus increasing the genetic diversity of the individual bacteria and improving their chances for survival. Bacteria in a biofilm are much less vulnerable to host defense systems such as cellular and humoral immune mechanisms and phagocytosis. Of great importance clinically is that bacteria in a biofilm have a markedly enhanced resistance to antimicrobial agents, being able to tolerate levels 10 to 1,000 times higher than the minimum inhibitory concentrations of genetically equivalent planktonic envirovars. Originally thought to be the result of poor penetration of the antibiotic molecules through the matrix, the primary reason for the resistance to antibiotics appears to be the decreased replicative and metabolic rates of bacteria living in a biofilm.[8,9] Bacteria in a

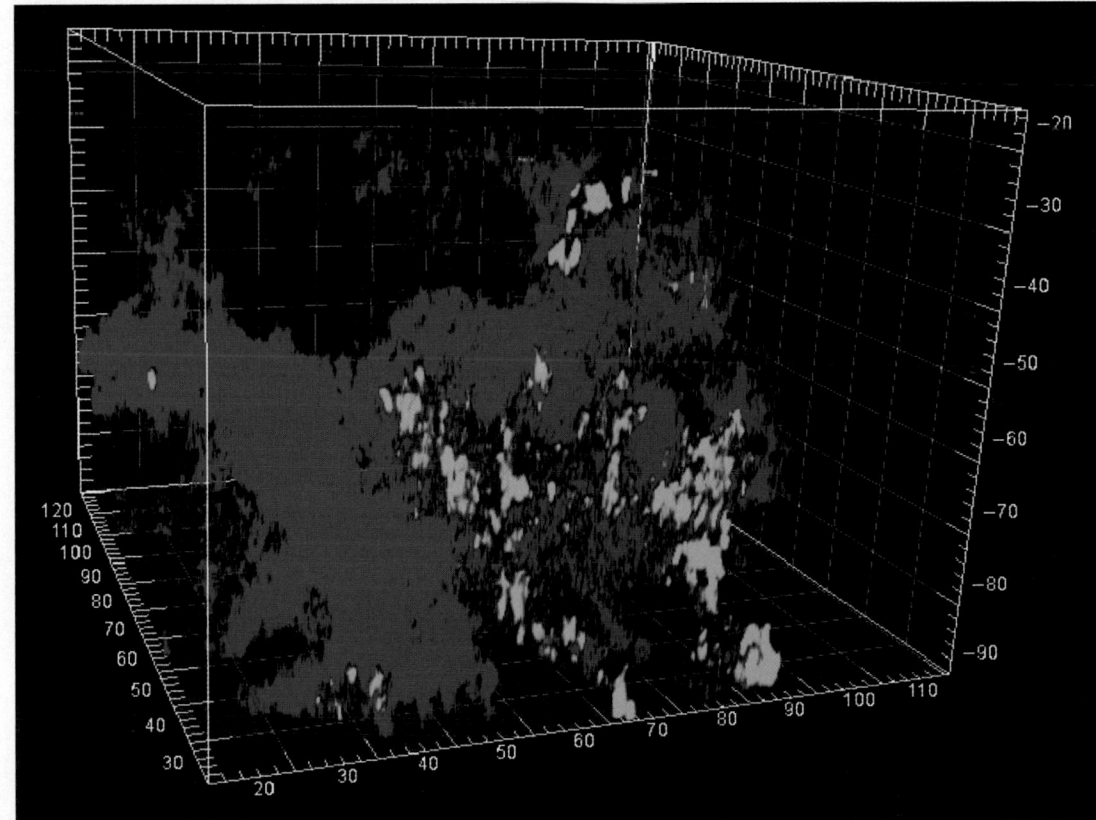

Figure 1 *Streptococcus pneumoniae* (serotype 23) biofilm grown in vitro. The biofilm was imaged by confocal microscopy with reflected light to show the extracellular polymeric substance (EPS) matrix (*blue*) and the BacLight Live/Dead (Invitrogen) kit to show live (*green*) and dead (red bacteria). The cells were viable and had produced voluminous quantities of EPS which anchored the biofilm cells to the glass substratum and to each other. Scale: Major divisions = 10 μm. (Image provided by Paul Stoodley, Laura Nistico, and Luanne Hall-Stoodley.)

Table 1 Properties of Biofilms

Multicellular bacterial communities	Highly resistant to antibiotics
Encased in a slime matrix	Highly resistant to host defenses
Complex intercellular communication systems	Display rapid phenotypic changes in response to environment
Large number of microenvironments	Difficult to culture planktonically
Differentiation of function	Utilize coordinate expression for toxins
Produce periodic planktonic showers	

biofilm have an enhanced opportunity to acquire a resistance phenotype through multiple mechanisms of genetic exchange, including plasmids; however, the phenomenon of antibiotic resistance due to the biofilm phenotype should be distinguished from the antibiotic resistance secondary to genotypic changes.

Planktonic Bacteria Have Held Center Stage for Too Long

We have been accustomed to studying planktonic bacteria, which is a phenotype where unorganized clonal collections of individual bacteria grow in liquid suspension or attached to culture plates in homogeneous colonies. This focus on studying planktonic bacteria has helped our understanding of acute infectious processes but fails to inform regarding chronic bacterial infections. Most of our current antimicrobial strategies have largely been developed to control acute systemic infections caused by planktonic bacteria. The fact that our basic understanding of bacteria has been based upon the study of the planktonic form, a form in which bacteria rarely exist, has provided a biased view of microbes, with profound implications for our understanding of the nature of infectious disease.

The Limitations of Culture

Another hindrance to a modern understanding of bacterial infections is thinking of culture results as a talisman. Our training has been that live bacteria are able to be grown in culture, thus we confuse the inability to grow bacteria from a specimen with proof that viable pathogens are absent. This confusion is particularly noticeable after several days of antibiotic treatment. Further, just because cultures can quantitatively assess the presence of pathogens, it does not mean that all bacteria in the specimen have been enumerated by culture. The ability to grow bacteria in culture is not the sine qua non of bacterial presence. There are at least four circumstances in which living bacteria are not able to be grown in culture: (1) slow-growing bacteria, such as *Mycobacterium tuberculosis*; (2) fastidious bacteria, such as *Treponema pallidum*; (3) bacteria stressed into a dormant viable but nonculturable state; and (4) bacteria in biofilms. Attached bacteria can be difficult to recover, and the bulk of bacteria in a biofilm is slow growing, thus biofilm bacteria are difficult to grow in vitro. Culturing a biofilm would yield only one colony per aggregate rather than one per bacterium; thus, the number of bacteria is often severely underestimated in the best of circumstances.

Biofilm Formation

It is important to understand that biofilms are not simply clusters of planktonic bacteria but are a markedly different phenotype; in fact within a biofilm there is phenotypic heterogeneity due to the plethora of microenvironments. Biofilm formation is an interplay among forces in the external environment such as shear stress and available nutrients and constitutive bacteria working in concert. Biofilm formation is a coordinated series of developmental events that include: (1) microbial attachment to a surface, although healthy biotic surfaces have a formidable array of antiattachment mechanisms, such as biochemical surfactants, epithelial exfoliation, phagocytosis, innate immunity, and other immune responses, thus mucosal surfaces are generally more resistant to biofilm formation than are abiotic surfaces; (2) after attachment, the bacteria begin to divide and form a monolayer some species then aggregate into microcolonies via twitch motility, which is a form of solid surface translocation dependent upon fimbriae or pili, and once the bacterial density is high enough, the bacteria begin producing an enclosing slimy matrix which hinders phagocytosis because of its sheer size; and (3) maturation into an aggregate structure that can be hundreds of cells thick, with intermittent dispersion of planktonic bacteria for formation of distant biofilms.

The bacteria communicate with one another through a series of processes called quorum sensing, which is a mechanism by which bacteria within a population secrete a signaling molecule, which, in a concentration-dependent fashion, serves as a coordinator of population activity.[5] As more bacteria congregate, the concentration of the signaling molecule increases until a "quorum" is sensed. Once the quorum is achieved, a series of "master switches" or sigma factors, up and down regulate specific bacterial genes, resulting in extensive changes in physiology including the coordinated production of toxins and other secreted molecules. Many different bacteria are known to use quorum sensing to control various aspects of their developmental process, including rate of bacterial division, incorporation of foreign DNA, formation and maintenance of biofilm structure, and virulence factors.

The Ancient History of Biofilms

Bacteria have been forming biofilms for over 3.25 billion years; thus, it is an ancient and markedly successful survival strategy and an integral element of the prokaryotic life cycle.[6] In some aquatic environments, biofilms contain over 99.99% of the bacteria present. Biofilms are key factors for surviving environmental hazards such as electromagnetic radiation, mechanical stressors such as shear, temperature fluctuation, and noxious chemical agents. Biofilms have been found in environments as diverse as hot springs in Yellowstone National Park, Antarctica, and subsurface sediments in deep ocean trenches. Evidence of ancient biofilms persists today in the form of stromatolites. Stromatolites are the most ancient macroscopic evidence of life that is our single best view into the emergence of life on earth. These intriguing fossils from "deep time" are laminated accretionary structures that were formed by biofilm bacteria capturing and precipitating particles in ancient seas. Given the primeval nature and survival advantages associated with biofilms, they are considered to be excellent biomarkers in the search for extraterrestrial life.

Industrial Biofilms

Biofilms are a major problem in industry (Table 2) and are commonly found at the interface between liquid and solid and also at air–liquid interfaces. Also known as biofouling, the industrial biofilm can have a broader group of constituents, including bacteria, algae, yeasts, and protozoa, as well as suspended solids and corrosion products. Biofouling can lead to contaminated water or petrochemical products, loss of product quality, formation of sludge, deterioration or physical plugging of pipe work and storage tanks, and degrading of sensors. Biofouling enhances microbial-influenced corrosion (MIC), which is the deterioration of metals, either directly or indirectly, by galvanic activity by microorganisms. A variety of bacteria and fungi comprise the microbial community found in aircraft fuel tanks. These tanks contain jet propellant-8 (JP-8), and the community has the potential to cause corrosion of the aluminum alloy.[10] Biofilms were found in the water lines of the space shuttle Columbia, and it has been recommended that all space station materials be carefully evaluated for possible degradability by biofilms before use.[11] The piping in active nuclear plants can be degraded by MIC, which requires the complete replacement of service water systems. Biofilms have also degraded the stone in ancient Mayan archeological sites in the Yucatan Peninsula of Mexico, as well as the Roman catacombs.[12,13]

Table 2 Industrial Processes and Sectors Affected by Biofilms

Petrochemical	Paper mills
Ships and marine structures	Food and beverage industry
Power generating	Brewery pasteurizers
Aircraft fuel systems	Milk processing plants
Water supply and distribution facilities	Mariculture
Heat exchangers and cooling towers	

BIOFILMS IN HUMAN DISEASE

Bacterial biofilms are now clearly recognized as a major cause of human disease, with the Centers for Disease Control estimating that greater than 60% of bacterial infections in the United States are biofilm related.[14] Understanding the unique aspects of a biofilm provides an explanation for paradoxical symptoms and signs in an ever-expanding list of diseases. Characteristics of a biofilm infection are: (1) a clinical presentation of a chronic infectious process with cycles of acute exacerbation in which antibiotic treatment results in the suppression of infection with remission of symptoms, only to be followed by recurrence, for example, recurrent otitis media, chronic osteomyelitis, and urinary tract infections (*vide infra*); (2) chronic sessile attachment to a surface acting as a nidus refractory to antimicrobial therapy, and if the biofilm is at a solid surface–fluid interface, such as the circulatory system, the gallbladder tract, or cerebrospinal fluid, there can be episodic acute systemic events from planktonic showering that can be controlled with antimicrobial therapy; (3) ineffective host defenses, with collateral tissue damage from "frustrated" phagocytes[7]; (4) Problematic diagnosis due to insufficient culturing or sampling techniques[15]; (5) chronic inflammatory response by the host, with the potential for stone formation; and (6) a milieu for the generation of resistant microorganisms, or a safe haven for bacteria to produce systemically acting substances, for example, endotoxins, exotoxins, enterotoxins, or superantigens.

Biofilms on Medically Related Implants

The concept that bacterial biofilm formation is important in human health is well established in regard to infected medical implants and cuts across all areas of medicine. Devices that have been shown to be subject to biofilm infection include urinary and central venous catheters, pacemakers and artificial heart valves, vascular grafts, sutures and mesh, hemodialysis and peritoneal dialysis catheters, gastrostomy and nasogastric tubes, penile and breast implants, intraocular and contact lenses, orthopedic implants such as joint prosthesis and fixation devices, intrauterine devices, biliary stents, and neurosurgical shunts and stimulators.[7,16] The biofilm paradigm explains the extreme difficulty encountered when attempting to eradicate prosthetic infections with conventional antimicrobial agents. Biofilms not only cause chronic localized infections but are also the nidus of planktonic "showers" that result in distal pathogen spread. The refractory nature of biofilms to conventional antimicrobial treatment now provides a rationale for the clinical dictum that the most effective treatment for line sepsis is to "pull the line," as once a prosthetic device is infected with a biofilm, it generally must be removed or replaced to effect a cure. Biofilms can also form in the dental water lines and channels of endoscopic instruments. These biofilms can be refractory to standard cleaning practices, with the potential of nosocomial infection.

The Role of Biofilms in Causing Human Disease

Among the first researchers to recognize the importance of biofilms in human health were those in the field of oral health; dental caries, gingivitis, periodontal disease, and plaque are caused by biofilms attached to the tooth enamel and the gingival mucosal. After dental diseases, perhaps the best-known non–device-related medical condition involving biofilms is cystic fibrosis (CF). CF pneumonia begins with an *H. influenzae* biofilm which is subsequently replaced by biofilms of the opportunistic pathogen *Pseudomonas aeruginosa* which makes cystic fibrosis refractory to treatment. Biofilm formation is implicated in many other chronic infections including infective endocarditis and cardiac valves, chronic prostatitis, Legionnaires' disease, biliary tract infections and gallstones, and kidney stones.[17,18] A particular problem in orthopedics, biofilm infections, such as chronic wound infections, necrotizing fasciitis and osteomyelitis, can involve either soft tissue or bone. Chronic urinary tract infections (UTIs) are also biofilm-related illnesses. Uropathogenic *Escherichia coli* can invade bladder epithelial cells and mature into biofilms, which create pod-like bulges on the bladder surface.[19] These pods explain the refractory nature of UTIs to antibiotic treatment and provide a reservoir for recurrent infection.

Biofilms in Public Health

Biofilms reside in drinking water distribution systems and are resistant to the effects of chlorine, which readily kills planktonic bacteria and those on the periphery of the biofilm but does not penetrate the depths of the biofilm. One example of this phenomenon occurred in April 1993 when an outbreak of cryptosporidiosis in Milwaukee sickened approximately 400,000 people and left 100 dead, generally those with immune systems weakened from AIDS or cancer. Biofilms growing in sand filters can be used to remove toxic contaminants and biodegradable molecules, a concept known as "biological stability" which is in essence a probiotics approach for drinking water.

Biofilms are important in the lifecycle of *Vibrio cholerae*, which forms biofilms in aquatic ecosystems such as coastal estuaries but appears to leave the biofilm mode once they are ingested. *Legionella pneumophilia* is the microorganism that causes Legionnaires' disease, a potentially lethal pneumonia. *Legionella* readily forms biofilms in cooling water towers, ventilation systems, respiratory care devices, hot tubs, hot water heaters, and fountains, where it can be dispersed as airborne water droplets and aspirated. *Mycobacterium*, including *M. tuberculosis*, the causative agent of tuberculosis, most likely forms biofilms.

Biofilms and Koch Postulates

Koch developed the following four postulates over one century ago to clarify the cause of acute bacterial illnesses.

1. The organism must be found in all animals suffering from the disease but not in healthy animals.
2. The organism must be isolated from a diseased animal and grown in pure culture.
3. The cultured organism should cause disease when introduced into a healthy animal.
4. The organism must be re-isolated from the experimentally infected animal.

While adherence to his postulates and the use of microbiological culture techniques have allowed us to control many acute infectious diseases, it is well recognized that there are exceptions to his rules. These include individuals who are asymptomatic carriers of pathogenic bacteria, individual susceptibility to infection, and polymicrobial infections. While his postulates are still useful, it is clear that the identification of single pathogens in pure culture is inadequate to explain chronic bacterial biofilm infections (Table 3).

Biofilms and Mucosal Disease

Biofilms and the host's reaction to them play a role in many mucosal diseases. Bacteria can play an important role as a barrier to pathogenic bacteria,[20] conversely, diseases of the gut, such as Crohn's disease and ulcerative colitis, may be the result of an aberrant immune response to intestinal bacteria in hosts that are genetically susceptible. While there is no direct proof that bacterial infections cause cancer, there is some suggestion that bacterial biofilms can influence the early stages of colon cancer. Biofilms are certainly known to add to the morbidity of patients with existing malignancies, particularly in the oral cavity. Both aerobic and anaerobic bacteria are found in greater numbers in ulcerated squamous cell carcinomas than on control mucosal, with over a third of neoplasms harboring *Candida* spp.[21]

BIOFILM DISEASES OF OTOLARYNGOLOGIC INTEREST

Biofilms in Otitis Media

The surge of interest in biofilms in otolaryngology grew out of an attempt to reconcile a series of molecular-based observations that conflicted with established dogma in the field of otitis media. While it was well established that acute otitis media (OM) was a bacterial process, chronic OM with effusion (OME) was thought to be a nonbacterial, inflammatory process based on several observations: cultures for the known pathogens of acute OM (*H. influenzae*, *S. pneumoniae*, and *Moraxella catarrhalis*) were only positive in 30 to 40% of OME specimens, and a wealth of inflammatory mediators were found in chronic effusions. Clinically, most antibiotics used achieved in vitro killing concentrations in

Table 3 Outdated Paradigms Regarding Our Understanding of Bacteria

Bacterium are free-living; each bacterium is a solitary organism	Bacteria do not have intercellular communication systems
Viable bacteria can be grown in culture	Sterile by culture is the same as "absence of bacteria"
Viable bacteria are continually dividing	Bacteria must be recovered as purified single isolates
All microorganisms of a population have the same genomic complement	Disease is caused by rapid planktonic growth
Bacterial resistance to antibiotics is genetically determined	

the middle ear, but chronic OME did not readily resolve with antibiotics. While it had long been recognized that bacteria could be identified on gram stain from chronic effusions that did not support microbial culture, this finding had been dismissed as a curiosity.

A series of studies challenged the established paradigm that OME was a nonbacterial process. Post and colleagues used polymerase chain reaction (PCR)-based assays for *H. influenzae*, *S. pneumoniae*, and *M. catarrhalis* and showed that in 97 OME specimens, while only 28 (28.9%) tested positive by both culture and PCR for the three main pathogens, 75 (77.3%) of the specimens were PCR positive for one or more of the three test organisms.[15] Thus, an additional 47 specimens (48%) were PCR positive, but culture negative, for these three bacterial species. In a second study using a reverse transcriptase PCT (RT-PCR) assay specific for *H. influenzae*, Rayner and colleagues showed that bacteria detected by PCR in middle-ear effusions are actively synthesizing mRNA, thus are viable, intact, and metabolically active.[22] Dingman and colleagues showed that the presence of endotoxin in chronic OME effusions was highly correlated with *H. influenzae* and *M. catarrhalis* organisms detected by the PCR, but sterile by culture.[23] These data suggested that the source of endotoxin was most likely bacteria detectable by PCR but undetectable by culture.

Chinchilla experiments demonstrated that raw DNA, and DNA from intact but heat-killed bacteria, does not persist in the middle-ear cleft in the presence of an effusion, but that live bacteria, while not culturable following antibiotic treatment, persist in a viable state for weeks.[24] Scanning electron microscopy (SEM) studies demonstrated that biofilms readily formed on middle-ear mucosa of chinchillas after transbullar inoculation of *H. influenzae* but not in controls, and confocal laser scanning microscopy (CLSM) indicated that the bacteria in the biofilms were viable.[18] In the cyno-mologus monkey model, Pseudomonas otorrhea is associated with biofilm formation.[25]

Most recently, biofilms have been directly detected on the mucosa of children undergoing tympanostomy and tube placement for OME and recurrent OM.[26] Using an array of techniques including cultures, PCR, fluorescence in situ hybridization (FISH), fluorescent immunostaining, and CLSM with bacterial live or dead staining, biofilms were detected in 46 of 50 specimens, while eight controls (from cochlear implant patients) were negative for biofilms. All 24 effusions that were tested by PCR were positive for

at least 1 OM pathogen (*H. influenzae*, *S. pneumoniae*, and *M. catarrhalis*) while only 6 (22%) of 27 effusions were culture positive for any pathogen, again showing the limitations of using culture results to make any definitive statement regarding the bacterial environment of the middle ear. One of the most surprising results of this study is that biofilms can be found in children with recurrent OM during periods of remission, suggesting that bacteria do not clear from the middle-ear space between acute episodes (Figure 2).

While OM results from an interplay of infectious, genetic, and environmental factors, these data, taken together, clearly demonstrate that biofilms are involved in middle-ear disease. Importantly, the biofilm paradigm integrates other observations regarding the pathogenesis of OM, that is, mucosal compromise from antecedent viral infections, the importance of eustachian tube function, and the fact that a variety of inflammatory mediators are present in OME. Inflammatory mediators, however, are not the engine that is driving the disease process but rather the result of a persistent bacterial presence.

The biofilm hypothesis also explains why the most effective treatment for OME is the placement of tympanostomy tubes. Tube placement is effective because: (1) reventilation of the middle-ear space increases the oxygen tension which promotes the regrowth of a ciliated epithelium and reduces the number of secretory cells; (2) it mechanically disrupts and debulks the biofilm; and (3) host middle-ear mucosal defenses are restored. These physiological changes promote biofilm clearance.

Biofilms in Cholesteatoma

A consistent feature of cholesteatoma is the persistence of infection that is highly resistant to antimicrobial agents. Bacterial biofilms have been shown to be present in cholesteatomas, a finding which helps explain the clinical observation that, in this setting, infection can only be eradicated with surgery. Chole and Faddis evaluated the keratin matrix of 24 human and 22 gerbiline cholesteatomas for evidence of biofilms using light and transmission electron microscopy.[27] They found regions with both gram-positive and gram-negative bacteria with the

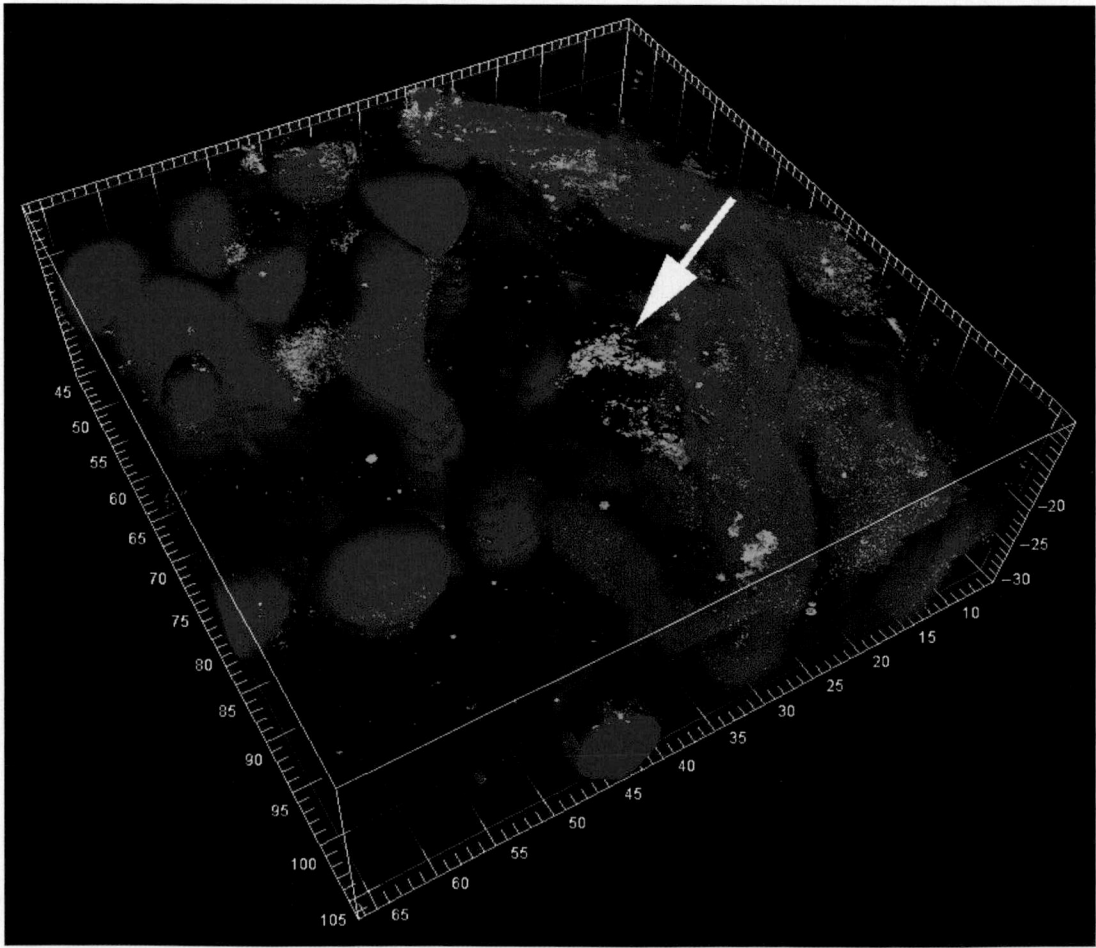

Figure 2 Biofilm bacteria (*green*) attached to the surface of a middle-ear mucosa of a patient diagnosed with recurrent otitis media. The BacLight Live/Dead kit (Invitrogen) showed that the bacteria were alive by the green staining. The nuclei of the host cells and fibrous tissue stained red with propidium iodide. Scale: Major divisions = 5 μm. (Image provided by Paul Stoodley, Laura Nistico, and Luanne Hall-Stoodley.)

characteristic ultrastructural appearance of biofilms in 16 of the 24 human specimens, and 21 of the 22 gerbil specimens.[27] The same laboratory demonstrated that strains of *P. aeruginosa* isolated from cholesteatoma are strongly adherent to keratinocytes, express quorum-sensing genes, and form biofilms in vitro, suggesting that these bacteria can contribute to biofilm formation in cholesteatoma.[28]

Biofilms in Adenoiditis

Biofilm formation is markedly increased on the mucosal surface area of adenoids removed from children with chronic rhinosinusitis when compared to adenoids removed from children with obstructive sleep apnea (OSA).[29] Using SEM, adenoids from patients with chronic rhinosinusitis (CRS) had a mean of 94.9% of their mucosal surface area covered with mature biofilms compared to 1.9% in adenoids removed from patients with OSA. The authors hypothesize that biofilms in the adenoids of CRS children may act as a bacterial reservoir and that mechanical removal of the adenoid-associated biofilms may explain the known clinical improvement in pediatric patients with CRS after adenoidectomy.

Biofilms in Tonsillitis

The presence of biofilms may underlie the pathophysiology of chronic tonsillitis and adenoiditis. Chole and Faddis used light microscopy and transmission electron microscopy (TEM) to examine 19 tonsils, removed either for a history of repeated infection or to relieve airway obstruction from hypertrophy.[30] Amorphous polysaccharide biofilm matrix and bacteria were seen within the tonsillar crypts of 11 of the 15 infected tonsils, and smaller clusters of bacteria were seen in 3 of the tonsils removed for hypertrophy.[30] In a more recent study, Kania and colleagues used CLSM with double fluorescent staining to examine 24 tonsils removed from children with a history of chronic or recurrent tonsillitis and found biofilms in 17 of the 24 (70.8%) specimens.[31] Biofilms were demonstrated in the majority of patients with chronic upper respiratory tract infections that had failed aggressive medical management.[32] *Streptococcus pyogenes* infections that fail to be resolved with antibiotic therapy could be related to biofilm formation.[33] While Pseudomonas biofilms have long been known to be present in the lungs of patients with cystic fibrosis, biofilms have also been demonstrated in patients with diffuse panbronchiolitis and bronchiectasia due to *P. aeruginosa* or *Klebsiella pneumoniae*.[34] In addition, Murphy and colleagues have demonstrated that chronic obstructive pulmonary disease is associated with *H. influenzae* and *P. aeruginosa* biofilms.[35]

Biofilms in Rhinosinusitis

Rhinosinusitis is a multifaceted group of diseases that most likely have a biofilm component. While CRS has a major inflammatory component, the mechanism(s) driving the inflammation are controversial. A variety of theories have been advanced, involving superantigens from *Staphylococcus aureus*, allergy, disorders of the innate immune system, or aberrant reaction to fungi; however, there is accumulating evidence that bacterial biofilms play some sort of role in the pathophysiology of CRS. There are certainly parallels between CRS and chronic otitis media, both being diseases of mucosally lined cavities connected to the nasopharynx, with similar resistance to antimicrobials and chronicity of course.

A variety of animal studies have been conducted to examine the relationship between CRS and biofilms. In a pioneering study, Perloff and Palmer, using a rabbit model of maxillary sinusitis, instilled *P. aeruginosa* and found mucosally based biofilms using SEM.[36] Using a sheep model, Wormald and colleagues found *S. aureus* biofilms in experimentally induced CRS.[37] The advantage of the larger animal is that the nasal cavities allow for endoscopic sinus surgery.

In human studies, biofilms were initially found on frontal sinus recess stents, and a growing number of studies have demonstrated the presence of biofilms in patients with CRS.[38] Earlier studies used SEM or TEM, but later studies have combined CLSM and FISH to speciate the bacteria isolated.[39] In these approaches FISH was used to determine that *H. influenzae* is the most predominate species forming biofilms in CRS patients. Bendouah and colleagues, investigating the in vitro biofilm-forming capacity of bacteria isolated from patients who had persistent CRS after functional endoscopic sinus surgery, found a positive correlation between the robustness of biofilms formation and unfavorable outcome.[40]

Biofilm Formation on Endotracheal Tubes, Trachcostomy Tubes and Voice Prostheses

Biofilms are readily demonstrated in the lumen of endotracheal tubes (ETT), with the degree of biofilm formation proportional to the length of time of intubation. ETT biofilms can lead to ventilator-associated pneumonia (VAP). Biofilms have been demonstrated on both the inner and outer surfaces of ETT in neonates, many with sterile culture results.[41] Biofilms readily form on tracheostomy tubes, and at least one study has concluded that there is no difference in susceptibility to *P. aeruginosa* and *Staphylococcus epidermidis* biofilms formation among tube materials, including polyvinyl chloride, silicone, stainless steel, and sterling silver.[42] Biofilms were recognized on silicone rubber voice prostheses over a decade ago, thus they are one of the most extensively studied otolaryngologic devices.[43] The prostheses, inserted in a nonsterile manner, in patients who have undergone total laryngectomy, quickly become covered with mixed biofilms of bacteria and yeast, mostly *Candida* species. The biofilm increases airflow resistance and rapidly degrades the rubber, necessitating frequent replacements. A number of strategies have been tried in an attempt to reduce biofilm formation, including modifying the surface properties of the prostheses, the administration of systemic antimicrobials, binding antimicrobial agents to the surface of the prosthesis, and using biosurfactants.[44] Interestingly, consumption of certain dairy products significantly reduced biofilm formation and increased the life of the prosthesis.

Biofilms on Facial Reconstruction Implants

Biofilm infections on implants used in facial reconstruction may result in delayed union or nonunion and can lead to removal of the implant with additional operations. Biofilms can form on bioimplant materials used in facial plastics such as titanium, silicone, and polytetrafluoroethylene (PTFE), whereas implants composed of PTFE with silver/chlorhexidine appeared more resistant to biofilm formation in an animal model.[45] Biofilms can also form on sutures.[46] Interestingly, Emery and colleagues were unable to demonstrate *S. aureus* biofilm formation on titanium or resorbable implants using an in vitro model, speculating that the absence of biofilm formation could be attributed to surface charge or polarity properties.[47] A study using SEM to examine biomaterials removed from 11 patients with persistent infections refractory to antimicrobial therapy and local wound care revealed adherent bacteria, often polymicrobial, but without frank biofilm formation.[48]

Biofilms on Tympanostomy Tubes

Robust biofilms are visualized on tubes removed from children with refractory posttympanostomy tube otorrhea, and removal of the tubes often results in clinical resolution.[49] It follows that a tube surface resistant to biofilm formation might decrease the incidence of otorrhea. Various parameters of tubes that have been manipulated include changing the surface morphology or surface energy to reduce bacterial attachment and adhesion and incorporation of antimicrobial agents into the tube material. While some studies show a variation in biofilm formation among different tube surfaces, the ideal material for tube construction has not yet been identified.

Biofilm Formation on Cochlear Implants

Biofilms were first recognized on the silicone outer surface of a cochlear implant internal receiver device and electrode array after explantation in 2003.[50] Cristobal and colleagues in the Wackym laboratory reported the clinical course of a child with chronic OM who underwent cochlear implantation and, after prolonged treatment with Floxin Otic (ofloxacin otic solution), she developed a secondary yeast infection with *Candida albicans* which extended from the middle ear to the auditory prosthesis.[50] Despite prolonged antifungal therapy, she required explantation of the device to clear her infection. In addition to the *C. albicans* grown in culture, they found SEM evidence of fungal biofilm on all aspects of the implanted device as evidenced by extracellular polymeric substance (EPS) in association with the yeast elements. Interestingly, there was no evidence of labyrinthitis or fibrosis of the cochlea at reimplantation (P. Ashley Wackym, personal communication, April 22, 2007).

Subsequently, it has become apparent that cochlear implants, like all other abiotic implantable devices, are subject to bacterial biofilm infection. Antonelli and colleagues compared the surfaces of implants removed from patients due to infection with those removed because of device failure, as well as with unimplanted devices.[51] They found bacterial biofilms on all implanted devices as evidenced by EPS but not on the unimplanted devices. They did, however, identify bacteria on the unimplanted devices suggesting that better sterilization techniques prior to surgery may reduce the infection rate. Similarly, Pawlowski and colleagues identified *S. aureus* biofilms on the receiver/stimulator device removed from a cochlear implant patient with infection that failed to resolve despite prolonged antibiotic therapy.[52] They reported that the entire surface was covered with EPS and embedded bacteria but that the biofilm was thickest in depressions on the device surface. They also identified polymorphonuclear leukocytes interspersed with the bacteria in the biofilm.

TECHNOLOGIES FOR THE STUDY OF BIOFILMS

Standard culture methods are not adequate to detect or enumerate bacteria in a biofilm; furthermore, culture results do not provide information regarding the complex ultrastructural aspects of a biofilm. Therefore, a suite of technologies have been developed to study biofilms. These include SEM, TEM, CLSM, and atomic force microscopy (ATM). Fixing specimens for SEM and TEM introduce drying artifacts, especially in the biofilm matrix. Another limitation is the reliance on bacterial morphology for speciation, which is nonspecific at best. CLSM can obtain 3-D reconstructions of intact, thick specimens without the need to fix and section the specimens. Images are obtained throughout the specimen at various depths throughout the Z-axis, reconstructed with a computer, and viewed on a monitor screen, rather than through an eyepiece, thus the CLSM is analogous to a computerized axial tomographic system. The focal plane is determined by using a laser to excite fluorescence in the sample; thus, fluorescent dyes must be used. Alternatively, bacteria can be engineered to produce their own fluorescence, using such molecules as green fluorescent protein. FISH can be used in a species-specific manner to identify bacteria in the specimen. Thus, CLSM combined with FISH provides the investigator with the capacity for noninvasive optical sectioning of intact specimens, with positive identification of the component bacteria.

ATM has also been used to study biofilms and the surfaces to which they adhere (Ehrlich and Avci, unpublished data). The atomic force microscope (AFM) does not obtain direct images but rather works by running an atomic tip over a surface, analogous to a phonograph needle running over a record. AFM can obtain images at the angstrom level, making it possible to study bacterial and surface interactions at the nanoscopic level, particularly in terms of bacterial adhesion and whether a biomaterial of interest attracts or repels bacteria.

TREATMENT AND PREVENTION OF BIOFILMS

Given the pervasive problem of biofilms in medicine and industry, there is tremendous interest in developing effective strategies to prevent or control biofilms. Overall antibiofilm strategies either attempt to develop a biofilm-resistant surface or have a bacteriacentric approach. The search for the "biofilm-resistant surface" has become a holy grail of materials engineering, but results to date have been disappointing. Considering that bacteria have been forming biofilms for over 3 billion years, there is little with which the bacteria have not dealt successfully. A great deal of effort has been expended modifying various physicochemical properties of the surface or using biosurfactants. Binding of antimicrobial agents to the surface is an attractive strategy but has the potential to develop resistant microorganisms. Various forms of energy have been applied to the surface to disrupt biofilms, including ultraviolet and bioelectric. Shearing forces on catheters can break off flocs of biofilm which are then disseminated distally, so strategies that decrease shear forces can reduce infectious complications associated with biofilms.

Approaches that focus on the bacteria have several strategies, including preventing initial bacterial attachment, interference with quorum sensing, or inducing the bacteria to return to the planktonic state. Targeted peptides or phages are being developed to kill biofilm bacteria. Chronic administration of antimicrobials to the patient induces the development of resistant strains, but prophylactic antibiotics in selected surgical procedures can kill the planktonic bacteria before they attach. Disruption of the biofilm matrix is an attractive treatment strategy, with the goals of releasing planktonic bacteria that are susceptible to antibiotic treatment or to induce detachment. Matrix disruption using recombinant human DNAase, an enzyme which selectively cleaves DNA, has been shown to be an effective strategy in the treatment of patients with cystic fibrosis.

Medical Treatments of Biofilms

Long-term use of low-dose macrolide antibiotics can be efficacious in some patients with diffuse panbronchiolitis and cystic fibrosis. This clinical effect is nonribosomal, as the doses used are well below the minimum inhibitory concentrations for *Pseudomonas* species. It is thought that low-dose macrolides are effective through both an immunomodulatory effect in which the host neutrophils are paralyzed thereby leading to a decrease in bystander damage from oxidative burst and an antibiofilm effect in which the macrolides suppress quorum-sensing associated genes and inhibit twitch motility.[53] Lactoferrin, an iron-chelating protein that is a component of the innate immune system, blocks biofilm development by *P. aeruginosa* by stimulating bacterial motility and thus preventing biofilm formation.[54]

Probiotics

One very interesting approach is the use of probiotics, or "beneficent bacteria," either to prevent pathogenic biofilm formation or to disrupt existing biofilms. Biofilms and humans have a long-standing symbiotic relationship, such that the average human has 10^{13} cells, and is home to 10^{14} bacteria. Biofilms are an integral part of the human oral cavity, gut and vagina, and the normal human flora serves as a barrier against pathogenic bacteria. Given that bacteria can form biofilms in the most hostile environments and can quickly develop new strains in response to environmental pressures, we will never defeat biofilms but should rather adapt their good characteristics to desired outcomes. We already take this approach when we ingest live culture yogurt or drink acidophilus milk. Such an approach has proven successful in such disparate arenas as preventing caries or Salmonella infections in chicken farms. In otolaryngology, alpha hemolytic streptococcus has been used in an attempt to prevent recurrences of acute OM and OME, as well as streptococcal pharyngitis, and "interfering" microorganisms help prevent recurrence of upper respiratory tract infections.[55]

CONCLUSIONS

Microbiologists now understand that biofilms are universal and are the preferred milieu for bacteria. Biofilms are an ancient strategy of bacteria and occur at every air- or aqueous–surface interface yet examined. Our previous narrow focus on planktonic bacteria, and culturability must be expanded to understand the complexities of biofilms and their profound differences from planktonic bacteria. The diagnostic, therapeutic, and preventive strategies that have served us so well in our fight against acute infections will not be effective against chronic biofilm diseases. Most bacterial infections are dependant upon attachment to tissue, but the distinctions among "bacterial attachment," "colonization," "commensalisms," and "infection" become blurred. Most likely, the distinctions are not absolute but rather more a matter of degree. We do not understand why some biofilm-associated microorganisms elicit disease, yet others do not. Pathogenesis appears to be as much related to the host inflammatory and immune responses as to the specific actions of the bacteria. Additionally, we need to understand bacteria and human health, as well as we understand bacteria and human disease.

REFERENCES

1. Whitchurch CB, Tolker-Nielsen T, Ragas PC, Mattick JS. Extracellular DNA required for bacterial biofilm formation. Science 2002;295:1487.

2. Moscoso M, Claverys JP. Release of DNA into the medium by competent *Streptococcus pneumoniae*: Kinetics, mechanism and stability of the liberated. DNA Mol Microbiol 2004;54:783–94.

3. Jurcisek JA, Bakaletz LO. Biofilms formed by nontypeable *Haemophilus influenzae* in vivo contain both dsDNA as well as type IV pilin protein. J Bacteriol 2007 Epub Feb 23.

4. Stoodley P, de Beer D, Lewandowski Z. Liquid flow in biofilm systems. Appl Environ Microbiol 1994;60:2711–6.

5. Davies DG, Parsek MR, Pearson JP, et al. The involvement of cell-to-cell signals in the development of a bacterial biofilm. Science 1998;280:295–8.

6. Hall-Stoodley L, Costerton JW, Stoodley P. Bacterial biofilms: From the environment to infectious disease. Nature Rev Microbiol 2004;2:95–108.

7. Ehrlich GD, Hu ZF, Post JC. Role for biofilms in infectious disease. In: Ghannoum M, O'Toole GA, editors. Microbial Biofilms. Washington, DC: ASM Press; 2004. p. 332–58.

8. Borriello G, Werner E, Roe F, et al. Oxygen limitation contributes to antibiotic tolerance of *Pseudomonas aeruginosa* in biofilms. Antimicrob Agents Chemother 2004;48:2659–64.

9. Abdi-Ali A, Mohammadi-Mehr M, Agha Alaei Y. Bactericidal activity of various antibiotics against biofilm-producing *Pseudomonas aeruginosa*. Int J Antimicrob Agents 2006;27:196–200.

10. McNamara CJ, Perry TD, Leard R, et al. Corrosion of aluminum alloy 2024 by microorganisms isolated form aircraft fuel tanks. Biofouling 2005;21:257–65.

11. Gu JD, Roman M, Esselman T, Mitchell R. The role of microbial biofilms in deterioration of space station candidate materials. Int Biodeterioration Biodegrad 1998;41:25–33.

12. Ortega-Morales O, Guezennec J, Hernandez-Duque G, et al. Phototrophic biofilms on ancient Mayan buildings in Yucatan, Mexico. Curr Microbiol 2000;40:81–5.

13. Albertano P, Urzi C. Structural interactions among epilithic cyanobacteria and heterotrophic microorganisms in Roman hypogea. Microb Ecol 1999;38:244–52.

14. Potera C. Forging a link between biofilms and disease. Science 1999;283:1837–9.

15. Post JC, Preston RA, Aul JJ, et al. Molecular analysis of bacterial pathogens in otitis media with effusion. JAMA 1995;273:1598–604.

16. Braxton EE, Jr, Ehrlich GD, Hall-Stoodley L, et al. Role of biofilms in neurosurgical device-related infections. Neurosurg Rev 2005;28:249–55.

17. Costerton W, Veeh R, Shirtliff M, et al. The application of biofilm science to the study and control of chronic bacterial infections. J Clin Invest 2003;112:1466–77.

18. Ehrlich GD, Veeh R, Wang X, et al. Mucosal biofilm formation on middle-ear mucosa in the chinchilla model of otitis media. JAMA 2002;287:1710–5.

19. Anderson GG, Palermo JJ, Schilling JD, et al. Intracellular bacterial biofilm-like pods in urinary tract infections. Science 2003;301:105–7.

20. Cummings JH. Dietary carbohydrates and the colonic microflora. Curr Opin Clin Nutr Metab Care 1998;1:409–14.

21. Nagy KN, Sonkodi I, Szoke I, et al. The microflora associated with human oral carcinomas. Oral Oncol 1998;34:304–8.

22. Rayner MG, Zhang Y, Gorry MC, et al. Evidence of bacterial metabolic activity in culture-negative otitis media with effusion. JAMA 1998;279:296–9.

23. Dingman JR, Rayner MG, Mishra S, et al. Correlation between presence of viable bacteria and presence of endotoxin in middle-ear effusions. J Clin Microbiol 1998;36:3417–9.

24. Post JC, Aul JJ, White GJ, et al. PCR-based detection of bacterial DNA after antimicrobial treatment is indicative of persistent, viable bacteria in the chinchilla model of otitis media. Am J Otolaryngol 1996;7:1–7.

25. Dohar JE, Hebda PA, Veeh R, et al. Mucosal biofilm formation on middle-ear mucosa in a nonhuman primate model of chronic suppurative otitis media. Laryngoscope 2005;115:1469–72.

26. Hall-Stoodley L, Hu FZ, Gieseke A, et al. Direct detection of bacterial biofilms on middle ear-mucosa of children with chronic otitis media. JAMA 2006;296:202–11.

27. Chole RA, Faddis BT. Evidence for microbial biofilms in cholesteatomas. Arch Otolaryngol Head Neck Surg 2002;128:1129–33.

28. Wang EW, Jung JY, Pashia ME, et al. Otopathogenic *Pseudomonas aeruginosa* strains as competent biofilm formers. Arch Otolaryngol Head Neck Surg 2005;131:983–9.

29. Coticchia J, Zuliani G, Coleman C, et al. Biofilm surface area in the pediatric nasopharynx: Chronic rhinosinusitis vs obstructive sleep apnea. Arch Otolaryngol Head Neck Surg 2007;133:110–4.

30. Chole RA, Faddis BT. Anatomical evidence of microbial biofilms in tonsillar tissues: A possible mechanism to explain chronicity. Arch Otolaryngol Head Neck Surg 2003;129:634–6.

31. Kania RE, Lamers GE, Vonk MJ, et al. Demonstration of bacterial cells and glycocalyx in biofilms on human tonsils. Arch Otolaryngol Head Neck Surg 2007;133:115–21.

32. Galli J, Ardito F, Calo L, et al. Recurrent upper airway infections and bacterial biofilms. J Laryngol Otol 2007;121:341–4.

33. Baldassarri L, Creti R, Recchia S, et al. Therapeutic failures of antibiotics used to treat macrolide-susceptible *Streptococcus pyogenes* infections may be due to biofilm formation. J Clin Microbiol 2006;44:2721–7.

34. Ohgaki N. Bacterial biofilm in chronic airway infection. Kansenshogaku Zasshi 1994;68:138–51.

35. Murphy TF, Brauer AL, Schiffmacher AT, Sethi S. Persistent colonization by *Haemophilus influenzae* in chronic obstructive pulmonary disease. Am J Respir Crit Care Med 2004;170:266–72.

36. Perloff JR, Palmer JN. Evidence of bacterial biofilms in a rabbit model of sinusitis. J Rhinol 2005;19:1–6.

37. Wormald PJ, Psaltis A, Ha K. A sheep model for the study of biofilms in sinusitis. In: Programs and abstracts of the 52nd Annual Meeting of the American Rhinologic Society; September 16, 2006; Toronto, ON, Canada.

38. Perloff JR, Palmer JN. Evidence of bacterial biofilms on frontal recess stents in patients with chronic rhinosinusitis. Am J Rhinol 2004;18:377–80.

39. Sanderson AR, Leid JG, Hunsaker D. Bacterial biofilms on the sinus mucosa of human subjects with chronic rhinosinusitis. Laryngoscope 2006;116:1121–6.

40. Bendouah Z, Barbeau J, Hamad WA, Desrosiers M. Biofilm formation by *Staphylococcus aureus* and *Pseudomonas aeruginosa* is associated with an unfavorable evolution after surgery for chronic sinusitis and nasal polyposis. Otolaryngol Head Neck Surg 2006;134:991–6.

41. Zur KB, Mandell DL, Gordon RE, et al. Electron microscopic analysis of biofilm on endotracheal tubes removed from intubated neonates. Otolaryngol Head Neck Surg 2004;130:407–14.

42. Jarrett WA, Ribes J, Manaligod JM. Biofilm formation on tracheostomy tubes. Ear Nose Throat J 2002;81:659–61.

43. Neu TR, Van der Mei HC, Busscher HJ, et al. Biodeterioration of medical-grade silicone rubber used for voice prostheses: A SEM study. Biomaterials 1993;14:459–64.

44. Rodrigues L, Banat IM, Teixeira J, Oliveira R. Strategies for the prevention of microbial biofilm formation on silicone rubber voice prostheses. J Biomed Mater Res B Appl Biomater 2006;81B:358–70.

45. Malaisrie SC, Malekzadeh S, Biedlingmaier JF. In vivo analysis of bacterial biofilm formation on facial plastic bioimplants. Laryngoscope 1998;108:1733–8.

46. Otten JE, Wiedmann-Al-Ahmad M, Jahnke H, Pelz K. Bacterial colonization on different suture materials—a potential risk for intraoral dentoalveolar surgery. J Biomed Mater Res B Appl Biomater 2005;74:627–35.

47. Emery BE, Dixit R, Formby CC, Biedlingmaier JF. The resistance of maxillofacial reconstruction plates to biofilm formation in vitro. Laryngoscope 2003;113:1977–82.

48. Nishioka GJ, Jones JK, Triplett RG, Aufdemorte TB. The role of bacterial-laden biofilms in infections of maxillofacial biomaterials. J Oral Maxillofac Surg 1988;46:19–25.

49. Post JC. Direct evidence of bacterial biofilms in otitis media. Laryngoscope 2001;111:2083–94.

50. Cristobal R, Edmiston CE, Jr, Runge-Samuelson CL, et al. Fungal biofilm formation on cochlear implant hardware after prophylactic antibiotic-induced fungal overgrowth within the middle ear. Ped Infect Dis J 2004;23:774–8.

51. Antonelli PJ, Lee JC, Burne RA. Bacterial biofilms may contribute to persistent cochlear implant infection. Otol Neurotol 2004;25:953–7.

52. Pawlowski KS, Wawro D, Roland PS. Bacterial biofilm formation on a human cochlear implant. Otol Neurotol 2005;26:972–5.

53. Tateda K, Standiford TJ, Pechere JC, Yamaguchi K. Regulatory effects of macrolides on bacterial virulence: Potential role as quorum-sensing inhibitors. Curr Pharm Des 2004;10:3055–65.

54. Singh PK, Parsek MR, Greenberg EP, Welsh MJ. A component of innate immunity prevents bacterial biofilm development. Nature 2002;417:552–5.

55. Roos K, Holm S. The use of probiotics in head and neck infections. Curr Infect Dis Rep 2002;4:211–6.

72

Development, Anatomy, and Physiology of the Larynx

Clarence T. Sasaki, MD,
Young-Ho Kim, MD, PhD,
Adam J. LeVay, MD

The human larynx is a complex organ that functions as a sphincter at the junction of the digestive and respiratory tracts and participates in the diverse roles of airway protection, respiration, and phonation. In his classic phylogenic observations, Negus prioritized three functions of the larynx.[1] In order of their priority, these are (1) protection of the lower airway, (2) respiration, and (3) phonation. To perform these roles, the internal and external structures of the larynx interact under precise neural control, producing in humans the most complex of laryngeal functions. Thus, the anatomy of the larynx reflects the specialization required by these multiple roles and is best understood in relation to its diverse physiologic behaviors.

EMBRYOLOGY

The larynx, trachea, and lungs begin to form during the fourth week of embryologic development (Figure 1). The respiratory diverticulum, also referred to as the laryngotracheal diverticulum, begins as a thickening on the ventral wall of the foregut lumen immediately caudal to the fourth branchial arch. The lining of this diverticulum is derived from the endoderm of the foregut and gives rise to the epithelial lining and glands of the larynx, trachea, and lungs. As the diverticulum elongates, it becomes invested by the splanchnic mesenchyme that will give rise to the cartilaginous and muscular structures of the lower respiratory organs. The caudal extent of the diverticulum begins to dilate by the end of the fourth week, giving rise to the primordial lung buds or bronchopulmonary buds.[3] Contrary to the notion proposed by His of an ascending tracheoesophageal septum, Zaw-Tun and Burdi demonstrated that the esophagus forms as a result of the continued ventrocaudal elongation of the respiratory

diverticulum as an outgrowth of the caudal aspect of the foregut.[2,4,5]

Larynx

As stated above, the epithelial lining of the larynx is derived from endoderm. The laryngeal carti-

lages are derived from the fusion of mesenchymal neural crest elements within the fourth and sixth branchial arches. The thyroid, cricoid, and arytenoid cartilages are hyaline cartilage, whereas the epiglottic, cuneiform, and corniculate cartilages are composed of elastic cartilage. The anlage of

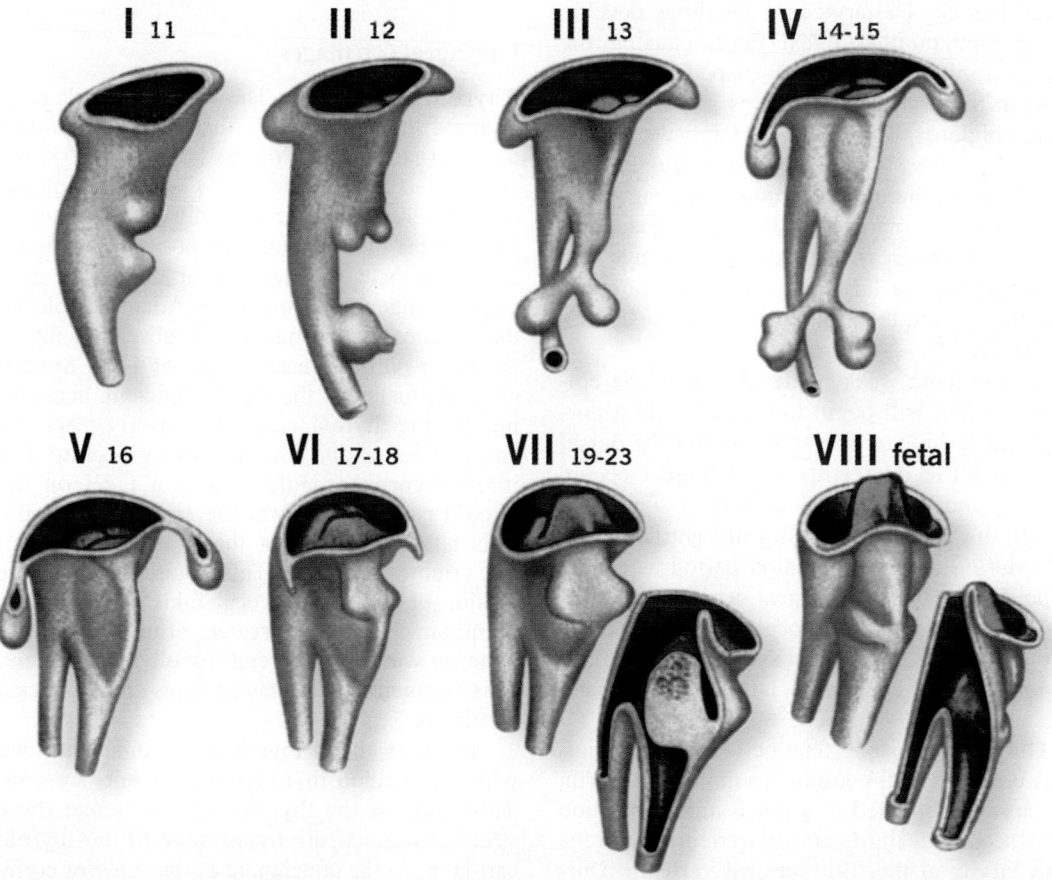

Figure 1 The development of the larynx in eight stages (I to VIII) as depicted by Holinger et al,[2] with corresponding Carnegie Institute embryologic stages (11 to 23). Salient points: I—the respiratory diverticulum develops from the ventral foregut; II—the formation of bronchopulmonary buds, III—elongation and formation of the infraglottis, carina, and bronchi; IV—the arytenoid swellings, developing epiglottis and the formation of the epithelial lamina; VII—recanalizaton of the epithelial lamina begins; VIII—laryngeal ventricles form. (Reprinted with permission from reference 2.)

the cricoid cartilage chondrifies bilaterally beginning from a single center in the ventral arch that proceeds toward the dorsal lamina. The arytenoids each chondrify from a single center, and each thyroid ala form froms two chondrification centers.[4] The epiglottis is derived from the hypobranchial eminence, which is a proliferation of mesenchyme in the ventral ends of the third and fourth branchial arches.

The cricothyroid muscle is derived from the fourth branchial arch and is, therefore, innervated by the superior laryngeal nerve. All other intrinsic laryngeal musculature is derived from the sixth branchial arch and is innervated by the recurrent laryngeal nerve.

The primitive pharyngeal floor, which is the site of origin of the respiratory diverticulum, becomes the glottis. Separating the primitive pharyngeal floor from the pharyngeal floor formed by the fourth branchial pouch is a segment of the foregut that will become the supraglottic portion of the larynx. The infraglottic portion of the larynx develops from the cephalic aspect of the respiratory diverticulum. As the foregut and respiratory diverticulum elongate in the coming weeks, the esophagus will lengthen, and the infraglottis will become separated from the carina by the developing trachea.[2]

Beginning in the sixth week, mesenchyme in the ventral portion of the developing larynx proliferates rapidly, causing eventual obliteration of the lumen and the creation of the epithelial lamina. The arytenoid swellings develop in the median pharyngeal floor, causing the laryngeal inlet to assume a T-shaped appearance between the arytenoid swellings and the developing epiglottis. The epithelial lamina will continue to enlarge in a ventral to dorsal fashion and almost obliterate the primitive laryngopharynx except for a narrow pharyngoglottic duct. In addition, between the arytenoid swellings and the epiglottis, the laryngeal cecum appears and descends toward the glottis ventral to the epithelial lamina.[3–5]

By the tenth week of development, the epithelial lamina will begin to recanalize in a dorsoventral fashion, which will connect the dorsal pharygoglottic duct with the laryngeal cecum ventrally and, when complete, link the supra- and infraglottic areas. The laryngeal ventricles also form during the recanalization period as caudal outpouchings of the laryngeal cecum, the lower lips of which form the vocal folds. Disruption of the recanalization process is believed to be responsible for congenital laryngeal webs and atresias.[6,7]

During the ensuing fetal period, the cartilaginous elements will continue to mature. At birth, the larynx is situated at a much higher position at the second or third cervical vertebrae than the adult larynx at the fifth cervical vertebra. During the first several years of life, the larynx will grow at an accelerated rate and the epiglottis will achieve its mature shape. The hyoid bone and larynx descend during growth and maturation, which is something unique to human beings and

necessary for the larynx to perform its complex functions described in the Physiology section.[8]

Trachea and Lungs

The endoderm lining the respiratory diverticulum caudal to the larynx forms the epithelium and glands of the trachea and lungs. The tracheal cartilages develop from the mesenchyme that surrounds the diverticulum. After the fourth week of development and the formation of the bronchopulmonary buds, further outpouchings develop and enlarge into the primordial pleural cavities. By the fifth week, the right and left bronchi develop. These will further subdivide into secondary and tertiary bronchi by the seventh week.[3]

Esophagus

The early stages of esophageal development are described above. The esophagus reaches it full length by the seventh week of development. It is lined by an endodermally derived epithelium that proliferates and obliterates the lumen. Subsequent recanalization is usually completed by the end of the embryonic period. The upper one-third of the esophageal musculature is striated and derived from the caudal branchial arch apparatus. The inferior one-third of the esophagus is composed of smooth muscle that develops from the surrounding splanchnic mesenchyme.[3]

ANATOMY

Laryngeal Cartilages

Thyroid Cartilage. The thyroid cartilage is a shield-shaped structure that serves to protect the internal anatomy of the larynx.[9–14] It is the largest cartilage of the larynx and is composed of two wings, the alae or laminae. The alae are fused in the midline and open posteriorly (Figure 2). In the male, the alae fuse at about 90°, making a laryngeal prominence or Adam's apple. In the female, this prominence is absent owing to the more oblique fusion angle of 120°. Superiorly, the fusion of the alae is deficient, accounting for the thyroid notch. Posteriorly, each ala has a superior and inferior horn or cornu. The inferior cornu articulates with a facet on the cricoid cartilage to form the cricothyroid joint. This is a synovial joint that allows rotation of the cricoid cartilage. This rotation varies the tension placed on the vocal folds. The superior cornu attaches to the greater cornu of the hyoid bone by way of the lateral thyrohyoid ligament. This ligament sometimes contains small triticeal cartilages.

The two lateral thyrohyoid ligaments, along with the median thyrohyoid ligament, are condensations of the thyrohyoid membrane; these structures attach the hyoid bone to the thyroid cartilage. At the attachment of the superior cornu to the ala of the thyroid cartilage, a protuberance called the superior tubercle is found. About 1 cm anterior and superior to this tubercle, the superior laryngeal artery and the internal branch of the superior laryngeal nerve and associated

lymphatics pierce the membrane to supply the supraglottic portion of the larynx. At this point, transcutaneous anesthesia of the internal branch can be performed. Running obliquely from the superior tubercle to the inferior tubercle (along the inferior margin of the thyroid cartilage) is a ridge called the oblique line, which serves as the attachment point for the thyrohyoid, sternothyroid, and inferior constrictor muscles.

The relationship of the surface anatomy to internal laryngeal anatomy merits consideration. Most important is the level of the true vocal folds in relation to the thyroid cartilage. An understanding of this relationship is crucial to performing supraglottic laryngectomy and phonosurgery (thyroplasty type I). In this regard, the midline vertical distance from the thyroid notch to the inferior border of the thyroid cartilage ranges from 20 to 47 mm in men and from 15.5 to 38 mm in women.[9,10] The anterior commissure is found at the midpoint between these landmarks. The posterior extent of the folds is anterior to the oblique line and is found in the middle third of this line.[4]

The thyroid cartilage is lined by a thick layer of perichondrium on all surfaces except the inner surface at the anterior commissure. At this point are attached five ligaments, which form the scaffolding for the corresponding laryngeal folds. From superior to inferior, they are the median thyroepiglottic ligament (median thyrohyoid fold), bilateral vestibular ligaments (vestibular folds or false folds), and bilateral vocal ligaments (vocal folds) (Figure 3).

The attachment of these ligaments penetrates the inner perichondrium, forming Broyle ligament. This ligament contains blood vessels and lymphatics and constitutes an important barrier to the spread of laryngeal neoplasms.

Cricoid Cartilage. The cricoid cartilage is a complete ring.[9–14] It is the only supporting structure that completely encircles the airway and serves as the major support for the functioning larynx. Its shape is classically described as that of a signet ring, with the anterior arch measuring 3 to 7 mm in height and the posterior lamina about 20 to 30 mm in height.[5–7] Its inferior border is nearly horizontal and is attached to the first tracheal cartilage by the cricotracheal ligament.

On the posterior surface of the cricoid, the posterior cricoarytenoid muscles are attached in depressions, which are separated by a midline vertical ridge. These muscles are the only abductors of the vocal folds. Attached to this midline vertical ridge are two fasciculi of longitudinal fibers of the esophagus.

Housed on the superior surface of the posterior lamina of the cricoid are the paired arytenoid cartilages. Posterior to anterior, the cricoid lamina slopes steeply downward to form the anterior arch of the cricoid. In the midline, between the superior portion of the arch and the inferior border of the thyroid cartilage is the cricothyroid membrane. It is this structure that must be incised in performing an emergent cricothyrotomy.

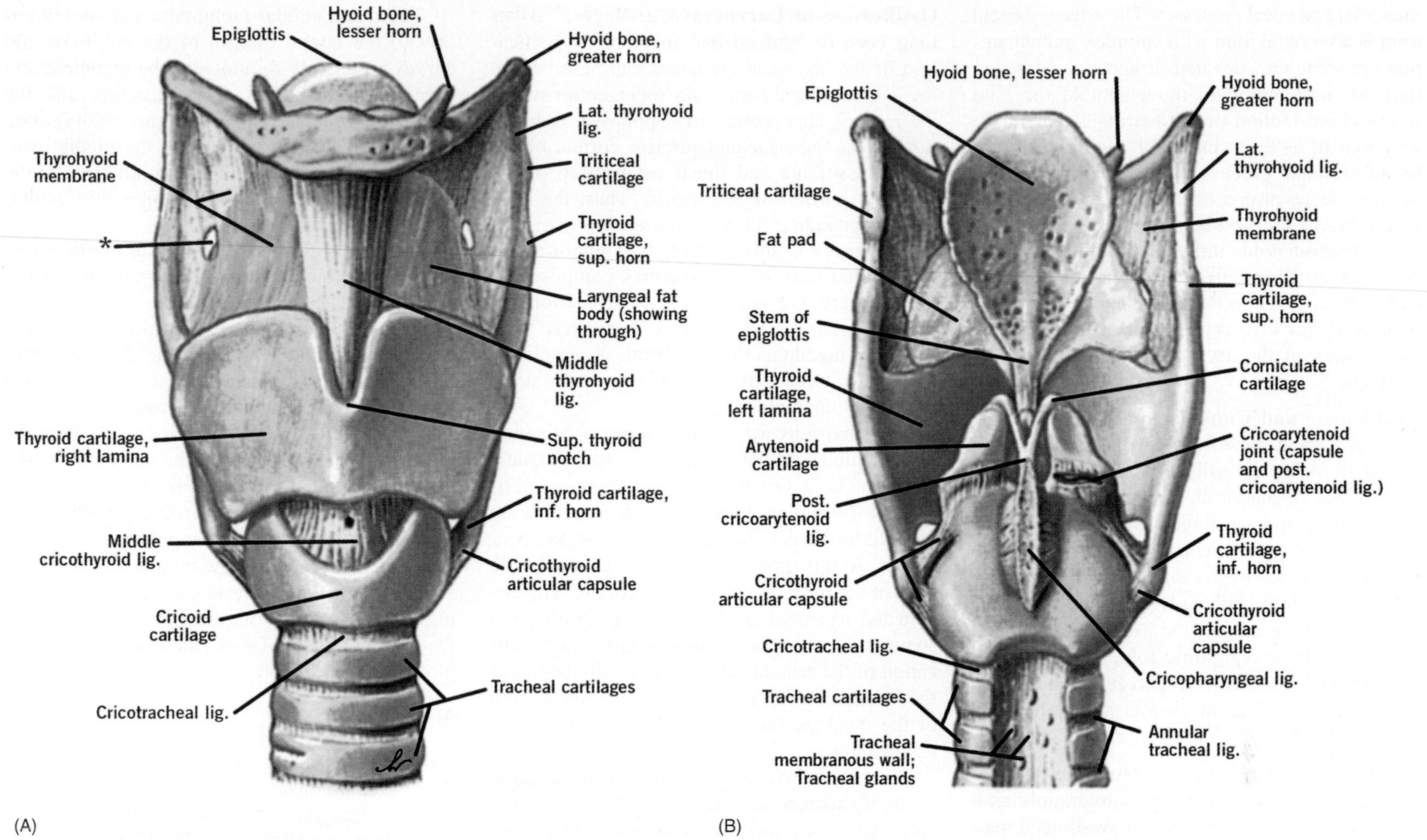

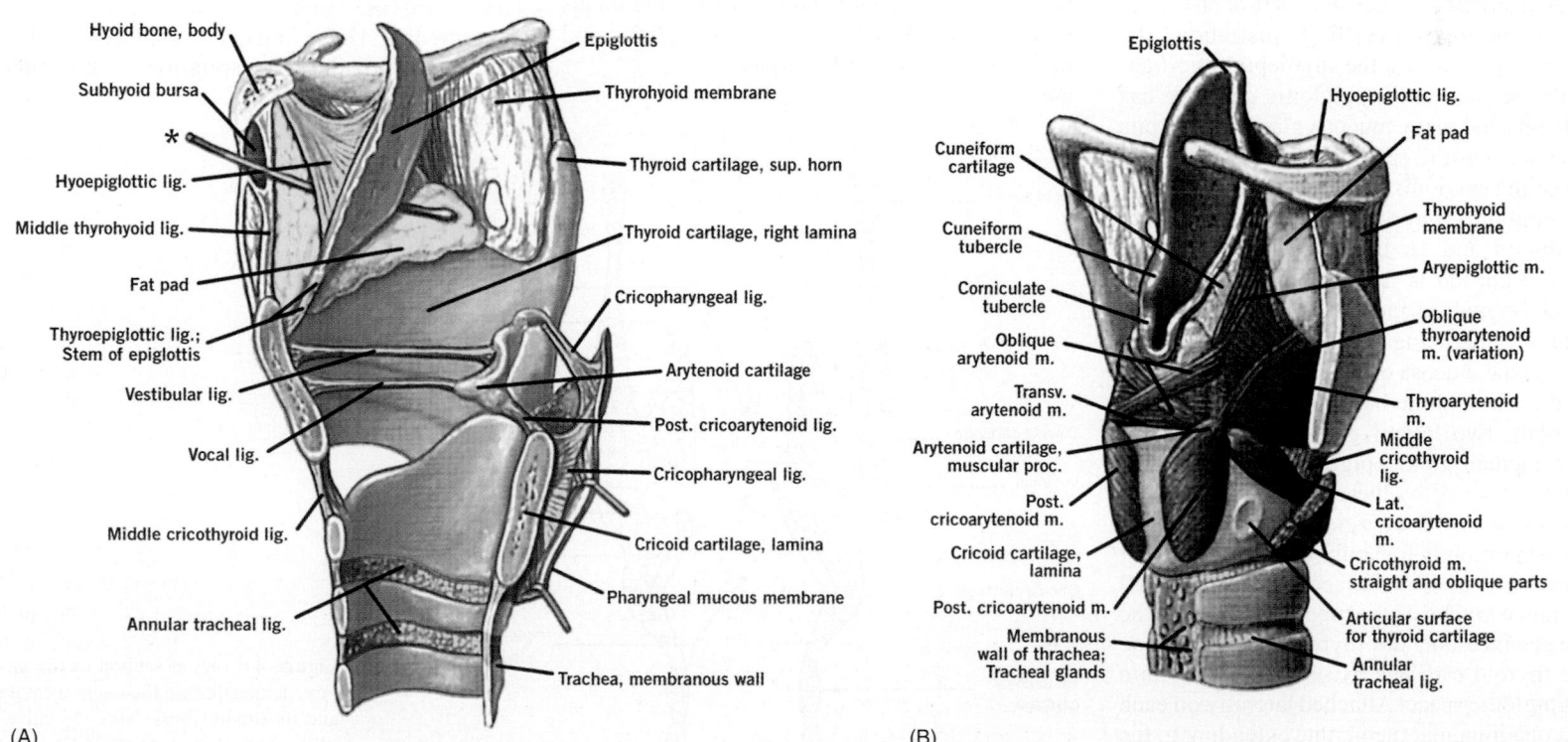

Figure 2 (A) Anterior view of the cartilages and ligaments of the larynx and hyoid bone. (B) Posterior view of the cartilages, ligaments, and articulations of the larynx and hyoid. *Passage for superior laryngeal nerve and vessels. (Reproduced with permission from reference 15.)

Arytenoid Cartilages. The arytenoids are paired cartilages that articulate with the posterosuperior portion of the cricoid cartilage.[9, 14] Movement of these cartilages and their attached vocal folds is involved in the diverse and complex functions of the larynx. Each arytenoid is roughly pyramidal in shape, giving it a base, an apex, and three sides. The base of the arytenoid provides the articular facet as well as the

Figure 3 (A) Sagittal view of the ligaments and articulations of the larynx. (B) Posterolateral view of the intrinsic musculature of the larynx. (Reproduced with permission from reference 15.)

muscular and vocal processes. The cricoarytenoid joint is a synovial joint with complex movements that are somewhat debated. It appears, however, that the most important movement of the joint is a rocking motion of the cartilage around the long axis of its facet. Laterally, the base forms a broad muscular process, and anteriorly, it forms the thinner vocal process. The anterolateral surface receives the vestibular ligament as well as the thyroarytenoid and vocalis muscles. The posterior surface receives muscular attachments, and to the medial surface is attached the prominent posterior cricoarytenoid ligament. Sitting at the apex of the arytenoid is the corniculate cartilage.

Corniculate and Cuneiform Cartilages. The corniculate and cuneiform cartilages are small, paired fibroelastic cartilages.[11] The corniculate, or cartilage of Santorini, is housed on the apex of the arytenoid cartilage. The cuneiform, or cartilage of Wrisberg, when present, is lateral to the corniculate cartilages and is embedded in the aryepiglottic fold. Although some feel that these cartilages are vestigial, they do appear to add rigidity to the aryepiglottic fold.[14] This rigidity augments the important rampart function of these folds, thus diverting swallowed matter laterally away from the larynx into the pyriform sinuses.

Epiglottis. The epiglottis contains a leaf-shaped elastic fibrocartilage that functions mainly as a backstop against the entrance of swallowed matter into the laryngeal aditus.[9–14] During swallowing, the larynx is raised anterosuperiorly. This action pushes the epiglottis against the base of the tongue, displacing it posteriorly over the laryngeal aditus. The epiglottis has two anterior attachments. Superiorly, it is attached to the hyoid bone by the hyoepiglottic ligament. Inferiorly at the stem or petiole, it is attached to the inner surface of the thyroid cartilage just above the anterior commissure by the thyroepiglottic ligament. The surface of the epiglottic cartilage has multiple pits and many mucous glands; these pits potentially allow the spread of cancer from one surface of the epiglottis to the other.

The epiglottis may arbitrarily be divided into a suprahyoid and an infrahyoid portion. The suprahyoid portion is free on both of its laryngeal and lingual surfaces, with the laryngeal mucosal surface being more adherent than the lingual. As the mucosa of the laryngeal surface is reflected back onto the base of the tongue, three folds result: two lateral glossoepiglottic folds and one median glossoepiglottic fold. The two depressions formed by these folds are known as the valleculae (*little depression* in Latin). The infrahyoid portion is free only on its laryngeal or posterior surface. This surface contains a small protuberance known as the tubercle. Between the anterior surface and the thyrohyoid membrane and the thyroid cartilage exists a fat pad within the preepiglottic space. Attached laterally on each side is a quadrangular membrane extending to the arytenoid and corniculate cartilages, constituting the aryepiglottic fold.

Ossification of Laryngeal Cartilages. It has long been recognized that incomplete ossification of the laryngeal cartilages can be mistaken for a foreign body on plain roentgenograms of the neck.[16] This particularly applies to ossification of the superior and inferior cornua of the thyroid cartilage and linear ossification of the posterior portion of the cricoid. Thus, the need for understanding the normal ossification pattern of the larynx is self-evident. It is important to realize that only those structures composed of hyaline cartilage will undergo ossification, ie, thyroid, cricoid, and arytenoid cartilages.[16,17] It should be noted that the hyoid bone is completely ossified at 2 years of age and is generally not a point of radiographic confusion.

The thyroid cartilage undergoes ossification in the male about the age 20 and in the female a few years later. Ossification begins posteroinferiorly on the lamina. It then extends anteriorly on the inferior border and superiorly at the posterior border. At this time, nuclei of ossification can be seen in the inferior and superior cornua. The cricoid and arytenoid cartilages undergo ossification somewhat later than the thyroid cartilage. Ossification of the cricoid cartilage generally begins at the inferior border, although the superior margin of the quadrate lamina may be an early site of ossification.

Neoplastic invasion of the laryngeal cartilages generally takes place in the ossified portion of the cartilage.[18] The incomplete ossification pattern may make it difficult to appreciate small areas of invasion.

Elastic Tissues

The elastic tissue of the larynx consists of two main parts: (1) the quadrangular membrane of the supraglottic larynx and (2) the thicker conus elasticus and vocal ligaments of the glottic and infraglottic portion of the larynx.

The quadrangular membrane attaches anteriorly to the lateral margin of the epiglottis and curves posteriorly to attach to the arytenoid and corniculate cartilages. This structure and the overlying mucosa constitute the aryepiglottic folds. Each fold forms part of the medial wall of each pyriform sinus. The inferior edge of the quadrangular membrane constitutes the vestibular ligaments.

The conus elasticus is a thicker elastic structure than the quadrangular membrane. It attaches inferiorly at the superior border of the cricoid cartilage. It then projects upward and medial to its superior attachments, the anterior commissure of the thyroid cartilage, and the vocal processes of the arytenoids. Between these superior attachments, the conus thickens to form the vocal ligament. Anteriorly, the conus forms the cricothyroid membrane, and in the midline, this membrane condenses to form the cricothyroid ligament (Figure 2–4).The superior extension of the conus (thyroglottic membrane) parallels the superior surface of the true vocal fold. Because it may normally be incomplete, it forms an imperfect barrier to the inferior extension of the transglottic cancers[14] (Figure 5).

Muscles

Extrinsic Muscles. The extrinsic muscles of the larynx are those muscles of the laryngohyoid complex that serve to raise, lower, or stabilize the larynx.[9–14] Those muscles that elevate the larynx are the thyrohyoid, stylohyoid, digastric, geniohyoid, mylohyoid, and stylopharyngeus. These muscles are important in the elevation and anterior displacement of the larynx during swallowing. They also help to suspend the larynx, via the hyoid bone, from the skull base and mandible. The principal depressors of the larynx are the omohyoid, sternothyroid, and sternohyoid. These muscles displace the larynx downward during inspiration. The middle

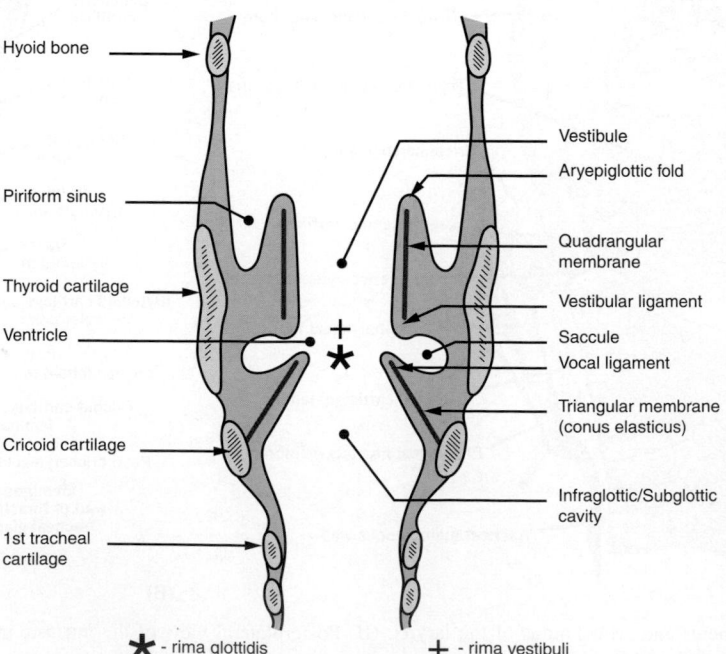

Figure 4 Coronal section of the larynx, demonstrating the internal cavity and its subdivisions. Note the valve-like nature of the true and false vocal folds. (Reproduced with permission from reference 19.)

Labels on figure: Hyoid bone; Piriform sinus; Thyroid cartilage; Ventricle; Cricoid cartilage; 1st tracheal cartilage; Vestibule; Aryepiglottic fold; Quadrangular membrane; Vestibular ligament; Saccule; Vocal ligament; Triangular membrane (conus elasticus); Infraglottic/Subglottic cavity

* - rima glottidis   + - rima vestibuli

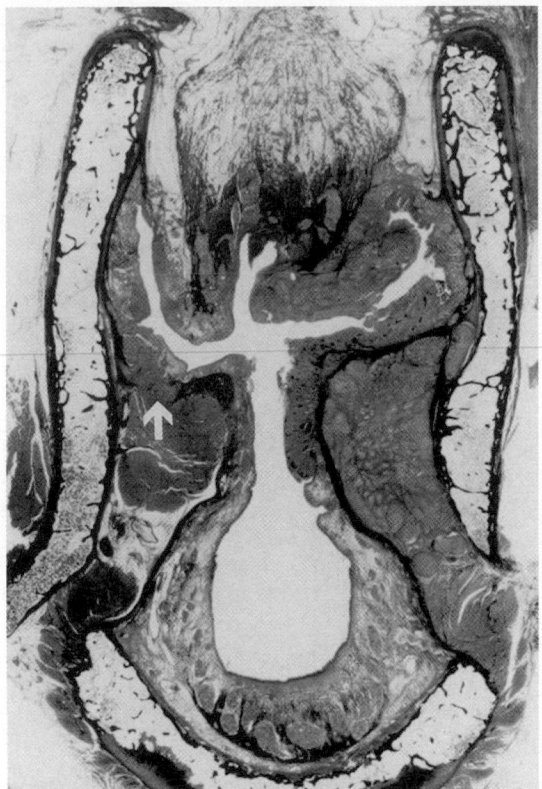 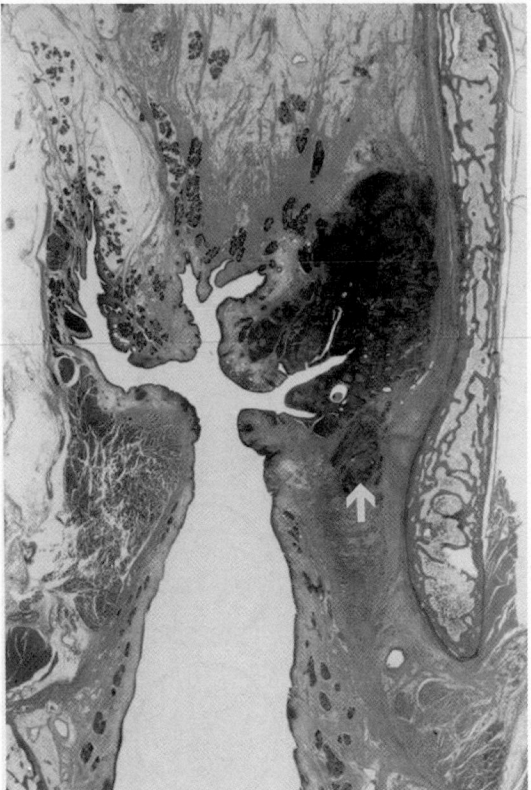

(A)   (B)

Figure 5 (A) The thyroglottic membrane may be naturally dehiscent (*arrow*). (B) Dehiscence in the thyroglottic membrane can allow transglottic cancer to extend inferiorly along the paraglottic space (*arrow*). (Courtesy of Dr. John A. Kirchner.)

constrictor, inferior constrictor, and cricopharyngeus muscles are also important extrinsic laryngeal muscles. The proper functioning of these muscles is crucial to the precisely timed swallowing reflex.

Intrinsic Muscles. The intrinsic muscles of the larynx are those muscles that are anatomically restricted to the larynx proper. They modify the size of the glottic opening along with the length and tension on the vocal folds. They consist of multiple adductors but only a single abductor. With the exception of the interarytenoid, the intrinsic muscles are paired, and these paired muscles appear to act synchronously (Figure 6).

Cricothyroid Muscle. The cricothyroid muscle is located on the external surface of the laryngeal cartilages. It is classically described as consisting of two bellies. The straight portion or pars recta attaches the lateral portion of the anterior part of the arch of the cricoid cartilage to the inferior border of the thyroid cartilage in a fairly vertical direction. The second belly, the pars obliqua, also from the anterolateral border of the cricoid arch, travels obliquely upward to insert on the anterior portion of the inferior cornu. When the right and left cricothyroid muscles contract, they rotate the cricoid at the cricothyroid joint. This action brings the anterior arch of the cricoid superiorly toward the inferior border of the thyroid laminae while displacing the posterior cricoid lamina (and the arytenoid cartilages) inferiorly. This inferior displacement increases the distance between the vocal processes and the anterior commissure;

the result of this action is to lower, stretch, and thin the vocal folds while bringing them into a paramedian position. The stretching of the vocal fold also sharpens the edge of the vocal fold and passively stiffens the component layers of the vocal fold (Figure 7). Biomechanically, this translates into a higher fundamental frequency produced by the vocal folds.

Posterior Cricoarytenoid Muscle. This muscle is the sole abductor of the vocal folds. It is seated in a depression on the posterior surface of the cricoid lamina, and its fibers run obliquely superior and lateral to attach onto the muscular process of the arytenoid cartilage. It is composed of two compartments: horizontal and vertical bellies. Contraction of these fibers brings the muscular process medial, posterior, and inferior while laterally rotating and elevating the vocal process. This action abducts, elongates, and thins the vocal folds while causing the vocal fold edge to be rounded. The stretching of the vocal fold leads to passive stiffening of its layers. The complex function of this muscle has been studied in the canine in which three distinct neuromuscular compartments are found. It is proposed that the vertical and oblique bellies normally cause vocal fold abduction during respiration, whereas the horizontal belly is primarily used to adjust the position of the vocal process during phonation.[22,23]

Lateral Cricoarytenoid Muscle. The lateral cricoarytenoid muscle is the main antagonist of the posterior cricoarytenoid. It attaches along the superior border of the cricoid cartilage and

sends fibers posteriorly to insert on the anterior portion of the muscular process. Contraction of this muscle brings the muscular process anterolaterally while adducting and lowering the vocal process. This results in adduction, elongation, and thinning of the vocal folds. The edge of the vocal fold becomes sharper, and its component layers are passively stiffened.

Interarytenoid/Aryepiglottic Muscle. The interarytenoid muscle is the only unpaired intrinsic muscle, consisting of two types of muscle fibers. The bulk of the muscle consists of transverse fibers passing from the posterior surface of one arytenoid cartilage to the posterior surface of the other. This muscle contracts to bring together the arytenoid cartilages, thus assisting in closing the posterior portion of the glottis. This does not significantly affect the mechanical properties of the vocal folds. Along with these transverse fibers are oblique fibers. These oblique fibers pass from the posterior portion of the arytenoid on one side to the apex of the arytenoid on the other side, thus crossing in the midline. Some fibers insert at the apex, whereas others travel along the quadrangular membrane. These fibers contract to narrow the laryngeal aditus. Those fibers traveling along the quadrangular membrane (thus the aryepiglottic fold) constitute the aryepiglottic muscle.

Thyroarytenoid Muscle. The thyroarytenoid muscle is classically divided into the thyroarytenoid internus and externus. These have the same attachments, but the internus lies deep or internal to the externus. In addition, the internus is more well developed than the externus. The thyroarytenoid externus arises from the anterior commissure and inserts onto the lateral surface of the arytenoid cartilage. It contracts to bring the vocal process and anterior commissure closer to each other, thus adducting the vocal folds. It also contracts to adduct the false cords. The externus sends a few slips of muscle fibers onto the quadrangular membrane to establish the thyroepiglottic muscle. This muscle, like the aryepiglottic muscle, acts to narrow the laryngeal inlet.

The thyroarytenoid internus or vocalis muscle attaches at the anterior commissure and inserts onto the vocal process, sending a few slips of fibers below the vocal ligament onto the conus elasticus. It contracts to adduct, shorten, thicken, and lower the vocal fold while rounding its edge. The body (muscle) of the vocal fold is actively stiffened, whereas the cover is passively slackened. Recently, immunohistochemical staining for myofibrillar adenosine triphosphatase reveals that the majority of fibers in internus are slow-twitch and those in externus fast-twitch, suggesting its unique human specialization for speech function.[24,25]

Internal Anatomy

The internal anatomy of the larynx consists of three compartments separated by two folds[9,10] (Figure 4). The three compartments are the

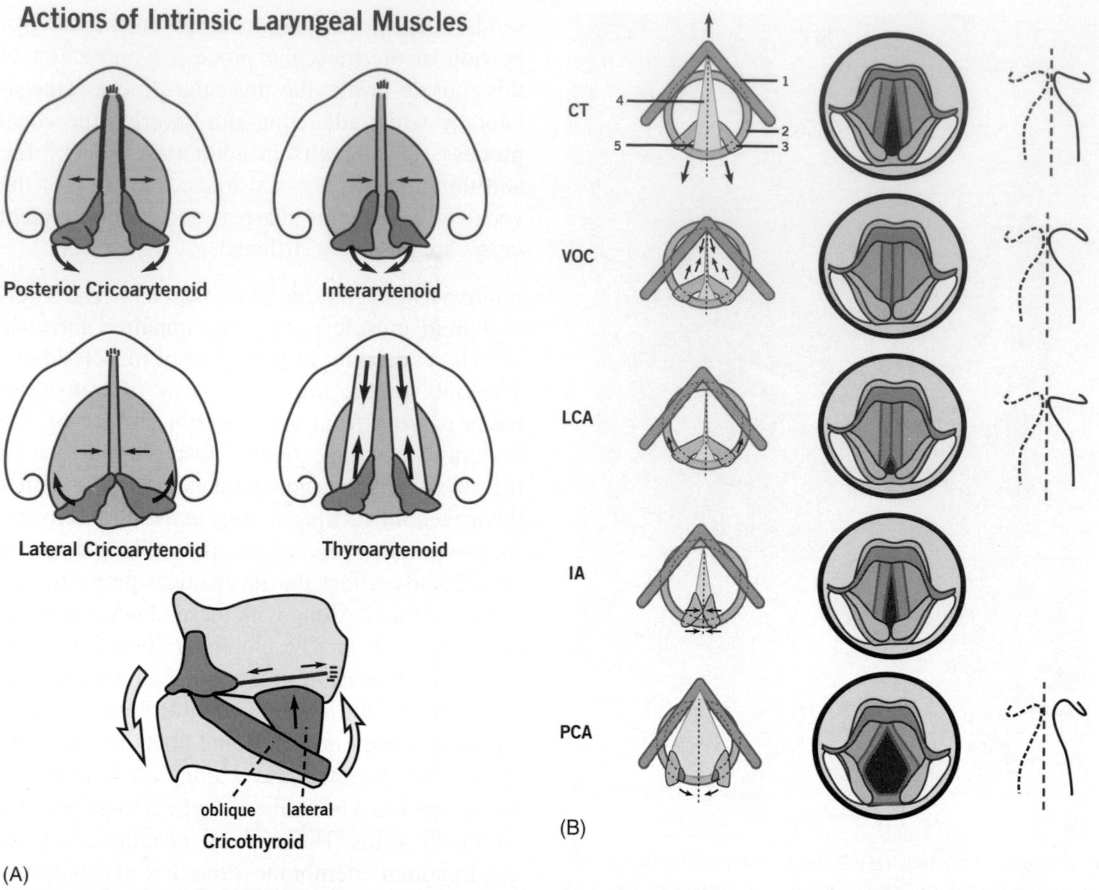

Actions of Intrinsic Laryngeal Muscles

Posterior Cricoarytenoid

Interarytenoid

Lateral Cricoarytenoid

Thyroarytenoid

oblique   lateral

Cricothyroid

(A)

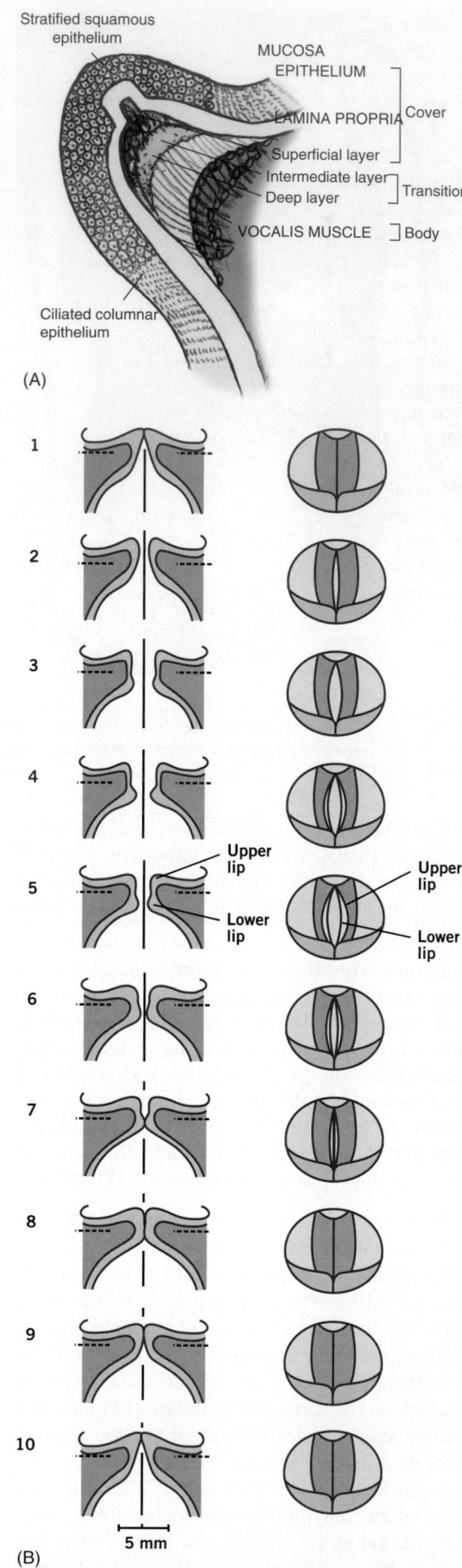

CT

VOC

LCA

IA

PCA

(B)

Figure 6 (A) The intrinsic muscles of the larynx and their actions. Heavy arrows indicate the direction of muscle action; fine arrows indicate the motion of vocal ligaments; and open arrows indicate the motion of cricoid and thyroid cartilages. (B) Schematic presentation of the function of the laryngeal muscles. The left column shows the location of the cartilages and the edge of the vocal folds when the laryngeal muscles are activated individually. The arrow indicates the direction of the force exerted. CT = cricothyroid muscle; IA = interarytenoid muscle; LCA = lateral cricoarytenoid muscle; PCA = posterior cricoarytenoid muscle; VOC = vocalis muscle; 1 = thyroid cartilage; 2 = cricoid cartilage; 3 = arytenoid cartilage; 4 = vocal ligament; 5 = posterior cricoarytenoid ligament. The middle column shows views from above. The right column presents contours of frontal sections at the middle of the membranous portion of the vocal fold. The dotted line shows a control, where no muscle is activated. (Reproduced with permission from reference 20.)

vestibule, ventricle, and infraglottic cavity. The false and true vocal folds separate the above compartments. These mucosa-lined compartments demarcate two spaces of importance: the preepiglottic space and the paraglottic space.

Vestibule. A laryngoscopic view of the larynx reveals the vestibule as that portion of the larynx from the tip of the epiglottis to the false vocal or vestibular folds. Thus, the vestibule is bound by the epiglottis anteriorly, the aryepiglottic folds laterally, and the arytenoid and corniculate cartilages with the interarytenoid muscle posteriorly. In the laryngoscopic view, the anterior commissure is frequently hidden by the protuberance of the epiglottis known as the tubercle. As previously discussed, the vestibular folds are formed by mucosa overlying the vestibular ligament (inferior border of the quadrangular membrane). The submucosa of the ventricle contains numerous seromucinous glands. The secretions produced by these exocrine glands provide both mechanical and immune (lysozyme) protection for the vocal folds.[26]

Ventricle. The ventricle or sinus of Morgagni is the small space between the false and

true vocal folds. The ventricle is often hidden during laryngoscopic examination of the larynx unless exposed by lateralization of the false vocal fold. At the anterior end of the ventricle is a diverticulum known as the laryngeal saccule. The saccule (of Hilton) is lined with mucous glands, which are thought to lubricate the vocal folds. Fibers of the thyroarytenoid muscle line the walls of the saccule and are thought to express mucus from the saccule when they contract. The size of the saccule is quite variable; however, it seldom extends above the superior border of the thyroid cartilage. Abnormal dilatation of the saccule results in an air-filled laryngocele that should be distinguished from a mucocele of the saccule (saccular cyst), which lacks free communication with the ventricle and thus is not air filled.[27] The vocal folds that form the inferior boundary of the ventricle are described in more detail below.

Infraglottic Cavity. The infraglottic cavity extends from the glottis down to the inferior border of the cricoid cartilage. Its lateral boundary is formed by the conus elasticus and walls of the cricoid cartilage.

Figure 7 (A) Schematic illustration showing the laryngeal structure of the adult vocal fold. (Reproduced with permission from reference 21.) (B) Coronal section showing the movement of the vocal folds during one vibratory cycle. (Reproduced with permission from reference 20. Copyright Urban & Fischer Verlag.)

Pyriform Sinus. Although the pyriform sinus is anatomically part of the hypopharynx, understanding its anatomy and its relationship to the larynx is essential. The pyriform sinus is a gutter formed by the aryepiglottic fold, arytenoid cartilage, and superior part of the cricoid cartilage medially and the thyrohyoid membrane and internal surface of the thyroid lamina laterally. Superiorly, it begins at the lateral glossoepiglottic fold. Inferiorly, the apex of the sinus blends with the esophageal inlet at about the superior border of the cricoid (Figure 8). Thus, cancer invasion of the apex implies the necessity of removing a portion of the cricoid if conservation laryngectomy is planned.[14] There are two important markings within the pyriform sinus. Anteriorly in the floor of the sinus, a small fold can be seen, which marks the course of the superior laryngeal nerve. This submucosal course of the nerve makes it possible to anesthetize the nerve topically in the pyriform sinus. The second, more variable landmark is the protrusion made into the sinus from the superior cornu of the thyroid cartilage. This smooth protrusion, which usually presents in the elderly, should not be confused with neoplasm.

Mucosa. The mucosa of the larynx is of two types: pseudostratified ciliated columnar cell (respiratory) epithelium and squamous cell epithelium. Much of the larynx is surfaced by respiratory epithelium; however, the superior portion of the epiglottis, upper portions of the aryepiglottic folds, and free edges of the vocal folds are surfaced by squamous cell epithelium. Beneath this covering epithelium is a variable basement membrane, and separating these two is a layer of loose fibrous stroma. It should be noted that this loose fibrous layer is absent on the true vocal folds as well as the laryngeal (posterior) surface of the epiglottis. The absence of this layer on the posterior surface of the epiglottis accounts for the more intense swelling of the lingual (anterior) surface of the epiglottis in inflammatory conditions of the larynx.

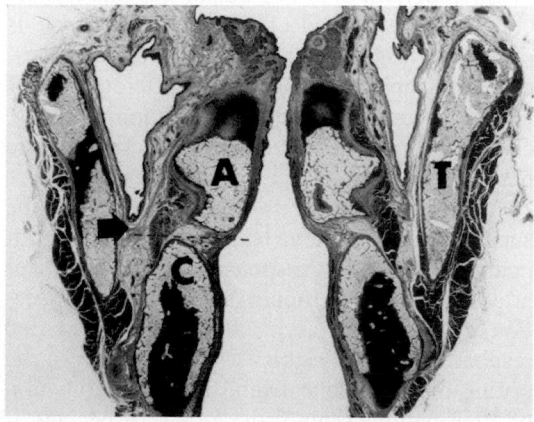

Figure 8 Coronal section through the human larynx, demonstrating the relationship of the cricoid cartilage (C) with the apex of the pyriform sinus (*arrow*). A = arytenoid cartilage; T = thyroid cartilage. (Courtesy of Dr John A. Kirchner.)

Preepiglottic Space. The preepiglottic space, as its name implies, lies anterior to the epiglottis, which serves as its posterior boundary. It is bound superiorly by the hyoepiglottic ligament and mucosa of the valleculae and inferiorly by the thyroepiglottic ligament. The anterior boundaries are the thyrohyoid membrane and the inner surfaces of the thyroid laminae. Laterally, the preepiglottic space opens in the paraglottic spaces. Cancer on the infrahyoid portion of the epiglottis can penetrate the epiglottis and gain access to the preepiglottic space.

Paraglottic Space. A paraglottic space, as its name implies, lies on each side of the glottis. This space lies above and below the true and false vocal folds and is important in the transglottic and extralaryngeal spread of neoplasms. Medially, the space is bound by the quadrangular membrane, ventricle, and conus elasticus. Laterally, it is bound by the perichondrium of the thyroid lamina and the cricothyroid membrane. Anterosuperiorly, the space opens in the posterior portion of the preepiglottic space. The mucosa of the pyriform sinus forms the posterior boundary. The relationships of this paraglottic space make it important in considering the spread of laryngeal cancer. Supraglottic cancer invading into this space may quickly extend extralaryngeally.

Vocal Folds

The anatomy of the vocal folds is complex and is thus considered separately. The vocal fold is considered the structure between the vocal process of the arytenoid and the anterior commissure. The vocal folds and the slit between them (rima glottidis) constitute the glottis. The glottis can be divided by a horizontal line between the tips of the vocal processes. This imaginary line divides the glottis into an intermembranous portion and an intercartilaginous portion. The anterior to posterior (length) ratio of the intermembranous portion to the intercartilaginous is 3:2; however, the ratio of cross-sectional areas defined by them is 2:3. Thus, owing to its more rectangular shape, the intercartilaginous portion is larger. Some have called this the respiratory portion of the rima.[11,28] The membranous or vibratory portion of the vocal folds consists of three well-defined structural layers. From superficial to deep, they are the epithelium, lamina propria (three layers), and vocalis muscle. Hirano divided these layers according to a body-cover concept (see Figure 7A).[28] The cover consists of the overlying epithelium and the gelatinous superficial layer of the lamina propria. The body consists of the vocalis muscle, which he likened to thick rubber bands. Between these exists a transition zone composed of the intermediate (elastic) and deep (collagenous) layers of the lamina propria. According to this concept, the vocal folds consist of a multilayered vibrator with increasing stiffness from the cover to the body. Thus, the cover is responsible for most of the vibratory action of the vocal folds. At the anterior and posterior ends of the vocal folds exist an anterior and a posterior macula flava, respectively.

These are essentially a thickening of the intermediate (elastic) layer of the lamina propria and are thought to function as "cushions" protecting the ends of the vocal folds from vibratory damage. It should be noted that the same body-cover concept does not apply to the larynx of children, because of the more homogeneous nature of the lamina propria. It is not until nearly the end of adolescence that the lamina matures into its adult form. In the senile larynx, the elastic layer and the vocalis muscle tend to atrophy, whereas the collagenous layer thickens. The cover becomes thickened and edematous secondary to changes in the superficial layer of the lamina, whereas the epithelium itself changes little.

The shape of the true and false vocal folds carries biomechanical significance. When seen in coronal section, both appear as valve-like structures, with the leaflets of the false folds pointing inferiorly and those of the true folds pointing superiorly (see Figure 4). Thus, the false folds passively impede egress of air, whereas the true folds impede its ingress. Working with cadaver larynges, Brunton and Cash demonstrated that the false folds offered a resistance equaling 30 mm Hg to the egress of air from below, whereas the true folds offered a resistance equaling 140 mm Hg to the ingress of air from above.[29] Both structures offered little resistance to the opposite flow of air; ie, they act as one-way valves.

Vessels

Arteries and Veins. The arterial supply to the larynx consists of the superior and inferior laryngeal arteries.[9–14] After the superior thyroid artery branches off the external carotid, it courses lateral to the laryngohyoid complex and gives off the superior laryngeal artery at approximately the level of the hyoid bone. This artery then runs anteromedially with the internal branch of the superior laryngeal nerve to enter the thyrohyoid membrane inferior to the nerve. It then enters the submucosa of the pyriform sinus and is distributed to intralaryngeal structures. The superior thyroid also gives off a cricothyroid branch that courses horizontally below the thyroid cartilage. The inferior laryngeal artery is a branch of the inferior thyroid artery that comes off the thyrocervical trunk branching from the subclavian artery. After coursing posterior to the cricothyroid joint with the recurrent laryngeal nerve, the artery enters the larynx by passing through a gap in the inferior constrictor muscle known as the Killian-Jamieson area. The artery is then distributed to the remainder of the internal larynx, making multiple anastomoses with the superior laryngeal artery. The venous supply parallels the arterial supply.

Lymphatics. An appreciation of the lymphatics of the larynx is prerequisite to understanding the spread of cancer of the larynx, as well as the operative procedures designed to eradicate the disease.[9–14,30] The lymphatics of the larynx are divided into superficial (intramucosal) and deep (submucosal) groups. The deep network is further divided into right and left halves, with little communication between them. These two halves can be further divided into supraglottic, glottic, and subglottic, with special consideration given to the ventricle in the supraglottic region. Although the superficial network is richly anastomotic throughout the larynx, it is the deep network that is important in the spread of cancer and will be given further consideration. The drainage of the supraglottic structures (aryepiglottic folds and false cords) follows the superior laryngeal and superior thyroid vessels. Thus, the lymphatics flow from the pyriform sinus through the thyrohyoid membrane to end primarily in the deep jugular chain around the carotid bifurcation. It should be noted that the epiglottis is a midline structure; thus, its lymphatic drainage is bilateral. The lymphatic drainage of the ventricle is different from the other supraglottic structures. Dye injected into the ventricle enters the paraglottic space and is quickly spread by the lymphatic system through the cricothyroid membrane and also into the ipsilateral lobe of the thyroid (justifying its resection in laryngectomy). The true vocal folds are devoid of lymphatics, accounting for the high curability of cancer localized to this structure. The subglottic larynx has two lymphatic drainage systems. One system follows the inferior thyroid vessels to end in the lower portion of the deep jugular chain of lymph nodes as well as the subclavian, paratracheal, and tracheoesophageal chains. The other system pierces the cricothyroid membrane. This system appears to receive lymphatics from both sides of the larynx and disseminate bilaterally to the middle deep cervical lymph nodes as well as the prelaryngeal (Delphian) lymph nodes.

PHYSIOLOGY

As previously stated, the three functions of the larynx in order of priority are (1) protection of the lower airway, (2) respiration, and (3) phonation.[1] A flawless performance of these functions requires an intact neuromuscular system to respond to both volitional and reflex signals presented to the larynx.

Innervation

The pattern of innervation to and from the larynx and the type and distribution of its receptors determine the functional capabilities of the larynx. The larynx is innervated by the superior and inferior laryngeal nerves. The superior laryngeal nerve leaves the nodose ganglion to pass between the carotid artery and the laryngohyoid complex. It divides into a larger internal and smaller external branch. The internal branch pierces the thyrohyoid membrane with the superior laryngeal artery and becomes the sensory supply to the ipsilateral supraglottic portion of the larynx, whereas the external branch innervates the cricothyroid and inferior constrictor muscles. The inferior laryngeal nerve originates from the recurrent laryngeal nerve and runs in the tracheoesophageal groove. It enters the larynx posterior to the cricothyroid

joint and classically divides into an anterior adductor and a posterior abductor branch. This branching, however, is quite variable, as is the muscular innervation from the branches.[5]

The receptors of the larynx can be divided into mucosal, articular, and myotatic. These receptors mediate much of the reflex activity of the larynx. The mucosal receptors respond to stimuli such as touch, mucosal deformation (mechanoreceptors), and liquids. The articular receptors are located in the joint capsule and respond to deformation of the capsule. The myotatic receptors respond to muscular stretch and appear to be most abundant in the vocalis muscle.[31]

Afferent System. The sensory innervation to the mucosa of the supraglottic portion of the larynx is carried by the internal branch of the ipsilateral superior laryngeal nerve, which is divided into three divisions. The superior division mainly supplies the mucosa of the laryngeal surface of the epiglottis, the middle division supplies the mucosa of the true and false vocal folds and the aryepiglottic fold, and the inferior division supplies the mucosa of the arytenoid, part of the subglottis, the anterior wall of the hypopharynx, and the upper esophageal sphincter.[32] The cricoarytenoid joint and thyroepiglottic ligament are both innervated by the internal branch of the superior laryngeal nerve. The inferior laryngeal nerve supplies the major portions of mucosa below the glottis as well as muscle spindles of intrinsic muscles. The external branch of the superior laryngeal nerve contains afferent fibers from the cricothyroid joint and from deep muscle receptors.

Histologic examination has revealed the presence of free nerve endings, Merkel cells, Meissner corpuscles, and taste buds scattered in the larynx. Mechanoreceptors are located either in the superficial mucosa or in the muscles and laryngeal joints. Some of them are spontaneously active, whereas others are silent until stimulated. The supraglottic portion of the larynx also has chemical and thermal sensors. A large number of taste buds populate the laryngeal surface of the epiglottis and extend caudally along the aryepiglottic folds, reaching peak density at the caudal extreme of the folds.[33,34] This sensory distribution facilitates the supraglottic portion of the larynx in its role of preventing foreign material from penetrating into the larynx.[35] These respond to a number of chemical stimuli and to water. The taste buds of the larynx tend to be most sensitive to the pH and tonicity of the stimulus. In this regard, the water receptors of the epiglottis appear to play a role in the production of prolonged apnea. When stimulated, they lead to a slowing of respiration with an increase in tidal volume. Chemoreceptors of the larynx are adapted to detect chemicals that are not salinelike in composition and can play an important role in modifying reflexes involved in the maintenance of upper airway patency.[34] It is important to note that this same response does not occur with saline. It is felt that the receptors may be responding to the washout of chloride ions.[31] Theoretically, this may be the

mechanism by which cold-steam mist assists the child with croup (slowing and deepening breathing, thus decreasing turbulent flow).[36] Interestingly, this response is more potent early in life. This apneic response has also been implicated in sudden infant death syndrome.[31] The vocal folds also have touch receptors that are more abundant posteriorly than anteriorly. The afferent impulses generated are delivered to the tractus solitarius through the ganglion nodosum.

Efferent System. The motor innervation is primarily through the inferior laryngeal nerve. This nerve innervates all the intrinsic muscles of the larynx except the cricothyroid, which is innervated by the external branch of the superior laryngeal nerve. Each nerve is responsible for the muscles on the ipsilateral side of the larynx, with the exception of the interarytenoid muscle. Thus, the only unpaired muscle of the larynx receives its innervation from both inferior laryngeal nerves. Injury to the recurrent laryngeal nerve leaves the injured vocal fold in the paramedian position, resulting from the adductor effect of the intact cricothyroid. Unilateral injury to the superior laryngeal nerve causes the posterior glottic opening to rotate to the paralyzed side, bowing the paralyzed vocal fold.[11,35] These changes in the larynx can be seen on laryngeal endoscopy.

Neurophysiology of Protective Function

The glottic closure reflex is a polysynaptic reflex that allows the larynx to protect the lower airway from penetration and aspiration. However, when exaggerated, this reflex accounts for the production of laryngospasm. Protective closure of the larynx occurs in three tiers. In the first tier, the laryngeal inlet is contracted by collapsing the aryepiglottic folds medially. The anterior and posterior gaps are filled by the epiglottic tubercle and the arytenoid cartilages, respectively. In the second tier, the false vocal folds are brought together. The final and most important tier occurs at the level of the true vocal folds. Because the valvular action of the true vocal folds resists ingress of material, they offer the most important level of protection. It should be noted that it is the thyroarytenoid or slips from this muscle that contract at each level of closure. This muscle is one of the fastest contracting of all striated muscles in the body. Classically, the afferent limb of this reflex occurs through stimulation of touch, chemical, or thermal receptors in the supraglottic portion of the larynx.[37]

Laryngospasm occurs when stimulation of the superior laryngeal nerve leads to a prolonged adductor response. This response is maintained well after the initiating stimulus is removed, and section of the superior laryngeal nerves abolishes the response. Clinically, this is typically seen in the setting of endotracheal intubation or extubation or after manipulation of the airway, especially if blood has contaminated the laryngeal inlet. The response is dampened in the face of barbiturates, hypercapnia, positive intrathoracic pressure, and severe hypoxia.[38]

Although not classically considered part of the protective reflex, reflex swallowing from stimulation of the superior laryngeal nerve may have protective functions. It has been shown that reflex swallowing occurs with application of hypotonic fluids to the supraglottic portion of the larynx, particularly the laryngeal surface of the epiglottis, glottis, and interior of the larynx. Although this is not the normal mechanism to initiate swallowing, it may serve to protect the larynx against fluid that enters the laryngeal inlet.[31]

Neurophysiology of Respiratory Function

It is intuitive that if the larynx is the sphincter to the lower airway for respiration to occur, the sphincter should actively open during inspiration. Also, the opening of the folds must be synchronous with, but slightly precede, the descent of the diaphragm. Through the work of many individuals, this observation is well supported.[35,39,40] The respiratory center of the medulla, with the help of higher central nervous system and peripheral input, maintains eupneic respiration. It drives the synchronous opening of the glottis and descent of the diaphragm during inspiration. The opening of the glottis is primarily through the action of the posterior cricoarytenoid. However, in hyperpneic conditions, the cricothyroid contracts rhythmically with the posterior cricoarytenoid.[39,40] The contraction of both these muscles increases the glottic aperture in both anteroposterior and horizontal dimensions. During phonation, the cricothyroid lengthens and passively adducts the vocal folds. However, during respiration, when contracted in concert with the posterior cricoarytenoid, the effect is to lengthen the open glottis, thus increasing the cross-sectional area for airflow. Understanding the role that the cricothyroid plays as an accessory muscle of inspiration underlies the rationale for superior laryngeal nerve section in the face of bilateral recurrent laryngeal nerve paralysis. Bilateral paralysis produces dyspnea, which will lead to cricothyroid contraction, further adducting the paralyzed folds. Unilateral superior laryngeal nerve section reduces glottic resistance by preventing full adduction.

The rhythmicity of the phrenic nerve and the posterior cricoarytenoid can be increased by hypercapnia and ventilatory obstruction. It is lessened by hypocapnia. The effect of ventilatory resistance on posterior cricoarytenoid activity has been extensively studied in the canine model. In this model, when ventilatory resistance is eliminated, so is the reflex abductor activity of the posterior cricoarytenoid. It is felt that the afferent limb of this reflex resides within the ascending vagus nerve and that the end-organ receptors are located within the thorax, although their precise location is unknown. The longer abductor activity is lost, the more difficult it is to reestablish.[41] This is the rationale for downsizing tracheostomy tubes (thus gradually increasing ventilatory load) prior to decannulation.

The role of the larynx in controlling expiration must also be considered. It is well known that the control of respiratory rate occurs primarily through variation of the expiratory phase. The time of expiration is dependent on the ventilatory resistance produced by the glottis. As discussed above, the cricothyroid contracting with the posterior cricoarytenoid will give the maximal glottic opening and hence the lowest ventilatory resistance. In this regard, cricothyroid contraction during expiration occurs when the critical subglottic pressure change of 30 cm H_2O/s is exceeded and continues as long as positive subglottic pressure is maintained. As expected, this threshold for activation is reduced in hypercapnia (allowing for quicker expiration and a faster respiratory rate) and increased in hypocapnia.[42]

Neurophysiology of Phonation

The complex mechanisms of phonatory control coordinate central and peripheral components.

Electromyographic investigation of the control of peripheral neuromuscular systems involved in phonation has demonstrated specific intrinsic and extrinsic muscle function in humans. Central mechanisms are less well understood, and their understanding often relies on animal models, from which the function in the unique phonatory systems of the human may only be inferred.

As a general model, the larynx, as a system, must respond to central commands from linguistic and motor centers. Signals are relayed to the motor cortex in the precentral gyrus and on to motor nuclei in the brainstem and spinal cord. These signals are transmitted to the respiratory, laryngeal, and articulatory muscles responsible for speech and voice production. These messages are influenced by the extrapyramidal system, including the cerebral cortex, cerebellum, and basal ganglia, exerting fine control of respiration, phonation, and articulation.[20]

Specific connectivity and the central control of brainstem motor neurons responsible for voluntary control of phonation remain illusive. Laryngeal reflexes, which are key to the coordination of respiration, phonation, and deglutition, are understood primarily from the research focused on respiration and deglutition.[31] Further, central projections to laryngeal mechanisms are not consistent across species and may differ

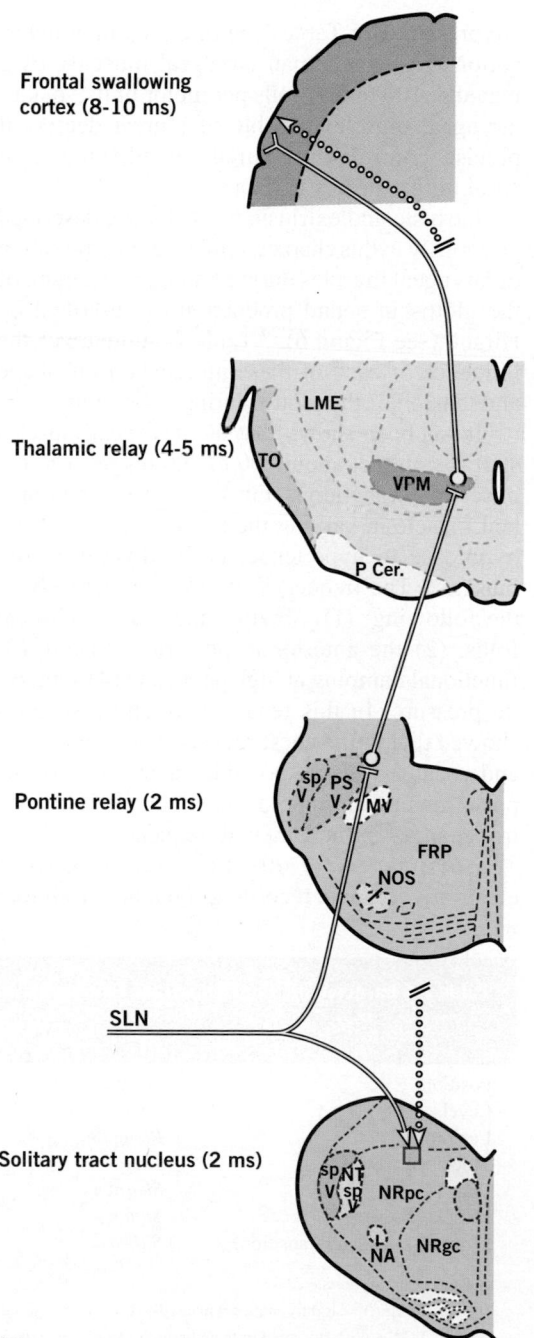

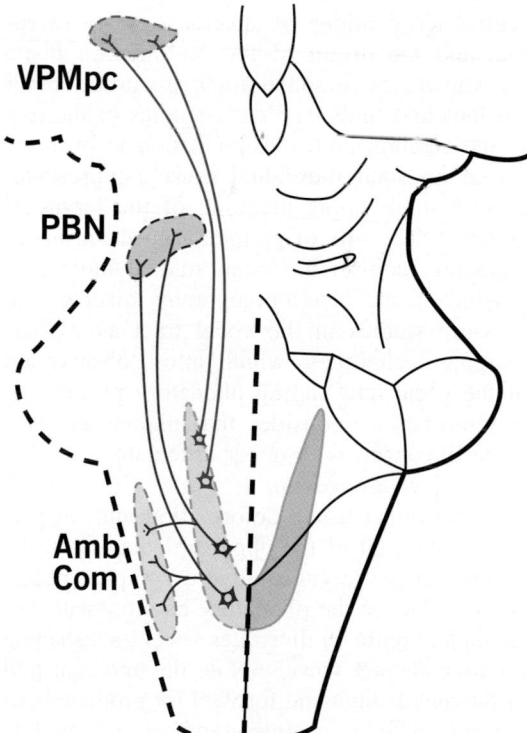

Figure 9 (A) Schematic illustration of fibers of the superior laryngeal nerve dividing into two branches, one going to the nucleus tractus solitarius, and the other to the parabrachial nuclei, where synapses are made with cells projecting to the thalamus. (Reproduced with permission from reference 43. Copyright Springer-Verlag.) (B) Schematic illustration of the projection of nucleus tractus solitarius cells. Rostral cells project directly to the thalamus, whereas more caudal cells project to the nucleus ambiguus (Amb Com) and parabrachial nuclei (PBN). (Reproduced with permission from reference 44.)

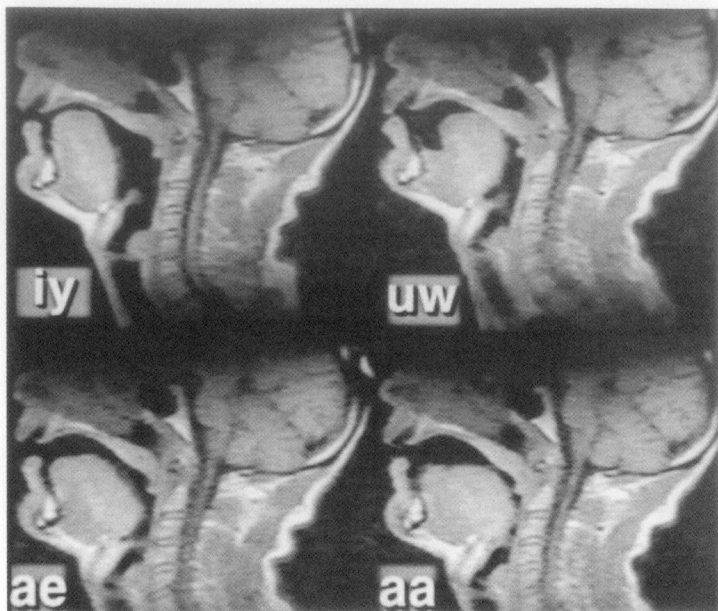

Table 1 Contraction Times in Milliseconds for Laryngeal Muscles by Species

Muscle	Dog	Cat	Human
		Subject	
Thyroarytenoid	14	21	35
	12.5	25	—
Posterior	30		
cricoarytenoid	44	22	—
Lateral			
cricoarytenoid	16	19	—
Cricothyroid	35	44	35

Figure 10 Magnetic resonance images of the vocal tract during sustained production of four vowels illustrate contrast in shape as viewed in sagittal section. (Courtesy of Carol Gracco, PhD.)

from nonhuman primates to humans as well. The nucleus tractus solitarius, periaqueductal gray matter, parabrachial nucleus, locus caeruleus, and ventromedial nucleus of the thalamus are all areas anatomically associated with the laryngeal system.[31] Figure 9 illustrates branching of the superior laryngeal nerve with central connectivity and projections of the nucleus tractus solitarius. However, specific mechanisms of control are not well defined. In some cases, the central terminations of specific sensory receptors and the origin of the motoneuron fibers are known, as in somatotopic organization for the face and limbs. To date, studies of the role of the cerebral cortex in phonation in primates reveal no such individual muscle representation or somatotopic mapping of the laryngeal system.[31] The role of peripheral mechanisms in phonatory control has been studied more successfully using electromyography, airflow, and pressure studies in the vocal tract as well as imaging techniques, which allow observation of the vocal tract during phonatory postures. It is important to consider that phonation takes place in concert with upper articulators, the lip, tongue, jaw, and velum.

Mechanical tissue deformation and, in particular, the pull of the upper articulators on the larynx via the laryngeal–hyoid complex necessarily influence the phonatory environment. For example, Figure 10 illustrates vocal tract shaping for four distinct vowels. Note the apparent pull of the tongue high and forward for production of /i/ (labeled "iy"), in contrast to posterior and low posture for /a/ (labeled "aa"). The consequent constriction or, conversely, the opening of the posterior part of the pharynx plays a key role in the acoustics of sound produced for each of these postures and influences laryngeal posturing for phonation.[45]

Electromyographic studies of specific muscle function indicate firing rates uniquely suited for fine control of laryngeal function. Contraction times for the intrinsic muscles in several species

are presented in Table 1. Further, the high innervation ratio for human laryngeal muscles, estimated at 100 to 200 cells per motor unit,[46] makes laryngeal muscles capable of a great degree of precise control as required for adjustment of speaking frequency and intensity.

Intrinsic and extrinsic musculature, described previously in this chapter, influence specific action of laryngeal muscles during phonatory shaping of the glottis in sound production as described by Hirano (see Figure 6).[20] Table 2 summarizes the influence of each of these muscles on the shape and tension of the glottis during phonation.

It has been shown that the laryngeal muscles start to contract about 100 to 200 ms prior to the onset of phonation.[47] Further, the most important muscle in varying the phonation style (from hypotense to hypertense) is the thyroarytenoid muscle.[48] The frequency of vibration depends on the following: (1) vibratory mass of both vocal folds, (2) the anterior to posterior tension, (3) functional damping at high pitch, and (4) subglottic pressure. In this regard, Gay and associates showed that in the chest register, the cricothyroid and vocalis, with the possible contribution of the posterior cricoarytenoid, most consistently control changes in fundamental frequency.[49]

Lovqvist and others later described electromyographic recordings obtained from four

intrinsic laryngeal muscles with simultaneous transillumination and acoustic signals.[50] The vocalis and lateral cricoarytenoid muscles were observed to participate in the control of both articulation and phonation. The interarytenoid muscle appeared to be involved only in articulatory adjustments. Activity in the cricothyroid was primarily related to changes in fundamental frequency. This muscle also showed an increase in activity for voiceless sounds. In addition, the vocalis muscle appeared to participate in glottal adduction without complete closure in voiceless clustered sounds, with the lateral cricoarytenoid and the interarytenoid playing no particular roles. Studies such as these underscore the complex interactive nature of laryngeal musculature in phonatory and articulatory interaction.

In considering the phonatory process, a variety of factors necessarily contribute to the acoustic product as defined in Table 3. The psychoacoustic parameters of pitch, loudness, quality, and fluctuation are correlated with acoustic qualities of fundamental frequency, amplitude, waveform, and acoustic spectrum. High-speed photography and observation of vocal fold vibration via videostroboscopic endoscopy reveal much about the behavior of the glottis during phonation.[20,51] The vibrations of the vocal folds are a passive phenomenon and represent the basis of the aerodynamic theory of sound production. Vibration of the vocal folds changes DC airflow to AC airflow, converting aerodynamic energy to acoustic energy. The mucosal wave produced by these vibrations has been captured on ultrahigh-speed photography by Hirano.[21] The vibratory cycle is described

Table 2 Characteristic Functions of the Laryngeal Muscles in Vocal Fold Adjustments

	CT	VOC	LCA	IA	PCA
Position	Paramed	*Adduct*	*Adduct*	*Adduct*	*Abduct*
Level	Lower	Lower	*Lower*	0	*Elevate*
Length	*Elongate*	*Shorten*	Elongate	(Shorten)	*Elongate*
Thickness	*Thin*	*Thicken*	Thin	(Thicken)	Thin
Edge	*Sharpen*	*Round*	Sharpen	0	Round
Muscle (body)	*Stiffen*	*Stiffen*	Stiffen	(Slacken)	Stiffen
Mucosa (cover and transition)	*Stiffen*	*Slacken*	Stiffen	(Slacken)	Stiffen

Adapted from reference 21.

0 = no effect; ( ) = slightly; italics = markedly; CT = cricothyroid muscle; IA = interarytenoid muscle; *LCA = lateral cricoarytenoid muscle*; PCA = posterior cricoarytenoid muscle; VOC = *vocalis muscle*.

Table 3 Parameters in the Peripheral Process of the Production and Perception of Voice

| Level | Parameters That Regulate Vibratory Pattern of Vocal Fold | | Parameters That Specify Vibratory Pattern | Parameters That Specify Sound Generated | |
	Physiologic	Physical	Physical	Acoustic	Psychoacoustic
Parameters	Neuromuscular control	(Primary)	Fundamental period	Fundamental frequency	Pitch
	Respiratory muscles	Expiratory force	Symmetry	Amplitude (intensity)	Loudness
			Periodicity		
	Laryngeal muscles	Vocal fold	Uniformity	Waveform	
		Position	Glottal closure	Acoustic spectrum	Quality
		Shape and size	Amplitude		
		Elasticity	Mucosal wave	Fluctuations	Fluctuations
		Viscosity	Speed of excursion		
	Articulatory muscles	State of vocal tract			
		(Secondary)	Glottal area waveform		
		Pressure drop across glottis			
		Volume velocity			
		Glottal impedance			

Adapted from reference 21.

as having three phases: opening, closing, and closed. By convention, the cycle is described as beginning with the vocal folds closed. Frames 1 to 5 (see Figure 7B) represent the opening phase. During this phase, subglottic pressure increases, forcing the vocal folds apart from an inferior to superior direction until the glottis opens, letting air escape and thus releasing subglottic pressure. As the elastic recoil of the vocal folds forces them back together, the portion of the vocal fold that was the last to open (superior portion) is the last to close. Thus, the vocal folds close from inferior to superior (frames 6 to 8). The folds then remain closed until the subglottic pressure

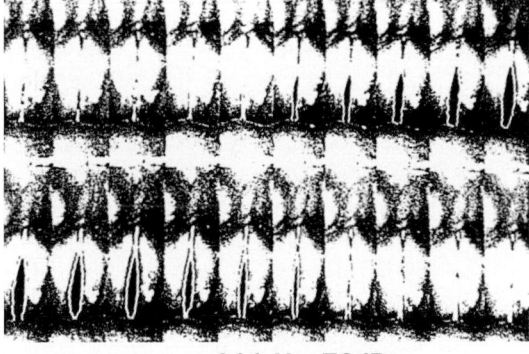

211 Hz, 72dB

(A)

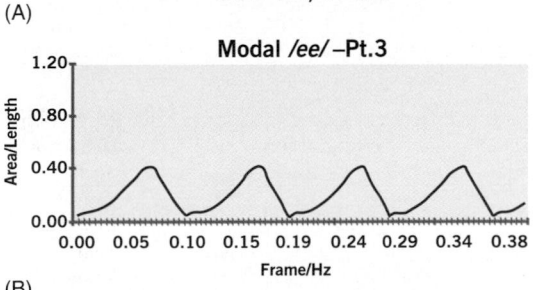

(B)

Figure 11 (A) Twenty frames of a glottal cycle are digitized. The glottal margin has been traced by computer. (B) Plot of the glottal area waveform (female, 211 Hz, 72 dB). (Adapted from reference 51. Copyright Lippincott Williams & Wilkins.)

builds up enough to force them open again. Anatomically, the movement of the mucosal wave depends on the soft and compliant lamina propria and a healthy layered structure. In extracting complex details of glottal area waveforms from videostrobolaryngoscopic recordings using modern computers and software (Figure 11), Woo demonstrated male and female differences as well as influences of pitch and loudness.[51] Women commonly demonstrate small posterior glottal gaps that seem to have no pathologic acoustic significance, whereas their glottal cycles have shorter closed phases than those of men. Mean peak glottal area is smaller in women, not only because of their smaller anatomic size but also because their higher frequency of vibration limits the lateral excursion of the vocal folds, thereby reducing the amplitude of vibration. As intensity increases, the closing phase becomes shorter and the closed period becomes longer, suggesting that the closing patterns of vocal folds are an especially important feature in normal and pathologic phonation. The coordination of higher cortical centers interacts with specific musculature in the vocal tract to produce acoustic products recognized as speech. The laryngeal contribution to this product continues to be revealed in basic studies of phonation as an interactive process.

REFERENCES

1. Negus VE. The Comparative Anatomy and Physiology of the Larynx. London: Heinemann; 1949.
2. Holinger LD, Lusk RP, Green CG. Pediatric Laryngology and Bronchoesophagology. Philadelphia: Lippincott-Raven; 1987.
3. Moore KL, Persaud TVN. The Developing Human: Clinically Orientated Embryology, 6th edition. Philadelphia: W.B. Saunders; 1998.
4. Zaw-Tun HA, Burdi AR. Reexamination of the origin and early development of the human larynx. Acta Anat 1985;122:163–84.
5. Henick DH. Three-dimensional analysis of murine laryngeal development. Ann Otol Rhinol Laryngol 1993;102:3–24.
6. Zaw-Tun HA. Development of congenital laryngeal atresias and clefts. Ann Otol Rhinol Laryngol 1988;97:353–8.
7. Pohunek P. Development, structure and function of the upper airways. Paediatr Respir Rev 2004;5:2–8.
8. Milczuk HA, Smith JD, Everts EC. Congenital laryngeal webs: Surgical management and clinical embryology. Int J Pediatr Otorhinolaryngol 2000;52:1–9.
9. Maue WM, Dickinson DR. Cartilages and ligaments of the adult larynx. Arch Otolaryngol 1971;94:432–9.
10. Meiteles LZ, Lin PT, Wenk EJ. An anatomic study of the external laryngeal framework with surgical implications. Otolaryngol Head Neck Surg 1992;106:235–40.
11. Hollinshead WH. Anatomy for Surgeons, Volume 1: The Head and Neck, 3rd edition. Philadelphia: JB Lippincott; 1982.
12. Spector GJ. Anatomy of the larynx. In: Ballenger JJ, editor. Diseases of the Nose, Throat, Ear, Head and Neck, 13th edition. Philadelphia: Lea & Febiger; 1985.
13. Hast MH. Anatomy of the larynx. In: English GM, editor. Otolaryngology, Volume 3. Philadelphia: JB Lippincott; 1993.
14. Sasaki CT, Driscoll BP, Gracco C. Anatomy and physiology of the larynx. In: Ballenger JJ, Snow JB, editors. Otorhinolaryngology Head and Neck Surgery, 15th edition. Baltimore, MD: Williams & Wilkins; 1996. p. 422–37.
15. Staubesand J, Taylor AN. Sabotta: Atlas of Human Anatomy, Volume 1, 11th edition. Baltimore, MD: Urban and Schwarzenberg; 1990.
16. Chamberlain WE, Young BR. Ossification (so-called "calcification") of normal laryngeal cartilages mistaken for foreign body. Am J Roentgen Rad Ther 1935;33:441–50.
17. Hately W, Evison E, Samuel E. The pattern of ossification in the laryngeal cartilages: A radiological study. Br J Radiol 1965;38:585–91.
18. Kirchner JA. What have whole organ sections contributed to the treatment of laryngeal cancer. Ann Otol Rhinol Laryngol 1989;98:661–6.
19. Cooper MH. Anatomy of the larynx. In: Blitzer A, Brin MF, Sasaki CT, et al, editors. Neurologic Disorders of the Larynx. New York: Thieme Medical Publishers; 1992.
20. Hirano M. Clinical Examination of Voice. New York: Springer-Verlag; 1981.
21. Hirano M. Phonosurgery: Basic and clinical investigations. Otologia (Fukuoka) 1975;21:239.
22. Sanders I, Jacobs I, Wu BL, Biller HF. The three bellies of the canine posterior cricoarytenoid muscle: Implications for understanding laryngeal function. Laryngoscope 1993;103:171–7.
23. Sanders I, Rao F, Biller HF. Arytenoid motion evoked by regional electrical stimulation of the canine posterior cricoarytenoid muscle. Laryngoscope 1994;104:456–62.
24. Han Y, Wang J, Fischman DA, et al. Slow tonic muscle fibers in the thyroarytenoid muscles of human vocal folds: a possible specialization for speech. Anat Rec 1999;256:146–57.
25. Sanders I. The microanatomy of the vocal folds. In: Rubin JS, Sataloff RT, Korovin GS, Gould WJ, editors. Diagnosis and Treatment of Voice Disorders. New York: Igaku-Shoin; 1995.
26. Gracco C, Kahane JC. Age-related changes in the vestibular folds of the human larynx: A histomorphometric study. J Voice 1989;3:204–12.

27. Holinger LD. Pharyngoceles, laryngoceles, and saccular cysts. In: English GM, editor. Otolaryngology, Volume 3. Philadelphia: JB Lippincott; 1993.

28. Hirano M. Phonosurgical anatomy of the larynx. In: Ford CN, Bless DM, editors. Phonosurgery: Assessment and Surgical Management of Voice Disorders. New York: Raven Press; 1991.

29. Brunton TL, Cash T. The valvular action of the larynx. J Anat Physiol 1883;17:363.

30. Johner CH. The lymphatics of the larynx. Otolaryngol Clin North Am 1970;3:439–51.

31. Garrett DJ, Larson CR. Neurology of the laryngeal system. In: Ford CN, Bless DM, editors. Phonosurgery: Assessment and Surgical Management of Voice Disorders. New York: Raven Press; 1991.

32. Sanders I, Mu L. Anatomy of human internal superior laryngeal nerve. Anat Rec 1998;252:646–56.

33. Anderson JW, Sant'Ambrogio FB, Mathew OP, Sant'Ambrogio G. Water-responsive laryngeal receptors in the dog are not specialized endings. Respir Physiol 1990;79:33–43.

34. Bradley RM. Sensory receptors of the larynx. Am J Med 2000;108:47–50.

35. Sasaki CT. Physiology of the larynx. In: English GM, editor. Otolaryngology, Volume 3. Philadelphia: JB Lippincott; 1993.

36. Sasaki CT, Suzuki M. The respiratory mechanism of aerosol inhalation in treatment of partial airway obstruction. Pediatrics 1977;59:689–94.

37. Sasaki CT, Suzuki M. Laryngeal reflexes in cat, dog and man. Arch Otolaryngol 1976;102:400–2.

38. Suzuki M, Sasaki CT. Laryngeal spasm: Neurophysiologic redefinition. Ann Otol Rhinol Laryngol 1977;86:150–7.

39. Suzuki M, Kirchner JA. The posterior cricoarytenoid as an inspiratory muscle. Ann Otol Rhinol Laryngol 1969;78:849–64.

40. Suzuki M, Kirchner JA, Murakami Y. The cricothyroid as a respiratory muscle. Its characteristics in bilateral recurrent laryngeal nerve paralysis. Ann Otol Rhinol Laryngol 1970;79:976–83.

41. Sasaki CT, Fukuda H, Kirchner JA. Laryngeal abductor activity in response to varying ventilatory resistance. Trans Am Acad Ophthalmol Otolaryngol 1973;77:403–10.

42. Sasaki CT. Electrophysiology of the larynx. In: Blitzer A, Brin MF, Sasaki CT, et al, editors. Neurologic Disorder of the Larynx. New York: Thieme Medical Publishers; 1992.

43. Car A, Jean A, Roman C. A pontine primary relay for ascending projections of the superior laryngeal nerve. Exp Brain Res 1975;22:197–210.

44. Beckstead RM, Morse JR, Rorgren R. The nucleus of the solitary tract in the monkey: Projections to the thalamus and brain stem nuclei. J Comp Neurol 1980;190:259–82.

45. Gracco C. Vocal Tract Imaging. New York: Biomedical Communications; 1994.

46. Kempster GB, Larson CR, Distler MK. Effects of electrical stimulation of cricothyroid and thyroarytenoid muscles on voice fundamental frequency. J Voice 1988;2:221–9.

47. Buchthal F, Faaborg-Anderson K. Electromyography of laryngeal and respiratory muscles: Correlation with phonation and respiration. Ann Otol Rhinol Laryngol 1964;73:118–23.

48. Hirano M, Koike Y, Joyner J. Style of phonation: An electromyographic investigation of some laryngeal muscles. Arch Otolaryngol 1969;89:902–7.

49. Gay T, Strome M, Hirose H, et al. Electromyography of the intrinsic laryngeal muscles during phonation. Ann Otol Rhinol Laryngol 1972;81:401–9.

50. Lovqvist A, McGarr N, Honda K. Laryngeal muscles and articulatory control. J Acoust Soc Am 1984;76:951–4.

51. Woo P. Quantification of videostrobolaryngoscopic findings–measurements of the normal glottal cycle. Laryngoscope 1996;106:1–27.

73

Assessment of Vocal Function

Christine M. Sapienza, PhD

Gayle E. Woodson, MD

Standard tests of voice assessment for patients with voice disorders are not analogous to the battery of audiometric tests that have evolved for assessing hearing loss. In audiology, the testing paradigm determines how well subjects can perceive specific sounds. In contrast, voice evaluation sets out to assess the performance of voluntary tasks, in which there is considerable performance variability, not only among subjects but also within the same person. A flexible instrument, the healthy human voice is able to produce a wide variety of "sounds." Even when a vocal task is tightly specified, with respect to pitch and loudness, the vocal quality can vary almost infinitely. Further, it is difficult to describe objectively and quantitatively the range of vocal qualities that a person can produce and perceive. Finally, there is great variation in the types of voice distortion that can be caused by a disorder, ranging from a perceived breathy voice quality to a strain, strangled voice quality. Thus, there is not a single parameter that can distinguish a normal from an abnormal voice, particularly when the alterations to the voice are only mildly or moderately distorted. Despite these problems, data in the literature support the use of certain vocal measures in managing patients with voice disorders. The diagnosis is based on the history and physical examination, while vocal function tests are used to quantify a voice disorder's severity and document treatment effectiveness.

Categories of voice assessment methods include perceptual assessment, quantitative analysis of acoustic signals, physiologic measurement of airflow and pressure, observation of the vibratory vocal fold movement during voicing tasks with videostroboscopy and patient's self-assessment (Table 1). There are some who believe that quantitative measures of vocal function are only relevant if they correlate with perceptual assessment; however, in most cases, it is unlikely that a strong correlation will exist between quantitative and qualitative measures because instrumental measures are focused on one component of the voice signal (frequency or intensity) while perceptual evaluation is influenced by multiple factors. Until further research is done to determine the specific components of the voice signal that strongly correlate with perception, each of the testing procedures should be considered separately but important facets of the assessment process.

PATIENT'S SELF-ASSESSMENT

The patient's self-assessment is the sine qua non in defining whether a voice disorder warrants treatment. As abnormal as a voice may sound to others, including clinicians, if it serves the patient's daily needs, it is an acceptable voice. Although there are general expectations of what a normal voice should sound like, it is important to realize that there is a broad spectrum of normal voice quality, even within age, gender, and ethnic categories. Patient's self-ratings of voice quality are subjective and can be influenced by the patient's mood and other intrinsic and extrinsic factors as well as their illness perception as described by Buck and colleagues.[1] A patient's responses lend insight about the desire to change the voice and can help the clinician realize the impact the voice disorder is having on the patient's quality of life. There are times in which the patient's insight does not match the severity of the voice disorder. This can be largely due to poor patient understanding, other cognitive deficits, or simply denial. Furthermore, patients are often not aware of how their voice sounds to others, and they may be acclimated to some level of dysfunction. On the other hand, a patient whose voice improves after treatment may not have an accurate recollection of what the voice was like before treatment, and thus may under- or overestimate the effectiveness of the treatment. Such inaccuracy of self-assessment is known as the *Rosenthal effect*.

Another issue in the patient's assessment of the effectiveness or efficacy of voice treatment is that individual expectations vary considerably. For example, a patient who has had a laryngectomy may be so happy to be able to speak at all that he or she will rate his or her voice favorably, even if it sounds hoarse and requires much physical effort. On the other hand, a patient whose occupation is vocally demanding can be quite dissatisfied with a subtle but functional change and thus his or her expectations are high, placing more demands on the clinician to produce a desired treatment effect. Despite these limitations, some methods for measuring patient's self-assessment are helpful.

Estimations of function as a percentage of normal have been used in assessing the results of botulinum toxin injections for spasmodic dysphonia.[2] Psychometrically standardized questionnaires have also been used to assess the emotional impact of spasmodic dysphonia as well as other voice disorders.[3] The Voice Handicap Index (VHI), developed by investigators at the Henry Ford Hospital, is a list of 30 questions that ask the patient to rate the frequency of specific consequences of the voice problem.[4] This is a relatively robust instrument statistically that has been validated in diverse voice disorders, although the number of persons used in the statistical validation could have included a larger sample. While the development of the VHI has proven to be one of the best advancements for producing a standardized questionnaire, users of the scale should look carefully at the population (including the age, gender, and cultural diversity) that was used to standardize the scale to make sure it matches the population they are assessing. The questions on the VHI address the impact on vocal function as well as quality of life. The original list was condensed to 10 questions (VHI-10) that seem to elicit the most important information about vocal dysfunction in general, and the shortened VHI has been translated into many languages.[5] A recent study has demonstrated that a subset of these questions is particularly relevant for performers with voice disorders.[6] Statistical analysis comparing the validity of the VHI-10 with the original

Table 1 Methods of Voice Assessment

Patient's self-assessment	Subjective	Voice quality and effort required
Perceptual assessment	Subjective	Voice quality
Acoustic analysis	Objective	Waveform mathematically described
	Subjective	Interpretation of spectrogram
Aerodynamic measures	Objective	Airflow and pressure
Stroboscopy	Subjective	Assessment of vocal fold vibration
Glottography	Objective	Precise timing of events in vibratory cycle

VHI was performed with 819 patients representing a wide spectrum of voice disorders, and the two were shown to be statistically comparable.

PERCEPTUAL ANALYSIS

The clinician forms an impression of a patient's vocal function during the interview, and the notation of this in the patient's record is the simplest form of perceptual analysis. More formalized and systematic assessment involves using standardized rating scales and attending to specific individual aspects of vocal quality. A recent study examined the reliability of two separate and routinely used scales [Consensus on Auditory Perceptual Evaluation of Voice (CAPE-V) and Grade, Roughness, Breathiness, Asthenia, Strain (GRBAS)] found that the differences between clinician-based and patient-based data are significant, as patients experience and consider dysphonia differently.[7] What that means is that the patient who fills out the VHI or VHI-10 will score their dysfunction differently than the clinician. However, the study also indicated that a clinician is consistent in rating regardless of the scale used. The GRBAS scale, which has been used faithfully, although without validation of its dimensions, rates five voice qualities, each on a five-point scale. The qualities include grade (severity), roughness, asthenia (thinness or lack of resonance), breathiness, and strain. Other perceptual assessment methods include paired comparison, visual analog scales, and direct magnitude estimation.[8] Eadie and Baylor indicated that either direct magnitude estimation or scales which use equal appearing interval scales were both appropriate selections for making auditory-perceptual judgments of pleasantness, but only the direct magnitude estimation scale was recommended for judging overall voice severity in those with voice disorders.[9]

Most recently, there has been much attention given to the development of a consistent rating scheme so that the recorded speech sample, elicitation techniques, and variables rated are identical across clinical settings. This process was guided by a consensus conference sponsored by the American Speech-Language-Hearing Association's (ASHA) Division 3: Voice and Voice Disorders and the Department of Communication Science and Disorders, University of Pittsburgh, held in 2002 in Pittsburgh. From that conference a consensus document/statement was produced by a working group subcommittee and entitled the CAPE-V.[10] More details about the development of the CAPE-V can be found at the URL http://www.asha.org. As stated in the consensus document, the CAPE-V is not intended to be used as the only means of determining the nature of the voice disorder such as is the case for rating scales in general. It is not to be used to the exclusion of other tests of vocal function and should be supplemented by visual examination of the larynx and other more objective means for quantifying vocal fold vibratory behavior.

When making judgments of voice production, the most reliable perceptual ratings are the result of blinded analysis of recorded samples.[11] This level of rigor is important for research purposes but is too time consuming and complex to be practical in most clinical situations. Therefore, most clinical ratings are unblinded. The aspects of voice, which are most commonly assessed, include pitch, loudness, and vocal quality. The first two can also be physically measured and can serve as some validation of the perceptual analysis. Vocal quality is essentially the esthetic impression that the voice invokes in the listener. Descriptive terms include such aspects as smoothness versus roughness, resonant versus thin, breathy versus full. Breathiness tends to correlate with increased airflow and appears to be cued by changes in the vowel spectrum. These changes are related to alterations in the intensity of aspiration noise and spectral slope of the harmonic energy.[12] Further research is needed to determine the acoustic correlates of voice qualities such as hoarseness.

VOCAL PERFORMANCE ASSESSMENT

The dynamic ranges of pitch and loudness have long been accepted as relevant parameters of vocal function, by singing teachers and clinicians alike. These ranges can be assessed with varying levels of rigor. The habitual pitch range is informally evaluated simply by listening to spontaneous speech during a patient's interview. A monotonous voice or one that lacks any variation in the pitch of the voice sounds as if it lacks emotional projection. The pitch range capacity of one's voice can be easily measured by having a patient match pitches on a keyboard. A healthy subject with no structural or functional problems with the vocal folds should be able to span two octaves. An octave is a doubling in pitch. To determine a patient's dynamic range in loudness, a simple sound level meter may be used. Dynamic range of loudness typically spans about 50 dB from 30 to 80 dB.

The objective correlates of pitch and loudness are frequency and intensity, respectively. One of the most common clinical tools that has been a mainstay in the clinic is the Visi-Pitch, which provides a computerized assessment of pitch and loudness by providing information about the fundamental frequency of the voice and the relative intensity of the voice. The Visi-Pitch is easy to use and can also provide patients with biofeedback, allowing them to match pitch and loudness targets using visual feedback. The Phonetogram is another formal process for defining the pitch and loudness range, by determining dynamic range for specified pitches throughout the frequency range (Figure 1). This is widely used in Europe and has been validated in several studies, but it is time consuming and fatiguing, and thus not widely use in the United States.[13]

One of the simplest performance measures to acquire is the maximum phonation time (MPT).

It can be acquired with a stopwatch, or even a wristwatch, simply asking the patient to take a deep breath and then phonate "ee" as long as possible at a comfortable pitch and loudness. It is also one of the most relevant and useful clinical tests. A multicenter study in Belgium several years ago compared several measures of vocal function and found that the MPT was the one test that was most often clinically useful. The average MPT for males ranges from 22 to 34 seconds, while for females, the ranges is from 16 to 25 seconds.[13] While a clinically useful measure, MPT data collection must consider patient fatigue and ensure that the directions for the task are consistent. Patients may not do the task as prescribed resulting in a high amount of performance variability. The clinician should ensure that the patient rests between MPT trials and is instructed to take a maximum inhalation prior to phonating on expiration. Phonation time will be diminished with glottal incompetence, as due to vocal fold paralysis or presbyphonia, and can also be decreased by decreased lung capacity. Sometimes excessive glottal closure, as in adductor spasmodic dysphonia, can prolong the MPT reserve, glottal incompetence, or submaximal effort. Pulmonary function testing is useful to clarify the cause of a low MPT. Lung function testing can be completed in the clinical setting using a digital spirometer; or, with more complex cases, patient referral to the pulmonary clinic is warranted to help identify the potential influence of lower airway disease on laryngeal function.

ACOUSTIC ANALYSIS

The sound of the human voice is not a pure tone, but like any complex waveform, it can be described mathematically as a sum of pure sine waves of varying frequency and amplitude (Figure 2). This is the basis for computerized acoustic analysis, which uses the waveform anaylsis to generate specific parameters. This process is objective and reproducible and would, therefore, seem to be the ideal approach for standardized testing of vocal function. However, there are a number of issues that limit applicability. Objective voice measures are relevant only if they correlate with differences in voice quality that can be perceived, and many parameters cannot. Conversely, some of the qualities that are easily perceived have not as yet been mathematically defined. But more significantly, most of the algorithms begin by identifying the fundamental frequency of the voice, and significantly hoarse voices are often so irregular that there is no fundamental frequency.

Over 10 years ago a document was put forth by the National Center for Voice and Speech (NCVS) in Iowa City with the intent of providing a standardized method for the use of acoustic analysis in the study of voice. Within the document, specific recommendations were made for the use of a standard set of test utterances to be used for voice recording and analysis, and a

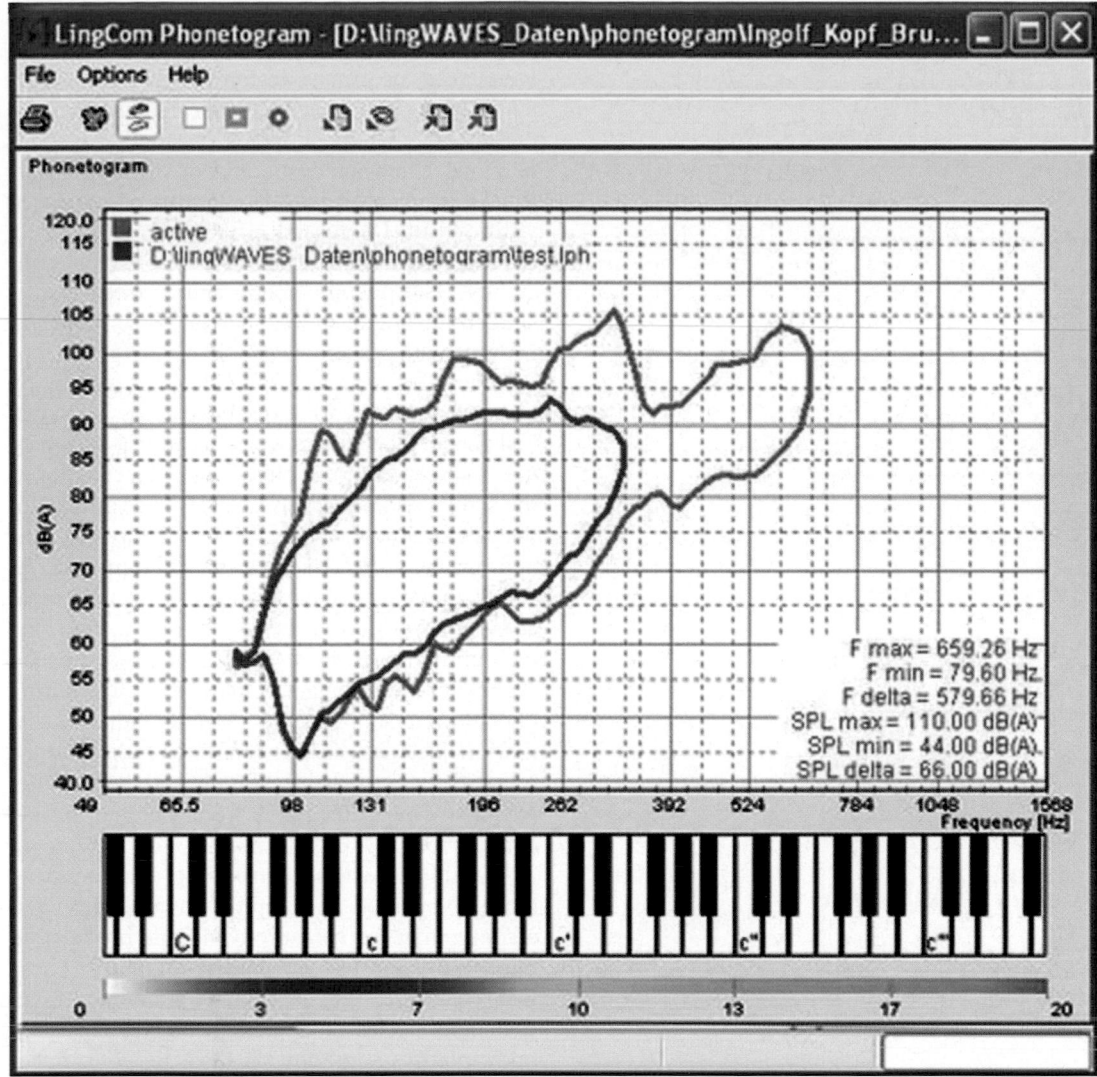

Figure 1 Phonetogram. The amplitudes of the loudest and softest possible phonation for a wide range of frequencies are displayed in an *x–y* plot. The keyboard depicted across the bottom is a handy reference to the pitch.

whenever computerized analysis is used, the raw waveform must be checked to assure adequate periodicity. If the voice is too irregular, none of the resultant analyses will be valid.

Harmonic to Noise Ratio. In common parlance, harmony means pitches that sound pleasing together. This is because harmonics frequencies are integer multiples of the fundamental frequency, and a sound that contains only a fundamental and harmonic frequencies will be smooth, with each sound cycle being identical. Frequencies that are not integer multiples will result in cycles that vary greatly in amplitude and shape, and if there is sufficient energy in nonharmonic frequencies, the sound becomes completely aperiodic, or noise. The harmonic to noise ratio of a sound reflects the amount of energy in f_0 and its harmonics divided by the energy in nonharmonic frequencies. A voice with a high harmonic to noise ratio is perceived as normal.

Perturbation Measures. An unstable voice has variations in the cycles of vocal fold vibration, in either pitch or loudness or both. This is perceived as *harshness*. Jitter is a parameter that reflects pitch instability, while shimmer measures differences in the amplitudes of neighboring cycles. Jitter is expressed in milliseconds or as a percentage of cycle length. Shimmer is expressed as a percentage of the mean amplitude. Although these measures have been used for many years, they have not proven to be clinically useful or relevant. The short-term variations in normal or near normal voices are frequently imperceptible, while in hoarse voices, the sound is too aperiodic to permit accurate derivation of perturbation measures.

Standard Deviation of the Fundamental Frequency. Standard deviation of the fundamental frequency (SDF_0) is a parameter that detects instability of the vocal signal over a longer sample than that used to calculate jitter. These fluctuations over longer cycles are more easily perceived, as fluctuating pitch. Pitch fluctuations are characteristic of motor control problems, as seen in neurologic disease and old age. It can also result from laryngeal pathology, such as scarring from surgery or radiation.

AERODYNAMIC ANALYSIS

Voice is sound: successive compressions and rarefactions of air created by the interplay of air exhaled by the lungs, and the valving activity of the larynx. Thus measurements of airflow and pressure can provide precise and objective indicators of vocal function. One can measure either steady state values, as indicators of glottal competence and vocal efficiency, or the rapid cycle-to-cycle changes that provide information about the vibratory capacity of the glottis. The airflow exiting the mouth and nose can be directly and easily measured using a facemask, usually in terms of liters per second. Mean airflow during a

workshop convened by the NCVS concluded that not all acoustic parameters were appropriate for all levels of voice severity.[14] Most acoustic measures are only valid for nearly periodic voices. Visual displays, such as spectrograms, are needed for more irregular voices. Acoustic analysis of any type is invalid for severely hoarse, aperiodic voices.

Spectral analysis performs a Fourier analysis of a sound and displays the amplitudes of all component frequencies, either as an *x–y* plot or as a "voice print" (Figure 3). The resulting image can be appreciated qualitatively. Harmonic components can clearly be identified as regularly spaced bands, while noise appears as continuous frequencies. Voice or pitch breaks are also well documented.[15] A broadband filter can be used to identify formant or peak frequencies. The formant structure is determined by the resonance of the upper vocal tract, which can be voluntarily altered to produce different vowels or vocal qualities. Thus, spectral analysis is highly influenced by the specific sound uttered, and a single utterance does not adequately characterize the overall quality of a subject's voice. Long-term average spectrum (LTAS) can provide spectral information from longer or multiple utterances,

even paragraphs. This provides a more accurate assessment of the voice. It has been used successfully to document improvement with treatment. However, the results can be markedly affected by the characteristics of the microphone or recording system. Thus, assessments from a given patient can only be compared if recorded with identical systems using identical settings.

Fundamental Frequency

The fundamental frequency (f_0) is the rate at which the vocal folds open and close. This is usually the slowest frequency obtained by Fourier analysis. The duration of one cycle of opening and closing is the fundamental period (T or $1/f_0$). The f_0 should be determined from a stable period of vocalization within a sustained vowel utterance. The sample to be analyzed should include at least 25 cycles or about 2 seconds, to be accurate. We can perceive pitch during connected speech. However, a computer requires sophisticated software and is still less accurate in tracking pitch during speech. The fundamental frequency is used as the basis for computing most other acoustic parameters. Unfortunately in severe dysphonia, the vibratory cycle is often aperiodic. Therefore,

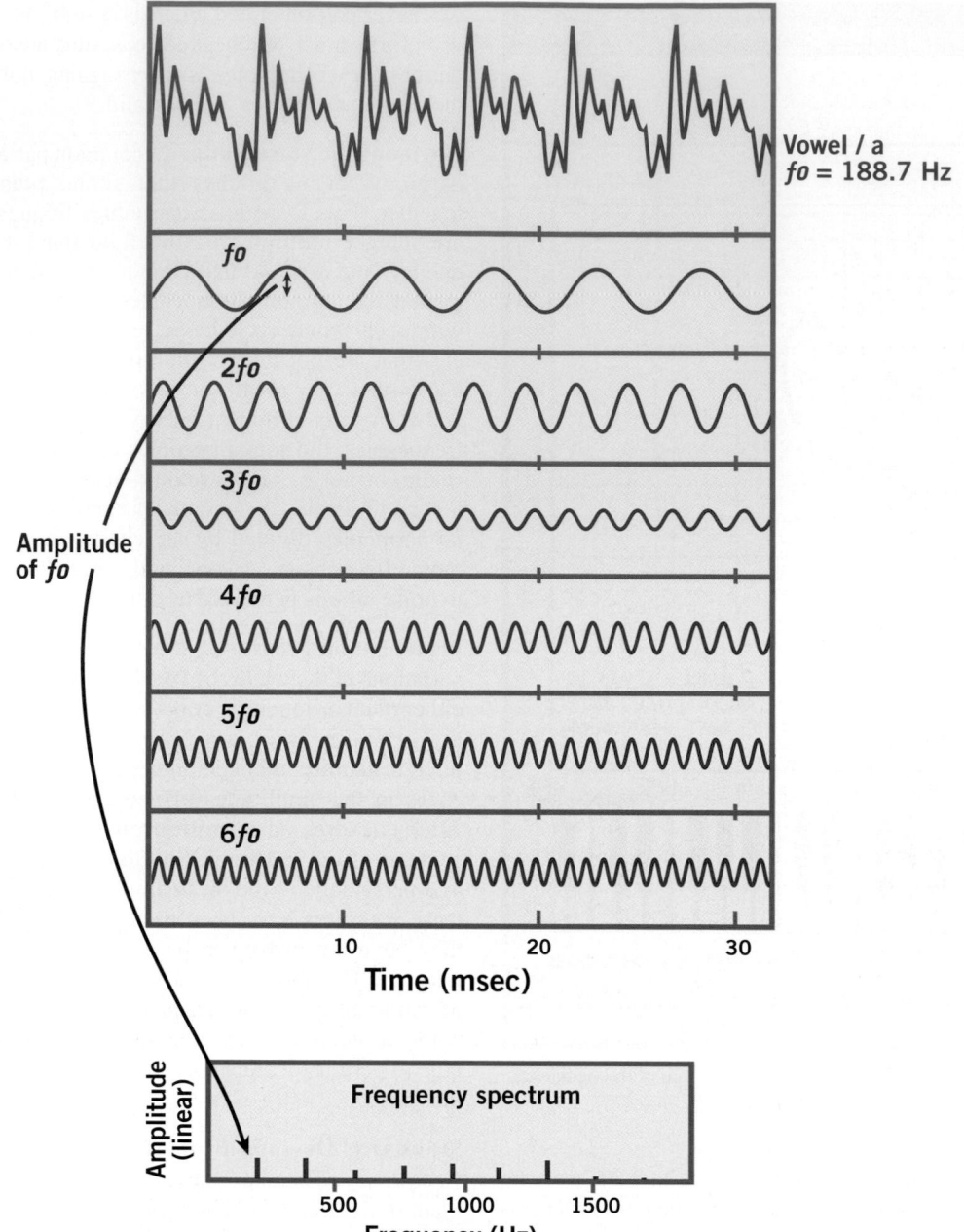

Figure 2 A complex sound wave can be mathematically described as a sum of sine waves of varying frequencies. Fourier analysis determines the amount of energy in each component signal.

It is higher in conditions of glottal incompetence, such as laryngeal paralysis, a mass deficit in the vocal fold, or a mass lesion that prevents glottal closure. It is lower with increased laryngeal resistance, such as adductor spasmodic dysphonia, muscle tension dysphonia, or vocal fold scarring. Laryngeal resistance can also be increased volitionally. Decreased airflow can also reflect reduced expiratory effort or pulmonary insufficiency. The pneumotachograph can also detect sudden airflow changes, such as voice breaks in patients with spasmodic dysphonia.

The pneumotachograph calculates airflow by measuring the pressure decrease across a known resistance. The resistance is usually a fine wire mesh screen, and the pressure produced prior to the screen and after the screen (P1-P2) allows for the calculation of airflow. It is crucial to select the appropriate pneumotachograph and transducer as stated above for the flow range to be validly measured and so that airflow will be detected with the minimal possible resistance. While some may argue that the facemask constrains airflow during phonation to some degree, research indicates that the full facemask in fact interferes little with the reliability of respiratory volume and did not alter frequency measures made from a glottal airflow waveform.[16]

While more time consuming and requiring more expensive and sophisticated equipment, airflow may be measured without obstructing outflow by the use of plethysmography. These techniques are more common to pulmonary function laboratories or clinics. A body box, called body plethysmography, is most reliable, but it requires a great deal of space. Indirect plethysmography uses induction coils. Both extrapolate expired airflow by detecting changes in chest volume and, therefore, do not obstruct airflow from the mouth and nose. Indirect plethysmography measures the summation of changes in the cross-sectional area within the thoracic and abdominal compartments and creates a weighted summation of these changes to provide a signal that is proportional to lung volume. Careful calibration is required, body movement artifact must be kept to a minimum, and interpretation may be subject to user error.

Another method of measuring airflow is the use of hot wire anemometry, which offers little resistance. The hot wire anemometer has a high frequency response but does not measure actual volume. Further, it can be distorted by turbulence and or changes in the ambient temperature.

Glottal Airflow

Airflow at the level of the glottis can be estimated by using a Rothenburg mask. This mask is circumferentially vented with multiple holes covered by fine wire mesh and uses a high frequency differential pressure transducer to measure airflow from the mouth and nose. The signal is processed by "inverse filtering," which is designed to subtract the resonant frequencies of the upper vocal tract.[17] The resultant waveform is considered to

sustained vowel can provide an estimate of glottal competence: a high flow is seen with poor glottal closure, whereas in a strained voice, such as adductor spasmodic dysphonia, airflow is low. However, measuring airflow without the context

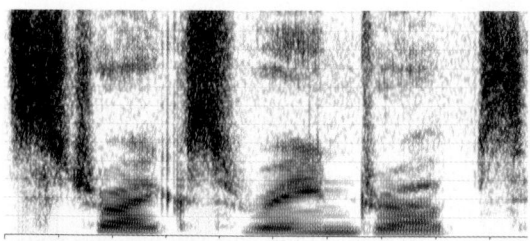

Figure 3 Spectrogram of a voice sample. The phrase "strikes raindrops" has been taken from a recording of a patient reading the Rainbow Passage, a standard reading task for voice analysis. The dark vertical bands are the "noise" of the "s" consonants, with energy in a continuous range of frequencies. The three striated segments are the three voiced consonants, with resonant frequencies represented by horizontal bands, and little or no noise between.

of pressure can be misleading. A decrease in phonatory airflow can indicate either an increase in laryngeal resistance or a decrease in expiratory effort. The driving force in phonation is subglottal pressure. Laryngeal resistance is a derived measure, calibrated from airflow and subglottal pressure, and usually expressed as centimeters of water per liter per second. Accurate measurement requires calibrated instruments, a standard protocol, and clear instructions to the subject.

Mean Phonatory Flow Rate

Mean phonatory flow rate has been one of the traditionally easier measures to collect and is the most common aerodynamic parameter to be reported on in the literature. Airflow usually is measured by a pneumotachograph, mounted in a full facemask. It should be measured during sustained phonation of a vowel at comfortable pitch and loudness, and normal mean phonatory airflow is about 200 cc/s.

reflect rapid airflow changes at the level of the glottis. Several derived values have been defined for use in assessing glottal function.[18]

Airflow Open Quotient. Clinically, the airflow open quotient (OQ = 20%) provides duration information about the length of time the glottis is open relative to the duration of the entire cycle of vocal fold vibration. Since glottal opening allows airflow to occur, this measure is useful for cases in which glottal closure is deemed inadequate or incomplete (hypofunctional vocal pathologies) or in cases where a high glottal resistance is suspected, that is, an obstruction, spasm, hyperfunction, or loud voice production.

Maximum Flow Declination Rate. Maximum flow declination rate can be used to define hypo- and hyperfunctional glottal configurations. Assuming no compensatory strategies exist, hypofunctional voice cases would predictably yield a low maximum flow declination rate value because of the disability in completely closing the vocal folds and the slowness in the return of the weakened vocal fold toward the midline. Maximum flow declination rate would be predictably higher in those with hyperfunctional voice disorders due to an increase in subglottal pressure and greater vibrational amplitudes. However, since those with hyperfunctional voice disorders can also have increased vocal fold stiffness, declination rates are not always predictable.

Peak Glottal Airflow. Peak glottal airflow relates to the maximum glottal area during vocal fold vibration. Increased stiffness, decreased mucosal wave, or any other pathological condition, which restricts the maximum displacement of the vocal folds, can alter the peak airflow during phonation.

Alternating Glottal Airflow. Changes in vocal fold tension and stiffness affect alternating airflow because the biomechanical changes to the vocal folds change the displacement of them during voicing. With increased stiffness of the vocal folds, alternating airflow typically decreases.

Minimum Glottal Airflow. Minimum glottal airflow relates to the amount of airflow through the glottis during the closed phase of vocal fold vibration. Theoretically, the higher the minimum airflow the more incomplete the glottal closure. This measure provides a way to document the hypofunctional component of vocal pathologies such as adductor vocal fold paralysis or other cases where there is glottal incompetence.

Subglottic Pressure

Subglottal pressure is the driving force for phonation. It results from expiratory effort against an upstream resistance. Subglottal pressure can increase because of greater expiratory effort or because laryngeal resistance increases. Unfortunately, subglottal pressure is difficult to measure directly in a clinical situation. Direct measure would require tracheal puncture. One can also

lower a solid-state pressure transducer between the vocal folds, but such a transducer interferes with glottal closure and phonation. Thus, subglottal pressure is estimated by measuring intraoral pressure as the subject repeats the syllable /pi/ at a rate of 1.5 syllables per second. The theory is that subglottal pressure and intraoral pressure are the same when the lips are sealed to form the consonant "P." The accuracy of the intraoral pressure in predicting subglottal pressure was developed by Smitheran and Hixon and has been validated for use in normal subjects.[19] However, it may not be accurate in the presence of pathology. An alternative approach to estimating subglottal pressure is to use an esophageal pressure transducer since intratracheal pressure is presumably equivalent to subglottic pressure and is transmitted transthoracically to the esophagus. This technique is not sensitive to rapid pressure changes in the airway.

Patients with disorders of voice or speech motor control often have difficulty in producing the precise repetition of syllables. Careful review of the literature will indicate that results of estimated subglottic pressure have only been reported for patients with a voice or speech disorder that is mild enough that they can produce the target rate. Subglottal pressures for comfortable effort level voice range from about 5 to 8 cm H_2O and increase with elevations in vocal loudness as well as rise slightly with increased fundamental frequency. Singers, because of their larger dynamic range, produce higher subglottal pressures during song production.

Laryngeal Resistance

Laryngeal resistance is calculated by dividing subglottic pressure by mean phonatory airflow rate. It varies greatly with vocal task and should always be measured at a standard pitch and loudness. Although it is a calculated parameter, it reflects the actual physical function of the larynx. Laryngeal resistance is low in glottal incompetence, such as in laryngeal paralysis or fixation, tissue deficit of the vocal fold, or in the presence of a mass lesion that prevents laryngeal closure. It is higher in glottal strain, as in spasmodic dysphonia or muscular tension dysphonia. It can be increased voluntarily, as one technique for increasing loudness. Laryngeal resistance is increased by vocal fold stiffness, as in patients with laryngeal scarring from surgery, trauma, or radiotherapy. Because so many factors can alter laryngeal resistance, this measure should always be interpreted in combination with patient history and laryngeal examination.

Laryngeal resistance can be used to calculate vocal efficiency, a measure of how much effort is required to generate a given level of sound. It is calculated by dividing the sound pressure level of the voice by a simultaneously determined laryngeal resistance. In fact, it reflects more than just glottic efficiency. The entire vocal tract, including the skull, chest, nasal cavity, and throat, can modulate the sound and thus has a consid-

erable influence on vocal efficiency. Recently, Grillo and Verdolini showed that laryngeal resistance but not vocal efficiency distinguished normal, pressed, resonant, and breathy voice qualities from one another further supporting the measure of laryngeal resistance as a useful method for examining vocal fold dynamics.[20]

As the vocal folds become stiffer, as with scarring or edema, greater pressure is required to induce oscillation of the vocal folds, and it becomes difficult to speak softly. The minimum pressure threshold for phonation (the minimum pressure that can produce a sound) is a relevant clinical measure.[21] An easier way to get a rough estimate of vocal fold stiffness is simply to measure the softest sound that can be produced.

PULMONARY FUNCTION TESTING

Those with voice disorders may have multiple reasons why breathing symptoms might be associated with their laryngeal condition. First, it may be that the patient has low muscular effort due to a primary disease process such as motor neuron disease. Second, it may be that the patient has a laryngeal disorder creating high laryngeal airway resistance. Cases such as adductor spasmodic dysphonia, muscle tension dysphonia, or other dynamic conditions resulting in increased glottal closed time can result in high laryngeal airway resistance, restricting airflow. Static laryngeal conditions, which result in high laryngeal airway resistance, include webbing, stenosis, abductor vocal fold paralysis, arytenoid joint dislocation, and others. Finally, the patient who presents with low laryngeal airway resistance and cannot control expiratory airflow may also complain of breathing symptoms. These cases of hypofunctional voice disorders include vocal fold paralysis or any other condition that limits the mobility of one or both vocal folds. In each of the conditions mentioned, the voice is often abnormal and the patient presents with a secondary complaint of breathing abnormality. This breathing abnormality is a sensation of breathlessness or dyspnea and is one of the most commonly perceived symptoms. Flow-volume loops and the measurement of forced inspiratory volumes are essential to document the severity of the problem and to track response to treatment. In clinical practice, pulmonary function testing should be available in the pulmonary function laboratory at the medical center, therefore preventing unnecessary duplication of services. These laboratories are equipped to maintain and calibrate the equipment correctly.

VOCAL FOLD MOVEMENT

Rapid oscillation of the vocal fold was first documented by high-speed motion picture photography. This required precise and expensive equipment, was only used in a few research laboratories, and was never available commercially for widespread use. Other techniques have been developed. Some are available clinically, whereas others remain research tools.

Videostroboscopy provides a slow motion image of vibration and is readily used as a clinical tool today. Keep in mind that the image acquired from videostroboscopy is not a true record of motion, but a composite that represents an average of motion over many cycles. There are many commercially available options for performing stroboscopy in the office. Stroboscopy can be qualitatively assessed, essentially as an extension of the physical examination. It can also be systematically analyzed, rating several measures. Stroboscopy is discussed in Chapter 83, "Laryngoscopy."

Glottographic measures are noninvasive techniques to track indirectly motion and contact of the vocal folds during phonation.[22,23] There are two forms of glottography, electroglottography (EGG) and photoglottography (PGG). They provide complementary information and are, therefore, more accurate and relevant when performed simultaneously. However, only EGG is commercially available.

EGG measures the electrical impedance between two plates on opposing sides of the neck over the thyroid cartilage, at the level of the vocal folds. A low-voltage, high-frequency current is passed between the plates. Impedance is highest when the glottis is open and decreases when the vocal folds come into contact. Impedance changes in proportion to the surface area of contact between the vocal folds. Impedance is highest during maximal glottic opening with minimal or no vocal fold contact. Impedance increases during the opening portion of the closed phase and decreases during the opening phase. Although changes in impedance are proportional to contact area, they cannot be calibrated to produce actual area measurements, since the contact area cannot be directly measured for calibration. Therefore, EGG is used to document the timing of vibration. Further, changes in distance between the edges of separated vocal folds do not affect impedance; therefore, EGG only provides information about the closed phase of the cycle. The filtered output of impedance is viewed and recorded as a waveform, termed "L_X." The L_X signal is less robust in obese individuals since impedance is measured against all neck tissue between the plates.

EGG is an effective tool for deriving f_0. L_X reflects events at the level of the glottis, without modulation of the waveform by the resonance of the upper vocal tract. Thus, the L_X waveform is much less complex than the acoustic signal, and the algorithm for deriving pitch is much simpler. The f_0 is a relevant measure in itself, and the signal can also be used to determine the frequency of a stroboscope during laryngeal stroboscopy.

Some useful parameters can be derived from EGG. The duration of the open and closed phases is easily extracted. In pressed phonation, the duration of the closed phase increases. With glottic insufficiency, the closed phase decreases and the open phase increases.

EGG can differentiate between modal and falsetto phonation, because there is a significant difference between these two registers in the thickness of the vocal folds and the duration of the closed phase. Vocal folds are thicker during modal phonation, and the mucosal wave progresses superiorly along the vibratory edge. Therefore, there is a "knee," or sharp turn in the L_X waveform at the onset of glottal closure in modal phonation when the inferior edges of the vocal folds begin to separate. During falsetto phonation, the vocal folds are thinner and tenser, and only the superior edges of the vocal folds come into contact. There is no mucosal wave, and the L_X waveform is less complex, nearly sinusoidal.

PGG measures light transmitted from the mouth or pharynx, through the larynx, and then through the soft tissues over the trachea. It does this by means of a photoelectric transducer placed on the skin over the trachea. This light can be supplied by as simple a mechanism as a flashlight in the mouth or transmitted through an endoscope. Minimal light is transmitted during glottic closure, and more light is transmitted as the vocal folds separate. Thus, PGG provides information about the open phase of the vibratory cycle and is complementary to EGG.[22,23]

As mentioned above, the two techniques provide the more useful information when performed simultaneously (Figure 4). With both measures, one can differentiate between the opening and closing phases of the total closed phase of the cycle. Flaccid vocal folds are quickly blown apart, resulting in a quick opening phase and then return to midline more slowly. In tight glottal closure, or with stiff vocal folds, the vocal folds are more difficult to open, resulting in a longer opening time. The edges then snap closed quickly. Opening and closing times can be quantified to derive the speed quotient, by dividing the opening time by the closing time. However, the different patterns are also easy to detect qualitatively on visual inspection of the waveform.

Recently, high-speed laryngeal imaging by digital video has been developed. The equipment is less unwieldy and is becoming commercially available. It is a promising new clinical tool for the assessment of voice disorders yet is still only available to those with expertise in its operation and interpretation. Sophisticated edge detection algorithms are required to track vocal fold movement accurately.

EQUIPMENT REQUIREMENTS

Many systems are commercially available for voice analysis, with varying degrees of complexity. A clinical practice is best served by the most user-friendly system, without complex assessment or calibration requirements. For research laboratories, off-the-shelf products generally lack the flexibility needed to modify software or to perform special tests. However, an audiotape recording system is an absolutely indispensable component of any voice laboratory. In patients treated for vocal problems, a voice recording is analogous to a photograph before cosmetic surgery. Voice recordings also are the substrate for acoustic voice analysis in clinical practice and research. An audio computer with the appropriate sound card selection may directly acquire input, but it is more efficient to record onto digital tape and select the samples to be analyzed post hoc. This also provides a means to archive the acquired recordings. It is essential that all components of the audio recording system, including microphones, amplifiers, and recorders, be of equal fidelity because any system is only as good as its poorest component.

Acoustic recordings must be made under controlled, standardized conditions, without background sound. The microphone should be at a standard distance to the mouth. The microphone's frequency response should be flat across both low and high frequencies. A standard reference tone should be used to calibrate recording levels,

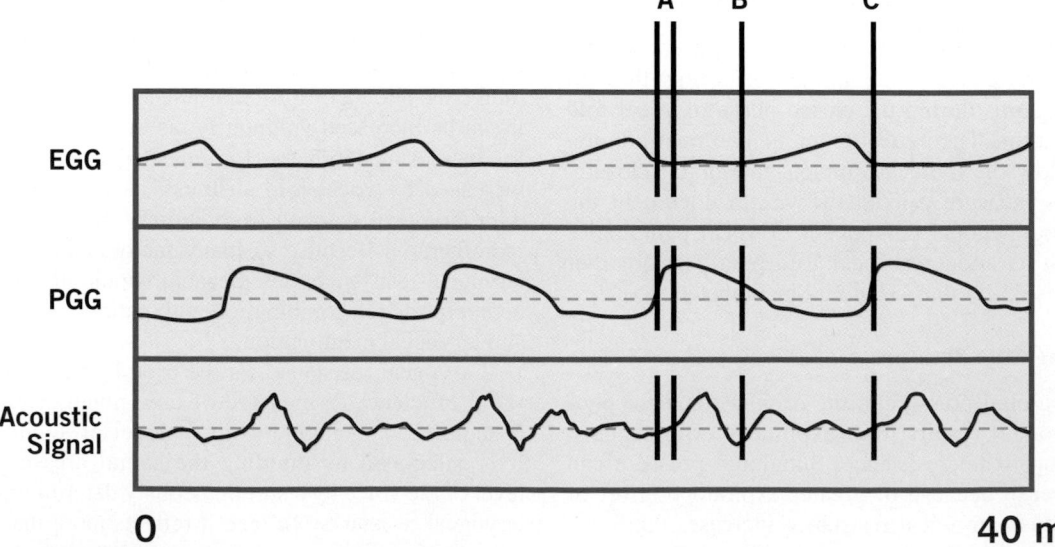

0   **40 ms.**

Figure 4 Simultaneous electroglottography (EGG), photoglottography (PGG), and acoustic signal of a short segment of a sustained vowel. The opening phase is between the two bars at A. From the second bar at A to B is the closing phase, and from B to C is the closed phase.

and the same protocol should be followed in each recording session, giving subjects the same instructions to utter the same speech samples at the same comfort levels.

Ideally, tests should be individually selected for each patient, depending on the disorder being evaluated, as not every parameter is relevant in every case. However, it is more efficient for each laboratory to define a core set of vocal function test which will be performed routinely on all subjects. Further, particularly in research laboratories, a parameter initially thought to be irrelevant may in fact demonstrate significant correlations to dysfunction. Therefore, the tests to be used can be selected to be appropriate for the majority of patients and subjects. Finally, a comprehensive voice laboratory must have a computer-based data acquisition system.

CONCLUSIONS

Although many techniques are available to assess vocal function and have been used frequently, most have not been validated. It is important to develop standards for voice assessment to permit documentation of dysfunction and response to treatment, and to allow valid clinical studies of treatment outcomes, thus developing the evidence our field needs to help justify our assessment and treatment plans. A standard voice battery is not actually a necessary goal since vocal quality is multidimensional and voice disorders vary greatly in types of distortion or dysfunction. A more achievable goal would be to develop consensus as to the relevant parameters for specific clinical voice disorders and to validate and standardize their use.

REFERENCES

1. Buck F, Drinnan M, Wilson J, Barnard IS. What are the illness perceptions of people with dysphonia: A pilot study. J Laryngol Otol 2007;121:31–9.
2. Brin MF, Blitzer A, Stewart C. Laryngeal dystonia (spasmodic dysphonia): Observations of 901 patients and treatment with botulinum toxin. Adv Neurol 1998;78:237–52.
3. Murry T, Cannito M, Woodson GE. Spasmodic dysphonia. Emotional status and botulinum toxin treatment. Arch Otolaryngol Head Neck Surg 1994;120:310–6.
4. Benninger MS, Ahuja AS, Gardner G, Grywalski C. Assessing outcomes for dysphonic patients. J Voice 1998;12:540–50.
5. Rosen CA, Lee AS, Osborne J, et al. Development and validation of the voice handicap index. Laryngoscope 2004;114:1549–56.
6. Rosen CA, Murry T. Voice handicap index in singers. J Voice 2000;14:370–7.
7. Karnell MP, Melton SD, Childes JM, et al. Reliability of clinician based (GRBAS and CAPE-V) and patient based (V-RQOL and IPVI) documentation of voice disorders. J Voice 2006, Jul 3 (Epub ahead of print).
8. Kreiman J, Gerratt BR, Kempster GB. Perceptual evaluation of voice quality: Review, tutorial, and a framework for future research. J Speech Hear Res 1993;36:21–40.
9. Eadie TL, Baylor CR. The effect of perceptual training on inexperienced listeners' judgments of dysphonic voice. J Voice 2006;20:527–44.
10. Consensus Auditory-Perceptual Evaluation of Voice (CAPE-V) ASHA Special Interest Division 3, Voice and Voice Disorders URL: http://www.asha.org/NR/rdonlyres/ C6E5F616-972F-445A-AA40-7936BB49FCE3/0/CAP-EVprocedures.pdf. Accessed May 15, 2007.
11. Gerratt BR, Kreiman J, Antonanzas-Barroso N, Berke GS. Comparing internal and eternal standards in voice quality judgments. J Speech Hear Res 1993;36:14–20.
12. Shrivastav R, Sapienza CM. Objective measures of breathy voice quality obtained using an auditory model. J Acoust Soc Am 2003;144:2217–24.
13. Heylen LG, Wuyts FL, Mertens FW, Pattyn JE. Phonetography in voice diagnoses. Acta Otorhinolaryngol Belg 1996;50:299–308.
14. Tietze IR. Workshop on acoustic voice analysis: Summary statement. Iowa City: National Center for Voice and Speech; 1995.
15. Rontal E, Rontal M, Rolnick MI. Objective evaluation of vocal pathology using voice spectrography. Ann Otol Rhinol Laryngol 1975;84:662–71.
16. Huber JE, Stathopoulos ET, Bormann LA, Johnson K. Effects of a circumferentially vented mask on breathing patterns of women as measured by respiratory kinematic techniques. J Speech Lang Hear Res 1998;41:472–8.
17. Rothenberg M. A new inverse-filtering technique for deriving the glottic air flow waveform during voicing. J Acoust Soc Am 1973;53:1632–45.
18. Holmberg EB, Hillman EB, Perkell JS. Glottal airflow and transglottal air pressure measurements for male and female speakers in soft, normal, and loud voice. J Acoust Soc Am 1988;84:511–29.
19. Smitheran JR, Hixon TJ. A clinical method for estimating laryngeal airway resistance during vowel production. J Speech Hear Disord 1981;46:138–46.
20. Grillo EU, Verdolini K. Evidence for distinguishing pressed, normal, resonant, and breathy voice qualities by laryngeal resistance and vocal efficiency in vocally, trained subjects. J Voice 2007; Mar 30 (Epub ahead of print).
21. Titze IR. Phonation threshold pressure: A missing link in glottal aerodynamics. J Acoust Soc Am 1992;91:2296–35.
22. Fourcin AJ, Abberton E. First applications of a new laryngograph. Med Biol Illus 1971;21:172–82.
23. Gerratt BR, Hanson DG, Berke GS, Precoda K. Photoglottography: A clinical synopsis. J Voice 1991;5:98–105.

74

Disorders of Speech and Language

Raymond D. Kent, PhD

The faculties of speech and language are the core behaviors of human communication, and disorders of these faculties can carry severe consequences that affect virtually every aspect of life. Speech is the oral expression of language, which, in turn, is the faculty for the reception, manipulation, and expression of symbols that carry meaning. The components of language include syntax (grammar), semantics (lexicon), phonology (sound patterns of words), and pragmatics (the way language is used socially). Language can be expressed orally (speech), manually (sign language), graphically (print or writing), or by other means, depending on culture and the sensorimotor and cognitive abilities of the individual. Worldwide, speech is the primary, and first-acquired mode of language. But so intimate is the association between speech and language in both learning and use that their division is not always sharp. Laypersons often do not distinguish speech and language and may be inclined to think of them as a single behavior. However, speech and language can be distinguished functionally and clinically, and they are recognized here as distinct but closely related behavioral domains.

Collectively, speech–language disorders occur with considerable frequency, with prevalence estimates generally ranging from 6 to 10% in the general population. There is considerable variance in the prevalence estimates for some disorders, owing largely to differing criteria for diagnosis, methodology (eg, screening or diagnostic techniques vs population surveys), and demographic characteristics (eg, age, socioeconomic status) of individuals studied. Many of these disorders are complex and behaviorally based, so that adequate assessment and diagnosis often requires a battery of tests or evaluation instruments. Furthermore, certain of these disorders in children (stuttering, language impairment, speech sound disorder) have a spontaneous or natural resolution as high as 60 to 80%, although the persistence of disorders into later childhood or adulthood can have severe effects on educational, vocational, and social achievements. Speech and language disorders may be associated with later-identified difficulties in reading and other cognitive achievements. For many of these disorders, males are affected more than females by ratios that average approximately 3:1 but sometimes higher, especially in disorders that persist beyond childhood. Clearly, male sex must be considered as a risk factor for communicative

disorders of many types, and this male vulnerability is observed in both children (speech sound disorder, developmental language impairment) and adults (aphasia related to stroke).

Disorders of speech and language can be classified as shown in Table 1, with a basic division by age in that childhood or developmental disorders are distinguished from adult or acquired disorders. Within each of these age categories, further divisions are made with regard to type or etiology of disorder. Unfortunately, a satisfactory etiologic taxonomy is not possible because some of the most frequently occurring communication disorders in children are of unknown or a complex multifactorial origin. Comorbidity is a complicating factor, as several of the disorders considered here have high rates of co-occurrence with other disorders. Specific comorbidities are identified in this chapter as the individual speech and language disorders are discussed. In adults, speech and language disorders usually are secondary to other conditions, such as a neurologic lesion, trauma, or various disease processes.

SPEECH–LANGUAGE DISORDERS IN CHILDHOOD

Developmental Milestones

Speech–language disorders in children reflect processes of disorder interacting with processes of development. The interaction of these two factors complicates the understanding of disorders and introduces challenges into considerations of epidemiology, diagnosis, and treatment. Assessment and management of childhood disorders require background knowledge of typical development in its anatomic, physiologic, and behavioral aspects.

Table 2 lists some of the major milestones in speech and language development along with

related milestones in the anatomic and physiologic development of the speech production system. Oral cavity and pharyngeal anatomy and physiology are discussed in Chapter 63, "Anatomy and Physiology of the Oral Cavity," and laryngeal development, anatomy, and physiology are discussed in Chapter 72, "Development, Anatomy and Physiology of the Larynx." It should be emphasized that there are large variations in developmental patterns even among typically developing children, and, therefore, milestones should be used advisedly. The pattern of milestones in Table 2 shows that speech and language are gradual accomplishments in childhood and that they involve an interaction of linguistic, phonetic, motor, sensory, and anatomic changes. A neonate's vocal tract anatomy resembles that of the chimpanzee or other nonhuman primate and is capable of rather limited sound production compared to the phonetic repertoire of adults. An elevated laryngeal position truncates the pharyngeal cavity and creates a velic-epiglottal apposition that may support nutrition (eg, breathing while sucking) but is unsuited to adult-like vocalizations that require reliable control of velopharyngeal function for nasal versus nonnasal sounds. The neonatal vocal folds are short and unlaminated (ie, the lamina propria is not evident). By the age of 2 years, a child's vocal tract anatomy is decidedly humanlike (with a well-defined oral and pharyngeal two-cavity morphology), and a child at this age typically has the capability to produce two-word utterances formed from about 20 different sounds. By the age of about 6 or 7 years, children have an overall mastery of the sounds in English, although errors may persist for a few sounds to be described later in this chapter. Maturation of the anatomic and physiologic aspects of speech production continues until the age of 16 or 18 years and includes several remarkable changes, including (a) lamination of the vocal

Table 1 Classification of Major Disorders of Speech and Language in Children and Adults

Disorders in Children	Disorders in Adults
Speech sound disorder or speech delay (also may be called phonological disorder or articulation disorder)	
Specific language impairment (SLI) or language impairment secondary to known causes	Aphasia
Dysarthria or motor speech disorder	Dysarthria
Structurally based disorders: craniofacial anomalies, including orofacial clefting	Structurally based disorders: residual effects of congenital anomalies; ablative surgery, trauma
Voice disorder	Voice disorder

Table 2 Milestones in Typical Development with an Emphasis on Speech and Language

Age	Speech–language Milestone	Anatomic or Physiologic Milestone
0–2 mo	Head turning to direction of sound source Vocalizations are largely cries or reflexive sounds	Larynx is positioned high in the neck (epiglottal-velic engagement) Vocal folds are 2–7 mm long and are not laminated
2–4 mo	Cooing vocalizations: vowel sounds occasionally accompanied by a consonant	Disengagement of epiglottis and velum, as larynx descends in neck (marking an essential transformation from a nonhuman primate anatomy to human anatomy)
4–6 mo	Single syllable babbles with expanding consonantal repertoire	Emergence of frontal incisors. Dental arcade serves as boundary for tongue actions during speech
6–9 mo	Babbling (repeated syllable babbling). First evidence of word comprehension and effects of auditory status on patterns of sound production. Hand banging typically evident	Capability for velopharyngeal closure during vocalizations enables nasal vs nonnasal sound contrasts
12–14 mo	Production of first words; auditory discrimination of speech sounds heavily favors ambient language	
15–18 mo	Vocabulary of 5–20 words, mostly nouns	Reliable occlusal pattern in jaw closure
20–24 mo	Two-word combinations; vocabulary of 150–200 words	
36–48 mo	Vowels typically mastered (except for r-colored vowel) Speech is at least 90% intelligible Vocabulary of about 1,000 words	Vocal ligament is formed by 48 mo Hypertrophy of nasopharyngeal tonsil Possible change in velopharyngeal valving
48–60 mo	Rapid vocabulary growth	
60–72 mo	All consonants are produced correctly at least 50% of the time	Larynx has descended to adult position Nasopharyngeal tonsil atrophies Permanent dentition emerges Cranium is nearly adult size

folds (essentially complete at about 12 years of age), (b) a sequence of hypertrophy and atrophy of the nasopharyngeal tonsil (adenoid) that occurs over a considerable span of childhood, (c) eruption of the primary dentition and its replacement by the secondary dentition, (d) development of an adult-like pattern of speech breathing (roughly acquired by about 7 years of age), and (e) growth of various tissues of the vocal tract according to their characteristic schedules (neural, somatic, lymphatic).[1] Speech as a motor skill basically parallels language in its development, such that refinements in both domains continue into adolescence.[1,2]

Speech Sound Disorders

Definition and Characteristics. These disorders pertain to errors in the production of speech sounds (lisping is a common example). They are also known as phonological or articulatory disorders, and opinion is divided regarding the more appropriate terminology. *Phonological disorder* emphasizes the linguistic aspects of speech production, whereas *speech disorder* emphasizes the articulatory-motor aspects. *Speech sound disorder* is a relatively neutral name for the classification and is used here without presumption as to etiology. Severe speech sound disorders can interfere with speech intelligibility and therefore pose a significant obstacle to effective communication.

The acquisition of speech sounds can be viewed as a process that extends from the cooing vocalizations produced during the first 2 or 3 months of life to more sophisticated speech marked by the phonetic mastery of sounds in the parent language. The age of phonetic mastery varies across children and across sounds. Most vowels are produced accurately by about 3 years of age (the r-colored vowel, as in the word *bird*, is an exception), but many consonants are not mastered until early school age. Table 3 shows data pertaining to consonant production in children and

includes the following: a graphemic symbol for the consonant sound, a keyword containing the sound in question (usually the first sound in the word except when the sound does not occur in a word initially), articulatory description based on the manner (how a sound is made) and place (where in the vocal tract a sound is made) of consonant production, frequency of occurrence of the sound as a percent of all consonants, cumulative percent frequency of occurrence, and typical age of mastery for the sound.[3,4] Several conclusions can be drawn: (1) Only about a dozen consonants account for 80% of all consonant productions, a conclusion that reflects large differences in the

Table 3 Summary of Information on Consonant Production in Children, Including Graphemic Symbol for the Consonant, Keyword Containing the Sound, Articulatory Description of Sound, Percentage Frequency of Occurrence of All Consonants, Cumulative Percentage Frequency, Age of Mastery of Consonants

Symbol	Keyword	Articulatory Description*	Percentage of All Consonants[†]	Cumulative Percentage[†]	Age of Mastery (Years)[‡]
N	No	Alveolar nasal	13	13	<3
T	Two	Alveolar stop, –vce	12	25	<3
D	Do	Alveolar stop, +vce	10	35	<3
R	Row	Palatal liquid	8	43	4–6
S	So	Alveolar fricative, –vce	6	49	3–5
Th (voiced)	This	Dental fricative, –vce	6	55	4–7
L	Low	Alveolar lateral	6	61	4–6
W	Woe	Labiovelar glide	5	66	<3
M	More	Bilabial nasal	5	71	<3
K	Cow	Velar stop, –vce	4	75	3–4
Z	Zoo	Alveolar fricative, +vce	4	79	5–7
H	How	Glottal fricative, –vce	3	82	<3
B	Bow	Bilabial stop, +vce	3	85	3–4
P	Pow	Bilabial stop, –vce	3	88	<3
G	Go	Velar stop, +vce	2	90	3–4
V	Vow	Labiodental fricative, +vce	2	92	4–6
F	Foe	Labiodental fricative, –vce	2	94	3
Ng	Wing	Velar nasal	2	96	3–6
Th (voiceless)	Thin	Dental fricative, +vce	1	97	5–6
Sh	She	Palatal fricative, –vce	1	98	4–5
Y	You	Palatal glide	1	99	3–4
J	Joe	Palatal affricate, +vce	<1	100	4–7
Ch	Chew	Palatal affricate, –vce	<1	100	4–5
Zh	Rouge	Palatal fricative, +vce	<1	100	4–6

*Place-manner description, with place of articulation indicated first and manner of articulation indicated second, and voicing indicated third, as relevant. Place refers to location in the vocal tract where articulatory constriction is formed. Manner refers to the way in which sound is formed. Voicing is shown as +vce for voiced or –vce for voiceless.

[†]Based on data in reference 3.

[‡]Based on data summarized in reference 4.

informational load of individual sounds; (2) The alveolar place of articulaton (involving the tongue tip and alveolar ridge) is very important in American English, accounting for about 50% of all consonant production; (3) Age of mastery varies markedly across consonants, with some consonants being accurately produced at 3 years or younger, but others at 6 years or older. This developmental pattern is highly important in assessment and treatment; (4) Among the last sounds to be mastered are the initial sounds in the keywords *thin*, *this*, *she*, *Joe*, *chew*, *so*, *zoo*, *low*, and *row*. Table 3 is relevant to understanding the effects on speech of various kinds of trauma or surgery on the oral tissues. Although speech is highly robust because of articulatory compensations, it can be difficult to overcome certain kinds of structural alteration (the tongue tip being particularly exercised in speech).

Epidemiology. The median prevalence estimates for speech sound disorders are in the range of 1 to 9%, with more recent estimates being in the range of 1 to 3%.[5–7] Males are affected more than females by a ratio of about 3:1. Peak prevalence occurs at around 5 years for males and around 3 to 4 years for females. The comorbidity profile of children with speech disorders includes co-occurrence with disorders of mental health, hearing, and respiration (especially asthma). General allergies also occurred with relatively high frequency among children with speech sound disorders. Not surprisingly, children who have speech sound disorders accompanied by respiratory disorders or allergies also have a high frequency of voice disorders.[5] Approximately 11 to 15% of children with persisting speech delay also have a language impairment.[6]

The severity of speech sound disorders ranges from mild (eg, distortion of a single sound, such as *s* as in *say* or *r* as in *ray*) to severe (multiple errors that interfere with speech intelligibility and effectiveness of communication). These errors may be termed as either disorder or delay.

Etiology. Speech sound disorders arise from several factors, including sensory impairment (hearing impairment is the most common), motor dysfunction, psychosocial problems, and the interaction of these factors. But for the majority of children who are classified as having a speech sound disorder, etiology is unknown or at least uncertain. Shriberg proposed a classification system that links characteristics of speech sound disorder with causal origins including genetic, hearing, motor-speech, and psychosocial factors.[8] In addition, speech disorders are likely to develop in certain medical conditions, including craniofacial anomalies (especially oral clefting), cerebral palsy, various congenital syndromes, and other developmental disabilities including autism. Neurogenic speech disorders occur especially in cerebral palsy, which has a prevalence of more than 2.0 per 1,000 live births, with speech impairment occurring in up to 80% of affected individuals.[9] As summarized in Table 4, chromosomes 3,

6, 7, and 15 have been related to speech sound disorder.[10–14] A disorder of particular interest in genetic studies is childhood apraxia of speech (also called developmental apraxia of speech), which is an often severe disorder affecting the organization and coordination of speech movements. It is classified as a childhood motor speech disorder and is suspected to result from subtle neurologic abnormalities that have not been identified. Speech sound disorders can also arise in children who are learning English as a second language, which is another reason why a complete history is important in determining etiology. Because some speech sound errors are related to a child's language background rather than to a disorder per se, it is appropriate to distinguish *disorder* from *difference*.

Assessment. The typical clinical assessment includes an articulation test that examines the proficiency of sound production. The term *speech* or *speech articulation* usually refers to the motoric expression of language through actions of the respiratory, laryngeal, and especially supralaryngeal (articulatory) systems. In contrast, *phonology* is a component of language that deals with the ways by which sounds are combined to form words. The articulation test can be accompanied by a variety of other tests, depending on the depth and scope of the communication disorder. Conversational samples can be analyzed with relatively simple but informative measures such as the percent of consonants correct (PCC). Because consonants carry a major part of the informational load in speech, they are of particular importance in gauging the effect of a speech sound disorder. Phonological assessment determines the error patterns for speech sounds as they combine to form words. This kind of assessment is based on the principle that certain error patterns occur across words; that is, they have a generality that is important to recognize in clinical assessment. For example, children may omit word-final consonants so that the word *nose* is produced as *no*, and the word *tooth* is produced as *too*. Recognition of these patterns occurring across several words is a primary motivation for phonological descriptions of speech sound errors. Deletion of final consonants is typical of young children in the early stages of word learning, but when this error pattern persists into later development, it can interfere greatly with intelligibility.

Speech sound errors are broadly categorized as omissions (deletions of the sound), substitutions (replacements of the sound by another phoneme, such as "t" for "s"), and distortions (modification of the sound). Generally speaking, the severity of error decreases across these three categories (omission being the most severe form of error). Patterns of speech sound errors can be complex, involving combinations of omission, substitution, and distortion in a given child. Speech articulation is considered relative to a child's overall language ability to arrive at a developmental assessment of communicative ability. Typically, several other tests or evaluations are performed

to determine if the status of a child's hearing, oral mechanism, or other factors contribute to the speech sound disorder. As noted previously, one form of speech sound disorder that can be especially severe is childhood apraxia of speech, a poorly understood disorder that appears to reflect exceptional difficulties in the coordination and positioning of the articulators.

Implications for Treatment. Behavioral treatments are tailored to a number of factors, including severity of the problem, etiology (if known), presence of accompanying disorders (eg, a language disorder), and characteristics of the child. Treatment is often based on consideration of information like that contained in Table 2. That is, sounds are targeted for treatment according to their expected, or normative, pattern of development, with treatment given first to deviant sounds that are acquired relatively early in normal development. Frequency of occurrence may also be considered, on the assumption that frequently occurring sounds contribute more to speech intelligibility than rarely occurring sounds. But other strategies have been proposed, including one approach that focuses on later acquired sounds in the belief that normalization of these sounds may induce normalization of deviant sounds that typically are acquired earlier. A number of different treatments have been described, ranging from emphasis on minimal sound contrasts (eg, the contrasts that distinguish the words *zip*, *sip*, *tip dip*) to language-based methods that emphasize overall communicative behavior. Particularly when a motor speech involvement is suspected, clinicians may use oral nonverbal exercises (nonspeech movements of the articulators), but, unless there is clear evidence of weakness, there is no evidence for the efficacy of these procedures and there are substantial theoretical arguments against their use.[15]

Phonological awareness is a concept that bears on both speech sound disorders and reading disorders. It is the ability to detect and manipulate sound segments in speech and to demonstrate access to the sound structure of language. Children are considered to demonstrate phonological awareness when they show the ability to recognize sounds independently of the words in which they occur. Phonological awareness is manifested in tasks such as sound detection, rhyming, alliteration, deleting sounds, and moving sounds within words or syllables. Phonological awareness is relevant to literacy in that a number of studies have linked phonological awareness to reading ability.[16] A link between phonological development and reading is a major direction of contemporary research in reading disorders. A connection between early phonological disorder and a later reading disorder would carry important implications for early intervention.

Specific Language Impairment

Definition and Characteristics. Specific language impairment (SLI) is diagnosed in children who have significant language deficits in the face of normal nonverbal intelligence, adequate educational opportunity, and intact sensorimotor abilities. Diagnosis is performed largely by exclusion insofar as careful clinical assessment rules out other conditions such as mental retardation, autism, hearing loss, craniofacial anomalies, or neurological disorders that may cause language impairments. Children with SLI often have a delay or deficit in using functional morphemes (such as the words *a*, *the*, *is*) and other grammatical morphemes (such as the elements marking plural forms or verb tense forms).

According to some sources, SLI is perhaps the most common impairment in childhood. Other sources question the validity of prevalence data because of variability in diagnostic criteria. Questions about their child's language development are among the most frequent that parents ask of medical specialists, especially pediatricians. It has been estimated that, at any given time, about 20% of parents have questions concerning their child's language.[17] Clearly, health specialists should be prepared to offer advice that is based on an understanding of language development and its disorders.

Table 4 Chromosomal and Loci Linkages with Major Types of Communication Disorders					
Chromosome	Language Disorder	Stuttering	Speech Disorder	Oral Clefting (Syndromic)	Oral Clefting (Nonsyndromic)
1				1q32–41, 1q	1p36, 1q41
2	X	X			2p13
3			X	3q27	
4					4p16, 1q31, 6p23
6			6p22		
7	7q31	X	7q31–FOXP2	7p	
9		X			
11				11q27	11q23
12		12q			
13	13q21	X			
14					14q24
15			15q14, 15q21		15q11
16	16q				
17					17q21
18		X			
19	19q				19q13
21		X			
22	X			22q11	
X				Xp22	

X = chromosomal involvement but with no further information on locus.

Epidemiology. Speech and language delay in children aged 2 to 4.5 years has a prevalence rate ranging from 5 to 8%, and language delay alone has reported prevalence rates of 2.3 to 19.0%.[18] The large variation in these figures is explained in part by inconsistencies in the criteria for diagnosis. Because SLI is diagnosed largely by exclusion, careful and thorough assessments are required for a confident diagnosis. Statistics on the persistence of these difficulties also vary considerably across studies, with figures ranging from 30 to 90% but mostly in the range of 40 to 60%.[18] Even if the midrange value of 50% is taken as an estimated persistence, then it is clear that a large number of children are affected by language disorder. The disorder is heterogeneous, and it has been concluded from one study that it represents four distinctive linguistic domains: (1) lexical-semantic abilities, (2) auditory conceptualization, (3) verbal sequential memory, and (4) speech production.[19] Such heterogeneity complicates epidemiologic studies and raises challenges for both assessment and treatment. SLI is comorbid with other communicative disorders, and it has been reported that approximately 5 to 8% of children with persisting SLI also have speech delay.[6]

Etiology. The etiology of SLI is not well established, although progress has been made in identifying genetic and environmental correlates. As shown in Table 4, language disorder has been linked to chromosomes 7, 13, 16, 19, and 22.[20–23] The most well known of the genetic factors is the *FOXP2* gene on chromosome 7, which has been described in the popular media as the "language gene." In fact, *FOXP2* is a transcription factor that influences the actions of several other genes, and chromosomes other than 7 have been associated with language abnormalities. One challenge in the genetic studies is to insure that the SLI

phenotype has been clearly established, which usually means extensive testing in language and related domains. There is evidence that SLI is associated with differences in brain morphology, particularly a small pars triangularis in the left hemisphere and a more rightward asymmetry of language regions.[24]

Several hypotheses have been advanced on the nature of the functional deficits in SLI. One proposal is that the difficulty that children have with grammatical morphology is related to a delay or difficulty in acquiring a specific underlying linguistic mechanism, such as the principle that verbs must be marked for tense and number (consider the contrasting verb forms in the three sentences *He goes fast*, *They go fast*, *They went fast*). Another hypothesis is that children with SLI have a poor short-term memory for speech sounds, which can be demonstrated in a task of nonsense-word repetition in which children are asked to repeat nonsense utterances. If the auditory representation for speech sounds is weakly developed, or fades quickly, this would hinder a child's efforts to learn and use language. A third hypothesis is that children with SLI experience a particular difficulty in auditory temporal processing for sounds that are brief or that change rapidly in their spectral properties (stop consonants fall in this category). The difficulty could be in the processing itself, in remembering the temporal order of auditory events, or both of these. This third proposal is considered further in the section "Implications for Treatment" in relation to an intervention called Fast ForWord. These different views of the nature of SLI hold different implications for both assessment and treatment. Another complicating factor is that the population of children diagnosed with SLI may actually consist of subpopulations who have somewhat different characteristics of language impairment.

Autistic spectrum disorders (ASD) are pertinent here both because of the role of speech–language symptoms in the identification of the disorder and because of the apparent increase in the prevalence of ASD, which has alarmed health-care and educational specialists, along with society in general. Epidemiological studies affirm that autism prevalence has been increasing, as shown by higher prevalences among younger birth cohorts.[25] Reasons for this increase are not known. One possibility is that the diagnosis of autism has been substituted for diagnoses of mental retardation and/or language impairment, but there are reasons to doubt this explanation.[25] ASD can be diagnosed as early as 2 years of age, and it is a life-long impairment in most individuals.

Assessment. As noted above, SLI is diagnosed largely by exclusion. If a child has a language impairment or delay that cannot be attributed to sensory disorder, cognitive limitations, social or educational deprivation, or other factors, then a diagnosis of SLI may be assigned. However, this does not mean that children diagnosed with SLI have no co-existing disorders. To the contrary, studies have shown that many children with SLI exhibit evidence of other co-occurring problems, such as motor difficulties.[26]

A thorough assessment considers the various components of language, including grammatical ability, vocabulary (both expressive and receptive), pragmatics, and phonology. Several tasks may be employed to gauge a child's language ability. Standardized tests are available, but some clinicians prefer nonstandardized tests for certain purposes. Table 2 lists several major milestones in language development, and these are useful as guidelines in assessing the status of a child's language development. However, these are only crude suggestions for assessment, and the complexities of language require intensive testing to determine the nature and severity of impairment. Formal screening instruments, which typically require no more than 10 minutes to perform, were reviewed by the United States (US) Preventive Services Task Force.[18] The summary recommendation was that the evidence was not sufficient to recommend for or against the use of these screening instruments in primary care to identify speech and language delay in children younger than 5 years of age.

Implications for Treatment. A variety of behavioral treatments have been described. Fey and colleagues describe general principles for treatment of grammatical deficits, which are common among children classified as having SLI.[27] It was concluded from a meta-analysis of treatments for language disorders in children that speech and language therapy may be effective for children with phonological or expressive vocabulary difficulties, but there was mixed evidence for the effectiveness of interventions for children with expressive syntax difficulties and little published evidence for the effectiveness of interventions for children with expressive vocabulary difficulties.[28] Randomized controlled trials on children younger than 5 years were reviewed by the US Preventive Services Task Force.[18] Although some positive outcomes were reported, the studies generally were limited by the lack of long-term outcomes, comparison data, and generalizability. One treatment that received considerable attention in the popular media is Fast ForWord, which is based on the manipulation of the acoustic properties of speech, particularly the dynamic aspects (formant transitions) that connect adjacent sounds. A randomized clinical trial did not show that this technique was associated with better outcomes than traditional language therapy or another computer-based method.[29]

Craniofacial Anomalies

Definition and Characteristics. Craniofacial anomalies are alterations of the normal or typical structure and appearance of the craniofacial system and are linked with a number of syndromic or nonsyndromic conditions. Congenital craniofacial anomalies are discussed in Chapter 70, "Congenital Anomalies of the Head and Neck." Craniofacial anomalies frequently affect the structures used in oral motor behaviors and can greatly compromise speaking and feeding abilities. Although surgery offers major benefits both functionally and aesthetically, there is clearly a need for behavioral treatments to ensure best outcomes. Craniofacial anomalies take a variety of forms, but the most common is orofacial clefting, which is discussed in more detail here.

Epidemiology. Clefting has a worldwide incidence of 1 in 700 and is the most common of the orofacial anomalies. Nonsyndromic, or isolated, clefting is distinguished from the clefting that occurs in syndromes (eg, velocardiofacial syndrome) or sequences (eg, Pierre Robin sequence). Cleft lip is associated with 171 syndromes, but only about 15% of cleft lip-cleft palate cases are syndromic.[30] Evidence indicates that the frequency of orofacial clefting is increasing.[31] The reasons for such an increase are not clear, but etiological factors considered next may be relevant to an eventual explanation.

Etiology. Embryologically, clefts of lip and palate almost always occur because the medial nasal process either fails to make contact, or maintain contact, with the lateral nasal and maxillary processes. Studies in developmental biology have shown that both genetics and environmental factors contribute to the etiology of clefting. Evidence points to an association between isolated clefting and genetic factors, as summarized in Table 4 (which also includes information on the genetic linkages for syndromic clefting).[31] Environmental factors include parental smoking, maternal nutrition (especially folic acid), maternal alcohol consumption, maternal obesity, and parental age.[32–36]

Assessment. Assessment begins with description of the cleft. As Eppley wrote, "A universally accepted classification scheme that fully encompasses, accurately describes, and integrates all the various types of orofacial and craniofacial clefts does not exist" (p. 101e).[30] Ultrasound examination of the fetus can detect clefting as early as 20 weeks of gestation. Early identification helps specialists to guide parents in preparing for special care in areas such as feeding (eg, a modified nipple for bottle feeding) and making decisions regarding medical and other treatment.

Implications for Treatment. Within the last three decades, palatal surgery has changed both in methods and timing. Newer methods, such as Furlow Z-plasty, have been introduced, and surgery is now often done at 10 to 11 months (as compared to 18 to 24 months before the 1980s).[37] Despite these advances, data indicate that the majority of preschoolers with cleft palate exhibit delays in speech sound development that require speech–language therapy.[37] Such therapy is typically directed to improve articulation ability and hence speech intelligibility. Children with clefting often have problems associated with the ear, nose, and voice.[38]

Childhood Fluency Disorders: Stuttering and Cluttering

Definition and Characteristics. Stuttering is a disorder of the flow of speech (fluency) and typically presents as repetitions of words or parts of words, prolongations of sounds, or blockages of speech. Although these disfluencies can occur occasionally in nearly all speakers, they become more severe in persons who stutter and can be associated with secondary characteristics (eg, facial grimacing) or avoidance of communicative situations. Cluttering is a much less common disorder characterized by a speech pattern that is rapid, dysrhythmic, and unorganized. It is possible for stuttering and cluttering to co-exist in the same child.

Disfluencies are normal during speech development, and many children exhibit stuttering-like behaviors, such as sound repetitions, during the age interval of 2 to 4 years. Because this is a period of rapid changes in speech, language, and other behaviors, disfluencies may be the result of trying to talk at a time when many demands are placed on a child who has limited but growing cognitive, linguistic, and motor resources. If stuttering is viewed as a disruption of a skilled motor behavior, it is interesting that no other motor behavior acquired during childhood has an equivalent vulnerability to its performance.

Epidemiology. Stuttering has a worldwide prevalence of 1% and a prevalence in the pediatric population of 5%.[39,40] Spontaneous and complete recovery occurs in about 60 to 80% of children who stutter, and a particular goal of research is to find ways of identifying that proportion of children who are not likely to recover spontaneously.[40] Males are more likely to stutter than females, with a male to female ratio of 2:1 for young children and 5:1 for adults.[41] Comorbidity with other speech disorders, language disorders, or non-speech–language disorders is estimated to be about 60%, with articulation and phonological disorders being the most frequently co-occurring disorders.[42]

Etiology. The etiology of stuttering is controversial, but the weight of evidence points to a multifactorial origin that includes genetic factors (Table 4), probably based on interactions among multiple genes, and with a likely sex difference in gene involvement.[43–45] A genetic influence has long been suspected because of familial patterns in stuttering and high rates of concordance in monozygotic twins. It appears that genetic influences interact with environmental variables to contribute to the etiology of developmental stuttering (which should be distinguished from acquired stuttering in adults, which usually has a neurogenic or psychogenic basis). Occasionally, stuttering-like behavior has been observed in connection with medications.[39] A neurogenic basis for developmental stuttering has long been suspected, and several hypotheses have been proposed on the neural correlates of stuttering. One of the most persistent of these is that stuttering is associated with anomalous hemispheric asymmetry, such that individuals who stutter have a greater degree of right hemisphere activation for speech. Little is known about the etiology of cluttering.

Assessment. Developmental stuttering is typically identified when the child is 3 to 5 years of age, and the major presenting symptom is the repetition of individual sounds or syllables. Stuttering is identified at an age when children are making rapid advances in speech and language abilities and when there are notable changes in emotional and personality traits. Various scales have been developed to quantify stuttering behaviors, but this remains an area of some controversy. The typical procedure is to count stuttering events or dysfluency types. Stuttering severity tends to be reduced under conditions such as choral reading or repeated reading of a passage, and these fluency-inducing conditions are sometimes used in assessments. A particular challenge is to determine which children who demonstrate stuttering-like behaviors are at risk for the disorder of stuttering. This is not an easy determination, but some guidelines have been described, mostly pertaining to the frequency of disfluencies and the child's reaction to these events.[39]

Implications for Treatment. Stuttering treatment has a long history that cannot be easily covered in any depth. The high rates of spontaneous recovery in developmental stuttering complicate efforts to demonstrate the efficacy of treatment outcome.[45] Another complication is that many treatments will lead to a reduction of stuttering in the short term but the benefits may not last. Reducing stuttering is not difficult as an immediate goal, given that a number of altered speaking situations (choral reading, speaking with altered auditory feedback) lead to fairly predictable reductions in stuttering.[45] A number of treatments have been introduced but few have been sufficiently examined in randomized clinical trials to formulate confident recommendations for clinical practice. The strongest evidence (in the form of randomized clinical trials) favors the Lidcombe method of stuttering therapy.[46] But clinical specialists endorse a number of different interventions that have been successful in their own practices but have not been evaluated in clinical trials. One of the commonly used approaches is to encourage an easy or relaxed phonation at the initiation of an utterance. Many clinicians also will try to reduce communicative pressures within the child's family or school, such as asking family members to reduce speaking rates.

Voice Disorders

Definition and Characteristics. A voice disorder is an abnormal voice quality, a definition that presumes an understanding of what constitutes normal voice (not an easy matter given the large variations in normal voices). Voice disorders in children are often identified perceptually and are characterized by terms such as hoarseness, roughness, and voice breaks. Auditory-perceptual assessment of voice disorders has generated a large literature, replete with arguments for and against the reliability and validity of this approach.

Epidemiology. Estimates of the prevalence of voice disorders in children range from 6 to 11%, depending on means of assessment and population under consideration.[39,47] Estimates based on parent report are about twice as high as estimates based on clinical evaluation.[47] The risk for dysphonia is greater for boys and for children with older siblings.[39]

Etiology. Voice disorders have several etiologies, with the most common being vocal fold nodule or polyp, laryngeal webbing, laryngitis,

juvenile papilloma, vocal fold paralysis, extrinsic or intrinsic trauma to the larynx, and velopharyngeal incompetence.[39] These conditions are discussed in Chapter 69, "Congenital Anomalies of the Larynx," Chapter 75, "Benign Laryngeal Lesions," and Chapter 80, "Laryngeal Paralysis."

Assessment. Although auditory-perceptual methods remain the standard method for the clinical assessment of voice, increasing use is being made of acoustic, aerodynamic, and imaging methods. Assessment of vocal function is discussed in Chapter 73, "Assessment of Vocal Function," Chapter 79, "Neurogenic Disorders of the Larynx," and Chapter 81, "Muscle Misuse Disorders of the Larynx."

Implications for Treatment. For many of these disorders, medical treatment or voice therapy is indicated, depending on etiology, severity, and patient characteristics. Surgery may be required to remove nodules, papillomas, or webs, and surgical reconstruction may be needed in the event of trauma. Laryngoplasty is a consideration in vocal fold paralysis. Several types of behavioral voice therapy may be appropriate. These include vocal rest, laryngeal manipulation, vocal exercises, and laryngeal hydration.[48,49] Medical treatments are discussed in other chapters of this section.

SPEECH AND LANGUAGE DISORDERS IN ADULTS

Adult Neurogenic Speech Disorders (Motor Speech Disorders)

Craniofacial Muscles. Because neuropathology is the basis of these disorders, it is pertinent to ask if the neurology of speech is the same as the neurology of arm or trunk movement. Although it is often assumed that the effect of neurologic disease or damage is essentially the same for the speech musculature as it is for the muscles of the trunk or limbs, recent studies show that the muscle fiber types of the craniofacial muscles are distinct from those in the limb and trunk muscles, generally showing considerable polymorphism.[50] In addition to muscle-fiber isoforms, such as type I and type II variants, the craniofacial muscles often contain hybrid fibers that coexpress two or more isoforms. Muscle-fiber composition varies within and across muscles in the craniofacial muscles, and the composition in humans differs from that in homologous muscles in nonhuman species.

This paragraph summarizes information on muscle fibers within different parts of the speech production system. The vocalis muscle compartment of the thyroarytenoid muscle contains a large population of slow tonic muscle fibers that do not exhibit a twitch contraction but rather have contractions that are prolonged, stable, precisely controlled, and fatigue resistant (properties that seem highly suited to the demands of phonation in human speech). The mandibular muscles contain at least four different isoforms of myosin heavy chain, have a continuous range

of contraction speeds, and have a high oxidative capacity (properties that are suited to variable dynamics and fatigue resistance). The tongue has a predominance of small type IIA fibers in its anterior portion (which has the capability for rapid movements) and a sizeable population of larger type I and type IM/IIC fibers in its posterior region (which is responsible for slower adjustments of tongue carriage). The palatal muscles also show considerable heterogeneity in muscle-fiber composition, with palatopharyngeus and uvula containing remarkable proportions of type II fibers, and levator and tensor veli palatini possessing mostly type I fibers. Like the other speech muscles just described, the palatal muscles also are fatigue resistant. In general, it can be said that the craniofacial muscles are unique in their genetic, developmental, functional, and phenotypical properties.[50]

Definition and Characteristics. Adult speech disorders usually appear in adults as acquired conditions secondary to neural trauma or disease. They occur as two general types, dysarthria and apraxia of speech (also known as verbal apraxia or dyspraxia). Dysarthria is a disorder of speech production associated with lesions to the central nervous system, peripheral nervous system, or both, and generally is accompanied by motor signs of weakness, paralysis, or incoordination. As shown in Table 5, the acquired dysarthrias in adults are further classified into seven major types identified through their auditory-perceptual features and interpreted in terms of classic neurology.[51,52]

Apraxia of speech is an isolated disorder of speech production characterized by difficulties in the sequencing or patterning of movements, but in the absence of motoric deficiencies in nonspeech movements performed by the same musculature. The responsible lesion is nearly always in the language-dominant hemisphere, especially in the frontal or parietal lobes, but occasionally in subcortical regions.[53] The disorder of childhood apraxia of speech, mentioned earlier in this chapter, was given its name because it was thought to share characteristics with the acquired disorder in adults. However, loss of praxis may be fundamentally different from a failure to develop praxis in the first place. Whether or not the terminology is apt, these terms are well established clinically and probably will continue to be used.

Epidemiology. Epidemiology of these disorders tracks that of the diseases with which they are associated. Most of these diseases are those of advancing age, especially stroke and the neurodegenerative diseases. Comorbidity is high among these neurogenic disorders. An individual patient may have aphasia along with dysarthria, or aphasia along with apraxia of speech.

Etiology. Neural lesion is either known or presumed. Table 5 depicts the clinicoanatomic relationships in general terms.[51–53] But it should be noted that even within a given dysarthria type, there can be quite different speech characteristics.

Table 5 Clinicoanatomic Relationships in Dysarthria

Type of Disorder	Typical Lesion(s) and Associated Diseases or Injuries
Ataxic dysarthria	Damage to the cerebellum or its outflow tracts
	Associated with Friedreich ataxia and other spinocerebellar degeneration syndromes, multiple sclerosis, Shy-Drager syndrome, olivopontocerebellar atrophy, posterior fossa surgery (especially in children)
Flaccid dysarthria	Damage to the motor neuron
	Associated with peripheral nervous system injury, myasthenia gravis, amyotrophic lateral sclerosis
Hypokinetic dysarthria	Damage to nigro-striatal pathway
	Associated with Parkinson disease, progressive supranuclear palsy, multiple system atrophy, Shy-Drager syndrome
Hyperkinetic dysarthria (with chorea)	Damage to basal ganglia
	Associated with Huntington disease
Hyperkinetic dysarthria (with dystonia)	Damage to basal ganglia
Spastic dysarthria	Bilateral damage to the pyramidal motor system
	Associated with amyotrophic lateral sclerosis, progressive supranuclear palsy, stroke (especially bilateral)
Spastic-flaccid dysarthria	Damage to pyramidal tract and ventral horn of spinal cord: upper and lower motor neuron damage
	Associated with amyotrophic lateral sclerosis
Apraxia of speech	Damage to the language-dominant hemisphere, especially in the frontal or parietal lobes, but occasionally in subcortical regions
	Associated with stroke

For example, in respect to flaccid dysarthria associated with peripheral nervous system damage, the speech abnormalities depend on the particular pattern of cranial nerve or spinal nerve injury.

Assessment. Auditory-perceptual assessment is the core method of assessment, often done in accord with the classic descriptions of dysarthria.[51,52] The original studies that delineated dysarthric types involved ratings of 38 different dimensions of speech-voice function and a subsequent identification of clusters of deviant dimensions that were associated with particular types of neural damage. Instrumental methods can provide valuable supplementary information; among the most commonly used are acoustic, aerodynamic, and kinematic descriptions.

Implications for Treatment. Because surgical or pharmacological treatments often do not lead to complete resolution of the speech disorder, behavioral treatments are commonly used. These treatments may focus on speech behavior, or they involve augmentative and alternative communication (AAC) systems. The latter are employed especially when the speech disorder is severe and when exacerbation is likely, as in the case of neurodegenerative diseases. Behavioral speech treatments may accompany or follow other treatments including pharmacotherapy, neurosurgery, or prosthodontics. The Lee Silverman Voice Training (LSVT), which emphasizes loudness or vocal effort in a systematic therapeutic program, was introduced to improve speech in patients with idiopathic Parkinson disease.[54] However, few satisfactory clinical trials have been reported to demonstrate the efficacy of treatment methods.[55]

Aphasia

Aphasia is an impairment of the cognitive systems that perform language resulting from focal brain damage or disease (typically cortical lesions, but subcortical lesions are occasionally involved). This definition is intended to exclude language impairments associated with diffuse brain damage, such as that in dementia. The focal nature of the neural damage invites hypotheses on clinicoanatomic relationships, and this issue has been a major topic of the literature on aphasia. The nature and severity of the impairment varies considerably, and there is controversy over the most appropriate classification of deficits in aphasia. One of the most well-established and frequently used systems is the Boston Diagnostic Aphasia Examination, which uses the classification summarized in Table 6.[56]

Epidemiology. Stroke is the main cause of aphasia, and the epidemiology of aphasia relates closely to the epidemiology of stroke. Aphasia is found in 21 to 38% of acute stroke patients and is linked with high morbidity, mortality, and expenditure.[57] The incidence of aphasia from first-ever ischemic stroke was estimated to be 43 of 100,000 inhabitants in a geographically defined population.[58]

Etiology. The primary risk factors for aphasia are advancing age and cardioembolism. Although aphasia usually is associated with stroke, it can result from other neuropathologies such as tumors or trauma. The responsible lesion is typically cortical (left hemisphere in the majority of cases), but aphasia can result from subcortical lesions, including those of the thalamus, putamen, and internal capsule.

Assessment. Several tests or test batteries have been developed for the assessment of aphasia, with the basic goal of classifying type and severity of aphasia. The classifications shown in Table 6 are frequently, but not universally, used.

Treatment. A number of pharmacological treatments for aphasia have been suggested, but the evidence favors only a modest benefit from amphetamine and the dopamine agonist piracetam.[59–62] Indications are that drug therapies used alone are less effective than drug therapies combined with behavioral speech–language treatment.[62] However, randomized clinical trials are needed to demonstrate the benefit of speech–language therapy.[57]

Structurally Based Speech Disorders

These disorders result from trauma, ablative surgery, or other factors that compromise the structural integrity of the speech production system. The effects on speech and voice depend on the extent of damage (eg, laryngectomy, glossectomy, mandibulectomy).

Epidemiology and Etiology. Epidemiology follows the responsible medical condition, making it difficult to offer a concise summary.

Assessment. The main objective in assessment is to identify the effects on speech of limitations in anatomy and physiology.

Treatment. Fortunately, a number of compensations permit adequate speech production even in individuals who have experienced serious alteration of the oral and laryngeal structures. Prosthetics can often restore a basic functionality that can be further enhanced by behavioral therapy.

Voice Disorder

Definition and Characteristics: Epidemiology. Few studies have been reported on the prevalence

Table 6 Features of Types of Aphasia for Several Tasks

Aphasic Syndrome	Conversational Speech	Auditory Comprehension	Auditory Speech Repetition	Confrontation Naming
Anomic	Fluent, empty	Good to mild impairment	Good	Severely impaired
Broca's	Nonfluent	Good	Abnormal	Abnormal
Wernicke's	Fluent, paraphasic	Abnormal	Abnormal	Abnormal
Conduction	Fluent, paraphasic	Good	Abnormal	Abnormal
Transcortical motor	Nonfluent	Good	Good	Abnormal
Transcortical sensory	Fluent, paraphasic echolalic	Severely impaired	Good	Abnormal
Mixed transcortical	Nonfluent with echolalia	Severely impaired	Good	Severely impaired

and risk factors for voice disorders in adults. But a recent report indicated a lifetime prevalence of a voice disorder to be 29.9%, with 6.6% of respondents indicating a current voice disorder.[63] Factors associated with chronic voice disorder were female sex, age of 40 to 59 years, patterns of voice use and demands, esophageal reflux, chemical exposures, and frequent colds or sinus infections.[63]

Etiology. See the earlier discussion of voice disorders in children and Chapters 75, 76, 79, 80, and 81.

Assessment. Discussion of the assessment of vocal function is found in Chapters 73, 79, and 81.

Implications for Treatment. Medical interventions are considered in Chapters 75, 76, 79, 80, and 81. Several behavioral interventions have been described, many of which are similar to those mentioned previously with respect to voice disorders in children.[64]

Dysphagia

Definition and Characteristics. Dysphagia is an impairment of deglutition and can affect any aspect or stage of this process. It often results from the neural and structurally based deficits considered above; and because dysphagia teams often include otolaryngologists, speech–language pathologists, and other specialists, it is mentioned in this chapter. Dysphagia is a critical concern in many medical conditions, and it may contribute to malnutrition, dehydration, aspiration pneumonia, and death. Less severe difficulties with swallowing can interfere with quality of life, including reduced pleasure in eating and reduced social interaction, particularly when eating is involved.

Epidemiology. Prevalence of dysphagia in the general population is difficult to estimate, and it may be more useful to consider dysphagia prevalence in specified populations: full-term infants (13.4%), individuals aged 87 years or more and still living in their homes (16%), individuals with traumatic brain injury (4.5 to 77.5%), individuals with stroke (19 to 80%), and individuals with Parkinson disease (18 to 81%).[64] Despite the wide variation in these estimates, it is safe to say that dysphagia occurs with considerable frequency, and it poses a major health issue to many at-risk populations.

Etiology. As noted in the preceding discussion of epidemiology, dysphagia is associated with various causes. Among the most frequently occurring are neural disorders that impair one or more of the stages of swallowing (oral preparation, oral transit, pharyngeal, or esophageal). Dysphagia also can result from trauma to the aerodigestive tract or from surgical procedures such as laryngectomy or pharyngolaryngectomy.

Assessment. Assessment can be accomplished with a number of methods. Patient complaint is not always a reliable indication of swallowing difficulties, as these problems may be insidious in

their development. Videofluoroscopic swallowing studies are useful to detect abnormalities in the different stages of swallow.

Implications for Treatment. Treatment is based on an understanding of the contributing factors, and a variety of surgical, pharmacologic, and behavioral interventions may be considered.

CONCLUSIONS

Disorders of speech and language are important considerations in functions of the stomatognathic, laryngeal, and auditory systems. Although prevalence estimates vary considerably, it is likely that these disorders have a prevalence of about 6 to 8% in the general population. These disorders may be of increasing concern because of the growing emphasis placed on communication for educational, vocational, and social pursuits in this digital age.

Epidemiologic and etiologic information is far from satisfactory for some of the most frequently occurring disorders. Multifactorial origins may underlie a large proportion of cases of specific language impairment, stuttering, speech sound disorders, and possibly craniofacial anomalies. As shown in Table 4, speech and language disorders are linked to loci on nearly all autosomes as well as the X sex chromosome. These complex genetic influences are matched by a tangle of environmental variables that affect the development of speech and language in children. Some of these disorders persist into adulthood, either in essentially the same form (eg, stuttering) or in different forms (such as a reading disorder that may be related to an earlier language disorder). High rates of comorbidity are observed for nearly all of the disorders. Co-occurrence of disorders can complicate diagnosis and treatment, but it may also provide insights into the etiology of these conditions.

REFERENCES

1. Kent RD, Hustad, KC. Speech production, development. In: Squire L, Albright T, Bloom F, et al, editors. Encyclopedia of Neuroscience. Oxford, UK: Elsevier, in press.
2. Grizzle KL, Simms MD. Early language development and language learning disabilities. Pediatr in Review 2005; 26:274–83.
3. Mader J. The relative frequency of English consonant sounds in words in the speech of children in grades one, two, and three. Speech Monogr 1954;21:294–300.
4. Smit AB, Hand L, Frelinger JJ, et al. The Iowa articulation norms project and its Nebraska replication. J Speech Hear Disord 1990;55:779–98.
5. Keating D, Turrell G, Ozanne A. Childhood speech disorders: Reported prevalence, cormorbidity and socioeconomic profile. J Paediatr Child Health 2001;37:431–36.
6. Shriberg LD, Tomblin JB, McSweeny JL. Prevalence of speech delay in 6-year-old children and comorbidity with language impairment. J Speech Lang Hear Res 1999; 42:1461–81.
7. Byles J. The epidemiology of communication and swallowing disorders. Adv Speech-Lang Pathol 2005;7:1–7.
8. Shriberg LD. Five subtypes of developmental phonological disorders. Clin Commun Disord 1994;4:38–53.
9. Odding E, Roebroeck ME, Stam JH. The epidemiology of cerebral palsy: Incidence, impairments and risk factors. Disabil Rehabil 2006;28:183–91.
10. Zeesman S, Nowaczyk MJ, Teshima K, et al. Speech and language impairment and oromotor dyspraxia due to

11. deletion of 7q31 that involves FOXP2. Am J Med Genet A 2006;140:509–14.
11. MacDermot KD, Bonora E, Sykes N, et al. Identification of FOXP2 truncation as a novel cause of developmental speech and language deficits. Am J Hum Genet 2005;76:1074–80.
12. Raskind WH, Igo RP, Chapman NH, et al. A genome scan in multigenerational families with dyslexia: Identification of a novel locus on chromosome 2q that contributes to phonological decoding efficiency. Mol Psychiatry 2005;10:699–711.
13. Stein CM, Millard C, Kluge A, et al. Speech sound disorder influenced by a locus in 15q14 region. Behav Genet 2006;36:858–68.
14. Stein CM, Schick JH, Gerry Taylor H, et al. Pleiotropic effects of a chomosome 3 locus on speech-sound disorder and reading. Am J Hum Genet 2004;74:283–97.
15. Clark HM. Neuromuscular treatments for speech and swallowing: A tutorial. Am J Speech Lang Pathol 2003; 12:400–15.
16. Smith BS, Simmons DC, Kameenui EJ. Synthesis of research on phonological awareness: Principles and implications for reading acquisition. Website on Phonological Awareness Resources and Links available at http://ca.geocities.com/phonological/.
17. Hall DMB, Elliman D. Health for All Children, 4th edition. Oxford: Oxford University Press; 2003.
18. US Preventive Services Task Force. Screening for speech and language delay in preschool children: Recommendation statement. Am Family Phys 2006;73,1605–10.
19. Van Weerdenburg M, Verhoeven L, van Balkom H. Towards a typology of specific language impairment. J Child Psychol Psychiatry 2006;47:176–89.
20. SLI Consortium (SLIC). Highly significant linkage to the SLI1f locus in an expanded sample of individuals affected by specific language impairment. Am J Hum Genet 2004; 74:1225–38.
21. Bartlet CW, Flax JF, Logue MW, et al. A major susceptibility locus for specific language impairment is located on 13q21. Am J Hum Genet 2002;71:45–55.
22. O'Brien EK, Zhang X, Nishimura C, et al. Association of specific language impairment (SLI) to the region of 7q31. Am J Hum Genet 2003;72:1536–43.
23. Shevell MI, Majnemer A, Webster RI, et al. Outcomes at school age of preschool children with developmental language impairment. Pediatr Neurol 2005;32:264–9.
24. Gauger LM, Lombardino LJ, Leonard CM. Brain morphology in children with specific language impairment. J Speech Lang Hear Res 1997;40:1272–84.
25. Newschaffer CJ, Falb MD, Gurney JG. National autism prevalence trends from United States special education data. Pediatr 2005;115:e277–82.
26. Hill EL. Non-specific nature of specific language impairment: A review of the literature with regard to concomitant motor impairments. Int J Lang Commun Disord 2001;36:149–71.
27. Fey ME, Long SH, Finestack, LH. Ten principles of grammar facilitation for children with specific language impairments. Am J Speech Lang Pathol 2003;12:3–15.
28. Law J, Garrett Z, Nye C. The efficacy of treatment for children with developmental speech and language delay/disorder: A meta-analysis. J Speech Lang Hear Res 2004;47:924–43.
29. Cohen W, Hodson A, O'Hare A, et al. Effects of computer-based intervention through acoustically modified speech (Fast ForWord) in a severe mixed receptive-expressive language impairment: Outcomes from a randomized controlled trial. J Speech Lang Hear Res 2005;48:715–29.
30. Eppley BL, van Aalst JA, Robey A, et al. The spectrum of orofacial clefting. Plast Reconstr Surg 2005;115:101e–14e.
31. Meyer KA, Williams P, Hernandez-Diaz S, Cnattingius S. Smoking and the risk of oral clefts: Exploring the impact of study designs. Epidemiology 2004;15:671–8.
32. Canfield MA, Collins JS, Botto LD, et al. National Birth Defects Prevention Network. Changes in the birth prevalence of selected birth defects after grain fortification with folic acid in the United States: Findings from a multi-state population-based study. Birth Defects Res A Clin Mol Teratol 2005;73:679–89.
33. Cedergren M, Kallen B. Maternal obesity and the risk for orofacial clefts in the offspring. Cleft Palate Craniofac J 2005;42:367–71.
34. Bille C, Skytthe A, Vach W, et al. Parent's age and the risk of oral clefts. Epidemiology 2005;16:311–6.
35. Warrington A, Vieira AR, Christensen K, et al. Genetic evidence for the role of loci at 19q13 in cleft lip and palate. J Med Genet 2006;43:e26 (ePub).
36. Olasoji HO, Ukiri OE, Yahaya A. Incidence and aetiology of oral clefts: A review. Afr J Med Med Sci 2005;34:1–7.
37. Hardin-Jones MA, Jones DL. Speech production of preschoolers with cleft palate. Cleft Pal-Craniofacial J 2005;42:7–13.
38. Hocevar-Boltezar I, Jarc A, Koxelj V. Ear, nose and voice problems in children with orofacial clefts. J Laryngol Otol 2006;120:276–81.

39. Baker BM, Blackwell PB. Identification and remediation of pediatric fluency and voice disorders. J Pediatr Health Care 2004;18:87–94.

40. Yairi E, Ambrose NG. Early childhood stuttering I. persistency and recovery rates. J Speech Lang Hear Res 1999;42:1097–112.

41. Ambrose N, Cox N, Yairi E. The genetic basis of persistence and recovery in stuttering. J Speech Lang Hear Res 1997;40:567–80.

42. Blood GW, Ridenour VJ, Qualls CD, Hammer CS. Co-occurring disorders in children who stutter. J Commun Disord 2003;36:427–48.

43. Riaz N, Steinberg S, Ahmad J, et al. Genomewide significant linkage to stuttering on chromosome 12. Am J Hum Genet 2005;76:647–51.

44. Suresh R, Ambrose N, Roe C, et al. New complexities in the genetics of stuttering: Significant sex-specific linkage signals. Am J Hum Genet 2006;78:554–63.

45. Saltuklaroglu T, Kalinowski J. How effective is therapy for childhood stuttering? Dissecting and reinterpreting the evidence in light of spontaneous recovery rates. Int J Lang Comm Dis 2005;40:359–74.

46. Jones M, Onslow M, Packman A, et al. Randomised controlled trial of the Lidcombe programme of early stuttering intervention. Brit Med J 2005;331:659 –61.

47. Carding PN, Roulstone S, Northstone K, Alspac Study Team. The prevalence of childhood dysphonia: A cross-sectional study. J Voice 2006;20:623–30.

48. Hersan R, Behlau M. Behavioral management of pediatric voice disorders. Otolaryngol Clin North Am 2000;33:1097–110.

49. Baker BM, Blackwell PB. Identification and remediation of pediatric fluency and voice disorders. J Pediatr Health Care 2004;18:87–94.

50. Kent RD. The uniqueness of speech among motor systems. Clin Ling Phon 2004;18:495–505.

51. Darley FL, Aronson AE, Brown JR. Differential diagnostic patterns of dysarthria. J Speech Hear Res 1969;12:249–69.

52. Darley FL, Aronson AE, Brown JR. Clusters of deviant speech dimensions in the dysarthrias. J Speech Hear Res 1969;12:462–96.

53. Ballard KJ, Granier JP, Robin DA. Understanding the nature of apraxia of speech: Theory, analysis and treatment. Aphasiology 2000;14:969–95.

54. Ramig LO, Sapir S, Countryman S, et al. Intensive voice treatment (LSVT) for patients with Parkinson's disease: A 2 year follow up. J Neurol Neurosurg Psychiatry 2001;71:493– 8.

55. Deane KH, Whurr R, Playford ED, et al. A comparison of speech and language therapy techniques for dysarthria in Parkinson's disease. Cochrane Database Syst Rev 2001;CD002814.

56. Goodglass H, Kaplan E. The Boston Diagnostic Aphasia Examination. Philadelphia: Lea and Febiger; 1983.

57. Hatfield B, Millet D, Cole J, et al. Characterizing speech and language pathology outcomes in stroke rehabilitation. Arch Phys Med Rehabil 2006;86:S61–72.

58. Engelter ST, Gostynski M, Papa S, et al. Epidemiology of aphasia attributable to first ischemic stroke: Incidence, severity, fluency, etiology, and thrombolysis. Stroke 2006;37:1379–84.

59. Berthier ML. Poststroke aphasia: Epidemiology, pathophysiology and treatment. Drugs Aging 2005;22:163–82.

60. Bakheit AM. Drug treatment of poststroke aphasia. Expert Rev Neurother 2004;4:211–7.

61. Greener J, Enderby P, Whurr R. Pharmacological treatment for aphasia following stroke. Cochrane Database Syst Rev 2001;CD000424.

62. de Boissezon X, Peran P, de Boysson C, Demonet JF. Pharmacotherapy of aphasia: Myth or reality? Brain Lang 2006; Sep 16; [Epub ahead of print].

63. Roy N, Merrill RM, Gray SD, Smith EM. Voice disorders in the general population: Prevalence, risk factors, and occupational impact. Laryngoscope 2005;115:1988–95.

64. Casper JK, Murry T. Voice therapy methods in dysphonia. Otolaryngol Clin North Am 2000;33:983–1002.

75

Benign Laryngeal Lesions

Michael M. Johns, MD
Shatul Parikh, MD

Benign laryngeal lesions are an increasingly commonly diagnosed cause of dysphonia.[1] Modern-day advances within the subspecialty field of laryngology have allowed otolaryngologists to become increasingly precise with their ability to diagnose and treat voice disorders. Prior to the advent of sophisticated office-based imaging, most vocal-fold lesions were diagnosed in the operating room. Innovative otolaryngologists, speech language pathologists, and voice scientists have developed preventive, diagnostic, and treatment modalities to improve the quality of life of those with dysphonia.

The gold standard for the diagnosis of benign vocal-fold lesions remains a thorough history and head and neck examination, followed by a subjective assessment of the voice and detailed imaging of the vocal folds. Despite the introduction of novel methods of visualizing vocal-fold vibration including high-speed photography, videokymography, photoglottography, and ultrasonography, laryngeal videostroboscopy remains the most practical and clinically useful tool in visualizing vocal folds. The equipment is relatively inexpensive, and the examination can be performed within an office setting either with flexible transnasal or rigid transoral endoscopy. Videostroboscopy allows for detailed evaluation of vocal-fold vibratory characteristics, mucosal wave and glottal closure. This detailed evaluation of the entire vocal fold allows for visualization of even subtle benign lesions.

PHONOTRAUMATIC VOCAL-FOLD LESIONS: NODULES, POLYPS, CYSTS

Etiology

The vocal folds are subject to mechanical stress during phonation. Vocal-fold vibration during phonation leads to impact stress during the collision of the vibratory surfaces. These stress forces have been analyzed, and it has been determined that maximal impact of stress occurs in the midmembranous vocal fold, the typical location for vocal nodules.[2] Vocal overuse in the form of excessive use, abuse, for example, yelling, and misuse, for example, vocal hyperfunction with excessive muscular tension, leads to undue mechanical stress resulting in trauma in this region. Repetitive trauma results in wound formation within the superficial layer of the

lamina propria and to a lesser extent the vocal-fold epithelium.[3,4] Vocal nodules are essentially calluses on the vocal fold. In contrast, a polyp is an outpouching of the epithelial cover, filled with mucoid or fibrous substance. Polyps may be pedunculated or sessile. Etiology of polyp formation is less clear, but often appears to be organization of a hematoma. When polypoid change involves the entire membranous fold, it is often referred to as Reinke edema. A cyst is an epithelial-lined mass. It is not clear whether cysts arise from trauma or from gradual enlargement of a congenital defect. A pseudocyst is an amorphous submucosal collection of fibrinoid material.

Diagnostic Principles

Vocal-fold nodules, polyps, and cysts can be differentiated on videostroboscopy, and the degree of dysphonia is associated with the extent of disruption of vocal-fold vibration.[4] Vocal-fold nodules are generally symmetric and always bilateral mass lesions of the vocal folds (Figure 1). They arise at the junction of the anterior and middle third of the vocal fold and tend to appear white to opaque and firm. They result in an hourglass closure glottal configuration and will affect vocal-fold mucosal wave and vibration variably, depending on their size and the degree of associated edema. Vocal-fold polyps are more translucent to red and are more commonly unilateral, although bilateral polyps may occur (Figure 2). The mucosal wave is generally present or increased with vocal-fold polyps. Vocal-fold cysts can be divided into two types: mucous retention cysts and squamous cell inclusion cysts. Mucous retention cysts usually arise below the

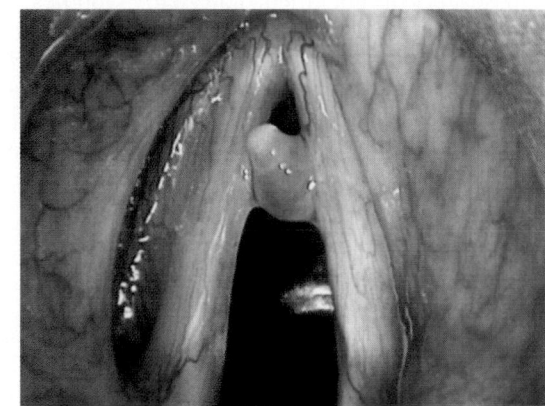

Figure 2 Posthemorrhagic polyp. Peduculated mass arising at the midmembranous vocal fold.

free margin of the glottis and are translucent collections of mucus likely arising from a plugged mucous gland duct. Squamous cell inclusion cysts appear as yellow fusiform masses within the lamina propria (Figure 3). Vocal-fold mucosal wave is affected variably depending on the size of the lesion. Small subepithelial lesions may not disrupt the mucosal wave, but larger lesions that extend to the vocal ligament distort vocal-fold pliability as they replace the superficial lamina propria (SLP). Optical coherence tomography (OCT) is a potentially new diagnostic tool for diagnosing phonotraumatic lesions.[5] This noncontact, noninvasive technology allows detailed imaging of the vocal fold by using cross-sectional images by means of backscattered light.

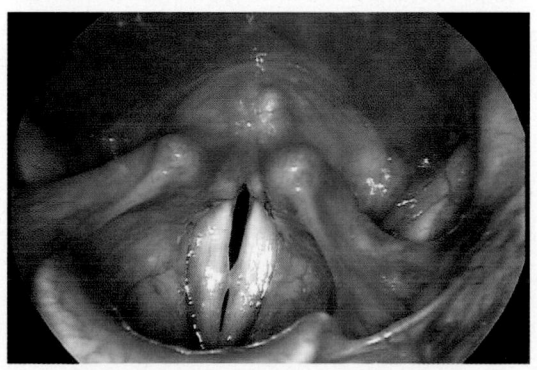

Figure 1 Vocal nodules. Generally bilateral, symmetric, midmembranous, and subepithelial vocal-fold lesions.

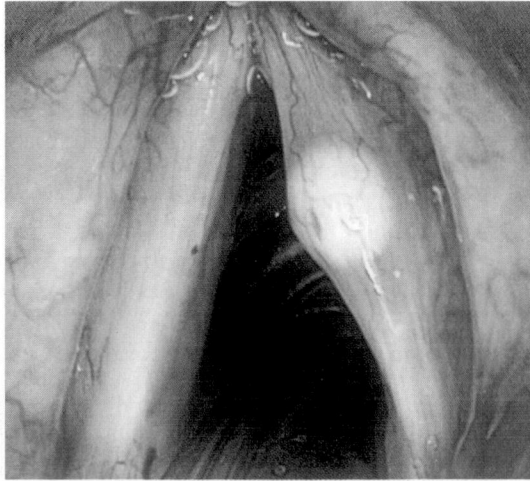

Figure 3 Vocal-fold cyst. Fusiform, epithelial-lined mass within vocal fold replacing the lamina propria.

Treatment Principles: Behavioral Intervention and Voice Therapy

The first-line treatment for lesions caused by phonotrauma, vocal-fold polyps, nodules, and cysts, is behavioral intervention with speaking and singing therapy. The primary goal of voice therapy is to maximize efficiency of phonation and to eliminate maladaptive vocal behaviors that exacerbate these masses. Additionally, patients should be treated for concomitant problems that contribute to mucosal friability, such as laryngopharyngeal reflux and poor vocal hygiene. Vocal nodules are responsive to voice therapy, and surgery is not often indicated. "Nodules" which persist after adequate therapy may actually prove to be cysts. In patients with vocal nodules, it has been concluded in one study that over a 4- to 6-month period of voice therapy patients experience significant perceptual improvements in voice and most have a reduction in the size of the nodules. Of note, the lesions did not disappear completely in any of the patients in this study. It must be kept in mind that adequate improvements in voice do not necessarily correlate with disappearance of the lesions.[6] Vocal-fold polyps and cysts are much less responsive to voice therapy although some patients may experience adequate improvement with voice therapy.

Treatment Principles: Surgical Intervention

When maximal behavior intervention does not achieve satisfactory improvements in voice, surgical treatment may be considered. The decision to pursue surgical management, however, should take into account multiple factors, including the patient's vocal impairment, type and location of the lesion, and willingness to accept surgical risk. Patients who do not have vocally demanding lifestyles or do not have significant functional impairment from their lesions may not warrant surgical intervention. Additionally, the probability of surgical success based on the lesion type and location should be considered. Patients with large pedunculated polyps have a high chance of significant vocal improvement with surgical resection with minimal scarring. On the contrary, vocal-fold cysts are more technically demanding to excise and have a higher chance of postoperative scarring based on their location and replacement of healthy SLP. Surgical intervention for vocal nodules should be reserved for select patients in whom appropriate behavioral intervention has been implemented and significant vocal incapacity remains and the patient is willing to accept the risk of vocal-fold scarring.

Significant improvement in laryngeal endoscopic microsurgical understanding, technique, and instrumentation has occurred over the past three decades, and refinements continue to be published in the medical literature. Nonetheless, endoscopic laryngeal microsurgery remains technically demanding. Even though operating through large microlaryngoscopes, there are significantly limited degrees of freedom of instrument movement. This problem, combined with long instruments and millimeter-sized pathology, makes endoscopic laryngeal microsurgery highly challenging.

The overall goal of surgical intervention for phonotraumatic lesions is careful removal of abnormal tissue with maximal preservation of normal SLP. Surgical techniques with these principles in mind are referred to as microflap, minimicroflap, or subepithelial resections.[7–9] The historical procedure of "vocal-fold stripping" does not play a role in modern endoscopic microlaryngeal surgery for benign vocal-fold lesions. Stripping the vocal fold of mucosa removes all the functional tissue required for healthy phonation and ensures a poor postoperative outcome.

The first important operative principle is patient positioning to optimize laryngeal exposure. Direct visualization of the entire membranous vocal fold to the anterior commissure using an adequately sized laryngoscope is a fundamental element for optimizing surgical success. Patient positioning in the "sniffing position" offers optimum laryngeal exposure for endoscopic microsurgery.[10] The sniffing position requires the neck to be flexed on the chest and the head being extended on the neck. A variety of suspension operating microlaryngoscopes are available that allow for binocular microscopic visualization of the larynx with the introduction simultaneously of instruments in each hand.

Once good exposure of the glottis is achieved with an appropriate laryngoscope in suspension, the surgeon should be sure to have comfortable, ergonomic seating with appropriate wrist and forearm support. Adequate arm and wrist support significantly improves microsurgical control and reduces fatigue. Specially designed operative chairs are made for this purpose, although adequate support can be achieved by stacking sheets on a mayo stand at the patient's head upon which the forearms can rest.

After adequate positioning, careful examination of the endolarynx is performed. Optimum examination initially includes the use of straight and angled telescopes. A 70° telescope is particularly useful for seeing the craniocaudal extent of lesions and for visualizing the ventricle and subglottis. The operating microscope can then be used at the highest power magnification for binocular visualization. Careful palpation with blunt microsurgical instruments gives the surgeon a sense of the lesion's character and helps identify the junction of normal and abnormal tissue.

An array of laryngeal microsurgical instrument sets are available that optimize surgical precision. The important principles in instrument selection are having instrument tips that are sufficiently small with a variety of functions to maintain control around small lesions and to maximize preservation of normal SLP. The surgeon should have a variety of microcannula for suction and blunt instruments for palpation. Micrograspers, microcups, and microscissors should be available in straight, up, right, and left configurations. Finally, sharp microsickle knives and blunt-angled microflap elevators are necessary.

The initial surgical incision can be made with a microsickle knife or microscissors. Placement should be at the precise junction of normal and abnormal tissue. Following the epithelial incision, blunt instruments and suction should be used to identify the junction between normal and abnormal tissue, preserving as much normal SLP deep to the lesion as possible. Human cadaver larynx investigations have determined that a natural plane of dissection occurs in the SLP of the vocal fold using semiblunt microdissectors.[11] Dissection is carried out within the SLP just around the abnormal subepithelial tissue, trying to disrupt as little healthy SLP and preserve healthy mucosa medially to redrape over the surgical defect. In the case of vocal-fold cysts, care must be taken not to rupture the cyst and excise the entire cyst wall to prevent recurrence.

The CO_2 laser can be a useful adjunctive tool in these procedures. Although some argue that the CO_2 laser leads to excessive thermal injury in the vocal fold, it must be remembered that lasers and cold microinstrumentation are simply tools. Maximizing preservation and minimizing disruption of healthy SLP are the overriding principles, and the care, knowledge, and experience of the surgeon drive surgical outcomes. Comparison of cold dissection technique versus microspot CO_2 laser-assisted dissection for surgical treatment of benign laryngeal lesions has been studied. It was found that there is no difference in clinical outcomes measured by acoustic analysis, airflow rates, videostroboscopic, and audio perceptual analysis in patients treated with either technique.[12]

With regard to postoperative care, voice rest is controversial. While many laryngologists advocate a period of 4 to 14 days of absolute voice rest following vocal-fold microsurgery, others feel that reduced voice use is preferable. It is difficult for patients to comply with absolute voice rest, and voice professionals may get "out of shape" without some voice use. Moreover, there may be less scarring with some vocal mobility. There are no clinical studies that can resolve this controversy.[13] In a study of wound healing following vocal-fold microsurgery in a canine model, it was found that longer healing times were necessary in the vocal-fold basement membrane zone in dogs that were allowed to phonate after surgery versus those on iatrogenic voice rest (recurrent laryngeal nerve resection).[14] Although extrapolation of these findings to humans may be difficult, the results imply that some voice rest may be beneficial following laryngeal microsurgery.

Outcomes of surgical intervention for benign laryngeal lesions have been extensively studied. Microsurgical excision has shown improved vocal function postoperatively in almost all patients as measured by patient perception, quality of life, videostroboscopy, and acoustic and aerodynamic measures.[1,7]

BENIGN NEOPLASMS

Recurrent Respiratory Papillomatosis

Etiology. Although recurrent respiratory papillomatosis (RRP) is a rare clinical entity, laryngeal papillomas are the most common benign laryngeal neoplasm.[15–17] RRP is caused by epithelial infection with the human papilloma virus (HPV). The disease process is clinically divided into an adult-onset and juvenile-onset form. In the juvenile onset the incidence in the United States is between 80 and 1,500 cases per 100,000 persons annually.[18] The means of transmission of HPV is unknown, although exposure to the virus is clearly required combined with host susceptibility. Maternal–fetal transmission in the juvenile form and sexual transmission in the adult form have been proposed.[19] While the juvenile-onset form has an equal female to male ratio, adult-onset disease has a male to female preponderance of 2:1.[15,20] RRP is considered to be adult onset if the patient presents older than 16 to 20 years.[21] In most pediatric studies, the diagnosis of RRP occurs 1 year after the start of symptoms. Most patients are firstborn, have young mothers, and come from families of low socioeconomic status.[19] The HPV 6 and 11 viral subtypes are most commonly found in RRP, though subtypes 16 and 18 have also been found. The latter two subtypes are associated with malignant degeneration.[21]

Diagnostic Principles. In the adult-onset form of the disease, the most common presenting symptom is dysphonia.[20] Children with RRP present with wide spectrum of laryngeal symptoms. Although pathologically indistinct lesions, a papilloma that presents as hoarseness in one child may present with stridor in another child depending on the location and bulk of the disease. Prior to definitive diagnosis of RRP, children are often mistakenly treated for having asthma, bronchitis, croup, epiglottitis, or gastroesophageal reflux. If the onset of stridor or dysphonia is gradually progressive, a neoplastic process should be considered. Although definitive diagnosis requires pathologic confirmation, RRP has a unique appearance on laryngoscopy. Lesions are exophytic, verrucous, and have characteristic pattern of vascular stippling (Figure 4). While the extent of the neoplasm can be estimated by

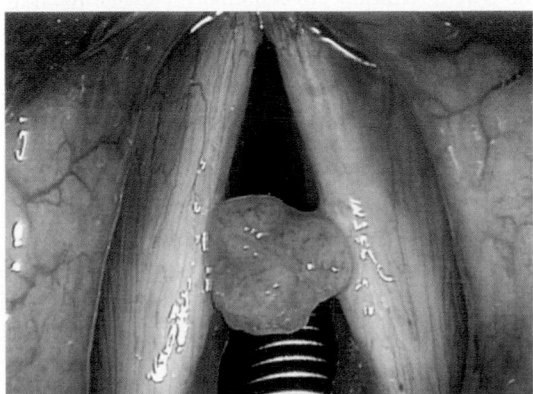

Figure 4 Papilloma. Exophytic, verrucous lesion with characteristic vascular stippling.

preoperative laryngeal imaging, careful examination in the operating room with the assistance of angled telescopes provides the most accurate assessment of disease severity.

Treatment Principles. Treatment success is determined by the ability to maintain an adequate airway and functional voice preservation. There has yet to be a surgical or medical treatment that has been shown to eradicate the disease in affected patients. Surgical treatment can occur via cold steel, CO_2 laser, or microdebrider excision.[22,23] These instruments are all simply tools, and the key to success lies in meticulous surgical technique. The preservation of voice with maintenance of the SLP is the important consideration. Additionally, resection should avoid the apposition of raw mucosal surfaces especially in the anterior commissure that may promote glottic webbing.

Traditionally, the CO_2 laser has been the surgical workhorse for patients with RRP.[16] These lasers are coupled to an operating microscope allowing precise vaporization of lesions. New scanning laser technology has allowed for increased precision and reduced thermal injury from the CO_2 laser. Currently, the technique most commonly used among pediatric otolaryngologists for excision of gross papilloma is the powered microdebrider.[24] This technique involves the use a small oscillating blade with a suction that allows papilloma to be drawn into the blade chamber and effectively sheared from its attachment. Several studies have shown improvement in operating time, patient postoperative pain, cost, and scarring when comparing microdebridement to CO_2 laser excision of RRP.[23] However, care must be taken to avoid injury to normal tissue, which can occur quickly and easily using this powered instrument, particularly at the glottal level.

Special precaution must be taken while treating disease at the anterior commissure to avoid raw opposing surfaces that can lead to the development of an anterior glottal web. Staged procedures several weeks apart to allow mucosalization of one side prior to surgery on the other can help prevent web formation.

Recent treatment advances in the field of RRP have emphasized the benefits of alternative technologies and medical therapies. Pulsed lasers (pulsed dye or pulsed KTP) with hemoglobin sensitivity have shown positive results in the operative and office-based treatment of RRP.[25–28] These types of lasers selectively coagulate the vascular stalk feeding the papilloma, causing it to blanch and eventually slough. Reported advantages include the avoidance of general anesthesia, reduced scarring, and the ability to treat the anterior commissure.

A variety of adjuvant therapies have been reported in the treatment of RRP. These include locally injected cidofovir (an antiviral agent), intravenous interferon-α, and oral indole-3-carbinol.[29–31] Varying degrees of success in treatment of RRP are reported, and use of these therapies has not been approved by the US Food

and Drug Administration, and their use is therefore off-label. Reports of carcinogenesis in animal models with cidofovir use necessitate more in-depth investigation. In patients with recalcitrant RRP or with progressive disease involving the tracheobronchial tree or pulmonary involvement, the benefit that these agents have may outweigh their risk to control spread of disease.

Currently, a quadrivalent (HPV types 6, 11, 16, 18) vaccine is available for reducing the risk of cervical cancer.[32] The availability of this vaccine could dramatically change the incidence of RRP. However, the vaccines effect on preexisting disease is unknown.

Granular Cell Tumor (Myoblastoma)

Historically, granular cell tumors were referred to in the literature as myoblastomas. Actually, these neoplasms arise from neural elements, more specifically Schwann cells. Granular cell tumors present in the head and neck region in 50% of cases. Approximately 10% of cases arise within the larynx. They present as a submucosal mass that most commonly arises at the junction of the vocal ligament and vocal process of the arytenoid cartilage. Surgical resection can be curative through an endoscopic or open approach. Pseudoepitheliomatous hyperplasia is a characteristic pathologic finding.[33]

Paraganglioma

Paragangliomas occur in the larynx infrequently. Their pathogenesis is similar to other chemodectomas that arise in the head and neck. They are the only head and neck neoplasm that shows a female preponderance. They most commonly arise from branches of the superior laryngeal nerve. They appear as a vascular submucosal mass. Diagnosis is confirmed with high-resolution computerized tomography, magnetic resonance imaging (MRI), or angiography. Characteristic salt and pepper appearance is found on MRI because of the vascular flow voids. Resection with consideration of organ preservation is important as these neoplasms are rarely malignant or metastasize. Depending on the size and extent or tumor, endoscopic or open resection can be considered. Preoperative embolization of these neoplasms has decreased intraoperative bleeding and facilitates total resection. Microscopically, these tumors show large polygonal cells with eosinophilic cytoplasm that cluster into islands or nests of cells known as Zellballen.[34,35]

Chondroma

The etiology of laryngeal chondroma is unclear. Cartilagenous neoplasms represent less than 1% of all laryngeal neoplasms.[36] Clinically, patients present with slowly progressive dyspnea, hoarseness, dysphagia, and stridor. Because chondromas are slow-growing lesions, symptoms can be present for years prior to the diagnosis. Physical examination can show a submucosal laryngeal mass, vocal cord immobility, and a narrowed subglottis. Vocal cord immobility is almost exclusively a sign of malignant transformation. Immobility may result from fixation of the cricoarytenoid joint, bulky disease, or involvement of the recurrent nerve. Although recurrence rates are high, treatment involves local excision with organ preservation via an open or closed approach. Chondroma is a benign cartilaginous neoplasm, encapsulated with a lobular growth pattern. Neoplastic cells resemble normal cells and produce the cartilaginous matrix.

LARYNGOCELES AND SACCULAR CYSTS

Etiology

The laryngeal saccule is a mucous gland-containing appendage that lies between the false vocal fold and the thyroid cartilage. It is an out-pouching of the laryngeal ventricle and extends as a sac posterolateral to the edge of the laryngeal surface of the epiglottis. The function of the saccule is unknown although it has been theorized that it may represent a vestigial air sac. Both laryngoceles and saccular cysts involve expansion of the saccule to form a mass. Laryngoceles by definition must have air contained within their lumen, while saccular cysts are strictly fluid-filled masses.

Laryngoceles contain air due to a patent communicate with the laryngeal lumen. Classification of laryngoceles depends on their location. They can be defined as internal, external, or combined. Internal laryngoceles are confined within the thyroid cartilage, external laryngoceles lie outside the cartilaginous laryngeal framework, and combined laryngoceles span both the inside and outside of the thyroid cartilage.

Saccular cysts are also classified according to their location: anterior and lateral. Anterior saccular cysts appear as rounded fluid-filled masses emanating from the anterior portion of the ventricle and extend medially into the lumen of the larynx (Figure 5). They are superior to the glottal level at or near the anterior commissure. They interfere with phonation or airway depending on their size. Lateral saccular cysts expand within the paraglottic space and appear similar to internal laryngoceles as a submucosal fullness in the ventricular fold.

Although the etiology of saccular masses is unclear, they result from abnormal dilation of the saccule. It has been suggested that those who routinely develop high transglottic pressures, for example, glass blowers or trumpet players, are at a higher risk of developing laryngoceles.[37,38] It is thought that saccular cysts arise secondary to obstruction of the saccular orifice as they have been found in patients with laryngeal carcinoma.[39] Congenital saccular cysts can occur in infants and present as a weak cry, stridor, or cyanosis.[40]

Diagnostic Principles

Patients with laryngoceles and saccular cysts report symptoms consistent with a laryngeal

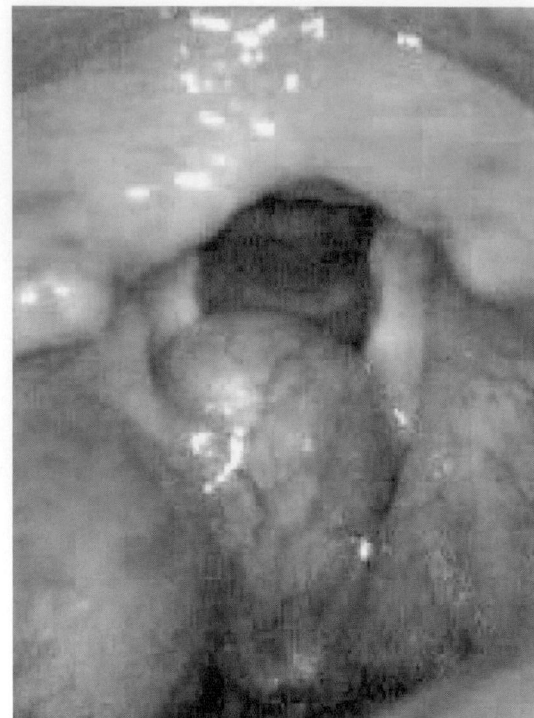

Figure 5 Anterior saccular cyst. Fluid-filled mass arising from the saccule and protruding into the laryngeal lumen.

mass: dysphonia, stridor, chronic cough, a neck mass, and occasionally dysphagia. Severity of symptoms depends on the size and location of the lesion. Small or nonobstructing lesions may be asymptomatic. The diagnosis is most commonly made by physical examination including transnasal or transoral laryngeal imaging and neck examination. In the case of anterior saccular cysts, a mass can be seen emanating from the vestibule to the laryngeal lumen while lateral saccular cysts and laryngoceles present as a submucosal mass in the false vocal fold. External and combined laryngoceles can present as a neck mass that enlarges with valsalva. Both laryngoceles and saccular cysts can become acutely infected to form a laryngopyocele or an infected saccular cyst. Superinfection can lead to rapid expansion and acute presentation with worsening symptoms, fever, and occasionally airway obstruction.

High-resolution computerized tomography (CT with 1 to 2.5 mm imaging sections) is a useful adjunctive tool diagnostically (Figure 6). The presence of air within the lesion differentiates laryngoceles from saccular cysts. The location and extent of the lesion can be accurately assessed with CT.

Treatment Principles

Although controversy exists in the literature as to the surgical management of laryngoceles and saccular cysts, most authors agree that surgery is the definitive management. Endoscopic treatment of these lesions involves either complete resection versus marsupialization. Complete resection via either an open or closed approach is the preferred methodology to prevent recurrence. Microsurgical or CO_2 laser–assisted endoscopic resection has shown to be curative for both

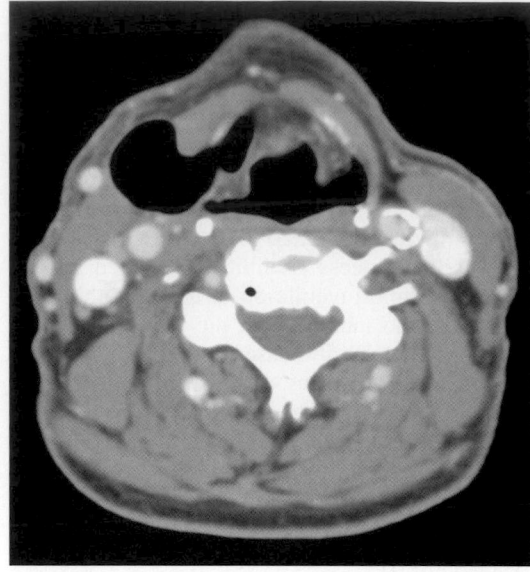

Figure 6 Combined laryngocele. Axial computed tomography showing air-filled dilation of the saccule extending through the thyrohyoid membrane into the neck.

laryngoceles and saccular cysts.[41,42] Open surgical management is necessary for external and large-combined laryngoceles or lateral saccular cysts that extend through the thyrohyoid membrane. Historically, it was felt that laryngofissure was necessary to remove these lesions. Internal laryngoceles and saccular cysts can be removed endoscopically with advanced instrumentation, visualization, and surgical technique. Combined laryngoceles can be removed through an external approach without performing laryngofissure. The lesion can be dissected through the often widened thyrohyoid membrane to their base and ligated without disrupting the thyroid cartilage.[42,43]

CONTACT GRANULOMAS

Etiology

Contact granulomas are benign lesions of the posterior glottis and vocal process. Synonyms are intubation granulomas, contact ulceration, and vocal process granulomas. These lesions can be thought of as a chronic nonhealing wound. They can be attributed to precipitating, for example, mechanical causes, and exacerbating factors, for example, laryngopharyngeal reflux (LPR) or vocal trauma. Mechanical causes include vocal trauma, for example, vocal hyperfunction and chronic chough, and nonvocal laryngeal trauma, for example, intubation injury.[44] Once an injury occurs to the thin mucosa and perichondrium overlying the cartilaginous portion of the glottis, ongoing trauma or irritation, for example, LPR, exacerbates the wound and prevents complete wound healing. An exuberant tissue response occurs, and a mature mass of acute and chronic inflammatory tissue develops.

Large tube size, intralaryngeal cuff placement, and blind traumatic intubation, and injury from movement of the larynx against the endotracheal tube have been implicated in the development of postintubation contact granulomas.[45] Although the length of intubation increases the likelihood of developing granuloma, patients incubated for periods as brief as 1 hour are found to have epithelial damage to the posterior glottis.[46] Infectious processes such as viral and bacterial upper respiratory infections can result in edematous and infected laryngeal mucosa, that is, further traumatized by accelerated laryngeal closure from reflex coughing and swallowing.

LPR is the most common cofactor exacerbating posterior laryngeal trauma and preventing wound healing.[47,48] Patients with LPR are also likely to develop vocally abusive behaviors such as chronic cough and throat clearing. In addition to LPR, speaking with excessive vocal hyperfunction is a common cofactor in development and persistence of laryngeal contact granulomas.[49] Objective assessments of patients with vocal hyperfunction and contact granulomas identified abnormally high vocal cord closure velocities and collision forces when compared to controls.[50]

Diagnostic Principles

Patients with contact granulomas commonly present with globus sensation, throat discomfort, odynophagia, and dysphonia. Dysphonia is often mild but is described by the patient as "huskiness."[47,51] Phonation requires increased effort, and patients complain of vocal fatigue. Globus sensation and throat pain can be localized to the greater horn of the thyroid cartilage, often on the involved side. Pain can also radiate to the ipsilateral ear. Airway obstruction with stridor is a less common presenting symptom.

A thorough history should include questions detailing circumstance surrounding the onset of symptoms, for example, intubation, upper airway infection, coughing, changing vocal demands. Investigation regarding caffeine use, alcohol use, poor eating habits, and other contributing factors to LPR is warranted. Palpation of the thyrohyoid region can often elicit discomfort. Endoscopic examination of the larynx frequently reveals a depressed ulcerated area or a bilobed heaped up lesion on the vocal process of the arytenoid cartilage (Figure 7). The bilobed lesion often articulates with the contralateral noninvolved vocal process in a "cup and saucer" fashion. The granuloma may appear sessile or pedunculated.

Treatment Principles

Classically appearing lesions with an appropriate history do not require biopsy for diagnosis. Patients with lesions that present in an atypical location or with an appearance worrisome for malignancy should undergo biopsy for diagnosis, particularly if the patient has risk factors for carcinoma. It should be emphasized, however, that surgery is not the first-line treatment for these lesions.[51] The treatment for laryngeal granuloma is directed at the cause. An antireflux regimen should be started on an empiric basis even for asymptomatic patients. Use of proton pump inhibitors in addition to diet and lifestyle modification for LPR has shown efficacy as a single modal-

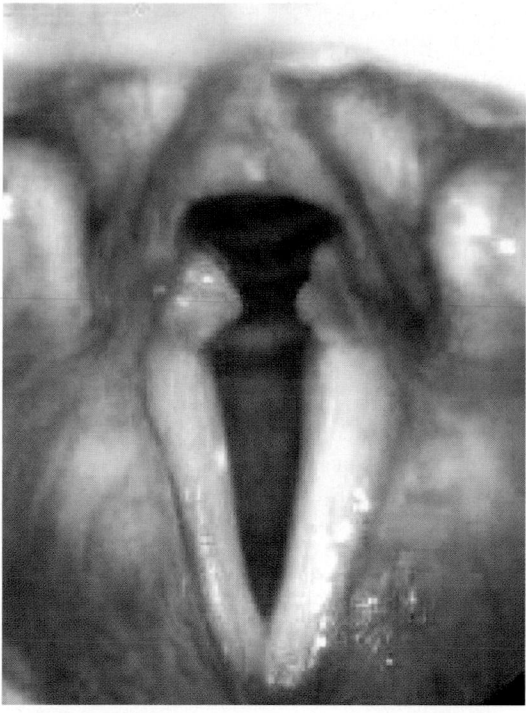

Figure 7 Contact granulomas. Bilateral, right larger than left, postintubation granulomas at the vocal processes.

ity treatment for contact granuloma.[48] Patients should be informed that healing can take months and close endoscopic follow-up is necessary. In the event of failure of outpatient management, the patient should be referred to a gastroenterologist for further workup, and other sources of ongoing vocal trauma should be investigated.[48] Voice therapy to reduce vocal effort, explosive speech, and hard glottal attack is efficacious in treatment and prevention of the disease.[52]

Surgery for vocal process granulomas results in a high recurrence rate.[47] Accepted indications for surgical management include airway obstruction and to rule out neoplasm. Persistent dysphonia despite maximal medical therapy is also an indication for surgery. Microsurgical resection involves amputation of the granuloma at its base maintaining the integrity of the underlying cartilage. Care should be taken operating in the posterior part of the glottis to minimize trauma and prevent scarring or injury to the cricoarytenoid joint. Postoperatively, patients may benefit from a short course of voice rest to promote healing. Injection of the laryngeal adductory musculature with botulinum toxin or corticosteroids is also a reported adjuvant treatment.[53] Inhaled topical corticosteroids are likely of limited benefit and can cause untoward side effects such as fungal laryngitis.[54]

SULCUS VOCALIS AND VOCAL-FOLD SCAR

Etiology

Sulcus vocalis and vocal-fold scarring are pathologic absence of the normal pliable vocal-fold epithelium and SLP. Theories for the congenital and acquired pathogenesis of sulcus vocalis have been presented. Sulcus vocalis is the migration

of the vocal-fold epithelium into the normally convex SLP or deeper.[55] The depression created by this migration can be focal or can extend the length of the vocal fold. Scar results from replaced SLP by disorganized collagen and extracellular matrix. Vocal-fold scarring is classified according to its underlying etiology: traumatic (blunt, penetrating, radiation, surgery, glottic carcinoma), iatrogenic (vocal cord surgery, prolonged intubation, tracheostomy), and inflammatory (inhalation injury, rheumatic diseases).[56]

Diagnostic Principles

Despite differences in etiology, patients with sulcus vocalis and vocal-fold scarring present similarly. Typical complaints are of dysphonia characterized by hoarseness, breathy voice quality, and vocal fatigue. Endoscopic findings for these two entities are also similar and include an asymmetric spindle-shaped glottic closure pattern, medial furrows or troughs at the glottic margin, and supraglottic hyperfunction. High-resolution videostroboscopic imaging with careful evaluation is most often necessary to identify these often subtle lesions. This examination will show disruption of mucosal wave with focal dynamic segments at the site of the lesion.

Treatment Principles

Treatment for sulcus vocalis and vocal-fold scarring should be directed at improving glottal efficiency and voice quality. It is essential to maximize the chance for healing by removing confounding aggravating factors. Strict control of laryngopharyngeal reflux may help to improve the overall laryngeal environment to assist in healing. Voice therapy should be instituted early to encourage optimum phonatory efficiency and cessation of maladaptive behaviors.[57] Patients should be encouraged to avoid smoking and other instigating irritants. Surgery may be considered when patients have failed maximal medical management. Surgical techniques include medialization thyroplasty, injection thyroplasty, local corticosteroid injection, fat or fascia implantation, and mucosal elevation and redraping.[55–57] The wide variety of described surgical options highlights the lack of an optimum treatment for this difficult problem.

REINKE EDEMA

Etiology

Reinke edema, also known as polypoid degeneration of the true vocal fold or "smokers polyps," occurs most commonly in women. Women present complaining of a deep voice and are often mistaken to be a man on the telephone. Patients are often heavy cigarette smokers who have vocally active lifestyles. Controversy exists regarding the role of hypothyroidism in the development of Reinke edema.[58–59] LPR has been proposed as an etiologic cofactor.[60] Large lesions can lead to stridor and airway obstruction.

Diagnostic Principles

Diagnosis is confirmed with endoscopy, which shows severely edematous, rounded, and yellow vocal folds (Figure 8). Videostroboscopy reveals vocal folds with increased mucosal wave amplitude, lowered fundamental frequency, and vibratory aperiodicity. Inspiratory phonation is a useful technique to draw the polypoid vocal folds into the lumen of the airway revealing the true size of the lesions.[61] Assessment of airway obstruction and degree of vocal incapacity helps direct treatment. Testing for hypothyroidism is warranted. The polypoid degeneration of the vocal folds appears histologically as the formation of excess lamina propria.[62]

Treatment Principles

Smoking cessation and management of hypothyroidism, if present, are the first step in the treatment of Reinke edema. With smoking cessation alone, patients with mild edema may have some improvement over time, supporting this as first line treatment.[63] Treatment for LPR, including lifestyle modification and pharmacotherapy, may be important in preventing disease progression as well. Surgical intervention should be reserved for patients who have airway obstruction or have failed conservative therapy. Patients wishing to undergo elective treatment for voice improvement should be counseled specifically about the risk of recurrence with ongoing smoking, vocal-fold scarring, vocal deterioration, and failure to improve the voice.

Surgical intervention follows the careful microsurgical principles described above for phonotraumatic lesions. Historically, surgical aspiration of these lesions was reported. However, the consistency of the polypoid tissue is similar to that of a grape, and subepithelial excision of redundant SLP with preservation of the vocal-fold cover for redraping is indicated. Again, vocal-fold stripping and removal of all functional SLP (overexcision) is to be avoided. Controversy exists regarding the role of staged procedures in treatment of bilateral disease to avoid the risk of a web and bilateral scarring.[64] Reported surgical techniques include cold excision, CO_2 laser excision, microdebridement, and hemoglobin-specific laser therapy (pulsed dye, pulsed KTP

lasers).[65–67] Regardless of tool used, attention to careful microsurgical principles and avoiding excessive excision are likely the most important factors in successful surgery.

SUMMARY

Benign laryngeal lesions are interesting and diverse forms of laryngeal pathology. Patients often report hoarseness as the common presenting symptom, and occasionally, airway obstruction or dysphagia. Careful history taking, physical examination, and thorough transnasal or transoral laryngeal endoscopy usually reveal the diagnosis. Prudent medical and surgical treatment often restores laryngeal function.

REFERENCES

1. Johns MM. Update on the etiology, diagnosis, and treatment of vocal fold nodules, polyps, and cysts. Curr Opin Otolaryngol Head Neck Surg 2003;11:456–61.
2. Titze IR. Mechanical stress in phonation. J Voice 1994;8:99–105.
3. Courey MS, Shohet JA, Scott MA, Ossoff RH. Immunohistochemical characterization of benign laryngeal lesions. Ann Otol Rhinol Laryngol 1996;105:525–31.
4. Gray SD, Hammond E, Hanson DF. Benign pathologic responses of the larynx. Ann Otol Rhinol Laryngol 1995;104:13–8.
5. Klein AM, Pierce MC, Zeitels SM, et al. Imaging the human vocal folds in vivo with optical coherence tomography: a preliminary experience. Ann Otol Rhinol Laryngol 2006;115:277–84.
6. Holmberg EB, Hillman RE, Hammarberg B, et al. Efficacy of a behaviorally based voice therapy protocol for vocal nodules. J Voice 2001;15:395–412.
7. Courey MS, Gardner GM, Stone RE, Ossoff RH. Endoscopic vocal fold microflap: A three-year experience. Ann Otol Rhinol Laryngol 1995;104:267–73.
8. Sataloff RT, Spiegel JR, Heuer RJ, et al. Laryngeal mini-microflap: A new technique and reassessment of the microflap saga. J Voice 1995;9:198–204.
9. Hochman, II, Zeitels SM. Phonomicrosurgical management of vocal fold polyps: The subepithelial microflap resection technique. J Voice 2000;14:112–8.
10. Hochman, II, Zeitels SM, Heaton JT. Analysis of the forces and position required for direct laryngoscopic exposure of the anterior vocal folds. Ann Otol Rhinol Laryngol 1999;108:715–24.
11. Gray SD, Chan KJ, Turner B. Dissection plane of the human vocal fold lamina propria and elastin fibre concentration. Acta Otolaryngol 2000;120:87–91.
12. Benninger MS. Microdissection or microspot CO_2 laser for limited vocal fold benign lesions: A prospective randomized trial. Laryngoscope 2000;110:1–17.
13. Behrman A, Sulica L. Voice rest after microlaryngoscopy: Current opinion and practice. Laryngoscope 2003;113:2182–6.
14. Zeitels SM, Hillman RE, Desloge R, et al. Phonomicrosurgery in singers and performing artists: Treatment outcomes, management theories, and future directions. Ann Otol Rhinol Laryngol Suppl 2002;190:21–40.
15. Lindeberg H, Elbrond O. Laryngeal papillomas: The epidemiology in a Danish subpopulation 1965–1984. Clin Otolaryngol Allied Sci 1990;15:125–31.
16. Strong MS, Vaughan CW, Cooperband SR, et al. Recurrent respiratory papillomatosis: Management with the CO_2 laser. Ann Otol Rhinol Laryngol 1976;85:508–16.
17. Jones SR, Myers EN, Barnes L. Benign neoplasms of the larynx. Otolaryngol Clin North Am 1984;17:151–78.
18. Armstrong LR, Preston EJ, Reichert M, et al. Incidence and prevalence of recurrent respiratory papillomatosis among children in Atlanta and Seattle. Clin Infect Dis 2000;31:107–9.
19. Kashima HK, Shah F, Lyles A, et al. A comparison of risk factors in juvenile-onset and adult-onset recurrent respiratory papillomatosis. Laryngoscope 1992;102:9–13.
20. Lindeberg H, Oster S, Oxlund I, Elbrond O. Laryngeal papillomas: Classification and course. Clin Otolaryngol Allied Sci 1986;11:423–9.
21. Capper JW, Bailey CM, Michaels L. Squamous papillomas of the larynx in adults. A review of 63 cases. Clin Otolaryngol Allied Sci 1983;8:109–19.
22. Zeitels SM, Sataloff RT. Phonomicrosurgical resection of glottal papillomatosis. J Voice 1999;13:123–7.
23. Pasquale K, Wiatrak B, Woolley A, Lewis L. Microdebrider versus CO_2 laser removal of recurrent respiratory papillomas: A prospective analysis. Laryngoscope 2003; 113:139–43.
24. Schraff S, Derkay CS, Burke B, Lawson L. American Society of Pediatric Otolaryngology members' experience with recurrent respiratory papillomatosis and the use of adjuvant therapy. Arch Otolaryngol Head Neck Surg 2004; 130:1039–42.
25. Zeitels SM, Akst LM, Burns JA, et al. Office-based 532-nm pulsed KTP laser treatment of glottal papillomatosis and dysplasia. Ann Otol Rhinol Laryngol 2006;115:679–85.
26. Franco RA, Jr., Zeitels SM, Farinelli WA, Anderson RR. 585-nm pulsed dye laser treatment of glottal papillomatosis. Ann Otol Rhinol Laryngol 2002;111:486–92.
27. Cohen JT, Koufman JA, Postma GN. Pulsed-dye laser in the treatment of recurrent respiratory papillomatosis of the larynx. Ear Nose Throat J 2003;82:558.
28. McMillan K, Shapshay SM, McGilligan JA, et al. A 585-nanometer pulsed dye laser treatment of laryngeal papillomas: Preliminary report. Laryngoscope 1998;108:968–72.
29. Shehab N, Sweet BV, Hogikyan ND. Cidofovir for the treatment of recurrent respiratory papillomatosis: A review of the literature. Pharmacotherapy 2005;25:977–89.
30. Avidano MA, Singleton GT. Adjuvant drug strategies in the treatment of recurrent respiratory papillomatosis. Otolaryngol Head Neck Surg 1995;112:197–202.
31. Rosen CA, Bryson PC. Indole-3-carbinol for recurrent respiratory papillomatosis: Long-term results. J Voice 2004; 18:248–53.
32. Villa LL, Costa RL, Petta CA, et al. Prophylactic quadrivalent human papillomavirus (types 6, 11, 16, and 18) L1 virus-like particle vaccine in young women: A randomised double-blind placebo-controlled multicentre phase II efficacy trial. Lancet Oncol 2005;6:271–8.
33. Ivatury R, Shah D, Ascer E, et al. Granular cell tumor of larynx and bronchus. Ann Thorac Surg 1982;33:69–73.
34. Del Gaudio JM, Muller S. Diagnosis and treatment of supraglottic laryngeal paraganglioma: Report of a case. Head Neck 2004;26:94–8.
35. Sanders KW, Abreo F, Rivera E, et al. A diagnostic and therapeutic approach to paragangliomas of the larynx. Arch Otolaryngol Head Neck Surg 2001;127:565–9.
36. Tiwari RM, Snow GB, Balm AJ, et al. Cartilagenous tumours of the larynx. J Laryngol Otol 1987;101:266–75.
37. de Vincentiis I, Biserni A. Surgery of the mixed laryngocele. Acta Otolaryngol 1979;87:142–51.
38. Holinger LD, Barnes DR, Smid LJ, Holinger PH. Laryngocele and saccular cysts. Ann Otol Rhinol Laryngol 1978; 87:675–85.
39. Micheau C, Luboinski B, Lanchi P, Cachin Y. Relationship between laryngoceles and laryngeal carcinomas. Laryngoscope 1978;88:680–8.
40. DeSanto LW, Devine KD, Weiland LH. Cysts of the larynx–classification. Laryngoscope 1970;80:145–76.
41. Frederick FJ. Endoscopic microsurgical excision of internal laryngocele. J Otolaryngol 1985;14:163–6.
42. Hogikyan ND, Bastian RW. Endoscopic CO_2 laser excision of large or recurrent laryngeal saccular cysts in adults. Laryngoscope 1997;107:260–5.
43. Baker HL, Baker SR, McClatchey KD. Manifestations and management of laryngoceles. Head Neck Surg 1982; 4:450–6.
44. Benjamin B, Croxson G. Vocal cord granulomas. Ann Otol Rhinol Laryngol 1985;94:538–41.
45. Ioannovich D. Bilateral polypoid granuloma of the larynx following endotracheal anesthesia; report of a case. AMA Arch Otolaryngol 1953;58:31–7.
46. Donnelly WH. Histopathology of endotracheal intubation. An autopsy study of 99 cases. Arch Pathol 1969; 88:511–20.
47. Ylitalo R, Ramel S. Extraesophageal reflux in patients with contact granuloma: A prospective controlled study. Ann Otol Rhinol Laryngol 2002;111:441–6.
48. Emami AJ, Morrison M, Rammage L, Bosch D. Treatment of laryngeal contact ulcers and granulomas: A 12-year retrospective analysis. J Voice 1999;13:612–7.
49. Koufman JA, Postma GN, Cummins MM, Blalock PD. Vocal fold paresis. Otolaryngol Head Neck Surg 2000; 122:537–41.
50. Hillman RE, Holmberg EB, Perkell JS, et al. Objective assessment of vocal hyperfunction: An experimental framework and initial results. J Speech Hear Res 1989; 32:373–92.
51. Ward PH, Zwitman D, Hanson D, Berci G. Contact ulcers and granulomas of the larynx: new insights into their etiology as

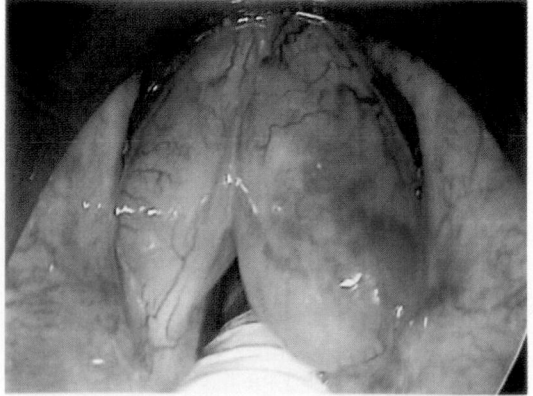

Figure 8 Reinke edema. Bilateral expansion of the superficial lamina propria.

a basis for more rational treatment. Otolaryngol Head Neck Surg 1980;88:262–9.

52. Bloch CS, Gould WJ, Hirano M. Effect of voice therapy on contact granuloma of the vocal fold. Ann Otol Rhinol Laryngol 1981;90:48–52.

53. Nasri S, Sercarz JA, McAlpin T, Berke GS. Treatment of vocal fold granuloma using botulinum toxin type A. Laryngoscope 1995;105:585–8.

54. Mehanna HM, Kuo T, Chaplin J, et al. Fungal laryngitis in immunocompetent patients. J Laryngol Otol 2004;118:379–81.

55. Dailey SH, Ford CN. Surgical management of sulcus vocalis and vocal fold scarring. Otolaryngol Clin North Am 2006; 39:23–42.

56. Benninger MS, Alessi D, Archer S, et al. Vocal fold scarring: Current concepts and management. Otolaryngol Head Neck Surg 1996;115:474–82.

57. Rosen CA. Vocal fold scar: Evaluation and treatment. Otolaryngol Clin North Am 2000;33:1081–6.

58. White A, Sim DW, Maran AG. Reinke's oedema and thyroid function. J Laryngol Otol 1991;105:291–2.

59. Lindeberg H, Felding JU, Sogaard H, Illum P. Reinke's oedema and thyroid function: A prospective study in 43 patients. Clin Otolaryngol Allied Sci 1987;12:417–20.

60. Toohill RJ, Kuhn JC. Role of refluxed acid in pathogenesis of laryngeal disorders. Am J Med 1997;103: 100S–6S.

61. Kothe C, Schade G, Fleischer S, Hess M. Forced inspiration: A laryngoscopy-based maneuver to assess the size of Reinke's edema. Laryngoscope 2003;113:741–2.

62. Lumpkin SM, Bennett S, Bishop SG. Postsurgical follow-up study of patients with severe polypoid degeneration. Laryngoscope 1990;100:399–402.

63. Hojslet PE, Moesgaard-Nielsen V, Karlsmose M. Smoking cessation in chronic Reinke's oedema. J Laryngol Otol 1990;104:626–8.

64. Desloge RB, Zeitels SM. Endolaryngeal microsurgery at the anterior glottal commissure: Controversies and observations. Ann Otol Rhinol Laryngol 2000;109:385–92.

65. Sant'Anna GD, Mauri M. Use of the microdebrider for Reinke's edema surgery. Laryngoscope 2000;110:2114–6.

66. Remacle M, Lawson G, Watelet JB. Carbon dioxide laser microsurgery of benign vocal fold lesions: Indications, techniques, and results in 251 patients. Ann Otol Rhinol Laryngol 1999;108:156–64.

67. Hirano S, Yamashita M, Kitamura M, Takagita S. Photocoagulation of microvascular and hemorrhagic lesions of the vocal fold with the KTP laser. Ann Otol Rhinol Laryngol 2006;115:253–9.

76

Laryngopharyngeal Reflux and Laryngeal Infections and Manifestations of Systemic Diseases

Kenneth W. Altman, MD, PhD
Jamie A. Koufman, MD

Inflammatory conditions in the larynx account for the majority of causes of laryngeal symptoms in patients presenting to the otolaryngologist, particularly because of the wide spectrum of diseases that result in inflammation. The term inflammation implies a local response to tissue injury, characterized by capillary dilation and leukocyte infiltration. Consequently, the typical symptoms include hoarseness, discomfort, and pain, while typical laryngeal signs include swelling and redness. The broad differential diagnosis of the causes of laryngitis is shown in Table 1, and includes predominantly laryngopharyngeal reflux, infections, autoimmune, and systemic disease. While each of these areas can be exhaustive in its depth and signs of laryngeal inflammation may be nonspecific, it is incumbent on the clinician to determine the root causes of the inflammation to affect successful treatment.

In adults, the most common cause of laryngitis is chronic laryngopharyngeal reflux (LPR), whereas in infants and children the most common cause is acute infection. Infectious conditions in the larynx may be subdivided into (1) pediatric versus adult patients, (2) viral, bacterial, fungal, and parasitic, (3) immunocompetent versus immunocompromised hosts, and (4) nongranulomatous versus granulomatous. Similarly autoimmune and systemic diseases affecting the larynx may manifest as granulomatous and nongranulomatous. These overlapping categories make the patient with laryngeal inflammation particularly challenging.

To add to this complexity, laryngeal inflammatory disorders are unusual in that often more than one causative factor or condition can be identified. For example, tobacco smoking results in inflammation that can progress to Reinke edema but also increases the likelihood of LPR which compounds the edema; both conditions are risk factors for the development of laryngeal carcinoma. Another example is the patient with autoimmune disease who may already be immune-suppressed or require immunosuppressive therapy; such a patient is more susceptible to typical and atypical infections. Systemic disease is also associated with exacerbation of LPR. These examples pay tribute to the multifactorial nature of laryngeal disorders. As more has been learned about the larynx, environmental influences, and the effects of systemic disorders on the larynx, imprecise diagnostic terms, such as *nonspecific laryngitis*, have appropriately begun to disappear from the otolaryngologic literature.

LARYNGOPHARYNGEAL REFLUX

LPR and gastroesophageal reflux disease (GERD) are highly prevalent in the general population, and the impact on health systems is growing dramatically. It has been estimated that 10% of Americans have heartburn daily, 20% weekly, and an additional 30 to 60% have it occasionally.[1,2] Furthermore, 10 to 50% of patients with laryngeal complaints have a GER-related underlying cause.[3] There has also been striking growth in disease or public/physician recognition, as the number of United States ambulatory care visits to all physicians for GERD increased from a rate of 1.7/100 in 1990 to 4.7/100 in 2001.[4]

The term reflux literally means back flow. Reflux of stomach contents into the esophagus is common, and many patients with GERD have symptoms such as heartburn and regurgitation related to inflammation of the esophagus by acid and digestive enzymes. When refluxed material escapes the esophagus and enters the pharynx and larynx, the event is termed LPR. Although the terms gastroesophageal reflux and laryngopharyngeal reflux are often used interchangeably, the latter is more specific. Laryngopharyngeal

Table 1 Inflammatory Disorders of the Larynx

I. Gastroesophageal (laryngopharyngeal) reflux disease
II. Pediatric laryngitis
  A. Acute (viral or bacterial) infections
    1. Laryngotracheitis (croup)
    2. Supraglottitis (epiglottitis)
    3. Diphtheria
  B. Noninfectious causes
    1. Spasmodic croup
    2. Traumatic laryngitis
III. Acute laryngeal infections of adults
  A. Viral laryngitis
    1. Common upper respiratory infection
    2. Laryngotracheitis
    3. Herpes simplex
  B. Bacterial laryngitis
    1. Supraglottitis
    2. Laryngeal abscess
    3. Gonorrhea
IV. Chronic (granulomatous) diseases
  A. Bacterial
    1. Tuberculosis
    2. Leprosy
    3. Scleroma
    4. Actinomycosis
    5. Tularemia
    6. Glanders
    7. Syphilis
  B. Mycotic (fungal)
    1. Candidiasis
    2. Blastomycosis
    3. Histoplasmosis
    4. Coccidiomycosis
    5. Aspergillosis
    6. Sporotrichosis
  C. Idiopathic
    1. Sarcoidosis
    2. Wegener granulomatosis
V. Allergic, immune, and idiopathic disorders
  A. Hypersensitivity reactions
    1. Angioedema
    2. Stevens-Johnson syndrome
  B. Immune and idiopathic disorders
    1. Infections of the immunocompromised host
    2. Rheumatoid arthritis
    3. Systemic lupus erythematosus
    4. Cicatricial pemphigoid
    5. Relapsing polychondritis
    6. Sjögren syndrome
    7. Amyloidosis
VI. Miscellaneous inflammatory conditions
  A. Parasitic infections
    1. Trichinosis
    2. Leishmaniasis
    3. Schistosomiasis
    4. Syngamosis
  B. Inhalation laryngitis
    1. Acute (thermal) injury
    2. Pollution and inhalant allergy
    3. Carcinogens
  C. Radiation injury
    1. Radiation laryngitis
    2. Radionecrosis
  D. Vocal abuse and misuse syndromes
    1. Vocal fold hemorrhage
    2. Muscle tension dysphonias
    3. Contact ulcer and granuloma

Table 2 Symptoms and Laryngeal Conditions Reported to Be Associated with Laryngopharyngeal Reflux

Symptoms	Conditions
Chronic dysphonia	Reflux laryngitis
Intermittent dysphonia	Subglottic stenosis
Vocal fatigue	Carcinoma of the larynx
Voice breaks	Endotracheal intubation injury
Chronic throat clearing	Contact ulcers and granulomas
Excessive throat mucus "Postnasal drip"	Posterior glottic stenosis Arytenoid cartilage fixation
Chronic cough	Paroxysmal laryngo-spasm
Dysphagia	Paradoxical vocal fold movement
Globus	Globus pharyngeus
Intermittent airway obstruction	Vocal nodules
Chronic airway obstruction	Polypoid degeneration
	Laryngomalacia
	Pachydermia laryngis
	Recurrent leukoplakia
	Sudden infant death syndrome

Table 4 Reflux Symptom Index

Within the Last Month, How Did the Following Problems Affect You?		Score*				
1. Hoarseness or a problem with your voice	0	1	2	3	4	5
2. Clearing your throat	0	1	2	3	4	5
3. Excess throat mucus or postnasal drip	0	1	2	3	4	5
4. Difficulty swallowing food, liquids, or pills	0	1	2	3	4	5
5. Coughing after you ate or after lying down	0	1	2	3	4	5
6. Breathing difficulties or choking episodes	0	1	2	3	4	5
7. Troublesome or annoying cough	0	1	2	3	4	5
8. Sensations of something sticking in your throat or a lump in your throat	0	1	2	3	4	5
9. Heartburn, chest pain, indigestion, or stomach acid coming up	0	1	2	3	4	5
						Total

*0 = no problem; 5 = severe problem.

reflux is the preferred term for use in otolaryngology because the patterns, mechanisms, and manifestations of LPR differ from classic GERD. The symptoms and laryngeal conditions of the patient with LPR are summarized in Table 2. Laryngopharyngeal reflux is also ubiquitous and pernicious in pediatric otolaryngology patients. The diagnosis may be particularly difficult to make because infants and children almost never complain of heartburn or other reflux symptoms. Physiologic barriers against the development of reflux and its adverse effects include the lower esophageal sphincter, esophageal peristalsis, the presence of saliva that buffers the refluxed contents, the mucus covering of the stomach–esophagus–larynx–pharynx, and the upper esophageal sphincter. A wide spectrum of diseases and medications may affect these physiologic barriers to GERD and LPR.[3]

The differences between the patient with typical GERD and the patient with LPR are as summarized in Table 3. Both have been associated with a wide spectrum of respiratory tract disease including chronic laryngitis, hoarseness, laryngeal carcinoma, globus sensation, cough and paradoxical vocal fold motion, laryngeal and subglottic stenosis, laryngomalacia, sudden infant death syndrome, sleep disturbance, recurrent laryngospasm, cricoarytenoid joint fixation, chronic rhinosinusitis, and asthma, among others.[5–8] The nine-item reflux symptom index (RSI) has been developed to quantify patient symptoms of LPR and evaluate treatment efficacy (Table 4). This outcome instrument has displayed excellent reproducibility and criterion-based validity.

Laryngeal Findings in Laryngopharyngeal Reflux

The impact of reflux on the larynx is multifold and includes both pathophysiologic and maladaptive behavioral changes. The direct effect of the acidic refluxate causes an immediate inflammatory response. Reflux contents of the stomach also includes pepsin, which is a proteolytic enzyme (digests protein) that is activated in acidic environments. As a result, there is autodigestion of the laryngeal mucosa with the effects of pepsin considered to be even more injurious than the acid. Pepsin likely persists on the mucosa with the potential for reactivation when it is exposed to subsequent episodes of reflux.[9]

Physical findings of LPR can range from mild, isolated edema, and/or erythema of the area of the arytenoid cartilages to diffuse laryngeal edema and hyperemia with granuloma formation and airway obstruction. The eight-item reflux finding score (RFS) has been developed to document the severity of the clinical findings of LPR (Table 5). Use of the RFS not only helps physicians identify subtle findings of reflux, it also assists in evaluating the severity of laryngeal tissue injury, as well as documenting treatment efficacy. The physical findings of LPR include edema, erythema, hypertrophy, formation of granuloma and granulation tissue, and thick mucus (Figure 1). Prominent are pseudosulcus vocalis and ventricular obliteration.

Pseudosulcus vocalis refers to a pattern of subglottic edema that extends from the anterior commissure to the posterior part of the larynx; it appears like a groove or sulcus. It can easily be differentiated from a true sulcus (sulcus vergeture), which is the adherence of the vocal fold epithelium to the vocal ligament secondary to the absence of the superficial layer of lamina propria. True sulcus is related to scarring of the vocal fold(s) in the phonatory striking zone. Whereas true sulcus stops at the vocal process and is in the midportion of the striking zone, pseudosulcus vocalis extends all the way to the back of the larynx.

Ventricular obliteration is a frequent finding that may be identified in up to 80% of patients with LPR. Swelling of the true and false vocal folds causes this space to become obliterated and thus poorly visualized. With partial ventricular obliteration, the space is reduced, and the false vocal fold edge is indistinct. With complete ventricular obliteration, the true and false folds appear to touch, and there is no true ventricular space.

Laryngeal erythema or hyperemia is a nonspecific finding that is dependent on the available endoscopic equipment. Subtle changes

Table 3 Differences between Typical Gastroesophageal Reflux Disease and Laryngopharyngeal Reflux

	GERD	LPR
Symptoms		
Heartburn and/or regurgitation	+++++	
Hoarseness, dysphagia, globus, etc	+	++++
Findings		
Endoscopic esophagitis	+++++	
Laryngeal inflammation	+	++++
Diagnostic yield (abnormality)		
Esophageal biopsy (inflammation)	+++++	
Abnormal esophageal radiography	++	—
Abnormal esophageal pH monitoring	+++++	
Abnormal pharyngeal pH monitoring	—	+++
Pattern of reflux		
Supine (nocturnal)	+++++	
Upright (daytime)	+	++++
Response to treatment		
Dietary/lifestyle modification	++	+
Histamine₂ antagonists*	+++	++
Proton pump inhibitors*	+++++++	

GERD = gastroesophageal reflux disease; LPR = laryngopharyngeal reflux.
*Assuming adequate dosage and duration of therapy.

Table 5 Reflux Finding Score (RFS)	
1. Subglottic edema	0 = absent, 2 = present
2. Ventricular obliteration	2 = partial, 4 = complete
3. Erythema/hyperemia	2 = arytenoids only, 4 = diffuse
4. Vocal fold edema	1 = mild, 2 = moderate, 3 = severe, 4 = polypoid
5. Diffuse laryngeal edema	1 = mild, 2 = moderate, 3 = severe, 4 = obstructing
6. Posterior commissure hypertrophy	1 = mild, 2 = moderate, 3 = severe, 4 = obstructing
7. Granuloma/granulation	0 = absent, 2 = present
8. Thick endolaryngeal mucus	0 = absent, 2 = present
	Total

in erythema are difficult to quantify and vary depending on the quality of the fiberscope, video monitor, and light source. True vocal fold edema is graded as mild (1 point) if only slight swelling exists and moderate (2 points) when it becomes more perceptible. Edema is graded as severe (3 points) when swelling of the cord becomes sessile. Finally, polypoid degeneration of the true vocal fold contributes 4 points to the RFS.

Diffuse laryngeal edema is judged by the size of the airway relative to the size of the larynx. It is graded as mild (1 point) to obstructing (4 points). Hypertrophy of the posterior commissure is another frequent finding of LPR. It is graded as mild (1 point) when there is a mustache-like appearance of the posterior commissure mucosa and moderate (2 points) when the posterior commissure mucosa is swollen enough to create a straight line across the back of the larynx. Posterior commissure hypertrophy (PCH) is graded as severe (3 points) when there is bulging of the posterior part of the larynx into the airway and obstructing (4 points) when a significant portion of the airway is obliterated. The final two items on the RFS are granuloma or granulation tissue formation and thick endolaryngeal mucus.

Ancillary Testing

Ambulatory 24-hour double-probe (simultaneous esophageal and pharyngeal) pH monitoring (pH-metry) is the current gold standard for the diagnosis of LPR.[10] The distal probe is placed 5 cm above the lower esophageal sphincter (LES), and the proximal probe is placed in the hypopharynx 1 cm above the upper esophageal sphincter (UES), just behind the laryngeal inlet (Figure 2). The traditional technique of probe placement is to place both the proximal and distal pH probes under manometric guidance. A manometer is inserted through the nasal cavity and advanced through the esophagus into the stomach. It is then slowly withdrawn, and the locations of the LES and UES are determined. The correct pH catheter is then chosen based on these measurements. An alternative technique involves placing the proximal probe just above the UES under direct fiberoptic visualization. The distance between the proximal and distal pH probes is fixed at 15 cm. This technique is easier, less time consuming, and less costly than using manometric guidance. Placement of the proximal probe above the UES can be performed accurately using this method. This technique, however, is unable to estimate precisely interprobe distances. Thus, the exact

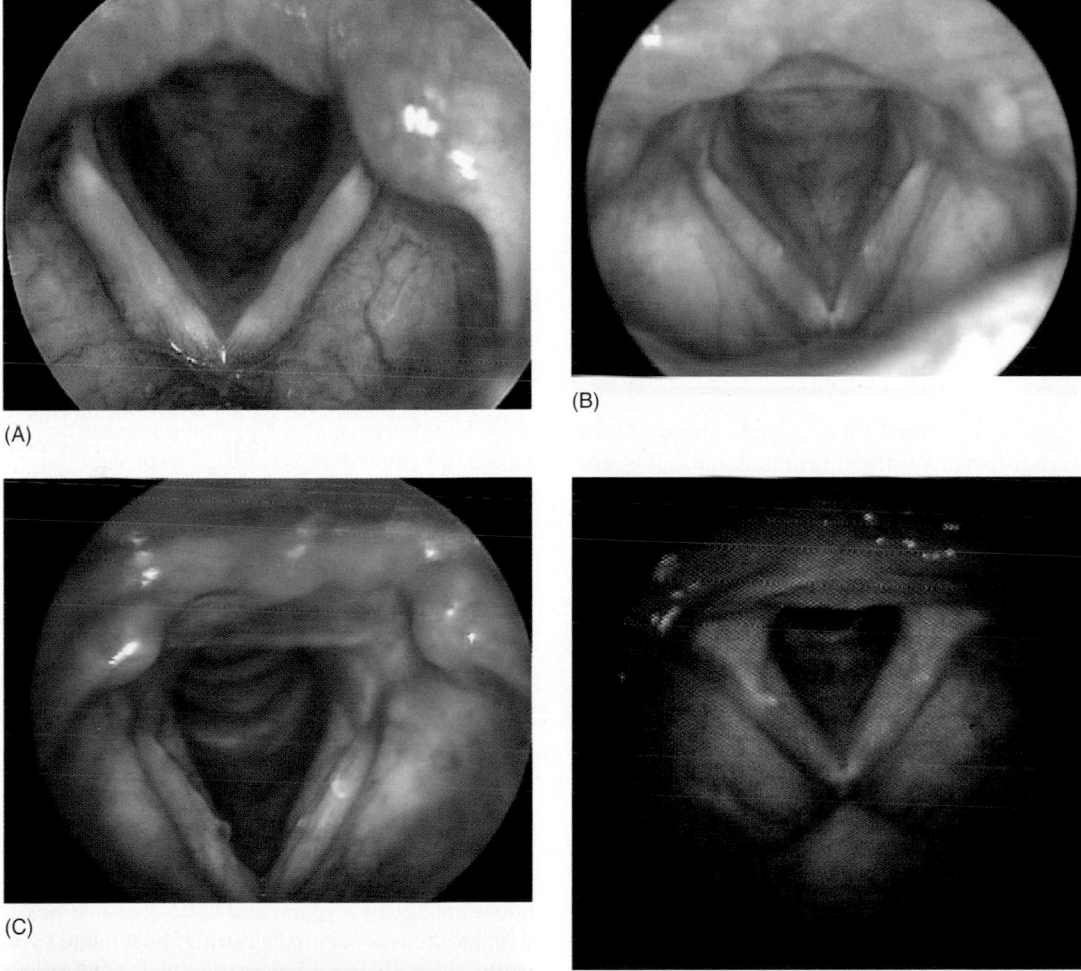

(A)

(B)

(C)

(D)

(E)

Figure 1 Findings of laryngopharyngeal reflux. (A) Mild bilateral pseudosulcus vocalis. Also present are mild posterior interarytenoid and vocal fold edema. (B) Moderate bilateral pseudosulcus vocalis. Notice that the subglottic edema extends past the vocal process. Also present are mild posterior commissure hypertrophy, mild vocal fold edema, and early vocal nodules. (C) Moderate pseudosulcus, posterior commissure hypertrophy, partial ventricular obliteration, and interarytenoid edema with erythema. Also noted is a right vocal hemorrhagic polyp. (D) Severe pseudosulcus, vocal fold edema with ventricular obliteration, posterior commissure hypertrophy with protrusion of posterior commissure into airway, and severe erythema. (E) Right vocal process granuloma.

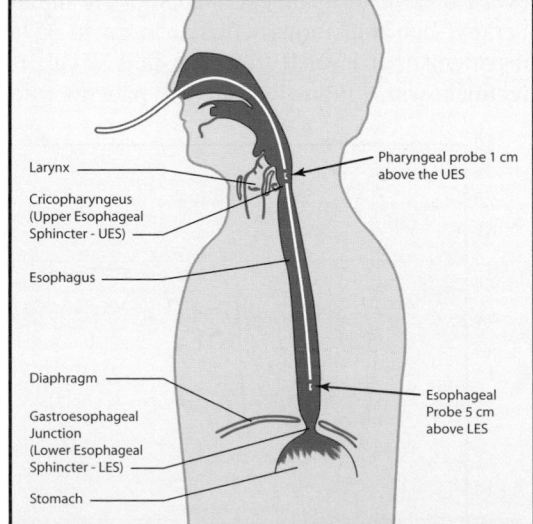

Figure 2 Technique of ambulatory 24-hour double-probe pH monitoring. The distal probe is placed 5 cm above the lower esophageal sphincter (LES), and the proximal (pharyngeal) probe is placed 1 cm above the upper esophageal sphincter (UES).

location of the distal probe is uncertain, and the esophageal data are often grossly inaccurate using this technique.

pH-metry has been available for many years, and standards (normal values) have been established in many laboratories.[3,11] In general, the most important parameter used to evaluate the presence of GERD at the distal probe is the percentage of time that the pH is less than 4. This measurement is usually recorded for time in the upright position, time in the supine position, and the total time of the study. For the upright period, the upper limit of normal is approximately 8.0%, and for the supine period, approximately 2.5%.[11] The proximal pharyngeal probe is placed behind the larynx just above the cricopharyngeus where it may accurately document episodes of LPR that may otherwise be missed in as many as 30 to 50% of patients (Figure 3).

Esophagitis has been demonstrated in 12% of patients with LPR, and Barrett metaplasia in an additional 7%.[12] While a barium esophagogram may be informative, the preferred adjunctive procedure is transnasal esophagoscopy (TNE).[13] This may be conveniently performed in an unsedated patient in the office setting as a diagnostic tool in the evaluation of reflux, globus, and dysphagia.

Treatment

There are three levels of antireflux treatment: level I—dietary and lifestyle modification plus antacids, level II—level I plus use of a histamine H2-receptor antagonist, for example, cimetidine, ranitidine, or famotidine, and level III—antireflux surgery, for example, fundoplication, or proton pump inhibitor (PPI) therapy, for example, omeprazole, esomeprazole, lansoprazole, pantoprazole, or rabeprazole. The details of each of the three levels are listed in Table 6.

Clinical experience with LPR suggests that treatment must be individualized, with the level of treatment depending on the severity of the patient's condition. For many patients with LPR, level I or level II treatment is appropriate initial therapy, but both forms will fail in up to 35% of patients.[14] If level II treatment fails, level III treatment with a PPI is indicated. In patients who

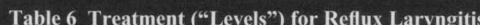

Table 6 Treatment ("Levels") for Reflux Laryngitis

Level I—Antireflux therapy (ART)
  A. Dietary modification
    1. No eating or drinking within 3 h of bedtime
    2. Avoid overeating or reclining right after meals
    3. No fried food; low-fat diet
    4. Avoid coffee, tea, chocolate, mints, and soda pop
    5. Avoid other caffeine-containing foods and beverages
    6. Avoid alcohol, especially in the evening
    7. Avoid other foods that cause you problems
  B. Lifestyle modification
    1. Elevate the head of the bed 4–6 in
    2. Avoid wearing tight-fitting clothing or belts
    3. If you use tobacco, quit!
  C. Liquid antacids qid (1 tablespoon 1 h after each meal and at bedtime)
Level II—Medication plus ART
  A. Level I (above), plus B or C (below)
  B. Initial treatment
    1. Histamine H2-receptor antagonists bid
  C. Escalation for treatment failures
    1. Increase histamine H2-receptor antagonist dose up to double-dose qid or
    2. Use a proton pump inhibitor (PPI)
Level III—Proton pump inhibitors or antireflux surgery
  A. Level I (above) minus antacids, plus B or C (below)
  B. Proton pump inhibitor bid (first dose in the morning, second at 5 pm; the duration of initial treatment should be 6 mo; large patients may require larger doses. Patient symptoms should improve by 2 mo)
  C. Antireflux surgery (fundoplication)

present with severe LPR or complications of LPR (laryngospasm, obstructing granuloma, subglottic stenosis, etc), initial treatment with twice-daily PPI is indicated.

While there is not a generally accepted "clinical pathway" for severe or complicated LPR patients, most laryngologists consider aggressive therapy with twice-daily PPI until resolution of symptoms to ensure complete resolution of tissue injury to the larynx and then scaling back to a lower maintenance dose by the time patients can make suitable lifestyle changes. Laryngeal reflux symptoms resolve sooner than the findings which may take 6 months or longer to reverse.[15]

If patients are still symptomatic at 2 months or if the laryngeal findings have not significantly improved by 6 months, repeat pH testing is indicated to ensure reasonably complete acid suppression (efficacy study). The failure of adequate acid suppression on twice-daily PPIs is significant, and a low threshold for obtaining an efficacy study on medication should be maintained. In some patients who face a lifetime of antireflux treatment or in patients who fail medical therapy, referral for a fundoplication is warranted.

Controversies in Laryngopharyngeal Reflux

There are many remaining controversies surrounding LPR that warrant further study of the etiology and pathophysiology, particularly as they pertain to the larynx. These controversies include variable correlation between pH probe findings in patients with substantial LPR symptoms,[16] abnormal laryngeal seromucinous secretions and decreased *MUC5AC* mucin gene expression seen in patients with chronic laryngitis associated with LPR,[9] the presence of pachydermia as a nonspecific finding associated with LPR,[17] some degree of a possible placebo effect with medical therapy,[18] and a high rate of failed endoscopic Nissen fundoplication surgery for symptoms of LPR.[19] One of the more recent and controversial discoveries pertaining to LPR is the demonstration of the H^+/K^+-ATPase (proton pump) in laryngeal seromucinous glands.[20] This proton pump has been previously noted only in the stomach as the source of hydrogen ions that form hydrochloric acid. The presence of the proton pump in the larynx may be an adaptive change to protect mucosal cells from an acidic environment, such as that from LPR and be an additional site of action of PPI pharmacotherapy. These controversies are playing an important role in our understanding of the LPR effects on the larynx, as well as appreciating the spectrum of treatment options.

VIRAL LARYNGEAL INFECTIONS

Viral Laryngotracheitis (Croup)

Viral laryngotracheitis is the most common laryngeal inflammatory disorder of childhood. Usually, this condition is self-limited, occurs in children under the age of 3 years, and has a seasonal peak, with most cases occurring during the winter. Typically, the child has a several day history of a viral upper respiratory infection with rhinitis, cough, and low-grade fever. Laryngotracheitis may be diagnosed as symptoms progress to include hoarseness, dyspnea, stridor, and a barking cough. The characteristic cough gives laryngotracheitis its common name, croup. Parainfluenza viruses (types 1, 2, and 3) account for more than half of croup cases. Other viruses frequently implicated in the disorder include rhinovirus, respiratory syncytial virus, and adenovirus. Less common causes of laryngotracheitis are influenza, measles, mumps, pertussis, and chickenpox.[21]

When airway obstruction is caused by laryngotracheitis, the stridor is characteristically

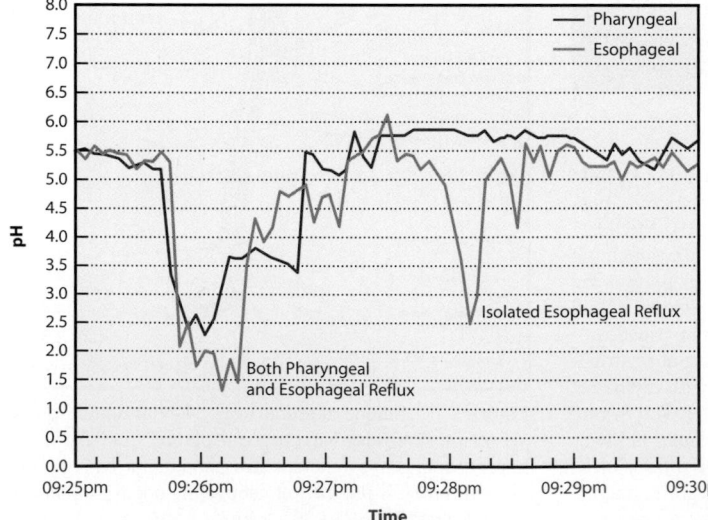

Figure 3 Example of an abnormal double-probe pH study. The blue tracing is the esophageal pH, and the red tracing is the pharyngeal pH. A combined esophageal and pharyngeal reflux event (pH <4) is demonstrated at 9:26. An isolated esophageal reflux event is demonstrated at 9:28.

inspiratory or biphasic. Although the diagnosis of laryngotracheitis is generally based on the history, examination of the larynx shows erythematous and edematous mucosa with normal vocal fold mobility. Radiographs reveal a narrowing of the subglottic lumen, the "steeple sign," and may be used to differentiate this condition from supraglottitis. Airway obstruction from inflammatory laryngeal edema is more common in children than in adults owing to the small size of the pediatric larynx. Equivalent amounts of mucosal swelling may result in critical narrowing and obstruction in a child, while causing only minimal symptoms in an adult. Table 7 demonstrates the more severe effect of glottic and subglottic inflammation in the pediatric population, showing the effects of 1 mm of edema on the cross-sectional (subglottic) area of a small neonate, an average child, and an adult male.

The need for inpatient hospitalization depends on the degree of airway obstruction. Treatment is aimed at decreasing laryngeal edema and preventing stasis and crusting of secretions within the airway. Therapy usually includes hydration, humidification of inspired air, and treatments with nebulized racemic epinephrine. Antipyretics, decongestants, and parenteral corticosteroids are often empirically administered to decrease airway inflammation. Artificial airway support, that is, intubation, is necessary in a relatively small proportion of patients with laryngotracheitis. When needed, however, intubation should be carried out by experienced personnel, preferably in the operating room, where maximum airway control can be achieved.

Secondary bacterial infection of the airway (membranous croup) may subsequently occur and is more serious and usually suspected when the patient experiences high temperature spikes and exudative, purulent drainage. The microorganisms most commonly involved are *Haemophilus influenzae, Staphylococcus aureus, Streptococcus pneumoniae, Moraxella catarrhalis,* and hemolytic streptococci. Antibiotic therapy is then indicated and is directed at the causative microorganisms.

Pediatric viral laryngotracheitis should be distinguished from spasmodic croup, or "false croup," which is a noninfectious form of laryngeal inflammation associated with a mild, chronic

intermittent, croup-like pattern. Spasmodic croup generally affects children 1 to 4 years of age and the afebrile child generally awakes at night with a barking cough, stridor, and mild dyspnea of sudden onset. Nocturnal attacks may occur as isolated events or recur over 2 to 3 nights, but generally the child is asymptomatic during the day and the episode subsides spontaneously. Although the cause of spasmodic croup remains uncertain, evidence suggests that extraesophageal reflux may frequently be the cause, so appropriate testing with 24-hour pH monitoring and antireflux therapy are often indicated.

Adult infectious croup is uncommon; when it does occur, it is quite similar to the laryngotracheitis seen in children. The viral prodrome lasts 1 to 7 days, followed by the development of a barking cough and sometimes inspiratory stridor. Throat cultures are usually negative. It has been reported that a relatively large proportion of adults with this syndrome require airway intervention.[22]

Viral Laryngitis

Acute viral laryngitis in adults is common and is generally less serious than in children because of the larger adult airway. Influenza and parainfluenza viruses, rhinoviruses, and adenoviruses are the most common causative agents although many other viruses have been implicated. Adult patients with viral laryngitis do not usually seek medical attention unless they are professional voice users, in which case, the laryngitis may be of great significance to the patient's ability to earn a living. Such patients present with symptoms of a generalized viral syndrome (low-grade fever, malaise, rhinitis) and hoarseness with voice breaks, episodic aphonia, and a lowering of pitch.[23]

Characteristically, the laryngeal mucosa is diffusely erythematous and edematous, especially over the true vocal folds. While newer antiviral medications may have some utility in reducing the duration and severity when administered in the first 24 hours of clinical infection, the disease is self-limited and treatment is usually centered on supportive care. In the professional vocalist, corticosteroids are sometimes used to reduce the vocal fold edema, particularly during the recovery phase. However, the physician's administration of such anti-inflammatory medications does

not imply that the vocalist with laryngitis can or should perform.

Herpes Simplex Virus

Herpes simplex infection is ubiquitous, may affect any age group, and, uncommonly, may infect the larynx. Most cases of herpetic laryngitis have been reported in young or debilitated patients. At the time of delivery, a neonate passing through the birth canal may contract genital herpes from a mother with active disease. Subsequent herpes infection in the infant may involve the upper airway and, if the larynx is involved, may cause acute airway obstruction. Adult laryngeal herpes is most commonly seen in the immunocompromised patient, although herpetic epiglottic infection causing airway obstruction in otherwise healthy adults has been reported.[24]

Herpes infection should be suspected whenever a patient presents with a painful vesicular mucosal eruption. After the vesicles rupture, ulceration and tissue necrosis may occur, and the surrounding inflammatory response may be intense. The diagnosis of a primary herpetic infection may be made by serologic testing; however, swab, culture, and polymerase chain reaction detection of viral deoxyribonucleic acid (DNA) are the most reliable diagnostic tests. Symptomatic treatment depends on the site of involvement; topical or systemic acyclovir or another specific antiherpetic medication may hasten recovery.

Human Papillomavirus

Human papillomavirus (HPV) results in epithelial changes and neoplastic growth in the upper aerodigestive tract; but, unlike most other viral infections, it does not present as an acute infection typified by a self-limited clinical course. It also may result in genital condyloma accuminatum. The predominant strains of HPV affecting the larynx are types 6 and 11, while more virulent types 16 and 18 have been implicated in higher risk of malignant degeneration.[25] Papillomatosis has also been implicated in immunocompromised and autoimmune disorders. Typical appearance of the papillomavirus lesion includes vascular ingrowth (stippling) and a cauliflower-like exophytic mass. This infection results in a neoplastic disease and is discussed in Chapter 75, "Benign Laryngeal Lesions."

BACTERIAL LARYNGEAL INFECTIONS

Bacterial Supraglottitis (Epiglottitis)

Acute supraglottitis is a life-threatening infection that is traditionally more common in children than adults. Since childhood immunization against type B *H. influenzae* has become commonplace, the disease is significantly less prevalent; and epidemiologic data suggest that nontype B *H. influenzae* is more frequent among vaccinated children.[26] Other microorganisms causing supraglottitis include *Streptococcus pyogenes, S. pneumoniae,* and *S. aureus.* The infection is

Table 7 Effect of 1 mm of Edema on the Cross-Sectional Area of the Subglottic Larynx in the Neonate, Child, and Adult (Area = πr^2*)			
	Neonate	Child	Adult
Normal			
Subglottic diameter (mm)	4	8	14
Subglottic radius (mm)	2	4	7
Subglottic area (mm^2)	12	48	147
Effect of 1 mm of edema			
Subglottic diameter (mm)	2	6	12
Subglottic radius (mm)	1	3	6
Subglottic area (mm^2)	3	27	108
Percent reduction of airway area	75	44	27

*For the sake of simplicity, for these calculations $\pi = 3$.

a true medical emergency. Children aged 2 to 4 years are the most frequently affected group, and cases are more frequent in the winter and spring months. The illness begins rapidly over 2 to 6 hours with the onset of fever, sore throat, and inspiratory stridor. The voice tends to be muffled, and there is no barking cough, as in croup. As the supraglottic structures become more edematous, airway obstruction develops.

The child is generally ill appearing, stridulous, sitting upright, and drooling because swallowing is painful. The diagnosis is usually based purely on the history and clinical findings. Examination of the epiglottis (in the emergency room) may precipitate airway obstruction and thus is not recommended. Lateral soft tissue radiographs may reveal the classic "thumb sign" of the edematous epiglottis with a dilated hypopharynx. Occasionally, the epiglottis itself is not enlarged, but the supraglottic region still appears hazy and indistinct owing to edema of other supraglottic structures. In severe cases, treatment should not be delayed to obtain radiographs.

The child should be transported to the operating room by the parents, an otolaryngologist, and an anesthesiologist to establish the diagnosis and secure an airway. Direct laryngoscopy usually will show the epiglottis to be swollen and cherry red, as are the aryepiglottic folds and the false vocal folds. The true vocal folds and subglottis typically appear to be normal or to be only minimally involved.

Treatment is directed at airway maintenance and then toward providing antimicrobial and supportive care. Drawing blood, starting intravenous lines, obtaining a rectal temperature, or otherwise disturbing the patient should be postponed until the airway is secured. In institutions without a highly skilled pediatric intensive care staff, a tracheostomy may be preferable to endotracheal intubation. Cultures of the epiglottis and blood are obtained after the airway is secured. Antimicrobial therapy is initiated against *H. influenzae* and group A streptococcus, and extubation is usually possible after 48 to 72 hours, at which time the edema has subsided sufficiently to allow an air leak around the endotracheal tube. Transnasal fiberoptic laryngoscopy is the most reliable and most commonly employed technique to ensure resolution of the edema before extubation. Differentiating acute epiglottitis from laryngotracheitis is not always easy, but it is of paramount importance. Some of the differentiating signs and symptoms are shown in Table 8.

In adults, supraglottitis is manifest by fever, sore throat, a muffled voice, dysphagia, and odynophagia. The onset of symptoms prior to presentation is typically longer than that seen in children (usually more than 24 hours). The diagnosis of supraglottitis is made by observing the swollen, bright-red epiglottis and/or supraglottic structures with fiberoptic laryngoscopy or a swollen epiglottis and dilated hypopharynx on a lateral neck radiograph.

In adults, the infectious cause is more likely group A streptococcus. The clinical course

Table 8 Some of the Distinguishing Characteristics of Laryngotracheitis (Croup) and Supraglottitis (Epiglottitis)

Feature	Croup	Epiglottitis
Age	Less than 3 yr	Over 3 yr
Onset	Gradual (d)	Rapid (h)
Cough	Barky	None
Posture	Supine	Sitting
Drooling	No	Yes
Radiograph	Steeple sign, narrowed subglottis	Thumb sign, enlarged epiglottis, dilated hypopharynx
Etiology	Viral	Bacterial
Treatment	Supportive (croup tent, corticosteroids)	Airway management (intubation or tracheostomy) and antibiotics

appears less severe, with less seasonal variation and airway compromise. Although one must never be complacent with management of the airway, conservative airway management in an intensive care setting is often successful, and tracheostomy is rarely required. Conservative measures include oxygenation, humidification, hydration, corticosteroids, and intravenous antibiotics. Bacterial supraglottitis should be distinguished from bacterial laryngeal seeding secondary to purulent rhinosinusitis ("rhinogenic laryngitis") or tracheobronchitis, as the latter are often far less severe than supraglottitis and rarely result in airway compromise.

In adults, there appear to be two relatively useful clinical predictors of the need to establish an airway. Patients who present to the emergency department less than 8 hours after the onset of a sore throat and patients who are drooling at presentation (in preference to swallowing because of severe odynophagia) almost always require airway intervention.

Laryngeal Abscess

Laryngeal abscess is a complication of perichondritis and a recognized sequela of bacterial laryngeal infection. Often the adult patient who develops a laryngeal abscess has a preexisting, predisposing laryngeal condition, such as prior irradiation for cancer. In the preantibiotic era, typhoid fever was a frequent cause and was usually fatal. Other less frequently associated infections include measles, scarlet fever, erysipelas, gonorrhea, syphilis, tuberculosis, and diphtheria. Laryngeal abscess may also be a complication of prolonged nasogastric or endotracheal intubation.[27]

The symptoms of laryngeal abscess are similar to those of supraglottitis. Localizing tenderness to palpation over the laryngeal framework is its hallmark. Fluctuance in the anterior neck, although uncommon, denotes necrosis of the thyroid cartilage. The diagnosis of laryngeal abscess may be made by computed tomographic scanning of the larynx and by fiberoptic or direct laryngoscopy.

When abscess is suspected and the patient's airway is marginal, a tracheostomy should be performed under local anesthesia prior to direct laryngoscopy. If the airway is not compromised, direct laryngoscopy, with laser-assisted incision and drainage of the abscess, may suffice as initial treatment. Granular mucosa should be removed,

and an attempt should be made to determine if necrotic cartilage is exposed within the endolarynx. Infection of the laryngeal framework can lead to severe laryngeal stenosis.

Gram stain and bacteriologic cultures of the abscess contents or necrotic debris should be obtained routinely, and the results should influence the choice of antibiotic. When necrotic cartilage is present, the combination of surgical debridement, prolonged parenteral antibiotic therapy, and hyperbaric oxygen therapy may enhance recovery and preserve laryngeal function. When all other alternatives have failed, laryngectomy may be considered.

Diphtheria

Worldwide, diphtheria is an uncommon laryngeal infection, although a report from India suggests that outbreaks still occur.[28] Laryngeal diphtheria is caused by *Corynebacterium diphtheriae* and generally affects children over the age of 5 years. A febrile illness of slow onset associated with sore throat and hoarseness is then followed by an inflammatory response in the mucous membranes, which results in a thick, grayish-green, plaque-like membranous exudate over the tonsils, pharynx, and laryngeal structures. This pseudomembrane may result in airway compromise, requiring establishment of a safe airway via a tracheostomy. Additional treatment consists of administering diphtheria antitoxin and penicillin or erythromycin to eradicate the microorganisms. Mortality results largely from the neuropathies that develop secondary to the diphtheria toxin. Even in the patient immunized against diphtheria, the disease may still occur but will tend to be mild.

Neisseria Gonorrhea

Gonorrhea is a sexually transmitted genital and sometimes oropharyngeal infection caused by the bacterum *Neisseria gonorrhoeae*. The genital infection may be asymptomatic, so carriers can unknowingly infect their sexual partners. Pharyngeal gonorrhea is transmitted by orogenital contact and is manifested as a diffuse and severe exudative pharyngitis that may directly or indirectly involve the larynx. The infection may produce a pseudomembranous inflammation, which may be confused with diphtheria or streptococcal pharyngitis. Diagnosis is made by culture and identification of the *N. gonorrhoeae* microorganism from swabs of the pharynx. Today, most cases of laryngopharyngeal gonorrhea are treated with a single intramuscular dose of ceftriaxone or a course of oral cefixime.

Tularemia

Tularemia, also called "rabbit fever" and "deer fly fever," is caused by the bacterium *Francisella tularensis*. It is found only in the northern hemisphere (Europe, Asia, and North America). Most cases occur from contact with rabbits or squirrels, but many other wild and domesticated animals have been reported to carry the disease. Transmission to humans can also occur by a bite from a tick or a deer fly, which are the intermediate hosts and insect vectors.

In humans, the most common portal of entry is through the skin or mucous membranes. Headache, myalgia, and malaise are common symptoms. Oropharyngeal tularemia, which occurs in approximately 1% of cases, produces an intense exudative pharyngitis associated with lymphadenopathy.[29] Diagnosis is made by serologic tests since the microorganisms are difficult to identify on culture or histologic examination. Treatment is with streptomycin or gentamicin for 7 to 10 days.

Glanders

At one time in history, glanders was "the plague of horses," and, secondarily, it affected humans. Today, glanders is rare around the world but still occurs in Asia, Africa, and South America. The disease is caused by infection by the bacterium *Pseudomonas mallei* (*Burkholderia mallei*). Transmission is still by contact with an infected horse or by inhalation or inoculation of contaminated material, and infected humans are almost exclusively horse handlers.[30] Infection by inoculation of broken skin causes systemic infection characterized by fever, malaise, prostration, pneumonia, and lymphadenopathy. Truly systemic (septicemic) involvement may be fatal. Infection by inhalation produces an intense, ulcerative mucopurulent granulomatous reaction in the mucous membranes of the aerodigestive tract and pneumonia. Treatment is with sulfonamides.

Tuberculosis

In 1900, laryngeal tuberculosis was very common, occurring in approximately half of patients with advanced pulmonary disease. With the discovery of effective antituberculous drugs, the incidence of both pulmonary and laryngeal tuberculosis rapidly declined. Nevertheless, tuberculous laryngitis remains one of the most common granulomatous diseases of the larynx, and, today, it is frequently unassociated with advanced active pulmonary disease. Because persons with laryngeal tuberculosis often have no simultaneous or previous pulmonary involvement, the clinical presentation may often be similar to that of a neoplastic process.[31] A biopsy is necessary to obtain an accurate diagnosis. Some of the distinguishing features of the most frequent laryngeal granulomatous conditions are shown in Table 9.

Table 9 Some Distinguishing Characteristics of Granulomatous Conditions That Affect the Larynx

Tuberculosis	Posterior third of larynx involved
Leprosy	Supraglottic involvement
Scleroma	Catarrhal stage; Mikulicz cells
Actinomycosis	Draining sinuses; sulfur granules
Syphilis	Painless ulcers; positive syphilis serology
Candidiasis	Leukoplakia-like lesions; identifiable on Gram stain
Blastomycosis	Painless ulcers; microabscesses
Histoplasmosis	Anterior laryngeal involvement; pseudocarcinoma
Coccidiomycosis	Painless abscesses; spores seen on histology
Sarcoidosis	Supraglottic swelling, nodules, granulomas
Wegener granulomatosis	Subglottic involvement; necrotizing vasculitis; pulmonary and/or renal involvement

Patients with laryngeal tuberculosis commonly present in their third to fourth decade of life with varying symptoms, including hoarseness, odynophagia, and otalgia. Respiratory obstruction may develop in later stages of the disease, and approximately one-quarter of patients with laryngeal tuberculosis have airway obstruction at the time of their initial presentation.

Laryngeal examination may reveal diffuse edema and hyperemic, hypertrophic mucosa involving the posterior third of the larynx, or the process may be diffuse including the true vocal folds with nodular and ulcerative lesions. In the nodular, ulcerative (later) stages, tuberculosis may easily be confused with laryngeal carcinoma.

The diagnosis is made by demonstrating typical caseating granulomas on histology and acid-fast staining microorganisms by smear and/or culture. Treatment with antituberculous drugs usually resolves both the pulmonary and the laryngeal disease. If tuberculous laryngitis is left untreated, cicatricial laryngeal stenosis with vocal fold fixation may develop, necessitating surgical correction or tracheostomy.

Leprosy (Hansen Disease)

Leprosy is caused by infection with the bacillus *Mycobacterium leprae*. The disease usually affects the skin and peripheral nerves but may affect other organ systems. Cutaneous nodules may become disfiguring and will eventually cause peripheral neural damage and muscular weakness. In 2000, 738,284 cases of leprosy were identified worldwide. In 1999, 108 cases were reported in the United States. Over one-third of the global cases are limited to India.[32]

The larynx is involved in approximately one-half of patients with leprosy, and it most consistently involves the epiglottis. As the disease progresses to involve the glottis, hoarseness develops, and later destruction of the cartilaginous laryngeal framework may occur, as

well as lepromatous nerve involvement, which may cause laryngeal paralysis and odynophagia. Direct laryngoscopy typically reveals a nodular, edematous supraglottis with ulceration, and biopsy reveals a chronic inflammatory cell infiltrate with foamy leprous cells that contain the bacillus *M. leprae* (Hansen bacillus). Nasal smears for the intracellular microorganisms may be diagnostic. Treatment consists of the long-term use of diaminodiphenylsulfone (dapsone). Tracheostomy may be required if laryngeal stenosis develops.

Scleroma

Scleroma, previously called "rhinoscleroma" because of its predilection for the nose, is a chronic infection caused by *Klebsiella rhinoscleromatis*. Scleroma remains endemic today in Europe, Mexico, Central America, South America, and Egypt, and may be found in immigrants to the United States. Laryngeal involvement has been reported in approximately 15 to 80% of cases.[33]

The disease has three distinct stages: (1) the catarrhal stage, characterized by persistent purulent rhinorrhea, with nasal crusting and obstruction; (2) the granulomatous stage, characterized by small, painless granulomatous nodules within the upper respiratory tract, including the larynx; and (3) the sclerotic stage, in which the glottis and subglottis are usually involved, and hoarseness and respiratory obstruction may develop. The progression through these three stages usually takes many years.

The diagnosis is made by isolating the microorganism from the tissues, although positive complement fixation and agglutination tests are highly suggestive. Foamy vacuolated histiocytes (Mikulicz cells) and bloated plasma cells with red birefringent inclusions (Russell bodies) are seen histologically.

Treatment consists of intravenous aminoglycosides, tetracycline, or cephalosporins. Laryngeal dilatation, endoscopic resection, and tracheostomy may be required during the sclerotic phase. Untreated rhinoscleroma may cause death owing to airway obstruction.

Actinomycosis

Cervicofacial actinomycosis is a chronic suppurative disease caused by the anaerobic bacterium *Actinomyces bovis* or *Actinomyces israelii*. Initial involvement of the cervical or mandibular region leads first to paralaryngeal and then to laryngeal disease. Pain is the most common initial manifestation, followed by hoarseness, cough, and, eventually, airway obstruction.

The larynx appears diffusely erythematous and swollen with draining sinuses; its consistency is firm and woody.[34] Diagnosis is made by identifying the typical "sulfur granules" in biopsy material and by culturing the microorganism. Long-term therapy with penicillin or tetracycline is effective. Stenosis and laryngeal fixation secondary to deep ulcerations and chondritis may develop if the disease is left untreated. Laryngeal dilatation, arytenoidectomy, or tracheostomy may be required.

Nocardia species of the Actinomyces family are soil saprophytes that are widely distributed throughout the world. Like other Actinomyces, Nocardia may infect humans by inhalation or through a break in the skin. Nocardiosis is characterized by diffuse microabscesses that, on histologic examination, show a neutrophilic predominance; sulfur granules are atypical. Aerodigestive tract involvement is common. The diagnosis is made by culture and isolation of the Nocardia microorganism, and treatment is with systemic sulfisoxazole.

Syphilis

Syphilis is a sexually transmitted spirochetal infection caused by *Treponema pallidum*. Syphilitic chancres do not usually involve the larynx, and, most commonly, the larynx becomes involved during the secondary and tertiary stages. However, tertiary syphilis may not develop until years after the initial infection. Diffuse erythematous papules, painless superficial ulcers, and cervical lymphadenopathy are seen during the secondary stage and generally clear without treatment within several weeks. Gumma formation during the tertiary stage can lead to laryngeal fibrosis, chondritis, and stenosis. Serologic tests for syphilis are diagnostic, and a lumbar puncture should be performed to rule out central nervous system involvement. Penicillin is still the treatment of choice.[35] Although rare, congenital syphilitic laryngitis can occur in infants born to mothers with syphilis. This diagnosis should be considered in the differential diagnosis of neonates with laryngeal stenosis.

FUNGAL LARYNGEAL INFECTIONS

Candidiasis

Among the risk factors for development of laryngeal candidiasis (usually infection by the species *Candida albicans*) are the use of corticosteroids and broad-spectrum antibiotics, diabetes, burns, alcoholism, endotracheal intubation, previous (viral or bacterial) laryngeal infection, and in patients who use corticosteroid inhalers.[36] In addition, inhaled corticosteroids in particulate form often used to treat pulmonary disease are increasingly recognized to cause laryngeal inflammation, leukoplakia and predispose to laryngeal candidiasis. This form of isolated laryngeal candidiasis has a distinctive appearance: intense, diffuse laryngeal erythema with an irregular, friable, white exudate (occurring most notably on the true vocal folds). The infection is superficial, and no ulceration or necrosis is seen (Figure 4). Oral nystatin suspension is often effective. More advanced laryngeal disease is associated with biofilm formation, encasing the *Candida* within a polysaccharide-rich extracellular matrix,[37] so an oral antifungal agent such as ketoconazole or fluconazole is sometimes necessary (in some cases for as long as several weeks).

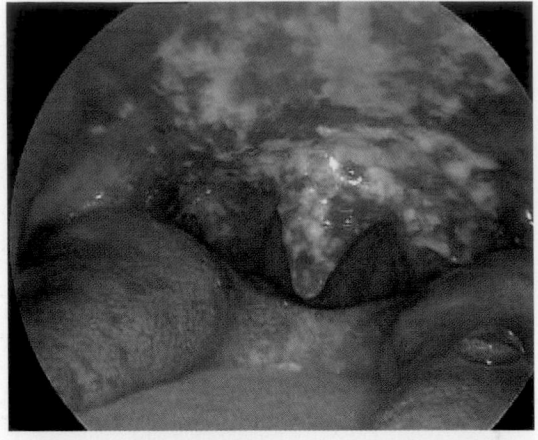

(A)

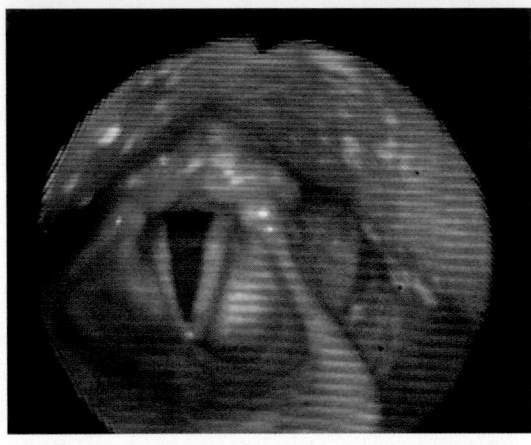

(B)

Figure 4 Candidiasis. (A) Oral thrush showing white patchy plaques surrounded by erythematous mucosa. (B) Laryngeal candidiasis in patient who had been using corticosteroid inhalers.

Candida biofilms are also common on indwelling medical devices, such as tracheotomy tubes, laryngeal voice prostheses, and nasogastric feeding tubes. Candidal esophagitis should be considered in a patient with laryngeal involvement and dysphagia.

In the immunocompromised patient, laryngeal candidiasis may be caused by local aerodigestive tract infection, which can subsequently give rise to locally invasive or widespread systemic candidiasis. When a patient presents with dysphagia and barium esophagography or transnasal esophagoscopy reveals *Candida* esophagitis, the clinician should suspect that the patient has acquired immunodeficiency syndrome (AIDS). Indeed, aerodigestive tract candidiasis may be the first presenting manifestation of AIDS.

Invasive *Candida* laryngitis in the immunocompromised host produces painful, ulcerative lesions and deep tissue necrosis and may progress rapidly. In addition to hoarseness, patients with this type of infection complain of sore throat, dysphagia, and odynophagia. Unlike other fungi, *Candida* species can easily be identified on Gram stain. Confirmation of the diagnosis is made by the histopathology and culture of biopsied tissue. Invasive laryngeal candidiasis is treated with parenteral amphotericin B and, when necessary, airway support.

Blastomycosis

North American blastomycosis is a granulomatous chronic pulmonary infection caused by the fungus *Blastomyces dermatitidis*. Laryngeal involvement occurs in 2 to 5% of cases, although primary laryngeal blastomycosis has been reported.[38] The microorganism is generally found in damp areas where decaying wood is present. Its distribution in the United States and Canada is concentrated around the Great Lakes and along the Mississippi, Ohio, and St. Lawrence rivers.

Patients typically present with multiorgan systemic involvement and severe hoarseness and cough when the larynx is involved. The microorganism produces erythematous, granular, mucosal lesions in the larynx, which progress to small, painless abscesses and ulcerations. Histologically, caseous necrosis with abundant acute inflammatory cells and microabscesses are seen, as well as giant cells in the surrounding tissue. Pseudoepitheliomatous hyperplasia is a characteristic change seen in the epithelial layer. The fungus in yeast form may be seen in the region of the microabscesses and is periodic acid–Schiff positive. Treatment is with long-term oral itraconazole, with amphotericin B being reserved for severe or recalcitrant cases. In the absence of treatment, progressive fibrosis with vocal fold fixation develops, as do pharyngocutaneous fistulae.

Histoplasmosis

Histoplasmosis is a systemic granulomatous mycotic disease caused by *Histoplasma capsulatum* and may involve the larynx (Figure 5). Nodular superficial granulomas that may ulcerate and become painful involve the anterior portions of the larynx and epiglottis. Esophageal involvement may occur (Figure 6). Histologic examination shows granulation tissue composed of plasma cells, microorganism-laden macrophages, lymphocytes, and giant cells, which may be confused with the granuloma of tuberculosis. Diagnosis is made by culture and the complement fixation test. Amphotericin B is the treatment of choice.

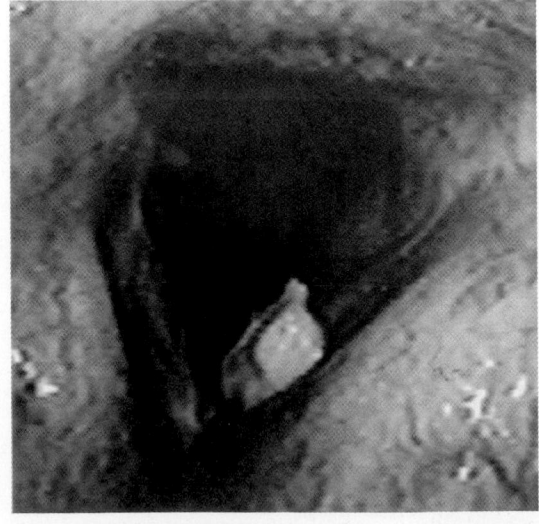

Figure 5 Histoplasmosis of the larynx. Note pedunculated lesion of the left true vocal fold.

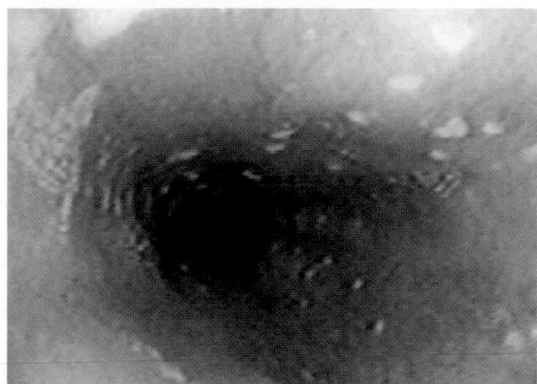

Figure 6 Diffuse esophageal histoplasmosis.

Laryngeal stenosis may develop when extensive ulceration leads to chondritis. In this instance, laryngeal dilatation, arytenoidectomy, or tracheostomy may be required to provide a safe airway.

Coccidioidomycosis

Coccidioidomycosis, also called "desert fever" (or "San Joaquin Valley fever" in the United States), is caused by the microorganism *Coccidioides immitis* which is found in desert soil. It is primarily a granulomatous pulmonary fungal infection that is endemic to the southwestern United States, Mexico, and central South America. Reportedly, 60% of people with this infection are asymptomatic; 40% develop a flu-like illness, and among those, 0.5% develop a systemic, disseminated, more severe form of the disease. Patients with the disseminated form may develop hoarseness, cough, and airway obstruction owing to laryngeal coccidioidomycosis.[39]

Laryngeal disease usually develops during the acute phase of the primary infection. Laryngeal involvement can, however, develop in patients who have had granulomatous lung disease for months or years. In addition to the laryngeal findings of intense, diffuse laryngeal erythema (with or without focal ulceration), most patients with *C. immitis* have cervical lymphadenopathy. Histology reveals caseating granulomas with multinucleated giant cells and pathognomonic, double-walled endospores. The diagnosis is made by serologic testing and biopsy of affected tissue. Treatment is with amphotericin B. When death occurs, it is usually owing to meningeal involvement.

Aspergillosis

Aspergillosis is generally an infection of immunocompromised patients, and respiratory tract involvement is common. When the larynx is involved, patients complain of hoarseness, dysphagia, and sometimes symptoms of airway obstruction. In the immunocompromised patient, *Aspergillus* infection is usually necrotizing, invasive, and associated with a poor prognosis. Despite aggressive antifungal treatment with amphotericin B and attempted wide surgical excision (including laryngectomy), most such patients with this infection die of progressive disease.

Sporotrichosis

Sporotrichosis, an uncommon fungal infection of the skin or airway, is caused by *Sporothrix schenckii* and occurs worldwide. The causative fungus is most commonly found in sphagnum moss and wood. People who work with wood usually get the cutaneous form of sporotrichosis, whereas most cases of laryngeal sporotrichosis occur in people working with the moss.

The more common cutaneous form of sporotrichosis causes granulomas in the subcutaneous layer of the skin and in regional lymph nodes. If the mucous membranes of the upper airway are damaged or abraded for any reason, inhalation of the fungus may result in laryngopharyngeal infection. Hoarseness and cough are the most common symptoms, and the lesions appear granulomatous. Diagnosis is made by biopsy and by culturing the microorganism. Oral potassium iodide is sufficient treatment for cases with superficial involvement; deep tissue involvement requires a course of amphotericin B therapy.[40]

PARASITIC LARYNGEAL INFECTIONS

Trichinosis

Trichinosis in humans is caused by ingesting meat contaminated with the helminthic roundworm *Trichinella spiralis*. Trichinosis is relatively common worldwide. About 30 cases occur each year in the United States. In the past, contaminated pork was the most common source of infection, but today, most cases are caused by eating feral meat, such as bear or wild boar. Humans are particularly susceptible to trichinosis infection. Soon after ingestion, the larvae penetrate the intestinal wall, where copulation and multiplication occur. The next generation of larvae enters the bloodstream and is distributed throughout the body, and finally enters and grows in skeletal muscle. The muscles of the diaphragm, eyes, tongue, chest, shoulders, and calves are often affected. Laryngeal involvement is uncommon.

In tissue, the larvae elicit an eosinophilic and lymphocytic inflammatory response. The severity of the clinical manifestations depends on the location and density of the larvae. The first symptoms occur within 2 days of ingestion. During the initial stage of infection, diarrhea, nausea, and malaise are common. During the muscle invasion stage (lasting 1 to 6 weeks), fever, weakness, skin rash, myalgia, muscle tenderness, and facial and periorbital edema are usually present. Some cases are complicated by urticaria, splinter hemorrhages, and angioedema. The primary symptom of laryngeal involvement is hoarseness. Trichinosis should be suspected by the history and eosinophilia. Diagnosis can be made by serologic testing and muscle biopsy. Treatment is with a 7-day course of thiabendazole. The disease can be prevented by cooking meat products to an internal temperature of 170°F.

Leishmaniasis

Leishmaniasis, although uncommon in the United States, is indigenous throughout the rest of the world. It is estimated that there are 1.5 to 2 million cases each year worldwide. The vast majority of the world's cases occur in India, Bangladesh, Nepal, Sudan, and Brazil. The organism infects rodents and dogs, and transmission to humans is usually from an animal, although the bite of an intermediate host, the sandfly, may cause the disease as well. Although there are several clinical forms of the disease, the mucocutaneous form, caused by *Leishmania braziliensis* and *Leishmania mexicana*, is the one that most commonly involves the airway. Espundia, the form caused by *L. mexicana*, is endemic in south-central Texas.

Usually, one or more skin lesions on the lower extremity begin as sores that slowly enlarge and ulcerate over a period of months. These untreated lesions seldom heal. Months or years later, metastatic lesions appear on the lips, nose, and pharynx. Leishmaniasis involves the larynx in approximately one-third of cases.[41]

Fever, anemia, weight loss, and hoarseness are common symptoms. As time passes, extensive soft tissue destruction may lead to grotesque facial disfiguration, as well as progression of the laryngeal disease. Examination of the larynx may reveal a localized, polypoid, inflammatory lesion or diffuse, granular, spongy mucosa. The lesions may be ulcerated, and airway obstruction may occur. These lesions are often mistaken for laryngeal cancer, tuberculosis, histoplasmosis, or blastomycosis.

Biopsy reveals a chronic granulomatous pattern, with a predominance of lymphocytic and histiocytic cells. The diagnosis can be made by identification of the parasite in biopsy specimens, but, in some cases, the parasites may be difficult to find. A specific agglutination test for leishmaniasis and the leishmaniasis skin test are diagnostic. The mucocutaneous form of leishmaniasis should be treated with antimonials for at least 30 days.

Schistosomiasis

Endemic in the tropics and subtropics, schistosomiasis ("bilharziasis" in Egypt) is widespread in 72 countries of the world and infects an estimated 5% of the world's population. It is the most prevalent helminthic infection in the world. There are three *Schistosoma* species parasitic in man: *S. mansoni*, *S. japonicum*, and *S. haematobium*. *Schistosoma mansoni* and *S. japonicum* inhabit the mesenteric veins; the eggs are found along the wall of the intestine and in the liver and are passed in the feces. *Schistosoma haematobium* invades the veins of the pelvic plexus, and the eggs are passed in the urine. Ectopic lesions occur in 18% of cases and may be found in any part of the body.

Humans contract schistosomiasis from water infested by cercariae, the microscopic infective stage. Cercariae penetrate the intact skin, and schistosomules form in the skin. After several days, the schistosomules migrate to the lungs and portal veins, where the male and female species mate. Weeks later, depending on the species and the time of transit, eggs are deposited in the infected organs. To complete the life cycle, organisms excreted by humans must contaminate water because the snail is the intermediate host. The cercariae grow in the soft tissue of the snail, and after 1 to 2 months, they are released back into the water, where they can again enter the human body.

Schistosomiasis in the aerodigestive tract is characterized by intense inflammatory granulomas around deposits of schistosome eggs. Granulomas may be as small as a pinhead or as large as an orange. Histologically, coagulation necrosis occurs around the egg deposits, and eosinophils, plasma cells, and lymphocytes predominate in the cellular response.[42] Patients with laryngeal schistosome granulomas present with hoarseness. The laryngeal lesion has the appearance of a pink–gray, cauliflower-like granuloma, with surrounding inflammation. The degree of surrounding fibrosis is determined by the egg density and the duration of the infection. Confirmation of the diagnosis is made by identification of parasitic ova in the urine or feces. Treatment is with antihelminthics.

Syngamosis

Syngamus laryngeus is a unique gapeworm indigenous to Brazil, Puerto Rico, Martinique, Trinidad, British Guyana, the West Indies, and the Philippines. It invades the upper respiratory tract of cattle, water buffalo, and (rarely) humans. Transmission to humans is believed to be through consumption of contaminated vegetables. Once ingested, the adult worms migrate to the larynx and upper trachea and firmly attach themselves to those mucosal surfaces. The primary symptoms of syngamosis are cough, a foreign body sensation in the throat, and, occasionally, hemoptysis. The diagnosis may be suspected if the patient coughs up worms in copula or if they are seen on laryngoscopy. Removal of the worms by direct laryngoscopy is the only known treatment.[43]

Table 10 Common Laryngeal Infections of the Immunocompromised Host

Viral
  Herpes simplex
  Herpes zoster
  Cytomegalovirus
  Papova (papilloma)
  Toxoplasmosis
Bacterial
  Tuberculosis
  Atypical mycobacteria
  Actinomycosis
Fungal
  Candidiasis
  Aspergillosis
  Histoplasmosis
  Coccidioidomycosis

Infections of the Immunocompromised Host

Immunocompromised patients, whether immunocompromised from diabetes, long-term corticosteroid therapy, chemotherapy, or AIDS, are at risk of developing opportunistic infections of the aerodigestive tract. The most commonly reported opportunistic infections that affect the larynx are shown in Table 10. Of those listed, laryngeal candidiasis, tuberculosis, and herpes infections are the most commonly encountered in patients with AIDS.

AUTOIMMUNE, ALLERGIC, AND IDIOPATHIC DISORDERS

Sarcoidosis

Sarcoidosis is a slowly progressive, rarely fatal, systemic granulomatous disease of unknown cause. The disease afflicts African Americans 10 times more commonly than whites. The lungs and skin are most commonly involved, and laryngeal sarcoidosis occurs in 1 to 5% of cases (with or without lung involvement).[44] When the skin of the nasal rim is affected, upper respiratory sarcoidosis involvement is seen in approximately 75% of cases.

Laryngeal sarcoid usually involves the supraglottic larynx and sometimes the subglottis but typically spares the true vocal folds (Figure 7). Characteristically, the entire supraglottis appears pale pink and massively edematous, sometimes obscuring visualization of the vocal folds. The turban-like appearance of the epiglottis is virtually pathognomonic. Less commonly, some laryngeal sarcoidosis patients present with a few discrete, sometimes hemorrhagic, nodules (up to 1 cm in diameter) on the epiglottis or other supraglottic structures.

Laryngeal sarcoidosis is a diagnosis of exclusion based primarily on finding noncaseating granulomas and diffuse edema with miliary nodules involving mainly the supraglottic structures and on excluding tuberculosis and fungal diseases. An elevated serum angiotensin converting enzyme (ACE) level may be found. The use of systemic and intralesional corticosteroids

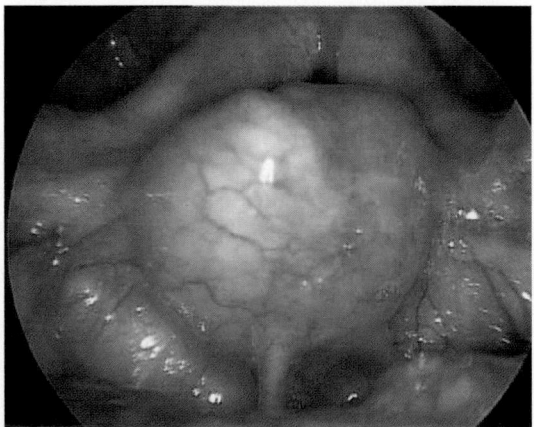

Figure 7 Sarcoidosis of epiglottis. Notice granulomatous epiglottic stub protruding posteriorly, with surrounding inflammation and airway compromise.

generally results in improvement or apparent resolution of the lesions. In severe cases, however, endoscopic dilatation and laser resection of involved supraglottic tissues, or tracheostomy, may be necessary for those patients with airway obstruction.

Wegener Granulomatosis

Wegener granulomatosis is characterized by necrotizing granuloma with vasculitis involving the upper respiratory tract, lungs, and kidneys. On presentation, its laryngeal involvement may resemble acute laryngitis, but the eventual development of granulomatous ulcers throughout the larynx may lead the clinician to suspect the diagnosis. Subglottic stenosis occurs in approximately 20% of cases and can lead to significant airway obstruction, requiring tracheostomy and surgical correction of the stenosis.[45] Diagnosis is based on typical histologic findings of necrotizing granulomas and vasculitis. The anticytoplasmic autoantibody test (C-ANCA) is highly specific for Wegener granulomatosis but may have low sensitivity in early disease. Recommended treatment includes cyclophosphamide with corticosteroids.

Hypersensitivity Reactions

The term hypersensitivity implies an overzealous response of the immune system to an antigenic stimulus. Hypersensitivity reactions include conditions such as allergic rhinitis, contact dermatitis, and urticaria, but these conditions do not produce life-threatening, obstructive edema within the airway. Anaphylaxis, an acute and profoundly life-threatening immune-mediated allergic response, is made up of a triad of clinical manifestations: (1) flushing, pruritus, and/or urticaria; (2) airway obstruction, for example, angioedema, laryngospasm, and/or bronchospasm; and (3) circulatory collapse, for example, shock.

Angioedema

Angioedema is an acute, allergic, histamine-mediated, inflammatory reaction characterized by acute vascular dilation and capillary permeability. In susceptible patients, angioedema can be precipitated by medications, food additives and preservatives, and by blood transfusions, infections, or insect bites. In addition, the condition may be associated with a coexisting connective tissue disorder. The hereditary form of angioedema is an autosomally dominant deficiency of C1 esterase inhibitor that leads to recurrent attacks of mucocutaneous edema.[46] An acquired form of C1 esterase deficiency has also been reported in patients with angioedema who have occult lymphoma.

Oral and laryngopharyngeal structures are frequently affected and with localized or general edema that may lead to airway obstruction, but it can also occur in other parts of the body. Diagnosis is made primarily from the history, although the offending agent may not be readily apparent. Treatment of both types of angioedema must be prompt and aggressive. Epinephrine, cortico-steroids, antihistamines, and aminophylline are the mainstays of therapy. If progressive airway obstruction develops, intubation or tracheostomy may be required. Chronic "pretreatment" of hereditary angioedema with danazol appears to elevate levels of functional C1 esterase inhibitor and to help prevent recurrent episodes.

Stevens-Johnson Syndrome

Stevens-Johnson syndrome is a mucocutaneous hypersensitivity reaction (at the severe end of the erythema multiforme spectrum) usually triggered by medications, for example, sulfonamides, phenobarbital, and carbamazepine. It is an acute febrile illness characterized by conjunctivitis, rash, and severe oropharyngeal mucositis. The mucosal and skin lesions rapidly progress to bullae formation and desquamation of the skin in sheets. The most severe form of this syndrome is called toxic epidermal necrolysis, and this variant may involve the larynx.[47] Diagnosis is made by biopsy, and treatment is primarily supportive, including tracheostomy when the airway is compromised. If death occurs, it usually owing to sepsis from bacterial superinfection.

Rheumatoid Arthritis

Rheumatoid arthritis is a systemic autoimmune disorder of unknown cause that can affect any organ in the body. The most common manifestation of rheumatoid arthritis is symmetric polyarthritis, but it can also cause inflammation in nonjoint structures, vasculitis, and pulmonary changes.[48] Rheumatoid arthritis may affect the larynx both directly and indirectly.

Rheumatoid involvement of the cricoarytenoid joints may cause hoarseness or airway obstruction. At postmortem examination, up to 87% of patients with rheumatoid arthritis have cricoarytenoid joint changes, but, based on laryngoscopy, only 17 to 33% of patients have clinical signs of laryngeal involvement, namely, posterior laryngeal inflammation and decreased arytenoid cartilage mobility.

Rheumatoid nodules may occur anywhere in the larynx or within the substance of the vocal fold itself, leading to hoarseness. The gross appearance of rheumatoid laryngeal nodules is variable. They may appear as white submucosal nodules, ulcerated friable polypoid lesions, or ill-defined masses deep within the substance of the vocal fold. Occasionally, unsuspected rheumatoid nodules are discovered during direct laryngoscopy by palpation of the nodule. Because the nodules lie within the substance of the vocal fold and may be inflamed, the vocal fold may be scarred after their removal. As a consequence, there may be persistent hoarseness following nodule removal.

Histologically, these lesions show a central area of fibrinoid necrosis surrounded by histiocytes, plasma cells, and lymphocytes. They can be highly vascularized and hyalinized and may have a fibrous capsule. Frequently, rheumatoid nodules of the larynx are misdiagnosed as pyogenic granulomas.

Rheumatoid arthritis, like other collagen vascular diseases, often involves the esophagus, causing esophageal dysmotility and reflux disease. Thus, patients with rheumatoid arthritis may have reflux laryngitis, but it is not known whether such reflux contributes to the arytenoid fixation. The choice of treatment for rheumatoid airway obstruction secondary to arytenoid cartilage fixation depends on the patient's overall medical condition. Since surgical rehabilitation of arytenoid cartilage function is not possible, endoscopic arytenoidectomy is usually the treatment of choice. Sometimes the rheumatoid arthritis so severely affects the neck that endoscopic exposure of the larynx is not possible. In such cases, an open surgical procedure or simply a tracheostomy may be performed.

Systemic Lupus Erythematosus

Lupus is a systemic, autoimmune disease that affects women more commonly than men and usually presents in the second and third decades of life. Patients with this condition may have autoantibodies to a variety of different tissues, and head and neck manifestations are common. Although the most common manifestations of lupus are arthritis, malar rash, and photosensitivity, up to 40% of patients have mucosal lesions of the aerodigestive tract as well.

The lesions may be varied, for example, petechiae, ulcerations, or raised nonulcerated lesions with erythematous borders. The palate and nose are commonly involved. Painless nasal septal perforations may occur. The larynx may also be involved by these mucosal lesions or, on occasion, by cricoarytenoid arthritis.[48]

Laryngeal involvement usually occurs at times of acute exacerbation of the systemic disease. Airway compromise is uncommon but does occur. Biopsy reveals a mononuclear cell infiltrate. Positive fluorescent antinuclear antibody tests are important for diagnosis and are a key part of American Rheumatism Association diagnostic criteria. Corticosteroids and symptomatic therapy are the treatment.

Cicatricial Pemphigoid

Pemphigus and pemphigoid are idiopathic, autoimmune epithelial disorders. There are several clinical variations; however, in common, they share subepithelial bullae inflammation. The primary distinctions between the two entities are the clinical patterns and histologic features: in pemphigus, there is suprabasilar separation (cantholysis), and in pemphigoid, the bullae are subepidermal. Different sites of involvement are believed to be the result of autoimmunity to distinct basement membrane antigens. Pemphigus and pemphigoid also may be associated with systemic lupus erythematosus. Of this group of uncommon bullous diseases, only cicatricial pemphigoid appears to involve the larynx with any frequency (9 to 20% of cases).

Cicatricial pemphigoid is a painful, unremitting, chronic inflammatory, vesiculobullous disease. Cicatricial formation may occur at any site of involvement, including the nose, nasopharynx, pharynx, larynx, and esophagus. Cicatricial pemphigoid affects women twice as often as men, and most patients are over 50 years of age. The oral cavity and eyes are most commonly involved; the aerodigestive tract is sometimes involved. The largest series in the otolaryngology literature reported 13 of 142 (9%) patients with laryngeal involvement, 3 of whom required airway intervention.[49] All 13 had involvement of other areas of the aerodigestive tract as well, but isolated laryngeal involvement has been reported. The primary symptom of laryngeal pemphigoid is severe odynophagia, and the most common findings are ulcers of the epiglottis and aryepiglottic folds.

Diagnosis is dependent on biopsy, which shows inflammatory subepithelial bullae surrounded by a mixed cellular inflammatory infiltrate. Immunofluorescent studies usually reveal linear deposition of immunoglobulins (IgG and IgM) along the basement membrane.[49] Long-term treatment is with the anti-inflammatory medication dapsone, with systemic corticosteroids and/or immunosuppressive therapy being reserved for dapsone treatment failures. Intralesional corticosteroids are ineffective. Stenosis of the larynx and other sites usually requires surgical intervention.

Relapsing Polychondritis

Relapsing polychondritis is a rare, idiopathic, generally progressive, autoimmune disease that causes inflammation of cartilage. It can mimic rheumatoid arthritis and sometimes occurs in patients with other autoimmune diseases, such as Sjögren syndrome, systemic lupus erythematosus, and psoriatic and rheumatoid arthritis.

Relapsing polychondritis occurs in all age groups, having a bell-shaped distribution and a peak incidence in the fourth decade. Although only 10% of patients present with respiratory tract involvement (larynx and trachea), more than 50% eventually develop such involvement, and 20% require tracheostomy. Of the 20 to 30% of patients who eventually die of the disease, most die of respiratory complications.[50]

This disease is characterized by episodes of inflammation with subsequent destruction of the cartilage of the ears, nose, and larynx. Most patients present with bilateral involvement of the ear cartilage, becoming red, swollen, and tender. With or without treatment, the condition may subside within 5 to 10 days. The next most common sites of involvement are the nose and the costal cartilages. Arthritis involving the large joints is also common. Laryngeal involvement is manifest by hoarseness, dyspnea, stridor, cough, and, sometimes, pain and hemoptysis. A clinical diagnosis is confirmed by cartilage biopsy although most patients with this disorder also have autoantibodies to type II collagen.

Histologically, the normal cartilage is replaced by an eosinophilic material, and acute and chronic infiltrates of lymphocytes and plasma cells are present. The usual basophilic appearance of the cartilage matrix is lost; lacunae are interrupted, and fibrous tissue replaces cartilage. As the disease progresses, fibrosis and chondronecrosis become marked.

Treatment includes corticosteroids and anti-inflammatory medications such as dapsone. Corticosteroid and immunosuppressive medications are used for patients with severe, recalcitrant, or rapidly progressive disease, especially when the larynx or other airway structures are involved. Tracheostomy may be necessary in the later stages of the disease.

Sjögren Syndrome

Sjögren syndrome is an idiopathic autoimmune disorder characterized by the clinical triad of xerostomia, that is, dry mouth, conjunctivitis sicca, that is, dry eyes, and rheumatoid arthritis. Patients with Sjögren syndrome have a relatively high incidence of developing lymphoma. There is also a "limited" form of the disease, occurring without the arthritis, called "sicca syndrome."

Although the cause (or causes) of these syndromes is unknown, both the limited and the full-blown forms have in common autoantibodies to glandular tissue in the eyes, nose, oral cavity, and laryngopharynx. In addition to the lacrimal glands and the major salivary glands, minor salivary and seromucinous glands are usually affected throughout the aerodigestive tract.

The diagnosis is made clinically using a Schirmer test to document the dryness of the eyes and by salivary gland biopsy. In the major salivary glands, the histologic picture demonstrates: (1) an intense lymphoid infiltrate, especially in periductal areas; (2) glandular atrophy; and (3) myoepithelial hyperplasia. Although the salivary glands are virtually always affected, biopsy of minor salivary gland tissue (lip biopsy) is usually sufficient to make the diagnosis. The histopathologic features seen in minor salivary glands are similar to those seen in the major salivary glands, although the myoepithelial hyperplasia is absent.

The seromucinous glands of the larynx may be involved, leading to inflammation of the larynx similar to that seen in the salivary glands. Clinically, this involvement produces edema, erythema, dryness, crusting, and, hence, chronic hoarseness. Laryngeal Sjögren syndrome, however, does not occur in isolation; that is, patients with laryngeal symptoms and signs of Sjögren syndrome also have other manifestations of the disease.[51]

In some cases, the mucosa of the posterior commissure appears so hypertrophic that the clinician must consider the possibility of tumor. The larynx in Sjögren syndrome usually exhibits intense erythema and hypertrophy of the posterior commissure with dry, tenacious mucus between the vocal folds. Biopsies of the larynx reveal histologic findings similar to those seen in the salivary glands. In addition, patients with Sjögren syndrome often have impaired esophageal function

and gastroesophageal reflux. Treatment is symptomatic, and antireflux and anti-inflammatory medications are sometimes prescribed.

Amyloidosis

Amyloidosis is a dysproteinemia in which a characteristic, amorphous, eosinophilic substance is deposited in the tissues of various organs. Amyloidosis is classified as being either "systemic" or "localized." The systemic types are familial, primary (with or without myeloma), and secondary (usually associated with chronic inflammatory disease). Primary amyloidosis has a 5-year survival of only 20%, with the patients dying of renal, central nervous system, or cardiac involvement.[52] The "localized" type of amyloidosis is almost never fatal and is the type that most commonly involves the larynx. Most cases of laryngeal amyloidosis occur in isolation, although simultaneous involvement of the trachea and, to a lesser extent, the bronchi occurs in about one-third of those cases.

On laryngoscopy, amyloidosis appears as diffuse mucosal thickening or subepithelial nodules, localized mainly to the anterior part of the subglottis. Patients are usually asymptomatic until the deposits involve the vocal folds or critically narrow the airway. When amyloidosis is suspected, biopsy specimens should be stained with Congo red, which, when viewed with polarized light, shows a pathognomonic apple green birefringence.

Laryngeal amyloidosis usually has a benign course. Symptomatic cases are best treated by endoscopic carbon dioxide laser excision of the lesions; laryngeal dilatation and tracheostomy are rarely necessary.

Inhalant Laryngeal Trauma and the Effects of Radiation

It is prudent to briefly discuss the effects of inhalant laryngeal trauma, as well as the effects of radiation. These conditions are often seen in otolaryngology practice and can predispose to edema, stasis of mucus secretions, and bacterial suprainfection. When nebulized radiolabeled acidic fog is inhaled and scanned, the density of aerosol deposit in the larynx is greater than in any other site in the aerodigestive tract. The size and anatomic configuration of the larynx (having the narrowest and most convoluted lumen of the upper airway) may explain this phenomenon. Perhaps for this reason, the larynx is especially susceptible to the effects of inhaled corticosteroids for treatment of asthma, tobacco smoke, dust, and other airborne environmental contaminants. Table 11 lists some of the commonly reported substances associated with acute and chronic inhalation injuries of the larynx.

Radiation therapy for laryngeal carcinoma, as well as for tumors in other head and neck sites, may deliver significant radiation doses to normal laryngeal tissue. The initial effects produce an intense inflammatory response, characterized by increased capillary permeability, edema,

Table 11 Causes of Inhalation Laryngitis (Substances Associated with Acute and Chronic Laryngeal Inflammation)

Acute inhalation injury	Steam
	Hot dry gases
	Smoke
Common allergens	Dust mites
	Animal danders
	Formaldehyde
	Mold
	Trees
	Grasses
	Weeds
	Dusts
Pollutants	Ozone
	Ammonia
	Chlorine
	Nitrous oxide
	Hydrogen disulfide
	Sulfur dioxide
	Carbon monoxide
	Sulfuric acid
	Hydrochloric acid
	Kerosene (heaters)
	Insecticides
	Dusts
	Pesticides
Known carcinogens	Tobacco
	Asbestos
	Radon
	Nickel
	Sulfuric acid
	Isopropyl oils
	Mustard gas

neutrophilic infiltration, vascular thrombosis, and obliteration of lymphatic channels. Patients undergoing radiation treatment complain of a globus sensation, dysphagia, odynophagia, dysphonia, and odynophonia, and are more likely to have exacerbation by LPR based on laryngeal sicca. Late tissue sequelae consist of degenerative changes and fibrosis in adipose, connective, and glandular tissues and a pronounced obliterative endarteritis of small blood vessels. Both the acute and chronic changes associated with radiation also predispose to bacterial suprainfection and LPR.

CONCLUSIONS

Laryngeal inflammation is the common theme linking the effects of LPR, infections and autoimmune/inflammatory diseases in the larynx. While it is imperative to identify the underlying causative diseases, these conditions tend to be further complicated by suprainfection and immune susceptibility.

REFERENCES

1. Castell DO, Wu WC, Ott DJ, editors. Gastroesophageal Reflux Disease, Pathogenesis, Diagnosis, Therapy. Mt. Kisko, NY: Futura; 1985. p. 1–324.
2. Locke GR, III, Talley NJ, Fett SL, et al. Prevalence and clinical spectrum of gastroesophageal reflux: A population-based study in Olmsted County, Minnesota. Gastroenterol 1997;112:1448–56.
3. Koufman JA. The otolaryngologic manifestations of gastroesophageal reflux disease (GERD): A clinical investigation

of 225 patients using ambulatory 24-hour pH monitoring and an experimental investigation of the role of acid and pepsin in the development of laryngeal injury. Laryngoscope 1991;10153:1–78.

4. Altman KW, Stephens RM, Lyttle CS, Weiss KB. Changing impact of gastroesophageal reflux in medical and otolaryngology practice. Laryngoscope 2005;115:1145–53.

5. Freije JE, Beatty TW, Campbell BH, et al. Carcinoma of the larynx in patients with gastroesophageal reflux. Am J Otolaryngol 1996;17:386–90.

6. Halstead LA. Role of gastroesophageal reflux in pediatric upper airway disorders. Otolaryngol Head Neck Surg 1999;120:208–14.

7. Altman KW, Simpson CB, Amin MR, et al. Cough and paradoxical vocal fold motion. Otolaryngol Head Neck Surg 2002;127:501–11.

8. Penzel T, Becker HF, Brandenburg U, et al. Arousal in patients with gastro-oesophageal reflux and sleep apnoea. Eur Respir J 1999;14:1266–70.

9. Johnston N, Bulmer D, Gill GA, et al. Cell biology of laryngeal epithelial defenses in health and disease: Further studies. Ann Otol Rhinol Laryngol 2003;112:481–91.

10. Koufman JA, Amin MR, Panetti M. Prevalence of reflux in 113 consecutive patients with laryngeal and voice disorders. Otolaryngol Head Neck Surg 2000;123:385–8.

11. Richter JE, Bradley LA, DeMeester TR, et al. Normal 24-hour pH values: Influence of study center, pH electrode, age, and gender. Dig Dis Sci 1992;37:849–56.

12. Koufman JA, Belafsky PC, Bach KK, et al. Prevalence of esophagitis in patients with pH-documented laryngopharyngeal reflux. Laryngoscope 2002;112:1606–9.

13. Postma GN, Cohen JT, Belafsky PC, et al. Transnasal esophagoscopy: Revisited (over 700 consecutive cases). Laryngoscope 2005;115:321–3.

14. Hanson DG, Kamel PL, Kahrilas PJ. Outcomes of antireflux therapy for the treatment of chronic laryngitis. Ann Otol Rhinol Laryngol 1995;104:550–5.

15. Belafsky P, Postma G, Koufman J. Laryngopharyngeal reflux symptoms improve before changes in physical findings. Laryngoscope 2001;11:979–81.

16. Yorulmaz I, Ozlugedik S, Kucuk B. Gastroesophageal reflux disease: Symptoms versus pH monitoring results. Otolaryngol Head Neck Surg 2003;129:582–6.

17. Hill RK, Simpson CB, Velazquez R, Larson N. Pachydermia is not diagnostic of active laryngopharyngeal reflux disease. Laryngoscope 2004;114:1557–61.

18. Steward DL, Wilson KM, Kelly DH, et al. Proton pump inhibitor therapy for chronic laryngo-pharyngitis: A randomized placebo-control trial. Otolaryngol Head Neck Surg 2004;131:342–50.

19. Spechler SJ, Lee E, Ahnen D, et al. Long-term outcome of medical and surgical therapies for gastroesophageal reflux disease. Follow-up of a randomized controlled trial. JAMA 2001;285:2331–8.

20. Altman KW, Waltonen JD, Hammer ND, et al. Proton pump expression in human laryngeal seromucinous glands. Otolaryngol Head Neck Surg 2005;133:718–24.

21. Cressman WR, Meyer CM. Diagnosis and management of croup and epiglottitis. Pediatr Clin North Am 1994;41:265–76.

22. Deeb ZE, Einhorn KH. Infectious adult croup. Laryngoscope 1990;100:455–7.

23. McNamara MJ, Pierce WE, Crawford YE, Miller LF. Patterns of adenovirus infection in the respiratory disease of naval recruits. A longitudinal study of two companies of naval recruits. Am Rev Respir Dis 1962;86:485–97.

24. D'Angelo AJ, Zwillenberg S, Olezszyk, et al. Adult supraglottis due to herpes simplex virus. J Otolaryngol 1990;19:179–81.

25. Moore CE, Wiatrak BJ, McClatchey KD, et al. High-risk human papillomavirus types and squamous cell carcinoma in patients with respiratory papillomas. Otolaryngol Head Neck Surg 1999;120:698–705.

26. Heath PT, Booy R, Azzopardi HJ, et al. Non-type b *Haemophilus influenzae* disease: Clinical and epidemiologic characteristics in the *Haemophilus influenzae* type b vaccine era. Pediatr Infect Dis J 2001;20:300–5.

27. Souliere CR, Kirchner JA. Laryngeal perichondritis and abscess. Arch Otolaryngol 1985;111:481–4.

28. Havaldar PV. Diphtheria in the eighties: Experience in a south Indian district hospital. J Indian Med Assoc 1992;90:155–6.

29. Everett ED, Templer JW. Oropharyngeal tularemia. Arch Otolaryngol 1980;106:237–8.

30. Wilkinson L. Glanders: Medicine and veterinary medicine in common pursuit of a contagious disease. Med Hist 1981;25:363–84.

31. Harney M, Hone S, Timon C, Donnelly M. Laryngeal tuberculosis: An important diagnosis. J Laryngol Otol 2000;114:878–80.

32. Soni NK. Leprosy of the larynx. J Laryngol Otol 1992;106:518–20.

33. Alfaro-Monge JM, Fernandez-Espinosa J, Soda-Morhy A. Scleroma of the lower respiratory tract: Case report and review of the literature. J Laryngol Otol 1994;108:161–3.

34. Nelson EG, Tybor AG. Actinomycosis of the larynx. Ear Nose Throat J 1992;71:356–8.

35. Musher DM. Syphilis, neurosyphilis, penicillin, and AIDS. J Infect Dis 1991;163:1201–6.

36. Tashjian LS, Peacock JE. Laryngeal candidiasis. Report of seven cases and review of the literature. Arch Otolaryngol 1984;110:806–9.

37. Chandra J, Zhou G, Ghannoum MA. Fungal biofilms and antimycotics. Curr Drug Targets 2005;6:887–94.

38. Reder PA, Neel IIB. Blastomycosis in otolaryngology: Review of a large series. Laryngoscope 1993;103:53–8.

39. Boyle JO, Coulthard SW, Mandel RM. Laryngeal involvement in disseminated coccidioidomycosis. Arch Otolaryngol Head Neck Surg 1991;117:433–8.

40. Remington PL, Vergeront JM, Stoebig JF, et al. Sporotrichosis in Wisconsin. Wis Med J 1983;82:25–7.

41. Marsden PD. Mucosal leishmaniasis ("espundia" Escomel, 1911). Trans R Soc Trop Med Hyg 1986;80:859–76.

42. Toppozada HH. Laryngeal bilharzia. J Laryngol Otol 1985;99:1039–41.

43. Weinstein L, Molavi A. Syngamus laryngeus infection (syngamosis) with chronic cough. Ann Intern Med 1971;74:577–80.

44. Neel HB, McDonald TJ. Laryngeal sarcoidosis: Report of 13 patients. Ann Otol Rhinol Laryngol 1982;91:359–62.

45. Lebovics RS, Hoffman GS, Leavitt RY, et al. The management of subglottic stenosis in patients with Wegener's granulomatosis. Laryngoscope 1992;102:1341–5.

46. Altman KW, Woodring AJ, Pappano JE. Angioedema presenting in the retropharyngeal space in an adult. Am J Otolaryngol 1999;20:136–8.

47. Wahle D, Beste DJ, Conley SF. Laryngeal involvement in toxic epidermal necrolysis. Otolaryngol Head Neck Surg 1992;107:796–9.

48. Campbell SM, Montanaro A, Bardana EJ. Head and neck manifestations of autoimmune disease. Am J Otolaryngol 1983;4:187–216.

49. Hanson RD, Olsen KD, Rogers RS. Upper aerodigestive tract manifestations of cicatricial pemphigoid. Ann Otol Rhinol Laryngol 1988;97:493–9.

50. McAdam LP, O'Hanlan MA, Bluestone C, Pearson CM. Relapsing polychondritis: Prospective study of 23 patients and a review of the literature. Medicine 1976;55:193–215.

51. Barrs DM, McDonald TJ, Duffy J. Sjögren's syndrome involving the larynx. Report of a case. J Laryngol Otol 1979;93:933–6.

52. Lewis JE, Olsen KD, Kurtin PJ, Kyle RA. Laryngeal amyloidosis: A clinicopathologic and immunohistochemical review. Otolaryngol Head Neck Surg 1992;106:372–7.

SUGGESTED READINGS

Ford CN. Evaluation and management of laryngopharyngeal reflux. JAMA 2005;294:1534–40.

Koufman JA. Laryngopharyngeal reflux 2002: A new paradigm of airway disease. Ear Nose Throat J 2002;81:2 31.

Pillsbury HC, Sasaki CT. Granulomatous diseases of the larynx. Otolaryngol Clin North Am 1982;15:539–51.

Richtsmeier WJ, Johns ME. Bacterial causes of granulomatous disease. Otolaryngol Clin North Am 1982;15:473–92.

Tami TA, Ferlito A, Rinaldo A, et al. Laryngeal pathology in the acquired immunodeficiency syndrome: Diagnostic and therapeutic dilemmas. Ann Otol Rhinol Laryngol 1999;108:214–20.

77

Trauma to the Larynx

Ricardo L. Carrau, MD
Bridget C. Hathaway, MD

BLUNT AND PENETRATING LARYNGEAL TRAUMA

Acute external trauma to the larynx is a rare occurrence because of the protection provided by the reflexive flexion of the neck along with the bony protection offered by the arch of the mandible and sternum anteriorly and the rigid cervical spine posteriorly. The reported incidence of acute laryngeal trauma is 1 per 5,000 to 137,000 emergency department visits per year in the United States, with an increased prevalence in younger populations.[1,2] Although the incidence of laryngotracheal trauma is low, <1% of blunt trauma and <5% of penetrating trauma, the consequences of mistreatment are severe. With its proximity to vital vascular, neural, and skeletal structures, a laryngeal injury can be overlooked. A high clinical suspicion is necessary in the setting of any neck trauma. Additionally, due to the increased incidence of long-term endotracheal intubation, iatrogenic laryngeal injury is becoming more common.

The larynx has multiple physiologic and mechanical functions that depend upon the integrity of the rigid and highly functional architecture of its framework.[3] Its rigid apparatus consists of the hyoid bone and the major cartilages of the larynx: the thyroid, cricoid, epiglottic, and paired arytenoid cartilages. Its soft tissue architecture comprises three important folds: the aryepiglottic fold, the vestibular fold, and the true vocal fold. These three folds, in association with their muscles, form a three-tiered sphincter allowing air exchange, while preventing passage of saliva and ingested material into the lower airway. Other laryngeal functions such as vocalization, although important, are secondary to respiration and airway protection from an evolutionary standpoint. Laryngeal fractures that heal improperly can result in chronic airway stenosis and deterioration of the sphincteric and phonatory functions of the larynx. Historically, the surgical repair of laryngeal fractures has involved the use of stitches or wire fixation of fragments, along with autologous cartilage grafts for large defects. Internal stents have been advocated as a technique to preserve the proper size and shape of the airway when extraluminal repair cannot ensure immediate restoration of a stable laryngeal framework.[4–6] Although these techniques may adequately align fracture fragments, they do not always restore the functional architecture of the larynx. The resulting asymmetry or loss of anteroposterior or lateral dimension of the larynx can lead to posttraumatic dysphonia, dysphagia, or inadequate airway. Even minimally displaced fractures cause changes in glottal resistance and sound pressure levels, resulting in phonatory alterations. Mechanical loads applied by the extralaryngeal and intralaryngeal muscles during swallowing and neck movements may bend wire fixation, causing angulation of fragments with subsequent loss of the reduction. Midline or paramedian fractures stabilized with wire fixation tend to heal in a flattened position with loss of the anteroposterior dimensions.[5] Metal alloy plating techniques, commonly used for the fixation of maxillofacial fractures, have been adapted to treat fractures of the laryngeal framework. The advantages of plate fixation for maxillofacial trauma equally apply to laryngeal trauma, and include stabilization across fracture lines and restoration of the premorbid architecture with immediate or accelerated restoration of function.

The mechanisms of external laryngeal injury are conceptually divided into blunt and penetrating trauma. Blunt injuries are most commonly the result of motor vehicle accidents, sports and assaults and include "clotheslining," crushing, and strangulation injuries. In the United States, the incidence of this type of injury is decreasing. This may be due to increased use of seat belts and front seat air bags. In the absence of a secured chest restraining belt, the driver is thrust forward during rapid deceleration while the neck is hyperextended. In this position, the bony protection afforded by the mandible is lost, exposing the larynx to crushing forces in an anteroposterior axis. In this situation the larynx may be compressed between a blunt object and the cervical spine.

Clothesline injuries occur when a patient encounters a fixed horizontal object, such as a line, rope, cable, or tree branch at high speed at neck level. This type of injury imparts a large amount of energy over a relatively small area, resulting in severe trauma.[7,8] Many of these injuries lead to immediate death due to laryngeal crush injury or separation of the cricoid cartilage from the larynx or trachea.

Strangulation injuries result from manual compression, garroting, or by hanging. Clinical findings may initially include hoarseness or abrasions on the neck skin. Later, within 12 to 24 hours, the injury may progress to marked edema of the larynx and subsequent loss of the airway. To avoid this progression in airway complications, initial management decisions are largely based on the magnitude of the force sustained to the anterior neck.

Unfortunately, in the United States and other countries, the incidence of penetrating trauma is increasing due to the rise in personal assaults. Penetrating trauma to the larynx includes such injuries as stab wounds, gunshot wounds, and impalements. Severity of injury from a gunshot wound depends on the firing range and the type of weapon used. Gunshots at close range are often fatal due to the intense energy imparted to the soft tissues. From a long range, the damage may be less critical. Low-velocity handguns impart a moderate blast effect injury on surrounding tissue. The bullet's erratic course in soft tissues makes initial assessment of the wound difficult. On the other hand, high-velocity weapons impart a significant amount of kinetic energy. In high-velocity injuries, the total extent of the injured area may not be clinically evident initially. Judicious debridement of surrounding tissue is advisable at the time of surgical repair. Knife injuries do not destroy tissue distant to the path of injury, and the course may be accurately estimated from the entrance and exit wounds.

Diagnosis

Otolaryngologic evaluation is essential for any patient suspected of suffering a laryngeal trauma. The signs and symptoms of external laryngeal trauma vary from obvious open fractures to subtle aberrations of laryngeal function. Clinical findings may include any subtle alterations in voice, dysphagia, odynophagia, subcutaneous crepitus, saliva leaking through an open wound, bruising of the anterior neck, loss of the thyroid cartilage prominence, and tenderness to palpation. Findings may help to elucidate the mechanism of injury when an adequate history is unavailable.

External examination of the neck may reveal loss of the thyroid prominence, an open fracture or laryngocutaneous fistula. The larynx should be palpated for any crepitance.[9] Tenderness to palpation, although not specific, is often present in significant injury. The skin of the neck may reveal contusions or abrasions from blunt trauma or a line pattern indicative of a strangulation injury.[10] Severity of symptoms does not always correlate with the severity of injury; patients with severe injury may have minimal or absent clinical findings. For this reason, a thorough evaluation is essential. Because any force to the neck sufficient to cause injury to the laryngeal framework has the potential to injure the cervical spine and other adjacent critical structures, initial management should follow current acute trauma life support (ATLS) protocols for patients with multiple traumas. The first priority is establishment of a secure airway. This is often difficult in an injured larynx that may present edema, lacerations, and bleeding. The difficulty is compounded by the fact that any flexion or extension of the neck must be avoided until a cervical spine injury has been excluded. If the airway has not been secured and the patient is in respiratory distress, tracheostomy is preferable to blind endotracheal intubation. An awake flexible fiberoptic intubation is a feasible alternative when skilled personnel and equipment are available. If the airway is stable, the first intervention should be a diagnostic flexible fiberoptic laryngoscopy (FFL) to evaluate the extent of the intraluminal injury and the adequacy of the airway.

The status of the laryngeal mucosa and any submucosal injuries are noted, including hematomas. If possible, phonatory and respiratory examination is performed to assess arytenoid cartilage range of motion. Partial mobility can help to distinguish between structural damage such as dislocation versus neural injury.

After the airway is stabilized, a high-resolution computed tomography (CT) scan of the larynx can be obtained to assess the integrity of the laryngeal framework.[10] The preferred system for classification of a laryngeal injury was proposed by Trone and colleagues[11] and later modified by Fuhrman and colleagues[12] (Table 1). Patients in class I are observed in a monitored setting for at least 24 hours with repeated flexible fiberoptic examinations of the airway every 8 hours. If the airway remains stable, the patients can be discharged the next day without any further intervention. Patients in class II through class V are treated surgically.

Table 1 Laryngotracheal Injury Classification

Class	Description of Injury
I	Minor endolaryngeal hematoma without detectable fracture
II	Edema, hematoma, minor mucosal disruption without exposed cartilage, nondisplaced fractures noted on computed tomographic scan
III	Massive edema, mucosal tears, exposed cartilage, cord immobility
IV	A class III injury with more than two fracture or massive trauma to laryngeal mucosa
V	Complete laryngotracheal separation

Management

A comprehensive clinical and radiologic examination determines the need for surgical or medical management of laryngeal trauma. Medical management is reserved for patients with a stable airway such as those who present with minor mucosal lacerations, minor nonexpanding hematoma or a single nondisplaced fracture of the thyroid cartilage with intact overlying mucosa.[13,14] Nonsurgical management includes close observation with continuous pulse oximetry, administration of humidified air, and head of bed elevation over 45°. The use of heliox (mixture of helium and 30 to 40% oxygen) is controversial because it may mask stridor, an important clinical sign of airway deterioration. Heliox, however, may be of use as a temporizing measure while securing the airway. Early administration of systemic corticosteroids may be advantageous although their onset of action may take hours. Further injury or compromised healing caused by laryngopharyngeal acid reflux can be minimized with proton pump inhibitors or high-dose H2 blockers.

Indications for an open repair of a laryngeal fracture include the presence of comminuted or displaced fractures, fracture of the median or paramedian parts of the thyroid alae, and cricoid cartilage fracture. Any fracture of the median or paramedian thyroid cartilage may result in loss of the anteroposterior dimension of the larynx; thus, an open repair is indicated. Any injury resulting in vocal fold paralysis, airway compromise requiring intubation or tracheostomy, or associated with an important injury to other areas of the neck is also best managed with surgical exploration.

Rationale for Plate Fixation

Injury to cartilage results in bleeding and inflammation, with activation of the wound-healing cascade. Cytokine release and the chemotaxis of inflammatory cells lead to deposition of scar tissue, which is primarily composed of type II collagen. Regeneration of cartilage tissue (primarily type I collagen and proteoglycans) by native chondrocytes commences simultaneously, but this process that can take up to 3 months.[15] Motion of fracture fragments increases bleeding, hematoma formation, inflammation, and the likelihood of infection, all of which promote scar formation as opposed to organized cartilage repair. Applying the principles of adaptation fixation, previously validated in craniomaxillofacial surgery, to laryngeal fractures optimizes the repair and regeneration of normal laryngeal cartilage.[16] Plating techniques are fundamentally different from wire or suture fixation. Traditionally, wire or sutures have been used to *approximate* the fracture fragments, whereas no attempt is made to prevent motion across the fracture line. Plated fragments are held in place by the interactions between the screw, the bone or cartilage, and the plate. Therefore, plates fix the fragments, leading to deposition of new cartilage or bone. The

interface of the screw and the bone or cartilage should be able to resist pullout and lateral torque forces. Ideally, two-point fixation should be used for fractures of the thyroid cartilage (either two straight plates or a box-shaped plate). The height of the cricoid cartilage does not allow for two-point fixation.

Surgical Technique

General anesthesia is induced after the airway is stabilized via endotracheal intubation or tracheostomy. Local anesthesia and sedation can be used in patients with no intraluminal injury and minimally displaced fractures (class II). The cervical incision is made in a transverse skin crease approximating the level of the cricothyroid membrane. Subplatysmal skin flaps are raised to the level of the hyoid bone superiorly and to the sternum inferiorly, thus exposing the entire larynx. The strap muscles are separated in the midline, revealing the thyroid and cricoid cartilages (Figures 1 and 2). The perichondrium is incised in the midline, and perichondrial flaps are raised to expose 1 to 2 cm of cartilage at both sides of the fracture lines. The surgical technique for the fixation of laryngeal fractures with adaptation plates is similar to the techniques used for fixation of the maxillofacial skeleton.[17] The most significant difference is the lack of rigidity of the laryngeal skeleton when the thyroid and cricoid cartilages are not completely ossified. To increase the screw-cartilage contact and pull out strength, a drill bit that is one size smaller than the bit appropriate for the screw size can be used. For example, it is customary to use a 1.1 mm drill bit for a 1.5 mm screw. Nonossified laryngeal cartilage, however, should be drilled with a 0.76 mm drill bit. Alternatively, an "emergency" screw may be used after drilling with the customary-sized drill bit. Emergency screws should only be used in patients in whom the drill hole has already been stripped. Currently, an integrated self-drilling, self-tapping screw, and plating system that does not require a drill hole is preferred and may be used regardless of the degree of calcification of the laryngeal framework. Obviating the need for a drill hole produces a tighter screw-tissue interface. One drawback is that the screwdriver has been designed to retain the screws; therefore, it requires significant lateral torque to disengage it from the screw after insertion. Any lateral torque applied to a screw in a nonossified cartilage may disrupt the screw-tissue interface; thus, to avoid stripping the screw hole, the surgeon must stabilize the screw head with an instrument before applying the lateral torque to disengage the screwdriver.

Fixation Techniques in Laryngeal Trauma

Paramedian fractures of the thyroid cartilage are best fixated with a four-hole "box-type" plate across the fracture (Figures 3 and 4). Midline fractures require additional attention because the plate must be conformed to

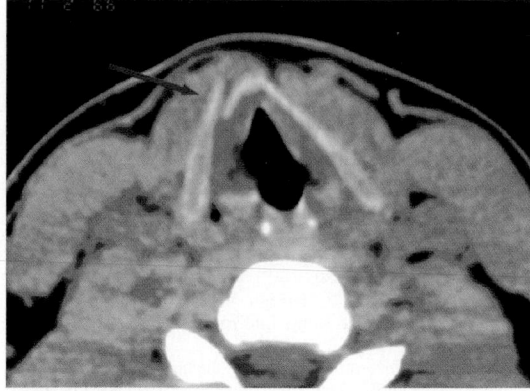

Figure 1 Computed tomographic scan depicting a fracture (*arrow*) of the thyroid cartilage.

the original curvature and angle of the thyroid cartilage (Figure 5–7). A four-point fixation of thyroid cartilage fractures is optimal; however, the height of the cricoid cartilage does not usually allow the application of more than a single straight plate. A single horizontal plate is generally adequate to preserve the structural integrity of the subglottic airway, the primary function of the cricoid cartilage. If significant mucosal injury exists, a thyrotomy which can be preplated should be performed, preferably through a midline or paramedian fracture line; and the intralaryngeal mucosa repaired primarily. Alternatively, if adequate visualization may be obtained with a rigid laryngoscope and a cervical spine injury has been ruled out, the lacerations are repaired endoscopically and the fractures are reduced and fixated transcervically. The goal of the repair is to cover all exposed cartilage while maintaining a patent lumen. Stenting is used only to prevent syncchiae when mucosal repair is not possible or to bolster mucosal flaps. Before closure of the thyrotomy, it is critical to reattach the vocal folds at the anterior commissure. After the fracture has been stabilized, the wound is closed in layers, a suction drain is placed, and a pressure dressing is applied. Patients who have not undergone tracheostomy are observed overnight and may be discharged the next day.

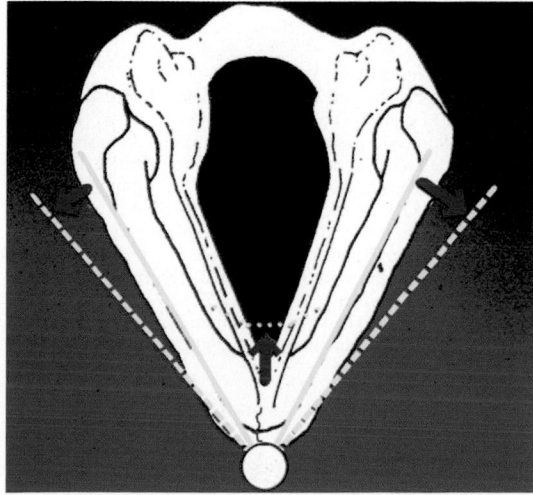

Figure 2 Schematic diagram of a median thyroid cartilage fracture and the force vectors leading to loss of anteroposterior dimension of the larynx.

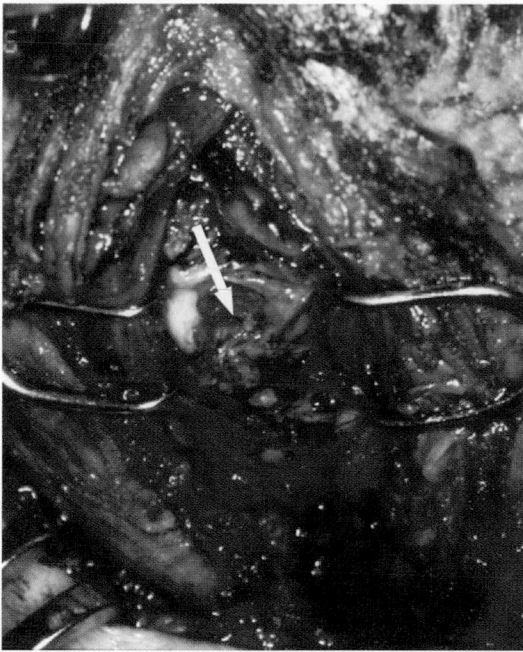

Figure 3 Transcervical approach using a horizontal incision, following a crease in the mid-neck. Subplatysmal dissection of the skin flaps facilitates the retraction of the skin flaps. The strap muscles have been dissected in the midline to expose the thyroid cartilage fracture (*arrow*).

IATROGENIC LARYNGEAL TRAUMA

Intubation

The incidence of laryngeal stenosis after prolonged or repeated intubation has been estimated to range from 3 to 8% for both adults and children.

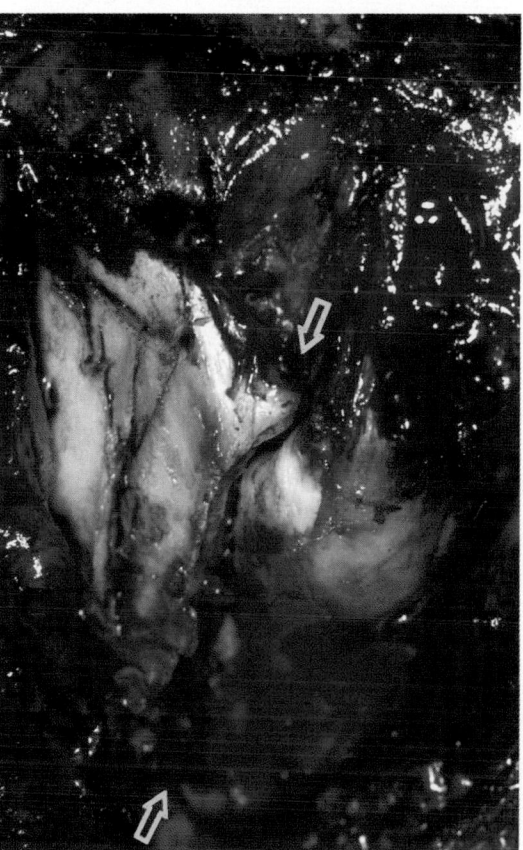

Figure 4 The perichondrium of the left thyroid ala has been elevated "en bloc" with the ipsilateral strap muscle. The paramedian fracture (*arrows*) is completely exposed.

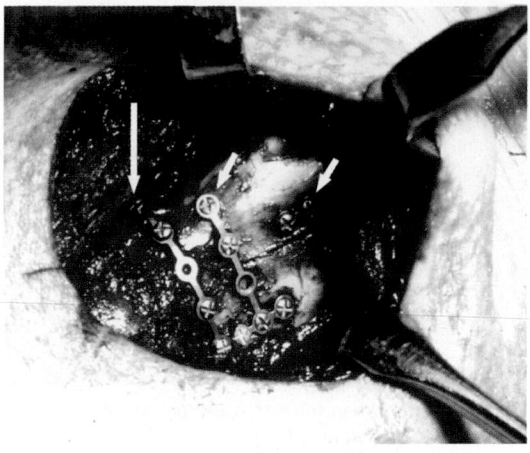

Figure 5 Two point fixation (*short arrows*) of a paramedian thyroid cartilage fracture and straight plate fixation of a cricoid fracture (*long arrow*).

Figures as high as 37% have been cited for low-birthweight neonates and those with respiratory distress syndrome.[18,19]

The causes of laryngeal stenosis after intubation are multifactorial. The mechanisms of injury most commonly associated with laryngotracheal intubation include, but are not limited to, duration of intubation, size of the tube, pressure and rubbing of the shaft against the larynx, repeated intubation, foreign body reaction to the tube, release of toxic substances used for sterilization, use of a stylet, route of intubation, nursing care, and anatomic differences between the genders.

Animal and clinical studies have correlated different intubation methods with clinical and histologic injury patterns. Nordin and Linholm, using a rabbit model, correlated the degree of damage with duration of intubation and cuff characteristics.[20] They concluded that the pressure of the cuff over the tracheal surface is more important than the duration of intubation. Since the microcirculation of the laryngeal mucosa stops at 30 mm Hg pressure, low-volume, high-pressure cuffs are more likely to cause ischemic injury than high-volume, low-pressure cuffs.

Whited, using a dog model, studied how the biomechanics of endotracheal tubes produce ulceration of the posterior glottis and circumferential injury of the subglottis and trachea.[21] He demonstrated that the inflammatory reaction progresses even after the tube is removed. Whited confirmed the findings of his animal study in a clinical prospective study that correlated the degree of injury with patterns and duration of intubation.[22] He found that patients intubated for 2 to 5 days had 0 to 2% incidence of chronic stenosis, those intubated for 5 to 10 days had a 4 to 5% incidence, and those with an indwelling tube for more than 10 days had a 12 to 14% incidence. He suggested that a tracheostomy may prevent laryngotracheal stenosis in patients who need endotracheal intubation for more than 10 days. Bryce also correlated duration of intubation with laryngeal injuries.[23] Lesions caused by repeated intubation were the most severe. This study suggested that perichondritis is the most significant factor for the development of stenosis.

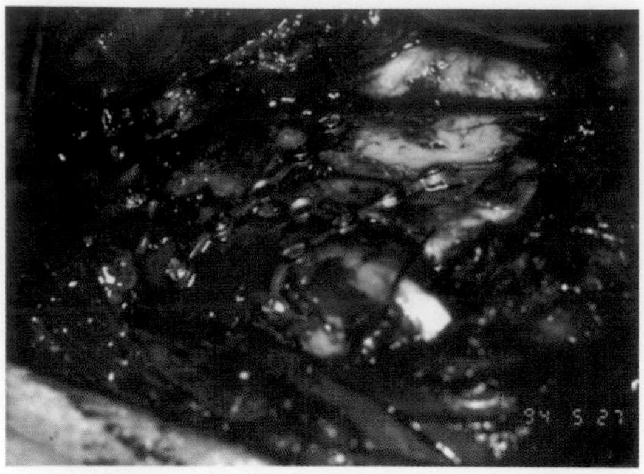

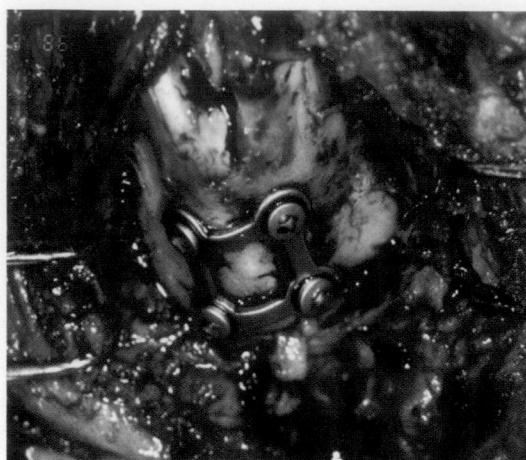

Figure 6 Paramedian fracture was reduced and stabilized with sutures to facilitate plating.

Figure 7 Median fracture reduced and fixed with a three-dimensional plate. Notice the bending of the plate to conform to the thyroid notch.

Age is another important factor influencing site and degree of stenosis. Neonates show a predisposition for subglottic involvement,[24] whereas adults are more prone to posterior commissure lesions.[18,19] Nevertheless, combined stenoses account for about one-third of all laryngeal stenoses at any age.

Tracheostomy

A high tracheostomy may be associated with glottic and subglottic injury. The type of incision and biomechanical factors related to the tracheostomy tube contribute to the development of stenosis.[25] Ideally, a tracheostomy should be performed through the third or fourth tracheal ring. A high tracheostomy through the first tracheal ring or the cricoid cartilage may lead to cricoid chondronecrosis with resultant fibrosis and stenosis.

Similarly, cricothyroidotomy has been associated with a higher incidence of laryngeal stenosis than has tracheostomy. The cricothyroid membrane ranges from 8 to 13 mm (average 9 mm) in adults.[26] Damage to the cricoid cartilage owing to introduction of microorganisms or direct trauma to the cartilage may lead to chondronecrosis. Tracheostomy tubes are poorly suited to intubate the subglottic larynx because of the lack of overlying soft tissue. In addition, the outer diameter of a number 6 Shiley tracheostomy tube is 10 mm, which is larger than the height of the cricothyroid membrane for a significant portion of the population.

Endoscopy

The effects of endoscopic instruments on the laryngeal airway reflect the care and skill of the operator. Rough handling of tissue, excessive biopsy of tissue, inadvertent or inaccurate laser ablation, and oversized instruments all promote tissue fibrosis and stenosis.

Nasogastric Intubation

Nasogastric tubes are often an unrecognized source of trauma. Nasogastric intubation produces inflammation owing to foreign body reaction to the tube, swallowing impairment with pooling of secretions, pressure necrosis, and gastropharyngeal reflux. All these factors play a role in the development of a postcricoid ulceration with resultant perichondritis. Healing leads to fibrosis and contracture. Trauma associated with the nasogastric tube may be synergistic with the trauma induced by an endotracheal tube.

HYOID FRACTURE

The hyoid is a U-shaped bone located in the superior part of the neck, well protected by the mandible. Given this location, fracture of the hyoid is relatively rare and usually associated with other cervical injuries. Hyoid fracture is often the result of a strangulation injury; however, other common mechanisms of blunt and penetrating trauma may be causative as well. Presenting symptoms may include dysphagia, odynophagia, or dyspnea. Physical examination may reveal swelling, neck crepitus, tenderness, or pain with movement of the neck. Diagnosis of hyoid fracture requires a high degree of clinical suspicion since the signs and symptoms are not unique to this injury. Diagnosis is confirmed with CT. Laryngoscopy is also indicated to assess associated mucosal injuries and airway swelling. Treatment is based on the severity of symptoms and clinical findings. Asymptomatic hyoid fractures may be observed. Significant soft tissue injuries, such as pharyngeal lacerations or skin lacerations, are sutured. Care is taken to remove small fragments of bone, and the remaining bone fragments may be fixed with wires.[27]

REFERENCES

1. Bent JP, III, Silver JR, Poribsky ES. Acute laryngeal trauma: A review of 77 patients. Otolarygol Head Neck Surg 1993;109:441–9.
2. Jewett BS, Shockley WW, Rutledge R. External laryngeal trauma analysis of 392 patients. Arch Olaryngol Head Neck Surg 1999;125:877–80.
3. de Mello-Filho FV, Carrau RL. The management of laryngeal fractures using internal fixation. Laryngoscope 2000;110:2143–6.
4. Lemay SR. Penetrating wounds of the larynx and cervical trachea. Arch Otolaryngol Head Neck Surg 1971;94:558–65.
5. Nahum AM, Siegel AW. Biodynamics of injury to the larynx in automobile collisions. Ann Otol Rhinol Laryngol 1967;76:781–5.
6. Schaefer SD. Laryngeal and esophageal trauma. In: Cummings CW, Flint PW, Haughey BH, Robbins KT, Thomas JR, Harker LA, Richardson MA, Schuller D, editors. Otolaryngology: Head and Neck Surgery, 4th edition. St. Louis: Mosby; 1998. p. 2090–2111.
7. Close DM. Traumatic avulsion of the larynx. J Laryngol Otol 1981;95:1157–8.
8. Schaefer SD. Acute management of external laryngeal trauma: A 27-year experience. Arch Otolaryngol Head Neck Surg 1992;118:598–604.
9. Stanley RB, Cooper DS, Florman SH. Phonatory effects of thyroid cartilage fractures. Ann Otol Rhinol Laryngol 1987;96:493–6.
10. Stanley RB, Hanson DG. Manual strangulation injuries of the larynx. Arch Otolaryngol 1983;109:344–7.
11. Trone TH, Schaefer SD, Carder HM. Blunt and penetrating laryngeal trauma: A 13-year review. Otolaryngol Head Neck Surg 1980;88:257–61.
12. Fuhrman GM, Stieg FH, III, Buerk CA. Blunt laryngeal trauma: Classification and management protocol. J Trauma Inj Infect Crit Care 1990;30:87–92.
13. Schaefer SD. The treatment of acute external laryngeal injuries. Arch Otolaryngol 1991;117:35–9.
14. Stanley RB, Cooper DS, Florman SH. Phonatory effects of thyroid cartilage fractures. Ann Otol Rhinol Laryngol 1987;96:493–6.
15. Silver FH, Glasgold AI. Cartilage wound healing. An overview. Otolaryngol Clin N Am 1995;280:847–64.
16. Lykins CL, Pinczower EF. The comparative strength of laryngeal fracture fixation. Am J Otolaryngol 1998;19:158–62.
17. Pou AM. Shoemaker. DL, Carrau RL, et al. Repair of laryngeal fractures using adaptation plates. Head Neck 1998;20:707–13.
18. Hawkins DB, Luxford MW. Laryngeal stenosis from endotracheal intubation: A review of 58 cases. Ann Otol Rhinol Laryngol 1980;80:454–8.
19. Whited RE. A retrospective study of laryngotracheal sequelae in long-term intubation. Laryngoscope 1984;94:367–77.
20. Nordin U, Linholm CE. The trachea and cuff-induced tracheal injury: An experimental study on causative factors and prevention. Acta Otolaryngol 1977;96:1–71.
21. Whited RE. A study of postintubation laryngeal dysfunction. Laryngoscope 1985;95:727–9.
22. Whited RE. A study of endotracheal tube injury to the subglottis. Laryngoscope 1985;95:1216–9.
23. Bryce DP. The surgical management of laryngotracheal injury. J Laryngol Otol 1972;86:547–87.
24. Papsidero HJ, Pashley NRT. Acquired stenosis of the upper airway in neonates. Ann Otol Rhinol Laryngol 1980;89:512–4.
25. Lulensky GC, Batsakis JG. Tracheal incision as a contributing factor to tracheal stenosis: An experimental study. Ann Otol Rhinol Laryngol 1975;84:781–6.
26. Caparosa RJ, Zavatsky AR. Practical aspects of the cricothyroid space. Laryngoscope 1957;67:577–91.
27. Dalati T. Isolated hyoid bone fracture: Review of an unusual entity. Int J Oral Maxillofac Surg 2005;34:449–52.

78

Airway Control and Laryngotracheal Stenosis in Adults

Brian B. Burkey, MD
Steven L. Goudy, MD
Sarah L. Rohde, MD

The successful management of the airway is of paramount importance. Airway control requires a logical and systematic approach guided by the principles of basic and advanced life support techniques and a working knowledge of relevant pharmacology. Most importantly, the physicians must possess a mastery of the anatomy and physiology of the upper aerodigestive tract. The airway surgeon is also uniquely responsible for the diagnosis and treatment of airway lesions such as laryngotracheal stenosis and arytenoid fixation.

ANATOMY

Successful airway intervention necessitates an understanding of the anatomy of the laryngotracheal complex. A detailed discussion of the anatomy of the larynx can be found in Chapter 72, "Development Anatomy and Physiology of the Larynx." The major cartilages of the larynx include the thyroid, cricoid, and paired arytenoids (Figure 1). The thyroid cartilage is a shield-shaped structure whose central prominence tends to be more acutely angled in men than in women. The position of the larynx varies between infants and adults. In infants, the cricoid cartilage is positioned at the level of the fourth cervical vertebra. The thyroid cartilage is often behind the hyoid and impalpable. The tip of the epiglottis then lies at the level of the dorsal surface of the soft palate. As the infant matures, the larynx gradually descends to its adulthood position with the cricoid cartilage at the level of the sixth vertebra.

The cricoid cartilage is the only complete ring of the airway, which accounts for the association between prolonged or traumatic endotracheal intubation and subglottic stenosis. The cricoid is composed of hyaline cartilage that often calcifies later in adult life. It is broader posteriorly and tapers to a smaller arch anteriorly, mimicking the shape of a signet ring. The thyroid and cricoid cartilages are attached anteriorly by the cricothyroid membrane.

The trachea begins at the lower border of the cricoid cartilage at the level of the sixth vertebra and extends to the upper border of the fifth thoracic vertebra, where it divides into the two bronchi. The trachea is composed of incomplete,

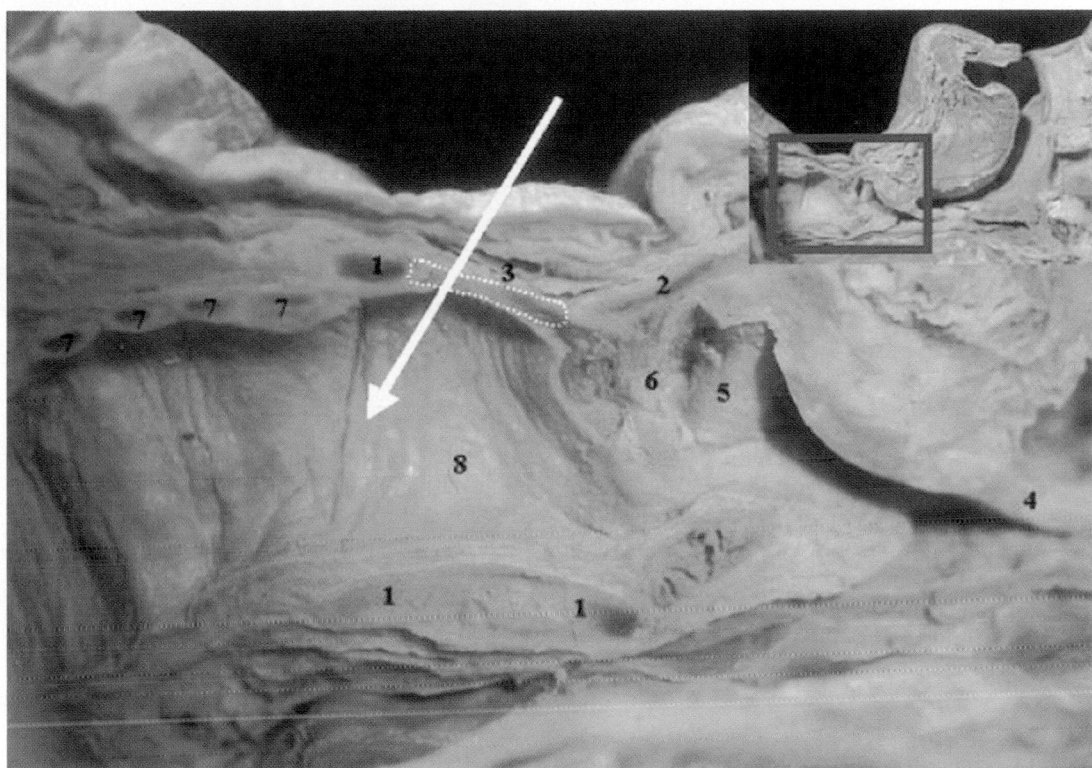

Figure 1 Sagittal section of the larynx. (Published with permission from reference 10.)

C-shaped "rings" of hyaline cartilage that are open posteriorly (pars membranosa) and connected here by fibroareolar connective tissue and smooth muscle fibers. The larynx and trachea are lined by pseudostratified, ciliated columnar epithelium interspersed with mucus-secreting cells, except at the glottis, which is lined with a stratified squamous cell epithelium. The trachea bifurcates at approximately the sternal angle. The right bronchus is wider, shorter, and more vertically oriented than the left bronchus. When using an open bronchoscope, one may most easily examine both bronchi by passing the instrument through the right side of the mouth, thus allowing the best view of the obliquely angled left bronchus while preserving visualization into the right bronchus.[1]

CLINICAL EVALUATION OF THE AIRWAY

The clinical evaluation of the airway must begin with a rapid assessment of the patient's ventilatory and respiratory status. A systematic evaluation of the patient based on advanced cardiac life support (ACLS) protocols should be used for each patient. Understanding the basic evaluation of the airway and using a diagnostic and therapeutic algorithm to secure an airway are necessary for treating these patients. Symptoms that indicate upper airway obstruction include hoarseness, dyspnea, stridor, restlessness, and drooling. Physical signs of a damaged airway include bloody sputum, subcutaneous emphysema, palpable laryngeal fractures, cyanosis, and suprasternal or intercostal retractions.

In evaluation of the nonemergent airway, a complete history, including prior history of trauma, previous intubations, and voice and swallowing complaints, should be obtained. The physician may then proceed with a diagnostic assessment of the upper aerodigestive tract. If the patient is seen in the clinic setting, a mirror indirect laryngoscopy may be performed to assess vocal fold mobility and possible lesions of the glottis and supraglottis. Perhaps the most

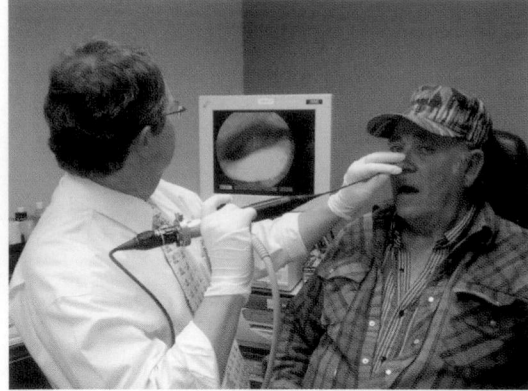

Figure 2 Flexible fiberoptic examination of the larynx with video documentation.

valuable study is an indirect fiberoptic examination via nasopharyngoscopy. This technique allows unparalleled visualization of the upper airway and larynx and may allow for video documentation in the clinic setting (Figure 2). A blood gas evaluation, chest X-ray, and airway radiographic evaluation via X-ray or computerized tomography (CT) may also be indicated.

MANAGEMENT OF THE EMERGENT AIRWAY

While management of the airway in the controlled environment of the operating room is usually straightforward, patients presenting in the emergency room pose unique problems such as cervical spine injuries, closed head injuries with the possibility of increased intracranial pressure, laryngotracheal disruption, airway hemorrhage, and facial injury. Supplemental oxygen is the simplest means of additional support and should be given almost universally to patients with airway distress. After this intervention, the clinician should evaluate for airway obstruction from foreign bodies such as displaced teeth or tongue and soft tissues collapse into the pharynx. Because of its efficacy and lack of cervical movement, jaw thrust is the most appropriate positioning.[2] Placement of an oropharyngeal airway or nasal trumpet may also aide in relieving soft tissue obstruction of the airway (Figure 3). An oropharyngeal airway displaces the tongue anteriorly, preventing soft tissue obstruction. A nasal trumpet is placed transnasally into the oropharynx relieving soft tissue obstruction at the level of the pharynx. Nasopharyngeal airways tend to be less stimulating than oral airways in the awake patient, but there is a small risk of epistaxis. Nasal airways should not be used in patients with known or suspected basilar skull fractures due to the risk of intracranial placement.[3]

The delivery of positive pressure ventilation may be achieved noninvasively using a facemask. Successful ventilation requires both an airtight mask and a patent airway. Without an airtight seal between the skin of the patient's face and the mask, sufficient pressure to inflate the lungs cannot be developed. Air leak is the most common problem in delivering facemask ventilation.

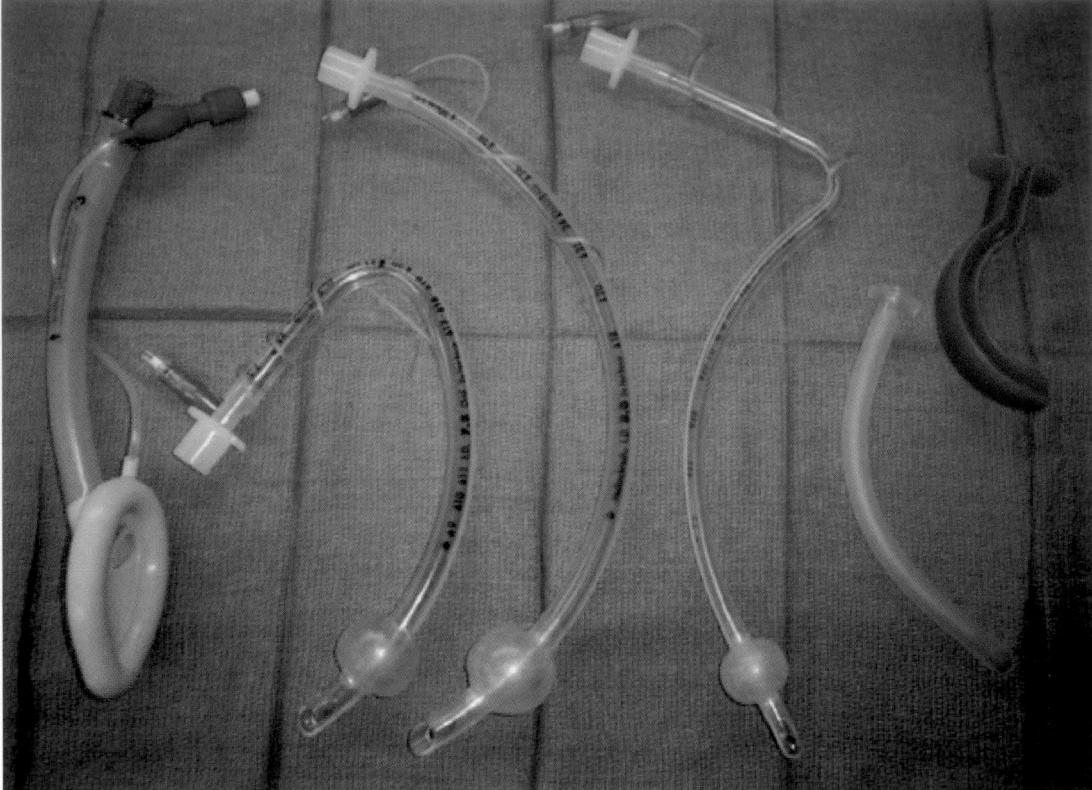

Figure 3 Photograph of an oral airway, nasal trumpet, laryngeal mask airway, and endotracheal tube.

An airtight seal may be achieved by using the thumb and index finger of one hand to secure the mask, that is, by pushing downward. The middle and ring finger are then used to grasp the mandible (and not the soft tissue of the chin) to extend the neck. The little finger is positioned under the angle of the jaw and thrusts it anteriorly. If an assistant is available to squeeze the ventilation bag, two hands may be used to secure an airtight seal. Signs of a successful seal and ventilation include a foggy mask, the rising of the chest with delivery of positive pressure, breath sounds on auscultation, a firm, full bag, and return of carbon dioxide on exhalation capnography.

A laryngeal mask airway (LMA) is a nondefinitive technique that may be employed to obtain a temporary airway for positive pressure ventilation. This device forms a seal over the larynx and provides a route for oxygen flow into the trachea. The LMA may also serve as a conduit for fiberoptic intubation. If a definitive airway is required, endotracheal intubation is the quickest and most successful option whenever possible. Endotracheal intubation allows ventilatory control with the ability to deliver high levels of oxygen as well as protecting against aspiration. Endotracheal intubation can be achieved though both oral and transnasal routes. In the case of head and neck trauma, oral intubation may be achieved while holding in-line cervical traction. Manual in-line immobilization is the optimal method of stabilization and results in significantly less cervical spine movement than stabilization in a cervical spine collar.[4]

The most common technique employed for oral intubation in the emergent setting is rapid sequence intubation (RSI). The first step is preoxygenation in which patients are administered 100% oxygen to produce a nitrogen washout. Preoxygenation is followed by administration of an induction agent to produce sedation and amnesia. A paralytic agent is also usually administered to provide muscle relaxation. In many situations, spontaneous ventilation may be of benefit; because once a patient's muscle tone is relaxed, the patient must be artificially ventilated. In the case that intubation is not successful, the medical professional must be prepared to establish a surgical airway. An assistant may hold cricoid pressure to prevent aspiration if the patient is unconscious. If a cervical spine injury is suspected, a second assistant maintains in-line stabilization during the procedure. If this technique is accomplished transnasally, a fiberoptic endoscope may also be placed inside an endotracheal tube to facilitate localization of the airway. The endotracheal tube can then be passed over the endoscope after the airway has been identified. Visualization of the airway with a fiberoptic endoscope may be obscured by the presence of blood and secretions.

A more invasive method of providing oxygenation to a patient who cannot be adequately ventilated or intubated is the technique of percutaneous transtracheal ventilation. This technique involves a caudally directed puncture of the cricothyroid membrane with a 14-guage intravenous catheter. Accidental placement of the catheter within the subcutaneous tissue will result in subcutaneous emphysema making further attempts at endotracheal intubation more difficult. After the catheter has been accurately placed into the trachea, the needle is removed and oxygen is provided via a jet ventilator, ventilating bag, or gas outlet of an anesthesia machine. It is important to realize that an adult cannot breathe through such a catheter and thus requires one of the above means of providing oxygen under pressure. Oxygen delivered under high pressures also poses the risk of pneumothorax. If there is an obstruction preventing the egress of air, a second catheter is necessary to prevent overinflation of the lungs and pneumothorax. Percutaneous transtracheal ventilation is merely a temporizing measure until a definitive surgical airway can be obtained, and there is little to recommend transtracheal puncture over cricothyroidotomy in adults.

CRICOTHYROIDOTOMY

If the airway cannot be controlled through endotracheal intubation or other medical maneuvers, a surgical airway must be obtained. Cricothyroidotomy is considered the preferred method of obtaining an emergent surgical airway. Chevalier Jackson condemned the procedure in 1921 because of the high rate of glottic and subglottic stenosis; however, over the past quarter century, multiple articles have reported the efficacy of the technique.[4] Indications for cricothyroidotomy include patients requiring emergent airway management that cannot be obtained through the oral or nasal route, for example, patients where manipulation of the neck is contraindicated, severe maxillofacial trauma, edema with inability to visualize the vocal cords, severe oropharyngeal or tracheobronchial hemorrhage, fracture of the base of skull, and supraglottic foreign body obstruction. Cricothyrotomy should not be performed when the landmarks cannot be palpated, as in the presence of tumor, hematoma, or other mechanical barrier, or before the age of 5 years, as the cartilaginous landmarks are not sufficiently distinct. The technique is also contraindicated in the presence of acute laryngeal pathology. Cricothyrotomy will not establish an airway when the trachea has been transected with retraction of the distal end into the mediastinum.[5–7]

The technique involves creation of an opening in the cricothyroid membrane followed by placement of a stenting tube. The procedure begins with identification of the cricothyroid space between the thyroid and cricoid prominences (Figure 4).[8] Local anesthesia may be infiltrated if time permits. The trachea is stabilized with the surgeon's nondominant hand. A horizontal incision is made over the middle third of the membrane and carried directly into the airway. The scalpel handle is inserted and rotated 90° or a dilating instrument may be inserted next to the scalpel to secure the airway opening. Mayo scissors may be used to enlarge the opening. Every effort is made not to damage the cricoid or thyroid cartilages. An endotracheal tube is then be placed through the cricothyroidotomy and directed distally into the trachea. It is best to have several sizes of endotracheal tubes available. Once the cuff has been inflated and the tube secured, ventilation is begun. Auscultation, bilateral chest rise, and the presence of end-tidal CO_2 should be utilized to confirm accurate placement. After

the airway has been secured, the patient should be taken to the operating room as soon as possible to convert the cricothyroidotomy to a formal tracheostomy because the endotracheal tube is not a stable airway.

While cricothyroidotomy has been utilized for long-term airway management, it is most useful in the emergency setting where an urgent surgical airway is needed. Cricothyroidotomy is usually faster and easier to perform than tracheostomy, especially in the hands of a nonsurgeon, as it requires little surgical skill other than knowledge of anatomy. Complications of cricothyroidotomy include hemorrhage, tube displacement, infection, vocal cord damage, subcutaneous emphysema, and the development of subglottic or tracheal stenosis.[9,10]

In 1995, Hawkins and colleagues reported a series of 5,603 consecutive adult trauma patients, of whom 66 required cricothyroidotomy. Three major complications, including hemorrhage, failure to obtain a surgical airway, and thyroid cartilage laceration, occurred in 2 patients.[11] No patient had significant clinical morbidity from the cricothyroidotomy. Cricothyroidotomy remains an important technique with low morbidity in patients needing emergent airway control.

TRACHEOSTOMY

Tracheostomies have been performed for over 2,000 years. Until a century ago, however, the procedure was essentially reserved for moribund patients due to high rates of morbidity and mortality. Attitudes toward tracheostomy changed in 1909, when Chevalier Jackson described the modern tracheostomy.[13] Jackson addressed the high rate of laryngeal and tracheal damage previously associated with tracheostomy in his landmark paper of 1921, "High Tracheostomy and Other Errors: The Chief Cause of Chronic Laryngeal Stenosis." In this paper, Jackson hypothesized that the unacceptably high rates of laryngeal and tracheal stenosis associated with tracheostomies were secondary to damage to the thyroid and cricoid cartilages incurred during the performance of "high" tracheostomies. Jackson instructed that tracheostomies be performed below the second tracheal ring, thereby avoiding these dreaded complications.[14] These teachings have been followed to the present day.

The relative indications for tracheostomy as outlined by the American Academy of Otolaryngology—Head and Neck Surgery include upper airway obstruction with stridor, air hunger, retractions, documented obstructive sleep apnea, bilateral vocal fold paralysis, previous neck surgery, throat trauma or irradiation to the neck, as well as, prolonged or expected prolonged intubation, inability of the patient to manage secretions, facilitation of ventilation support, inability to intubate, and as an adjunct to manage head and neck surgery or significant head and neck trauma.

Technique

A tracheostomy is generally begun with a horizontal skin incision approximately midway

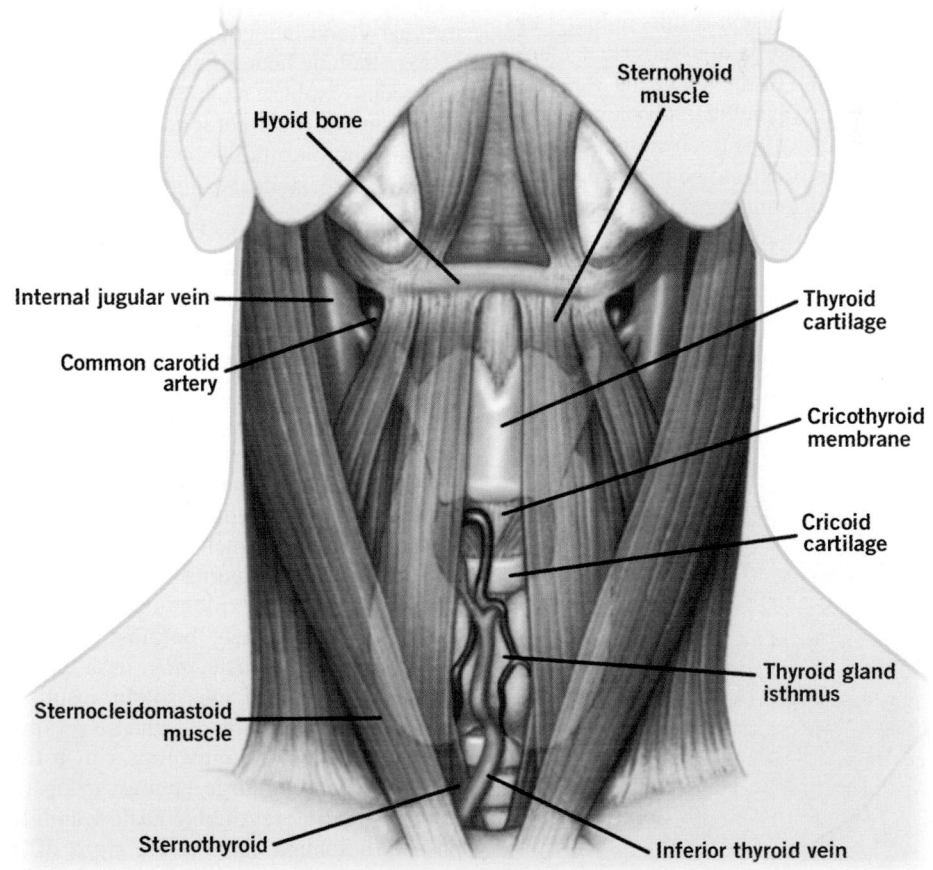

Figure 4 Landmarks of the neck. (Published with permission from reference 8.)

between the sternal notch and the cricoid cartilage. The incision is carried down through the skin, subcutaneous tissue, and platysma to the level of the strap muscles. After identification of the strap muscles, dissection is begun in the vertical plane. The strap muscles are separated in the midline and retractors are used to pull the muscles laterally revealing the thyroid isthmus. The cricoid cartilage is identified by palpation, and a cricoid hook is used to pull the trachea superiorly. The isthmus of the thyroid gland is dissected off the trachea in a bloodless fascial plane just superficial to the trachea. The isthmus is transected and suture ligated, if necessary. The fine fascia overlying the trachea is carefully separated.

While horizontal and vertical incisions into the tracheal wall have been proposed, an inferiorly based Bjork flap consisting of the second and third tracheal rings is a superior option for adults. Following Jackson's principles, a horizontal incision is made above either the second or third tracheal ring and then carried inferiorly on the lateral aspects with Mayo scissors to fashion an inferiorly based flap. The space between the rings may be calcified in older patients. The Bjork flap is sewn to the subcutaneous tissue of the inferior skin margin with absorbable suture (Figure 5). The Bjork flap makes recannulation easier in the event of accidental extubation but does lead to a slightly increased risk of tracheocutaneous fistula. For this reason, a horizontal H-incision based on the second or third tracheal ring or the removal of an anterior section of a single tracheal ring may be preferable in patients who are expected to require a tracheostomy for only a short period of time. The Bjork flap is contraindicated in children because it results in high rates of tracheocutaneous fistula and subglottic stenosis. A vertical incision of the trachea is preferred, along with carefully labeled and secured stay sutures on either side of the tracheal incision.

When a tracheostomy is to be permanent or of long duration, the surrounding skin may be surgically defatted and sutured to create a tracheostoma circumferentially. This technique is useful in obese patients, in whom a semipermanent tracheostoma is less prone to maceration or the formation of granulation tissue as the skin directly abuts the respiratory mucosa of the trachea. The

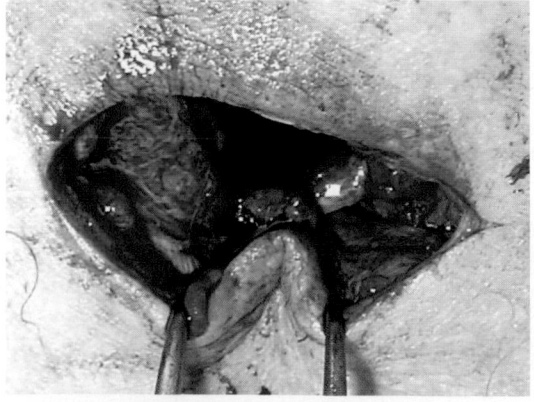

Figure 5 Intraoperative photograph of the creation of an inferiorly based Bjork flap.

creation of a semipermanent tracheostoma also serves to decrease the length of the tracheostomy tract facilitating removal and reinsertion of the tracheostomy tube.

After the tracheostomy has been secured, a reinforced endotracheal tube may be inserted while the operation is finished or the desired tracheostomy tube may be placed. Correct placement of the tube should be verified using end-tidal CO_2 measurement, the presence of bilateral breath sounds and chest rise. Finally, the tracheostomy incision should never be tightly closed because leakage of air around the tube will be trapped below the skin, leading to subcutaneous emphysema, pneumomediatstinum, pneumothorax, or infection. Instead, the incision should be loose around the tube to allow passive egress of air from the trachea. A post-tracheostomy chest X-ray is often advisable to detect possible complications of trapped air, and in children, such X-ray is mandatory.[15]

For a patient who is intubated and in the intensive care unit, tracheostomy may be performed as an open procedure at the bedside. This avoids the costs associated with the operating room, and equipment is less expensive than that required for percutaneous tracheostomy. Disadvantages of performing an open bedside tracheostomy may include lack of adequate lighting, surgical assistance, and inferior equipment. Just as with percutaneous tracheostomy, patients with unfavorable anatomy are not candidates for open bedside tracheostomy.

Complications of Tracheostomy

Complications of tracheostomy are often divided into early and late complications. Early complications include hemorrhage, pneumothorax, subcutaneous emphysema, tube obstruction, and tube displacement. Late complications include infection, aspiration, granuloma formation, laryngeal or subglottic stenosis, and tracheo-innominate artery fistula.

Early Complications. Mild bleeding is the most common early complication of tracheostomy, occurring in about 5% of cases. The hemorrhage usually results from venous oozing from either the soft tissues or the incised thyroid tissue. Mild bleeding can generally be controlled by raising the head of the patient to decrease venous pressure or by placing hemostatic gauze over oozing areas. Major hemorrhage is unusual and most often involves a branch of the superior thyroid artery. Arterial bleeding is an indication for immediate surgical exploration.

Tube obstruction is the most common cause of ventilatory insufficiency in a post-tracheostomy patient and most often results from a mucous plug. Dried mucus and secretions in and around the tracheostomy tube can form crusts that may become large enough to obstruct the lumen of the tube. Audible airflow and difficulty passing a suction catheter are signs of impending tube obstruction. Adequate humidification, irrigation, frequent suctioning, and cleaning of

the inner cannula help to reduce the risk of plugging and tube obstruction. If the tracheostomy tube becomes obstructed, first the inner cannula should be removed. If removal of the inner cannula fails to relieve the obstruction, the patient and care staff should be instructed to remove the entire tube. It is mandatory to have a same size and the next smaller size tracheostomy tubes available at the bedside.

Displacement of the tracheostomy tube or dislocation of the tube from the tracheal lumen poses a considerable risk in the postoperative period. Displacement of the tracheostomy tube is most likely to occur in the early postoperative period before a stable tract has matured between the tracheal lumen and the skin. Displacement most often occurs due to the tube being inadequately secured. Excessive tension applied to the tube from the ventilatory apparatus also poses a risk of tube dislodgement.

Tracheostomy tube replacement in the early postoperative period and during the first tube change should be done under direct vision. Blind reinsertion poses the risk of creating a false passage for the tube. If reinsertion cannot be accomplished, the airway may be reestablished by oral endotracheal intubation.

Subcutaneous emphysema results from the forced entrance of air into the fascial planes of the neck, usually resulting from closing the tracheostomy incision too tightly. Tube obstruction or displacement can also lead to escape of air into the fascial planes. Crepitus and soft tissue swelling can involve the neck, face, and upper torso. Minor amounts of subcutaneous emphysema usually resolve spontaneously without significant sequelae, while massive amounts may progress to pneumomediastinum and pose increased risk of infection through bacterial contamination. A flexible scope inserted through the tracheostomy tube is a valuable means of confirming that the tube is actually in the lumen of the trachea.

Pneumothorax occurs in less than 5% of tracheostomies and can result from damage to the pleural apices during dissection that veers away from the midline. Pneumothorax may also be caused by excessively forceful ventilation that prevents passive exhalation of air, leading to alveolar rupture and the entrance of air into the pleural space. Air can also enter the pleural space or mediastinum via a misplaced tracheostomy tube. A pneumothorax may become apparent due to respiratory distress or be detected by decreased breath sounds on auscultation of the chest, but this complication is usually asymptomatic and noted incidentally on the postoperative chest X-ray. A small pneumothorax can be expectantly observed with serial chest radiographs, while a large or symptomatic pneumothorax may require a chest tube for lung re-expansion.

Late Complications. Innominate artery erosion is perhaps the most dreaded post-tracheostomy complication and, although rare, results in only a 10 to 25% survival rate. Tracheo-innominate fistula most commonly occurs at the tip of the tracheostomy tube, and causes include inappropriately low tracheostomy, erosion from a high-pressure cuff, movement of the tube, and infection. Innominate artery erosion is often heralded by a sentinel bleed. Rapid peristomal bleeding, even when it resolves, should trigger a fiberoptic examination of the tracheostoma, with the tracheostomy tube removed to rule out innominate artery involvement. When massive bleeding does occur, the tracheostomy tube should be rapidly replaced with a longer endotracheal tube in order to allow oxygenation while digital pressure is applied between the anterior trachea and the manubrium to compress the innominate artery. Placement of an orotracheal tube allows better access through the stoma for digital pressure. The patient must be taken immediately to the operating room for median sternotomy and innominate artery ligation, with a coordinated thoracic surgery-otolaryngology team. Many surgeons feel the Bjork flap technique lessens the risk of this potentially fatal complication.

While bacterial colonization of the trachea and peristomal area is unavoidable, significant infections occur rarely. Local cellulitis can generally be managed with local cleansing measures and topical antibiotics. Uncontrolled local infection can lead to such serious complications as mediastinitis, peristomal tissue loss, or tracheo-innominate fistula. Local infection that does not respond to aggressive wound care should be treated with systemic antibiotics.

Dysphagia and aspiration following tracheostomy is often overlooked. Tracheostomies have been shown to decrease the protective glottic closure reflexes of both the true and false vocal cords. Loss of this protective mechanism predisposes the tracheostomized patient to aspiration and concomitant pneumonia. Prophylactic measures include a soft, solid diet and a somewhat upright position during feeding. While inflating the tracheostomy tube cuff can afford temporary airway protection, hyperinflation of the cuff actually causes exacerbated aspiration due to compression of the esophagus. Consultation with a speech and swallowing therapist is advisable for any patient who requires a tracheostomy.

Granulation tissue may form in the peristomal area due to chronic mucosal and skin irritation, which may be exacerbated by an inadequately fixed or improperly sized tracheostomy tube. Granulation tissue may also form inside the tracheal lumen. Early and small granulomas may be managed with local debridement. Mature, fibrotic lesions generally require endoscopic laser excision.

Tracheostomies may contribute to subglottic stenosis by causing chronic irritation to the tracheal mucosa while also providing a route of bacterial contamination that causes increased inflammation in the damaged area. This inflammation may result in the formation of scar tissue and subsequent subglottic or tracheal stenosis. Gastroesophageal reflux is also felt to increase the risk of subglottic stenosis by providing additional mucosal irritation that contributes to

granulation and scar tissue formation. When a patient requires mechanical ventilation, tracheostomy tube cuff pressure must be checked at regular intervals. If the cuff pressure is higher than the tracheal mucosal capillary filling pressure, the mucosa will slough leading to chondritis and stenosis. The risk of subglottic stenosis underscores the importance of minimizing extraneous motion of the tracheostomy tube, managing gastroesophageal reflux, and decannulation when the tracheostomy is no longer required for airway support.

Percutaneous Tracheostomy

While percutaneous tracheostomy was first described in 1955, it has experienced a resurgence in popularity after its reintroduction by Ciaglia and colleagues in 1985.[16] The technique involves the transcervical insertion of a guidewire into the airway followed by blunt dilation of the guidewire tract. The tracheostomy tube is then inserted over the guidewire using a modified Seldinger technique. The advantage of percutaneous tracheostomy is that it can be performed at the bedside in the intensive care unit eliminating the potential risks associated with transport of a critically ill patient to the operating room. Relative advantages also include the time- and cost-saving aspects of the procedure.

Initial concern over the safety of the technique has been tempered by increased use of bronchoscopy, allowing direct visualization of airway entry, and newer commercially available kits using a single dilator, lessening manipulation of the trachea, and allowing the procedure to be performed more quickly. Visualization of the guidewire insertion, dilation, and tracheostomy tube placement may be achieved using a flexible bronchoscope inserted through the endotracheal tube at the time of the procedure. Improved visualization with bronchoscopy decreases airway complications by preventing improper placement of the guidewire into the subcutaneous tissue or the esophagus. The proper level of tracheostomy placement may also be confirmed with airway visualization at the time of the procedure.

Percutaneous dilational tracheostomy is an elective procedure and should not be performed in an emergency setting. Proper patient selection is crucial to successful outcomes. Patients undergoing percutaneous tracheostomy should have easily palpable surgical landmarks to avoid damage to the thyroid or cricoid cartilage. Patients who are difficult to intubate or obese have documented or suspected cervical spine injury and have a neck mass or infection, and those with an inability to extend the neck are not generally considered candidates for the procedure. Additionally, patients requiring high positive end expiratory pressures should be considered carefully. Percutaneous tracheostomy is contraindicated in pediatric patients.

Technique. Percutaneous tracheostomy is most often performed in the intensive care unit (ICU) setting under deep intravenous sedation. The patient should have continuous monitoring with

nursing and respiratory staff at the bedside. Additionally, since a percutaneous tracheostomy must sometimes be converted to a standard open tracheostomy, a surgical tracheostomy tray should be present at the time of the procedure, and the operator should be able to perform a standard tracheostomy.

After placing a shoulder roll to extend the patient's neck, the thyroid and cricoid cartilages, as well as the hyoid and suprasternal notch, are palpated. Local anesthesia with epinephrine is infiltrated into the surgical area, and an approximately 2 cm horizontal incision is made midway between the cricoid cartilage and suprasternal notch. Using blunt dissection, the pretracheal plane is identified and the thyroid isthmus is swept inferiorly or superiorly.

A bronchoscope is then passed through the endotracheal tube. After the cuff is deflated, the endotracheal tube is withdrawn to the level of the subglottis taking care not to extubate the patient. The light from the bronchoscope serves as an additional guide for placement of the tracheostomy.

Next, the surgeon passes the needle through the anterior tracheal wall under direct visualization. The guidewire is inserted, the needle withdrawn, and the tract dilated. The tracheostomy tube is inserted over an introducer. The tube should be sutured and secured with tracheostomy ties. After securing the tracheostomy tube and verifying placement, the bronchoscope and endotracheal tube are withdrawn.

Advantages, Disadvantages, and Complications. As the popularity of percutaneous tracheostomy has increased over the last two decades, debates on the precise indications for percutaneous tracheostomy and the possible advantages over conventional surgical tracheostomy have ensued. A meta-analysis of prospective trials comparing percutaneous and open tracheostomy in critically ill patients performed by Freeman and colleagues found no difference with respect to the overall complication rate between the two techniques.[17] Percutaneous tracheostomy was, however, found to have a lower incidence of peristomal bleeding and postoperative infection. Antonelli and colleagues performed a prospective, randomized trial with 1-year double-blind follow-up comparing the two techniques. The study found no difference in the complication rates between the two procedures at the time of 1-year follow-up.[18]

Percutaneous dilational tracheostomy is most often performed at the bedside in the ICU, decreasing complications associated with transport of a critically ill patient to the operating room. Although percutaneous tracheostomy has been shown to save an average of 5 to 10 minutes, the clinical implications of this time savings are likely limited. More importantly, because the procedure is performed in the ICU, operating room personnel and facilities are not necessary and patient charges are reduced.[19]

Compared to open tracheostomy, percutaneous tracheostomy results in a narrow, dilated tract rather than a formal stoma. The narrow tract results in an increased rate of tube displacement and difficult tube reinsertion with percutaneous tracheostomy as compared to an open tracheostomy. An additional disadvantage of percutaneous tracheostomy is the risk of tracheal or subglottic stenosis due to cartilage damage incurred during the procedure. Unlike soft tissue, cartilage is rigid and incapable of conforming to the shape of the dilator. The progressive dilations performed during percutaneous tracheostomy put the tracheal cartilages at high risk for crush injury during the procedure. Damaged cartilage poses a risk of scar tissue formation and subsequent tracheal or subglottic stenosis. The risk of cartilage damage is minimized by bronchoscopic guidance during the procedure ensuring proper placement of the tracheostomy. Overall, with proper patient selection and adequate training, percutaneous tracheostomy is a safe and efficient alternative to open tracheostomy.

LARYNGEAL AND TRACHEAL STENOSIS IN THE ADULT

Laryngotracheal stenosis (LTS) is, in adults, challenging to manage. The diagnosis and evaluation of these lesions requires a complete mastery of the anatomy and function of the upper aerodigestive tract. The multiplicity of stenotic lesions in the adult larynx and trachea requires unique strategies for management and careful individualization of treatment. LTS is an unfortunate complication of diseases and therapies.

Etiology

The list of causes of laryngotracheal stenosis is extensive. Historically, the majority of adult LTSs result either from external trauma or prolonged endotracheal intubation; however, sequela of intubation has become the number one cause. External trauma causes cartilage damage and mucosal disruption with hematoma formation. The resulting hematoma organizes and leads to collagen deposition and scar tissue formation through the healing process. This scar may eventually contract leading to the development of stenosis. Endotracheal intubations can cause mucosal damage through pressure necrosis and direct injury resulting from the pressure of the endotracheal tube or cuff. Mucosal ulceration also leads to chondritis and healing with collagen deposition and fibrosis, leading to eventual scar formation. Lesions from endotracheal intubation are usually located in the posterior glottis where the tube most often contacts mucosa or in the trachea where the cuff or tube tip may cause mucosal damage. Damage related to the cuff has been significantly reduced by the development of low-pressure, high-volume cuffs. The duration of intubation, amount of tube movement, the tube size, and the presence of gastroesophageal reflux all may contribute to the development of LTS. Patient specific disease processes may also contribute to the development of LTS. Patients with diabetes mellitus, congestive heart failure, and a history of stoke or tuberculosis have an increased incidence of laryngeal injury from intubation. Benign and malignant neoplasms, collagen vascular infections, fungal disease, and inflammatory conditions all may cause LTS without a history of trauma or previous intubation.[20]

Classification

Since areas of LTS are so variable in their size, consistency, and location, a rigid classification scheme is essentially impossible; and, for this reason, multiple staging systems exist. Although introduced as a staging system for subglottic stenosis, the Myer-Cotton system remains the most widespread classification system in use. The classification system separates obstruction into four categories: Grade I, less than 50% lumen obstruction; Grade II, 50 to 70% obstruction; Grade 3, 71 to 99% obstruction; and Grade IV, complete obstruction without a detectable lumen.[21] Regardless of the classification system used, it is important for the surgeon to describe and document the lesion in a way that is widely understandable and reproducible. Photodocumentation when available aids in documenting the lesion and preparing for future surgical intervention.

In 1992, McCaffrey developed a classification system based on 72 cases of LTS. In this system, Stage 1 lesions are confined to the subglottis or trachea and are less than 1 cm long. Stage 2 lesions are subglottic and longer than 1 cm but do not extend into the glottis or trachea. Stage 3 lesions involve the upper trachea but do not involve the glottis. Stage 4 lesions involve the glottis with fixation or paralysis of one or both vocal folds. McCaffrey found the above system to be highly predictive for successful decannulation, with 90% of Stages 1 and 2 patients, 70% of Stage 3 patients, and 40% of Stage 4 patients achieving successful decannulation.[22,23]

The general description of LTS in adults begins with the anatomic location of the lesion. Stenotic areas are first described by their origin in the glottis, subglottis, trachea, or a combination of the above areas. Stenotic segments may be further described as anterior, posterior, or circumferential in nature. Posterior glottic stenosis always involves impaired vocal fold abduction, due to soft tissue contracture or actual fixation of the cricoarytenoid joints. The size and length of the stenotic area are critical in classifying the lesion as well. The quality of the lesion, soft versus fibrous, and any associated vocal fold motion impairment should also be noted. This quantitative, reproducible method offers the most consistent technique for describing laryngotracheal stenosis.

Diagnostic Assessment

The evaluation of the patient with LTS must begin with a meticulous history and physical examination. Since most cases of LTS result from laryngotracheal trauma or endotracheal intubation, the timing of the predisposing incident should be recorded. Any previous airway evaluations or attempts at repair should also be noted. The patient should be questioned regarding the onset, duration, and severity of symptoms such as exercise intolerance, disruption of lifestyle, and tracheostomy dependence. Patients who require a tracheostomy should be questioned as to how often and the duration that the tracheostomy tube can be plugged. Symptoms of aspiration, voice change, or dysphagia may indicate glottic involvement.

The entire upper aerodigestive tract must be carefully examined in a patient with suspected LTS. Indirect laryngoscopy and flexible fiberoptic laryngoscopy provide critical information regarding the supraglottic airway and mobility of the true vocal folds. In extreme abduction, areas of subglottic stenosis may be visible using these techniques. Video documentation offers a valuable method of treatment planning and patient education. Although imaging studies such as airway radiographs, computerized tomography, and magnetic resonance imaging occasionally provide useful information, the most valuable diagnostic assessment stems from examination of the patient endoscopy.

After the patient has been examined by indirect laryngoscopy and flexible fiberoptic techniques, open endoscopy evaluation under general anesthesia should be performed in all patients with symptomatic airway abnormalities. Direct objective measurement and documentation of the diameter and length of the stenotic areas are critical steps in the management of patients with these lesions. Measurement of the diameter of stenotic segments is best evaluated by passing a telescope, with a known diameter, that just fits through the stenotic area. Alternatively, an uncuffed endotracheal tube may be used. It should be noted, however, that the endoscope or tube will compress soft tissue and can temporarily dilate the lumen, so that the actual dimensions are usually overestimated. Measurement of stenosis length may be performed by placing the endoscope at the distal end of the stenotic segment and marking the instrument at the incisors. The endoscope is then withdrawn to the proximal aspect of the stenosis and remarked. The length of the stenosis may then be directly measured on the endoscope.

Treatment of Laryngotracheal Stenosis

The goal of treating the patient with LTS is to reconstruct an adequate airway, while preserving phonation and airway protection. Operative intervention ranges from outpatient endoscopic procedures to major open airway reconstruction, including laryngotracheoplasty, cricotracheal resection, and tracheal resection. Many patients require multiple procedures to treat this severe and challenging disease process.

Medical Treatment. Most surgeons who treat LTS recommend the use of antibiotics, local or systemic corticosteroids, and H2 antagonists or proton pump inhibitors when treating mild or acute subglottic injuries. Treatment of underlying disease processes such as inflammation, infection, and autoimmune processes may lessen the degree of stenosis in appropriate cases. In mature areas of laryngotracheal scarring, these medical treatments are unlikely to result in significant clinical improvement. In the treatment of glottic stenosis, static enlargement of the glottis impairs vocal function, to varying degrees.

Endoscopic Treatment. Some areas of LTS are amenable to endoscopic treatment techniques such as laser vaporization and dilation, excision using a microtrapdoor technique, or serial dilation with radial incisions of the stenotic segment. Regardless of the technique used, the most common cause of failure is restenosis. A corticosteroid may be injected into the stenotic area, or mitomycin-C may be applied to the lesion under endoscopic guidance to inhibit recurrent scar formation. Lasers allow the precise treatment of tissue throughout the airway while avoiding external incisions and provide an excellent method of cutting, coagulating, or vaporizing tissue. Hemostasis may be achieved and perioperative edema is often less with the use of lasers due to smaller amounts of tissue thermal damage compared to electrocautery.

The ideal laser for any particular patient depends on the type of tissue and lesion that requires treatment. Due to the precision, that is, the small spot size of the carbon dioxide (CO_2) laser, it remains the instrument of choice in the endoscopic management of LTS. While the CO_2 laser is precise, it is not a good instrument for coagulation and can only be used to coagulate vessels up to 0.5 mm in size. If the area of stenosis is felt to be particularly vascular, a laser with better hemoglobin absorption, such as KTP or Nd:YAG, would be recommended. One further disadvantage of the CO_2 laser is that it lacks a good fiberoptic delivery system and must generally be controlled via a micromanipulator system mounted on a microscope.

Laser ablation of areas of LTS is a useful technique that may be combined with dilation of the stenotic segment or placement of an intraluminal stent. Laser ablation is most successful in the management of early lesions composed mostly of granulation tissue that have not yet evolved into a mature scar. Stenotic segments less than 1 cm in length may also be addressed with this method. The microtrapdoor technique is used to debulk stenotic areas confined to a single quadrant of the airway. This technique is somewhat more technically demanding than simple ablation of the stenosis. The procedure begins by performing an incision on the superior aspect of the stenotic shelf (Figure 6). Once the incision has been made, a microelevator is used to elevate a mucosal flap over the area of scar tissue. The laser may by used to vaporize the underlying scar tissue forming the stenosis. Once the scar tissue has been adequately ablated, the flap is repositioned into its correct anatomic location. The laser may be defocused and milli-

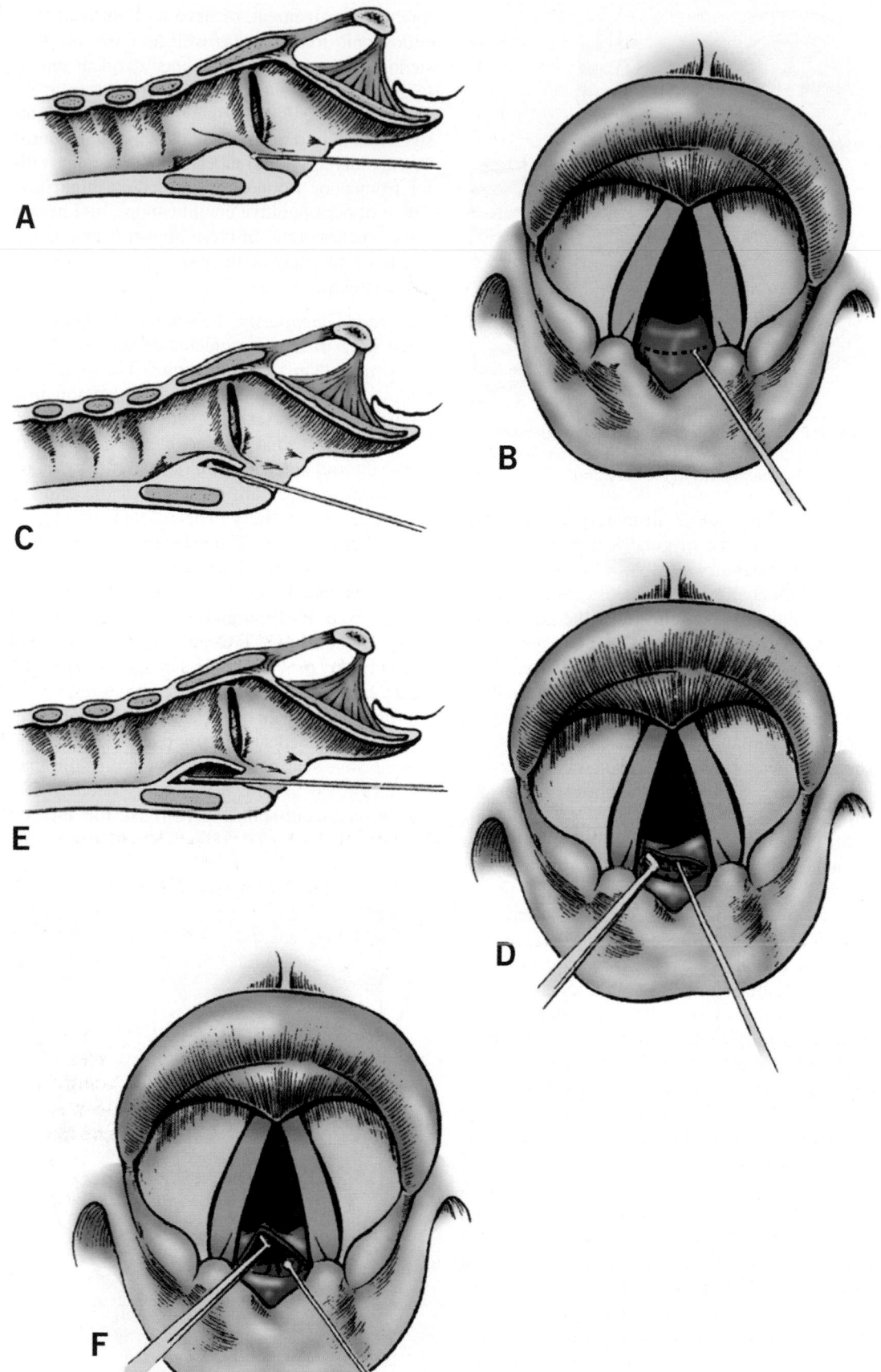

Figure 6 Microtrapdoor technique for debulking stenotic areas. (Published with permission from reference 26.)

watt power settings used to weld the edges of the incision back together.[24]

Areas of circumferential stenosis may be addressed endoscopically by making radial incisions in the scar tissue with a laser and dilating the treated area with a bronchoscope or other dilating instrument. The laser is used to create radial incisions in the scar tissue in four to six areas (Figure 7). The laser may be coupled to a ventilating bronchoscope if the patient is not tracheostomy dependent. The incisions break up the circumferential scar band and leave islands of intact mucosa. The areas of intact mucosa are critical to prevent circumferential denuded areas

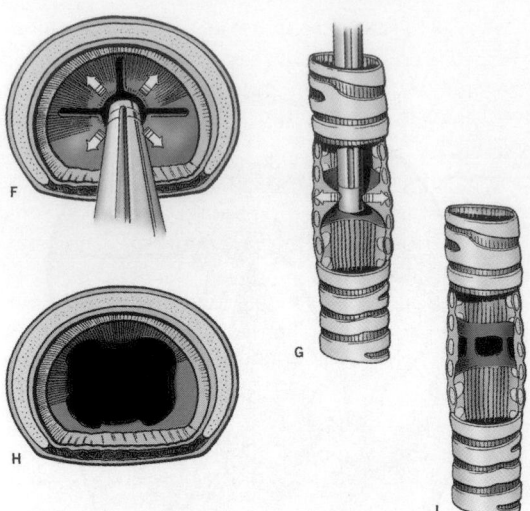

Figure 7 Laser-assisted radial incision and dilation technique for treating tracheal or subglottic stenosis. (Published with permission from reference 26.)

of mucosa that would ultimately reform scar tissue similar to the original lesion or possibly create a narrower airway.[25,26]

Local applications of corticosteroids or mitomycin-C may be used with any of the endoscopic techniques in an attempt to prevent the reformation of scar. Corticosteroids have long been known to affect the healing process and inhibit scar formation primarily through their ability to suppress the inflammatory process. At this time, however, there remains no clear evidence supporting the use of intraoperative local corticosteroid injection.

Mitomycin-C is an antineoplastic antibiotic that acts as an alkylating agent inhibiting cell division, protein synthesis, and fibroblast proliferation. Mitomycin-C has been used successfully in ophthalmologic procedures to decrease scar formation and restenosis; however, at this time the local use of mitomycin-C in LTS is still controversial. Rahbar and colleagues published the results of a multicenter prospective trial aiming to evaluate the efficacy and safety of the topical application of mitomycin-C in the prevention and treatment of airway stenosis. Over an average follow-up period of 18 months, 14 of 15 patients (93%), ranging in age from 2 to 78 years, showed a significant improvement in their airway.[27] A retrospective review of 55 patients by Ubell and colleagues showed only 1 suspected complication in 93 applications. The patient in question suffered from diffuse inflammation and possible fungal infection, ultimately requiring a tracheostomy.[28] Although many trials point to promising initial results for application of mitomycin-C, ultimately additional studies are needed to estimate better the risks and benefits of its use.

Open Surgical Treatment. Severe areas of laryngotracheal stenosis that do not respond to endoscopic techniques require an open surgical procedure. Open techniques attempt either to excise the stenotic segment and anastomose the airway or to augment the circumference of the stenotic segment with transplanted tissue. Stenoses that are longer than 1 cm have glottic or extensive

tracheal involvement, or have no improved with endoscopic treatment, as well as near-complete stenoses are candidates for open surgical repair. In patients with diabetes or severe systemic illnesses, for example, systemic lupus erythematosus, rheumatoid arthritis, open approaches must be considered with great care. Such patients suffer from poor wound healing, have a high incidence of perioperative complications, and have a lower success rate. In these high-risk patients, a tracheostomy may be the most prudent choice of management.[29]

Laryngotracheoplasty. Laryngotracheoplasty is often used to repair segments of subglottic stenosis more than 1 cm in length.[30] The procedure begins with a transverse cervical incision in a natural skin crease at the level of the cricoid cartilage. Subplatysmal flaps are elevated superiorly to the thyroid notch and inferiorly to the sternum. The strap muscles are separated in the midline and retracted laterally. The thyroid isthmus is divided and ligated. The anterior cricoid ring is divided vertically with a knife or saw. The incision is extended superiorly and inferiorly based on the exact location and extent of the stenosis (Figure 8). The goal is to open the entire stenotic segment. To prevent voice damage, the incision is not extended to the anterior commissure unless this area is involved by the stenosis. If the cricoid cannot be opened sufficiently due to calcification or extensive scaring, a posterior cricoid split may be performed to gain the mobility needed. If a posterior cricoid split is performed, the surgeon

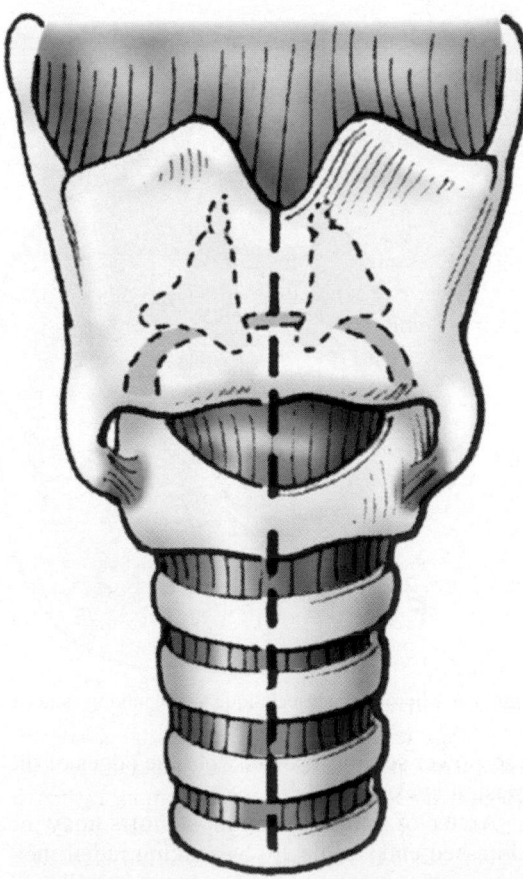

Figure 8 Vertical splitting of the thyroid cartilage during laryngotracheoplasty. (Published with permission from reference 30.)

must be careful not to damage the underlying esophagus. While it is tempting to remove scar tissue at this point in the procedure, the surgeon must remember that the goal of the procedure is to open the area of stenosis widely rather than to remove tissue. Resection of scar tissue and mucosa risks scar regeneration and recurrent stenosis in the postoperative period. Submucosal resection of scar tissue, however, is generally safe and does not increase the risk of restenosis. A posterior graft, if it must be used, is placed next. Posterior grafts usually contain a flange that is tucked behind the posterior lamina of the cricoid cartilage bilaterally to prevent extrusion into the airway. An airway stent, if one is to be placed, is inserted after placement of the posterior cricoid graft. Placing an airway stent requires one to leave a tracheostomy in place while healing occurs. The anterior cartilage graft is generally cut in a fusiform or boat-shaped fashion with beveled edges to prevent the graft from slipping into the airway. The graft is sutured into place while taking great care to ensure the sutures remain extraluminal. The strap muscles are reapproximated in the midline, and the platysma and skin are closed over a passive drain to allow air egress. The success rate of primary laryngotracheal reconstruction in adults is in the 60 to 70% range.[31]

Cartilage grafts for laryngotracheoplasty may be harvested from the costal cartilage or from nasal septal cartilage. Costal cartilage is the most commonly used source for grafts. The fifth or sixth costal cartilage is harvested with the anterior perichondrium intact. The grafts are carved to the appropriate shape with the perichondrium facing the airway lumen. The hyoid bone may also be harvested through the existing cervical incision and used as an interposition graft, which offers the advantage of avoiding a second operative area. The central portion of the hyoid bone between the lesser cornua may be used as a free graft and fixed into place. The hyoid bone has also been used as a pedicled graft based inferiorly on the sternohyoid muscle.[32] In children, the outer table of the thyroid cartilage taken from the lateral edge may be used as a graft.

Tracheal Resection and Anastomosis. Areas of cervical tracheal stenosis up to about 5 cm can generally be excised and the trachea reanastomosed primarily, providing that it is not in close proximity to the carina. Sternotomy may be needed if the lesion is intrathoracic. A suprahyoid laryngeal release may be required to allow for closure under minimal tension. When performing this procedure, the surgeon must keep in mind the age and body habitus of the patient. Old patients tend to have calcifications between tracheal rings, resulting in decreased tracheal elasticity. Patients with large, thick necks and older patients with cervical kyphosis also tend to lack tracheal mobility.

Prior to the procedure, the patient is positioned with the neck hyperextended on a shoulder roll. If a tracheostomy is present, the skin of the tracheostomy site is included in the incision planning and is excised. After a transverse skin incision has been made, subplatysmal flaps are raised superiorly to the thyroid cartilage and inferiorly to the manubrium. The strap muscles are separated in the midline and retracted laterally. The thyroid isthmus is divided and ligated if necessary. The area of stenosis is located and can be confirmed endoscopically. Care is taken to preserve the lateral blood supply to the trachea proximal and distal to the site of stenosis. The dissection around the area of stenosis must proceed directly on the trachea to prevent injury to the recurrent laryngeal nerves. The esophagus is identified and carefully dissected away from the membranous trachea. The trachea may then be incised above and below the stenotic segment. The endotracheal tube is placed transorally into the distal tracheal segment. The closure always begins posteriorly. Vicryl sutures are placed in an extraluminal fashion through the perichondrium of the proximal and distal tracheal segments (Figure 9). The neck is flexed prior to tying the sutures. Additional sutures may be placed around a tracheal ring above and below the site of anastomosis to decrease tension on the closure. The strap muscles are reapproximated in the midline. The platysma and skin are closed after placement of a passive drain to allow the egress of air.

It is essential to minimize the tension on the closure after tracheal reanastamosis. Surgical techniques that decrease tension include mobilization of the trachea through blunt anterior and posterior dissection and release of the suprahyoid muscular attachments. A cardiothoracic surgeon may also perform a division and reattachment of a bronchus, which allows further superior mobility of the distal trachea, although this is rarely necessary. Positioning maneuvers such as neck flexion also decrease tension on the site of anastamosis. Some surgeons place a stitch between the chin and manubrium (Grillo stitch) to prevent patients from extending the neck during the postoperative period. The patient may be extubated at the conclusion of the procedure or remain intubated overnight and extubated on the first postoperative day at the discretion of the surgeon. Multiple studies show operative success, defined by decannulation, in excess of 90%.[33]

Complications of laryngotracheal resection and anastomosis include subcutaneous

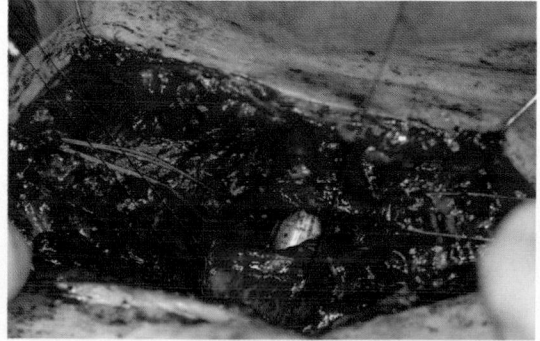

Figure 9 Intraoperative photograpgh after excision of a stenotic tracheal segment. Sutures have been placed but not tied.

emphysema, pneumomediastinum, mediastinitis, hematoma formation, abscess, wound dehiscence, cellulitis, reintubation or prolonged intubation, tracheitis, pleural effusion or pneumonia, and tracheocutaneous fistula, in addition to anastomotic complications including granulation tissue formation, stenosis, and separation. In a review by Wright and colleagues of 901 patients undergoing tracheal resection, predictors of anastomotic complications were reoperation, diabetes, resections greater than or equal to 4 cm, laryngotracheal resection, need for tracheostomy before the operation, and age 17 years or younger.[34] Anastomotic complications, while uncommon, may require multiple additional airway procedures including multiple dilations, temporary tracheostomy, permanent T-tube, and reoperation. Overall, tracheal resection in the hands of a skilled surgeon has a high success rate with low mortality.

Additional Open Techniques. Several new techniques have recently been described and applied in the treatment of segmental tracheal stenosis. Cryopreserved, irradiated tracheal homograft transplantation has been used to treat patients with tracheal stenosis. This technique requires the harvest of tracheal tissue from donor cadavers within 24 hours of death. The grafts are placed in a –70°C chamber prior to irradiation to 25,000 Gy and then stored at –70°C until transplantation. Kunachak and colleagues reported that three of four patients treated with this technique were successfully decannulated and display a near-normal tracheal lumen with histologic evidence of normal respiratory epithelium at the graft site.[35]

The technique of microvascular-free tissue transfer has been applied to the challenging problem of laryngotracheal stenosis. Esclamado and Carroll reported the use of a fibular osseocutaneous-free flap in the reconstruction of a complex LTS.[36] At this point, the usefulness of free tissue transfer appears to be limited to a subset of complex cases not amenable to more conventional surgical techniques.

CRICOARYTENOID JOINT FIXATION

The cricoarytenoid joint is a synovial joint formed by the articulation of the arytenoid cartilages with the posterosuperior aspect of the cricoid cartilage. The vocal process of the arytenoid cartilage is usually free to rotate in three dimensions to allow proper apposition of the true vocal folds. This normal mobility of the arytenoids can be impaired by several factors. First, dislocation of the arytenoid cartilage may occur due to external trauma or intubation. The arytenoids may be dislocated either anteriorly or posteriorly, with anterior dislocation being slightly more common due to the force vector exerted by the blade of a laryngoscope. Several inflammatory disorders such as rheumatoid arthritis and gout may also involve the cricoarytenoid joint and result in fixation of the joint. With cricoarytenoid arthri-

tis, the patient generally presents with symptoms of stridor and dyspnea with a variable degree of dysphonia. The dysfunction results from a fixed position of the vocal folds in a paramedian position and the inability to create normal apposition or abduction of the vocal folds. Other causes include denervation of the larynx, Wegener granulomatosis, previous laryngeal operations, and caustic ingestion.[37]

In the patient with suspected cricoarytenoid joint dysfunction, the differential diagnosis includes denervation, dislocation, or fixation due to an inflammatory condition. A history of trauma should always be carefully elicited in this group of patients. The proper location and mobility of the cricoarytenoid joint is best assessed under general anesthesia by gently rocking the arytenoid cartilage. An electromyelogram of the intrinsic laryngeal musculature can determine if the immobility is due to denervation or is secondary to fixation of the joint. Bilateral arytenoid cartilage fixation bears resemblance to bilateral recurrent laryngeal nerve paralysis, and the two conditions may be difficult to distinguish clinically.[38]

The treatment of cricoarytenoid joint dysfunction must be carefully individualized to the patient and the disease process. A patient with an inflammatory disorder should be treated medically with the aid of a rheumatologist. Stable patients that are able to phonate, breathe, and swallow without aspiration may be safely observed. Unstable patients or patients who are not improved with medical and rehabilitative strategies must be treated surgically. Patients with inadequate ventilation may undergo a tracheostomy, which would likely result in an excellent voice due to the paramedian position of the vocal folds. Patients that wish to be decannulated can be offered a cordotomy or arytenoidectomy; however, the patient must be counseled that this will result in an inferior voice.

A CO_2 laser endoscopic posterior partial transverse cordotomy can sometimes provide an adequate airway and allow decannulation in a patient whose true vocal folds are in a paramedian position, cannot be abducted, and prevent adequate airflow through the glottis. The cause of the medialized vocal folds may be either bilateral cricoarytenoid joint fixation or bilateral vocal fold paralysis. The procedure of laser cordotomy involves excising a transverse wedge of tissue from the posterior portion of the vocal fold just anterior to the vocal process of the arytenoid cartilage. The technique may also be performed bilaterally. Sequelae of the procedure include granulation or scar tissue formation at the site of the cordotomy, possible need for a repeat procedure, and decreased voice quality.

Excision or lateralization of the arytenoid cartilage is a second option for providing for improved patency of the airway when the vocal folds are adducted and airflow through the glottis is inadequate. The arytenoid cartilage may be removed surgically, and the true vocal fold sutured laterally to improve the airway. Likewise, an endoscopic laser partial arytenoidectomy may be performed. The goal of both techniques, as with posterior transverse laser cordotomy, is to improve airflow through the posterior part of the glottis while minimally affecting the anterior two-thirds of the glottis, which is largely responsible for phonation. Another option is to split the posterior cricoid plate and interpose a cartilage plate to increase the diameter of the posterior glottis. This is particularly useful in patients with concomitant subglottis stenosis. None of these techniques are ideal, and the choice of technique used should be tailored to the individual patient.

CONCLUSIONS

The successful management of the airway requires a complete understanding of the anatomy and function of the upper aerodigestive tract. A systematic and progressive algorithm must be employed in cases of airway distress. Several options exist for the management of patients that require a surgical airway, and the correct technique must be individually matched to the clinical situation.

LTS poses a formidable challenge to the airway surgeon due to variability in both the location and degree of stenosis. Stenosis segments must be carefully evaluated prior to treatment planning. Treatment must be individualized to the patient taking into account the cause and structure of the lesion as well as the health status of the patient.

REFERENCES

1. Kharasch M, Graff J. Emergency management of the airway. Crit Care Clin 1995;11:53–66.
2. Rodricks MB, Deutschman CS. Emergent airway management. Indications and methods in the face of confounding conditions. Crit Care Clin 2000;16:389–409.
3. Walls RM. Airway management in the blunt trauma patient: How important is the cervical spine? Can J Surg 1992;35:27–30.
4. Brantigan CO, Grow JB. Cricothyroidotomy: Elective use in respiratory problems requiring tracheostomy. J Thorac Cardiovasc Surg 1976;71:72–80.
5. Grande CM, Stene JK, Berhard WN. Airway management: Considerations in the trauma patient. Crit Care Clin 1990;6:37–59.
6. Walls RM. Management of the difficult airway in the trauma patient. Emerg Med Clin North Am 1998;16:45–61.
7. Burkey BB, Esclamado R, Morganroth M. The role of cricothyroidotomy in airway management. Clin Chest Med 1991;12:561–71.
8. Heffner JE. The technique of tracheotomy and cricothyroidotomy. When to operate–and hoe to manage complications. J Crit Ill 1995;10:561–8.
9. Einarsson O, Rochester CL, Rosenbaum S. Airway management in respiratory emergencies. Clin Chest Med 1994;15:13–34.
10. Boon JM, Abrahams PH, Meiring JH, Welch T. Cricothyroidotomy: A clinical anatomy review. Clin Anat 2004;17:478–86.
11. Hawkins ML, Shapiro MB, Cue JI, Wiggins SS. Emergency cricothyroidotomy: A reassessment. Am Surg 1995;61:52–5.
12. Advanced Trauma Life Support for Doctors, 6th edition. Chicago: American College of Surgeons; 1997.
13. Jackson C. Tracheostomy. Laryngoscope 1909;18:285–90.
14. Jackson C. High tracheostomy and other errors: The chief cause of chronic laryngeal stenosis. Surg Gynecol Obstet 1921;32:382–98.
15. Smith DK, Grillone GA, Fuleihan N. Use of postoperative chest x-ray after elective adult tracheostomy. Otolaryngol Head Neck Surg 1999;120:848–51.
16. Ciaglia P, Firsching R, Syneic C. Elective percutaneous dilational tracheostomy: A new simple bedside procedure; preliminary report. Chest 1985;87:715–9.
17. Freeman BD, Isabella K, Lin N, Buchman TG. A meta-analysis of prospective trials comparing percutaneous and surgical tracheostomy in critically ill patients. Chest 2000;118:1412–8.
18. Antonelli M, Michetti V, Di Palma A, et al. Percutaneous translaryngeal versus surgical tracheostomy: A randomized trial with 1-yr double-blind follow-up. Crit Care Med 2005;33:1015–20.
19. Kearney PA, Griffen MM, Ochoa JB, et al. A single-center 8-year experience with percutaneous dilational tracheostomy. Ann Surg 2000;231:701–9.
20. Volpi D, Lin PT, Kuriloff DB, Kimmelman CP. Risk factors for intubation injury of the larynx. Ann Otol Rhinol Laryngol 1987;96:684–6.
21. Myer CM, IIIrd, O'Connor DM, Cotton RT. Proposed grading system for subglottic stenosis based on endotracheal tube sizes. Ann Otol Rhinol Laryngol 1994;103:319–23.
22. McCaffrey TV. Classification of laryngotracheal stenosis. Laryngoscope 1992;102:1335–40.
23. McCaffrey TV. Management of laryngotracheal stenosis on the basis of site and severity. Otolaryngol Head Neck Surg 1993;109:468–73.
24. Dedo HH, Sooy CD. Endoscopic laser repair of posterior glottic, subglottic, and tracheal stenosis by division or microtrapdoor flap. Laryngoscope 1984;94:445–50.
25. Duncavage JA, Ossoff RH, Toohill RJ. Carbon dioxide laser management of laryngeal stenosis. Ann Otol Rhinol Laryngol 1985;94:565–9.
26. Coleman JA, Van Duyne JA, Ossoff RH. Laser treatment of lower airway stenosis. Otol Clin North Am 1995;28:771–83.
27. Rahbar R, Shapshay SM, Healy GB. Mitomycin: Effects on laryngeal and tracheal stenosis, benefits, and complications. Ann Otol Rhinol Laryngol 2001;110:1–6.
28. Ubell ML, Ettema SL, Toohill RJ, et al. Mitomycin-C application in airway stenosis surgery: Analysis of safety and costs. Otol Head Neck Surg 2006;134:403–6.
29. Lorenz RR. Adult laryngotracheal stenosis: Etiology and surgical management. Curr Opin Otol Head Neck Surg 2003;11:467–72.
30. Duncavage JA, Koriwchak MJ. Open surgical techniques for laryngotracheal stenosis. Otol Clin North Am 1995;28:785–95.
31. Lano CF, Duncavage JA, Reinisch L, et al. Laryngotracheal reconstruction in the adult: A ten year experience. Ann Otol Rhinl Laryngol 1998;107:92–7.
32. Ward PH, Canalis R, Fee W. Composite hyoid sternohyoid muscle grafts in humans. Its use in reconstruction of subglottic stenosis and the anterior tracheal wall. Arch Otolaryngol 1977;103:531–4.
33. Grillo HC, Mathisen DJ, Ashiku SK, et al. Successful treatment of idiopathic laryngotracheal stenosis by resection and primary anastomosis. Ann Otol Rhinol Laryngol 2003;112:798–800.
34. Wright CD, Grillo HC, Wain JC, et al. Anastomotic complications after tracheal resection: Prognostic factors and management. J Thorac Cardiovasc Surg 2004;128:731–9.
35. Kunachak S, Kulapaditharom B, Vajaradul Y, Rochanawutanon M. Cryopreserved, irriadiated tracheal homograft transplantation for laryngotracheal reconstruction in human beings. Otolaryngol Head Neck Surg 2000;122:911–6.
36. Esclamado RM, Carroll WR. Repair of a complete glottic-subglottic stenosis with a fibular osseocutaneous free flap. Arch Otolaryngol Head Neck Surg 1997;23:877–9.
37. Gacek RR, Gacek MR, Montgomery WW. Evidence for laryngeal paralysis in cricoarytenoid joint arthritis. Laryngoscope 1999;109:279–83.
38. Eckel HE, Wittekindt C, Klussmann JP, et al. Management of bilateral arytenoid cartilage fixation versus recurrent laryngeal nerve paralysis. Ann Otol Rhinol Laryngol 2003;112:103–8.

79

Neurogenic Disorders of the Larynx

Christy L. Ludlow, PhD
Steven A. Bielamowicz, MD

Normal speech requires the complex integration of peripheral and central motor control mechanisms. The voice component of speech requires (1) neural control of the intrinsic and extrinsic laryngeal muscles to shape the glottis, and (2) a steady stream of airflow from the respiratory system to support regular, symmetric, and synchronous vibration of the vocal folds. Speech production requires the coordination of laryngeal function with pharyngeal shape as well as tongue, lip and jaw position, and articulation. Thus, the central nervous system must coordinate the respiratory, phonatory, and speech mechanisms to produce normal phonation during speech.

EFFECTS OF SPEECH ON LARYNGEAL VIEW DURING ENDOSCOPY

The larynx does not function in isolation from other structures in the vocal tract. Muscles shaping the pharynx and oral cavity, particularly those controlling the tongue, lip, and jaw, alter laryngeal tension as they change vocal tract posture. In normal speech, the vocal tract moves rapidly between different target shapes for specific speech sounds.

Valving at the glottis, velum, tongue, lips, and jaw amplifies certain harmonics of the fundamental frequency of vocal fold vibration, based on the posture and shape of the vocal tract. Depending upon the shape of the vocal tract, harmonics of certain resonant frequencies are amplified resulting in sound energy in formants. The frequency regions of the formants are responsible for the vowel sounds. In high vowel sounds such as /i/ or "ee," the posture of the tongue is high and forward exerting tension from the tip to the base of tongue. Coupling between the hyoid bone and suspended thyroid cartilage distributes tension to extrinsic and intrinsic laryngeal musculature that may tilt the thyroid cartilage. During /i/, the pharyngeal cavity is large, making conditions for airflow different than for production of /a/ or "ah" which is characterized by a constricted pharyngeal cavity because of the low and posterior placement of the tongue.

These differences in pharyngeal constriction also affect videoendoscopy; the vowel /i/ allows a better view of the larynx because the tongue is forward and high, opening the pharynx

and bringing the epiglottis forward. In contrast, during /a/ the larynx is much less visible because the tongue is back and consequently the epiglottis covers the larynx, providing a more obstructed view of the larynx.

MULTIDIMENSIONAL ASPECTS OF VOICE FUNCTION AND DISORDERS

Pharyngeal and/or laryngeal constriction can produce turbulence in airflow, in the case of neurogenic disorders. In these disorders, reduced vocal fold adduction can produce glottal insufficiency and inefficient voice production leading to a disturbance in vocal quality and durability of sound production. The acoustic product is thus affected by changes in constriction and air pressures in the pharynx and oral cavity. Both peripheral and central neurogenic disorders may alter the voice by changing the configuration of the larynx and vocal tract. In functional voice disorders, changes in vocal tract tension can also alter voice to a similar degree as in neurogenic voice disorders. Abnormalities in vocal tract tension due to voluntary or involuntary muscle contractions occur in neurogenic and/or functional voice disorders. The origins of these disorders may be traumatic, neoplastic, vascular, infectious, degenerative, or idiopathic. They are often present in conjunction with disease processes that alter not only the laryngeal musculature but also lip, tongue, and jaw control and other motor systems such as respiration.

In addition to the degree of motor impairment, the diagnostic process must also take into account the body's capacity for reorganization and compensation that may alter the perceived severity of speech disturbance. Perceptual voice parameters such as pitch, loudness, voice quality, and their variability, may help to characterize neurogenic and functional voice disorders. Quantification of acoustic and perceptual characteristics of voice and speech may be useful based on a variety of instrumental techniques.[1] Computer-assisted quantification of the acoustic product may be a valuable adjunct to the perceptual parameterization of voice, however the two are not synonymous. Measures based on pressure and flow transduction during phonation provide information about the functional relationship between the respiratory and phonatory

systems. Further, the use of diagnostic imaging techniques, including rigid and flexible fiberoptic videoendoscopy, allows observation of laryngeal and pharyngeal movement. Flexible fiberoptic examination is required when the voice disorder occurs more during connected speech, such as in spasmodic dysphonia (SD). Stroboscopic examination is useful in assessing the vibratory characteristics of the vocal folds. High-speed photography, ultrasound, videofluoroscopy, and magnetic resonance (MR) are other imaging tools that have value in the diagnostic protocol.[2,3] Use of electromyography (EMG) accompanied by magnetic stimulation of the laryngeal nerve may be valuable in differentiating peripheral and central neurogenic dysfunction.[4] The goal of instrumental and perceptual techniques has been to characterize vocal fold movement control in terms of timing, speed, and accuracy of movement of vocal tract structures and to quantify these parameters for the documentation of the status and progression of disease for therapeutic purposes.

NEUROGENIC DISORDERS

Dysphonia can appear as the first sign of neurogenic disease while the other speech symptoms (dysarthria) may only become evident as the disease progresses. Therefore, caution should be used in treatment of neurogenic voice symptoms until it can be assured that the laryngeal disorder is focal and not part of a progressive neurodegenerative disease. For example, what may initially appear to be a unilateral idiopathic vocal fold paralysis might later progress to become a vocal fold paralysis as part of a peripheral neuropathy,[5] early unilateral effects of Parkinson disease with bowing in one vocal fold[6] or multiple systems atrophy.[7] A unilateral thyroplasty could be detrimental if bilateral vocal fold paralysis developed due to a peripheral neuropathy or neurological disease subsequently resulting in airway compromise. For this reason, a complete neurological examination is important before planning intervention in these disorders.

Functionally, neurogenic disorders resulting in dysphonia may be divided into the following categories:

1. Consistent neurogenic voice disorders are characterized by constant vocal quality,

loudness or pitch deviations during speech, and sustained vowels. Examples include flaccid dysarthria, due to lower motor neuron disease such as amyotrophic lateral sclerosis, progressive supranuclear palsy, a peripheral neuropathy or laryngeal nerve injury. These can produce paralysis or paresis of the adductor and/or abductor muscles, causing asymmetries in movement. On the other hand, tension in the vocal fold may be altered when either the cricothyroid muscle or the thyroarytenoid muscles are affected as both contribute to vocal fold tension.

2. Spastic dysarthria, including dysphonia, is associated with upper motor neuron disease involving the corticobulbar tracts. For example, spasticity of the vocal tract, including the vocal folds, may be seen in multiple sclerosis.

3. Nonrhythmically fluctuating neurogenic voice disorders are most common. These are characterized by unpredictable, irregular variations in quality, loudness, and pitch during speech. Sustained vowel production may accentuate irregularities in some cases. Ataxic, choreic, and dystonic dysphonias, including spasmodic dysphonia, display this type of irregularity.

4. Rhythmically, fluctuating neurogenic voice disorders include palatopharyngolaryngeal myoclonus and essential voice tremor. These dysphonias are marked by regular or rhythmic fluctuations in voice, pitch, and loudness.

5. Neurogenic voice disorders associated with loss of volitional control of voice production, including apraxia of phonation, respiration or speech, and akinetic mutism, usually follow a cerebrovascular accident or cortical injury. In addition, paroxysmal neurogenic voice disorders exhibit bursts of dysphonic voice, as in Gilles de la Tourette syndrome.

6. Fluctuating vocal fold paralysis can occur in myasthenia gravis mimicking a vocal fold paralysis.

Upper Motor Neuron Disorders

Upper motor neuron diseases which affect the voice include Parkinson disease and related syndromes. Parkinsonism is a pathophysiologic state reflecting failure of the nigrostriatal dopaminergic neuronal system due to degeneration or destruction of the substantia nigra. This can occur by depleting neuronal dopamine, inhibiting its synthesis, or blocking the striatal dopamine receptors. The basal ganglia modulate cortical control via the thalamus. Neural activity at the cortex, in turn, controls the lower motor neurons. Hence, damage to the basal ganglia can release inhibition of nerve impulses affecting the lower motor neurons, resulting in rigidity and reduced rate of movement (bradykinesia).

Hypophonia in Parkinson Disease. Although parkinsonism can be described as a syndrome of diverse origins, distinct syndromes are identified by specific clinical features, although differentiation is often difficult. Parkinson disease occasionally can be familial, and genetic predisposition can be both Mendelian or a complex interaction of a genetic predisposition with environmental factors. Onset is typically in the sixties or later, but the disease may appear as early as the mid-thirties. Rare cases have been reported as early as 15 years of age.

Reduced loudness and breathy vocal quality, referred to as hypophonia, are the hallmark of voice disorders in early Parkinson disease. An essential feature is a voice quality that fades into breathiness in contextual speech. The patient may have difficulty with production of glottal stops or voice onset after voiceless consonants such as /s/. For this reason, persons with early onset of Parkinson disorder may have similar voice symptoms to abductor spasmodic dysphonia.[6] A reduced range and speed of vocal fold movement, particularly on the more affected side, is often identified. Distinctions between voiceless and voiced sounds become reduced due to impaired ability to produce glottal stops to mark word boundaries. In later stages of the disease, the patient may be unable to produce phonation even with instruction. In advanced disease, severe "on-off" drug-related phenomena may occur, during which patients may experience breathy voice followed by periods of propulsive speech with strained quality. Vocal fold imaging studies in Parkinson disease often illustrate incomplete glottic closure during voicing along with bowing of the vocal folds.[6] Asymmetries have also been demonstrated in vocal fold closure as well as thinning of the vocal fold mucosa and vocal fold bowing.

Patients can increase voice intensity on demand, and voice therapy aimed at increasing vocal intensity can improve speech intelligibility and voice when combined with dopaminergic enhancement therapy.[8] Focus on upper articulator (lip, tongue, and jaw) movement produces little in the way of increased intelligibility for this population. Percutaneous collagen has been used to improve the breathy hypophonia of Parkinson disease in persons with vocal fold bowing and glottic insufficiency,[9] especially in the patient with early symptoms. Collagen therapy does not, however, improve overall speech intelligibility in patients with preexisting dysarthria producing speech intelligibility and articulatory precision problems.

Progressive Supranuclear Palsy. Progressive supranuclear palsy (PSP) is a rare degenerative neurological disorder characterized by supranuclear ophthalmoplegia, complaints of falling backward, nuchal dystonia in extension, moderate axial dystonia, pseudobulbar palsy, difficulty in swallowing, dysarthria, bradykinesia, masked facies, nonspecific changes in personality, lability, sleep disturbance, and performance decrements on various neuropsychological tasks. PSP may be differentiated from Parkinson disease in that supranuclear ophthalmoplegia is characteristic of PSP and the tremor present in parkinsonism is typically absent in PSP. Patients with PSP may have voice symptoms similar to those in parkinsonism, with the possible exception of vocal tremor. Dysphagia is a major problem for these patients. Hypophonia is present, with unilaterally reduced vocal fold range and speed of movement. The associated dysarthria may include palilalia (uncontrolled syllable repetition) and oral motor rigidity.

Multiple Systems Atrophy. Multiple systems atrophy is another disease which is included as a Parkinson plus syndrome. This is a rare degenerative movement disorder with lesions in the cerebellum, brainstem, and basal ganglia. Three clinical variants are recognized: (1) spinocerebellar degeneration (olivopontocerebellar atrophy or OPCA); (2) progressive autonomic failure (Shy-Drager syndrome); and (3) atypical parkinsonism (striatonigral degeneration). OPCA is characterized by progressive cerebellar ataxia, and coordination of the laryngeal muscles is affected as in ataxic dysarthria. One sees loss of muscle coordination (dyssynergia), loss of ability to gauge range of motion (dysmetria), and tremor during voluntary movement (intention tremor). The degree of laryngeal impairment depends upon the severity of the ataxia. Dysphonia may take one of several forms: sudden bursts of loudness, irregular increases in pitch and loudness, or coarse voice tremor.

In Shy-Drager syndrome, voice symptoms typical of Parkinson disease are present, along with progressive autonomic dysfunction. The principal distinguishing features of this disease is autonomic dysfunction, including loss of bowel and bladder control as well as erectile dysfunction. Voice may be more severely affected due to reduced range and speed of adduction and abduction of the vocal folds. Speech is slowed with a reduction in vocal intensity, an absence of glottal stops and poor voicing contrasts. Patients may also be predisposed to laryngospasm. The most prominent laryngeal feature is airway compromise secondary to bilateral abductor paresis, and patients often require tracheostomy in the late stages of the disease. Voice treatment for these syndromes largely depends on the stage of disease and may include compensatory strategies as well as supportive nonverbal communication alternatives in end stages.

Pseudobulbar Palsy. Pseudobulbar palsy results from neuronal loss above the level of the nucleus ambiguus involving the corticobulbar tracts bilaterally. It can occur with vascular and degenerative lesions involving the cortical motor areas bilaterally, vascular lesions and tumors of the internal capsule or brainstem, degenerative lesions involving the entire corticobulbar tract system, or infections. Dysphonia associated with these types of lesions is characterized by strained strangled, harsh voice, likely the result of hyperadduction of true and false vocal folds. This is thought to occur from inhibition of excitation of vagal nuclei. Some persons have a breathy voice with vocal fold asymmetry.

Multiple Sclerosis. Multiple sclerosis (MS) is a progressive demyelinating disorder, having sensory and motor impairments, some cognitive problems, spasticity, and tremor. Although one of the most common causes of ataxia, patients with MS usually have evidence of central nervous system disease outside the cerebellum and its pathways. For example, optic nerve and corticospinal tract involvement are usually present. Dysarthria, tremor, and decomposition of movement are frequently associated with gait and limb ataxia in MS.

Essential features include staccato speech and harsh voice quality with intermittent hyperadduction of the vocal folds. Spasticity and tremor may affect all or some regions of the vocal tract, thereby reducing speech intelligibility and making speech effortful. Breathy voice and vocal fold movement asymmetry are common findings. Depending on the systems involved, voicing may or may not be affected in some stages of this disease. Given the predominant ataxia that may influence speech motor systems, voicing is characteristic of other ataxic dysarthrias (due to cerebellar degeneration). A principal feature of the natural history of MS is repeated acute neurological deficits with recovery in the relapsing–remitting phase followed by chronic progressive loss in the secondary progressive stage.

Myoclonus. Myoclonus is a sudden, brief, jerking involuntary movement of the involved muscles that occurs in a rhythmic fashion. The distribution may be focal, multifocal, or generalized, with the presentation spontaneous, active, and stimulus-sensitive. The source of the neural discharge may be cortical, brainstem, or spinal. Four main pathophysiologic categories of myoclonus have been described: cortical, subcortical, cortical-subcortical and spinal. These differ in the location of neurons involved in producing myoclonus. Sometimes these jerks are produced in response to external stimuli but most occur both at rest and during purposeful movements. In some patients, the symptoms can be volitionally suppressed for short time periods.

Palatal myoclonus is focal affecting the movements of the palate either unilaterally or bilaterally at 1.5 to 3 Hz. It is frequently accompanied by synchronous movements of adjacent muscles such as the pharynx, tongue, larynx and occasionally by synchronous movement of the extraocular muscles, face, neck, or diaphragm. When the soft palate is involved, abrupt, rhythmic, anteroposterior, and vertical movements are present. This rhythmic activity can open and close the eustachian tubes, thereby producing a clicking sound transmitted to the middle ear. The clicking sound is the most disturbing feature of this illness and can result in a severe inability to initiate sleep. The constant clicking sounds can be treated by injection of the tensor veli palatini muscles with small dosages of botulinum toxin A.[10] Movements are often present during sleep and may occur without the patient's knowledge. Myoclonus may be idiopathic or may be seen in association with stroke, MS, brainstem tumors, closed head injury, or metabolic encephalopathy. Pathology affecting the inferior olivary nuclei may be the origin of palatal myoclonus. When the pharynx and larynx are involved, rhythmic

adductor movements of the vocal folds and gross upward and downward movements of the larynx cause momentary and rhythmic phonatory interruptions. Voicing deficits are not often perceived during connected speech but will be apparent on vowel prolongation.

Lower Motor Neuron Disorders: Amyotrophic Lateral Sclerosis

Amyotrophic lateral sclerosis (ALS), a motor neuron disease, may produce a mixed dysarthria because of both upper motor neuron involvement and some lower motor neuron involvement, particularly in the late stages of the disease (flaccid-spastic paralysis). ALS is a degenerative disease of the corticobulbar tracts and lower motor neuron nuclei. The speech and voice symptoms may vary depending on the predominance of spastic or flaccid components. Flaccid symptoms present as hypoadduction of one or both vocal folds and pooling of saliva in the pyriform sinuses on laryngeal examination. Voicing is characterized by breathy, hypernasal quality with reduced intensity range. A "wet" phonation is the result of poor management of secretions due to flaccidity. Dysphagia is common. If spastic components prevail, voicing will be strained and harsh because of hyperadduction of the true and false vocal folds. A mixed form of dysphonia may result in voicing characterized by both flaccid and spastic components.

ALS occurs in the fifth to seventh decade of life and may present with primarily pyramidal tract signs or lower motor neuron signs of progressive muscular atrophy. Fasciculations are more common in the pyramidal tract form. When the disease affects the brainstem rather than the spinal cord, it may progress more rapidly. Speech symptoms may be the first signs in the bulbar type. Facial muscle weakness, palatal weakness, lip, tongue, and jaw weakness with tongue fasciculations are predominant and cause poor speech intelligibility. Voicing is weak and breathy because of flaccidity of the vocal folds.

Myasthenia Gravis. Myasthenia gravis is a disorder of acetylcholine transfer at the neuromuscular junction, characterized by weakness and fatigability of striated muscle. Muscle contraction, dependent on stimulation of the motor end plate by acetylcholine, is weakened or reduced by the reduction of acetylcholine receptors. This disorder causes a flaccid dysphonia, characterized by breathy, weak phonation. Sometimes stridor can develop with bilateral abductor muscle weakness. The voice intensity range is reduced, and sustained effort causes progressive weakness. This disorder may affect phonation (larynx), resonation (velum), and articulation (lip, tongue, and jaw), and these systems may be affected separately or serially as the disease progresses. The larynx is less frequently affected, whereas the extraocular muscles are usually the first affected. Dysphagia can be severe.[11] This and other early disorders of neurogenic origin may present with reduced movement range and speed of the vocal folds on

laryngoscopic examination and are often mistaken for psychogenic voice disorders. Flaccid dysphonia may be an early symptom of neurogenic disease.

Wallenberg Syndrome. Occlusion of the posterior–inferior cerebellar artery may produce infarction of the lateral medulla, resulting in Wallenberg syndrome, also known as lateral medullary syndrome. The medial and descending vestibular nuclei are usually included in the zone of infarction consisting of a wedge of the dorsolateral medulla just posterior to the olive. This syndrome is marked by dysarthria and dysphagia, ipsilateral impairment of pain and temperature sensation on the face, and contralateral loss of pain and temperature in the trunk and extremities. Major symptoms include vertigo, nausea, vomiting, intractable hiccupping, ipsilateral facial pain, and diplopia. Unilateral vocal fold paralysis and flaccid dysphonia occur when the nucleus ambiguus or corticobulbar tracts leading to the nucleus ambiguus are affected. If the paralysis does not completely resolve, a medialization laryngoplasty can provide improvement in both voice and some of the swallowing difficulties. However, many of these patients also have a central loss of swallowing patterning because of their brainstem lesions.

Postpolio Syndrome. Of the 250,000 survivors of the poliomyelitis epidemics, approximately 25% experience progressive muscle weakness known as postpolio syndrome (PPS). Patients with PPS who complain of swallowing difficulties are at risk for laryngeal dysfunction. This syndrome is characterized by the new onset of progressive muscle weakness, fatigue, and pain. This may occur 30 to 40 years after the initial infection with polio. Electrodiagnosis of neuronal dropout or axonal loss in these patients is consistent with neurogenic change. Patients with previous bulbar symptoms show evidence of neural degeneration. The course of this disease is variable. In some cases, patients may develop progressive vocal fold involvement leading to bilateral vocal fold paralysis and acute respiratory distress. Polio patients with swallowing complaints require a thorough laryngeal and voice assessment to evaluate for coexistent laryngeal pathology in addition to identifying appropriate therapy for dysphagia.

Disorders of the Peripheral Nervous System

The recurrent laryngeal nerves (RLNs) and external branches of the superior laryngeal nerves (SLNs) supply motor innervation to the laryngeal muscles, providing support for fine laryngeal control, as described in Table 1. The conduction velocity is high, estimated to be 50 m/s. Although the innervation ratio of fibers per motor unit in the human larynx is unknown, the laryngeal muscles are somewhat unique in that single muscle fibers have multiple neuromuscular junctions from the same nerve fiber.[12] Multiple innervations per fiber would support an ability to control precisely the laryngeal muscles during phonation for parameters such as fundamental frequency.

Table 1 Characteristic Functions of the Laryngeal Muscles in Vocal Fold Adjustments

Vocal Fold	CT	VOC	LCA	IA	PCA
Position	Paramed	*Adduct*	*Adduct*	*Adduct*	*Abduct*
Level	Lower	Lower	*Lower*	0	*Elevate*
Length	*Elongate*	*Shorten*	Elongate	(Shorten)	*Elongate*
Thickness	*Thin*	*Thicken*	Thin	(Thicken)	Thin
Edge	*Sharpen*	*Round*	Sharpen	0	Round
Muscle (body)	*Stiffen*	*Stiffen*	Stiffen	(Slacken)	Stiffen
Mucosa (cover and transition)	*Stiffen*	*Slacken*	Stiffen	(Slacken)	Stiffen

Reproduced with permission from reference 1.

0 = no effect; ( ) = slightly; italics = markedly; CT = cricothyroid; IA = interarytenoid; PCA = posterior cricoarytenoid; LCA = lateral cricoarytenoid; VOC = vocalis.

Lesions of the tenth cranial nerve at any point along its pathway from the nucleus ambiguus in the brainstem to the musculature cause paresis or paralysis of the laryngeal muscles resulting in dysphonia or even aphonia. The extent of vocal fold weakness and the degree of dysphonia depend upon degree of neural injury and the location of the lesion along this pathway.

EVALUATION OF VOICE FUNCTION

Clinical evaluation of dysphonia includes diagnostic procedures to determine the cause of the voice disorder, the degree of phonatory deficit, and the prognosis for recovery of function. Based on these assessments, therapeutic recommendations may involve behavioral, medical, or surgical treatment. The most effective treatment plan often includes a multidisciplinary approach, using complementary techniques. For example, patients who present with vocal fold polyp may require microflap removal. To optimize outcomes, preoperative voice therapy is often used to provide education on vocal hygiene and resonant voice techniques. Some diagnostic parameters measure the degree and nature of vocal impairment to determine appropriate intervention. Monitoring the patient's progress throughout treatment is essential to achieve a successful outcome. Because phonosurgery does not always result in a normal voice, the speech-language pathologist or laryngologist must decide whether difficulties in ease of phonation are structurally or behaviorally based. This is best accomplished with a combination of instrumental and perceptual tests.

Videostroboscopy

The importance of adequate visualization of the larynx during phonation and respiration cannot be overstated. These observations are easily made using laryngeal videostroboscopy, which allows viewing of the vibratory characteristics of the vocal folds, as well as opening and closing gestures. A description of vibratory characteristics of the vocal folds should include basic information about the (1) symmetry of bilateral movements, (2) regularity of vibration, (3) degree of glottal closure, (4) mucosal wave amplitude, (5) mucosal wave excursion, (6) adynamic regions, and (7) the opening-closing pattern of the glottis during the most closed phase.

Acoustic and Perceptual Measures

Perceptual assessment and acoustic objective measures are also useful in documenting progress and success of treatment. Measures of frequency and intensity characteristics of phonation should include fundamental frequency mean, vocal range, measures of vocal intensity, and vibration periodicity. Fundamental frequency is the acoustic correlate of pitch, measured in Hertz (Hz). Intensity, measured in decibels (dB), is the acoustic correlate of loudness. The range in each of these parameters reflects the flexibility of laryngeal dynamics available to the subject. Instrumental assessment of these factors as well as noise and harmonic structure in the voice signal is now available in a variety of computer-based systems designed specifically for voice analysis. Measures of the irregularity in frequency and intensity of the voice signal, also known as perturbation measures, may be useful in monitoring vocal performance in normal voices but often cannot be accurately used in dysphonia because of tracking difficulties for an abnormal signal. Jitter refers to cycle-to-cycle variation in time or period of vibration (frequency). Shimmer refers to variation in amplitude from cycle to cycle (intensity). Harmonics-to-noise ratio is often used to assess the degree of energy contained in harmonics of the fundamental frequency compared to turbulent noise between harmonics present during phonation. These values are thought to reflect abnormalities or asymmetries in mass, neural control, tension, and biomechanical characteristics of the vocal folds.

Aerodynamic Measures

Some measure of airflow or volume velocity is useful in determining how rapidly the air passes through the glottis. Mean airflow may be obtained from averaged measures over several glottal cycles. Mean airflow rates are useful in documenting change following phonosurgery, especially in surgical management of vocal fold paresis. Preoperative airflow is high and may return to normal after surgery. These measures are made using a pneumotachograph connected to a facemask placed over the face during voice production and, thus, provide indirect measure of laryngeal airflow.

Subglottal pressure is important for vocal fold vibration and for modulation of vocal intensity. Subglottal pressure may be measured indirectly by a pressure transducer placed in the oral cavity.[13] During production of sound "p" requiring lip closure, the vocal tract is a closed tube with equal pressure throughout. Pressure measured in the oral cavity reflects pressure beneath the glottis. In a related measure, glottal resistance is calculated by dividing subglottal pressure by mean airflow. Glottal resistance increases with vocal intensity and is thought to be low in cases of RLN paralysis. Phonation threshold pressure is the lowest subglottal pressure that a person can use to achieve phonation, and as such can be used as a measure of vocal fold stiffness.[14] These and other quantifiable measures are currently routinely used in the evaluation of voice deficits including vocal fold paralysis. The acquisition of self-perceptual and objective data is key in the treatment program of patients with neurogenic voice disorders.

Neurophysiological Measures of Voice and Laryngeal Function

Electromyographic (EMG) evaluation is a useful adjunct in the assessment of neuromuscular disorders and is often used in prognostic judgments about patients with those disorders. Electrical silence, fibrillation potentials, polyphasic potentials, high-amplitude potentials, and percentage of normal potentials are the basis for interpretation of such examinations. EMG may be useful in differentiating a variety of voice disorders: peripheral and central vocal fold paralysis, functional disorders and arytenoid joint fixation[15] (Table 2). Others have suggested the use of neuromyographic assessment that involves the direct stimulation of a laryngeal nerve in conjunction with the use of EMG to monitor resulting muscle activity. During this examination, the contraction of laryngeal muscles is monitored with EMG while the skin surface is stimulated in the area of the SLN. Transcranial magnetic stimulation over the mastoid can produce an action potential in the RLN as it emits from the skull, allowing measurement of the muscles response latency in the thyroarytenoid muscle.[16] This technique can also invoke a response in the efferent branch of the superior laryngeal nerve producing a response in the cricothyroid muscle. This is one means of obtaining an early estimate of the type and degree of laryngeal nerve injury. Compared with standard EMG, this technique may offer some advantage in monitoring the reinnervation of paralyzed laryngeal muscles following different reinnervation techniques.

LARYNGEAL PARALYSIS AND ASPIRATION

Vocal fold paralysis alone, rarely, results in aspiration unless the patient has a wide glottal gap. When vocal fold paralysis occurs in conjunction with other motor or sensory dysfunction, the combination may significantly impair the protective function of the larynx, leading to aspiration. Neurogenic causes of aspiration may include cerebrovascular accidents, degenerative

Table 2 Electromyographic Patterns in Relation to the Duration of Vocal Fold Paralysis

Muscle	Duration EMG	0–2 W	2 W–1 M	1–2 M	2–3 M	3–6 M	6–12 M	12 M+	Total
VOC	S	0	3	1	1	2	3	6	16
	F	1	3	11	5	6	0	5	31
	P	0	0	0	1	4	2	0	7
	H	0	0	1	0	0	0	0	1
	N or n	3	3	15	2	5	4	3	35
	Total	4	9	28	9	17	9	14	90
LCA	S	1	2	0	0	3	2	3	11
	F	1	6	7	7	8	0	4	33
	P	0	0	0	3	6	5	1	15
	H	0	0	1	0	1	1	0	3
	N or n	2	8	25	5	9	6	13	68
	Total	4	16	33	15	27	14	21	130
PCA	S	0	2	0	0	3	2	6	13
	F	0	5	11	7	4	0	4	31
	P	0	0	0	1	0	3	0	4
	H	0	0	1	0	0	0	0	1
	N or n	2	3	14	4	5	7	9	44
	Total	2	10	26	12	12	12	19	93

From reference 1.

F = fibrillation potentials; H = high-amplitude potentials; LCA = lateral cricoarytenoid; M = months of paralysis; n = normal potentials reduced in number; N = normal potential normal in number; P = polyphasic potentials; PCA = posterior cricoarytenoid; S = electrical silence; VOC = vocalis; W = weeks of paralysis.

When two or more different patterns were observed within a given muscle, the categorization in this table was made according to the following rule: F + S → F, P + x → P (x = any pattern), H + x → H, n + S and/or F → n, N + S and/or F → N.

diseases, neuromuscular disorders, peripheral nerve disorders, intracranial neoplasms, and anoxic or traumatic brain injury.

Evaluation of the patient with aspiration begins with a thorough history and physical examination and requires a multidisciplinary evaluation. The history should elicit information about associated neurological symptoms. These may suggest a generalized neurogenic disorder. In addition, information regarding baseline pulmonary status is critical, as this will dictate a patient's tolerance of minor or moderate aspiration. Physical examination should include a general physical examination, a detailed neurological examination, as well as a thorough evaluation of cranial nerve function. Other testing should include a modified barium swallow to evaluate the oral and pharyngeal phase of swallowing using contrast material of different consistencies (thin liquids, semi-solids, and solid food) performed with the guidance of a speech-language pathologist.

Nonsurgical management of the patient with aspiration usually consists of discontinuing oral intake and providing alternative methods of alimentation. Enteral alimentation is preferable and short-term feeding is usually provided by a nasogastric feeding tube. For long-term feeding, however, a gastrostomy or jejunostomy is usually preferred. Attention should also be given to pulmonary toilet. Tracheostomy may be helpful in caring for patients with copious secretions; however, the presence of a tracheostomy may also contribute to problems with aspiration.[17] Specific surgical treatment of the patient with significant aspiration and vocal fold paralysis includes a variety of procedures to medialize the vocal fold discussed in Chapter 80, "Laryngeal Paralysis." Patients in whom recovery of function is expected, procedures that are temporary or reversible are indicated, such as Cymetra or collagen injections.

For permanent difficulties with severe aspiration, other surgical techniques aim to separate the upper digestive tract from the upper respiratory tract.[18] Unfortunately, patients undergoing such procedures frequently lose the ability to phonate and may also require a permanent tracheostomy. Such procedures can be performed with low morbidity, and some of these procedures are at least theoretically reversible should function return.

Narrow-field laryngectomy remains the oldest and one of the most effective surgical treatments of aspiration. Tracheoesophageal puncture can be used to restore phonation. Reluctance by the patient to sacrifice their larynx has led to the development of other procedures to close the larynx. Montgomery described a glottic closure technique in which the true and false vocal cords were approximated. Closure was improved by Sasaki and associates with the interposition of a sternohyoid muscle flap.[19] This procedure was extremely effective but did not permit phonation, which was sometimes possible with supraglottic laryngeal closure methods. Since first being described in 1972, the epiglottic flap closure technique has undergone certain modifications, including intentionally leaving an opening posteriorly to permit phonation.[20] Successful reversal of this procedure with an endoscopic approach has been reported.[21] Biller and colleagues have also described a supraglottic closure technique with vertical laryngoplasty intended for use in patients undergoing total glossectomy.[22] This method also permits speech.

Efforts to devise a procedure that is completely reversible have led to the development of different endolaryngeal stents. Weisberger and Huebsch used a solid Silastic stent in conjunction with a tracheostomy[23] whereas Eliachar and Nguyen devised vented silicone stents that permit phonation.[24] Advantages of stenting include the use of the endoscopic approach and ease of reversibility. However, successful control of aspiration has not been uniform and long-term use of stents carries the risk of endolaryngeal injury, limiting their utility.

Tracheoesophageal diversion was developed by Lindeman with the goal of controlling aspiration definitively while preserving the larynx and RLNs and thus the potential for reversal. In this procedure, the trachea is divided at the level of the fourth or fifth ring. The proximal trachea is anastomosed to the esophagus; whereas the distal trachea is anastomosed to the skin. Thus, aspirated secretions are diverted back into the gastrointestinal tract. In the modified laryngotracheal separation procedure, the proximal segment is instead closed as a blind pouch.[25] Both techniques have provided good control of aspiration, and both have been successfully reversed. Because no current method is completely satisfactory, investigations continue in an attempt to find a safe, effective means of controlling aspiration without disrupting respiratory or phonatory function. One possibility for the future may be implantable electronic systems now being developed in animals that can produce tight glottic closure or hyolaryngeal elevation during swallowing.

SPASMODIC DYSPHONIAS

The spasmodic dysphonias (SDs) include *adductor* SD (uncontrolled closing of the vocal folds), *abductor* SD (prolonged vocal fold opening after voiceless sounds extending into vowels), or *vocal fold tremor* (modulations in phonatory pitch and loudness most evident during prolonged vowels). These disorders are characterized by involuntary changes in the ability to maintain voicing during speech either because of intermittent glottal catches (voice breaks) in the adductor type or breathy breaks due to prolonged vocal fold abductions in the abductor type. Only speech is affected; singing is less affected, and emotional expression (laughter and cry) and shout are unaffected. As the disorder progresses during the first 2 years, it may progress from only affecting vowel production during speech to interfering with other tasks or postures such as singing and speaking using falsetto. In mild to moderate forms of SD, patients may have uncontrolled spasms affecting only the speaking voice, with normal singing and falsetto phonation.

Onset often follows an upper respiratory infection, laryngeal injury or inflammation, a period of excessive voice use, or occupational or emotional stress. Increased effort is one of the major patient complaints along with loss of control and an increased difficulty with prolonged voice use or stress. Onset is characteristically between 30 and 50 years of age, and 60 to 80% of those affected are women. Characteristics include

1. Symptoms are specific to a particular task, gesture, or posture of the larynx (vowels and glottal stops in adductor SD and voice onset after voiceless consonants in abductor SD);
2. Symptoms are action induced, that is, they appear only with voluntary movement and are not usually apparent at rest;
3. Symptoms become worse with prolonged speaking, practice, or performance;
4. Onset is usually gradual, often following an upper respiratory infection, laryngeal inflammation or injury, or a stressful period;
5. Reflexive and emotional aspects of vocal function are unaffected, such as coughing, crying, shouting, and laughing;
6. In professional voice users, the symptoms may appear with heavy professional schedules or following injury.

In some patients, particularly those with abductor SD, some degree of vocal fold asymmetry may be apparent only during speech.[26]

Movement abnormalities occur when the patient attempts specific gestures such as phonation of vowels or voice initiation after glottal stops in adductor SD, or for initiation of voice after voiceless consonants (such as s, h, f, t, k) in abductor SD, or on prolonged vowels in a speaking voice in vocal tremor. The etiology of these disorders is unclear at this time. In some individuals, these disorders occur in persons with a family history of dystonia; however, this occurrence is rare.

Diagnosis and Assessment

Diagnosis and management of patients with SDs is best accomplished by a voice team including an otolaryngologist, a speech pathologist, a neurologist, and, in some cases, a psychiatrist. Because these movement disorders affect the larynx, diagnosis depends upon observing the vocal folds during speech and nonspeech gestures. In addition, the larynx must be visualized to rule out other disorders which could account for the symptoms. The laryngologist rules out vocal fold nodules, polyps, carcinoma, cysts, contact ulcers, inflammation (laryngitis), vocal fold paresis, or paralysis using fiberoptic laryngoscopy. A neurological examination is necessary to rule out amyotrophic lateral sclerosis, Parkinson disease, or supranuclear palsy, which can all produce vocal fold movement abnormalities. Some patients may also have concomitant focal dystonias such as writer's cramp or blepharospasm. Many patients may have some degree of laryngeal tremor in addition to spasmodic hyperadduction or hyperabduction. These patients are usually included as a subtype of the spasmodic dysphonias and may have a more severe disorder.

An extensive history, a trial of voice therapy, and a psychosocial interview may be needed to rule out psychogenic dysphonia. Patients may have psychosocial reactions as a result of their voice disorder, confounding the ability to differentiate idiopathic SD from psychogenic disorders through history and interview. For example, many patients will no longer use the telephone and avoid social gatherings as a result of having a speech disorder. Voice disorders have not been found to produce mental illness, however.

Tasks to Be Examined during Fiberoptic Laryngoscopy

Both speech and nonspeech tasks must be sampled to identify (1) movement control abnormalities during vocal fold abduction (opening) and adduction (closing) in speech and (2) movement during nonspeech items such as respiration, sniffing, throat clearing, whistling, and singing. This is in contrast to paradoxical vocal fold movement disorder (PVFMD) where vocal fold abnormalities may only appear during inspiratory breathing but not speaking.

Fiberoptic laryngoscopy is useful in evaluating patients with dysphonia associated with neurological disorders for vocal fold movement during speaking. Usually, stroboscopy is less helpful because patients with tremor or spasms do not have regular phonatory cycles that can be tracked from the contact microphone or electroglottographic signal. Further, in patients with other functional voice disorders, such as muscular tension dysphonia, the severe signal aperiodicity similarly interferes with tracking of the stroboscopy light source, rendering stroboscopic interpretation meaningless. The emerging use of kymography and eventually high-speed video will be particularly useful for examining vocal fold vibration in such patients, as these techniques do not rely on signal periodicity.[2,3]

Speech Testing

Voice symptoms should be compared during following three tasks to discriminate between adductor spasmodic dysphonia, abductor spasmodic dysphonia, and vocal tremor:

1. Prolonged vowel phonation usually manifests tremor if it is present. Prolonged vowel production is affected only in the more severe forms of adductor and abductor SD.
2. Production of sentences in which most sounds are voiced and contact glottal stop at word boundaries, for example, "We mow our lawn all year" and "We eat eels every day," are usually most difficult and demonstrate frequent breaks or voice arrest in adductor spasmodic dysphonia.
3. Production of sentences with voiceless consonants (s, t, p, k, h), for example, "She speaks pleasingly," "Keep Tom at the party," "When he comes home we'll feed him," are usually most difficult in abductor spasmodic dysphonia. Sentences with predominantly voiced sounds are much easier to produce and smoother for these patients.

Electromyography

The laryngeal muscle activation abnormalities differ greatly across patients and can account for the wide variety of symptoms. The laryngeal muscles should be examined using laryngeal electromyography to determine which muscles contain spasms concurrent with a patient's voice symptoms during speech. In adductor SD, the thyroarytenoid is the most often affected muscle. In abductor SD, spasms can be seen either in the cricothyroid or the posterior cricoarytenoid muscles as well as asymmetries in thyroarytenoid muscle activation during speech. In others, no spastic activity is identifiable and the thyroarytenoid muscle is inactive during vowels, that is, a "negative dystonia."

In vocal tremor, a variety of muscles can be involved. Most often the thyroarytenoid is affected, but other muscles including the strap muscles can be affected including the thyrohyoid, the sternothyroid, and in some patients with abductor tremor, either the cricothyroid or posterior cricoarytenoid, or both. By using a concentric EMG electrode connected to an amplifier with a dual channel storage oscilloscope, one channel for the EMG and another for the speech waveform, at a slow sweep speed, quick identification can be made of the muscles having spasms during voice breaks.

For the thyroarytenoid and lateral cricoarytenoid muscles, items to be examined for spasmodic bursts concurrent with voice breaks include prolonged "ee," repeated "ee," and all voiced sentences such as "We mow our lawn all year." When examining abductor SD, while recording from the cricothyroid or posterior cricoarytenoid, speech should include "see-see-see," "pea-pea-pea," "he-he-he," "Kathy took a potato," and "Keep Tom at the party." Muscles with bursts of activity before and during voice breaks can be considered for injection with botulinum toxin injection.

Treatment

In the last 20 years, the following treatments have been used for managing symptoms of patients with adductor spasmodic dysphonia.

Voice Therapy. Voice therapy can assist mildly affected patients but may not have long-lasting effects. When uncertain of the diagnosis of a patient's voice disorder, a trial of voice therapy is recommended. Usually within three sessions, a speech pathologist experienced in voice therapy will report whether or not voice therapy might be beneficial for a patient. Voice therapy may also be helpful after botulinum toxin injection by prolonging the benefit period.[27]

Recurrent Laryngeal Nerve Section. Dedo[28] first described unilateral removal of a short segment of the RLN below the thyroid isthmus for the treatment of adductor SD in 1976. The procedure resulted in an initial dramatic reduction or elimination of voice spasms, but symptoms may recur in up to 64% of cases.[29] Recurrence of symptoms has been attributed to reinnervation of the operated side based on electromyographic and histological studies. Those patients failing surgery may still respond to botulinum toxin injections. Due to the high rate of symptom recurrence, the permanent alteration in laryngeal function, and the requirements for subsequent medialization surgery in some patients with excessive breathiness, RLN section is less preferred to botulinum toxin injections at the present time.

Recurrent Laryngeal Nerve Avulsion. Netterville and his colleagues[30] proposed a more extensive removal of the recurrent nerve in an effort to reduce the risk of reinnervation into the distal stump of the sectioned recurrent laryngeal nerve. After mobilization of the ipsilateral thyroid lobe, all branches of the RLN are identified, traced, and avulsed from their muscular insertions deep to the cricopharyngeus muscle. The total length of RLN removed averages 9 cm, in contrast to an average of 2 cm reported in previous RLN section studies. Long-term follow-up, 3 to 7 years, on 18 patients following recurrent laryngeal nerve avulsion revealed that 16 patients (89%) were free of SD symptoms at 3 years.[31] Two of these patients, however, later developed recurrent spasms following medialization laryngoplasty for treatment of a breathy voice. Thus, an overall success rate of 78% (14/18) was reported for this series which compares favorably to long-term recurrence rates for the more limited RLN section. Weed and colleagues recommend that RLN avulsion be reserved for patients who do not benefit from or do not tolerate botulinum toxin injections and for patients who have failed prior RLN section.[31]

Selective Laryngeal Adductor Denervation Reinnervation. Berke and colleagues published preliminary results with selective bilateral denervation of the laryngeal adductor muscles in an attempt to achieve a permanent bilateral adductor weakness that mimics the transient effects of botulinum toxin injection.[32] This procedure involves bilateral section of the adductor RLN branches to the thyroarytenoid and lateral cricoarytenoid muscles while preserving the natural innervation of the posterior cricoarytenoid muscle. In addition, the distal thyroarytenoid branches are reinnervated using branches of the ansa cervicalis nerve. The aim of this directed reinnervation is to prevent unwanted reinnervation by RLN efferents and to preserve adductor muscle tone.

The study presented 1- to 5-year follow-up on 21 patients with adductor SD who underwent the procedure. In general, symptoms and overall severity of SD improved from moderate to severe ratings preoperatively to mild to absent ratings postoperatively. All patients experienced severe vocal fold bowing and breathiness in the early postoperative period that improved after 3 to 6 months. Aspiration of greater than 2 weeks duration was noted in 2 patients, one of whom required hospitalization for aspiration pneumonia. Additional treatments (botulinum toxin, voice therapy, collagen injection, thyroarytenoid myotomy) were also performed in several patients to enhance the postoperative voice result. These authors have subsequently published an analysis of the long-term results of these procedures.[33] The average follow-up was 49 months. A total of 83 patients filled out pre- and postoperative Voice Handicap Index (VHI) scores with an improvement from 36 to 13. Eighty-three percent

of the subjects showed improvement in the VHI. Perception evaluation of voice samples after surgery revealed voice breaks in 26% of the subjects. The authors report promising results with normal conversational voice intensity, good inflection in most patients, and patient satisfaction of 91%.

Botulinum Toxin. This approach was developed in 1987 and has been evaluated using unilateral or bilateral thyroarytenoid injections in adductor spasmodic dysphonia.[34] Significant voice improvement occurs in 70% of patients for up to 3 months, followed by gradual symptom return over a 1- to 3-month period. Patients are usually treated three to four times per year. Difficulties associated with this treatment include the wide variability of dosing response. Whereas the average patient receiving a bilateral injection is treated with a total of 4 units, patients may receive from 0.375 units up to 12 units. In patients receiving unilateral treatments, dosing may vary from 0.25 units up to 30 units. Identifying the ideal dosing is by trial and error.

The most commonly used method of injection is the percutaneous EMG-guided approach through the cricothyroid membrane. The injection needle is Teflon coated except for the bared tip which serves as a monopolar electromyographic electrode when the bared hub is connected to an EMG amplifier. This allows monitoring of the needle tip into active muscles, avoiding areas of dennervation. Placing the medication at the site of active units within the muscle is the optimal treatment location.

To approach the thyroarytenoid (TA) muscle percutaneously, the needle is angled superiorly and slightly laterally to approximate the vocalis portion of the TA muscle. However, the needle tip can easily be placed more posteriorly than intended, medial to the lateral cricoarytenoid (LCA) muscle. From this, it is apparent that posteriorly placed injections may dennervate portions of the LCA and cricothyroid (CT) muscles, in addition to the TA either by direct injection of these muscles or by diffusion across fascial planes. This could account for the variability in response that is often seen (1) among patients and (2) in the same patient from consecutive EMG-guided injections several months apart, although the same technique and dosages are used.

Two approaches have been used, either large unilateral injections producing unilateral vocal fold paresis or small bilateral injections which do not alter vocal fold mobility.[35] The long-term effects of repeated needle insertion and repeated dennervation by botulinum toxin on laryngeal

muscles are as yet unknown. Muscle biopsies in blepharospasm patients treated repeatedly with botulinum toxin injection have demonstrated significant muscle scarring and atrophy.[36] Similar changes in both thyroarytenoid muscles could have long-term effects on airway protection.

The disadvantage of the unilateral injection approach is that a large dosage of toxin must be administered, and immobility of the injected fold often results. An advantage of the bilateral approach is that much smaller dosages of botulinum toxin can be used, reducing the cost, and effective symptom control can be obtained without any observable change in range of motion. Partial dennervation seems to be effective in reducing the degree of hyperadduction, resulting in less interference with phonation. The disadvantages are that injections and needle insertions are performed on both sides of the larynx. With repeated injections over many years, damage might result to both sides of the larynx. A few patients lose symptom control over a period of many years with continued injections, although the mechanisms for the loss of benefit is not clear.[37] Some of these patients may be managed by switching injection sides and beginning treatment in a previously noninjected muscle resulting in the return of symptom control. Other injection techniques which utilize visualization of the vocal folds rather than electromyography to guide placement of the injection needle include the indirect laryngoscopic peroral method, a transcartilaginous method, as well as injection using a flexible catheter through a channeled laryngoscope. The usual dosages used by each technique are presented in Table 3.

Within 5 days of TA muscle botulinum toxin injection, the numbers of breaks in phonation on vowels are reduced, the presence of voice roughness or hoarseness is reduced on spectrographic analyses, and speech rate is increased.[39] Patients' subjective reports include a reduction in speech effort and tension, reduced numbers of breaks, and greater voice control. Two major side effects are reported, breathiness and swallowing difficulties. These side effects do not occur in all patients; however, they are dose-dependent affects.

Botulinum toxin injections have been employed in abductor spasmodic dysphonia in both the CT and the posterior cricoarytenoid muscles. Only about two-thirds of persons with abductor SD are benefited and to a lesser degree than those with adductor SD following TA muscle injections.[44] The effects of vocal tremor on voice production can also be reduced by

Table 3 Usual Dosages Used for Unilateral and Bilateral Injection of the Thyroarytenoid Muscle in Adductor Spasmodic Dysphonia

Injection Technique	EMG Guided[38]	Peroral[41]	Transcartilaginous[42]	Endoscopic[43]
Unilateral (units)	15[39]	2.5		6
Bilateral (units per side)	2.5[40]	2.5	2	2

EMG = electromyography.
Superscript numbers indicate references.

botulinum toxin injection; however, the outcome is less predictable and not all persons with vocal tremor are benefited.[45] In those patients with tremor affecting only the vocal folds and involving just the TA muscles, this treatment can be as effective as in adductor spasmodic dysphonia. However, many patients with this disorder have involvement of the strap muscles and have limited benefit even when these additional muscles are injected. Great care should be exercised with strap muscle injections due to significant concerns over aspiration symptoms.

MUSCULAR TENSION DYSPHONIA

Muscular tension dysphonia was first described by Morrison and his colleagues[46] as dysphonia resulting from increased muscular tension in the larynx and neck associated with (1) palpably increased phonatory muscle tension in the paralaryngeal and suprahyoid muscles, (2) elevation of the larynx in the neck on increasing vocal pitch, (3) an open posterior glottic chink between the arytenoid cartilages on phonation, and (4) variable degrees of mucosal changes such as vocal nodules or chronic laryngitis. These patients are thought to have a high level of anxiety and may have learned an abnormal pattern of laryngeal muscle use.

Not infrequently patients with voice tremor or adductor SD also present with muscular tension dysphonia making diagnosis difficult, particularly in patients with more severe symptoms. Such patients may also have medial hyperadduction of the supraglottic structures. It is unclear whether this additional muscular tension is part of the SD or tremor disorder or the result of the patient using a compensatory strategy to prevent instability during vocal fold vibration for speech. In some patients, the muscular tension dissipates following injection of botulinum toxin whereas in others, voice therapy may be a helpful adjunct in alleviating some of this tension following botulinum toxin injection.

The distinction between muscular tension dysphonia and adductor SD can be the degree to which the abnormal laryngeal posture is used consistently for voice production (Table 4). In muscular tension dysphonia and other variants of vocal misuse, the abnormal vocal fold positioning seen on fiberoptic videoendoscopy is consistent regardless of the type of speech. In the spasmodic dysphonias, the abnormalities are intermittent depending upon the voicing gesture required and contain irregular rapid adductor or abductor movements causing intermittent voice breaks on particular types of speech sounds, vowels in adductor SD, and prolonged voiceless consonants in abductor SD. In benign essential tremor, these intermittent voice breaks are regular, usually around 5 Hz. However, in some of the more extreme forms of spasmodic dysphonia and/or muscular tension dysphonia, the differentiation can be difficult because the spasmodic involuntary movement abnormalities may be difficult to identify when patients have extreme muscular tension. Whenever a possibility of either diagnosis exists, a trial of voice therapy by a speech pathologist experienced in treatment of these disorders is recommended, before considering botulinum toxin. Muscle tension dysphonia is also discussed in Chapter 81, "Muscle Misuse Disorders of the Larynx".

Table 4 Movement Characteristics Observed during Fiberoptic Laryngoscopy in Various Types of Laryngeal Movement Disorders

Task	Movement Examined	Adductor SD	Abductor SD	Tremor Adductor	Tremor Abductor	Paradoxical Vocal Fold Movement Disorder	Muscular Tension Dysphonia
Deep inhalation	Abduction range	Normal abduction	May be increased	Normal	May have tremor	Vocal fold adduction	Normal
Prolonged vowel "ee"	Adduction for voice	Normal or intermittent hyperadductions	Normal	Repetitive hyperadductions (5 Hz)	Repetitive abductions (5 Hz)	Normal	Constant hyperadduction
Throat clear three times	Adduction	Normal	Normal	Normal	Normal	Normal	Normal
Whisper	Vocal fold partial abduction	May have hyperadduction	May have increased abduction	Normal	May have tremor	Normal	May have constant adduction
Whistling	Vocal fold abduction and adduction	Normal	Normal	Normal	Normal	Normal	Normal
Repeated and quick sniffs	Speed of abduction	Normal	May be increased in range	Normal	May have tremor on abduction	Adduction on sniff	Normal
Alternating between sniff and vowel "ee"	Speed and range of abduction and adduction	Intermittent hyperadduction on vowel	Normal	Tremor on vowel	Tremor on vowel	May have hyperadduction on sniff	Constant hyperadduction on vowel
Rapid repetition of vowel "ee" six times	Phonation offset owing to glottal stop	Prolonged glottal stops	Normal	Tremor on vowel	Tremor on vowel	Normal	Constant hyperadduction with anteroposterior squeeze
Rapid repetition of "see" six times	Speed of abduction and adduction	Normal or intermittent adductions on vowel	Prolonged abductions during "s"	Adductor tremor on vowel	Abductor tremor on vowel	Normal	Constant hyperadduction
Ascending and descending glides	Controlled lengthening and shortening of folds	Normal or intermittent adductions on low end	Normal	Adductor tremor on low end	Abductor tremor	Normal	Constant hyperadduction
Sentences: "We eat eels every day"	Glottal stops in sentences	Prolonged glottal stops	Normal	Adductor tremor	Abductor tremor	Normal	Constant hyperadduction
"The waves were rolling along"	Constant voicing in sentences	Intermittent spasms in vowels	Normal	Adductor tremor	Abductor tremor	Normal	Constant hyperadduction
"He will keep the keys"	Voiceless consonants in sentences	Normal	Prolonged voiceless consonants "he," "k"	Adductor tremor	Abductor tremor	Normal	Constant hyperadduction

SD = spasmodic dysphonia.

PARADOXICAL VOCAL FOLD MOVEMENT

Paradoxical vocal fold movement (PVFM) is the adduction of the vocal folds during the inspiratory phase of respiration producing impaired inspiratory airflow and stridor. These patients have normal vocal fold movement during speech yet have breathing difficulties on inspiration during connected speech. This disorder may be categorized as (1) an idiopathic focal dystonia or part of Meige syndrome[47]; (2) associated with or masquerading as asthma[48]; (3) exercise-induced stridor[49]; (4) psychogenic[50]; and, (5) associated with laryngopharyngeal reflux.[51] Most cases of PVFM have been reported as psychogenic. In such cases, the symptoms abate following psychotherapy and speech therapy.

The first presentation of PVFM as a focal laryngeal dystonia specific to inspiration suggested that in some patients this is not psychogenic, but rather due to involuntary spasmodic bursts in the thyroarytenoid muscle.[47] Patients with a focal dystonia report that the symptoms are not present during sleep, but that the symptoms are often present during the daytime and may become exacerbated by exercise and stress. Some success with bilateral thyroarytenoid injection of botulinum toxin has been reported in selected cases not responsive to speech therapy, psychotherapy, and pharmacology.[52]

Patients with Meige syndrome, an orofacial dyskinesia, can develop pharyngeal spasms producing intermittent airway obstruction, either because of pharyngeal constriction or obstruction at the epiglottis. Again, the symptoms are absent during sleep, almost always present during the day, but are exacerbated by stress.

Patients with chronic asthma can have laryngeal vocal fold adduction during asthmatic attacks.[48] However, the underlying pathophysiology has been hypothesized as either psychological overlay, a learned response, or a dystonic reaction following many years of inhalant use for disease management. Exercise-induced asthma has also been reported to have a laryngeal adduction component.[49]

Loughlin and Koufman have suggested that gastroesophageal reflux is a common cause of paroxysmal laryngospasms.[51] Patients presented with intermittent, sudden-onset, noisy obstructed breathing, that some termed choking episodes. These attacks of stridor often occurred following a meal, after the start of exercise, or after bending over. Sometimes they occurred at night. The number of reported episodes can range from twice a day to twice a year. These attacks usually last a few minutes. All complained of symptoms of reflux such as a lump in the throat, chronic throat clearing, cough, intermittent hoarseness, and difficulty swallowing. All responded well to life style modification and omeprazole 20 mg b.i.d.

REFERENCES

1. Hirano M. Clinical Examination of Voice. New York: Springer-Verlag Wien 1981. p. 1–98.
2. Qiu Q, Schutte HK. A new generation videokymography for routine clinical vocal fold examination. Laryngoscope 2006;116:1824–8.
3. Yan Y, Chen X, Bless D. Automatic tracing of vocal-fold motion from high-speed digital images. IEEE Trans Biomed Eng 2006;53:1394–400.
4. Rodel RM, Olthoff A, Tergau F, et al. Human cortical motor representation of the larynx as assessed by transcranial magnetic stimulation (TMS). Laryngoscope 2004;114:918–22.
5. Dyck PJ, Litchy WJ, Minnerath S, et al. Hereditary motor and sensory neuropathy with diaphragm and vocal cord paresis. Ann Neurol 1994;35:608–15.
6. Hanson DG, Gerratt BR, Ward PH. Cinegraphic observations of laryngeal function in Parkinson's disease. Laryngoscope 1984;94:348–53.
7. Hanson DG, Ludlow CL, Bassich CJ. Vocal fold paresis and Shy-Drager syndrome. Ann Otol Rhinol Laryngol 1983;92:85–90.
8. Ramig LO, Countryman S, O'Brien C, et al. Intensive speech treatment for patients with Parkinson's disease: Short- and long-term comparison of two techniques. Neurology 1996;47:1496–504.
9. Berke GS, Gerratt B, Kreiman J, Jackson K. Treatment of Parkinson hypophonia with percutaneous collagen augmentation. Laryngoscope 1999;109:1295–9.
10. Bryce GE, Morrison MD. Botulinum toxin treatment of essential palatal myoclonus tinnitus. J Otolaryngol 1998;27:213–6.
11. Kluin KJ, Bromberg MB, Feldman EL, Simmons Z. Dysphagia in elderly men with myasthenia gravis. J Neurol Sci 1996;138:49–52.
12. Perie S, Guily JL, Callard P, Sebille A. Innervation of adult human laryngeal muscle fibers. Neurol Res 1997;149:81–6.
13. Smitheran JR, Hixon TJ. A clinical method for estimating laryngeal airway resistance during vowel production. J Speech Hear Disord 1981;46:138–46.
14. Titze IR. Phonation threshold pressure: A missing link in glottal aerodynamics. J Acoust Soc Am 1992;91:2926–35.
15. Kotby MN, Fadly E, Madkour O, et al. Electromyography and neurography in neurolaryngology. J Voice 1992;6:159–87.
16. Sims S, Yamashita T, Rhew k, Ludlow CL. An evaluation of the use of magnetic stimulation to measure laryngeal muscle response latencies in normal subjects. Otolaryngol Head Neck Surg 1996;114:761–7.
17. Nash M. Swallowing problems in the tracheotomized patient. Otolaryngol Clin North Am 1988;21:701–9.
18. Eibling DE, Snyderman CH, Eibling C. Laryngotrachcal separation for intractable aspiration: A retrospective review of 34 patients. Laryngoscope 1995;105:83–5.
19. Sasaki CT, Milmoe G, Yanagisawa E, et al. Surgical closure of the larynx for aspiration. Arch Otolaryngol Head Neck Surg 1980;106:422–3.
20. Vecchione TR, Habal MB, Murray JE. Further experiences with the arytenoid-epiglottic flap for chronic aspiration pneumonia. Plas Reconstr Surg 1975;55:318–23.
21. Strome M, Fried MP. Rehabilitative surgery for aspiration: A clinical analysis. Arch Otolaryngol Head Neck Surg 1983;109:809–11.
22. Biller HF, Lawson W, Baek SML. Total glossectomy: A technique of reconstruction eliminating laryngectomy. Arch Otolaryngol 1983;109:69–73.
23. Weisberger C, Huebsch SA. Endoscopic treatment of aspiration using a laryngeal stent. Otolaryngol Head Neck Surg 1982;90:215–22.
24. Eliachar I, Nguyen D. Laryngotracheal stent for internal support and control of aspiration without loss of phonation. Otolaryngol Head Neck Surg 1990;103:837–40.
25. Lindeman RC, Yarington CT, Sutton D. Clinical experience with the tracheoesophageal anastomosis for intractable aspiration. Ann Otol Rhinol Laryngol 1976;85:609–12.
26. Cyrus CB, Bielamowicz S, Evans FJ, Ludlow CL. Adductor muscle activity abnormalities in abductor spasmodic dysphonia. Otolaryngol Head Neck Surg 2001;124:23–30.
27. Murry T, Woodson GE. Combined-modality treatment of adductor spasmodic dysphonia with botulinum toxin and voice therapy. J Voice 1995;9:460–5.
28. Dedo HH. Recurrent laryngeal nerve section for spastic dysphonia. Ann Otol Rhinol Laryngol 1976;85:451–459.
29. Aronson AE, Desanto LW. Adductor spasmodic dysphonia: Three years after recurrent nerve section. Laryngoscope 1983;93:1–8.
30. Netterville JL, Stone RE, Rainey C, et al. Recurrent laryngeal nerve avulsion for treatment of spastic dysphonia. Ann Otol Rhinol Laryngol 1991;100:10–4.
31. Weed DT, Jewett BS, Rainey C, et al. Long-term follow-up of recurrent laryngeal nerve avulsion for the treatment of spastic dysphonia. Ann Otol Rhinol Laryngol 1996;105:592–601.
32. Berke GS, Blackwell KE, Gerratt RR, et al. Selective laryngeal adductor denervation-reinnervation: A new surgical treatment for adductor spasmodic dysphonia. Ann Otol Rhinol Laryngol 1999;108:227–31.
33. Chhetri DK, Mendelsohn AH, Blumin JH, Berke GS. Long-term follow-up results of selective laryngeal adductor denervation-reinnervation surgery for adductor spasmodic dysphonia. Laryngoscope 2006;116:635–42.
34. Blitzer A, Brin MF, Stewart CF. Botulinum toxin management of spasmodic dysphonia (laryngeal dystonia): A 12-year experience in more than 900 patients. Laryngoscope 1998;108:1435–41.
35. Bielamowicz S, Stager SV, Badillo A, Godlewski A. Unilateral versus bilateral injections of botulinum toxin in patients with adductor spasmodic dysphonia. J Voice 2002;16:117–23.
36. Borodic GE, Ferrante R. Effects of repeated botulinum toxin injections on orbicularis oculi muscle. J Clin Neuro-opthal 1992;12:121–7.
37. Smith ME, Ford CN. Resistance to botulinum toxin injections for spasmodic dysphonia. Arch Otolaryngol Head Neck Surg 2000;126:533–5.
38. NIH concensus development conference statement: Clinical use of botulinum toxin. Arch Neruol 1991;48:1294–8.
39. Ludlow CL, Naunton RF, Sedory SE, et al. Effects of botulinum toxin injections on speech in adductor spasmodic dysphonia. Neurology 1988;38:1220–5.
40. Blitzer A, Brin MF, Fahn S, Lovelace RE. Localized injections of botulinum toxin for the treatment of focal laryngeal dystonia (spastic dysphonia). Laryngoscope 1988;98:193–7.
41. Ford CN, Bless DM, Lowery JD. Indirect laryngoscopic approach for injection of botulinum toxin in spasmotic dysphonia. Otolaryngol Head Neck Surg 1990;103:752–8.
42. Green DC, Berke GS, Ward PH, Gerratt BR. Point-touch technique of botulinum toxin injection for treatment of spasmotic dysphonia. Ann Otol Rhinol Laryngol 1992;101:883–7.
43. Rhew K, Fredler DA, Ludlow CL. Technique for injection of botulinum toxin through the flexible nasolaryngoscope. Otolaryngol Head Neck Surg 1994;111:787–94.
44. Bielamowicz S, Squire S, Bidus K, Ludlow CL. Assessment of posterior cricoarytenoid botulinum toxin injections in patients with abductor spasmodic dysphonia. Ann Otol Rhinol Laryngol 2001;110:406–12.
45. Warrick P, Dromey C, Irish JC, et al. Botulinum toxin for essential tremor of the voice with multiple anatomical sites of tremor: A crossover design study of unilateral versus bilateral injection. Laryngoscope 2000;110:1366–74.
46. Morrison MD, Rammage LA, Belisle GM, et al. Muscular tension dysphonia. J Otolaryngol 1983;12:302–6.
47. Marion MH, Klap P, Perrin A, Cohen M. Stridor and focal laryngeal dystonia. Lancet 1992;339:457–8.
48. Christopher KL, Wood R, Eckert RC, et al. Vocal-cord dysfunction presenting as asthma. New Engl J Med 1983;306:1566–70.
49. Hurbis CG, Schild JA. Laryngeal changes during exercise and exercise-induced asthma. Ann Otol Rhinol Laryngol 1991;100:34–7.
50. Craig T, Sitz K, Squire E, et al. Vocal cord dysfunction during wartime. Mil Med 1992;157:614–6.
51. Loughlin CJ, Koufman JA. Paroxysmal laryngospasm secondary to gastroesophageal reflux. Laryngoscope 1996;106:1501–5.
52. Grillone GA, Blitzer A, Brin MF, et al. Treatment of adductor laryngeal breathing dystonia with botulinum toxin type A. Laryngoscope 1994;24:30–2.

80

Laryngeal Paralysis

Lucian Sulica, MD

Paralysis of one or both vocal folds may compromise any of the important physiologic functions of the larynx, that is, breathing, swallowing, and voicing. Individuals with laryngeal hemiparesis typically complain of a broad range of symptoms reflecting variable degrees of glottic insufficiency. The most prominent of these are breathy dysphonia and dysphagia, particularly for liquids. Breathlessness while speaking and breathlessness during physical activity may also be present. When both vocal folds are involved, patients generally complain of symptoms of glottic obstruction like stridor and dyspnea. The distinction in symptoms between unilateral and bilateral paralysis arises from the two essentially opposed valving tasks of the larynx: glottic opening for respiration, and glottic closure for airway protection, thoracic stabilization during effortful activity, and phonation.

The first important clinical task in the evaluation of an individual with vocal fold motion impairment is to identify and treat the cause, if possible. In the majority of cases, vocal fold immobility or hypomobility is caused by disease or injury of the peripheral laryngeal nerves. Less commonly, laryngeal paralysis results from central nervous system damage. Rarely, mechanical factors may result in cricoarytenoid fixation, usually after prolonged intubation or other obvious laryngeal trauma.

Effective and rational management of symptoms follows the search for the cause of paralysis. Some cases of paralysis resolve or at least improve symptomatically, without intervention, whereas others require treatment. Distinguishing between these two groups remains a challenge, and many otolaryngologists consequently choose to delay treatment, sometimes despite considerable patient disability, until the possibility of spontaneous recovery is judged remote. In patients with unilateral paralysis, a variety of procedures are available to alleviate symptoms in almost any clinical situation, regardless of prognosis. Temporary and permanent injection medialization, medialization laryngoplasty, arytenoid cartilage repositioning surgery, and reinnervation procedures have all been used with varying degrees of success. On the other hand, treatment options in bilateral immobility are less satisfactory, occasionally requiring the sacrifice of some voice quality to establish an adequate airway.

PATHOPHYSIOLOGIC CONCEPTS

In the majority of cases, laryngeal paralysis is the result of peripheral nerve damage, typically from a variety of mechanical traumas. Although the superior laryngeal nerve may or may not be affected (and in fact, may be affected alone, a clinical situation which will not be reviewed here), the fibers of the recurrent nerve at least must be involved to cause gross vocal fold immobility.

Generally speaking, mild pressure on a peripheral nerve produces segmental demyelination and impairs axonal transport, the degree and severity of the conduction block being proportional to the severity of the injury. Remyelinization over a preserved axon usually restores nerve conduction and function. Injuries which interrupt the axon, such as nerve section or severe crush, produce wallerian degeneration along the entire length of the nerve distal to the injury beginning within 24 hours of injury. Functional recovery depends on preservation of neural conduits for axonal regeneration. The basal lamina of the original nerve fibers may be preserved in a severe crush injury (axonotmesis), and proximal axonal sprouts may reach the appropriate muscle. If the nerve is transected (neurotmesis), the proportion of nerve fibers that find their way to the original target is low and inversely proportional to the size of the gap between proximal and distal segments.

Regeneration of the recurrent nerve is more problematic than that of most peripheral nerves, because it carries a mixed population of adductor and abductor fibers. Furthermore, laryngeal paralysis turns out to be a heterogeneous condition according to many clinical criteria, for example, symptoms, vocal fold position, and electromyographic evidence of the degree of nerve damage.[1–2] Unless due to severe trauma like transection, each case differs from the next in degree of neural impairment, and features a mix of injury types among its nerve fibers. This latter aspect is a principal reason why the Seddon classification of nerve injury, reviewed in the previous paragraph, is not entirely useful or satisfactory in vocal fold paralysis.

In addition, both human and animal studies have shown that the larynx has a strong propensity for reinnervation.[2–4] In fact, reinnervation appears to be the rule rather than the exception, even after deliberate recurrent nerve section, as was formerly done for the treatment of spasmodic dysphonia.[5,6] A paralyzed vocal fold is thus only sometimes, and perhaps quite rarely, a denervated vocal fold.

In many cases, however, vocal fold reinnervation is dysfunctional and does not yield physiologic motion. This neural dysfunction extends beyond traditional notions of synkinesis, in which co-contraction of adductor and abductor fibers produces no net vocal fold motion; after all, such perfectly balanced antagonism is an extremely improbable outcome of a largely random process. Dysfunctional reinnervation may also result when nerve regrowth is appropriate but inadequate, which may result in decreased force of contraction, loss of motor unit specificity, increased muscle fatigue, and possibly also in changes in neural organization peripherally and centrally.[7] The complex, highly specialized nature of the laryngeal neuromotor system leaves many ways in which reinnervation may miscarry.

Vocal fold innervation has traditionally been conceptualized as an all-or-none phenomenon, with paralysis or, more precisely, absence of motion, resulting from a lack of neural input. This view is clearly oversimplified and inaccurate. Vocal fold paralysis is probably best considered as a continuum of neurogenic dysfunction encompassing partial denervation, complete denervation, and variable degrees and patterns of reinnervation.

This has at least two important clinical implications. First, differing degrees and patterns of innervation probably account for variability in the position of the paralyzed vocal fold. For most of the last century, vocal fold position was thought to reveal the site or type of lesion, beliefs that have no physiologic basis and, moreover, have been invalidated by careful clinical and laboratory work.[8–10] Terms like "paramedian" and "cadaveric" carry no topodiagnostic significance, and are useful as mere descriptive conventions, if at all. Further, it is now clear that notions of discrete "abductor" or "adductor paralysis" also have no physiologic validity.

Second, the natural tendency for reinnervation may account for the general trend for the voice to improve over time in unilateral vocal fold paralysis. Reinnervation likely acts to restore or preserve muscle bulk and tone, increasing the vocal fold's mass and resistance to airflow, occasionally to the point that phonatory glottic closure is restored and conversational voice sounds normal although the vocal fold itself remains immobile (Figure 1). This explanation, well supported by electrophysiologic evidence,[1,2] is probably closer to reality than the notion of gradual contralateral compensation.

CAUSES OF LARYNGEAL PARALYSIS

Most sources of nerve injury fall into three broad categories: damage from surgical operation or other trauma; compromise from a range of medical conditions; and dysfunction due to factors yet to be completely identified, designated "idiopathic." The relative frequency of causes of unilateral laryngeal paralysis varies considerably, both among and within these broad categories (Table 1). Differences result from demographic and epidemiologic features of populations from which case series are drawn, as well as differences specific to the reporting institution. For example, an unusually high proportion of cases due to malignancy in a Scotch series reflects the high incidence of lung cancer in that country.[11] Because reports tally causes in relative incidences, unusual distributions may skew the relative frequency of other causes and create inaccurate impressions. The relatively high incidence of idiopathic unilateral paralysis in two Japanese series,[12,13] for example, is more likely the consequence of a low prevalence of mediastinal malignancy than any heretofore unrecognized virus tending to cause laryngeal paralysis.

Despite such variability, it is possible to draw some conclusions regarding unilateral laryngeal paralysis.[24] In the vast majority of cases, laryngeal paralysis is caused by a peripheral neuropathy rather than a central nervous system process. In most series, laryngeal paralysis tends to affect men more often than women, probably reflecting the underlying gender distribution of thoracic malignancy. Uniformly, the left vocal fold is affected more often than the right, in approximately a 60:40 ratio or greater, due to the greater length and more profound descent into the thorax of the left recurrent laryngeal nerve and its

consequent greater vulnerability to disease and surgery. Left-sided paralysis is more likely to be related to malignancy, although the possibility of malignant causation in right-sided paralysis should not be discounted.[24]

Iatrogenic sources of injury have multiplied over time. In addition to thyroidectomy, still a main source of iatrogenic laryngeal paralysis, anterior approach to the cervical spine, carotid endarterectomy, and various cardiac and thoracic procedures have all become significant sources of laryngeal nerve injury (Table 2). Table 3 shows composite data for incidences of laryngeal paralysis, including information regarding permanent and temporary paralysis where available, from several recent series. Recurrent nerve damage from the cuffed endotracheal tube was recognized in the 1960s and early 1970s and continues to account for instances of vocal fold immobility which are demonstrably neural in origin and not the result of cricoarytenoid joint disruption.

A number of neurogenic conditions remain important albeit unusual causes of laryngeal paralysis (many are discussed in Chapter 79, "Neurogenic Disorders of the Larynx"). In contrast to other causes, some of these may be through a central mechanism. Vocal fold paralysis may appear in the wake of a stroke, almost always in conjunction with other deficits. Lateral

medullary infarct (Wallenberg syndrome) is a well-known complex of neural injury featuring vocal fold paralysis, dysphagia, vertigo, ataxia, Horner syndrome, and hemifacial sensory deficit and/or pain. The vocal fold paralysis tends to improve with time, although measures may be needed in the short term to prevent aspiration. The vocal fold paralysis of Arnold-Chiari malformation tends to be bilateral and is important to recognize promptly because it is reversible with timely hindbrain decompression. Charcot-Marie-Tooth disease and its variants are a heterogeneous group of hereditary motor and sensory neuropathies which may involve the laryngeal nerves. Neural compromise of the vocal fold appears to evolve slowly but relentlessly and is usually bilateral, although it may be asymmetric. Vocal fold paralysis may also evolve as a complex of bulbar deficits resulting in dysphagia, dysphonia, and

Table 1 Causes of Unilateral Vocal Fold Paralysis

Study	Year	N	Tumor	Trauma	Idiopathic	Other
Laccourreye and colleagues[14]	2003	325	9%	75%	12%	—
Loughran and colleagues[11]	2002	77	52%	22%	12%	5% intubation
Yumoto and colleagues[15]	2002	422	19%	33%	22%	8% intubation
Ramadan and colleagues[16]	1998	98	32%	30%	16%	11% intubation
Benninger and colleagues[17]	1998	280	25%	35%	20%	8% intubation
Bruggink and colleagues[18]	1998	215	25%	43%	18%	—
Yamada and colleagues[13]	1983	519	17%	12%	41%	11% intubation
Tucker[19]	1980	210	22%	42%	14%	—
Hirose[12]	1978	600	7%	37%	41%	2% intubation
Parnell and Brandenburg[20]	1970	100	32%	32%	10%	11% medical
Clerf[21]	1953	299	38%	20%	12%	9% medical
Work[22]	1941	183	14%	39%	23%	15% medical
Smith and colleagues[23]	1933	173	27%	16%	17%	36% medical

Adapted with permission from reference 24.

Table 2 Operations and Procedures Which Place Laryngeal Nerves at Risk

Cervical surgery

- Thyroidectomy or parathyroidectomy
- Anterior approach to the cervical spine
- Carotid endarterectomy
- Implantation of vagal nerve stimulator
- Cricopharyngeal myotomy/repair of Zenker diverticulum

Thoracic procedures

- Pneumonectomy and pulmonary lobectomy
- Repair of thoracic aortic aneurysm
- Coronary artery bypass graft
- Aortic valve replacement
- Esophageal surgery
- Tracheal surgery
- Mediastinoscopy
- Thymectomy
- Ligation of persistent ductus arteriosus
- Cardiac and pulmonary transplant

Other surgery

- Skull base surgery
- Brainstem surgery or neurosurgery which requires brainstem retraction

Other medical procedures

- Central venous catheterization
- Endotracheal intubation

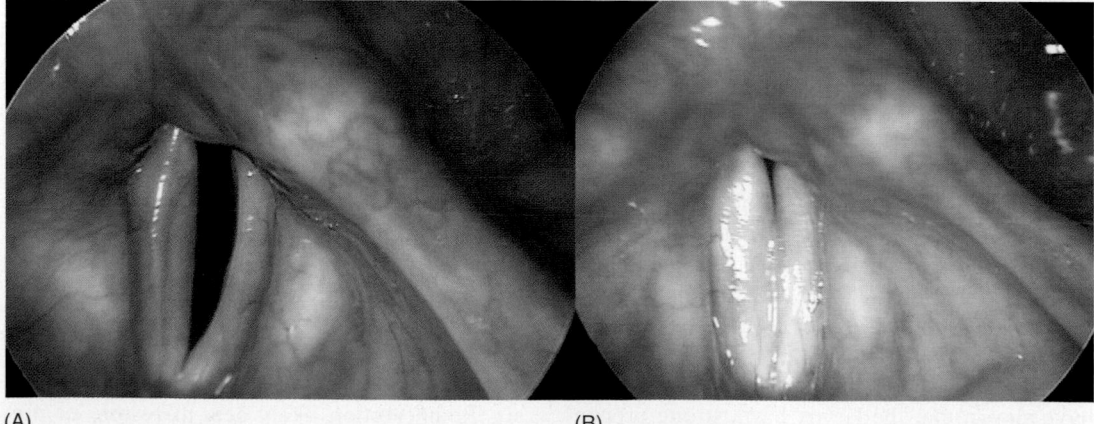

(A)   (B)

Figure 1 Reinnervation may improve vocal fold closure, even when motion does not return. (A) Photograph on the left is the best phonatory closure in a patient with left vocal fold paralysis some 4 weeks after carotid endarterectomy. (B) Photograph on the right is the same patient 3 months later. The left vocal fold has regained substantial tone and bulk.

Table 3 Incidences of Vocal Fold Paralysis after Operations: Composite Data from Recent Series

Surgery Type	Temporary Paralysis	Permanent Paralysis	Overall
Thyroidectomy (A)	1.0–5.1%	0.4–2.9%	1.0–8.6%
AACS	3.0–20.8%	0.3–6.6%	
Carotid endarterectomy (B)	1.0–7.1%	0.2–4.0%	
Pneumonectomy or lobectomy			6.7–31%
CABG			0.7–1.9%
Esophagectomy (C)			15–45%

Adapted with permission from reference 24.

AACS = anterior approach to the cervical spine; CABG = coronary artery bypass graft; A = incidences expressed as number of patients/operations rather than nerves at risk, series from 1990 to present; B = series from 1990 to present; C = 10 to 27% of these are bilateral.

dysarthria in postpolio syndrome, a degenerative condition seen many decades after the acute disease, and also as part of multisystem atrophy, a degenerative parkinsonian condition. In the latter disease, laryngeal dysfunction may contribute to mortality by creating respiratory obstruction. Laryngeal paresis and paralysis may also figure in oculopharyngeal dystrophy and inclusion body myositis.

The most striking trend over time is the decreasing proportion of vocal fold paralysis due to nonmalignant medical conditions. Historically, aortic aneurysm, largely due to syphilitic arteritis, tuberculous lymphadenopathy, and several other infectious diseases occurred with greater frequency and accounted for a larger proportion of cases. Vocal fold paralysis was also related to a series of infectious diseases that have become rare or nonexistent, for example, diphtheria, puerperal fever, typhus and particularly typhoid fever, as well as complications of untreated infectious disease that have become uncommon since the advent of antibiotics, like pleuritis, massive mediastinal lymphadenopathy, and pericardial effusion.

Of interest, the incidence of idiopathic paralysis had remained approximately unchanged over the past century, unaffected by the introduction and refinement of computed tomography (CT) and magnetic resonance imaging (MRI). The relationship between idiopathic laryngeal paralysis and infectious disease has long been apparent. Based on serologies, laryngeal paralyses have been attributed to Lyme borreliosis, herpes zoster and simplex, Epstein-Barr virus, and even the West Nile virus. Moreover, several sources document a transient increase in the number of cases of idiopathic laryngeal paralysis in the wake of the Hong Kong flu in the winter of 1969 to 1970 in both England and Japan. Even though direct causation remains to be established, these clinical relationships are convincing. However, they still do not explain many cases of vocal fold paralysis in which serologies are normal and there is no history of antecedent viral disease.

UNILATERAL VOCAL FOLD PARALYSIS

Clinical Evaluation

History. Most frequently, patients with unilateral laryngeal paralysis complain of hoarseness and hypophonia. These can range from subtle vocal fatigue, most pronounced when speaking loudly or over background noise to obvious, near-total aphonia. These symptoms are generally directly proportional to the degree of glottic insufficiency that varies from affected individual to individual.

Patients with unilateral laryngeal paralysis may also report dysphagia, also due to glottic insufficiency, although less often than voice complaints. Frank aspiration has been reported in 18 to 38% of patients with vocal fold paralysis,[25–27] although it is more likely to occur in certain clinical situations. Dysphagia-related complaints are more frequent in patients with "high" vagal injury, affecting both superior and recurrent laryngeal nerves, which adds hemilaryngeal anesthesia, piriform sinus atony, and cricopharyngeal muscle hyperfunction to glottic insufficiency from the immobile vocal fold. Situations in which laryngeal anesthesia exists alongside other cranial nerve deficits, as in jugular foramen syndromes, after stroke and after skull base surgery probably also carry increased dysphagia risk. Operations which affect pulmonary reserve, as do most thoracic procedures, appear to carry a higher risk of aspiration, and age may be an independent risk factor.[28]

Sometimes, patients will demonstrate a characteristically "wet" vocal quality, arising from pooled secretions which interfere with phonation. By definition, such secretions have at least penetrated into the laryngeal introitus; these patients should attract the otolaryngologist's attention as being at risk for aspiration. More subtle symptoms include laryngospasm resulting from reaction to unexpected penetration or aspiration. This may occur in patients with surprisingly small degrees of glottic insufficiency and reasonably good voice quality.

Occasionally, patients may complain of shortness of breath, particularly during phonation or physical activity. Careful questioning will reveal that this is not obstructive dyspnea but rather breathlessness that results from excessive air escape during voicing, or from compromise of thoracic fixation (Valsalva) maneuver during effortful activity. An airflow loop will inevitably reveal an extrathoracic obstruction; this, plus a lack of insight into laryngeal physiology, may lead the physician directly away from measures to medialize the vocal fold, restore glottic function, and relieve these symptoms.

When the onset of symptoms immediately follows an operation that places the laryngeal nerves at risk, no further search for cause is necessary. In other patients, the inquiry should be made regarding smoking history, the most recent chest imaging, and antecedent illness. A review of systems should focus on illnesses likely to affect the larynx. Relevant factors include neurogenic symptoms like weakness, tremor, and dysarthria; pulmonary symptoms suggestive of tuberculosis or malignancy; and exposure to neurotoxic agents like solid tumor chemotherapy (vincristine, vinblastine, and cisplatin) and organophosphates found in pesticides. Unilateral vocal fold immobility is rarely mechanical in nature, but the possibility should not be dismissed in patients in whom the symptoms appear in the wake of clearly traumatic intubation, external trauma, or in the presence of arthralgias or known inflammatory joint disease.

Physical Examination. The examination of a patient with laryngeal paralysis should include careful palpation of the neck for lymphadenopathy or thyroid enlargement. The remaining cranial nerves should be systematically evaluated, with special attention to the spinal accessory and hypoglossal nerves, which share the jugular foramen with the vagus. Finally, other branches of the vagus should be examined. The presence of ipsilateral tongue deviation, palate droop or Horner syndrome should raise the suspicion of a base of skull lesion.

The larynx itself should be examined across a variety of laryngeal tasks. Flexible transnasal laryngoscopy probably offers a more accurate impression of laryngeal function than rigid techniques, as the tongue traction necessary for the latter introduces some artificial biomechanical factors which may be misleading. Any debate about the superiority of one or the other means of examination is somewhat academic, however; there is nothing to prevent evaluation by both techniques.

A hypomobile vocal fold may sometimes be surprisingly difficult to appreciate; in such cases, asking the patient to alternate sustained vowel phonation and sniffing (the so-called "eee-sniff" maneuver) should bring any asymmetry into stark evidence. The examiner should take care not to be mislead by small amounts of vocal fold motion which may be caused by the interarytenoid muscle still partially innervated from the contralateral nerve, by an intact cricothyroid muscle, or even by passive lateral displacement of the arytenoid cartilage on the paralyzed side by its pair during adduction. This last is known as the "jostle sign," described by Chevalier Jackson in the 1930s, and when present offers unambiguous evidence against cricoarytenoid joint fixation.

We have seen that the position of the paralyzed vocal fold carries no significance with respect to the site of the injury or prognosis. Nevertheless, careful examination can reveal features which may inform clinical care. Occasionally, increasing tension and length of the paralyzed vocal fold upon raising the pitch of the voice may suggest an intact superior laryngeal nerve, although the absence of such motion should not be taken as proof positive of superior nerve compromise. Sometimes, patients may take advantage of intact cricothyroid muscle function to improve voice projection by increasing vocal fold resistance to exhaled air during phonation (Figure 2); this phenomenon, which also inevitably raises pitch, results in a characteristic voice described as "paralytic falsetto."

The presence of supraglottic hyperfunction during phonatory effort, which sometimes obstructs the view of the vocal folds, should raise the possibility of glottic insufficiency. The ventricular folds serve as an accessory valving mechanism which tends to be engaged without deliberate effort when the vocal folds do not close effectively.[29] Maneuvers such as humming or sighing can serve to relax the ventricular folds (Belafsky and colleagues have used the term "unloading the larynx" to describe this) to permit a more thorough evaluation of glottic closure.

Vocal fold adduction and abduction do not take place in two dimensions; the folds tend to abduct in a cephalad direction (into the ventricles) and adduct caudally. Thus, a paralyzed vocal fold may not rest in the same plane as its partner. Such three-dimensional judgments are difficult to make on laryngoscopy, but height mismatch is important to identify, as simple medial displacement of the paralyzed fold may not suffice for good apposition during phonation.

Asymmetry of the arytenoids, with displacement of the cartilage on the paralyzed side forward into the laryngeal introitus (a so-called "prolapsed arytenoid") is not a rare finding in laryngeal paralysis (Figure 3). This is not a sign of cricoarytenoid dislocation. The presence of a prolapsed arytenoid does, however, suggest profound denervation with loss of muscular support for the cartilage. In addition, it strongly suggests a height and tension mismatch between the vocal folds. These are all factors which argue for an arytenoid stabilization procedure, discussed further below, should surgical rehabilitation be contemplated.

The incidence of cricoarytenoid dislocation has been the subject of much debate. Experimental

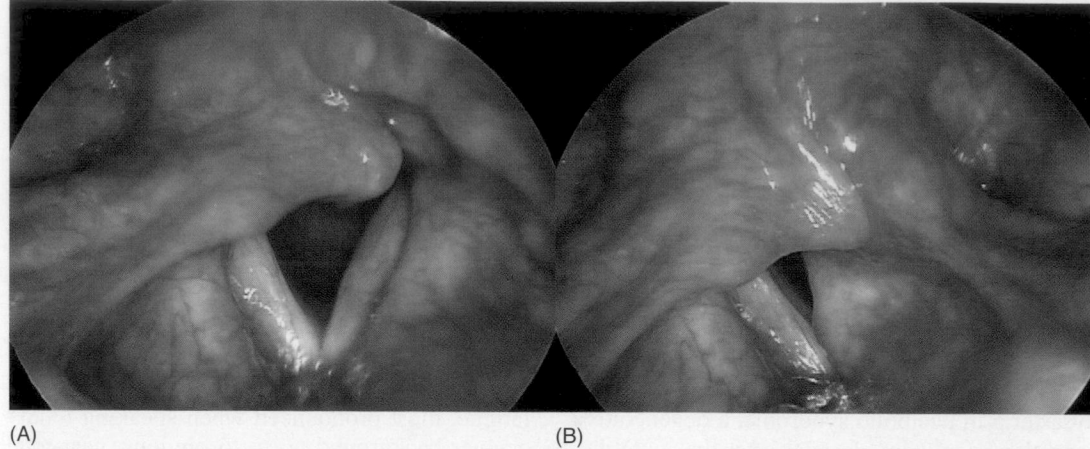

(A)   (B)

Figure 3 Photograph of idiopathic right vocal fold paralysis confirmed with electromyography. (A) The right arytenoid is prolapsed into the laryngeal introitus. (B) In adduction, the right arytenoid cartilage interferes with the opposite cartilage and impedes closure. Rehabilitation without arytenoid cartilage repositioning surgery would likely be suboptimal.

study has shown the cricoarytenoid joint to be strikingly robust and resistant to disruption.[30–32] Most laryngologists agree that a problem-free intubation is extraordinarily unlikely to cause a joint injury and that joint injuries usually follow obvious trauma, be it from intubation or external sources. The presence of arytenoid edema and erythema and the absence of a jostle sign are suggestive of cricoarytenoid joint injury and should prompt further investigation, in which electromyography may be of special utility.

In hemilaryngeal paralysis, the glottal gap may be of two principal configurations. It may be essentially spindle-shaped, involving principally the membranous portion of the vocal fold, or V-shaped, marked by greater distance between the vocal processes of the arytenoid cartilage. This latter configuration is called a posterior gap; the term does not refer to the absolute distance between vocal processes (Figure 4). The presence of a posterior gap argues in favor of an arytenoid stabilization procedure for rehabilitation because implant medialization alone, or injection augmentation for that matter, is notoriously poor at correcting this deficit.

Although there is no single metric of severity of symptoms of vocal fold paralysis, several simple clinical tools may help grade features of the history and examination. These are important to understand, even if for no other reason than to aid in interpretation of the copious literature in this area. The Voice Handicap Index (VHI) and the Voice Related Quality of Life (VRQOL) are standardized and validated patient-completed self-rating scales which measure various aspects of vocal disability. The Consensus Auditory Perceptual Evaluation-Voice (CAPE-V) and its antecedent Grade, Roughness, Breathiness, Asthenia, Strain (GRBAS) scale, are perceptual scales which are completed by the health-care professional based on voice quality. The maximum phonation time (MPT) is the longest duration of sustained vowel phonation (typically an /i/) which the patient can sustain. Times in excess of 20 seconds are normal in adults, and the MPT is approximately inversely proportional to the degree of glottic insufficiency. The s/z ratio compares the maximum phonation time of unvoiced (/s/) and voiced (/z/) and sounds. Under normal circumstances, the duration of the unvoiced sound should be approximately equal to that of the voiced (the s/z ratio should be 1.0), but when glottic insufficiency is present, the duration that the voiced sound can be sustained decreases (the s/z ratio tends to increase).

Supplementary Investigations. Fundamentally, diagnostic testing in addition to the history and physical examination is intended to uncover occult causes of vocal fold paralysis. In cases temporally related to an operation that places the vocal folds at risk, no additional workup is required. In others, malignancy is the principal pathology not to be overlooked. Imaging of the entire course of the affected laryngeal nerves is obligatory. This includes the mediastinum and the pulmonary apex, even when the paralysis is right-sided; it should be recalled that the right-sided nerve loops underneath the subclavian artery.

Although some authors have suggested that routine radiography may be adequate to image the chest, Glazer and colleagues have demonstrated a sobering rate of false negatives.[33] This, plus

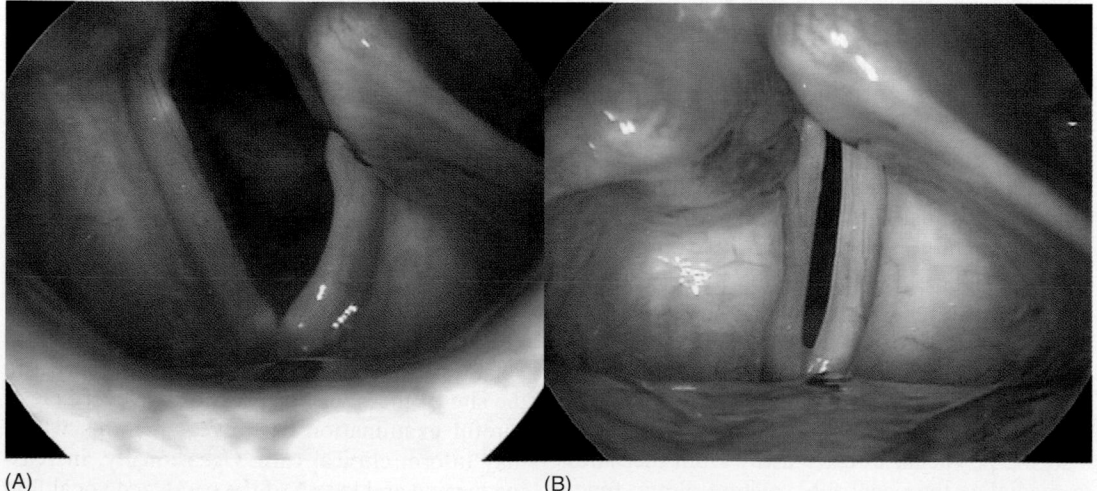

(A)   (B)

Figure 2 Photographs of left vocal fold paralysis in a patient following anterior approach to the cervical spine. Comparison of left vocal fold tension during quiet respiration (A) and phonation (B) suggests that the superior laryngeal nerve is intact.

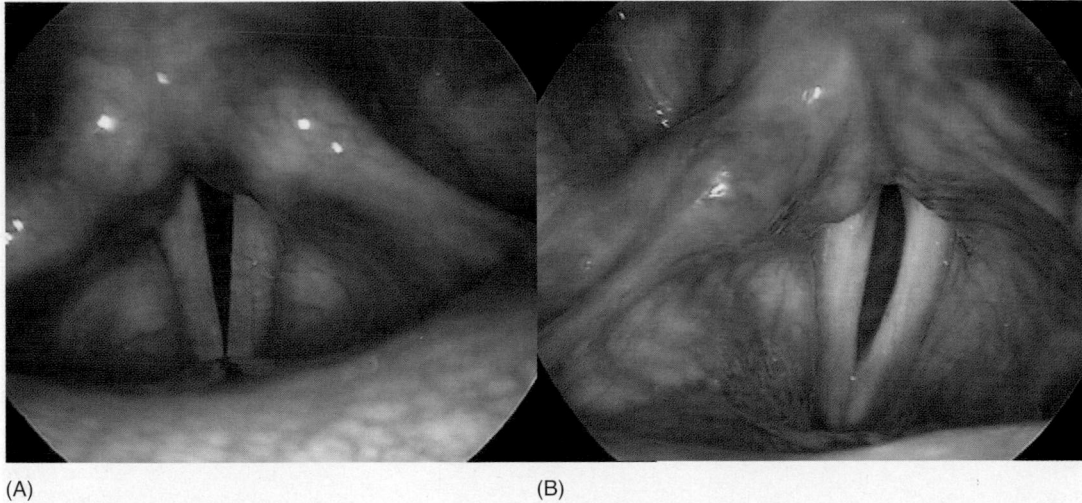

(A)   (B)

Figure 4 (A) Left vocal fold paralysis following thyroidectomy deomonstrates a posterior gap. Compare with the case in Figure 3, which also demonstrates a posterior gap. (B) Left vocal fold paralysis from malignant mediastinal lymphadenopathy with good closure at the vocal process.

the need to image the neck, has made CT from base of skull through the arch of the aorta or the right subclavian, as appropriate, the minimum recommended study for laryngeal paralysis. In cases where a "high vagal" paralysis is suspected according to criteria reviewed earlier, MRI may offer a more reliable means of imaging the skull base or central nervous system.

A recent survey has suggested that otolaryngologists continue to obtain serologic tests in most cases of vocal fold paralysis.[34] Systematic examination has demonstrated a 0% yield for serologic tests in 84 patients.[35] Moreover, the serologic tests that are ordered are inconsistent with the frequencies of the causes of laryngeal paralyses; rheumatoid factor and Lyme titers, the most frequently ordered serologic tests are for diseases that are exceptionally rare in all published series of vocal fold paralyses. In light of this information, serologic testing is probably useless unless there is clinical suspicion of a specific underlying illness. Modified barium swallow is useful if a question of aspiration exists. The potential of morbidity related to dysphagia is a key element in determining the need for treatment.

Laryngeal Electromyography. Laryngeal electromyography (LEMG) measures the integrity of laryngeal innervation with percutaneous needle electrodes. It can provide unambiguous evidence of denervation and reinnervation, yet its utility in cases of vocal fold paralysis has been hotly debated. Its detractors have claimed that it is "subjective" and unreliable. In fact, LEMG might be better described as "qualitative," requiring interpretation. In this respect, it does not differ from laryngoscopy and stroboscopy, except inasmuch as training and familiarity has allowed otolaryngologists to use these latter modalities more comfortably in everyday practice. In fact, LEMG exceeds both of these in its ability definitively and objectively to contribute to the diagnosis of vocal fold paralysis, as opposed to immobility.

The practical clinical difficulty in the use of LEMG for prognosis has been that the appearance of electromyographic signs of reinnervation does

not always lead to a return of vocal fold function, for pathophysiologic reasons reviewed earlier. Therefore, experience with LEMG for prognosis in patients with vocal fold paralysis has been uneven, depending heavily on criteria used for "good" prognosis. The broader these criteria are, the more false positives, and the more restrictive, the more false negatives. The available literature suggests that LEMG may be more useful as a predictor of poor outcome (Table 4), principally because these signs, namely fibrillations and fasciculations revealing an absence of reinnervation, offer no physiologic ambiguities. The subject remains open for further investigation. For now, it is clear that LEMG offers a reliable way to distinguish neurogenic from mechanical vocal fold immobility and may offer variable prognostic information when used less than 6 months from the onset of paralysis. While LEMG, when used circumspectly, may offer further refinement in making treatment decisions for patients with vocal fold paralysis, it is not essential to the standard of care, which has relied on treatment delays of 6 to 12 months to resolve uncertainty about prognosis.

Treatment

Decisions regarding therapeutic intervention for glottic insufficiency from unilateral vocal fold paralysis are guided by concerns regarding morbidity from dysphagia and aspiration, the patient's own perception of the severity of the vocal disability, and expectations and assumptions about the eventual outcome without treatment. In

turn, outcome expectations are influenced by the apparent cause of the paralysis and the time that has elapsed since onset.

Observation. Patients with hemilaryngeal paralysis, especially of short duration, may simply be observed. Factors favoring observation include

1. no evidence of aspiration,
2. certainty that the injured laryngeal nerve(s) is (are) intact,
3. minimal vocal disability and/or minimal vocal demand,
4. good functional prognosis, and
5. comorbidites or other medical factors which discourage or prevent intervention.

Voice and swallowing therapy may be used as needed during the observation period. There is no convincing clinical evidence that voice therapy is useful to relieve symptoms or affect the course of vocal fold paralysis. As with many interventions for this condition, the natural tendency of glottic insufficiency to improve over time makes it difficult to evaluate efficacy. Nevertheless, a skilled voice therapist may offer patients reassurance and insight into their condition and may help prevent or reverse harmful compensatory behaviors.

The presence of severe dysphagia, history of aspiration pneumonia, or observed aspiration during clinical evaluation (either radiologic or endoscopic) effectively trumps other factors and demands intervention.

Injection Augmentation. Patients may opt for temporary relief of their symptoms, even when eventual recovery is expected. This is accomplished by injection of an absorbable bulking substance into the paralyzed fold to improve the glottic insufficiency. Such substances include various collagen and hyaluronic acid preparations, micronized human dermis, autologous fat, and carboxymethylcellulose-glycerine gel. Factors favoring injection augmentation include

1. dysphagia,
2. high degree of vocal disability or high vocal demand,
3. functional prognosis is good or indeterminate,
4. relatively small glottic gap (<2 to 3 mm),
5. no posterior glottic gap, and
6. short life expectancy (less than the expected duration of the injectate).

Injection augmentation may be performed via direct laryngoscopy in the operating room, or perorally or transcutaneously under topical

Table 4 Laryngeal Electromyography and Prognosis in Vocal Fold Paralysis of Less than 6 Months Duration			
Study	N	Accurate Prediction of Recovery	Accurate Prediction of No or Impaired Recovery
Munin and colleagues[36]	31	80%	80%
Sittel and colleagues[37]	111	13%	94%
Gupta and Bastian[38]	18	70%	75%
Hirano and colleagues[39]	29	63%	80%
Parnes and Satya-Murti[40]	18	80%	100%

Adapted with permission from reference 24.

anesthetic or superior laryngeal nerve block in the office, provided the patient is cooperative and committed. Office use is a major advantage of the technique. Selection of the substance to be injected depends on the surgeon's evaluation of its tissue properties, experience and, probably in no small part, preference.

Injection augmentation is usually regarded as temporary since the abandonment of polytetrafluoroethylene polymer (Polytef, Teflon) because of well-known adverse tissue response. Calcium hydroxylapatite particle paste has been recently introduced as a durable injectable with effect exceeding 1 year, and possibly permanent, although its relatively recent introduction leaves the latter claim unsubstantiated at present. This product may reopen the possibility of using injection as a definitive treatment for paralytic glottic insufficiency. In considering this treatment option, otolaryngologists should not forget the lessons of polytetrafluoroethylene polymer, however: the larynx tends to punish careless use (such as superficial injection or overinjection) of nonbiodegradable materials.

Injection augmentation has inherent limitations. It will not effectively reposition the arytenoid cartilage to rectify a height discrepancy or close a posterior glottal gap. It is not ideal for large glottic gaps. Most injection substances require overinjection to allow for reabsorption, rendering fine adjustment of vocal fold position virtually impossible. In addition, should the injectate infiltrate into an unintended site (typically the superficial layers of the vocal fold), impairing mucosal phonatory vibration, corrective intervention is challenging Patients may have to await natural resolution over weeks to months. It should be noted that no substance, not even low viscosity hyaluronic acid preparations, is ideally suited for use in the lamina propria; all currently available substances will stiffen this tissue. The proper location of the injection is within the thyroarytenoid muscle at the mid- and posterior portions of the membranous vocal fold (Figure 5).

Framework Surgery. Laryngeal framework surgery is generally reserved for treatment of glottic insufficiency from unilateral paralysis which is not expected to improve. Factors favoring a framework approach are following:

1. dysphagia,
2. high degree of vocal disability or high vocal demand,
3. poor functional prognosis,
4. relatively large glottic gap (>2 to 3 mm),
5. posterior glottic gap, and
6. life expectancy is not shortened.

In its simplest and most common form, framework surgery consists of the medialization thyroplasty, the insertion of an implant, made of silicone, formed polytetrafluoroethylene (Gore-Tex), formed calcium hydroxylapatite, or other biologically inert material, into the paraglottic space to displace the paralyzed vocal fold

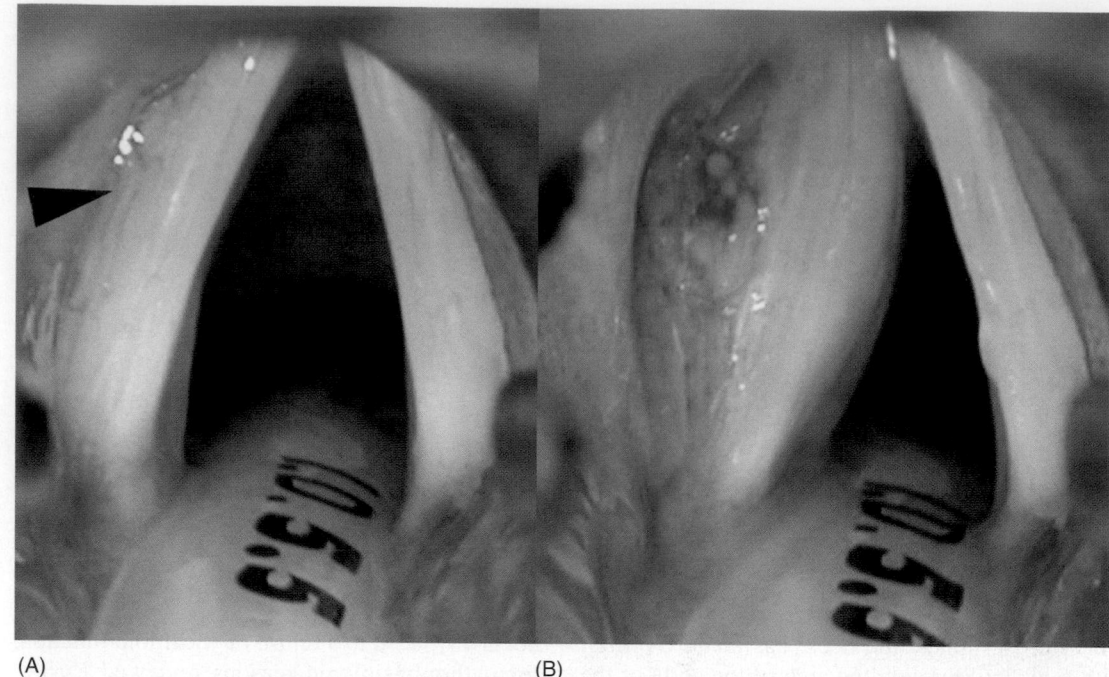

(A) (B)

Figure 5 Injection of autologous fat at direct laryngoscopy. (A) In most cases, vocal fold injection should not be placed anterior or medial to point indicated by the arrowhead. (B) Note that autologous fat requires substantial overinjection compared to other injectable materials.

medially (Figure 6).[43] Typically, this operation is performed under a local anesthetic, with or without additional intravenous sedation. This allows the surgeon, guided by patient phonation and endoscopic visualization, to size and position the implant for optimal correction of the patient's glottic insufficiency without functional restriction of the airway.[41–42] The critical anatomic task is to identify the level of the vocal fold in relation to the thyroid lamina so that the thyroid cartilage aperture through which the implant is inserted can be placed appropriately. Medialization via thyroplasty, in contrast to injection, is precise, predictable, and durable. Often considered more aggressive treatment than injection, medialization thyroplasty under local anesthesia can be safer and better suited to high-risk patients than injection under general anesthesia.

Serious complications include airway obstruction and perforation into the laryngeal lumen. Necessarily, medialization narrows the airway and, in combination with postoperative edema and

hematoma, can cause airway obstruction. For this reason, many surgeons prefer to observe patients in the hospital for one night following the procedure. Some 0.6 to 1.1% of patients undergoing medialization thyroplasty have been reported to require intubation or tracheostomy in the immediate postoperative period.[44–45] Perforation of the laryngeal mucosa increases the likelihood of infection and subsequent extrusion of implanted material. Perforation typically takes place in the delicate ventricular mucosa, which lies close to the thyroid lamina, or anteriorly where there is little soft tissue cover.

The most common "complication," however, is suboptimal voice outcome. This is typically due to technical factors, and revision rates of 5.4 to 14%, to even as high as 33% when adjunctive procedures such as fat injection are included, have been reported.[44–46] Common causes of poor voice result include persistent posterior gap, undermedialization and implant malposition, generally in too anterior or too superior a position (Figure 7).

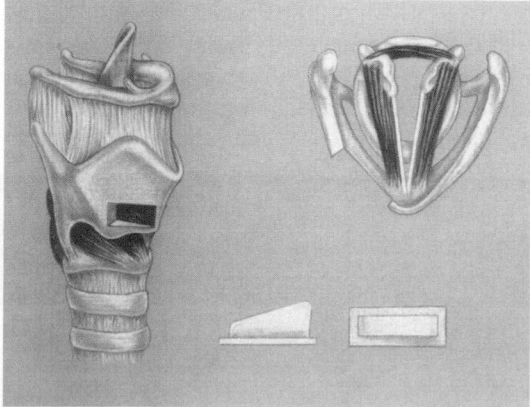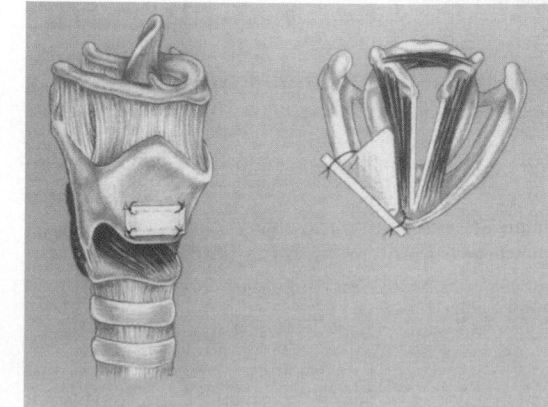

Figure 6 In medialization laryngoplasty, a medialization shim of biologically inert material is inserted into the paraglottic space through a thyroid cartilage window to displace the vocal fold toward the midline. (Published with permission from reference 43.)

Arytenoid cartilage repositioning procedures may be added to medialization thyroplasty when there is a flaccid, poorly supported arytenoid cartilage or a posterior gap (see Figures 2 and 3). This configuration is notoriously difficult to remedy with thyroplasty alone. Arytenoid repositioning surgery is designed to internally rotate and/or suspend the arytenoid cartilage in physiologic phonatory position. Most commonly, the muscular process of the arytenoid cartilage is

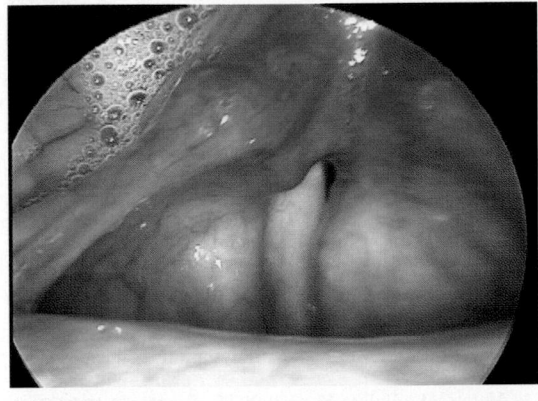

(A)

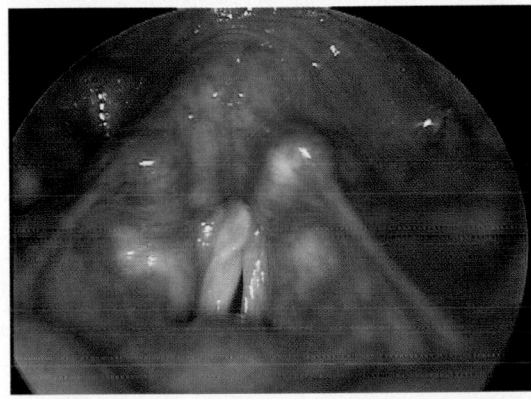

(B)

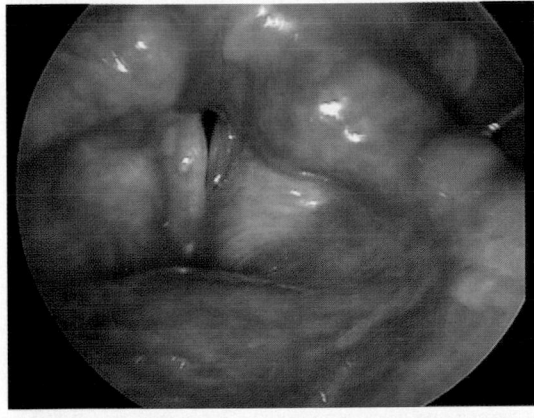

(C)

Figure 7 Suboptimal outcomes of medialization laryngoplasty. (A) Superior malposition of implant in this patient with left vocal paralysis after irradiation of a glomus tumor causes the ventricular fold to obscure the vocal fold, which is not well adducted. This is not supraglottic hyperfunction. (B) Inadequate medialization of the left vocal fold in a patient with idiopathic paralysis results in persistent midfold glottic insufficiency and compensatory supraglottic hyperfunction. (C) Inadequate arytenoid cartilage medialization in this patient with idiopathic right vocal fold paralysis does not close the posterior gap. Note supraglottic hyperfunction on the left side.

approached through the inferior constrictor muscle and around the back of the thyroid lamina. A nonabsorbable suture is passed through the muscular process and secured to the thyroid lamina so as to exert anterolateral traction on the muscular process and thus rotate the vocal process medially and slightly caudally; this is known as arytenoid adduction.[47] Adduction arytenoidopexy, a less common approach, involves opening the cricoarytenoid joint capsule and suturing the arytenoid in optimal position directly to the crest of the cricoid cartilage.[48]

These procedures are technically challenging and more time consuming than thyroplasty alone and have a higher incidence of complications, largely because edema or bleeding into the paraglottic space can cause airway obstruction. Despite these problems, for the experienced phonosurgeon, arytenoid procedures are an essential adjunct to medialization thyroplasty in achieving an optimal voice outcome.

Reinnervation. Reinnervation using nearby nerves (both the ansa cervicalis and the hypoglossal have been studied[49]) would seem to be an attractive and logical approach to vocal fold paralysis. It is subject to the same limitations as spontaneous recovery, however. Because of the complex innervation of the vocal fold muscles, reinnervation generally improves the bulk and tone of vocal fold muscle but will not restore physiologic motion. Reinnervation is ideally suited when the vocal fold is known to be completely denervated. In fact, in patients in whom the nerve has been sectioned and the section is recognized during surgery, immediate reanastomosis, or reinnervation if tension-free reanastomosis is not possible, is the treatment of choice. However, when considering reinnervation later in the course of paralysis, the surgeon should be reasonably confident that he or she is not depriving the vocal fold of existing reinnervation by sectioning a partially recovered recurrent nerve to use the distal stump. In addition, the patient must be counseled that symptom improvement may take weeks or months. For this reason, reinnervation has sometimes been combined with other rehabilitation techniques.

The armamentarium of procedures to remedy unilateral laryngeal paralysis is flexible and effective enough so that, given an understanding of the underlying pathophysiology, as well as the advantages, disadvantages and technical requirements of each procedure, meaningful symptomatic relief can be offered to nearly every patient.

BILATERAL VOCAL FOLD PARALYSIS

Virtually any condition that can cause unilateral laryngeal paralysis may affect both recurrent laryngeal nerves to cause bilateral paralysis. Thyroidectomy remains the leading surgical cause[50]; both nerves are also at risk at esophagectomy, tracheal resection, thymectomy, and other mediastinal procedures. Similarly, tracheal, esophageal, and thyroid malignancies may compromise both nerves. Neurogenic disorders

tend to involve both nerves. Amyotrophic lateral sclerosis, postpolio syndrome, Charcot-Marie-Tooth neuropathy, Arnold-Chiari malformation, and Guillain-Barre syndrome have been documented causes of bilateral paralysis. Some bilateral laryngeal paralyses are idiopathic, attributed to the same infectious agents as unilateral paralysis.

A clinician encountering bilateral vocal fold immobility should consider the possibility of joint fixation or posterior glottic scar, particularly when the condition follows intubation. In such cases the vocal folds are not denervated but merely appear to be paralyzed because of mechanical limitation. Careful inspection, sometimes requiring operative laryngoscopy, radiologic investigation, and/or electromyography should be used to clarify the diagnosis, as mechanical limitations may occasionally be correctible.

Patients with bilateral vocal fold paralysis typically complain of dyspnea, noisy breathing, and exercise intolerance. The severity of these respiratory symptoms is inversely proportional to the size of the glottic aperture between the two immobile vocal folds. Respiratory noise is worse on inspiration, as negative pressure pulls the denervated vocal folds into closer approximation and causes greater airway restriction. Voice, while not entirely normal, may not be greatly altered, and swallowing is usually not affected.

When bilateral vocal fold paralysis is acute, symptoms may be dramatic and even life threatening. The typical situation is unexpected respiratory distress after extubation from thyroid surgery, and, in such a patient, securing an adequate airway is the only consideration. In progressive cases, as found in certain neurogenic diseases, patients may compensate as the paralysis becomes more dense and may tolerate unexpectedly small glottic airways. Occasionally, the clinician may be surprised to discover bilateral vocal fold paralysis in relatively asymptomatic patients; close questioning about noisy inspiration or limitations in physical activity may suggest that paralysis has been present for some time.

Investigation includes radiologic imaging in the manner of unilateral vocal fold paralysis, with special emphasis on the mediastinum and infralaryngeal part of the neck, where the recurrent nerves are in close proximity, as well as the central nervous system. The degree of airway obstruction may be quantified using a flow-volume loop. Bilateral paralysis typically shows a variable (rather than fixed) extrathoracic obstruction, as the vocal folds will passively adduct during inspiration and abduct with positive expiratory air pressure.

Treatment is guided by the degree of airway limitation; except in situations of acute airway distress, the patient may be the best judge of the functional disability. Tracheostomy is frequently performed emergently and may be a reasonable treatment option for the long term as well, as it provides an adequate airway with minimal compromise of phonation and deglutition. However, patients often prefer to avoid the inconveniences of tracheostomy if possible. Other treatment options include lateralization of one vocal fold or removal of one arytenoid cartilage or vocal fold tissue to enlarge the glottic aperture. Effort is made to preserve the membranous vocal fold to the greatest extent possible, but voice and sometimes swallowing may be adversely affected. These procedures are destructive and irreversible, so that any reasonable possibility of spontaneous improvement should be excluded before they are considered.

VOCAL FOLD PARESIS

A sophisticated understanding of underlying pathophysiology clearly reveals that vocal fold paralysis is not an all-or-none phenomenon, as it has been commonly conceptualized for the last century. It should come as no surprise that paresis or incomplete paralysis in which some gross vocal fold mobility is preserved exists alongside paralysis as a clinical entity. The symptoms of paresis differ only in degree from paralysis, whether unilateral or bilateral. In place of constant breathy hypophonia, for instance, the patient with hemiparesis may complain of voice difficulty only after speaking for some time or at high intensity. In place of inspiratory stridor, the patient may complain only of changes in exercise tolerance. Diagnosing paresis may be extremely challenging because preserved vocal fold mobility may lull the examiner into overlooking subtle glottic insufficiency or limitations in abduction. Perhaps the most difficult task is distinguishing paresis from innocent asymmetries in vocal fold motion, which are probably present in many individuals. Stroboscopy may occasionally be helpful. Decrease in muscular tone affects the amplitude and frequency of the mucosal wave during phonation. When glottic closure appears essentially normal under continuous light, stroboscopic examination may help identify subtle asymmetries in vocal fold tension. LEMG undoubtedly holds considerable potential in diagnosing paresis, but it must be used with as much judgment as laryngoscopy. That laryngeal paresis exists as a clinical entity is beyond doubt. Its incidence, impact, and treatment are currently being elucidated, however.

CONCLUSIONS

Laryngeal paralysis usually results from peripheral nerve injury of one or more laryngeal nerves, and results in clinically significant changes in phonation, swallowing and respiration. Often thought of as an all-or-none phenomenon, laryngeal paralysis represents a spectrum of nerve injury and reinnervation, which accounts for the variability in its clinical presentation. Investigation is aimed at discovering underlying causes. Because of the strong laryngeal propensity to reinnervation, paralysis tends to improve over time, and sometimes resolves spontaneously. When it does not, numerous surgical options are available to remedy dysphonia and dysphagia from the glottic insufficiency of unilateral laryngeal paralysis. Respiratory restriction from bilateral paralysis is a greater challenge, however, since surgical measures are destructive, irreversible, and stand to impact voice and swallowing adversely.

REFERENCES

1. Bielamowicz S, Stager SV. Diagnosis of unilateral recurrent laryngeal nerve paralysis: Laryngeal electromyography, subjective rating scales, acoustic and aerodynamic measures. Laryngoscope 2006;116:359–64.
2. Blitzer A, Jahn AF, Keidar A. Semon's law revisited: An electromyographic analysis of laryngeal synkinesis. Ann Otol Rhinol Laryngol 1996;105:764–9.
3. Woodson GE. Spontaneous laryngeal reinnervation after recurrent nerve or vagus nerve injury. Ann Otol Rhinol Laryngol 2007;116:66–8.
4. Zealear DL, Hamdan Al, Rainey CL. The effects of denervation on posterior cricoarytenoid muscle physiology and histochemistry. Ann Otol Rhinol Laryngol 1994;103:780–8.
5. Aronson AE, DeSanto LW. Adductor spastic dysphonia: Three years after recurrent laryngeal nerve resection. Laryngoscope 1983;93:1–8.
6. Netterville JL, Stone RE, Rainey C, et al. Recurrent laryngeal nerve avulsion for treatment of spastic dysphonia. Ann Otol Rhinol Laryngol 1991;100:10–4.
7. Zealear DL, Billante CR. Neurophysiology of vocal fold paralysis. Otolaryngol Clin North Am 2004;37:1–23.
8. Woodson GE. Configuration of the glottis in laryngeal paralysis I: Clinical study. Laryngoscope 1993;103:1227–34.
9. Woodson GE. Configuration of the glottis in laryngeal paralysis II: Animal experiments. Laryngoscope 1993;103:1235–41.
10. Koufman JA, Walker FO, Joharji GM. The cricothyroid muscle does not influence vocal fold position in laryngeal paralysis. Laryngoscope 1995;105:368–72.
11. Loughran S, Alves C, MacGregor FB. Current aetiology of unilateral vocal fold paralysis in a teaching hospital in the West of Scotland. J Laryngol Otol 2002;116:907–10.
12. Hirose H. Clinical observations on 600 cases of recurrent laryngeal nerve paralysis. Auris Nasus Larynx 1978;5:39–48.
13. Yamada M, Hirano M, Ohkubo H. Recurrent laryngeal nerve paralysis. A 10-year review of 564 patients. Auris Nasus Larynx 1983;10:S1–S15.
14. Laccourreye O, Papon JF, Kania R, et al. Paralyses laryngeés unilatérales: Données épidemiologiques at évolution thérapeutique. Presse Med 2003;32:781–6.
15. Yumoto E, Minoda R, Hyodo M, Yamagata T. Causes of recurrent laryngeal nerve paralysis. Auris Nasus Larynx 2002;29:41–5.
16. Ramadan HH, Wax MK, Avery S. Outcome and changing cause of unilateral vocal cord paralysis. Otolaryngol Head Neck Surg 1998;118:199–202.
17. Benninger MS, Gillen JB, Altman JS. Changing etiology of vocal fold immobility. Laryngoscope 1998;108:1346–50.
18. Bruggink TP, van der Rijt AJ, van den Broek P. Cause, diagnosis and course in 215 patients with vocal cord paralysis [in Dutch]. Ned Tijdschr Geneeskd 1995;139:570–4.
19. Tucker HM. Vocal cord paralysis – 1979: Etiology and management. Laryngoscope 1980;90:585–90.
20. Parnell FW, Brandenburg JH. Vocal cord paralysis: A review of 100 cases. Laryngoscope 1970;80:1036–45.
21. Clerf LH. Unilateral vocal cord paralysis. J Am Med Assoc 1953;151:900–3.
22. Work WP. Paralysis and paresis of the vocal cords: A statistical review. Arch Otolaryngol 1941;34:267–80.
23. Smith AB, Lambert VF, Wallce HL. Paralysis of the recurrent laryngeal nerve: A survey of 235 cases. Edinburgh Med J 1933;40:344–54.
24. Sulica L, Cultrara A, Blitzer A. Vocal fold paralysis: Causes, outcomes and clinical aspects. In: Sulica L, Blitzer A, editors. Vocal Fold Paralysis. Heidelberg: Springer; 2006. p. 33–54.
25. Tabaee A, Murry T, Zschlommer A, Desloge RB. Flexible endoscopuic evaluation of swallowing with sensory testing in patients with unilateral vocal fold immobility: Incidence and pathophysiology of aspiration. Laryngoscope 2005;115:565–9.
26. Bhattacharyya N, Kotz T, Shapiro J. Dysphagia and aspiration with unilateral vocal fold immobility: Incidence, characterization, and response to surgical treatment. Ann Otol Rhinol Laryngol 2002;111:672–9.
27. Heitmiller RF, Tseng E, Jones B. Prevalence of aspiration and laryngeal penetration inpatients with unilateral vocal fold motion impairment. Dysphagia 2000;15:184–7.
28. Baron EM, Soliman AM, Gaughan JP, et al. Dysphagia, hoarseness and unilateral true vocal fold motion impairment following anterior cervical diskectomy and fusion. Ann Otol Rhinol Laryngol 2003;112:921–6.
29. Belafsky PC, Postma GN, Reulbach TR, et al. Muscle tension dysphonia as a sign of underlying glottic insufficiency. Otolaryngol Head Neck Surg 2002;127:448–51.
30. Paulsen FP, Jungmann K, Tillman BN. The cricoarytenoid joint capsule and its relevance to endotracheal intubation. Anesth Analg 2000;90:180–5.
31. Paulsen FP, Rudert HH, Tillman BN. New insights into the pathomechanism of postintubation arytenoid subluxation. Anesthesiology 1999;91:659–66.
32. Wang RC. Three-dimensional analysis of cricoarytenoid joint motion. Laryngoscope 1998;108:1–17.
33. Glazer HS, Aronberg DJ, Lee JKT, Sagel SS. Extralaryngeal causes of vocal fold paralysis: CT evaluation. AJR 1983;141:527–31.
34. Merati AL, Halum SL, Smith TL. Diagnostic testing for vocal fold paralysis: Survey of practice and evidence-based medicine review. Laryngoscope 2006;116:1539–52.
35. Terris DJ, Arnstein DP, Nguyen HH. Contemporary evaluation of unilateral vocal fold paralysis. Otolaryngol Head Neck Surg 1992;107:84–90.
36. Munin MC, Rosen CA, Zullo T. Utility of laryngeal electromyography in predicting recovery after vocal fold paralysis. Arch Phys Med Rehabil 2003;84:1150–3.
37. Sittel C, Stennert E, Thumfart WF, et al. Prognostic value of laryngeal electromyography in vocal fold paralysis. Arch Otolaryngol Head Neck Surg 2001;127:155–60.
38. Gupta SR, Bastian RW. Use of laryngeal electromyography in prediction of recovery after vocal cord paralysis. Muscle Nerve 1993;16:977–78.
39. Hirano M, Nozoe I, Shin T, Maeyama T. Electromyography for laryngeal paralysis. In: Hirano M, Kirchner JA, Bless DM, editors. Neuroalaryngology: Recent Advances. San Diego: Singular Publishing; 1991. p. 232–48.
40. Parnes SM, Satya-Murti S. Predictive value of laryngeal electromyography in patients with vocal cord paralysis of neurogenic origin. Laryngoscope 1985;95:1323–6.
41. Isshiki N, Okamura H, Ishikawa T. Thyroplasty type I (lateral compression) for dysphonia due to vocal cord paralysis or atrophy. Acta Otolaryngol 1975;80:465–73.
42. Netterville JL, Stone RE, Luken ES, et al. Silastic medialization and arytenoid adduction: The Vanderbilt experience. A review of 116 phonosurgical procedures. Ann Otol Rhinol Laryngol 1993;102:413–24.
43. Bielamowicz S. Perspectives on medialization laryngoplasty. Otolaryngol Clin North Am 2004;37:139–60.
44. Weinman EC, Maragos NE. Airway compromise in thyroplasty surgery. Laryngoscope 2000;110:1082–5.
45. Rosen CA. Complications of phonosurgery: Results of a national survey. Laryngoscope 1998;108:1697–703.
46. Anderson TD, Spiegel JR, Sataloff RT. Thyroplasty revisions: Frequency and preduictive factors. J Voice 2003;17:442–8.
47. Woodson GE. Arytenoid repositioning surgery. In: Sulica L, Blitzer A, editors. Vocal Fold Paralysis. Heidelberg: Springer; 2006. p. 177–85.
48. Zeitels SM, Hochman I, Hillman RE. Adduction arytenoidopexy: A new procedure for paralytic dysphonia with implications for implant medialization. Ann Otol Rhinol Laryngol 1998;173:2–24.
49. Paniello RC. Laryngeal reinnervation. In: Sulica L, Blitzer A, editors. Vocal Fold Paralysis. Heidelberg: Springer; 2006. p. 189–202.
50. Goding G. Bilateral vocal fold immobility. In: Sulica L, Blitzer A, editors. Vocal Fold Paralysis. Heidelberg: Springer; 2006. p. 237–48.

81

Muscle Misuse Disorders of the Larynx

Linda Rammage, PhD
Murray Morrison, MD
Hamish Nichol, MBChir

Traditionally, voice disorders have been classified as "organic or structural" or "functional or psychogenic" based on the nature of the assumed primary etiological factor(s). Such a simplistic classification system does little to delineate the complex, multifactorial nature of disorders of the larynx and, taken literally, could lead us to believe that one of two primary treatment pathways should be followed for a given individual. The term "muscle misuse disorder" refers to the broad spectrum of dysfunctional patterns that contribute to or cause voice problems, chronic cough, paradoxical vocal fold movements, and other symptoms that can be associated with muscle hypertonicity and/or asynchrony of movement patterns affecting laryngeal function.

The term "misuse" implies that the psychomotor system involved in voluntary muscle activity is providing the wrong commands with respect to the degree of muscle tonus required to perform a motor act, the specific muscles that need to be involved for a particular movement, or the coordination among muscle systems that allows for efficient and effective movement patterns. Although voluntary muscles can be controlled at a conscious level, it is largely at a subconscious level that inappropriate patterns of movement are acquired, through repetitive maladaptive gestures or postures, responses to environmental stimuli or anatomical changes, or psychological mechanisms such as defense or inhibition of the expression of emotions.

CAUSES OF MUSCLE MISUSE DISORDERS OF THE LARYNX

The larynx is susceptible to dysfunction related to muscle hypertonicity and/or asynchrony of movements through the voluntary and autonomic nervous systems. A number of physiological factors result in the larynx being a target organ for muscle misuse patterns.

First, the evolutionary and developmental patterns of the larynx reinforce its primary life-preserving function of airway protection, manifested by its multilayer folding structure which creates a complex and dynamic valve system in the respiratory tract.[1]

Second, the larynx, pharynx, and esophagus form an embryologically related neuromuscular tube that is controlled by both voluntary and involuntary systems. Not surprisingly, nonspeech functions such as swallowing, breath-holding, and coughing have both voluntary and involuntary system involvement. Voice production for speech is a psychomotor act that is the result of complex interactions among multiple systems in the central nervous system and in peripheral structures. Speech involves contributions from cognitive, linguistic, emotional, neuromotor, respiratory, phonatory, resonance, and articulatory systems. Some aspects of vocal communication may be associated with significant contributions from high-level cognitive control while others may be considered more primal. For example, an "involuntary" scream or cry is regulated by a psychomotor command with focal activity in the limbic system and periaqueductal gray matter in the brainstem. Although this type of vocal response can be considered primal, full vocal expression of basic emotions such as fear, anger, and grief can effectively be inhibited by higher central nervous system (CNS) commands. One of the most effective ways to inhibit free vocal expression is to maintain a higher level of tone in muscles that would need to be involved in the act of crying out, laughing, screaming, etc. Through a variety of executive functions, the psychomotor system can produce tonic levels in the peripheral muscles in multiple systems involved in speech production: those of respiration, phonation, resonance, and articulation. Examples of this type of muscle pattern misuse include jaw clenching (to inhibit "biting someone's head off/chewing someone out") and breath-holding at the abdominal/laryngeal levels (to inhibit screaming, shrieking, or crying). It is worth noting that these executive cognitive-emotional functions are not fully developed until after puberty and so are not operational in infants and young children to the extent that they are in adults. Certain neurological and psychiatric conditions may also disrupt or enhance the tendency to repress the vocal expression of emotions through these sophisticated cognitive-emotional programs.

Third, the nonspeech functions of the face, articulators, larynx, pharynx, and esophagus may interfere with voluntary muscle activity required for vocal communication. For example, the rhythmic vertical movements of the larynx during respiration may not coincide with the desired laryngeal level required for optimal resonance during vocal productions. Or, after swallowing, if the tongue does not return to its neutral position, it may result in inappropriate resonance and/or articulation patterns for vocal communication or performance.

There are also a number of individual factors that may make certain individuals more susceptible to muscle misuse patterns in the larynx. Both intellectual and emotional elements of thought are influenced by an individual's personality and style, and these set the postural and muscle tonus patterns required to deliver an utterance with the appropriate pragmatic intent. The neuromotor activities associated with vocal communication require sophisticated coordination. Some individuals appear to execute the complex motor acts with relative ease, whereas other individuals struggle to coordinate the movements between the various systems that must work together to produce energetic, fluent, and dynamic speech phrases.

Individual anatomical and health issues may play a role in the ease with which one coordinates the various muscle systems for natural and free vocal acts. The influence of gastroesophageal reflux (GER) on laryngeal function is described in Chapter 76, "Laryngopharyngeal Reflux, Infections, and Manifestations of Systemic Diseases." Reflex hypertonicity in the larynx due to GER can interfere with normal tonicity required to initiate and sustain appropriate phonatory patterns.[2] Normal developmental and aging changes can cause compensatory muscle misuses in the vocal tract that result in poor adaptation. The pubescent boy whose larynx grows quickly may adapt to the changing acoustic and kinesthetic feedback by misusing muscles to maintain a high laryngeal posture and a glottal posture that produces falsetto register. A senescent man may react to the gradually rising natural fundamental frequency (f_0) of his thinning, aging vocal folds by adopting an abnormally low laryngeal posture, and a glottal posture that compresses the vocal folds in anterior-posterior and/or lateral directions to increase adduction and superior-inferior contact of the vocal folds.

Social, domestic, and/or occupational demands for some individuals result in a heavy vocal "dose."[3] The need to vocalize at high intensities for extended periods of time due to poor acoustic conditions, occupational demands, and/or psychosocial expectations is frequently associated with changes in speech breathing, articulation, and laryngeal muscle tension.

EVALUATION OF INDIVIDUALS WITH MUSCLE MISUSE DISORDERS OF THE LARYNX

We find it helpful to evaluate muscle misuse disorders of the larynx within a framework that encompasses four basic realities that can influence muscle use at different levels of the vocal tract.[4,5] The model represents four broad areas, or "platforms," of human function that, at any given time, are exerting a variable influence on muscle tonus and coordination for vocal communication and performance and primary laryngeal functions: lifestyle, emotion, reflux, and technique (a-LERT). A primary or secondary lesion or other disease process can be superimposed on the four core platforms (Figure 1). A distinct lesion on the vocal fold(s) or a neurological disease affecting muscle tonus/coordination will always be depicted as potentially influencing or interacting with the four core platforms. More specifically, pathologic processes that effect changes in anatomic relationships will inevitably lead to adjustments in laryngeal posture and muscle use in an effort to compensate for the anatomic or physiologic aberration.

The a-LERT model assumes that any of the four basic platforms could cause laryngeal disorders and that all play an etiologic role in every patient's symptoms if only to a minor degree. Individual platform components may be predisposing, precipitating, or perpetuating factors. We will use the a-LERT format to present evaluation strategies and techniques for individuals with muscle misuse disorders of the larynx.

During the history taking process, significant time is spent exploring both health and lifestyle profiles. The in-person interview is expedited by information obtained on a patient intake questionnaire, provided in advance for completion by the patient or guardian (Figure 2). The intake profile also serves to provide some indication which of the interdisciplinary team members may need to be present during the initial evaluation.

Lifestyle and Environment

An individual's occupational, domestic, and recreational activities, and the environments in which vocal demands are met may contribute to or cause muscle misuse patterns, which may be associated with primary or secondary vocal fold lesions such as nodules, hemorrhagic lesions, polyps, or Reinke edema.

The environmental conditions under which one lives and works need to be described to identify potential stimulants to muscle misuse. A common cause of occupational voice disorders characterized by muscle misuse is frequent voice use in poor acoustic conditions. High ambient noise levels, poor signal-to-noise ratios, and reverberation times that are too short or too long are the most common acoustic conditions that contribute to reduced speech intelligibility and cause individuals to raise their voices above a comfortable and efficient loudness level and to change muscle patterns in the respiratory system, larynx, and articulatory system. The Lombard reflex, which predicts an increase in speech intensity in the presence of background noise, is largely responsible for changes in speech breathing, vocal intensity, and f_0.[6–8] The *vocal dose* is a useful way of documenting vocal demand.[3] Measures of voice dosimetry that include both phonation time and intensity are used in some settings in an attempt to quantify vocal dose, with portable voice accumulator devices.[9] Such measures of acoustical power over time may provide a good estimation of vocal dose.

Although documentation of acoustic environment for vocal use is impractical from the laryngologist's office, initial questioning about ambient noise, reverberation (or "echo"), room size, building construction features (eg, floor surface, ceiling surface, ceiling height, windows, "open-plan" features, indoors, or outdoors) will suggest whether further steps need to be taken to assess the acoustic environment.

Some individuals are exposed to high levels of toxins and/or odors they perceive to be noxious. In certain individuals, these types of airborne stimulants can trigger hypertonic responses in the larynx, known as *irritable larynx syndrome*, which will be discussed in greater detail later in the text. Question patients about multiple chemical sensitivities, "allergies," or hypersensitivity to odors. Sometimes having a patient elaborate on reactions to a specific odor will reveal a sensory memory that is associated with a significant psychological event. It is often also the case that individuals who are concerned that a particular odor represents a noxious agent in the environment will have an exaggerated reaction in the airway, and environmental testing may need to be completed to allow for reassurance or environmental corrections.

Individuals who work in environments that are extremely dry or humid may also exhibit airway hypersensitivities resulting in a variety of muscle misuse patterns in the larynx. Finally, individuals who are frequently exposed to viral contaminants may be more susceptible to muscle misuse problems in the larynx. Public school teachers are frequent targets for this environmental hazard.

It is important to consider personality features and occupational, domestic, and social activities when exploring voice use patterns with each patient. Some individuals may not appreciate the extent of their daily voice use and may need to be assigned a task to record voice use and conditions, with the help of an external observer if necessary, to reach an appreciation of their vocal demands. It is necessary to identify that nonspeech vocal activities, such as yelling, screaming, throat clearing and coughing, or imitation of mechanical noises are associated with muscle misuse in the larynx and, additionally, that they can induce trauma that may cause voice changes or trigger other laryngeal symptoms. It may also be necessary to consider sociolinguistic influences on vocal activity and acoustic targets. Attempts to match vocal intensity, pitch or quality of parents, peers, or media personalities may result in chronic misuse of muscles to emanate a particular vocal style. Listen for breathy voice, vocal roughness from glottal fry use, or inappropriate pitch, all of which may be subconsciously mediated by a desire to make a particular vocal impression.

Other lifestyle factors that affect laryngeal health, such as smoking, excessive caffeine or alcohol intake, hydration, and fitness should all be explored to gain a full appreciation of the potential influences on laryngeal muscle use.

Emotion

Emotions are a normal human function. Everyone experiences psychological stressors due to external and internal demands, and a variety of coping

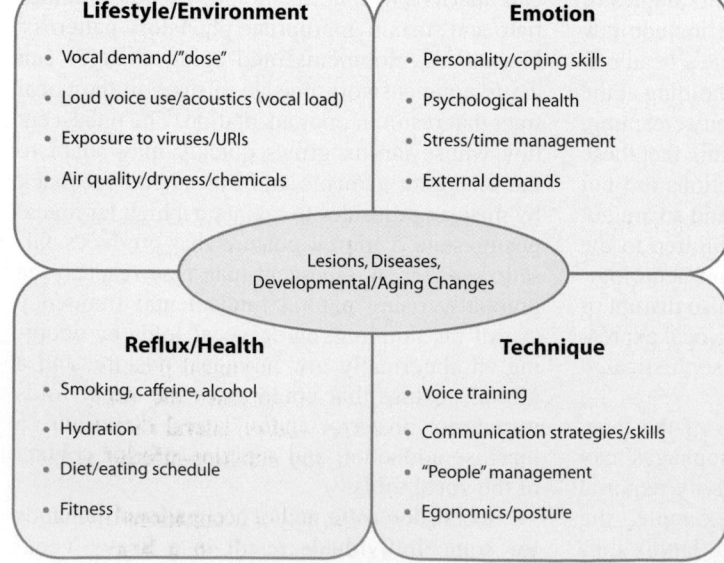

Figure 1 The a-LERT model for evaluation of individuals with muscle misuse disorders of the larynx.

PVCRP

PROVINCIAL VOICE CARE RESOURCE PROGRAM
Linda A. Rammage, PhD, S-LP(C), Director

PACIFIC VOICE CLINIC. INC
Murray D. Morrison, MD, FRCSC, Director

www.pvcrp.com

Diamond Health Care Centre
Vancouver General Hospital
2775 Laurel Street
Vancouver, BC   V5Z 1M9

Phone: 604-875-4204
Fax: 604-875-5382

PLEASE PROVIDE THE FOLLOWING INFORMATION AS ACCURATELY AND COMPLETELY AS POSSIBLE:

NAME: _____   TODAY'S DATE: _____

DATE OF BIRTH: _____   AGE: _____   SEX: M or   F

Tel: Res:_____   Work/Cell:_____   Email: _____

OCCUPATION(S) (list all **current** & seasonal occupations)   # YEARS   Full-Time or Part-Time (specify %)

1) _____   _____   _____   _____ - _____

2) _____   _____   _____   _____ - _____

3) _____   _____   _____   _____ - _____

REASON FOR VISIT: Describe Symptoms in order of Importance: How Long?

Symptom #1: _____ ;   _____

Symptom #2: _____ ;   _____

Symptom #3: _____ ;   _____

Other Concerns: _____

_____

Work days missed due to throat/voice problems:_____   When? _____

MEDICATIONS AND DOSAGE: _____

_____

ALLERGIES, INCLUDING DRUG ALLERGIES: _____

SURGERIES, SERIOUS ILLNESSES, INJURIES AND HOSPITALIZATIONS (descriptions and dates):

_____

_____

_____ **(Please turn over)**

(A)

mechanisms may be observed. Some coping styles are more adaptive than others, and some contribute to laryngeal problems.[10] Personality and psychological health characteristics may contribute to maladaptive coping styles. The motor system activity associated with vocal communication and other laryngeal functions cannot be considered in isolation from emotional influences. Under some conditions, emotional reactions can and frequently do contribute to muscle misuse patterns through mechanisms of the voluntary and involuntary muscle systems and through the sympathetic nervous system. For example, misuse of muscles in the respiratory system and larynx may result in a quiet and monotone voice, which is commonly identified as a sign of depression. Feeling a "lump in

the throat" and associated dysphonia is associated with hypertonicity in the pharyngeal constrictor muscles, which may result from gastroesophageal reflux, unexpressed fear, or both. Voice disorders may be caused by dry mucosa in the vocal tract, which is sometimes caused by an anxiety response of the sympathetic nervous system.

Psychological or personality disorders and unresolved emotional conflicts can result in chronic physical conditions that contribute to dysphonia or other laryngeal muscle misuse symptoms.[11] The voluntary muscle system is by far the most common physical mechanism through which psychological factors contribute to muscle misuse in the larynx and its suspensory system. We use the words "tense" and "uptight" to refer

to the body's reaction to psychological stressors. When these factors are the primary cause of a laryngeal problem, a variety of muscle misuse patterns and subsequent dysphonia features may be observed. Certain patterns of muscle misuse affecting laryngeal posture are associated more frequently with psychological stressors, conflict, or psychiatric disorders. The classification system for muscle misuse disorders of the larynx is presented in section "Classification of Laryngeal Muscle Misuse Patterns."

Most of the information about a patient's psychological status is obtained by listening attentively to his or her verbal response to open-ended questions, listening to changes in voice or other laryngeal symptoms, watching for changes in facial expression or body posture, and probing gently as indicated by any cues to pursue issues that may provide insight into relationships between emotions and the laryngeal disorder. More specifically, in the history, seek evidence of

- a traumatic event around the onset of the dysphonia;
- difficulties in communicating with significant others;
- suppression of significant amounts of negative emotion, such as sadness or anger;
- abusive relationships in childhood or later;
- narcissistic preoccupation with voice;
- overt anxiety or depression;
- potential primary or secondary gain factors (*primary gain* is the benefit of reduced anxiety about some internal stressor, such as concern about a potentially life-threatening illness, by focusing on the laryngeal problem; *secondary gain* is benefit from external sources enjoyed by the person with the laryngeal problem, such as not having to go to work in an unpleasant environment).

Most people will agree that their voice difficulty gets worse at times of high stress. It is helpful to ask which stressors seem to affect the voice most noticeably and which stressors are current because this may direct the interview to the source of psychologically based muscle misuse.

The inclusion of a psychiatrist or psychologist who is knowledgeable about muscle misuse disorders on the voice clinic team expedites identification of prevailing personality or psychological factors that are contributing to laryngeal dysfunction. The American Psychiatric Association has provided a standardized protocol for differential diagnosis of recognized disorders of psychological and personality function: the Diagnostic and Statistical Manual (DSM) of Mental Disorders. The current version is DSM-IV-TR.[12] The text includes advisories that it is intended for diagnostic use by mental health specialists, and that its use by individuals who are not trained in mental health evaluation should be as a reference tool to obtain information, not to make specific diagnoses.

Personality tests can provide helpful supplements to the interview, for example, the NEO

FAMILY HISTORY OF SERIOUS ILLNESSES, AND SPEECH AND HEARING PROBLEMS:

_____

_____

PLEASE ESTIMATE YOUR **DAILY SERVINGS** OF THE FOLLOWING:

_____ Water   _____ Herbal tea, Juice (non-caffeinated/non-alcoholic beverages)

_____ Caffeinated Coffee   _____ Caffeinated Tea   _____ Caffeinated Soft Drinks

_____ Chocolate   _____ Beer   _____ Wine   _____ Spirits

Do you smoke?   **Yes** or **No**   If **no**, are you a former smoker?   **Yes** or **No**

If you are a **former** smoker, when did you stop smoking? _____

If **you currently smoke** please indicate your daily consumption:

_____ Cigarettes   _____ Cigars   _____ Pipe   _____ Other
                                                                  (medicinal or recreational)

PLEASE CHECK IF YOU HAVE EVER HAD:

____ Anxiety Disorder	____ Headaches (Chronic)	____ Neck or Back Injury
____ Asthma	____ Head Injury	____ Neurological Disease
____ Arthritis	____ Hearing Problems	____ Post-Nasal Drip
____ Breathing Problems	____ Heartburn	____ Psychiatric Disorder
____ Chronic Fatigue	____ Hiatal Hernia	____ Severe Snoring
____ Chronic Cough/Choking	____ Hoarseness	____ Sleep Disorder
____ Depression	____ Irritable Bladder	____ Swallowing Problem
____ Diabetes	____ Irritable Bowel	____ Throat Clearing
____ Dramatic Weight Gain / Loss	____ Lump in Throat Sensation	____ Thyroid Problem
____ Eating / Digestive Disorder	____ Mutiple Chemical Sensitivity	____ TMJ Disorder
____ Fibromyalgia	____ Nose or Sinus Problems	____ Tremor
		____ Total Voice Loss

When was your last hearing test? _____   Result? _____

Does your voice change with your emotions? (describe): _____

_____

Do you use your voice in your occupation, or in performance? (describe): _____

_____

Do your symptoms change with the amount and type of voice use? (describe): _____

_____

(B)

Figure 2 (A and B) Patient intake questionnaire.

Five-Factor Personality Inventory[13] or inventories to identify depression, anxiety or other common symptoms of psychological dysfunction, such as the Million Behavioural Inventory[14] or the Beck Depression Inventory.[15]

Patients' self-evaluation inventories include items intended to identify the psychological impact of a laryngeal disorder. Chronic and unexplained symptoms of dysphonia, cough, globus pharyngeus, or laryngospasm may themselves become psychological stressors that perpetuate or exacerbate muscle misuse in the anatomic region associated with the symptom. The Voice Handicap Index[16] and the Voice-Related Quality of Life inventory[17] probe the psychosocial impact of a voice problem.

Look for signs of muscle misuse in the face, which can reveal prevailing emotions, both conscious and subconscious. Psychological mechanisms may result in the misuse of facial muscles to inhibit emotional expression, particularly in persons suppressing the urge to cry in sorrow, shout in anger, or scream in fear (Figure 3). Freedom of speech and voice movements can be jeopardized by tension in the muscles of the upper, middle, and lower facial areas.

Emotional distress aggravates most laryngeal disorders by adding muscle misuse to a system that may already be hypertonic. Even in the presence of a primary neuromuscular disorder, such as laryngeal dystonia, the voice may be normal when an individual is relaxed, and symptomatic when he or she is experiencing emotional distress. Vocally abusive behaviors may be associated with aggressive or attention-seeking personality characteristics. Certain psychopathological conditions identified in the DSM IV-TR, such as schizophrenia, obsessive-compulsive disorder, or Gilles de la Tourette syndrome may also lead an individual to misuse the voice by yelling, screaming, cursing, using inappropriate pitch or voice registers, or producing noncommunicative vocal gestures such as throat clearing, moaning, grunting, or coughing. A few researchers have investigated statistical relationships between vocal abuse–based voice disorders and personality or psychological characteristics.[18–24] This research suggests strong relationships between psychobehavioral characteristics and the incidence of vocal fold lesions that are secondary to vocal abuse and muscle misuse, sometimes in combination with reflux. Common behavior patterns associated with these secondary lesions in children include aggression, tension, frustration, argumentative behavior, poor coping skills, and disobedience. It is helpful to ask significant others, parents, guardians or teachers, about an individual's behavior patterns, as a patient may not have full insight into features that are perceived by others as pathological or dysfunctional.

Gastroesophageal Reflux and Associated Medical Conditions

GER, retrograde movement of gastric contents into the esophagus, is a transient, usually postprandial event that occurs undetected and without symptoms several times a day in healthy individuals. Relaxation of the lower esophageal sphincter (LES) is thought to be a normal adaptive function that relieves pressure on the stomach after eating to enhance the digestive process. Gastroesophageal reflux disease (GERD) is characterized by a broad spectrum of clinical presentations from heartburn to ulcerative esophagitis.

GERD is an important cause of both chronic laryngitis and muscle misuse in the larynx. The mechanism through which GER can cause muscle misuse in the larynx has been described both theoretically and through study of a porcine model and reflects the primary life-preserving role of the larynx in protecting the airway.[2] GERD seems to increase laryngeal, pharyngeal, and esophageal muscle tone; accompanying symptoms include postnasal drip, globus, and the feeling of a need to clear the throat. Habitual throat clearing contributes to vocal abuse and hoarseness. An irritated esophagus reflexly affects the muscles of the pharynx and larynx, causing them to be hypertonic; the resulting muscle misuse contributes to wear-and-tear injury.

Technique and Vocal Skill

Motor learning theory tells us that both adaptive skills and maladaptive motor patterns become programmed through repetition and feedback and that the CNS codes change with time to accept the frequently reinforced patterns and associated

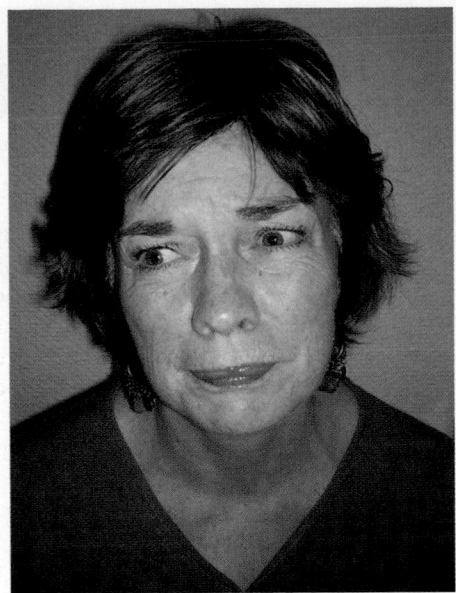

(A)

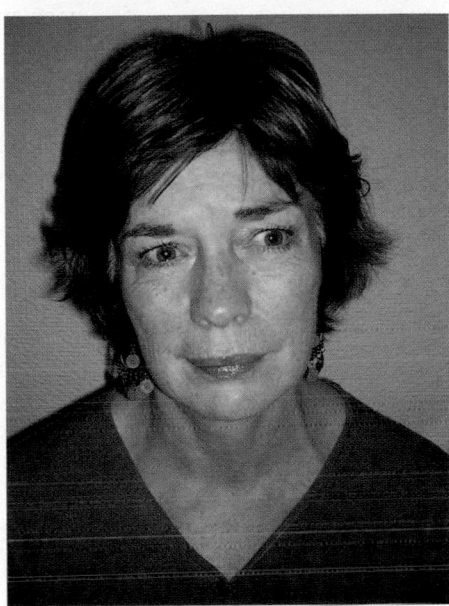

(B)

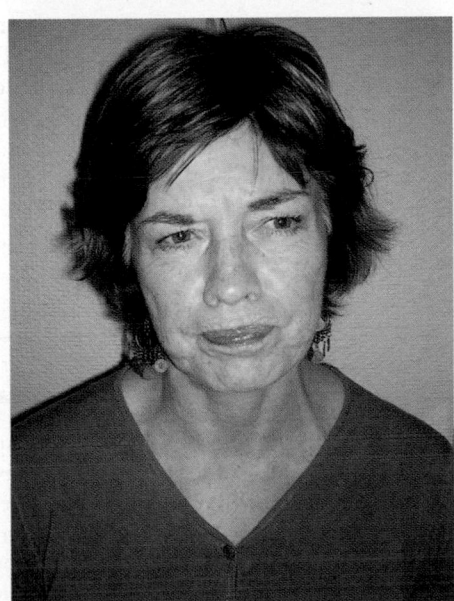

(C)

Figure 3 Muscle misuse patterns in the face in chronic repression of the vocal expression of emotions: (A) anxiety, (B) grief, and (C) anger.

kinesthetic, visual, and/or acoustic manifestations as normal technique.[25–28] Physical trauma or disease processes can precipitate or perpetuate muscle misuse, as can developmental and aging changes. Whiplash injuries sometimes result in long-term "splinting" of neck, shoulder, throat, and jaw muscles, which contributes to muscle misuse voice disorders. Body alignment, linguistic competence and comfort, communication strategies and pragmatics are among many factors influencing the neuromuscular commands that orchestrate complex muscle patterns for vocal communication.

Inquire about degree and type of vocal training and specific skills that were acquired through the programs. Consider linguistic competence, general cognitive level, and communication style of the patient throughout the evaluation. Is he or she comfortable using the primary language required to conduct his or her daily activities? Does the individual listen attentively; take turns; ask appropriate questions at appropriate times; treat others with respect; and hear well? Or does he or she seem distracted or impatient; interrupt frequently; and perseverate on issues? Does the individual speak at a normal rate; quickly; slowly? It is difficult for someone who speaks quickly, holds his or her breath while waiting to speak, or whose message is unfocused and language disorganized to coordinate the component systems for speech.

Good body posture is essential to healthy vocal production. Poor posture is often related to both technique and unhealthy ergonomic support. Ask about ergonomics in various life situations, particularly with respect to furniture and electronic props, such as computer keyboards, screens, and telephones. Some typical postural misuses may be observed in the clinical setting, depending on the type of furniture provided. You should observe informally first, then ask the patient to stand or adjust sitting posture depending on what you observe.

During conversation and a variety of vocal tasks, look for signs of

- head and neck extension, a commonly observed misuse resulting in "jaw jut," or exaggerated neck flexion, sometimes seen in individuals with globus pharyngeus;
- collapsed shoulder and rib-cage position with increased cervical lordosis;
- clenched jaw and jaw restriction during speech;
- static facial postures around the eyes, and "perma-smile" with minimal lip movement during speech; and
- strap muscle activity, especially omohyoid action with speech.

During conversation and a variety of vocal tasks, listen for signs of

- vocal tension and strain, pitch breaks, phonation breaks;
- inappropriate pitch (registration) or loudness;
- rough voice quality due to glottal fry use;
- diplophonia, typically related to asymmetry in structure or tension of the vocal folds;
- breathy voice quality;

- inappropriate resonance focus, hypernasality, hyponasality, cul-de-sac resonance with a backed tongue posture, inappropriate juvenile resonance with fronted tongue posture;
- audible inhalation with laryngeal friction or stridor; and
- variability in any of the perceptual acoustic features with changes in posture, conversation topic, or vocal task.

During conversation and a variety of vocal tasks, palpate for signs of

- inappropriate speech breathing movements: exaggerated thoracic cage activity during inhalation or vocalization; limited or no abdominal excursion during inhalation;
- hypertonic activity in suprahyoid, thyrohyoid, cricothyroid, and inferior pharyngeal constrictor muscles; and
- crepitus, bulging, or limited movement around the temporomandibular joint.

During conversation and a variety of stimulability tasks, observe improvement in muscle misuse symptoms and voice with appropriate diagnostic therapy techniques (Table 1).

The evaluation of vocal technique continues as the laryngoscopic examination is conducted. The glottal and supraglottal shapes or postures that are noted on indirect laryngoscopy have been used traditionally to classify patterns of muscle misuse. A typical example is hyperadduction of the false vocal folds, historically referred to as "dysphonia plica ventricularis."

Signs of organic change secondary to misuse may complicate the clinician's diagnostic task. Symmetrical bilateral vocal nodules are mucosal changes known to be secondary to vocal overuse and muscle misuse. Nodules often can be identified with a laryngeal mirror and, if assignment of a diagnosis is based solely on this readily identified clinical sign, it seems logical to label the disease process "vocal nodules." Such an approach to classification focuses on organic pathology, often out of context with an individual's habitual voice use patterns and may bias a clinician to focus on the organic change when planning treatment for patients. If instead, the primary etiology (misuse of muscles) is implied in the diagnostic classification, as in the descriptive term *muscle misuse dysphonia with secondary vocal nodules*, then management will more likely be directed appropriately toward reducing chronic dysfunctional muscle use.

CLASSIFICATION OF LARYNGEAL MUSCLE MISUSE PATTERNS

Our current classification of laryngeal muscle misuse patterns includes six postures, observable during phonation, often seen in combination.

Laryngeal Isometric Pattern

The laryngeal isometric pattern is most commonly seen in untrained occupational and professional voice users including singers, teachers, actors,

Table 1 Facilitation Techniques for Diagnostic and Symptomatic Therapy*

Technique	Indications	Contraindications
Adduction (forced): pushing; pulling; cough	Incomplete vocal fold closure in conversion aphonia	Do not use if mucosal edema or erythema is present
Articulation exaggeration; increased orality	Hypernasality; restricted jaw/tongue/lip movements	
Auditory masking during phonation	Incomplete vocal fold closure in conversion dysphonia; low intensity	
Breathy-flow phonation (increase MFR)	Lateral compression of vocal folds and/or false folds; aggressive glottal attacks	Do not use with laryngeal isometric
Chanting (decrease intonation and stress)	Muscle misuses resulting in pitch and/or phonation breaks	
Chewing with phonation	General tension in supralaryngeal muscles	Do not use in individuals with TMJ dysfunction
Character voices/impersonation (eg, opera singer, puppet voices)	Inappropriate pitch, resonance, monotonicity, monointensity	
Coordinated voice onset	Most laryngeal muscle misuse patterns; poor speech breathing; aggressive glottal attacks	
Distraction: eg, hum while walking, turning pages, shaking head	General muscle and postural misuse; psychological feed-forward mechanisms restricting voice range	
Inhalation phonation	Supraglottal compression; incomplete vocal fold closure; laryngeal dysfluency	Do not use if paradoxical vocal fold movements are present
Intonation increase	Monotonicity; inappropriate pitch	
Jaw movements during syllable repetition	Muscle misuse in lower face; restricted jaw movements; distraction	
Loudness change	Inappropriate loudness level; lateral glottic compression ($\downarrow$ loudness); asthenia ($\uparrow$ loudness)	Do not use exaggerated loudness if mucosal edema is present
Lower lung volume change: breathe out; "Hm!, UmHm"	Laryngeal isometric; inappropriate speech breathing; breath-holding	
Manipulation (eg,):		
Increase thyrohyoid space	Tense T–H; A–P compression	Clinician should be trained in laryngeal manipulation techniques by a qualified manual therapist
Depress larynx	Tense suprahyoids; high larynx	
Hold tongue forward	Tense tongue; backed carriage	Beware of TMJ dysfunction
Hold jaw open	Lower facial tension; poor orality	
Movements in upper body: head-nods; shoulder rolls	General muscle/postural misuse; distraction	
Pitch change	Inappropriate pitch; incomplete adduction in conversion disorder; bowed vocal folds	
Posture adjustments:	Distraction	Do not use if patient has neck/spine injuries
Head position		
Drop forward	Jaw jut; upper back/neck tension	
Drop back	Tense laryngeal suspensory muscles	
Supine position	General postural misuse	
Lean forward, neck flexed	Inappropriate speech breathing	
Register change: eg, falsetto, glottal fry	Incomplete glottal closure; tense cricothyoid muscles	
Resonance focus adjustment:		
Forward: humming-buzzing	Harsh/rough/breathy quality; poor glottal closure; poor projection	
Backed: "covering"	Fronted tongue posture; thin sound	
Siren imitation/howling/etc	Pitch range restrictions; register break	
Speech rate change	Rapid or excessively slow speech; inappropriate speech breathing; laryngeal/supralaryngeal tension	
Spontaneous phonation: extend cough, laugh, /mhm/, /hm/!	Incomplete glottal closure in conversion disorder; falsetto in adolescent transitional disorder	Do not use cough if mucosal edema is present
Taunting-teasing (ngya ngya ng-ngya-ya!)	Incomplete glottal closure; laryngeal isometric; poor resonance	
Tongue position change	Cul-de-sac resonance (front tongue)	
	Immature resonance (back tongue)	
Trills: extend voiced lip or tongue trills	Restricted pitch range; register breaks	
Voice mode change: singing to speaking; chanting to speaking; speaking to singing	Laryngeal dysfluencies; inappropriate resonance focus	
Yawn-sigh phonation	Restricted speech breathing movements; supralaryngeal compression	Beware of TMJ dysfunction with exaggerated yawn
		Do not use with laryngeal isometric or bowed vocal folds

*These techniques are used in various combinations for the purpose of diagnostic therapy, often during laryngoscopy with flexible fiberoptics to observe changes in laryngeal and supralaryngeal postures and vocal symptoms. Techniques that result in symptom reduction may be developed further during voice therapy.

media personnel, and sales representatives. It represents a generalized increase in muscle tension throughout the larynx and in paralaryngeal structures.[29] A key feature is sustained hypertonicity of the posterior cricoarytenoid muscle (PCA) which may create a posterior glottal chink (PGC)[29,30] (Figure 4). The etiology usually includes a combination of poor vocal technique, extensive and extraordinary voice use demands, and interacting or secondary psychological

factors. Anxiety is most commonly identified; and, in some cases, the diagnosis of generalized anxiety disorder is made based on criteria listed in the DSM-IV-TR.[12]

Other forms of muscle misuse may accompany the laryngeal isometric pattern. Disease of the vocal fold mucosa, most commonly bilateral symmetrical nodules (in prepubertal males and females) or chronic Reinke edema (in postpubertal males), often is identified as a component to

the diagnosis and generally assumed to be secondary to the specific pattern of muscle misuses associated with the laryngeal isometric posture.

The laryngeal isometric pattern frequently is associated with palpable increases in suprahyoid muscle tension on phonation particularly in higher pitch ranges during singing and during high vowels and phoneme transitions in connected speech. Elevation of the larynx in the neck and mandible extension may be observed as the

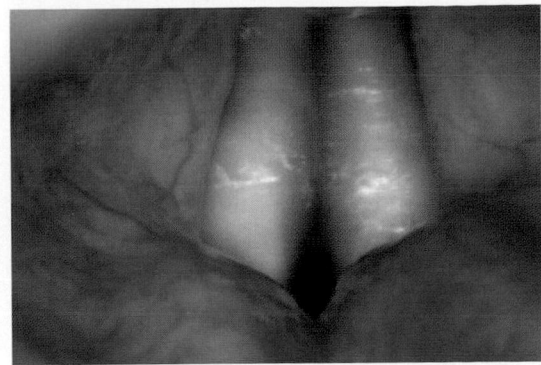

Figure 4 The laryngeal isometric posture.

patient ascends a sung scale. "Jaw jut" describes the frequently seen posture that results from simultaneous extension of the neck and mandible. During transnasal fiberoptic endoscopy, correction of the inappropriate laryngeal posture may be elicited with nasalization or humming, relaxation of supralaryngeal muscles (by palpation or head, tongue, or jaw movements), and during "coordinated voice onsets" on spontaneous utterances such as "Hm!"[5,31]

Lateral Compression

Lateral compression is a dysfunctional pattern and is a type of tension fatigue syndrome in which the larynx tends to be hyperadducted in a side-to-side direction. It may exist at the glottal level, the supraglottal level, or both. The glottal form usually is related to technical errors, but sometimes acute anxiety states may be identified. By contrast, supraglottal compression (or *plica ventricularis*) is often associated with ongoing psychogenic factors.

Subtype A: Glottal Compression. Speech associated with hyperadduction of the vocal folds typically is characterized by a harsh or strident voice quality and aggressive voice onsets, that is, glottal compression (*glottal attacks*) (Figure 5). Phonation is associated with high laryngeal resistance that explains why patients complain of vocal fatigue and discomfort at the end of a working day. In some situations, an organic illness such as an upper respiratory infection triggers the problem, but persistent hoarseness remains many weeks after the viral illness has resolved. Koufman and Blalock have used the term "habituated hoarseness" to note this relationship.[32]

Lateral compression of the vocal folds generally is accompanied by incoordinate breathing, which requires that the larynx functions as a valve to control expiratory airflow. Laryngoscopy with stroboscopy will show a prolonged closed phase, reduced vibratory amplitude, and suppression of the mucosal wave in persons with lateral glottal compression. Associated ventricular fold adduction may be seen to a limited degree. It may be important to differentiate between primary glottal level compression and primary supraglottal compression because relegation of a patient to the supraglottal contraction category may carry a stronger inference of psychogenic etiology.[5,11] During transnasal fiberoptic endoscopy, reduction in the lateral compression may be seen during more relaxed phonation, with a greater emphasis on speech-breathing and flow phonation.

Subtype B: Supraglottal Adduction. The supraglottal adduction pattern is characterized by movement of the ventricular folds toward the midline (Figure 6). It is associated with hypoadduction or hyperadduction of the true vocal folds. The status of the true vocal folds can be difficult to identify if the supraglottal adduction is extreme and occluding view of the true vocal folds.

A supraglottal compression pattern is sometimes compensatory for glottal incompetence, such as that created by sulcus vocalis, senile atrophy of the vocal folds, or vocal fold paralysis. In some cases, it may contribute to dysphonia; in other cases, adduction and phonation of the ventricular folds may contribute a desired (if not ideal) sound source. In some rare instances, supraglottal adduction may be intentional, when an individual uses the ventricular folds as a voice source. This might be trained in individuals who have congenital or acquired glottal incompetence that cannot be adequately treated with surgery.

In our experience, the lateral supraglottal compression pattern seen on laryngoscopy in patients who do not have glottal incompetence is usually associated with unresolved psychological conflict.[11] Conscious or unconscious repression of anger or sadness is common in depressed patients, and primary or secondary gain may be accrued from the voice disorder. Therapy approaches must combine correction of specific misuses with a careful evaluation and management of the psychological factors. It is in this area that the advantages of a joint approach within

a multidisciplinary voice clinic, encompassing laryngology, speech pathology, and psychiatry or psychology, are most obvious. During transnasal fiberoptic endoscopy, some relaxation of the supraglottal larynx may be elicited during imitation of a sigh, yawn, breathy voice, or inhalation phonation. Watch carefully for the patient's response to improved voice. A denial or negative reaction to improved voice, and inability to reproduce the better sound, may be an indication of psychological gain factors and/or malingering.

Anteroposterior Supraglottal Compression

Koufman and Blalock have presented a voice type labeled "Bogart–Bacall syndrome," in which patients exhibit a tension-fatigue dysphonia with phonation at the bottom of their vocal dynamic ranges, that is, anteroposterior (A–P) supraglottal compression.[32] They have reduced space between the epiglottis and the arytenoid prominences in the anteroposterior direction during phonation (Figure 7). It is commonly seen in association with the laryngeal isometric pattern. Hypertonicity in the thyrohyoid muscles is typically noted in conjunction with the A–P constriction. Individuals using this posture complain of effortful voice and rapid fatigue when speaking at a low pitch, but they are able to talk more clearly and freely at a higher pitch. This kind of voice can be "put on" by those wishing to get a particular effect of authority or sultriness; as a result it is often present in the speech of vocal performers. Singers may exhibit a similar A–P contraction pattern on phonation in association with tense pharyngolaryngeal postures. This pattern may be used to achieve a particular resonance quality, an example of which is native North American throat singing, but in other singers it may be unintentional and secondary to technical error. Some singing teachers are beginning to use transnasal flexible videolaryngoscopy with their students to provide instant visual feedback that enables them to avoid or create this contraction pattern.

This laryngoscopic pattern is not readily seen with mirror examination or with the rigid telescope because the tongue pull may extend the aryepiglottic length. Transnasal fiberoptic examination during connected speech or singing is the most effective way to demonstrate this misuse. Elicitation of slow glissando pitch glides may effect some release of the A–P constriction.

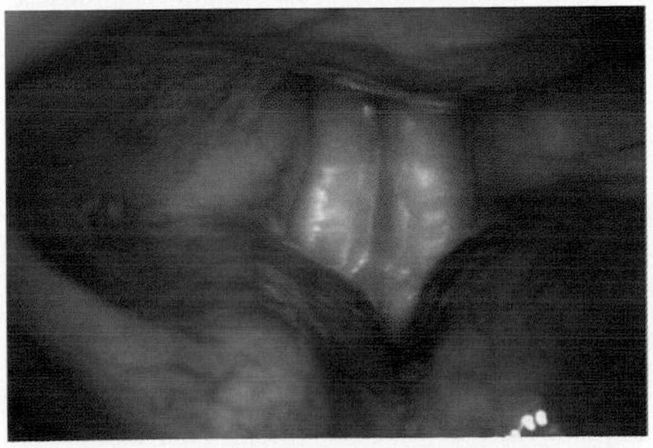

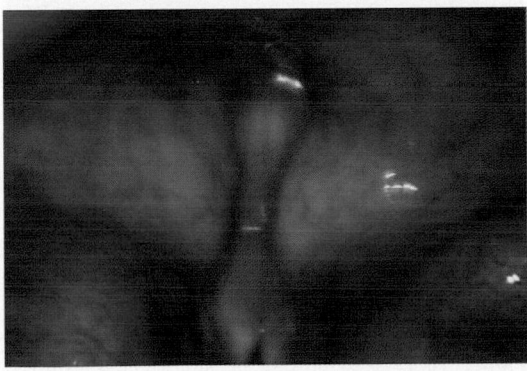

Figure 5 Lateral compression at the glottal level.

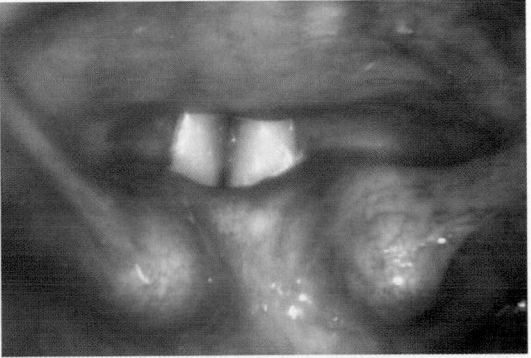

Figure 6 Lateral compression at the supraglottal level.

Figure 7 Anteroposterior compression.

Incomplete Adduction in Conversion Reaction Dysphonia

The psychological stressor or conflict that leads to a conversion reaction has produced such psychological distress that a physical symptom such as aphonia is more bearable to the person.[10,11] The type of psychological stressors and resulting muscle misuse pattern differ from those associated with other muscle misuse voice problems. In conversion disorder, the misuse may be beyond the patient's awareness, hence the typical *belle indifference* affect and facial expression. The vocal folds have full movement and can adduct normally for cough or other types of vegetative phonation such as laughter, but they stop short of sufficient adduction for voicing, and thus breathiness or a harsh whisper is the common perceptual feature (Figure 8). Generalized hypertonicity can be identified in the larynx; when sound does come out, it is usually high pitched and harsh or breathy. Forced adduction, distraction, glottal fry, or high pitches may elicit vocal fold approximation during diagnostic therapy, in which case the successful technique is used to initiate therapy in the absence of unresolved psychological gain factors that may affect motivation to achieve a normal voice.

Bowed Vocal Folds Associated with Psychogenic Dysphonia

In older patients, presbyphonia is associated with loss of muscle bulk and tone, as well as weakening and fragmentation of elastin and collagen fibers. This often results in a bowed glottal closure configuration. This so-called *senile atrophy* is not necessarily the principal dysphonia factor in patients who have bowed vocal folds (Figure 9). Occasionally, patients who appear to have a psychogenic dysphonia will phonate with a bowed glottis but may resume normal phonation and laryngoscopic appearance after voice therapy, psychotherapy, or both. This may also represent one of the forms of dysphonia in "habituated hoarseness" that follows an upper respiratory tract infection or other organic trigger.[11] During the fiberoptic laryngoscopic examination, normal approximation of the vocal folds may be elicited with pitch change (typically elevated pitch); humming or vowel resonance; coordinated voice onset ("Hm!"); inhalation phonation; or glottal fry.

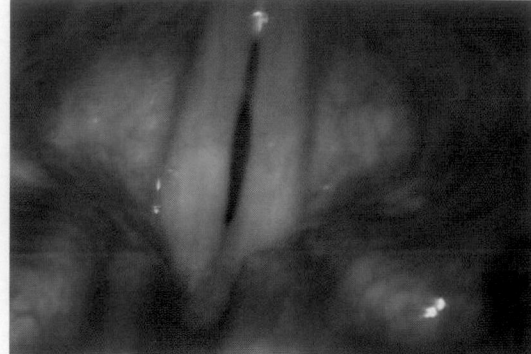

Figure 9 Bowed vocal folds due to muscle misuse.

Falsetto Register in Adolescent Transitional Voice Disorder

Normal adolescent voice change during puberty is often accompanied by pitch breaks, register breaks, and a degree of embarrassment. Psychological factors may lead to inhibition of the transitional event and establishment of perpetual falsetto phonation.[33] Laryngoscopy reveals laryngeal hypertonicity, and the cartilaginous glottis may be hyperadducted, restricting phonation to the anterior membranous part of the vocal folds (Figure 10). The larynx generally is elevated by suprahyoid muscle contraction so it approximates the hyoid bone or base of tongue. Downward traction on the thyroid cartilages sometimes results in modal register phonation at a pitch that is more representative of the adult male voice. During the fiberoptic laryngeal examination, more appropriate phonation may be elicited with a cough or throat clear; glottal fry register; effort closure; loud phonation; or coordinated voice onset ("Hm!").

Muscle Misuse Laryngeal Disorders in the Elderly

Certain voice changes are a normal part of the aging process and should not be considered disordered, but it is important for the voice clinician to recognize and understand these, to be in a position to help out when problems develop. It seems that there are two primary altered states in the larynx that develop with aging. One, which predominates in women, is a thickened, chronically edematous larynx, resulting in a naturally lower f_0 that may be below the typical "gender-ambiguous" f_0 around 160 Hz,

sometimes with accompanying dysphonic features. In the other altered state, atrophic changes predominate. These patients, most of them men, develop a higher f_0 which may be above the gender-ambiguous f_0, and thin voice timbre. Other age-related changes, such as reduced vital capacity, elasticity in structures of the chest wall, and strength in articulators, can contribute to altered speech and voice dynamics and muscle misuse patterns.[34-36] Additionally, changes in the neurological system, cognitive functioning, and peripheral hearing may contribute to muscle misuse compensations. Neurogenic disorders of the larynx are discussed in Chapter 79, "Neurogenic Disorders of the Larynx." Benign essential tremors tend to emerge in middle age or later, as do some neural events and degenerative disorders, such as cerebrovascular accidents (CVAs) and Parkinson disease. Medical and surgical procedures used to treat disorders common to the elderly, such as cardiovascular disease, may result in peripheral nerve damage, most commonly to the left recurrent laryngeal nerve during cardiac surgery or intubation injuries in the larynx during general anesthesia. Presbyacusis may play a role in voice changes as self-monitoring becomes more difficult. Finally, in older patients, loneliness or separation from family, loss of independence, and other lifestyle changes may lead to adjustment disorders with depression and anxiety, which may contribute to muscle misuse affecting the larynx.

The aging process in the male larynx involves muscle atrophy and loss of elasticity. The normal voice effect is increased pitch and "thinning" of the vocal tone. Attempts to compensate for these changes usually result in glottal fry phonation, increased laryngeal effort, and rapid vocal fatigue. Indirect laryngoscopy reveals apparent shortening and bowing of the true vocal folds. The vocal folds may adduct more efficiently if lengthening can be achieved with a higher pitched voice.

A more masculine-sounding voice in women (particularly those who have smoked for many years), caused by Reinke edema and polypoid degeneration, may be socially unacceptable. Those women who attempt to correct the pitch change by compensatory muscle misuse may develop lateral glottal and supraglottal compression and increased vocal effort. Phonation becomes easier and clearer when the patient is encouraged to allow the vocal tone to drop to a more natural range that is consistent with the age-related mucosal changes.

How far do these changes have to go before they cease to be normal? The answer usually rests with the individual patient's physical and psychological reaction to the changes and the ease and effectiveness with which he or she is communicating. A change in vocal image is often at the core of an individual's concern. When the older woman's voice is so low in pitch that she is addressed as "sir" on the phone, she may consciously or subconsciously make muscular adjustments to raise the pitch. This tactic may work to a point, but soon the dysphonic voice

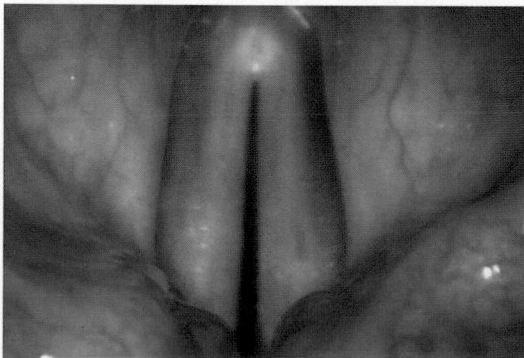

Figure 8 Hypoadduction in conversion dysphonia or aphonia.

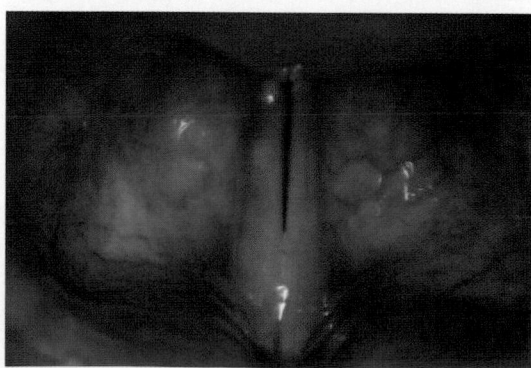

Figure 10 Falsetto posture in adolescent transitional voice disorder (ATVD).

resulting from muscle misuses associated with the attempted compensations is a greater problem than the natural changes causing the low pitch. Similarly, the old man with an easily tiring "glottal fry" phonation and bowed vocal folds may be suffering more from his subconscious attempt to drive the vocal pitch down to the male range than from the muscle atrophy, fragmented collagen, and weakened elastin of his larynx.

The Irritable Larynx Syndrome

In the irritable larynx syndrome, laryngeal spasm is triggered by a sensory stimulus. The laryngospasm might produce airway obstruction, often called "vocal cord dysfunction" or "paradoxical vocal cord motion." Obstruction during inspiration rather than expiration is a helpful cue in differential diagnosis, as this does not fit the typical profile for asthma. Laryngeal spasm can cause episodes of cough, a sense of a lump in the throat (globus), or voice difficulties, manifest as episodes of tight, strained, spasmodic voice.[29,33] The irritable larynx syndrome (ILS) was initially defined in 1999 as "hyperkinetic laryngeal dysfunction resulting from an assorted collection of causes in response to a definitive triggering stimulus."[37] We hypothesized that some or several processes had altered brainstem control of laryngeal sensory-motor processes so that abnormal muscle tension or spasm occurred in response to what would otherwise be a normal sensory stimulus. Inclusion criteria for the ILS are episodic laryngospasm and/or dysphonia with or without globus or chronic cough, visible or palpable evidence of tension or tenderness in laryngeal muscles, and a definite symptom-triggering stimulus. The scoring system for extralaryngeal muscular tension, estimated by palpation, has been previously published.[38]

The overreaction to normal sensory stimuli may be postviral or a somatoform disorder related to anxiety, depression, or posttraumatic stress disorder (PTSD). ILS is often part of a bigger clinical picture that includes irritable bowel, fibromyalgia, migraine headache, and other clinical conditions that might be lumped together as central hypersensitivity disorder (CHD). Causes of CHD may include personality predisposition, life traumas (PTSD), chronic pathologic stress, immune disorder, infections, and others. The presence of significant GER seems to play a role in development of throat (ILS) symptoms in patients with CHD.

MANAGEMENT OF MUSCLE MISUSE DISORDERS OF THE LARYNX

The management program is informed by patients' a-LERT profiles and any complicating lesion, disease process or other physiologic changes. In some individuals, reflux may play a major role in predisposing, precipitating, and/or perpetuating the hypertonicity, and an appropriate level of reflux management is designated as a priority. Other forms of treatment, such as psychotherapy or voice therapy may be less effective if reflux symptoms are not minimized first. In other cases, reflux may not appear to contribute significantly to muscle misuse patterns, and focus for management may be primarily on changing specific aspects of lifestyle, technique and/or approaches to coping with emotions and personality characteristics.

Voice Therapy

Voice therapy programs are managed by speech-language pathologists with an expertise in disorders of the larynx. Programs may take any of a number of formats. In cases where psychological factors appear to be minimal, attention will be given to patient education, insight and modification of any relevant lifestyle and environmental factors that are contributing to muscle misuse. Suggestions may be made about modifying the acoustic environment, using voice amplification systems, or changing people management styles, for example, using nonvocal approaches to behavioral management in the public school classroom.

For patients in whom muscle misuse in the larynx is associated with general body posture misuses, voice rehabilitation will include a comprehensive hierarchical motor relearning program for body alignment, appropriate use of muscles around the head, neck and shoulders, and specific adjustments and exercises for tongue, jaw and facial muscles. If dysphonia is associated with the muscles misuse problem, motor relearning activities will be introduced to improve speech breathing and voice onset, resonance, vocal flexibility, vocal dynamics and meaningful speech phrasing. This type of comprehensive program is often provided in a group format, which can offer time and financial efficiencies to a number of individuals needing similar instruction and mutual support. Self-evaluation inventories are used at various stages to help clinician and patient chart progress and document areas that need more intense focus. A self-help guidebook is used in our clinic to provide specific direction for practice.[31]

Group therapy is not recommended for individuals who may have significant psychological factors contributing to their muscle misuse disorder, who are reserved about working with others, who have difficulties attending and turn-taking, or other personality features that might reduce the benefit for themselves or others. Individual programs of voice therapy and psychotherapy should be coordinated to ensure appropriate ordering of treatment. In instances where psychological gain factors, personality disorder, or psychological illness are impinging on a patient's motivation to participate fully in a voice therapy program, it should be deferred until the psychological issues are managed.

Symptomatic therapy may be used to deal with short-term, specific symptoms of muscle misuse. Specific techniques may be identified during the evaluation that result in improved function, and these can be shaped into more appropriate muscle function for speech, relaxation, or the laryngeal valve system. For example, a 15-year-old boy with adolescent transitional voice disorder is using the posture for falsetto during speech. By manually releasing the larynx down and/or initiating a cough or glottal fry, modal register may be produced. The patient can take on the responsibility of lowering his larynx and practicing the designated voice onset technique. Once he can consistently initiate his voice in modal register, he is encouraged to sustain the tone, using any combination of kinesthetic feedback to reinforce appropriate muscle use patterns. Once tone can be extended reliably in the modal register, articulatory movements can be introduced to allow for speech sequences. Any combination of facilitation techniques may be used in a similar way to assist a patient with conversion dysphonia, assuming psychological factors have been identified and resolved. The support of a family member or friend during therapy can be reinforcing and help the patient adjust to the dramatic difference that is typically experienced rapidly.

Manual therapy, specific manipulation of hypertonic muscles, is used both as primary and adjuvant therapy for some individuals with muscle misuse disorders of the larynx. The techniques often involve release of large muscle sets first, followed by more manipulation of specific paralaryngeal and laryngeal muscles.[39] This type of management requires a thorough understanding of anatomy, indications and contraindications, and specific techniques for effective and safe application, and training should be sought from an experienced manual practitioner.

In addition to the various techniques used in comprehensive and symptomatic therapy, a variety of holistic approaches to body realignment, relaxation, and fitness may serve as adjuvant therapy. Patients with muscle misuse disorders of the larynx often experience benefit from participating in programs of yoga, Alexander technique, Feldenkrais, massage therapy, acupuncture, and various approaches to aerobics and fitness.

Principles of Psychological Intervention

In cases where it is clear that psychological factors play a definitive role in the etiology of an individual's muscle misuse disorder, the mental health professional is advised to proceed with caution to avoid instilling skepticism in the patient who may be unaware of or unwilling to accept this aspect of the diagnostic profile. Begin by asking patients to state their understanding of the cause of their symptoms. It is astonishing how frequently intelligent patients respond to this request with something as simplistic as, "My stomach makes too much acid," immediately after the team has explained that all four a-LERT factors are relevant. After correcting this misunderstanding, it is possible to continue the discussion with some hope of receptivity and collaboration.

Despite Descarte's apparent separation of mind and body in his well-known comment, "Cogito ergo sum," we are indeed *unitary organisms*: thought, emotion, and bodily action are all united. A thought that evokes no emotion gives rise to no impulse to action. A thought that does evoke emotion elicits the impulse to action. It is not possible to act without the use of muscles. In those situations in which an individual has long been suppressing the impulse to express emotionally charged sounds, muscles of the vocal mechanism will be compromised, hence the need for voice therapy and psychotherapy.

Management of Compensatory Muscle Misuse Problems Due to Aging Changes

Management of voice problems that are compensatory to aging changes and their complications may include assisting the individual to accept the natural pitch associated with his or her senescent structure, followed by voice therapy to reduce muscle misuse and facilitate use of the natural pitch range. In patients in whom compensatory misuse is an attempt to control other anatomic and physiologic processes, such as benign essential tremor (BET) with or without dystonic spasms, additional strategies should be considered. Individuals with BET typically compensate by adopting a laryngeal posture that stabilizes the hyperkinetic laryngeal movement. In doing so, they usually increase the A–P and lateral compression of the vocal folds, decrease the pitch, and increase the vocal tremor and/or spasms. Adjusting to a higher f_0 range allows for a less muscular and more aerodynamic mode of phonation, reducing the tremor and spasms.

Management Program for Irritable Larynx Syndrome

Based on the belief that ILS is related to a hypersensitive reaction to normal sensory stimuli, we treat patients using a three-level strategy.

Level 1. Minimize sensory stimuli, for example, reflux, odors. When the patients are aware that they have spasm symptoms on exposure to airborne irritants such as perfume or car exhaust, they can be more attentive to avoiding exposure, such as being able to make their workplace "scent-free." Since it is likely that GER is a strong sensory stimulant of laryngeal muscle tension, it makes sense to minimize reflux as much as possible. Most ILS patients stay on protein pump inhibitors in the long term, in addition to lifestyle and diet measures.

Level 2. Reprogram the malhabituated central response. Voice therapy and training in relaxed throat breathing can be helpful in reprogramming motor behavior. Specific exercises, repeated many times a day, such as sniffing or pursed lips breathing can help to take the brainstem focus away from the larynx.[40] Cognitive behavioral therapy, with a skilled psychotherapist, may be most effective. This gives the patient the opportunity to understand the background of symptom causation as well as ways in which they can let go of the need to continue the course they are on.

Level 3. Use neuropsychotropic medication if indicated. Selective serotonin reuptake inhibitors (SSRIs) and combined serotonin and norepinephrine reuptake inhibitors, such as venlafaxine, are the most frequently used preparations. Tricyclic antidepressants, more frequently used in chronic pain and fibromyalgia, have a mouth- and throat-drying side effect that is sometimes a problem for those with throat symptoms. Baclofen, a centrally acting spasmolytic drug, and gabapentin, an antiepileptic, may also be effective.

Other treatment modalities such as botulinum toxin (Botox) injection into the vocal folds might be employed in selected patients. Considerable benefit can be achieved through regular and progressively increasing exercise. Being in better shape makes all the parts of the body work better, and the benefits of regular production of endorphins probably exceed those of exogenous medication.

RESPONSIBILITY OF THE PATIENT AND VOICE-CARE PROFESSIONALS

Patients who are successful in rehabilitation programs are those who own their problem and assume ultimate responsibility for their rehabilitation. Barriers to acceptance of the diagnosis and responsibility to participate in a rehabilitation program include poor understanding of the nature of their dysfunction, psychological gain factors, untreated or untreatable psychological or personality disorders, mistrust of the referring health practitioner and/or therapist, and stories of success or failure of other individuals in therapy. To best prepare a patient for acceptance of the problem and solution(s), it is critical to ensure that he or she fully understands the multifactorial etiology of muscle misuse disorders, which justifies a multifaceted rehabilitation program. Once the patient understands the problem, it is helpful to offer immediately a suggestion for an initial treatment step that requires commitment by the individual. The task should be chosen carefully so that it has maximum impact on dominant symptoms without imposing an excessive burden on the patient. For some individuals, this may involve initial steps to minimize reflux. In others, it might be a simple postural adjustment suggestion, such as "Check your chin level ten times each day in a mirror, and lower it if it is tilted up or protruding." Providing this simple initial step empowers the patient, by placing immediate responsibility for carrying out the necessary changes on the individual with the problem.

For patients in whom environmental factors are clearly contributing to muscle misuse, the professional team offers suggestions and support for environmental change. In instances where it is clear that uncontrollable ambient noise is interfering with normal voice function, it is important to provide support in the form of letters to employers explaining the problem and the need for solutions to be sought. These solutions may include having the acoustics assessed by an acoustical engineer, moving the patient to a different job or location, changing his or her vocal schedule, changing the room acoustics, and providing appropriate voice amplification devices. Provide written recommendations or prescriptions to employers or third-party insurers as required to support the necessary environmental and/or job status changes. Often, institutions require that the chief signatory be a physician, but cosignatories including the speech–language pathologist, psychologist, psychiatrist, and other relevant members of the team may be helpful.

CONCLUSIONS

Muscle misuse disorders of the larynx are caused by a combination of factors and may be associated with other overlying lesions, diseases or anatomical changes related to development or aging. Identification of each of the etiological factors contributing to an individual's voice disorder is imperative for the most descriptive clinical profile to be developed and for the most effective management to be planned.

ACKNOWLEDGMENT

The authors wish to thank Shelagh Davies, MSc, for her contributions.

REFERENCES

1. Fink BR, Demarest RJ. Laryngeal Biomechanics. Cambridge: Harvard University Press; 1978. p. 1–112
2. Gill C, Morrison MD. Esophagolaryngeal reflex in a porcine animal model. J Otolaryngol 1997;27:76–80.
3. Titze IR, Svec, JG, Popolo PS. Vocal dose measures: Quantifying accumulated vibration exposure in vocal fold tissues. J Sp Lang Hear Res 2003;46:919–32.
4. Morrison MD. A Pathophysiological Model of Dysphonia. Proceed XVI World Congr Otolaryngol. Bologna: Monduzzi Editore; 1997. p. 1649–55.
5. Rammage L, Morrison M, Nichol H, et al. Management of the Voice and Its Disorders. San Diego: Singular-Thomson Learning; 2001.
6. Lombard E. Le signe de l'élévation de la voix. Annales Maladies Oreilles Larynx Nez Pharynx. 1911;37:101–19.
7. Summers WV, Pisoni DB, Bernacki RH, et al. Effects of noise on speech production: Acoustic and perceptual analyses. J Acoust Soc Am 1988;84:917–28.
8. Winkworth AL, Davis PJ. Speech breathing and the Lombard effect. J Sp Lang Hear Res 1997;37:535–56.
9. Buekers R. Voice dosimetry. In: Dejonkere PH, editor. Occupational Voice: Care and Cure. The Hague: Kugler Publications; 2001. p. 21–8.
10. Egger J, Friedl W, Freidrich G. Functional dysphonia: Personality and coping behavior in stressful situations. In: Zapotoczky HG, Wenzel T, editors. The Scientific Dialogue: From Basic Research to Clinical Intervention. Amsterdam: Swets and Zeitlinger; 1990.
11. Rammage LA, Nichol H, Morrison MD. The psychopathology of voice disorders. Hum Commun Canada 1987;11:21–5.
12. DSM-IV-TR Diagnostic and Statistical Manual of Mental Disorders. American Psychological Association; 2000.
13. Costa PT, Jr, McCrae RR. Revised NEO Personality Inventory (NEO PI-R™) and NEO Five-Factor Inventory (NEO-FFI). PAR, Inc; 1992.
14. Million T. Million Behavioural Inventory. Minnetonka, MN: National Computer Systems, Inc; 1981.
15. Beck AT. Beck Depression Inventory. San Antonio, Texas: Psychological Corp; 1978.
16. Jacobson BH, Johnson A, Grywalski C, et al. The voice handicap index (VHI): Development and validation. Am J Sp Lang Pathol 1997;6,66–70.
17. Hogikjan N, Sethuraman G. Validation of an instrument to measure voice-related quality of life (V-RQOL). J Voice 1999;13:557–69.
18. Green G. The interrelationships between vocal and psychological characteristics. A literature review. Austral J Hum Comm Dis 1988;16:31–43.
19. Green G. Psycho-behavioural characteristics of children with vocal nodules: WPBIC ratings. J Sp Hear Dis 1989;54:306–12.

20 Mans EJ, Kuhn AG, Lamprecht-Dinnesen A. Psychosomatic findings in patients with vocal cord contact granulomas: Initial results. Head Neck Surg 1992;40:346–51.

21 McHugh-Munier C, Scherer KR, Lehmann W, Scherer U. Coping strategies, personality, and voice quality in patients with vocal fold nodules and polyps. J Voice 1997;11:452–61.

22 Toohill RJ. The psychosomatic aspects of children with nodules. Arch Otolaryngol 1975;101:591–5.

23 Wilson FB, Lamb MM. Comparison of personality characteristics of children with and without vocal nodules on Rorschach protocol interpretation. Acta Symbolica 1973;5:43–55.

24 Yano J, Ichimura K, Hoshino T, Nozue M. Personality factors in the pathogenesis of polyps and nodules of the vocal cords. Auris Nasus Larynx 1982;9:105–10.

25 Adams JA. A closed-loop theory of motor learning. J Motor Behav 1971;3:111–49.

26 Adams JA. Use of the model's knowledge of results to increase the observer's performance. J Hum Mov Studies 1987; 12:89–98.

27 Schmidt RA. A schema theory of discrete motor skill learning. Psychol Rev 1975;82:225–60.

28 Schmidt RA. Motor Control and Learning. Champaign, IL: Human Kinetic Publishers; 1988.

29 Morrison MD, Rammage LA, Belisle G, et al. Muscular tension dysphonia. J Otolaryngol 1983;12:302–6.

30 Belisle G, Morrison MD. Anatomic correlation for muscle tension dysphonia. J Otolaryngol 1983;12:319–21.

31 Rammage L. Vocalizing with Ease: A Self-Improvement Guide. Vancouver: Pacific Voice Clinic; 1997.

32 Koufman JA, Blalock PD. Classification and approach to patients with functional voice disorders. Ann Otol Rhinol Laryngol 1982;91:372–7.

33 Morrison MD, Rammage LA. Muscle misuse voice disorders: Description and classification. Acta Otolaryngol 1993;113:428–34.

34 Kahane JC. Anatomic and physiologic changes in the aging peripheral speech mechanism. Aging: Communication Processes and Disorders. New York: Grune & Stratton; 1981. p. 21–45.

35 Linville SE. The sound of senescence. J Voice 1996; 10:190–200.

36 Sataloff RT, Rosen DC, Hawkshaw M, Spiegel JR. The three ages of voice: The aging adult voice. J Voice 1997:11:156–60.

37 Morrison MD, Rammage LA, Emami AJ. The irritable larynx syndrome. J Voice 1999;13:447–55.

38 Angsuwaransee T, Morrison MD. Extrinsic laryngeal muscular tension in patients with voice disorders. J Voice 2002;16:333–43.

39 Lieberman J. Principles and techniques of manual therapy: Application in the management of dysphonia. In: Harris T, Harris S, Rubin JS, Howard DM, editors. The Voice Clinic Handbook. London: Whurr Publishers Ltd; 1998. p. 91–138.

40 Blager FB. Breathing Exercises for Cough: Pursed Lips Breath. Denver, CO: National Jewish Medical and Research Center; 2005.

82

Imaging of the Larynx, Trachea and Esophagus

Albert L. Merati, MD
Lacey Washington, MD

Clinical laryngology continues to include radiological evaluation as an important adjunct to the hands-on assessment of patients. In contrast to the paranasal sinuses and recesses of the tympanic cavity, however, the mucosal surfaces of the larynx, trachea and esophagus are readily accessible for examination in the office setting.[1] As a result, relatively fewer *anatomical* imaging studies are used in laryngology compared to some disciplines within otorhinolaryngology head and neck surgery. In contrast, the modified barium swallow (MBS) or video swallow is the most common *dynamic* imaging study used in this field. In this chapter, the upper aerodigestive tract will be divided into three anatomical sections: larynx, trachea and esophagus. Most of this chapter is devoted to imaging related to the larynx; indeed, some topics span several organs (such as the MBS and the discussion of airway stenosis) and are reviewed in additional sections.

The importance of history and physical examination is emphasized; interpretation of imaging studies is often useless or misleading without this information. An example of this arose recently with positron emission tomography (PET) scans[2]; a number of patients undergoing PET scans for detection or surveillance of malignancy were found to have suspicious uptake in their larynx contralateral to their known vocal fold paralysis. While understandably alarming for potential occult carcinoma causing this increased signal, 15 of the 17 patients were found to have "false-positive" studies; the enhanced uptake was felt to reflect the increased metabolic activity of the compensating vocal fold musculature and not from occult laryngeal cancer. Although this is a dramatic example, it suffices to say that patients are better served by the marriage of clinical and radiographic information.

LARYNX

Computed tomography (CT) continues to be the principal modality for imaging of the larynx. The first clinical work regarding CT evaluation of laryngeal disease emerged in 1977.[3] This early paper from Mancuso and colleagues dealt with carcinoma of the larynx and the potential role of CT in the care of these patients; over three decades later, the evaluation of suspected malignancy continues to be one of the principal indications for CT imaging of the larynx. Indeed, the clinical frontiers of laryngeal imaging involve the use of intraoperative CT scanning to follow tumor excision by the transoral laser approach.[4] Generally speaking, the larynx may be imaged for intrinsic disease as well as for invasion by extralaryngeal neoplasms, such as thyroid cancer. Other common uses for laryngeal imaging include the evaluation of vocal fold paralysis without an obvious precipitating cause, acute external trauma as well as in the assessment of airway stenosis.

Normal Radiographic Anatomy of the Larynx

While the fine structure of the vibrating vocal folds cannot be detailed with standard radiographic imaging techniques, CT imaging of the larynx allows for precise assessment of the framework of the larynx and the hyolaryngeal complex (larynx and hyoid bone). The epiglottis, preepiglottic space, aryepiglottic folds, false vocal folds, true vocal folds, arytenoid cartilages, cricoarytenoid joints, thyroid cartilage, cricoid cartilage, and the paraglottic musculature can all be easily identified on CT imaging (Figure 1).

The thyroid cartilage is not perfectly symmetrical; this may be somewhat misleading when investigating trauma to the larynx. Hirano and colleagues dissected 20 larynges and found that most, if not all, had some asymmetrical features.[5] Interestingly, there was one directional trend with a greater number of the specimens from older subjects revealing some medial rotation of the right thyroid lamina and corresponding lateral rotation of the left thyroid lamina. The clinical significance of this asymmetry is not known.

Structural Abnormalities of the Larynx: Benign Masses, Trauma, and Stenosis

Benign Masses. Some congenital laryngeal masses, such as the thyroglossal duct cyst (TGDC), are intimately associated with the hyolaryngeal complex. TGDC can present early in life as a painless midline neck mass overlying the thyroid notch. The mean age at presentation in one series was 21.5 years.[6] If the mass is higher in the neck, that is, the submental space, the differential diagnosis favors other masses, such as a ranula or dermoid cyst.

CT may be helpful in differentiating among the benign midline masses; in reality, however, the diagnosis is easily made clinically and imaging studies are confirmatory. In addition to their characteristic location, their smooth rounded appearance on radiographic images supports the diagnosis of TGDC. If atypical features, such as irregular shape or a thick wall, are present, the possibility of carcinoma arising in TGDC should be considered. In a review from the University of Utah, carcinoma was found in 6 of 6 TGDCs with soft tissue elements within the cysts on imaging whereas 3 of 18 with benign appearing cysts contained carcinoma.[7] These usually had a peripherally based mass within the cyst; calcifications were also present in the malignancies which provided CT imaging an advantage in evaluating these patients (Figure 2).

Laryngoceles are uncommon and interesting laryngeal abnormalities in which the air-filled laryngeal ventricle is enlarged into the false vocal fold and supraglottis, that is, internal laryngocele (Figure 3); in some cases, the sac extends beyond the confines of the larynx out through the thyrohyoid membrane, that is, external laryngocele (Figure 4). Whereas the internal laryngocele typically presents with hoarseness, sense of fullness, or throat clearing, an external laryngocele will manifest as a variable neck mass with or without the other laryngeal symptoms of an internal laryngocele.

Glazer and colleagues advocated CT in the evaluation of a suspected laryngocele in the 1980s.[8] CT has remained the imaging modality of choice for this clinical condition. The utility of radiography depends on its ability to confirm the diagnosis of internal versus external laryngocele; although the diagnosis is clinically straightforward in most cases, CT is useful in delineating the extent of the laryngocele and, therefore, in surgical planning. Small, internal laryngoceles may be treated endoscopically with marsupialization[9,10] (removal of the false vocal fold to open the sac into the aditus of the larynx). Traditionally, the external laryngoceles have been treated with open resection.[11] The laryngocele may have fluid in it; if this becomes infected, it may represent a surgical emergency as swelling and inflammation may compromise the airway (Figure 5).

Laryngeal Stenosis. The management of airway stenosis represents one of the great ongoing challenges in laryngology. Imaging, particularly in the form of CT, has been advocated for assessing the diseased airway both at the site of stenosis and

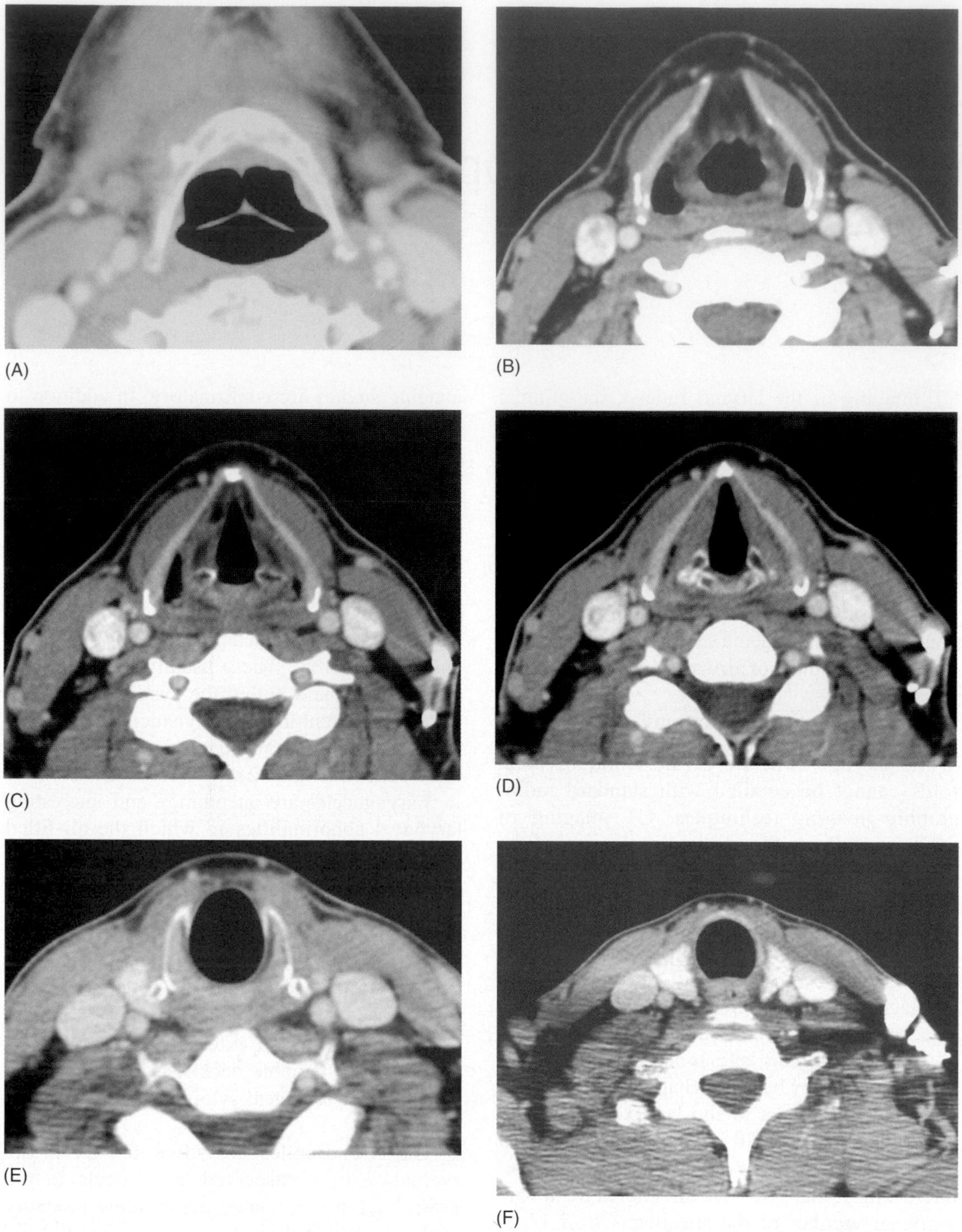

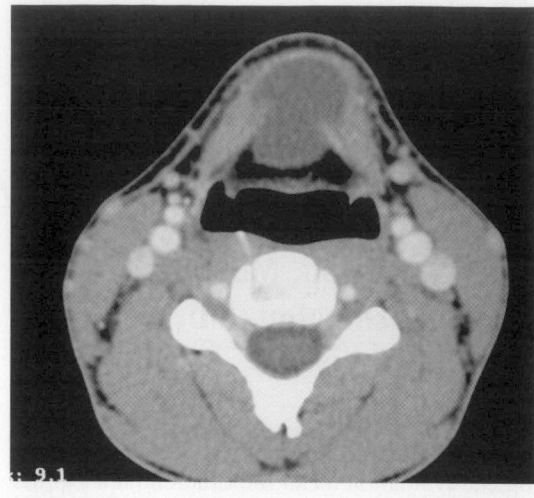

Figure 2 Computed tomography of thyroglossal duct cyst positioned over the anterior prominence of the thyroid cartilage. (Published with permission, copyright © 2007 M.A. Michel, MD.)

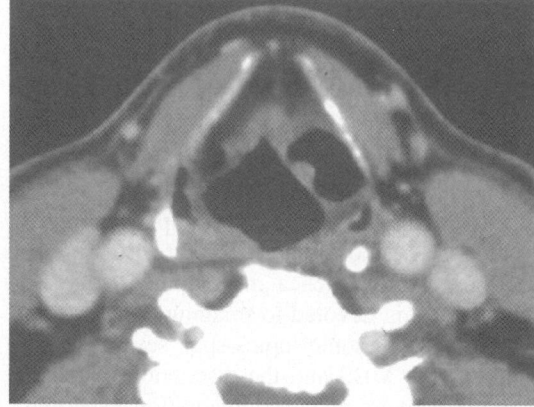

Figure 3 Computed tomography of left internal laryngocele. This sac is modestly distended with air. The normal, undistended pyriform sinuses are seen bilaterally lateral to the aryepiglottic folds and supraglottic structures. (Published with permission, copyright © 2007 M.A. Michel, MD.)

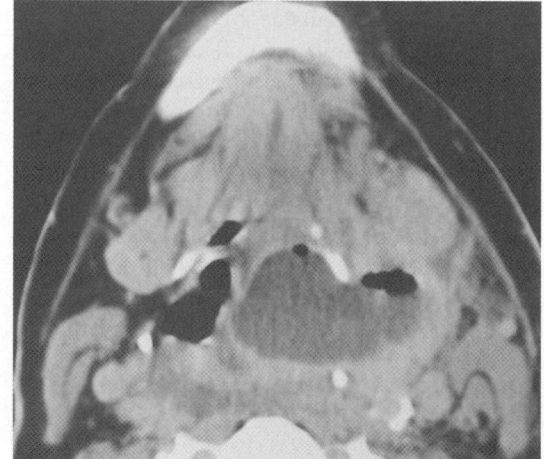

Figure 4 Computed tomography of an external laryngocele. The external elements of the laryngocele are emerging laterally through the left aspect of the thyrohyoid membrane. The sac is partially filled with air as well as fluid. (Published with permission, copyright © 2007 M.A. Michel, MD.)

Figure 1 Normal laryngeal anatomy on computed tomography (CT) scanning. (A) Laryngeal CT at the level of the hyoid and epiglottis. The midline glossoepiglottic fold can be seen in this cut. (B) At the level of the aryepiglottic folds, the thyroid cartilage comes into view. The paired pyriform sinuses are present just lateral to each aryepiglottic fold. (C) At the level of the false vocal folds, the bodies of the arytenoid cartilages are seen on each side. The relative lucency in the anterior portion of each false vocal fold represents the laryngeal ventricle. In this view, less of the pyriform sinus is seen than in superior cuts. The pyriform sinus approaches its apex at the level of the true vocal folds below. (D) At the level of the true vocal folds, the facet of the cricoarytenoid joint is seen, as is the most superior central portion of the posterior lamina of the cartilage. (E) The cricoid cartilage, though a complete ring, has a limited vertical dimension anteriorly. It may appear to be incomplete in all except a few cuts of a laryngeal CT. The cartilages seen just posterolateral to the cricoid are the inferior cornua of the thyroid cartilage. The recurrent laryngeal nerve lies in close proximity to this cricothyroid articulation on either side. (F) At the level of the trachea, the relationship between the anterolateral cartilaginous trachea and its membranous posterior wall is seen. The cervical esophagus is in direct apposition to this aspect of the trachea. Usually, the cervical esophagus is devoid of luminal air. Distension of the esophagus with air in this region may represent distal obstruction or a swallowing artifact. (Published with permission, copyright © 2007 M.A. Michel, MD.)

distal to it. A typical example of this might occur when a clinician obtains a CT scan to evaluate the subglottis and trachea in a patient with glottic stenosis; whereas the subglottis and trachea can certainly be viewed in the routine clinical setting with modest risk,[1] the presence of glottic compromise is a relative contraindication to endoscopy. In other words, it may be unwise to traverse a 5 mm airway with a 4 mm endoscope in the outpatient setting unless absolutely necessary.

The clinical history associated with airway stenosis can be helpful in characterizing the extent of the obstruction and understanding its cause,[12] whereas most patients with airway stenosis have had some endolaryngeal or external trauma, some have no history of intubation or external injury.

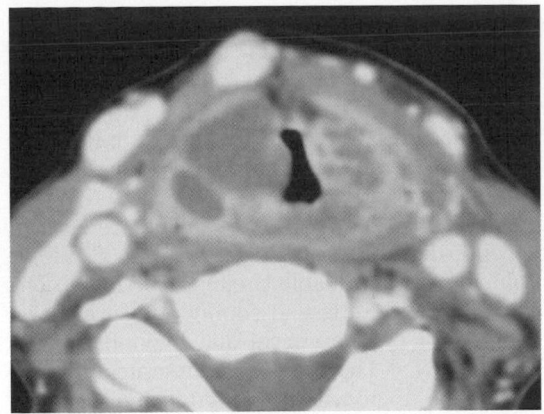

Figure 5 Computed tomography of infected bilateral mucopyocoeles. This patient had 2 weeks of progressive odynophagia and shortness of breath. She weighed only 77 lb when she was evaluated in the emergency department.

These patients without known cause are most often women. Within the larynx, stenosis can be differentiated into supraglottic, glottic, and subglottic (Figure 6). As many as 40% of patients have more than one site of stenosis.[12]

Imaging of laryngeal stenosis is executed, for the most part, with noncontrast CT. The variable nature of the radiographic appearance limits the diagnostic information obtained from CT imaging. In one review from the Massachusetts General Hospital,[13] many different configurations were noted in a series of idiopathic laryngeal stenoses; these included an hourglass-shaped airway in 53% of patients and an eccentric airway in the other 47% of patients. The superior and inferior margins of the stenotic area were smooth in 60% of patients and irregular and lobulated in the remainder. Interestingly, no evidence of calcification or ossification was seen in this series of patients without a history of mechanical trauma, that is, no intubation or external trauma.

Carretta and colleagues provided an interesting comparison between endoscopic and radiographic evaluation of airway stenosis in their evaluation of postintubation laryngeal and laryngotracheal stenosis.[14] In a prospectively evaluated series of 12 preoperative airway patients, their spiral CT imaging findings were compared to both flexible and rigid bronchoscopic assessment of the airway. While all three modalities correctly indicated the presence or absence of subglottic involvement in 92, 83, and 83%, respectively, CT did poorly in predicting the length of the stenosis at the time of open surgery. Rigid and flexible bronchoscopy were accurate 83 and 92% of the time, with only 3 of 12 cases (25%) having a correct preoperative measurement of the length of the stenosis. This is an important limitation as stenosis length is an important negative predictive factor in airway surgery. Because this study was small and limited to patients undergoing open surgery, caution must be taken before applying these findings to airway patients in general. Furthermore, the negative predictive value of CT imaging in the detection of additional areas of stenosis has not been described.

Three-dimensional (3-D) reconstruction of airway imaging is an exciting frontier in laryngology. While the elegance and attractiveness of the images cannot be denied, their actual clinical utility over and above airway endoscopy and routine CT imaging has not been proven.

Trauma. Arytenoid cartilage dislocation is an uncommon entity in which the arytenoid cartilage is dislodged from its complex perch on the facet of the cricoarytenoid joint; it is almost always associated with intubation although it may occur with external trauma. Patients complain of unilateral throat pain, hoarseness, and ipsilateral otalgia in some cases.[15] CT has been advocated to assess the position of the arytenoid cartilage in relation to the cricoid (Figure 7). The differential diagnosis to consider in these patients is acute vagal neuropathy from intubation or injury from the operative procedure itself. Laryngeal electromyography may be helpful in assessing mechanical, that is, dislocation, versus neural impairment of cricoarytenoid joint motion. Mechanical disruption of the cricothyroid articulation, also resulting in pain and hoarseness, has also been described along with its imaging features.[16]

External Trauma. It is estimated that 1 in 23,000 emergency room admissions includes the diagnosis of blunt or penetrating laryngeal trauma.[17] It is far less common than endolaryngeal injury related to intubation. Once again, CT imaging is the diagnostic procedure of choice in the case of

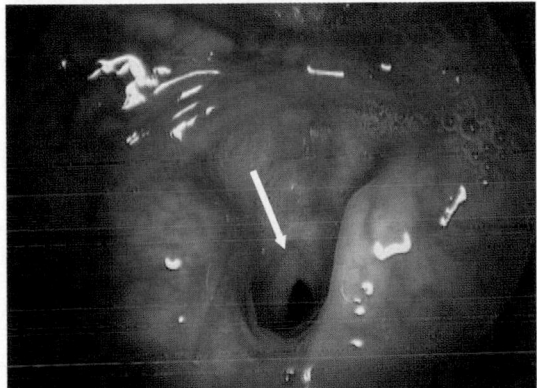

(A)

(B)

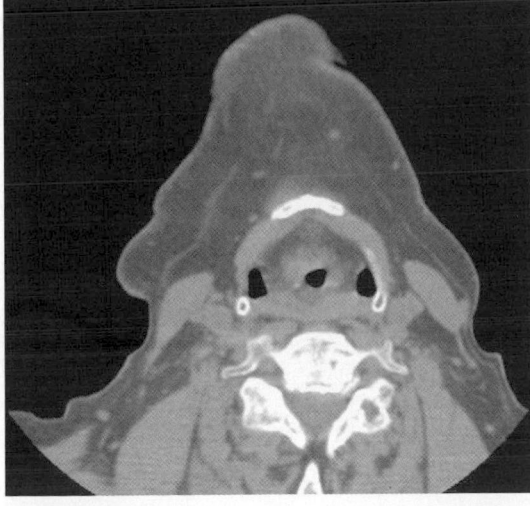

(C)

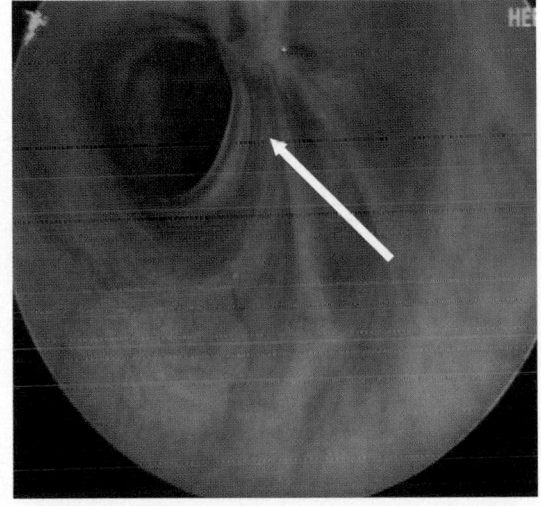

(D)

Figure 6 (A) Endoscopic view of supraglottic stenosis. The arrow points to cicatricial stenosis at the level of the false vocal folds. The true vocal folds are below this level and out of view. (B) Endoscopic view of subglottic stenosis: this patient's radiograph is seen in Figure 6D. The arrow indicates the approximate "center" of the normal airway. Her airway is about 5 mm in diameter at the time of this photograph. (C) Computed tomography of the same patient in Figure 6A. Note the airway obstruction above the level of the body of the arytenoid cartilage, the presence of the hyoid bone, and air in the pyriform sinus. (D) CT of the same patient in Figure 6B. Her subglottic stenosis is eccentric; it is entirely confined in the cricoid.

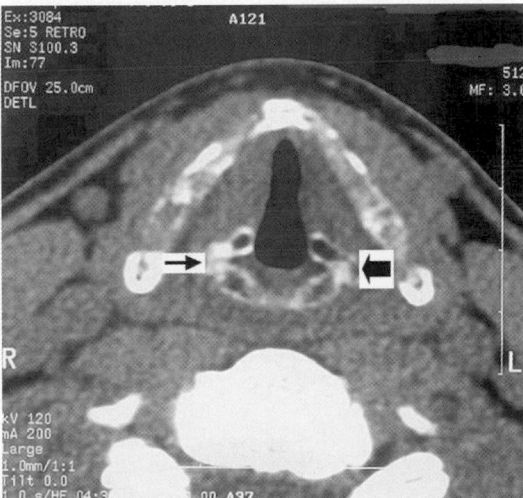

Figure 7 Computed tomography image of an arytenoid cartilage dislocation. Thick arrow on the left indicates obliterated joint space. Thin arrow on the right points to normal joint size and configuration. (Published with permission, copyright © 2007 A. Rubin, MD.)

suspected laryngeal trauma.[18] If blunt anterior cervical trauma is suspected, the airway, breathing, and circulation, that is, "ABCs," and the cervical spine receive the first considerations. This critical paradigm of trauma care impacts radiological investigation. If the injured patient is in distress, there may not be time for radiographic imaging. A surgical airway or, in some instances, intubation precedes imaging; once the airway is secure, the surgeons may explore the neck, including the laryngeal framework, or stop the procedure at that point and obtain the radiographic investigations. If, on the other hand, a patient is not in distress, the managing physician has the luxury of pursuing CT scanning for the suspected injury. Airway management depends on sensible, conservative clinical assessment; a modest laryngeal injury in an otherwise compromised patient, for example, systemic injury, anticipated difficult intubation, and/or mental status changes, may mandate an urgent surgical airway, in contrast to some severe isolated laryngeal injuries in a slender, cooperative patient which may allow for prompt radiographic investigation prior to surgery.

An example of external laryngeal trauma is seen in Figure 8. Characteristics of cartilaginous fractures include disruption of the continuity of the thyroid ala or the cricoid ring. Few scholarly comparisons have been made to detail the respective roles of laryngoscopy and radiographic imaging; as noted above, the clinical environment may impact this greatly. Many fractures result in extravisceral air; this represents air escaping into the soft tissues of the neck. If the injury is in the airway, particularly below the vocal folds, this may result in a great deal of gas escape into the soft tissues (Figure 9); a simple supraglottic or pharyngeal injury is less likely to result in air trapping in soft tissue. Scaglione and colleagues noted that CT imaging may be advantageous even in suspected minor mucosal injuries;[19] in these cases, the presence of a small amount of air was indicative of perforation and not simple mucosal laceration. Goudy and colleagues reported on a series of patients with air in the neck on CT scan; the location of the injury was found to be laryngotracheal in 37% of the cases, with a smaller amount originating from the hypopharynx (27%), oropharynx (16%), and the esophagus (5%).[20] The

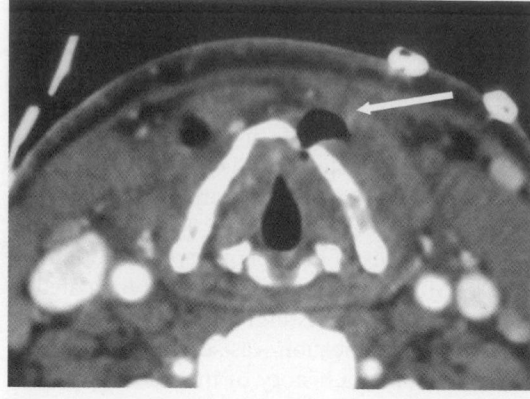

Figure 9 Computed tomography of a thyroid lamina fracture with air escape into the soft tissues of the neck (*arrow*). (Published with permission, copyright © 2007 M.A. Michel, MD.)

source of the injury was not located in 15% of patients. Recently, ultrasound has been studied in the laboratory as a potential tool for the assessment of laryngeal injury following trauma.[21] This rapid, noninvasive mode of imaging could theoretically allow for airway examination without moving the patient from the trauma room to the radiology department. For the time being, however, CT remains the dominant imaging tool to complement clinical assessment of laryngeal injury.

Malignant Neoplasms of the Larynx

Squamous Cell Carcinoma. Squamous cell carcinoma of the larynx continues to be a major source of morbidity and mortality. Laryngeal cancer has, remarkably, become more deadly since the early 1990s, the only solid neoplasm in which the 5-year survival rate has fallen in the past 10 years.[22] It is believed by many that this decline is related to the trend away from total laryngectomy as a principal component of treatment for advanced neoplasms. Radiography is used in the care of laryngeal cancer patients for two main objectives: initial staging and subsequent tumor surveillance. Recently, PET combined with CT scanning has become popular in surveillance.[23] MRI is useful in these patients as well, particularly in assessing cartilage invasion.

The vast majority of laryngeal malignancies are squamous cell carcinoma. Of these, the majority arise in the glottis, with the bulk of the remainder being supraglottic in origin.[24] Primary subglottic carcinomas are rare, comprising less than 2% of laryngeal malignancies.

Initial Staging. Many of the clinical staging parameters are related to the absolute size (in maximal dimension) of the primary tumors and their metastases. For example, a supraglottic tumor smaller than 2 cm is categorized as a T1. An otherwise similar tumor measuring 2.5 to 3 cm in size is a T2, carrying significant prognostic impact to the patient. With the advent of CT imaging, the calculated volume of the primary tumor has been found to be a potent predictor of local control in both glottic and supraglottic primaries. Mancuso and colleagues, in an important prospective series published in 1999, demonstrated that local control was 89% in tumors less than 6 cc volume; in tumors larger than 6 cc, the

local control rate at 2 years was 52% when primary radiotherapy was used as the principal treatment.[25] The initial tumor size also had an impact on maintaining laryngeal function. Mendenhall and colleagues, in a major review from the University of Florida, concluded that although the initial T category was the single most potent predictor of local control in head and neck cancer in general, the CT-derived determination of tumor volume was a valuable predictor of local control for both glottic and supraglottic primaries, but not for oropharyngeal and hypopharyngeal malignancy.[26] The inter- and intrarater reliability of this approach was reported by Mukherji and colleagues in 2005.[27] In this study, clinicians were found to have high intraclass correlation in determining the tumor volume present in a series of supraglottic carcinomas. In contrast, Hoorweg and colleagues studied 55 patients in whom the interrater reliability of tumor volume calculation, cartilage invasion, and cartilage sclerosis were found to have significant clinical variation.[28]

Gordin and colleagues have reported on their experience with combined PET/CT scanning in the diagnosis of laryngeal cancer.[23] In their series or 42 patients, they recorded a 96% positive predictive value for combined PET/CT as compared with 76% for PET scan alone or 48% for CT alone. As access to PET technology becomes more widespread, these promising figures will likely continue to impact the care of laryngeal cancer patients. In the Gordin and colleagues study, in 25 (59%) of their 42 patients, PET/CT studies resulted in an important clinical management decision.

Cartilage Invasion. Imaging if often the only preoperative indicator of cartilaginous invasion by malignancy, either from primary laryngeal carcinoma or extralaryngeal, that is, invasion by a nonlaryngeal carcinoma, for example, thyroid carcinoma (Figure 10). As noted above, cartilage invasion is an important prognostic indicator for survival and resistance to primary radiotherapy. CT scanning depends on multiple criteria to enhance the positive predictive value for the detection of cartilage invasion. Although the presence of tumor on both sides of the cartilage (understandably) is the single best indicator

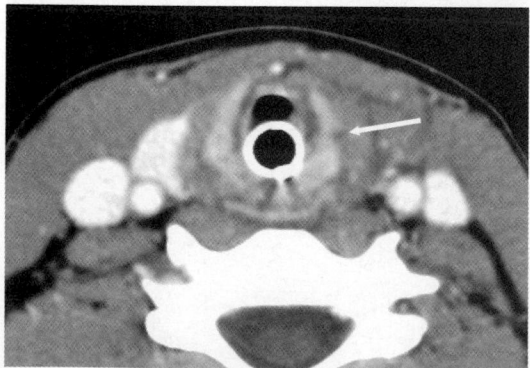

Figure 8 Computed tomography of a cricoid cartilage fracture (endotracheal tube in place). Arrow points to discontinuity of the left aspect of the cricoid cartilage. (Published with permission, copyright © 2007 M.A. Michel, MD.)

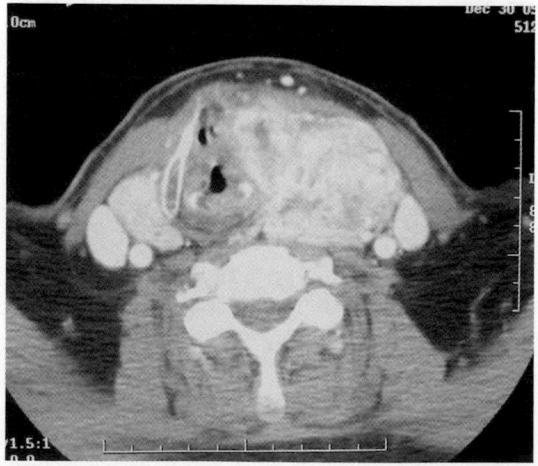

Figure 10 Computed tomography of a massive anaplastic carcinoma of the thyroid invading the larynx. (Published with permission, copyright © 2007 M.A. Michel, MD.)

of cartilage invasion,[29,30] other features are also important. The presence of tumor adjacent to nonossified cartilage as well as the obliteration of marrow space are specific but not sensitive signs of invasion of the arytenoid or cricoid cartilage.[30] In this study, however, this finding was not a specific indicator when considering the thyroid cartilage. In a major review, Becker concluded that the detection of cartilage invasion with CT "greatly depended on the appropriate use of individual and combined CT criteria."[31] MRI has been advocated by several authors over CT scanning because of its high negative predictive value.[31,32] As a matter of practicality, however, CT is still the most common modality used; in the future, the role of combined PET/CT imaging may further refine the clinical management practice for this important clinical question.

Surveillance. Although the larynx, or what is left of it, is technically easy to examine following cancer treatment, the interpretation of clinical findings is often more challenging. The following discussion focuses on the follow-up of patients treated nonoperatively as well as the detection of second primaries.

The significance of surveillance with regard to a *second primary* is illustrated in a comprehensive study by McGuirt and colleagues in which 377 surviving patients with nontotal laryngectomy were examined for metachronous lesions. Five percent of the patients who survive more than 3 years developed second primary cancers in the larynx. The likelihood of a new laryngeal cancer was lower in the patients who were originally treated with radiotherapy (4.3%) compared to the rate seen in surgical patients (9.2%). Patients with earlier stage malignancies are more likely, paradoxically, to develop second malignancies as they are more likely to survive their first malignancy.

Often, the clinician is faced with a painful and dysfunctional larynx following radiation with or without chemotherapy; the larynx may be swollen and its endoscopic appearance significantly distorted. Detection of recurrence or metachronous lesions is understandably difficult in this situation. Hermans and colleagues from Belgium reported on a series of 66 patients who underwent CT before and after definitive radiotherapy for laryngeal cancer.[33] The study included a minimum of 2-year follow-up of these patients; the likelihood of local failure was found to be well-stratified by assignment of the posttreatment scans into three grades:

1. local changes without a focal mass,
2. focal mass with maximal 1 cm diameter and or asymmetric obliteration of laryngeal tissue planes, or
3. the presence of a focal mass with a maximal diameter equal to or greater than 1 cm or an estimated posttreatment tumor volume reduction of less than 50%.

In 12 of 29 patients with local failure, "grade 3" findings were present a median of 5.5 months before the clinical examination indicated failure,

a much higher rate than in the first two, more favorable grades.

PET imaging has been advocated for over 10 years as a useful examination when faced with the question of recurrent carcinoma versus chondroradionecrosis following radiation therapy.[34,35] Terhaard published a remarkable prospective series of 75 patients (both laryngeal and pharyngeal primaries) evaluated before and after radiotherapy with a mean follow-up time of nearly 2 years.[36] Of the 27 initially negative PET scans following treatment, there were no positive biopsies at that time nor over the following 1-year period. The first PET scan was truly positive in 34 of 48 patients; in 12 of 14 patients with false-positive results, that is, biopsy negative for recurrence, subsequent PET scans demonstrated decreased uptake, thus raising the specificity and sensitivity of the PET scans to 97 and 82%, respectively. They concluded that PET imaging should be the first study when recurrence is suspected following radiation for cancer of the larynx or pharynx. If the PET scan is negative, no biopsy is needed; if the PET scan is positive but the biopsy is negative, decreased fluorodeoxyglucose uptake measured in a follow-up scan is indicative that local failure is unlikely.

Even in the absence of tumor, CT may be helpful in characterizing the status of the irradiated larynx. Chondroradionecrosis (Figure 11) is a painful and frustrating byproduct of laryngeal radiation in which the cartilage framework of the larynx becomes nonviable. Laryngeal function, including voice, swallowing, and airway, can be affected. Although hyperbaric oxygen has been recommended for treatment, many patients undergo laryngectomy for the removal of a painful and dysfunctional larynx. The principal goal of imaging in cases of suspected chondroradionecrosis will be detection of viable carcinoma in the larynx; that having been said, there are some helpful but nonspecific CT characteristics of chondroradionecrosis,[37,38] such as arytenoid

cartilage sloughing, collapse or fragmentation of the thyroid cartilage, or the presence of gas bubbles around the laryngeal framework.

Other Malignancies. Although uncommon overall, imaging is particularly helpful in identifying and determining the extent of nonepithelial malignant neoplasms, such as chondrosarcoma. These rare neoplasms comprise only a small percentage of laryngeal malignancies. Most arise in the cricoid cartilage; surgical removal is the treatment of choice. Imaging, particularly with CT, can distinguish between varieties of epithelial-derived neoplasms and these cartilaginous neoplasms (Figure 12). A review of CT findings in chondrosarcoma was published by Wippold and colleagues in 1993.[39] In this paper, the authors noted that coarse or stippled calcification within the neoplasm was the most helpful radiologic finding and was universally present in their 10 patients with chondrosarcoma. Eight of 10 patients had both endolaryngeal and extralaryngeal growth patterns. Other neoplasms do occur in the larynx, including neuroendocrine carcinomas, basilosquamous malignancies, and soft tissue sarcomas.

Inflammatory Disorders

Acute laryngeal inflammation ranges from the routine, such as viral laryngitis accompanying an upper respiratory infection, to the life threatening, such as epiglottitis. It is uncommon for imaging to be performed for the clinical extremes of these problems; for example, when a patient is in marked distress, management is focused on relief of airway obstruction. In less severe situations, a soft tissue plain lateral radiograph of the neck may be obtained by the emergency department physician. In the patient with suspected epiglottitis, the classic "thumb print" sign can be seen. The clinical impression made by the patient on the physician will be dominated by the history and endoscopic examination, if it is possible to perform laryngoscopy on the patient.

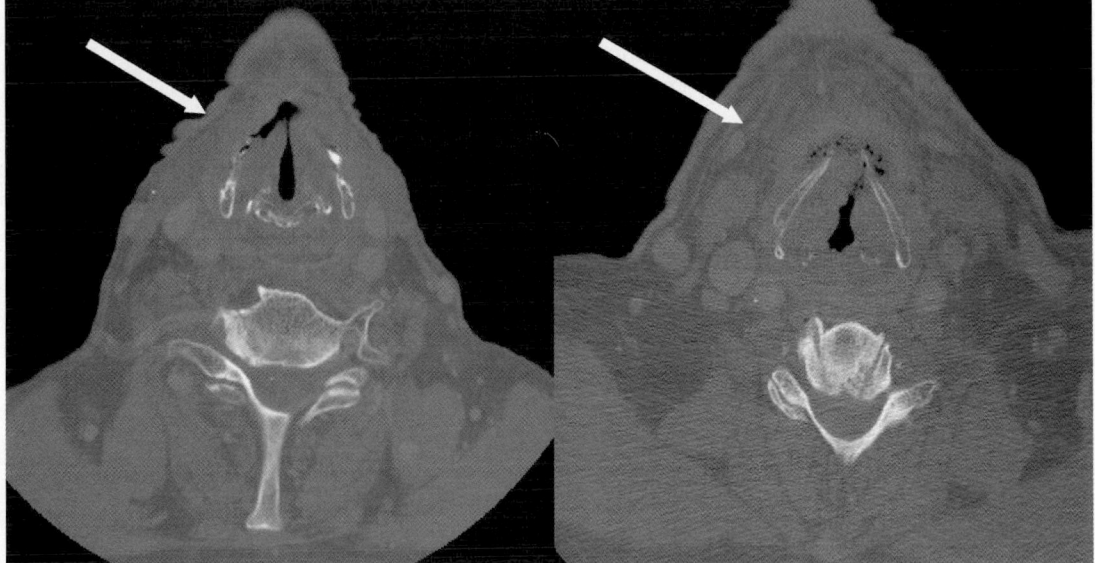

Figure 11 Computed tomography of a laryngeal chondroradionecrosis following therapeutic irradiation. Note air is present in the cartilage remnant in the image (on the *left*). In a different patient (on the *right*), persistent tumor was identified. (Published with permission, copyright © 2007 L. Ginsberg, MD.)

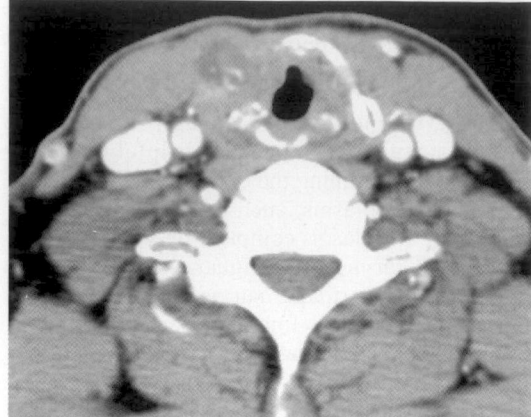

Figure 12 Computed tomography of a laryngeal chondrosarcoma of the right thyroid ala. (Published with permission, copyright © 2007 M.A. Michel, MD.)

Atypical chronic laryngeal inflammation, often infectious in nature, may be the subject of imaging. Laryngeal tuberculosis, although rare, may be endoscopically confused with carcinoma of the larynx due to the irregular appearance of the mucosa and chronic symptoms such as hoarseness and cough. In two review papers from the last decade, mycobacterial infection of the larynx was studied and noted to have several suggestive features that may help to distinguish it from malignancy.[40,41] Laryngeal tuberculosis is more likely to demonstrate bilateral abnormalities, diffuse thickening of the epiglottic-free margin, and the absence of submucosal or preepiglottic space involvement when compared to laryngeal malignancy. In addition, cartilage destruction was not seen in any patients with tuberculosis in these series. It would be hard to imagine deferring a biopsy of the laryngeal abnormality despite a high clinical suspicion of mycobacterial disease. The supportive radiographic information may be helpful in alerting the clinician to handle the sampled tissue with caution and directing appropriate cultures in addition to histopathological examination.

While the management of other challenging laryngeal conditions, including Wegener granulomatosis and sarcoidoisis, often includes imaging, the specific CT findings usually do not add to the information gathered from the endoscopic examination.[42]

Vocal Fold Paralysis

Vocal fold paralysis continues to generate a great deal of discussion in laryngology; the radiographic evaluation of these patients does not, however, focus on the larynx itself but rather on extralaryngeal structures along the course of the vagus nerve and its branches. That is not to say that the larynx is devoid of interesting findings in vocal fold paralysis; several diagnostic features, such as medial position and thickening of the aryepiglottic fold, hypopharyngeal dilation, and ventricular dilation, all on the involved side, have been established as characteristic findings[43] (Figure 13). Occasionally, unusual causes of mechanical impairment of vocal fold and arytenoid motion will be detected, as shown in Figure 14.

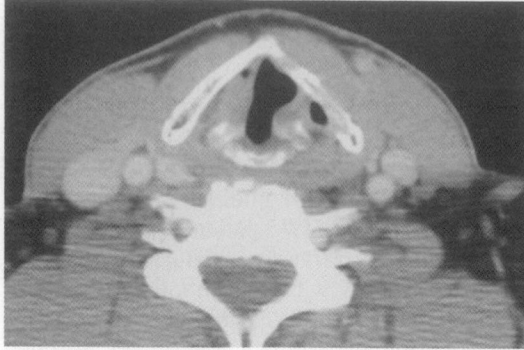

Figure 13 Computed tomography of the larynx of a patient with idiopathic left vocal fold paralysis. (Published with permission, copyright © 2007 M.A. Michel, MD.)

Nonetheless, the principal motivation for clinicians pursuing imaging related to vocal fold paralysis is to evaluate for a possible neoplastic cause. It is not clear what is the likelihood of detecting an otherwise occult neoplasm with radiography along the course of the laryngeal nerves. A recent publication from Finland has found that 9 of 34 patients in the "noniatrogenic" category harbored neoplasia, including those secondary to goiters and chest malignancies. Overall, the relative incidence of neoplasia as the cause of vocal fold paralysis has declined in the past few years, with more cases of idiopathic and iatrogenic neuropathy.[44–47] Nonthyroid surgical procedures, such as anterior approaches to the cervical spine, have surpassed thyroid surgery as the dominant cause of iatrogenic vocal fold paralysis.

The debate between advocates of plain chest radiography (CXR) and CT with regard to imaging of "idiopathic" vocal paralysis has died down in the past few years. This matter has not been settled because of the advent of any thorough investigation or even a major retrospective study; it is a matter of practicality. It has been argued that CXR should be used as screening based on

its relatively low cost and high yield (upward of 50% in some series).[48] Proponents of CT imaging, on the other hand, cite several important studies, including the Glazer and colleagues study in which 27 of 33 patients had positive CT scans.[49] This high incidence of abnormal findings in the Glazer and colleagues study is well above that seen in otolaryngology practice; the potent message of the paper is that 13 (72%) of the 18 of the patients with left-sided vocal fold paralysis with aortopulmonary masses on CT scan had a normal appearing mediastinum on CXR. The mean size of the chest mass in the negative CXR–positive CT group was 2.3 cm. In contrast, the smallest lesion detected in the positive CXR group was 3.8 cm.

Despite these conflicting views, in practical terms a normal CXR would likely be followed by a CT to evaluate the chest further in a patient with an otherwise unexplained vocal fold paralysis; by the same token, a positive CXR would also mandate a CT for more detailed characterization of the thoracic lesion. This commonly employed logic renders the CXR less useful, regardless of the scientific evidence supporting this approach.

With regard to MRI, there is not much evidence for or against this modality in the evaluation of vocal fold paralysis; several papers report on a small number of MRI evaluations for the evaluation of "idiopathic" vocal fold paralysis.[50,51] Although the yield for MRI in these retrospective papers was high, the absolute numbers (6 of 10 patients having abnormalities detected on their MRI examinations) are quite small and preclude significant conclusions. While MRI is useful in related clinical conditions, such as in the detection of recurrent laryngeal nerve involvement by thyroid cancer,[52] it has a high false-positive rate in patients with lower risk,[53] limiting its role in many practices.

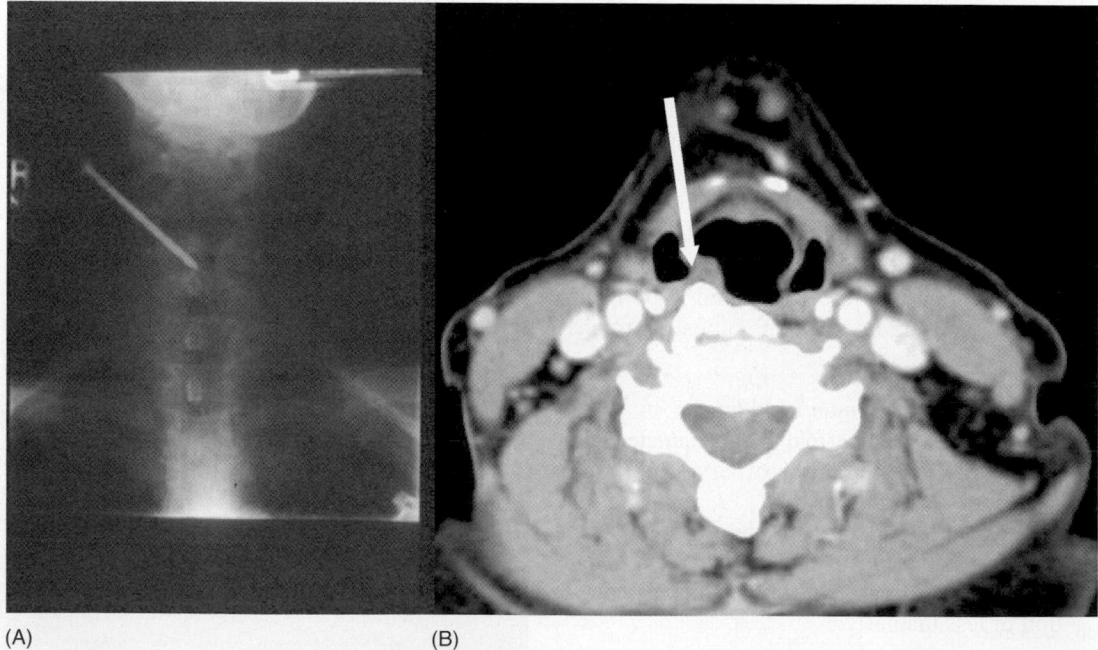

(A) (B)

Figure 14 Some unusual causes of vocal fold paralysis. (A) A plain radiograph of the neck reveals a nail gun injury to the right side of the larynx. (B) Computed tomography of a patient with right vocal fold immobility in whom an osteophyte was noted to be growing into the area just lateral to the right artytenoid cartilage.

TRACHEA

The trachea (formerly *tracheia arteria*, Greek for rough artery) harbors relatively few neoplasms compared to the larynx or the lungs. CT is the imaging modality of choice for the vast majority of tracheal disorders.[54,55] Most imaging of the trachea is by CT, either for the evaluation of stenosis or malignant invasion.

The normal trachea is composed of 14 to 22 C-shaped rings of cartilage with a membranous posterior segment. The cross-sectional diameter of the trachea approaches 20 mm in some adults. Global airway physiology is dependent on respiratory mechanics, in addition to the "baseline" cross-sectional area, as the trachea lies partially in the neck and partially in the chest; it is thus subject to the thoracic negative pressure necessary for normal inspiration. Conversely, the trachea is also subject to compressive force from expiration. This dynamic quality is exploited in radiographic examination of patients with suspected tracheomalacia.

Tracheal Stenosis

As noted in the section on laryngeal stenosis, imaging may be helpful in characterizing the length of the stenotic segment as well as in detecting secondary lesions. Plain radiography (Figure 15) may be revealing; however, if the clinician suspects extramural compression by a thyroid lesion or a vascular ring, CT imaging will provide superior information (Figure 16). The radiological findings are generally not exclusive to any one cause, although, as noted above, patients with no history of mechanical injury, that is, no intubation or external trauma, are less likely to have calcification or ossification on their studies.[13] While this is a retainable clinical "pearl," it is unlikely to supersede the patient's history of an intensive care unit stay or an incision on their

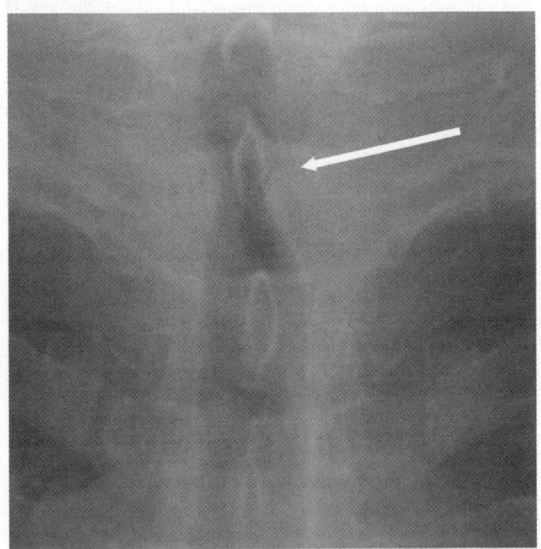

Figure 15 Postero-Anterior (PA) radiograph tracheal stenosis, as most commonly seen following intubation or tracheostomy. It shows smooth narrowing of the tracheal air column (*arrow*) a few centimeters below the level of the larynx. The narrowing of the tracheal air column is readily evident although detailed characterization is limited.

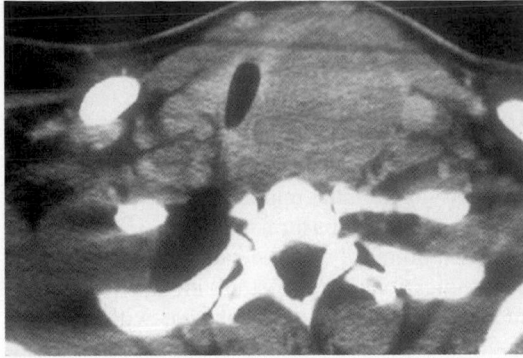

Figure 16 Computed tomography of compression and displacement of the cervical trachea by a massive goiter. The tracheal air column is displaced from the prevertebral area.

neck. Improvements have been achieved in the past few years with the advent of helical CT scanning. In this modality, rapid image acquisition has significantly reduced respiratory and cardiac motion artifact in airway studies; prior to this, 3-D reconstructions of airway lesions were put together from multislice images taken from different breath-holds. In a significant early paper, Whyte and colleagues reported on 25 patients who underwent helical CT and multiplanar reconstruction and compared these findings to plain tomography and bronchoscopy for evaluation of central airway obstruction.[56] The helical CT with reconstruction accurately demonstrated both the site and severity of stenoses with a sensitivity of 93% and a specificity of 100%. Interestingly, the one false-negative study was in a patient with tracheomalacia. The patients (often debilitated and dyspneic) are required to hold their breath for 15 to 45 seconds, a potential limitation to this technique.

The next phase of imaging in airway evaluation for stenosis is referred to as "virtual endoscopy" by its proponents.[57] In this, the collected data from the 3-D airway assessment are synthesized into video format with a tour through the airway. The overall contribution of virtual endoscopy to clinical care is not known for tracheal stenosis. A still image from the 3-D reconstruction is seen in Figure 17.

Neoplasms Affecting the Trachea

Primary neoplasms of the trachea are rare; when they do occur, more are likely to be malignant than benign.[58] Squamous cell carcinoma (SCC) accounts for about 50% of tracheal malignancies, adenoid cystic carcinoma for 30%, adenocarcinoma for 10%, and the remainder of the principal cell types for 10%. There are few imaging distinctions among these cell types, other than their local behavior and what is known about their natural history. Patients with SCC of the trachea are certainly at risk of a synchronous or metachronous SCC in the larynx or lungs.

CT images of adenoid cystic carcinomas may feature submucosal growth and a resultant "thickened" appearance to the trachea.[59] Computed tomography is particularly useful in determining the extent of tumor extension into

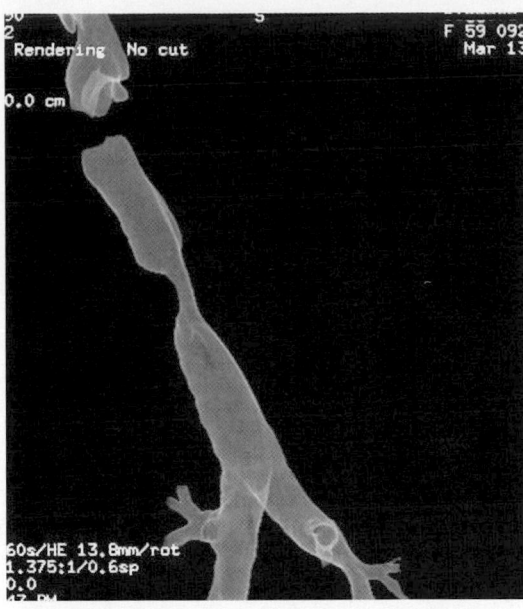

Figure 17 Three-dimensional reconstruction of computed tomography of tracheal stenosis. The presence of normal trachea above and below the stenosis is particularly helpful in these patients, as is the determination of the length of the stenosis.

the mediastinum. Other tumors, such as mucoepidermoid carcinomas, are believed to feature more "endoluminal" growth patterns but no one of these findings is consistent enough to be diagnostic.[60] Although quite rare, carcinoid tumors have dependable CT findings which may assist in the diagnostic process. Carcinoid tumors, derived from neuroendocrine cells, tend to arise in central bronchi and not in the trachea. When they are seen on CT scan, however, they feature high contrast enhancement due to the vascularity of the tumor. Other paratracheal masses, such as a tracheocele, may be detected on CT imaging. They are characterized by air in a paratracheal mass. In some cases, the tract connecting the air sac to the trachea can be seen on CT (Figure 18). If the tracheocele becomes fluid filled, it may be more difficult to distinguish it from other paratracheal masses.

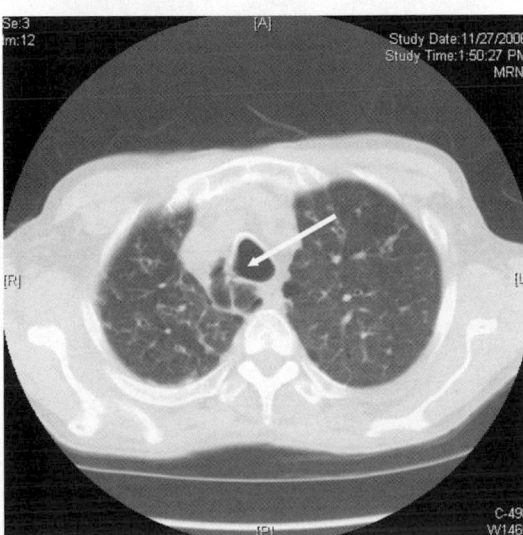

Figure 18 Computed tomography image at lung window settings in a patient with a tracheocele and severe diffuse bronchiectasis, demonstrating a bubbly airspace along the right posterior tracheal wall with a small tract communicating with the tracheal lumen (*arrow*).

Tracheomalacia

Tracheomalacia typically presents with dyspnea on exertion or chronic cough. It may be congenital or acquired following prolonged intubation. It is believed that the endotracheal tube cuff pressure destabilizes the cartilaginous trachea. On clinical examination, the endoscopic appearance of the trachea may be normal; the ideal clinical imaging to supplement awake or even sedated endoscopy would be dynamic CT. In this modality, both end inspiratory and end expiratory CTs are taken of the trachea. The dynamic change in the tracheal configuration is noted in comparing the two images; Boiselle and Ernst described as the expiratory "frown sign" which was found in over one-half of their patients[61] (Figure 19). In their study, the images of patients with bronchoscopically proven malacia were reviewed in a blinded manner. During inspiration, 16 of 17 patients had normal configuration; on expiration, all of the patients demonstrated some degree of abnormality, the "frown sign" being the most common, seen in 9 of 17 patients. They also suggested that the presence of this finding may aid in the detection of tracheomalacia in patients who inadvertently breathe during CT scans.

ESOPHAGUS

Imaging of the upper esophageal sphincter (UES) area and esophagus is directed at both form and function; important structural abnormalities can be detected by contrast radiography (such as the barium esophagram), CT, and even by endoscopically guided ultrasound. Dysphagia is a major clinical issue, and aspiration is a common cause of morbidity and mortality. More patients die each year of aspiration pneumonia complicating stroke than the head and neck cancers combined.[62]

Dynamic Evaluation of Swallowing

The standard examination for the investigation of pharyngeal and upper esophageal function is the modified barium swallow (MBS), also known commonly as the video swallow study. The indications for this study include the assessment of patients with dysphagia, with or without suspected aspiration. In addition to providing structural and dynamic information about the area, this study provides an opportunity for a speech-language pathologist to assess the impact of postural maneuvers, swallowing strategies, and choices of ingested material in an attempt to guide the patient toward idealized safe oral intake if at all possible. Contrast entering the aditus of the larynx but not passing inferior to the vocal folds is referred to as penetration. If the ingested material enters the subglottis or trachea, aspiration has occurred. Other key findings on the MBS include a description of hyolaryngeal movement, base of the tongue propulsion, and upper esophageal sphincter opening, including timing, degree of opening, and duration (Figure 20).

Martin-Harris and colleagues reviewed a series of 608 MBS studies and noted that only 10% were classified as "normal," whereas aspiration occurred in 32% of patients, swallowing abnormalities without aspiration occurred in 57%.[63]

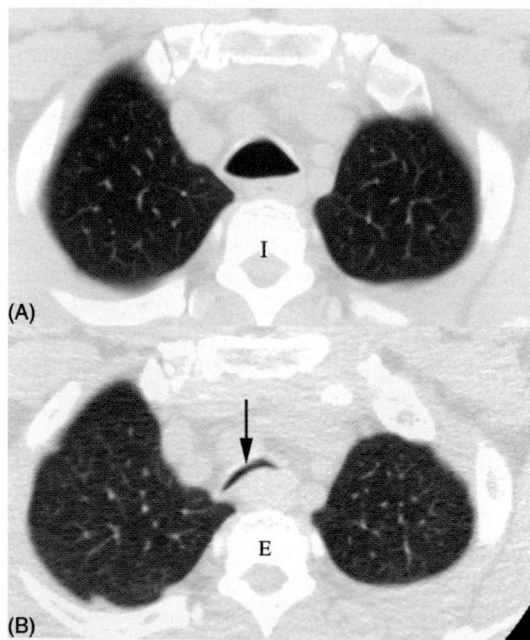

Figure 19 Computed tomography of the chest. Note the "frown sign" on expiration (*black arrow* in lower figure). Patient is a middle-aged male with chronic cough. (A) In the upper film, taken at inspiration, a normal tracheal lumen is seen. (B) Dynamic collapse of the trachea is seen in the expiratory film. (Published with permission, copyright © 2007 P.M. Boiselle, MD.)

Department of Otolaryngology and Communication Sciences
Center for Communication and Swallowing Disorders

Froedtert & MEDICAL COLLEGE

VIDEOFLUOROSCOPIC SWALLOW STUDY
WORK SHEET

Name: _____ Date: _____

Date of Birth: _____ MR#: _____

Tape #: _____ SS: _____ Unit Input: _____ Unit Output: _____

Referring Physician: _____

CHIEF SWALLOWING COMPLAINT: _____
_____

Barriers: ——— ☐ Comprehension ☐ Behavior ☐ Fatigue ☐ Pain ☐ Postural issues

Trach: ——— ☐ No ☐ Yes (type) _____ ☐ Tracheostoma

Primary feeding method: ——— ☐ Oral ☐ NG ☐ G-Tube ☐ J-Tube

Current diet: ——— ☐ General ☐ Mechanical soft ☐ Pureed ☐ Thickened liquids

Method of taking pills: ——— _____

Dentition: ——— ☐ Own teeth ☐ Dentures (U / L) ☐ Partials (U / L) ☐ Edentulous

Contrast: ——— ☐ Gastrograffin ☐ Thin barium ☐ Thickened liquid ☐ Applesauce
☐ Pudding ☐ Paste ☐ Cookie ☐ Barium tablet ☐ Barium capsule

Position: ——— ☐ Standing ☐ Sitting ☐ Semi-reclined

View: ——— ☐ Lateral ☐ AP ☐ Oblique

KEY FOR SEVERITY RATING: **T** = TRACE **M** = MILD **MOD** = MODERATE **S** = SEVERE

ORAL PREPARATORY/ORAL	(COMMENTS)	SEVERITY RATING
POOR BOLUS REDUCTION: _____		
POOR BOLUS FORMATION: _____		
PROLONGED BOLUS PREPARATION: _____		
PROLONGED ORAL TRANSIT TIMES: _____		
LABIAL LEAKAGE: _____		
ORAL RESIDUE: _____		
SERIAL SWALLOWS: _____		
POOR TONGUE PALATE CONTACT: _____		
EXTRAVASATION: _____		

(A)

VIDEOFLUOROSCOPIC SWALLOW STUDY
WORK SHEET (CONTINUED)

KEY FOR SEVERITY RATING: T = TRACE   M = MILD   MOD = MODERATE   S = SEVERE

PHARYNGEAL	(COMMENTS)	SEVERITY RATING
DELAYED OR ABSENT SWALLOW:		
POOR BASE OF TONGUE/PHARYNGEAL WALL CONTACT:		
NASAL REFLUX:		
POOR PHARYNGEAL CONTRACTION:		
POOR HYOLARYNGEAL EXCURSION:		
POOR EPIGLOTTIC RETROVERSION:		
ARYTENOID-EPIGLOTTIC CONTACT:		
VALLECULAR RESIDUE: LEFT RIGHT BILATERAL		
PYRIFORM SINUS RESIDUE: LEFT RIGHT BILATERAL		
DIFFUSE HYPOPHARYNGEAL RESIDUE:		
PENETRATION: BEFORE DURING AFTER LIQUID (THIN / THICK) PUREED SOLID		
ASPIRATION: BEFORE DURING AFTER LIQUID (THIN / THICK) PUREED SOLID		
COUGH RESPONSE: SPONTANEOUS DELAYED STRONG WEAK		
DECREASED UPPER ESOPHAGEAL SPHINCTER (UES) OPENING:		
DECREASED DURATION OF UES OPENING:		
EXTRAVASATION/FISTULA:		

ESOPHAGEAL (PER RADIOLOGIST)	(COMMENTS)	SEVERITY RATING
DYSMOTILITY:		
DIVERTICULUM:		
REFLUX:		

VOCAL QUALITY POST SWALLOWING: _____   PENETRATION/ASPIRATION SCALE RATING: _____

STRATEGIES/EFFECTIVENESS

1. _____
2. _____
3. _____
4. _____

DIET RECOMMENDATIONS: _____

THERAPY/STRATEGY RECOMMENDATIONS: _____

(B)

Figure 20 Videofluoroscopic swallow study work sheet: (A) page 1 and (B) page 2.

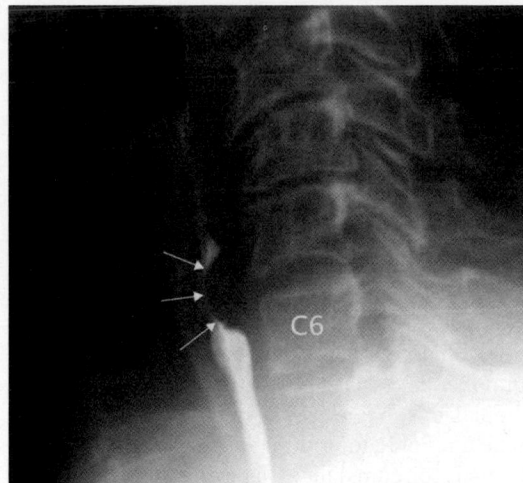

Figure 21 Lateral view of a modified barium swallow. Note the cricopharyngeal bar (*arrows*) on an image taken during a swallow.

bar are more complex than simple mechanical impedance. Dantas and colleagues from the Medical College of Wisconsin studied a small group of dysphagic patients with CP bars and compared their pharyngeal and UES manometry to a group of controls.[66] They noted that whereas this group of patients with CP bars demonstrated normal peristalsis and flow rates across the sphincter, as well as normal duration of opening, there were several important abnormalities noted. The subjects with CP bars had reduced maximal dimensions of UES opening and increased resulting intrabolus pressure in the pharynx upstream of the sphincter. They suggested that the underlying pathogenesis of the bar reflected reduced muscle compliance.

Endoscopic Evaluation of Swallowing versus Modified Barium Swallow

The advent of the flexible endoscopic evaluation of swallowing (FEES) study with[67] and without sensory testing[62] in the 1990s had some advocates predicting the demise of the MBS. In this valuable procedure, the patient is "fed" while a flexible nasopharyngoscope is in place. With the addition of laryngopharyngeal sensory testing, this purely endoscopic approach may have significant benefit in the care of stroke patients to give one important example.[62] Proponents of this approach have pointed out several key advantages over standard MBS; first of all, endoscopic examination can take place at the bedside. The sensory testing that accompanies the FEES examination (in some cases) does not depend on a cooperative patient. In addition, the examination can take place at the bedside or in the clinic at the time of the initial examination and does not require transportation to the radiography site. Wu and colleagues compared MBS to FEES testing in 28 patients with dysphagia.[67] They found that the effectiveness of the cough reflex and determination of velopharyngeal incompetence were underreported on MBS in 1 of 3 subjects. Premature oral spillage into the pharynx was better detected on MBS; in general, however, even other familiar MBS findings such as aspiration, penetration, and

Clinical management was influenced in over 80% following the MBS, mostly by the initiation of referrals to specialists, the institution of compensatory strategies and dietary changes, as well as the recommendation for swallowing therapy. The authors concluded that "the low percentage of normal studies coupled with the high percentage of change in measurable variables indicate high clinical utility for the modified barium swallow study." This important study supported the belief that the MBS should be viewed as more than just a method for detecting the presence or absence of aspiration. Some concern has been raised over the possibility that the subjective nature of the test leads to variability in test results. In one study

of normal volunteers, some variation was noted among experienced clinicians in their interpretation of MBS findings; the differences did not, however, reach statistical significance.[64]

Certain specific MBS findings deserve further comment, such as the enigmatic cricopharyngeal (CP) bar. This common and conceptually embraceable radiographic finding does indeed have clinical significance (Figure 21). It is associated with the manometric high-pressure zone of the UES.[65] This function alone makes the CP bar an important area to examine during MBS studies. The functional UES is about 1 cm in length and moves rostrally with swallowing. Interestingly, the changes implied by the presence of a pharyngeal stasis were all slightly more likely to be detected during FEES than MBS.

A major prospective paper from Aviv studied 126 subjects prospectively and followed them for 1 year.[68] The MBS and FEES with sensory testing studies were equivalent in guiding behavioral and dietary management in a series of outpatients with dysphagia in terms of their ability to avoid pneumonia and further morbidity from aspiration. The overall familiarity with MBS and its ability to detect UES dysfunction as well as allowing for more objective assessment of response to postural maneuvers has kept MBS in the forefront of clinical dysphagia assessment. FEES continues to be a reliable tool in the clinic or at the bedside in many circumstances as well. Unfortunately, despite excellent clinical research and promising initial data, enthusiasm for the laryngopharyngeal sensory testing component of the endoscopic swallowing evaluation has not expanded into general practice.

Structural and Inflammatory Disorders

Zenker Diverticulum. Discussion of this disorder is properly included with the hypopharynx as its origin is above the UES. The presence of a "sac" containing contrast extending past the cricopharyngeal muscle, usually on the left side, is the classic finding in Zenker diverticulum (Figure 22). These may be treated with open surgery or by endoscopic techniques.[69–71] Radiographic assessment is often, but not always, performed following surgical treatment. The initial examination may be for the detection of a "leak" or extravasation of contrast from the hypopharynx into the soft tissues of the neck or the mediastinum. It is important to note that there are several other findings which may be of note on these "leak" studies. Regardless of the mode of surgical treatment, it is not uncommon to detect a remnant of the Zenker diverticum sac; this is an important item to communicate to the patient and the radiologist and speech–language pathologist

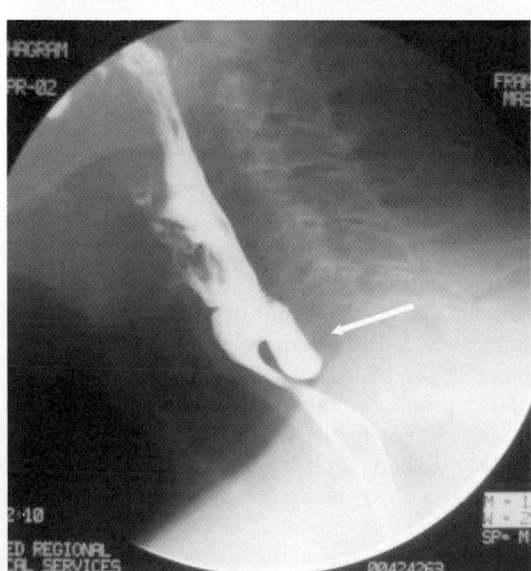

Figure 22 Modified barium swallow. A Zenker diverticulum (*arrow*) is seen on the lateral view. The structure between the sac and the native esophagus is composed mostly of the cricopharyngeus muscle.

reporting on the study. Jaramillo and colleagues reported on a series of Zenker diverticula treated with endoscopic stapling; 15 of the 32 patients were restudied 2 years postoperatively.[72] All 15 who underwent postoperative MBS had evidence of a persistent pouch; indeed, of the 12 with both pre- and postoperative studies, only 4 of the 12 showed any decrease in the size of the pouch. Twelve of the 15 patients surveyed were satisfied with the results of their procedure. There was no correlation between symptomatic outcome and pouch persistence.

Tsikoudas and colleagues investigated the association between radiological findings and outcomes in endoscopic stapling of Zenker diverticula.[73] Interestingly, when examined retrospectively, an association between pouch configuration and clinical outcome was noted. In short sacs with a broad angle between the sac and the native esophagus, there was a higher incidence of perioperative complications, both technical and medical. Zenker sacs with long necks and large pouches were associated with a higher rate of revision surgery.

Reflux. Few topics in laryngology and bronchoesophagology generate as much disagreement as gastroesophageal and laryngopharyngeal reflux. Generally, radiographic studies are not used as the first line of investigation for these disorders; nonetheless, contrast examinations of the esophagus may be helpful in some patients both in the assessment for reflux as well as for the detection of peptic complications. Ambulatory pH monitoring[74,75] and impedance testing[76,77] continue to be the dominant quantitative tests for reflux; esophagoscopy, either traditional transoral sedated or by transnasal awake technique[78–80] continues to be the definitive test for the assessment of esophageal mucosal disease, including inflammation and injury from reflux as well as neoplastic disorders.

Esophagitis, resulting from peptic injury of the esophagus, can be readily detected in the double (barium and air) contrast esophagram; when used in combination with single-contrast views, the sensitivity approaches 90%.[81] This sensitivity does, however, result in a notable rate of false-positives.[82] The most common finding of reflux esophagitis on these studies is a finely nodular or granular appearance with poorly defined radiolucencies due to edema and inflammation of the mucosa (Figure 23). These reflux-associated findings typically occur in the area immediately superior to the gastroesophageal junction.

Strictures and the Schatzki Ring. Contrast esophagography is useful in distinguishing between neoplasia and luminal narrowing of the esophagus, as in the case of stricture. These are often peptic in nature, although they may also be associated with other disorders, such as collagen vascular diseases and radiation injury (Figure 24). In symptomatic lower esophageal concentric narrowing, that is, Schatzki ring, if the lumen is compromised to a maximum diameter of 13 mm, dysphagia is almost always present; in contrast, a lumen of 20 mm rarely results in swallowing

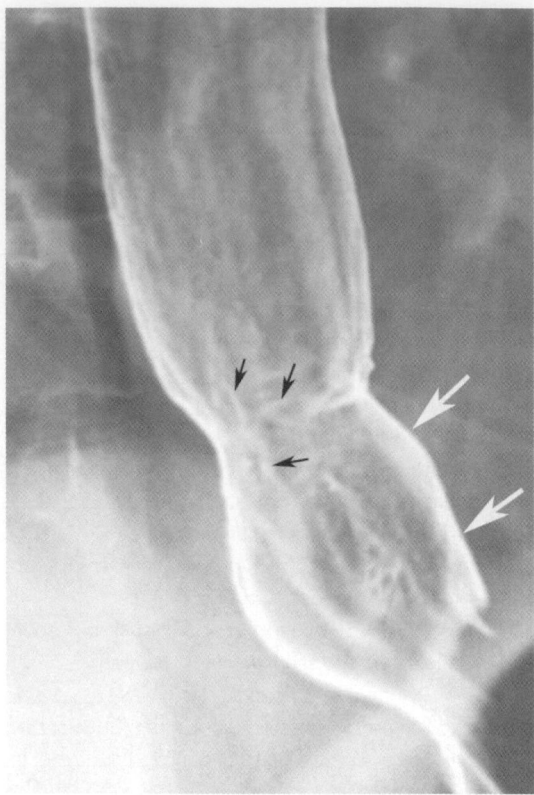

Figure 23 Barium esophagram. Reflux esophagitis with small linear ulcers (*black arrows*) in distal esophagus just above hiatal hernia (*white arrows*). (Image courtesy of M. Levine, MD.)

complaints.[83] Esophagography may be superior to endoscopy in some cases of lower rings.

Neoplasia. Benign tumors, such as leimyoma, represent the minority (20%) of esophageal neoplasia.[84] They have some characteristic imaging features on contrast esophagography; they are smooth and submucosal and form a broad angle with the native esophagus when viewed in

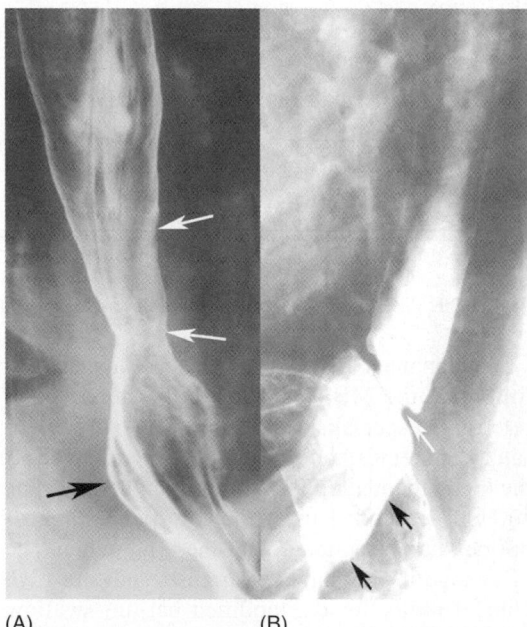

Figure 24 (A) Double contrast esophagram demonstrating a tapering stricture (*white arrows*) just above the gastroesophageal junction (*black arrow*). (B) A short-segment lower esophageal ring (Schatzki ring) is seen (*white arrow*). (Published with permission, copyright © 2007 M. Levine, MD.)

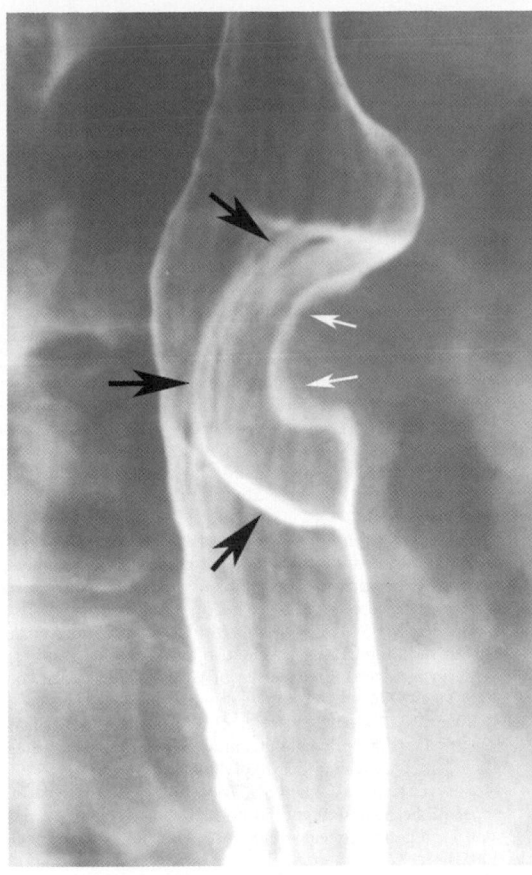

Figure 25 Smooth submucosal mass in the midesophagus consistent with a leiomyoma (*white and black arrows*). (Published with permission, copyright © 2007 M. Levine, MD.)

profile, depending on where the tumor is based (Figure 25). Computed tomography reveals much of the same structural description; one review noted that leiomyomata mostly featured eccentrically elevated filling defects with homogeneous low or isoattenuation.[85] Interestingly, the same study noted that the plain chest radiographs were

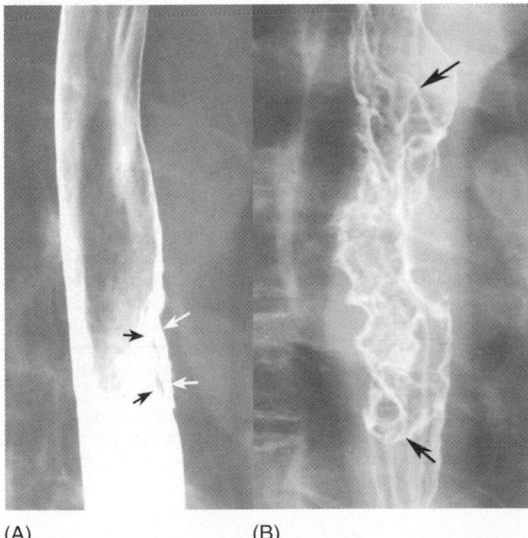

Figure 26 Double contrast esophagography. (A) This irregular mass proved to be an early esophageal carcinoma (*black and white arrows*). (B) An advanced infiltrating carcinoma with irregular narrowing, mucosal nodularity, ulceration, and shelf-like margins (*black arrows*) in the midesophagus. (Published with permission, copyright © 2007 M. Levine, MD.)

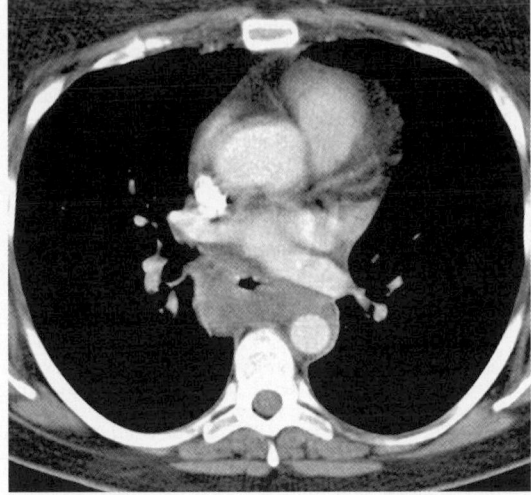

Figure 27 Computed tomography of a carcinoma of the esophagus. Note the irregular borders and infiltrative growth.

also able to detect the esophageal leiomyoma in all 12 subjects.

The incidence of esophageal carcinoma continues to increase; particularly Barrett-associated adenocarcinoma of the distal esophagus and gastroesophageal junction. While endoscopic surveillance of at-risk patients continues to dominate the clinical management of suspected esophageal malignancy, there is an ongoing role for contrast esophagography in these patients. Indeed, double-contrast esophagography has a sensitivity comparable to that of endoscopy (>95%) in the detection of esophageal carcinoma.[86] The esophagographic appearance of early lesions has been described as the appearance of plaque-like lesions with focal irregularity. More advanced lesions demonstrate marked irregularity (Figure 26). The extraesophageal extension of carcinoma is better demarcated by CT imaging (Figure 27). A mass arising in the area of radiographically detectable peptic injury, such as a distal stricture may represent adenocarcinoma arising in association with preexisting Barrett metaplasia.[84]

Endoscopic ultrasound (EUS) is a relatively new technology that adds information to the clinical diagnosis of mucosal tumors and their submucosal extent. This approach has demonstrated great sensitivity and accuracy; Holden and colleagues reported on 15 patients with esophageal carcinoma near the gastroesophageal junction staged by EUS and CT.[87] When the pathological depth of tumor invasion was measured from the surgical pathology specimen, EUS was far more accurate than CT, with 87% of lesions properly staged by EUS compared to 40% by CT. An example of an EUS of esophageal cancer invading the aortic wall is see in Figure 28. Periesophageal lymph node assessment is also significantly more accurate with EUS than CT (73% vs 33%). Even obstructing lesions that prevent the probe from passing may be accurately categorized.

CONCLUSIONS

Imaging will continue to be a tremendous tool for clinicians dealing with disorders of the larynx,

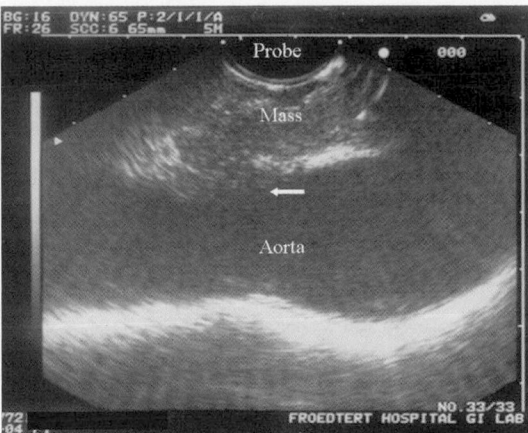

Figure 28 Linear endoscopic ultrasound (EUS) scan showing an esophageal cancer invading into the aortic wall (*arrow*). This tumor is categorized T4. The aortic wall invasion was found with EUS; and, hence, the tumor was considered unresectable. (Published with permission, copyright © 2007 K. Dua, MD.)

Trachea and Esophagus. Marriage of advancing endoscopic technology such as "chip-tip" cameras and robotic surgery may reconfigure the precise role of radiology in these disciplines. The dominant modality for structural imaging in laryngology and bronchoesophagology continues to be CT, with and without contrast. Whereas these radiographic investigations add only a modest amount to the surface endoscopic information, the ability to assess deep structures and their association with pathological changes, such as thyroid cartilage invasion by laryngeal malignancy, continues unrivaled except perhaps by surgical exploration with its inherent morbidity.

REFERENCES

1. Simpson CB, Amin MR, Postma GN. Topical anesthesia of the airway and esophagus. Ear Nose Throat J 2004;83:2–5.
2. Lee M, Ramaswamy MR, Lilien DL, Nathan CA. Unilateral vocal cord paralysis causes contralateral false-positive positron emission tomography scans of the larynx. Ann Otol Rhinol Laryngol 2005;114:202–6.
3. Mancuso AA, Hanafee WN, Juillard GJ, et al. The role of computed tomography in the management of cancer of the larynx. Radiology 1977;124:243–4.
4. Stieve M, Schwab B, Haupt C, et al. Intraoperative computed tomography in otorhinolaryngology. Acta Otolaryngol 2006;126:82–7.
5. Hirano M, Kurita S, Yukizane K, Hibi S. Asymmetry of the laryngeal framework: A morphologic study of cadaver larynges. Ann Otol Rhinol Laryngol 1989;98:135–40.
6. Josephson GD, Spencer WR, Josephson JS. Thyroglossal duct cyst: The New York Eye and Ear Infirmary experience and a literature review. Ear Nose Throat J 1998;77:642–4, 646–7, 651.
7. Glastonbury CM, Davidson HC, Haller JR, Harnsberger HR. The CT and MR imaging features of carcinoma arising in thyroglossal duct remnants. AJNR Am J Neuroradiol 2000;21:770–4.
8. Glazer HS, Mauro MA, Aronberg DJ, et al. Computed tomography of laryngoceles. AJR Am J Roentgenol 1983;140:549–52.
9. Martinez Devesa P, Ghufoor K, Lloyd S, Howard D. Endoscopic CO$_2$ laser management of laryngocele. Laryngoscope 2002;112:1426–30.
10. Dursun G, Ozgursoy OB, Beton S, Batikhan H. Current diagnosis and treatment of laryngocele in adults. Otolaryngol Head Neck Surg 2007;136:211–5.
11. Myssiorek D, Madnani D, Delacure MD. The external approach for submucosal lesions of the larynx. Otolaryngol Head Neck Surg 2001;125:370–3.
12. Poetker DM, Ettema SL, Blumin JH, et al. Association of airway abnormalities and risk factors in 37 subglottic stenosis patients. Otolaryngol Head Neck Surg 2006;135:434–7.

13. Bhalla M, Grillo HC, McLoud TC, et al. Idiopathic laryngotracheal stenosis: Radiologic findings. AJR Am J Roentgenol 1993;161:515–7.

14. Carretta A, Melloni G, Ciriaco P, et al. Preoperative assessment in patients with postintubation tracheal stenosis: Rigid and flexible bronchoscopy versus spiral CT scan with multiplanar reconstructions. Surg Endosc 2006;20:905–8.

15. Rubin AD, Hawkshaw MJ, Moyer CA, et al. Arytenoid cartilage dislocation: A 20-year experience. J Voice 2005;19:687–701.

16 Sataloff RT, Rao VM, Hawkshaw M, et al. Cricothyroid joint injury. J Voice 1998;12:112–6.

17. Kandogan T, Olgun L, Gultekin G, et al. External laryngeal trauma. Swiss Med Wkly 2003;133:372.

18. Schaefer SD. Use of CT scanning in the management of the acutely injured larynx. Otolaryngol Clin North Am 1991;24:31–6.

19. Scaglione M, Romano L, Grassi R, et al. Diagnostic approach to acute laryngeal trauma: Role of computerized tomography. Radiol Med (Torino) 1997;93:67–70.

20. Goudy SL, Miller FB, Bumpous JM. Neck crepitance: Evaluation and management of suspected upper aerodigestive tract injury. Laryngoscope 2002;112:791–5.

21. Moriwaki Y, Sugiyama M, Fujita S, et al. Application of ultrasonography for blunt laryngo-cervical-tracheal injury. J Trauma 2006;61:1156–61.

22. Hoffman HT, Porter K, Karnell LH, et al. Laryngeal cancer in the United States: Changes in demographics, patterns of care, and survival. Laryngoscope 2006;116:1–13.

23. Gordin A, Daitzchman M, Doweck I, et al. Fluorodeoxyglucose-positron emission tomography/computed tomography imaging in patients with carcinoma of the larynx: Diagnostic accuracy and impact on clinical management. Laryngoscope 2006;116:273–8.

24. Hunt JP, McWhorter AJ. Malignant neoplasms of the larynx. In: Merati AL, Bielamowicz SA, editors. Textbook of Laryngology. San Diego: Plural Publishing; 2007. p. 323–50.

25. Mancuso AA, Mukherji SK, Schmalfuss I, et al. Preradiotherapy computed tomography as a predictor of local control in supraglottic carcinoma. J Clin Oncol 1999;17:631–7.

26. Mendenhall WM, Morris CG, Amdur RJ, et al. Parameters that predict local control after definitive radiotherapy for squamous cell carcinoma of the head and neck. Head Neck 2003;25:535–42.

27. Mukherji SK, Toledano AY, Beldon C, et al. Interobserver reliability of computed tomography-derived primary tumor volume measurement in patients with supraglottic carcinoma. Cancer 2005;103:2616–22.

28. Hoorweg JJ, Kruijt R, Heijboer RJ, et al. Reliability of interpretation of CT examination of the larynx in patients with glottic laryngeal carcinoma. Otolaryngol Head Neck Surg 2006;135:129–34.

29. Fernandes R, Gopalan P, Spyridakou C, et al. Predictive indicators for thyroid cartilage involvement in carcinoma of the larynx seen on spiral computed tomography scans. J Laryngol Otol 2006;120:857–60.

30. Becker M, Zbaren P, Delavelle J, et al. Neoplastic invasion of the laryngeal cartilage: Reassessment of criteria for diagnosis at CT. Radiology 1997;203:521–32.

31. Becker M. Neoplastic invasion of laryngeal cartilage: Radiologic diagnosis and therapeutic implications. Eur J Radiol 2000;33:216–29.

32. Duflo S, Christian M, Guelfucci B, et al. Comparison of magnetic resonance imaging with histopathological correlation in laryngeal carcinomas. Ann Otolaryngol Chir Cervicofac 2002;119:131–7.

33. Hermans R, Pameijer FA, Mancuso AA, et al. Laryngeal or hypopharyngeal squamous cell carcinoma: Can follow-up CT after definitive radiation therapy be used to detect local failure earlier than clinical examination alone? Radiology 2000;214:683–7.

34. McGuirt WF, Greven KM, Keyes JW, Jr, et al. Laryngeal radionecrosis versus recurrent cancer: A clinical approach. Ann Otol Rhinol Laryngol 1998;107:293–6.

35. McGuirt WF, Greven KM, Keyes JW, Jr, et al. Positron emission tomography in the evaluation of laryngeal carcinoma. Ann Otol Rhinol Laryngol 1995;104:274–8.

36. Terhaard CH, Bongers V, van Rijk PP, Hordijk GJ. F-18-fluoro-deoxy-glucose positron-emission tomography scanning in detection of local recurrence after radiotherapy for laryngeal/pharyngeal cancer. Head Neck 2001;23:933–41.

37. De Vuysere S, Hermans R, Delaere P, Marchal G. CT findings in laryngeal chondroradionecrosis. JBR-BTR 1999;82:16–8.

38. Hermans R, Pameijer FA, Mancuso AA, et al. CT findings in chondroradionecrosis of the larynx. AJNR Am J Neuroradiol 1998;19:711–8.

39. Wippold FJ, Smirniotoplous JG, Moran CJ, Glazer HS. Chondrosarcoma of the larynx: CT features. Am J Neuroradiology. 1993;14(2):453–9.

40. Kim MD, Kim DI, Yune HY, et al. CT findings of laryngeal tuberculosis: Comparison to laryngeal carcinoma. J Comput Assist Tomogr 1998;180:463–9.

41. Moon WK, Han MH, Chang KH, et al. Laryngeal tuberculosis: CT findings. AJR Am J Roentgenol 1996;166:445–9.

42. Ferretti GR, Calaque O, Reyt E, et al. CT findings in a case of laryngeal sarcoidosis. Eur Radiol 2002;12:739–41.

43. Chin SC, Edelstein S, Chen CY, Som PM. Using CT to localize side and level of vocal cord paralysis. AJR Am J Roentgenol 2003;180:1165–70.

44. Benninger MS, Gillen JB, Altman JS. Changing etiology of vocal fold immobility. Laryngoscope 1998;108:1346–50.

45. Ishman SL, Halum SL, Patel NJ, et al. Management of vocal paralysis: A comparison of adult and pediatric practices. Otolaryngol Head Neck Surg 2006;135:590–4.

46. Merati AL, Halum SL, Smith TL. Diagnostic testing for vocal fold paralysis: Survey of practice and evidence-based medicine review. Laryngoscope 2006;116:1539–52.

47. Merati AL, Shemirani N, Smith TL, Toohill RJ. Changing trends in the nature of vocal fold motion impairment. Am J Otolaryngol 2006;27:106–8.

48. Altman JS, Benninger MS. The evaluation of unilateral vocal fold immobility: Is chest x-ray enough? J Voice 1997;11:364–7.

49. Glazer HS, Aronberg DJ, Lee JK, Sagel SS. Extralaryngeal causes of vocal cord paralysis: CT evaluation. AJR Am J Roentgenol 1983;141:527–31.

50. Ramadan HH, Wax MK, Avery S. Outcome and changing cause of unilateral vocal cord paralysis. Otolaryngol Head Neck Surg 1998;118:199–202.

51. Terris DJ, Arnstein DP, Nguyen HH. Contemporary evaluation of unilateral vocal cord paralysis. Otolaryngol Head Neck Surg 1992;107:84–90.

52. Takashima S, Takayama F, Wang J, et al. Using MR imaging to predict invasion of the recurrent laryngeal nerve by thyroid carcinoma. AJR Am J Roentgenol 2003;180:837–42.

53. Liu AY, Yousem DM, Chalian AA, Langlotz CP. Economic consequences of diagnostic imaging for vocal cord paralysis. Acad Radiol 2001;8:137–48.

54. Boiselle PM, Ernst A. Recent advances in central airway imaging. Chest 2002;121:1651–60.

55. Holbert JM, Strollo DC. Imaging of the normal trachea. J Thorac Imaging 1995;10:171–9.

56. Whyte RI, Quint LE, Kazerooni EA, et al. Helical computed tomography for the evaluation of tracheal stenosis. Ann Thorac Surg 1995;60:27–30; discussion 30–21.

57. Rodel R, Rodenwaldt J, Hommerich CP. Inner surface imaging of laryngeal and tracheal stenosis by spiral-CT: Role of a new diagnostic procedure. Laryngorhinootologie 2000;79:584–90.

58. Mark EJ. Imaging of the larynx and trachea. In: Grillo HC, editor. Surgery of the Trachea and Bronchi. Hamilton: BC Decker; 2004. p. 103–60.

59. Cleveland RH, Nice CM, Jr, Ziskind J. Primary adenoid cystic carcinoma (cylindroma) of the trachea. Radiology 1977;122:597–600.

60. Heitmiller RF, Mathisen DJ, Ferry JA, et al. Mucoepidermoid lung tumors. Ann Thorac Surg 1989;47:394–9.

61. Boiselle PM, Ernst A. Tracheal morphology in patients with tracheomalacia: Prevalence of inspiratory lunate and expiratory "frown" shapes. J Thorac Imaging 2006;21:190–6.

62. Aviv JE, Sacco RL, Mohr JP, et al. Laryngopharyngeal sensory testing with modified barium swallow as predictors of aspiration pneumonia after stroke. Laryngoscope 1997;107:1254–60.

63. Martin-Harris B, Logemann JA, McMahon S, et al. Clinical utility of the modified barium swallow. Dysphagia 2000;15:136–41.

64. Lof GL, Robbins J. Test-retest variability in normal swallowing. Dysphagia 1990;4:236–42.

65. Kahrilas PJ, Dodds WJ, Dent J, et al. Upper esophageal sphincter function during deglutition. Gastroenterology 1988;95:52–62.

66. Dantas RO, Cook IJ, Dodds WJ, et al. Biomechanics of cricopharyngeal bars. Gastroenterology 1990;99:1269–74.

67. Wu CH, Hsiao TY, Chen JC, et al. Evaluation of swallowing safety with fiberoptic endoscope: Comparison with videofluoroscopic technique. Laryngoscope 1997;107:396–401.

68. Aviv JE. Prospective, randomized outcome study of endoscopy versus modified barium swallow in patients with dysphagia. Laryngoscope 2000;110:563–74.

69. Nyrop M, Svendstrup F, Jorgensen KE. Endoscopic CO_2 laser therapy of Zenker's diverticulum—experience from 61 patients. Acta Otolaryngol Suppl 2000;543:232–4.

70. Chang CW, Burkey BB, Netterville JL, et al. Carbon dioxide laser endoscopic diverticulotomy versus open diverticulectomy for Zenker's diverticulum. Laryngoscope 2004;114:519–27.

71. Chang CY, Payyapilli RJ, Scher RL. Endoscopic staple diverticulostomy for Zenker's diverticulum: Review of literature and experience in 159 consecutive cases. Laryngoscope 2003;113:957–65.

72. Jaramillo MJ, McLay KA, McAteer D. Long-term clinico-radiological assessment of endoscopic stapling of pharyngeal pouch: A series of cases. J Laryngol Otol 2001;115:462–6.

73. Tsikoudas A, Eason D, Kara N, et al. Correlation of radiologic findings and clinical outcome in pharyngeal pouch stapling. Ann Otol Rhinol Laryngol 2006;115:721–6.

74. Merati AL, Lim HJ, Ulualp SO, Toohill RJ. Meta-analysis of upper probe measurements in normal subjects and patients with laryngopharyngeal reflux. Ann Otol Rhinol Laryngol 2005;114:177–82.

75. Meyer TK, Olsen E, Merati A. Contemporary diagnostic and management techniques for extraesophageal reflux disease. Curr Opin Otolaryngol Head Neck Surg 2004;12:519–24.

76. Aslam M, Bajaj S, Easterling C, et al. Performance and optimal technique for pharyngeal impedance recording: A simulated pharyngeal reflux study. Am J Gastroenterol 2007;102:33–9.

77. Kawamura O, Aslam M, Rittmann T, et al. Physical and pH properties of gastroesophagopharyngeal refluxate: A 24-hour simultaneous ambulatory impedance and pH monitoring study. Am J Gastroenterol 2004;99:1000–10.

78. Saeian K, Staff DM, Vasilopoulos S, et al. Unsedated transnasal endoscopy accurately detects Barrett's metaplasia and dysplasia. Gastrointest Endosc 2002;56:472–8.

79. Postma GN. Transnasal esophagoscopy. Curr Opin Otolaryngol Head Neck Surg 2006;14:156–8.

80. Postma GN, Cohen JT, Belafsky PC, et al. Transnasal esophagoscopy: Revisited (over 700 consecutive cases). Laryngoscope 2005;115:321–3.

81. Creteur V, Thoeni RF, Federle MP, et al. The role of single and double-contrast radiography in the diagnosis of reflux esophagitis. Radiology 1983;147:71–5.

82. Koehler RE, Weyman PJ, Oakley HF. Single- and double-contrast techniques in esophagitis. AJR Am J Roentgenol 1980;135:15–9.

83. Ott DJ, Chen YM, Wu WC, et al. Radiographic and endoscopic sensitivity in detecting lower esophageal mucosal ring. AJR Am J Roentgenol 1986;147:261–5.

84. Levine MS, Rubesin SE. Diseases of the esophagus: Diagnosis with esophagography. Radiology 2005;237:414–27.

85. Yang PS, Lee KS, Lee SJ, et al. Esophageal leiomyoma: Radiologic findings in 12 patients. Korean J Radiol 2001;2:132–7.

86. Levine MS, Chu P, Furth EE, et al. Carcinoma of the esophagus and esophagogastric junction: Sensitivity of radiographic diagnosis. AJR Am J Roentgenol 1997;168:1423–6.

87. Holden A, Mendelson R, Edmunds S. Pre-operative staging of gastro-oesophageal junction carcinoma: Comparison of endoscopic ultrasound and computed tomography. Australas Radiol 1996;40(3):206–12.

83

Laryngoscopy

Mark S. Courey, MD
Fredrick C. Roediger, MD

Laryngoscopy, that is, viewing of the larynx, can be accomplished by two basic methods. These are grouped into either indirect or direct techniques. Indirect laryngoscopy uses mirrors, glass prisms, fiberoptic glass rods, or microchip cameras to view the larynx and hypopharynx with the patient's head and neck in a neutral position. The image obtained from indirect laryngoscopy is viewed after it has been reflected and/or transmitted by one of the previously mentioned systems (Figure 1). Direct laryngoscopy, on the other hand, is performed with the neck flexed forward while the head is extended on the atlanto-occipital joint. The tongue is displaced either laterally or anteriorly. This position affords a direct line-of-sight for visualization through an open mouth to the larynx (Figure 2).

It is critical to understand that any manner of viewing the larynx which is not accomplished through direct line-of-sight and requires bending the image through glass fibers or reflecting the image with mirrors or prisms is considered an indirect technique. Prior to the development of fiberoptic technology, this distinction was clear. Fiberoptic techniques transfer light and the image along flexible glass fibers. Therefore, by the historical definition, fiberoptic techniques for laryngoscopy are indirect techniques. With improvements in image and light transfer, the miniaturization of charge coupled device (CCD) cameras placed at the end of the flexible scope, and the development of instrumentation which may be used through side channels on the flexible endoscope, the larynx can be indirectly viewed

and manipulated. These indirect flexible techniques are gaining popularity among the current generation of laryngologists due the relative ease of performance and enhanced patient comfort. Some surgeons may elect to consider "fiberoptic" laryngoscopy an entirely different form of indirect laryngoscopy and may have valid arguments for this point.

Both the direct and indirect forms of laryngoscopy have advantages and disadvantages for viewing and intervening in laryngeal processes. The purpose of this chapter is to discuss the technical aspects of each form of laryngoscopy. The forms will be discussed as indirect rigid laryngoscopy, indirect flexible laryngoscopy, and direct rigid laryngoscopy.

HISTORY AND INSTRUMENT DEVELOPMENT

A review of the development of indirect and direct laryngoscopy is complicated due to discrepancies throughout historical records. However, the concept of viewing the larynx, mainly

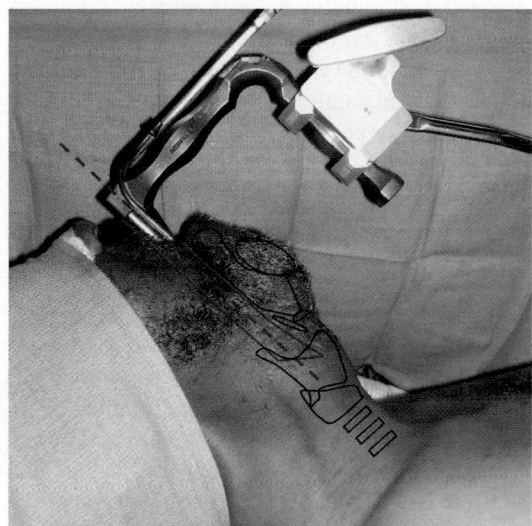

Figure 2 During direct laryngoscopy, the anterior part of the tongue and the base part of the tongue are compressed by the laryngoscope. In this example a tubular laryngoscope is used with a Lewy suspension apparatus. The neck is flexed on the chest while the head is extended. Variable degrees of flexion, extension and displacement of the tongue allow the creation of a direct line of sight (*red line*) between the examiner and the patient's larynx. The larynx is represented schematically in black.

for the purpose of placing "tubes" for ventilatory support, was introduced by Hippocrates and reported intermittently by various physicians throughout the Middle Ages and into the eighteenth century. History is replete with descriptions from physicians of innovative instruments developed to view the various cavities of the human body. Commonly, these tubed instruments used curved mirrors and lenses to focus and reflect light from the sun, candles, or gas lamps. This light, which was largely inadequate by today's standards, was shone into the body cavity. Instruments were adapted to distend the cavity or soft tissues so that the region could be viewed in a direct line-of-sight, that is, direct endoscopy. In other descriptions, mirrors were employed to reflect the image around an angle back to the observer, that is, indirect endoscopy.

Development of Indirect Mirror Laryngoscopy

In 1829, Guy Babington was most likely the first physician to present an instrument designed entirely for the purpose of viewing the larynx.[1] Babington's instrument, termed a "glottiscope," consisted of an oblong mirror mounted on a handle which was designed to be held against the palate, while the tongue was retracted with a spatula. The mirror reflected both light and image. The technique, due to complexity and limited patient tolerance, was not adopted by other physicians. It was not until 1855, when Manuel Garcia, a music teacher, used a series of mirrors to reflect light and image to view his own larynx that attention was directed to the practice of indirect laryngoscopy. Garcia is therefore credited with inventing indirect mirror laryngoscopy. Garcia reported his observations to the Royal College of Surgeons, but initial reviews were guarded. The technique of indirect mirror laryngoscopy was adopted by Turck, a physician in Vienna, who studied its use in cadavers. Turck's systematic evaluation of the clinical technique, developed by Garcia, provided the scientific validation required for the process to continue in patients. Turck's findings were reported to the Vienna Imperial Society of Medicine in 1857. Czmerak, a student of Turck's, pursued the technique and improved on applicability by developing a head mirror which reflected artificial light. This obviated the clinician's dependence

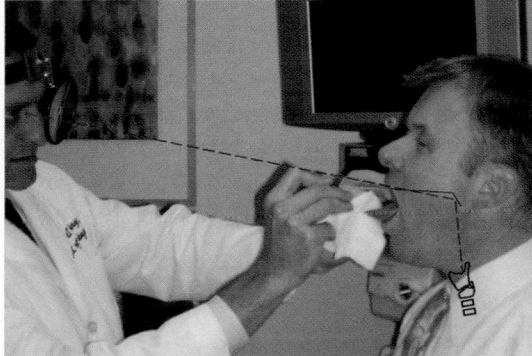

Figure 1 During indirect laryngoscopy, a mirror can be used to reflect light into the larynx from an external light source. In this case a head mirror was used to reflect light from over the patient's right shoulder. The image is then reflected back to the examiner from the mirror (*red line*).

on sunlight and further popularized the practice of indirect mirror laryngoscopy.[2]

Development of Direct Laryngosocpy

Again, from Hippocrates and throughout the Middle Ages, multiple surgeons reported designing instruments to view body cavities with direct line-of-sight visualization. Many of these instruments were long tubes designed to look into the urethra, bladder, uterus, and esophagus. Viewing of the larynx was primarily considered as the larynx needed to be passed to enter the trachea. However, in 1852 Horace Green designed a bladelike instrument specifically to view the larynx. Green reported his experiences with the excision of laryngeal lesions using this instrument in one hand and a curved forceps in the other. Due to the difficult nature of the technique and poor patient tolerance, without anesthesia, Green's reports were also viewed skeptically by the medical community.[1] Green lost credibility and, therefore, most of the credit for developing or popularizing direct laryngoscopy is given to Alfred Kirstein.[3]

In the 1890s, working with a tubed esophagoscope modified from a urethroscope,[2] Kirstein noted that if the scope intended for the esophagus accidentally slipped into the larynx and trachea, an excellent view could be obtained. Therefore, in 1895 Kirstein began developing a reproducible method to view the larynx directly.[3] Initially, Kirstein used a 25 cm tubed esophagoscope with the upper incisors serving as a fulcrum. This allowed Kirstein to displace the base of the tongue and epiglottis anteriorly with the tip of the scope. In addition, Kirstein used an electrical light source fixed to the proximal end of the scope. The light was reflected down the scope with a 90° prism. Worried about pressure placed on the upper incisors, Kirstein made adjustments to his original tubelike laryngoscope. By eliminating the posterior aspect of the esophagoscope, Kirstein created bladelike instruments that resembled the laryngoscopes used by anesthesiologists for intubation today. In addition, Kirstein designed one type of blade that was developed to expose the larynx by lifting the tongue base from the vallecula rather than lifting the epiglottis directly. The tip on this scope was thickened to reduce the likelihood of injury to the mucosa of the vallecula and appears similar to the Macintosh blade in use today.

Kirstein's practice of direct laryngoscopy was termed "autoscopy." Historical accounts depict Kirstein performing "autoscopy" from in front of the patient with the patient leaning forward[4] and from behind the patient with the neck flexed on the chest and the atlanto-occipital joint extended.[3] It is probable that Kirstein performed direct laryngoscopy in either position to improve on the technique. What is important is that Kirstein recognized that extreme extension of the neck was not required for the procedure, and he reported that "the body must be placed in such a position that an imaginary continuation

of the laryngotracheal tube would fall within the opening of the mouth…"[3]

Gustov Killian learned about Kirstein's technique of direct laryngoscopy at a meeting in 1895 and realized the potential. In 1912, Killian was the first to report suspension laryngoscopy. The advantage of the technique was that it permitted bimanual manipulation of laryngeal structures.[5] This was a new concept as prior surgeons, such as Green and Kirstein, stabilized the bladelike laryngoscope with one hand and operated with the other. In his suspension system, Killian used the bladelike laryngoscopes designed by Kirstein to reduce pressure on the upper incisors. The system provided excellent visualization and was reported by Lynch and others in the United States for use during the resection of laryngeal lesions.[6]

The cumbersome nature of the Killian and Lynch suspension systems provided the stimulus for other surgeons such as Samuel Roberts and Robert Lewy to work on developing a system that was easier to use. This development occurred during the middle of the twentieth century. One fundamental difference between the Killian suspension system and the "newer" system developed by Roberts and Lewy was that the "newer" laryngoscope stabilizer system was designed for use with tubular laryngoscopes.[7] This led Roberts to use the upper incisors as a partial fulcrum as was originally described by Kirstein. In an attempt to simplify the process of suspension laryngoscopy further and to reduce pressure on the upper incisors, Lewy reevaluated patient positioning. The standard practice during the time was that most rigid direct endoscopy was performed under local anesthesia. Cocaine had been introduced in the 1880s. The procedure often started with the patient sitting and the head and neck extended. As the endoscope was introduced, the patient was reclined. This required two assistants. One assistant stabilized the shoulders and upper torso, and one stabilized the head while the physician controlled the endoscope. Even if the patient was positioned supine to start the case, one assistant was still required to stabilize the shoulders in case of coughing, while still another controlled the head. By starting with the head on the operating table, Lewy was able to eliminate the need for a second assistant (Figure 3A). Lewy claimed that with his "laryngoscope stabilizer" device, direct suspension laryngoscopy could be accomplished with atlanto-occipital extension and variable degrees of flexion of the neck on the chest[8] (Figure 3B). The results were that with tubular laryngoscopes the upper incisors were often used as a partial fulcrum. Lewy recognized this and cautioned against applying undue pressure as should all laryngologists teaching residents techniques of bimanual suspension microlaryngoscopy. In addition, at the time that Lewy was practicing, most tubular laryngoscopes were narrow and provided inadequate binocular visualization. Therefore, Lewy described modifications of the "new" suspension system for use with open or bladelike laryngoscopes for a larger field of visualization. These devices incorporated a Jennings

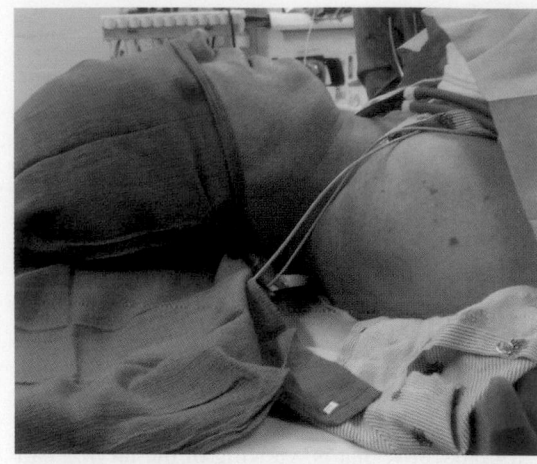

(A)

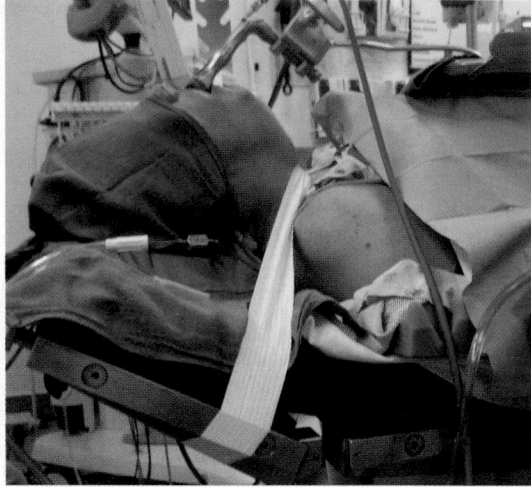

(B)

Figure 3 (A) During direct laryngoscopy, the procedure is begun with the patient's head at the top of the operating table. The patient is placed in a neutral position with the head on a cushion ring (doughnut) for stabilization. A shoulder role is not needed as the neck will be flexed to help with alignment of the larynx. (B) To obtain exposure the neck is flexed on the chest while the head is extended on the neck. This is accomplished by lifting with the laryngoscope as the tubular blade is inserted. The headpiece of the operating room table is also flexed to maintain support for the patient's head. The tongue is compressed and care is taken not to use the upper incisor teeth as a fulcrum. After exposure is obtained, tape is used across the neck to depress the larynx posteriorly for better exposure of the anterior aspect of the larynx.

type mouth gag to hold the upper incisors out of the field of view. Ultimately, the Lewy "suspension" system has become the most popular system in use today. When combined with appropriate head positioning and attention to pressure on both the upper incisors and the soft tissue over the mandible, the system can be used with relative ease to provide stabilization for suspension laryngoscopy in the majority of patients.

Advances with Light Delivery Systems

The practice of both indirect and direct laryngoscopy has also been influenced by the development of adequate lighting. Today, surgeons take the phenomena of adequate light for granted. It is amusing to hear ourselves asking our assistant to turn down the light intensity when we think that our historical counterparts worked by sun light, candlelight, or dim electric light produced by the original light bulbs of the late nineteenth and early twentieth centuries.

During the development of laryngoscopy, one area of debate revolved around the use of proximal or distal lighting. Before electricity was harnessed, light for endoscopy was only available from external sources. Therefore, by necessity light came from the proximal end of the endoscope, and it was required that the light be focused down the endoscope shaft. With relative short laryngoscopes, this was possible, but difficult. For anyone performing esophagoscopy or bronchoscopy, one can readily appreciate the difficulty in reflecting and focusing and external proximal light source down a long tubular endoscope. Many types of focusing lenses were introduced. The equivalent experience today is obtained when the surgeon attempts to focus the CO_2 laser and the helium-neon aiming beam down the bronchoscope for CO_2 laser bronchoscopy. Regardless, when electrical lighting was developed, Kirstein originally proposed placing a light at the proximal end of the laryngoscope. This practice of using a source of proximal illumination was also continued by Killian and Lynch who used electric headlamps during suspension laryngoscopy.

In 1904, Chevalier Jackson proposed distal illumination through the use of miniature light bulbs placed at the end of a long carrier. The light carrier was fitted in a second tube alongside or inside the lumen of the endoscope. These light bulbs were small, and the electric current used to supply energy was often erratic. Commonly, bulbs needed to be replaced multiple times throughout one case as they would fail. However, as frail as the systems of distal illumination may have been, the principle of distal illumination for laryngoscopy and bronchoscopy was introduced and continued by other surgeons, many of whom had spent time with Jackson in his clinic.[1]

Improvements in distal illumination awaited the development of the principle of fiberoptic light transmission. This discovery revolutionized all forms of endoscopy and was advanced by multiple scientists. Baird, in 1927 identified the concept that glass fibers can transmit light. This led to the development of the "clad fiber." Essentially the transmission of light down a glass fiber occurs through internal refraction. Glass fibers are produced from glass with a high refractive index. These fibers are surrounded by glass with a lower refractive index. Light is transmitted along the high refractive index core. If these glass fibers are arranged haphazardly light only is transmitted. When the fibers are aligned in a parallel manner, they can transmit an image.[9]

In the early 1960s, the understanding of fiberoptic light transmission and technology was developed to permit replacing light carriers in rigid endoscopes with fiberoptic technology. Clad fibers were surrounded by a hard metal carrier and formed a fiberoptic carrier of small diameter which was placed through the second channel in the endoscope. The light was supplied distally. It was not a source of heat. Originally, light sources were standard 150 W electric bulbs. This was still an improvement over the small distal bulb. Later, halogen and xenon sources were developed to improve distal light delivery further.

Indirect Rigid Laryngoscpy: The Hopkins Rod

In the 1950s Harold Hopkins, a physics professor in England, developed the rod-lens optical system which transmitted an image or light through an elongated lens. The lens was essentially a short, 1 mm long, glass fiber. In a rigid rod-lens system, a series of these glass rod lenses are placed within a tube. The ends of each lens are ground precisely to provide a highly refractive surface and a small airspace between each lens allows transmission to the next lens in the series (Figure 4). The image is transmitted from lens to lens to the proximal end of the instrument. If a prism is placed at the distal end of the rod or telescope, the image is reflected through an angle prior to transmission. The optics produced by the original rod lenses were probably inferior to the image from standard lenses at the time; however, Karl Storz recognized the potential of these types of systems. In the late 1950s or early 1960s, Storz was also introduced to the concept of fiberoptic light transmission through clad fibers and patented the idea of the rod-lens optical system combined with fiberoptic glass light transmission. With time and refinements in production techniques, the quality of rod-lens production improved. This enhanced the resolution of image which was transmitted[10] (Figures 5A and B). The Hopkins rod was first introduced for indirect rigid laryngoscopy in the 1960s but took nearly 10 years to gain acceptance.[11] The typical rod-lens telescope contains between 2 and 20 rod lenses each approximately 1 mm in length and thousands of glass fibers around the lens system for illumination.

Indirect Flexible Laryngoscopy

The concept and practice of indirect flexible laryngoscopy was originally developed based on fiberoptic light and image transmission but currently encompasses both flexible endoscopy performed with traditional fiberoptic technology and flexible endoscopy accomplished with miniaturized CCDs small enough to be passed through the oral and nasal cavity.

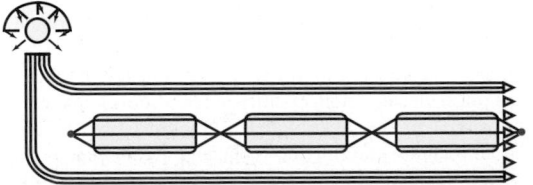

Figure 4 Schematic representation of rod-lens telescope. Light is supplied externally and is represented at the upper left of the image. The light is transmitted through fiberoptic clad fibers on the outside of the telescope. Individual lenses in the middle of the endoscope are aligned to transmit the image.

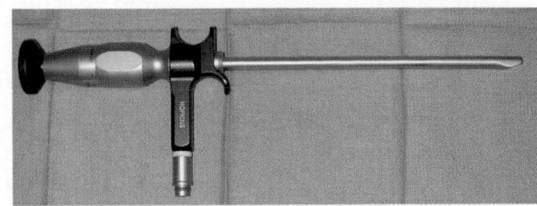

(A)

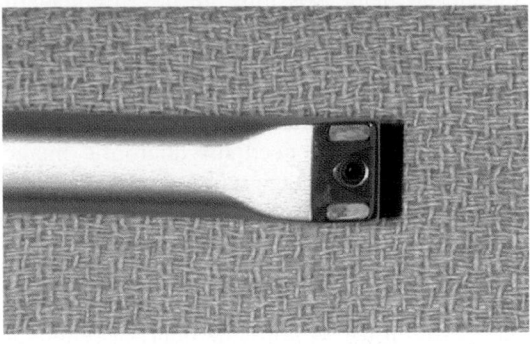

(B)

Figure 5 (A) A contemporary rod-lens endoscope with a 70° viewing angle (Storz, Germany). Light is supplied through a fiberoptic cable connected to the scope on the bottom left. Visualization is through the eyepiece on the far left while the smaller end at the right is placed in the patient's oral cavity. A camera with a c-mount can be attached to the eyepiece for photodocumentation. (B) Close-up of the distal end of the rod-lens endoscope. The round lens in the middle of the scope is for image transfer. The oblong openings on either side are for light transmission through the fiberoptic light carriers.

Due to technical limitations in clad fiber production, the development of traditional flexible "fiberoptic" endoscopes with resolution adequate for image transmission lagged behind the development of the rod-lens image transmission system and the development of the fiberoptic light transmission system. For image transmission, the clad fibers needed to be arranged in parallel, flexible, and small enough to bend through the endoscope. Resolution is dependent on fiber diameter and number. Scopes with greater numbers of smaller fibers produce higher resolution images than scopes with few numbers of larger fibers. Theoretically, clad fibers of 5 μ diameter would provide the greatest resolution. Production technology has not yet reached this ideal. Therefore, resolution with flexible fiberoptic endoscopes has not reached that of current rod-lens image transmission systems.

In spite of limitations in resolution, flexible fiberoptic image transmission was explored for bronchoscopy and esophagoscopy and originally introduced for laryngoscopy in 1968 by Sawashima and Hirose.[12] Clinical trials were reported from England in 1975 which demonstrated that the indirect flexible laryngoscopy, even with limited resolution, permitted adequate diagnosis of laryngeal pathology.[13] This trial demonstrated that indirect flexible laryngoscopy was technically easy to perform, easy to teach to young practitioners, and well tolerated by patients. These revelations led to an explosion in the application of flexible endoscopic techniques for visualization of the larynx. Simultaneous refinements in production methods for traditional fiberoptic technology resulted in improved resolution in smaller diameter endoscopes and further popularized the technique of indirect flexible laryngoscopy.

Desire for further improvement in resolution, similar to that produced with rod-lens systems, along with advances in computer technology fueled and made possible the development of computerized videoendoscopy systems. In computerized indirect flexible endoscopy, a miniature CCD, a digital computer chip camera, is placed at the end of a flexible endoscope (Figure 6A and B). This eliminates the need for fiberoptic image transmission as the image is transferred electronically from the chip at the distal end of the endoscope to a processing unit outside of the patient. This information is decoded and projected on a monitor for viewing. Fiberoptic light transmission is still utilized to provide light for illumination of the body cavity. By eliminating fiberoptic image transmission, degradation of scope resolution due to fiber breakage is not a problem.

The original systems, produced in the middle 1980s, included chips that were too large to be placed transnasally. The technology resulted in an improvement in image resolution which practitioners considered useful.[1] Therefore, as the ability to produce computer chips small enough to pass the nasal cavity developed in the late 1990s, systems were designed specifically for laryngoscopy. These fiber systems have approached external diameter sizes comparable to adult fiberscopes and have improved resolution over traditional

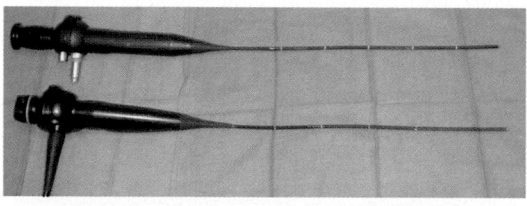

(A)

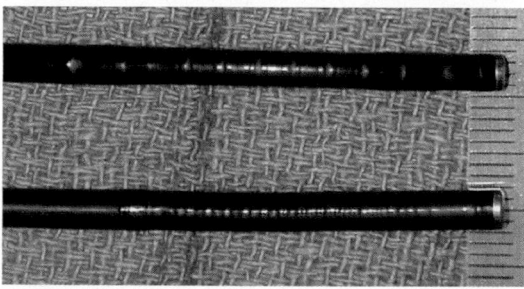

(B)

Figure 6 (A) Comparison of a traditional fiberoptic flexible endoscope (Karl Storz, Germany) above with a distal chip endoscope (Olympus ENF-V2, Japan) below. Both flexible endoscopes are manufactured with similar outer diameter. The proximal hand piece of the distal chip fiberoptic scope has an integrated camera. This improves image transmission; however, the image cannot be rotated to obtain a straight view of the larynx if introduction of the endoscope creates rotation. A camera can be attached to the eyepiece of the traditional fiberoptic scope. (B) A close-up of the distal end of both endoscopes against a ruler with millimeter markings demonstrates the diameter of both endoscopes.

fiberoptic systems, but controlled clinical trials comparing accuracy in diagnosis of the systems have not been undertaken. In addition, resolution and light transfer from videoendoscopy systems has still not reached that achieved from available rod-lens systems. Therefore, the gold standard for laryngeal imaging remains the rod-lens system (Figure 7A and B).

Ease of use and practitioner's familiarity with the technique which results in improved perceived patient comfort have popularized indirect flexible endoscopy in the clinic setting. Currently, prototype videoendoscopes with working side ports and at lengths facilitating laryngoscopy are being produced (Figure 8). These scopes have advantages in the clinic setting. They allow laryngeal manipulation for biopsy with forceps or brush

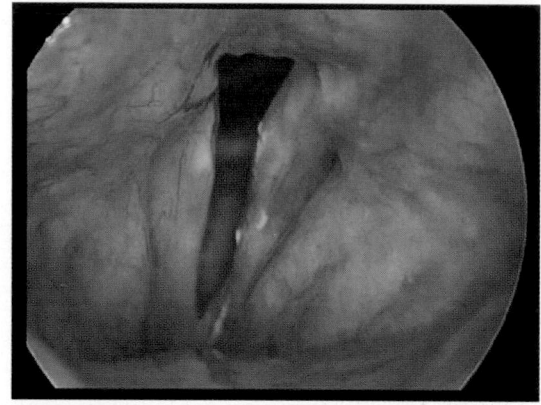

(A)

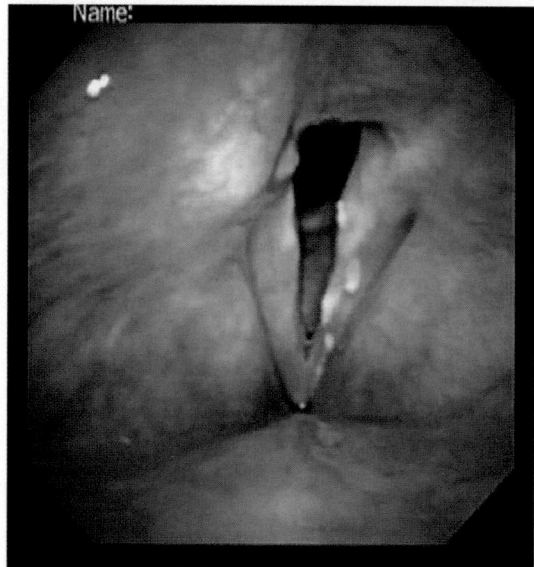

(B)

Figure 7 (A) Image taken through a 70° rod-lens endoscope with an Olympus-processing unit and remote camera head. Captured as MPEG 2 video. Still image captured and converted to JPEG format. Resolution quality provides visualization of microcirculation of the vocal folds. (B) Image taken with an Olympus ENF-V2 distal chip endoscope (Olympus, Japan). Again captured as MPEG 2 video and converted to a JPEG image. Resolution approaches the quality of the previous image. However, the vocal fold microcirculation is not visible. In both images illumination was obtained with the Storz Pulsar Strobsocopic Light Source (Storz, Germany). Intensity was set at 56% of maximum for Figure 7A and 100% of maximum for Figure 7B.

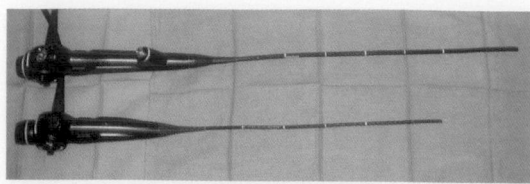

(A)

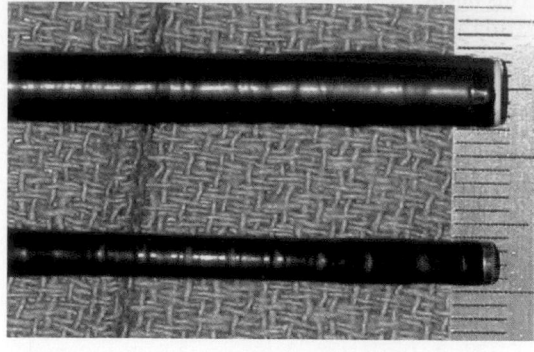

(B)

Figure 8 (A) Prototype distal chip laryngoscope with 2 mm side channel for instrumentation and suction. The endoscope is 10 cm longer than standard fiberoptic scope, but shorter than esophagoscopes which facilitates manipulation within the larynx. In this photograph, the standard distal chip endoscope (Olympus ENF-V2) is placed next to the channeled laryngoscope for comparison. (B) Close-up of the distal ends of the endoscopes with a ruler allows comparison of diameter.

and ablation of disease with laser fibers. These instruments are all passed through the side channel on the laryngoscope. These techniques can be used without general anesthesia and may prove to have a significant role in the future for patient management. However, we need to remember that the original endoscopists performed rigid endoscopy without local or general anesthesia. The techniques can be mastered but are not easy. In a similar manner, intervening in the larynx of an awake patient is not always an easy technique to master even with flexible endoscopes.

ANESTHESIA

Laryngoscopy can be performed with or without anesthesia. Anesthesia can be local or general, and it is accepted that improvements in techniques of general anesthesia have revolutionized the performance of direct laryngoscopy. The original endoscopists did not have anesthesia available. Cocainization came about in the 1880s. Ether was used for general anesthesia in the later part of the nineteenth century.[14] Our ability to support the respiration of sedated and paralyzed patients developed in the middle and later half of the twentieth century.[15] Endotracheal tube technology improved through the 1970s allowing the production of smaller outer diameter tubes for intubation. Use of these newer endotracheal tubes enhances intervention in the larynx because the tubes occupy less space in the airway lumen and permit a greater work area. In addition, the newer tubes permit safer application of laser energy because they are produced of flame-resistant materials.[16] Improvements in patient's O_2 and

CO_2 monitoring have made apneic and jet ventilation techniques for general anesthesia more acceptable to surgeons. Jet ventilation for maintenance of oxygenation can be accomplished with the jet ventilation catheter above or below the larynx. With these techniques, either no catheter or only a small catheter is placed in the larynx. This allows the surgeon to work easily in the posterior aspect of the glottis or in the subglottis for extended periods while the patient's oxygen supply is maintained.

With regard to indirect laryngoscopy, anesthesia is not usually required for either mirror or rod-lens techniques. For patients with a hypersensitive gag reflex, topical anesthesia to the palate and posterior pharynx (benzocaine 20%) may be helpful to reduce sensation of instrumentation. Topical anesthesia may be used in the nasal cavity (pontocaine 2%) for comfort when passing a fiberscope or videoendoscope through the nasal cavity. This is not absolutely required, but it is helpful in most patients to reduce the burning sensation that may be associated with irritation of the septal and turbinate mucosa. In spite of adequate nasal anesthesia, some patients may complain of pharyngeal irritation or exhibit a hyperactive gag reflex. In this instance, topical anesthesia to the oropharynx may be helpful. It is critical that these agents be avoided in patients with known hypersensitivity to local anesthetic agents.

If laryngeal instrumentation is planned during indirect flexible laryngoscopy, most patients will require topical anesthesia. This can usually be accomplished with lidocaine 4% dripped through the side channel of the laryngoscope directly on to the vocal folds. Alternatively, lidocaine can be aerosolized and inhaled. Finally, for some sensitive patients, blocking of the superior laryngeal nerve with injection of lidocaine may be necessary. Superior laryngeal nerve bocks can be accomplished by injecting the internal branch of the nerve as it courses through the neck just inferior to the greater horn of the hyoid bone and deep to the thyrohyoid membrane. Lidocaine 1% with 2 to 4 mL bilaterally is usually sufficient.

CURRENT PRACTICE OF OFFICE INDIRECT LARYNGOSCOPY

Indirect mirror laryngoscopy is considered part of the complete head and neck examination. The mirrors used for laryngeal examination were modified from dental mirrors. They are produced in various sizes, but the #10 size mirror is most commonly used. The mirror should be heated to prevent fogging. Heating has been accomplished in the past with various techniques including small flames from gas burners and more recently electric devices which heat ceramic beads. These electric bead warmers can be turned on at the beginning of clinic. Heat is transferred to the beads, and the mirror is submersed in the beads for a few seconds. The mirror should be tested on the back of the examiner's hand to be certain that it will not burn the palate on insertion. Once the mirror

has been inserted into the patient, it should not be inserted back into the bead warmer for rewarming as this may lead to contamination of the beads. The examination is begun with the examiner placing the patient and him- or herself in a comfortable position. This can be accomplished with the examiner seated or standing in front of the patient with the examiner's shoulders slightly above the patient's. Light can be reflected into the patient's mouth with a head mirror or directly from a headlight. The patient's tongue is retracted by grasping the tip gently with a gauze sponge (Figure 1).

Indirect laryngoscopy can also be performed with a rod-lens telescope (Figure 9). In a study comparing mirror laryngoscopy with indirect rod-lens laryngoscopy, patient tolerance of the rod-lens was significantly better than that of mirror laryngoscopy (83% vs 52%).[17] Examination sensitivity was equal between the techniques. As with indirect mirror laryngoscopy, the indirect rod-lens laryngoscopy starts by the examiner placing the patient and him- or herself in a comfortable position either seated or standing with the patient's shoulders slightly below the level of the examiner's. The light comes from the end of the endoscope; therefore, headlights are not required. The tip of the endoscope should be warmed to prevent fogging. Electric bead warmers lead to early deterioration of the optical system. Therefore, it is preferable that the rod-lens scopes be warmed with hot water. Hot water for the purpose of warming the endoscopes can be kept in the room in a thermos and poured into individual cups for use with each patient. The tongue tip is held lightly with gauze and retracted gently. The examiner balances the scope on the top of his index finger to avoid touching the tongue and stimulating the glossopharyngeal nerve. Under direct visualization, the scope is inserted into the oropharynx until the desired view is obtained. A camera head can be attached to the eyepiece of the endoscope, and the examination can be viewed and recorded from a monitor if desired.

Indirect flexible laryngoscopy is performed with both standard fiberscopes as well as

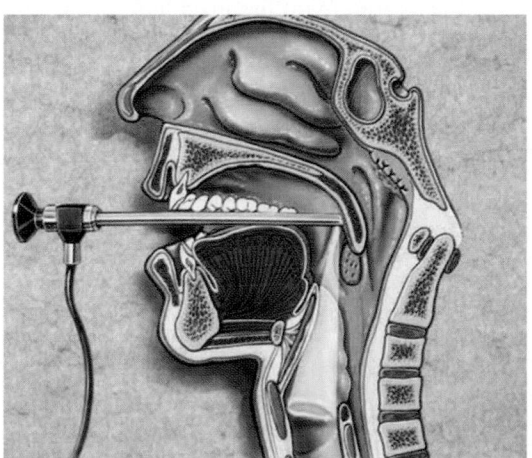

Figure 9 Schematic representation of the path of the rod-lens telescope when positioned in the patient's oral cavity and pharynx.

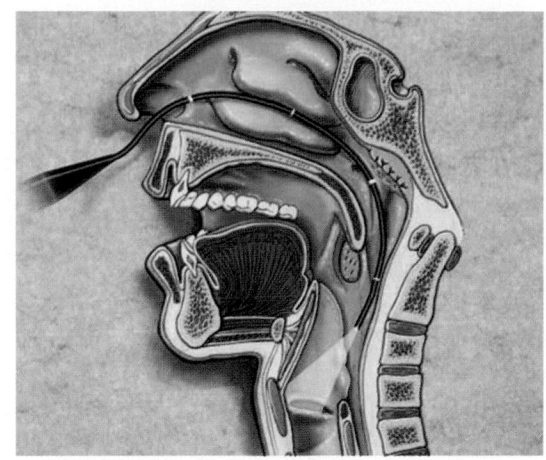

Figure 10 Schematic representation of a fiberscope passed through the nasal cavity, nasopharynx, oropharynx, and hypopharynx. The scope may be passed through either the middle or inferior meatus in the nasal cavity. The endoscope is passed along the posterior wall of the pharynx which allows a posterior to anterior view of the larynx during phonation.

videoendoscopes in a similar manner (Figure 10). Many examiners topically decongest and anesthetize the nasal cavity after visual inspection to determine the larger side. The patient should be seated comfortably leaning forward with the forearms resting on the thighs. The patient's neck is flexed forward with the head extended at the atlanto-occipital joint. Under direct visualization, the scope is passed through the nasal cavity into the nasopharynx, into the oropharynx, and into the desired position in the hypopharynx.

Interpreting Results from Office Indirect Laryngoscopy

The purpose of laryngoscopy is to view laryngeal and pharyngeal anatomy and function. With any of the three previous techniques described, the examiner can observe vocal fold abduction and adduction as well as pharyngeal wall motion to determine the functional status of the muscles and their innervation from cranial nerve X.[18] In addition, indirect laryngoscopy can be used to inspect the mucosal surfaces for benign or malignant lesions and the status of the airway lumen. Typically the patient is asked to phonate with the vowel sound /i/. This results in flattening of the tongue base and allows better visualization of the larynx. The valleculae and pyriform sinuses are visualized and inspected for mucosal lesions and pooling of secretions. Pooling of secretions in a vallecula is indicative of tongue weakness while pooling of secretions in the pyriform sinus is indicative of pharyngeal wall weakness.[19] The esophageal inlet is inspected and pooling of secretions in this region may be indicative of a structural lesion in the esophagus. Next the aryepiglottic folds, false vocal folds, and arytenoids are inspected. Vocal fold abduction and adduction is observed by asking the patient to alternate between phonation of the vowel /i/ and inhalation. High-pitched phonation of the vowel /i/ allows observation of lateral pharyngeal wall function. The lateral pharyngeal

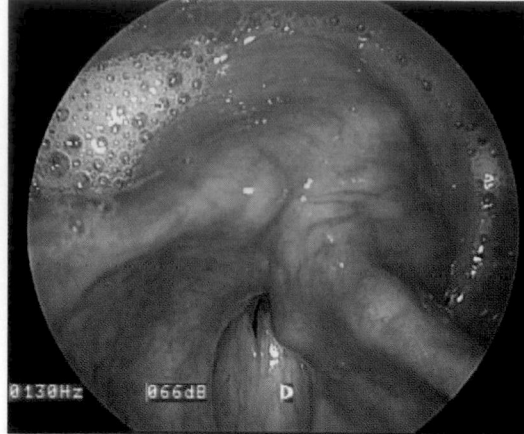

(A)

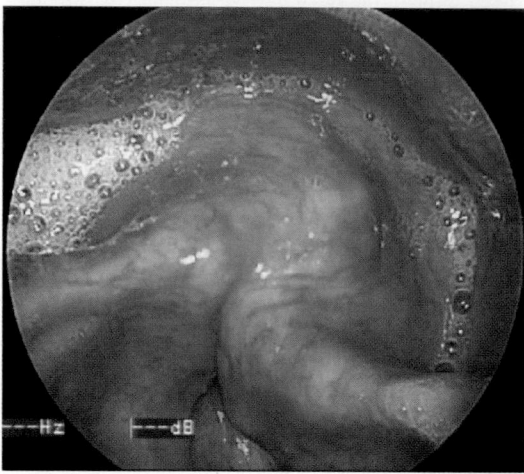

(B)

Figure 11 (A) During phonation at modal pitch, the lateral pharyngeal walls maintain a relaxed posture. In this patient with pharyngeal weakness from prior resection of CN X and XII at the skull base on the right, pooling of secretions in the pyriform sinus as well as vallecula is greater on the right. This is indicative of weakness. The image as captured with a camera on a 700 rod-lens telescope. (B) The patient is asked to phonate with a high-pitched /i/. The left pharyngeal wall, with intact innervation, contracts and partially covers over the pyriform sinus. The right side remains flaccid.

walls should contract and bulge toward the midline with this maneuver. Failure of contraction is indicative of either muscular weakness or loss of nerve function (Figure 11A and B). If the flexible endoscope is used, base of tongue strength can be assessed by having the patient say words such as "Paul" and "tall." In patients with intact tongue strength, the base of the tongue will nearly approximate the posterior pharyngeal wall (Figure 12A and B).

LARYNGEAL STROBOSCOPY

Indirect laryngoscopy is an excellent tool to evaluate pharyngeal and laryngeal function in breathing, swallowing, and speech production. Vocal fold adduction and abduction as well as pharyngeal wall motion can be readily observed. In addition, vocal fold mucosal lesions can be evaluated for characteristics indicative of malignancy. Voice production and voice quality, however, are

determined by vocal fold vibratory characteristics.[20] During voice production the vocal folds vibrate between 80 and 800 times each second. The human eye can only resolve five distinct images each second. Therefore, with steady state light sources, the vocal folds appear to stand still in an adducted position while the patient is phonating. Vocal fold vibration can be observed with either high speed cinematography in which film captures individual still frames 2,000 to 4,000 times each second or through the application of stroboscopy.[21] In stroboscopy, a bright xenon light flash is used to illuminate the larynx for a fraction of a microsecond. The image of the vocal folds at the instant in time is captured by the human retina and persists for 0.2 seconds. The light is then flashed repetitively and another image captured when the vocal folds are in a different position. The process is repeated. A microphone is used to sense vocal fold vibration rate so that the flashing of the strobe light can be synchronized with the frequency of vocal fold vibration. If the light is flashed in phase with the rate of vocal fold vibration, the vocal folds appear to stand still as the same point in the vibratory cycle is sampled repetitively. If the light is flashed slightly out of phase with the vibratory rate, a montage of images is collected which provide an apparent slow motion view of vocal fold vibration.

For complete evaluation, vocal fold vibratory characteristics should be observed at multiple phonatory frequencies. At low and modal pitch frequencies, the vocal folds have large vibratory patterns. As the phonatory frequency increases, due to increased vocal fold tension, the vibratory patterns become smaller possibly because vibration is only occurring within the most superficial portion of the mucosa. Observing stroboscopy at high frequencies of phonation allows the examiner to observe the supple nature of the vocal fold mucosa. If the mucosa is stiff on one vocal fold, then the vibratory patterns will be further reduced comparatively. At low frequencies of vibration, these mucosal differences may not be as apparent.

Originally, laryngeal stroboscopy was performed by reflecting the strobe light off of the laryngeal mirror. With the invention of rod-lens systems, it became possible to attach the stroboscopic light source to the endoscope. Examiners used an indirect rod with either a 90° or a 70° prism at the end. The fiberoptic delivery systems in the rod-lens improved light delivery and when combined with the rod optical system, the resolution of the scopes was enhanced over the traditional mirror systems. With the 90° endoscope, the examiner must place the scope higher on the oropharynx or toward the soft palate. This keeps the endoscope off of the base of the tongue but may stimulate gagging by touching the palate. With a 70° endoscope, the scope is placed closer to the base of the tongue. This is probably the preferred method or scope by most endoscopists.

Stroboscopy may also be viewed through flexible endoscopes. However, due to both

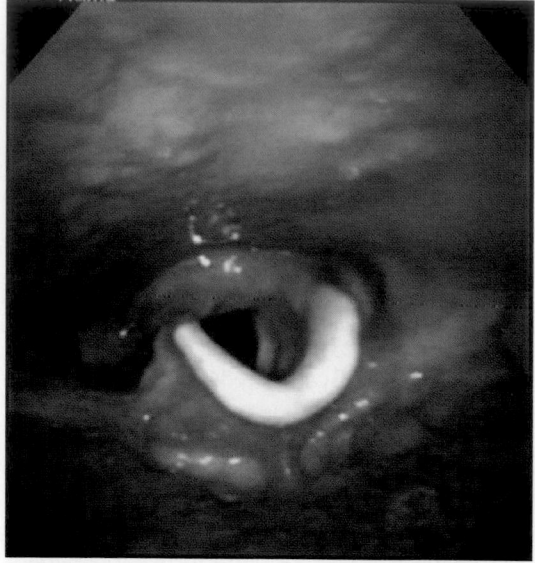

(A)

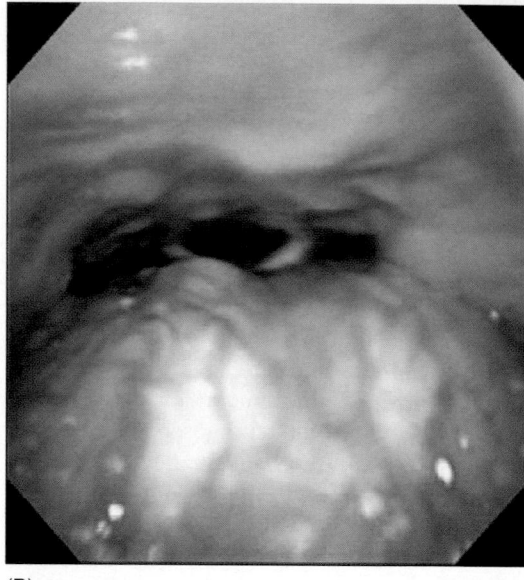

(B)

Figure 12 (A) This image is obtained through a fiberoptic distal chip scope (Olympus ENF-V2, Japan). At rest, the base of the tongue is in a neutral position. (B) While voicing "Paul," the base of the tongue contracts and approaches the posterior pharyngeal wall indicative of normal base of the tongue innervation.

reduced light and image transfer ability of fiberoptic systems, the resolution is reduced when compared to that obtained with rod-lens systems. Both light and image carrying are important for optical resolution. Flexible endoscopes for transnasal use are smaller in diameter than rod-lens telescope. Therefore, the number of light fibers is reduced. As mentioned previously, the ability to obtain image resolution is also dependent on fiber size. While technology is improving, fiber size is limited and the overall number of optical fibers is also limited by the size of the endoscope. With videoendoscopes, resolution is limited in part by the number of illuminating fibers in the scope as well as the primary resolution capabilities of the distal chip camera. While these systems are approaching the resolution capabilities of the rod-lens endoscopes, they are not yet the same.

RECORDING SYSTEMS

With the use of indirect endoscopes, the ability to attach a camera over the eyepiece of the scope is simplified. This provides the opportunity to record the examination for playback, review, and consultation. Examinations may be compared within and among patients. This provides a significant advantage when trying to determine the relevance of a lesion or laryngeal or pharyngeal defect in creating the patient's problem. Serial examination can be stored for direct comparison rather than needing to rely on the physician's memory and notes. Images can be recorded as still pictures or as video files. The images or files can be stored in the patient chart or electronically in a database system. Thanks to the work of some innovative individuals, who recognized the need, true relational databases for video storage and retrieval are currently available. These systems convert the video image to an MPEG 2 format. This is the standard format used in today's DVD technology and movie industry. It provides excellent resolution for video images while the files are small enough to be moved easily through the database system. By encoding the data to provide security for patient records according to the United States Health Insurance Portability and Accountability Act (HIPAA) guidelines, the information can be shared over the Internet from multiple sites. It is possible to record information from several data acquisition sites, store them to a server in a different site, and review the data in yet another site. The speed with which this occurs is dependent on the bandwidth of Internet access. Within one office or one university campus, it is usually possible to allow this transfer to occur in real time.

OFFICE SURGERY

Office surgery has always been possible with direct and indirect laryngoscopy. Historically, those who began with these techniques did so in their offices without the aid of general anesthesia. The procedures were not easy. With the advent and improvement of general anesthetic techniques, direct endoscopy has moved into the operating room. Surgical procedures are still performed in the office but usually under indirect techniques. Some trained surgeons may choose to use a mirror to view the larynx. The patient can retract the tongue. This will allow the surgeon to hold the mirror with one hand and a curved instrument to reach the glottis with the other. Alternatively, the mirror can be replaced with a rod-lens telescope.[22] In addition, a video camera can be attached to the end of the rod telescope so the procedure can be viewed and recorded on a video monitor if desired. Using these techniques, injection laryngoplasty can be accomplished with a curved needle of sufficient length, and laryngeal biopsy can be accomplished.

Visualization can also be accomplished with a flexible scope placed through the nasal cavity.

With this technique, an assistant can position and stabilize the endoscope. If a video monitor setup is employed, the surgeon can view the larynx on the monitor and use both hands for patient and laryngeal manipulation. In this manner, the surgeon can control the patient's tongue during peroral techniques.[23] If the goal of the procedure is to inject the larynx, either transoral or percutaneous techniques can be utilized. For percutaneous techniques, the surgeon can stabilize the larynx in the neck with one hand and pass the needle, either through the cricothyroid membrane, the thyrohyoid membrane, or transcartilagenously, with the other hand.[24] Observing on the video monitor allows the surgeon to verify needle placement during the procedure as well as position of the injected substance.

TECHNIQUES OF DIRECT LARYNGOSCOPY

As mentioned earlier, direct laryngoscopy is most commonly undertaken in the operative room with the assistance of general anesthesia or heavy sedation with local anesthesia. Direct laryngoscopy for the purpose of biopsy or injection can be accomplished by either technique. Some surgeons prefer local with sedation specifically for injection laryngoscopy as this method allows the patient to phonate at times during the procedure to aid in determining the degree of medialization.[25] For these types of procedures, a monocular tubular laryngoscope of the Holinger variety is most commonly used. These monocular scopes are designed to be placed on the side of the mouth along the floor. The tongue is displaced to the opposite side of the oral cavity and oropharynx from which the laryngoscope is introduced. Most surgeons prefer to place the endoscope in the right gutter. The surgeon uses their left hand to distract the maxilla. By pulling on the maxilla, the atlanto-occipital joint is extended. The neck can be placed in variable degrees of flexion as required or desired by the surgeon. The fingers on the surgeon's left hand are also used to distract and protect the lips so the lips are not inadvertently pinched between the endoscope and the teeth (Figure 13). The endoscope itself is held in the surgeon's right hand.

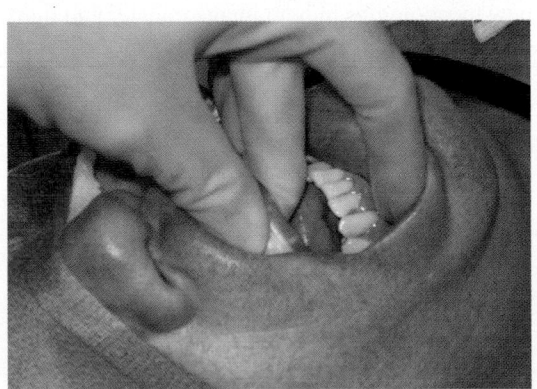

Figure 13 Hand position used to protect the patient's lips and teeth during insertion of the laryngoscope. A disposable tooth guard of heavy plastic is used to protect the teeth.

The scope is advanced with the vector of force upward on the mandible. The patient's head can be lifted off the bed. The head is resupported by adding pillows or flexing the headpiece of the operating table upward. The surgeon can support his or her hand by resting the ipsilateral elbow in the operating table. Commonly, maxillary dentition is protected with a tooth guard. Tooth guards can be purchased inexpensively and used as disposable items for each patient. Alternatively, individualized custom-molded teeth protectors can be used for each patient. Some surgeons find this preferable for patients who may need repeated endoscopy for surveillance of disease. If the maxilla is edentulous, then a folded gauze sponge to protect the gum is usually sufficient. One sponge can be moistened and placed between the lip and maxillary ridge. A second sponge can then be placed over the lip and first gauze sponge to hold it in place. If biopsy or injection is required, most surgeons will switch hands so that they are holding the positioned scope with their left hand and manipulation can be accomplished with their right hand.

Suspension laryngoscopy is most often performed under general anesthesia with the patient deeply sedated or paralyzed to avoid movement. This technique affords the surgeon excellent control during delicate surgical interventions in which precision is required to achieve reliable outcomes. Patient position starting with the head on or off the operating table has been previously discussed. The key to obtaining laryngeal exposure is to utilize both the atlanto-occipital joint and the neck positioning until the desired view is obtained. Most commonly this is through atlanto-occipital extension and variable degrees of neck flexion. If the surgeon starts with the neck in a neutral position, flexion or extension can be added as needed. Tubular laryngoscopes for suspension laryngoscopy are designed to accommodate binocular vision. Therefore, they are wider than endoscopes used for direct laryngoscopy without suspension. Binocular microlaryngoscopes are made with either a straight distal tip as the original esophagoscopes used for laryngoscopy or with a flared distal tip similar to the tip originally produced by Kirstein on his bladelike laryngoscope. If a flared distal tip scope is used, the posterior aspect of the proximal opening needs to be eliminated or flared in the opposite direction to allow adequate visualization of the anterior commissure of the larynx. In addition, the binocular scopes are designed to be placed over the patient's tongue, rather than along the floor of the mouth. The tongue is displaced anteriorly (see Figure 2).[26,27]

Once the scope is in position, a suspension apparatus is used. These suspension devices are either the Killian gallows type or the Lewy type. As long as the surgeon takes care not to use the maxillary teeth as a fulcrum for the endoscope, suspension can be accomplished with either system. During suspension, pressure is placed on the tongue or on the inside of the mandible. Patients need to be warned about pressure in these regions

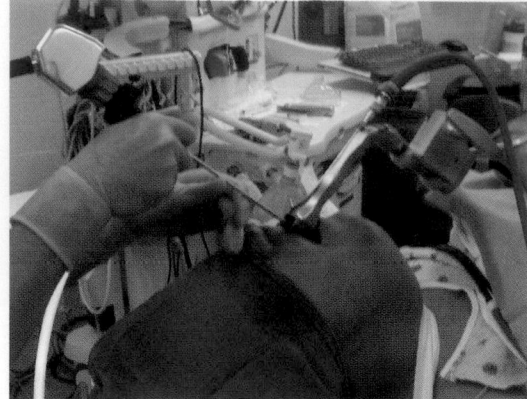

Figure 14 The patient has been stabilized in suspension with the Lewy suspension device. The larynx is inspected with a 0° rod-lens telescope and photographed.

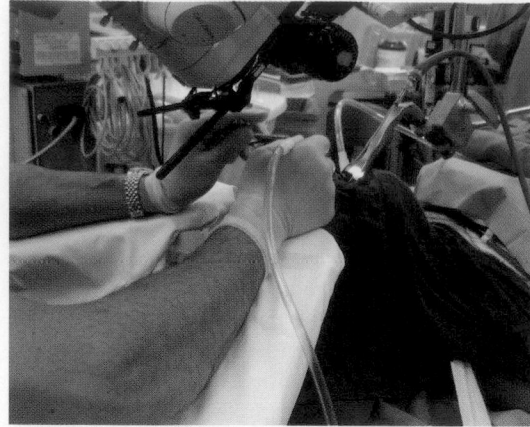

Figure 15 Bimanual manipulation is possible. Arm support is used to stabilize the surgeon's forearms. Two instruments can be inserted simultaneously allowing bimanual manipulation.

as excessive prolonged pressure on the tongue can result in temporary paresthesias or an alteration in taste.[28] Reports of permanent changes can be found in the literature, but most of the changes are self-limiting and most likely result from pressure on cranial nerves IX and XII or the lingual nerve. The anterior angle of the mandible is most often the limiting site for exposure of the larynx. As the endoscope is inserted in a patient with a narrow mandibular arch, the endoscope rubs on the inner surface of the mandible. This can cause ulceration on the inner surface of the mandible. The lateral mandibular incisors as well as the premolars are at risk for injury from the endoscope. To obtain exposure in these challenging patients, multiple endoscopes are available which are produced in variable widths. The Pilling Company, Fort Washington, Pennsylvania has produced a scope which is as narrow as possible but still allows binocular vision.[29]

Once stabilization has been applied, the surgeon is able to operate with both hands. If a narrow scope has been placed, room for bimanual manipulation will be limited. Therefore, ideally, the largest scope possible should be placed. After exposure and prior to surgical intervention, it is often helpful to inspect the larynx with rod-lens telescopes. These are produced with a variety of angles, from 0° to 120°, to allow visualization of the recesses of the laryngeal ventricles or the under surface of the vocal folds. With telescopic endoscopy, laryngeal lesions can be precisely mapped, and the surgical intervention designed to remove only the lesion and reduce injury to surrounding uninvolved tissues. For visual documentation, a camera can be attached to the eyepiece of the rod-lens telescope[30,31] (Figure 14). Next, a binocular operating microscope may be used to view the larynx under magnification. This enhances surgical precision. The surgeon can use a Mayo stand, or specialized chairs with armrests can be used to support his or her arms. Once again, this technique reduces unwanted movement and also improves surgical techniques. Multiple instruments can be used through the laryngoscope to facilitate surgical intervention (Figure 15).

CONCLUSIONS

Laryngoscopy has been performed since ancient times but was developed as a distinct clinical intervention in the middle of the nineteenth century. There are two basic forms, direct and indirect. These forms are categorized by the method of viewing the larynx. In indirect laryngoscopy, a mirror, prism, or flexible fiberoptic rod is used to transfer the image of the larynx back to the observer. The patient's head and neck are maintained in a relatively neutral position. In direct laryngoscopy, the patient's head and neck are positioned so that the larynx can be viewed directly through a long rigid tube.

Fiberoptic light delivery technology has improved our ability to view the larynx. The principle of fiberoptic light transmission is now used routinely to transfer light through smaller channels to the distal end of the endoscope without an internal source of heat. This has resulted in better illumination and better resolution of the laryngeal image. Resolution has also been improved through rod-lens technology, advances in fiber production technology for fiberoptic image carrying fibers, and advances in CCD production technology which have resulted in microchip cameras small enough to be placed at the distal end of a flexible endoscope.

Improvement in image resolution due to the new technologies in both image transfer and light delivery has resulted in rapid advances in our capability to perform office procedures. Rather than using indirect rigid laryngoscopy or direct laryngoscopy techniques in the office, many surgeons are using indirect flexible laryngoscopy, either with a fiberscope or a videoendoscope to guide their interventions. Finally, direct rigid laryngoscopy, with or without suspension, continues to allow the finest control over patient movement and enhances precision in surgical intervention. Suspension direct microlaryngoscopy remains the gold standard against which results from other techniques must be judged.

REFERENCES

1. Marsh BR. Historic development of bronchoesophagology. Otolaryngol Head Neck Surg 1996;114:689–716.
2. Goldman JL, Roffman JD. Indirect laryngoscopy. Laryngoscope 1975;85:530–3.
3. Hirsch NP, Smith GB, Hirsch PO. Alfred Kirstein. Pioneer of direct laryngoscopy. Anaesthesia 1986;41:42–5.
4. Zeitels SM. Premalignant epithelium and microinvasive cancer of the vocal fold: The evolution of phonomicrosurgical management. Laryngoscope 1995;105:1–51.
5. Zeitels SM, Burns JA, Dailey SH. Suspension laryngoscopy revisited. Ann Otol Rhinol Laryngol 2004;113:16–22.
6. Lynch RC. Suspension laryngoscopy and its accomplishments. Ann Otol Rhinol Laryngol 1915;24:429–46.
7. Roberts SE. A self-retaining dual distal lighted laryngoscope with screw driven fulcrum lift. Laryngoscope 1952;62:215–21.
8. Lewy RB. New instruments: A changing view of endoscopic instruments and methods for accurate direct observation of the larynx and per oral laryngeal surgery. Acta Otolaryngol 1956;46:80–6.
9. Miller RA. Endoscopic instrumentation: Evolution, physical principles and clinical aspect. Br Med Bull 1986;42:223–5.
10. Linder TE, Simmen D, Stool SE. Revolutionary inventions in the 20th century. The history of endoscopy. Arch Otolaryngol Head Neck Surg 1997;123:1161–3.
11. Andrews AH, Gould WJ. Laryngeal and nasopharyngeal indirect telescope. Ann Otol Rhinol Laryngol 1977;86:627.
12. Sawashima M, Hirose H. New laryngoscopic technique by use of fiber optics. J Acoust Soc Am 1968;43:168–9.
13. Williams GT, Farquharson IM, Anthony J. Fibreoptic laryngoscopy in the assessment of laryngeal disorders. J Laryngol Otol 1975;89:299–316.
14. Bergman NA. Michael Faraday and his contributions to anesthesia. Anesthesiology 1992;77:812–6.
15. Somerson SJ, Sicilia MR. Historical perspectives on the development and use of mechanical ventilation. AANA J 1992;60:83–94.
16. Ossoff RH. Laser safety in otolaryngology—head and neck surgery: Anesthetic and educational considerations for laryngeal surgery. Laryngoscope 1989;99:1–26.
17. Barker M, Dort JC. Laryngeal examination: A comparison of mirror examination with a rigid lens system. J Otolaryngol 1991;20:100–3.
18. Tabeen A, Murry T, Zschommler A, Desloge RB. Flexible endoscopic evaluation of swallowing with sensory testing in patients with unilateral vocal fold immobility: Incidence and pathophysiology of aspiration. Laryngoscope 2005;115:565- -9.
19. Murray J, Langmore SE, Ginsberg S, Dostie A. The significance of accumulated oropharyngeal secretions and swallowing frequency in predicting aspiration. Dysphagia 1996;11:99–103.
20. Jiang J, Lin E, Hanson DG. Vocal fold physiology. Otolaryngol Clin North Am 2000;33:699–718.
21. Hertegard S. What have we learned about laryngeal physiology from high-speed digital videoendoscopy? Curr Opin Otolaryngol Head Neck Surg 2005;13:152–6.
22. Mortensen M, Woo P. Office steroid injections of the larynx. Laryngoscope 2006;116:1735–9.
23. Tai SK, Chu Py Chang SY. Transoral laryngeal surgery under flexible laryngovideostroboscopy. J Voice 1998;12:233–8.
24. Green DC, Berke GS, Ward PH, Gerratt BR. Point-touch technique of botulinum toxin injection for the treatment of spasmodic dysphonia. Ann Otol Rhinol Laryngol 1992;101:883–7.
25. Lewy RB. Experience with vocal cord injection. Ann Otol Rhinol Laryngol 1976;85:440–50.
26. Jako GJ. Laryngoscope for microscopic observation, surgery, and photography. The development of an instrument. Arch Otolaryngol 1970;91:196–9.
27. Benjamin B. A new adult microlaryngoscope. Ann Otol Rhinol Laryngol 1986;95:207.
28. Tessema B, Sulica L, Yu GP, Session RB. Tongue paresthesia and dysgeusia following operative microlaryngoscopy. Ann Otol Rhinol Laryngol 2006;115:18–22.
29. Weed DT, Courey MS, Ossoff RH. Microlaryngoscopy in the difficult surgical exposure: A new microlaryngoscope. Otolaryngol Head Neck Surg 1994;110:247–52.
30. Benjamin B. Digital photography of the larynx. Ann Otol Rhinol Laryngol 2002;111:603–8.
31. Yanagisawa E, Yanagisawa R. Laryngeal photography. Otolaryngol Clin North Am 1991;24:999–1022. Erratum in: Otolaryngol Clin North Am 1992;25:ix.

84

Bronchology

Marshall E. Smith, MD
Mark R. Elstad, MD

Bronchology refers to the diagnosis and treatment of diseases of the large airways—the trachea and bronchi. The tracheobronchial tree comprises critical anatomical passages in which disease may affect health at any age, infant to elderly. Although the importance of these structures has been recognized for centuries, bronchology as a discipline began only 110 years ago. Advances in treatment have depended on the development of tools to examine the tracheobronchial tree, that is, bronchoscopes. The history of bronchology is largely the history of bronchoscopy. The utility of bronchoscopy will be well demonstrated in the discussion of airway disorders and their management. There have also been advances in other areas. For example, through image processing of computerized tomography (CT) scans of the airway a "virtual bronchoscopy" can be reconstructed with images and video which simulate the visual perspective of bronchoscopy.

APPLIED AIRWAY ANATOMY/ PHYSIOLOGY

A knowledge of the anatomy of the pharynx and larynx is crucial to any airway endoscopist and is discussed in detail in Chapter 72, "Development, Anatomy and Physiology of the Larynx."

The trachea extends from the cricoid cartilage to the bifurcation into the right and left bronchi. Its length averages 10 cm in women and 12 cm in men. The average anteroposterior diameter is 13 mm, and the transverse diameter is 18 mm. The anterior wall is formed by approximately 18 incomplete C-shaped rings of cartilage, and the posterior membranous wall contains the trachealis muscle. Approximately one-third of the trachea is in the neck, and two-thirds are in the mediastinum. The airway is lined by respiratory epithelium containing a prominent basement membrane and numerous goblet cells. The length and position of the trachea vary with changes in position of the head and neck. The trachea is midline in the neck and deviates slightly to the right at the level of the aortic arch which compresses its left lateral wall.

The right bronchus averages 2.5 cm in length and has six to eight cartilages. It bifurcates at an angle of 25° lateral to the trachea. The right upper lobe branches into apical, posterior, and anterior segmental bronchi. After the right upper lobe bronchus takeoff, the right bronchus continues as the bronchus intermedius. The anteromedial aspect of this bronchus opens into the right middle lobe bronchus which contains medial and lateral segmental bronchi. The short right lower lobe bronchus divides into five segmental bronchi. The typical configuration is the superior segmental bronchus followed by the medial, anterior, lateral, and posterior basal segmental bronchi.

The left bronchus bifurcates from the trachea at 45°, a sharper angle than the right bronchus takes. The average length of the left bronchus is 5 cm. It divides into the left upper and lower lobe bronchi. The upper lobe bronchus opens into the inferior lingular division (superior and inferior segmental bronchi) and the superior upper lobe division (typically an apical posterior and an anterior segmental bronchi). The left lower lobe bronchus divides into the superior segmental bronchi followed by the anteromedial, lateral, and posterior basal segmental bronchi. This nomenclature is summarized in Table 1. A visual comparison of external and endobronchial views of the tracheobronchial structures is seen in Figure 1.

For interventional bronchoscopists and those performing advanced diagnostic procedures, it is critically important to understand the relationship of vascular, lymph, and other structures to endobronchial anatomy. When doing interventional procedures such as laser and mechanical resection, one can be within millimeters of large and vascular structures, the injury of which is potentially lethal. The posterior aspect of the trachea and the esophagus is joined by the so-called "party wall." The aortic arch compresses the distal third of the left anterolateral trachea wall. The superior vena cava and azygous vein lay adjacent to the right anterolateral wall of the distal trachea. On the right, the right pulmonary artery lays directly anterior to the right and right upper lobe bronchi. The left and left upper lobe bronchi are in close association with the aorta and the left pulmonary artery. Lymph nodes are closely related to the trachea, carina, right and left bronchi, and airways in the hila.

Heffner suggested that the compliant and noncylindrical structure of the trachea, comprising incomplete cartilaginous rings, allows for more than simple conduit function.[1] Enlargement of the lumen during inspiration may allow sufficiently decreased airflow velocity at the periphery of the air column so as not to impede the normal egress of the mucociliary blanket. In

Table 1 Nomenclature and Numbering System Commonly Used for the Segmental Anatomy of the Lungs				
Lung	Lobes	Division	Segments	Number
Right	Upper		Apical	B1
			Anterior	B2
			Posterior	B3
	Middle		Lateral	B4
			Medial	B5
	Lower		Superior	B6
			Medial basal	B7
			Anterior basal	B8
			Lateral basal	B9
			Posterior basal	B10
Left	Upper	Superior	Apical posterior	B1–2
			Anterior	B3
		Inferior (lingula)	Superior	B4
			Inferior	B5
	Lower		Superior	B6
			Anteromedial	B7–8
			Lateral	B9
			Posterior	B10

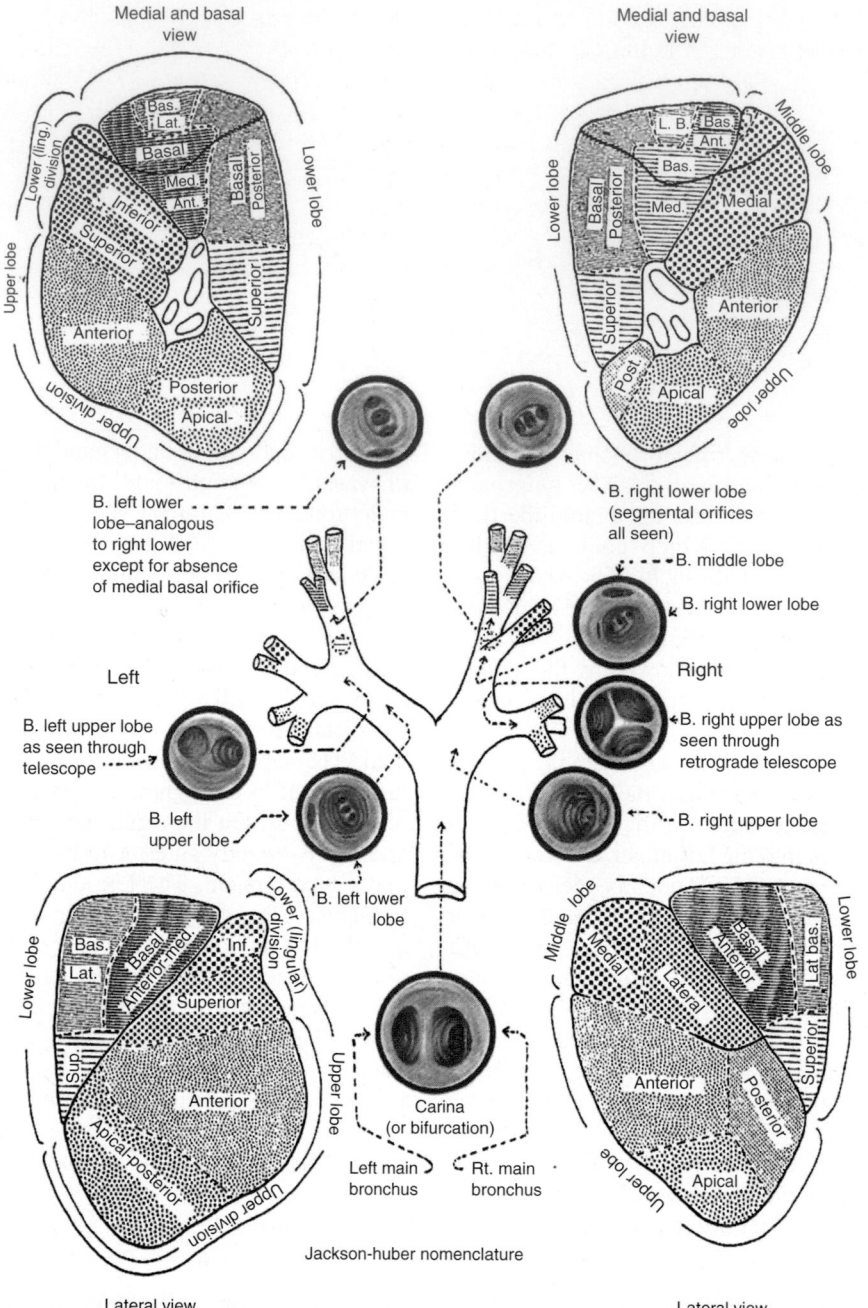

Figure 1 Drawings of the pulmonary segments, and the lobar bronchi and their segmental branches. The bronchial views are seen from the perspective of supine position. (From Jackson and Jackson, 1950.)

ing lesions in the middle or distal trachea. The best treatment options for congenital tracheal stenosis include tracheoplasty repair via median sternotomy. The slide tracheoplasty technique is currently the procedure of choice for lesions judged favorable for repair.

Other anomalies of the vascular arch can compress and obstruct the airway. These include double aortic arch, right aortic arch with left ligamentum arteriosum, and pulmonary sling. These develop from abnormalities in formation of the major vessels during embryogenesis. The innominate artery may also cause compression of the trachea in infants due to its origin to the left of the midline (Figure 3). With growth, usually by 3 years of age, it moves away from the trachea to the right. Pulsatile anterior tracheal compression narrows the trachea lumen in the shape of a teardrop. When vascular compression of the airway is suspected on bronchoscopy, the anatomy of the great vessels should be delineated with magnetic resonance imaging (MRI) or chest CT with contrast. The lesions are repaired by cardiothoracic surgery, with the capability for cardiac bypass a necessity.

Tracheomalacia or bronchomalacia refers to narrowing of the trachea or bronchi without extrinsic compression or internal stenosis. In infants it presents as inspiratory and/or expiratory stridor, wheezing, retractions that may be associated with feeding difficulties, cyanotic spells, or pneumonia. The pathophysiology of this condition may relate to excessive compressibility of the tracheobronchial tree during respiration in concert with intrathoracic pressure changes associated with respiration. Chest radiographs may show airway collapse depending on the phase of respiration when the radiograph is taken. Bronchoscopy of this condition demonstrates collapse of the posterior and anterior walls of the airway during spontaneous respiration. Other airway lesions may be associated with tracheomalacia or bronchomalacia such as extrinsic vascular compression or tracheoesophageal fistula. In the neonatal period, continuous positive airway pressure may be used to manage this condition until the structures grow

contrast, compression of the lumen at the beginning of a cough contributes to the increased driving pressure and increased airflow velocity that promote mucus expulsion; the abrupt noise of the cough results from suddenly increased airflow turbulence. Normal airflow in the trachea is laminar; masses or stenoses obstructing the lumen cause turbulent airflow evidenced as stridor.

AIRWAY DISORDERS AND DISEASES

Diseases of the airway affect all ages. They can be divided into congenital, infectious, inflammatory, neoplastic, and traumatic causes.

Congenital anomalies of the larynx are discussed in Chapter 69, "Congenital Anomalies of the Larynx." Tracheal atresia or agenesis is usually

fatal at birth unless the infant has a coexisting tracheoesophageal or bronchoesophageal fistula through which to maintain ventilation. In the tracheobronchial tree, congenital stenosis that narrows and obstructs the airway occurs in various forms. Mild forms include thin membranes or webs. More severe forms include segmental stenosis, funnel-shaped tracheal stenosis, or long-segment stenosis. In the more severe forms, the cartilaginous rings of the trachea are fused to create complete rings like the cricoid cartilage, with absence of membranous trachea (Figure 2). Long-segment tracheal stenosis may be accompanied by aberrant left pulmonary artery, also known as pulmonary artery sling. The diagnosis is made by bronchoscopy. Endoscopic repair of these anomalies are generally not successful. Tracheostomy is often not helpful for obstruct-

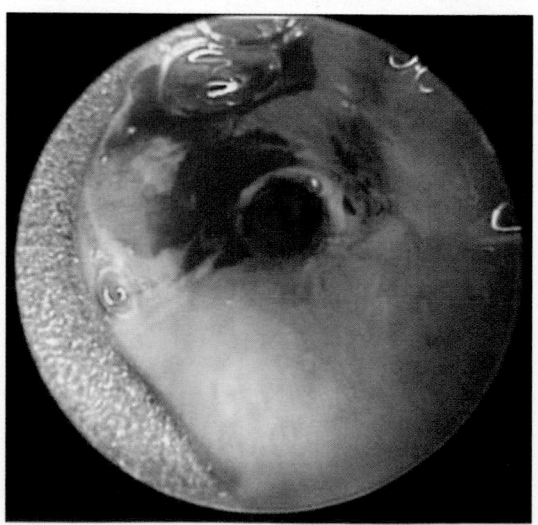

Figure 2 Congenital tracheal stenosis in a 2-month-old infant.

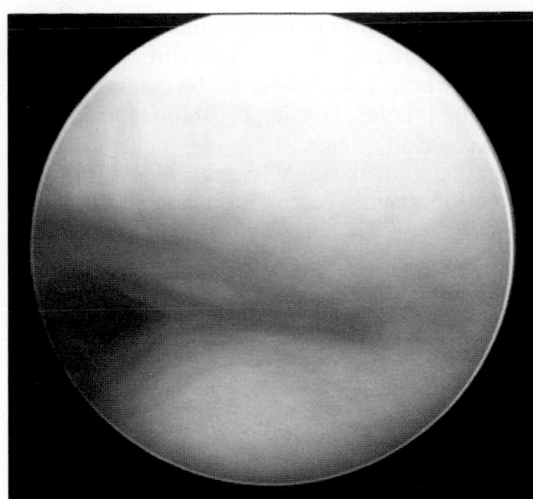

Figure 3 Innominate artery compression of the trachea in a 6-month-old infant.

and avoid more invasive treatment. In severe cases, tracheostomy and mechanical ventilation may be required.

Other congenital diseases that affect the bronchi include webs, atresia, immotile cilia syndrome, cystic fibrosis, and syndromes of abnormal cartilage formation (see below).

Infectious

A variety of viral, bacterial (including mycobacterial), and fungal infections can cause tracheobronchial disease. Acute bronchiolitis is a viral disease of the respiratory tract that occurs in children under 2 years of age. The respiratory syncytial virus (RSV) causes more than 50% of cases; other viral pathogens include influenza, parainfluenza, and adenovirus. Following a viral prodrome, patients develop respiratory distress characterized by wheezing cough, dyspnea, tachypnea, and cyanosis. Treatment is generally supportive, including O_2 supplementation. In severe cases that require intubation, bronchoscopy may be helpful to suction secretions and facilitate extubation.

Bacterial tracheitis may occur as a complication of a viral respiratory tract infection. It can cause life-threatening sudden airway obstruction due to thick tenacious mucus and mucosal edema that obstruct the large airways, especially in younger children. It is usually caused by *Staphylococcus aureus*, although *Moraxella catarrhalis* and *Hemophilus influenzae* can also be pathogens. Management involves intubation in severe cases, bronchoscopy to clear secretions and obtain cultures, antimicrobial therapy, and supportive care.

Pneumonias are usually divided into three groups: community acquired, nosocomial, and ventilator-acquired. Initial management includes appropriate empiric antibiotic therapy directed toward common pathogens based on the type of pneumonia and the patient's immune status. Cultures, obtained when patients have inadequate response despite standard therapy, are often obtained from expectorated material, which may be contaminated by oropharyngeal flora. Bronchoscopy allows directed aspiration of secretions directly from the tracheobronchial tree and has proven to be of benefit in immunocompromised patients.[2] Proper disassembly and cleaning of equipment between patients and proper specimen collection techniques must be used to prevent contamination. Bronchoalveolar lavage and bronchoscopic protected specimen brushing can retrieve specimens adequate for quantitative analysis. Bronchoscopy is indicated for lung abscesses unresponsive to postural drainage and chest physiotherapy to rule out an underlying carcinoma or foreign body and to obtain secretions for culture.

Bronchiectasis, irreversible dilatation of the bronchial tree, most commonly presents with chronic purulent sputum production and hemoptysis. Bronchiectasis may be postinflammatory, obstructive, or congenital. Stasis of secretions leads to infections that damage the bronchial walls, resulting in further dilatation and distortion. Infectious causes include RSV, pertussis, rubella, and tuberculosis. Obstructive lesions include tumors, foreign bodies, extrinsic compression, and impacted mucus. Congenital causes include bronchial webs and atresia, immotile cilia syndrome, cystic fibrosis, and syndromes associated with abnormal cartilage formation such as Williams-Campbell syndrome (absence of annular bronchial cartilage distal to the first division of the bronchi) and Mounier-Kuhn syndrome (congenital tracheobronchomegaly).[3] High-resolution CT is a useful imaging modality in suspected bronchiectasis.

Fungal infections of the lungs may create *mycetomas*. These aggregates are usually due to *Aspergillus* species and may develop in immunosuppressed patients. Diagnosis is generally made by chest radiographs or chest CT scan. Serum precipitin levels are usually elevated. Bronchoscopy is indicated for directed culture sampling or for evaluation of hemoptysis or progressive disease. Aspergillomas can cause life-threatening hemoptysis by erosion into bronchial arteries with 26% mortality. Surgical resection provides definitive treatment but is associated with high morbidity and mortality.

Mycobacterium tuberculosis is a bacillus transmitted by inhalation of infected airborne droplets. It is highly contagious. The highest incidence in the United States occurs among immigrants. Pulmonary symptoms include cough, chest pain, and hemoptysis. Other symptoms include chills, fever, night sweats, loss of appetite, and loss of weight. Diagnosis is usually based on skin-test reactivity to purified protein derivative of tuberculin, chest radiograph, and histologic or culture identification of the acid-fast bacillus. Bronchoscopy with bronchoalveolar lavage and/or biopsy has a high yield and should be considered in high risk patients who have negative sputum cultures, or who cannot produce adequate sputum samples. The therapy for tuberculosis involves four first-line antibiotics, including isoniazid (INH), rifampin (RMP), pyrazinamide (PZA), and ethambutol (EMB) or streptomycin. Tuberculosis in children is usually contracted from adults and adolescents in the household rather than from other children in day care or school; congenital infection is rare. The presentation of primary pediatric tuberculosis may be subtle, including erythema nodosum and nonspecific constitutional symptoms.[4] As tuberculin skin testing may be negative in 40% of these children, chest radiography demonstrating hilar and paratracheal lymphadenopathy is important in the diagnostic process. If young children cannot provide sputum specimens, three morning gastric aspirate specimens may be obtained. Children, especially those younger than 6 years of age, have a more rapid progression of disease from inoculation to dissemination; they are treated immediately from the time of exposure until the incubation period has passed and repeat diagnostic tests are negative. The principal drugs used to treat pediatric tuberculosis also include EMB, INH, PZA, and RMP; pyridoxine is given to infants to prevent nervous system complications of INH therapy. *M. tuberculosis* in children is rarely contagious. *Nontuberculous mycobacterial* diseases encompass all *Mycobacterium* species other than *M. tuberculosis*. *Mycobacterium avium-intracellulare* complex is the most common nontuberculous mycobacterial disease and is treated principally with clarithromycin, azithromycin, RMP, and EMP. *Mycobacterium kansasii* is the most virulent of the nontuberculous mycobacterial pathogens and is treated with INH, RMP, and EMB.

Inflammatory

Interstitial Lung Disease. Interstitial lung disease encompasses a wide variety of pulmonary diseases characterized by diffuse parenchymal opacities. Although more than 160 causes have been reported, pneumoconiosis, drug-induced disease, and hypersensitivity pneumonitis account for over 80% of cases. A thorough history can elucidate patient exposure to a large variety of injurious inorganic dusts such as coal, carbon black, asbestos, or talc; chemicals such as polyvinyl chloride, sulfur dioxide, or ammonium; pharmacologic agents such as cyclophosphamide, methotrexate, certain anticonvulsants, and beta-blocking agents, etc; and radiation therapy. Open or thoracoscopic lung biopsy, considered the gold standard for diagnosis, is not always a viable option in the elderly or patients whose respiratory status is significantly compromised; less invasive bronchoscopy with transbronchial lung biopsy may provide useful information.[5]

Sarcoidosis. Sarcoidosis is a nonnecrotizing granulomatous disease of unknown etiology, more common in African-Americans.[6] Patients most commonly present with nonproductive cough and dyspnea; head and neck manifestations include cervical adenopathy, uveitis or episcleritis, parotid swelling, nasal obstruction, neuropathies such as facial palsy and sudden sensorineural hearing loss, epiglottic swelling, and nasal mucosal edema. Ninety to 95% of patients with sarcoidosis have an abnormal finding on chest radiography, most commonly hilar adenopathy. Occasionally, endobronchial granulomas or stenoses occur. Elevated serum angiotensin converting enzyme levels appear to correlate with the activity of the disease but should not be used in isolation. Laboratory studies may also reveal elevated liver enzymes, particularly aspartate aminotransferase and alkaline phosphatase, elevated erythrocyte sedimentation rate, eosinophilia, hypercalcemia, and hypergammaglobulinemia. Fiberoptic bronchoscopy with transbronchial biopsy is the invasive procedure of choice for diagnosis; bronchoalveolar lavage is investigational. Corticosteroids are the mainstay of therapy. Pediatric sarcoidosis is rare and presents with fatigue and lethargy.[7]

Idiopathic Pulmonary Fibrosis. Idiopathic pulmonary fibrosis is a chronic fibrosing interstitial pneumonia of unknown etiology associated with the histologic appearance of "usual" interstitial pneumonia. This diffuse parenchymal disease occurs almost exclusively in adults, usually over 50 years of age, who present with slowly progressive dyspnea and nonproductive cough. Rales, particularly at the lung bases, are noted on auscultation in 80% of patients; fever is rare, and the disease is limited to the lungs. Characteristic abnormal findings on chest radiograph include asymmetric, bilateral, peripheral areas of reticular opacification. High-resolution CT is not diagnostic but can help determine prognosis; a fibrotic appearance portends a worse prognosis than a predominantly ground-glass appearance. Diagnosis is usually presumptive, based on clinical criteria; bronchoscopy and laboratory evaluation may be indicated to exclude other pulmonary diseases. Open or thoracoscopic lung biopsy is generally obtained to establish a histologic diagnosis; bronchoalveolar lavage is investigational. Although corticosteroids are standard therapy, no clear evidence exists proving that corticosteroids or any other available treatment is efficacious.[8]

Relapsing Polychondritis. Relapsing polychondritis manifests with acute, recurrent, progressive inflammation and degeneration of cartilage and connective tissue, including that within the tracheobronchial tree, affecting men and women in equal numbers. Serious airway manifestations occur in about one-half of patients with relapsing polychondritis; bronchoscopy is useful to identify and quantify inflammation, stenosis, or dynamic collapse of the tracheobronchial tree. Bronchoscopic stent placement may be required to maintain airway patency.[9]

Wegener's Granulomatosis. Wegener's granulomatosis is a necrotizing granulomatous vasculitis, affecting both the upper and lower part of the respiratory tract and the kidneys. The introduction of flexible fiberoptic bronchoscopes has revealed tracheobronchial involvement in more than half of patients with Wegener's granulomatosis.[10]

Neoplastic

Benign Neoplasms and Tumor-like Masses. Although some neoplasms occurring within the trachea and bronchi are histologically benign, they may still cause airway obstruction. Recurrent respiratory papilloma has a predilection for the larynx, but the trachea and bronchi may be involved by disseminated disease (Figure 4).

Traumatic granulomas may occur at sites of repeated mucosal trauma, such as the carina or bronchi in patients with endotracheal or tracheostomy tubes undergoing repeated mechanical suctioning. Granulation tissue can also develop within the tracheal lumen at the superior margin of a tracheostoma; initially, the tissue is soft and friable; overtime, it may become fibrotic. In patients with *tracheopathia osteochondroplastica*, multiple submucosal nodules, consisting of cartilage and lamellar bone, can be seen projecting into the lumen of the tracheobronchial tree. Right middle lobe collapse is a common finding. The differential diagnosis of multiple nodular lesions of the tracheobronchial tree include papillomatosis, amyloidosis, and sarcoidosis.[11] If the lesions cause airway obstruction, they can be excised bronchoscopically. Other reported benign lesions of the trachea or bronchi include inflammatory pseudotumors, plasma cell granulomas, fibrous histiocytomas, fibrolipomas, histiocytosis X, hamartomas, intratracheal ectopic thyroid tissue, pleomorphic adenomas, fibromas, fibrous histiocytomas, hemangiomas, hemangiopericytomas, paragangliomas, peripheral nerve sheath tumors, granular cell tumors, and leiomyomas.[1]

Malignant Neoplasms. Bronchogenic carcinoma, often referred to as "lung cancer," is the most common malignancy in the United States. Long-term tobacco use is the single greatest risk factor for developing lung cancer; approximately 87% of all cases of lung cancer are attributable to tobacco use. Additional environmental factors, particularly exposure to asbestos and radon, increase the risk of lung cancers in smokers. The risk of a nonsmoker developing lung cancer is 1% or less of that of a smoker.[12] The symptoms of lung cancer are nonspecific; the most common symptom is cough; other pulmonary symptoms include dyspnea, hemoptysis, chest pain, and manifestations of paraneoplastic syndromes. Chest radiograph may demonstrate a lung consolidation, atelectasis, infiltrate, or a solid nodule; CT of the chest with contrast often provides better definition of the lesion and is useful for assessing disease recurrence, persistence, or response to treatment. Bronchoscopy has emerged as an integral tool for the diagnosis and staging of

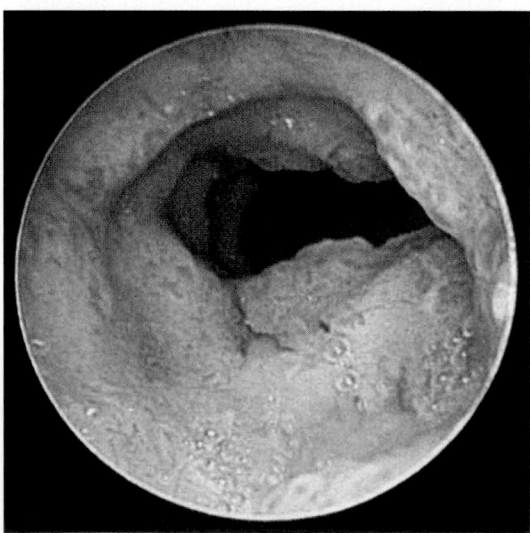

Figure 4 Tracheal papillomata in a 12-year-old boy.

lung cancer and may obviate the need for open biopsy. Bronchoscopy provides direct visualization of central lesions and can be combined with bronchoalveolar lavage, brushings, or biopsy to increase the diagnostic yield. Transbronchial aspiration of mediastinal lymph nodes can be performed to stage disease. Bronchogenic carcinomas are divided histologically into non–small cell cancers, including squamous cell carcinoma, adenocarcinoma, and large cell carcinoma, and small cell cancers. Surgery is the primary treatment modality for non–small cell cancer; radiation therapy and chemotherapy are reserved for advanced cases and cancers not amenable to surgical resection. Small cell cancer is noted for rapid growth and early development of widespread metastases; although it is extremely sensitive to radiation and chemotherapy, 5-year survival is only 3 to 8% and recurrence is common.[12] Only approximately 4% of primary lung neoplasms are not bronchogenic carcinomas. Bronchial *carcinoid* is a neuroendocrine neoplasm comprising approximately 2% of primary lung neoplasms. This reddish, polypoid, endobronchial mass often presents with obstructive symptoms. As the neoplasms arise from Kulchitsky cells, part of the amine precursor uptake and decarboxylation (APUD) system, they may secrete hormones such as adrenocorticotrophic hormone, antidiuretic hormone, gastrin, somatostatin, calcitonin, and growth hormone. Carcinoid tumors are categorized as typical, which is relatively benign and is treated with conservative resection, or atypical, also referred to as neuroendocrine carcinoma, which is more aggressive and often has metastasized widely by the time of diagnosis. Aggressive local resection with lymph node dissection is recommended for locoregional disease; chemotherapy is indicated when distant metastases are present. Five-year survival is about 60% and is dependent on the histologic subtype.[13] Other malignant neoplasms of the trachea or bronchi include spindle cell, oat cell, and adenoid cystic carcinomas (Figure 5); adenocarcinomas; mucoepidermoid carcinomas; malignant melanomas; sarcomas; lymphoreticular neoplasms; and malignancies invading the trachea or bronchi from adjacent structures.[1]

Traumatic

Acquired stenosis of the tracheobronchial tree may result from thermal inhalation, chemical burns, or from intubation (Figure 6). Pressure necrosis from an endotracheal or tracheostomy tube or their attached cuffs may result in healing by cicatrization, resulting in a spectrum of lesions.[14] Management of acute stenosis is controversial; some authorities advocate cautious dilatation, and the topical application of mitomycin-C shows promising early results. The use of a laser to enlarge the airway lumen may ultimately cause more scarring and stricture formation, although it may be indicated for highly selected lesions. A tracheostomy or T tube may be used for temporary or long-term management; definitive treatment involves surgical resection, expansion, and/or reconstruction. Flow volume curves are of little practical use in the management of severe

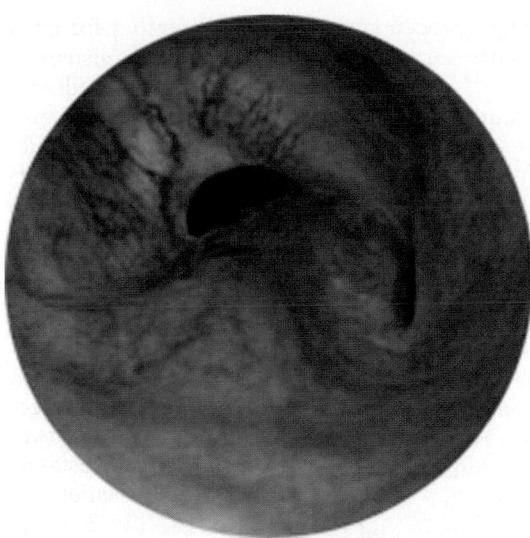

Figure 5 Adenoid cystic carcinoma of the trachea in a 37-year-old man.

tracheal stenosis.

Burn Injuries

Inhalation injury is defined as aspiration of superheated gases, steam, hot liquids, or noxious products of incomplete combustion. Early diagnosis is important but can be difficult, and there is no standard method for quantifying severity of inhalation injury.[15] History and physical examination may underestimate the severity of injury that may affect pulmonary function severely in a delayed fashion. Thermal or chemical inhalation can produce significant edema and mucosal necrosis of the trachea and bronchi and may cause stenosis.[16] Clinical findings include facial, oropharyngeal or nasal burns, singed vibrissae, carbonaceous sputum, wheezing, rales, rhonchi, and hoarseness. Arterial blood gas may indicate hypoxemia, hypercapnia, and the presence of carboxyhemoglobin. Chest radiography is generally not helpful in the early stages of interstitial lung injury. Bronchoscopy is the gold standard diagnostic tool for assessment of degree and extent of inhalation injury. Cytology or biopsy may also be done. However, bronchoscopy is not utilized routinely because history and clinical examination are adequate for management of most situa-

tions. Mucous plugs due to the cellular debris and mucus from inhalation injury can obstruct the airway of children. These have been successfully managed with respiratory treatments of aerosolized heparin/N-acetylcystine.[17]

RIGID BRONCHOSCOPY

History

Gustav Killian is known as the father of bronchoscopy.[18] He used a modified esophagoscope and then practiced examination of the airway in corpses, in patients with tracheostomies, and finally on a volunteer. In 1897, a Black Forest farmer had aspirated a piece of bone while eating his soup. Listening to his breathing, Killian heard a wheezing noise in the farmer's right lung. Killian used a head mirror as light source and forceps through his bronchoscope to remove the bone splinter, which was 11 mm long and 3 mm thick. He became famous for his expertise in removing foreign bodies, including beans, buttons, coins, and a tin whistle.

In May 1898, about 1 year after his initial experiments, Killian described some basic facts of modern bronchoscopy: "The bronchial tubes are elastic, mildly flexible and can be dilated. It is hence possible under local anesthesia to carefully insert the instruments from the bifurcation into the different sites and to view the small branches."

In Philadelphia, Chevalier Jackson made the next important advancement in 1904.[19] He produced a bronchoscope with a small light bulb at its distal end and incorporated a suction device. The main emphasis of this method was the retrieval of foreign bodies. Further technical advances in rigid bronchoscopy came through the development of rod lens optical telescopes in the 1960s and video camera technology.

Indications/Contraindications

The original use of rigid bronchoscopes was therapeutic, for foreign body removal. This continues to be an important application. Rigid bronchoscopy was the sole means or airway examination until the 1960s when the flexible bronchoscope was introduced. This was embraced by pulmonologists, yet not as rapidly by surgeons trained in rigid bronchoscopy. The flexible bronchoscope was quickly considered to be superior and expected to replace rigid bronchoscopy. However, over the last quarter century the utility of rigid bronchoscopy has been appreciated more. This is related to the introduction of new treatment modalities that are best used with the rigid bronchoscope. These include laser therapy, dilation of stenosis, stent placement, and brachytherapy. Rigid bronchoscopy is the treatment of choice for airway foreign body removal, laser procedures for tumors of the airway, dilation of stenosis and strictures, stent placement, and evaluation of massive hemoptysis.

Rigid bronchoscopy is contraindicated in patients with a difficult upper airway that can-

not be instrumented with a straight rigid scope. This includes patients with severe neck kyphosis who cannot tolerate neck extension, cervical spine instability, Class II malocclusion, trismus, mandibular hypoplasia, macroglossia. Rigid bronchoscopy is not possible in these cases. In patients with a tracheostomy, the rigid bronchoscope may be passed through the tracheostome.

Techniques: General, Specific, and New

When originally performed by Killian, topical anesthesia was used for rigid bronchoscopy. After Sigmund Freud's experiments with cocaine in 1883, it was found to be an excellent topical anesthetic. This paved the way for many applications in peroral endoscopy, including bronchoscopy. Now, general anesthesia methods have improved so that it is typically used to perform rigid bronchoscopy. Anesthesiologists now commonly employ techniques of total intravenous anesthesia or deep plane insufflation of inhaled agents by spontaneous ventilation, supplemented by propofol. The position of the patient is supine, rather than the upright position employed by Killian. Suspension tracheoscopy may be used with jet ventilation.[20] This technique allows both hands to be free to use instruments and visualize the airway through an operating microscope.

Equipment and Personnel. Rigid bronchoscopy is usually performed in the operating room. An operating room that has equipment for surgical endoscopy is preferred. The increasing use of optical rod lens telescopes in surgical endoscopy has helped to familiarize operating room personnel with endoscopes, including the rod lens telescopes that have been used in rigid bronchoscopy since the 1960s. Video cameras, light sources, and monitors that are conveniently located throughout the operating room allow the nursing staff and anesthesiologists to view the examination. This allows much greater cooperation and communication in management of the airway between members of the team. The room has equipment that is dedicated to bronchoscopy with a variety of bronchoscope sizes, optical lens telescopes, suction catheters and instruments, grasping forceps, biopsy forceps, and laser if needed. Commonly used lasers in bronchoscopy include the KTP and YAG lasers with fiberoptic capability, Argon laser, and CO_2 laser.

Techniques. Before performing rigid bronchoscopy, the plan of airway management is discussed with the anesthesiologists. The endoscopist has an idea of what is to be looked for, the risk of airway obstruction relating to both the disease process and the intervention. The safety of rigid bronchoscopy lies in the simultaneous control of and examination of the airway. The patient is taken to the operating room and placed in supine position on the table. Sedation and anesthesia are induced by the anesthesiologist, usually with intravenous infusion of propofol. The patient may be intubated by the anesthesiologist and turned over to the bronchoscopist or mask ventilated until insertion of the bronchoscope. The latter method is preferred in cases of known airway

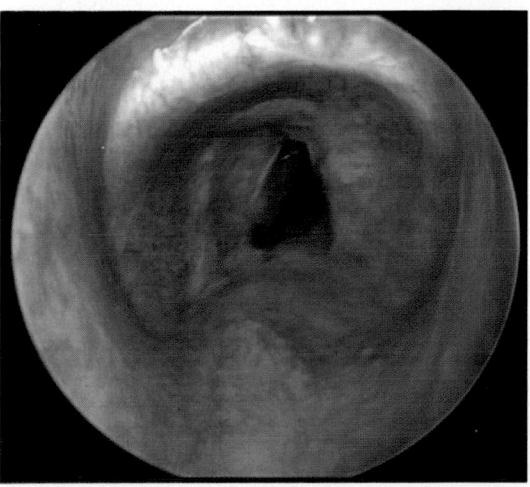

Figure 6 Tracheal stenosis in a 48-year-old man with prolonged intubation for chemical asphyxiation and burns.

obstruction. If the patient has not received neuromuscular blockade, 3 to 5 mL of 4% topical lidocaine is sprayed into the larynx and trachea to reduce coughing. Anesthesiologists frequently choose to administer propofol and remifentanil in a total intravenous anesthesia technique for these cases. The operating table is turned 90° to facilitate examination by the bronchoscopist at the head of the bed and positioning of the scrub nurse and equipment tray. At this time, direct laryngoscopy is performed with a straight laryngoscope blade, and pass a 0° rod lens telescope through the larynx and to inspect briefly the airway under magnification. A rigid bronchoscope is then passed through the larynx and into the trachea, and the anesthesiologist connects the breathing circuit to the bronchoscope to ventilate the lungs. Adequacy of ventilation is confirmed prior to proceeding with the examination. The tracheobronchial tree is examined by passing the bronchoscope to the carina, the right bronchus, and left bronchus. The segmental and subsegmental bronchial openings are visualized. Because the left bronchus makes a more acute angle from the trachea, the head is rotated to the right to pass the bronchoscope down the left side. If an examination of the distal bronchial segments is needed beyond the view through the rigid bronchoscope, a flexible bronchoscope may be passed through the rigid scope. Interventions taken after the diagnostic process are completed and are discussed below. At the completion of the procedure, the patient may be mask ventilated or intubated until emergence from general anesthesia.

Complications

Rigid bronchoscopy is a procedure that has both great therapeutic potential and risk of major complications. Because the instruments are metal and the soft tissue of the airway is elastic and pliable, the possibility of injury exists. This can lead to perforation of the airway which can cause pneumomediastinum, pneumothorax, hemorrhage of the great vessels into the airway, and esophageal injury. These serious complications may cause respiratory compromise, mediastinitis, or death. In the airway that is unprotected in an anesthetized patient, aspiration of secretions can cause pneumonia. Edema of the larynx and subglottis can be created or worsened by rigid bronchoscopic manipulation. This may cause airway obstruction requiring intubation or tracheostomy.

FLEXIBLE FIBEROPTIC BRONCHOSCOPY

Definition

Flexible bronchoscopy is an invasive procedure used to examine the tracheobronchial tree and, in addition, the nasal passages, pharynx, and larynx. It has both diagnostic and therapeutic applications for lung and airway disorders. Flexible bronchoscopy is most commonly performed in an endoscopy suite but may also be performed in the operating room, at the bedside, in the clinic, or in other locations. Indeed, flexible bronchoscopy has been safely performed on climbers with high-altitude pulmonary edema in a tent on Denali (Mt. McKinley, Alaska) at 4,200 m.[21]

History

A prototype flexible fiberoptic bronchoscope was developed by Dr Shigeto Ikeda in the mid-1960s and used for a series of clinical trials. The fiberscope, which became commercially available in 1967, rapidly caught on and transformed the practice of pulmonary medicine. In 1987 Dr Ikeda introduced a prototype video bronchoscope that transmitted an improved image to a high-definition monitor and allowed processing of the digitized image.

Indications

The flexible bronchoscope is used for both diagnosis and therapy. Guidelines for flexible bronchoscopy are reviewed in detail elsewhere.[22] Table 2 compares flexible and rigid bronchoscopy with respect to advantages, disadvantages, and indications. Diagnostic indications include the evaluation of lung masses and infiltrates, selected cases of pneumonia, hemoptysis, endobronchial lesions, airway stenosis or malacia, mediastinal lymphadenopathy, cough, wheezing, or stridor. Diagnostic procedures include airway inspection, bronchial wash, bronchoalveolar lavage, bronchial brush, endobronchial biopsy, transbronchial biopsy, transbronchial needle aspiration, endobronchial ultrasound, and autofluorescence bronchoscopy.

Therapeutic indications may include pulmonary toilet, foreign body aspiration, airway obstruction by tissue, stenosis or malacia, or difficult intubation. Therapeutic procedures include suctioning, laser ablation, balloon dilation, photodynamic therapy, intraluminal radiation, and stent placement. As discussed below, many therapeutic procedures are more efficiently performed using the rigid bronchoscope.

Contraindications and Risks

Many consider the inability to oxygenate the patient adequately to be the only true contraindication to bronchoscopy. The risk of complications is increased in patients with an unstable cardiac status, respiratory failure, or bleeding diathesis (if biopsy is performed), and these conditions are often considered relative contraindications. More importantly, one should treat these conditions prior to bronchoscopy if possible and pay particular attention to their management during bronchoscopy.

Equipment and Personnel

All of the necessary equipment should either be out in the room or readily available. For typical cases in a hospital setting, this includes patient monitoring equipment (oxygen saturation, blood pressure, heart rhythm), resuscitation and airway management supplies, suction, bronchoscopes of different sizes, video processor and monitor, biopsy forceps, cytology brushes, needle aspiration catheters, bronchoalveolar lavage supplies, and fluoroscopy.

Flexible bronchoscopy is most often performed by an operator who is dedicated to the endoscopic aspect of the procedure and two other personnel. One person, typically a registered nurse in our institution, administers medications and monitors sedation. A second person assists the bronchoscopist with specimen handling and other technical duties.

Techniques

In a bronchoscopy suite or operating room setting, the patient is positioned appropriately (the supine position is most commonly used),

Table 2 Comparison of Flexible and Rigid Bronchoscopy

Factors	Rigid Bronchoscopy	Flexible Bronchoscopy
Advantages	Large size working channel (larger tools, larger suction, shorter procedures)	General anesthesia not required
	More ventilation options (circuit or jet)	Training in rigid bronchoscopy not required
	Greater number of interventions	
Disadvantages	Requires general anesthesia	Less airway control unless intubated
	Airway injury from rigid tube	Limited number of interventions
Indications		
Airway obstruction	Compromised airway	Noncompromised airway
	Respiratory distress	No respiratory distress
	Treatment > diagnosis	Diagnosis > treatment
Cancer	Treatment > diagnosis	Diagnosis > treatment
Hemoptysis	Massive	Nonmassive
	Diagnosis and treatment	Diagnosis > treatment
Foreign body	All pediatric cases	Often first procedure in adults
	Adults if flexible unsuccessful or unlikely to be successful	Not used in children
Parenchymal lung disease	Rarely used	Diagnosis
Mediastinal adenopathy	Rarely used	Diagnosis

monitors are attached, and vital signs are taken. Intravenous access is obtained, and supplemental oxygen is supplied by nasal cannula or facemask. If sedation is used, slow titration is started immediately. Numerous approaches to moderate or "conscious" sedation are used. We most commonly use an infusion of a fixed combination of propofol and remifentanil as the rapid onset and short duration of action of these drugs are excellent for this procedure. A topical anesthetic (lidocaine and/or cocaine) is applied to the nasal passages and pharynx.

After appropriate sedation is reached, the bronchoscope is passed either through the nares (preferred) or an oral bite block. Careful examination of the nasal passages, pharynx, and larynx is considered an important component of bronchoscopy, and particular attention is paid to the appearance and function of the vocal folds. After traversing the larynx, a complete airway examination is performed using topical lidocaine, and titration of sedation as indicated.

Following inspection, the diagnostic and/or therapeutic procedures are performed. It is critically important that the order of various procedures is considered prior to the bronchoscopy and modified as needed. We generally perform the high yield and low-risk procedures first and progress toward those with lower yields in the event that the bronchoscopy has to be terminated.

In our outpatient airway disorder clinic, we routinely perform flexible laryngoscopy, tracheoscopy, and esophagoscopy on unsedated patients sitting upright in a chair. With a flexible fiberoptic laryngoscope, the trachea down to the carina and the proximal bronchi can be seen in most patients. This is a simple, safe, and effective way to evaluate central airway problems.[23] For laryngoscopy and tracheoscopy, topical anesthesia is atomized in the nasal passages and transorally. A lubricated laryngoscope is passed through the nares, pharynx, larynx, and into the distal trachea. Careful examination is performed and recorded. A similar technique is used for transnasal or transoral esophagoscopy. We find that the vast majority of our patients tolerate the procedure well and that, in many cases, it obviates the need for scheduling additional visits to the endoscopy suite.

Complications

Diagnostic flexible bronchoscopy is a safe procedure. Mortality is rare with a reported death rate of 0 to 0.04%. Major complications such as significant bleeding, respiratory depression, pneumothorax, arrhythmias, and cardiac arrest occur in <1% of cases.

THERAPEUTIC BRONCHOSCOPY

Although bronchoscopy is most frequently used for diagnostic indications, the bronchoscope was initially invented for foreign body retrieval. Bronchoscopy by otolaryngologists is typically done with the rigid instrument. However, a recent survey of members of the American College of Chest Physicians noted that 99% of bronchoscopies in the United States by pulmonologists were performed with the flexible instrument and that only 8% of pulmonologists use the rigid bronchoscope.[24] Pulmonologists generally lack training in rigid bronchoscopy, and surgeons generally lack training in flexible bronchoscopy. However, there is no doubt that the rigid bronchoscope is an invaluable tool for those performing therapeutic bronchoscopy. It is our opinion that many of the therapeutic procedures listed below are performed more efficiently and safely with the rigid bronchoscope. In our practice, we routinely use suspension laryngoscopes, rigid and flexible bronchoscopes, and rigid and flexible esophagoscopes. Having all of these tools available allows one to choose the correct tool for the task at hand. The interventional procedures discussed below have recently been reviewed in detail and extensively referenced in guidelines published by the American College of Chest Physicians.[25]

Laser Therapy

Lasers (light amplification of stimulated emission of radiation) interact with endobronchial tissue to cause vaporization, coagulation, and hemostasis. The lasers most commonly used for endobronchial therapy are the neodymium:yttrium–aluminum–garnett (Nd:YAG), carbon dioxide (CO_2), and potassium titanyl phosphate (KTP) lasers. The Nd: YAD and KTP laser light can be transmitted through flexible fibers. A flexible guide for CO_2 laser delivery has also become available recently. We use the CO_2 laser, which has precise cutting but minimal hemostatic properties, primarily for benign lesions in the larynx, subglottis, for example, subglottic stenosis and proximal trachea. The Nd:YAG laser, which provides deeper tissue penetration and superior photocoagulation and hemostasis, is used for malignancies and lesions in the trachea and bronchi. The KTP laser is used most often for benign lesions in the more distal airways.

Although the laser therapy can be performed through either rigid or flexible instruments, we prefer use of the rigid bronchoscope for most patients because it is faster, safer, and more versatile in the performance of other techniques, for example, stenting. Nd:YAG laser therapy is a safe and effective tool for relieving endobronchial obstruction due to malignant tumors. In central lesions involving the trachea, right and left bronchi, or the bronchus intermedius, the recannulization rates are greater than 90%. Serious complications of laser therapy include death, airway perforation, hemorrhage, pneumothorax, pneumomediastinum, and myocardial infarction. Complications may be minimized by careful patient selection, careful consideration of the characteristics of the airway lesion, and meticulous technique.

Electrocoagulation

Electrocautery uses high-frequency electric current to destroy tissue. These devices require grounding the device, the patient, and the bronchoscope to complete the circuit. A snare device using electrocautery is particularly useful for removing pedunculated lesions. Argon plasma coagulation (APC) is a relatively newer form of noncontact electrocoagulation. Argon plasma formed at the tip of a probe is used to transmit electric current to the nearest grounded tissue and thereby cause coagulation. Coagulation depth of 2 mm is typically achieved. This is quite useful for providing hemostasis with little risk of perforating the airway. It is an excellent tool for controlling hemoptysis from the surface of lesions; however, laser therapy is generally more effective for debulking large masses.

Airway Dilation

Airways may be dilated using the rigid bronchoscope barrel, Pilling dilators, or "angioplasty" balloon catheters. Airway dilation (bronchoplasty) may be used as sole therapy but is most often used in combination with other procedures. For example, when there is subtotal occlusion of a right or left bronchus by tumor, we will frequently use bronchoplasty to provide a visual "path" for laser resection. In patients with central airway stenosis, bronchoplasty is frequently followed by stenting. For endoscopic therapy of subglottic stenosis, we often use radial incisions with a CO_2 laser followed by balloon bronchoplasty.[26] The major potential complication is airway disruption.

Airway Stents

The first dedicated airway stent, the Montgomery T-tube, was introduced in 1965. Dumon introduced the first dedicated endoluminal airway stent in 1990.[27] Currently, there are two main categories of endobronchial stents; fixed tube (silicone) and self-expanding (wire mesh). Fixed tube stents are typically placed using a rigid bronchoscope. In comparison to self-expanding stents, they are relatively easy to remove and reposition and cause minimal irritation to the airway. We prefer silicone stents for most applications.[28] Self-expanding stents may be either covered or uncovered. Compared to fixed tube stents, self-expanding metallic stents may be placed using a flexible bronchoscope and have a larger internal/external diameter ratio. However, granulation tissue is a more common complication and these stents can be difficult or impossible to remove.[29,30] The Polyflex stent is a hybrid design that uses a self-expanding polyester mesh imbedded in silicone. The Polyflex stent is placed using a rigid bronchoscope but has the property of easy removal similar to the tube stents.

Airway stents are used for obstruction by benign or malignant disorders. They are best suited for extrinsic compression or endoluminal tumor although they can be used for malacia. Stents are frequently used in combination with other therapies such as laser resection or radiation. There are now many studies that demonstrate impressive results using stents for malignant airway obstruction. Interventional bronchoscopists should have significant experience using all of the major stent types to ensure that the appropriate stent is selected for a given lesion. Occasionally, combined stenting of the airway and the gastrointestinal tract is required as shown in Figure 7. Anecdotally, we have seen numerous problems resulting from inexperienced bronchoscopists attempting to use self-expanding stents for benign disease. It is our practice only rarely to use metallic stents for benign central airway obstruction. The US Food and Drug Administration has issued a warning regarding the use of metallic stents in benign tracheobronchial disease.[31]

Intraluminal Radiation

Intraluminal radiation (brachytherapy) is most commonly delivered to the airway using a transnasal catheter that is placed in the airway using the bronchoscope. One is able to deliver therapeutic doses of radiation to airway tumor, with minimal dose being supplied to the normal surrounding tissues, using this technique. The after-

loading catheter is advanced across the area to be treated through the working channel of the flexible bronchoscope. The bronchoscope is withdrawn over the catheter using fluoroscopy to maintain position of the catheter. Then the position of the catheter is confirmed both bronchoscopically and radiographically. The patient is then transferred to radiation oncology for dosimetry and after loading of the radioactive source. The catheter is withdrawn immediately after the treatment. Typical regimens deliver three fractions at weekly intervals. Intraluminal radiation is most commonly used for palliation of malignant airway obstruction (Figure 8). Occasionally, it may be used for carcinoma in situ or early stage lung cancer in patients who are not candidates for surgery. In addition, there are occasional uses in nonmalignant disease such as endobronchial amyloidosis.[32]

Photodynamic Therapy

Photodynamic therapy (PDT) involves infusion of a photosensitizer, preferential retention of the photosensitizer by malignant cells, activation of

the photosensitizer by nonthermal laser light, and finally removal of necrotic tissue. Most typically, porfimer sodium (Photophrin) is injected intravenously 48 to 72 hours before light is applied through a flexible fiber. Subsequent bronchoscopy is often required 1 to 3 days later for debridement of necrotic tumor. Although PDT is effective in selective cases of endobronchial malignancies, it is our opinion that Nd:YAG and mechanical resection are more efficient in the majority of patients with obstruction of the central airways. However, PDT can be performed using a flexible bronchoscope without general anesthesia and may be more easily delivered to the peripheral airways, for example, the upper lobes. Another indication is early stage lung cancer of the airways in patients who are not surgical candidates. Skin photosensitivity for a period of time of up to 6 weeks can be a problem if patients are unable to stay out of the sun, and massive hemoptysis has been reported.

Cryotherapy

Cryotherapy uses a flexible cryoprobe to repeatedly freeze and thaw tissue causing tumor cell death. It may be used for both benign and malignant obstruction. Its major advantages include cost and relative safety. As the maximal effects are delayed, it is not as useful as other modalities for treatment of severe obstruction. In addition, it often requires follow-up bronchoscopy exposing the patient to additional procedures.

Microdebrider

Microdebriders are used by a variety of specialties including otolaryngology for laryngeal surgery. The device has a rotating blade at the tip of a hollow tube that is connected to suction for trapping and removing debris. In selected cases, it allows rapid debridement of obstructing airway lesions. As there is no coagulation of tissue, there is the potential for significant bleeding, but this has not been an issue in the reported series or in our experience. The relatively short length of the instruments commercially available limits use to the more proximal airways.

Anesthesia and Ventilation

Every detail of the approach to airway management, anesthesia, and ventilation is extremely important in the care of patients with central airway obstruction.[33] One must be prepared for virtually any airway emergency. We generally use intravenous agents for induction and maintenance of anesthesia because we find induction to be smoother; we often interchange open, for example, suspension laryngoscopes, and closed, for example, rigid bronchoscope, circuits, and the patients have fewer postoperative symptoms. We find the combination of propofol and remifentanil to be ideal and use specific muscle relaxants based on the time required for the procedure.

Ventilation can be managed using either a closed (the rigid bronchoscope is connected to

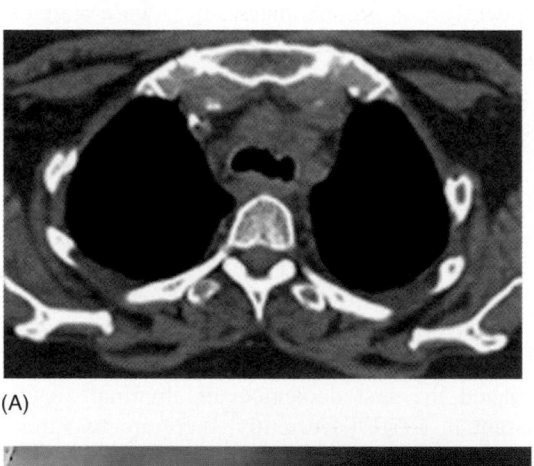

(A)

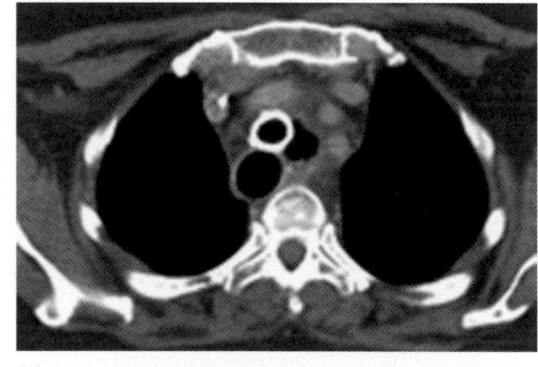

(B)

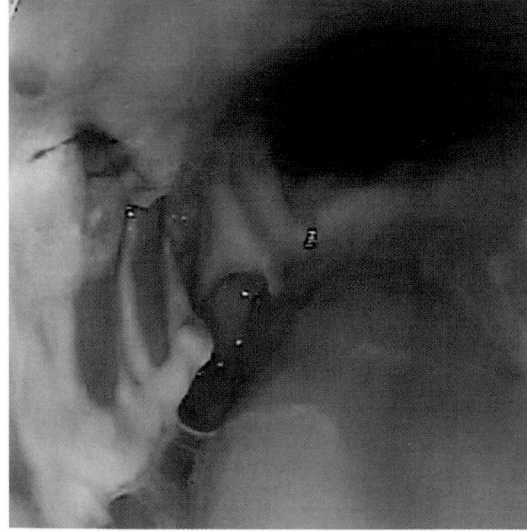

(C)

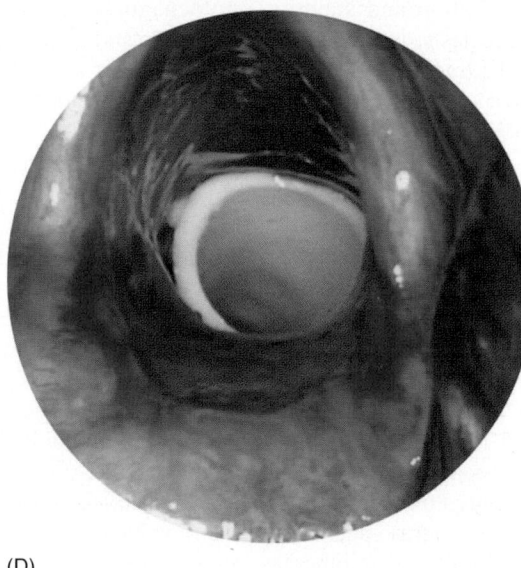

(D)

Figure 7 Combined tracheal and esophageal stenting for malignant tracheoesophageal fistula. This 60-year-old female developed symptoms suggesting a tracheoesophageal fistula during her initial course of chemotherapy for a diffuse mediastinal large B cell lymphoma. A CT scan (A) suggested a large communication between the trachea and the esophagus. Bronchoscopy and esophagoscopy confirmed a 5 cm defect in the left posterolateral aspect of the mid to distal trachea (C) directly communicating with the esophagus. A self-expanding plastic stent placed in the esophagus sealed the fistula but impinged on the airway lumen. Thus, a silicone stent was placed in the trachea. Follow-up CT scan (B) shows the radiopaque tracheal stent, the radiolucent esophageal stent, and a pocket of air in the mediastinum. The upper limb of the tracheal stent is seen through the larynx (D). The patient did well postoperatively, completed chemotherapy without further complications, and appears to be in remission.

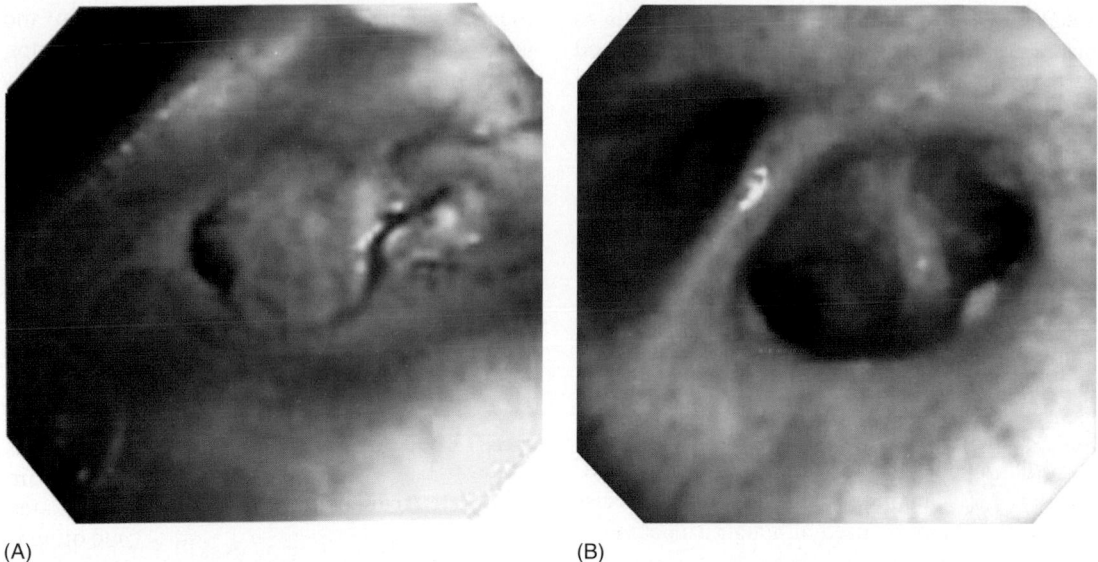

(A)   (B)

Figure 8 Treatment of localized squamous cell carcinoma using intraluminal radiation therapy (brachytherapy). This 57-year-old male smoker had a history of multiple recurrent squamous cell carcinomas over a period of 8 years. Initially he was treated with a right upper lobectomy and then a left upper lobectomy. Later he was noted to have carcinomas in both the right and left lower lobe bronchi that were treated with photodynamic therapy because he was no longer a surgical candidate. Bronchoscopic follow-up 1 year after photodynamic therapy revealed squamous cell carcinoma in the right lower lobe (A). He was then treated with intraluminal radiation, and follow-up at 1 year showed no evidence of cancer in specimens from biopsy of the still abnormal looking mucosa (B).

Foreign Body Removal

Foreign bodies in the airway are common and occasionally life threatening. They may present acutely and be obvious or chronically and be occult. The diagnosis requires a high index of suspicion and a low threshold for performing bronchoscopy. Radiographs may at times be useful but are not a sensitive test. If the history is suggestive of foreign body aspiration, one must not be dissuaded from performing bronchoscopy because of unremarkable imaging.

Bronchoscopy is the "gold standard" for the diagnosis of an airway foreign body and the most useful therapeutic tool. Either the flexible or the rigid bronchoscope may be used depending on the clinical situation. At our institution, we prefer using the rigid bronchoscope for many of these procedures. When we use the flexible bronchoscope as the initial tool, we do not hesitate to progress to general anesthesia and the rigid bronchoscope. A variety of removal devices should be available including forceps, baskets, and balloons. Complications of bronchoscopy for foreign body removal are infrequent, although great care to protect the airway is warranted. On rare occasions thoracotomy may be required.

Life-Threatening Hemoptysis

Bronchoscopy plays a role in the diagnosis and therapeutic approach to the management of patients with life-threatening hemoptysis. Although less than 5% of patients with hemoptysis are classified as "massive," acutely fatal bleeds have been reported in up to one-third of these patients. We favor an aggressive approach to airway management, diagnosis, and

the anesthesia circuit) or an open system (jet ventilation). In most patients for whom the rigid bronchoscope is used, we start with the closed system because it is easier to monitor the adequacy of ventilation. We do not hesitate to use jet ventilation in individual patients. When working through a suspension laryngoscope, we either use intermittent ventilation with an endotracheal tube or jet ventilation. Problems related to inadequate ventilation, inadequate oxygenation, or dynamic hyperinflation must be anticipated as they may develop quickly.

Central Airway Obstruction

Central airway obstruction may result from a long list of malignant and "benign" processes.[33] Bronchogenic carcinoma is the most commonly encountered malignant cause. Complications resulting from endotracheal and tracheostomy tubes are the most common nonmalignant causes. An algorithm for the management of central airway obstruction is presented in Figure 9.

Signs and symptoms of central airway obstruction may include dyspnea, wheezing, cough, and hoarseness. Dyspnea occurs when there is a significant increase in the work of breathing. Physical examination, pulmonary functions testing, and imaging techniques such as conventional radiographs may provide useful information. CT scans using new imaging protocols often provide more information; however, bronchoscopy remains the diagnostic "gold standard."

The diagnostic and therapeutic approach, using bronchoscopy and other means, depends on the clinical urgency, the cause, and the anatomical details including the location and nature (extrinsic compression, intraluminal exophytic tumor, etc). In certain cases, we proceed directly to rigid bronchoscopy with plans for immediate

therapy. In others, we will perform flexible bronchoscopy for more detailed analysis prior to planning the therapeutic approach.

Exophytic endobronchial lesions are often managed with a combination of dilation, laser and mechanical resection, and/or APC. Extrinsic compressing lesions are typically managed using a combination of dilation and stenting. In nonemergent cases, a variety of additional therapies may be useful as outlined in Figure 9.

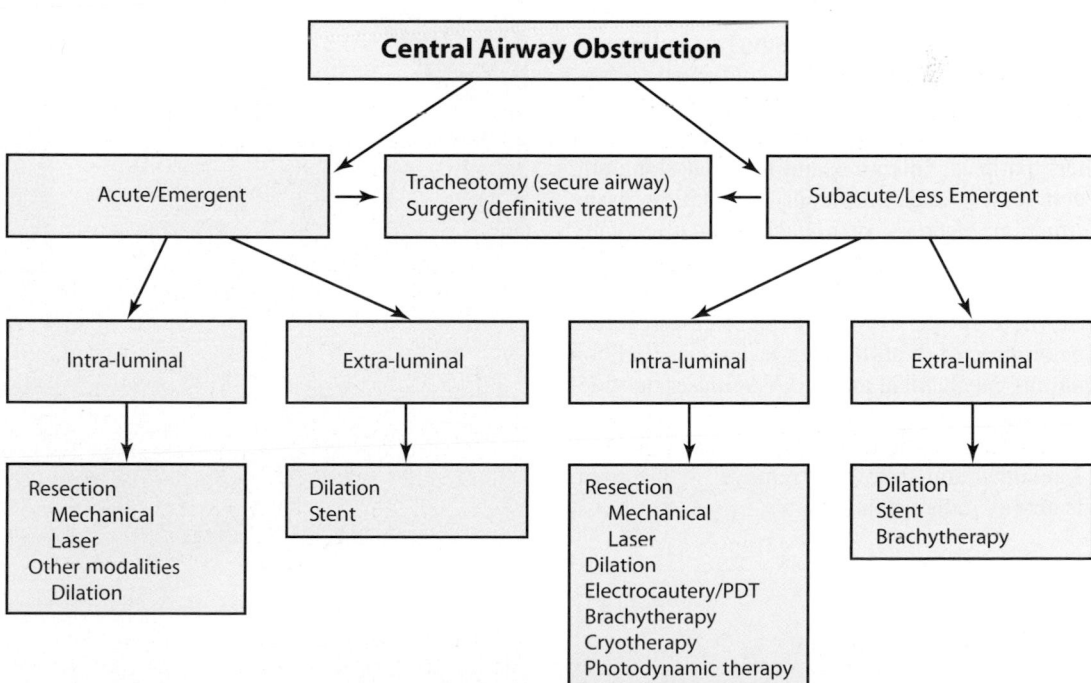

Figure 9 Algorithm for the management of central airway obstruction. The algorithm focuses on endoscopic interventional procedures, but surgical intervention is always considered. Tracheostomy may be the procedure of choice for securing the airway in severe proximal obstruction, and surgical curative resection is preferred when possible. Obstruction of the central airways often presents as a medical emergency. As a result, the initial intervention must frequently be done prior to complete characterization of the lesion or, in the case of malignancy, histopathological diagnosis. A multidisciplinary approach allows the use of a combination of modalities as is often required for the best outcome.

intervention because of the unpredictable course in such patients.

Localization is accomplished by combining history, physical examination, and imaging studies with bronchoscopy. Either the flexible bronchoscope, in the intubated patient, or the rigid bronchoscope may be used. Although there are no studies directly comparing the safety and yield of these two procedures, we favor the rigid bronchoscope because the larger lumen allows improved suctioning capacity and, therefore better airway clearance.

After localization a decision is made regarding therapeutic intervention. Bronchoscopic therapies include airway blockade, topical therapies, and laser coagulation. Other therapies include arteriography and embolization and surgical resection.

Endobronchial Lung Volume Reduction

Lung volume reduction surgery has been shown to be effective for symptom palliation in selected patients with emphysema. Unfortunately, the surgery has a high morbidity and mortality rate. Intrabronchial valve treatment for emphysema uses one-way valves implanted in appropriate airways to cause lung volume reduction and other physiologic changes achieved by lung volume reduction surgery. Valves are placed into the upper lobe airways using a flexible bronchoscope. A recent multicenter trial demonstrated acceptable safety and improvements in health-related quality of life.[34] Further studies of this promising technique are ongoing.

Airway Complications of Lung Transplantation

Lung transplantation has become relatively common in patients with end-stage lung disease in disorders such as chronic obstructive pulmonary disease, pulmonary fibrosis, and cystic fibrosis. Airway complications are significant clinical problems that occur on average in 15% of these patients. Infection and mucosal sloughing occur early, and exuberant granulation tissue formation, stenosis, or malacia may occur later on. Combinations of granulation tissue, stenosis, and malacia are handled in a manner similar to elsewhere in the airway. Typical cases require one or more of the following techniques (balloon dilation, mechanical and Nd:YAG laser debridement, and airway stenting). It is not uncommon that stenting can be temporary, for example, 6 to 12 months, and following removal of the stent, the airway remains patent.

NEWER PROCEDURES

Endobronchial Ultrasound

Endobronchial ultrasound (EBUS) uses a miniature probe that can be inserted through the working channel of a flexible bronchoscope. A fluid-filled balloon surrounds a rotating piezoelectric crystal allowing an ultrasound view of the airway. The penetration depth allows visualization of the airway wall layers as well as mediastinal and paratracheal lymph nodes and peripheral lung lesions. This technique can be used for visualization of the airway, guiding transbronchial needle aspiration, and assessing airway anatomy to guide other therapeutic procedures. EBUS with transbronchial needle aspiration is emerging as a safe and accurate means for staging lung cancer.

Navigational Systems

A variety of navigational systems have been used to supplement direct vision of the airways through the bronchoscope. Traditionally, fluoroscopy has been used for guiding transbronchial biopsies. CT scanning, which allows more precise localization, may be used although it is cumbersome. EBUS is discussed above. Most recently, a navigational system has been developed that uses previously acquired CT images coupled with an electromagnetic field around the patient's chest to localize an endoscopic tool with a microsensor. Preliminary studies have suggested that, although time intensive, this technology may improve accuracy in biopsy of peripheral lung lesions.

Autofluorescence Bronchoscopy

Autofluorescence bronchoscopy was developed to differentiate normal from malignant tissue. This technique uses a blue light for illumination. Images are captured and manipulated in a way that normal tissue appears green and abnormal tissue appears reddish brown. Abnormal tissue that is discovered can be biopsied during autofluorescence inspection or under white light. It is proposed that this technique can increase the yield of fiberoptic bronchoscopy for the detection of dysplasia, carcinoma in situ, and early invasive cancers.

Bronchial Thermoplasty

Bronchial thermoplasty uses a catheter that can be delivered through a flexible bronchoscope to coagulate bronchial tissue using controlled therapeutic radiofrequency. It is suggested that this can reduce the amount of airways smooth muscle and may benefit selected patients with asthma.

ADDITIONAL TOPICS

Pediatric Bronchoscopy

Bronchoscopy is a critical skill for evaluation and treatment of airway disorders in children. It has saved the lives of many children who aspirated foreign bodies (Figure 10). Pediatric rigid bronchoscopes with rod–lens telescopes have been available since the early 1970s and have made a large improvement in ability to examine the small airways in children. The smallest rigid bronchoscope available (Karl Storz, size 2.5 mm about 3.3 mm outer diameter) will fit nearly all premature newborns, and the smallest flexible fiberoptic laryngoscope or bronchoscope is 2 mm diameter. This is useful for examination of the airway of an intubated infant with a 3.0 or 3.5 mm inner diameter endotracheal tube. Common indications for bronchoscopy in children include congenital stridor, postextubation stridor, cough, hemoptysis, suspected foreign body aspiration, difficult pneumonia, and aspiration of retained

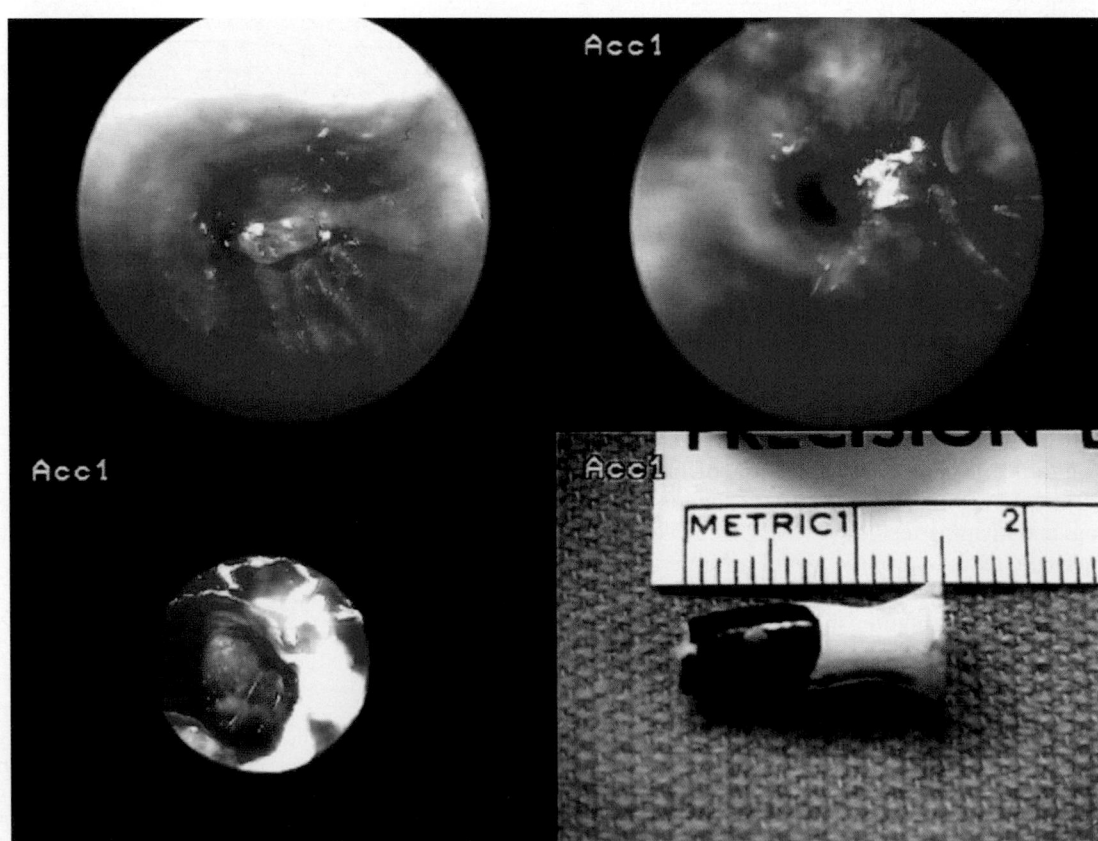

Figure 10 Aspirated broken wooden golf tee removed from the airway of a 20-month-old child.

secretions. Regarding anesthesia techniques for bronchoscopy in children, changes have occurred. In 1950, Jackson and Jackson reported, "In infants and young children we use no anesthetic, general or local."[35] Due to advances in pediatric anesthesia since the 1970s, rigid bronchoscopy at children's hospitals is now always done with general anesthesia. Rapid acting inhalational anesthetics are employed that create a deep plane of anesthesia with the child breathing spontaneously.

Training and Teaching Bronchoscopy

Bronchoscopy is mainly practiced by pulmonologists, otolaryngologists, thoracic surgeons, and anesthesiologists. In the last group, bronchoscopy skills are learned exclusively to perform fiberoptic intubation or confirm endotracheal tube placement. The other specialists learn bronchoscopy to manage the variety of medical conditions discussed in this chapter. It is important to have systematized training in bronchoscopy as part of the residency educational curriculum. This includes didactic lectures, practice on nonhuman models and simulators[36] and animal laboratories. Bronchoscopy on dogs was used by Chevalier Jackson to teach for many years. Video technology now greatly facilitates teaching because the student and teacher can observe the examination together. In fiberoptic bronchoscopy, clinical training on patients who are intubated may start first, then move to sedation and bronchoscopy of unintubated patients. Rigid bronchoscopy in the operating room is learned on both pediatric and adult patients. Through residency training, experience in the variety of disease processes assessed by bronchoscopy is essential to gaining familiarity with managing patients. A survey of pulmonologists found that over 60% responded that over 50 bronchoscopies in training are needed to become competent in flexible bronchoscopy.[24] For otolaryngology residents, additional training in bronchoscopy is also available in fellowships in surgical head and neck oncology, laryngology, and pediatric otolaryngology. For pulmonologists who desire skills beyond diagnostic flexible bronchoscopy, additional training in interventional pulmonary medicine is available at a few centers in the United States.

REFERENCES

1. Heffner DK. Diseases of the trachea. In: Barnes L, editor. Surgical Pathology of the Head and Neck, Volume 1. New York: Dekker; 1985. p. 437–531.
2. Broughton WA, Middleton RM, Kirkpatrick MB, Bass JB. Bronchoscopic protected specimen brush and bronchoalveolar lavage in the diagnosis of bacterial pneumonia. Infect Dis Clin North Am 1991;5:437–52.
3. Stanford W, Galvin JR. The diagnosis of bronchiectasis. Clin Chest Med 1988;9:691–9.
4. Powell DA, Hunt WG. Tuberculosis in children: An update. Adv Pediatr 2006;53:279–322.
5. Bourke SJ. Interstitial lung disease: Progress and problems. Postgrad Med J 2006;82:494–9.
6. Cox CE, Davis-Allen A, Judson MA. Sarcoidosis. Med Clin North Am 2005;89:817–28.
7. Fauroux B, Clement A. Paediatric sarcoidosis. Paediatr Respir Rev 2005;6:128–33.
8. King TE, Costabel U, Cordier J, et al. Idiopathic pulmonary fibrosis: Diagnosis and treatment. International consensus statement. Am J Respir Crit Care Med 2000;161:646–64.
9. Herrington HC, Weber SM, Andersen PE. Modern management of laryngotracheal stenosis. Laryngoscope 2006;116:1553–7.
10. Daum TE, Specks U, Colby TV, et al. Tracheobronchial involvement in Wegener's granulomatosis. Am J Respir Crit Car Med 1995;151:522–6.
11. Prince JS, Duhamel DR, Levin DL, et al. Nonneoplastic lesions of the tracheobronchial wall: Radiologic findings with bronchoscopic correlation. Radiographics 2002;22:S215–30.
12. Strauss GM, Rathore R. Lung cancer. In: Crapo JD, Glassroth JL, Karlinsky JB, King TE, editors. Baum's Textbook of Pulmonary Diseases, 7th edition. Philadelphia: Lippincott Williams & Wilkins; 2004, p. 787–858.
13. Kruklitis RJ, Vachani A, Morgolis ML. Solitary pulmonary nodule and lung tumors other than bronchogenic carcinoma. In: Crapo JD, Glassroth JL, Karlinsky JB, King TE, editors. Baum's Textbook of Pulmonary Diseases, 7th edition. Philadelphia: Lippincott Williams & Wilkins; 2004, p. 859–82.
14. Grillo HC, Donahue DM. Postintubation tracheal stenosis. Semin Thorac Cardiovasc Surg 1996;8:370–80.
15. Paul S, Bueno R. The burned trachea. Chest Surg Clin N Am 2003;13:343–8.
16. Saffle JR. What's new in general surgery: Burns and metabolism. J Am Coll Surg 2003;196:267–89.
17. Desai MH, Mlcak R, Richardson J, et al. Reduction in mortality in pediatric patients with inhalation injury with aerosolized heparin/N-acetylcystine therapy. J Burn Care Rehabil 1998;19:210–2.
18. Becker HD, Marsh BR. History of the rigid bronchoscope. In: Bolliger CT, Mathur PN, editors. Interventional Bronchoscopy. Progress in Respiratory Research, Volume 30. Basel: Karger; 2000. p. 22–30.
19. Boyd AD. Chevalier Jackson: The father of American bronchoesophagology. Ann Thorac Surg 1994;57:502–5.
20. Ossoff RH, Duncavage JA, Dere H. Microsubglottoscopy: An expansion of operative microlaryngoscopy. Otolaryngol Head Neck Surg 1991;104:842–8.
21. Grissom CK, Albertine KH, Elstad MR. Alveolar haemorrhage in a case of high altitude pulmonary oedema. Thorax 2000;55:167–9.
22. British Thoracic Society guidelines on diagnostic flexible-bronchoscopy. Thorax 2001;56:i1–21.
23. Hogikyan ND. Transnasal endoscopic examination of the subglottis and trachea using topical anesthesia in the otolaryngology clinic. Laryngoscope 1999;109:1170–3.
24. Prakash UB, Offord KP, Stubbs SE. Bronchoscopy in North America: The ACCP survey. Chest 1991;100:1668–75.
25. Ernst A, Silvestri GA, Johnstone D, et al. Interventional pulmonary procedures: Guidelines from the American College of Chest Physicians. Chest 2003;123:1693–717.
26. Shapshay SM, Valdez TA. Bronchoscopic management of benign stenosis. Chest Surg Clin N Am 2001;11:749–68.
27. Dumon JF. A dedicated tracheobronchial stent. Chest 1990;97:328–32.
28. Kurrus JA, Gray SD, Elstad MR. Use of silicone stents in the management of subglottic stenosis. Laryngoscope 1997;107:1553–8.
29. Eller RL, Livingston WJ, III, Morgan CE, et al. Expandable tracheal stenting for benign disease: Worth the complications? Ann Otol Rhinol Laryngol 2006;115:247–52.
30. Lunn W, Feller-Kopman D, Wahidi M, et al. Endoscopic removal of metallic airway stents. Chest 2005;127: 2106–12.
31. FDA public health notification: Complications from metallic tracheal stents in patients with benign airway disorders. Issued: July 29, 2005, http://www.fda.gov/cdrh/safety/072905-tracheal.html.
32. Kurrus JA, Hayes JK, Hoidal JR, et al. Radiation therapy for tracheobronchial amyloidosis. Chest 1998;114:1489–92.
33. Ernst A, Feller-Kopman D, Becker HD, Mehta AC. Central airway obstruction. Am J Respir Crit Care Med 2004;169:1278–97.
34. Wood DE, McKenna RJ, Jr, Yusen RD, et al. A multicenter trial of an intrabronchial valve for treatment of severe emphysema. J Thorac Cardiovasc Surg 2007;133:65–73.
35. Jackson C, Jackson CL. Bronchoesophagology. Philadelphia: WB Saunders; 1950. p. 59.
36. Ost D, De Rosiers A, Britt EJ, et al. Assessment of a bronchoscopy simulator. Am J Respir Crit Care 2001;164:2248–55.

SUGGESTED READING

Willems LNA. Pulmonary Interventional Medicine. Lung Biology in Health and Disease, Volume 189. Beamis JF, Mathur P, Mehta AC, editors. New York: Marcel Dekker; 2004. p. 689.

85

Esophagology

Gregory N. Postma, MD,

Melanie W. Seybt, MD,

Catherine J. Rees, MD

Esophagology is the study of the normal anatomy and physiology of the esophagus as well as the diseases and disorders that arise or involve the esophagus. In particular, congenital anomalies, infectious and inflammatory processes, disorders of motility, systemic diseases affecting the esophagus, trauma and neoplasms of the esophagus and treatment of patients with these processes are the central focus of esophagology. The field has been revolutionized by the development of rigid and flexible esophagoscopes and highly informative imaging permitting a wide array of diagnostic and therapeutic options.

ANATOMY

The esophagus is a conduit between the pharynx and the stomach. Measuring approximately 25 centimeters long, it is continuous with the pharynx at the level of the sixth cervical vertebra and passes through the diaphragm at the level of the tenth thoracic vertebra. It has been subdivided into three portions: the cervical, thoracic and abdominal. The cervical portion extends from the cricopharyngeus to the suprasternal notch. The thoracic portion extends from the suprasternal notch to the diaphragm, and the abdominal portion continues to the gastric cardia.

Histologically, the esophagus has four concentric layers. The innermost layer is the mucosa, and the mucosa changes from squamous cell epithelium to columnar cell epithelium at the gastroesophageal junction (GEJ). This junction has been termed the 'Z line' or squamocolumnar junction (SCJ). The second layer, the submucosa, surrounds the mucosa. The third layer is muscular and is divided into two portions, with the inner muscular fibers arranged in a circular fashion and the outer fibers oriented longitudinally. The proximal one-third of the esophagus consists primarily of striated muscle. Smooth muscle predominates in the distal portion, and there is a transition zone of both striated and smooth muscle at approximately the level of the aortic arch. The adventitial layer is the fourth and outermost layer. Unlike the remainder of the gastrointestinal tract, no serosa layer is present in the esophagus.

The upper esophageal sphincter (UES) is more aptly described as the pharyngoesophageal segment (PES). This 2 to 4 cm high pressure zone consists of the cricopharyngeus muscle, the inferior pharyngeal constrictor muscle, and the proximal striated muscle of the upper cervical esophagus. The cricopharyngeus is tonically contracted at rest and is innervated by branches of the vagus nerve. The sling-shaped muscle attaches bilaterally to the cricoid lamina. During swallowing, the cricopharyngeus muscle relaxes and is pulled open by the anterior and superior motion of the larynx and hyoid bone. Aside from allowing passage of food and liquid into the esophagus during deglutition, the cricopharyngeus also plays a role in eructation and preventing refluxate from entering the pharynx.

The lower esophageal sphincter (LES) is an anatomic and physiologic high pressure zone between the esophageal body and the stomach. It is made of up of circular and oblique muscle fibers that are contiguous with the circular muscle of the esophagus. The diaphragm also contributes to this high pressure zone. The LES relaxes during swallowing to allow passage of the bolus from the esophagus into the stomach. The SCJ is normally located at the same level as the gastroesophageal junction (GEJ), which is best identified by the termination of the gastric rugae in the esophagus and the point where the linear blood vessels of the esophagus end. When more than two centimeters of gastric rugae is present proximal to the level of the diaphragm (observed by a constriction of the lumen during a sniff maneuver on endoscopy), a sliding hiatal hernia is present. Sliding hiatal hernias are commonly observed in adults undergoing barium esophogram and increase the risk of gastroesophageal reflux. The much less common, and more serious, paraesophageal hernia occurs when part of the stomach herniates into the thorax along side the esophagus, but the gastric cardia remains in the native position.

There are three areas of constriction in the normal esophagus that can be visualized on fluoroscopy and endoscopy. The level of the cricopharyngeus is the narrowest portion of the esophagus, located at approximately the sixth cervical vertebra. The second narrowing is approximately 25 cm from the incisors where the aortic arch and left bronchus cross the esophagus. This area along the UES and the LES are three natural esophageal constrictions and are the most common sites of foreign body impaction.

Lymphatic drainage of the esophagus contains little barrier to spread. The lymphatic drainage of the upper third is to the deep cervical lymph nodes, the middle third is to the superior and posterior mediastinal lymph nodes, and the lower third to lymph nodes along the left gastric vessels and celiac artery. However, the esophageal lymphatics are all densely interconnected. Esophageal carcinoma can spread throughout the length of the esophagus via the lymphatics and may have lymph nodal involvement several centimeters away from the primary lesion.

ESOPHAGOSCOPY

The ability to visualize the esophagus was pioneered by laryngologists such as Chevalier Jackson who described the use of rigid esophagoscopy for examination, dilation, removal of foreign bodies, and biopsy. Fiberoptic lighting systems were later added to improve visualization. The next major advance was the development of flexible endoscopy by Hirschowitz et al in 1958.[1] Today, flexible esophagoscopy is usually performed by gastroenterologists and requires patient sedation. First reported by Herrmann and Recio in 1997, transnasal esophagoscopy (TNE) has emerged as a new technology available for unsedated esophagoscopy.[2] In 1994, Reza Shaker, a gastroenterologist, published the first report of an unsedated transnasal esophagogastroduodenoscopy (EGD).[3] Although initially met with little enthusiasm by the gastroenterology community, interest continued to grow among otolaryngologists. The use of TNE in North America became popular after the publication of Aviv et al's work in 2001.[4]

Rigid Esophagoscopy

Rigid esophagoscopy is often used by otolaryngologists for foreign body removal and dilation and as part of head and neck cancer staging. Rigid esophagoscopy is superior in the evaluation of the postcricoid region and cervical esophagus, where insufflation is difficult to achieve for flexible esophagoscopy, whereas flexible esophagoscopy is best for visualizing the distal esophagus and GEJ. Although rigid esophagoscopy can be performed with topical anesthesia and conscious sedation, most surgeons use general anesthesia in the modern era.

In the supine position, the neck should be kept in the neutral position, and the maxillary teeth and gums should be protected. The rigid esophagoscope is typically held in the left hand between the thumb and index finger. The remaining fingers of the left hand are used to control the mouth and prevent resting of the endoscope on the teeth. Following the palate, uvula, and posterior pharyngeal wall, the endoscope is passed through the mouth to the postcricoid region. The endoscope is held at approximately a 90-degree angle to the long axis of the patient, and the angulation is changed so that the endscope is roughly parallel to the esophagus by the time the tip reaches the postcricoid region. The larynx is lifted anteriorly to expose the inlet of the esophagus and the posterior bulge formed by the cricopharyngeus muscle. The right (dominant) hand is used only for changing the angle of the endoscope and should not be used to advance the endoscope. The endoscope should be advanced only with the left thumb and index finger to prevent excessive pressure. The esophagoscope is advanced only when the lumen is clearly visualized to decrease the risk of perforation. The endoscope is passed gently to the GEJ, and the esophagus is completely examined as the endoscope is withdrawn, taking care to examine the entire circumference of the esophagus along its whole length. This examination is best performed with the aid of a rigid telescope through the esophagoscope. Biopsies, if necessary, should be performed after the entire esophagus has been examined.

Transnasal Esophagoscopy

The introduction of distal chip and high-quality fiberoptic esophagoscopes now allows the esophagus to be easily examined in the office using only topical anesthesia, and this has produced a major change in otolaryngologic practice. Advances in optics as well as the placement of a working channel in a thin endoscope have given endoscopists the ability to examine the entire esophagus, larynx and trachea in unsedated patients using the technique of TNE. A working channel in the endoscope allows for biopsies, either cup or brush, as well as laser use.[5,6]

Esophageal indications for TNE include dysphagia, recalcitrant reflux symptoms, odynophagia, screening for Barrett esophagus (BE), and long standing reflux disease. Extraesophageal indications are somewhat controversial but in our practice include globus pharyngeus, chronic cough, cervical dysphagia, head and neck cancer, asthma and moderate to severe laryngopharyngeal reflux (LPR).

TNE is a safe, well tolerated, and easily learned procedure. In the largest consecutive series published, Postma et al reported that the unsedated examination was well tolerated and that abnormal findings were present in over 50% of the patients.[7] The patient population for this series consisted of patients with extraesophageal

reflux symptoms, not gastroesophageal reflux disease (GERD) or "heartburn." Complications in these 700 patients included six cases of self-limited epistaxis and two vagovagal episodes. Additional studies, such as those of Andrus et al, confirmed that TNE is a safe and effective tool for patient evaluation.[8] Wilkins and Gillies reported that 95% of patients tolerated examination with an ultra thin endoscope introduced transorally through an appliance.[9] No case of esophageal perforation has been reported with TNE.[10]

A complete TNE involves examination of the entire length of the esophagus. This includes a retroflexed view of the GEJ and gastric cardia. The question of whether a full EGD should be performed has been addressed by a study conducted by Wildi et al.[11] In their report, when patients were classified by symptoms, patients without daily abdominal pain, nausea, or a history of gastric or duodenal ulcer were unlikely to have major pathology of the stomach or duodenum. They concluded that esophagoscopy was sufficient for use in the patient without those complaints.

To visualize the entire esophagus, the transnasal esophagoscope should be of sufficient length to allow for a retroflexed view of the GEJ and the gastric cardia (at least 60 cm). The diameter should be small enough to allow for easy placement through the nasal cavity. Channels for air insufflation, suction and working, i.e., for the passage of biopsy instruments, are also standard parts of the transnasal esophagoscope or sheath.

When possible, the patient should not eat or drink for three hours before the procedure; however, a recent meal is not a contraindication to TNE. Adequate nasal anesthesia and decongestion are vital to performing the procedure successfully. The patient is sitting upright across from the endoscopist. The patient's more patent nasal cavity is first sprayed with 1:1 oxymetazoline (0.05%) and lidocaine (4%) and is gently packed with a cotton pledget soaked in the same mixture.[7] Two sprays of 20% benzocaine (Hurricane) are occasionally administered to the oropharynx. The transnasal esophagoscope (VE-1530, Pentax Precision Instrument Corporation, Orangeburg, New York) is lubricated and introduced into the naris. The transnasal esophagoscope is passed along the floor of the nose or between the middle and inferior turbinates. Next, the head is slightly flexed toward the chest as the endoscope is passed toward the cricopharyngeus muscle. The patient is asked to swallow, and the endoscope is gently advanced into the esophagus. Gentle suctioning and air insufflation are used as needed, and the instrument is advanced only when the lumen is visualized.

The instrument is advanced into the distal esophagus for a view of the GEJ and SCJ, or Z-line (Figure 1). Close examination of this area may detect esophageal lesions such as BE or adenocarcinoma. The endoscope is advanced and retroflexed to view the gastric cardia. Using air insufflation and irrigation, the mucosa of the entire esophagus is examined while the transnasal esophagoscope is withdrawn. When mucosal

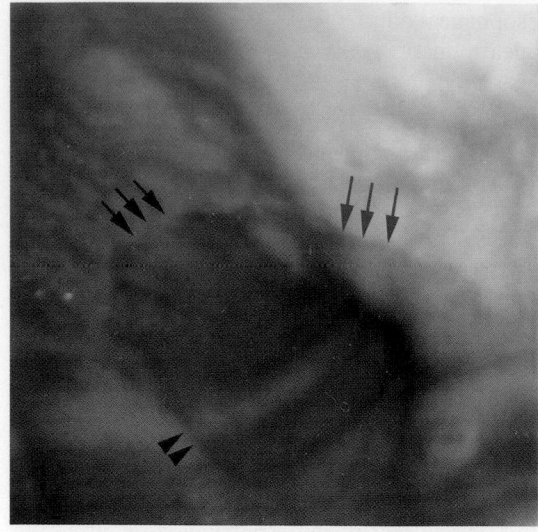

Figure 1 Normal squamocolumnar junction (blue arrows). The termination of the linear esophageal mucosal vessels from above (black arrows) and the gastric rugae from below (black arrowheads) delineate the gastroesophageal junction.

lesions or irregularities are appreciated, biopsy forceps are passed through the working channel, and multiple biopsies under direct vision are obtained.

TNE has been demonstrated to be equal to "conventional" sedated esophagoscopy with regard to diagnostic sensitivity and specificity and equal or superior in patient tolerance and preference. In a randomized cross-over study by Jobe et al, 121 patients underwent office-based TNE and traditional sedated esophagoscopy, comparing the histological detection of BE, dysplasia, and biopsy size.[12] Both procedures accurately detected Barrett metaplasia and dysplasia; however, over 70% of patients in the study reported a preference for the unsedated TNE over conventional endoscopy for future surveillance. While there was significantly more minor anxiety and discomfort associated with unsedated TNE, there was no difference in overall self-rated patient tolerability between the two modalities. In a prospective trial by Thota et al comparing sedated versus unsedated esophagoscopy, patients were randomized to either unsedated transnasal or transoral esophagoscopy prior to a second sedated transoral esophagoscopy.[13] Results of this study indicate that the transnasal approach was better tolerated (initial discomfort and choking sensation) except with respect to pain. Additionally, 93% of the transnasal and 91% of the transoral patients were willing to have the unsedated procedure again. The diagnostic accuracy of the unsedated approaches with a smaller endoscope was equivalent to those of the standard larger endoscope, which required sedation. In addition, new brush biopsy methodology may represent an improved technique to increase diagnostic accuracy,[14] but further trials are needed.

Transnasal Esophagoscopy Procedures

In addition to diagnostic visualization, procedures that can be performed with the transnasal esophagoscope include biopsy, laser use, esophageal dilation, and secondary tracheoesophageal puncture (TEP). The placement of a wireless pH telemetry capsule with unsedated TNE has also been reported by Belafsky et al.[15]

Patients with malignancies of the head and neck often have comorbidities that make panendoscopy under general anesthesia a high risk activity. An unsedated TNE and biopsy alleviates these concerns. In a prospective study, patients underwent a TNE with biopsy followed by a standard panendoscopy under general anesthesia. Findings were congruent between the two modalities.[16] This suggests that in selected patients panendoscopy can be performed in the clinic, thereby avoiding the time, risks and costs of the procedure under general anesthesia.

Traditional methods of evaluating dysphagia have included barium esophagram and modified barium swallow. While these diagnostic modalities may allow for the detection of strictures, they do not provide a description of the epithelium of the esophagus and can be a source of aspiration in patients with impaired swallowing function. Esophagoscopy can detect areas of narrowing as well as provide direct mucosa evaluation. With unsedated TNE, the peristaltic wave of a swallow can be followed by having the patient ingest an item such as a Tylenol capsule and follow its path through the esophagus. This can provide a rough estimate of esophageal motility.

When strictures are detected, it is possible to treat selected patients with use of unsedated TNE. After standard TNE anesthesia, the patient swallows 4% viscous lidocaine. A guide wire can then be positioned just in front of the endoscope and advanced to the stricture. After the transnasal esophagoscope is advanced to or past the stricture under direct visualization, the guide wire is placed through the stricture. Alternatively, the guidewire can be passed through the working channel of the esophagoscope. The endoscope is removed over the guidewire and reintroduced alongside it through the nose. A concentric radial expansion balloon is placed over the guidewire, and the stricture is dilated, using the transnasal esophagoscope for visualization throughout the entire procedure.[17]

For postlaryngectomy patients, it is usually appropriate to place a TEP in an unsedated. A catheter or the prosthesis itself can be inserted at this time. In addition, air insufflation may be useful to insert a dislodged or difficult-to-replace TEP device.[18]

Tissue excision or ablation can be accomplished with use of the transnasal esophagoscope scope by placing a laser through the working channel. Lasers such as the pulsed dye laser, KTP, thulium, or gold laser have been used to remove lesions such as recurrent respiratory papillomas, granulomas and recurrent leukoplakia in the office without sedation. Patient tolerance of this unsedated procedure has been reported to be high.[19]

Complications of Esophagoscopy

The most serious complication of both rigid and flexible esophagoscopy is esophageal perforation.

Perforation is higher with rigid esophagoscopy and most often occurs in the setting of esophageal carcinoma or during procedures such as dilation. The importance of gentle technique and refraining from forcing the endoscope past a stricture or lesion cannot be over-emphasized. Bleeding in the esophageal lumen should alert the surgeon to the possibility of perforation. In the event of a possible perforation, the procedure should be aborted and broad-spectrum antibiotics should be initiated. If possible, a nasogastric tube or small feeding tube can be placed under direct visualization. The patient is awakened from general anesthesia and monitored for signs of perforation, including subcutaneous emphysema, fever, tachycardia, and chest pain. Chest x-ray should be performed. When the patient is able, a gastrograffin esophagram is obtained to evaluate for perforation. Small proximal esophageal injuries can be treated with nasogastric tube, antibiotics, and nothing to eat or drink by mouth. Large injuries in the cervical esophagus should be repaired surgically.[20] Thoracic esophageal injuries require assessment and intervention by a thoracic surgeon. Some authors have recommended more conservative treatment of esophageal perforation with computed tomography-guided drainage of leaks and control of sepsis.[21]

More common complications of esophagoscopy include aspiration and injuries to teeth or the mucosa of the oral cavity and pharynx. Aspiration may occur during rigid esophagoscopy, especially with severe esophageal phase dysphagia or an obstructing foreign body. Standard anesthesia practices to limit aspiration risk, such as rapid sequence induction, should be considered in these cases. During rigid esophagoscopy, injuries to teeth and lacerations of the tongue or pharynx can result from improper technique.

During TNE, epistaxis is a rare and usually self-limited complication. Treatment of epistaxis with nasal packing or cautery is almost never necessary, and the bleeding usually resolves with topical oxymetazoline and nasal pressure. As with unsedated flexible laryngoscopy, vagovagal episodes can also occur during TNE.

CINEFLUOROSCOPIC EVALUATION OF THE ESOPHAGUS

The most useful radiologic examination of the esophagus is the contrast esophagram using cinefluoroscopy. This differs from the standard "modified barium swallow" in that the oropharyngeal phase of deglutition is not completely evaluated. The esophagram provides a more detailed evaluation of the esophagus than the full upper gastrointestinal series. Barium is usually used for videofluoroscopic examination, although in the setting of suspected esophageal perforation or pharyngocutaneous fistula, gastrograffin is preferred because it is water-soluble. When aspiration is strongly suspected, barium is preferred over gastrograffin.

The first phase of the esophagram is perormed with the patient standing in the anterior-posterior

view. A single large bolus of barium is ingested, and it is followed from the mouth to the stomach. The single swallow is useful to assess esophageal motility, since rapid repetitive swallowing inhibits peristalsis. Primary peristalsis is triggered by the swallow, and normal secondary peristalsis occurs in response to distal esophageal reflux or residual bolus. Tertiary contractions are non-peristaltic abnormal contractions commonly seen in the elderly population and in the presence of dysmotility. After the initial swallow, the patient is asked to ingest barium rapidly through a drinking straw. This maneuver is performed to dilate the esophagus and aids in evaluation of strictures, webs, rings, or hiatal hernia. Mucosal relief films, with the esophagus slightly collapsed, may help to identify mucosal lesions, such as esophagitis or carcinoma. A 13 mm barium tablet or marshmallow can be used to identify levels of obstruction, since this is the amount of esophageal lumen narrowing usually required to produce dysphagia. The esophagram is repeated in a right-anterior-oblique position (simulating a prone position) to negate the effects of gravity on bolus transit. Finally, many clinicians place the patient in the supine position and proceed with rapid water drinking and maneuvers to increase intrabdominal pressure, such as a leg lift. This "water siphon" test increases the esophagram's sensitivity for detecting reflux. However, even with this maneuver, the esophagram is neither sensitive nor specific for diagnosing GERD.

CONGENITAL ANOMALIES OF THE ESOPHAGUS

The most common congenital anomalies of the esophagus are esophageal atresia and tracheoesophageal fistula (TEF). Esophageal atresia occurs in 1 in 3000 to 5000 births. Other less common congenital lesions include stenosis, duplications and cysts.[22]

Esophageal atresia and TEF often occur together. The most common situation (over 80%) is distal TEF and proximal esophageal atresia. Atresia with no TEF is the next most common variant. TEF without atresia (H-type) is the most common of the remaining types and may have subtle symptoms, presenting later in childhood. Symptoms include respiratory distress, regurgitation, aspiration and drooling and frequently present early in life. More than half of infants with esophageal atresia have serious comorbid defects such as cardiac anomalies. Prompt surgical repair is indicated for esophageal atresia and TEF.

Congenital esophageal muscosal webs or muscular hypertrophy can cause symptomatic narrowing of the esophagus. Esophageal duplications can take many forms and may present as a neck mass or dysphagia. *Dysphagia lusoria* is induced by vascular anomalies involving the aortic root. Complete vascular rings encircling the esophagus include double aortic arch and variants caused by a right aortic arch and left ligamentum arteriosum and/or left subclavian artery. Incomplete rings include a retroesophageal aberrant right subclavian artery (i.e., *arteria lusoria*) and abnormal left pulmonary artery. These vascular anomalies may be seen on fluoroscopy and endoscopy, and arteriography or computed tomography confirm the diagnosis.

ESOPHAGITIS

Esophagitis may cause heartburn, dysphagia and/or odynophagia, or it may be incidentally noted on esophagoscopy. The many causes of esophagitis include gastroesophageal reflux, foreign bodies (e.g., pills), infection, allergy, caustic injury, and radiation therapy.

Infectious Esophagitis

Infectious esophagitis is most commonly caused by *Candida albicans*. While frequently seen in immunocompromised patients (e.g., human immunodeficiency virus infection, diabetes mellitus, and corticosteroid use), candidal esophagitis may also occur in immunocompetent individuals. The appearance is characterized by yellowish punctuate mucosal plaques, which may coalesce as the infection progresses (Figure 2). The diagnosis is confirmed by endoscopic biopsy, and treatment includes topical and systemic antifungal agents.

Viral esophagitis is most commonly due to herpes virus and cytomegalovirus. Endoscopy reveals multiple, shallow ulcerations, sometimes forming a large series of ulcers. Human immunodeficiency virus may also cause an ulcerative esophagitis. Diagnosis is made with biopsy of the ulcers, preferably at the rim and the central portion.

Pill-Induced Esophagitis

Pill-induced esophagitis is caused by prolonged contact of the esophageal mucosa with medication resulting in inflammation and ulceration of the epithelium. This may occur in patients with normal esophageal motility.[23] The cause of the esophageal injury may be due to direct caustic effects, alteration of esophageal pH, accumulation

of toxic levels of drugs within the esophagus, or induction of reflux.[24] The most common "offenders" are doxycycline, tetracycline, clindamycin, ascorbic acid, quinidine, potassium chloride, and alendronate.

Eosinophilic Esophagitis

Eosinophilic esophagitis is an uncommon disorder being recognized more frequently. This probable allergic disorder is most commonly seen in children but is now being recognized more frequently in adults. Adults usually present with chronic dysphagia for solids, food impaction, strictures, or refractory gastroesophageal reflux symptoms.[25] Endoscopic findings include single or multiple "rings" or corrugations (esophageal trachealization), a thin esophagus, proximal esophageal stenosis, and small white vesicles or exudate resembling candida esophagitis. The diagnosis is confirmed by biopsy demonstrating > 20 eosinophils per high-powered field. Treatment options include topical corticosteroids (such as fluticasone spray ingested orally) and other antiallergy medications, such as montelukast. The esophageal mucosa may be exquisitely friable in eosinophilic esophagitis. Even during careful endoscopy, superficial lacerations are common, so dilation should be approached with caution.

Reflux Esophagitis

Reflux esophagitis is caused by abnormal exposure of the esophageal mucosa to gastric and/or duodenal contents. The exact mechanism of gastroesophageal reflux has not been thoroughly elucidated, but it is likely related to transient relaxations of the LES allowing passage of gastric contents into the esophagus. Symptoms of reflux esophagitis include pyrosis and dysphagia, although it may be asymptomatic. It is characterized by areas of mucosal slough or erythema which are well demarcated from adjacent normal mucosa and termed mucosal breaks. Chronic esophageal reflux may result in development of mucosal bridges secondary to repeated episodes of inflammation and healing, leading to scar formation and possible strictures. Signs of reflux esophagitis may be noted on cinefluoroscopy. Other tests, such as ambulatory pH monitoring, are useful for diagnosing GERD, but the presence of esophagitis can only be confirmed with endoscopy. Numerous classification systems based on the severity of endoscopic findings have been developed. The Los Angeles classification based on the number and size of mucosal breaks is currently the most generally accepted system.[26]

Nonerosive GERD may be treated with behavioral modifications, antacids, and H2-receptor blockers such as ranitidine. Erosive esophagitis is usually treated with a once-daily proton pump inhibitors in addition to behavioral modifications. Endoscopy is rarely indicated in routine esophagitis promptly responding to therapy. However, it is the practice of many clinicians to confirm the

resolution of esophagitis with endoscopy after appropriate treatment if symptom resolution is slow, incomplete or if symptoms have been present for more than three to five years. Endoscopy after treatment of esophagitis is also useful to evaluate for BE, which may not be apparent in untreated esophageal inflammation.

Barrett Esophagus

BE is the metaplastic replacement of squamous cell epithelium of the esophagus with specialized columnar cell intestinal epithelium that extends proximal to the GEJ. This condition predisposes to esophageal adenocarcinoma, which has one of the fastest growing malignancy rates in the United States and England. Endoscopic findings of BE include finger like projections or islands of salmon-pink mucosa that extend beyond the squamocolumnar transition of the GEJ (Figure 3). The diagnosis can only be made with biopsy, which will show intestinal metaplasia with goblet cells. Biopsies are also important to evaluate for dysplasia. Low-grade dysplasia should be followed closely and does not greatly increase the risk of malignancy over nondysplastic BE. However, high-grade dysplasia is typically treated as esophageal adenocarcinoma. Currently, experts in BE disagree about how frequently the esophagus should be screened for high-grade dysplasia and adenocarcinoma in patients with biopsy-proven BE or low-grade dysplasia.

STRICTURES, WEBS AND RINGS

Narrowing of the esophageal lumen becomes symptomatic when the normal 20 mm lumen is reduced to about 13 mm. Narrowing of the lumen is evaluated with cinefluoroscopy (including a 13 mm barium tablet or marshmallow) and endoscopy. Strictures may result from peptic injury in the distal esophagus, postradiation injury, or caustic ingestion. Less common causes include prior esophageal trauma. Treatment is serial dilation with bougie, balloon, or Savary dilators. The most

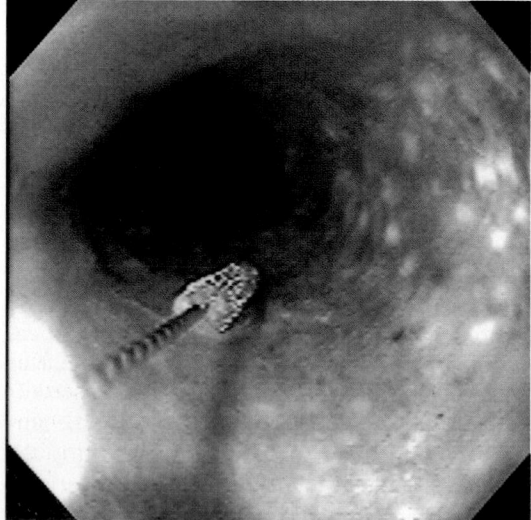

Figure 2 Candida esophagitis. There are isolated yellow, tan plaques on the esophageal mucosa.

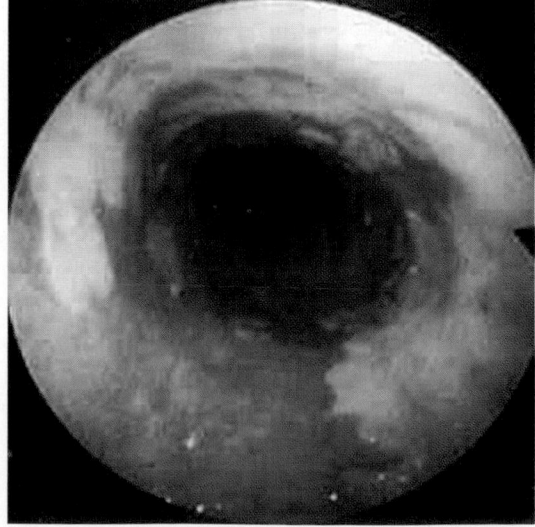

Figure 3 Barrett esophagus. Note the area of columnar cell epithelium extending into squamous cell epithelium.

dreaded complication of dilation is esophageal perforation, and the safety of the procedure may be improved by using a soft flexible guidewire.

Esophageal webs are thin bands consisting of squamous cell mucosa. Webs may be congenital, idiopathic, or associated with diverticula. These can often be treated successfully with a single dilation. A common type of cervical esophageal web is associated with iron deficiency anemia in Scandinavian women and is termed Plummer-Vinson or Paterson-Kelly syndrome.

There are two major types of esophageal rings: A and B. The A-ring is a muscular hypertrophy occurring at the most proximal aspect of the LES. A-rings are frequently incidental findings. Dilation is not likely to improve symptomatic A-rings, and treatment often entails endoscopic botulinum toxin injection. B-rings, or Schatzki rings, occur at the SCJ and are typically associated with a hiatal hernia and gastroesophageal reflux. The proximal aspect is lined with squamous cell epithelium, and the distal aspect is composed of columnar cell epithelium. Schatzki ring can be treated with endoscopic dilation and frequently recur.

ESOPHAGEAL DIVERTICULA

Esophageal diverticula, or outpouchings of the lumen, include pharyngoesophageal (Zenker) diverticulum, midesophageal diverticulum, and epiphrenic diverticulum. Many esophageal diverticula are asymptomatic; the most common presenting symptoms are dysphagia and regurgitation. The diagnosis of esophageal diverticulum is most readily made with cinefluoroscopy.

Midesophageal diverticula are found in the middle third of the esophagus and are likely caused by traction from mediastinal disease or scarring, such as tuberculosis. These are usually asymptomatic and do not require treatment. Epiphrenic, or distal esophageal, diverticula cause large volume regurgitation and dysphagia, when symptomatic. They are pulsion diverticula strongly associated with esophageal motility disorders. If symptomatic, they are treated with surgery directed at both the diverticulum and the underlying motility disorder.

Zenker diverticulum is the most commonly encountered esophageal diverticulum and is the most likely to be symptomatic. The outpouching occurs between the inferior pharyngeal constrictor muscle and the cricopharyngeus, in an area called Killian dehiscence. This pulsion diverticulum likely results from cricopharyngeal dysfunction and is frequently associated with gastroesophageal reflux and esophageal motility disorders.[27] Spontaneous regurgitation of undigested food is the most common symptom, although a Zenker diverticulum may also present with dysphagia, aspiration, cough, halitosis, or weight loss. Zenker diverticula are much more common in the elderly population. Rarely, they are associated with carcinoma of the esophagus or fistula formation.

Zenker diverticula frequently require treatment. Small diverticula may be treated with open or endoscopic cricopharyngeal myotomy alone. Classic surgical therapy is open diverticulectomy with cricopharyngeal myotomy. A left lateral cervical approach is used to expose the diverticulum, which can be excised with the aid of a stapling device or using excision and meticulous closure of the resulting pharyngoesophageal defect. Open cricopharyngeal myotomy is usually performed over an esophageal dilator with a scalpel. Great care must be taken to incise the entire length of the cricopharyngeus muscle and proximal esophageal musculature without entering the lumen. Many surgeons recommend excising a strip of the cricopharyngeus muscle to prevent recurrence. Diverticulopexy, with repositioning of the diverticulum to a more superior position so that it drains by gravity, is an option for large diverticula in poor surgical candidates.

Over the past decade, the endoscopic approach has become the standard of care. Endoscopic Zenker diverticulostomy, also called the Dohlman procedure, has been refined since its original description in the 1960s. A bivalved diverticuloscope, such as the Weerda, is used to expose the common wall between the diverticulum and the esophagus, which contains the cricopharyngeus muscle. Either a gastrointestinal stapling device (preferably) or the carbon dioxide laser is used to divide this wall.[28,29] This technique does not result in the removal of the diverticulum but instead eliminates the retention of food in the diverticulum by opening it to the esophageal lumen and divides the muscle which produces the outpouching. Therefore, fluoroscopy will still appear abnormal after the procedure. In a series of 159 endoscopic staple diverticulostomies, the procedure was successfully completed in 94%, with 98% of subjects reporting symptom improvement.[29] The most common complications in this series were chipped teeth and postoperative fever. The recurrence rate was 11.8% after an average of 33 months. The endoscopic approach has a lower complication rate than the open approach with an equivalent success rate. Other advantages of the endoscopic procedure include shorter operating times, shorter hospital stays and more rapid return to normal diet. The endoscopic approach is standard in most institutions, with the open approach reserved for patients in whom the endoscopic approach failed, most commonly because of low-lying diverticula or an inadequate hypopharyngeal opening. Flexible endoscopic-assisted diverticulostomy has recently been suggested as an alternative for diverticula that cannot be exposed with rigid endoscopes.[30]

ESOPHAGEAL MOTILITY DISORDERS

Motility disorders of the esophagus, which may present as dysphagia, reflux symptoms not responding to treatment, regurgitation, or chest pain, are best evaluated with esophageal manometry. Cinefluoroscopy and esophagoscopy may be normal in many individuals with motility disorders. Primary esophageal motility disorders include ineffective esophageal motility (IEM), hypertensive LES, diffuse esophageal spasm (DES), nutcracker esophagus, and achalasia.

Manometry and Impedance

Esophageal body and LES manometry can be performed with solid state or perfusion catheters, usually passed into the esophagus and stomach through the nose. Manometry assesses contraction pressures and peristaltic coordination at multiple sites in the esophagus (more than 30 sites using high resolution manometry). The resting pressure of the LES and the degree of LES relaxation are also assessed. Many manometry systems incorporate impedance testing as well. Impedance measures bolus transit throughout the esophagus by detecting changes in electrical current across electrodes. Impedance testing permits differentiation of retrograde and anterograde bolus flow and detection of all types of reflux, including weakly acid or alkaline reflux.[31] Manometry may also be used in the evaluation of the PES and pharyngeal muscle dysfunction. Individuals with a hypertonic cricopharyngeus muscle or one that fails to relax may benefit from the injection of botulinum toxin or division of the muscle in an analogous manner to a hypertensive LES.

Ineffective Esophageal Motility and Hypertensive Lower Esophageal Sphincter

IEM is common in people with GERD, although it is not clear that IEM is directly caused by GERD. The diagnosis is made by the observation of > 30% of swallows with low amplitude (< 30 mm Hg) peristaltic contractions. Patients with IEM may have a normal esophagram. The primary therapies for patients with IEM are behavioral modifications and pharmacologic treatment for GERD. Patients with severe IEM may respond to bethanechol.[32]

A hypertensive LES is diagnosed if manometry reveals LES resting pressure greater than 45 mm Hg. Typically, the hypertensive LES relaxes completely and is associated with either normal or ineffective esophageal body peristalsis. Treatment includes endoscopic injection of botulinum toxin into the LES, surgical myotomy, or smooth muscle relaxants.

Diffuse Esophageal Spasm and Nutcracker Esophagus

DES is diagnosed by the presence of high amplitude simultaneous nonperistaltic contractions.[33] Dysphagia and atypical, i.e., noncardiac, chest pain are common symptoms of DES. Cinefluoroscopy may show the classic "corkscrew" appearance of the simultaneous esophageal contractions. Treatment may be medical or surgical, including myotomy, botulinum toxin injections, calcium channel blockers, nitrates, and smooth muscle relaxants. If present, GERD should also be treated in patients with DES.

In contrast to DES, the high amplitude contractions seen in nutcracker esophagus are peristaltic. Cinefluoroscopy is usually normal in the setting of nutcracker esophagus. The symptoms are similar to DES, and smooth muscle relaxants and antireflux therapy may be useful treatments.

Achalasia

Achalasia is characterized by absent esophageal peristalsis and absent relaxation of the LES. Slowly progressive dysphagia may be accompanied by weight loss as the disease progresses. The etiology of this disorder is unknown. Classic signs of achalasia on fluoroscopy include a dilated esophagus with minimal or no contractions and a tapered "bird's beak" appearance where the distal esophagus meets the contracted LES. Manometry reveals nonperistaltic low amplitude contractions and incomplete LES relaxation. Endoscopy must be performed to exclude an obstructing carcinoma at the GEJ (pseudoachalasia). Patients with achalasia are treated with LES botulinum toxin injections, pneumatic dilation of the LES, or surgical myotomy.[34]

Systemic Diseases Affecting the Esophagus

Many connective tissue disorders and systemic diseases may affect the esophagus. Scleroderma is surprisingly common and involves the smooth muscle of the esophagus, while the proximal striated muscle remains unaffected. The LES may be incompetent in scleroderma, leading to profound gastroesophageal reflux. Inflammatory myopathies, such as dermatomyositis, involve the proximal striated muscle of the esophagus and the UES, leaving the distal esophagus and LES unaffected. Systemic lupus erythematosis can also cause esophageal dysmotility. Diabetes mellitus can lead to autonomic dysfunction affecting both esophageal motility and gastric emptying. Hypothyroidism may cause reversible esophageal dysmotility.

ESOPHAGEAL TRAUMA

Esophageal Perforation

Esophageal perforation is usually iatrogenic from esophagoscopy with or without dilation. Perforation is most common in narrow strictures or esophageal cancer. In eosinophilic esophagitis, the esophageal mucosa is extremely friable and susceptible to laceration. While these injuries are usually superficial, great care should be taken during esophagoscopy and dilation in patients with eosinophilic esophagitis. Blind placement of nasogatric or feeding tubes has also been associated with hypopharyngeal and esophageal perforation.[35] Other causes of perforation include blunt and penetrating chest and cervical trauma, esophageal foreign bodies, or acute esophageal necrosis. Progression or treatment of mediastinal neoplasms, such as lymphoma, may result in esophageal perforation with or without tracheoesophageal fistula. A rare transmural perforation of the distal esophagus, known as Boerhaave

syndrome, is frequently associated with forceful emesis. Unlike Mallory-Weiss tear, hematemesis is not common with Boerhaave syndrome.

Foreign Body Ingestion

Ingestion of foreign bodies may account for up to 1,500 deaths a year in the United States, and the pediatric age group is most commonly affected.[36] Foreign bodies typically become lodged in the normal anatomic constrictions of the esophagus, especially at the level of the cricopharyngeus. Since the party wall between the trachea and esophagus is thin and deformable, esophageal foreign bodies often present with respiratory distress, in addition to drooling and dysphagia. By far, coins are the most common foreign bodies to become lodged in the esophagus; other commonly ingested items are large food boluses and toys. Hot dog pieces are especially dangerous and may completely obstruct the adjacent trachea leading to death. Button batteries may appear as coin-shaped objects on radiographs but should be treated as surgical emergencies. Batteries cause rapid necrosis of the esophageal mucosa by strong alkali injury and should be removed immediately before severe esophageal injury and perforation ensue. Impaction of a food bolus in a child, especially when recurrent, should alert the surgeon to the possibility of eosinophilic esophagitis.

Foreign body ingestion should be evaluated promptly with thorough history and chest radiographs. The addition of lateral films can help clarify the location of the foreign body (trachea versus esophagus) and provide clues to the presence of multiple foreign bodies (Figure 4). Coins and batteries are well visualized on plain films, but toys and food boluses may not be seen. Some clinicians use contrast esophagography to demonstrate esophageal foreign bodies. Evaluation for an esophageal foreign body requires endoscopy.

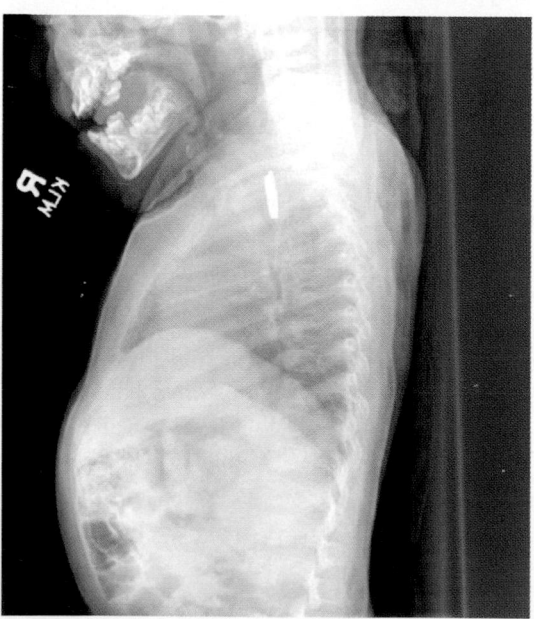

Figure 4 Double esophageal foreign body. Lateral chest radiograph showing two overlapping coins lodged in the proximal port of the esophagus.

Esophageal foreign bodies are best managed with rigid endoscopy under general anesthesia although reports have suggested that flexible endoscopic removal or pushing the foreign body into the stomach with a bougie may be acceptable for coins.[37,38] Rigid endoscopy provides the benefit of a protected airway, and limits the risk of converting an esophageal foreign body to a laryngotracheal foreign body during extraction. Optical forceps provide excellent visualization of the foreign body and firm control of the object. An impacted distal food bolus can sometimes be managed by carefully pushing it into the stomach. A full evaluation of the esophagus is recommended after retrieval of the foreign body to evaluate for multiple foreign bodies, esophageal injury, and underlying esophageal disorders, e.g., stricture or eosinophilic esophagitis. Since up to 25% of esophageal coins will pass spontaneously, chest x-ray should be repeated prior to general anesthesia if more than two hours have passed since the original film.[39] Some clinicians also utilize gastrointestinal motility agents, such as glucagon, in an attempt to promote passage of the object into the stomach before surgery.

Complications of esophageal foreign bodies are rare but may be serious. Chronic foreign bodies may cause esophageal perforation, severe inflammation with resultant stricture, or tracheoesophageal fistula. Button batteries and sharp foreign bodies (such as safety pins) may rapidly lead to these complications. The potential complications of esophagoscopy, such as perforation or aspiration, also apply to esophageal foreign body extraction.

Caustic Ingestion

Ingestion of caustic substances is a common problem although federally regulated labeling of hazardous materials has decreased the incidence of accidental ingestion. Caustic ingestion occurs most commonly in small children or suicidal adults. In the case of children, the volume ingested is usually small, as children are deterred by the foul taste of most toxic substances. The exposure volume may be significantly higher in adults with intentional ingestion.

The history and identification of the ingested substance are most important when evaluating a patient with caustic ingestion. Alkali substances (pH > 7) include lye and laundry detergents. Alkali ingestion leads to liquefaction necrosis with deep esophageal injuries. Acidic substances with pH < 7 (e.g., battery fluid) cause corrosive injury which is frequently limited to the mucosa. Household bleaches usually have a pH around 7. While bleaches may irritate esophageal mucosa, permanent sequelae are uncommon. Hair relaxer is another commonly ingested substance in the pediatric population, with a pH of 11.2 to 11.9. Hair relaxer does not appear to cause serious or permanent esophageal sequelae.[40] Liquid caustic ingestions have the potential to affect a greater area of the aerodigestive tract, and solid caustics (such as solid lye) tend to cause more localized injury. Thermal injuries are also possible from hot ingestions.

Evaluation of patients with caustic ingestion should include a careful examination of the entire upper aerodigestive tract. Oral and pharyngeal injuries are common, especially with acid ingestion (acidic substances are especially foul-tasting and stimulate gagging and retching). Attempts to neutralize the substance are usually misguided and may result in further injury to the esophageal mucosa. There may be some benefit from water or milk ingestion to dilute the substance. Gastric lavage and emetics are strictly contraindicated in caustic ingestion.

If the ingested substance is believed to be injurious, or if it is unknown, endoscopy is indicated.[41] The amount of damage may be underestimated if endoscopy is performed too early (less than 12 hours). Therefore, endoscopy is best performed 24 to 48 hours after injury. Any further delay significantly increases the risk of perforation during esophagoscopy, and esophagography should be considered. Due to its small caliber of the endoscope and the ability to perform it without sedation, TNE is a good option for evaluation of injuries due to caustic ingestion. In cases of suspected perforation, flexible esophagoscopy of any type is contraindicated.

Injuries are graded on esophagoscopy according to the extent of mucosal injury. Grade 1 injuries are superficial and do not usually lead to permanent sequelae. These injuries do not usually require treatment. Grade 2 injuries are transmucosal and have a high risk of stricture formation. Grade 3 injuries are transmural and are at high risk for perforation and strictures, almost always requiring surgical intervention. Circumferential injuries are more likely to lead to late complications. If possible, nasogastric tubes should be placed during endoscopy in the setting of transmucosal or transmural injuries to allow esophageal rest and prevent acute complete stricture. The administration of corticosteroids to prevent strictures is highly controversial and should be avoided for grade 1 or 3 injuries. In grade 2 injuries, some authors have suggested that corticosteroids decrease stricture formation, but other studies have refuted this.[42,43] Antibiotics should be reserved for cases with clear evidence of perforation or secondary infection. Antireflux therapy may be of some benefit in preventing strictures.

Aside from the acute risk of perforation, caustic ingestion (grade 2 and 3 injury) can lead to serious long-term complications. The most common is stricture formation, which often requires serial endoscopic dilation or surgical resection. A history of caustic ingestion predisposes the patient to a much higher risk of esophageal squamous cell carcinoma throughout life as well.

Esophageal Bleeding

Hematemesis of bright red blood is a gastrointestinal emergency. The most common cause of upper gastrointestinal bleeding is ulcerative disease of the stomach or duodenum. Esophageal causes of hemorrhage include varices, Mallory-Weiss tear, esophagitis, and neoplasms. Rare causes of bleeding are aortoesophageal fistula or acute esophageal necrosis.[44] TNE is contraindicated in acute hematemesis.

Esophageal varices are most commonly associated with portal hypertension as a result of cirrhosis of the liver. On endoscopy, these varices typically appear as tortuous blue or white submucosal lesions. Endoscopic sclerotherapy or clipping or systemic drugs, such as vasopressin or somatostatin, are frequently used for acute variceal bleeding although uncontrolled life-threatening bleeds may require balloon tamponade. Asymptomatic varices seen upon endoscopy are a serious finding since such patients often present with life threatening hematemesis that can be avoided with beta-blockers or surgical shunts.

Mallory-Weiss tear occurs at the gastric cardia or GEJ and is the result of prolonged retching, often associated with alcoholism and binge drinking. This tear usually involves only the mucosa. The bleeding stops spontaneously in 90%. Treatment options for life-threatening active bleeding include endoscopic clipping, electrocautery, or injection of saline with epinephrine.

BENIGN ESOPHAGEAL NEOPLASMS

Benign neoplasms of the esophagus are rare and usually slow-growing and asymptomatic. Dysphagia is the most common symptom that ensues and is dependent on the size and location of the mass.

Leiomyomas are intramural and represent 60 to 70% of benign esophageal neoplasms. These are generally found in the distal esophagus, where smooth muscle predominates. These neoplasms typically occur as a single mass and can be difficult to visualize on endoscopy. An intact layer of mucosa is usually present over the neoplasm. Most are discovered incidentally. Enucleation at thoracotomy is an effective treatment for large symptomatic leiomyomas.

Esophageal cysts are the second most common benign mass. These intramural masses are often congenital. As with leiomyomas, most esophageal cysts are asymptomatic. Acute inflammation may result in growth and the subsequent development of symptoms. On esophagoscopy, the cyst may appear as a blue, smooth, round mass beneath an intact layer of mucosa. Enucleation and excision at thoracotomy are effective treatment options.

Fibrovascular polyps are intraluminal lesions that are found in the upper esophagus or the postcricoid region. Generally pedunculated, they can grow to "giant" proportions. Laryngeal obstruction with subsequent asphyxiation by a regurgitated fibrovascular polyp is a well-described cause of death.[45] Therefore, surgical excision by cervical esophagotomy is the typical treatment although some of these lesions may be removed successfully endoscopically. There is typically a

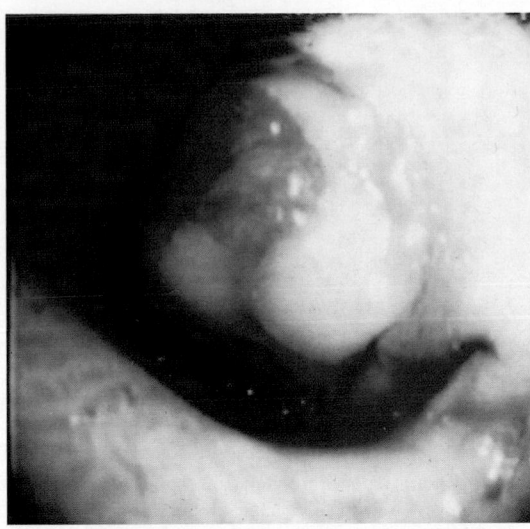

Figure 5 Inflammatory pseudotumor. Note the pedunculated mucosal covered mass in the distal third of the esophagus.

large vessel in the stalk of the polyp that must be addressed during resection.

Inflammatory pseudotumors appear as polypoid masses. Although they may appear malignant, they are not comprised of neoplastic cells but contain fibrous and granulation tissue. Often located in the middle or distal parts of the esophagus, they are frequently associated with mucosal ulcers (Figure 5).

Single or multiple papillomas may be present in the esophagus. Both human papilloma virus and mucosal irritation have been implicated. Malignant change may occur in large papillomas. Snare cautery may be used for endoscopic excision.

MALIGNANT ESOPHAGEAL NEOPLASMS

The vast majority of esophageal neoplasms are malignant. While fluoroscopy may suggest the presence of malignant neoplasms, the most sensitive method of detecting esophageal cancer is endoscopy with biopsy. Barium esophagram should not be used to "rule out" malignancy. Most symptoms of esophageal carcinoma are nonspecific and include weight loss, vomiting, and mild hematemesis. With rare exception, all patients with solid food dysphagia should be evaluated for esophageal carcinoma by esophagoscopy. Unfortunately, dysphagia does not usually occur until the esophageal lumen is narrowed to 13 mm, so patients with esophageal carcinoma often present at a late stage. More than half of patients with esophageal malignancies have distant metastases at the time of diagnosis.

Squamous cell carcinoma of the esophagus has been traditionally considered the most common malignancy of the esophagus, but this is changing. Among cancers, the incidence of adenocarcinoma of the esophagus is the fastest growing in America and is now greater than its squamous cell counterpart.[46] Squamous cell carcinomas appear most commonly in the middle

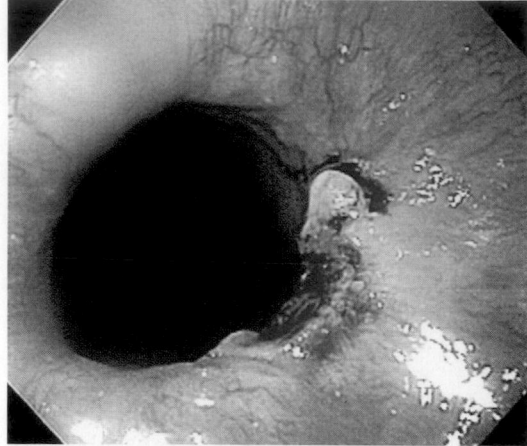

Figure 6 Early adenocarcinoma of esophagus. Note the subtle elevation of the esophageal mucosa relative to surrounding tissue at the gastroesophageal junction.

third of the esophagus, with the lesion often friable and notable for an area of central ulceration with raised edges. Adenocarcinoma is almost always found in the distal third of the esophagus, and an area of BE is commonly seen adjacent to the neoplasm. On esophagoscopy, adenocarcinoma may appear as a mucosa-covered nodule or as an ulcerative mass with esophageal obstruction in more advanced cases (Figure 6).

As mentioned earlier, esophageal malignancies may spread throughout the length of the esophagus from any primary site because of the lymphatic network. Therefore, the entire esophagus is usually treated regardless of the primary location in the esophagus. Primary surgical therapy, usually with total esophagectomy and gastric pull-up or colonic interposition, is the traditional mainstay of esophageal carcinoma treatment, with chemotherapy and radiotherapy used for lesions that invade the muscularis or deeper. In the presence of distant metastases, palliation with esophageal stents is usually the only treatment offered. Survival from adenocarcinoma has improved somewhat in recent years, presumably from earlier diagnosis. In a study of 263 patients undergoing surgery for esophageal adenocarcinoma, Portale et al, reported a 46.5 to 50.4% overall five-year survival.[47] The most important predictor of survival in esophageal carcinoma is stage.

REFERENCES

1. Hirschowitz BI, Curtiss LE, Peters CW, et al. Demonstration of a new gastroscope "the fiberscope." Gastroenterology 1958;35:50–3.
2. Herrmann, IF, Recio SA. Functional pharyngoesophagoscopy: a new technique for diagnostics and analyzing deglutition. Oper Tech Otolaryngol Head Neck Surg 1997;8:163–7.
3. Shaker R. Unsedated transnasal pharyngoesophagogastroduodenoscopy (t-EGD). Gastrointest Endosc 1994;40:346–8.
4. Aviv JE, Takoudes T, Ma G, et al. Office-based esophagoscopy – a preliminary report. Otolaryngol Head Neck Surg 2001;125:170–5.
5. Glaws WR, Etzkorn KP, Wenig BL, et al. Comparison of rigid and flexible esophagoscopy in the diagnosis of esophageal disease: diagnostic accuracy, complications and cost. Ann Otol Rhinol Laryngol 1996;104:262–6.
6. Saeian K, Staff DM, Vasilopoulos S, et al. Unsedated transnasal endoscopy accurately detects Barrett's metaplasia and dysplasia. Gastrointest Endosc 2002;56:472–8.
7. Postma GN, Cohen JT, Belafsky PC, et al. Transnasal esophagoscopy: revisited (over 700 consecutive cases). Laryngoscope 2005;115:321–3.
8. Andrus JG, Dolan RW, Anderson TD. Transnasal esophagoscopy: a high yield diagnostic tool. Laryngoscope 2005;115:993–6.
9. Wilkins T, Gillies RA. Office-based unsedated ultrathin esophagoscopy in a primary care setting. Ann Fam Med 2005;3:126–30.
10. Halum SL, Postma GN. Office-based examinations in laryngology. In: Merati AL, Bielamowicz SA, editors. Textbook of laryngology. Abingdon, United Kingdom: Plural Publishing; 2007. p.135–45.
11. Wildi SM, Glenn TF, Wolson RF, et al. Is esophagoscopy alone sufficient for patients with reflux symptoms? Gastrointest Endosc 2004;59:349–54.
12. Jobe BA, Hunter JG, Chang EY, et al. Office-based unsedated small-caliber endoscopy is equivalent to conventional sedated endoscopy in screening and surveillance for Barrett's esophagus: a randomized and blinded comparison. Am J Gastro 2006;101:2693–2703.
13. Thota PN, Zuccaro G Jr. Vargo JJ 2nd, et al. A randomized prospective trial comparing unsedated esophagoscopy via transnasal and transoral routes using a 4 mm video endoscope with conventional endoscopy with sedation. Endoscopy 2005;37:559–65.
14. Halum SL, Postma GN, Bates DD, et al. Incongruence between histologic and endoscopic diagnoses of Barrett's esophagus using transnasal esophagoscopy. Laryngoscope 2006;116:303–6.
15. Belafsky PC, Allen K, Castro-Del Rosario L, et al. Wireless pH testing as an adjunct to unsedated transnasal esophagoscopy: the safety and efficacy of transnasal telemetry capsule placement. Otolaryngol Head Neck Surg 2004;131:26–8.
16. Postma GN, Bach KK, Belafsky PC, et al. The role of transnasal esophagoscopy in head and neck oncology. Laryngoscope 2002;112:2242–43.
17. Rees CJ, Belafsky PC. Chronic esophageal stricture with Barrett's esophagus. Ear Nose Throat J 2007;86:88.
18. Belafsky PC, Postma GN, Koufman JA. Replacement of a failed tracheoesophageal puncture (TEP) under direct vision. Ear Nose Throat J 2001;80:862.
19. Rees C, Halum S, Wijewickrama R, et al. Patient tolerance of in-office pulsed dye laser treatments to the upper aerodigestive tract. Otolaryngol Head Neck Surg 2006;134:1023–7.
20. Eroglu A, Can Kurkcuogu I, Karaoganogu N, et al. Esophageal perforation: the importance of early diagnosis and primary repair. Dis Esophagus 2004;17:91–4.
21. Vogel SB, Rout WR, Martin TD, et al. Esophageal perforation in adults: aggressive, conservative treatment lowers morbidity and mortality. Ann Surg 2005;241:1016–21.
22. Achildi O, Grewal H. Congenital anomalies of the esophagus. Otolaryngol Clin North Am 2007;40:219–44.
23. Kikendall JW. Pill-induced esophageal injury. Gastroenterol Clin North Am 1991;20:835–46.
24. Chami TN, Nikoomanesh P, Katz PO. An unusual presentation of pill-induced esophagitis. Gastrointest Endosc 1995;45:263–5.
25. Potter JW, Saeian K, Staff D, et al. Eosinophilic esophagitis in adults: an emerging problem with unique esophageal features. Gastrointest Endosc 2004;53:355–61.
26. Lundell LR, Dent J, Bennett, JR, et al. Endoscopic assessment of esophagitis: clinical and functional correlates and further validation of the Los Angeles classification. Gut 1999;45:172–80.
27. Sasaki CT, Ross DA, Hundal J. Association between Zenker's diverticulum and gastroesophageal reflux disease: development of a working hypothesis. Am J Med 2003;115 Suppl 3A:169S–171S.
28. Maune S. Carbon dioxide laser diverticulostomy: a new treatment for Zenker diverticulum. Am J Med 2003;115 Suppl 3A:172S–174S.
29. Chang CY, Payyapilli RJ, Scher RL. Endoscopic staple diverticulostomy for Zenker's diverticulum: a review of literature and experience in 159 cases. Laryngoscope 2003;113:957–65.
30. Altman JI, Genden EM, Moche J. Fiberoptic endoscopic-assisted diverticulotomy: a novel technique for the management of Zenker's diverticulum. Ann Otol Rhinol Laryngol 2005;114:347–51.
31. Hirano I, Richter JE, and the Practice Parameters Committee of the American College of Gastroenterology. ACG practice guidelines: esophageal reflux testing. Am J Gastroenterol 2007;102:668–85.
32. Agrawal A, Hila A, Tutuian R, et al. Bethanechol improves smooth muscle function in patients with severe ineffective esophageal motility. J Clin Gastroenterol 2007;41:366–70.
33. Tutuian R, Castell DO. Esophageal motility disorders (distal esophageal spasm, nutcracker esophagus, and hypertensive lower esophageal sphincter): modern management. Curr Treat Options Gastroenterol 2006;9:283–94.
34. Lopushinksy SR, Urbach DR. Pneumatic dilation and surgical myotomy for achalasia. JAMA 2006;296:2227–33.
35. Metheny NA, Meert KL, Clouse RE. Complications related to feeding tube placement. Curr Opin Gastroenterol 2007;23:178–82.
36. Webb WA. Management of foreign bodies in the upper GI tract. Gastroenterology 1988;94;204–16.
37. Gmeiner D, von Radhen BH, Meco C, et al. Flexible versus rigid endoscopy for treatment of foreign body impaction in the esophagus. Surg Endosc 2007 Mar 29;[Epub ahead of print].
38. Dahshan AH, Kevin Donovan G. Bougienage versus endoscopy for esophageal coin removal in children. J Clin Gastroenterol 2007;41:454–6.
39. Waltzman ML, Baskin M, Wypij D, et al. A randomized clinical trial of the management of esophageal coins in children. Pediatrics 2005;116:614–9.
40. Aronow SP, Aronow HD, Blanchard T, et al. Hair relaxers: a benign caustic ingestion? J Pediatr Gastroenterol Nutr 2003;36:120–5.
41. Poley JW, Steyerberg EW, Kuipers EJ, et al. Ingestion of acid and alkaline agents: outcome and prognostic value of early upper endoscopy. Gastroinest Endosc 2004;60:372–7.
42. Howell JM, Dalsey WC, Hartsell FW, et al. Steroids for the treatment of corrosive esophageal injury: a statistical analysis of past studies. Am J Emerg Med 1992;10:421–5.
43. Pelclova D, Navratil T. Do corticosteroids prevent oesophageal stricture after corrosive ingestion? Toxicol Rev 2005;24:125–9.
44. Wu J, Chan FK. Esophageal bleeding disorders. Curr Opin Gastroenterol 2004;20:386–90.
45. Carrick C, Collins KA, Lee CJ, et al. Sudden death due to asphyxia by esophageal polyp: two case reports and review of asphyxial deaths. Am J Forensic Med Pathol 2005;26:275–81.
46. Conio M, Blanchi S, Lapertosa G, et al. Long-term endoscopic surveillance of patients with Barrett's esophagus. Incidence of dysplasia and adenocarcinoma: a prospective study. Am J Gastroenterol 2003;98:1931–9.
47. Portale G, Hagen JA, Pmeters JH, et al. Modern 5-year survival of resectable esophageal adenocarcinoma: single institution experience with 263 patients. J Am Coll Surg 2006;202:588–96.

ADDITIONAL READING:

Castell DO, Richter JE, editors. The esophagus. 4th edition. Philadelphia: Lippincott Williams and Wilkins; 2004.

86

Sleep Medicine and Surgery

B. Tucker Woodson, MD

Pharyngeal resistance is normally a minor component of upper-airway resistance during wakefulness. During sleep, however, pharyngeal resistance increases. The sequence of increasing resistance, persistent respiratory effort, hypoventilation, and obstruction ultimately lead to snoring and sleep apnea. The starting point of sleep disordered breathing is a structurally small or vulnerable upper airway.[1] At its center is inspiratory flow limitation which is a biologic marker of airway obstruction. This disorder's intricate pathology remains inadequately understood and is a complex interaction of structural and physiologic factors. Understanding this complexity is critical to successful treatment and advanced care of the patient with a medical and surgical sleep disorders.

PREVALENCE

Snoring and sleep apnea are common disorders. Accurate determinations of the prevalence of sleep apnea and snoring are confounded by varied definitions of disease and by age, ethnicity, and gender effects.[2] Occasional snoring is common. A community-based study demonstrated 80% of subjects snored at least 10% of the night and 20% snored for greater than 50% of the night. Habitual frequent or "always" snoring affects more than 21% of men and 8% of women. Sleep apnea is estimated to affect 34 to 60% of habitual snorers when defined by having symptoms of fatigue and observed apneas. Estimates of snoring in children range from 3 to 12%.[3]

Sleep apnea, defined using polysomnography plus symptoms of sleepiness, has a prevalence in a United States population of middle-aged employed adults of 4% in men and 2% in women. Based on polysomnography only (apnea-hypopnea index [AHI] greater than 15 events/h), the prevalence of was 9% in men and 4% in women. The risk of developing sleep-disordered breathing is affected by obesity but does not require it. Obesity, aging, smoking, and postmenopausal status alter the incidence of snoring and presumably sleep apnea. Few data exist about prevalence of other less common forms of sleep-disordered breathing including central sleep apnea syndromes and obesity hypoventilation, that is, Pickwickian syndrome. Data suggest that milder forms of sleep apnea may progress to more severe sleep apnea.

Obstructive sleep apnea (OSA) is common in children, and the polysomnographically documented incidence of the disorder is often stated to be 1 to 2% of the US general population. The range varies from 1 to 10%; however, in some populations, such as obese Asian children, 33% have OSA. Habitual snoring occurs in 3 to 12% of Asian children.[4] Relative risk is increased with obesity, lymphoid hyperplasia, cough, inflammatory airway disease, and abnormal patterns of craniofacial development. Sleep apnea in children is discussed further in Chapter 66, "Sleep Apnea in Children."

SYMPTOMS

The two primary symptoms of sleep-disordered breathing are snoring and manifestations of sleepiness.[5] Other major symptoms of sleep apnea are listed in Table 1. Since the primary symptoms are common in the population, symptoms poorly predict disease. Clinical impression has only 60% sensitivity and specificity in identifying patients with sleep apnea in a sleep clinic population.

Incorrectly considered by some as the primary motivating complaint of sleep apnea, sleepiness is a common complaint in the population and has many differing descriptions. These include fatigue, daytime impairment, depression, change in mood, poor long- or short-term memory, decreased executive function, and increased risk of accidents. Unfortunately, none of these symptoms alone predict apnea, although all may have major impact on the patient and disease severity. Snoring is also common and is a frequent complaint. As with sleepiness, alone it is poorly predictive of disease. A more significant marker of disease is observed apneas by others. Since apnea has significant health concerns, patients with higher risk such as serious cardiovascular disease, atrial fibrillation, poorly controlled hypertension, and others warrant further evaluation. In lower-risk populations, screening has a less certain role. Currently, symptom-based algorithms with high sensitivity have unacceptably low specificity, and algorithms with high specificity, that is, few false-negatives, have low sensitivity. Women may present with different symptoms than men for the same level of disease with fatigue being more common and snoring, snorting, and gasping being less common.[6,7] Premenopausal women with OSA are, as a group, more obese than control males with similar levels of disease.

Children present symptomatically distinct from adults.[8] Snoring and restless sleep are

Table 1 Symptoms of Sleep Apnea in Adults and Children	
Symptoms and Signs	
Adults	Children
Major symptoms	Major symptoms
Chronic and loud snoring	Noisy breathing (snoring)
Gasping or choking episodes during sleep	Mouth breathing
Excessive daytime sleepiness	Agitated sleep
Personality changes or cognitive difficulties related to fatigue	Nocturnal awakenings
Sleepiness during driving or other activities requiring alertness	Learning difficulties
Other symptoms	Abnormal daytime behavior
Morning headaches	Hard to wake up and daytime fatigue
Sexual dysfunction	Other symptoms
Restless sleep	Persistent enuresis
Diaphoresis	Sleepwalking with or without night terrors
Recent weight gain	Failure to thrive
Worsening of habitual snoring	Repeated upper respiratory infections
Signs	
Obesity	Signs
Conditions associated with decreased upper airway size	Obesity
Systemic hypertension	Enlarged tonsils (grade 3 or 4)
Pulmonary hypertension and cor pulmonale (rarely)	Enlarged adenoid (adenoid index > 0.5)
	Increased Mallampati score
	High-arched palate
	Allergic rhinitis

common. Sleepiness is infrequently presented as hypersomnolence and usually with symptoms of inattention, behavior disorders, impulsivity, and poor school performance. Ancillary symptoms and signs such as growth retardation and enuresis are not specific. Although snoring, mouth breathing, and tonsil hypertrophy have high sensitivity, specificity may be low.[9] Hypersomnolence and witnessed apneas are highly specific in the snoring child in predicting an abnormal sleep study but have low sensitivity. Diagnosis is further confounded by uncertainty about the accuracy of routine polysomnography in identifying sleep apnea.

MORBIDITY AND MORTALITY

OSA is associated with hypertension and increased risks of cardiovascular disease including cardiac dysrhythmias, recurrence of atrial fibrillation, stroke, and myocardial infarction.[10–12] Mortality is increased in OSA, likely from increased vascular disease. The absolute risk of cardiovascular disease in OSA populations is still significantly influenced by obesity, smoking, alcohol use, and genetic factors. The thresholds of clinically significant risks are unclear and likely differ among disorders. Mortality has been associated with an apnea index (AI) of greater than 20 apneas/h and is reduced in patients treated successfully with nasal continuous positive airway pressure (CPAP), uvulopalatopharyngoplasty (UPPP) or tracheostomy. It is estimated that an AHI of 15 events/h is associated with sleep impairment and that an AHI of 20 to 30 events/h may be associated with hypertension. Motor vehicle accident rates may increase seven times with sleep apnea.[13] Absolute risk of impairment may be increased with OSA but is not independent of insufficient sleep, shift work, drug and alcohol use, exposure risk, and other medical disorders. Identifying and treating OSA in the sleepy individual may not eliminate risk. Care should be used with using any single measure as a disease threshold. Mean AHI of populations evaluated for disease risk are often two to three times the lower threshold. Thresholds also do not account for comorbidities, which combined with apnea may pose significant health risks. Although an AHI of 15 events/h without symptoms of excessive sleepiness or significant oxygen desaturation is a common polysomnographic definition of sleep apnea in adults, it should be viewed as only a useful benchmark.

PATHOPHYSIOLOGY

Upper airway collapse results from abnormal structure, ventilatory control, and sleep physiology. A structurally small upper airway increases pharyngeal resistance. Loss of airway muscle tone is both due to changes in sleep and ventilatory control. Airway obstruction leads to progressive increases in ventilatory effort, causing arousal through stimulation of airway and chest wall mechanoreceptors. Arousals and sleep disruption produce neurocognitive disorders

and create breathing instability but also augment cyclic (periodic) obstruction. As such, arousal is both an effect and cause of apnea.

The pharynx and supraglottis are the sites of obstruction. Obstruction may occasionally occur due to overt pathology but obstruction is most often due to structure that is normal but structurally disproportionate. Due to this structure, the pharynx is vulnerable to obstruction under certain conditions particularly during the sleep state. There are a multitude of causes of this instability. A fundamental cause relates to the unique property of the human airway having the larynx in the neck (Figure 1). This is in contrast to other mammals where the larynx is close to the skull base. Human cranial development results in skull-base angulation and associated changes in facial and airway form. These include a longer soft tissue supralaryngeal airway (pharynx), a shorter and more vertically oriented maxilla, posterior maxillary constriction, and a vulnerable soft tissue upper airway with the loss of muscle tone. In humans, the combination of a soft tissue supralaryngeal airway, decreased airway size, and changes in physiology associated with sleep ultimately cause sleep apnea events. The "syndrome" of OSA is the pathophysiologic cascade resulting from these events.

Many variables affect the sleep-apnea airway. Anatomy, tissue mass, body position, negative inspiratory pressure, airflow velocity, muscle tone, ventilatory drive, tissue adhesive forces, and sleep physiology may contribute. Integrating such a complex process can be difficult. One method to understand and quantify the process is to use a balance of forces model (Figure 2). This model first defines the upper-airway transmural pressure ($P_{tm} = P_{tissue} - P_{luminal}$) and then divides the forces that act on the airway as those promoting stability or collapse. An increased transmural pressure (P_{tm}) enlarges the airway, and decreased P_{tm} collapses the airway. Anatomy, muscle tone, tissue elastic forces, surface adhesive forces, and vascular volume are tissue forces (P_{tissue}). Intraluminal airway pressure and flow are luminal forces ($P_{luminal}$). The balance between the two determines airway patency. No single factor determines obstruction.

Initial theories describing sleep apnea conceived that the upper airway at rest was patent. Collapse occurred from negative airway pressure during inspiration. Later it was realized that subatmospheric intraluminal pressures was not needed to obstruct the airway during sleep and that just a decrease or loss of muscle tone could lead to obstruction. Muscle tone does not differ significantly in individuals with sleep apnea compared to normal individuals. The larger magnitude loss of muscle tone in sleep-disordered breathing is a consequence of a loss of augmented waking muscle tone needed to compensate for a structurally small airway. Physiologic changes are critical in causing sleep apnea but are secondary for most, not primary.

Obesity

Obesity increases the risk and severity of OSA and the severity of hypoxemia during sleep. Obesity effects metabolism, ventilation, and lung volume to worsen apnea. Leptin and various inflammatory obesity-related cytokines may increase CO_2 response, and central ventilatory sensitivity augments the tendency toward periodic breathing and increases airway instability. Fat distribution around the neck has long been postulated without evidence to compromise the airway.

The relationship of obesity and sleep apnea is bidirectional. A shared etiology is also supported. The metabolic syndrome of obesity, hyperinsulinemia, and hypertension is often associated with sleep apnea. Treatment reduces this association. Population data demonstrate both shared and unshared genetic linkage of obesity and apnea each to one another and support an

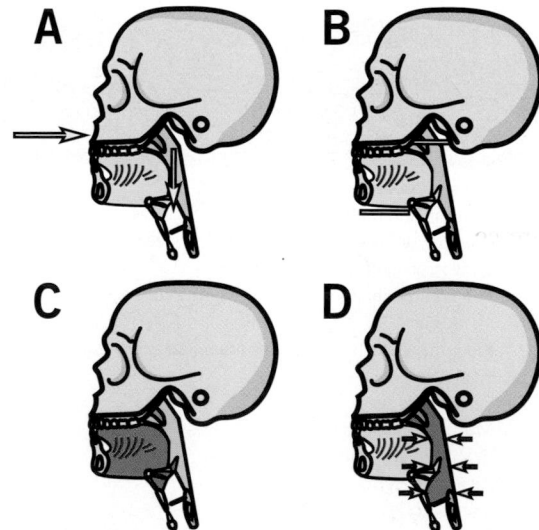

Figure 1 Human nasomaxillary development effects on upper airway risk factors for sleep apnea are shown. (A) Skull-base angulation is associated with a decreased maxillary and mandibular projection and laryngeal descent. (B) Posterior maxillary constriction. (C) Increased vertical height of the tongue with the tongue compromising the anterior pharyngeal wall. (D) A vulnerable soft tissue pharyngeal airway requiring muscular compensation for stability.

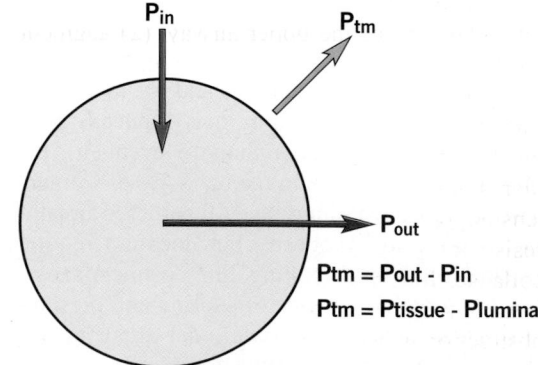

Figure 2 A method to model multiple forces acting on the airway is shown. The resultant force, that is, transmural pressure (P_{tm}), on the upper airway is the difference between collapsing and dilating pressures ($P_{tm} = P_{out} - P_{in}$). As P_{tm} increases, the airway enlarges, and as P_{tm} decreases, the airway collapses. P_{tm} may also be described as the difference in tissue forces (P_{tissue}) and luminal forces ($P_{luminal}$) ($P_{tm} = P_{tissue} - P_{luminal}$).

interrelated origin. Sleep apnea may also contribute to obesity due to behavior factors related to sleepiness.

Craniofacial Characteristics

The upper airway's bony and cartilaginous framework ultimately determine its size, shape, and compliance. The framework of the airway is highly variable. Differences exist between individuals, ethnic groups, and gender. Nonetheless, a generalized constellation of abnormalities are observed in sleep apnea. Craniofacial variables associated with OSA include: increased distance of the hyoid bone from the mandibular plane, decreased mandibular and maxillary projection, increased vertical length of the lower anterior part of the face, increased vertical length of the posterior airway, and increased cervical angulation. A fundamental abnormality in OSA is related to posterior maxillary positioning and relates to patterns of maxillary growth and development.

Facial structure interacts with obesity to create apnea risk. In the Wisconsin Cohort, a population-based study, two-thirds of the AHI was explained by a combination of facial structure and obesity.[14] In nonobese subjects, facial structure explains AHI alone. Individuals with normal craniofacial structures generally require morbid obesity to display OSA. Those with severe facial structural abnormalities may demonstrate severe OSA without any obesity. Increased tongue size has been associated with both OSA and obesity.

Nose

Nasal obstruction contributes to the presence and severity of OSA. Population and experimental studies associate nasal obstruction and nasal allergies with both sleep apnea and snoring. Obstructive nasal aberrations demonstrate greater positional dependence and increased obstruction in OSA patients compared to normals. The cause of this is unresolved but may result from both structural and physiologic medical disorders including vasomotor instability and increased inflammation. Nasal blockage may (1) reduce nasal afferent reflexes which help to maintain muscular tone of the upper airway, (2) augment the tendency for mouth opening which destabilizes the lower pharyngeal airway (by posterior rotation, vertical opening, and inferior displacement of the hyoid), (3) reduce humidification, increase mucus viscosity, and increase surface tension forces, and (4) increased upstream airway resistance predisposing to downstream airway collapse. Improving nasal airflow is critical in treating snoring and sleep apnea. Treating nasal obstruction may have significant impact on other sleep disorders including central sleep apnea and insomnia.

Pharyngeal Soft Tissues

The soft tissue conduit is not only the site of collapse and obstruction but in many is also a site of pathology. Contributions to apnea differ among individuals and ethnic groups. Nonetheless, there is strong familial aggregation of apnea, and, in some populations, this has been linked to soft-tissue abnormalities. Genetic studies have demonstrated inheritability of abnormal lateral wall size and tongue size in apnea populations.[15] Such abnormalities are more common in African Americans versus Caucasians and Asian populations in whom skeletal abnormalities are more common. Soft tissue abnormalities include a longer and wider soft palate, larger tongue, smaller oropalatal airspace, a posteriorly placed epiglottis, and smaller posterior airspace. Abnormalities may not only relate to tissue volume but cross-sectional shape as well. The airway in apneics may be more elliptical than circular, a property which increases airway surface area and frictional resistance.

Physiology

Lung volume affects pharyngeal upper airway size during both wake and sleep. Increased lung volume increases pharyngeal size. Decreased lung volume reduces airway size and increases pharyngeal collapse. Effects are asymmetric with decreases in normal functional residual capacity (FRC) having larger effects on airway size than increases in FRC. Effect of lung volume on the pharynx is likely thoracic traction, commonly, referred to as "tracheal tug."[16] Lung volume interacts with the mediastinum, intrathoracic pressures, and the trachea to change pharyngeal size and stiffness independent of neuromuscular activity. Passive tracheal traction increases longitudinal tension on the pharyngeal wall which stabilizes the pharyngeal airway. Starting at a normal resting lung volume, increases have small changes on pharyngeal volume; however, decreases in lung volume (such as during sleep) have much greater effects on the pharynx. Factors, such as obesity, which reduce lung volume below a normal FRC may have significant effects on airway collapse, and conversely, interventions which prevent this (such as positional therapy) may significantly improve airway function.

Vascular Volume

Soft tissues surrounding the airway and neck are composed of muscle, connective tissue, fat, lymphoid tissue, salivary and thyroid tissue, extracellular space, and arterial and venous blood volume. Of all these, only the venous blood volume is compressible under pressures of effective nasal CPAP. The vascular lateral pharyngeal walls are the structures mostly affected by nasal CPAP. Vascular blood volume causes a decrease in pharyngeal airway size of the patient with OSA by elevating the legs and by venous compression stockings. Effects are mediated through changes in central venous blood volume. Blood volume is altered in hypertension and other disorders, but its link to OSA is unknown.

Airway Resistance

Changes in inspiratory and expiratory resistance increase during sleep and are hallmarks defining patients who are normal, nonsnoring and snoring, and have OSA. Whereas, flow limitation is not observed in normal nonsnoring individuals, snorers demonstrate inspiratory flow limitation, and sleep apneics demonstrate both inspiratory and expiratory flow limitation. The end result is either normal ventilation (normals), airway flutter (snorers), and airway obstruction (apneics).

In normal ventilation, inspiration is associated with activation of airway dilator muscles. Normal levels of negative intraluminal pressures will not affect airway stability. With increased airway resistance, decreased muscle tone, or increased airway compliance, negative inspiratory pressure collapses the airway. When collapse leads to the situation where increasing negative pressure does not increase airflow, the state of airflow limitation is defined. Principles of a Starling resistor (if negative inspiratory pressure exceeds the closing pressure of the airway wall, the airway collapses) apply, and snoring and airway flutter may occur. When flow limitation progresses to occur in both inspiration and expiration, collapse likely leads to obstructive apnea. At end expiration, the airway is at its smallest and most vulnerable to collapse due to loss of both muscle tone and airway positive pressure and when the upper airway is at its most risk of abnormal resistance effects.

Normally in wake, phasic augmentation of airway muscles occurs and is dependent on negative pressure sensitive mechanoreceptors located in the nasal, pharyngeal, and laryngeal airway. The reflex controlling this activation may have increased latency in patients who snore or have sleep apnea which makes their airway at risk of collapse with application of negative pressure.[17] This reflex is also decreased with the acute onset of sleep (at the alpha theta transition) during stage I and stage II nonrapid eye movement (non-REM) sleep (but not stage 3 or stage 4 non-REM sleep). This critically important event destabilizes the airway in patients with snoring or sleep apnea. It also explains relative airway stability despite high negative airway pressure in non-REM stage III or stage IV sleep.

The "apneic" event is a process that begins several breaths prior to the scored event during sleep. In OSA, a phasic pattern of airway collapse is observed with each ventilatory cycle (Figure 3). Preceding an apneic event, progressive collapse occurs. This collapse is during expiration, presumably due to loss of muscle tone.[18] When critical size and airway pressure are reached, increased resistance, flow limitation, and inspiratory collapse are observed. This results in increasingly negative airway pressures and arousal. The process then repeats.

Sites of Obstruction

No single site of obstruction exists in sleep apnea. Hypotonic and manometric methods demonstrate the most frequent site of primary obstructions in the retropalatal segment.[19] Sites and areas of obstruction both differ among individuals and in the same individual during sleep and varying

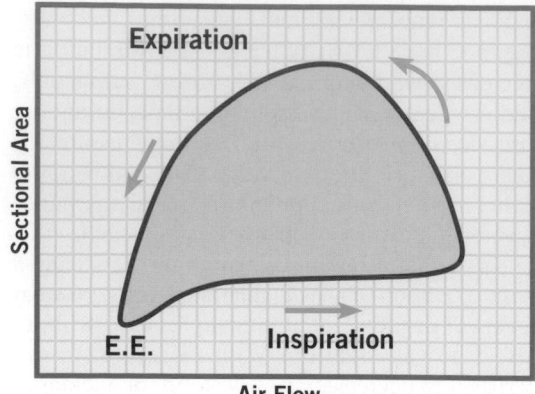

Figure 3 Effects of the ventilatory cycle on cross-sectional area is shown. During inspiration, activation of phasic airway dilator muscles increases airway size but is countered by increasing negative pressure. Early expiration is associated with loss of negative luminal pressure, addition of positive pressure, and loss of phasic muscle dilation resulting in additional increases in airway size. In later expiration, the airway collapses and is associated with loss of muscle tone, decreased "tracheal tug" and lung volume, and decreased positive pressure. At end expiration (EE), the airway is at its smallest and most vulnerable to obstruction.

body position and sleep state. Studies suggest that an isolated palatal level of obstruction occurs in approximately 20% of adults with hypopharyngeal obstruction occurring alone in another 10%. Combined levels of obstruction occur in 70% or more.

Sleep

Fatigue, hunger, and thirst are universal human experiences, and sleep, food, and drink are universal human requirements. Without them in sufficient quantity and quality, life and health cannot be maintained. Disorders of sleep are related to significant economic costs.[20] Sleep is composed of two distinct states: rapid eye movement (REM) and non-REM sleep. Sleep is actively generated within the brain and is regulated by both homeostatic and circadian processes. Inadequate sleep results in the primary symptom of hypersomnolence, excessive daytime sleepiness (EDS).

Sleep Stages. In clinical practice, these states are arbitrarily defined using electroencephalography (EEG), electrooculography, and electromyography. REM and non-REM sleep have multiple physiological differences and differ from each other as much as from wakefulness. The restorative nature of sleep is determined by the duration of sleep, the pattern of the sleep cycle, and sleep continuity. Abnormalities in these, by intrinsic or extrinsic factors, disrupt homeostatic sleep and lead to EDS.

Sleepiness is the result of the homeostatic sleep drive (process S) and the "biological clock" (process C) interacting with extrinsic and intrinsic sleep factors to create a level of wake and sleepiness. Intrinsic medical disorders include sleep apnea, limb movement disorders, narcolepsy, and other sleep-related disease. The homeostatic sleep drive is the biologic drive to sleep resulting from prolonged wakefulness. In the late afternoon, the homeostatic drive to sleep is countered by the circadian drive that increases and promotes wakefulness. Disorders such as jet lag, sleep phase advancement, and sleep phase delay result from mismatch of circadian rhythm and sleep homeostasis. Lack of adequate sleep increases "sleep debt." Sleep decreases homeostatic sleep drive. If sleep is adequate in duration (approximately 8 h in adults) and quality, process S sleepiness is normalized. Following normal sleep, upon awakening, an individual should feel refreshed and sleepiness should be absent. During periods of wakefulness, sleepiness indicates that sleep drive is increased.

Unless countered, this sleep drive (process S) would rapidly result in an overwhelming drive to sleep. Activation of the circadian rhythm counters the sleep drive. The circadian rhythm is an oscillating biologic rhythm of approximately one day's length. The circadian drive is a wakefulness promoter and counters sleepiness. The circadian rhythm originates from a small group of neurons in the suprachiasmatic nucleus and is reprogrammed (entrained) every day by external time stimulants (zeitbigers). The most important of these is exposure to bright light.

Sleep Stages: Rapid Eye Movement and Non-rapid Eye Movement. Sleep is divided into REM and non-REM sleep states. Non-REM is further divided into multiple sleep stages. The progression of non-REM through REM sleep stages is referred to as the sleep cycle, and progression through different sleep stages repeats several times during a sleep period. REM periods cycle approximately every 90 minutes after sleep onset. Each REM period usually becomes longer during sleep resulting in greater amounts of REM in the second half of the night. Often sleep is terminated following the last REM of the sleep cycle. Electroencephalographically, the brain is active during REM sleep. It is more similar to wake than non-REM sleep. Eye movements have a characteristic rapid oscillating pattern (REM). There is virtual paralysis of skeletal (but not diaphragm or eye) muscles, decreased arousal threshold, loss of temperature regulation, more vivid dreaming, nocturnal penile tumescence, and autonomic instability with both hyperventilation and hypoventilation, and fluctuating heart rate and blood pressure. Loss of skeletal muscle tone contributes to increased airway collapse in REM compared to non-REM sleep. The combination of decreased muscle tone which also reduces the lungs FRC, and longer apneas from a change in arousal may result in markedly worse oxygen desaturations during REM sleep. For this reason, it is important to assess sleep apnea severity and treatment success accurately and to observe REM sleep during sleep diagnostic testing.

REM latency is the time to the onset of the first REM and is usually 90 minutes in middle-aged adults. REM latency is shortened following withdrawal of REM suppressant drugs (such as alcohol), in depression and intrinsic sleep disorders, in certain cases of circadian sleep disorders (jet lag, shift work), and following acute resolution of severe sleep fragmentation (such as occurs with severe sleep apnea). Sudden and transient increase in REM sleep duration may occur (REM rebound). If significant underlying lung or cardiac disease is present, REM mediated hypoventilation may occur. REM-related sleep apnea is worse in the second half of sleep.

Non-REM sleep predominates adult sleep (75 to 80%) and is divided into four stages (I, II, III, and IV). Brain activity, respiratory rate, heart rate, and arousal thresholds are decreased in non-REM sleep. Muscle tone to the upper-airway muscles is present but is decreased. Sensitivity to CO_2 is decreased, resulting in decreased ventilation and slight hypercarbia during non-REM sleep.

Stage I sleep (5 to 10% normal sleep) is a transitional sleep. Patients awoken in stage I may actually describe a drowsy wakefulness and deny sleep. Stage I is increased by disorders that fragment sleep or when sleeping in an unfamiliar environment (first night effect in the sleep laboratory). Stage II, is a consolidated sleep and comprises 40 to 50% of total sleep time. Spontaneous arousals are less frequent than in stage I. The EEG is a synchronized low frequency low voltage signal marked by sleep spindles and K complexes. Stage III and IV sleep, referred to as slow-wave sleep due to the presence of low frequency high voltage waves on the EEG, contributes less than 10% of adult sleep time. Slow-wave sleep represents the most consolidated non-REM sleep. It may be this association rather than the absolute level of slow-wave sleep that links it to the refreshing quality of sleep. Stage III and IV sleep is necessary for the secretion of growth hormones during sleep and decreases with aging. In addition, stage III and IV sleep is reduced with sleep apnea and most disorders that disrupt sleep.

Sleep efficiency (total sleep/total time in bed ×100, expressed as a percent) decreases with age, insomnia, or any condition that impairs initiating or maintaining sleep. Sleep latency is shortened in sleepy individuals. Arousals are transient awakenings (3 to 15 seconds) during sleep. Arousals may be spontaneous but are often the result of an external environmental stimulus such as noise, apneic event, periodic leg movement, or stimulus to swallow. Arousals fragment normal sleep and increase the amount of lighter stages of sleep. Sleep fragmentation may also occur with aging, alcohol, and drugs.

POLYSOMNOGRAPHY

The goals of sleep testing are to (1) establish the correct diagnosis, (2) establish disease severity, and (3) initiate or direct appropriate treatment. Evaluation of sleep with overnight polysomnography is the consensus standard of comparison. It may measure sleep, respiration, leg movements, esophageal pH, video, and other physiologic parameters in a technician attended environment. The complexity of testing varies with some studies done nonattended, and others only measuring limited cardiorespiratory signals. Polysomnography is primarily indicated for the diagnosis of sleep-disordered breathing. Many sleep disorders are diagnosed by careful history and physical examination.

Respiratory Events

Ventilatory events are classified into three basic physiologic types: obstructive, central, or mixed apneas based on respiratory effort and airflow (Figure 4). Apneas (complete loss of airflow) and hypopneas (partial decrease in airflow) must last at least 10 seconds in adults. Events in which airflow is reduced and effort continues imply upper-airway obstruction. Central events are characterized by no measured respiratory effort. Mixed events demonstrate an initial central component followed by an obstructive component. These are a variant of obstructive apnea. Although the definition of physiologic apnea is conceptually straightforward, the pathologic process is more complex.

The initial manifestations of obstructive apnea include snoring, hypoxemia, asphyxia, and arousal. Increasing ventilatory effort trigger arousals and not the associated hypoxemia. Since central apneas have no ventilatory effort, arousals do not occur unless asphyxia is extreme. Hypopneas may be central or obstructive and are variably defined.[21] Common criteria include a 30% decrease in airflow and a 4% oxygen desaturation. Definitions incorporating 3%, 2%, 1%, or no desaturations with or without an associated EEG arousal are also used. Multiple methods of measuring effort are used including strain gauges, electrical impedance, or even esophageal pressures which measure intrathoracic pleural pressures. Some hypopneas have been classified into a separate category. Respiratory-related arousals demonstrate some indication of obstructed breathing but are not apneas, hypopneas, and may not demonstrate oxygen desaturations.[22]

The AI is the number of apnea events/h of sleep and when combined with the hypopnea index results in the AHI which is the most common metric used to describe disease severity. The respiratory disturbance index includes the AHI and respiratory-related arousals.

The prevalence sleep-disordered breathing varies age, gender, and population studied. Consensus has defined a normal AHI for the adult population as less than five events/h and in children as an index of less than one event/h. Although widely applied, these thresholds are arbitrary; and, given the changing methods and definitions of polysomnography and improving understanding of sleep apnea, may not accurately define abnormality. An AHI of less than 15 events/h is likely mild apnea, 15 to 30 events/h defines moderate apnea, and greater than 30 events/h currently defines severe OSA. However, the AHI is an imprecise metric of severity. These thresholds are likely better descriptors of epidemiologic prevalence and may not describe actual sleep apnea morbidity. In children, an AI of one is considered abnormal. Defined events are only a marker of blockage to breathing in this population, and various more sensitive techniques may identify aberrations including abnormal capnography, flow limitation with arousals, and abnormal esophageal pressure measurements.[23]

Oxygen desaturation with events is primarily affected by obesity (altering FRC and total body oxygen stores) and the duration of events. Desaturation is independent of AHI. Other contributing factors to desaturation include underlying pulmonary disease, pulmonary hypertension, pulmonary or arterial venous vascular shunts, patent foramen ovale, or ductus arteriosus. Desaturation unexplained by length of events or obesity may warrant further evaluation for these diseases. Desaturations below 60% have been associated with severe cardiac dysrhythmias.

Accurate interpretation of sleep study results requires knowledge of: (1) the methods of measurement and the parameters monitored, (2) the duration and time of day of the study, (3) sleep quality including presence or absence of sleep, sleep stages, REM latency, and sleep efficiency, (4) baseline and minimal oxygen saturation levels, (5) apneic events, and relationship of ventilatory events to REM/non-REM sleep and body position, (6) cardiac rate and rhythm, (7) limb and motor movements, and (8) patients clinical presentation. No single number such as the AHI is adequate. Sleep-disordered breathing and apnea are widespread in the population, and they often coexist with other disease.

The diagnosis of OSA does not require traditional measures of sleep. Testing of sleep for breathing disorders may be done by measuring different physiologic metrics without sleep.[24] The use of polysomnography should be to obtain the best available information to care for patients. Limited sleep testing is not a standardized method and may measure different physiologic variables and measure them with different tools. Comparison of devices is often biased and is influenced by multiple factors including risk of disease in the population studied, arbitrary AHI thresholds, and the testing environment. How well these exclude apnea in lower-risk patient groups or determine accurate disease severity is uncertain. For example, pulse oximetry may demonstrate a high false-negative rate of up to 30%. Many devices may function to identify a threshold of five or 15 events/h in normal or severe apnea populations but may be an inaccurate guide to severity (a measure that may be more critical to surgically treated patients than to medically treated patients). Using these tools to make clinical decisions requires an understanding of the device in use.

Split-Night Polysomnography

Some diagnostic sleep studies are performed and followed by a therapeutic study for nasal CPAP titration. A split-night diagnostic and therapeutic sleep study permits the diagnosis of OSA and a trial of nasal CPAP in a single night of testing. This approach is successful in titrating nasal CPAP in up to 78% of patients. Split-night studies save resources, expense, and patient time but may underestimate necessary CPAP pressures in mild sleep apnea without observed REM sleep (when apnea may be more severe and require higher pressures). Split-night studies have become a standard of care but may be inadequate for some patients.

HYPERSOMNOLENCE/SLEEPINESS

Sleepiness is a cardinal symptom of many sleep disorders. It is variably defined with subjective sleepiness described as a state of fatigue, tiredness, personality changes, increased automatic behavior, impairment in executive functioning, decreased motor skills, and lack of alertness. Acute and chronic sleepiness may present differently due to chronic adaptation. Impaired perception, environment, age, gender, and behavior modification all affect symptoms, and directed questioning about symptoms in passive activities requiring sustained attention may be needed.

Sleepiness may also be described by the propensity to fall asleep, propensity to stay awake, or vigilance. Sleepiness may be subjectively or objectively measured.[25] The Epworth sleepiness scale was developed as a population measure (Table 2). The propensity or tendency to fall asleep is objectively measured by the multiple sleep latency test (MSLT). This test is a series of five scheduled daytime naps with latency to

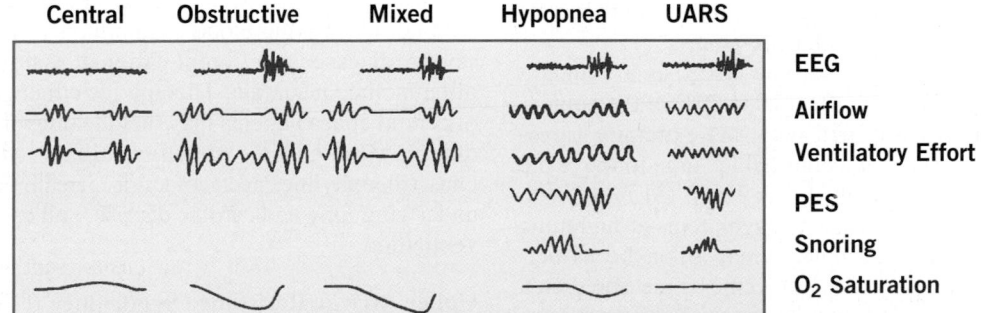

Figure 4 Diagram of ventilatory events during sleep is depicted. Apnea is defined by airflow, and central and mixed apneas are further defined by ventilatory effort. Using traditional sleep study methods, changes in effort may not be appreciated, and more sensitive methods, such as esophageal pressure (PES), have been used to define other sleep disordered breathing events. Hypopneas have variably defined reductions in airflow (30 to 50%) with or without oxygen desaturations (or arousals). RERA (respiratory-related arousals) have no defined change in measured airflow or oxygen desaturation but are associated with crescendo snoring, increased effort and arousal. Common snoring findings and oxygen desaturation patterns are also depicted for events. UARS = upper airway resistance syndrome.

Table 2 The Epworth Sleepiness Score*

Activity	No Chance of Dozing	Slight Chance of Dozing	Moderate Chance of Dozing	High Chance of Dozing
Sitting and reading	0	1	2	3
Watching television	0	1	2	3
Sitting inactive in a public place	0	1	2	3
As a passenger in a car for an hour without a break	0	1	2	3
Lying down in the afternoon when circumstances permit	0	1	2	3
Sitting and talking to someone	0	1	2	3
Sitting quietly after lunch without alcohol	0	1	2	3
In a car, while stopped for a few minutes in traffic	0	1	2	3
Total				

*This evaluation has eight domains and are self-reported by the patient. An Epworth sleepiness score (ESS) score of greater than 10 is often considered abnormal; however, there is a wide range of variability and overlap among individuals. Scores of greater than 15 are definitely abnormal and scores of 5 or less are likely normal.

stage I sleep (and REM latency) measured. A sleep latency of less than 8 minutes indicates marked sleepiness equivalent to narcoleptics. Nonpathologic is greater than 10 minutes with normal greater than that. REM sleep during two naps is considered diagnostic of narcolepsy if no other sleep disorder is present (sleep deprivation, severe OSA, sleep phase delay). MSLT is usually indicated to diagnose narcolepsy or if daytime sleepiness needs to be evaluated objectively (such as commercial drivers). An alternative method of assessing sleepiness is the maintenance of wakefulness test. This test measures the propensity to stay awake by asking the patient to stay awake lying down in a quiet darkened room for 20 or 40 minute nap periods. Acceptable values are greater than 20 minutes. Normal values vary by laboratory and locality.

DISORDERS OF SLEEP

Snoring and sleep apnea are common reasons to seek medical care due to concerns about snoring, sleepiness, risks of hypertension, and cardiovascular disease, but patients presenting with these complaints are at risk of other sleep disorders as well. Thirty-one to fifty-five percent of individuals undergoing polysomnography are diagnosed with other sleep disorders. The actual prevalence is likely higher.

Hypersomnolence is not unique to OSA. Sleep deprivation and insomnia are common. Insomnia is the complaint of inadequate or poor-quality sleep and has variable presentation including EDS, difficulty falling asleep or maintaining sleep. Insomnia may be classified as primary, acute situational, secondary to medical, chronic psychiatric, or other causes. Insomnia or anxiety complicates medical treatment of sleep-disordered breathing and may coexist with snoring and OSA.

Narcolepsy is uncommon but not rare (prevalence similar to multiple sclerosis) presenting with symptoms of excessive daytime somnolence and with a possible quadruplet of classic symptoms. These include sleep attacks, cataplexy (a sudden, brief loss of muscle tone with extreme emotion or laughter that is virtually pathognomonic for narcolepsy), sleep paralysis, and hypnagogic/hypnopompic hallucinations (vivid dreams intruding into wakefulness). These symptoms conceptually represent intrusion of REM-related phenomena into wakefulness. Sleep paralysis and hypnagogic hallucinations may occur independently or with other disorders with severe sleepiness, namely obstructive sleep apnea syndrome (OSAS) or sleep deprivation. In narcolepsy, a short nap often refreshes in contrast to severe OSAS in which a nap is minimally refreshing. Symptoms onset for narcolepsy is common in late adolescence or early adulthood. Narcolepsy may be familial. The HLA-DBQ12 antigen is more common in some but not all populations of narcoleptics. Decreased cerebrospinal fluid levels of the neuropeptide hypocretin has been observed. Classic symptoms including cataplexy are diagnostic for narcolepsy. In cataplexy-negative cases, MSLT may be used. Treatment includes stimulant medications, behavioral modification, prophylactic naps (for EDS), and tricyclic antidepressants, serotonin reuptake inhibitors, or gabahydroxybuturate for cataplexy. Narcoleptics commonly also manifest other disorders sleep including sleep apnea, limb movements, insomnia, and depression.

Restless leg syndrome (RLS) is a common disorder that may affect 10 to 20% of the population. It is associated with: (1) extremity paresthesias, (2) an "uncontrollable" urge to move the extremities (usually lower legs), (3) relief with movement, (4) worsened symptoms at nighttime (circadian linked). RLS may often be associated with periodic leg movements measured on a sleep study. RLS may be associated with insomnia or hypersomnia. The cause of the disorder is a central nervous system loss of descending inhibition of a spinal motor neuron activity; the inhibition is mediated through dopaminergic neurons. It has been associated with decreased transport of iron across the blood-brain barrier. Iron is a necessary cofactor in dopamine metabolism (dopamine decarboxylase). RLS is more common in the elderly as it is associated with symptoms of insomnia. A familial form also occurs often in younger individuals and is more often associated with hypersomnolence. Periodic limb movement disorder (PLMD) presents with repetitive stereotypical flexion extension movements during sleep that are 5 to 90 seconds apart with or without arousals and sleep fragmentation. PLMD often occurs independently of RLS and is often asymptomatic and does not require treatment. Due to the association with iron transport, RLS and PLMD warrant screening for anemia and iron replacement may be beneficial, especially if ferritin levels are low or low normal (45 µg/mL). Drug therapy may include dopaminergic agonist drugs, opioids, benzodiazepams, or gabapentin. These either act directly on dopamine centers or help consolidate sleep and reduce insomnia. Both disorders are worsened with caffeine and alcohol.

Multiple drugs (beta blockers), alcohol, and sedatives contribute to sleepiness. Some disrupt sleep architecture and decrease respiratory muscle tone (worsening upper-airway patency and sleep apnea). Regular snorers may convert to apnea, and apnea may become more severe. Sedatives may dangerously decrease arousal thresholds and increase event duration, elevating CO_2 levels and worsening of oxygen desaturation during apneic events.

Central Sleep Apnea

Central sleep apnea syndromes are uncommon. Central sleep apnea may be idiopathic or secondary to congestive heart failure, brainstem lesions, or high altitude. Central sleep apnea often has two presentations based on daytime blood gases. Patients who hypoventilate during wakefulness may present with symptoms of morning headaches and sleepiness. Respiratory failure and cor pulmonale occur. Obesity hypoventilation, neuromuscular weakness, abnormal chest wall compliance, or primary alveolar hypoventilation may be present. Ondine curse is a severe central sleep apnea syndrome that features normal ventilation during wakefulness but apnea and hypoventilation with sleep onset. Central sleep apnea patients with normal waking blood gas findings have less severe disease and complications. Symptoms often include insomnia. Therapy for either group of central apnea patients may include bilevel ventilation, nasal CPAP, oxygen, ventilatory stimulants (theophyline, acetazolamide), treatment of underlying lung and cardiac disease, and assisted ventilation.

Upper Airway Resistance Syndrome

Upper airway resistance syndrome (UARS) is associated with increased ventilatory effort, arousal, sleep fragmentation, and symptoms of EDS. Apneas and hypopneas are not present with increased upper-airway resistance during sleep causing the clinical symptoms. UARS is associated with smaller upper airways and elevated upper-airway resistance compared to normals. Resistance is equal to those who snore suggesting the primary pathology is closely linked with a lower arousal threshold which makes the individual more prone to sleep disruption.

Snoring

Snoring is a form of a Starling resistor. When negative inspiratory pressure exceeds the closing pressure of the airway wall, the airway collapses. The closed upper airway is then exposed to the pressure of the nasopharynx or oral cavity that is greater than the closing pressure, opening the airway. When the process oscillates, flutter results and creates snoring. Vibratory tissues may include the palate, uvula, and lateral pharyngeal walls or less commonly from the lower oropharynx or epiglottis. The noise is low frequency (50 to 1,000 Hz); and the acoustic characteristics are determined primarily by the stiffness of pharyngeal tissues. Snoring has been shown to be an independent contributor to sleepiness and in epidemiologic studies has been associated with increased risks of strokes and other morbidity.

When circadian drive begins to decrease in the evening, sleepiness increases, and the likelihood of falling asleep (propensity to sleep) increases. Sleep onset usually occurs while this drive decreases. The circadian drive is linked to core body temperature, and both are lowest in the early morning (acrophase is about 1 hour prior to awakening). It is at this time of day that the impact of a residual sleep debt (Process S) is greatest. The incidence of sleep-related motor vehicle accidents increases at this time.

UPPER AIRWAY EVALUATION

Upper airway evaluation identifies structural abnormalities contributing to snoring and sleep apnea. It identifies patients at risk and those who might benefit from surgery and provides information needed for selecting appropriate surgical procedures. Little data compares methods of evaluation. Fujita defined three types of upper-airway obstruction (Figure 5). These included: Type I, upper pharyngeal obstruction at the palate; Type II, combined upper pharyngeal and base of the tongue at the palate and the base of the tongue; and Type III, hypopharyngeal or base of the tongue. Moore developed a base of the tongue classification initially based on cephalometry but also useful with endoscopy that defines three general patterns of hypopharyngeal narrowing (Figure 6). Although conceptually useful, neither has been validated. Cephalometry has not been utilized clinically to screen for patients and has limited use in selecting individuals for palatopharyngoplasty. An inferiorly positioned hyoid bone (MP-H [cephalometric measurement from the plane of the mandible to the most anterior and superior point on the body of the hyoid bone] greater than 21 mm) had been associated with poor palatopharyngoplasty results. The Mallam-

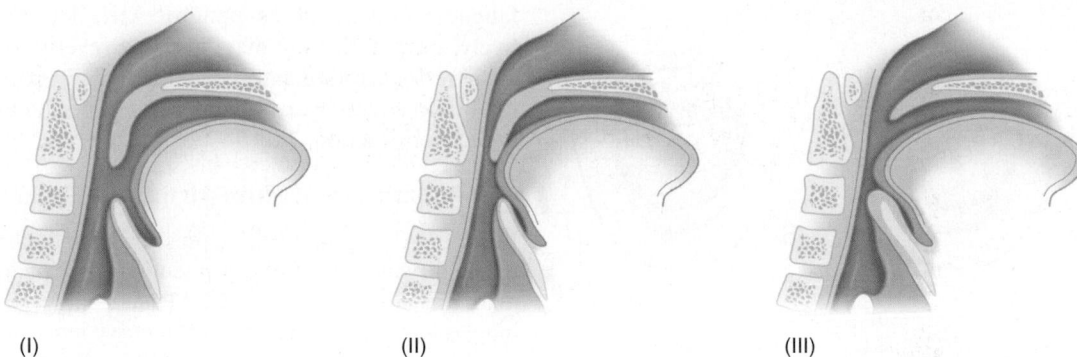

Figure 5 Fujita classification is shown demonstrating Type I, upper pharyngeal obstruction, Type II, combined upper pharyngeal and base of tongue obstruction, and Type III, hypopharyngeal or base of tongue obstruction (Type III).

pati classification is most widely used (Figure 7). As the patient opens the mouth as widely as possible without protruding the tongue, in Type I the palliative tonsils, uvula, and free margin of the palate can be seen; in Type II, the free margin of the soft palate and the base of the uvula are visible, in Type III, the soft palate but not its free margin is seen; and in Type IV, only the hard palate is in view.

Müller Maneuver

The Müller maneuver is used widely to predict UPPP success. It is a reverse Valsalva maneuver performed with a fiberoptic scope visualizing the pharynx. At end expiration, the patient inspires against a closed mouth and nares and airway collapse is subjectively or objectively assessed. Although retrospective studies suggested that collapse in the hypopharyngeal region of less than 25% was associated with improved UPPP outcomes, prospective studies have not confirmed this.[26] The Müller maneuver has little positive predictive value. Collapse of the airway on the Müller maneuver of greater than 50% at the base of the tongue is a negative predictor for UPPP success (5 to 10%). Physiologically, the Müller maneuver fails to correlate with manometry or endoscopy during sleep. The Müller maneuver does not relate anatomy or structure, and no data suggest it is useful in predicting outcomes of any procedure except UPPP failure.

Friedman Staging

The Friedman staging system defines three stages based on: (1) tonsil size (1 to 4+), (2) a modifi-

cation of the Mallampati classification (1 to 4+, see Figure 7), (3) presence or absence of severe obesity (> or < BMI [body mass index] of 40 kg/M²), and (4) major craniofacial abnormalities.[27] The Friedman staging system identifies patients at risk for apnea who present with symptoms of snoring. It also demonstrates both positive and negative predictive value with UPPP outcomes.

Friedman staging groups tonsil size as "favorable" (tonsil grades 3 and 4, large tonsils) or "unfavorable" (tonsil grades 1 and 2, small tonsils). The modified Mallampati classification is "favorable" (Types I and II, visualizing the free margin of the soft palate) and "unfavorable" (Types III and IV, free margin of palate not visible) on examination (Figure 7).

MEDICAL TREATMENT OF OBSTRUCTIVE SLEEP APNEA SYNDROME

Treatment objectives of OSAS include (1) elimination of obstruction and snoring, (2) decreasing morbidity (cardiovascular and sleep), and (3) decreasing mortality. Treatment is dependent on OSAS severity, the desired outcome, and confounding medical conditions. No single treatment is appropriate for all patients. Treatment interventions include: elimination or amelioration predisposing factors, attention to medical causes, and use of drugs, nasal CPAP, oral appliances, and reconstructive surgery.

Positional therapy, weight loss, sleep hygiene, nasal interventions, avoiding sedatives and alcohol, increasing exercise, and smoking cessation

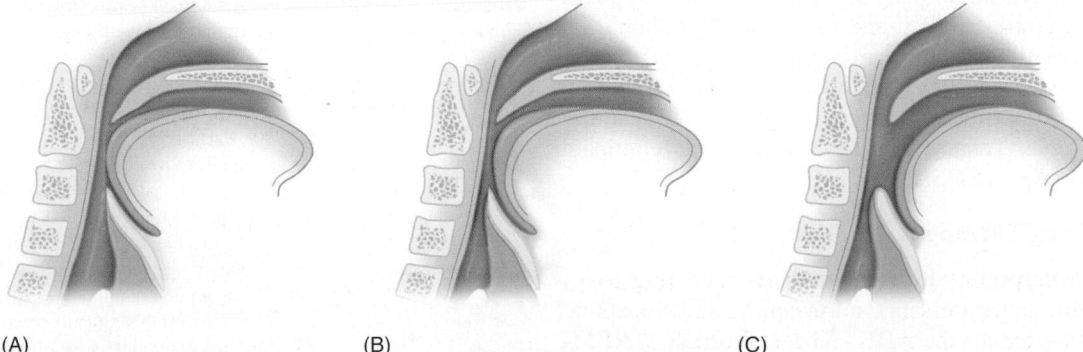

Figure 6 Moore tongue classification. This classification has three general patterns of hypopharyngeal obstruction. (A) Proximal. (B) Combined and retroepiglottic. (C) Retroepiglottic obstruction.

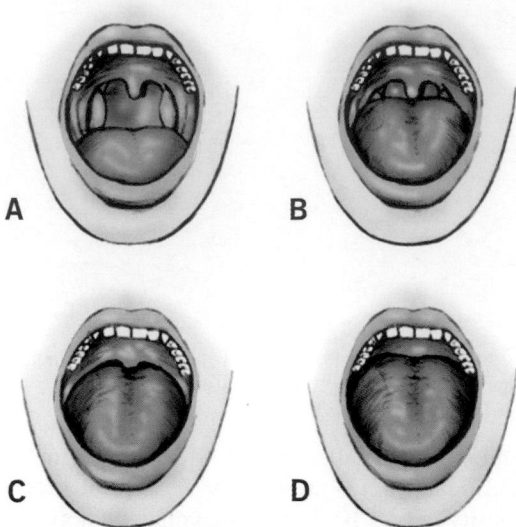

Figure 7 Modified Mallampati classification. The method is performed with the patient leaving the tongue in the mouth (not protruding) and can be repeated for consistency. (A) In Type I, the palatine tonsils, uvula and free margin of the palate are readily visible. (B) In Type II, the free margin of the soft palate and the base of uvula are only visible. (C) In Type III, the soft palate is visible but the free margin of the palate is not visible. (D) In Type IV, neither the soft palate or free margin of the soft palate are visible and only the hard palate can be seen. Modified Mallampati most commonly reflects differences in tongue size and not palatal length.

may be used. Elevating the head of bed may be a critical intervention for OSA; and, for snoring, lateral (on the side) sleeping may be helpful. A multitude of snore pillows, alarms, or proprietary mechanical devices have been described to assist in side sleeping, but therapy is undependable.

Behavioral weight loss is seldom successful in long-term treatment of OSA (less than 3%). Nonetheless, weight control is vital to prevent worsening or recurrence of OSA. Bariatric surgery may be a successful apnea treatment. However, OSA may recur even in patients who do not regain weight, and long-term follow-up is needed.

Medical Causes and Treatment

Hypothyroidism, Marfan syndrome, acromegaly, and congestive heart failure may contribute to OSAS in a small subset of patients. Routine laboratory screening for these conditions without symptoms has no role. Treatment of them may reduce OSA, and these disorders should be considered in appropriate patients. Heart failure may not only become worse with OSA but may also contribute to it by making periodic breathing worse. Treatment of heart failure may eliminate or improve OSA.

Drug Therapy

Protryptyline hydrochloride (nonsedating tricyclic antidepressant), mirtazapine, and fluoxetine may reduce the AHI.[28] These also reduce REM-related apnea by decreasing REM sleep. Antidepressants may independently reduce daytime

fatigue even without lessening of AHI. Alternatively, oxygen therapy may diminish severity of oxygen desaturation and reduce periodic breathing in some individuals but does not correct anatomical obstruction.

Nasal Continuous Positive Airway Pressure

Nasal CPAP applies positive pressure to open the upper airway acting like a pneumatic splint to maintain airway patency. CPAP also increases lung volume (potentially improving oxygen saturation) and reduces tone to upper-airway muscles at therapeutic pressures. Variants of nasal CPAP are available to address specific patient needs or preferences (Table 3). CPAP levels may vary depending on sleep state, body weight, head and body position, nasal patency, and sedative use. The effective pressure to prevent collapse is pressure applied during expiration when the airway is most vulnerable to collapse. CPAP pressure is most often individually titrated in the sleep laboratory by a technician with occasional empiric adjustments as symptoms and signs warrant (persistent snoring, sleepiness, movement, worsened central apnea, etc).

Nasal CPAP objectively reduces the respiratory disturbance, EDS, hypertension, and other morbidity associated with OSA.[29] However, even a single night without the use of nasal CPAP may result in worsening of many of the symptoms and daytime sleepiness of OSAS. Rarely is it associated with severe complications. CPAP use requires a correct pressure setting, a comfortable mask, tolerance, and patient compliance. It is common to refit masks; change heated and cool humidification; add chin straps, nasal prongs, or better-fitting face masks to improve use. Nasal CPAP may contribute to rhinitis, nasal obstruction, mask discomfort and leak, excessive pressures, claustrophobia, eustachian tube dysfunction, and noise.

Clinical effectiveness requires nightly use. Many factors influence patient tolerance and compliance. Verbal reports of compliance range from 50 to 70%. Objective studies demonstrate lower compliance rates. Although 70% of patients utilize CPAP for 20 minutes on five of seven nights (70%), only 50% of patients use CPAP for

4 hours a night. Patient compliance may be higher in patients with more severe disability.[30] Compliance patterns with CPAP are established early in the course of treatment and may be improved by regular encouragement from the physician. The pattern of use as early as 3 weeks has been correlated to subsequent compliance. Multiple evidence based studies have demonstrated CPAP effectiveness. Effectiveness is not universal and has not been established in patients with milder disease and in those without abnormal daytime sleepiness. Despite these limitations, nasal CPAP is widely considered first line therapy for OSAS in many adult patients.

Other Continuous Positive Airway Pressure Devices

Bilevel nasal CPAP is a device that applies a higher inspiratory than expiratory pressure with each independently adjusted. Changes in pressure are usually triggered by the patient's ventilatory efforts. Although initially advocated to improve CPAP use by lowering the sensation of expiratory load, this has not been demonstrated for most CPAP failures. Bilevel pressure is used primarily as a ventilatory device in individuals who hypoventilate during sleep or in other complex patients. Lower expiratory pressures may improve patient tolerance especially if pressure differences required are greater than 6 cm H_2O.

A variety of CPAP machines have been developed to minimize patient intolerance. Several types of variable pressure nasal CPAP machines exist. "Ramped" CPAP devices may start with low CPAP pressures, which gradually increase during sleep onset. Auto-titrating CPAP "smart machines" self-titrate the pressure based on the machine's constantly monitoring for signs of airway collapse or obstruction. Other variable pressure CPAP machines adjust the pressure across the ventilatory cycle so that pressure is dropped at the end of inspiration and the beginning of expiration, and it is increased for the end of expiration and the beginning of inspiration. While awake, these machines act to improve patient comfort and tolerance.

Table 3 Options for Continuous Positive Airway Pressure for Sleep-Disordered Breathing	
Nasal CPAP	Applies positive pressure to open the upper airway acting like a pneumatic splint to maintain airway patency
"Ramped" CPAP	Starts with low CPAP pressures and gradually increase during sleep onset
Auto-titrating CPAP	Self-titrates the pressure based on the machine's ability constantly to monitor for airway collapse or obstruction
Expiratory pressure relief and CPAP	Applies lower pressure at end inspiration and early expiration
Bilevel nasal CPAP	Applies a higher inspiratory than expiratory pressure with each independently adjusted by the patient's ventilatory efforts or may be set by clinician
Oral appliances	Mandibular repositioning devices use teeth to protrude mandible forward to open the airway. Tongue-retaining devices do not use dentition but use a suction bulb that pulls the tongue forward theoretically to open the airway. Both require enlarging the retropalatal and retroglossal airway for effectiveness for OSA

CPAP = continuous positive airway pressure.

Oral Appliances

Oral appliances are classed as mandibular repositioning devices or tongue-retaining devices.[31] They act effectively primarily by advancing the mandible forward and enlarging both the retropalatal and retroglossal airway. Individual clinical responses are variable, but a significant reduction in respiratory disturbance, snoring, and morbidity of OSA have been observed. Sixty to eighty percent of patients will note a decrease in snoring. Patient compliance is required for successful therapy. Adequate dentition is required for use. Some patients may report discomfort or changes in teeth, gums, and temporomandibular joints with their use.

SURGERY

Surgery to treat the patient with sleep apnea and snoring effectively reduces obstruction and collapse by (1) bypassing the upper airway, (2) reconstructing soft tissues, (3) reconstructing skeletal structure, or (4) augmenting the effects of other procedures. Multiple procedures have been described for sleep-disordered breathing (Table 4). Surgery indirectly treats sleep by improving ventilation via changing airway size, shape, or collapsibility. Successful responders are defined as having a 50% improvement in apnea or AHI. Unfortunately, scant data exist to define thresholds of OSAS.[33]

Anesthetic Considerations

Sleep apnea patients may have unique preoperative, intraoperative, and postoperative care problems.[32,33] Difficulty with intubation and extubation occurs related to facial structural or ventilatory control. High-risk patients include, but are not limited to, patients with severe obesity, poor pulmonary reserve, pharyngeal tissue redundancy, hypoxemia, excessive narcotic use, multiple airway surgical procedures, and excessive sleepiness.[34] Controversy exists as to the appropriateness of outpatient surgery and the need for intensive postoperative monitoring.[34] Postoperative management can be assisted in many cases with the use of nasal CPAP. Rarely

tracheostomy is required. Objective monitoring to include pulse oximetry has been advocated; however, it is critical to realize that oximetry does not measure hypoventilation especially when assessed on an intermittent basis or when low-flow oxygen is in use. Close nursing observation is necessary in the perioperative period. Symptoms of respiratory insufficiency and hypercarbia may include increased pulse and respiratory rate, elevated blood pressure, and agitation or restlessness. Studies suggest that stimulating environments of the hospital provide a degree of activity and that risk may increase in quiet and unobserved areas. Risk is elevated with sedation, dehydration (increasing tenacious secretions), and higher doses of narcotics. Postoperative interventions for apnea patients who have airway and nonairway surgery may include nasal airways, nasal CPAP, patient positioning (head of bed), adequate hydration, corticosteroids, and other nonnarcotic pain medication. Patients with sleep apnea are also at elevated risk due to significant comorbidities of hypertension, cardiac and pulmonary disease, and obesity.

Tracheostomy

Tracheostomy reduces the morbidity and mortality associated with sleep apnea. Obesity, a short neck, a low larynx, and the inability to extend the neck may make tracheostomy more difficult. To address wound problems, "skin-flap" tracheostomy techniques have been described, which include debulking fatty tissue to create an epithelialized stoma and reduce complications. Since the airway in wakefulness is patent, tracheostomies may be occluded during wakefulness and opened only during sleep. Due to the psychosocial implications, risks of stenosis, infection, and other potential complications, tracheostomy is often unacceptable. The procedure is indicated for severe OSAS, complicated airway management, perioperative airway safety and in patients too ill for other procedures or therapies.

Nasal Surgery

The nose contributes 70% of upper-airway resistance in adult humans and is a segment with the greatest upper-airway resistance during wake-

fulness. A patent nasal airway is important for successful medical and surgical treatment.[35] A paradox has been described; although nasal obstruction is a risk factor for OSA, treatment of it does not necessarily affect the risk. The paradox is at least partially explained by two factors. Symptomatic nasal obstruction is poorly correlated with abnormal resistance and structure, making correct diagnosis difficult. Additionally, many treatments applied for sleep apnea have been uni-dimensional, only partially addressing the nasal abnormality. Effective treatment of the nose for OSA requires accurate diagnosis and comprehensive treatment.

Understanding nasomaxillary development provides insight into treating the nasal airway in sleep apnea. In humans this development has consisted of progressive shortening of the nasal maxillary complex and elongation of the pharyngeal airway. A smaller maxilla narrowed the retromaxillary space but also reduced the volume of the nasal cavity. Population-based studies measurements associate a smaller maxilla with patients with sleep apnea. As the defining structure of sleep apnea, this small maxilla predisposes to chronic nasal abnormalities. The abnormality, therefore, in patients with sleep disordered breathing is not necessarily traditionally identified on clinical examination (such as septal deviation, polyps, markedly hypertrophic turbinates) but is a naturally small nasal cavity.

Tonsillectomy and Adenoidectomy

Adenotonsillectomy is the treatment of choice for OSA in children. Traditionally, it has been considered highly effective but with actual efficacy uncertain. In uncomplicated pediatric patients, meta-analysis of level 4 evidence (case series) demonstrated that tonsillectomy and adenoidectomy reduced AHI by an average of 13.9 events/h and normalized AHI in 80% of patients. Outcomes vary by population and are affected by airway and facial structure, obesity, nasal abnormalities, allergies, and underlying medical conditions.[36] Factors predictive of postoperative elevated AHI, in uncomplicated pediatric patients include enlarged inferior turbinates, deviated nasal septum, Mallampati Types of III and IV, and retropositioned mandibles. Persistent airway inflammatory disease has been identified in other groups and responds successfully to anti-inflammatory therapies including topical nasal corticosteroids and leukotriene inhibitors.[37] Adenotonsillectomy has demonstrated significant improvements in behavior and school performance independent of final AHI levels.[38]

Pediatric patients with sleep apnea may represent an at risk population for sleep apnea independent of hypertrophic tonsils and adenoids. Associated anatomical problems include disproportionate facial growth and development. Identifying and correcting these abnormalities while facial growth and development are still malleable may be critical. A family history of sleep apnea

Table 4 Selected Surgical Treatment Options for Sleep-Disordered Breathing	
	Surgical
Nose	Septoplasty, turbinate surgery, polypectomy, nasal valve repair
Nasopharynx	Adenoidectomy
Upper pharynx	Tonsillectomy, uvulopalatopharyngoplasty, uvulopalatoplasty, other palatopharyngoplasties
Lower pharynx	Midline glossectomy, lingualplasty, radiofrequency ablation
	Lingual tonsillectomy
	Epiglottoplasty and removal of obstructive supralaryngeal tissues
	Limited mandibular osteotomies and genioglossus advancement
	Inferior sagittal osteotomy
	Hyomandibular and hyolaryngeal suspension
	Suspension suture
Nonsegmental	Maxillomandibular advancement, bariatric surgery
Bypass upper airway	Tracheostomy

associated with findings of a high-arched palate, long faces, or retrognathic mandible may warrant orthodontic assessment and treatment to correct the airway independent of any dental problems. Ancillary treatment of facial growth, nasal structure, and nasal inflammatory disease is commonly needed in addition to tonsillectomy and adenoidectomy. These problems are discussed in Chapter 66, "Sleep Apnea in Children."

Removal of nonhypertrophic tonsils is generally ineffective in adults. Removal of tonsils in adults is commonly a part of other pharyngoplasty procedures.

Palatopharyngoplasty (Uvulopalatopharyngoplasty)

UPPP was first described by Fujita. The procedure removes distal soft palate, the faucial tonsils, uvula, and redundant mucosa from the anterior and posterior tonsillar pillars. The posterior pillar is then sutured anteriorly, and the mucosa is approximated. Multiple variations of the technique have been described. Effectiveness for sleep apnea is not related to symptomatic reduction in snoring, instead is associated with increases in pharyngeal airway size in the retropalatal airway segment. UPPP is generally combined with other surgical procedures to treat other airway sites. The procedure may be contraindicated in patients with velopharyngeal insufficiency (VPI), submucous cleft palate, or a nonpalatal level of obstruction and in patients whose speech or swallowing may be at special risk. Aggressive resection of the palate with UPPP techniques has demonstrated no improvement in success but does increase the risk of VPI. Side effects of UPPP include mucosal dryness, sensation of oropharyngeal tightness or phlegm, pharyngeal dysphagia, and severe postoperative pain. Velopharyngeal stenosis and insufficiency are rare but serious complications.

Both controlled and randomized studies demonstrate UPPP is effective in treating physiologic measures of sleep and respiration, quality of life, risk of motor vehicle accidents, cardiovascular risks, and mortality.

Failure of UPPP includes persistent obstruction at the retropalatal airway segment or obstruction in other pharyngeal airway sites.[39] More effective treatment of the palate with reconstructive procedures and with treatment of the hypopharynx improves outcomes.[40] Historical success rates of UPPP have included reduction in snoring in 90%, sleepiness in 84%, and reduction in AHI to less than 20 events/h in 30 to 40%. Using the Friedman staging system outcomes can be better stratified. (Stage 1 = 70% success, stage 2 = 40% success, and stage 3 = 10% success). Traditional UPPP is most useful in individuals with massive tissue redundancy of the pharynx that requires excision and enlarged tonsils. Avoidance of excessive removal of distal soft palate is important to prevent incompetence between the soft palate and tongue, worsening possible nasal CPAP tolerance by increasing possible mouth leak.

Complications and side effects of palatopharyngoplasty are common. Major complications are rare and include acute respiratory distress, VPI, rhinolalia, nasopharyngeal stenosis, and hemorrhage. Respiratory distress and fatality with UPPP are rare. Minor degrees of transient nasopharyngeal reflux are common but usually self-limiting (less than 6 months). Nasopharyngeal stenosis may be minimized by mucosal sparing surgery, avoiding simultaneous adenoidectomy and meticulous wound and surgical technique. Other more minor complications are more common and include impaired mucous clearing, sneezing, and abnormal pharyngeal sensations.

Reconstructive Palatopharyngoplasty

Several methods of UPPP and palatopharyngoplasty (PPP) have now been described and compared to more traditional methods using evidence-based medicine. These surgical techniques differ from traditional UPPP in reconstructing the soft and hard tissue framework of the palate and not modifying mucosa and tonsil. Described techniques include lateral pharyngoplasty, expansion sphincteroplasty, and palatal advancement. Lateral pharyngoplasty exposes and plicates the lateral pharyngeal wall muscles and superior constrictor proximal to the free margin of the soft palate.[41] The advancement is then covered with a laterally based palatal mucosal flap (Figure 8). Expansion sphincteroplasty exposes, isolates, and divides the palatopharyngeus muscle on the pharyngeal wall and uses this muscle as a sling to advance and open the soft palate and pharynx

(Figure 9). Palatal advancement removes distal hard palate to advance the soft palate anteriorly and superiorly (Figure 10).

Other Palatal Procedures

Multiple palatal procedures have been advocated to treat primary snoring. Most have shown short-term effectiveness. Since primary snoring is not an isolated disorder and may represent a benign point in time of a progressive upper-airway disease, conservative treatments with the least side effects and complications should be considered first, if possible.

Laser assisted uvulopalatoplasty (LAUP) using the carbon dioxide laser is hemostatic surgery of the palate and can be performed under local anesthesia.[42] The palate, velum, and uvula could be resected with healing by secondary intent. Two vertical trenches in the soft palate lateral to the uvula of variable width and length at free margin of the distal part of the soft palate are created and the uvula reduced. The operation may be single stage or "titrated" to improvement in snoring or appearance of velopharyngeal dysfunction. LAUP is associated with severe pain and common complaints of pharyngeal dryness. Serious complications are infrequent. Palatal scarring initially increases tension and reduces snoring but long-term data (5 years) suggest recurrence of snoring is common. Airway narrowing may occur and worsen sleep apnea. Effectiveness for sleep apnea has not been demonstrated in clinical trials. Alternatives to the use of lasers have also been described. Various

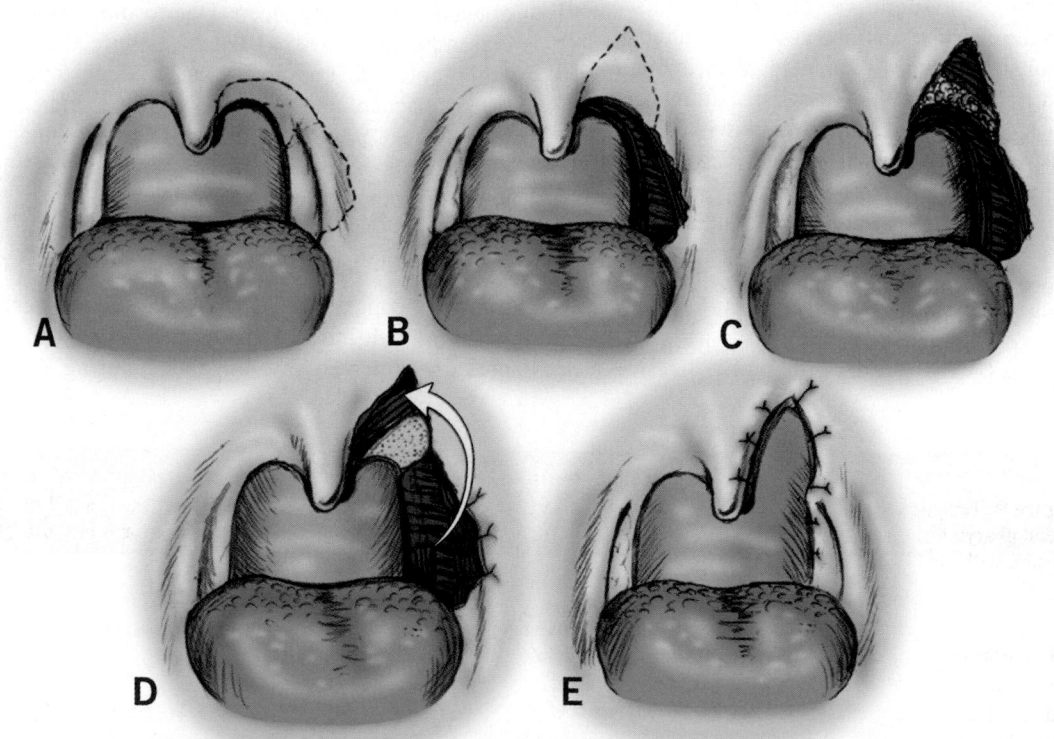

Figure 8 A method of a lateral pharyngeal wall flap is shown. This flap allows closure of lateral wall defect after advancement using mucosa from the dorsal palate. (A) and (B) A ventral triangle of mucosa, submucosal and periuvular fat is removed. (C) Dorsal palatal mucosa is left intact. (D) Dorsal mucosa is incised parallel to the uvula, that is, "uvula lengthening," to create a laterally based flap. (E) Final closure is shown.

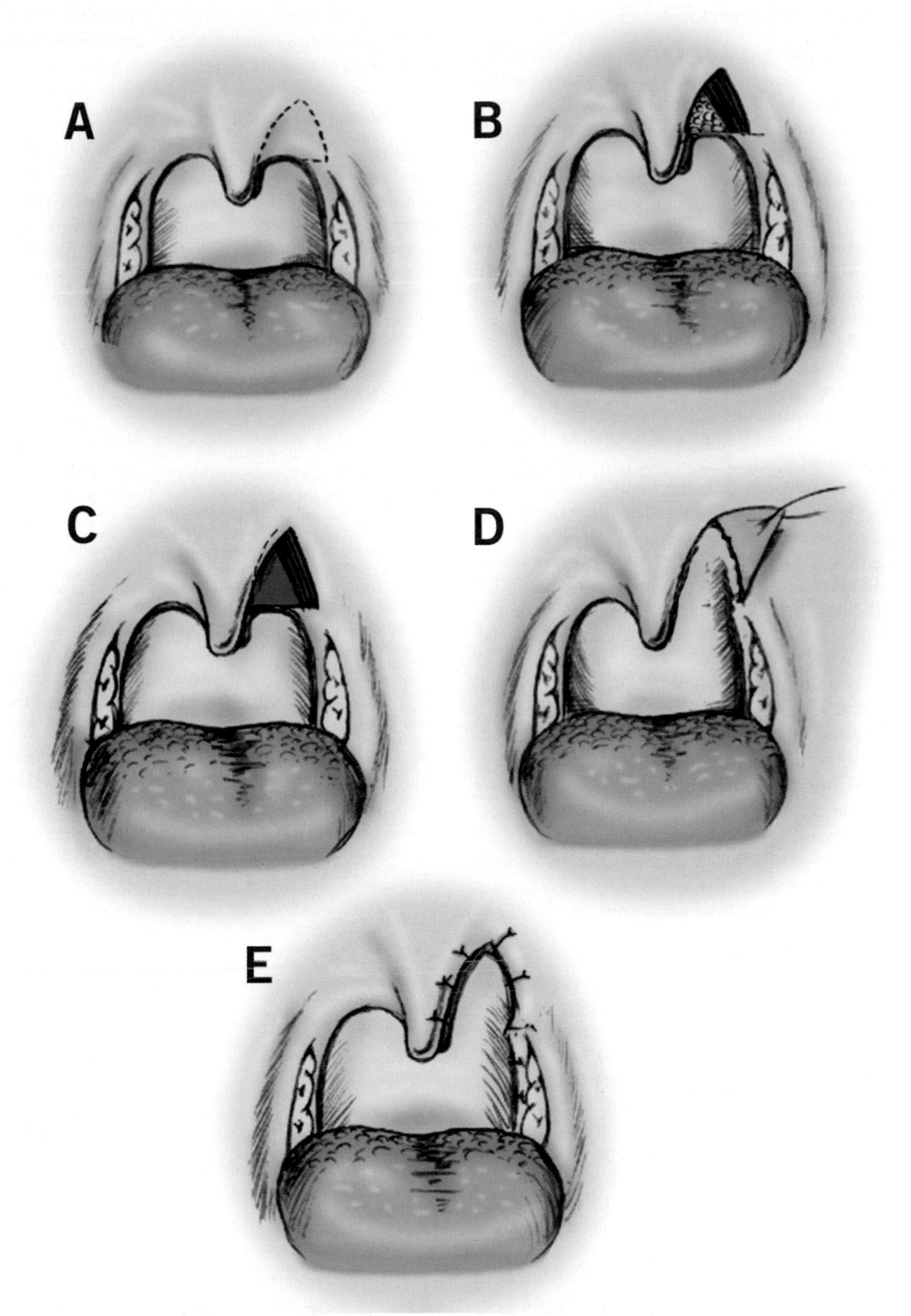

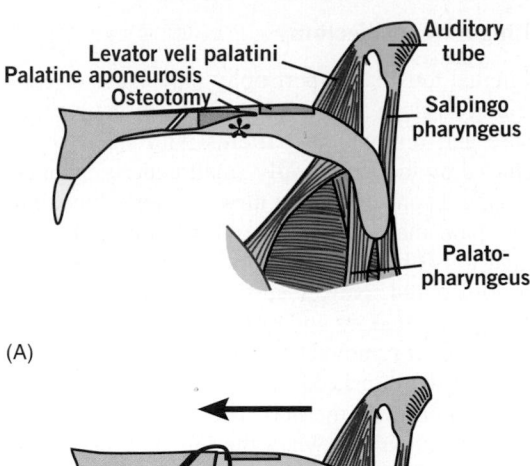

(A)

Figure 10 Diagram of palatal advancement pharyngoplasty. (A) A posterior osteotomy is performed (cross-hatched) leaving a 1 to 2 mm rim of bone. Proximal drill holes are placed in the hard palate lateral to septum and medial to the inferior turbinates. The osteotomy is separated from the posterior nasal septum and lateral tendinolysis is performed (not shown). (B) Sutures are placed through palatal drill holes and around the palatal osteotomy and and into the tensor aponeurosis laterally and the palate advanced enlarging the pharyngeal isthmus.

Figure 9 Technique of expansion sphincteroplasty. (A) through (C) The palatopharyngeus muscle is exposed on the lateral pharyngeal wall. (D) The muscle is then freed and rotated to pull the palate anteriorly, superiorly and laterally. (E) Closure with lateral pharyngoplasty flap is shown.

less expensive tools for cutting and ablation have been used to shorten the palate, remove mucosa, reduce the uvula and direct healing by secondary intension, and all likely create scar and reduce snoring with variable effectiveness. Failure may be from persistent flow limitation, softening of scar, or flutter at nonpalatal airway sites. All patients seeking snoring operations should be cautioned both about the risk of recurrence of snoring and the possible later development of overt sleep apnea.

To avoid the extensive thermal damage created by the laser to all three layers of the soft palate and chronic inflammation, ulceration, and loss of seromucinous glands, alternative approaches to create palatal stiffening have been developed. Techniques using ablational radiofrequency demonstrate less pain for treatment of snoring compared to the laser. Sclerotherapy agents create scar in the mucosa of the soft palate and have been used to treat patients with primary snoring.[43] Agents are injected into the submucosa of the soft palate creating scar and tissue slough. The procedure has less pain than laser, and long-term results for snoring are better than 70% with few major complications. Alternatively, palatal implants have been developed and are effective for the treatment of primary snoring, in selected populations

Base of Tongue Soft Tissue Techniques

Obstruction at the base of the tongue level is surgically challenging. Multiple techniques have been used.[44] These include partial glossectomy, ablational glossectomy, mandibular advancement, maxillary advancement, limited mandibular osteotomies, tongue suspension, hyoid suspension, lingual tonsillectomy, and supraglottoplasty.

Radiofrequency ablation of the base of the tongue can be performed in the office-based setting.[45] The procedure is performed under local or general anesthesia either alone or in combination with other pharyngeal procedures. Complications including tongue abscess, infection (cellulitis), tongue weakness, changes in speech and swallowing, and acute airway edema and obstruction are rare. Randomized, blinded, controlled, and uncontrolled studies of radiofrequency ablation have demonstrated effectiveness in reducing the severity and improving the disease specific quality of life. Effectiveness has also been demonstrated in longer-term studies. Alone these procedures rarely definitively relieve the patient of OSA and must be combined with other procedures that reconstruct other segments of the upper airway.

Lingual Tonsillectomy

Lingual tonsillar hypertrophy may cause or contribute to sleep apnea. Historically, difficult exposure and removal in patients with sleep apnea caused by the structurally small underlying anatomy and concerns about airway edema, bleeding, and pain made the threshold to remove the lingual tonsil high. Only in more severe cases was it considered. Newer surgical techniques combining endoscopes and excisional radiofrequency allow easier removal of lingual tonsil tissue. This reduces the threshold of removal and provides a lower morbidity method of enlarging the hypopharyngeal airway when the lingual tonsil is the cause of the problem.

Midline Glossectomy/Lingualplasty

Midline glossectomy and lingualplasty are partial glossectomies to enlarge the lower pharyngeal airway and treat OSA. In severe OSAS following UPPP failure, lingualplasty reduces AHI to less than 20 events/h in 70% of patients. Using laser, complication rates approach 25% and included bleeding, severe odynophagia, tongue edema, and taste changes. For this reason, more aggressive glossectomy techniques have been uncommonly performed. Because these procedures directly involve the airway in patients with preexisting airway risk, risk was considered high and a perioperative tracheostomy historically was often performed resulting in major morbidity for the procedure. Newer technologies allow aggressive glossectomy with atraumatic excision not requiring tracheostomy and even allowing outpatient surgery in selected patients (Figure 11).

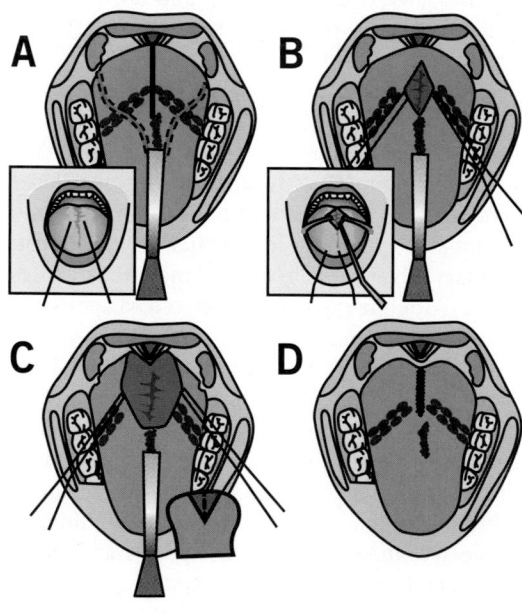

Figure 11 A method of posterior midline glossectomy is depicted. (A) A traction suture is placed, the location of midline incision is marked, and relative position of the lingual artery and the dorsum of the tongue is identified using ultrasound. (B) and (C) The midline incision is deepened and widened and carried back toward the valleculae. (D) Closure is shown.

Maxillofacial Surgery

Maxillofacial surgery for OSA is to enlarge the airway by advancing the skeletal support of the soft tissues which surrounds the airway. Maxillofacial operations with or without combined ancillary soft tissue procedures have been demonstrated to provide results of greater than 90% success even in obese populations.

Limited Mandibular Osteotomies and Genioglossus Advancement with Hyoid Myotomy. The anterior wall of the lower part of the pharynx is the tongue. The genioglossus and geniohyoid muscles and the hyoid bone contribute to determining the position of the tongue. By advancing the insertion of the genioglossus muscle, geniohyoid muscle, or hyoid bone, the characteristics of the tongue can be altered. Multiple osteotomy techniques to capture the genioglossus insertion and advance the genioglossus muscle have been described including a bicortical rectangular osteotomy of the mentum, sliding genioplasties, and split sliding ramus osteotomies. Osteotomies may alter dentition and innervation with paresthesias not uncommon. Major complications or tooth damage requiring restorative surgery, however, are rare.

Hyoid movement may stabilize the hypopharyngeal airway. The hyoid may be suspended anteriorly and superiorly to the mandible or anteriorly and inferiorly to the thyroid cartilage. Hyoid myotomy may be performed with other operations such as UPPP or genioglossal advancement. Hyoid myotomy is performed through neck skin incision. Fascia lata or suture may be used for mandibular suspension. Thyrohyoid suspension has been described with suture or wire. Controlled studies are lacking.

Mandibular and Bimaxillary Advancement. Mandibular advancement techniques may markedly enlarge the lower pharyngeal airway. Procedures have been described as "telegnathic" in contrast to traditional orthognathic surgery. Aggressive advancement is required in sleep apnea compared with orthodontic treatment. Dentition may limit advancement in traditional techniques, and orthodontic methods alone may be inadequate to maintain a normal bite. Maxillary advancement is then required. Cosmetic changes occur and may limit application.

Bimaxillary advancement is indicated in patients who have significant maxillomandibular deficiency, morbid obesity, and OSAS and when other forms of more conservative treatment have failed. Bimaxillary surgery may retain preoperative dentition and does not require orthodontic treatment. As part of a staged protocol, bimaxillary surgery for severe OSAS has a greater than 90% success rate. Ancillary procedures such as partial glossectomy, genioglossus advancement, and palatopharyngoplasty are often required in severe apnea. In lower-risk patients, segmental operations are often performed initially, and maxillomandibular advancement is performed as a second step. In higher-risk patients or patients with maxillofacial deformities, repair

may be performed as a primary procedure. Complications of tissue relapse are uncommon with modern rigid fixation. Facial paresthesia, change in occlusion, and temporomandibular joint dysfunction are more common complications.

Maxillary Expansion. Maxillary constriction with and without crossbite can be treated with maxillary expansion. Rapid maxillary expansion may be performed orthodontically and nonsurgically in children prior to closure of palatal sutures. Both short- and long-term studies demonstrate benefit in reducing the severity of OSA and in improving nasal resistance.

REFERENCES

1. Isono S, Remmers JE, Tanaka A, et al. Anatomy of the pharynx in patients with obstructive sleep apnea and in normal subjects. J Appl Physiol 1997;82:1319–26.
2. Brietzke SE, Katz ES, Roberson DW. Can history and physical examination reliably diagnose pediatric obstructive sleep apnea/hypopnea syndrome? A systematic review of the literature. Otolaryngol Head Neck Surg 2004;131:827–32.
3. Young T, Palta M, Dempsey J, et al. The occurrence of sleep-disordered breathing among middle-aged adults. N Engl J Med 1993;328:1230–5.
4. Ng DK, Kwok K, Cheung JM, et al. Prevalence of sleep problems in Hong Kong primary school children. Chest 2005;128:1315–23.
5. Chaska B, Millman RP, Phillips BA, et al. Sleep Apnea: Is Your Patient at Risk? Bethesda, MD: National Center for Sleep Disorders Research, National Heart, Lung, and Blood Institute; 1995. p. 1–10.
6. Baldwin CM, Kapur VK, Holberg CJ, et al. Associations between gender and measures of daytime somnolence in the Sleep Heart Health Study. Sleep 2004;27:305–11.
7. Svensson M, Lindberg E, Naessen T, Janson C. Risk factors associated with snoring in women with special emphasis on body mass index: A population based study. Chest 2006;129:933–41.
8. Chervin R, Dillon J, Bassetti C, et al. Symptoms of sleep disorders, inattention, and hyperactivity in children. Sleep 1997;20:1185–92.
9. Wong ML, Sandham A, Ang PK, et al. Craniofacial morphology, head posture, and nasal respiratory resistance in obstructive sleep apnoea: An inter-ethnic comparison. Eur J Orthod 2005;27:91–7.
10. McArdle N, Riha R, Vennelle M, et al. Sleep-disordered breathing as a risk factor for cerebrovascular disease: A case-control study in patients with transient ischemic attacks. Stroke 2003;34:2916–21.
11. Shahar E, Whitney C, Redline S, et al. Sleep-disordered breathing and cardiovascular disease: Cross-sectional results of the Sleep Heart Health Study. Am J Respir Crit Care Med 2001;163:19–25.
12. Dincer HE, O'Neill W. Deleterious effects of sleep-disordered breathing on the heart and vascular system. Respiration 2006;73:124–30.
13. Barbe F, Sunyer J, de la Pena A, et al. Effect of continuous positive airway pressure on the risk of road accidents in sleep apnea patients. Respiration 2007;74:44–9.
14. Dempsy JA, Skatrud JB, Jacques AJ, et al. Anatomical determinates of sleep disordered breathing across the spectrum of clinical and non-clinical subjects. Chest 2002;122:40–51.
15. Schwab RJ, Pasirstein M, Kaplan L, et al. Family aggregation of upper airway soft tissue structures in normal subjects and patients with sleep apnea. Am J Respir Crit Care Med 2006;173:453–63.
16. Rowley JA, Permutt S, Willey S, et al. Effect of tracheal and tongue displacement on upper airway airflow dynamics. J Appl Physiol 1996;80:2171–8.
17. Malhotra A, Pillar G, Fogel RB, et al. Pharyngeal pressure and flow effects on genioglossus activation in normal subjects. Am J Respir Crit Care Med 2002;165:71–7.
18. Morrell MJ, Arabi Y, Zahn B, Badr MS. Progressive retropalatal narrowing preceding obstructive apnea. Am J Respir Crit Care Med 1998;158:1974–81.
19. Morrison DL, Launois SH, Isono S, et al. Pharyngeal narrowing and closing pressures in patients with obstructive sleep apnea. Am Rev Respir Dis 1993;148:606–11.
20. Hillman DR, Murphy AS, Antic R, Pezzullo L. The economic cost of sleep disorders. Sleep 2006;29:299–305.

21. Tsai WH, Flemons WW, Whitelaw WA, Remmers JE. A comparison of apnea-hypopnea indices derived from different definitions of hypopnea. Am J Respir Crit Care Med 1999;159:43–8.

22. Douglas NJ. Upper airway resistance syndrome is not a distinct syndrome. Am J Respir Crit Care Med 2000;161:1413–6.

23. Uliel S, Tauman R, Greenfeld M, Sivan Y. Normal polysomnographic respiratory values in children and adolescents. Chest 2004;125:872–8.

24. Chesson AL, Berry RB, Pack A. Practice parameters for the use of portable monitoring devices in the investigation of suspected obstructive sleep apnea in adults. Sleep 2003;26:907–13.

25. John MW. Sleepiness in different situations measured by the Epworth sleepiness scale. Sleep 1994;17:703–10.

26. Katsantonis GP, Maas CS, Walsh JK. The predictive efficacy of the Mueller maneuver in uvulopalatopharyngoplasty. Laryngoscope 1989;99:677–80.

27. Friedman M, Ibrahim H, Bass L. Clinical staging for sleep-disordered breathing. Otolaryngol Head Neck Surg 2002;127:13–21.

28. Veasey S, Guilleminault C, Strohl KP, et al. Medical therapy for obstructive sleep apnea: A review by the medical therapy for obstructive sleep apnea task force of the standards of practice committee of the American Academy of Sleep Medicine. Sleep 2006;29:1036–44.

29. Gay P, Weaver T, Loube D, Iber C. Evaluation of positive airway treatment for sleep related breathing disorders in adults: A review of the positive airway pressure task force of the standards of practice committee of the American Academy of Sleep Medicine. Sleep 2006;29:381–401.

30. Barnes M, Houston D, Worsnop CJ, et al. A randomized controlled trial of continuous positive airway pressure in mild obstructive sleep apnea. Am J Respir Crit Care Med 2002;165:773–80.

31. Ferguson KA, Cartwright R, Rogers R, Schmidt-Nowara W. Oral appliances for snoring and obstructive sleep apnea: A review. Sleep 2006;29:244–62.

32. Hillman DR, Platt PR, Eastwood PR. The upper airway during anaesthesia. Br J Anaesth 2003;91:31–9.

33. Powell NB, Riley RW, Guilleminault C. Rationale and indications for surgical treatment in obstructive sleep apnea syndrome. Oper Tech Otolaryngol Head Neck Surg 1991;2:87–90.

34. Mickelson SA, Hakim I. Is postoperative intensive care monitoring necessary after uvulopalatopharyngoplasty? Otolaryngol Head Neck Surg 1998;119:352–6.

35. Sugiura T, Noda A, Nakata S, et al. Influence of nasal resistance on initial acceptance of continuous positive airway pressure in treatment for obstructive sleep apnea syndrome. Respiration 2007;74:56–60.

36. Guilleminault C, Li K, Quo S, Inouye RN. A prospective study on the surgical outcomes of children with sleep-disordered breathing. Sleep 2004;27:95–100.

37. Goldbart AD, Goldman JL, Veling MC, Gozal D. leukotriene modifier therapy for mild sleep-disordered breathing in children. Am J Respir Crit Care Med 2005;172:364–70.

38. Mitchell RB, Kelly J. Long-term changes in behavior after adenotonsillectomy for obstructive sleep apnea in children. Otolaryngol Head Neck Surg 2006;134:374–8.

39. Isono I, Shimada A, Tanaka A, et al. Effects of uvulopalatopharyngoplasty on collapsibility of the retropalatal airway in patients with obstructive sleep apnea. Laryngoscope 2003;113:362–7.

40. Friedman M, Ibrahim H, Lee G, Joseph NJ. Combined uvulopalatopharyngoplasty and radiofrequency tongue base reduction for treatment of obstructive sleep apnea/hypopnea syndrome. Otolaryngol Head Neck Surg 2003;129:611–21.

41. Cahali MB. Lateral pharyngoplasty: A new treatment for obstructive sleep apnea hypopnea syndrome. Laryngoscope 2003;113:1961–8.

42. Littner M, Kushida CA, Hartse K, et al. Practice parameters for the use of laser-assisted uvulopalatoplasty: An update for 2000. Sleep 2001;24:603–19.

43. Brietzke SE, Mair EA. Injection snoreplasty: Extended follow-up and new objective data. Otolaryngol Head Neck Surg 2003;128:605–15.

44. Kezirian EJ, Goldbery AN. Hypopharyngeal surgery in obstructive sleep apnea: An evidence based medicine review. Arch Otolaryngol Head Neck Surg 2006;132:206–13.

45. Woodson BT, Steward DL, Weaver EM, Javaheri S. A randomized trial of temperature-controlled radiofrequency, continuous positive airway pressure, and placebo for obstructive sleep apnea syndrome. Otolaryngol Head Neck Surg 2005;132:630–5.

Molecular Biology of Squamous Cell Carcinoma

Carter Van Waes, MD, PhD

Head and neck squamous cell carcinoma (HNSCC) is the most common cancer that affects both human communication and survival. It accounts for 90% of the cancers arising in the upper aero digestive tract, making it the most common type of cancer and cause of cancer deaths among patients with head and neck cancer. It accounts for over 40,000 new cancer cases and 11,000 deaths annually in the United States.[1] Despite progress in refinement of surgery, radiation, and chemotherapeutic approaches that have enhanced organ preservation, there has been little improvement in survival of patients with HNSCC over the past 25 years.[1] Recent advances in determining the identity and function of molecular events involved in the pathogenesis of HNSCC have provided a foundation for development of new methods for screening, prevention, and therapy.

Progress in understanding the molecular biology of HNSCC has been made possible through advances in technology that have permitted detection and mapping of alterations in sequence of deoxyribonucleic acid (DNA) and expression of genes throughout the human genome.[2] Initially, cytogenetic analysis using special stains and fluorescence in situ hybridization (FISH) with probes for specific genes enabled detection of gross chromosomal abnormalities and altered gene copy number. Comparative genomic hybridization (CGH) is a newer technique that allows genome wide identification and quantification of genetic alterations. Using these methods, certain abnormalities such as deletions, amplifications, and translocations have been detected in certain chromosomal regions with increased frequency in HNSCC and other cancers. In some cases, these abnormalities have led to the identification of specific genes whose deletion, amplification, or truncation is involved in development of cancer. DNA polymorphism analysis is another important tool made possible by identification of differences in DNA sequence fragments between individuals at chromosomal locations throughout the genome. With this method, different-size DNA fragments cut by enzymes from the DNA contributed by each parent are identified with electrophoresis, allowing the detection of two copies (alleles) in normal cells from the patient. In cancer cells, loss of one marker, called a loss of heterozygosity (LOH), has been used to detect nearby alterations in DNA. DNA microsatellite and LOH analyses have permitted the detection and mapping of molecular alterations in DNA that were too small to be detected by cytogenetic analysis, thereby resulting in finer maps and detection of additional submicroscopic DNA abnormalities.[2] Further mapping and sequencing of these regions have been made possible by development of methods for cloning large fragments of chromosomal DNA and methods for high throughput DNA sequencing, resulting in the positional cloning of many of the mapped genes. The complete determination of the sequence and location of genes in the human genome from high throughput DNA sequencing has rapidly resulted in the identification of genes associated with abnormalities detected by genomic methods.

The identification of the sequence and isolation of genes have enabled studies of global alterations in expression of messenger ribonucleic acid (mRNAs) using complementary DNA microarrays in tumor cell lines and tissue and verification by quantitative reverse transcription-polymerase chain reaction (RT-PCR) methods.[3] Determination of the mRNA sequence for the transcriptome and predicted protein sequence of the proteome has facilitated the use of quantitative RT-PCR and mass spectroscopy to identify sequences of multiple mRNAs and proteins which are aberrantly expressed in tumor specimens, serum, and saliva. The development of antibodies to many of the proteins and phosphorylated activated proteins has enabled immunostaining in multiple specimens in tissue microarrays (TMAs) and semiquantitation of hundreds of proteins in tumor extracts or sera serially diluted and spotted on slides, called reverse phase microarrays. All of these different types of microarrays provide the capability to compare simultaneously and detect differences among hundreds or thousands of different mRNAs or proteins in samples from normal and malignant tissue and body fluids. Studies to determine the relative expression and function of genes in the cell are leading to a better understanding of the molecular pathways and programs involved in the pathogenesis of cancer and their potential usefulness for molecular diagnosis and therapy. As a result of these advances, prevention and treatment of HNSCC will increasingly involve use of molecular assays for prediction of prognosis and response to therapy and targeted prevention and therapy using molecular medicine, radiation, and surgery.

CRITICAL MOLECULAR EVENTS IN THE DEVELOPMENT OF CANCER

Tumor development following exposure to carcinogenic agents involves molecular changes that affect key cellular functions necessary for malignant behavior.[4] These changes include overriding the normal program for cell differentiation and death to those favoring an increase in cell proliferation and life span.[4,5] Malignant tumor progression involves additional changes that result in establishment of a blood supply, migration, invasion, and metastasis within the host environment of the patient.

Weinberg has shown that molecular alteration in expression or function of at least three genes is required to alter important cellular functions and cause transformation and tumor development from normal human cells under experimental conditions.[5] One important requirement for neoplastic transformation and tumor formation is an increase in cell proliferation. He showed that increased cell-cycle progression and proliferation can result from activation of a signaling kinase called Ras. Ras may be activated by viral infection, mutation, or by upstream signal activation due to overexpression of growth factors or receptors, such as epidermal growth factor receptor (EGFR). Growth factor receptors and Ras are potent activators of the mitogen activated protein kinases (MAPKs), transcription factor activator protein-1 (AP-1), and genes involved in cell-cycle entry and proliferation, such as cyclin D1. However, Ras activation and increased proliferation alone are not sufficient as such cells eventually undergo programmed cell death or reach the end of their life span, undergoing "crisis." Additional alterations, leading to inactivation of tumor suppressor genes that encode proteins such as p14ARF, p16INK4a, or p53, are needed.[5,6] These proteins are all components of a key damage pathway that when activated induces cell-cycle arrest, repair of damaged DNA, or cell death when DNA cannot be repaired.[6] Thus, inactivation or loss of p14ARF, p16INK4a, or p53 may result in continuous replication of cells with DNA mutations and damage and further changes in the expression and function of additional genes, leading to further increases in malignant behavior. Alteration of one or more oncogenes leading to activation of other signal transcription factor pathways, such as nuclear factor kappa B (NF-κB) and signal transduction and activator transcription factor (STAT-3), has been shown to alter the balance between life and death of cancer cells.[7] Alterations in expression of certain genes, including decrease in p53 regulated proteins p21 and Bax and increase in NF-κB and STAT-3 regulated proteins such and BCL-2 and BCL-XL, have been shown to be important in preventing programmed cell death of cancer cells. A third requirement for cancer development is an increase in cell life span, or immortalization.[5] Even basilar layer stem cells from which the epithelia arise normally stop proliferating and reach the end of their life in a finite number of cell divisions. The life-span limit of normal cells has been shown to be associated with a gradual shortening of the telomeres, which are the ends of chromosomes. In contrast, cancer cells do not exhibit shortening of the telomeres, and this has been found to be attributable to increased expression of an enzyme called telomerase.[5]

Thus, when genes provide an important regulatory brake and their loss promotes cancer development, they are termed tumor suppressor genes; whereas, when the abnormal expression of genes "turns on" transformation and growth, these genes have been called oncogenes. Genes that suppress cancer that when lost cause cancer include p53 and retinoblastoma (Rb). Genes expressed by viruses, such as E6 and E7, are called viral oncogenes. Mutated genes such as the signal kinase Ras are termed cellular oncogenes. An accumulation of alterations in the expression of different combinations of tumor suppressor genes and oncogenes may result in increased proliferation and life span and decreased cell death, leading to progressive formation of premalignant and malignant lesions.

PATHOLOGIC AND MOLECULAR CHANGES DURING DEVELOPMENT OF HEAD AND NECK SQUAMOUS CELL CARCINOMA

Pathologic Events during Tumor Development

The development of HNSCC involves a series of progressive pathologic changes in behavior of cells in squamous cell mucosa and underlying stroma of the upper aerodigestive tract, as illustrated in Figure 1A. Cells injured by exposure to physical or viral agents may undergo irreversible damage and cell death or undergo repair and survive. The surviving cells often acquire increased cellular resistance and proliferate and migrate, healing the area of injury. With repeated injury, increased numbers of cells may accumulate to produce a thickened epithelium, termed hyperplasia. With repeated exposure to mutagenic agents, irreversible genetic mutations and epigenetic changes may occur with changes in cell behavior that include a partial- or full-thickness increase in proliferating and morphologically atypical cells called dysplasia or carcinoma in situ (CIS), respectively. Dysplasia and CIS lesions are premalignant. Migration through the basement membrane into the stroma is the hallmark of invasive carcinoma, which is the stage of malignant tumor development. Hyperplasia, dysplasia, or CIS may be accompanied by hyperkeratinization, which may be visible clinically as leukoplakia. Dysplasia, CIS, or microinvasive carcinoma is accompanied by a progressive increase in inflammation, vascularity, and proliferation of fibrous stroma, which may be visible clinically as induration and vascular erythema, called erythroplasia.

Molecular Carcinogenesis

Development of HNSCC has been associated with repeated exposure to and injury by chemical carcinogens contained in tobacco and alcohol[8] or chronic infection by human papillomavirus

Tumor Development

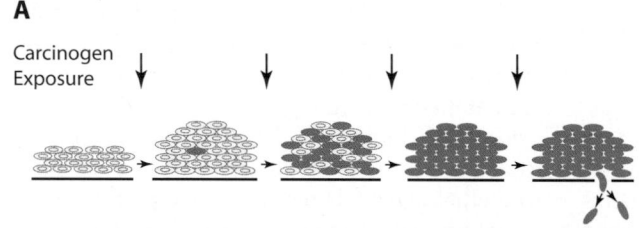

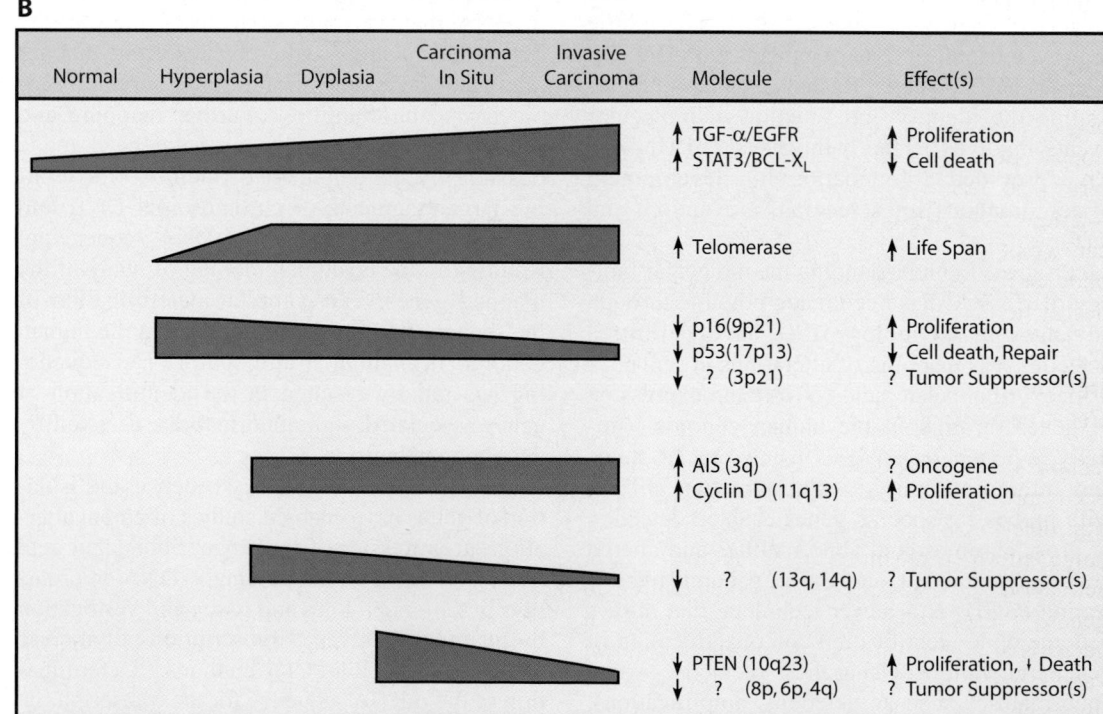

Figure 1 Model of histopathologic and molecular changes with development and progression of head and neck squamous cell carcinoma (HNSCC). (A) Histopathologic changes during tumor development of HNSCC occur following repeated carcinogen exposure, as described in the text. (B) Molecular alterations with tumor development. p14/16 = protein 14 and 16 kDa; p53 = protein 53 kDa; FHIT = fragile histidine triad; RAR = retinoic acid receptor; RASSF1 = Ras associated domain family1; PTEN = phosphatase and tensin homolog deleted on chromosome 10; CSMD1 = cub sushi multiple domains1; Rb = retinoblastoma; p40AIS = activated in squamous carcinoma; IL = interleukin; TNF = tumor necrosis factor; NF-κB = nuclear factor-kappa B; TGF = transforming growth factor; EGFR = epidermal growth factor receptor; AP = activator protein; STAT = signal transducers and activators of transcription; BCL-XL = BCL-XLong; GRO1 = growth regulated oncogene1; MMP = matrix metalloproteinase; PDGF = platelet derived growth factor; VEGF = vascular endothelial growth factor; eIFs = eukaryotic translation initiation factors.

(HPV)[9] or Epstein-Barr virus.[10] Several physical and viral causative agents associated with the development of HNSCC can cause defined molecular changes that result in malignancy. Worldwide, tobacco and alcohol products are the leading risk factors for development of HNSCC. Tobacco contains aromatic hydrocarbons that can cause DNA damage, most commonly resulting in G:C to T:A base-pair transversions and G:C to A:T base-pair transitions.[11] Alcohol appears to increase the risk when used in combination with tobacco. Other physical agents that appear to contribute to the incidence of HNSCC at specific subsites can cause DNA damage. The increased incidence of lip and skin cancer in regions nearer the equator such as in Australia and the southwestern United States is associated with sun exposure. The ultraviolet spectrum in sunlight can cause thymidine dimer formation, resulting in C to T base transitions.[11]

Certain viruses have been associated with HNSCC, and these viruses can commandeer vital cellular control pathways and cause DNA disruption on integration. HPV types 16 and 18, which are the subtypes that cause most cervical carcinomas in women, have been shown to be prevalent in oropharyngeal carcinomas, including nonsmokers.[9] Cells infected with HPVs express proteins encoded by viral genes called E6 and E7 that can inactivate the tumor suppressor proteins p53 and Rb, which help regulate cell proliferation and death. Epstein-Barr virus has been associated with nasopharyngeal carcinoma, particularly in Asia.[10] It encodes viral proteins such as LMP-1 (latent membrane protein-1) that activate NF-κB, a signal and DNA transcription factor, that promotes expression of genes involved in cell survival and proliferation of epithelia and lymphocytes.[12] Epstein-Barr virus also carries a gene homologous to human interleukin-10 (IL-10), an immune hormone that can suppress development of cytotoxic T-lymphocyte immunity, which is needed for immune destruction of cancer cells.

Genetic and Epigenetic Changes during Development of Head and Neck Squamous Cell Carcinoma

Changes in gene expression and function can occur through genetic mechanisms, such as mutation, deletion, or amplification of genes, or through epigenetic mechanisms, such as inactivation or activation of the regulatory promoter regions of genes.[2,5,8] Methylation of the promoter region of genes is an important epigenetic cause of inactivation and underexpression of genes in cancers in which mutations are not found. Conversely, aberrant activation of signal transcription factors is an important cause of overexpression of genes that are not genetically amplified by duplication of multiple copies. There is evidence for frequent genetic or epigenetic alteration of several important tumor suppressor genes and oncogenes during development of HNSCC.[13] These may lead to inactivation or activation of important signal pathways and transcription factors important in regulation of expression of a wider set of genes and the malignant phenotype (Figure 1B).

Tumor Suppressor Genes in Development of Head and Neck Squamous Cell Carcinoma

A locus on the short (p) arm of chromosome 9 located at 9p21 has been found to exhibit LOH at an early stage during the development of hyperplasia.[13] The 9p21 locus has been found to encode overlapping genes that encode proteins called p14ARF and p16INK4a, and this locus is found to be inactivated in the majority of HNSCC by homozygous deletion, mutation, or by methylation of the regulatory promoter region.[14] The p14ARF protein is an important activator of the p53 pathway and repressor of the NF-κB pathway during programmed cell death,[15] so its loss may be an important early event in dysfunction of both the p53 and NF-κB pathways, which are altered in dysplastic and malignant squamous cell epithelia.[16,17] The p16INK4a protein is a cyclin-dependent kinase called CDKN2/MTS-1/INK4A that normally inhibits cell-cycle progression. Thus, genetic or epigenetic alteration of this locus can result in loss of p14ARF protein causing decreased programmed cell death, and loss of p16INK4a, causing increased proliferation. Consistent with this, re-expression of p16 in HNSCC cells by gene transfer suppresses cell growth in vitro.[18] Re-expression of p14ARF has been shown to repress NF-κB mediated prosurvival gene expression and promote cell death in other cell lines.[15]

Chromosome 17p13 encodes the p53 gene, which is itself altered with relatively low frequency in dysplasia and CIS, but with increased frequency in ~50% of primary carcinomas.[13] Alternatively, HPV infection and E6 expression have been shown to inactivate p53, presumably at an earlier stage, particularly in oropharyngeal SCC.[9] As described above, a variety of functions have been attributed to the p53 gene, which is thought to mediate tumor suppression by cell-cycle arrest and DNA repair or induction of cell death when damage is irreversible.[19] Tumor suppressor p53 may also repress the activation of prosurvival genes by NF-κB, through competition for a transcriptional co-factor called CBP/p300.[20] Thus loss of p53 can lead to dysfunction of mechanisms by which cancer cells undergo repair or cell death, as well as promote activation of prosurvival pathways.

Chromosome 3p is altered with increasing frequency with the development of dysplasia in HNSCC,[13] lung,[21] and esophageal carcinomas[22] and contains at least three putative loci. Several genes on the 3p arm have been implicated as tumor suppressors, including genes fragile histidine triad (FHIT), retinoic acid receptor-beta (RAR-β), and Ras associated domain family-1 (RASSF1).[22] These genes have variously been implicated in checking proliferation and migration, and hence their loss can contribute to proliferation, invasion, and tumorigenesis.

LOH involving chromosomes 8p is observed later, in association with invasive HNSCC, and a locus on chromosome 8p23 is associated with poor prognosis.[23] The putative tumor suppressor gene at the chromosome 8p23 locus has been identified and is a large transmembrane protein called cub sushi multiple domains 1 (CSMD1).[24] Another gene that infrequently undergoes mutations which results in loss of function maps to the chromosome 8p21 region in HNSCC and is a p53 regulated growth inhibitory gene that is a member of the tumor necrosis factor-related apoptosis-inducing ligand (TRAIL) family.[25]

LOH at chromosome 10q23 is detected with intermediate frequency in primary HNSCC and has been found to reflect deletion or inactivation of a gene called phosphatase and tensin (PTEN) homologue deleted on chromosome 10.[26] PTEN functions in the inactivation of Akt, also known as protein kinase B. Akt plays an important role in activation of transcription factor NF-κB and co-activator CBP/p300m transcription of prosurvival genes,[27] and activation of molecular target of rapamycin (mTOR), important in translation of proteins, such as angiogenesis factor, vascular endothelial growth factor (VEGF).[28] Early activation of Akt by autocrine stimuli such as EGFR and cytokine receptors, and later by loss of PTEN, could lead to increased survival and growth of HNSCC and other cancers.

Several other important chromosomal alterations are observed with variable frequency in HNSCC. Chromosome 13q21 has been shown to exhibit increasing LOH with CIS and invasive carcinoma.[13] This region encodes the retinoblastoma gene, another tumor suppressor gene. However, mutation of the retinoblastoma gene occurs relatively infrequently in the HNSCC studied, indicating the possible presence of another gene at this location.

Tumor Oncogenes in Development of Head and Neck Squamous Cell Carcinoma

A locus alteration on the long (q) arm of chromosome 11 located at 11q13 in increasing frequency during the CIS stage[13] is associated with amplification of a cell-cycle regulatory protein called cyclin D1.[29] Alternatively, cyclin D1 may be overexpressed as a result of transcriptional activation by NF-κB.[30] Cyclin D1 is required for progression of cells through the cell cycle, thereby stimulating squamous cells to proliferate. Inhibition of cyclin D1 results in inhibition of growth of HNSCC in vitro.

On chromosome 3q, amplification of a homologue of p53 was identified, and this protein, designated p40AIS (amplified in squamous cell carcinoma), was found to occur with high frequency in HNSCC and lung squamous cell carcinoma.[31] p40AIS is a short splice variant of a related p53 family member called ΔNp63, and both lack the tumor suppressor function of p53. Expression of AIS was found to promote growth of rat cells in soft agar and in mice, indicating that it may play an early role in transformation as an oncogene. Increased p40 expression appeared to be correlated with loss of p53, and p40 may interact and inhibit normal p53 function. Subsequently ΔNp63 has recently been shown to promote survival of a subset of HNSCC by binding and inhibiting p73, another proapoptotic p53 family member.[32] ΔNp63 also regulates expression of integrin α6β4 and extracellular matrix protein laminin 5,[33] shown to be important markers of poor prognosis and mediators of cell adhesion of HNSCC.[34]

Early activation of telomerase has been detected in HNSCC. Mao and colleagues reported that although telomerase is not detected in normal mucosa, increased telomerase activity is detected with the development of squamous hyperplasia, dysplasia, and invasive carcinoma.[35] Califano and colleagues have also shown that increased telomerase activity may be detected in dysplasia and invasive carcinoma and, with lower sensitivity, in shed cells in oral rinses from patients.[36] The increased expression of telomerase observed in HNSCC is consistent with the requirement for immortalization of cancer cells in a study of carcinogenesis by Weinberg.[5]

In summary, HNSCCs have been found to accumulate a series of genetic or epigenetic changes during the cytopathologic stages of tumor development. The functions of the affected genes identified to date are consistent with the changes required for the development of cancer, namely genes involved in regulation of cell-cycle progression and proliferation and cell death and life span. The occurrence of multiple events at different stages in individual cancers from different patients suggests that different combinations of several key genes affecting cell-cycle progression and proliferation, cell life span, and cell death can contribute to the common histopathologic stages of tumor development observed in HNSCC.

ABERRANT ACTIVATION OF SIGNALING, GENE TRANSCRIPTION, AND PROTEIN TRANSLATION IN HEAD AND NECK SQUAMOUS CELL CARCINOMA

The genetic or epigenetic changes in HNSCC can lead to altered activation of several signaling and transcription factor pathways that in turn regulate many of the several hundred genes and proteins altered in cancer. These common pathways explain why most cancers show aberrant activation of certain gene programs involved in cell proliferation, survival, migration, and angiogenesis. As important common pathways, they may also prove to be most useful markers for molecular diagnosis and targets for therapy. The accumulation of molecular changes in expression or activation of several key growth factors, cytokines, receptors, or their downstream signaling and transcription factors with cytopathologic changes that occur during the stages of tumor development of HNSCC are shown in Figures 1 and 2.

Aberrant Activation of the NF-κB Pathway in Head and Neck Squamous Cell Carcinoma

NF-κB is a signal transcription factor found to play an important role in aberrant gene expres-

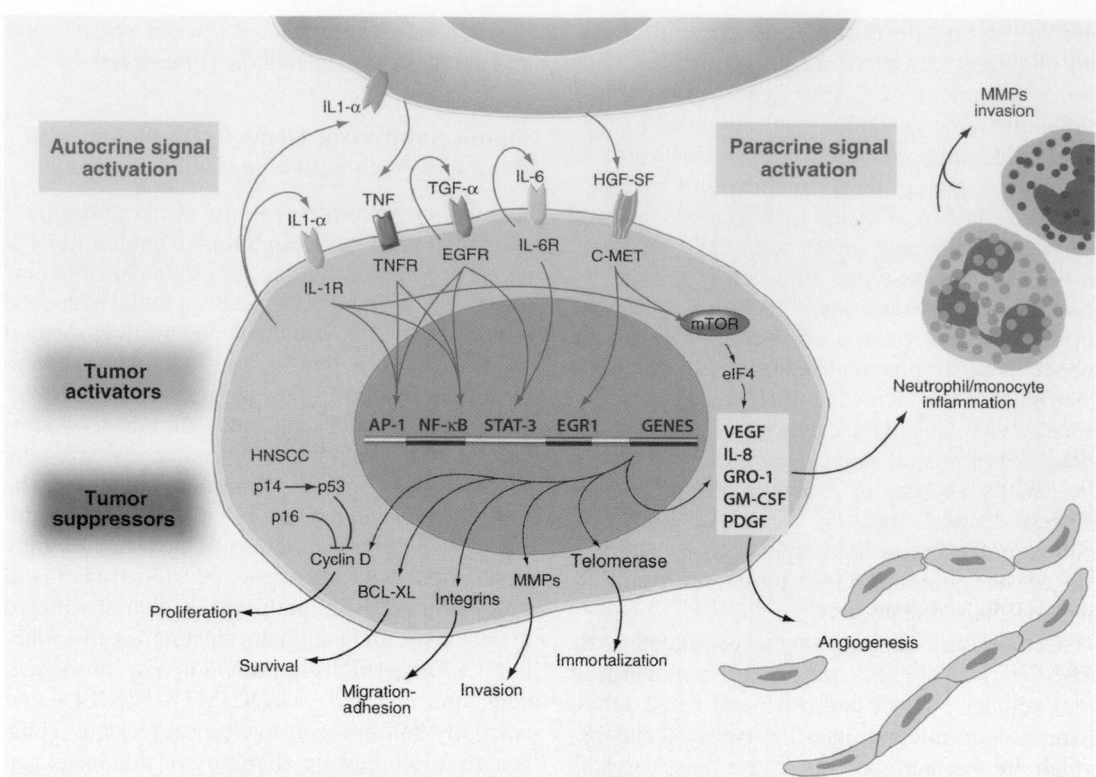

Figure 2 Autocrine and paracrine factors that act as tumor activators and tumor suppressors that affect tumor development and progression of head and neck squamous cell carcinoma (HNSCC). Factors produced by tumor and host cells provide autocrine and paracrine stimuli that activate signal receptors, transcription factors and genes. Genes activated by transcription factors cause cellular changes in HNSCC that lead to tumor development and host inflammatory and angiogenesis responses that promote malignant tumor progression and metastasis. IL = interleukin; TNF = tumor necrosis factor; TGF = transforming growth factor; EGFR = epidermal growth factor receptor; HGF-SF = hepatocyte growth factor-scatter factor; AP = activator protein; NF-κB = nuclear factor-kappa B; STAT = signal transducers and activators of transcription; EGR = early growth response; p14/16 = protein 14 and 16 kDa; p53 = protein 53 kDa; BCL-XL = BCL-XLong; MMP = matrix metalloproteinase; GRO = growth-regulated oncogene; VEGF = vascular endothelial growth factor; GM-CSF = granulocyte-macrophage-colony stimulating factor; PDGF = platelet derived growth factor.

sion and the malignant phenotype of SCC.[30] NF-κB is inducible by nicotine and chemicals contained in tobacco and betel nut, two of the most important carcinogenic agents that promote development of HNSCC.[37,38] Increased nuclear activation of NF-κB has been shown to occur in premalignant dysplastic lesions and ~85% of HNSCC, indicating that it is an early event, and strong immunostaining is associated with the increased rate of malignant progression of dysplasia and decreased survival in patients with HNSCC.[17] NF-κB was found to be constitutively activated in HNSCC cell lines and tumor, suggesting that further events contribute to sustained activation.[17,30] Thus far, expression and autocrine activation by IL-1α and tumor necrosis factor (TNF) have been implicated in activation of NF-κB in HNSCC.[39,40] EGFR appears to contribute weakly to constitutive activation of NF-κB pathway.[41] Activation of NF-κB via the PI3K, Akt, and CK2 kinases appears to be important in signal activation of these pathways in HNSCC.[41,42] By cDNA microarray profiling, NF-κB was found to directly or indirectly regulate ~60% of the genes aberrantly expressed with malignant progression in a murine SCC model,[43] and genes from a 99 gene signature subset from that study were shown to group with genes aberrantly expressed in microarray gene profile found in tumor specimens from patients at high risk for malignant progression.[44] NF-κB

regulates key genes involved in cell proliferation (cyclin D1), survival (BCL-XL), migration and invasion matrix metalloproteinase 9 (MMP9), and angiogenesis (IL-8, GRO1) in cancer (see Figure 1B). Confirming this, blocking NF-κB activation inhibits these genes and cell proliferation, survival, angiogenesis, and tumorigenesis of SCC.[43] Recently, NF-κB mediated activation of one of the cytokines, IL-6, has been shown to be an important activator of STAT3, also important in cell survival.[45]

Overexpression of Transforming Growth Factor α, Epidermal Growth Factor Receptor, and Activation of the MAPK-AP-1 and STAT3 Pathways in Head and Neck Squamous Cell Carcinoma

Another of the early alterations in signaling identified in the development of HNSCC is overexpression of the EGFR and one of its stimulatory factors, transforming growth factor-α (TGF-α)[46] (see Figures 1B and 2). Over 90% of HNSCCs overexpress EGFR and TGF-α.[46] Increased expression of TGF-α and EGFR has been detected in tumor cells and mucosa from patients with HNSCC, when compared with normal mucosa from controls, indicating that TGF-α and EGFR expression may be an early event in carcinogenesis of HNSCC.[46] Increased expression of both TGF-α and EGFR occurs with progression to carcinoma (see Figure 1B). EGFR and TGF-α appear to be overexpressed owing to transcriptional activation of the genes for this receptor and ligand in most HNSCC. Patients with carcinomas expressing higher levels of these factors have been shown to have a shortened disease-free survival, independent of cervical lymph node stage.

Production of TGF-α and expression of EGFR establish a potential autocrine signal pathway for continuous stimulation of proliferation of squamous cells, and the importance of TGF-α and EGFR expression in the growth of HNSCC has been established. Inhibition of either TGF-α or EGFR expression or function using antisense oligonucleotides[47,48] or pharmacologic inhibitors in combination with radiation[49,50] was found to decrease the proliferation and growth of HNSCC cells in vitro and of xenografts in mice in vivo. The effects of EGFR activation may be mediated through several signal transcription factor pathways, which include Ras, MAPK, or ERK that activate transcription factor AP-1[41] and STAT3.[51] EGFR activation of STAT3 inhibits HNSCC cells from undergoing cell death (apoptosis) and stimulates proliferation. The cytokine IL-6 regulated by NF-κB has been reported to be another important factor in STAT3 activation.[45] Thus, overexpression of EGFR appears to be one of several factors contributing to MAPK and STAT3 activation, the increase in proliferation, and the decrease in cell death involved in HNSCC tumorigenesis.

Increased Activation of the Hepatocyte Growth Factor and cMET Pathway in Head and Neck Squamous Cell Carcinoma

Murine and human SCC have been shown to express a receptor/oncogene cMET, which binds the hepatocyte growth factor (HGF), also known as the scatter factor, owing to its ability to induce separation and spreading of epithelial and endothelial cells.[52,53] Consistent with this, increased responsiveness to HGF and cMET activation has been implicated in increased angiogenesis and metastasis of murine and human HNSCC. HGF/cMET activation amplifies the induction of the PI3K and Akt pathway by other growth factors and cytokines[52] and also activates another transcription factor, EGR-1.[54] The platelet derived growth factor (PDGF) and VEGF involved in angiogenesis have been shown to be among the important targets of the HGF-cMET-EGR-1 signaling.[54]

Molecular Target of Rapamycin Pathway

The cytokine and growth factor induced activation of PI3K-Akt kinases activates another important target, mTOR, that is important in activating kinases and proteins that enhance protein translation in HNSCC.[55] Activation of several targets has been associated with activation or Akt and/or mTOR. One of these, eIF4 (elongation initiating factor), has been shown to be a marker in most HNSCC. This protein has been implicated in enhancing translation of angiogenesis factors such as VEGF.[56] Although inhibition of mTOR by rapamycin has little effect on HNSCC lines in vitro, such inhibition sensitizes HNSCC cells to apoptosis and reduces angiogenesis in vivo in animal models.[57]

In summary, HNSCC exhibits loss of tumor suppressors p14ARF, p16INK4a, and p53 and activation of ligand–receptor pairs which are tumor activators that modulate a network of signal pathways that regulate expression of target genes and proteins that mediate the phenotypic features of the malignant phenotype (see Figure 2). This includes autocrine activation by IL-1R, TNFR, and EGFR, which contribute to activation of the MAPK-AP-1, PI3K-NF-κB, and Akt-mTOR pathway; EGFR and IL-6R which contribute to STAT3 activation; and cMET which contributes to PI3K and EGR1 pathways. Groups of genes, predominantly regulated by one or a combination of the factors AP-1 and NF-κB (cyclinD, MMPs, IL-8), NF-κB and STAT3 (BCL-XL), AP-1, EGR1, and mTOR (VEGF) are key molecular mediators of cell proliferation, survival, invasion, and angiogenesis.

Molecular Mediators of Tumor Progression and Metastasis of Squamous Cell Carcinoma

The stages of cancer involve progressive tumor invasion and metastasis, which are the stages that ultimately affect vital functions and cause death in patients. Figures 1A and 2 highlight some of the intermediate and late histopathologic and molecular events associated with tumor progression and metastasis. Development of invasive carcinoma is associated with focal dissolution of the basement membrane and extracellular matrix (ECM), detachment, and migration of cells into the submucosal tissue. HNSCCs that exhibit a streaming pattern of small clusters of cells through the ECM are associated with more aggressive behavior and poor prognosis.[58] Tumor progression to a size that becomes visible and has an effect on adjacent structures requires an increase in supply of oxygen and nutrients and removal of waste. Folkman established the concept that new blood vessel formation is critical in cancer.[59] Enlargement of tumors to a size beyond 0.5 cm exceeds the range for diffusion of oxygen from existing vessels and necessitates new blood vessel formation, called neoangiogenesis. Such new vessel formation has been demonstrated in all cancers and is commonly associated with an increase in inflammatory cells. Increased vessel density and inflammation within tumors have been associated with more rapid growth, metastasis, and a decrease in prognosis, suggesting that the increase in vessels may somehow relate to increased access for metastasizing cancer cells. Invasion of the lymphatics and blood vessels and circulation of cells are necessary for regional and distant spread of HNSCC.

Growth of the tumor epithelia and angiogenesis is also accompanied by increased infiltration of inflammatory cells and proliferation of fibrous stroma. Several studies have suggested that tumor cells that induce host inflammatory and stromal cell responses grow, invade, and metastasize more rapidly. Chen and colleagues have shown that during progression, squamous cell carcinomas undergo additional changes needed for growth and metastasis that depend on the host.[60] Young and colleagues have shown that inflammatory cells infiltrating human and murine squamous cell carcinomas are one of the host components that promote growth and metastasis.[61] These inflammatory cells bear a stem cell marker called CD34 and appear to differentiate into granulocytes and the endothelial cells that form new blood vessels. Young[62] and Pekarek and colleagues[63] have shown that the granulocytes promote increased growth and metastasis. Granulocytes from the host can release growth factors[63] and proteases[64] that stimulate growth and invasion of tumor cells. Squamous cell carcinomas also induce proliferation of stromal fibroblasts. Fibroblasts also secrete factors, such as HGF, and ECM substances, that can promote growth.[65] The establishment of metastases requires cell arrest and vessel formation in a new location. HNSCC shows a predilection for metastases to the lymphatics, lungs, liver, and bone marrow, suggesting that the cells and substrate of the reticuloendothelial system provide a favorable environment for arrest and formation of squamous cell carcinoma metastases.

Molecules Involved in Cell Adhesion, Migration, and Invasion by Head and Neck Squamous Cell Carcinoma

HNSCCs exhibit alterations in expression of a repertoire of cell adhesion molecules and ECM substances that function in attachment and migration. Increased expression of cell adhesion molecules called integrins has been detected in HNSCC by Van Waes and colleagues.[66] The integrins are heterodimers comprising α and β subunits that form a superfamily of cell surface receptors involved in cell–cell and cell–ECM adhesion and recognition. The integrin $\alpha6\beta4$, $\alpha2\beta1$, and $\alpha3\beta1$ heterodimers are normally expressed among proliferating layers of squamous cell epithelium but are expressed in suprabasilar layers of many squamous cell carcinomas in association with increased proliferation and immortalization that occur during early tumor development.[66] Increased suprabasilar expression of $\alpha6\beta4$, as detected by monoclonal antibody A9, was found to be correlated with a poorer prognosis in a prospective study of 80 patients with HNSCC.[67] Expression of integrin $\alpha6\beta4$ has been shown to promote aggressive tumor behavior.[68] The $\alpha6\beta4$, $\alpha2\beta1$, and $\alpha3\beta1$ integrins have been found to be receptors for ECM laminin, and $\alpha2\beta1$, and $\alpha3\beta1$ integrins also bind to collagen. HNSCCs secrete the basement membrane component laminin in vitro and in situ, and blockade of $\alpha6\beta4$, $\alpha2\beta1$, and $\alpha3\beta1$ completely inhibits attachment of HNSCC to laminin and collagen.[69] Monoclonal antibody to the $\alpha6$ integrin has also been shown to reduce binding to activated endothelial cells. Thus, HNSCCs exhibit constitutive alterations in expression of a repertoire of integrin cell adhesion molecules, and expression of integrin $\alpha6\beta4$ in particular is linked with aggressive tumor behavior.

Increased expression and activation of enzymes involved in remodeling of the ECM have been detected in HNSCC and are associated with increased invasiveness and pathogenicity. The MMPs comprise a family of proteases that digest ECM, which are upregulated in HNSCC (see Figures 1 and 2). HNSCC exhibits increased expression of urokinase-type plasminogen activator (uPA) and uPA receptor as well as the MMPs membrane-type MMP-1, collagenase 1, stromelysin 1, and gelatinase B.[70] Expression of these factors and invasiveness appear to be inducible by EGF or scatter factor (SF).[70–72] Invasion of EGF- or SF-stimulated cells is completely suppressed by recombinant and synthetic MMP inhibitors.[70] These studies suggest that MMPs may be more important than the plasminogen activator–plasmin system in mediating EGF- or SF-induced tumor cell invasion of interstitial matrix barriers. Inflammatory cells infiltrating tumors also can express MMPs. MMP-9 may be expressed by host-derived neutrophils, macrophages, and mast cells attracted to the tumor site. MMP-9 expressed by bone marrow derived cells appears to promote malignant tumor progression of squamous cell carcinoma in vivo.[73]

Cytokine and Growth Factors Involved in Inflammation and Angiogenesis in Head and Neck Squamous Cell Carcinoma

The demonstration of the role of host inflammatory and angiogenesis responses in the development and progression of squamous cell carcinoma has led to efforts to identify the molecules involved. HNSCC have been found to express a number of cytokines and growth factors that mediate inflammatory and angiogenesis responses (see Figures 1 and 2). SCC produces a repertoire of factors in vitro and in situ that include IL-1α, IL-6, IL-8, granulocyte-macrophage colony-stimulating factor (GM-CSF), growth-regulated oncogene-α (GRO-α), and VEGF.[74,75] Tumor fibroblasts have been shown to produce SF/ HGF.[65] IL-6, IL-8, GRO-α, VEGF, and HGF are of sufficient stability and are produced at high enough concentrations that increased concentrations have been detected in the serum of patients.[52,76] Decreasing cytokine levels were associated with therapeutic response, while increasing levels were related to progression of recurrence.[76]

IL-1 is a cytokine that can regulate NF-κB activation and expression of several of the other factors detected in SCC.[32,77] IL-1 can serve as an autocrine factor to stimulate HNSCC to produce IL-6, IL-8, GM-CSF, and VEGF and as a paracrine factor to stimulate the production of HGF by stromal fibroblasts (see Figure 2). In addition, IL-1 has important systemic regulatory effects as an important mediator of acute-phase reactions, increased catabolic state and cachexia often observed in patients with aggressive HNSCC.[77] IL-1 and IL-6 both can have direct effects as

autocrine or paracrine factors that can stimulate proliferation of HNSCC cells.[39,78]

IL-8 and GRO-α are both members of a related family of chemoattractant and proliferative factors that contain a cysteine-X-cysteine (C-X-C) amino acid motif. IL-8 and GRO-α have been shown to serve as chemoattractants for neutrophils, monocytes, and endothelial cells, which are major constituents of the inflammatory response in HNSCC (see Figure 2). Loukinova and colleagues have shown that expression of the murine homologues of GRO-α and IL-8 promote aggressive growth and metastases, angiogenesis, and inflammatory cell infiltration in squamous cell carcinoma.[75] The aggressive pattern of growth is reversed in knockout mice deficient in C-X-C receptor 2, the receptor for the chemokine. These results provide direct evidence that tumor factors and the host response induced by them are critical in tumor progression and metastasis of squamous cell carcinoma. Kitadai and colleagues have shown that IL-8 has similar effects on growth of other histologic types of human tumors as xenografts in mice.[79] Young and colleagues have shown that GM-CSF produced by squamous cell carcinoma may also play a role in the activity of CD34 progenitors of granulocytes and endothelium, which they reported are associated with metastasis.[61] VEGF also promotes angiogenesis and stimulates expression of $\alpha v\beta3$ and $\alpha v\beta5$ integrin heterodimers that are involved in migration of endothelial cells during angiogenesis. Inhibition of αv integrins inhibits tumorigenesis of SCC in mice.[80]

MOLECULAR DIAGNOSIS OF HEAD AND NECK SQUAMOUS CELL CARCINOMA

Progress in the determination of molecular mechanisms involved in the pathogenesis of development and progression of HNSCC, together with sensitive molecular assay methods, has expanded opportunities for use of molecular diagnosis in patients with HNSCC. Using PCR-based methods for amplification of DNA, LOH of specific markers associated with HNSCC has been shown to occur in biopsy specimens of lesions prior to development of invasive malignancy.[2] Mutant p53 detected in surgical margins from patients has been shown to predict positive margins and sites of future recurrence.[81] Overexpression of telomerase and mutant p53 has been detected in tissue biopsies as well as in saliva,[35] opening possibilities for screening. Microsatellite and methylated DNAs, which are markers for inactivated tumor suppressor genes, have been detected in blood[82,83] and may eventually be useful for diagnosis and detection of recurrence. Using DNA microarray, quantitative RT-PCR or immunoassays, overexpression of cytokines and angiogenesis factors has been demonstrated in blood and saliva and examined as markers for diagnostic prediction of response, recurrence, and survival.[76,84] These studies have established the feasibility of using molecular methods to screen patients for diagnosis, prognosis, and detection of recurrence. Further understanding of the "anatomy" of activation of pathways and target genes, as in Figure 2, will eventually offer the possibility of determining

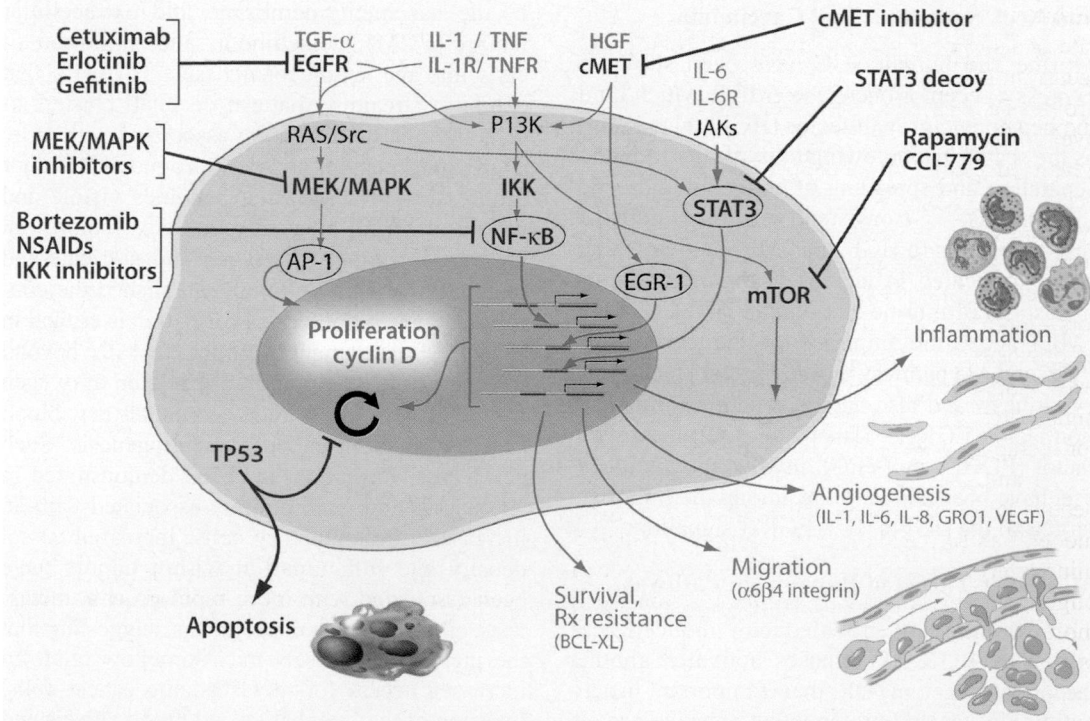

Figure 3 Investigational agents for molecular targeting in HNSCC. Epidermal growth factor receptor (EGFR) monoclonal antibody cetuximab is approved, and tyrosine kinase inhibitors erlotinib and gefitinib are under United States Food and Drug Administration (FDA) investigation for treatment of HNSCC. Agents targeting mitogen extracellular signal-regulated kinase and mitogen activated protein kinases (MAPKs) are of interest for inhibiting transcription factor Activator Protein-1 (AP-1). Proteasome inhibitor bortezomib, nonsteroidal anti-inflammatory drugs (NSAIDs) and inhibitor kpa B kinase (IKK) are under investigation for therapy or prevention of cancer. Metastasis (MET) oncogene receptor inhibitors, signal transducer and activator transcription (STAT) factor and molecular target of rapamycin (mTOR) are under FDA investigation for treatment of HNSCC.

susceptibility or resistance of HNSCC to different therapies.

Microarray analysis of gene expression has revealed clusters of genes that group together, associated with malignant potential, decreased prognosis, recurrence, and resistance to drugs such as cisplatinum.[44,85-87] Gene programs related to malignant potential and clinical outcome include those associated with immortalization of HNSCC observed in cell culture, and epithelial-mesenchymal transition (EMT) and NF-κB, associated with high-risk prognostic group among patients with HNSCC. To date, these studies have been most useful in generating hypotheses about important functions of genes and identifying most unique as potential markers for study using more direct and quantitative methods.

MOLECULAR THERAPY AND PREVENTION OF HEAD AND NECK SQUAMOUS CELL CARCINOMA

The determination of molecular mechanisms involved in pathogenesis of development and progression of HNSCC has enabled the development and testing of a few specific molecular therapies. Chemoprevention using inhibitors of several of these pathways are also under investigation. Figure 3 summarizes some of the targets and agents under investigation.

Identification of the role of EGFR in HNSCC and other cancers led to testing of therapy with receptor antibody inhibitors, small molecule inhibitors, and DNA antisense sequence to the target gene. The anti-EGFR antibody cetuximab (Erbitux) was found to have an ~13% response rate as a second-line single agent in patients with recurrent HNSCC and, with concurrent radiation, provides an ~10 to 15% enhancement in survival over radiotherapy alone in patients with locally advanced disease.[88] As a result, cetuximab has been approved for these indications. The EGFR tyrosine kinase inhibitor gefitinib showed limited response rates in patients with recurrent HNSCC. The relatively limited activity of EGFR inhibitors alone together with evidence for activation of downstream intermediates and of other pathways important in the malignant phenotype has highlighted the need to investigate other targets for therapy.

Xi and colleagues have shown that STAT3 decoys inhibit growth of HNSCC in a xenograft model,[89] and clinical trials are under way to determine safety in patients and effects of expression of oligonucleotides on tumor gene expression. Small molecule inhibitors of the proteasome, such as bortezomib (Velcade), can inhibit activation of the NF-κB pathway and are under study in patients with HNSCC.[90] Early results of the first study to combine bortezomib with radiation, conducted in patients with HNSCC, showed that bortezomib can inhibit NF-κB and prosurvival target genes, and induce apoptosis in tumor biopsies postdrug infusion.[90] Bortezomib is a first-in-class proteasome inhibitor that was initially approved for multiple myeloma.[91] This agent may also inhibit

turnover of tumor suppressor p53 and its target gene p21, which inhibit proliferation. Nonsteroidal anti-inflammatory drug (NSAID) inhibitors of cyclooxygenase, which affect prostaglandin synthesis and NF-κB activation, are of interest for chemoprevention of HNSCC. A study of topical rinse with NSAID ketorolac showed no effect versus placebo in a randomized study of patients with leukoplakia.[92] Natural compounds that inhibit NF-κB activation, such as curcumin from the spice tumeric (a major seasoning component of curry), are under investigation for chemoprevention.[93] Recent evidence that TNF inhibitors and targeting the inhibitor-κB kinase can block NF-κB activation may make possible use of agents with greater specificity and lower toxicity than proteasome or NSAIDs with broad activities.[40,42]

Preclinical laboratory and animal studies with mTOR inhibitors have shown promise and have led to initiation of clinical trials. Rapamycin induced apoptosis and tumorigenesis in HNSCC xenograft studies.[57] A rapamycin precursor CI-779 has also been of interest. Inhibitors of Ras and MAPK have shown antiproliferative activity in HNSCC cells, and MET and PI3K inhibitors are the subject of preclinical drug development. Inhibitors of NF-κB, STAT3, MAPK, PI3K, and mTOR may be most useful together in combinations when molecular diagnostics and suitable agents make such studies feasible.

REFERENCES

1. Jemal A, Murray T, Ward E, et al. Cancer statistics. CA Cancer J Clin 2005;55:10–30
2. Sidransky D. Emerging molecular markers of cancer. Nat Rev Cancer 2002;2:210–9
3. Khan J, Saal LH, Bittner ML, et al. Expression profiling in cancer using cDNA microarrays. Electrophoresis 1999;20:223–9.
4. Hanahan D, Weinberg RA. The hallmarks of cancer. Cell 2000;100:57–70.
5. Hahn WC, Weinberg RA. Rules for making human tumor cells. N Engl J Med 2002;347:1593–603.
6. Lowe SW, Sherr CJ. Tumor suppression by Ink4a-Arf: Progress and puzzles. Curr Opin Genet Dev 2003;13:77–83.
7. Redell MS, Tweardy DJ. Targeting transcription factors for cancer therapy. Curr Pharm Des 2005;11:2873–87.
8. Sidransky D. Molecular genetics of head and neck cancer. Curr Opin Oncol 1995;7:229–33.
9. Gillison ML, Koch WM, Capone RB, et al. Evidence for a causal association between human papillomavirus and a subset of head and neck cancers. J Natl Cancer Inst 2000; 92:709–20.
10. Niedobitek G. Epstein-Barr virus infection in the pathogenesis of nasopharyngeal carcinoma. Mol Pathol 2000; 53:248–54.
11. Ostwald C, Gogacz P, Hillmann T, et al. p53 mutational spectra are different between squamous-cell carcinoma of the lip and the oral cavity. Int J Cancer 2000;88:82–6.
12. Yoshizaki T. Promotion of metastasis in nasopharyngeal carcinoma by Epstein-Barr virus latent membrane protein-1. Histol Histopathol 2002;17:845–50.
13. Califano J, van der Riet P, Westra W, et al. Genetic progression model for head and neck cancer: Implications for field cancerization. Cancer Res 1996;56:2488–92.
14. Reed AL, Califano J, Cairns P, et al. High frequency of p16 (CDKN2/MTS-1/INK4A) inactivation in head and neck squamous cell carcinoma. Cancer Res 1996;56:3630–3.
15. Rocha S, Garrett MD, Campbell KJ, et al. Regulation of NF-kappaB and p53 through activation of ATR and Chk1 by the ARF tumour suppressor. Embo J 2005;24:1157–69.
16. Gorgoulis V, Rassidakis G, Karameris A, et al. Expression of p53 protein in laryngeal squamous cell carcinoma and dysplasia: Possible correlation with human papillomavirus infection and clinicopathological findings. Virchows Arch 1994;425:481–9.

17. Zhang PL, Pellitteri PK, Law A, et al. Overexpression of phosphorylated nuclear factor-kappa B in tonsillar squamous cell carcinoma and high-grade dysplasia is associated with poor prognosis. Mod Pathol 2005;18:924–32.
18. Liggett WH, Jr, Sewell DA, Rocco J, et al. p16 and p16 beta are potent growth suppressors of head and neck squamous carcinoma cells in vitro. Cancer Res 1996;56:4119–23.
19. Sidransky D, Hollstein M. Clinical implications of the p53 gene. Annu Rev Med 1996;47:285–301.
20. Webster GA, Perkins ND. Transcriptional cross talk between NF-kappaB and p53. Mol Cell Biol 1999;19:3485–95.
21. Lerman MI, Minna JD. The 630-kb lung cancer homozygous deletion region on human chromosome 3p21.3: Identification and evaluation of the resident candidate tumor suppressor genes. The International Lung Cancer Chromosome 3p21.3 Tumor Suppressor Gene Consortium. Cancer Res 2000;60:6116–33.
22. Kuroki T, Trapasso F, Yendamuri S, et al. Allele loss and promoter hypermethylation of VHL, RAR-beta, RASSF1A, and FHIT tumor suppressor genes on chromosome 3p in esophageal squamous cell carcinoma. Cancer Res 2003;63:3724–8.
23. Scholnick SB, Haughey BH, Sunwoo JB, et al. Chromosome 8 allelic loss and the outcome of patients with squamous cell carcinoma of the supraglottic larynx. J Natl Cancer Inst 1996;88:1676–82.
24. Scholnick SB, Richter TM. The role of CSMD1 in head and neck carcinogenesis. Genes Chromosomes Cancer 2003;38:281–3.
25. Pai SI, Wu GS, Ozoren N, et al. Rare loss-of-function mutation of a death receptor gene in head and neck cancer. Cancer Res 1998;58:3513–8.
26. Okami K, Wu L, Riggins G, et al. Analysis of PTEN/MMAC1 alterations in aerodigestive tract tumors. Cancer Res 1998;58:509–11.
27. Madrid LV, Mayo MW, Reuther JY, Baldwin AS, Jr. Akt stimulates the transactivation potential of the RelA/p65 Subunit of NF-kappa B through utilization of the Ikappa B kinase and activation of the mitogen-activated protein kinase p38. J Biol Chem 2001;276:18934–40.
28. Amornphimoltham P, Patel V, Sodhi A, et al. Mammalian target of rapamycin, a molecular target in squamous cell carcinomas of the head and neck. Cancer Res 2005; 65:9953–61.
29. Okami K, Reed AL, Cairns P, et al. Cyclin D1 amplification is independent of p16 inactivation in head and neck squamous cell carcinoma. Oncogene 1999;18:3541–5.
30. Chang AA, Van Waes C. Nuclear factor-KappaB as a common target and activator of oncogenes in head and neck squamous cell carcinoma. Adv Otorhinolaryngol 2005; 62:92–102.
31. Hibi K, Trink B, Patturajan M, et al. AIS is an oncogene amplified in squamous cell carcinoma. Proc Natl Acad Sci U S A 2000;97:5462–7.
32. Rocco JW, Leong CO, Kuperwasser N, et al. p63 mediates survival in squamous cell carcinoma by suppression of p73-dependent apoptosis. Cancer Cell 2006;9:45–56.
33. Carroll DK, Carroll JS, Leong CO, et al. p63 regulates an adhesion programme and cell survival in epithelial cells. Nat Cell Biol 2006;8:551–61.
34. Van Waes C, Kozarsky KF, Warren AB, et al. The A9 antigen associated with aggressive human squamous carcinoma is structurally and functionally similar to the newly defined integrin alpha 6 beta 4. Cancer Res 1991;51:2395–402.
35. Mao L, El-Naggar AK, Fan YH, et al. Telomerase activity in head and neck squamous cell carcinoma and adjacent tissues. Cancer Res 1996;56:5600–4.
36. Califano J, Ahrendt SA, Meininger G, et al. Detection of telomerase activity in oral rinses from head and neck squamous cell carcinoma patients. Cancer Res 1996;56:5720–2.
37. Tsurutani J, Castillo SS, Brognard J, et al. Tobacco components stimulate Akt-dependent proliferation and NFkappaB-dependent survival in lung cancer cells. Carcinogenesis 2005;26:1182–95.
38. Ni WF, Tsai CH, Yang SF, Chang YC. Elevated expression of NF-kappaB in oral submucous fibrosis--Evidence for NF-kappaB induction by safrole in human buccal mucosal fibroblasts. Oral Oncol 2006.
39. Wolf JS, Chen Z, Dong G, et al. IL (interleukin)-1alpha promotes nuclear factor-kappaB and AP-1-induced IL-8 expression, cell survival, and proliferation in head and neck squamous cell carcinomas. Clin Cancer Res 2001; 7:1812–20.
40. Jackson-Bernitsas DG, Ichikawa H, Takada Y, et al. Evidence that TNF-TNFR1-TRADD-TRAF2-RIP-TAK1-IKK pathway mediates constitutive NF-kappaB activation and proliferation in human head and neck squamous cell carcinoma. Oncogene 2007;26:1385–97.
41. Bancroft CC, Chen Z, Yeh J, et al. Effects of pharmacologic antagonists of epidermal growth factor receptor, PI3K and

MEK signal kinases on NF-kappaB and AP-1 activation and IL-8 and VEGF expression in human head and neck squamous cell carcinoma lines. Int J Cancer 2002;99:538–48.

42. Yu M, Yeh J, Van Waes C. Protein kinase casein kinase 2 mediates inhibitor-kappaB kinase and aberrant nuclear factor-kappaB activation by serum factor(s) in head and neck squamous carcinoma cells. Cancer Res 2006;66:6722–31.

43. Loercher A, Lee TL, Ricker JL, et al. Nuclear factor-kappaB is an important modulator of the altered gene expression profile and malignant phenotype in squamous cell carcinoma. Cancer Res 2004;64:6511–23. Erratum in: Cancer Res 2004;64:8130–2.

44. Chung CH, Parker JS, Ely K, et al. Gene expression profiles identify epithelial-to-mesenchymal transition and activation of nuclear factor-{kappa}B signaling as characteristics of a high-risk head and neck squamous cell carcinoma. Cancer Res 2006;66:8210–8.

45. Squarize CH, Castilho RM, Sriuranpong V, et al. Molecular cross-talk between the NFkappaB and STAT3 signaling pathways in head and neck squamous cell carcinoma. Neoplasia 2006;8:733–46.

46. Grandis JR, Melhem MF, Gooding WE, et al. Levels of TGF-alpha and EGFR protein in head and neck squamous cell carcinoma and patient survival. J Natl Cancer Inst 1998;90:824–32.

47. Grandis JR, Chakraborty A, Zeng Q, et al. Downmodulation of TGF-alpha protein expression with anti-sense oligonucleotides inhibits proliferation of head and neck squamous carcinoma but not normal mucosal epithelial cells. J Cell Biochem 1998;69:55–62.

48. He Y, Zeng Q, Drenning SD, et al. Inhibition of human squamous cell carcinoma growth in vivo by epidermal growth factor receptor antisense RNA transcribed from the U6 promoter. J Natl Cancer Inst 1998;90:1080–7.

49. Bonner JA, Raisch KP, Trummell HQ, et al. Enhanced apoptosis with combination C225/radiation treatment serves as the impetus for clinical investigation in head and neck cancers. J Clin Oncol 2000;18:47S–53S.

50. Milas L, Mason K, Hunter N, et al. In vivo enhancement of tumor radioresponse by C225 antiepidermal growth factor receptor antibody. Clin Cancer Res 2000;6:701–8.

51. Grandis JR, Drennnig SD, Zeng Q, et al. Constitutive activation of Stat3 signaling abrogates apoptosis in squamous cell carcinogenesis in vivo. Proc Natl Acad Sci U S A 2000; 97:4227–32.

52. Dong G, Chen Z, Li ZY, et al. Hepatocyte growth factor/scatter factor-induced activation of MEK and PI3K signal pathways contributes to expression of proangiogenic cytokines interleukin-8 and vascular endothelial growth factor in head and neck squamous cell carcinoma. Cancer Res 2001;61:5911–8.

53. Dong G, Lee TL, Yeh NT, et al. Metastatic squamous cell carcinoma cells that overexpress c-Met exhibit enhanced angiogenesis factor expression, scattering and metastasis in response to hepatocyte growth factor. Oncogene 2004; 23:6199–208.

54. Worden B, Yang XP, Lee TL, et al. Hepatocyte growth factor/scatter factor differentially regulates expression of proangiogenic factors through Egr-1 in head and neck squamous cell carcinoma. Cancer Res 2005;65:7071–80.

55. Nathan CA, Amirghahari N, Abreo F, et al. Overexpressed eIF4E is functionally active in surgical margins of head and neck cancer patients via activation of the Akt/mammalian target of rapamycin pathway. Clin Cancer Res 2004;10:5820–7.

56. Nathan CA, Franklin S, Abreo FW, et al. Expression of eIF4E during head and neck tumorigenesis: Possible role in angiogenesis. Laryngoscope 1999;109:1253–8.

57. Amornphimoltham P, Patel V, Sodhi A, et al. Mammalian target of rapamycin, a molecular target in squamous

58. Truelson JM, Fisher SG, Beals TE, et al. DNA content and histologic growth pattern correlate with prognosis in patients with advanced squamous cell carcinoma of the larynx. The Department of Veterans Affairs Cooperative Laryngeal Cancer Study Group. Cancer 1992;70:56–62.

59. Folkman J. Fighting cancer by attacking its blood supply. Sci Am 1996;275:150–4.

60. Chen Z, Smith CW, Kiel D, Van Waes C. Metastatic variants derived following in vivo tumor progression of an in vitro transformed squamous cell carcinoma line acquire a differential growth advantage requiring tumor-host interaction. Clin Exp Metastasis 1997;15:527–37.

61. Young MR, Wright MA, Lozano Y, et al. Increased recurrence and metastasis in patients whose primary head and neck squamous cell carcinomas secreted granulocyte-macrophage colony-stimulating factor and contained CD34+ natural suppressor cells. Int J Cancer 1997;74:69–74.

62. Young MR. Chemokines and cancer. Arch Pathol Lab Med 2000;124:642.

63. Pekarek LA, Starr BA, Toledano AY, Schreiber H. Inhibition of tumor growth by elimination of granulocytes. J Exp Med 1995;181:435–40.

64. Itoh T, Tanioka M, Matsuda H. Experimental metastasis is suppressed in MMP-9-deficient mice. Clin Exp Metastasis 1999;17:177–81.

65. Tamura M, Arakaki N, Tsubouchi H, et al. Enhancement of human hepatocyte growth factor production by interleukin-1 alpha and -1 beta and tumor necrosis factor-alpha by fibroblasts in culture. J Biol Chem 1993;268:8140–5.

66. Van Waes C, Surh DM, Chen Z, et al. Increase in suprabasilar integrin adhesion molecule expression in human epidermal neoplasms accompanies increased proliferation occurring with immortalization and tumor progression. Cancer Res 1995;55:5434–44.

67. Wolf GT, Carey TE, Schmaltz SP, et al. Altered antigen expression predicts outcome in squamous cell carcinoma of the head and neck. J Natl Cancer Inst 1990;82:1566–72.

68. Rabinovitz I, Mercurio AM. The integrin alpha 6 beta 4 and the biology of carcinoma. Biochem Cell Biol 1996; 74:811–21.

69. Van Waes C, Surh DM, Chen Z, Carey TE. Inhibition of integrin mediated cell adhesion of human head and neck squamous cell carcinoma to extracellular matrix laminin by monoclonal antibodies. Int J Oncol 1997;11:457–64.

70. Rosenthal EL, Johnson TM, Allen ED, et al. Role of the plasminogen activator and matrix metalloproteinase systems in epidermal growth factor- and scatter factor-stimulated invasion of carcinoma cells. Cancer Res 1998;58:5221–30.

71. Hanzawa M, Shindoh M, Higashino F, et al. Hepatocyte growth factor upregulates E1AF that induces oral squamous cell carcinoma cell invasion by activating matrix metalloproteinase genes. Carcinogenesis 2000;21:1079–85.

72. O-charoenrat P, Modjtahedi H, Rhys-Evans P, et al. Epidermal growth factor-like ligands differentially up-regulate matrix metalloproteinase 9 in head and neck squamous carcinoma cells. Cancer Res 2000;60:1121–8.

73. Coussens LM, Tinkle CL, Hanahan D, Werb Z. MMP-9 supplied by bone marrow-derived cells contributes to skin carcinogenesis. Cell 2000;103:481–90.

74. Chen Z, Malhotra PS, Thomas GR, et al. Expression of proinflammatory and proangiogenic cytokines in patients with head and neck cancer. Clin Cancer Res 1999;5:1369–79.

75. Loukinova E, Dong G, Enamorado-Ayalya I, et al. Growth regulated oncogene-alpha expression by murine squamous cell carcinoma promotes tumor growth, metastasis, leukocyte infiltration and angiogenesis by a host CXC

receptor-2 dependent mechanism. Oncogene 2000;19: 3477–86.

76. Druzgal CH, Chen Z, Yeh NT, et al. A pilot study of longitudinal serum cytokine and angiogenesis factor levels as markers of therapeutic response and survival in patients with head and neck squamous cell carcinoma. Head Neck 2005;27:771–84.

77. Chen Z, Colon I, Ortiz N, et al. Effects of interleukin-1alpha, interleukin-1 receptor antagonist, and neutralizing antibody on proinflammatory cytokine expression by human squamous cell carcinoma lines. Cancer Res 1998; 58:3668–76.

78. Hong SH, Ondrey FG, Avis IM, et al. Cyclooxygenase regulates human oropharyngeal carcinomas via the proinflammatory cytokine IL-6: A general role for inflammation? FASEB J 2000;14:1499–507.

79. Kitadai Y, Takahashi Y, Haruma K, et al. Transfection of interleukin-8 increases angiogenesis and tumorigenesis of human gastric carcinoma cells in nude mice. Br J Cancer 1999;81:647–53.

80. Van Waes C, Enamorado-Ayala I, Hecht D, et al. Effects of the novel alphav integrin antagonist SM256 and cis-platinum on growth of murine squamous cell carcinoma PAM LY8. Int J Oncol 2000;16:1189–95.

81. Koch WM, Brennan JA, Zahurak M, et al. p53 mutation and locoregional treatment failure in head and neck squamous cell carcinoma. J Natl Cancer Inst 1996;88:1580–6.

82. Nawroz H, Koch W, Anker P, et al. Microsatellite alterations in serum DNA of head and neck cancer patients. Nat Med 1996;2:1035–7.

83. Sanchez-Cespedes M, Esteller M, Wu L, et al. Gene promoter hypermethylation in tumors and serum of head and neck cancer patients. Cancer Res 2000;60:892–5.

84. St John MA, Li Y, Zhou X, et al. Interleukin 6 and interleukin 8 as potential biomarkers for oral cavity and oropharyngeal squamous cell carcinoma. Arch Otolaryngol Head Neck Surg 2004;130:929–35.

85. Akervall J, Guo X, Qian CN, et al. Genetic and expression profiles of squamous cell carcinoma of the head and neck correlate with cisplatin sensitivity and resistance in cell lines and patients. Clin Cancer Res 2004;10:8204–13.

86. Hunter KD, Thurlow JK, Fleming J, et al. Divergent routes to oral cancer. Cancer Res 2006;66:7405–13.

87. Ginos MA, Page GP, Michalowicz BS, et al. Identification of a gene expression signature associated with recurrent disease in squamous cell carcinoma of the head and neck. Cancer Res 2004;64:55–63.

88. Cohen EE. Role of epidermal growth factor receptor pathway-targeted therapy in patients with recurrent and/or metastatic squamous cell carcinoma of the head and neck. J Clin Oncol 2006;24:2659–65.

89. Xi S, Gooding WE, Grandis JR. In vivo antitumor efficacy of STAT3 blockade using a transcription factor decoy approach: Implications for cancer therapy. Oncogene 2005; 24:970–9.

90. Van Waes C, Chang AA, Lebowitz PF, et al. Inhibition of nuclear factor-kappaB and target genes during combined therapy with proteasome inhibitor bortezomib and reirradiation in patients with recurrent head-and-neck squamous cell carcinoma. Int J Radiat Oncol Biol Phys 2005;63:1400–12.

91. Richardson PG, Mitsiades C, Hideshima T, Anderson KC. Bortezomib: Proteasome inhibition as an effective anticancer therapy. Annu Rev Med 2006;57:33–47.

92. Mulshine JL, Atkinson JC, Greer RO, et al. Randomized, double-blind, placebo-controlled phase IIb trial of the cyclooxygenase inhibitor ketorolac as an oral rinse in oropharyngeal leukoplakia. Clin Cancer Res 2004;10:1565–73.

93. Aggarwal BB, Shishodia S. Molecular targets of dietary agents for prevention and therapy of cancer. Biochem Pharmacol 2006;71:1397–421.

Mechanisms of Immune Evasion of Head and Neck Cancer

Brian R. Gastman, MD
Aaron H. D. Wood, MD

Immune evasion by cancerous cells is a key part of the carcinogenesis process. Cells displaying altered malignant phenotypes are prime targets for destruction by the host immune system unless they develop methods to avoid or block immune attacks. The phenomenon of tumor immune evasion exhibits both passive and active components. Passive components involve tumor becoming inconspicuous to the immune system, as well as becoming resistant to immune-mediated killing through manipulation of the tumor's homeostatic molecular machinery. The active components of evasion consist of tumors directly inducing cell death or dysfunction of immune effector cells or recruiting the host's normal immunosuppressive mechanisms to induce an inferior and ultimately inadequate immune response.[1] These active evasion strategies have, in addition to local tumor and immune cell effects, global immune consequences for the host as well. Reports of opportunistic infections are abundant in patients with various cancers, especially hematopoietic malignancies. Furthermore, immunocompromised patients, due to HIV or organ transplantation, are much more susceptible to acquire cancers of many types. By becoming more inconspicuous, less vulnerable, and more virulent to the immune system, cancers can grow essentially unchecked until they lead to inevitable devastating consequences for the patient.

On the other hand, clinicians can use these immune system changes caused by malignant cells as tools to diagnose and prognosticate the advancement of cancer. For example, normal T cell activity requires the T cell receptor (TCR) to function through a variety of supportive molecules. It had been shown that patients with cancer frequently have decreased expression of the TCR molecule zeta, with resultant reduced signaling through this receptor. Others and we have now shown that this can be explained in part by tumors activating cell death machinery within T cells, causing cleavage of the zeta molecule.[2] Importantly, zeta loss has now been shown to be important in prognosis in a variety of cancers.[3] The ability to monitor these types of molecular changes within host immune cells and tumors has improved our understanding of the behavior of malignant disease. More importantly, understanding the various tumor immune evasion strategies can provide guidance during the development

and implementation of current and future selective cancer treatment modalities.

TUMOR IMMUNE ESCAPE VIA INVISIBILITY

One of the most straightforward methods by which tumors evade immune attack in patients with head and neck cancer is by avoiding immune recognition in the first place. Preventing recognition allows tumors to thwart the induction of an antitumor immune response or, failing that, to avoid an effective antitumor cytotoxic attack. Because host cytotoxic cells must recognize tumor antigens within the correct molecular "context," a tumor can sidestep the immune system by downregulating its expression of targeted antigens, reducing levels of context-supplying molecules, or preventing effective antigen exposure to secondary lymphatic organs, where recognition occurs (Figure 1). Attack by cytotoxic T cells

or natural killer (NK) cells is prevented by loss of tumor-associated antigens (TAAs), downregulation of tumor human leukocyte antigen Class I (HLAI) or costimulatory molecule expression, downregulation of NK-activating ligands, and upregulation of NK inhibiting ligands, or immune ignorance caused by physical separation of tumor and effector cells.

Compared to infectious agents such as viruses, tumors have the advantage of having developed from the host's own cells, thereby inheriting significant protection against attack through immune self-tolerance. The presence of self-tolerance means that tumors potentially express few antigen targets by which the innate or adaptive immune responses can distinguish neoplastic cells from adjacent normal cells. Nevertheless, intact host immune responses against tumor neoantigens or overexpressed normal proteins have been demonstrated.[4] The result is that many tumors either modify the expression of these recognized antigens or downregulate the processing

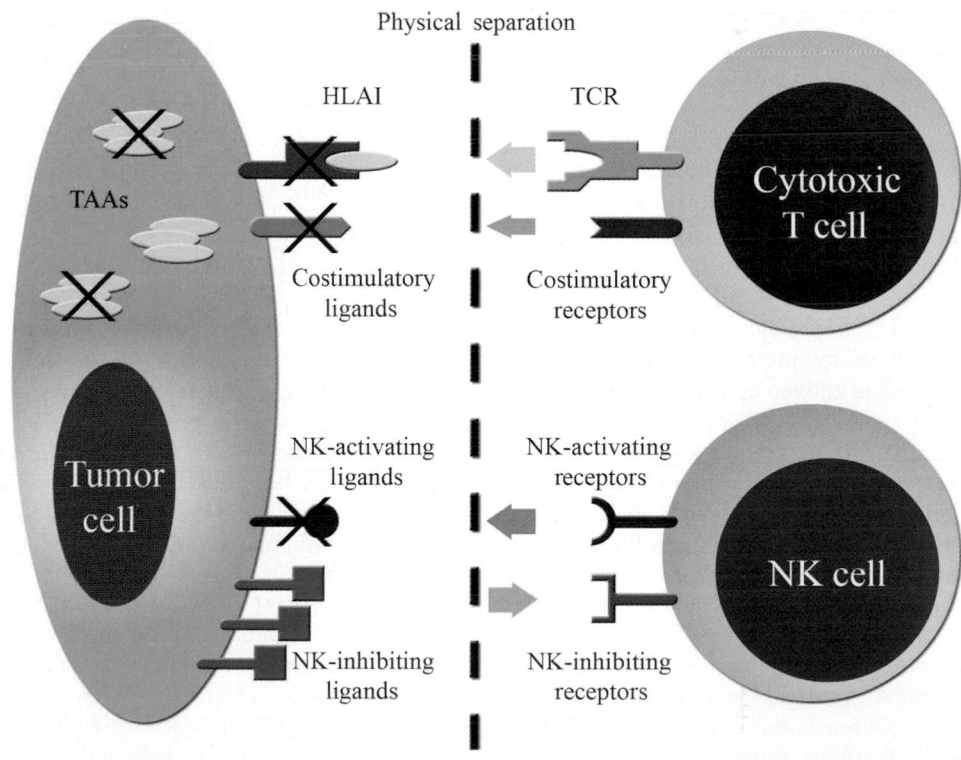

Figure 1 Tumor invisibility. Attack by cytotoxic T cells or natural killer (NK) cells is prevented by (1) loss of tumor-associated antigens (TAAs), (2) downregulation of tumor HLA Class I (HLAI) or costimulatory molecule expression, (3) downregulation of NK-activating ligands, (4) upregulation of NK-inhibiting ligands, or (5) immune ignorance caused by physical separation of tumor and effector cells.

machinery required for antigen presentation to immune effector cells.

TUMOR-ASSOCIATED ANTIGEN LOSS

Native tumors consist of a heterogeneous population of malignant cells expressing variable levels of cellular proteins. Several different categories of cancer protein antigens have been identified that can induce cytotoxic T lymphocyte (CTL) responses in vitro and in vivo. These TAAs fall into five groups: (1) "cancer testis" (CT) antigens, expressed in multiple malignancies and normal testis, (2) melanocyte differentiation antigens, (3) point mutations of normal genes, such as the tumor suppressor p53, (4) self antigens that are overexpressed in malignant tissues, and (5) viral antigens.[5] Although tumors presumably benefit from producing these various oncogenic products, in the setting of T cell attack, individual tumor cells that can downregulate these TAAs and survive have a significant advantage. The result is a tumor "immunoselected" to evade host immunity. Indeed, repeated biopsies of metastatic melanoma have shown that TAA loss correlates with tumor progression. Residual tumors following vaccination with TAA peptides have also shown decreased levels of corresponding TAA expression.[6] The presence of TAA-specific immune effector cells has little impact on these adapted cancers, and they can grow aggressively.

HLA CLASS I LOSS

One of the most well-characterized methods of tumor antigen loss is alteration in the cellular expression of the major histocompatability complex (MHC) Class I proteins, also referred to as HLAI. Classical HLAI molecules, required for CD8[+] T cell recognition of antigens, are found on nearly all human cells. The loss of HLAI has a profound effect on the ability of these cytotoxic T cells to recognize a tumor antigen, become activated, and attack tumor cells. Seven HLAI loss phenotypes have been described, involving everything from loss of a single HLAI allele to a total loss of all HLAI expression. Tumors can display these phenotypes by altering one or more of the steps involved in antigen breakdown, processing, and loading onto HLA molecules.[7] Downregulation of HLAI levels in a human tumor relative to a normal tissue was first described in 1977. Since then, numerous investigators have found a high percentage of HLAI loss in multiple human solid tumors, including squamous cell carcinoma of the head and neck (SCCHN). For example, Cabrera and colleagues showed loss of HLAI in 70% of laryngeal carcinomas.[8] Another survey of SCCHN found 15% HLAI loss in primary tumors and 40% in metastasis, suggesting that HLAI loss correlates with tumor aggressiveness.[9]

Although downregulation of HLA Class I may help a tumor cell evade T cell cytotoxic attack, tumor cells must also contend with host NK cell surveillance. Classically, NK cells were understood to detect and eliminate cells that failed to express the "self" identifying protein HLA1. This NK targeting of "missing self" cells appears incompatible with successfully growing HLA1-negative tumors, suggesting that neoplasms must employ additional methods to inhibit NK cell function. Although still an area of ongoing investigation, it appears that NK cell cytotoxicity is controlled by a balance between stimulation of activating and inhibitory receptor populations on the surface of NK cells. There is recent evidence that some tumor-bearing patients express either abnormally low levels of activating receptors, on their NK cells or low levels of ligands, to these receptors on tumor cells. Theoretically, tumor-induced activation of NK inhibitory receptors, may also protect cancers from NK attack.[10]

IMMUNE IGNORANCE

Tumors that express adequate levels of tumor antigens and HLA molecules can still avoid immune attack if the signals that these proteins represent never reach T cells in sufficient amounts to stimulate an antigen-specific response. This phenomenon is termed immune ignorance and is distinct from T cell anergy or deletion in that T cells capable of responding to tumor antigen in vitro are present in the host but fail to react to the tumor in vivo. These T cells act as if they do not "see" the nearby tumor cells at all. Immune ignorance is primarily a feature of solid tumors located in the periphery, which shed relatively a few antigen-expressing malignant cells to the lymph nodes, where the cellular immune response is initiated. Any cells that do metastasize wall themselves off from nearby T cells in these nodes by producing an isolating matrix coat. These geographical barriers prevent potentially reactive circulating T cells from encountering sufficient levels of the tumor antigen they recognize for full activation, rendering them "ignorant" of the tumor's presence.[11]

COSTIMULATORY RECEPTOR LOSS

Once a host adaptive immune response is induced, either from normal tumor cell death causing shedding of TAAs or from TAA vaccination, tumors may still prevent antigen-specific CD8[+] T cell destruction by modifying the expression of costimulatory molecules on their surface. Costimulation is essential for activated CD8[+] cytotoxic T lymphocytes (CTLs) to exhibit efficient cytotoxicity, as CD8[+] cells whose TCRs interact with HLA1 in the absence of the "second signal" of costimulation are quickly rendered anergic. Squamous cell carcinomas have been found universally to lack the potent costimulatory proteins CD80 and CD86, while dramatic loss of similar molecules CD40 and intercellular adhesion molecule-1 (ICAM-1) has been demonstrated as well.[12,13] As the latter costimulator is also a cell adhesion molecule, tumor ICAM-1 loss may contribute to tissue invasion in addition to immune evasion. T cell anergy from lack of costimulation can be a significant barrier to effective natural induction or tumor vaccine therapy, as development of a large population of antigen-specific T cells will produce no significant CTL effect at the tumor site.

TUMOR IMMUNE ESCAPE VIA APOPTOSIS CONTROL

Although many human malignancies are masters of molecular disguise, they need not simply hide from the immune system. Tumors can also evade host immunity by making intracellular molecules that block cytotoxic attacks or by attacking their attackers. This is accomplished through manipulation of the normal cellular machinery responsible for the phenomenon of programmed cell death (PCD), also known as apoptosis. Apoptosis is a conserved and self-regulating pathway, operative in all eukaryotic cells. It occurs during embryonic development and is essential for successful organogenesis and the crafting of complex multicellular tissues. The evolutionary advent of differentiated cell types may have necessitated controlling cell death as well as division to keep neighboring cells interdependent and insure the proper balance of each cell lineage. For instance, apoptosis is responsible for negative selection of nonreactive leukocyte precursors and autoreactive T lymphocytes. Without this, process of immune cell selection, T cell-mediated autoimmunnity would ensue. Apoptosis also operates in adult organisms to maintain normal cellular homeostasis. This is especially critical in the removal of precancerous and virally infected cells. Gain- and loss-of-function models of genes in the core apoptotic pathways indicate that the violation of this cellular homeostatic process can lead to the development of a wide range of human diseases, including cancer. Clinically, there is now strong evidence that insufficient apoptosis can manifest as cancer or autoimmunity, while accelerated cell death is evident in acute and chronic degenerative diseases, immunodeficiency, and infertility.

Apoptotic Family of Molecules

Within the various groups of molecules responsible for apoptotic control, there are a few key protein families. Although many molecules have an apoptotic role, the Caspase, Bcl-2, and IAPs (inhibitors of apoptosis) families are the major arbiters of this phenomenon. Also of importance are the death-receptor families and mitochondrial-based molecules, by which the two main pathways of classic apoptosis are initiated.

Caspases, a group of cysteine proteases related to mammalian ICE (interleukin-1 beta converting enzyme), play a crucial role in apoptosis. These enzymes appear to be involved in both the initial signaling events and the downstream proteolytic cleavages that characterize the apoptotic phenotype. In addition, cleavage of cellular proteins can change their function and cause the phenotypic changes seen in PCD. For instance, caspase-cleaved proteins are responsible for plasma membrane blebbing, cellular breakage into "apoptotic bodies," the dissolution of cellular integrity and cellular packaging, disruption of macromolecule synthesis, and termination of survival signals. Predictably, these changes lead to the general destruction of the cell.

The apoptosis-inhibiting molecule Bcl-2 (B-cell leukemia/lymphoma 2) was first discovered as a proto-oncogene in follicular lymphomas. It is the prototype of a large family of proteins, with both anti- and proapoptotic members, that share Bcl-2 homology (BH) domains. Unlike caspases, which have no antiapoptotic counterpart, it is the ratio of these anti- to proapoptotic Bcl-2 family members that determines a cell's fate. This may be related to their separate antagonizing functions or to the ability of the two types of family members to heterodimerize. Antiapoptotic family members, such as Bcl-2, Bcl-XL, and Bcl-w, have been found to be overexpressed in a variety of solid tumors. As would be expected, proapoptotic molecules, like Bax, Bim, and Bak, have been shown to be significantly downregulated in a host of malignancies.

Numerous mechanisms for the functions of the Bcl-2 family have been proposed. Anti-apoptotic members may function as an antioxidant or redox-regulating protein, as recent data implicate Bcl-2 in the general adaptation to oxidative stress. Bcl-2 and Bcl-XL also protect against mitochondrial outer membrane permeabilization. Both pro- and antiapoptotic Bcl-2 molecules have been suggested to be channel-forming proteins that are incorporated into lipid membranes to control the movement of other important PCD regulators. The pore-producing ability of proapoptotic molecules, such as Bax and Bak, appears to be essential for the release of apoptogenic molecules from the mitochondria, initiating the intrinsic apoptosis pathway (discussed below).

IAPs are the third intracellular family of apoptosis-related molecules. Their most well-described mechanism of action involves binding to and inhibiting caspase activity. IAPs are therefore potentially involved at several points in multiple apoptosis pathways.

Two Pathways to Apoptosis

All of the previously described PCD control molecules function within two major apoptotic pathways.[14] The extrinsic pathway is initiated at the cell surface through a variety of prodeath receptors belonging to the tumor necrosis factor (TNF) receptor family. The intrinsic pathway is initiated at the level of an organelle, proto-typically the mitochondria. Ultimately, both the pathways converge on the so-called downstream caspases, which function to cleave the majority of molecules necessary to complete the PCD process. It is likely that neither pathway is independent of the other, with extrinsic/intrinsic crosstalk required for a complete death signal (Figure 2).

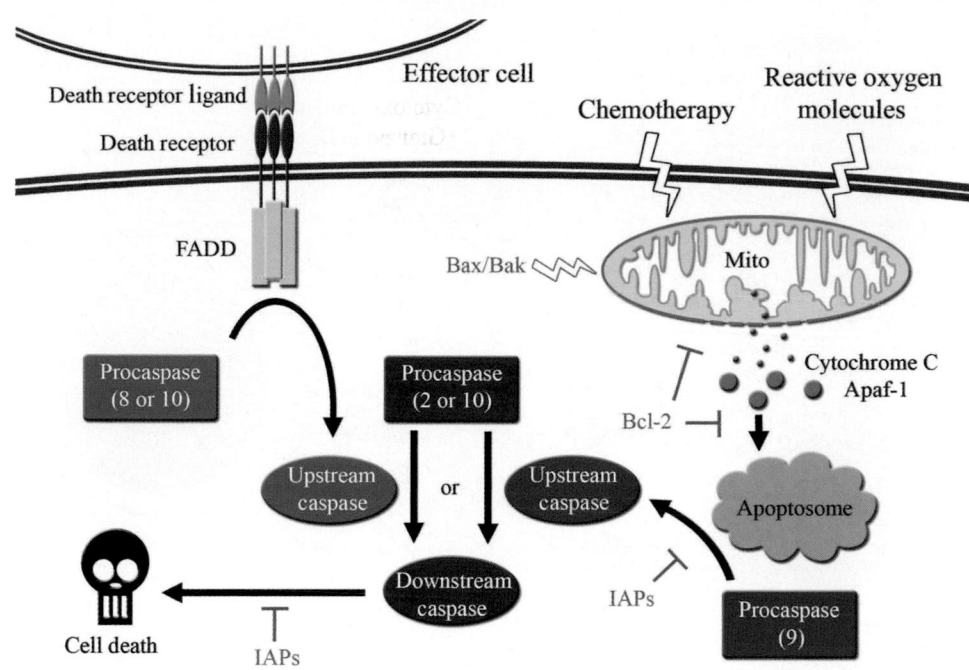

Figure 2 Apoptosis pathways. Extrinsic and intrinsic pathways of apoptosis converge upon common downstream caspases to initiate cell death. FADD = Fas-associated death domain molecules; IAPs = inhibitors of apoptosis; Mito = mitochondrion.

The extrinsic apoptotic pathway begins when cell death receptors, such as Fas, TRAIL-R1-4 (TNF-related apoptosis-inducing ligand-R1-4), and TNF-R1, bind to their corresponding ligands and form tri-molecular complexes at the cell surface. These complexes recruit adapter molecules such as FADD (Fas-associated death domain) that then activate "upstream" caspases, such as caspase-8 and -10, which cleave and activate the downstream caspases that finally kill the cell. Death receptor–ligand interactions have been shown to be important in immune system development, homeostasis, and function. Various studies have focused on manipulating either receptors or ligands in a variety of disorders. For example, inhibition of Fas prevents rejection in a mouse transplant model, as transplanted cells gain resistance to the corresponding Fas-Ligand (FasL) on host immune effector cells.[15]

The intrinsic pathway is initiated in the mitochondria, where numerous apoptogenic proteins, such as cytochrome c, reside. The pathway progresses in two steps. Initially, breakdown of the inner mitochondrial membrane diffusion barrier frees cytochrome c from the unraveling cristae to the intermitochondrial space. Following this, cytochrome c is released into the cytosol via pores in the mitochondrial outer membrane. This second step requires the proapoptotic Bcl-2 family proteins Bak and Bax, while cristae remodeling is regulated by a protease PARL (presenilin-associated rhomboid-like protein) and its target hetero-oligomer OPA1 (dominant optic atrophy gene). Ultimately cytochrome c combines with other proteins to form the apoptosome (an oligomer of procaspase-9, Apaf-1, dATP, and cytochrome c). It is the apoptosome that activates the upstream caspase, casepase-9, which in turn cleaves the downstream caspases of the common pathway.

Additionally, other mitochondrial apoptogenic molecules can move throughout the cell and cause various variations of cell death and dysfunction besides classic apoptosis.

Apoptosis in Tumor Cytotoxic Resistance

Because immune effector cells require their targets to express intact apoptotic machinery for effective cytotoxicity, modification of even a few PCD mediators will cause molecules normally toxic to target cells to become ineffective. For instance, others and we have shown the importance of mitochondria in granzyme B-mediated apoptosis. Granzyme B, a serine protease transferred from cytotoxic T cells into their targets, directly activates the mitochondrial apoptotic pathway. Recent data have shown that upregulation of Mcl-1 (a mitochondrial-associated anti-apoptotic Bcl-2 molecule) can inhibit granzyme B in vitro.[16] Granzyme B also shows significant homology to endogenous caspases, and common caspase inhibitors will inhibit granzyme B as well.

Successful cancers display a multitude of similar resistances to PCD due to modification of various pathway components (Figure 3). To control the extrinsic pathway, tumors may downregulate the expression of death receptor complex members, upregulate levels of death receptor inhibitors, or qualitatively and quantitatively modify the expression of associated caspases and their inhibitors.[17] The loss or mutation of extrinsic and intrinsic pathway caspases have been reported widely in cancer. A variety of natural caspases inhibitors are upregulated in cancerous cells as well. For example, the expression of the IAP *Survivin* has been shown to be critical in colorectal and lung cancer growth,

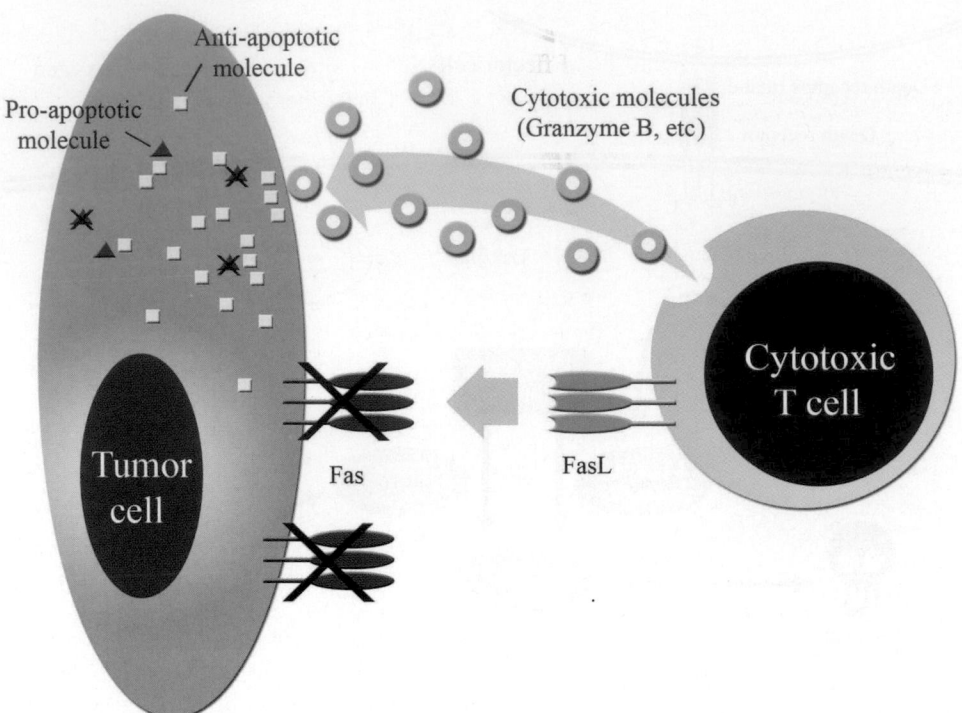

Figure 3 Tumor apoptosis resistance. T cell attack by either cytotoxic molecules or death receptors (FasL) is prevented by (1) downregulation of tumor Fas molecules, (2) upregulation of intracellular anti-apoptotic molecules, or (3) downregulation of intracellular pro-apoptotic molecules.

although specific links to immune evasion have yet to be identified.[18] Alternatively, both tumors and associated suppressor cells produce anti-inflammatory cytokines and soluble factors such as transforming growth factor beta (TGF$_\beta$), interleukin 10 (IL-10), phosphatidylserine (sPS), and prostaglandin E_2 (PGE$_2$) that induce a shift in the tumor cell ratio of pro- to antiapoptotic Bcl-2 type molecules[1] (Table 1). Significantly, these immune escape mechanisms can make cancer cells insensitive to other apoptosis-inducing events such as low oxygen environments, chemotherapy, and radiation therapy.[19] These studies suggest that our inability to develop adequate chemotherapies for many cancers may be a direct result of production of apoptosis-resistant malignant cells by normal immune selection pressure.

Apoptosis in Tumor Immune Counterattack

Beyond simply avoiding or resisting immune attack, cancer can actually co-opt the immune system's apoptotic weaponry. Tumors employ both membrane-bound and soluble mediators of PCD to produce immune cell dysfunction or death, both in the tumor microenvironment and systemically (Figure 4).

This ability is normally restricted to "immune privileged" tissues, such as ocular tissue and Sertoli cells of the testis, which mediate their unique immune exclusion through expression of the death protein, Fas-Ligand (FasL). Membrane-bound FasL activates Fas on the surface of immune effector cells during cell-to-cell contact, causing degradation of the TCR zeta chain and ultimately apoptosis of threatening T cells. This mechanism has been utilized in transplantation studies to immune-protect allografts through forced expression of FasL on the transplanted cells. Unfortunately, FasL and other death-inducing ligands such as TRAIL can also mediate immune evasion of malignancies, with tumor-induced apoptosis of T cells (TIAT) demonstrated in a variety of different cancer types.[20,21] Furthermore, FasL can be cleaved from the tumor cell surface by metalloproteases to form soluble FasL (sFasL), which demonstrates systemic as well as local immune killing ability.[22]

Along with cell death receptors, tumors can express other inhibitory receptors that access the PCD pathway. In particular, the costimulatory molecule B7-H1 has been recently shown to induce TIAT upon ligation with either Programmed Death 1 (PD-1) or, more likely, another as-yet-undefined receptor on activated T cells. B7-H1 has been found constitutively expressed at high levels on the surface of over 60% of head and neck squamous cell carcinomas, and antibody blockade of tumor B7-H1 protects CD8$^+$ T cell from apoptosis in murine SCCHN models.[23]

Tumors need not actually kill cytotoxic effector cells, as the same anti-inflammatory cytokines and soluble factors (TGF$_\beta$, IL-10, sPS, and PGE$_2$) that protect malignant cells from apoptosis also inhibit antigen presenting cell (APC) maturation, T cell induction and proliferation, and T cell effector function.[1] Tumors also secrete metalloproteases that cleave Fas from tumor cell membranes to form sFas, which competitively inhibits Fas on CTL. Similarly, the NK ligand MICA can be solubilized (sMICA) to cause inhibition and downregulation of the activating NKG2D receptor, blunting the innate immune system's ability to attack cancerous cells (Table 1).

TUMOR IMMUNE ESCAPE VIA INDIRECT SUPPRESSION OF CELLULAR IMMUNITY

In addition to direct inactivation or destruction of cytotoxic effector cells, tumors recruit several populations of host immune cells with immunosuppressive functions. These suppressive cells can be generally grouped together as either T regulatory cells (T$_{regs}$) or myeloid suppressor cells (MSCs). These suppressors normally function to blunt potentially overaggressive host immune responses to inflammation and infection. In the setting of cancer, however, they have been found to prevent both effective tumor surveillance and effective immunotherapy. Importantly, these effects can be measured both within the tumor microenvironment and systemically (Figure 4).

T Regulatory Cells in Indirect Suppression

T$_{regs}$, classically identified as CD4$^+$CD25$^+$FOXP3$^+$ expressing cells, normally make up 5 to 10% of peripheral CD4$^+$ T cells in humans and play an important part in peripheral tolerance of effector T cells to self antigens.[24] Increased numbers of several different subtypes of T$_{regs}$ have been found in many different human cancers, including cancers of the head and neck, both as tumor infiltrating lymphocytes (TILs) and as peripheral blood lymphocytes (PBLs).[25] T$_{reg}$ populations have also been shown to correlate with tumor stage in gastric and esophageal cancers.[26] It appears that malignancy predominantly increases the number of active T$_{regs}$ rather than increasing each cell's suppressive activity.[24]

Cancers display several different methods for producing expanded T$_{reg}$ populations. Precise delineation of these methods has been somewhat limited by the lack of reliable cell surface markers distinguishing T$_{reg}$ subtypes; nevertheless, in vitro and mouse in vivo evidence suggests potential mechanisms likely active in cancer patients. Tumor secretion of local growth factors and cytokines such as VEGF, TGF$_\beta$, and IL-10 can prevent dendritic cell (DC) maturation and result in myeloid DCs that stimulate the expansion and activation of thymus-derived natural T$_{regs}$.[24] These cytokines and immature DCs can also convert normal T cells into CD4+ (T$_R$1-type) T$_{regs}$ or CD8$^+$ T$_{regs}$, both within the tumor microenvironment and in tumor-draining lymph nodes.[27,28] Finally, T$_{regs}$ may be recruited to the tumor site by cancer cells expressing chemokine ligands such as macrophage-derived chemokine CCL22.[29]

As T$_{regs}$ accumulate in the patient with tumor, they cause both antigen-specific and nonspecific suppression of the host immune system. T$_{regs}$, like tumors, can produce TGF$_\beta$ and IL10, cytokines which suppress the activation and function of antigen presenting cells (APCs), NK cells, and effector T cells.[30] In addition, T$_{regs}$ can directly kill T cells and APCs through release of cytotoxic granzyme B and perforin or expression of FasL.[31] Since T$_{regs}$ express IL-2 receptors at much higher levels than other T cells, it has been suggested that

Table 1 Soluble Factors Contributing to Tumor Immune Evasion

Soluble Factors	Origin	Function
Interleukin 10 (IL-10)	• Tumor • MSCs • T_{regs} • Stroma	• Inhibits CTL and NK function • Inhibits DC maturation • Stimulates tumor anti-apoptotic molecule levels • Stimulates IDO/ARG1 activity in MSCs • Induces T_{regs}
Transforming growth factor β (TGFβ)	• Tumor • MSCs • T_{regs}	• Inhibits CTL and NK function • Inhibits DC maturation • Stimulates VEGF/PGE$_2$/IL-10/IL-4 production by stroma • Stimulates ARG1 activity in MSCs • Induces T_{regs}
Interleukin 4 (IL-4)	• Tumor • MSCs • Stroma	• Increases tumor anti-apoptotic molecule levels • Inhibits DC maturation • Stimulates tumor growth • Stimulates ARG1 activity in MSCs • Induces T_{regs}
Interleukin 13 (IL-13)	• Tumor	• Inhibits DC maturation • Stimulates ARG1 activity in MSCs • Stimulates TGFβ release from MSCs • Induces T_{regs}
Phosphatidylserine (sPS)	• Tumor	• Inhibits inflammatory cytokine production • Inhibits DC maturation • Stimulates IL-10/ TGFβ/PGE$_2$ production by tumors and MSCs
Prostaglandin E$_2$ (PGE$_2$)	• Tumor • Stroma	• Inhibits inflammatory cytokine production • Inhibits DC HLAI and HLAII expression
Vascular endothelial growth factor (VEGF)	• Tumor • Stroma	• Inhibits DC maturation • Stimulates angiogenesis • Recruits MSCs and stimulates iNOS function
Granulocyte-monocyte colony-stimulating factor (GM-CSF)	• Tumor	• Inhibits CTL function • Recruits MSCs and stimulates iNOS function
Colony stimulating factor-1 (CSF-1)	• Tumor	• Inhibits DC maturation • Recruits MSCs
CC-type chemokine ligand 22 (CCL22)	• Tumor	• Recruits T_{regs}
Soluble Fas ligand (sFasL)	• Tumor	• Mediates CTL counterattack • Blocks and downregulates tumor Fas
Soluble Fas (sFas)	• Tumor	• Causes CTL FasL blockade
Soluble MICA (sMICA)	• Tumor	• Blocks and downregulates NKG2D receptor on NK cells
Matrix metalloproteases (MMPs)	• Tumor • MSCs	• Cleaves FasL/Fas/MICA from tumor cells • Cleaves VEGF from stroma
Indoleamine 2,3-dioxygenase (IDO)	• MSCs	• Depletes extracellular tryptophan (inhibiting CTL function)

T_{regs} outcompete effector T cells for this important growth factor, especially within the tumor microenvironment where T_{regs} vastly outnumber effector T cells.[32] Finally, T_{regs} constitutively express the costimulatory receptor inhibitor CTLA-4, which blocks costimulation of effector T cells and induces anergy. CTLA-4 can also induce APCs to produce the enzyme IDO (Indoleamine 2,3-dioxygenase), locally depleting essential tryptophan and suppressing T cell activation.[33]

Myeloid Suppressor Cells in Indirect Suppression

MSCs, like T_{regs}, are a group of normally occurring immune regulatory cells co-opted by malignancies to avoid immune attack. MSCs include undifferentiated myeloid cells, macrophages, dendritic cells, and granulocytes that exhibit immature cell surface markers such as CD34 and can be differentiated into functional APCs in vitro.[34] Human cancer MSCs were first identified in head and neck tumors.[35] They are concentrated at the tumor site, where they mediate local immunosuppression primarily through enzymatic factors. These cells may also be present throughout lymphoid tissues and contribute to the global immunosuppression of malignancy. Mouse studies suggest that MSCs mediate a reversible block of effector T cells function rather than destruction or anergy, as surgical removal of tumor and its associated MSCs restores tumor-specific T cell function. Prognostically, clinical studies have shown an association between MSC accumulation in tumor with disease stage and duration.[36]

MSCs are induced by various tumor secreted cytokines, in particular IL-10, VEGF, IL-6, IL-13, CSF-1, and high-dose GM-CSF. These factors block maturation of MSCs and stimulate them to suppress effector T cells, stimulate T_{regs}, and encourage tumor growth. MSCs in the tumor microenvironment express inducible nitric oxide synthase (iNOS), which suppresses T cell proliferation and induces T cell apoptosis by producing high levels of superoxide and nitric oxide. MSCs also target T cell cytotoxic function though the enzyme Arginase 1 (ARG1), which depletes the amino acid L-arginine required for T cell zeta chain expression, IL-2 receptor function, and IFN^γ (interferon-gamma) production.[37] Moreover, ARG1 induces iNOS expression, and the two enzymes work synergistically. MSCs have been shown to further assist tumor growth and invasion through production of matrix metalloproteases that stimulate angiogenesis and facilitate tissue invasion.[38] The end result is increasingly robust tumor growth and an immunosuppressive environment that predictably frustrates systemic anticancer therapies.

STRATEGIES TO ADDRESS TUMOR IMMUNE EVASION IN CANCER THERAPY

Immune-based therapies are a promising new line of treatment for cancer, treatment that is potentially much more tumor-specific than the traditional modalities of surgery, chemotherapy, and radiotherapy. Current immunotherapy includes both active strategies that seek to induce and support a robust host antitumor response and passive administration of tumor targeted cytotoxic cells or antibodies. Some encouraging clinical responses have now been reported and, as these tailored therapies are improved with genetic engineering, their effectiveness will likely greatly increase.[39] Successfully using any of these methods will require therapies that address the central problem of tumor immune evasion described previously, that is, immunotherapy must make cancer more visible, more vulnerable, and less virulent to the immune effectors that target malignant cells both within the tumor microenvironment and throughout the patient's body.

Because of immunoselective pressure, malignancies tend to downregulate TAAs targeted by immunotherapy. One method for limiting this escape is to target TAAs vital to cancer growth and survival, forcing cancerous cells to pay a price for antigen loss. This strategy is, by definition, limited to TAAs of known function. However, the presence of alternate intracellular pathways within tumor cells may still allow downregulation of individual "vital" TAAs. Targeting multiple TAAs at the same time is likely to be more successful, which has stimulated an extensive search for novel TAA targets. An intriguing alternative is the use of gene therapy to force TAA expression by tumor cells, potentially bypassing internal gene suppression mechanisms.

The discovery of tumor-specific effector T cells in cancer patients showed that the host immune system has the theoretical potential to treat malignancies. On the other hand, the presence of self-tolerance and the fact that tumors are poor antigen presenting cells prevent most patients with established cancers from achieving immune-mediated cures. Tumor vaccines attempt to sidestep these limitations by providing TAA

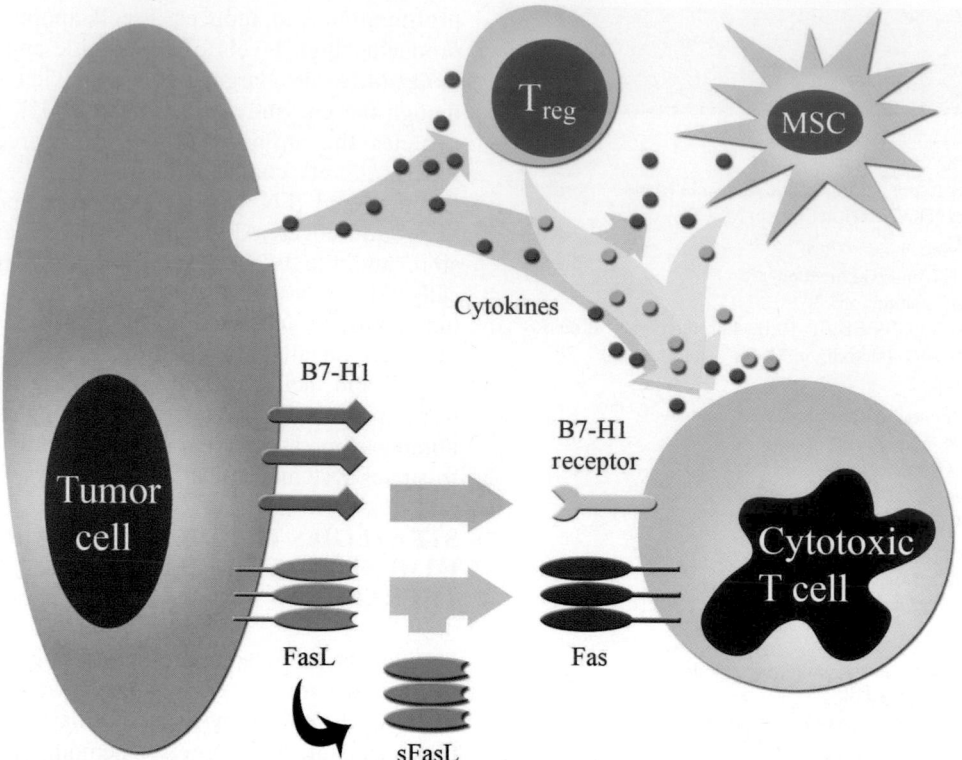

can cause direct cell death of cancer, as well as improve the potency of both nonspecific NK cells and tumor-specific cytotoxic T cells. The ability of these activated cells to destroy both tumors and tumor-associated vasculature has been clearly demonstrated in animals; however, the results in humans have been disappointing.[39,44] In addition, the clinical application of cytokine therapy may be limited by the unacceptable systemic side effects. Consequently, methods to improve clinical efficacy and reduce side-effect profiles are key to future use of cytokine-based therapies. Transfection of tumors with cytokine genes may help focus cytokine action at the tumor site. Manipulation of cytokine structure also shows promise. Certain cytokine molecules can be linked to bacterial toxins to poison tumors expressing high levels of specific cytokine receptors. Furthermore, as the cytokines components responsible for producing side effects become more defined, they could be removed to decrease these specific effects. Other components that improve cytotoxic activity or protect immune cells might be enhanced to optimize their effectiveness and allow them to survive in the harsh tumor microenvironment.

The tumor microenvironment actively induces apoptosis of immune effector cells. It is, therefore, vital to protect effector cells, whether induced or administered, from attack. Many studies have confirmed that cytokine therapy, in addition to having antitumor effects, also reduces the susceptibility of immune effector cells to undergo apoptosis.[45] These cytokines upregulate factors that inhibit caspases and downregulate pro-apoptotic Bcl-2 family members.[46] Less studied are strategies, such as RNA interference, that reduce tumor virulence through decreasing tumor expression of death-inducing ligands such as FasL or B7-H1. By reducing these immune-killing molecules, most likely several concurrently, the process of cancer "counter attack" can be thwarted, and the balance of cytotoxicity can be shifted in favor of the immune system.

Strategies of immune protection are particularly potent when combined with adoptive T cell therapy. Because the T cells are activated and expanded ex vivo, immunologists can tailor these lymphocytes to improve tumor recognition, as well as their resistance to tumor-induced apoptosis. Although most work to date has used patients' own T cells, derived from either TILs or PBLs, it is now known that lymphocytes taken from patients with advanced cancer are functionally compromised due to the general immunosuppressive state of malignancy.[1] Furthermore, they often exhibit limited persistence after adoptive transfer due to poor proliferation and rapid deletion. Tumor recognition and cytolytic function can be augmented through genetic engineering strategies that provide the T cells with high expression of TAA-specific TCR molecules or block intracellular inhibitory pathways. Lymphocyte persistence is improved with cytokine stimulation of proliferation and could also benefit from genetically engineered overexpression of anti-apoptotic molecules, such as Bcl-2 or IAPs.[47] Finally, pro-apoptotic

Figure 4 Tumor direct and indirect counterattack. Direct attack of cytotoxic T cells by tumor utilizes inhibitory cytokines, costimulatory molecules (B7-H1), and membrane-bound or soluble death receptor ligands (FasL or sFasL). Indirect attack occurs when tumors produce soluble factors that recruit or induce regulatory T cells (T_{regs}) or myeloid suppressor cells (MSCs). These suppressor cells then contribute their own cytokines to an effector counterattack.

targets in an optimized immunogenic format. By providing host APCs with tumor antigens in an inflammatory context, vaccines can overcome immune ignorance, allowing induction of endogenous effector T cells. Alternatively, vaccination with activated, TAA-peptide-loaded DCs prevents immune escape due to tumor downregulation of HLA Class I molecules, as DCs express high levels of TAA-presenting HLAI. The structure of these HLA-restricted peptides can also be modified, producing "heteroclitic" peptides that exhibit enhanced binding to the TCRs of low-affinity T cells.[40] Finally, gene therapy can re-establish tumor immunogenicity by forced re-expression of downregulated proteins in the HLAI pathway of tumor cells.

Vaccination has been shown to induce successfully functional tumor-specific cytotoxic cells in a variety of malignancies. However, the lack of a costimulatory signal at the tumor site can still prevent efficient killing. To address this, expression of costimulatory molecules, such as B7, has been induced in several carcinomas and sarcomas.[41] In addition, squamous cell carcinoma and melanoma xenograph models have shown that costimulatory signals can be provided by infusing agonist antibodies specific for human T cell costimulatory receptors.[42] Engineered antibodies that recognize multiple targets represent a third alternative. Each "bi-specific" antibody binds both a TAA and a T cell activation molecule, such as CD3, and provides a novel method of cytotoxic targeting combined with T cell stimulation at the tumor cell surface.[43]

Suppressive cells co-opted by cancers have been found to be potent obstacles to immuno-

therapy. T_{regs} and MSCs work together to create an immunosuppressive cytokine environment in the host, and strategies directed at reversing these effects are vital for successful treatment. Control of T_{reg} number and function has been attempted through numerous methods: blocking chemokine-mediated T_{reg} trafficking to tumor sites, removing stimulation provided by both MSCs and mature DCs, decreasing available IL-2, blocking CTLA-4 molecules expressed on T_{regs}, and depleting T_{regs} with low-dose cyclophosphamide or CD25-targeted toxins.[24] It is clear from the toxic autoimmune redponses induced by many of these methods that selective depletion of T_{reg} subsets is preferable. This will require further investigation into the markers and behavior that characterize different T_{reg} populations in patients with tumors. To address MSC immunosuppression, investigators have targeted the enzymes ARG1 and iNOS with inhibitory drugs such as nitroaspirins. In addition, MSCs can be forced to mature into functional APCs by stimulatory cytokines, all-trans retinoic acid (ATRA), or Vitamin D_3. Forced maturation is a potentially powerful strategy, as refinements of this method would produce mature APCs ideally placed to capture and present TAAs to effector cells for a robust tumor-specific immune response.[34]

Immunotherapy must also address innate tumor resistance to immune attack. Alerting malignant tissues to make them more susceptible to chemotherapy and radiotherapy have been extensively studied. Similar strategies can be used to make cancer cells more susceptible to cytotoxic immune effector cells. Administration of exogenous cytokines, especially IL-2, 7, and 12, molecules might be reduced with novel small molecule inhibitors and RNA interference strategies prior to transfer into tumor-bearing patients.[48–50]

CONCLUSIONS

The human immune system and programmed cell death machinery may prevent the vast majority of abnormal cells from ever becoming life-threatening malignancies; however, those cells that do survive to establish growing tumors are masters of immune evasion. The multiple pressures of innate and adaptive host immunity produce cancers that are weakly immunogenic, resistant to cytotoxic attack, and capable of twisting normal immune defenses to their own ends. In particular, tumors use components of the homeostatic apoptosis pathways to evade destruction and mount a counterattack against effector cells that enter their microenvironment. The challenge of immunotherapy is to tip successfully the balance in this "arms race" toward immune activation and potency without producing unacceptable levels of autoimmune disease or inflammatory side effects. Current immune modalities such as vaccination, cytokine administration, and adoptive lymphocyte transfer have produced some promising clinical results to date. The addition of novel molecular and genetic strategies has the potential to increase treatment specificity and effectiveness even more. In the future, combinations of these therapies will allow clinicians to attack a cancer from multiple sides at once while protecting and enhancing immune cells tailored to that tumor's particular methods of immune evasion.

REFERENCES

1. Kim R, Emi M, Tanabe K, Arihiro K. Tumor-driven evolution of immunosuppressive networks during malignant progression. Cancer Res 2006;66:5527–36.
2. Gastman BR, Johnson DE, Whiteside TL, Rabinowich H. Caspase-mediated degradation of T cell receptor zeta-chain. Cancer Res 1999;59:1422–7.
3. Reichert TE, Day R, Wagner EM, Whiteside TL. Absent or low expression of the zeta chain in T cells at the tumor site correlates with poor survival in patients with oral carcinoma. Cancer Res 1998;58:5344–7.
4. Lee PP, Yee C, Savage PA, et al. Characterization of circulating T cells specific for tumor-associated antigens in melanoma patients. Nat Med 1999;5:677–85.
5. Jager D, Jager E, Knuth A. Immune responses to tumour antigens: Implications for antigen specific immunotherapy of cancer. J Clin Pathol 2001;54:669–74.
6. Khong HT, Restifo NP. Natural selection of tumor variants in the generation of "tumor escape" phenotypes. Nat Immun 2002;3:999–1005.
7. Garcia-Lora A, Algarra I, Garrido F. MHC class I antigens, immune surveillance, and tumor immune escape. J Cell Physiol 2003;195:346–55.
8. Cabrera T, Lopez-Nevot MA, Gaforio JJ, et al. Analysis of HLA expression in human tumor tissues. Cancer Immunol Immunother 2003;52:1–9.
9. Ferris RL, Hunt JL, Ferrone S. Human leukocyte antigen (HLA) class I defects in head and neck cancer: Molecular mechanisms and clinical significance. Immunol Res 2005;33:113–33.
10. Bottino C, Moretta L, Moretta A. NK cell activating receptors and tumor recognition in humans. Curr Top Microbiol Immunol 2006;298:175–82.
11. Ochsenbein AF. Immunological ignorance of solid tumors. Springer Semin Immunopathol 2005;27:19–35.
12. Zheng P, Sarma S, Guo Y, Liu Y. Two mechanisms for tumor evasion of preexisting cytotoxic T cell responses: Lessons from recurrent tumors. Cancer Res 1999;59:3461–7.

13. Viac J, Schmitt D, Claudy A. CD40 expression in epidermal tumors. Anticancer Res 1997;17:569–72.
14. Gastman BR. Apoptosis and its clinical impact. Head Neck 2001;23:409–25.
15. Taylor MA, Chaudhary PM, Klem J, et al. Inhibition of the death receptor pathway by cFLIP confers partial engraftment of MHC class I-deficient stem cells and reduces tumor clearance in perforin-deficient mice. J Immunol 2001;167:4230–7.
16. Han J, Goldstein LA, Gastman BR, et al. Degradation of Mcl-1 by granzyme B: Implications for Bim-mediated mitochondrial apoptotic events. J Biol Chem 2004;279:22020–9.
17. Gastman BR, Johnson DE, Whiteside TL, Rabinowich H. Tumor-induced apoptosis of T lymphocytes: Elucidation of intracellular apoptotic events. Blood 2000;95:2015–23.
18. LaCasse EC, Baird S, Korneluk RG, MacKenzie AE. The inhibitors of apoptosis (IAPs) and their emerging role in cancer. Oncogene 1998;17:3247–59.
19. Kim R, Tanabe K, Uchida Y, et al. Current status of the molecular mechanisms of anticancer drug-induced apoptosis. The contribution of molecular-level analysis to cancer chemotherapy. Cancer Chemother Pharmacol 2002; 50:343–52.
20. Gastman BR, Atarshi Y, Reichert TE, et al. Fas ligand is expressed on human squamous cell carcinomas of the head and neck, and it promotes apoptosis of T lymphocytes. Cancer Res 1999;59:5356–64.
21. Song E, Chen J, Ouyang N, et al. Soluble Fas ligand released by colon adenocarcinoma cells induces host lymphocyte apoptosis: An active mode of immune evasion in colon cancer. Br J Cancer 2001;85:1047–54.
22. Hallermalm K, De Geer A, Kiessling R, et al. Autocrine secretion of Fas ligand shields tumor cells from Fas-mediated killing by cytotoxic lymphocytes. Cancer Res 2004;64:6775–82.
23. Strome SE, Dong H, Tamura H, et al. B7-H1 blockade augments adoptive T cell immunotherapy for squamous cell carcinoma. Cancer Res 2003;63:6501–5.
24. Zou W. Regulatory T cells, tumour immunity and immunotherapy. Nat Rev Immunol 2006;6:295–307.
25. Schaefer C, Kim GG, Albers A, et al. Characteristics of CD4+CD25+ regulatory T cells in the peripheral circulation of patients with head and neck cancer. Br J Cancer 2005;92:913–20.
26. Kono K, Kawaida H, Takahashi A, et al. CD4(+)CD25 high regulatory T cells increase with tumor stage in patients with gastric and esophageal cancers. Cancer Immunol Immunother 2006;55:1064–71.
27. Dhodapkar MV, Steinman RM. Antigen-bearing immature dendritic cells induce peptide-specific CD8(+) regulatory T cells in vivo in humans. Blood 2002;100.174–7.
28. Chen W, Jin W, Hardegen N, et al. Conversion of peripheral CD4+CD25−naive T cells to CD4+CD25+ regulatory T cells by TGF-beta induction of transcription factor Foxp3. J Exp Med 2003;198:1875–86.
29. Curiel TJ, Coukos G, Zou L, et al. Specific recruitment of regulatory T cells in ovarian carcinoma fosters immune privilege and predicts reduced survival. Nat Med 2004; 10:942–9.
30. O'Garra A, Vieira P. Regulatory T cells and mechanisms of immune system control. Nat Med 2004;10:801–5.
31. Grossman WJ, Verbsky JW, Barchet W, et al. Human T regulatory cells can use the perforin pathway to cause autologous target cell death. Immunity 2004;21:589–601.
32. von Boehmer H. Mechanisms of suppression by suppressor T cells. Nat Immun 2005;6:338–44.
33. Fallarino F, Grohmann U, Hwang KW, et al. Modulation of tryptophan catabolism by regulatory T cells. Nat Immun 2003;4:1206–12.
34. Serafini P, Borrello I, Bronte V. Myeloid suppressor cells in cancer: recruitment, phenotype, properties, and mechanisms of immune suppression. Semin Cancer Biol 2006; 16:53–65.
35. Pak AS, Wright MA, Matthews JP, et al. Mechanisms of immune suppression in patients with head and neck cancer: presence of CD34(+) cells which suppress immune functions within cancers that secrete granulocyte-macrophage colony-stimulating factor. Clin Cancer Res 1995; 1:95–103.
36. Almand B, Resser JR, Lindman B, et al. Clinical significance of defective dendritic cell differentiation in cancer. Clin Cancer Res 2000;6:1755–66.
37. Bronte V, Serafini P, Mazzoni A, et al. L-arginine metabolism in myeloid cells controls T-lymphocyte functions. Trends Immunol 2003;24:302–6.
38. Yang L, DeBusk LM, Fukuda K, et al. Expansion of myeloid immune suppressor Gr+CD11b+ cells in tumor-bearing host directly promotes tumor angiogenesis. Cancer Cell 2004;6:409–21.

39. Eigentler TK, Caroli UM, Radny P, Garbe C. Palliative therapy of disseminated malignant melanoma: A systematic review of 41 randomised clinical trials. Lancet Oncol 2003;4:748–59.
40. Slansky JE, Rattis FM, Boyd LF, et al. Enhanced antigen-specific antitumor immunity with altered peptide ligands that stabilize the MHC-peptide-TCR complex. Immunity 2000;13:529-38.
41. Chen L, Ashe S, Brady WA, et al. Costimulation of antitumor immunity by the B7 counterreceptor for the T lymphocyte molecules CD28 and CTLA-4. Cell 1992;71:1093–102.
42. Wilcox RA, Flies DB, Zhu G, et al. Provision of antigen and CD137 signaling breaks immunological ignorance, promoting regression of poorly immunogenic tumors. J Clin Invest 2002;109:651–9.
43. Daniel PT, Kroidl A, Kopp J, et al. Immunotherapy of B-cell lymphoma with CD3x19 bispecific antibodies: Costimulation via CD28 prevents "veto" apoptosis of antibody-targeted cytotoxic T cells. Blood 1998;92:4750–7.
44. Jackaman C, Bundell CS, Kinnear BF, et al. IL-2 intratumoral immunotherapy enhances CD8+ T cells that mediate destruction of tumor cells and tumor-associated vasculature: A novel mechanism for IL-2. J Immunol 2003; 171:5051–63.
45. Waldmann TA. The biology of interleukin-2 and interleukin-15: Implications for cancer therapy and vaccine design. Nat Rev Immunol 2006;6:595–601.
46. Eaton D, Gilham DE, O'Neill A, Hawkins RE. Retroviral transduction of human peripheral blood lymphocytes with Bcl-X(L) promotes in vitro lymphocyte survival in pro-apoptotic conditions. Gene Ther 2002;9:527–35.
47. Oltersdorf T, Elmore SW, Shoemaker AR, et al. An inhibitor of Bcl-2 family proteins induces regression of solid tumours. Nature 2005;435:677–81.
48. Soutschek J, Akinc A, Bramlage B, et al. Therapeutic silencing of an endogenous gene by systemic administration of modified siRNAs. Nature 2004;432:173–8.
49. Ryan AE, Shanahan F, O'Connell J, Houston AM. Addressing the "Fas counterattack" controversy: Blocking fas ligand expression suppresses tumor immune evasion of colon cancer in vivo. Cancer Res 2005;65:9817–23.
50. Gastman BR, Yin XM, Johnson DE, et al. Tumor-induced apoptosis of T cells: Amplification by a mitochondrial cascade. Cancer Res 2000;60:6811–7.

SUGGESTED READINGS

Balkwill F, Mantovani A. Inflammation and cancer: Back to Virchow? Lancet 2001;357:539–45.
Good description of the suppressive tumor microenvironment, including cytokines and myeloid suppressor cells.

Blattman JN, Greenberg PD. Cancer immunotherapy: A treatment for the masses. Science 2004;305:200–5.
Review of current and possible future tumor immunotherapies.

Immunity to tumors, Chapter 17. In: Abbas A, Lichtman A, editors. Cellular and Molecular Immunology 5th edition. Philadelphia: Saunders Publishing;2005p. 391–410.
An excellent introduction to basic tumor immunosurveillance and evasion.

Gastman BR. Apoptosis and its clinical impact. Head Neck 2001;23:409–25.
Review of apoptotic mechanisms and their impact on head and neck cancers.

Pardoll D. T cells and tumours. Nature 2001;411:1010–2.
Description of mechanisms of immune induction and ignorance in patients with tumors.

Rathmell JC, Thompson CB. Pathways of apoptosis in lymphocyte development, homeostasis, and disease. Cell 2002;109:S97–107.
Review of extrinsic and intrinsic apoptotic pathways.

Sakaguchi S, Sakaguchi N, Asano M, et al. Immunologic self-tolerance maintained by activated T cells expressing IL-2 receptor alpha-chains (CD25). Breakdown of a single mechanism of self-tolerance causes various autoimmune diseases. J Immunol 1995;155:1151–64.
Article that stimulated resurgence of interest in T regulatory cells as key suppressive influences on cellular immunity.

Whiteside, TL. Immune suppression in cancer: Effects on immune cells, mechanisms and future therapeutic intervention. Semin Cancer Biol 2006;16:3–15.
Review of tumor escape mechanisms and therapies to restore immune competence.

Zhang X, Strome SE. B7-H1-targeted immunotherapy for head and neck cancer. Expert Opin Biol Ther 2004; 4:1577–83.
Review of costimulatory molecule function in tumor immunity and immunotherapy.

89

Molecular Diagnostic Approaches to Head and Neck Cancer

Ian M. Smith, MD
Joseph A. Califano, MD

Each year approximately 40,000 people in the United States and 500,000 people worldwide are diagnosed with head and neck squamous cell carcinoma (HNSCC). Despite significant improvements in the past few decades in the treatment of this disease, the 5-year survival rate has remained essentially unchanged at 50%. HNSCC continues to be a treatment challenge because of an advanced stage at presentation and a high rate of disease recurrence. Early stage at diagnosis continues to be the strongest factor in predicting survival. Coupled with emerging biomedical technologies, there has been a large push to develop early screening and noninvasive diagnostic tests for HNSCC.

These molecular diagnostic approaches are often based on the developing understanding of the genetic and epigenetic alterations and viral agents that have been implicated in the tumorigenesis of head and neck neoplasms. Efforts have been focused at leveraging these advances in our understanding of tumor molecular biology into relevant applied management.

Investigators have analyzed body fluids and margins for the presence of cancer cells. Improved molecular characterization of primary tumors, surgical margins, and body fluids may allow clinicians to detect and treat earlier lesions, predict a tumor's response to treatment, tailor treatment to specific molecular alterations, and ultimately improve clinical outcomes related to HNSCC.

To date, many biomarkers have been studied that show promise: human papilloma virus (HPV) positivity, p53, cyclin D1, p16, cyclooxygenase-2 (Cox-2), epidermal growth factor (EGF), and vascular endothelial growth factor (VEGF). This chapter presents the findings on potential molecular biomarkers for HNSCC and discusses their benefits and limitations to being employed for the practicing head and neck surgeon.

Molecular diagnostic approaches can be organized in one of three ways (Figure 1): by tissue compartment, for example, saliva or serum, or by various detection methods specific for finding deoxyribonucleic acid (DNA), ribonucleic acid (RNA), or protein. This chapter will address the most relevant approaches to molecular diagnosis in head and neck cancer based primarily on molecular biologic targets, for example, p53,

p16, and HPV, with some specific attention paid to novel technologies being developed.

CANCER PROGRESSION MODEL

Most molecular approaches to diagnosis are rooted in the head and neck cancer progression model derived from Fearon and Vogelstein's description of colon cancer progression.[1] This theory states that cancer results from multiple accumulated, progressively transforming genetic alterations in a clonal population cells. This hypothesis is based on several principles, including: (1) neoplasms are caused by tumor-suppressor gene inactivation and/or protooncogene activation; (2) there is a defined order of genetic and epigenetic events causing the development of a tumor phenotype; and (3) net accumulation of alterations rather than a specific order of events determines the malignant phenotype.[2,3]

Within this context, genetic and epigenetic lesions can be classified as early or late. Early genetic changes offer the ability to diagnose molecularly, treat, and follow premalignant lesions before the patient develops cancer. In particular, dysplastic leukoplakic lesions can be stratified for their ability to develop into cancer.[4,5] Later lesions tend to have more specificity with regard to tumor diagnosis. The common clinical lesions that may reflect a premalignant state leading to HNSCC are leukoplakia, erythroplakia, oral lichen planus, and submucous fibrosis. These lesions are found either proceeding or synchronously with HNSCC. They are variable in their malignant potential as well as their genetic

background and may be associated with varied histological evidence of dysplasia.

HNSCC is highly correlated with environmental exposures such as cigarette smoke or smokeless tobacco, and most theories concerning the etiology of HNSCC are derived from accumulated heritable changes that are inflicted by DNA damaging, carcinogenic exposures. Ultimately, survival rates are highly dependent on stage at presentation, so early diagnosis should lead to improved overall survival of those with head and neck cancer.

EARLY DETECTION AND SCREENING

HNSCCs have a tendency toward late-stage presentation. This is because these growing neoplasms are often asymptomatic. Taken as a whole, the noted exception is that of laryngeal lesions which can often arise on the vocal folds and cause hoarseness which often leads to an earlier medical presentation, as well as anterior oral cavity lesions that may be easily visualized by the patient or primary care medical or dental professionals. Other head and neck cancers will present with dysphagia, odynophagia, or a mass, symptoms associated with late-stage presentation. While the proposed molecular model of cancer progression is new, cancers have long been noted to arise from premalignant precursors. This chapter will cover areas of investigation in molecular diagnostics, which include tests that may be adapted to screen high-risk populations without previous symptoms or findings, and the development of tests that may be used

Diagnostic categories

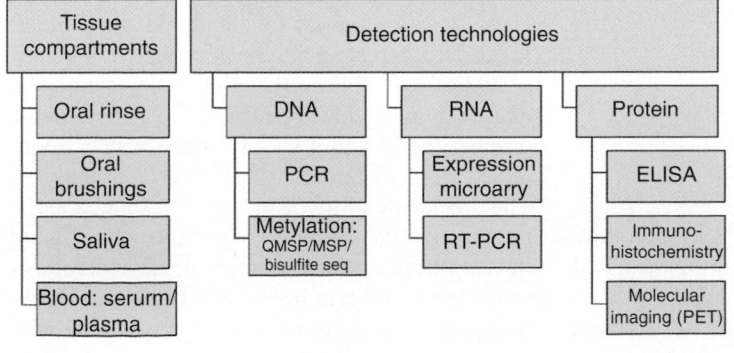

Figure 1 Classifications of diagnostic and screening studies in head and neck squamous cell carcinoma (HNSCC). Studies can be classified based on tissue compartment, for example, saliva, scrapings, rinses, or blood, as well as by detection means, for example, deoxyribonucleic acid (DNA)-bases polymerase chain reaction (PCR), or targets, for example, p53, human papilloma virus (HPV), p16.

for detection of occult, persistent, or recurrent disease in patients who have already been diagnosed with HNSCC.

Issues with Molecular Detection

Molecular assays for disease can be divided into two uses: population-based screening tests and molecular detection. Population-based screening tests do benefit from well-outlined risk factors including tobacco and alcohol use but suffer because of the difficulty in producing tests with adequate sensitivity so that they are useful in detection and adequate specificity not to generate large numbers of false positives in the setting of low incidence. Molecular detection strategies studied to date include molecular margin detection, detection of nodal metastasis, and disease surveillance after treatment. These techniques require reasonable sensitivity over and above the current guidelines for disease surveillance, physical examination, and imaging.

Tests developed in the laboratory for molecular diagnosis must be validated in clinical trails. To date few of the approaches for molecular screening and diagnosis have been taken to clinical trails with the notable exceptions of tests for loss of heterozygosity (LOH) used for prognosis and toluidine blue as a detection means.

Sample Collection

Unlike other fields where screening approaches have worked with more traditional clinical pathology approaches, such as cytology, head and neck cancer diagnosis still relies on physical examination, imaging, and biopsy. Much controversy exists regarding the application of oral cytology, but this technique generally suffers from low specificity. However, many types of clinical samples exist for testing patients. Samples for screening and diagnostic studies can come from various sources and be collected in a variety of fashions. Efforts to use fractions of the blood for molecular diagnosis will be discussed in this chapter. Studies utilize either blood plasma, the liquid component of blood, or the serum, blood plasma in which clotting factors, for example, fibrin, have been removed.

From the oral cavity, several collection methods exist. Salivary rinses refer to sample collection in which a patient simply expels their saliva and oral liquid into a specimen cup. Saliva can be isolated from centrifugation or can be drawn from salivary duct cannulation. Oral rinses are commercially available liquids that patients swish and then spit into a cup. Oral brushings can be made from commercially available cytology kits in which a patient's oral mucosa, particularly an area of interest can be brushed which yields markedly more cells.

Human Papilloma Virus

Over the past few years, the body of literature implicating the HPV in the carcinogenesis of HNSCC has been building. HPV has long been a well-characterized primary cause of cervical cancer that has yielded one of the most effective forms of cancer screening, early detection, and increased cure rates. HPV is now recognized as a likely cause of head and neck cancer.[6] There are numerous subtypes of this virus (>120), but most have not been shown to be carcinogenic. HPV subtypes 16 and 18 are the best-studied subtypes, but the majority of evidence in head and neck cancer has implicated HPV subtype 16 as an etiologic agent.

HPV contains two key proteins E6 and E7 that have the potential to transform human cells. These viral oncogenes have been shown to inactivate two crucial human tumor-suppressor genes p53 (E6) and retinoblastoma protein (pRb or E7). This inactivation results in loss of cell-cycle control, impaired cell differentiation, increased mutations, and chromosomal instability.[7]

Overall in HNSCC, HPV genomic DNA can be detected by real-time PCR-based methods in 26% of all cancers.[8] However in head and neck cancer, this virus has a predilection for the lingual and palatine tonsils of the oropharynx. Data looking at only the subset of the oropharynx suggest 50% or more of these tumors are HPV positive.

Interestingly HPV-associated cancers have been shown to have increased survival and outcomes. Schwartz and colleagues found HPV 16–positive patients had significantly reduced mortality and disease-specific mortality compared with HPV 16–negative patients after adjustment for age, stage, treatment, smoking, alcohol, education, and comorbid disease.[9]

New studies show promising molecular screening approaches that have increased sensitivity for detection. Real-time PCR of HPV-associated DNA is now the standard for detection at low thresholds. However, employment of these technologies as screening tests suffers from low sensitivity.[10] Zhao and colleagues studied the utility of saliva screening for HPV and found that in a cohort of patients with HNSCC with a 45.6% incidence of tumor HPV positivity only 57% of the positive patients with tumor had detectable saliva rinse HPV16 which resulted in a sensitivity of 32.6% for the saliva rinse test for head and neck cancer. Depending on the threshold for HPV16 positivity in the assay, specificity only increased slightly, from 97.2 to 98.7% at the higher cutoff and the authors conclude that >99% specificity would be required for population-cased screening.[11]

HPV seropositivity has also been an intriguing risk-factor for the development of head and neck cancer, and the largest study examining HPV 16 seropositivity found an odds ratio of 2.2 for developing head and neck cancer in a cohort of 292 patients followed in a screening study who had eventually developed HNSCC, 50% of the oropharyngeal and 14% of tongue cancers contained HPV-16 DNA, according to PCR analysis. The diagnostic utility is again poor, related to the number of HPV seropositive patients who will not develop head and neck cancer or have seropositivity from any number of other sources. Technologies such as competitive PCR coupled with mass spectrometry have promise to yield more specificity compared to real-time PCR, detecting with accuracy a single copy of DNA, but the issue of false-positive nonpathologic detection of HPV remains.[12] In a case-control study examining HPV16 in the saliva, 19% of head and neck cancer patients (201 total) were saliva-positive, and 10% of control subjects (333 total) were positive, with an odds ratio of 2.6.[13] While the utility in population-based screening is still being evaluated, HPV positivity may eventually play a role in disease monitoring and surveillance.

Microsatellite Instability

Microsatellite instability (MSI) is an additional molecular alteration discovered initially in colon cancer[14] that has been found in head and neck cancer. MSI refers to alterations in copy number of small repeats of a short nucleotide motif, that is, usually one to five nucleotides long. For example, a mononucleotide repeat might be a stretch of 17 adenines and the most common microsatellite in humans is a dinucleotide repeat of cytosine and adenine, which occurs in tens of thousands of locations in our genome. In MSI, these areas are aberrantly replicated leading to expansion or contraction of the specific area. In colon cancer, MSI has been linked to errors in DNA replication and DNA repair enzymes.[15] After their discovery, efforts were made to utilize microsatellite alterations to detect cancer cell DNA in a background of normal cells. Microsatellite analysis can reveal either MSI or LOH in a given amplified microsatellite repeat locus (Figure 2). Head and neck cancers have been found to have MSI at a variety of loci in the genome.[16]

For screening and diagnostic purposes, these tumor-specific alterations have been found in the saliva and plasma of patients with these changes. A specific subset of alterations was initially reported in the serum of 29% of patients with HNSCC.[17] Subsequently, these alterations were studied in the saliva samples of patients with HNSCC in a screening feasibility study to detect tumor-specific genetic alterations in exfoliated oral mucosal cell samples from 44 patients with HNSCC and 43 healthy control subjects. Their results showed that LOH or MSI of at least one marker was detected in 38 (86%) of 44 primary tumors with identical alterations found in the saliva samples in 35 of these 38 patients (92% of those with markers; 79% overall). MSI was detectable in the saliva in 24 (96%) of 25 patients in whom MSI was present in the tumor, and LOH was identified in the test sample in 19 (61%) of 31 patients. No microsatellite alterations were detected in any of the samples from the healthy control subjects.[18]

These tests are just now starting to be clinically available from pathology services. The ability to detect microsatellite changes in the background of blood or saliva can reduce markedly the sensitivity of these tests[19] and has resulted in significant limitations on the widespread adoption of the technology.

Microsatellite Instability

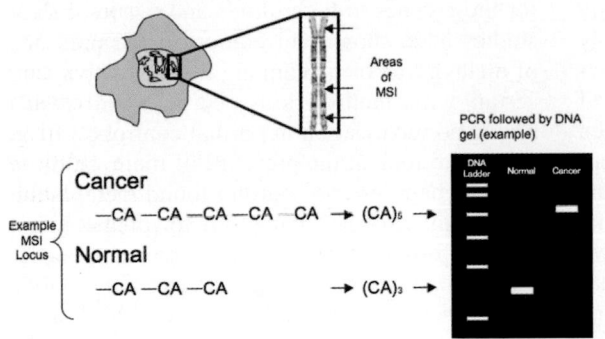

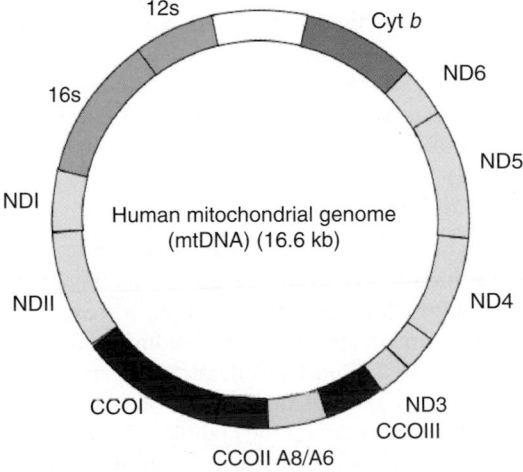

Figure 2 Microsatellite instability (MSI) in cancer, example coding sequence, and example diagnostic DNA gel. Areas of MSI have been noted in many places in the genome. On a given chromosome, one area can be tested with specifically designed primers that flank the area. Differences in the lengths of the products are seen by the distance of migration on the gel. PCR = polymerase chain reaction; DNA = deoxyribonucleic acid; CA = cytosine and adenine.

p53

p53 is a powerful tumor-suppressor gene found altered in many cancers and the inherited Li-Fraumeni cancer syndrome of cancer susceptibility.[20] p53 is a transcription factor, that is, binds to a gene's promoter and upregulates transcription of mRNA, that is activated in normal cells for a variety of reasons when DNA has been damaged. p53 induces cell-cycle arrest in response to DNA damage, as well as either DNA repair activation or activation of apoptosis, depending on the context of the DNA injury (Figure 3).

Mutations, specifically missense, in p53 have been found in many human cancers and are present in around 50% of head and neck cancers. Detecting these mutations in body fluids in patients with HNSCC has been the subject of a variety of studies. Early efforts used plaque hybridization approaches to identify known p53 mutation in salivary rinses from patients with corresponding p53 mutation in primary HNSCC in five of seven patients.[21,22]

Other approaches involve the observation that patients with cancer often generate p53 antibodies. Investigators have found that 27% (7/26) of patients with oral squamous cell carcinoma had circulating antibodies against p53 in the serum by enzyme-linked immunosorbent assay (ELISA).[23] Additionally, in a study of 126 patients with oral SCC and 80 control patients, assaying for p53 autoantibodies in the serum with surveillance over 5 years using ELISA, 18.6% of the patients with primary cancer and 50% of the patients with recurrent cancer had p53 autoantibodies detected, versus none of the sera in the controls. In addition, these p53-positive patients had noticeably poorer prognosis ($p < .005$), and overall survival rate at 5 years of the p53-positive group was 24% (half that of the p53-negative group).[24] Clinical utilization of p53 protein detection strategies and p53 mutation detection strategies for screening has not seen implementation although efforts continue to be made to link treatment response to p53 mutation.

Mitochondria

Mitochondria are the source of aerobic energy to meet a cell's demands for adenosine triphosphate (ATP). Mitochondria are critically involved in the pathway and regulation of apoptosis, site of oxidative phosphorylation, generation of free radicals, and source of cellular energy in rapidly dividing cells using increased energy. Their role in tumorigenesis has been hypothesized in head and neck cancer. Mitochondria have their own genome (Figure 4) that includes genes encoding for the electron transport chain [nicotinamide adenine dinucleotide (NADH), cytochrome c, and cytochrome c oxidase], ATP synthase, and protein synthesis. Mitochondrial DNA (mtDNA) also has the benefit of having a much higher copy number making it easier for detection studies. As a screening tool, Fliss and colleagues found detectable mitochondrial mutations by PCR in 67% (six of nine) saliva samples from patients with head and neck cancer that corresponded to mutations found in tumors.[25]

One additional change in mitochondria has been noted in that the overall content of mitochondrial DNA increases as a proposed compensation for general mitochondrial dysfunction that has been conclusively demonstrated to increase with increasing degrees of mild, moderate, to severe dysplasia and finally carcinoma.[26] This change was further detected in the saliva when multivariate analysis of the saliva of patients with head and neck cancer versus screening patients showed a significant and independent association of HNSCD diagnosis, age, and smoking with increasing mtDNA/nuclear DNA for cytochrome C oxidase I (Cox I) and Cox II.[27]

CD44

The soluble adhesion molecule CD44 has been implicated in the pathogenesis of head and neck cancer. It is an attractive molecular alteration for molecular diagnosis because of its cell-surface location and its availability for clinically employable approaches such as ELISA. In an important study of 81 patients with head and neck cancer and 20 controls, the levels of soluble CD44 standard (sCD44st), soluble CD44 variant 5 (sCD44v5), sCD44v6, soluble intercellular adhesion molecule (sICAM-1), and soluble vascular cell adhesion molecule (sVCAM-1) were considered before and after treatment of HNSCC.[28] This group found that levels of all five of these markers were significantly higher in the HNSCC group than those of the control group. Coupled

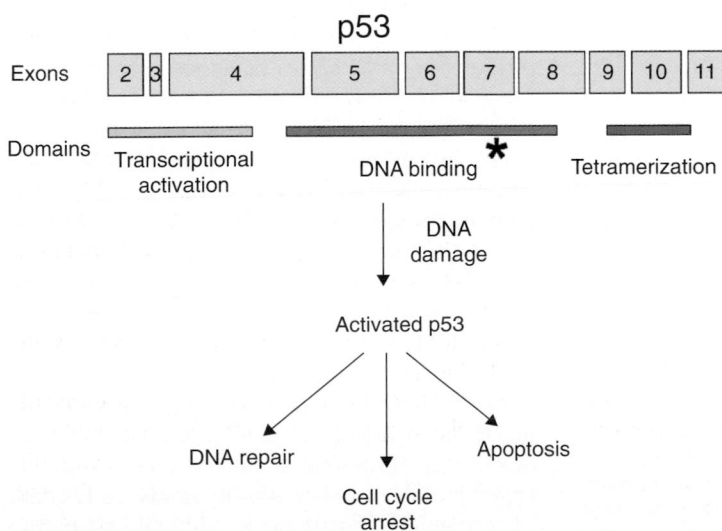

Figure 3 Function of the transcription factor and human cancer tumor-suppressor gene p53. DNA damage from a variety of source leads to a tetramerization and activation of p53 that causes activation of DNA repair, arrest of the cell cycle, and activation of apoptosis. In head and neck cancers, missense mutations can occur at almost any point in the coding sequence, but the majority are in the DNA binding domain.

Mitochondrial genome

Human mitochondrial genome (mtDNA) (16.6 kb)

Figure 4 Map of the human mitochondrial genome. Shown here are the seven subunits of nicotinamide adenine dinucleotide [reduced form] (NADH) dehydrogenase-coenzyme Q oxidoreductase (ND), one unit of the coenzyme Q-cytochrome c oxidoreductase (Cyt b), and three subunits of cytochrome c oxidase (CCO), and two subunits of ATP synthase (A), and the protein synthesis genes (12S and 16S). Not shown are the genes for the 22 transfer RNAsn(RNAs). mtDNA = mitochondrial DNA.

with this was the finding that sCD44st, sCD44v5, sCD44v6 median serum level was significantly diminished after treatment. However, a separate group considering CD44 isoforms in the serum utilized ELISA to show that, "there was no significant difference between the serum levels of sCD44v6 in HNSCC and healthy smokers. Nor was there a correlation between the serum level of sCD44v6 and UICC (International Union Against Cancer) stage, TNM stage or histologic grading."[29]

Epidermal Growth Factor Receptor

HNSCC have been shown to have upregulated EGF pathways. These growth factors fit within the molecular tyrosine-kinase family of cell-surface receptors that have been implicated in the pathogenesis of many forms of cancer. EGF receptor (EGFR) overexpression is observed in 42 to 80% of head and neck cancers.[30] In fact in a meta-analysis of eight trials, seven trials showed a poorer outcome for patients with EGFR overexpression.[31] Promising clinical trials of tyrosine kinase inhibitors such as cetuximab have demonstrated the role these signaling pathways play in the treatment of head and neck cancer.[32] Recently, overexpression of EGFR has been used to find immunomagnetic cell enrichment in combination with RT-PCR for the detection of circulating head and neck tumor cells. This technique was successful in finding one cancer cell per 10^5 total leukocytes 77.8% of the time.[33]

Vascular Endothelial Growth Factor

VEGF is also a promising serum biomarker. A group at the University of Michigan studied the utility of measuring serum VEGF levels via ELISA in a group of controls versus patients with cancer of the larynx and found that for the healthy control group the level was 47.83 ± 0.13 pg/mL, compared with the mean s-VEGF level of 317.22 ± 25.46 pg/mL in the cancer patients. This elevation was statistically significant ($p < .001$), and in a univariate analysis, elevated s-VEGF correlated with poor Karnofsky performance status for all patients with advanced laryngeal carcinoma ($p < .008$).[34]

Methylation

Heritable alterations in head and neck cancer have broadened from the early understanding of changes such as gene mutation, for example, missense or deletion, LOH, genomic deletions, amplifications, and translocations to epigenetic changes. Epigenetics is the study of DNA alterations that do not affect the coding of bases but do affect the regulation of genes. Examples of these changes that are inherited by cells in a clonal fashion include promoter hypermethylation, acetylation, and histone modifications. By far the most useful to date and best studied of these in HNSCC is gene promoter hypermethylation. This phenomenon takes place in the regulatory units of the genome (the promoters) in areas called CpG islands. CpG (cytosine-guanine dinucleotides)

can be modified at the 5′ carbon of the carbon ring of cytosine (Figure 5), by the addition of a methyl group from s-adenyl methionine (SAM) by the DNA methyl-transferase enzyme family (DNMT). Although this phenomenon was initially shown to be the cause of X-chromosome inactivation and genetic imprinting, inactivation of tumor-suppressor genes in this manner has been increasingly shown to play a role in tumorigenesis. This keeps with the basic principles of the Knudson two-hit hypothesis which suggests that tumor-suppressor genes are inactivated by two separate hits to a gene's alleles. Methylation has been shown to be sufficient to cause a "hit" to one allele in many cases. Once both alleles have been silenced, the cell undergoes changes in its phenotype that are more malignant, for example, cell-cycle alterations, inhibition of apoptosis. Tumors have been shown to preferentially shed DNA, and one large advantage of methylation is its ready use for screening, as DNA is stable in the blood or saliva, and small levels of methylation can be detected by sophisticated means, including bisulfite sequencing, quantitative or standard methylation-specific PCR (Figure 6) in a background of other DNA products.

Early molecular biology work in head and neck cancer on methylation examined a panel of four putative tumor-suppressor genes whose inactivation was associated with a cancer phenotype. These genes, p16, MGMT (methylguanine-DNA methyltransferase), GST-π (glutathione-S-transferase Pi), and DAPK (death-associated protein kinase) exhibited significant promoter hypermethylation in at least one of the four genes in 42% of primary tumors.[35] Other genes epigenetically silenced include RASSF1A,[36] hMLH1 (DNA mismatch repair gene),[37] E-cadherin,[38] and recently, a group has found that HNSCC shows promoter hypermethylation of STAT1 (signal transduction and activator transcription factor 1).[39] Other genes being studied include ATM (ataxia-telangectasia).[40]

Methylation

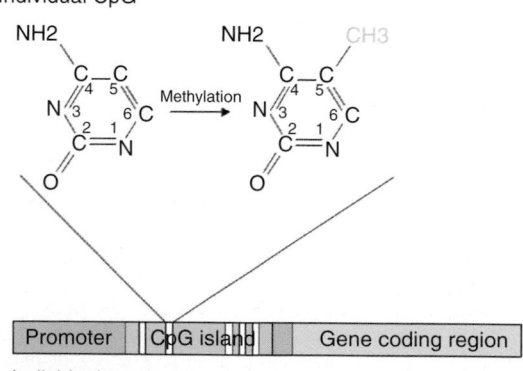

Individual CpG

Figure 5 Cytosine-guanine dinucleotide (CpG) methylation. Individual CpG shown within the context of a CpG island that is found in the promoter segment of a gene upstream from the transcription start site. Methylation performs a gene silencing function through alterations in tertiary structure, direct binding of methylation-sensitive promoters and repressors, and activation of the deacetylation complexes.

Once these molecular changes were identified, screening for these hypermethylated promoters was undertaken in the laboratory. In screening for these genes in body fluids and tissues, recent studies have shown correlation in the presence of methylation of p16 among tumors, saliva, and serum with methylation-specific PCR (MSP) noting no methylation in normal controls.[41] In an attempt to look at the presence of methylation in premalignant lesions, a group found methylation in the oral rinses of patients with premalignant lesions corresponded to that of reported cancer oral rinse methylation rates; and p16 and MGMT were observed to be methylated with MSP in 44 and 56% of the oral samples, respectively. To date it has been difficult to develop assays with sufficient sensitivity (HNSCC tumors are heterogeneous in their genetic changes) and specificity (normal cells may have methylated alleles) for clinical application.

Gene Expression Microarray

Expression microarrays utilize a small silicon chip embedded with thousands of gene-specific oligonucleotides to study the simultaneous mRNA expression of many genes in a sample. This technology affords an unmatched ability to compare large numbers of gene expressions in many samples to establish differences in gene expression patterns between, for example, tumor tissues and normal tissues. In the field of molecular diagnostics, scientists have used this technology to create a gene expression signature that can differentiate normal aerodigestive mucosa from HNSCC. One of the prominent examples for the use of gene expression microarray in clinical oncology is from the breast cancer literature where gene expression array clustering analysis has a proven efficacy in determining treatment effects and prognosis proven in clinical trials. In head and neck cancer, this approach has been employed for screening and diagnosis. These techniques have been applied to saliva and blood serum to look for early detection markers. Despite the inherent advantages of this technique, the inherent instability of RNA in the blood or saliva makes these techniques tenuous.

Efforts to examine the mRNA expression differences in the saliva have been promising. A group at the University of California Los Angeles (UCLA) found 1,679 genes had differing expression levels in saliva of patients with HNSCC and controls ($p < .05$). These potential salivary RNA biomarkers were interleukin-8 (IL8), IL-B, dual specificity phosphatases (DUSP1), hemagglutin 3 (HA3), orinthine decarboxylase antizyme 1 (OAZ1), S100P, and SAT, and in combinations yielded sensitivity (91%) and specificity (91%) in distinguishing squamous cell carcinoma.[42] These findings have yet to be validated in an independent set, and recent results have brought up questions about the efficacy of this technique. A recent feasibility study concluded: "The combination of (a) a minimal microarray signal, which was unaffected by RNase treatment, (b) the presence of a conventional RT-PCR

Strategies for methylation analysis

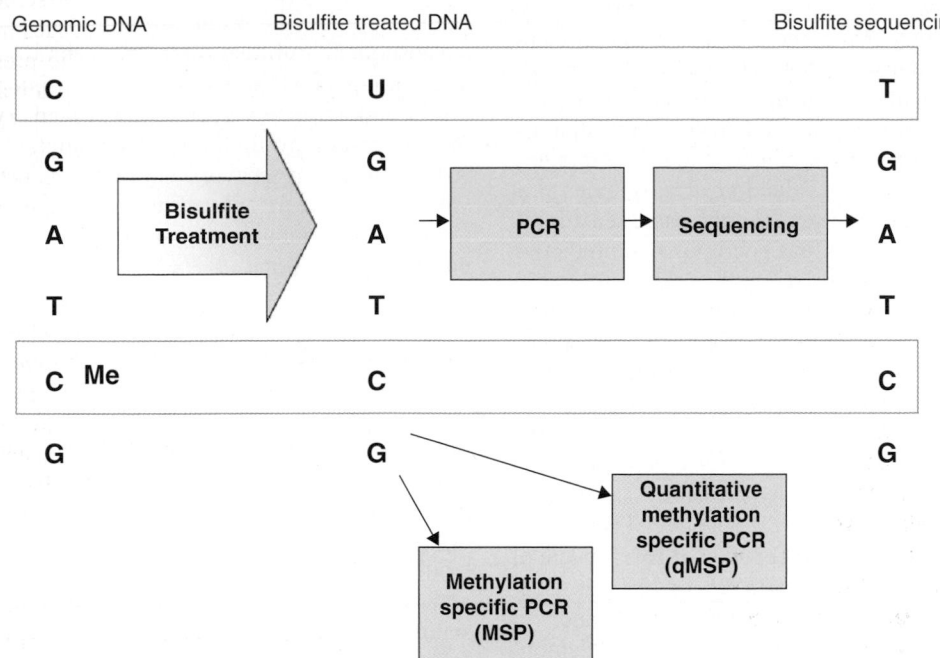

Figure 6 Bisulfite treatment. Bisulfite treatment is the foundation for technologies that assess promoter and CpG island methylation status. Methylated cytosine residues are protected from the bisulfite reaction, and changes from cytosine to thymine can be seen in unmethylated bases. Methylated cytosines can be differentiated from unmethylated ones in this manner. After bisulfite treatment, methylation can be studied by bisulfite sequencing, methylation-specific PCR (MSP) which uses primers specific to methylated versus unmethylated CpGs, and quantative MSP (does the same with real-time PCR).

housekeeper product in both RNase-treated and no-RT saliva samples, (c) the absence of a conventional RT-PCR housekeeper product in DNase-treated conditions, and (d) the absence of a RNA-specific RT-PCR product shows that any microarray or RT-PCR signal in the saliva must arise from genomic DNA, not RNA. Thus, saliva extracts do not support messenger RNA expression studies."[43]

Proteomic Approaches

Beyond expression microarray, new proteomic techniques that compare protein expression between cancer and normal tissues promise the possibility of identifying in the blood or saliva, new markers that would be amenable to clinical tests in the form of ELISAs. Techniques include two-dimensional SDS-PAGE (sodium dodecyl sulfate-polyacrylamide gel electrophoresis) that separate proteins based on size, charge, and isoelectric point, also the improvements of mass spectrography and SELDI-TOF (surface-enhanced laser desorption and ionization time-of-flight) mass spectrometry as well as MALDI-TOF (matrix-assisted laser desorption ionization time-of-flight) mass spectrometry techniques that look at large numbers of proteins. These techniques are in the category of "proteomic," a study of whole-genome protein expression in a sample. Protein-based microarray technologies with chips embedded with a library of known antibodies (>10,000 is now possible) are also available to look at widespread protein expression in a sample.

These proteomic techniques have just recently been applied in the field of head and neck cancer research. The most recognized and promising study is from Soltys and colleagues, which implemented SELDI-TOF mass spectrometry to look at the plasma of patients with head and neck cancer (57 vs 52 controls). In this study, they generated a total of 37,356 data points representing the protein profile for each sample, and from these two groups significant differences in protein expression were isolated to 65 specific SELDI-TOF peaks.[44] This study also included a blinded "validation set" of 57 cancer patients and 52 normal controls, with an attempt to predict from the plasma if the patient has cancer based on this "discovery pattern." These results were promising and showed correct identification of 39 of 57 patients with HNSCC and 40 of 52 noncancer controls, a sensitivity of 68% and specificity of 73%. Interestingly, their model tended to overpredict cancer in control smokers. These types of high-throughput molecular marker discovery techniques will be critical for finding diagnostic and predictive detectable changes in the blood or saliva.

In addition, a group at the University of Pittsburgh recently used simultaneous testing using a multiplexed immunobead-based panel to assay in the serum 60 biomarkers simultaneously in 116 patients with HNSCC before treatment, 103 patients successfully treated, and 117 smoker controls. The highest diagnostic power was composed of 25 biomarkers, including EGF, EGFR, IL-8, TPA (tissue plasminogen activator) inhibitor-1, α-fetoprotein, MMP-2 (matrix metalloproteinase-2), MMP-3, IFN-α (interferon-α), IFN-γ, IFN-inducible protein-10, regulated on activation

normal T-cell expressed and secreted (RANTES), macrophage inflammatory protein-1 α, IL-7, IL-17, IL-1 receptor-α, IL-2 receptor, granulocyte colony-stimulating factor, mesothelin, insulin-like growth factor binding protein 1, E-selectin, cytokeratin-19, VCAM, and cancer antigen-125. This study had a remarkable sensitivity of 84.5% and specificity of 98%, and 92% of patients in the active disease group correctly classified from a cross-validation serum set. This is extremely promising data that suggests that utilizing many markers in tandem may enable adequate sensitivity and specificity for molecular detection.[45]

These technologies do have difficulties producing reproducible results in validation sets, but there are significant signs that this type of approach will eventually afford new molecular markers that could be used in diagnosis and prognosis of HNSCC.

MOLECULAR IMAGING

Radiological imaging has recently joined the array of molecular techniques being employed to diagnose head and neck cancer. Radiologists now offer molecular-based physiologic and functional imaging that boasts an ability to improve the diagnosis and staging of head and neck cancer. Of these techniques, combined positron emission tomography-computed tomography (PET-CT) imaging or conventional PET has been the most utilized in the clinic. PET works by detecting gamma radiation emitted from a tracer that is designed to be a biological component that will undergo specific interactions. By far the most commonly used tracer is fluorodeoxyglucose (18FDG) which is a molecular marker, an analog of part of the glucose pathway, and this produces signal most strongly in cells metabolizing large amounts of glucose.[46] This tracer is also the most commonly used imaging tracer in the diagnosis and staging of HNSCC; and, while sensitivity is often excellent, this technology has many false positives caused often times by benign inflammation. Yet in the clinical setting, PET scans are now routinely used to define the extent of primary disease, the presence of lymph nodal spread, and distant metastasis. PET is also routinely used for follow-up, to assess response to chemotherapy or radiation therapy, and to detect disease spread.

In addition to this typical use, PET scientists now offer more advanced tracers that can molecularly target specific epitopes. Researchers are working on utilizing PET tracers that bind to the VEGF receptor that has been shown to be upregulated in HNSCC. Researchers have also used DNA precursors, which are incorporated into DNA during repair or division, which identify areas of cell proliferation. Imidazole agents can identify areas under hypoxic conditions. PET scans are already quite sensitive, but improvements in molecular targeting of tracers will invariably lead to improved diagnostic capabilities that will be used by physicians in the clinic.

PREMALIGNANT PROGRESSION

Molecular diagnostics also encompasses the prediction of which premalignant lesions will become cancer. Diagnosis of oral premalignant lesions is currently based on clinical information: histopathologic features, lesion site, and staging. Many recent advances in the diagnosis and prediction of malignant progression have been made.

Loss of Heterozygosity

Recently, promising advances in molecular methods offer to change the evaluation and diagnosis of oral premalignant lesions and squamous cell carcinoma (Figure 7). Early changes in HNSCC include LOH at two specific chromosome sites (sites 3p14 and 9p21).[47] These changes are correlated to clinical outcome, with a study of 48 oral squamous cell carcinomas (OSCCs) showing that patients with allelic imbalance (AI) at 3p24-26, 3p13, and 9p21 having a 25-times increase in their mortality rate.[48] Increased frequencies of AI at more loci ($p = .002$), without consistent patterns, were found in the three grades of dysplasia: mild, moderate, and severe that developed into cancer (39 cases) compared with case-matched dysplastic lesions that did not progress into cancer. Interestingly, many lesions developed in a different site which advocates for the theory of field cancerization, that is, genetic changes caused by mutagens that produce a field effect.[49] Rosin and colleagues studied 116 patients with premalignant lesions for LOH at 19 microsatellite loci on 7 chromosome arms (3p, 4q, 8p, 9p, 11q, 13q, and 17p), and found that individuals with LOH at 3p and/or 9p and additional losses (on 4q, 8p, 11q, or 17p), showed 33-fold increases in relative cancer risk.[4] This technique also shows promise for monitoring frequently patients with oral lesions with cell cytology showing the same LOH noted in primary biopsies.[50]

Toluidine Blue

The primary nonmolecular tools use vital tissue staining with toluidine blue (TB) and exfoliative cytology. Toluidine blue is a metachromatic dye that stains mtDNA. The use of TB to stain premalignant lesions in the clinical office has been a promising new advance in the diagnosis of head and neck cancer. Studies employing toluidine blue for evaluation of suspicious oral lesions have demonstrated impressive sensitivity, low false negatives and good positive predictive values. This stain is used in the oral cavity to differentiate dysplasia from carcinoma, and clinical studies are in progress to affirm its widespread application. From a molecular diagnostic point of view, this technology was recently compared to a panel of loci that have known LOH in head and neck neoplasms. The study considered 39 biopsy specimens (14 hyperplastic, 25 dysplastic), 14 of which were TB-negative. TB-positive samples had a higher frequency of LOH (panel of 10 microsatellite loci on 3p, 9p, or 17p was used) than TB-negative cases at 3p ($p = .013$) and 17p ($p = .049$). More TB-positive samples demonstrated LOH at multiple arms (>2 arms, $p = .015$), which was found to be associated with markedly increased cancer risk. An additional study considering TB-stained lesions found that all of the patients with SCC or carcinoma in situ cases showed LOH, but more than one-half (59%, 13 of 22) of the normal epithelia also harbored LOH in at least one marker.[51]

Aneuploidy

In 2001, Sudbo and colleagues published an impressive study in the *New England Journal of Medicine* evaluating the prognostic value of chromosomal copy changes, that is, aneuploidy, in HNSCC.[52] His group found a substantial link between cancer progression in premalignant lesions and chromosomal aneuploidy. This assessment was impressive and ground breaking, but this publication has recently been the source of considerable controversy, with a subsequent publication in the same journal questioning the validity of one of the primary figures,[53] and ultimately a retraction printed because of an oversight group finding fabrication of data. At this time, further work is being conducted to validate if there is any promise of the effect of chromosomal aneuploidy on the progression of premalignant lesions.

SURGICAL MARGINS AND LYMPH NODES

Surgical margins and lymph nodes are an area requiring the development of molecular methods for the detection and diagnosis of head and neck cancer. Methods that detect residual disease would be helpful in reducing local recurrences and regional metastasis and lead to improved staging and better outcomes. Several studies have been conducted in this area, and they use many of the techniques and targets discussed previously, for example, p53, VEGF, cyclin D1, methylation. In a study of surgical margins and lymph nodes, negative surgical margins were positive based on p53 mutation in 13 of 25 cases, and negative lymph nodes actually harbored a mutation in 6 of 28 cases.[54] Differentiating at surgical margins which lesions are genetically identical to the primary lesion in contrast to separate lesions that are part of an overall field effect, for example, genetic changes affecting a large area of tissue caused by tobacco smoke, have complicated this field greatly. In a small study that wished to address this, 61% of lesions studied that had recurred appeared to be part of a field effect cancerization which underscores the importance of close follow-up for these patients and the difficulty in relying on molecular means at the margin of a resection to diagnose direct cancer extension in the absence of histological proof.[55]

Other techniques used for molecular margin analysis include methylation detection strategies: quantitative MSP (QMSP) to look for promoter methylation in operative margins during resection and a pilot study doing this found methylation at the margins in 50% of cases where the primary tumor was also methylated.[56] Additional work looking at immunohistochemical expression of p53 and the proto-oncogene eIF4E (4E) found a significant difference in the disease-free interval between patients with 4E-positive and 4E-negative margins ($p = .003$), but not significant with p53 multivariate analysis.[57] These results give promise that molecular detection at the margin will eventually prove to have prognostic significance and possibly guide surgical management.

Molecular detection of occult tumor cells in lymph nodes is made easier by the facts that there is no background of field cancerization nor the genetic changes of dysplastic lesions to confound the molecular results. This field does struggle with

Loss of Heterozygosity

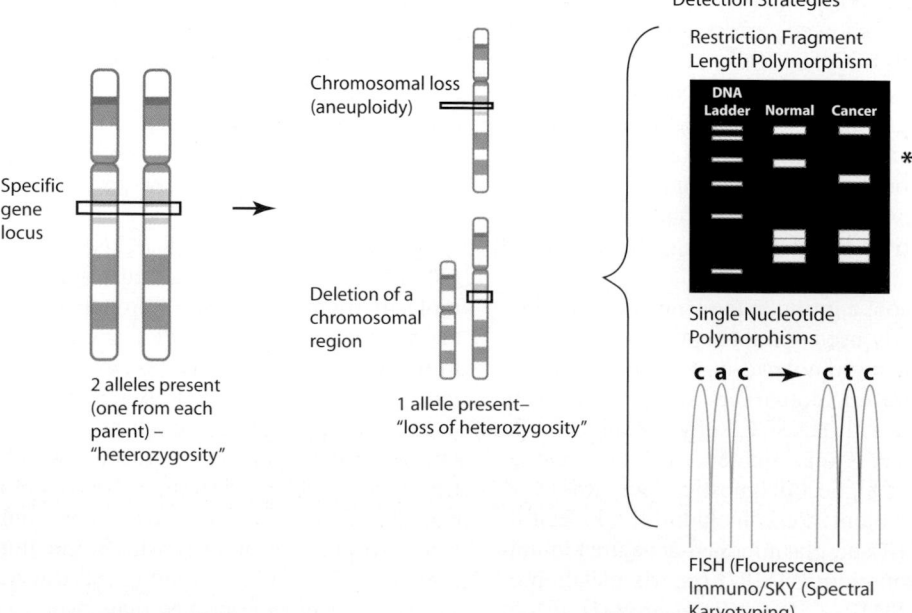

Figure 7 Loss of heterozygosity.

trying to show that there is a survival difference or staging difference for micrometastasis, as well as the type of detection molecular analysis that lymph nodes avail in the setting of grossly negative nodes. In the M.D. Anderson Cancer Center retrospective study considering selective neck dissection failures, they found selective neck dissection was definitive if all the nodes are negative based on standard pathological assessment; but, if the node was invaded with cancer, postoperative radiation offered benefit.[58] Efforts to find micrometastasis considered whether p53 mutations could be detected in lymph nodes and found that 5 of 33 (15%) nodes examined showed metastases by light microscopy, but 11 of 33 (33%) were found to be tumor positive with molecular diagnosis.[59]

Other work on squamous cell carcinoma antigen (SCCA) mRNA expression in 198 histologically metastasis-negative lymph nodes found SCCA mRNA expression in 37 (18.7%) by nested PCR and micrometastatic foci were found in 9 of these nodes (4.6%), with additional sectioning.[60] Other subsequent studies have considered the MUC1 gene, E48, cytokeratin 14 (CK14), CK20 primarily using RT-PCR. Each study has been shown to uncover successfully patients with negative lymph nodes; but because clinical management of head and neck cancer dictates that patients with even a slight risk of nodal metastasis based on tumor site and staging receive therapy that treats the nodal basins of the neck with either radiation therapy or surgical node dissection; this increased fidelity in finding regional lymph nodal disease has not translated to improved regional control or survival changes.

CONCLUSIONS

Molecular diagnosis of head and neck cancer remains in the preclinical stages. To date, few advances have made it into the clinic. At present, there are many diagnostic markers and diagnostic techniques that show promise. Indeed, technologies, such as, mRNA expression arrays, proteomic approaches (protein microarrays, SELDI/MALDI-TOF mass spectrometry), molecular imaging techniques (PET), RT-PCR, quantitative DNA PCR, QMSP, ELISA, all offer hope in detecting molecular changes in head and neck cancer. Changes studied include the detection of inactivation (LOH), mutations (p53, p16, cyclin D1, VEGF), expression levels, protein levels, and presence of methylation. These techniques will be applied in six areas: screening high risk patients for disease, predicting malignant progression, improvements in staging and prediction of outcome, therapy selection, adequate margin assessment, and diagnosis of metastases to lymph nodes.

Many lessons have been learned over the last few years. Studies must perform rigorous multivariate analyses. To reach significance, often times multiple markers are needed. In every case, these diagnostic markers obtained through statistical analysis of one set of patients must be validated in new cohorts. These targets require the design of prospective clinical studies to validate and prove efficacy. There is considerable reason for optimism that, in the near future, novel molecular markers will exist that will assist in the diagnosis of patients uninvasively and predict clinical course and response to therapy.

REFERENCES

1. Fearon ER, Vogelstein B. A genetic model for colorectal tumorigenesis. Cell 1990;61:759–67.
2. Califano J, van der Riet P, Westra W, et al. Genetic progression model for head and neck cancer: Implications for field cancerization. Cancer Res 1996;56:2488–92.
3. Ha PK, Benoit NE, Yochem R, et al. A transcriptional progression model for head and neck cancer. Clin Cancer Res 2003;9:3058–64.
4. Rosin MP, Cheng X, Poh C, et al. Use of allelic loss to predict malignant risk for low-grade oral epithelial dysplasia. Clin Cancer Res 2000;6:357–62.
5. Zhang L, Cheung KJ, Jr, Lam WL, et al. Increased genetic damage in oral leukoplakia from high risk sites: Potential impact on staging and clinical management. Cancer 2001;91:2148–55.
6. Schwartz SM, Daling JR, Doody DR, et al. Oral cancer risk in relation to sexual history and evidence of human papillomavirus infection. J Natl Cancer Inst 1998;90:1626–36.
7. Munger K, Howley PM. Human papillomavirus immortalization and transformation functions. Virus Res 2002; 89:213–28.
8. Kreimer AR, Clifford GM, Boyle P, Franceschi S. Human papillomavirus types in head and neck squamous cell carcinomas worldwide: A systematic review. Cancer Epidemiol Biomarkers Prev 2005;14:467–75.
9. Schwartz SR, Yueh B, McDougall JK, et al. Human papillomavirus infection and survival in oral squamous cell cancer: A population-based study. Otolaryngol Head Neck Surg 2001;125:1–9.
10. Ha PK, Pai SI, Westra WH, et al. Real-time quantitative PCR demonstrates low prevalence of human papillomavirus type 16 in premalignant and malignant lesions of the oral cavity. Clin Cancer Res 2002;8:1203–9.
11. Zhao M, Rosenbaum E, Carvalho AL, et al. Feasibility of quantitative PCR-based saliva rinse screening of HPV for head and neck cancer. Int J Cancer 2005;117:605–10.
12. Yang H, Yang K, Khafagi A, et al. Sensitive detection of human papillomavirus in cervical, head/neck, and schistosomiasis-associated bladder malignancies. Proc Natl Acad Sci U S A 2005;102:7683–8.
13. Smith EM, Ritchie JM, Summersgill KF, et al. Human papillomavirus in oral exfoliated cells and risk of head and neck cancer. J Natl Cancer Inst 2004;96:449–55.
14. Ionov Y, Peinado MA, Malkhosyan S, et al. Ubiquitous somatic mutations in simple repeated sequences reveal a new mechanism for colonic carcinogenesis. Nature 1993;363:558–61.
15. de la Chapelle A. Microsatellite instability. N Engl J Med 2003;349:209–10.
16. El-Naggar AK, Hurr K, Huff V, et al. Microsatellite instability in preinvasive and invasive head and neck squamous carcinoma. Am J Pathol 1996;148:2067–72.
17. Nawroz H, Koch W, Anker P, et al. Microsatellite alterations in serum DNA of head and neck cancer patients. Nat Med 1996;2:1035–7.
18. Spafford MF, Koch WM, Reed AL, et al. Detection of head and neck squamous cell carcinoma among exfoliated oral mucosal cells by microsatellite analysis. Clin Cancer Res 2001;7:607–12.
19. Coulet F, Blons H, Cabelguenne A, et al. Detection of plasma tumor DNA in head and neck squamous cell carcinoma by microsatellite typing and p53 mutation analysis. Cancer Res 2000;60:707–11.
20. Baker SJ, Fearon ER, Nigro JM, et al. Chromosome 17 deletions and p53 gene mutations in colorectal carcinomas. Science 1989;244:217–21.
21. Boyle JO, Mao L, Brennan JA, et al. Gene mutations in saliva as molecular markers for head and neck squamous cell carcinomas. Am J Surg 1994;168:429-32.
22. Koch WM, Boyle JO, Mao L, et al. p53 gene mutations as markers of tumor spread in synchronous oral cancers. Arch Otolaryngol Head Neck Surg 1994;120:943–7.
23. Warnakulasuriya S, Soussi T, Maher R, et al. Expression of p53 in oral squamous cell carcinoma is associated with the presence of IgG and IgA p53 autoantibodies in sera and saliva of the patients. J Pathol 2000;192:52–7.
24. Hofele C, Schwager-Schmitt M, Volkmann M. Prognostic value of antibodies against p53 in patients with oral squamous cell carcinoma—five years survival rate. Laryngorhinootologie 2002;81:342–5.
25. Fliss MS, Usadel H, Caballero OL, et al. Facile detection of mitochondrial DNA mutations in tumors and bodily fluids. Science 2000;287:2017–9.
26. Kim MM, Clinger JD, Masayesva BG, et al. Mitochondrial DNA quantity increases with histopathologic grade in premalignant and malignant head and neck lesions. Clin Cancer Res 2004;10:8512–5.
27. Jiang WW, Masayesva B, Zahurak M, et al. Increased mitochondrial DNA content in saliva associated with head and neck cancer. Clin Cancer Res 2005;11:2486–91.
28. Kawano T, Yanoma S, Nakamura Y, et al. Evaluation of soluble adhesion molecules CD44 (CD44st, CD44v5, CD44v6), ICAM-1, and VCAM-1 as tumor markers in head and neck cancer. Am J Otolaryngol 2005;26:308–13.
29. Andratschke M, Chaubal S, Pauli C, et al. Soluble CD44v6 is not a sensitive tumor marker in patients with head and neck squamous cell cancer. Anticancer Res 2005;25:2821–6.
30. Ford AC, Grandis JR. Targeting epidermal growth factor receptor in head and neck cancer. Head Neck 2003; 25:67–73.
31. Lothaire P, de Azambuja E, Dequanter D, et al. Molecular markers of head and neck squamous cell carcinoma: Promising signs in need of prospective evaluation. Head Neck 2006;28:256–69.
32. Hartig F, Pechlaner C. Cetuximab plus radiotherapy for head and neck cancer. N Engl J Med 2006;354:2187.
33. Tong X, Yang L, Lang JC, et al. Application of immunomagnetic cell enrichment in combination with RT-PCR for the detection of rare circulating head and neck tumor cells in human peripheral blood. Cytometry B Clin Cytom 2007 [Epub ahead of print].
34. Teknos TN, Cox C, Yoo S, et al. Elevated serum vascular endothelial growth factor and decreased survival in advanced laryngeal carcinoma. Head Neck 2002;24:1004–11.
35. Sanchez-Cespedes M, Esteller M, Wu L, et al. Gene promoter hypermethylation in tumors and serum of head and neck cancer patients. Cancer Res 2000;60:892–5.
36. Dong SM, Sun DI, Benoit NE, et al. Epigenetic inactivation of RASSF1A in head and neck cancer. Clin Cancer Res 2003;9:3635–40.
37. Liu K, Zuo C, Luo QK, et al. Promoter hypermethylation and inactivation of hMLH1, a DNA mismatch repair gene, in head and neck squamous cell carcinoma. Diagn Mol Pathol 2003;12:50–6.
38. Hasegawa M, Nelson HH, Peters E, et al. Patterns of gene promoter methylation in squamous cell cancer of the head and neck. Oncogene 2002;21:4231–6.
39. Xi S, Dyer KF, Kimak M, et al. Decreased STAT1 expression by promoter methylation in squamous cell carcinogenesis. J Natl Cancer Inst 2006;98:181–9.
40. Ai L, Vo QN, Zuo C, et al. Ataxia-telangiectasia-mutated (ATM) gene in head and neck squamous cell carcinoma: Promoter hypermethylation with clinical correlation in 100 cases. Cancer Epidemiol Biomarkers Prev 2004;13:150–6.
41. Nakahara Y, Shintani S, Mihara M, et al. Detection of p16 promoter methylation in the serum of oral cancer patients. Int J Oral Maxillofac Surg 2006;35:362–5.
42. Li Y, St John MA, Zhou X, et al. Salivary transcriptome diagnostics for oral cancer detection. Clin Cancer Res 2004;10:8442–50.
43. Kumar SV, Hurteau GJ, Spivack SD. Validity of messenger RNA expression analyses of human saliva. Clin Cancer Res 2006;12:5033–9.
44. Soltys SG, Le QT, Shi G, et al. The use of plasma surface-enhanced laser desorption/ionization time-of-flight mass spectrometry proteomic patterns for detection of head and neck squamous cell cancers. Clin Cancer Res 2004; 10:4806–12.
45. Linkov F, Lisovich A, Yurkovetsky Z, et al. Early detection of head and neck cancer: Development of a novel screening tool using multiplexed immunobead-based biomarker profiling. Cancer Epidemiol Biomarkers Prev 2007;16:102–7.
46. Kutler DI, Wong RJ, Kraus DH. Functional imaging in head and neck cancer. Curr Oncol Rep 2005;7:137–44.
47. Mao L, Lee JS, Fan YH, et al. Frequent microsatellite alterations at chromosomes 9p21 and 3p14 in oral premalignant lesions and their value in cancer risk assessment. Nat Med 1996;2:682–5.
48. Partridge M, Emilion G, Pateromichelakis S, et al. The prognostic significance of allelic imbalance at key chromosomal loci in oral cancer. Br J Cancer 1999;79:1821–7.
49. Partridge M, Pateromichelakis S, Phillips E, et al. A case-control study confirms that microsatellite assay can identify

patients at risk of developing oral squamous cell carcinoma within a field of cancerization. Cancer Res 2000;60:3893–8.

50. Rosin MP, Epstein JB, Berean K, et al. The use of exfoliative cell samples to map clonal genetic alterations in the oral epithelium of high-risk patients. Cancer Res 1997;57:5258–60.

51. Guo Z, Yamaguchi K, Sanchez-Cespedes M, et al. Allelic losses in OraTest-directed biopsies of patients with prior upper aerodigestive tract malignancy. Clin Cancer Res 2001;7:1963–8.

52. Sudbo J, Kildal W, Risberg B, et al. DNA content as a prognostic marker in patients with oral leukoplakia. N Engl J Med 2001;344:1270–8.

53. Curfman GD, Morrissey S, Drazen JM. Expression of concern: DNA content as a prognostic marker in patients with oral leukoplakia. N Engl J Med 2001;344:1270–8 and Sudbo J et al. the influence of resection and aneuploidy on mortality in oral leukoplakia. N Engl J Med 2004;350:1405–13. N Engl J Med 2006;354:638.

54. Brennan JA, Mao L, Hruban RH, et al. Molecular assessment of histopathological staging in squamous-cell carcinoma of the head and neck. N Engl J Med 1995;332:429–35.

55. Tabor MP, Brakenhoff RH, Ruijter-Schippers HJ, et al. Genetically altered fields as origin of locally recurrent head and neck cancer: A retrospective study. Clin Cancer Res 2004;10:3607–13.

56. Goldenberg D, Harden S, Masayesva BG, et al. Intraoperative molecular margin analysis in head and neck cancer. Arch Otolaryngol Head Neck Surg 2004;130:39–44.

57. Nathan CA, Amirghahri N, Rice C, et al. Molecular analysis of surgical margins in head and neck squamous cell carcinoma patients. Laryngoscope 2002;112:2129–40.

58. Byers RM, Clayman GL, McGill D, et al. Selective neck dissections for squamous carcinoma of the upper aerodigestive tract: Patterns of regional failure. Head Neck 1999;21:499–505.

59. Partridge M, Li SR, Pateromichelakis S, et al. Detection of minimal residual cancer to investigate why oral tumors recur despite seemingly adequate treatment. Clin Cancer Res 2000;6:2718–25.

60. Hamakawa H, Fukizumi M, Bao Y, et al. Genetic diagnosis of micrometastasis based on SCC antigen mRNA in cervical lymph nodes of head and neck cancer. Clin Exp Metastasis 1999;17:593–9.

90

Imaging of the Oral Cavity, Pharynx, Salivary Glands and Neck

Robert E. Morales, MD
Adam E. Flanders, MD

Imaging plays a major role in the work-up of patients with head and neck diseases. The modalities commonly utilized for the radiologic evaluation of the neck include computed tomography (CT), magnetic resonance imaging (MRI), and combined positron emission tomography with computed tomography (PET-CT). The role of the radiologic evaluation is to determine the extent of a lesion, identify associated findings and characterize these findings to stage the lesion or develop a differential diagnosis.

In evaluating the extent of a mass, the portions of the lesion "hidden" beneath the skin or mucosal surface are of particular importance as these areas are difficult to assess by clinical examination. In addition to the lesion's dimensions and extent, critical imaging features such as osseous invasion or perineural spread must be assessed. Finally, a fundamental understanding of anatomic landmarks and spaces is essential as the resultant information may alter surgical approach or therapeutic management.

The identification of lymphadenopathy is paramount to the complete imaging interpretation. Reactive or neoplastic lymph nodes should be identified. These include enlarged lymph nodes or lymph nodes of any size that have necrosis. The margins of the lymph nodes also need to be evaluated for extranodal extension. The adjacent fat planes surrounding the primary lesion are also studied for the presence of tumor infiltration or edema. Extensive edema with overlying skin thickening usually suggests an infectious/inflammatory process although occasionally a neoplastic process can cause lymphatic obstruction resulting in a similar appearance.

The imaging evaluation of head and neck disease is not complete without a full description of the intrinsic imaging features such as density or signal intensity of a process on CT or (MRI), respectively. This includes a description of the internal architecture and composition including the presence of calcification, necrosis, cyst formation, or prominent vascularity. Imaging margins adjacent to or surrounding a process offer clues regarding growth characteristics. Irregular, infiltrative margins often suggest a more aggressive or rapidly growing lesion. When a process abuts an osseous structure, erosion of the bone is a feature more suggestive of rapid expansion whereas bone remodeling with a sclerotic margin often suggests slow growth.

This chapter will summarize the imaging approach to the various regions including the nasopharynx, oropharynx, larynx and hypopharynx, oral cavity, salivary glands, and the suprahyoid portion of the neck. There is emphasis on the anatomic approach to the involved spaces and a focus on particular anatomic landmarks that aid in description of a lesion or in developing a differential diagnosis. Where appropriate, the imaging characteristics of some of the more common lesions will be described.

SUPRAHYOID PORTION OF THE NECK

The anatomic junction of the oropharynx and hypopharynx is at the level of the pharyngoepiglottic fold. The hyoid bone is located at approximately the same level, and it divides the neck functionally, as well as anatomically, into two distinct parts: the suprahyoid and infrahyoid portions. The three layers of the deep cervical fascia merge at the hyoid bone, functionally dividing it into these two regions.[1] The suprahyoid portion of the neck extends from the skull base to the hyoid bone and surrounds the nasopharynx and oropharynx and includes the deep spaces. These spaces consist of the prestyloid parapharyngeal space, the poststyloid parapharyngeal space (carotid space), the pharyngeal mucosal space of the nasopharynx and oropharynx, the parotid space, the masticator space, the retropharyngeal space, and the prevertebral space. In general, MRI is the modality of choice when evaluating suprahyoid neck lesions. The superior soft tissue contrast and multiplanar capability provided with MRI enable better evaluation of intracranial extension by perineural spread, in this anatomically complex region, or via direct skull base invasion.[2] However, for osseous assessment of the skull base, particularly the cortex, CT imaging should also be added. MR imaging is also less prone to extensive artifact from dental hardware.

The key to developing a differential diagnosis regarding a mass in the suprahyoid portion of the neck is to identify the anatomic space from which the lesion has originated. Identifying the space of origin of a small lesion is easy; however, when the lesion is large, the distortion of the regional anatomy can make localization difficult. In the suprahyoid portion of the neck, one visual indicator which aids in the identity of the space of origin is the direction of displacement of the prestyloid parapharyngeal fat.[1] The prestyloid parapharyngeal space is a useful imaging landmark because it is composed primarily of fat, and it is located in the central position relative to the surrounding anatomic spaces. Fat is markedly low in attenuation on CT and high in signal on T1-weighted MRI. Because of the unique imaging features of fat, normal anatomic structures and lesions remain distinct from the parapharyngeal fat. Since essentially all the other deep spaces of the suprahyoid portion of the neck abut the prestyloid parapharyngeal space, large masses in those spaces will usually displace the parapharyngeal fat.

On cross-sectional imaging, the prestyloid parapharyngeal fat is triangular in shape (Figure 1). In three-dimensions, the space is

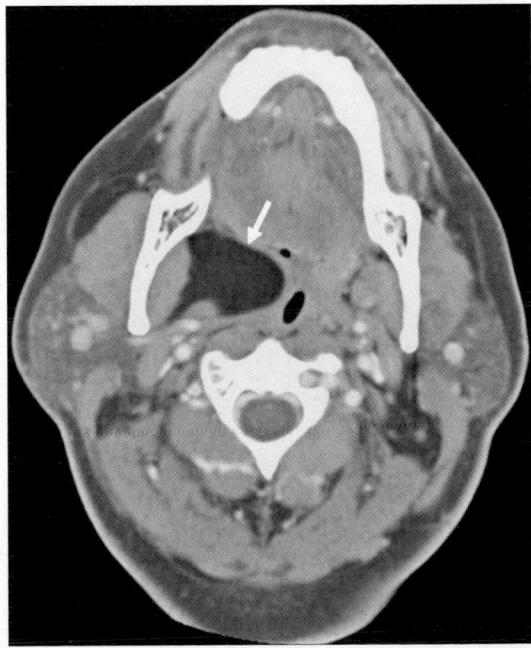

Figure 1 Axial CT with contrast. The triangular shape of the prestyloid parapharyngeal space fat is accentuated by the presence of a lipoma (*arrow*).

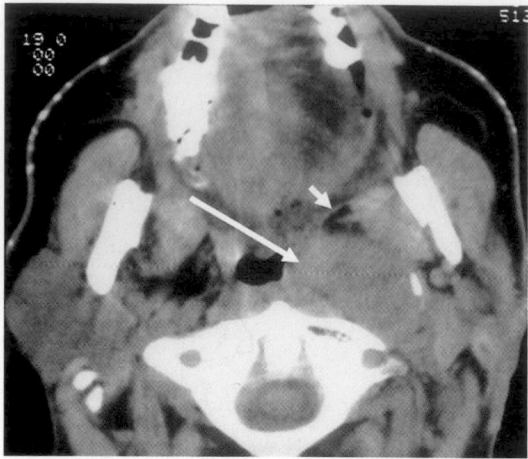

Figure 2 Axial CT with contrast. The fat of the prestyloid parapharyngeal space (*short arrow*) is displaced anteriorly by a glomus vagale within the poststyloid parapharyngeal space (*long arrow*).

pyramidal in shape with its widest portion and base at the level of the skull base and its apex approximately at the level of the hyoid bone. In general, a lesion within the poststyloid parapharyngeal space displaces the prestyloid parapharyngeal fat anteriorly (Figure 2). A lesion within the masticator space displaces the fat posteriorly (Figure 3). A lesion within the pharyngeal mucosal space displaces the fat laterally (Figure 4), and a lesion within the parotid space displaces the fat medially (Figure 5).

The anatomic space in which a lesion originates provides clues to its identity. A differential diagnosis can be formulated by first considering lesions that can derive from normal structures contained

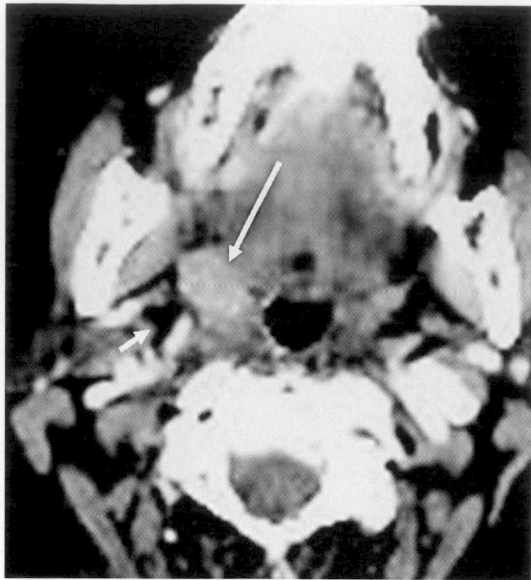

Figure 4 Axial CT with contrast. The fat of the prestyloid parapharyngeal space (*short arrow*) is displaced laterally by a tonsillar mass (*long arrow*).

within the space. For example, in the complex poststyloid parapharyngeal space, the traversing structures include the internal carotid artery, the internal jugular vein, cranial nerves IX through XII, the sympathetic chain, and lymph nodes. From these structures, carotid pseudoaneurysm (Figure 6), jugular vein thrombosis, schwannomas, paragangliomas, and lymphadenopathy can occur. Once the vascular are excluded, the primary diagnosis of a mass in the poststyloid parapharyngeal space is often limited to schwannomas and paragangliomas. Schwannomas are typically

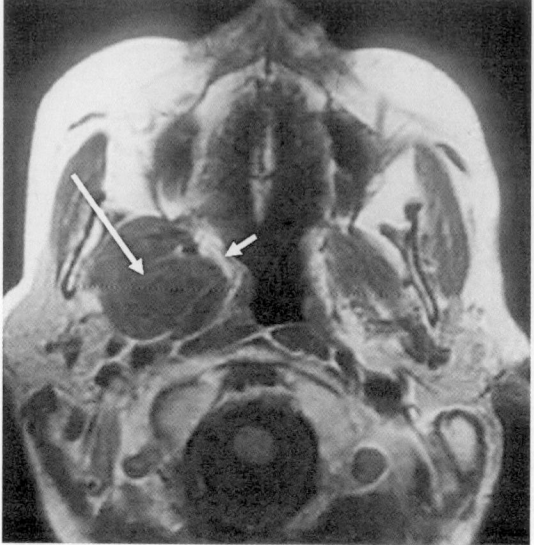

Figure 5 Axial T1-weighted MRI. The fat of the prestyloid parapharyngeal space (*short arrow*) is displaced medially by a pleomorphic adenoma (*long arrow*) of the deep portion of the parotid gland.

well circumscribed and have areas of high signal on T2-weighted images and strong enhancement. They often displace the carotid artery anteriorly as they follow the course of the involved cranial nerve (Figure 7). The marked vascularity of glomus tumors provides a distinctive appearance on MRI ("salt and pepper") attributed to flow voids and prominent enhancement within the lesion (Figure 8).

Another relatively common diagnostic dilemma is distinguishing between a deep parotid lesion and a prestyloid parapharyngeal lesion. Intrinsic lesions to the prestyloid parapharyngeal space are relatively uncommon. Ectopic salivary gland tissue, however, can be present throughout the head and neck and can be a source of neoplastic transformation. A parotid space mass displaces the prestyloid parapharyngeal fat medially. Other imaging features that suggest a deep parotid mass include an indistinct fat plane adjacent to the parotid gland, extension through the stylomandibular notch or a tissue margin which abuts the retromandibular vein (Figure 9).

Masticator space pathology is principally derived from the mandible and muscles of mastication. Odontogenic infections (see Figure 3) are the most common lesions with sarcomas of the bone and soft tissues occurring less often. Cranial nerves, course throughout the neck, and schwannomas can be found in the masticator space, arising from the branches of the trigeminal nerve and virtually anywhere within the neck. The clinical presentation, regarding signs and symptoms of possible infection, is essential to accurate interpretation of imaging studies of this region.

Although the most common malignant neoplasm of the pharyngeal mucosal space is squamous cell carcinoma (SCC), other lesions in this space also need to be considered. Rests of salivary gland tissue are common throughout much of the neck, particularly along the mucosal surfaces, so salivary gland neoplasms are occasionally encountered. The lymphoid tissue of

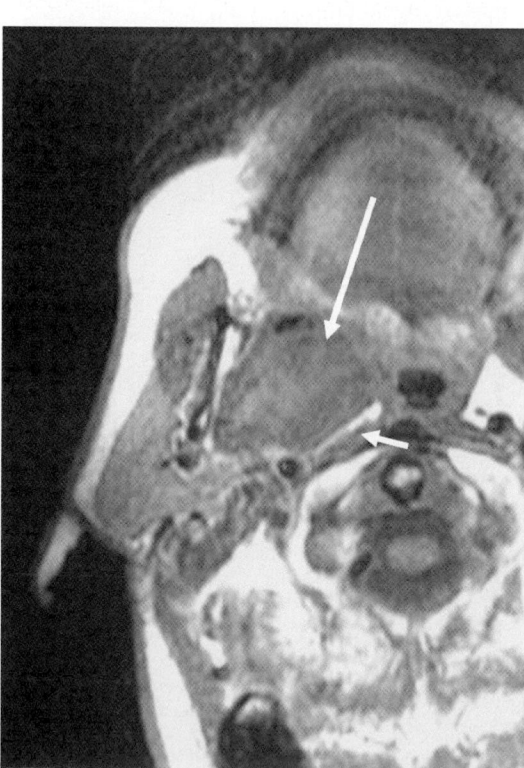

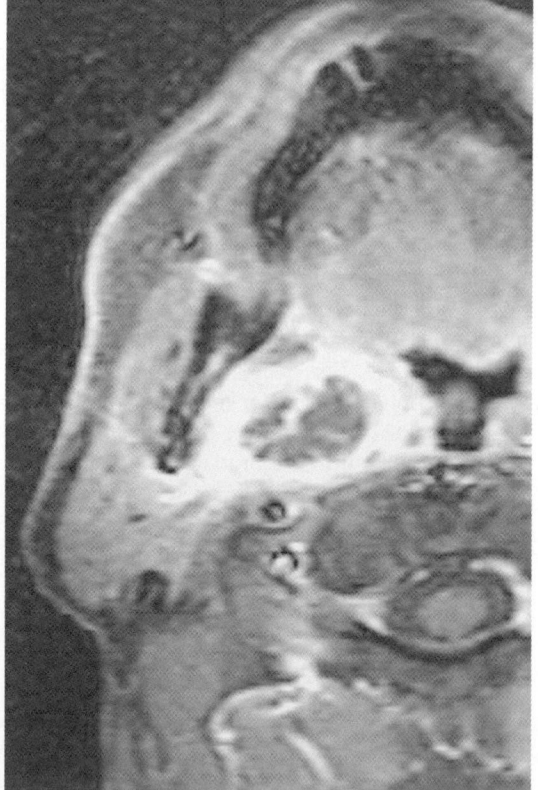

(A)   (B)

Figure 3 Axial T1-weighted MRI (A) and axial T1-weighted MRI with contrast and fat-saturation (B). The fat of the prestyloid parapharyngeal space (*short arrow*) (A) is displaced posteriorly by an abscess within the masticator space (*long arrow*) (A).

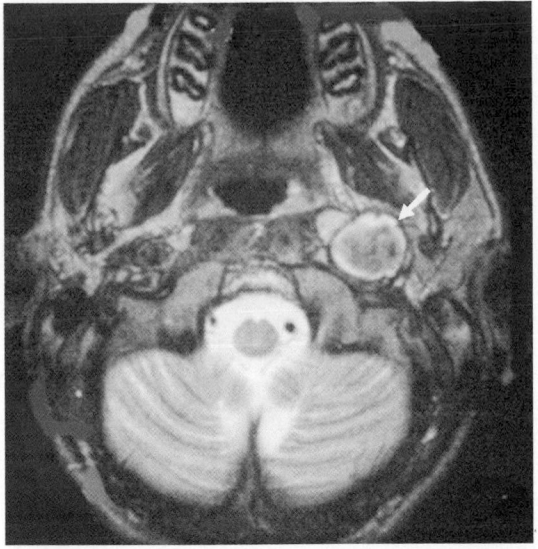

(A)

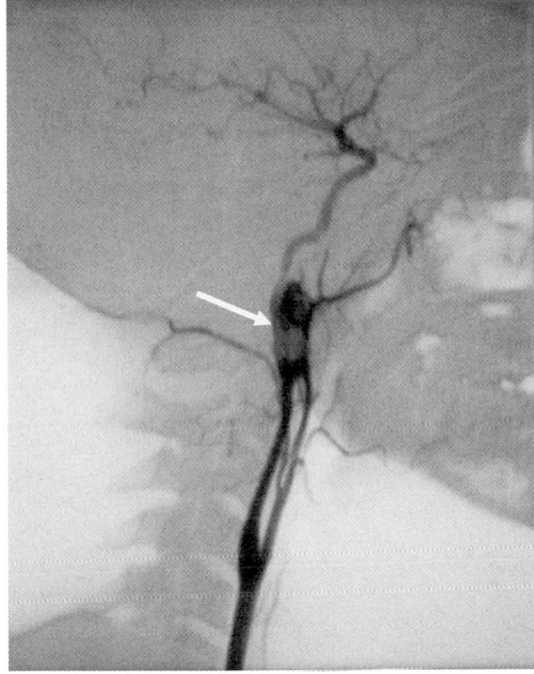

(B)

Figure 6 Axial T2-weighted MRI (A) and conventional arteriogram (B). Complex signal is identified within a carotid pseudoaneurysm (*arrows*) (A, B) representing a combination of thrombus of different ages and a partially patent lumen.

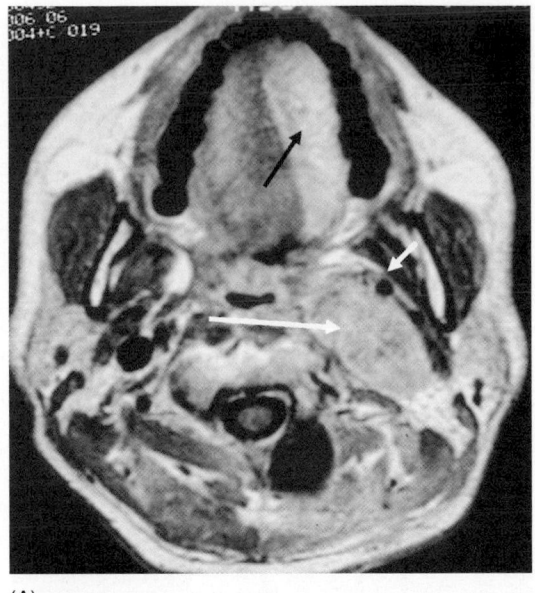

(A)

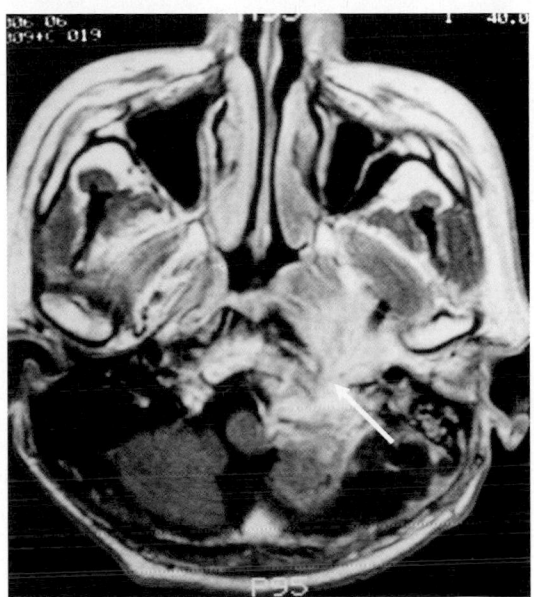

(B)

Figure 7 Axial T1-weighted MRI with contrast. A schwannoma of the hypoglossal nerve (cranial nerve XII) (*long arrow*) (A) displaces the prestyloid parapharyngeal fat and carotid artery anteriorly (*short arrow*) (A) and extends through the hypoglossal canal (*arrow*) (B) into the posterior fossa. Note the atrophy of the left side of the tongue with fat replacement (*black arrow*) (A).

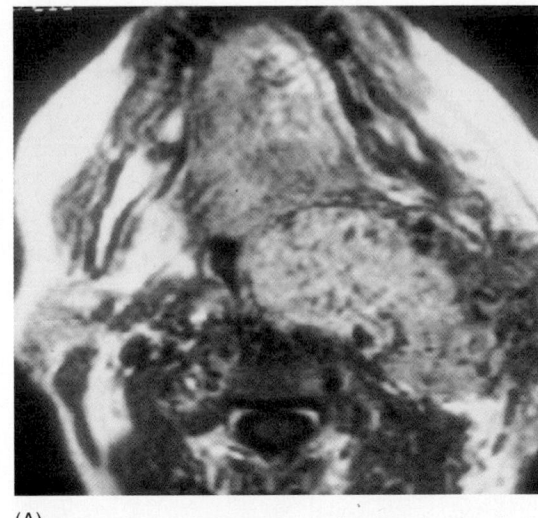

(A)

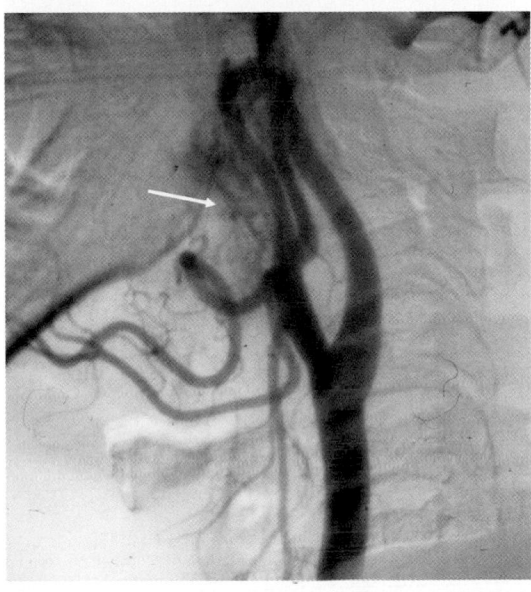

(B)

Figure 8 Axial T1-weighted MRI with contrast (A) and conventional arteriogram (B). The characteristic "salt and pepper" appearance of large paragangliomas is demonstrated with the low signal "pepper" representing arterial flow voids of this vascular mass (glomus vagale) (A). The prominent vessels (*arrow*) are easily identified on the conventional arteriogram (B).

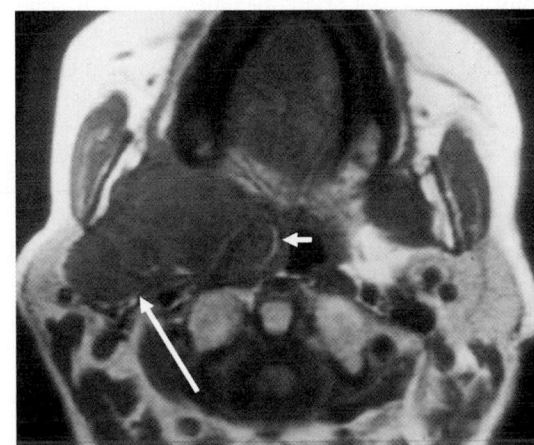

Figure 9 Axial T1-weighted MRI. A deep parotid pleomorphic adenoma is identified markedly displacing the prestyloid parapharyngeal fat medially (*short arrow*) and extending through the stylomandibular notch (*long arrow*). There is no identifiable fat plane between the lesion and the parotid gland.

Waldeyer ring is part of the pharyngeal mucosal space. Therefore, lymphoma and adenoidal hyperplasia, in addition to peritonsillar abscess formation or other infection, are additional processes that occur in this location.

Another important anatomic landmark in the suprahyoid neck region is the longus colli and capitis muscle complex, which is part of the prevertebral portion of the perivertebral space. These muscles form the boundary between the retropharyngeal space and the prevertebral space. Inflammatory changes and abscess formation within the retropharyngeal space often originates from mucosal space infections and retropharyngeal adenopathy, causing posterior displacement of these muscles. Alternatively, disease processes within the prevertebral space often extend from

the spine, causing anterior displacement of the muscles. Finally, a potential space exists (otherwise known as "the danger space") that can serve as a route of spread of infection into the mediastinum (Figure 10).

Nasopharyngeal carcinoma originating from the overlying pharyngeal mucosal space can invade the prevertebral fascia, the skull base, or extend intracranially via perineural spread. Yousem and colleagues reviewed the imaging evaluation of resectability criteria for head and neck cancer.[3] Extension to the prevertebral fascia is one of the criteria for a T4b category. Although Hsu and colleagues found that preservation of the high signal within the retropharyngeal fat stripe on T1-weighted images is highly consistent with a lack of invasion and fixation of the

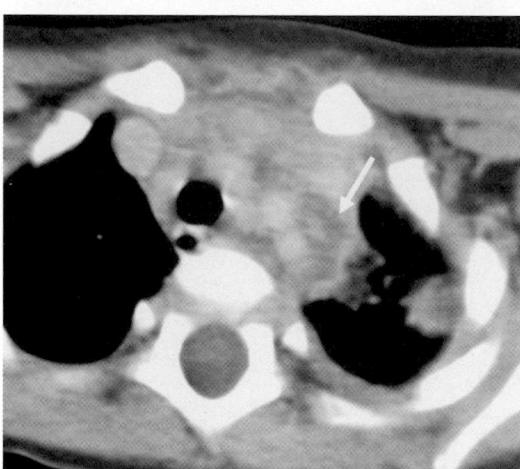

(A)

(B)

Figure 10 Axial CT with contrast. Edema versus early abscess formation is identified within the retropharyngeal space, located in front of the longus colli/capitis muscles (*arrows*) (A), with spread of infection into the mediastinum (*arrow*) (B).

tumor to the prevertebral fascia and prevertebral muscles, Lovener and colleagues found that the radiologic suggestion of invasion was not nearly as reliable.[3–5] They concluded that surgical endoscopic assessment should remain the standard of care to detect invasion, whereas the observation that preservation of the fat plane, however, is a useful indicator for lack of fixation.[3,5] Xie and colleagues found that MRI was more sensitive to skull base invasion than CT.[3,6] MR imaging is also essential for the evaluation of perineural spread of tumor. Although CT imaging may demonstrate widening of the neural foramen, MRI is far superior at visualizing actual thickening and enhancement of the affected nerve (Figure 11).

LARYNX AND HYPOPHARYNX

The larynx and hypopharynx are primarily better evaluated with CT as motion of the respiratory structures often degrades MRI due

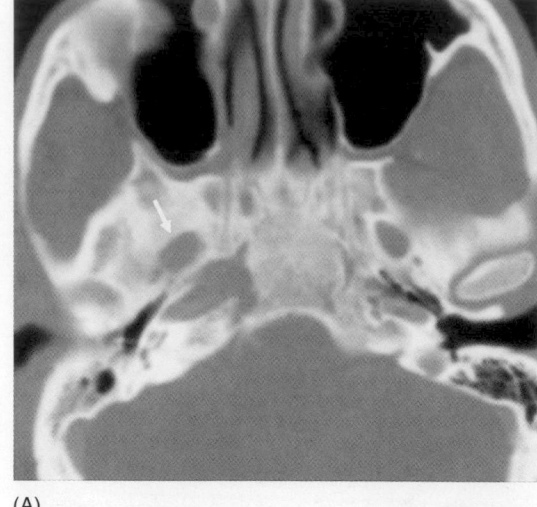

(A)

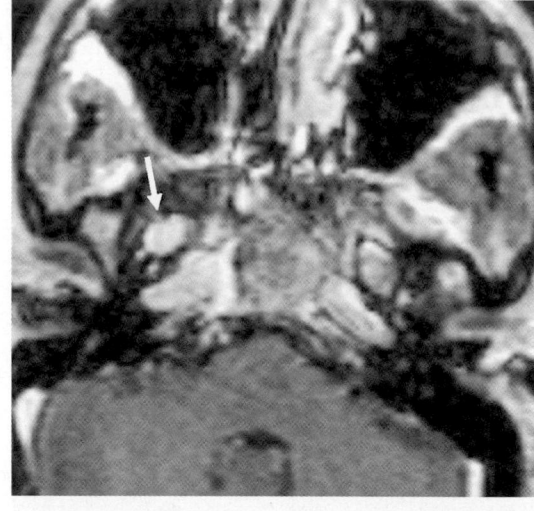

(B)

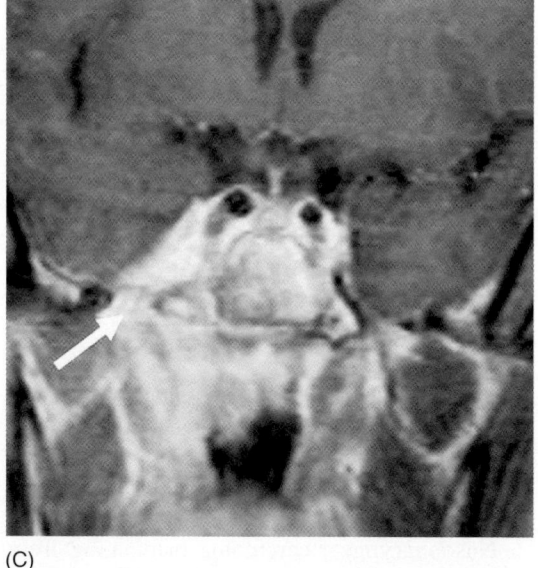

(C)

Figure 11 Axial CT (*bone window*) (A), axial T1-weighted MRI with contrast (B), coronal T1-weighted MRI with contrast and fat-saturation (C). Nasopharyngeal carcinoma with perineural spread along cranial nerve V-3 as evidenced by foramen ovale widening on CT imaging (*arrow*) (A) with loss of a well defined cortical margin and visualization of nerve thickening and enhancement on MRI (*arrows*) (B, C).

to longer inherent scanning times. This region is less complex anatomically and is bordered by prominent fat planes that facilitate visualization

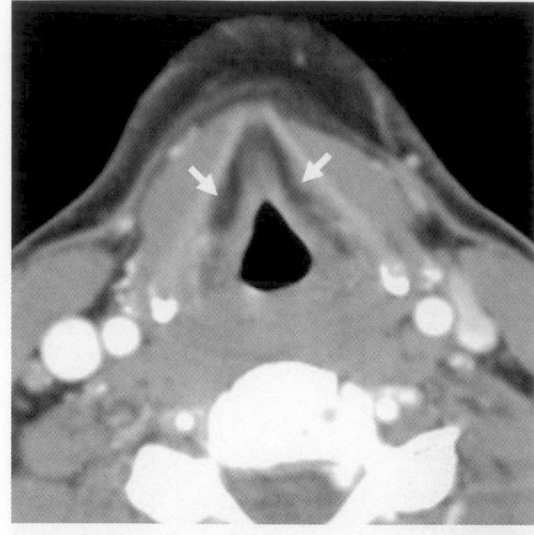

(A)

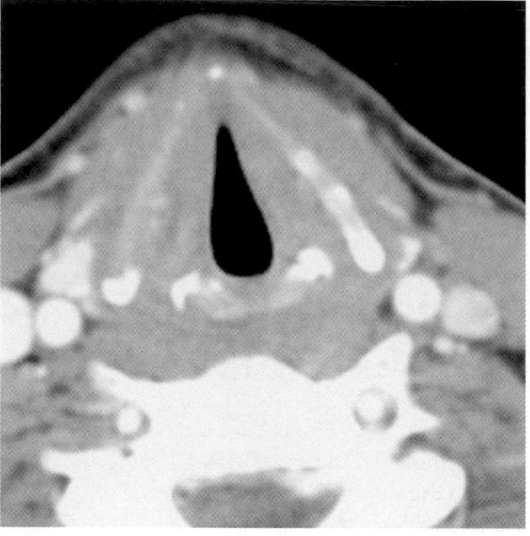

(B)

Figure 12 Axial CT with contrast. Paraglottic fat is identified submucosally (*arrows*) at the level of the "false cords" (A) and supraglottic larynx with no identifiable submucosal fat at the level of the "true cords" (B).

of anatomic structures on CT. Staging of laryngeal and hypopharyngeal SCC is one of the major indications for the evaluation of this region. Staging on an imaging study is not accurate without a description of the clinical findings obtained on physical examination. Imaging can greatly assist the evaluation of the primary lesion by defining the size of the lesion and extent of spread into the subcutaneous tissues and adjacent subsites, detecting erosion of the laryngeal cartilages and identifying associated adenopathy.

Most laryngeal neoplasms originate in the mucosal surface. A mucosal lesion may be difficult to visualize radiographically when it is small. On imaging studies, it is identified by the presence of a nodular enhancing tissue that distorts the mucosal surface. Submucosal extension is represented by extension of soft tissue into the underlying submucosal fat or other structures. Loss of fat or other soft tissue planes in this region is helpful in demarcating spread of neoplasm and provides important information regarding staging of the neoplasm and surgical approach,

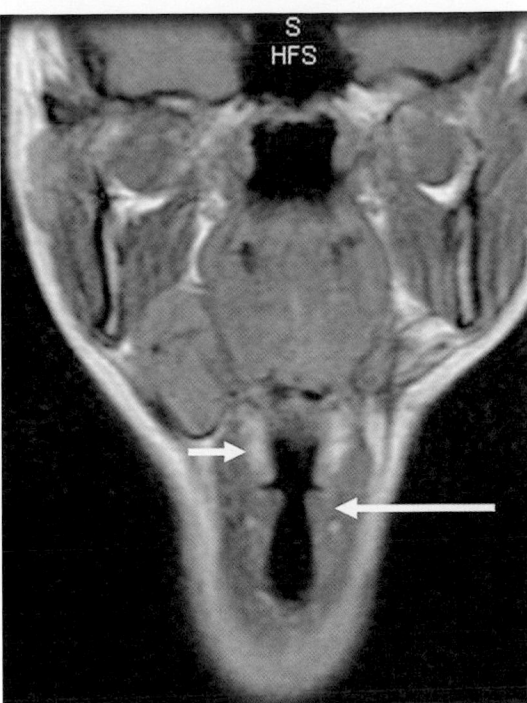

Figure 13 Coronal T1-weighted MRI without contrast. The high signal fat (*short arrow*) sharply demarcates the supraglottic larynx above the laryngeal ventricle with the glottis (*long arrow*) clearly seen inferior to the ventricle.

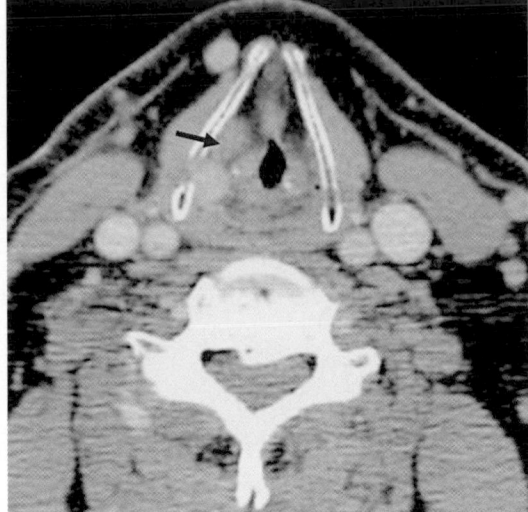

(A)

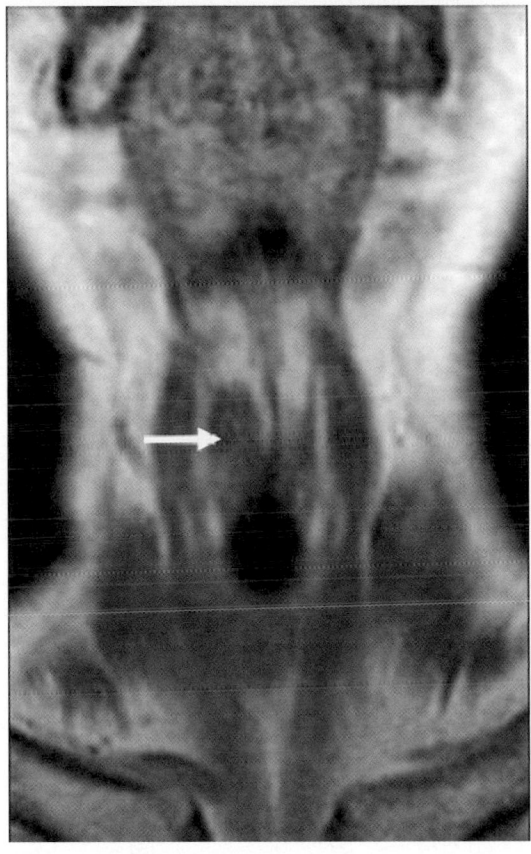

(B)

Figure 14 Axial CT with contrast (A), Coronal T1-weighted MRI without contrast (B). Recurrent fibrosarcoma of the hypopharynx is identified extending into the paraglottic fat (*arrows*) (A, B).

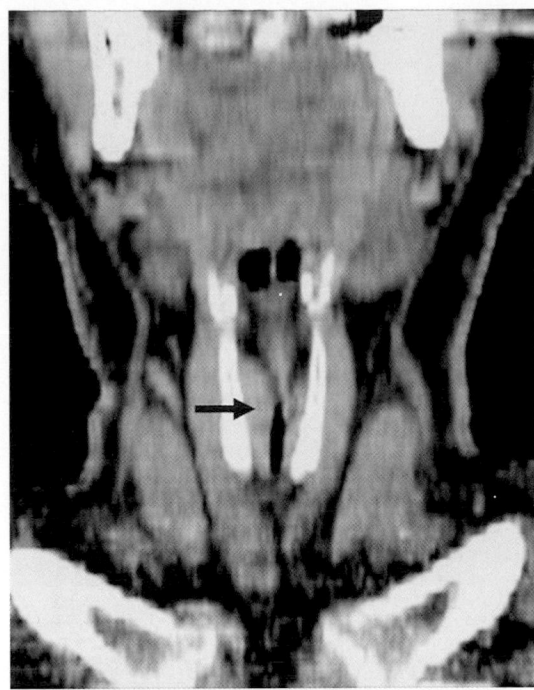

Figure 15 Coronal CT reconstruction. Same patient as Figure 14 with recurrent fibrosarcoma extending into the right paraglottic fat (*arrow*), from its origin within the pyriform sinus.

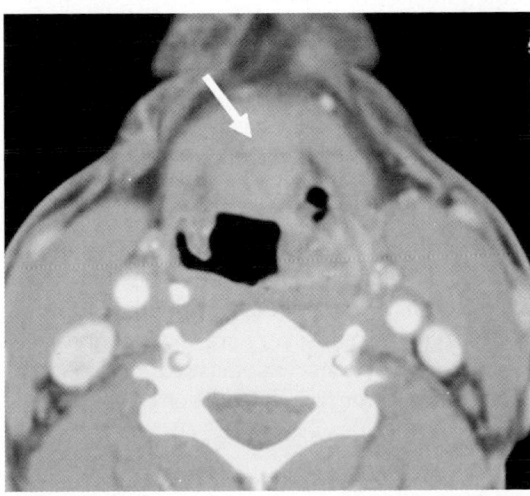

Figure 16 Axial CT with contrast. Supraglottic carcinoma with extensive infiltration into the preepiglottic fat (*arrow*) and also involvement of the left aryepiglottic fold.

particularly when the tumor invades the paraglottic and preepiglottic fat. Fat serves as natural contrast against the higher density on CT and lower signal on MRI of infiltrating tumor.

The paraglottic fat is a useful landmark in distinguishing the supraglottic larynx from the soft tissue characteristically found at the level of the glottis (Figure 12). Coronal T1-weighted images are particularly helpful in evaluating for transglottic spread of carcinoma by displaying the supraglottic, glottic, and subglottic regions simultaneously with the supraglottic larynx demarcated by the extensive submucosal paraglottic fat (Figure 13). Pyriform sinus lesions that spread into the paraglottic fat can also be visualized in this manner (Figure 14). Current multidetector CT scanners acquire images that are 1 mm in thickness or less resulting in isotropic datasets, which can be reformatted into any imaging plane without inherent loss in resolution. As a result, coronal CT reconstructions can also be helpful in a similar fashion to coronal T1-weighted MR images (Figure 15). Extension of a lesion into the preepiglottic fat has important clinical staging implications and, therefore, will affect the type of surgical management (Figure 16). Lovener and colleagues found an accuracy rate of 90% with MRI evaluation of preepiglottis space invasion with attention to the high intensity fat signal on T1-weighted images in the axial and sagittal planes.[7]

Another critical imaging finding which has impact on staging and treatment is the identification of laryngeal cartilage erosion (Figure 17). Cortical invasion of only the inner margin of the thyroid cartilage is the principal criterion for a categorization of laryngeal SCC as T3, whereas invasion of the entire cartilage is considered category T4. Compared to MRI CT evaluation of thyroid

cartilage invasion has a higher specificity but lower sensitivity, whereas MRI is more sensitive but with lower specificity. The mean accuracy of CT for thyroid cartilage invasion is approximately 75 to 80%, and the mean accuracy of MRI is 80 to 85%.[3] Nishiyama and colleagues found that single photon emission computed tomography may have an accuracy approaching 90% in detecting cartilaginous invasion.[8]

Chondrification/ossification of the thyroid cartilage can be irregular; however, it is usually symmetric[9] (Figure 18). An important imaging feature associated with glottic carcinoma is

sclerosis of the arytenoid cartilage (Figure 19). When this is seen on the side of a known glottic carcinoma, it usually is indicative of tumor extension up to the perichondrium, and this finding has been shown to represent true neoplastic infiltration of the cartilage approximately 50% of the time.[10] One must also be aware, that arytenoid cartilage sclerosis can occur normally, in the absence of a carcinoma, particularly in women, in whom it is more common on the left side.[11]

Evaluation for a source of vocal cord paresis is also a common indication for imaging evaluation. If the left vocal cord is paretic, imaging should extend from the posterior fossa and skull base to just below the aortic arch to assess the entire course of the left recurrent laryngeal nerve as it travels around the aortic arch. At this location the nerve is susceptible to compression, particularly by lymphadenopathy in the aorto-pulmonic

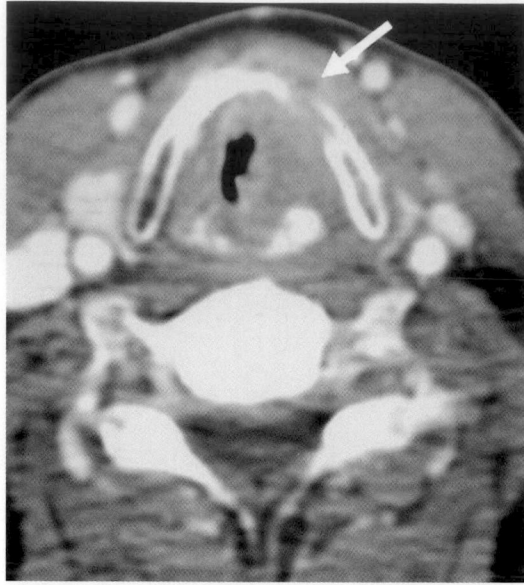

(A)

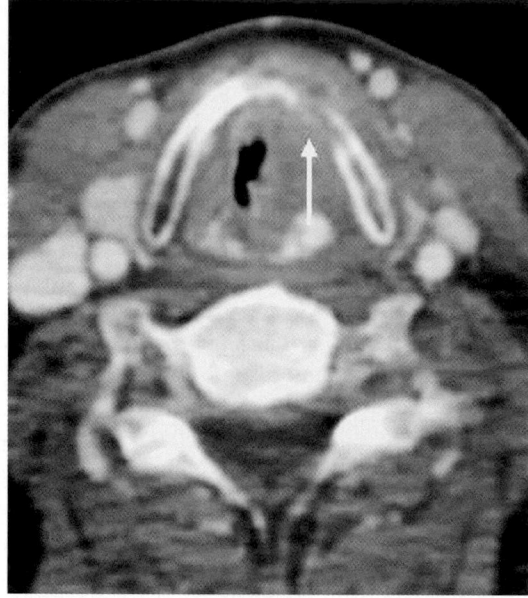

(B)

Figure 17 Axial CT with contrast (A), bone window (B). Laryngeal carcinoma with erosion of the left thyroid lamina better seen on bone window (*arrow*), with extension into the strap muscles well seen on soft tissue window (*arrow*).

window of the mediastinum (Figure 20). The inferior aspect of the right recurrent laryngeal nerve passes under the subclavian artery; and, therefore, imaging of the mediastinum is not required to evaluate the complete course of this structure. When there are other associated cranial neuropathies, a more proximal lesion is suggested. Secondary imaging findings that suggest cranial nerve dysfunction at the level of the skull base include unilateral tongue atrophy with fat infiltration (from hypoglossal nerve dysfunction) and atrophy of the sternocleidomastoid muscle (from spinal accessory nerve dysfunction) (Figure 21).

ORAL CAVITY

Lesions within the oral cavity are often small when detected on physical examination and do

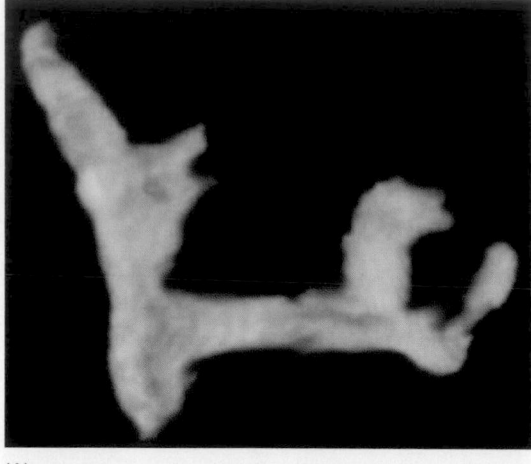

(A)

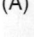

(B)

Figure 18 3D CT reconstructions of right (A) and left (B) thyroid laminae. Although there is incomplete ossification of the laminae in this 60-year-old male bilaterally, it is symmetric.

not always require imaging evaluation. However, CT and MRI play an important role in answering specific questions. These include determining the degree of submucosal extension of a lesion, particularly within the tongue, evaluating for possible invasion into the adjacent osseous structures, and detecting perineural spread of tumor. The tumor can spread along the palatine nerves into the pterygopalatine fossa to involve cranial nerve V2 or along cranial nerve V3 if there is violation of the inferior alveolar canal of the mandible or masticator space. Imaging also allows for the assessment of extension of the lesion into the sublingual or submandibular spaces.

Masses within the tongue are usually much better demonstrated on MRI. The submucosal extent of the affected side and involvement of the contralateral part of the tongue are particularly well demonstrated on coronal imaging (Figure 22). Coronal imaging is also particularly useful to evaluate for extension of a lesion or

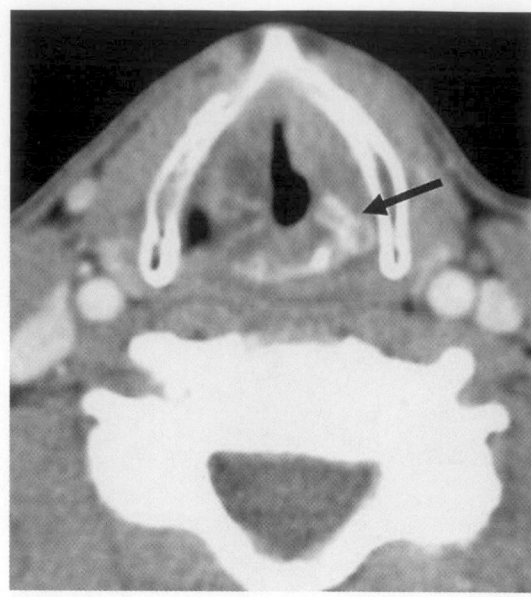

Figure 19 Axial CT with contrast. There is sclerosis of the left arytenoid cartilage (*arrow*) associated with glottic carcinoma on that side.

inflammatory process from the sublingual to the submandibular space. The mylohyoid muscle, which forms the anatomic boundary between these two spaces, is easily visible, particularly on coronal imaging or reconstructions (Figures 23 and 24). Ranulas and sublingual space infections (Ludwig angina) are relatively common lesions in this area. The distinction between ranula and

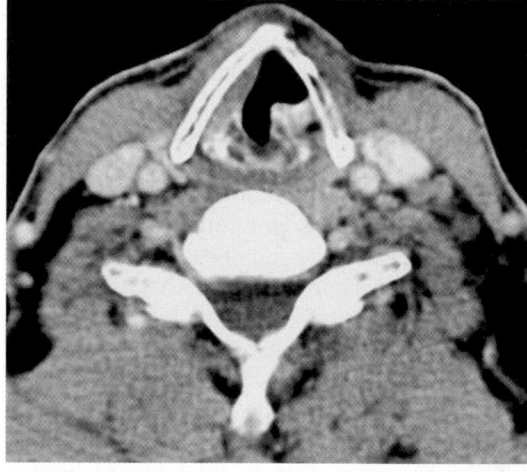

(A)

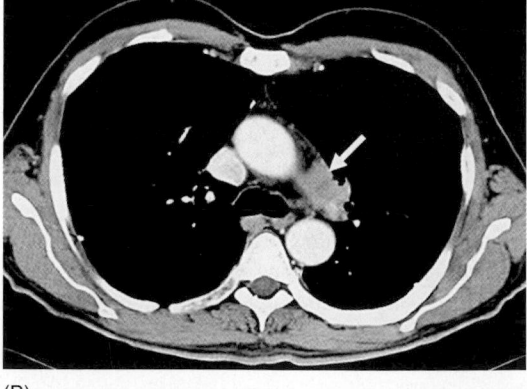

(B)

Figure 20 Axial CT with contrast. Left vocal cord paresis is identified (A) in a patient with mediastinal adenopathy at the level of the aortic arch (*arrow*) (B).

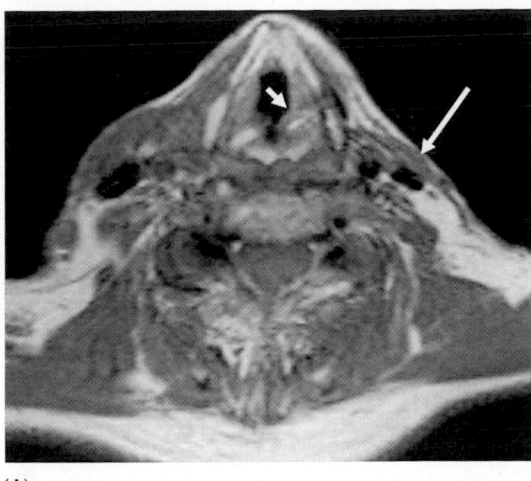

(A)

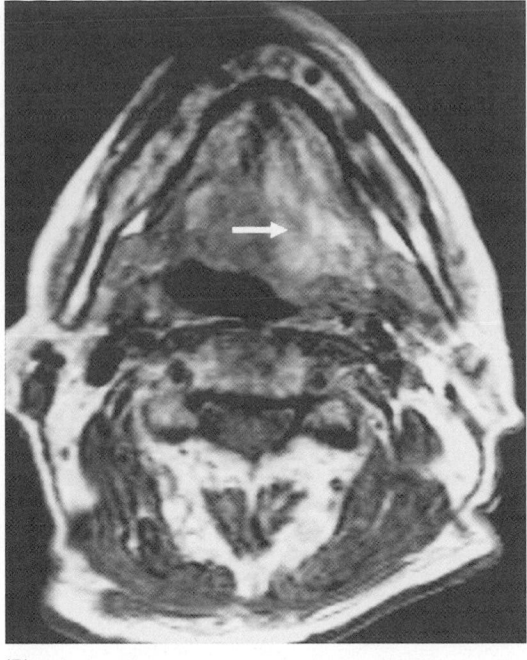

(B)

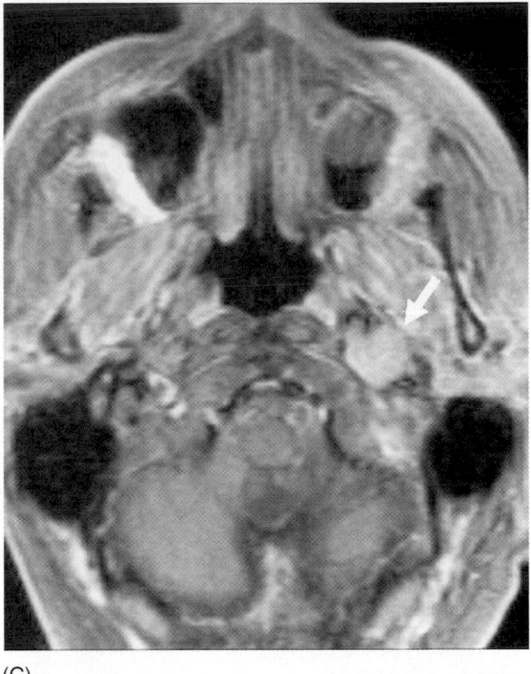

(C)

Figure 21 Axial T1-weighted MRI without contrast (A, B) and with contrast and fat-saturation (C). Left vocal cord paralysis (*short arrow*) (A) with left sternocleidomastoid muscle atrophy (*long arrow*) (A) and left tongue atrophy with fat infiltration (*arrow*) (B) suggest proximal mass with cranial nerve X, XI, and XII involvement. A hypoglossal schwannoma (*arrow*) (C) in the poststyloid parapharyngeal space is identified.

abscess or superinfection is made clinically, however, in general, radiologic clues of infection include an enhancing wall, infiltration of the surrounding fat planes with edema, and thickening of the overlying skin (Figure 25).

Identification of osseous erosion or invasion in the evaluation of malignancies is of particular importance (Figure 26). As in other areas, MR imaging is more sensitive to detection of bone invasion while CT remains more specific. Bolzoni and colleagues reported a sensitivity of 93%, specificity of 93%, and accuracy of 93% using MRI in the detection of mandibular erosion from oral or oropharyngeal SCC.[12] Imaizumi and colleagues found that CT had greater specificity (88%) compared

to MRI (54%) in detecting mandibular invasion by SCC.[13] An early study evaluating the utility of PET-CT for mandibular invasion by Babin and colleagues reported this modality to be 100% sensitive and 83% specific.[3,14]

SALIVARY GLANDS

This section will focus on some of the important imaging concepts regarding the salivary glands. Other superficial, palpable lesions will also be included as occasionally patients come to imaging to determine whether a palpable mass represents a primary salivary gland lesion, an adjacent lymph node or other superficial mass. Imaging can be helpful in characterizing the lesion

identified by the patient or on physical examination. In younger patients, palpable masses are often of cystic origin (Figure 27). These cystic masses have characteristic imaging appearances; however, they can be complicated by superimposed infections or congenital anomalies, such as residual thyroid tissue within a thyroglossal duct cyst. Masses within the superficial soft tissues or within the salivary glands are most appropriately evaluated with MRI where they can be most accurately characterized by studying their signal

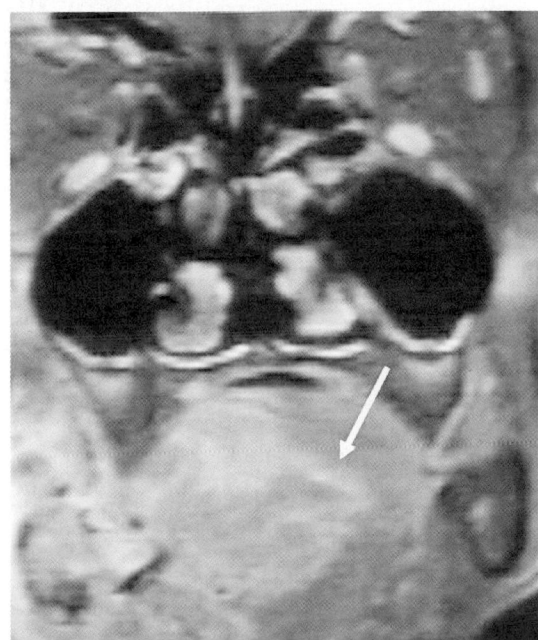

Figure 22 Coronal T1-weighted MRI with contrast and fat-saturation: squamous cell carcinoma of the tongue clearly crossing the midline (*arrow*).

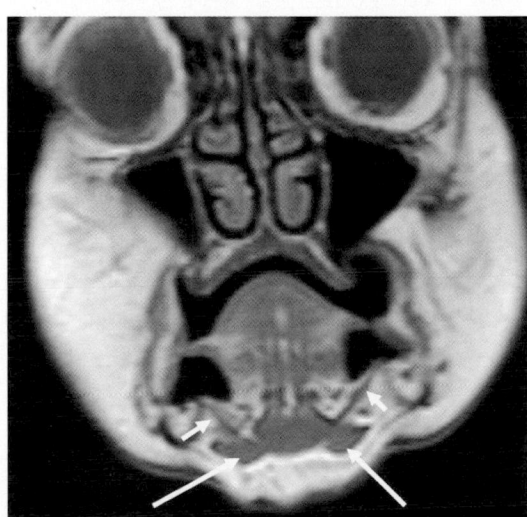

Figure 23 Coronal T1-weighted MRI without contrast. The mylohyoid muscle (*short arrows*) is clearly identified coursing between both sides of the mandible separating the sublingual from the submandibular space with the anterior belly of the digastric muscles (*long arrows*) directly beneath its inferior surface.

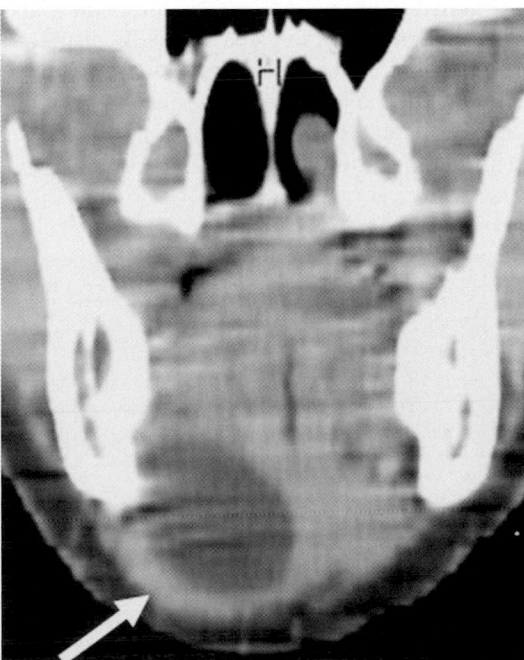

Figure 24 Coronal CT reconstruction. A dermoid within the sublingual space is identified above the mylohyoid (*arrow*) with no evidence of extension into the submandibular space. A ranula would have a similar appearance, but the lower density of this lesion is consistent with a dermoid.

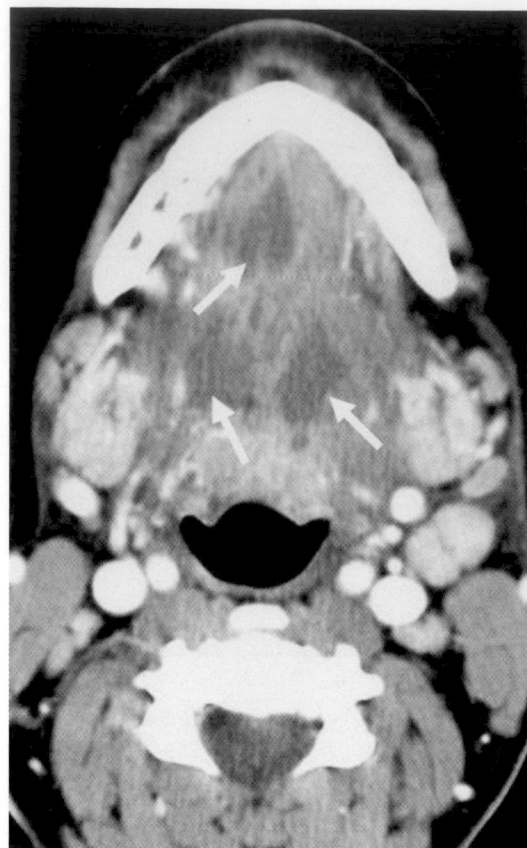

Figure 25 Axial CT with contrast. Phlegmon or early abscess formation within the sublingual space consistent with Ludwig angina.

characteristics and enhancement patterns. Infections, however, should be initially evaluated with CT imaging.

It is often difficult to discriminate lymphadenopathy from an intrinsic submandibular gland mass on physical examination alone. Imaging is extremely useful in making this distinction. Extrasalivary lesions are separated from the gland by a fat plane, and the gland is usually displaced by the lesion. Intrinsic salivary lesions are inseparable from the gland with normal salivary tissue surrounding much, if not all, of the mass. A

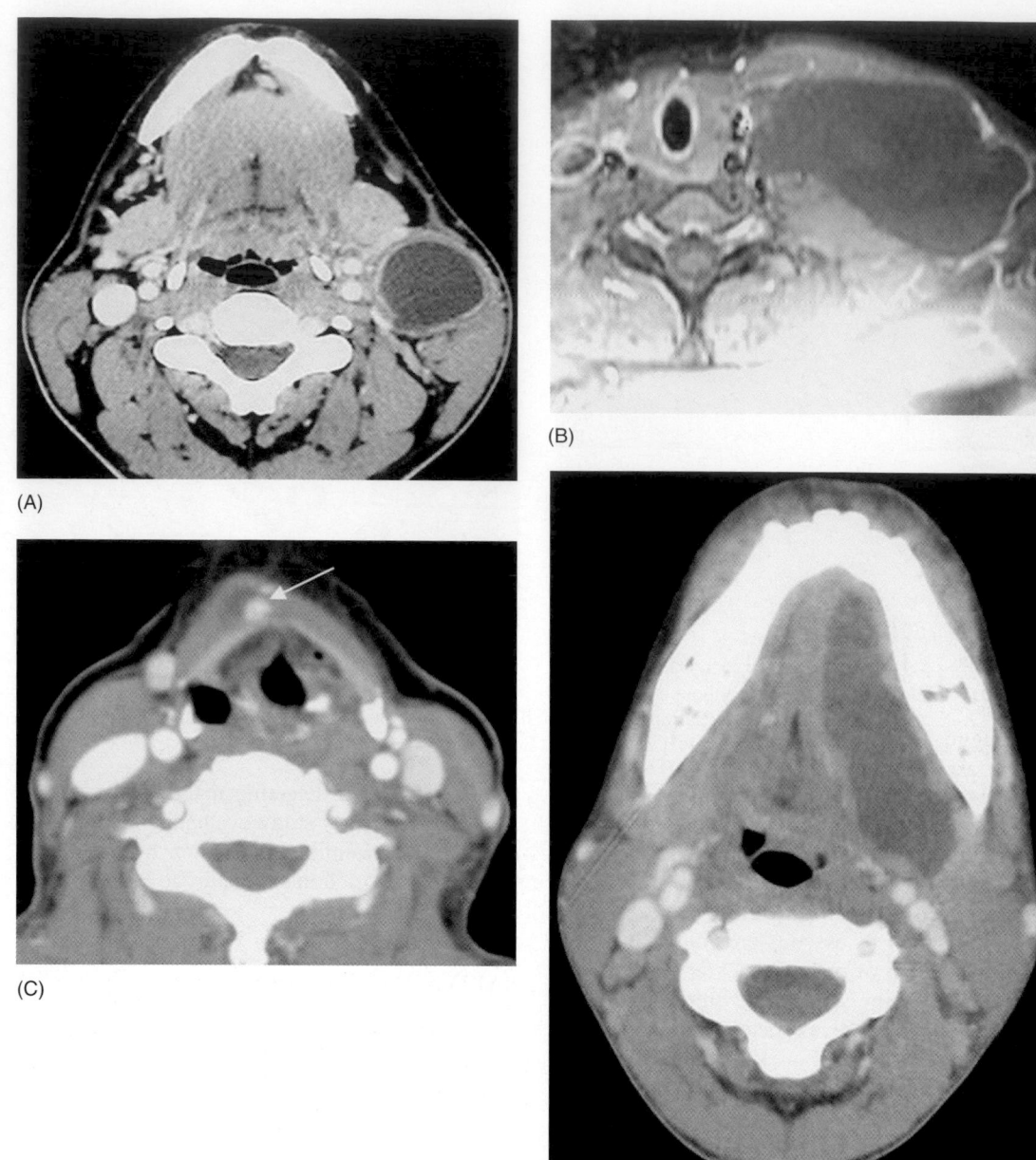

Figure 27 Axial CT with contrast (A, C, D) and axial T1-weighted with contrast and fat-saturation MRI (B). Type II branchial cleft cyst (A), cystic hygroma/lymphangioma (B), thyroglossal duct cyst with thyroid tissue (*arrow*) (C), and ranula (D).

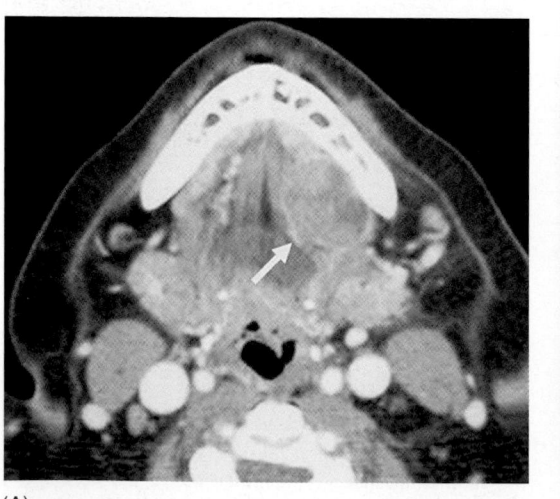

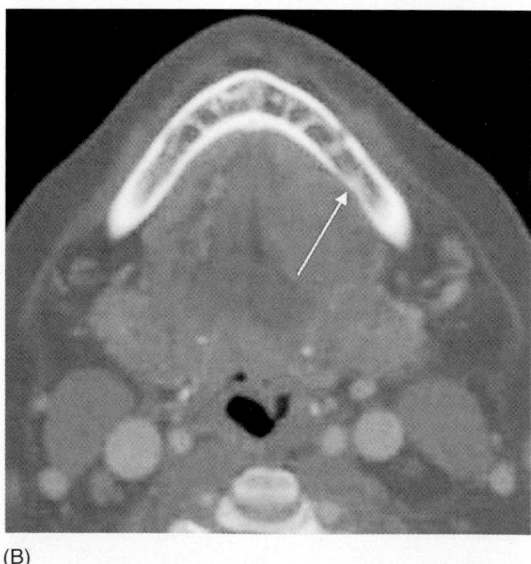

Figure 26 Axial CT with contrast (A) and bone window (B). Adenocarcinoma of the sublingual gland (*arrow*) (A) with cortical erosion of the mandible (*arrow*) (B) identified on bone window.

helpful anatomic landmark is a prominent branch of the facial vein that is consistently identified along the lateral margin of the submandibular gland. This vein will be seen coursing around an intrinsic submandibular gland mass, as it expands the gland, while the vein will often course between the gland and adjacent adenopathy (Figure 28).

While virtually all intrinsic salivary gland masses are managed with surgical resection, there are imaging findings that may suggest the diagnosis preoperatively. In general, parotid masses which demonstrate high signal intensity on T2-weighted MR images are more likely to be benign; pleomorphic adenoma is the prototypical example of this feature (Figure 29). Most primary salivary gland carcinomas such as mucoepidermoid carcinoma demonstrate lower signal intensity on T2-weighted MR images (Figure 30). Another important imaging characteristic is the definition of the lesion margin as benign masses typically demonstrate sharp, well-circumscribed

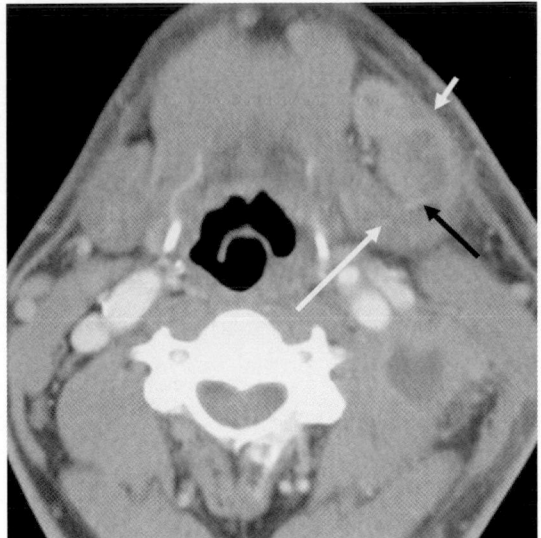

Figure 28 Axial CT with contrast. Submandibular lymphadenopathy (*short arrow*) is identified separated from the submandibular gland (*long arrow*) by a fat plane as well as a consistently identified branch of the facial vein (*black arrow*) along the lateral margin of the gland.

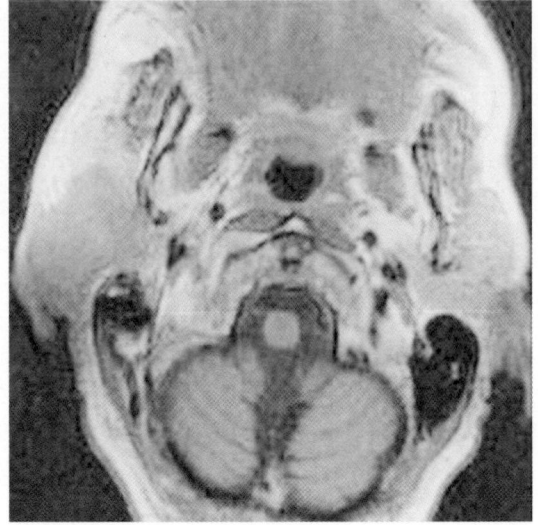

(A)

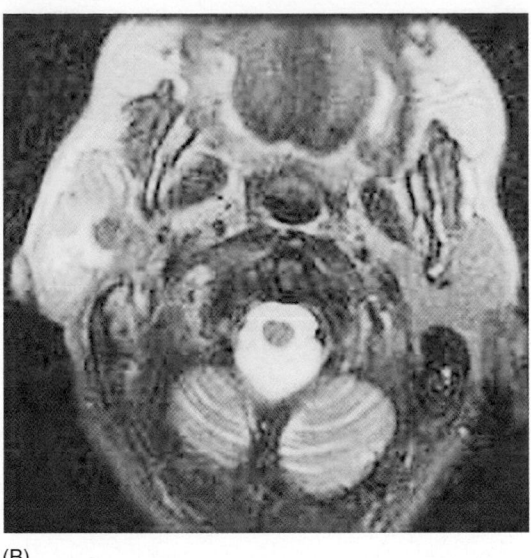

(B)

Figure 30 Axial T1-weighted (A) and T2-weighted (B) MRIs. Mucoepidermoid carcinoma of the right parotid with somewhat irregular margins and lower signal intensity on the T2-weighted image.

margins, whereas irregular, infiltrative margins suggest malignancy. When parotid gland lesions are bilateral or multiple, consideration should be given to Warthin tumors (especially in elderly males), lymphoepithelial cysts (in HIV-positive patients), metastatic or inflammatory lymphadenopathy, and Sjögren syndrome. Clinical history is essential in separating these entities. The triad of multiple bilateral parotid lesions, prominent soft tissue in the nasopharynx and lymphadenopathy is highly suggestive of HIV infection (Figure 31).

Nonpalpable superficial parotid lesions can be biopsied easily under ultrasound guidance and deep parotid lesions are amenable to biopsy with CT guidance (Figure 32). Ultrasound is also particularly useful in characterizing masses throughout the neck, with regard to determining their cystic or vascular nature and in evaluating for lymphadenopathy. In general, regarding any palpable or superficial mass throughout the neck, unless

it has unequivocal benign imaging features suggestive of a lipoma or hemangioma (Figure 33), it is managed with biopsy or complete surgical resection.

Contrast-enhanced CT is the most appropriate initial imaging study to evaluate patients with head and neck infections. CT can be used to distinguish a superficial cellulitis from a true abscess. CT is also useful in determining the source of the infection such as in secondary superficial cellulitis from sinusitis, periapical abscess formation from endodontal disease (Figure 34), or sialoadenitis secondary to sialolithiasis (Figure 35). Although MRI can be used to diagnosis an abscess, it is less useful in determining the source of infection.

Evaluation for lymphadenopathy is a major indication for neck imaging. CT is the usual modality of choice if detection of pathologic lymph nodes is the only clinical question since it is more accurate in detecting necrosis in nodes of normal size.[2] The imaging criteria for pathologic adenopathy often vary from institution to

institution.[2,15] In general, level I and jugulodigastric lymph nodes are considered to be pathologic if they are larger than 1.5 cm in long axis, and level II to VI nodes are considered to be pathologic if greater than 1 cm in long axis. Retropharyngeal and intraparotid lymph nodes should be considered pathologic at an even smaller size. Any lymph node that demonstrates central necrosis should also be considered pathologic. Other criteria that should suggest malignant infiltration until proven otherwise include groups of three or more borderline in size lymph nodes, any lymph node with calcification in a patient with papillary carcinoma of the thyroid and any lymph node in a patient with mucocutaneous malignant melanoma if it has different imaging characteristics from nodes on the contralateral side.[16]

NEW TECHNIQUES

CT and MRI techniques continue to improve, and their use in specific clinical situations

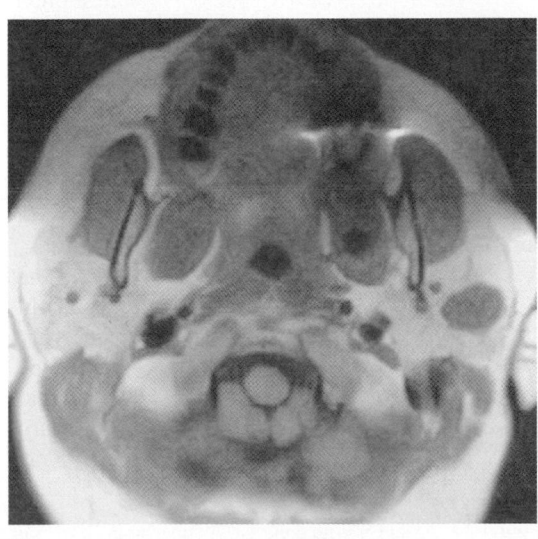

(A)

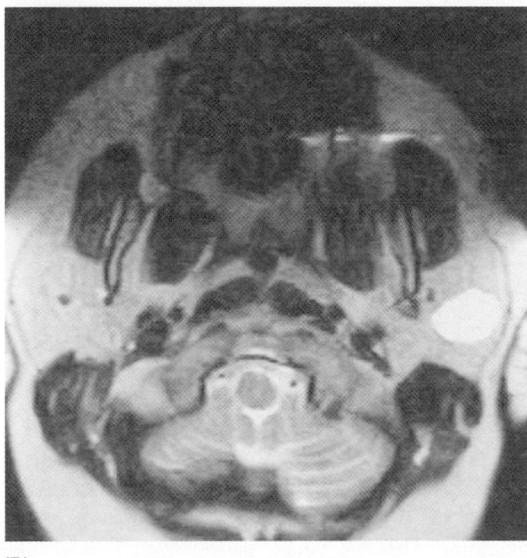

(B)

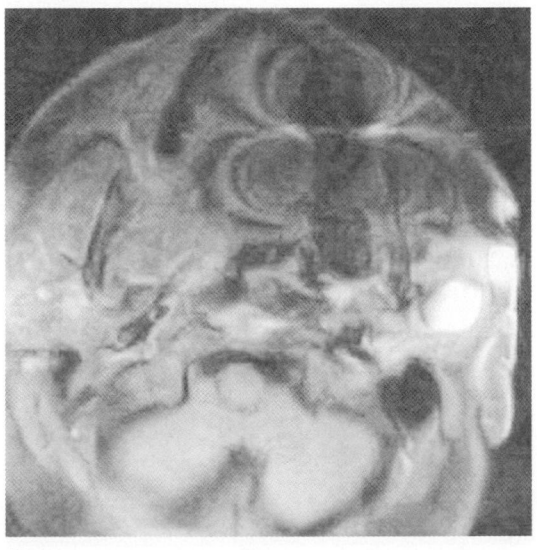

(C)

Figure 29 Axial T1-weighted (A), T2-weighted (B), and T1-weighted MRIs with contrast and fat-saturation (C). A pleomorphic adenoma is identified within the superficial left parotid that shows well-circumscribed margins and marked high signal on the T2-weighted image simulating a cyst, however, the solid nature of the lesion is confirmed by diffuse enhancement.

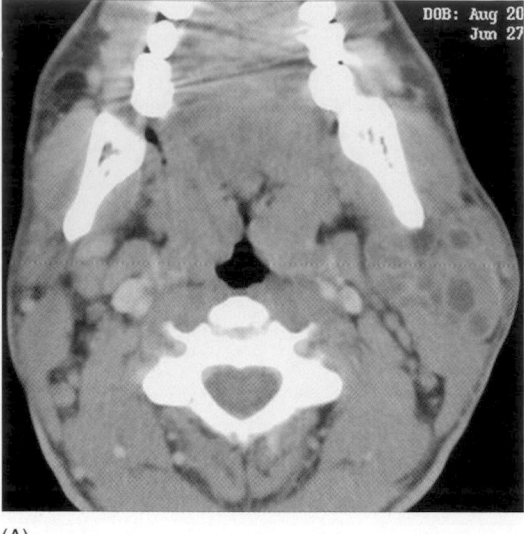

(A)

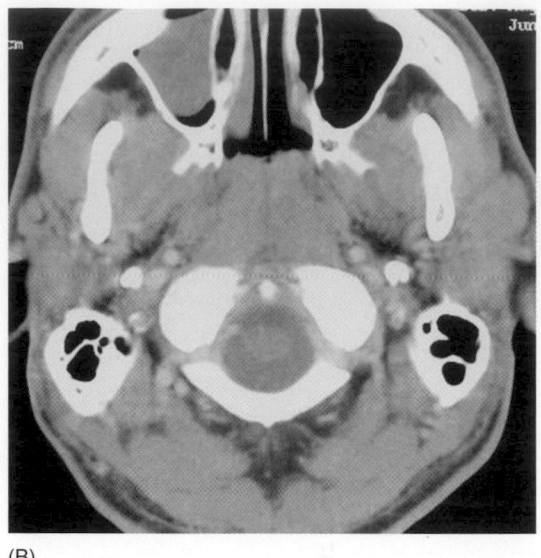

(B)

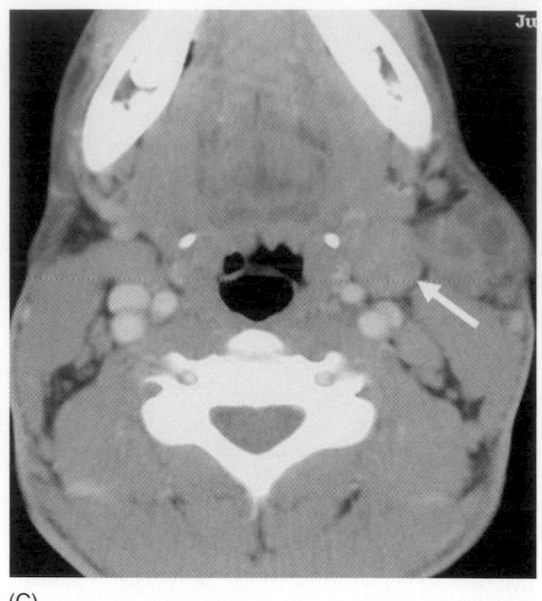

(C)

Figure 31 Axial CT with contrast. The combination of parotid cystic lesions (A) with prominent soft tissue within the nasopharynx (B) and lymphadenopathy (*arrow*) (C) is highly suggestive of HIV infection.

continues to be evaluated. As illustrated above, prior studies have evaluated the utility of these modalities in evaluating osseous erosion. In general, MRI tends to be more sensitive than CT in this application but CT findings generally have a higher specificity. CT is particularly valuable in evaluating cortical bone for invasion. With the advent of multidetector CT scanner, isotropic (volumetric) CT datasets and sub-second data acquisitions, the entire head and neck region can be scanned in seconds instead of minutes. This improved temporal resolution can be exploited to "capture" contrast in the arterial phase and provide a three-dimensional arteriographic-like image of the vascular anatomy (CT angiography). The axial "raw data" images are evaluated similar to standard neck CT images but are much more numerous and are obtained such that peak contrast enhancement is present within the

arterial lumen. Multiplanar reconstructions can be performed in any plane to visualize a segment of interest from any perspective (Figure 36). This has particular value in planning surgical resection around critical vascular structures. For example, Yousem and colleagues found a 100% positive predictive value for vascular invasion when tumor encases the carotid artery by more than 270º.[17]

The capability to obtain three-dimensional information on CT and MRI has led to the development of techniques to study tumor volumes as opposed to the traditional methods of estimating tumor size by utilizing calculations solely based on longest dimensions in three planes. Mukherji and colleagues reviewed the clinical applications and technique of this procedure, citing multiple studies that have shown how calculation of gross

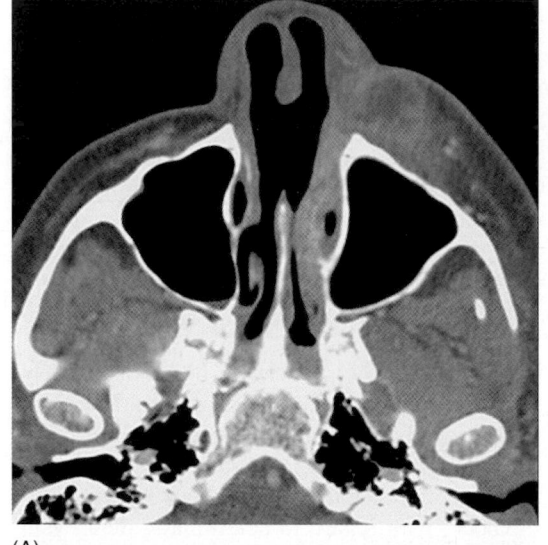

(A)

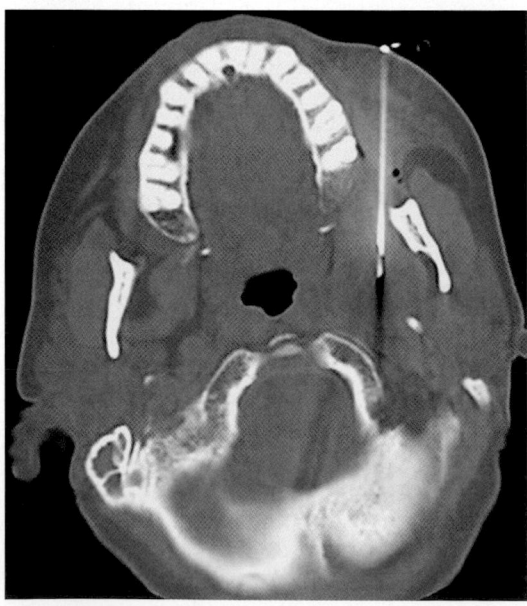

Figure 32 Axial CT bone window. CT-guided biopsy of a pleomorphic adenoma within the deep parotid utilizing coaxial technique.

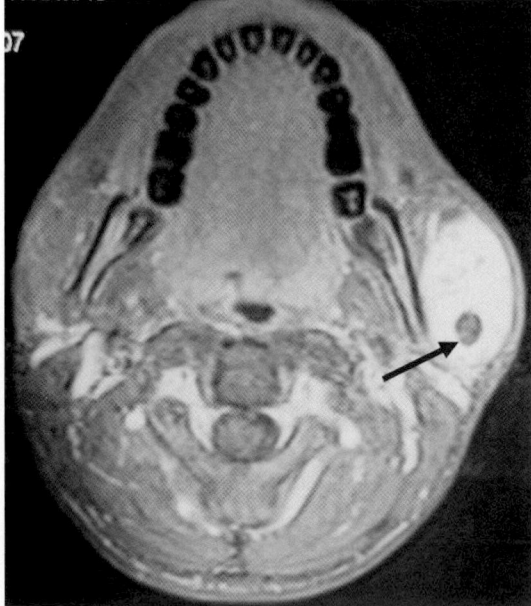

Figure 33 Axial T1-weighted with contrast and fat-saturation MRI. A young patient with a markedly enhancing lesion that extends into the parotid gland and masseter muscle. The large phlebolith (*arrow*) is highly suggestive of hemangioma.

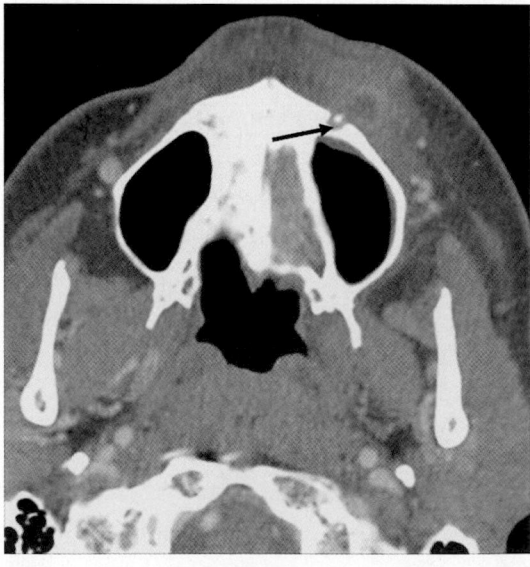

(B)

Figure 34 Axial CT with contrast. A superficial abscess is identified (A) extending from a periapical abscess within the maxilla (*arrow*) (B) with cortical breakthrough along the buccal cortex.

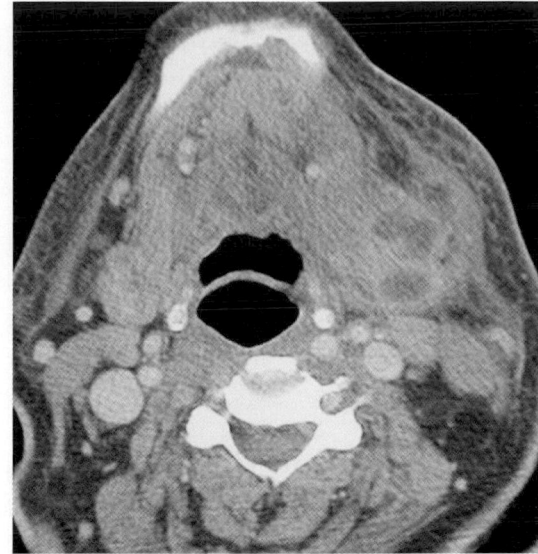

(A)

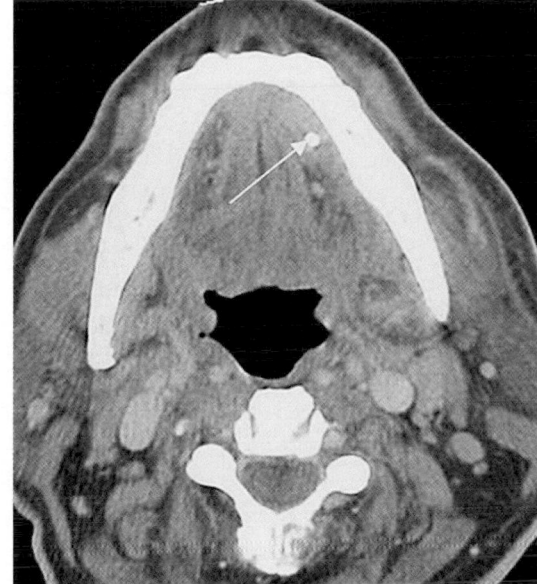

(B)

Figure 35 Axial CT with contrast. A small calculus is identified within the distal part of Wharton duct (*arrow*) (B) with associated sialoadenitis and intraglandular abscess formation (A).

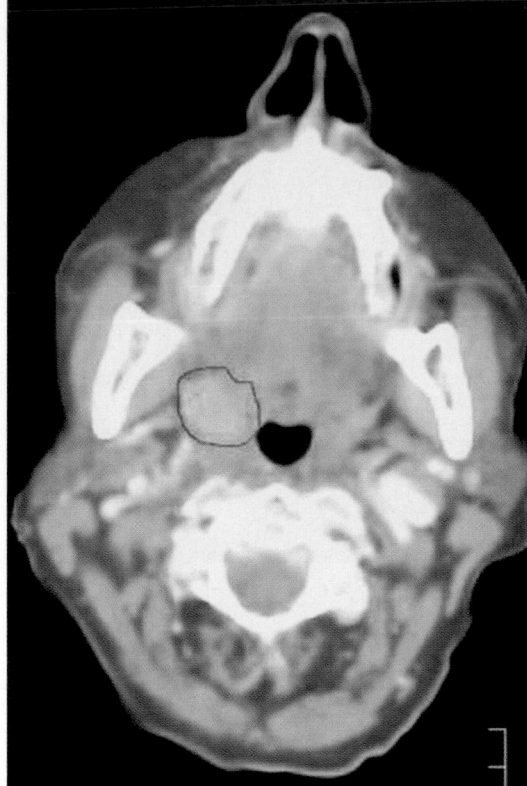

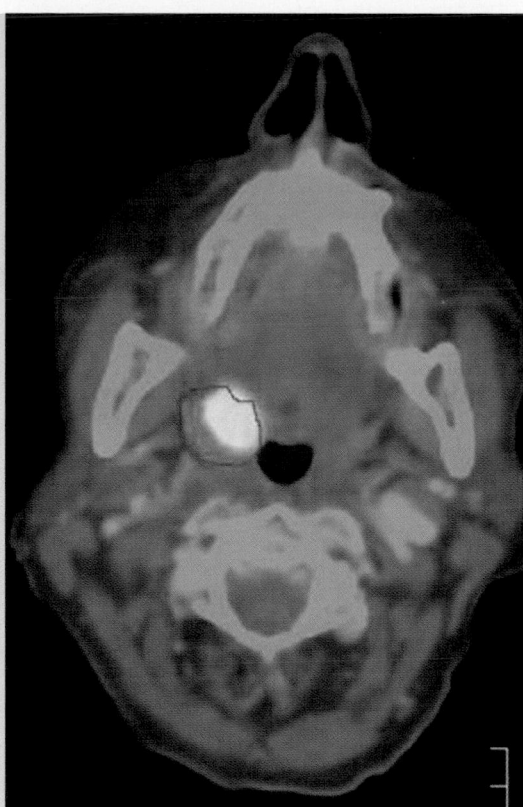

Figure 37 Axial CT with contrast (*left*), PET-CT fusion (*right*). The digitally fused image (*right*) unites the anatomic spatial resolution of CT with the physiologic information of PET in this presumed tonsillar carcinoma.

tumor volume is extremely useful in predicting local control of SCC at different head and neck subsites.[18] This information can be integrated into the treatment plan by identifying patients at higher risk of local recurrence after nonsurgical organ-preservation therapy. In addition, this technology may be proved as useful in identifying patients who may be benefited from earlier

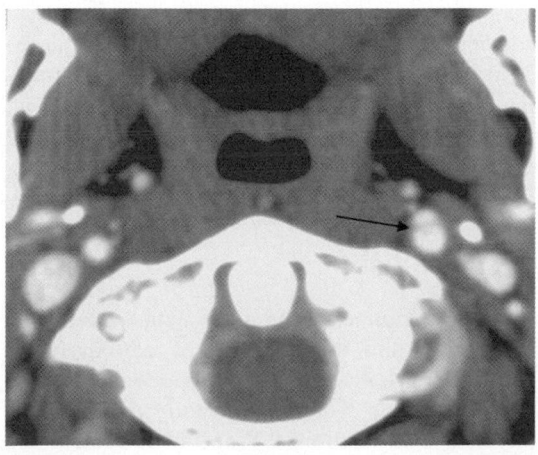

(A)

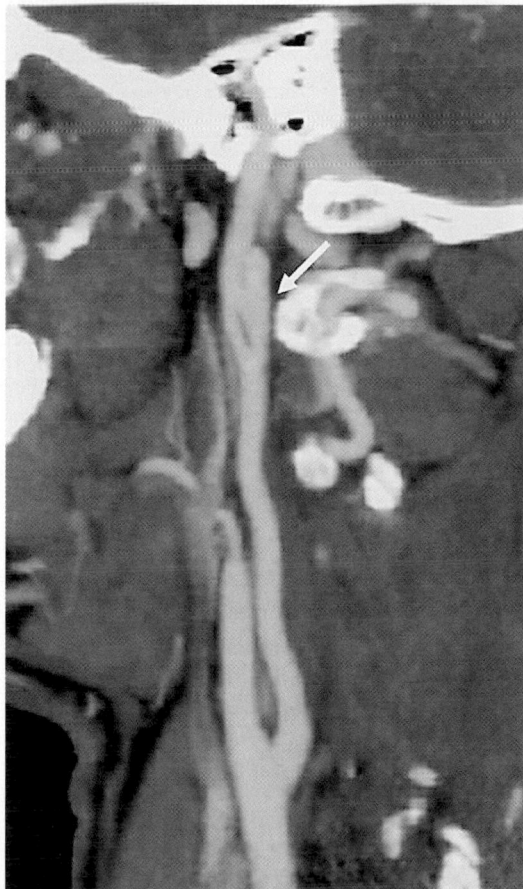

(B)

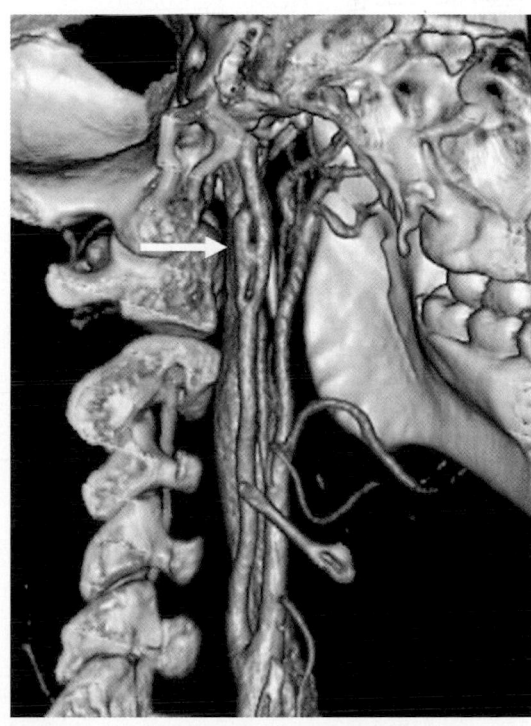

(C)

Figure 36 Axial computed tomography angiography (CTA) (A), sagittal multiplanar reconstruction (B), three-dimensional reconstruction (C). The axial image (A) demonstrates the intimal flap (arrow) within the internal carotid artery, but the full extent and morphology of the pseudoaneurysm is much better depicted on the reconstructed images (*arrows*) (B, C).

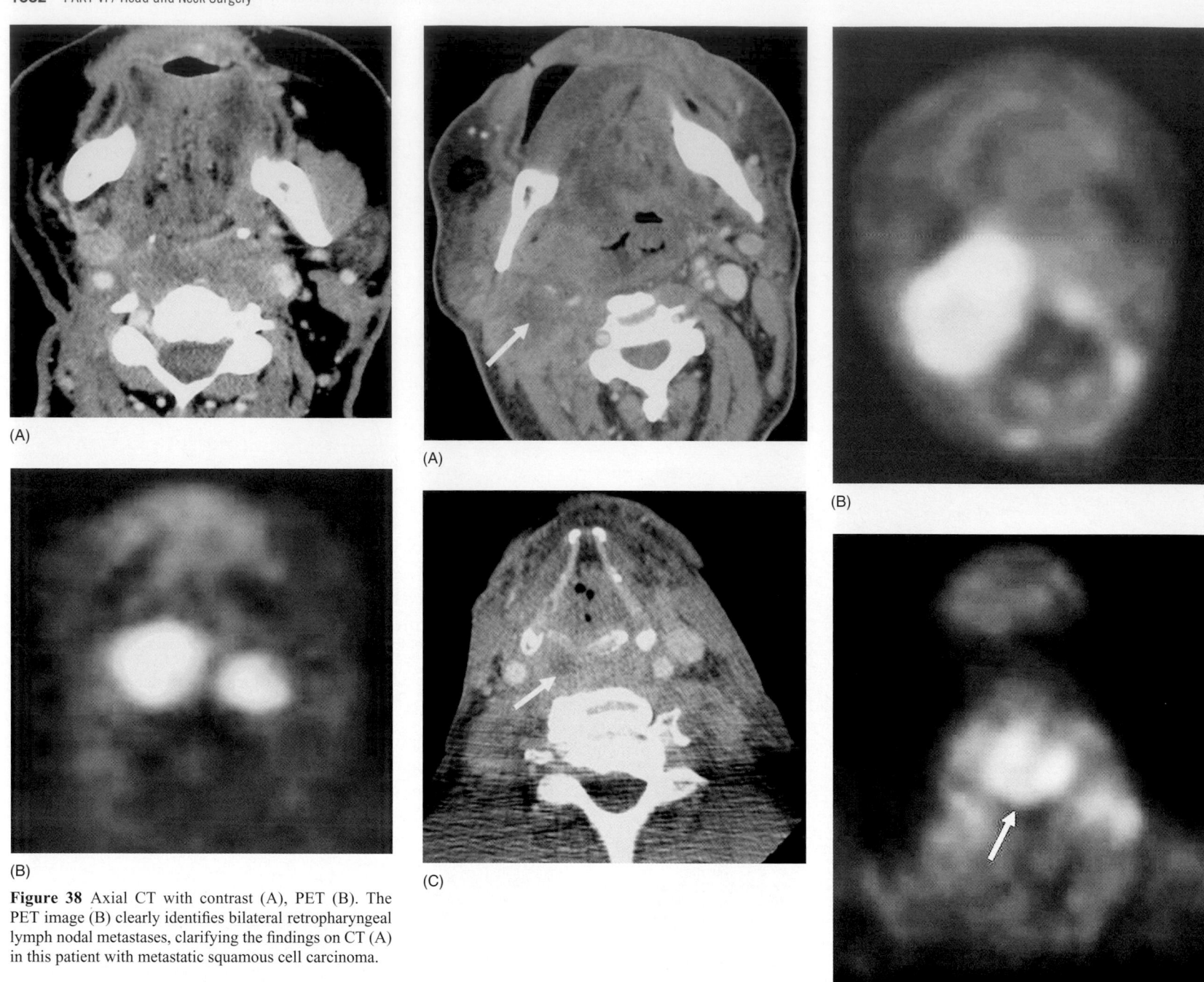

(A)

(B)

(C)

(D)

Figure 38 Axial CT with contrast (A), PET (B). The PET image (B) clearly identifies bilateral retropharyngeal lymph nodal metastases, clarifying the findings on CT (A) in this patient with metastatic squamous cell carcinoma.

Figure 39 Axial CT with contrast (A, C), PET (B, D). The necrotic lymph node is clearly demonstrated on CT (*arrow*) (A) and PET imaging (B) in this patient with metastatic hypopharyngeal squamous cell carcinoma. However, the PET study (D) also highlights the local recurrence within the postcricoid region of the hypopharynx (*arrows*) (C, D).

surveillance for recurrence, the addition of adjuvant chemotherapy or perhaps earlier surgical intervention.[18]

PET is an important imaging method for estimating the physiologic activity of a lesion. PET exploits the intrinsic radiation from a radionuclide tracer that is labeled to a compound, which is taken up in greater proportion in neoplastic tissue compared to the surrounding normal tissues. Multiple tracers are available; however, 2-fluoro-2-deoxy-D-glucose is most commonly utilized. Glucose utilization is increased in tumor cells and has been suggested to be related to the malignant potential of the lesion.[19] Moreover, protein synthesis and amino acid transport are also elevated in tumor cells. These observations have led to the evaluation of the efficacy of PET in determining the aggressiveness of a lesion and predicting long-term outcomes for patients with head and neck cancer.[19] Previously, this technique was limited by inherently low spatial resolution and poor anatomic detail. Fusion of PET and CT or MR data has greatly improved the

ability to localize anatomically areas of abnormal physiologic activity (Figure 37). PET-CT is particularly useful in detecting recurrence in the treated patient in whom postsurgical and radiation therapy changes distort the normal anatomic relationships. The combination of PET with the high-resolution spatial anatomic data provided by CT or MRI ensures improved reliability in differentiating tumor recurrence and lymphadenopathy from posttreatment scarring and inflammation (Figures 38 and 39). PET has some known inherent limitations including compromised sensitivity for neoplasms with slow growth rate, large intrinsic mucinous components, large portion that spreads superficially or large area of central necrosis.[20] Additionally, the identification of a lesion is also particularly problematic if it is

adjacent to structures of normally high 2-fluoro-2-deoxy-D-glucose uptake. Finally, as in all imaging modalities, there are technical factors that can result in poor image quality if optimization is not consistently utilized.

CONCLUSIONS

Imaging continues to be an essential tool in the evaluation and management of patients with head and neck diseases as it provides supplemental information that is not readily available on physical examination. CT and MRI remain the foundation of imaging evaluation with combined PET-CT imaging proving more and more useful in answering specific clinical questions.

REFERENCES

1. Harnsberger HR, Osborn AG. Differential diagnosis of head and neck lesions based on their space of origin. 1. The suprahyoid part of the neck. AJR 1991;157:147–54.

2. Scanlon M, Lovener LA. Head and neck I. In: Pretorius SE, Solomon JA, editors. Radiology Secrets, 2nd edition. Philadelphia, PA: Elsevier Mosby; 2006. p. 388–93.

3. Yousem DM, Gad K, Tufano RP. Resectability issues with head and neck cancer. AJNR Am J Neuroradiol 2006;27:2024–36.

4. Hsu WC, Loevner LA, Karpati R, et al. Accuracy of magnetic resonance imaging in predicting absence of fixation of head and neck cancer to the prevertebral space. Head Neck 2005;27:95–100.

5. Loevner LA, Ott IL, Yousem DM, et al. Neoplastic fixation to the prevertebral compartment by squamous cell carcinoma of the head and neck. AJR Am J Roentgenol 1998;170: 1389–94.

6. Xie CM, Liang BL, Wu PH, et al. Spiral computed tomography (CT) and magnetic resonance imaging (MRI) in assessment of the skull base encroachment in nasopharyngeal carcinoma {in Chinese}. Ai Zheng 2003;22:729–33.

7. Lovener LA, Yousem DM, Montone KT, et al. Can radiologists accurately predict preepiglottic space invasion with MR imaging? AJR Am J Roentgenol 1997;169:1681–7.

8. Nishiyama Y, Yamamoto Y, Yokoe K, et al. Superimposed dual-isotope SPECT using 99mTc-hydroxymethylene diphosphonate and 201 Tl-chloride to assess cartilage invasion in laryngohypopharyngeal cancer. Ann Nucl Med 2004;18:527–32.

9. Maiorana CR, Obuchowski AM, Strome SE, Morales RE. Evaluation of normal patterns of ossification of the thyroid cartilage by multidetector CT imaging utilizing 3D reconstructions. ASNR Proc 2006;159.

10. Munoz A, Ramos A, Ferrando J, et al. Laryngeal carcinoma: Sclerotic appearance of the cricoid and arytenoid cartilage: CT-pathologic correlation. Radiology 1993;189:433–7.

11. Schmalfuss IM, Mancuso AA, Tart RP. Arytenoid cartilage sclerosis: Normal variations and clinical significance. AJNR Am J Neuroradiol 1998;19:719–22.

12. Bolzoni A, Cappiello J, Piazza C, et al. Diagnostic accuracy of magnetic resonance imaging in the assessment of mandibular involvement in oral-oropharyngeal squamous cell carcinoma: A prospective study. Arch Otolaryngol Head Neck Surg 2004;130:837–43.

13. Imaizumi A, Yoshino N, Yamada I, et al. A potential pitfall of MR imaging for assessing mandibular invasion of squamous cell carcinoma in the oral cavity. AJNR Am J Neuroradiol 2006;27:114–22.

14. Babin E, Hamon M, Benateau H, et al. Interest of PET/CT scan fusion to assess mandible involvement in oral cavity and oropharyngeal carcinomas{in French}. Ann Otolaryngol Chir Cerivofac 2004;121:235–40.

15. Harnsberger HR. Handbook of Head and Neck Imaging, 2nd edition. St. Louis, MO: Mosby-Year Book; 1995.

16. Mafee MF. Imaging of the oral cavity, pharynx, larynx, trachea, salivary glands and neck. In: Snow JB, Ballenger JJ, editors. Ballenger's Otorhinolaryngology Head and Neck Surgery, 16th edition. Philadelphia,: BC Decker; 2002. p. 1353–91.

17. Yousem DM, Hatabu H, Hurst RW, et al. Carotid artery invasion by head and neck masses: Prediction with MR imaging. Radiology 1995;195:715–20.

18. Mukherji SK, Schmalfuss IM, Castelijns J, Mancuso AA. Clinical applications of tumor volume measurement for predicting outcome in patients with squamous cell carcinoma of the upper aerodigestive tract. AJNR Am J Neuroradiol 2004;25:1425–32.

19. Lindholm P, Lapela M, Leskinen S Minn H. PET canning of head and neck cancer. In: Mukherji SK, Castelijns JA, editors. Modern Head and Neck Radiology. Berlin: Springer-Verlag; 2000. p. 87–105.

20. Fukui MB, Blodgett TM, Snyderman CH, et al. Combined PET-CT in the head and neck: Part 2. Diagnostic uses and pitfalls of oncologic imaging. Radiographics 2005;25:913–30.

91

Targeted Therapeutic Approaches to Head and Neck Cancer

Stephen Y. Lai, MD, PhD
Jennifer R. Grandis, MD

Head and neck squamous cell carcinoma (HNSCC) accounts for more than 500,000 new cases projected annually worldwide, representing the sixth most common cancer in the developed world. In the United States, approximately 45,000 new cases will be diagnosed, and the majority will present as locoregionally advanced disease (stage III/IV).[1] Despite advances in surgery, radiation oncology, and medical oncology, overall survival for HNSCC patients has not improved in decades. An increased understanding of the molecular mechanisms governing the etiology and progression of HNSCC is providing a foundation for the development of targeted therapeutics. Targeted therapeutics are directed at known molecular targets that are relatively specific for tumor cells. Unlike standard radiation therapy and chemotherapy agents, targeted therapeutics are less likely to have systemic cytotoxic effects and are predicted to have minimal associated toxicities. The relative ease of access to the mucosa of the head and neck region also permits direct delivery of therapeutic agents.

A RATIONAL APPROACH TO MOLECULAR TARGETING

Specific pathways relevant to the development or progression of HNSCC serve as the basis for identifying relevant therapeutic targets. These targets include growth factor receptors, intracellular signal transduction molecules, nuclear transcription factors, and other related proteins. The challenge in molecular therapy involves distinguishing those proteins that are differentially expressed in HNSCC cells as compared to their normal counterparts. A number of criteria distinguishes specific cellular proteins for therapeutic targeting:

1. *Increased expression/activity of the therapeutic target:* Growth factor/cytokine receptor subunits or intracellular signaling molecules that have increased expression and/or activity within cancer cells may represent potential targets. The higher level of expression in cancer cells, as compared to normal tissues, provides improved selectivity of the therapeutic molecule for the tumor.
2. *Poor clinical outcome associated with the therapeutic target:* Expression or overexpression of the therapeutic targets is usually associated with tumors that have poor clinical outcome. This finding supports the contribution of a specific signaling pathway/target in tumor progression.
3. *Preclinical inhibitor studies demonstrate antitumor effects:* Preclinical studies of small molecular inhibitors against a particular target should demonstrate antitumor effects, such as decreased proliferation and/or increased apoptosis. Typically, these antitumor effects are associated with downregulation of the target molecule.

Preclinical and Clinical Studies

Upon identification of a potential targeted therapeutic agent, rigorous preclinical and clinical studies must be performed before a novel drug becomes a valid treatment option. Initial studies are performed in vitro, usually with cell lines derived from tumors. Investigators of HNSCC are fortunate as there are a vast number of cell lines available for preclinical studies.[2] In vitro studies examine the ability of a particular agent to inhibit tumor proliferation or to promote programmed cell death (apoptosis). These studies also demonstrate the sensitivity of tumor cells to the agent and determine whether antitumor effects are evoked at reasonably low concentrations. The selectivity or therapeutic index of a particular agent is determined by comparing its effects on tumor and normal cells. Additionally, these studies may explore the molecular mechanisms of an agent by measuring the expression and activity of signaling proteins related to the targeted molecule.

If a candidate agent demonstrates sufficient antitumor activity, preclinical testing moves forward to animal studies. In HNSCC, the model system involves human cancer cells grown in mouse hosts. Human xenograft tumors within immunocompromised mice are treated with a candidate agent, and the antitumor effects are measured. These studies often assess the ability of an agent to prevent tumor initiation or inhibit tumor growth. These studies are less than ideal as the behavior of human tumor cells within a mouse host does not always replicate tumor behavior within humans. Additionally, toxic side effects of a drug in humans may often not be detected in a mouse model. Nevertheless, this model represents the best experimental system that is currently available. An agent that has demonstrated antitumor effects in both cell lines and animal models without significant toxic effects may be promoted for testing in humans.

The evaluation of a potential therapeutic agent in humans involves three separate levels or phases. Phase I clinical trials are designed to assess the safety of a particular agent. A candidate agent is given to a small number of patients at various doses, including the presumed therapeutic dose, to evaluate toxic side effects. Dosage usually begins at a low level that is typically determined by any information available from animal studies. In a series of patients, dose levels are increased incrementally until the drug begins to induce unacceptable toxicities. Thus, a therapeutic window and maximum tolerated dose (MTD) are determined through dose escalation to guide further testing. With an acceptably low toxicity profile, a candidate agent will move to a phase II trial with a larger number of patients. Phase II trials continue not only to monitor treatment toxicities but also assess treatment efficacy. If a candidate agent demonstrates efficacy against certain types of cancer in a phase II trial, a phase III trial may be undertaken. A phase III trial typically involves many more patients than phase I or II trial and compares a treatment with a novel agent with standard treatment. These studies need to be carefully designed and conducted to determine if the measured clinical responses are statistically significant. The licensing of a candidate agent for a specific disease indication by the United States Food and Drug Administration (FDA) usually depends upon the demonstration of a therapeutic benefit that is greater than the existing standard of care.

Imatinib: A Molecular Targeting Therapy Success Story

The development of imatinib (STI-571; Gleevac) for the treatment of chronic myeloid leukemia (CML) demonstrates successful development of a targeted therapy.[3,4] CML is caused by reciprocal translocation of chromosomes 9 and 22, resulting in the formation of the constitutively active tyrosine kinase BCR-ABL. This chromosomal defect is present in more than 95% of CML patients. Imatinib was identified as a low-molecular weight antagonist of BCR-ABL that targeted the catalytic cleft of the BCR-ABL tyrosine kinase. By 1996, imatinib was found to inhibit the growth of CML cells in vitro while not affecting normal bone marrow cells. Initial clinical trials began in 1998 and demonstrated disease remissions in all of the 31 treated patients with CML. Within 4 years, 6,000 patients had been enrolled in imatinib clinical trials, and imatinib was approved by the FDA in 2002 as first-line treatment for CML. Imatinib is a shining example of rational drug design which has dramatically altered the treatment of patients with CML and represents a vastly superior alternative to any other available treatment regimen.

HEAD AND NECK SQUAMOUS CELL CARCINOMA THERAPEUTIC TARGETS

Overview

While there has not been a success story as dramatic as imatinib in the treatment of HNSCC, a number of approaches to identifying targeted therapeutic agents may significantly improve our current ability to treat HNSCC patients. This chapter will focus on a number of developing strategies that target different facets of HNSCC disease progression (Table 1). The epidermal growth factor receptor (EGFR) has emerged as an attractive therapeutic target in HNSCC and other cancers. A number of different approaches have been directed at the inhibition of EGFR ligand-binding and tyrosine kinase activity. Some progress has been made in the development of targeted therapeutics directed at EGFR in HNSCC. In 2006, FDA approval of cetux-

imab for HNSCC treatment represented the first new agent for this disease in nearly one-half century.

Although the development of approaches to other molecular targets may not be similarly advanced, they hold tremendous promise for improvements in the treatment of HNSCC patients. EGFR-associated signaling molecules, for example, Src or signal transduction and activator of transcription factor 3 (STAT3), have been targeted in preclinical models. G-protein–coupled receptors (GPCR), such as the bradykinin receptor, also appear to be an important target as they can activate EGFR and its signaling pathways in HNSCC. As HNSCC tumors rapidly increase in size, they must adapt to an environment low in oxygen and nutrients. Tumors initiate blood vessel formation (angiogenesis) and receive more oxygen and nutrients. Interference of vascular endothelial growth factor receptor (VEGFR) signaling that promotes angiogenesis is under active investigation. Additionally, the hypoxic environment itself may represent an effective means of selectively targeting HNSCC cells. Finally, p53 is the most commonly mutated gene in human cancer and frequently mutated in HNSCC.[5,6] Attempts to target p53-mutant HNSCC cells are under active investigation.

Epidermal Growth Factor Receptor

The human epidermal receptor (HER) family consists of four closely related transmembrane receptors: HER-1/EGFR, HER-2, HER-3, and HER-4. These receptors are structurally similar, but unique characteristics determine ligand-binding specificity and signaling properties.[7] Activation of the EGFR signaling complex occurs with oligomerization of the various receptor subunits. The specific signaling complex that is assembled depends upon the activating ligand

and the relative expression of the different HER family receptor subunits on the cell surface.

EGFR is a widely expressed 170 kDa protein composed of 1,186 amino acid residues and approximately 40 kDa of N-linked oligosaccharide. The receptor subunit consists of an extracellular ligand-binding domain, a transmembrane domain, an intracellular tyrosine kinase domain and additional receptor regulatory motifs and critical tyrosine residues within the cytoplasmic tail.[7] Binding of ligand by the extracellular portion of the receptor results in receptor oligomerization, activation of the receptor tyrosine kinase and autophosphorylation of several C-terminal tyrosine residues (Figure 1). These phosphorylated tyrosine residues serve as docking sites for cytoplasmic signal transduction molecules. Signaling pathways activated by EGFR include the Ras/mitogen-activated protein kinase (MAPK) and phosphatidylinositol-3 kinase (PI3K) pathways. Other important signaling molecules that interact with EGFR include Src kinase and STAT factors, including STAT3 and STAT5. Activation of these signaling pathways leads to cell proliferation, differentiation, alterations in cell adhesion and migration, enhanced survival and differentiation.

Different members of the HER family of receptors are known to be upregulated in a variety of different tumor types.[8] EGFR is commonly overexpressed in HNSCC and increasing levels of expressing of EGFR and the ligand, transforming growth factor-alpha (TGF-α), are associated with worse patient prognosis and disease recurrence.[9,10] Overexpression of EGFR appears to be a relatively early event as expression levels increase with the increasing severity of dysplasia in premalignant lesions.[11] Furthermore, EGFR-dependent signaling pathways are activated in HNSCC and drive cellular functions critical for HNSCC disease progression, including proliferation and antiapoptosis. These findings demonstrate a significant role for EGFR in HNSCC pathogenesis that is similar to the role of EGFR in colorectal and nonsmall cell lung cancer.[12] The critical role of EGFR in cancer was solidified when the oncogene v-erbB was identified as a truncated form of EGFR.[13] Mendelsohn and colleagues proposed EGFR blockade to inhibit tumor growth.[14,15]

Preclinical studies soon demonstrated that monoclonal antibodies against EGFR could enhance the effects of standard chemotherapy in preclinical tumor models.[16] Additionally, these inhibitors also had radiosensitizing effects.[17] Several strategies have been developed to interfere with EGFR activity. Selective compounds were developed that targeted EGFR either through blockade of the extracellular ligand-binding region of EGFR or inhibition of the intracellular tyrosine kinase domain. Conjugated toxins that target EGFR are in preclinical development. Additionally, gene therapy strategies are being evaluated to decrease the expression of EGFR in HNSCC cells. These approaches, related compounds and their clinical status are described below.

Table 1 Therapeutic Targets in Head and Neck Squamous Cell Carcinoma

General Target	Specific Target	Type of Agent	Example(s)
Growth factor receptors	EGFR	Monoclonal antibody	Cetuximab
			Nimotuzumab
			Matazumab
			Panitumumab
			806 (anti-EGFRvIII)
		Tyrosine kinase inhibitor	Erlotinib
			Genfitinib
			EKB-659
			CI-1033
			Lapatinib (EGFR + HER2)
			Vanitinib (EGFR + VEGFR2)
		Toxin conjugates	*Diphtheria*
			Pseudomonas
		Gene therapy	EGFR antisense
	GPCR	Small molecule	CU201
	VEGFR	Gene therapy	VEGF antisense
		Monoclonal antibody	Bevacizumab
Signal transduction molecules	Src	Small molecule	Dasatinib
	STAT3	Antisense oligonucleotide	
		Binding site decoy	
Cell cycle regulator	p53	Adenovirus	ONYX-015
Hypoxia		Small molecule	Tirapazmine (TPZ)

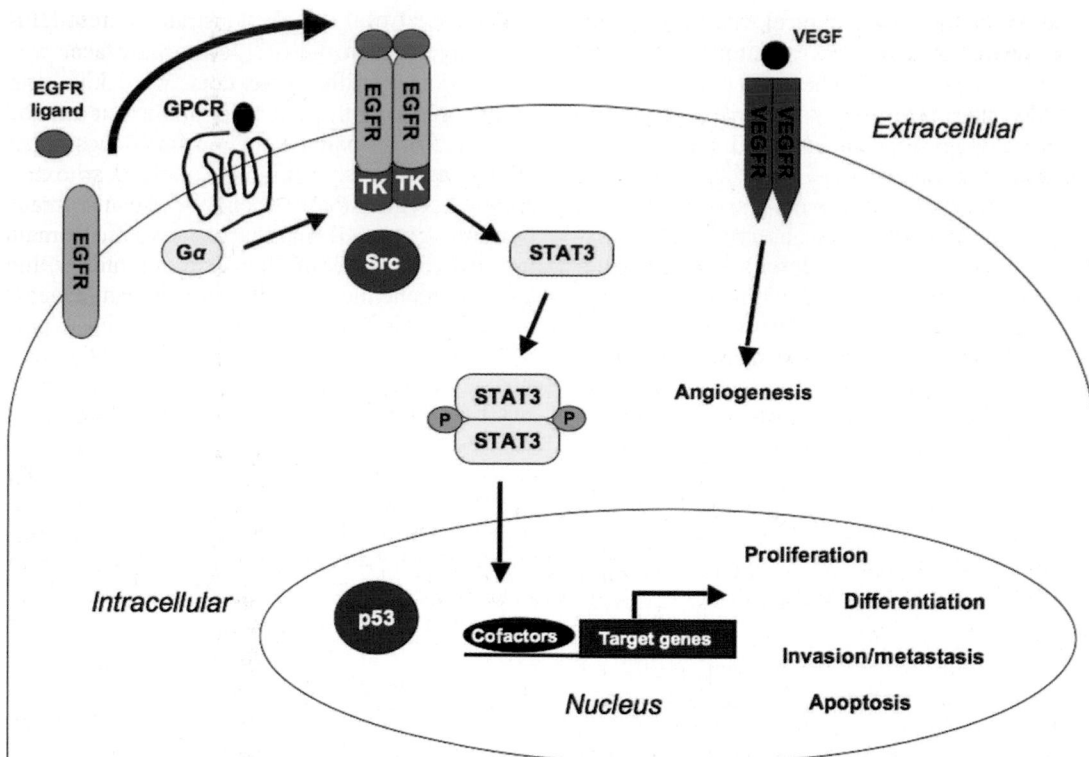

Figure 1 Therapeutic targets in head and neck squamous cell carcinoma (HNSCC). The schematic illustration highlights growth factor receptors and their associated downstream signaling molecules that are potential targets for molecular therapy. The epidermal growth factor receptor (EGFR) can be activated by its ligand, for example, transforming growth factor-alpha (TGF-α), or by transactivation via a G-protein–coupled receptor (GPCR). The vascular endothelial growth factor receptor (VEGFR) is critical for tumor angiogenesis. Novel therapeutic agents are being investigated for intracellular signaling molecules, including Src kinase and the transcription factors, p53 and signal transduction and activator transcription factor 3 (STAT3), which are important in HNSCC disease progression.

Antibodies: Targeting the Epidermal Growth Factor Receptor Extracellular Ligand-Binding Region

A number of anti-EGFR monoclonal antibodies are in clinical trials for a variety of human epithelial malignancies, including HNSCC (see Table 1). These antibodies have a number of potentially important differences, including their structure and target EGFR epitope. These differences may influence their efficacy and toxicity.

Cetuximab. Cetuximab (Erbitux; IMC-225) is a chimeric monoclonal antibody that is approximately 65% human (35% murine). Cetuximab targets the extracellular domain of EGFR to prevent binding by its natural ligands.[18,19] In preclinical studies, cetuximab demonstrated enhanced cytotoxicity with a number of chemotherapy agents, for example, cisplatin and doxorubicin, and radiation.[20] Several phase II and III trials with patients with HNSCC have demonstrated the efficacy of cetuximab in combination with chemotherapy or radiotherapy.[21] In a phase III trial, Burtness and colleagues treated 117 patients with either cetuximab/cisplatin or placebo/cisplatin. There was no significant difference in overall or progression-free survival, but objective response was higher in the cetuximab/cisplatin group ($p = .03$).[22]

Originally developed for colon carcinoma, cetuximab was approved by the FDA for the treatment of unresectable HNSCC in combination with radiation therapy and as a monotherapy for the treatment of platinum-based therapy-resistant HNSCC. A critical phase III study by Bonner and colleagues demonstrated the effectiveness of cetuximab in combination with radiation therapy.[23] In this multicenter, international trial, 424 patients with stage III/IV HNSCC without prior chemotherapy exposure were randomized for treatment with cetuximab and radiation therapy or radiation therapy alone. Tumor sites were oropharynx (60%), larynx (25%), and hypopharynx (15%). Patients with oral cavity and nasopharyngeal tumors were not enrolled. These investigators demonstrated a statistically significant improvement in the median duration of locoregional control from 14.9 to 24.4 months ($p = .005$). Three-year survival was similar increased from 44% with radiation therapy alone to 57% with the addition of cetuximab ($p = .02$). Except for grade 3/4 skin reactions, the incidence of toxicity did not increase with the addition of cetuximab. Although cetuximab and radiation therapy is more effective than radiation therapy alone, assessment of radiation therapy/cetuximab versus concurrent chemoradiation still needs to be performed. Additionally, perhaps the addition of cetuximab to concurrent chemotherapy may prove to be more effective than currently available treatment regimens. Clinical trials to address these issues are currently in progress.

Other Epidermal Growth Factor Receptor Antibodies. Nimotuzumab (h-R3; TheraXIM) is a humanized monoclonal antibody that has an order of magnitude lower affinity for EGFR ($KD = 10^{-9}$ M) as compared to other anti-EGFR antibodies. In a phase I/II trial combining nimotuzumab with radiation therapy for patients with locally advanced HNSCC, patients tolerated combination treatment without suffering skin toxicities.[24] Survival was best at higher antibody dose levels, and further clinical exploration is continuing.

Matazumab (EMD7200) is an anti-EGFR antibody adapted to recognize human EGFR with potent cell-mediated cytotoxicity against HNSCC in vitro.[25] A phase I study demonstrated partial response to matazumab in 5 of 22 patients with diverse malignancies, including 2 of 4 patients with HNSCC. Responding patients were treated for up to 18 months without cumulative toxicity.[26]

Panitumumab (rHuMAb-EGFr) is a fully human anti-EGFR antibody. Without any mouse immunoglobulin domains present, panitumumab may be less likely to elicit host responses leading to infusional allergic reactions. Clinical studies in colorectal cancer have demonstrated significant activity of panitumumab as a single agent with increased progression-free survival.[27] Current studies are underway to determine if the addition of panitumumab to standard first-line therapy for metastatic colorectal cancer will improve progression-free and overall survival of these patients. Unlike cetuximab, matazumab, and nimotuzumab which are based on a human IgG_1 framework, panitumumab is constructed on an IgG_2 framework. Classically, the IgG_1 isotype mediates antibody-dependent cell-mediated cytotoxicity (ADCC) by natural killer (NK) cells and macrophages. Thus, the ability of panitumumab to mediate this potentially important immune function is under current investigation. Phase I clinical trials of panitumumab in combination with chemoradiation therapy in patients with HNSCC are underway.

The chimeric monoclonal antibody 806 targets the EGFRvIII mutant (del2-7).[28] Additionally, 806 binds the amplified wild-type EGFR in tumor cells but not in normal tissue.[29] In preclinical studies, antibody 806 was reactive with a high proportion of differentiated epithelial cancers of the lung and HNSCC.[30] Phase I trials are currently in progress.[31]

Tyrosine Kinase Inhibitors

Small molecule inhibitors of the intracellular tyrosine kinase domain of EGFR are also under clinical evaluation (see Table 1). These inhibitors competitively inhibit adenosine triphosphate (ATP) binding to EGFR, preventing autophosphorylation.[31] The currently available tyrosine kinase inhibitors (TKIs) are 4-anilinoquinazolines, 4-[ar(alk)ylamino]pyridopyrimidines, and 4-phenylaminopyrrolo-pyrimidines. Two oral agents that have shown promising antitumor effects are erlotinib (OSI-774; Tarceva) and gefitinib (ZD1839; Iressa).

Erlotinib. Erlotinib is a quinazoline derivative that reversibly inhibits the EGFR tyrosine kinase by targeting the ATP-binding pocket. Preclinical studies demonstrated inhibition of tumor growth through cell cycle arrest and apoptosis.[32]

A phase III trial demonstrated the additional of erlotinib with gemcitabine significantly improved survival rates in patients with advanced pancreatic cancer.[33] A phase III trial in patients with advanced nonsmall cell lung cancer (NSCLC) demonstrated an increase in overall survival (6.7 months vs 4.7 months; $p < .001$).[34] Erlotinib was granted approval by the FDA for pancreatic cancer and second-line treatment for patients with locally advanced or metastatic NSCLC.

In patients with HNSCC, clinical trials have investigated the efficacy of erlotinib as monotherapy or in combination with chemotherapy. A phase II study of patients ($n = 115$) with advanced HNSCC demonstrated an overall response rate of 4.3% alone.[35] Disease stabilization, median overall survival, and 1-year survival rates were comparable to current palliative chemotherapy regimens. Although the response rate was lower than chemotherapy, toxicity due to erlotinib was favorable compared to conventional therapies. A more recent phase II study of erlotinib in combination with cisplatin and docetaxel demonstrated impressive interim results in patients with advanced/recurrent HNSCC.[36] In 19 patients, 16 patients demonstrated partial response and 3 patients demonstrated complete disease regression in the head and neck region. The regimen was well tolerated with only one grade 3 rash and one grade 4 febrile neutropenia.

Gefitinib. Gefitinib is an anilinoquinazoline that competes with ATP for its binding site on the intracellular domain of the receptor.[37,38] In preclinical studies, gefitinib was effective in blocking EGFR activity and suppressing the growth of cell lines overexpressing HER.[39] In 2003, the FDA granted accelerated approval of gefitinib as a third-line monotherapy for advanced NSCLC. However, two subsequent phase III trials did not demonstrate increased survival in patients with NSCLC who were treated with gefitinib in combination with two separate chemotherapy regimens.[40,41] Approximately 10% of patients with NSCLC demonstrate a rapid and dramatic clinical response to gefitinib.[42] Activating mutations near the ATP-binding pocket of the tyrosine kinase domain appear to increase kinase activity in response to EGF and increase sensitivity to inhibition by gefitinib. Unlike NSCLC, there is little evidence of activating mutations of EGFR in HNSCC.[35]

In HNSCC, gefitinib has been employed as a monotherapy and in combination with standard chemotherapy. A phase II trial in patients with HNSCC with gefitinib monotherapy demonstrated an observed response rate of 10.6% and a disease control rate of 53%.[43] In combination with docetaxel and cisplatin in patients with recurrent/metastatic HNSCC, treatment with gefitinib resulted in a 62.5% overall response and a median progression-free survival of 5.1 months.[44] Additionally, simultaneous targeting of EGFR by gefitinib in combination with cetuximab is being evaluated.[45] The clinical future of gefitinib remains uncertain, given the negative results from the NSCLC phase III trials and the accompanying pulmonary toxicity.

Within a number of clinical trials in different types of malignancies, investigators have noted an interesting correlation between clinical benefit and the intensity of the characteristic acneiform or maculopapular rash caused by anti-EGFR therapy.[46] In HNSCC, the correlation between rash intensity and improved response rates as well as survival has been observed with cetuximab,[22,23] gefitinib,[43] and erlotinib.[35] This intriguing observation requires additional confirmation and should be cautiously evaluated. Although the skin rash may be a surrogate marker for tumor response to an EGFR inhibitor, the rash may signal some other global biological factor, for example, immune status.[47]

Other Epidermal Growth Factor Receptor Tyrosine Kinase Inhibitors. A number of other TKIs are currently under investigation. EKB-569 is an irreversible inhibitor of EGFR.[48] CI-1033 targets all four EGFR family members by binding covalently to a cysteine residue near the ATP-binding site.[49] EGFR and HER2 are frequently coexpressed in HNSCC, and EGFR: HER2 heterodimers may be more potent in their signaling than EGFR homodimers.[50] Lapatinib (GW572016) is a dual inhibitor of EGFR and HER2 tyrosine kinase activity.[51] Finally, vanitinib (ZD6474) is a competitive inhibitor of EGFR and the vascular endothelial growth factor receptor 2 (VEGFR2) tyrosine kinase activities that have demonstrated antiangiogenesis activity in preclinical studies.[52]

OTHER EPIDERMAL GROWTH FACTOR RECEPTOR TARGETING STRATEGIES

Toxin Conjugates

The bacterial toxins of *Pseudomonas* or *Diphtheria* have been conjugated to EGFR-specific ligands, for example, TGF-α, or EGFR-specific monoclonal antibodies.[53,54] The ligand or the antibody binds to EGFR, resulting in the internalization of the toxic conjugate which mediates cytotoxic effects. This strategy has demonstrated antitumor effects in HNSCC cell lines and tumor xenografts,[55,56] but no clinical trials have been initiated to evaluate safety and efficacy in patients with HNSCC.

Gene Therapy

Given the increased expression of EGFR in HNSCC, efforts to decrease EGFR expression have been investigated. Antisense oligonucleotides complement a portion of the mRNA of the target protein. The single-stranded oligonucleotide binds to the mRNA, resulting in a disruption in translation and activates ribonuclease (RNase) H, resulting in the cleavage of the targeted mRNA.[57] Treatment with EGFR antisense oligonucleotides demonstrated a significant decrease in HNSCC cell growth in vitro.[58] An EGFR antisense gene was developed from the oligonucleotides and repeated intratumoral administration resulted in growth inhibition within a murine xenograft model system.[59] The authors

led a phase I trial that demonstrated that intratumoral injection of the EGFR antisense gene was safe, and no significant toxicities were noted and we are preparing these data for publication. Additionally, 5 of 17 patients demonstrated significant clinical responses, including 2 patients who had complete regression of their tumor at the injection site. A phase II trial that achieves dual targeting of EGFR by combining intratumoral EGFR antisense gene therapy with cetuximab and radiation therapy is in development.

Src FAMILY KINASE INHIBITORS

Activation of the Src family kinases appears to be important in HNSCC development and progression. Src family kinases are activated downstream of EGFR, STAT3, and STAT5.[60] Src family kinases are key intermediates in the transactivation of EGFR by G-protein–coupled receptors (GPCRs).[61] Although imatinib has dramatically altered the treatment and prognosis of patients with CML, the evidence of emerging resistance to imatinib led to the development of other potential therapies.[62,63] Dasatinib (BMS-354825) was identified as an oral agent with activity against BCR-ABL and a number of Src kinase family members, including Src, c-KIT, platelet-derived growth factor receptor (PDGFR), and ephrin A receptor kinases. Preclinical studies have demonstrated decreased invasion and increased apoptosis in HNSCC and NSCLC cell lines following dasatinib treatment.[64] A clinical trial employing cetuximab and dasatinib is currently being developed at our institution.

SIGNAL TRANSDUCER AND ACTIVATOR OF TRANSCRIPTION FACTORS

The signal transducer and activator of transcription (STAT) factors are activated upon phosphorylation by Janus kinases (JAKs) or tyrosine kinase receptors such as EGFR.[65] STATs can form homodimers or heterodimers that translocate to the nucleus to form transcription complexes. STAT3 is persistently activated in many human cancers and is critical for tumorigenesis in HNSCC.[66,67]

Strategies to target STAT3 include decreasing STAT3 levels, reducing tyrosine phosphorylation of STAT3, and interfering with STAT3 recruitment to receptor complexes and to promoter sites. AG-490 and JSI-124 (cucurbitacin I) are inhibitors that demonstrate selective inhibition of JAKs resulting in decreased STAT3 activity.[68] Introduction of antisense oligonucleotides into tumors in a mouse HNSCC xenograft model resulted in decreased STAT3 activity and increased apoptosis.[69] Another promising approach has been the use of a STAT3 decoy composed of a double-stranded oligonucleotide based upon the STAT3 response element within the c-fos promoter.[70] The STAT3 decoy successfully binds activated STAT3, inhibits proliferation and induces apoptosis.[71] The development of clinical trials is currently in progress.

G-PROTEIN–COUPLED RECEPTORS

G-protein–coupled receptors (GPCRs) are ubiquitously expressed in epithelial cells. Stimulation of HNSCC cells by GPCR ligands, such as lysophosphatidic acid (LPA) and thrombin results in activation of EGFR.[72] Additionally, stimulation of the gastrin-releasing peptide (GRP) receptor activates EGFR and modulates HNSCC growth and invasion.[73] Activation of GPCRs by prostaglandin E2 and bradykinin release EGFR ligands and transactivate EGFR through Src-mediated activation of matrix metalloproteinases.[61,74] Preclinical studies with the bradykinin antagonist CU201 demonstrated growth inhibition in HNSCC cells, and additive inhibitory effects were noted when CU201 was used in combination with erlotinib. Similar findings with CU201 have also been reported in lung cancer cells.[75]

VASCULAR ENDOTHELIAL GROWTH FACTOR RECEPTOR

The formation of new blood vessels is necessary for tumors to continue to grow and/or to metastasize. Vascular endothelial growth factor (VEGF) is crucial for vessel formation and is induced under hypoxic conditions.[76] Overexpression of VEGF within HNSCC specimens has been associated with increased recurrence and decreased survival.[77] Antisense VEGF transfection decreases VEGF secretion from HNSCC cells and decreases endothelial cell proliferation and migration, but clear antitumor effects were not demonstrated.[78,79] Preclinical data suggest a synergistic role of antiangiogenesis agents with radiation.[80] Bevacizumab, a monoclonal antibody developed to recognize human VEGF, has demonstrated potent antitumor activity in preclinical studies.[81] In a phase III study in patients with previously untreated colorectal cancer, the addition of bevacizumab to standard chemotherapy increased survival.[82] Phase I and phase II clinical trials of bevacizumab in combination with concurrent chemoradiation or with erlotinib in patients with HNSCC are currently in progress.[83] Additionally, combined targeting of EGFR and VEGFR is in progress. A phase I evaluation of erlotinib and bevacizumab in patients with HNSCC is underway as well as the evaluation of a dual EGFR/VEGFR inhibitor, AEE788.[84,85]

p53 TRANSCRIPTION FACTOR

The level and activity of the p53 transcription factor increases in response to cellular stress and DNA damage, leading to cell cycle arrest or apoptosis.[86] The loss of the tumor-suppressor p53 gene is a critical event in the genetic progression from normal mucosa to invasive cancer.[87,88] Attempts to restore the p53 gene were among the first goals of cancer gene therapy. ONYX-015 is an adenovirus lacking the E1B-55kd gene, theoretically permitting replication only in p53-deficient cells.[89] Thus, ONYX-015 should only replicate in and lyse p53-deficient cells. In a phase II trial, intratumor injection in recurrent HNSCC led to a 13% response rate as monotherapy and a 63% response rate (27% complete responses) when combined with cisplatin and 5-fluorouracil.[90,91] In the chemoprevention setting, topical application of ONYX-015 in a mouthwash has demonstrated some efficacy in the treatment of premalignant oral dysplasia.[92] Despite early success, progress has been slowed with recent questions regarding the selectivity of ONYX-015.[93] ONYX-015 has now been licensed for therapeutic use in China, but the virus is unlikely to be used as a therapeutic agent in Western countries without complete understanding of its selectivity for cancer cells.

HYPOXIA

HNSCCs that demonstrate regions of decreased oxygenation or hypoxia are associated with worse patient prognosis.[94] Poorly oxygenated tumors are less likely to respond to surgery, radiation therapy, and/or chemotherapy.[95,96] The adverse conditions within hypoxic regions of tumors may select for cells that are more resistant to standard therapy and behave more aggressively.[97] Additionally, hypoxic cells are relatively radioresistant, requiring a larger radiation dose to achieve an equivalent log-kill as cells in normal oxygen conditions.

Tirapazimine (TPZ; SR-4233) is a benzotrazine compound that exhibits differential cytotoxicity for hypoxic cells.[98] In anaerobic conditions, TPZ is reduced to form a highly reactive radical species capable of inducing DNA single- and double-strand breaks. Preclinical studies demonstrated an additive effect when TPZ was used in combination with radiation or cisplatin. TPZ has been developed to improve the efficacy of radiation and chemotherapy in HNSCC. Phase I and II trials in patients with locally advanced HNSCC employed conventional fractionated radiation therapy with cisplatin and TPZ.[99,100] The 3-year failure-free survival rate was 69% which represented an improvement over historical controls with similar advanced stage disease. These trials demonstrated acceptable toxicity profiles, and two phase III trials are currently in progress to determine whether TPZ and cisplatin-based chemoradiation therapy is superior to cisplatin-based chemoradiation therapy.[101] The initial trial enrolled 880 patients and is currently in the follow-up phase. A confirmatory trial, TFACE (tirapazamine radiation and cisplatin evaluation), has an enrollment target of 550 patients.

CONCLUSIONS AND FUTURE DIRECTIONS

Given the advances in knowledge regarding carcinogenesis and related signaling pathways, the evolution of novel therapies has begun to accelerate. Successful efforts have led to substantial improvements in treatment of diseases like CML with imatinib. Efforts are underway to identify similar agents for HNSCC. The combination of targeted therapies with standard cytotoxic treatments may improve disease response and survival for our patients. The effect of combining molecular therapies that target the same signaling pathway at different points or different signaling pathways simultaneously is unknown and will be explored. Finally, with the multitude of potential targeted agents, the development of methods for target validation and rapid estimates of efficacy are as important identifying potential targets. Both tumor and patient heterogeneity contribute to therapeutic response. As the number of potential therapeutic agents increases, specific approaches will be more effective against certain tumors. Identifying critical biomarkers that demonstrate these differences may predict the effectiveness of a particular targeted agent, leading to personalized medicine. Additionally, these biomarkers may also provide insight regarding the intensity of therapy required, thus preventing unnecessary toxicity or side effects from certain treatments.

REFERENCES

1. Jemal A, Siegel R, Ward E, et al. Cancer statistics, 2006. CA Cancer J Clin 2006;56:106–30.
2. Lin CJ, Grandis JR, Carey TE, et al. Head and neck squamous cell carcinoma cell lines: Established models and rationale for selection. Head Neck 2007;29:163–88.
3. Ren R. Mechanisms of BCR-ABL in the pathogenesis of chronic myelogenous leukaemia. Nat Rev Cancer 2005;5:172–83.
4. Sawyers CL. Making progress through molecular attacks on cancer. Cold Spring Harb Symp Quant Biol 2005;70:479–82.
5. Bartek J, Bartkova J, Vojtesek B, et al. Aberrant expression of the p53 oncoprotein is a common feature of a wide spectrum of human malignancies. Oncogene 1991;6:1699–703.
6. Koch WM, Brennan JA, Zahurak M, et al. p53 mutation and locoregional treatment failure in head and neck squamous cell carcinoma. J Natl Cancer Inst 1996;88:1580–6.
7. Kalyankrishna S, Grandis JR. Epidermal growth factor receptor biology in head and neck cancer. J Clin Oncol 2006;24:2666–72.
8. Hynes NE, Lane HA. ERBB receptors and cancer: The complexity of targeted inhibitors. Nat Rev Cancer 2005;5:341–54.
9. Rubin Grandis J, Melhem MF, Barnes EL, et al. Quantitative immunohistochemical analysis of transforming growth factor-alpha and epidermal growth factor receptor in patients with squamous cell carcinoma of the head and neck. Cancer 1996;78:1284–92.
10. Rubin Grandis J, Melhem MF, Gooding WE, et al. Levels of TGF-alpha and EGFR protein in head and neck squamous cell carcinoma and patient survival. J Natl Cancer Inst 1998;90:824–32.
11. Rubin Grandis J, Tweardy DJ, Melhem MF. Asynchronous modulation of transforming growth factor alpha and epidermal growth factor receptor protein expression in progression of premalignant lesions to head and neck squamous cell carcinoma. Clin Cancer Res 1998;4:13–20.
12. Baselga J, Arteaga CL. Critical update and emerging trends in epidermal growth factor receptor targeting in cancer. J Clin Oncol 2005;23:2445–59.
13. Downward J, Yarden Y, Mayes E, et al. Close similarity of epidermal growth factor receptor and v-erb-B oncogene protein sequences. Nature 1984;307:521–7.
14. Masui H, Kawamoto T, Sato JD, et al. Growth inhibition of human tumor cells in athymic mice by anti-epidermal growth factor receptor monoclonal antibodies. Cancer Res 1984;44:1002–7.
15. Mendelsohn J. Growth factor receptors as targets for antitumor therapy with monoclonal antibodies. Prog Allergy 1988;45:147–60.

16. Baselga J, Norton L, Masui H, et al. Antitumor effects of doxorubicin in combination with anti-epidermal growth factor receptor monoclonal antibodies. J Natl Cancer Inst 1993;85:1327–33.
17. Balaban N, Moni J, Shannon M, et al. The effect of ionizing radiation on signal transduction: Antibodies to EGF receptor sensitize A431 cells to radiation. Biochim Biophys Acta 1996;1314:147–56.
18. Goldstein NI, Prewett M, Zuklys K, et al. Biological efficacy of a chimeric antibody to the epidermal growth factor receptor in a human tumor xenograft model. Clin Cancer Res 1995;1:1311–8.
19. Herbst RS, Kim ES, Harari PM. IMC-C225, an anti-epidermal growth factor receptor monoclonal antibody, for treatment of head and neck cancer. Expert Opin Biol Ther 2001;1:719–32.
20. Bonner JA, Raisch KP, Trummell HQ, et al. Enhanced apoptosis with combination C225/radiation treatment serves as the impetus for clinical investigation in head and neck cancers. J Clin Oncol 2000;18:47S–53S.
21. Egloff AM, Grandis J. Epidermal growth factor receptor-targeted molecular therapeutics for head and neck squamous cell carcinoma. Expert Opin Ther Targets 2006;10:639–47.
22. Burtness B, Goldwasser MA, Flood W, et al. Phase III randomized trial of cisplatin plus placebo compared with cisplatin plus cetuximab in metastatic/recurrent head and neck cancer: An Eastern Cooperative Oncology Group study. J Clin Oncol 2005;23:8646–54.
23. Bonner JA, Harari PM, Giralt J, et al. Radiotherapy plus cetuximab for squamous-cell carcinoma of the head and neck. N Engl J Med 2006;354:567–78.
24. Crombet T, Osorio M, Cruz T, et al. Use of the humanized anti-epidermal growth factor receptor monoclonal antibody h-R3 in combination with radiotherapy in the treatment of locally advanced head and neck cancer patients. J Clin Oncol 2004;22:1646–54.
25. Bier H, Hoffmann T, Haas I, et al. Anti-(epidermal growth factor) receptor monoclonal antibodies for the induction of antibody-dependent cell-mediated cytotoxicity against squamous cell carcinoma lines of the head and neck. Cancer Immunol Immunother 1998;46:167–73.
26. Vanhoefer U, Tewes M, Rojo F, et al. Phase I study of the humanized antiepidermal growth factor receptor monoclonal antibody EMD72000 in patients with advanced solid tumors that express the epidermal growth factor receptor. J Clin Oncol 2004;22:175–84.
27. Wainberg Z, Hecht JR. Panitumumab in colon cancer: A review and summary of ongoing trials. Expert Opin Biol Ther 2006;6:1229–35.
28. Sok JC, Coppelli FM, Thomas SM, et al. Mutant epidermal growth factor receptor (EGFRvIII) contributes to head and neck cancer growth and resistance to EGFR targeting. Clin Cancer Res 2006;12:5064–73.
29. Panousis C, Rayzman VM, Johns TG, et al. Engineering and characterisation of chimeric monoclonal antibody 806 (ch806) for targeted immunotherapy of tumours expressing de2-7 EGFR or amplified EGFR. Br J Cancer 2005;92:1069–77.
30. Jungbluth AA, Stockert E, Huang HJ, et al. A monoclonal antibody recognizing human cancers with amplification/overexpression of the human epidermal growth factor receptor. Proc Natl Acad Sci U S A 2003;100:639–44.
31. Astsaturov I, Cohen RB, Harari P. Targeting epidermal growth factor receptor signaling in the treatment of head and neck cancer. Expert Rev Anticancer Ther 2006;6:1179–93.
32. Moyer JD, Barbacci EG, Iwata KK, et al. Induction of apoptosis and cell cycle arrest by CP-358,774, an inhibitor of epidermal growth factor receptor tyrosine kinase. Cancer Res 1997;57:4838–48.
33. Moore MJ. Brief communication: A new combination in the treatment of advanced pancreatic cancer. Semin Oncol 2005;32:5–6.
34. Shepherd FA, Rodrigues Pereira J, Ciuleanu T, et al. Erlotinib in previously treated non-small-cell lung cancer. N Engl J Med 2005;353:123–32.
35. Soulieres D, Senzer NN, Vokes EE, et al. Multicenter phase II study of erlotinib, an oral epidermal growth factor receptor tyrosine kinase inhibitor, in patients with recurrent or metastatic squamous cell cancer of the head and neck. J Clin Oncol 2004;22:77–85.
36. Kim E, Kies M, Sabichi A, et al. Phase II study of combination cisplatin, docetaxel and erlotinib in patients with metastatic/recurrent head and neck squamous cell carcinoma (HNSCC). J Clin Oncol 2005;23:5546.
37. Sirotnak FM, Zakowski MF, Miller VA, et al. Efficacy of cytotoxic agents against human tumor xenografts is markedly enhanced by coadministration of ZD1839 (Iressa), an inhibitor of EGFR tyrosine kinase. Clin Cancer Res 2000;6:4885–92.
38. Barker AJ, Gibson KH, Grundy W, et al. Studies leading to the identification of ZD1839 (IRESSA): An orally active, selective epidermal growth factor receptor tyrosine kinase inhibitor targeted to the treatment of cancer. Bioorg Med Chem Lett 2001;11:1911–4.
39. Moasser MM, Basso A, Averbuch SD, et al. The tyrosine kinase inhibitor ZD1839 ("Iressa") inhibits HER2-driven signaling and suppresses the growth of HER2-overexpressing tumor cells. Cancer Res 2001;61:7184–8.
40. Giaccone G, Herbst RS, Manegold C, et al. Gefitinib in combination with gemcitabine and cisplatin in advanced non-small-cell lung cancer: A phase III trial–INTACT 1. J Clin Oncol 2004;22:777–84.
41. Herbst RS, Giaccone G, Schiller JH, et al. Gefitinib in combination with paclitaxel and carboplatin in advanced non-small-cell lung cancer: A phase III trial–INTACT 2. J Clin Oncol 2004;22:785–94.
42. Lynch TJ, Bell DW, Sordella R, et al. Activating mutations in the epidermal growth factor receptor underlying responsiveness of non-small-cell lung cancer to gefitinib. N Engl J Med 2004;350:2129–39.
43. Cohen EE, Rosen F, Stadler WM, et al. Phase II trial of ZD1839 in recurrent or metastatic squamous cell carcinoma of the head and neck. J Clin Oncol 2003;21:1980–7.
44. Belon J, Irigoyen I, Rodriguez Y, et al. Preliminary results of a phase II study to evaluate gefitinib combined with docetaxel and cisplatin in patients with recurrent and/or metastatic squamous-cell carcinoma of the head and neck. J Clin Oncol 2005;23:5563.
45. Baselga J, Schoffski P, Rojo F, et al. A phase I pharmacokinetic (PK) and molecular pharmacodynamic (PD) study of the combination of two anti-EGFR therapies, the monoclonal antibody (MAb) cetuximab (C) and the tyrosine kinase inhibitor (TKI) gefitinib (G), in patients (pts) with advanced colorectal (CRC), head and neck (HNC) and non-small cell lung cancer (NSCLC). Proc Am Soc Clin Oncol 2006;24:122s.
46. Tang PA, Tsao MS, Moore MJ. A review of erlotinib and its clinical use. Expert Opin Pharmacother 2006;7:177–93.
47. Perez-Soler R, Saltz L. Cutaneous adverse effects with HER1/EGFR-targeted agents: Is there a silver lining? J Clin Oncol 2005;23:5235–46.
48. Erlichman C, Hidalgo M, Boni JP, et al. Phase I study of EKB-569, an irreversible inhibitor of the epidermal growth factor receptor, in patients with advanced solid tumors. J Clin Oncol 2006;24:2252–60.
49. Baselga J, Hammond LA. HER-targeted tyrosine-kinase inhibitors. Oncology 2002;63:6–16.
50. Grandis JR, Sok JC. Signaling through the epidermal growth factor receptor during the development of malignancy. Pharmacol Ther 2004;102:37–46.
51. Spector NL, Xia W, Burris H, III, et al. Study of the biologic effects of lapatinib, a reversible inhibitor of ErbB1 and ErbB2 tyrosine kinases, on tumor growth and survival pathways in patients with advanced malignancies. J Clin Oncol 2005;23:2502–12.
52. Ciardiello F, Caputo R, Damiano V, et al. Antitumor effects of ZD6474, a small molecule vascular endothelial growth factor receptor tyrosine kinase inhibitor, with additional activity against epidermal growth factor receptor tyrosine kinase. Clin Cancer Res 2003;9:1546–56.
53. Schmidt M, Wels W. Targeted inhibition of tumour cell growth by a bispecific single-chain toxin containing an antibody domain and TGF alpha. Br J Cancer 1996;74:853–62.
54. Shinohara H, Morita S, Kawai M, et al. Expression of HER2 in human gastric cancer cells directly correlates with antitumor activity of a recombinant disulfide-stabilized anti-HER2 immunotoxin. J Surg Res 2002;102:169–77.
55. Azemar M, Schmidt M, Arlt F, et al. Recombinant antibody toxins specific for ErbB2 and EGF receptor inhibit the in vitro growth of human head and neck cancer cells and cause rapid tumor regression in vivo. Int J Cancer 2000;86:269–75.
56. Thomas SM, Zeng Q, Epperly MW, et al. Abrogation of head and neck squamous cell carcinoma growth by epidermal growth factor receptor ligand fused to *Pseudomonas* exotoxin transforming growth factor alpha-PE38. Clin Cancer Res 2004;10:7079–87.
57. Coppelli FM, Grandis JR. Oligonucleotides as anticancer agents: From the benchside to the clinic and beyond. Curr Pharm Des 2005;11:2825–40.
58. Rubin Grandis J, Chakraborty A, Melhem MF, et al. Inhibition of epidermal growth factor receptor gene expression and function decreases proliferation of head and neck squamous carcinoma but not normal mucosal epithelial cells. Oncogene 1997;15:409–16.
59. He Y, Zeng Q, Drenning SD, et al. Inhibition of human squamous cell carcinoma growth in vivo by epidermal growth factor receptor antisense RNA transcribed from the U6 promoter. J Natl Cancer Inst 1998;90:1080–7.
60. Xi S, Zhang Q, Dyer KF, et al. Src kinases mediate STAT growth pathways in squamous cell carcinoma of the head and neck. J Biol Chem 2003;278:31574–83.
61. Zhang Q, Thomas SM, Xi S, et al. SRC family kinases mediate epidermal growth factor receptor ligand cleavage, proliferation, and invasion of head and neck cancer cells. Cancer Res 2004;64:6166–73.
62. Kantarjian HM, Talpaz M, O'Brien S, et al. Dose escalation of imatinib mesylate can overcome resistance to standard-dose therapy in patients with chronic myelogenous leukemia. Blood 2003;101:473–5.
63. Gorre ME, Mohammed M, Ellwood K, et al. Clinical resistance to STI-571 cancer therapy caused by BCR-ABL gene mutation or amplification. Science 2001;293:876–80.
64. Johnson FM, Saigal B, Talpaz M, et al. Dasatinib (BMS-354825) tyrosine kinase inhibitor suppresses invasion and induces cell cycle arrest and apoptosis of head and neck squamous cell carcinoma and non-small cell lung cancer cells. Clin Cancer Res 2005;11:6924–32.
65. Darnell JE, Jr, Kerr IM, Stark GR. Jak-STAT pathways and transcriptional activation in response to IFNs and other extracellular signaling proteins. Science 1994;264:1415–21.
66. Bromberg JF, Wrzeszczynska MH, Devgan G, et al. Stat3 as an oncogene. Cell 1999;98:295–303.
67. Grandis JR, Drenning SD, Chakraborty A, et al. Requirement of Stat3 but not Stat1 activation for epidermal growth factor receptor- mediated cell growth In vitro. J Clin Invest 1998;102:1385–92.
68. Leeman RJ, Lui VW, Grandis JR. STAT3 as a therapeutic target in head and neck cancer. Expert Opin Biol Ther 2006;6:231–41.
69. Grandis JR, Drenning SD, Zeng Q, et al. Constitutive activation of Stat3 signaling abrogates apoptosis in squamous cell carcinogenesis in vivo. Proc Natl Acad Sci U S A 2000;97:4227–32.
70. Leong PL, Andrews GA, Johnson DE, et al. Targeted inhibition of Stat3 with a decoy oligonucleotide abrogates head and neck cancer cell growth. Proc Natl Acad Sci U S A 2003;100:4138–43.
71. Xi S, Gooding WE, Grandis JR. In vivo antitumor efficacy of STAT3 blockade using a transcription factor decoy approach: Implications for cancer therapy. Oncogene 2005;24:970–9.
72. Gschwind A, Hart S, Fischer OM, et al. TACE cleavage of proamphiregulin regulates GPCR-induced proliferation and motility of cancer cells. Embo J 2003;22:2411–21.
73. Lui VW, Thomas SM, Zhang Q, et al. Mitogenic effects of gastrin-releasing peptide in head and neck squamous cancer cells are mediated by activation of the epidermal growth factor receptor. Oncogene 2003;22:6183–93.
74. Thomas SM, Bhola NE, Zhang Q, et al. Cross-talk between G-protein–coupled receptor and epidermal growth factor receptor signaling pathways contributes to growth and invasion of head and neck squamous cell carcinoma. Cancer Res 2006;66:11831–9.
75. Chan DC, Gera L, Stewart JM, et al. Bradykinin antagonist dimer, CU201, inhibits the growth of human lung cancer cell lines in vitro and in vivo and produces synergistic growth inhibition in combination with other antitumor agents. Clin Cancer Res 2002;8:1280–7.
76. Smith BD, Smith GL, Carter D, et al. Prognostic significance of vascular endothelial growth factor protein levels in oral and oropharyngeal squamous cell carcinoma. J Clin Oncol 2000;18:2046–52.
77. Kyzas PA, Cunha IW, Ioannidis JP. Prognostic significance of vascular endothelial growth factor immunohistochemical expression in head and neck squamous cell carcinoma: A meta-analysis. Clin Cancer Res 2005;11:1434–40.
78. Nakashima T, Hudson JM, Clayman GL. Antisense inhibition of vascular endothelial growth factor in human head and neck squamous cell carcinoma. Head Neck 2000;22:483–8.
79. Riedel F, Gotte K, Hormann K, et al. Antiangiogenic therapy of head and neck squamous cell carcinoma by vascular endothelial growth factor antisense therapy. Adv Otorhinolaryngol 2005;62:103–20.
80. Mauceri HJ, Hanna NN, Beckett MA, et al. Combined effects of angiostatin and ionizing radiation in antitumour therapy. Nature 1998;394:287–91.
81. Mordenti J, Thomsen K, Licko V, et al. Efficacy and concentration-response of murine anti-VEGF monoclonal antibody in tumor-bearing mice and extrapolation to humans. Toxicol Pathol 1999;27:14–21.
82. Hurwitz H, Fehrenbacher L, Novotny W, et al. Bevacizumab plus irinotecan, fluorouracil, and leucovorin for metastatic colorectal cancer. N Engl J Med 2004;350:2335–42.

83. Chen HX. Expanding the clinical development of bevacizumab. Oncologist 2004;9:27–35.

84. Traxler P, Allegrini PR, Brandt R, et al. AEE788: A dual family epidermal growth factor receptor/ErbB2 and vascular endothelial growth factor receptor tyrosine kinase inhibitor with antitumor and antiangiogenic activity. Cancer Res 2004;64:4931–41.

85. Vokes E, Cohen E, Mauer A, et al. A phase I study of erlotinib and bevacizumab for recurrent or metastatic squamous cell carcinoma of the head and neck (HNC). J Clin Oncol 2005;23:501s.

86. Vousden KH. p53: Death star. Cell 2000;103:691–4.

87. Nees M, Homann N, Discher H, et al. Expression of mutated p53 occurs in tumor-distant epithelia of head and neck cancer patients: A possible molecular basis for the development of multiple tumors. Cancer Res 1993;53:4189–96.

88. Shin DM, Kim J, Ro JY, et al. Activation of p53 gene expression in premalignant lesions during head and neck tumorigenesis. Cancer Res 1994;54:321–6.

89. Bischoff JR, Kirn DH, Williams A, et al. An adenovirus mutant that replicates selectively in p53-deficient human tumor cells. Science 1996;274:373–6.

90. Nemunaitis J, Khuri F, Ganly I, et al. Phase II trial of intratumoral administration of ONYX-015, a replication-selective adenovirus, in patients with refractory head and neck cancer. J Clin Oncol 2001;19:289–98.

91. Khuri FR, Nemunaitis J, Ganly I, et al. a controlled trial of intratumoral ONYX-015, a selectively-replicating adenovirus, in combination with cisplatin and 5-fluorouracil in patients with recurrent head and neck cancer. Nat Med 2000;6:879–85.

92. Rudin CM, Cohen EE, Papadimitrakopoulou VA, et al. An attenuated adenovirus, ONYX-015, as mouthwash therapy for premalignant oral dysplasia. J Clin Oncol 2003;21:4546–52.

93. Rothmann T, Hengstermann A, Whitaker NJ, et al. Replication of ONYX-015, a potential anticancer adenovirus, is independent of p53 status in tumor cells. J Virol 1998;72:9470–8.

94. Brizel DM, Sibley GS, Prosnitz LR, et al. Tumor hypoxia adversely affects the prognosis of carcinoma of the head and neck. Int J Radiat Oncol Biol Phys 1997;38:285–9.

95. Becker A, Hansgen G, Bloching M, et al. Oxygenation of squamous cell carcinoma of the head and neck: Comparison of primary tumors, neck node metastases, and normal tissue. Int J Radiat Oncol Biol Phys 1998;42:35–41.

96. Janssen HL, Haustermans KM, Balm AJ, et al. Hypoxia in head and neck cancer: How much, how important? Head Neck 2005;27:622–38.

97. Semenza GL. Targeting HIF-1 for cancer therapy. Nat Rev Cancer 2003;3:721–32.

98. Koch CJ. Unusual oxygen concentration dependence of toxicity of SR-4233, a hypoxic cell toxin. Cancer Res 1993;53:3992–7.

99. Rischin D, Peters L, Hicks R, et al. Phase I trial of concurrent tirapazamine, cisplatin, and radiotherapy in patients with advanced head and neck cancer. J Clin Oncol 2001;19:535–42.

100. Rischin D, Peters L, Fisher R, et al. Tirapazamine, cisplatin, and radiation versus fluorouracil, cisplatin, and radiation in patients with locally advanced head and neck cancer: A randomized phase II trial of the Trans-Tasman Radiation Oncology Group (TROG 98.02). J Clin Oncol 2005;23:79–87.

101. Brizel DM, Esclamado R. Concurrent chemoradiotherapy for locally advanced, nonmetastatic, squamous carcinoma of the head and neck: Consensus, controversy, and conundrum. J Clin Oncol 2006;24:2612–7.

92

Chemoradiation for Head and Neck Cancer

Rob McCammon, MD
Changhu Chen, MD
Mohan Suntha, MD
David Raben, MD

Radiotherapy has long played a role in the treatment of head and neck squamous cell carcinoma (HNSCC). Early-stage disease at sites such as the laryngeal glottis and base of tongue have frequently been treated successfully with radiotherapy alone. Historically, more advanced cancers were addressed by surgery as the primary modality with postoperative radiation therapy when indicated. However, tremendous strides have been made in the realm of radiotherapy and chemotherapy such that organ preservation is now the rule rather than the exception in many head and neck sites. In instances when surgery is indicated, advances have also been made in the delivery of postoperative combined modality therapy. Moreover, recent times have been witness to exciting progress in the characterization of molecular features of HNSCC with subsequent development of biologic agents targeting specific pathways responsible for tumor growth and dissemination. In spite of this progress, failure rates in locally advanced HNSCC remain high regardless of treatment modality, underscoring the need for continued research.

HISTORY OF RADIATION THERAPY

The advent of therapeutic radiation followed closely on the heels of the discovery of X-rays by Roentgen in November of 1895. In fact, within months of the discovery of the "New Light," at least one visionary had already performed palliative "roentgentherapy" on a patient with recurrent breast cancer.[1] Since those pioneering days, more than a century of experience has been attained in the treatment of cancer with radiation.

The introduction of megavoltage radiotherapy delivered via a linear accelerator, or "linac," marked the dawn of the modern radiation era. The ability to generate high-energy photons enabled practitioners to effectively treat not only superficial lesions but also deep-seated tumors. The introduction of computed tomography (CT) has made possible three-dimensional 3-D conformal radiotherapy. Planning CT scans are now frequently merged, that is, fused, with diagnostic CT, magnetic resonance imaging (MRI), and/or positron emission tomography (PET) datasets to improve target delineation. Improvements in patient immobilization with the use of thermoplastic masks and other similar devices have allowed for reduction in uncertain margins and enabled better overall treatment accuracy. More recently, the integration into clinical practice of multileaf collimators (MLCs) has facilitated design and delivery of radiation fields with complex shapes, obviating the use of heavy and cumbersome manually cut blocks in most instances (Figure 1). Perhaps even more exciting is the use of intensity modulated radiation therapy (IMRT), which utilizes inverse planning to generate true "dose painting" to treat tumor and areas at risk for microscopic spread, while sparing critical normal structures, most notably salivary tissue. Inverse planning refers to the process by which an idealized radiation dose distribution is first defined, and an iterative computer algorithm is subsequently employed to optimally achieve that distribution. In IMRT, the overall beam intensity is defined by many smaller beams known as "beamlets." The radiation intensity of each beamlet is carefully controlled by frequent changes in the overall conformation of the larger beam. Each conformation is known as a segment; a typical head and neck IMRT plan is composed of 50 to 100 or more segments. A broader discussion of stereotactic radiosurgery and radiotherapy is found in Chapter 36, "Stereotactic Radiosurgery and Radiotherapy."

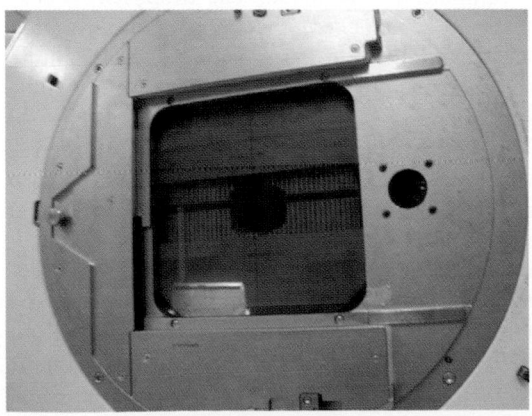

Figure 1 Multileaf collimators (MLCs) within the head of a linear accelerator.

PRETREATMENT EVALUATION

Prior to embarking upon radiotherapy for HNSCC, it is essential that patients undergo a multidisciplinary evaluation. This includes consultation with the following: (1) dentistry to provide fluoride trays and other prophylaxis for serviceable teeth or extraction of poor dentition, (2) nutrition to educate the patient and institute measures to minimize weight loss and deconditioning during treatment, and (3) speech therapy in anticipation of future issues with speech and swallowing. Given the significant acute mucosal toxicity attendant to concurrent chemoradiation, prophylactic gastric tube placement is frequently performed at the outset, usually via a percutaneous endoscopic gastrostomy (PEG). Baseline endocrinologic evaluation is also prudent in view of the potential thyroid or pituitary dysfunction related to treatment of certain head and neck sites.

RADIATION TREATMENT PLANNING

The initial step in the treatment planning process is the "simulation." Today, this is almost exclusively performed on a CT simulator. Patients are typically positioned supine for head and neck treatments, and immobilization is achieved with a thermoplastic mask (Figure 2). Images through the anatomic area of interest are then obtained at 3 to 5 millimeter intervals. Reference marks are made on the thermoplastic mask to reproduce day-to-day patient setup. Axial images from the CT simulation are utilized to identify tumor volumes and involved or potentially involved nodal regions, as well as critical organs at risk such as the spinal cord, salivary glands, and true vocal cords. The physician "contours" these volumes, and radiation fields are then placed by trained dosimetrists, under the guidance of the radiation oncologist, to encompass the contoured volumes. While the specifics of the radiotherapy plan vary widely based on the primary site and stage of disease, a typical initial non-IMRT field arrangement for treatment of a primary tumor and the regional lymphatics employs laterally opposed 4 to 10 MV beams matched to a low

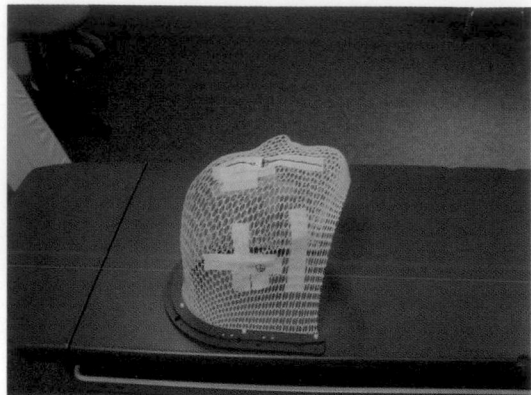

Figure 2 Thermoplastic mask.

anterior–posterior field. Due to the low threshold for potential damage to the spinal cord, doses above approximately 45 to 50 Gray (Gy) to that organ are considered unacceptable. Therefore, "off cord" lateral fields in which the posterior border of the field lies anterior to the spinal cord, for example, at the midvertebral body in the sagittal plane, are initiated prior to reaching the tolerance dose. To adequately treat potentially involved lymph nodes lying in the region posterior to the "off cord" fields, electron fields ("posterior electron strips") are utilized. Electron therapy deposits dose superficially compared to photons, with rapid dose fall-off at depth. The lymph nodes of interest are located relatively close to the surface and receive the prescribed dose, but the spinal cord, a deep structure in the sagittal plane, is essentially spared. Finally, a 3-D "boost" field is designed to encompass only areas of gross tumor and a margin to account for setup uncertainty and internal anatomic motion. The delivery of definitive doses of radiation has, at times, been limited by the risk of normal tissue damage. Given the anatomic proximity of vital structures, tumors of the head and neck present a significant therapeutic challenge. Standard beam arrangements and treatment planning techniques are able to achieve uniform dose delivery throughout the entire anatomic region. The ability to deliver a homogeneous dose to a tumor-bearing region is desirable; however, it proves to be a disadvantage in terms of dose delivered to surrounding critical structures. The advent of CT-based planning has allowed treating physicians to gain a better understanding of the potential toxicities of radiation therapy according to the dose delivered to these structures. Recent advances such as IMRT have clearly improved the ability to safely deliver effective total doses of radiation to HNSCC while simultaneously decreasing the risk of untoward side effects. IMRT also allows for delivery of a "synchronous integrated boost" in which modifications to treatment fields such as off-cord laterals and posterior electron strips are unnecessary (Figure 3). It is not uncommon for IMRT and conventional (3-D conformal) fields to be planned in combination. One example of this approach is the use of IMRT to the primary tumor and upper neck matched to a conventional low anterior–posterior field.

RATIONALE FOR COMBINED CHEMOTHERAPY AND RADIATION

A litany of evidence has been attained in the clinic demonstrating enhanced tumor control with the addition of concurrent chemotherapy to radiation (Table 1). A clear rationale exists for this marriage of modalities in that chemotherapy and radiotherapy can combine in an additive, or even supra-additive fashion to enhance tumor kill by multiple mechanisms. Prior to garnering clinical experience in concurrent chemoradiotherapy, data were obtained in the laboratory to suggest treatment synergy. In general, the goal of adding concurrent chemotherapy to radiation is to improve the therapeutic ratio. That is, the addition of a drug has a differential effect on tumor and normal tissue: while the dose-response curve is shifted to the left for both tumor and normal tissue, the magnitude of the shift is greater for the tumor[2] (Figure 4). Therefore, at a given level of normal-tissue injury, a greater likelihood of tumor control is achievable. Various techniques are available to measure the effects of chemotherapy and radiotherapy either in vivo or in vitro. In vitro methods entail subjecting cells in culture to various treatments to assess response. Examples of in vivo methods include simple tumor growth measurements, tumor cure (TCT_{50}) assays, dilution assays, and lung colony assays.[3]

Although cell survival curves generated by the various laboratory assays demonstrate the effect of combined modality treatment, they say nothing regarding its mechanism. The possible interactions of combined chemotherapy and radiation were promulgated by Steel in a classic paper.[4] The conceptual cornerstones of the interaction were spatial cooperation and toxicity independence, referring to the targeting of different anatomic sites by the respective modalities without overlapping toxicity. While providing a rationale for combined treatment, the original framework outlined by Steel did not propose a direct interaction of the modalities on common tissues nor provide an explanation for the supra-additive effect on tumors when delivered in combination. Decades of subsequent research have helped elucidate the interaction of chemotherapy and radiation, although much remains incompletely understood. The proposed mechanisms by which chemotherapy is radiosensitizing are numerous, and it is instructive to examine the more commonly utilized agents in HNSCC individually.

Cisplatin has been administered more frequently with radiotherapy than any other agent in HNSCC. The water-soluble drug is converted intracellularly to its active agent, which subsequently reacts with nuclear DNA to form inter-strand and intrastrand crosslinks. Crosslink formation triggers a cascade involving signaling pathways, checkpoint activation, DNA repair activity, and apoptosis.[5] Several mechanisms have been proposed to account for the synergy of cisplatin and radiation (Figure 5), but the

explanation given most currency is that cisplatin inhibits repair of radiation-induced DNA damage. Other mechanisms have been inferred, including: enhanced formation of toxic platinum intermediates via radiation-induced free radicals, increased permanence of DNA damage by way of cisplatin mediated free electron scavenging, increased cellular uptake of cisplatin in the presence of radiation, and cell-cycle disruption.

5-Fluorouricil (5-FU) is another agent frequently administered in HNSCC. The drug is converted to its cytotoxic form by multiple pathways resulting in depletion of thymidine 5′-monophosphate and thymidine 5′-triphosphate with subsequent derangement of DNA synthesis and repair. The combination of 5-FU and radiation can clearly be synergistic, although the exact mechanism eludes our full understanding. It has been proposed that the linchpin of the interaction derives from rapid progression of cells through S-phase (when they are relatively resistant to radiation) due to presence of the drug.[6] Other studies have suggested that 5-FU synergizes with radiation by eliminating the radiation-induced G2 cycle arrest, thereby reducing the overall time for sublethal damage repair or directly inhibiting repair of DNA double-strand breaks from radiation.

Taxanes have proven to be potent radiosensitizers with resultant use in treating cancers of various sites, including the head and neck, esophagus, lung, breast, bladder, pancreas, and female urogenital systems. The success of taxanes in combination with radiotherapy highlights the influence of the cell cycle on radiation sensitivity, as first described by Terasima and Tolmach nearly half a century ago.[7] Generally speaking, cells are most radiosensitive in G2 and M phases, whereas they are most radioresistant in S phase. Therefore, any agent that promotes the accumulation of cells in the sensitive phase of the cell cycle and/or selectively eradicates cells in the resistant phase will optimally combine with radiotherapy. Taxanes, which bind to $\widetilde{\beta}$-tubulin and thereby increase polymerization to promote

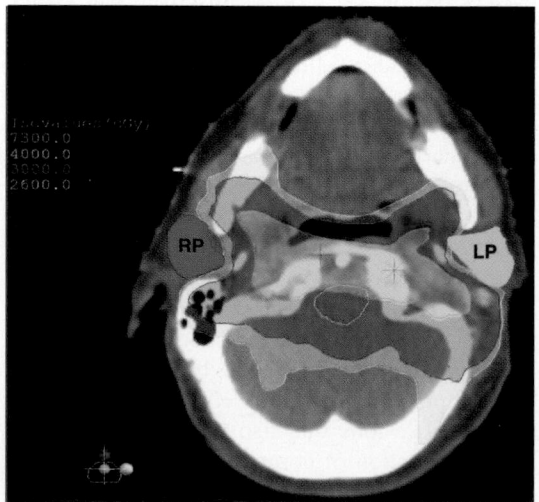

Figure 3 IMRT dose distribution on an axial image demonstrating parotid sparing.
RP = right parotid; LP = left parotid.

Table 1 Randomized Trials of Chemoradiotherapy versus Radiotherapy for Head and Neck Squamous Cell Carcinoma

Study Reference	Number of Patients Assessed	Primary Site	Experimental Design/ Fractionation	Drugs	Local Control or Progression-Free Survival (Experimental versus Control)	Overall Survival (Experimental versus Control)
Intergroup 0099, 2003	147	NP	Concurrent/QD	Concurrent cisplatin; adjuvant cis+5-FU q3 weeks	24% versus 69% (PFS) at 3 yr ($p < .001$)	47% versus 78% ($p = .005$)
Hong Kong (Chan), 2005	350	NP	Concurrent/QD	Cisplatin weekly	60.2% versus 52.1% (PFS) at 5 yr ($p = .16$)	70.3% versus 58.6% ($p = .049$)
RTOG 9111, 2003	547	L	(i) Induction (ii) Concurrent/QD	(i) Cisplatin +5-FU q3 weeks (ii) Cisplatin q3 weeks	(i) 61% versus (ii) 78% ($p = .003$) versus 56% (LC) ($p < .001$) at 2 yr	(i) 76% versus (ii) 74% versus 75% (NS)
GORTEC 94-01, 2004	226	OP	Concurrent/QD	Carboplatin+5-FU q3 weeks	47.6% versus 24.7% (LC) at 5 yr ($p = .002$)	22.4% versus 15.8% ($p = .05$)
German multicenter, 1998	270	OC, OP, L, HP	Concurrent/split course	Cisplatin+5-FU q3 weeks	36% versus 17% (LC) at 3 yr ($p < .004$)	48% versus 24% ($p < .0003$)
Duke University, 1998	116	OC, OP, L, HP	Concurrent/hyperfractionated	Cisplatin+5-FU q5 weeks +adjuvant	70% versus 44% (LC) at 3 yr ($p = .01$)	55% versus 34% ($p = .07$)
Head and Neck Intergroup (Adelstein), 2003	295	OC, OP, L, HP	(i) Concurrent/QD (ii) Concurrent/split course	(i) Cisplatin q3 weeks (ii) Cisplatin +5-FU q3 weeks		(i) 37% versus (ii) 27% versus 23% at 3 yr ($p = .014$ between (i) and control)
SAKK (Swiss), 2004	224	OC, OP, L, HP	Concurrent/hyperfractionated	Cisplatin q4 weeks	51% versus 33% (LC) at 5 yr ($p = .039$)	46% versus 32% ($p = .15$)
Jeremic and colleagues, 2000	130	OC, OP, L, HP	Concurrent/hyperfractionated	Daily cisplatin	50% versus 36% (LC) at 5 yr ($p = .041$)	46% versus 25% ($p = .0075$)
EORTC 22931	334	OC, OP, L, HP	Postoperative concurrent/QD	Cisplatin q3 weeks	82% versus 69% (LC) at 5 yr ($p = .07$)	53% versus 40% ($p = .02$)
RTOG 9501	459	OC, OP, L, HP	Postoperative concurrent/QD	Cisplatin q3 weeks	78% versus 67% (LC) at 3 yr ($p = .01$)	56% versus 47% ($p = .09$)
Bachaud and colleagues, 2004	83	OC, OP, L, HP	Postoperative concurrent/QD	Cisplatin weekly	70% versus 55% at 5 yr ($p < .05$)	36% versus 13% ($p = .01$)

OC = oral cavity; OP = oropharynx; L = larynx; HP – hypopharynx; NP = nasopharynx; QD = once daily.

stable microtubule generation, arrest cells in the radiosensitive G2/M phases.

CHEMORADIATION CLINICAL TRIALS

One of the seminal studies evaluating the feasibility of organ preservation in the treatment of head and neck cancer was the Department of Veterans Affairs Laryngeal Cancer Study Group trial (VALSG).[8] This phase III multicenter trial randomized medically operable patients with resectable stage III or IV laryngeal SCC to either conventional laryngectomy and postoperative radiation or induction chemotherapy followed by radiation. Patients in the induction chemotherapy arm received two cycles of cisplatin and 5-FU prior to assessment of tumor response. Responders went on to a third cycle of chemotherapy followed by definitive radiotherapy to a dose of 66 to 76 Gy. Nonresponders underwent laryngectomy. The results revealed no difference between the two arms in estimated 2-year overall survival at a median follow-up of 33 months. Moreover, the larynx was preserved in 64% of patients in the nonsurgical arm. The trial included quality of life studies and functional assessments regarding communication, swallowing, and eating. At 6, 12, and 24 months, the patients with a preserved larynx reported better communication scores, although there was no statistical difference in swallowing function.

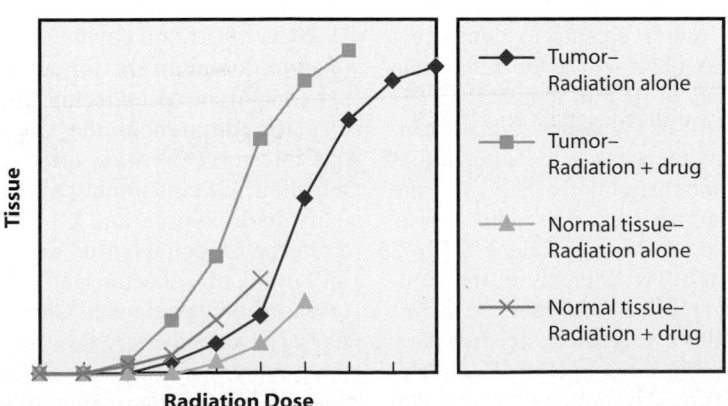

Figure 4 The effect of the addition of chemotherapy to radiation on both tumor control and normal tissue damage. Note that the improvement in tumor control when drug is added exceeds the increase in normal tissue damage; ie, the therapeutic ratio is improved.

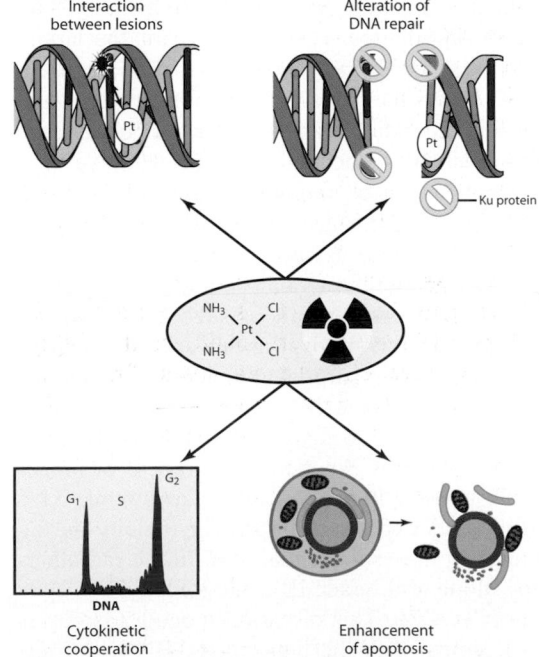

Figure 5 Proposed interactions of radiation and cisplatin. (Published with permission from reference 5.)

A study of similar design to the VA trial was conducted by the European Organization for Research and Treatment of Cancer (EORTC) in patients with locally advanced HNSCC of the hypopharynx.[9] Patients were randomized to either immediate surgery and postoperative radiation or induction chemotherapy followed by definitive radiation. In contrast to the VA trial, immediate surgery was deferred only in those patients who had a complete response to induction chemotherapy. Like the VA trial, the chemotherapy regimen in the EORTC trial was cisplatin and 5-FU for three cycles. Organ preservation in chemotherapy responders was 64%, virtually identical to that seen in the VA trial. Although there was an apparent initial survival advantage in the nonsurgical arm at 3-year follow-up (57% vs 43%), there was no statistically significant difference noted at 5 years (30% in the induction chemotherapy arm vs 35% in the surgery arm). Nevertheless, the organ-preservation approach was heralded as the new standard of care against which future treatment regimens would be judged.

In an effort to better delineate the exact contribution of the chemotherapy to radiation in the treatment of HNSCC, as well as the optimal treatment sequencing, the Radiation Therapy Oncology Group (RTOG) conducted a randomized trial, RTOG 91–11.[10] This three-arm trial randomized 547 patients with resectable stage III and IV SCC of the glottic or supraglottic larynx to radiotherapy alone, induction chemotherapy (cisplatin/5-FU as per the VA trial) followed by radiation, or concurrent chemoradiation (cisplatin 100 mg/m^2 on days 1, 22, 43). Patients with T1 primaries or large-volume T4 disease were excluded. The primary endpoint was larynx preservation. Radiation to gross disease was 70 Gy in 35 fractions; all patients received elective treatment to the entire neck to a minimum of 50 Gy. The results clearly demonstrated that laryngx preservation was improved in the concurrent chemoradiotherapy compared to the other two arms to a statistically significant degree. To wit: at 2 years, the larynx was preserved in 88% of patients in the concurrent arm, 75% in the induction chemotherapy arm, and 70% in the radiotherapy alone arm. Likewise, the improvement in locoregional control at 2 years in the concurrent chemoradiotherapy arm reached statistical significance as compared to the other two arms (78% in the concurrent arm vs 61% in the induction arm vs 56% in the radiotherapy alone arm). As a result of successful surgical salvage, overall survival rates were similar in all three arms. Not surprisingly, acute toxicity was worse in the concurrent chemoradiation arm, predominately due to increased mucositis. Overall, 77% of patients experienced a grade 3 or higher acute toxicity in the concurrent arm, while 51% of patients experienced a similar toxicity during radiation in the sequential arm. In the radiotherapy alone arm, grade III acute toxicity was even lower at 47%. This disparity in acute toxicity is in keeping with the majority of HNSCC trials comparing concurrent with sequential chemoradiotherapy or radiotherapy alone. Long-term

speech and swallowing function was also monitored; notably, 23% of patients in the concurrent arm were limited to swallowing only soft foods or liquids 1 year following treatment, and 3% were completely feeding tube dependent. In contrast, only 9% of patients assigned to induction chemotherapy were limited to soft foods and liquids at 1 year, and all patients maintained some degree of swallowing. Among patients assigned to radiotherapy alone, 18% of patients described swallowing dysfunction at 1 year, including 3% unable to swallow even liquids. By 2 years, however, there was no significant difference in swallowing function among the cohorts. There were no differences between the three arms vis-a-vis speech at either 12- or 24-month follow-up.

Despite the fact that many trials combining chemotherapy and radiation have been conducted in the last four decades, the absolute survival benefit associated with combined modality therapy has historically remained poorly defined. To better define the potential advantage of cytotoxic therapy, four large meta-analyses have been performed comparing chemotherapy (administered neoadjuvantly, concurrently, or adjuvantly) plus radiation versus radiation alone.[11–14] The primary endpoint in each analysis was overall survival. Among the four reports, three were literature-based,[12–14] and one updated actual patient data for the meta-analysis.[11] The total number of cases included in each analysis ranged from 4,292 (from 28 trials) to 10,741 (63 trials). The median followup for all patients varied from 2 years to as long as 6.8 years. Despite significant differences in the databases analyzed, the four meta-analyses reached similar conclusions. The results of each study confirmed a small but reproducible survival benefit favoring the addition of chemotherapy. The magnitude of the benefit ranged from an absolute survival advantage of 2.8 to 6.5%. The study by Pignon and colleagues identified an overall survival advantage at both 2 and 5 years of 4%.[11] All four studies noted that the survival benefit was greatest when chemotherapy was administered concurrently with radiation. The magnitude of this benefit varied from 8 to 12% in the four analyses.

The benefit of adding concurrent chemotherapy to radiotherapy has been demonstrated in other site-specific trials. For instance, one of the most marked improvements to concurrent chemoradiation was observed in the Intergroup 0099 trial.[15] This phase III trial randomized 193 patients with stage III or IV nasopharyngeal cancer without distant metastases to either radiation alone or chemoradiation, of which 147 were evaluable for primary analysis. The radiation was delivered on a once per day schedule at 1.8 to 2 Gy per fraction to 70 Gy. Patients in the combined modality arm received cisplatin 100 mg/m^2 on days 1, 22, and 43; following radiation they received an additional three cycles of adjuvant cisplatin 80 mg/m^2 on day one and 5-FU 1,000 mg/m^2 on days 1 through 4, every 4 weeks. A striking difference was seen in progression-free and overall survival between the two arms. The

3-year progression free survival (PFS) rates were 24% and 69% ($p < .001$) in the radiotherapy alone and chemoradiotherapy arms, respectively; overall survival was 47% versus 78% ($p = .005$) at the same interval. In fact, the outcomes were so disparate that the data activated an early stopping rule. Acute toxicity was dramatic, however; and only 62% of patients received all three cycles of concurrent chemotherapy. Moreover, one-third of patients in the combined modality arm received no adjuvant chemotherapy, with an additional 11% receiving less than the full three cycles. Additional nasopharynx trials have demonstrated comparable outcomes with the delivery of fewer cycles of chemotherapy[16] as well as other regimens such as weekly cisplatin.[17] The French Head and Neck Oncology and Radiotherapy Group conducted a randomized trial in stage III and IV SCC of the oropharynx comparing conventionally-fractionated radiotherapy alone with the same radiotherapy and concurrent 5-FU and carboplatin given every 3 weeks for three cycles, with 5-year outcomes published in an updated report.[18] Five-year overall survival, disease-free survival, and locoregional control rates were 22% and 16% (log-rank $p = .05$), 27% and 15% ($p = .01$), and 48% and 25% ($p = .002$), in the concurrent chemoradiotherapy and radiotherapy alone arms, respectively.

Many chemotherapeutic agents are active in HNSCC, and several clinical trials have been conducted to assess the optimal combination of agents in concert with radiotherapy. Early trials primarily employed agents such as bleomycin and methotrexate.[19] In fact, the first trial conducted by the RTOG following its inception in 1968 evaluated the sequential addition of methotrexate to radiotherapy in advanced head and neck cancer. Later, the use of cisplatin and 5-FU, known to be active in the metastatic setting, gained currency. Agents known to synergize with radiation, such as mitomycin or hydroxyurea, have also been frequently used. Taxanes, known to be potent radiosensitizers, have become a widely utilized component of HNSCC treatment.

RTOG 97-03 was a multicenter trial in which three different chemotherapy doublets were examined prospectively when given with concurrent radiotherapy.[20] This phase II trial assigned 241 patients with stage III or IV (M0) HNSCC of the oral cavity, oropharynx, or hypopharynx to one of the following three regimens: (1) concurrent radiotherapy plus low-dose daily cisplatin throughout the course and continuous infusion (CI) 5-FU for the final 10 days of radiation, (2) concurrent radiotherapy plus twice daily hydroxyurea and CI 5-FU; chemoradiotherapy was delivered on an alternating 1-week on/1-week off schedule, and (3) low-dose weekly cisplatin and paclitaxel with concurrent radiation. The radiotherapy dose was identical in the three arms, with the only difference in fractionation being the alternating split-course regimen assigned to patients in arm 2. All three arms were found to be feasible, with less than ten percent of patients having unacceptable deviations from treatment or incomplete chemotherapy. Overall, grade 4 or higher toxicity was seen in 18, 29, and 23% of patients in arms 1, 2, and 3. The most common toxicity was mucosal in nature. While not designed to directly compare the efficacy of the respective regimens, it bears mentioning that estimated 2-year disease-free survival and overall survival rates were 38.2% and 57.5% for arm 1, 48.6% and 69.4% for arm 2, and 51.3% and 66.6% for arm 3.

POSTOPERATIVE CHEMORADIOTHERAPY FOR LOCALLY ADVANCED HEAD AND NECK SQUAMOUS CELL CARCINOMA

Surgery continues to be the primary treatment of HNSCC in certain situations. Certainly, primary resection remains the standard of care in oral cavity SCC. Moreover, advanced disease in which significant bone or deep cartilage invasion is present suggests that organ preservation is unattainable and is best addressed surgically. Nevertheless, radiotherapy is commonly indicated following resection of advanced disease. Historically, adjuvant radiation therapy was delivered without concurrent chemotherapy, as evidenced by the control arms in the VALSG and EORTC trials mentioned previously. However, two recent trials examining the postoperative treatment of advanced HNSCC have established adjuvant chemoradiotherapy as the standard of care in selected patients.

RTOG 95-01 was a phase III trial in which patients with high-risk resected HNSCC were randomized to conventionally fractionated radiotherapy to 60 to 66 Gy with or without concurrent cisplatin (100 mg/m^2 days 1, 22, and 43).[21] "High-risk" was defined as any of the following features: positive margins, two or more positive lymph nodes, or evidence of involved nodal extracapsular extension (ECE). A total of 459 patients with HNSCC of the oral cavity, oropharynx, larynx, or hypopharynx were treated; at a median follow-up of 46 months, there was a statistically significant improvement in locoregional failure rate (3-year estimate 22% vs 33%, $p = .01$) and disease-free survival (47% vs 36%, $p = .04$) in the combined modality arm. While overall survival was higher in the combined modality arm, the difference did not reach statistical significance (56% vs 47%, $p = .09$). Eligibility for the EORTC 22931 trial was somewhat different, requiring any of the following: tumor within 5 mm of the surgical margin, ECE, clinical involvement of level 4 or 5 lymph nodes (limited to oral cavity and oropharynx primaries), perineural involvement, or vascular embolism[22] (Figure 6). Three hundred and thirty-four patients were enrolled and randomized to 66 Gy of radiation at conventional fractionation with or without cisplatin as in the RTOG trial. Again, locoregional control (LRC) and disease-free survival (DFS) were significantly improved in the concurrent chemoradiotherapy arm (5-year estimate, 82% vs 69% $p = .007$ for LRC; 47% vs

36% $p = .04$ for DFS). Additionally, the improvement in overall survival in the combined arm reached statistical significance (53% vs 40%, $p = .02$). A subsequent combined retrospective subgroup analysis of the two trials suggested that the addition of concurrent cisplatin to postoperative radiotherapy was most beneficial to patients with either ECE or positive margins. In fact, when neither risk factor was present, there appeared to be no significant advantage to combined postoperative treatment (EORTC 22931, $p = .33$; RTOG 9-501; $p = .78$).[23]

A prospective trial conducted at MD Anderson Cancer Center revealed the importance of timely postoperative treatment of patients with HNSCC.[24] Patients were stratified into low, intermediate, or high risk groups based on a variety of surgical-pathologic features, for example, oral cavity site, mucosal margin status, nerve invasion, >1 involved node or nodal region, >3 cm node, ECE, and >6-week delay prior to treatment. The presence of ECE alone or clusters of two or more other features qualified patients for high-risk status, whereas single other features met the threshold for intermediate risk. Low-risk patients, defined as those with no adverse tumor features, received no postoperative radiotherapy. Intermediate risk patients received 57.6 Gy at 1.8 Gy per fraction over 6.5 weeks. High-risk patients received 63 Gy at 1.8 Gy per fraction over either a standard 7-week course or an accelerated 5-week course. No concurrent chemotherapy was delivered. Outcomes were poorest among the high-risk patients in spite of the delivery of an escalated radiation dose. There was a nonstatistically significant trend toward improved locoregional control and overall survival in the accelerated (5 weeks) high-risk arm as compared to the standard (7 weeks) high-risk arm. Moreover, there was a significant decrement in locoregional control and survival for patients in whom the overall treatment time, that is, date of surgery to date of radiotherapy completion, was protracted. Among patients treated in less than 11 weeks, LRC was 76% and overall survival (OS) was 48%, whereas those treated in 11 to 13

weeks LRC was 62% and OS was 27%. Patients treated in greater than 13 weeks fared even more poorly, with LRC of 38% and OS of 25%.

INDUCTION CHEMOTHERAPY IN LOCALLY ADVANCED HEAD AND NECK SQUAMOUS CELL CARCINOMA

Many trials have been conducted in the past three decades comparing local therapy (surgery or radiotherapy alone) with or without induction chemotherapy. With few exceptions,[25] outcomes were not improved by induction therapy. Furthermore, several trials, including RTOG 91-11, have demonstrated improved outcomes in patients randomized to concurrent rather than sequential treatment, establishing the former regimen as the standard organ-preserving approach in locally advanced disease. However, the development of new cytotoxic agents such as the taxanes, as well as the relative increase in the rate of distant recurrences in patients treated with concurrent chemoradiotherapy, has fomented a resurgent interest in induction chemotherapy. Recent trials have established the superiority of the intensified triplet regimen of cisplatin, 5-FU, and a taxane over the combination of cisplatin and 5-FU in the induction setting.[26,27] Ongoing research will compare concurrent chemoradiation with or without induction chemotherapy. At least three trials are enrolling patients to such a regimen: the Southwest Oncology Group (SWOG) 0427 trial, the Paradigm Trial spearheaded by investigators at the Dana–Farber Cancer Center, and the DeCIDE Trial at the University of Chicago.[28]

INTRA-ARTERIAL CHEMOTHERAPY AND RADIATION

The concurrent application of chemotherapy and radiation is often associated with an increase in acute toxicity including mucositis and leukopenia. The incidence of these toxicities often restricts patient selection for concurrent combined modality treatment. Another approach to the delivery of chemotherapy involves the regional infusion of the primary tumor with a cytotoxic agent. Intra-arterial (IA) delivery of chemotherapy has a therapeutic advantage over intravenous administration as a result of the higher drug concentrations that can be achieved in the tumor. Advances in the field of interventional radiology now make it possible to infuse selectively chemotherapy into head and neck subsites without significant catheter-related side effects. Cisplatin is ideally suited as a cytotoxic agent delivered intra-arterially with radiation in that it has a proven role as a radiosensitizer and has systemic effects that can be mitigated by the addition of sodium thiosulfate. Single institution trials have been conducted combining IA supradose cisplatin with conventional[29] and hyperfractionated[30] radiotherapy (so called RADPLAT) with promising response rates. Based on these experiences, the RTOG conducted a prospective feasibility trial

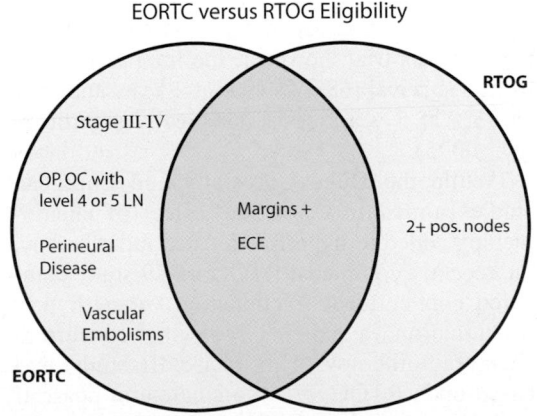

Figure 6 Eligibility criteria in EORTC 22931 and RTOG 95-01. (Published with permission from reference 23.) OP = oropharynx; OC = oral cavity; LN = lymph nodes; ECE = extracapsular extension.

of concurrent radiation and intra-arterial chemotherapy. RTOG 96-15 enrolled 67 patients with HNSCC of the oral cavity, oropharynx, hypopharynx, or larynx.[31] T4 disease was required for eligibility. The radiation was 70 Gy in 35 daily fractions employing a shrinking field technique. Patients received IA cisplatin at 150 mg/m^2 on days 1, 8, 15, and 22 of radiation. Response rates were high, with 80% of patients experiencing a complete response; 2-year estimated local control and overall survival rates were 57% and 63%, respectively. Grade 4 or higher acute toxicity was low (14%) in "experienced" centers, defined as those having treated ten or more patients previously with RADPLAT, whereas over half of all patients treated at "inexperienced" centers incurred a grade 4 (47%) or 5 (4%) toxicity.

ALTERED FRACTIONATION OF RADIATION THERAPY

While much attention has been given to combining chemotherapy and radiation in the treatment of HNSCC, there has also been avid interest in investigating the impact of altered radiation fractionation regimens on tumor control. Altered fractionation purports to improve the therapeutic ratio by exploiting the differential response of tumor cells and late responding normal tissues to fractionated radiation. For instance, hyperfractionation entails the delivery of a higher total dose of radiation via an increased number of fractions, as compared to conventional fractionation, with a smaller dose delivered per fraction. Accelerated fractionation refers to the delivery of a conventional dose in an accelerated fashion. The impetus behind accelerated fractionation is the notion, borne out by laboratory and clinical evidence, that HNSCC cells undergo accelerated repopulation approximately 3 to 4 weeks into radiation therapy. This phenomenon is so pronounced that it has been suggested that there is a need for a dose increment of 0.6 Gy each day to compensate just for repopulation after the 4-week mark of radiotherapy.[32]

Several clinical trials have compared various radiation fractionation schemes in HNSCC. RTOG 90-03 was a four-arm radiation only trial designed to compare three altered fractionation regimens against standard once daily fractionation.[33] This prospective phase III trial enrolled 1,113 patients with stage III–IV SCC of the oral cavity, non-base of tongue (BOT) oropharynx, supraglottic larynx, and stage II–IV SCC of the BOT and hypopharynx. The control arm was 70 Gy in 35 fractions delivered once daily. The second arm was treated with pure hyperfractionation in a regimen widely employed previously at the University of Florida: 1.2 Gy two times per day to a total of 81.6 Gy (78 fractions) over 7 weeks. Arm three received an accelerated course of 1.6 Gy two times per day to a total dose of 67.2 Gy in 42 fractions over 6 weeks, which included a 2-week break at 38.4 Gy, a regimen popularized at Massachusetts General Hospital. The

final arm employed accelerated fractionation via concomitant boost, a regimen conceptualized at MD Anderson Cancer Center, in which patients received 1.8 Gy to a large field daily for 6 weeks with the addition of a reduced field boost treatment of 1.5 Gy on each of the final 12 days of the course. In those arms in which twice daily radiation was delivered, a 6-hour interfraction interval was mandatory to allow for normal tissue repair of sublethal damage. Although there was no difference in overall survival between the various treatment arms, improved LRC was observed in the pure hyperfractionation and concomitant boost cohorts. Specifically, 2-year LRC was 54.4% in the hyperfractionation arm ($p = .045$), 54.5% in the concomitant boost arm ($p = .05$), and 46.0% in the standard arm. A significant improvement in LRC was not seen in the split-course regimen. The hyperfractionation and concomitant boost arms also yielded improved disease-free survival, but the improvement did not meet statistical significance.

A trial conducted at Duke University Medical Center compared hyperfractionated radiotherapy alone with hyperfractionation plus concurrent cisplatin and 5-FU.[34] One hundred twenty-two patients with similar eligibility to the RTOG 90-03 trial were randomized to either radiation alone to a total dose of 75 Gy at 1.25 Gy twice daily or twice daily radiation of 1.25 Gy to a reduced dose of 70 Gy with 5 days of cisplatin 12 mg/m^2 and 5-FU 600 mg/m^2 in weeks 1 and 6 of treatment. Most patients in both arms also received adjuvant cisplatin and 5-FU for two additional cycles. Improved LRC was observed in the combined modality arm (70% at 3 years vs 44% in the radiation alone arm, $p = .01$). Disease-free and overall survival also appeared to be better in the combined arm, but the difference was not statistically significant. While mucositis rates were comparable between the two arms, there was a higher rate of feeding tube dependence as well as sepsis in the combined arm. A similarly designed European trial was conducted in locally advanced HNSCC using low-dose (6 mg/m^2) daily cisplatin without a radiation dose reduction in the concurrent arm.[35] The results mirrored the Duke University study in that the addition of concurrent chemotherapy clearly improved outcome without significantly increased radiation-associated toxicity. In this trial, however, the improvement in overall survival (68% vs 49% at 2 years and 46% vs 25% at 5 years) was statistically significant ($p = .0075$).

While the Duke University and European studies aimed to assess the effect of chemotherapy added to hyperfractionated radiotherapy, the recently completed RTOG 01-29 study compared conventional fractionation versus hyperfractionation in patients receiving concurrent chemoradiotherapy. This phase III study was based upon RTOG 99-14, a single-arm phase II trial that established the feasibility of concurrent concomitant boost radiotherapy and cisplatin.[36] RTOG 01-29 randomized patients with selected stage III-IV SCC of the oral cavity, oropharynx,

larynx, or hypopharynx to conventionally fractionated radiotherapy (70 Gy in 35 fractions) and concurrent cisplatin (100 mg/m^2 on days 1, 22, and 43) versus concomitant boost radiation and the same chemotherapy (days 1 and 22 only). The eagerly anticipated results have not yet been published, although a successor trial, RTOG 05-22, has already opened and will compare concurrent chemoradiotherapy with or without cetuximab [an antibody to epidermal growth factor receptor (EGFR)] in the definitive setting. Notably, conventional fractionation will not be permitted in the RTOG 05-22 trial; investigators will be allowed to treat patients with either the concomitant boost approach as in RTOG 90-03 and RTOG 01-29, or IMRT with delivery of six treatments per week [www.astro.org]. The IMRT fractionation scheme is adapted from the Danish Head and Neck Cancer Study Group (DAHANCA), which published the results of a phase III trial in which patients with locally advanced HNSCC were randomized to 5 versus 6 weekly radiation treatments.[37] The total dose and dose per fraction were identical in the two arms; the only difference being the delivery of a second daily treatment once per week in the accelerated arm, that is, six total treatments per week as opposed to five. Patients with glottic primaries received radiotherapy alone, whereas those with nonglottic primaries also received the hypoxic radiosensitizer nimorazole. At 5 years, there was a statistically significant improvement in LRC (70% vs 60%, $p = .0005$), primary tumor control (76% vs 64%, $p = .001$), voice preservation (80% vs 68%, $p = .01$), and disease-specific survival (73% vs 66%, $p = .01$) in the accelerated arm.

MOLECULAR BIOLOGIC TARGETS

The understanding of cellular and molecular pathways responsible for tumorigenesis and malignant tumor behavior has grown exponentially in recent years. The cellular processes characteristic of all cancer cells were elegantly described by Hanahan and Weinberg in a seminal thesis to include: (1) autonomy in growth signaling, (2) evasion of apoptosis, (3) lack of responsiveness to growth inhibitory signaling, (4) limitless replication, (5) angiogenesis, and (6) invasion and metastasis.[38] In particular, the concepts of autonomy in growth signaling and angiogenesis have impelled intense research with subsequent development of clinically useful therapeutic agents that interfere with various growth-related signaling cascades.

The EGFR is a 170 kD membrane-spanning glycoprotein consisting of an extracellular ligand-binding domain, a transmembrane domain, and an intracellular cytoplasmic protein domain with tyrosine kinase activity.[39] EGFR is a member of the human epidermal receptor (HER) family of receptor tyrosine kinases, which includes EGFR (HER1, erbB1), HER2 (neu, erbB2), HER3 (erbB3), and HER4 (erbB4). The HER family responds to an assortment of growth factors to mediate various cell signaling pathways involved in growth and proliferation. EGFR is present in most epithelial tissues and is expressed in many solid tumors. Although there are six known ligands for EGFR, tumor growth factor-alpha (TGF-α) and EGF are the two thought to contribute most to malignant behavior.[40] Upon binding of ligand, the EGFR forms homo- or heterodimers with resultant autophosphorylation and receptor tyrosine kinase activity. This initiates intracellular signaling cascades involving multiple pathways including Ras/MAPK, phosphatidylinositol-3′-OH (PI3) kinase, and signal transduction and activator of transcription (STAT)-3 (Figure 7). In nonmalignant tissue, regulation of EGFR activity results in controlled growth and other vital cellular functions. In tumor, EGFR is either overexpressed or aberrant, for example, manifesting constitutively activated tyrosine kinase function, and contributes to the malignant phenotypic characteristics of proliferation, angiogenesis, metastasis, and evasion of apoptosis.

Agents that target EGFR are particularly appealing in HNSCC for several reasons. First, the expression of EGFR or other members of the erbB family is more prevalent in head and neck tumors than any other solid tumor (Table 2).[41] In fact, EGFR messenger RNA and protein are frequently overexpressed in dysplastic and even histologically normal head and neck mucosa in patients with HNSCC, insinuating a role in carcinogenesis.[42] Also, EGFR overexpression has been shown to be an independent poor prognos-

tic factor in HNSCC.[43] The correlation between EGFR expression and adverse outcome was first posited more than a decade ago, but subsequent early studies further evaluating the correlation yielded inconsistent results. More recently, Ang and colleagues reviewed tumor specimens from the RTOG 90-03 trial for EGFR expression via immunohistochemistry (IHC).[44] Although approximately 95% of specimens had detectable EGFR expression, there was a wide range to the degree of expression. Contrary to several previous studies, there was no apparent correlation between tumor stage, nodal stage, or stage grouping and the degree of EGFR expression. However, there was a striking correlation between high EGFR expression and poor disease-free and

overall survival independent of T and N stage. It is important to note that the examined specimens were limited to those patients randomized to the control, that is, conventionally fractionated, arm of the trial. Patterns of relapse were examined in the context of variable EGFR expression in the same study. While there was no apparent correlation with distant metastases, LRC was markedly diminished in patients with high EGFR expression. This is in keeping with preclinical data, which strongly suggests that high EGFR expression renders tumor cells radioresistant in cell culture and animal xenografts. Recent data presented at the American Society of Clinical Oncology (ASCO) 2006 meeting also suggested a strong trend ($p = .057$) toward decreased disease-free survival in HNSCC patients with high-polysomy or EGFR gene amplification by fluorescence in situ hybridization (FISH).[45] Hence, it appears that effecting EGFR inhibition has the potential to decrease tumor radioresistance and thereby improve outcomes in patients with HNSCC.

One manifestation of increased EGFR-associated radioresistance is the finding that patients with tumors demonstrating high level EGFR expression appear to benefit particularly from accelerated radiotherapy. Bentzen and colleagues retrospectively reviewed outcomes according to EGFR expression in a series of patients with HNSCC previously treated on a prospective randomized protocol comparing continuous hyperfractionated accelerated radiotherapy (CHART), in which patients are treated three times daily, with conventional once-daily fractionation.[46] Patients with relatively high EGFR expression (greater than the median for the study) had a statistically significant improvement in LRC in the CHART arm, whereas patients with relatively low EGFR expression did not seem to benefit from the accelerated course. A similar analysis was performed on the submitted tissue from three previous prospective trials conducted by the DAHANCA group in which patients with supraglottic larynx primaries were treated with definitive radiotherapy and a hypoxic radiosensitizer over 9.5, 6.5, or 5.5 weeks.[47] IHC staining for EGFR as well as E-cadherin was performed

Table 2 Epidermal Growth Factor Receptor (EGFR) Overexpression in Tumors. Note High Degree of Overexpression in Head and Neck Tumors Relative to Other Sites and Histologies. (Adapted from Reference 41.)

EGFR overexpression in tumors

Tumor type	Percentage of tumors overexpressing EGFR	Reference
Colon	25–77%	23,48
Head and neck	80–100%	23,51,52
Pancreatic	30–50%	23,53
Nonsmall cell lung carcinoma	40–80%	23,54–56
Breast	14–91%	57–60
Renal carcinoma	50–90%	23,61
Ovarian	35–70%	23
Glioma	40–63%	23
Bladder	31–48%	23

EGFR: epidermal growth factor receptor.

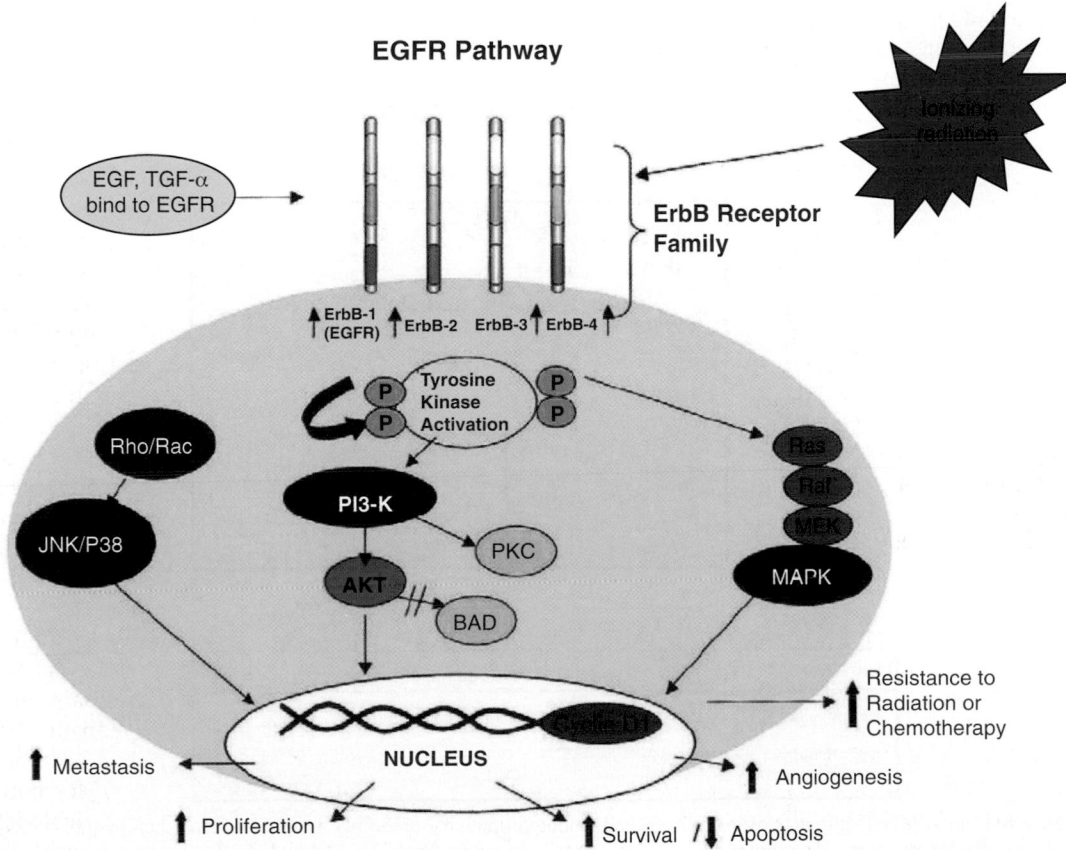

Figure 7 Possible mechanisms underlying responses to epidermal growth factor receptor (EGFR) inhibition.

on the submitted tissue. E-cadherin is a protein on the cellular membrane involved in cell–cell adhesion; decreased E-cadherin is postulated to diminish adhesion, promote tumor invasion and metastasis, and prevent terminal cell differentiation. Patients tumors with high EGFR and low E-cadherin expression were found to have better tumor control rates when treatment was accelerated over 5.5 weeks as opposed to 6.5 or 9 weeks.

The targeting of EGFR has led to a rapid expansion of clinical investigations in recent years evaluating the utility of this approach. There are several classes of molecular-targeted agents designed to arrest EGFR-mediated pathways. Monoclonal antibodies were among the first agents designed to inhibit EGFR activity. They achieve EGFR blockade by targeting the ligand-binding domain of the receptor. Cetuximab (C-225, Erbitux, ImClone Systems/Bristol Myers Squibb) is farthest along in clinical development in HNSCC, although a host of other agents are in phase I–III trials. The small-molecule tyrosine kinase inhibitors (TKIs) are another category of agents targeting EGFR. These quinazoline- or pyrimidine-based molecules interrupt the intracellular signal transduction cascade downstream of EGFR-ligand binding. Four general categories of small-molecule TKIs exist: reversible EGFR-specific, irreversible EGFR-specific, reversible pan-HER, and irreversible pan-HER. Two reversible EGFR-specific agents in particular, gefitinib (ZD1839, Iressa, Astra-Zeneca) and erlotinib (OSI 774, Tarceva, Genentech), have been the basis of several phase II and III clinical trials in multiple solid tumors. Novel categories of agents in earlier stages of clinical development include antisense oligonucleotides directed against EGFR mRNA and EGFR ligand-toxin or immunotoxin conjugates which pair an EGFR-tropic moiety with a cellular toxin.

A multitude of HNSCC clinical trials incorporating agents targeting EGFR have been conducted in the recent past or are currently underway, although relatively few results have been published at this time. As described above, EGFR expression clearly has prognostic value; however, its utility as a predictive marker for response to EGFR blockade is considerably murkier. Interestingly, the development of the acneiform rash frequently observed in patients receiving EGFR blockade appears to serve as a surrogate marker of response to EGFR inhibition.[48] Recent preclinical studies suggest that a transition from an epithelial to mesenchymal phenotype may also predict response to EGFR inhibitors.[49]

The results of a landmark trial affirming a role for EGFR inhibition in locally advanced HNSCC were recently reported.[50] This randomized multicenter trial enrolled 413 patients with stage III or IV (M0) SCC of the oropharynx, larynx, or hypopharynx to either definitive radiotherapy alone or radiotherapy plus weekly cetuximab. More than half of the enrolled patients had an oropharyngeal primary; approximately 75% had stage IV disease. The

radiotherapy was either conventional once-daily treatment, hyperfractionation with twice daily treatment throughout the course, or accelerated radiotherapy via concomitant boost. IMRT was not permissible, but the selection of one of the three regimens was at the treating physician's discretion. In the end, the majority (59%) of patients were treated with the concomitant boost approach. No patient received planned cytotoxic chemotherapy. In the combined modality arm, a cetuximab loading dose of 400 mg/m^2 was delivered 1 week prior to radiotherapy and weekly dosing was 250 mg/m^2 during concurrent treatment. The results revealed a significant improvement in LRC, progression-free survival, and overall survival in the radiotherapy plus cetuximab arm. The median duration of LRC was improved from 14.9 months in the radiotherapy alone arm to 24.4 months in the combined arm ($p = .005$). At a median follow-up of 54 months, overall survival was 49.0 months versus 29.3 months respectively in the combined modality and radiotherapy alone arms ($p = .03$) (Figure 8).[50] Progression-free survival was similarly improved. Moreover, the combined treatment was well tolerated with no significant difference in mucositis rates between the two arms, a result that starkly contrasts the markedly increased acute mucosal toxicity typical of concurrent chemoradiation. Patients in the combined arm frequently experienced the acneiform rash that is characteristic of EGFR blockade, but it rarely exceeded grade 2 in severity. Subgroup analysis suggested that patients with an orpharyngeal primary and those treated with hyperfractionation or concomitant boost treatment benefited the most from the addition of cetuximab. It is important to emphasize that the subgroup data should be interpreted cautiously since the trial was not powered for such analysis. Interestingly, the results in the combined arm compare favorably with previ-

ously published concurrent chemoradiotherapy data, although one obvious limitation of the trial was the absence of a chemoradiation arm. This will be addressed, in part, by the aforementioned RTOG 05-22 trial that will randomize patients in the definitive setting to chemoradiotherapy with or without cetuximab. A pilot study of concurrent radiotherapy, full-dose cisplatin, and cetuximab in the definitive setting was recently reported.[51] Previous phase I studies reinforced the safety of such a combination, but the study in question was stopped early because of adverse events, including two toxic deaths. Nevertheless, the outcomes were very encouraging from an efficacy standpoint with 3-year progression-free and overall survival rates of 56% and 75%, respectively.

Building upon the above work, preliminary reports of several trials combining radiotherapy, cytotoxic chemotherapy, and EGFR inhibition were presented at the 2006 ASCO meeting. A small series of patients treated with cisplatin, infusional 5-FU, and cetuximab (weeks 1, 4, and 7) alternating with radiotherapy and cetuximab (weeks 2 to 3, 5 to 6, and 8 to 10) was presented by Merlano and colleagues.[52] Kies and colleagues presented a series of 41 patients treated on a phase II protocol of induction cetuximab with paclitaxel and carboplatin prior to either surgery and postoperative radiotherapy, radiotherapy alone, or chemoradiotherapy depending on response.[53] A complete response to induction treatment was witnessed in 83% of patients, and no patient experienced less than a partial response. This regimen is also emblematic of the resurgent interest in exploring a role for induction treatment in organ preservation approaches to locally advanced HNSCC.

Progress in clinical trials utilizing small-molecule TKIs in locally advanced HNSCC is also evident in several recent presentations.

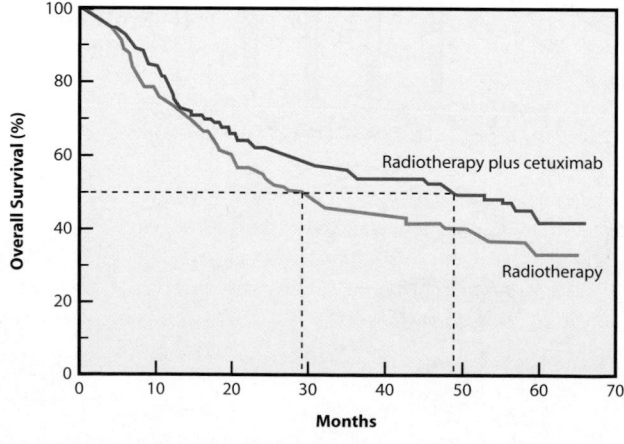

No. at Risk							
Radiotherapy	213	162	122	97	73	47	22
Radiotherapy plus cetuximab	211	177	136	116	98	61	24

Figure 8 Kaplan-Meier estimates of overall survival among all patients randomly assigned to radiotherapy plus cetuximab or radiotherapy alone. The dotted lines indicate median survival times. Hazard ratio for radiation plus cetuximab versus radiation alone was 0.74 (95% confidence interval, 0.57 to 0.97; $p = .03$). (Adapted from reference 50.)

Investigators from the Minnie Pearl Cancer Center reviewed initial results of their series of patients treated with induction gefitinib (250 mg per oral daily), taxotere, and carboplatin followed by concurrent radiotherapy, taxotere, and gefitinib.[54] Progression-free survival was 68% and overall survival was 86% at 1 year, without unexpected toxicity. A recently conducted multi-institutional phase II trial led by investigators at the University of Colorado Cancer Center randomized patients with locally advanced HNSCC in the definitive setting to concurrent radiotherapy, cisplatin, and either 250 mg daily gefitinib, 500 mg daily gefitinib, or placebo. The results have yet to be reported, although the trial has completed accrual. The use of pre- and post-concurrent erlotinib has also been explored in the definitive radiotherapy setting in two recently reported phase I trials.[55,56] Agents which target multiple receptors in the HER family are also in clinical development. One such agent, lapatanib (Tykerb), is a small-molecule TKI with activity against both EGFR and ErbB-2 (Her-2). A recent series of 17 patients treated in the definitive setting with radiotherapy, lapatanib, and cisplatin revealed the regimen to be well tolerated and will serve as the foundation for subsequent investigation.[57] Anti-angiogenesis approaches are also being investigated in view of the utility of bevacizumab (Avastin) in other disease sites. A recently reported feasibility trial consisting of every-other week radiotherapy with concurrent bevacizumab, hydroxyurea, and 5-FU demonstrated encouraging survival rates in high-risk patients, some of which were undergoing retreatment, and will be further pursued in a phase III setting.[58] Toxicity included a fatal esophageal tumor bed bleed and a fatal carotid artery rupture, underscoring the importance of proceeding cautiously with such a combination in a clinical trial setting.

The RTOG has also investigated the combination of chemoradiotherapy and EGFR blockade in the postoperative setting. RTOG 02-34, a two arm phase II trial, has nearly completed accrual of over 200 patients following surgery for locally advanced HNSCC with high-risk pathologic features including positive surgical margins, two or more involved lymph nodes, or evidence of ECE, that is, identical eligibility criteria as RTOG 95-01. All patients receive radiotherapy and concurrent cetuximab and are randomized to either concurrent weekly cisplatin or docetaxel. The results are eagerly anticipated and will form the basis for a future phase III trial.

ADDITIONAL PROGNOSTIC/PREDICTIVE MARKERS AND RADIOPROTECTORS IN HEAD AND NECK SQUAMOUS CELL CARCINOMA

Yet another avenue of research in HNSCC relates to the fairly recent recognition of human papillomavirus (HPV) as an etiologic factor in a subset of HNSCC. The number of identified HPV serotypes is in excess of one hundred, with multiple low-risk constituents, for example, 6 and 11, implicated in the development of benign oral hyperproliferative lesions such as papillomas and warts. High-risk HPV serotypes, for example, 16, 18, 31, and 35, on the other hand, are thought to contribute to the malignant transformation of head and neck epithelium, particularly in the oropharynx. Among the oncogenic serotypes, HPV16 is responsible for greater than 90% of all HPV-associated HNSCC.[59] Evidence to support the causal role of HPV in a subset of HNSCC abounds. Case-control studies demonstrate a markedly elevated odds-ratio for developing oropharyngeal SCC in those who are seropositive for high-risk HPV. Moreover, in HPV-positive tumors, the virus is integrated and transcriptionally active in the cell nuclei, whereas it is absent in adjacent normal tissue. High-risk HPV produces the oncoproteins E6 and E7, which render the tumor-suppressor genes p53 and pRb functionally inactive. Several epidemiologic and clinical features distinguish HPV-positive from HPV-negative HNSCC. The stereotypical patient with an HPV-positive tumor is a young male or female without a significant alcohol or tobacco history presenting with a poorly differentiated or basaloid SCC of the lingual or palatine tonsils. While it is highly unlikely that the typical risk factors for HNSCC are protective against the development of HPV-positive tumors, the data regarding the carcinogenic interplay of HPV and tobacco and alcohol are inconsistent, with some studies that suggest a synergism and others that do not. As is the case in cervix cancer, high-risk sexual behavior is believed to predispose patients to HPV-positive HNSCC. For the head and neck oncologist, the ramifications of the increased awareness of HPV-associated oropharyngeal cancer are numerous. First, the recognition of high-risk HPV in nodal biopsies of patients with occult primary disease clearly guides further diagnostic work-up and treatment toward the tonsillar region. Furthermore, the preponderance of data supports the notion that patients with HPV-positive tumors are ideal candidates for organ preservation in that HPV-positive tumors tend to be particularly radiosensitive. Finally, and most importantly, a vaccine approved by United States Food and Drug Administration against HPV16 exists and serves as a promising method of primary prevention of HPV-positive tumors at many sites. However, much additional time and research will be needed to assess its full role in that regard.

While a vast array of research aimed at improving patient outcomes in HNSCC has been conducted in recent decades, significant effort has also been undertaken to minimize treatment-associated toxicity. IMRT is a quantum leap forward in terms of preservation of salivary function. Preceding the conceptualization of IMRT by several decades was the notion that thiol-containing compounds could potentially lessen radiation-induced damage by way of free radical scavenging. The United States Army examined thousands of possible radioprotectors for military applications before recognizing amifostine (WR-2721, Ethyol, Medimmune Oncology) as the most promising agent, in part due to its tolerable side effect profile (primarily nausea, vomiting, and hypotension) and dense accumulation in epithelial tissue. Several small early trials suggested amelioration of mucosal and salivary gland toxicity in irradiated patients given amifostine. Additional investigation revealed apparent protection against cisplatin-induced nephrotoxicity. More recently, a randomized phase III trial of intravenous amifostine versus placebo was conducted in patients receiving radiotherapy for HNSCC.[60] Patients receiving amifostine experienced less acute and chronic xerostomia than those receiving placebo. Specifically, the grade 2 and higher acute xerostomia rates were 78% and 51% ($p < .0001$); chronic xerostomia rates were 57% and 34% respectively ($p = .002$). Mucositis rates were unchanged, and disease outcomes did not appear to differ, suggesting that the protection conferred by amifostine did not extend to mucosal tissue or, more importantly, the tumor.

A recent small randomized, placebo controlled phase III trial evaluating the role of L-alanyl-L-glutamine supports its nascent role in mucositis prevention in patients receiving head and neck radiotherapy.[61] Thirty-two patients undergoing chemoradiotherapy received either the IV drug or placebo; statistically significant reductions in mucositis, severe mucositis (greater than 4 and higher), pain scores, and feeding tube reliance were observed in the arm receiving the study drug. The results will likely provide the impetus for a larger confirmatory trial before L-alanyl-L-glutamine becomes a component of the radiation oncologist's armamentarium.

Another potentially protective agent generating interest is recombinant human keratinocyte-growth factor (palifermin). Palifermin is hypothesized to minimize the mucosal toxicity associated with radiotherapy by providing both a cellular growth stimulus as well as a direct cytoprotective effect. Preclinical data are strongly suggestive of a protective benefit, and there is an established role for palifermin in patients receiving stem-cell transplant conditioning regimens and other mucositis-inducing chemotherapeutic combinations. However, a previously conducted trial in patients receiving concurrent chemoradiation failed to demonstrate efficacy. Subsequent dose-response data led investigators to conclude that the lack of benefit derived from underdosing of the study drug. The RTOG is therefore conducting a phase III trial (RTOG 04-35) which randomizes patients undergoing chemoradiotherapy to either palifermin at the escalated dose (180 µg/kg weekly for up to eight doses) or placebo. A secondary endpoint will be disease outcome given concerns that administration of a growth factor during treatment will be counterproductive from the standpoint of tumor control, although such a finding has not been observed in previous preclinical or clinical experience with palifermin.

FUTURE DIRECTIONS

It is an exciting time to be a head and neck oncologist. HNSCC continues to pose an enormous challenge with immense room for improvement in terms of maximizing patient outcome while simultaneously minimizing treatment toxicity. However, practitioners cast an optimistic eye toward the development and selection of an ever-expanding array of targeted therapies which take aim at the myriad of cell pathways and processes that run amok in HNSCC. While the application of targeted therapies may in time lead to a sea change regarding the use of cytotoxic chemotherapy, its role today is primarily as an adjuvant to the hard-won concept of concurrent chemoradiation. New technologies such as IMRT and imaging modalities such as PET- and MRI-fusion will continue to be developed in an effort to deliver more accurate and less toxic radiotherapy. The optimal use of accelerated fractionation and hyperfractionation will be better understood as accrued trial data matures. Also, the resurgent interest in induction therapy prior to chemoradiotherapy holds promise and will be explored in ongoing and future trials.

REFERENCES

1. Del Regato JA. Radiological Oncologists: The Unfolding of a Medical Specialty. Reston, VA: Radiology Centennial Inc.; 1993. p. 1–2.
2. Hall EJ, Giaccia AJ. Dose response relationships for model normal tissues, Chapter 18. Radiobiology for the Radiologist, 6th edition. Philadelphia: Lippincott Williams & Wilkins; 2006. p. 303–26.
3. Hall EJ, Giaccia AJ. Model tumor systems, Chapter 20. Radiobiology for the Radiologist, 6th edition. Philadelphia: Lippincott Williams & Wilkins; 2006. p. 349–62.
4. Steel GG. Exploitable mechanisms in combined radiotherapy-chemotherapy: The concept of additivity. Int J Radiat Oncol Biol Phys 1979;5:85–91.
5. Wilson GD, Bentzen SM, Harari PM. Biologic basis for combining drugs with radiation. Semin Radiat Oncol 2006;16:2–9.
6. Davis MA, Tang HY, Maybaum J, et al. Dependence of fluorodeoxyuridine-mediated radiosensitization on S phase progression. Int J Radiat Oncol Biol Phys 1995;67:509–17.
7. Terasima T, Tolmach LJ. Changes in X-ray sensitivity of HeLa cells during the division cycle. Nature 1961;190:1210–1.
8. The Department of Veterans Affairs Laryngeal Cancer Study Group. Induction chemotherapy plus radiation compared with surgery plus radiation in patients with advanced laryngeal cancer. N Engl J Med 1991;324:1685–90.
9. Lefebvre J-L, Chevalier D, Luboinski B, et al. Larynx preservation in pyriform sinus cancer: Preliminary results of a European Organization for Research and Treatment of Cancer Phase III Trial. J Natl Cancer Inst 1996;88:890–9.
10. Forastiere AA, Goepfert H, Maor M, et al. Concurrent chemotherapy and radiotherapy for organ preservation in advanced laryngeal cancer. N Engl J Med 2003;349:2091–8.
11. Pignon JP, Bourhis J, Domenge C, et al. Chemotherapy added to locoregional treatment for head and neck squamous-cell carcinoma: Three meta-analyses of updated individual data. MACH-NC collaborative group. Meta-analysis of chemotherapy on head and neck cancer. Lancet 2000;355:949–55.
12. Stell PM, Rawson NS. Adjuvant chemotherapy in head and neck cancer. Br J Cancer 1990;61:779–87.
13. Munro AJ. An overview of randomized controlled trials of adjuvant chemotherapy in head and neck cancer. Br J Cancer 1995;71:83–91.
14. El-Sayed S, Nelson N. Adjuvant and adjunctive chemotherapy in the management of squamous cell carcinoma of the head and neck region. A meta-analysis of prospective and randomized trials. J Clin Oncol 1996;14:838–47.
15. Al-Sarraf M, LeBlanc M, Giri PG, et al. Chemoradiotherapy versus radiotherapy in patients with advanced nasopharyngeal cancer: Phase III randomized Intergroup study 0099. J Clin Oncol 1998;16:1310–7.
16. Cheng SH, Jian JJ, Tsai SYC, et al. Long-term survival of nasopharyngeal carcinoma following concomitant radiotherapy and chemotherapy. Int J Radiat Oncol Biol Phys 2000;48:1323–30.
17. Chan AT, Leung SF, Ngan RK, et al. Overall survival after concurrent cisplatin-radiotherapy compared with radiotherapy alone in locoregionally advanced nasopharyngeal carcinoma. J Natl Cancer Inst 2005;97:536–9.
18. Denis F, Garaud P, Bardet E, et al. Final results of the 94–01 French Head and Neck Oncology and Radiotherapy Group randomized trial comparing radiotherapy alone with concomitant radiochemotherapy in advanced-stage oropharynx carcinoma. J Clin Oncol 2004;22:69–76.
19. Fu KK, Phillips TL, Silverberg IJ, et al. Combined radiotherapy and chemotherapy with bleomycin and methotrexate for advanced inoperable head and neck cancer: Update of a Northern California oncology group randomized trial. J Clin Oncol 1987;5:1410–18.
20. Garden AS, Harris J, Vokes EE, et al. Preliminary results of radiation therapy oncology group 97–03: A randomized phase ii trial of concurrent radiation and chemotherapy for advanced squamous cell carcinomas of the head and neck. J Clin Oncol 2004;22:2856–64.
21. Cooper JS, Pajak TF, Forastiere AA, et al. Postoperative concurrent radiotherapy and chemotherapy for high-risk squamous-cell carcinoma of the head and neck. N Engl J Med 2004;350:1937–44.
22. Bernier J, Domenge C, Ozsahin M, et al. Postoperative irradiation with or without concomitant chemotherapy for locally advanced head and neck cancer. N Engl J Med 2004;350:1945–52.
23. Bernier J, Cooper JS, Pajak TF, et al. Defining risk levels in locally advanced head and neck cancers: A comparative analysis of concurrent postoperative radiation plus chemotherapy trials of the EORTC (#22931) and RTOG (# 9501). Head Neck 2005;27:843–50.
24. Ang KK, Trotti A, Brown BW, et al. Randomized trial addressing risk features and time factors of surgery plus radiotherapy in advanced head-and-neck cancer. Int J Radiat Oncol Biol Phys 2001;51:571–8.
25. Domenge C, Hill C, Lefebvre JC, et al. Randomized trial of neoadjuvant chemotherapy in oropharyngeal carcinoma. GETTEC. Br J Cancer 2000;83:1594–8.
26. Vermorken J, Remenar E, van Herpen C, et al. Standard cisplatin/infusional 5-fluorouracil (PF) vs docetaxel (T) plus PF (TPF) as neoadjuvant chemotherapy for nonresectable locally advanced squamous cell carcinoma of the head and neck (LA-SCCHN): A phase III trial of the EORTC Head and Neck Cancer Group (EORTC #24971) (abstr 5508). Proc Am Soc Clin Oncol 2004;22:490.
27. Hitt R, Lopez-Pousa A, Rodriguez M, et al. Phase III study comparing cisplatin (P) and 5-fluorouracil (F) versus P,F and paclitaxel (T) as induction therapy in locally advanced head & neck cancer (LAHNC) (abst 1997). Proc Am Soc Clin Oncol 2003;22:496.
28. Gibson MK, Forastiere AA. Reassessment of the role of induction chemotherapy for head and neck cancer. Lancet Oncol 2006;7:565–74.
29. Robbins KT, Kumar P, Wong FSH, et al. Targeted chemoradiation for advanced head and neck cancer: Analysis of 213 patients. Head Neck 2000;22:687–93.
30. Spring PM, Valentino J, Arnold SM, et al. Long-term results of hyperfractionated radiation and high-dose intraarterial cisplatin for unresectable oropharyngeal carcinoma. Cancer 2005;104:1765–71.
31. Robbins KT, Kumar P, Harris J, et al. Supradose intra-arterial cisplatin and concurrent radiation therapy for the treatment of stage IV head and neck squamous cell carcinoma is feasible and efficacious in a multi-institutional setting: Results of radiation therapy oncology group trial 9615. J Clin Oncol 2005;23:1447–54.
32. Withers HR, Taylor JM, Maciejewski B. The hazard of accelerated tumor clonogen repopulation during radiotherapy. Acta Oncol 1988;27:131–46.
33. Fu KK, Pajak TF, Trotti A, et al. A Radiation Therapy Oncology Group (RTOG) phase III randomized study to compare hyperfractionation and two variants of accelerated fractionation to standard fractionation radiotherapy for head and neck squamous cell carcinomas: First report of RTOG 9003. Int J Radiat Oncol Biol Phys 2000;48:7–16.
34. Brizel DM, Albers ME, Fisher SR. Hyperfractionated irradiation with or without concurrent chemotherapy for locally advanced head and neck cancer. N Engl J Med 1998;338:1798–804.
35. Jeremic B, Shibamoto Y, Milicic B, et al. Hyperfractionated radiation therapy with or without concurrent low-dose daily cisplatin in locally advanced squamous cell carcinoma of the head and neck: A prospective randomized trial. J Clin Oncol 2000;18:1458–64.
36. Ang KK, Harris J, Garden AS, et al. Concomitant boost radiation plus concurrent cisplatin for advanced head and neck carcinomas: Radiation therapy oncology group phase II trial 99-14. J Clin Oncol 2005;23:3008–15.
37. Overgaard J, Hansen HS, Specht L, et al. Five compared with six fractions per week of conventional radiotherapy of squamous-cell carcinoma of head and neck: DAHANCA 6 and 7 randomised controlled trial. Lancet 2003;362:933–40.
38. Hanahan D, Weinberg RA. The hallmarks of cancer. Cell 2000;100:57–70.
39. Carpenter G. Receptors for epidermal growth factor and other polypeptide mitogens. Annu Rev Biochem 1987;56:881–914.
40. Laskin JJ, Sandler AB. Epidermal growth factor receptor: A promising target in solid tumours. Cancer Treat Rev 2004;30:1–17.
41. Herbst RS, Shin DM. Monoclonal antibodies to target epidermal growth factor receptor-positive tumors. Cancer 2002;94:1593–1611.
42. Raben D, Biano C, Milas L, et al. Targeted therapies and radiation for the treatment of had and neck cancer: Are we making progress? Semin Radiat Oncol 2004;14:139–52.
43. Rubin Grandis J, Melhem MF, Gooding WE, et al. Levels of TGF-alpha and EGFR protein in head and neck squamous cell carcinoma and patient survival. J Natl Cancer Inst 1998;90:824–32.
44. Ang KK, Berkey BA, Tu X, et al. Impact of epidermal growth factor receptor expression on survival and pattern of relapse in patients with advanced head and neck carcinoma. Cancer Res 2002;62:7350–6.
45. Chung CH, Ely K, Carter J, et al. High gene copy number of epidermal growth factor receptor by fluorescence in situ hybridization is frequent in head and neck squamous cell carcinomas and associates with worse recurrence-free survival. J Clin Oncol (ASCO Ann Mtg Proc, Part I) 2006;5502.
46. Bentzen SM, Atasoy BM, Daley FM, et al. Epidermal growth factor receptor expression in pretreatment biopsies from head and neck squamous cell carcinoma as a predictive factor for a benefit from accelerated radiation therapy in a randomized controlled trial. J Clin Oncol 2005;23:5560–7.
47. Eriksen JG, Steiniche T, Overgaard J, et al. The role of epidermal growth factor receptor and E-cadherin for the outcome of reduction in the overall treatment time of radiotherapy of supraglottic larynx squamous cell carcinoma. Acta Oncol 2005;44:50–8.
48. Perez-Soler R, Saltz L. Cutaneous adversed effects with HER1/EGFR-Targeted agents: Is there a silver lining? J Clin Oncol 2005;23:5235–46.
49. Thomson S, Buck E, Petti F, et al. Epithelial to mesenchymal transition is a determinant of sensitivity of non-small-cell lung carcinoma cell lines and xenografts to epidermal growth factor receptor inhibition. Cancer Res 2005;65:9455–62.
50. Bonner JA, Harari PM, Giralt J, et al. Radiotherapy plus cetuximab for squamous-cell carcinoma of the head and neck. N Eng J Med 2006;354:567–78.
51. Pfister DG, Su YB, Kraus DH, et al. Concurrent cetuximab, cisplatin, and concomitant boost radiotherapy for locoregionally advanced, squamous cell head and neck cancer: A pilot phase II study of a new combined-modality paradigm. J Clin Oncol 2006;24:1072–8.
52. Merlano MC, Numico G, Colantonio I, et al. AlteRCC phase I-II trial: Alternating radiotherapy and chemotherapy plus cetuximab in advanced head and neck cancer (HNC). J Clin Oncol (ASCO Ann Mtg Proc, Part I) 2006;15515.
53. Kies MS, Garden AS, Holsinger C, et al. Induction chemotherapy (CT) with weekly paclitaxel, carboplatin, and cetuximab for squamous cell carcinoma of the head and neck (HN). J Clin Oncol (ASCO Ann Mtg Proc, Part I) 2006:5520.
54. Doss HH, Greco FA, Meluch AA, et al. Induction chemotherapy + gefitinib followed by concurrent chemotherapy/radiation therapy/gefitinib for patients (pts) with locally advanced squamous carcinoma of the head and neck: A phase I/II trial of the Minnie Pearl Cancer Research Network. J Clin Oncol (ASCO Ann Mtg Proc, Part I) 2006:5543.
55. Savvides P, Agarwala SS, Greskovich J, et al. Phase I study of the EGFR tyrosine kinase inhibitor erlotinib in combination with docetaxel and radiation in locally advanced squamous cell cancer of the head and neck (SCCHN). J Clin Oncol (ASCO Ann Mtg Proc, Part I) 2006;5545.
56. Herchenhorn D, Dias FL, Ferreira CG, et al. Phase I/II study of erlotinib combined with cisplatin and radiotherapy for

locally advanced squamous cell carcinoma of the head and neck (SCCHN). J Clin Oncol (ASCO Ann Mtg Proc, Part I) 2006;5575.

57. Harrington KJ, Bourhis J, Nutting CM, et al. A phase I, open-label study of lapatinib plus chemoradiation in patients with locally advanced squamous cell carcinoma of the head and neck (SCCHN). J Clin Oncol (ASCO Ann Mtg Proc, Part I) 2006;5553.

58. Seiwert TY, Haraf J, Cohen EE, et al. A phase I study of bevacizumab (B) with fluorouracil (F) and hydroxyurea (H) with concomitant radiotherapy (X) (B-FHX) for poor prognosis head and neck cancer (HNC). J Clin Oncol (ASCO Ann Mtg Proc, Part I) 2006;245:530.

59. Fakhry C, Gillison ML. Clinical implications of human papillomavirus in head and neck cancers. J Clin Oncol 2006;24:2606–11.

60. Brizel DM, Wasserman TH, Henke M, et al. Phase III randomized trial of amifostine as a radioprotector in head and neck cancer. J Clin Oncol 2000;18:3339–45.

61. Cerchietti LG, Navigante AH, Lutteral MA, et al. Double-blinded, placebo-controlled trial on intravenous L-alanyl-L-glutamine in the incidence of oral mucositis following chemoradiotherapy in patients with head-and-neck cancer. Int J Radiat Oncol Biol Phys 2006;65:1330–7.

93

Immunotherapy for Head and Neck Cancer

Andrei I. Chapoval, PhD
Dan H. Schulze, PhD
Scott E. Strome, MD

The term head and neck cancer embraces all malignances that arise in the head or neck region (in the skin, nasal cavity, sinuses, lip, mouth, salivary glands, throat, larynx lymph nodes, or thyroid gland). According to recent National Cancer Institute estimates that there will be 40,500 newly diagnosed head and neck cancer cases and approximately 11,000 deaths in 2006 in the United States,[1] and approximately 900,000 new cases and 240,000 deaths worldwide. Squamous cell carcinoma (SCC) represents more than 90% of all head and neck tumors. Standard therapy for advanced head and neck squamous cell carcinoma (HNSCC) includes surgery, radiotherapy, and chemotherapy. Despite available treatment options, disease recurs locally in about 40% of the cases and nearly 25% of patients develop distant metastases. Both successful surgical and medical therapy of HNSCC can result in severe cosmetic, speech, and swallowing defects, which negatively impact quality of life. Hence, the development of alternative therapies capable of improving disease-free survival and eliminating tumors not suitable for organ-sparing approaches are warranted.

Based on promising new data in both HNSCC and other histological tumor types, the possibility of developing immunotherapeutic approaches as a treatment option for HNSCC has gained interest. For example, adaptive transfer of native or genetically modified tumor-specific T lymphocytes is an effective approach to treat metastatic, immunogenic melanoma.[2,3] Moreover, it is well documented that infiltration of head and neck tumors with T lymphocytes and/or natural killer (NK) cells correlated with both better locoregional control and a longer survival rate of head and neck cancer patients.[4,5] It has also been reported that regression of HNSCC in mice can be induced by activated T lymphocytes.[6] In addition, spontaneous regression of head and neck tumors was observed in humans,[7] suggesting that this is an immune mediated process.[8] Therefore, it is conceivable that the immune system could potentially control head and neck cancer development, and immunotherapy may be effective for the treatment of patients with HNSCC. Cellular-based therapies provide unique tumor specificity, the ability to detect and destroy micrometastases, and the potential to develop prolonged antitumor memory. In this chapter, we discuss current developments in human head and neck cancer immunotherapy including: passive immunotherapy (antibody based and adoptive T-cell transfer) and active immunotherapy [dendritic cells (DCs) based vaccine, cytokine immunotherapy and costimulation-based immunotherapy].

MECHANISTIC GOAL OF CANCER IMMUNOTHERAPY

The primary goal of cancer immunotherapy is to utilize the effector mechanisms of immunity to detect and destroy tumor targets. This can be achieved in two ways: by passive transfer of antitumor effectors generated *in vitro* or by inducing an antitumor immune response *in vivo* utilizing various vaccine approaches. Both methods have been tested in animal models and in patients with HNSCC with varied degrees of success.

Passive cancer immunotherapy can be logically divided into two categories: antibody-based immunotherapy and cell-transfer therapy. Antibody-based cancer immunotherapy became a reality after the development of techniques which made possible production large quantities of antigen specific antibodies (Abs).[9] The basic premise of Abs-based immunotherapy is that tumor cells express on their surface antigens (Ags) that distinguish them from normal cells. Abs can specifically bind to tumor Ags, triggering multiple immune responses that result in tumor cell lysis.

Cell-transfer therapy relies on expanding autologous tumor-reactive killer CD8+ T lymphocyte populations *in vitro* to large cell numbers for injection back into the patient. CD8+ T lymphocytes are routinely expanded in the presence of anti-CD3 monoclonal antibodies, which act as surrogate Ags, and interleukin-2 (IL-2), a T-cell growth factor. The target tumor Ag for this method of immunotherapy should be a processed protein presented by human leukocyte antigen (HLA), also known as major histocompatibility complex (MHC) protein. In contrast to Abs that react only with Ag expressed on the tumor cell surface, T lymphocytes can recognize processed Ag expressed inside or on the surface of tumor cells.

The term active cancer immunotherapy combines various vaccine approaches including the utilization of peptide vaccine, dendritic cell vaccines, costimulation-based therapy, and cytokine therapy. These methods seek to boost the patient's own immune response against cancer *in vivo*. Many of the vaccine approaches that are currently being investigated for the treatment of cancer seek to optimize the activation of T-cells that can specifically recognize tumor Ags presented in the context of HLA (MHC) molecules resulting in the eliminating of Ag positive tumor cells *in vivo*. Recent advances in immunology bring additional optimism for the development of more effective antitumor vaccines for treatment of head and neck cancer.

CHALLENGES FOR IMMUNOTHERAPY OF HEAD AND NECK CANCER

One of the major challenges of HNSCC immunotherapy is the impaired immune response in patients with HNSCC and the ability of HNSCC to avoid immune surveillance. Detailed mechanisms of immunosupression in patients with HNSCC are described in Chapter 88, "Mechanisms of Immune Evasion of Head and Neck Cancer." Here, we briefly outline possible mechanisms that permit HNSCC to avoid immune responses. It has been demonstrated that HNSCC cells completely or partially lose expression of HLA (MHC) molecules that makes this malignancy virtually invisible to T lymphocytes. Another mechanism by which HNSCC cells can circumvent immune responses is by expressing Fas ligand, which can destroy T-cells that attack neoplasms. Additionally, HNSCC can also inhibit immune cell function by producing inhibitory factors such as tumor growth factor beta (TGF-β) and IL-10.

PASSIVE IMMUNOTHERAPY OF HEAD AND NECK CANCER

Antibody-Based Immunotherapy

Monoclonal antibodies (mAb) which specifically bind to tumor surface antigens may result in tumor cell death by the following mechanisms: (1) antibody dependent cellular cytotoxicity

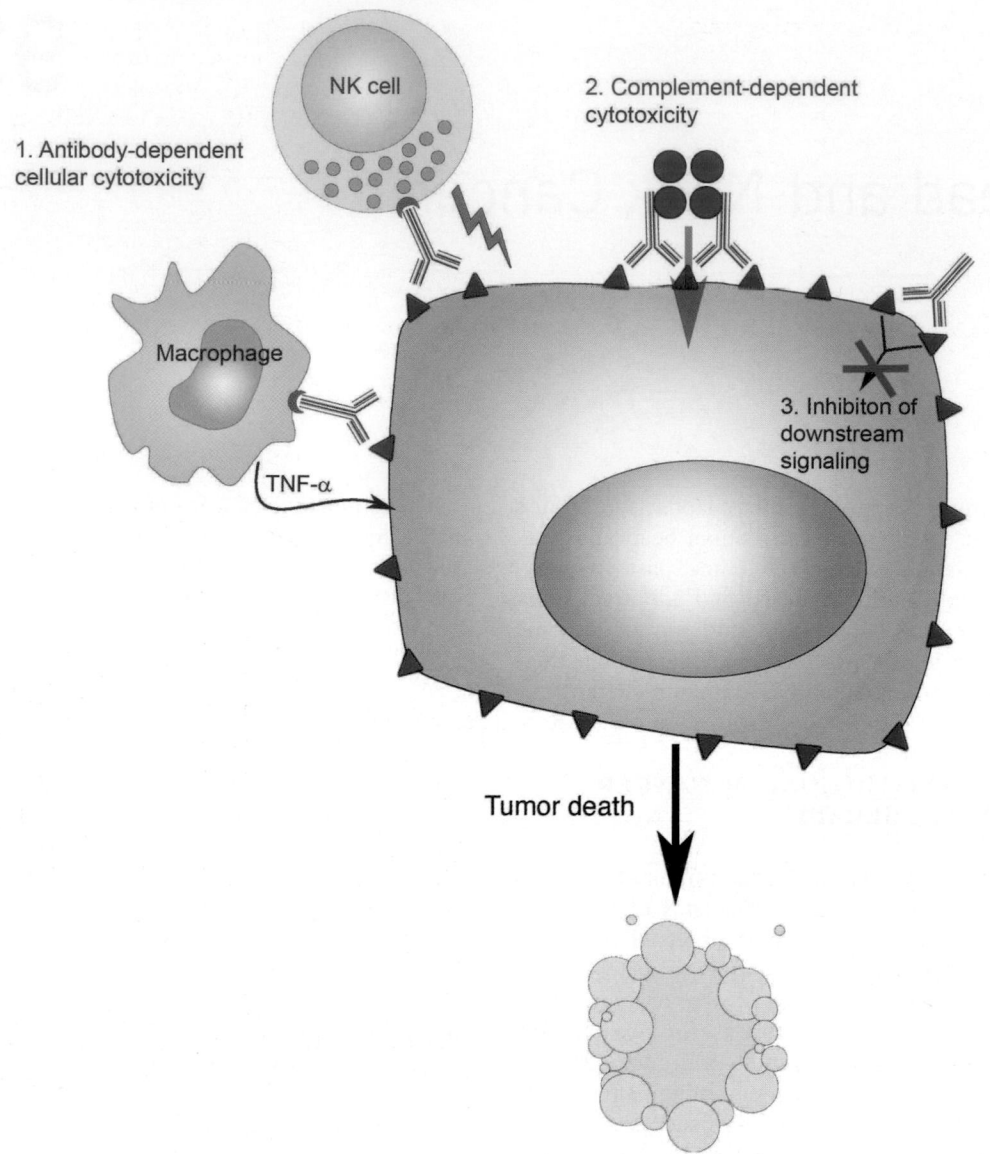

Figure 1 Mechanisms of antibody-based immunotherapy. Tumor-specific antibodies can kill tumor cells by (1) inducing antibody-dependent cellular cytotoxicity of natural killer cells and macrophages expressing Fc receptors, (2) complement-mediated lysis, (3) directly by inhibiting signaling of growth factor receptors.

(ADCC) mediated by NK cells or macrophages; (2) activation of the complement system; and (3) blocking the receptors that are essential for proliferation and survival of tumor cells (Figure 1).

Cancer cells often express developmental antigens that are not normally seen on mature cell types. For example, Her-2/neu, a protein proto-oncogene, was shown to be overexpressed on various types of cancer including squamous cell carcinoma. *In vitro* studies with human HNSCC cell lines showed that combined treatment with anti-Her-2 mAb and irradiation inhibited proliferation of Her-2 expressing HNSCC lines.[10] The results of other recent studies indicate that mAb specific for Her-2 can induce ADCC of Her-2 expressing SCC cell lines.[11] While it was shown that anti-Her-2 mAb were effective in treatment of patients with breast cancer,[12] this approach has not been tested in patients with HNSCC.

Another promising antibody target for HNSCC immunotherapy may be CD44, a cell adhesion molecule. While CD44 is widely expressed in normal tissues, the expression of an abnormal CD44 variant 6 (CD44v6) has been

related to aggressive behavior of various tumor types and was shown to be elevated on the cell surface of HNSCC.[13] The therapeutic potential of anti-CD44v6 mAb was confirmed in nude mice bearing human HNSCC xenografts.[13] Radiolabeled mAb directed against the CD44v6 antigen provided promising antitumor effects in phase I trials in patients with inoperable HNSCC.[14,15]

The epidermal growth factor receptor (EGFR) is expressed on the majority of, if not all, HNSCCs,[16] which makes it an ideal target for Ab-based immunotherapy. Cetuximab is a human-murine chimeric monoclonal Ab that binds to the extracellular domain of EGFR and is currently used for the treatment of patients with locally advanced HNSCC. Cetuximab is an example of an Ab that blocks signaling through the receptor essential for survival and proliferation of tumor cells (see Figure 1, Step 3). Binding EGFR to its ligand TGF-α induces a signaling cascade that results in tumor cell growth, invasion, angiogenesis, and metastases. Cetuximab blocks the interaction of EGFR with TGF-α and that prevents tumor pathogeneseis. In a Phase III clinical trial,

117 patients with advanced head and neck cancer treated with cisplatin plus cetuximab demonstrated an improved response rate when compared to those that were treated with cisplatin alone.[17] But treatment with cisplatin plus cetuximab did not significantly improve survival. A separate randomized study (involving 424 patients) comparing radiotherapy alone with radiotherapy plus cetuximab demonstrated that radiation plus antibody is superior to radiotherapy alone, increasing both the duration of locoregional disease control and survival.[18] These data suggest that cetuximab mAb in combination with radiotherapy can be used for treatment of patients with NHSCC, however, additional studies are required to improve the therapeutic efficacy of cetuximab combined with radio- or chemotherapy.

Recently, it was found that 42% of HNSCCs express a mutant form of EGFR (EGFRvIII) that results in ligand-independent activation of EGFR signaling pathway that causes tumor growth. This observation may explain the limited clinical response to EGFR-targeted therapy and suggest that the antitumor efficacy of EGFR targeting strategies may be enhanced by the addition of EGFRvIII-specific blockade.[19]

Additionally, the immunoglobulin Fc receptor polymorphism should be taken into consideration when Ab treatment is used for HNSCC immunotherapy. It was shown that the differential affinity for the IgG binding of polymorphic alleles of the human Fc receptor can influence the effectiveness of antibody immunotherapy. For example, in human Fc Gamma R IIIA (CD16) having a valine at 158 amino acid position binds to antibody better than CD16 having phenylalanine at the same position. This polymorphism was associated with a reduced response in patients with B cell malignancies treated with rituximab, an anti-CD20 human IgG1 mAb.[20] Similarly, a polymorphic change from histidine to arginine at amino acid position 131 of the human Fc Gamma R IIa (CD32) results in reduced IgG binding affinity and therapeutic effectiveness of neuroblastoma treatment with anti-GD2 antibody.[21] These results may be explained by variable ability of NK cells and macrophages expressing polymorphic variants of Fc receptors to bind to Ab and mediate ADCC.

Alternative methods for Ab-based immunotherapy include the use of recombinant bispecific Ab which can recognize a T-cell co-receptor like CD3 and tumor-associated antigens, for example, carcinoembryonic antigen (CEA), pan-epithelial homotypic cell adhesion molecule (EpCAM), HER2/neu, CD19, resulting in selective retargeting of cytotoxic T lymphocytes (CTLs) to tumor cells and the induction of cytotoxic effects. Such bispecific Ab represent a way to arm unique tumor specificity to the CTLs. A bispecific Ab that retarget CD3+ T lymphocytes to tumor cells expressing EpCAM membrane protein were shown to kill SCC *in vitro* experiments.[22]

Adoptive T-Cell Transfer

In general, adoptive T-cell transfer is accomplished by harvesting cells from the peripheral

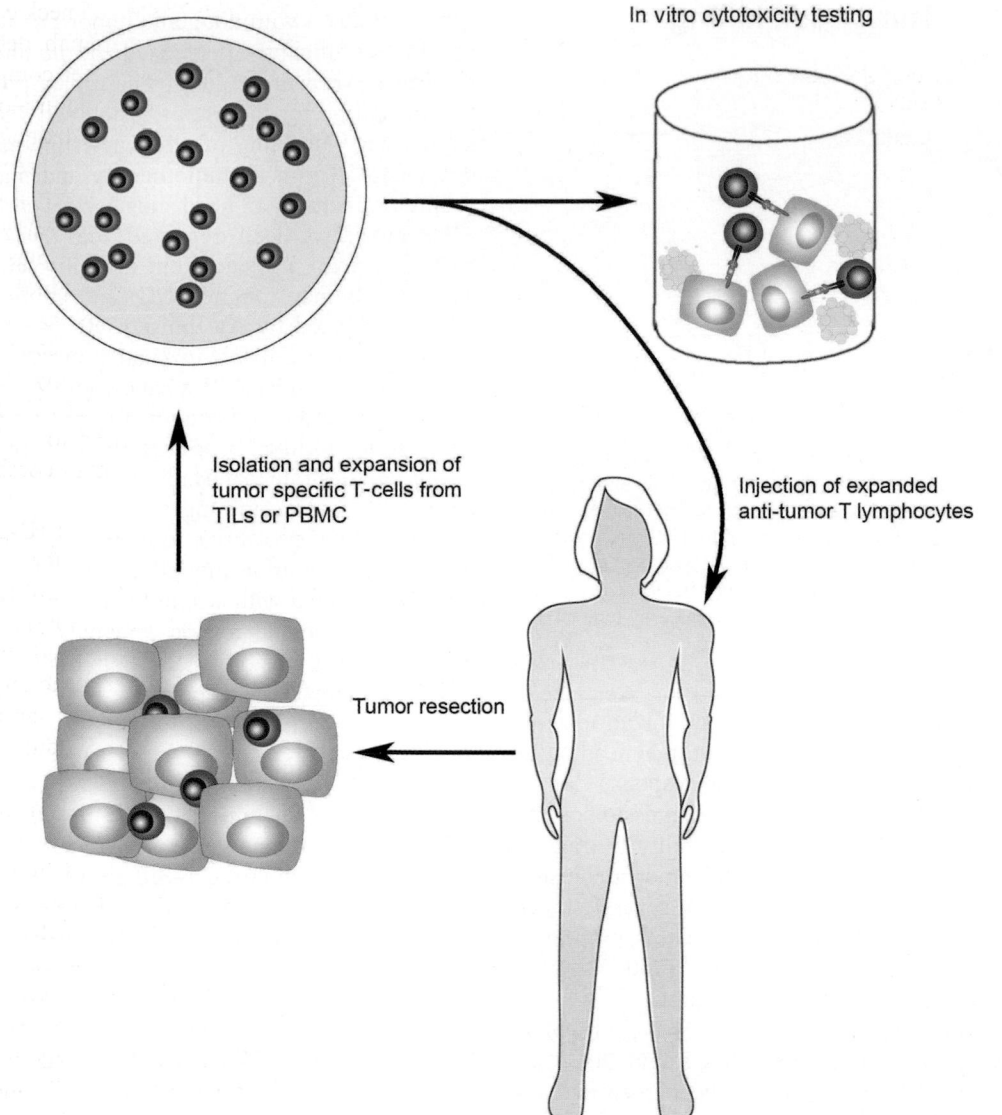

In vitro cytotoxicity testing

Isolation and expansion of
tumor specific T-cells from
TILs or PBMC

Injection of expanded
anti-tumor T lymphocytes

Tumor resection

Figure 2 Adoptive T-cell transfer. Tumor-specific T-cells can be isolated from tumor-infiltrating lymphocytes (TILs) or peripheral blood mononuclear cells (PBMCs) of patients with cancer. Isolated T-cells are then expanded using high doses of IL-2. The cells are successively selected for their ability to kill autologous or allogenic HLA-matched tumor cell lines. Tumor reactivity of expanded cells is validated before adoptive transfer.

blood, tumor sites, or draining lymph nodes of the patient. Then depending on the application and technology, effector cells expanded in a specific or nonspecific fashion are infused back into the tumor-bearing host (Figure 2).

The benefits of adoptive T-cell transfer immunotherapy are best seen in treatment of patients with melanoma.[23] However, a single clinical trial that involved only 6 HNSCC patients showed no clinical response to adoptively transferred T lymphocytes.[24] In these studies, T lymphocytes obtained from primary draining lymph nodes after immunization with autologous tumor cells were activated and expanded *in vitro* using an anti-CD3/IL-2 protocol. Anti-CD3-activated vaccine-primed T lymphocytes secreted elevated levels of interferon-gamma (IFN-γ) and granulocyte-macrophage colony-stiumlating factor (GM-CSF) in response to autologous tumor cells but not to allogenic (antigenically distinct) tumors, suggesting tumor specific immune response. These cells were then infused back into the patient with the concomitant administration of IL-2. Though no significant clinical response was observed,

these studies indicate that immune response can be achieved in head and cancer patients who are believed to be severely immunosuppressed. In another clinical trial 15 patients with unresectable squamous cell carcinoma of the head and neck were successfully treated with T-cell immunotherapy.[25] These studies demonstrated that adoptive immunotherapy is a technically feasible and safe treatment with low toxicity and may provide therapeutic activity in patients with unresectable HNSCC.

Oncogenic human papillomavirus (HPV) has been shown to be a risk factor for development of HNSCC. HPV infection has been detected in approximately 30% of SCCs located in all head and neck sites. HPV infection promotes p53 degradation that disrupts the tumor suppressor function of p53 and may result in tumor development. HPV infected tumor cells express highly immunogenic viral proteins. Immunization of patients with cervical carcinoma, a disease more frequently associated with HPV, with HPV derived peptides were shown to induce a significant antitumor immune response. Methods

for rapid enrichment of HPV-specific polyclonal T-cell populations for adoptive immunotherapy of cervical cancer are described.[26] Recently, it was shown that HPV-specific T-cells derived from peripheral blood mononuclear cells (PBMC) of patients with oropharyngeal and laryngeal HNSCC were able to recognize and kill HPV+ SCC cells.[27] It is conceivable that HPV-specific T lymphocytes can be used for adoptive T-cell therapy of HNSCC. This will require strict selection criteria for patients eligible for HPV therapy which should include the type of HPV infection and MHC haplotype of HNSCC patients.

ACTIVE IMMUNOTHERAPY OF HEAD AND NECK CANCER

The goal of active immunotherapy is to generate antitumor T-cell responses in patients with cancer *in vivo* through the development of potent antitumor vaccines. Tumor antigens are a prerequisite for non–cell-based cancer vaccine immunotherapy. So far, over 1,000 different tumor Ags including Mart-1, gp100, and NY-ESO-1 have been identified, mainly from melanoma. Tumor associated Ags can be divided into several groups: tumor-specific Ags (usually viral Ags), differentiation Ags [cancer-testis (CT) Ags], mutated normal proteins (β-catenin, caspase 8, mutated p53) and Ags overexpressed by tumors (ERb2b, p53). Based on the evidence of tumor specific Ags, existing experimental and clinical cancer vaccine follow two general directions: (1) immunization with unique identified tumor Ags; or (2) use of undefined tumor-derived products (Figure 3).

Peptide-Based Antitumor Vaccine

The recent identification of tumor-associated antigens, presented as peptides in the context of appropriate HLA molecules, which are targeted by antitumor CTL has opened the way to cancer vaccine utilizing peptide epitopes for stimulation the tumor-specific CTL. Many HNSCC express mutated or overexpress wild type p53 (wt-p53), a protein involved in cell-cycle regulation and in apoptosis. A number of investigators have identified a subset of T lymphocytes in peripheral blood of patients with HNSCC which are able to recognize and lyse HNSCC cell lines over expressing p53.[28,29] These results led to the development of preclinical models that demonstrated efficacy in tumor rejection in mice immunized with DCs pulsed wt-p53 peptide.[30] Based on the encouraging preclinical data, a Phase I study utilizing DCs pulsed with wt-p53 was initiated at the University of Pittsburgh for treatment HNSCC patients. In the final part of this study, patients will be immunized with HLA A*0201-restricted wt-p53 peptides loaded onto autologous, mature DCs. The study is designed to monitor the immunological status and observe tumor response in subjects after vaccine administration. As mentioned above, nearly 30% of head and neck tumors are associated with HPV infection which results in p53

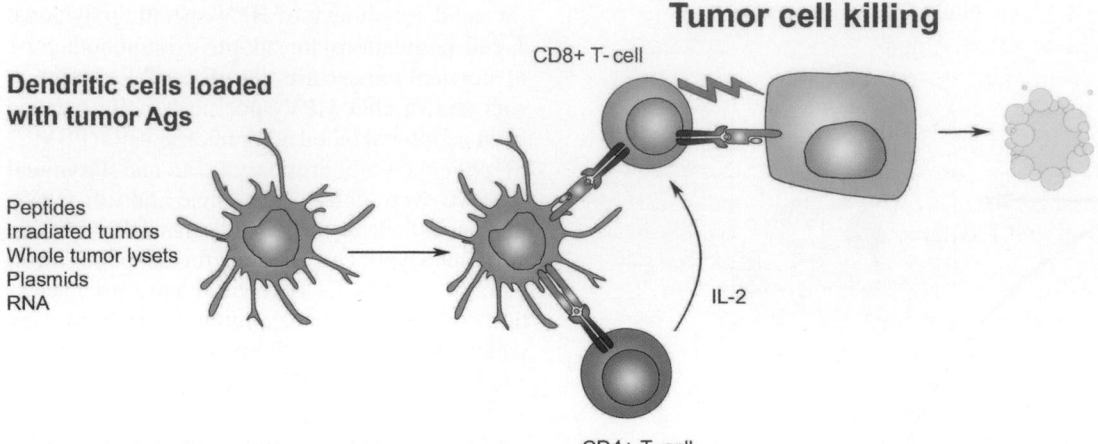

Tumor cell killing

Figure 3 Antitumor vaccines. Dendritic cells (DCs) can be loaded with various tumor Ags (peptide, whole tumor lysets, plasmids encoding tumor Ag, and tumor-derived RNA) *in vitro*. Alternatively, Ags can be injected into patients with cancer in formulation providing favorable condition for Ags uptake by DCs. Ags are processed by DCs and presented in the context of HLA class I for CD8+ killer T lymphocytes or HLA class II for CD4+ helper T lymphocytes. CD4+ helper T lymphocyte secrete cytokines, for example, IL-2, that are necessary for optimal activation of CD8+ killer T-cell. Activated CD8+ killer T lymphocytes migrate to tumor site where they recognize tumor Ags presented by tumor HLA class I molecules and kill malignant cells.

degradation. Therefore, it is conceivable that p53 negative tumors from HPV positive patients may not respond to p53 vaccine treatment. As an alternative, it is possible to supplement p53 vaccine with HPV-derived peptides to induce immune response to HPV Ags in p53-negative tumors.[27]

We have recently identified that HNSCCs express significant levels of MAGE-A1 and MAGE-A3 Ags which are CT Ags from multiple myeloma cells and have also been found in a variety of other cancers, including melanoma and renal cell carcinoma.[31] MAGE-3 peptide-based vaccine was used for treatment of melanoma, however, a single peptide vaccine has shown only limited therapeutic responses.[32] One of the promising approaches of peptide-based cancer immunotherapy is a "Trojan" peptide vaccine that allows the use of multiple T-cell epitopes in a single construct. Recently several investigators, including our research team, have identified a high prevalence of MAGE-A3 and HPV 16 on HNSCC and characterized several putative cytolytic and helper epitopes.[31] Additionally, we have developed a novel method to enhance the immune response to therapeutic peptide vaccines using "Trojan" complexes composed of CD4 and CD8 T-cell epitopes connected by protease cleavable linkers. Using murine T-cell epitopes, it was shown that the "Trojan" peptide vaccine can generate MHC: peptide complexes and is capable of inducing a substantial immune response in vaccinated mice.[33] Based on these observations, a Phase I clinical trial, led by S E Strome, is ongoing at the University of Maryland to define the feasibility and safety of MAGE-A3/HPV 16 Trojan peptides vaccine for the treatment of HNSCC.

Whole Tumor Cell Vaccines

Because only a small number of HNSCC specific Ags have been identified, whole tumor cells or their products may provide a more plausible alternative as a source of immunogen for HNSCC immunotherapy. However, immunization with tumor cells alone does not result in a meaningful therapeutic antitumor immune response due to lack of costimulatory molecule expression on the tumor cell surface and their inability to process and present adequate levels of tumor associated Ags. To overcome this problem, several strategies utilizing powerful Ag-presenting properties of DCs loaded with tumor cell products were tested *in vitro* and in animal models.[34–36]

O-Sullivan and colleagues have prepared vaccine by transfecting DNA-fragments from KLN205 SCC cell line into bone marrow derived mature DCs.[35] Subcutaneous injection of DC transfected with DNA from the KLN205 tumor but not from non-crossreactive B16 melanoma prolonged the survival of mice bearing SCC. As determined by ELISPOT assay mice immunized with transfected DCs show the activation of cell-mediated immunity against SCC. Preclinical data from the University of Pittsburgh also indicates that DNA encoding tumor associated Ags delivered by apoptotic SCC cell line to DC can induce significant antitumor immune response ex vivo.[36] Moreover, it was shown that DCs preincubation with apoptotic and necrotic but not live SCC induced maturation of DCs which is essential for the generation of optimal antitumor immune response. Therefore, SCC can not only provide the crucial Ag load to the DCs but also increase their Ag presenting functions.

Another tumor cell immunotherapy approach utilizes the fusion of DCs with tumor cells. The fusion products retain the antigen-presenting properties of the DCs and can present protein antigens carried by the parent tumor cell. The cell fusion is usually done by exposure of cells to electric field stimulation which creates reversible membrane breakdown required for the fusion of different cell types. Vaccines prepared by this method were shown to be effective in treatment of tumors expressing model Ags (β-galactosidase). Immunization of mice bearing established pulmo-

nary metastases with allogenic tumor-DC fusion vaccine significantly decreased the number of metastases seen in the lung. These data provide the foundation for the use of fusion cell vaccine approaches consisting of allogeneic tumors and syngeneic DCs in immunotherapy and may be useful for treatment of head and neck cancer.[34]

It has also been reported that DCs can be pulsed with a lysate from a tumor cell line Tca8113 (human tongue SCC) and autologous T-cells activated by Ag; pulsed DCs were able to lyse Tca8113 cells *in vitro* and diminish tumor growth in nude mice.[37] We have compared three methods of tumor preparation for DC priming: irradiation, boiling, or freeze-thaw lysis. Our results demonstrate that irradiated tumor provides the most effective priming of DCs for the generation of local protective immunity in a poorly immunogenic murine model for SCC.[38] Therefore, DCs loaded with whole tumor cell product can induce immune response against HNSCC, but the clinical feasibility of whole tumor-based vaccine remains to be determined.

Cytokine Immunostimulation

Cytokines play an important role in generating and sustaining immune responses in general. IL-2, a cytokine essential for T-cell growth, has been used to activate antitumor T and NK cells both *in vitro* and *in vivo*. Injections of IL-2 were shown to cause increased antitumor responses, especially in immunogenic tumors such as melanoma and renal cancer. Other cytokines such as IFN-α, IL-12, and GM-CSF have also been used as natural adjuvants to boost the antitumor immune responses in cancer patients (Figure 4).

A preliminary trial of nonrecombinant IFN-α in patients with HNSCC was performed in 1991.[39] This trial demonstrated low-level toxicity and potent antitumor activity.[39] A subsequent Phase II trial in 71 patients with HNSCC indicated that low- but not high-dose IFN-α was well tolerated.[40] Clinical benefits of a low concentration of INF-α were overall unimpressive. However, 2 of 29 patients treated with a high concentration of IFN-α had a complete response and 7 had stable disease. The duration of survival in patients who received high doses of IFN-α correlated with a high level of NK activity.[40]

In a series of clinical trials, IL-2 was successfully used to improve immune function of patients with head and neck cancer.[41–43] The local administration of recombinant human IL-2 to patients with HNSCC demonstrated a statistically significant increase in disease-free survival as well as increased overall survival.[41] The improved clinical response after administration of recombinant IL-2 was associated with increased numbers of activated T lymphocytes and NK cells.

In a Phase II clinical trial, a natural cytokine mixture including IL-2 was administered before conventional therapy, that is, surgery followed by radiotherapy, of patients with HNSCC. In this trial, about 42% overall response rate was observed in the IL-2-treated group.[43] Natural IL-2

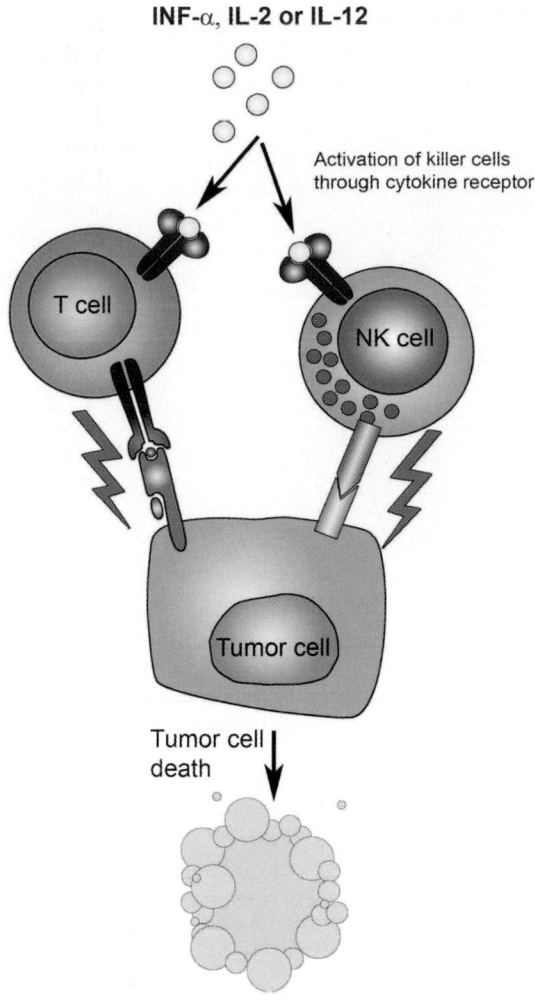

INF-α, IL-2 or IL-12

Activation of killer cells through cytokine receptor

T cell

NK cell

Tumor cell

Tumor cell death

Figure 4 Cytokine immunostimulation. T lymphocytes and natural killer (NK) cells express cytokine receptors upon contact with tumor Ags. Cytokine injected into patients with cancer activate lymphocytes expressing specific receptors and induce tumor-cell killing.

administration resulted in an augmented number of CD4+ T lymphocytes infiltrating tumors. The highest densities of CD4+ T-cell infiltrates were detected in the responders to cytokine treatment. In addition, it was demonstrated that an increased number of CD11c+ DCs were present at the tumor–stroma interface of patients responding to cytokine treatment.[43] The presence of T lymphocytes and DCs in the tumor site suggests an active immune response against the tumor in patients treated with IL-2.

Because systemic therapy with IL-2 is often associated with significant toxicity, local IL-2 gene therapy also has been explored by several groups. It was shown that in vivo delivery of IL-2 encoded plasmid into orthotopic murine head and neck tumors induced antitumor immunity and significantly inhibited tumor growth. A randomized, dose-escalation, phase I study shows that IL-2 nonviral gene therapy for head and neck cancer is safe and well tolerated when administered by direct intratumoral injections up to six times over a 28-day period.[42] These results indicate that IL-2-based gene immunotherapy may be a promising treatment for HNSCC.

An interesting way of IL-2 delivery for HNSCC treatment was tested in vitro by another group of head and neck surgeons. They have

covalently linked IL-2 to surgical suture which made it an effective immune stimulant. The suture material resulted in IL-2 induced proliferation of normal donor and HNSCC patients' lymphocytes.[44] The IL-2 induced production of IL-12 and IFN-γ, which can either directly inhibit tumor cell growth or potentiate the antitumor activity of NK and T lymphocytes. The clinical use of functionally active cytokines incorporated into surgical suture may be beneficial for manipulation the immune system in head and neck cancer patients.

IL-12 is a cytokine with a wide range of biological activities and has effects on both the innate and adaptive immune system. It has been shown that IL-12 can increase antitumor activity of NK and T lymphocytes. A phase II study of the administration of recombinant human IL-2 (rhIL-12) to patients with HNSCC before surgery to evaluate the immune effects on the primary tumor and regional lymph nodes was performed. After therapy with rhIL-12, an increase number of NK cells in peripheral blood and in tumors was observed.[5] In addition, patients treated with rhIL-12 showed increased production of IFN-γ which indicated an active immune response against tumors.

All phase I clinical trials for therapeutic use of cytokines, that is, natural or recombinant IL-2, IL-12, and IFN-α, in patients with HNSCC evaluated toxicity of cytokines and were not designed to answer the question of efficacy or to test the restoration of immune cell function in patients with cancer. Therefore, additional advanced clinical trials are required to assess the clinical outcome of cytokine immunostimulation of patients with HNSCC.

Costimulation-Based Immunotherapy

Perhaps, one of the most important recent discoveries relevant to cancer immunotherapy is the elucidation of the roles of various costimulatory molecules in antitumor immune response (Figure 5, #1). In particular, it has been demonstrated that cytotoxic T lymphocyte antigen-4 (CTLA-4), a receptor of B7-1 and B7-2 ligands, functions as a negative regulator of T-cell activation (Figure 5, #2). It has been convincingly shown that in vivo antibody-mediated blockade of the CTLA-4 expressed on T lymphocytes can greatly augment antitumor immune responses both in animal models and in patients with cancer. In fact, a fully humanized anti-CTLA-4 mAb (MDX-010) has been developed and is being tested for the immunotherapeutic treatment of a number of human malignancies including, but not limited to, melanoma, ovarian cancer, and carcinoma of the prostate. The patients treated with anti-CTLA-4 mAb demonstrated significant antitumor immunity, sometimes resulting in either partial or total disease regression.[45] Although CTLA-4 blockade was well tolerated, mild autoimmune-like responses including vitiligo dermatitis, enterocolitis, hepatitis, uveitis, and hypophysitis were observed in patients with metastatic melanoma and renal cancer.[46] Based on the promising data on therapy of other can-

cers, anti-CTLA-4 immunotherapy may also be applied for treatment of HNSCC. However, there is no preclinical or clinical data on effects of CTLA-4 for treatment of HNSCC.

4-1BB (CD137) is a member of the TNF receptor superfamily of costimulatory molecules and is expressed upon activation on the surface of T-cells, B-cells, DCs, and NK cells. Stimulation of 4-1BB by its natural ligand (4-1BBL) or agonistic Ab potentiates the antitumor immune response in vivo, either through direct stimulation of tumor-reactive T lymphocytes (Figure 5, #2) or indirectly through activation of the regulatory properties of NK cells and DCs. Introduction of the 4-1BBL gene into murine SCC cell line efficiently elicited antitumor immune responses in syngeneic mice that resulted in the development of specific immunity against wild-type SCC tumors.[47] Therefore, immunotherapy utilizing the 4-1BB costimulatory pathway could be applied for treatment of head and neck cancer. One of the advantages of 4-1BB-based cancer immunotherapy is that agonistic anti-4-1BB may enhance antitumor immunity while minimizing autoimmunity. Unlike what has been observed after injection of anti-CTLA-4 mAb which stimulated the development of mild autoimmune reactions,[46] anti-4-1BB mAbs have been shown to abrogate autoimmune manifestations in the mouse lupus model.[48] Moreover, a recent report indicates that the combination of anti-CTLA-4 and anti-4-1BB mAb dramatically augmented antitumor immunity while reducing autoimmune effects.[49]

B7-H1 ligand, a cell-surface glycoprotein belonging to the B7 family, is expressed on activated DC, epithelial and endothelial cells. Programmed death-1 protein (PD-1) is a specific receptor expressed on activated T lymphocytes that binds B7-H1 ligand. Engagement of the PD-1 receptor by B7-H1 inhibits proliferation, cytokine production and induces apoptosis of activated T lymphocytes (Figure 5, #3). Recently, it was shown that many tumors including HNSCC express B7-H1.[50] Tumor-associated B7-H1 increased the apoptosis of T-cells interacting with tumors and antibody against B7-H1 inhibited T-cells in vitro.[51] Therefore, it was postulated that B7-H1 may contribute to the evasion of tumor immunity in vivo. To verify the role of B7-H1 in HNSCC, the authors established a murine SCCVII cell line that was transfected with B7-H1. Combined with the adoptive transfer of activated tumor-specific T-cells, the injections of blocking anti-B7-H1 mAb significantly promote the survival of mice bearing B7-H1-expressing SCCVII tumors as compared to adoptive T-cell therapy alone.[50] Interestingly eight different human HNSCC tissue samples were positive for B7-H1.[51] A more recent report confirms that many human oral SCC cell lines constitutively express B7-H1, and its expression is further up regulated by IFN-γ.[52] This implies that altering interactions of tumor-B7-H1 with PD-1 on tumor infiltrating lymphocytes by recombinant fusion protein or neutralizing antibodies (Figure 5, #3) may have a great potential for benefit in immunotherapy of oral SCC.

(1) Resting T-cell
express CD28

(2) Activated tumor specific T-cell
express CTLA-4 and 4-1BB

(3) Tumor specific T-cell in tumor site
express PD-1

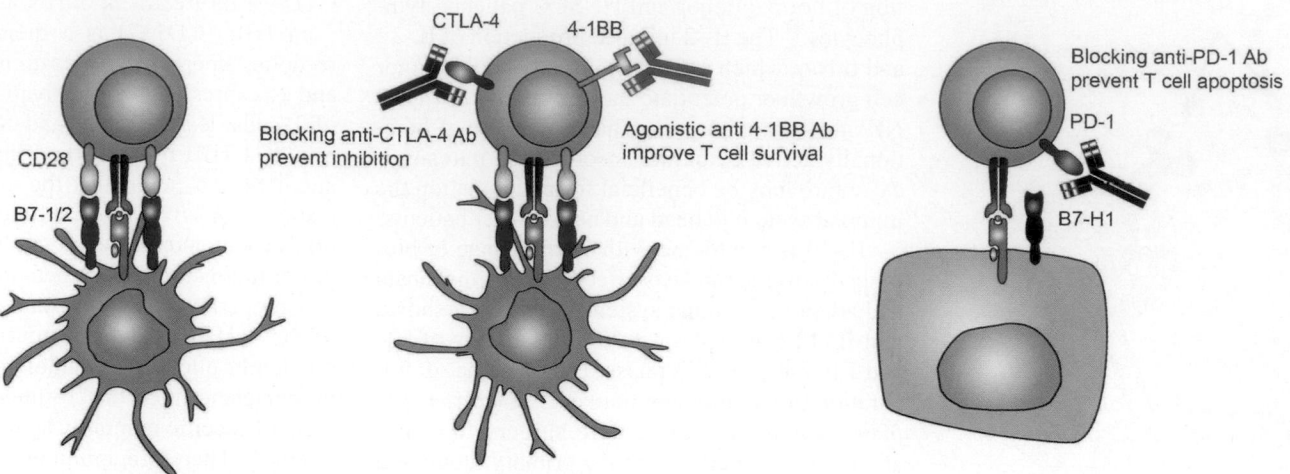

Figure 5 Costimulation-based immunotherapy. Dendritic cells can present tumor Ags to T lymphocytes. (1) The optimal activation of tumor specific T-cells requires the interaction of T-cell antigen receptor (TCR) with HLA/Ags complex and costimulation by contact of B7-1/2 ligands with CD28, a costimulatory receptor constitutively expressed on T lymphocytes. (2) Activated T-cells express CTLA-4 (a CD28 homolog). Blocking anti-CTLA-4 mAb can prevent CTLA-4 mediated T-cell inhibition. Activated T lymphocytes also express 4-1BB costimulatory molecule. Agonistic anti-4-1BB mAb improve survival of activated antitumor T lymphocytes. (3) B7-H1 is expressed by some tumor cells that induces antitumor T-cell apoptosis through a programmed death-1 protein (PD-1) dependent pathway. Blockade of the interaction between tumor associated B7-H1 and PD-1 expressed on antitumor T-cell prevent T-cell apoptosis

CONCLUSIONS

It is clear that the immune system plays critical roles in tumor development and cancer immunosurveillance. It is also widely accepted that immunity may play a pivotal role in future cancer therapy. The immune system can recognize and destroy tumor cells that present unique antigens. However, most malignant cells possess various approaches that can evade the immune system's attack on tumor cells. HNSCC can avoid immune cells through downregulation of HLA antigens and production of immuno-inhibitory molecules. The challenges for HNSSC immunotherapy are to understand the molecular mechanisms in play between HNSCC cells and the immune system and then to design novel approaches that can tip the balance in favor of the immune system in its fight against HNSCC cells.

REFERENCES

1. Jemal A, Siegel R, Ward E, et al. Cancer statistics, 2006. CA Cancer J Clin 2006;56:106–30.
2. Dudley ME, Wunderlich JR, Robbins PF, et al. Cancer regression and autoimmunity in patients after clonal repopulation with antitumor lymphocytes. Science 2002;298:850–4.
3. Morgan RA, Dudley ME, Wunderlich JR, et al. Cancer regression in patients after transfer of genetically engineered lymphocytes. Science 2006;314:126–9.
4. Badoual C, Hans S, Rodriguez J, et al. Prognostic value of tumor-infiltrating CD4+ T-cell subpopulations in head and neck cancers. Clin Cancer Res 2006;12:465–72.
5. van Herpen CM, van der Laak JA, de Vries IJ, et al. Intratumoral recombinant human interleukin-12 administration in head and neck squamous cell carcinoma patients modifies locoregional lymph node architecture and induces natural killer cell infiltration in the primary tumor. Clin Cancer Res 2005;11:1899–909.
6. Mandpe AH, Tsung K, Norton JA. Cure of an established nonimmunogenic tumor, SCC VII, with a novel interleukin 12-based immunotherapy regimen in C3H mice. Arch Otolaryngol Head Neck Surg 2003;129:786–92.
7. Oya R, Ikemura K. Spontaneous regression of recurrent squamous cell carcinoma of the tongue. Int J Clin Oncol 2004;9:339–42.

8. Patel A, Halliday GM, Barnetson RS. CD4+ T lymphocyte infiltration correlates with regression of a UV-induced squamous cell carcinoma. J Dermatol Sci 1995;9:12–9.
9. Kohler G, Milstein C. Continuous cultures of fused cells secreting antibody of predefined specificity. Nature 1975;256:495–7.
10. Uno M, Otsuki T, Kurebayashi J, et al. Anti-HER2-antibody enhances irradiation-induced growth inhibition in head and neck carcinoma. Int J Cancer 2001;94:474–9.
11. Mimura K, Kono K, Hanawa M, et al. Trastuzumab-mediated antibody-dependent cellular cytotoxicity against esophageal squamous cell carcinoma. Clin Cancer Res 2005;11:4898–904.
12. Sawaki M, Ito Y, Tada K, et al. Efficacy and safety of trastuzumab as a single agent in heavily pretreated patients with HER-2/neu-overexpressing metastatic breast cancer. Tumori 2004;90:40–3.
13. Verel I, Heider KH, Siegmund M, et al. Tumor targeting properties of monoclonal antibodies with different affinity for target antigen CD44V6 in nude mice bearing head-and-neck cancer xenografts. Int J Cancer 2002;99:396–402.
14. Colnot DR, Quak JJ, Roos JC, et al. Phase I therapy study of 186Re-labeled chimeric monoclonal antibody U36 in patients with squamous cell carcinoma of the head and neck. J Nucl Med 2000;41:1999–2010.
15. Borjesson PK, Postema EJ, Roos JC, et al. Phase I therapy study with (186)Re-labeled humanized monoclonal antibody BIWA 4 (bivatuzumab) in patients with head and neck squamous cell carcinoma. Clin Cancer Res 2003;9:3961 S–72S.
16. Hynes NE, Lane HA. ERBB receptors and cancer: The complexity of targeted inhibitors. Nat Rev Cancer 2005;5:341–54.
17. Burtness B, Goldwasser MA, Flood W, et al. Phase III randomized trial of cisplatin plus placebo compared with cisplatin plus cetuximab in metastatic/recurrent head and neck cancer: An Eastern Cooperative Oncology Group study. J Clin Oncol 2005;23:8646–54.
18. Bonner JA, Harari PM, Giralt J, et al. Radiotherapy plus cetuximab for squamous-cell carcinoma of the head and neck. N Engl J Med 2006;354:567–78.
19. Sok JC, Coppelli FM, Thomas SM, et al. Mutant epidermal growth factor receptor (EGFRvIII) contributes to head and neck cancer growth and resistance to EGFR targeting. Clin Cancer Res 2006;12:5064–73.
20. Treon SP, Hansen M, Branagan AR, et al. Polymorphisms in FcgammaRIIIA (CD16) receptor expression are associated with clinical response to rituximab in Waldenstrom's macroglobulinemia. J Clin Oncol 2005;23:474–81.
21. Cheung NK, Sowers R, Vickers AJ, et al. FCGR2A polymorphism is correlated with clinical outcome after immunotherapy of neuroblastoma with anti-GD2 antibody and granulocyte macrophage colony-stimulating factor. J Clin Oncol 2006;24:2885–90.

22. Gronau SS, Schmitt M, Thess B, et al. Trifunctional bispecific antibody-induced tumor cell lysis of squamous cell carcinomas of the upper aerodigestive tract. Head Neck 2005;27:376–82.
23. Gattinoni L, Powell DJ, Jr, Rosenberg SA, Restifo NP. Adoptive immunotherapy for cancer: Building on success. Nat Rev Immunol 2006;6:383–93.
24. Chang AE, Li Q, Jiang G, et al. Generation of vaccine-primed lymphocytes for the treatment of head and neck cancer. Head Neck 2003;25:198–209.
25. To WC, Wood BG, Krauss JC, et al. Systemic adoptive T-cell immunotherapy in recurrent and metastatic carcinoma of the head and neck: A phase 1 study. Arch Otolaryngol Head Neck Surg 2000;126:1225–31.
26. de Jong A, van der Hulst JM, Kenter GG, et al. Rapid enrichment of human papillomavirus (HPV)-specific polyclonal T-cell populations for adoptive immunotherapy of cervical cancer. Int J Cancer 2005;114:274–82.
27. Albers A, Abe K, Hunt J, et al. Antitumor activity of human papillomavirus type 16 E7-specific T-cells against virally infected squamous cell carcinoma of the head and neck. Cancer Res 2005;65:11146–55.
28. Albers AE, Ferris RL, Kim GG, et al. Immune responses to p53 in patients with cancer: Enrichment in tetramer+ p53 peptide-specific T-cells and regulatory T-cells at tumor sites. Cancer Immunol Immunother 2005;54:1072–81.
29. Asai T, Storkus WJ, Mueller-Berghaus J, et al. In vitro generated cytolytic T lymphocytes reactive against head and neck cancer recognize multiple epitopes presented by HLA-A2, including peptides derived from the p53 and MDM-2 proteins. Cancer Immun 2002;2:3–17.
30. Mayordomo JI, Loftus DJ, Sakamoto H, et al. Therapy of murine tumors with p53 wild-type and mutant sequence peptide-based vaccines. J Exp Med 1996;183:1357–65.
31. Kienstra MA, Neel HB, Strome SE, Roche P. Identification of NY-ESO-1, MAGE-1, and MAGE-3 in head and neck squamous cell carcinoma. Head Neck 2003;25:457–63.
32. Hersey P, Menzies SW, Coventry B, et al. Phase I/II study of immunotherapy with T-cell peptide epitopes in patients with stage IV melanoma. Cancer Immunol Immunother 2005;54:208–18.
33. Lu J, Higashimoto Y, Appella E, Celis E. Multiepitope Trojan antigen peptide vaccines for the induction of antitumor CTL and Th immune responses. J Immunol 2004;172:4575–82.
34. Lee WT, Shimizu K, Kuriyama H, et al. Tumor-dendritic cell fusion as a basis for cancer immunotherapy. Otolaryngol Head Neck Surg 2005;132:755–64.
35. O-Sullivan I, Ng LK, Martinez DM, et al. Immunity to squamous carcinoma in mice immunized with dendritic cells transfected with genomic DNA from squamous carcinoma cells. Cancer Gene Ther 2005;12:825–34.
36. Whiteside TL, Gambotto A, Albers A, et al. Human tumor-derived genomic DNA transduced into a recipient cell

induces tumor-specific immune responses ex vivo. Proc Natl Acad Sci U S A 2002;99:9415–20.

37. Wang Z, Hu Q, Han W, et al. Effect of dendritic cell vaccine against a tongue squamous cell cancer cell line (Tca8113) in vivo and in vitro. Int J Oral Maxillofac Surg 2006;35: 544–50.

38. Strome SE, Voss S, Wilcox R, et al. Strategies for antigen loading of dendritic cells to enhance the antitumor immune response. Cancer Res 2002;62:1884–9.

39. Vlock DR, Johnson J, Myers E, et al. Preliminary trial of nonrecombinant interferon alpha in recurrent squamous cell carcinoma of the head and neck. Head Neck 1991;13: 15–21.

40. Vlock DR, Andersen J, Kalish LA, et al. Phase II trial of interferon-alpha in locally recurrent or metastatic squamous cell carcinoma of the head and neck: Immunological and clinical correlates. J Immunother Emphasis Tumor Immunol 1996;19:433–42.

41. De Stefani A, Forni G, Ragona R, et al. Improved survival with perilymphatic interleukin 2 in patients with resectable squamous cell carcinoma of the oral cavity and oropharynx. Cancer 2002;95:90–7.

42. O'Malley BW, Jr, Li D, McQuone SJ, Ralston R. Combination nonviral interleukin-2 gene immunotherapy for head and neck cancer: From bench top to bedside. Laryngoscope 2005;115:391–404.

43. Timar J, Ladanyi A, Forster-Horvath C, et al. Neoadjuvant immunotherapy of oral squamous cell carcinoma modulates intratumoral CD4/CD8 ratio and tumor microenvironment: A multicenter phase II clinical trial. J Clin Oncol 2005;23: 3421–32.

44. Shibuya TY, Kim S, Nguyen K, et al. Covalent linking of proteins and cytokines to suture: Enhancing the immune response of head and neck cancer patients. Laryngoscope 2003;113:1870–84.

45. Phan GQ, Yang JC, Sherry RM, et al. Cancer regression and autoimmunity induced by cytotoxic T lymphocyte-associated antigen 4 blockade in patients with metastatic melanoma. Proc Natl Acad Sci U S A 2003;100:8372–7.

46. Sanderson K, Scotland R, Lee P, et al. Autoimmunity in a phase I trial of a fully human anti-cytotoxic T-lymphocyte antigen-4 monoclonal antibody with multiple melanoma peptides and Montanide ISA 51 for patients with resected stages III and IV melanoma. J Clin Oncol 2005;23:741–50.

47. Mogi S, Sakurai J, Kohsaka T, et al. Tumour rejection by gene transfer of 4-1BB ligand into a CD80(+) murine squamous cell carcinoma and the requirements of co-stimulatory molecules on tumour and host cells. Immunology 2000;101:541–7.

48. Foell J, Strahotin S, O'Neil SP, et al. CD137 costimulatory T-cell receptor engagement reverses acute disease in lupus-prone NZB x NZW F1 mice. J Clin Invest 2003;111: 1505–18.

49. Kocak E, Lute K, Chang X, et al. Combination therapy with anti-CTL antigen-4 and anti-4-1BB antibodies enhances cancer immunity and reduces autoimmunity. Cancer Res 2006;66:7276–84.

50. Strome SE, Dong H, Tamura H, et al. B7-H1 blockade augments adoptive T-cell immunotherapy for squamous cell carcinoma. Cancer Res 2003;63:6501–5.

51. Dong H, Strome SE, Salomao DR, et al. Tumor-associated B7-H1 promotes T-cell apoptosis: A potential mechanism of immune evasion. Nat Med 2002;8:793–800.

52. Tsushima F, Tanaka K, Otsuki N, et al. Predominant expression of B7-H1 and its immunoregulatory roles in oral squamous cell carcinoma. Oral Oncol 2006;42:268–74.

94

Nutrition of the Patient with Head and Neck Cancer

Laurence J. DiNardo, MD

Elizabeth G. Miller, RD

About 30 to 50% of all patients with head and neck cancer are malnourished even before treatment starts.[1] Four factors are generally responsible for calorie and protein malnutrition in these individuals. First, the tumor itself may present a barrier to deglutition through obstruction or pain. Second, tumor metabolism remains constant despite changes in nutritional status. Consequently, starvation responses such as lipolysis are not used by tumor cells, and glucose is continuously derived from protein catabolism. Third, recent evidence suggests that cancer cachexia may be induced by catabolic factors secreted by tumor cells.[2] Finally, tumor treatment may induce anorexia through discomfort, obstruction, and loss of taste. Accelerated radiotherapy has been associated with grade 3 to 4 reactions necessitating nasogastric (NG) or percutaneous gastrostomy feedings in 26% of patients with a median weight loss of 4.1 kg.[3] Difficulties are not limited to high-dose, large-field radiation treatments. A significant decrease in body mass index (BMI) has been observed in 80% of patients undergoing radiation therapy for early laryngeal carcinoma despite dietetic consultation and protein/calorie supplementation.[4] Further, it has been shown that poor performance status, advanced stage disease, and a history of smoking identified those at high risk for requiring enteral feedings during definitive radiation therapy.[5] Unfortunately, swallowing difficulties are not limited to the duration of treatment. Shiley and colleagues found that 31% of patients successfully treated for advanced oropharyngeal carcinoma with chemoradiation therapy required feeding tubes 1 year later.[6] Tables 1 to 3 list the possible consequences of cancer treatment—surgery, radiation, and chemotherapy—that may impact a patient's nutritional status.[1]

Conversely, complications resulting from modern, aggressive treatment regimens for head and neck cancer are exacerbated by poor nutrition. Patients receiving accelerated fraction radiation therapy, chemoradiation, or extended

Table 1 Surgery-Related Nutritional Consequences

Negative nitrogen balance
Interference with mastication
Aglutition
Dysphagia
Aspiration

Table 2 Radiation-Related Nutritional Consequences

Mucositis
Xerostomia
Odynophagia
Dysgeusia, ageusia
Dysosmia
Dental caries
Osteoradionecrosis

resection with free flap reconstruction are particularly at risk. Preoperative weight loss of greater than 10% has been identified as the most prominent nutrition-related factor in the development of postoperative complications.[7] In addition, preoperative weight loss of greater than 5% has been associated with higher mortality rates for men with head and neck cancer.[8]

Recent work has identified relationships among immune function, nutritional status, and postoperative wound infection. Malnourished patients with head and neck cancer demonstrate a significantly lower human leukocyte antigen (HLA)-DR expression on monocytes than well-nourished, matched controls.[9] Theoretically, this places these patients at a higher risk for postoperative infection. Intervention with immune-enhancing formulas has resulted in a significant decrease in the incidence of postoperative infectious complications.[10]

NUTRITION SCREENING AND ASSESSMENT OF NUTRITIONAL STATUS

Two steps are indicated to ensure the appropriate level of nutrition intervention and follow-up: screening and assessment. Nutrition screening is used to detect the possibility of nutrition risk

Table 3 Chemotherapy-Related Nutritional Consequences

Nausea
Vomiting
Diarrhea
Cheilosis, glossitis
Pharyngitis
Esophagitis
Anorexia

and whether or not nutrition follow-up is needed. Ongoing nutrition screening is indicated to determine if at any point during treatment a patient may need a more detailed evaluation due to progressive nutritional decline. Nutrition assessment is more comprehensive than screening; it includes intervention and ongoing follow-up.

Usually, nutritional status will be negatively affected in individuals diagnosed with head and neck cancer. Nutrition intervention in the patient with head and neck cancer should be initiated prior to tumor treatment and should continue even after the treatment has ended.[11] Study has found that there is a role for dietary intervention to improve the survival of laryngeal and hypopharyngeal cancer patients.[12] Swallowing difficulties are common prior to treatment and can continue after therapy. Early and intensive nutritional intervention is helpful in minimizing weight loss, maintaining functional status and quality of life, and in overall maintenance of nutritional status. In the head and neck cancer patient population, simply maintaining weight may be the most appropriate and achievable goal.[13]

The initial nutritional assessment includes anthropometric, biochemical, clinical, and dietary history data.

Anthropometric Measurements

The percentage of weight loss (% wt loss) that a patient has experienced is the most common estimate of malnutrition. The patient's usual body weight (UBW) is defined as his or her weight 6 months prior to the assessment. Actual or current body weight is then measured. The % wt loss is calculated as follows:

$$\% \text{ wt loss} = \frac{(\text{UBW} - \text{current wt})}{\text{UBW}} \times 100$$

Severe malnutrition is defined as greater than 10% weight loss in 6 months.[14]

A patient's height is needed to allow determination of ideal body weight (IBW), percent IBW (% IBW), and additional anthropometric measurements. IBW may be determined using reference values for a given height and frame size[15] or by the Hamwi method[16]:

- For men: 106 lb for the first 5 ft, with an additional 6 lb for each inch over 5 ft;
- For women: 100 lb for the first 5 ft, with an additional 5 lb for each inch over 5 ft.

Percent IBW is then calculated as follows:

$$\% \text{IBW} = \frac{\text{actual (current) wt}}{\text{IBW}} \times 100$$

The extent of malnutrition is then estimated as follows[14]:

- Mild malnutrition = 80 to 90% IBW
- Moderate malnutrition = 70 to 79% IBW
- Severe malnutrition = <69% IBW

Another method for assessing weight status is by determination of BMI:

$$\text{BMI} = \frac{\text{wt (kg)}}{\text{ht}^2}(m)$$

Once calculated, the patient's BMI is compared to reference values:

- Underweight: BMI <18.5
- Adequate weight: BMI = 18.5 to 24.9
- Overweight: BMI = 25 to 29.9
- Obese: BMI > 30

Further assessment of a patient's nutritional status using anthropometric data can be performed through measurement of triceps skinfold thickness and midarm muscle circumference using skinfold calipers and a measuring tape. These determine the adequacy of a patient's fat and somatic protein or skeletal muscle status. Given inconsistency in measurements among clinicians and the influence of hydration on results, as well as time constraint, these are now uncommonly performed tests. Body fat, lean body mass, and total body water can be calculated from bioelectrical impedance analysis and may be used as a bedside measurement of a patient's fluid status.[17]

Biochemical Assessment

Assessment of laboratory data comprises another facet of the nutritional status evaluation. The serum proteins that are often used to assess nutritional status include albumin, transferrin, and prealbumin or transthyretin. Each have different synthesis rates and half-lives; therefore, these parameters vary in their reflection of alterations in nutritional status.

The general availability of albumin measurement renders it a useful test. It reflects visceral protein status. Since it has a long half-life of approximately 20 days, however, it does not detect early protein deficiency. Various levels of depletion have been defined[14]:

- Adequate = >3.5 g/dL
- Mild depletion = 2.7 to 3.5 g/dL
- Moderate depletion = 2.1 to 2.6 g/dL
- Severe depletion = <2.1 g/dL

Albumin is influenced by many nonnutritional variables, including hydration status, liver or renal disease, sepsis, trauma, surgery, and congestive heart failure, as well as infusion of albumin, fresh frozen plasma, or whole blood. Unfortunately, this necessitates cautious interpretation of albumin values.

In protein-calorie malnutrition from cancer-related cachexia, there appears to be an insufficient supply of amino acids for liver protein synthesis, resulting in a decline in serum albumin. A decline in serum albumin is correlated with cachexia and is a predictor of mortality. In patients with cancer, postoperative complications are more frequent with serum albumin <3.0 g/dL. Decreased tube feeding tolerance has also been observed with a serum albumin <2.5 g/dL.

Transferrin is more useful than albumin as a measure of visceral protein status. Owing to its relatively short half-life (8 days), it is more sensitive to short-term changes in nutrient intake. The degree of malnutrition relative to serum transferrin levels is as follows:

- Adequate = 200 to 400 mg/dL
- Mild malnutrition = 180 to 200 mg/dL
- Moderate malnutrition = 160 to 180 mg/dL
- Severe malnutrition = <160 mg/dL

As with albumin, transferrin can be impacted by nonnutritional variables. Levels may be increased with iron deficiency anemia, some malignancies, acute hepatitis, oral contraceptive use, and pregnancy. Levels may be decreased with chronic infection, cancer, iron overload, liver disease, and protein-losing enteropathy. Despite its shorter half-life, transferrin is not as commonly used as albumin or prealbumin in evaluating malnutrition and visceral protein status.

Prealbumin, also named transthyretin or thyroxine-binding globulin, has a half-life of 2 to 3 days and therefore has replaced the transferrin assay in many institutions. Its shorter half-life makes it a sensitive indicator of visceral protein status. It is most useful when assessing a patient for acute changes in nutritional status and short-term response to nutritional support through weekly measurements. Assessment of visceral protein status based on the serum transthyretin value is estimated as follows:

- Adequate = 18 to 42 mg/dL
- Mild depletion = 13 to 17 mg/dL
- Moderate depletion = 8 to 12 mg/dL
- Severe depletion = ≤7 mg/dL

Prealbumin levels are also impacted by nonnutrition factors. Levels can be increased with renal dysfunction, dehydration, and blood transfusions. Levels may be decreased by stress, surgery, inflammation, cirrhosis, hepatitis, and hyperthyroidism.

Retinol-binding protein, with a half-life of 10 hours, measures acute protein deprivation or minor stress. Normal values range from 2.6 to 7.6 mg/dL.

Evaluation of immune function can also provide information relevant to the patient's nutritional status and serves as a predictor of postoperative complications. In the past, intradermal antigen challenge for the detection of delayed hypersensitivity was used as a measure of immune competence. It has fallen out of favor owing to its lack of specificity. Total lymphocyte count (TLC) is currently the most frequently employed test of immune status in the patient with head and neck cancer. It is calculated as follows[7]:

TLC = [% lymphocytes × white blood count (WBC)]100

Immune competence is then evaluated as follows[14]:

- Adequate immunocompetence = > 1,800 mm^3
- Mild depletion = 1,500 to 1,800 mm^3
- Moderate depletion = 900 to 1,500 mm^3
- Severe depletion = < 900 mm^3

The use of TLC as an indicator of nutritional status is limited since marked changes can occur in the WBC and differential counts on a day-to-day basis. Also, numerous nonnutrition-related factors can alter the value, such as severe stress, infection, corticosteroid therapy, cancer, renal failure, surgery, and cancer treatments such as radiation therapy and chemotherapy.

Several parameters have been combined to create the prognostic nutritional index (PNI), which has been defined by various formulas.[7] An example:

PNI = [0.14 × alb(g/dL)] + [0.03 × % IBW] + [0.73 × TLC(10^9/mm^3)] − 8.90

A correlation between the PNI and surgical risk in patients with head and neck cancers has been observed. A value less than 1.31 is considered below normal.

CLINICAL DATA AND DIETARY HISTORY

The physical examination is an important component of the nutritional status assessment. Physical findings that imply vitamin, mineral, and protein-calorie deficiencies and excesses are listed in Table 4. However, most of the physical findings are not specific for individual nutrient deficits and must be considered together, along with diet history, anthropometric data, and laboratory results.

A diet history is used to identify underlying risks for nutrition depletion or excess. Causes include inadequate intake, compromised metabolism (altered absorption, decreased use, or increased losses), and heightened requirements for nutrients. Patients with the characteristics included in Table 5 have increased susceptibility for nutritional problems.[18]

The diet history of the patient with head and neck cancer should include questions about alcohol consumption. When alcohol is substituted for good nutrition, malnutrition owing to inadequate nutrient intake occurs. Alcoholic persons are prone to develop malabsorption of nutrients owing to inflammation of the gastrointestinal tract. Altered absorption or metabolism of thiamin, folic acid, pyridoxine, vitamin A, vitamin B$_{12}$, sodium, potassium, magnesium, calcium, phosphorus, zinc, and selenium can result. Long-term alcoholism can also induce cirrhosis, with the potential development of ascites and/or hepatic encephalopathy. Glucose intolerance may

Table 4 Physical Findings and Associated Nutrient Deficiencies/Excesses

Finding	Deficiency	Excess
Hair and nails		
Transverse hair depigmentation	Protein	
Sparse hair	Protein, biotin, zinc	Vitamin A
Corkscrew hair	Vitamin C	
Transverse nail ridging	Protein	
Skin		
Scaling	Vitamin A, zinc, fatty acids	Vitamin A
Cellophane appearance	Protein	
Cracking dermatitis	Protein	
Follicular hyperkeratosis	Vitamins A, C	
Petechiae	Vitamin C	
Purpura	Vitamins C, K	
Pigmentation, desquamation of sun-exposed areas	Niacin	
Yellow pigmentation-sparing sclerae		Carotene
Eyes		
Papilledema		Vitamin A
Night blindness	Vitamin A	
Perioral		
Angular stomatitis	Riboflavin, pyridoxine, niacin	
Cheilosis	Riboflavin, pyridoxine, niacin	
Oral		
Atrophic lingual papillae	Riboflavin, niacin, folate, vitamin B_{12}, protein, iron	
Glossitis	Riboflavin, niacin, pyridoxine, folate, vitamin B_{12}	
Hypogeusia, hyposmia	Zinc	
Swollen, retracted, bleeding gingiva	Vitamin C	
Neurologic		
Headache		Vitamin A
Drowsiness, lethargy, vomiting		Vitamins A, D
Dementia	Niacin, vitamin B_{12}, folate	
Confabulation, disorientation	Thiamin	
Ophthalmoplegia	Thiamin, phosphorus	
Peripheral neuropathy	Thiamin, pyridoxine, vitamin B_{12}	Pyridoxine
Tetany	Calcium, magnesium	
Others		
Parotid enlargement	Protein (consider bulimia)	
Heart failure	Thiamin, phosphorus	
Hepatomegaly	Protein	Vitamin A
Edema	Protein, thiamin	
Poor wound healing, decubitus ulcers	Protein, vitamin C, zinc	

be observed in alcoholics secondary to pancreatic inflammation or injury.

Commonly used methods for obtaining a diet history include the 24-hour recall, a 1- to 7-day food intake record, and a food frequency questionnaire. A number of computer programs allow rapid estimation of nutrient intake based on these records or questionnaires. It is important to remember that in the course of the complete medical history, information elicited from the patient

Table 5 Patients at High Risk for Nutritional Deficits

Underweight: less than 80% standard and/or recent loss greater than 10% usual body weight

Poor intake: anorexia, nothing by mouth more than 5 d

Protracted nutrient loss: malabsorption, enteric fistulae, draining abscesses or wounds, renal dialysis

Hypermetabolic state: sepsis, fever, extensive burn, or trauma

Chronic alcohol/drug use: corticosteroids, antimetabolites, immunosuppressants

Impoverishment, isolation, advanced age

in all of the areas noted in Table 6 will aid in identifying possible nutrient deficits not gathered from the dietary recall.[18]

ASSESSMENT OF NUTRITIONAL NEEDS

The assessment of nutritional needs must include calorie, protein, lipid, vitamin, mineral, and water requirements. Calorie and protein needs vary depending on several factors: (1) a patient's current nutritional status, (2) whether the need is for maintenance or repletion, (3) whether a patient is at risk for refeeding syndrome, and (4) whether a patient is in a catabolic state. Adults' daily calorie requirements are estimated at 30 to 35 kilocalories per kilogram (kcal/kg) of body weight, with the lower end of needs being the initial aim if a patient is at refeeding risk.[19] Usually, as many as 10 kcal/kg body weight may be added to regain lost weight and compensate for surgical stress. The Harris-Benedict equation was derived to estimate more accurately a patient's basal energy expenditure (BEE), the energy expended at rest.[20]

For men:
$$BEE = 66.47 + [13.75 \times wt\,(kg)] + [5.0 \times ht\,(cm)] - [6.76 \times age\,(yr)]$$
For women:
$$BEE = 665.10 + [9.56 \times wt\,(kg)] + [1.85 \times ht\,(cm)] - [4.68 \times age\,(yr)]$$

In general, to calculate the total calorie need of a patient with head and neck cancer, the BEE is multiplied by a stress and activity factor totaling 1.3 to 1.5, with the higher number used for sepsis or other hypermetabolic states. If weight gain or nutritional repletion is desired, approximately 500 to 1,000 calories/d is added to the total calorie need. Since these calculations are estimates and not based on actual measurement of caloric expenditure, frequent monitoring of a patient's response to the nutrition regimen is required. It has been found through experience that calorie need for maintenance is as high as 35 to 40 kcal/ kg.

Acceleration in protein turnover and derangements in protein metabolism have been observed in patients with cancer. In contrast to simple starvation, protein use increases when a patient with cancer is under metabolic stress. Protein needs are usually calculated based on actual or adjusted body weight. The approximate protein need can then be adjusted based on the degree of protein depletion and metabolic stress factors. Under normal conditions with no stress, protein requirements are estimated at 1.0 g/kg/d. For the well-nourished, mildly stressed patient with cancer the protein need may only be 1.2 g/kg/d. However, with mild to moderate depletion along with metabolic stress, up to 1.5 g/kg/d may be necessary. If a patient with head and neck cancer undergoes surgery with reconstruction, protein needs for healing may be up to 2.0 g/kg/d. The amount of protein provided may require further adjustments if renal or liver disease is present.

The best method to determine if protein needs are met in the malnourished patient is by monitoring for gradual weight gain and positive nitrogen balance. In the well-nourished patient, weight maintenance and nitrogen equilibrium are the goals. Weekly serial monitoring of a patient's prealbumin or transthyretin level is another method for tracking protein supplementation.

Ideally, ≤30% of nonprotein calories should be derived from fat. The appropriate administration of essential fatty acids helps to blunt the insulin response by decreasing the need for infusions rich in glucose. Deriving calories from fat also has a protein-sparing effect.[21] Using greater amounts of fat in combination with less glucose is especially important in patients with diabetes mellitus in whom fat can provide as much as 60% of nonprotein calories.

Although recommended daily doses of vitamins, minerals, and trace elements exist,[22] requirements for nutritionally depleted patients with cancer have not been established. It is recommended that patients requiring prolonged parenteral nutrition receive regular doses of multivitamins and trace elements. Research indicates that the zinc status may be less than adequate in up to 50% of patients with head and neck cancer.[23]

Table 6 Nutrition History Survey

Mechanism of Deficiency	History	Deficiency to Suspect
Inadequate intake	Alcoholism	Calories, protein, thiamin, niacin, folate, pyridoxine, riboflavin
	Avoidance of fruit, vegetables, grains	Vitamin C, thiamin, niacin, folate
	Avoidance of meat, dairy products, eggs	Protein, vitamin B_{12}
	Constipation, hemorrhoids, diverticulosis	Dietary fiber
	Isolation, poverty, dental disease, food idiosyncrasies	Various nutrients
	Weight loss	Calories, other nutrients
Inadequate absorption	Drugs (especially antacids, anticonvulsants, cholestyramine, laxatives, neomycin, alcohol)	Varies, dependent on drug
	Malabsorption (diarrhea, weight loss, steatorrhea)	Vitamins A, D, and K; calories; protein; calcium; magnesium; zinc
	Parasites	Iron, vitamin B_{12} (fish tapeworm)
	Pernicious anemia	Vitamin B_{12}
	Surgery	Vitamin B_{12} (if distal ileum), iron, others as in malabsorption
	Gastrectomy	
	Intestinal resection	
Decreased utilization	Drugs (especially anticonvulsants, antimetabolites, oral contraceptives, isoniazid, alcohol)	Varies, dependent on drug
	Inborn errors of metabolism (by family history)	Various nutrients
Increased losses	Alcohol abuse	Magnesium, zinc
	Blood loss	Iron
	Paracentesis (ascitic, pleural)	Protein
	Diabetes, uncontrolled	Calories
	Diarrhea	Protein, zinc, electrolytes
	Draining abscesses, wounds	Protein, zinc
	Nephrotic syndrome	Protein, zinc
	Peritoneal dialysis or hemodialysis	Protein, water-soluble vitamins, zinc
Increased requirements	Fever	Calories
	Hyperthyroidism	Calories
	Physiologic demands (infancy, adolescence, pregnancy, lactation)	Various nutrients
	Surgery, trauma, burns, infection	Calories, protein, vitamin C, zinc
	Tissue hypoxia	Calories (inefficient utilization)
	Cigarette smoking	Vitamin C, folate

Moreover, it has also been suggested that zinc supplementation aids in decreasing the impact of radiation therapy on taste loss and recovery.[24] More definitive guidelines likely to evolve as knowledge is gained regarding the role of vitamins, minerals, and trace elements in critically ill patients. Experimental evidence exists in mice, for example, which demonstrates increased survival in endotoxin shock with the administration of vitamin D analogues.[25]

There has been recent interest regarding the impact of antioxidants on cancer, cancer treatments, and treatment-related side effects. Results of a clinical trial conducted by the United States National Cancer Institute have shown that the use of vitamin E supplementation is not of help to patients with Stage I or II head and neck cancer, either in reducing the severity of radiation-induced side effects or as a chemoprevention agent.[26] Research is underway to evaluate the impact of fruit and vegetable extracts on patients with Stages I through IVB head and neck cancer.

NUTRITIONAL SUPPORT

Whenever possible, nutritional support should be provided through the enteral route. The use of an intact gastrointestinal tract is not only more cost effective, safer, and more practical than parenteral nutrition, it also maintains the integrity of the gut mucosal barrier and immune function.[27] In addition, no survival advantage or reduction in treatment toxicity has been demonstrated with the routine administration of total parenteral nutrition in cancer patients.[28] Moreover, while perioperative enteral feeding decreases infection rates, parenteral nutrition does not demonstrate this advantage.[29]

Oral alimentation should always be considered first. Simple interventions such as the eradication of oral candidiasis or the treatment of mucositis may facilitate oral intake. Nutrition counseling and provision of nutritional supplements can further support oral intake in patients with head and neck cancer. Nutritious liquid formulas can be taken by mouth when other foods cannot be tolerated. The administration of appetite stimulants such as megestrol acetate has been advocated in patients with cancer-related anorexia or cachexia. The risk of side effects such as adrenal suppression, hyperglycemia, and thromboembolic events must be considered with this medication.[30] However, if surgery, radiation, or chemotherapy side effects prevent a patient from taking oral liquids, nutritional support can be provided via a feeding tube. Despite the ability to take some oral nutrition, the seriously malnourished patient should be considered for early feeding tube placement owing to the impending side effects of cancer therapy. A review of patients with head and neck cancer who were treated with radiation therapy found that early initiation of enteral nutrition lowered the need for treatment breaks and possibly led to enhanced treatment efficacy.[31]

TYPES AND SELECTION OF FEEDING TUBES

Enteral feeding involves the administration of nutrient solutions through a tube into the upper gastrointestinal tract. There are two major routes for tube placements: those entering the gastrointestinal tract via the nose [nasogastric (NG) and nasointestinal] and those entering the gastrointestinal tract through the abdominal wall (gastrostomy, duodenostomy, jejunostomy). Occasionally, a feeding may be given through a tube inserted in the mouth (orogastric) or esophagus (cervical esophagostomy).

The timing and type of enteral tube feeding are largely dependent on the anticipated duration of nutritional supplementation. Placement of a pliable red rubber or Dobbhoff tube for feeding is preferred if short-term nutritional support is expected. NG tube feeding should be restricted to short-term use owing to nasopharyngeal and laryngeal irritation as well as potential for necrosis of the nasal alae.

With the placement of an NG tube, the patient can be weaned quickly from intravenous hydration after surgery, receive adequate nutrition postoperatively, and have access for medications. If there is difficulty transitioning to complete oral intake, then the patient is considered for placement of a percutaneous endoscopic gastrostomy (PEG), which is more appropriate for long-term feeding. If it is anticipated that the patient will require long-term tube feeding postoperatively, a PEG tube can be placed intraoperatively. Intraoperative PEG tube placement has been associated with fewer complications than preoperative insertion.[32] Open or laparoscopic gastrostomy tube placement is considered in cases for which PEG placement is not feasible. When definitive radiation or chemoradiation therapy is the preferred treatment for oropharyngeal or hypopharyngeal tumors, pretreatment gastrostomy tube placement should be strongly considered.

Intestinal feedings are indicated when gastric reflux results in aspiration, with depressed gastric motility and emptying, with significant pulmonary disease, or when ulcer disease, cancer, or surgery involves the stomach. Tube feeding into the intestine may be provided via a nasointestinal tube, PEG-jejunostomy, or a surgical jejunostomy tube. If a patient is dependent on a feeding jejunostomy tube for medication administration, an 8 French tube or larger should be used to prevent clogging.

TUBE FEEDING FORMULAS

Numerous oral and tube feeding solutions are available. Some are intended for general nutrition; others are designed to meet specific metabolic or clinical needs. Occasionally, blenderized foods can be used for the provision of adequate nutrition by oral or feeding tube routes.

The majority of patients with head and neck cancer is administered commercially available polymeric formulas. Polymeric formulas consist of macronutrients in the form of isolates of intact protein, fats, and carbohydrate polymers. In most of these solutions, protein makes up 12 to 20% of total calories; carbohydrates, 40 to 60%; and fats, 30 to 40%. In the standard formulas, the ratio of nonprotein calories to nitrogen is approximately 150:1. In the high-nitrogen formulas, this ratio is much lower, approximately 75:1. Table 7 provides an overview of these formulas.

Polymeric formulas contain whole proteins isolated from casein, whey, lactalbumin, and egg white. The source of carbohydrate is usually glucose polymers from starch and its hydrolysates. The fats are from vegetable sources. Essential vitamins and minerals are present in sufficient amounts so that 100% of the United States Recommended daily allowance for each nutrient is met through a daily intake of 1,500 to 2,000 calories of the formula. The amounts of minerals such as sodium and potassium vary greatly, allowing for adjustment based on requirements.

Polymeric formulas are lactose free with a caloric density between 1 and 2 cal/mL. The higher-calorie formulas allow for more calories in a smaller volume and are therefore suitable for patients requiring fluid restriction. These high-osmolality formulas often are best initiated at half strength and advanced as tolerated to full strength while maintaining appropriate hydration. Modified, more costly, polymeric formulas have been devised to suit the needs of patients with renal failure, liver failure, and diabetes.

Monomeric formulas require less digestion than do regular foods or polymeric solutions. They are suitable for patients with impaired digestion. These formulas are rarely used in patients with head and neck cancer with the exception of extremely low-fat preparations administered in the presence of a chylous fistula. Formulas with medium-chain triglycerides are also useful in the presence of a chyle leak since they enter the systemic circulation without passing through the thoracic duct.

TUBE FEEDING ADMINISTRATION

With an NG tube, placement in the stomach must be verified prior to each feeding and the head of the patient's bed elevated. Initiation of bolus feeding may range from 100 to 200 mL every 3 to 4 hours, with the final feeding provided to the patient no later than 11:00 pm. Feedings should be administered by gravity drip over 30 to 60 minutes. Advancement of feedings by 50 to 100 mL

every shift (8 hours) or daily are performed as tolerated, and residuals are monitored until the tube feeding volume goal is attained.

Initiation of tube feeding through a surgically placed gastric tube is similar to NG tube feeding except a delay of as much as 48 hours after insertion is required to allow for maturation of the stoma and return of bowel function.

After PEG or percutaneous radiologic gastrostomy feeding tube placement, feeding can often be initiated within 12 hours. If bowel sounds are present, continuous delivery of water at 50 mL/h can begin within a few hours of insertion.

If water is tolerated, feeding is initiated using a full-strength, isotonic formula infused at 50 mL/h. Residuals should be monitored every 4 hours, and feeding is advanced as with an NG or gastric tube.

Feeding into the intestine requires an intermittent or continuous pump-assisted delivery of formula since bolus amounts and hyperosmolarity can lead to diarrhea. After placement of a nasointestinal (nasoduodenal or nasojejunal) tube, feedings are administered over a 12- to 24-hour period and should be started at an isotonic level (300 mOsm) or at a low rate (10 to 15 mL/h). The rate of infusion may be increased every 8 to 24 hours as tolerated until the desired volume is reached. The rate and concentration of the formula should not be increased simultaneously.

Administration of formula through a feeding jejunostomy tube is identical to a nasointestinal feeding tube except feeding initiation may not begin for 12 to 24 hours after tube placement. With a PEG/jejunostomy, initiation is the same as for a PEG except a continuous infusion of formula is required.

FEEDING TUBE COMPLICATIONS

Tube Clogging

If a feeding tube becomes clogged, any enteral solution remaining in the tube should be withdrawn. To remove any obstruction, the following steps are attempted: (1) inject 5 mL of warm water into the tube and clamp for 5 minutes. Flush with water until tube is cleared; if the tube remains clogged, then (2) inject a bolus (20 to 30 cc) of air to dislodge the clog. If the air seems to free the obstruction, follow it with 30 to 50 mL of warm water, cola, or cranberry juice to cleanse the tube. If the tube remains clogged, (3) crush one 324 mg sodium bicarbonate tablet. Mix the powder with the contents of one pancrelipase (Cotazym or Viokase) capsule and 5 mL of sterile water. Inject the alkalinized enzyme mixture into the tube and clamp it for 5 minutes. Flush the tube with water until clear. If the aforementioned techniques fail, the tube should be replaced.

Table 7 Comparison and Components of Selected Polymeric Enteral Formulas

Product	Manufacturer	Cal/mL	Protein (g/L)	Osmolality (moSm/kg)	Nonprotein Cal:N Ratio
Isocal	Mead Johnson	1.06	34	270	168
Isocal HN	Mead Johnson	1.06	44	270	125
Isocal HN Plus	Mead Johnson	1.2	54	400	114
Boost	Mead Johnson	1.01	43	610–670	125
Boost Plus	Mead Johnson	1.52	61	630–670	134
Ensure	Ross	1.06	37.2	555	153
Ensure Plus	Ross	1.5	54.9	690	146
Ensure Plus HN	Ross	1.5	62.6	650	125
Isosource	Novartis	1.2	43	490	149
IsosourceHN	Novartis	1.2	53	490	115
Nutren 1.0	Nestle	1.0	40	300–350	134
Nutren 1.5	Nestle	1.5	60	430–530	134
Nutren 2.0	Nestle	2.0	80	720	134
Osmolite	Ross	1.06	37.1	300	153
Osmolite HN	Ross	1.06	37.1	300	153
Osmolite HN Plus	Ross	1.2	55.5	360	110
Resource Plus	Novartis	1.5	55	600	148
Deliver 2.0	Mead Johnson	2.0	75	640	144
Two-Cal HN	Ross	2.0	83.5	690	125
Promote	Ross	1.0	62.5	340	75
Replete	Nestle	1.0	62.4	300–350	75
Boost with Fiber	Mead Johnson	1.06	46	480	120
Ultracal	Mead Johnson	1.06	45	360	124
Ultracal HN Plus	Mead Johnson	1.2	54	370	114
Compleat Modified	Novartis	1.07	43	300	131
Isosource 1.5 Cal	Novartis	1.5	68	650	116
Jevity	Ross	1.06	44.3	300	125
Jevity Plus	Ross	1.2	55.5	450	110
Nutren 1.0 with Fiber	Nestle	1.0	40	310–370	134
Probalance	Nestle	1.2	54	350–450	114
Promote with Fiber	Ross	1.0	62.5	380	75
Replete with Fiber	Nestle	1.0	62.5	310–390	77

Formula–Drug Interactions

Formula–drug interactions resulting in delayed or diminished drug absorption are outlined in Table 8.[33] In addition, physical incompatibilities between enteral formulas and medications may result in tube obstruction, as detailed in Table 9.[34]

Diarrhea

Diarrhea is defined as an increase in the quantity and/or frequency of bowel movements. Diarrhea has been reported to occur in approximately 30% of patients receiving tube feeding.[35] However, tube feeding itself is often not the cause.[36] Potential causes of diarrhea include (1) an inappropriate rate of formula infusion, (2) impaired functional capacity of the gastrointestinal tract, (3) hypoalbuminemia, (4) the concurrent use of antibiotics and other medications, (5) altered bacterial flora, and (6) enteral formula contamination.

The healthy gastrointestinal tract can handle intermittent feedings of as much as 500 mL given over 10 to 15 minutes. This feeding method has routinely been used with success in patients with dysphagia owing to cancer of the head and neck.[35] If diarrhea occurs, slower delivery of intermittent feedings or a change in the tube feeding product to one that is isotonic or contains fiber may be helpful.

Enteral nutrition-related diarrhea is often secondary to an osmotic effect, which is the result of the small intestine's inability to absorb specific nutrients. This condition is frequently associated with a decline in intestinal blood flow and absorptive capacity. Hypoalbuminemia, which is associated with poor water absorption by the colon, can also contribute to diarrhea. This is observed in patients with edema and fluid overload. Switching the enteral solution to a more calorie-dense product (1.5 to 2.0 cal/mL) will decrease free water intake and may help correct fluid balance. When serum albumin is severely low, intravenous infusion of albumin may be indicated to correct fluid balance and promote protein repletion.

The diarrhea resulting after tolerance to an enteral formula has been achieved may be attributable to bacterial overgrowth. This overgrowth is often caused by long-term antibiotic use. If suspected, stool cultures for *Clostridium difficile* should be performed and the patient treated with oral vancomycin or metronidazole as indicated. The use of a fiber-containing formula has been helpful in correcting loose stools in these cases. Antidiarrhea medications should be used with caution if an infectious cause of diarrhea is suspected.

Another potential cause of diarrhea is fecal impaction in which loose stool can leak around the area of impaction until the bowel is cleared. Medications, especially antacids, can also induce diarrhea and should be considered.

Refeeding Syndrome

Refeeding syndrome is a serious metabolic disturbance that may occur with the initiation of aggressive nutrition support in a patient with severely depleted nutrition stores. Significant compartmental shifts in phosphorus, magnesium, and potassium can be induced. These shifts, as well as sodium retention with resultant expansion of the extracellular space and associated increased circulatory demands, may prove disastrous.

Hypophosphatemia is potentially the most serious single consequence in refeeding syndrome.[37] In starvation, there is a slowing of the overall metabolic rate and, in particular, glucose oxidation. The need for phosphorus is low. When carbohydrates and glucose are reintroduced, this need dramatically rises and may surpass the rate at which phosphorus can be mobilized from bone. Cardiopulmonary failure and death may occur within days of feeding a previously starved but stable patient.

In patients at risk for refeeding syndrome, normal levels of phosphorus, potassium, and magnesium should be present prior to initiating nutrition support. Calorie repletion begins at less than 50% of need and is advanced over the course of a week to a goal of 30 cal/kg/d or less. If adequate renal and hepatic function exists, 1.5 g of protein/kg/d can also be administered. A daily multivitamin, mineral supplement, thiamine (100 mg/d), and selenium (50 μg/d) are recommended. Careful monitoring of vital signs, weight, and input and output, as well as electrolytes, is necessary during nutrition support of at-risk individuals.

PARENTERAL NUTRITION

Parenteral nutrition is the intravascular administration of carbohydrates, protein, fat, vitamins, and minerals. Total parenteral nutrition involves nutrient administration into the superior vena

Table 9 Mediations Incompatible with Enteral Nutritional Formulas

Product	Incompatibility/Interaction
Vitamin B elixir	Forms large particle clumping
Brompheniramine elixir	Forms adhesive gelatinous material
Brompheniramine phenylpropanolamine elixir	Enteral food breakdown
Calcium glubionate syrup	Adhesive gelatinous mass created
Chlorpromazine concentrate	Granulation occurs at point of mixing
Doxepin liquid	Feeding separates slightly with no clogging
Ferrous sulfate elixir	Completely gels and clogs feeding tubes
Guaifenesin expectorant	Viscous precipitate forms
KCl 10% and 20% liquid	Incompatible at mixing interface
KCl syrup	Enteral products become viscous and gelatinous
Lithium syrup	Enteral products form granular film
Medium-chain triglyceride oil	Immiscible with enteral products
Methenamine mandelate suspension forte	Mixture becomes gelatinous
Metoclopramide	Some feedings form thin granular formulation
Opium liquid	Separation, globular particle formation
Phosphosoda	Results in heavy or granular feedings
Pseudoephedrine syrup	Viscous gelatinous mass forms on mixing
Sucralfate	Solidifies formula
Thioridazine solution	Granule formation
Zinc sulfate capsules	May induce gelatinous or hard mass formation

Table 8 Significant Drug–Nutrient Interactions

Medications	Interaction	Possible Outcome
Antibiotics		
Tetracycline	Decreased bioavailability with milk and dairy products	Treatment failure
Quinolones(ciprofloxacin/ norfloxacin)	Decreased bioavailability with milk and dairy products	Treatment failure
Azithromycin	Decreased bioavailability with food	Treatment failure
Antifungal		
Itraconazole	Increased bioavailability with food	Possible treatment failure if not administered with meals
Antiviral		
Didanosine	Food decreases bioavailability	Treatment failure
Indinavir		
Saquinavir	Food increases bioavailability	Increased antiviral activity if administered with meals
Warfarin	Vitamin K–rich foods antagonize the anticoagulant effect	Decreased anticoagulation
Cyclosporin	Food and grapefruit juice increase plasma levels	Possible toxicity, lower doses may be efficacious
Alendronate	Food decreases bioavailability	Treatment failure

cava, thereby allowing for the infusion of hypertonic solutions. Hyperalimentation solutions typically contain 25% glucose given at a gradually increasing infusion rate toward a goal of 5 mg glucose/kg/min.

Insulin requirements must be closely monitored. Amino acids are administered in 2.5 to 5.0% solutions in sufficient quantity to ensure positive nitrogen balance. The remainder of noncarbohydrate calories is derived from fat emulsions. Peripheral partial nutrition supplements enteral feeding with the administration of a 10% glucose solution, amino acids, and fat emulsion through a peripheral vein.

Complications from parenteral nutrition are significantly higher than for enteral feeding and include sepsis, hyperglycemia, hypoglycemia, hyperlipidemia, hepatic dysfunction, electrolyte imbalance, and thrombophlebitis. The indications for parenteral nutrition in the head and neck patient are limited to gastrointestinal dysfunction or intractable aspiration of tube feedings. Occasionally, total parenteral nutrition is used to treat a chyle fistula not responsive to medium-chain triglyceride formulas.

CONCLUSIONS

Several factors conspire to induce malnutrition in the head and neck patient. It is necessary to identify and quantify nutritional deficits to replete losses adequately. Enteral feeding is desired with a functioning gastrointestinal tract, and various maneuvers exist to use an intact gut better. Nutrition repletion should be carefully monitored to allow the patient the potential benefits of increased treatment tolerance and perhaps improved survival.

REFERENCES

1. van Bokhorst-de van der Schueren MA, van Leeuwen A, Kuik D, et al. The impact of nutritional status on the prognosis of patients with advanced head and neck cancer. Cancer 1999;86:519–27.

2. Todorov P, Cariuk P, McDevitt T, et al. Characterization of cancer cachectic factor. Nature 1996;379:739–42.

3. Allal AS, Maire D, Becker M, Dulguerov P. Feasibility and early results of accelerated radiotherapy for head and neck carcinoma in the elderly. Cancer 2000;88:648–52.

4. Collins MM, Wight RG, Partridge G. Nutritional consequences of radiotherapy in early laryngeal carcinoma. Ann R Coll Surg Engl 1999;81:376–81.

5. Mangar S, Slevin N, Mais K, Sykes A. Evaluating predictive factors for determining enteral nutrition in patients receiving radical radiotherapy for head and neck cancer: A retrospective review. Radiother Oncol 2006;78:152–8.

6. Shiley SG, Harfunani CA, Skoner JM, et al. Swallowing function after chemoradiation for advanced stage oropharyngeal cancer. Otolaryngol Head Neck Surg 2006;134:455–9.

7. van Bokhorst-de van der Schueren MA, van Leeuwen PA, Sauerwein HP, et al. Assessment of malnutrition parameters in head and neck cancer and their relation to postoperative complications. Head Neck 1997;19:419–25.

8. Ursule G, Kyle. The patient with head and neck cancer. In: Bloch AS, editor. Nutrition Management of the Cancer Patient. Boston: Jones & Bartlett Publishers; 1990. p. 55.

9. van Bokhorst-De van der Schuer MA, von Blombergvan der Flier BM, Riezebos RK, et al. Differences in immune status between well-nourished and malnourished head and neck cancer patients. Clin Nutr 1998;17:107–11.

10. Snyderman CH, Kachman K, Molseed L, et al. Reduced postoperative infections with an immune-enhancing nutritional supplement. Laryngoscope 1999;109:915–21.

11. Larsson M, Hedelin B, Johansson I, et al. Eating problems and weight loss for patients with head and neck cancer: A chart review from diagnosis until 1 year after treatment. Cancer Nurs 2005;28:425–35.

12. Dikshit RP, Boffeta P, Bouchardy C, et al. Lifestyle habits as prognostic factors in survival of laryngeal and hypopharyngeal cancer: A multicentric European study. Int J Cancer 2005;117:992–5.

13. Isenring FA, Capra S, Bauer JD. Nutrition intervention is beneficial in oncology outpatients receiving radiotherapy to the gastrointestinal or head and neck area. Br J Cancer 2004;91:447–52.

14. Gottschlich MM, Matarese LE, Shronts EP. Nutrition Support Dietetics Core Curriculum, 2nd edition. Washington, Dc: American Society of Parenteral Nutrition; 1993.

15. Metropolitan Life Insurance Company. Height and frame size vs body weight. January–June: Statistical Bulletin, 1983.

16. Hamwi GJ. Therapy: Changing dietary concepts. In: Donowski TS, editor. Diabetes Mellitus: Diagnosis and Treatment. New York: American Diabetes Association; 1964. p. 55.

17. Scheltinga MR. Bioelectrical impedance analysis (BIA): A bedside method for fluid measurement. Studies of the bodies electrical impedance in various models of health and disease [thesis]. Amsterdam: Vrije Universiteit; 1992.

18. Heimburger DC, Weinsier RL. Nutritional assessment. Handbook of Clinical Nutrition, 3rd edition. St. Louis, Mo: Mosby-Year Book, 1997. p. 183.

19. National Academy of Sciences. Recommended Dietary Allowances. Washington, DC: US Government Printing Office; 1974.

20. Cerra FB. Surgical Nutrition. St. Louis, MO: CV Mosby; 1984.

21. Nordenstrom J, Askanazi J, Elwyn DH, et al. Nitrogen balance during total parenteral nutrition: Glucose vs fat. Ann Surg 1983;197:27–33.

22. Gallagher-Allred C. Vitamin and mineral requirements. In: Krey SH, Murray RL, editors. Dynamics of Nutrition Support. Norwalk, CT: Appleton-Century-Crofts; 1986.

23. Prasad A, Beck F, Doerr T, et al. Nutritional and zinc status of head and neck cancer patients: An interpretive review. J Am Coll Nutr 1998;17:409–18.

24. Ripamonti C, Zecca E, Brunelli C, et al. A randomized controlled clinical trial to evaluate the effects of zinc sulfate on cancer patients with taste alterations caused by head and neck irradiation. Cancer 1998;82:1938–45.

25. Horiuchi H, Nagata I, Komoriya K. Protective effect of vitamin D3 analogues on endotoxin shock in mice. Agents Actions 1991;33:343–8.

26. Bairati I, Meyer F, Gelinas M, et al. A randomized trial of antioxidant vitamins to prevent secondary primary cancers in head and neck cancer patients. J Natl Cancer Inst 2005;97:481–8.

27. Mercadante S. Parenteral versus enteral nutrition in cancer patients: Indications and practice. Support Care Cancer 1998;6:85–93.

28. Klein S, Kinney J, Jeejeebhoy K, et al. Nutrition support in clinical practice: Review of published data and recommendations for future research directions. Am J Clin Nutr 1997;66:683–706.

29. Gramlich L, Kichian K, Pinilla J, et al. Does enteral nutrition compared to preenteral nutrition result in better outcomes in critically ill adult patients? A systematic review of the literature. Nutrition 2004;20:843–8.

30. Loprinzi CL, Kugler JW, Sloan JA, et al. Randomized comparison of megestrol acetate versus dexamethasone versus fluoxymesterone for the treatment of cancer anorexia/cachexia. J Clin Oncol 1999;17:3299–306.

31. Colasanto JM, Prasad P, Nash MA, et al. Nutritional support of patients undergoing radiation therapy for head and neck cancer. Oncology 2005;19:371–9; discussion 380–2, 387.

32. Raynor EM, Williams MF, Martindale RG, Porubsky ES. Timing of percutaneous endoscopic gastrostomy tube placement in head and neck cancer patients. Otolaryngol Head Neck Surg 1999;120:479–82.

33. Huey L, Way J. Medication administration via enteral access tubes. Patient Care News. Sherwood Medical Company; 1997. p. 2–3.

34. Guenter PA, Settle RG, Perlmutter S, et al. Tube feeding related diarrhea in acutely ill patients. JPEN J Parenter Enteral Nutr 1991;15:277–80.

35. Edes TE, Waek BE, Austin JL. Diarrhea in tube-fed patients: Feeding formula not necessarily the cause. Am J Med 1990;88:91–3.

36. Shike M, Berner YN, Gerdes H, et al. Percutaneous endoscopic gastrostomy and jejunostomy for long-term feeding in patients with head and neck cancer. Otolaryngol Head Neck Surg 1989;101:549–54.

37. Crook MA, Collins D, Swaminathan R. Severe hypophosphatemia related to refeeding. Nutrition 1996;12:538–9.

95

Neoplasms of the Anterior Skull Base

Lawrence J. Marentette, MD

Becky L. Massey, MD

Robert M. Kellman, MD

Walter Dandy, a neurosurgeon at Johns Hopkins Hospital, described the first anterior craniofacial resection in 1941.[1] His procedure involved an anterior craniotomy with the resection of an orbital tumor and the adjacent ethmoid sinuses. Alfred Ketcham and colleagues, in 1963, described the anterior craniofacial resection for paranasal sinus tumors in 19 patients.[2] His subsequent paper reported the results of 32 patients with a 10-year follow-up. Although the long-term survival improved to 61%, the complication rate was 80%. All of these procedures involved frontal lobe retraction which can lead to encephalomalacia and neurologic impairment. In the 1960s, the principles of craniofacial surgery were introduced and began to serve as the basis for skull base surgery. Tessier described various periorbital osteotomies for the correction of orbital hypertelorism.[3] Based on these principles, Raveh in 1983 developed the technique of the subcranial approach initially for patients with craniobasilar trauma.[4] This approach involved the removal of a portion of the frontal bone exposing the anterior cranial fossa along with the glabella and attached nasal bones, thus allowing a direct path to the skull base without frontal lobe retraction. He and his colleagues expanded this approach in 1993 to anterior skull base tumor surgery.[5] Obwegeser in 1985 described various malar and mandibular osteotomies to gain access to the infratemporal fossa.[6] He also described the dissection in the temporal fat pad, during a coronal exposure, to preserve the temporal branches of the facial nerve.

Today, advances in surgical technique, chemotherapy, and radiation therapy have led to improved survival for patients with skull base tumors. Diagnostic advances in magnetic resonance imaging (MRI), computerized tomography (CT), and positron emission tomography (PET) now allow surgeons to delineate the exact margins of the tumor, improving surgical selection of patients. In spite of these advances, however, patients often present with advanced disease as a result of minimal symptoms in the early stages of their disease process.

EVALUATION

Symptoms

Anterior skull base neoplasms are rare. These neoplasms originate from the paranasal sinuses and orbits below, the intracranial contents above and rarely in and from the bone of the cranial base. Symptoms may be vague, and the patients are often diagnosed with sinusitis. Significant delay in diagnosis may occur until attempts at medical treatment for sinusitis fail or additional symptoms present prompting an imaging study.

Common symptoms and signs in patients with anterior skull base neoplasms can be conveniently divided into early and late (Table 1). Symptoms of early skull base neoplasms may be minimal, making early diagnosis difficult. Early symptoms and signs include epistaxis, nasal obstruction, and foul smelling nasal discharge. The presence of new onset, unilateral symptoms is one of the most important indicators that helps to differentiate neoplastic from inflammatory sinonasal disease. Epistaxis is generally moderate to severe in patients with poorly differentiated neoplasms such as squamous cell carcinoma or sinonasal undifferentiated carcinoma. Well differentiated neoplasms such as esthesioneuroblastoma, may only develop nasal obstruction.

Late symptoms and signs include paresthesias, proptosis, olfactory impairment, pain on opening the mouth, hearing loss, and malocclusion. Paresthesias may result from the neoplasm invading the branches of the trigeminal nerve. The first division of the trigeminal nerve (cranial nerve V1) is often involved as a result of invasion by a neurotropic cutaneous squamous cell carcinoma. The

second division (V2) may be involved in maxillary carcinomas and sarcomas. The third division (V3) is frequently involved by neoplasms arising in the infratemporal fossa. Neoplasms that exhibit neurotropism, commonly adenoid cystic carcinoma, develop retrograde spread and may invade the pterygopalatine ganglion, then follow the nerve of the pterygoid canal to the geniculate ganglion and produce facial paralysis. Proptosis results from tumor invasion into the orbit and can be an early sign in patients with lacrimal gland neoplasms or a late sign with undifferentiated carcinoma. Patients presenting with anosmia usually have bilateral involvement of the nasal cavities or may have an olfactory grove meningioma with no intranasal findings. The late symptoms include neck mass as a result of lymphatic metastasis. Pain on opening the mouth may be a late presenting symptom as a result of erosion of the posterior portion of the maxilla with extension of the neoplasm into the pterygoid muscles. Unilateral conductive hearing loss can result from the neoplasm extending posteriorly into the nasopharynx causing eustachian tube obstruction. Malocclusion may be a late complaint resulting from maxillary neoplasms extending inferiorly into the alveolar ridge causing displacement of the dentition.

Physical Findings

On physical examination, a nasal mass can often be readily seen either with anterior rhinoscopy or endoscopic evaluation. The finding of a friable mass is indicative of a poorly or undifferentiated malignant neoplasm. There may be restriction of the extraocular muscles, in particular the medial rectus, as a result of invasion of the neoplasm through the lamina papyracea. The extraocular muscle dysfunction may also result from retrograde spread of the tumor into a cavernous sinus. Paresthesias of the second division of the trigeminal nerve occur when the neoplasm involves the maxilla. Paresthesias of the third division of the trigeminal nerve often occur with involvement of the infratemporal fossa as a result of neoplastic invasion in the retromaxillary space. These patients will also present with pain on opening the mouth. Facial paralysis in a patient with facial paresthesias results from spread of the neoplasm along the trigeminal nerve with a jump lesion

---

Table 1 Symptoms and Signs of Skull Base Neoplasms

Early
   Epistaxis
   Nasal obstruction
   Nasal discharge
Late
   Proptosis
   Impaired extraocular movement
   Parasthesia
   Anosmia
   Hearing loss
   Malocclusion
   Neck mass

to the facial nerve. Epiphora is a late finding in patients with nasal cavity neoplasms but an early sign in patients with ethmoid sinus carcinoma invading the lacrimal fossa and the medial portion of the orbit.

Imaging

A CT scan is important in evaluating the extent of anterior skull base neoplasms and in particular delineating areas of bone destruction. With soft tissue windows the extent of the tumor can be delineated but may not be distinguishable from secretions in the paranasal sinuses from ostial obstruction by the neoplastic mass. MRI has proven invaluable for evaluating the soft tissue extent of the neoplasm and also invasion of the dura and brain parenchyma. Combined axial and coronal T1- and T2-weighted images with gadolinium will clearly identify areas of tumor enhancement and also possible brain edema which is seen on the T2 image. Retained sinus secretions will appear hyperintense on the T2 image (Figure 1). With any question or orbital involvement, fat saturation technique is important to delineate the mass from orbital fat. This is accomplished by eliminating the fat signal on the gadolinium enhanced T1 image (Figure 2). CT angiography or MR angiography has been helpful in evaluating any vascular involvement by the neoplasm and is a much less invasive method than conventional angiography. Angiography is still helpful, particularly in vascular lesions that will require preoperative embolization, such as juvenile nasopharyngeal angiofibroma.

Existing Medical Records and Other Data

An important part of the patient's overall evaluation is the careful review of earlier medical records from the referring physician. The patient should bring actual scans in addition to reports to be reviewed by the skull base surgeon as well as office records indicating the duration of symptoms and other findings as well as potential comorbid factors.

Prior biopsies should be reviewed at a tertiary care center; and, if necessary, additional staining techniques should be performed to confirm the diagnosis. The definitive diagnosis may depend on the immunohistochemical profile of the neoplasm. Often, a diagnosis of esthesioneuroblastoma is changed to sinonasal undifferentiated carcinoma after immunostaining.

Appropriate consultations with the neurosurgeon, reconstructive surgeon, and radiation and medical oncologists should be initiated preoperatively to optimize patient care and offer participation in clinical trials.

Special Testing

In some instances, it may be necessary to resect the internal carotid artery to achieve tumor extirpation. If this is the case, a balloon test occlusion is warranted to evaluate the potential for a stroke. The catheter is inserted via the femoral artery into the internal carotid artery and inflated.

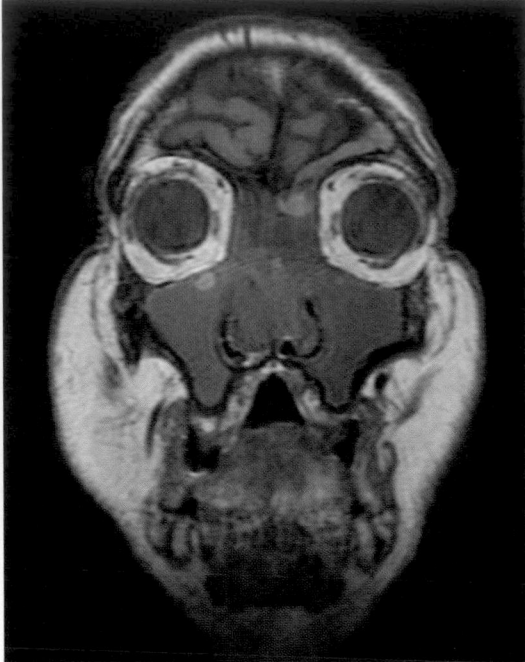

(A)

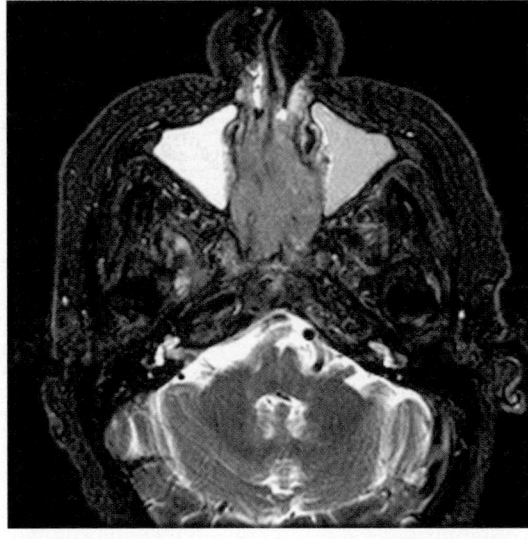

(B)

Figure 1 Inspissated secretions distinguished from tumor. (A) T1-weighted coronal magnetic resonance imaging (MRI) with contrast enhancement. Opacification of the maxillary sinuses is difficult to distinguish from tumor. (B) T2-weighted axial MRI shows hyperintensity in maxillary sinuses consistent with inspissated mucus. (Published with permission, copyright © 2007 B.L. Massey, MD.)

The patient is evaluated for any changes in his or her neurologic status. If the patient becomes hemiparetic or aphasic, the balloon is deflated and the catheter is immediately withdrawn. If the patient can tolerate balloon test occlusion for 15 to 20 minutes, the surgeon may proceed with a carotid resection. However, up to 22% of patients who pass the balloon test occlusion may have delayed ischemic complications.

PATHOLOGY

Benign Neoplasms

A variety of benign neoplasms occur in the anterior skull base and may cause significant

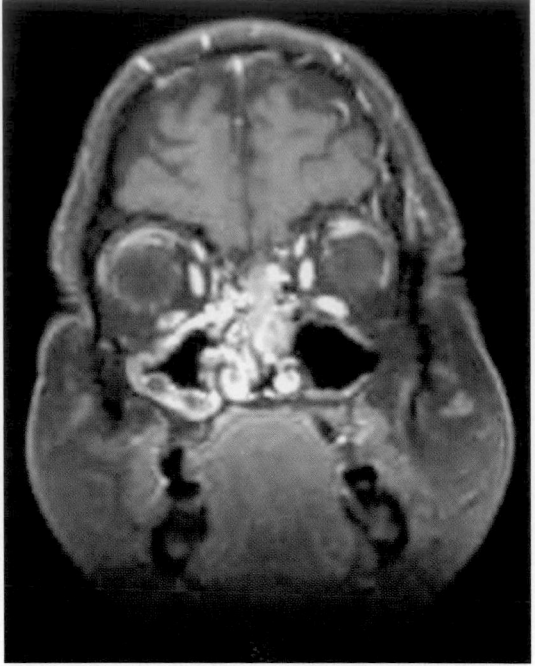

Figure 2 Coronal T1-weighted magnetic resonance imaging with fat saturation shows an esthesioneuroblastoma involving the left ethmoid sinus. (Published with permission, copyright © 2007 B.L. Massey, MD.)

disability from compression of critical structures. Growth rates are variable, and symptoms may not occur until the neoplasm has obtained large size. Observation and limited resection are possible for many patients. The most common benign lesions are listed in Table 2. Benign sinonasal neoplasms are discussed in Chapter 51, "Endoscopic Surgery of the Skull Base, Orbits, and Benign Sinonasal Neoplasms."

Osseous and Fibroosseous Tumors

Many osteomas, chrondromas, and fibroosseous tumors may remain asymptomatic or may produce symptoms which vary with site and growth rate of the tumor. Osteomas occur most often in the frontal sinus and are rarely symptomatic. Fibrous dysplasia is more common in women and may cause cosmetic deformity. In those with asymptomatic tumors found incidentally, surgery may be recommended to establish a definitive diagnosis. Intervention may also be needed in those with pain, obstruction of frontoethmoid outflow leading to mucocele, and cranial nerve dysfunction due to foraminal compression.

Table 2 Benign Anterior Skull Base Neoplasms
Chondroma
Craniopharyngioma
Fibrous dysplasia
Inverted papilloma
Juvenile nasopharyngeal angiofibroma
Lymphangioma
Meningioma
Neurofibroma
Ossifying fibroma
Osteoma
Osteoblastoma
Schwannoma

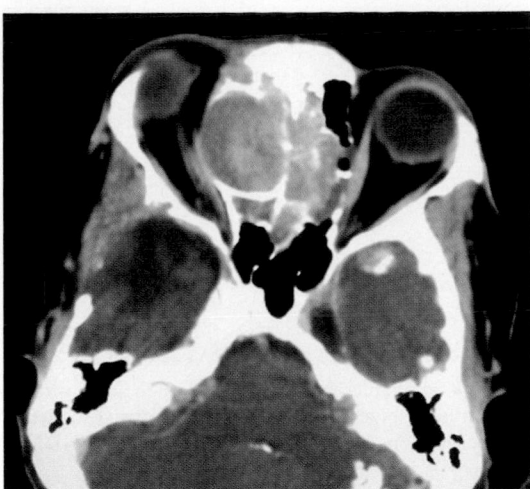

Figure 3 Sinonasal schwannoma. Axial contrast enhanced computed tomography. (Published with permission, copyright © 2007 B.L. Massey, MD.)

Nerve Sheath Neoplasms

Peripheral nerve sheath neoplasms of the sinonasal tract are rare. Sinonasal schwannomas represent only 4% of head and neck schwannomas.[7] Schwannomas of the sinonasal tract are most common in the ethmoid sinuses where they are thought to originate from sensory branches of the trigeminal nerve and autonomic nerves. Unlike other head and neck schwannomas, sinonasal schwannomas are typically not encapsulated and may have surface ulceration.[8] Schwannomas may grow to large size and may involve the orbit, skull base, and intracranial cavity by pushing rather than invading the surrounding tissue (Figure 3). Neurofibromas of the skull base are rare even in those with neurofibromatosis.

Malignant Neoplasms

Paranasal sinus cancers are the most common malignancies to involve the anterior skull base. Paranasal sinus malignancies account for only 3% of head and neck cancers, and the annual incidence is approximately one to three cases per 100,000 people. Those with skull base involvement represent an even smaller group. There is no high level evidence to prove optimal therapy, and most patients are treated with surgery followed by adjuvant radiotherapy. Early symptoms of paranasal sinus and skull base malignancies including nasal obstruction and epistaxis may be difficult to distinguish from benign sinonasal complaints. Late signs including proptosis, diploplia, and cranial neuropathy occur after extensive local invasion and should prompt evaluation for malignancy. A diverse group of epithelial and nonepithelial malignant neoplasms with variable biologic aggressiveness may occur and are listed in Table 3. The more common tumors are described.

Squamous Cell Carcinoma. Squamous cell carcinoma (SCC) is the most common malignant neoplasm of the paranasal sinuses. Most paranasal SCCs arise in the maxillary sinuses and skull base involvement occurs late and in advanced disease (Figure 4). Primary SCC arising in the ethmoid sinus is less common, but its likelihood

Table 3 Malignant Anterior Skull Base Neoplasms
Adenoid cystic carcinoma
Basaloid carcinoma
Chondrosarcoma
Chordoma
Esthesioneuroblastoma
Fibrosarcoma
Hemangiopericytoma
Lymphoma
Malignant fibrous histiocytoma
Osteosarcoma
Rhabdomyosarcoma
Malignant schwannoma
Sinonasal melanoma
Sinonasal undifferentiated carcinoma
Squamous cell carcinoma

of invading the skull base is high. Primary SCC of the frontal or sphenoid sinuses is rare. SCC of the nasal cavity may extend directly to the skull base. Males are affected twice as often as females, which is believed to be due to greater occupational exposure to carcinogens. Multiple studies have evaluated risk factors for sinonasal malignancy. While nickel refining is most often cited as a risk for SCC, asbestos, formaldehyde and textile industry exposure have also been implicated.[9,10] As in other head and neck SCC, tobacco use is a known risk factor.[11] The role of chronic inflammatory sinus disease as a risk factor for SCC is controversial. Treatment for paranasal SCC is usually primarily surgical with adjuvant radiotherapy for all except small tumors. The incidence of regional metastases is less than 10%, and the clinically negative neck is typically not treated. While prognosis for SCC remains poor with 5-year survival less than 50%, outcomes for adenocarcinoma and esthesioneuroblastoma are much better.

Adenocarcinoma. Adenocarcinoma accounts for a third of paranasal sinus malignancies. Adenocarcinoma arises from the glandular elements of the sinonasal epithelium or from

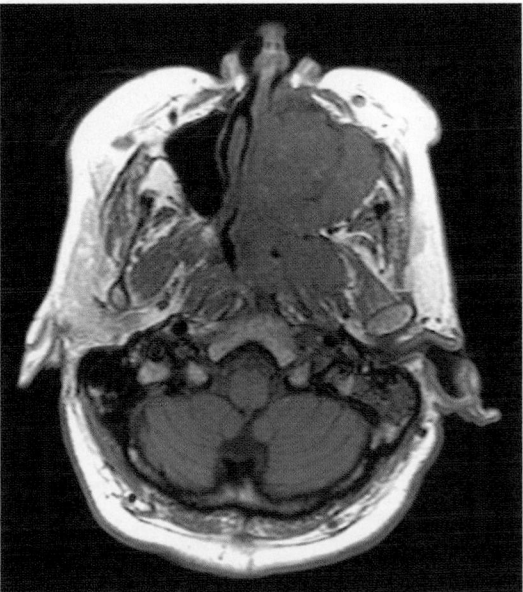

Figure 4 Axial T 1-weighted magnetic resonance imaging. Left maxillary sinus squamous cell carcinoma with extension to the skull base. (Published with permission, copyright © 2007 B.L. Massey, MD.)

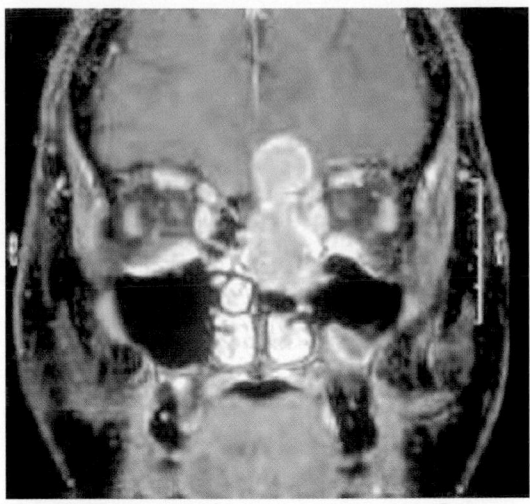

Figure 5 Adenocarcinoma with intracranial extension. T1-weighted coronal magnetic resonance imaging with contrast enhancement. (Published with permission, copyright © 2007 B.L. Massey, MD.)

minor salivary tissue. Occupational exposure in woodworkers to both wood dust and chemicals, such as formaldehyde, used in wood preservation is a well-documented risk factor for sinonasal adenocarcinoma.[12] Adenocarcinomas commonly arise in the upper nasal cavity and ethmoid sinuses affecting the anterior skull base by direct extension (Figure 5). Adenocarcinomas are classified by grade based on glandular architecture and cytopathologic features. Comparison of biologic behavior is difficult due to low incidence and variable classification systems in the literature. In general, low-grade adenocarcinomas have more glandular differentiation, fewer nuclear pleomorphism and less locoregional metastases. Treatment is surgical with adjuvant radiation therapy. In contrast to SCC, 5-year survival from adenocarcinoma approaches 80%.

Adenoid Cystic Carcinoma. Adenoid cystic carcinoma is the most common malignancy occurring in the minor salivary tissue in the sinonasal mucosa adjacent to the skull base. Adenoid cystic carcinoma comprises approximately 10% of paranasal sinus malignancies and affects the skull base by direct extension and/or perineural spread. Adenoid cystic carcinoma usually presents as a slow growing mass with early perineural involvement. Adenoid cystic carcinoma has three subtypes: tubular, cribriform, and solid. Tumor grade is determined by percentage of solid growth pattern and nuclear pleomorphism. Higher grade is associated with distant metastases and poorer survival. Perineural invasion and submucosal spread are common in both low and high grades leading to a high rate of local recurrence with considerable morbidity at the skull base. Involvement of the skull base leads to poorer prognosis, and en bloc resection with negative margins is difficult. Adenoid cystic carcinoma is indolent with delayed distant metastases frequent, but regional lymph nodal metastasis is uncommon. Treatment is surgical with adjuvant radiation therapy. Proton beam radiotherapy has been used for gross residual disease at the skull base with encouraging results.[13] Chemotherapy is not recommended outside of a clinical trial.

Lymphoma. Lymphoma. occurring in the sinonasal regional is typically non-Hodgkin lymphoma. Lymphomas of B-cell, T-cell, T/Natural Killer (NK)-cell types may occur and have distinct biologic behavior. Surgical intervention is typically limited to biopsy. Definitive diagnosis of lymphoma subtype often requires advanced immunostaining for cell markers. Treatment is typically local radiotherapy with possible adjuvant chemotherapy with distinct differences in response rates between the subtypes. T-cell lymphomas have good response to treatment except those that also stain for NK markers. Sinonasal T/NK-cell lymphoma is an aggressive, destructive lesion formally known as lethal midline granuloma. Sinonasal T/NK-cell lymphoma presents as an angiodestructive mass causing nasal obstruction with foul odor and associated tissue necrosis. There is believed to be an association with the Epstein-Barr virus. Destruction of the nasal septum is common, and skull base destruction may be impressive with leptomeningeal spread (Figure 6).

Esthesioneuroblastoma. Esthesioneuroblastoma, or olfactory neuroblastoma, is a neural crest derived neoplasm arising directly from the olfactory neuroepithelium. Esthesioneuroblastoma is a rare neoplasm accounting for 3% of intracranial tumors and 6% of sinonasal tumors. In 1997, approximately 1,000 cases of esthesioneuroblastoma had been reported.[14] Bimodal peaks of incidence occur at the second and sixth decades. There are no clear racial or ethnic predilections or known risk factors.

Esthesioneuroblastoma may be limited to the upper nasal vault but most commonly involves the cribriform plate allowing direct intracranial extension. Like other sinonasal neoplasms, esthesioneuroblastoma often presents with unilateral nasal obstruction and epistaxis. Headache, diplo-

plia, proptosis, and cranial nerve deficits appear as orbital and intracranial invasion occur. Anosmia occurs when both sides of the upper nasal cavity or the entire cribriform plate are replaced by the neoplasm. Esthesioneuroblastoma grows slowly and may have extensive submucosal spread. Intracranial extension occurs as the neoplasm spreads through the cribriform foramina and with overt cribriform destruction (Figure 7). Extension through the perforating vessels of the lamina papyracea allows direct access to the orbit. Cervical lymph node metastases occur in approximately 20% of patients with esthesioneuroblastomas but may not be apparent at the initial diagnosis. Local recurrences are common, and long-term follow-up is necessary.

Esthesioneuroblastoma usually presents as a mass centered in the superior part of a nasal cavity. Microscopically, esthesioneuroblastoma is

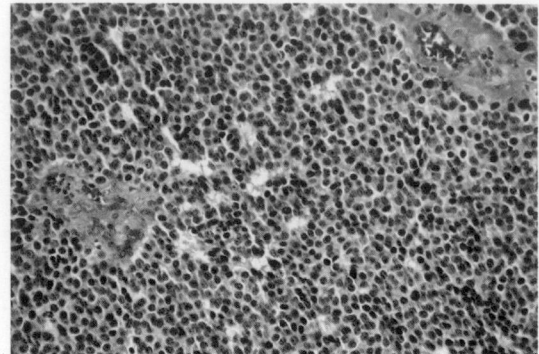

Figure 8 Photomicrograph of an esthesioneuroblastoma. Small, round, blue cells with rosette pattern. (Published with permission, copyright © 2007 B.L. Massey, MD.)

composed of small, blue round cells that must be differentiated from similarly appearing neoplasms including lymphoma, melanoma, neuroendocrine carcinoma, rhabdomyosarcoma, and sinonasal undifferentiated carcinoma. In low-grade esthesioneuroblastoma, histopathologic evaluation shows small, round cells arranged in a pseudorosette pattern (Figure 8). In high-grade esthesioneuroblastoma, there is more nuclear pleomorphism, and rosettes are not common. Immunohistochemistry is necessary to distinguish it from sinonasal undifferentiated carcinoma which carries a much more ominous prognosis.

Despite its rarity, esthesioneuroblastoma has a number of staging systems. The American Joint Commission on Cancer (AJCC) staging system and the Kadish staging system (Table 4) are most commonly used.[15] Although it has been replaced by the AJCC staging system, the Kadish system introduced in 1976 is often used to provide adjunct information. Esthesioneuroblastoma has the best prognosis of all paranasal sinus malignant neoplasms with 5-year survival from 80 to 100%.[16,17] Morbidity associated with surgical treatment and from local recurrence remains high.

Given the low incidence of esthesioneuroblastoma, adequately powered studies comparing different treatment regimens are not available. The treatment for esthesioneuroblastoma remains dynamic and controversial. There are several, single institution studies reporting excellent outcomes with variable combinations of surgery, radiation, and chemotherapy. Treatment protocols between institutions lack uniformity. Craniofacial resection has been the accepted standard at most institutions. The treatment approach reported by the MD Anderson Cancer Center includes craniofacial resection with adjuvant radiation.[18] Craniofacial resection with adjuvant radiation for positive margins has been reported from the Johns Hopkins group.[19] The single institutional experience reported from

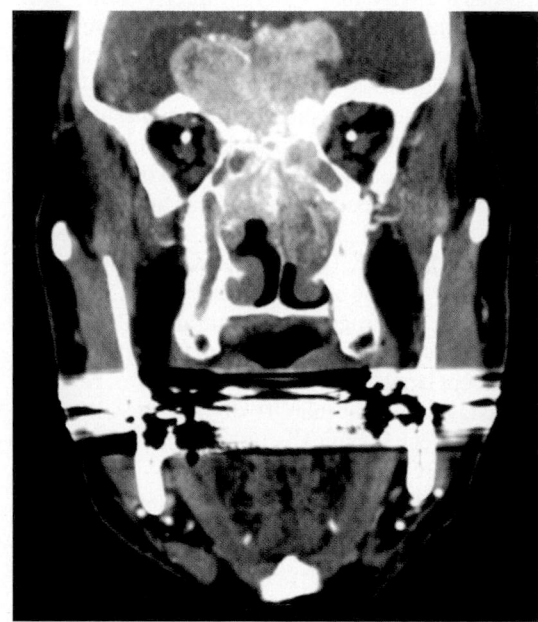

(A)

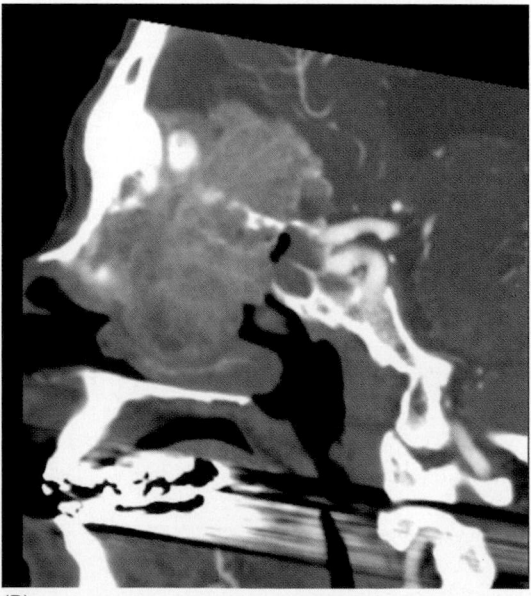

(B)

Figure 7 (A) Coronal and (B) sagittal computed tomography imaging of esthesioneuroblastoma with intracranial involvement. (Published with permission, copyright © 2007 B.L. Massey, MD.)

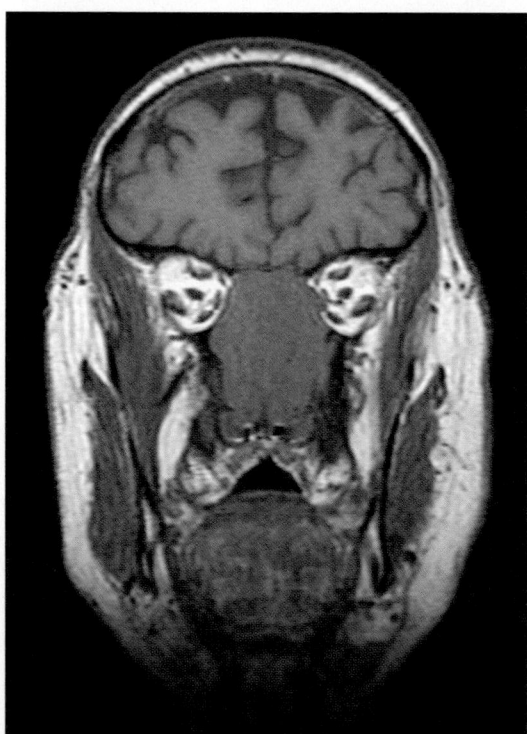

Figure 6 Magnetic resonance imaging of a sinonasal lymphoma. (Published with permission, copyright © 2007 B.L. Massey, MD.)

Table 4 Kadish Staging System	
A	Tumor limited to nasal cavity and paranasal sinuses
B	Tumor extension to orbit
C	Tumor extension to brain

Adapted from reference 15.

the University of Virginia advocates preoperative radiation or chemoradiation therapy followed by craniofacial resection.[20–22] Endoscope-assisted cranial facial resection has become more popular to limit facial and degloving incisions. For more limited neoplasms, endoscopic resection alone is becoming more commonly attempted. Despite the variety of treatment approaches, outcomes do not appear to be significantly different.[23]

Sinonasal Undifferentiated Carcinoma. Sinonasal undifferentiated carcinoma (SNUC) is an uncommon, highly aggressive neoplasm of unknown etiology. It is rare with only 100 reported cases.[24] It often presents as a rapidly enlarging mass with considerable extension to the orbital and intracranial contents (Figure 9). SNUC is associated with poor long-term survival making correct tissue diagnosis critical. SNUCs are hypercellular proliferations with prominent necrosis lacking squamous, glandular, and neuroendocrine features. Chemotherapy is typically used in an induction or primary role. Aggressive surgery and radiation therapy have been associated with decrease symptoms and modest increase in short-term survival. Multiple institutional reports with few patients per report suggest occasional patients with long-term survival.[25,26] Despite aggressive multimodality therapy, 5-year survival is poor.

Staging. The AJCC tumor, regional lymph node metastasis, and distant metastasis (TNM) staging system is most commonly used to stage paranasal sinus cancers.[27] Maxillary sinus cancers that reach the skull base structures are advanced and represent T4 disease. Most tumors with skull base involvement are of nasal cavity or ethmoid sinus origin. There are specific T category guidelines for ethmoid and nasal cavity neoplasms (Table 5) and most patients present with at least a T3 tumor.[28]

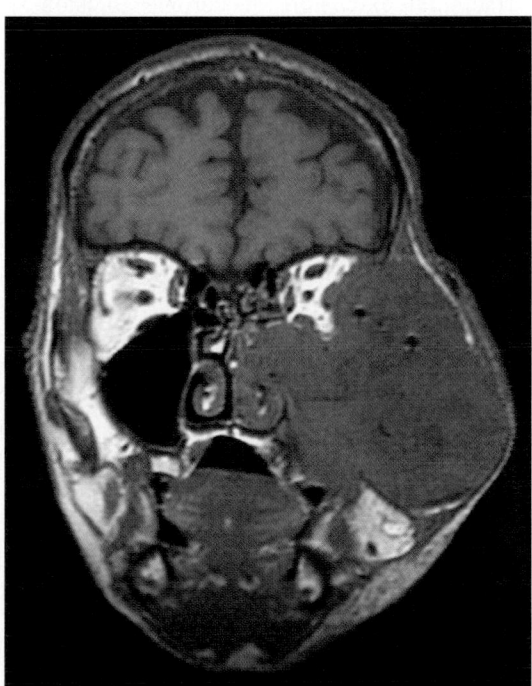

Figure 9 Coronal T 1-weighted magnetic resonance imaging of a sinonasal undifferentiated carcinoma. (Published with permission, copyright © 2007 B.L. Massey, MD.)

Table 5 American Joint Commission on Cancer Tumor System Category for Nasal Cavity and Ethmoid Sinus*

T1	Tumor restricted to one site, with or without bone invasion
T2	Tumor involves two subsites or extends to adjacent region in nasoethmoid complex
T3	Tumor extends to medial wall or orbital floor, maxillary sinus, palate or cribriform plate
T4a	Invades orbit, skin, minimal extension to anterior cranial fossa or pterygoid plates
T4b	Invades orbital apex, dura, brain, middle cranial fossa or clivus

Adapted from reference 27.

*Maxillary sinus tumors invading cribriform plate T4.

SURGICAL MANAGEMENT

Craniofacial Resection

The standard surgical approach for patients with anterior skull base neoplasms is the craniofacial resection. This procedure involves the combined services of otolaryngology and neurosurgery. It is typically performed with a coronal incision in combination with a transfacial incision. Through the coronal incision, the neurosurgeon exposes the frontal bone. As part of the exposure, an anteriorly based pericranial flap is elevated to be employed in the reconstruction of the skull base defect. After the exposure, a bifrontal craniotomy is performed providing access to the anterior cranial fossa. The olfactory grooves are dissected bilaterally to allow retraction of the frontal lobes, thus gaining access to the orbital roof, cribriform plate, fovea ethmoidalis, and planum sphenoidale back to the sphenoid wing and anterior clinoid processes (Figure 10). From below, a lateral rhinotomy is performed or a Weber-Ferguson incision is utilized, if more access is needed to expose the mid-facial skeleton (Figure 11). At this time, the nasal bones may be cut and retracted; and, if necessary, osteotomies of the anterior face of the maxilla may be made and the anterior aspects of the maxilla may be removed. These steps allow wide access to the nasal cavity and the nasal vault up to the cribriform plate as well as the floor of the anterior skull base. The neoplasm is resected in a combined fashion with cuts being made from above in the base of the anterior cranial fossa and below in affected areas, thus allowing the specimen to be removed. This degree of exposure also allows the surgeon to obtain wide margins around the lesion accurately. The pericranial flap is inset along the floor of the skull base to seal the nasal cavity from the intracranial compartment. In patients with larger skull base defects or orbital exenteration, reconstruction with vascularized tissue decreases complications. The craniotomy is closed in a standard fashion; and, if possible the anterior maxilla and nasal bones may be replaced and secured with fixation plates. The two major advantages of this approach are wide exposure of the anterior skull base and exposure of the entirety of the nasal cavity and paranasal

sinuses. However, it has the disadvantage of prolonged frontal lobe retraction which can lead to frontal encephalomalacia and permanent neurological deficits. In many patients, the disadvantage of facial incisions is avoided with endoscopic assisted craniofacial resection.

Subcranial Approach

The subcranial approach is derived from craniofacial surgery for congenital and traumatic deformities. The degree of exposure of the anterior skull base dictates the location of the osteotomies. This approach involves a coronal incision with dissection carried down not only over the frontal bone but the nasal bones, medial canthal ligament areas, and if necessary, the orbital rim of the zygoma, exposing the arch and the body. The supraorbital and supratrochlear neurovascular bundles are dissected from their foramina or notches and preserved. As originally described, the frontal bone segment and nasal bones were removed as a single unit. This can be modified into a two-step procedure. A bifrontal craniotomy is performed with this procedure as well. After removal of the bone flap, additional osteotomies are created in the region of the nasoglabellar complex. These osteotomies extend vertically through the remainder of the frontal bone, down along the nasal bones and across the dorsum of the nose. An osteotomy is made from the intracranial aspect of the frontal bone through the orbital roofs and anterior to the crista galli thus allowing the removal of what is termed the frontal bar. At this point, the anterior fossa may be approached directly with minimal or no retraction of the frontal lobes. In patients with benign tumors, olfaction may be preserved on the contralateral side avoiding anosmia. The anterior cranial base defect is reconstructed with the anteriorly based pericranial flap. The flap measures approximately 15 cm in length and can extend posteriorly to the anterior clinoid processes. Care must also be taken to close all openings in the dura to ensure a water-tight seal. Any dural dehisences above the nasal cavity will result in cerebrospinal fluid (CSF) rhinorrhea. The nasoglabellar complex is repositioned and secured laterally to the frontal bone with microplates. The frontal bone flap is replaced and secured in position with fixation plates and screws (Figure 12).

Le Fort I Osteotomy

The Le Fort I osteotomy provides excellent access to the nasal cavity and nasopharynx and is particularly useful in patients presenting with juvenile nasopharyngeal angiofibroma. The procedure is started utilizing a sublabial approach extending between the first molars of the maxillae. A subperiosteal dissection exposes the faces of the maxillae with care taken to preserve the infraorbital nerves. The dissection proceeds around the lateral buttress to the pterygomaxillary fissure. The mucosa of the floor of the nose and the inferior meatus is elevated to avoid laceration during

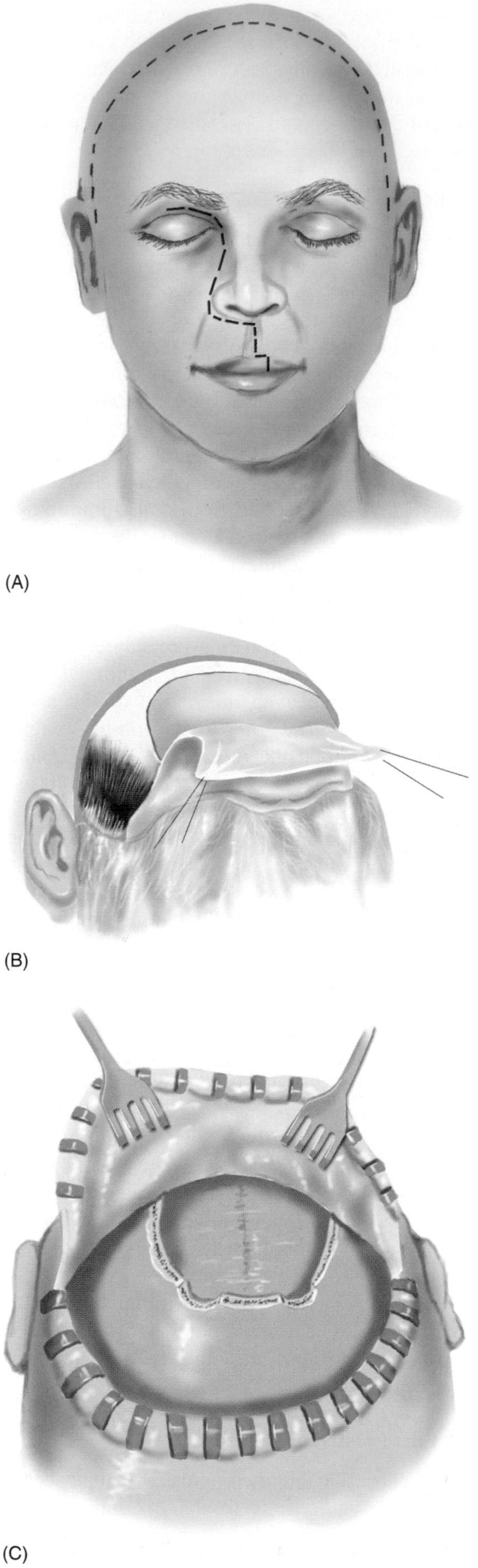

(A)

(B)

(C)

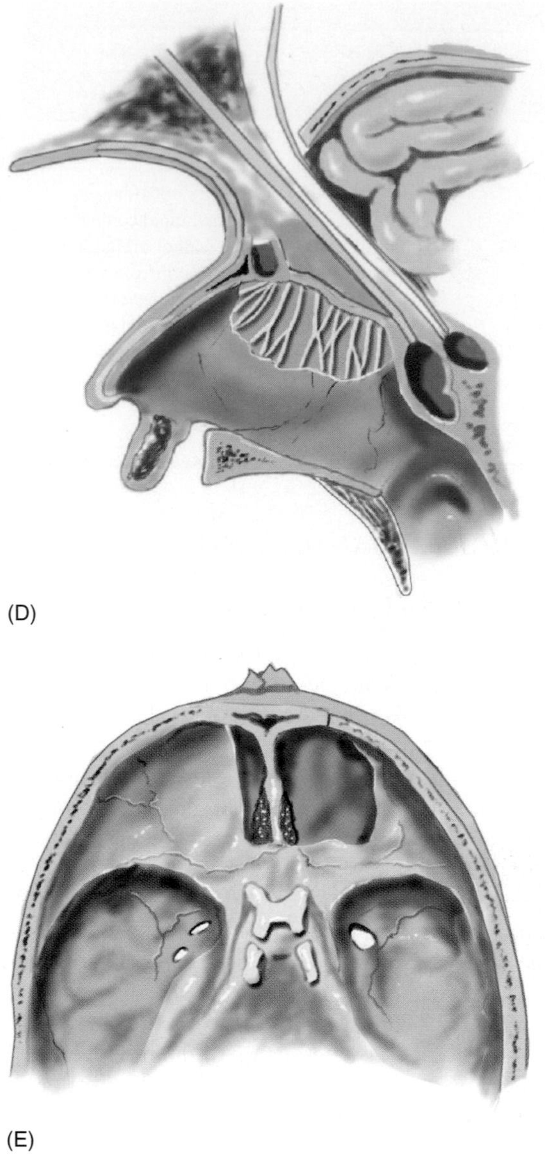

(D)

(E)

Figure 10 Craniofacial resection: intracranial exposure. (A) Bicoronal and lateral rhinotomy incisions, (B) bicoronal flap elevation with harvest of pericranial flap, (C) bifrontal craniotomy, (D) sagittal view of retraction of frontal lobes, (E) view of exposed anterior skull base from above. (Published with permission, copyright © 2007 P.A. Wackym, MD.)

The nasal septum is disengaged from the floor of the nose with an osteotome. The surgeon should have a finger in the nasopharynx while making this osteotomy to avoid injury to the cervical spine. The final osteotomies are made with a curved pterygomaxillary osteotome through the pterygomaxillary fissure to disjoin the maxillary tuberosity from the anterior surface of the pterygoid plates. The surgeon must place a finger medial to the tuberosity to ensure that the osteotome has completely traversed the fissure. All osteotomies are checked for completeness, and the maxillae are gently downfractured either with a bone hook or with maxillary spreaders. Pterygoid plate fractures can result from incomplete osteotomies which may cause laceration of the internal carotid artery in the foramen lacerum. The maxillae are retracted in its downfractured position while tumor extirpation proceeds. The maxillae should be released from the retractors about every 15 to 20 minutes to ensure the viability of their blood supply. If at any time during the procedure, the gingiva becomes white or purple; vascular compromise has occurred, and the maxillae must be replaced immediately. Following tumor removal, the maxillae are replaced; and, utilizing the predrilled holes in the bone, fixation plates are applied to restore the presurgical occlusion. The incision is closed in a two-layer fashion with absorbable sutures.

Transzygomatic Approach

This approach is useful to access the postzygomatic space and, when combined with lateral mandibular osteotomies, the infratemporal fossa. The transzygomatic approach aids in removal of extensive tumors involving the maxilla, infratemporal fossa, and the anterior skull base such as a juvenile nasopharyngeal angiofibroma with intracranial extension. A coronal incision is made with the pretragal portion extending below the zygomatic articulation with the temporal bone on the surgical side. As the dissection proceeds on the lateral aspect of the skull, the superficial temporal fat pad is encountered. An incision is made in the superficial layer of the deep temporal fascia with the dissection continuing inferiorly on the undersurface of the fascia. Avoiding extensive dissection in the fat pad can minimize temporal wasting. This preserves the temporal branches of the facial nerve. The periosteum on the superior aspect of the arch is incised, and a subperiosteal dissection exposes the entire zygoma. Osteotomies are then designed to provide the necessary access for tumor removal. These may include only the arch or the entire zygoma for more extensive exposure. If a total malar osteotomy is performed in conjunction with a craniotomy, the osteotomy through the body of the zygoma should be placed lateral to the zygomaticofacial nerve. This will avoid the maxillary sinus and prevent the potential for CSF rhinorrhea. The zygoma remains pedicled on the masseter muscle, preserving its blood supply. If the infratemporal fossa must be accessed, various

the osteotomy. To preserve the patient's presurgical occlusion, fixation plates are contoured to the medial and lateral buttresses of the maxillae, and holes are predrilled into the maxillae through the plate so that at the end of the procedure the maxillae are replaced into their presurgical posi-

tion. After this has been accomplished, an osteotomy is made across the faces of the maxillae including the medial and lateral buttresses with care taken to avoid tooth roots. The osteotomy must extend more than 5 mm above the apices of the teeth and passes through the inferior meatus.

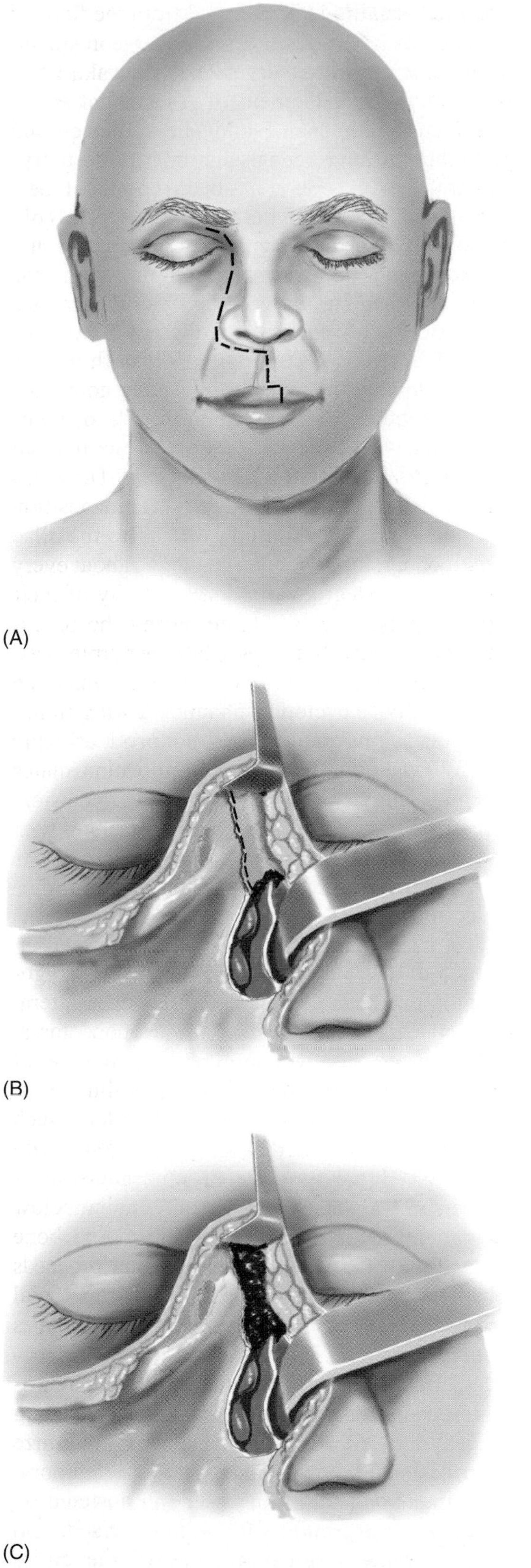

(A)

(B)

(C)

Figure 11 Craniofacial resection: transfacial exposure. (A) Lateral rhinotomy or Weber-Ferguson incision, (B) nasomaxillary osteotomy, (C) exposure and removal of neoplasm en bloc. (Published with permission, copyright © 2007 P.A. Wackym, MD.)

osteotomies are made in the lateral portion of the mandible to access the pterygoid muscles and the deeper structures. If access to the lateral part of the infratemporal fossa is required the coronoid process may be sectioned and retracted superiorly pedicled on the temporalis tendon. For more extensive exposure, the condylar neck may be

(A)

(B)

(C)

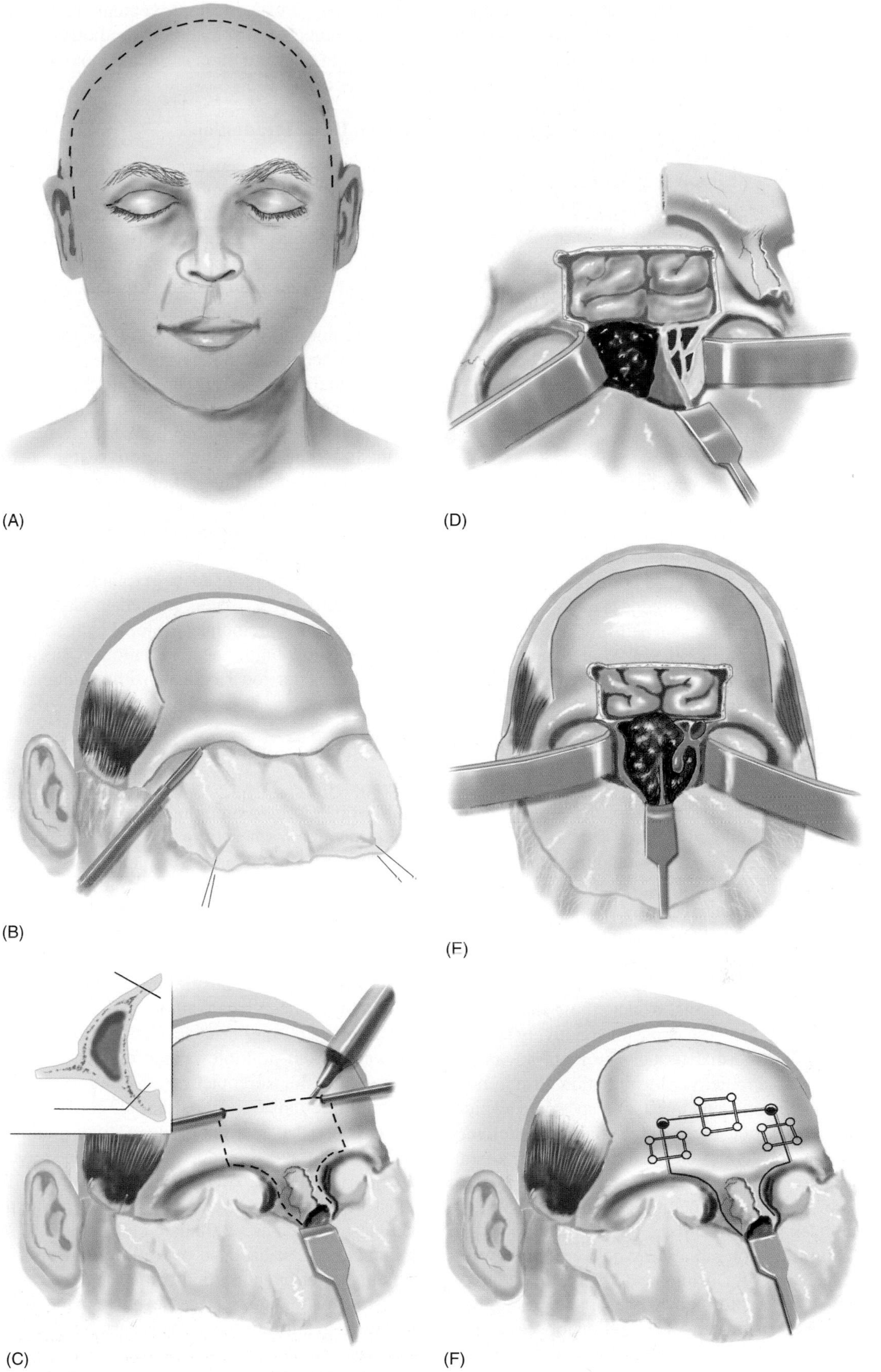

Figure 12 Subcranial approach. (A) Bicoronal incision, (B) Bicoronal exposure and mobilization of supratrochlear and supraorbital neurovascular bundles, (C) frontal bone and nasal bones removed as one unit, (D) removal of frontal bone segment included frontal bar, (E) tumor exposed without retracting frontal lobes, and (F) replacement of bone flap after pericranial flap is placed. (Published with permission, copyright © 2007 P.A. Wackym, MD.)

transected and the ramus of the mandible may be sectioned above the antilingular prominence and retracted superiorly. At the conclusion of the procedure, the osteotomies are stabilized with internal fixation.

(D)

(F)

(F)

Endoscopic Resection

With the improvement in endoscopic instrumentation and the routine availability of image guidance systems in the last decade, transnasal, transoral, and trans-sinus endoscopic techniques have become more popular. Endocopic-assisted craniofacial resection allows excellent visualization while avoiding facial incision. The boundaries for transnasal endoscopic resection alone are expanding, and good outcomes are reported in appropriately selected patients. Some surgeons advocate replacing virtually all "open" procedures with endoscopic techniques. However, there remain cases that we believe are better approached via an open craniofacial resection, and the complete surgeon today should be familiar with all the means necessary to provide access and exposure for both resection of these challenging neoplasms and postoperative reconstruction.

RADIATION THERAPY

In most malignant neoplasms of the skull base, there is a role for radiotherapy. Radiation therapy (RT) is most often delivered as adjuvant therapy in skull-based malignant neoplasms. Despite improvements in disease control, RT can have significant complications due to radiation-induced injury to the brain, visual pathway, and remaining skull base supportive tissue. Modern advances in RT technology may allow improvements in radiation delivery to tumor tissue and may decrease devastating complications such as radiation-induced retinopathy and optic neuropathy.

Intensity Modulated Radiation Therapy

Intensity modulated radiation therapy (IMRT) is an advanced form of three-dimensional (3-D) conformal radiotherapy. The patient, initially, undergoes a treatment planning CT scan, and the data from this scan is fed into a computer. The software reconstructs the targeted area in three dimensions that allow the radiation oncologist and radiation physicist to determine the dose of radiation to the neoplasm while relatively sparing surrounding normal tissue. The main advantage is being able to deliver the radiation dose in non-uniform beam densities that may spare critical structures while maintaining high dose delivery to the gross tumor volume. Prior to the treatment, the patient has a mask fabricated specifically to his or her facial structure. During the treatment, the mask is worn, and the head is fixed in a rigid position. Photon radiation is delivered from a linear accelerator. During the delivery, the radiation beams are conformed to the precise configuration of the neoplasm with collimator leaves that adjust the targeting area to the irregular shape of the tumor. The leaves may be adjusted to alter the specific dose from any given beam to the target area, so that radiation aimed at the neoplasm may have different doses for each beam. This technique has proved to be useful in treating patients with neoplasms in the anterior fossa, so that the radiation may be delivered to a neoplasm close to vital structures such as the optic nerve, pituitary or spinal cord while minimizing radiation that would damage these structures. While

studies may not show improvement in disease control compared to conventional radiotherapy, a decrease in early radiation associated toxicity has been demonstrated.[29]

Proton Beam Irradiation

Although proton beam irradiation therapy is a type of external beam radiation, it differs in that protons rather than photons are used in treating the patient with a neoplasm. Proton irradiation can be delivered in a conformal fashion so that the beam can be altered to the irregular shape of the neoplasm and to minimize or avoid radiating adjacent normal tissue. When protons are delivered to a neoplasm, the entrance dose into adjacent normal tissue is low, however, the protons themselves release high doses of radiation when they strike the neoplasm which is referred to as the Bragg peak. After the protons exit the neoplasm, there is a minimal, if any, dose delivered to normal tissue deep to the neoplasm. Proton irradiation is effective in patients with chordomas or chondrosarcomas, and the uses of this therapy are continuing to be expanded. Proton beam irradiation has been studied in skull base adenoid cystic carcinoma. Proton beam irradiation may allow higher dose radiation to the skull base with better local control without changing overall survival.[30]

Stereotactic Radiosurgery

Stereotactic radiosurgery is a type of radiation which is delivered in a single dose in a one-time treatment setting. During this procedure, the patient undergoes a planning CT scan and those data are fed into a computer that uses software to determine the area of the tumor in three dimensions. Following treatment planning, a head frame is secured to the patient's skull using pins. The positioning of this is determined by CT scan localization. Radiation, either from cobalt 60 or linear accelerator sources, is delivered from multiple beams to focus on the tumor site. In stereotactic radiosurgery, there are multiple radiation ports that all converge on the tumor so that adjacent tissue receives minimal radiation dosage; however, the tumor receives a tumoricidal dose. Stereotactic radiosurgery is most often used in treating benign intracranial neoplasms, such as vestibular schwannomas and meningiomas. It has also proved quite useful in treating arteriovenous malformations (AVMs). The role in malignant disease has expanded in not only treating primary malignant neoplasms, but also intracranial metastatic lesions. The approximate upper limit diameter of neoplasms can be treated with this modality is approximately 3 cm. After treatment, the neoplasm may either shrink or remain stable. However, with ongoing follow-up MRI scans, neoplasms usually are noted to cease their growth. In response to radiosurgery, AVMs develop thickening in their walls and usually cease to grow. Stereotactic radiosurgery is discussed in Chapter 36, "Stereotactic Radiosurgery."

CHEMOTHERAPY

Generally speaking, surgery has been the mainstay for the management of resectable anterior skull base neoplasms, and chemotherapy and radiotherapy have been used primarily in an adjuvant role. An exception has been reported in 1997 by Bhattacharyya and colleagues in which 8 of 9 patients with esthesioneuroblastoma treated with cisplatin and etoposide had complete responses and were then treated with 68 Gray (Gy) of stereotactic fractionated proton therapy.[31] Although lack of recurrence was reported, the patients were only followed for a mean of 14 months (range 2 to 26 months). Most commonly, esthesioneuroblastoma is treated with surgical resection followed by adjuvant RT adding chemotherapy in selected cases. Chemotherapy regimens may include cisplatin and etoposide, as well as vincristine, cyclophosphamide, and doxorubicin. However, one group reported excellent results using preoperative RT for Kadish stage A and B tumors and preoperative chemotherapy and RT for Kadish stage C tumors.[32] Chemotherapy generally included cyclophosphamide and vincristine with occasional addition of doxorubicin. Only 5 of 30 patients developed complications from chemotherapy. The majority of patients (64%) had Kadish stage C.[33]

Squamous cell carcinomas and adenoid cystic carcinomas are generally treated using surgical resection and postoperative RT. Postoperative RT is used for chordomas and sarcomas when complete resection is not possible although the quantitative benefits are not entirely clear.

SNUC is a particularly aggressive lesion with a poor prognosis. Although postoperative RT is commonly employed, we have had some increased success with induction chemotherapy-RT using a SCC protocol followed by surgical resection.

In an interesting recent report from MD Anderson Cancer Center in 2007, the survivals of patients with all paranasal sinus carcinomas treated with RT (with or without surgery and/or chemotherapy) were evaluated by decade.[33] No improvement in survival was noted, but complications of treatment have decreased significantly.

Certainly, most surgeons today would treat unresectable carcinoma with combined chemotherapy and RT for palliative intent, hoping for an occasional unexpected cure.

Samant and colleagues used intra-arterial cisplatin with concomitant RT followed by planned organ-sparing surgical resection for advanced paranasal sinus cancer.[34] After a median follow-up of 53 months, actuarial overall survival at 2 and 5 years was 68% and 53%, respectively. Chemoradiation is discussed in Chapter 92, "Chemoradiation for Head and Neck Cancer."

COMPLICATIONS

Although fairly uncommon today, craniofacial resection carries with it a risk of mortality in the perioperative period. Fortunately, with modern skull base surgery and anesthesia techniques, death as a direct result of treatment is infrequent. Of the more common complications of craniofacial resection, the most feared has always been infection since this can quickly lead to meningitis, cerebritis, and cerebral abscess. Better methods for reconstructing the skull base using living tissue (locoregional flaps and free flaps) have resulted in better segregation of the nose and sinuses from the anterior cranial fossa, minimizing the occurrence of infection. Other complications include pneumocephalus, hematoma (intradural or epidural), cerebral contusion, edema and/or stroke, as well as cranial nerve injuries, particularly anosmia, since this may be completely unavoidable when resecting neoplasms involving the cribriform plate. CSF leaks occur as well although these are also minimized by improved flap reconstructions.

The use of lumbar spinal drainage to prevent CSF leakage is controversial, and the lumbar drains pose their own nontrivial risks, including particularly excessive CSF drainage, that may lead to increased pneumocephalus. The drains can also be a source of infection and meningitis.

Pneumocephalus is an expected finding in the early postoperative period. As the reconstructed skull base heals, separation of the nasal cavity from the intracranial cavity prevents further collection, and the intracranial air is resorbed. Airtight closure of the skull base reconstruction, nasal packing, and avoidance of nose blowing decrease troublesome pneumoncephalus. CSF leak may create a ball-valve phenomenon that predisposes to tension pneumocephalus. Tension pneumocephalus is uncommon, but it must be identified early and managed, or it can be devastating. Any postoperative patient who develops a change in sensorium should have an immediate CT. Percutaneous aspiration and airway diversion can relieve tension pneumocephalus. Prophylactic tracheostomy was commonly used in the past to avoid pneumocephalus but is no longer employed routinely by most surgeons. The use of tracheostomy is controversial, but we would generally advocate using it only for intractable pneumocephalus.

Orbital complications may include diplopia, visual loss, change in eye position, telecanthus, and epiphora. Wound complications may occur as well, including infection, hematoma, or fistula.

Patients may complain of nasal crusting and foul odor. This may require frequent debridement by the surgeon. Aggressive nasal irrigations may prove helpful. Systemic complications generally relate to complications of craniotomy, particularly diabetes insipidus and hemodynamic instability.

Late complications include encephalocele, wound complications, and cosmetic alterations such as enophthalmos, telecanthus, nasal deformity, forehead deformity, and scar prominence including alopecia. Bone flap resorption and necrosis is more likely when postoperative RT is used. Skull base osteoradionecrosis is often difficult to distinguish from tumor recurrence.

REFERENCES

1. Dandy WE. Orbital Tumor: Results Following Transcranial Operative Attack. New York: Oskar Piest; 1941. p. 168.
2. Ketcham AS, Wilkins RH, Van Buren JM, Smith RR. A combined intracranial facial approach to the paranasal sinuses. Am J Surg 1963;106:689–703.
3. Tessier P, Guiot G, Rougerie J. Osteotomies cranio-naso-orbito-facialeshypertelorisme. Ann Chir Plast 1967;12:103–18.
4. Raveh J. Das einzeitge vorgehan bei der widerherstellung von fronto-basal-mittelgesichtsfracturen modifikatinen und behandlungsmodalitaeten. Chirurgie 1983;54:385–93.
5. Raveh J, Laedrach K, Speiser M, et al. The subcranial approach for fronto-orbital and anterior–posterior skull base tumors. Arch Otolaryngol Head Neck Surg 1993;119:385–93.
6. Obwegeser HL. Temporal approach to the TMJ, the orbit, and the retromaxillary-infracranial region. Head Neck Surg 1985;7:185 99.
7. Hillstrom RP, Zarbo RJ, Jacobs JR. Nerve sheath tumors of the paranasal sinuses: Electron microscopy and histopathologic diagnosis. Otolaryngol Head Neck Surg 1990; 102:257–63.
8. Buob D, Wacrenier A, Chevalier D, et al. Schwannoma of the sinonasal tract: A clinicopathologic and immunohistochemical study of 5 cases. Arch Pathol Lab Med 2003;127:1196–9.
9. Luce D, Leclerc A, Begin D, et al. Sinonasal cancer and occupational exposures: A pooled analysis of 12 case-control studies. Cancer Causes Control 2002;13:147–57.
10. Sunderman FW, Morgan LG, Andersen A, et al. Histopathology of sinonasal and lung cancers in nickel refinery workers. Ann Clin Lab Sci 1989;19:44 50.
11. Zhu K, Levine RS, Brann EA, et al. Case-control study evaluating the homogeneity and heterogeneity of risk factors between sinonasal and nasopharyngeal cancers. Int J Cancer 2002;99:119–23.
12. Wolf J, Schmezer P, Fengel D, et al. The role of combination effects on the etiology of malignant nasal tumours in the woodworking industry. Acta Otolaryngol Suppl 1998;535:1–16.
13. Pommier P, Liebsch NJ, Deschler DG. Proton beam radiation therapy for skull base adenoid cystic carcinoma. Arch Otolaryngol Head Neck Surg 2006;132:1242–9.
14. Broich G, Pagliari A, Ottaviani F. Esthesioneuroblastoma: A general review of the cases published since the discovery of the tumour in 1924. Anticancer Res 1997;17:2683–706.
15. Kadish S, Goodman M, Wang CC. Olfactory neuroblastoma: A clinical analysis of 17 cases. Cancer 1976;37:1571–6.
16. Bilsky MH, Kraus DH, Strong EW, et al. Extended anterior craniofacial resection for intracranial extension of malignant tumors. Am J Surg 1997;174:565–8.
17. Bentz BG, Bilsky MH, Shah JP, et al. Anterior skull base surgery for malignant tumors: A multivariate analysis of 27 years of experience. Head Neck 2003;25:515–20.
18. Diaz EM, Johnigan RH, Pero C, et al. Olfactory neuroblastoma: The 22-year experience at one comprehensive cancer center. Head Neck 2005;27:138–49.
19. Resto VA, Eisele DW, Forastiere A, et al. Esthesioneuroblastoma: The Johns Hopkins experience. Head Neck 2000;22:550–8.
20. Oskouian RJ, Jane JA, Dumont AS, et al. Esthesioneuroblastoma: Clinical presentation, radiological, and pathological features, treatment, review of the literature, and the University of Virginia experience. Neurosurg Focus 2002;12:e4.
21. Levine PA, Gallagher R, Cantrell RW. Esthesioneuroblastoma: Reflections of a 21-year experience. Laryngoscope 1999;109:1539–4.
22. Levine PA, Debo RF, Meredith SD, et al. Craniofacial resection at the University of Virginia (1976–1992): Survival analysis. Head Neck 1994;16:574–7.
23. Sandeep PD, Bared A, Casiano RR. Surgical outcomes and safety of transnasal endoscopic resection for anterior skull base tumors. Otolaryngol Head Neck Surg 2007;136:920–7.
24. Mendenhall WM, Mendenhall CM, Riggs CE, Jr, et al. Sinonasal undifferentiated carcinoma. Am J Clin Oncol 2006;29:27–31.
25. Enepekides DJ. Sinonasal undifferentiated carcinoma: An update. Curr Opin Otolaryngol Head Neck Surg 2005;13:222–5.
26. Ejaz A, Wenig BM. Sinonasal undifferentiated carcinoma: Clinical and pathologic features and a discussion on classification, cellular differentiation, and differential diagnosis. Adv Anat Pathol 2005;12:134–43.
27. American Joint Committee on Cancer Staging Manual, 6th edition. New York, NY: Springer-Verlag; 2002.
28. Lee CH, Hur DG, Roh HJ, et al. Survival rates of sinonasal squamous cell carcinoma with the new AJCC staging system. Arch Otolaryngol Head Neck Surg 2007;133:131–4.
29. Daly ME, Chen AM, Bucci MK, et al. Intensity-modulated radiation therapy for malignancies of the nasal cavity and paranasal sinuses. Int J Radiat Oncol Biol Phys 2007;67:151–7.
30. Pommier P, Liebsch NJ, Deschler DG, et al. Proton beam radiation therapy for skull base adenoid cystic carcinoma. Arch Otolaryngol Head Neck Surg 2006;132:1242–9.
31. Bhattacharyya N, Thornton AF, Joseph MP, et al. Successful treatment of esthesioneuroblastoma and neuroendocrine carcinoma with combined chemotherapy and proton radiation: Results in 9 cases. Arch Otolaryngol Head Neck Surg 1997;123:34–40.
32. Loy AH, Reibel JF, Read PW, et al. Esthesioneuroblastoma: Continued follow-up of a single institution's experience. Arch Otolaryngol Head Neck Surg 2006;132:134–8.
33. Chen AM, Daly ME, Bucci MK, et al. Carcinomas of the paranasal sinuses and nasal cavity treated with radiotherapy at a single institution over five decades: Are we making improvement? Int J Radiat Oncol Biol Phys 2007;67:151–7.
34. Samant S, Robbins KT, Vang M, et al. Intra-arterial cisplatin and concommitant radiation therapy followed by surgery for advanced paranasal sinus cancer. Arch Otolaryngol Head Neck Surg 2004;130:948–55.

96

Neoplasms of the Nasopharynx

Randall L. Plant, MD

ANATOMY

The superior border of the nasopharynx is the sphenoid bone, the inferior border is the free border of the soft palate, the posterior border comprises the clivus and first two cervical vertebrae, and the anterior border occurs at the choanae. Several key anatomic structures situated along the perimeter of the nasopharynx play an important role in the presentation and the prognosis of juvenile nasopharyngeal angiofibromas (JNAs) and nasopharyngeal carcinoma (NPC). The eustachian tube enters into the nasopharynx through a defect in the lateral wall of pharyngeal fascia known as the sinus of Morgagni. The posterior portion of the cartilaginous eustachian tube forms a ridge in the lateral nasopharynx called the torus tubaris. The recess posterior to the torus tubaris, called the fossa of Rosenmuller, is a frequent site of NPC. The foramen lacerum lies within the nasopharynx, serving as a route of perivascular tumor spread to the middle cranial fossa, the cavernous sinus, and the adjacent cranial nerves (CNs) III, IV, V1, V2, and VI. Other foramina adjacent to the nasopharynx include the foramina ovale and rotundum, the carotid canal, the jugular foramen, and the superior orbital fissure.

The pharyngobasilar fascia surrounding the nasopharynx provides an initial barrier to tumor spread. Passage of the eustachian tube through this fascia allows spread of tumor into the parapharyngeal region and the cavernous sinus.[1]

The nasopharynx has an extensive bilateral lymphatic drainage system, accounting for the high rate of neck involvement at initial presentation; up to one-half of all patients with NPC have cervical node metastasis at the time of diagnosis.[2] The lymphatic system drains anterior to posterior toward the midline into the parapharyngeal and retropharyngeal lymph nodes. Lymphatic drainage also occurs into the deep posterior cervical chain near the mastoid tip and down along the jugulodigastric chain.

JUVENILE NASOPHARYNGEAL ANGIOFIBROMA

JNAs are benign, highly vascular lesions that occur almost exclusively in adolescent males. The lesions are locally expansile, usually growing in a pushing fashion but also possess the ability to infiltrate local structures. They are rare, representing only about 0.05% of all head and neck tumors, but are the most common benign neoplasms of the nasopharynx.

Epidemiology and Etiology

The site of origin of JNAs is felt to be at the junction of the sphenoidal process of the palatine bone and the pterygoid process of the sphenoid bone, just superior to the sphenopalatine foramen. The main blood supply to JNAs is the ipsilateral internal maxillary artery, usually its distal branches, that is, sphenopalatine or vidian artery. There can be contributions from internal carotid artery branches, that is, mandibular artery and inferolateral trunk, in nearly 50% of cases. Other arteries may become prominent after embolization.[3,4]

Presentation

JNAs are slow-growing neoplasms that can reach large size before detection. Patients with them most commonly present with nasal complaints such as nasal obstruction and recurrent epistaxis. With lateral growth, the neoplasms can erode into the pterygoid plates and extend into the infratemporal fossa via the pterygomaxillary fissure.

Intracranial extension can occur in 20 to 35% of the patients in whom most spread into the middle cranial fossa, the pituitary fossa, and the anterior cranial fossa.

Histology

JNAs are unencapsulated neoplasms consisting of endothelially lined vascular spaces and fibrous connective tissue. The nasopharyngeal surface is lined by mucosa, giving the tumor a deceptively nonvascular appearance.[5] The precise histogenesis of JNAs has been subject to debate, particularly as to whether they are of angiomatous or fibromatous origin. Recent electron micrograph studies have shown that the tumor consists of an actively proliferating part and a relatively nonactive part, with a transitional zone in between. The actively proliferating part contains hyperplastic capillaries and vascular sinuses that lack muscular components (Figure 1). This tissue, seen primarily at the periphery of the neoplasm, consists of a bicellular combination of epithelial cells and pericytes. Toward the central portion of the lesion, the neoplasm is in more of a reactive state with a higher component of fibrous tissue. These findings indicate that JNA may arise as a reactive process or defective development rather than a neoplastic proliferation. In origin it,

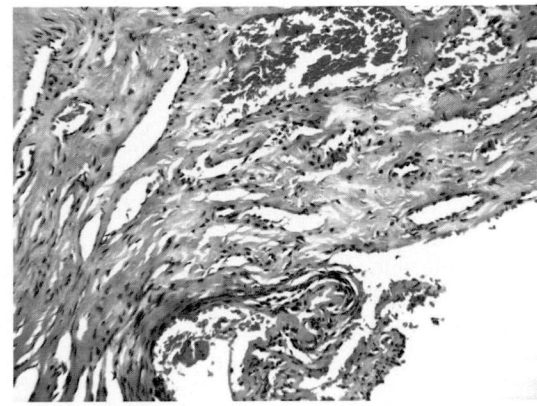

Figure 1 Photomicrograph of a juvenile nasopharyngeal angiofibroma showing numerous vascular spaces varying in size and contour. The spaces are lined by a single layer of endothelial cells. Some of the spaces are elongated and distended with erythrocytes.

therefore, is similar to vascular hamartomas and other hemangiomatous processeses.[6]

Immunohistochemical staining has shown the presence of transforming growth factor ß-1 in JNA. This polypeptide is associated with fibroblast proliferation and angiogenesis and was found in both endothelial and stromal tissue of angiofibromas.[7] Elevated levels of other types of growth factor, including vascular endothelial growth factor (VEGF), fibroblast growth factor, and the proliferation marker Ki67 have been found in JNA endothelium and stroma. Tumor angiogenesis may be promoted when androgens such as testosterone stimulate the secretion of these growth factors.[8] Although JNAs have increased expression of androgen receptors, administration of the androgen blocker flutamide does not produce a significant decrease in size of these tumors.[9]

Advanced JNAs have increased expression of the proto-oncogene *C-MYC*. Overexpression of *C-MYC* may interact with androgen receptor genes and the cytoplasmic protein ß-catenin to induce cell and tumor growth.[10]

Evaluation

Both contrast-enhanced computed tomography (CT) scans and magnetic resonance imaging (MRI) are useful for evaluation of JNAs and their relationship with important adjacent structures. As with most other tumors, CT scans typically provide more information about bone erosion, and MRI is most useful for assessment of soft tissue structures. On CT scans, infratemporal involvement may produce a thinning and anterior bowing of the posterior wall of the maxillary paranasal sinus. Other signs of tumor erosion include displacement of the hard palate, erosion of the medical pterygoid plate, and orbital fissure enlargement.[11] MRI has shown accuracy in detecting erosion of the pterygoid process, and is especially useful for evaluating extension into the pterygomaxillary and infratemporal fossae.[4] MRI can help determine whether intracranial tumors are intradural or extradural. For follow-up studies, MRI has the advantage of avoiding radiation exposure to what is usually a young patient population.

Angiography can be performed preoperatively to define and embolize the feeding vessels. Embolization is usually done within a day or two of the operative date.

Although the combination of clinical presentation, appearance on imaging studies, and risk of bleeding typically precludes the need for biopsy, some clinicians feel that tissue diagnosis is useful to rule out other lesions. Differential diagnosis includes NPC, rhadomyoscarcoma, Kaposi sarcoma, neovascularized inflammatory polyps, teratomas, hemangiomas, and lymphoproliferative disorders.[3]

Staging

Many different staging systems have been proposed for JNAs; Table 1 shows two recent recommendations. The classification by Close and colleagues has used a staging system from Fisch and modified it to account for involvement of the cavernous sinus.[12] However, preoperative classification based on radiological assessment of cavernous sinus involvement may overestimate the stage.[13] The Radkowski and colleagues' staging system has taken a system proposed by Sessions and modified it to emphasize the importance of extension posterior to the pyerygoid plates and erosion of the skull base.[5]

Treatment

Surgery remains the primary treatment option for JNAs. Multiple external surgical approaches have been used for JNA, including lateral rhinotomy, transpalatal, transantral, and midface degloving approaches, along with a LeFort I osteotomy or medial maxillectomy as needed for additional exposure. Drawbacks of these external approaches include facial scarring and epiphora from a lateral rhinotomy and risk of palatal fistula from the transpalatal approach. There are some concerns that external approaches with extensive osteotomies may have an effect on bony growth in young patients, though some authors feel these concerns are overstated.[11]

Certain JNAs can be resected using endoscopic surgery as a stand-alone procedure or in conjunction with open techniques.[4,14–17] Endoscopy allows multiangled view of the mass and adjacent structures, eliminates the need for skin or mucosal incisions, and minimizes disruption of bony structures. JNAs are typically expansile and less densely attached to adjacent tissue, so they and their feeding vessels can often be retracted into the surgical field. Endoscopic approaches were first used for lower-stage JNAs, with involvement of the pterygopalatine or infratemporal fossa initially considered contraindications for this technique. However, higher-stage neoplasms have now been resected with endoscopes although it is still not considered appropriate when there is involvement of the orbit or the middle cranial fossa.

Preoperative embolization of the tumor is recommended in almost all cases when an endoscopic approach is to be used. Open procedures without embolization had an average blood loss of 1,250 mL in one series, with embolization the loss dropped to 425 mL, and using endoscopic approaches and embolization the loss dropped to 225 mL.[17] Preservation of the blood supply to the temporalis muscle is important in cases in which a temporalis muscle flap may be used for reconstruction.[18]

The surgeon must also be prepared to convert to an open procedure if necessary. During resection, methods for hemostasis include bipolar or monopolar cautery and YAG laser. Depending on the tumor location, a partial middle turbinectomy may be required. The maxillary antrostomy is enlarged, anterior and posterior ones are performed, and the posterior maxillary wall is removed to expose the pterygomaxillary fossa. At this point, the sphenopalatine artery and the descending palatine artery can be clipped. Use of a suction Freer elevator may facilitate dissection of the tumor.[15] If necessary, lateral exposure can be improved using a Caldwell–Luc approach through the anterior face of the maxilla.

Giant angiofibromas or those with intracranial involvement may require skull-base surgery with a combined otolaryngology–neurosurgery team. For example these cases may require infratemporal/middle fossa, craniofacial, or anterior subcranial approaches.[19]

Close and colleagues described successful resection of JNAs involving the cavernous sinus using either an extracranial transpalatal or midface degloving approach or intracranially via a frontotemporal or lateral infratemporal craniotomy.[12] In their series, all tumors involved only the medial or inferiomedial portion of the cavernous sinus, and none had massive invasion. None of the tumors invaded the dura, and dural invasion by JNAs in general is felt to be rare.[20] Bales and colleagues used a craniofacial approach with lateral rhinotomy and craniotomy to resect JNAs in the cavernous sinus and intracranial extension.[11] This approach avoids disruption of the middle ear and eustachian tube that can occur with infratemporal approaches.

The risk of recurrence is increased when there is evidence on imaging of invasion into the vidian canal and the sphenoid bone. Careful exploration of the basosphenoid bone may reveal invagination of tumor into the cancellous portion of the sphenoid bone. This bone, as well as the pterygoid plates and the clivus, should be drilled out to remove all remaining tumor and reduce the likelihood of recurrence.[13,21]

Radiation therapy has been used for tumors with intracranial extension, for tumors considered unresectable due to their proximity to structures such as the optic nerve, or for tumors receiving extensive supply from the internal carotid artery. Tumor dosages range from 36 to 40 Gray (Gy) and recurrence rates from this treatment have been 10 to 15%. Presence of radiographic abnormalities after radiation therapy is not uncommon and may represent chronic inflammation rather than persistence of tumor. Further treatment, is therefore, considered necessary only if there are recurrent symptoms or new changes on imaging studies.[22,23]

NASOPHARYNGEAL CANCER

Epidemiology

NPC occurs with widely variable rates throughout the world. The disease is especially common among ethnic Chinese in and around the Guangdong province of China, in certain regions of southeast Asia, northern Africa, and among the Inuit (Eskimo) population of Alaska. Within China, the risk decreases in the more northern portions of the country. Average age-adjusted incidence rates per 100,000 population are 0.75 among the general US population, 8.4 among the Alaska Native population and range as high as 20 to 30 in certain regions near Hong Kong.[24] The

Stage	Close and Colleagues[12] System	Radkowski and Colleagues[5] System
I	Nasopharynx and nasal cavity, no bone destruction	(A) Tumor limited to nose or nasopharyngeal vault (B) Extension into ≥ sinuses
II	Extension into pterygomaxillary fossa, maxillary, ethmoid or sphenoid sinuses with bone destruction	(A) Minimal extension into pterygomaxillary fossa (B) Full occupation of pterygomaxillary fossa with or without erosion of orbital bones (C) Posterior to pterygoid plates
III	(A) Medial cavernous sinus with or without infratemporal fossa or orbit (B) Medial and inferior cavernous sinus, floor middle cranial fossa, intratemporal fossa, orbit	(A) Erosion of skull base, minimal intracranial (B) Erosion of skull base, extensive intracranial with or without cavernous sinus
IV	Optic chiasm, pituitary fossa, massive invasion of cavernous sinus	

Table 1 Staging Systems Used for Juvenile Angiofibroma

peak incidence for NPC in the Chinese population occurs in the 45- to 54-year age group although it continues to rise with age for the Alaskan Native and the average US population (Figure 2). Residents from these regions who have migrated to low-risk countries experience a decline in their risk of acquiring NPC.[24]

Infection with the Epstein–Barr virus (EBV) is a known risk factor for a wide variety of lymphoid neoplasms, including NPC, endemic Burkitt lymphoma, certain types of Hodgkin's disease, nasal T-cell lymphoma, and posttransplantation lymphoproliferative neoplasm. The virus has a special affinity for human lymphocytes of the upper respiratory tract.[25] In situ hybridization studies have shown the presence of EBV-encoded RNA (EBER) within the nuclei of all three variants (undifferentiated, nonkeratinizing, and squamous cell) of NPC cells,[26] although it more often correlated with the undifferentiated variant.[27] This modality for detection is powerful because it is not affected by infected lymphocytes in the surrounding tissue. Latent EBV infection has also been found within preinvasive lesions. The EBV DNA in these lesions is a single clonal form, suggesting that EBV infection occurs prior to and may be an initiating event in malignant transformation.[28]

Cellular infection with EBV can be lytic, eventually leading to cell death, or latent. In the presence of latent EBV infections, several different types of proteins are typically expressed. Nasopharyngeal cells produce latent membrane protein-1 (LMP1) and EBV nuclear antigen-1 (EBNA1). LMP1 is known to have oncogenic properties, including inhibition of differentiation, downregulation of epithelial markers, and activation of cell growth factors.[29]

NPC, particularly the undifferentiated variant, contains high levels of the oncogene *Bcl-2*.[29] Expression of this gene is believed to trigger tumor progression and improve protection for neoplastic cells. The tumor suppressor gene *p53* is overexpressed in NPC, but the impact of this finding is controversial.[30] It is generally felt that abnormal expression of the gene does not alone lead to the malignant transformation of nasopharyngeal epithelium. Rather it is felt that overexpression of

the gene may arise from nonmutational processes that develop in the course of tumor progression.[25] The clinical response of NPC to radiotherapy is not influenced by the presence or absence of expression of *p53*.[31]

High consumption of salted fish and other preserved food, especially during childhood, has also been shown to be associated with higher rates of NPC. Salted fish have been shown to contain carcinogenic nitrosamines and EBV-activating substances. However, it is uncertain if the proportion of NPC cases due to consumption of preserved food alone is significant in endemic regions.[32] Changes in diet, in particular decreases in intake of salted fish among young children, may be having an effect on rates of NPC: the average annual incidence of NPC in Hong Kong has fallen by about 35% between 1973 and 1977 and 1993 and 1997.[24] Among Chinese residents in Malaysia, NPC was found to be associated with high consumption levels of salted fish, salted eggs, beer, and pork or beef liver and with low consumption of cabbage, oranges or tangerines, and shrimp.[33]

Tobacco smoking is an independent risk factor for NPC although the magnitude of the effect is less than seen in other parts of the upper aerodigestive tract. Heavy smokers have two to four times the risk of developing NPC compared to nonsmokers. High alcohol consumption has not been shown to be a risk among Chinese although a correlation was seen in some studies from the United States. Industrial exposure to formaldehyde and wood dust has also been shown to increase the risk of NPC.[24]

In endemic regions, there appears to be an underlying genetic predisposition to development of NPC. In these areas, the rate of NPC involvement by first-degree relatives ranges from 5.8 to 19%. This familial version of NPC does not differ clinically from nonfamilial NPC.[34]

Presentation

Early signs and symptoms of NPC are both subtle and nonspecific, and the nasopharynx is a difficult area to examine for primary care physicians. As a result, NPC is often diagnosed at a later stage than other head and neck malignancies. Due to its rich lymphatic supply and its relative inaccessibility, in many cases cervical metastases are present on initial presentation.[2] Unlike other head and neck malignancies, there is no relationship between primary tumor size and the presence of cervical lymph nodal disease.[1] Eustachian tube dysfunction from infiltration into the levator veli palatini results in formation of serous otitis media in about 40% of patients, and its presence should warrant careful examination of the nasopharynx in any individual from the endemic regions.[35] Other symptoms related to the nasal cavity include epistaxis and nasal obstruction, seen in about 35% of patients as initial presentation.[36]

Incidence of neurological signs and symptoms at initial presentation ranges from 13 to 25% and most often results from CN involvement rather than extension of the tumor into the cranial cavity.

Tumor can extend along natural routes of spread through the foramen lacerum, the jugular foramen, or the hypoglossal canal. Infiltration along these routes normally precedes bone erosion. The most commonly involved CNs are CN V and VI, followed by III and IV.[37] Clinical manifestations of CN involvement include partial or complete ophthalmoplegia, facial pain or paralysis, and dysphagia. Horner syndrome can develop due to tumor compression of the cervical sympathetic chain. Headaches are seen in about one-third of patients, usually indicating some sort of deep spread into the skull base. The most common sites for distant spread are the bone, lung, and liver.[38]

Evaluation

As with most neoplasms in nonvisible regions, an accurate history and physical examination and high degree of suspicion are crucial for early diagnosis of NPC. The clinician should examine the nasopharynx with Hopkins rod telescopes or flexible nasopharyngoscope. In tumors with submucosal spread, the nasopharynx can be normal despite extensive destruction of the underlying structures. A careful neurological examination should also be performed for assessment of CN abnormalities. Biopsies of the nasopharynx can often be done under local anesthesia in the office with the use of flexible or rigid endoscopes with sensitivities and specificities of greater than 95%.[39] If there are problems with patient tolerance or risk of bleeding, the biopsy should be performed in the operating room. The neck should also be thoroughly examined since cervical lymph node involvement is so common, and fine-needle aspiration should be performed on suspicion nodes.

Imaging studies are crucial to define the full extent of tumor spread (Figures 3 and 4). MRI with gadolinium enhancement is superior to CT scanning for distinguishing tumor from soft tissue, assessing lymph nodal metastases, and detecting perineural spread of tumor and bone marrow involvement. However, CT imaging is better for detecting early signs of skull-base bone erosion and other bony destruction. Accurate imaging is also necessary to define the tumor volumes to be treated during radiation therapy. CT imaging most commonly shows a mildly enhancing mass in the lateral pharyngeal recess, often with metastatic nodal disease in the neck. Presence of lateral extension into the parapharyngeal and masticator space helps distinguish NPC from benign processes. There can also be posterior extension through the deep cervical fascia into the carotid space and subsequent intracranial extension. Tumor can pass through the defect at the entry point for the eustachian tube in the lateral pharyngobasilar fascia and travel in a retrograde fashion along V3 to the cavernous sinus. Nearly one-third of patients will have caudal extension, sometimes submucosal, along the lateral pharyngeal wall, and anterior and posterior tonsillar pillars.[1]

T1-weighted MRI images show a mass that is hypointense or isointense to muscle, with obliteration of the normal fat pad at the skull

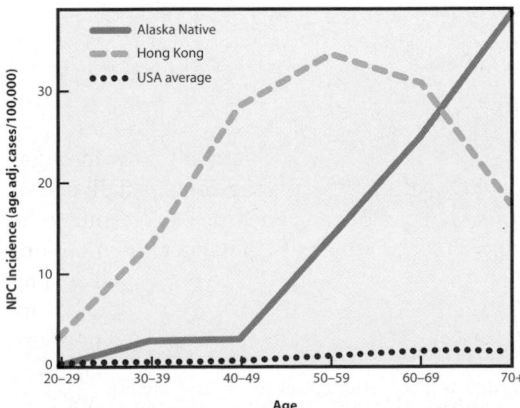

Figure 2 Graph showing incidence of nasopharyngeal cancer for different populations and age distributions. NPC = nasopharyngeal carcinoma.

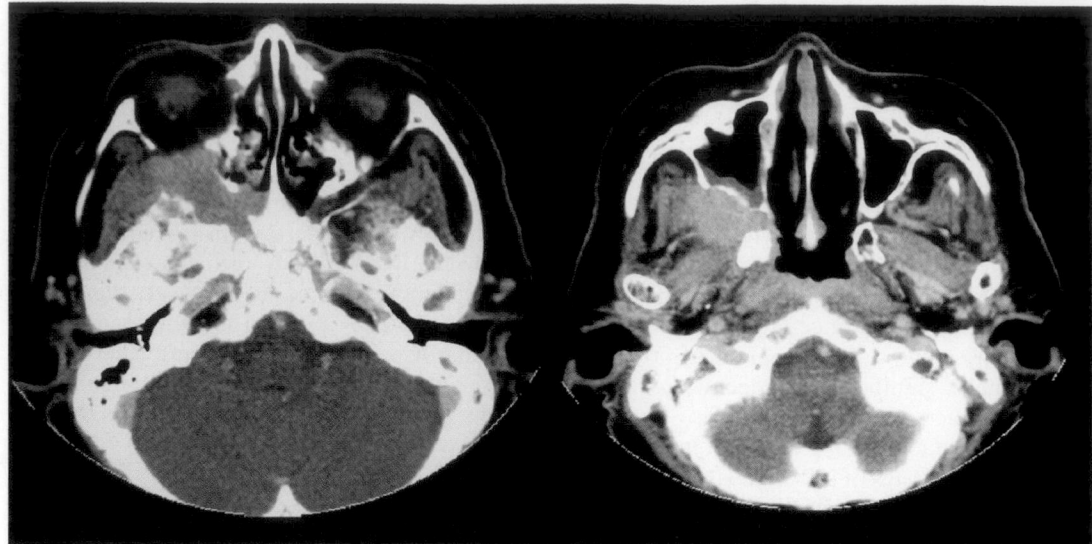

Figure 3 Computed tomography with contrast showing a nasopharyngeal carcinoma involving the posterior aspect of the right orbit and the submucosal region of the posterolateral part of the nasopharynx, with extension into the medial aspect of the middle cranial fossa and osseous destruction of the posterolateral wall of the right maxillary sinus.

base foramina. Skull-base lesions also produce abnormally low signal intensity. T2-weighted imaging shows moderate hyperintensity when compared to muscle. Contrast-enhanced T1 imaging shows mild homogeneous enhancement of the nasopharyngeal mass. Retropharyngeal nodes often are better seen with MRI than with CT.[40]

Distant metastases are not uncommon in NPC. The combination of chest X-ray, bone scan, and liver ultrasound has allowed detection of distant spread in 5% of patients with N2 disease and 14% of patients with N3 disease.[41] Patients presenting with advanced stage disease should, therefore, be evaluated for metastasis. PET scans using (18)F-fluorodeoxyglucose have been shown to be valuable in detecting distant spread, especially in individuals with N2 or N3 disease.[42,43] Scanning with PET is more sensitive than scintigraphy in locating spread to bones.[44]

Histology

NPC is a squamous cell cancer originating in the epithelial lining of the nasopharynx. The World Health Organization (WHO) has subdivided NPC into two groups, keratinizing and nonkeratinizing. The keratinizing variant, classified as WHO type 1, is similar to squamous cell cancer seen in other parts of the upper aerodigestive tract. Microscopic examination shows intercellular bridges and keratinization (Figure 5). This variant is also typically associated with a desmoplastic reaction. It is graded as well, moderately, or poorly differentiated and typically has poorer overall survival than nonkeratinizing types although the risk of metastasis is lower.[45,46]

The nonkeratinizing variant is further divided into differentiated (WHO type 2) and undifferentiated (WHO type 3, sometimes called WHO type 2b) carcinoma. WHO type 2 carcinoma makes up about 12% of all NPC. One sees a growth pattern similar to transitional cell cancer of the bladder, with stratified cells sharply delineated from the surrounding stroma (Figure 6).

The undifferentiated form of nonkeratinizing NPC (WHO type 3) is the most common throughout the world and accounts for almost

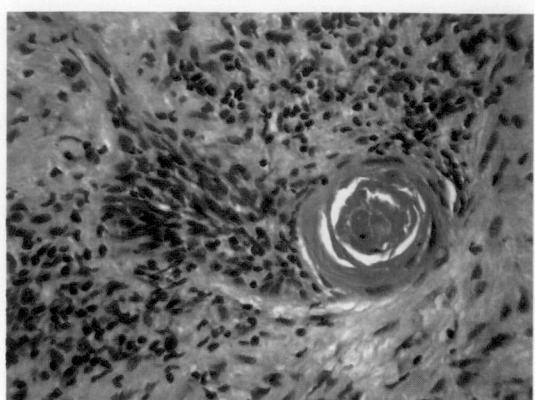

Figure 5 Photomicrograph of World Health Organization (WHO) type 1 nasopharyngeal carcinoma, showing nests of pavement-like cells with enlarged pleomorphic and mildly hyperchromatic nuclei with altered nucleus/cytoplasm ratios. A keratin pearl is demonstrated.

all nasopharyngeal malignancies in endemic regions (Figure 7A and B). Tumor cells are uniform with round to oval vesicular nuclei and prominent nucleoli. In addition to the malignant epithelial cells, one also sees a prominent infiltrate of nonneoplastic lymphoid tissue. Although the term "lymphepithelioma" is sometimes used to describe the nonkeratinizing variant, this term is incorrect since the tumor originates entirely from epithelial tissue and the lymphoid component typically is an associated benign process. The malignant tissue can occur in a nested, syncytial pattern, known as the Regaud type, or it can have a diffuse growth pattern without cohesion and known as the Schmincke type. Since a desmoplastic reaction is often absent, the latter pattern can be difficult to differentiate from lymphoma without the aid of immunohistochemistry. NPC can be distinguished from non-Hodgkin lymphoma by its reactivity with cytokeratin and its lack of reactivity with leukocyte common antigen (LCA).[47]

Staging

The heterogeneous nature of NPC is also reflected in two distinct staging systems used to describe extent of disease (Table 2). In endemic regions, the Ho system was felt to better describe the disease and its clinical course.[48] Most nonendemic regions use a TNM staging system

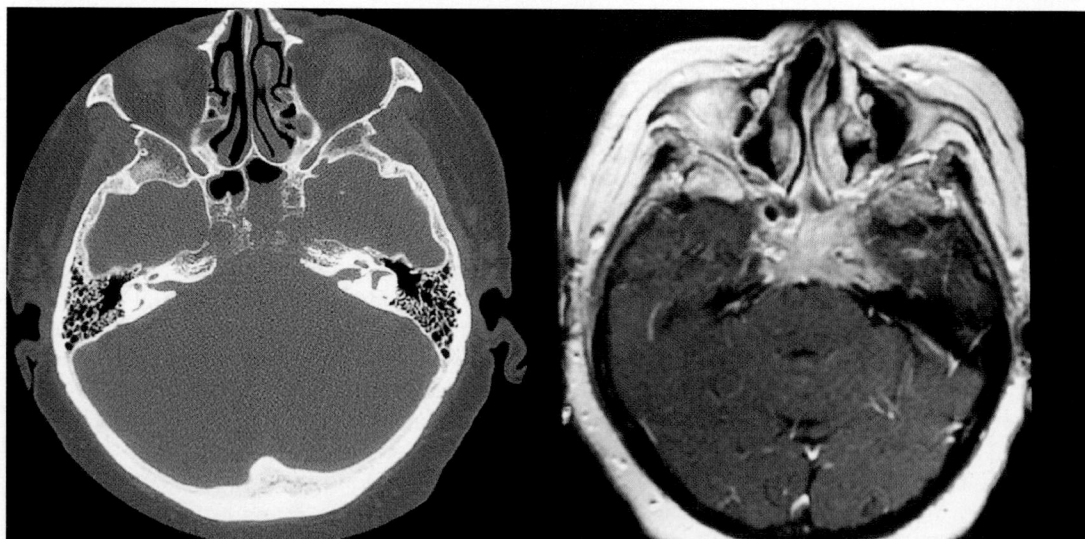

Figure 4 Computed tomography and magnetic resonance imaging scans with contrast showing a mildly enhancing mass in the posterior part of the nasopharynx eroding into the clivus and left sphenoid sinus.

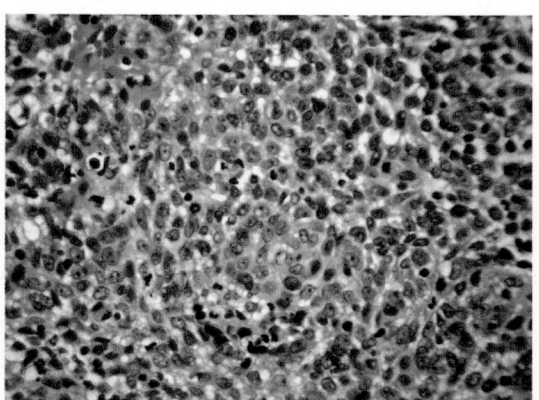

Figure 6 Photomicrograph of World Health Organization (WHO) type 2 nasopharyngeal carcinoma, showing absence of keratinization, with cylindrical spindle-shaped cells in a growth pattern similar to transitional cell carcinoma of the bladder.

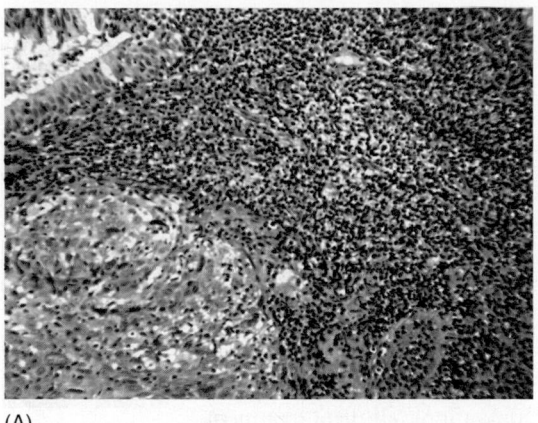
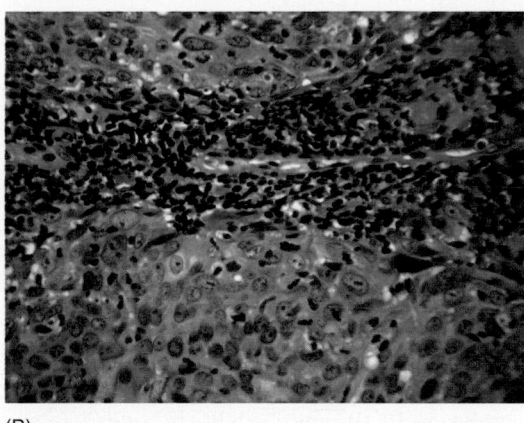

(A)   (B)

Figure 7 Photomicrographs of WHO type 3 nasopharyngeal carcinoma, showing atypical cells surrounded by dense infiltrates of lymphocytes and plasma cells. (A) The neoplastic cells have large oval to irregular vesicular nuclei, variably prominent nucleoli, and cytoplasm with indistinct boundaries. (B) There are scattered mitotic figures and no evidence of keratinization or distinct intercellular bridges.

developed by the American Joint Committee on Cancer/International Union Against Cancer (AJCC/UICC).[49] To help reduce discrepancies between the systems, the fifth edition of the AJCC/UICC system incorporated some of the features of Ho system (see Table 2). The major difference between the Ho system and previous AJCC/UICC was in evaluation of the neck. The Ho system bases the N status only on the location of neck nodes, with no consideration to their number or size. Older AJCC/UICC systems were based only on size and laterality, similar to other head and neck cancer sites. The newest AJCC/UICC system now takes location into account and judges nodes only as to whether they are larger or smaller than 6 cm. For T status, the key difference is that the Ho system does not have a T4 level and instead divides level T3 into four subsets, one of which the AJCC/UICC system classifies as T4. Compared to the 1988 AJCC system, the 1997 staging considers tumor confined to the nasopharynx, whether one side or two, to be T1. Invasion to bony structures classifies tumor as T3 instead of T4. The new T4 status now includes, in addition to intracranial extension and CN involvement, extension of tumor into the infratemporal fossa, hypopharynx, or orbit.

The AJCC/UICC staging system has been shown to be superior to the Ho system both in producing an even distribution of patients across different stages and in predicting cancer recurrence and death from cancer.[50,51] Closer analysis of outcomes has shown that better prognosis might be achieved if the N status were modified to include a subset of patients with nodes less than 3 cm. In addition, patients with T2a disease under the current system are classified as stage II although their prognosis is similar to those in stage I.[50,52] However, the distinction between T2a and T2b depends on whether or not there is parapharyngeal space involvement, and the precise boundaries of this space are not uniformly defined. Stratification of parapharyngeal space into an advanced region, defined as extension across a line drawn from the lateral pterygoid plate to the styloid process, has been shown to be a better predictor of survival that parapharyngeal space invasion alone.[36]

Treatment

Due to its anatomic location and its tendency to present in an advanced stage, surgical resection is seldom possible for NPC. Both of the non-keratinizing forms of the tumor (WHO type 2 and type 3) are radiosensitive, and radiotherapy, therefore, comprises the main component of treatment. Treatment targets for radiation therapy are based on the original extent of the tumor, regardless of any regression that may have occurred with neoadjuvant chemotherapy. Most centers now electively treat all the cervical lymphatics in N0 disease because of the high incidence of cervical metastasis.[53]

Treatment is usually given in 1.8 to 2 Gy daily fractions. T1 and T2 lesions are treated to 65 Gy, with boosts to 70 to 76 Gy for T3 and T4 lesions. Spinal cord dosage should not exceed 45 Gy. Best outcomes have occurred with a total dosage of about 75 Gy, delivered within 12 weeks.[54] Local control rates as high as 98% can be achieved with conventional radiotherapy in Stage I disease and Stage II disease without neck involvement.[55] Brachytherapy has been used to help improve outcomes in NPC. Although treatment protocols are not standardized, most studies have shown at least some improvement in local control, without major increases in toxicity.[56]

For more advanced tumors, the high incidence of locoregional and distant failures has led to a combined approach using chemotherapy in conjunction with radiotherapy. Addition of chemotherapy can enhance the effect of radiotherapy by serving as a radiosensitizing agent for tumor tissue and can also reduce systemic micrometastasis. One of the key questions is

Table 2	Staging Systems Used for Nasopharyngeal Carcinoma		
	AJCC/UICC Au and Colleagues[50]	Ho[48]
T category		
T1	Confined to nasopharynx	Confined to nasopharynx
T2	Nasal cavity or oropharynx	Nasal fossa, oropharynx, parapharynx, muscles/nerves below base of skull
	(A) Without parapharyngeal extension	
	(B) With parapharyngeal extension	
T3	Invasion of bony structures, paranasal sinuses	(A) Bone below base of skull
		(B) Bone at base of skull
		(C) Cranial nerve
		(D) Orbit, intratemporal fossa, laryngopharynx
T4	Cranial nerve, intracranial extension, orbit, hypopharynx, infratemporal fossa	
N category		
N1	Unilateral, ≤6 cm, above the supraclavicular fossa	Upper neck (above skin crease just below the thyroid notch)
N2	Bilateral, ≤6 cm, above the supraclavicular fossa	Midneck (between N1 and supraclavicular fossa)
N3	(A) >6 cm	Supraclavicular fossa, or involvement of skin
	(B) Extension to supraclavicular fossa	
M category		
M0	No distant metastasis	No distant metastasis
M1	Distant metastasis	Distant metastasis or nodal metastasis below the clavicle
Stage group		
I	T1 N0 M0	T1 N0 M0
II	(A) T2a N0 M0	T2 N0 M0, T1 or T2 N1 M0
	(B) T2b N0 M0, T1 N1 M0	
	T2a or T2b N1 M0	
III	T1 or T2a or T2b N2 M0,	T3 N0 or N1 M0,
	T3 N0 or N1 or N2 M0	T1 or T2 or T3 N2 M0
IV	(A) T4 N0 or N1 or N2 M0	Any T N3 M0
	(B) Any T N3 M0	
	(C) Any T Any N M1	
V		Any T Any N M1

what timing of chemotherapy produces the highest beneficial effect. Many previous trials showed improved disease control and disease-free survival with combined treatment, but it was not until the Intergroup Study 0099 that an improvement in overall survival was also seen.[57] That particular randomized trial compared results of stage III and IV patients from North America who received radiotherapy alone with similar patients who received both concurrent and adjuvant chemotherapy. Both arms received 35 to 39 treatments of 1.8 to 2.9 Gy/d of radiotherapy. The chemotherapy arm received in addition cisplatin (100 mg/m²) on days 1, 22, and 43 of the radiation therapy and three courses of postradiation chemotherapy (cisplatin and fluorouracil) spaced 4 weeks apart. The 3-year survival for the radiotherapy was 47%, and it was 78% in the combined treatment arm. Rates of locoregional recurrence and distant metastasis were also lower in the chemoradiotherapy (CRT) arm. Results at 5 years continued to show significant improvements for the combined treatment protocol. The improved survival was seen with combined therapy despite poor overall compliance with chemotherapy: only 55% of those scheduled to receive all courses of adjuvant therapy actually completed the treatment.

Several aspects of the Intergroup 0099 raised questions as whether the improved overall survival rates could be duplicated, especially for those patients from endemic regions. Nearly 25% of the patients in the Intergroup Study 0099 patients had WHO type 1 NPC, a much different distribution than seen in endemic regions. Also, the survival rate for the radiotherapy-alone treatment arm in the Intergroup 0099 study was also particularly poor when compared to other studies, increasing the relative beneficial effects of concurrent chemotherapy.[58]

Lin and colleagues studied the role of concurrent CRT in a randomized sample of Taiwanese patients. They stratified patients into low and high risk based on neck lymph node status. Patients in the study arm received combined cisplatin (20 mg/m²) and fluorouracil, both delivered as continuous 96-hour infusions, on weeks 1 and 5. Unlike the Intergroup 0099 study, no adjuvant or neoadjuvant chemotherapy was used. The combination of a substantially lower chemotherapy dose combined with continuous infusion substantially decreased its morbidity and improved compliance, such that 94% of the patients in the CRT arm completed their full regimen. The addition of concurrent chemotherapy significantly improved overall survival for patients in the low-risk group. However, no difference in survival was seen in high-risk patients. These patients often died of distant metastases, indicating that the elimination of adjuvant therapy may have increased the risk of micrometastasis.[59,60]

Chan and colleagues compared concurrent chemotherapy and radiotherapy with radiotherapy alone in 350 patients in Hong Kong.[61] Unlike the two previously cited studies, their protocol included patients with stage II disease, as well as

stage III and stage IV. The chemotherapy protocol consisted of weekly infusions of cisplatin (40 mg/m²) during the radiation therapy, with no neoadjuvant or adjuvant chemotherapy. Patients with persistent cancer in the nasopharynx also received intracavitary brachytherapy. The overall 5-year survival for all patients receiving combined treatment was significantly better that the radiation therapy arm (70% vs 59%, p = .049). However, there was no difference in survival among those patients with T1 or T2 disease.

Wee and colleagues followed a protocol similar to the Intergroup 0099 study on patients with stage II, III, and IV NPC in Singapore and found improved survival with CRT.[62] All of their patients had WHO type 2 or type 3 histology. Compliance with chemotherapy was problematic. Due primarily to toxicity problems, only 71% and 59% of the patients received complete concurrent and adjuvant chemotherapy treatments, respectively. CRT patients had significantly higher incidences of toxicity than the radiotherapy alone group, most notably with oropharyngeal mucositis (48% vs 32%), anorexia (22% vs 4%), and neutropenia (14% vs 0%). However, overall 3-year survival was 80% for CRT patients and 65% for the radiotherapy arm.

Not all trials have demonstrated these improved survival rates with concurrent CRT. Lee and colleagues randomized patients with WHO type 2 and type 3 NPC to receive either radiotherapy or combined treatment identical to that in the Intergroup 0099 study.[63] All of their patients had either N2 or N3 neck disease. They found no difference in distant control or overall survival in the combined arm, though locoregional control was higher in this group (92% vs 82%). Improved radiotherapy techniques may have narrowed the survival advantage usually seen with chemotherapy: In their trial, over 50% of their patients received radiation therapy based on 3-D techniques, instead of less accurate 2-D techniques used in earlier studies.

Kwong and colleagues showed a trend toward improvement in overall survival with CRT, although the difference was not statistically significant.[64] They randomized patients into four groups: radiation therapy with and without adjuvant chemotherapy, and concurrent chemotherapy and radiation therapy with and without adjuvant chemotherapy. Using factorial analysis, they were able to determine the effectiveness of concurrent CRT and of adjuvant therapy. The chemotherapy protocol consisted of oral UFT (a fluorouracil prodrug consisting of uracil and tegafur) used for concurrent treatment and a combination of cisplatin, fluorouracil, methotrexate, vincristine, and bleomycin for adjuvant treatment. Toxicity to adjuvant chemotherapy was high, with 65% of the patients developing a grade 3 or 4 toxic reaction.

Baujat and colleagues performed a meta-analysis of the effect on event-free survival and overall survival of adding chemotherapy to radiation therapy.[65] The authors were able to obtain individual patient data files from eight

randomized clinical trials comparing the two types of treatment. Their results showed a significant improvement in both event-free survival and overall survival with addition of chemotherapy. The hazard ratio for 5-year event-free survival was 54% in the radiotherapy groups and 63% in the combined CRT groups. The timing of the chemotherapy was not significant for this parameter. For 5-year overall survival, the hazard ratio was 18% lower for the combined group, resulting in a statistically significant increase in survival (56% for radiotherapy, 62% for combined treatment). Concurrent CRT showed better results than neoadjuvant or adjuvant treatment.

To reduce problems with toxicity, newer chemotherapeutic agents have been used to treat patients with NPC. Zhang and colleagues used oxaliplatin, a new analog of platinum that has fewer gastrointestinal side toxicities than cisplatin and less myelosuppression than carboplatin, in a phase III study comparing radiotherapy versus concurrent CRT. Oxaliplatin was given weekly for 6 weeks, and 97% of patients were able to complete the entire course of chemotherapy. Patients in the CRT arm had significantly better overall survival, relapse-free survival, and metastasis-free survival.[66]

Improvements in radiotherapy have also narrowed the advantages seen with concurrent treatment. In particular, 3-D conformal radiation therapy (3DCRT) and intensity-modulated radiation therapy (IMRT) allow higher dose delivery to the tumor with reduced damage to adjacent structures such as the spinal cord, brain stem, and the parotid glands.[67] Both techniques allow finer control of dose distribution such that the planned treatment volume conforms to the tumor anatomy.

IMRT offers several distinct advantages that allow better dosimetry in treatment of NPC. In particular, IMRT allows adjustment of intensities within individual beams, called "beamlets." For example, the intensity at tumor boundaries can be increased to account for edge effects that, in 3DCRT, require extension of radiation fields into surrounding tissue. IMRT allows both concave and convex isodose curves that can more accurately curve around critical nontumor structures. More homogeneous dosage within the target volumes can also be achieved with IMRT. Field shaping is done with computer controlled multileaf collimaters (MLCs), eliminating the need for other shielding devices (Figure 8). 3DCRT uses a "forward planning" model in which the doses are calculated after the beam parameters have been specified. In contrast, IMRT uses an "inverse planning" model in which the dosage curves are defined and the treatment software designs beam parameters to produce these curves. The nasopharynx is also well suited for IMRT techniques since there is little motion in that structure during treatment and it is centrally located.[68] Stereotactic radiosurgery and radiotherapy is discussed in Chapter 36, "Stereotactic Radiosurgery and Radiotherapy."

There are several different methods for delivering IMRT. The static multileaf collimation technique uses standard MLCs and irregular

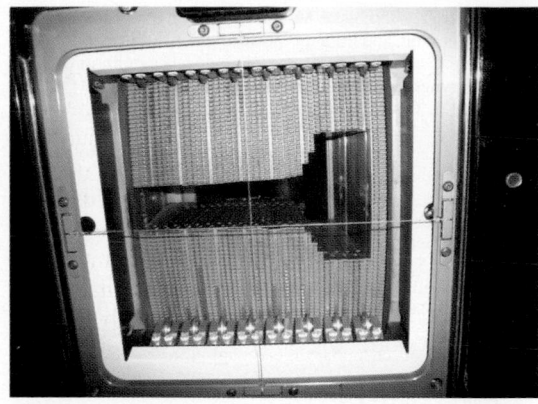

Figure 8 Multileaf collimator used in intensity modulated radiation therapy.

fields to produce a nonuniform distribution of radiation energy. A second technique, known as dynamic multileaf collimation, also uses conventional MLCs but the leaves move during the actual treatment. In a third technique, known as tomotherapy, the linear accelerator is rotated around the patient while the collimators are opened and closed depending on the trajectory of the beam. A fourth technique uses physical filters, usually made out of metal, to produce a nonuniform fluence distribution.[68]

To date, there have been no randomized studies comparing control rates for using IMRT to those achieved with 2DRT or 3DCRT. However, nonrandomized retrospective studies tend to show higher survival than seen with historic techniques. Lee and colleagues treated 67 patients with NPC using three different methods for delivering IMRT.[69] Fifty of these patients received concurrent chemotherapy using the Intergroup 0099 protocol, and 26 patients received brachytherapy. With a median follow-up of 31 months, there was only one locoregional failure. Mucositis requiring feeding tube placement occurred in 22% of the patients, and there was a high incidence of skin reaction. However, xerostomia was reduced, with only 1 of 41 patients reporting Grade 2 xerostomia at 24 months.[69]

Kam and colleagues treated 63 newly diagnosed patients with NPC in Hong Kong with IMRT.[70] Nineteen of the 36 patients with advanced stage disease also received either neoadjuvant or concurrent CRT. After 3 years, the local relapse-free survival rate and overall survival rate were 92% and 90%, respectively. Four patients, all of whom had T3 or T4 disease, recurred locoregionally, and 13 patients had distant metastases.

Wolden and colleagues used IMRT in treating 74 patients (65% WHO type 3) at Memorial Sloan-Kettering Cancer Center in New York.[71] Patients with stage II, III, and IV disease also received concurrent and adjuvant chemotherapy according the Intergroup 0099 protocol. The 3-year local control rate was 91%, compared with a historic rate of about 79% for those patients treated with non-IMRT techniques. The overall survival rate was 83%, with distant metastases the prominent form of failure.

The parotid-sparing properties of IMRT were directly measured by Hsiung and colleagues.[72]

The maximal excretion ratio (MER) from the gland was calculated both before and after treatment using quantitative salivary scintigraphy. Patients receiving IMRT had a drop in their MER from 53% down to 23% 9 months after treatment, compared with historic posttreatment MER of 0.6% in patients who had previously been treated using conventional techniques.

Treatment Side Effects. Toxicities of some degree to either radiotherapy alone or combined with chemotherapy are common. Over one-half or more of patients suffer some degree of problem such as leukopenia, vomiting, skin reaction, or mucositis.[59] With several exceptions, the incidence of higher-grade toxicities is low. Mucositis is the most common severe side effect, with grade 3 or higher toxicities occurring in 25 to 65% of patients. Rates are higher, although not always with statistical significance, in patients receiving combined treatment. When severe, a feeding tube may be necessary to maintain nutrition.

Severe leukopenia is usually not a major problem during concurrent chemotherapy, and its frequency (~5%) matches that seen in radiotherapy alone. However, during adjuvant therapy the incidence of grade 3 or 4 toxicity rises to 30 to 57%. Rates of severe skin reaction are roughly comparable in both combined therapy and radiotherapy and range from 10 to 30%.[57,59,64,73] Although seldom life threatening, xerostomia is a chronic problem after treatment, affecting up to 75% of patients. New radiation therapy techniques such as IMRT have been shown to reduce its incidence.[53]

Hypothalamic–pituitary dysfunction, temporal lobe necrosis, and other forms of intracranial radiation injury have been seen in small numbers of patients. Pituitary hypofunction is associated with abnormal levels of serum thyroxin, cortisol, or prolactin. Retinopathy has been noted in some patients, as well as vitreous hemorrhage and ischemic neuropathy.[54]

Patients treated for NPC have an increased risk of developing otitis media with effusion due to deterioration in eustachian tube function. Placement of ventilation tubes can in some cases worsen the situation by aggravating the inflammatory process. In these patients, better results may be obtained with myringotomy, even if repeated, and local treatment.[74]

Combined chemotherapy and radiation therapy or radiation therapy alone can produce significant ototoxic effects.[75] In a follow-up study of 132 patients treated with radiotherapy for NPC of whom 52 also received neoadjuvant cisplatin, 24% of the patients experienced a 15 dB or greater sensorineural hearing loss. Rates were significantly higher in older male patients, with sensorineural loss in 17% of patients 30 to 50 years old and 37% of patients older than 50. The administration of neoadjuvant chemotherapy did not increase the risk for SNHL. Forty-seven percent of the patients developed serous otitis, and this was found to be a risk factor for SNHL.[76] In a more recent study in which 22 patients

received combined therapy using conformal radiation therapy, SNHL was found in 57% of the ears. Exposure of the ear to greater than 48 Gy increased the risk of developing hearing loss, but the effect of cisplatin on hearing loss was variable.[77]

Serological Markers of NPC

A variety of serologic markers based on serum antibodies or tumor DNA have been detected and proposed as possible tools for screening for NPC and monitoring patients following treatment. Patients with NPC develop elevated levels of a wide variety of antibodies to various EBV antigens, including viral capsid antigen (VCA), early antigen (EA), a protein of the early replicating phase, and nuclear antigen (EBNA1). Prospective studies have shown that the cumulative risk of NPC in a Taiwanese male population is significantly higher for those individuals who tested positive for either antibodies for EBVCA or EBV-specific DNase, and substantially greater for those who tested positive for both.[78]

Serology for EA IgA has been found highly specific for NPC, but it has a sensitivity of only 70 to 80%. In contrast, VCA IgA is much more sensitive for NPC but less specific, suggesting that the optimal screening based in immunofluorescence would be achieved by tandem detection of antibodies to EA and VCA.[78–80]

With polymerase chain reaction techniques, circulating EBV DNA can be detected in the serum of NPC patients. The actual mechanism for release of DNA into the circulation is not known but is believed to be related to cell death.[81] This DNA, usually in fragmented form, has been found in over 95% of individuals with NPC but only 7% of controls. In those controls without NPC but with detectable EBV DNA, the levels are much lower than in seropositive patients with NPC. EBV DNA concentrations are also lower or nondetectable in patients who have a complete remission following radiotherapy.[82] Patients with high levels of EBV DNA prior to treatment are more likely to relapse following treatment and to have lower overall survival. PCR has also been used to detect the *LMP1* gene and the *EBNA1* gene from nasopharyngeal swab samples.[83] This technique had a sensitivity of 91% and a specificity of 98% in detecting NPC among 437 Taiwanese patients. However, the sample population chosen for the study may not have been representative since the prevalence of NPC was high (16%). Nasopharyngeal swabbing and detection of these two genes also was valuable in detecting recurrences following treatment. In one study, 11 of 12 patients with positive tests for both genes had recurrence, and all but one of 72 patients who were negative for the gene testing remained free of disease.[84]

Management of the Neck

One of the principal roles for surgery in NPC is management of the neck after definitive radiotherapy or CRT. Recurrent disease often occurs in the upper neck nodes and is frequently more extensive than appreciated on clinical examination.[85] There is a high incidence of extracapsular spread and infiltration into adjacent structures such as the sternocleidomastoid muscle, the spinal accessory nerve, or the internal jugular vein. Isolated clusters of tumor cells have been detected lying within fat or fibrous tissue in 35% of neck specimens. Radical neck dissection is, therefore, considered necessary for control of disease in this setting.[86]

Recurrence

Local recurrence rates in recent concurrent chemotherapy/radiation therapy trials have ranged around 10 to 20%. In a large review of 2,915 patients treated initially for nonmetastatic NPC between 1996 and 2000, the local recurrence rate with or without synchronous regional failure or distant metastasis was 11% (recurrence was defined as the presence of disease more than 24 weeks after completion of radiotherapy).[87] In 82% of these patients, the T-classification at recurrence was the same as the initial T stage. Two hundred of these patients were given salvage treatment of some sort, most often radiotherapy (79%), but also surgery (11%) and chemotherapy (9%). Multivariate analysis showed that the initial T-stage most accurately predicted overall survival, with limited benefit for those initially staged as T3 or T4.[87]

In certain cases, surgical resection of recurrent tumor at the primary site has been performed. Chang and colleagues reported 2-year survival rates of 94, 75, and 82%, for tumors at recurrence staged as T1, T2, and T3, respectively.[88] Facial translocation approach, in some performed in conjunction with a craniotomy, was used. Attempt to acheive surgical salvage was contraindicated if there was extensive intradural invasion or cavernous sinus involvement. Fee and colleagues have used intraoral, transpalatal, and sublabial approaches to recurrent carcinomas with 5-year survivals of 73 and 40% for rT1 and rT2 disease, and 14 and 0% for rT3 and rT4 disease.[89] Hsu and colleagues tailored their approach to recurrent disease to the site and stage of the recurrence, with transpalatal approaches for limited disease and transmaxillary and transmandibular for more extensive disease. They consider CN involvement to be an absolute contraindication for surgery.[90]

Chemotherapy has been used for salvage treatment, either alone or in conjunction with radiotherapy. Response rates of about 60 to 75% have been achieved, occasionally associated with a high incidence of toxicity.[91,92]

Surveillance

Endoscopic examination with rigid endoscopes is more sensitive and specific than CT scans and has better positive and negative predictive value. Accuracy is not as high with flexible scopes but still roughly comparable and less expensive than CT imaging.[93] Nevertheless, approximately one-third of the tumors are not visible on endoscopic examinations,[94] and some studies have shown that the overall sensitivity of endoscopy in predicting persistent disease is only 40%. Tumor necrosis can continue after completion of radiation therapy, such that biopsies taken too soon (within 10 weeks of treatment conclusion) may be falsely positive. There is a false-negative rate of about 60% with posttreatment biopsies from a single site; multiple biopsies are therefore important.[95]

Prognosis

In a review of treatment outcomes of 2,687 patients treated at five oncology centers in Hong Kong, multivariate analysis showed that the presenting stage was consistently the most significant factor for survival.[73] Nodal failure was predicted by the presenting N status, and distant failure was predicted by the T and N categories. Male gender and increased age were associated with higher rates of disease progression and distant failure. In this group, treated between 1996 and 2000, the 5-year disease-specific survival was 92% for stage I, 87% for stage II, 79% for stage III, and 65% for stage IV. The overall 5-year disease-specific survival for all patients was 80%; the similar figure for patients treated at these same institutions between 1976 and 1985 was 52%, indicating a true improvement in tumor control.[73]

In addition to clinical attributes, other biomarkers have been investigated for their predictive strength. NPC expresses high levels of two proteins that inhibit cell apoptosis, survivin and livin. Patients with low levels of survivin expression have better overall survival and disease-free survival than those with high expression.[96]

EBV antigens expressed on NPC cells membranes, such as latent membrane protein-2, can be used as targets for cell therapy techniques. In this technique, peripheral blood mononuclear cells are harvested and transformed to produce autologous EBV-specific cytotoxic T-lymphocytes. When transfused back into patients with progressive chemotherapy- and radiotherapy-resistant NPC, a partial response was seen in 2 of 10 patients and disease stabilization occurred in 4 of 10.[97]

REFERENCES

1. Mukherji SK. Head and Neck Imaging. In: Som PM, Curtin HD, editors. St. Louis, MO: Mosby; 2003. p. 1478–84.
2. Farias TP, Dias FL, Lima RA, et al. Prognostic factors and outcome for nasopharyngeal carcinoma. Arch Otolaryngol Head Neck Surg 2003;129:794–7.
3. Scholtz AW, Appenroth E, Kammen-Jolly K, et al. Juvenile nasopharyngeal angiofibroma: Management and therapy. Laryngoscope 2001;111:681–7.
4. Nicolai P, Berlucchi M, Tomenzoli D, et al. Endoscopic surgery for juvenile angiofibroma: When and how. Laryngoscope 2003;113:775–82.
5. Radkowski D, McGill T, Healy GB, et al. Angiofibroma: Changes in staging and treatment. Arch Otolaryngol Head Neck Surg 1996;122:122–9.
6. Liang J, Yi Z, Lianq P. The nature of juvenile nasopharyngeal angiofibroma. Otolaryngol Head Neck Surg 2000;123:475–81.
7. Dillard DG, Cohen C, Muller S, et al. Immunolocalization of activated transforming growth factor b-1 in juvenile nasopharyngeal angiofibroma. Arch Otolaryngol Head Neck Surg 2000;126:723–5.
8. Brieger J, Wierzbicka M, Sokolov M, et al. Vessel density, proliferation, and immunolocalization of vascular endothelial growth factor in juvenile nasopharyngeal angiofibroma. Arch Otolaryngol Head Neck Surg 2004;130:727–31.
9. Labra A, Chavolla-Magana R, Lopez-Ugalde A, et al. Flutamide as a peroperative treatment in juvenile angiofibroma with intracranial invasion: Report of 7 cases. Otolaryngol Head Neck Surg 2004;130:466–9.
10. Schick B, Wemmert S, Jung V, et al. Genetic heterogeneity of the MYC oncogene in advanced juvenile angiofibroma. Cancer Genet Cytogenet 2006;164:25–31.
11. Bales C, Kotapka M, Loevner LA, et al. Craniofacial resection of advanced juvenile nasopharyngeal angiofibroma. Arch Otolaryngol Head Neck Surg 2002;128:1071–8.
12. Close LG, Schaefer SD, Mickey BE, et al. Surgical management of nasopharyngeal angiofibroma involving the cavernous sinus. Arch Otolaryngol Head Neck Surg 1989;115:1091–5.
13. Danesi G, Panizza B, Mazzoni A, et al. Anterior approaches win juvenile nasopharyngeal angiofibromas with intracranial extension. Otolaryngol Head Neck Surg 2000;122:277–83.
14. Roger G, Huy PT, Froelich P, et al. Exclusively endoscopic removal of juvenile nasopharyngeal angiofibroma. Arch Otolaryngol Head Neck Surg 2002;128:928–35.
15. Wormald PJ, Van Hasselt A. Endoscopic removal of juvenile angiofibromas. Otolaryngol Head Neck Surg 2003;129: 684–91.
16. Mair EA, Battiata A, Casler JD. Endoscopic laser-assisted excision of juvenile nasopharyngeal angiofibromas. Arch Otolaryngol Head Neck Surg 2003;129:454–9.
17. Pryor SG, Moore EJ, Kasperbauer JL. Endoscopic versus traditional approaches for excision of juvenile nasopharyngeal angiofibroma. Laryngoscope 2005;115:1201–07.
18. Carrau RL, Snyderman CH, Kassam AB, et al. Endoscopic and endoscopic-assisted surgery for juvenile angiofibroma. Laryngoscope 2001;111:483–7.
19. Donald PJ, Enepikedes D, Boggan J. Giant juvenile nasopharyngeal angiofibroma. Arch Otolaryngol Head Neck Surg 2004;130:882–6.
20. Jones G, DeSanto L, Bremer J, et al. Juvenile angiofibromas: Behavior and treatment of extensive residual tumors. Arch Otolaryngol Head Neck Surg 1986;112:1191–3.
21. Howard DJ, Lloyd G, Lund V. Recurrence and its avoidance in juvenile angiofibroma. Laryngoscope 2001;111:1509–11.
22. Lee JT, Chen P, Safa A, et al. The role of radiation in the treatment of advanced juvenile angiofibroma. Laryngoscope 2002;112:1213–20.
23. McAfee W, Morris C, Amdur R, et al. Definitive radiotherapy for juvenile nasopharyngeal angiofibroma. Am J Clin Oncol 2006;29:168–70.
24. Yu MC, Yuan J-M. Epidemiology of nasopharyngeal cancer. Cancer Biol 2002;12:421–9.
25. Burgos JS. Involvement of the Epstein–Barr virus in the nasopharyngeal carcinoma pathogenesis. Med Oncol 2005;22:113–21.
26. Pathmanathan R, Prasad U, Chandrika G, et al. Undifferentiated, nonkeratinizing, and squamous cell carcinoma of the nasopharynx. Variants of Epstein-Barr virus-infected neoplasia. Am J Pathol 1995;146:1355–67.
27. Nakao K, Mochiki M, Nibu K, et al. Analysis of prognostic factors of nasopharyngeal carcinoma: Impact of in situ hybridization for Epstein–Barr virus encoded small RNA 1. Otolaryngol Head Neck Surg 2006;134:639–45.
28. Pathmanathan R, Prasad U, Sadler R, et al. Clonal proliferations of cells infected with Epstein-Barr virus in preinvasive lesions related to nasopharyngeal carcinoma. N Engl J Med 1995;333:693–8.
29. Vasef MA, Ferlito A, Weiss LM. Nasopharyngeal carcinoma, with emphasis on its relationship to Epstein-Barr virus. Ann Otol Rhinol Laryngol 1997;106:348–56.
30. Agaoglu F, Dizdar Y, Dogan O, et al. p53 overexpression in nasopharyngeal carcinoma. In Vivo 2004;18:555–60.
31. Ho K-Y, Kuo W-R, Chai C-Y, et al. A prospective study of p53 expression and its correlation with clinical response of radiotherapy in nasopharyngeal carcinoma. Laryngoscope 2001;111:131–6.
32. Yuan J-M, Wang XL, Xiang YB, et al. Preserved food in relation to risk of nasopharyngeal carcinoma in Shanghai, China. Int J Cancer 2000;85:358–63.
33. Armstrong RW, Imrey PB, Lye MS, et al. Nasopharyngeal carcinoma in Malaysian Chinese: Salted fish and other dietary exposures. Int J Cancer 1998;77:228–35.
34. Loh KS, Goh BC, Lu J, et al. Familal nasopharyngeal carcinoma in a cohort of 200 patients. Arch Otolaryngol Head Neck Surg 2006;132:82–5.
35. Sham JST, Wei WI, Lau SK, et al. Serous otitis media: An opportunity for early recognition of nasopharyngeal carcinoma. Arch Otolaryngol Head Neck Surg 1992;118:794–7.

36. Yeh S-A, Tang Y, Lui C-C, et al. Treatment outcomes and late complications of 849 patients with nasopharyngeal carcinoma treated with radiotherapy alone. Int J Radiat Oncol Biol Phys 2005;62:672–9.

37. Chang J, Lin C, Chen T, et al. Nasopharyngeal carcinoma with cranial nerve palsy: The importance of MRI for radiotherapy. Int J Radiat Oncol Biol Phys 2005;63:1354–60.

38. Wei WI, Sham JST. Nasopharyngeal carcinoma. Lancet 2005;365:2041–54.

39. Waldron J, Van Hasselt C, Wong K. Sensitivity of biopsy using local anesthesia in detecting nasopharyngeal carcinoma. Head Neck 1992;14:24–7.

40. Hudgins PA. Squamous cell carcinoma, nasopharynx. In: Harnsberger HR, Davidson HC, Wiggins RH, et al, editors. Diagnostic Imaging: Head and Neck. Salt Lake City, UT: Amirsys; 2004. p. III-1-16–9.

41. Kumar M, Lu J, Loh K, et al. Tailoring distant metastatic imaging for patients with clinically localized undifferentiated nasopharyngeal carcinoma. Int J Radiat Oncol Biol Phys 2004;58:688–93.

42. Yen T, Chang J, Ng S, et al. The value of 18F-FDG PET in the detection of stage M0 carcinoma of the nasopharynx. J Nucl Med 2005;46:405–10.

43. Chang J, Chan S, Yen T, et al. Nasopharyngeal carcinoma staging by (18)F-fluorodeoxyglucose emission tomography. Int J Radiat Oncol Biol Phys 2005;62:501–7.

44. Liu F, Chang J, Wang H, et al. (18F)fluorodeoxyglucose positron emission tomography is more sensitive than skeletal scintigraphy for detecting bone metastasis in endemic nasopharyngeal carcinoma at initial staging. J Clin Oncol 2006;24:599–604.

45. Reddy SP, Raslan WF, Gooneratne S, et al. Prognostic significance of keratinization in nasopharyngeal carcinoma. Am J Otolaryngol 1995;16:103–8.

46. Koukourakis MI, Whitehouse RM, Giatromanolaki A, et al. Predicting distant failure in nasopharyngeal cancer. Laryngoscope 1996;106:765–71.

47. Wenig BM. Head and neck. In: Weidner N, Cote RJ, Suster S, Weiss LM, editors. Modern Surgical Pathology. Philadelphia: WB Saunders; 2003. p. 168–71.

48. Ho J. Stage classification of nasopharyngeal carcinoma: A review. IARC Sci Publ 1978;20:99–113.

49. Greene FL, Page DL, Fleming ID, et al. AJCC Cancer Staging Handbook. New York: Springer; 2002. p. 47–59.

50. Au J, CK L, Foo W, et al. In-depth evaluation of the AJCC/UICC 1997 staging system of nasopharyngeal carcinoma: Prognostic homogeneity and proposed refinements. Int J Radiat Oncol Biol Phys 2003;56:413–26.

51. Chua DTT, Sham JST, Wei WI, et al. The predictive value of the 1997 American Joint Committee on Cancer stage classification in determining failure patterns in nasopharyngeal carcinoma. Cancer 2001;92:2845–55.

52. Lee A, Au J, Teo P, et al. Staging of nasopharyngeal carcinoma: Suggestions for improving the current UICC/AJCC staging system. Clin Oncol 2004;16:269–76.

53. Chao KSC, Ozyigit G. Nasopharynx. In: Chao KSC, Ozyigit G, editors. Intensity Modulated Radiation Therapy for Head and Neck Cancer. Philadelphia: Lippincott Williams & Wilkins; 2003. p. 68–84.

54. Chao KSC, Perez CA. Nasopharynx. In: Perez CA, Brady LW, Halperin EC, Schmidt-Ullrich RK, editors. Principles and Practice of Radiation Oncology. Philadelphia: Lippincott Williams and Wilkins; 2004. p. 918–60.

55. Chua D, Sham J, Kwong D, et al. Treatment outcome after radiotherapy alone for patients with Stage I-II nasopharyngeal carcinoma. Cancer 2003;98:74–80.

56. Thiagarajan A, Lin K, Tiong CE, et al. Sequential external beam radiotherapy and high-dose-rate intracavitary brachytherapy in T1 and T2 nasopharyngeal carcinoma: An evaluation of long-term outcome. Laryngoscope 2006;116:938–43.

57. Al-Sarraf M, LeBlanc M, Giri PGS, et al. Chemotherapy versus radiotherapy in patients with advanced nasopharyngeal cancer: Phase III randomized Intergroup Study 0099. J Clin Oncol 1998;16:1310–7.

58. Chow E, Payne D, O'Sullivan B, et al. Radiotherapy alone in patients with advanced nasopharyngeal cancer: Comparison with an intergroup study. Is combined modality treatment really necessary? Radiother Oncol 2002;63:269–74.

59. Lin J-C, Jan J-S, Hsu C-Y, et al. Phase III study of concurrent chemoradiotherapy versus radiotherapy alone for advanced nasopharyngeal carcinoma: Positive effect on overall and progression-free survival. J Clin Oncol 2003;21:631–7.

60. Lin J-C, Liang W-M, Jan J-S, et al. Another way to estimate outcome of advanced nasopharyngeal carcinoma- Is concurrent chemoradiotherapy adequate? Int J Radiat Oncol Biol Phys 2004;60:156–64.

61. Chan ATC, Leung SF, Ngan RKC, et al. Overall survival after concurrent cisplatin-radiotherapy compared with radiotherapy alone in locoregionally advanced nasopharyngeal carcinoma. J Natl Cancer Inst 2005;97:536–9.

62. Wee J, Tan EH, Tai BC, et al. Randomized trial of radiotherapy versus concurrent chemoradiotherapy followed by adjuvant chemotherapy in patients with American Joint Committee on Cancer/International Union against cancer stage III and IV nasopharyngeal cancer of the endemic variety. J Clin Oncol 2005;23:6730–8.

63. Lee AWM, Lau WH, Tung SY, et al. Preliminary results of a randomized study on therapeutic gain by concurrent chemotherapy for regionally-advanced nasopharyngeal carcinoma: NPC-9901 Trial by the Hong Kong Nasopharyngeal Cancer. J Clin Oncol 2005;23:6966–75.

64. Kwong DLW, Sham JST, Au GKH, et al. Concurrent and adjuvant chemotherapy for nasopharyngeal carcinoma: A factorial study. J Clin Oncol 2004;22:2643–53.

65. Baujat B, Audry H, Bourhis J, et al. Chemotherapy in locally advanced nasopharyngeal carcinoma: An individual patient data meta-analysis of eight randomized trials and 1753 patients. Int J Radiat Oncol Biol Phys 2006;64:47–56.

66. Zhang L, Peng P-J, Lu L-X, et al. Phase III study comparing standard radiotherapy with or without weekly oxaliplatin in treatment of locoregionally advanced nasopharyngeal carcinoma: Preliminary results. J Clin Oncol 2005;23:8461–8.

67. Cheng J, Chao K, Low D. Comparison of intensity modulated radiation therapy treatment techniques for nasopharyngeal cancer. Int J Cancer 2001;96:126–31.

68. Mohan R, Low D, Chao KSC, et al. Intensity-modulated radiation treatment planning, quality assurance, delivery, and clinical application. In: Perez CA, Brady LW, Halperin EC, Schmidt-Ullrich RK, editors. Principles and Practice of Radiation Oncology. Philadelphia: Lippincott Williams & Wilkins; 2004. p. 314–36.

69. Lee N, Xia P, Quivey JM, et al. Intensity-modulated radiotherapy in the treatment of nasopharyngeal carcinoma: An update of the UCSF experience. Int J Radiat Oncol Biol Phys 2002;53:12–22.

70. Kam M, Teo P, Chau R, et al. Treatment of nasopharyngeal carcinoma with intensity-modulated radiotherapy: The Hong Kong experience. Int J Radiat Oncol Biol Phys 2004;60:1440–50.

71. Wolden S, Chen W, Pfister D, et al. Intensity-modulated radiation therapy for nasopharynx cancer: Update of the Memorial Sloan-Ketering experience. Int J Radiat Oncol Biol Phys 2006;64:57–62.

72. Hsiung CY, Ting HM, Huang HY, et al. Parotid-sparing intensity modulated radiotherapy (IMRT) for nasopharyngeal carcinoma: Preserved parotid function after IMRT on quantitative salivary scintigraphy and comparison with historical data after conventional radiotherapy. Int J Radiat Oncol Biol Phys 2006;66:454–61.

73. Lee AW, Sze WM, Au JS, et al. Treatment results for nasopharyngeal carcinoma in the modern era: The Hong Kong Experience. Int J Radiat Oncol Biol Phys 2005;61:1107–16.

74. Young Y-H, Lin K-L, Ko J-Y. Otitis media with effusions with nasopharyngeal carcinoma, postirradiation. Arch Otolaryngol Head Neck Surg 1995;121:765–8.

75. Wang L, Kuo W, Ho K, et al. A long term study on hearing status in patients with nasopharyngeal carcinoma after radiotherapy. Otol Neurotol 2004;25:168–73.

76. Kwong D, Wei W, Sham J, et al. Sensorineural hearing loss in patients treated for nasopharyngeal carcinoma: A prospective study of the effect of radiation and cisplatin treatment. Int J Radiat Oncol Biol Phys 1996;36:281–9.

77. Chen W, Jackson A, Budnick A, et al. Sensorineural hearing loss in combined modality treatment of nasopharyngeal carcinoma. Cancer 2006;106:820–9.

78. Chien YC, Chen JY, Liu MY, et al. Serologic markers of Epstein-Barr virus infection and nasopharyngeal carcinoma in Taiwanese men. N Engl J Med 2001;345:1877–82.

79. Low W-K, Leong J-L, Goh Y-H, et al. Diagnostic value of Epstein-Barr viral serology in nasopharyngeal carcinoma. Otolaryngol Head Neck Surg 2000;123:505–7.

80. Hsu MM, Hsu WC, Sheen TS, et al. Specific IgA antibodies to recombinant early and nuclear antigens of Epstein-Barr virus in nasopharyngeal carcinoma. Clin Otolaryngol 2001;26:334–8.

81. Chan KCA, Lo YMD. Circulating EBV DNA as a tumor marker for nasopharyngeal carcinoma. Cancer Biol 2002;12:489–96.

82. Lo Y, Chan L, Chan A, et al. Quantitative and temporal correlation between circulating cell-free Epstein-Barr virus DNA and tumour recurrence in nasopharyngeal cancer. Cancer Res 1999;59:5452–5.

83. Hao S-P, Tsang N-M, Chang K-P, et al. Molecular diagnosis for nasopharyngeal carcinoma: Detecting LMP-1 and EBNA by nasopharyngeal swab. Otolaryngol Head Neck Surg 2004;131:651–4.

84. Hao S-P, Tsang N-M, Chang K-P. Monitoring tumor recurrence with nasopharyngeal swab and latent membrane protein-1 and Epstein-Barr nuclear antigen-1 gene detection in treated patients with nasopharyngeal carcinoma. Laryngoscope 2004;114:2027–30.

85. Wei WI, Ho WK, Cheng AC, et al. Management of extensive cervical nodal metastasis in nasopharyngeal carcinoma after radiotherapy. Arch Otolaryngol Head Neck Surg 2001;127:1457–62.

86. Yen KL, Hsu L-P, Sheen T-S, et al. Salvage neck dissection for cervical recurrence of nasopharyngeal cancer. Arch Otolaryngol Head Neck Surg 1997;123:725–9.

87. Yu KH, Leung SF, Tung SY, et al. Survival outcome of patients with nasopharyngeal carcinoma with first local failure: A study by the Hong Kong nasopharyngeal carcinoma study group. Head Neck 2005;27:397–405.

88. Chang K-P, Hao S-P, Tsang N-M, et al. Salvage surgery for locally recurrent nasopharyngeal carcinoma- A 10-year experience. Otolaryngol Head Neck Surg 2004;131:497–502.

89. Fee WE, Moir MS, Choi EC, et al. Nasopharyngectomy for recurrent nasopharyngeal cancer. Arch Otolaryngol Head Neck Surg 2002;128:280–4.

90. Hsu M-M, Ko J-Y, Sheen T-S, et al. Salvage surgery for recurrent nasopharyngeal carcinoma. Arch Otolaryngol Head Neck Surg 1997;123:305–9.

91. Poon D, Yap S, Cheung Y, et al. Concurrent chemoradiotherapy in locoregionally recurrent nasopharyngeal carcinoma Int J Radiat Oncol Biol Phys 2004;59:1312–8.

92. Chua DTT, Sham JST, Au GKH. Induction chemotherapy with cisplatin and gemcitabine followed by reirradiation for locally recurrent nasopharyngeal carcinoma. Am J Clin Oncol 2005;28:464–71.

93. Chao S-S, Loh K-S, Tan LK. Modalities of surveillance in treated nasopharyngeal cancer. Otolaryngol Head Neck Surg 2003;129:61–4.

94. Chua D, Sham J, Kwong D, et al. Locally recurrent nasopharyngeal carcinoma: Treatment results for patients with computerized tomography assessment. Int J Radiat Oncol Biol Phys 1998;41:379–86.

95. Kwong D, Nicholls J, Wei W, et al. Correlation of endoscopic and histologic findings before and after treatment for nasopharyngeal carcinoma. Head Neck 2001;23:34–41.

96. Xiang Y, Yao H, Wang S, et al. Prognostic value of survivin and livin in nasopharyngeal carcinoma. Laryngoscope 2006;116:126–30.

97. Comoli P, Pedrazzoli P, Maccario R, et al. Cell therapy of stage IV nasopharyngeal carcinoma with autologous Epstein-Barr virus-targeted cytotoxic T lymphocytes. J Clin Oncol 2005;23:8942–9.

97

Neoplasms of the Oral Cavity

Dennis H. Kraus, MD
Mark G. Shrime, MD

The list of neoplasms involving the oral cavity is extensive, including neoplasms of the minor salivary glands and neoplasms of lymphatic tissue and epidermoid tissue, that is, squamous cell carcinoma. Given that over 90% of neoplasms of the oral cavity are of the latter variety, they will serve as the focus of this chapter. Neoplasms of the oral cavity have significant effects on respiration, deglutition, and speech. The propensity for locoregional recurrence of cancers of the oral cavity often necessitates multimodality therapy. Consequently, appropriate treatment planning should be undertaken by a multidisciplinary team including the following specialties: head and neck surgical oncology, radiation oncology, medical oncology, prosthodontics, and speech-language pathology.

ANATOMY

The oral cavity is composed of distinct anatomic subsites. Malignancy arising at different subsites varies in behavior; as a result, recognition of this anatomic classification allows for prognostic evaluation and appropriate treatment planning.

Oral Cavity

The oral cavity is defined as the region from the skin–vermilion junction of the lips to the junction of the hard and soft palate superiorly and to the line of the circumvallate papillae inferiorly. Laterally, the oral cavity ends at the anterior face of the palatoglossal pillar. The various subsites of the oral cavity are illustrated in Figure 1,[1] specifically the lips, the buccal mucosa, the upper and lower alveolar ridges with their attached gingiva, the retromolar trigone, the hard palate, the floor of the mouth, and the anterior two-thirds of the tongue.

The upper and lower lips begin at the junction of the skin with the vermilion border. The lips connect laterally at the oral commissure and form the anterior boundary of the oral cavity. Sensory innervation to the lower lip is provided by the mental branch of the mandibular division of the fifth cranial nerve as it exits the mandible at the mental foramen. This nerve may serve as an important pathway for spread of malignancy into the body of the mandible. Sensory innervation to the upper lip is provided by the infraorbital branch of the maxillary division of the fifth cranial nerve as it exits the infraorbital foramen

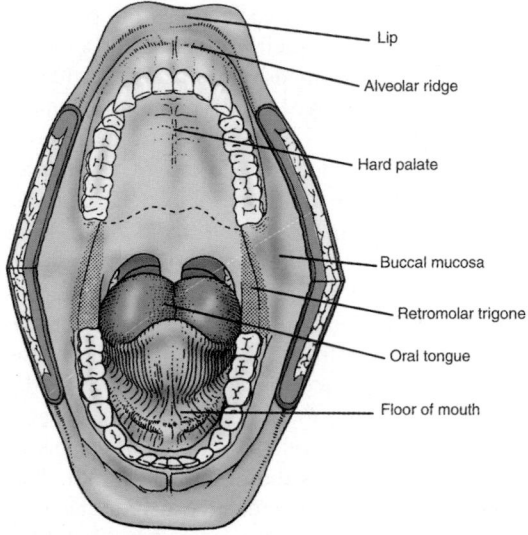

Figure 1 Anatomic sites of the oral cavity. (Adapted from reference 1.)

in the maxilla. This may provide a pathway for perineural spread of malignancy.

The buccal mucosa includes the mucosal lining of the inner surface of the cheeks and lips, extending from the line of contact of the opposing lips to the line of attachment of the mucosa of the upper and lower alveolar ridges and the pterygomandibular raphé. The buccal mucosa forms the lateral limit of the oral cavity. Neoplasms of the buccal mucosa may penetrate past the lamina propria into the deeper structures of the cheek, including the buccal fat pad and the buccinator muscle, or through the skin.

The upper alveolus and its attached gingival mucosa constitute the dental surface of the maxilla, extending from the gingivobuccal sulcus laterally to the hard palate medially. The posterior border of this mucosa is the pterygopalatine arch, which serves as the superior border of the retromolar trigone (see below). Cancer of the upper alveolar ridge may extend superiorly to involve the floor of the nasal cavity or the lower aspect of the antrum of the maxilla.

The lower alveolar ridge refers to the mucosa-covered alveolar process of the mandible, extending from the line of attachment of mucosa on the inferior gingivobuccal sulcus laterally to the line of free mucosa at the floor of the mouth medially. Posteriorly, the alveolar gingiva extends to the ascending ramus of the mandible. The mucosa of the upper and lower alveolar ridges is tightly

adherent to bone; treatment of cancers at these subsites necessitates treatment of the bony mandible and maxilla as well.

The retromolar trigone is the triangular stretch of mucosa extending from the level of the distal surface of the upper and lower third molars to attach to the hamulus of the medial pterygoid process of the sphenoid bone. The mucosa of the retromolar trigone is tightly adherent to the underlying tendon between the buccinator and superior pharyngeal constrictor muscles and is separated from the periosteum of the ascending ramus of the mandible by the buccal fat pad. Neoplasms in this region frequently invade the mandible. The site of entry of the inferior alveolar nerve into the mandibular foramen places the nerve at risk for involvement by neoplasms of the retromolar trigone. Pain from this site may be referred to the ipsilateral ear due to sensory innervation of the retromolar trigone by branches of the ninth cranial nerve. This referred otalgia is common in cancers of the oral cavity.

The hard palate is the semilunar area within the upper alveolar ridge that includes the palatine processes of the maxillary bone and the horizontal processes of the palatine bones bilaterally. It extends from the medial surfaces of the maxillary alveolar ridge to the posterior edge of the palatine bone and forms the roof of the oral cavity. The descending palatine arteries and the anterior, middle, and posterior palatine nerves are transmitted through the palatine foramina which lie laterally near the junction of the hard and soft palate. Similarly, the incisive canal, located anteriorly at the midline junction of the palatine processes of the maxillary bone, transmits the nasopalatine nerves and branches of the maxillary division of the trigeminal nerve. The mucosa at this subsite is also tightly adherent to the bone, often necessitating treatment of the underlying maxillary bone in cancers of the hard palate. In addition, the palatine and incisive foramina serve as potential routes of spread of cancer from the hard palate to the pterygopalatine fossae and the skull base.

The floor of the mouth is the semilunar space over the mylohyoid and hyoglossus muscles, extending from the inner surface of the lower alveolar ridge to the undersurface of the anterior two-thirds of the tongue. Its posterior boundaries are the bases of the palatoglossal pillars. The floor of the oral cavity is divided into two sides by the lingual frenulum and contains the openings of the ducts from the submandibular and sublingual salivary glands. The lingual nerve provides sensory innervation to the floor of the mouth and may act as a conduit for neoplasm extension. Direct extension from the floor of the mouth to the mandible or to the tongue is not uncommon; likewise, the submandibular ducts may serve as routes for neoplasm spread. Because both the lingual nerve and the auriculotemporal nerve, which provides sensation to portions of the auricle, the external auditory canal, and the tympanic membrane, are branches of the mandibular division of the fifth cranial nerve, cancer of the floor of mouth may present with referred pain to the ipsilateral ear.

The oral tongue includes the freely mobile anterior two-thirds of the tongue, extending anteriorly from the linea terminalis at the circumvallate papillae to the undersurface of the tongue at the junction of the floor of the mouth. It is composed of four areas: the tip, the lateral borders, the dorsum, and the nonvillous ventral surface of the tongue. The posterior one-third of the tongue and the lingual tonsils are considered part of the oropharynx. The hypoglossal nerve provides motor innervation to the tongue; general somatic afferents from the tongue are carried along the lingual nerve while special sensory afferents are carried along the chorda tympani branch of the facial nerve. As with the floor of the mouth, cancers of the oral tongue may present with referred pain to the ipsilateral ear due to involvement of the mandibular branch of the trigeminal nerve.

Lymphatics

Lymph nodes in the neck are grouped into various levels for ease of description.[2] Although multiple staging systems have been proposed, the accepted staging system is illustrated in Figure 2.[3] Level I contains the submental and

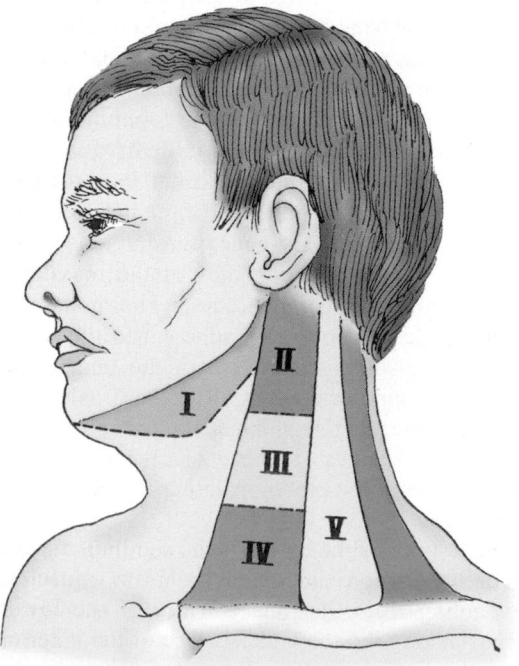

Figure 2 Cervical lymph node levels. (Adapted from reference 3.)

submandibular triangles, bounded by the posterior belly of the digastric muscle posteriorly, the midline of the neck anteriorly, the hyoid bone inferiorly, and the body of the mandible superiorly. Level I is subdivided into levels I_A and I_B. The former comprises the fibrofatty lymphatic packet between the midline of the neck medially and the anterior belly of the digastric laterally and the inferior edge of the mandible superiorly and the hyoid bone inferiorly. Level I_B contains the lymph nodes between the two bellies of the digastric muscle. Levels II, III, and IV contain the lymphatics in the anterior cervical chain, running along the sternocleidomastoid muscle (SCM). The posterior limit of these three levels is the posterior border of the SCM; their anteromedial border is the vertical line formed by the lateral borders of the strap musculature. Level II contains the upper jugular lymph nodes and extends from the level of the skull base superiorly to the inferior border of the hyoid bone inferiorly. Level III contains the middle jugular lymph nodes, extending from the inferior border of the hyoid bone superiorly to the inferior border of the cricoid cartilage inferiorly. Level IV contains the lower jugular lymph nodes, extending from the inferior border of the cricoid cartilage superiorly to the superior border of the clavicle inferiorly. As with level I, level II is subdivided into levels II_A and II_B. The superior border of level II_A is the base of the skull. This lymph node packet extends inferiorly to the horizontal plane defined by the inferior border of the hyoid bone; the anterior border is the stylohyoid muscle and the posterolateral border is defined by the spinal accessory nerve. Level II_B extends from the skull base to the inferior border of the hyoid bone. The nodes in this level extend anteriorly from the eleventh cranial nerve to the lateral border of the sternocleidomastoid posteriorly.

Level V contains lymph nodes in the posterior triangle, bounded by the anterior border of the trapezius posteriorly, the posterior border of the SCM anteriorly, and the clavicle inferiorly. Level V is subdivided into levels V_A and V_B. Both levels are constrained anteriorly and posteriorly by the same limits as level V; level V_A extends from the skull base superiorly to the horizontal plane demarcated by the lower border of the cricoid cartilage inferiorly. Level V_B extends from this horizontal plane to the superior border of the clavicles inferiorly. Level VI contains all the lymphatics in the central portion of the neck. This level extends from the inferior border of the hyoid bone superiorly to the suprasternal notch inferiorly. The lateral borders of this level are defined by the common carotid arteries. Although not widely accepted, a designation of level VII has been assigned to lymphatics within the anterior mediastinum.[1]

Metastasis to regional lymph nodes occurs in a predictable, sequential fashion. Regional lymph nodes at highest risk for metastases from primary squamous cell cancer of the oral cavity include those at levels I, II, and III, known collectively as the supraomohyoid triangle.[4] In addition, neoplasms of each anatomic subsite

have their own predictable first-echelon lymph nodes; these regional lymphatic metastatic patterns are summarized in Table 1. Nodal metastasis of squamous cell cancer of the lip is uncommon but tends to involve adjacent submental and submandibular nodes initially, followed by ipsilateral jugular nodes. Neoplasms of the buccal mucosa also tend to spread first to submental and submandibular nodes prior to metastasizing to the remainder of the anterior jugular chain. Cancers of the upper and lower alveolar ridges involve buccinator, submandibular, jugular, and occasionally retropharyngeal nodes; metastases, however, are uncommon. Likewise, neoplasms of the hard palate do not commonly metastasize to regional lymph nodes, but when lymphatic metastasis occurs it usually involves the buccinator, submandibular, jugular, and retropharyngeal nodes. Lymphatics from the retromolar trigone drain to the upper jugular nodes as well as to the retropharyngeal and intraparotid lymphatic beds. The first echelon of lymphatic drainage from the floor of the mouth is the submandibular and jugular lymph node packet. Finally, lymphatics of the tongue involve submental, submandibular, and jugular nodes. Most regional metastases are ipsilateral; however, lesions of the midline of the lip, the floor of mouth, or the tongue, will not uncommonly spread to both sides of the neck.

EPIDEMIOLOGY

In the United States, an estimated 30,990 cases of squamous cell cancer of the oral cavity and oropharynx are expected in 2006. This incidence has been slowly declining in both men and women, but the disease still affects men more than twice as often as women. Five thousand deaths due to oral cavity cancer occur per year, representing approximately 1% of the cancer mortality in the United States.[5] As with incidence, death rates have been declining over the last 25 years, with rapid declines seen within the last decade. Worldwide, the incidence of oral cavity and oropharyngeal cancer increases 10-fold,[6] with significant changes in its relative proportional incidence. In parts of India and Southeast Asia, oral cavity and oropharyngeal cancer represent greater than 30% of all cancers, likely related to geographic differences in tobacco and other carcinogen consumption.

ETIOLOGY

The majority of patients with cancer of the oral cavity have a significant history of tobacco and alcohol consumption. Both tobacco and alcohol contribute independently to the development of cancer of the oral cavity.[7] However, their combined effects are synergistic, rather than simply additive, in the development of oral cancer. This multiplicative effect of smoking and alcohol abuse is shown in Figure 3,[8] which demonstrates a 35-fold increase in the risk of cancer for men who smoke two or more packs of cigarettes and consume more than four alcoholic drinks per day.[9]

Table 1 Primary Echelon Lymphatic Drainage of Oral Cavity Cancers by Subsite		
Subsite	At-Risk Lymphatics	Comments
Lip	I_A, I_B, II, III	Midline lesions metastasize bilaterally
Buccal mucosa	I_A, I_B	
Alveolar ridges and gingiva	I_B, II, III	Also buccinator and retropharyngeal nodes
Hard palate	I_B, II, III	Also buccinator and retropharyngeal nodes
Retromolar trigone	II	Also parotid and retropharyngeal nodes
Floor of mouth	I_B, II, III	Midline lesions metastasize bilaterally
Tongue	I_A, I_B, II, III, IV	Midline lesions metastasize bilaterally

As previously mentioned, the geographic differences in carcinogen consumption may explain the higher proportion of cancers arising in the oral cavity worldwide. In Southeast Asia, cultural practices such as "reverse smoking," in which the lit end of the cigarette is held within the mouth, have been shown to produce dysplastic changes in the hard palate. Similarly, betel, a compound chewed regularly throughout Southeast Asia and the western Pacific basin, has been implicated in oral carcinogenesis. Composed of the nut of the areca palm (*Areca catechu*), the leaf of the betel pepper (*Piper betle*), and lime (calcium hydroxide), and occasionally mixed with tobacco, betel is chewed for its mild psychoactive effects. Other common practices in Southeast Asia include bidi smoking (tobacco rolled within a betel leaf) and the consumption of paan, a quid composed of the *Piper betle* leaf, the areca nut, lime, sweeteners, and sometimes tobacco. This quid is placed in the mouth and sucked or chewed over several hours, thereby remaining in contact with the oral mucosa for a significant amount of time.[10]

Tobacco need not be smoked to be carcinogenic. For example, chronic snuff dipping, in which smokeless tobacco is placed in the gingivobuccal sulcus and retained, has been associated with a nearly 50-fold increase in cancers of the

gum and buccal mucosa. Pipe and cigar smoking have also been linked to cancer of the oral cavity.[10–12] The deleterious effects of these initiators and promoters of carcinogenesis may be partially reversible; smoking cessation is associated with a sharply reduced risk of cancer, particularly for those who have quit for periods greater than 10 years.[9]

The mechanisms through which alcohol induces cancer development are less well characterized. The increased risk of cancer of the oral cavity associated with frequent use of alcohol-containing mouthwashes suggests that the etiology involves topical exposure, although this association is controversial.[10,11,13] Because alcohol has never been shown to be carcinogenic in either in vitro or animal studies; the specific mechanism responsible for alcohol-induced carcinogenesis has yet to be identified, but promotion of cellular proliferation has been implicated. Other possible mechanisms proposed include enhancement of the metabolism of other carcinogens or the development of nutritional deficiencies, specifically in vitamins A and B_2, which themselves promote neoplastic changes in oral mucosa.[10,14]

Viral infection has also been correlated with the development of head and neck cancer. Human papillomavirus (HPV) is a well-established cause for benign recurrent oral and laryngeal papillomas. Genetic DNA sequences of HPV type 16 have been detected in squamous cell cancers of the tongue, tonsil, and pharynx, and the presence of HPV in the oral cavity has been associated with an almost fourfold increased risk of cancer, independent of exposure to tobacco and alcohol.[15,16] However, other population-based studies have not implicated sexual transmissibility for oral cavity cancer.[11] The human immunodeficiency virus does appear to confer an increased risk for neoplasia. Squamous cell carcinoma in patients infected with HIV appears additionally to assume an accelerated course; cancers in HIV-infected patients who concomitantly abuse tobacco and/or alcohol occur at an earlier age and result in a significantly poorer disease-specific survival when compared with non-HIV-infected patients.[17]

Poor socioeconomic status, neglected oral hygiene, and recurrent trauma from ill-fitting dentures have also been implicated in the development of oral cavity cancer.[11,15] Outdoor occupations requiring prolonged exposure to ultraviolet radiation pose a greater risk of carcinoma of the lower lip[10]; UV radiation may itself

be synergistic with the nitrosamines contained in tobacco in effecting DNA damage.[18]

PATHOLOGY

Slaughter and colleagues first proposed the theory of "field cancerization," a concept predicated on the notion that carcinogen-induced cytologic changes occur throughout the mucosal lining of the upper aerodigestive tract, resulting in the persistent risk for multiple primary cancers, despite the removal of overt neoplasm.[19] This theory is supported by the threefold increase in the rate of second primary neoplasms in patients with oral cancer. The risk of second primary neoplasms in patients with squamous cell cancer of the oral cavity is approximately 4% annually. Both tobacco and alcohol consumption contribute independently to the risk of second primary neoplasms, with the effects of smoking more pronounced than those of alcohol, and with beer consumption potentially more detrimental than the consumption of other alcohols.[20] The risk of developing subsequent primary neoplasms in patients who cease smoking after control of the first cancer is one-sixth that of those who continue to smoke. These subsequent primary malignancies are described as *simultaneous* if diagnosed at the same time as the primary neoplasm, *synchronous* if diagnosed within 6 months of the primary neoplasm, or *metachronous* if diagnosed later than 6 months after the primary neoplasm.

Molecular Events

The development of malignant neoplasms appears to be the result of multiple, accumulated genetic alterations which must occur in the correct sequence for cancer to develop. This progression of genetic events was first described in colorectal neoplasmigenesis and a similar model has since been established for head and neck cancer.[21] Microsatellite-based genetic analysis of chromosomal alterations has demonstrated that recurrent premalignant lesions arise from a common clonal progenitor with subsequent outgrowth of clonally divergent populations.[22] Phenotypically benign mucosa in the upper aerodigestive tract, therefore, may harbor foci of clonal, preneoplastic cells that are genetically related to cancers at other sites. This observation may explain the incidence of local recurrence following complete surgical resection of cancers in the oral cavity.

Genetic alterations in the progression to carcinogenesis include activation of proto-oncogenes and the inactivation of neoplasm suppressor genes. Among the latter, p53, p16, MGMT (a DNA-repair protein), and death-associated protein kinase (DAP-K), a putative metastasis suppressor, have all been implicated.[23] Activation of proto-oncogenes and inactivation of neoplasm suppressors may occur by altered methylation of their promoter sequences,[23] or by loss of heterozygosity at their respective loci.[24]

p53 is a neoplasm suppressor that plays an important role in either initiating apoptosis or

		Smoking (cigarette equivalents/day)			
		0	< 20	20-39	40+
Alcohol (oz/day)	0	1.00	1.52	1.43	2.43
	< 0.4	1.40	1.67	3.18	3.25
	0.4-1.5	1.60	4.36	4.46	8.21
	1.6+	2.33	4.13	9.59	15.5

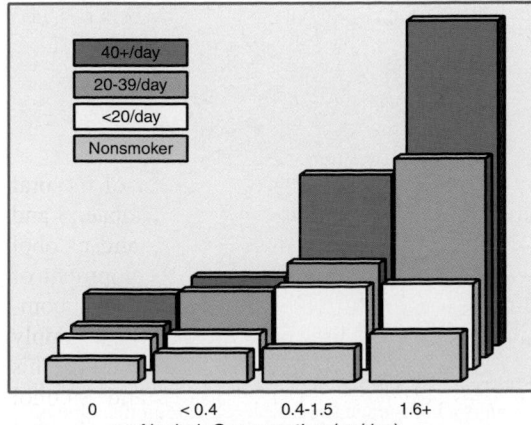

Figure 3 Multiplicative effects of smoking and alcohol abuse on the development of oral cancer. (Adapted from reference 8.)

arresting cell growth in the presence of genetic damage to permit DNA repair. Mutations in and subsequent inactivation of the *p53* neoplasm suppressor gene may result in accumulation of DNA damage and uncontrolled cellular growth. It has been shown that the incidence of *p53* mutations increases throughout the progression from premalignant lesions to invasive carcinomas. A history of tobacco and alcohol use is associated with a high frequency of *p53* mutations in patients with squamous cell cancer of the head and neck, providing an important link between these etiologic factors and the molecular progression to carcinogenesis.[25] In this light, previous reports have examined pathologic specimens in patients undergoing surgery for squamous cell cancer of the head and neck for *p53* mutations: among neoplasm resection margins and regional lymph nodes initially judged to be negative for cancer, a substantial number contain *p53* mutations identical to the mutations found in the primary neoplasm, lending credence to the concept of field cancerization.[26] These patients demonstrate an increased risk of local recurrence.

Precancerous Lesions

Akin to the progression of genetic events leading to phenotypic malignancy, various precancerous lesions can affect the oral cavity with the potential for malignant degeneration.[27] *Leukoplakia* describes a white patch in the oral cavity that does not rub off. Approximately 10% of these lesions will display squamous cell carcinoma (either in situ or invasive) on histology.[28] *Oral lichen planus*, which may be mistaken for leukoplakia, is a white, lacy, striated lesion of unknown etiology that most commonly occurs on the buccal mucosa. Malignant change in oral lichen planus is rare.

Erythroplakia (the term *erythroplasia*, often incorrectly used interchangeably with erythroplakia, describes a similar-appearing lesion located specifically on the penis) appears as a red, slightly raised, granular lesion in the oral cavity and oropharynx. In contrast to the low incidence of cancer in patients with leukoplakia, up to 90% of patients with erythroplakia will display concurrent or subsequent malignancy. Mutations of *p53* and instances of DNA aneuploidy have been demonstrated in erythroplakic lesions, and minimal size of the lesions does not preclude invasiveness, mandating biopsy at the time of clinical suspicion.[29]

Oral submucous fibrosis is a precancerous lesion predominantly seen in people from the Indian subcontinent. It is a chronic disease of the oral mucosa characterized by inflammation and progressive fibrosis of the lamina propria and deeper connective tissues. Bands of oral submucous fibrosis can be found in the posterior portion of the oral cavity in milder cases; anterior bands are more commonly found in cases of increasing severity. The malignant transformation frequently associated with oral submucous fibrosis is likely multifactorial in origin, but its presence

alone confers a 19-fold increased risk for the development of oral cancer.

Histopathology

Morphologically, squamous cell carcinoma can be classified according to its growth patterns: exophytic, infiltrative, and ulcerative. The latter type is the most common in the oral cavity and demonstrates a proclivity for rapid invasion.

Histologically, squamous cell cancer may be classified into five types: keratinizing, nonkeratinizing, spindle cell, basaloid squamous, and verrucous. Keratinizing types generally arise from ectoderm, tend to be ulcerative or exophytic, have a lower tendency for submucosal spread, and have infiltrating margins (Figure 4). The nonkeratinizing cancers typically arise from endoderm, spread submucosally, and have "pushing" or noninfiltrative, margins. Spindle cell carcinoma is rare, demonstrating spindle-shaped mesenchymal cells resembling highly anaplastic sarcoma admixed with components of epidermoid carcinoma (Figure 5). Basaloid squamous carcinoma is also a rare variant with high-grade features (Figure 6).

Verrucous carcinoma was initially described by Ackerman as a slowly growing exophytic or warty neoplasm in the oral cavity[30] (Figure 7). It is a well-differentiated variant of squamous cell carcinoma and has the histologic appearance of keratinized epithelium arranged in long, papillomatous folds. Like the nonkeratinizing subtype, verrucous carcinoma has "pushing" margins. It typically affects the buccal mucosa of elderly patients with a history of tobacco exposure or poor oral hygiene. True verrucous carcinoma has an astoundingly low metastatic potential. As a result, wide surgical excision is the recommended treatment, although irradiation may be considered in selected patients.[27,31] However, there have been controversial reports of anaplastic transformation of verrucous carcinoma in patients treated with radiation therapy. In addition, recurrence of verrucous carcinoma tends to be in the form of less differentiated cancers,

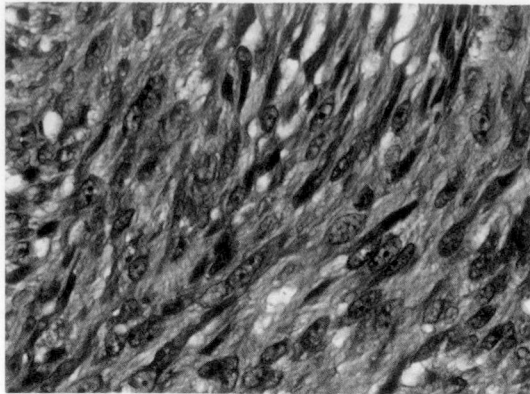

Figure 5 Sarcomatoid or spindle cell squamous cell carcinoma, resembles a sarcoma and no longer resembles an epithelial tumor.

likely from foci of these less-differentiated subtypes that have been observed coexisting within verrucous lesions.[27]

MECHANISMS OF CANCER SPREAD

Local Spread

Primary neoplasms of the oral cavity spread along tissue planes of least resistance, initially extending superficially along mucosa. As lesions enlarge, deeper structures may become involved, including the submucosa, underlying muscle, cartilage, or bone. Frequently, microscopic neoplasm extends in irregular, finger-like projections as far as 1 cm beyond palpable neoplasm margins.[26] This insidious microscopic course of squamous cell carcinoma may provide an additional mechanism for local recurrence in the presence of apparently negative surgical margins.

Primary neoplasm may also track along the course of nerves and vessels and spread outside the oral cavity, sometimes in a discontinuous fashion. The negative prognostic implications of perineural invasion include spread to the base of the skull, making the neoplasms less amenable to surgical resection and intensive radiotherapy, and discontinuous spread, making adequate margins difficult to establish. Microvascular spread has

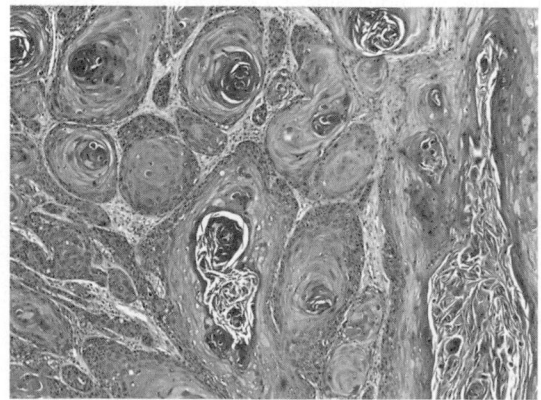

Figure 4 Invasive squamous cell carcinoma is considered to be well, moderately, or poorly differentiated based upon the extent of cytoplasmic keratinization, keratin pearl formation, and morphological resemblance to squamous epithelium. The more difficult it is to appreciate that the invasive carcinoma is squamous in origin, the less well differentiated it is.

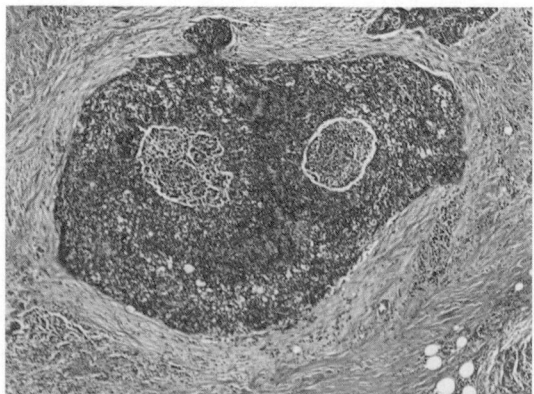

Figure 6 By definition, basaloid squamous cell carcinoma is a high-grade squamous cell carcinoma. One often sees areas of central necrosis and cystic change. The cells are hyperchromatic, angular, and basophilic, and there can also be areas of keratinization and keratin pearl formation.

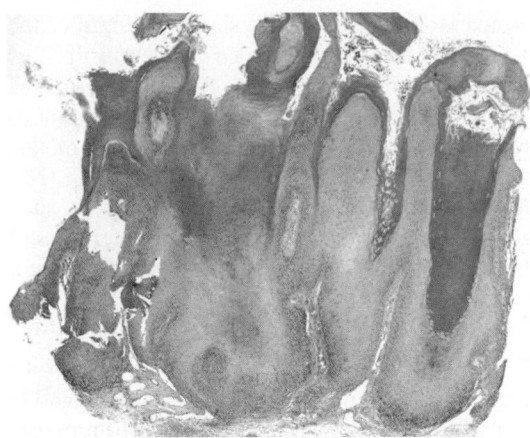

Figure 7 Verrucous squamous cell carcinoma is considered to be a well-differentiated squamous cell carcinoma, which grows with a broad pushing base and is considered to not have any cytological atypia. This entity is considered to not have metastatic potential.

also been correlated with higher rates of locoregional recurrence.

Regional Spread

Prevalence of metastases to regional lymphatics is predicated upon neoplasm size, location, depth of invasion, and the density of lymphatics at the primary site. Previous surgery, radiation, or inflammation may result in aberrant lymphatic drainage secondary to fibrosis of lymphatic channels. The metastatic potential of primary neoplasms of the lip, alveolar ridge, and hard palate is significantly less than that of neoplasms arising elsewhere in the oral cavity, due to a paucity of lymphatic drainage at these sites. Over all, the 5-year survival of patients with cervical metastases is approximately 50% that of those without.[32] In patients with metastases to the neck, extracapsular spread of carcinoma in cervical lymph nodes portends a poor prognosis, as do an increased number of involved nodes and the spread of neoplasm to lymph nodes more inferiorly located within the neck.[33]

Although up to 20% of patients who succumb to head and neck cancer develop metastases to distant sites, only 4% of these have distant spread without antecedent locoregional failure. Treatment efforts have therefore concentrated on locoregional control of the disease.

Distant Spread

Distant metastases from cancers of the oral cavity generally do not occur until the disease is advanced. Distant metastases typically first involve the lungs, followed by the liver, then by bone. Surveillance computed tomography (CT) of the chest, therefore, is often employed as part of the routine follow-up of a patient treated for squamous cell carcinoma of the oral cavity.[34]

Positron emission tomography (PET) with [21]F- fluorodeoxyglucose has been shown to be beneficial in the follow-up of patients with head and neck cancer. PET scanning following the completion of therapy (2 to 6 months after surgery or chemoradiation) has been shown to provide an accurate assessment of the patient's response to therapy and is able to detect locoregional and distant recurrence earlier than conventional imaging.[35]

CANCER OF THE ORAL CAVITY IN YOUNG ADULTS

Squamous cell carcinoma of the oral cavity tends to affect patients around the sixth decade of life, but there is evidence of an increasing incidence in younger adults, specifically cancers of the oral tongue and palatine tonsils.[36] The biologic behavior of cancer in the oral cavity in the younger adult population presents a topic of significant debate. Although molecular differences in tumor biology have not been demonstrated in these younger patients, there is some indication that these neoplasms require more aggressive treatment: patients younger than 40 years of age with squamous cell carcinoma of the tongue demonstrate higher rates of local recurrence. However, these rates have not been shown to translate to poorer survival.[37,38] It should be noted that studies on either side of this debate tend to be retrospective reviews of relatively small patient groups in light of the infrequent nature of this disease.

OTHER MALIGNANT NEOPLASMS OF THE ORAL CAVITY

Other malignancies affecting the oral cavity besides squamous cell cancer include Kaposi sarcoma, extranodal non-Hodgkin lymphoma, mucosal melanoma, and minor salivary gland cancers.

Kaposi sarcoma is a common manifestation of AIDS and clinically presents as a nonpruritic, violaceous macule on the mucosa of the upper aerodigestive tract. These neoplasms grow slowly and are amenable to radiation, laser excision, cryotherapy, or intralesional injections of vinblastine.

Extranodal non-Hodgkin lymphoma may present as a painless mass along the palate or gingiva or as an asymptomatic enlargement of one tonsil. Treatment is similar to that of non-Hodgkin lymphoma elsewhere in the body.

Mucosal melanoma of the head and neck is rare, representing only 3% of all melanomas. Its mortality, however, is significant when compared with mortality of the nonmucosal type. The palate is the most common site of involvement in the oral cavity, with intralesional lymphatic and vascular invasion frequently seen. Surgical excision is recommended, although the ultimate prognosis is typically poor, owing to frequent distant dissemination.[39,40]

Adenoid cystic carcinoma is the most common minor salivary gland neoplasm of the oral cavity, although mucoepidermoid carcinoma and adenocarcinoma are also present in this region. As with other regions, the incidence of minor salivary cancer in the oral cavity is increased following therapeutic irradiation. Treatment protocols are similar to those for primary salivary cancers.[5]

EVALUATION

History and Physical Examination

The first step in the evaluation of a patient with cancer of the oral cavity is a thorough history and a comprehensive examination of the head and neck. The patient should be questioned about symptoms of dysphagia, odynophagia, dysarthria, globus sensation, difficulty breathing, hemoptysis, otalgia, weight loss, and other constitutional symptoms. An especially important component of the complete history, given the aforementioned risk factors for oral cavity cancer, is an adequate social history: the patient should be asked about the consumption of tobacco and alcohol, about occupational, sexual, and avocational exposures (including sunlight), and about previous exposure to radiation.

During the comprehensive examination of the head and neck, the oral cavity should be thoroughly assessed. Pigmentation changes or ulcerations of the oral mucosa, the state of dentition, and an evaluation for trismus should all be undertaken. A thorough examination includes both visual inspection and palpation of all subsites in the oral cavity for mucosal lesions and masses. Bimanual palpation is particularly useful in the evaluation of the buccal surfaces and the floor of the mouth. Tongue mobility should be assessed, and palpation of the base of the tongue should not be neglected. Somatosensory function of the lower two divisions of the trigeminal nerve should be evaluated for symmetry. The patient's neck should be palpated for masses, with palpable masses assessed for size, location, consistency, mobility, and tenderness. Other factors which also require attention, namely tumor size, bleeding, pain, and interference with speech, breathing, or eating, should not be overlooked.

The necessity for a systematic, comprehensive approach to the history and physical examination cannot be overemphasized. It has been shown that a delay in diagnosis for a primary neoplasms of the oral cavity is greatest when the neoplasm is located in the floor of the mouth and shortest when the neoplasm is on the tongue. In addition, the concept of field cancerization implies that finding one lesion in the oral cavity does not preclude the existence of others.

Imaging and Pathologic Evaluation for Regional Metastases

Clinical assessment of regional nodal metastases is not infallible. It may be difficult to appreciate lymphadenopathy in patients with a short, stout neck, in patients with fibrotic changes secondary to previous radiotherapy, and at sites, such as the parapharyngeal or retropharyngeal spaces, typically inaccessible by routine physical examination. Although there is no substitute for a systematic, comprehensive examination of the neck, imaging techniques provide valuable supplemental information regarding the status of regional lymph nodes. The sensitivity of CT and magnetic resonance imaging (MRI) for nodal metastasis is between 80 and 90%, but recent studies have implied that clinical examination may be more efficient than CT at the identification of cervical metastases.[41] Although the actual diagnosis of malignancy cannot be made on imaging, there are certain characteristic changes apparent on CT and MRI that suggest the presence of carcinoma. These include rim enhancement, central necrosis, a nodal size of ≥1 cm, and a round shape suggest carcinoma within a neck node.

PET has a sensitivity of approximately 85% and a specificity of approximately 99% in the evaluation of the node-positive neck, but only a 67% sensitivity and 85% specificity in the evaluation of the clinically negative neck (Figure 8).[42] It cannot be relied on as a sole diagnostic modality. A combined strategy involving clinical examination and imaging is therefore indicated. However, because both physical examination and imaging are techniques prone to false-positive and false-negative errors, pathologic confirmation by fine-needle aspiration (FNA) is commonly employed for any suspicious neck mass. FNA is a highly sensitive procedure with minimal morbidity that allows cytologic examination of a mass in the head and neck. Repeat FNA should be considered following an initial nondiagnostic FNA. Open neck biopsy is a procedure with limited applications and should be considered only when both the surgeon and the patient are prepared to proceed immediately with a neck dissection if indicated.

Imaging Evaluation of the Mandible

CT and MRI provide useful adjuvant information regarding soft tissue and bony invasion of advanced oral cavity neoplasms, particularly with extension toward the nasal cavity, maxillary sinus, parapharyngeal space, and larynx. Optimal radiologic evaluation of mandibular involvement by cancer, however, remains controversial.

Patterns of spread within the mandible include direct extension through the cancellous bony trabeculae and along the inferior alveolar nerve.[43] Panoramic radiographs are helpful in the evaluation of gross mandibular invasion but cannot resolve minimal cortical invasion. The utility of CT scans may be limited owing to the presence of irregular dental sockets and artifacts (Figure 9). Dedicated CT reconstructions of the mandible (DentaScans, see Figure 9) may obviate some of this artifact, but their utility is controversial.[44] In addition, clinical evaluation is valuable in determining the extent of bony invasion and therefore the optimal method of mandibular resection.

Endoscopy

Endoscopic examination may be performed both in the office and in the operating room. Diagnostic nasopharyngoscopy is a simple in-office procedure, routinely employed for the detection of malignancies throughout the upper aerodigestive tract; it is critical in the follow-up of patients with tumors of the head and neck. However, endoscopic examination under anesthesia provides the most thorough inspection of the primary neoplasm and evaluation for second primary neoplasms, as well as the ability to biopsy suspicious sites. The oropharynx, hypopharynx, and larynx should be examined in a systematic fashion. The routine use of both esophagoscopy and bronchoscopy is controversial owing to the low yield of simultaneous carcinoma of the lung or esophagus, especially in the absence of clinical or radiographic findings.[45]

Staging

Staging systems for cancer provide a standardized measurement for the extent of disease. Staging allows for the estimation of prognosis, provides assistance with treatment planning, provides a framework for the evaluation of treatment effectiveness, and promotes a uniform

comparison of results. The staging system of the American Joint Committee on Cancer for cancers of the oral cavity is given in Table 2. This TNM staging categorizes tumors based on the extent of the primary tumor (T), the extent of nodal metastasis (N), and the presence of distant disease (M). While of utmost importance, patient factors, such as comorbidities, and molecular characteristics of the tumor are not incorporated into the current staging system.

Sentinel Lymph Node Biopsy

In an effort to improve accuracy of staging and to guide further treatment, the technique of lymphoscintigraphy and sentinel lymph node biopsy have recently been applied to cancers of the oral cavity. This technique, adopted from the melanoma literature, involves injection of a radiocolloid marker into the primary tumor with subsequent timed scintigraphy of the neck; the first-echelon node specific to the particular tumor is thereby identified. In theory, that particular node could be removed and histologically examined. If tumor is found in that node, a complete neck dissection would then be undertaken; if the node is clear of tumor, no further treatment of the neck would be indicated. Unfortunately, the data regarding this technique are sparse. Although initial reports put the negative predictive value of a sentinel node for carcinoma elsewhere in the neck as high as 100%,[46] more recent studies have reported a false-negative rate up to 33%.[47] Further prospective, randomized studies are required before establishing this technique as useful in the armamentarium of the head and neck surgeon.

TREATMENT

In general, early-stage lesions in the oral cavity may be treated by either surgery or radiation with comparable results, and more advanced

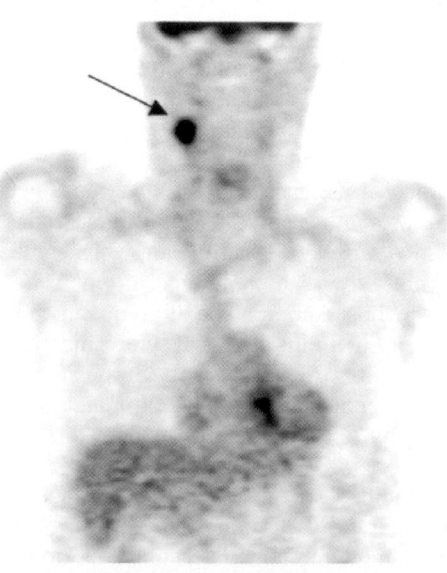

(A)

(B)

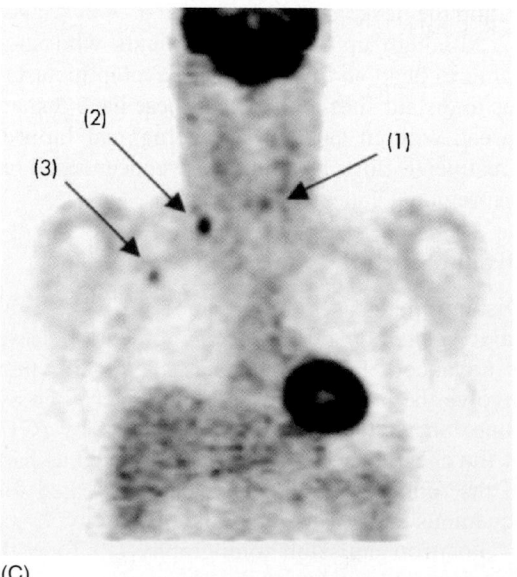

(C)

Figure 8 (A) A positron emission tomographic (PET) scan demonstrating carcinoma of the floor of the mouth and lower alveolar ridge (1), with a second primary at the base of the tongue (2). (B) A PET scan demonstrating cervical lymph node metastasis (*arrow*) in a patient with cancer of the oral cavity. Normal 18-fluorodeoxyglucose (FDG) uptake is noted in the brain, myocardium, and liver. (C) A PET scan demonstrating FDG uptake in paratracheal (1), supraclavicular (2), and axillary (3) lymph nodes in a patient with cancer of the oral cavity, suspicious for nodal metastases. Normal FDG uptake in noted in the brain, myocardium, and liver.

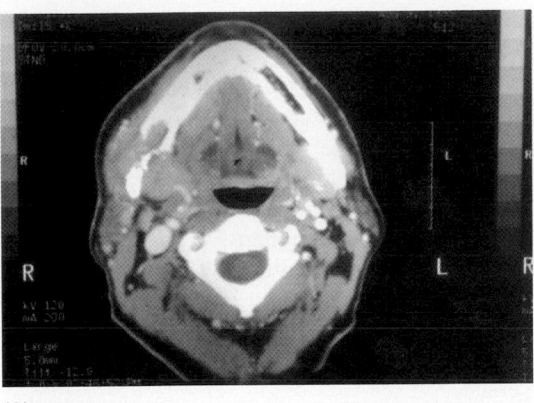 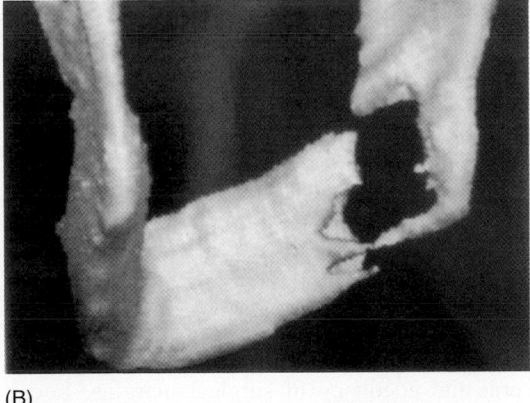

(A)   (B)

Figure 9 (A) Axial computed tomographic (CT) scan of the neck demonstrating mandibular invasion from oral cavity carcinoma. (B) Three-dimensional reformatted CT scan of the mandible demonstrating bony invasion in the same patient.

cancers are best approached with combined therapy. The proclivity of these tumors for locoregional failure, however, mandates recognition of the specific prognostic factors associated with each case. Tailoring the most appropriate therapy involves consideration of patient characteristics, including motivation and comorbidities; physician resources, including experience and facilities; and tumor presentation, including location, grade, and extent of disease.

Furthermore, the optimization of aesthetic form and preservation of proper functions of speech, respiration, and deglutition must be reconciled with tumor eradication.

Surgery

In light of the comparable results for early-stage lesions treated with either surgery or radiation therapy, factors in favor of surgical resection include the ability to stage local invasion and the avoidance of the sequelae of radiotherapy, namely xerostomia and osteoradionecrosis. The primary limitation of surgery, however, involves functional impairment, particularly when resection involving the mandible or a large portion of the tongue is necessary.

Surgical Approaches. Different approaches to the oral cavity exist, depending on tumor location and extent. Peroral excision is suitable for small lesions of the oral cavity. A cheek flap, however, may be constructed for larger lesions. A visor flap may be used for anterior lesions in the oral cavity if one wishes to avoid external facial incisions, but this is done at the expense of bilateral mental nerve sacrifice.

Carcinomas arising at or extending to the posterior portion of the oral cavity may require a mandibulotomy for adequate exposure. A paramedian mandibulotomy with paralingual extensions, that is, a mandibular swing, illustrated in Figure 10,[48] offers more versatility and less morbidity than a mandibulotomy through a lateral approach. Placing the mandibulotomy anterior to the mental foramen preserves the integrity of the inferior alveolar nerve and may exclude the osteotomy from portals typically employed for adjuvant external beam radiation.

The mandible should be spared in the absence of bony invasion. Oncologically, there is no benefit from removal of a portion of the mandible simply to keep the contents of a neck dissection in continuity with the primary resection. Functionally, resection of the anterior arch of the mandible results in significant disability, including drooling and interference with eating, in direct relation to the amount of bone removed. Aesthetically, this may also result in a significant recession of the pogonion, leading to what is known as an "Andy Gump" deformity.

Instances of bony invasion by tumor, however, mandate resection of that portion of the

Table 2 American Joint Committee on Cancer Staging of Lip and Oral Cavity Cancers	
Primary tumor (T)	
T_X	Primary tumor cannot be assessed
T_0	No evidence of primary tumor
T_{is}	Carcinoma in situ
T_1	Tumor 2 cm or less in greatest dimension
T_2	Tumor more than 2 cm but not more than 4 cm in greatest dimension
T_3	Tumor more than 4 cm in greatest dimension
T_4 (lip)	Tumor invades adjacent structures, eg, through cortical bone, inferior alveolar nerve, floor of mouth, skin of face
T_4 (oral cavity)	Tumor invades adjacent structures, eg, through cortical bone, into the deep (extrinsic) muscles of the tongue, into the maxillary sinus, into the skin; superficial erosion of bone or tooth socket by a gingival primary is not sufficient to classify as T_4
Regional lymph nodes (N)	
N_X	Regional lymph nodes cannot be assessed
N_0	No regional lymph node metastases
N_1	Metastases in a single ipsilateral lymph node, no greater than 3 cm in greatest dimension
N_2	Metastasis in a single ipsilateral lymph node, >3 cm but no greater than 6 cm in greatest dimension; or in multiple ipsilateral lymph nodes, no greater than 6 cm in greatest dimension; or in bilateral or contralateral lymph nodes, no greater than 6 cm in greatest dimension
N_{2a}	Metastasis in a single ipsilateral lymph node, >3 cm but no greater than 6 cm in greatest dimension
N_{2b}	Metastasis in multiple ipsilateral lymph nodes, no greater than 6 cm in greatest dimension
N_{2c}	Metastasis in bilateral or contralateral lymph nodes, no greater than 6 cm in greatest dimension
N_3	Metastasis in any lymph node more than 6 cm in greatest dimension
Distant metastases (M)	
M_X	Distant metastasis cannot be assessed
M_0	No distant metastasis
M_1	Any distant metastasis

Stage grouping

	T_1	T_2	T_3	T_4
N_0	I	II	III	IV_A
N_1	III	III	III	IV_A
N_2	IV_A	IV_A	IV_A	IV_A
N_3	IV_B	IV_B	IV_B	IV_B
M_1	IV_C	IV_C	IV_C	IV_C

Adapted from the American Joint Committee on Cancer Staging Manual, 6th edition.

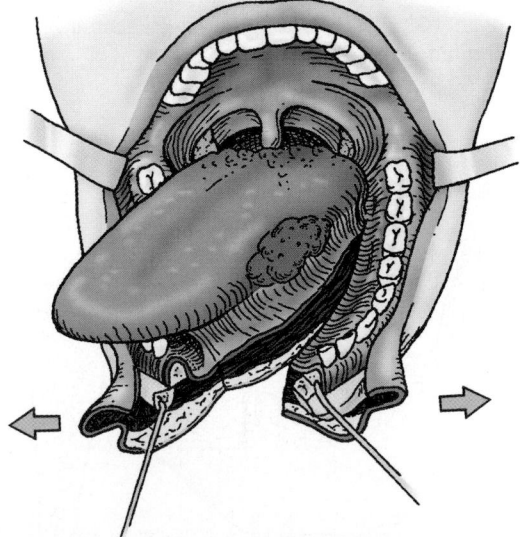

Figure 10 Paramedian mandibulotomy for resection of carcinoma of the posterior part of the tongue. (Adapted from reference 48.)

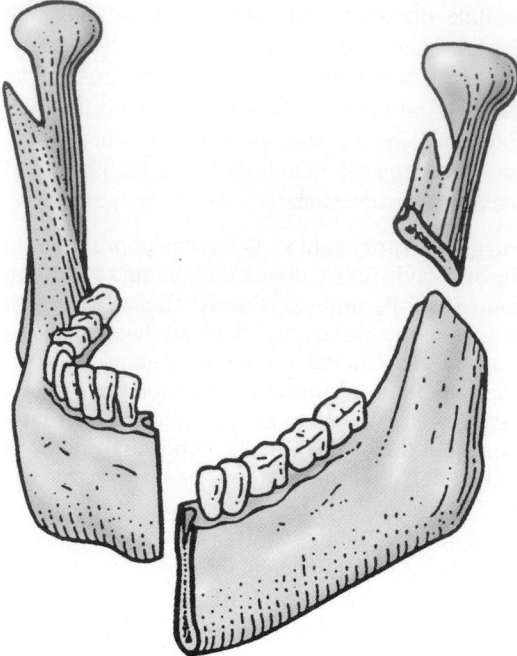

Figure 11 Segmental mandibulectomy. (Adapted from reference 49.)

mandible.[44] Segmental mandibulectomy is illustrated in Figure 11.[49] The amount of bone to be resected is predicated upon the location and extent of bony involvement. Marginal mandibulectomy has been recommended for lower gingival cancers if the erosive bony defects do not extend beyond the inferior alveolar canal or if they are confined to a superficial area of alveolar bone (Figure 12). Rim (superior marginal) mandibulectomy may be effective for carcinomas of the mandibular alveolus provided at least 1 cm of bone inferiorly can be preserved, thereby decreasing the chance of mandibular fracture. It is the authors' objective opinion that the use of marginal mandibulectomy has dramatically decreased as a consequence of the availability of bone incorporating free flap reconstruction. The ability to replace the mandible with free tissue transfer from the fibula and iliac crest has reduced the need for marginal mandibulectomy, thus the use of the free flap has reduced the significant risk of secondary fracture when marginal mandibulectomy is employed.

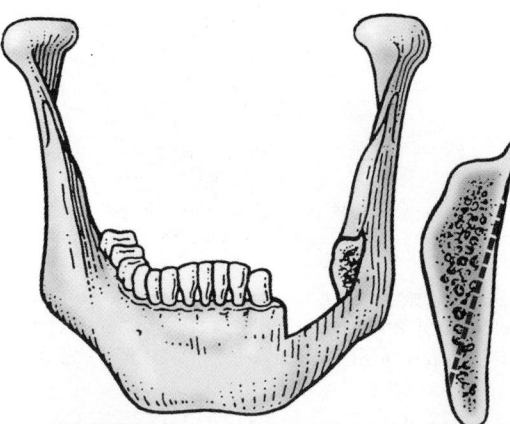

Figure 12 Marginal mandibulectomy. (Adapted from reference 49.)

Cancers of the hard palate often require an inferior maxillectomy. The same principles should be followed for the maxilla as are for the mandible: as little bone as needed should be removed to maintain a balance between functional outcome and oncologic result. However, the rehabilitation of hard palate defects with the use of prosthodontics, in addition to free tissue transfer, is significantly easier than that of mandibular defects.

Surgical Margins. An important concept in the management of cancers of the oral cavity concerns the adequacy of surgical margins. Local recurrence in patients with positive surgical margins following resection may be as high as four times that following resection with negative margins.[50] Furthermore, local recurrence rates and 5-year survival rates of patients with "close" surgical margins (less than 5 mm) are comparable to those with microscopically positive margins.[51] In that light, it is critical to ensure the resection of adequate margins at the time of surgery. It should be remembered, however, that oral cavity margins shrink approximately 30 to 50% from the in situ measurement by the surgeon to the final pathologic evaluation after formalin fixation.

Radiation Therapy

An environment high in oxygen provides an ideal setting for therapeutic radiation, leading to the generally favorable radioresponsiveness of most early-stage head and neck cancers; invasion of bone or deep muscle, therefore, portends a poorer response to radiotherapy.

Modalities for primary radiation include wide-field or intensity-modulated external beam radiation therapy, interstitial implantation, that is, brachytherapy, or a combination of modalities. Definitive radiotherapy shares comparable results with surgical treatment for early-stage oral cancers and is therefore preferred for early-stage lesions in patients in whom surgical management is contraindicated. The dosage of radiation depends upon the extent of disease and the tolerance of surrounding normal tissues to radiation injury. In general, definitive radiotherapy may be delivered with doses of 60 to 65 Gy over 6 weeks for smaller tumors, with larger tumors requiring up to 70 Gy delivered over 7 weeks.

Improvement continues in the mode of radiation delivery. Hyperfractionation or accelerated fractionation with boosts is more effective than traditional radiation therapy in unresectable head and neck cancers; this added benefit, however, does not approach the added benefit obtained with concomitant chemotherapy and radiation therapy.[52,53] Interstitial brachytherapy has also been employed effectively for carcinoma of the oral cavity.[32] Intensity-modulated radiation therapy may increase the amount of radiation delivered to the tumor itself while sparing the surrounding normal tissues, such as the major salivary glands and the mandible, leading to a

potential decrease in xerostomia and osteoradionecrosis, respectively.[54]

In addition to the side effects of mucositis and xerostomia, major complications of definitive radiotherapy to the oral cavity include osteoradionecrosis, pathologic mandibular fractures, and mucosal ulcerations. The risk of osteoradionecrosis necessitates comprehensive dental care prior to the initiation of radiotherapy. The adjuvant use of hyperbaric oxygen, either prophylactically or for treatment of mandibular osteoradionecrosis, although commonly practiced, remains controversial.[55,56]

Combined Therapy

A combination of surgery and chemoradiation is recommended for advanced cancers of the oral cavity in light of the high propensity for locoregional failure. Although neoadjuvant, ie, preoperative, radiotherapy has been used in the past, the current standard of care for combined modalities is surgery followed by adjuvant radiotherapy with or without chemotherapy.[57] Indications for adjuvant radiotherapy include multiple positive nodes, extracapsular lymph node extension, and positive margins of resection, as well as Stage III or IV primary disease (Table 3). Adjuvant radiation therapy has been shown to improve locoregional control in the presence of extracapsular spread or positive resection margins, but it should not be construed as a panacea for inadequate operations: it does not appear to decrease the risk of local recurrence in patients with positive margins to a level similar to comparable patients with negative margins not treated with radiotherapy.

The addition of chemotherapy improves overall and disease-free survival, especially when undertaken concomitant with radiation therapy.[58,59] It should be noted, however, that these concomitant chemoradiation regimens hold a significant increase in morbidity and up to a 5% mortality rate when compared with adjuvant radiotherapy alone.

The ideal timing of postoperative radiotherapy with or without chemotherapy is 6 weeks following surgery. For Stage III and IV squamous cell cancer of the head and neck, locoregional recurrence is 5.5% when adjuvant radiotherapy is initiated within 6 weeks of surgery, but 31.5% when adjuvant therapy is delayed for more than 6 weeks.[60] This increase in nodal recurrence is observed whether the nodal metastases were initially confined to a single nodal level or whether multiple levels were involved and is not abrogated by higher doses of radiation.

Table 3 Indications for Postoperative Radiation Therapy

Multiple positive regional nodes
Extracapsular lymph node extension
Positive margins on surgical resection
Stage III or IV primary disease

Chemotherapy

As with radiation, chemotherapy can be delivered either prior to (*neoadjuvant*), following (*adjuvant*), or simultaneous with (*concomitant*) definitive treatment. Neoadjuvant chemotherapy has not been shown to confer a survival advantage.[61] Adjuvant cisplatin and 5-fluorouracil (5-FU) following postoperative radiotherapy decreases the incidence of distant metastases but confers no difference in 4-year locoregional control, overall survival, or disease-free survival.[52] As discussed above, however, concomitant chemoradiation has been shown to be effective in improving overall survival and progression-free survival in patients with advanced head and neck squamous cell cancers. The price paid for this improved survival is an increase in mucositis and hematopoetic toxicity. Chemotherapy is also frequently employed in the palliation of advanced head and neck cancer not amenable to other primary methods of treatment.

Chemoprevention

Recent efforts to expand the armamentarium of treatments for cancer of the oral cavity have included the investigation of chemopreventive agents.[28,62,63] As the genetic events leading to carcinogenesis are further elucidated, attempts are being made to identify potential agents that can prevent DNA damage or enhance DNA repair. A prospective randomized trial demonstrated effective treatment of oral leukoplakia with a 6-month trial of isotretinoin (13-*cis*-retinoic acid), with significant reduction in lesion size and reversal of dysplasia. However, withdrawal of treatment led to relapse within 3 months in over half the population. A follow-up study on a 1-year course of isotretinoin after primary treatment for squamous cell cancer of the oral cavity, oropharynx, and larynx demonstrated no significant difference at 32 months in local, regional, or distant recurrences between the treated and untreated groups. Other studies of chemoprevention in oral cavity cancer have involved the use of beta-carotenes, alpha-tocopherol, and ascorbic acid. Similarly, no randomized, prospective trial has demonstrated any long-term benefit with the use of these agents. Initial animal studies in the topical application of cyclooxygenase-2 inhibitors appear promising, but no human trials have proven as optimistic. Because the response to chemopreventive agents may include genetic alterations not readily apparent phenotypically, a number of investigations continue.

Management of the Neck

An issue of ongoing controversy concerns the management of the neck in patients without clinical evidence of regional nodal metastases (the N_0 neck). As stated earlier, lymphatic metastases from primary tumors of the oral cavity occur in a predictable fashion through sequential spread. Although previous surgery or irradiation may result in aberrant lymphatic drainage, there are well-established first-echelon lymph nodes for each primary tumor site. In light of the propensity for various sites within the oral cavity to spread to regional lymphatics and the high risk of nodal recurrence, and in light of the fact that pathologic evidence of micrometastases has been observed on gross sections in up to one-third of elective neck dissection specimens, what constitutes the ideal approach to the N_0 neck?

Elective Neck Dissection. It has been previously reported that, despite the data quoted above, elective neck dissection offers no survival advantage compared with observation alone.[64] However, in patients at risk for neck metastasis, failure tends to be from advanced nodal disease, despite close follow-up; because elective neck dissection has been shown to improve locoregional control, it may therefore impact positively on the quality of patients' survival. Recognizing that some sites of the oral cavity have a decreased propensity for spread to regional lymphatics, specifically hard palate, alveolar ridge, and nonmidline aspects of the lip, the risk of regional failure with primaries of the oral cavity at most subsites is sufficiently high to warrant elective treatment of the neck.

Elective neck dissection is not without its complications. First described by Crile in 1906[65] and popularized by Martin and colleagues,[66] the radical neck dissection is associated with significant morbidity due to sacrifice of the spinal accessory nerve, the SCM muscle, and the internal jugular vein. Significant compromise of shoulder function results from the loss of the spinal accessory nerve, and cosmetic deformity from the removal of the SCM. Removal of the internal jugular vein risks significant edema of the face and occasional central nervous system deficits, particularly following bilateral neck dissection or when radiotherapy is employed.

In light of this morbidity, there has been a trend toward selective neck dissection, based on the aforementioned predictable pattern of lymph node metastases. A selective lymphadenectomy clearing nodal levels I, II, and III (so-called "supraomohyoid neck dissection," or SOHND) is traditionally recommended for N_0 patients with primary squamous cell cancers of the oral cavity. While some have also advocated the use of the SOHND in N_1 necks without evidence of extracapsular spread, concerns of skip metastases to inferior cervical nodes at levels III or IV in the absence of demonstrable involvement at levels I and II may limit these recommendations.[67] Clearing level IV during a SOHND adds little in terms of operative time and may reduce the approximately 5% incidence of isolated level IV metastases from tumors of the oral cavity. However, dissection of level IV places the patient at a slightly increased risk for postoperative chyle leakage. For primary tumors of the oral cavity, the risk of involvement of level V is minimal and is therefore not routinely included in the selective lymphadenectomy of N_0 necks for oral cavity primaries.

Elective Neck Irradiation. The theoretical advantages of treating the N_0 neck with surgical lymphadenectomy include the ability to obtain pathologic staging information, the preparation of donor and recipient vasculature for microvascular reconstruction when indicated, and the avoidance of morbidity associated with radiotherapy. However, no significant differences in regional recurrence have been demonstrated following treatment of the N_0 neck with either elective neck irradiation or elective neck dissection.[64] The modality chosen to address the clinically negative neck, therefore, may largely be influenced by the philosophy of the treating physician. As a general rule, however, the treatment modality chosen for the primary carcinoma of the oral cavity is employed concurrently to address the risk of occult regional metastases.

Therapeutic Neck Dissection. For the clinically positive neck, the traditional surgical procedure of choice has been the comprehensive neck dissection, with preservation of the spinal accessory nerve, and, increasingly, the internal jugular vein and SCM, in cases without gross involvement of these anatomic structures by tumor. The continuing evolution of a more selective approach to the neck, however, has included the clinically positive neck as well. Comprehensive neck dissections with preservation of all three major structures discussed above may be performed for the N_1, N_{2a}, and N_{2b} neck when technically feasible. A more selective neck dissection may be acceptable for N_1 disease without extracapsular extension, particularly when the single involved node is in level I. In patients in whom the primary tumor has been treated with radiotherapy, the neck is often included in the radiation portals as well; in these N-positive patients, a postradiation neck dissection is often planned as a staged procedure. There is some evidence, however, that the neck may be followed with serial CT, thereby obviating unnecessary neck dissections in patients with a complete response to therapy.[63] The role of PET scans in the follow-up of these patients is under investigation.

SPECIFIC SITES IN THE ORAL CAVITY

Lip

Squamous cell carcinoma of the lip, by virtue of its location, tends to present at a relatively early stage. The lower lip is affected more commonly, presumably secondary to sunlight exposure. Origins at the oral commissure occur in fewer than 1% of cases.

Comparable cure rates have been reported for small carcinomas of the lip using either surgery or radiation therapy, but the former is the treatment of choice in most instances owing to its lower morbidity and better cosmetic results. Advantages of surgery over irradiation include the ability to assess tumor margins and rapid rehabilitation. Lesions of up to one-third of the lip length may be resected with primary closure, and a number of options exist for flap reconstructions of larger defects. Specifically, a lip-switching procedure, that is, the Abbé–Estlander flap, may be employed for defects between one-third and one-half the length of the lip. This involves mobilizing a portion of uninvolved opposite lip, rotating it to fill the defect in the involved lip while keeping it attached to its blood supply. In a staged fashion, the attachment to the uninvolved lip is divided. The Karapandzic flap, a bilateral rotation/advancement flap may be used for even larger defects involving greater than half the lip length.

Metastases from carcinoma of the lip are uncommon (7 to 16%) except in advanced lesions, recurrent lesions, or lesions arising at the oral commissure. When lymphatic spread arises from midline lip lesions, bilateral lymph node metastases are common. Depth of invasion is an important prognostic factor for regional lymph node metastases, particularly for lesions greater than 2 mm in thickness.[69] Other prognostic factors include size of tumor, histologic grade, and subsite.

Overall survival rates are approximately 90% when surgery is used for stages I and II, and surgery plus adjuvant chemoradiation is used for stages III and IV. Survival estimations in most studies, however, may be skewed by the exceedingly high proportion of patients who present with stage I disease. Surgical salvage for local recurrence is successful in over 70% of cases. Survival rates for each subsite in the oral cavity are summarized in Table 4. Despite the relatively low incidence of nodal metastasis in tumors at this site, mortality in patients with regional lymphadenopathy is significantly higher than patients with N_0 necks, leading some authors to advocate elective lymphadenectomy in all patients with squamous cell carcinoma of the lip.[70]

Buccal Mucosa

Cancers of the buccal mucosa are characteristically locally aggressive, spreading to the adjacent gingiva and involving the retromolar trigone or pterygoid region in up to one-third of cases. The intraoperative photograph in Figure 13 depicts an advanced squamous cell cancer of the right buccal mucosa extending to the skin. Surgical resection is recommended for stage I and II tumors, with combination therapy employing both surgery and chemoradiotherapy for stages III and IV. Using this treatment modality, 5-year survival rates have been reported at 77% for stage I, 65% for stage II, 27% for stage III, and 18% for stage IV. Unfortunately, treatment of tumors of the buccal mucosal is difficult given the significant functional deficit their surgical

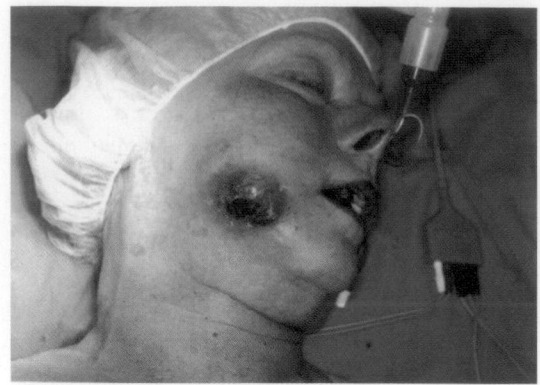

Figure 13 Advanced-stage squamous cell carcinoma of the right buccal mucosa penetrating through the skin.

excision often engenders. Myriad reconstructive methods have been attempted, including skin grafting, microvascular free tissue transfer, local flap advancement, and even healing by secondary intention; each has its attendant morbidities.

Alveolar Ridges

Carcinomas of the alveolar ridge typically present with soreness or pain in the gum, ulceration with intraoral bleeding, loosening of teeth, or ill-fitting dentures.[71] Patients tend to present with symptoms within 3 months of onset. Cancer of the upper alveolar ridge may extend superiorly to involve the floor of the nasal cavity or maxillary sinus. Carcinoma of the alveolar ridge, however, more commonly arises from the lower alveolus, and these cancers may spread along the course of the inferior alveolar nerve toward the skull base.

Based on 2-year survival rates, marginal mandibulectomy has been demonstrated to be an oncologically sound procedure for stage I and II disease of the lower alveolus. Marginal mandibulectomy is contraindicated, however, if the mandible is enveloped by tumor, if there is tumor invasion through the cortical plate, or if there has been recent tooth extraction in proximity to the tumor. The use of adjuvant radiotherapy or chemoradiotherapy is advocated, as with other cancers of the oral cavity, for instances of inadequate surgical margin, perineural invasion, extensive nodal metastases, or extracapsular extension within nodal metastases. It should be noted, however, that regional metastases to cervical lymphatics are uncommon from carcinoma of the alveolar ridge.

Carcinoma of the upper alveolar ridge is treated in a similar manner to that of the lower

ridge, with single-modality therapy recommended for stage I and II disease. There is no equivalent of the marginal mandibulectomy in the maxilla however, and en bloc resection is recommended for all tumors, including resection of involved teeth and hard palate when necessary. Using surgery as primary modality with the addition of postoperative radiotherapy or chemoradiotherapy for advanced lesions, the following 5- year survival rates have been demonstrated: 77% for stage I, 70% for stage II, 42% for stage III, and 24% for stage IV.

Retromolar Trigone

Cancers of the retromolar trigone, like those of the lower gingiva, are often associated with chewing tobacco.[72] Branches of the glossopharyngeal nerve provide sensory innervation to the retromolar trigone, so patients with carcinoma of this region may present with pain referred to the ipsilateral ear. Numbness in the distribution of the inferior alveolar nerve is an ominous sign for invasion of the mandible and perineural extension. Trismus may result from invasion of the pterygoid musculature. Direct extension into the pterygopalatine fossa may also lead to disease at the skull base. The proximity of the structures of the oropharynx to the retromolar trigone also places them at risk for involvement by direct extension. The tight adherence of mucosa to underlying structures often necessitates resection of the ascending portion of the mandible. Using a protocol of surgery with or without chemoradiation therapy, 5-year disease-free survival rates are 83% for stages I to III combined and 61% for stage IV. There has been some discussion of radiation therapy alone for cancers of the retromolar trigone given the difficulty in surgical access to this portion of the oral cavity, but removing surgery from the treatment protocol drastically reduces the survival.[72]

Hard Palate

Although relatively rare in the United States, carcinoma of the hard palate is more prevalent in areas in which the practice of reverse smoking is more common.[73,74] The heat generated from holding the lit end of the cigarette near the hard palate has been demonstrated to result in malignant transformation. Presenting symptoms of cancer of the hard palate include pain, bleeding, altered speech, or improperly fitting dentures. Biopsy may be necessary to distinguish carcinoma of the hard palate from other mimicking entities such as necrotizing sialometaplasia. There is, unfortunately, often a confounding delay in presentation of patients with cancer of the hard palate: at presentation, over half have had symptoms for at least 12 weeks, and over one-third wait at least 6 months before seeking treatment.

For early-stage lesions, no difference has been demonstrated between radiation or surgery as single-modality treatments, so selection of therapy should be based on the anatomic location

Table 4 Five-Year Survival Rates by Oral Cavity Subsite*				
Site	Stage I	Stage II	Stage III	Stage IV
Alveolar ridge	77%	70%	42%	24%
Buccal mucosa	77%	65%	27%	18%
Floor of mouth	95%	86%	82%	52%
Hard palate	92%	43%	37%	17%
Lip		90%		
Oral tongue	90%	72%	54%	34%
Retromolar trigone		83%		61%

*After appropriate treatment as described in the text.

and extent of the disease, the presence of second primaries, and associated patient comorbidities.[73] Surgery followed by adjuvant radiotherapy is recommended for advanced-stage disease, which may extend into the nasal cavity through the incisive foramen or may approach the skull base via the greater palatine foramina. Because of the paucity of cases, 5-year survival rates have been reported in a limited fashion. Overall survival with optimal treatment is 92% for stage I, 43% for stage II, 37% for stage III, and 17% for stage IV tumors.

Regional lymphatic drainage from the hard palate is sparse; metastases to cervical lymph nodes are relatively uncommon.

Floor of the Mouth

By virtue of their location, cancers of the floor of the mouth often remain undetected until they progress to advanced disease.[50] Bulky tumors affect normal speech and deglutition, and patients may also complain of pain referred to the ipsilateral ear from tumor involvement of the lingual nerve. Advanced tumors may also invade the tongue or mandible by direct extension. As a result, an aggressive surgical paradigm for the management of these neoplasms is warranted. Regardless of stage, local recurrence is 13% in patients who undergo complete resection with histologically negative margins.

Second primary neoplasms are particularly common in cancers of the floor of the mouth. In addition, elective treatment of the neck is warranted owing to the significant incidence of occult nodal metastases, even with T_1 lesions. Patients with high-stage primary cancers are at increased risk for advanced nodal metastases: approximately one-third of patients with T_4 tumors present with N_3 disease. The risk of contralateral nodal metastases is significant with these primaries, and multiple levels are often involved.

Primary therapy includes surgery with the addition of postoperative chemoradiation for stage III and IV disease and allows for survival rates of 95% for stage I, 86% for stage II, 82% for stage III, and 52% for stage IV. Of note, postoperative radiation therapy does not seem to affect overall survival significantly; it does, however, decrease the rate of regional but, interestingly, not local recurrence. Figure 14 illustrates the surgical management of a patient with biopsy-proven squamous cell cancer of the floor of the mouth invading the ventral surface of the oral tongue. The patient underwent resection of the lesion at the floor of the mouth, extending to the ventral surface of the tongue, with concomitant marginal mandibulectomy, tracheostomy, and bilateral SOHND. Repair of the surgical defect was accomplished with the use of a radial forearm free tissue transfer.

Oral Tongue

The most common presenting symptoms and signs for carcinoma of the oral tongue include localized pain with the presence of an ulcer, frequently on

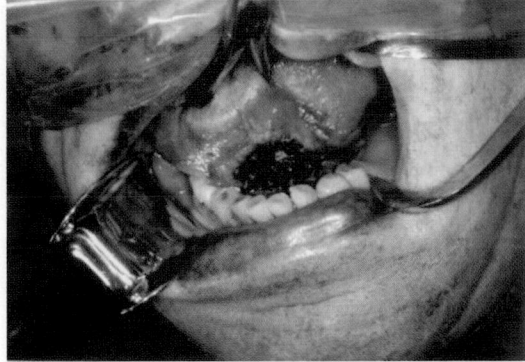

(A)

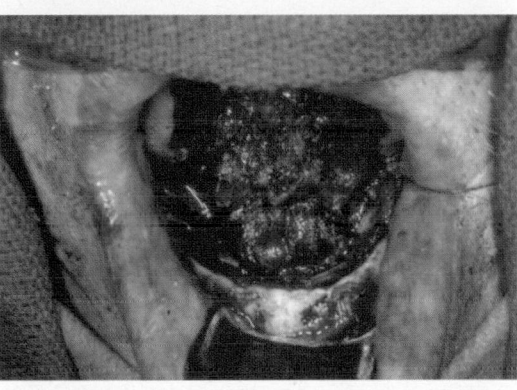

(B)

(C)

Figure 14 (A) Floor of the mouth carcinoma presenting as an ulcerated lesion extending onto the ventral surface of the oral tongue. (B) Surgical specimen demonstrating en bloc resection of the lesion at the floor of the mouth and ventral surface of the oral tongue, in continuity with marginal mandibulectomy. (C) Surgical defect following tumor resection. Reconstruction was accomplished using a radial forearm free flap reconstruction.

the middle one-third of the tongue, dysarthria or glossodynia with eating.[32,75,76] As with cancers of the floor of the mouth, primary neoplasms on the oral tongue may present with referred pain in the ipsilateral ear, owing to involvement of the lingual nerve. Second primary neoplasms are also common in cancers of the tongue, occurring in approximately one-quarter of patients.

There are no reported differences in the rate of locoregional control or survival between surgery and irradiation for T_1 and T_2 lesions. Surgical resection is typically employed for these early-staged tumors, whereas combined modalities are indicated for higher-staged tumors. Occult metastases in regional lymphatics are common in carcinoma of the oral tongue, particularly when the

depth of the primary tumor is greater than 4 mm. Other risk factors for occult metastasis include the presence of perineural or perivascular invasion, infiltrating-type margins, poorly differentiated primary tumors, and T_2 stage. The rates of locoregional control and survival are improved with elective neck dissection, even for T_1 and T_2 tumors. Selective neck dissection is adequate treatment for the N_0 neck: no differences in survival or locoregional control have been demonstrated in patients undergoing comprehensive or selective neck dissections.

Improvements in the observed rates of overall 5-year survival have been attributed to a more aggressive approach to the neck in patients with early-stage tumors and the addition of postoperative radiotherapy or chemoradiotherapy in patients with advanced-stage disease. Reported 5-year survival rates with these modalities are 90% for stage I, 72% for stage II, 54% for stage III, and 34% for stage IV. Overall, significant improvement in 5-year disease-free survival is seen with the following parameters: clear margins, clinical T_1 or T_2 disease, clinical stages I or II disease, lack of nodal metastases (or T_1N_1 patients), and postoperative radiotherapy for patients with close or positive margins. The increasing use of mandible-sparing procedures and selective, rather than comprehensive, neck dissection may result in improved quality of life in the survivors, as well.

RECONSTRUCTION OF THE ORAL CAVITY

Following the resection of cancers of the oral cavity, reconstruction of the defect must be individualized based on the extent of the defect and the availability of reconstructive techniques. Selected small, intraoral defects may be closed primarily or covered with a local flap, a split-thickness skin graft, or acellular dermis. They may also be allowed to heal by secondary intention. Larger defects require more complex flap reconstruction. A number of factors affect the type of reconstruction used. These include tumor extent and location, patient comorbidities, surgeon experience and/or preference, and the anticipated postoperative dysfunction in respiration, deglutition, or speech.

A variety of reconstructive techniques is available for defects in the oral cavity. Two key reconstructive techniques deserve mention: pedicled flaps and microvascular free tissue transfer.

The pectoralis major myocutaneous flap provides well-vascularized soft tissue for the reconstruction of the oral cavity. It is a pedicled flap, receiving its blood supply from the pectoral branch of the thoracoacromial artery and can be used, with or without an attached skin paddle, for the reconstruction of both intraoral and external defects. Its reliable vascularity, proximity to the head and neck, and availability for harvest while the patient is in the supine position has led to its wide acceptance for reconstruction of head and neck defects. The flap, however, has several disadvantages in intraoral reconstruction: its skin-paddle contains nonglabrous tissue; its soft tissue bulk may be inappropriate for smaller defects; and it has a limited arc of rotation.

Microvascular free tissue transfer has revolutionized head and neck reconstruction, providing flaps and their nutrient vessels from such disparate sites as the fibula, the scapula, the iliac crest, the rectus muscle, and the radial forearm to repair complex defects with uniformly perfused tissue. The fibula, radial forearm, and anterolateral thigh flaps are most frequently used in the reconstruction of intraoral defects, the latter two for predominantly soft-tissue reconstruction and the former for reconstructions requiring bone.

The fibula free flap is an osteomyocutaneous flap based on the peroneal artery and its two attendant peroneal veins. It has the benefit of being able to provide significant bone stock for mandibular defects, even allowing for postoperative dental implantation. Its drawback is its relatively short pedicle and occasionally unreliable skin paddle, the survival of which is often more operator-dependent than that of other flaps. Because the blood supply to the fibula is both endosteal and periosteal, osteotomies are possible, allowing the reconstructive surgeon the ability to contour the bone to the ablative defect.

The radial forearm free flap is an extremely reliable fasciocutaneous flap based on the radial artery and its attendant venae comitantes. It has also been described as an osteomyocutaneous flap, with the inclusion of the radius and/or the palmaris longus (absent in 10 to 15% of patients). The advantages of the radial forearm flap include the fact that the skin in the region is thin, pliable, and relatively hairless. In addition, the flap is relatively easy to harvest and the pedicle is long; this allows for versatility in the use of this reconstructive method. Disadvantages are minor and are usually limited to donor-site morbidity, for example, scarring and often some degree of carpal weakness.

The anterolateral thigh free flap is a fasciocutaneous flap based on the descending branch of the lateral femoral circumflex artery and its vein. Unlike many flaps used in head and neck reconstruction, this can be made sensate with the inclusion of the lateral femoral cutaneous nerve. It has a long pedicle length and provides more bulk than the radial forearm flap, allowing for improved reconstruction of larger defects. Its drawback, however, is that the vascular anatomy to the anterior thigh is more often variable, making this flap more difficult to use.

Mandibular defects may be successfully reconstructed with composite bone flaps, including the free fibula and the iliac crest osteomyocutaneous flaps. Such vascularized composite flaps provide reliable bone stock for optimal aesthetic contour and masticatory function. Figure 15 illustrates the surgical management of a patient with biopsy-proven squamous cell cancer of the floor of the mouth, involving the anterior part of the mandible and the anterior part of the tongue. The patient underwent resection of the floor of

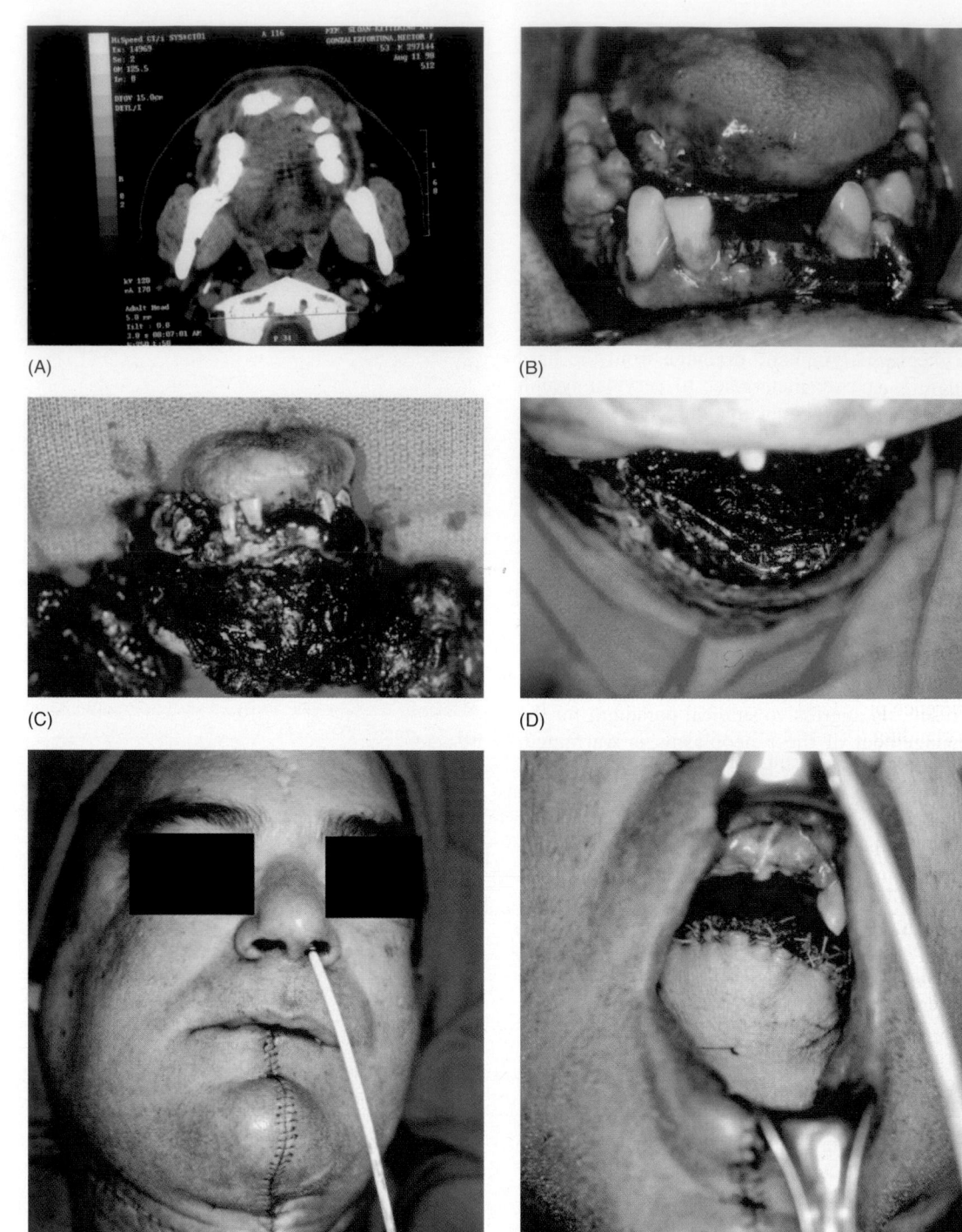

(A) (B) (C) (D) (E) (F)

Figure 15 (A) Axial computed tomographic scan of the neck demonstrating extensive squamous cell carcinoma of the floor of the mouth. (B) Tumor extended through the dental alveoli of the anterior parts of the mandibles, as well as into the anterior portion of the oral tongue. (C) Surgical specimen demonstrating en bloc segmental mandibular resection. (D) Reconstruction of the anterior parts of the mandibles using contoured fibular free flap. (E) Closure of the midline lip split incision. (F) Soft tissue reconstruction of the oral cavity using radial forearm free flap.

the mouth, subtotal glossectomy, segmental mandibulectomy, tracheostomy, and bilateral selective neck dissections incorporating nodal levels I through IV. Mandibular reconstruction was accomplished with the use of two flaps: a fibula for bone stock and a radial forearm for the provision of soft tissue coverage.

Reconstruction of the maxilla presents a unique situation. Maxillary defects may be reconstructed with vascularized osteomyocutaneous flaps (fibula, iliac crest, and scapula have all been used), which allow for improved orodental rehabilitation

and an overall increase in the quality of life.[77] However, surgeon experience and patient comorbidities may interfere with optimal results for this technique. As a result, reconstruction is often accomplished simply with prosthodontia, without significant decrease in patient benefit.

SALVAGE SURGERY

There is a dictum in the treatment of cancers of the head and neck: the first intervention is the best opportunity for cure. That is, recurrent squamous cell cancer is significantly more difficult to treat than a primary tumor, with the rate of success of salvage therapy hovering around one-third, even in patients with low-stage initial tumors.[78–85] Overall, anywhere from one-quarter to one-half of patients with squamous cell cancer of the oral cavity suffer a recurrence; local recurrences predominate (58%), followed by locoregional (27%), and distant recurrences (16%), with some patients suffering recurrence at more than one site.

Strategies for the treatment of recurrent oral cavity squamous cell cancer vary. All modalities are employed, including salvage surgery, chemotherapy, radiation therapy (with or without brachytherapy), and combinations of the above. Often, treatment is dictated by the size and site of the recurrence as well as the type of therapy previously employed.

The success of salvage therapy depends on a number of tumor, patient, and treatment factors. Patients with more advanced primary tumors tend to do worse, as do patients recurring fewer than 6 months after their initial definitive treatment. The site of recurrence also appears to affect postrecurrence prognosis, with locoregional recurrence portending the worst prognosis, followed by local recurrence, and then by nodal recurrence alone; there is some evidence, however, that recurrence in the neck portends a worse prognosis overall. Younger patients appear to have a better survival.

Finally, the type of salvage therapy undertaken appears to be significant in overall survival, with patients undergoing salvage surgery enjoying significantly longer survival time than those undergoing other treatment modalities. Despite this finding, the overall cure rate with salvage surgery has not been found to be significantly higher than that seen with other treatment modalities. The numbers in most studies are small, care must be taken in interpreting these statistical trends.

Other poor prognostic indicators include the use of a neck dissection and the employment of radiotherapy in the primary treatment, although these variables may only be markers for biologically more aggressive disease, rather than being true, independent variables. Although counterintuitive, overall survival and success of salvage do *not* depend on the size of the recurrence; stage of recurrence is important only insofar as it renders a patient not a candidate for salvage surgery and not as an independent variable.

Unfortunately, only about one-third of patients who recur are candidates for salvage surgery. Surgical salvage should be limited to the resection of visible, gross tumor. Re-resection of the primary site in the absence of evidence of local recurrence leads to an increase in the morbidity of the salvage therapy without an increase in its benefits.

Median survival after recurrence of squamous cell carcinoma of the oral cavity is 9 months, emphasizing the need for disease control with primary therapy.

CONCLUSIONS

Carcinomas of the oral cavity are disparate in presentation and in therapy. As with most carcinomas in the head and neck, tobacco and alcohol abuse are significant risk factors contributing to genetic changes in both normal and malignant tissue that are just beginning to be elucidated. These genetic changes provide an overall "cancerization" to the entire mucosa, predisposing patients to second primary neoplasms. Treatment generally involves single-modality therapy (either radiation or surgery) for early-stage carcinomas and combined therapy (generally surgery followed by concomitant chemoradiation therapy) for larger neoplasms. Neck metastases are common but vary with site and stage of the primary tumor; their presence portends a significant decrease in survival. Rehabilitation may be managed with prosthetic devices or reconstruction of surgical defects, pedicled rotation flaps, or free tissue transfer.

REFERENCES

1. Alvi A, Myers EN, Johnson JT. Cancer of the oral cavity. In: Myers EN, Suen JY, editors. Cancer of the Head and Neck, 3rd edition. Philadelphia: WB Saunders; 1996. p. 321
2. Robbins KT, Clayman G, Levine PA, et al. Neck dissection classification update. Arch Otolaryngol Head Neck Surg 2002;128:751–8.
3. Alvi A, Myers EN, Johnson JT. Cancer of the oral cavity. In: Myers EN, Suen JY, editors. Cancer of the Head and Neck, 3rd edition. Philadelphia: WB Saunders; 1996. p.322.
4. Shah JP. Patterns of cervical lymph node metastasis from squamous carcinomas of the upper aerodigestive tract. Am J Surg 1990;160:405–9.
5. American Cancer Society. Cancer Facts and Figures 2006. Available at http://www.cancer.org/downloads/STT/CAFF-2006PWSecured.pdf. Accessed January 1 2007.
6. Sudbø J. Novel management of oral cancer: A paradigm of predictive oncology. Clin Med Res 2004;2:233–42.
7. Altieri A, Bosetti C, Gallus S, et al. Wine, beer and spirits and risk of oral and pharyngeal cancer: A case-control study from Italy and Switzerland. Oral Oncol 2004;40:904–9.
8. Larson DL. Management of the mandible. In: Close LG, Larson DL, Shah JP, editors. Essentials of Head and Neck Oncology. New York: Thieme Medical Publishers; 1998.
9. Blot WJ, McLaughlin JK, Winn DM, et al. Smoking and drinking in relation to oral and pharyngeal cancer. Cancer Res 1988;48:3282–7.
10. Johnson N. Tobacco use and oral cancer: A global perspective. J Dent Educ 2001;65:328–39.
11. Fernandez Garrote L, Herrero R, Ortiz Reyes R, et al. Risk factors for cancer of the oral cavity and oro-pharynx in Cuba. Br J Cancer 2001;85:46–54.
12. Henley SJ, Thun MJ, Chao A, Calle EE. Association between exclusive pipe smoking and mortality from cancer and other diseases. J Natl Cancer Inst 2004;96:853–61.
13. Carretero-Pelaez MA, Esparza-Gomez GC, Figuero-Ruiz E, Cerero-Lapiedra R. Alcohol-containing mouthwashes and oral cancer. Critical analysis of the literature. Med Oral 2004;9:116–23.
14. Ogden GR. Alcohol and oral cancer. Alcohol 2005;35:169–73.
15. Rosenquist K. Risk factors in oral and oropharyngeal squamous cell carcinoma: A population-based case-control study in southern Sweden. Swed Dent J Suppl 2005;179:1–66.
16. Scully C. Oral cancer, the evidence for sexual transmission. Br Dent J 2005;199:203–7.
17. Singh B, Balwally AN, Shaha A, et al. Upper aerodigestive tract squamous cell carcinoma. The human immunodeficiency virus connection. Arch Otolaryngol Head Neck Surg 1996;122:639–43.
18. Chuang C-H, Hu M-L. Synergistic DNA damage and lipid peroxidation in cultured human white blood cells exposed to 4-(methyl-nitrosamino)-1-(3-pyridyl)-1-butanone and ultraviolet A. Environ Mol Mutagen 2006;47:73–81.
19. Slaughter DP, Southwick HW, Smejkal W. "Field cancerization" in oral stratified squamous epithelium: Clinical implications of multicentric origin. Cancer (Phila) 1953;6:963–8.
20. Day GL, Blot WJ, Shore RE, et al. Second cancers following oral and pharyngeal cancers: Role of tobacco and alcohol. J Natl Cancer Inst 1994;86:131–7.
21. Ha PK, Benoit NE, Yochem R, et al. A transcriptional progression model for head and neck cancer. Clin Cancer Res 2003;9:3058–64.
22. Califano J, Westra W, Meininger G, et al. Genetic progression and clonal relationship of recurrent premalignant head and neck lesions. Clin Cancer Res 2000;6:347–52.
23. Rosas SL, Koch W, da Costa Carvalho MdG, et al. Promoter hypermethylation patterns of p16, O6-methylguanine-DNA-methyltransferase, and death-associated protein kinase in tumors and saliva of head and neck cancer patients. Cancer Res 2001;61:939–42.
24. Huang M-F, Chang Y-C, Liao P-S, et al. Loss of heterozygosity of p53 gene of oral cancer detected by exfoliative cytology. Oral Oncol 1999;35:296–301.
25. Brennan JA, Boyle JO, Koch W, et al. Association between cigarette smoking and mutation of the p53 gene in squamous cell carcinoma of the head and neck. N Engl J Med 1995;332:712–7.
26. Brennan JA, Mao L, Hruban RH, et al. Molecular assessment of histopathological staging in squamous cell carcinoma of the head and neck. N Engl J Med 1995;332:429–35.
27. Neville BW, Day TA. Oral cancer and precancerous lesions. CA Cancer J Clin 2005;52:195–215.
28. Lodi G, Sardella A, Bez C, et al. Interventions for treating oral leukoplakia. Cochrane Database Systematic Rev 2004;3: Art No: CD001829.pub001822.
29. Reichart PA, Philipsen HP. Oral erythroplakia—a review. Oral Oncol 2005;41:551–61.
30. Steffen C. The man behind the eponym: Lauren V. Ackerman and verrucous carcinoma of Ackerman. Am J Dermatopathol 2004;26:334–41.
31. Spiro RH. Verrucous carcinoma, then and now. Am J Surg 1998;176:393–7.
32. Sessions DG, Spector GJ, Lenox J, et al. Analysis of treatment results for oral tongue cancer. Laryngoscope 2002;112:616–25.
33. Ferlito A, Rinaldo A, Devaney K, et al. Prognostic significance of microscopic and macroscopic extracapsular spread from metastatic tumor in the cervical lymph nodes. Oral Oncol 2002;38:747–51.
34. Ferlito A, Buckley JG, Rinaldo A, Mondin V. Screening tests to evaluate distant metastases in head and neck cancer. ORL J Otorhinolaryngol Relat Spec 2001;63:208–11.
35. Juweid ME, Cheson BD. Positron-emission tomography and assessment of cancer therapy. N Engl J Med 2006;354:496–507.
36. Shiboski CH, Schmidt BL, Jordan RCK. Tongue and tonsil carcinoma: Increasing trends in the US population ages 20-44 years. Cancer 2005;103:1843–9.
37. Friedlander PL, Schantz SP, Shaha A, et al. Squamous cell carcinoma of the tongue in young patients: A matched-pair analysis. Head Neck 1998;20:363–8.
38. Pitman KT, Johnson JT, Wagner RL, Myers EN. Cancer of the tongue in patients less than forty. Head Neck 2000;22:297–302.
39. Lengyel E, Gilde K, Remenar E, Esik O. Malignant mucosal melanoma of the head and neck—a review. Pathol Oncol Res 2003;9:7–12.
40. Mendenhall WM, Amdur RJ, Hinerman RW, et al. Head and neck mucosal melanoma. Am J Clin Oncol 2005;28:626–30.
41. Freire ARS, Lima ENP, Almeida OP, Kowalski LP. Computed tomography and lymphoscintigraphy to identify lymph node metastases and lymphatic drainage pathways in oral and orpharyngeal squamous cell carcinomas. Eur Arch Otorhinolaryngol 2003;260:148–52.
42. Wax MK, Myers LL, Gona JM, et al. The role of positron emission tomography in the evaluation of the N-positive neck. Otolaryngol Head Neck Surg 2003;129:163–7.
43. Brown JS, Lowe D, Kalavrezos N, et al. Patterns of invasion and routes of tumor entry into the mandible by oral squamous cell carcinoma. Head Neck 2002;24:370–83.
44. Genden EM, Rinaldo A, Jacobson A, et al. Management of mandibular invasion: When is a marginal mandibulectomy appropriate? Oral Oncol 2005;41:776–82.
45. Davidson J, Gilbert R, Irish J, et al. The role of panendoscopy in the management of mucosal head and neck malignancy—a prospective evaluation. Head Neck 2000;22:449–55.
46. Taylor RJ, Wahl RL, Sharma PK, et al. Sentinel node localization in oral cavity and oropharynx squamous cell cancer. Arch Otolaryngol Head Neck Surg 2001;127:970–4.
47. Akmansu H, Oguz H, Atasever T, et al. Evaluation of sentinel node in the assessment of cervical metastases from head and neck squamous cell carcinomas. Tumori 2004;90:596–9.
48. Larson DL. Management of the mandible. In: Close LG, Larson DL, Shah JP, editors. Essentials of Head and Neck Oncology. New York: Thieme Medical Publishers; 1998. p. 196.

49. Alvi A, Myers EN, Johnson JT. Cancer of the oral cavity. In: Myers EN, Suen JY, editors. Cancer of the Head and Neck, 3rd edition. Philadelphia: WB Saunders; 1996.

50. Hicks WL, Loree TR, Garcia RI, et al. Squamous cell carcinoma of the floor of the mouth: A 20-year review. Head Neck 1997;19:400–5.

51. Spiro RH, Guillamondegui O, Paulino AF, Huvos AG. Pattern of invasion and margin assessment in patients with oral tongue cancer. Head Neck 1999;21:408–13.

52. Budach W, Hehr T, Budach V, et al. A meta-analysis of hyperfractionated and accelerated radiotherapy and combined chemotherapy and radiotherapy regimens in unresected locally advanced squamous cell carcinoma of the head and neck. BMC Cancer 2006;6:28–39.

53. Fu KK, Pajak TF, Trotti A, et al. A radiation therapy oncology group (RTOG) phase III randomized study to compare hyperfractionation and two variants of accelerated fractionation to standard fractionation radiotherapy for head and neck squamous cell carcinomas: First report of RTOG 9003. Int J Radiat Oncol Biol Phys 2000;48:7–16.

54. Eisbruch A. Intensity-modulated radiation therapy in the treatment of head and neck cancer. Nat Clin Pract Oncol 2005;2:34–39.

55. Annane D, Depondt J, Aubert P, et al. Hyperbaric oxygen therapy for radionecrosis of the jaw: A randomized, placebo-controlled, double-blind trial from the ORN96 study group. J Clin Oncol 2004;22:4893–900.

56. Teng MS, Futran ND. Osteoradionecrosis of the mandible. Curr Opin Otolaryngol Head Neck Surg 2005;13:217–21.

57. Palme CE, Gullane P, Gilbert R. Current treatment options in squamous cell carcinoma of the oral cavity. Surg Oncol Clin N Am 2004;13:47–70.

58. Bernier J, Domenge C, Ozsahin M, et al. Postoperative irradiation with or without concomitant chemotherapy for locally advanced head and neck cancer. N Engl J Med 2004;350:1945–52.

59. Cooper JS, Pajak TF, Forastiere AA, et al. Postoperative concurrent radiotherapy and chemotherapy for high-risk squamous cell carcinoma of the head and neck. N Engl J Med 2004;350:1937–44.

60. Vikram B, Strong EW, Shah JP, Spiro RH. Elective postoperative radiation therapy in stages III and IV epidermoid carcinoma of the head and neck. Am J Surg 1980;140:580–4.

61. Umeda M, Komatsubara H, Ojima Y, et al. Lack of survival advantage in patients with advanced, resectable squamous cell carcinoma of the oral cavity receiving induction chemotherapy with cisplatin (CDDP), docetaxel (TXT) and 5-fluorouracil (5FU). Kobe J Med Sci 2004;50:189–96.

62. Mulshine JL, Atkinson JC, Greer RO, et al. Randomized, double-blind-placebo-controlled phase IIB trial of the cyclo-oxygenase inhibitor ketorolac as an oral rinse in oropharyngeal leukoplakia. Clin Cancer Res 2004;10:1565–73.

63. Sood S, Shiff SJ, Yang CS, Chen X. Selection of topically applied non-steroidal anti-inflammatory drugs for oral cancer chemoprevention. Oral Oncol 2005;41:562–7.

64. Layland MK, Sessions DG, Lenox J. The influence of lymph node metastasis in the treatment of squamous cell carcinoma of the oral cavity, oropharynx, larynx, and hypopharynx: N_0 versus N+. Laryngoscope 2005;115:629–39.

65. Crile GW. Excision of cancer of the head and neck with special reference to the plan of dissection based on one hundred and thirty-two operations. JAMA 1906;47:1780–6.

66. Martin H, DelValle B, Ehrlich H, Cahan WG. Neck dissection. Cancer 1951;4:441–9.

67. Byers RM, Weber R, Andrews T, et al. Frequency and therapeutic implications of "skip metastases" in the neck from squamous carcinoma of the oral tongue. Head Neck 1997;19:14–9.

68. Liauw SL, Mancuso AA, Amdur RJ, et al. Postradiotherapy neck dissection for lymph node-positive head and neck cancer: The use of computed tomography to manage the neck. J Clin Oncol 2006;24:1421–7.

69. Stein A, Tahan S. Histologic correlates of metastasis in primary invasive squamous cell carcinoma of the lip. J Cutan Pathol 1994;21:16–21.

70. Zitsch RP, Lee BW, Smith RB. Cervical lymph node metastases and squamous cell carcinoma of the lip. Head Neck 1999;21:447–53.

71. Overholt SM, Eicher SA, Wolf P, Weber R. Prognostic factors affecting outcome in lower gingival carcinoma. Laryngoscope 1996;106:1335–9.

72. Mendenhall WM, Morris CG, Amdur RJ, et al. Retromolar trigone squamous cell carcinoma treated with radiotherapy alone or combined with surgery. Cancer 2005;103:2320–5.

73. Evans JF, Shah JP. Epidermoid carcinoma of the palate. Am J Surg 1981;142:451–5.

74. Yorozu A, Sykes AJ, Slevin NJ. Carcinoma of the hard palate treated with radiotherapy: A retrospective review of 31 cases. Oral Oncol 2001;37:493–7.

75. Byers RM, El-Naggar AK, Lee Y-Y, et al. Can we detect or predict the presence of occult nodal metastases in patients with squamous cell carcinoma of the oral tongue? Head Neck 1998;20:138–44.

76. Sparano A, Weinstein G, Chalian A, et al. Multivariate predictors of occult neck metastasis in early oral tongue cancer. Otolaryngol Head Neck Surg 2004;131:472–6.

77. Genden EM, Okay D, Stepp MT, et al. Comparison of functional and quality-of-life outcomes in patients with and without palatomaxillary reconstruction. Arch Otolaryngol Head Neck Surg 2003;129:775–80.

78. Keski-Sandtti H, Atula T, Tornwall J, et al. Elective neck treatment verus observation in patients with T_1/T_2 N_0 squamous cell carcinoma of oral tongue. Oral Oncol 2006;42:96–101.

79. Urashima Y, Nakamura K, Kunitake N, et al. Is glossectomy necessary for late nodal metastases without clinical local recurrence after initial brachytherapy for N_0 tongue cancer? A retrospective experience in 111 patients who received salvage therapy for cervical failure. Jpn J Clin Oncol 2006;36:3–6.

80. Lin YC, Hsiao JR, Tsai ST. Salvage surgery as the primary treatment for recurrent oral squamous cell carcinoma. Oral Oncol 2004;40:183–9.

81. Kowalski LP. Results of salvage treatment of the neck in patients with oral cancer. Arch Otolaryngol Head Neck Surg 2002;128:58–62.

82. Schwartz GJ, Mehta RH, Wenig BL, et al. Salvage treatment for recurrent squamous cell carcinoma of the oral cavity. Head Neck 2000;22:34–41.

83. Llewelyn J, Mitchell R. Survival of patients who needed salvage surgery for recurrence after radiotherapy for oral carcinoma. Br J Oral Maxillofac Surg 1997;35:424–8.

84. Yuen AP, Wei WI, Lam LK, et al. Results of surgical salvage of locoregional recurrence of carcinoma of the tongue after radiotherapy failure. Ann Otol Rhinol Laryngol 1997;106:779–82.

85. Sun LM, Leung SW, Su CY, Wang CJ. The relapse patterns and outcome of postoperative recurrent tongue cancer. J Oral Maxillofac Surg 1997;55:827–31.

98

Neoplasms of the Oropharynx and Hypopharynx

Amy Anne D. Lassig, MD; Theodoros N. Teknos, MD; Douglas B. Chepeha, MD, MPH

The upper aerodigestive tract is divided into anatomical sites in which the behavior of the types of neoplasms varies. The oropharynx and hypopharynx represent pharyngeal conduits for respiration and alimentation and are important regions for the origin of malignancy in the head and neck. The oropharynx lies just beyond the oral cavity and connects the oral cavity to the nasopharynx, hypopharynx, and larynx. As such, it is somewhat out of immediate view but can be well visualized on physical examination. The hypopharynx is less accessible to easy visual inspection in the office, requiring indirect mirror examination or flexible nasopharyngoscopy for evaluation, and as such is an anatomical region that is not well known by nonotolaryngologists. The hypopharynx connects the oropharynx to the cervical esophagus below but also shares space with the glottic and supraglottic structures. Malignancies of the oropharynx and hypopharynx are uncommon relatively to all of those arising elsewhere in the body; oropharyngeal cancers make up approximately 1% of new cancers diagnosed each year and hypopharyngeal cancers occur even less commonly. Nevertheless, oropharyngeal neoplasms comprise 10 to 20% of all head and neck cancers and approximately 9,000 new cases are reported each year. Hypopharyngeal neoplasms, on the other hand, represent about 5 to 10% of all new head and neck malignancies registered each year.

Although oropharyngeal and hypopharyngeal neoplasms largely comprise squamous cell carcinoma, the causes and behaviors of these lesions vary by site. The treatment paradigms for neoplasms of the oropharynx and hypopharynx have evolved significantly over the past decades, and a multidisciplinary approach is paramount to these therapies. Multiple modalities including surgery, radiation, and chemotherapy are available for treating these lesions with the balance shifting toward organ preservation programs in more recent years. Basic science and clinical research protocols continue to search for the development of treatment plans which provide the greatest survival and lowest morbidity and mortality. Despite the advances in chemoradiation treatments, surgical therapy continues to be a necessary part of the treatment of these malignancies, and the ability to perform radical resection in these sites is essential to the practice of head and neck surgery. Likewise, the necessity of performing complex reconstructions of the oropharynx and hypopharynx has not diminished. In the end, clinicians in

many disciplines must work well together to recognize and treat malignancies of the oropharynx and hypopharynx optimally and to provide these patients with the best achievable quantity and quality of life.

OROPHARYNX

Anatomy and Physiology

The oropharynx lies at the junction of the oral cavity with the remainder of the upper

aerodigestive tract, including the nasopharynx, hypopharynx, and supraglottis. Form and function in this region are highly intertwined, resulting in important challenges for the physician treating patients with neoplasms in this area. The oropharynx is made up of several anatomic subsites including the tonsillar complexes, the soft palate, the base of tongue and the pharyngeal wall. These structures lie within fascial and muscular compartments that are important to the understanding of patterns of spread of the neoplasms (Figure 1).

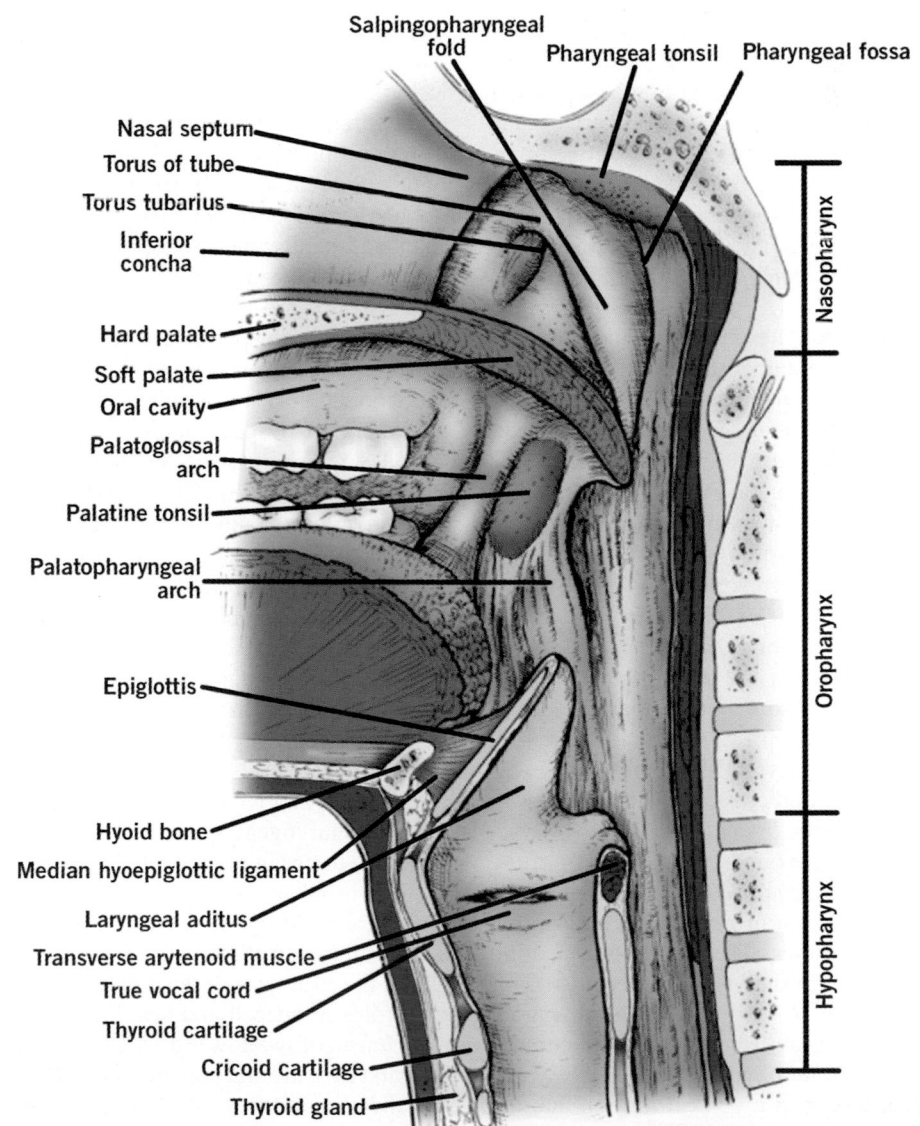

Figure 1 Illustration showing the sagittal anatomy of the oropharynx in relationship to the nasopharynx and hypopharynx.

The anterior border of the oropharynx is marked by the edge of the soft palate superiorly and the superior aspect of the hyoid bone inferiorly. The circumvallate papillae define the anterior edge of the base of tongue, and the anterior insertions of the anterior pillars mark the anterior aspect of the tonsillar complex. The posterior border of the oropharynx is delimited by the posterior pharyngeal wall, and likewise the lateral border is bounded by the lateral pharyngeal walls and tonsillar complexes. The soft palate indicates the level of the superior limit of the oropharynx, and the inferior extent is marked by the pharyngoepiglottic folds and valleculae, both considered part of the oropharynx.

The tonsillar complexes are a set of bilateral structures abutting the posterior aspect of the oral cavity. They are comprised of an anterior tonsillar pillar and posterior tonsillar pillar with intervening capsule-encased tonsillar lymphoid tissue. The palatoglossus muscle underlies the anterior pillar and the palatopharyngeous underlies the posterior pillar to create a muscular sling for the palatine tonsils. These structures are contiguous with the soft palate. The palatine tonsils represent lymphoid tissue of the Waldeyer ring and are a common site of origin for both lymphoid and epithelial malignancy. The vascular supply to the region includes the tonsillar branch of the facial artery, the tonsillar branch of the lingual artery, the ascending pharyngeal artery, and branches of the greater and lesser palatine arteries. Lymphatic drainage from the tonsillar fossae primarily includes retropharyngeal lymph nodes as well as levels II, III, and IV lymph nodes. Contralateral drainage can also occur with malignant neoplasms.

The base of tongue represents the posterior third of the tongue and is demarcated anteriorly by the circumvallate papillae and sulcus terminalis. The base of the tongue is comprised of intrinsic tongue musculature covered by squamous cell mucosa and submucosa. The lingual tonsils, another lymphoid tissue component of the Waldeyer ring, are located within the base of tongue. Bilateral lingual arteries serve as the vascular supply to the base of the tongue. The cranial nerve (CN) XII, hypoglossal nerve, allows for motor innervation. CN IX, the glossopharyngeal nerve, allows for sensory innervation. Lymphatic vessels from the base of tongue drain primarily to lymph nodes in levels II, III, and IV. Lymphatic structures often cross the midline to result in bilateral lymphatic drainage.

The soft palate extends posteriorly from the hard palate and is comprised of the palatine aponeurosis, an extension of hard palate periostium, with attached muscles. The tensor veli palatini, innervated by the third division of CN V (trigeminal nerve), forms a sling around the pterygoid hamulus and inserts onto the palatine aponeurosis. The levator veli palatini, innervated by CN X, the vagus nerve, inserts in a vertical fashion into the palatine aponeurosis and elevates the palate. The uvula hangs inferiorly at the posterior aspect of the soft palate and is comprised of uvular muscle covered by mucosa and submucosa. Minor salivary glands are also present within the soft palate mucosa and submucosa and can give rise to benign and malignant neoplasms. The sensory innervation of the soft palate is provided by the glossopharyngeal nerve and the second division of CN V. The vascular supply is primarily from branches of the internal maxillary artery via the descending palatine artery. Lymphatic drainage from the soft palate primarily involves the level II and retropharyngeal lymph nodes, and drainage can be bilateral.

The posterior pharyngeal wall is comprised of mucosa overlying submucosa, musculature, and fascial layers. Immediately deep to the mucosa and submucosa lies the superior and, more inferiorly, the middle constrictor muscles. Deep to these muscles is the buccopharyngeal fascias followed by the alar and then the prevertebral fascia. The prevertebral musculature overlies the vertebral column. Potential spaces lie between these structures. The retropharyngeal space lies between the buccopharyngeal fascia and the alar fascia, and the danger space lies between the alar and prevertebral fascias. These fascial layers are important barriers to spread of malignant processes originating within the oropharynx. Once these barriers have been violated and the prevertebral musculature is involved with tumor, the lesion is no longer considered resectable. Lymphatic drainage of the posterior pharyngeal wall is to retropharyngeal lymph nodes as well as lymph nodes at levels II, III, and IV.

Just as the posterior pharyngeal wall is surrounded by muscular layers, fascial barriers, and potential spaces, the remainder of the oropharyngeal subsites are as well. Deep to mucosa and submucosa, the superior and middle pharyngeal constrictors form a muscular tube surrounding the structures of the oropharynx. Laterally, the parapharyngeal space abuts the oropharynx, a complex region that can be invaded by oropharyngeal malignancies. The parapharyngeal space is an inverted pyramid extending from the skull base superiorly to the greater cornu of the hyoid bone inferiorly. The lateral boundary of the space includes the deep lobe of the parotid gland, a portion of the mandible, and the medial pterygoid muscle. The pterygomandibular raphe marks the anterior aspect of the space and the prevertebral fascia the posterior. Important structures including the great vessels, CNs IX to XII, the sympathetic chain, and lymphatics are contained within the parapharyngeal space and can be compromised by tumor in the region.

The oropharynx plays many critical physiologic roles. At the most basic level, it serves as a respiratory and alimentary conduit. Also importantly, the structures of the oropharynx play complex roles in speech and swallowing. The basic mechanism of swallow is divided into four phases. The first two, the oral preparatory and oral phases, are under voluntary control, and the last two, the pharyngeal and esophageal phases, are involuntary. The oral preparatory phase makes the food ready for swallowing. The oral phase moves the food from the oral cavity to the oropharynx. During the pharyngeal phase, the food bolus is rapidly propelled through the pharynx to the esophagus. This pharyngeal phase involves glottic protection, velopharyngeal closure, tongue base retraction, constrictor contraction, and cricopharyngeal muscle relaxation. The final phase of swallowing is the esophageal, during which foodstuff travels from the cervical esophagus into the stomach.

The oropharyngeal structures are critical to this process. During the preparatory and oral phases of swallowing, the soft palate is raised and slightly anterior to allow food to remain within the oral cavity and to keep the nasal airway open. The soft palate is also essential to the propagation of the swallowing mechanism during the oral phase, as the tongue elevates to abut the palate and push food particles posteriorly. The soft palate also serves as the anatomic separator of the oral cavity and oropharynx from the nasal cavity and nasopharynx. This separation is essential to the mechanism of swallowing, during which elevation of the palate allows for velopharyngeal competence, preventing the reflux of foodstuff into the nasopharynx. The base of tongue is also essential to swallow; it serves to initiate the pharyngeal phase of swallow by thrusting posteriorly to abut the posterior pharyngeal wall which then contracts to propel the bolus as the process continues.

In addition to swallowing, the oropharyngeal structures are also essential to speech. The oropharyngeal structures create a compliant conduit for airflow and are also important to modifying resonance of phonation. Most important in this role, the soft palate allows air passage in the nasal and oral cavities to be separate and creates a controlled volume of airflow, thus preventing hypernasal speech. This is important as all phonemes in the English language, except for m, n, and ng, are produced via airflow through the oral cavity, requiring concurrent velopharyngeal closure. In addition, the oropharyngeal structures assist in the articulation portion of speech production. The soft palate plays an important role in this function. By contracting to abut the posterior pharyngeal wall during speech, explosive consonants, such as p, b, g, d, and t, can be created. Other structures within the oropharynx contribute to the spincteric velopharyngeal competency and include the palatoglossus and palatopharyngeus as well as the superior constrictor.

Histopathology

The oropharyngeal portion of the upper aerodigestive tract is lined primarily by stratified squamous cell epithelium. This is most commonly nonkeratinized but can become keratinized in response to irritation. The region where the soft palate contacts the posterior pharyngeal wall marks the superior limit of the oropharynx and is called Passavant ridge. This is the location of the transition from pseudostratified ciliated columnar or respiratory epithelium of the nasal tissues to stratified squamous cell epithelium. Lymphoepithelial tissues are also located in the oropharynx as part of the Waldeyer ring. These tissues are found predominantly in the pharyngeal, palatine, and lingual tonsils. In addition, minor salivary glands are scattered throughout the mucosa and submucosa of the oropharynx in the soft palate, base of tongue, tonsillar pillars, and retromolar trigone.

The most common malignancy of the oropharyngeal structures is squamous cell carcinoma, comprising greater than 90% of neoplasms. These lesions are more commonly keratinizing, but nonkeratinizing ones are also quite common. Multiple other carcinomas also occur, however, and include adenosquamous, baseloid, and spindle cell squamous cell carcinoma as well as verrucous carcinoma. Adenosquamous and baseloid variants are rare but more aggressive variants of squamous cell carcinoma. Spindle cell variant of squamous cell carcinoma contains spindle cells coexisting with squamous cells within the neoplasm, and is also termed sarcomatoid carcinoma. This lesion generally behaves more aggressively with a higher propensity for local recurrence and distant spread. Verrucous carcinoma is marked by papillomatous fronds of well-differentiated squamous cells. These tumors advance locally but generally do not metastasize. They are not radiosensitive, and the treatment is wide excision. In addition to variants of squamous cell carcinoma, precursor lesions to squamous cell carcinoma also occur within the oropharynx. Leukoplakia and erythroplakia are less common in the oropharynx than in the oral cavity. These lesions can undergo malignant transformation to become a squamous cell carcinoma, with this occurring more commonly in an erythroplakic lesion. Finally, the concept of field cancerization must be mentioned with regard to squamous cell carcinoma of the upper aerodigestive tract. This idea, put forth by Slaughter in 1953, suggests that for a number of patients, multifocal areas of precancerous change surround diagnosed cancers. Such "field cancerization" significantly affects diagnosis and treatment planning in the region. Recent work by Braakhuis and colleagues suggests that field cancerization and second primary neoplasms occur along a continuum of disease.[1] The mechanism of this process continues to be clarified through the ongoing study of molecular carcinogenesis.

Other types of neoplasms also occur within the oropharynx, originating from the various histological cells and structures that comprise the tissues. Benign processes such as papilloma, pyogenic granuloma, and pseudoepithelialomatous hyperplasia occur in the oropharynx and can imitate malignant neoplasms. Papilloma, of course, can undergo malignant transformation to squamous cell carcinoma, but this occurs in less than 5% of lesions. Minor salivary glands give rise to benign and malignant neoplasms, with the balance tipped toward malignant lesions such as adenoid cystic carcinoma, mucoepidermoid carcinoma, adenocarcinoma, and acinic cell carcinoma. The most common minor salivary gland malignancy is adenoid cystic carcinoma. This neoplasm occurs as tubular, cribriform, and solid growth patterns and is characterized by frequent perineural and hematogenous spread. Treatment is wide excision with postoperative radiation. Mucoepidermoid carcinoma is the second most common minor salivary gland malignancy and is histologically graded as low, intermediate, and high. Treatment is wide excision, frequently with added neck dissection for larger lesions with suspicious or positive cervical metastases, followed by postoperative radiation for aggressive features. Lymphoma commonly occurs in the Waldeyer ring structures, and the palative tonsils are the most frequent site of extra-nodal non-Hodgkin lymphoma within the head and neck. Treatment is with chemotherapy and radiation, and the role of the surgeon is only in tissue diagnosis. Lymphoepithelial carcinoma is a malignant neoplasm of the oropharynx which has both lymphoid and epithelial characteristics. This is a poorly differentiated, nonkeratinized neoplasm histologically identical to World Health Organization (WHO) Type III nasopharyngeal carcinoma. This tumor frequently presents in patients younger than typical patients with squamous cell carcinoma and is known to be quite radiosensitive. True sarcomas can occur within the oropharynx but are quite uncommon.

Etiology and Epidemiology

Squamous cell carcinoma of the oropharynx like other malignancies is thought to result from multiple genetic alterations which result in unregulated cell proliferation and an unchecked cell cycle. These genetic changes can result from multiple environmental exposures as well as inherited defects. Once altered, these cancer cells proliferate and evade the natural process of apoptosis. The result is a tumor which may locally, regionally, or distantly metastasize. The immune system is a critical player in this process and at present great interest lies in understanding this interaction. It is known that patients with immune system deficiencies resulting from inherited defects, medications (transplant or other immunosuppression), or illness (such as HIV) are at a significant disadvantage in the battle against these neoplasms.

As with most subsites of the upper aerodigestive tract, squamous cell carcinoma of the oropharynx most frequently occurs in relation to tobacco and alcohol exposure. These substances act as carcinogens individually in a dose-dependent manner. When considered separately, tobacco smoke is a greater risk factor. When used together, however, alcohol and tobacco have a synergistic cancer-causing effect and are thought to be causative in 80 to 90% of oropharyngeal cancers. Use of other substances can also be causative or contributory in squamous cell carcinoma of the oropharynx. A combination of betel leaves and the areca nut commonly consumed in India and Southeast Asia, betel quid is a risk factor for oropharynx and upper aerodigestive tract squamous cell carcinoma. In addition, maté products largely consumed in South America have been found to increase independently the risk of squamous cell carcinoma of the oral cavity and oropharynx.[2]

Viral infection has also been shown to be associated with squamous cell carcinoma of the upper aerodigestive tract. Human papilloma virus (HPV), initially implicated in cervical cancer, has been more recently thought to also induce a viral carcinogenesis within the upper aerodigestive tract, most often in the oropharynx at the palatine and lingual tonsillar subsites. At these locations HPV is responsible for a sizeable proportion of cancers. HPV DNA has been found in 45 to 100% of all tonsillar neoplasms and is thought to be causative in greater than 50%.[3] HPV 16 is by far the most common HPV type in oropharyngeal cancer, inducing carcinogenesis via oncogenes E6 and E7. A recent case-control study found that oropharyngeal squamous cell carcinoma is strongly associated with oral HPV infection and HPV seropositivity, completely independent of alcohol and tobacco use. This study concluded that the mechanism of carcinogenesis is likely entirely different than alcohol or tobacco induced tumors, and that HPV tumors are likely sexually acquired.[4] HPV-positive squamous cell carcinoma is more likely to occur in younger patients. These cancers portend an improved prognosis, particularly in patients with high viral load, and single institution work from the University of Michigan indicates that these tumors are more likely to respond to organ preservation therapy. In the future, HPV vaccines may play an important role in the prevention and treatment of oropharyngeal squamous cell carcinoma.

The epidemiology of squamous cell carcinoma of the oropharynx has identified the greatest risk factors, tobacco and alcohol use. There are approximately 5,000 new cases of oropharyngeal neoplasms diagnosed each year in the United States.[5] The incidence of squamous cell carcinoma of the oropharynx is 2 per 100,000 persons in the United States.[6] The United States National Cancer Institute Surveillance Epidemiology and End Results (SEER) database reports an incidence of 10.5 per 100,000 for oral cavity and pharynx neoplasms combined. It continues to be more common in men than in women, and the incidence is higher in African–American men than in Caucasian. The overall incidence of squamous cell carcinoma and the mortality from it have decreased minimally over the last 30 years. Most squamous cell carcinomas of the oropharynx are diagnosed in persons older than 45 and are most common between the ages of 60 and 80. The most common site of malignancy in the oropharynx is the tonsil.

Clinical Manifestations and Mechanisms of Spread

Squamous cell carcinoma of the oropharynx presents with a variety of symptoms depending on the subsite of the primary neoplasm. These neoplasms are often asymptomatic initially and frequently evade examination by the untrained eye. Thus, these neoplasms may be locally advanced at the time of diagnosis. Additionally, 15 to 75% may have evidence of cervical lymph nodal metastases at the time of presentation, and the presence of such adenopathy decreases survival by approximately 50%. Such regional metastases are typically predictable in nature, occurring in the primary echelon lymph nodes for the oropharynx in levels II and III and the retropharynx. Approximately 5 to 10% have distant metastases on initial evaluation.

Symptoms of oropharyngeal malignancy include sore throat, otalgia, odynophagia, and globus sensation. As the neoplasm progresses and adjacent structures become involved, symptoms such as dysphagia, dysarthria, and trismus may develop. Difficulty in swallowing often leads to weight loss, malnutrition, and weakness. Once symptoms are present, the neoplasms are often at a quite advanced stage.

The tonsillar fossae and tonsils are the most common locations for squamous cell carcinoma in the oropharynx, comprising approximately 75% of oropharyngeal neoplasms. Small, early neoplasms are often asymptomatic and can present with a neck mass in approximately 25% of neoplasms. With growth of the neoplasm, frequently dysphagia and odynophagia as well as otalgia and hemoptysis occur. These neoplasms are often exophytic, originating in the tonsil itself and extending onto the anterior tonsillar pillar. Tonsillar squamous cell carcinomas often extend onto other subsites of the oropharynx, frequently onto the base of tongue and less often the posterior pharyngeal wall. These neoplasms also often advance anteriorly into the oral cavity especially to the retromolar trigone and buccal mucosa. As these tumors continue to enlarge, they can invade deeply to involve the mandible as well as nervous structures such as the CN IX, the lingual nerve, and the inferior alveolar nerve. This invasion can result in jaw pain, loose teeth, dysphagia, and dysesthesias. Further growth of the neoplasm can result in pterygoid muscle invasion, typically medial then lateral. This results in trismus and discomfort. Locoregional cervical metastases also occur as the neoplasm progresses and greater than 65% of patients with tonsillar squamous cell carcinoma present with adenopathy at diagnosis.

Base of tongue neoplasms, like tonsillar cancers, often present at an advanced stage. Early symptoms for these lesions include throat discomfort, however, lesions are often difficult to visualize, especially by the nonotolaryngologist. Base of tongue neoplasms are often submucosal and thus only deep oropharyngeal palpation reveals their location. These lesions tend to be aggressive and are more likely to be less differentiated. These lesions spread to involve the glossotonsillar sulcus, tonsillar fossa and pillars, soft palate, and retromolar trigone. Deeper invasion can occur along the intrinsic muscles of the tongue and advanced neoplasms can involve the mandible and pterygoid muscles or the supraglottic larynx. Cervical metastases can occur early, even in small neoplasms, and more than 60% of patients diagnosed with a base of tongue neoplasm have evidence of adenopathy at presentation. In addition, approximately 20% of patients with base of tongue neoplasms have evidence of

bilateral lymphatic spread. The aggressive behavior of base of tongue neoplasms is quite distinct from the behavior of oral tongue lesions, and the resulting poorer outcomes reflect this. Increased difficulty achieving local control in these lesions results in a higher rate of distant metastases.

Squamous cell carcinoma of the lateral and posterior pharyngeal walls is much less common than primary lesions of the tonsils or base of tongue. Like these neoplasms, however, this location can be quite difficult to visualize. As a result, lesions in this area can be quite advanced at diagnosis, and cervical adenopathy is the presenting sign in 20% of patients. Patients also often present with sore throat as well as dysphagia and odynophagia. As these neoplasms enlarge, weight loss, dysphonia, and otalgia are common complaints. These neoplasms often spread to oropharyngeal structures but can extend superiorly into the nasopharynx and inferiorly into the hypopharynx. Once these neoplasms traverse the barriers of muscle and fascia surrounding the pharynx, particularly posteriorly, or have significant superior extension, their resectability comes into question.

Squamous cell carcinoma of the soft palate comprises approximately 15% of oropharyngeal neoplasms. Contrary to other subsites, these lesions are more easily visualized on physical examination and often present with symptoms earlier in their course. Pain and odynophagia are frequent presenting symptoms. As these lesions progress, they can extend along the soft palate to the tonsillar structures and retromolar trigone or anteriorly along the hard palate. These lesions become more worrisome with superior extension into the nasopharynx. Rates of cervical metastases are less common than in other subsites of the oropharynx, but lymphatic drainage can be bilateral and retropharyngeal lymph nodes are included.

Diagnosis and Work-Up

The diagnosis and work-up of oropharyngeal malignancies should be completed in an expeditious manner as with any other malignancy. The first step is to perform a complete history including previous evaluation and treatment of the neoplasm as well as comorbidities which affect suitability for treatment. A thorough physical examination follows the history. A full head and neck evaluation is performed with attention particularly to the oropharynx and adjacent anatomic sites. Direct illuminated inspection should be performed in these areas followed by palpation. The neck should be evaluated for evidence of regional metastases. Attention should also be given to examination findings consistent with advanced disease such as trismus, bony invasion, cutaneous involvement, CN deficits, or signs of unresectable disease. Flexible fiberoptic nasopharyngoscopy should be performed to complete the evaluation of the primary neoplasm as well as to evaluate the remainder of the upper aerodigestive tract.

Radiologic evaluation should next be completed. Computed tomography (CT) scanning of the neck with contrast is extremely helpful in

delineating the extent of the primary neoplasm, the presence of regional metastases, and the status of surrounding structures. Magnetic resonance imaging (MRI) scanning is helpful in patients in whom further soft tissue delineation is needed. Findings such as CN or dural enhancement in advanced disease are reliably revealed by MRI, and thus this study can be helpful when resectability is in question. Positron emission tomography (PET) studies have more recently become much more widely used in the evaluation of head and neck malignancy. This is not routinely used in the work-up of a new known primary oropharyngeal malignancy but can be helpful in delineating questionable sites of distant or regional metastases. PET is much more useful in posttreatment surveillance and treatment decisions, and the role of this scan is still being delineated. Panorex can be useful at times for mandibular and dental evaluation, but this is often not necessary as CT scans give adequate bony information.

Evaluation for pulmonary metastases or synchronous primaries must be performed prior to initiation of treatment. Our center routinely orders a chest CT, as multiple studies to date show this to be highly sensitive for this work-up. A chest radiograph, however, is generally acceptable as well, although patients with high-risk disease features should be screened with CT.[7] Although useful, a chest CT is not a perfect screening tool for distant metastases; thus, several centers have evaluated the use of PET as a screening tool for distant metastases, and some suggest its combination with chest CT will likely give the most accurate assessment.[8]

Laboratory and medical work-up should be completed to evaluate the patient's general health as well as fitness for surgery, anesthesia, or other treatments (chemotherapy and radiation). Routine laboratory tests, such as a basic metabolic panel and complete blood count, should be obtained. Some recommend a screening liver function panel as an indicator of metastatic disease and to indicate hepatic health in a population with frequent alcohol abusers. An EKG should be included in the work-up. Other outstanding medical problems should be evaluated as indicated.

The diagnostic work-up proceeds with staging endoscopy under general anesthesia. Direct laryngoscopy and esophagoscopy are performed to delineate the primary neoplasm and to evaluate for any synchronous second primary neoplasms. Bronchoscopy is often not performed due to the accuracy of thoracic CT but can be helpful in visualizing small endotracheal lesions. The oral cavity, oropharynx, surrounding structures, and cervical region should be palpated to determine the extent of disease. Tattoo of the neoplasm is then performed with India Ink to mark the area for future surveillance. Biopsies of the neoplasm and any surrounding regions of concern should be completed after the visual inspection is complete. This may include tonsillectomy for presumed tonsillar primary. The primary tumor tissue is necessary for a diagnosis even if a previous fine-needle aspiration (FNA) of a cervical lymph node is positive for carcinoma. When biopsying, lesions that are potentially lymphoma should be sent to pathology fresh (not fixed in preservative) for evaluation. Once the evaluation is complete, the neoplasm should be staged and documented on a neoplasm diagram for the permanent medical record. As treatment planning proceeds a speech and swallowing evaluation can be helpful in assessment and future treatment. Also, a dental evaluation should be carried out as well if dental health is in question and surgery or radiation to the teeth and jaw are upcoming.

Staging and Prognosis

Oropharyngeal squamous cell carcinoma is staged with the American Joint Committee on Cancer (AJCC) system[9] (Table 1). The tumor itself is categorized to give a T value. This categorization is based on size, involvement with adjacent sites, and finally involvement of areas which indicate advanced disease or poorer prognosis. Cervical lymph adenopathy is likewise categorized to give a lymph nodal or N stage. Again this is based on size and location (Table 2). Finally an M, or metastasis, value is given based on the presence or absence of metastasis (see Table 2). These three evaluations are put together to create a TNM label for each patient as well as a stage for each patient (Table 3). In general, any evidence of nodal disease will cause patients to be considered at least stage III. T4 neoplasms and more bulky lymphadenopathy will fall into Stage IV, with T4b considered unresectable.

Distant metastases are thought to occur in approximately 5 to 10% of patients at presentation and impart a poor prognosis. Lung, liver, and bone are the most common sites of distant metastases. Over the course of the disease, distant metastases will occur in 15 to 20% of patients with oropharyngeal squamous cell carcinomas and are more common in patients who present with advanced disease, have low neck or multiple levels of neck lymphadenopathy, have high histologic grade and those who have local or regional recurrences.[10] In general for the oropharynx, approximately 20 to 30% of patients with neoplasms larger than T1 and who are clinically N0 will have evidence of occult regional metastatic disease. The presence of such cervical metastases is thought to decrease survival by approximately 50%. Five-year survival rates for patients with squamous cell carcinoma of the

Table 1	American Joint Committee on Cancer Tumor Categorization of Oropharyngeal Squamous Cell Carcinoma
T1	Tumor 2 cm or less in greatest dimension
T2	Tumor more than 2 cm but not more than 4 cm in greatest dimension
T3	Tumor more than 4 cm in greatest dimension
T4a	Tumor invades the larynx, deep/extrinsic muscle of tongue, medial pterygoid muscle, hard palate, or mandible
T4b	Tumor invades lateral pterygoid muscle, pterygoid plates, lateral nasopharynx, or skull base or encases carotid artery

Table 2	American Joint Committee on Cancer Categorization of Lymph Node and Metastasis of Oropharyngeal Squamous Cell Carcinoma[8]
Nx	Regional lymph nodes cannot be assessed
N0	No regional lymph node metastasis
N1	Metastasis in a single ipsilateral lymph node, 3 cm or less in greatest dimension
N2	Metastasis in a single ipsilateral lymph node, more than 3 cm but not more than 6 cm in greatest dimension, or in multiple ipsilateral lymph nodes, none more than 6 cm in greatest dimension, or in bilateral or contralateral lymph nodes, none more than 6 cm in greatest dimension
N2a	Metastasis in a single ipsilateral lymph node more than 3 cm but not more than 6 cm in greatest dimension
N2b	Metastasis in multiple ipsilateral lymph nodes, none more than 6 cm in greatest dimension
N2c	Metastasis in bilateral or contralateral lymph nodes, none more than 6 cm in greatest dimension
N3	Metastasis in a lymph node more than 6 cm in greatest dimension
Mx	Distant metastasis cannot be assessed
M0	No distant metastasis
M1	Distant metastasis

oropharynx are 57% for Stage I disease and 54% for Stage II disease. Patients with higher stages at diagnosis have a worse prognosis, with 5-year survival rates for Stage III disease of 43% and of Stage IV disease of 30%.

Treatment

General Approach. The treatment for squamous cell carcinoma of the oropharynx has evolved significantly over the last quarter century. The concept of organ preservation has changed the treatment paradigm such that surgical therapy is often no longer the first-line treatment. Radiation and chemotherapy have taken the forefront in many centers with surgery left for salvage of treatment failures. The end result is that the technical challenges of surgery in this region are all the greater. With these changes, a multidisci-

Table 3	American Joint Committee on Cancer TNM Staging of Oropharyngeal Squamous Cell Carcinoma[8]
Stage 0	Tis N0 M0
Stage I	T1 N0 M0
Stage II	T2 N0 M0
Stage III	T3 N0 M0
	T1 N1 M0
	T2 N1 M0
	T3 N1 M0
Stage IVa	T4a N0 M0
	T4a N1 M0
	T1 N2 M0
	T2 N2 M0
	T3 N2 M0
	T4a N2 M0
Stage IVb	T4b Any N M0
	Any T N3 M0
Stage IVc	Any T Any N M1

plinary approach to treating head and neck cancer has become paramount. Otolaryngologists, medical oncologists, radiation oncologists, dentists, nurses, speech pathologists, and others must work in concert as a team to care for these patients with complicated problems.

Organ Preservation. The idea of preserving native structures within the upper aerodigestive tract while treating malignancy in the area has been an attractive goal in the recent history of head and neck cancer. This is particularly important in the oropharynx as the defects in speech and swallowing resulting from surgical resection can be significant. Over the last century, radiation has been used in many forms in the treatment of malignancy of the head and neck. During the 1980s, radiation was combined with chemotherapy, and the era of organ preservation began. Prior to this chemotherapy had been an adjunct for palliation; but, with the use and development of platinum-based agents, treatment results changed. The combination of cisplatin with 5-fluorouracil allowed chemotherapy to be used for curative intent. Early studies of such protocols focused on laryngeal cancer, including the landmark US Veterans Administration Laryngeal Cancer Clinical Trial published in 1991 which showed no significant survival difference between patients undergoing induction chemotherapy [5-fluorouracil (5-FU) and cisplatinum] and radiation versus surgical resection and radiotherapy.[11] Since that time, multiple studies have emerged evaluating and endorsing organ preservation treatments in the head and neck and in the oropharynx specifically. This treatment continues to evolve and advance. Chemotherapy regimens and agents continue to be developed and studied in the treatment of squamous cell carcinoma of the head and neck. Likewise, radiation therapy protocols continue to be studied and modified for optimum results. Intensity modulated radiation therapy has been recently developed to aid in dosing radiation therapy. This method aims to give maximum dose to neoplasm but a lesser dose to lower risk, functional surrounding structures, such as the parotid glands, and pharyngeal constrictors, to help minimize complications and side effects.[12] Fractionation schemes of radiation therapy including accelerated fractionization and hyperfractionization continue to be studied to determine the most effective regimen with the least morbidity. As the understanding of the molecular mechanisms of carcinogenesis and response to treatment continue to unfold, organ preservation therapy will continue to evolve and improve. For example, recent single institution work from the University of Michigan indicates that good response to organ preservation therapy and improved prognosis are indicated by low EGFR and high p16 expression in oropharyngeal tumors. Ongoing scientific study at the basic science and translational levels are essential to forward progress in organ preservation and treatment success, and over time these discoveries make their way from bench top to bedside.

Treatment Plan. Oropharyngeal malignancies can be treated by radiation, chemotherapy, and surgical resection. Treatment decisions must be based on neoplasm site and stage as well as patient desires and comorbidities. In the majority of cases, our group prefers to avoid surgical resection as the primary means of treating oropharyngeal malignancies. Surgical treatment of the primary neoplasm at this site can result in significant morbidity. In addition, as cervical metastases tend to occur early in oropharyngeal squamous cell carcinomas, the neck must be addressed and treated even at an early stage. Treatment of the neck often must include the retropharyngeal nodal basin which is not well addressed with standard neck dissection. Despite these factors, surgical resection can be an appropriate method of treating oropharyngeal neoplasms, particularly when a tumor is unresponsive to induction chemotherapy or after failure of primary chemotherapy and radiation protocols.

Early-stage oropharyngeal neoplasms which are T1 or T2 primaries with little or no nodal disease (N0 or N1) can be treated by definitive radiation therapy. With evidence of nodal disease, however, consideration is given to adding chemotherapy to the regimen, although this is not absolutely necessary with only N1 disease. With such organ preservation treatment, residual or recurrent disease is treated by surgical resection. Early-stage neoplasms of the oropharynx can also be treated with wide excision of the primary neoplasm with treatment of the neck including unilateral or bilateral neck dissection. Evidence of nodal disease in the neck dissection specimen requires treatment with postoperative radiation. High-risk features from the surgical resection include extracapsular extension of the nodal disease as well as close or positive margins on the primary resection. These patients should be treated with chemotherapy and radiation therapy postoperatively. Other risk indicators such as perineural or vascular invasion and multiple positive nodes also argue for postoperative treatment with both chemotherapy and radiation therapy, however, the benefit of adding chemotherapy is still being determined.[13–15] New agents are constantly being evaluated to add to therapy and improve survival. Cetuximab is one such agent and functions as an antiepidermal growth factor receptor antibody; it has been shown to be beneficial in recurrent or metastatic squamous cell carcinoma of the head and neck.[16,17]

More advanced stage neoplasms of the oropharynx are best treated by combined chemotherapy and radiation therapy. This is typically completed in a concurrent fashion; however, induction chemotherapy continues to be investigated and is promising. Evidence of neoplasm response after such induction indicates that a successful outcome with organ preservation therapy is more likely. With poor response to induction chemotherapy, the likelihood of successful cure with primary chemotherapy and radiation is lower and in these patients, some groups proceed to surgical resection at that time. Evidence of nodal disease is common at presentation in advanced T-category oropharyngeal malignancies, and residual nodal disease must be addressed post treatment. For patients with significant pretreatment nodal burden, many proceed with a planned neck dissection after the completion of chemotherapy and radiation therapy, despite the response to treatment. Our center has recently used the cutoff of evidence of a 3 cm lymph node pretreatment in planning a posttreatment neck dissection. This is an area of current investigation, however, and PET scanning has taken the forefront in the discussion. In patients with complete response to therapy, the role of planned posttreatment neck dissection versus monitoring the neck, particularly with PET scan, is still being debated.

For advanced oropharyngeal neoplasms, some centers continue to pursue primary surgical resection with postoperative radiation or postoperative combined radiation and chemotherapy for high-risk features as described above. Approaches to such surgical resection are described below. These approaches are also applicable to patients who have evidence of residual or recurrent disease after treatment with chemotherapy and radiation therapy.

Surgical Treatment. There are numerous approaches to surgical resection of oropharyngeal neoplasms. The approach taken is dependent on many variables including the size of the primary neoplasm, the location of the neoplasm and access to that location, involved structures, previous treatment, other necessary procedures, and the skills and comfort of the operating surgeon. Tracheostomy is a necessary accompaniment to surgical resection of most neoplasms of the oropharynx, unless the primary is small. This is typically performed at the outset of the procedure and allows resection without hindrance from the endotracheal tube. Adequate exposure of the neoplasm for resection can be difficult but is a necessity to achieve wide, negative margins. After surgical resection is complete, the next challenge is reconstruction of the area.

Small primary neoplasms of the oropharynx can be resected with an intraoral approach. Typically a mouth gag such as a Crow-Davis, McIver, or Dingman is used to allow for visualization of the neoplasm and surrounding structures. Tonsillectomy by standard means can be considered for resection of a small tonsillar primary. Small T1 lesions of the soft palate can likewise be widely excised without difficulty with an intraoral approach. Base of tongue and pharyngeal wall lesions can be excised transorally if they are small as well. Such resections can be performed by cold dissection or with cautery but are frequently accomplished with a laser.

Interest in CO_2 laser resection has increased in recent years with interest in organ preservation. The CO_2 laser is ideal in its precision for ablating neoplasm as well as its hemostatic properties. Transoral and endoscopic approaches have been used with success by a number of groups which report successful functional and oncologic results. Recently Pradier and colleagues presented the use of CO_2 laser in Stage III and IV squamous cell carcinoma of the head and neck with adjuvant radiotherapy.[18] With this treatment, they had equivalent success to surgery followed by radiotherapy with respect to survival and locoregional control, and they reported diminished operative morbidity.[2] Such results will continue to be investigated over time, and the role of laser treatment will continue to be developed. In addition, fiberoptic capabilities for this laser are being developed at present which will continue to increase its ease in use.

Open approaches to the oropharynx are more frequently used for lesions that are moderate to large in size. These approaches are combined with surgical treatment for the neck and require cervical incisions. Typically, neck dissection is performed prior to resection of the primary neoplasm. Operative and incision planning is important for appropriate access, optimum cosmesis, and well-vascularized skin flaps. This is particularly important in the posttreatment neck where vascularity is already compromised, and in such cases it is particularly important to ensure that important structures such as the common carotid artery are not left at risk under repairs with vertical limbs or trifurcations. Frequently a lip split incision is necessary to achieve sufficient access to oropharyngeal structures. This incision is best designed as a midline extension of a unilateral apron incision used for unilateral neck dissection. The midline limb of the incision should contain several z angulations to break up the incision visually and ensure accurate reapproximation of skin flaps at the completion of the operation. This should continue up to the vermillion border, and this border should be appropriately marked preoperatively. Methylene blue is also used to mark the midline at the superior and inferior extent of the exposed surgical field and used to mark planned incisions. If bilateral neck dissections are planned, the apron incision can also be extended up the midline to perform a lip split. Alternatively, a visor flap can be raised and folded over the mandible for access.

The lateral pharyngotomy approach is a means of resecting neoplasms of the inferolateral oropharynx. An incision in the pharynx is planned which spans from the hypoglossal nerve superiorly to the superior laryngeal nerve inferiorly. A vertical pharyngotomy is made, and the thyroid cartilage ala is retracted. This allows visualization and resection of neoplasms at the posterolateral base of tongue as well as the lateral pharyngeal wall. A Connell-type mucosal inverting stitch is used for closure of the pharyngotomy site.

A second open approach to neoplasms of the oropharynx is a pharyngotomy via the transhyoid route (Figure 2). This allows exposure and resection of midline base of tongue, posterior pharyngeal wall, and some neoplasms of the inferior aspect of the lateral pharyngeal wall. Planning for this approach, with immediately preresection direct laryngoscopy, is especially important as the site of the pharyngotomy should be carefully chosen to avoid violating the neoplasm.

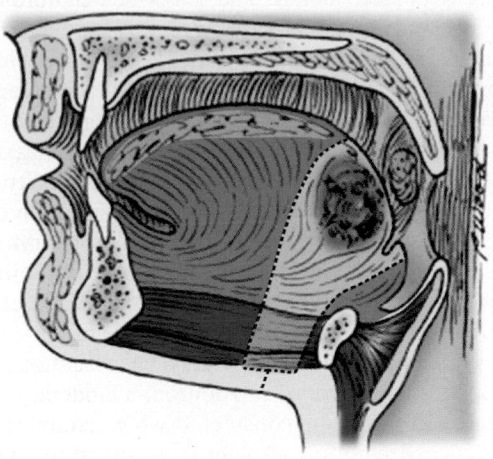

Figure 2 Transhyoid resection of oropharyngeal tumor. This transhyoid pharyngotomy approach is particularly useful for resection of base of tongue tumors.

The primary neoplasm is resected once neck dissection is completed. Suprahyoid musculature is divided from the hyoid as in a laryngectomy. The vallecula is entered at an oncologically sound site away from the neoplasm. The pharyngotomy is extended to visualize the lesion and bring it into the operative site. Dissection proceeds around the neoplasm. Release of the digastric and stylohyoid muscles allows greater exposure if necessary and rarely this approach is combined with a lateral pharyngotomy for even wider exposure. Care must be taken to preserve the hypoglossal nerve if uninvolved in neoplasm as well as the ipsilateral lingual artery. If the ipsilateral lingual artery must be ligated during the resection, the contralateral lingual artery must be preserved to preserve arterial inflow to the tongue. Generally, the transhyoid pharyngotomy approach can be closed primarily. The advantages of this approach include avoidance of a lip split or mandibulotomy, but disadvantages include difficult exposure of the neoplasm which extends superiorly or anteriorly.

The approach which allows greatest exposure of oropharyngeal malignancies is the mandibulotomy with mandibular swing and lip split. In preparation for mandibulotomy, the midline lip-splitting soft tissue cuts are made. The midline lip-splitting cut is extended through the musculature and mucosa into the oral cavity. The incision then makes a 90° turn to extend horizontally along the mandibular alveolus. Care is taken to preserve an adequate cuff of alveolar mucosa to allow for closure. Once the soft tissue cuts are made, the bony mandibular split is planned in a parasymphaseal location. A reconstruction plate that is 2.0 or larger is bent to the location and attached in the usual manner. Once the mandibular plate is appropriately fitted and attached, it is removed and carefully set aside. The bony mandibulotomy can now be made. Care is taken to preserve the mental nerve, and a stair-step mandibulotomy is used to allow for greatest bony stability. Tooth extraction may be necessary along the site of osteotomy.

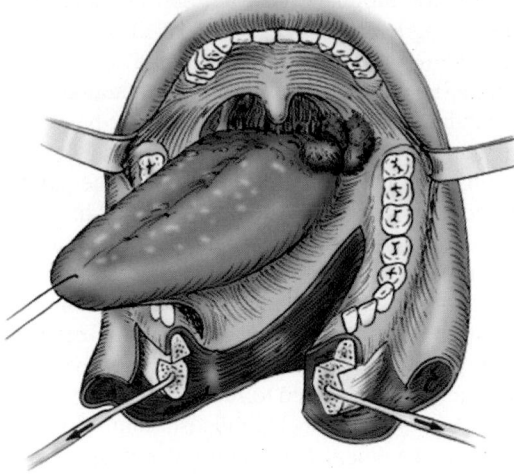

Figure 3 Mandibulotomy for access to oropharyngeal tumor and subsequent resection.

Once the mandibulotomy is complete, the mandible is opened and reflected laterally (Figure 3). Soft tissue dissection then proceeds posteriorly to expose the neoplasm. The neoplasm is widely excised. Reconstruction of the area is planned based on the resulting defect. As this approach allows the greatest exposure of the area, the resulting defect can be quite sizeable and generally requires a pedicled or free flap for reconstruction. The mandibular bone is then plated as planned previously.

Because oropharyngeal malignancies can invade bone also, mandibulotomy can be necessary for the resection of the neoplasm. Physical examination findings such as loose teeth, neoplasm fixation to bone, and diminished sensation in the CN V3 distribution can indicate mandibular involvement with the neoplasm. CT scanning, particularly with bony windows, and panorex imaging can confirm this and indicate the need for bony resection. If bony invasion is minimal and tooth roots, bone marrow, or the inferior alveolar canal are not involved, a rim mandibu-

lectomy will be adequate. Otherwise, a segmental mandibulectomy and composite resection will be necessary (Figure 4). Just as in mandibulotomy for neoplasm access, the mandible should be pre-plated with a 2.0 or larger reconstruction plate. Once bony resection is complete, frozen section margins can be sent of the marrow, periosteum, and inferior alveolar nerves. Reconstruction must then be completed as will be described below.

Reconstruction. Reconstruction of oropharygeal defects often is not simple because of the complex integration of form and function in this region. Reconstruction varies by the site of the defect and extent of surrounding tissue involved as well as by the size of the tissue loss. Each defect is considered individually to obtain the best end result. In addition to defect considerations, patient characteristics must be considered when choosing reconstruction. This includes functional needs, available donor sites, comorbidities, and tolerance of anesthetic. As with other reparative tasks, the reconstructive ladder is a useful tool in thinking about methods of repair. The tool allows one to consider the closure and repair of surgical defects from the most simple to the most complex.

The reconstructive ladder begins with a region of open tissue after neoplasm resection, and the most basic means of reconstruction along the ladder are suitable for small, simple defects. The first means of reconstruction begins with healing by granulation or secondary intention, which of course requires no further surgical intervention. This method can be used in the oropharynx for simple tissue defects. Healing by secondary intention allows granulation tissue to fill a small defect with sensate tissue that is generally not tethered. This would be appropriate for a small defect at the soft palate, tongue base, or pharyngeal wall but should not be used in areas in continuity with the neck, adjacent to important structures,

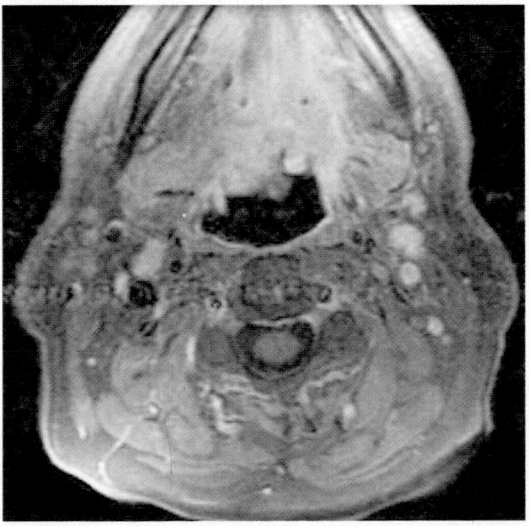
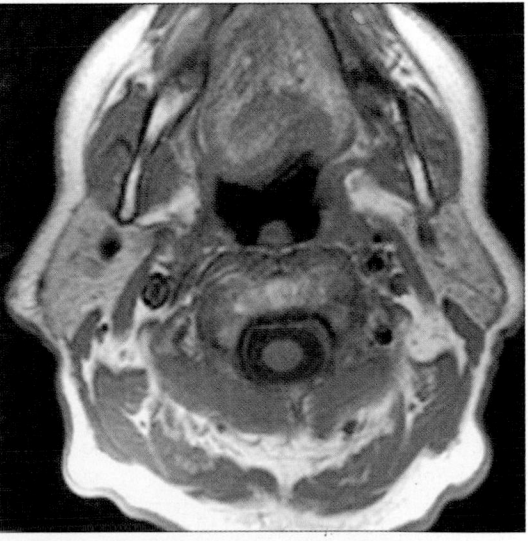

(A) (B)

Figure 4 Magnetic resonance imaging (MRI) showing bone marrow involvement with squamous cell carcinoma necessitating a composite resection. (A) Axial T1-weighted, gadolinium enhanced and with fat saturation image demonstrates an enhancing squamous cell carcinoma involving the left base of tongue with extension across the midline, (B) axial T1-weighted precontrast image shows early bone marrow involvement of the left mandible which will require a composite resection for tumor extirpation.

or overlying bone. Healthy tissue is required for adequate granulation and thus, patients with poor vasculature or tissue health will achieve a less optimum result from this method. Similarly, primary closure can be used on small defects within the oropharynx which have sufficient tissue laxity for reapproximation. Benefits of this method also include sensate tissue but tethering of structures can occur which may result in functional defects. Healthy tissue is also a requisite for primary closure.

The next step along the ladder's progression is the skin graft. For oropharyngeal defects, a split-thickness graft is generally used. A split-thickness skin graft is appropriate for some small- and intermediate-sized defects and is often harvested from the lateral aspect of the thigh using a dermatome. Skin grafts are most useful in regions that are not highly mobile or subject to tensile forces, as the graft must remain adherent for inosculation and graft take. Areas that can be skin grafted include the soft palate and pharyngeal wall. Typically split-thickness skin grafts will not heal well to exposed bony surfaces. The graft is traditionally secured with a bolster, but Dermabond (octyl-2-cyanocrylate) and overlying sutures are also a successful means of immobilization.

The reconstructive ladder proceeds to local flaps for reconstruction of moderate-sized defects. Tissue health including things such as history of past radiation, nutritional status and vascularity are also important for this type of tissue rearrangement. Common types of local flaps used to

reconstruct oropharyngeal defects include a posterior tongue flap. This portion of tongue can be divided and pedicled posteriorly and rotated into a tonsillar or palatal defect. The vascularity is dependable; however, the patient may have significant speech and swallowing functional defects resulting from fixation of the tongue. The palatal island flap is useful in the oropharynx. This local flap is based on the greater palatine artery and is a rotation flap comprised of the mucosa, submucosa, and periostium overlying the hard palate. This tissue is rotated into a small- or medium-sized tonsillar pillar or soft palate defect with good results. Another local flap used to reconstruct oropharyngeal defects is the buccal mucosal flap. This flap is an advancement flap of buccal mucosa which can cover small defects of the retromolar trigone, tonsillar pillar, and soft palate.

Regional flaps are the next means of reconstructing oropharyngeal defects. These flaps historically were the workhorse means of reconstructing larger oropharyngeal defects prior to the era of free tissue transfer. Such pedicled regional flaps are still used today for reconstruction of the oropharynx and include the pectoralis major flap, deltopectoral flap, and latissimus dorsi flap. The pectoralis major flap is a myocutaneous pedicled flap based on the pectoral branch of the thoracoacromial artery. The pectoralis major flap can be used to reconstruct the tonsillar region, base of tongue, and soft palate but generally reaches no further superiorly than the top of the oropharynx. These flaps are reliable and allow for a large myocutaneous paddle to be rotated into place in a single stage. The donor-site morbidity is relatively mild from a functional standpoint but can be less than ideal from a cosmetic standpoint, particularly for a woman. These flaps are insensate and can be less than optimum for three-dimensional filling of a large defect due to their tether to the chest. As a result functional outcomes for speech and swallowing can be less than ideal.

The latissimus dorsi pedicled regional flap can be used to reconstruct oropharyngeal defects. This flap is based on the thoracodorsal artery off of the circumflex scapular system. This flap is a reliable, myocutaneous flap that can be used in a single stage. Intraoperative positioning may add operative time to the procedure, but the donor-site morbidity is mild. Difficulties with the flap are due to inadequate reach to oropharyngeal defects and lack of ability to create an optimum three-dimensional reconstruction due to the long rotational pedicle. The latissimus dorsi muscle can also be used as a free tissue transfer as will be later discussed with the subscapular system free tissue transfer.

The deltopectoral flap is another pedicled regional flap used to reconstruct oropharyngeal defects. This flap is based on perforators from the intercostal arteries, particularly the first two, off of the internal mammary artery. This flap was popularized in the 1960s for head and neck reconstruction. It has been used for reconstructing mucosal pharyngeal defects. This flap can be raised in a single stage but delaying it allows for

greater pedicle length. The donor-site morbidity is minimal. The reconstructive result from this flap in the oropharynx is marginal and thus this flap is typically not a first choice for such reconstruction.

Free tissue transfer represents the last rung on the reconstructive ladder and for many patients is the gold standard today for reconstruction of moderate and large defects of the oropharynx. As with smaller defects in the oropharynx, the choice of free flap depends on the details of the defect. Defects may require soft tissue only or bony reconstruction. Bulk may be necessary to help restore function. In addition, availability of donor sites must be considered when choosing a means of free tissue transfer reconstruction. Soft tissue flaps of the subscapular system will be discussed during the segment on free tissue bony reconstruction.

For defects that require only soft tissue reconstruction and require little bulk, the radial forearm fasciocutaneous free tissue transfer is an ideal choice. This flap is based on the radial artery, venae comitantes, and cephalic vein and is a reliable method of free tissue reconstruction (Figures 5 and 6). Vascularity of the hand and distal forearm is tested preoperatively with the Allen test to ensure that the ulnar artery will be adequate via the superficial palmar arch. The donor morbidity is typically minor, but a skin graft is typically required for closure. The forearm flap is especially useful in palatal and pharyngeal wall reconstruction due to its pliability and flexibility. It can also be used for smaller defects of the tonsillar fossa and base of tongue that do not require significant bulk.

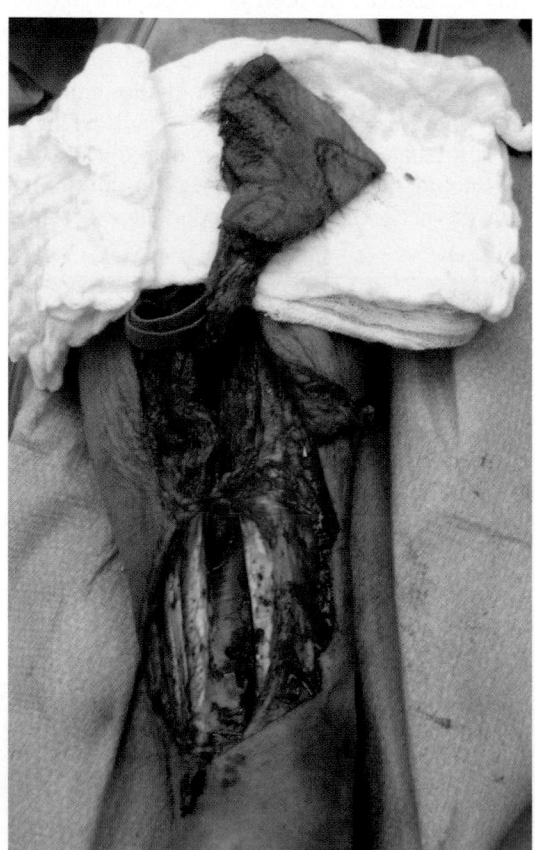

Figure 5 Photograph of harvesting the radial forearm free tissue transfer for reconstruction of oropharyngeal defect. Elevation of the radial forearm free tissue transfer prior to reconstruct a tonsillar and palate defect.

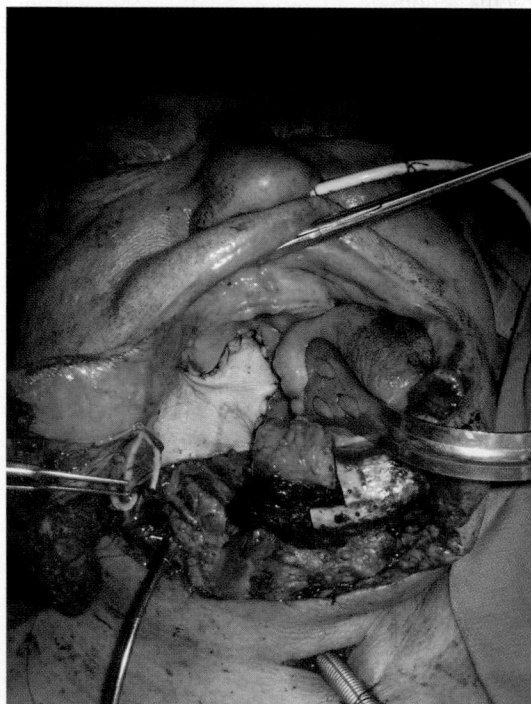

Figure 6 Photograph of a radial forearm free tissue transfer inset into oropharynx. The radial forearm free tissue transfer is well suited to reconstruct many tonsillar and hemi-soft palate defects, with additional tissue available to reconstruct small adjacent defects of the base of tongue and retromolar trigone.

When more bulk is required, the lateral arm fasciocutaneous flap is a good choice. This flap is based on the posterior radial collateral artery a branch of the profunda brachii and a paired venous system. Harvest of the posterior radial collateral artery with this flap can be completed without concern for the residual arterial inflow to the arm. The donor site can frequently be closed with a linear approximation of the wound margins without use of a skin graft. This flap works well for moderate to large defects of the base of tongue and tonsillar region. It can be used for large palatal and pharyngeal defects as well. The flap allows for adequate bulk in regions where the volume of the reconstruction is important to the functional result.

The anterolateral thigh free tissue transfer is another fasciocutaneous flap which allows for bulk in oropharyngeal reconstruction. The anterolateral thigh is based on the descending branch of the lateral femoral circumflex artery which is found surrounded by the vastus lateralis, rectus femoris, and tensor fascia latae. This flap allows for nice bulk of reconstruction in the oropharynx especially for large defects of the base of tongue and tonsil, and the donor-site morbidity is relatively minor. This flap can, however, be technically difficult to harvest, and at times perforators adequate for cutaneous paddle arterial inflow can be difficult to find.

In a situation where significant bulk is necessary for adequate soft tissue reconstruction, the rectus abdominus free flap is a good choice. This musculocutaneous flap is based on the deep inferior epigastric artery and vein; however the superior epigastric vessels can be used as well. There is no opportunity for sensory nerve transfer. The rectus abdominous is quite reliable, and harvest is not technically demanding. Significant bulk can be provided by this flap which is useful in large defects including those of the tongue. The donor-site morbidity is typically mild but can include an ileus in the immediate postoperative period or a ventral hernia during the recovery.

Advanced malignancies of the oropharynx can invade mandibular bone as previously described. In such instances, a composite resection is necessary and bony reconstruction is needed. The bony resection nearly always results in a lateral defect only. The principle of the reconstructive ladder exists for replacing mandibular bone. The lowest rung on the ladder is to do nothing—not replace the bone or reapproximate the mandible and allow the jaw to "swing." The second option on this reconstructive ladder would be to plate the jaw and primarily close the bony defect. This is only an option in an edentulous patient. Following the reconstructive ladder up, the next option is reconstructing the mandible in anatomic position with a reconstructive bar and covering the defect with a pedicled or free flap of soft tissue. Again, this may only be used in an edentulous patient, as the mastication forces generated by a person with teeth will almost certainly result in fracture of the bar. Reconstruction of the mandible could also be completed by a free bone graft plated in the region.

Healing of such nonvascularized tissue is often difficult adjacent to saliva and in the microbial environment of the upper digestive tract, particularly in patients undergoing radiation. The gold standard and last rung on the reconstructive ladder is to reconstruct the mandible with a vascularized free tissue transfer which includes bone.

The first option for vascularized bone in this situation is a fibular free flap. This flap is an osteocutaneous free tissue transfer based on the peroneal artery and its venae comitantes. Up to 25 cm of bone can be harvested from this nonweight-bearing bone while still preserving the integrity of the knee and ankle joints. Fasciocutaneous perforators supply the skin paddle of this flap which is best centered at the mid- to lower-third of the fibula. Although useful, this skin paddle typically cannot adequately reconstruct a large, bulky soft tissue defect in the oropharynx. It is also less reliable than the bony transplant with a rate of loss of 5 to 10%. Osteotomies can be nicely used to recreate the shape of the mandible with the bony portion of this flap. This bony reconstruction is reliable and can allow the placement of osseointegrated implants to the bone at a later date. Donor-site morbidity can include weakness of dorsiflexion of the great toe and edema. Ambulation is possible within the first postoperative week.

The iliac crest free tissue transfer represents another alternative for bony reconstruction of the mandible in oropharyngeal defects. This flap is based on the deep circumflex artery and its venae comitantes and can reconstruct composite defects resulting from oropharyngeal malignancies. Up to 16 cm of bone can be harvested from the crest, which can be both osteocutaneous and osteomusculocutaneous if the internal oblique is included. This flap can nicely reconstruct a mandibular segment and works well for later dental implants. It is technically easier to maneuver if the internal oblique is included. Donor-site morbidity can include ventral hernias which can be prevented by careful postharvest closure as well as postoperative ileus.

Another choice for vascularized bone in reconstruction of the oropharynx is the scapular free flap. This versatile flap is based on the subscapular system which can supply multiple variations of free tissue reconstruction. The resulting free tissue transfer can be fasciocutaneous, osteocutaneous, and musculocutaneous as well as combinations of these to result in the scapular, parascapular, latissimus, and serratus free flaps. The subscapular system begins with the subscapular artery, a branch of the axillary artery. This divides into the circumflex scapular artery and the thoracodorsal artery. The circumflex scapular artery supplies the periosteum of the lateral border of the scapula as well as the scapular and parascapular surrounding soft tissue. The thoracodorsal artery sends branches to the latissimus dorsi, serratus anterior, and scapular tip in the form of the angular artery, as well as supplying the surrounding soft tissue.

As a result of the diverse tissue and branching vascular supply surrounding the scapula, multiple flaps can be designed for various reconstructive needs. Parascapular fasciocutaneous flaps based on the circumflex scapular artery as well as musculocutaneous flaps based on the thoracodorsal artery can nicely fill soft tissue defects of the oropharynx. Bony defects up to 10 cm from a composite resection and their adjacent soft tissue defects can be reconstructed with a scapular osteocutaneous flap or with a scapular tip osteocutaneous flap, from the angular branch, allowing for longer pedicle length. These flaps supply both good quality bone for the mandible and bulky soft tissue for large tissue deficits. Finally, complex composite defects of intraoral and intrapharyngeal soft tissue, bone, and cutaneous soft tissue can be reconstructed by utilizing the entire subscapular system by using a bony scapular segment with two soft tissue paddles or one large folded paddle. The benefits of the scapular region free tissue transfers are versatility and ability to reconstruct a large complex defect with one pedicle. The downside includes a lateral decubitus or semidecubitus position for harvest which prevents two-team surgery. Patient morbidity can include shoulder pain and mild dysfunction.

Rehabilitation

The treatment for oropharyngeal squamous cell carcinoma is not an innocuous or easy endeavor. After chemotherapy and radiation therapy treatment, dysphagia and xerostomia are the most frequent complaints. This can result in gastric tube dependence, reliance on a soft or liquid diet, and aspiration. Patients also complain of sore throat and dysgusia. These symptoms typically evolve and improve over the first year posttreatment, but attention must be given to rehabilitation, especially through work with a speech pathologist. Likewise, surgical treatment in the area frequently results in dysphagia and dysarthria, depending on the location and size of the primary neoplasm, resection, and type of reconstruction. Again, the speech pathologist is essential to assisting the patient and training the patient to use functional methods to cope with these difficulties. Behavior modification is also important to treatment response and recovery. Because tobacco use has been shown to diminish the effectiveness of treatment, patients must be strongly instructed and assisted in smoking cessation.[19,20] Nutritional status is similarly important in tolerating treatment and recovery, and support in this regard is also essential.[21] Finally, patients with oropharyngeal malignancies must be followed closely for recurrence and metastases once treatment is complete. Physical examination, although often difficult due to edema and posttreatment change, is the primary means to do this and should address the primary site as well as the neck. Typically a schedule of return visits of every 6 to 8 weeks year one, every 2 to 3 months year two, every 3 to 4 months year three, every 4 to 6 months year four, and yearly starting in year five. Once patients have reached the 2-year mark posttreatment, the likelihood of local or regional recurrence diminishes significantly and distant metastases are of more concern. Patients should also be followed for distant metastases with a chest X-ray 6 months and then 1 year posttreatment, then yearly from there. TSH should be drawn as well on the same schedule to evaluate for posttreatment hypothyroidism.

HYPOPHARYNX

Anatomy and Physiology

The hypopharynx is a continuation of the upper aerodigestive tract from the oropharynx. It is comprised of three subsites which are the lateral and posterior pharyngeal wall, postcricoid region, and paired pyriform sinuses (Figure 7). The hypopharynx begins superiorly with the posterior pharyngeal wall at the level of the hyoid bone. Here it abuts the inferior-most point of the oropharynx. The posterior pharyngeal wall continues inferiorly to the level of the lowest point of the postcricoid region. This is marked by the inferior-most aspect of the cricoid cartilage, and it is here that the pharynx becomes the cervical esophagus. The lateral border of the hypopharynx is the mucosa covering the thyroid cartilage. The anterior border of the hypopharynx comprises several structures which are not themselves part of the hypopharynx: the epiglottis, the laryngeal aditus, the aryepiglottic folds, the arytenoids, and cricoarytenoid joints. Sitting just posterior to the cricoarytenoid joints and cricoid cartilage with

their attached muscles, is the postcricoid region. This comprises mucosa and submucosa overlying the cartilaginous ring of the cricoid and the posterior muscles of the larynx. At the inferior-most point of the postcricoid region and inferior pharyngeal constrictor, lays the cricopharyngeus muscle or upper esophageal sphincter. This lies just deep to the submucosa at the lowest point of the hypopharynx, inserting onto the cricoid cartilage. The pyriform sinuses are outpouchings of mucosa just lateral to the glottis proper, and they open posteriorly into the pharynx. They are funnel-shaped with the inferiorly oriented apex lying approximately at the level of the base of the cricoarytenoid joint. The superior border is marked by the pharyngoepiglottic fold. The medial wall of the pyriform sinus is adjacent to the aryepiglottic fold, false vocal fold, true vocal fold, arytenoids, and cricoid cartilage. The lateral wall of the pyriform sinus is contiguous with the lateral pharyngeal wall and is bounded by the thyroid cartilage and thyrohyoid membrane.

As in the oropharynx, the pharyngeal wall, pyriform sinus walls, and postcricoid tissue are comprised of mucosa and submucosa. Minor salivary glands are also present, scattered throughout the region. Deep to the posterior pharyngeal wall and lateral walls of the pyriform sinuses, lays the inferior constrictor muscle, and then the pharyngobasilar fascia. In the region immediately posterior to the hypopharynx, the same relationships regarding the alar fascia and prevertebral fascia are present as in the oropharynx. This results in a retropharyngeal space, danger space, and pre-

vertebral space that are in continuity with those above. Abutting the hypopharynx laterally are the great vessels as well as lymphatic and neural structures just external to the visceral space. The thyroid gland typically is located just inferior to the lowest point of the hypopharynx.

The hypopharynx has a varied neurovascular supply. The arterial inflow stems from the external carotid system in the form of the ascending pharyngeal and the superior thyroid arteries as well as from the inferior thyroid artery off the thyrocervical trunk from the subclavian system. The venous drainage pattern parallels this in the form of the pharyngeal venous plexus. The sensory supply to the hypopharynx is provided by the CN IX as well as the internal branch of the superior laryngeal nerve, from the vagus nerve. Motor innervation of the muscles of the hypopharynx, the inferior pharyngeal constrictor, and the cricopharyngeus, is provided by the pharyngeal plexus, comprised of CNs IX and X. Extensive submucosal lymph channels are evident in the hypopharynx, making regional metastases a prominent feature of carcinomas in this site. The lymphatic drainage of the hypopharynx has been mapped to lymph nodes in levels II, III, and IV, as well as retropharyngeal lymph nodes. Metastases to level I and level V lymph nodes are uncommon, however, level V is more likely to be involved if level IV nodes are positive. More inferior nodal basins can also be involved including the paratracheal, paraesophageal, and level VI lymph nodes. Bilateral drainage can occur especially with primary neoplasms at the medial pyriform aspect of the sinus.

The hypopharynx, like the oropharynx, serves as a respiratory and alimentary conduit. The hypopharyngeal structures are important players in the process of swallowing. The hypopharynx is primarily involved in the pharyngeal phase of swallowing, during which a food bolus travels from the oropharynx, through the hypopharynx, and into the cervical esophagus. During this phase, laryngeal elevation and glottic protection occur as do velopharyngeal closure and base of tongue propagation of the food bolus. As the food transits, the pharyngeal walls of the hypopharynx contract to clear food deposits from the pharynx and pyriform sinuses. At the completion of the pharyngeal phase of swallowing, the pharyngeal pressure continues to increase from the contraction of the pharyngeal constrictors and the tonic contraction of the cricopharyngeus is released. The food bolus then passes through the upper esophageal sphincter into the cervical esophagus.

Histopathology

Mucosa in the hypopharynx comprises stratified squamous cell epithelium. Similar to the oropharynx, this is typically nonkeratinized but can become keratinized in response to irritation. As a result, squamous cell carcinoma is by far the most common neoplasm found in the hypopharynx and is most frequently keratinizing. All variants of this malignancy have been found within the

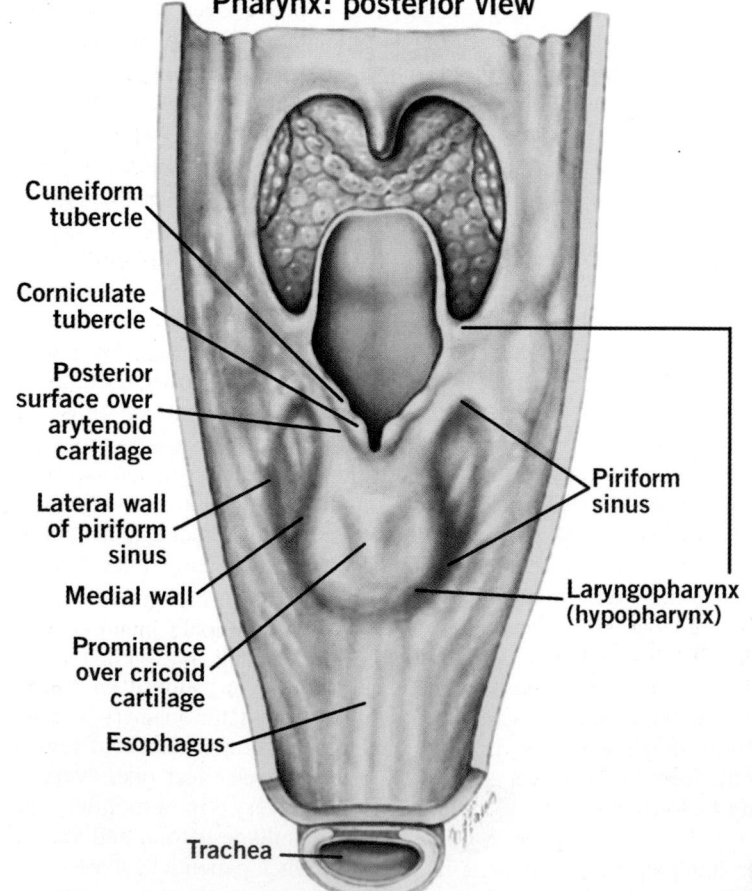

Pharynx: posterior view

Cuneiform tubercle

Corniculate tubercle

Posterior surface over arytenoid cartilage

Lateral wall of piriform sinus

Medial wall

Prominence over cricoid cartilage

Esophagus

Trachea

Piriform sinus

Laryngopharynx (hypopharynx)

Figure 7 Anatomy of the hypopharynx.

hypopharynx including verrucous, baseloid, adenosquamous, and spindle cell.

In addition, lymphoepithelial neoplasms have been found in the hypopharynx as have lymphomas. Adenocarcinomas originating from glandular structures native to the hypopharynx or from ectopic gastric tissue have also been found in the hypopharynx. Papilloma, secondary to HPV, and other benign lesions can be present in the hypopharynx. Precursor lesions to squamous cell carcinoma such as leukoplakia and erythroplakia can also occur in the hypopharynx, but are uncommonly seen especially since these lesions are frequently asymptomatic. Minor salivary gland neoplasms of a benign and malignant nature can also occur in this location. Sarcomas can also arise in the hypopharynx.

Etiology and Epidemiology

Malignancy of the hypopharynx is not a common illness, and this cancer comprises less than 1% of all malignancies. The incidence of squamous cell carcinoma of the hypopharynx is 0.7 per 100,000 persons in the United States as recorded in the SEER database. At present this malignancy is more common in men in all subsites; however, historically it was more common in women in the postcricoid region. The most common site of hypopharyngeal malignancy in the United States is the pyriform sinus; however, in other parts of the world including the Middle East, the postcricoid region is more common. This is thought to be secondary to differences in diet.

Squamous cell carcinoma of the hypopharynx is associated with tobacco and alcohol exposure. Similar to the oropharynx, tobacco is more strongly causative, yet these two substances act synergistically when consumed together. Although HPV has been found in hypopharyngeal squamous cell carcinomas and it may play a part in carcinogenesis in this site, there is no evidence that the viral carcinogenesis that is so prominent in the oropharynx occurs in a similar manner in the hypopharynx. Laryngopharyngeal reflux is thought to play a carcinogenic role, particularly in postcricoid carcinoma. Patients with the Plummer–Vinson syndrome have a high risk of developing hypopharyngeal carcinoma. This syndrome occurs primarily in women and is comprised of a constellation of webbing of the esophagus and hypopharynx, iron-deficiency anemia, dysphagia, and weight loss. Also known as Paterson–Kelly syndrome, it is thought to result in squamous cell carcinoma just proximal to a web because of chronic irritation in this region. Plummer–Vinson syndrome is now more widely recognized and treated than in prior generations, resulting in a decreased incidence of hypopharyngeal carcinoma in this group.

Pathophysiology and Mechanisms of Spread

Squamous cell carcinoma of the hypopharynx most commonly occurs in the pyriform sinus. Particularly when the medial wall of the sinus is involved, these neoplasms may invade deeply into glottic and supraglottic structures. The false vocal fold, arytenoid, and aryepiglottic fold may be involved. The cricoarytenoid joint or true vocal cord may be involved and result in vocal fold paresis or paralysis. With further extension, these cancers can involve the preepiglottic and paraglottic spaces as well. Lesions originating at the lateral wall of the pyriform sinus often spread to the posterior pharyngeal wall but can involve the thyroid cartilage or the thyroid gland.

Malignancy arising from the posterior pharyngeal wall is likely to spread longitudinally along the pharyngeal wall, superiorly to the oropharynx and inferiorly to the cervical esophagus. These lesions can also invade deeply into the retropharyngeal space or prevertebral muscles. Squamous cell carcinoma of the postcricoid region frequently invades into the cricoid cartilage and posterior glottic musculature, including the posterior cricoarytenoid muscles. All lesions of the hypopharynx may have significant submucosal spread, even with normal appearing mucosa, and this must be considered if primary surgical treatment is being performed. Skip lesions can result from this spread pattern necessitating wider margins (2 to 3 cm) during surgical resection as well as frozen section margins at that time.

Because regional lymphatic channels are so rich in the tissues surrounding the hypopharynx, lymph node metastases are common in hypopharyngeal squamous cell carcinoma. T1 to T2 lesions have evidence of lymphadenopathy at presentation in approximately one-half of patients, but greater than three-quarters of patients with primary neoplasms larger than T2 have evidence of lymphadenopathy at presentation. Approximately 40% of patients have evidence of occult micrometastases in the clinically N0 neck after neck dissection.[22] Regional metastases are evident in the contralateral neck at presentation in greater than 15%, and occult positive nodes are present at a greater rate than this, nearly 50% in some studies.[23] Five-year survival rates for all-comers with hypopharyngeal cancer are 25 to 40%.

Clinical Manifestations

Patients with squamous cell carcinoma of the hypopharynx often present with advanced disease, and this unfortunately affects prognosis. The hypopharynx is not amenable to examination by nonotolaryngologists as it requires indirect mirror evaluation or nasopharyngoscopic examination. In addition, early symptoms of hypopharyngeal malignancy can be vague, and their significance can be missed. Patients often present with dysphagia, voice change, sore throat, or globus sensation. A neck mass is not infrequently the first sign of a hypopharyngeal cancer, with approximately 25% of patients with this malignancy presenting this complaint. As the disease progresses, otalgia often becomes a prominent feature and weight loss is evident. Regional lymphatic spread continues and more than two-thirds of patients have evidence of palpable neck metastases at presentation to the otolaryngologist. Likewise,

distant metastatic disease and second primary malignancies are more common in hypopharyngeal malignancies than in most other sites in the upper aerodigestive tract. As a result, signs and symptoms such as hemoptysis, dyspnea, hematuria, and jaundice should alert the physician to the possibility of more widespread disease.

Diagnosis and Work-Up

The process of diagnosis and work-up of a hypopharyngeal malignancy is largely similar to that of oropharyngeal malignancies. A thorough history must be obtained including risk factors such as alcohol and tobacco use or Plummer–Vinson syndrome. Other medical comorbidities and all previous treatments must be ascertained. A physical examination is completed which includes an indirect mirror examination as well as flexible fiberoptic nasopharyngoscopy. Large exophytic lesion are easily visualized with these examinations, and many invasive carcinomas can show evidence of vocal fold weakness. Smaller lesions may be less obvious on in-office examination, but have evidence of secretions pooling in the postcricoid region or pyriform sinuses as well as edema and erythema of laryngeal and hypopharyngeal structures. The neck is thoroughly examined for any adenopathy. After the examination, the neoplasm should be staged as well as possible.

The work-up should proceed with diagnostic imaging as well as panendoscopy with biopsy in the operating room. A CT scan of the neck is extremely helpful in evaluating and staging these lesions, particularly with regard to extent of primary neoplasm and evidence of regional lymphatic spread. If cartilaginous invasion is in question or further soft tissue delineation is necessary, MRI scanning can be helpful. The chest must also be evaluated for metastatic disease, and a CT scan of the thorax is the study of choice for this. A chest radiograph is also acceptable but provides less information. The patient then undergoes operating room endoscopy. Direct laryngoscopy, esophagoscopy, and biopsy are completed under general anesthesia, and formal staging is completed in this setting. During this evaluation close attention must be given to detecting a second primary malignancy in the upper aerodigestive tract; the oral cavity is a common site for this to occur with a hypopharyngeal squamous cell carcinoma. Some continue to recommend bronchoscopy as part of the operative endoscopy for the diagnosis of a second primary, however, CT scanning of the thorax is more sensitive for detecting a primary pulmonary malignancy. Once operative evaluation, radiographic imaging, and staging have been completed, the patient optimally should be presented to a multidisciplinary neoplasm board for treatment planning.

Staging and Prognosis

Squamous cell carcinoma of the hypopharynx is staged with the AJCC system[9] (Table 4). This begins with evaluation of the primary neoplasm,

Table 4   American Joint Committee on Cancer Tumor Categorization of Hypopharyngeal Squamous Cell Carcinoma[9]

T1	Tumor limited to one subsite of hypopharynx and 2 cm or less in greatest dimension
T2	Tumor invades more than one subsite of hypopharynx or an adjacent site, or measures more than 2 cm but not more than 4 cm in greatest diameter without fixation of hemilarynx
T3	Tumor more than 4 cm in greatest dimension or with fixation of hemilarynx
T4a	Tumor invades thyroid/cricoid cartilage, hyoid bone, thyroid gland, esophagus, or central compartment soft tissue
T4b	Tumor invades prevertebral fascia, encases carotid artery, or involves mediastinal structures

to which a T value is assigned. This categorization is based on size, involvement with adjacent sites, and finally involvement of areas which indicate advanced disease or poorer prognosis. Regional lymphatic spread is likewise staged to give a nodal or N category. This is also determined by size and location of nodal disease. Lastly, depending on the presence or absence of metastasis, an M category, is given. These three assessments are put together to create a TNM label for each patient as well as a stage of disease (see Tables 2 and 3). In general, any evidence of nodal disease will cause patients to be considered at least stage III. T4 neoplasms and more bulky lymphadenopathy will fall into Stage IV, with T4b considered unresectable. Positive nodal disease in level V portends a poor prognosis, and contralateral nodal disease is likewise an adverse risk factor. Due to the high frequency of advanced primary neoplasm, extensive regional metastases, and relatively increased incidence of distant metastases and concurrent second primary neoplasms, outcomes in hypopharyngeal squamous cell carcinoma are some of the worst of all head and neck malignancies. Unfortunately, these outcomes have improved by only small degrees over recent decades. The most recent AJCC survival statistics show 5-year survival for squamous cell carcinoma of the hypopharynx to be 41% in Stage I disease and 36% in Stage II disease. More frequently patients present with Stage III and IV disease, which have 5-year survival rates of 36% and 10%, respectively.

Therapy

General Approach. The general approach to treating squamous cell carcinoma of the hypopharynx has changed significantly over the last several decades. Previously a malignancy treated primarily by surgical extirpation, hypopharyngeal squamous cell cancer is now often treated with organ preservation protocols. As most of this patient population present with advanced disease, few of these neoplasms meet criteria for conservation surgical procedures. Thus, typically the primary attempts at organ preservation are achieved through chemotherapy and radiother-

apy as the initial treatment. If the end result of organ preservation therapy is residual or recurrent disease, then radical surgery is performed and frequently requires free tissue transfer reconstruction. Of course, resectability and the absence of distant metastatic disease must be ensured prior to such extensive surgical procedures.

Organ Preservation. The idea of organ preservation in treatment of squamous cell carcinoma of the hypopharynx has evolved to prominence over the last 20 years. Radiation therapy for such lesions is not a novel idea, however, this treatment alone is only successful in small primary neoplasms. In the late 1980s and early 1990s interest in preserving the laryngeal and pharyngeal structures grew. Trials specific to hypopharyngeal malignancies built on previous and ongoing studies of organ preservation in the head and neck, such as those mentioned in the oropharynx section. A trial conducted by the (European Organization for Research and Treatment of Cancer) EORTC in the early 1990s showed favorable results comparing induction chemotherapy followed by radiation to surgical treatment followed by radiation in treatment of hypopharyngeal squamous cell carcinoma.[24] A subsequent randomized clinical trial of patients with resectable hypopharyngeal neoplasms compared treatment with induction chemotherapy followed by surgery then postoperative radiation with induction chemotherapy followed by radiation alone (surgery was used for salvage). In this study, patients who underwent all three modalities (chemotherapy, surgery, and radiation) had improved survival over chemotherapy and radiation but of course did not have organ preservation.[25] Another study assessed hyperfractionated radiation therapy and its use in combination with concurrent chemotherapy for advanced head and neck tumors.[26] In this study the combined chemotherapy and radiation therapy regimen produced improved survival. The Radiation Therapy Oncology Group (RTOG) 91-11 (year and number of study initiated in that year) trial evaluated induction chemotherapy with radiation therapy, concurrent chemotherapy and radiation therapy, and radiation therapy alone for advanced laryngeal cancer.[27] Results indicated better locoregional control, laryngeal preservation, and rate of distant metastases with concurrent chemotherapy and radiation therapy but similar overall survival in induction and concurrent regimens. Similar studies are ongoing in a continued search to determine the most effective and least morbid treatment for squamous cell carcinoma of the hypopharynx and other upper aerodigestive tract sites.

Treatment Plan. Just as in oropharyngeal malignancy, treatment recommendations for hypopharyngeal malignancy vary based on T classification and nodal burden. Small lesions in the hypopharynx are less frequently diagnosed than advanced but can be treated with less aggressive regimens. Early T-category tumors (T1 or T2) without evidence of nodal disease are preferably treated with primary radiation therapy. Conservation laryngopharyngeal surgery is also considered stan-

dard of care for these lesions and should include bilateral selective neck dissection. In T1 lesions with N1 nodal disease, radiation therapy can still be considered the definitive therapy. If nodal disease persists posttreatment, a neck dissection should be performed. For T1N1 lesions being treated with primary surgical therapy, consideration should be given to performing a modified neck dissection instead of a selective. Poor prognostic features in the specimen (close margins, extracapsular spread from lymph nodes) should prompt postsurgical chemotherapy and radiation therapy, however, features such as multiple positive nodes, perineural invasion, or vascular invasion should typically be treated with postoperative radiation therapy alone.

For more advanced lesions of the hypopharynx, more aggressive treatment regimens are necessary in an attempt at cure. For stage III or IV squamous cell carcinoma of the hypopharynx, several treatment plans are considered standard of care. At our center, organ preservation protocols prevail, and this occurs by two primary mechanisms. The first occurs with induction chemotherapy, off-protocol or on-protocol as part of a clinical trial (in which case the exact procedure and agents may vary somewhat). Patients receive induction chemotherapy for two cycles and then undergo operative endoscopy to evaluate neoplasm response. Neoplasm tattoo and pretreatment documented staging assist in this evaluation. Evidence of complete response or partial response at the primary site allows patients to continue in the organ preservation protocol with a third cycle of chemotherapy followed by definitive radiation therapy or concomitant chemoradiation. For patients with nodal disease larger than 3 cm pretreatment, a planned posttreatment neck dissection is performed after therapy. For patients who achieve less than partial response at the primary site after induction chemotherapy, surgical salvage is then performed. This includes extirpation of the primary neoplasm, bilateral neck dissection, and necessary reconstruction, typically with free tissue transfer. Patient survival and laryngeal preservation rates are excellent with protocols using single-cycle induction for chemoradiation therapy for selection while utilizing early salvage surgery.[28] With regards to laryngeal preservation rates alone, however, there is no proven difference between induction and concurrent chemoradiation regimens.

Similar to induction chemotherapy regimens, patients can also be treated with concurrent chemotherapy and radiation therapy. The same principles apply to lack of response or recurrent disease as with induction chemotherapy in that patients are then treated with salvage surgery which is often quite technically challenging. Likewise, the same regimen applies for planned neck dissection posttreatment. As described in the oropharynx section, the criteria for proceeding with planned posttreatment neck dissection continue to change, and the role of PET in this regard continues to be evaluated.

Surgical therapy is also considered the standard of care for Stage III and IV hypopharyngeal cancer. At many centers this may be the first choice in treatment of these patients. This typically includes total laryngectomy with partial or total pharyngectomy and bilateral neck dissections followed by reconstruction. At our center, patients with T4a carcinomas of the hypopharynx have been treated via organ preservation protocols with success rates comparable to surgical therapy. This has not been universal at other centers, however, and as a result, many head and neck specialists recommend surgical therapy for T4a disease. This issue will no doubt continue to be studied via protocols in coming years so that the question of the viability of this approach is answered definitively.

Surgical Resection. Surgical treatment of hypopharyngeal malignancies can be used to treat small as well as advanced or recurrent primary disease. For small T1 or T2 neoplasms, consideration can be given to primary conservation surgery as described above. Unfortunately, however, these small primary neoplasms are few and far between. Patients with such small neoplasms must be evaluated as to their suitability to undergo conservation surgery. Factors such as comorbidities and performance status, particularly with regard to pulmonary disease, are important in patient selection for these procedures. Laryngeal subsite involvement and overall extent of disease are also important. Small lesions solely involving the lateral or posterior pharyngeal wall are amenable to primary resection, often via an endoscopic approach. A CO_2 laser is frequently used for this type of approach, and several groups have reported treatment success with this approach.

Suprahyoid and lateral pharyngotomy approaches can be used for open resection of small lesions of the pharyngeal wall. Lesions of the pyriform sinus and postcricoid region can also be evaluated for conservation surgery. Small lesions of the pyriform sinus may be resectable by partial laryngopharyngectomy if the apex is not involved, the interarytenoid region is free, vocal fold motion is preserved, and there is no evidence of cartilaginous invasion. Primary neoplasms of the postcricoid region are nearly impossible to resect with conservation of structures because of the close proximity of this subsite to many laryngeal structures. Larger primary neoplasms of the hypopharynx typically require total laryngectomy with partial or total pharyngectomy (Figure 8). Neoplasms of the larynx are discussed in Chapter 99, "Neoplasms of the Larynx."

Regardless of the evidence of nodal disease and the T category of the primary neoplasm, patients undergoing primary surgical treatment for hypopharyngeal squamous cell carcinoma should undergo neck dissection at the time of surgical extirpation due to the extensive regional lymphatics in the region. At least unilateral neck dissection should be performed including attention to retropharyngeal lymph nodes; but depending on the location and size of the primary neoplasm,

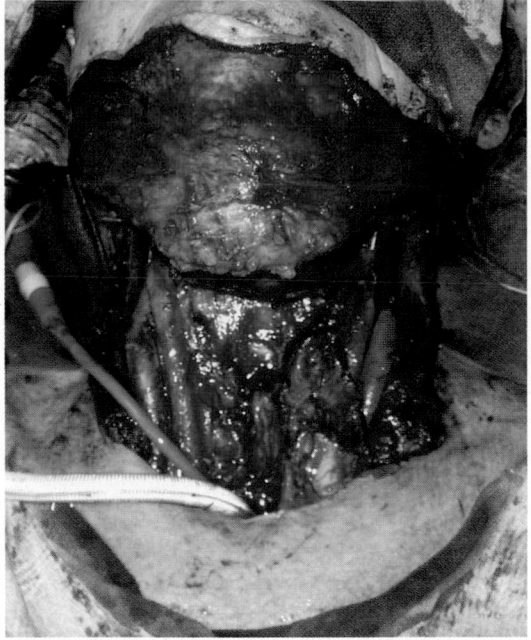

Figure 8 Photograph of laryngopharyngectomy in progress. Note the appearance of the neck during laryngopharyngectomy after removal of the specimen and ready for reconstruction.

bilateral neck dissection may be necessary. The type of neck dissection performed, selective versus modified radical or radical, is determined by the disease status at presentation. Levels I to V should be addressed in all cases.

Reconstruction. As in reconstruction after resection of oropharyngeal malignancies, in selecting a means of rebuilding it is useful to consider the options in a stepwise fashion from simplest to most complex, that is, to reconstruct defects that range from partial to subtotal to total pharyngectomy. Previous treatment effects on tissue vascularity and healing must be considered, as the rate of hypopharyngocutaneous fistulas with free flap closure of hypopharyngeal defects created by surgical salvage of previously chemoradiated tissue is around 20%.[29]

For small defects of the pharyngeal wall, healing by secondary intention, primary closure, or a skin graft may be acceptable. For larger defects that are subtotal, a pedicled flap such as the pectoralis major or latissimus dorsi can be used for reconstruction (see Figure 9). Similarly, vascularized free tissue can be used in such situations. The radial forearm free flap is an excellent choice in this location. Depending on the extent of the subtotal defect, the anterior lateral thigh free flaps and the temporoparietal fascial flaps could also be considered. For a total laryngectomy with partial or subtotal pharyngectomy defect, the radial forearm is again an ideal choice for a partially tubed reconstruction in this area.

When resection of the primary neoplasm requires total laryngopharyngectomy, a tubed reconstruction is necessary to build a neopharynx. This could be done with a pedicled flap, but a better result is obtained using free vascularized tissue. Such a free flap must have available

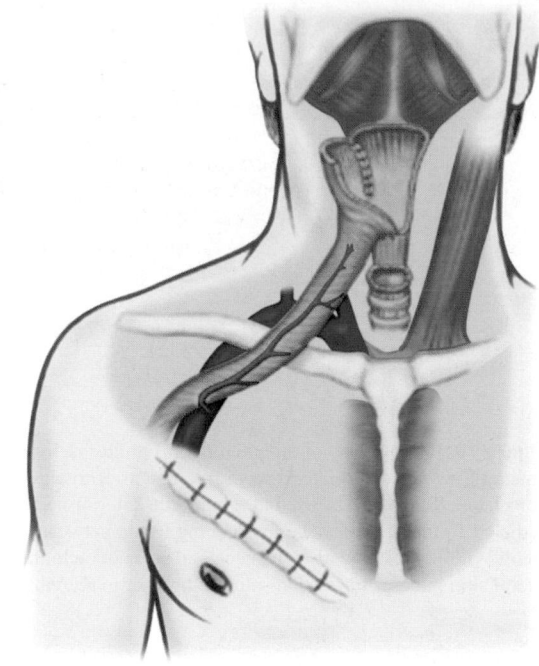

Figure 9 Pectoralis major flap used to reconstruct a partial hypopharyngeal defect.

vessels for vascular anastamoses, should be thin and pliable enough to reconstruct the pharynx, and should cover vital structures such as the carotid artery that are at high risk of exposure. Our first choice for this reconstruction is a tubed radial forearm free flap, an extremely reliable flap, which is pliable enough to nicely recreate a pharynx. If increased bulk is needed, particularly if cutaneous tissue must be reconstructed, the anterior lateral thigh free tissue transfer works well in this reconstruction (Figure 10). Such free fasciocutaneous flaps have been found to decrease fistula rates to 20% for hypopharyngeal reconstruction and also work well if the defect extends into the oropharynx.

Free jejunal grafts can also be used to create a tubed neopharynx. This free visceral transfer is supplied by a single mesenteric artery and vein, often from the second arcade. This flap requires the assistance of a general surgeon for harvest and bears the added risk of major abdominal surgery. The flap is susceptible to ischemia. Strictures occur in about 10% of patients causing dysphagia, which can also result from peristalsis. The voice produced can be "wet" which is improved with postoperative radiation. In cases where the extirpated tissue is inferior to the cricopharyngeus muscle, gastric interposition is necessary to keep the resection oncologically sound while making reconstruction technically possible. This flap is pedicled on the gastroepiploic vessels and is frequently complicated by leak, fistula, or reflux disease. The gastro-omental free tissue transfer is one other option for reconstructing a neopharynx. This involves the harvest of the greater curvature of the stomach with the right gastroepiploic artery. This provides nice great vessel coverage and a lower fistula rate but again involves the complications of abdominal surgery.

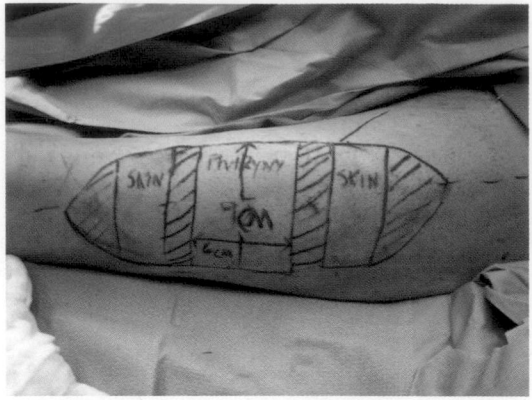
(A)

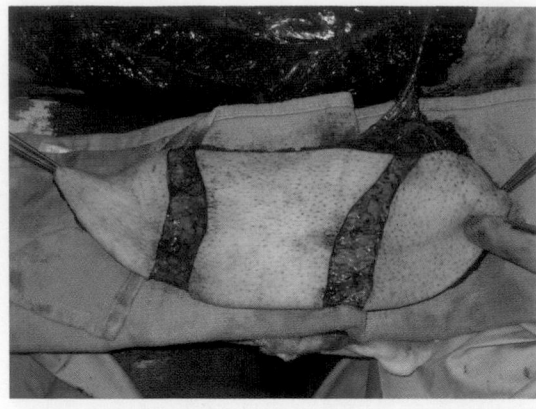
(B)

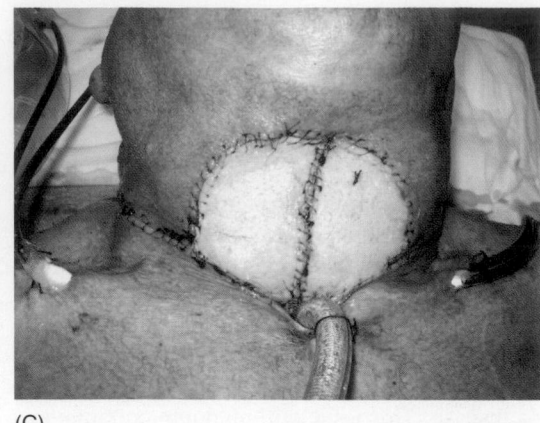
(C)

Figure 10 Photographs of an anterolateral thigh fasciocutaneous free flap being formed into a tube to reconstruct a laryngopharyngectomy defect and a cutaneous defect. (A) This image shows the anterolateral thigh free flap prior to elevation. The central portion measuring 9 by 6 cm will be formed into a tube to reconstruct the neopharynx. The two lateral portions labeled skin will be used to rebuild the anterior neck skin and will remain in continuity with the tubed central portion. (B) This image shows the free tissue transfer harvested and pedicled from the thigh. The intervening tissue between the central neopharynx tissue and lateral skin paddles has been de-epithelialized. This is necessary as these intervening segments will be located within the neck and will not be lining a mucosal or cutaneous surface. (C) This image shows the anterolateral thigh free tissue transfer inset into the neck. The two lateral skin paddles have been sutured together to recreate the anterior neck skin. The tubed central portion of the flap lies just deep to these skin paddles.

Rehabilitation

The treatment for squamous cell carcinoma of the hypopharynx is difficult, and the morbidity is not insignificant. After organ preservation techniques, weak voice, sore throat, dysphagia, and xerostomia are frequent complaints. Patients may have to limit themselves to a soft or liquid diet, may aspirate, and may depend on tube feedings for nutrition. This can result in gastric tube dependence, reliance on a soft or liquid diet, and aspiration. Surgical therapy at times preserves swallowing function but limits voice production. This occurs if results are not optimal with partial procedures or if total laryngectomy is performed and the patient has difficulty with tracheoesophageal speech or use of an electrolarynx. Work with a speech pathologist is critical, particularly during the first year posttreatment when the body and mechanisms of adaptation are heavily evolving. The speech pathologist plays an essential role in assisting the patient and training the patient to use functional methods to cope with these alterations in speech and swallowing. Similar to other squamous cell carcinomas of the head and neck, modification of unhealthful behaviors is also important to treatment response and recovery. Strong nutritional supplementation and abstinence from tobacco and alcohol predict a better prognosis for long-term survival.

Finally, just as with oropharyngeal malignancies, patients with squamous cell carcinoma of the hypopharynx must be followed closely for recurrence and metastases once treatment is complete. The primary means to evaluate patients is through a thorough physical examination of the head and neck region, with particular attention to the primary site and the neck. This can be difficult to accomplish because posttreatment tissue alteration in the form of edema and erythema is frequently significant. Patients should be monitored closely on a schedule which is spaced out as patients get farther from therapy. Return visits are scheduled approximately every 6 to 8 weeks during the first year, every 2 to 3 months during the second year, every 3 to 4 months during the third year, every 4 to 6 months during the fourth year, and once a year starting in the fifth year. A significant landmark for patients is that of reaching 2 years posttreatment without recurrence. Once this is achieved, the incidence of local or regional recurrence diminishes significantly, and distant metastases are of more concern. A chest X-ray is typically ordered 6 months and then 1 year after the completion of treatment, and then once a year subsequently. Thyroid function should be assessed on the same schedule to assess for hypothyroidism after surgical or chemoradiation in the area.

COMPLICATIONS

As in all sites of upper aerodigestive tract malignancy, complications can occur after the treatment of squamous cell carcinoma of the oropharynx and hypopharynx. In addition to the aforementioned side effects of surgical treatment, chemotherapy, and radiation therapy, complications of these treatments can occur. Wound infections or abscesses can occur requiring treatment with antibiotics or drainage. Dysphagia and strictures can result in esophageal obstruction, dehydration, or malnutrition with weight loss. Aspiration may result from both organ preservation therapy and conservation surgical therapy. This may be complicated by recurrent pneumonias. Fistulae may occur in the setting of poor wound healing and as a sign of residual or recurrent malignancy. Hemorrhage can occur during or after treatment. This can be minor or life threatening as in a carotid artery blowout. Airway obstruction can occur secondary malignancy or posttreatment changes and can require emergency treatment with a tracheostomy if severe. Osteoradionecrosis and chondroradionecrosis can occur after treatment of both oropharyngeal and hypopharyngeal malignancies with radiation therapy. This can result in fractures and or tissue loss which potentially require later free tissue transfer to rehabilitate the patient.

Although the current management for cancer of the oropharynx or hypopharynx has many complications that are severe and require extensive treatment, the average patient is still better served by the therapy compared to the alternative of not undergoing therapy.

CONCLUSIONS

Neoplasms of the oropharynx and hypopharynx are challenging lesions for the treating physician and the patient. Although largely squamous cell carcinomas, the management of these lesions in not one-sided and requires a complex understanding of the anatomy, physiology, and disease processes in the area. Management involves complex organ preservation therapies, radical operations, and intricate reconstructions. Multidisciplinary teams of otolaryngologists, radiation and medical oncologists, dentists, speech pathologists, nurses, and other specialists must be assembled to treat patients with these malignancies appropriately. In addition, strong partnerships must be created between treating physicians and basic scientists to continue to understand these diseases better at a molecular level. The acquisition of this knowledge brings better treatment regimens, more advanced protocols, and improvements in morbidity and mortality. Most importantly, research on squamous cell carcinoma of the oropharynx and hypopharynx allows the clinician to meet the challenge of the twenty-first century: to bridge not only the gaps in survival but also to improve on the equally important outcomes which are essential to the quality of a patient's life.

REFERENCES

1. Braakhuis BJM, Tabor MP, Leemans R, et al. Second primary tumors and field cancerization in oral and oropharyngeal cancer: Molecular techniques provide new insights and definitions. Head Neck 2002;24:198–206.
2. Goldenberg D. Mate': A risk factor for oral and oropharyngeal cancer. Oral Oncol 2002;38:646–9.
3. Dahlstrand HM, Dalianis T. Presence and influence of human papillomaviruses (HPV) in tonsillar cancer. Adv Cancer Res 2005;93:59–89.

4. D'Souza G, Kreimer AR, Viscidi R, et al. Case-control study of human papilloma virus and oropharyngeal cancer. N Engl J Med 2007: 356: 1944–56.

5. Greenlee RT, Hill-Harmon MB, Murray T, et al. Cancer statistics, 2001. Ca J Clin 2001;51:15–36.

6. SEER Cancer Statistics Review, 1975–2003. National Cancer Institute. April, 2006.

7. De Bree R, Deurloo EE, Snow GB, Leemans CR. Screening for distant metastases in patients with head and neck cancer. Laryngoscope 2000;110:397–401.

8. Brouwer J, de Brèe R, Hoekstra OS, et al. Screening for distant metastases in patients with head and neck cancer: Is chest computed tomography sufficient? Laryngoscope 2005;115:1813–7.

9. American Joint Committee on Cancer, Cancer Staging Manual, 6th edition; 2002.

10. Garavello W, Ciardo A, Spreafico R, Guini RM. Risk factors for distant metastases in head and neck squamous cell carcinoma. Arch Otolaryngol Head Neck Surg 2006;132:762–6.

11. Department of Veterans Affairs Laryngeal Cancer Study Group. Induction chemotherapy plus radiation compared with surgery plus radiation in patients with advanced laryngeal cancer. N Engl J Med 1991;324:1685–90.

12. Feng FY, Kim HM, Lyden TH, et al. Intensity-modulated radiotherapy of head and neck cancer aiming to reduce dysphagia: early dose-effect relationships for the swallowing structures. Int J Radiat Oncol Biol Phys. 2007; 68(5): 1289–98.

13. Bernier J, Domenge C, Ozsahin M, et al. Postoperative irradiation with or without concomitant chemotherapy for locally advanced head and neck cancer. N Engl J Med 2004;350:1945–52.

14. Cooper JS, Pajak TF, Forastiere AA, et al. Postoperative concurrent radiotherapy and chemotherapy for high-risk squamous-cell carcinoma of thc head and neck. N Engl J Med 2004;350:1937–44.

15. Bernier J, Cooper JS, Pajuk TF, et al. Defining risk levels in locally advanced head and neck cancers: A comparative analysis of concurrent postoperative radiation plus chemotherapy trials of the EORTC (#22931) and RTOG (#9501). Head Neck 2005;27:843–50.

16. Burtness B, Goldwasser MA, Flood W, et al. Phase III randomized trial of cisplatin plus placebo versus cisplatin plus antiepidermal growth factor-receptor antibody cetuximab in metastatic/recurrent head and neck cancer. J Clin Oncol 2005;23:8646–54.

17. Balsega J, Trigo JM, Bourhis J, et al. Phase II multicenter study of the antiepidermal growth factor receptor monoclonal antibody cetuximab in combination with platinum-based chemotherapy in patients with platinum-refractory metastatic and/or recurrent squamous cell carcinoma of the head and neck. J Clin Oncol 2005;23:5568–77.

18. Pradier O, Christiansen H, Schmidberger H, et al. Adjuvant radiotherapy after transoral laser microsurgery for advanced squamous carcinoma of the head and neck. Int J Radiat Oncol Biol Phys 2005;63:1368–77.

19. Schnoll RA, Zhang B, Rue M, et al. Brief physician-initiated quit-smoking strategies for clinical oncology settings: A trial coordinated by the Eastern Cooperative Oncology Group. J Clin Oncol 2003;21:355–65.

20. Gritz ER, Carr CR, Rapkin D, et al. Predictors of long-term smoking cessation in head and neck cancer patieints. Cancer Epidemiol Biomarkers Prev 1993;2:261–70.

21. Colasanto JM, Prasad P, Nash MA, et al. Nutritional support of patients undergoing radiation therapy for head and neck cancer. Oncology 2005;19:371–82.

22. Ferlito A, Shaha A, Buckley JG, Rinaldo A. Selective neck dissection for hypopharyngeal cancer in the clinically negative neck: Should it be bilateral? Acta Otolaryngol 2001;121:329–35.

23. Buckley JG, MacLennan K. Cervical node metastases in laryngeal and hypopharyngeal cancer: A prospective analysis of prevalence and distribution. Head Neck 2000;22: 380–5.

24. Lefebrvre JL, Chevalier D, Luboinski B, et al. Larynx preservation in pyriform sinus cancer: Preliminary results of a European Organization for Research and Treatment of Cancer phase III study. J Natl Cancer Inst 1996;13:890–9.

25. Beauvillain C, Mahe' M, Bourdin S, et al. Final results of a randomized trial comparing chemotherapy plus radiotherapy with chemotherapy plus surgery plus radiotherapy in locally advanced resectable hypopharyngeal carcinomas. Laryngoscope 1997;107:648–55.

26. Brizel DM, Albers ME, Fisher SR, et al. Hyperfractionated irradiation with or without concurrent chemotherapy for locally advanced head and neck cancer. N Engl J Med 1998;338:1798–1804.

27. Forastiere AA, Goepfert H, Maor M, et al. Concurrent chemotherapy and radiotherapy for organ preservation in advanced laryngeal cancer. N Engl J Med 2003;349: 2091–8.

28. Urba S, Wolf G, Eisbruch A, et al. Single-cycle induction chemotherapy selects patients with advanced laryngeal cancer for combined chemoradiation: a new treatment paradigm. J Clin Oncol 2006;24:593–8.

29. Teknos TN, Myers LL, Bradford CR, Chepeha DB. Free tissue reconstruction of the hypopharynx after organ preservation therapy: analysis of wound complications. Laryngoscope. 2001;111(7):1192–6

99

Neoplasms of the Larynx

Marshall Strome, MD
C. Arturo Solares, MD

Laryngeal carcinomas are prevalent in heavy smokers, tend to have a relatively early presentation, and with the exception of supraglottic malignancies, are less likely to metastasize early to the adjacent lymph nodes. Importantly, because of the shortened time from symptom evolution to diagnosis, tumors confined to the laryngeal framework have a substantially better prognosis. Early detection relates to the effectiveness of the American Cancer Society's campaign regarding early warning signs for malignancy which include persistent hoarseness and the ease of in-office endoscopic examination.

In the last decade, significant changes have occurred in the management of patients with advanced laryngeal malignancies. Prospective randomized studies have shown that a more conservative approach, that is, laryngeal preservation with chemoradiation therapy, as the initial treatment is feasible. Partial or total laryngectomy is reserved for cases of recurrent or persistent disease. Unfortunately, salvage surgery, following chemoradiation, results in increased surgical morbidity, including decreased voice quality following restorative measures and dysphagia. These issues need continued thought. Nevertheless, quality-of-life studies suggest that preservation of the larynx is a worthwhile goal and objective.

This chapter reviews the current knowledge in the diagnosis and treatment of laryngeal cancer and future directions in the management of this disease.

ETIOLOGY

Tobacco is the most acknowledged and preventable risk factor for the development of laryngeal cancer, being a documented covariable in 90 to 95% of these malignancies. The risk of malignancy rises as the use of tobacco increases.[1] Other factors increasing the carcinogenic potential of tobacco include hand-rolling cigarettes and use of dark tobacco.[2–4] The risk of developing laryngeal cancer decreases with time after smoking cessation. Thus, tobacco acts as a promoter and an initiator in carcinogenesis. A French study showed that people who smoked more than one packet of cigarettes a day have a risk that is 13 times higher than that of nonsmokers, and those who drink more than 1.5 L of wine per day have a risk that

is 34 times higher of developing head and neck cancer. Additional smoking risk is attributed to early age of onset and duration.[3] Alcohol is an independent risk factor and a significant covariable for laryngeal carcinoma. The combination of alcohol and smoking results in more than an additive risk.[3,5]

Mate, a Latin American tea that contains high levels of phenols, has been shown to increase the relative risk for laryngeal cancer in people who consume more than 1.5 L/d.[4] Other factors that have been linked to laryngeal cancer are occupational exposure to asbestos, nickel compounds, and certain mineral oils. Glass-wool has been associated with an increased mortality in a study from Italy.[6] Laryngopharyngeal reflux has also been linked to laryngeal cancer in some series.[7,8]

The genetics of head and neck cancer is an area of ongoing research. Aneuploidy accompanies the progression from dysplasia to malignancy.[9] Some of the chromosomal alterations associated with laryngeal carcinogenesis include 9p21 early in the process, 17p13.1, 3p25, and 3p14.2 in the intermediate events, and 8p21.3-p22 in the later stages of the process.[10] Alterations in the *p16* gene that acts in cell-cycle regulation have also been linked to laryngeal cancer.[11] Overexpression of p53 is noted in some laryngeal squamous cell carcinomas, and it likely plays an important role in an early stage of malignant transformation.[12] The activation of a proto-oncogene in 11q13 amplifies the oncogene cyclin D1, which activates cell wall progression and is associated with tumor invasion.[13] These are just some of the most relevant genetic alterations linked with laryngeal cancer.

The human papilloma virus (HPV) has been detected in head and neck squamous cell carcinoma, but the specific role of HPV in laryngeal cancer is not clear. Almadori and colleagues reported that one-third of laryngeal tumors had evidence of HPV DNA.[14] The presence of HPV DNA may not represent causality and perhaps only a small subset of laryngeal cancer is directly related to HPV. Moreover, there are conflicting opinions relative to the prognostic implications of HPV. While some studies suggest that detectable HPV may represent a biologically distinct subset of tumors with poor prognosis,[15] others report that patients with detectable HPV have improved survival rates.[16]

Smoking cessation and reduced alcohol consumption are the most effective means of preventing the development and recurrence of laryngeal cancer. A toxin-free work environment is also important. Genetics and susceptibility to cancer are difficult to separate from lifestyle and the environment and thus more difficult to influence in a preventive fashion. Patient education is paramount in cancer prevention.

EPIDEMIOLOGY

It was estimated that 9,510 people in the United States would learn that they have cancer of the larynx in 2006, according to the National Cancer Institute. Although this figure has not changed significantly in the last four decades, the male/female incidence of laryngeal cancer has dropped from 15:1 to less than 5:1 in 2004.[17] This statistical change in the United States has been hypothesized to be a result of women obtaining an equal place in the toxic work environment and participating in what had become an acceptable act: public cigarette smoking. The time between these behavioral changes, that is, since World War II, and the recent gender statistics on cancer of the larynx may represent the duration of exposure needed for malignancy to evolve.

DIAGNOSIS

Early recognition of malignancies of the larynx is crucial. Any patient with hoarseness lasting longer than 4 weeks should be evaluated by an otolaryngologist. Other symptoms of laryngeal carcinoma are hemoptysis, halitosis, and the so-called hot potato voice. A thorough laryngeal examination is essential. While mirror examination suffices in some patients, in others evaluation with a telescope or flexible laryngoscope is required. Patients with a strong gag reflex, or patients whose local anatomy prohibits complete examination of the entire intrinsic larynx, in particular, the anterior commissure, require supplemental examination. The pyriform sinuses should be free of secretions when the examination is performed so that the mucosa is clearly visualized. Vocal cord mobility is assessed and recorded, because it has major implications in staging and management.

Cancers of the supraglottic larynx generally present later due to a paucity of early symptoms. Dysphagia, otalgia, and odynophagia should raise suspicion. Often, these symptoms are managed medically before referral for endoscopy. Airway obstruction with no apparent voice change may represent the presenting sign of a large supraglottic or subglottic lesion. The latter can present as refractory asthma without voice change, and referral may be indicated by a flow volume loop showing upper airway obstruction patterns in a patient with known asthma.

An office video endoscopic laryngeal assessment is outpatient state of the art. Replaying the video will often reveal subtleties not initially seen. With good topical anesthesia, outpatient endoscopic biopsies are easily obtained. With transnasal esophagoscopy (TNE) becoming increasingly available and outpatient flexible bronchoscopy established, is there still the need for an inpatient assessment of disease extent? For limited pathology, there is a shift toward outpatient (office) settings. Advanced stage tumors, we believe, still warrant a traditional exploratory evaluation. In the operating room, fixation of the vocal cord is differentiated from arytenoid cartilage fixation by palpation and can help stage the disease. The laryngeal probe permits assessment of extension into the ventricle. Telescopes can be used to assess the subglottic extent and visualize better the anterior commissure. The operating microscope also affords enhanced visualization. It is important to obtain appropriate biopsy specimens from varied sites to help in management planning.

Imaging studies are of paramount importance in the management of laryngeal malignancies as they may aid in the selection of the most appropriate therapeutic modality. Critical factors in the evaluation of laryngeal images include tumor volume, cartilaginous invasion, spread across supraglottic-glottic-subglottic boundaries, infiltration of preepiglottic, paraglottic, and pharyngeal planes, and nodal disease. Magnetic resonance imaging (MRI) offers greater sensitivity to cartilaginous invasion than computed tomography (CT) but has a higher false-positive rate. Thin-section CT with multiplanar capability is competitive with direct coronal MRI and benefits from high specificity.[18] CT and MRI modalities are complementary and should be used judiciously in the preoperative planning. Ideally, these studies should be completed prior to operative endoscopy and before biopsy. Lastly, radiologic evaluation of the chest helps to rule out metastasis or second primary malignancies. Chest CT scan is widely believed to be superior to simple chest X-rays for this purpose, but the available literature does not support this notion.[19] More recently, positron emission tomography (PET) has emerged as a part of the imaging armamentarium in laryngeal cancer,[20,21] but further experience will be required before widespread use of this technology can be recommended.

The need for a biopsy to confirm the diagnosis cannot be overemphasized. The gross appearance of several benign conditions, for example, fungal laryngitis, sarcoidosis, tuberculosis, or Wegener granulomatosis may mimic malignancy. Biopsies should be judicious but must include sufficient tissue volume to ensure the correct diagnosis. Small suspicious lesions should be completely excised with a limited border of healthy laryngeal submucosa to afford depth of invasion evaluation. Frozen sections are usually taken to prevent the need for a repeat endoscopy due to inadequate sampling. Educating the patient is paramount prior to proceeding with definitive management.

Staging is important, enabling standardization of patient populations and permitting comparisons between institutional series. TNM staging is necessary for patient discussion, tumor board consideration, and ultimately therapeutic delivery. It is required by institutions managing cancer patients and maintaining a tumor registry (Joint Commission on Accreditation of Healthcare Organizations [JCAHO] requirement). Table 1 outlines the staging of laryngeal cancer.

APPROACH TO LARYNGEAL CANCER

The main goal of therapy is the eradication of cancer. Quality of life research shows that cancer cure is the main determinant of quality of life outcomes. Patients usually adapt well to lifestyle modifications resulting from treatment sequelae.[22] Secondary objectives include voice quality and adequate swallowing. Tumor considerations, patient issues, and institutional factors all play a role in the decision-making process.

Tumor

Over 90% of laryngeal cancer is of the squamous cell type. Important tumor parameters include mobility of the vocal cords, anterior commissure involvement, depth of cord invasion, T classification, tumor location, that is, glottic versus supraglottic, and proximity of a supraglottic lesion to the anterior commisure. Exophytic tumors tend to respond better to radiation than endophytic tumors and have a more favorable prognosis.[23] The degree of differentiation has been correlated with metastatic potential, poorly differentiated tumors being more aggressive.

Patient

Occupational demands, mental and health status, and patient tolerances are germane in formulating a

---

Table 1   TNM Categorization for Laryngeal Cancer

Tumor (T)

Supraglottis

T1: Tumor limited to one subsite* of supraglottis with normal vocal cord mobility

T2: Tumor invades mucosa of more than one adjacent subsite* of supraglottis or glottis or region outside the supraglottis (eg, mucosa of base of tongue, vallecula, medial wall of pyriform sinus) without fixation of the larynx

T3: Tumor limited to larynx with vocal cord fixation and/or invades any of the following: postcricoid area, preepiglottic tissues

T4: Tumor invades through the thyroid cartilage, and/or extends into soft tissues of the neck, thyroid, and/or esophagus

Glottis

T1: Tumor limited to vocal cord(s) (may involve anterior or posterior commissure) with normal mobility

T1a: Tumor limited to one vocal cord

T1b: Tumor involves both vocal cords

T2: Tumor extends to supraglottis and/or subglottis, and/or with impaired vocal cord mobility

T3: Tumor limited to the larynx with vocal cord fixation

T4: Tumor invades through the thyroid cartilage and/or to other tissues beyond the larynx (eg, trachea, soft tissues of neck, including thyroid, pharynx)

Subglottis

T1: Tumor limited to the subglottis

T2: Tumor extends to vocal cord(s) with normal or impaired mobility

T3: Tumor limited to larynx with vocal cord fixation

T4: Tumor invades through cricoid or thyroid cartilage and/or extends to other tissues beyond the larynx (eg, trachea, soft tissues of neck, including thyroid, esophagus)

Regional lymph nodes (N)

NX: Regional lymph nodes cannot be assessed

N0: No regional lymph node metastasis

N1: Metastasis in a single ipsilateral lymph node, 3 cm or less in greatest dimension

N2: Metastasis in a single ipsilateral lymph node, more than 3 cm but not more than 6 cm in greatest dimension, or in multiple ipsilateral lymph nodes, none more than 6 cm in greatest dimension, or in bilateral or contralateral lymph nodes, none more than 6 cm in greatest dimension

N2a: Metastasis in a single ipsilateral lymph node more than 3 cm but not more than 6 cm in greatest dimension

N2b: Metastasis in multiple ipsilateral lymph nodes, none more than 6 cm in greatest dimension

N2c: Metastasis in bilateral or contralateral lymph nodes, none more than 6 cm in greatest dimension

N3: Metastasis in a lymph node more than 6 cm in greatest dimension

Distant metastasis (M)

MX: Distant metastasis cannot be assessed

M0: No distant metastasis

M1: Distant metastasis

*Subsites include the following: ventricular bands (false cords); arytenoids; suprahyoid epiglottis; infrahyoid epiglottis; aryepiglottic folds (laryngeal aspect).

tailored therapeutic regimen. The medical status is critical, with pulmonary function being of particular importance. Voice quality is becoming less of an issue when considering radiation therapy versus judicious laser ablation, yet it merits in-depth discussion with professional voice users. For many, the time disparity between these treatment modalities as well as differences in morbidity are leading more to consider surgical alternatives for early-stage laryngeal malignancy.

Institution

A multidisciplinary approach with input from all parties is state-of-the-art management for laryngeal cancer. This requires well-trained head and neck surgeons, medical oncologists, and radiotherapists who meet regularly at a multidisciplinary conference. This approach avoids the potential bias of a given discipline recommending a specific regimen to the relative exclusions of others. Supporting services should include speech and swallowing therapists, restorative dentistry, psychology/psychiatry, and physical and occupational therapists.

Surgical Treatment

The choice of a surgical approach depends on the tumor size and location. For early laryngeal cancer, there are the traditional partial procedures. However, today, endoscopic surgery is playing an ever-increasing role. In the majority of patients with advanced disease, if surgery is chosen, the treatment remains total laryngectomy, with partial laryngeal surgery reserved for selected patients. In advanced lesions, extirpation of the primary tumor must be accompanied by management of the neck, with an appropriate lymphadenectomy as a primary modality of therapy. A brief description of the traditional surgical procedures follows acknowledging the trend toward newer approaches.

Vertical Partial Laryngectomy. This technique involves removal of the majority of the ipsilateral thyroid cartilage, the true and false vocal cords, and limited subglottic mucosa (Figure 1). It is indicated for tumors that arise on the true vocal cord with limited involvement of the anterior commissure. The defect can be allowed to heal spontaneously or it can be reconstructed with the epiglottis. Another alternative is the rotation of a pedicled muscle flap beneath retained perichondrium. A temporary tracheostomy is most often performed but is not universally felt to be requisite. Anterior commissure involvement dictates a frontolateral or extended vertical partial laryngectomy. Contraindications to this procedure include posterior commissure involvement, subglottic extension of more than 10 mm, and potential pulmonary reserve issues. Voice quality is not as good as that achieved with radiation or an endoscopic resection. Endoscopic CO_2 laser techniques have, for the most part, replaced this procedure in our institution as a primary modality; rather, it is performed in selected patients after radiation failure.

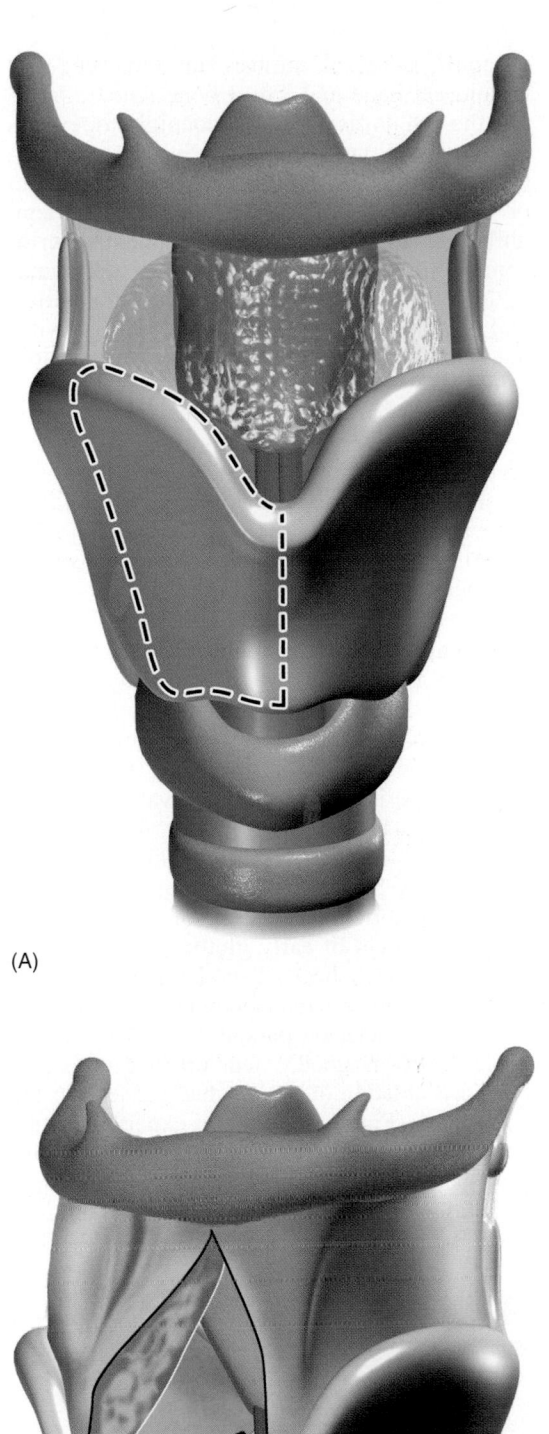

(A)

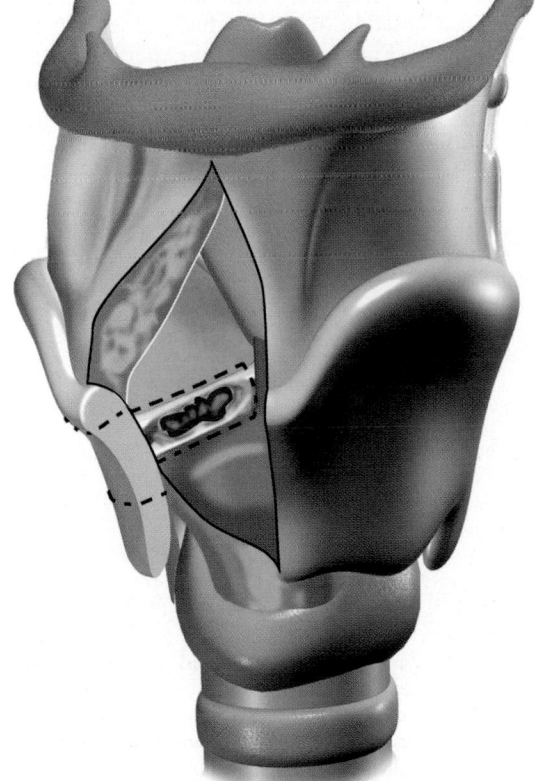

(B)

Figure 1 Diagrammatic representation of a vertical partial laryngectomy. (A) External view showing the resection of the thyroid ala. (B) Schematic representation of the tumor visualization after a midline thyrotomy. (Reprinted with permission. Copyright © 2004. The Cleveland Clinic Foundation. All rights reserved.)

Supraglottic Laryngectomy. This technique involves the removal of the epiglottis, thyrohyoid membrane, preepiglottic space, upper half of the thyroid cartilage, and the false vocal folds (Figure 2). We preserve the hyoid bone when

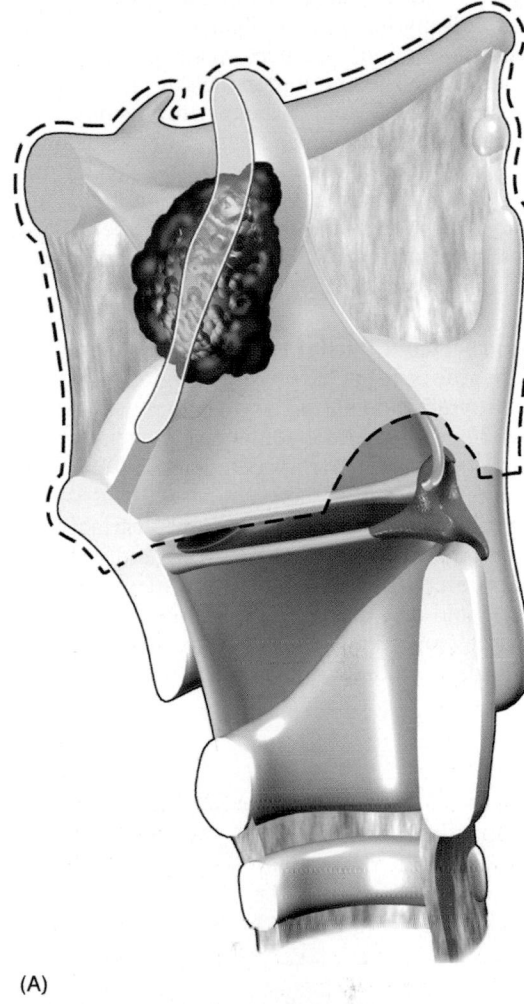

(A)

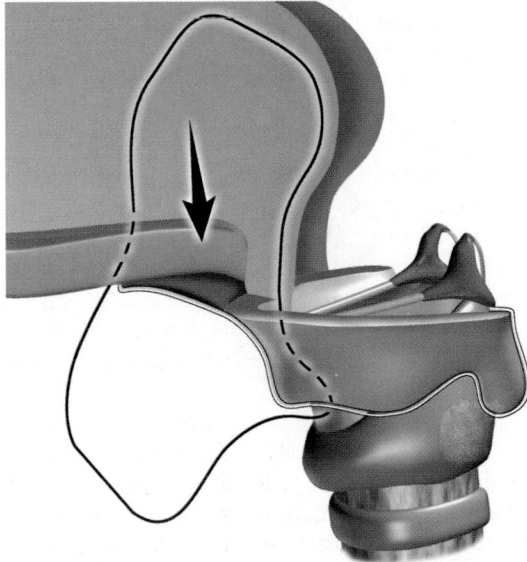

(B)

Figure 2 Diagrammatic representation of the laryngeal cuts and reconstruction in a supraglottic partial laryngectomy. (A) External view outlining the resection. (B) Schematic representation of the reconstruction. (Reprinted with permission. Copyright © 2004. The Cleveland Clinic Foundation. All rights reserved.)

feasible from an oncologic perspective. This technique is suitable for T1 and T2 tumors of the laryngeal surface of the eqiglottis and false vocal cords. The inferior margin only needs to be 2 to 3 mm above the vocal folds. Closure is achieved by approximating the thyroid cartilage remnant to the hyoid bone with three sutures placed 1 cm apart. Patients require a temporary tracheostomy. For infrahyoid tumors, ipsilateral or bilateral neck dissections are performed. Contraindications related to the tumor include involvement of the interarytenoid space, pyriform sinus apex, anterior commissure, and significant invasion of the preepiglottic space. Also, FEV1 greater than 50% is a requirement in some institutions.[24] In our institution, this procedure, like the vertical partial laryngectomy, has taken a secondary role to endoscopic laryngeal surgery.

Supracricoid Partial Laryngectomy with Cricohyoidopexy or Cricohyoidoepiglottopexy. In the supracricoid partial laryngectomy with cricohyoidopexy or cricohyoidoepiglottopexy operation, the whole thyroid cartilage and the paraglottic spaces are resected (Figures 3 and 4). The cricoid cartilage, the hyoid bone, variably the epiglottis and, at least, one arytenoid cartilage are preserved. The preservation of one mobile arytenoid unit results in physiologic speech and swallowing. Maintenance of the cricoid cartilage affords decannulation. For closure, three submucosal 0-Vicryl sutures circumscribe the cricoid cartilage and hyoid bone with or without the epiglottis (cricohyodoepiglottopexy vs cricohyoidopexy). These procedures are indicated for bilateral T1 glottic carcinomas with or without anterior commissure involvement, unilateral T1 glottic carcinomas with anterior commissure involvement, T1 glottic carcinomas with multiple areas of dysplasia, and unilateral or bilateral T2 glottic tumors with or without impaired vocal cord mobility. In addition, selected T3 glottic carcinomas may be amenable to this approach if the ipsilateral arytenoid is mobile and the preepiglottic space is not involved. This procedure can be performed successfully after radiation failure. Contraindications include poor pulmonary reserve, posterior commissure involvement, and subglottic extension below 10 mm.

Endoscopic Resection. Endoscopic surgery for vocal fold malignancies is accomplished with CO_2 laser linked to the operating microscope. A new hollow core fiber that allows for the transmission of CO_2 laser energy (OmniGuide Corporation) is currently being evaluated at our institution. The use of CO_2 laser for the management of laryngeal malignancies was first described by Strong.[25] Vaughan and colleagues, in 1978, reported on the use of CO_2 laser for the management of early glottic cancer.[26] Since then, there have been several reports supporting its role in the management of early glottic cancer in selected patients.[27–29] The reported voice quality is good.[30] Our practice is to perform cryoablation of the residual tissue after the resection[31] (Figure 5). In our experience, this serves two purposes, first it theoretically allows for a better tumor control, but it also decreases collagen deposition and increases hyaluron,

leading to increased pliability and improved vocal function.[32]

Selected supraglottic tumors can also be approached endoscopically. Vaughan and colleagues first described the use of CO_2 laser for debulking of supraglottic tumor,[26] but it was Davis and colleagues who first described a technique for transoral CO_2 laser resection of the supraglottis.[33] Since 1979, Steiner has been using a transoral CO_2 laser technique to resect supraglottic tumors successfully.[34] Initially early-stage tumors were resected, but more recently, there have been reports of advanced supraglottic tumors being resected endoscopically. The advantages of the endoscopic technique include a more rapid recovery of swallowing and speech, a limited need for tracheostomy, and a decreased hospital stay. The procedure is performed using a bivalved laryngoscope specially designed for the operation. The resection is accomplished by midline splitting and resection of the suprahyoid epiglottis, followed by a split of the infrahyoid epiglottis with evaluation of the extent of invasion of the tumor at this point. The specimen is removed and subjected to frozen section control. The preepiglottic space is included in the specimen and is often infiltrated. The resection may require removal of all tissue to the inner perichondrium of the thyroid cartilage and thyrohyoid membrane. False cords are also resected when indicated. We currently favor this approach.

Total Laryngectomy. The total laryngectomy procedure involves the removal of the entire larynx, as well as the hyoid bone and cricoid cartilage. An appropriate neck dissection is usually performed. This procedure is usually indicated for selected Stage III and IV disease. In the current

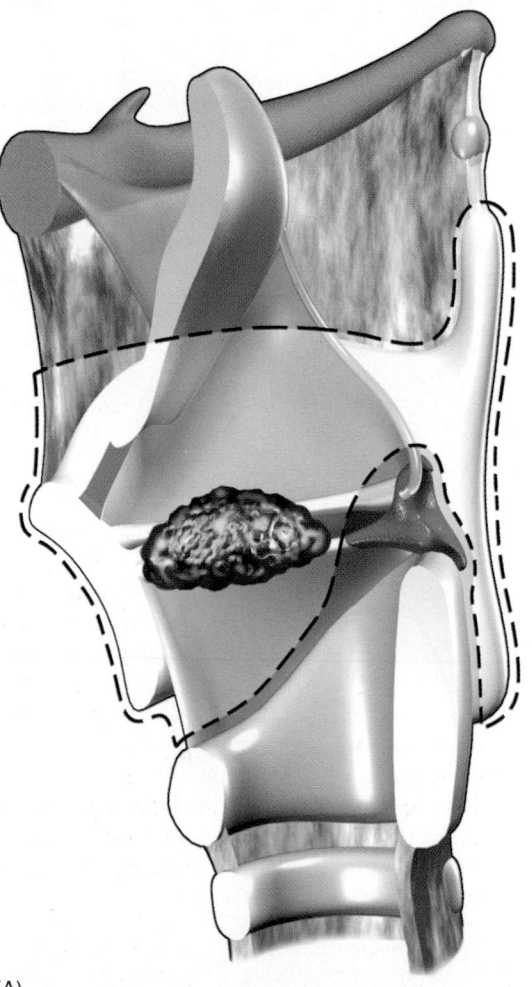

(A)

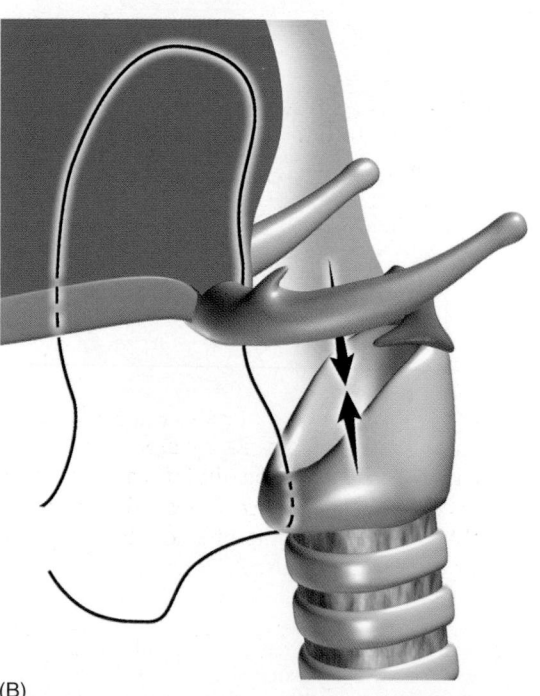

(B)

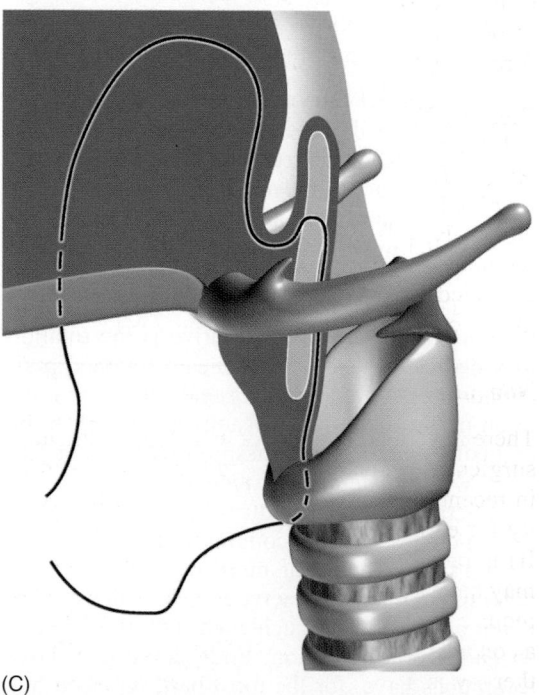

(C)

Figure 3 Diagrammatic representation of the laryngeal cuts and reconstruction in a supracricoid partial laryngectomy. (A) External view outlining the resection. (B) Schematic representation of the reconstruction when the epiglottis is resected (cricohyoidopex), or (C) when it is preserved (cricohyoidoepiglottopexy). (Reprinted with permission. Copyright © 2004. The Cleveland Clinic Foundation. All rights reserved.)

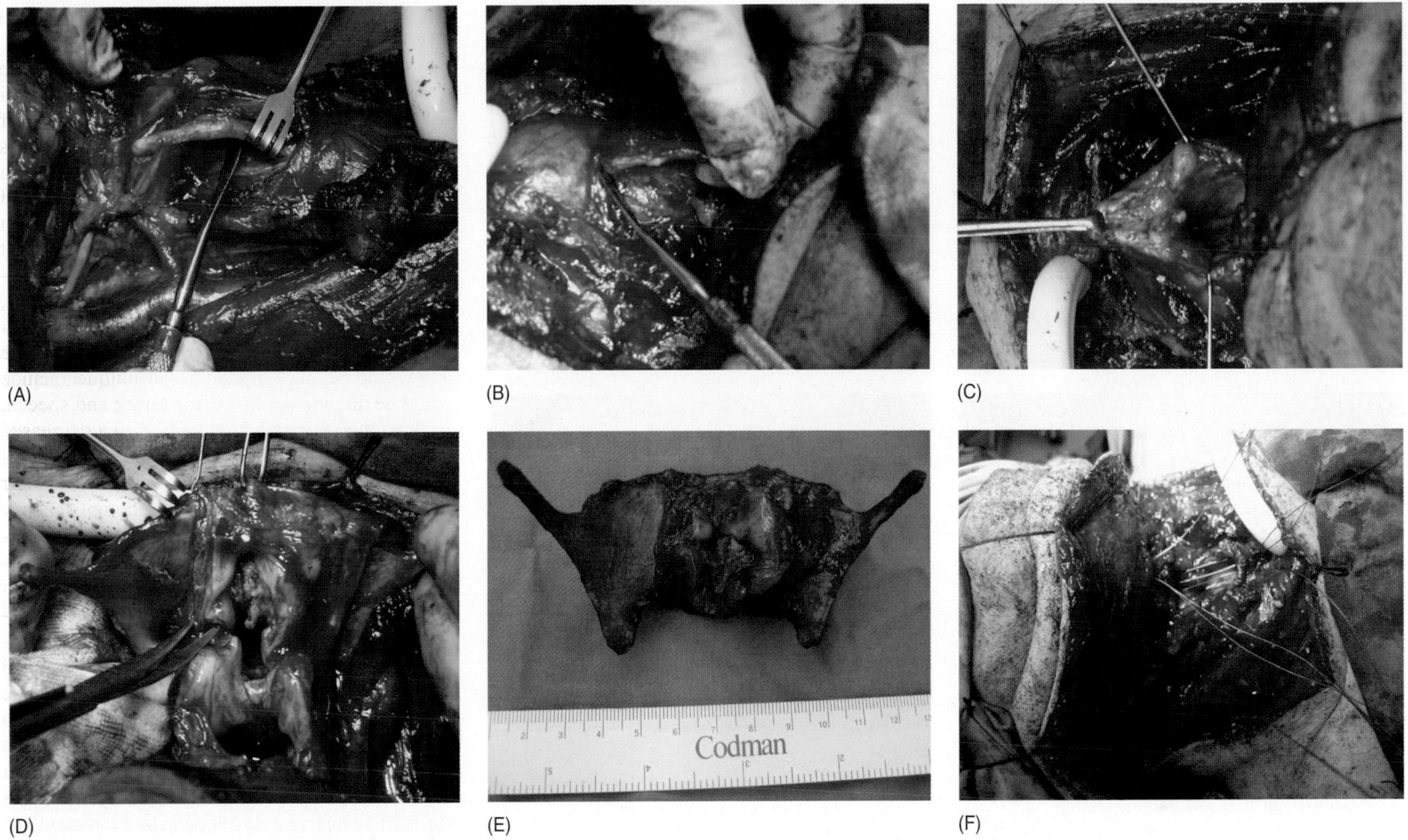

Figure 4 Intraoperative view during a supracricoid laryngectomy showing (A) the dissection of the constrictor muscles of the thyroid cartilage, (B) dislocation of the cricoarytenoid joint to protect the recurrent laryngeal nerve, (C) the larynx being entered, (D) removal of the specimen, (E) the specimen, and (F) repair of the laynx. (Published with permission, copyright © 2007 Scott Coman, MBBS.)

era of conservation therapy, this procedure is usually performed for chemoradiation failures, or when conservation therapy is contraindicated as in the case of extensive cartilage involvement. In our practice, total laryngectomy is rarely performed as a primary treatment modality.

Elective Neck Dissection. The nodal groups at risk for occult spread in laryngeal cancer are levels II, III, and IV.[35] Levels I and V are rarely involved. Therefore, when the neck is treated electively, a lateral neck dissection is all that is required. Paratracheal nodes (level VI) should be dissected in cases of advanced glottic and subglottic cancer.[36])

Nonsurgical Treatment

There have been significant advances in the nonsurgical management of head and neck cancer in recent years. The primary nonsurgical modality for early-stage laryngeal cancer (stages I and II) is radiation therapy. Chemoradiation therapy may have a role in bulky T2 tumors which would require a total laryngectomy but is otherwise not a consideration for early disease. Chemoradiation therapy is generally used in laryngeal preservation for advanced tumors. The concept of laryngeal preservation for advanced laryngeal cancer had its basis in the Veterans Affairs Laryngeal

Cancer Study Group (VA study).[37] In this study, 332 patients with stage III to IV laryngeal carcinoma were randomized to either induction chemotherapy with cisplatin and fluorouracil followed by radiation therapy in those with more than 50% decrease in tumor size, or total laryngectomy followed by radiation therapy. Patients in the chemotherapy group underwent total laryngectomy if their tumor did not decrease by more than 50% or if they had persistent disease following radiation therapy. The laryngeal preservation rate was 66% at 5 years with no difference in survival between the chemoradiation and surgery groups.[37] At 12 years, 61% of patients in the chemoradiation group still had their larynx, and their survival rates were similar to those of the surgical arm.[38]

In addition to survival, speech, swallowing, pain, and cosmetic deformity are important to consider when evaluating the efficacy of organ preservation therapy. At 2-year follow-up in the VA study cohort, the chemoradiation group had better objective speech, with only 2 patients (1%) requiring tracheostomy.[39] However, at 10 years, there were no differences between the chemoradiation group and the surgical group in their speech and swallowing abilities as reported by the patients.[40] Interestingly, the chemoradiation patients had better quality of life scores than the laryngectomy patients, and

this was related to freedom from pain; better emotional well-being scores, and lower levels of depression, and not to laryngeal preservation. Although this study did not report significant swallowing dysfunction, it has been detailed in other publications.[41,42]

The National Cancer Institute Cooperative Trials Head and Neck Intergroup (R 91-11) conducted a randomized, three-arm trial to determine whether radiation therapy alone with surgical salvage was superior to either induction chemotherapy followed by radiation therapy or concurrent chemoradiation therapy. Five hundred and forty-seven patients were enrolled, of which 497 patients were ultimately included in the final analysis. The median follow-up was 36 months. At the 2-year mark, no survival benefit was noted in either group. Interestingly, laryngectomy-free survival was greater in the concurrent chemoradiation group (66%) than in the induction chemotherapy (59%) or radiation-alone (53%) groups. Laryngeal preservation was achieved in 88% of patients in the chemoradiation group which was significantly better that the other two groups. The rate of distant control was similar in both chemotherapy groups. It is important to mention that in this study, treatment-related mortality rates ranged between 3 and 5% among all groups which is higher than the expected surgical

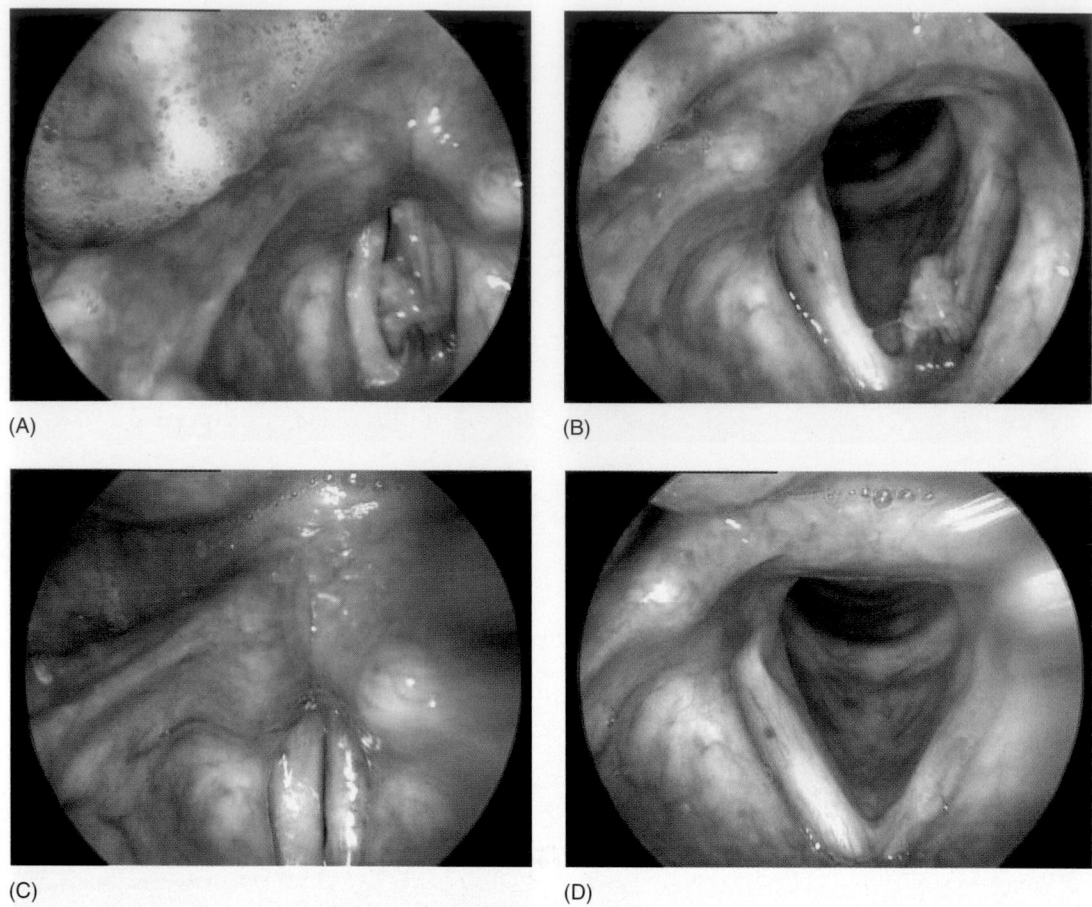

(A) (B)

(C) (D)

Figure 5 Pre- (A and B) and postoperative (C and D) images of a patient who underwent CO_2 laser resection and cryoablation. (Published with permission, copyright © 2007 Marshall Strome, MD.)

mortality of 1%. In addition, more than 40% of tumors were T2 or T3 without vocal cord fixation and therefore were amenable to conservation laryngeal surgery. Lastly, swallowing was particularly affected in the chemoradiation therapy group; 23% of patients were still on a soft diet at 1 year, and 3% had no ability to swallow at all. At 2 years, 15% of patients in all three groups had a diet limited to soft foods.[43] Unfortunately, this study did not include an arm consisting of patients who had undergone surgery, that is, partial laryngeal surgery with an appropriate neck dissection, followed by radiation therapy.

Weber and colleagues analyzed the survival, locoregional control, and complications after salvage total laryngectomy in the Radiation Therapy Oncology Group (RTOG) 91-11 study. The need for total laryngectomy was less common in the chemoradiation therapy group. In addition, patients who required salvage surgery had a poorer survival than those who did not. The incidence of complications after salvage surgery was no different among all three groups. However, one-third of the patients who required salvage surgery after chemoradiation therapy developed pharyngocutaneous fistulas.[44]

A phase II study was conducted at the University of Michigan using a single cycle of induction chemotherapy to identify patients who responded with more than 50% reduction in tumor volume. Patients who responded to induction chemotherapy underwent chemoradiation therapy. Nonresponders underwent total laryngectomy. Adjuvant chemotherapy was available to patients who completed chemoradiation. The overall survival rate was 85% and functional laryngeal preservation was achieved in 71% of the patients, with a median follow-up of 30 months. Laryngectomy-free survival was 62% at 2 years and 58% at 3 years. This nonrandomized study showed significantly improved survival rates when compared with historical controls.[45]

There are no prospective, randomized trials on the use of chemotherapy as a single modality for the management of laryngeal cancer. Laccourreye and colleagues retrospectively analyzed the local recurrence rates in 35 patients with glottic cancer treated with cisplatin and fluoracil alone. Of 231 patients, 77 achieved complete clinical response with this induction chemotherapy regimen, and 35 of these 77 were treated with chemotherapy alone for cure. Five-year actuarial survival and local control rates in this group were 88.6% and 64.8%, respectively. Salvage treatment for local recurrence in this group yielded a 100% local control and larynx preservation rate. Patients with tumors originating from sites other that the glottis had worse survival and failure rates than those patients with glottic cancer. Although local recurrences were found in about one-third of patients with T1 to T3 disease, there were no disease-related deaths and no patient required a total laryngectomy.[46] The role of chemotherapy alone will need to be determined in the years to come. At present, chemotherapy is given concurrently with radiation.

RADIATION OR CHEMORADIATION THERAPY AND SURGERY

Combined radiation therapy and surgery began in the early 1960s. Initial studies compared patients who received preoperative radiation followed by planned surgical resection with historical controls.[47–49] Increased survival rates were demonstrated in these early studies. The primary advantage of preoperative radiotherapy was theorized to be that well-oxygenated unoperated tissue had a better vascular supply, making delivery more effective than radiotherapy to an operated field. In addition, the field and extent of radiotherapy would be more limited because this modality could be directly applied to the tumor site.

Postoperative radiation gained general acceptance in the late 1970s. The advantage of postoperative radiotherapy was that it enabled surgeons to establish the pathologic extent of disease, true status of cervical nodes, and status of the surgical margins. Studies showed a significant improvement in lymph node control with postoperative versus preoperative radiotherapy.[50] The perceived disadvantages were the need for a larger radiation port and possible delay in the radiotherapy if wound healing was not adequate. Vikram noted the need to deliver postoperative radiotherapy within 7 weeks of the operative procedure. In 7 of 10 patients to receiving postoperative radiotherapy within 7 weeks of surgery, no signs of recurrence developed. In 11 patients in whom the initiation of postoperative radiotherapy was delayed, 3 had regional or local tumor recurrence.[51] A more recent retrospective study on 420 patients with oropharyngeal and hypopharyngeal malignancies failed to support Vikram's findings. This study could not demonstrate that radiotherapy started more than 6 weeks postoperatively affected survival and showed that the status of the margins and N stage were the predictors of locoregional recurrence.[52]

Two prospective randomized studies were designed to determine whether preoperative or postoperative radiotherapy was more advantageous. The largest study was performed between 1973 and 1975 under the direction of the RTOG.[53] Patients with carcinoma of the supraglottic larynx and hypopharynx were randomly assigned to receive preoperative radiation of 50 Gy or postoperative radiation of 60 Gy. Patients with oral cavity or oropharynx lesions were randomly assigned to preoperative radiation, postoperative radiation, or definitive radiation therapy (65 to 70 Gy). Surgery was reserved for salvage if residual disease was present 6 weeks after the completion of irradiation. Three hundred and twenty patients were accessed in follow-up, and the median follow-up was 60 months. Based on results in 277 patients across all four regions combined, locoregional control was significantly better for the patients assigned to receive postoperative radiation therapy (65%) than in those assigned to receive preoperative radiation therapy (48%, $p = .04$). This was due to a higher rate of both persistent and recurrent local and regional disease in the preoperative group. Survival was also better in the postoperative group (38%) compared with the preoperative group 33%, but the difference was not statistically significant ($p = .10$).[53] A 10-year follow-up study showed that locoregional control was significantly better for 141 postoperative radiation therapy patients than for 136 preoperative radiation therapy patients ($p = .04$), but absolute survival was not affected ($p = .15$).[54] When the analysis was restricted to supraglottic larynx primaries (60 postoperative radiation therapy patients vs. 58 preoperative radiation therapy patients), the difference for locoregional control was highly significant ($p = .007$), but survival was comparable in both groups ($p = .18$). When looking at only the supraglottic larynx, 78% of locoregional failures occurred in the first 2 years. Thirty-one percent (18 of 58) of preoperative patients experienced local failures within 2 years versus 18% (11 of 60) of postoperative patients. After 2 years, distant metastases and second primaries became the predominant failure pattern, especially in postoperative radiation therapy patients. This shift in the late failure pattern along with the increased number of unrelated deaths negated any advantage in absolute survival for postoperative radiation therapy patients. The rates of severe surgical and radiation therapy complications were similar between the two arms. This study concluded that given an increased incidence of late distant metastases and secondary primaries, additional therapeutic intervention would be required beyond surgery and postoperative irradiation to impact significantly upon survival.[54]

Recently, reports on the successful use of postoperative chemoradiation therapy in head and neck tumors with high-risk features have been published. Cooper and colleagues reported the results of a phase III trial on postoperative chemoradiation versus radiation alone.[55] This study was supported by the RTOG, Eastern Cooperative Oncology Group (ECOG), and the Southwest Oncology Group (SWOG). Four hundred and fifty-nine patients with head and neck cancer who were noted to have high-risk features, that is, two or more positive lymph nodes, extracapsular spread, and/or positive margins, were randomized to either postoperative radiation or radiation plus cisplatin. Roughly, 20% of patients in either group had laryngeal malignancies. The conclusion was that concurrent postoperative chemoradiation therapy improved the rates of local and regional control and disease-free survival. Importantly, the combined treatment increased adverse effects.[55] In a similar study conducted by the European Organization for Cancer Research (EORTC), the benefit of postoperative chemoradiation therapy in advanced head and neck cancer was demonstrated.[55]

TREATMENT OUTCOMES

Premalignant Lesions and Carcinoma In Situ

The laryngeal pathology of squamous cell epithelium progresses through five categories: hyperkeratosis, hyperkeratosis with atypia, carcinoma in situ (CIS), superficially (micro) invasive carcinoma, and invasive carcinoma. Lesions that show atypia and CIS can be managed with local excision with clear margins. We follow these lesions monthly for 6 months with video stroboscopy and then at 2-month intervals for the first year. Lesions in this category are superficial to the basement membrane. Differentiation between severe hyperkeratosis with atypia and CIS is often difficult. The significance of this differentiation is more academic than clinical as these lesions are managed in a similar manner.

Voice quality following surgical excision is dependant on the amount of tissue removed and the location of the tumor. Anterior commissure involvement and resection results in a decreased voice quality.[56] Generally, voice outcomes are good with both surgery and radiation therapy.

Precancerous lesions and CIS should be managed surgically because radiation therapy will fail in 1 out of 10 patients. Successful surgical results are obtained when the entire lesion is resected with clear margins. This is best achieved with CO_2 laser surgery. The need for rebiopsy and close surveillance for many years is discussed with the patient. We believe that radiation therapy should be reserved for those patients with a high anesthesia risk or those who do not wish to have repeated surgical procedures. Smoking cessation and antireflux therapy are of paramount importance for a successful outcome.

LARYNGEAL CANCER

Glottic Cancer

Squamous cell carcinoma of the glottis is usually well to moderately differentiated and presents at an early stage (T1 to T2). It is rarely associated with locoregional metastasis. This differs from supraglottic or laryngopharyngeal disease and is thought to be due to sparse submucosal lymphatics in the glottis. Symptoms usually appear early as most carcinomas originate on or near the phonatory surface of the vocal folds. Early-stage disease can be managed with radiotherapy or conservation surgery without the need for elective neck management. The surgical cure rates for T1 to 2 lesions reported in the literature range between 92 and 100%.[57–59] Reexcision is required in 10 to 50% of patients, with an average of two procedures per patient.[58] Surgical salvage can be done by reexcision, partial or total laryngectomy. Glottal function can be preserved in 92 to 100% of patients.[57–59] Voice quality following laser resection is comparable to radiation therapy results in selected cases.[60] In our experience, the addition of cryotherapy significantly improves the voice quality, even when a cordectomy is performed.[31] Local control rates for T1 to T2 lesions with radiation therapy are between 77 and 89% and as low as 70% for T2 lesions.[61–64] Local cure by radiotherapy for glottic tumors, which almost always matches tumor-free survival, has not changed since 1974.[65] Surgical salvage includes partial laryngeal surgery and total laryngectomy with voice preservation rates around 75%.[66–68]

No clear advantage between surgery and radiotherapy has been noted in the literature for early glottic malignancy. Therefore, patients must be thoroughly counseled and involved in decision-making. Surgery is more successful for lesions with subglottic extension and impaired cordal mobility. Postradiation edema lasting for longer than 3 months has a 43% association with persistent or recurrent disease and requires follow-up by endoscopy and imaging.[69]

Tumor site is of importance in considering the varied therapeutic options. Middle third of vocal fold lesions are easiest to cure and respond well to radiotherapy, endoscopic laser resection, or open cordectomy. Surgical cure rates approach 100% for such lesions excised with good margins, while radiation therapy cure rates approach 95%. Radiation failures may be caused by unrecognized deep invasion. Endoscopically removed lesions are carefully observed via video laryngoscopy, with reexcision or radiotherapy used for recurrence. Radiation is a viable alternative to surgery, but recurrent disease or second primaries may not be amenable to conservation surgery. The anterior commissure is always of concern regarding radiotherapy.[70]

Hypomobility of the vocal fold is associated with reduced cure rates after radiation therapy.[70] Harwood and De Boer noted that impaired cord mobility resulted in lower control rates in T2 lesions, and they suggested the classification be divided into T2a and T2b on the basis of mobility.[72] In this analysis, a 77% local control rate was noted for the former category versus 51% in the latter.[72] In 1996, McLaughlin and colleagues reported an 11% recurrence rate for T2a lesions and a 26% recurrence rate for T2b lesions.[73] Surgery salvaged six of nine T2b radiation failures.

T2 and early T3 lesions of the glottis have more recently been managed by supracricoid laryngectomy with cricohyoidoepiglottopexy. This operation was championed in Europe in the late 1970s. Reports of this surgery performed in the United States began to enter the American literature in the early 1990s. The operation requires resection of the entire thyroid cartilage and paraglottic space. The cricoid cartilage, the hyoid bone, much of the epiglottis, and at least one arytenoid cartilage are preserved. A study of 36 patients reported satisfactory deglutition, phonation, and 100% decannulation with a 5% local recurrence rate.[74] Sixty-one percent of the patients had been pretreated with chemotherapy.[74] In a current series of 17 patients, 9 (53%) were able to resume eating a normal diet and 6 additional patients had moderate dysphagia. Voice quality was limited in range and intensity but was not equal to that of supraglottic laryngectomy.[75] A total laryngectomy with tracheoesophageal puncture with or without postoperative radiotherapy is another option for T3 glottic cancer and may be the best alternative in some patients, that is, poor pulmonary reserve, poor chemoradiation candidates. The locoregional control rates with this approach range from 65 to 77% in some studies.[76]

With the advent of chemoradiation therapy protocols, primary surgery for advanced laryngeal cancer is less common. Although there is no survival benefit demonstrated in recent studies, functional laryngeal preservation has been demonstrated.

Supraglottic Cancer. In managing supraglottic cancer, consideration of the neck is requisite. Early supraglottic (epiglottic) tumors, which are suprahyoid, can be grossly excised endoscopically with the CO_2 laser. Suprahyoid lesions rarely involve the preepiglottic space or regional neck nodes in contrast to infrahyoid lesions. Cancer can traverse the foramina of the elastic epiglottic cartilage. There have been reports of excellent results with endoscopic laser treatment of selected supraglottic carcinomas; however, infrahyoid tumors are less favorable. A need for a repeat laryngoscopy with biopsy is common. Following endoscopic resection, the neck can be addressed in a staged fashion. Separating neck dissection from the endoscopic resection of the primary seems to enhance swallowing and usually precludes the need for a temporary tracheostomy. Improved local control has been reported when postoperative radiation is included in the management.[77,78] The resumption of an oral diet, often in 1 to 2 weeks, can be attributed to base of tongue integrity and arytenoid mobility. Complications of the procedure include failure to eradicate the tumor and early postoperative bleeding, which can be fatal.

Ambrosch and colleagues reported 48 untreated patients with early supraglottic cancer (12 T1N0 and 36 T2 N0) who underwent primary transoral laser excision with a median follow-up time of 55 months.[79] The 5-year local control rate was 100% for T1 and 89% for T2 lesions. The ultimate local control rate with voice preservation, including patients who underwent successful salvage procedures after local recurrence, was 97% for T2 tumors. Only 5 patients died of tumor related issues. The 5-year recurrence-free rate and 5-year overall survival rates were 83% and 76%, respectively. No patients had symptomatic aspiration. Reports on the management of more advanced malignancies are still sparse.[78,80–82] Experience with laser supraglottic laryngectomy has been increasing in the United States.[83] At the moment, this technique requires continued evaluation and larger series to determine efficacy. It is operator dependent, and there is a steep learning curve. However, earlier and better deglutition, a limited need for tracheostomy, the potential to delay neck dissection, and, in some centers, the potential to reduce the dose of postoperative radiotherapy make it, at present, a meaningful option. At this time, it is more cost effective than traditional open supraglottic laryngectomy and appears to compare favorably in tumor control.

The preepiglottic space can be invaded in up to 50% of infrahyoid squamous cell carcinoma.

CT and physical examination are not uniformly helpful in detection. The relationship between preepiglottic space invasion and metastasis to the lateral part of the neck is unclear but metastasis has a reported incidence of up to 50%, even for early tumors.[84] Metastases to either side of the neck can occur because the preepiglottic space has bilateral lymphatic drainage. It is acknowledged that invasion of the preepiglottic space is associated with a poorer prognosis.

Limited supraglottic tumors, defined as T1 to T3 (because the preepiglottic space invasion upstages the lesion), can be managed with an open supraglottic laryngectomy if the vocal cords are mobile. Limited arytenoid involvement and lateral extension to the medial aspect of the pyriform sinus are not contraindications to partial surgery. With the advent of transoral laser surgery, we believe this approach will fall out of favor. Extended supraglottic laryngectomies are associated with increased difficulty in deglutition. Also, these more aggressive tumors often require postoperative radiation. Extended resections that allow preservation of voice and airway can include removal of the vallecula and base of the tongue up to the level of the circumvallate papilla. Despite reconstruction, this surgical magnitude affects swallowing; and, when combined with radiotherapy, rehabilitation can be challenging.

The acknowledged risks for open extirpation of supraglottic malignancies, aspiration and altered deguttion, make patient selection critical. Young, motivated patients with good pulmonary reserve fare best. Minimal aspiration always occurs but, for the most part, is readily tolerated. However, those with chronic pulmonary disease and reduced ciliary clearance are at greater risk for pneumonia. Most still believe the ability to walk a flight of stairs is important in clearing patients for surgery.

Those failing therapeutic full course radiation for supraglottic lesions are at increased risk because of the inability to detect submucosal extent of the persistent carcinoma. Occasionally, when the original tumor configuration is completely understood and evaluation of the recurrent lesion is favorable, partial laryngeal surgery may be warranted. The morbidity for salvage surgery is increased due to wound healing issues, persistent edema, and pharyngeal dysfunction from radiation fibrosis.

Contraindications to supraglottic laryngectomy include thyroid cartilage invasion and anterior commissure involvement. Anterior commissure involvement portends thyroid cartilage invasion.

Radiotherapy, for the most part, is less effective than supraglottic laryngectomy in controlling supraglottic cancer.[85,86] Over a 10-year period, 166 cases of stage I and II supraglottic carcinoma were treated for cure.[86] Sixty-six were treated with surgery, and 100 were treated with radiation. Surgery resulted in a local recurrence of 5%. On the other hand, a 23% local failure rate was observed with radiotherapy, but the

data suggested that hyperfractionation may yield results comparable to those of surgery. Local control after salvage was achieved in all except one surgical patient and in half of the radiation failures, resulting in an overall control rate of 98 and 89% for surgery and radiation, respectively. Most head and neck cancer centers agree that surgery is a better alternative for most supraglottic tumors if conservation laryngeal surgery is planned. When advanced disease requires a total laryngectomy, chemoradiation therapy is an alternative. In the RTOG 91-11 study, 68% of the treated tumors were supraglottic tumors. Although, laryngeal preservation was feasible, it was not without significant sequelae, including a higher treatment-related mortality than primary surgery.[43]

Subglottic Cancer. Subglottic cancer is unusual. Shaha and Shah reported that only 1% of 2,180 laryngeal cancers were located 1 cm below the vocal folds.[87] The clinical presentation is usually airway obstruction. Not infrequently, the carcinomas are initially misdiagnosed as lower airway in origin. True subglottic lesions arise below the conus elasticus (1 cm below the free edge of the true vocal cord) and spread locally to invade the cricoid cartilage and thyroid gland with lymphatic spread to lower deep jugular lymph nodes, the Delphian node (prelaryngeal), and the paratracheal nodes.[88] Management requires total laryngectomy because invasion of the laryngeal framework is common.[89] Ipsilateral thyroidectomy and paratracheal node dissection are essential. Positive paratracheal nodes and extensive invasion requires postoperative radiotherapy to include the superior mediastinum to prevent stomal recurrence.

FUTURE DIRECTIONS

There is continued evolution in the surgical management of laryngeal cancer.

Robotic Laryngeal Surgery

Hockstein and colleagues, from the University of Pennsylvania, reported that it was feasible to use the daVinci robot system for laryngopharyngeal surgery following studies with a human mannequin and a cadaver model.[90,91] Later, this group reported the first transoral robotic supraglottic laryngectomy in a canine model.[92] This work demonstrated that bleeding could be readily controlled with this technology. Monopolar cautery was used to perform the surgery, a technique thought to produce greater thermal injury than with an appropriately used CO_2 laser. Recently, OmniGuide (Boston, MA) developed a hollow core fiber that affords transmission of CO_2 laser energy through flexible instruments.[93] We coupled this technology to the daVinci Surgical Robot system to determine if the combined modalities would prove to be efficacious in the management of supraglottic laryngeal lesions. We conducted cadaveric dissections and animal studies demonstrating the utility of this technology.

Subsequently, a 74-year-old woman presenting with a large supraglottic malignancy had an endoscopic tumor excision, successfully, with this technology. The patient was able to swallow without difficulty on postoperative day 5. Follow-up endoscopic examination at 1 month showed no evidence of residual laryngeal tumor. Robotic CO_2 laser supraglottic laryngectomy was attempted in 2 additional patients; but adequate exposure could not be attained, and traditional approaches were utilized. Clearly, the daVinci Surgical Robot coupled with CO_2 laser technology can be used in selected instances for extirpation of supraglottic neoplasms. However, further development of this technology is needed for a greater applicability in the future.[94]

Adjuvant Cryotherapy after Laser Resection of Early Glottic Cancer

Based on our data inferring that adjunctive cryoablative therapy improved postoperative vocal outcomes in patients with early stage glottic carcinoma treated with laser resection, a prospective study was implemented to evaluate the vocal outcomes of patients managed with the combined modalities.[31] Twenty patients with early stage glottic carcinoma were evaluated. The mean follow-up was 32.6 months. The primary outcome measures were disease free survival as well as subjective and objective measures of posttreatment vocal quality. Serial videolaryngostroboscopy was performed in all instances. The extent of the resection was graded, and three professional observers reviewed the videos in a blinded manner. The extent of the resection was graded according to the criteria of the European Laryngological Society Working Committee (ELSWC). Five patients had a Type I cordectomy, 8 had a Type II, 5 had a Type III, and 2 had a Type IV. One patient failed locally which gave an overall mean disease-free follow-up of 32.6 months (range, 3 to 93 months). CO_2 laser resection and cryoablative therapy were associated with a significant improvement in subjective voice quality ($p < .0005$). Long-term dysphonia was uniformly improved vis-à-vis the pretreatment condition, even among patients with the most advanced disease undergoing the widest resections. Posttreatment web formation was not noted among four patients with anterior commissure involvement. Based on this initial study we concluded that endoscopic laser laryngeal surgery performed in conjunction with cryotherapy for early-stage glottic carcinoma yielded excellent primary site control while improving subjective and objective measures of voice quality. Combined laser surgery and cryotherapy is a possible alternative to radiation therapy for selected patients with early-stage glottic carcinoma who desire curative therapy while optimizing vocal outcomes.

LARYNGEAL TRANSPLANTATION

The first successful composite human laryngeal transplantation was performed in our department on January 4, 1998.[95] The recipient, a 40-year-old male, had sustained a crush injury to his larynx 20 years earlier, rendering him aphonic. Multiple prior attempted reconstructive efforts had failed. The donor was a 40-year-old male who had succumbed to a ruptured cerebral aneurysm. The primary consideration for laryngeal extirpation in the United States is cancer. Laryngeal transplantation in patients treated for malignancy would carry an unacceptably high risk of recurrent or second malignancy if conventional treatment with corticosteroids and calcineurin inhibitors were needed for immunosuppression.

Transplantation after tumor ablative surgery will only be possible when immunosuppression does not increase the risk of tumor recurrence. Everolimus is an immunosuppressive agent that has shown early evidence of potent antitumor activity. Our recent data lead us to conclude that everolimus can inhibit the in vivo growth of squamous cell carcinoma. Its antiproliferative and immunosuppressive capabilities make it attractive as a stand alone therapeutic modality or a partner in a dual treatment protocol.[96,97]

REFERENCES

1. Rothman KJ, Cann CI, Flanders D, Fried MP. Epidemiology of laryngeal cancer. Epidemiol Rev 1980;2:195–209.
2. De Stefani E, Oreggia F, Rivero S, Fierro L. Hand-rolled cigarette smoking and risk of cancer of the mouth, pharynx, and larynx. Cancer 1992;70:679–82.
3. Andre K, Schraub S, Mercier M, Bontemps P. Role of alcohol and tobacco in the aetiology of head and neck cancer: A case-control study in the Doubs region of France. Eur J Cancer B Oral Oncol 1995;31B:301–9.
4. De Stefani E, Correa P, Oreggia F, et al. Risk factors for laryngeal cancer. Cancer 1987;60:3087–91.
5. Guenel P, Chastang JF, Luce D, et al. A study of the interaction of alcohol drinking and tobacco smoking among French cases of laryngeal cancer. J Epidemiol Community Health 1988;42:350–4.
6. Bertazzi PA, Zocchetti C, Riboldi L, et al. Cancer mortality of an Italian cohort of workers in man-made glass-fiber production. Scand J Work Environ Health 1986;12:65–71.
7. Cammarota G, Agostino S, Rigante M, et al. Preliminary laryngeal examination during magnifying upper gastrointestinal video endoscopy in two patients with reflux symptoms. Endoscopy 2006;38:287.
8. Qadeer MA, Colabianchi N, Strome M, Vaezi MF. Gastroesophageal reflux and laryngeal cancer: Causation or association? A critical review. Am J Otolaryngol 2006;27:119–28.
9. Zatterstrom UK, Wennerberg J, Ewers SB, et al. Prognostic factors in head and neck cancer: Histologic grading, DNA ploidy, and nodal status. Head Neck 1991;13:477–87.
10. Yoo WJ, Cho SH, Lee YS, et al. Loss of heterozygosity on chromosomes 3p, 8p, 9p and 17p in the progression of squamous cell carcinoma of the larynx. J Korean Med Sci 2004;19:345–51.
11. Temam S, Benard J, Dugas C, et al. Molecular detection of early-stage laryngopharyngeal squamous cell carcinomas. Clin Cancer Res 2005;11:2547–51.
12. Luo K, Wang Z, Wang N, et al. Effect of expression of p53 in squamous cell carcinoma of larynx and mucosa adjacent to tumor on the biological behavior. Lin Chuang Er Bi Yan Hou Ke Za Zhi 2005;19:405–8.
13. Okami K, Reed AL, Cairns P, et al. Cyclin D1 amplification is independent of p16 inactivation in head and neck squamous cell carcinoma. Oncogene 1999;18:3541–5.
14. Almadori G, Cadoni G, Cattani P, et al. Human papillomavirus infection and epidermal growth factor receptor expression in primary laryngeal squamous cell carcinoma. Clin Cancer Res 2001;7:3988–93.
15. Clayman GL, Stewart MG, Weber RS, et al. Human papillomavirus in laryngeal and hypopharyngeal carcinomas:

16. Sisk EA, Soltys SG, Zhu S, et al. Human papillomavirus and p53 mutational status as prognostic factors in head and neck carcinoma. Head Neck 2002;24:841–9.
17. Jemal A, Tiwari RC, Murray T, et al. Cancer statistics, 2004. CA Cancer J Clin 2004;54:8–29.
18. Yousem DM, Tufano RP. Laryngeal imaging. Magn Reson Imaging Clin N Am 2002;10:451–65.
19. Tan L, Greener CC, Seikaly H, et al. Role of screening chest computed tomography in patients with advanced head and neck cancer. Otolaryngol Head Neck Surg 1999;120:689–92.
20. Zinreich SJ. Imaging in laryngeal cancer: Computed tomography, magnetic resonance imaging, positron emission tomography. Otolaryngol Clin North Am 2002;35:971–91.
21. Gordin A, Daitzchman M, Doweck I, et al. Fluorodeoxyglucose-positron emission tomography/computed tomography imaging in patients with carcinoma of the larynx: Diagnostic accuracy and impact on clinical management. Laryngoscope 2006;116:273–8.
22. Deleyiannis FW, Weymuller EA, Jr, Coltrera MD, Futran N. Quality of life after laryngectomy: Are functional disabilities important? Head Neck 1999;21:319–24.
23. Thompson LD, Wenig BM, Heffner DK, Gnepp DR. Exophytic and papillary squamous cell carcinomas of the larynx: A clinicopathologic series of 104 cases. Otolaryngol Head Neck Surg 1999;120:718–24.
24. Beckhardt RN, Murray JG, Ford CN, et al. Factors influencing functional outcome in supraglottic laryngectomy. Head Neck 1994;16:232–9.
25. Strong MS. Laser excision of carcinoma of the larynx. Laryngoscope 1975;85:1286–9.
26. Vaughan CW, Strong MS, Jako GJ. Laryngeal carcinoma: Transoral treatment utilizing the CO2 laser. Am J Surg 1978;136:490–3.
27. Bocciolini C, Presutti L, Laudadio P. Oncological outcome after CO2 laser cordectomy for early-stage glottic carcinoma. Acta Otorhinolaryngol Ital 2005;25:86–93.
28. Ossoff RH, Sisson GA, Shapshay SM. Endoscopic management of selected early vocal cord carcinoma. Ann Otol Rhinol Laryngol 1985;94:560–4.
29. Peretti G, Nicolai P, Piazza C, et al. Oncological results of endoscopic resections of Tis and T1 glottic carcinomas by carbon dioxide laser. Ann Otol Rhinol Laryngol 2001;110:820–6.
30. Lopez Llames A, Nunez Batalla F, Llorente Pendas JL, et al. Laser cordectomy: Oncologic outcome and functional results. Acta Otorrinolaringol Esp 2004;55:34–40.
31. Knott PD, Milstein CF, Hicks DM, Abelson TI, Byrd MC, Strome M. Vocal outcomes after laser resection of early-stage glottic cancer with adjuvant cryotherapy. Arch Otolaryngol Head Neck Surg. 2006;132:1226-30.
32. Knott PD, Byrd MC, Hicks DG, Strome M. Vocal fold healing after laser cordectomy with adjuvant cryotherapy. Laryngoscope 2006;116:1580–4.
33. Davis RK, Shapshay SM, Strong MS, Hyams VJ. Transoral partial supraglottic resection using the CO2 laser. Laryngoscope 1983;93:429–32.
34. Steiner W. Results of curative laser microsurgery of laryngeal carcinomas. Am J Otolaryngol 1993;14:116–21.
35. Candela FC, Shah J, Jaques DP, Shah JP. Patterns of cervical node metastases from squamous carcinoma of the larynx. Arch Otolaryngol Head Neck Surg 1990;116:432–5.
36. Ferlito A, Silver CE, Rinaldo A, Smith RV. Surgical treatment of the neck in cancer of the larynx. ORL 2006;62:217–225.
37. The Department of Veterans Affairs Laryngeal Cancer Study Group. Induction chemotherapy plus radiation compared with surgery plus radiation in patients with advanced laryngeal cancer. N Engl J Med 1991;324:1685–90.
38. Wolf G. Chemotherapy for laryngeal cancer. In: Ferlito A, editor. Diseases of the Larynx. London: Arnold Publishers; 2000. p. 709–25.
39. Hillman RE, Walsh MJ, Wolf GT, et al. Functional outcomes following treatment for advanced laryngeal cancer. Part I–Voice preservation in advanced laryngeal cancer. Part II–Laryngectomy rehabilitation: The state of the art in the VA System. Research Speech-Language Pathologists. Department of Veterans Affairs Laryngeal Cancer Study Group. Ann Otol Rhinol Laryngol Suppl 1998;172:1–27.
40. Terrell JE, Fisher SG, Wolf GT. Long-term quality of life after treatment of laryngeal cancer. The Veterans Affairs Laryngeal Cancer Study Group. Arch Otolaryngol Head Neck Surg 1998;124:964–71.
41. Smith RV, Kotz T, Beitler JJ, Wadler S. Long-term swallowing problems after organ preservation therapy with concomitant radiation therapy and intravenous hydroxyurea:

Initial results. Arch Otolaryngol Head Neck Surg 2000;126:384–9.

42. Eisbruch A, Lyden T, Bradford CR, et al. Objective assessment of swallowing dysfunction and aspiration after radiation concurrent with chemotherapy for head-and-neck cancer. Int J Radiat Oncol Biol Phys 2002;53:23–8.

43. Forastiere AA, Goepfert H, Maor M, et al. Concurrent chemotherapy and radiotherapy for organ preservation in advanced laryngeal cancer. N Engl J Med 2003;349:2091–8.

44. Weber RS, Berkey BA, Forastiere A, et al. Outcome of salvage total laryngectomy following organ preservation therapy: The Radiation Therapy Oncology Group trial 91-11. Arch Otolaryngol Head Neck Surg 2003;129:44–9.

45. Wolf GT, Bradford CR, Urba S, et al. Immune reactivity does not predict chemotherapy response, organ preservation, or survival in advanced laryngeal cancer. Laryngoscope 2002;112:1351–6.

46. Laccourreye O, Veivers D, Bassot V, et al. Analysis of local recurrence in patients with selected T1-3N0M0 squamous cell carcinoma of the true vocal cord managed with a platinum-based chemotherapy-alone regimen for cure [discussion 21–2]. Ann Otol Rhinol Laryngol 2002;111:315–21.

47. Goldman JL, Roffman JD. Combined pre-operative irradiation and surgery for advanced cancer of the larynx and laryngopharynx. A 14-year correlative statistical and histopathological study. Can J Otolaryngol 1975;4:251–64.

48. Kirchner JA, Owen JR. Five hundred cancers of the larynx and pyriform sinus. Results of treatment by radiation and surgery. Laryngoscope 1977;87:1288–303.

49. Ogura JH, Mallen RW. Partial laryngopharyngectomy for supraglottic and pharyngeal carcinoma. Trans Am Acad Ophthalmol Otolaryngol 1965;69:832–45.

50. Arriagada R, Eschwege F, Cachin Y, Richard JM. The value of combining radiotherapy with surgery in the treatment of hypopharyngeal and laryngeal cancers. Cancer 1983;51:1819–25.

51. Vikram B. Importance of the time interval between surgery and postoperative radiation therapy in the combined management of head and neck cancer. Int J Radiat Oncol Biol Phys 1979;5:1837–40.

52. Bastit L, Blot E, Debourdeau P, et al. Influence of the delay of adjuvant postoperative radiation therapy on relapse and survival in oropharyngeal and hypopharyngeal cancers. Int J Radiat Oncol Biol Phys 2001;49:139–46.

53. Kramer S, Gelber RD, Snow JB, et al. Combined radiation therapy and surgery in the management of advanced head and neck cancer: Final report of study 73-03 of the Radiation Therapy Oncology Group. Head Neck Surg 1987;10:19–30.

54. Tupchong L, Scott CB, Blitzer PH, et al. Randomized study of preoperative versus postoperative radiation therapy in advanced head and neck carcinoma: Long-term follow-up of RTOG study 73-03. Int J Radiat Oncol Biol Phys 1991;20:21–8.

55. Cooper JS, Pajak TF, Forastiere AA, et al. Postoperative concurrent radiotherapy and chemotherapy for high-risk squamous-cell carcinoma of the head and neck. N Engl J Med 2004;350:1937–44.

56. Sittel C, Eckel HE, Eschenburg C. Phonatory results after laser surgery for glottic carcinoma. Otolaryngol Head Neck Surg 1998;119:418–24.

57. Nguyen C, Naghibzadeh B, Black MJ, et al. Carcinoma in situ of the glottic larynx: Excision or irradiation? Head Neck 1996;18:225–8.

58. Myers EN, Wagner RL, Johnson JT. Microlaryngoscopic surgery for T1 glottic lesions: A cost-effective option. Ann Otol Rhinol Laryngol 1994;103:28–30.

59. Thomas JV, Olsen KD, Neel HB, III, et al. Recurrences after endoscopic management of early (T1) glottic carcinoma. Laryngoscope 1994;104:1099–104.

60. McGuirt WF, Blalock D, Koufman JA, et al. Comparative voice results after laser resection or irradiation of T1 vocal cord carcinoma. Arch Otolaryngol Head Neck Surg 1994;120:951–5.

61. Franchin G, Minatel E, Gobitti C, et al. Radiotherapy for patients with early-stage glottic carcinoma: Univariate and multivariate analyses in a group of consecutive, unselected patients. Cancer 2003;98:765–72.

62. Le QT, Fu KK, Kroll S, et al. Influence of fraction size, total dose, and overall time on local control of T1-T2 glottic carcinoma. Int J Radiat Oncol Biol Phys 1997;39:115–26.

63. Jones AS, Fish B, Fenton JE, Husband DJ. The treatment of early laryngeal cancers (T1-T2 N0): Surgery or irradiation? Head Neck 2004;26:127–35.

64. Bron LP, Soldati D, Zouhair A, et al. Treatment of early stage squamous-cell carcinoma of the glottic larynx: Endoscopic surgery or cricohyoidoepiglottopexy versus radiotherapy. Head Neck 2001;23:823–9.

65. Fletcher GH, Jessee RH. The place of irradiation in the management of the primary lesion in head and neck cancers. Cancer 1977;39:862–7.

66. Makeieff M, Venegoni D, Mercante G, et al. Supracricoid partial laryngectomies after failure of radiation therapy. Laryngoscope 2005;115:353–7.

67. Ganly I, Patel SG, Matsuo J, et al. Results of surgical salvage after failure of definitive radiation therapy for early-stage squamous cell carcinoma of the glottic larynx. Arch Otolaryngol Head Neck Surg 2006;132:59–66.

68. Yiotakis J, Stavroulaki P, Nikolopoulos T, et al. Partial laryngectomy after irradiation failure. Otolaryngol Head Neck Surg 2003;128:200–9.

69. Ichimura K, Sugasawa M, Nibu K, et al. The significance of arytenoid edema following radiotherapy of laryngeal carcinoma with respect to residual and recurrent tumour. Auris Nasus Larynx 1997;24:391–7.

70. Maheshwar AA, Gaffney CC. Radiotherapy for T1 glottic carcinoma: Impact of anterior commissure involvement. J Laryngol Otol 2001;115:298–301.

71. Fein DA, Mendenhall WM, Parsons JT, Million RR. T1-T2 squamous cell carcinoma of the glottic larynx treated with radiotherapy: A multivariate analysis of variables potentially influencing local control. Int J Radiat Oncol Biol Phys 1993;25:605–11.

72. Harwood AR, DeBoer G. Prognostic factors in T2 glottic cancer. Cancer 1980;45:991–5.

73. McLaughlin MP, Parsons JT, Fein DA, et al. Salvage surgery after radiotherapy failure in T1-T2 squamous cell carcinoma of the glottic larynx. Head Neck 1996;18:229–35.

74. Laccourreye H, Laccourreye O, Weinstein G, et al. Supracricoid laryngectomy with cricohyoidopexy: A partial laryngeal procedure for selected supraglottic and transglottic carcinomas. Laryngoscope 1990;100:735–41.

75. Bron L, Pasche P, Brossard E, et al. Functional analysis after supracricoid partial laryngectomy with cricohyoidoepiglottopexy. Laryngoscope 2002;112:1289–93.

76. Sessions DG, Lenox J, Spector GJ, et al. Management of T3N0M0 glottic carcinoma: Therapeutic outcomes. Laryngoscope 2002;112:1281–8.

77. Pradier O, Christiansen H, Schmidberger H, et al. Adjuvant radiotherapy after transoral laser microsurgery for advanced squamous carcinoma of the head and neck. Int J Radiat Oncol Biol Phys 2005;63:1368–77.

78. Davis RK, Kriskovich MD, Galloway EB, III, et al. Endoscopic supraglottic laryngectomy with postoperative irradiation. Ann Otol Rhinol Laryngol 2004;113:132–8.

79. Ambrosch P, Kron M, Steiner W. Carbon dioxide laser microsurgery for early supraglottic carcinoma. Ann Otol Rhinol Laryngol 1998;107:680–8.

80. Iro H, Waldfahrer F, Altendorf-Hofmann A, et al. Transoral laser surgery of supraglottic cancer: Follow-up of 141 patients. Arch Otolaryngol Head Neck Surg 1998;124:1245–50.

81. Motta G, Esposito E, Testa D, et al. CO2 laser treatment of supraglottic cancer. Head Neck 2004;26:442–6.

82. Rudert HH, Werner JA, Hoft S. Transoral carbon dioxide laser resection of supraglottic carcinoma. Ann Otol Rhinol Laryngol 1999;108:819–27.

83. Zeitels SM. Surgical management of early supraglottic cancer. Otolaryngol Clin North Am 1997;30:59–78.

84. Zeitels SM, Vaughan CW, Domanowski GF. Endoscopic management of early supraglottic cancer. Ann Otol Rhinol Laryngol 1990;99:951–6.

85. Sessions DG, Lenox J, Spector GJ. Supraglottic laryngeal cancer: Analysis of treatment results. Laryngoscope 2005;115:1402–10.

86. Spriano G, Antognoni P, Piantanida R, et al. Conservative management of T1-T2N0 supraglottic cancer: A retrospective study. Am J Otolaryngol 1997;18:299–305.

87. Shaha AR, Shah JP. Carcinoma of the subglottic larynx. Am J Surg 1982;144:456–8.

88. Harrison DF. The pathology and management of subglottic cancer. Ann Otol Rhinol Laryngol 1971;80:6–12.

89. Harrison DF. Laryngectomy for subglottic lesions. Laryngoscope 1975;85:1208–10.

90. Hockstein NG, Nolan JP, O'Malley BW, Jr, Woo YJ. Robot-assisted pharyngeal and laryngeal microsurgery: Results of robotic cadaver dissections. Laryngoscope 2005;115:1003–8.

91. Hockstein NG, Nolan JP, O'Malley BW, Jr, Woo YJ. Robotic microlaryngeal surgery: A technical feasibility study using the daVinci surgical robot and an airway mannequin. Laryngoscope 2005;115:780–5.

92. Weinstein GS, O'Malley BW, Jr, Hockstein NG. Transoral robotic surgery: Supraglottic laryngectomy in a canine model. Laryngoscope 2005;115:1315–9.

93. Devaiah AK, Shapshay SM, Desai U, et al. Surgical utility of a new carbon dioxide laser fiber: Functional and histological study. Laryngoscope 2005;115:1463–8.

94. Solares CA, Strome M. Transoral robotic assisted CO_2 laser supraglottic laryngectomy: experimental and clinical data. Laryngoscope 2007;117:817–820.

95. Strome M, Stein J, Esclamado R, et al. Laryngeal transplantation and 40-month follow-up. N Engl J Med 2001;344:1676–9.

96. Khariwala SS, Kjaergaard J, Lorenz R, et al. Everolimus (RAD) inhibits in vivo growth of murine squamous cell carcinoma (SCC VII). Laryngoscope 2006;116:814–20.

97. Khariwala SS, Knott PD, Dan O, et al. Pulsed immunosuppression with everolimus and anti-alphabeta T-cell receptor: Laryngeal allograft preservation at six months. Ann Otol Rhinol Laryngol 2006;115:74–80.

100

Diseases of the Salivary Glands

Rodney J. Taylor, MD
Jeffrey S. Wolf, MD

There are three paired major salivary glands in the human: parotid, submandibular, and sublingual. These glands drain via ducts into the oral cavity. Saliva from the parotid gland enters the oral cavity adjacent to the second maxillary molar tooth via Stensen duct. The submandibular gland duct, known as Wharton duct, opens into the anterior part of the floor of the mouth. Multiple sublingual ducts enter Wharton duct or may drain separately into the floor of the mouth. The minor salivary glands individually drain through the mucosa of the oral cavity and pharynx.

Histologically, salivary glands are composed of acinar and ductal cells. The organization of the glands is 80% acinar, 15% ducts, with the remaining percentage comprised of nerves, connective tissues, and blood vessels. The composition of saliva differs depending on the gland: the sublingual glands secrete mucous saliva, the parotid glands secrete serous saliva, and submandibular glands secrete both mucous and serous saliva. Saliva is 99% water and contains electrolytes, urea, lipids, amino acids, and proteins including digestive and other enzymes and immunoglobulins.

The primary secretion of saliva occurs in the acinar region of the glands where protein production and water secretion occurs. The initial saliva secreted in the acinus is hypotonic and as the saliva travels down the branching ducts, the secretions are modified by both protein secretion and salt reabsorption by ductal cells. The final saliva product that enters the oral cavity is isotonic.

The neural control of saliva production is a complex interaction of the sympathetic and parasympathetic nervous systems. Secretion of saliva occurs in response to both alpha- and beta-adrenergic stimulation as well as parasympathetic stimulation. There is a basal or resting flow of saliva as well as an inducible flow in response to stimulation which may increase 10 to 20 times over basal flow. Over a 24-hour period, 1 to 1.5 L of saliva are secreted.

ANATOMY

The parotid gland is located on the face between the ramus of the mandible and the mastoid process. The medial surface of the gland is surrounded by the musculature that originates on the styloid process. The gland has two "lobes" that are artificially divided by the facial nerve, the lateral lobe being significantly larger than the deep lobe. The parotid duct traverses the surface of the masseter muscle and crosses anterior to the ramus of the mandible one-finger's breadth below the zygomatic arch. It turns medially to penetrate the buccinator muscle at the level of the second maxillary molar tooth.

The parotid is innervated by the glossopharyngeal nerve. The fibers begin in the inferior salvitory nucleus and travel with cranial nerve (CN) IX through the jugular foramen. Jacobson nerve travels back into the skull via the inferior tympanic canaliculus into the middle ear. The nerve penetrates the roof of the tympanic cavity into the middle cranial fossa. It forms in part the lesser petrosal nerve which exits the skull at the foramen ovale where it synapses in the otic ganglion. The parasympathetic fibers join with the auriculotemporal nerve (V_3) and enter the parotid gland with this nerve. The sympathetic fibers travel with the branches of the external carotid artery from the sympathetic ganglia to gland.

The submandibular gland occupies the majority of the submandibular triangle in the neck. It is located superior to the digastric tendon and against the mylohyoid and hyoglossus muscles. Like the parotid, it is composed of two lobes: a superficial lobe that is superficial to the mylohyoid and a deep lobe that extends behind the posterior part of the mylohyoid. In nonobese patients, the gland can usually be easily palpated in the neck. Wharton duct arises in the deep lobe of the submandibular gland and courses between the hyoglossus and the mylohyoid. It extends to the papilla on the floor of mouth lateral to the lingual frenulum. The duct passes underneath (medial) to the lingual nerve.

The submandibular gland is innervated by secretomotor fibers of the facial nerve which originate in the superior salvitory nucleus. They exit as the nervus intermedius and travel with CN VII until the descending portion of the nerve. The fibers then exit as the chorda tympani through the middle ear deep to the malleus and superficial to the incus and exit via the petrotympanic fissure. The chorda tympani joins the lingual branch of V_3 and travels along the floor of mouth where parasympathetic fibers descend and synapse in the submandibular ganglion and enter the gland. The sympathetic fibers accompany the arterial blood supply.

The sublingual duct is closely associated with the distal half of Wharton duct and is located between the mylohyoid and hyoglossus muscles. The sublingual glands are innervated by parasympathetic fibers from the submandibular ganglion and the sympathetic fibers accompany its arterial supply.

SALIVA FUNCTIONS

There are many functions of saliva. The alpha amylase in saliva initiates digestion of starches into maltose. Saliva assists with taste perception as food dissolves in it and is carried to the pore of the taste bud. Perhaps most importantly, the wetness of saliva allows for lubrication of food into a slick bolus that is easily transported to the oropharynx. The flow of saliva can whisk away food debris that remains in the oral cavity, which is important for oral hygiene and the protection of the teeth. Lysozyme in saliva prevents overgrowth of oral microbes. Immunoglobulins in the saliva play an important immune role. In some nonhuman animals, evaporation of saliva during panting acts as a cooling mechanism.

INFLAMMATORY DISEASES OF THE SALIVARY GLANDS

Viral Infections

The best-known viral infection of the salivary glands is mumps. Mumps is a paramyxovirus infection and is transmitted by respiratory droplets. Inflammation of the parotid glands (parotitis) occurs in 40% of patients with the mumps. After a prodrome of nonspecific viral symptoms, patients may develop parotitis or infection at other sites: the testes, pancreas, eyes, ovaries, central nervous system, joints, or kidneys. The swollen parotid glands may be tender but are not typically erythematous or warm. Chewing and eating often exacerbates the pain associated with viral parotitis. Less commonly, submandibular and sublingual glands may also be involved.

Although it is typically a clinical diagnosis, mumps virus can be isolated from nasopharyngeal swabs, urine, blood, and fluid from buccal cavity typically from 7 days before up until 9 days after the onset of parotitis. Serious complications are uncommon but can include sensorineural hearing loss often unilateral, meningoencephalitis (1.5% mortality), pancreatisis, and orchitis.

Clinical mumps has become uncommon in communities where universal immunization with the measles, mumps, and rubella vaccine is practiced.

There are other acute viral parotid infections. Viruses such as parainfluenza, influenza, coxsackie, ECHO, and choriomeningitis virus may also cause parotitis.[1] In patients with human immunodeficiency virus (HIV), adenovirus and cytomegalovirus can cause parotitis.[2] The management of most cases of viral parotitis is supportive therapy.

HIV infection is associated with benign lymphoepithelial cysts of the parotid and possible glandular malfunction (Figure 1). It is unknown whether the HIV-associated parotid disease is caused by the virus itself or related to progressive lymphadenopathy associated with HIV. HIV-associated salivary disease may occur early in HIV disease when CD4 levels are within the normal range and this may be the initial presenting sign of HIV infection.[3] Up to 20% of children with HIV will have salivary gland involvement.

Histologically, these glands are composed of multiple adjacent cysts. They contain lymphocytes and macrophages in a serous yellow fluid with cholesterol centers.[4,5] There may be many features of HIV-related salivary gland disease including dry eyes, xerostomia, and arthralgia.[6] The lymphoid infiltration that occurs in some patients is known as "diffuse infiltrative lymphocytosis syndrome." It shares clinical features with Sjögren syndrome; however, it differs in that the predominant infiltrating cells are CD8 positive T cells as compared to CD4 in Sjögren syndrome.[7] Diffuse infiltrative lymphocytosis syndrome may be a favorable prognostic marker in HIV disease.[8]

Most HIV-infected patients with parotid gland benign lymphoepithelial cysts can be treated with observation and antiretroviral medication. For others, who are symptomatic or more concerned about their cosmetic appearance, sclerotherapy or repeated needle aspiration may offer a reasonable option. Radiation therapy and surgery should be reserved for select cases.[9] There is concern for underlying Kaposi sarcoma and lymphoma in these cysts, which have been reported in up to 10% of patients.[7,10]

Bacterial

Acute bacterial infections of the salivary glands carried an 80% mortality rate in the nineteenth century.[11] Among prominent persons to die of this disease was the twentieth president of the United States, James Garfield.[12] In the antibiotic era, the mortality of bacterial parotitis and parotid abscess has decreased dramatically.

There are many potential causes of bacterial sialadenitis. It is hypothesized that retrograde contamination from oral bacteria as well as stasis of salivary flow has import in the pathogenesis of acute suppurative lymphadenitis. Most commonly dehydration or obstruction from calculi leads to static salivary flow. Diseases, conditions, and medications that cause dehydration or decreased salivary flow are thus potential causative agents of sialadenitis. Traditionally, abdominal surgery, in which patients are on nothing by mouth (NPO) or third-spacing fluid postoperatively, may facilitate salivary gland infections. Chronic debilitating diseases such as liver or renal failure, malnutrition, and HIV infection are associated with higher incidence of sialadenitis. Bulimia and cystic fibrosis are also associated with acute bacterial salivary gland infections. Any conditions that lead to xerostomia, including Sjögren syndrome, and prior radiation as well as medications that cause xerostomia predispose patients to acute salivary gland infections. Certain occupations such as glass blowing and trumpet playing increase the risk of sialadenitis by both mechanical trauma to the ducts as well as retrograde contamination.[13]

The populations most at risk of sialadenitis are people at the extremes of the age range, with the elderly population at the greatest risk. In addition to the decreased salivary quantity in the elderly, chronic debilitating illness can further contribute to dehydration and poor nutritional states.[14] Patients with psychiatric conditions such as depression, anorexia nervosa, and bulimia are at increased risk of bacterial sialadenitis.

Although an acute infection can occur in any salivary gland, the major glands are more likely to become infected, especially the parotid. The parotid gland is at increased risk because it produces serous saliva which does not contain the quantity of mucins, glycoproteins, or antibodies that the more mucous secreting glands, that is, submandibular and sublingual glands do.[15,16]

The pathogenic microorganism most commonly responsible for acute suppurative parotitis is *Staphylococcus aureus*. This is followed in frequency by *Streptococcus pyogenes* (Group A beta hemolytic *Streptococcus*), *S. pneumoniae*, and *Hemophilus influenzae*. Other microorganisms, such as gram-negative and anaerobic bacteria, can be found in salivary gland infections, but this is relatively uncommon. Immunosuppressed patients may have unusual microorganisms such as *Salmonella* species.[17] The clinical presentation of patients with acute sialadenitis includes pain and edema over the involved gland. It is unilateral 90% of the time.[11] Stensen or Wharton ducts may be edematous or erythmatous, and purulent material may be expressed by massaging the affected gland.

Patients may present with bacterial sepsis which is more common with parotid sialadenitis. Patients with acute parotitis may appear toxic and can progress to develop multiorgan system failure. The diagnosis of acute bacterial sialadenitis is predominantly clinical. With the exception of patients with abscesses, diagnostic imaging is not typically needed in acute sialadenitis (Figure 2). Laboratory testing may reveal a leukocytosis with predominance of neutrophils.[12] The differential diagnosis of acute sialadenitis includes other infections such as actinomycosis,[18] cat scratch disease (CSD),[19] and dental infections. Also included in the differential are autoimmune and inflammatory diseases such as Sjögren syndrome[20,21] and Wegener granulomatosis,[22] and neoplasms such as lymphomas.[23]

The treatment of acute bacterial sialadenitis is hydration, warm compresses, and improved oral hygiene. Sialogogues function to increase salivary flow and along with salivary gland massage may improve clearance of the bacterial infection. Antibiotic therapy is needed and geared toward the treatment of gram positives and anaerobic bacteria. Augmented penicillins such as amoxicillin with clavulanic acid, ampicillin with sulbactam, and beta-lactams with anti-staphylococcal coverage are the primary treatment.

Neonatal Sialadenitis

Neonatal suppurative sialadenitis usually occurs in the parotid glands with a higher incidence in preterm and male neonates. Like bacterial parotitis in adults, it is usually caused by *S. aureus*; however, *Escherichia coli* and *Pseudomonas* species have also been reported.[24] Data suggest that risk factors may include cytomegalovirus infection and maternal methyldopa use.[25] This usually presents as fever, anorexia, and failure to gain weight. The glands may be unilaterally or bilaterally edematous, and the overlying skin may

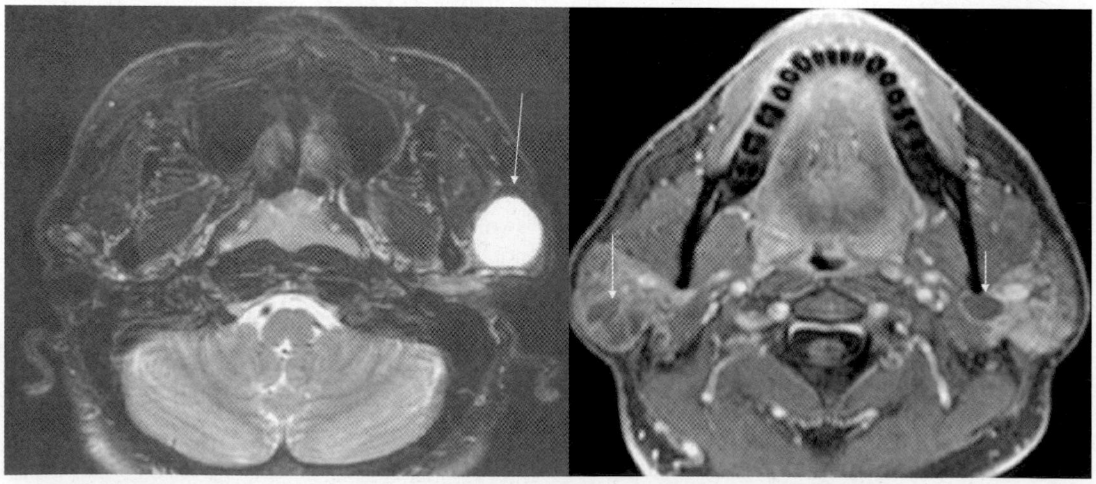

Figure 1 Lymphoepithelial cysts in the parotid gland of patients with HIV. The left side of the figure contains a T2-weighted image of a cyst in the left parotid (*arrow*). Note the intensity of the cyst on T2. The right side of the figure is a T1-weighted image of bilateral parotid cysts (*arrows*).

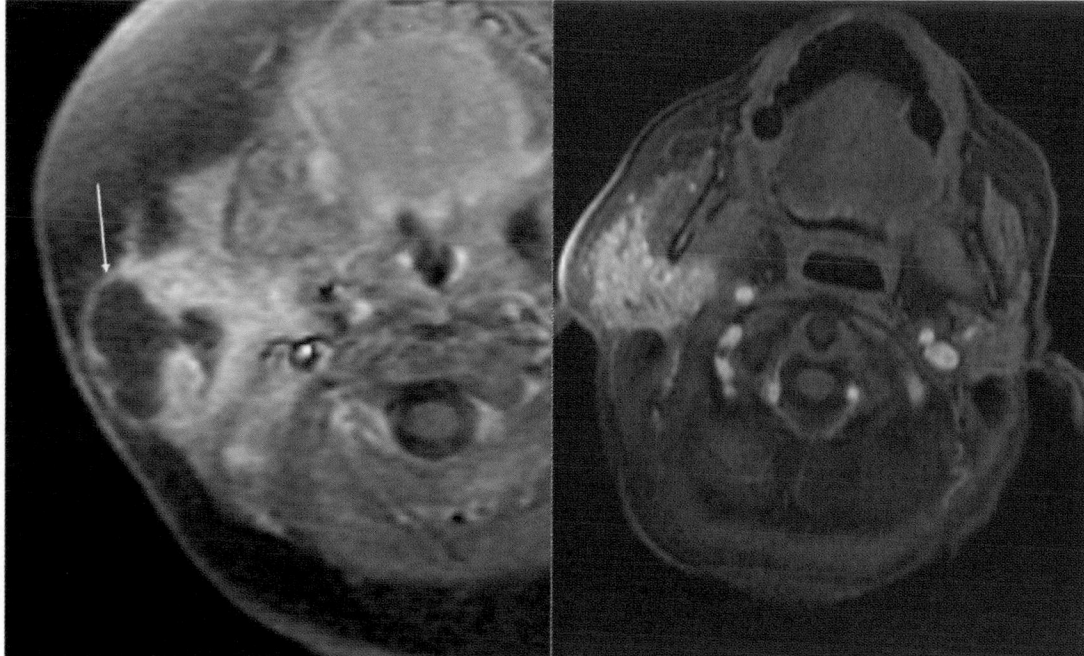

Figure 2 Bacterial sialadenitis of the parotid gland. Bacterial sialadenitis can progress to a frank abscess (*left*), but most commonly imaging will show enlargement of the gland with acute inflammation (*right*).

become erythematous. Diagnosis is clinical with fine-needle aspiration (FNA) to collect purulent material for culture. Open drainage procedures are reserved for patients in whom clinical improvement does not occur or a frank abscess forms.[24]

Recurrent Parotitis of Childhood

Recurrent parotitis (RP) of childhood is of unknown etiology and is thought to be probably immune mediated.[26] Although it is rare, it is second to mumps as the most common inflammatory salivary gland disorder in children. It has a biphasic age distribution with peaks at 3 and 10 years. Children suspected of this disease should be screened for Sjögren and immune deficiency syndromes.[27] Signs and symptoms at presentation include recurrent episodes of glandular swelling, pain after a meal, fever, and malaise. The diagnosis is mostly clinical, and ultrasound can confirm this diagnosis. Treatment is supportive with hydration, gland massage, and sialogogues. Antibiotics are not beneficial in the treatment of this disease.[26]

Chronic Sialadenitis

Chronic sialadenitis is a localized condition of the salivary glands that is characterized by repeated episodes of painful inflammation that results in parenchymal degeneration and replacement of the gland by fibrous tissue. The average age of onset is the sixth decade, and patients with this disease have a history of acute sialadenitis. The repeated episodes of sialadenitis are thought to be caused by chronic obstruction of the ducts, ductal dilation, or decreased salivary flow. Over time, irreversible changes in the glandular architecture result in ectasia of the ducts and inflammatory and fibrous infiltration. Historically, treatment has been difficult and has included duct ligation, removal of the gland, and tympanic neurectomy.

More recent treatment options include partial gland removal with duct preservation and intraductal infusion of penicillin or saline.[28,29]

Sialolithiasis

Salivary calculi may present as isolated events or in the setting of chronic sialadenitis. It is typically a disease of the sixth through ninth decades of life and may be largely responsible for the development of chronic sialadenitis.

Salivary calculi are usually composed of hydroxyapatite $[Ca_5(PO_4)_3(OH)]$ combined with cations such as magnesium, ammonia, and zinc. Frequently organic material, such as protein and mucopolysaccharides, is also found in stones,

and some stones are composed entirely of organic material.[30]

The etiology of stone formation has yet to be elucidated but may include a variety of factors such as salivary stasis, ductal narrowing, the presence of a nidus from trauma, or inflammation, and the absence of natural crystallization inhibitors such as myoinositol hexaphosphate.[30] Eighty percent of salivary duct stones occur in the submandibular duct (Figure 3), 19% occur in Stensen duct (Figure 4), and 1% occurs in the sublingual ducts.[31,32] This differential among glands is thought to be due to the viscosity of mucous saliva.[12,33]

The presentation of sialolithiasis consists of postprandial pain and edema. It may be a colicky type of pain with a classic crescendo pattern. The stone may be palpable along a duct. This is accomplished with a bimanual examination of the floor of mouth in patients with submandibular stones. Parotid stones present more of a challenge because the stones may be small, the buccal fat pad may make palpation more difficult, and 80% of parotid stones are radiolucent.[34] Contrast studies can be helpful for identification of radiolucent stones associated with proximal duct dilation. Trauma to the duct from pressure may lead to fistula formation between the duct and the gland parenchyma. Ultrasound, magnetic resonance sialography (MRS) and digital subtraction sialography have been used with some success in diagnosing radiolucent stones.[35–38] Recently sialoendoscopy has been utilized to diagnose and treat submandibular and parotid stones.[39]

Initial management of calculi is conservative and supportive. Nonsteroidal antiinflammatory medications, warm compresses, and sialogogues may be useful especially in the face of a nonobstructing stone. Stones near the ductal orifice can be "milked" out of the orifice, but most

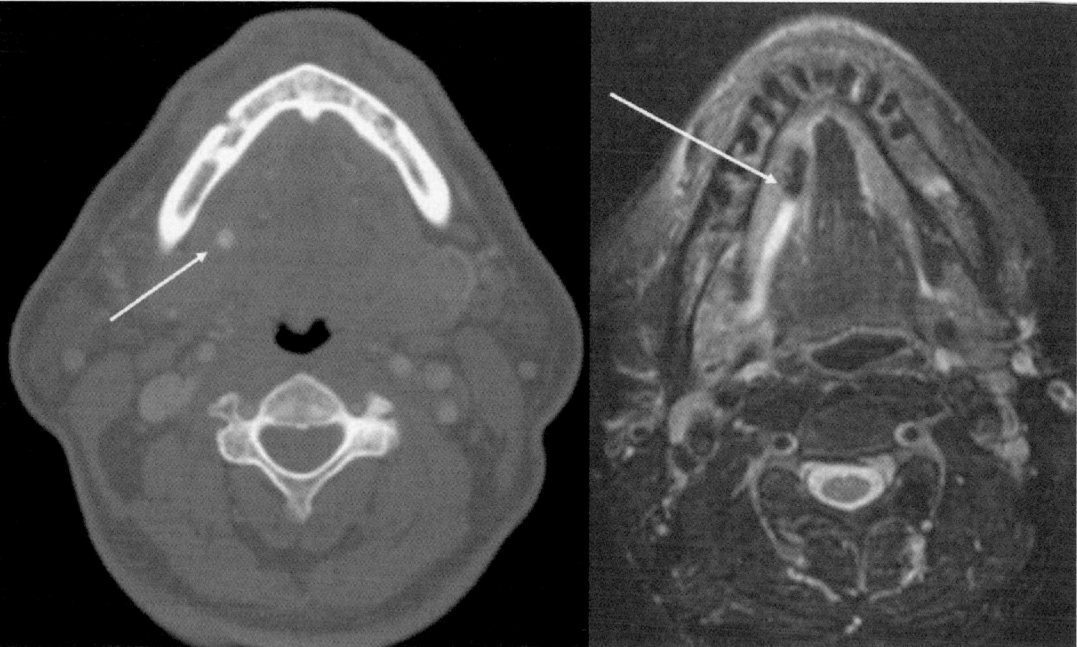

Figure 3 Sialolithiasis of the submandibular gland. The left side of the figure demonstrates a radiointense density on CT of a submandibular stone (*arrow*). The T2-weighted MRI on the right reveals a hypodense obstructing stone (*arrow*) with proximal dilation of the Wharton duct.

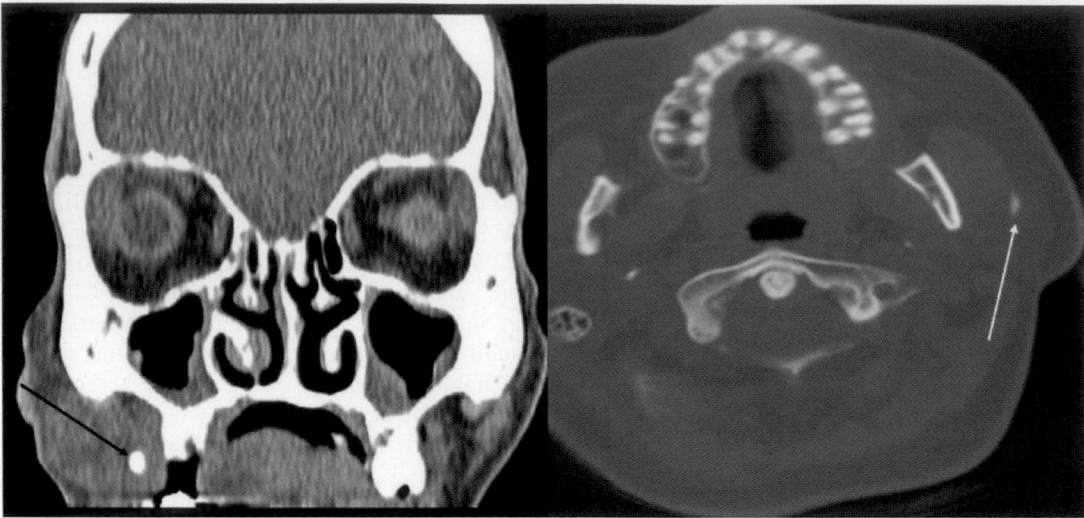

Figure 4 Sialolithiasis of the parotid glands. Only 20% of parotid stones are radiopaque. The arrows indicate opaque parotid stones in both coronal (*left*) and axial (*right*) planes on CT scan.

require sialolithotomy. Occasionally, sialodocho-plasty will be required to remove a stone. More "state-of-the-art" ways to remove stones include sialoendoscopy with basket retrieval and litho-tripsy.[35,39]

GRANULOMATOUS SALIVARY GLAND DISEASES

Nontuberculous mycobacterial infections are most common in children 2 to 3 years of age. They usually present with an enlarging neck mass. These infections most frequently involve lymph nodes that are within or adjacent to the parotid and submandibular glands and will com-monly have sinus tracts to the skin. The overlying skin may be discolored. The diagnosis is largely clinical and may require excluding other diseases. Tissue histopathology is usually nonspecific, and myobacterial cultures usually take up to 6 weeks for the results. FNA biopsy can be used to make the diagnosis and is preferred over incisional biopsy. Imaging is nonspecific and reveals asym-metric adenopathy with contiguous low-density ring-enhancing masses.[40] The treatment of choice is usually excision, which usually results in the most rapid resolution of the disease.[41]

Tuberculosis involves the salivary glands less commonly than cervical lymph nodes. These patients will have painless indolent enlargement of the parotid or submandibular glands. These infections are usually in lymph nodes within the glands rather than actual parenchymal disease. Other than the enlarged glands, the patient may be asymptomatic without constitutional signs or facial nerve involvement. Although skin testing may lead to suspicion of tuberculosis, diagno-sis of glandular involvement is usually made by excisional biopsy of the gland. More recently, polymerase chain reaction (PCR) techniques have has been described as a diagnostic modality for this disease.[42] Antituberculous chemotherapy is needed to treat systemic disease.

Actinomycosis of the salivary glands is rare and has been most commonly described in the parotid gland.[43–45] Most cases are odontogenic and are thought to spread retrograde along sali-vary ducts. Actinomycosis occurs predominantly in immunocompetent individuals, and patients present with painless enlargement of the involved gland. Causative microorganisms are bacteria of low pathogenicity and cause disease only in the setting of antecedent tissue injury, such as dental work. The disease process is character-ized by the formation of induration of tissues and draining sinuses that discharge "sulfur gran-ules." Diagnosis is usually made through culture of *Actinomyces* species (*Actinomyces israelii, A. bovis, A. naelsundi*) from clinical specimens, or microscopic visualization of gram-positive, non-acid-fast, thin, branching filaments in cytologic specimens. Penicillin is the drug of choice and is usually administered for 2 to 12 months. Surgical therapy is often indicated for curettage of bone, resection of necrotic tissue, excision of sinus tracts, and drainage of soft tissue abscesses. The prognosis for treated infection is excellent.

CSD is a type of granulomatous lymphadeni-tis that may involve the salivary glands. Greater than 90% of patients have a history of expo-sure to cats. Approximately 70 to 90% of CSD cases occur in the fall and early winter months. This seasonality is presumed to be due to a mid-summer rise in kitten births accompanied by increased flea infestation. In most children and adolescents, swollen lymph nodes are the main symptom of the disease, and the illness often is mild. About one-third of patients with CSD have generalized symptoms. These include fever, headache, odynophagia, fatigue, loss of appetite, headache, rash, and malaise. In the United States, about 22,000 cases are diagnosed annually, most of them in people under the age of 21. With sali-vary involvement, the patients will present with edematous glands or masses within the salivary gland. The skin over these swollen lymph nodes may become warm and red, and occasionally the lymph nodes drain purulent material. The causative agent is *Bartonella henselae*, and the serologic test for CSD is positive in 90% of the

patients.[46] PCR techniques expedite the diagno-sis. Elevated serum titers can be found 1 to 3 weeks after the onset of the illness. The titers con-tinue to rise for the first 8 weeks and then gradu-ally decrease over the next several months.[47] The disease is usually self-limited, but for persistent cases as well as immunocompromised patients, antibiotics may be needed. Typical first-line treat-ment for CSD is azithromycin or rifampin.

Tularemia is an insect-borne disease that may involve the parotid gland. The most com-mon hosts in the United States are ticks and the cottontail rabbit. After an incubation of 3 to 4 days, a papule forms at the site of cutaneous transmission. Involved lymph nodes may enlarge and drain, and the infected patients may develop fever, myalgias, malaise, or headache. The caus-ative microorganism *Franciscella tularensis* is difficult to isolate form the blood, and the diagno-sis is most commonly made with serologic tests. The treatment is with aminoglyosides and fluoro-quinolones.

Toxoplasmosis is caused by *Toxoplasma gondii* and is usually contracted by exposure to domestic cats. Humans can become infected with *T. gondii* by ingesting either material contami-nated with infectious oocysts or tissue cysts con-tained in raw or undercooked meat from another intermediate host. The parotid gland may be involved through intraparotid lymph nodes. Most cases of toxoplasmosis in the immunocompetent host are subclinical or benign. The most severe symptoms occur in the congenitally acquired form and in immunocompromised hosts. In the severe and disseminated cases, patients will also develop myalgia, anorexia, necrotizing encepha-litis, pneumonitis, hepatosplenomegaly, and myo-carditis. The diagnosis of toxoplasmosis is usually made by immunoglobulin M (IgM) immunofluo-rescent antibody (IFA) test. An IgM-IFA titer of 1:160 or greater or an IgM enzyme-linked immu-nosorbent assay (ELISA) titer of 1:256 or greater is considered diagnostic of recently acquired *T. gondii* infection. The treatment consists of a com-bination of pyrimethamine and a sulfonamide (or clindamycin) in immunocompetent adults.[48]

SALIVARY NEOPLASMS

Benign and malignant salivary neoplasms encom-pass as broad and diverse a histologic spectrum as found in any organ system (Table 1). Although they are relative rare, their range of clinical behavior is wide.

Pathogenisis of Benign Salivary Gland Neoplasms

The salivary gland unit and its component cell types provide the basis for understanding the development of the array of neoplasms of the salivary glands. The multicellular theory postu-lates that the multiplicity of cell types in normal salivary glands have the potential to give rise to any of the numerous neoplasms occurring within the salivary glands. Evidence for this is based on

Table 1 United States Armed Forces Institute of Pathology Classification of Salivary Gland Neoplasms

Benign
- Pleomorphic adenoma
- Warthin tumor
- Basal cell adenoma
- Myoepithelioma
- Canalicular adenoma
- Oncocytoma
- Cystadenoma
- Sebaceous adenoma
- Ductal papillotas
    Sialadenoma papilliferum
    Inverted ductal papilloma
    Lymphadenoma
- Intraductal papilloma

Malignant
- Adenocarcinomas
    Acinic cell adenocarcinoma
    Basal cell adenocarcinoma
    Clear cell adenocarcinoma
    Cystadenocarcinoma
    Sebaceous adenocarcinoma
    Lymphadenocarcinoma
    Adenoid cystic carcinoma
    Mucinous adenocarcinoma
- Malignant mixed tumor
    Carcinoma ex mixed tumor
    Metastasizing mixed tumor
    Carcinosarcoma
- Carcinomas
    Squamous cell carcinoma
    Mucoepidermoid carcinoma
    Adenosquamous carcinoma
    Epithelial-myoepithelial carcinoma
    Oncocytic carcinoma
    Salivary duct carcinoma
    Myoepithelial carcinoma
- Others
    Mesenchymal tumors
    Lymphomas
- Metastatic tumors

DNA studies which have demonstrated that basal duct cells, luminal cells at all levels of the duct system, myoepithelial cells, and acinar cells are all capable of aberrant proliferation.[49] In contrast, the semipluripotential bicellular theory proposes that stem cells in the intercalated duct and excretory duct give rise to the variety of neoplasms that are observed.[50]

Incidence

Salivary gland neoplasms comprise approximately 3 to 4% of head and neck neoplasms. They most commonly present in the fifth to sixth decades with malignant tumors presenting approximately a decade later than benign neoplasms. Spiro reviewed the largest series, which included 2,807 salivary gland neoplasms over a 35-year period. The parotid gland represents the most common site (70%), followed by the minor salivary glands (22%), and the submandibular gland (8%). Other large series show a similar anatomic distribution, with approximately 70% of all tumors being benign.[51] Nagler and Laufer reviewed 245 patients with salivary gland neoplasms and found that 73.5% were benign and

68% occurred in the parotid gland with pleomorphic adenoma representing the most frequent histopathologic type (76%).[52]

Genetic Alterations

Although the precise genetic sequences leading to tumorigenesis are not known, increasingly genetic alterations are being discovered that are associated with several neoplasms. The range of alterations include loss of heterogosity, chromosomal rearrangements, point mutations, and monosomy or polysomy. El-Nagar and colleagues reported that 4 of 11 pleomorphic adenomas (36.4%) had allele loss on the long arm of chromosome 8.[53] Others have shown that overexpression of pleomorphic adenoma gene 1 (*PLAG1*) proto-oncogene in vivo and in transgenic mice produces the growth of both pleomorphic and malignant salivary neoplasms following reciprocal chromosomal translocations involving 8q12.[54–56] The association of p53 in the tumorigenesis of malignant salivary gland neoplasms appears to be modest with less than 15% of malignant neoplasms having alterations in *p53* tumor suppressor gene.[57–59]

Enviromental Factors

Prior exposure to ionizing radiation is associated with a higher risk of developing both benign and malignant salivary gland neoplasms. A population-based study of atomic bomb survivors who were followed by the Radiation Effects Research Foundation (RERF) in Hiroshima and Nagasaki, Japan, demonstrated that individuals who were exposed as a result of the atomic bomb had a higher rate of benign and malignant neoplasms, particularly mucoepidermoid carcinoma (MEC).[60] Additionally, those having received radiation to the head and neck demonstrated a 2.6-fold increase in benign salivary neoplasms and a 4.5-fold increase in malignant salivary tumors. There was a dose-response observed with Warthin tumor and mucoepidemoid carcinoma representing the most common benign and malignant neoplasms respectively.[61–63]

Epstein–Barr virus (EBV) has been shown to be associated with lymphoepithelial and undifferentiated salivary malignancies and has a higher incidence in the Eskimo and Chinese individuals.[64,65] Histologically, the neoplasms resemble lymphoepithelial nasopharygeal carcinoma. These neoplasms, however, are quite rare, and the impact of EBV in salivary malignancies is thought to be small.

As with other benign and malignant neoplasms, tobacco exposure has been associated with increased incidence of salivary gland neoplasms. It is believed that tobacco-specific N-nitrosamines may concentrate in salivary tissue and underlie the association with salivary neoplasms and tobacco exposure. Warthin tumors have shown the highest association with tobacco exposure; there is a dose relationship between tobacco and synchronous or metachronous Warthin tumors.[66–68]

Clinical Evaluation

Typically, patients with salivary gland neoplasms will present with a painless, unilateral mass. Benign neoplasms are slow growing and tend to have longer duration of symptoms. Rapid change in size may be the result of obstruction of Stensen duct causing sudden enlargement or may arise from cystic degeneration. Accelerated growth in a longstanding neoplasm is a warning of possible malignancy arising from a pleomorphic neoplasm. Malignant neoplasms occurring in the parotid gland are frequently painless but may be associated with pain and facial weakness. Benign neoplasms of the submandibular gland are generally painless. Malignant submandibular neoplasms may invade the lingual and hypoglossal nerves, mandible, floor of mouth and tongue, and such involvements are hallmarks of advance disease. Symptoms arising from neoplasms of minor salivary glands depend on their location; intraorally, the first signs may be poorly fitting of dentures, loose teeth, and malocclusion.

A comprehensive head and neck examination should be performed to assess the extent of the neoplasm. Intraoral examination may reveal bulging of the pharyngeal wall arising from deep lobe involvement of the parotid gland or from a minor salivary neoplasm in the parapharyngeal space. Cranial neuropathies may indicate neural involvement from adenoid cystic carcinoma (ACC). Careful examination of the neck may reveal cervical lymph node metastasis of a high-grade malignant neoplasm. Dermatological examination of the scalp and face is crucial and may confirm a cutaneous malignancy. Other sites of involvement from minor salivary gland neoplasms include the palate, lacrimal gland, sinonasal tract, and larynx.

Radiographic Evaluation

Routine imaging is not essential for small neoplasms involving the superficial part of the parotid gland. However, for large neoplasms, submandibular and minor salivary neoplasms, neoplasms involving the parapharygeal space and those suspicious for malignancy, imaging is recommended to assess the extent of involvement of adjacent vital structures. A high-resolution computed tomography (CT) with contrast or magnetic resonance imaging (MRI) with gadolinium provides excellent characterization of neoplasms in the context of the local anatomy. The strength of CT is its ability to delineate fat planes and vascular structures, as well as demonstrate bone involvement. Its disadvantage is that it gives exposure to ionizing radiation and may be compromised by dental artifact; furthermore, it distinguishes inflammation from neoplastic processes less well. Prestyloid tumors of the parapharyngeal space can be easily identified by CT with location of the carotid artery and medial displacement of the parapharyngeal fat pad.[69] Also, studies have shown that low-grade and benign neoplasms appear as well-demarcated, homogeneous lesions on CT in contrast to high-grade lesions which appear as infiltrative and ill-defined.[70]

MRI provides superior soft tissue detail without ionizing radiation; however, its high expense, sensitivity to motion, poor osseous detail, and contraindication for patients with implants are limiting factors. Fat, muscle, nerves, and other soft tissue structures have more clearly differing enhancement characteristics, which provides a mechanism for better soft-tissue detail. MRI is superior in its ability to delineate involvement of the pterygoid musculature, dural involvement of extensive skull-base lesions, and perineural involvement.[71,72] Both imaging modalities can effectively identify nodal metastasis. Indeed, for extensive neoplasms with suspected bony involvement, MRI and CT may complement each other in the diagnostic work-up. Presently, positron emission tomography (PET) has not proven sufficiently accurate for routine utilization.[71]

Cytologic Evaluation

FNA has emerged as a safe, accurate tool in the work-up of patients with salivary gland neoplasms. Certainly, the experience of the cytopathologist has an impact on the accuracy for the various histologic subtypes which may be challenging even for the expert cytopathologist. There is some debate regarding the indications for FNA. Many believe it is not warranted when the result will not change the management. Supporters feel that when a malignancy is diagnosed, it permits better preoperative planning and counseling for the patient. In some instances, it may preclude surgical intervention by detecting nonneoplastic processes or secondary involvement from metastatic spread. Baccoto and colleagues reviewed 841 FNAs collected over a 16-year period to assess their overall accuracy.[73] The overall accuracy was 97%; the sensitivity to the presence of a neoplasm 98%, and the specificity for absence of a neoplasm 98%. Heller and colleagues reviewed 169 consecutive patients presenting at a tertiary academic medical center who had FNAs performed for salivary gland masses who also went on to surgical resection.[74] Eleven percent of the samples were not adequate for evaluation; the FNA diagnosis of malignant or suspicious lesion had positive and negative predictive values of 84% and 77%, respectively. Half of the 10 patients with false-negative FNA results were found to have low-grade lymphoma on the final histologic evaluation. FNA diagnosis of a benign neoplasm had positive and negative predictive values of 83% and 88%, respectively. A cytopathologic diagnosis of a nonneoplastic lesion was predictive in only 47% of cases. Others have reported accurate diagnosis of malignant tumors whereas the diagnosis of nonparotid neoplasms may be less accurate and the overall accuracy may be less in nontertiary less experienced centers, ranging from 44 to 88%.[75–77]

Histologic Types of Benign Neoplasms

Pleomorphic Adenoma. Pleomorphic adenoma (benign mixed tumor) is by far the most common histologic subtype of all of the salivary glands neoplasms, and represents approximately 70% of parotid neoplasms, and three-quarters of all benign neoplasms.[51,78,79] Pleomorphic adenoma is believed to derive from a pluripotential reserve cell of the intercalated duct that gives rise to both epithelial cells and stromal producing myoepithelial cells. The stromal component may vary and can be myxoid, chondroid, or osteoid. Generally, there is a thin capsule with pseudopod extension of the neoplasm through the capsule. For this reason, enucleation leads to unacceptable recurrence rates and risk of neoplasm spillage. Most neoplasms (nearly 90%) occur in the superficial lobe, and a wide cuff of normal parotid tissue or superficial parotidectomy is the recommended treatment. Neoplasms that extend to or originate in the deep lobe require a total parotidectomy. For those that arise in the submandibular gland, complete excision of the gland is also recommended. Observation of pleomorphic adenomas is not recommended in young or healthy individuals because of the risk of malignant transformation. Although the risk is small early on, it increases to 10% for neoplasms present for greater than 15 years.[80]

Warthin Tumor. Warthin tumor is the second most common benign salivary gland neoplasm and occurs almost exclusively in the parotid gland. It is also referred to as papillary cystadenoma lymphomatosum. Warthin tumors represent 10% of parotid tumors and are bilateral 10% of the time; there is a strong male predominance and an association with tobacco exposure.[68,81] Most commonly, these neoplasms are located near the angle of the mandible, occurring in the tail of the parotid. Microscopically, these neoplasms are characterized by papillary epithelium with a lymphoid stroma projecting into cystic spaces with a double layer of oncocytic cuboidal cells. It is believed that these tumors arise from ectopic ductal epithelium in intraparotid lymph nodes.[78] Superficial parotidectomy is the recommended treatment for complete excision and avoidance of recurrence.

Basal Cell Adenoma. Basal cell adenoma is the most commonly occurring monomorphic adenoma and occurs most commonly in the upper lip. These are usually well-capsulated, slow-growing lesions that may also occur in the parotid gland. Microscopically, several growth patterns may be observed, and confusion with the solid growth pattern of adenoid cytic carcinoma may arise. Generally, basal cell adenomas will have a more visible capsule, lack invasion and perineural spread, and has rows of peripheral palisading cells with a thick basement membrane. Complete excision with a margin of normal tissue is the recommended treatment.

Myoepithelioma. Myoeptitheliomas are derived from the myoepithelial contractile cells that line the ductal unit. As with most benign salivary neoplasms, they are well demarcated and have a thin capsule histologically. The cells are homogeneous and polygonal in shape but sometimes may have a spindle appearance.[82] Sciubba and Brannon reviewed 23 cases in which 70% demonstrated a spindle cell type, 17% a plasmatoid cell type, and the remainder mixed. Twelve of 23 were in the parotid, while 22% each were found in both the submandibular gland and minor salivary glands. There was no observed difference in clinical behavior based upon cell type. These neoplasms tend to have an innocuous clinical course with complete excision being the treatment of choice.

Canalicular Adenoma. Canalicular adenoma is an uncommon, clinically nonaggressive tumor that classically occurs in the elderly and involves the minor salivary glands of the oral cavity, the upper lip being the most prevalent site.[83] They may have the cystic appearance of a mucocele and at times are multifocal.[84] Histologically, these neoplasms are well circumscribed and lack any destructive features; occasionally they may be uncapsulated. The cells are aligned in parallel rows in a canalicular-fashion. Complete excision is the treatment of choice.

Oncocytoma. Oncocytomas are benign neoplasms that occur in all of the major as well as minor salivary glands with the parotid being most common site. A painless, slow-growing mass in a middle-aged adult is the typical presentation. The cell of origin is the mitochondrial-rich oncocyte. These tumors are encapsulated and granular in appearance microscopically, owing to the abundant mitochondrial content. The lack of lymphoid component readily distinguishes it from a Warthin tumor. These tumors may cause diagnostic challenges with other neoplasms comprised of clear cells, such as MEC, acinic cell carcinoma, "clear cell" oncocytoma, epithelial-myoepithelial carcinoma, clear cell adenocarcinoma, and metastatic renal cell carcinoma.[85] When they are found in minor salivary glands, they may assume a clinically more aggressive behavior and infiltrate local structures. Although rare, malignant oncocytic carcinoma does exist and should be distinguished from its benign counterpart. Surgical excision is the recommended treatment for benign oncocytomas.[86]

Oncocytic Papillary Cystadenoma. Oncocytic papillary cystadenoma is a rare lesion and has been described most frequently in the larynx but has been seen in the nasopharynx and oral cavity. It usually occurs in the supraglottis in the elderly and may present with hoarseness or upper airway obstruction.[87] The pathogenesis of the lesion is debatable, and some question if it is a true neoplasm or a process of metaplasia–hyperplasia from the ductal epithelium. They are painless, solitary masses that present with hoarseness when involving laryngeal structures and may be confused for other cystic laryngeal structures.[88] These tumors histologically are similar to Warthin tumors, but they lack a lymphoid matrix. Treatment is surgical excision.

Sebaceous Adenoma. Sebaceous adenomas are uncommon and usually asymptomatic. Sebaceous glands are commonly present in parotid and submandibular glands. The neoplasms are classified as sebaceous lymphadenoma or sebaceous adenoma. Histopathologic observations strongly suggest that sebaceous lymphadenomas arise from sebaceous glandular rests in a lymph node in a fashion similar to that of a Warthin tumor.[89,90] The two adenomas have a low recurrence potential, and surgical excision is recommended.

Ductal Papillomas. The term ductal papilloma is used to identify a group of three rare benign papillary salivary gland tumors known as inverted ductal papilloma, sialadenoma papilliferum, and intraductal papilloma. They represent adenomas with unique papillary features and arise from the salivary gland duct system. Brannon and colleagues described 19 cases: 13 inverted ductal papillomas, 3 sialadenoma papilliferums, and 3 intraductal papillomas.[91] Collectively, these 19 ductal papillomas occurred most commonly in the sixth to eighth decade of life, with a male predominance. The sialadenoma papilliferums presented as papillary lesions clinically. The inverted ductal papillomas and intraductal papillomas appeared as submucosal nodules. The lip and the palate were the most common locations for inverted ductal papilloma and sialadenoma papilliferum, respectively. The sites for the three intraductal papillomas were the parotid papilla of the Stensen duct, the upper lip, and the buccal mucosa. With light microscopy, inverted ductal papillomas appeared to arise from the excretory ducts near the mucosal surface, whereas intraductal papillomas appeared to arise from the excretory ducts at a deeper level. Sialadenoma papilliferum had a more complex histology, with a biphasic growth pattern of exophytic papillary and endophytic components.[92] Sialadenoma papilliferum has a recurrence rate of 10 to 15% and seems to assert a more significant biological behavior than inverted ductal papilloma and intraductal papilloma. Surgical excision is recommended.

Histologic Types of Malignant Neoplasms

Just as is the case with their benign counterparts, there is a wide variety of histologic types of malignant neoplasms. The broad categories include carcinomas, adenocarcinomas, malignant mixed neoplasms, lymphomas, and metastatic. Malignant neoplasms account for less than 15% of all salivary neoplasms; hence they are even more rare than benign salivary neoplasms. Several malignant histologic types are more frequent and emphasis will be placed on them. The location in the salivary subunit in which the neoplasm originates is believed to correlate with its clinical aggressiveness with those of the excretory duct behaving more aggressively than neoplasms from the intercalated duct region.[93] Advanced-stage neoplasms generally are associated with a worse survival. Tables 2 and 3 describe American Joint Committee on Cancer TNM categorization and TNM staging, respectively.

Mucoepidermoid Carcinoma. Mucoepidermoid carcinoma (MEC) is the most common malignancy of the salivary glands; the parotid gland represents the most common site accounting for 70% of these neoplasms. It is the second most common malignancy of the submandibular glands following ACC. MEC is the most common salivary malignancy of childhood. For

Table 2 American Joint Committee on Cancer TNM Categorization of Major Salivary Gland Malignant Neoplasms

Tx	Primary tumor cannot be assessed
T0	No evidence of primary tumor
T1	Tumor ≤2 cm
T2	Tumor >2 cm ≤4 cm
T3	Tumor >4 cm or extraparenchymal extension
T4a	Tumor invades skin, mandible, ear canal, or facial nerve
T4b	Tumor invades skull base, pterygoid plates, or encases carotid artery
Nx	Regional lymph nodes cannot be assessed
N0	No regional lymph nodes
N1	Metastasis in a single ipsilateral lymph node ≤3 cm
N2a	Metastasis in a single ipsilateral lymph node 3 to 6 cm
N2b	Metastasis in multiple ipsilateral lymph nodes <6 cm
N3	Metastasis in lymph node >6 cm
Mx	Distant metastasis cannot be assessed
M0	No distant metastsis
M1	Distant metastasis

minor salivary neoplasms, the palate and buccal mucosa are the most frequent sites. Patients may present with a range of symptoms, including a painless, slow-growing mass to a rapidly enlarging mass and cervical metastasis, with or without facial nerve paralysis. The biological behavior is related to histologic grade of the neoplasm. Well-differentiated (low grade) neoplasms have a low propensity for local invasion and metastasis, while poorly differentiated (high grade) neoplasms may be locally aggressive with regional and distant metastases (DM). Moderately differentiated (intermediate grade) neoplasms have a tendency for local recurrence but metastasize uncommonly. Histologically low-grade neoplasms have more mucinous cells (>50%) while high-grade neoplasms may have a paucity of mucinous cells that may only be detected by immunohistochemical markers. A US Armed Forces Institute of Pathology (AFIP) review of 234 MECs demonstrated that 75% of patients were neoplasm free at 5 years, but clinical features associated with metastasis or death were advanced age, neoplasm size, and preoperative symptoms. Histopathologic features

Table 3 American Joint Committee on Cancer TNM Staging System of Major Salivary Gland Malignant Neoplasms

Stage I	T1N0M0
Stage II	T2N0M0
Stage III	T3N0M0
	T1N1M0
	T2N1M0
	T3N1M0
Stage IVA	T4aN0M0
	T1N2M0
	T2N2M0
	T3N2M0
	T4N2M0
Stage IVB	T4b, any NM0
	Any TN3M0
Stage IVC	Any T, any NM1

that are associated with poor outcome were cystic component less than 20%, four or more mitotic figures per 10 high-power fields, neural involvement, necrosis, and anaplasia.[94]

Adenoid Cystic Carcinoma. Billroth is credited for first describing this intriguing neoplasm with unique features, but the term "adenoid cystic carcinoma," which describes its histologic appearance was not coined until 1953. ACC is the second most common salivary malignancy with most series reporting the majority occurring in the submandibular gland and minor salivary glands.[95,96] Some of the hallmarks of ACC are its slow growth with lengthy presentation and its propensity for perineural spread. A painless growth is the most common presentation with neural deficits depending on the site of involvement, including unilateral tongue weakness, facial paralysis, and trigeminal nerve distribution symptoms.

Three main histologic subtypes based upon neoplasm architecture are recognized, which correlate with prognosis and clinical behavior: cribiform, tubular, and solid. The cribiform pattern has a glandular architecture with the classic features of a "Swiss cheese" appearance where cells are arranged in clusters and are separated by oval spaces. The tubular pattern demonstrates elongated tubular structures that have a central lumen and also show a glandular architecture. The solid pattern is characterized by high cellularity with sheets of cells with little evidence of glandular architecture. Any given neoplasm may have elements of all of the patterns, which leaves the pathologist with the challenge of deciding which pattern predominates. Patients with neoplasms with the solid pattern predominating have the worst prognosis while those with the cribiform pattern have the best. Those with tubular pattern have an intermediate prognosis.[97]

ACC is renowned for its tendency for both local and distant recurrence that may occur following definitive treatment. ACC has a strong proclivity for neurotropism and perineural spread, with a tendency for tracking along major neural structures. Skip lesions are common and are seen in most of these neoplasms, although it is believed that perineural spread occurs along the path of least resistance and is microscopically contiguous with the primary neoplasm. Garden and colleagues reported on the 30-year experience at MD Anderson Cancer Center with 198 salivary and lacrimal ACCs; 62% occurred in minor salivary glands, 21% in the submandibular gland, and the remaining among parotid and lacrimal glands.[95] Among these patients, perineural spread was found in 69%, with named nerves involved 28% of the time. DM was the most common site of failure (37%), but skull base and neck recurrences were also frequently observed. Microscopic disease and involvement of named nerves lead to worse prognosis, but with postoperative radiation, locoregional control was improved.

Cervical metastases are uncommon for ACC while distant failure occurs frequently, often years after treatment. Patients may survive for protracted periods even in the presence of local and DM. Most recurrences occur in the first 5 years but recurrences occur commonly 20 years later and more. Common sites of hematagenous distant spread include lung (70%), bone, and liver. Because of frequent late failure, actual survival rates have been difficult to assess. Initial extent of disease was the dominant prognostic factor with advanced age and duration of symptoms also associated with poor outcome.[98] Patients with advanced disease at presentation and those with neoplasms located in the submandibular region and sinonasal tract had worse outcomes.[96]

Fordice and colleagues reviewed 160 patients at MD Anderson Cancer Center with ACC during the 20 years between 1977 and 1996, with 140 treated with surgery and postoperative radiation therapy. The average age was 49.5 years. Combined treatment yielded an 85% locoregional freedom from relapse, and disease-specific survival at 5, 10, and 15 years was 89, 67.4, and 39.6%, respectively. Thirty-five patients (21.9%) had DM as the only site of failure. Perineural invasion of major nerves, positive margins at surgery, and solid histological features were associated with increased treatment failures. Four or more symptoms present at diagnosis, positive lymph nodes, solid histology, and perineural invasion of major nerves were associated with increased mortality from the neoplasm.[97]

Spiro and colleagues reviewed 196 previously untreated, patients with ACC treated at Memorial Sloan-Kettering Cancer Institute with minimum 10-year follow-up to evaluate the factors contributing to DM.[99] Variables assessed for their impact on DM included age, gender, site, size, node status, stage, grade, and locoregional treatment failure. Treatment failure occurred in a total of 122 of 196 determinate patients (62%), 74 (38%) of whom had DM, which was usually associated with locoregional recurrence (51 patients), but DM was the only indication of failure in 23 whose primary neoplasm was controlled. Of the 74 patients with known DM, the lung was recorded as the only involved site in 50 patients, lung was involved in addition to other sites in 17, bone metastases alone occurred in 5, and the remaining 2 developed disseminated disease. Disease-free intervals varied from 1 month to 19 years (median 36 months) and exceeded 10 years in 9 of 113 patients (8%) with adequate information about treatment failure. Survival with DM was less than 3 years in 54%, but more than 10 years in 10% (maximum 16 years). The only significant factors influencing survival were the size of the primary neoplasm ($p < .0000$), local or neck recurrence ($p = .0006$), and the presence of nodal involvement ($p = .02$).[99]

Acinic Cell Carcinoma. Acinic cell carcinoma accounts for approximately 6 to 8% of salivary gland malignancies, with 81 to 97% occurring in the parotid gland and it is the second most common pediatric salivary gland malignancy.[100–102] It commonly presents as a painless parotid mass, with facial weakness being rare. It has a

3% chance of occurring bilaterally, second only to Warthin neoplasm in that regard. It tends to have a benign biological course and has the best overall outcome of all salivary gland malignancies. Rarely, a more aggressive form occurs.

There are several histologic subtypes that do not generally correlate with survival. They include: solid, microcystic, papillary cystic, and follicular with the majority of cancers displaying multiple cell types. The intercalated duct or reserve cells of the terminal duct are believed to be sites of origin. Acinic cell carcinoma may have morphologic features similar to other clear cell carcinomas, such as MEC, epithelial-myoepithelial carcinoma, oncocytoma, and renal cell carcinoma. Rarely, there is a form of acinic cell carcinoma that is dedifferentiated with a more aggressive biological activity and worse prognosis; it usually has a higher rate of mitotic activity, nuclear atypia. and solid growth pattern.[103,104] Spiro and colleagues reviewed 67 patients treated over a 30-year period, and patients with small neoplasms without local invasion did extremely well. However, larger, more extensive neoplasms had a much worse survival.[102] Cure rates for the entire series were 76, 63, and 55% at 5, 10, and 15 years, respectively. Cervical lymph node metastases occurred in 16% of the patients, and DM in 12%. Hoffman and colleagues evaluated 1,353 cases registered in the National Cancer Data Base for the years 1985 to 1995.[105] Five-year disease-specific survival was 91.4%. Worse survival was associated with high grade ($p < .0001$), age greater or equal to 30 years ($p = .0055$), and the presence of metastatic disease ($p < .0001$). Although acinic cell carcinoma usually has a favorable course, rarely an aggressive form occurs.

Adenocarcinoma. It is important to clarify that because malignancies arising in the salivary ductal unit are technically termed adenocarcinomas, adenocarcinoma not otherwise specified (nos) refers to a salivary malignancy that is generally high grade, has a high rate of metastases, and has a poor survival. They frequently have the morphologic features of adenocarcinomas of the breast and lung. They represent 1 to 9% of salivary malignancies,[106] and they occur in minor salivary glands most commonly (68%), followed by the parotid gland (28%) and submandibular gland (8%). The prognosis of adenocarcinoma nos was among the worse of any histologic type with a 10-year survival of 55%; locoregional recurrences and DM were common.[107]

Polymorphous Low-Grade Adenocarcinoma. Distinct from other adenocarcinomas, polymorphous low-grade adenocarcinoma (PLGA) has a much more benign clinical course. It was first described in 1983 and has a strong propensity for minor salivary glands, although it infrequently occurs in the parotid gland as well. It has also been termed terminal duct carcinoma and is thought to be derived from the intercalated duct region of the salivary unit. The palate and buccal mucosa are the most common sites.[93] Its tendency for perineural spread sometimes causes diagnostic confusion with ACC. PLGA frequently presents

as an incidental finding on examination: painless mass or change in denture fit.

One hundred sixty-four patients with PGLA were reviewed at the AFIP and evaluated for prognostic factors.[108] There was a 2:1 female to male predominance, and ages ranged from 23 to 94 years (average, 57.6 years). Most presented clinically with a palatal mass that ranged in size from 0.4 to 6 cm (average, 2.2 cm). The neoplasms were characterized by a polymorphous growth pattern, with individual neoplasms demonstrating solid, ductotubular, cribiform, trabecular, and single-file growth. Neurotropism was seen frequently. With a mean follow-up of 115.4 months after presentation, 97.6% of all patients were either alive or had died without evidence of recurrent disease after treatment with surgical excision alone.[108,109] Batsakis and Luna reported 69 patients with PGLA who demonstrated a 12% recurrence after surgery and a 10% rate of metastases and one death.[93] PGLAs may infrequently recur and metastasize, but they are characterized by a favorable clinical course with surgical excision as the treatment of choice. There is no established benefit of radiation therapy for patients with this disease.

Salivary Duct Carcinoma. Salivary ductal carcinoma (SDC) is among the most aggressive behaving salivary malignancies. It accounts for approximately 1% of salivary gland malignancies and generally occurs in the parotid gland. Histologically, it is high grade and similar to mammary ductal carcinoma; mitoses are frequent, and DM is the rule. Lewis and colleagues reviewed 26 cases of SDC treated at the Mayo Clinic from 1960 to 1989.[110] The population consisted of 22 men and 4 women (mean age, 66 years). SDC involved the parotid 88% and the submandibular gland 12% of the cases. Only 21% were diploid and 79% were nondiploid. Local recurrence occurred in 35%, and DM developed in 62%. The 5-year survival was only 30% with 77% of the patients dying of the neoplasm at a mean interval of 3 years after diagnosis. Batsakis and Luna reported on 30 patients, of whom 55% had local recurrences while both regional and DM were found in 66%.[93] Despite treatment with radical parotidectomy, neck dissection and postoperative radiation, survival was dismal.

Malignant Mixed Neoplasm. Malignant mixed neoplasm is an umbrella term that encompasses carcinoma ex-pleomorphic adenoma (CXPA), carcinosarcoma, metastasizing mixed neoplasm (MZMT). These constitute 3 to 12% of all salivary gland malignancies.[63,111,112] CXPA is by far the most common of the malignant mixed neoplasms. Malignant degeneration may occur in any benign neoplasm; but, because pleomorphic adenoma is the most prevalent salivary gland neoplasm, CXPA most commonly arises from it. It typically presents as a rapidly enlarging mass in the setting of a preexisting lesion. Up to 5 years from presentation, the risk of malignant degeneration is 1.5%; however, after 15 years the risk increases to 9.5%. For those patients with recurrent pleomorphic adenoma, the risk of malignant degeneration is 7 to 10%.[113,114] Depth of invasion into adjacent tissue has an important impact on survival and recurrence. Tortoledo and colleagues reported in their series of 40 patients that depth of invasion <8 mm yielded a 5-year survival of 100% compared to 50% for those with >8 mm of invasion.[112] When depth of invasion was >6 mm, recurrence was as high as 70% compared to only 16.5% when depth of invasion was <6 mm.[112,113]

Carcinosarcoma or true malignant mixed neoplasms are extremely rare and contain two malignant components (carcinoma and sarcoma), as opposed to CXPA which only contains one malignant component (carcinoma). These neoplasms have an aggressive biological behavior. The carcinoma component is most commonly either squamous cell carcinoma (SCC) or adenocarcinoma, while the sarcomatous portion is most commonly chondrosarcoma followed by fibrosarcoma.[115,116] The long-term survival is poor being less than 20% at 15 years.[111]

MZMT too are extremely rare. In this instance, both the primary and metastatic neoplasms have a completely benign morphology. The most common cause is multiple local recurrences with eventual metastases to lung and bone. Wenig and colleagues reported 11 cases from the AFIP.[117] Primary sites included the parotid gland (8 cases), submandibular gland (2 cases), and the nasal septum (1 case). At least two recurrences generally occurred prior to identification of metastases. The metastases were discovered from 6 to 52 years following the occurrence of the primary neoplasm. Metastases were identified in bone, lung, regional lymph nodes, skin, kidney, retroperitoneum, oral cavity, pharynx, calvaria, and central nervous system.[117] While some advocate excising accessible DM, this is not uniformly accepted; and despite their benign appearance, patients may ultimately succumb to their disease.[117–119]

Squamous Cell Carcinoma. Primary salivary SCC accounts for 1 to 2% of salivary malignancies. It is important to exclude synchronous or prior history of cutaneous or mucosal SCC. It must also be distinguished from high-grade MEC. Flynn and colleagues reviewed 40 parotid neoplasms originally classified as SCC but upon careful review only eight were primary SCC arising from the salivary gland; cutaneous metastases or high-grade MECs were the most frequently assigned misdiagnoses.[120] The parotid gland is the most common primary site, followed by the submandibular gland. The usual presentation is a firm painless mass, either with or without facial paralysis. Cervical metastases are frequently present. The largest series described of primary SCC includes 50 patients over a 30-year span; the main limitation to the interpretation of the study is the lack of routine use of postoperative radiotherapy.[121] Cervical metastases were present in 46% of patients. Five-year survival was 24% for patients with parotid lesions and 20% for those with submandibular neoplasms. As with other malignant salivary gland neoplasms, advanced stage and pain as a presenting symptom were ominous findings. Locoregional recurrence

was the most common site of failure in primaries both in the parotid (51%) and in the submandibular (67%) glands.[121] This is an aggressive malignancy where radical parotidectomy, neck dissection, and postoperative radiotherapy are recommended.

Lymphoma. Salivary gland lymphoma may be a localized or systemic disease and most often affects the parotid gland and rarely the submandibular gland. It comprises 4.7% of extranodal lymphoma and 1.7% of salivary gland neoplasms. Although non-Hodgkin B-cell lymphoma is most prevalent, all forms of lymphoma may be observed. They may also be associated with benign lymphoepithelial lesions both in the presence or absence of Sjögren syndrome. Patients with Sjögren disease have 44-fold increased risk of developing primary lymphomas of the salivary glands over the general population; and their lymphomas are biologically more aggressive.[122]

Patients with primary salivary lymphoma fare better than those with systemic disease, and those with primary Hodgkin lymphoma do better than those with non-Hodgkin lymphoma, 5-year survivals of 90% and 48%, respectively.[123–126] Clinical stage of disease did affect survival. The worse prognosis is for the patient with concurrent Sjögren syndrome who have a mean survival of less than 3 years.[127]

Sarcoma. Sarcomas arising in the salivary glands are extremely uncommon.[128,129] The two most common types were malignant schwannoma and fibrosarcoma, but a diverse group has been described: malignant fibrous histiocytomas, neurosarcomas, rhabdomyosarcomas, fibrosarcomas, and osteosarcomas. Auclair and colleagues reported 42 patients with sarcoma; 17 experienced recurrences, 16 developed metastases (most commonly to lung), and 15 died of disease.[128] The mean time until death following treatment was 2.4 years. Treatment generally included surgery followed by radiation. Prognosis was based on neoplasm grade and size. For large neoplasms, prognosis is poor, despite aggressive surgical resection and radiation therapy.

SURGICAL MANAGEMENT

For benign parotid neoplasms, a superficial parotidectomy is the treatment of choice to avoid recurrence. Simple enucleation without an adequate cuff of normal tissue for benign neoplasms such as pleomorphic adenomas leads to an unacceptably high rate of recurrence.[114] For a benign neoplasm of the submandibular gland, complete excision of the entire submandibular gland is the recommended treatment. Treatment of benign minor salivary gland neoplasms requires wide resection of the anatomic site where they occur.

For malignant parotid neoplasms, a total parotidectomy is recommended with preservation of the facial nerve, whenever possible. When there is complete encasement of the facial nerve or its branches, sacrifice of the involved portions of the nerve is required. When the extratemporal portion of the facial nerve is sacrificed, primary repair with

a cable graft is desired, irrespective of the need for postoperative radiotherapy. For malignant submandibular neoplasms, complete excision of the submandibular gland is the minimum therapy. Because of the proximity of the mandible, a marginal or segmental mandibulectomy may be necessary. The extent of resection of minor salivary neoplasms depends on the anatomic site involved. Frequently, neoplasms of the palate and nasal cavity require a maxillectomy. In general, high-grade neoplasms should be resected with wide margins.

Lymphadenectomy

Whenever there is clinically positive regional adenopathy, a therapeutic neck dissection is performed as part of definitive treatment. For instances of high-grade malignancies, for example, high-grade mucoepidermoid, adenocarcinoma, or SCC, an elective neck dissection is recommended for optimal regional control. For low-grade neoplasms, for example, acinic cell carcinoma, low-grade MEC, PLGA, without radiographic or clinical adenopathy, elective dissection of the neck is not indicated.

RADIATION

While surgical excision is the first-line therapy for parotid neoplasms, radiotherapy has an important role in the postoperative setting for high-risk malignant neoplasms, presence of cervical metastasis, recurrent disease, and unresectable disease.[130] Postoperative radiotherapy has been demonstrated to improve locoregional control, although the impact on survival and DM may be less clear. Armstrong and colleagues compared 46 matched-pairs with malignant parotid neoplasms, one group treated with complete surgical resection whereas the other was treated with surgical excision and postoperative radiotherapy.[131] The 5-year locoregional control for stage III and IV neoplasms in the surgery with postoperative radiotherapy versus surgery alone was 51% versus 17%, respectively; and 5-year survival was 51% versus 10%, respectively. Garden and colleagues reviewed 160 patients with malignant minor salivary neoplasms treated with complete surgical resection with postoperative radiotherapy at MD Anderson Cancer Center. Locoregional recurrence occurred in only 14% of patients; DM occurred in 27%, and 10-year overall survival was 65%.[132]

It is believed that additional benefit may be gained using fast neutron therapy rather than conventional photon radiotherapy for advanced ACC. Douglas and colleagues reviewed 151 patients treated at the University of Washington who had either unresectable disease or gross residual disease (GRD) after an attempted surgical extirpation.[133] The 5-year actuarial locoregional control rate for the 151 patients with GRD was 57%; the 5-year actuarial overall survival rate was 72%; and the 5-year actuarial cause-specific survival rate was 77%. Eight patients with microscopic disease had 100% locoregional control. The prognostic factors associated with worse outcome were skull base involvement and surgical biopsy versus gross resection. For locoregional control, others have confirmed the promising results of fast neutron therapy, but benefits on DM and consequently long-term survival have not been established.[134,135] Furthermore, severe long-term toxicities such as osteoradionecrosis, deafness, cerebral necrosis, and other cranial neuropathies must be considered.

COMPLICATIONS OF TREATMENT

Complications that may occur with salivary gland surgery include postoperative hemorrhage, seroma, infection, sensory deficit, and skin necrosis, but the most debilitating complication is facial nerve paralysis from injury during parotid surgery. Whether inadvertent or planned, facial nerve section results in a cosmetic and functional deformity that requires rehabilitation. Certainly, temporary facial nerve paresis related to neurapraxia may result even when the nerve is preserved and able to be stimulated at low voltage at the conclusion of the operation. Gaillard and colleagues reviewed 131 patients in whom a superficial parotidectomy or total parotidectomy with nerve preservation was performed.[136] On the first postoperative day, there was a 42.7% incidence of nerve dysfunction, in whom 100% resolved by 6 months. The most common injury was of one branch (48%), with the marginal mandibular branch being the one most commonly affected. Total parotidectomy was associated with an increased incidence of early dysfunction, but there was complete resolution at the end of a 6-month period. When other factors such as the patient's age, smoking, size of lesion, histology of lesion, and duration of surgery were considered, only the age of the patient had a significant impact on long-term facial nerve weakness in those patients in whom the marginal mandibular branch was the nerve that was most commonly affected.[137] When the facial nerve is severed, primary tension-free anastamosis is recommended whenever possible. Otherwise, a cable graft should be performed with the possible donor-nerves including the greater auricular, sural, or antebrachial cutaneous. Other options include hypoglossal transposition and free tissue transfers. Static repair with facial slings, gold weight, and lid-shortening procedures are also important options depending on patient factors. Details of the surgical management of facial paralysis are discussed in Chapter 34, "Facial Paralysis."

Frey syndrome or gustatory sweating is a sequela of parotidetomy that has wide clinical variation. It is hypothesized to be the result of severed postganglionic parasympathetic nerve fibers reestablishing connection with sweat glands located in the dermis. Linder and colleagues, in a prospective study, demonstrated that 43% of patients were clinically symptomatic at 1 year.[138] The Minor starch-iodine test is performed to demonstrate gustatory sweating and they found it to be positive in 96% of patients at

1 year. Whereas most patients are not markedly disturbed, a few patients (5 to 10%) suffer from severe gustatory sweating.[138] Intraoperatively, several techniques may be used to reduce Frey syndrome, such as placement of dermis-fat grafts, muscle interpositional grafts, or acellular dermis under the skin flap.[139,140] Conservative treatment for patients with severe symptoms include botulinum injection; however, the efficacy is reduced over time.[141] Topical glycopyrrolate and antiperspirants offer less invasive and less predictable relief.

REFERENCES

1. Brill SJ, Gilfillan RF. Acute parotitis associated with influenza type A: A report of twelve cases. N Engl J Med 1977;296:1391–2.
2. Brook I. Diagnosis and management of parotitis. Arch Otolaryngol Head Neck Surg 1992;118:469–71.
3. de Vries EJ, Kapadia SB, Johnson JT, Bontempo FA. Salivary gland lymphoproliferative disease in acquired immune disease. Otolaryngol Head Neck Surg 1988;99:59–62.
4. Ioachim HL, Ryan JR. Salivary gland lymphadenopathies associated with AIDS. Hum Pathol 1988;19:616–7.
5. Ryan JR, Ioachim HL, Marmer J, Loubeau JM. Acquired immune deficiency syndrome–related lymphadenopathies presenting in the salivary gland lymph nodes. Arch Otolaryngol 1985;111:554–6.
6. Yeh CK, Fox PC, Ship JA, et al. Oral defense mechanisms are impaired early in HIV-1 infected patients. J Acquir Immune Defic Syndr 1988;1:361–6.
7. Chapple ILC, Hamburger J. The significance of oral health in HIV disease. Sex Transm Infect 2000;76:236–43.
8. Katz MH, Mastrucci MT, Leggott PJ, et al. Prognostic significance of oral lesions in children with perinatally acquired human immunodeficiency virus infection. Am J Dis Child 1993;147:45–8.
9. Dave SP, Pernas FG, Roy S. The benign lymphoepithelial cyst and a classification system for lymphocytic parotid gland enlargement in the pediatric HIV population. Laryngoscope 2007;117:106–13.
10. Ioachim HL, Cooper MC, Hellman GC. Lymphomas associated with the acquired immune deficiency syndrome (AIDS): A study of 35 cases. Cancer Detect Prev Suppl 1987;1:557–65.
11. Hemenway WG, English GM. Surgical treatment of acute bacterial parotitis. Postgrad Med 1971;50:114–9.
12. Raad II, Sabbagh MF, Caranasos GJ. Acute bacterial sialadenitis: A study of 29 cases and review. Rev Infect Dis 1990;12:591–601.
13. Saunders HF. Wind parotitis. N Engl J Med 1973;289:698.
14. Lundgren A, Kylen P, Odkvist LM. Nosocomial parotitis. Acta Otolaryngol, 1976;82:275–8.
15. McQuone SJ. Acute viral and bacterial infections of the salivary glands. Otolaryngol Clin North Am 1999;32:793– 811.
16. Tabak LA, Levine MJ, Mandel ID, Ellison SA. Role of salivary mucins in the protection of the oral cavity. J Oral Pathol 1982;11:1–17.
17. Knee TS, Ohl CA. Salmonella parotitis with abscess formation in a patient with human immunodeficiency virus infection. Clin Infect Dis 1997;24:1009–10.
18. Bartels LJ, Vrabec DP. Cervicofacial actinomycosis. Arch Otolaryngol 1978;104:705–8.
19. Earle AS, Wolinsky E. Cat scratch disease with involvement of intra-parotid lymph nodes. Case report. Plast Reconstr Surg 1978;61:917–9.
20. Bradus RJ, Hybarger P, Gooding GA. Parotid gland: US findings in Sjögren syndrome. Work in progress. Radiology 1988;169:749–51.
21. Hemenway WG. The parotid gland in Mikulicz disease and Sjögren's syndrome. Ann Otol Rhinol Laryngol 1960;69:849–68.
22. Ah-See KW, McLaren K, Maran AG. Wegener's granulomatosis presenting as major salivary gland enlargement. J Laryngol Otol 1996;110:691–3.
23. Sente M, Canji V, Dukic Z. Lymphoma of the parotid salivary gland. Med Pregl 1998;51:77–81.
24. Spiegel R, Miron D, Sakran W, Horovitz Y. Acute neonatal suppurative parotitis: Case reports and review. Pediatr Infect Dis J 2004;23:76–8.
25. Todoroki Y, Tsukahara H, Kawatani M, et al. Neonatal suppurative parotitis possibly associated with congenital
26. Leerdam CM, Martin HC, Isaacs D. Recurrent parotitis of childhood. J Paediatr Child Health 2005;41:631–4.
27. Fazekas T, Wiesbauer P, Schroth B, et al. Selective IgA deficiency in children with recurrent parotitis of childhood. Pediatr Infect Dis J 2005;24:461–2.
28. Antoniades D, Harrison JD, Epivatianos A, Papanayotou P. Treatment of chronic sialadenitis by intraductal penicillin or saline. J Oral Maxillofac Surg 2004;62:431–4.
29. Nouraei SA, Ismail Y, McLean NR, et al. Surgical treatment of chronic parotid sialadenitis. J Laryngol Otol 2006;14:1–5.
30. Grases F, Santiago C, Simonet BM, Costa-Bauza A. Sialolithiasis: Mechanism of calculi formation and etiologic factors. Clin Chim Acta 2003;334:131–6.
31. Blatt IM. Studies in sialolithiasis. III. Pathogenesis, diagnosis and treatment. South Med J 1964;57:723–9.
32. Blatt IM, Denning RM, Zumberge JH, Maxwell JH. Studies in sialolithiasis. I. The structure and mineralogical composition of salivary gland calculi. Ann Otol Rhinol Laryngol 1958;67:595–617.
33. McAnally T. Parotitis: Clinical presentations and management. Postgrad Med 1982;71:87–93, 97–9.
34. Suleiman SI, Hobsley M. Radiological appearances of parotid duct calculi. Br J Surg 1980;67:879–80.
35. Andretta M, Tregnaghi A, Prosenikliev V, Staffieri A. Current opinions in sialolithiasis diagnosis and treatment. Acta Otorhinolaryngol Ital 2005;25:145–9.
36. Heverhagen JT, Kalinowski M, Rehberg E, et al. Prospective comparison of magnetic resonance sialography and digital subtraction sialography. J Magn Reson Imaging 2000;11:518–24.
37. Kalinowski M, Heverhagen JT, Rehberg E, et al. Comparative study of MR sialography and digital subtraction sialography for benign salivary gland disorders. AJNR Am J Neuroradiol 2002;23:1485–92.
38. Varghese JC, Thornton F, Lucey BC, et al. A prospective comparative study of MR sialography and conventional sialography of salivary duct disease. AJR Am J Roentgenol, 1999;173:1497–503.
39. Nahlieli O, Baruchin AM, Librus H, London D. Salivary gland endoscopy: A new technique for diagnosis and treatment of sialolithiasis. Harefuah 1997;132:693–5, 743.
40. Robson CD, Hazra R, Barnes PD, et al. Nontuberculous mycobacterial infection of the head and neck in immunocompetent children: CT and MR findings. AJNR Am J Neuroradiol 1999;20:1829–35.
41. Mandell DL, Wald ER, Michaels MG, Dohar JE. Management of nontuberculous mycobacterial cervical lymphadenitis. Arch Otolaryngol Head Neck Surg 2003;129:341–4.
42. Kim YH, Jeong WJ, Jung KY, et al. Diagnosis of major salivary gland tuberculosis: Experience of eight cases and review of the literature. Acta Otolaryngol 2005;125:1318–22.
43. Oostman O, Smego RA. Cervicofacial actinomycosis: Diagnosis and management. Curr Infect Dis Rep 2005;7:170–4.
44. Stewart AE, Palma JR, Amsberry JK. Cervicofacial actinomycosis. Otolaryngol Head Neck Surg 2005;132:957–9.
45. Volante M, Contucci AM, Fantoni M, et al. Cervicofacial actinomycosis: Still a difficult differential diagnosis. Acta Otorhinolaryngol Ital 2005;25:116–9.
46. Smith DL. Cat-scratch disease and related clinical syndromes. Am Fam Physician 1997;55:1783–9, 1793–4.
47. Case records of the Massachusetts General Hospital. Weekly clinicopathological exercises. Case 1-1998. An 11-year-old boy with a seizure. N Engl J Med 1998;338:112–9.
48. Wong SY, Remington JS. Biology of Toxoplasma gondii. AIDS 1993;7:299–316.
49. Dardick I, Byard RW, Carnegie JA. A review of the proliferative capacity of major salivary glands and the relationship to current concepts of neoplasia in salivary glands. Oral Surg Oral Med Oral Pathol 1990;69:53–67.
50. Batsakis JG, Regezi JA, Luna MA, el-Naggar A. Histogenesis of salivary gland neoplasms: A postulate with prognostic implications. J Laryngol Otol 1989;103:939–44.
51. Spiro RH. Salivary neoplasms: Overview of a 35-year experience with 2,807 patients. Head Neck Surg 1986;8:177–84.
52. Nagler RM, Laufer D. Neoplasms of the major and minor salivary glands: Review of 25 years of experience. Anticancer Res 1997;17:701–7.
53. el-Naggar AK, Hurr K, Kagan J, et al. Genotypic alterations in benign and malignant salivary gland neoplasms: Histogenetic and clinical implications. Am J Surg Pathol 1997;21:691–7.
54. Declercq J, Van Dyck F, Braem CV, et al. Salivary gland neoplasms in transgenic mice with targeted PLAG1 proto-oncogene overexpression. Cancer Res 2005;65:4544–53.
55. Queimado L, Lopes C, Du F, et al. Pleomorphic adenoma gene 1 is expressed in cultured benign and

malignant salivary gland neoplasm cells. Lab Invest 1999; 79:583–9.
56. Zhao XD, Yang WJ, Wang L, et al. Development of salivary gland neoplasms in pleomorphic adenoma gene 1 transgenic mice. Zhonghua Yi Xue Yi Chuan Xue Za Zhi 2003;20:390–5.
57. Felix A, El-Naggar AK, Press MF, et al. Prognostic significance of biomarkers (c-erbB-2, p53, proliferating cell nuclear antigen, and DNA content) in salivary duct carcinoma. Hum Pathol 1996;27:561–6.
58. Kiyoshima T, Shima K, Kobayashi I, et al. Expression of p53 neoplasm suppressor gene in adenoid cystic and mucoepidermoid carcinomas of the salivary glands. Oral Oncol 2001;37:315–22.
59. Lazzaro B, Cleveland D. p53 and Ki-67 antigen expression in small oral biopsy specimens of salivary gland neoplasms. Oral Surg Oral Med Oral Pathol Oral Radiol Endod 2000;89:613–7.
60. Saku T, Hayashi Y, Takahara O, et al. Salivary gland neoplasms among atomic bomb survivors, 1950–1987. Cancer 1997;79:1465–75.
61. Land CE, Saku T, Hayashi Y, et al. Incidence of salivary gland neoplasms among atomic bomb survivors, 1950–1987. Evaluation of radiation-related risk. Radiat Res 1996; 146:28–36.
62. Modan B, Chetrit A, Alfandary E, et al. Increased risk of salivary gland neoplasms after low-dose irradiation. Laryngoscope 1998;108:1095–7.
63. Spitz MR, Batsakis JG. Major salivary gland carcinoma. Descriptive epidemiology and survival of 498 patients. Arch Otolaryngol 1984;110:45–9.
64. Nagao T, Ishida Y, Sugano I, et al. Epstein–Barr virus-associated undifferentiated carcinoma with lymphoid stroma of the salivary gland in Japanese patients. Comparison with benign lymphoepithelial lesion. Cancer 1996;78:695–703.
65. Tsai CC, Chen CL, Hsu HC. Expression of Epstein–Barr virus in carcinomas of major salivary glands: A strong association with lymphoepithelioma-like carcinoma. Hum Pathol 1996;27:258–62.
66. Hoffmann D, Rivenson A, Amin S, Hecht SS. Dose-response study of the carcinogenicity of tobacco-specific N-nitrosamines in F344 rats. J Cancer Res Clin Oncol 1984;108:81–6.
67. Peter Klussmann J, Wittekindt C, Florian Preuss S, et al. High risk for bilateral Warthin neoplasm in heavy smokers–review of 185 cases. Acta Otolaryngol 2006;126:1213–17.
68. Vories AA, Ramirez SG. Warthin's neoplasm and cigarette smoking. South Med J 1997;90:416–8.
69. Som PM, Sacher M, Stollman AL, et al. Common neoplasms of the parapharyngeal space: Refined imaging diagnosis. Radiology 1988;169:81–5.
70. Bryan RN, Miller RH, Ferreyro RI, Sessions RB. Computed tomography of the major salivary glands. AJR Am J Roentgenol 1982;139:547–54.
71. Yousem DM, Kraut MA, Chalian AA. Major salivary gland imaging. Radiology 2000;216:19–29.
72. Miller FR, Wanamaker JR, Lavertu P, Wood BG. Magnetic resonance imaging and the management of parapharyngeal space neoplasms. Head Neck 1996;18:67–77.
73. Boccato P, Altavilla G, Blandamura S. Fine needle aspiration biopsy of salivary gland lesions. A reappraisal of pitfalls and problems. Acta Cytol 1998;42:888–98.
74. Cohen EG, Patel SG, Lin O, et al. Fine-needle aspiration biopsy of salivary gland lesions in a selected patient population. Arch Otolaryngol Head Neck Surg 2004;130:773–8.
75. Zbaren P, Nuyens M, Loosli H, Stauffer E. Diagnostic accuracy of fine-needle aspiration cytology and frozen section in primary parotid carcinoma. Cancer 2004;100:1876–83.
76. Stewart CJ, MacKenzie K, McGarry GW, Mowat A. Fine-needle aspiration cytology of salivary gland: A review of 341 cases. Diagn Cytopathol 2000;22:139–46.
77. Pitts DB, Hilsinger RL, Jr, Karandy E, et al. Fine-needle aspiration in the diagnosis of salivary gland disorders in the community hospital setting. Arch Otolaryngol Head Neck Surg 1992;118:479–82.
78. Batsakis JG. Neoplasms of the Major Salivary Glands, Volume 1. Baltimore MD: Willams & Wilkins; 1979.
79. Ito FA, Ito K, Vargas PA, et al. Salivary gland neoplasms in a Brazilian population: A retrospective study of 496 cases. Int J Oral Maxillofac Surg 2005;34:533–6.
80. Seifert G. Histopathology of malignant salivary gland tumours. Eur J Cancer B Oral Oncol 1992;28B:49–56.
81. Yoo GH, Eisele DW, Askin FB, et al. Warthin's neoplasm: A 40-year experience at The Johns Hopkins Hospital. Laryngoscope 1994;104:799–803.
82. Sciubba JJ, Brannon RB. Myoepithelioma of salivary glands: Report of 23 cases. Cancer 1982;49:562–72.
83. Daley TD. The canalicular adenoma: Considerations on differential diagnosis and treatment. J Oral Maxillofac Surg 1984;42:728–30.
84. Harmse JL, Saleh HA, Odutoye T, et al. Recurrent canalicular adenoma of the minor salivary glands in the upper lip. J Laryngol Otol 1997;111:985–7.
85. Ellis GL. Clear cell neoplasms in salivary glands: Clearly a diagnostic challenge. Ann Diagn Pathol 1998;2:61–78.
86. Gray SR, Cornog JL, Jr, Seo IS. Oncocytic neoplasms of salivary glands: A report of fifteen cases including two malignant oncocytomas. Cancer 1976;38:1306–17.
87. Brandwein M, Huvos A. Laryngeal oncocytic cystadenomas. Eight cases and a literature review. Arch Otolaryngol Head Neck Surg 1995;121:1302–5.
88. Friedman L, Patel M, Steinberg J, Hardy D. CT appearance of an oncocytic papillary cystadenoma of the larynx. J Comput Assist Tomogr 1990;14:322–4.
89. Batsakis JG, el-Naggar AK. Sebaceous lesions of salivary glands and oral cavity. Ann Otol Rhinol Laryngol 1990; 99:416–8.
90. Gnepp DR, Brannon R. Sebaceous neoplasms of salivary gland origin. Report of 21 cases. Cancer 1984;53:2155–70.
91. Brannon RB, Sciubba JJ, Giulani M. Ductal papillomas of salivary gland origin: A report of 19 cases and a review of the literature. Oral Surg Oral Med Oral Pathol Oral Radiol Endod 2001;92:68–77.
92. Fantasia JE, Nocco CE, Lally ET. Ultrastructure of sialadenoma papilliferum. Arch Pathol Lab Med 1986;110:523–7.
93. Batsakis JG, Luna MA. Low-grade and high-grade adenocarcinomas of the salivary duct system. Ann Otol Rhinol Laryngol 1989;98:162–3.
94. Goode RK, Auclair PL, Ellis GL. Mucoepidermoid carcinoma of the major salivary glands: Clinical and histopathologic analysis of 234 cases with evaluation of grading criteria. Cancer 1998;82:1217–24.
95. Garden AS, Weber RS, Morrison WH, et al. The influence of positive margins and nerve invasion in adenoid cystic carcinoma of the head and neck treated with surgery and radiation. Int J Radiat Oncol Biol Phys 1995;32:619–26.
96. Spiro RH, Huvos AG, Strong EW. Adenoid cystic carcinoma: Factors influencing survival. Am J Surg 1979;138:579–83.
97. Fordice J, Kershaw C, El-Naggar A, Goepfert H. Adenoid cystic carcinoma of the head and neck: Predictors of morbidity and mortality. Arch Otolaryngol Head Neck Surg 1999;125:149–52.
98. Spiro RH, Huvos A. Stage means more than grade in adenoid cystic carcinoma. Am J Surg 1992;164:623–8.
99. Spiro RH. Distant metastasis in adenoid cystic carcinoma of salivary origin. Am J Surg 1997;174:495–8.
100. Colmenero C, Patron M, Sierra I. Acinic cell carcinoma of the salivary glands. A review of 20 new cases. J Craniomaxillofac Surg 1991;19:260–6.
101. O'Brien CJ, Soong SJ, Herrera GA, et al. Malignant salivary neoplasms–analysis of prognostic factors and survival. Head Neck Surg 1986;9:82–92.
102. Spiro RH, Huvos AG, Strong EW. Acinic cell carcinoma of salivary origin. A clinicopathologic study of 67 cases. Cancer 1978;41:924–35.
103. Perzin KH, LiVolsi VA. Acinic cell carcinomas arising in salivary glands: A clinicopathologic study. Cancer 1979;44:1434–57.
104. Piana S, Cavazza A, Pedroni C, et al. Dedifferentiated acinic cell carcinoma of the parotid gland with myoepithelial features. Arch Pathol Lab Med 2002;126:1104–5.
105. Hoffman HT, Karnell LH, Robinson RA, et al. National Cancer Data Base report on cancer of the head and neck: Acinic cell carcinoma. Head Neck 1999;21:297–309.
106. Spiro RH, Huvos AG, Strong EW. Adenocarcinoma of salivary origin. Clinicopathologic study of 204 patients. Am J Surg 1982;144:423–31.
107. Wahlberg P, Anderson H, Biorklund A, et al. Carcinoma of the parotid and submandibular glands–a study of survival in 2465 patients. Oral Oncol 2002;38:706–13.
108. Castle JT, Thompson LD, Frommelt RA, et al. Polymorphous low grade adenocarcinoma: A clinicopathologic study of 164 cases. Cancer 1999;86:207–19.
109. Evans HL, Luna MA. Polymorphous low-grade adenocarcinoma: A study of 40 cases with long-term follow up and an evaluation of the importance of papillary areas. Am J Surg Pathol 2000;24:1319–28.
110. Lewis JE, McKinney BC, Weiland LH, et al. Salivary duct carcinoma. Clinicopathologic and immunohistochemical review of 26 cases. Cancer 1996;77:223–30.
111. Spiro RH, Huvos AG, Strong EW. Malignant mixed neoplasm of salivary origin: A clinicopathologic study of 146 cases. Cancer 1977;39:388–96.
112. Tortoledo ME, Luna MA, Batsakis JG. Carcinomas ex pleomorphic adenoma and malignant mixed neoplasms. Histomorphologic indexes. Arch Otolaryngol 1984; 110:172–6.
113. Olsen KD, Lewis JE. Carcinoma ex pleomorphic adenoma: A clinicopathologic review. Head Neck 2001;23:705–12.
114. Phillips PP, Olsen KD. Recurrent pleomorphic adenoma of the parotid gland: Report of 126 cases and a review of the literature. Ann Otol Rhinol Laryngol 1995;104:100–4.
115. Kwon MY, Gu M. True malignant mixed neoplasm (carcinosarcoma) of parotid gland with unusual mesenchymal component: A case report and review of the literature. Arch Pathol Lab Med 2001;125:812–5.
116. Stephen J, Batsakis JG, Luna MA, et al. True malignant mixed neoplasms (carcinosarcoma) of salivary glands. Oral Surg Oral Med Oral Pathol 1986;61:597–602.
117. Wenig BM, Hitchcock CL, Ellis GL, Gnepp DR. Metastasizing mixed neoplasm of salivary glands. A clinicopathologic and flow cytometric analysis. Am J Surg Pathol 1992;16:845–58.
118. Hoorweg JJ, Hilgers FJ, Keus RB, et al. Metastasizing pleomorphic adenoma: A report of three cases. Eur J Surg Oncol 1998;24:452–5.
119. Klijanienko J, El-Naggar AK, Servois V, et al. Clinically aggressive metastasizing pleomorphic adenoma: Report of two cases. Head Neck 1997;19:629–33.
120. Flynn MB, Maguire S, Martinez S, Tesmer T. Primary squamous cell carcinoma of the parotid gland: The importance of correct histological diagnosis. Ann Surg Oncol 1999; 6:768–70.
121. Shemen LJ, Huvos AG, Spiro RH. Squamous cell carcinoma of salivary gland origin. Head Neck Surg 1987;9:235–40.
122. Batsakis JG Regezi JA. Selected controversial lesions of salivary tissues. Otolaryngol Clin North Am 1977;10:309–28.
123. Batsakis JG. Primary lymphomas of the major salivary glands. Ann Otol Rhinol Laryngol 1986;95:107–8.
124. Gleeson MJ, Bennett MH, Cawson RA. Lymphomas of salivary glands. Cancer 1986;58:699–704.
125. Hyman GA, Wolff M. Malignant lymphomas of the salivary glands. Review of the literature and report of 33 new cases, including four cases associated with the lymphoepithelial lesion. Am J Clin Pathol 1976;65:421–38.
126. Wolvius EB, van der Valk P, van der Wal JE, et al. Primary non-Hodgkin's lymphoma of the salivary glands. An analysis of 22 cases. J Oral Pathol Med 1996;25:177–81.
127. Nime FA, Cooper HS, Eggleston JC. Primary malignant lymphomas of the salivary glands. Cancer 1976;37:906– 12.
128. Auclair PL, Langloss JM, Weiss SW, Corio RL. Sarcomas and sarcomatoid neoplasms of the major salivary gland regions. A clinicopathologic and immunohistochemical study of 67 cases and review of the literature. Cancer 1986;58:1305–15.
129. Luna MA, Tortoledo ME, Ordonez NG, et al. Primary sarcomas of the major salivary glands. Arch Otolaryngol Head Neck Surg 1991;117:302–6.
130. Bell RB, Dierks EJ, Homer L, Potter BE. Management and outcome of patients with malignant salivary gland neoplasms. J Oral Maxillofac Surg 2005;63:917–28.
131. Armstrong JG, Harrison LB, Spiro RH, et al. Malignant neoplasms of major salivary gland origin. A matched-pair analysis of the role of combined surgery and postoperative radiotherapy. Arch Otolaryngol Head Neck Surg 1990;116:290–3.
132. Garden AS, Weber RS, Ang KK, et al. Postoperative radiation therapy for malignant neoplasms of minor salivary glands. Outcome and patterns of failure. Cancer 1994;73:2563–9.
133. Douglas JG, Laramore GE, Austin-Seymour M, et al. Treatment of locally advanced adenoid cystic carcinoma of the head and neck with neutron radiotherapy. Int J Radiat Oncol Biol Phys 2000;46:551–7.
134. Huber PE, Debus J, Latz D, et al. Radiotherapy for advanced adenoid cystic carcinoma: Neutrons, photons or mixed beam? Radiother Oncol 2001;59:161–7.
135. Potter R, Prott FJ, Micke O, et al. Results of fast neutron therapy of adenoid cystic carcinoma of the salivary glands. Strahlenther Onkol 1999;175:65–8.
136. Gaillard C, Perie S, Susini B, St Guily JL. Facial nerve dysfunction after parotidectomy: The role of local factors. Laryngoscope 2005;115:287–91.
137. Mra Z, Komisar A, Blaugrund SM. Functional facial nerve weakness after surgery for benign parotid neoplasms: A multivariate statistical analysis. Head Neck 1993;15:147– 52.
138. Linder TE, Huber A, Schmid S. Frey's syndrome after parotidectomy: A retrospective and prospective analysis. Laryngoscope 1997;107:1496–501.
139. Govindaraj S, Cohen M, Genden EM, et al. The use of acellular dermis in the prevention of Frey's syndrome. Laryngoscope 2001;111:1993–98.
140. Harada T, Inoue T, Harashina T, et al. Dermis-fat graft after parotidectomy to prevent Frey's syndrome and the concave deformity. Ann Plast Surg 1993;31:450–2.
141. Laccourreye O, Akl E, Gutierrez-Fonseca R, et al. Recurrent gustatory sweating (Frey syndrome) after intracutaneous injection of botulinum toxin type A: Incidence, management, and outcome. Arch Otolaryngol Head Neck Surg 1999;125:283–6.

101

Diseases of the Thyroid and Parathyroid Glands

Jan L. Kasperbauer, MD
Bryan McIver, MB, PhD

Diseases of the thyroid and parathyroid glands are common and, as with all glands, may present with syndromes related to excessive function, reduced function, hyperplasia, and neoplasia. The majority of patients with abnormal tests of thyroid function suffer from primary thyroid diseases, most commonly hypothyroidism as a result of autoimmune destruction of the thyroid gland or hyperthyroidism as a result of Graves disease, toxic multinodular goiter, or destructive thyroiditis. However, many other factors, both exogenous and endogenous, may affect thyroid function, and these conditions must be considered in the differential diagnosis of thyroid disease.

Disorders of the parathyroid gland include hyperfunction related to parathyroid hyperplasia or adenoma formation; and hypofunction as a result of autoimmune mediated or iatrogenic destruction of the glands. Although parathyroid hyperplasia and adenomas are common, malignant transformation of the parathyroid gland is a rare event. In contrast, thyroid neoplasms, both benign and malignant, are the most frequent endocrine tumors, and thyroid cancer is the most frequently diagnosed and most frequently fatal endocrine malignancy.

Diffuse hyperplasia of the thyroid gland may occur physiologically, for example, during pregnancy; as a result of iodine deficiency; in response to elevated levels of thyrotropin, thyroid stimulating hormone (TSH), or stimulation by thyrotropin antibodies in Graves disease; or as a result of reduced efficiency of thyroid hormone production (dyshormonogenesis). Nodular thyroid disease is also common, mainly the result of hyperplastic processes, including the nodular hyperplasia of multinodular goiter and asymmetric goiter development in glands affected by autoimmune thyroid disease. Nodular hyperplasia may follow prolonged or repeated episodic diffuse hyperplasia, as seen in so-called nodular Graves disease, or it may arise *de novo* as a multinodular goiter. Although hyperplastic nodules may present as an apparently solitary nodule, more detailed assessment (with ultrasound or on pathologic evaluation) typically reveals hyperplastic changes within the remainder of the gland.

Neoplasia of the thyroid gland is also common, including solitary or multiple adenomas and carcinomas of various histologic types: papillary, follicular, Hürthle cell, medullary, and anaplastic. Solitary thyroid nodules are usually neoplastic nodules, most commonly follicular adenomas. An adenoma to carcinoma sequence is suspected, though not proven, to underlie the development of follicular thyroid carcinoma (FTC), while the more common papillary thyroid carcinoma (PTC) almost certainly arises with no pre-existing benign stage. Both PTC and FTC are derived from thyroid follicular cells, the source of both thyroid hormone and thyroglobulin, a useful tumor marker in these diseases. Medullary thyroid carcinoma (MTC) arises instead from the thyroid C-cells, whose main protein product, calcitonin, is a similarly useful marker of residual MTC in the postoperative patient. The deadly anaplastic thyroid carcinoma (ATC) arises in most cases as a dedifferentiated form of either PTC or FTC.

Treatment of nodular thyroid disease remains surgical, with few medical options for therapy. The management of thyroid cancer requires surgical excision of the disease, extirpation of the thyroid gland, and removal of regional lymph nodes where appropriate. Solitary neoplastic nodules are also treated surgically because the exclusion of malignancy currently requires histologic analysis and therefore mandates excisional biopsy in the form of thyroid lobectomy but also because of the suspected adenoma to carcinoma sequence. Surgery remains an excellent, if now infrequently exercised option, for management of both Graves disease and toxic multinodular goiter although medical treatment, particularly radioactive iodine, is now used in most cases, at least in North America.

Surgery is the mainstay of management for adenomatous nodules of the parathyroid glands and for significant autonomous multigland hyperplasia (primary or tertiary hyperparathyroidism). Medical treatments are effective for secondary hyperparathyroidism caused by vitamin D deficiency or failure of vitamin D activation in renal insufficiency; the increasingly aggressive management of vitamin D deficiency in renal failure seems likely to change the spectrum of renal bone disease in the future. New calcimimetic agents are also becoming available for medical management of primary hyperparathyroidism, but the chronic use of such agents is generally limited to situations where surgery is either ineffective or deemed inappropriate because of a patient's comorbidities.

THYROID DISEASES

Hyperplastic and Inflammatory Diseases of the Thyroid Gland

Iodine Deficiency and Excess. Worldwide, the most frequent cause of hyperplastic goiter and of thyroid dysfunction remains iodine deficiency, causing endemic goiter and Cretinism.[1,2] Lesser degrees of iodine deficiency, common even in the developed world, may also contribute to the development of multinodular goiter through its impact on thyroid gland hyperplasia,[3] while altering the spectrum of thyroid cancer toward the more aggressive follicular phenotype.[4] Excessive iodine intake may also trigger thyroid disease, and in the United States this is seen increasingly in the context of cardiac arrhythmia treated with amiodarone, a potent antiarrhythmic agent, which contains large amounts of inorganic iodide.[5] The drug may also have a direct impact on the deiodination of thyroid hormones, altering triiodothyronine (T3) bioavailability and complicating the interpretation of thyroid function tests.[5]

Iodine Deficiency. Goiter, with or without thyroid dysfunction, affects an estimated 190 million people worldwide,[6] the result of dietary iodine deficiency, which causes "endemic goiter." An estimated 800 million people worldwide are at risk for iodine deficiency disorders, based on the population median adult iodine intake of less than 100 µg/d, compared to the recommended daily intake of at least 150 µg/d.[2]

Endemic goiter, associated with hypothyroidism, remains a leading cause of mental retardation, through its impact on the developing fetus and neonate, in whom neurological development, growth, and a number of other developmental processes are dependent on maternal and neonatal thyroid hormone production.[7] Cretinism, the most extreme form of iodine deficiency disorder (IDD), is associated with irreversible mental retardation, deafness, growth retardation, and other developmental abnormalities. This clinical condition is likely to represent the extreme end of a spectrum of IDDs, which nevertheless may affect large segments of the population at risk for IDDs in more subtle, less well-recognized forms.[8]

Under conditions of severe iodine deficiency (intake of less than 25 µg elemental iodine per day for adults), insufficient iodination of thyroglobulin occurs to meet the needs of thyroidal production of thyroid hormones. As a consequence, thyroid hormone levels fall, thyrotropin or thyroid-stimulating hormone (TSH) concentrations rise and the thyroid gland is subjected to a growth stimulus that causes thyroid enlargement and goiter.[9] Initially, the enlargement takes the form of diffuse hyperplasia. However, the gland may be exposed to varying degrees of growth stimulation over many years, so that ultimately a more nodular appearance becomes common, resembling the multinodular goiter seen more commonly in North America.

A number of factors other than iodine deficiency may contribute to the development of endemic goiter, including selenium deficiency, which commonly coexists with iodine deficiency, and the consumption of a variety of goitrogenic substances in foodstuffs.[1,10] These substances include lithium, which interferes with iodine retention within the thyroid, and a variety of organic molecules that interfere with iodine organification, including thiocyanates, phthalates, and "goitrin" (L-5-vinyl-2-thiooxazolidone). These substances may be present in water, milk, cassava, millet, onions, seaweeds, and grasses, and may contribute to endemic goiter even in regions where iodine sufficiency would otherwise be expected, such as coastal China and parts of India.[11,12]

Pregnancy, during which the demands on the maternal thyroid increase substantially, exacerbates the state of iodine depletion, worsening maternal hypothyroidism and goiter, and subsequent pregnancies may occur in the face of more severe iodine deficiency, with increasingly severe consequences on subsequent offspring.[13]

Successful iodine supplementation programs have been implemented in a number of endemic goiter areas, including much of the United States and parts of Europe.[14] These programs have all but eliminated endemic goiter in these countries, although arguably at a cost of an increased incidence of autoimmune thyroid disease, including thyrotoxicosis and hypothyroidism.[15]

However, iodine deficiency remains a widespread problem, despite intensive efforts to implement similar iodine supplementation programs among developing-country populations who remain at risk for IDDs.[15] A variety of largely social and political hurdles remains in the way of universal iodine sufficiency.

Iodine Excess. In contrast to iodine deficiency, iodine excess is a disease of developed countries, reflecting the consequences of iodine supplementation in a population previously deficient in iodine, the impact of individual choice or medical necessity. Arguably the most important, and certainly the most common cause of significant iodine excess in the USA is the use of the antiarrhythmic agent amiodarone (Cardarone). Amiodarone is a di-iodinated benzo-furanate derivative, which contains 75 mg of iodine per 200 mg tablet, of which at least 10% (7.5 mg) is liberated as free iodine during drug metabolism. This compares to normal average daily iodine intakes of between 220 and 450 µg in Western Europe and

North America and reflects a more than 20-fold increase in iodine exposure.[16] Chronic treatment causes at least a 40% increase in sustained plasma and urinary iodide, and the drug's fat solubility ensures a long biological half-life, with increased urinary iodide excretion detected many months after drug withdrawal.[17]

A large intake of iodine from amiodarone, or any other source, causes an acute inhibition of production and release of thyroid hormone from the thyroid, the so-called "Wolff-Chaikoff effect."[18] This may last a few weeks to a few months and can cause a transient fall in the concentrations of circulating T3 and thyroxine (T4). In addition, amiodarone (but not other sources of iodine) inhibits the hepatic deiodinase, the source of most of the circulating T3 in humans. This action is specific for amiodarone and may reflect the close structural similarity between thyroid hormone and amiodarone, resulting in a competitive inhibition of the enzyme. As a result of these actions, the TSH rises in the face of falling T3, while T4 remains relatively normal because of reduced deiodination and therefore reduced T4 clearance. These changes may transiently cause symptomatic hypothyroidism but are rarely severe.

As the acute response to iodine loading fades, the normal thyroid recovers its capacity to produce and secrete thyroid hormone under the control of TSH. However, the high iodine availability results in a higher proportion of thyroid hormone released in the form of T4, while the amiodarone-induced block on T4 to T3 conversion is maintained. This causes a fall in the circulating T3 concentrations, a rise in circulating T4 concentrations, and a normal TSH, and a different "normal range" for thyroid function has been suggested for otherwise healthy patients receiving treatment with amiodarone.[19]

Among patients with underlying thyroid disease, excessive iodine intake may have additional effects on thyroid function, which can result in both hypo- and hyperthyroidism. The reported rates of each of these depend on the prevailing iodine intake in the population under study, and presumably the underlying prevalence of autoimmune or nodular thyroid disease. In populations with low or marginal iodine intakes, hyperthyroidism may affect up to 10% of patients receiving excessive iodine supplementation, while hypothyroidism occurs in around 5% of these individuals.[20,21] In contrast, in areas with adequate or high iodine intakes, as in the United States, hyperthyroidism in response to iodine excess is substantially less common, at around 2%, while hypothyroidism is frequent, affecting up to 20% of patients treated with amiodarone or other sources of excess iodine.[17]

In iodine depleted populations, chronic nodular hyperplasia is a common finding, with the development of autonomous function of the thyroid gland in many of these individuals. Iodine loading of autonomously functioning glands results in hyperthyroidism, a reflection of increased substrate for the production of thyroid hormone, known as the "Jod–Basedow phenomenon."[22]

The precise mechanism of this phenomenon remains obscure, but it may reflect the unmasking of latent hyperthyroidism by iodine supplementation, causing the rates of thyrotoxicosis to rise dramatically.[23]

Because of the high rates of iodine-induced thyroid disease initial assessment and ongoing monitoring should be undertaken routinely for patients receiving amiodarone, or other chronic high dose iodine supplementation. Prior to initiating amiodarone, a clinical assessment for evidence of underlying thyroid disease and measurement of TSH and thyroid peroxidase (TPO) antibodies should be undertaken. Patients with evidence of hyperthyroidism should be considered for definitive therapy typically with the radioactive iodine isotope (I-131) before the initiation of amiodarone if possible. Patients with a high TSH or positive TPO antibodies are at particularly high risk for the development of iodine-induced hypothyroidism and should be monitored more closely as a consequence. During treatment with amiodarone, all patients should have regular thyroid screening, including twice-yearly measurement of TSH (every 3 months in patients with positive baseline tests), with T3 measurement as a follow-up if the TSH becomes suppressed.[17]

It has been stated that a patient should "earn their amiodarone," implying that treatment with this toxic drug should be used as a last resort, after all other options have failed. Increasingly, however, amiodarone is being used at an early stage because of its remarkable efficacy. Alternatives should certainly be considered when thyrotoxicosis arises as a complication. In all cases of amiodarone-induced thyroid disease, the first consideration in treatment is whether the amiodarone might be withdrawn.

Withdrawal of amiodarone may effectively eliminate the thyroid complications of the drug in some cases, while the use of corticosteroids and antithyroid drugs may prove beneficial, hastening recovery after amiodarone withdrawal.[24] However, the thyrotoxicosis may prove self-perpetuating, so that even withdrawal of the amiodarone may not always be effective in resolving the problem. In addition, the long half-life of amiodarone, caused by its high lipid solubility, and the high iodine-load that even short-term treatment makes drug withdrawal alone a slow and uncertain treatment, suitable only for mild to moderate disease.[19]

Thiourea drugs, including propylthiouracil (PTU) and methimazole may be used to impair iodine organification and improve the thyrotoxicosis. However, this approach is often only slowly and incompletely effective, particularly if the amiodarone is continued, since the high iodine load may overcome the effect of the PTU.[24] High doses may be required, with the possibility of significant toxicity, including hepatic and bone marrow effects. Sodium- or potassium-perchlorate and lithium have also both been used to promote iodide flux from the thyroid gland, and these drugs may accelerate recovery from the iodine-loading effect.[25] Toxicity and intolerable side effects are significant problems, and once again the efficacy of this approach is questionable if the amiodarone must be continued. Radioactive iodine is largely ineffective in amiodarone-induced thyrotoxicosis because of the low-iodine uptakes, the result of iodine loading.

Ultimately, the treatment of choice for iodine-induced thyrotoxicosis that does not respond to more conservative measures is surgical resection of the thyroid gland, followed by thyroid hormone replacement.[26,27] Although many patients who are receiving amiodarone are at high surgical risk because of underlying heart disease, improvements in general anesthesia and monitoring techniques, as well as improvements in surgical techniques, have made thyroid surgery even in this group of patients a relatively safe procedure, with reported mortality rates of <5%.[27] This definitive approach should be considered for all patients with persistent symptomatic or progressive amiodarone-induced thyrotoxicosis, particularly those for whom withdrawal from the amiodarone is not an option.

Hyperthyroidism and Thyrotoxicosis. Hyperthyroidism and thyrotoxicosis are common and important endocrine disorders that result from several distinct pathologic conditions of the thyroid gland, or from overt or covert ingestion of thyroid hormone. The incidence of overt and subclinical hyperthyroidism among adults is between 0.05 and 0.1% per year in the United States, with an estimated prevalence of ~1.2% and a female to male ratio of approximately 3:1.[28]

The term thyrotoxicosis is generally reserved to describe the clinical syndrome that results from elevated levels of T4 and T3 in the circulation. Hyperthyroidism, on the other hand, describes a state of increased production and release of thyroid hormones from the thyroid gland, which may or may not lead to thyrotoxicosis.

The most common cause of hyperthyroidism, responsible for almost two-thirds of cases, is Graves disease, an autoimmune process of the thyroid that also exhibits extrathyroidal manifestations.[29] Autonomously functioning nodules within a multinodular goiter become more common with age, often causing mild thyrotoxicosis, which may be manifested by atypical symptoms. Solitary autonomous thyroid nodules, almost always benign, are infrequent causes of hyperthyroidism. Inflammatory conditions of the thyroid, resulting in damage to the gland (thyroiditis), may also induce the release of thyroid hormone with consequent thyrotoxicosis. Although this might occur at any age, it is seen most frequently among young women in the postpartum phase. Overtreatment with thyroid hormone (either deliberately or accidentally) will also, of course, result in thyrotoxicosis in the absence of hyperthyroidism.

The majority of the symptoms and many of the signs of thyrotoxicosis are independent of the underlying cause (Table 1). In many cases, however, certain clinical features will point to the cause. These include most importantly, the size and shape of the thyroid gland and the presence of extrathyroidal features of Graves disease.

Table 1 Major Clinical Findings in Hyperthyroidism	
Symptom (%)	Sign (%)
Nervousness (99)	Tachycardia (100)
Increased sweating (91)	Goiter (95)
Hypersensitivity to heat (89)	Skin changes (97)
Palpitations (89)	Tremor (97)
Weight loss (85)	Thyroid bruit (77)
Tachycardia (82)	Eye signs (71)
Dyspnea (75)	Atrial fibrillation (10)
Eye complaints (54)	
Diarrhea (23)	
Anorexia (9)	

Adapted from reference 30.

Confirming the diagnosis biochemically is rarely complex, and determining the underlying cause is straightforward in most cases. The treatment of thyrotoxicosis is effective but is most commonly directed toward destruction of the thyroid gland and rarely addresses the cause of the hyperthyroidism. In consequence, the majority of patients so treated require lifelong replacement of thyroid hormone, and all patients require lifelong monitoring of thyroid function.

Neonatal Hyperthyroidism. The transplacental passage of TSH-receptor antibodies (TRAb), from a mother with Graves disease, can rarely result in significant neonatal hyperthyroidism, the result of "vertical transmission" of maternal Graves disease to the baby, both in utero and postpartum during breastfeeding.[31] Typically, the neonate exhibits goiter, lid retraction without exophthalmos, irritability, low birthweight, poor feeding, and "failure to thrive." Treatment is supportive, with occasional use of antithyroid drugs. Because the condition is self-limiting, definitive treatment is rarely required, with surgery reserved only for life-threatening thyrotoxicosis and obstructive goiter.[30]

Pediatric Hyperthyroidism. Approximately one per million young children and three per million adolescents are diagnosed with hyperthyroidism per year, with 95% of cases due to Graves disease. Symptoms include the usual spectrum of symptoms that affect adults, including weight loss, palpitations, tremor, and hyperactivity. In addition, however, behavioral difficulties, deteriorating performance at school and difficulties with socialization are common features of thyrotoxicosis in childhood.[32] Treatment options are identical to those in adults, discussed below, although it is common for endocrinologists to avoid the use of radioactive iodine, in an effort to minimize exposure to ionizing radiation, with its theoretical risks of carcinogenesis and fertility changes. Consequently, first-line treatment is typically administered in the form of antithyroid drugs, with surgery as the first-line option for "definitive" therapy.[33]

Graves Disease. Graves disease is an autoimmune disease of the thyroid and certain other extrathyroidal tissues, most notably the eyes and skin. The hyperthyroidism manifested by these patients is the result of autoantibodies against the TSH receptor, which mimic the effects of TSH on thyroid cells, thereby stimulating autonomous production of T4 and T3. The alteration of immune function that leads to the production of these antibodies is complex, involving the interaction of B- and T cells in the production of antibodies against several autoantigens in addition to the TSH receptor.[29] TSH receptor antibodies are detectable in the serum of almost all patients with Graves disease and may be used clinically in making the diagnosis. Lymphocytic infiltrates are commonly seen in the thyroid gland of patients with this condition. A considerable overlap in histologic appearance between Graves disease and Hashimoto disease (autoimmune thyroiditis) exists, with only the presence of hypertrophic follicles characterizing the former.[29] It is not surprising then, that some patients with Graves disease undergo spontaneous remission, or develop hypothyroidism in the long term. This may result from autoimmune destruction of the gland, or from the production of TSH receptor-blocking antibodies, which may also be seen in Hashimoto disease or autoimmune atrophic hypothyroidism.[34]

Lymphocytic infiltrates are also seen in the extraocular muscles of patients with Graves ophthalmopathy (though not in the subcutaneous tissues of patients with dermopathy), emphasizing the systemic nature of the autoimmune process.[35] It remains unclear what links these apparently separate manifestations of the disease although the search for common antigens continues. There is also an association between Graves disease and the other organ-specific autoimmune syndromes, including pernicious anemia, diabetes mellitus, vitiligo, Addison disease, and myesthenia gravis.[36] These associations support the hypothesis that autoimmunity is the result of a subtle but generalized immune system abnormality.

The most sensitive and specific test to distinguish Graves disease from silent thyroiditis, postpartum thyroiditis, or exogenous thyrotoxicosis is the measurement of iodine uptake. This test is performed after the oral ingestion of a fixed small dose (usually 1 to 5 mCi) of radioactive iodine. Quantification of the iodine uptake is commonly performed after 6 to 24 hours, by detection of the gamma emissions over the neck at that time. The normal thyroid gland retains approximately 8 to 20% of the administered iodine at 24 hours. In cases of Graves disease, iodine uptake is increased, often dramatically. Similarly, multinodular goiter and solitary hot nodules usually exhibit increased iodine uptake. In contrast, postpartum thyroiditis, silent thyroiditis, and exogenous thyrotoxicosis all result in reduced iodine uptake, either because of gland injury or as a result of TSH suppression.[29]

Antibodies against the thyrotropin receptor are the proximate cause of Graves disease, and act by binding to, and so stimulating, the TSH receptor, mimicking the action of TSH itself. These antibodies are detectable in 95 to 98% of patients with Graves disease and are absent in all but a tiny minority of patients with other causes of thyrotoxicosis.[37] Although less specific and less sensitive than measurement of radioactive iodine uptake, these assays are useful particularly when radioactive iodine uptake cannot be measured. In addition to pregnancy and breastfeeding, previous imaging, for example, computed tomography (CT) scanning, or treatment with iodine-containing drugs, for example, amiodarone, may interfere with the measurement of iodine uptake. Measurement of TSH-receptor antibody concentrations provides a useful alternative means to confirm a diagnosis of Graves disease.[38]

TPO antibodies are also commonly found in the serum of patients with autoimmune thyroid disease.[39] However, the finding of TPO antibodies is relatively nonspecific, and may be positive in as many as 10% of women of childbearing age.[28] Since postpartum thyroiditis is more likely in women with positive TPO antibodies, this test is not useful in distinguishing Graves disease from postpartum thyroiditis. Ultrasound of the thyroid gland can be helpful to exclude multinodular goiter or a solitary nodule. In Graves disease, the gland may also be enlarged and hypervascular.[40] In general, thyroid biopsy is also not regarded as a useful tool in this context.

Except in the mildest cases, treatment of thyrotoxicosis can be expected to improve the patient's symptoms and quality of life and to reduce the likelihood of complications. Symptomatic benefit can be achieved by the use of adrenergic beta-receptor blocking agents, which improve tachycardia, tremor, and sweating, reflecting the sympathetic overactivity common in thyrotoxicosis.[29,41] Nonselective beta-blockers, for example, propranolol, have a significant advantage over more cardioselective agents in this context. Patients with severe thyrotoxicosis may be extremely resistant and require high doses to achieve symptomatic improvement and control of the heart rate. Starting doses of 40 to 80 mg three times daily are usual, titrated upward according to the heart-rate response. Propranolol may have some inhibitory action on the deiodinase system, slowing the rate of T4 to T3 conversion, but it is likely that this is of minimal, if any, benefit in the treatment of thyrotoxicosis.[42] Propranolol is generally regarded as safe for use in pregnancy and lactation. It should be used with extreme caution in patients with asthma or coincident heart disease. The drug can be continued during the more definitive treatment of the patient's thyroid disease and can be weaned gradually as the symptoms remit.

Three treatment options are available for the management of Graves disease. All three are generally safe and effective, but each has unique advantages and disadvantages, and no one treatment can be regarded as better than any other, except in unusual circumstances.

Thyroidectomy for Graves Disease. The first effective therapy for Graves disease, which became available around the turn of the twentieth century, was surgical removal of the thyroid gland. A number of medical and surgical advances in the late 1800s and early 1900s, most prominently the appropriate preoperative correction of thyrotoxicosis and reduction of gland vascularity, made this surgery safe. Modern anesthetic techniques and careful preoperative preparation have lowered the mortality rates for this surgery virtually to zero, at least among young people without other significant illnesses.[43]

Under rare circumstances, in which the patient's life is at risk, preoperative preparation with beta-blockers alone (administered intravenously) has been shown to be possible.[44,45] While this approach lowers the anesthetic risk, however, the risk of significant bleeding from a highly vascular thyroid gland remains high. More commonly, and probably more safely, patients first are rendered euthyroid, most often with antithyroid drugs. Ten to 14 days prior to surgery, the antithyroid drugs are withdrawn, and potassium iodide (Lugol iodine solution) is commenced. This treatment, pioneered by Henry Plummer of the Mayo Clinic, maintains a block on thyroid hormone production and release (the Jod–Basedow phenomenon) and decreases the vascularity of the gland, improving the safety of the surgical procedure.[45,46]

In addition to the potential complications of any surgical procedure (scarring, infection, and hemorrhage), thyroidectomy may be associated with injury to the parathyroid glands and the recurrent laryngeal nerves, as discussed in detail below. Total or near-total thyroidectomy is not necessary in the management of Graves disease, and subtotal thyroidectomy (leaving 10 to 30% of the gland in situ) is recommended in many centers, reducing further the risk of these specific surgical complications.[47] Some surgeons attempt to leave sufficient thyroid tissue in place to render the patient euthyroid without thyroid hormone replacement therapy. This increase in the probability of surgical treatment failure is probably unnecessary in the era of sensitive thyroid function tests and accurate thyroid hormone replacement therapy, and is usually futile, since the majority of patients will go on to develop thyroid failure in the future, from progressive autoimmune thyroid gland destruction.[48]

Although rarely the treatment of first choice, surgery remains a viable treatment option for carefully selected patients. It remains the fastest and most certain means to achieve euthyroidism.

Radioactive Iodine. By far the most widely used treatment for Graves disease in North America, radioactive iodine is a safe and effective, nonsurgical means of thyroid ablation. Now in use for almost 60 years, this treatment option has proven to be well tolerated and predictable.[29] Because of the high iodine-concentrating capacity of the thyroid gland, particularly in Graves disease, the vast majority of ingested radioactive iodine is concentrated within the thyroid gland or excreted through the urine within 12 to 24 hours. This minimizes total body exposure to radiation although detectable uptake also occurs in salivary glands, gastric mucosa, colon, and bladder.[49] Nevertheless, concerns about carcinogenesis have not been substantiated, at least in the doses used for the treatment of thyrotoxicosis, in several large case series.[50] Despite this objective evidence of safety and a long track record of simplicity and efficacy, concerns about the long-term safety of radioactive isotopes remain the single most frequent reason given by patients (and physicians) in selecting other modalities of therapy.

I-131 is used for the treatment of patients with Graves disease, and acts principally as a beta-particle emitter. Iodine-123, which is a better, albeit more expensive, isotope for imaging, is a gamma-emitter, and these gamma-waves fail to interact adequately with tissue and, therefore, do not cause significant tissue injury. The beta particles released from I-131, however, generate superoxide radicals within the thyroid cell, causing double-strand deoxyribonucleic acid (DNA) breaks and resulting in apoptosis and gland involution.

Initially after treatment with radioactive iodine, thyroid hormone synthesis and release are impaired as the thyroid follicular cell responds to injury. Thyroid follicles are later disrupted, and there is often a temporary worsening of thyrotoxicosis, as previously synthesized thyroid hormone is released from thyroglobulin stored within the follicle.[51] Thereafter, thyroid hormone is cleared with its usual 7-day half-life, and the patient is rendered euthyroid and subsequently hypothyroid.

Permanent hypothyroidism is the expected and accepted outcome of treatment with radioactive iodine in most centers.[52] Depending on the dose used, between 60 to 95% of patients will be rendered permanently hypothyroid within 2 to 3 months of a single treatment dose. A small number of patients experience primary treatment failure, requiring a subsequent repeat dose. A small proportion of patients may experience temporary hypothyroidism within a few weeks of treatment followed by recurrent thyrotoxicosis as the thyroid remnant recovers. Both of these treatment failure types are minimized by use of adequate doses of I-131.[53]

In most centers in the United States, some form of dosimetry is used to calculate a suitable initial dose of I-131. Most commonly, this is based on some estimate of thyroid gland weight, assessed clinically or by ultrasound. A planned dose of between 100 and 200 μCi/g of gland weight can be administered, which takes into account the avidity of the gland for iodine. In a few centers worldwide, dosimetry has been abandoned in favor of a single fixed dose for all patients. Most commonly this dose is between 10 and 30 mCi (lower in countries with low iodine intakes), and is expected to render approximately 80 to 90% of patients hypothyroid with a single treatment dose. There is little evidence to favor one approach over the other.

Attempts to titrate the dose carefully to render the patient euthyroid, not requiring thyroid hormone replacement therapy, have generally been disappointing and have the disadvantage of leaving many patients thyrotoxic for prolonged periods. These efforts are often doomed for the same reason that "titrated surgery" is ineffective, namely, the progressive destruction of the gland remnant by the underlying autoimmune process. Once again, this approach is hard to justify when thyroid hormone replacement therapy is so straightforward in the majority of cases.

There remain concerns about the impact of radioactive iodine treatment on the natural history of Graves ophthalmopathy.[54,55] Considerable controversy has taken place over this subject, which remains under debate,[56] but in most centers patients with significant ophthalmopathy are either guided toward alternative treatments, or offered coverage with corticosteroids following their treatment with radioactive iodine.[57]

Radioactive iodine can be safely administered even to most patients who are allergic to topical iodine. However, it is absolutely contraindicated in pregnancy and breastfeeding.[58] In the first trimester of pregnancy, radioactive iodine treatment has been associated with increased rates of spontaneous abortion. Beyond the twelfth week of pregnancy, when the fetal thyroid is capable of concentrating iodine, radioactive iodine would render the fetus hypothyroid.[59] Similarly, radioactive iodine is concentrated in breast milk and would likely injure the infant's thyroid gland. A negative pregnancy test is mandatory prior to treatment with I-131, in all women of childbearing potential. There is no proven teratogenic effect in either males or females at any age, but pediatric endocrinologists have been reluctant to use radioactive iodine in patients under the age of 18 because of concerns on future fertility.[60]

Antithyroid Drugs. The thiourea group of drugs, for example, PTU, methimazole (MMZ), and carbimazole (CBZ), inhibit the intrathyroidal organification of iodine, so reducing iodine retention within the gland and impairing synthesis of thyroid hormone.[61] The gland becomes iodine deficient, and initially, under continued stimulation of the TSH receptor by TSH receptor antibodies, increases the proportion of T3 to T4 secreted. Thereafter, T3 secretion is also impaired, and thyroid hormone levels fall peripherally, with resolution of thyrotoxicosis.[62] PTU, perhaps more so than the other drugs in this group, also inhibits the peripheral conversion of T4 to T3, which may accelerate the return to euthyroidism.[63]

Administered orally, these drugs are rapidly absorbed and inhibit the release of thyroid hormones from the gland almost immediately. Resolution of hyperthyroidism occurs quickly, limited only by the plasma half-life of the thyroid hormones. In any case, return to normal of plasma thyroid hormone levels is expected within 3 to 4 weeks, although suppression of the pituitary thyrotroph may delay a return to normal of the TSH by some weeks.

Antithyroid drugs effectively treat the thyrotoxicosis caused by Graves disease, toxic multinodular goiter, or an autonomously functioning thyroid nodule. They are ineffective in the treatment of thyrotoxicosis resulting from silent or postpartum thyroiditis, in which the release of preformed thyroid hormone is the cause of thyroid hormone excess.

Since both multinodular goiter and autonomous thyroid nodules have a low likelihood of spontaneous remission, the use of antithyroid drugs in these contexts is rarely justified and more definitive therapy, either in the form of surgery or radioactive iodine, is generally recommended. However, the situation in Graves disease is rather different. Spontaneous remissions may occir, even in untreated patients. Between 30 and 50% of patients with Graves disease, treated with antithyroid drugs, may remain in long-term remission once those drugs are withdrawn.[64] Patients maintained in the euthyroid state using these drugs, exhibit an increasing probability of long-term remission with increasing duration of antithyroid drug treatment, up to at least 18 to 24 months.[64] Longer-term treatment appears to offer little additional benefit.

Rapid and profound falls in TRAb concentrations have been reported during drug treatment of Graves disease, and both the rate of fall and the final level of TRAb prior to discontinuation of drug therapy predict the likelihood of relapse.[65] Other, more subtle changes in immune system function have also been reported during drug treatment of Graves disease, and several in vitro studies have also suggested a possible immunomodulatory role for these drugs.[66]

Traditionally, treatment is initiated with a high dose of PTU (300 to 600 mg three times daily) or methimazole (40 to 80 mg daily), and the dose is then gradually reduced over a period of several months to a low maintenance dose. Treatment is continued for 12 to 24 months, with thyroid function being monitored at approximately 3-month intervals, and the dose adjusted to maintain thyroid hormones and TSH within their respective normal ranges. Following discontinuation of medication, close monitoring is required to detect early evidence of relapse.

Because of the suggestion of an immunomodulatory effect of these drugs, several controlled trials were undertaken in the 1980s to assess the impact of so-called combination therapy. Consisting of continued high-dose PTU accompanied by thyroid hormone, this treatment was designed either simply to prevent hypothyroidism during PTU treatment (a "block and replace" regimen), or specifically to maintain a suppressed TSH during (and after) antithyroid drug therapy, in an effort to "keep the thyroid asleep."[64,67,68] Despite an exciting positive initial report from a group of Japanese investigators, all other studies have proven disappointing, with no long-term benefit to the patient, and some potential side effects from both the PTU and the thyroid hormone.[64] Such combination therapies appear to have no major role in the management of patients with Graves disease.

Antithyroid drugs are generally well tolerated, with few side effects except for their impact on thyroid function. True drug allergy is infrequent, resulting in an urticarial rash in 5 to 10% of patients. Patients who are allergic to one of this group of drugs may tolerate one of the others, although cross-allergy is well recognized. Less common, and much more serious, is the potential for agranulocytosis, a sometimes irreversible bone marrow dyscrasia that results in a reduced white cell count (neutropenia) and susceptibility to infection.[69] Most commonly this presents with a bacterial pharyngitis. Immediate cessation of the drug therapy may permit bone marrow recovery, but trials of granulocyte colony stimulating factor have proven disappointing for the most serious cases.[70] This potentially life-threatening complication is reported to occur with an incidence of approximately 1 per 1,000 to 1 per 5,000 and appears to be idiosyncratic, being clearly related neither to dose nor duration of therapy.[71] Abnormalities of liver function are relatively common, and rare cases of drug-induced hepatitis have been reported.[71] Regular monitoring of liver function studies and CBC are routinely practiced, though of uncertain utility in detecting pre-symptomatic liver or bone marrow dysfunction.

Use of these drugs in pregnancy and lactation is relatively safe. PTU crosses the placental barrier less freely than CBZ or MMZ and is the drug of choice during pregnancy.[72] Reports of aplasia cutis, a defect of scalp skin maturation, exist for CBZ and MMZ, but this appears to be less of a problem with PTU.[73] However, because these drugs do enter the fetal and infant circulation and affect thyroid function, the use of the lowest possible dose of these drugs is recommended in pregnancy and lactation.[72]

Extrathyroidal Manifestations of Graves Disease. In addition to thyrotoxicosis, Graves disease is frequently associated with a number of extrathyroidal manifestations, including ophthalmopathy, dermopathy, and acropachy.[29,74] These features of the disease are distinct components of a multiorgan autoimmune process so that, although they are seen most commonly in association with thyrotoxicosis, these phenomena can occur independently, and their time course in relationship to the development of thyrotoxicosis may be quite variable. It was recognized many years ago that the eye changes of "exophthalmic goiter" can precede the symptoms of hyperthyroidism by months, or sometimes years, but most commonly become apparent coincident with the development of thyrotoxic symptoms or within the following 6 to 12 months.[75] Similarly, Graves dermopathy often first becomes apparent some time after the onset of thyrotoxicosis.[76]

There remains substantial controversy over the impact of thyrotoxicosis itself on the development and progression of extrathyroidal features of Graves disease. It has been argued that the presence of a source of thyroid antigens (the thyroid itself) sustains the autoimmune process in other organs, and that complete removal or ablation of the thyroid might result in immunomodulation of the systemic process, though not all authors agree.[77] A parallel argument holds that the increased release of thyroidal antigens, following administration of radioactive iodine, can exacerbate the extrathyroidal autoimmune process, antithyroid drugs or surgery might prove beneficial, either by removing the source of the antigen (surgery) or by decreasing the release of this antigen into the systemic circulation (antithyroid drugs).[78] Similarly, hypothyroidism in the aftermath of incomplete thyroid ablation may increase thyroid autoantigen release, and there is some evidence that a rise of TRAb levels and worsening of ophthalmopathy can occur in this situation.[79]

The evidence for each of these lines of reasoning is often weak or contradictory, and the practical implications for management of patients are not entirely "evidence based." Nevertheless, some anecdotal and observational data suggest that treatment of thyrotoxicosis with radioactive iodine is associated with a mild to moderate worsening of established ophthalmopathy, especially when hypothyroidism is permitted to ensue.[79] Whether such changes are clinically relevant in most cases remains in dispute. Many groups however, avoid this treatment for such patients, or use concurrent treatment with corticosteroids to minimize proinflammatory changes.[77] Others prefer to use higher ablative doses of radioactive iodine, ensuring prompt treatment with thyroxine to avoid hypothyroidism. Careful avoidance of postradioactive iodine hypothyroidism is important, particularly in patients with preexisting eye changes.[80]

Ophthalmopathy. The ophthalmologic features are the result of inflammatory changes within the orbital space, causing edema and, therefore, enlargement of both muscle and fat.[81] Orbital fibroblasts involved in this process lay down extracellular glycosaminoglycans that contribute to increased retro-orbital pressure. This swelling causes anterior protrusion of the globe (exophthalmos), impaired lymphatic and venous drainage resulting in periorbital edema, and imbalance of retro-ocular muscle function, which causes diplopia and strabismus.[81] Lid retraction and lid-lag are the result of the exophthalmos, involvement of the levator palpebrae superioris muscle in the inflammatory process, and possibly an increase in sympathetic muscle tone caused by the thyrotoxic state. Finally, muscle fibrosis and permanent deposition of glycosaminoglycans, may result in irreversible changes, causing permanent exophthalmos, diplopia, and lid retraction, even when the inflammatory changes resolve. Up to 50% of patients with Graves disease have some evidence for ophthalmopathy at the time of diagnosis of Graves disease, though in only around 20% of patients is it clinically overt, and only a small minority develop sight threatening changes.

Dermopathy. The characteristic lesions of Graves dermopathy occur on the lower extremities, most frequently on the anterior lower third of the shin or on the dorsum of the foot. This condition is relatively uncommon, affecting less than 5% of patients with Graves disease. The lesion is typically well demarcated, nodular, raised, brawny rather than edematous, dusky, and discol-ored. They blanch to pressure and are nonpitting to pressure. The skin overlying them is pitted and described as *peu d'orange* (literally "skin of the orange"), an accurate description of its appearance and texture. In most cases these lesions are asymptomatic, but pruritis and mild discomfort may occur and ulceration has been described.[76] In more extreme cases, the dermopathy may become diffuse, occasionally even resembling elephantiasis. Although the lower extremity anatomic distribution is characteristic, dermopathy is recognized to occur at other sites, particularly if there is a history of local trauma (the Koebner phenomenon), including the upper extremities, shoulders, trunk, face, and ears. Histologically, the findings are of subcutaneous infiltration with mucinous material consisting of extracellular glycosaminoglycans, found most prominently in a perivascular distribution.[82,83] The normal collagen matrix is distorted, but the overlying epidermis is often normal. The pathogenesis of the condition is unknown, but it is seen rarely in the absence of ophthalmopathy and occurs most frequently in patients with high circulating levels of TRAbs. There are data from in vitro studies that implicate serum factors, but it remains unclear whether these represent circulating autoantibodies (presumably to a cross-reacting antigen) or perhaps more likely some other factors that trigger a fibroblast response.[84]

Acropachy. Soft tissue swelling also characterizes the thickened extremities of thyroid acropachy, the least common manifestation of Graves disease, affecting fewer than 1% of patients. Swelling and clubbing of the digits is associated with subperiosteal new bone formation and fibrosis of the marrow space. The overlying skin is often pigmented. Histologic findings are virtually identical to those seen in Graves dermopathy.[85]

Evaluation and Treatment of Ophthalmopathy. Unilateral eye changes mandate exclusion of a retro-ocular mass lesion. Both carcinoma (most commonly metastatic) and lymphoma have been described as possible causes of unilateral exophthalmos, and the increased retro-orbital pressure arising in these conditions impedes venous and lymphatic drainage and mimics the periorbital edema of Graves disease.[86] Anterior protrusion of the globe results in apparent lid retraction, with secondary conjunctival inflammatory changes and exposure keratitis. Nevertheless, even in a patient with no prior history of thyrotoxicosis, Graves disease is one of the most common causes of exophthalmos, even when it is unilateral. In such cases of euthyroid Graves eye disease, thyrotropin receptor and TPO antibodies are commonly detectable, even when thyroid function is normal, and many such patients will eventually go on to develop thyrotoxicosis.[87]

A detailed ophthalmologic examination is mandatory in the care of Graves patients to document lid placement, proptosis, ocular mobility and alignment, and visual function. CT scanning of the orbits is the investigation of choice in all cases of Graves eye disease and will defini-tively exclude a mass lesion. In addition, specific features of Graves disease will be identified, most prominently swelling of the muscle bodies and increased retro-orbital fat volume.[88] CT scanning is, of course, essential if decompressive surgery is being considered.

Symptomatic therapy can be effective, particularly in mild or moderate ophthalmopathy, in which mild exposure keratitis and conjunctival irritation predominate. Lid retraction may result in failure of eye closure, particularly during sleep, resulting in dry, gritty, irritated eyes, with discomfort and photophobia. The frequent use of artificial tears during the day, and nonmedicated ophthalmic ointment at night, along with tinted spectacles or sunglasses may go a long way to resolving mild symptoms. Periorbital edema is largely a cosmetic issue, and will often resolve although incompletely as the inflammation settles and venous drainage improves. The use of cold compresses may provide some symptomatic relief.

If lid retraction remains after resolution of any acute inflammatory changes, a relatively minor lid-lengthening procedure can be easily performed. Similarly, minor cosmetic procedures to remove redundant skin, left in the aftermath of periorbital edema, can improve the appearance. Such interventions are generally delayed for at least 12 to 24 months after the development and stabilization of Graves ophthalmopathy, to ensure that any acute inflammatory changes have completely resolved.[81]

More aggressive ophthalmopathy, particularly with severe exophthalmos, exposure keratitis, and conjunctival ulceration, or features of optic nerve compression (manifested by altered color vision, reduced visual acuity, or visual field changes), requires more active acute management. In extreme cases, emergency decompression surgery is indicated to preserve sight.[77] More commonly, high-dose corticosteroids (prednisone 60 mg/d or equivalent) are used initially, reserving surgery for nonresponders or for patients who develop recurrent severe ophthalmopathy at unacceptably high maintenance doses of corticosteroid. Systemic corticosteroids abrogate the inflammatory process, decrease orbital swelling, improve lymphatic and venous drainage, and rapidly relieve optic-nerve compression.[77]

Short courses of corticosteroids are also commonly used as an adjunct to therapy with radioactive iodine, particularly in patients with established mild or moderate ophthalmopathy, to attempt to minimize any posttherapy exacerbation.[89] The known side effects of prednisone may outweigh the benefits in many cases, particularly if the ophthalmopathy is mild.

Even in severe ophthalmopathy, long-term treatment with corticosteroids is generally regarded as an unacceptable risk, because of the high doses required to maintain control of the eye changes. If symptoms and signs fail to resolve, or if they recur when the corticosteroid dose is reduced, alternative therapy is generally recommended, particularly in the form of decompressive surgery.[77]

For many years, the longer-term treatment of choice in moderate to severe ophthalmopathy in which sight is not actively threatened has been orbital radiotherapy.[77] The observation that radiation therapy might be beneficial was made incidentally in patients receiving pituitary irradiation administered as treatment for Graves disease at a time when the condition was thought to originate from pituitary oversecretion. Once the pathogenesis of Graves disease was understood, a re-analysis of the radiation fields showed that a substantial dose was being administered to the orbit, and specific orbital radiotherapy became popular.

Despite its popularity and widespread use, few clinical trials of this modality existed until recently. Somewhat surprisingly to many proponents of the technique, several large randomized controlled trials have shown only minimal improvement in clinical symptom scores in patients receiving orbital radiotherapy compared to a sham control.[90] A carefully controlled randomized double-blind trial, performed by Gorman and colleagues,[91] in which each patient served as his or her own control, and radiotherapy was administered to a single orbit, showed no significant change in any objective measurement of severity following radiotherapy. While this study remains highly controversial, there seems little doubt that orbital radiotherapy is far less effective than previously assumed and that previous apparent improvements might simply have reflected spontaneous resolution of the underlying disease process in many cases.

Orbital decompression is being used increasingly and, in experienced hands, carries an excellent outcome even in severe ophthalmopathy.[92] By removal of the medial, inferior, lateral, and occasionally superior walls of the orbit, the orbital contents are allowed to herniate into adjacent cavities. By increasing the space available for the swollen orbital contents, pressure reduction is achieved, globe position is improved, and improvement is seen in venous drainage with resolution of the secondary changes. A proportion of these patients will develop postoperative diplopia, even when no diplopia existed prior to decompression. While appropriate prism lenses improve visual function, most patients with diplopia will require surgical correction to restore conjugate gaze. This procedure is generally delayed for some months to allow complete resolution of the inflammatory process and is often combined with lid lengthening and other cosmetic procedures.[77,92]

Plummer Disease (Toxic Multinodular Goiter). In contrast to our understanding of the pathogenesis of Graves disease, toxic multinodular goiter remains something of an enigma. A number of factors, including childhood iodine deficiency and unknown genetic factors may be responsible for the development of nodular hyperplasia of the thyroid gland. In contrast to autonomously functioning solitary toxic adenomas, whose etiology may lie in activating mutations of the TSH receptor, the generalized hyperplasia of the gland seen in multinodular goiter remains unexplained, with no recognized genetic influences.[3,93] Whatever the trigger, progressive hyperplasia results in an increasingly enlarged and nodular gland, which, in many cases, becomes autonomously functional.

Disruption of the normal follicular architecture, with microfollicles, sheets of follicular cells, and isolated islands of cells, makes iodine trapping less efficient, resulting in the production of less iodinated forms of thyroid hormone.[94] Consequently, as autonomy develops progressively, patients may develop gradual onset of "T3-toxicosis." Typically, a suppressed TSH is associated with a normal level of T4, leading to a diagnosis of "subclinical hyperthyroidism," despite what may often be significant clinical features, including a significant risk of thyrotoxic bone disease (exacerbating osteoporosis) and atrial fibrillation.[95] Measurement of T3 typically reveals the degree of thyrotoxicosis which may be severe, particularly in older patients. Iodine excess contributes to the development of thyrotoxicosis by overcoming the relative inefficiency of iodine trapping exhibited by these goiters, so that severe thyrotoxicosis may result from iodine exposure, for example after administration of iodine-containing contrast material for an angiogram or CT scan.[96]

Treatment of toxic multinodular goiters is identical to that of Graves disease, with the exception that antithyroid drugs will only be effective while they are administered, with little chance of spontaneous remission, except in cases that have been triggered by iodine exposure.[97] Iodine uptake, measured as a 24-hour uptake, is often normal or only slightly elevated because of the inefficiency of iodine trapping.[94] Consequently, effective treatment with I-131 requires higher administered doses. Stimulation with recombinant TSH (rTSH) may overcome this problem, and the treatment of toxic multinodular goiter increasingly is being performed with radioactive iodine rather than surgery.[98,99]

Hypothyroidism. Hypothyroidism, resulting primarily from autoimmune destruction of the thyroid gland, is among the most common of endocrine diseases, affecting 1 to 1.5% of all women and up to 0.5% of men.[100] Several community-based surveys show an increasing prevalence with age in both sexes, reaching over 12% among women over the age of 70.[100–102] Many more individuals of both sexes develop subclinical disease, and some evidence of autoimmune thyroiditis can be found at autopsy in 45% of women and 20% of men in the United States.[103]

The diagnosis of hypothyroidism is generally straightforward, both clinically and biochemically, and treatment with oral thyroid hormone replacement is simple and well tolerated. The widespread availability of sensitive TSH assays, and the broad range of L-thyroxine (T4) doses produced by several manufacturers have made accurate dose titration possible. However, there remains controversy about the dose of thyroid hormone required for replacement therapy, the use of T4 alone or in combination with T3, the need for dose adjustment during pregnancy or intercurrent illness, and the treatment of patients with subclinical hypothyroidism.[104]

Transient hypothyroidism, seen most often as postpartum thyroiditis, is increasingly being recognized and may be associated with adverse maternal and fetal outcomes, including postpartum depression.[105] Treatment with thyroid hormone may be offered to symptomatic patients but may only be required for a short time. Such patients are at increased risk for the development of permanent hypothyroidism in later life, and screening of these individuals may be justified.[106]

Hypothyroidism most often is caused by decreased production of thyroid hormone because of disease of the thyroid gland termed *primary hypothyroidism*. Far less common is *secondary hypothyroidism*, caused by reduced pituitary TSH secretion, the presentation of which is often dominated by other features of the pituitary disease. In primary hypothyroidism, symptoms are almost exclusively the result of a fall in circulating thyroid hormone concentrations.

Primary hypothyroidism may be caused by damage or destruction of thyroid tissue, or by interference with thyroid hormone synthesis (Table 2). By far the most common cause is autoimmune thyroiditis, of either atrophic or goitrous type, commonly known as Hashimoto disease.

The symptoms of hypothyroidism are broad ranging but may be quite nonspecific, particularly in mild forms of the disease (Table 3). Because many of these symptoms are frequent in the population even in the absence of thyroid disease and hypothyroidism is so common, it is frequently the case that a patient complaining of fatigue (for example) may be found to have abnormal laboratory tests for thyroid function. It is tempting to assume that the thyroid dysfunction is the cause of the symptoms. However, particularly when

Table 2 Causes of Hypothyroidism
Thyroid tissue destruction
Atrophic thyroiditis
Hashimoto thyroiditis
External beam irradiation
Radioactive iodine therapy
Thyroidectomy
Infiltrative diseases (amyloidosis)
Thyroid tissue injury
Postpartum thyroiditis
Silent thyroiditis
Subacute thyroiditis
Thyroid hormone synthesis defect
Iodine deficiency and excess
Antithyroid drugs
Dyshormonogenesis
Central hypothyroidism
Pituitary disease
Hypothalamic disease
Generalized resistance to thyroid hormone

Adapted from reference 107.

Table 3 Symptoms and Signs of Hypothyroidism

Neuropsychiatric
  Fatigue
  Lethargy
  Sleepiness
  Mental impairment
  Depression
  Slow speech
  Bradykinesia
  Hyporeflexia
  Delayed relaxation of the reflexes
  Paresthesiae, especially carpal tunnel syndrome
Thermoregulatory
  Cold intolerance
  Hypothermia
Dermatologic
  Dry skin
  Decreased perspiration
  Nonpitting edema (myxedema)
Metabolic
  Weight gain
  Decreased appetite
  Hyperlipidemia
  Glucose intolerance
Cardiovascular
  Bradycardia
  Cool extremities
Gastrointestinal
  Constipation
Hormonal
  Menstrual disturbances
  Galactorrhea
Miscellaneous
  Arthralgia
  Hoarseness
  Normochromic normocytic anemia

laboratory testing shows only borderline abnormalities, that appropriate consideration should be given to alternative explanations of the patient's symptoms.

Treatment of Hypothyroidism. The mainstay of treatment for patients with hypothyroidism for the last century has been oral thyroid hormone replacement.[104] Initially available as an extract of animal thyroid, synthetic T4 and T3 have become widely available in the last 30 years. The total daily secretion of thyroxine from a healthy thyroid gland is proportional to body mass, but typically thyroid hormone is not prescribed on a microgram per kilogram basis. Instead, patients with uncomplicated primary hypothyroidism most often receive a small initial dose of approximately 50 µg daily, and the dose is increased at intervals of 4 to 6 weeks to a full replacement dose of approximately 100 to 150 µg/d. Patients with preexisting symptomatic coronary artery disease or poorly controlled atrial or ventricular arrhythmias should begin treatment more cautiously because of the increased myocardial oxygen requirements induced by thyroid hormone, and its transient proarrhythmic effect.[108] Starting doses of 12.5 to 25 µg/d are used commonly, with gradual increases, guided by the TSH response. The final achieved dose should be the same, however.

Because of the long half-life of thyroxine (~87 days), it is possible to administer thyroxine once

weekly, and at least one study has demonstrated satisfactory control of both biochemical and clinical parameters using such an approach.[109] More traditionally, thyroxine is administered once daily. If patients forget to take a dose, then the subsequent dose can safely be doubled, or the dose simply omitted, without any major adverse impact on thyroid hormone concentrations or thyrotropin response.[110,111]

The long thyroxine half-life and the relatively slow response of the pituitary thyrotroph to changes in circulating thyroid hormone concentration make frequent adjustments of thyroid hormone dose undesirable.[110] Changes in thyroxine dose more frequent than every 2 to 3 months may result in overcompensation, with the risk of symptomatic hyperthyroidism from overtreatment, and apparently unstable dose requirements.

Although rare allergies have been reported to the inert ingredients of specific thyroxine preparations, the drug is otherwise without side effects, except for the impact of over- or under-replacement. Excessive dosing is associated with symptoms of thyrotoxicosis, while inadequate treatment allows persistent hypothyroidism. Occasionally, particularly if the dose is changed rapidly, patients experience concurrent symptoms of both under- and overreplacement; but almost always this will be a transient phenomenon. The goal should be to achieve stable thyroid hormone concentrations.

Other causes of altered dose requirements include patient noncompliance and erratic thyroxine absorption. This arises only infrequently in patients with extensive small bowel disease and malabsorption.[112] More commonly, other drugs, minerals, or food supplements are responsible, either by increasing thyroxine metabolism, for example, phenytoin, or by interfering with intestinal absorption, for example, cholestyramine, ferrous sulfate, calcium carbonate. Ideally, thyroxine should be taken along with no other medication, preferably on an empty stomach prior to breakfast.

Following the initiation and stabilization of treatment with thyroxine, repeat thyroid function testing is recommended after approximately 3 months, a further 6 months, and then annually. Hypothyroidism in some patients may be gradually progressive, and dose requirements often change over the first few months of treatment. Thereafter, only minor and gradual changes in thyroid hormone dose are required in most patients, with a slight reduction necessary with aging. As noted below, pregnancy is also associated with significant alterations in thyroid hormone metabolism, and careful monitoring is justified. The clinical conditions most often requiring altered thyroxine dosing are shown in Table 4.

Most patients with long-standing hypothyroid symptoms notice an improvement with thyroxine replacement within 2 to 3 weeks of starting treatment. Weight reduction, cardiovascular symptoms, changes in metabolic parameters, and many of the neuropsychiatric symptoms improve quite rapidly, while structural changes including

Table 4 Conditions Often Requiring Adjustment of
Thyroxine Dose

Increased dose requirement
  Other drugs used concurrently
    Phenytoin
    Caramezepine
    Rifampicin
    Cholestyramine
    Sucralfate
    Ferrous sulfate
    Calcium carbonate
    Amiodarone
  Pregnancy
  Recent onset of hypothyroidism
  Recent I-131 treatment for Graves disease
  Small bowel malabsorption
Decreased dose requirement
  Aging

Adapted from reference 110.

skin and hair changes, hoarseness, and anemia take longer to resolve.

Optimal thyroid hormone replacement would correct all of the symptoms of hypothyroidism without causing side effects, and in the majority of patients this can be achieved with the dose between 100 and 200 µg of L-thyroxine daily. Replacement therapy can be monitored accurately with the use of TSH measurement, and restoration of TSH to within the normal range is usually accepted as the goal of therapy.[113] However, a proportion of patients fails to achieve complete correction of hypothyroid symptoms when their TSH lies within the normal range, and many patients report a symptomatic benefit from slight over treatment with thyroxine.[110] It has long been argued that thyroid hormone replacement with thyroxine alone, without replacing the thyroidal component of T3 production, leaves patients relatively T3 deficient.[114,115] Certainly, treatment with doses of thyroxine sufficient to restore the TSH to midnormal range is associated with free-thyroxine concentrations toward the upper limit of normal and triiodothyronine concentrations in the lower half of the normal range.[110] Whether this has any significant impact on target organs remains unclear.

Overtreatment with thyroxine may also be associated with adverse outcomes, and the risks of atrial fibrillation and postmenopausal osteoporosis are both increased by subclinical hyperthyroidism.[116,117] Similarly, nocturnal heart rate, circulating liver enzyme concentrations, and serum cholesterol all show similar, though less marked, changes with thyroid hormone-induced TSH-suppression as they do in thyrotoxicosis.[118] How significant these changes really are remains unclear at this time, and some studies suggest that asymptomatic TSH suppression with exogenous thyroxine, carries no excess morbidity or mortality. Nevertheless, optimal replacement of thyroxine should probably be regarded as that dose required to eliminate symptoms, while maintaining a TSH in the lower half of the normal range, with free thyroxine at, or slightly above, the upper limit of normal, and a T3 concentration well within its normal range.[113]

Although the majority of patients treated with thyroxine for autoimmune thyroid disease experience complete resolution of symptoms, a significant minority continues to exhibit symptoms and signs compatible with mild hypothyroidism. Most often the lingering symptoms include fatigue and lethargy, cold intolerance, dry skin, and difficulty losing weight.[119] Although definitive evidence is lacking, these symptoms have been blamed on persistent tissue hypothyroidism.

In normal health, the thyroid gland itself is the source of approximately 20% of circulating T3, while the remainder is produced by deiodination of thyroxine in the liver and, to a lesser extent, the kidney.[120] The regulation of this process depends on the rate of T4 transport across the hepatocyte membrane.[121] Following destruction of the thyroid gland by autoimmune disease, surgery or radioactive iodine, all circulating T3 must be derived from exogenous thyroid hormone. As a result, patients treated with thyroxine alone often exhibit somewhat reduced circulating T3 concentrations, and the typical profile in such a patient is for normal TSH, free thyroxine in the upper half of the normal range, and a low-normal or even frankly reduced T3 concentration.[108]

One important study addressed this issue of apparent persistent hypothyroid symptoms in patients receiving thyroid hormone, by comparing replacement using T4 alone with a combination of T4 and T3.[122] This randomized, double-blind, placebo-controlled crossover trial included 33 patients receiving thyroxine treatment for Hashimoto thyroiditis or thyroid cancer. Participants were randomized to treatment with either thyroxine alone (plus placebo), or a slightly reduced dose of thyroxine supplemented with triiodothyronine. After 5 weeks, patients were converted to the other treatment arm for another 5 weeks. The patients receiving combined T4 and T3 treatment exhibited higher circulating T3 concentrations, an increase in some biochemical markers of thyroid hormone action, and a small but significant improvement in several psychometric parameters, most importantly feelings of fatigue, depression, and hostility. This study has led to a clamor for conversion to the combined therapy, or the use of thyroid hormone extracts that contain T3 as well as T4. While a small minority of patients do appear to gain some benefit from this approach, the benefits are often transitory and probably reflect the pharmacologic impact of transient excessive T3 dosing. Several subsequent studies have shown no significant benefit of combination therapy for these patients.[123]

Such combinations do have possible adverse affects, and treatment with T3 is associated in many patients with transient thyrotoxic symptoms, including palpitations, tremor, and sleep disturbance. Nevertheless, combinations of T4 and T3 are becoming increasingly popular in the management of such patients, particularly those with persistent hypothyroid symptoms. It is worth remembering that such combinations were the mainstays of treatment for many years prior to the introduction of synthetic L-thyroxine and that their use is associated with adequate control of biochemical parameters. For patients who wish it, who are willing to tolerate the possible side effects, the use of both T4 and T3, or a mixture of the two hormones, for example, Armour Thyroid™, is an acceptable alternative to the more usual treatment with thyroxine alone.

Subclinical Hypothyroidism. Most commonly the result of early chronic autoimmune thyroid disease or of inadequate thyroid hormone treatment, subclinical hypothyroidism is defined as an elevated TSH concentration (usually between 5.0 and 10.0 mU/L), with normal thyroid hormone concentrations, in the absence of symptoms of hypothyroidism.[124] The condition often is identified incidentally during biochemical screening for nonspecific symptoms, most commonly fatigue, cold intolerance, and weight gain. Almost all of the symptoms of hypothyroidism (see Table 3) are quite nonspecific and may arise for a variety of nonthyroid reasons. Nevertheless, it is common for the thyroid to "take the blame" for these nonspecific symptoms. Both patient and physician may be disappointed when the symptoms fail to improve after adequate thyroid hormone replacement.

Weight gain of more than 3 to 5 kg is unusual even in quite profound hypothyroidism, and progressive weight gain over many years is not consistent with relatively mild thyroid failure. While tiredness and fatigue may be caused by hypothyroidism, the failure of these to improve when taking thyroid hormone implies that they are likely to have an alternative cause. While a trial of therapy with thyroid hormone may well be justified in patients with mild hypothyroidism, it is important to ensure that alternative causes of the symptoms are considered.

In the presence of mildly elevated TSH, positive thyroid antibodies imply that a patient has autoimmune thyroid disease. A 20-year follow-up study in the North of England demonstrated that over 50% of women with positive thyroid antibodies and a TSH greater than 6 mU/L, would go on to develop overt hypothyroidism, a rate of over 4% per year.[100] Such patients probably warrant thyroxine replacement even in the absence of significant symptoms, because of the likely future need for this treatment.

Subclinical hypothyroidism is accompanied by changes in target organs, which may be reversible. Changes in auditory acuity, left ventricular function, and capillary permeability have all been reported although it is not clear whether these changes justify treatment with thyroid hormone.[125,126] Similarly, changes in lipid profiles are common in overt hypothyroidism, and subclinical hypothyroidism has been suggested as a risk factor for atherosclerosis.[125] The evidence for this is weak, however, and patients with truly subclinical hypothyroidism (TSH less than 10.0 mU/L and no symptoms) do not exhibit hyperlipidemia. Nor does treatment to restore the TSH to normal significantly affect lipid profiles.[127] As yet, there is no adequate clinical trial assessing the impact of treatment of subclinical hypothyroidism.

It is, therefore, reasonable to consider treatment with thyroxine for patients discovered to have subclinical hypothyroidism as a result of autoimmune thyroid disease. However, those patients should not be led to expect a dramatic resolution of all of their symptoms, and the "trial and error" nature of the treatment should be discussed fully. Other contributory causes for the patient's symptoms also require evaluation.

Autoimmune Hypothyroidism. Hashimoto thyroiditis was originally defined on the basis of characteristic pathologic features, including lymphocytic infiltrates, germinal centers, reduced follicle size, and oxyphilic follicular cells (Hürthle cells). Clinically, patients have a goiter and may become hypothyroid although circulating antibodies and the goiter may predate thyroid gland failure, sometimes by years.[128]

The goiter is firm and slightly irregular, with the surface texture described as bosselated. These surface irregularities represent areas of hyperplasia within the gland; and, in some cases, one or more of these regions may enlarge and become a clinically detectable thyroid nodule. Such "hyperplastic nodules" are the most common cause of thyroid nodules in patients (especially women) with autoimmune thyroid disease. These nodules are often poorly defined clinically and may be "cool" or "warm" on isotope scanning, which is therefore not a reliable technique in this setting. Ultrasound examination often reveals a poorly defined nodule, which is isoechoic or hypoechoic, and contiguous with the remainder of the gland. Fine-needle aspiration biopsy (FNAB) reveals thyroid follicular cells but may also show Hürthle cells, which can be easily misinterpreted as indicating a Hürthle cell neoplasm, so leading to unnecessary surgery. Lymphocytes may also be identified, consistent with autoimmune thyroid disease. Occasionally, lymphocytic infiltration is marked, and low-grade lymphoma may occasionally be suspected. A core biopsy or even an open biopsy may rarely be necessary to exclude this diagnosis.[129]

Thyroid nodules developing as a hyperplastic response in thyroid autoimmunity may appear and grow rapidly, mimicking thyroid cancer. They will resolve spontaneously in many cases with simple observation. Treatment of hypothyroidism, with consequent reduction of TSH, may speed their resolution. Suppression of TSH is not justified, however, as there is no indication that this approach is any more effective than simply treating the hypothyroidism.[130]

Secondary (Central) Hypothyroidism. Pituitary or hypothalamic disease may reduce or destroy the capacity of the pituitary to manufacture and secrete TSH in response to falling thyroxine levels, leading to secondary hypothyroidism. The clinical features of secondary hypothyroidism are usually dominated by symptoms of the underlying pituitary or hypothalamic disease process and by failure of other pituitary hormones. Most

Table 5 Causes of Secondary (Central) Hypothyroidism

Pituitary lesions
  Tumors
    Pituitary adenoma
    Craniopharyngioma
    Metastatic tumor
  Ischemia
    Postpartum necrosis (Sheehan syndrome)
    Diabetes mellitus
    Shock
  Internal carotid artery aneurysm
  Iatrogenic
    External beam irradiation
    Pituitary surgery
  Infection
    Tuberculosis
    Syphilis
    Other bacterial
  Sarcoidosis
  Histiocytosis
  Hemachromatosis
  Lymphocytic hypophysitis (autoimmune)
  Idiopathic
Hypothalamic lesions
  Tumors
    Craniopharyngioma
    Meningioma
    Metastatic tumors
  Trauma
  Ischemia
  Sarcoidosis
  Histiocytosis
  Congenital
  Idiopathic

Adapted from reference 131.

often, the diagnosis is made incidentally during evaluation of hypopituitarism. Nevertheless, management of thyroid status in hypopituitarism is an important aspect of treating these patients. Recognized causes of secondary hypothyroidism are shown in Table 5.

Measurement of circulating TSH has become the principal method used to assess the adequacy of thyroid hormone replacement. In central hypothyroidism, this is not reliable, and concentration of circulating thyroid hormones provides the only useful information. Titration of thyroid hormone under these conditions is more complex, but in general optimal replacement is signaled by a free-T4 at the upper limit of its normal range, with a T3 lying well within the normal range. The temptation to reduce thyroid hormone dose in response to a suppressed TSH must be resisted.

Transient Hypothyroidism. The majority of patients who develop hypothyroidism require lifelong treatment with thyroxine. However, transient hypothyroidism is increasingly recognized and may cause symptomatic or asymptomatic changes in thyroid hormone concentrations for a few weeks, months, or even years.[132,133]

Occasionally, spontaneous remission of hypothyroidism associated with autoimmune thyroiditis may occur, and there are several case reports of patients with long-standing hypothyroidism whose thyroid function returns to normal,

or who go on to develop thyrotoxicosis secondary to Graves disease.[134] The majority of such cases almost certainly developed hypothyroidism as a result of blocking antibodies, binding to the TSH receptor and preventing its activation by TSH. A shift in the antibody epitope spectrum, perhaps triggered by pregnancy or intercurrent infection, may cause the development of stimulating antibodies, and consequently Graves disease.

Transient hypothyroidism may also be seen following treatment of Graves disease either with surgery, or with radioactive iodine. Incomplete surgical removal of the gland (subtotal thyroidectomy or lobectomy) leaves sufficient tissue in situ to permit regrowth of the gland under the trophic stimulation of TSH receptor antibodies.[33] Similarly, the use of low doses of radioactive iodine may result in incomplete ablation of the thyroid, and regrowth of the thyroid remnant is possible. Recurrence of the hyperthyroidism may occur although a few patients do maintain euthyroid status.[135]

More commonly, transient hypothyroidism reflects reversible injury to the thyroid gland by an inflammatory process, or by external factors, including goitrogens and iodine (Table 6). Of these, the most common are silent thyroiditis and postpartum thyroiditis, which are related conditions.

SILENT AND POST-PARTUM THYROIDITIS. Silent and post-partum thyroiditis are related, autoimmune-mediated, transient inflammatory diseases of the thyroid. The acute or subacute inflammation causes damage and disruption of the thyroid follicles, release of pre-formed thyroid hormone, and later hypothyroidism during gland repair and recovery. Return of normal thyroid function occurs in the majority (>90%) of cases after 3–6 months.

Although postpartum thyroiditis is normally transient, the risk of transient postpartum thyroid-

Table 6 Causes of Transient Hypothyrodism

Spontaneous
  Autoimmune thyroid disease
    Blocking antibodies against the TSH receptor
    Transplacental passage of blocking antibodies
    (neonatal hypothyroidism)
  Silent thyroiditis
  Postpartum thyroiditis
Iatrogenic
  Treatment of Graves disease
    Antithyroid drugs
    Subtotal thyroidectomy
    Low-dose radioactive iodine
  Goitrogens
    Lithium
    Cassava beans
  Thiocyanates (environmental toxin)
  Iodine loading (Wolff–Chaikov effect)
    Treatment with amiodarone
    Use of Betadine in surgical procedures
    (especially gynecologic)
    Iodine containing contrast material in
    CT scanning

itis is increased 100-fold in patients with positive TPO antibodies, and a significant proportion of patients develop persistent autoimmune hyper- or hypothyroidism.[136]

During the thyrotoxic phase, postpartum thyroiditis can be distinguished from Graves disease on the basis of radioactive iodine uptake, since the uptake in postpartum thyroiditis will be low. This reflects the gland injury, with release of preformed thyroid hormone. Alternatively, measurement of TSH receptor antibodies can be used to distinguish these two conditions, avoiding exposure to radioactive iodine. This is particularly important if the patient is still breastfeeding. This thyrotoxic phase is often brief and not severe and may go unnoticed by patient and physician, particularly in the early weeks following the birth of a baby.[132]

Thyrotoxicosis rarely lasts more than a few weeks and is followed in the majority of cases by more prolonged and often symptomatic hypothyroidism. It is during this hypothyroid phase that postpartum depression may first come to light.[132] The distinction between transient and permanent hypothyroidism depends on the history, and there are no diagnostic tests to distinguish between them. The uptake of iodine will be low in both cases, and TPO antibodies are commonly positive in both. In postpartum thyroiditis, hypothyroidism gradually results over a period of 4 to 6 months, and rarely lasts longer than 8 to 12 months in total.

Treatment of the hypothyroidism may be considered if symptoms are sufficiently troublesome.[137] The goal should be to achieve a low-normal TSH, as outlined earlier. Because the hypothyroidism will almost certainly prove transient, a gradual supervised dose reduction, guided by thyroid function testing, is appropriate.

In less severe cases, where the symptoms of hypothyroidism are mild, it is reasonable simply to observe thyroid function until spontaneous resolution. The management of silent thyroiditis follows the same lines but is less likely to require temporary thyroid hormone treatment.

Riedel Thyroiditis. Riedel thyroiditis is the least common form of thyroiditis with an operative incidence of 0.06% (37 cases in 57,000 thyroidectomies).[138] The typical age of presentation is between 30 and 50 years with women affected more commonly than men (4:1). This disease is a chronic fibro-inflammatory process which produces a stony hard, painless thyroid mass with potential fibrotic extension into adjacent tissues. The fibrotic process often generates tracheal compression, laryngeal distortion, and pharyngeal and esophageal narrowing. The picture of a rock-hard thyroid mass with associated dyspnea, hoarsness, stridor, or dysphagia raises obvious concern for malignancy.

Functional studies are not helpful in the diagnosis as most patients remain euthyroid although both hypothyroidism and hyperthyroidism have been reported.[139,140] Other laboratory investigations are nonspecific including sedimentation rate and antithyroid antibodies, while imaging features lack diagnostic characteristics. Radionuclide imaging reveals findings similar to other forms of thyroiditis with a heterogeneous or low uptake. Ultrasonography reveals a homogenously hypoechoic pattern and magnetic resonance imaging (MRI) reveals a hypointense appearance on T1- and T2-weighted images.[141] CT is the most useful imaging technique demonstrating a variable (normal to hypodense) appearance of the thyroid gland with direct extension, infiltration, and encasement of adjacent structures.

Fine needle aspiration is frequently nondiagnostic due to an acellular specimen and the diagnosis will often require an open biopsy. Diagnostic criteria include: (1) grossly visible fibro-inflammatory process involving all or a portion of the thyroid gland; (2) gross and/or histological evidence of extension into adjacent structures; (3) absence of granulomatous reaction; and (4) absence of neoplasm.[139] The characteristic cellular infiltrate progresses from lymphocytes, plasma cells, neutrophils, and eosinophils to a dense fibrous infiltration with hyalinization. It is the extension of the dense hyalinized fibrous tissue, which obliterates tissue planes, that renders safe resection nearly impossible. Based on the clinical history, imaging and benign FNAB, patients who have airway obstructive lesions should undergo a decompressive isthmusectomy only.

The relative rarity of Riedel thyroiditis has precluded any clinical trials to guide medical management. Glucocorticoids and tamoxifen have been reported to provide benefit. Typically glucocorticoids are used as first-line therapy with a variable rate and duration of response. These drugs are often used as first-line therapy because of the progressive perithyroidal infiltration and fibrosis with potentially life-threatening destruction of local structures. In some instances dramatic responses to glucocorticoids have been described as well as lasting benefit even after their withdrawal, while several case reports have suggested subjective and objective improvement in response to tamoxifen, in glucocoriticoid resistant cases.[142,143]

Riedel thyroiditis is most likely to represent a variant of idiopathic multifocal fibrosclerosis, a suggestion supported by its association with retroperitoneal fibrosis, sclerosing cholangitis, mediastinal fibrosis, and orbital pseudotumor.[144] Multifocal fibrosclerosis is a disorder apparently related to a plasma cell infiltrate that expresses high levels of IgG4.[145] Biopsy studies reveal T- and B-cell infiltrates with the plasma cells consistently expressing IgG4. The IgG4 plasma cells are diminished in number with glucocorticoid therapy, and elevated serum levels of IgG4 are not consistently identified.

Suppurative Thyroiditis. Acute suppurative thyroiditis (AST) is an uncommon disorder, perhaps because the gland is difficult for bacterial access because of fibrous encapsulation of the gland and represents a hostile environment for

bacterial growth because of the high iodine concentration and highly oxidizing state. The most common predisposing factor associated for AST is the persistence of an embryologic connection of the gland to the upper aerodigestive tract via a fourth pharyngeal pouch remnant or a thyroglossal duct remnant. Therefore, it is not uncommon for the onset of AST to follow an upper respiratory or oral infection, especially with lingual involvement. Fourth pharyngeal pouches are only found on the left side. If the right side is the primary site involved, an alternative underlying cause should be considered. In adults, thyroid abnormalities such as goiter or nodular disease may become infected by hematogenous or lymphatic routes, and direct inoculation has also been reported. Bacterial microorganisms are the most common source of AST although fungi, viruses, and parasites have been implicated rarely. The bacterial microorganisms most frequently associated with AST include staphylococcal and streptococcal species.[146]

Symptoms and findings that suggest the development of AST include fever, neck swelling, pain, and leukocytosis. Regional inflammation may also prompt pharyngeal and laryngeal swelling with resultant odynophagia and dysphonia. In young children lethargy can be a finding in the early stage of abscess formation. Suspicion of a neck abscess should prompt radiological evaluation with both ultrasound and CT scanning providing useful information. A pharyngeal pouch should be considered as a source even in young adults and therefore a barium swallow or CT scanning performed after the administration of oral contrast should be performed. The authors prefer to have these studies completed when the neck is not acutely infected since the regional edema at the time of acute inflammation can obstruct the pouch tract. Thyrotoxicosis is generally not associated with AST, although a few case reports exist of thyrotoxicosis in association with AST, due to the disruption of follicles and the release of preformed thyroid hormone.[147]

Treatment involves supportive care, appropriate antibiotic therapy, drainage of the abscess, and closure of any pharyngeal connection. Closure of this connection requires exposure of the piriform sinus mucosa near the cricothyroid articulation. Identification and preservation of the recurrent nerve is necessary and often the thyroid lobe will be sufficiently involved that a significant portion of the lobe must be removed.[148]

Nonthyroidal Illness (the "Euthyroid Sick Syndrome"). Abnormalities of thyroid hormone concentrations, without evidence of intrinsic thyroid or pituitary gland disease, are seen frequently in a wide variety of nonthyroidal illnesses, including infections, trauma, myocardial infarction, major surgery, malignancy, inflammatory conditions, and starvation.[149] Following recovery from the underlying illness, the thyroid function normalizes, and the "euthyroid sick syndrome" was so named because the abnormalities seem to represent a response to the underlying illness,

rather than an abnormality of the thyroid gland itself. The implicit assumption that the patient is therefore euthyroid has led to recommendations to avoid testing the pituitary–thyroid axis during intercurrent illness, and among the majority of hospitalized patients. Whether these patients are truly euthyroid remains unproven, however, and some studies have shown evidence of hypothyroidism at least in some tissues in these patients.[150] Because of these uncertainties, the preferred term for this condition remains "nonthyroidal illness" (NTI).

A variety of patterns of thyroid hormone and TSH concentrations have been reported in NTI, reflecting both the type of illness and its severity. Three patterns of thyroid function are recognized: low T3 syndrome; low T3 and low T4; and low TSH.

Low T3 Syndrome. This is the most common form of NTI, most often resulting from acute illness. The serum T3 concentration falls rapidly within 30 minutes to 24 hours of the onset of the causative illness, and the degree of fall reflects the severity of the disease process.[151,152] Reverse-T3 (rT3) rises as T3 falls, reflecting altered activity of hepatic de-iodinase, the source of around 80% of T3 in humans.

Low T3 and Low T4 Syndrome. With more severe and more prolonged illness, total T4 concentrations fall over 24 to 48 hours. Once again, the degree of fall in T4 correlates with mortality in a number of conditions.[149,151,152] Free thyroxine concentrations are variable, perhaps reflecting an impact of NTI on the assays used to measure free-T4. The fall in T4 reflects a fall in thyroid-binding globulin and, in some cases at least, the presence of an unidentified inhibitor of T4 binding. Transient elevations in free-T4 are seen in some NTI as a result.[153]

Low TSH Syndrome. In the most severe or prolonged forms of NTI, and prominent in cases of starvation and malnutrition, TSH concentrations fall despite the low T4 and T3 concentrations. The TSH response to exogenous thyrotropin releasing hormone (TRH) is blunted within 24 hours of onset of NTI, while TSH pulsatility and the normal nocturnal TSH surge are both impaired, suggesting an effect of NTI on both the pituitary and hypothalamus.[154] During the recovery from NTI, TSH may transiently rise to levels above normal.

A number of possible mediators of NTI have been suggested, most promisingly some of the known mediators of the inflammatory response, particularly members of the interleukin family. Interleukins and tumor necrosis factor-alpha (TNF-α) mimic almost all of the features of NTI, including reduced thyroid hormone and TSH concentrations, a blunted TSH response to TRH injection and impaired thyroid hormone de-iodination.[155,156] In addition, TNF-α concentrations show a close correlation with T3 concentrations in a number of studies of NTI.[151,157] However, the precise role of these and other potential mediators of NTI remains speculative.

Whatever the precise mechanism, the triggers for NTI are well recognized. Starvation and malnutrition appear to be particularly potent causes of abnormal TRH and TSH secretion, and altered hypothalamic control seems likely to play a major role.[158] In premenopausal women, other evidence of hypothalamic dysfunction is provided by the presence of secondary amenorrhea, caused by hypogonadotropic hypogonadism, which is an almost universal accompaniment to prolonged NTI.

The challenge remains to determine whether the patients are euthyroid. A suppressed TSH indicates thyrotoxicosis only when the hypothalamic and pituitary feedback mechanism is intact. Hypothalamic or pituitary disease, including tumors, infarction, and trauma, may disrupt this mechanism, and the discovery of apparently "inappropriate" TSH suppression requires further assessment.

Our limited ability to determine thyroid status at a tissue level remains one of the major barriers to understanding the impact of NTI. Several tissue-specific markers of thyroid hormone action are directly correlated with T3 concentrations in NTI, suggesting that at least some tissues experience true "hypothyroidism."[150,159] It remains unknown whether this tissue hypothyroidism is protective or destructive.

The vast majority of patients with NTI who recover from their underlying illnesses experience prompt recovery also of the hypothalamic-pituitary–thyroid axis. No specific therapy is indicated for their thyroid status. Few human studies have been performed of thyroid hormone replacement in NTI. In a small number of patients in a medical intensive care unit, with NTI caused by a variety of underlying illnesses, intravenous T4 resulted in a more prolonged suppression of TSH and delayed the rise in T3 during recovery from illness, perhaps impairing the recovery of the thyroid axis.[160] Because of the impairment of the hepatic deiodinase discussed above, restoration of T3 concentration to normal would probably require administration of T3 rather than T4. A double-blind, placebo-controlled, prospective study of 142 patients undergoing coronary artery bypass surgery confirmed improved cardiac output and lower systemic vascular resistance, but no difference was seen in outcomes.[161] In contrast, intravenous T3 in 211 patients undergoing high-risk coronary artery surgery had no impact on any hemodynamic variable and failed to alter the need for postoperative inotropic support, time in intensive care, or time to hospital dismissal.[162] In summary, no convincing evidence exists of therapeutic benefit from the administration of thyroid hormone to patients with NTI. Further trials are certainly justified and necessary but will be large and difficult to perform.[149]

Pituitary TSH-Secreting Adenoma and the Syndrome of Thyroid Hormone Resistance. While laboratory testing of the pituitary-thyroid axis is well developed and highly reliable, there are times when the pattern of thyroid function tests remains confusing. One common anomaly is the finding of a combination of elevated TSH with normal thyroid hormone measurements, or normal TSH with elevated thyroxine concentrations. The most common cause of a pattern of this type is intermittent administration of L-thyroxine, most often the result of variable compliance. Because TSH takes some time to respond to changes in thyroid hormone concentrations, a patient who takes L-thyroxine intermittently may exhibit persistently elevated TSH, reflecting their true thyroid status, but have normal or even elevated thyroid hormone concentrations in the hours following ingestion of the hormone.

The possibility of a laboratory error should also be considered in the setting of test results that do not appear to be compatible. Each of the thyroid hormones is measured routinely by immunologically based assays, and all are prone to error if binding between the antibody and the analyte is altered. One common example is the presence in the serum of antimouse antibodies, which can interfere with the binding of TSH to the mouse monoclonal antibodies used in many commercial TSH assay systems. In a two-site assay, this can result in spuriously elevated TSH measurements.[163]

Among patients who have not previously been treated with thyroid ablation, a pattern of this type should raise the question of a TSH-secreting pituitary adenoma, a rare cause of secondary hyperthyroidism. This condition causes increased thyroidal production of thyroid hormones, driven by TSH stimulation. The majority of these cases are associated with TSH values within or close to the normal range, but higher concentrations are occasionally seen. However, these patients often exhibit signs and symptoms of thyroid hormone excess, rather than of hypothyroidism. Nevertheless, the possibility of a TSH-secreting pituitary adenoma should be considered in the differential diagnosis of any patient with a goiter, elevated thyroid hormone concentrations, and an inappropriately detectable or elevated TSH.[164] Management of this condition requires treatment of the hyperthyroidism, followed by definitive treatment of the pituitary tumor, either surgically or by radiotherapy.

Thyroid hormone action is thought to be entirely dependent on the binding of T3 to its receptor within the cell, with consequent alteration in the affinity of the receptor for its DNA-binding sites. Consequently, the laboratory findings of a normal TSH in the setting of elevated thyroid hormone concentrations, or an elevated TSH in the face of normal thyroid hormone, suggest the possibility of thyroid hormone resistance syndrome implicating a defective cellular response to T3.[165,166]

Abnormalities of the T3 receptor have been described, in which ligand (T3) binding is impaired, reducing T3 sensitivity.[167] These abnormalities result in variable degrees of resistance to thyroid hormone, and reflect inherited germ-line mutations of the T3-receptor gene. Homozygous nonsense mutations, resulting in a nonfunctional T3 receptor, are probably lethal in utero, and it is the heterozygous mutations that have largely been described in humans. The severity of the disease correlates with the degree of inhibition of thyroid hormone binding in laboratory assays.[168]

Resistance to thyroid hormone may be generalized resistance the thyroid hormone (GRTH), isolated only to the pituitary, that is, pituitary resistance to thyroid hormone (PRTH), or peripheral tissue resistance to thyroid hormone (PTRTH).[168] By far the most common, although still exceptionally rare, is GRTH, and the mechanism by which PRTH and PTRTH might arise remains unclear, since the same gene is responsible for the thyroid hormone receptor in all tissues, including the pituitary. Nevertheless, several distinct clinical entities have been described and remain largely to be explained. The diagnosis of GRTH should be considered in patients with a history of goiter with elevated thyroid hormone concentrations but lack thyrotoxic symptoms or signs. If the goiter is treated by thyroid ablation, the development of hypothyroid signs and symptoms despite apparently normal or elevated thyroid hormone concentrations is suggestive of GRTH.

Confirmation of the diagnosis can be made in most cases by sequencing of the thyroid hormone receptor.[169] In the meantime, exclusion of other causes of elevated TSH with normal thyroid hormone concentrations is required. Many laboratories are capable of screening patient serum for antimouse antibodies to exclude the rare case of inaccurate TSH measurements. Imaging of the pituitary by MRI scanning should be performed to exclude a TSH-secreting pituitary adenoma. The majority of these are detectable on MRI scanning although tiny microadenomas have been reported rarely.[170]

Neoplastic (Nodular) Thyroid Disease

Benign Thyroid Nodules. Thyroid nodules are common. Nodules can be detected by careful palpation in almost 10% of the general population in North America and in up to 60% either by high-resolution ultrasound or in autopsy studies.[171,172] In contrast, clinically significant thyroid cancer is rare, being diagnosed in only around 1 in 10,000 individuals in the United States each year, a prevalence of less than 0.1%.[173] As is the case for most thyroid disease, thyroid nodules are found more frequently in women (approximately 5:1 ratio), and the incidence rises with age, particularly after the age of around 45 years.

The discovery of a thyroid nodule mandates the exclusion of malignancy, and professional guidelines recommend a FNAB as a first-line investigation for this purpose.[174,175] The vast majority (>75%) of clinically detected thyroid nodules are benign on fine-needle biopsy, making their excision optional.[176] As a result, many patients live with persistent thyroid nodularity. This can make both patient and physician uncomfortable, sometimes leading to a desire to intervene by medical therapy in an effort to shrink the nodule.

Suppression of thyroid nodules with thyroid hormone was first used in the 1950s, and there are numerous studies addressing the efficacy of this approach, with somewhat contradictory findings.[177] Many of the studies are limited by technical inadequacy, failing to define the pathologic process that causes the nodule and estimating, rather than measuring, the size of the nodule. In addition, these studies have included a broad range of nodule types and sizes, both solitary and multiple, and a wide array of thyroid hormone treatment and TSH targets. Consequently, this area of the field is confused.

For nonfunctional, or minimally functional nodules, radioactive iodine offers little chance of benefit, although there is an increasing trend toward the use of radioactive iodine in the management of both toxic and nontoxic multinodular goiter, the latter following stimulation of uptake of iodine with injections of recombinant human TSH (rhTSH).[178] While goiter volume reduction is likely using this approach, there is a high risk of developing hypothyroidism.[178] Radioactive iodine treatment is not suitable for management of solitary nodules, unless they are "hot nodules," causing thyrotoxicosis (and TSH suppression).

In contrast, the surgical approach to benign nodular thyroid disease is well established, effective, and generally safe. The surgical technique is described later, along with risks and precautions.

Thyrotropin Regulation of Thyroid Cell Growth. Thyroid follicular cells depend on the trophic effect of TSH (thyrotropin) for maintenance of gland volume, and perhaps number of cells.[179] TSH acts via a cell surface receptor, the TSH receptor, and activates both the cyclic adenosine monophosphate (cAMP)-dependent and inositol-tri-phosphate pathways.[180] The second messenger systems are responsible both for the increased metabolic activity (thyroid hormone synthesis and release) and the maintenance of cell growth and division.[181] In the absence of TSH, induced either by exogenous thyroid hormone or by pituitary insufficiency, the normal thyroid undergoes atrophy, exhibiting a reduction in extracellular volume (decreased colloid content) and cell mass (reduced cell volume and apoptosis). Suppression of gland volume can be achieved with thyroid hormone, which acts by reducing pituitary TSH secretion, via the pituitary-hypothalamic negative feedback mechanism.[182]

While the normal thyroid decreases in volume with thyroid hormone suppression, the response of a thyroid nodule is less predictable. That response is determined by the dependence of that nodule on TSH for continued growth. Consequently, some nodules cannot be expected to respond to thyroid hormone suppression, while others may be exquisitely sensitive to a reduction in TSH concentration.[183]

Pathology of Thyroid Nodules. The majority of thyroid nodules are benign. However, this classification includes a broad range of pathologic processes, including solitary adenomas, adenomatous (hyperplastic) nodules within a multinodular gland, thyroid (colloid) cysts, and regenerative nodules within a gland involved by Hashimoto disease.

Solitary Benign Follicular Adenoma. Activating mutations of the TSH receptor gene have been described in a proportion of these nodules.[184] These mutations are somatic rather than germ-line. The TSH receptor in this context functions autonomously, in the absence of interaction with its ligand (TSH). Constitutive activation of the second messenger system within the cell results in development of a truly autonomous, often hyperfunctioning nodule. Ultimately, the nodule will cause excess thyroid hormone production, with consequent suppression of TSH and downregulation of the remaining thyroid tissue. In the presence of a thyroid nodule and a suppressed TSH, a thyroid scan should be performed to assess the function of the nodule.[185] "Hot" nodules, almost never malignant, can be treated by radioactive iodine rather than surgery, with a high likelihood of success in eliminating the nodule and leaving the remaining thyroid tissue intact, with long-term euthyroidism.[186]

Other follicular adenomas may be premalignant, and therefore warrant excision in their own right.[185] In any case, FNA cannot reliably distinguish follicular adenoma from carcinoma, and all such lesions should be surgically excised.

Thyroid Cysts. The cause of most thyroid cysts remains obscure. In most cases, they show the histologic features of a simple cyst, with proteinaceous cyst fluid surrounded by a simple cuboidal epithelium. The colloid cyst, by far the most common benign cyst of the thyroid gland, contains material that closely resembles the colloid within a normal thyroid follicle. Less often, a cyst forms in association with a thyroid carcinoma, most often papillary carcinoma, which may form only a small solid nodule on the wall of the cyst.[187] Distinguishing a benign from a malignant cyst can sometimes be challenging, since both can reaccumulate fluid. Multiple ultrasound-guided biopsy efforts may be required, and biopsy-indeterminate cysts which continue to reaccumulate have an incidence of malignancy between 10 and 30%, and so warrant surgical excision.[188]

Benign Adenomatous Nodule. These nodules are nonclonal, arising from a group of follicular cells rather than from a single cell that has undergone neoplastic transformation.[189] The stimulus for the growth of such a nodule is unclear, but in many cases, the serum TSH concentration in these patients is normal, and the follicular cells that make up the nodule are likely sensitive to TSH. Lowering circulating TSH with thyroid hormone may be worthwhile for such a nodule, although it is difficult to know a priori whether any individual nodule is likely to respond to such an approach.

Regenerative Nodule. Perhaps the commonest cause of thyroid nodules, particularly in young women, is Hashimoto disease.[190] In response to the inflammatory process and chronic destruction of the parenchyma, the thyroid's capacity to secrete thyroid hormone is reduced. TSH begins to rise, and there is increasing evidence that a TSH even in the upper normal range may represent early thyroid failure among patients with Hashimoto disease.[100] TSH stimulates growth of the remaining thyroid cells. However, it is not always possible for the entire gland to respond, particularly in the presence of intraglandular fibrosis. A situation analogous to the hepatic cirrhosis arises. In most cases, a "micronodular" pattern develops, creating the classic clinical features of a bosselated goiter. In a few cases however, a "macronodular" pattern develops, with the development of a discrete nodule within the gland. Sometimes these nodules can grow rapidly, and they are clearly under the regulation of TSH or of TSH-receptor antibodies. It is for this group of patients that thyroid hormone suppression is most likely to be of benefit, and a trial of thyroxine treatment is certainly justified in this context before proceeding to surgical excision.[177]

Follicular Cell Derived Thyroid Carcinoma. *Follicular Carcinoma and Papillary Carcinoma.* Differentiated thyroid carcinoma (DTC) is the most common group of endocrine malignancies, with an estimated annual incidence in the United States of around 30,000 cases, resulting in approximately 1,500 deaths each year.[191] The vast majority of these (85 to 95%) are sporadic follicular cell derived thyroid carcinomas (FCDTCs), either of papillary or follicular histotype, while only 2 to 5% represent the C-cell derived medullary carcinoma (MTC),[192,193] which can develop as part of the multiple endocrine neoplasia syndrome type 2 (MEN-2).[194]

Although they represent less than 2% of clinically diagnosed human malignancies, DTC kills prematurely more patients than all other endocrine malignancies combined.[191] Nevertheless, with a crude mortality rate of only around 7%, the vast majority of patients with DTC, are either cured or live with cancer, often for many years. However, the recurrence rates after apparent surgical cure of the primary tumor range from 10 to 35%. Depending on histotype and stage at diagnosis, the neoplasm may sometimes recur many years after the initial, apparently successful, treatment.[195]

Thyroid carcinomas have a wide range of malignant potential, ranging from the incidentally discovered papillary microcarcinoma, which probably has no impact on long-term survival,[196] to the almost universally lethal anaplastic thyroid carcinoma, with a median life expectancy of only a few months.[197]

There have been many studies designed to identify factors that predict outcome among patients with DTC. Unfortunately, there have been no randomized, prospective trials of thyroid cancer management, largely because of the relative rarity of the neoplasm, its generally slow clinical course with long survivorship, and the difficulty and expense of mounting large multicenter studies over prolonged periods. Nevertheless, a great deal of information is available from large retrospective reviews from a number of centers, and this information should influence the management of the patient with DTC.[175]

The primary treatment of newly diagnosed DTC is surgical. Nevertheless, several options exist for the postoperative (adjuvant and long-term) management of these patients, and there exists a broad range of opinion regarding the appropriate use of these therapeutic modalities. Similarly, there remains considerable controversy regarding the frequency of follow-up and the techniques best employed to detect recurrent disease.

The therapeutic goals for the primary treatment of DTC are clear. First, we should seek to avoid, or reduce to a minimum, cause-specific mortality from the cancer. Second, it is important to prevent postoperative tumor recurrence. And third, we should avoid treatment-induced morbidity whenever possible.[175,198]

Tumor Classification. FCDTCs commonly retain many of the features of the parent cell type, including follicle formation and a capacity to concentrate iodine, to manufacture and secrete thyroglobulin and on occasion even to produce thyroid hormone.[199,200] The cells that comprise these neoplasms often express TSH receptors on their surface, and may respond to TSH stimulation by both increased uptake of iodine and an increased rate of growth, suggesting that they retain many of the differentiated functional features of their presumed tissue of origin.[201,202] Histologically, two major types of FCDTC are recognized: PTC and FTC.[203] Each also has a number of subtypes (Table 7), which may have distinct growth patterns and possible clinical implications.

PTC is named for its characteristic histologic architecture of papilliform growth but also exhibits characteristic cytological features, including large, clear nuclei with nuclear grooving and "signet ring" nuclei, the result of asymmetrical chromatin aggregation.[176] Despite its name, PTC may exhibit a predominantly follicular growth pattern ("follicular variant" of PTC), a subtype that previously was classified as FTC, but which should now be classified as PTC based on its cytological features.[204]

Psammoma bodies, microscopic extracellular structures of concentric calcified layers, are of uncertain origin, occur in around 75% of PTC, and are pathognomonic of the disease.[204] They can often be recognized on preoperative ultrasound, as internal calcified densities, with a characteristic "sparkling" appearance.[205] The nuclear features and occasionally the presence of psammoma bodies frequently permit a firm diagnosis of PTC to be made on cytologic analysis of FNA material.[206]

FTC displays a more solid growth pattern, within a fibrous capsule, with formation of irregular follicular structures, surrounded by epithelial cells of rather bland, uniform appearance, which exhibit none of the nuclear features that characterize PTC.[204] The degree of cellular and nuclear atypia is variable, with no clear distinction between benign and malignant follicular neoplasms.[207] This distinction is made solely on the basis of invasion, either of the capsule or of blood vessels, by the carcinoma, a feature that cannot be ascertained from FNA and requires surgical removal of the suspect nodule for recognition.

The Hürthle cell variant of FTC [also known as Hürthle cell carcinoma (HCC), or as oncocytic or oxyphilic FTC] is the commonest "atypical" FTC, comprising up to 25% of all FTC and may warrant its own classification, distinct from FTC.[208] Histologically, HCC differs from typical FTC only in the proportion of oncocytes within the tumor. These cells are characterized by a granular acidophilic cytoplasm, the result of the presence of large numbers of densely packed mitochondria.[204] Oncocytes represent >75% of the cells in HCC, which may also exhibit a rather more trabecular growth pattern than typical FTC.

Tall cell, columnar cell, and diffuse sclerosing variants of PTC, as well as the insular and clear cell variants of FTC, may have biological and clinical features distinctly different from the more typical neoplasms. Reports have been published of more frequent regional lymph node involvement, higher recurrence rates, more frequent distant metastases, and possibly higher mortality rates in these subtypes.[209] However, all of these studies are limited by a lack of uniform criteria for histologic diagnosis, by ascertainment bias, and by the small numbers of cases reported.

Most authors accept that the insular variant of FTC is a less well-differentiated tumor, with a consequently adverse prognosis.[210–213]

However, even for HCC, the most common of the neoplastic variants, controversy persists regarding the clinical implications of this diagnosis, with some authors reporting a worse prognosis,[214,215] whereas others see no significant difference in outcome between HCC and FTC when tumor stage is taken into account.[216] Recurrence rates are higher for HCC than for FTC, particularly within the thyroid bed and adjacent regional lymph nodes, arguably justifying a separate diagnostic category.[217]

A great deal of progress has been made in the last quarter century regarding the molecular pathogenesis of thyroid cancer in general, and PTC in particular, with the identification of causative oncogenes in the majority of cases.[218] These findings are summarized in Table 8.

Management of Differentiated Thyroid Carcinoma. The primary management of DTC is surgical. Postoperative management of patients with newly diagnosed and treated DTC should include staging and risk assessment. The goal of this approach is to permit accurate prognostication for an individual patient being treated for DTC and to allow individualization of postoperative surveillance and the extent of adjunctive therapy.

American Joint Committee on Cancer and International Union Against Cancer Staging. The pathological Tumor-Node-Metastasis (pTNM) classification system of the American Joint Committee on Cancer (AJCC) and International Union Against Cancer (IUCC)[220] is applicable to patients with tumors of all types, providing a convenient shorthand method to describe the extent of the tumor in an individual patient. This scheme is recommended for use also with patients with thyroid carcinomas.[175] Using this system, the tumor is assessed according to the size and extent of the primary tumor mass, the presence (N1) or absence (N0) of lymph node metastases, and the presence (M1) or absence (M0) of distant metastases (Table 9). Whereas the prognosis for many tumor types is determined largely or exclusively by the anatomical extent of disease, described efficiently by the pTNM classification, and the

---

Table 7 Histological Classification of Differentiated Thyroid Carcinomata

Follicular cell derived
  Papillary carcinoma
    Follicular variant
    Oncocytic papillary thyroid carcinoma
    Tall cell
    Columnar
    Diffuse sclerosing
  Follicular carcinoma
    "Typical" (nonoxyphilic)
    Hürthle cell carcinoma (oxyphilic)
    Insular
    Clear cell
C cell derived
  Medullary carcinoma

Table 8 Summary of Genetic and Epigenetic Alterations in Thyroid Cancer*

Type of Genetic Alterations	Prevalence of Occurrence (%)	
	PTC	FTC
BRAF mutation	45	0
Ras mutation	15	40
RET/PTC rearrangements	20	0
RASSFLA methylation[†]	20	60
Pax8/PPARg rearrangement	0	40

Adapted from reference 219.

*Shown is the prevalence of various genetic and epigenetic alterations in the two most common thyroid malignancies, papillary thyroid cancer (PTC) and follicular thyroid cancer (FTC). The prevalence of each alteration shown here represents the overall prevalence reported in the literature for sporadic thyroid cancers in adult patients.

[†]Methylation level at ≥50% of total *RASSFLA* alleles.

Table 9 Definition of TNM Classification (VIth Edition)

Category	Definition
Primary tumor (T)*	
TX	Primary tumor cannot be assessed
T0	No evidence of primary tumor
T1	Tumor 2 cm or less in its greatest dimension, limited to the thyroid
T2	Tumor more than 2 cm but not more than 4 cm in greatest dimension limited to the thyroid
T3	Tumor more than 4 cm in its greatest dimension limited to the thyroid or any tumor with minimal extrathyroidal extension (eg, extension to sternothyroid muscle or perithyroid soft tissues)
T4a[†]	Tumor of any size extending beyond the thyroid capsule to invade subcutaneous soft tissues, larynx, trachea, esophagus, or recurrent laryngeal nerve
T4b[†]	Tumor invades prevertebral fascia or encases carotid artery or mediastinal vessels
Regional lymph nodes (N)‡	
NX	Regional lymph nodes cannot be assessed
N0	No regional lymph node metastasis
N1	Regional lymph node metastasis
N1a	Metastasis to level VI (pretracheal, paratracheal, and prelaryngeal/Delphian lymph nodes)
N1b	Metastasis to unilateral, bilateral, or contralateral cervical or superior mediastinal lymph nodes
Distant metastasis (M)	
MX	Distant metastasis cannot be assessed
M0	No distant metastasis
M1	Distant metastasis

*All categories may be subdivided: (I) solitary tumor, (II) multifocal tumor (the largest determines the classification).

[†]All anaplastic carcinoma are considered T4 tumors: T4a—intrathyroidal anaplastic carcinoma (surgically resectable); T4b—extrathyroidal anaplastic carcinoma (surgically unresectable).

‡Regional lymph nodes are the central compartment, lateral cervical, and upper mediastinal lymph nodes.

Staging	T	N	M
Papillary or follicular under 45 years			
Stage I	Any T	Any N	M0
Stage II	Any T	Any N	M1
Papillary or follicular 45 years and older			
Stage I	T1	N0	M0
Stage II	T2	N0	M0
Stage III	T3	N0	M0
	T1	N1a	M0
	T2	N1a	M0
	T3	N1a	M0
Stage IVA	T4a	N0	M0
	T4a	N1a	M0
	T1	N1b	M0
	T2	N1b	M0
	T3	N1b	M0
	T4	N1b	M0
Stage IVB	T4b	Any N	M0
Stage IVC	Any T	Any N	M1
Medullary carcinoma			
Stage I	T1	N0	M0
Stage II	T2	N0	M0
Stage III	T3	N0	M0
	T1	N1a	M0
	T2	N1a	M0
	T3	M1a	M0
Stage IV A	T4a	N0	M0
	T4a	N1a	M0
	T1	N1b	M0
	T2	N1b	M0
	T3	N1b	M0
	T4	N1b	M0
Stage IV B	T4b	Any N	M0
Stage IV C	Any T	Any N	M1
Anaplastic carcinoma*			
Stage IV A	T4a	Any N	M0
Stage IV B	T4b	Any N	M0
Stage IV C	Any T	Any N	M1

Any anaplastic carcinomas are considered Stage IV.

success of resection, thyroid tumors of follicular cell origin are unique, in that their prognosis is most strongly influenced by patient age at diagnosis. As a result, the AJCC/UICC staging system takes into account patient age for defining stage for FCDTC.

In this staging system, all patients under the age of 45 with FCDTC have Stage I disease unless they have evidence of distant metastases, which makes them Stage II. More advanced stages are restricted to patients over the age of 45, with locally invasive tumors (Stage IVA or IVB), or with evidence of nodal (Stage III or IVA) or distant (Stage IVC) metastases.

The pTNM system is the most widely accepted tool to describe the extent of disease for staging in thyroid carcinoma, and this and its associated AJCC staging scheme, are recommended for general use by the American Thyroid Association (ATA), American Association of Clinical Endocrinologists (AACE), and the National Comprehensive Cancer Network (NCCN). The AJCC stage correlates well with outcome of FCDTC, in both retrospective[220,221] and prospectively collected data,[192] with Stage I and II disease exhibiting a less than 1% overall mortality at 5 years. In contrast, more advanced stages of disease, limited to those patients over the age of 45 with locally invasive or metastatic disease, carries a less favorable prognosis, with Stage IVC (metastatic) disease exhibiting a 5-year mortality in excess of 50% in both PTC and FTC.[222]

Despite its simplicity and utility, however, the AJCC Stage does not provide all the information a clinician may need to classify a patient with DTC adequately, and to assist in making therapeutic decisions. It does not take account of several additional prognostic variables and may, therefore, risk misclassification of some patients.

Clinicopathological Prognostic Schemes for Follicular Cell Derived Thyroid Carcinoma. Among patients with FCDTC, age at initial treatment, tumor size, the presence of extrathyroidal invasion, and the presence of distant metastases at diagnosis are the most important risk factors for recurrence and for cause-specific mortality.[223] All of these are included in the AJCC Staging system detailed above. However, unlike almost any other cancer type, the presence of lymph node metastases in PTC has little influence on cause-specific mortality from this disease although it increases significantly the risk of locoregional recurrence.[224,225]

Several other factors, not included in the AJCC staging scheme, have also been shown to be prognostic variables, in multivariate analysis. These include tumor grade in PTC; extent of microinvasion of capsule or of blood vessels in FTC; DNA aneuploidy in HCC and PTC; delay to initial surgical intervention; and completeness of surgical resection of the primary tumor.[226] These prognostic factors are not of equal importance in predicting mortality or recurrence, with the most predictive factors generally being regarded as the presence of distant metastases, the age of the patient, and the extent of the tumor.

Several prognostic systems have been developed, that include a number of these variables, weighted according to their importance in predicting outcomes, in multivariate analyses, of retrospectively analyzed large cohorts of patients.

All of these schemes permit classification of patients with FCDTC (particularly PTC, the most common type) into low-, medium-, and high-risk groups, accurately predicting long-term outcome for these patients. The use of one or other of these schemes is recommended by the ATA to assist in predicting outcome and deciding initial and long-term management of the disease.[175]

Each of the prognostic schemes includes a slightly different group of variables, weighted in slightly different ways. However, all have certain features in common, and all include both tumor and patient variables, emphasizing the likely importance of host–tumor interaction in the behavior of this group of cancers. Almost all of the schemes accept the importance of the patient's age as an important (probably the most important) variable predicting outcome. The size of the primary tumor, its histologic type, the presence of extrathyroidal invasion, and the presence of distant metastases are almost universally included. Hay and colleagues[223] also found the completeness of the achieved surgical resection to be an important independently predictive variable, of both recurrence and cause-specific mortality.

At the Mayo Clinic we use the _m_etastases, _a_ge, _c_ompleteness of surgical excision, local _i_nvasion and tumor _s_ize (MACIS) score, which is named for its predictive variables.[223] This numeric score can be calculated using the formula detailed in Table 10. The MACIS equation generates a single score for patient classification, which has proven to be a reliable predictor of outcome over a 20-year period in these patients.

A MACIS score of <6.0, representing the lowest risk group, carries a less than 1% cause-specific 20-year mortality risk from PTC and encompasses more than 80% of patients presenting with PTC to our institution. A score of between 6.0 and 6.9 has an 11% 20-year mortality; scores of between 7.0 and 7.9 have a mortality rate of 44%; and scores of 8.0 and over (fortunately, a rare occurrence, affecting less than 5% of this group of patients) have a predicted mortality of 76% at 20 years.

Many of the other clinicopathologic prognostic schemes provide a similar rapid, accurate assessment of a patient's risk group category. While the choice of prognostic scheme remains a matter more of preference than of science, we and others commend the use of one or another of the schemes in addition to the AJCC/UICC classification. Classification allows accurate identification of the majority (80 to 85%) of patients with FCDTC at low risk of mortality. These patients can be reassured and managed with less inten-

sive intervention. More intensive follow-up and perhaps more aggressive adjuvant therapy can be targeted to the higher-risk patients, the small minority who are most likely to benefit from a more aggressive management strategy.

Predicting Disease Recurrence. As outlined above, recurrence of FCDTC is considerably more likely than death. Recurrences carry significant physical and psychological morbidity and increase the likelihood of subsequent mortality.[227,228] Recurrences are largely predictable and follow the patterns of spread seen at the time of diagnosis. These vary with histotype, with PTC exhibiting early spread to and frequent recurrence in regional lymph nodes, and less frequently distant spread, principally to the lungs and later to skeleton.[217] The Hürthle cell variant of FTC follows a similar pattern although perhaps more frequently exhibiting distant metastases.[229] Typical nonoxyphilic FTC, however, less often involves lymph nodes, spreading preferentially by a hematogenous route to lungs, bones and brain.[229] Metastatic spread to other organs also occurs although all of these are rare.

Local recurrence within the thyroid bed occurs mainly ipsilateral to the primary tumor site, as a result of incomplete surgical resection, local invasiveness of the primary tumor, or failure of adjunctive therapy to destroy persistent microscopic tumor deposits. Local recurrence at sites other than the thyroid bed may result from unrecognized local spread of the tumor outside the thyroid remnant or multifocal tumor that has been incompletely resected.[202]

Regional recurrence occurs more frequently in lymph nodes in the central compartment, often as a result of incomplete initial surgical exploration and resection. These nodes are involved in up to 40 to 60% of patients with PTC at the time of diagnosis,[217] and adequate primary surgery should include their resection through a formal sixth compartment node dissection.[175] Jugular nodes may also commonly be the site of regional recurrence, presumably as a result of unrecognized micrometastases, present at the time of the original diagnosis. Adequate assessment of the jugular chain nodes is essential prior to primary surgery, using ultrasound.[175]

The development of distant metastases, fortunately, is rare in FCDTC but heralds a poor prognosis for older patients, with cause-specific mortality rates of up to 60% at 10 years in Stage IV disease.[202] By contrast, the presence of distant metastases, particularly micrometastases in the lungs, in young patients need not signal an imminent demise, with long-term survivorship

being the norm,[230] justifying their classification as Stage II disease.

The risk factors for the development of distant metastatic disease in PTC largely mirror those already established for mortality, with the age of the patient, the size of the tumor, and the presence of local invasion or incomplete surgical resection dominating the picture. In addition, however, the involvement of lymph nodes with PTC, particularly those in the jugular chains, at the time of diagnosis, substantially increases the risk of future regional recurrences, but its role in the development of distant spread remains controversial.[231] For FTC, the presence of angioinvasion of the primary tumor, and possibly of extensive capsular invasiveness, substantially increase the subsequent risk of developing distant metastases.[232,233]

Postoperative Adjuvant Therapy. Two major forms of adjuvant therapy are commonly used following surgical treatment of FCDTC: radioactive iodine and thyroid hormone suppression of TSH.[202] Unfortunately, the widespread availability of radioactive iodine (in the form of I-131), its ease of use, and perhaps misconceptions regarding its efficacy have resulted occasionally in complacency regarding the initial surgical treatment of these tumors, on the basis that "radioactive iodine will get whatever we miss." We believe that the importance of the primary surgical procedure cannot be overstated, and that the long-term outcome for the patient depends largely on the adequacy of that procedure, particularly for patients at higher-than-average risk of death or recurrence.

No such systemic modalities of treatment are currently available to reduce the risk of recurrence in the postoperative management of MTC, the treatment of which initially lies entirely in the hands of the surgeon. The adequacy of the primary surgical resection, including accurate, effective lymph node sampling, is therefore even more important in this form of DTC. Patients with MTC who undergo thyroidectomy will, of course, require thyroid hormone replacement therapy.

Thyroid Hormone. The suppression of TSH by administration of supraphysiologic doses of thyroid hormone in the postoperative thyroid cancer patient, is probably the most widely used adjuvant therapy for FCDTC.[202] In use for nearly half a century, this treatment is based on the belief that suppression of TSH removes an essential growth factor for cells of thyroid follicular origin, so slowing or preventing altogether the re-growth of the cancer.[201]

Without doubt, many thyroid cancer cell lines of both rat[179] and human[234] origin grow more rapidly in media supplemented with TSH, and are growth inhibited when the growth medium is stripped of TSH, and other probably growth factors, by charcoal stripping. There is also anecdotal evidence that at least a proportion of thyroid nodules, eventually proven to be malignant, can shrink somewhat during thyroid hormone suppressive therapy.[235] However, firm evidence that

Table 10 Prognostic Factors in Thyroid Cancer: Metastasis, Age, Completeness of Resection, Invasion, and Size (MACIS) Score Calculation

Score 3.1 (if Age < 40 Yr) or 0.08 × Age (if age = 40 yr)	Percent Survival for 20 Yr by MACIS Score
+0.3 × tumor size (cm maximum diameter)	<6 = 99%
+1 (if completely resected)	6–6.99 = 89%
+1 (if locally invasive)	7–7.99 = 56%
+3 (if distant spread)	>8.00 = 24%

TSH-suppressive therapy is truly effective in the postoperative management of DTC is hard to obtain, in the absence of any randomized prospective trials.

Initially, the goal of TSH suppression therapy was to attain an absent response to intravenous TRH administration, assessed on a first-generation TSH radioimmunoassay, consistent with essentially complete suppression of the pituitary thyrotrope.[236] With the development of more sensitive TSH assays in the 1980s, it became possible simply to maintain an undetectable TSH, measured using a sensitive (second-generation) immunometric TSH assay,[237] with a lower limit of detection of around 0.1 mU/L. Over the last decade, since the advent of "ultra-sensitive" TSH assays (third and fourth generation), with lower limits of detection of 0.01 mU/L, 0.001 mU/L, or less, it has become possible to titrate the dose of thyroid hormone in the majority of patients to achieve levels of TSH within prespecified ranges.[238] Unfortunately, a paucity of data makes decision-making about the "desirable range" for TSH largely speculative at the present time.

The changes in our ability to measure TSH concentrations over the last quarter century, as well as changes in the surgical and other nonsurgical practices over the same time period, complicate our interpretation of the retrospective data that forms the basis of our current understanding of DTC management. The majority of patients treated for DTC in the last quarter century have undergone surgery extensive enough that thyroid hormone replacement was necessary to avoid hypothyroidism. Comparisons in long-term retrospective studies between patients treated with thyroid hormone and those not treated, therefore, become comparisons between patients operated on in the middle years of the last century by what would now be regarded by most as inadequate surgery, with those treated by more extensive surgery in the last few decades, who also have received thyroid hormone replacement or suppression.

Not surprisingly, therefore, univariate analyses of thyroxine therapy show decreases in cancer-related deaths,[239,240] and a decreased recurrence rate of both PTC and FTC.[241,242] This effect may be confined to older patients,[243] who are likely to represent more advanced stage disease, and the apparent beneficial effect is reduced or even eliminated when patients with PTC are stratified according to their tumor stage.[244,245] However, a recent retrospective, multicenter study of 683 patients, stratified by NTCTCS stage, who had been treated and followed at 14 institutions over a 10-year period, did show a significantly reduced risk of disease progression (defined as cause-specific mortality or recurrence) in Stage III and IV patients with FCDTC, treated with suppressive doses of thyroid hormone. No such difference in outcome was observed in Stage I and II patients.[246]

The use of supraphysiological doses of thyroid hormone may, however, carry some risk of adverse consequences. A small proportion of patients experience hyperthyroid symptoms of tremor, anxiety, sleep disturbance, heat intolerance, and palpitations which can be intolerable and can sometimes require reductions in thyroid hormone dosage.

More worrying is the possible impact of TSH suppression on bone turnover,[247] especially in postmenopausal women, with an increased risk of osteoporosis in older women treated with suppressive doses of thyroid hormone.[248] The danger of this is probably negligible in premenopausal women although it remains unclear whether estrogen replacement after menopause is equally protective. The possible impact of TSH suppression on bone health in men remains unknown.[249]

A suppressed TSH is also a risk factor for the development of atrial fibrillation (AF), with its consequent increased risk of cerebrovascular events. It has been estimated that such a finding increases the odds ratio for the development of AF by three fold over baseline.[250] This finding was based on prospectively collected data from the Framingham cohort and did not distinguish between endogenous and exogenous sources of thyroid hormone as the cause of the suppressed TSH. Since T3 is the active hormone at the cardiac level, and since T3 concentrations are somewhat lower for any given concentration of TSH when exogenous thyroxine is the source of thyroid hormone excess, the actual risk may be somewhat lower than indicated from the Framingham data. Nevertheless, the potential for significant morbidity exists and may not be balanced by an improvement in outcome of the FCDTC, at least for Stage I and II patients.

Our approach to the use of thyroid hormone suppression of TSH in patients with FCDTC, is in keeping with the recent guidelines of both the AACE[251] and ATA.[175] These suggest a stratified approach, according to both AJCC stage and patient risk as assessed by one of the clinicopathological prognostic schemes. In patients at low risk (MACIS score less than 6.0, or AJCC Stage 1 PTC), whose life expectancy is essentially normal and whose lifetime risk of recurrence is less than 5%,[223] we aim to maintain the serum TSH at or just below the lower limit of the normal range (0.1 to 0.3 mU/L in our laboratory, whose normal range is 0.3 to 5.0 mU/L). Since the risk of tumor recurrence in these low-risk patients falls to less than 1% in the 20 years beyond the first 5 postoperative years, we would subsequently permit the TSH to rise into the lower third of the normal range. This strategy avoids the potential morbidity associated with long-term TSH suppression. Life-long monitoring of thyroid hormone status, by annual measurement of serum TSH concentration, is recommended.

Patients at intermediate risk of tumor recurrence include those patients with PTC whose MACIS score lies between 6.0 and 6.9, AJCC Stages I and II, or Stage III with only lymph node metastases and patients with minimally invasive FTC. These groups almost certainly warrant rather more aggressive management than the low-risk patients, and we aim to maintain the TSH in the subnormal range, without achieving frank hyperthyroidism. Our goal in this setting is a TSH concentration below 0.1 mU/L and ideally in the range between 0.05 and 0.1 mU/L.

Attempts to maintain virtually complete TSH suppression (TSH <0.05 mU/L) are reserved for high-risk patients, including those with widely invasive FTC or HCC, or PTC with MACIS scores over 7.0, Stage IV disease or Stage III disease with local extrathyroidal invasion. These patients may experience hyperthyroid symptoms when TSH suppression is achieved although this may prove to be transient. The potential for morbidity must be recognized, and these patients warrant screening and monitoring of bone density, at least in postmenopausal women, with appropriate prophylactic and therapeutic management of this bone disease.[248]

Radioactive Iodine Therapy. The majority (75% or more) of FCDTC retain the capacity to take up and significantly concentrate iodine although frequently rather less efficiently than normal thyroid tissue.[202] This residual differentiated function permits radioactive isotopes of iodine to be used for both the detection and treatment of residual thyroid follicular cells.

Administered orally, iodine isotopes are absorbed rapidly and reliably from the upper gastrointestinal tract, circulate transiently in the blood stream, and are concentrated in tissues that express a functional sodium-iodide transporter (NIS).[252] These include normal and cancerous thyroid tissue, salivary gland, breast, stomach, and colon.[252,253] The NIS is also expressed in the kidney which transports as well as filters iodine,[254] and circulating iodine is excreted rapidly through the urine and stool.[255] The uptake of iodine into both normal and cancerous thyroid tissue is dependent on TSH, the result of upregulation of expression and possibly increased function of NIS.[256]

Radioactive isotopes of iodine (I-131, I-123) emit γ rays,[257] which can be detected using an appropriate detection apparatus (a gamma-camera), thus permitting imaging of iodine concentrating tissues, and thereby the detection of residual or metastatic thyroid tissue, provided there has been sufficient prior stimulation with TSH. This technique of whole body scanning, following TSH stimulation resulting from the induction of hypothyroidism, has become the mainstay of postoperative surveillance in North America[195] and will be discussed later.

Although γ rays are of high energy, their tissue absorption is low, and the majority of these particles fail to interact with the cell in which the iodine is concentrated or with surrounding tissue.[257] While this is ideal for imaging purposes, treatment of residual thyroid carcinoma with radioactive iodine depends on β particle emission, the major emitted particle released by the decay of I-131.[257] These moderately high-energy β particles travel only short distances, on average around 0.5 cm before interacting with surrounding tissue, and result in ionization and the generation of superoxide radicals, which cause DNA damage, including double-strand DNA breaks.[258] This activates the p53 pathway (commonly intact in differentiated thyroid carcinoma) and leads to apoptosis of the affected cell.[259] Since cancer cells often lack efficient mechanisms to repair double-strand DNA breaks,[260] there is theoretical reason to believe that residual thyroid cancer cells might be more susceptible to the effects of β irradiation than the surrounding normal tissue although no in vitro or clinical evidence yet exists to support this.

Radioiodine Remnant Ablation. Postoperative ablation of the thyroid remnant by treatment with 30 to 100 mCi of I-131 is often used to "complete" the initial surgical treatment in FCDTC.[261] Defined as "the destruction of residual, macroscopically normal thyroid tissue following thyroidectomy," there remains controversy about the optimal dose required to achieve this. Most North American centers use between 30 and 75 mCi, values which have some theoretical and experimental support.[262–264]

Most often, radioactive iodine is administered 4 to 6 weeks after surgery, with the patient in a hypothyroid state, to maximize TSH-stimulated iodine uptake, and whole-body iodine retention.[265] Some authorities advocate a low-iodine diet during preparation for I-131 treatment and scanning,[266,267] although there remains skepticism regarding its efficacy. Hypothyroidism may be achieved by avoiding thyroid hormone replacement therapy postoperatively and waiting for at least 4 weeks for endogenous hormone concentrations to fall. Alternatively, initial substitution for 4 weeks with T3 (Cytomel), followed by 2 weeks of withdrawal can be used, and may shorten the duration of symptomatic hypothyroidism. Oral I-131 administration, most often in an outpatient setting, follows confirmation of a serum TSH elevated to at least 30 mIU/L, and a negative serum pregnancy test in women of childbearing potential.

There is little doubt that even quite substantial remnants of normal thyroid tissue can be eliminated by this approach.[264] Whether small amounts of residual thyroid carcinoma are also eliminated by these remnant ablative doses is uncertain, since carcinoma cells may be several orders of magnitude less efficient than normal follicular cells in the accumulation of iodine.[231] Many groups regard remnant ablation as a necessary first step before proceeding, at a later date, to higher-dose treatment of known residual (or recurrent) disease.

Elimination of the postsurgical remnant may carry two theoretical advantages. First, it may destroy residual normal thyroid tissue, making subsequent neck and whole-body scans easier to interpret, since areas of more subtle uptake, for example, in metastatic tumor within regional lymph nodes, might otherwise be overshadowed. Second, it may simplify interpretation of serum thyroglobulin (Tg) concentrations, since residual normal thyroid tissue will otherwise contribute, to some degree, to the production of Tg,[195] particularly in the stimulated state, that is, with elevated TSH.

Does remnant ablation with I-131 improve the outcomes for patients with thyroid carcinoma?

Unfortunately, few data are extant with which to address this vexing question, and this "absence of data fuels strongly held opinions on both sides of the debate."[268] No randomized trials have been reported of radioactive iodine therapy; and, to our knowledge, none are in progress. Our understanding of the risks and benefits of this widely used therapeutic approach is based entirely on observational, retrospectively analyzed, nonrandomized studies.

In low-risk patients, with small intrathyroidal papillary tumors (pT1-2, stage I disease), I-131 ablation yields no detectable benefit either on cause-specific survival, or on the risk of recurrent disease, provided the primary surgery is adequate.[196,269] Even in those patients with regional nodal involvement, I-131 does not further improve the already low risk of either death or recurrence in these otherwise low-risk patients.[241,270,271] It is, of course, extremely difficult for any adjunctive therapy to improve on survival rates that approach 100% and even more difficult to prove any such benefit, in view of the low overall risk of recurrence and the long (essentially normal) life-expectancy of this group of patients.

The possible benefit of such ablation in higher risk patients, without evidence of residual disease, continues to stimulate heated debate in national and international meetings and in numerous publications. These arguments are largely fueled by apparently contradictory data from a few major centers. On the one hand are data from Mazzaferri's group, showing that 30-year recurrence rates, in patients with tumors larger than 1.5 cm, were halved (from 38 to 16%) in the 350 patients who received ablation with I-131, compared to the 802 who did not.[239] Similarly, cause-specific 30-year mortality rates fell from 8 to 3%, with no deaths observed in patients who received I-131 in whom there was no evidence of residual disease. This view is shared by DeGroot[272] and by the MD Anderson Cancer Center group.[273]

On the other hand are data from our institution, reported by Hay and colleagues,[202,274] which have failed to show any significant benefit of "routine" I-131 ablation in patients with adequate primary surgery, including selective node dissection, in whom no evidence of residual disease was detected. Analysis of a total of 1,542 patients with PTC, treated at the Mayo Clinic, of similar stage to those reported by Mazzaferri and colleagues, showed recurrence rates (16.6% vs 19.1%; *p* = .89) and mortality rates (5.9% vs 7.8%; *p* = .43) that were no different with or without I-131 remnant ablation.[202] These data have recently received support from a large, prospectively collected data-set, in which patients with tumors up to 4 cm, including both local invasion and cervical nodal involvement, though without distant metastatic spread, showed no evidence of benefit from I-131 remnant ablation. Indeed, the authors concluded that remnant ablation provided no benefit "and may actually be harmful" to these low risk patients.[271]

The recurrence rates reported in this Mayo Clinic study, and in others from the now over

2,000 patients accumulated by Hay and his colleagues,[274] are considerably lower than those reported from several other institutions, even in the absence of routine I-131 ablation. This almost certainly reflects the completeness of surgical excision of the primary tumor, achieved in this highly specialized surgical center, and emphasizes the importance of the primary surgery in determining outcome. It should be noted, however, that the surgical procedure of choice here remains a *near*-total thyroidectomy, and that these low rates of recurrent disease and mortality have been achieved while maintaining low rates of permanent hypoparathyroidism and recurrent laryngeal nerve injury (2% and 1%, respectively, for near-total thyroidectomy).[275]

It may be that I-131 ablation has proven useful in other studies because of the presence of unrecognized residual disease, almost certainly within regional lymph nodes, the site of the majority of recurrences in several studies.[202] With adequate preoperative assessment (using ultrasound), and careful intraoperative exploration of these affected nodes, the rate of later recurrence can almost certainly be reduced substantially. The ATA cancer management guidelines, published in 2006, support the *selective* use of I-131 ablation in low-risk patients with PTC.[175]

Although long-term data suggest that ablative doses of I-131 are safe and are not associated with significant side effects or carcinogenic risk,[202,276] the financial cost and inconvenience to the patient may outweigh any potential benefit, at least in low-risk patients, who have undergone adequate primary surgery. This group represents over 80% of patients with PTC at our institution,[277] and consequently, we strongly favor highly selective use of I-131 remnant ablation as adjunctive therapy following adequate primary surgery. Rather, we reserve its use for those patients at moderate or high-risk of tumor recurrence (based on postoperative risk assessment), who will require follow-up by isotope scans and stimulated Tg concentrations and who may need treatment for residual or recurrent disease. Since FTC, and particularly its Hürthle-cell variant, appears to carry somewhat higher risks for recurrent and metastatic disease than PTC, we favor the use of I-131 ablation and treatment in the majority of these patients.

Radioiodine Therapy for Local Residual Disease. In contrast to the controversies surrounding routine remnant ablation, outlined above, there is widespread agreement that treatment with I-131 can be effective for the elimination or control of residual disease in some patients. Approximately 75 to 85% of FCDTCs concentrate iodine appreciably when sufficiently stimulated by TSH, and adequate doses of orally administered I-131 can induce apoptosis in these cells and in surrounding tissue in a radius of up to 2 mm.[278]

Microscopic residual disease is likely to remain after resection of locally invasive (pT4) tumors, even if adequate clearance of gross residual disease is achieved surgically. This may be detected histologically, as tumor presence at the surgical margin at the time of the initial resection, even in some tumors initially thought to be contained within the thyroid. Such microscopic disease substantially increases the risk of true PTC thyroid-bed recurrence and of cause-specific mortality at least in older (Stage III) patients.[279] Similarly, invasive Hürthle-cell variant of FTC is more likely to recur within the thyroid bed and can prove difficult or impossible to eradicate.[280]

Both local recurrence and 20-year cause-specific survival rates in patients with microscopic residual disease were improved by either I-131 and/or external beam irradiation, in a multicenter review from North America.[244] Traditionally, treatment of residual disease is a two-step process, with a relatively low dose (30 to 75 mCi) administered for ablation, and a higher treatment dose (100 to 200 mCi) given, at a later date, for treatment. There is no empirical evidence that this approach is superior to administration of therapeutic doses on the first occasion, and this is now often the preferred approach for high-risk patients. It does have the drawback, however, that a significant thyroid remnant may overshadow the presence of subtler uptake in extrathyroidal tissues and mask the presence of residual disease on the posttherapy scan.

A few patients present with locally advanced disease, which makes complete surgical resection difficult or impossible, and a small number of these patients have gross residual disease in the neck despite an optimal surgical procedure.[223] We advocate an aggressive primary surgical approach for these patients, including partial resection of trachea or esophagus, if necessary, to achieve local control.[202] When this is not possible, the presence of gross residual disease is an independent risk factor for both recurrence and cause-specific mortality.[223]

Radioactive iodine provides a therapeutic option in this setting, and divided doses of up to 500 mCi may be necessary in an attempt to achieve local control. Some groups advocate even higher total doses of I-131, guided by dosimetry studies, to achieve the maximum dose possible, to a point just short of bone marrow toxicity.[281] Consequences of high-dose I-131 therapy include significant lifelong xerostomia, dysphagia, bone marrow suppression, and increasingly realistic risks of secondary malignancy, including leukemia, lymphoma, transitional cell bladder carcinoma, and colon carcinoma[282] (Table 11).

Unfortunately, dosimetry is fraught with a number of significant problems, making it prone to substantial error in predicting the radiation dose received by tumor tissue in response to a dose of I-131.[283] The estimated volume of the residual or recurrent tumor to be treated is, at best, only an approximation. The uptake of iodine may vary from one area of residual tumor to another and, indeed, may be heterogeneous within a single focus of recurrence. Additionally, the effective half-life of I-131 may vary substantially between patients, and even within a single patient, between the tracer and the therapeutic dose. And finally, the use of a prior tracer dose of I-131, necessary to calculate dosimetry, may result in "stunning" of the tumor tissue,[284] and decrease the uptake of a subsequent therapeutic dose.[285] Nevertheless, dosimetry remains a controversial tool in the administration of therapeutic I-131 and is used only by a minority of endocrinologists and nuclear medicine specialists.

Recurrent FCDTC, even in the presence of gross residual disease, is often slow-growing, may be alternatively treated (in rare selected cases) by external beam irradiation, and may be amenable to local control by intermittent repeat surgical neck exploration.[202,286] High-dose I-131 therapy is of unproven efficacy, beyond that of more standard doses (<500 mCi), and has significant associated morbidity; and dosimetry may be unreliable, as noted above. We prefer, therefore, to pursue alternative approaches once total doses of administered I-131 exceed approximately 500 to 800 mCi.

Radioiodine Therapy for Metastatic Disease. As outlined above, metastatic FCDTC may concentrate iodine in up to 80% of cases, and TSH can stimulate this uptake. Treatment with I-131 is, therefore, used widely to treat distant metastases, whether they are present at the time of the original diagnosis or appear at a later time.

In the treatment of microscopic pulmonary metastases, I-131 appears effectively to minimize further growth, and possibly induce regression, at least in children and young adults.[230] This approach may lower the serum Tg concentration and reduce or eliminate iodine trapping although the chest X-ray may never return entirely to normal and later recurrences remain a possibility.[287] Whether I-131 improves survival in these cases remains unproven but seems likely, and certainly long-term survival is expected in younger patients with PTC, treated with adequate surgery and I-131, even when presenting with pulmonary metastatic disease.[288]

There are also numerous anecdotal reports and case series showing significant shrinkage of pulmonary and other distant metastases in older patients after effective I-131 treatment.[261] Once again, however, there are no prospective data showing an improvement in survival with this treatment. Larger metastases (over ~1 cm in maximum diameter) appear to be significantly less responsive to I-131, perhaps because of the limited tissue penetration of the emitted beta-particles.[289] Hypoxia within these larger tumor masses also induces relative radioresistance, possibly by limiting the production of superoxide radicals, so reducing the impact of radioactivity on tissue injury.[290]

Initial enlargement of treated metastases occurs commonly in response to the trophic effect of the elevation of TSH necessary to induce iodine trapping and due to the edema that occurs in response to effective tumor tissue injury.[290] Such enlargement can cause significant problems from a space-occupying effect, particularly in critical locations such as within the central nervous system and close to the spinal cord.[291] Prophylactic corticosteroid administration may be helpful, and the use of exogenously administered recombinant human TSH (rhTSH) (rather than thyroid hormone withdrawal) has been suggested as an alternative approach to stimulate iodine uptake, while avoiding the growth stimulation of more prolonged elevations in TSH concentrations.[292]

It should also be noted that the whole body retention of iodine is lower after the use of rhTSH than after thyroid hormone withdrawal, however, since hypothyroidism decreases renal I-131 clearance, increasing its effective biological half-life. This effect does not occur with rhTSH; and, therefore, more attention to dosimetry may be necessary when treating after rhTSH use.[293] The efficacy of I-131 therapy after rhTSH stimulation has not been evaluated, and it currently represents an unlicensed use of this product, except for compassionate use in selected patients.

Alternative therapeutic modalities, including surgery and localized external beam irradiation, may also play a role in the management of metastases from FCDTC, and I-131 should be viewed as merely one component of a multimodal therapeutic approach.

There is no role for the use of radioactive iodine in the treatment of medullary thyroid carcinoma, since these tumors do not express NIS and are incapable of iodine accumulation. Rare mixed FTC/MTC tumors may concentrate I-131, although it is not known whether such treatment alters the long-term outcome.[294]

External Beam Irradiation as Adjunctive Therapy for Follicular Cell-Derived Thyroid Carcinoma. The use of external beam irradiation for thyroid cancer is an unresolved management issue, and the current available information is not high-level data. Several retrospective studies report benefit for patients with differentiated thyroid cancer who receive external beam irradiation.[295–298]

Patient selection has in general included pT4 lesions, gross residual disease, microscopic residual disease, or advanced neck disease. Factors that limit firm comparisons and conclusions include: small numbers of patients treated, variable dosage and delivery techniques, and quality of detection methods to establish local and regional recurrence. Regardless, the identified benefit is limited to improved local regional control in papillary thyroid cancer (no benefit has been identified for follicular thyroid carcinoma). Unfortunately, neither overall survival nor cause specific survival is improved. The decision-making must balance the benefit of local regional

Table 11 Reported Complications of High-Dose Therapy with I-131	
Salivary glands	Xerostomia
Lung	Pneumonitis
	Pulmonary fibrosis
Bone marrow	Bone marrow suppression/aplasia
	Leukemia
Bladder	Transitional cell carcinoma of bladder

control and the morbidity of irradiation. The general side effects of external beam irradiation include xerostomia, skin and soft tissue fibrosis, and telangiectasia formation. Irradiation of the larynx will generate variable degrees of edema and risk of chondritis.

Chondroradionecrosis, fortunately rare, is a challenging problem that may respond to corticosteroids, antibiotics, and hyperbaric oxygen therapy but can relentlessly progress and require laryngopharyngectomy.

Consistently, the most important factor in local and regional control is the completeness of resection (no residual disease vs microscopic residual disease vs gross residual disease). Conservation surgery of the larynx, trachea, pharynx, and esophagus is complex but can address invasive disease while preserving voice, swallowing, and avoidance of a tracheostomy.[299,300] Rarely does one need to consider a laryngopharyngectomy. The impact radiation therapy has on wound healing significantly increases the risk of wound breakdown, specifically in areas in direct contact with saliva (pharynx and esophagus) or in tissues composed largely of cartilage (larynx, subglottis, and trachea). Segmental tracheal resection in the setting of prior surgery and irradiation likely should not be considered. Therefore, prior to the administration of external beam irradiation, it should be determined that further surgery is not an option. Once it is determined that surgery is not an option (based risk or patient preference), the potential for retreatment with radioactive iodine should be established. Noniodine-avid disease with evidence of progression warrants consideration of external beam irradiation. It is not clear that all patients with residual disease warrant treatment with external beam irradiation. The clinical behavior (growth rate, invasive characteristics) of the tumor and the age of the patient should be considered.

Postoperative Surveillance and Follow-Up. After apparently successful initial therapy, recurrence rates range from 10 to 35% in most series of FCDTC, with rather higher rates observed in MTC, as detailed above. Although the majority of such recurrences occur within the first 5 to 10 postoperative years,[288] recurrences have been reported as long as 25 years after apparently successful primary treatment.[301] Long-term follow-up for these tumors is therefore necessary. Many of the recurrences are easily amenable to treatment, particularly if detected early, before vital structures are compromised,[217] and some form of sensitive surveillance is therefore desirable to detect such recurrences before they become clinically apparent.

The vast majority of patients with PTC, however, are at low-risk of recurrence, and these patients are even less likely to succumb to their disease. Follow-up surveillance must therefore involve negligible risk, minimal morbidity or discomfort, and must be financially responsible. We believe that such follow-up should be tailored to the patients' level of risk, with high-risk patients being offered more intensive assess-

ment, directed to the likely sites of recurrence, while low-risk patients should be reassured and offered much less intensive (and less expensive) follow-up. The clinical staging and risk assessment schemes detailed above provide a logical and accurate basis for determining an appropriate follow-up strategy.

Anatomic Evaluation. The majority of recurrences of FCDTC and MTC occur in regional lymph nodes in the neck or thyroid bed. Ultrasound examination, using modern high-resolution 10 MHz transducers, permits accurate anatomical evaluation of the postoperative neck, and should be the imaging modality of choice for postoperative surveillance for locoregional recurrence.[217] Tumor deposits as small as 2 mm can be detected within the thyroid bed, and tumor deposits of a similar size within lymph nodes may also be reliably detected. Recurrent PTC, in particular, may exhibit ultrasonographic features that are highly characteristic, with intralesional calcifications that result in multiple tiny bright echos within the tumor deposit.[205] Lymph node architecture is also a highly sensitive marker of nodal metastases, which result in enlargement, rounding, and loss of the normally visible, hyperechoic hilar structures. Ultrasound has a major added advantage over other imaging modalities, in that ultrasound-guided FNA can be undertaken reliably, providing cytologic confirmation of the presence of metastatic cancer.[302] The only limitation of this technique is the need for a skilled and dedicated thyroid ultrasonographer since the technique is highly operator dependant. Nevertheless, in our experience, ultrasound is by far the most sensitive and specific method of surveillance of the postoperative neck, permitting detection of small tumor deposits at a stage well before other currently available, more expensive, anatomical imaging methods. The technique is more sensitive than the more widely used radioactive iodine scanning and is better for the detection of thyroid bed and neck nodal recurrences, the site of the majority of recurrences in DTC of all types.

MRI and CT scanning are also widely used to assess the postoperative neck. CT scanning is usually performed without contrast, since the iodine loading from the contrast material otherwise obviates the subsequent use of radioactive iodine therapy for at least 8–12 weeks, until the iodine load can be cleared.[302] While either of these techniques can be used to detect recurrences in the neck, their resolution is less good than ultrasound, in part because thyroid carcinoma exhibits similar spin-decay kinetics and similar X-ray density to other soft-tissue structures in the neck. The minimum detectable size of recurrent tumor deposits within the neck using these techniques is around 0.5 to 1.0 cm. These techniques are also substantially more expensive than ultrasound.

Spiral CT scanning (without contrast) may be useful to detect the pulmonary metastases that may occur rarely in DTC. However, although the lung and mediastinum represent the most frequent distant metastatic sites for DTC of all types, the majority of patients are at low-risk of this event,

and a chest X-ray may be sufficient on a routine basis, to exclude pulmonary metastases, in the majority of low-risk patients.[302] In higher-risk patients, radioactive iodine scanning may prove even more useful than CT scanning, since it also provides evidence regarding the possible future treatment of the detected disease with I-131.

Functional Evaluation Isotope Scanning. Functional scanning with radioactive iodine (I-131 or I^{123}) remains the most widespread, and often the only, postoperative surveillance undertaken in many centers. Although less efficient than normal thyroid, the majority of (~80%), but not all, FCDTCs retain the capacity to concentrate iodine and its isotopes.[303] Use of a gamma-camera permits visualization of the neck within 24 hours of ingestion of oral I-131 or I^{123}, while whole body scanning requires clearance of the physiologically accumulated gastrointestinal and renal iodine and, therefore, requires 48 to 72 hours between administration of the isotope and imaging. Positive imaging demonstrates functional thyroid tissue and implies that it may be amenable to destruction with the beta-emitter I-131. It must be noted again, however, that not all functional thyroid tissue is amenable to such treatment, whose efficacy depends on achieving an adequate intralesional dose of I-131, without inducing systemic toxicity.

Whole-body scanning is commonly performed using doses of 1 to 5 mCi I-131, although a variety of larger doses has also been used. Recently, several reports have demonstrated a "stunning" effect of doses above around 3 mCi, resulting in reduced uptake of subsequent I-131 doses,[284] thereby perhaps diminishing the potential efficacy of treatment with radioiodine following such a scan. The cause of this stunning effect remains in doubt, although it likely results from follicular cell injury, and might represent either reduced activity of NIS, increased iodide leak from the cell, or both. Consequently, we recommend the use of I-131 tracer doses of 3 mCi or less, for diagnostic whole-body scanning purposes. Alternatively, though more expensive, the use of I-123 for the scan appears to eliminate stunning, almost certainly a beta-particle effect, but it may not significantly improve the quality of whole-body imaging.[285]

Follicular cell iodide concentration is a TSH-dependent process, both in normal and malignant tissue. Preparation for scanning has traditionally required withdrawal of thyroid hormone therapy for several weeks, to allow high levels of endogenous TSH to develop, thus stimulating uptake. Serum TSH concentrations of over 30 mU/L are recommended for scanning and treatment purposes. During the withdrawal of thyroid hormone, which lasts 4 weeks or more, patients will develop hypothyroidism, with all its attendant morbidity, and efforts to mitigate against this, by conversion to T3 (Cytomel) prior to thyroid hormone withdrawal, are incompletely effective.[304] In addition, a small number of patients are unable to mount an adequate endogenous TSH response because of hypopituitarism or may be particularly sensitive to the effects of hypothyroidism because of various nonthyroidal illnesses.[305] Purified bovine TSH administered by injection was used in the past to stimulate I-131 uptake in these patients, for both scanning and treatment purposes.[306]

More recently, genetic engineering has permitted the large-scale production of recombinant human thyrotropin (rhTSH), and this is now approved for human diagnostic, but not therapeutic, use by the US Food and Drug Administration (FDA). Several large studies have now been completed comparing withdrawal scans with rhTSH-stimulated scans. Clearly, patients experience considerably fewer hypothyroid symptoms during rhTSH-stimulation, when compared to withdrawal scanning, and patients report higher quality of life scores during the days prior to the scan.[293] The use of rhTSH, which must be administered by intramuscular injection, is not entirely without side effects of its own, but these are relatively minor for most patients.[307]

The recommended dose of rhTSH is two injections on consecutive days, with the second injection administered 24 hours prior to ingestion of the iodine isotope.[308] This process requires some logistical organization, since the whole process of rhTSH administration followed by scanning, requires approximately 5 days to complete. While avoiding the symptoms of hypothyroidism that most patient find unpleasant, and some find intolerable, rhTSH fails to trigger urinary iodine retention; and the effective biological half-life of I-131 is therefore somewhat lower for rhTSH than for withdrawal scans. This results in rather lower whole-body iodide retention and so marginally poorer quality scans.[308] This may be compensated for by using higher tracer isotope doses (raising concerns about stunning) or by prolonging the acquisition time in "count-poor" scans, and under these circumstances the detection rate of metastatic disease approaches that of the withdrawal scan.[309] In carefully controlled, blinded studies of hormone withdrawal versus rhTSH-stimulated scans, a small number of "discordant" scans have been reported, with rather more areas of uptake missed following rhTSH-stimulation than after withdrawal scanning in the same patients.[308] The addition of stimulated Tg measurements to the scan itself improves the identification rate of patients with residual or recurrent disease to levels similar to withdrawal scanning.[309] It has been argued that few treatment decisions would be altered by this minimal difference in sensitivity, but the approach remains a trade-off of sensitivity for symptom minimization.

Except in a compassionate use setting, rhTSH is not currently approved for treatment with radioiodine, since the difference in renal iodide clearance may make such treatment less effective. Studies of the use of rhTSH for I-131 therapy are underway, however, and it has already been used in a small number of patients with hypopituitarism, who are unable to mount an endogenous TSH rise with conventional hormone withdrawal.[310]

The precise role for rhTSH-stimulated radioiodine scanning in the routine postoperative follow-up of patients with DTC remains unclear at this time. While the small difference in sensitivity may have minimal clinical impact, the inability to follow a positive scan immediately by administration of therapeutic radioiodine remains a significant hurdle to its widespread use. For high-risk patients, in whom therapy with I-131 is felt likely to be required, withdrawal scanning seems more appropriate, to allow treatment to follow immediately. In low-risk patients, isotope scanning is not typically advocated. Intermediate-risk patients who might best benefit from this new approach remain to be clearly defined. It has yet to be determined whether the additional cost and logistical complexity involved in reducing the hypothyroid symptoms for most of these patients is justifiable.

Other Functional Scans. A variety of other isotopic scanning approaches have been assessed in thyroid cancer detection. The most promising of these is positron emission tomography (PET) scanning which depends on the tumor metabolism of fluorodeoxyglucose tracer and provides a combination of functional and anatomical imaging.[311] The precise sensitivity and specificity of this technique for the detection of recurrent thyroid carcinoma continues to be assessed, but there is evidence that its main utiltiy is in the assessment of iodine-scan negative, thyroglobulin positive tumors, and more aggressive variants of the disease.[312]

Octreotide scanning, using isotope labeled octreotide and traditional gamma-camera imaging, will identify tumors expressing the appropriate receptor.[313] It may be a useful adjunctive method for the detection of residual and recurrent medullary thyroid carcinoma, and there are reports that FCDTC may sometimes express the somatostatin receptor.[314] At present, however, it has no role to play in the routine management of FCDTC, and this study is even more expensive than PET scanning.

Tumor Markers. Serum Tg is a highly specific product of the thyroid follicular cell and is detectable in the circulation of patients with residual normal or abnormal thyroid tissue.[199] In the athyreotic patient, following surgery, an elevated or rising Tg concentration is a highly specific and sensitive marker of recurrent FCDTC. Because Tg may be produced by residual normal thyroid tissue following surgery and even after I-131 thyroid remnant ablation, it should be recognized that a low stable level of Tg might not indicate residual disease.[286] Similarly, a few tumors, particularly those that are high grade and less well differentiated, may not produce large amounts of Tg, making a recurrence without elevated Tg a possibility.[315] Nevertheless, measurement of serum Tg is an invaluable component of a comprehensive surveillance program, allowing detection of early recurrent disease in the majority of such patients and identifying some patients who might benefit from more aggressive anatomical imaging.

Tg production and secretion into the circulation are TSH-dependent,[199] and Tg concentrations will increase following withdrawal of thyroxine therapy, or following stimulation with rhTSH.[307] However, the majority of patients with clinically significant recurrent disease will have a rise in Tg levels even when on suppressive thyroxine therapy, and it is not clear that TSH-stimulated Tg measurement is worthwhile in the majority of patients at low risk of recurrent disease. Radioactive iodine remnant ablation will lower basal and stimulated Tg concentrations by ablating a postsurgical thyroid remnant. However, this ablation is often incomplete, even with relatively high doses of I-131, and the Tg concentration may remain detectable even in this setting.[316] While we generally use a serum Tg concentration greater than 5 ng/mL (while on suppressive thyroxine therapy) as a trigger for further investigation, it is not uncommon for patients with Tg concentrations of 5 to 20 ng/mL to have no anatomic or functional evidence of disease and to have stable, nonprogressive Tg levels.

One potential drawback to the widespread use of this tumor marker is the temptation it provides, to treat a low-risk patient aggressively, in a misguided attempt to eliminate "every last molecule of thyroglobulin." There is no evidence that this is beneficial to such patients, either in terms of survival, or of later development of clinically relevant, recurrent disease.[286] A low detectable but stable serum Tg concentration may still be consistent with long-term recurrence-free survival in low-risk PTC. The measurement of serum Tg is complicated in as many as 20% of patients, by the presence of circulating anti-Tg antibodies, as a result of autoimmune thyroiditis.[199] Depending on the assay, these antibodies may artificially raise or lower the measured Tg concentration and complicate its interpretation. All assays should incorporate screening for anti-Tg antibodies, and their presence should lead to caution in interpretation of the result. Since autoantibody titers may wax and wane, even long-term trends in Tg concentrations may not reliably reflect the underlying growth of thyroid tissue in these patients.

To avoid this interference, there have been several recent attempts to substitute measurement of circulating messenger RNA for Tg (Tg-mRNA), rather than measuring the protein itself.[317–319] Tg-mRNA may circulate within "sloughed" thyroid cells, or as a "naked" mRNA molecule,[318] and can be detected using highly sensitive techniques of reverse transcription and polymerase chain reactions (RT–PCR). This technique can be qualitative, or quantitative. Although the latter is a more complex and costly undertaking, it is likely to prove preferable, since again, low levels of circulating Tg-mRNA may be analagous to low stable concentrations of Tg, and may not herald the presence of significant recurrent disease. Without doubt, RT–PCR permits extremely sensitive detection of circulating Tg-mRNA in patients with recurrent FCDTC. Whether it is predictive of recurrence and how it should be used in the postoperative surveillance of these patients, remain uncertain at this time. It may, however, in the future provide an alternative approach to Tg measurement, at least for patients who exhibit interfering anti-Tg antibodies.

Calcitonin, the normal product of thyroidal C cells, provides a similar highly sensitive and specific marker for postoperative monitoring in MTC.[320] Elevated concentrations are seen consistently in patients with nodal or metastatic recurrence, and a rising concentration over time predicts disease that may be progressing.[321] Antibodies do not represent a significant problem for this assay, which is both reliable and predictive. Once again, however, a significant proportion of patients may live for many years or even decades with elevated calcitonin concentrations derived from relatively stable and non or slowly progressive disease, most commonly within cervical lymph nodes.[322]

Carcinoembryonic antigen (CEA) also provides a sensitive, though rather less specific, marker for neuroendocrine tumor progression, including MTC.[277] The combination of a rising CEA and stable or falling calcitonin in a patient with known MTC may herald a de-differentiation of the tumor and predict more rapid progression and a fatal outcome.[323]

Combining the available postoperative therapeutic and surveillance options in an optimal and cost-effective manner, continues to challenge patient and physician alike and is the substrate for heated debate at every regional, national, and international endocrine meeting. As stated elsewhere in this chapter, the appropriate management of these patients must take certain fundamentals into account, recognizing the natural history of the disease and the wide range of malignant potential, which is largely predictable.

We use the tumor histology, clinical stage and MACIS prognostic score to place the patient into one of several risk groups. Adjunctive therapy with radioiodine remnant ablation, radioiodine therapy, and the TSH goals of suppressive thyroid hormone therapy are determined on the basis of the individual patient's risk, both of mortality and of recurrence of the disease. Similarly, the intensity of follow-up and the modalities of assessment are based both on the risk of recurrence and on the natural history of progression and spread of the disease. In the absence of prospective randomized clinical trials, this strategy strives to balance the risks of disease recurrence with the costs and morbidity of both treatment and follow-up, while avoiding both under- and overtreatment of individuals with this disease.

The majority of patients with PTC, who represent most patients in the United States with FCDTC, are at minimal risk of cancer-related mortality and at low risk of recurrence following adequate surgery. Adequate surgical treatment alone is curative in this majority, and adjunctive therapies can rarely be of additional benefit. Similarly, postoperative surveillance for this group of patients should be inexpensive, noninvasive, and carry negligible morbidity. Postoperative

therapy in these patients should consist of TSH suppression to the lower limit of normal but not necessarily below the normal range. In this group of patients with PTC, with MACIS scores less than 6, radioactive iodine remnant ablation or treatment has no routine role to play. Subsequent surveillance in this group of patients should take the form of careful neck examination by palpation and high-resolution ultrasound, serum Tg (measured while taking thyroid hormone), at 3 to 6 months postoperatively and at annual intervals for 3 to 5 years. Thereafter, annual clinical assessment and serum Tg measurement may be sufficient for this group, whose subsequent risk of developing recurrent disease is almost zero.

Intermediate-risk patients, representing older patients, those with FTC, and those with more extensive disease, require rather more aggressive management. Also in this group might be included those patients with extensive cervical nodal metastases, whose risk of mortality remains low but whose risk of regional recurrence within cervical lymph nodes is rather higher. In this smaller group of patients, we recommend thyroid remnant ablation with outpatient doses of I-131 (30 to 75 mCi), and thyroid hormone suppression to achieve TSH concentrations marginally below the normal range. Posttherapy surveillance also needs to be rather more aggressive and prolonged, with thyroid hormone withdrawal stimulated radioiodine whole-body scans at 6 to 12 weeks postoperatively (prior to remnant ablation), and on one or perhaps two annual return visits thereafter. This group of patients may be suitable candidates in the near future, for rhTSH stimulated isotope scans, after remnant ablation, to avoid the morbidity of annual thyroid hormone withdrawal. In addition, neck ultrasound at 3 to 6 months postoperatively and annually for at least 5 years is indicated, as well as annual chest X-ray, and measurements of serum Tg both on and off thyroid hormone therapy, at the times of hormone withdrawal for whole body scanning.

Patients at the highest risk of recurrent PTC, with MACIS score of 7 and above, including elderly patients, with locally invasive disease or large primary tumors, probably warrant still more aggressive therapy. We recommend either one- or two- stage treatment with I-131, in the form of ablation of the thyroid remnant, if present, at 6 postoperative weeks, followed by treatment dose I-131, of 100 to 200 mCi, a few months later, preferably with a posttherapy scan. Thyroid hormone suppression should also be more aggressive, with the goal of achieving TSH suppression, without inducing symptomatic hyperthyroidism. Surveillance with neck ultrasound, withdrawal isotope whole-body scans, and stimulated Tg measurements are undertaken at 3 to 6 postoperative months and at annual intervals for at least 5 years. For the majority of these patients, rhTSH stimulated whole body scanning is not indicated in the first few years, in view of the high chance that treatment with I-131 will be necessary to deal with residual or recurrent disease. After one or two negative scans, and in the absence of other

evidence of recurrent disease, rhTSH stimulated scans may be appropriate for subsequent follow-up. For patients with FTC and high-risk features (vascular invasion, extrathyroidal invasion, large tumor, and older patients), an assessment for distant metastatic disease may also be worthwhile, including CT scan examination of the chest and abdomen and diphosphonate whole-skeleton bone scintigraphy.

The most aggressive I-131 therapy should be reserved for patients either with unresectable disease, who may benefit from postoperative external beam irradiation as well as I-131 or with distant metastases at diagnosis, who may require several treatment doses with I-131 over a relatively prolonged time course. It should be noted, however, that young patients with PTC, presenting with Stage II disease and pulmonary metastases, carry a generally favorable prognosis and may live for many decades with persistent anatomical evidence of disease, which may be nonprogressive.

Older FCDTC patients with distant metastases may also live for many years, and surgical debulking of solitary metastatic deposits in anatomically threatening locations has proven to be effective palliation.[202] External beam irradiation to focal bony deposits may also reduce local symptoms, and reduce the risk of pathologic fracture.[295] Radioiodine in moderately high dosage may rarely be of additional benefit in treating tumors that concentrate I-131, although the acute enlargement which may be caused by TSH stimulation and by the edema precipitated by I-131 induced injury, can cause increases in local compressive symptoms. This may be a significant problem in certain sites, particularly the brain and spinal cord.[291]

SUMMARY

FCDTC is the most common of the endocrine malignancies, representing almost 2% of all reported human cancers, and is responsible for more deaths than all other endocrine malignancies combined. Nevertheless, the vast majority of patients with this disease are destined to be cured or to live with their disease for many years, and these patients have an essentially normal life expectancy. Thyroid carcinoma, however, exhibits one of the widest ranges of malignant potential of any known cancer, making management of these patients complex. Fortunately, clinical, surgical, and pathologic features allow accurate disease staging and prognostication for individual patients, rapidly and with minimal effort. This staging process should influence all aspects of the management of these patients, and should determine the aggressiveness of postoperative therapy and surveillance for recurrent disease. This process permits the identification of low-risk individuals, whose primary treatment can be limited simply to surgery, and whose follow-up requirements are simple, noninvasive, and inexpensive. Similarly, higher risk patients can be targeted for progressively more aggressive management with radioactive iodine, thyroid hormone suppression and other modalities. These higher risk patients also warrant more active and more frequent surveillance for recurrent disease.

Effective postoperative adjunctive therapy is available for patients who require it, and recurrent local and metastatic disease is amenable to both surgical and medical intervention. Even in the rare patient with advanced and progressive disease, useful palliative therapies can often extend life and improve its quality for many years.

Anaplastic Thyroid Carcinoma. Anaplastic thyroid carcinoma (ATC) is arguably the most aggressive human malignancy, presenting a stark contrast to the usually indolent behavior of the more common differentiated forms of thyroid carcinoma. Most often presenting as a rapidly growing goiter, the majority of anaplastic carcinomas are regarded as inoperable by the time of diagnosis because of extensive local invasion into the structures of the neck. Almost half of all patients diagnosed with ATC have evidence of metastatic spread of the tumor at the time of diagnosis, making a surgical cure impossible, even when the disease in the neck makes surgery technically feasible.[324] Unfortunately, these tumors are poorly responsive to traditional postoperative adjunctive therapies of external beam irradiation and chemotherapy. As a result, most patients with ATC are essentially untreatable, and death ensues rapidly from progressive locally invasive disease involving major structures in the neck or from the rapid and inexorable growth of distant metastases in multiple sites.

Of the approximately 1,500 deaths per year attributed to thyroid cancer annually in the United States, almost half result from anaplastic carcinoma although it represents less than 5% of all clinically recognized cancers of the thyroid gland.[325,326] Most studies of ATC show cause-specific mortality rates of 70 to 95% with a median survival of less than 6 months, and only a tiny proportion of patients with long-term survival.[327–329]

Our understanding of the pathogenesis of these rare tumors is improving slowly although much remains unknown. However, advances in our understanding of these tumors cannot yet be translated into improved clinical management, and the prospects for such knowledge-based therapies seem remote. In the meantime, the optimal approach to treatment of patients presenting with ATC remains a subject of debate. Thyroid surgery, radiation, and chemotherapy may have only limited roles in the majority of these patients, for many of whom palliation may be the best available option. Novel therapeutic approaches are desperately needed for this horrific disease.

Clinical Presentation. The typical presentation of a patient with ATC is with a rapidly enlarging, often painful neck mass, seen commonly in the context of a preexisting goiter or apparently benign thyroid nodule. In a series of 134 patients presenting to our institution over 50 years, 97% presented in this way, with a small minority being detected as a result of symptomatic distant metastases.[324] The rate of growth of a neck mass resulting from ATC is often terrifying with anecdotal reports suggesting a doubling in size in as little as a few weeks.

As they grow, these tumors aggressively invade local tissues, tracking along and destroying fascial planes. It is often difficult to distinguish the primary neck mass from nodal metastases, which are also common, being present in virtually all patients at diagnosis.[324] The primary tumor and its nodal metastases may form a single extensive mass, the extent of which may be almost impossible to define, even with modern imaging procedures. Examination reveals a solid, almost stony mass, which may encase and invade the trachea and larynx and distort local structures. The average size of the resected tumors in the Mayo Clinic series was almost 7 cm whereas many of the unresectable tumors were estimated to be much larger (unpublished data). Consequently, an overall tumor size of 10 to 20 cm is not uncommon, often only a few weeks after the initial discovery of a thyroid nodule, reflecting the almost explosive growth of ATC.

CT scanning reveals a large heterogeneous mass, distortion of the tissue planes, and extensive local infiltration. As the tumor extends beyond the thyroid gland, laryngeal fixation and esophageal invasion occur, causing dysphagia. Tracheal deviation, compression and invasion lead to stridor and dyspnea, while involvement of the recurrent laryngeal nerves causes hoarseness and dysphonia. The massive goiter may lead to thoracic outlet compression, resulting in a positive Pemberton sign. Infiltration of the skin causes necrosis, while growth of the tumor around and through the site of a tracheostomy has been described, with consequent respiratory compromise. Pain, reflecting aggressive local infiltration, is a prominent feature in the late stages of the disease.[324] Involvement of the great veins of the neck can cause superior vena cava syndrome, while invasion of the carotid artery may result in massive hemorrhage, sometimes precipitating death.

If the patient survives the local disease, death is likely to occur from rapidly progressive distant metastases, most often pulmonary, mediastinal, skeletal, or cerebral. Distant metastases are detected at some stage of the illness in the majority of patients (80%), and in almost half of patients, evidence of metastases can be found at the time of the original diagnosis.[324] In many cases, however, a search for metastases is not undertaken, because the obvious lethality of the primary tumor makes further evaluation pointless.

For most patients the mode of death involves local invasion, a painful and merciless process. For those lucky enough to gain control over the primary tumor, death almost always ensues rapidly either from respiratory failure, as a result of pulmonary metastases, or from brain metastases.

Demographics. In studies published before the early 1980s, ATC was thought to represent as much as 10 to 20% of all thyroid cancers.[330,331] Over the last two decades, with the advent of more sophisticated immunologic techniques in histopathology, it has been increasingly recognized that the majority of small cell "anaplastic" tumors are in fact primary non-Hodgkin lymphoma of the thyroid.[332–334] Others represent de-differentiated medullary carcinoma[334] or "insular" variants of follicular carcinoma.[335] These tumors carry a better prognosis than anaplastic carcinoma, and lymphoma in particular, may show an excellent response to radiation and chemotherapy.[334,335] True ATC, by modern histologic criteria, represents a diminishing proportion of thyroid carcinoma in the Western world.[192]

In recent studies, ATC represents between 1 and 3% of thyroid carcinoma in both clinical series and national surveys.[193,324,329] The estimated annual incidence of ATC should therefore lie between 200 and 600 cases in the United States. Consequently, ATC may represent as much as 50% of the overall thyroid cancer mortality, a total of approximately 1,500 deaths in 2002.[191]

The median age at diagnosis is between 60 and 70 years in most series although patients as young as 40 may be diagnosed with this disease.[324] There is a female preponderance of approximately 1.5:1, less than the female excess seen in other forms of thyroid cancer.[193,324,329,333,336–341] There may be an association between low iodine intake and the development of ATC, perhaps through its effect on endemic goiter, and this might explain the falling incidence of ATC in the Western world.[338] However, iodine supplementation has not yet been shown clearly to lower the incidence of ATC.[342]

Nevertheless, ATC is thought often to arise in the context of a preexisting goiter or thyroid nodule. In at least a proportion of cases, coexisting DTC, follicular adenomas or multinodular goiters have been reported although the precise frequency of this occurrence remains uncertain, ranging from 25 to almost 80% in various studies.[324,336,339] In the Mayo Clinic series, fewer than 5% of patients had a prior history of treated differentiated thyroid carcinoma (DTC). However, a further 20% of patients had coincidentally noted DTC on pathologic examination of surgically resected ATC, often seen in close association with the ATC. A further 20% of patients had one or more benign thyroid nodules or a goiter, bringing the total number of patients with preexisting thyroid disease to almost 50%, a proportion that almost certainly underestimates its true prevalence, given the difficulty of evaluating nonsurgically treated patients with ATC.[324]

Pathology. Most true anaplastic cancers are so-called "large cell tumors," which exhibit giant cells, spindle shaped cells, or cells resembling osteoclasts.[343] Cytologic and nuclear atypia are common, and cells may be multinucleated, with frequent mitotic figures, suggesting a rapid rate of cell division.[343] Vascular tissue can be detected within these tumors, suggesting that angiogenesis is activated.[344,345] However, extensive necrosis is also seen, with continued tumor growth around blood vessels and the periphery of the tumor mass,[343] while expression of vascular endothelial growth factor, a major determinant of neoangiogenesis, is lower in ATC than in differentiated thyroid carcinomas.[346]

As previously noted, it is now recognized that as many as 25% of tumors previously classified as ATC, in fact represent other thyroid cancer types, often with a better prognosis.[333,343] In particular, so-called "small cell" ATC often stains for lymphocyte markers, while being negative for keratin or thyroglobulin.[347,348] These tumors are now classified as thyroid lymphoma and should be treated accordingly.[343] Immunohistochemical and other stains for calcitonin and amyloid also distinguish poorly differentiated medullary thyroid carcinoma from true ATC, while poorly-differentiated ("insular") follicular carcinoma can be recognized by careful histological examination.[349]

True ATC stains positively in most cases for cytokeratin, confirming an epithelial origin, but only a minority stains positively for thyroglobulin.[334,350] Many, perhaps most, ATC arise in the context of preexisting benign or malignant thyroid disease, and a step-wise process of "de-differentiation" from thyroid carcinoma has been proposed, during which sequential genetic changes lead to progressively more aggressive biological behavior, ultimately resulting in the anaplastic phenotype.[351]

As a result of these data, it has been claimed that ATC always arises in the context of preexisting differentiated thyroid carcinoma and that it represents a de-differentiated form of FCDTC. Although this is an attractive hypothesis, it remains unproven. It is important to recall that small foci of papillary carcinoma may be found commonly

at autopsy in patients without clinical evidence of thyroid cancer,[352] while follicular adenomas and other benign thyroid nodules affect a substantial proportion of patients in the age group most commonly affected by ATC.[353,354] Consequently, the coexistence of differentiated cancer or adenomas in the thyroid of patients with anaplastic cancer may be nothing more than coincidence. Nevertheless, the intimate coexistence of differentiated and undifferentiated carcinoma, in some patients, supports the hypothesis that at least a proportion of ATC may be derived from preexisting differentiated thyroid carcinoma.

Unfortunately, the concept that an inadequately treated papillary thyroid carcinoma in a young patient might de-differentiate and "become anaplastic" continues to be used to justify aggressive surgical and post-surgical management for patients with otherwise low-risk thyroid tumors.[355] It is sobering to note that, in the recently reported Mayo Clinic series, only 6 of the 134 patients (4.5%) had previously been diagnosed with differentiated thyroid cancer.[324] Furthermore, fewer than 5 patients have been documented to develop ATC after treatment for differentiated thyroid cancer, out of a total experience of over 2,000 patients managed for this disease at Mayo Clinic, and followed for an average of more than 20 years (personal communication, Dr Ian D. Hay). Patients who have been successfully treated for DTC should be reassured that the risk of anaplastic transformation is negligible.

Pathogenesis and Etiology. The precise pathogenesis of ATC remains unknown. The rarity of the tumor has limited experimental study to small numbers of specimens, and the majority of studies are based on data derived from cell lines, which may not completely reflect the behavior of the tumor itself.

In many cases, differentiated thyroid carcinoma is seen in close proximity to the anaplastic tumor, which in some cases forms marely a "focus" of ATC within an otherwise differentiated carcinoma.[356,357] This close proximity is consistent with the hypothesis that ATC arises from preexisting DTC, although clear evidence for this concept remains scant.

Aneuploidy is seen commonly in ATC, as it is in FTC, and its Hürthle cell variant,[358,359] adding support to the hypothesis that ATC may be derived from FTC. However, the most common cancer type seen in association with ATC is the papillary histotype, itself most often euploid.[324,360] The *RET/PTC* gene rearrangements, known to be the cause of a proportion of PTC, may also be present in a proportion of ATC,[361] a finding that is consistent with the derivation of ATC as a de-differentiated form of PTC (Figure 1).

Mutations and expression changes of the p53 tumor suppressor gene are found commonly in ATC, in contrast to findings in differentiated thyroid carcinoma, where such mutations are rare.[362] The rate of such mutations is increased in vitro by radiation exposure,[363] although p53 mutations alone are insufficient to cause transformation to ATC, since biallelic loss is required to inactivate the p53 tumor suppressor gene fully. The combination of *RET/PTC* rearrangements and p53 inactivation in mice is sufficient to induce anaplastic thyroid carcinoma in a mouse model.[364] As is the case in almost all other tumor types in which p53 mutations are seen, these mutation events appear to be sporadic but are made more likely by a high cell-turnover state. Presumably, this explains at least in part the association between the anaplastic thyroid carcinoma and preexisting benign as well as malignant thyroid disease. In cell lines derived from ATC, re-expression of wild-type p53 is sufficient to induce apoptosis, decrease the rate of cell division, and restore some differentiated

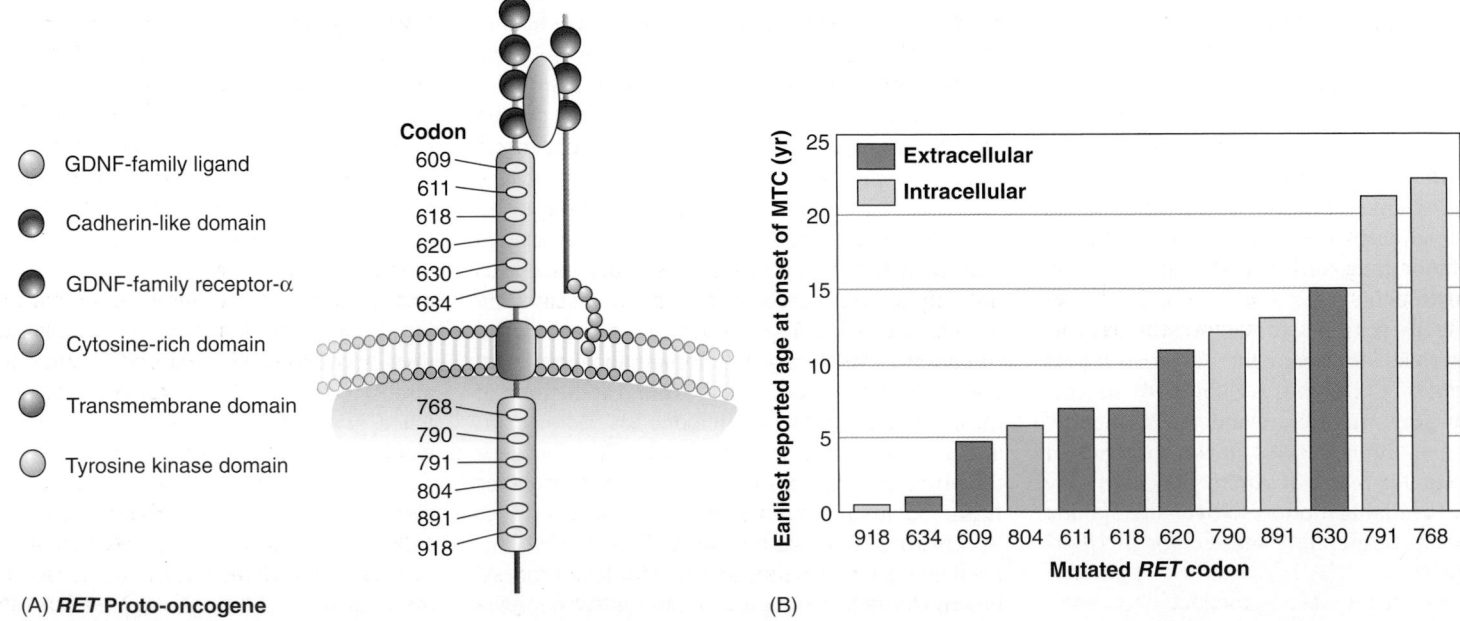

Figure 1 (A) Structure of rearranged during transfection (*RET*) proto-oncogene. (B) The earliest reported age at the onset of medullary thyroid carcinoma (MTC), according to the *RET* mutation. GDNF = glial cell-derived neurotrophic factor. (Published with permission, Cote GJ. Gagel RF. Lessons learned from the management of a rare genetic cancer. N Engl J Med 2003;349:1566–8. Copyright 2003 Massachusetts Medical Society. All rights reserved.)

follicular cell functions, including thyroglobulin expression.[365]

Little additional information is available on the molecular pathogenesis of this tumor, but the advent of gene expression array techniques, which provide the capability to probe expression of many thousands of genes simultaneously, raises the likelihood that more answers will be forthcoming in the next few years. This knowledge will be essential if we are to begin to improve our treatment options for ATC.

Prognosis and Staging. A number of moderately large retrospective studies of ATC have been published over the last decade, documenting the almost universal lethality of the tumor when the diagnosis is confirmed by modern histologic criteria.[193,324,329,333,336,338–341,349,366–368] Unfortunately, those few cases of ATC previously reported as curable are perhaps more likely to have represented thyroid lymphoma, and the survival rate for ATC in modern series is depressingly small.[324]

Because of the extremely high mortality rates, it is difficult to identify any relevant prognostic factors, and such factors in any case would be unlikely to improve our ability to manage individual patients with this disease. The reported median life expectancy in most modern studies ranges from 3 to 12 months, with almost 25% of patients surviving less than one month.[324] Only around 10% of patients survive more than 1 year from the time of diagnosis, and true long-term survivors, apparently cured of their disease, are a rarity.

Even among patients diagnosed with a small anaplastic focus within an otherwise differentiated thyroid carcinoma, outcomes are extremely poor, with 7 out of 8 patients dying of their disease an average of only 11 months from diagnosis in one study.[367] One report of 17 patients with small anaplastic foci within differentiated thyroid carcinoma showed improved long-term outcome following complete tumor resection, compared with larger ATCs.[336] Perhaps not surprisingly, small tumor size may be associated with a more favorable prognosis, at least in some studies.[329,369,370]

Nevertheless, death results in almost all cases of ATC, from continued growth of unresectable tumor in the neck or from the growth of distant metastases in vital structures including the lung and brain. Small tumor size (<5 to 6 cm) and an absence of metastases at the time of diagnosis appear to favor long-term survival although the majority of patients still fare poorly.[329,341] Presumably, these rare instances represent patients with tumors, caught at an early stage, in whom resection has the opportunity to be curative.

Few patients with ATC are fortunate enough to be diagnosed at an early stage, with fewer than 20% of patients with tumors being less than 5 cm in maximum dimension in most series.[324,339] Of the 15 (11%) of patients with "small" tumors in the Mayo Clinic series, only half were free from distant metastases at the time of diagnosis and were felt to have been completely resected following surgery. It was from among these 8 patients (6%) that all four long-term (>24 months) survivors

were derived, suggesting that adequate resection of truly localized disease, may provide the only real opportunity for "cure" of this disease, at the present time. Even in this optimal setting, however, the 2-year survival was only 50%.

Patient age, the most important risk factor in differentiated thyroid carcinoma, appears to have little bearing on outcome of ATC,[193,329,367] with young patients faring equally poorly as older individuals. Similarly, patient gender has no detectable influence on outcome, whereas the presence of lymph node metastases and perhaps also distant metastases are so frequent that their impact on outcome becomes impossible to measure.[324,339,370] As a consequence of the bleak outlook for virtually all patients with this disease, ATC are classified by the WHO as Stage IV disease, regardless of the tumor size, nodal status, presence of metastases, or age of the patient.[207]

Treatment

Surgery The discovery of a large, rapidly growing, malignant mass in the neck fuels an almost irresistible desire, in both patient and physician, to seek a surgical solution. In many cases however, such surgery proves impossible; and, at best, a debulking procedure can be offered. In the Mayo Clinic series, fewer than 30% of patients were deemed to have "surgically curable" disease; and, of those, only 25 (19% of the total) achieved apparently "complete resection" following the operation,[324] figures that closely resemble those of other large institutional series.

Surgical resection significantly prolongs survival, compared to that following biopsy alone or biopsy and tracheostomy from a median of 3 weeks to 3.5 months from diagnosis.[324] However, it remains unclear whether this improvement is truly the result of the surgical resection or merely reflects the less advanced stage of the disease among patients with "resectable" tumor, compared to those more advanced tumors that are not amenable to surgery. Indeed, outcomes differ little between disease that is "completely resected" during surgery, with a median survival of 4.0 months, and that in which "gross residual disease" is left behind by the surgeon, with a median survival of 2.3 months, a difference that is not statistically different (p = .3).[324] Even among patients with apparently complete surgical resection, local recurrence in the neck occurred in over one-third (37%), although this recurrence was unlikely to be the cause of the patient's death.[324]

The extent of the primary surgery, beyond resection of the primary tumor and local involved lymph nodes, is probably of little relevance, and the arguments that still rage about the appropriate extent of surgery for differentiated thyroid carcinoma have little bearing on the management of ATC. There has been no demonstrable advantage to more extensive surgery in ATC.[324,336,339,370]

Nevertheless, patients in whom local control of the disease can be achieved surgically gain both slightly prolonged survival and, arguably more worthwhile, are less likely to die as a result of direct invasion of the upper aerodigestive

tract, at least when external beam irradiation is administered postoperatively.[324] Without doubt, an improved "quality of death" is a worthwhile goal, but this should not encourage surgeons to undertake inappropriately heroic surgery. Our view, and that of many other centers, is that debulking surgery should be offered to patients with ATC only when such surgery can reasonably be expected effectively to debulk the tumor without threatening major vital structures. Even then, however, such surgery is most often likely to be palliative rather than curative.

External Beam Irradiation. When surgery is deemed impossible, external beam irradiation is used frequently, in an effort to gain some control locally of the disease. Although often regarded as "second best," in fact radiotherapy may offer similar outcomes to surgery. Of the 29 patients (22%) in the Mayo Clinic series treated with external beam irradiation as primary treatment of ATC, median survival was 2.3 months, comparing favorably with the outcome of surgical resection, with a 3.5 month median survival, a difference that was not statistically significant.[324] External beam irradiation is most commonly delivered in a fractionated dose of up to 20 Gray (Gy), over 4 to 6 weeks, however, so that much of the patient's remaining life expectancy is involved in receiving this treatment. More aggressive radiotherapy protocols, including hyperfractionated radiation, with a total dose of 35 to 45 Gy, have not yielded demonstrably better outcomes, but are associated with increased toxicity.[371] Side effects of radiation are common and well recognized, including dysphagia, xerostomia and skin burns, whereas higher-dose treatments may also result in neutropenia and cervical myelitis.[371]

Radiation therapy may play an adjunctive role following primary surgical resection of ATC. In the Mayo Clinic series, complete or near-complete resection of the primary tumor was achieved in 54 patients. Local recurrence within the neck was documented in 20 of these patients (37%), after a median of 2.5 months, a rate that was no different, whether or not the patient underwent postoperative radiotherapy. However, the time to develop that local recurrence was slightly longer, 5 months versus 3 months, ensuring that a greater proportion of treated patients died from complications of metastatic disease, rather than locally progressive disease in the neck.[324]

Radiotherapy may also be used to treat local recurrences or metastatic disease, particularly in the skeleton and brain. However, such treatment should certainly be regarded as end-of-life palliation, since in only a single patient in the Mayo Clinic series was a local recurrence or a metastatic deposit demonstrated to decrease in size following such radiotherapy.[324] In the majority of patients experiencing local recurrence after initial effective surgery, death ensued rapidly, with a median survival following local recurrence of a mere 66 days. There was no difference in survival between those patients whose recurrence was treated with external beam irradiation and those treated conservatively (p = .44).

Chemotherapy. Because ATC is so often metastatic by the time of diagnosis, systemic therapy will be essential to achieve a cure in the majority of patients. At present, however, there are no proven systemic therapies available for the treatment of ATC. Because the tumor does not concentrate iodine, radioactive iodine plays no role in its management. Similarly, there is no evidence of TSH responsiveness, so that TSH-suppression, used commonly in the postoperative management of differentiated thyroid carcinoma, is of no possible benefit.[372]

No evidence exists of benefit from chemotherapy alone in the management of ATC, but "multimodal therapy," including surgical debulking, followed by chemotherapy and external beam irradiation, has gained some acceptance as a viable treatment scheme for patients with ATC. This has largely been based on small pilot studies and case reports,[373,374] but the largest study to date included 37 patients with ATC.[341] Combination treatment was feasible in only 14 of these patients, largely because of the previously noted difficulties achieving useful surgical debulking. Among these 14 patients, treated with aggressive surgery, doxorubicin and radiation, survival was significantly prolonged, to a median of eight months.[341] Unfortunately, other studies have been less promising, with a reduction in survival duration observed for patients receiving combination treatment with preoperative doxorubicin and hyperfractionated radiotherapy in one retrospective study.[328]

In the Mayo Clinic series, 13 patients since 1980 were treated with debulking surgery and postoperative radiotherapy and radio-sensitizing chemotherapy with doxorubicin. The median survival among these patients did not differ ($p = .32$) from the group as a whole, suggesting that such a combined approach was no more effective than surgery alone in the management of patients with ATC. Despite that, a greater proportion of long-term (>1 year) survivors was seen in this group ($n = 3$), a rate of 23%, compared with less than 10% in the group as a whole. Although not statistically significant ($p = .19$), this result may justify further study in selected patients.

Newer chemotherapeutic agents might also prove beneficial. Paclitaxel has been shown to inhibit the growth of ATC cell in vitro and in xenografted nude mice,[375] while a combination of paclitaxel, 5-fluorouracil and radiation therapy was shown to induce a useful preoperative clinical response in one patient with a large ATC, who showed "no evidence of viable tumor" at subsequent thyroidectomy.[376] Antiangiogenic therapy, using thalidomide, is also currently under evaluation, whereas redifferentiation therapy, using gene therapy approaches based on the reintroduction of the p53 tumor suppressor gene may ultimately provide a novel therapeutic opportunity.

Novel approaches, using alternative chemotherapeutic agents in the short term and gene therapy approaches in the long term, are desperately needed for this almost universally lethal disease. These therapies will require clinical trials, and the rarity of ATC makes such clinical trials difficult to organize, fund, and complete. Without them, however, the outlook for patients with ATC remains grim.

Summary. ATC is among the most aggressive of human malignancies, and death by choking, aspiration, or hemorrhage is almost universal if surgical resection cannot be achieved. Extensive surgery does not seem to carry any benefit beyond debulking, and placement of a tracheostomy followed by external beam radiation may be almost as effective in many cases. Postoperative radiotherapy may delay local recurrence but does not prevent or delay death from the disease. More aggressive combination treatments, including chemotherapy, remain disappointing in the majority of patients, with no clear impact on survival.

Nevertheless, a small proportion of patients do survive, and an occasional patient may live disease-free for decades. Good prognostic factors seem to include the absence of metastatic disease at the time of presentation, small tumor size, complete or almost complete tumor resection, and postoperative radiotherapy, with or without chemotherapy. For patients with ATC to survive long-term, the disease must therefore be diagnosed early, before metastatic spread has occurred, and treated aggressively. For the majority of patients, who exhibit metastatic disease or extensive invasive disease within the neck at the time of diagnosis, the most humane approach may be to protect the airway, to treat with radiotherapy, and to ensure adequate end of life care.

Unfortunately, our ability to treat ATC lags far behind our capacity to diagnose it, and we have seen no improvement in outcome in this disease in over one-half century.[197] Surgery alone is insufficient to extend life, and more aggressive management provides no clear additional benefit in the majority of patients. New approaches to the management of this disease are desperately needed.

Thyroid Lymphoma and Secondary Malignancies of the Thyroid Gland.

Thyroid Lymphoma. Primary lymphoma of the thyroid is rare, representing a mere 1% of thyroid malignancy, and only around 2 to 3% of lymphomas.[377,378] As discussed above, thyroid lymphoma may easily be confused with small cell anaplastic carcinoma although modern histologic methods, including immunostaining for epithelial and lymphoid markers have simplified the diagnosis considerably.[343] Nevertheless, the clinical presentation is easily mistaken for that of ATC, with rapid growth of the tumor, involvement of lymph nodes, and symptoms of local compression.

The majority of thyroid lymphomas are B-cell non-Hodgkin lymphoma, which may arise in association with Hashimoto thyroiditis.[379] Presumably the development of lymphoid tissue within the thyroid gland in Hashimoto disease provides the substrate in which the lymphoma arises, and rates of thyroid lymphoma are estimated to be as much as 80-fold higher among patients with Hashimoto disease.[378] Nevertheless, lymphoma remains a rare complication of Hashimoto disease.

Unlike ATC, effective systemic treatment is available for thyroid lymphoma and there remains little role of surgery as primary treatment for this condition. As is the case for all lymphomas, the prognosis depends largely on the extent of disease at the time of diagnosis.

Clinical Presentation and Diagnosis. The presentation of thyroid lymphoma closely resembles that of ATC, with a rapidly growing thyroid mass, often arising on a background of a longstanding benign goiter or Hashimoto disease. In contrast to ATC, however, the goiter is often painless, but it may still be associated with hoarseness, stridor, dysphagia, dyspnea, and thoracic outlet obstruction as a result of compression of surrounding structures. The gland may be fixed to adjacent structures, in part the result of fibrosis. Lymphadenopathy is common in the neck and may be present elsewhere, depending on the stage of the disease. Destruction of the thyroid gland may occur with consequent hypothyroidism in a proportion of patients although many patients have preexisting thyroid failure as a result of Hashimoto disease.

Presumably beçause of its association with Hashimoto's disease, the majority of patients are female with a female to male ratio of approximately 3:1.[377,378,380,381] As is the case for other non-Hodgkin lymphomas, thyroid lymphoma most often presents between the ages of 60 and 80 years, an age range that overlaps extensively with that of ATC.

The distinction between thyroid lymphoma and ATC can usually be made on FNAB, but open biopsy is still sometimes required to distinguish lymphoma from Hashimoto disease. That distinction depends on identifying the monoclonal cell proliferation characteristic of lymphoma, which produces a restricted set of immunoglobulin light chains, in contrast to the polyclonal features of inflammatory thyroid disease. Staining for immunoglobulin light chains is straightforward using immunohistochemistry but takes both time and tissue, sometimes delaying the diagnosis and requiring a core biopsy or even an open biopsy in some cases[379] although modern molecular techniques may render this unnecessary in the future.[382]

Pathology and Staging. The vast majority of thyroid lymphomas are B-cell derived non-Hodgkin lymphomas.[379,381] The tumor cells are uniform, forming sheets of cells that displace and destroy the normal thyroid parenchyma. Nuclear atypia is less commonly seen than in ATC, but mitotic figures are frequent, consistent with the rapid growth of this tumor.[383] As already noted, thyroid lymphoma is thought to be monoclonal, and a restricted set of immunoglobulin light chains helps to confirm the diagnosis.

The staging of lymphoma is currently based on the extent of disease.[384] Stage I represents intrathyroidal disease, without other manifestations; Stage II is disease confined to the thyroid and cervical lymph nodes; Stage III involves both sides of the diaphragm; and Stage IV is defined as disseminated lymphoma, often including the bone marrow.

The prognosis of thyroid lymphoma is determined principally by disease stage, with 5-year survival rate of 80% for Stage I , 50% for Stage II, and 35% for Stages III and IV.[381] Recurrence after initial successful therapy may occur in up to 30% patients with of Stage I and II disease, usually within the first 3 to 5 years, raising the question of whether a systemic approach to treatment might be justified even in apparently localized disease.[385] The prognosis is also influenced by the extent of local disease, with worse prognosis for large primary tumors (>10 cm), for patients exhibiting local compressive symptoms in the neck, and for those with mediastinal involvement, reflecting direct extension of the primary tumor.[386]

Treatment. Like other forms of lymphoma, the treatment of thyroid lymphoma should probably be tailored to the stage of the disease. Surgery, chemotherapy, and external beam irradiation all may have a role to play in the management of this disease. However, in most patients with advanced lymphoma, surgery should be restricted to whatever biopsy is necessary for diagnosis since the benefits of surgical resection of the thyroid gland are probably minimal. One exception, of course, is protection of the airway, and a tracheostomy should certainly be considered for patients with significant airway obstruction.

Stage I lymphoma, limited to the thyroid, represents a minority of thyroid lymphomas, and a surgical approach to this localized disease has been advocated by same.[381] However, it is likely that the alternative treatments of chemotherapy and radiotherapy are equally effective.[387] Chemotherapy also has the theoretical advantage of treating undetectable systemic lymphoma, which may reduce the risk of later relapse. This theory remains unproven but attractive to some. Nevertheless, there remains a strong case for surgical debulking, particularly of bulky disease localized to the neck (Stage I and Stage II) since the risk of relapse is closely correlated to the extent of residual disease in the neck. Improved survival has been documented following surgical resection,[388] and the combination of surgical debulking followed by external beam irradiation leads to an excellent rate of remission, approaching 90% in Stage I and Stage II disease.[381]

Unfortunately, moderately high rates of relapse have been reported following apparently successful localized treatment for Stage I and Stage II disease, with up to 30% of patients suffering a systemic relapse after apparently successful initial therapy.[385] Consequently, chemotherapy with cyclophosphamide, vincristine, doxorubicin, methotrexate, and prednisone, in various combinations, has been recommended, even for apparently well-localized disease.[385] This approach has not yet been tested formally in a clinical trial, and our approach remains one of localized treatment for localized disease, after an extensive staging process, while chemotherapy is reserved for patients with Stage III or Stage IV disease, or for those who suffer a relapse.

For Stage III and IV disease, the surgical role should probably be limited to biopsy alone and protection of the airway, and treatment should be focused on systemic chemotherapy, as outlined above, with irradiation of bulky deposits, including the thyroid gland.[381]

Thyroid Metastases. Metastatic spread to the thyroid gland, of nonthyroid malignancy may occur in up to 25% of widely metastatic malignancies[389] although most studies suggest a rather lower rate, closer to 5%.[352,390] Some malignancies are particularly likely to involve the thyroid, including melanoma, breast, renal clear-cell, lung, and squamous cell carcinoma of the head and neck.[390]

Clinically important metastases are less common, however, probably affecting fewer than 1% of patients with disseminated malignancy. Much more commonly, the possibility of thyroid metastasis presents a diagnostic dilemma, in a patient with a known malignancy who is discovered incidentally to have a thyroid nodule.[391] Fortunately, FNA is generally a reliable method to distinguish primary from secondary malignancies in the thyroid.[392] When diagnostic confusion remains, thyroglobulin and calcitonin immunostaining can often clarify the situation. The exception is in the case of an undifferentiated malignancy, when the distinction between a primary ATC and a metastatic deposit of undifferentiated carcinoma can be difficult or impossible. A careful search for other sites of metastases and for the primary neoplasm may provide the answer; but, in the case of possible ATC, the treatment for the (presumed) primary neoplasm must not be inappropriately delayed while searching for a possible alternative site of origin.

The treatment of metastases in the thyroid should be determined by the nature of the primary neoplasm and the presence or absence of other metastases. Surgical resection of solitary thyroid metastases may improve the prognosis, at least for some neoplasm types, including breast and renal carcinoma.[391,393]

Medullary Carcinoma of Thyroid Gland and the Multiple Endocrine Neoplasia Syndrome Type 2. MTC develops from parafollicular C cells which are of neural crest origin and make up approximately 1% of thyroid cells. These cells are present throughout the gland but are concentrated in the posterior and lateral upper third of the gland, the most common site of medullary cancer. Parafollicular C cells produce calcitonin that serves as a tumor marker and is associated with the endocrine symptoms (pain, flushing, and diarrhea) that are often associated with MTC. Approximately 5 to 10% of thyroid cancers are medullary and sporadic MTC accounts for 75% with familial forms accounting for the remainder.

MTC generally presents as a slow growing firm thyroid nodule. On histologic examination, amyloid may be found in one-third of the cases. C-cell hyperplasia is a precursor to MTC most commonly seen in hereditary forms. Lymph node metastases are common and may be widely distributed at diagnosis independent of tumor size.[394]

Approximately 50 to 80% of patients with MTC presenting with a thyroid nodule have lymph node metastases at the time of diagnosis, and the distribution of lymph node metastases can be wide spread. Central compartment nodes are the most frequent sites involved, but all areas of the neck and mediastinum may be involved. The contralateral neck may be involved in up to 50%. Distant metastases must also be considered and may be difficult to identify due to small size and lack of unique imaging characteristics. The lungs, liver, bone, brain, and soft tissue may be affected by hematogenous metastases.[395]

Surgery remains the primary mode of therapy for MTC due to the lack of impact on survival by either radiation or standard chemotherapeutic agents. Ideally the initial surgery would be scaled to address the primary neoplasm and nodal metastases appropriately. Preoperative imaging of the neck with ultrasound and CT imaging are useful in identifying nonpalpable adenopathy and atypically located nodal metastases. A preoperative calcitonin level is useful to correlate with postoperative levels. In general a total thyroidectomy, central compartment and ipsilateral neck dissection should be planned for MTC that presents with a palpable thyroid mass. Preoperative identification of bilateral adenopathy by ultrasound or computed tomography should prompt bilateral neck dissections.

Calcitonin levels are a key element in postoperative surveillance of MTC. Levels typically drop quickly after resection and usually reach baseline in 72 hours. Delayed decreases have been noted. In patients presenting with palpable disease, 50% will have persistent evidence of biochemical disease.[396] Asymptomatic or borderline elevation of calcitonin presents a dilemma since radiographic quantification of disease can be challenging and individuals may do well for long periods of time. New elevations in calcitonin level, onset or recurrence of symptoms, and the development of a neck mass should prompt a metastatic work up of the neck, chest, and abdomen keeping in mind the not infrequent inability to accurately image metastatic disease (low sensitivity and significant false positive rate).

Adjuvant treatments to this point remain lacking. Since C cells do not concentrate iodine, I-131 is not useful.[397] A retrospective review of 73 patients deemed to be at high risk for local recurrence (microscopic residual disease, extraglandular extension, or lymph node involvement) demonstrated that those patients who received external beam irradiation had a significantly higher locoregional relapse-free rate (86% at 10 years vs 52%, $p = .049$).[398] However, it remains difficult to balance the morbidity of external beam irradiation (xerostomia, neck fibrosis, increased difficulty with revision surgery) with the known high rate of late recurrence.

Primary prognostic factors for MTC include age and disease stage at time of diagnosis. Post-thyroidectomy calcitonin level is an indicator of prognosis for both local recurrence and long-term survival.[399] Importantly, overall survival is strikingly higher than disease free survival. In general, at 5 years, the overall survival rate varies according to clinical stage: 98% for Stages I and II, 73% for Stage III, 40% for Stage IV, and overall rates ranging 80 to 85%. At 10 years, the survival rates are consistently 70 to 80%. A recent Mount Sinai Hospital study showed 5-, 10-, and 20-year overall survival rates as 97, 88, and 84%, respectively. However, disease-free survival rates were lower at 97, 74, and 29% at 5, 10, and 20 years.[399]

Perhaps there is no better example of molecular medicine impacting the care of surgical patients than in the management of hereditary MTC. Specific germ-line point mutations on chromosme 10q11.2 in the RET (rearranged during transformation) proto-oncogene (a membrane bound tyrosine kinase receptor) result in activation of the associated tyrosine kinase. These autosomal dominant mutations are associated with abnormal development of cells derived from the neural crest (parathyroid, chromaffin cells of the adrenal medulla, thyroid parafollicular C cells, and enteric autonomic plexus) and generate the clinical findings associated with multiple endocrine neoplasia type 2 (MEN2). Three clinically distinct forms of MEN2 exist with all three demonstrating MTC as a common and often earliest clinical feature; MEN2A, MEN2B, and familial medullary thyroid cancer (FMTC). In patients with FMTC, only the thyroid gland is involved. MEN2A is characterized by the potential development of pheochromocytomas (50%) and hyperparathyroidism (30%). Other uncommon manifestations of MEN 2A include cutaneous lichen amyloidosis and Hirschsprung disease. MEN2B has unique features in addition to MTC including mucosal neuromatosis, intestinal ganglioneuromatosis, and a marfanoid habitus but does not include hyperparathyroidism.

The RET proto-oncogene ligand is glial cell derived neurotrophic factor, and RET activation requires the formation of a multimeric receptor complex that includes GDNF as ligand and a glycosylphosphatidyl inositol-anchored protein termed GDNF receptor that functions as coreceptor. Missense mutations in the extracellular cytosine rich domain frequently involve one of six highly conserved cysteines (codons 609, 611, 618, and 620 in exon 10 and codons 630 and 634 in exon 11). These mutations activate the tyrosine kinase receptor by ligand-independent dimerization and cross-phosphorylation. Point mutations at condons 609, 618, and 620 may exert a dual effect with resultant loss of kinase function (Hirschsprung disease) and gain in kinase function (FMTC, MEN2A, or MEN2B).

The majority of MEN2A cases have germline missense RET mutations involving codons 609, 611, 618, and 620 in exon 10 and codons 630 and 634 in exon 11. In patients with FMTC, RET mutations are mainly detected in the same six codons as for MEN 2A and also in codon 768 (exon 13), or in codon 891 (exon 15), which lies in the intracellular region (Figure 1).

The majority of MEN2B mutations involve codon 918 in RET exon 16, which lies within the intracellular RET tyrosine kinase domain. This mutation appears to alter the substrate specificity of the RET tyrosine kinase. Several studies have identified the presence of RET mutations in sporadic MTC (codons 918 and 768) and pheochromocytoma (codon 918) tumor tissues but not in constitutional DNA from the same patient (Table 12).

Presently, the morbidity and mortality of MEN2A, MEN2B, and FMTC are primarily associated with MTC because the identification and management of pheochromocytomas has advanced significantly. In MEN2B, MTC typically is more aggressive than in MEN2A or FMTC. Patients develop C cell hyperplasia, transformation to MTC as well as metastatic disease on a much earlier time line. Guidelines for the timing of total thyroidectomy and area VI nodal dissection have evolved [400] formulated on the concept that molecular identification of individuals in whom a solid organ cancer will develop provides the opportunity to prevent the development of cancer or foster early treatment by gland/organ removal prior to disease identification. For this approach to be successful, there must be a clear correlation of the mutation and the development of disease, and the gland or organ must be expendable. Ideally the procedure to remove the organ should not carry excessive risk and there should exist mechanisms to closely monitor disease.[401]

Total thyroidectomy and area VI node dissection for MEN2A, MEN2B, and FMTC should be considered at an age that would precede malignant transformation and metastasis. For many of the identified mutations, guidelines have been developed. The challenge can arise when mutations which have not been characterized are identified. Counseling patients in this setting is difficult. An additional consideration in MEN2A is the management of the parathyroid disease which occurs in 30% of the patients and is managed in a fashion similar to MEN1.

MEN2 consensus summary statements follow[400]:

1. MEN2 has distinctive variants. MEN2A and MEN2B are the MEN2 variants with the greatest syndromic consistency.
2. FMTC is the mildest variant of MEN2. To avoid missing a diagnosis of MEN2A with its risk of pheochromocytoma, physicians should diagnose FMTC only from rigorous criteria.
3. Morbidity from pheochromocytoma in MEN2 has been markedly decreased by improved recognition and management. The preferred treatment for unilateral pheochromocytoma in MEN2 is laparoscopic adrenalectomy.
4. Hyperparathyroidism (HPT) is less intense in MEN2 than in MEN1. Parathyroidectomy should be the same as in other disorders with multiple parathyroid tumors.
5. The main morbidity from MEN2 is MTC. MEN2 variants differ in aggressiveness of MTC, in decreasing order as follows: MEN2B > MEN2A > FMTC.
6. MEN2 carrier detection should be the basis for recommending thyroidectomy to prevent or cure MTC. This carrier testing is mandatory in all children at 50% risk.
7. Compared with *RET* mutation testing, immunoassay of basal or stimulated CT results in more frequent false positive diagnoses and delays of the true positive diagnosis of the MEN2 carrier state. However, the CT test still should be used to monitor the tumor status of MTC. It can be the first index of persistent or recurrent disease.
8. *RET* germline mutation testing has replaced CT testing as the basis for carrier diagnosis in MEN2 families. When performed rigorously, it reveals a *RET* mutation in over 95% of MEN2 index cases.
9. The *RET* codon mutations can be stratified into three levels of risk from MTC. These three categories predict the MEN2 syndromic variant, the age of onset of MTC, and the aggressiveness of MTC.
10. Detailed recommendations about aggressiveness of interventions for MTC are derived from knowledge about the specific *RET* codon mutated and/or from a clear familial pattern.
11. Thyroidectomy should be performed before age 6 months in MEN2B, perhaps much earlier, and before age 5 years in MEN2A. Policies about central lymph node dissection at initial thyroidectomy are controversial and may differ among the MEN2 variants.

Table 12 Multiple Endocrine Neoplasia Type 2 and Its Clinical Variants or Syndromes

Syndrome	Characteristic Features
MEN2A	MTC
	Adrenal medulla (pheochromocytoma)
	Parathyroid glands
FMTC	MTC
MEN2A with cutaneous lichen amyloidosis	MEN2A and a pruritic cutaneous lesion located over the upper back
MEN2A or FMTC with Hirschsprung disease	MEN2A or FMTC with Hirschsprung disease
MEN2B	MTC
	Adrenal medulla (pheochromocytoma)
	Intestinal and mucosal ganglioneuromatosis
	Characteristic habitus, marfanoid

12. Testing (in blood leukocytes) for germline *RET* mutation should be performed in all cases with apparently isolated and nonfamilial (ie, sporadic) MTC or with apparently isolated and nonfamilial pheochromocytoma. A germline mutation is found only occasionally, but such a discovered mutation is important.

13. Tests (in tumor tissue) for somatic *RET* mutation in sporadic MTC or in sporadic pheochromocytoma are generally not recommended for clinical use.

14. Periodic screening for tumors in MEN2 carriers is based upon the MEN2 variant, as characterized by the *RET* codon mutation and by manifestations in the rest of the family.

SUMMARY

MTC is uncommon, representing only a minority of thyroid cancers. However, its involvement in the various genetically determined syndromes noted above, and rapid advances in our understanding of the mechanism of both familial and sporadic disease have led to significant improvements in our ability to detect the disease early, and even to identify and treat individuals before the onset of the malignant transformation in some cases. Sporadic MTC remains a challenge, because of the absence of effective systemic therapy and the disease remains essentially incurable once it has spread beyond the thyroid gland. However, rapid advances in small-molecule targeted therapies hold out the promise for more effective chemotherapeutic agents in the near future.

PARATHYROID GLAND DISEASES

Parathyroid Gland Neoplasia

Primary hyperparathyroidism (PHPT) is one of the most common endocrine syndromes, especially in postmenopausal women, in whom it reaches a prevalence of 2 to 3%.[402] PHPT has an expected incidence of 1 in every 500 women and 1 in every 2,000 men older than 40 years of age[403] and is usually a sporadic disorder. Sporadic PHPT results from a single parathyroid adenoma in 80 to 85% of cases, multiglandular hyperplasia in 15 to 20% of cases, and carcinoma in less than 1% of cases.[404]

In a minority of cases (<10%), PHPT is part of hereditary syndromes, namely, multiple endocrine neoplasia types 1 and 2A (MEN1 and MEN2A), hyperparathyroidism-jaw tumor (HPT-JT) syndrome, or familial isolated hyperparathyroidism (FIHP). Hereditary HPT-JT is an autosomal dominant disease that has recently been mapped to chromosomal region 1q21–q32 (*HRPT2*).[405] The syndrome is characterized by fibro-osseous tumors of the jaws, parathyroid adenomas, and rarely parathyroid carcinoma. Renal abnormalities may also develop including Wilm tumors, hamartomas, and polycystic kidney disease.

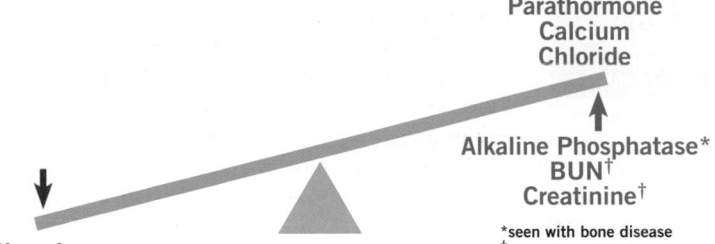

Serology of 1° Hyperparathyroidism

Parathormone
Calcium
Chloride

Alkaline Phosphatase*
BUN†
Creatinine†

*seen with bone disease
†seen with renal disease

Phosphorus

Figure 2 Illustration of the key serology manifestations of primary hyperparathyroidism. (Copyrighted and used with permission of Mayo Foundation for Medical Education and Research.)

Diagnosis of Primary Hyperparathyroidism. PHPT is diagnosed by persistent hypercalcemia in the presence of inappropriately normal or elevated levels of PTH (Figure 2). The modern clinical profile of asymptomatic PHPT is a disorder in which there are neither signs nor symptoms typically associated with hypercalcemia or parathyroid hormone excess. Prior to the advent of the automated serum screening chemistry panel, the clinical profile was characterized by hypercalcemic symptoms, kidney stones, overt bone disease, or neuromuscular dysfunction. Importantly, not all patients with PHPT have hypercalcemia each time serum calcium levels are measured. Some may have elevated ionized calcium or even completely normal calcium levels. As PTH is incorporated in evaluation for skeletal health, a group of patients with an elevated PTH with normal calcium levels has been identified (normocalcemic PHPT). Potential causes of secondary elevations of PTH need to be ruled out, particularly low calcium intake due to a gastrointestinal disorder, renal insufficiency, vitamin D deficiency (as defined by serum levels of 25-hydroxyvitamin D <20 ng/mL), or hypercalciuria of renal origin.

The target organs of parathyroid hormone, the kidneys and skeleton, require evaluation in patients diagnosed with PHPT. The skeleton is best evaluated by bone densitometry using dual energy X-ray absorptiometry. As kidney stones are still the most common complication of PHPT, a baseline assessment with renal ultrasound and/or abdominal X-rays is reasonable. Twenty-four-hour urinary calcium measurement can be useful not only in helping to distinguish between PHPT and FHH, but also in giving a general measure of the renal burden for handling calcium.[406]

PHPT may be associated with neuropsychological disturbances. Complaints include weakness and easy fatigability (in the absence of overt muscular weakness), depression, intellectual weariness, and increased sleep requirement. In addition, some centers have reported on patient-related outcome variables in PHPT that can negatively influence estimates of quality of life. Improvement in some of these indexes may be noted after successful parathyroidectomy, but it is not possible at this time to predict which patients will benefit.[407–409]

A typical laboratory investigation for a patient with probable hyperparathyroidism includes serum calcium (total), phosphorus, alkaline phosphatase, PTH, vitamin D, and 24-hour urine collection for calcium. Additional information from the patient's history should also consider other causes of hypercalcemia/hyperparathyroidism including parathyroid malignancy, medications (lithium, thiazide diuretics), milk alkali syndrome, and hypervitaminosis D.

Familial hypocalciuric hypercalcemia is an autosomal dominant disorder characterized by modest elevation of the serum calcium concentration that is generally asymptomatic, relative hypocalciuria, and parathyroid hormone (PTH) levels that are not suppressed by the hypercalcemia and are inappropriately normal. This condition can be identified by the low urinary calcium losses, in contrast to high losses seen in primary hyperparathyroidism. Measurement of a fractional calcium excretion provides the best way to rule out FHH, prior to surgery for presumed primary hyperparathyroidism. FHH is associated with heterogeneous inactivating mutations in the calcium-sensing receptor (*CASR*) gene located at chromosome 3q13.3-21. The CASR protein, encoded by six exons of the gene, is a G protein-coupled receptor well expressed in parathyroid and renal tubule cells. About 100 inactivating mutations in the *CASR* that cause a decreased sensitivity to extracellular calcium, impairing the ability to respond to normo- and hypercalcemia by appropriately inhibiting PTH secretion and renal calcium reabsorption have been described in patients with FHH and/or neonatal severe hyperparathyroidism (NSHPT). The most common are missense mutations.[410] The recent finding of inactivating mutations of the *MEN1*, CASR, and *HRPT2* genes in FIHP families suggests that at least some kindreds may represent a variant of these syndromes.[411–413]

Treatment. Surgery is the only definitive treatment for hyperparathyroidism. Patients with complications of hyperparathyroidism (severe bone disease, fractures, renal stones, or overt neuromuscular dysfunction) should undergo parathyroidectomy. Management of asymptomatic patients is guided by consensus guidelines most recently modified in 2002.[410] The guidelines for selection of asymptomatic patients for surgery are outlined in Table 13. It should be noted that the any individual under the age of 50 should be considered for parathyroidectomy regardless

Table 13 Guidelines for Parathyroid Gland Surgery in Asymptomatic Primary Hyperparathyroidism

Measurement	Guidelines
Serum calcium (above upper limit of normal)	1.0 mg/dL
24-Hour urinary calcium	>400 mg
Creatinine clearance	Reduced by 30%
Bone mineral density	t-score < −2.5 at any site
Age	<50 yr

of other measurements related to the risk of renal or bone disease developing over time. The measurements recommended are aimed at identification of target organ disease with the goal of treating individuals before renal or bone disease develops. Surgery is also indicated in patients for whom medical surveillance is neither desired nor possible.[410]

Patients who qualify for observation should then be monitored for the development of renal or bone disease over time. Table 14 presents recommendation for the appropriate measurements and timing of the evaluations.

Secondary Hyperparathyroidism. Secondary hyperparathyroidism is an adaptive increase in the production of parathyroid hormone in response to a known clinical stimulus, usually via hypocalcemia and hyperphosphatemia. The most common cause is chronic renal failure. Other causes are vitamin D deficiency, calcium deficiency, malabsorption, and low serum magnesium. The parathyroid glands show hyperplastic changes resembling those of primary chief cell hyperplasia. These are not treated surgically unless parathyroid hormone secretion has become autonomous.

Tertiary Hyperparathyroidism. Tertiary hyperparathyroidism is apparently autonomous parathyroid hyperfunction on a background of known secondary hyperparathyroidism. Most cases result from diffuse or nodular chief cell hyperplasia affecting multiple glands, but about 5% of patients have adenomas; carcinoma may occur on rare occasions.

Multiple Endocrine Neoplasia Type 1. MEN1 is a hereditary syndrome characterized by the development of multiple endocrine neoplasms frequently involving the parathyroid, pancreatic islets, and pituitary. It is important to note that tumors may develop in other nonendocrine sites (Table 15).

MEN1 is an autosomal dominant familial disorder with current evidence supporting a tumor suppressor role of menin, the MEN1 gene, located on chromosome 11q13, product. Patients with a mutated nonfunctional gene are thought to develop disease when the nonmutated allele is lost [loss of heterozygosity (LOH)]. Over 400 mutations of the menin gene have been identified. Multiple functions have been suggested for menin largely based on animal studies. These include: regulation of gene transcription by affecting histone methyl transferases and histone deacetylases, regulation of cell proliferation via cyclin-dependent kinases, and augmenting transforming growth factor beta (TGF-β)-induced inhibition of cell cycle progression, promoting apoptosis possibly via caspase 8, and regulation of genomic instability by associating with various DNA repair genes. The precise mechanism by which menin fosters tumor development has yet to be determined.

The information obtained from genetic testing for MEN1 is not clearly as helpful in patient counseling as it is for MEN2 as outlined in Table 16.

Parathyroid Tumors in Multiple Endocrine Neoplasia Type 1. Although MEN1 is an uncommon diagnosis, MEN1 HPT accounts for 2 to 4% of HPT, HPT is the most common endocrine abnormality in MEN1 and is typically the first clinical expression of the disease. The onset of HPT in MEN1 occurs at 20 to 25 years of age, approximately 30 years earlier than sporadic HPT. HPT in MEN1 reaches nearly 100% penetrance by age 50 years. In contrast to sporadic primary HPT, there is an equal male to female ratio of disease. HPT in MEN1 must be considered multiglandular since most patients have tumors in three or all four glands.

The clinical diagnosis is established in a patient with primary HPT and either a pituitary tumor or an islet cell tumor. Genetic counseling should be provided to patients and offered to family members. Laboratory studies documenting

PTH, serum calcium, and 24-hour urine calcium are consistent with primary HPT. In suspected carriers, annual calcium determinations beginning at age 20 should promote identification of disease prior to the loss of bone mass which can occur as early as 35 years of age in patients with MEN1 and HPT. The indications for parathyroidectomy in children with MEN1 have not been determined. In adults, hypercalcemia increases gastrin secretion from gastrinomas, and effective parathyroidectomy will lower gastrin release. However, pharmacotherapy for Zollinger–Ellison syndrome (ZES) is so successful that ZES plus HPT is not an indication for parathyroidectomy in MEN1.

Treatment is not indicated until clinical or biochemical evidence of disease is identified. The specific procedure performed for MEN1 HPT is controversial and requires consideration of the morbidity of the effects of HPT balanced against the risks of surgery, postoperative hypoparathyroidism, and the likely recurrence of HPT.[414] This has led to the traditional recommendations for a subtotal parathyroidectomy (3.5 glands) with transcervical near total thymectomy for the initial operation or total parathyroidectomy with transcervical near total thymectomy and autotransplantation. Subtotal parathyroidectomy with transcervical near-total thymectomy is the commonest initial neck operation performed in patients with MEN1. Parathyroid cryopreservation is wise due to the 5 to 10% risk of hypoparathyroidism. Total parathyroidectomy with autograft provides similar results.[415]

Recurrent HPT is a significant problem since 50% of MEN1 patients with a "successful" parathyroidectomy will develop recurrent HPT within 8 to 12 years.[416] Placement of the autograft at distant sites facilitates imaging in the setting of recurrent HPT. To prevent late recurrence, another alternative is total parathyroidectomy followed by life-long treatment with vitamin D analogs, a challenging endocrinologic problem. Relatively unexplored is the opportunity to utilize intraoperative PTH measurement to stratify the procedure, especially given the potential to avoid hypoparathyroidism.[417,418]

It is important to note that MEN1 generates significant morbidity through hormone excess (PTH, gastrin, others) and malignant tumors (gastrinoma, islet cell tumors, foregut carcinoid). The care of patients with MEN1 relies on several principles. In contrast to MEN2, surgery has not been shown to prevent or cure MEN1 related cancer. Surgery does play a role in the management of hormonal excess for PTH and insulin. Medications manage most other tumor-related symptoms. HPTH develops at least 90% of patients with MEN1, and the preferred parathyroid operation in the HPTH of MEN1 is subtotal parathyroidectomy (with or without autograft) including a transcervical, near-total thymectomy performed simultaneously. Parathyroid tissue can be cryopreserved to retain the possibility of subsequent autograft. It is not clear whether parathyroid surgery should be performed for different indications in MEN1 than in sporadic HPT.[400]

Table 14 Management Guidelines for Patients with Asymptomatic Primary Hyperparathyroidism Who Do Not Undergo Parathyroid Surgery

Measurement	Guidelines
Serum calcium	Biannually
24-hour urinary calcium	Not recommended*
Creatinine clearance	Not recommended*
Serum creatinine	Annually†
Bone density	Annually, three sites: lumbar spine, hip, forearm
Abdominal X-ray (± ultrasound)	Not recommended*

Adapted from reference 410.

*Except at the time of the initial evaluation.

†If the serum creatinine concentration suggests a change in the creatinine clearance, when the Cockcroft-Gault equation is applied, further, more direct, assessments of the creatinine clearance are recommended.

Table 15 Multiple Endocrine Neoplasia Type 1

Endocrine Features	Nonendocrine Features (NF)
Parathyroid adenoma (90%)	Lipomas (30%)
Entero-pancreatic tumor	Facial angiofibromas (85%)
Gastrinoma (40%)	Collagenomas (70%)
Insulinoma (10%)	
NF including pancreatic polypeptide (20%)	Rare, may be innate, endocrine or nonendocrine
	features
Other: glucagonoma, VIPoma, somatostatinoma, etc (2%)	
Foregut carcinoid	
Thymic carcinoid NF (2%)	Pheochromocytoma (<1%)
Bronchial carcinoid NF (2%)	Ependymoma (1%)
Gastric enterochromaffin-like tumor NF (10%)	
Anterior pituitary tumor	
Prolactinoma (20%)	
Other: GH + PRL, GH, NF (each 5%)	
ACTH (2%), TSH (rare)	
Adrenal cortex NF (25%)	

Parathyroid Carcinoma. Parathyroid carcinoma is identified in less than 5% of patients with HPT. De Quevain provided the first description of parathyroid carcinoma in 1904 in a patient who presented with a nonfunctioning lesion.[419] In 1933, Sainton and Millot[420] described the first functioning parathyroid carcinoma. These patients have significant elevations in calcium and parathyroid hormone levels, are frequently symptomatic, often have renal or bone disease, and may present with a neck mass. In one study of 43 patients, 15 (35%) presented with polydipsia or polyuria, 11 (26%) with myalgias or arthralgias, 7 (16%) with weight loss, and 4 (9%) with nephrolithiasis; three patients (7%) were asymptomatic at presentation. At initial presentation 45% had a palpable neck mass. The mean serum calcium and serum phosphorus levels were 14.6 mg/dL and 2.3 mg/dL, respectively. Parathyroid hormone levels were elevated in 21 of 21 patients (mean elevation, 10.2 times upper limit of normal). Complications included nephrolithiasis in 56%, bone disease in 91% and both nephrolithiasis and bone disease in 53%.[421]

The primary histologic features attributed to parathyroid carcinoma include (1) uniform sheets of cells arranged in a lobulated fashion with intervening fibrous trabeculae; (2) capsular and/or vascular invasion; and (3) the presence of mitotic figures, which should be differentiated clearly from those observed in endothelial cells.[422] Unfortunately, these findings are not uniformly present and can also be found in benign parathyroid adenomas. At the initial operation, the local histologic findings that support malignancy include invasion of local tissues, perineural invasion, and vascular invasion. Regional nodal metastasis is confirmation of malignancy but is rare, distant metastases being more common.

The key molecular mechanisms responsible for the development of parathyroid cancer have not been established. The *HRPT2* gene, associated with the HPT-JT syndrome, has been suggested to contribute to the development of sporadic parathyroid carcinoma.[408,423,424] The *HRPT2* gene encodes a 531 amino acid protein, parafibromin.[425] Parafibromin is primarily located in the nucleus and downregulates the expression of cyclin D1. Mutations inactivating parafibromin have been identified in 77% of sporadic parathyroid carcinomas corresponding with the loss of immunoreactivity in most. A recent study investigating the correlation of parafibromin immunostaining and *HRPT2* mutations and LOH found that loss of parafibromin staining had a sensitivity of 100%, greater than that of *HRPT2* mutations and LOH. However, the finding of LOH or mutation was more specific.[426] Although parathyroid carcinoma is rare, in patients in whom the differentiation from atypical adenoma and carcinoma is in question, immunostaining for parafibromin holds promise.

Hypercalcemia is the primary source of morbidity and mortality in parathyroid cancer. In patients with undetectable or unresectable disease, medical management of hypercalcemia becomes of primary importance. Calcimimetic agents provide an important adjunct to conventional treatment of hypercalcemia[427] in addition to the conventional treatment of hypercalcemia (IV fluids, diuretics, and antiresorptive agents). Surgical management is focused on complete resection. Clinical and radiologic features guide the resection. A comprehensive soft tissue resection should be accomplished and may include the strap muscles, fascia, and fat in the adjacent nodal areas. The removal of adjacent nodal areas is not aimed at the removal of nodes but to provide additional soft tissue margins if there is direct extension into those areas. The role of adjuvant radiation is not well defined but may provide improved local control in patients at high risk.[421,428,429] Many patients may require re-explorations for carcinoma in the neck and mediastinum. Revision surgery does provide an effective option for control of hypercalcemia. Intraoperative PTH monitoring may be of benefit in assessing surgical "cure." No cytotoxic regimen with proven efficacy is currently available for patients with parathyroid carcinoma.

Patients with parathyroid carcinoma are few, and prognostication is difficult. Long-term follow-up is necessary, and PTH and calcium levels serve as markers for disease recurrence. Survival drops off significantly between 5 and 10 years, from approximately 80% at 5 years to 50 to 70% at 10 years. (The American college of Surgeons National Cancer Data Base survey reports overall 5- and 10-year survival rates of 85% and 49%.)[430]

Hypoparathyroidism. *Aplasia or Hypoplasia.* Hypoparathyroidism due to congenital absence or hypoplasia of the parathyroid glands typically is diagnosed neonatally and may be associated with several genetic abnormalities. The triad of hypoparathyroidism, thymic hypoplasia, and recurrent infections was initially termed the DiGeorge syndrome, described in 1965. Velocardiofacial syndrome and conotruncal anomaly-face syndrome are two separate syndromes which include the component of aplasia or hypoplasia of the parathyroid glands. A common element in 90% of these syndromes is microdeletion on chromosome 22q11.[431] Currently, all three syndromes are included in single genetic classification, chromosome 22q11 deletion syndrome. The acronym CATCH 22 has been used to summarize the major components of these syndromes (cardiac defects, abnormal facies, thymic aplasia, cleft palate, and hypocalcemia). Associated abnormalities of the third and fourth pharyngeal pouches are common; these include conotruncal defects of the heart in 25%, velopharyngeal insufficiency in 32%, cleft palate in 9%, renal anomalies in 35%, and aplasia of the thymus with severe immunodeficiency in 1%. The specific cardiac anomalies are conotruncal defects (tetralogy of Fallot, truncus arteriosus, double-outlet right ventricle, subarterial ventricular septal defect) and branchial arch defects (coarctation of the aorta, interrupted aortic arch, right aortic arch). Congenital airway anomalies such as tracheomalacia

Table 16 Contrasts between *MEN1* and *RET* Germline Mutation Tests

Test Feature	*MEN1* Gene	*RET* Gene
Information to patient and physician	Yes	Yes
Guides intervention to prevent cancer	No	Yes
Guides intervention to cure cancer	No	Yes
Recommended for child	Maybe	Yes
Chromosomal locus of gene	11q13	10cen
Mutation type to cause tumor	Inactivate	Activate
Genotype/phenotype correlation	No	Yes
Mutation test shortcuts	No	Yes
False negative rule	10–20%	2–5%

and bronchomalacia are sometimes present. The characteristic facial features associated with this syndrome have been described as prominent nose with hypoplastic nasal alae, midface hypoplasia, minor auricular anomalies, and micrognathia. This syndrome occurs in 1 per 7,500 newborns and is the most common contiguous gene deletion syndrome.[432] Most cases arise de novo, and approximately 25% are inherited from a parent. This syndrome has also been reported in a small number of patients with a deletion of chromosome 10p13, in infants of diabetic mothers, and in infants born to mothers treated with retinoic acid for acne early in pregnancy.

Hypocalcemia in chromosome 22q11 deletion syndrome most frequently manifests during the neonatal period[431,433] probably due to the interruption of the active transport of calcium from the mother to the fetus and an insufficient intake of calcium in the first few days of life. Hypocalcemia occurs in 60% of affected patients and is transitory in the majority. A spectrum of hypocalcemia may develop ranging from hypocalcemia to normal PTH levels and normal calcium.[434–437] Late onset hypocalcemia presents at times of calcemic stress (cardiac surgery and medication related altered vitamin D metabolism) and accounts for diagnosis in late adolescence and adults.[438] The majority of asymptomatic adults are identified as parents of affected children.

Autoimmune Polyendocrinopathy Related Hypoparathyroidism. Autoimmune hypoparathyroidism can occur as an isolated clinical abnormality, as part of autoimmune polyendocrinopathy syndrome 1 (APS-1) or, less commonly, as part of APS-2.[439] APS-1 most commonly comprises mucocutaneous candidiasis, hypoparathyroidism, and Addison disease. APS-2 includes two or more of the following: Addison disease, Graves disease, autoimmune thyroiditis, type 1 diabetes mellitus, primary hypogonadism, myasthenia gravis, or celiac sprue.

APS-I, also known as autoimmune polyendocrinopathy–candidiasis–ectodermal dystrophy (APECED), is a rare autosomal recessive disorder caused by defects in the autoimmune regulator (*AIRE*) gene on chromosome 21.[440,441] The disorder is manifested as chronic mucocutaneous candidiasis (100%), hypoparathyroidism (79%), and Addison disease (72%). All three elements are expressed in 51% of patients. Mucocutaneous candidiasis is often the earliest presenting symptom (during childhood) followed by hypoparathyroidism and Addison disease. Not all elements of the syndrome may be expressed, and the onset of hypoparathyroidism and Addison disease may be quite delayed requiring long-term follow-up. Dysfunction of other glands may be identified as well.[442] Gonadal failure (60% in women, 14% in men) and hypoplasia of the dental enamel (77%) were also frequent findings. Ectodermal dystrophy (pitted nails, keratopathy, and enamel hypoplasia) are not attributable to hypoparathyroidism and enamel hypoplasia may develop before or after the onset of hypoparathyroidism.[443] Recurrent

candidiasis commonly affects the mouth and nails and, less frequently, the skin and esophagus.

A target antigen for the autoantibodies found in autoimmune hypoparathyroidism was described by Li and colleagues.[444] It was noted that 56% of 25 patients, 17 with APS-1, reacted to the extracellular domain of a membrane-associated antigen of 120 to 140 kDa, which was identified as the calcium-sensing receptor. Similar results have been documented in patients with non-APS autoimmune hypoparathyroidism.

Iatrogenic Hypoparathyroidism. Hypoparathyroidism occurs most commonly as a complication of thyroid surgery and has been reported to occur transiently in up to 30% of cases and permanently in up to 4% of cases.[445–450] In a large prospective study of 5,846 patients, multivariate logistic regression analysis identified the extent of thyroidectomy (total thyroidectomy), site of ligation of the inferior thyroid artery (proximal vs peripheral), and number of identified parathyroid glands as significantly associated with the development of permanent hypoparathyroidism. Transient hypoparathyroidism was found to be associated with Graves disease, female gender, site of arterial ligation, and extent of surgery.[451] It is clear that preservation of well-vascularized parathyroid glands (two or more) should minimize this complication.

Identification of patients at risk of postoperative hypocalcemia has traditionally relied on serial determination of serum calcium levels (6-to 12-hour intervals) and close observation for the development of symptoms or signs of hypocalcemia. Postoperative hypocalcemia may develop 24 to 48 hours after thyroidectomy and prompts observation in the hospital to monitor the potential development of hypocalcemia. The introduction of rapid PTH measurement and the economic pressure for early dismissal has fostered the use of rapid PTH measurement to identify patients at risk for symptomatic hypocalcemia.[452] This study identified an 80% sensitivity and 100% specificity for a postoperative level (at the time of wound closure) of less than 10 pg/mL for the development of symptomatic hypocalcemia. Further increase sensitivity to 88% was noted when the rapid PTH was measured in the postanesthesia care unit (PACU).[453] Close observation and initiation of calcium and vitamin D supplements immediately after surgery for patients at risk are warranted (greater than 75% decrease or a level less than 12 pg/mL). A suggested starting regimen is 500 to 1,000 mg calcium carbonate (Os-Cal, GlaxoSmithKline, Research Triangle Park, NC) orally four times daily and 0.25 µg calcitriol (Rocaltrol, Roche Pharmaceuticals, Nutley, NJ) orally twice daily, which should be titrated as necessary by monitoring serial calcium levels. The development of tetany should be treated with intravenous calcium gluconate via a central line. This avoids the risk of calcium-related tissue necrosis should a peripheral line infiltrate during intravenous calcium administration. In this study, patients with PACU rapid PTH levels 12 pg/mL

or more or a 75% or lesser decline in PACU rapid PTH had a low risk of hypocalcemia. These patients should nonetheless still be counseled on symptoms of hypocalcemia and instructed to report for follow-up evaluation if these occur.

THYROID GLAND SURGERY

Modern thyroid surgery traces it origins to the work of Emil Theodor Kocher, who in 1909 received the Nobel Prize for his contributions to medicine, physiology, and surgery. As Professor of Surgery in Bern (1872–1917), Kocher contributed more than any other surgeon to the development of safe thyroidectomy and the science of thyroid surgery. His results for goiter surgery were remarkable for the time, with overall mortality in more than 2,000 cases a remarkable 4.5% and by the end of the nineteenth century for simple goiter that mortality rate was 2%. Following Kocher came several surgeons who pioneered advances in the art of thyroid surgery. Identification of the role of the parathyroid glands, establishing the importance of preserving the recurrent laryngeal nerve, employing preoperative iodine in patients with Graves disease, and advancing the role of subtotal thyroidectomy in advanced thyrotoxic patients were problems faced by subsequent surgeons and physicians. Halsted, Mayo, Crile, Lahey, and Dunhill all played prominent roles in the development of modern thyroid surgery.

Surgery for diseases of the thyroid gland requires understanding of the anatomy of the mediastinum and neck as well as the embryology of the branchial apparatus and laryngopharyngeal physiology. This knowledge must be integrated with an understanding of the pathophysiology of the specific disease process affecting the thyroid gland. The preceding sections of the chapter outline the diseases of the thyroid gland and the role surgery has in each. This section will review the key steps in a standard thyroidectomy, consider specific indications for thyroidectomy, intraoperative PTH monitoring, wound drainage, nerve monitoring, and review specific issues in thyroid surgery.

Steps in Standard Surgery of the Thyroid Gland

Consent. Informed consent for thyroid surgery requires a discussion addressing the risks of the type of anesthesia (general vs sedation with local anesthesia), incisions, the consequences of the absence of thyroid tissue, the risk of injury to neck structures, removal of area VI, VII, and lateral nodes, extension of surgery based on intraoperative findings, convalescence, hospital stay, and follow-up.

Preoperative Preparation. Patients are instructed to avoid aspirin for 7 days and nonsteroidal anti-inflammatory medications for at least 2 days. Patients on Coumadin are appropriately bridged to heparin if indicated. A prothrombin time international normalized ratio (INR) is determined prior to surgery in patients receiving Coumadin or heparin therapy.

In the operating room, the patient is anesthetized and intubated. An endotracheal tube with implanted wire electrodes can be placed to facilitate recurrent and vagal nerve monitoring. In patients with historical office examination or imaging evidence of tracheal or esophageal invasion, esophagoscopy, laryngoscopy, and tracheoscopy facilitate operative planning. The author consistently places a Maloney bougie in the esophagus. This facilitates identification of the esophagus and the tracheoesophageal groove as well as providing anterior displacement of the laryngotracheal complex. This anterior displacement provides greater separation of the larynx and trachea from the prevertebral space aiding in the identification of the structures in the tracheoesophageal groove.

Positioning. The patient is placed supine with neck extension accomplished by a shoulder roll (Figure 3). Appropriate support of the occiput must be maintained. In patients with severe rheumatoid arthritis, flexion and extension views of the cervical spine should be obtained to assess stability. Patients with Down syndrome may also have cervical spine abnormalities.

Skin Preparation. For patients who will undergo postoperative I-131 therapy, it is advisable to avoid Betadine since significant iodine absorption may occur.[454]

Thyroidectomy. Performing a thyroidectomy involves a skin incision of appropriate size to

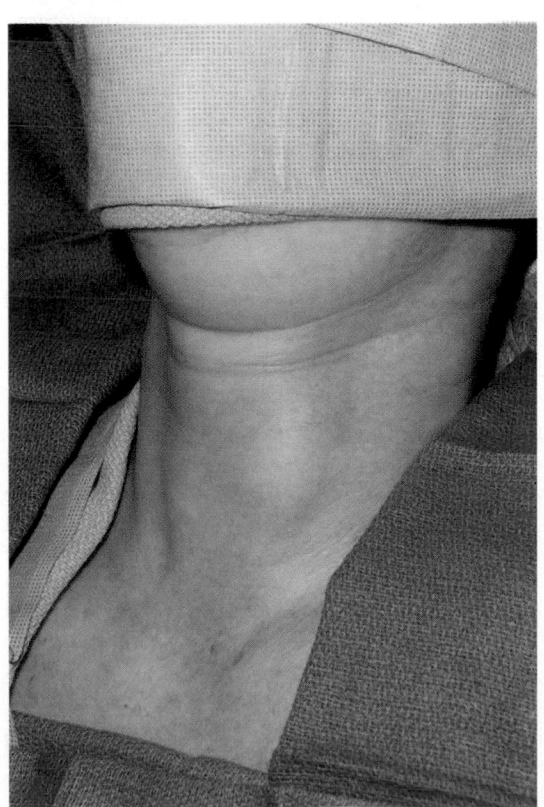

Figure 3 Patient positioned and prepared for standard thyroidectomy (left thyroid mass). (Copyrighted and used with permission of Mayo Foundation for Medical Education and Research.)

address the clinically expected pathology. This may be a limited incision or an incision of sufficient length to allow bilateral lymph node dissections as far superior as area II and as far posterior as area V. Laterally the platysma will provide a superficial landmark for flap elevation. Medially, the platysma is absent and the plane of dissection is superficial to the anterior jugular veins. Typically flap elevation is extended to the level of the anterior superior edge of the thyroid cartilage and inferiorly to the sternum. The strap muscles are identified and separated in the midline, exposing the isthmus and area VI.

Evaluation of the extent of the thyroid pathology should be ongoing during the course of the procedure. Elevation or division of the sternohyoid and sternothyroid musculature provides exposure of the anterior surface of the thyroid lobes. Identification and ligation of the middle thyroid vein are followed by the mobilization of the lateral border of the thyroid gland superiorly and inferiorly. At this point, the inferior parathyroid gland could be seen and, if noted, preserved. The superior pole of the thyroid is then isolated allowing identification of the external branch of the superior laryngeal nerve and ligation of the superior thyroid artery and vein. Dissection of the inferior pole then facilitates mobilization of the gland anteriorly. The recurrent nerve can be identified in several locations. The cricothyroid articulation is a consistent landmark rarely obscured by thyroid disease. The recurrent nerve will enter the larynx just posterior and superior to the joint. Alternatively, identification of the recurrent nerve in the tracheoesophageal groove after elevation of the thyroid lobe medially may require dissection and mobilization of fat. Palpation of the nerve and location of the inferior thyroid artery provide clues to finding the nerve. At this point review of the location of the parathyroid glands is followed by ligation of the inferior thyroid artery and associated veins, taking care to preserve blood supply to the parathyroids if not limited by thyroid pathology.

Once the parathyroid glands and the recurrent nerve have been identified, the thyroid lobe can be elevated off the trachea which requires division of the ligamentous attachments of the thyroid gland to the trachea (Berry ligament) located near the junction of the trachea and cricoid cartilage (Figure 4). The size of the lobe, the presence of gland inflammation, and the proximity of the nerve to the Berry ligament influence the difficulty of this dissection and the ability to remove all thyroid tissue. Careful use of vessel clips or fine suture ligature is favored over bipolar cautery. The surgeon should be aware of the potential for the presence of a pyramidal lobe and include this tissue in the resection. When the thyroid resection is performed for malignancy, the fat and lymph nodes located between the recurrent nerves laterally and from the superior border of the thyroid cartilage to the sternal notch are removed again preserving the inferior parathyroid gland (level VI dissection).

Once the thyroidectomy is completed, the wound is examined for the quality of hemostasis.

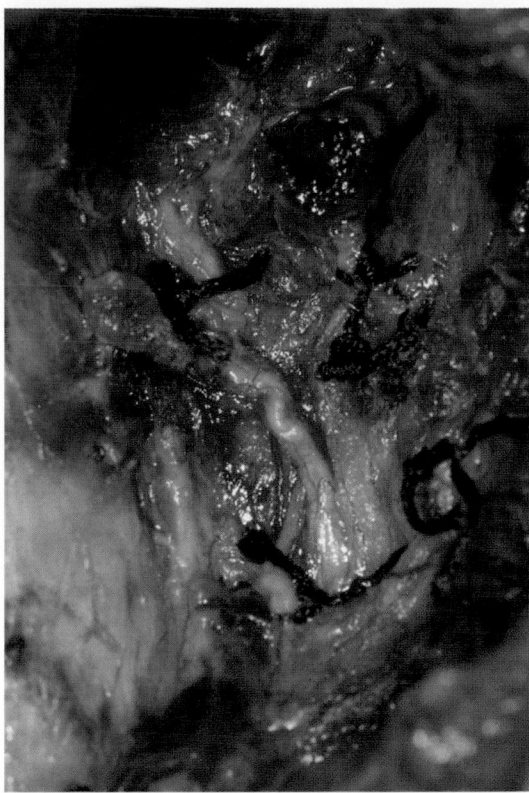

Figure 4 Close-up view of the bed of the left lobe of the thyroid gland demonstrating an intact recurrent nerve, suture ligature of adjacent vasculature, and a vascularized parathyroid gland. (Copyrighted and used with permission of Mayo Foundation for Medical Education and Research.)

Any concern regarding the stability or integrity of hemostasis should be assessed by combining a temporary increase in venous pressure, by the application of positive pressure via the endotracheal tube, with irrigation and wound inspection prior to closure. The need for routine drain placement following thyroid surgery has been scrutinized for some time.[455] The populations studied generally included routine thyroidectomy and occasionally parathyroid procedures. The incidence of hematoma formation, length of hospital stay, volume of fluid in the operative cavity based on ultrasound examination whether using passive versus active drainage or high versus low vacuum were documented and were not found to be significantly different between patients with or without drains. One study found that drains prompted a longer hospital stay.[456] Therefore, routine drainage of thyroid or parathyroid operative site is not necessary. The surgeon must evaluate the wound and integrate the extent of the surgical cavity and the risk of bleeding on an individual basis. Formal nodal dissections involving areas II, III, IV, or V should prompt consideration of routine drainage.

Minimally Invasive Video-Assisted Thyroidectomy. The development of videolaparoscopic abdominal surgery fostered the formation and application of minimal access techniques to other surgical procedures. In minimally invasive video-assisted thyroidectomy (MIVAT), application of endoscopic viewing of the thyroid bed via a small incision has been completed in large series of patients[457] and studied in a randomized fashion.[458–461]

Three elements facilitate performance of the thyroidectomy via limited access: improved visualization with angled telescopes, hemostasis with the harmonic scalpel, and an additional assistant for retraction or holding the scope. Limited access has less flexibility to manage problematic bleeding, large masses and address adenopathy and therefore requires careful patient selection. An example of guidelines for patient selection include the following: thyroid nodule less than 35 mm in largest diameter, ultrasound estimated thyroid gland volume less than 20 mL, no thyroiditis, no prior neck surgery, and no history of radiation. Malignancies other than low-risk papillary thyroid cancer, presence of enlarged lymph nodes, and goiters greater than 20 mL are considered contraindications to MIVAT. Benefits confirmed include less pain and improved cosmesis. An issue yet to be resolved is the efficiency and efficacy of central compartment node dissection.[462]

Harmonic Scalpel (HS). The HS is an instrument that uses vibration at 55.5 kHz, that is, mechanical action, to cut and coagulate tissue simultaneously and generates minimal lateral thermal tissue damage, less smoke formation, no neuromuscular stimulation, and no electrical energy to or through the patient. Multiple studies have identified various advantages compared to standard methods.[463–465] The primary advantage is the ability to effectively coagulate the vasculature encountered in routine thyroid surgery with decreased access thus facilitating minimal access surgery and decreased operating time (10 to 35%) when compared to standard techniques. Other reported benefits include decrease drainage and less pain. The importance of decreased drainage is uncertain since the need for drain placement in routine thyroid surgery has not been supported by large studies. Whether decreased pain will be further substantiated and found to be clinically significant remains to be determined. One disadvantage is the cost associated with the disposable instrument.[466] When using the instrument, one must appreciate that the functional end of the instrument retains heat and accurate exit from the wound cavity is necessary after activation.

Complications of Thyroidectomy. Complications of surgery for thyroid diseases have been noted and scrutinized since the inception of thyroid surgery. Abu al-Qasim, Islam's legendary medieval surgeon, is credited with performing the first goiter excision in which the patient just avoided exsanguination, as recorded in his surgical tome, "Al-Tasrif," in 952 AD. The concern regarding the safety of thyroid surgery in the mid-nineteenth century was characterized by the opinion of Diffenbach in Germany who in 1848 condemned such surgery to be, "one of the most thankless, most perilous undertakings which, if not altogether prohibited, should at least be restricted," dismissing such operations as "foolhardy performances" (Dieffenbach JF. Die

Operative Chirurgie II. Leipzig: FA Brockhaus; 1848. p. 331). The position of Liston in 1846 was similarly pessimistic suggesting one "could not cut the thyroid gland out of the living body in its sound condition without risking the death of the patient from haemorrhage. It is a proceeding by no means to be thought of"(Liston R, Mutter TD. Lectures on the operations of surgery and on diseases and accidents requiring operations. Philadelphia: Lea Blanchard; 1846. p. 318). In 1866 Gross also denounced thyroid surgery as "horrid butchery deserving of rebuke and condemnation," and that "no honest and sensible surgeon would ever engage in it" (Gross SD. A System of Surgery, 4th edition. Philadelphia: Lea Febiger; 1866. p. 394). Fortunately, pioneers in the field of thyroid surgery persevered, and today thyroid surgery is considered safe and effective.

As with any surgical procedure involving a skin incision and formation of a surgical wound or cavity, potential exists for hemorrhage into the wound and postoperative wound infection. The incidence of wound infections typically occurs in less than 1% of cases. This seems to be independent of whether antibiotic prophylaxis or antibiotic prophylaxis and subsequent antibiotic therapy are administered.[467] Hemorrhage is similarly uncommon, occurring in less than 2% of patients and noted at a higher rate in bilateral procedures than in unilateral procedures. Hemorrhage is a particularly worrisome complication due to the potential for airway obstruction. If noted, emergent airway evaluation and drainage are required.

Hypocalcemia is the most common complication following thyroid surgery occurring in 10 to 33% of patients, and the highest rates of hypocalcemia are associated with total thyroidectomy.[467–469] Hypocalcemia is related to transient hypoparathyroidism in the vast majority of cases (>95%). Preservation of the vascular pedicle to the parathyroid glands provides the best insurance of avoiding permanent hypocalcemia. The number of parathyroid glands necessary to maintain normal serum calcium levels has not been determined. During thyroidectomy, if the parathyroid glands are anatomically well separated from the thyroid in the parathyroid capsule, the surgeon may easily preserve them without significant manipulation. In contrast, if they are attached to the thyroid capsule, as is often the case, they must be accurately separated, and pericapsular ligature of the branches of the inferior thyroid artery must be carefully executed. The posterolateral branch of the superior thyroid artery should be ligated only after having determined that it does not supply the superior parathyroid gland.[470] A devascularized parathyroid gland is minced and reimplantated in a muscle body and localized with a nonabsorbable suture.

Early identification of patients at risk for postoperative hypocalcemia would facilitate institution of vitamin D and calcium therapy in appropriate individuals. Because the onset of symptomatic hypocalcemia tends to occur 24 to 48 hours after resection, early dismissal places

patients dismissed within 24 hours at risk of developing symptoms in a nonhospital setting. Recent studies provide strong support that intraoperative parathyroid hormone levels can provide this stratification.[468,469] The results of these studies suggest that patients with decreases of 75% or greater from baseline PTH at either ten or 20 minutes postresection should be considered for administration of calcium and vitamin D.

Laryngeal nerve injury is perhaps the most frustrating complication following thyroid surgery due to the impact on the patient's quality of life. Identification of either recurrent nerve injury or injury of the external branch of the superior laryngeal nerve requires careful laryngeal postoperative examination. Postoperative nerve injury in a large study from Italy was noted in 3.4% of 14,934 patients.[467] This accounted for 22% of the noted complications. As expected, when both lobes of the thyroid were manipulated, a greater number of laryngeal nerve injuries were identified. Approximately half of the injuries were permanent. At least one large series supports the routine identification of the recurrent laryngeal nerve to minimize nerve injury.[471]

Laryngeal nerve monitoring may be employed to aid the surgeon in nerve identification and preservation as well as provide some estimate of postoperative vocal fold mobility. Nerve monitoring in thyroid surgery focuses on recurrent laryngeal nerve with muscle activity identified by hook wire electrodes placed in the vocal fold, electrodes imbedded in an endotracheal tube, a paddle placed in the postcricoid region, or a finger placed in the region of the arytenoid cartilage. Regardless of the method of monitoring, anatomical knowledge and a principled approach to the procedure are required as each monitoring system has limitations and potential for system failure. It is not clear whether the use of a nerve monitoring system decreases the rate of nerve injury.[472] The potential benefits of nerve monitoring should be balanced with the costs. Some data exist to support utility of predicting postoperative recurrent nerve function with nerve stimulation and palpation of arytenoid cartilage motion.[473,474] Altenatively, others conclude that the sensitivity and specificity were insufficient to be useful.[475] The low percentage of patients with postoperative nerve injury following routine thyroid surgery requires that a large population be studied to determine whether nerve monitoring in some form will provide a significant reduction in nerve injury or be sufficiently accurate to differentiate temporary versus permanent vocal fold dysfunction. A selected group of patients undergoes nerve monitoring by one of the authors (JLK), specifically patients in whom risk of nerve injury is particularly high, such as advanced malignancy, large benign lesions, or revision surgery, with the goal of facilitating nerve identification in challenging operative fields.

Well-Differentiated Follicular Cell Derived Thyroid Cancer: Extent of Thyroidectomy. The principles and concepts driving surgical decision-making for well-differentiated FCDTC are plagued by high-level data deprivation, and debate ensues based on large retrospective studies. Data support improved cause-specific mortality and recurrence with a transition from lobectomy to near total or total thyroidectomy.[476] This issue has come into greater scrutiny in part due to the earlier identification of thyroid carcinomas due to the routine use of ultrasonography. The earlier identification has likely prompted the increased incidence noted for thyroid cancer recently.[191] In this group of patients, one must keep in mind the behavior of PTC, which is usually a slow growing, indolent tumor. As noted elsewhere in this chapter, reliable prognostic indicators exist to predict the outcome in PTC in particular. Some authorities recommend performing a total thyroidectomy in all patients because of advantages such as removing contralateral microscopic disease, improving the specificity of serial postoperative thyroglobulin measurements, allowing radioactive iodine to be administered to ablate residual thyroid tissue and treat residual cancer, and possibly decreasing the recurrence rate and increasing survival. A near-total or total thyroidectomy may not hold an advantage over lobectomy in low- or high-risk patients, however, and lobectomy generates less risk of recurrent laryngeal nerve injury and postoperative hypocalcemia.[477] In the United States, most patients are treated with a near-total or total thyroidectomy. It is likely that in Stage I disease the extent of thyroid surgery does not impact survival.[272]

SUMMARY

To optimize the quality of care for the patient with thyroid cancer, the pre-operative assessment, surgical approach, adjuvent therapy and post-operative surveillance should involve an integrated, consistent team-based approach. These authors find that patients with thyroid cancer are best managed with an initial near-total thyroidectomy, central neck dissection for those patients with PTC, Hürthle cell variant FTC or MTC, and more extensive compartmental node dissection guided by pre-operative ultrasound findings. This approach also characterizes the surgical management recommended by several professional organizations in recently published guidelines for the management of thyroid cancer.

Substernal Goiter. A challenging problem in a small population of patients with multinodular goiter is extension of the disease into the mediastinum (Figures 5 and 6). Symptomatic patients often present with dyspnea, dysphagia, choking, and hoarseness. The following issues require consideration in this group of patients: risk of malignancy, correlation of the mass with tracheal or esophageal obstruction, and risk of resection. In general the risk of malignancy in multinodular goiter is low (17%),[478] however, the techniques that facilitate the stratification of risk of malignancy (ultrasound and FNA) are not readily applicable to the substernal extension of

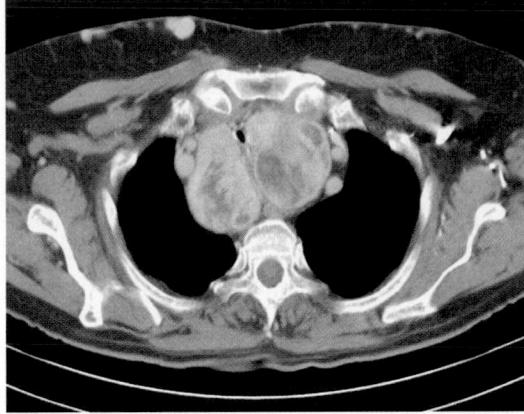

Figure 5 Computed tomography shows the substernal extention of multinodular goiter generating tracheal compression and airway obstruction. (Copyrighted and used with permission of Mayo Foundation for Medical Education and Research.)

the goiter. CT does demonstrate the extent of the goiter, adjacent vascular anatomy, and distortion of the tracheal and esophageal lumen. CT is not as sensitive as ultrasound in identification of features suggesting malignancy. Correlation of the radiographic finding with symptoms can be facilitated by functional studies. Pulmonary function studies[479] and a video swallow study with an esophagram will assess compromise of tracheal and esophageal patency.

Those patients with substernal goiter and symptoms that correlate with functional studies should be offered surgical removal. The procedure should be coordinated with a thoracic surgeon available in case a thoracotomy would be required. Office fiberoptic tracheoscopy facilitates evaluation of the airway diameter and dynamics. This information promotes a safer endotracheal anesthesia, facilitates fiberoptic intubation guiding the endotracheal tube past the tracheal deformity, allows the patient to maintain spontaneous respiration until intubated, and can be performed in an upright position during intubation in those patients whose dyspnea is exacerbated in a supine position.

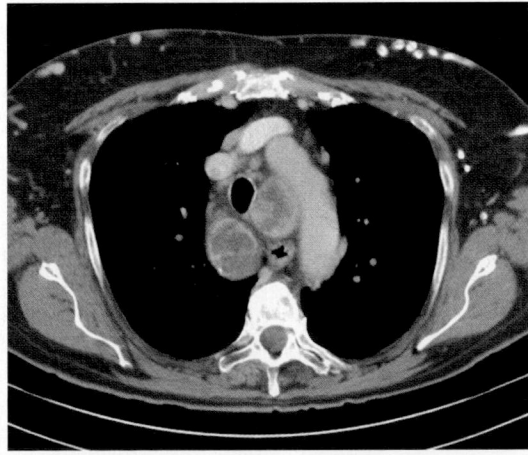

Figure 6 Computed tomography shows the inferior extent of the substernal goiter shown in Figure 5. This goiter was successfully removed through the neck and the patient did not require a tracheostomy. (Copyrighted and used with permission of Mayo Foundation for Medical Education and Research.)

The procedure requires some modifications from standard thyroid surgery. A larger incision is required to allow egress of the mass, the strap muscles will likely require division, and identification of the recurrent nerves and parathyroid glands may be more challenging (Figures 7 and 8). Nerve monitoring may be of help not only to identify the nerve but also to detect stretch induced nerve stimulation. Identification of the nerve near the cricothyroid articulation may be technically easier when the substernal extension and goiter size prevent rotation of the gland anteromedially, limiting access to the tracheoesophageal groove. The need for a thoracotomy is rare as most cases can be elevated into the neck. A suspicion of malignancy, prior surgery, and previous external beam irradiation increase the potential need for a sternotomy. The sternotomy can be limited to the upper one-third of the sternum and is generally well tolerated by the patient. Drain placement should be considered routine. Tracheomalacia is rarely a problem and can preliminarily be assessed by fiberoptic examination on extubation which would also allow evaluation of vocal fold mobility. Extubation over an airway exchange catheter is a safe option.

Conservation and Reconstructive Surgery of the Larynx, Pharynx, Trachea, and Esophagus in Advanced Thyroid Cancer. It is indeed fortunate for patients with thyroid cancer and for the head and neck surgeon that the majority of thyroid carcinomas are PTCs. This provides a patient population which, in the vast majority of cases, will likely survive the cancer being treated but may unfortunately mute the suspicion of aggressive disease. Ideally, the patient's initial surgery should be the only procedure required in the thyroid bed with a goal of microscopically free margins. Therefore, an appropriate preoperative evaluation combined with a surgeon or surgical team skilled should result in complete resection of the disease and preservation of voice and swallowing. To accomplish this goal, skills in conservation and reconstructive surgery of the larynx, trachea, pharynx, and esophagus are invaluable.

Characteristic symptoms and findings which should prompt investigation of invasive and aggressive disease and require an advanced surgical skill set include the following: pain

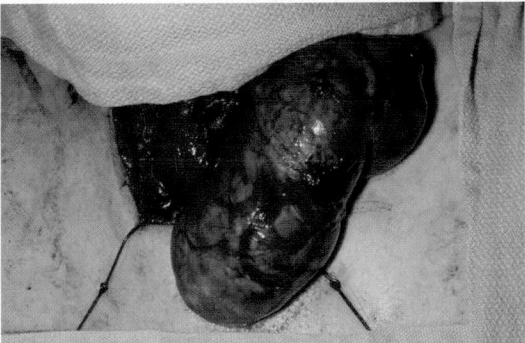

Figure 7 The goiter is advanced onto the neck. (Copyrighted and used with permission of Mayo Foundation for Medical Education and Research.)

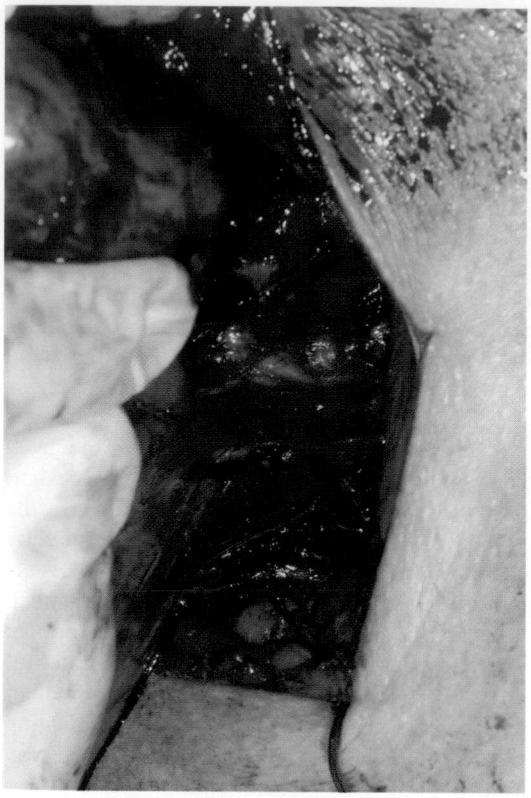

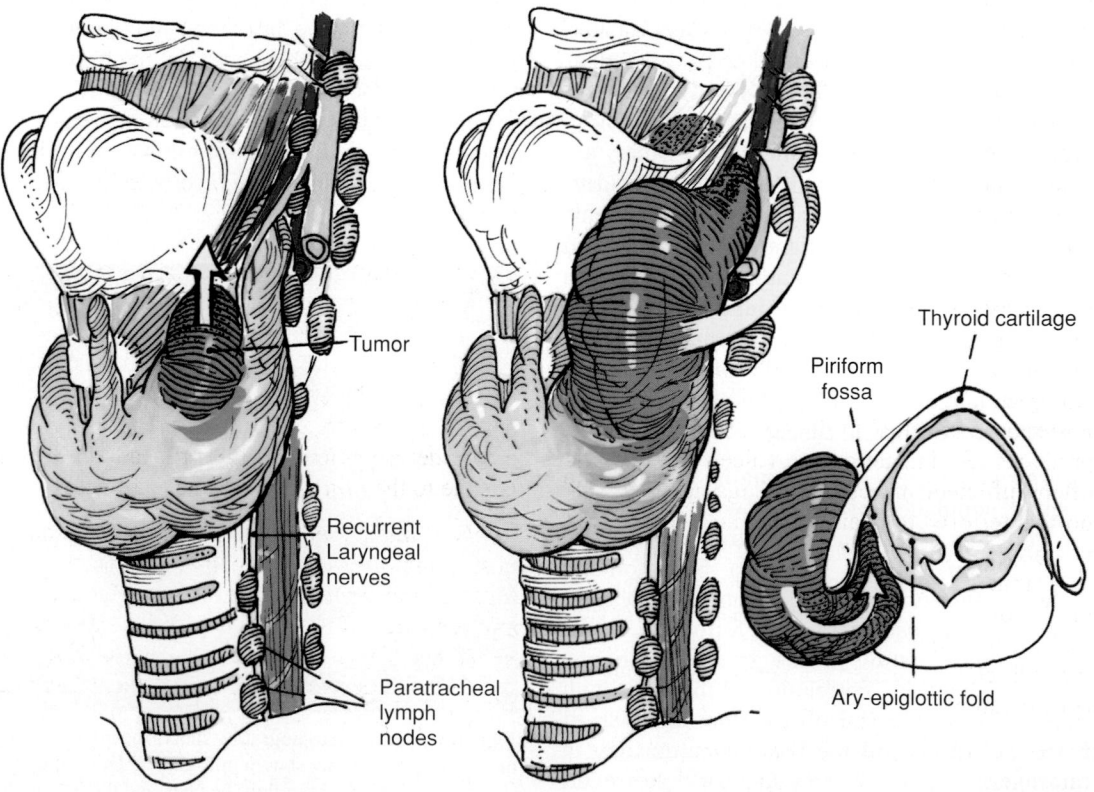

Figure 8 Identification and preservation of the recurrent nerve during removal a substernal goiter. (Copyrighted and used with permission of Mayo Foundation for Medical Education and Research.)

(perineural invasion, mucosal ulceration), rapid growth (higher grade tumor), dysphagia (compression or invasion of the pharynx or esophagus), dysphonia (vocal fold paralysis, tumor volume altering laryngeal anatomy), hemoptysis or bloody secretions (tumor invasion through airway or digestive tract mucosa), and large tumor volume in the thyroid or neck.

The assessment of cancer invasion of the larynx and trachea is best evaluated by direct examination combined with CT or MRI imaging. Direct examination of the larynx is facilitated by fiberoptic examination. By topically anesthetizing the supraglottis, glottis, and upper trachea, an excellent view of the airway mucosa from the epiglottis to the carina can be obtained in the office. With the advent of transnasal esophagoscopy, the cricopharygeal region and esophagus can also be examined in an office setting. Findings of importance include luminal narrowing, aberrant submucosal vasculature, mucosal ulceration, and intralumenal tumor mass. Radiographic studies provide information regarding tumor volume, mediastinal extension, and can identify intraluminal tumor but are not as sensitive as direct examination in identification of invasion. In our experience the most consistently useful study is a high-resolution (64 slice) CT scan. The use of iodine-containing contrast material creates some difficulty with post-operative treatment and imaging with radioactive iodine, but clearance of that iodine load is typically complete within 8–12 weeks, following which radioactive iodine can be administered in the usual way. Although MRI may provide better soft tissue information,

motion of the airway related to respiration frequently degrades images. Ultrasound imaging is not useful in the evaluation of aerodigestive tract invasion and cannot evaluate the extent of mediastinal disease.

Sites of Invasion. Sites of early extracapsular invasion of thyroid cancer include the upper three tracheal rings, the anterior and lateral border of the cricoid cartilage, posterior inferior aspect of the thyroid cartilage, the recurrent laryngeal nerve, and on the left the esophagus. As cancer volume expands, extention into the cricothyroid, retrotracheal, and retropharyngeal space developes. The perichondrium and cartilage provide a relatively strong barrier to tumor extension into the airway lumen while natural gaps in continuity or loss of cartilaginous integrity from shave resections may provide access to the lumen or the cartilaginous space. The nonstructural factors determining invasion are not well defined but likely involve interactions between the immune system and tumor derived cytokines and angiogenic factors.

The surgical approach to upper aerodigestive tract invasion by thyroid cancer is guided by the concepts of conservation surgery but requires an approach based on the pathway of invasion that is different from mucosally derived aerodigestive tract cancer. Knowledge of laryngeal anatomy and physiology and experience with mucosal malignancies provide the essential grasp of the structural requirements and resection limits allowing organ preservation. For example, knowledge of partial laryngeal surgery (partial vertical, supraglottic, and supracricoid laryngectomy) will

vastly impact the ability to approach complete resection of invasive thyroid cancer with voice and swallowing preservation. Thus, the need to consider a laryngopharyngectomy is a rare event even in advanced cancers. Options for conservation surgery are limited, however, by external beam irradiation due to its effect on tissue vascularity. Although conservation surgery can be considered after external beam radiation, there is a much greater risk of chondritis and wound breakdown.

Invasion of the pharynx and esophagus is much less common than invasion of the larynx, cricoid cartilage, and trachea. When the invasion is limited to the muscular coat, a myectomy preserving mucosal integrity is practical. When mucosa is invaded, the potential for a salivary fistula is established and the tolerance of primary closure is site dependent. The hypopharynx has a greater surface area and a larger defect can be closed primarily while resections at the level of the cricopharyngeus or upper cervical esophagus are more likely to result in some degree of stenoisis. In this setting, preoperative planning for reconstruction of the defect helps limit the tendency to fail to resect disease.[299,300]

Larynx and Pharynx. The attachment of the strap musculature to the oblique line of the thyroid cartilage positions a superior-lobe neoplasm directly adjacent to the perichondrium of the thyroid alae. Laryngeal invasion can occur through cartilaginous perforations following blood vessels or can reach the piriform sinus by extending posteriorly and medially to the thyroid ala (Figures 9 and 10).

Figure 9 An upper pole tumor with superiorly directed growth meets resistance at the oblique line. Subsequent growth extends posteriorly and invades through the pharyngeal constrictors to begin to fill the piriform sinus. (Copyrighted and used with permission of Mayo Foundation for Medical Education and Research.)

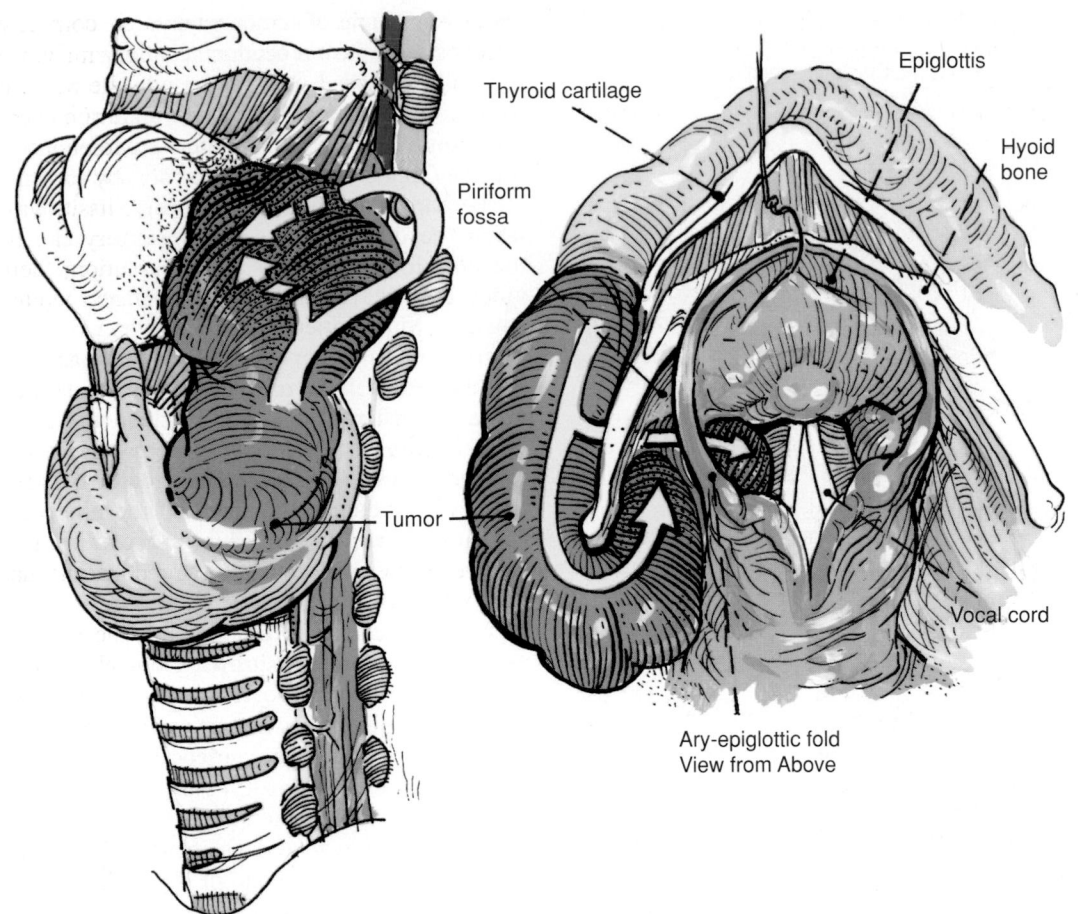

Figure 10 This figure demonstrates routes of invasion into the larynx and pharynx by tumor in the upper pole of the left thyroid lobe. Direct invasion through the thyroid ala reaches the anterior part of the piriform sinus or the paraglottic space of the larynx. When the tumor extends posteriorly to the thyroid ala, it accesses the posterior part of the piriform sinus and has proximity to the prevertebral fascia. (Copyrighted and used with permission of Mayo Foundation for Medical Education and Research.)

Growth of tumor superiorly from the isthmus superior to the cricoid cartilage can extend into the subglottis via the cricothyroid space. There are relatively few structural barriers in this area until the conus elasticus is reached.

Extension within the paraglottic space, can progress easily from the upper border of the cricoid to the pre-epiglottic fat, aryepiglottic fold and piriform sinus due to a lack of a structural boundry (Figure 11). Access can occur via a lateral thyrotomy with or without resection of cartilage. Resection of a thyroid ala with preservation of laryngeal mucosa will generate deviation of the anterior commisure and alter vocal fold tension generating a hoarse voice. Tumor extention posterior and medial to the thyroid ala generally produces less impact on the voice since there is often sufficient muscular and ligamentous support anteriorly to maintain a more functional position of the vocal folds. Resection of piriform sinus mucosa is generally well tolerated. Dysphagia becomes a consideration when the resection extends onto the posterior pharyngeal wall. Pharyngeal reconstruction then becomes a necessary consideration.

Cricoid Cartilage and the Hypopharynx. Cricoid cartilagenous and adjacent hypopharyngeal invasion by thyroid cancer presents greater challenges for functional preservation than adjacent sites. This relates to the key role the cricoid cartilage

plays in serving as the foundation of the larynx and the transition from the generous surface area of the piriform sinus region to the limited surface area of the cricopharyngeal region. The posterior part of the cricoid cartilage supports the thyroid and arytenoid cartilages and provides the origin of the posterior cricoarytcnoid muscle. Resections in this area are necessarily intimate with the recurrent nerve and readily impact arytenoid function and the position of arytenoid and thyroid cartilages with potential airway narrowing. Mucosal resections in this area of a limited extent can be tolerated. Based on the residual lumen, one should expect a need for augmentation of the lumen at the time of resection or dilatation of a post-surgical stenosis. The optimal flap to consider is a microvascular free radial forearm flap due to the thin pliable tissue available.

Trachea and Esophagus. Tracheal invasion is most commonly identified in the anterior two-thirds of the tracheal circumference due to the approximation of the thyroid gland to this area of the trachea (Figures 12 and 13). The surface area involved will determine the required resection. If limited in extent, a wedge resection and primary closure without resecting the posterior wall of the trachea may be all that is involved. When the defect requires mobilization of the trachea for closure, a segmental resection with primary closure is utilized. Extention of the resection into

the subglottis generates a greater risk of glottic edema, and the need for a tracheostomy is significantly increased.

On the left side, posterior extension generates potential for esophageal involvement. Tumor can fill the potential space between the trachea and esophagus and potentially invade both structures. With esophageal muscle involvement only, a myectomy preserving intact mucosa is completed. This resection should not generate significant symptoms of dysphagia, but patients may note pharyngeal reflux similar to that following a cricopharyngeal myotomy. When mucosa is involved to a limited extent, primary closure can be accomplished. The team should be prepared for a radial forearm microvascular free flap reconstruction.

Occasionally, tumor will insinuate between the trachea and esophagus with an opening developing in the posterior wall of the trachea and a defect in the trachea (Figures 14 and 15). If small in diameter, primary closure with interposition of a muscle flap should promote healing and prevention of a tracheoesophageal fistula. Larger defects are best managed with a microvascular free flap (Figures 16 and 17).

Lymph Nodes. Lymph nodes with extracapsular extension of tumor can be the source of invasive thyroid cancer (Figure 18). When the larynx, pharynx, trachea, or esophagus is involved, principles outlined above will generally facilitate successful management. As disease extends farther inferiorly, the surgical team should be prepared to improve access and vascular control with a partial sternotomy (Figure 19).

A well-prepared surgical team should rarely need to consider a laryngopharyngectomy when treating advanced thyroid cancer unless significant posterior cricoid and interarytenoid invasion are not amenable to preservation of the larynx. Replacement of large areas of hypopharyngeal mucosa would generate a risk of aspiration due to the loss of sensate mucosa. Comorbidities must be considered when aspiration may be generated. For example, limited aspiration that may resolve with swallowing therapy would likely be tolerated by an individual with normal pulmonary reserve but could be life threatening in a patient with severe chronic obstructive pulmonary disease.

Anaplastic Thyroid Carcinoma. Surgery for ATC should be considered for two primary reasons, obtaining tissue for diagnosis and palliation.[197,480] Often, FNA will establish the diagnosis, but not infrequently cases occur where the cytology does not clarify whether a high-grade lymphoma, high-grade metastatic lesion or ATC is present (Figure 20). In that setting, an open biopsy is indicated. The issue of whether a tracheostomy should be performed should be individualized. If there are significant comorbidities and evidence of metastasis, consideration should be given to avoiding a tracheostomy as the challenge of caring for a tracheostomy may significantly detract from the patient's quality of life. Often

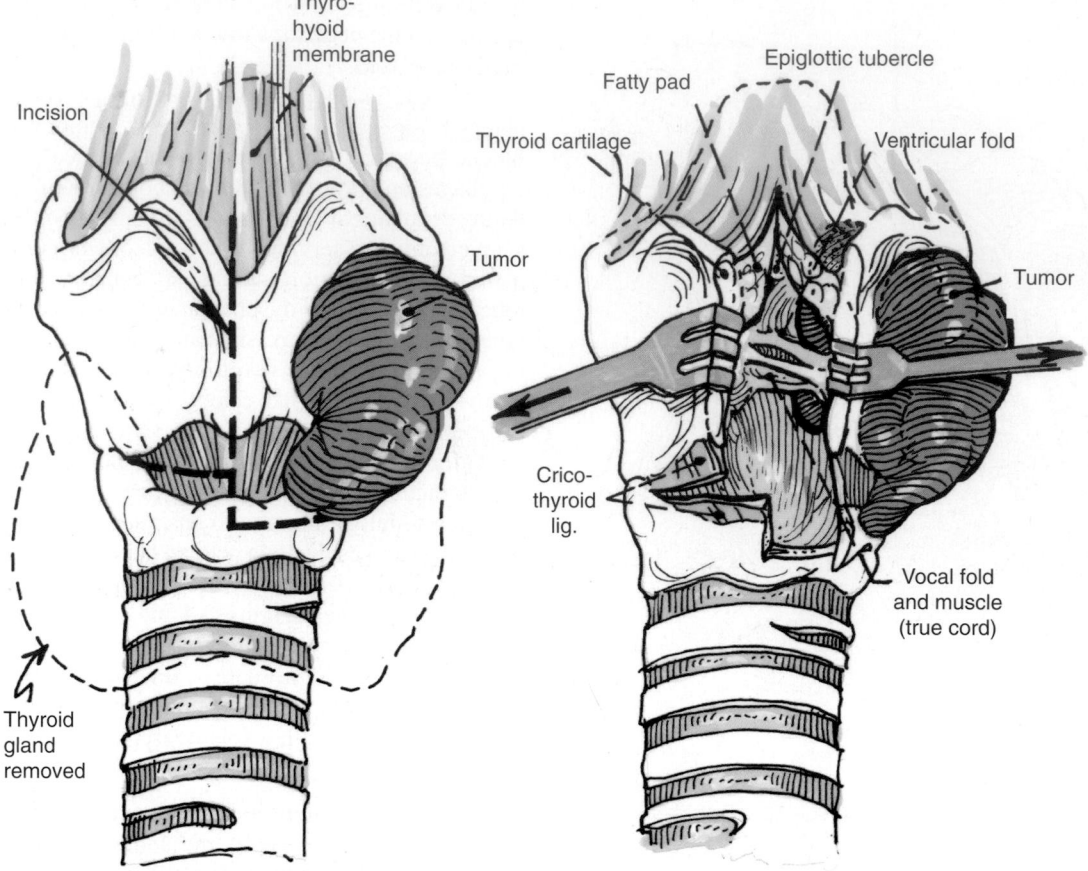

Figure 11 Residual/recurrent thyroid cancer invading the upper border of the cricoid cartilage and the thyroid ala with extension into the paraglottic space. This figure illustrates the ligamentous structures of the larynx which can facilitate preservation of the airway and voice if not involved by cancer. This figure also demonstrates the outside-in pathway of invasion. (Copyrighted and used with permission of Mayo Foundation for Medical Education and Research.)

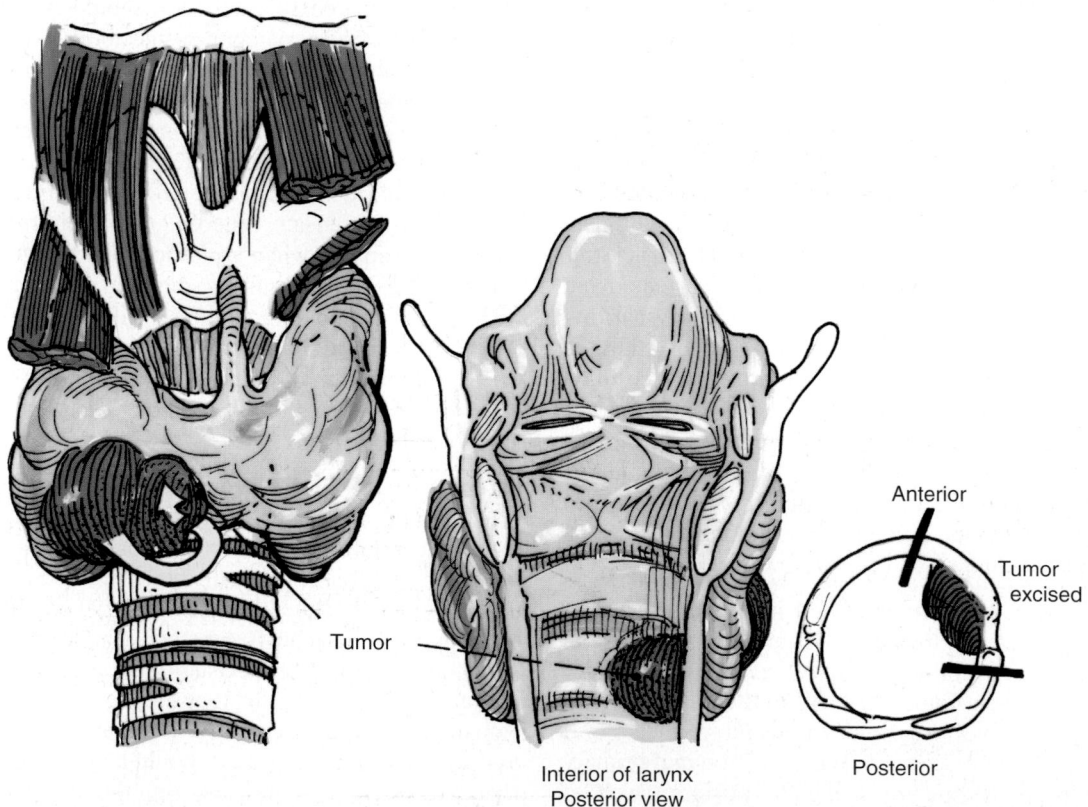

Figure 12 The primary tumor has invaded the anterior–lateral wall of the trachea and an excision of approximately one fourth the circumference of the trachea is pictured. In this case, a fusiform excision oriented transversely would facilitate primary closure. (Copyrighted and used with permission of Mayo Foundation for Medical Education and Research.)

the large volume of tumor renders creation of a tracheostomy site a procedural challenge, and the site will be seeded with high-grade cancer cells likely to enlarge promptly. High-quality hospice care should be able to facilitate a graceful end of life even in the setting of airway obstruction.

Perhaps the most challenging situation is when the diagnosis has been established, and the decision required is whether surgery provides benefit, particularly in younger healthy pateints. Most patients who survive ATC have small primary tumors identified at the time of resection of an initial papillary or follicular carcinoma and undergo postoperative chemoradiation. Resectability or unresectability may be difficult to define or establish. Resection should be undertaken with the understanding that the procedure is palliative and that residual microscopic disease is likely locally or regionally. For example, a 44-year-old father of three children has a large thyroid and neck mass recently biopsy-confirmed as ATC. His tumor is growing out the biopsy site in his neck lateral to the sternocleidomastoid muscle. The tumor has not encased the common carotid artery, and the prevertebral space and the esophagus appear normal. No metastatic disease was noted on PET/CT imaging. This patient was offered resection to reduce local and regional disease and alter his mode of death. Postoperatively, his voice and swallowing were normal and he underwent chemoradiation. Within 6 months abdominal metastases occurred and proved to be the cause of death. The goal of preventing gross cervical disease creating a wound care problem and death by asphyxiation was accomplished.

Controversies in Thyroid Surgery

Extent of Lymph Node Dissection for Papillary Thyroid Cancer. As previously discussed, PTC has a high incidence of lymph node metastasis (40 to 60%). Spreading from the thyroid gland, the central and lateral lymph node compartments on the side of the thyroid tumor represent the first echelons of lymphatic drainage. The opposite lateral and the mediastinal lymph node compartments then follow suit.[481] Despite the recognized sequence of lymphatic dissemination, discontinuous lymphatic spread or skip metastasis is not uncommon in node-positive papillary thyroid cancer. However, in stark contrast to other head and neck cancers, nodal metastasis does not have an impact on survival in low-risk groups. This generates two approaches to the scope of nodal dissection for low-risk PTC. One approach is to accept the nodal persistence or recurrence rate and perform neck dissection when these metastatic nodes become clinically evident. Alternatively, nodal dissections of variable extent can be part of the initial procedure. Arguments for the more conservative approach include the lack nodal dissection positively impacting survival and the morbidity of the surgical procedure. Also, some would anticipate radioactive iodine to provide an opportunity to eliminate nodal disease. Proponents for nodal dissection argue that

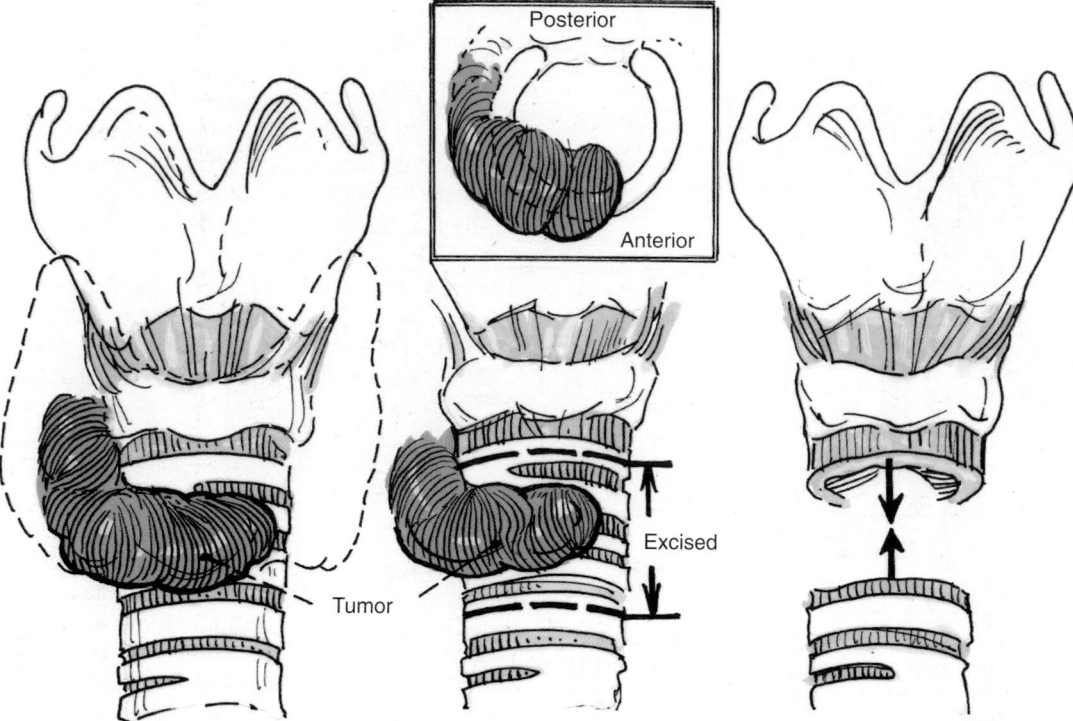

Figure 13 Recurrent/residual thyroid cancer adjacent to the lower lateral part of the cricoid cartilage and invading the upper tracheal rings. Resection and primary anastomosis of the trachea performed due to the amount of tracheal involvement. (Copyrighted and used with permission of Mayo Foundation for Medical Education and Research.)

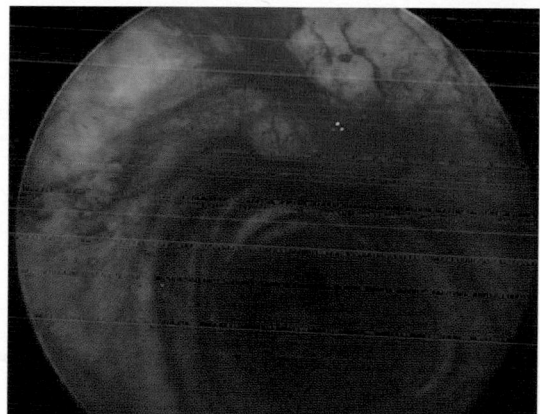

Figure 14 Endoscopic image of papillary thyroid cancer demonstrating submucosal invasion. (Copyrighted and used with permission of Mayo Foundation for Medical Education and Research.)

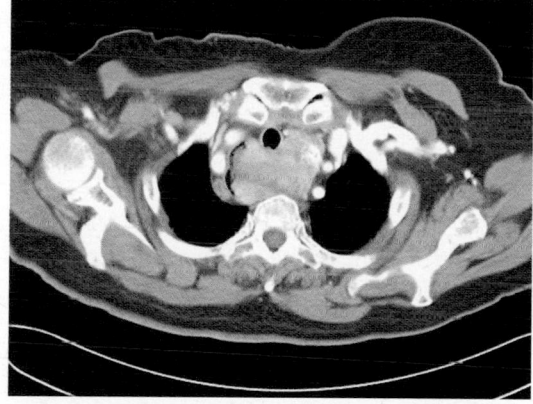

Figure 16 Computed tomography image demonstrating posterior extention of thyroid cancer with esophageal invasion. (Copyrighted and used with permission of Mayo Foundation for Medical Education and Research.)

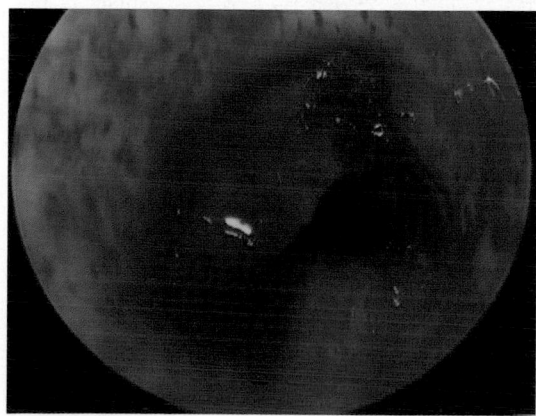

Figure 15 Endoscopic view of gross tracheal invasion by papillary thyroid cancer. (Copyrighted and used with permission of Mayo Foundation for Medical Education and Research.)

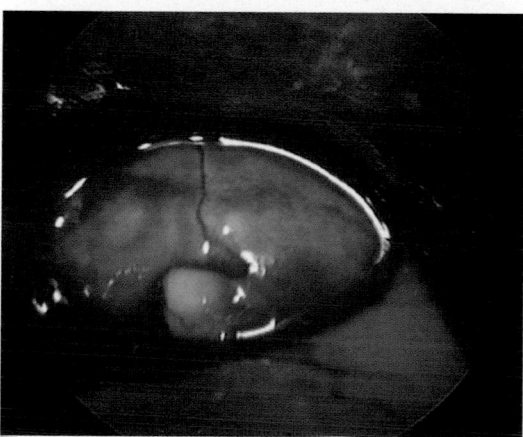

Figure 17 Endoscopic image of esophageal lumen invasion by thyroid cancer. (Copyrighted and used with permission of Mayo Foundation for Medical Education and Research.)

nodal dissections carry minimal morbidity and provide the opportunity for a patient to avoid further treatment.

Technological advances have impacted these decisions as well.[482] The consistent use of high-resolution ultrasound and increasingly sensitive thyroglobulin detection provides identification of much smaller tumor volumes in both the primary and recurrent setting. To provide a greater degree of efficiency for the patient and facilitate follow-up, a total thyroidectomy combined with an area VI nodal dissection is a reasonable initial treatment. This is based on the inability of the ultrasound to image the nodes posterior to the thyroid gland effectively, and this dissection would treat the most likely sites of nodal metastases. Frozen section information can also be used to expand the scope of surgery. Preoperative identification of suspicious nodes in the neck (either by clinical examination or ultrasound) should be addressed with a compartmental dissection.

PARATHYROID GLAND SURGERY

Surgical Anatomy

The normal location of the parathyroid glands is the foundation for surgical management of hyperparathyroidism (Figures 21 and 22). The study by Akerström[483] remains a useful guide to the location and number of parathyroid glands. This was an autopsy study of 503 unselected cases in which the tissues were dissected from the base of the tongue to the diaphragm. Gross and histological characteristics were characterized as was the number and location. The shape of the gland was described as oval, bean, or spherical in 83% of cases. An elongated shape was noted in 11%. Bilobed and multilobulated glands were noted in 5 and 1% of cases, repectively. Four parathyroid glands were found in 84%, more than four glands were identified in 13%, and only three glands were found in 3%. In cases in which only three glands were identified, the lower weight of the parathyroids suggested a gland had been missed. Supernumerary glands were classified as three types: supernumerary rudimentary glands were small nubbins closely approximated to a normal-sized gland (2%), supernumerary split glands appeared divided (6%), and a proper supernumerary gland weighed more than 5 mg and was located well away from the other four glands (5%). In the cases of proper supernumerary glands; 18 had five glands, 3 had six glands, 1 had seven glands, 1 had eight glands, and 1 had eleven glands.

The locations of the superior parathyroid glands were correlated to the intersection of the recurrent laryngeal nerve and the inferior thyroid artery. Eighty percent of the superior parathyroid glands were located within an area 2 cm in diameter centered approximately 1 cm above the intersection of the nerve and artery. The glands were commonly found in the fascial fibers on the posterior edge of the thyroid gland. Occasionally the normal superior gland was located inferiorly (4%), in some cases obscured by the artery, nerve,

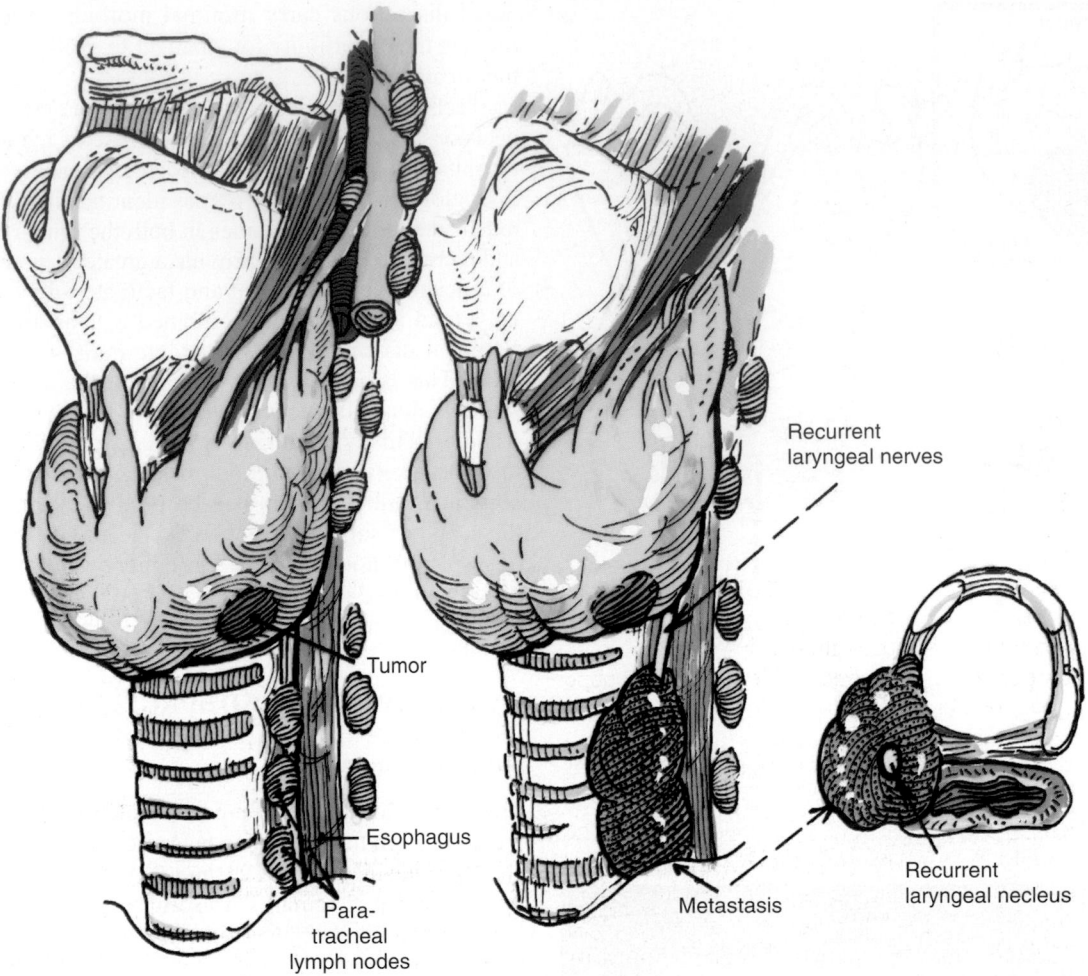

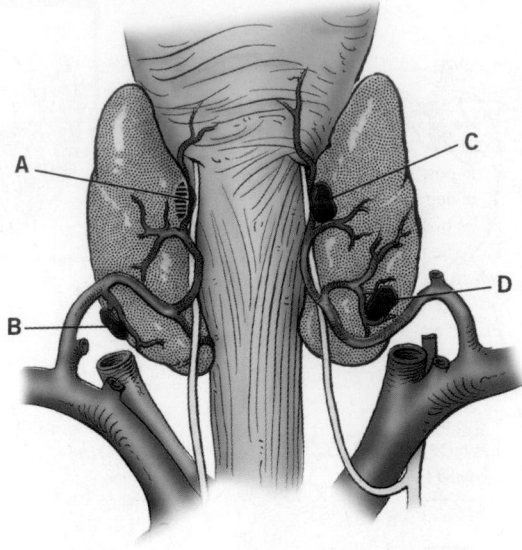

Figure 21 Diagram depicting the "normal" location of the parathyroid glands in relation to the inferior thyroid arteries and recurrent laryngeal nerves (posterior view). (Copyrighted and used with permission of Mayo Foundation for Medical Education and Research.)

Figure 18 An occult thyroid cancer in the left lower pole is the primary site for metastasis to the area VI lymph nodes in the tracheoesophageal groove. The extracapsular spread invades the posterior part of the lateral wall of the trachea, encases the recurrent laryngeal nerve, and invades the esophageal musculature. (Copyrighted and used with permission of Mayo Foundation for Medical Education and Research.)

with the thyrothymic ligament or in the cervical portion of the thymic glands (26%). In 2%, the inferior parathyroid was located in the mediastinal portion of the thymus, and 0.2% was found below the thymus in the mediastinum. The embryologic origin of the inferior parathyroid from the third pharyngeal pouch and its association with the thymus gland (also a third pharyngeal pouch

or the tubercle of Zuckerkandl. Rarely was the superior gland located higher in the neck. Ectopic locations were detected in 1% with identification in the retroesophageal or retropharyngeal space. True intrathyroidal glands were rare, and typically noted in cases of goiter in which the gland

was hidden in the nodules and could often be dissected along a fascial cleavage plane.

The majority of the inferior parathyroid glands (61%) were associated with the posterior, inferior, or lateral surface of the lower pole of the thyroid gland (below the inferior thyroid artery). Inferiorly displaced glands were commonly associated

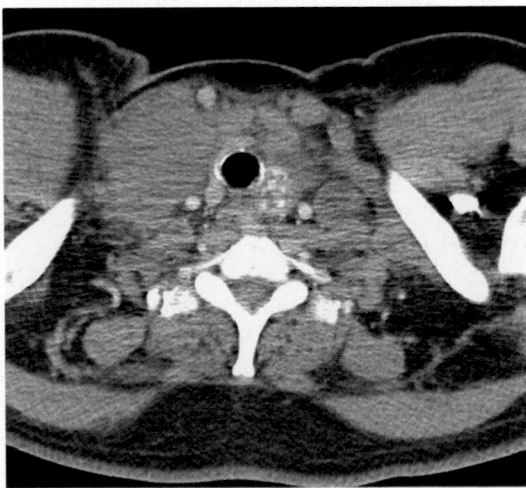

Figure 19 Magnetic resonance imaging demonstrating advanced recurrent thyroid cancer with mediastinal disease and intravascular invasion of the left brachiocephalic vein. (Copyrighted and used with permission of Mayo Foundation for Medical Education and Research.)

Figure 20 Computed tomography image of an anaplastic thyroid cancer. Note the large right thyroid mass with indistinct borders. (Copyrighted and used with permission of Mayo Foundation for Medical Education and Research.)

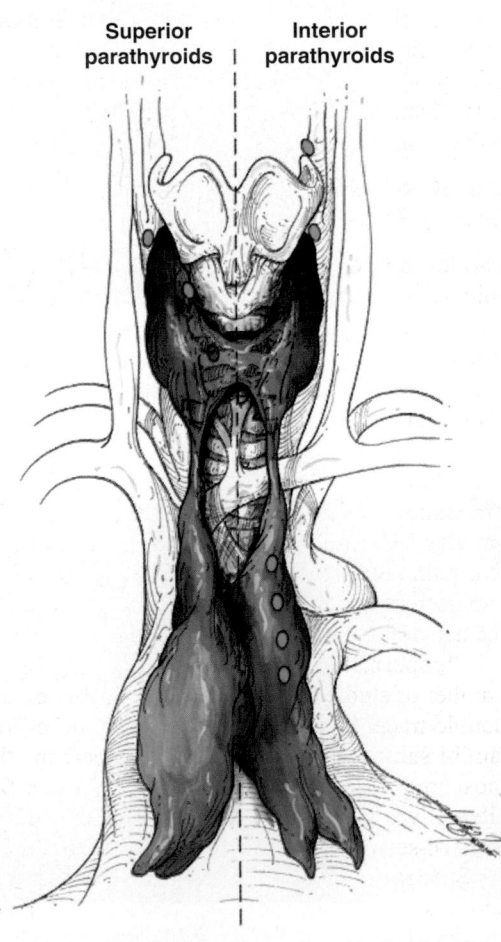

Figure 22 Distribution of parathyroid glands. (Copyrighted and used with permission of Mayo Foundation for Medical Education and Research.)

Table 17 Results of Intraoperative PTH Monitoring in Patients with 1HPT

Result*	Overall (n = 1,302)	Overall, Excluding Reoperations (n = 1,106)	Primary Bilateral Exploration (n = 498)	Minimal Access Parathyroidectomy (n = 610)	Multiglandular Disease (n = 165)
True positive	1,162 (89.2%)	994 (90%)	402 (81%)	594 (97%)	95 (58%)
True negative	106 (8.1%)	83 (8%)	75 (15%)	8 (1%)	65 (39%)
False positive	12 (0.9%)	8 (1%)	4 (1%)	4 (1%)	0 (0%)
False negative	22 (1.7%)	21 (2%)	17 (3%)	4 (1%)	5 (3%)
Sensitivity	98%	98%	96%	99%	95%
Specificity	90%	91%	95%	67%	100%
Positive predictive value	99%	99%	99%	99%	100%
Negative predictive value	83%	80%	82%	67%	93%
Accuracy	97%	97%	96%	99%	97%

*True positive, IOPTH criteria met and patient cured, true negative, did not meet IOPTH criteria and additional disease identified: false positive. IOPTH criteria met and patient not cured; false negative, did not meet IOPTH criteria, no additional disease identified, and patient cured.

Adapted from reference 494.

derivative) accounts for the distribution from the region of the greater cornu of the hyoid (a third arch derivative) into the mediastinum.

Symmetrical positioning of superior and inferior contralateral glands was noted to occur in 60% of cases. However, both superior glands were found above the intersection on inferior thyroid artery and the recurrent laryngeal nerve and the inferior parathyroid gland below this level occurred in 53%. When asymmetric positioning was noted, the most common finding was the lower gland located in the thymus. It should be kept in mind that the majority of the inferior and superior parathyroid glands were closely associated with the thyroid capsule. These findings should be kept in mind when attempting to identify parathyroid glands. Additionally, the embryologic origin of the inferior parathyroid gland results in the potential for the inferior gland to be located high in the neck.

Parathyroid Gland Surgery: General Principles

Parathyroid surgery for sporadic hyperparathyroidism has evolved from a standard four-gland exploration to minimal access procedures. This transition has been dependent on improved localization of adenomas (preoperative and intraoperative) and intraoperative confirmation of cure by rapid PTH analysis. Compared with four-gland exploratory procedures, directed procedures result in less cervical dissection, a smaller surgical incision, decreased postoperative pain, an earlier discharge from the hospital, and decreased cost; many patients may also avoid the use of general anesthesia.[484-486]

Preoperative localization may involve a number of studies. Imaging with a single-session double-tracer 99 mTc-pertechnetate/99 mTc-Sestamibi subtraction scintigraphy[487] is perhaps the most frequent nuclear medicine study used, but alternatives exist, for example, simultaneous 123I-99 mTc-sestamibi subtraction SPECT imaging.[488]

Successful minimal access or directed procedures are dependent on accurate localizing studies. In patients with double adenomas and four-gland parathyroid hyperplasia, as well as in patients with thyroid nodules and thyroiditis, pre-

operative sestamibi scintigraphy is less accurate and often does not detect the abnormal parathyroid gland(s). Single gland disease can also be difficult to image on sestamibi imaging if the adenoma is small in volume and located in the upper position. Adenomas with a higher percentage of oxyphil cells are more readily imaged.[489]

The limited anatomic detail available from SPECT images has prompted the pursuit of other imaging techniques. Ultrasound has been confirmed to contribute preoperative localization and may be combined with sestamibi scanning.[487,490,491] An additional potential benefit of a preoperative ultrasound is the identification of any associated thyroid pathology that could be addressed under the same anesthetic. Sestamibi imaging and ultrasonography may still be inadequate for preoperative localization in patients with a history of previous neck surgery, in patients with coexisting thyroid disease (eg, thyroid nodules or Hashimoto thyroiditis), and in patients with an unfavorable body habitus (eg, obesity, short neck, or kyphosis). These challenges foster new imaging modalities, such as four-dimensional CT to be applied to parathyroid adenomas.[492] The application of more detailed imaging information will continue to impact minimally invasive parathyroid surgery.[493]

Radioguided minimal access parathyroidectomy includes a 99 mTc-Sestamibi injection preoperatively to facilitate intraoperative localization of the adenoma with a hand held gamma counter. Typical preoperative studies are completed including localizing studies. The incision and dissection are similar with the dissection directed by intraoperative measurement of radioactivity. Decrease in radioactivity subsequent to resection is used to document cure. For example, ten minutes (alternate times have been used) before the beginning of the surgical procedure 37 MBq of 99 mTc-Sestamibi is injected intraveneously. Prior to surgical incision, the patient's neck is scanned with a collimated gammaprobe to identify the maximum activity count area corresponding to the anticipated parathyroid adenoma. A transverse neck incision is appropriately placed. The gammaprobe is repeatedly inserted through a 2 to 2.5 cm skin incision guiding the direction of

the dissection. Radioactivity is measured keeping the gammaprobe on the presumed parathyroid adenoma, thyroid gland and background. After removal of the target tissue, radioactivity is measured to evaluate success of parathyroid surgery. Intraoperative PTH (ioPTH) measurement is sometimes added to the procedure to assess cure.

Accurate ioPTH measurement is a key element in minimally invasive parathyroidectomy. Initially introduced in 1998, practical applicability required reduction in the 1 hour processing. Currently, the test can be completed in as little as 15 minutes and measures the active component of PTH (1–84 or intact-PTH). The site and timing of the blood draw for ioPTH sampling has been debated as has the appropriate postresection level to confirm cure. In general the same site should

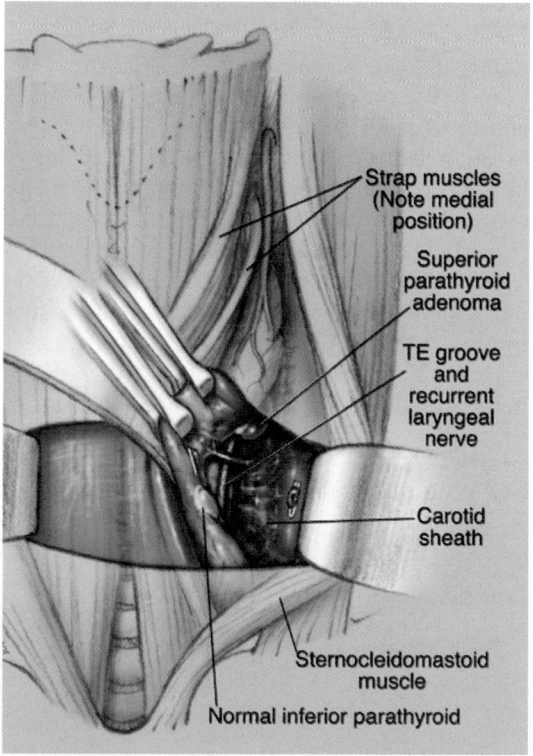

Strap muscles (Note medial position)

Superior parathyroid adenoma

TE groove and recurrent laryngeal nerve

Carotid sheath

Sternocleidomastoid muscle

Normal inferior parathyroid

Figure 23 Diagram demonstrating exposure of the recurrent laryngeal nerve, superior parathyroid adenoma, and normal inferior parathyroid gland. (Copyrighted and used with permission of Mayo Foundation for Medical Education and Research.)

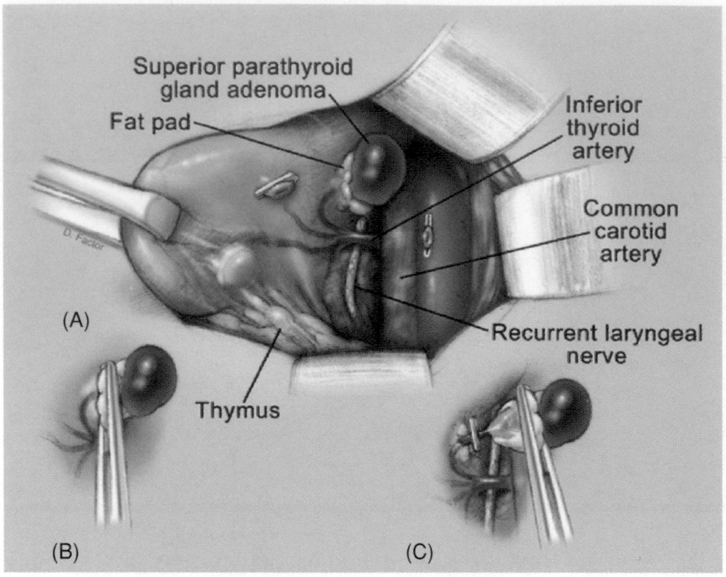

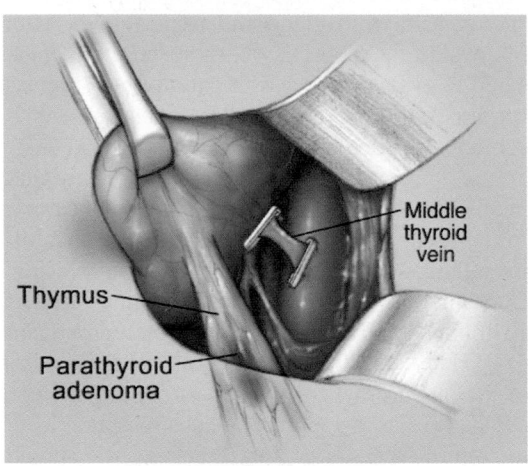

Figure 24 Isolation of a superior parathyroid adenoma demonstrating careful isolation and control of vasculature. a: exposure of superior parathyroid adenoma; b: careful mobilization of the parathyroid gland on its pedicle; c: application of a vascular clip, securing the pedicle. (Copyrighted and used with permission of Mayo Foundation for Medical Education and Research.)

Figure 25 Parathyroid adenoma located in the thymus. (Copyrighted and used with permission of Mayo Foundation for Medical Education and Research.)

provide the pre- and postexcision blood sample, and most studies suggest a 50% fall from preexcision levels and the postexcision level should be in the normal range. Table 17 presents the outcomes from a large center demonstrating accuracy of greater than 95%.

Currently minimal access parathyroidectomy has supplanted routine four-gland exploration. When four-gland exploration is necessary, localization techniques utilized for minimal access surgery have been applied to

facilitate gland identification,[495] and ioPTH has been employed to assess removal of sufficient parathyroid tissue in secondary and tertiary hyperparathyroidism.[494]

In summary, parathyroid surgery has and continues to evolve with several options available to assess cure and facilitate minimal access surgery rapidly. Local expertise and resource availability will influence practice since ioPTH is not uniformly available and radiographic expertise varies. The best practice will continue to evolve with technological advances.

Parathyroidectomy. Consent. Informed consent for parathyroid surgery requires a discussion addressing the risks of the type of anesthesia (general vs sedation with local anesthesia), incisions, the risk of injury to neck structures, extension of surgery based on intraoperative findings, possible recurrent hypercalcemia, convalescence, hospital stay, and follow-up.

Preoperative Preparation. Patients are instructed to avoid aspirin for 7 days and nonsteroidal antiinflammatory medications for at least 2 days. Patients on Coumadin are appropriately bridged to heparin if indicated. An INR is determined prior to surgery in patients receiving Coumadin or heparin therapy.

In the operating room, the patient is anesthetized and intubated if a general anesthetic is

planned. Laryngeal mask anesthesia is an option and has been employed to facilitate visualization of the vocal folds in response to nerve stimulation. Alternatively, an endotracheal tube with implanted wire electrodes can be placed to facilitate recurrent and vagal nerve monitoring.

Positioning. Positioning of the patient is the same as in thyroid gland surgery.

Procedure. Following routine skin preparation and antibiotic prophylaxis, the incision is planned. The incision should be placed to provide exposure to the site suggested by preoperative localization studies with the flexibility to access adjacent areas and be incorporated for bilateral exposure if necessary. An incision 2 cm in length lateral to the midline at the approximate level of the lower border of the cricoid cartilage will typically provide sufficient access. When the adenoma is expected in the location of the superior parathyroid gland, an approach lateral to the sternohyoid and sternothyroid muscles but medial to the omohyoid muscle facilitates exposure posterior to the thyroid gland and to the region of the tracheoesophageal groove. If the adenoma is suspected to be in the location of the inferior gland, an approach medial to the sternohyoid and sternothyroid muscles is used.

After elevation of skin flaps and mobilization of the musculature, the lateral border of the thyroid gland is identified and inspected, and the carotid sheath structures are identified (Figures 23 and 24). An ioPTH can be obtained from the jugular vein or a peripheral site followed by systematic examination of the anticipated location of the adenoma (superior vs inferior to the inferior thyroid artery). This process should involve identification of the recurrent nerve unless the adenoma is obvious with minimal dissection. If not identified after thorough examination, the carotid sheath, tracheoesophageal groove, and superior thymus should be examined (Figure 25). If unable to identify an adenoma, consideration of a false positive localization study should be considered and the opposite side explored in a similar systematic fashion. If an adenoma is still unable to be identified, consideration should be given to an ectopic parathyroid (Figure 26). Removal of a thyroid lobe on the side where normal parathyroid tissue is not identified should be considered. Preoperative imaging may provide clues to this ectopic location as well.

Intraoperative cytology and/or conventional frozen sections merely confirm tissue type rather than functional status and are of limited benefit in minimal access parathyroidectomy.[496] However, the surgeon must be alert to features that suggest parathyroid carcinoma. This may be suspected preoperatively, but the classic clinical picture is not always seen. A thick fibrous capsule around the gland with adhesion to and/or overt infiltration of adjacent tissues including the thyroid gland should prompt consideration of parathyroid carcinoma, and frozen section analysis should be performed. If a parathyroid hyperplasia

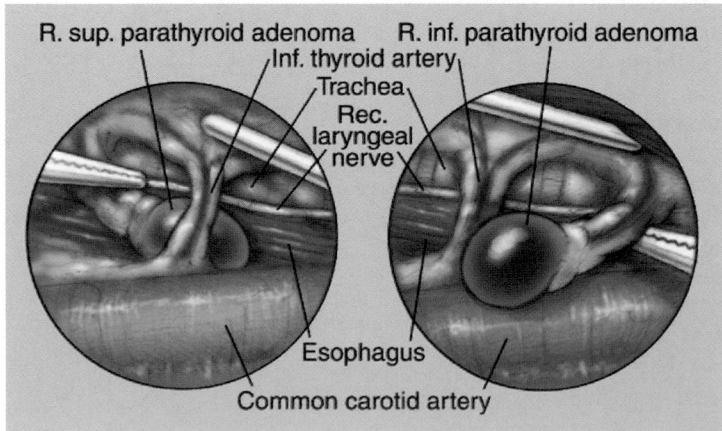

Figure 26 Diagram demonstrating potential overlapping sites of superior and inferior parathyroid adenomas and the potential for superior parathyroid adenomas to be deep to the inferior thyroid artery. (Copyrighted and used with permission of Mayo Foundation for Medical Education and Research.)

or adenoma has undergone previous hemorrhage or degeneration, this can induce a potentially misleading dense irregular fibrotic capsule, possibly with "pseudoinvasion," but this is usually accompanied by hemosiderin deposition, which is absent in carcinomas. This is in contrast to an adenoma, which has a smooth thin capsule, making dissection easy.

CONCLUSIONS

Patients with diseases of the thyroid and parathyroid glands benefit from integrated care by physicians with a broad knowledge base including the anatomy, physiology and pathophysiology of the thyroid gland, parathyroid glands, and aerodigestive tract. This chapter presents information that reflects many current principles followed in an integrated academic practice. Clearly change should be expected as higher-quality data are obtained, further advances in molecular medicine become applicable, new technology is developed, and cost contraints rise.

REFERENCES

1. Vanderpas J. Nutritional epidemiology and thyroid hormone metabolism. Ann Rev Nutr 2006;26:293–322.
2. Andersson M, Takkouche B, Egli I, et al. Current global iodine status and progress over the last decade towards the elimination of iodine deficiency. Bull World Health Org 2005;83:518–25.
3. Georgopoulos NA, Sykiotis GP, Sgourou A, et al. Autonomously functioning thyroid nodules in a former iodine-deficient area commonly harbor gain-of-function mutations in the thyrotropin signaling pathway. Eur J Endocrinol 2003;149:287–92.
4. Feldt-Rasmussen U. Iodine and cancer. Thyroid 2001;11:483–6.
5. Basaria S, Cooper DS. Amiodarone and the thyroid. Am J Med 2005;118:706–14.
6. Lamberg BA. Endemic goitre–iodine deficiency disorders. Ann Med 1991;23:367–72.
7. Lazarus JH. Thyroid disease in pregnancy and childhood. Minerva Endocrinol 2005;30:71–87.
8. Delange F. The role of iodine in brain development. Proc Nutr Soc 2000;59:75–9.
9. Obregon MJ, Escobar del Rey F, Morreale de Escobar G. The effects of iodine deficiency on thyroid hormone deiodination. Thyroid 2005;15:917–29.
10. Zimmermann MB, Kohrle J. The impact of iron and selenium deficiencies on iodine and thyroid metabolism: Biochemistry and relevance to public health. Thyroid 2002;12:867–78.
11. Aramrattana A, Limpijarnkit L, Leelapat P, et al. Difference in goiter rates between two areas in Mae Hong Son Province despite an equally sufficient iodine supply. J Med Assoc Thailand 2002;85:831–8.
12. Chandra AK, Mukhopadhyay S, Lahari D, Tripathy S. Goitrogenic content of Indian cyanogenic plant foods their in vitro anti-thyroidal activity. Indian J Med Res 2004;119:180–5.
13. Kung AW, Lao TT, Chau MT, et al. Goitrogenesis during pregnancy and neonatal hypothyroxinaemia in a borderline iodine sufficient area. Clin Endocrinol 2000;53:725–31.
14. Angermayr L, Clar C. Iodine supplementation for preventing iodine deficiency disorders in children. Cochrane Database of Systematic Reviews 2004:CD003819.
15. Delange F, Lecomte P. Iodine supplementation: Benefits outweigh risks. Drug Safety 2000;22:89–95.
16. Martino E, Bartalena L, Bogazzi F, Braverman LE. The effects of amiodarone on the thyroid. Endocr Rev 2001;22:240–54.
17. Trip MD, Wiersinga W, Plomp TA. Incidence, predictability, and pathogenesis of amiodarone-induced thyrotoxicosis and hypothyroidism. Am J Med 1991;91:507–11.
18. Markou K, Georgopoulos N, Kyriazopoulou V, Vagenakis AG. Iodine-Induced hypothyroidism. Thyroid 2001;11:501–10.

19. Pollak PT, Bouillon T, Shafer SL. Population pharmacokinetics of long-term oral amiodarone therapy. Clin Pharmacol Ther 2000;67:642–52.
20. Delange F, Lecomte P. Iodine supplementation: Benefits outweigh risks. Drug Saf 2000;22:89–95.
21. Weetman AP, Bhandal SK, Burrin JM, Robinson K, McKenna W. Amiodarone and thyroid autoimmunity in the United Kingdom. BMJ 1988;297:33.
22. Woeber KA. Iodine and thyroid disease. Med Clin N Am 1991;75:169–78.
23. Livadas DP, Koutras DA, Souvatzoglou A, Beckers C. The toxic effect of small iodine supplements in patients with autonomous thyroid nodules. Clin Endocrinol 1977;7:121–7.
24. Broussolle C, Ducottet X, Martin C, et al. Rapid effectiveness of prednisone and thionamides combined therapy in severe amiodarone iodine-induced thyrotoxicosis. Comparison of two groups of patients with apparently normal thyroid glands. J Endocrinol Invest 1989;12:37–42.
25. Erdogan MF, Gulec S, Tutar E, et al. A stepwise approach to the treatment of amiodarone-induced thyrotoxicosis. Thyroid 2003;13:205–9.
26. Farwell AP, Abend SL, Huang SK, et al. Thyroidectomy for amiodarone-induced thyrotoxicosis. JAMA 1990;263:1526–8.
27. Gough J, Gough IR. Total thyroidectomy for amiodarone-associated thyrotoxicosis in patients with severe cardiac disease. World J Surg 2006;30:1957–61.
28. Hollowell JG, Staehling NW, Flanders WD, et al. Serum TSH, T(4), and thyroid antibodies in the United States population (1988 to 1994): National Health and Nutrition Examination Survey (NHANES III). J Clin Endocrinol Metab 2002;87:489–99.
29. McIver B, Morris JC. The pathogenesis of Graves disease. Endocrinol Metab Clin N Am 1998;27:73–89.
30. Zimmerman D. Fetal and neonatal hyperthyroidism. Thyroid 1999;9:727–33.
31. Radetti G, Zavallone A, Gentili L, et al. Foetal and neonatal thyroid disorders. Minerva Pediatr 2002;54:383–400.
32. Roth C, Scortea M, Stubbe P, et al. Autoimmune thyreoiditis in childhood—epidemiology, clinical and laboratory findings in 61 patients. Experimental Clin Endocrinol Diabetes 1997;105:66–9.
33. Bergman P, Auldist AW, Cameron F. Review of the outcome of management of Graves disease in children and adolescents. J Paediatr Child Health 2001;37:176–82.
34. De Moraes AV, Pedro AB, Romaldini JH. Spontaneous hypothyroidism in the follow up of Graves hyperthyroid patients treated with antithyroid drugs. South Med J 2006;99:1068–72.
35. Bleeker GM. Changes in the orbital tissues and muscles dysthyroid ophthalmopathy. Eye 1988;2:193–7.
36. Dittmar M, Kahaly GJ. Polyglandular autoimmune syndromes: Immunogenetics and long-term follow-up. J Clin Endocrinol Metab 2003;88:2983–92.
37. Rees Smith B, McLachlan SM, Furmaniak J. Autoantibodies to the thyrotropin receptor. Endocr Rev 1988;9:106–21.
38. Takasu N, Oshiro C, Akamine H, et al. Thyroid-stimulating antibody and TSH-binding inhibitor immunoglobulin in 277 Graves patients and in 686 normal subjects. J Endocrinol Invest 1997;20:452–61.
39. Mariotti S, Caturegli P, Piccolo P, et al. Antithyroid peroxidase autoantibodies in thyroid diseases. J Clin Endocrinol Metab 1990;71:661–9.
40. Saleh A, Cohnen M, Furst G, et al. Differential diagnosis of hyperthyroidism: Doppler sonographic quantification of thyroid blood flow distinguishes between Graves disease and diffuse toxic goiter. Experimental Clin Endocrinol Diabetes 2002;110:32–6.
41. Streetman DD, Khanderia U. Diagnosis and treatment of Graves disease. Ann Pharmacother 2003;37:1100–9.
42. Geffner DL, Hershman JM. Beta-adrenergic blockade for the treatment of hyperthyroidism. Am J Med 1992;93:61–8.
43. Alsanea O, Clark OH. Treatment of Graves disease: The advantages of surgery. Endocrinol Metab Clin N Am 2000;29:321–37.
44. Langley RW, Burch HB. Perioperative management of the thyrotoxic patient. Endocrinol Metab Clin N Am 2003;32:519–34.
45. Feek CM, Sawers JS, Irvine WJ, et al. Combination of potassium iodide and propranolol in preparation of patients with Graves disease for thyroid surgery. New Engl J Med 1980;302:883–5.
46. Plummer H, Boothby W. The value of iodin in exophthalmic goiter. J Iowa State Med Soc 1924;xiv:66–73.
47. Schussler-Fiorenza CM, Bruns CM, Chen H. The surgical management of Graves disease. J Surg Res 2006;133:207–14.

48. Chi SY, Hsei KC, Sheen-Chen SM, Chou FF. A prospective randomized comparison of bilateral subtotal thyroidectomy versus unilateral total and contralateral subtotal thyroidectomy for Graves disease. World J Surg 2005;29:160–3.
49. Metso S, Jaatinen P, Huhtala H, et al. Long-term follow-up study of radioiodine treatment of hyperthyroidism. Clin Endocrinol 2004;61:641–8.
50. Ron E, Doody MM, Becker DV, et al. Cancer mortality following treatment for adult hyperthyroidism. Cooperative Thyrotoxicosis Therapy Follow-up Study Group. JAMA 1998;280:347–55.
51. Vijayakumar V, Nusynowwitz ML, Ali S. Is it safe to treat hyperthyroid patients with I-131 without fear of thyroid storm? Ann Nuclear Med 2006;20:383–5.
52. Tavintharan S, Sundram FX, Chew LS. Radioiodine (I-131) therapy and the incidence of hypothyroidism. Ann Acad Med Singapore 1997;26:128–31.
53. Peters H, Fischer C, Bogner U, et al. Radioiodine therapy of Graves hyperthyroidism: Standard vs. calculated 131iodine activity. Results from a prospective, randomized, multicentre study. Eur J Clin Invest 1995;25:186–93.
54. Kung AW, Yau CC, Cheng A. The incidence of ophthalmopathy after radioiodine therapy for Graves disease: Prognostic factors and the role of methimazole. J Clin Endocrinol Metab 1994;79:542–6.
55. Tallstedt L, Lundell G, Torring O, et al. Occurrence of ophthalmopathy after treatment for Graves hyperthyroidism. The Thyroid Study Group. New Engl J Med 1992;326:1733–8.
56. Sridama V, DeGroot LJ. Treatment of Graves disease and the course of ophthalmopathy. Am J Med 1989;87:70–3.
57. Bartalena L, Marcocci C, Bogazzi F, et al. Use of corticosteroids to prevent progression of Graves ophthalmopathy after radioiodine therapy for hyperthyroidism. New Engl J Med 1989;321:1349–52.
58. Green HG, Gareis FJ, Shepard TH, Kelley VC. Cretinism associated with maternal sodium iodide I 131 therapy during pregnancy. Am J Dis Child 1971;122:247–9.
59. Lloyd RD, Tripp DA, Kerber RA. Limits of fetal thyroid risk from radioiodine exposure. Health Phys 1996;70:559–62.
60. Krassas GE, Laron Z. A questionnaire survey concerning the most favourable treatment for Graves disease in children and adolescents. Eur J Endocrinol 2004;151:155–6.
61. Raby C, Lagorce JF, Jambut-Absil AC, et al. The mechanism of action of synthetic antithyroid drugs: Iodine complexation during oxidation of iodide. Endocrinol 1990;126:1683–91.
62. Wenzel KW, Lente JR. Syndrome of persisting thyroid stimulating immunoglobulins and growth promotion of goiter combined with low thyroxine and high triiodothyronine serum levels in drug treated Graves disease. J Endocrinol Invest 1983;6:389–94.
63. Kampmann JP, Hansen JM. Clinical pharmacokinetics of antithyroid drugs. Clin Pharmacokinet 1981;6:401–28.
64. Abraham P, Avenell A, Watson WA, et al. Antithyroid drug regimen for treating Graves hyperthyroidism.[update in Cochrane Database Syst Rev. 2005;(2):CD003420; PMID: 15846664][update of Cochrane Database Syst Rev. 2003;(4):CD003420; PMID: 14583975]. Cochrane Database of Systematic Reviews 2004:CD003420.
65. Okamoto Y, Tanigawa S, Ishikawa K, Hamada N. TSH receptor antibody measurements and prediction of remission in Graves disease patients treated with minimum maintenance doses of antithyroid drugs. Endocrine J 2006;53:467–72.
66. Volpe R. The immunomodulatory effects of anti-thyroid drugs are mediated via actions on thyroid cells, affecting thyrocyte-immunocyte signalling: A review. Curr Pharmaceut Design 2001;7:451–60.
67. Hashizume K, Ichikawa K, Sakurai A, et al. Administration of thyroxine in treated Graves disease. Effects on the level of antibodies to thyroid-stimulating hormone receptors and on the risk of recurrence of hyperthyroidism. New Engl J Med 1991;324:947–53.
68. McIver B, Rae P, Beckett G, et al. Lack of effect of thyroxine in patients with Graves hyperthyroidism who are treated with an antithyroid drug. New Engl J Med 1996;334:220–4.
69. Dai WX, Zhang JD, Zhan SW, et al. Retrospective analysis of 18 cases of antithyroid drug (ATD)-induced agranulocytosis. Endocr J 2002;49:29–33.
70. Tajiri J, Noguchi S. Antithyroid drug-induced agranulocytosis: How has granulocyte colony-stimulating factor changed therapy? Thyroid 2005;15:292–7.
71. Werner MC, Romaldini JH, Bromberg N, et al. Adverse effects related to thionamide drugs and their dose regimen. Am J Med Sci 1989;297:216–9.

72. Atkins P, Cohen SB, Phillips BJ. Drug therapy for hyperthyroidism in pregnancy: Safety issues for mother and fetus. Drug Safety 2000;23:229–44.

73. Chattaway JM, Klepser TB. Propylthiouracil versus methimazole in treatment of Graves disease during pregnancy. Ann Pharmacother 2007;41:1018–22.

74. Weetman AP. Extrathyroidal complications of Graves disease. Quar J Med 1993;86:473–7.

75. Bartley GB, Fatourechi V, Kadrmas EF, et al. Chronology of Graves ophthalmopathy in an incidence cohort. Am J Ophthalmol 1996;121:426–34.

76. Fatourechi V, Pajouhi M, Fransway AF. Dermopathy of Graves disease (pretibial myxedema). Review of 150 cases. Medicine 1994;73:1–7.

77. Wiersinga WM. Management of Graves ophthalmopathy. Nature Clin Pract Endocrinol Metab 2007;3:396–404.

78. Marcocci C, Marino M, Rocchi R, et al. Novel aspects of immunosuppressive and radiotherapy management of Graves ophthalmopathy. J Endocrinol Invest 2004; 27:272–80.

79. Bartalena L, Tanda ML, Piantanida E, et al. Relationship between management of hyperthyroidism and course of the ophthalmopathy. J Endocrinol Invest 2004;27:288–94.

80. Perros P, Kendall-Taylor P, Neoh C, et al. A prospective study of the effects of radioiodine therapy for hyperthyroidism in patients with minimally active Graves ophthalmopathy. J Clin Endocrinol Metab 2005;90:5321–3.

81. Garrity JA, Bahn RS. Pathogenesis of Graves ophthalmopathy: Implications for prediction, prevention, and treatment. Am J Ophthalmol 2006;142:147–53.

82. Fatourechi V. Pretibial myxedema: Pathophysiology and treatment options. Am J Clin Derm 2005;6:295–309.

83. Prabhakar BS, Bahn RS, Smith TJ. Current perspective on the pathogenesis of Graves disease and ophthalmopathy. Endocr Rev 2003;24:802–35.

84. Daumerie C, Ludgate M, Costagliola S, Many MC. Evidence for thyrotropin receptor immunoreactivity in pretibial connective tissue from patients with thyroid-associated dermopathy. Eur J Endocrinol 2002;146:35–8.

85. Fatourechi V, Ahmed DD, Schwartz KM. Thyroid acropachy: Report of 40 patients treated at a single institution in a 26-year period. J Clin Endocrinol Metab 2002; 87:5435–41.

86. Soroudi AE, Goldberg RA, McCann JD. Prevalence of asymmetric exophthalmos in Graves orbitopathy. Ophthal Plast Reconstr Surg 2004;20:224–5.

87. Khoo DH, Eng PH, Ho SC, et al. Graves ophthalmopathy in the absence of elevated free thyroxine and triiodothyronine levels: Prevalence, natural history, and thyrotropin receptor antibody levels. Thyroid 2000;10:1093–100.

88. Bahn RS, Garrity JA, Bartley GB, Gorman CA. Diagnostic evaluation of Graves ophthalmopathy. Endocrinol Metab Clin N Am 1988;17:527–45.

89. Marcocci C, Bartalena L, Tanda ML, et al. Graves ophthalmopathy and 131I therapy. Quart J Nuclear Med 1999; 43:307–12.

90. Bartalena L, Marcocci C, Gorman CA, et al. Orbital radiotherapy for Graves ophthalmopathy: Useful or useless? Safe or dangerous? J Endocrinol Invest 2003;26:5–16.

91. Gorman CA, Garrity JA, Fatourechi V, et al. A prospective, randomized, double-blind, placebo-controlled study of orbital radiotherapy for Graves ophthalmopathy.[see comment][erratum appears in Ophthalmology 2004; 111:1306]. Ophthalmology 2001;108:1523–34.

92. Kasperbauer JL, Hinkley L. Endoscopic orbital decompression for Graves ophthalmopathy. Am J Rhinol 2005; 19:603–6.

93. Krohn K, Fuhrer D, Bayer Y, et al. Molecular pathogenesis of euthyroid and toxic multinodular goiter. Endocrine Rev 2005;26:504–24.

94. Rapoport B, Niepomniszcze H, Bigazzi M, Hati R, DeGroot LJ. Studies on the pathogenesis of poor thyroglobulin iodination in non-toxic multinodular goiter. J Clin Endocrinol Metab 1972;34:822–30.

95. Vitti P, Rago T, Tonacchera M, Pinchera A. Toxic multinodular goiter in the elderly. J Endocrinol Invest 2002; 25:16–8.

96. van der Molen AJ, Thomsen HS, Morcos SK. Contrast Media Safety Committee ESoUR. Effect of iodinated contrast media on thyroid function in adults. Eur Radiol 2004; 14:902–7.

97. van Soestbergen MJ, van der Vijver JC, Graafland AD. Recurrence of hyperthyroidism in multinodular goiter after long-term drug therapy: A comparison with Graves disease. J Endocrinol Invest 1992;15:797–800.

98. Cohen O, Ilany J, Hoffman C, et al. Low-dose recombinant human thyrotropin-aided radioiodine treatment of large, multinodular goiters in elderly patients. Eur J Endocrinol 2006;154:243–52.

99. Albino CC, Mesa CO, Jr, Olandoski M, et al. Recombinant human thyrotropin as adjuvant in the treatment of multinodular goiters with radioiodine. J Clin Endocrinol Metab 2005;90:2775–80.

100. Vanderpump MP, Tunbridge WM, French JM, et al. The incidence of thyroid disorders in the community: A twenty-year follow-up of the Whickham Survey. Clin Endocrinol 1995;43:55–68.

101. Diez JJ, Molina I, Ibars MT. Prevalence of thyroid dysfunction in adults over age 60 years from an urban community. Exp Clin Endocrinol Diabetes 2003;111:480–5.

102. Bagchi N, Brown TR, Parish RF. Thyroid dysfunction in adults over age 55 years. A study in an urban US community. Arch Intern Med 1990;150:785–7.

103. Okayasu I, Hara Y, Nakamura K, Rose NR. Racial and age-related differences in incidence and severity of focal autoimmune thyroiditis. Am J Clin Pathol 1994;101: 698–702.

104. Weetman AP. Controversy in thyroid disease. J Royal Coll Phys London 2000;34:374–80.

105. Lucas A, Pizarro E, Granada ML, et al. Postpartum thyroiditis: Epidemiology and clinical evolution in a nonselected population. Thyroid 2000;10:71–7.

106. Lazarus JH. Clinical manifestations of postpartum thyroid disease. Thyroid 1999;9:685–9.

107. Braverman LE, Utiger RD.In: Werner SC, Ingbar SH, Editors. The Thyroid, 6th edition, Philadelphia: Lippincott; 1986.

108. Toft AD. Thyroxine therapy[erratum appears in N Engl J Med 1994;331:1035]. New Engl J Med 1994;331:174–80.

109. Grebe SK, Cooke RR, Ford HC, et al. Treatment of hypothyroidism with once weekly thyroxine. J Clin Endocrinol Metab 1997;82:870–5.

110. Toft AD. Thyroxine therapy. N Engl J Med 1994; 331:174–80.

111. Leslie PJ, Toft AD. The replacement therapy problem in hypothyroidism. Baillieres Clin Endocrinol Metab 1988; 2:653–69.

112. d'Esteve-Bonetti L, Bennet AP, Malet D, et al. Gluten-induced enteropathy (coeliac disease) revealed by resistance to treatment with levothyroxine and alfacalcidol in a sixty-eight-year-old patient: A case report. Thyroid 2002; 12:633–6.

113. American Association of Clinical Endocrinologists medical guidelines for clinical practice for the evaluation and treatment of hyperthyroidism and hypothyroidism. Endocr Pract 2002;8:457–69.

114. Smith RN, Taylor SA, Massey JC. Controlled clinical trial of combined triiodothyronine and thyroxine in the treatment of hypothyroidism. British Med J 1970;4:145–8.

115. Taylor S, Kapur M, Adie R. Combined thyroxine and triiodothyronine for thyroid replacement therapy. British Med J 1970;2:270–1.

116. Dorr M, Volzke H. Cardiovascular morbidity and mortality in thyroid dysfunction. Minerva Endocrinol 2005; 30:199–216.

117. Franklyn JA, Sheppard MC. Thyroxine replacement treatment and osteoporosis. BMJ 1990;300:693–4.

118. Toft AD, Boon NA. Thyroid disease and the heart. Heart 2000;84:455–60.

119. Saravanan P, Chau WF, Roberts N, et al. Psychological well-being in patients on 'adequate' doses of l-thyroxine: Results of a large, controlled community-based questionnaire study. Clin Endocrinol 2002;57:577–85.

120. van Doorn J, Roelfsema F, van der Heide D. Concentrations of thyroxine and 3,5,3'-triiodothyronine at 34 different sites in euthyroid rats as determined by an isotopic equilibrium technique. Endocrinology 1985;117:1201–8.

121. Vos RA, De Jong M, Bernard BF, et al. Impaired thyroxine and 3,5,3'-triiodothyronine handling by rat hepatocytes in the presence of serum of patients with nonthyroidal illness. J Clin Endocrinol Metab 1995;80:2364–70.

122. Bunevicius R, Kazanavicius G, Zalinkevicius R, Prange AJ, Jr. Effects of thyroxine as compared with thyroxine plus triiodothyronine in patients with hypothyroidism. New Engl J Med 1999;340:424–9.

123. Escobar-Morreale HF, Botella-Carretero JI, Escobar del Rey F, Morreale de Escobar G. REVIEW: Treatment of hypothyroidism with combinations of levothyroxine plus liothyronine. J Clin Endocrinol Metab 2005;90:4946–54.

124. Fatourechi V. Subclinical thyroid disease. Mayo Clinic Proc 2001;76:413–6; quiz 416–7.

125. Sawka AM, Fatourechi V. Subclinical thyroid dysfunction and the heart. Ann Intern Med 2003;139:866; author reply 866–7.

126. Fatourechi V. Mild thyroid failure [subclinical hypothyroidism]: To treat or not to treat? Compr Ther 2002;28:134–9.

127. Danese MD, Ladenson PW, Meinert CL, Powe NR. Clinical review 115: Effect of thyroxine therapy on serum lipoproteins in patients with mild thyroid failure: A quantitative review of the literature. J Clin Endocrinol Metab 2000;85:2993–3001.

128. Sato A, Aizawa T, Koizumi Y, et al. Ten-year follow-up study of thyroid function in euthyroid patients with simple goiter or Hashimoto's thyroiditis. Intern Med 1995; 34:371–5.

129. MacDonald L, Yazdi HM. Fine needle aspiration biopsy of Hashimoto's thyroiditis. Sources of diagnostic error. Acta Cytol 1999;43:400–6.

130. Sdano MT, Falciglia M, Welge JA, Steward DL. Efficacy of thyroid hormone suppression for benign thyroid nodules: Meta-analysis of randomized trials. Otolaryngol Head Neck Surg 2005;133:391–6.

131. Pinchera, Martino and Faglia. In: Werner SC, Ingbar SH, editors. The Thyroid, 6th edition, Philadelphia: Lippincott; 1986.

132. Lazarus JH. Thyroid disorders associated with pregnancy: Etiology, diagnosis, and management. Treat Endocrinol 2005;4:31–41.

133. Ross DS. Syndromes of thyrotoxicosis with low radioactive iodine uptake. Endocrinol Metab Clin N Am 1998; 27:169–85.

134. Lu R, Burman KD, Jonklaas J. Transient Graves hyperthyroidism during pregnancy in a patient with Hashimoto's hypothyroidism. Thyroid 2005;15:725–9.

135. Sawers JS, Toft AD, Irvine WJ, et al. Transient hypothyroidism after iodine-131 treatment of thyrotoxicosis. J Clin Endocrinol Metab 1980;50:226–9.

136. Sarvghadi F, Hedayati M, Mehrabi Y, Azizi F. Follow up of patients with postpartum thyroiditis: A population-based study. Endocrine 2005;27:279–82.

137. Fatourechi V. Demystifying autoimmune thyroid disease. Which disorders require treatment? Postgrad Med 2000; 107:127–34.

138. Hay ID. Thyroiditis: A clinical update. Mayo Clinic Proc 1985;60:836–43.

139. Schwaegerle SM, Bauer TW, Esselstyn CB, Jr. Riedel's thyroiditis. Am J Clin Pathol 1988;90:715–22.

140. de Lange WE, Freling NJ, Molenaar WM, Doorenbos H. Invasive fibrous thyroiditis (Riedel's struma): A manifestation of multifocal fibrosclerosis? A case report with review of the literature. Quart J Med 1989;72:709–17.

141. Perez Fontan FJ, Cordido Carballido F, Pombo Felipe F, et al. Riedel thyroiditis: US, CT, and MR evaluation. J Comp Assist Tomogr 1993;17:324–5.

142. Few J, Thompson NW, Angelos P, et al. Riedel's thyroiditis: Treatment with tamoxifen. Surgery 1996;120:993–8; discussion 998–9.

143. Vaidya B, Harris PE, Barrett P, Kendall-Taylor P. Corticosteroid therapy in Riedel's thyroiditis. Postgrad Med J 1997;73:817–9.

144. Heufelder AE, Hay ID. Evidence for autoimmune mechanisms in the evolution of invasive fibrous thyroiditis (Riedel's struma). Clin Invest 1994;72:788–93.

145. Neild GH, Rodriguez-Justo M, Wall C, Connolly JO. Hyper-IgG4 disease: Report and characterisation of a new disease. BMC Medicine 2006;4:23.

146. Dunham B, Nicol TL, Ishii M, Basaria S. Suppurative thyroiditis. Lancet 2006;368:1742.

147. Sicilia V, Mezitis S. A case of acute suppurative thyroiditis complicated by thyrotoxicosis. J Endocrinol Invest 2006; 29:997–1000.

148. Seki N, Himi T. Retrospective review of 13 cases of pyriform sinus fistula. Am J Otolaryngol 2007;28:55–8.

149. McIver B, Gorman CA. Euthyroid sick syndrome: An overview. Thyroid 1997;7:125–32.

150. Hennemann G, Docter R, Krenning EP. Causes and effects of the low T3 syndrome during caloric deprivation and non-thyroidal illness: An overview. Acta Medica Austriaca 1988;15:42–5.

151. Karga H, Papaioannou P, Venetsanou K, et al. The role of cytokines and cortisol in the non-thyroidal illness syndrome following acute myocardial infarction. Eur J Endocrinol 2000;142:236–42.

152. Opasich C, Pacini F, Ambrosino N, et al. Sick euthyroid syndrome in patients with moderate-to-severe chronic heart failure. Eur Heart J 1996;17:1860–6.

153. Tikanoja SH, Joutti A, Liewendahl BK. Association between increased concentrations of free thyroxine and unsaturated free fatty acids in nonthyroidal illnesses: Role of albumin. Clinica Chimica Acta 1989;179:33–43.

154. Kabadi UM. Thyrotropin dysregulation during a non-thyroidal illness: Transient hypothalamic hypothyroidism? J Endocrinol Invest 2001;24:178–82.

155. Boelen A, Kwakkel J, Platvoet-ter Schiphorst M, et al. Interleukin-18, a proinflammatory cytokine, contributes to the pathogenesis of non-thyroidal illness mainly via the central part of the hypothalamus-pituitary-thyroid axis. Eur J Endocrinol 2004;151:497–502.

156. Wolf M, Hansen N, Greten H. Interleukin 1 beta, tumor necrosis factor-alpha and interleukin 6 decrease nuclear

thyroid hormone receptor capacity in a liver cell line. Eur J Endocrinol 1994;131:307–12.
157. Chopra IJ, Sakane S, Teco GN. A study of the serum concentration of tumor necrosis factor-alpha in thyroidal and nonthyroidal illnesses. J Clin Endocrinol Metab 1991;72:1113–6.
158. Lechan RM, Fekete C. Feedback regulation of thyrotropin-releasing hormone (TRH): Mechanisms for the nonthyroidal illness syndrome. J Endocrinol Invest 2004; 27:105–19.
159. Lim CF, Docter R, Krenning EP, et al. Transport of thyroxine into cultured hepatocytes: Effects of mild non-thyroidal illness and calorie restriction in obese subjects. Clin Endocrinol 1994;40:79–85.
160. Brent GA, Hershman JM. Thyroxine therapy in patients with severe nonthyroidal illnesses and low serum thyroxine concentration. J Clin Endocrinol Metab 1986;63:1–8.
161. Klemperer JD, Klein I, Gomez M, et al. Thyroid hormone treatment after coronary-artery bypass surgery. N Engl J Med 1995;333:1522–7.
162. Bennett-Guerrero E, Jimenez JL, White WD, et al. Cardiovascular effects of intravenous triiodothyronine in patients undergoing coronary artery bypass graft surgery. A randomized, double- blind, placebo- controlled trial. Duke T3 study group. JAMA 1996;275:687–92.
163. Despres N, Grant AM. Antibody interference in thyroid assays: A potential for clinical misinformation. Clin Chemistry 1998;44:440–54.
164. Smallridge RC, Czervionke LF, Fellows DW, Bernet VJ. Corticotropin- and thyrotropin-secreting pituitary microadenomas: Detection by dynamic magnetic resonance imaging. Mayo Clinic Proc 2000;75:521–8.
165. Bernal J, Refetoff S, DeGroot LJ. Abnormalities of triiodothyronine binding to lymphocyte and fibroblast nuclei from a patient with peripheral tissue resistance to thyroid hormone action. J Clin Endocrinol Metab 1978; 47:1266–72.
166. Refetoff S, Degroot LJ, Barsano CP. Defective thyroid hormone feedback regulation in the syndrome of peripheral resistance to thyroid hormone. J Clin Endocrinol Metab 1980;51:41–5.
167. Beck-Peccoz P, Chatterjee VK, Chin WW, et al. Nomenclature of thyroid hormone receptor beta gene mutations in resistance to thyroid hormone. First workshop on thyroid hormone resistance, July 10–11, 1993, Cambridge, UK. J Endocrinol Invest 1994;17:283–7.
168. Olateju TO, Vanderpump MP. Thyroid hormone resistance. Ann Clin Biochem 2006;43:431–40.
169. Florkowski CM, Brownlie BE, Croxson MS, et al. Thyroid hormone resistance: The role of mutational analysis. Intern Med J 2006;36:738–41.
170. Smallridge RC. Thyrotropin-secreting pituitary tumors. Endocrinol Metab Clin N Am 1987;16:765–92.
171. Tan GH, Gharib H. Thyroid incidentalomas: Management approaches to nonpalpable nodules discovered incidentally on thyroid imaging. Ann Intern Med 1997;126:226–31.
172. Sampson RJ, Woolner LB, Bahn RC, Kurland LT. Occult thyroid carcinoma in Olmsted County, Minnesota: Prevalence at autopsy compared with that in Hiroshima and Nagasaki, Japan. Cancer 1974;34:2072–6.
173. Greenlee RT, Murray T, Bolden S, Wingo PA. Cancer statistics, 2000. Ca: A Cancer J Clin 2000;50:7–33.
174. Goellner JR, Gharib H, Grant CS, Johnson DA. Fine needle aspiration cytology of the thyroid, 1980 to 1986. Acta Cytol 1987;31:587–90.
175. Cooper DS, Doherty GM, Haugen BR, et al. Management guidelines for patients with thyroid nodules and differentiated thyroid cancer. Thyroid 2006;16:109–42.
176. Cersosimo E, Gharib H, Suman VJ, Goellner JR. "Suspicious" thyroid cytologic findings: Outcome in patients without immediate surgical treatment. Mayo Clin Proc 1993; 68:343–8.
177. Csako G, Byrd D, Wesley RA, et al. Assessing the effects of thyroid suppression on benign solitary thyroid nodules. A model for using quantitative research synthesis. Medicine 2000;79:9–26.
178. Silva MN, Rubio IG, Romao R, et al. Administration of a single dose of recombinant human thyrotrophin enhances the efficacy of radioiodine treatment of large compressive multinodular goitres. Clin Endocrinol 2004;60:300–8.
179. Li X, Lu S, Miyagi E, et al. Thyrotropin prevents apoptosis by promoting cell adhesion and cell cycle progression in FRTL-5 cells. Endocrinology 1999;140:5962–70.
180. Metcalfe RA, Findlay C, Robertson WR, et al. Differential effect of thyroid-stimulating hormone (TSH) on intracellular free calcium and cAMP in cells transfected with the human TSH receptor. J Endocrinol 1998;157:415–24.
181. Medina DL, Santisteban P. Thyrotropin-dependent proliferation of in vitro rat thyroid cell systems. Eur J Endocrinol 2000;143:161–78.
182. Chin WW, Carr FE, Burnside J, Darling DS. Thyroid hormone regulation of thyrotropin gene expression. Rec Prog Horm Res 1993;48:393–414.
183. Gharib H, Mazzaferri EL. Thyroxine suppressive therapy in patients with nodular thyroid disease. Ann Intern Med 1998;128:386–94.
184. Russo D, Arturi F, Suarez HG, et al. Thyrotropin receptor gene alterations in thyroid hyperfunctioning adenomas. J Clin Endocrinol Metab 1996;81:1548–51.
185. Fagin JA. Molecular genetics of human thyroid neoplasms. Ann Rev of Med 1994;45:45–52.
186. Nodules AATFoT. American Association of Clinical Endocrinologists and Associazione Medici Endocrinologi medical guidelines for clinical practice for the diagnosis and management of thyroid nodules. Endocr Pract 2006; 12:63–102.
187. Hatabu H, Kasagi K, Yamamoto K, et al. Cystic papillary carcinoma of the thyroid gland: A new sonographic sign. Clin Radiol 1991;43:121–4.
188. Hammer M, Wortsman J, Folse R. Cancer in cystic lesions of the thyroid. Arch Surg 1982;117:1020–3.
189. Krohn K, Emmrich P, Ott N, Paschke R. Increased thyroid epithelial cell proliferation in toxic thyroid nodules. Thyroid 1999;9:241–6.
190. Gharib H. Single thyroid nodule. Curr Ther Endocrinol Metab 1997;6:112–7.
191. Jemal A, Siegel R, Ward E, et al. Cancer statistics, 2007. CA: A Cancer J Clin 2007;57:43–66.
192 Hundahl SA, Fleming ID, Fremgen AM, Menck HR. A National Cancer Data Base report on 53,856 cases of thyroid carcinoma treated in the US, 1985–1995. Cancer 1998; 83:2638–48.
193. Gilliland FD, Hunt WC, Morris DM, Key CR. Prognostic factors for thyroid carcinoma. A population-based study of 15,698 cases from the Surveillance, Epidemiology and End Results (SEER) program 1973–1991. Cancer 1997; 79:564–73.
194. O'Riordain DS, O'Brien T, Weaver AL, et al. Medullary thyroid carcinoma in multiple endocrine neoplasia types 2A and 2B. Surgery 1994;116:1017–23.
195. Mazzaferri EL. An overview of the management of papillary and follicular thyroid carcinoma. Thyroid 1999;9:421–7.
196. van Heerden JA, Hay ID, Goellner JR, et al. Follicular thyroid carcinoma with capsular invasion alone: A nonthreatening malignancy. Surgery 1992;112:1130–6; discussion 1136–8.
197. McIver B, Hay ID, Giuffrida DF, et al. Anaplastic thyroid carcinoma: A 50-year experience at a single institution. Surgery 2001;130:1028–34.
198. Thyroid Carcinoma Task F. AACE/AAES medical/surgical guidelines for clinical practice: Management of thyroid carcinoma. American Association of Clinical Endocrinologists. American College of Endocrinology. Endocr Pract 2001;7:202–20.
199. Spencer CA, LoPresti JS, Fatemi S, Nicoloff JT. Detection of residual and recurrent differentiated thyroid carcinoma by serum thyroglobulin measurement. Thyroid 1999; 9:435–41.
200. Maxon HR. Detection of residual and recurrent thyroid cancer by radionuclide imaging. Thyroid 1999;9:443–6.
201. Williams ED. Mechanisms and pathogenesis of thyroid cancer in animals and man. Mutat Res 1995;333:123–9.
202. Grebe SK, Hay ID. The role of surgery in the management of differentiated thyroid cancer. J Endocrinol Invest 1997; 20:32–5.
203. Hedinger C, Williams ED, Sobin LH. The WHO histological classification of thyroid tumors: A commentary on the second edition. Cancer 1989;63:908–11.
204. Rosai J, Carcangui ML, DeLellis RA. Tumors of the Thyroid Gland Atlas of Tumor Pathology. Washington D.C.: Armed Forces Institute of Pathology; 1992.
205. Ahuja AT, Chow L, Chick W, et al. Metastatic cervical nodes in papillary carcinoma of the thyroid: Ultrasound and histological correlation. Clin Radiol 1995;50:229–31.
206. Gharib H. Fine-needle aspiration biopsy of thyroid nodules: Advantages, limitations, and effect. Mayo Clin Proc 1994; 69:44–9.
207. Hedinger CE. Histological typing of thyroid tumors. In: Hedinger CE, editor. International Histological Classification of Tumours. Berlin: Springer-Verlag; 1988. p. 22–3.
208. Grebe SK, Hay ID. Follicular thyroid cancer. Endocrinol Metab Clin N Am 1995;24:761–801.
209. Rosai J, Saxen EA, Woolner L. Undifferentiated and poorly differentiated carcinoma. Semin Diagn Pathol 1985; 2:123–36.
210. Marchesi M, Biffoni M, Biancari F, et al. Insular carcinoma of the thyroid. A report of 8 cases. Chirurgia Italiana 1998; 50:73–5.
211. Hassoun AA, Hay ID, Goellner JR, Zimmerman D. Insular thyroid carcinoma in adolescents: A potentially lethal endocrine malignancy. Cancer 1997;79:1044–8.
212. Rodriguez JM, Parrilla P, Moreno A, et al. Insular carcinoma: An infrequent subtype of thyroid cancer. J Am Coll Surg 1998;187:503–8.
213. Pilotti S, Collini P, Mariani L, et al. Insular carcinoma: A distinct de novo entity among follicular carcinomas of the thyroid gland. Am J Surg Pathol 1997;21:1466–73.
214. Samaan NA, Schultz PN, Haynie TP, Ordonez NG. Pulmonary metastasis of differentiated thyroid carcinoma: Treatment results in 101 patients. J Clin Endocrinol Metab 1985;60:376–80.
215. Ruegemer JJ, Hay ID, Bergstralh EJ, et al. Distant metastases in differentiated thyroid carcinoma: A multivariate analysis of prognostic variables. J Clin Endocrinol Metab 1988;67:501–8.
216. Har-El G, Hadar T, Segal K, et al. Hurthle cell carcinoma of the thyroid gland. A tumor of moderate malignancy. Cancer 1986;57:1613–7.
217. Grebe SK, Hay ID. Thyroid cancer nodal metastases: Biologic significance and therapeutic considerations. Surg Oncol Clin N Am 1996;5:43–63.
218. Fagin JA. Genetics of papillary thyroid cancer initiation: Implications for therapy. Trans Am Clin Climatol Assoc 2005;116:259–69; discussion 269–71.
219. Lang BH, Lo CY, Chan WF, et al. Staging systems for papillary thyroid carcinoma: A review and comparison. Ann Surg 2007;245:366–78.
220. Xing M, Coteen Y, Mambo E et al. Early occurrence of RASSF1A hypermethylation and its mutual exclusion with BRAF mutation in thyroid tumorigenesis. Cancer Res 2004;64:1664–8
221. Brierley JD, Panzarella T, Tsang RW, et al. A comparison of different staging systems predictability of patient outcome. Thyroid carcinoma as an example. Cancer 1997; 79:2414–23.
222. Loh KC, Greenspan FS, Gee L, et al. Pathological tumor-node-metastasis (pTNM) staging for papillary and follicular thyroid carcinomas: A retrospective analysis of 700 patients. J Clin Endocrinol Metab 1997;82:3553–62.
223. Farley DR, Eberhardt NL, Grant CS, et al. Expression of a potential metastasis suppressor gene (nm23) in thyroid neoplasms. World J Surg 1993;17:615–20; discussion 620–1.
224. Sanders LE, Cady B. Differentiated thyroid cancer: Reexamination of risk groups and outcome of treatment. Arch Surg 1998;133:419–25.
225. McConahey WM, Hay ID, Woolner LB, et al. Papillary thyroid cancer treated at the Mayo Clinic, 1946 through 1970: Initial manifestations, pathologic findings, therapy, and outcome. Mayo Clin Proc 1986;61:978–96.
226. Dean DS, Hay ID. Prognostic indicators in differentiated thyroid carcinoma. Cancer Control 2000;7:229–39.
227. Niederle B, Roka R, Schemper M, et al. Surgical treatment of distant metastases in differentiated thyroid cancer: Indication and results. Surgery 1986;100:1088–97.
228. Vassilopoulou-Sellin R, Schultz PN, Haynie TP. Clinical outcome of patients with papillary thyroid carcinoma who have recurrence after initial radioactive iodine therapy. Cancer 1996;78:493–501.
229. Dinneen SF, Valimaki MJ, Bergstralh EJ, et al. Distant metastases in papillary thyroid carcinoma: 100 cases observed at one institution during 5 decades. J Clin Endocrinol Metab 1995;80:2041–5.
230. Samuel AM, Rajashekharrao B, Shah DH. Pulmonary metastases in children and adolescents with well-differentiated thyroid cancer. J Nucl Med 1998;39:1531–6.
231. Grebe SK, Hay ID. Prognostic factors and management in thyroid cancer--consensus or controversy? West J Med 1996;165:156–7.
232. Jorda M, Gonzalez-Campora R, Mora J, et al. Prognostic factors in follicular carcinoma of the thyroid. Arch Pathol Lab Med 1993;117:631–5.
233. Sanders LE, Silverman M. Follicular and Hurthle cell carcinoma: Predicting outcome and directing therapy. Surgery 1998;124:967–74.
234. Zielke A, Hoffmann S, Plaul U, et al. Pleiotropic effects of thyroid stimulating hormone in a differentiated thyroid cancer cell line. Studies on proliferation, thyroglobulin secretion, adhesion, migration and invasion. Exp Clin Endocrinol Diabetes 1999;107:361–9.
235. Gharib H, Mazzaferri EL. Thyroxine suppressive therapy in patients with nodular thyroid disease. Ann Intern Med 1998;128:386–94.
236. Hoffman DP, Surks MI, Oppenheimer JH, Weitzman ED. Response to thyrotropin releasing hormone: An objective criterion for the adequacy of thyrotropin suppression therapy. J Clin Endocrinol Metab 1977;44:892–901.
237. Bayer MF, Kriss JP, McDougall IR. Clinical experience with sensitive thyrotropin measurements: Diagnostic and therapeutic implications. J Nucl Med 1985;26:1248–56.
238. Pujol P, Daures JP, Nsakala N, et al. Degree of thyrotropin suppression as a prognostic determinant in differentiated

thyroid cancer. J Clin Endocrinol Metab 1996; 81:4318–23.
239. Mazzaferri EL. Papillary and follicular thyroid cancer: Aselective approach to diagnosis and treatment. Annu Rev Med 1981;32:73–91.
240. Szanto J, Ringwald G, Karika Z, et al. Follicular cancer of the thyroid gland. Oncology 1991;48:483–9.
241. Young RL, Mazzaferri EL, Rahe AJ, Dorfman SG. Pure follicular thyroid carcinoma: Impact of therapy in 214 patients. J Nucl Med 1980;21:733–7.
242. Mazzaferri EL, Young RL, Oertel JE, et al. Papillary thyroid carcinoma: The impact of therapy in 576 patients. Medicine 1977;56:171–96.
243. Cunningham MP, Duda RB, Recant W, et al. Survival discriminants for differentiated thyroid cancer. Am J Surg 1990;160:344–7.
244. Simpson LO. The etiopathogenesis of premenstrual syndrome as a consequence of altered blood rheology: A new hypothesis. Med Hypotheses 1988;25:189–95.
245. Staunton MD. Thyroid cancer: A multivariate analysis on influence of treatment on long-term survival. Eur J Surg Oncol 1994;20:613–21.
246. Cooper DS, Specker B, Ho M, et al. Thyrotropin suppression and disease progression in patients with differentiated thyroid cancer: Results from the National Thyroid Cancer Treatment Cooperative Registry. Thyroid 1998; 8:737–44.
247. Toivonen J, Tahtela R, Laitinen K, et al. Markers of bone turnover in patients with differentiated thyroid cancer with and following withdrawal of thyroxine suppressive therapy. Eur J Endocrinol 1998;138:667–73.
248. Franklyn JA, Betteridge J, Daykin J, et al. Long-term thyroxine treatment and bone mineral density [see comments]. Lancet 1992;340:9–13.
249. Nguyen TT, Heath H 3rd, Bryant SC, et al. Fractures after thyroidectomy in men: A population-based cohort study. J Bone Miner Res 1997;12:1092–9.
250. Sawin CT, Geller A, Wolf PA, et al. Low serum thyrotropin concentrations as a risk factor for atrial fibrillation in older persons. N Engl J Med 1994;331:1249–52.
251. Hay ID, Feld S, Garcia M. AACE clinical practice guidelines for the management of thyroid carcinoma. Endocr Pract 1997;3:60–71.
252. Ajjan RA, Kamaruddin NA, Crisp M, et al. Regulation and tissue distribution of the human sodium iodide symporter gene. Clin Endocrinol (Oxf) 1998;49:517–23.
253. Spitzweg C, Joba W, Eisenmenger W, Heufelder AE. Analysis of human sodium iodide symporter gene expression in extrathyroidal tissues and cloning of its complementary deoxyribonucleic acids from salivary gland, mammary gland, and gastric mucosa. J Clin Endocrinol Metab 1998; 83:1746–51.
254. Wen C, Iuanow E, Oates E, et al. Post-therapy iodine-131 localization in unsuspected large renal cyst: Possible mechanisms. J Nucl Med 1998;39:2158–61.
255. Hays MT. Colonic excretion of iodide in normal human subjects. Thyroid 1993;3:31–5.
256. Filetti S, Bidart JM, Arturi F, et al. Sodium/iodide symporter: A key transport system in thyroid cancer cell metabolism. Eur J Endocrinol 1999;141:443–57.
257. Feinendegen LE. Contributions of nuclear medicine to the therapy of malignant tumors [editorial]. J Cancer Res Clin Oncol 1993;119:320–2.
258. Rydberg B. Clusters of DNA damage induced by ionizing radiation: Formation of short DNA fragments. II. Experimental detection. Radiat Res 1996;145:200–9.
259. Mallya SM, Sikpi MO. Requirement for p53 in ionizing-radiation-inhibition of double-strand- break rejoining by human lymphoblasts. Mutat Res 1999;434:119–32.
260. Daza P, Schubler H, McMillan TJ, et al. Radiosensitivity and double-strand break rejoining in tumorigenic and nontumorigenic human epithelial cell lines. Int J Radiat Biol 1997;72:91–100.
261. Maxon HRd, Smith HS. Radioiodine-131 in the diagnosis and treatment of metastatic well differentiated thyroid cancer. Endocrinol Metab Clin N Am 1990;19:685–718.
262. Vermiglio F, Violi MA, Finocchiaro MD, et al. Short-term effectiveness of low-dose radioiodune ablative treatment of thyroid remnants after thyroidectomy for differentiated thyroid cancer. Thyroid 1999;9:387–91.
263. Johansen K, Woodhouse NJ, Odugbesan O. Comparison of 1073 MBq and 3700 MBq iodine-131 in postoperative ablation of residual thyroid tissue in patients with differentiated thyroid cancer. J Nucl Med 1991;32:252–4.
264. Bal C, Padhy AK, Jana S, et al. Prospective randomized clinical trial to evaluate the optimal dose of 131 I for remnant ablation in patients with differentiated thyroid carcinoma. Cancer 1996;77:2574–80.
265. M'Kacher R, Legal JD, Schlumberger M, et al. Biological dosimetry in patients treated with iodine-131 for differentiated thyroid carcinoma. J Nucl Med 1996;37:1860–4.
266. Beierwaltes WH. The treatment of thyroid carcinoma with radioactive iodine. Semin Nucl Med 1978;8:79–94.
267. Maxon HR, Thomas SR, Boehringer A, et al. Low iodine diet in I-131 ablation of thyroid remnants. Clin Nucl Med 1983;8:123–6.
268. Dunn JT. Thyroid suppression and medical ablation for differentiated thyroid cancer. Arch Otolaryngol Head Neck Surg 1986;112:1207–9.
269. Mazzaferri EL. Papillary thyroid carcinoma: Factors influencing prognosis and current therapy. Semin Oncol 1987; 14:315–32.
270. Grant CS, Hay ID, Ryan JJ, et al. Diagnostic and prognostic utility of flow cytometric DNA measurements in follicular thyroid tumors. World J Surg 1990;14:283–9; discussion 289–90.
271. Jonklaas J, Sarlis NJ, Litofsky D, et al. Outcomes of patients with differentiated thyroid carcinoma following initial therapy. Thyroid 2006;16:1229–42.
272. DeGroot LJ, Kaplan EL, Straus FH, Shukla MS. Does the method of management of papillary thyroid carcinoma make a difference in outcome? World J Surg 1994;18:123–30.
273. Samaan NA, Schultz PN, Hickey RC, et al. The results of various modalities of treatment of well differentiated thyroid carcinomas: A retrospective review of 1599 patients. J Clin Endocrinol Metab 1992;75:714–20.
274. Hay ID, Thompson GB, Grant CS, et al. Papillary thyroid carcinoma managed at the Mayo Clinic during six decades (1940–1999): Temporal trends in initial therapy and long-term outcome in 2444 consecutively treated patients. World J Surgery 2002;26:879–85.
275. Flynn MB, Lyons KJ, Tarter JW, Ragsdale TL. Local complications after surgical resection for thyroid carcinoma. Am J Surg 1994;168:404–7.
276. Franklyn JA, Maisonneuve P, Sheppard M, et al. Cancer incidence and mortality after radioiodine treatment for hyperthyroidism: A population-based cohort study. Lancet 1999;353:2111–5.
277. Hay ID, Klee GG. Thyroid cancer diagnosis and management. Clin Lab Med 1993;13:725–34.
278. Hufner M, Stumpf HP, Grussendorf M, et al. A comparison of the effectiveness of 131I whole body scans and plasma Tg determinations in the diagnosis of metastatic differentiated carcinoma of the thyroid: A retrospective study. Acta Endocrinol (Copenh) 1983;104:327–32.
279. Hay ID. Nodular thyroid disease diagnosed during pregnancy: How and when to treat. Thyroid 1999;9:667–70.
280. Khafif A, Khafif RA, Attie JN. Hurthle cell carcinoma: A malignancy of low-grade potential. Head Neck 1999; 21:506–11.
281. Van Nostrand D, Neutze J, Atkins F. Side effects of "rational dose" iodine-131 therapy for metastatic well-differentiated thyroid carcinoma. J Nucl Med 1986;27:1519–27.
282. Rubino C, de Vathaire F, Dottorini ME, et al. Second primary malignancies in thyroid cancer patients. British J Cancer 2003;89:1638–44.
283. Reynolds JC. Percent 131I uptake and post-therapy 131I scans: Their role in the management of thyroid cancer. Thyroid 1997;7:281–4.
284. Park HM, Park YH, Zhou XH. Detection of thyroid remnant/ metastasis without stunning: An ongoing dilemma. Thyroid 1997;7:277–80.
285. Yaakob W, Gordon L, Spicer KM, Nitke SJ. The usefulness of iodine-123 whole-body scans in evaluating thyroid carcinoma and metastases. J Nucl Med Technol 1999; 27:279–81.
286. Grebe SKG, Hay ID. Management of differentiated thryoid cancer. Curr Opin Endocrinol Diabetes 1995;2:449–54.
287. Sisson JC, Giordano TJ, Jamadar DA, et al. 131-I treatment of micronodular pulmonary metastases from papillary thyroid carcinoma. Cancer 1996;78:2184–92.
288. Zimmerman D, Hay ID, Gough IR, et al. Papillary thyroid carcinoma in children and adults: Long-term follow-up of 1039 patients conservatively treated at one institution during three decades. Surgery 1988;104:1157–66.
289. Hoie J, Stenwig AE, Kullmann G, Lindegaard M. Distant metastases in papillary thyroid cancer. A review of 91 patients. Cancer 1988;61:1–6.
290. Hockel M, Schlenger K, Mitze M, et al. Hypoxia and radiation response in human tumors. Semin Radiat Oncol 1996;6:3–9.
291. Datz FL. Cerebral edema following iodine-131 therapy for thyroid carcinoma metastatic to the brain. J Nucl Med 1986;27:637–40.
292. Chiu AC, Delpassand ES, Sherman SI. Prognosis and treatment of brain metastases in thyroid carcinoma. J Clin Endocrinol Metab 1997;82:3637–42.
293. Sherman SI, Ringel MD, Smith MJ, et al. Augmented hepatic and skeletal thyromimetic effects of tiratricol in comparison with levothyroxine. J Clin Endocrinol Metab 1997;82:2153–8.
294. Hales M, Rosenau W, Okerlund MD, Galante M. Carcinoma of the thyroid with a mixed medullary and follicular pattern: Morphologic, immunohistochemical, and clinical laboratory studies. Cancer 1982;50:1352–9.
295. Brierley JD, Tsang RW. External radiation therapy in the treatment of thyroid malignancy. Endocrinol Metab Clin N Am 1996;25:141–57.
296. Chow SM, Law SC, Au SK, et al. Changes in clinical presentation, management and outcome in 1348 patients with differentiated thyroid carcinoma: Experience in a single institute in Hong Kong, 1960–2000. Clin Oncology 2003;15:329–36.
297. Farahati J, Reiners C, Stuschke M, et al. Differentiated thyroid cancer. Impact of adjuvant external radiotherapy in patients with perithyroidal tumor infiltration (stage pT4). Cancer 1996;77:172–80.
298. Tsang RW, Brierley JD, Simpson WJ, et al. The effects of surgery, radioiodine, and external radiation therapy on the clinical outcome of patients with differentiated thyroid carcinoma. Cancer 1998;82:375–88.
299. Czaja JM, McCaffrey TV. The surgical management of laryngotracheal invasion by well-differentiated papillary thyroid carcinoma. Arch Otolaryngol Head Neck Surg 1997;123:484–90.
300. Kasperbauer JL. Locally advanced thyroid carcinoma. Ann Otol Rhinol Laryngol 2004;113:749–53.
301. Viswanathan K, Gierlowski TC, Schneider AB. Childhood thyroid cancer. Characteristics and long-term outcome in children irradiated for benign conditions of the head and neck. Arch Pediatr Adolesc Med 1994;148:260–5.
302. Hopkins CR, Reading CC. Thyroid and parathyroid imaging. Semin Ultrasound CT MR 1995;16:279–95.
303. Grunwald F, Menzel C, Bender H, et al. Redifferentiation therapy-induced radioiodine uptake in thyroid cancer. J Nucl Med 1998;39:1903–6.
304. Denicoff KD, Joffe RT, Lakshmanan MC, et al. Neuropsychiatric manifestations of altered thyroid state. Am J Psychiatry 1990;147:94–9.
305. Ringel MD, Ladenson PW. Diagnostic accuracy of 131I scanning with recombinant human thyrotropin versus thyroid hormone withdrawal in a patient with metastatic thyroid carcinoma and hypopituitarism. J Clin Endocrinol Metab 1996;81:1724–5.
306. Robbins J. Pharmacology of bovine and human thyrotropin: An historical perspective. Thyroid 1999;9:451–3.
307. Meier CA, Braverman LE, Ebner SA, et al. Diagnostic use of recombinant human thyrotropin in patients with thyroid carcinoma (phase I/II study). J Clin Endocrinol Metab 1994;78:188–96.
308. Ladenson PW, Braverman LE, Mazzaferri EL, et al. Comparison of administration of recombinant human thyrotropin with withdrawal of thyroid hormone for radioactive iodine scanning in patients with thyroid carcinoma. N Engl J Med 1997;337:888–96.
309. Haugen BR, Pacini F, Reiners C, et al. A comparison of recombinant human thyrotropin and thyroid hormone withdrawal for the detection of thyroid remnant or cancer. J Clin Endocrinol Metab 1999;84:3877–85.
310. Masiukiewicz US, Nakchbandi IA, Stewart AF, Inzucchi SE. Papillary thyroid carcinoma metastatic to the pituitary gland. Thyroid 1999;9:1023–7.
311. Wang W, Macapinlac H, Larson SM, et al. [18F]-2-fluoro-2-deoxy-D-glucose positron emission tomography localizes residual thyroid cancer in patients with negative diagnostic (131)I whole body scans and elevated serum thyroglobulin levels. J Clin Endocrinol Metab 1999;84:2291–302.
312. Wang W, Larson SM, Fazzari M, et al. Prognostic value of [18F]fluorodeoxyglucose positron emission tomographic scanning in patients with thyroid cancer. J Clin Endocrinol Metab 2000;85:1107–13.
313. Krausz Y, Rosler A, Guttmann H, et al. Somatostatin receptor scintigraphy for early detection of regional and distant metastases of medullary carcinoma of the thyroid. Clin Nuclear Med 1999;24:256–60.
314. Wilson CJ, Woodroof JM, Girod DA. First report of Hurthle cell carcinoma revealed by octreotide scanning. Ann Otol Rhinol Laryngol 1998;107:847–50.
315. Westbury C, Vini L, Fisher C, Harmer C. Recurrent differentiated thyroid cancer without elevation of serum thyroglobulin. Thyroid 2000;10:171–6.
316. Sisson JC, Thompson NW, Giordano TJ, et al. Serum thyroglobulin levels after thyroxine withdrawal in patients with low-risk papillary thyroid carcinoma. Thyroid 2000; 10:165–9.
317. Tallini G, Ghossein RA, Emanuel J, et al. Detection of thyroglobulin, thyroid peroxidase, and RET/PTC1 mRNA

transcripts in the peripheral blood of patients with thyroid disease. J Clin Oncol 1998;16:1158–66.

318. Ringel MD, Ladenson PW, Levine MA. Molecular diagnosis of residual and recurrent thyroid cancer by amplification of thyroglobulin messenger ribonucleic acid in peripheral blood. J Clin Endocrinol Metab 1998;83:4435–42.

319. Ringel MD, Balducci-Silano PL, Anderson JS, et al. Quantitative reverse transcription-polymerase chain reaction of circulating thyroglobulin messenger ribonucleic acid for monitoring patients with thyroid carcinoma. J Clin Endocrinol Metab 1999;84:4037–42.

320. Smith SA, Gharib H, Goellner JR. Fine-needle aspiration. Usefulness for diagnosis and management of metastatic carcinoma to the thyroid. Arch Intern Med 1987; 147:311–2.

321. Chi DD, Moley JF. Medullary thyroid carcinoma: Genetic advances, treatment recommendations, and the approach to the patient with persistent hypercalcitoninemia. Surg Oncol Clin N Am 1998;7:681–706.

322. van Heerden JA, Grant CS, Gharib H, et al. Long-term course of patients with persistent hypercalcitoninemia after apparent curative primary surgery for medullary thyroid carcinoma. Ann Surg 1990;212:395–400.

323. Mendelsohn G, Wells SA, Jr, Baylin SB. Relationship of tissue carcinoembryonic antigen and calcitonin to tumor virulence in medullary thyroid carcinoma. An immunohistochemical study in early, localized, and virulent disseminated stages of disease. Cancer 1984;54:657–62.

324. McIver B, Hay ID, Giuffrida DF, et al. Anaplastic thyroid carcinoma: A 50-year experience at a single institution. Surgery 2001;130:1028–34.

325. Ain KB. Anaplastic thyroid carcinoma: A therapeutic challenge. Semin Surg Oncol 1999;16:64–9.

326. Jemal A, Thomas A, Murray T, Thun M. Cancer statistics, 2002. CA Cancer J Clin 2002;52:23–47.

327. Ain KB. Anaplastic thyroid carcinoma: A therapeutic challenge. Semin Surg Oncol 1999;16:64–9.

328. Nilsson O, Lindeberg J, Zedenius J, et al. Anaplastic giant cell carcinoma of the thyroid gland: Treatment and survival over a 25-year period. World J Surg 1998;22:725–30.

329. Tan RK, Finley RK, 3rd, Driscoll D, et al. Anaplastic carcinoma of the thyroid: A 24-year experience. Head Neck 1995;17:41–7.

330. Heitz P, Moser H, Staub JJ. Thyroid cancer: A study of 573 thyroid tumors and 161 autopsy cases observed over a thirty-year period. Cancer 1976;37:2329–37.

331. Christensen SB, Ljungberg O, Tibblin S. Thyroid carcinoma in Malmo, 1960-1977. Epidemiologic, clinical, and prognostic findings in a defined urban population. Cancer 1984;53:1625–33.

332. LiVolsi VA, Brooks JJ, Arendash-Durand B. Anaplastic thyroid tumors. Immunohistology. Am J Clin Pathol 1987; 87:434–42.

333. Holting T, Moller P, Tschahargane C, et al. Immunohistochemical reclassification of anaplastic carcinoma reveals small and giant cell lymphoma. World J Surg 1990; 14:291–4.

334. Samaan NA, Ordonez NG. Uncommon types of thyroid cancer. Endocrinol Metab Clin N Am 1990;19:637–48.

335. Tobler A, Maurer R, Hedinger CE. Undifferentiated thyroid tumors of diffuse small cell type. Histological and immunohistochemical evidence for their lymphomatous nature. Virchows Arch A Pathol Anat Histopathol 1984;404:117–26.

336. Demeter JG, De Jong SA, Lawrence AM, Paloyan E. Anaplastic thyroid carcinoma: Risk factors and outcome. Surgery 1991;110:956–61.

337. Levendag PC, De Porre PM, van Putten WL. Anaplastic carcinoma of the thyroid gland treated by radiation therapy. Int J Radiat Oncol Biol Phys 1993;26:125–8.

338. Bakiri F, Djemli FK, Mokrane LA, Djidel FK. The relative roles of endemic goiter and socioeconomic development status in the prognosis of thyroid carcinoma. Cancer 1998; 82:1146–53.

339. Venkatesh YS, Ordonez NG, Schultz PN, et al. Anaplastic carcinoma of the thyroid. A clinicopathologic study of 121 cases. Cancer 1990;66:321–30.

340. Hadar T, Mor C, Shvero J, et al. Anaplastic carcinoma of the thyroid. Eur J Surg Oncol 1993;19:511–6.

341. Kobayashi T, Asakawa H, Umeshita K, et al. Treatment of 37 patients with anaplastic carcinoma of the thyroid. Head Neck 1996;18:36–41.

342. Pettersson B, Coleman MP, Ron E, Adami HO. Iodine supplementation in Sweden and regional trends in thyroid cancer incidence by histopathologic type. Int J Cancer 1996;65:13–9.

343. Rosai J, Saxen EA, Woolner L. Undifferentiated and poorly differentiated carcinoma. Semin Diag Pathol 1985; 2:123–36.

344. Herrmann G, Schumm-Draeger PM, Muller C, et al. T lymphocytes, CD68-positive cells and vascularisation in thyroid carcinomas. J Cancer Res Clin Oncol 1994;120:651–6.

345. Belletti B, Ferraro P, Arra C, et al. Modulation of in vivo growth of thyroid tumor-derived cell lines by sense and antisense vascular endothelial growth factor gene. Oncogene 1999;18:4860–9.

346. Huang SM, Lee JC, Wu TJ, Chow NH. Clinical relevance of vascular endothelial growth factor for thyroid neoplasms. World J Surg 2001;25:302–6.

347. Wolf BC, Sheahan K, DeCoste D, et al. Immunohistochemical analysis of small cell tumors of the thyroid gland: An Eastern Cooperative Oncology Group study. Human Pathol 1992;23:1252–61.

348. Shvero J, Gal R, Avidor I, et al. Anaplastic thyroid carcinoma. A clinical, histologic, and immunohistochemical study. Cancer 1988;62:319–25.

349. Carcangiu ML, Steeper T, Zampi G, Rosai J. Anaplastic thyroid carcinoma. A study of 70 cases. Am J Clin Pathol 1985; 83:135–58.

350. Miettinen M, Franssila KO. Variable expression of keratins and nearly uniform lack of thyroid transcription factor 1 in thyroid anaplastic carcinoma. Hum Pathol 2000; 31:1139–45.

351. Fagin JA. Molecular genetics of human thyroid neoplasms. Annu Rev Med 1994;45:45–52.

352. Mortensen JD, Woolner LB, Bennett WA. Secondary malignant tumors of the thyroid gland. Cancer 1956;9:306–10.

353. Brander A, Viikinkoski P, Nickels J, Kivisaari L. Thyroid gland: US screening in middle-aged women with no previous thyroid disease. Radiology 1989;173:507–10.

354. Hintze G, Windeler J, Baumert J, et al. Thyroid volume and goitre prevalence in the elderly as determined by ultrasound and their relationships to laboratory indices. Acta Endocrinol (Copenh) 1991;124:12–8.

355. Stephenson BM, Wheeler MH, Clark OH. The role of total thyroidectomy in the management of differentiated thyroid cancer. Curr Opin Gen Surg 1994:53–9.

356. van den Brekel MW, Hekkenberg RJ, Asa SL, et al. Prognostic features in tall cell papillary carcinoma and insular thyroid carcinoma. Laryngoscope 1997;107:254–9.

357. Demeter JG, De Jong SA, Lawrence AM, Paloyan E. Anaplastic thyroid carcinoma: Risk factors and outcome. Surgery 1991;110:956–61.

358. Jonasson JG, Hrafnkelsson J. Nuclear DNA analysis and prognosis in carcinoma of the thyroid gland. A nationwide study in Iceland on carcinomas diagnosed 1955–1990. Virchows Arch 1994;425:349–55.

359. Salmon I, Gasperin P, Remmelink M, et al. Ploidy level and proliferative activity measurements in a series of 407 thyroid tumors or other pathologic conditions. Hum Pathol 1993;24:912–0.

360. Wallin G, Backdahl M, Tallroth-Ekman E, et al. Co-existent anaplastic and well differentiated thyroid carcinomas: A nuclear DNA study. Eur J Surg Oncol 1989;15:43–48.

361. Sheils OM, O'Leary JJ, Sweeney EC. Assessment of ret/PTC-1 rearrangements in neoplastic thyroid tissue using TaqMan RT-PCR. J Pathol 2000;192:32–6.

362. Vecchio G, Santoro M. Oncogenes and thyroid cancer. Clin Chem Lab Med 2000;38:113–6.

363. Fogelfeld L, Bauer TK, Schneider AB, et al. p53 gene mutations in radiation-induced thyroid cancer. J Clin Endocrinol Metab 1996;81:3039–44.

364. La Perle KM, Jhiang SM, Capen CC. Loss of p53 promotes anaplasia and local invasion in ret/PTC1-induced thyroid carcinomas. Am J Pathol 2000;157:671–7.

365. Moretti F, Farsetti A, Soddu S, et al. p53 re-expression inhibits proliferation and restores differentiation of human thyroid anaplastic carcinoma cells. Oncogene 1997; 14:729–40.

366. Passler C, Scheuba C, Prager G, et al. Anaplastic (undifferentiated) thyroid carcinoma (ATC). A retrospective analysis. Langenbecks Arch Surg 1999;384:284–93.

367. Junor EJ, Paul J, Reed NS. Anaplastic thyroid carcinoma: 91 patients treated by surgery and radiotherapy. Eur J Surg Oncol 1992;18:83–8.

368. Levendag PC, De Porre PM, van Putten WL. Anaplastic carcinoma of the thyroid gland treated by radiation therapy. Int J Rad Oncol Biol Phys 1993;26:125–8.

369. Kobayashi S, Yamadori I, Ohmori M, et al. Anaplastic carcinoma of the thyroid with osteoclast-like giant cells. An ultrastructural and immunohistochemical study. Acta Pathol Jpn 1987;37:807–15.

370. Staunton MD. Thyroid cancer: A multivariate analysis on influence of treatment on long-term survival. Eur J Surg Oncol 1994;20:613–21.

371. Simpson WJ. Anaplastic thyroid carcinoma: A new approach. Can J Surg 1980;23:25–7.

372. Thomas CG, Jr. Role of thyroid stimulating hormone suppression in the management of thyroid cancer. Semin Surg Oncol 1991;7:115–9.

373. Kim JH, Leeper RD. Treatment of anaplastic giant and spindle cell carcinoma of the thyroid gland with combination Adriamycin and radiation therapy. A new approach. Cancer 1983;52:954–7.

374. Kim JH, Leeper RD. Treatment of locally advanced thyroid carcinoma with combination doxorubicin and radiation therapy. Cancer 1987;60:2372–5.

375. Ain KB, Tofiq S, Taylor KD. Antineoplastic activity of taxol against human anaplastic thyroid carcinoma cell lines in vitro and in vivo. J Clin Endocrinol Metab 1996; 81:3650–3.

376. Sweeney PJ, Haraf DJ, Recant W, et al. Anaplastic carcinoma of the thyroid. Ann Oncol 1996;7:739–44.

377. Pledge S, Bessell EM, Leach IH, et al. Non-Hodgkin's lymphoma of the thyroid: A retrospective review of all patients diagnosed in Nottinghamshire from 1973 to 1992. Clin Oncol 1996;8:371–5.

378. Pedersen RK, Pedersen NT. Primary non-Hodgkin's lymphoma of the thyroid gland: A population based study. Histopathology 1996;28:25–32.

379. Matsuzuka F, Miyauchi A, Katayama S, et al. Clinical aspects of primary thyroid lymphoma: Diagnosis and treatment based on our experience of 119 cases. Thyroid 1993;3:93–9.

380. Junor EJ, Paul J, Reed NS. Primary non-Hodgkin's lymphoma of the thyroid. Eur J Surg Oncol 1992;18:313–21.

381. Pyke CM, Grant CS, Habermann TM, et al. Non-Hodgkin's lymphoma of the thyroid: Is more than biopsy necessary? World J Surg 1992;16:604–9.

382. Matsuzuka F, Fukata S, Kuma K, et al. Gene rearrangement of immunoglobulin as a marker of thyroid lymphoma. World J Surg 1998;22:558–61.

383. Derringer GA, Thompson LD, Frommelt RA, et al. Malignant lymphoma of the thyroid gland: A clinicopathologic study of 108 cases. Am J Surg Pathol 2000;24:623–39.

384. Pasieka JL. Anaplastic cancer, lymphoma, and metastases of the thyroid gland. Surg Oncol Clin N Am 1998;7:707–20.

385. Doria R, Jekel JF, Cooper DL. Thyroid lymphoma. The case for combined modality therapy. Cancer 1994;73:200–6.

386. Skarsgard ED, Connors JM, Robins RE. A current analysis of primary lymphoma of the thyroid. Arch Surg 1991;126:1199–203.

387. Briggs JH, Algan O, Miller TP, Oleson JR. External beam radiation therapy in the treatment of patients with extranodal stage IA non-Hodgkin's lymphoma. Am J Clin Oncol 2002;25:34–7.

388. Rosen IB, Sutcliffe SB, Gospodarowicz MK, et al. The role of surgery in the management of thyroid lymphoma. Surgery 1988;104:1095–9.

389. Silverberg SG, Vidone RA. Carcinoma of the thyroid in surgical and postmortem material. Analysis of 300 cases at autopsy and literature review. Ann Surg 1966;164:291–9.

390. Shimaoka K, Sokal JE, Pickren JW. Metastatic neoplasms in the thyroid gland: Pathological and clinical findings. Cancer 1962;15:557–9.

391. Ivy HK. Cancer metastatic to the thyroid: A diagnostic problem. Mayo Clin Proc 1984;59:856–9.

392. Lin JD, Huang BY. Comparison of the results of diagnosis and treatment between solid and cystic well-differentiated thyroid carcinomas. Thyroid 1998;8:661–6.

393. McCabe DP, Farrar WB, Petkov TM, et al. Clinical and pathologic correlations in disease metastatic to the thyroid gland. Am J Surg 1985;150:519–23.

394. Moley JF, DeBenedetti MK. Patterns of nodal metastases in palpable medullary thyroid carcinoma: Recommendations for extent of node dissection. Ann Surg 1999;229:880–7.

395. Fialkowski EA, Moley JF. Current approaches to medullary thyroid carcinoma, sporadic and familial. J Surg Oncol 2006;94:737–47.

396. Quayle FJ, Moley JF. Medullary thyroid carcinoma: Including MEN 2A and MEN 2B syndromes. J Surg Oncol 2005;89:122–9.

397. Saad MF, Guido JJ, Samaan NA. Radioactive iodine in the treatment of medullary carcinoma of the thyroid. J Clin Endocrinol Metab 1983;57:124–8.

398. Brierley J, Tsang R, Simpson WJ, et al. Medullary thyroid cancer: Analyses of survival and prognostic factors and the role of radiation therapy in local control. Thyroid 1996;6:305–10.

399. Clark JR, Fridman TR, Odell MJ, et al. Prognostic variables and calcitonin in medullary thyroid cancer. Laryngoscope 2005;115:1445–50.

400. Brandi ML, Gagel RF, Angeli A, et al. Guidelines for diagnosis and therapy of MEN type 1 and type 2. J Clin Endocrinol Metab 2001;86:5658–71.

401. Skinner MA, Moley JA, Dilley WG, et al. Prophylactic thyroidectomy in multiple endocrine neoplasia type 2A. New Engl J Med 2005;353:1105–13.

402. Adami S, Marcocci C, Gatti D. Epidemiology of primary hyperparathyroidism in Europe. J Bone Mineral Res 2002;17:N18–23.

403. Wermers RA, Khosla S, Atkinson EJ, et al. Incidence of primary hyperparathyroidism in Rochester, Minnesota, 1993–2001: An update on the changing epidemiology of the disease. J Bone Mineral Res 2006;21:171–7.

404. Marx SJ. Hyperparathyroid and hypoparathyroid disorders. New Engl J Med 2000;343:1863–75.

405. Teh BT, Farnebo F, Kristoffersson U, et al. Autosomal dominant primary hyperparathyroidism and jaw tumor syndrome associated with renal hamartomas and cystic kidney disease: Linkage to 1q21-q32 and loss of the wild type allele in renal hamartomas. J Clin Endocrinol Metab 1996;81:4204–11.

406. Hendy GN, D'Souza-Li L, Yang B, et al. Mutations of the calcium-sensing receptor (CASR) in familial hypocalciuric hypercalcemia, neonatal severe hyperparathyroidism, and autosomal dominant hypocalcemia. Human Mutat 2000;16:281–96.

407. Carpten JD, Robbins CM, Villablanca A, et al. HRPT2, encoding parafibromin, is mutated in hyperparathyroidism-jaw tumor syndrome. Nature Genetics 2002;32:676–80.

408. Howell VM, Haven CJ, Kahnoski K, et al. HRPT2 mutations are associated with malignancy in sporadic parathyroid tumours. J Med Genet 2003;40:657–63.

409. Warner J, Epstein M, Sweet A, et al. Genetic testing in familial isolated hyperparathyroidism: Unexpected results and their implications. J Med Genet 2004;41:155–60.

410. Bilezikian JP, Potts JT, Jr, Fuleihan Gel H, et al. Summary statement from a workshop on asymptomatic primary hyperparathyroidism: A perspective for the 21st century. J Clin Endocrinol Metab 2002;87:5353–61.

411. Roman S, Sosa JA. Psychiatric and cognitive aspects of primary hyperparathyroidism. Curr Opin Oncol 2007; 19:1–5.

412. Coker LH, Rorie K, Cantley L, et al. Primary hyperparathyroidism, cognition, and health-related quality of life. Ann Surg 2005;242:642–50.

413. Perrier ND, Coker LH, Rorie KD, et al. Preliminary report: Functional MRI of the brain may be the ideal tool for evaluating neuropsychologic and sleep complaints of patients with primary hyperparathyroidism. World J Surg 2006;30:686–96.

414. Arnalsteen LC, Alesina PF, Quiereux JL, et al. Long-term results of less than total parathyroidectomy for hyperparathyroidism in multiple endocrine neoplasia type 1. Surgery 2002;132:1119–24.

415. Lakhani VT, You YN, Wells SA. The multiple endocrine neoplasia syndromes. Ann Rev Med 2007;58:253–65.

416. Malone JP, Srivastava A, Khardori R. Hyperparathyroidism and multiple endocrine neoplasia. Otolaryngol Clin N Am 2004;37:715–36.

417. Tonelli F, Spini S, Tommasi M, et al. Intraoperative parathormone measurement in patients with multiple endocrine neoplasia type I syndrome and hyperparathyroidism. World J Surg 2000;24:556–62.

418. Lee CH, Tseng LM, Chen JY, et al. Primary hyperparathyroidism in multiple endocrine neoplasia type 1: Individualized management with low recurrence rates. Ann Surg Oncol 2006;13:103–9.

419. Quevain FD. Parastruma maligna aberrata. Dtsch Z Chir 1904;100:334–52.

420. Sainton P, Millot J. Malegne du´n adenoma parathyroidiene eosinophile; au cours dune de Recklinghausen. Ann Anat Pathol (Paris) 1933;10:813.

421. Wynne AG, van Heerden J, Carney JA, Fitzpatrick LA. Parathyroid carcinoma: Clinical and pathologic features in 43 patients. Medicine 1992;71:197–205.

422. DeLellis RA. Parathyroid carcinoma: An overview. Adv Anat Pathol 2005;12:53–61.

423. Shattuck TM, Valimaki S, Obara T, et al. Somatic and germ-line mutations of the HRPT2 gene in sporadic parathyroid carcinoma. New Engl J Med 2003;349:1722–9.

424. Cetani F, Pardi E, Borsari S, et al. Genetic analyses of the HRPT2 gene in primary hyperparathyroidism: Germline and somatic mutations in familial and sporadic parathyroid tumors. J Clin Endocrinol Metab 2004;89:5583–91.

425. Rubin MR, Silverberg SJ. HRPT2 in parathyroid cancer: A piece of the puzzle. J Clin Endocrinol Metab 2005; 90:5505–7.

426. Cetani F, Ambrogini E, Viacava P, et al. Should parafibromin staining replace HRTP2 gene analysis as an additional tool for histologic diagnosis of parathyroid carcinoma? Eur J Endocrinol 2007;156:547–54.

427. Collins MT, Skarulis MC, Bilezikian JP, et al. Treatment of hypercalcemia secondary to parathyroid carcinoma with a novel calcimimetic agent. J Clin Endocrinol Metab 1998;83:1083–8.

428. Chow E, Tsang RW, Brierley JD, Filice S. Parathyroid carcinoma–the Princess Margaret Hospital experience. Int J Rad Oncol Biol Phys 1998;41:569–72.

429. Clayman GL, Gonzalez HE, El-Naggar A, Vassilopoulou-Sellin R. Parathyroid carcinoma: Evaluation and interdisciplinary management. Cancer 2004;100:900–5.

430. Lumachi F, Basso SM, Basso U. Parathyroid cancer: Etiology, clinical presentation and treatment. Anticancer Res 2006; 26:4803–7.

431. Driscoll DA. Molecular and genetic aspects of DiGeorge/velocardiofacial syndrome. Meth Molec Med 2006; 126:43–55.

432. Goodship J, Cross I, LiLing J, Wren C. A population study of chromosome 22q11 deletions in infancy. Arch Dis Child 1998;79:348–51.

433. McDonald-McGinn DM, Kirschner R, Goldmuntz E, et al. The Philadelphia story: The 22q11.2 deletion: Report on 250 patients. Genet Counsel 1999;10:11–24.

434. Cuneo BF, Driscoll DA, Gidding SS, Langman CB. Evolution of latent hypoparathyroidism in familial 22q11 deletion syndrome. Am J Med Genet 1997;69:50–5.

435. Weinzimer SA. Endocrine aspects of the 22q11.2 deletion syndrome. Genet Med 2001;3:19–22.

436. Taylor SC, Morris G, Wilson D, et al. Hypoparathyroidism and 22q11 deletion syndrome. Arch Dis Child 2003; 88:520–2.

437. Greig F, Paul E, DiMartino-Nardi J, Saenger P. Transient congenital hypoparathyroidism: Resolution and recurrence in chromosome 22q11 deletion. J Pediatrics 1996; 128:563–7.

438. Maalouf NM, Sakhaee K, Odvina CV. A case of chromosome 22q11 deletion syndrome diagnosed in a 32-year-old man with hypoparathyroidism. J Clin Endocrinol Metab 2004;89:4817–20.

439. Manz B, Scholz GH, Willgerodt H, et al. Autoimmune polyglandular syndrome (APS) type 1 and candida onychomycosis. Eur J Derm 2002;12:283–6.

440. Buzi F, Badolato R, Mazza C, et al. Autoimmune polyendocrinopathy-candidiasis-ectodermal dystrophy syndrome: Time to review diagnostic criteria? J Clin Endocrinol Metab 2003;88:3146–8.

441. Heino M, Scott HS, Chen Q, et al. Mutation analyses of North American APS-1 patients. Human Mutat 1999; 13:69–74.

442. Ahonen P, Myllarniemi S, Sipila I, Perheentupa J. Clinical variation of autoimmune polyendocrinopathy-candidiasis-ectodermal dystrophy (APECED) in a series of 68 patients. New Engl J Med 1990;322:1829–36.

443. Walls AW, Soames JV. Dental manifestations of autoimmune hypoparathyroidism. Oral Surg Oral Med Oral Pathol 1993;75:452–4.

444. Li Y, Song YH, Rais N, et al. Autoantibodies to the extracellular domain of the calcium sensing receptor in patients with acquired hypoparathyroidism. J Clin Invest 1996; 97:910–4.

445. Demeester-Mirkine N, Hooghe L, Van Geertruyden J, De Maertelaer V. Hypocalcemia after thyroidectomy. Arch Surg 1992;127:854–8.

446. Glinoer D, Andry G, Chantrain G, Samil N. Clinical aspects of early and late hypocalcaemia afterthyroid surgery. Eur J Surg Oncol 2000;26:571–7.

447. Falk SA, Birken EA, Baran DT. Temporary postthyroidectomy hypocalcemia. Arch Otolaryngol Head Neck Surg 1988;114:168–74.

448. Bourrel C, Uzzan B, Tison P, et al. Transient hypocalcemia after thyroidectomy. Ann Otol Rhinol Laryngol 1993;102:496–501.

449. Adams J, Andersen P, Everts E, Cohen J. Early postoperative calcium levels as predictors of hypocalcemia. Laryngoscope 1998;108:1829–31.

450. Hundahl SA, Cady B, Cunningham MP, et al. Initial results from a prospective cohort study of 5583 cases of thyroid carcinoma treated in the United States during 1996. U.S. and German Thyroid Cancer Study Group. An American College of Surgeons Commission on Cancer Patient Care Evaluation Study. Cancer 2000;89:202–17.

451. Thomusch O, Machens A, Sekulla C, et al. The impact of surgical technique on postoperative hypoparathyroidism in bilateral thyroid surgery: A multivariate analysis of 5846 consecutive patients. Surgery 2003;133:180–5.

452. Richards ML, Bingener-Casey J, Pierce D, et al. Intraoperative parathyroid hormone assay: An accurate predictor of symptomatic hypocalcemia following thyroidectomy. Arch Surg 2003;138:632–5.

453. McLeod IK, Arciero C, Noordzij JP, et al. The use of rapid parathyroid hormone assay in predicting postoperative hypocalcemia after total or completion thyroidectomy. Thyroid 2006;16:259–65.

454. Tomoda C, Kitano H, Uruno T, et al. Transcutaneous iodine absorption in adult patients with thyroid cancer disinfected with povidone-iodine at operation. Thyroid 2005;15:600–3.

455. Pothier DD. The use of drains following thyroid and parathyroid surgery: A meta-analysis. J Laryngol Otology 2005;119:669–71.

456. Ahluwalia S, Hannan SA, Mehrzad H, et al. A randomised controlled trial of routine suction drainage after elective thyroid and parathyroid surgery with ultrasound evaluation of fluid collection. Clin Otolaryngol 2007;32:28–31.

457. Miccoli P, Berti P, Frustaci GL, et al. Video-assisted thyroidectomy: Indications and results. Langenbecks Arch Surg 2006;391:68–71.

458. Lombardi CP, Raffaelli M, Princi P, et al. Safety of video-assisted thyroidectomy versus conventional surgery. Head Neck 2005;27:58–64.

459. Miccoli P, Elisei R, Materazzi G, et al. Minimally invasive video-assisted thyroidectomy for papillary carcinoma: A prospective study of its completeness. Surgery 2002;132:1070–3.

460. Bellantone R, Lombardi CP, Bossola M, et al. Video-assisted vs conventional thyroid lobectomy: A randomized trial. Arch Surg 2002;137:301–4.

461. Miccoli P, Berti P, Raffaelli M, et al. Comparison between minimally invasive video-assisted thyroidectomy and conventional thyroidectomy: A prospective randomized study. Surgery 2001;130:1039–43.

462. Kitagawa W, Shimizu K, Akasu H, Tanaka S. Endoscopic neck surgery with lymph node dissection for papillary carcinoma of the thyroid using a totally gasless anterior neck skin lifting method. J Am Coll Surg 2003;196:990–4.

463. Siperstein AE, Berber E, Morkoyun E. The use of the harmonic scalpel vs conventional knot tying for vessel ligation in thyroid surgery. Arch Surg 2002;137:137–42.

464. Cordon C, Fajardo R, Ramirez J, Herrera MF. A randomized, prospective, parallel group study comparing the Harmonic Scalpel to electrocautery in thyroidectomy. Surgery 2005;137:337–41.

465. Miccoli P, Berti P, Dionigi GL, et al. Randomized controlled trial of harmonic scalpel use during thyroidectomy. Arch Otolaryngol Head Neck Surg 2006;132:1069–73.

466. Ortega J, Sala C, Flor B, Lledo S. Efficacy and cost-effectiveness of the UltraCision harmonic scalpel in thyroid surgery: An analysis of 200 cases in a randomized trial. J Laparoendoscopic Adv Surg Tech Part A 2004; 14:9–12.

467. Rosato L, Avenia N, Bernante P, et al. Complications of thyroid surgery: Analysis of a multicentric study on 14,934 patients operated on in Italy over 5 years. World J Surg 2004;28:271–6.

468. Higgins KM, Mandell DL, Govindaraj S, et al. The role of intraoperative rapid parathyroid hormone monitoring for predicting thyroidectomy-related hypocalcemia. Arch Otolaryngol Head Neck Surg 2004;130:63–7.

469. Di Fabio F, Casella C, Bugari G, et al. Identification of patients at low risk for thyroidectomy-related hypocalcemia by intraoperative quick PTH. World J Surg 2006;30:1428–33.

470. Olson JA, Jr, DeBenedetti MK, Baumann DS, Wells SA, Jr. Parathyroid autotransplantation during thyroidectomy. Results of long-term follow-up. Ann Surg 1996;223:472-8; discussion 478–80.

471. Thomusch O, Machens A, Sekulla C, et al. Multivariate analysis of risk factors for postoperative complications in benign goiter surgery: Prospective multicenter study in Germany. World J Surg 2000;24:1335–41.

472. Yarbrough DE, Thompson GB, Kasperbauer JL, et al. Intraoperative electromyographic monitoring of the recurrent laryngeal nerve in reoperative thyroid and parathyroid surgery. Surgery 2004;136:1107–15.

473. Randolph GW, Kobler JB, Wilkins J. Recurrent laryngeal nerve identification and assessment during thyroid surgery: Laryngeal palpation. World J Surg 2004;28:755–60.

474. Tomoda C, Hirokawa Y, Uruno T, et al. Sensitivity and specificity of intraoperative recurrent laryngeal nerve stimulation test for predicting vocal cord palsy after thyroid surgery. World J Surg 2006;30:1230–3.

475. Chan WF, Lo CY. Pitfalls of intraoperative neuromonitoring for predicting postoperative recurrent laryngeal nerve function during thyroidectomy. World J Surg 2006; 30:806–12.

476. Wartofsky L, Sherman SI, Gopal J, et al. The use of radioactive iodine in patients with papillary and follicular thyroid cancer. J Clin Endocrinol Metab 1998;83:4195–203.

477. Haigh PI, Urbach DR, Rotstein LE. Extent of thyroidectomy is not a major determinant of survival in low- or high-risk papillary thyroid cancer. Ann Surg Oncol 2005;12:81–9.

478. Netterville JL, Coleman SC, Smith JC, et al. Management of substernal goiter. Laryngoscope 1998;108:1611–7.

479. Stephenson BM, Shandall AA, Griffith GH. Peak expiratory flow in the detection of retrosternal goitre. Ann Royal Coll Surg Engl 1991;73:215–8.

480. Are C, Shaha AR. Anaplastic thyroid carcinoma: Biology, pathogenesis, prognostic factors, and treatment approaches. Ann Surg Oncol 2006;13:453–64.

481. Machens A, Hinze R, Thomusch O, Dralle H. Pattern of nodal metastasis for primary and reoperative thyroid cancer. World J Surg 2002;26:22–8.

482. Stulak JM, Grant CS, Farley DR, et al. Value of preoperative ultrasonography in the surgical management of initial and reoperative papillary thyroid cancer. Arch Surg 2006;141:489–94.

483. Akerstrom G, Malmaeus J, Bergstrom R. Surgical anatomy of human parathyroid glands. Surgery 1984;95:14–21.

484. Goldstein RE, Blevins L, Delbeke D, Martin WH. Effect of minimally invasive radioguided parathyroidectomy on efficacy, length of stay, and costs in the management of primary hyperparathyroidism. Ann Surg 2000;231:732–42.

485. Sosa JA, Udelsman R. Minimally invasive parathyroidectomy. Surg Oncol 2003;12:125–34.

486. Udelsman R. Six hundred fifty-six consecutive explorations for primary hyperparathyroidism. Ann Surg 2002; 235:665–70.

487. Rubello D, Piotto A, Medi F, et al. 'Low dose' 99mTc-Sestamibi for radioguided surgery of primary hyperparathyroidism. Eur J Surg Oncol 2005;31:191–6.

488. Neumann DR, Esselstyn CB, Jr, Go RT, et al. Comparison of double-phase 99mTc-sestamibi with 123I-99mTc-sestamibi subtraction SPECT in hyperparathyroidism. AJR. Am J Roentgenol 1997;169:1671–4.

489. Stephen AE, Roth SI, Fardo DW, et al. Predictors of an accurate preoperative sestamibi scan for single-gland parathyroid adenomas. Arch Surg 2007;142:381–6.

490. Krausz Y, Lebensart PD, Klein M, et al. Preoperative localization of parathyroid adenoma in patients with concomitant thyroid nodular disease. World J Surg 2000;24:1573–8.

491. Berri RN, Lloyd LR. Detection of parathyroid adenoma in patients with primary hyperparathyroidism: The use of office-based ultrasound in preoperative localization. Am J Surg 2006;191:311–4.

492. Rodgers SE, Hunter GJ, Hamberg LM, et al. Improved preoperative planning for directed parathyroidectomy with 4-dimensional computed tomography. Surgery 2006; 140:932–40.

493. Grant CS, Thompson G, Farley D, van Heerden J. Primary hyperparathyroidism surgical management since the introduction of minimally invasive parathyroidectomy: Mayo Clinic experience. Arch Surg 2005;140:472–8.

494. Richards ML, Grant CS. Current applications of the intraoperative parathyroid hormone assay in parathyroid surgery. Am Surgeon 2007;73:311–7.

495. Lal A, Bianco J, Chen H. Radioguided parathyroidectomy in patients with familial hyperparathyroidism. Ann Surgical Oncology 2007;14:739–43.

496. Johnson SJ, Sheffield EA, McNicol AM. Best practice no 183. Examination of parathyroid gland specimens. J Clin Pathol 2005;58:338–42.

Index